W9-DCM-957

Nursing Care Plans

Procedures

Drug Guides

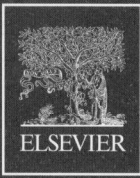

Maternal-Child

NURSING

Emily Slone McKinney, MSN, RN, C

Baylor University Medical Center

Dallas, Texas

Susan Rowen James, RN, PhD (c)

Associate Professor

Division of Nursing Studies

Curry College

Milton, Massachusetts

Sharon Smith Murray, MSN, RN, C

Professor, Health Professions

Golden West College

Huntington Beach, California

Jean Weiler Ashwill, MSN, RN

Director of Undergraduate Student Services

School of Nursing

University of Texas at Arlington

Arlington, Texas

Maternal-Child

NURSING

SECOND EDITION

With 588 Illustrations

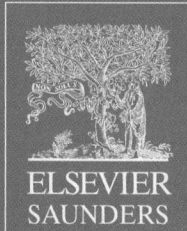

ELSEVIER
SAUNDERS

ELSEVIER
SAUNDERS
An Imprint of Elsevier

11830 Westline Industrial Drive
St. Louis, Missouri 63146

MATERNAL-CHILD NURSING

NOTICE

Nursing is an ever-changing field. Standard safety precautions must be followed, but as new research and clinical experience broaden our knowledge, changes in treatment and drug therapy become necessary or appropriate. Readers are advised to check the product information currently provided by the manufacturer of each drug to be administered to verify contraindications. It is the responsibility of the licensed prescriber, relying on experience and knowledge of the patient, to determine dosages and the best treatment for each individual patient. Neither the publisher nor the editor assumes any liability for any injury and/or damage to persons or property arising from this publication.

Previous editions copyrighted 2000

ISBN-13: 978-0-7216-0699-6
ISBN-10: 0-7216-0699-7

Executive Editors: Michael Ledbetter/Loren Wilson
Senior Developmental Editors: Lisa P. Newton/Nancy O'Brien
Publishing Services Manager: Catherine Jackson
Senior Project Manager: Celeste Clingan
Designer: Julia Dummitt

Printed in China

Last digit is the print number: 9   8   7   6   5   4

DEDICATION

To Michael, my love, support, and faithful friend.
To our daughters, Cathy and Amy.
To my late parents, Juanita and Charles Slone, who
gave me life, faith, and understanding of others.

Emily Slone McKinney

To the women in my family—mothers, sisters, and
daughters—whose unique talents, individual pursuits,
and constant encouragement have greatly influenced my
view of nursing care. And, as always, to my husband,
Bob, with love.

Susan Rowen James

To my husband, Skip, and my children
Vicki, Holly, and Shannon;
to my grandchildren Marina, Nicholas, and Giovanni;
and to my mother, Clare, with gratitude for all
your love, patience, and encouragement.

Sharon Smith Murray

To my husband, Vince, for his love and friendship.
To my grandchildren, Avery, Liam, Katie, Patrick,
Charlie, and Andrew, who make growth and develop-
ment come alive and continually amaze me.

Jean Weiler Ashwill

CONTRIBUTORS

Madoka Armstrong, MSN, RN, CS, PMHNP
Psychiatric Mental Health Nurse Practitioner
The Holiner Psychiatric Group
Dallas, Texas

Virginia Benepe, RNC, CDE, CPN
Driscoll Children's Hospital
Corpus Christi, Texas

Karen Samper Bernardy, RN, MSN
Conyers, Georgia

Cam Brandt, RN, MS
Education Coordinator
Cook Children's Health Care System
Fort Worth, Texas

Debra L. Calligaro-Wharton, RN, MS
Dallas, Texas

Dolores Clark, RN, MSN, FNP, CPNP
Pediatric Nurse Practitioner
Cook Children's Physician Network
Fort Worth, Texas

Wrennah L. Gabbert, RN, MSN, CPNP, FNP-C
Professional Specialist, Nursing Department
Angelo State University
San Angelo, Texas

Melissa A. Saffarrans LeMoine, RN, MSN, CPNP
Pediatric Nurse Practitioner
Cook Children's Physicians Network
Fort Worth, Texas

Mary Mallory, MSN, PNP, ACRN, BC, APRN
Department of Pediatrics
University of Texas Southwestern Medical School
Dallas, Texas

Gwendolyn T. Martin, RN, MS, CNS, CPN
Assistant Clinical Professor
Texas Woman's University
Dallas, Texas

Sharon M. McLeod, MS, CCLS, CTRS
Clinical Director II, Division of Child Life and
    Recreational Therapy
Cincinnati Children's Hospital Medical Center
Cincinnati, Ohio

Patricia Newcomb, RN, CPNP, PhD
Assistant Professor
Harris School of Nursing
Texas Christian University
Fort Worth, Texas

Tracey Carnes Pickering, RN, MHA
Cook Children's Medical Center
Fort Worth, Texas

Sharon Ransom, RN, MHA, CPN
Education Coordinator
Cook Children's Health Care System
Fort Worth, Texas

James Riddel, RN, CPNP
Pediatric Nurse Practitioner
Children's Hospital, Oakland
Oakland, California

Jennifer Walsh Treseler, RN, MSN
Clinical Coordinator, Pulmonary Division
Children's Hospital
Boston, Massachusetts

Kathleen White, RN, MSN, CPNP
Nursing Faculty, Tarrant County College
Pediatric Nurse Practitioner
Cook Children's Health Care System
Fort Worth, Texas

REVIEWERS

Jessica L. Alexander, BSN, MN
Assistant Professor
Mississippi University for Women
Columbus, Mississippi

Darlene Nebel Cantu, RNC, MSN
Quality Manager
St. Luke's Hospital
Faculty, Department of Nursing Education
San Antonio College of Nursing Department
San Antonio, Texas

Traudel B. Cline, MSN, RN
Milwaukee Area Technical College
Milwaukee, Wisconsin

Darlene Del Prato, MS, RNC
Faculty
St. Joseph's Hospital
Syracuse, New York

Amy Zlomek Hedden, RN, MS, NP
California State University, Bakersfield
Bakersfield Family Medical Center
Bakersfield, California

Jill Janke, RNc, ANP, DNSc
Professor
University of Alaska Anchorage
Anchorage, Alaska

Ronnette Chereese Langhorne, MS, RN
Instructor, Department of Nursing
Norfolk State University
Norfolk, Virginia

Barbra Manning, RN, MSN
Instructor/Level Coordinator
Northwest Mississippi Community College
Senatobia, Mississippi

Debra Migues, RN, MSN, ICCE
Associate Professor
Louisiana College
Pineville, Louisiana

Donna L. Miller, RN, MSN, CPNP
Instructor, Department of Nursing
Thomas Jefferson University
College of Health Professions
Methodist Hospital School of Nursing
Philadelphia, Pennsylvania

Virginia Bradford Pearson, RN, MSN
Instructor
University of Southern Mississippi
College of Nursing
Hattiesburg, Mississippi

Anne Rentfro, MSN, RN
Associate Professor
University of Texas at Brownsville and
Texas Southmost College
Brownsville, Texas

PREFACE

Children are a precious gift. Some of the most satisfying nursing roles involve helping families bring their children into the world, being a resource as they rear them, and supporting families during times of illness. In addition to providing care to young families as they bear and raise children, nurses play a crucial role in women's health care from the teen years through postmenopausal life. The second edition of *Maternal-Child Nursing* is written to provide a foundation for care of these individuals and their families to the nursing student or the nurse entering maternity and women's health nursing or nursing of children from another area of nursing.

Maternal-Child Nursing builds on two successful texts to combine maternity, women's health, and nursing of children. *Nursing Care of Children: Principles and Practice*, 2nd edition, by Susan Rowen James and Jean Weiler Ashwill and *Foundations of Maternal-Newborn Nursing*, 3rd edition, by Sharon Smith Murray, Emily Slone McKinney and Trula Myers Gorrie form the foundation of this text.

Maternal-Child Nursing, 2nd edition, emphasizes evidence-based nursing care throughout. The scientific base of maternal-newborn, women's health, and nursing care of children is demonstrated in the narrative and features in which the nursing process is applied. Physiological and pathophysiological processes are presented so the reader can understand why problems occur and the reasons behind nursing care. Current references, many of them from Internet sources for maximum timeliness, provide the reader with the latest information that applies to the clinical area. National standards and guidelines, such as those from the Association of Women's Health, Obstetric, and Neonatal Nurses (AWHONN); Society of Pediatric Nurses (SPN); and American Nurses Association (ANA), are used when they apply.

Maternal-newborn, women's health, and nursing of children may be practiced in a wide variety of settings. Where appropriate, our text discusses care of clients in settings as diverse as acute and chronic care facilities, the community, schools, and the home. Methods to ease transition among facilities and improve continuity of care are highlighted when appropriate.

Legal and ethical issues add to the complexity of practice for today's nurse. Discussion of nurses' legal obligations when providing health care to women, newborns, and children optimizes care for all clients in each group. Legal topics include such areas as Standards of Care, informed consent, and refusal of treatment. Ethical principles and decision making are discussed in the first chapter of the text. Ethical issues, such as care of babies born at a very early gestation or nursing care at the end of life, are discussed in appropriate chapters.

Nursing students have time demands from work, family, and community activities in addition to their nursing education. A significant number of nurses use English as a second language. With those realities in mind, we have written a text to effectively convey necessary information that focuses on critical elements and that is concise without the use of unnecessarily complex language.

Important terms are defined at the beginning of each chapter for ready access as the student studies the chapter.

Concepts

Several conceptual threads are woven into our book. The *family* is a concept that is incorporated throughout our book as a vital part of maternal-child nursing care and nursing care of women. Family considerations appear in every step of the nursing process. The family may be the conventional mother-father-child arrangement or might be a single-parent or multigenerational family. We consider several types of family styles as we present nursing care. We sometimes ask the reader to use critical thinking to examine personal assumptions and biases about families while studying.

Without *communication*, nursing care would be inadequate and sometimes unsafe. Teaching effective communication skills is incorporated into several features of the text as well as into the main narrative. Highlighted text within the narrative contains communication cues to give tips about verbal and nonverbal communication with clients and their families. Children are not little adults and nowhere is this more true than when communicating with them. Therefore, communicating with children is presented in a separate chapter to supplement information given in other nursing of children chapters.

Health promotion is obvious in chapters covering normal childbearing and child rearing, but we also incorporate it into the chapters covering various disorders. Health promotion during illness may be as simple as reminding the reader that a technology-laden woman in labor is still having a baby, a usually normal process, and thus needs human contact. Sick children need activities to promote their normal growth and development as much as they need the technology and procedures that return them to physical wellness. This edition of *Maternal-Child Nursing* contains health promotion boxes in each of the developmental chapters. The goal of these boxes is to highlight anticipatory guidance appropriate for an infant or child's developmental level according to the schedule of well visits recommended by the American Academy of Pediatrics.

Teaching is closely related to health promotion. Teaching is an expected part of nursing care to help clients and their families maintain health or return to health after illness or injury. Several features discussed later help the reader provide better teaching to clients in an understandable form.

Cultural diversity characterizes nursing practice today as the lines between individual nations become more blurred. The nurse must assess for unique cultural needs and incorporate them into care as much as possible to promote acceptance of nursing care by the client. Cultural influences are examined in many ways in our text, including critical thinking exercises to help the student "think outside the box" of his or her own culture.

Growth and development are concepts that appear throughout the book. We cover physical growth and development as the child is conceived and matures before birth and throughout childhood, and as the woman matures through the childbearing years and into the climacteric. Specific chapters in the nursing of children section focus on growth and development issues, including anticipatory guidance, specific to each age group from infancy through adolescence.

Advocacy is emphasized in our text. Whether it is advocacy for a woman or family to be informed about their rights or advocacy for child and adult victims of violence, the concept is incorporated in relevant places.

Features

Maternal-newborn and women's health nursing care differs from nursing care of children and their families in several important respects. Because of this fact, some features in the text appear in one part but not in the other, often with references to the chapter containing related content. Other features appear in both parts of the text.

Visual appeal characterizes many features in the text. Beautiful illustrations and photographs convey developmental or clinical information, capturing the essence of care for maternity, newborn, women's health, and child clients.

LEARNING OBJECTIVES

Learning objectives provide direction for the reader to understand what is important to glean from the chapter. Many objectives ask that the learner use critical thinking and apply the nursing process—two crucial components of professional nursing—to care of clients with the conditions discussed in that chapter. Other features within the chapters reinforce these two components of care.

NURSING PROCESS

Several methods help the learner use the nursing process in care of maternal-newborn, women's health, and child clients. Steps of the nursing process include doing assessment; formulating nursing diagnoses after analysis of the assessment data; planning care; providing nursing interventions; and evaluating the nursing interventions, expected outcomes or goals, and appropriateness of nursing diagnoses as care proceeds. We address these steps in different ways in our book, often varying with whether the nursing process is discussed in the maternal-newborn, women's health, or the nursing of children section. The varied approaches show the student that there is more than one way to communicate the nursing process. These different approaches to the nursing process also provide teaching tools to meet the needs of students' varied learning styles.

In the maternal-newborn and women's health section, the nursing process is presented in two ways. Nursing care is first presented as a *text discussion* that would apply to a typical client with the condition. In addition, a *nursing care plan* that applies to a client created in a specific scenario is constructed for many common conditions. This technique helps the student see individualization of nursing care. Many nursing care plans list *additional nursing diagnoses to consider* encouraging the reader to reflect on client needs other than the obvious needs. The approach of scenario-based care plans is especially useful for showing learners how to apply the nursing process in dynamic conditions such as labor and birth.

In the nursing care of children section, the nursing process is applied to care of the most common childhood conditions by a blend of a text discussion similar to the maternal-newborn and women's health section and a generic rather than scenario-based nursing care plan. The student thus has the benefit of seeing typical nursing diagnoses, expected outcomes, and interventions with their rationales discussed in a manner similar to standard care plans the learner may encounter in clinical facilities. The evaluation step of the nursing process provides sample questions the nurse would need to answer to determine whether the expected outcomes were achieved and whether further actions or revisions of nursing care are needed. The application of the nursing process in the nursing care of children provides a framework for the nursing instructor to help students individualize nursing care for their specific clients based on a generic plan of care. *Maternal-Child Nursing* demonstrates not only the use of nursing process when caring for acutely ill children but also emphasizes its application when providing care in the community setting. Community-based use of the nursing process applies to many nursing specialties, including those in both sections of this updated edition of *Maternal-Child Nursing*.

CRITICAL THINKING EXERCISES

Critical thinking is encouraged in multiple ways in *Maternal-Child Nursing*, but specific Critical Thinking exercises present typical client scenarios or other real-life situations and ask the reader to solve nursing care problems that are not always obvious. We use the exercises to help the student learn to identify the answer, choose the best interventions, or determine possible meanings or importance of signs and symptoms. Answers are provided at the end of the chapter so the student can check his or her solutions to these problems.

CRITICAL TO REMEMBER

Students always want to know, "Will this be on the test?" The authors cannot answer that question, but Critical to Remember boxes provide a condensed summary of very important information needed to provide safe care.

WANT TO KNOW BOXES

Because teaching is an essential part of nursing care, we give students teaching guidelines for common client needs in terms that most lay people can understand. The Want to Know boxes provide sample answers for questions that clients are most likely to ask, such as when to go to the birth center or methods of managing diet and insulin requirements for type 1 diabetes at home.

CLINICAL REFERENCE PAGES

Clinical Reference pages provide a resource for the reader when studying conditions affecting children. This feature provides the reader with basic information related to a group of disorders and includes a compact review of related anatomy and physiology; differences between children and adults in the system being studied; commonly used drugs, lab values, and diagnostic tests; and procedures that apply to the conditions discussed in that chapter.

PATHOPHYSIOLOGY BOXES

Also present in many chapters in the nursing care of children are pathophysiology boxes. These boxes give the reader a brief overview of how the illness occurs. The boxes provide a scientific basis for understanding the therapeutic management of the illness and its nursing care.

PHOTO STORIES

"A picture is worth a thousand words" applies to the photo stories that appear in the nursing care of children section. Photo stories help the reader see well-child checks and assessments of growth and development. Some photo stories take the reader through the experience of care for a specific condition.

PROCEDURES

Clinical skills are presented in procedures throughout the text. Procedures related to maternal-newborn and women's health are presented in the chapters to which they apply. Because many procedures are common to care of children with a variety of health conditions, they are covered in a chapter devoted to procedures, Chapter 37.

DRUG GUIDES

Drug information may be presented in two ways: tables for related drugs used in the care of various conditions and drug guides for specific common drugs. Drug guides provide the nurse with greater detail for commonly encountered drugs in maternity and women's health care and in care of children with specific pharmacological needs.

KEY CONCEPTS

Key concepts summarize important points of each chapter. They provide a general review for the material just presented to help the reader identify areas in which more study is needed.

Appendixes

Eight appendixes in the back of the book provide a reference source for both the reader and the teacher. Some appendixes apply to maternal-newborn, women's health, and nursing of children. Others apply to a single specialty. Additional important information that relates to drug ingestion during pregnancy and lactation appears in Appendix B. Appendix I, Resources for Health Care Providers and Families, can be found on this book's Evolve website at http://evolve.elsevier.com/McKinney/mat-ch/

Ancillaries

Materials that complement *Maternal-Child Nursing* include:

The *Maternal-Child Nursing CD-ROM*: This interactive CD is included with the text. This CD includes NCLEX-style review questions; nursing skills outlines, and an audio glossary.

Instructor's Resource CD-ROM: Four separate teacher support programs are available on a single CD-ROM or from this book's Evolve website: (a) a full instructor's manual in the most common word processing formats; (b) a computerized test bank using the ExamView program; (c) PowerPoint slides, containing a combination of lecture slides and selected images from the text, and (d) an image collection in a variety of downloadable formats.

Virtual Clinical Excursions workbook/CD-ROM package: A groundbreaking learning tool guides the student through a computer-generated virtual clinical environment and helps the student apply textbook content to "virtual clients" in that environment. The clinical simulations and workbook represent the next generation of research-based learning tools that promote critical thinking and meaningful learning.

The *Study Guide for Maternal-Child Nursing*: This student study aid provides learning exercises, supplemental classroom and clinical activities, and multiple-choice review questions to reinforce material addressed in the text.

Evolve Learning Resources

Weblinks for both instructor's and students allows access to information and resources based on topics covered in this edition of *Maternal-Child Nursing*.

The *Instructor's Online Resource* includes the Instructor's Manual, Test Bank, Image Collection and PowerPoint Lecture slides.

Evolve Course Management System (CMS):

- The CMS is available to instructors upon adoption of the second edition of *Maternal-Child Nursing*.

- Instructors and students will have **full access** to a comprehensive suite of communication and organization tools, including discussion boards, e-mail, chat rooms, calendars, address books, task organizers, and more.

- Instructors will have **exclusive access** to the course management tools that allow them to customize their course content, build online tests, create assignments, enter grades, post announcements, manage student groups, and much more.

Acknowledgments

Many people in addition to the authors made the second edition of *Maternal-Child Nursing* a reality. Michael Ledbetter and Loren Wilson, Executive Editors, recognized the success of the first edition of *Maternal-Child Nursing* and worked with the authors to identify new teaching and learning techniques and supplements. Lisa Newton and Nancy O'Brien, Senior Developmental Editors, have been particularly helpful with keeping the publication process going smoothly. Mary Parker and Charlene Ketchum, Editorial Assistants, helped us many times with various details required to bring the project and its ancillaries to fruition. Celeste Clingan, Senior Project Manager, graciously ensured that production proceeded in a smooth and timely fashion.

Our acknowledgments would not be complete without thanking the many contributors to the nursing of children section. Many of them have been involved with both *Maternal-Child Nursing* and *Nursing Care of Children* from the beginning. Their willingness and commitment to keeping current in their practice and giving us the benefit of their experience is most appreciated. We would like to thank Ainat Koren, PhD, for her able and thorough assistance with research for several of the chapters in the nursing of children section of the text.

CONTENTS

MATERNITY NURSING CARE

PEDIATRIC NURSING CARE

49 The Child with an Integumentary Alteration, 1361

50 The Child with a Musculoskeletal Alteration, 1402

51 The Child with an Endocrine or Metabolic Alteration, 1448

APPENDIXES

1

Foundations of Maternity and Child Health Nursing

LEARNING OBJECTIVES

After studying this chapter, you should be able to:

◎ Describe the historical background of maternity and child health care.

◎ Compare current settings for childbirth both within and outside the hospital setting.

◎ Identify trends that led to the development of family-centered maternity and pediatric care.

◎ Describe issues that affect perinatal and child health nursing, including cost containment, outcomes management, home care, and advances in technology.

◎ Discuss trends in maternal, infant, and childhood mortality rates.

◎ Identify some of the effects of poverty and violence on children and families.

◎ Apply theories and principles of ethics to ethical dilemmas.

◎ Discuss ethical conflicts that the nurse may encounter in maternal and pediatric nursing practice.

◎ Relate how major social issues, such as poverty and access to health care, affect maternal-child nursing.

◎ Describe the legal basis for nursing practice.

◎ Identify measures used to defend malpractice claims.

◎ Identify current trends in health care and their implications for nursing.

DEFINITIONS

advocacy Speaking or arguing in support of a policy or a person's rights.

antepartum Term that refers to the period of pregnancy before the onset of labor.

bioethics Rules or principles that govern right conduct, specifically those that relate to health care.

case management A practice model that uses a systematic approach to identify specific client needs and to manage client care to ensure optimal outcomes.

deontologic theory Ethical theory that holds that the right course of action is the one dictated by ethical principles and moral rules.

ethical dilemma A situation in which no solution seems completely satisfactory.

ethics Rules or principles that govern right conduct and distinctions between right and wrong.

infant mortality rate Number of deaths per 1000 live births that occur within the first 12 months of life.

intrapartum Term that describes the time of labor and childbirth.

lactation Secretion of milk from the breasts; also describes the time when a child is breast-fed.

malpractice Negligence by a professional person.

maternal mortality rate Number of maternal deaths from childbirth and the complications of pregnancy, childbirth, and the puerperium (the first 42 days after the end of the preg-

nancy) per 100,000 live births. New criteria add deaths after 42 days to the total if pregnancy aggravated a disease that existed before pregnancy or developed during pregnancy and the disease subsequently led to the woman's death.

morbidity Ratio of sick to well persons in a defined population.

negligence Failure to act in the way a reasonable, prudent person of similar background would act in similar circumstances.

neonatal mortality rate Number of deaths per 1000 live births that occur before 28 days of life.

nurse practice acts Laws that determine the scope of nursing practice in each state.

postpartum Term that denotes the first 6 weeks after childbirth.

standard of care Level of care that can be expected of a professional. This level is determined by laws, professional organizations, and health care agencies.

standardized procedures Procedures determined by nurses, physicians, and administrators that allow nurses to perform duties usually part of the medical practice.

utilitarian theory Ethical theory that holds that the right course of action is the one that produces the greatest good.

WIC A Special Supplemental Food Program for Women, Infants, and Children that provides nutritious food and nutrition education to low-income pregnant and postpartum women and their children.

To better understand contemporary maternity and pediatric nursing, the nurse needs to understand the history of these fields, trends and issues affecting contemporary practice, and the ethical and legal frameworks within which maternity and pediatric nursing care is provided.

HISTORICAL PERSPECTIVES

Maternity Nursing

Major changes in maternity care occurred in the first half of the twentieth century as childbirth moved out of the home and into a hospital setting. Rapid change continues as health care reform attempts to control the rising cost of care while advances in expensive technology accelerate. Despite changes, health care professionals attempt to maintain the quality of care.

"Granny" Midwives

Before the twentieth century, childbirth usually occurred in the home with the assistance of a "granny," or lay, midwife whose training came through an apprenticeship with a more experienced midwife. Physicians were involved in childbirth only if there were serious problems.

Although many women and infants fared well when a lay midwife assisted with birth in the home, maternal and infant death rates resulting from childbearing were high. The primary causes of maternal death were postpartum hemorrhage, postpartum infection, also known as *puerperal sepsis* (or "childbed fever"), and toxemia, a hypertensive disorder of pregnancy now known as *preeclampsia* (National Heart, Lung, and Blood Institute, 2001). The primary causes of infant death were prematurity, dehydration from diarrhea, and contagious diseases.

Emergence of Medical Management

In the late nineteenth century, technologic developments that were available to physicians but not to midwives led to a decline in home births and an increase in physician-assisted hospital births. Important discoveries that set the stage for a change in maternity care included:

- The discovery by Semmelweis that puerperal infection could be prevented by hygienic practices
- The development of forceps to facilitate birth
- The discovery of chloroform, which was used to control pain during childbirth
- The use of drugs to initiate labor or to increase uterine contractions
- Advances in operative procedures, such as cesarean birth

By 1960, 90% of all births in the United States occurred in hospitals. Maternity care became highly regimented. All antepartum, intrapartum, and postpartum care was managed by physicians. Lay midwifery became illegal in many areas, and nurse-midwifery was not well established. The woman had a passive role in childbirth, as the physician "delivered" her baby. Nurses' primary functions were to assist the physician and to follow prescribed medical orders after childbirth. Teaching and counseling were not valued nursing functions at that time.

Unlike home births, early hospital births hindered bonding between parents and infant. During labor, the woman often received medication, such as "twilight sleep," a combination of a narcotic and scopolamine, that provided pain relief but left her disoriented, confused, and heavily sedated. Because of this practice and because little was known of the importance of early contact between parents and child, many mothers did not see the infant for several hours after the delivery. The father was relegated to a waiting area and was not allowed to see the mother until some time after birth.

Despite the technologic advances and the move from home birth to hospital birth, maternal and infant mortality declined, but slowly. The slow decline was caused primarily by problems that could have been prevented, such as poor nutrition, infectious diseases, and inadequate prenatal care. These stubborn problems remained because of inequalities in health care delivery. Whereas affluent families could afford comprehensive medical care that began early in the pregnancy, poor families had very limited access to care or to information about childbearing. Two concurrent trends—federal involvement and consumer demands—led to additional changes in maternity care.

Government Involvement in Maternal-Infant Care

The high rates of maternal and infant mortality among indigent women provided the impetus for federal involvement in maternity care. The Sheppard-Towner Act of 1921 provided funds for state-managed programs for mothers and children. Although this act was later repealed, it set the stage for future allocation of federal funds. Today the federal government supports several programs to improve the health of mothers, infants, and young children (Box 1-1). Although projects supported by government funds partially solved the problem of maternal and infant mortality, the *distribution* of health care remained unequal. Most physicians practiced in urban or suburban areas where the affluent could afford to pay for medical services, but women in rural or inner city areas had difficulty obtaining care. The distribution of health care services is a problem that persists today.

The ongoing problem of providing health care for poor women and children left the door open for nurses to expand their roles, and programs emerged to prepare nurses for advanced practice (see Chapter 2).

Impact of Consumer Demands on Health Care

In the early 1950s, consumers began to insist on their right to be involved in the health care they received. Pregnant women wanted a greater voice in their health care. They wanted information about planning and spacing their children, and they wanted to know what to expect during pregnancy. The father, siblings, and grandparents wanted to be part of the extraordinary events of pregnancy and childbirth. Parents began to insist on active participation in decisions about how their child would be born.

A growing consensus among child psychologists and nurse researchers, moreover, indicated that the benefits of early, extended parent-newborn contact far outweighed the risk of infection. Parents began to insist that their infant remain with them, and the practice of separating the well infant from the family was abandoned.

Development of Family-Centered Maternity Care

Family-centered maternity care is the term used to describe safe, quality care that recognizes and adapts to both the physical and psychosocial needs of the family, including those of the newborn. The emphasis is on fostering family unity while maintaining physical safety.

BOX 1-1
Federal Projects for Maternal-Child Care

Program	Purpose
Title V of Social Security Act	Provides funds for maternal-child health programs
National Institute of Health and Human Development	Supports research and education of personnel needed for maternal and child health programs
Title V Amendment of Public Health Service Act	Established the Maternal and Infant Care (MIC) projects to provide comprehensive prenatal and infant care in public clinics
Title XIX of Medicaid program	Provides funds to facilitate access to care by pregnant women and young children
Head Start	Provides educational opportunities for low-income children of preschool age
National Center for Family Planning	A clearinghouse for contraceptive information
Women, Infants, and Children (WIC) program	Provides supplemental food and nutrition information
Healthy Start	Enhances community development of culturally appropriate strategies designed to decrease infant mortality and causes of low birth weights
Individuals with Disabilities (PL 94-142)	Provides for free and appropriate education of all disabled children
National School Lunch/Breakfast Program	Provides nutritionally appropriate free or reduced-price meals to students from low-income families

---

The basic principles of family-centered care are as follows:

- Childbirth is usually a normal, healthy event in the life of a family.
- Childbirth affects the entire family, and restructuring of family relationships is required.
- Families are capable of making decisions about care, provided that they are given adequate information and professional support.

Family-centered care greatly increased the responsibilities of nurses. It is no longer enough for nurses to provide only physical care and to assist physicians. Nurses now assume a major role in teaching, counseling, and supporting families in their decisions.

Current Settings for Childbirth

As family-centered maternity care has emerged, settings for childbirth have changed to meet the needs of new families.

Traditional Hospital Setting

In hospitals of the past, labor often took place in a functional hospital room, often occupied by several laboring women. When birth was imminent, the mother was moved to a delivery area similar to an operating room. After giving birth, the mother was transferred to a recovery area for 1 to 2 hours of observation and then taken to the postpartum unit, which resembled a standard hospital room. The infant was moved to the newborn nursery when the mother was transferred to the recovery area. Mother and infant were reunited when the mother was settled in the postpartum unit. Beginning in the 1970s, the father or another significant support person could usually remain with the mother throughout labor, birth, and recovery.

Although birth in a traditional hospital setting was safe, the setting was impersonal and uncomfortable. Having to move from room to room, especially during late labor, was a major disadvantage. Each move was uncomfortable for the mother, disrupted the family's time together, and often separated the parents from the infant. Because of these disadvantages, hospitals began to devise settings that were more comfortable and that facilitated family participation.

Labor, Delivery, and Recovery Rooms. Today most hospitals offer alternative settings for childbirth. The most common is the labor, delivery, and recovery (LDR) room. In an LDR room, labor, birth, and early recovery from childbirth occur in one setting. Furniture has a less institutional appearance but can be quickly converted into the setup needed for birth. A typical LDR room is illustrated in Figure 1-1.

During labor, the woman's significant others are allowed to remain with her. Once she has given birth, the mother typically remains in the LDR room for 1 to 2 hours, after which she is transferred to the postpartum unit. The infant often stays with the mother throughout her stay in the LDR room. When the mother is transferred to the postpartum unit, the infant may be transferred to the nursery or may remain with the mother.

The major advantages of LDR rooms are that the setting is more comfortable and the family can remain with the mother. Disadvantages include the routine (rather than selective) use of technology, such as electronic fetal monitoring and the administration of intravenous fluids.

Labor, Delivery, Recovery, and Postpartum Rooms. Some hospitals offer rooms that are similar to LDR rooms in layout and in function, but the mother is not transferred to a postpartum unit. She and the infant remain in the labor, delivery, recovery, and postpartum (LDRP) room until discharge. The father or another primary support person is encouraged to stay with the mother and infant, and many facilities provide beds so they can stay through the night.

Birth Centers

Free-standing birth centers provide maternity care outside the hospital setting to low-risk women during pregnancy, birth, and postpartum. Most provide gynecologic services such as annual checkups and contraceptive counseling. Both

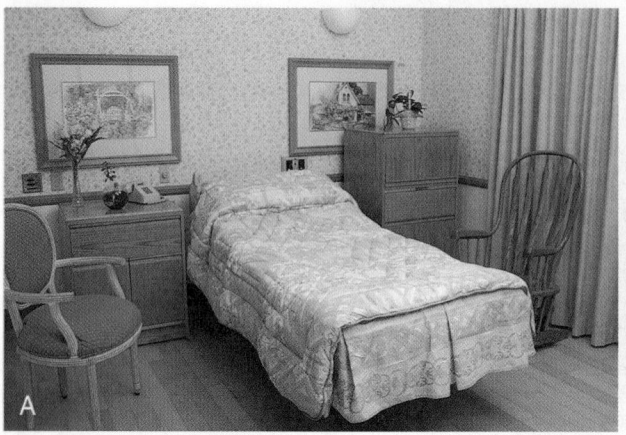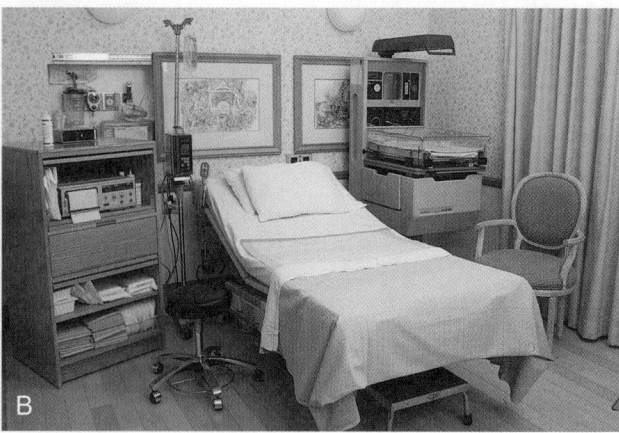

Figure 1-1 A typical labor, delivery, and recovery room. Home-like furnishings *(A)* can be adapted quickly to reveal needed technical equipment *(B)*.

the mother and infant continue to receive follow-up care during the first 6 weeks. This may include help with breast-feeding problems, a postpartum examination at 4 to 6 weeks, family planning information, and examination of the new-born. Care is often provided by certified nurse-midwives (CNM) who are registered nurses with advanced preparation in midwifery.

Birth centers are less expensive than acute-care hospitals, which provide advanced technology that may be unnecessary for low-risk clients. Moreover, women who want a safe, home-like birth in a familiar setting with staff they have known throughout their pregnancies express a very high rate of satisfaction.

The major disadvantage is that most free-standing birth centers are not equipped for obstetric emergencies. Should unforeseen difficulties develop during labor, the woman must be transferred by ambulance to a nearby hospital to the care of a backup physician who has agreed to perform this role. Some families do not feel that the very short stay after birth, often less than 12 hours, allows enough time to detect very early complications in mother and infant.

Home Births

In the United States, only a small number of women have their babies at home. Because malpractice insurance for mid-wives attending home births is expensive and difficult to obtain, the number of midwives who offer this service has decreased greatly.

Home birth provides the advantages of keeping the family together in their own environment throughout the childbirth experience. Bonding with the infant is unimpeded by hospital routines, and breast-feeding is encouraged. Women and their support person have a sense of control because they actively plan and prepare for each detail of the birth.

Giving birth at home also has disadvantages. Women who plan a home birth must be screened carefully to make sure that they have a very low risk for complications. If transfer to a nearby hospital becomes necessary, the time required may be too long in an emergency. Other problems of home birth include the need for the parents to provide a setting and adequate supplies for the birth. Moreover, the mother must take care of herself and the infant without the immediate help she would have in a hospital setting.

Nursing of Children

The nursing care of children has been influenced by factors similar to those affecting maternity care. Children have not always enjoyed the valued position that they hold in most families today. Historically, in times of economic or social instability, children have been viewed as expendable. In societies in which the struggle for survival is the central issue and only the strongest survive, the needs of children are secondary. The well-being of children in the past depended on the economic and cultural conditions of the society. At times, parents have viewed their children as property and children have been bought and sold, beaten, or, in some cultures, sacrificed in religious ceremonies. At times, infanticide has been a routine practice. Conversely, in other instances, children have been highly valued and their birth considered a blessing. Historically viewed by society as miniature adults, children in the past received the same remedies as adults and, during illness, were cared for at home by family members, just like adults.

Societal Changes

On the North American continent, as European settlements expanded during the seventeenth and eighteenth centuries, children were valued as assets to the community because of the desire to increase the population and to share the work to be done. Public schools were established, and the courts began to view children as minors and to protect them accordingly. Devastating epidemics of smallpox, diphtheria, scarlet fever, and measles took their toll on children in the eighteenth century. Children often died of these virulent diseases within 1 day.

The high mortality rate in children led some physicians to examine common child-care practices. In 1748 William Cadogan's "Essay Upon Nursing" discouraged unhealthy child-care practices, such as swaddling infants in three or four layers of clothing and feeding them thin gruel within hours after birth. Instead, Cadogan urged mothers to breast-feed their infants and identified certain practices that were thought to contribute to childhood illness. Unfortunately, despite the efforts of Cadogan and others, child-care practices were slow to change. Later in the eighteenth century, the health of children improved with certain advances such as inoculation against smallpox.

In the nineteenth century, with the flood of immigrants to eastern American cities, infectious diseases flourished as a result of crowded living conditions, inadequate and unsanitary food, and harsh working conditions for men, women, and children. Twelve- and fourteen-hour workdays were common for children working in factories, whose earnings were essential to the survival of the family. The most serious child health problems during the nineteenth century were caused by poverty and overcrowding. Infants were fed contaminated milk, sometimes from tuberculosis-infected cows. Milk was carried to the cities and purchased by mothers with no means to refrigerate it. Infectious diarrhea was a common cause of infant death.

During the late nineteenth century, conditions began to improve for children and families. Lillian Wald initiated public health nursing at Henry Street Settlement House in New York City, where nurses taught mothers in their homes. In 1889 a milk distribution center opened in New York City to provide uncontaminated milk to sick infants.

Hygiene and Hospitalization

The discoveries of scientists, such as Pasteur, Lister, and Koch, who proved that bacteria caused many diseases, supported the use of hygienic practices in hospitals and foundling homes. Hospitals began to require personnel to wear uniforms and to limit contact among children in the wards. In an effort to prevent infection, hospital wards were closed to visitors. Because parental visits were noted to cause distress, particularly when parents had to leave, parental visitation was considered to be emotionally stressful to hospitalized children. In an effort to prevent such emotional distress and the spread of infection, parents were prohibited from visiting hospitalized children. As hospital care focused on preventing disease transmission and curing physical diseases, the emotional health of hospitalized children received little attention.

During the twentieth century, as knowledge about nutrition, sanitation, bacteriology, pharmacology, medication, and psychology increased, dramatic changes in child health occurred. In the 1940s and 1950s, medications such as penicillin and corticosteroids and vaccines against many communicable diseases saved the lives of tens of thousands of children. Technologic advances in the 1970s and 1980s, which led to more children surviving conditions that had previously been fatal (e.g., cystic fibrosis), resulted in an increasing number of children living with chronic disabilities. An increase in societal concern for children brought about the development of federally supported programs designed to meet their needs, such as school lunch programs, the Special Supplemental Program for Women, Infants and Children (WIC), and Medicaid (see p. 3), under which the Early Periodic Screening, Diagnosis, and Treatment program was implemented.

Development of Family-Centered Child Care

Family-centered child health care was born out of the recognition that the emotional needs of hospitalized children usually were unmet. Parents were not involved in the direct care of their children. Children were often unprepared for procedures and tests, and visiting was severely controlled and even discouraged.

Family-centered care is based on a philosophy that recognizes and respects the pivotal role of the family in the lives of both well and ill children. It strives to support families in their natural caregiving roles and promotes healthy patterns of living at home and in the community. Finally, parents and professionals are viewed as equals in a partnership committed to excellence at all levels of health care.

In health care settings that have a family-centered philosophy, families are given choices, provide input, and are given information that is understandable by them. The family is respected, and its strengths are recognized.

The Association for the Care of Children's Health (ACCH), an interdisciplinary organization, was founded in 1965 to provide a forum for sharing experiences and common problems and to foster growth in children who must undergo hospitalization. Today the organization has broadened its focus on child health care to include the community and the home.

Through the efforts of ACCH and other organizations, increasing attention has been paid to the psychologic and emotional effects of hospitalization during childhood. In response to greater knowledge about the emotional effects of illness and hospitalization, hospital policies and health care services for children have changed. Twenty-four-hour parental visitation and sibling visitation policies and home care services have become common. The psychologic preparation of children for hospitalization and surgery has become standard nursing practice. Many hospitals have established child life programs to help children and their families cope with the stress of illness. Shorter hospital stays, home care, and day surgery have also helped to minimize the emotional impact of hospitalization and illness on children.

CURRENT TRENDS IN MATERNITY AND CHILD HEALTH CARE

In the past few years the government, insurance companies, hospitals, and health care providers have made a concerted effort to reform health care delivery in the United States and to control rising costs. This trend has involved a change in where and how money is spent. In the past, most of the health care budget was spent in acute care settings, where the facility charged for services after the services were provided. Because hospitals were paid for whatever materials and services they provided, they had no incentive to be efficient or cost-conscious.

Cost Containment

One way in which those paying for health care have attempted to control costs is by shifting to a *prospective* form of payment. In this arrangement, clients no longer pay whatever charges the hospital decides on for service provided. Instead, a fixed amount of money is agreed to in advance for necessary services for specifically diagnosed conditions. Any of several strategies may be used to contain the cost of services.

Diagnosis-Related Groups

Diagnosis-related groups (DRGs) are a method of classifying related medical diagnoses based on the amount of resources that are generally required by the client. This method became a standard in 1987, when the federal government set the amount of money that would be paid by Medicare for each DRG. If the facility delivers more services or has greater costs than what it will be reimbursed for by Medicare, the facility must absorb the excess costs. Conversely, if the facility delivers the care at less cost than the payment for that DRG, the facility keeps the remaining money. Health care facilities working under this arrangement benefit financially if they can reduce the client's length of stay and thereby reduce the costs for service. Although the DRG system originally applied only to Medicare clients, most states have adopted the system for Medicaid payments, and many insurance companies use a similar system.

Managed Care

Health insurance companies also examined the cost of health care and instituted a health care delivery system that has been called *managed care*. Examples of managed care organizations are health maintenance organizations (HMOs), point of service plans (POSs), and preferred provider organizations (PPOs). HMOs provide relatively comprehensive health services for persons enrolled in the organization for a set fee or premium. Similarly, PPOs are groups of health care providers who agree to provide health services to a specific group of clients at a discounted cost. When the client needs medical treatment, managed care includes strategies such as payment arrangements and preadmission or pretreatment authorization to control costs.

Capitated Care

Capitation may be incorporated into any type of managed care plan. In a pure capitated care plan, the employer (or government) pays a set amount of money each year to a network of primary care providers. This amount might be adjusted for age and sex of the client group. In exchange for access to a guaranteed client base, the primary care providers agree to provide general health care and to pay for all aspects of the client's care, including laboratory work, specialist visits, and hospital care.

Capitated plans are of interest to both employers and the government because they allow a predictable amount of money to be budgeted for health care. Clients do not have unexpected financial burdens from illness. However, clients lose most of their freedom of choice regarding who will provide their care. Providers can lose money (1) if they refer too many clients to specialists, who may have no restrictions on their fees, (2) if they order too many diagnostic tests, or (3) if their administrative costs are too high. Some health care providers and consumers fear that cost constraints might affect treatment decisions.

Effects of Cost Containment

Prospective payment plans have had major effects on maternity care, primarily in relation to the length of stay. Mothers who have a normal vaginal birth are typically discharged from the hospital at 48 hours, and mothers who give birth by cesarean section leave at 96 hours. Many mothers and infants developed problems with shorter lengths of stay, sometimes called "drive-through deliveries," that were mandated under early prospective pay arrangements. The problems often required disruptive readmission and more expensive treatment than might have been needed if the problem had been identified early. As a result, many states passed legislation requiring a minimum 48-hour length of stay for vaginal births and 4 days for cesarean births, unless the woman and her health care provider choose an earlier discharge time. Some insurance plans use a compromise, in which the woman who elects to leave 24 hours after vaginal birth is provided one or more home visits by a nurse to check on her status and that of her baby.

Reduced lengths of stays have also affected caregivers, particularly nurses. Since the mid-1990s, nurses have become increasingly concerned with meeting the needs of families who leave the hospital a short time after the birth of an infant. Nurses find it especially difficult to provide adequate information about self-care and infant care when the mother is still recovering from childbirth.

Concerns related to managed care and the care of children include financial disincentives to provide appropriate pediatric referrals; delays in treatment authorization; obstacles to access of specialty care, particularly for chronically ill persons; the unique vulnerability of developing children that requires comprehensive health promotion as well as prompt episodic care; and concerns about profit limiting health care access for vulnerable families (Center for the Future of Children, 1998).

Managed care, provided appropriately, can increase access to a full range of health care providers and services, but it must be closely monitored. Child health nurses serve as child advocates in the areas of preventive, acute, and chronic care. The teaching timelines for preventive and home care have been shortened drastically, and the call to "begin teaching the moment the child enters the health care system" has taken on a new meaning. Parents and other caregivers are being asked to do procedures at home that were once done by professionals in a hospital setting. Systems must be in place to monitor compliance, understanding, and the total care of the child. Assessment and communication skills need to be keen, and the nurse must be able to work with specialists in other disciplines.

Case Management

Case management is a practice model that uses a systematic approach to identify specific clients and to manage care collaboratively to ensure optimal outcomes through access to the best available resources (Alfaro-LeFevre, 2004). In this model, a case manager or case coordinator, who focuses on both quality and cost outcomes, coordinates the services needed by the client and family. Inherent to case management is the coordination of care by all members of the health care team. The guidelines established in 1995 by the Joint Commission on the Accreditation of Healthcare Organizations require an interdisciplinary, collaborative approach to client care. This concept is at the core of case management. Nurses who provide case management evaluate client needs, establish needs documentation to support reimbursement, and may be part of long-term care planning in the home or a rehabilitation facility.

Clinical Practice Guidelines

The Agency for Healthcare Research and Quality (AHRQ), a branch of the United States Public Health Service, is actively sponsoring research in health issues facing women. From research generated through this agency as well as others, evidence can be accumulated to guide the best clinical practices. Priority women's health issues for the AHRQ include disparity of care among women in racial minorities, rural women's health needs, and health care for women with chronic illness and disabilities. Other major areas for ongoing research include women's cardiovascular disease, breast and cervical cancer, hysterectomy and alternatives, domestic violence, human immunodeficiency virus (HIV) and acquired immunodeficiency syndrome (AIDS) in women, and reproductive concerns (Agency for Healthcare Research and Quality [AHRQ], 2001, 2002). For detailed information, see the website at www.ahcpr.gov.

Clinical practice guidelines are an important tool in developing guidelines for safe, effective care. AHRQ has developed several guidelines related to adult and child care (AHRQ, 2003). Guidelines for the following areas of child health have been released: acute pain management, sickle cell disease, management of cancer pain, and otitis media with effusion. Continued research and sharing of information in this area are needed to ensure quality case management.

Outcomes Management

The determination to lower health care costs while maintaining the quality of care has led to a clinical practice model called *outcomes management*. This is a systematic method to identify client outcomes and to focus care on interventions that will accomplish the stated outcomes for specific case types, such as the woman who has just given birth or the child with asthma. The planning tools used by the health care team to identify and meet stated outcomes are *clinical pathways*. Other names for clinical pathways include *critical* or *clinical paths*, *care paths*, *care maps*, *collaborative plans of care*, *anticipated recovery paths*, and *multidisciplinary action plans*.

Clinical Pathways

Clinical pathways are standardized, interdisciplinary plans of care devised for clients with a particular health problem. Clinical pathways identify client outcomes, specify time lines to achieve those outcomes, direct appropriate interventions and sequencing of interventions, include interventions from a variety of disciplines, promote collaboration, and involve a comprehensive approach to care. Although the concept of clinical pathways is not new, it has only recently been widely accepted as the use of case management has become widespread in various health care settings. The purpose, as in managed care and case management, is to provide quality care while controlling costs.

Clinical pathways can be used in settings other than the hospital. Home health agencies use clinical pathways, which may be developed in collaboration with hospital staff.

Facilities differ in how they use clinical pathways. For instance, they may be used for change-of-shift reports to indicate information about length of stay, individual needs, and priorities of the shift for each client. They may also be used for documentation of the client's nursing care plan and his or her progress in meeting the desired outcomes. Many pathways are particularly helpful in identifying families that need follow-up care (see pp. 266-267 for an example of a clinical pathway).

Variances. Deviations, often called *variances*, may occur, either in the time line or in the expected outcomes. A variance is the difference between what was expected and what actually happened. A variance may be positive or negative. A positive variance occurs when a client progresses faster than expected and is discharged sooner than planned. A negative variance occurs when progress is slower than expected, outcomes are not met within the designated time frame, and the length of stay is prolonged.

Students' Use of Clinical Pathways. Clinical pathways are guidelines for care. Although a pathway provides insight into the scheduling of assessments and care, it is not meant to teach nursing skills and procedures. One purpose of this book is to provide ample information so that students can *use* clinical pathways in a clinical setting. This involves teaching *why and how to perform assessments* and interpreting the significance of the data obtained. Moreover, the book emphasizes ways of providing information, care, and comfort for clients and their families as they progress along a clinical pathway.

HOME CARE

Home nursing care has experienced dramatic growth since 1990. Advances in portable technology, such as infusion pumps for the administration of intravenous nutrition or subcutaneous medications and various monitoring devices, allow nurses to perform complicated procedures in the home. In addition, consumers often prefer home care because of decreased stress on the family when the client is able to remain at home rather than be separated from the family support system because of the need for hospitalization.

Home care services may be provided in the form of telephone calls, home visits, information lines, and lactation consultations, among others. Infants with congenital anomalies, such as cleft palate, may need care that is adapted to their condition. Moreover, increasing numbers of technology-dependent infants and children are now cared for at home. The numbers include those needing ventilator assistance, total parenteral nutrition, intravenous medications, apnea monitoring, and other device-associated nursing care.

Nurses must be able to function independently within established protocols and must be confident of their clinical skills when providing home care. They should be proficient at interviewing, counseling, and teaching. They often assume a leadership role in coordinating all the services a family may require, and they frequently supervise the work of other care providers.

A model for community care of children is the school-based health center. Many school districts in the United States are putting full-service health centers in school buildings as new schools are built or older schools renovated. School-based health centers provide immediate medical treatment for schoolchildren, one-on-one health counseling, well-child care, immunizations, health education in the classroom, collaboration with school personnel, and other support services (Rienzo, Button, & Wald, 2000; Shuler, 2000). A major goal for school-based health centers is to address physical and psychosocial health barriers to learning, including increasing access to appropriate health care. Some school-based health centers are independent, and some are operated by hospitals. Many are used in off-hours to provide health care to uninsured adults and adolescents.

HEALTH INSURANCE

The number of uninsured children in the United States is beginning to decrease because of concerted efforts brought about by the Federal Government's commitment to providing health care access to children (United States Department of Health and Human Services [USDHHS], 2000). About 92% of children have some form of health insurance, either privately or publicly funded. Public health insurance for children is provided primarily through Medicaid or the State Children's Health Insurance Program, but it is also provided through Medicare and the Tricare Standard. The number of children younger than 18 years covered by private health insurance decreased from 74% in 1987 to 64% in 2002. During the same period, the proportion of children covered by public health insurance increased from 19% to 27% (Centers for Disease Control and Prevention [CDC], 2003a). The Centers for Disease Control and Prevention (CDC, 2003a) reports a significant

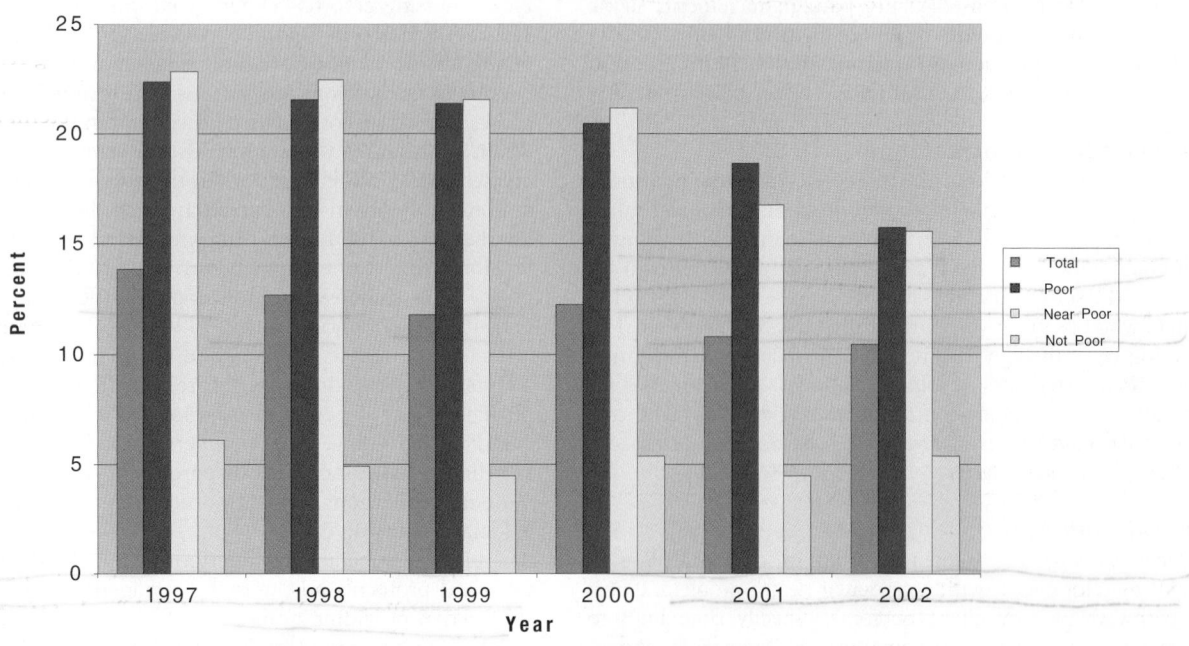

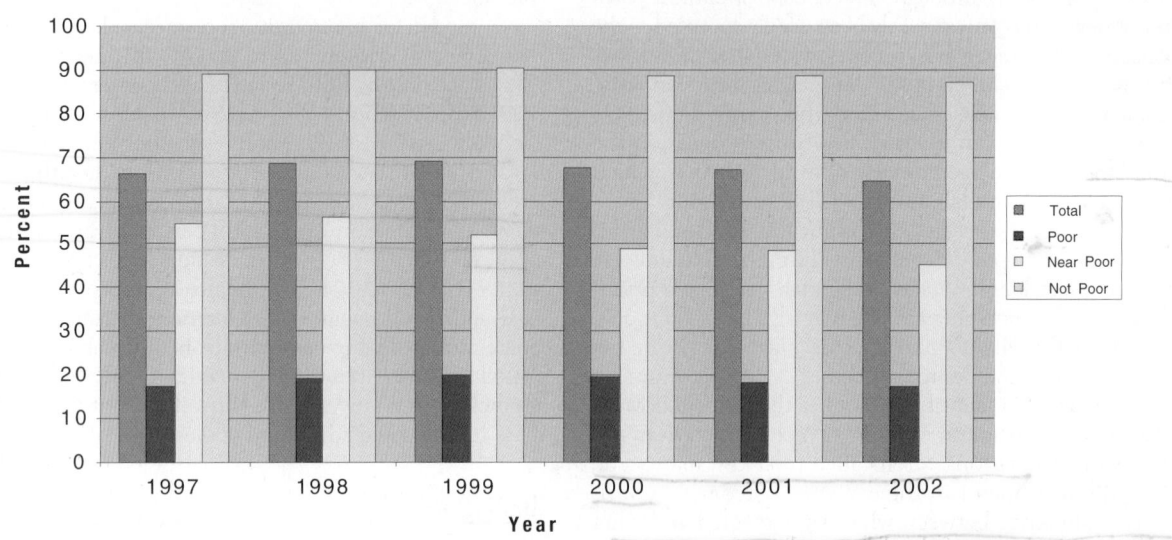

Figure 1-2 Percentage of children under 18 years of age with no health insurance and with private health insurance, by family income. (From Centers for Disease Control and Prevention, National Center for Health Statistics. *National Health Interview Survey, 2002.*)

decrease in private health insurance coverage for children whose families are classified as near poor or not poor (Fig. 1-2). Hispanic children are less likely to have health insurance than either white or African-American children (USDHHS, 2000).

Children in the United States remain uninsured for any of the following reasons (Sochalski, 1999):

- Most uninsured children live in families whose income is less than twice the federal poverty level.
- The parent's employer does not provide private health insurance, despite the fact that the parent is employed full time.
- Children who are ethnic minorities are less likely to be insured.

- Welfare reform has resulted in larger numbers of children not eligible for Medicaid benefits because of the welfare-to-work initiatives.
- Parents leaving welfare rolls are more likely to find low-paying jobs that do not provide insurance.
- Welfare administrators are not conscientious about informing families in the welfare-to-work program that their children are still eligible for Medicaid benefits.

Besides the obvious implication of not having health insurance—the inability to pay for health care during illness—there is another very important effect on children and adults who are not insured: they are less likely to receive preventive care such as prenatal care or immunizations. This places them at increased risk for preventable illnesses, and, because preventive health care is a learned behavior, these children are more likely to become adults who are less healthy. Complications of pregnancy or illness are more likely to be severe if they occur, and the fetus is more likely to be born prematurely or with a low birth weight. Therefore the lack of health insurance for adults and children is likely to cost society more.

Another issue related to health insurance and adolescents is the recently executed Health Insurance and Portability Accountability Act (HIPAA) regulations. Because HIPAA regulations do not supercede state regulations regarding confidentiality under certain circumstances (e.g., substance abuse, contraceptive education and access), states might be more likely to enact more privacy restrictions that would adversely affect confidentiality for adolescent health services. The consequence could be increased reluctance on the part of adolescents to access services they need (Maradiegue, 2002).

HEALTH CARE ASSISTANCE PROGRAMS

Many programs, some funded privately, others by the government, assist in the care of mothers, infants, and children. The supplemental food program known as the WIC program, which was established in 1972, provides supplemental food supplies to low-income women who are pregnant or breast-feeding and to their children up to the age of 5 years. The WIC program has long been heralded as a cost-effective program that not only provides nutritional support but also links families with other services, such as prenatal care and immunizations.

Medicaid's Early and Periodic Screening, Diagnosis, and Treatment Program was developed to provide comprehensive health care to Medicaid recipients from birth to 21 years of age. The goal of the program is to prevent health problems before they become severe. This program pays for well-child examinations and for the treatment of any medical problems diagnosed during such checkups.

Public Law 99-457 is part of the Individuals With Disabilities Act that provides financial incentives to states to establish comprehensive early intervention services for infants and toddlers with or at risk for developmental disabilities. Services include screening, identification, referral, and treatment. Although this is a federal law and entitlement, each state bases coverage on its own definition of developmental delay. Thus coverage may vary from state to state. Some states provide care for at-risk children.

The Healthy Start Program, begun in 1991, is a major initiative to reduce infant deaths in communities with disproportionately high infant mortality rates. Strategies used include reducing the number of high-risk pregnancies, reducing the number of low-birth-weight and preterm births, improving birth-weight-specific survival, and ameliorating specific causes of postneonatal mortality.

The March of Dimes, long an advocate for improving the health of infants and children, has launched a 5-year campaign to reduce the devastating toll that prematurity takes on the population. Between 1981 and 2001, the incidence of prematurity increased 27 percent, often resulting in perma-nent health or developmental problems for survivors of early birth (www.modimes.org/prematurity).

The March of Dimes prematurity campaign involves:

- Identifying causes of preterm birth by funding research
- Educating families about prevention and early identification of preterm labor before it results in preterm birth
- Helping health care providers learn how to reduce the incidence of preterm delivery

STATISTICS ON MATERNAL, INFANT, AND CHILD HEALTH

Statistics are important sources of information about the health of groups of people. They may also be an indication of the value a society places on health care and the kind of health care available to the people. The newest statistics about maternal, infant, and child health for the United States can be obtained from the National Center for Health Statistics (www.cdc.gov/nchs).

Maternal and Infant Mortality

Throughout history, women and infants have had high death rates, especially around the time of childbirth. Infant and maternal mortality rates began to fall when the health of the general population improved, basic principles of sanitation were put into practice, and medical knowledge increased. A further large decrease was a result of the widespread availability of antibiotics, improvements in public health, and better prenatal care in the 1940s and 1950s. Today, mothers seldom die in childbirth and the infant mortality rate is falling, although the rate of change has slowed for both. Racial inequality of maternal and infant mortality rates continues, with nonwhite groups having higher mortality rates than white groups.

Maternal Mortality

In 2001 the maternal mortality rate was 9.9 per 100,000 live births for all women in the United States. African-American women are more likely to die from birth-related causes than white women. The maternal mortality rate for African-American women is 24.7, whereas for white women it is 7.2 (Arias, et al, 2003). The rate is higher if compared with previous years because deaths that were aggravated by pregnancy are now included, even if they occur more than 42 days after the end of pregnancy.

Infant Mortality

Between 1950 and 1990, infant mortality dropped from 29.2 to 9.2 deaths per 1000 live births. In 2001 the infant mortality rate (death before the age of 1 year) was 6.8 per 1000 live births, the lowest ever recorded in the United States. Moreover, the neonatal mortality rate (death before 28 days of life) dropped to 4.5 deaths per 1000 live births. The fall in infant mortality is attributed to better neonatal care and to public awareness campaigns such as the "Back to Sleep" campaign to reduce the occurrence of sudden infant death syndrome (Anderson & Smith, 2003; Freid, et al., 2003).

Although infant mortality rates in the United States have declined overall, rates have declined faster for whites than for non-Hispanic African-American infants. The mortality rate in 2001 for white infants was 5.7. For African-American infants the rate was 14.0 (Anderson & Smith, 2003). Figure 1-3

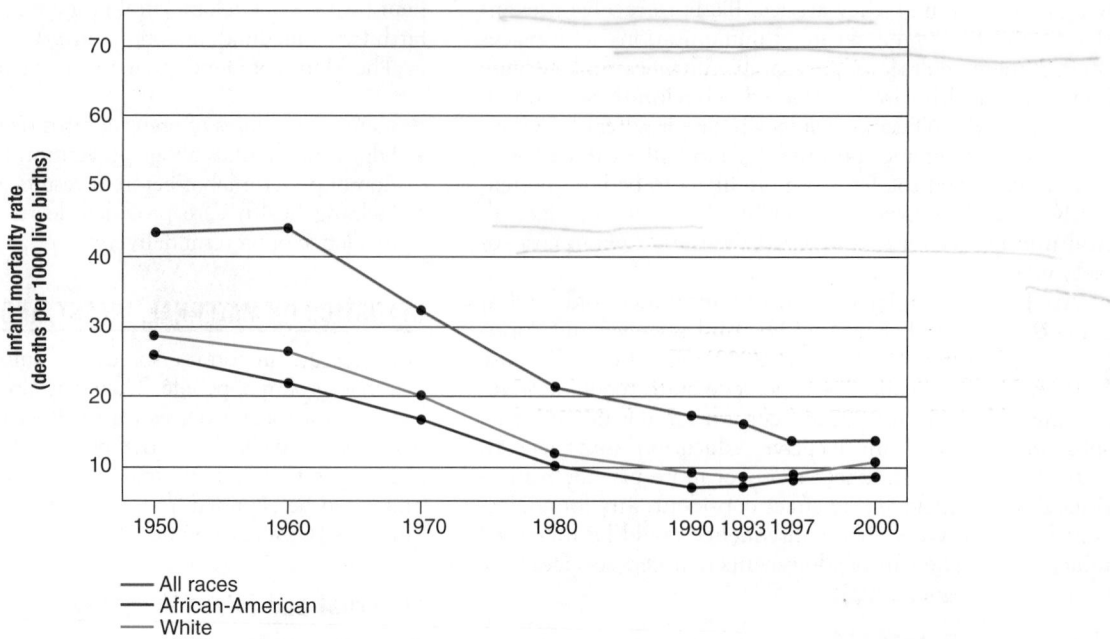

Figure 1-3 Infant mortality rates from 1950 to 2000 based on deaths before 1 year per 1000 live births. (From Centers for Disease Control and Prevention. (2002d). Infant mortality statistics from the 2000 period linked birth/infant death data set. *National Vital Statistics Reports, 50*(12). Retrieved June 16, 2003, from www.cdc.gov/nchs/data/nvsr/nvsr50/nvsr50_12.pdf.)

BOX 1-2
Infant Mortality Rates for Selected Countries (Based on 1999 Data)

Country	Infant Mortality (per 1000 Live Births)
Hong Kong	3.1
Japan, Sweden	3.4
Singapore	3.5
Finland	3.7
Norway	3.9
Denmark	4.2
France	4.3
Austria	4.9
Germany, Spain	4.5
Czech Republic, Switzerland	4.6
Belgium	4.9
Scotland	5
Italy	5.1
Netherlands	5.2
Canada	5.3
Ireland, New Zealand	5.5
Portugal	5.6
Australia, Israel	5.7
England and Wales	5.8
Greece	6.2
Northern Ireland, Cuba	6.4
United States	7.1

From Freid, V.M., Prager, K., MacKay, A.P., and Xia, H. (2003). *Health, United States, 2003, with trends in the health of Americans.* Hyattsville, MD: National Center for Health Statistics.

compares the rates of infant mortality for all races and for whites and African-Americans since 1950.

Racial Disparity for Mortality. The racial differences in both maternal and infant mortality rates are obvious when rates for African-Americans are compared with those for other races. Much of the racial disparity for infant mortality is attributable to premature (born before 37 weeks) and low-birth-weight infants (below 2500 g), both more common among African-American infants. Premature and low-birth-weight infants have a greater risk for short-term and long-term health problems as well as death (Anderson & Smith, 2003).

Poverty is an important factor. Proportionally more non-whites than whites are poor in the United States. Poor people are less likely to be in good health, to be well nourished, or to get the health care they need. Obtaining care becomes vital during pregnancy and infancy, and lack of care is reflected in the high mortality rates in all categories.

International Infant Mortality. One would expect that a nation such as the United States would have one of the lowest infant mortality rates when compared with other developed countries. The most recent year for which comparative international data on infant mortality are available is 1999, slightly older than data for the United States only. These data show that the mortality rate in the United States is 28th (Box 1-2) (Freid, Prager, MacKay, & Xia, 2003). International rankings are difficult to compare because countries differ in how and when they compute statistics, but the numbers show the need for improvement in the United States.

The major reasons for the poor U.S. showing are (1) unequal access to health care for women of different socioeconomic levels and (2) excess low birth weight and premature infants. Congenital anomalies, sudden infant death syndrome, problems related to pregnancy complications, and respiratory distress syndrome are also leading causes of infant mortality.

Adolescent Pregnancy

United States adolescent birth rates have fallen to an historic low in 2001. The rate has decreased from 62.1 per 1000 in 1991 to 43 per 1000 teenagers 15 to 19 years old in 2002. The lower adolescent birth rate reflects a lower overall birth rate and in the teen population because the population is rising. Births to younger African-American teenagers 15 to 17 years old have fallen more rapidly than other groups, from 86.7 per 1000 (1991) to 40 per 1000. The birth rate to the youngest mothers of all races, age 10 to 14 years, is now at the lowest ever, 0.7 per 1000 mothers in this youngest age-group (Martin, Hamilton, Sutton, et al, 2003). These rates are nearing the *Healthy People 2010* target rates for females 15 to 17 years old of 43 per 1000 girls (*Healthy People 2010* Online Documents, 2000).

Childhood Mortality

Death rates for children have significantly declined over the past 20 years. Table 1-1 shows the leading causes of death in children. Although death rates attributed to unintentional injury have also dropped, accidents are still the leading cause of death in children ages 1 to 19 years. Homicide is the fourth leading cause of death for children ages 1 to 14 years and the second leading cause for children older than 14 years (Anderson, 2003). Other common causes of death in children include cancer and chronic lower respiratory diseases. Self-inflicted injury is a leading cause of death in the adolescent population.

Morbidity

Morbidity describes illness. The morbidity rate is the ratio of sick to well persons in a population and is presented as the number of ill persons per 1000 population. This term is used in reference to acute and chronic illness as well as disability. Because morbidity statistics are collected and updated less frequently than mortality statistics, it is difficult to present current data in all areas of pediatrics.

Respiratory tract–related illnesses are the leading cause of morbidity in children. Children experience an average of six respiratory tract infections per year. Infectious diseases are the most common cause of school absenteeism (Feigin & Cherry, 1998). Statistics regarding morbidity related to particular disorders are presented throughout this book as the disorders are discussed.

The Youth Risk Behavior Surveillance System has identified categories of health risk behaviors among youth that contribute to increased morbidity: tobacco use; unhealthy dietary behaviors; inadequate physical activity; alcohol and other drug use; sexual behaviors that may result in HIV infection, other sexually transmitted diseases, and unintended pregnancies; and behaviors that result in intentional injuries (violence, suicide) and unintentional injuries (motor vehicle crashes) (CDC, 2002a).

There is a link between children living in poverty and poorer health outcomes. Children who live in families of higher income and higher education have a better chance of being born healthy and remaining so. Access to health care, the health behaviors of parents and siblings, and exposure to environmental risks are among the factors contributing to the disparity in children's health (National Institute of Child

TABLE 1-1 Death Rates (per 100,00): Ten Leading Causes of Death by Age-Group

Cause	1-4 Years	5-14 Years	15-24 Years
All causes	32.6	18.5	80.7
Accidents	11.7	7.3	35.5
Motor vehicle	4.2	4.3	27
All other	7.6	2.9	8.5
Congenital anomalies	3.1	1	1.1
Malignant neoplasms	2.6	2.6	4.3
Homicide and legal intervention	2.1	0.9	12.5
Diseases of the heart	1.1	0.6	2.4
Pneumonia and influenza	0.6	0.2	0.5
Human immunodeficiency virus infection	—	—	0.5
Septicemia	0.6	—	—
Benign neoplasms	0.4	0.3	—
Cerebrovascular diseases	0.3	0.2	0.5
Suicide	—	0.7	10.1
Chronic lower respiratory disease	—	0.3	0.5
All other causes	9.5	4.4	12.8

Data from a table of deaths and death rates for the 10 leading causes of death in specified age-groups: United States, preliminary data for 2000. Centers for Disease Control and Prevention. (2001). Deaths: Preliminary data for 2000. *National Vital Statistics Reports, 49*(12). Retrieved on July 9, 2003, from www.cdc.gov/nchs.

Health and Human Development [NICHHD], 1998; Velsor-Friedrich, 2003).

ETHICAL PERSPECTIVES ON MATERNAL AND CHILD NURSING

Maternal-child nurses often struggle with ethical and social dilemmas that affect families. Nurses must know how to approach these issues in a knowledgeable and systematic way.

Ethics and Bioethics

Ethics involves determining the best course of action in a certain situation. Ethical reasoning is the analysis of what is morally right and reasonable. *Bioethics* is the application of ethics to health care. Ethical behavior for nurses is discussed in various codes, such as the American Nurses Association Code for Nurses. Ethical issues have become more complex as developing technology has allowed more options in health care. These issues are controversial because there is lack of agreement over what is right or best and because moral support is possible for more than one course of action.

Ethical Dilemmas

An ethical dilemma is a situation in which no solution seems completely satisfactory. Opposing courses of action may seem equally desirable, or all possible solutions may seem undesirable. Ethical dilemmas are among the most difficult situations in nursing practice. Finding solutions involves applying ethical theories and principles and determining the burdens and benefits of any course of action.

> ## BOX 1-3
> ### Ethical Principles
>
> - _Beneficence_. One is required to do or promote good for others.
> - _Nonmaleficence_. One must avoid risking or causing harm to others.
> - _Autonomy_. People have the right to self-determination. This includes the right to respect, privacy, and the information necessary to make decisions.
> - _Justice_. All people should be treated equally and fairly regardless of disease or social or economic status.

Ethical Theories

Two major theories guide ethical decision making. Few people use one theory exclusively. Instead, they make decisions by examining both theories and trying to determine which one is more appropriate for the circumstances.

Deontologic Theory. The deontologic approach determines what is right by applying ethical principles and moral rules. It does not vary the solution according to individual situations. One example is the rule "life must be maintained at all costs and in all circumstances." Strictly used, the deontologic approach would not consider the quality of life or weigh the use of scarce resources against the likelihood that the life maintained would be near normal.

Utilitarian Theory. The utilitarian theory approaches ethical dilemmas by analyzing the benefits and burdens of any course of action to find one that will result in the greatest amount of good. With this theory, the appropriate actions may vary according to the situation. It is a pragmatic approach concerned with the consequences of actions more than the actual actions themselves. In its simplest form, this is an end-justifies-the-means approach. If the outcome is positive, the method of arriving at that outcome is less important.

Ethical Principles

Ethical principles are also important in solving ethical dilemmas. Four of the most important principles are beneficence, nonmaleficence, autonomy, and justice. Although principles guide decision making, in some situations it may be impossible to apply one principle without encountering conflict with another. In such cases, one principle may outweigh another in importance.

For example, treatments designed to do good may also cause some harm. A cesarean birth may prevent permanent harm to a fetus in distress. However, the surgery that saves the fetus also harms the mother, causing pain, temporary disability, and possible financial hardship. Both mother and health care providers may decide that the principle of beneficence outweighs the principle of nonmaleficence. A third possibility is that if the mother does not want surgery, the principles of autonomy and justice must also be considered. Is the mother's right to determine what happens to her body more or less important than the right of the fetus to fair and equal treatment (Box 1-3)?

Solving Ethical Dilemmas

Although using a specific approach does not guarantee a right decision, it provides a logical, systematic method for going through the steps of decision making.

Decision making in ethical dilemmas may seem straightforward, but it may not result in answers agreeable to everyone. Many agencies, therefore, have bioethics committees to formulate policies for ethical situations, provide education, and help make decisions in specific cases. The committees include a variety of professionals such as nurses, physicians, social workers, ethicists, and clergy members. The client and family also participate, if possible. A satisfactory solution to ethical dilemmas is more likely to occur when a variety of people work together.

Ethical dilemmas may also have legal ramifications. For example, although the American Medical Association has stated that anencephalic organ donation is ethically permissible, it may be illegal. In many states, the legal criteria for death include both cardiopulmonary and brain death.

Ethical Issues in Reproduction

Reproductive issues often involve conflicts in which a woman behaves in a way that may cause harm to her fetus or that is disapproved of by some or most members of society. Conflicts between a mother and fetus occur when the mother's needs, behavior, or wishes may injure the fetus. The most obvious instances are those involving abortion, substance abuse, or a mother's refusal to follow the advice of caregivers. Health care workers and society in general may respond to such a woman with anger rather than support. The rights of both mother and fetus must be examined, however.

Elective Abortion

Abortion was a volatile legal, social, and political issue even before the _Roe v. Wade_ decision by the U.S. Supreme Court in 1973. Before that time, states could prohibit abortion, making the procedure illegal. In _Roe v. Wade_, the court stated that abortion was legal anywhere in the United States and that existing state laws prohibiting abortion were unconstitutional because they interfered with the mother's constitutional right to privacy. The Supreme Court decision stipulated that (1) a woman could obtain an abortion at any time during the first trimester, (2) the state could regulate abortions during the second trimester only to protect the woman's health, and (3) the state could regulate or prohibit abortion during the third trimester, except when the mother's life might be jeopardized by continuing the pregnancy.

For many, a woman's constitutional right to privacy conflicts with a fetus's right to life. The Supreme Court did not rule, however, on when life begins. This omission provokes debate between those who believe life begins at conception and those who believe life begins when the fetus is viable, or capable of living outside the uterus. Those who believe life begins at conception may be opposed to abortion at any time during pregnancy. Those who believe life begins when the fetus can survive if born (currently about 24 weeks of gestation) may oppose abortion after that time. Nurses need to be knowledgeable about past Supreme Court decisions related to abortion and about the conflicting beliefs that divide society on this issue.

Conflicting Beliefs About Abortion. Perhaps no issue creates greater division or incites more powerful emotions among Americans than that of elective abortion. The issue recurs in every presidential campaign in the United States. Some people believe abortion should be illegal at any time because it deprives the fetus of life. In contrast, others believe that women have the right to control their reproductive

---

CRITICAL THINKING EXERCISE 1-1

The parents of an infant with anencephaly state that they would like to donate the organs from their dying infant to another infant who might live as a result. They feel that in this way their own infant will live on as a part of another baby. Although these transplants have been performed in the past, they are not currently performed because of the ethical concerns involved.

1. What is the deontologic view of this decision?
2. How does the opposing ethical view differ?
3. What ethical principles are involved? If such transplants became routine, what potential problems might arise?

---

function and that political discussion of reproductive rights is an invasion of the most private decisions of women.

Belief That Abortion Is a Private Choice. At the heart of political action to keep abortion legal is the conviction that women have the right to make decisions about their reproductive function on the basis of their own ethical and moral beliefs and that the government has no place in these decisions.

In 1999 the rate of legal abortion was 25.6 for every 100 live births, down from its high of 35.9 per 100 live births in 1980. Girls younger than 15 years had the highest abortion rate, 70.9 for every 100 live births (Freid, et al., 2003). Advocates of the legal right to abortion point out that abortion, either legal or illegal, has always been a reality of life and will continue to be so, regardless of legislation or judicial rulings. Advocates express concern about the unsafe conditions that accompany illegal abortion, citing the deaths that occurred as a result of illegal abortions performed before the *Roe v. Wade* decision.

Belief That Abortion Is Taking a Life. Many people believe that legalized abortion condones taking a life and feel morally bound to protect the lives of fetuses. Persons opposed to abortion have demonstrated their commitment by organizing to become a potent political force. They have willingly been arrested for civil disobedience when they attempted to prevent admissions to clinics where abortions are performed.

Legal Aspects of **Roe v. Wade.** Abortion has been a complex legal issue since 1973, and the U.S. Supreme Court has made major decisions that affect abortion law since that time. Some decisions have strengthened the original *Roe v. Wade* ruling, and others have weakened it. Because nurses should know about the legal history of abortion, some of these decisions are enumerated in the accompanying box. Legislation introduced in 1995 banning late-term abortions received a presidential veto because it did not provide an exception for when the mother's health is at risk. In late 2003, a new president signed a bill that banned late-term abortions into law. The late-term abortion bill was challenged immediately in court and will almost certainly come before the Supreme Court at some time (Box 1-4).

Implications for Nurses. As health care professionals, nurses are involved in the conflict between differing beliefs about abortion. Nurses have several responsibilities that cannot be ignored. First, they must be informed about the complexity of the abortion issue from a legal and ethical standpoint and know the exact regulations and laws in their state. Second, they must realize that, for many, abortion is an ethical dilemma that results in confusion, ambivalence, and personal distress.

BOX 1-4
Supreme Court Decisions on Abortion Since
Roe v. Wade

- *1976:* States cannot give a husband veto power over his wife's decision to have an abortion.
- *1977:* States do not have an obligation to pay for abortions as part of government-funded health care programs (considered by abortion rights advocates to be unfair discrimination against poor women who are unable to pay for an abortion).
- *1979:* Physicians have broad discretion in determining fetal viability, and states have leeway to restrict abortions of viable fetuses.
- *1979:* States may require parental consent for minors seeking abortions as long as an alternative, such as the minor getting a judge's approval, is also available.
- *1989:* Upheld a Missouri law barring abortions performed in public hospitals and clinics or performed by public employees. Also required physicians to conduct tests for fetal viability at 20 weeks of gestation.
- *1990:* States may require notification of both parents before a person younger than 18 years has an abortion. A judge can authorize the abortion without parental consent.
- *1992:* Validated Pennsylvania law imposing restrictions on abortions. The restrictions upheld include the following:
  —A woman must be told about fetal development and alternatives to abortion.
  —She must wait at least 24 hours after this explanation before having an abortion.
  —Unmarried women younger than 18 years must obtain consent from their parents or a judge.
  —Physicians must keep detailed records of each abortion, subject to public disclosure.
  —Struck down only one requirement of the Pennsylvania law: that a married woman must inform her husband before having an abortion.
- *1993:* Rescinded the so-called *gag rule,* which restricted the counseling that health care professionals (with the exception of physicians) could provide at federally funded family planning clinics.
- *1995:* Upheld a ruling that states cannot withhold state funds for abortions in case of pregnancies resulting from rape or incest or when the mother's life is in danger.
- *2000:* Struck down a Nebraska law making late-term abortions illegal. The Court held that the law placed undue burden on the pregnant woman because there was no provision for late abortion to protect the woman's health.

Next, they must also recognize that the issue is not a dilemma for many but is a fundamental violation of the personal or religious views that give meaning to their lives. Finally, it is essential that nurses acknowledge the sincere convictions and the strong emotions of people on all sides of the issue.

Personal Values. Nurses respond to abortion in ways that illustrate the complexity of the issue and the ambivalence that it often produces. For instance, some nurses have no objection to participating in abortions. Others do not assist with abortions but may care for women after the procedure. Some nurses assist with a first-trimester abortion but may object to later abortions. Many nurses are comfortable assisting in abortion if the fetus has severe anomalies but are uncomfortable in other circumstances. Some nurses feel that they could not provide care before, during, or after an abortion but that they are bound by conscience to try to dissuade a woman from the decision to abort.

Professional Obligations. Nurses have no obligation to support a position with which they disagree. Many states have laws that allow nurses to refuse to assist with the procedure if abortions violate ethical, moral, or religious beliefs. Nurses are obligated, however, to disclose this information before they are employed in an institution that performs abortions. It would be unethical for a nurse to withhold this information until assigned to care for a woman having an abortion and then refuse to provide care. As always, nurses must respect the decisions of women who look to nurses for care. If nurses feel that they are not able to provide compassionate care because of personal convictions, they must inform a supervisor so that appropriate care can be arranged.

Mandated Contraception

The availability of long-term contraceptives has led to speculation about whether certain women should be forced to use them. In fact, long-term contraception has been used as a condition of probation, allowing women accused of child abuse to avoid jail terms. Legislative efforts have been made to require women who receive public assistance to use long-term contraception.

Some feel that forced contraception is a way to prevent additional births to women considered unsuitable parents and a way to decrease government expenses for dependent children. This punitive approach to social and ethical problems, however, does not provide long-term solutions. In addition, coercing the poor to use birth control to limit the money spent supporting them is questionable both legally and ethically.

Such a practice would interfere with a woman's constitutional rights to privacy, to reproduction, to refusal of medical treatment, and to freedom from cruel and unusual punishment. Contraceptives may pose health risks to the woman. Other methods of limiting unwanted pregnancies, such as access to free or low-cost information on family planning, are more appropriate.

Fetal Injury

If a mother's actions cause injury to her fetus, the question of whether she should be restrained or prosecuted has both legal and ethical implications. In some instances, courts have issued jail sentences to women who have caused or who may cause injury to the fetus. This response punishes the woman and places her in a situation in which she cannot further harm the fetus. In other cases, women have been forced to undergo cesarean births against their will when physicians have testified that such a procedure was necessary to prevent injury to the fetus.

The state has an interest in protecting children, and the Supreme Court has ruled that a child has the right to begin life with a sound mind and body. Many states have laws requiring the reporting of evidence of prenatal drug exposure, which is considered child abuse. Women have been charged with negligence, involuntary manslaughter, delivering drugs to a minor, and child endangerment.

Yet forcing a woman to behave in a certain way because she is pregnant violates the principles of autonomy, self-determination of competent adults, bodily integrity, and personal freedom. Because of fear of prosecution, this practice could impede health care during pregnancy instead of advancing it. Women are unlikely to seek prenatal care or treatment for substance abuse unless they feel safe.

The punitive approach to fetal injury also raises the question of how much control the government seeking to protect the fetus should have over a pregnant woman. Laws could be passed mandating fetal testing, the use of tocolytics for preterm labor, intrauterine surgery, or even the foods a pregnant woman eats. It could be hard to decide just how much control should be allowed in the interests of fetal safety.

Fetal Therapy

Fetal therapy is in its early phases but may become more widespread as techniques improve. Although intrauterine blood transfusions are relatively standard practice in some areas, most fetal surgery is not yet routine.

The risks and benefits of surgery for major fetal anomalies must be considered in every case. Even if surgery is successful, the fetus may not survive, may have other serious problems, or may be born prematurely. The mother may need weeks of bed rest and a cesarean delivery. Yet in spite of the risks, successful surgery may result in the birth of an infant who could not otherwise have survived.

Parents need help in balancing the potential risks to the mother with the best interests of the fetus. There is a danger that they might feel pressured to have surgery or other fetal treatment they do not understand. As with any situation involving informed consent, women need adequate information before making a decision. They should understand whether procedures are still experimental, what the chances of success are, and what alternatives are available.

Issues in Infertility

Infertility Treatment. Perinatal technology has found ways for some infertile couples to bear children (see Chapter 10). There are many happy results from such practices when infertile couples are finally able to give birth, but infertility therapy has also raised many ethical questions.

Concerns include the high cost and overall low success of some treatments. Because the costs are usually not covered by insurance, their use is limited to the affluent. The high price of research on techniques that will benefit only a few has also been questioned. Some think that the money should be spent on research that will help a greater number of people. Even with high-technology treatments, many infertile couples will never give birth. Success rates for these procedures are still low. Also, when treatment is successful, the risk of multiple births and premature infants is higher, leading to newborn complications and expensive care associated with preterm birth.

Other ethical concerns focus on the fate of unused embryos. Should they be frozen for later use by the woman or someone else, or could they be used in genetic research? Who should make these decisions? In multiple pregnancies with more fetuses than can be expected to survive intact, reduction surgery may be used to destroy one or more fetuses for the benefit of those remaining. The ethical and long-term psychologic implications of this procedure are also controversial.

Assisted reproductive techniques now allow even postmenopausal women to become mothers. What are the ethical implications of giving birth to children who may very well be orphaned at an early age? Should the age and health of the parents be a factor in determining whether this treatment is offered? Should the risk these women face for developing complications that might result in low-birth-weight infants be considered?

Surrogate Parenting. In surrogate parenting, a woman agrees to bear an infant for another woman. Cases in which the surrogate mother has wanted to keep the child have been controversial. There are no standard regulations governing these cases, which are decided on an individual basis. Ethical concerns involve who should be a surrogate mother, whether she should have a role after birth, and who should make these decisions. Screening of parents as well as surrogates may be necessary to determine whether they are suitable for their roles. But who should do the screening? Should it be left to the private interests of those involved, or should the government become involved?

Ethical Concerns in Child Health Nursing

Cessation of Treatment. The decision to cease treatment is an ethical situation that is always difficult and seems to be compounded when the client is an infant or child. Children who would have died in the past can now have their lives extended through the use of life support. Parents must be involved in the decision-making process immediately and informed about available options. Laws in some states permit parents to provide advance directives for their minor children. When older children are involved, their views are considered.

In this age of resource allocation, debate centers on how to manage critical care resources. Many believe that these decisions should not be made at the bedside. The American Academy of Pediatrics, in its statement entitled *Ethics and the Care of Critically Ill Infants and Children* (1996), encouraged society to engage in a thorough debate about the economic, cultural, religious, social, and moral consequences of imposing limits on which patients should receive intensive care.

Terminating Life Support. Decisions to terminate life support systems continue to present gut-wrenching ethical and legal situations to nurses, especially when an infant or child is involved. Contrary to the common belief that such decisions should be determined by what is termed *quality of life*, the legal system plays a major role in this area of health care.

Frequently, parents become attached to a primary care nurse and request that the nurse participates in the decision as to whether to terminate life support for their child. A nurse might be faced with such a situation in the neonatal intensive care unit (NICU) with a teenage parent of a premature infant with a congenital defect or in a chronic care oncology unit with a terminally ill child. Ethical decisions may need to be made concerning the extremely low birth weight newborn or for the newborn born at the edge of viability.

In such instances a team conference should be arranged with the parents, primary nurse, physician, and a hospital staff attorney who is knowledgeable about applicable laws in that particular state. Problems may arise when there is a discrepancy among what families, physicians, and nurses think is best.

The issue of when first to discuss with adolescents the idea of cardiopulmonary resuscitation, mechanical ventilation, and do-not-resuscitate (DNR) orders is always sensitive.

Adolescents who have reached majority age must give consent if they are of sound mind. In most states, minority status ends at the age of 18 years.

SOCIAL ISSUES

Nurses are exposed to many social issues that influence health care and often have legal or ethical implications. Some of the issues that affect maternity and child health care include poverty, homelessness, access to care, and allocation of funds.

Poverty

Poverty is an underlying factor in problems such as inadequate access to health care and homelessness and is a major predictor for unmet health needs in children (Newacheck, Hughes, Hung, Wong, & Stoddard, 2000). The number of children living in households with cash incomes below the poverty level has stayed around 20% since 1981. Children younger than 6 years are more often found in families with incomes below the poverty line than are older children. Children in female-headed households are more likely to be living in poverty (Forum on Child and Family Statistics, 2000).

Poverty becomes a health issue because it affects access to health care and decreases opportunities linked with health promotion. Poverty rates in the United States are geographic. The southern and western portions of the country have disproportionately more of the nation's poor population.

Nurses can play a role in meeting the health care needs of mothers and their infants and children by recognizing the adverse effect of poverty on health and identifying poverty as a practice concern. Several goals in the *Healthy People 2010* goals (USDHHS, 2000) have implications for maternal-child nurses:

- To reduce the infant mortality rate to no more than 4.5 per 1,000 live births and the childhood mortality rate to 18.6 per 100,000 for children 1 to 4 years old and 12.3 per 100,000 for children 5 to 9 years old; to similarly reduce the rate of adolescent deaths.
- To reduce the incidence of low birth weight to no more than 5% of live births and the incidence of very low birth weight to 0.9% of live births.
- To ensure that 90% of all pregnant women receive prenatal care in the first trimester of pregnancy.
- To achieve and maintain effective vaccination coverage levels for universally recommended vaccines to 90% of children from 19 to 35 months of age and increase routine vaccination coverage for adolescents.
- To reduce vaccine-preventable diseases as follows: (1) measles, mumps and rubella to zero cases; and (2) pertussis in children younger than 7 years to no more than 2000 cases per year.
- To increase to 100% the proportion of persons with health insurance.

Poverty tends to breed poverty. In poor families, children may leave the educational system early, making them less likely to learn skills necessary to obtain good jobs. Childbearing at an early age is common and interferes with education and the ability to work. The cycle of poverty (Fig. 1-4) may continue from one generation to another as a result of hopelessness and apathy.

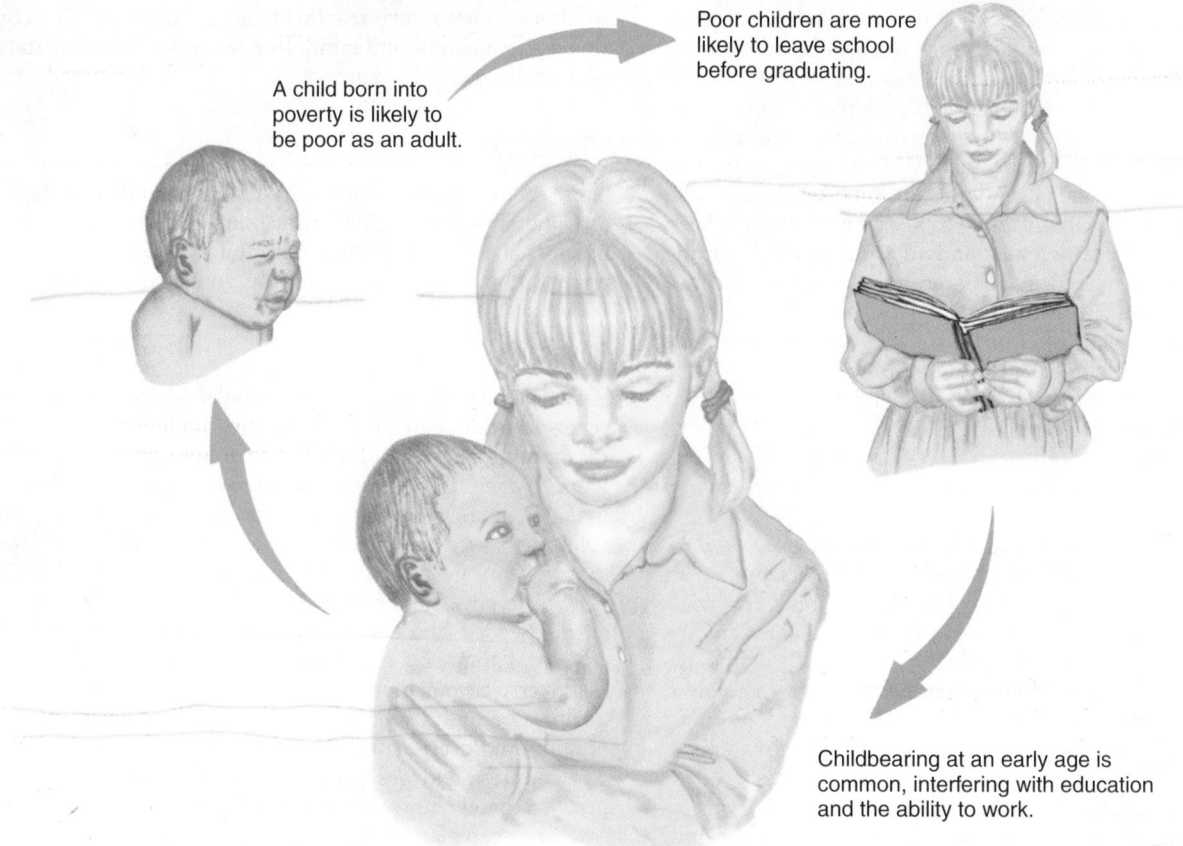

A child born into poverty is likely to be poor as an adult.

Poor children are more likely to leave school before graduating.

Childbearing at an early age is common, interfering with education and the ability to work.

Figure 1-4 The cycle of poverty.

Homelessness

Families, 84% of which are composed of single women and their children, are the fastest-growing group of homeless people. Some homeless women are substance abusers. Both homeless women and their children are poorly nourished and are exposed to tuberculosis, HIV infection, and sexually transmissible diseases. Rape and assault are problems, with a high rate of pregnancy among homeless girls. Infants born to homeless women are subject to low birth weight and having a greater likelihood of neonatal mortality (National Resource Center on Homelessness and Mental Illness, 2003a).

Pregnancy and birth, especially among teenagers, are important causes contributing to homelessness. Adolescent mothers are more likely to be single mothers and poor. Pregnancy interferes with a woman's ability to work and may decrease her income to the point at which she loses her housing. Without child care or a home address, she may have less chance of obtaining and keeping employment. In addition, her children are more likely to be sick because of inadequate food and shelter. Without money to pay for insurance or early health care, there is an increased chance that children will need hospitalization.

Federal funding has provided assistance with shelter and health care for homeless people. The homeless, however, have the same difficulties in obtaining health care as other poor people because of lack of transportation, inconvenient hours, and lack of continuity of care.

Access to Health Care

Even people with incomes above the poverty level may not be able to pay for health care. The working poor have jobs but receive wages that barely meet their day-to-day needs. They have little opportunity to save for emergencies such as serious illness. In 2001, 16.2% of the population younger than 65 years in the United States had no health insurance; this figure includes 11% of children younger than 18 years (Freid, et al., 2003). Millions of others have limited insurance and would not be able to survive financially should serious illness occur. People without insurance seek care only when absolutely necessary. Health maintenance and illness prevention may seem costly and unnecessary to them. Some receive no health care during pregnancy until they arrive at the hospital for birth.

A decline in private, employer-paid insurance coverage has decreased the number of privately insured American children. This decline has had a tremendous impact on the low-income worker who does not have employer-paid coverage and cannot afford individually purchased insurance. Although Medicaid has expanded its coverage and the State Children's Health Insurance Program (SCHIP) has enrolled many children of marginal income, some children still live in households whose families cannot afford to purchase private insurance and have not accessed public insurance programs. A recent federal initiative has begun to address this issue through community-wide publication of the Medicaid and SCHIP benefits and intense efforts to enroll children via schools and pediatricians' offices.

Prenatal Care in the United States

Prenatal care is widely accepted as an important element in improving the health of mothers and infants. In 2001, 83.4% of mothers had prenatal care in the first trimester of pregnancy. In the same year, 3.7% of mothers had prenatal care that began during the third trimester or did not have prenatal care. Poor prenatal care often occurs because care is not easily available (Freid, et al., 2003).

Lack of access to care contributes to the infant mortality rate and the large number of low-birth-weight infants born each year in the United States. Because preterm infants form the largest category of those needing intensive care, millions of dollars could be saved each year by ensuring adequate prenatal care. Even a small improvement in an infant's birth weight decreases complications and hospital time.

In some situations, women can obtain prenatal care but choose not to do so. These women may not understand the importance of the care or may deny they are pregnant. Some have had such unsatisfactory past experiences with the health care system that they avoid it as long as possible. Others want to hide substance use or other habits from disapproving health care workers. Language and cultural differences also play a part in whether a woman seeks prenatal care. Although these are not access issues as such, they must be addressed to improve health care.

Government Programs for Health Care: Medicaid

Having health insurance coverage, often employer-sponsored, often determines whether a person will seek care early. A major government program that increases access to health care for those not having private health insurance is Medicaid. Medicaid covered 22.9% of the U.S. population younger than 65 years in 2000. Medicaid provides health care for the poor, aged, and disabled, with pregnant women and young children especially targeted. Medicaid is funded by both the federal and the state governments. The states administer the program and determine which services are offered. Although there is variation among the states in just how poor one must be to qualify for assistance, all women at less than 133% of the current federal poverty level for income are eligible for perinatal care.

Medicaid has a number of problems. It often takes weeks for a client to go through the process to become eligible. The woman must fill out lengthy, complicated forms, provide documentation of income, and then wait for determination of eligibility. If a woman is not already enrolled at the beginning of her pregnancy, she is unlikely to finish the process in time to receive early prenatal care. Medicaid criteria may deny payment for some services that are routinely provided to those who hold private insurance. Welfare reforms instituted in 1996 made it more difficult for legal immigrants to become eligible for Medicaid. The Balanced Budget Act of 1997 resolved some of these issues, but foreign-born, non-English-speaking people find it excessively difficult to navigate the system of application (Truong & Ferguson, 2003).

Some physicians and dentists are unwilling to care for Medicaid clients who are likely to be at high risk. Many are especially unwilling if reimbursement is slow and less than that paid by other insurers. With their continual concern about malpractice suits, physicians may be less inclined to accept high-risk, lower-paying clients. Because only 1 in 5 children receiving Medicaid assistance obtain needed preventive dental care, access to dental care has been identified as a major priority for American children (Mouradian, Wehr, & Crall, 2000). In addition, maternal periodontal disease is emerging as a contributing factor to prematurity, with its adverse effects on the child's long-term health.

Greater restrictions on private insurance are blurring the distinction between private and public health coverage. Many private health plans have restrictions such as prequalification for procedures, drugs the plan covers, and services that will be covered at all. Persons with employer-sponsored health insurance often find that they must change providers each year because the available plans change, possibly impacting the provider-client relationship negatively.

Allocation of Health Care Resources

In 2001 the United States spent $1.4 trillion on health care. This amount is 13.3 percent of the gross domestic product—a larger percentage than any other major industrialized country (Freid, et al., 2003). Expenditures climb every year although the rate of growth slowed somewhat during the 1990s. However, the large population of "baby boomers," born from 1946 through 1964, are expected to need more health care dollars as they age.

Reforming health care delivery and financing is a complex area of national concern. How to provide care for the poor, the uninsured or underinsured, and those with long-term care needs are some areas that must be addressed. In addition, major acute care facilities often deal with greater financial burdens because of the growing numbers of uninsured clients presenting for treatment who are often very ill or severely injured. Escalating liability costs are another drain on health care dollars, leading some states to enact legislation that places a cap on awards for damages in malpractice cases.

Care Versus Cure

One problem to be addressed is whether the focus of health care should be on preventive and caring measures or on cure of disease. Medicine has traditionally centered more on treatment and cure than on prevention and care. Yet prevention not only avoids suffering but is also less expensive than treating diseases once they are diagnosed.

The focus on cure has resulted in technologic advances that have enabled some people to live longer, healthier lives. Financial resources are limited, however, and the costs of expensive technology must be balanced against the benefits obtained. Indeed, the cost of one organ transplant would pay for the prenatal care of many low-income mothers, possibly preventing the births of many low-birth-weight infants who may suffer disability throughout life.

In addition, quality-of-life issues are important in regard to technology. Neonatal nurseries are able to keep very-low-birth-weight babies alive because of advances in knowledge. Some of these infants go on to lead normal or near-normal lives. Others gain time but not quality of life. Families and health care professionals face difficult decisions about when to treat, when to terminate treatment, and when suffering outweighs the benefits.

Health Care Rationing

Modern technology has had a great impact on health care rationing. Some might argue that such rationing does not exist, but it occurs when some people have no access to care and there is not enough money for all people to share equally in the technology available. Health care is also rationed when it is more freely given to those who have money to pay for it than to those who do not.

Many questions will need answers as the costs of health care increase faster than the funds available. Is health care a fundamental right? Should a certain level of care be guaranteed to all citizens? What is that basic level of care? Should the cost of treatment and its effectiveness be considered when one is deciding how much government or third-party payers will cover? Nurses will be instrumental in finding solutions to these vital questions.

Violence

In today's society, women and children are the victims and sometimes the perpetrators of violence. Violence is not only a social problem but also a health problem. Acts of violence can include child abuse, domestic abuse, and murder. Children who live in an environment of violence feel helpless and ineffective. These children have difficulty sleeping and show increased anxiety and fearfulness. They may perpetuate the violence they see in their homes when they are adults because they have known nothing else in family relationships.

Although violent crimes among children have decreased over the past decade, violence in schools continues to rise, and for many children it is a daily stressor. Experts in the field of education have cited socioeconomic disparity, language barriers, diverse cultural upbringing, lack of supervision and behavioral feedback, domestic violence, and changes within the family as possible causes for the increased violence. Traditional approaches to aggressive behavior in the school, such as suspension, detention, and being sent to the principal's office, have been ineffective in changing behavior and serve only to exclude the student from education, leading to an increased dropout rate. Nurses must educate themselves on the issue of violence and, in turn, work with schools and parents to combat the problem. In addition, they should not ignore the child who is afraid to go to school or is having other school-related problems.

Children and adolescents are also exposed to violence via television, movies, video games, and youth-oriented music. Nurses should make this issue a part of anticipatory guidance. Parents should be encouraged to monitor their children's media exposure and limit their children's television viewing to 2 hours or less per day.

The American Academy of Pediatrics encourages clinicians to be concerned about adolescents who display aggressive or acting-out behaviors, such as lying, stealing, temper outbursts, vandalism, excessive fighting, and destructiveness. It further recommends that health care providers promote the responsibility of every family to create a gun-safe home environment. This includes asking about the presence of guns in the home at every well visit and counseling children,

parents, and relatives on the importance of firearm safety and the dangers of having a gun, especially a handgun.

Nurses working with children should ask them about violence in their school, home, or neighborhood, and whether they have had any personal experience with violent behavior. In some cases it may be necessary to contact parents, human resource departments, police, or other authorities to protect children and adolescents who are either in violent situations or at risk for violence.

LEGAL ISSUES

The legal foundation for the practice of nursing provides safeguards for health care and sets standards by which nurses can be evaluated. Nurses need to understand how the law applies specifically to them. When nurses do not meet the standards expected, they may be held legally accountable.

Safeguards for Health Care

Three categories of safeguards determine how the law views nursing practice: (1) state nurse practice acts, (2) standards of care set by professional organizations, and (3) rules and policies set by the institution employing the nurse. Additional information about nursing responsibilities is presented in Chapter 2.

Nurse Practice Acts

Every state has a nurse practice act that determines the scope of practice for registered nurses in that state. Nurse practice acts define what the nurse is and is not allowed to do in caring for clients. Some parts of the law may be very specific. Others are stated broadly enough to permit flexibility in the role of nurses. Nurse practice acts vary from state to state, and nurses must be knowledgeable about these laws wherever they practice.

In 1998 the National Council of State Boards of Nursing initiated a nurse licensure compact program. A nurse licensure compact allows a nurse who is licensed in one state to practice nursing in another participating state without having to be licensed in that state. Nurses must comply with the practice regulations in the state in which they practice. Since 1998, thirteen states have become participants in the nurse licensure compact program (National Council of State Boards of Nursing, 2003).

Laws relating to nursing practice also delineate methods, called *standard procedures* or *protocols*, by which nurses may assume certain duties commonly considered part of medical practice. The procedures are written by committees of nurses, physicians, and administrators. They specify the nursing qualifications required for practicing the procedures, define the appropriate situations, and list the education required. Standard procedures allow for changing the role of the nurse to meet the needs of the community and to reflect expanding knowledge.

Standards of Care

Courts have generally held that nurses must practice according to established standards and health agency policies, although these standards and policies do not have the force of law. Standards of care are set by professional associations and describe the level of care that can be expected from practitioners. For example, perinatal nurses are held to the specialty standards published by the Association of Women's Health, Obstetric, and Neonatal Nurses (AWHONN, www. awhonn.org). The Society of Pediatric Nurses is the primary specialty organization that sets standards for pediatric nurses. See Chapter 2 for additional information about professional organizations for maternity and pediatric nurses.

Other regulatory bodies, such as the Occupational Safety and Health Administration (OSHA), the Food and Drug Administration (FDA), and the Centers for Disease Control and Prevention (CDC), also provide guidelines for practice. Accrediting agencies, such as the Joint Commission on Accreditation of Healthcare Organizations and the Community Health Accreditation Program, give their approval after visiting facilities and observing whether standards are being met in practice. Governmental programs such as Medicare, Medicaid, and state health departments require that their standards are met for the facility to receive reimbursement for services.

Agency Policies

Each health care facility sets specific policies, procedures, and protocols that govern nursing care. All nurses should be familiar with those that apply in the facilities in which they work. Nurses are involved in writing nursing policies and procedures that apply to their practice and in reviewing or revising them regularly.

Accountability

Nursing accountability involves a knowledge of current laws. Accountability in child health nursing requires special consideration because the nurse must be accountable to the family as well as the child.

In 1984 the subject of disabled infants was addressed by the Child Abuse Amendments and delegated to state child protective agencies to investigate allegations of denial of necessary medical care. These regulations come into play when caring for children with symptoms of AIDS.

Both federal and state legislative bodies have addressed the issue of child abuse. Considerable variation exists among state laws in the investigative authority and procedures granted to child protective workers. When child abuse is suspected, issues often arise as to whether a health care provider may investigate the home situation and obtain relevant records.

A recent issue pertaining to nursing accountability is inadequate hospital staffing as a result of budget cuts. A nurse has a duty to communicate concerns about staffing levels immediately through established channels. A nurse will not be excused from responsibility (e.g., late medication administration or injury resulting from inadequate supervision of a client), just as a hospital will not be excused for insufficient staffing because of budget cuts.

Accountability also involves competency. If a nurse is not competent to perform a nursing task (e.g., to administer a new chemotherapeutic drug), or if a client's status worsens to the point at which the care needs are beyond the nurse's competency level (e.g., a client requiring hemodynamic monitoring), the nurse must immediately communicate this fact to the nursing supervisor or physician. The fact that a client's transfer to the intensive care unit (ICU) was requested but denied because the ICU was at full capacity is an insufficient defense in a charge of nursing negligence. In addition, the fact that a call was placed to a physician but there was no return call is no excuse for harm caused to a client be-

cause of delayed treatment. The nurse has an obligation to pursue needed care through the established chain of command at the facility.

Malpractice

Negligence is failure to perform the way a reasonable, prudent person of similar background would act in a similar situation. Negligence may consist of doing something that should not be done or failing to do something that should be done.

Malpractice is negligence by professionals, such as nurses or physicians, in the performance of their duties. Nurses may be accused of malpractice if they do not perform according to established standards of care and in the manner of a reasonable, prudent nurse with similar education and experience. Four elements must be present to prove negligence. They are duty, breach of duty, damage, and proximate cause.

Prevention of Malpractice Claims

Malpractice awards have escalated in both number and amount of awards to plaintiffs, resulting in high malpractice insurance for all health care providers. In addition, more health care workers practice defensively, accumulating evidence that they are acting in the client's best interest. For example, nurses must be careful to include detailed data when they chart. This responsibility is especially important in perinatal nursing because this is the area in which most lawsuits occur.

There are many reasons why perinatal nurses may become defendants in lawsuits. Complications are usually unexpected because parents view pregnancy and birth as normal. The birth of a child with a problem is a tragic surprise, and they may look for someone to blame. Although very small preterm infants now survive, some have long-term disabilities that require expensive care for the child's lifetime. Statutes of limitations vary in different states, but plaintiffs often have more than 20 years for lawsuits that involve a newborn. Therefore the period during which a malpractice suit may be filed is longer.

Prevention of claims is sometimes referred to as *risk management* or *quality assurance*. Although it is not possible to prevent all malpractice lawsuits, nurses can help defend themselves against malpractice judgments by following guidelines for informed consent, refusal of care, and documentation; acting as a client advocate; working within accepted standards and the policies and procedures of the facility; and maintaining their level of expertise.

Informed Consent. When clients receive adequate information, they are less likely to file malpractice suits. Informed consent is an ethical concept that has been enacted

---

> ! **CRITICAL** TO REMEMBER
> #### Elements of Negligence
>
> *Duty.* The nurse must have a duty to act or give care to the client. It must be part of the nurse's responsibility.
> *Breach of Duty.* A violation of that duty must occur. The nurse fails to conform to established standards for performing that duty.
> *Damage.* There must be actual injury or harm to the client as a result of the nurse's breach of duty.
> *Proximate Cause.* The nurse's breach of duty must be proved to be the cause of harm to the client.

BOX 1-5
Types of Advance Directives

Living Will	• Written document that directs withholding or withdrawing life-sustaining treatment if the client's condition is terminal. • Must be witnessed and/or notarized. Eligible witnesses may be specified by state law. • May provide some immunity from civil and criminal actions and from actions by licensing boards of the health care provider if the provider abides by the client's wishes.
Durable Power of Attorney for Health Care	• Written and witnessed document in which the client appoints an agent to make decisions for him or her about treatment options if the client is unable to do so. The client may be well for this document to be executed. • Many states do not allow a health care provider to serve as a witness. • May provide some immunity from civil and criminal actions and from actions by licensing boards of the health care provider if the provider abides by the client's wishes.
Medical Directive	• Allows the client to appoint a surrogate decision maker. • Often allows the client to provide instructions about care ahead of time. • Not based on state statutes, and protections for the client (right to cancel the directive; restrictions on allowed witnesses) and health care providers (immunity from legal action) may not exist.

Modified from Brent, N. J. (2001). *Nurses and the law: A guide to principles and applications* (2nd ed.). Philadelphia: Saunders.

into law. Clients have the right to decide whether to accept or reject treatment options as part of their right to function autonomously. To make wise decisions, they need full information about treatments offered. Without proper informed consent, assault and battery charges can result.

The law mandates what procedures require informed consent. The law mandates what to inform about as "risks" specific to each procedure. Nurses must be familiar with those procedures requiring consent.

Competence. Certain requirements must be met before consent can be considered informed. The first requirement is that the client be competent, or able to think through a situation and make rational decisions. A client who is comatose or severely mentally retarded is incapable of making such decisions. Minors are not allowed to give consent; however, children should have procedures explained to them in terms

CRITICAL TO REMEMBER
Requirements of Informed Consent

- Client's competence to consent
- Full disclosure of information
- Client's understanding of information
- Client's voluntary consent

appropriate for their age. In most states, minority status for informed consent ends at the age of 18 years.

A client who has received drugs that impair ability to think is temporarily incompetent. In these cases, another person is appointed to make decisions for the client if the client has not specified that person in advance.

Most states allow some exceptions for parental consent in cases involving emancipated minors. An *emancipated minor* is a minor child who has the legal competency of an adult because of circumstances involving marriage, divorce, parenting of a child, living independently without parents, or enlistment in the armed services. Legal counsel may be consulted to verify the status of the emancipated minor for consent purposes.

Most states allow minors to obtain treatment for drug or alcohol abuse or sexually transmitted diseases and to have access to birth control without parental consent. At present, laws governing adolescent abortion vary widely from state to state.

Client information about advance directives such as a living will, durable power of attorney for health care, and an alternate decision maker for the client must be assessed upon admission to the health care facility (Box 1-5). Assessment for existence of advance directives is often part of a nursing admission assessment. The client who has not made advance directives must be offered the opportunity to make these choices.

Full Disclosure. The second requirement is that of full disclosure of information, including what are the treatment's purpose and the expected results. The risks, side effects, and benefits as well as other treatment options must be explained to clients. The client must also be informed as to what would happen if no treatment were chosen.

For example, the National Childhood Vaccine Injury Act mandates that explanations about the risks of communicable diseases and the risks and benefits associated with immunizations should be given to all parents to enable them to make informed decisions about their child's health care. Parents need to know the common side effects and what to do in an emergency if any occur. The law stipulates that children injured by the vaccine must go through the administrative compensation system (funds from an excise tax levied on the vaccines) and reject an award before attempting to sue in a civil suit either the manufacturer or the person who gave the vaccine. Furthermore, the law mandates certain record-keeping and reporting requirements for nurses.

Understanding of Information. The client must comprehend information about proposed treatment. Health professionals must explain the facts in terms the person can understand. Nurses must be client advocates when they find that a client does not fully understand a treatment or has questions about it. If it is a minor point, the nurse may be able to explain it. Otherwise, the nurse must inform the physician so that the client's misunderstandings can be clarified.

Throughout hospitalization and discharge preparations, considerations should be given to those who do not understand the prevailing language and to the hearing impaired. Foreign language and sign language interpreters must be obtained when indicated. Provision for those who cannot read any language or adults with a low education level must be considered as well.

Voluntary Consent. Clients must be allowed to make choices voluntarily without undue influence or coercion from others. Although others can give information, the client alone, or the parent in the case of a child, makes the decision. Clients should not feel pressured to choose in a certain way or feel that their future care depends on their decision.

Children cannot legally consent for treatment or participation in research. However, children should give voluntary assent for research participation. Assent involves the principles of competence and full disclosure. Children should have the implications of the research (risks and benefits) explained in a way that is appropriate for their cognitive development. In general, children older than 7 years are cognitively capable of giving assent (Lindeke, Hauck, & Tanner, 2000).

The Committee on Pediatric Emergency Medicine has recently issued a policy regarding consent for emergency medical services for children and adolescents. The policy recommends that every effort be made to secure consent from a parent or legal guardian, but emergency treatment should not be denied if there are problems obtaining the consent (Committee on Pediatric Emergency Medicine, 2003).

Refusal of Care

Sometimes clients decline treatment, including hospitalization, offered by health care workers. Clients may refuse treatment when they believe that the benefits of treatment do not outweigh the burdens of the treatment or the quality of life they can expect after that treatment. Clients have the right to refuse care, and they can withdraw agreement to treatment at any time. When a person makes this decision, a number of steps should be taken.

First, the physician or nurse should establish that the client understands the treatment and the results of refusal. The physician, if unaware of the client's decision, should be notified by the nurse. The nurse documents on the chart the refusal, explanations given to the client, and notification of the physician. If the treatment is considered vital to the client's well-being, the physician discusses the need with the client and documents the discussion. Opinions by other physicians may be offered to the client as well.

Clients may be asked to sign a form indicating that they understand the possible results of rejecting treatment. This measure is to prevent a later lawsuit in which a client claims lack of knowledge of the possible results of a decision. If there is no ethical dilemma, the client's decision stands.

Refusal of care by a pregnant woman involves the life of the fetus, however, sometimes resulting in legal actions. One example is a woman's refusal of a cesarean birth, even though her refusal is likely to cause grave harm to the fetus. Outcomes of legal actions have been divided, some upholding the mother's right to refuse treatment and others ordering a treatment despite the mother's objections (Brent, 2001). Court action is avoided if possible, however, because it places the client, family, and caregiver in adversarial positions. In addition, it invades the client's privacy

and interferes with her autonomy and right to informed consent.

When parents refuse to give consent for what is deemed necessary treatment of a child, the state may be petitioned to intervene. The court may place the child in the temporary custody of the government or a private agency. The nurse may be asked to witness such a transaction when physicians act in cases of emergencies, such as a life-saving blood transfusion for a child despite parental objections based on religious beliefs.

Adoption

Nurses may care for infants involved in adoptions. The nurse may need to consult with the birth parents, adoptive parents, social workers, obstetrician, or pediatrician to determine the various rights of the child, birth parents, and adoptive parents (e.g., in matters concerning visitation rights, informed consent, or discharge planning).

In open adoptions, the birth mother may opt to room in with the baby during hospitalization. The birth mother and adoptive parents typically have had contact before the delivery and have an informal agreement regarding shared responsibility for the baby. The birth parent may even participate in discharge planning because she may have extended rights to visit the child after adoption.

Issues may develop as to the state of mind of the birth mother at the time of relinquishing parental rights (which cannot occur until after birth, unlike the relinquishment of the birth father's rights). State laws vary as to the legal time period necessary (1 day to several weeks after the birth of the child) before a birth mother can lawfully relinquish her rights to the child.

Some state laws allow the birth mother to relinquish her rights immediately after birth. In such cases, the nurse has the responsibility of protecting the birth mother and child to ensure that the birth mother is not coerced into making a decision while under the effects of medication. Factual documentation of such circumstances may be requested if the birth mother later asserts her rights to the child, claiming "undue influence" or "coercion."

Birth fathers have the same rights as the birth mother. Unless the birth father relinquishes his legal rights to the child, he may later assert his rights to the child after attachment has occurred with the adoptive parents. This situation may occur if the birth mother denies knowledge of the father's identity.

Documentation

Documentation, whether on paper or electronic media, is the best evidence that a standard of care has been maintained. All information recorded about a client should reflect that standard of care. This information includes nurses' notes, electronic fetal monitoring records, flow sheets, and any other data in the client record. In many instances, notations on hospital records are the only proof that care has been given. When documentation is not present, juries tend to assume that care was not given. Although documentation is not listed as a step in the nursing process, it is an integral part of the process.

Documentation must be specific and complete. Nurses are unlikely to be able to recall situations that happened years in the past and, if sued, must rely on their documentation to explain their care. Documentation must show that the standards of care and facility policies and procedures in effect at the time of the incident were met. Documentation must demonstrate that appropriate client assessment and continued monitoring, problem identification and provision of correct interventions, and communication of changes in client status to the primary care provider were done. If the nurse believes that the primary care provider has responded inappropriately, the nurse must refer the provider response through the appropriate chain of command for the facility and document the notification.

Documenting Discharge Teaching. Because of brief hospital stays, discharge teaching is essential to ensure that new parents know how to take care of themselves and their infants and that parents know how to care for their child. Nurses must document the teaching they perform as well as the client's understanding of that teaching. It is important to include information about the parents' degree of understanding of the teaching. The nurse should also note the need for reinforcement and how that reinforcement was provided. If follow-up home care is planned, teaching can be continued at home and documented on forms by the home care nurse.

Documenting Incidents. A type of documentation used in risk management is the *incident report*, often called a *quality assurance, occurrence,* or *variance report*. The nurse completes a report when something occurs that might result in legal action, such as in injury to a client or a departure from the expectations in the situation. The report warns the agency's legal department that there may be a problem. It also helps identify whether changing processes within the system might reduce the risk for similar incidents in the future. They are not intended to be punitive if an error was made. Incident reports are not a part of the client's chart and should not be referred to on the chart. Documentation of the incident on the chart should be restricted to the same type of factual information about the client's condition that would be recorded in any other situation.

The Nurse as Client Advocate

Malpractice suits may be brought if nurses fail in their role of client advocate. Nurses are ethically and legally bound to act as the client's advocate. This means that the nurse must act in the client's best interests at all times. When nurses feel that the client's best interests are not being served, they are obligated to seek help for the client from appropriate sources. This usually involves taking the problem through the chain of command established at the facility. The nurse consults a supervisor and the client's physician. If the results are not satisfactory, the nurse continues through administrative channels to the director of nurses, hospital administrator, and chief of the medical staff, if necessary. All nurses should know the chain of command for their workplaces.

In seeking help for clients, nurses must document their efforts. For example, if a postpartum woman experiences excessive bleeding, the nurse documents what was done to control the bleeding. The nurse also documents each time the physician was called about the problem, what information was given the physician, and the response received. When nurses cannot contact the physician or do not receive adequate instructions, they should document their efforts to seek instruction from others, such as the nursing supervisor or chief of medical staff for the specialty. They should also complete an incident report. It is essential that they continue in their efforts until the client receives the care needed.

Maintaining Expertise

Maintaining expertise is another way for nurses to prevent malpractice liability. To ensure that nurses maintain their expertise to provide safe care, most states require proof of continuing education for renewal of nursing licenses. Nursing knowledge changes rapidly, and it is essential that all nurses keep current. Incorporating new information learned by attending classes or conferences and reading nursing journals can help nurses perform the way a reasonably prudent peer would perform. Journals provide information from nursing research that may be important in updating nursing practice. It is important for all nurses to analyze research articles to determine whether changes in client care are indicated.

Employers often provide continuing education classes for their nurses. Many workshops and seminars are available on a wide variety of nursing subjects. Membership in professional organizations, such as state branches of the American Nurses Association or specialty organizations such as AWHONN and the Society of Pediatric Nurses, gives nurses access to new information through publications as well as nursing conferences and other educational offerings.

Maintaining expertise may be a concern when nurses "float" or are required to work with clients who have needs different from those of their usual clients. In these situations, the employer must provide orientation and education so that the nurse can perform care safely in new areas. Nurses who work outside their usual areas of expertise must assess their own skills and avoid performing tasks or taking on responsibilities in areas in which they are not competent. Many nurses learn to provide care in two or three different areas and are floated only to those areas. This system meets the need for flexible staffing while providing safe client care.

CURRENT TRENDS AND THEIR LEGAL AND ETHICAL IMPLICATIONS

Recent health care changes have affected the way nurses give care and may have legal and ethical implications as well. These changes result from efforts to lower health care costs. Two of special concern are the use of unlicensed assistive personnel and early discharge.

Use of Unlicensed Assistive Personnel

In an effort to reduce health care costs, many agencies have increased the use of unlicensed assistive personnel to perform direct client care and have decreased the number of nurses who supervise them. An unlicensed person may be trained to do everything from housekeeping tasks to drawing blood and performing other diagnostic testing to giving medications, all in the same day. This practice raises grave concerns about the quality of care clients receive when the nurse is responsible for the care of more clients but must rely on unlicensed persons to perform much of the care formerly provided by professionals. At the same time, use of an expert nurse for housekeeping and other mundane, but necessary, unit tasks is inefficient and detracts from available time for patient care. A balanced approach is needed when incorporating unlicensed assistive personnel into a unit's work.

Nurses must be aware of their legal responsibilities in these situations. They must know that the nurse is always responsible for client assessments and must make the critical judgments that are necessary to ensure client safety. Nurses must know what each unlicensed person caring for clients is able to do and must supervise them closely enough to ensure that they perform delegated tasks competently. More information about the use of unlicensed personnel is available in a position statement at www.awhonn.org.

Concerns About Early Discharge

Clients are discharged from the hospital quickly, usually no later than 48 hours after vaginal birth and often with minimal recovery from illness or surgery. Health care professionals are concerned about the ability of women to care for themselves or their infant or child when discharge occurs very early. Women may be exhausted from a long labor or complications and unable to take in all the information that nurses attempt to teach before discharge. Once home, many women must care for other children as well, often without family members or friends to help them.

While in the birth or acute care facility, professionals may detect indications of complications that may not be apparent to lay people. Mothers at home may not recognize the developing signs of serious maternal or neonatal infection or of jaundice, and care may be delayed until the illness is severe.

There may be legal issues if a client develops a complication after early discharge.

Dealing With Early Discharge

Nurses must establish ways of helping clients who go home soon after birth or parents who must take their child home when only slightly less ill or very soon after surgery. New teaching tactics may be necessary, with more teaching taking place during pregnancy when the mother's physical needs do not interfere with her ability to assimilate new knowledge. Parent teaching can be done before actual admission of a child for surgery. If a child is admitted when acutely ill, parent teaching begins almost immediately after admission. Nurses can take advantage of any "teachable moment" to provide clients with the information they need to better care for themselves.

Careful documentation and notification of the primary care provider are essential when abnormal findings develop so that clients are not discharged inappropriately. Methods of follow-up such as home visits, phone calls, or return visits by the families to the birth facility for nursing assessments in the first 24 to 48 hours after discharge have become increasingly important. Nursing case managers are often involved to identify and advocate for the best avenues for care and to facilitate extension of stay if the client's condition warrants.

KEY CONCEPTS

- Maternity and child health care in the United States have changed because of technologic advances, increasing knowledge, government involvement, and consumer demands.
- Family-centered maternity and child health care, based on the principle that families can make decisions about health care if they have adequate information, have greatly increased the autonomy of families and the responsibility of nurses.
- Prospective payment plans such as preferred provider organizations (PPOs) or health maintenance organizations (HMOs) control health care costs by negotiating reduced charges with providers such as facilities and physicians and by restricting client access to any provider of choice.
- Capitated plans are those in which a group of providers agrees to provide all services for a client for a set annual fee. If the client requires more costly care, the provider network pays those added charges. If the client requires less care than the annual fee, the network keeps the remaining money.
- Case management and outcomes management have resulted in new tools to reduce the length of stay for mothers and infants in the birth facility. Preparation for continuation of care at home begins as soon as the mother or child enters the health care system.

- Clinical pathways are interdisciplinary guidelines for assessments and interventions designed to accomplish the identified outcomes in the shortest time.
- Home care of clients has increased because of the need to control costs and because of the availability of portable technology.
- The number of uninsured adults and children continues to be excessive, reducing their chances of receiving preventive health care and increasing the costs of the late care they often seek.
- Infant and maternal mortality rates have declined dramatically in the past 50 years; however, the United States continues to rank well below other developed nations, and infant mortality rates still vary widely across ethnic groups.
- Accidents are the leading cause of death in children ages 1 to 19 years.
- Nurses must examine their beliefs and come to a personal decision about abortion before they are faced with the situation in their own practice. Nurses are obligated to share objections related to abortion care with their employer before the need to provide that care arises.
- Punitive approaches to ethical and social problems may prevent clients from seeking care, particularly preventive care.
- Poverty is a major social issue that leads to questions about allocation of health care re-

sources, access to care, government programs to increase health care to indigent women and children, and health care rationing.
- To give informed consent, the client must be competent, receive full information, understand that information, and consent voluntarily. The parents usually give consent for a minor child, although adolescents may be able to consent to their own treatment related to sexually transmitted diseases, contraception, and alcohol and drug abuse.
- Nurses are accountable for their practice and must be acquainted with laws, standards of care, and agency policies and procedures that affect their practice.
- Nurses can help defend malpractice claims by following guidelines for informed consent, refusal of care, and documentation and by maintaining their level of expertise.
- Documentation is the best evidence that the standard of care was met in client care. Therefore nurses must ensure that their documentation accurately reflects the care given.
- The nurse is the professional who decides what tasks may safely be delegated to unlicensed assistive personnel. In making such decisions, the nurse is guided by recommendations of the state licensing board, standards of care, and agency policy.

ANSWERS to Critical Thinking Exercise 1-1

1. The deontologic view is that it is wrong to take organs necessary for life from one human being to give to another, even when the donor cannot survive. This view disapproves of aggressive treatment necessary to maintain perfusion of the organs until a recipient is located because treatment does not help the dying infant and may increase suffering. This concern invokes the principle of nonmaleficence.

2. The utilitarian view is that anencephalic infants cannot survive but that their organs

could provide great benefit to other infants (beneficence). Because this family feels strongly that helping other infants allows good to come from their own tragedy, the greatest good would be for an organ transplant.

3. Potential problems include the possibility that transplants might someday be required, even against the parents' will (and might deny them autonomy). A woman might be forced to carry a pregnancy to term so that the organs can be harvested, even if the par-

ents would rather terminate the pregnancy. If anencephalic infants are used for organ donation, perhaps people with profound mental retardation or in persistent vegetative states might be placed in the same situation. Choosing infants to benefit would also be a concern, involving principles of justice. An overriding concern would be determining who would make the decisions necessary.

REFERENCES and READINGS

Agency for Healthcare Research and Quality. (2001). AHRQ Publication No. 012-PO12: Program brief: Women's health highlights. Rockville, MD: Author. Retrieved July 13, 2003, from www.ahcpr.gov/research/womenh1.htm.

Agency for Healthcare Research and Quality. (2002). AHRQ Publication No. 02-MO17: Health care for women. Rockville, MD: Author. Retrieved July 13, 2003, from www.ahcpr.gov/news/focus/focwomen.htm.

Agency for Healthcare Research and Quality. (2003). Clinical practice guidelines. Retrieved July 9, 2003, from www.ahrq.gov.

Alfaro-LeFevre, R. (2004). Critical thinking in nursing: A practical approach (3rd ed.). Philadelphia: Saunders.

American Academy of Pediatrics and American College of Obstetricians and Gynecologists. (2002). Guidelines for perinatal care (5th ed.). Elk Grove Village, IL, and Washington, DC: Author.

Anderson, R.N., & Smith, B.L. (2003). Deaths: Leading causes for 2001. National Vital Statistics Reports, 52(10). Hyattsville, MD: National Center for Health Statistics. Retrieved February 5, 2004, from www.cdc.gov/nchs/nvsr/nvsr52/nvsr52_09.pdf.

Arias, E., Anderson, R.N., Hsaing-Ching, K., Murphy, S.L., Kochanek, K.D. (2003). Deaths: Final data for 2001. National Vital Statistics Reports, 52(3). Hyattsville, MD: National Center for Health Statistics. Retrieved February 5, 2004, from www.cdc.gov/nchs/nvsr/nvsr52/nvsr52_03.pdf.

Association of Women's Health, Obstetric, and Neonatal Nurses. (2000). The role of unlicensed assistive personnel in the nursing care for women and newborns (Position statement). Retrieved June 23, 2003, from www.awhonn.org.

Association of Women's Health, Obstetric, and Neonatal Nurses. (2003). Standards for professional nursing practice in the care of women and newborns (6th ed.). Washington, DC: Author.

Badura, M. (1999). The Healthy Start Program: Mobilizing to reduce infant mortality and morbidity. Journal of Pediatric Nursing, 14(4), 263-265.

Bragadottir, H. (2000). Children's rights in clinical research. Journal of Nursing Scholarship, 32(2), 179-184.

Brent, N.J. (2001). Nurses and the law: A guide to principles and applications (2nd ed.). Philadelphia: Saunders.

Center for the Future of Children. (1998). The future of children: Children and managed health care (Vol. 8, No. 2). Los Altos, CA: David and Lucille Packard Foundation.

Centers for Disease Control and Prevention. (2002a). Chartbook on trends in the health of Americans. Author.

Centers for Disease Control and Prevention. (2002b). Deaths: Final data for 2000. National Vital Statistics Reports, 50(15). Retrieved June 16, 2003, from www.cdc.gov/nchs/data/nvsr/nvsr50/nvsr50_15.pdf.

Centers for Disease Control and Prevention. (2002c). Infant mortality statistics from the 2000 period linked birth/infant death data set. National Vital Statistics Reports, 50(12). Retrieved June 16, 2003, from www.cdc.gov/nchs/data/nvsr/nvsr50/nvsr50_12.pdf.

Centers for Disease Control and Prevention. (2002d). Surveillance and research: Abortion surveillance, 1999. Retrieved June 16, 2003, from www.cdc.gov/nccdphp/drh/surv_abort99.htm.

Centers for Disease Control and Prevention. (2003a). Early release of selected estimates based on data from the 2002 National Health Interview Survey. Retrieved July 9, 2003, from www.cdc.gov/nchs/.

Centers for Disease Control and Prevention. (2003b). Youth risk behavior surveillance— United States. Retrieved July 9, 2003, from www.cdc.gov.

Chamberlain, L. (1999). States offering different approaches to CHIP. Infectious Diseases in Children, 12(10), 51-54.

Committee on Pediatric Emergency Medicine. (2003). Consent for emergency medical services for children and adolescents. Pediatrics, 111(3), 703-706.

Daley, M. (1999). Head Start: Program and legislative update. Journal of Pediatric Nursing, 14(3), 186-188.

Daltzell, M.D. (2002). Has capitation weathered the storm? Managed Care Magazine (July 2002). Retrieved June 23, 2003, from www.managedcaremag.com/archives/0207/0207.capitationstorm.html.

Doolittle, D. (1998). Welfare reform: Loss of supplemental security income (SSI) for children with disabilities. Journal of Society of Pediatric Nurses, 3(1), 33-44.

Driscoll, K.M. (1998). Legal aspects of perinatal care. In C. Kenner, J.W. Lott, & A.A. Flandermeyer (Eds.), Comprehensive neonatal nursing: A physi-

ologic perspective (pp. 32-45). Philadelphia: Saunders.

Feigin, R., & Cherry, J. (1998). Textbook of pediatric infectious diseases. Philadelphia: Saunders.

Feinberg, E., Swartz, K., Zaslavsky, A., Gardner, J., & Walker, D. (2002). Family income and the impact of a children's health insurance program on reported need for health services and unmet health need. Pediatrics, 109(2), e29.

Freid, V.M., Prager, K., MacKay, A.P., & Xia, H. (2003). Chartbook on trends in the health of Americans. Health, United States, 2003. National Center for Health Statistics.

Forum on Child and Family Statistics. (2000). America's children 2000: Indicators of children's well-being. Retrieved July 9, 2003, from www.childstats.gov.

Heymann, S., & Earle, A. (1999). The impact of welfare reform on parents' ability to care for their children's health. American Journal of Public Health, 89(4), 502-505.

Horns, K.M. (2002). Medication errors: Analysis not blame. Journal of Obstetric, Gynecologic, and Neonatal Nursing, 31(3), 347-354.

Janssen, P.A., Klein, M.C., Harris, S.J., Soolsma, J., & Seymour, L.C. (2000). Single room maternity care and client satisfaction. Birth, 27(4), 235-243.

Koniak-Griffin, D. (1999). Strategies for reducing the risk of malpractice litigation in perinatal nursing. Journal of Obstetric, Gynecologic, and Neonatal Nursing, 28(3), 291-299.

Laganá, K. (2000). The "right" to a caring relationship: The law and ethic of care. Journal of Perinatal and Neonatal Nursing, 14(2), 12-24.

Lindeke, L., Hauck, M., & Tanner, M. (2000). Practical issues in obtaining child assent for research. Journal of Pediatric Nursing, 15(2), 99-104.

Lobar, S., Phillips, S., & Simunek, L. (1997). Legal issues in nonrelated infant adoption: Nursing implications. Journal of Society of Pediatric Nurses, 2(3), 116-124.

Longo, H. (1999). SBCHs help to provide immediate treatment to school children. Infectious Diseases in Children, 12(10), 11, 22.

Malkin, J.D., Garber, S., Broder, M.S., & Keeler, E. (2000). Infant mortality and early postpartum discharge. Obstetrics and Gynecology, 96(2), 183-188.

Maradiegue, A. (2002). The health insurance portability and accountability act and adolescents. Pediatric Nursing, 28(4), 417-421.

March of Dimes. Perinatal profiles: Statistics for monitoring state maternal and infant health. Retrieved

June 17, 2003, from peristats.modimes.org/ataglance/us.pdf.

Martin, J.A., Hamilton, B.E., Sutton, P.D., Ventura, S.J., Menacker, F., & Munson, M.L. (2003). Births: Final data for 2002. *National Vital Statistics Reports, 52*(10). Hyattsville, MD: National Center for Health Statistics. Retrieved February 5, 2004, from www.cdc.gov/nchs/data/nvsr/nvsr52/nvsr52_10.pdf.

Mouradian, W., Wehr, E., & Crall, J. (2000). Disparities in children's oral health and access to dental care. JAMA: *the Journal of the American Medical Association, 284*(20), 2625-2631.

National Council of State Boards of Nursing. (2003). *Just the facts: Nurse licensure compact.* Retrieved July 9, 2003, from www.ncsbn.org.

National Heart, Lung, and Blood Institute. (2001). *Report of the working group on research on hypertension during pregnancy.* National Institutes of Health: Bethesda, MD. Retrieved July 12, 2003, from www.nhlbi.nih.gov/resources/hyperten_pret/index.html.

National Institute of Child Health and Human Development. (1998). *America's children: Key national indicators of well-being.* Hyattsville, MD: Author.

National Resource Center on Homelessness and Mental Illness. (2003a). *What about the needs of children who are homeless?* Retrieved June 17, 2003, from www.nrchmi.com/facts/facts_question_5.asp.

National Resource Center on Homelessness and Mental Illness. (2003b). *Who is homeless?* Retrieved June 17, 2003, from www.nrchmi.com/facts/facts_question_2.asp.

Rienzo, B., Button, J., & Wald, K. (2000). Politics and the success of school-based health centers. *Journal of School Health, 70*(8), 331-337.

Ritley, D., & Porter, J. (2001). Exploring advanced directives in the OB setting. *AWHONN Lifelines 5*(5), 10-12.

Shuler, P. (2000). Evaluating student services provided by school-based health centers: Applying the Shuler Nurse Practitioner Practice Model. *Journal of School Health, 70*(8), 348-352.

Simpson, K.R., & Chez, B.F. (1999). Professional and legal issues. In K.R. Simpson & P.A. Creehan (Eds.). AWHONN's perinatal nursing (2nd ed., pp. 21-49). Philadelphia: Lippincott.

Sochalski, J. (1999). Improving access to health care for children. *Journal of Society of Pediatric Nurses, 4*(4), 147-154.

Truong, E., & Ferguson, S. (2003). Welfare reform at the crossroads: Pediatric nurses bridging the gap between self-sufficiency and health. *Journal of Pediatric Nursing, 18*(1), 60-63.

United States Department of Health and Human Services (USDHHS). (2000). *Healthy People 2010 online documents.* Retrieved June 17, 2003, from www.healthypeople.gov/document/html/objectives/09-07.htm.

United States Department of Health and Human Services, Centers for Medicare & Medicaid Services (2002). Medicaid eligibility. Retrieved June 17, 2003, from www.hhs.gov.

Velsor-Friedrich, B. (2000). Healthy People 2000/2010: Health appraisal of the nation and future objectives. *Journal of Pediatric Nursing, 15*(1), 54-59.

Velsor-Friedrich, B. (2003). Federally sponsored insurance programs for children: The State Children's Health Insurance Program. *Journal of Pediatric Nursing, 18*(2), 134-136.

Wertz, R., & Wertz, D. (1992). *Lying-in: A history of childbirth in America* (2nd ed.). New Haven, CT: Yale University Press.

Wilder, M.A. (2000). Ethical issues in the delivery room: Resuscitation of extremely low birth weight infants. *Journal of Perinatal and Neonatal Nursing, 14*(2), 44-57.

Woodring, B. (1998). *Standards and guidelines for pre-licensure and early professional education for the nursing care of children and their families* (Rev. ed.). Denver, CO: Society of Pediatric Nurses.

Yoos, H.L., Kitzman, H., Olds, D.L., & Overacker, I. (1995). Child-rearing beliefs in the African-American community: Implications for culturally competent pediatric care. *Journal of Pediatric Nursing, 10*(6), 343-353.

Yudkowsky, B., & Tang, S. (1997). Children at risk: Their health insurance status by state. *Pediatrics, 99*(5), e2.

2

The Nurse's Role in Maternity and Pediatric Nursing

◆ LEARNING OBJECTIVES

After studying this chapter, you should be able to:

◎ Explain roles the nurse may assume in maternity and pediatric nursing practice.

◎ Explain the roles of nurses with advanced preparation for maternity and pediatric nursing practice.

◎ Explain the incorporation of critical thinking into nursing practice.

◎ Describe the steps of the nursing process and relate them to maternity and pediatric nursing.

◎ Explain issues surrounding use of complementary and alternative therapies.

◎ Discuss the importance of nursing research in clinical practice.

◆ DEFINITIONS

advocacy Speaking or arguing in support of a policy or a person's rights.

ambiguity (ambiguous) Lack of clarity or certainty; having more than one meaning.

assumptions Beliefs taken for granted without examination.

baseline data Information that describes the status of the client before treatment begins.

bias A prejudice that sways the mind.

cesarean birth Surgical birth of the fetus through an incision in the abdominal wall and uterus.

delegated nursing interventions Physician-prescribed nursing actions that require nursing judgment because nurses are accountable for correct implementation. See also *independent nursing interventions.*

fetus The developing baby from 9 weeks after conception until birth. In everyday practice, the term is often used to describe a developing baby during pregnancy, regardless of age.

independent nursing interventions Nurse-prescribed actions used in both nursing diagnoses and collaboratively addressed problems. See also *delegated nursing interventions.*

inference The act of drawing a conclusion or making a deduction.

judgment An opinion.

nursing diagnosis A clinical judgment about individual, family, or community responses to actual or potential health problems or life processes.

reflection Meditation, attentive consideration.

skepticism Doubt in the absence of conclusive evidence.

suspend To delay or to bring to a stop temporarily.

validate To make certain that the information collected during assessment is accurate.

As nursing care changed from the category-specific care of the mother, newborn, or child to family-centered care, maternity and pediatric nursing entered a new era of autonomy and independence. Nurses today must be able to communicate with and teach effectively clients of many ages and levels of development and education. They must be able to think critically and use the nursing process to develop a plan of care that meets the unique needs of each client and family. They are expected to use current research to solve problems and to collaborate with other health care providers.

THE ROLE OF THE PROFESSIONAL NURSE

The professional nurse has a responsibility to provide the highest quality care to every client. The American Nurses Association (ANA) Code of Ethics for Nurses (Box 2-1) provides guidelines for ethical and professional behavior. The code emphasizes the nurse's accountability to the client, the community, and the profession. The nurse should understand the implications of this code and strive to practice accordingly. Professional nurses have a legal obligation to know and understand the standard of care imposed on them. It is critical that nurses maintain competence and a current knowledge base in their areas of practice.

Standards of practice describe the level of performance expected of a professional nurse as determined by an authority in the practice. For example, perinatal nurses are held to the standards published by the Association of Women's Health, Obstetric, and Neonatal Nurses (AWHONN). AWHONN recently published the sixth edition of its *Standards for Professional Nursing Practice in the Care of Women and Newborns* (Association of Women's Health, Obstetric, and Neonatal Nurses [AWHONN] 2003) to guide practice and shape institutional guidelines.

The ANA and the Society of Pediatric Nurses formed a task force to develop *Standards of Care and Standards of Professional Performance for Pediatric Nurses*. Nurses who care for children in all clinical settings can use these standards and *The SPN/ANA Guide to Family Centered Care* as guides for practice. Other standards of practice for specific clinical areas, such as pediatric oncology nursing or emergency nursing, are available from nursing specialty groups.

As health care moves to family-centered and community-based health services, all nurses should expect to care for children, adolescents, and their families. *Standards and Guidelines for Pre-licensure and Early Professional Education for the Nursing Care of Children and Their Families* has been developed by academic and clinical educators to meet this need. These published standards are stated in the form of 11 goals, based on issues central to the health of children and their families. The issues are child, family, and societal areas; clinical problems; and care delivery (Woodring, 1998).

Maternity and pediatric nurses function in a variety of roles, including those of care provider, teacher, collaborator, researcher, advocate, and manager.

Care Provider

The nurse provides direct nursing care to women, infants, children, and their families in times of childbearing, illness, injury, recovery, and wellness. Nursing care is based on the nursing process. The nurse obtains health histories, assesses client needs, monitors growth and development, performs health-screening procedures, develops comprehensive plans of care, provides treatment and care, makes referrals, and evaluates the effects of care. Nursing of children is especially based on an understanding of the child's developmental stage and is aimed at meeting the child's physical and emotional needs at that level. Developing a therapeutic relationship with and providing support to clients and their families are essential components of nursing care. Maternity and pediatric nurses practice family-centered care, embracing diversity in family structures and cultural backgrounds. These nurses strive to empower families, encouraging them to participate in their care and the care of their child.

Teacher

Education is an essential role of today's nurse. Client teaching begins early, before and during a woman's prenatal care, and continues through her recovery from childbirth (Fig. 2-1). Nurses who care for children prepare them for procedures, hospitalization, or surgery, using knowledge of growth and development to teach children at various levels of understanding.

BOX 2-1
ANA Code of Ethics for Nurses

1. The nurse, in all professional relationships, practices with compassion and respect for the inherent dignity, worth, and uniqueness of every individual, unrestricted by considerations of social or economic status, personal attributes, or the nature of health problems.
2. The nurse's primary commitment is to the patient, whether an individual, family, group, or community.
3. The nurse promotes, advocates for, and strives to protect the health, safety, and rights of the patient.
4. The nurse is responsible and accountable for individual nursing practice and determines the appropriate delegation of tasks consistent with the nurse's obligation to provide optimum patient care.
5. The nurse owes the same duties to self as to others, including the responsibility to preserve integrity and safety, to maintain competence, and to continue personal and professional growth.
6. The nurse participates in establishing, maintaining, and improving health care environments and conditions of employment conducive to the provision of quality health care and consistent with the values of the profession through individual and collective action.
7. The nurse participates in the advancement of the profession through contributions to practice, education, administration, and knowledge development.
8. The nurse collaborates with other health professionals and the public in promoting community, national, and international efforts to meet health needs.
9. The profession of nursing, as represented by associations and their members, is responsible for articulating nursing values, for maintaining the integrity of the profession and its practice, and for shaping social policy.

Families need information as well as emotional support so that they can cope with the anxiety and uncertainty of a child's illness. Nurses teach family members how to provide care, watch for important signs, and increase the child's comfort. They also work with new parents and parents of ill children so that the parents are prepared to assume responsibility for care at home after the child has been discharged from the hospital.

Education is essential for promotion of health. The nurse applies principles of teaching and learning to change the behavior of family members. Nurses motivate women, children, and families to take charge of and make responsible decisions about their own health. For teaching to be effective, it must incorporate the family's values and health beliefs.

Nurses caring for children and families play an important role in the prevention of illness and injury through education and anticipatory guidance. Teaching about immunizations, safety, dental care, socialization, and discipline is a necessary component of care. Nurses offer guidance to parents with regard to child-rearing practices and preventing potential problems. They also answer questions about growth and development and

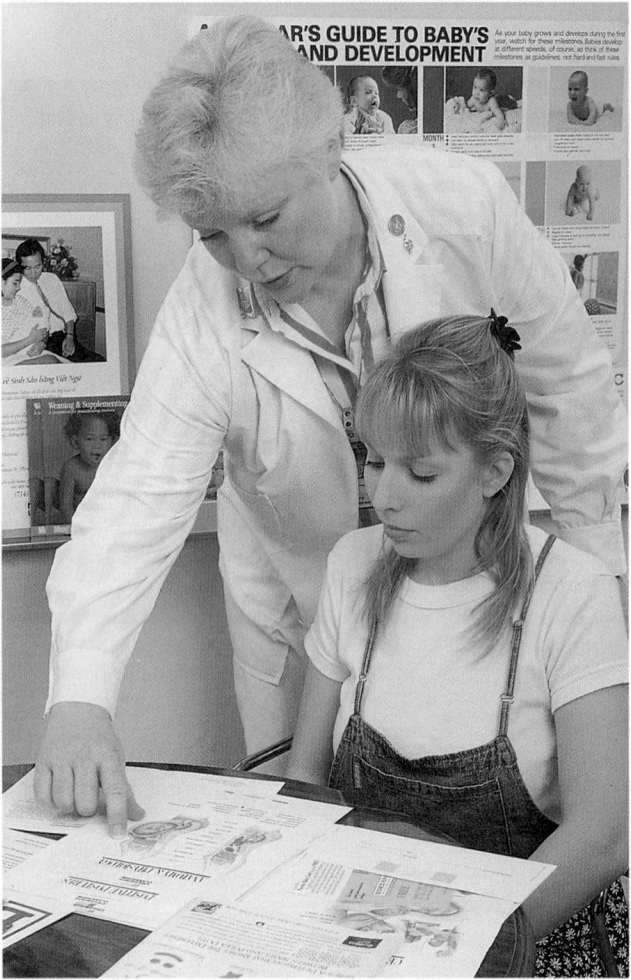

Figure 2-1 In the prenatal clinic, the nurse teaches a woman one-on-one.

assist families in understanding their children. Teaching often involves providing emotional support and counseling to children and families.

Factors Influencing Learning

A number of factors influence learning at any age. These factors include:

- *Developmental level.* Teenage parents often have very different concerns than older parents. Developmental level also influences whether a person learns best by reading printed material, using computer-based materials, watching videos, participating in group discussions, play, or other means. When teaching children, teaching must be adapted to the child's developmental level rather than the child's chronologic age.
- *Language.* The ability to understand the language in which teaching is done determines how much the family learns. Families for whom English is not their primary language may not understand idioms, nuances, slang terms, informal usage of words, or medical words. An interpreter for the deaf may be necessary for the client who is hearing impaired.
- *Culture.* People tend to forget or disregard content with which they disagree. The nurse's teaching can be most effective if cultural considerations are weighed and incorporated into the education.

- *Previous experiences.* Parents who have other children may need less education about pregnancy care or infant and child care. They may, however, have additional concerns about meeting the needs of several children and about sibling rivalry.
- *Physical environment.* The nurse must consider privacy when discussing sensitive issues such as adolescent sexuality or domestic violence. A group discussion, on the other hand, may prompt participants to ask questions of concern to all members of the group, such as the experiences they can expect in labor.
- *Organization and skill of the teacher.* The teacher must determine the objectives of the teaching, develop a plan to meet the objectives, and gather all materials before teaching. The nurse must determine the best way to present the material for the intended audience. A summary of the information is helpful when concluding a teaching session.

Principles of Teaching and Learning

Applying the following principles will help nurses become effective teachers in the childbearing setting:

- Real learning depends on the readiness of the family to learn and the relevance of the content.
- Active participation increases learning. Whenever possible, the learner should be involved in the educational process and not act as a passive listener or viewer. A discussion format in which all can participate stimulates more learning than a straight lecture.
- Repetition of a skill increases retention and promotes a feeling of competence.
- Praise and positive feedback are powerful motivators for learning. They are particularly important when the family is trying to master a frustrating task, such as breast-feeding an unresponsive infant.
- Role modeling is an effective method for demonstrating behavior. Nurses must be aware that their behavior is scrutinized carefully at all times and that it may be copied later.
- Conflicts and frustration impede learning, and they should be recognized and resolved for learning to progress.
- Learning is enhanced when teaching is structured to present simple tasks before more complex material. For instance, the nurse teaches how to care for the umbilical cord, which is simple, before teaching how to bathe and shampoo the newborn, which is more difficult for inexperienced parents.
- A variety of teaching methods is necessary to maintain interest and to illustrate concepts. Posters, videos, and printed materials supplement lectures and discussion. Models may be especially useful for teaching family planning or the processes of labor.
- Information is retained better when it is presented in small segments over a period of time. Short hospital stays do not support this practice, making follow-up care particularly important for some clients.

Collaborator

Nurses collaborate with other members of the health care team, often coordinating and managing the client's care. Care is improved by an interdisciplinary approach as nurses work together with dietitians, social workers, physicians, and others.

Managing the transition from a hospital or any other acute care setting to the client's home or another facility involves discharge planning and collaboration with other health care professionals. The trend toward home care makes collaboration increasingly important. The nurse must be knowledgeable about community resources, appropriate home care agencies for the type of client or problem, and financial resources. Cooperation and communication are essential as clients, including parents of children, are encouraged to participate in their care.

Researcher

Nurses contribute to their profession's knowledge base by systematically investigating theoretic or practice issues in nursing. Nursing does much more than simply "borrow" scientific knowledge from medicine and basic sciences. Nursing generates and answers its own questions based on research of its unique subject matter. The responsibility for research within nursing is not limited to nurses with graduate degrees. It is important that all nurses apply research findings to their practice, rather than basing care decisions merely on intuition or tradition. Evidence-based practice is no longer just an ideal but an expectation of nursing practice. Nurses can contribute to the body of professional knowledge by demonstrating an awareness of the value of nursing research and assisting in problem identification and data collection. Nurses should keep their knowledge current by networking and sharing research findings at conferences, by publishing, and by evaluating research journal articles.

Advocate

An advocate is one who speaks on behalf of another. As the health care environment becomes increasingly complex, care can become impersonal. The wishes and needs of children and families are sometimes discounted or ignored in the effort to treat and to cure. As the health professional who is closest to the client, the nurse is in an ideal position to humanize care and to intercede on the client's behalf. As an advocate, the nurse considers the family's wishes in planning and implementing care. The nurse informs families of treatments and procedures, ensuring that the families are involved directly in decisions and activities related to their care. The nurse must be sensitive to the values, beliefs, and customs of families.

Nurses must be advocates for health promotion for vulnerable groups such as children or victims of domestic violence. Nurses can promote the rights of children and families by participating in groups dedicated to the welfare of children and families, such as professional nursing societies, parent support groups, religious organizations, and voluntary organizations. Through involvement with health care planning on a political or legislative level and by working as consumer advocates, nurses can initiate changes for better quality health care. Nurses possess unique knowledge and skills and can make valuable contributions in developing health care strategies to ensure that all clients receive optimal care.

Manager of Care

As a result of the decreased length of stay in acute care facilities, nurses often are not able to provide total direct client care. Instead, they delegate concrete tasks, such as giving a bath or taking vital signs, to others. As a result, nurses spend more time teaching and supervising nonlicensed personnel, planning and

coordinating care, and collaborating with other professionals and agencies. Moreover, nurses are expected to understand the financial squeeze resulting from cost-containment strategies and to contribute to their institutions' economic viability. At the same time, they must continue to act as client advocates and to maintain a standard of care.

ADVANCED PREPARATION FOR MATERNITY AND PEDIATRIC NURSES

The increasing complexity of care and a focus on cost containment have led to a greater need for nurses with advanced preparation. Advanced practice nurses may practice as certified nurse-midwives, nurse practitioners, or clinical nurse specialists, among other possibilities. Advanced practice nurses may also work as nurse administrators, nurse educators, and nurse researchers. Preparation for advanced practice involves obtaining a master's or doctoral degree.

Certified Nurse-Midwives

Certified nurse-midwives (CNMs) are registered nurses who have completed an extensive program of study and clinical experience. They must pass a certification test administered by the American College of Nurse-Midwives. CNMs are qualified to provide complete care during pregnancy, childbirth, and the postpartum period in uncomplicated pregnancies. They provide information about preventive measures and preparation for normal pregnancy and childbirth. They spend a great deal of time counseling and supporting the childbearing family. The CNM also provides gynecologic services as well as family planning and counseling.

Despite the proven effectiveness of nurse-midwives, for many years they were restricted in the scope and location of their practice. In 1970, however, many of these restrictions were alleviated when the American College of Obstetricians and Gynecologists, together with the Nurses Association of the American College of Obstetricians and Gynecologists— now known as the *Association of Women's Health, Obstetric, and Neonatal Nurses*—issued a joint statement that admitted nurse-midwives as part of the health care team. In 1981 Congress authorized Medicaid payments for the services of CNMs. This measure has greatly increased use of nurse-midwives, particularly by health maintenance organizations (HMOs), in birthing centers, and in some hospitals.

Nurse Practitioners

Nurse practitioners are advanced practice nurses who work according to protocols and provide many primary care services that were once provided only by physicians. Most nurse practitioners collaborate with a physician, but, depending on their scope of practice and their individual state's board of nursing mandates, they may work independently and prescribe medications. Nurse practitioners provide care for specific groups of clients in a variety of settings (primary care facilities, schools, acute care facilities, rehabilitation centers). They may address occupational health, women's health, family health, and the health of the elderly or the very young.

Women's health nurse practitioners provide wellness-focused, primary, reproductive, and gynecologic care over the life span but do not usually manage care of women during birth. Common responsibilities include performing well-woman examinations, screening for sexually transmitted diseases, and providing family planning services. Some hospitals employ women's health nurse practitioners to assess and screen women who present to obstetric triage units, many of whom have non-obstetric problems.

Pediatric nurse practitioners use advanced skills to assess and treat well and ill children according to established protocols. The health care services they provide range from physical examinations and anticipatory guidance, to the treatment of common illnesses and injuries. It is becoming more common for newborn nurseries and some children's hospital specialty units to be staffed by pediatric or neonatal nurse practitioners.

Family nurse practitioners are prepared to provide care for people of all ages. They may care for women during uncomplicated pregnancies and provide follow-up care for the mother and infant after childbirth. Unlike certified nurse-midwives, they do not assist with childbirth. They diagnose and treat clients holistically, with a strong emphasis on prevention.

School nurse practitioners receive education and training that is similar to that of pediatric nurse practitioners. However, because of the setting in which they practice, the school nurse practitioner receives advanced education in managing chronic illness, disability, and mental health problems in a school setting, as well as skills required to communicate effectively with students, teachers, school administrators, and community health care providers. School nurse practitioners expand the traditional role of the school nurse by providing on-site treatment of acute care problems and providing extensive well-child examinations and services (Brindis et al., 1998).

Clinical Nurse Specialists

Clinical specialists are registered nurses who, through study and supervised practice at the graduate level (master's or doctorate), have become expert in the care of childbearing families or pediatric clients. Four major subroles have been identified for clinical nurse specialists: expert practitioner, educator, researcher, and consultant. These professionals often function as clinical leaders, role models, client advocates, and change agents. Unlike nurse practitioners, clinical nurse specialists are not prepared to provide primary care. An emerging role in the provision of high quality health care to children, however, is an advanced practice nurse whose role combines the practice of the clinical nurse specialist and the pediatric nurse practitioner. Found primarily in tertiary settings, this advanced practice nurse provides cost-effective care for chronically ill, critically ill, and disabled children in acute care settings (Teicher, Crawford, Williams, Nelson, & Andrews, 2001).

IMPLICATIONS OF CHANGING ROLES FOR NURSES

As nursing care has changed, so also have the roles of maternity and pediatric nurses with both basic and advanced preparation. Nurses now work in a variety of areas. Although they previously worked almost exclusively in the hospital setting, many now provide home care and community-based care. Some of the settings for care of maternity and pediatric clients include:

- Acute care settings: general hospital units, intensive care units, surgical units, postanesthesia care units, emergency care facilities, and on board emergency transport craft
- Clinics and physicians' offices
- Home health agencies
- Schools
- Rehabilitation centers and long-term care facilities
- Summer camps and day care centers
- Hospice programs and respite care programs
- Psychiatric centers

Therapeutic Communication

Therapeutic communication is a skill nurses must have to carry out the many roles expected within the profession. Therapeutic communication, unlike social communication, is purposeful, goal directed, and focused. Although it may seem simple, therapeutic communication requires conscious effort and considerable practice.

Guidelines for Therapeutic Communication

Therapeutic communication requires flexibility and cannot depend on a particular set of learned techniques. Certain guidelines, however, may prove helpful.

- A calm setting that provides privacy, reduces distractions, and minimizes interruptions is essential.
- Interactions should begin with introductions and clarification of the nurse's role. The nurse might say, "My name is Claudia Lyall. I am here to complete the discharge teaching that was started yesterday." This introduction acknowledges the nurse's purpose and sets the stage for a discussion of the client's concerns about what happens when the family is discharged from the hospital.
- Therapeutic communication should be focused because it is directed toward meeting the needs expressed by the family. Beginning the interaction with an open-ended question, such as "How do you feel about going home today?" is one method of focusing the interaction. It may also be necessary to redirect the conversation. For instance, the nurse might say, "Thanks for showing me the beautiful pictures of the baby. I understand you are having a bit of trouble getting him to nurse."
- Nonverbal behaviors may communicate more powerful messages to the client than the spoken word. For example, facial expressions and eye movements can confirm or contradict what is said. Repetitive hand gestures, such as finger tapping or twirling a lock of hair, may indicate frustration, irritation, or boredom. Body posture, stance, and gait can convey energy, depression, or discomfort. Voice tone, pitch, rate, and volume may indicate joy, anger, or fear. Communicating with a young child may require that the nurse sit or squat to get to the child's level. Grooming also conveys messages about the nurse's self-image.
- Active listening requires that the nurse attend to what is being said as well as to the nonverbal clues. Attending behaviors that convey the nurse's interest and a sincere desire to understand include the following:
  —Eye contact, which signals a readiness to interact.
  —Relaxed posture, with the upper portion of the body inclined toward the client.
  —Encouraging cues, such as nodding, leaning closer, and smiling. Verbal cues include "Uh huh, go on," "Tell me about that," or "Can you give me an example?"
  —Touch, which can be a powerful response when words would break a mood or fail to convey the depth of feeling experienced between the woman and the nurse.

—Cultural differences influence communication. In some cultures, such as Chinese and Southeast Asian, prolonged eye contact is considered confrontational. People from Middle Eastern or Native American cultures are sometimes uncomfortable with touch and would be disturbed by unsolicited touching.

—Clarifying communication involves a unique process of the listener receiving the message as the sender intended. It may be necessary for the nurse to ask questions if the meaning of a statement is unclear. For instance, the nurse might say, "I'm not sure I understand."

—Emotions are part of communication, and nurses must often reflect feelings that are expressed verbally or nonverbally. The nurse might suggest, "You looked forward to delivery in a birth center and are disappointed that you needed a cesarean birth?"

Therapeutic Communication Techniques

Therapeutic communication involves responding as well as listening, and nurses must learn to use responses that facilitate rather than block communication. These facilitative responses, often called *communication techniques*, focus on both the content of the message and the feeling that accompanies the message. Communication techniques include clarifying, reflecting, being silent, questioning, and directing. A brief review of these and other communication techniques can be found in Box 2-2. In addition to being aware of effective communication techniques, nurses must be aware of blocks to communication. These are listed with examples and alternatives in Table 2-1. Chapter 32 describes in more detail methods of communicating with pediatric clients and their families.

Critical Thinking

In recent years critical thinking has received widespread attention in nursing. Clearly, nurses must be concerned with the development of critical thinking skills, which are needed not only to pass the National Council Licensure Examination (NCLEX) but also to function clinically.

Definitions

Unlike undirected thinking, during which the mind wanders freely, critical thinking is controlled and directed toward finding solutions or forming opinions. To do this effectively, people must gain insight into their own thought processes. This process means analyzing one's own thinking thoroughly. It includes recognizing and acknowledging specific habits and responses that can interfere with productive thinking.

Critical thinking is based on reason rather than on preference or prejudice. Moreover, critical thinking seeks to examine feelings so that one can understand how emotions affect thinking. Last but not least, critical thinking requires that one suspend judgment until there is adequate evidence to support inferences or conclusions.

The Purpose of Critical Thinking

The purpose of critical thinking is to identify and then to overcome habits or impulses that can result in poor decisions or inappropriate actions. The primary purpose of critical thinking in nursing is to help nurses make the best clinical judgments. The process begins when nurses realize that it is not enough to accumulate a fund of knowledge from texts and lectures. They must also be able to *apply* the knowledge to specific clinical situations and thus to reach conclusions that provide the most effective care in each situation.

In addition to acquiring knowledge and learning to apply that knowledge, nurses must also examine their own thought processes for flaws that can lead to inaccurate conclusions or poor judgments. Although this examination requires a great deal of self-analysis, a series of steps makes the process easier. Critical thinking exercises are presented throughout this book to help students develop skill in critical thinking and applying knowledge.

Steps in Critical Thinking

A series of steps may help clarify how critical thinking is learned. These steps may be called the *ABCDEs* of critical thinking. They include recognition of *assumptions*, an examination of personal *biases*, analysis of how much pressure one has for *closure*, examination of how one collects and analyzes *data*, and evaluation of how *emotions* and *environmental factors* may interfere with one's ability to think critically.

A. Recognizing Assumptions. *Assumptions* are ideas, beliefs, or values that are taken for granted. Assumptions may lead to unexamined thoughts, unsound actions, or stereotyping. For instance, consider the consequences of the following assumptions: "Anyone who wants a job can get one." "Teenagers don't listen." "Every woman wants a baby." "Children should be seen but not heard."

When attempting to identify assumptions, it may be helpful to make a list of everything known about a specific situation. Then each item on the list should be analyzed to determine which is true, which could be true, and which is either untrue or lacks enough evidence to determine whether it is true or not.

B. *Examining Biases*. *Biases* are prejudices that sway an individual toward a particular conclusion or course of action on the basis of personal theories or stereotypes. Biases are based on unexamined beliefs, and many are widespread. Some examples are "fat people are lazy," "women are bad drivers," and "men are insensitive."

People are often biased toward those of different races, religions, or life-styles. When faced with a predisposition to judge a person or a group of persons, it may be wise to ask oneself (or a co-worker) a series of questions: "Why do you think that?" "What if this person were a different client?" "What if there were different circumstances?" "What might someone who disagrees say?" "What is influencing my thinking?"

C. *Analyzing the Need for Closure*. Many people look for immediate answers and experience anxiety until a solution is found for any problem. They have very little tolerance for doubt or uncertainty, sometimes called *ambiguity*. As a result, they feel pressure to come to a decision, or to reach *closure*, as early as possible. This is one of the most important aspects of critical thinking because those who feel pressure to come to an early decision or to find a quick solution often do so with insufficient data.

To overcome the pressure to reach an early conclusion, a conscious effort must be made to suspend judgment. This is sometimes called *reflective skepticism*. The first step is to acknowledge the anxiety that postponing decisions creates. The next step involves deliberately waiting to make a decision.

People who jump to conclusions often stop with one answer. To overcome this tendency, they should always look for a second right answer. They could also imagine the problem from the perspective of someone else. They might also

BOX 2-2
Communication Techniques

Definition	Examples
Clarifying Clearing up or following up to understand both content and feelings expressed, to check the accuracy of how the nurse perceives the message.	"I'm confused about your plans. Could you explain?" "Tell me what you mean when you say you don't feel like yourself." "Are you saying that _____?" "Can you tell me more about _____?"
Paraphrasing Restating in words other than those used by the client what the client seems to express; this is a form of clarification.	EXAMPLE NO. 1 Client: "My boyfriend won't even come into the room for the birth. I am furious with him." Nurse: "You want him with you, and you are angry because he won't be here?" EXAMPLE NO. 2 Client: "My baby cries all of the time. We aren't getting any sleep." Nurse: "You are feeling exhausted, and it seems like your baby cries a great deal? Can you tell me what a typical day is like?"
Reflecting Verbalizing comprehension of what the client said and what the client seems to be feeling. It is important to link content and feeling and to reflect the client as a mirror reflects a person. The opinion, values, and personality of the nurse should not be in the reflected image.	EXAMPLE NO. 1 Client: "I don't know what to do. My husband doesn't think a cesarean is needed, but the doctor says the baby is showing some stress." Nurse: "You're confused and frightened because they don't agree?" EXAMPLE NO. 2 Client (woman in early labor): "It was my husband's idea for me to become pregnant. I wasn't too excited about it at first." Nurse: "I'll bet the dad will be a pushover as a father." The nurse's statement reflects the nurse's opinion and fails to acknowledge the mother's statement. A better response might be: "Your husband was more excited early in the pregnancy than you?"
Silence Waiting and allowing time for the client to continue. Verbal communication need not be constant.	The nurse waits quietly for the client to continue.
Structuring Creating guidelines or setting priorities.	"You said you don't know how to take care of the baby and also that you are afraid of getting pregnant again. What should we talk about first?"
Pinpointing Calling attention to differences or inconsistencies in statements.	Nurse talking to an 8-year-old child: "You said you didn't want your mother to spend the night with you, but you cry every night after she leaves. It can be scary being alone. I will sit with you, and we can talk about asking your mother to stay tomorrow night."
Questioning Eliciting information directly; using open-ended questions to avoid "yes" or "no" answers and to prevent controlling the answers.	"How do you feel about being pregnant?" instead of "Are you happy to be pregnant?" "Will you tell me how you feel about your brother being very sick?" instead of "Are you frightened because your brother is very sick?"
Directing Using nonverbal responses or succinct comments to encourage the client to continue.	Nodding. "Um mm." "You were saying." "Please go on."
Summarizing Reviewing the main themes or issues that were discussed	"You had two major concerns today." "We have talked about breast-feeding and how to bathe the baby today."

ask a series of questions, such as "What alternatives do we have?" "What else might work?" "What information supports this?" "What effect would that have?" "Is there good evidence to support that decision?" "Is there reason to doubt that evidence?"

Unlike those who feel pressure for closure, some people can tolerate a great deal of doubt and uncertainty. They are comfortable with data collection and analysis but feel uncomfortable making decisions. They may delay coming to a decision for as long as possible. Failure to make a decision in the

TABLE **2–1** Behaviors That Block Communication

Behavior	Example	Alternative
Conveying lack of interest	Looking away, fidgeting	Attending behaviors such as eye contact, nodding
Conveying sense of haste	Checking the time, standing near the door	Sitting at bedside
Closed posture	Arms crossed over chest, holding clipboard in front of body	Leaning forward with arms relaxed
Interrupting, finishing sentences	Woman: "I'm not sure how _____." Nurse: "We will have a bath demonstration later."	"Go on _____." "You were saying _____."
Providing false reassurance	"You're going to be okay."	"I sense you are concerned about how to care for the baby. I will help you give the bath today."
Inappropriate self-disclosure	To woman in labor: "I was in labor 12 hours, then had a cesarean."	"What concerns you most about labor?"
Giving advice	"You should _____." "If I were you, I would _____."	"How do you feel about that?" "What do you think is most important?"
Failure to acknowledge comments or feelings	Mother: "Being a parent is hard work. I never have time for myself." Nurse: "It is going to get worse before it gets better. Parenting is hard work."	"Parenting is hard work. Let's talk about some ways that you might get a break."

clinical area may have serious consequences for clients and their families. Several questions may help overcome the tendency to put off coming to a decision. Some of these questions are "What signs indicate something is wrong?" "Do I need to do something about it?" "How much time do I have?" "What happens if I don't do something about this?" "What could happen if I do?" "What should I do first?" "What resources can help me?" This step might also be called *priority setting*; it is one of the most important aspects of critical thinking.

D. *Managing Data.* Expertise in collecting, organizing, and analyzing data involves developing an attitude of *inquiry* and learning to live with questions. Questions to ask for data management include "Why?" "What if?" "What else?" "Is this relevant?" "How does it relate to that?" "How can I organize the data?" "Does it form patterns?" "What can I infer from those patterns?"

Collecting Data. To obtain complete data, one must develop skill in verbal communication. Asking open-ended questions elicits more information than asking questions that require only a one-word answer. Follow-up questions are often needed to clarify information or to pursue a particular train of thought.

Validating Data. Information that is unclear or incomplete should be validated. This process may involve rechecking physical signs, collecting additional information, or determining whether a perception is accurate. For instance, the comment "You seem uncomfortable" may result in the client's denying or acknowledging discomfort.

Organizing and Analyzing Data. Data are more useful when organized into patterns or clusters. The first step is to separate data that are relevant from data that may be interesting but that are not related to the current situation.

The next step is to compare one's data with expected norms to determine what is within the expected range (normal) and what is not within the expected range (abnormal). Abnormal results provide cues that can be grouped or clustered so that conclusions can be made. For example, grouping all data that may indicate excessive bleeding, such as pulse rate, blood pressure, amount of visible bleeding, and skin color, may make the information more meaningful. Organizing data into clusters often reveals that additional data are needed before a decision can be reached.

E. *Evaluating Other Factors.* A variety of *emotions* and *environmental factors* can influence critical thinking. For instance, the clinical area is often a noisy, fast-paced, hectic environment with time limitations and distractions that make calm reflection and reasoning difficult. Moreover, fatigue may reduce one's ability to concentrate at the end of a trying 12-hour shift. The nurse may desperately want to reassure anxious parents about their sick child. Inexperienced nurses and students may lack confidence in their knowledge and experience. As a result, they often feel anxious, which can reduce their ability to think critically.

Many nurses, both experienced and inexperienced, have a strong need to protect their self-image. As a result, they become very defensive when they have said or done something wrong. This response is a serious barrier to critical thinking and requires that all health care professionals learn to acknowledge mistakes and to feel comfortable with constructive criticism.

Extreme emotions, such as anger or frustration, impede critical thinking by narrowing the focus to only data that support the intense feeling. For example, people who are extremely frustrated may repeat the perceived cause of their frustration over and over and may be unable to move on to other information so the problem can be addressed.

The first step in dealing with factors or emotions that impede thinking is to recognize and acknowledge them. To develop critical thinking skills, one must learn to admit mistakes and become comfortable saying, "I was wrong." Asking for assistance, verification, or validation is wise when fatigue is a problem or when lack of confidence creates anxiety.

It is essential for the person who experiences intense frustration or anger to recognize the emotions and their impact on rational thought. It may be helpful to ask a trusted colleague to point out when signs of these emotions, such as repetitive vehement comments, occur. Some people use other methods of control, such as visualizations, a series of breathing exercises, or, when possible, a brief, self-imposed "time-out" from the precipitating situation.

BOX 2-3
Developing Individualized Nursing Care Through the Nursing Process

Although the nursing process is the foundation for maternal-child nursing, initially it is a challenging process to apply in the clinical area. It requires proficiency in focused assessments of the client as well as the ability to analyze data on and plan nursing care for individual clients and families. It may be helpful to pose questions at each step of the nursing process.

Assessment
1. Were there data that were not within normal limits or expected parameters? For example, the client states that she feels "dizzy" when she tries to ambulate.
2. If so, what else should be assessed? (What else should I look for? What might be related to this symptom?) For instance, what are the blood pressure, pulse, skin color, temperature, and amount of lochia if the client feels "dizzy"?
3. Did the assessment identify the cause of the abnormal data? What are the prepregnancy and current hemoglobin and hematocrit values? What was her estimated blood loss (EBL) during childbirth?
4. Are there other factors? What medication is the client taking? How long has it been since she has eaten? Is the environment a related factor (crowded, warm, unfamiliar)? Is she reluctant to ask for assistance?

Analysis
1. Are adequate data available to reach a conclusion? What else is needed? (What do you wish you had assessed? What would you look for next time?)
2. What is the major concern? (On the basis of the data, what are you worried about?) The client who is "dizzy" may fall as she ambulates to the bathroom or she may drop her new baby. Or her dizziness may be a clue that a new complication is developing.
3. What might happen if no action is taken? (What might happen to the client if you do nothing?) She may suffer an injury or a complication.
4. Is there a NANDA-approved diagnostic category that reflects your major concern? How is it defined? Suppose that during analysis you decide the major concern is that the client will faint and suffer an injury. What diagnostic category most closely reflects this concern? Risk for Injury? Definition: "The state in which an individual is at risk for harm because of a perceptual or physiologic deficit, a lack of awareness of hazards, or maturational age."

5. Does this category and definition fit this client? Is she at greater risk for a problem than others in a similar situation? Why? What are the additional risk factors?
6. Is this a problem that nurses can manage independently? Is collaboration with other health professionals such as medicine needed?
7. If the problem can be managed by nurses, is it an actual nursing diagnosis (defining characteristics are present), a risk nursing diagnosis (risk factors are present), or possible problem (you have a hunch and some data, but not enough)?

Planning
1. What outcomes are desired? That the client will remain free of injury during hospital stay? That she will demonstrate position changes that reduce the episodes of vertigo?
2. Would the outcomes be clear, specific, and measurable to anyone reading them?
3. What nursing interventions should be initiated and carried out to accomplish these goals or outcomes?
4. Are your written interventions specific and clear? Would another nurse know your planned interventions clearly enough to complete them after you leave? Are action verbs used (*assess, teach, assist*)? After you have written the interventions, look them over. Do they define exactly what is to be done (when, what, how far, how often)? Will they prevent the client from suffering an injury?
5. Are the interventions based on sound rationale? For instance blood loss during birth may be excessive, which results in hypotension that is aggravated when the client stands suddenly.

Implementing Nursing Interventions
1. What are the expected effects of the prescribed intervention? Are there potential adverse effects? What are they?
2. Are the interventions acceptable to the client and family?
3. Are the interventions clearly written so that they can be carefully followed?

Evaluation
1. What is the status of the client right now?
2. What were the goals and outcomes? Are they specific? Can they be measured?
3. Compare the current status of the client with the stated goals and outcomes.
4. What should be done now?

NANDA, North American Nursing Diagnosis Association.

THE NURSING PROCESS IN MATERNITY AND PEDIATRIC CARE

The nursing process is the foundation for all nursing. The nursing process consists of five distinct steps: (1) assessment, (2) nursing diagnosis, (3) planning, (4) implementation of the plan (interventions), and (5) evaluation. Despite the apparent complexity of the process, the nurse soon learns to use the steps of the nursing process in order when caring for clients (Box 2-3).

In maternal-newborn nursing, the nursing process must be adapted to a population that is generally healthy and that is experiencing a life event that holds the potential for growth as well as for problems. Much maternal-newborn nursing activity is devoted to assessing and diagnosing client strengths and healthy functioning and to supporting adaptive responses. This focus differs somewhat from providing care for clients who are ill.

Pediatric nursing, including care of a newborn, presents another problem for many nursing students. Whereas use of the nursing process when caring for adults may involve only the client, in caring for infants and children it must involve their family as well. Therefore it is common for planning and interventions to state what the parent is expected to do or to specify interventions such as teaching a parent. The involvement of a third party (the family) may be different to the nursing student who has applied the nursing process only to care of adults in the past.

Assessment

Nursing assessment is the systematic collection of relevant data to determine the client's and family's current health status, coping patterns, needs, and problems. The data collected include not only physiologic data but also psychologic, social, and cultural data relevant to life processes. Nurses must assess the belief systems, available support, perceptions, and plans of other family members in an effort to provide the best nursing care.

During the assessment phase, three activities take place: collecting data, grouping findings, and writing the nursing diagnoses. Data can be collected through interview, physical examination, observation, review of records, and diagnostic reports, as well as through collaboration with other health care workers and the family. Two levels of nursing assessment are used to collect comprehensive data: (1) screening, or database, assessment; and (2) focused assessments.

Screening Assessment

The screening, or database, assessment is usually performed during the initial contact with the client. Its purpose is to gather information about all aspects of the client's health. This information, called *baseline data,* describes the client's health status before interventions begin. It forms the basis for identifying both strengths and problems. An example of baseline data would be the information in a woman's prenatal record.

A variety of methods may be used to organize the assessment. For example, information may be grouped according to body systems. Assessment can also be organized around nursing models that are based on nursing theory, such as Roy's adaptation model, Gordon's Functional Health Patterns, NANDA's Human Response Patterns, or Orem's self-care deficit theory.

Focused Assessment

A focused assessment is used to gather information that is specifically related to an actual health problem or a problem that the client or family is at risk for acquiring. A focused assessment is often performed at the beginning of a shift and centers on areas relevant to the client's diagnosis and current status. For example, the nurse would perform a focused assessment of the respiratory system several times during the child's hospitalization for the child with acute asthma.

Nursing Diagnosis

The data gathered during assessment must be analyzed to identify problems or potential problems. Data are validated and grouped in a process of critical thinking so that cues and inferences can be determined. The nurse identifies client responses to actual or potential health problems and to normal life processes. The nursing diagnosis provides a basis for nursing accountability for client interventions and outcomes.

There are three types of nursing diagnoses. An *actual nursing diagnosis* describes a human response to a health condition or life process affecting an individual, family, or community. It is supported by defining characteristics (manifestations, signs and symptoms) that can be clustered in patterns of related cues or inferences. *Risk nursing diagnoses* describe human responses to health conditions or life processes that may develop in a vulnerable individual, family, or community. They are supported by risk factors that contribute to increased vulnerability. *Wellness nursing diagnoses* describe human responses to levels of wellness in an individual, family, or community that have a potential for enhancement to a higher state.

Each nursing diagnosis is a concise term or phrase that represents a pattern of related cues or signs and symptoms. One problem that nurses often encounter is writing nursing diagnoses that nursing actions cannot address. For example, a medical diagnosis, such as pyloric stenosis, cannot be treated by a nurse. It is appropriate, however, to say that there are nursing actions that can decrease the fluid volume deficit associated with pyloric stenosis.

A nursing diagnosis consists of two sections joined by the phrase "related to." The statement begins with the client's response to the current problem and then describes the causative factor or factors. An example is *Interrupted Family Processes* related to *the diagnosis of a child with cancer.* The causative factors can be physiologic, psychologic, sociocultural, environmental, or spiritual. They assist the nurse in identifying nursing interventions as planning takes place.

Planning

The nurse next plans care for problems that were identified during assessment and are reflected in the nursing diagnoses. During this step, nurses set priorities, develop goals or outcomes that state what is to be accomplished by a certain time, and plan interventions to accomplish those goals.

Setting Priorities

Setting priorities includes (1) determining what problems need immediate attention (i.e., life-threatening problems) and taking immediate action; (2) determining whether there are potential problems that call for a physician's orders for diagnosis, monitoring, or treatment; and (3) identifying actual nursing diagnoses, which take precedence over at-risk diagnoses. For clients with many health and psychosocial problems, a realistic number of nursing diagnoses must be chosen.

Establishing Goals and Expected Outcomes

Although the terms *goals* and *outcome criteria* are sometimes used interchangeably, they are different. Generally, broad goals do not state the specific outcome criteria and are less measurable than outcome statements. If broad goals are developed, they should be linked to more specific and measurable outcome criteria. For example, if the goal is that the parents will demonstrate effective parenting by discharge, *outcome criteria* that serve as evidence might be prompt, consistent responses to infant signals and competence in bathing, feeding, and comforting the infant.

Certain rules should be followed when writing outcomes:

- Outcomes should be stated in client terms. This wording identifies who is expected to achieve the goal (the woman, infant or child, or family).
- Measurable verbs must be used. For example, "identify," "demonstrate," "express," "walk," "relate," and "list" are

verbs that are observable and measurable. Examples of verbs that are difficult to measure are "understand," "appreciate," "feel," "accept," "know," and "experience."

- A time frame is necessary. When is the person expected to perform the action? After teaching? By 1 day after hospitalization? Before discharge?
- Goals and outcomes must be realistic and attainable by nursing interventions only.
- Goals and outcomes are worked out in collaboration with the client and family to ensure their participation in the plan of care.

Implementation

Implementation is the action phase of the nursing process. Once the goals and desired outcomes are developed, it is necessary to select nursing interventions that will help the client meet the established outcomes. During this phase, the nurse is constantly evaluating and reassessing to determine that the interventions remain appropriate. As the client's condition changes, so does the plan of care.

The type of nursing interventions implemented depends on whether the nursing diagnosis was an actual, risk, or wellness diagnosis. Nursing interventions for actual nursing diagnoses are aimed at reducing or eliminating the causes or related factors. Interventions for risk nursing diagnoses are aimed at (1) monitoring for onset of the problem, (2) reducing or eliminating risk factors, and (3) preventing the problem. For a wellness nursing diagnosis, interventions focus on supporting the individual's or family's coping mechanisms and promoting a higher level of wellness.

Nursing interventions in care plans or protocols are most easily implemented if they are specific and spell out exactly what should be done. A well-written nursing intervention is specific: "Provide 200 ml of fluid (water or juice of choice) every 2 hours while the woman is awake." Vague interventions, such as "assist with breast-feeding," do not provide specific steps to follow.

Evaluation

The evaluation determines how well the plan worked or how well the goals or outcomes were met. To evaluate, the nurse must assess the status of the client and compare the current status with the goals or outcome criteria that were developed during the planning step. The nurse then judges how well the client is progressing toward goal achievement and makes a decision. Should the plan be continued? Modified? Abandoned? Are the problems resolved or the causes diminished? Is another nursing diagnosis more relevant?

The nursing process is dynamic, and evaluation frequently results in expanded assessment and additional or modified nursing diagnoses and interventions. Nurses are cautioned not to view lack of goal achievement as a failure. Instead, it is simply time to reassess and to begin the process anew.

Collaborative Problems

In addition to nursing diagnoses, which describe problems that respond to independent nursing functions, nurses must also deal with problems that are beyond the scope of independent nursing practice. These are sometimes termed *collaborative problems*—physiologic complications that usually occur in association with a specific pathologic condition or treatment.

Nurses monitor to detect the onset of the complication and collaborate with physicians to manage changes in client status. Both physician-prescribed and nursing-prescribed interventions are necessary to minimize complications (Carpenito, 2002).

Planning

It is inappropriate to identify client-centered goals for a collaborative problem because the goals cannot be achieved by independent nursing action. Collaborative problems should reflect the nurse's responsibility in situations requiring physician-prescribed interventions. The nurse's responsibility includes (Carpenito, 2002):

- Monitoring for signs of complications
- Managing the complications with nursing- and physician-prescribed interventions

Interventions

Nursing interventions for collaborative problems include (1) performing frequent assessments to monitor the status of the client and detect signs and symptoms of complications, (2) communicating with the physician when signs and symptoms of complications are noted, (3) performing physician-prescribed interventions, including standing orders and protocols, to prevent or correct the complication, and (4) performing nursing interventions described in the standards of care or policy and procedure manuals.

Evaluation

Although client-centered goals or outcomes are not developed for collaborative problems, the nurse collects data, compares the data with established norms, and judges whether the data are within normal limits. If the data are not within normal limits, the nurse consults with the physician for additional direction and implements physician-prescribed interventions as well as nursing interventions.

COMPLEMENTARY AND ALTERNATIVE MEDICINE

Today's nurse will likely encounter clients who use complementary and alternative medicine (CAM). Complementary and alternative medicine can be defined as those systems, practices, interventions, modalities, professions, therapies, applications, theories, or claims that are currently not an integral part of the dominant or conventional medical system in North America (American College of Obstetricians and Gynecologists, 1999). The therapies may be used instead of conventional medical therapy (alternative therapy) or used in addition to conventional medical therapy (complementary therapy). Integrative medicine combines conventional medical therapies with CAM therapies that have substantial evidence as to their safety and effectiveness.

A major concern in the use of CAM is safety. Clients who use these techniques may delay needed care by a conventional health care provider, or they may take herbal remedies or other substances that are toxic when combined with conventional medications or when taken in excess. Adverse effects of CAM therapies may be unknown for the fetus or children. Safety and effectiveness of botanical or vitamin therapies are often unregulated. Thus people may take in variable amounts of active ingredients from these substances. Some clients do not consider these therapies to be medicine and may not report them to their conventional health care provider, setting the stage for interactions between conventional medications and CAM therapies that have pharmacologic properties. Many people may not consider some of these therapies "alternative" at all because the therapy is mainstream in their culture.

Nurses may find that their professional values do not conflict with many of the CAM therapies. Nursing as a profession supports a self-care and preventive approach to health care in which the individual bears much of the responsibility for his or her health. Nursing practice has traditionally emphasized a holistic, or body-mind-spirit, model of health that fits with CAM. Nurses already practice CAM therapies such as therapeutic touch fairly widely. The rising interest in CAM provides opportunity for nurses to participate in research related to the legitimacy of these treatment modalities.

The National Center for Complementary and Alternative Medicine, a division of the National Institutes of Health, has a website (nccam.nih.gov/) to provide a source of information and classification of the therapies.

NURSING RESEARCH

As nursing and the health care system change, nurses will be challenged to demonstrate that what they do improves client outcomes and is cost-effective. To meet this challenge, nurses must participate in research and encourage the utilization of research. With the establishment of the National Institute of Nursing Research as a member of the National Institutes of Health (www.nih.gov/ninr), nurses now have an infrastructure in place to ensure that nursing research is supported and that a group of well-prepared nurse researchers will be educated.

The amount of clinically based nursing research conducted is increasing rapidly as nurse researchers strive to develop an independent body of knowledge that demonstrates the value of nursing interventions. The Association of Women's Health, Obstetric, and Neonatal Nurses has an ongoing commitment to develop and disseminate evidence-based practice guidelines through the association's Research-Based Practice Program. Implementation of evidence-based guidelines promotes application of the best available scientific evidence for nursing care rather than care based on tradition alone (AWHONN, 2003).

Although students and inexperienced nurses may not participate in research projects, they must take advantage of the knowledge obtained by the research team. Professional journals are the best sources of new information that can help nurses provide improved care and demonstrate that what they do makes a difference in client outcomes.

KEY CONCEPTS

- Maternal-newborn and pediatric nurses function in a variety of roles, including care provider, teacher, collaborator, researcher, advocate, and manager.
- The care settings in which maternity and pediatric nurses may practice include acute care settings, clinics, physicians' offices, home health agencies, schools, rehabilitation centers, summer camps, day care centers, and hospices.
- Registered nurses with advanced education are prepared to provide primary care for women and children as certified nurse-midwives and nurse practitioners.
- Clinical nurse specialists function as educators, researchers, and consultants to provide in-depth interventions for many problems encountered in maternity and pediatric care.
- Nurses must be adept at communicating and at removing blocks to communication to meet their responsibilities as educators and counselors.
- A primary responsibility of nurses is to provide information to childbearing families and to children and their families; nurses must know the principles of teaching and learning to fulfill the role of educator.
- Nurses must learn to think critically by examining their own thought processes for flaws that can lead to inaccurate conclusions or poor clinical judgments.
- The nursing process begins with assessment and includes analysis of data that may result in nursing diagnoses. Nursing diagnoses are problems that nurses are legally accountable for identifying and managing independently.
- Collaborative problems are usually physiologic complications that require both physician-prescribed and nurse-prescribed interventions.
- Nurses must consider the impact of complementary and alternative therapies when assessing the client and planning care.
- Professional journals are the best sources of information about scientifically sound research projects that demonstrate the effectiveness of nursing interventions.

REFERENCES and READINGS

Ackley, B.J., & Ladwig, G.B. (2002). *Nursing Diagnosis Handbook: A guide to planning care* (5th ed.). St. Louis: Mosby.

Alfaro-LeFevre, R. (2003). *Critical thinking and clinical judgement* (3rd ed.). Philadelphia: Saunders.

American Academy of Pediatrics. (2001). The role of the school nurse in providing school health services. *Pediatrics, 108*(5), 123-125.

American College of Obstetricians and Gynecologists. (1999). *Complementary and alternative medicine* (ACOG Committee Opinion No. 227, November 1999). Washington, DC: Author.

American Nurses Association. (2001). *Code of ethics for nurses: Major provisions*. Retrieved August 12, 2003, from www.nursingworld.org/ethics/chcode.htm.

American Nurses Association and Society of Pediatric Nurses. (2003). *The scope and standards of pediatric nursing practice*. Washington, DC: American Nurses Publishing. (PNP #23).

Angelini, D.J. (1999). Obstetric triage and advanced practice nursing. *Journal of Perinatal and Neonatal Nursing, 13*(4), 1-12.

Association of Women's Health, Obstetric, and Neonatal Nurses (AWHONN). (2003). *Standards for professional nursing practice in the care of women and newborns* (6th ed.). Washington, DC: Author.

Arnold, E., & Boggs, K. (1999). *Interpersonal relationships: Professional communication skills for nurses* (3rd ed.). Philadelphia: Saunders.

Barnsteiner, J., Wyatt, J., & Richardson, V. (2002). What do pediatric nurses do? Results of the role delineation study in Canada and the United States. *Pediatric Nursing, 28*(2), 165-171.

Beal, J.A. (2000). A nurse practitioner model of practice in the neonatal intensive care unit.

REFERENCES and READINGS

MCN: *American Journal of Maternal-Child Nursing, 25*(6), 18-24.

Brindis, C., Sanghvi, R., Melinkovich, P., Kaplan, D., Ahlstrand, D., & Phibbs, S. (1998). Redesigning a school health workforce for a new health care environment: Training school nurses as nurse practitioners. *Journal of School Health, 68*(5), 179-184.

Brucker, M.C. (2000). Nurse-midwifery: Yesterday, today, and tomorrow. MCN: *American Journal of Maternal-Child Nursing, 25*(1), 322-326.

Capitulo, K.L. (1998). The rise, fall, and rise of nurse-midwifery in America. MCN: *American Journal of Maternal-Child Nursing, 21*(6), 314-321.

Carpenito, L.J. (2002). *Handbook of nursing diagnosis* (9th ed.). Philadelphia: Lippincott.

Curran, L. (2002). The women's health nurse practitioner: Evolution of a powerful role. *AWHONN Lifelines, 6*(4), 332-337.

Davies, B.L. (2002). Sources and models for moving research evidence into clinical practice. *Journal of Obstetric, Gynecologic, and Neonatal Nursing, 31*(5), 558-562.

Lewandowski, L., & Tesler, M. (Eds.). (2003). *Family-centered care: Putting it into action: The SPN/ANA guide to family-centered care.* Washington, DC: American Nurses Publishing. (FCC #23).

Lewis, J.A. (2000). Advanced practice in maternal/child nursing: History, current status, and thoughts about the future. MCN: *American Journal of Maternal-Child Nursing, 25*(6), 327-330.

Longo, H. (1999). SBCHs help to provide immediate treatment to school children. *Infectious Diseases in Children, 12*(10), 11, 22.

National Center for Complementary and Alternative Medicine. (2002). *What is complementary and alternative medicine (CAM)?* Retrieved June 28, 2003, from nccam.nih.gov/health/whatiscam/.

Roberts, J. (2001). Challenges and opportunities for nurse-midwives. *Nursing Outlook, 49*(5), 213-216.

Roux, G.M., Haas, P., & Sandefur, J.A. (1998). Advanced practice nursing: Two NPs reflect on their roles & responsibilities. *AWHONN Lifelines, 2*(2), 39-42.

Rubenfeld, M.G., & Scheffer, B.K. (1995). *Critical thinking in nursing: An interactive approach.* Philadelphia: Lippincott.

Sams, L., & DeGeorges, K.M. (1998). Seize the evidence and the opportunity. *AWHONN Lifelines, 2*(3), 15-17.

Selekman, J., & Woodring, B. (2002). The changing dynamics of pediatric pre-licensure education. *Pediatric Nursing, 28*(4), 367-372.

Simpson, K.R., & Knox, E. (1999). Strategies for developing an evidence-based approach to perinatal care. MCN: *American Journal of Maternal-Child Nursing, 24*(3), 122-131.

Teicher, S., Crawford, K., Williams, B., Nelson, B., & Andrews, C. (2001). Emerging role of the pediatric nurse practitioner in acute care. *Pediatric Nursing, 27*(4), 387-390.

Ward, S. (1998). Caring and healing in the 21st century. MCN: *American Journal of Maternal-Child Nursing, 23*(4), 210-215.

Woodring, B. (1998). *Standards and guidelines for pre-licensure and early professional education for the nursing care of children and their families* (Rev. ed.). Denver, CO: Society of Pediatric Nurses.

Youngblut, J.M., & Brooten, D. (2000). Moving research into practice: A new partner. *Nursing Outlook, 48*(2), 55-56.

The Childbearing and Child-Rearing Family

After studying this chapter, you should be able to:

◎ Explain the importance of family when caring for maternity and pediatric clients.

◎ Describe different family structures and their impact on family functioning.

◎ Differentiate between healthy and dysfunctional families.

◎ List internal and external coping behaviors used by families when they face a crisis.

◎ Compare Western cultural values with those of other cultural groups.

◎ Describe the effect of cultural diversity on nursing practice.

◎ Describe common styles of parenting that nurses may encounter.

◎ Explain how variables in parent and child may affect their relationship.

◎ Discuss the use of discipline in a child's socialization.

◎ Evaluate the effects of an ill child on the family.

⬙ DEFINITIONS

coping Efforts directed toward managing and solving various problems, events, and stressors.

culture The sum of values, beliefs, and practices of a group of people that are transmitted from one generation to the next.

discipline The structure an adult sets for a child's life, designed to allow the child to appropriately interact socially in the real world; the training expected to produce a specific type or pattern of behavior.

egocentric Preoccupied with one's own interests and needs.

ethnic Pertaining to religious, racial, national, or cultural group characteristics, especially speech patterns, social customs, and physical characteristics.

ethnicity Condition of belonging to a particular ethnic group; also refers to ethnic pride.

ethnocentrism The opinion that the beliefs and customs of one's own ethnic group are superior to those of others.

family Two or more emotionally involved people living in close proximity and having reciprocal obligations with a sense of commonness, caring, and commitment (Friedman, 1998).

fatalism The belief that events are predestined.

nuclear family A family consisting of a two-generation relationship of parents and children, living together and more or less isolated from other close relatives.

stress Any situation or condition, positive or negative, requiring adjustment on the part of the individual, family, or group.

No factor influences a person as profoundly as the family. Families protect and promote children's growth, development, health, and well-being until the children reach maturity. A healthy family provides children with love, affection, and a sense of belonging and nurtures feelings of self-esteem and self-worth. Children need stable families to grow into happy, functioning adults. Family relationships continue to be important during adulthood. Family relationships influence, positively or negatively, people's relationships with others. Family influence continues into the next generation as a person selects a mate, forms a new family, and often rears children.

For nurses in maternity and pediatric practice, the whole family is the client. The nurse cares for the client in the context of a dynamic family system, rather than caring for just a woman, an infant, or a child. The nurse is responsible for supporting families and encouraging healthy coping patterns as families experience the crisis of birth, illness, or even changes of aging.

THE FAMILY AND NURSING CARE

Family structures in the United States are changing. The number of families with children that are headed by a married couple has declined, and the number of single-parent families has increased. In addition, roles have changed within the family. Whereas the role of provider was once almost exclusively assigned to the father, both parents now may be providers, and many fathers are active in nurturing and disciplining their children.

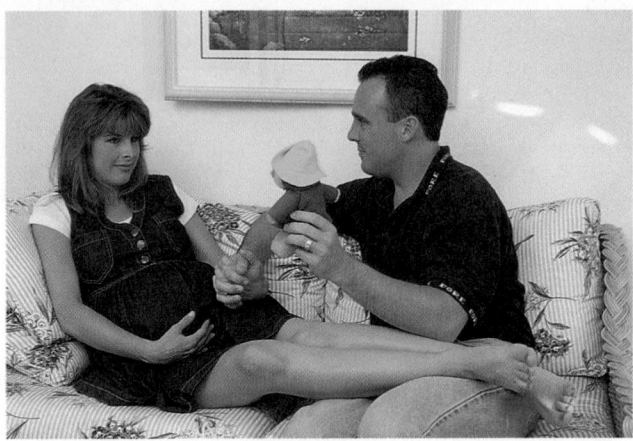

Figure 3-1 Traditional, two-parent families typically have the resources to prepare for childbirth and the needs of infants.

Types of Families

Family types are sometimes categorized into three groups: traditional, nontraditional, and high-risk. Nontraditional and high-risk families often need care that differs from the care needed by traditional families. Different family structures can produce varying stressors. For example, the single-parent family has as many demands placed on it for resources, such as time and money, as the two-parent family. There is only one parent, however, to meet these demands.

Traditional Families

Traditional families (also called nuclear families) are headed by two parents who view parenting as the major priority in their lives and whose energies are not depleted by many stressful conditions, such as poverty, illness, or substance abuse. Generally, traditional families are motivated to learn all they can about pregnancy, childbirth, and parenting (Fig. 3-1). Traditional families can be single-income or dual-income families. Today, the family structure that comprises two married parents and their children represents only 69% of families with children, down from 87% in 1970 (Fields & Casper, 2001).

Single-income families in which one parent, usually the father, is the sole provider are a minority among households in the United States. Most two-parent families depend on two incomes, either to make ends meet or to provide nonessentials that they could not afford on one income. One or both parents must often travel as a work responsibility. Dependence on two incomes has created a great deal of stress on parents, subjecting them to many of the same problems that single-parent families face. For instance, reliable, competent child care is a major issue and has increased the stress traditional families experience. A high consumer debt load gives them less cushion for financial setbacks such as job loss. It may be difficult for parents in these families to have the time and flexibility to attend to the requirements of both their careers and their children.

Nontraditional Families

The growing number of nontraditional families includes single-parent families, blended families, adoptive families, unmarried couples with children, multigenerational families, and homosexual parent families (Fig. 3-2).

Single-Parent Families. Millions of families are now headed by a single parent, most often the mother, who not only must function as homemaker and caregiver but also is often the major provider for the family's financial needs. Divorce is the most common cause of single-parent families, although childbirth among unmarried women is also a major contributor. Widowhood of the parent sometimes occurs as well. The proportion of families with children that are headed by a single mother is now 26%, while single father families, once rare, now comprise 5% of this group.

Single-parent families headed by a woman are more likely to have an income below the poverty level (34%) than those headed by a man (16%) (Fields & Casper, 2001). Single parents may feel overwhelmed by the prospect of assuming all child-rearing responsibilities and may be less prepared for illness or loss of a job than two-parent families.

Blended Families. Blended families are formed when single, divorced, or widowed parents bring children from a previous union into their new relationship. Many times the couple desires children with each other, creating a contemporary family structure commonly described as "yours, mine, and ours." These families must overcome differences in parenting styles and values to form a cohesive blended family. Differing expectations of children's behavior and development as well as differing beliefs about discipline often cause family conflict. Financial difficulties can result if one parent is obligated to pay child support from a previous relationship.

Adoptive Families. People who adopt a child may have problems that biologic parents do not face. Biologic parents have the long period of gestation and the gradual changes of pregnancy to help them adjust emotionally and socially to the birth of a child. An adoptive family, both parents and siblings, is expected to make these same adjustments suddenly when the adopted child arrives. Adoptive parents may add pressure to themselves by having an unrealistically high standard for themselves as parents. Additional issues with adoptive families may include possible lack of knowledge of the child's biologic health history, the difficulty assimilating if the child is adopted from another country, and the question of when and how to tell the child about being adopted. Adoptive parents as well as biologic parents need information, support, and guidance to prepare them to care for the infant or child and to maintain their own relationship.

Multigenerational Families. The multigenerational or extended family includes members from three or more generations living under one roof. This family structure is becoming increasingly common in the United States. Elderly parents may live with their adult children, or in some cases adult children return to their parents' home, either because they are unable to support themselves or because they want the additional support that the grandparents provide for the grandchildren. The latter arrangement has given rise to the term *boomerang* families. Extended families are vulnerable to generational conflicts and may need education and referral to counselors to prevent disintegration of the family unit.

Grandparents or other older family members, because of the inability of the parents to care for the children, now head a growing number of households with children. The strain of raising children a second time may cause tremendous physical, financial, and emotional stress.

Same-Sex Parent Families. Although families headed by same-sex parents are proportionately uncommon, they are recognized increasingly in the United States. The children in such families may be the offspring of previous heterosexual unions, or they may be adopted children or children conceived by an artificial reproductive technique such as in vitro fertilization. This couple may face many challenges from a community that is unaccustomed to alternative life-styles. The children's adaptation depends on the parents' psychologic adjustment, the degree of participation and support from the absent biologic parent, and the degree of community support.

Communal Family. Communal families include groups of people who have chosen to live together as an extended family group. Their relationship to each other is motivated by social value or financial necessity, rather than by kinship. Their values are often spiritually based and may be more liberal than the traditional family. Traditional family roles may not exist.

Characteristics of Healthy Families

In general, healthy families are able to adapt to changes that occur in the family unit. Pregnancy and parenthood create some of the most powerful changes that a family experiences.

Healthy families exhibit some common characteristics that provide a framework for assessing how all families function:

- Members of healthy families communicate openly with one another to express their concerns and needs.
- Healthy families remain flexible in role assignment so that if one person is unable to complete the usual tasks, another member offers assistance.
- Adults in healthy families agree on the basic principles of parenting so that there is minimal discord about such things as discipline and sleep schedules.
- Healthy families are adaptable and are not overwhelmed by changes that occur in the home and in relationships as a result of childbirth and parenthood.
- Members of healthy families volunteer assistance without waiting to be asked.

FACTORS THAT INTERFERE WITH FAMILY FUNCTIONING

Factors that interfere with the family's ability to provide for the needs of its members include lack of financial resources, absence of adequate family support, birth of an infant who needs specialized care, an ill child, unhealthy habits such as smoking or abuse of other substances, and inability to make mature decisions that are necessary to provide care for the children.

High-Risk Families

All families encounter stressors, but some factors add to the usual stress experienced by a family. The nurse must consider the additional needs of the family with a higher risk for being dysfunctional. Examples of these high-risk families are those experiencing marital conflict and divorce, those with adolescent parents, families affected by violence against one or more of the family members, those involved with substance abuse, and families with an ill child.

Marital Conflict and Divorce

Although divorce is traumatic to children, research has shown that living in a home filled with conflict is even more traumatic. Divorce can be the outcome of many years of unresolved family conflict. It can result in disputes over child custody, visitation, and child support; changes in housing, life-style, cultural

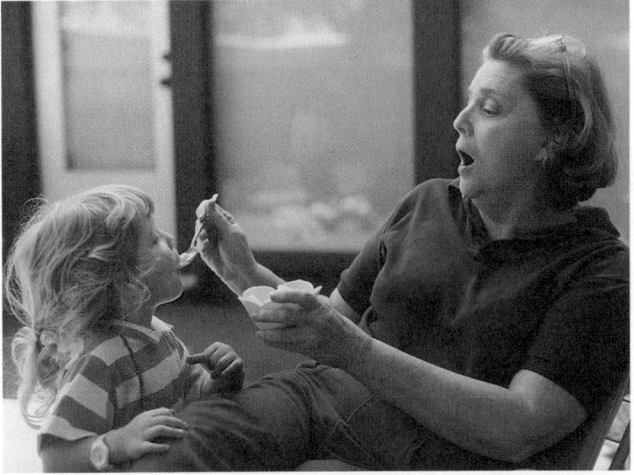

Busy parents may rely on grandparents for child care or for an additional measure of love and attention for their children. Some grandparents raise grandchildren because of their own children's inability to do so.

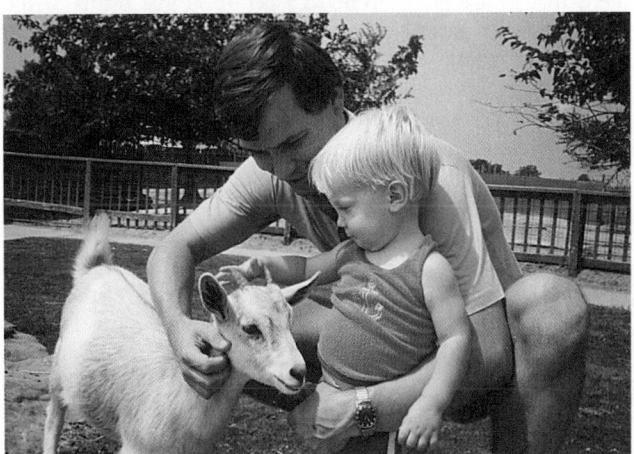

Fathers are the primary child care providers in a growing number of families. Fathers who are not the primary caregivers often participate more actively in caring for their children than the fathers of previous generations.

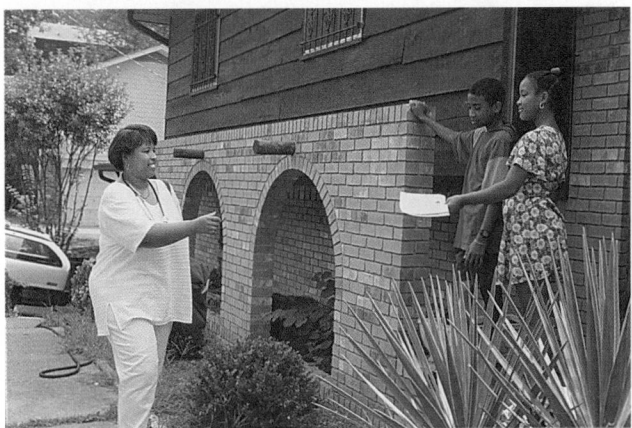

A single parent often experiences financial and time constraints. Children in single-parent families are often given more responsibility to care for themselves and younger siblings.

Figure 3-2 The nurse caring for a child needs to know the child's family structure and the identity of the child's primary caregiver. This background becomes the context in which the nurse provides care. If family support is a concern, the nurse can provide information about local community resources. For example, in some communities, after-school programs and "warm lines" can help self-care children with schoolwork and alleviate loneliness and fear for some children.

expectations, friends, and extended family relationships; diminished self-esteem; and changes in the physical, emotional, or spiritual health of the child and other family members.

Divorce is loss that needs to be grieved. The conflict and divorce may affect children, and young children may be unable to verbalize their distress. Nurses can help children through the grieving process with age-appropriate activities such as therapeutic play (see Chapter 35). Principles of active listening (see Chapter 2) are valuable for both adults and children to help them express their feelings. Nurses can also help newly divorced or separated parents through listening, encouragement, and referrals to support groups or counselors.

Adolescent Parenting

The pregnancy rate for teenagers in the United States remains higher than in other developed countries, although it has declined recently. **In 2002 in the United States, 43 per 1000 live babies were born to teenagers between the ages of 15 and 19 years.** Adolescent birth rates vary by race. Births to white teens in this age-group were 28.5 per 1000 live births, while 68.3 per 1000 were to black teens. Birth rates for Hispanic teens 15 to 19 years old were 83.4 per 1000 live births. Teen pregnancy rates vary by state as well (Martin et al, 2003).

Teenage parenting often has a negative impact on the health and social outcomes of the entire family. Adolescent girls are at increased risk for a number of pregnancy complications such as hypertension or fetal growth restriction. Those who become parents during adolescence are unlikely to attain a high level of education and as a result are more likely to be poor and often homeless. The father of the child often does not contribute to the economic or psychologic support of his children. Children of adolescent parents have a higher mortality rate and are more likely to suffer violence and neglect. Moreover, the cycle of teen parenting and economic hardship is more likely to be continued because children of adolescent parents are themselves more likely to become teenage parents. Chapter 25 provides additional information about adolescent childbearing.

Violence

Violence is a constant stressor in some families. Violence can occur in any family of any socioeconomic or educational status. Women who suffer physical or emotional abuse frequently have poorer pregnancy outcomes than women who are not abused (see Chapter 25). Their children endure the psychologic pain of seeing their mother victimized by the man who is supposed to love and care for her. In addition, because of the role models they see in the adults, these children may repeat the cycle of violence when they are adults and become abusers or victims of violence themselves.

Abuse of the child may also be physical or emotional, or the abuse may be in the form of neglect (see Chapter 53). Often, one child in the family is the target of abuse or neglect, while others are given proper care. As in adult abuse, children who witness abuse are more likely to repeat that behavior when they are parents themselves because they have not learned constructive ways to deal with their stress or to discipline children.

Substance Abuse

Substance abuse can adversely affect the health of the child before birth. The infant may suffer direct effects of the abused substances or may experience adverse effects from the mother's inadequate diet or lack of prenatal care during pregnancy (see Chapter 30).

Parents who abuse drugs or alcohol may also neglect their children. Obtaining and using the substance or substances have a stronger pull on the parents than does care of their children. In addition, their children are more likely to live in poverty and to be homeless because so much money is spent maintaining the parent's substance habit.

The child may be the substance abuser in the home. The drug habit can lead a child into unhealthy friendships and may result in criminal activity to maintain the habit. School achievement is likely to plummet, and the older adolescent may drop out of school. Both children and adults can die as a result of their drug activity, either as a direct effect of the drugs or from associated criminal activity or risk-taking behaviors.

Child With Special Needs

When a child is born with a birth defect or has an illness that requires special care, the family is under additional stress. In most cases, their initial reactions of shock and disbelief gradually resolve into acceptance of the child's limitations. However, the parents' grieving may be chronic as they repeatedly see other children doing things that their child cannot and perhaps will not ever do.

These families often suffer financial hardship. Health insurance benefits may quickly reach their maximum. Even if the child has public assistance for health care costs, the family often experiences a fall in income because one parent must remain home with the sick child rather than work outside the home.

Strains on the marriage and the parents' relationships with their other children are inevitable under these circumstances. Parents have little time or energy left to nurture their relationship with each other, and divorce may add yet another strain to the family. Siblings may resent the parental time and attention required for care of the ill child yet feel guilty if they express their resentment.

The outlook is not always pessimistic in these families, however. If the family learns skills to cope with the added demands imposed on it by this situation, there is potential for growth in maturity, compassion, and strength of character. See Chapter 36 for more information about families that have children with special needs.

HEALTHY VERSUS DYSFUNCTIONAL FAMILIES

Family conflict is unavoidable. It is a natural result of a perceived unequal exchange or an imbalance in the use of resources by individual members. Conflict should not be viewed as bad or disruptive, because it is the management of the conflict, not the conflict itself, that may be problematic. Conflict can produce growth and improved family functioning if the outcome is resolution as opposed to dissolution or continued conflict. Three ingredients are required to resolve conflict:

1. Open communication
2. Accurate perceptions about the nature and degree of conflict
3. Constructive efforts to resolve the conflict, such as willingness to consider the view of the other, consider alternate solutions, and compromise

Dysfunctional families have problems in any one or a combination of these areas. They tend to become trapped in patterns in which they maintain conflicts rather than resolve them. The conflicts create stress, and the family must cope with the resultant stress.

BOX 3-1
Coping Strategies of Families

Internal Coping Strategies
- Reliance on the family group
- Use of humor
- Greater sharing of feelings, thoughts, time, and activities
- Controlling the meaning of the problem (reframing)
- Making the event less important (normalizing)
- Joint problem solving
- Role flexibility

External Coping Strategies
- Seeking information
- Increasing links to the community
- Using social support systems (e.g., family, friends, experts, co-workers, professional services)
- Seeking spiritual support

Data from Friedman, M., Svavarsdottir, E., & McCubbin, M. (1998). Family stress and coping processes: Family adaptation. In M. Friedman. *Family nursing research, theory and practice* (4th ed.). Stamford, CT: Appleton & Lange.

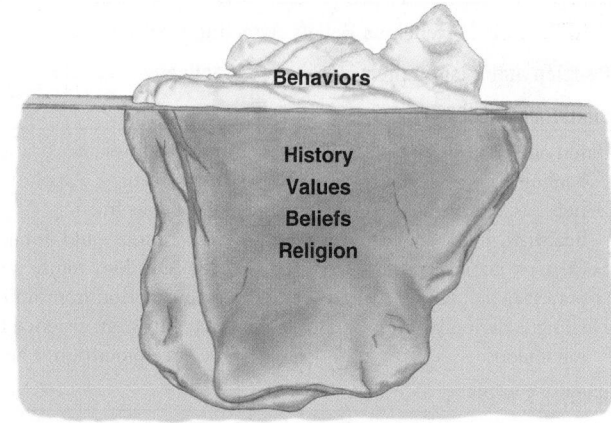

Figure 3-3 Visible and hidden layers of culture are like the visible and submerged parts of an iceberg. Many cultural differences are hidden below the surface.

Coping With Stress

When viewing the family as a balanced system that has interrelationships both internally and externally, stressors are viewed as forces that change the balance in the system. Families respond to stressors according to the relative strengths of their relationships, availability of external resources to assist with coping, cultural background, and perceptions of the seriousness of the stressors (Box 3-1) (Friedman, 1998). Some families are able to mobilize their strengths and resources, thus effectively adapting to the stressors. Other families fall apart.

Nurses can help families cope with stress by helping each family identify its strengths and resources. Feeley and Gottlieb (2000) identified four internal family strengths:

1. Traits such as optimism or resilience
2. Financial and other assets
3. Capabilities and skills of family members
4. Less defined qualities, such as motivation

Feedback to families as they use their strengths gives families a different and more positive assessment of their abilities to cope. Nurses can help families develop and use strengths by helping them (Feeley & Gottlieb, 2000):

- See how a strength that has been helpful in other situations can be used to help the current problem
- Turn a deficit into a strength
- Increase their knowledge or skill

In addition to helping families identify strengths and use them to their advantage, nurses help families identify and mobilize appropriate community resources.

Coping Strategies

Some families adjust quickly to extreme crises, whereas other families become chaotic with relatively minor crises. Family functional patterns that existed before the crisis are probably the best indicators of how the family will respond to a crisis.

Family coping strategies can be divided into internal (intrafamilial) and external (extrafamilial).

CULTURAL INFLUENCES ON MATERNITY AND PEDIATRIC NURSING

Culture is the sum of the beliefs and values that are learned, shared, and transmitted from generation to generation by a particular group. Cultural values guide the thinking, decisions, and actions of the group, particularly in pivotal events such as birth, reaching sexual maturity, and death. *Ethnicity* is the condition of belonging to a particular group that shares race, language and dialect, religious faiths, traditions, values, and symbols, as well as food preferences, literature, and folklore. Cultural beliefs and values vary among different groups, and nurses must be aware that individuals often believe their cultural values and patterns of behavior are superior to those of other groups. This belief, termed *ethnocentrism*, forms the basis for many conflicts that occur when people from different cultural groups have frequent contact.

Nurses must be aware that culture is composed of visible and invisible layers that could be said to resemble an iceberg (Fig. 3-3). The observable behaviors can be compared with the visible tip of the iceberg. The history, beliefs, values, and religion are not observed, but they are the hidden foundation on which behaviors are based and can be likened to the large, submerged part of the iceberg. To comprehend cultural behavior fully, one must seek knowledge of the hidden beliefs that behaviors express.

Religious beliefs often have a strong influence on families as they face the crisis of illness. Specific beliefs about the causes, treatment, and cure of illness are important for the nurse to know to empower the family to deal with the immediate crisis. Table 3-1 describes how some religious beliefs affect health care.

Implications of Cultural Diversity for Nurses

Many immigrants and refugees are relatively young, which means that nurses in most localities will provide care for culturally diverse childbearing and child-rearing families. To provide effective care, nurses must be aware that culture is among the most significant factors that influence birth and parenthood, health and illness.

TABLE **3-1** Religious Beliefs Affecting Health Care

Religion and Basic Beliefs	Practices
CHRISTIAN SCIENCE	
Based on scientific system of healing. Beliefs based on Bible, science, and health with key to scriptures. Seek to overcome evil through prayer, belief, and Christian acts. Healing is divinely natural, not miraculous.	*Birth:* Use physician or midwife during childbirth. No baptism ceremony. *Dietary practices:* Alcohol and tobacco are considered drugs and are not used. Coffee and tea may also be declined. *Death:* Autopsy and donation of organs are usually declined. *Health care:* May refuse medical treatment. View health in a spiritual framework. Seek exemption from immunizations, but obey legal requirements. When Christian Science believer is hospitalized, parent or client may request that a Christian Science practitioner be notified to come.
JEHOVAH'S WITNESS	
Believe in God and Son Jesus Christ. Expected to follow the example of Jesus Christ in daily living. Expected to preach house to house about the good news of God. Bible is doctrinal authority. No distinction made between clergy and laity.	*Baptism:* No infant baptism. Baptism by immersion of adults. *Dietary practices:* Use of tobacco and alcohol discouraged. *Death:* Autopsy decided by persons involved. Burial and cremation acceptable. *Birth control and abortion:* Use of birth control is a personal decision. Abortion opposed based on Exodus 21:22-23. *Health care:* Blood transfusions not allowed. May accept alternatives to transfusions, such as use of non-blood plasma expanders, careful surgical technique to minimize blood loss, and use of autologous transfusions. Nurses should check unconscious clients for identification that states that the person does not want a transfusion. Jehovah's Witnesses are prepared to die rather than break God's law. Respect the health care given by physicians, but look to God and His laws as the final authority for their decisions.
THE CHURCH OF JESUS CHRIST OF LATTER-DAY SAINTS (MORMON)	
Restorationism: True church of Christ ended with the first generation of apostles but was restored with the founding of Mormon Church. Articles of faith: Mormon doctrine states that individuals are saved if they are obedient to God's divine ordinances (faith, repentance, baptism by immersion and laying on of hands, observance of Lord's Supper on Sunday). Word of God can be found in the Bible, Book of Mormon, Doctrine, and Covenants, Pearl of Great Price, and current revelations. Christ will return to rule in Zion, located in America.	*Baptism:* By immersion. Considered essential for the living and the dead. If a child older than 8 is very ill, whether baptized or unbaptized, a member of the church's priesthood should be called. *Holy Communion:* Hospitalized client may desire to have a member of the church's priesthood administer the sacrament. *Anointing of the sick:* Mormons frequently are anointed and given a blessing before going to the hospital and after admission by laying on of hands. *Dietary practices:* Tobacco and caffeine are not used. Mormons eat meat (limited) but encourage the intake of fruits, grains, and herbs. *Death:* Prefer burial of the body. A church elder should be notified to assist the family. *Birth control and abortion:* Abortion is opposed unless the life of the mother is in danger. Only natural methods of birth control are recommended. Other means are used only when the physical or emotional health of the mother is at stake. *Other practices:* Believe in the healing power of "laying on of hands." Cleanliness is very important. Believe in healthy living and adhere to health care requirements. Families are of great importance, so visiting should be encouraged. The church maintains a welfare system to assist those in need.

Data from Carson, V.B. (1989). *Spiritual dimensions of nursing practice* (pp. 100-102). Philadelphia: Saunders; Betz, C.L., Hunsberger, M., & Wright, S. (1994). *Family-centered nursing care of children* (2nd ed., pp. 2230-2236). Philadelphia: Saunders.

Western Cultural Beliefs

Nursing practice in the United States is based largely on Western beliefs. Nurses must recognize that these beliefs may differ significantly from those of other societies and that the differences may cause a great deal of conflict.

Leininger (1978) identified seven dominant Western cultural values. These values greatly influence the thinking and action of nurses in the United States but may not be shared by their clients.

1. *Democracy* is a cultural value not shared by families who believe that elders or other higher authorities in the group make decisions. Fatalism, or a belief that events and results are predestined, may also affect health care decisions.
2. *Individualism* conflicts with the values of many cultural groups in which individual goals are subordinated to the greater good of the group.
3. *Cleanliness* is an American "obsession" viewed with amazement by many.

TABLE **3-1** Religious Beliefs Affecting Health Care—cont'd

Religion and Basic Beliefs	Practices
ROMAN CATHOLIC	
Beliefs based on Bible, apostolic tradition, and contemporary revelation.	*Baptism:* Infant baptism by affusion (sprinkling of water on head). Original sin is believed to be "washed away." If death is imminent or a fetus is aborted, anyone can perform the baptism by sprinkling water on the forehead, saying "I baptize thee in the name of the Father, Son, and Holy Spirit." *Anointing of the sick:* Encouraged for anyone who is ill or injured. Always done if prognosis is poor. *Dietary practices:* Fasting and abstinence from meat optional during Lent. No meat on Ash Wednesday and on Fridays during Lent strongly encouraged. Children and ill adults exempt from all fasting. *Death:* Organ donation permitted.
HINDUISM	
Belief in reincarnation and Karma, Yoga. Nonviolent approach to living. Various deities worshipped: Vishnu, Shiva, Ganesh, Surya, Durgam, Shati. Congregation worship is not customary.	*Dietary practices:* Dietary restrictions vary according to sect. *Death:* Death rituals specify practices and who can touch corpse. *Other practices:* Oppose artificial insemination. Circumcision is observed by ritual.
ISLAM	
Sunni (90%), Shiite (10%). Belief in one god. Based on the teaching of Muhammad. Five Pillars of Islam. Compulsory prayers are said at dawn, noon, afternoon, after sunset, and after nightfall.	*Dietary practices:* Prohibit eating pork and the use of alcohol. Fast during Ramadan (ninth month of Muslim year). *Death:* Oppose autopsy and organ donation. Death ritual prescribes the handling of corpse by only family and friends.
JUDAISM	
Beliefs are based on the Old Testament, the Torah, and the Talmud, the oral and written laws of faith. Belief in one god who is approached directly. Believe Messiah is still to come. Believe Jews are God's chosen people.	*Circumcision:* A symbol of God's covenant with Israel. Done on eighth day after birth. *Bar Mitzvah:* Ceremonial rite of passage for boys (approximately 13 years of age) into manhood. *Death:* Remains are washed according to rite by members of the Ritual Burial Society. Burial occurs as soon as possible.

4. *Preoccupation with time*, which is measured by health care professionals in minutes and hours, is a major source of conflict with those who mark time by different standards, such as seasons or body needs.
5. *Reliance on machines and equipment* may intimidate families who are not comfortable with technology.
6. *The belief that optimal health is a right* is in direct conflict with beliefs in many cultures in the world in which health is not a major emphasis or even an expectation.
7. *Admiration of self-sufficiency and financial success* may conflict with the beliefs of other societies that place less value

on wealth and more value on less tangible things such as spirituality.

Cultural Influences on the Care of Specific Groups

To provide the best care for all clients, the nurse should know common cultural beliefs and practices that influence nursing care. Because communication is an essential component of nursing assessment and teaching, the nurse must understand cultural influences that may form barriers to communicating with people from another culture.

Asian-Americans

Asian-Americans have origins in many areas, such as the Far East, Southeast Asia, or the Philippines . Their roots are not only in their country of origin but their ethnic viewpoint. Asian-Americans comprise 4.2% of the U.S. population (Barnes & Bennett, 2002).

In Asian-American culture, the family is highly valued and often consists of many generations that remain close to each other. The elders of the family are highly respected. Self-sufficiency and self-control are highly valued. Asian-Americans place a high value on "face," or honor and may be unwilling to do anything that causes another to "lose face." When medication or therapy is recommended, they seldom say no. They may accept the prescription or medication sample but not take the medicine, or they may agree to undergo a procedure but not keep the appointment. Stoicism may make pain assessment difficult. Herbal medicines and practices such as acupressure may play an important part in healing for these people.

Language is the greatest barrier to health care for those from Southeast Asia (Mattson, 1995). Besides the national languages of Vietnam, Cambodia, and Laos, numerous languages are spoken within subgroups in each country. People from Southeast Asia speak softly and avoid prolonged eye contact, which they consider rude.

Hispanics

Hispanics, also called *Latinos*, include those whose origin is Mexico, Central and South America, and Puerto Rico. This group is now the fastest growing population in the United States. Half of all U.S. Hispanic residents reside in two states, California and Texas (Guzman, 2001).

Men are usually the head of household and considered strong (macho). Women are the homemakers. Hispanics usually have a close extended family and place a high value on children.

Hispanics tend to be polite and gracious in conversation. Preliminary social interaction is particularly important, and Hispanics may be insulted if a problem is addressed directly without taking time for "small talk." This is counter to the value of "getting to the point" for many white people in the United States and may cause frustration for the client as well as for the health care worker.

There is a strong association between religion and health. The *curandero*, a folk healer, may be consulted for health care before an American health care worker is consulted.

African-Americans

African-Americans comprise 12.9% of the U.S. population and have increased faster than the overall population (McKinnon, 2001). African-Americans are often part of a close extended family, although many heads of household are single women. They have a sense of loyalty to their people and community, but they sometimes distrust the majority group.

African-Americans sometimes use a communication style that may cause conflict when they seek health care. They may use idioms, colloquial expressions, or speech patterns that are unfamiliar to health care workers. Nurses must often clarify what is being said to avoid misunderstandings and enhance teaching.

The black minister is highly influential, and religious rituals, such as prayer, are frequently used. Illness may be seen as the will of God.

Native Americans

Native Americans include American Indians and Alaska Natives. This group makes up 1.5% of the total U.S. population. Many who consider themselves Native Americans are of mixed race. The largest American Indian tribal groups include Cherokee, Navajo, Latin American Indian, Choctaw, Sioux, and Chippewa. The largest tribe among Alaska Natives are the Eskimos (Ogunwole, 2002).

Native Americans may consider a willful child to be strong and a docile child to be weak. They have close family relationships, and respect for their elders is the norm. Native Americans may consider health to be a state of harmony with nature and may believe that supernatural influences have a great impact on health and illness. Native Americans may highly respect a medicine man, who they believe to be given power by supernatural forces. The use of herbs and rituals is part of the medicine man's curative practice.

Middle Easterners

Middle Eastern immigrants come from several countries, including Lebanon, Syria, Saudi Arabia, Egypt, Turkey, Iran, and Palestine. Islam is the dominant, and often the official, religion in these countries; its followers are known as *Muslims*. The man is typically the head of the household in Muslim families. Muslim women often prefer a female health care provider because of laws of modesty. Many Muslim women keep their head, arms to the wrists, and legs to the ankles covered. Islam requires believers to kneel and pray five times a day, at: dawn, noon, afternoon, after sunset, and after nightfall. Muslims do not eat pork and do not use alcohol. Many are vegetarians.

Communication in these countries is elaborate, and obtaining health information may be difficult because Islam dictates that family affairs should be kept within the family. Personal information is shared only with personal friends, and the health assessment must be done gradually. When interpreters are used, they should be of the same country and religion, if possible, because of regional differences and hostilities. Because Islamic society tends to be paternalistic, it is wise to ask the husband's permission or opinion when family members need health care.

Cross-Cultural Health Beliefs

More than 100 different ethnocultural groups reside in the United States, and numerous traditional health beliefs are observed among these groups. For example, definitions of health are often culturally based. People of Asian origin may view health as the balance of yin and yang. Those of African or Haitian origin may define health as harmony with nature. Those from Mexico, Central and South America, and Puerto Rico often see health as a balance of hot and cold.

Traditional Methods of Preventing Illness

The traditional methods of preventing illness rest in the person's ability to understand the cause of a given illness in their culture. These causes may include:

- Agents such as hexes, spells, or the evil eye, which may strike a person (often a child) and cause injury, illness, or misfortune
- Phenomena such as soul loss or accidentally provoking envy, jealousy, or hate of a friend or acquaintance
- Environmental factors such as bad air, and natural events such as solar eclipses

Practices to prevent illness developed from beliefs about the cause of illness. One must avoid those known to transmit hexes and spells. Elaborate methods are used to prevent inciting envy or jealousy of others and to avoid the evil eye. Protective or religious objects, such as amulets with magic powers or consecrated religious objects (talismans), are frequently worn or carried to prevent illness. There are also numerous food taboos and traditional combinations that are prescribed in traditional belief systems to prevent illness. For instance, people from many ethnic backgrounds eat raw garlic to prevent illness. Those of African origin may consume nonfood substances such as starch to make labor easier.

Traditional Practices to Maintain Health

A variety of traditional practices are used to maintain health. For instance, wearing proper clothing, such as a scarf, may prevent drafts and thus maintain the health of a woman who is pregnant and believes she must avoid cool air. Mental and spiritual health are maintained by activities such as silence, meditation, and prayer. Many people view illness as punishment for breaking a religious code and adhere strictly to religious morals and practices to maintain health.

Traditional Practices to Restore Health

Traditional practices to restore health often conflict with Western medical practice. Some of the most common practices include the use of natural substances, such as herbs and plants, to treat illness. Religious charms, holy words, or traditional healers may be tried before an individual seeks a medical opinion. Wearing religious medals, carrying prayer cards, and performing sacrifices are other practices used to treat illness.

A variety of substances may be ingested for the treatment of illnesses. The nurse should try to identify what the woman or child is taking and to determine whether the active ingredient may alter the effects of prescribed medication. In the case of a pregnant woman, the effects of the traditional substance on the developing fetus must be considered as well.

Dermabrasion, the rubbing or irritation of the skin to relieve discomfort, is a common health care practice. The most popular form is *coining*, in which an area is covered with an ointment and the edge of a coin is rubbed over the area. All dermabrasion methods leave marks resembling bruises or burns on the skin and may be mistaken for signs of physical abuse.

Cultural Assessment

All health care professionals must develop skill in performing a cultural assessment so they can understand the meaning of health and illness in the cultural groups they encounter. The following questions might be considered in making such an assessment:

- What is the family's ethnic affiliation?
- Is childbearing viewed as a normal process, a time of vulnerability, or a state of illness?
- What are the prescribed practices, customs, or rituals related to diet, activity, or behavior during pregnancy and childbirth or illness?
- What maternal restrictions or precautions are necessary during pregnancy, childbirth, and after birth? Are women exempted from any religious practices at this time?

- Who provides support during pregnancy, childbirth, and parenthood?
- What are the prescribed practices and restrictions related to care of the newborn?
- Who in the family hierarchy makes health care decisions?
- How is time marked—in minutes and hours, or by seasons and body needs?
- How does the family view life and death? Are predestination and fatalism among the family's beliefs?
- How can health care professionals be most helpful?

After such an assessment, plans for care should show respect for cultural differences and traditional healing practices. Additional cultural information is presented throughout this book relating to specific areas in maternity and child health care.

PARENTING

Parenting implies the commitment of an individual or individuals to provide for the physical and psychosocial needs of a child. Many believe that parenting is the most difficult and yet rewarding experience an individual can have. Many parents assume this important job with little education in parenting or child rearing. If the parents themselves have had good parents as role models and seek resources, the transition to parenting is made easier. Nurses are in a good position to provide parents with information on effective parenting skills through many venues, such as formal classes, anticipatory guidance at well-child checkups, or role modeling.

Parenting Styles

Three major parenting styles have been identified in the literature. These categories, while discussed in general here, are being viewed with increasing skepticism as researchers recognize that parenting styles work in different ways in different cultures. For example, the authoritative parenting style may not work effectively for parents of inner-city children. These parents may more frequently use authoritarian-style parenting techniques because strict obedience to rules may keep the child safer in an urban environment.

Authoritarian parents have rules. They expect obedience from the child without any questioning about the reasons behind the rule. They also expect the child to accept the family beliefs and principles without question. Give and take is discouraged.

Children raised with this style of parenting can be shy and withdrawn because of a lack of self-confidence. If the parents are somewhat affectionate, the child may be sensitive, submissive, honest, and dependable. If affection has been withheld, however, the child may exhibit rebellious, antisocial behavior.

Authoritative parents tend to show respect for the opinions of each of their children by allowing them to be different. Although there are rules in the household, the parents permit discussion if the children do not understand or agree with the rules. The parents make it clear to the children that although they (the parents) are the ultimate authority, some negotiation and compromise may take place. This style of parenting tends to result in children who have high self-esteem and are independent, inquisitive, happy, assertive, and highly interactive.

Permissive parents have little or no control over the behavior of their children. If any rules exist in the home, they are inconsistent and unclear. Underlying reasons for rules may be given, but the children are generally allowed to decide whether they will follow the rule and to what extent. Limits are not set, and discipline is inconsistent. The children learn that they can get away with any behavior. Role reversal occurs: the children are more like the parents, and the parents are like the children.

Children who come from this type of home are typically disrespectful, disobedient, aggressive, irresponsible, and defiant. They tend to be insecure because of a lack of guidelines to direct their behavior. These children tend to be creative and spontaneous.

Regardless of the primary parenting style, parenting is more effective when parents are able to adjust their parenting techniques according to the child's developmental level and when parents are involved and interested in their children's activities and friends.

Parent-Child Relationship Factors

Relationships between parents and children are bi-directional, with the parent's behavior affecting the child and the child's behavior affecting the parenting. The parents' age, experience, and self-confidence affect the quality of the parent-child relationship, the stability of the marital relationship, and the interplay between the child's individualism and the parents' expectations of the child.

Parental Characteristics

Parenting is multidimensional. Simpson (2001) described five positive parenting tasks for parenting adolescents. Each of these five tasks is a parenting skill that exemplifies parenting regardless of the child's developmental stage.

1. Emotional availability (loving and connecting)
2. Control (guiding and limiting)
3. Monitoring (being informed)
4. Modeling (decision making and consultation)
5. Providing (maintaining a supportive physical, emotional, and social environment)

In addition, parents who have had previous experience with children, whether through younger siblings, a career, or raising previous children, bring an element of experience to the art of parenting. Self-confidence and age can also be factors in a person's ability to parent. How an individual was parented has a major impact on how he or she will assume the role. The strength of the parents' relationship also affects their parenting skills as does the presence or absence of support systems. Support can come from the family or community. Peer groups can provide an arena for parents to share experiences and solve problems. Parents with more experience are often an important resource for new parents.

Characteristics of the Child

Characteristics that may affect the parent-child relationship include the child's physical appearance, sex, and temperament. At birth, the infant's physical appearance may not meet the parents' expectations, or the infant may resemble a disliked relative. As a result, the parent may subconsciously reject the child. If the parents desired a baby of a particular sex, they may be disappointed. If parents are not given the opportunity to talk about this disappointment, they may reject the infant. See Chapter 21 for additional information about bonding and attachment.

Temperament and Parental Expectations

Temperament can be described as the way individuals behave, or their behavioral style. Several researchers have studied temperament. Chess and Thomas (1996) developed three temperament categories based on nine characteristics of temperament they identified in children.

1. *Easy:* These children are even-tempered, predictable, and regular in their habits. They react positively to new stimuli.
2. *Difficult:* These children are highly active, irritable, moody, and irregular in their habits. They adapt slowly to new stimuli and often express intense negative emotions.
3. *Slow to warm up:* These children are inactive, moody, and moderately irregular in their habits. They adapt slowly to new stimuli and express mildly intense negative emotions.

There has been some objection to the term *difficult* because it tends to have a negative connotation. That is the term established in temperament research, however, and it is important that parents recognize that a "difficult" child is very normal. As is true for other characteristics such as appearance, the parent-child relationship is likely to have less conflict if the child's temperament meets the parents' expectations.

Discipline

Children's behavior challenges most parents. The manner in which parents respond to a child's behavior has a profound effect on the child's self-esteem and future interactions with others. Children learn to view themselves in the same way that the parent views them. Thus if parents view their children as wild, the children begin to view themselves as wild, and soon their actions consistently reinforce their self-image. In this way, the children will not disappoint the parents. This pattern is called a *self-fulfilling prophecy* and is a cyclic process.

Discipline refers to the system of teaching and nurturing that prepares children to achieve competence, self-control, self-direction, and caring for others (Howard, 1996). Discipline is designed to teach a child how to function effectively within society. It is the foundation for self-discipline. The primary goal of a parent should be to help the child feel lovable and capable. This goal is best accomplished by the parent setting limits to enhance a sense of security until the child can incorporate the family's values and is capable of self-discipline.

When a child is in the health care system, the nurse has the opportunity to aid in the socialization of the child to some degree. Through both formal instruction and informal role modeling, the nurse can help the parent learn how to discipline a child effectively. Box 3-2 lists ways in which a parent or nurse can facilitate children's socialization and increase their self-esteem.

Dealing With Misbehavior

A child's misbehavior may be defined as behavior outside the norms of acceptance within the family. Misbehavior stretches the limits of tolerance in all parents, even the most patient parent. A parent's response to the child's misbehavior can have minor consequences such as short-term frustration, or major consequences such as child abuse. To prevent these negative consequences, the nurse can help teach parents various strategies for effective discipline. There are three essen-

> ### BOX 3-2
> *Effective Discipline for Positive Socialization and Self-Esteem*
>
> - Attend promptly to an infant's and young child's needs.
> - Provide structure and consistency for young children.
> - Give positive attention for positive behavior; use praise when deserved.
> - Listen.
> - Set aside time every day for one-on-one attention.
> - Demonstrate appreciation of the child's unique characteristics.
> - Encourage choices and decision making, and allow the child to experience consequences of mistakes.
> - Model respect for others.
> - Provide unconditional love.

tial components of effective discipline (American Academy of Pediatrics, 2003):

1. A positive, supportive, loving relationship between the parent(s) and child
2. Use of positive reinforcement strategies to increase desired behaviors
3. Removing reinforcement or applying punishment to reduce or eliminate undesired behaviors. Using time out or other alternatives, rather than spanking or other forms of physical punishment when punishment is needed

Punishment is the application of a negative stimulus to reduce or eliminate a behavior. Punishment can be in the form of a verbal statement, or it can be of a corporal nature that involves some form of physical pain or restriction of activities to emphasize a point. The American Academy of Pediatrics discourages the use of spanking or other forms of physical punishment (American Academy of Pediatrics, 2003).

Redirection. Redirection is a simple and effective method in which the parent removes the problem and distracts the child with an alternative activity or object. This method is helpful with infants through preadolescents.

Reasoning. Reasoning involves explaining why a behavior is not permitted. Younger children lack the cognitive skills and developmental abilities to comprehend reasoning fully. For example, a 4-year-old may better understand that he will have to spend time in his room if he breaks his brother's toy rather than understanding the concept of respecting the property of others.

When this technique is used with older children, it is important to focus on the behavior and not the child. The child should not be made to feel guilt and shame, because these feelings are counterproductive and can damage the child's self-esteem. The parent can focus on the behavior most effectively by using "I" rather than "you" messages.

A "you" message is one that criticizes children and uses guilt in an attempt to get them to change their behavior. An example of a "you" message is "Don't take your little sister's toys away and make her cry. You're being a bad boy!"

By contrast, an "I" message focuses on the misbehavior by explaining its effect on others. An example of an "I" message is "Your little sister cries when you take her toys away because she doesn't know that you will give them back to her."

Time-Out. Time-out is a method to remove the attention given to a child who is misbehaving. The child is placed in a nonstimulating environment where the parent can observe unobtrusively. For example, a chair could be placed facing a wall in a hall or bathroom. The child is told to sit on the chair for a predetermined time, usually 1 minute per year of age. If the child cries or fights, the timing is not begun until the child is quiet. The use of a kitchen timer with a bell is effective because the child knows when the time begins and when it has elapsed. At that time, the child is permitted to get up. After the child has calmed and the time is completed, it may be appropriate to discuss the behavior that prompted the time-out at a level appropriate to the child's age.

Consequences. This technique helps children learn the direct result of their misbehavior and can be used with toddlers through adolescents. If children must deal with the consequences of their behavior and the consequences are meaningful to them, they are less likely to repeat the behavior. There are three categories of consequences:

1. *Natural:* Consequences that occur spontaneously. For example, a child loses a favorite toy after leaving it outside and the parent does not replace it.
2. *Logical:* Consequences that are directly related to the misbehavior. For example, when two children are fighting over a toy, the parent removes the toy from both of them for a day.
3. *Unrelated:* Consequences that are imposed purposely. For example, a child comes in late for dinner and, as a consequence, is not allowed to watch TV that evening.

Some parents have difficulty allowing their children to face the consequences of their actions. When parents choose to deny their children this experience, they lose an important opportunity to teach responsibility for one's actions.

Behavior Modification. The behavior modification technique of discipline rewards positive behavior and ignores negative behavior. This technique requires parents to choose selected behaviors, preferably only one at a time, that they desire to stop. They choose others that they want to encourage. The basic technique is useful for any age from toddlerhood through adolescence. For a young child, the selected positive behaviors are marked on a chart and explained to the child. For an older child, a contract can be written. The negative behaviors are kept in mind by the parents but are not recorded where the child can see them. A system of rewards is established. Stickers or stars on a chart for young children and tokens for older children are effective ways to record the behaviors. Children should receive a predetermined reward (e.g., a movie, book, or outing) after they successfully perform the behavior a set number of times. This system should continue for several months until the behavior becomes a habit for the child. Children gain a sense of mastery and actually enjoy the process, often viewing it as a game.

Negative behaviors are simply ignored. If the parent refuses to give the child attention for the behavior, the child soon gives up that strategy. Consistency is the key to success for this technique, and many parents find this method difficult to enforce. Parents need to be warned that children frequently test the seriousness of this attempt by increasing their negative behavior soon after the parents begin ignoring it. If this technique is to be successful, the parents need to ignore the negative behavior every time.

Corporal Punishment. Corporal punishment usually takes the form of spanking. It is highly controversial and should be discouraged. The problems cited when corporal punishment is used include:

- The decrease in misbehavior is short term.
- Children learn that violence is acceptable.
- Children become accustomed to the pain, so some parents may feel that more severe pain is needed.
- Parents may experience rage and lose control, causing harm to the child.

Because of the negative consequences of spanking and because it is no more effective than other methods of discipline,

! CRITICAL TO REMEMBER

Corporal Punishment as Discipline

Corporal punishment can lead to child abuse if the disciplinarian loses control. It can also lead to false accusations of child abuse by either the child or other adults. Because of the high cost and low benefit of this form of punishment, parents should think seriously before using it.

the American Academy of Pediatrics (1998) recommends that parents be encouraged and assisted in developing methods of discipline other than spanking.

KEY CONCEPTS

- Traditional families may be single-income or dual-income families. Two-income families are much more common at present.
- Nontraditional family structures may require nursing care that is different from that required by traditional families. These families may include single-parent, blended, adoptive, multigenerational (extended), and homosexual parent families.
- High-risk families have additional stressors that affect their functioning. Some high-risk families include families headed by adolescents; families affected by marital discord or divorce, violence, or substance abuse; or families with a severely or chronically ill member.

- All families experience stress. It is how the family deals with stress that is important.
- Identifying healthy versus dysfunctional family patterns can help the nurse implement effective strategies to care for the child and the family.
- Clients during health and illness are cared for within the framework of their family and their culture.
- Traditional cultural beliefs may be used to prevent illness, maintain health, and restore health.
- Differing cultural beliefs and expectations between the health care provider and the family can create conflict.

- The effects of an ill child on a family may include fear, helplessness, anxiety, role confusion, and general stress on the parents. The siblings of the ill child may experience confusion, anger, resentment, and guilt.
- A knowledge of generally effective, healthy internal and external coping strategies can help the nurse offer the family specific suggestions for coping.
- The nurse can help parents learn effective discipline methods by teaching and role modeling.

REFERENCES and READINGS

American Academy of Pediatrics Committee on Community Health Services. (1997). Health care for children of immigrant families. *Pediatrics, 100*(1), 153-156.

American Academy of Pediatrics Committee on Psychosocial Aspects of Child and Family Health. (1998). Guidance for effective discipline. *Pediatrics, 101*(4), 723-728. (2003). *Just the facts.....effective discipline.* Retrieved from www.aap.org

Ateah, C. (2003). Disciplinary practices with children: Parental sources of information, attitudes, and educational needs. *Issues in Comprehensive Pediatric Nursing, 26*(2), 89-101.

Banks, J. (2002). Childhood discipline: Challenges for clinicians and parents. *American Family Physician, 66*(8), 1447-1452.

Banks-Wallace, J. (1999). Storytelling as a tool for providing holistic care for women. *MCN: American Journal of Maternal-Child Nursing, 24*(1), 20-24.

Barnes, J.S., & Bennett, C.E. (2002). *The Asian population: Census 2000 brief.* Washington, DC: U.S. Census Bureau. Retrieved from www.census.gov/prod/2002pubs/c2kbr01-16.pdf. 7/3/2003.

Bear, G., Minke, K., & Thomas, A. (1997). *Children's needs II: Development, problems and alternatives.* Bethesda, MD: National Association of School Psychologists.

Bowen, M. (1976). Theory in the practice of psychotherapy. In P.J. Guerin (Ed.). *Family therapy theory and practice* (pp. 42-89). New York: Gardner Press.

Callister, L.C. (2001). Culturally competent care of women and newborns: Knowledge, attitude, and skills. *Journal of Obstetric, Gynecologic, and Neonatal Nursing, 30*(2), 209-215.

Centers for Disease Control and Prevention. (2001). *New CDC report tracks trends in teen births from 1940-2000.* Retrieved July 3, 2003, from www.cdc.gov/nchs/releases/01facts/teenbirths.htm.

Centers for Disease Control and Prevention. (2002). Births: Final data for 2001. *National Vital Statistics Reports, 51*(2). Retrieved June 17, 2003, from www.cdc.gov/nchs/data/nvsr/nvsr51/nvsr51_02.pdf.

Cesario, S.K. (2001). Care of the Native American woman: Strategies for practice, education, and research. *Journal of Obstetric, Gynecologic, and Neonatal Nursing, 30*(1), 13-19.

Chess, S., & Thomas, A. (1996). *Temperament theory and practice.* New York: Brunner/Mazel.

Cohen, F. (1984). Coping. In J.D. Matarazzo, S. Weiss, J. Herd, & S. Weiss (Eds.). *Behavioral health: A handbook of health enhancement and disease prevention* (pp. 261-274). New York: Wiley.

D'Avanzo, C.E., & Geissler, E.M. (2003). *Cultural health assessment* (3rd ed.). St. Louis: Mosby.

Davis, R.E. (2001). The postpartum experience for Southeast Asian women in the United States. *MCN: American Journal of Maternal-Child Nursing, 26*(4), 208-213.

Feeley, N., & Gottlieb, L. (2000). Nursing approaches for working with family strengths and resources. *Journal of Family Nursing, 6*(1), 9-24.

Fields, J., & Casper, L.M. (2001). *America's families and living arrangements: March 2000.* Current Population Reports P20-537. Washington, DC: U.S. Census Bureau. Retrieved June 29, 2003, from www.census.gov/prod/2001pubs/p20-537.pdf.

Friedman, M. (1998). *Family nursing: Theory, research and practice.* Stamford, CT: Appleton & Lange.

Gross, D., & Garvey, C. (1997). Scolding, spanking, and time out revisited. *American Journal of Maternal Child Nursing, 22*(4), 209-213.

Guzman, B. (2001). *The Hispanic population: Census 2000 brief.* Washington, DC: U.S. Census Bureau. Retrieved July 3, 2003, from www.census.gov/prod/2001pubs/c2kbr01-3.pdf.

Hackworth, S. (1998). Grandparents raising grandchildren. *Contemporary Pediatrics, 15*(9), 75-83.

Hanson, S. (2001). *Family health care nursing: Theory, practice, and research* (2nd ed.). Philadelphia: Davis.

Howard, B. (1996). Advising parents on discipline: What works. *Pediatrics, 98*(4), 809-815.

Hutchinson, M.K., & BaqiAziz, M. (1994). Nursing care of the childbearing Muslim family. *Journal of Obstetric, Gynecologic, and Neonatal Nursing, 23*(9), 767-772.

Katz, A. (2002). Where I come from we don't talk about that: Exploring sexuality among Blacks, Asians, and Hispanics. *AWHONN Lifelines, 6*(6), 533-536.

Lamberg, L. (1996). Nationwide study of health and coping among immigrant children and families. *Journal of the American Medical Association, 276*(18), 1455-1456.

Leininger, M. (1978). *Transcultural nursing: Concepts, theories, practices.* New York: Wiley.

Levine, M., Carey, W., & Crocker, A. (1999). *Developmental-behavioral pediatrics.* Philadelphia: Saunders.

Logsdon, M.C. (2000). Helping hands: Exploring the cultural implications of social support during pregnancy. *AWHONN Lifelines, 4*(6), 29-32.

Martin, J.A., Hamilton, B.E., Sutton, P.D., Ventura, S.J., Menacker, F., & Munson, M.L. (2003). Births: Final data for 2002. *National Vital Statistics Reports, 52*(10). Hyattsville, MD: National Center for Health Statistics, 2003.

Mattson, S. (1995). Culturally sensitive perinatal care for Southeast Asians. *Journal of Obstetric, Gynecologic, and Neonatal Nursing, 24*(4), 335-342.

Mattson, S. (2000a). Providing culturally competent care: Strategies and approaches for perinatal clients. *AWHONN Lifelines, 4*(5), 37-39.

Mattson, S. (2000b). Striving for cultural competence: Providing care for the changing face of the U.S. *AWHONN Lifelines, 4*(3), 48-52.

Mattson, S. (2000c). Working toward cultural competence: Making the first steps through cultural assessment. *AWHONN Lifelines, 4*(4), 41-43.

McKinnon, J. (2001). *The Black population: Census 2000 brief.* Washington, DC: U.S. Census Bureau. Retrieved July 3, 2003, from www.census.gov/prod/2001pubs/c2kbr01-5.pdf.

Mrazek, D., Mrazek, P., & Klinnert, M. (1995). Clinical assessment of parenting. *Journal of the American Academy of Child and Adolescent Psychiatry, 34*(3), 272-282.

Nance, T.A. (1995). Intercultural communication: Finding common ground. *Journal of Obstetric, Gynecologic, and Neonatal Nursing, 24*(3), 249-255.

Nicholson, B.C., Janz, P.C., & Fox, R.A. (1998). Evaluating a brief parental-education program for parents of young children. *Psychological Report, 82*(3 Pt. 2), 1107-1113.

Ogunwole, S.U. (2002). *The American Indian and Alaska Native Population: Census 2000 brief.* Washington, DC: U.S. Census Bureau. Retrieved July 3, 2003, from www.census.gov/prod/2002pub/c2kbr01-15.pdf.

Ottani, P.A. (2002). Enhancing global similarities: A framework for cross-cultural nursing care. *Journal of Obstetric, Gynecologic, and Neonatal Nursing, 31*(1), 31, 33-38.

Pawel, J. (2001). Tools for building self-esteem. *The Brown University Child and Adolescent Behavior Letter, 17*(4), S1.

Riordan, J., & Gill-Hopple, K. (2002). Breastfeeding care in multicultural populations. *Journal of Obstetric, Gynecologic, and Neonatal Nursing, 30*(2), 216-223.

Simpson, A. (2001). *Raising teens: A synthesis of research and a foundation for action.* Boston, MA: Center for Health Communication, Harvard School of Public Health.

Spector, R.E. (1995). Cultural concepts of women's health and health-promoting behaviors. *Journal of Obstetric, Gynecologic, and Neonatal Nursing, 24*(3), 241-245.

Ventura, S.J., Mathews, T.J., & Hamilton, B.E. (2002). Teenage births in the United States: Trends, 1991-2000, an update. *National Vital Statistics Reports, 50*(9). Hyattsville, MD: National Center for Health Statistics.

4

Health Promotion for the Developing Child

After studying this chapter, you should be able to:
- Define terms related to growth and development.
- Discuss principles of growth and development.
- Describe various factors that affect growth and development.
- Discuss the following theorists' ideas about growth and development: Piaget, Freud, Erikson, and Kohlberg.
- Discuss theories of language development.
- Identify methods used to assess growth and development.
- Describe the classifications and social aspects of play.
- Explain how play enhances growth and development.
- Identify health-promoting activities that are essential for the normal growth and development of infants and children.
- Discuss recommendations for scheduled vaccines.
- Discuss the components of a nutritional assessment.
- Discuss the etiology and prevention of childhood injuries.

◆ DEFINITIONS

cephalocaudal Progression from head to toe.

chronologic age Age in years.

developmental age Age based on functional behavior and ability to adapt to the environment; does not necessarily correspond to chronologic age.

dramatic play Play in which children act out roles and experiences that may have happened to them, that they fear will happen to them, or that they have observed happening to someone else.

familiarization play Use of materials that are commonly associated with health care situations in creative and playful activities.

growth spurts Brief periods of a rapid increase in growth rate.

heredity Transmission of genetic characteristics from parent to offspring.

learning Behavior changes that occur as a result of both maturation and experience with the environment.

nutrients Foods that supply the body with elements necessary for metabolism.

proximodistal Progression from the center outward or from the midline to the periphery.

recommended dietary allowance (RDA) Recommendations for the average amounts of nutrients that should be consumed daily by healthy people in the United States.

regression Appearance of behavior more appropriate to an earlier stage of development; often used to cope with stress or anxiety.

symbolic play Use of games and interactions that represent an issue or concern to be addressed.

Humans grow and change dramatically during childhood and adolescence. Normal growth and development proceed in an orderly, predictable pattern that establishes a basis for assessing an individual's abilities and potential. Nurses provide health care teaching and anticipatory guidance about the growth and development of children in many settings, such as newborn nurseries, emergency departments, community clinics and health centers, and pediatric inpatient units.

OVERVIEW OF GROWTH AND DEVELOPMENT

Nurses frequently are the members of the health care team whom parents approach. Parents are often concerned that their children are not progressing normally. Nurses can reassure parents about normal variations in development and can also identify problems early so that developmental delays can

be addressed as soon as possible. Nurses who work with ill children must have a clear understanding of how children differ from adults and from each other at various stages. This awareness is essential to allow nurses to create developmentally appropriate plans of care to meet the needs of their young clients.

Definition of Terms

Although the terms *growth* and *development* often are used together and interchangeably, they have distinct definitions and meanings. Growth generally refers to an increase in the physical size of a whole or any of its parts or an increase in the number and size of cells. Growth can be measured easily and accurately. For example, any observer can see that an infant grows rapidly during the first year of life. This growth can be

BOX 4-1
Stages of Growth and Development

The following stages and age-groupings refer to stages of childhood growth and development:

Newborn	Birth to 1 month
Infancy	1 month to 1 year
Toddlerhood	1 to 3 years
Preschool age	3 to 6 years
School age	6 to 11 or 12 years
Adolescence	11 or 12 to 21 years

! CRITICAL TO REMEMBER

Patterns of Growth and Development

Although heredity determines each individual's growth rate, the normal pace of growth of all children falls into four distinct patterns:

1. A rapid pace from birth to 2 years
2. A slower pace from 2 years to puberty
3. A rapid pace from puberty to approximately 15 years
4. A sharp decline from 16 years to approximately 24 years, when full adult size is reached

measured readily by determining changes in weight and length. The difference in size between a newborn and a 12-month-old is an obvious sign of the remarkable growth that occurs during the first year of life.

Development is a more complex and subtle concept. Development is generally considered a continuous, orderly series of conditions that leads to activities, new motives for activities, and patterns of behavior.

Another definition of development is an increase in function and complexity that occurs through growth, maturation, and learning—in other words, an increase in capabilities. The process of language acquisition provides an example of development. The use of language becomes increasingly complex as the child matures. At 10 to 12 months of age, a child uses single words to communicate simple desires and needs. By age 4 to 5 years, complete and complex sentences are used to relate elaborate tales. Language development can be measured by determining vocabulary, articulation skill, and word use.

Maturity and learning also affect development. *Maturation* is the physical change in the complexity of body structures that enables a child to function at increasingly higher levels. Maturity is programmed genetically and may occur as a result of several changes. For example, maturation of the central nervous system depends on changes that occur throughout the body, such as an increase in the number of neurons, myelinization of nerve fibers, lengthening of muscles, and overall weight gain.

Learning involves changes in behavior that occur as a result of both maturation and experience with the environment. Predictable patterns are observed in learning, and these patterns are sequential, orderly, and progressive. For example, when learning to walk, babies first learn to control their heads, then to roll over, next to sit, then to crawl, and finally to walk. The child's muscle mass and nervous system must grow and mature as well.

These examples show how complex and interrelated the processes of growth, development, maturation, and learning are. Children must be monitored carefully to ensure that these complicated events and activities unfold normally. Wide variations occur as children grow and develop. Each child has a unique rate and pattern of development, although parameters are used to identify abnormalities. Nurses must be familiar with normal parameters so that delays can be detected early. The earlier that delays are discovered and intervention initiated, the less dramatic their effect will be.

Stages of Growth and Development

To simplify analysis and discussion of the complex processes and theories related to growth and development, researchers and theorists have identified stages or age-groupings. These stages serve as reference points in describing various features of growth and development (Box 4-1). Chapters 5 through 8 discuss the physical growth and cognitive, emotional, language, and motor development specific to each stage.

Parameters of Growth

Statistical data derived from research studies of large groups of children provide health care professionals with information about how children normally grow. Throughout infancy, childhood, and adolescence, growth occurs in bursts separated by periods when growth is stable or consistent.

Weight, height, and head circumference are parameters that are used to monitor growth. They should be measured at regular intervals during childhood. The weight of the average term newborn is approximately $7^1/_2$ to 8 lb (3.4 to 3.6 kg). Male infants are usually slightly heavier than female infants. Usually, the birth weight doubles by 6 months of age and triples by 1 year of age. Between 2 and 3 years of age, the weight quadruples. Slow, steady weight gain during childhood is followed by a growth spurt during adolescence.

The average newborn is approximately 20 inches (50 cm) long, with an average increase of approximately 1 inch (2.54 cm) per month for the first 6 months, followed by an increase of approximately 1/2 inch (1.27 cm) per month for the remainder of the first year. The child gains 3 inches (7.6 cm) per year from age 1 through 7 years and then 2 inches (5 cm) per year from age 8 through 15 years. Boys generally add more height during adolescence than do girls. Body proportion changes are shown in Figure 4-1.

Head circumference indicates brain growth. The normal occipital-frontal circumference of the term newborn head is 13 to 14 inches (33 to 35.5 cm). Average head growth occurs according to the following pattern: 4.8 inches (12 cm) during the first year; 1 inch (2.5 cm) during the second year; 1/2 inch (1.2 cm) per year from 3 to 5 years; and 1/2 inch (1.2 cm) per year from 5 years until puberty. The average adult head circumference is approximately 21 inches (53 cm).

Dentition, the eruption of teeth, also follows a sequential pattern. Primary dentition usually begins to emerge at approximately 6 to 8 months. Most children have 20 teeth by

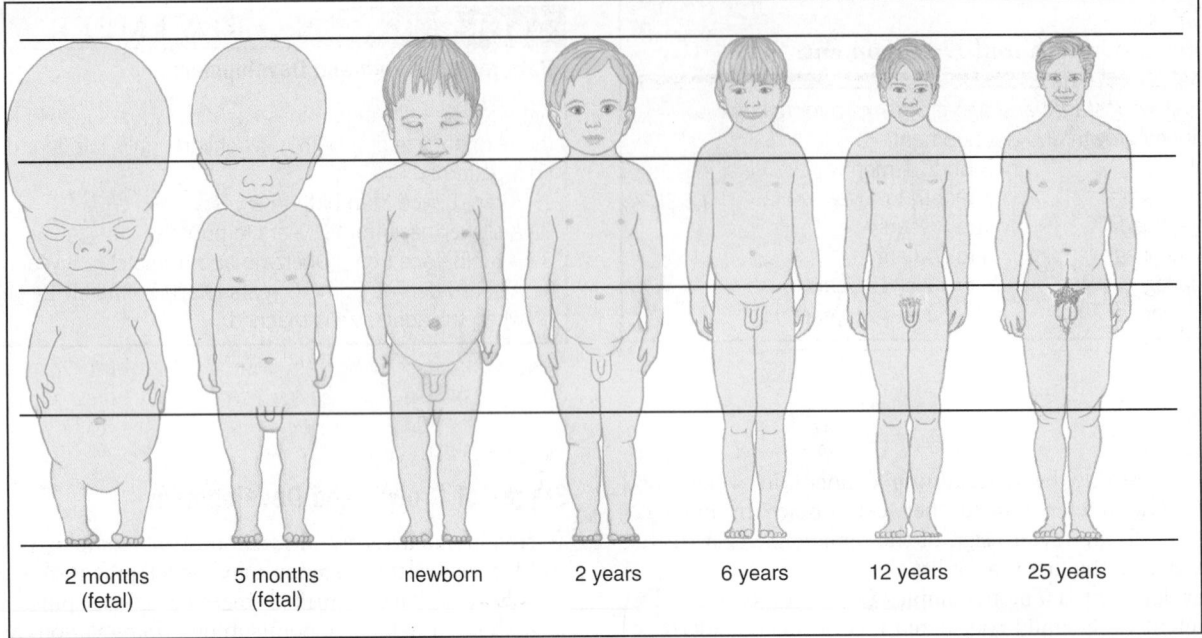

Figure 4-1 Changes in body proportions with growth.

age 2½ years. Permanent teeth, 32 in all, erupt beginning at approximately age 6 years, accompanied by the loss of primary teeth (see Chapter 33). Although some parents place importance on eruption of the teeth as a sign of maturation, dentition is not related to the level or rate of development.

PRINCIPLES OF GROWTH AND DEVELOPMENT

Patterns of Growth and Development

Growth and development are directional and follow predictable patterns. The first direction of growth is *cephalocaudal*, or proceeding from head to tail (or toe). This means that structures and functions originating in the head develop before those in the lower parts of the body. At birth the head is large, a full one fourth of the entire body length; the trunk is long; and the arms are longer than the legs. As the child matures, the body proportions gradually change; and by adulthood the legs have increased in size from approximately 38% to 50% of the total body length (see Fig. 4-1).

Directional growth and development are illustrated further by myelinization of the nerves, which begins in the brain and spreads downward as the child matures (Box 4-2). Growth of the myelin sheath and other nerve structures contributes to cephalocaudal development, which is illustrated by an infant's ability to raise the head before being able to sit and to sit before being able to stand.

A second directional aspect of growth and development is *proximodistal*, which means progression from the center outward, or from the midline to the periphery. The growth and branching pattern of the respiratory tract illustrates this concept. The trachea, which is the central structure of the respiratory tree, forms in the embryo by 24 days of gestation. Branching and growth outward occur in the bronchi, bronchioles, and alveoli throughout fetal life and infancy. Alveoli, which are the most distal structures of the system, continue to grow and develop in number and function until middle childhood.

Growth and development follow patterns, one of which is general to specific. As a child matures, activities become less generalized and more focused. For example, a newborn's response to pain is usually a whole-body response, with flailing of the arms and legs even if the pain is in the abdomen. As the child matures, the pain response becomes more localized to the stimulus. An older child with abdominal pain guards the abdomen.

Another pattern is the progression of functions from simple to complex. This pattern is easily observed in language development. A toddler's first sentences are formed simply, using only a noun and a verb. By age 5 years, the child constructs detailed stories using many complex modifiers.

The rate of growth is not constant as the child matures. *Growth spurts*, alternating with periods of slow or stagnant growth, are observed throughout childhood. Spurts are frequently seen as the child prepares to master a significant developmental task, such as walking. An increase in growth around a child's first birthday may promote the neuromuscular maturation needed for taking the first steps.

All facets of development (cognitive, motor, emotional, language) normally proceed according to these patterns. Knowledge of these concepts is useful when determining how a child's development is progressing and when comparing a child's development with normal patterns.

Mastery of developmental tasks is not static or permanent, and developmental stages do not always correlate with chronologic age. Children progress through developmental stages at varying rates within normal limits and may master developmental tasks only to regress to earlier levels when ill or stressed. Also, people can struggle repeatedly with particular developmental tasks throughout life, even though they have achieved more advanced levels of development.

Directional Patterns of Growth and Development

Cephalocaudal Pattern (Head to Toe)
Examples
- Head initially grows fastest (fetus), then trunk (infant), then legs (child).
- Infant can raise the head before sitting and can sit before standing.

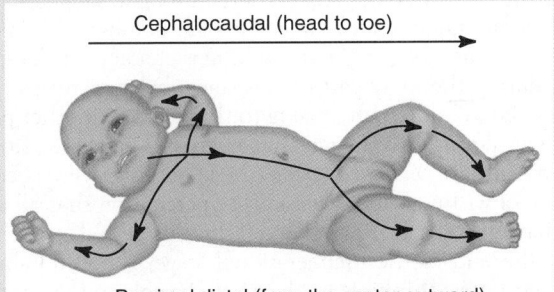

Cephalocaudal (head to toe)

Proximal distal (from the center outward)

Proximodistal Pattern (From the Center Outward)
Examples
- In the respiratory system, the trachea develops first in the embryo, followed by branching and growth outward of the bronchi, bronchioles, and alveoli in the fetus and infant.
- Motor control of the arms comes before control of the hands, and hand control comes before finger control.

Critical Periods

After birth, critical or sensitive periods exist for optimal growth and development. Similar to times during embryologic and fetal life, in which certain organs are formed and are particularly vulnerable to injury, critical periods are blocks of time during which children are ready to master specific developmental tasks. Children can master tasks outside these critical periods, but some tasks are learned more easily during particular periods.

Many factors affect a child's sensitive learning periods, such as injury, illness, and malnutrition. For example, the sensitive period for learning to walk seems to be during the latter part of the first year and the beginning of the second year. Children seem to be driven by an irresistible urge to practice walking and display great pride as they succeed. If a child is immobilized, for instance for the treatment of an orthopedic condition from age 10 months to 18 months, the child may have difficulty learning to walk. The child can learn to walk, but the task may be more difficult than for other children.

Factors Influencing Growth and Development

Genetics
One factor that greatly influences a child's growth and development is genetics. Genetic potential is affected by many factors. Environment influences how and to what extent particular genetic traits are manifested. Genetic influences on development are discussed in Chapter 9.

Environment
The environment is a significant determinant of growth and developmental outcome, both before and after birth. Examples of prenatal environmental factors include maternal smoking, alcohol intake, and disease, such as diabetes. Socioeconomic status, interpersonal relationships, and environmental hazards are only a few factors that affect children both before and after birth. Environmental factors that affect children are discussed in each individual growth-and-development chapter.

Culture
Culture is the way of life of a people, including their habits, beliefs, language, and values. It is a significant factor influencing children as they grow toward adulthood.

When gathering data, nurses must recognize how the common family structures and traditional values of various groups affect children's performance on assessment tests. The child's cultural and ethnic background must be considered when assessing growth and development. Standard growth curves and developmental tests do not necessarily reflect the normal growth and development of children of various cultural groups. Growth curves for children of various racial and cultural backgrounds are increasingly available. Nurse researchers and others conduct studies to determine the effectiveness of measurement tools for culturally diverse populations. In addition, culturally sensitive instruments are being developed to gather data to determine appropriate nursing interventions. To provide quality care to all patients, nurses must consider the effect of culture on children and families (see Chapter 3).

Nutrition
Because children are growing constantly and need a continuous supply of nutrients, nutrition plays an important role throughout childhood. For optimal growth and adequate energy, children need to obtain a variety of nutrients in amounts necessary to meet the recommended daily allowances for age and body size (Story, Holt, & Sofka, 2002). Good nutritional status is also needed for normal function of hormones, especially growth factor and sex hormones.

Health Status
Overall health status plays an important part in the growth and development of children. At the cellular level, inherited or acquired disease can affect the delivery of nutrients, hormones, or oxygen to organs and also can affect organ growth and function. Disease states that affect growth and development include digestive or malabsorption disorders, heart defects, and metabolic diseases.

Family
A child is an inseparable part of a family. Family relationships and influences are major determinants of how children grow and progress. Because of the special bond and influence of the family on the child, there can be no separation of child from family in the health care setting. For example, to diminish anxiety in a child, nurses sometimes attempt to reduce parental anxiety, which may then reduce the stress on the child. Nursing care of children involves nursing care of the whole family and requires skill in dealing with both adults and children.

Nurses might reduce parental anxiety about an ill child by saying "Your child is in the best place possible here at the hospital. You brought him in at just the right time so that we can help him."

Family structures are in a constant state of change, and these dynamic states influence how children develop. Within the family, relationships change because of marriage, birth, divorce, death, and new roles and responsibilities. Societal forces outside the family, such as economics, population shifts, and migration, change how children are raised. These forces cause changes in family structures and the outcomes of child rearing that must be considered when planning nursing care for children. The family is discussed in Chapter 3.

Parental Attitudes. Parental attitudes affect growth and development. Growth and development continue throughout life, and parents have stage-related needs and tasks that affect their children. Superimposed on these developmental issues are other factors influencing parental attitudes: educational level, childhood experiences, financial pressures, marital status, and available support systems. Parental attitudes are also affected by the child's temperament, the child's unique way of relating to the world. Different temperaments affect parenting practices and whether a child's unique personality traits develop into assets or problems.

Child-Rearing Philosophies. Child-rearing philosophies, shaped by myriad life events, have an effect on how children grow and develop. For example, well-educated, well-read parents often provide their children with extra stimulation and opportunities for learning, beginning at a young age. This enrichment includes extra parental attention and interaction—not necessarily expensive toys. Generally, development progresses best when enriched opportunities for learning are provided.

Other parents may not recognize the need to provide a rich learning environment at home, may not have time, or may not value this type of parenting. Children of these parents may not progress at the same rate as those raised in a more enriching atmosphere.

A significant point for parents to remember is that children must be ready to learn. If motor and neurologic structures are not mature, no amount of added stimulation will produce new behavior. The result of an overzealous approach toward accomplishing a specific task is frustration for both child and parent. For example, a child who is 6 months old will not be able to walk alone, no matter how much time and effort the parent expends. However, at 12 to 14 months, a child usually is ready to begin walking and will do so with ease if given opportunities to practice.

THEORIES OF GROWTH AND DEVELOPMENT

Many theorists have attempted to organize and classify the complex phenomena of growth and development. No single theory can adequately explain the wondrous journey from infancy to adulthood. However, each theorist contributes a piece of the puzzle. Theories are not facts but merely attempts to explain human behavior. Table 4-1 compares and contrasts theories discussed in the text. The chapters on each age-group provide further discussion of these theories.

Piaget's Theory of Cognitive Development

Jean Piaget (1896-1980), a Swiss theorist, made major contributions to the study of how children learn. His complex theory provides a framework for understanding how thinking during childhood progresses and differs from adult thinking. Like other developmental theorists, Piaget postulated that as children develop intellectually, they pass through progressive stages. The ages assigned to these periods are only averages.

During the sensorimotor period of development, infant thinking seems to involve the entire body. Reflexive behavior is gradually replaced by more complex activities. The world becomes increasingly solid through the development of the concept of *object permanence,* which is the awareness that objects continue to exist even when they disappear from sight. By the end of this stage, the infant shows some evidence of reasoning.

During the period of preoperational thought, language becomes increasingly useful. Judgments are dominated by perception and are illogical, and thinking is characterized, especially during the early part of this stage, by egocentrism. In other words, children are unable to think about another person's viewpoint and believe that everyone perceives situations as they do. *Magical thinking* (the belief that events occur because of wishing) and *animism* (the perception that all objects have life and feeling) characterize this period.

At the end of the preoperational stage, the child shifts from egocentric thinking and begins to be able to look at the world from another person's view. This shifting enables the child to move into the period of concrete operations, where the child is no longer bound by perceptions and can distinguish fact from fantasy. The concept of time becomes increasingly clear during this stage, although far past and far future events remain obscure. Although reasoning powers increase rapidly during this stage, the child cannot deal with abstractions or socialized thinking.

Normally, adolescents progress to the period of formal operations. In this period the adolescent proceeds from concrete to abstract and symbolic, and from self-centered to other-centered. How the adolescent understands and perceives the world is affected by this period (Ford & Coleman, 1999).

Nursing Implications of Piaget's Theory

Although other developmental theorists have disputed Piaget's theories, especially the ages at which cognitive changes occur, his work provides a basis for learning about and understanding cognitive development. Piaget's theory is especially significant to nurses as they develop teaching plans of care for children. Piaget believed that learning should be geared to the child's level of understanding and that the child should be an active participant in the learning process. For health teaching to be effective, nurses must understand the different cognitive abilities of children at various ages. Nurses also must know how to engage children in the learning process with developmentally appropriate activities. Because illness and hospitalization are often frightening to children, especially toddlers and preschoolers, nurses must understand the cognitive basis of fears related to treatment and be able to intervene appropriately (see Chapter 35).

Freud's Theory of Psychosexual Development

Sigmund Freud (1856-1939) developed theories to explain psychosexual development. His theories were in vogue for many years and provided a basis for other theories. Freud postulated that early childhood experiences provide unconscious motivation for actions later in life. According to Freudian theory, certain parts of the body assume psychologic significance as foci of sexual energy. These areas shift from one part of the body to another as the child moves through different

TABLE **4-1** Theories of Growth and Development

	Piaget's Periods of Cognitive Development	Freud's Stages of Psychosexual Development	Erikson's Stages of Psychosocial Development	Kohlberg's Stages of Moral Development
Infancy	**Period 1 (birth-2 yr): Sensorimotor Period**	**Oral Stage**	**Trust vs. Mistrust**	**Stage 0 (0-2 yr): Naïveté and Egocentrism**
	Reflexive behavior is used to adapt to the environment; egocentric view of the world; development of object permanence.	Mouth is a sensory organ; infant takes in and explores during oral passive substage (first half of infancy); infant strikes out with teeth during oral aggressive substage (latter half of infancy).	Development of a sense that the self is good and the world is good when consistent, predictable, reliable care is received; characterized by hope.	No moral sensitivity; decisions are made on the basis of what pleases the child; infants like or love what helps them and dislike what hurts them; no awareness of the effect of their actions on others. "Good is what I like and want."
Toddlerhood	**Period 2 (2-7 yr): Preoperational Thought**	**Anal Stage**	**Autonomy vs. Shame and Doubt**	**Stage 1 (2-3 yr): Punishment-Obedience Orientation**
	Thinking remains egocentric, becomes magical, and is dominated by perception.	Major focus of sexual interest is anus; control of body functions is major feature.	Development of sense of control over the self and body functions; exerts self; characterized by will.	Right or wrong is determined by physical consequences: "If I get caught and punished for doing it, it is wrong. If I am not caught or punished, then it must be right."
Preschool Age		**Phallic or Oedipal/Electra Stage**	**Initiative vs. Guilt**	**Premorality or Preconventional Morality, Stage 2 (4-7 yr): Instrumental Hedonism and Concrete Reciprocity**
		Genitals become focus of sexual curiosity; superego (conscience) develops; feelings of guilt emerge.	Development of a can-do attitude about the self; behavior becomes goal-directed, competitive, and imaginative; initiation into gender role; characterized by purpose.	Child conforms to rules out of self-interest: "I'll do this for you if you do this for me"; behavior is guided by an "eye for an eye" orientation. "If you do something bad to me, then it's OK if I do something bad to you."
School Age	**Period 3 (7-11 yr): Concrete Operations**	**Latency Stage**	**Industry vs. Inferiority**	**Morality of Conventional Role Conformity, Stage 3 (7-10 yr): Good-Boy or Good-Girl Orientation**
	Thinking becomes more systematic and logical, but concrete objects and activities are needed.	Sexual feelings are firmly repressed by the superego; period of relative calm.	Mastering of useful skills and tools of the culture; learning how to play and work with peers; characterized by competence.	Morality is based on avoiding disapproval or disturbing the conscience; child is becoming socially sensitive.

Continued

TABLE **4-1** Theories of Growth and Development—cont'd

	Piaget's Periods of Cognitive Development	Freud's Stages of Psychosexual Development	Erikson's Stages of Psychosocial Development	Kohlberg's Stages of Moral Development
School Age (cont'd)				***Stage 4 (begins at about 10-12 yr): Law and Order Orientation***
				Right takes on a religious or metaphysical quality. Child wants to do duty, show respect for authority, and maintain social order; obeys rules for their own sake.
Adolescence	***Period 4 (11 yr-Adulthood): Formal Operations***	***Puberty or Genital Stage***	***Identity vs. Role Confusion***	***Morality of Self-Accepted Moral Principles, Stage 5: Social Contract Orientation***
	New ideas can be created; situations can be analyzed; use of abstract and futuristic thinking; understands logical consequences of behavior.	Stimulated by increasing hormone levels; sexual energy wells up in full force, resulting in personal and family turmoil.	Begins to develop a sense of "I"; this process is life-long; peers become of paramount importance; child gains independence from parents; characterized by faith in self.	Right is determined by what is best for the majority; exceptions to rules can be made if a person's welfare is violated; the end no longer justifies the means; laws are for mutual good and mutual cooperation.
Adulthood			***Intimacy vs. Isolation***	
			Development of the ability to lose the self in genuine mutuality with another; characterized by love.	

stages of development. Freud's work may help to explain normal behavior that parents may confuse with abnormal behavior, and it also may provide a good foundation for sex education.

Freud believed that during infancy, sexual behavior seems to focus around the mouth, the most erogenous area of the infant body (oral stage). Infants derive pleasure from sucking and exploring objects by placing them in their mouths. During early childhood, when toilet training becomes a major developmental task, sensations seem to shift away from the mouth and toward the anus (anal stage). Psychoanalysts see this period as a time of holding on and letting go. A sense of control or autonomy develops as the child masters body functions.

During the preschool years, interest in the genitalia begins (phallic stage). Children are curious about anatomic differences, childbirth, and sexuality. Children at this age often ask many questions, freely exhibit their own sexual organs, and want to peek at those of others. Children often masturbate, sometimes causing parents great concern. Although it is not universal, a phenomenon described by Freud as the Oedipus complex in boys and the Electra complex in girls is seen in preschool children. This possessiveness of the child for the opposite-sex parent, marked by aggressiveness toward the same-sex parent, is considered normal behavior, as is a heightened interest in sex. To resolve these disturbing sexual feelings, the preschooler identifies with or becomes more like the same-sex parent. The superego (an inner voice that reprimands and evokes guilt) also develops. The superego is similar to a conscience (S. Freud, 1923/1960).

Freud describes the school-age period as the latency stage, when sexuality plays a less prominent role in the everyday life of the child. Best friends and same-sex peer groups are influential in the school-age child's life. Younger school-age children often refuse to play with children of the opposite sex, whereas prepubertal children begin to desire the companionship of opposite-sex friends.

During adolescence, interest in sex again flourishes as children search for identity (genital stage). Under the influence of fluctuating hormone levels, dramatic physical changes, and shifting social relationships, the adolescent develops a more adult view of sexuality. Adolescents' cognitive skills are not fully developed, however, and they often make questionable judgments about sexual matters and may have questions and

TABLE **4-1** Theories of Growth and Development—cont'd

	Piaget's Periods of Cognitive Development	Freud's Stages of Psychosexual Development	Erikson's Stages of Psychosocial Development	Kohlberg's Stages of Moral Development
Adulthood, cont'd			**Generativity vs. Stagnation**	**Stage 6: Personal Principle Orientation**
			Production of ideas and materials through work; creation of children; characterized by care.	Achieved only by the morally mature individual; few people reach this level; these people do what they think is right, regardless of others' opinions, legal sanctions, or personal sacrifice; actions are guided by internal standards; integrity is of utmost importance; may be willing to die for their beliefs.
			Ego Integrity vs. Despair	**Stage 7: Universal Principle Orientation**
			Realization that there is order and purpose to life; characterized by wisdom.	This stage is achieved by only a rare few; Mother Teresa, Gandhi, and Socrates are examples; these individuals transcend the teachings of organized religion and perceive themselves as part of the cosmic order, understand the reason for their existence, and live for their beliefs.

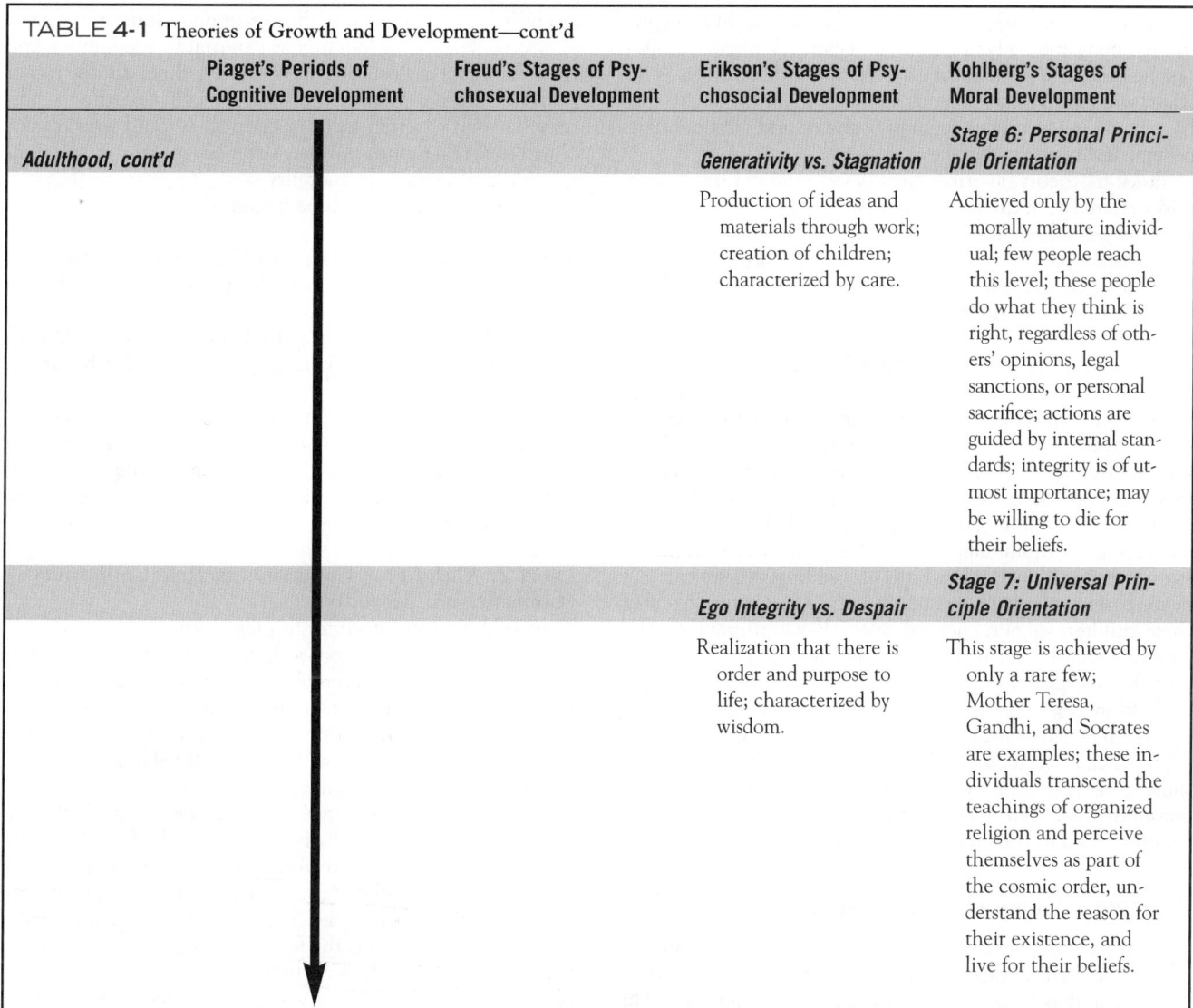

concerns about their behavior and feelings (A. Freud, 1974; Litt & Martin, 1999).

Nursing Implications of Freud's Theory

Both children and parents may have questions and concerns about normal sexual development and sex education. Nurses must understand normal sexual growth and development to help parents and children form healthy attitudes about sex.

Erikson's Psychosocial Theory

Born in 1902, Erik H. Erikson, inspired by the work of Sigmund Freud, proposed a popular theory about child development. He viewed development as a lifelong series of conflicts affected by social and cultural factors. Each conflict must be resolved for the child and adult to progress emotionally. How individuals address the conflicts varies widely. According to Erikson, however, unsuccessful resolution leaves the individual emotionally disabled.

Each of eight stages of development has a specific central conflict or developmental task. These eight tasks are described in terms of a positive or negative resolution. The ac-

tual resolution of a specific conflict lies somewhere along a continuum between a perfect positive and a perfect negative.

The first developmental task is the establishment of trust. The basic quality of trust provides a foundation for the personality. If an infant's physical and emotional needs are met in a timely manner through warm and nurturing interactions with a consistent caregiver, the infant begins to sense that the world is trustworthy. The infant begins to develop trust in others and a sense of being worthy of love. Through successful achievement of a sense of trust, the infant can move on to subsequent developmental stages.

According to Erikson, unsuccessful resolution of this first developmental task results in a sense of mistrust. If needs are consistently unmet, acute tension begins to appear in children. During infancy, signs of unmet needs include restlessness, fretfulness, whining, crying, clinging, physical tenseness, and physical dysfunctions, such as vomiting, diarrhea, and sleep disturbances. All children exhibit these signs at times. If these behaviors become personality characteristics, however, unsuccessful resolution of this stage is suspected.

The toddler's developmental task is to acquire a sense of autonomy rather than a sense of shame and doubt. A positive resolution of this task is accomplished by the ability to control the body and body functions, especially elimination. Success at this stage does not mean that the toddler, even as an adult, will exhibit autonomous behavior in all life situations. In certain circumstances, feelings of shame and self-doubt are normal and may be adaptive.

Erikson's theory describes each developmental stage, with crises related to individual stages emerging at specific times and in a particular order. Likewise, each stage is built on the resolution of previous developmental tasks. During each conflict, however, the child spends some energy and time resolving earlier conflicts (Erikson, 1963).

Nursing Implications of Erikson's Theory

In stressful situations, such as hospitalization, children, even those with healthy personalities, evoke defense mechanisms that protect them against undue anxiety. *Regression,* a behavior used frequently by children, is a reactivation of behavior more appropriate to an earlier stage of development. This defense mechanism is illustrated by a 6-year-old boy who reverts to sucking his thumb and wetting his pants under increased stress, such as illness or the birth of a sibling. Nurses can educate parents about regression and encourage them to offer their children support, not ridicule. They can provide constructive suggestions for stress management and reassure parents that regression normally subsides as anxiety decreases.

Erikson's main contribution to the study of human development lies in his outline of a universal sequence of phases of psychosocial development. His work is especially relevant to nursing because it provides a theoretic basis for much of the emotional care that is given to children. The stages are further discussed in the chapters on each age-group.

Kohlberg's Theory of Moral Development

Lawrence Kohlberg (1927-1987), a psychologist and philosopher, described a stage theory of moral development that closely parallels Piaget's stages of cognitive development. He discussed moral development as a complicated process involving the acceptance of the values and rules of society in a way that shapes behavior. This cognitive-developmental theory postulates that although knowing what behaviors are right and wrong is important, it is much less important than understanding and appreciating why the behaviors should or should not be exhibited (Bear, Richards, & Gibbs, 1997).

Guilt, an internal expression of self-criticism and feeling of remorse, is an emotion closely tied to moral reasoning. Most children 12 years old or older react to misbehavior with guilt. Guilt helps them realize when their moral judgment fails.

Building on Piaget's work, Kohlberg studied boys and girls from middle- and lower-class families in the United States and other countries. He interviewed them by presenting scenarios with moral dilemmas and asking them to make a judgment. His focus was not on the answer but on the reasoning behind the judgment (Kohlberg, 1964). He then classified the responses into a series of levels and stages, as described below.

Level 1: Premorality (Preconventional Morality)

The child demonstrates acceptable behavior because of fear of punishment from a superior force, such as a parent. At this stage of cognitive and moral development, children cannot reason as mature members of society. They view the world in a selfish, egocentric way, with no real understanding of right or wrong. They view morality as external to themselves, and their behavior reflects what others tell them to do, rather than an internal drive to do what is right. In other words, they have an external locus of control. A child who thinks, "I will not steal money from my sister because my mother will spank me" illustrates premorality.

Within this level are three stages:

- Stage 0 (0 to 2 years): The infant has no awareness of right or wrong and does not consider the effect of actions on others.
- Stage 1 (2 to 3 years): The child obeys rules to avoid punishment and acts to avoid displeasing those who are in power.
- Stage 2 (4 to 7 years): The child conforms to rules to obtain rewards or have favors returned. This type of behavior coincides with Piaget's preconceptual stage of cognition, in which thinking is dominated by perception and egocentrism.

Level 2: Morality of Conventional Role Conformity (Conventional Morality)

The child conforms to rules to please others. The child still has an external locus of control, but a concern for social order begins to emerge and replace the more egocentric thinking of the earlier stage. The child has an increased awareness of others' feelings. In the child's view, good behavior is that which those in authority will approve. If behavior is not acceptable, the child feels guilty.

Within this level are stage 3 (7 to 10 years), in which conformity occurs to avoid disapproval or dislike by others, and stage 4 (10 to 12 years), in which the child has more concern with society as a whole. In these stages, emphasis is on obeying laws to maintain social order. This level of moral reasoning develops as the child shifts the focus of living from the family to peer groups and society as a whole. As the child's cognitive capacities increase, an internal sense of right and wrong emerges and the individual is said to have developed an internal locus of control. Along with this internal locus of control comes the ability to consider circumstances when judging behavior.

Level 3: Morality of Self-Accepted Moral Principles (Postconventional Morality)

The person focuses on individual rights and principles of conscience during this stage. There is an internal locus of control. Concern about what is best for all is uppermost, and persons step back from their own viewpoint to consider what rights and values must be upheld for the good of all. Because abstract thinking abilities are necessary for this type of reasoning, this level is not attained until adolescence. Some individuals never reach this point. Within this level is stage 5, in which conformity occurs because individuals have basic rights and society needs to be improved. The adolescent in this stage gives as well as takes and does not expect to get something without paying for it. In stage 6, conformity is based on universal principles of justice and occurs to avoid self-condemnation (Colby, Kohlberg, & Kauffman, 1987; Feldman, 1998; Kohlberg, 1964).

Only a few morally mature individuals achieve stage 6. These people, committed to a moral idea, live and die for their principles.

Kohlberg believes that children proceed from one stage to the next in a sequence that does not vary, although some people may never reach the highest levels. Even though children are raised in different cultures and with different experiences, he believes that all children progress according to his description.

Nursing Implications of Kohlberg's Theory

To provide anticipatory guidance to parents about expectations and discipline of their children, nurses must be aware of how moral development progresses. Parents are often distraught because their young children apparently do not understand right and wrong. For example, a 6-year-old girl who takes money from her mother's purse does not show remorse or seem to recognize that stealing is wrong. In fact, she is more concerned about her punishment than about her misdeed. With an understanding of normal moral development, the nurse can reassure the concerned parents that the child is showing age-appropriate behavior.

THEORIES OF LANGUAGE DEVELOPMENT

Human language has a number of characteristics that are not shared with other species of animals that communicate with each other. Human language has meaning, provides a mechanism for thought, and permits tremendous creativity.

Because language is such a complex process and involves such a vast number of neuromuscular structures, brain growth and differentiation must reach a certain level of maturity before a child can speak. Language development closely parallels cognitive development and is discussed by most cognitive theorists as they explain the maturation of thinking abilities. The process of how language develops remains a mystery, however.

Passive, or receptive, language is the ability to understand the spoken word. Expressive language is the ability to produce meaningful vocalizations. In most people, the areas in the brain responsible for expressive language are close to motor centers in the left cerebral area that control muscle movement of the mouth, tongue, and hands. Humans use a variety of facial and hand movements as well as words to convey ideas.

Crying is the infant's first method of communication. These vocalizations quickly become distinct and individual and accurately convey such states as hunger, diaper discomfort, pain, loneliness, and boredom. Vowel sounds appear first, as early as 2 weeks of age, followed by consonants at approximately 5 months of age.

By age 2 years, children have a vocabulary of roughly 300 words and can construct simple sentences. By age 4 years, children have gained a sense of correct grammar and articulation, but several consonants, including "l" and "r," remain difficult to pronounce. For example, the sentence "The red and blue bird flew up to the tree" might be pronounced by the preschooler as "The wed and boo bud fwew up to the twee!"

The language of school-age children is less concrete and much more articulate than that of the preschooler. Between the ages of 5 and 10 years, children begin to understand the structure of language. By 12 years, the child has many of the cognitive and linguistic skills of adults (Kelly & Sally, 1999).

Infants learn much of their language from their parents. Children who are raised in homes where verbalization is encouraged and modeled tend to display advanced language skills. Also, in infancy, receptive ability (the understanding of language) is more developed than expressive skill (the actual articulation of words). This tendency persists throughout life and is important to realize when caring for children. In clinical situations, nurses must communicate what is happening to their young clients, using simple, age-appropriate words, even though the child may not verbalize understanding. Language development is discussed in more depth in chapters on each age-group.

ASSESSMENT OF GROWTH

Because growth is an excellent indicator of physical well-being, accurate assessments must be made at regular intervals so that patterns of growth can be determined. Trained individuals using calibrated equipment and proper techniques should perform growth measurement. Methods of obtaining accurate measurements in children are described in Chapter 33. To minimize the chance of error, data should be collected on children under consistent conditions on a routine basis and values should be recorded and plotted on growth charts immediately.

Standardized growth charts allow an individual child's growth (height, weight, head circumference) to be compared with statistical norms. The most commonly used growth charts are those developed by the National Center for Health Statistics. Separate charts are available for boys and girls. One set of charts is used for children from birth to 36 months, and another set is used for children ages 2 years to 20 years (see Appendix E).

Because height and weight are the best indicators of growth, these parameters are measured, plotted on growth charts, and monitored over time at each well visit. Brain growth can also be monitored by measuring infant frontal-occipital circumference at intervals and plotting the values on growth charts. It is important to relate head size to weight because larger babies have bigger heads. These measurements are routinely performed during the first 2 years of life.

Body mass index (BMI), which is a function of both height and weight, is an important measure of growth and overall nutritional status in children older than two years. Child health professionals increasingly use BMI when assessing growth, and BMI charts are included in the most recent versions of charts available from the National Center for Health Statistics.

Growth rate is measured in percentiles. The area between any two percentiles is referred to as a *growth channel*. Childhood growth normally progresses according to a pattern along a particular growth channel. Deviations from normal growth patterns may suggest problems. Any change of more than two growth channels indicates a need for more in-depth assessment.

Recognition of abnormal growth patterns is an important nursing function. The earlier that growth disorders are detected, diagnosed, and treated, the better the long-term prognosis.

ASSESSMENT OF DEVELOPMENT

Assessment of development is a more complex process than assessment of growth. To assess developmental progress accurately, nurses must gather data from many sources, including observations and interviews, physical examinations, interactions with the child and parents, and various standardized assessment tools.

Observation is a valuable method most often used to obtain information about a child's developmental age (level of functioning). By watching a child during daily activities, such as eating, playing, toileting, and dressing, nurses gather a great deal of assessment data. Observation of the child's problem-solving abilities, communication patterns, interaction skills, and emotional responses can yield valuable information about the child's level of development. Similarly, interviews and physical examinations can provide much information about how the child functions.

In addition to these sources of data, many standardized assessment tools are available for nurses and other health care professionals to use for developmental assessment. Developmental assessment should be part of a newborn's assessment and of every well-child examination, for several reasons. One reason is that parents want to know how their child compares with others and whether development is normal, especially if they experienced a difficult pregnancy or have developmentally delayed children. Developmental assessment tends to allay fears. Another reason is that abnormal development must be discovered early to facilitate optimal outcomes through early intervention.

Newborn Assessment

Two newborn screening tools are the Brazelton Neonatal Behavior Assessment Scale and the New Ballard Score which are described in Chapter 22.

Pre-Screening Assessments

The American Academy of Pediatrics has issued a policy statement regarding developmental screening for all children, which emphasizes the importance of detecting early delays and referring for early intervention (American Academy of Pediatrics [AAP], 2001). Depending on the screening method used, developmental screening can take up to 30 minutes to administer—time not often available in a busy pediatric office or well clinic. Many providers have elected to do multilevel screening, first using a pre-screening assessment tool and then administering (or referring for administration) a more comprehensive developmental assessment. Studies have suggested that parent concern is an important predictor of actual developmental delay in children (AAP, 2001; Glascoe, 1999; Glascoe & Shapiro, 2003). Some of the newer pre-screening tools based on parent concerns, such as the Parents' Evaluation of Developmental Status (PEDS) and the Ages and Stages Questionnaires, have been found to be reliable and valid for detecting developmental delay (AAP, 2001; Glascoe, 1999; Glascoe & Shapiro, 2003). These screening tools are organized around major developmental areas (language, cognitive, social, behavioral, and motor. They are given to parents to complete in the office or clinic waiting room, take only 5 to 10 minutes to do, and are considered to be predictive for delay. The Prescreening Developmental Questionnaire (PDQ II) is organized according to categories in the Denver Developmental Screening Test II. It is an objective measure of development and also is relatively easy and quick to administer (Frankenburg, 2002). Regardless of the screening method chosen, the AAP recommends periodic developmental screening for all young infants and children as part of well-child care (AAP, 2001).

Denver Developmental Screening Test II

The most widely used screening tool for infants and young children is the Denver Developmental Screening Test II (DDST-II; see Appendix F). The DDST-II provides a clinical impression of a child's overall development and alerts the user to potential developmental difficulties.

The DDST-II, designed to be used with children between birth and 6 years of age, assesses development based on the performance of a series of age-appropriate tasks. There are 125 tasks or items arranged in four functional areas:

1. Personal-social (getting along with others, caring for personal needs)
2. Fine motor (eye-hand coordination, problem-solving skills)
3. Language (hearing, using, and understanding language)
4. Gross motor (sitting, jumping)

Items for rating the child's behavior are also included at the end of the test.

The test form is arranged with age scales across the top and bottom (see Appendix F for a sample test form). After calculating the child's chronologic age (age in years), the test administrator draws an age line on the form. Each of the 125 tasks or items is arranged on a shaded bar depicting at which ages 25%, 50%, 75%, and 90% of the children in the research sample completed that particular item. The examiner assesses the child using the items clustered around the age line. The directions must be followed exactly during administration of the test. A score for performance on each item is recorded according to the following scale: pass (P), fail (F), no opportunity (NO), and refusal (R). At the completion of the test, the screener scores test behavior ratings (located at the bottom left of the form).

Interpretation of the test is based first on individual items and then on the test as a whole. Individual items are considered as "advanced, normal, caution, delayed, or no opportunity." Reliability and validity of the test can be altered if the child is not feeling well or is under the influence of medications. Parental presence and input as to whether the child is behaving as usual is desired.

The results of the test can be used to identify a child's developmental age and how a child compares with others of the same chronologic age. This information can be used to alert health care providers to potential problems. To ensure that the results are accurate, only individuals who are trained to administer the test in a standardized manner should perform testing. Training is obtained through study of the testing manual, review of the accompanying videotape, and supervised practice with children of various ages.

Although the DDST-II is widely used, it is a screening test only, not an intelligence quotient (IQ) test. It is not a definitive predictor of future abilities, and it should not be used to determine diagnostic labels. It is, however, a useful tool for noting problems, validating hunches, monitoring development, and providing referrals.

Implications for Nurses

To ensure the child's best performance, nurses must first establish rapport and create a comfortable screening environment. The test should be administered in a comfortably warm room with the child dressed but with restrictive clothing and shoes removed. Test materials should be located where the child can easily reach them. Only materials that are being used immediately for testing should be available to the child. All other materials should be out of sight. Young children may be held, but they should be able to rest their elbows on the testing table to manipulate objects.

Nurses should avoid making prejudgments about how a child will perform on the tests based on the child's or the parents' physical appearance. It is important to avoid being misled by a child's charm, facial features, small or large size, handicap, or oddly shaped head. Children should be given every opportunity to perform to the best of their ability.

As the testing progresses, it is important to avoid causing unnecessary worry in parents. Doubts should not be expressed until the screener is certain that the child should be seen for further evaluation. The slightest suggestion of concern, which may be communicated by even a casual facial expression, can create unnecessary worry and diminished trust. The role of the nurse is to gather valid assessment data, determine deviations from normal, make appropriate referrals, and provide support. Diagnosing developmental delay is a function of other health care professionals.

At the completion of the DDST-II, the nurse should ask the parents if the child acted in a normal and expected manner. If the parent responds negatively, the evaluation should be rescheduled. When explaining the results, emphasis should be placed on the items the child passed, those items the child failed but was not expected to pass, and finally those items the child failed and was expected to pass. Answer the parent's questions, and if indicated, refer for additional developmental testing.

NURSE'S ROLE IN PROMOTING OPTIMAL GROWTH AND DEVELOPMENT

Nurses are particularly concerned with preventing disease and promoting health. One aspect of preventive care is providing anticipatory guidance or basic information for parents about normal growth and development as their child approaches different age levels.

Brazelton (1992) describes "touchpoints" as predictable times during which health care professionals can reach into a family system and, through supportive help, diminish or prevent problems. These points generally occur just before a growth or developmental spurt in which the child's behavior changes and the parents' normal modes of handling behavior do not work. During these periods the child becomes difficult to understand. The nurse can anticipate these predictable periods, which also provide a window of opportunity to offer information about normal growth and development as well as practical interventions to prevent problems characteristic of that age. Age-appropriate topics for anticipatory guidance are discussed in depth in the chapters on specific age-groups.

DEVELOPMENTAL ASSESSMENT

Nursing care for children is not complete without addressing the developmental issues that are unique to each child. Because children grow and change rapidly, the nurse must use knowledge of theories of growth and development to create plans of care for both healthy and ill children. Assessment data are collected from a variety of sources, categorized, and analyzed with a theoretic knowledge base and clinical experience. A list of strengths and problems related to growth and development is generated. Nursing diagnoses are formulated with individualized goals, interventions, and evaluation to address specific problems that are related to, but differ from, physiologic and psychosocial needs.

Interview

During the initial interview, the nurse asks questions about the child's cognitive, language, motor, and emotional development. The parents' emotional state, level of education, and culture must be considered when information is gathered. The nurse might use the following questions and statements when interviewing the parents of a 4-year-old child:

- What does your child like to do at home?
- Does your child know the days of the week?
- Describe your child's typical day.
- Does your child attend preschool?
- Can your child throw a ball, ride a tricycle, climb?
- Can your child draw pictures, color them?
- How effective is your child's use of language?
- How did your child's development progress during infancy and toddlerhood?

The nurse also assesses the child's ability to think through situations and to communicate verbally. In addition, how the child interacts with other children and adults can be a measure of cognitive abilities. The number, type, length, appropriateness, and correct use of words and sentences are also noted. Careful observation of the child in a variety of situations, including play, provides valuable information about cognitive development.

A child's stage of emotional development can be assessed in a number of ways. From Erikson's theory, it is expected that the major conflict of a 4-year-old would be developing a sense of initiative rather than a sense of guilt. If the child is hospitalized, however, regressive behaviors might be exhibited if the anxiety of hospitalization becomes overwhelming. Questions directed to the parents, such as those that follow, could help validate inferences about the child's psychosocial development:

- What types of play activities does your child like best?
- How does your child get along with other children? With adults?
- How does your child usually handle stressful situations?
- What do you do to help your child cope with problems?
- How does your child's ability to cope compare with your other children?
- Is the behavior exhibited your child's usual behavior?

The nurse can also obtain valuable information from careful observation of a child who is hospitalized. The nurse should note how the child deals with pain, intrusive procedures, and separation from parents.

Play

Although play is not work in the traditional sense, it is the work of children. Play is those tasks, done to amuse oneself, that have behavioral, social, or psychomotor rewards. To

Administering the Denver Developmental Screening Test II

TeVonte ("T") is visiting the clinic for preventive health care shortly after his third birthday. The nurse will administer a Denver Developmental Screening Test II (DDST-II) to evaluate his development in each of four areas: personal-social, fine motor–adaptive, language, and gross motor.

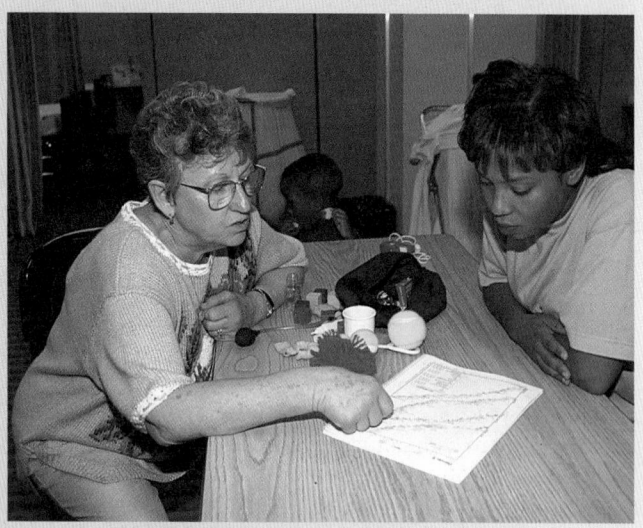

Before beginning T's DDST-II screening test, the nurse explains its purpose to his mother, Monifa Lee. The test assesses the child's performance of various age-appropriate tasks. The nurse emphasizes to the mother that the DDST-II is not an IQ test but rather compares her child's development with that of other children of the same age.

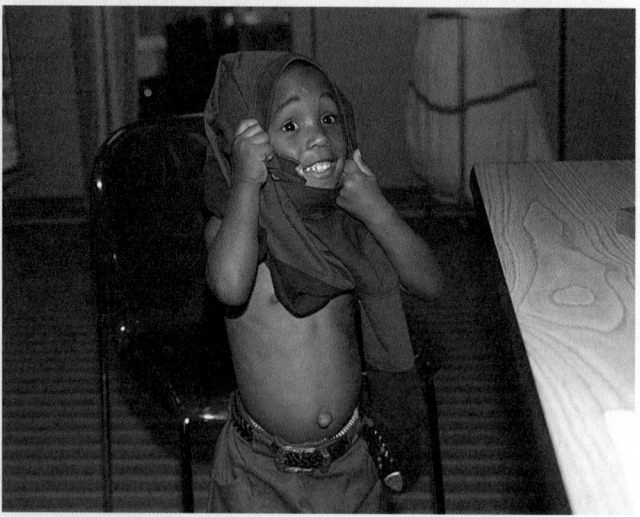

After verifying T's age, the nurse begins the test with personal-social items. After helping him remove his shirt, the nurse asks T to put it back on. T pulls the shirt over his head and then slips each arm into a sleeve.

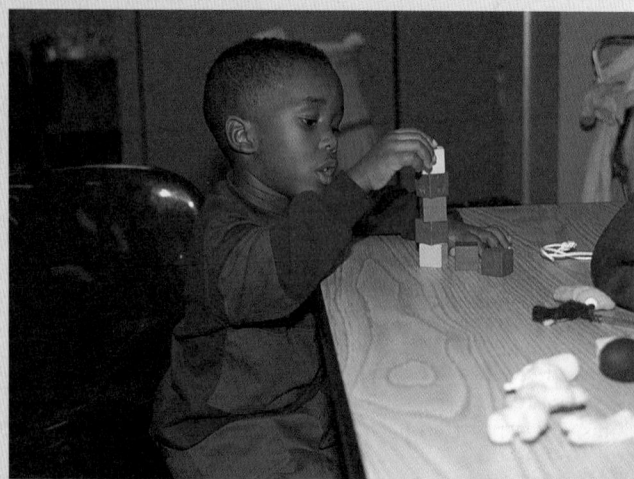

Colored cubes are used to evaluate T's ability to name colors and to build a tower. T is building a tower of eight blocks, which allows the tester to evaluate his fine motor–adaptive development.

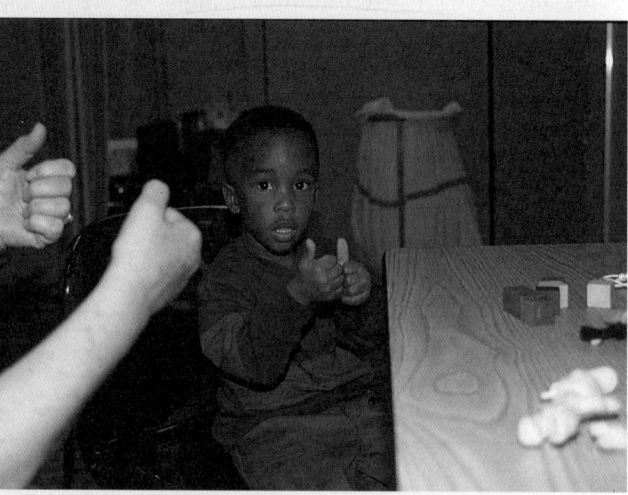

The nurse shows T how to wiggle his thumbs. T passes this part of the test because he keeps his fists closed and wiggles only his thumbs.

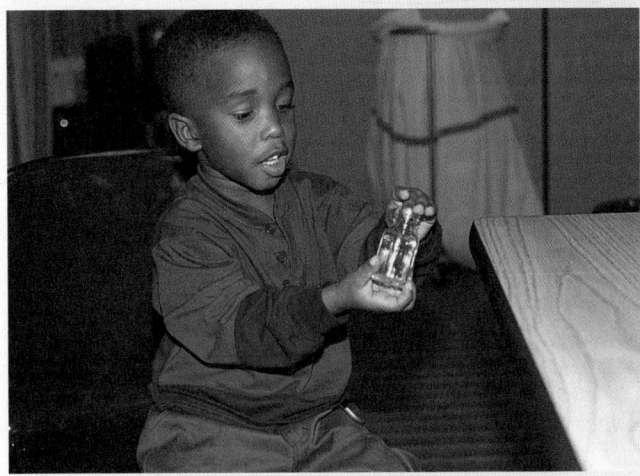

T plays with a raisin in a jar as part of the fine motor screening. The nurse observes to see whether T will pick up the raisin using his thumb and forefinger. T is really more interested in eating the raisin!

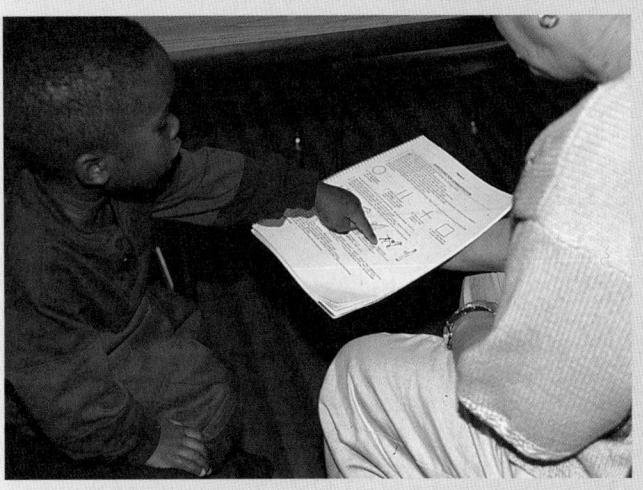

As she administers the DDST-II, the nurse evaluates T's speech, which is completely understandable, as it should be at his age. An additional part of the language test is to identify at least four of the pictures printed in the test manual. T correctly names the dog as well as other objects.

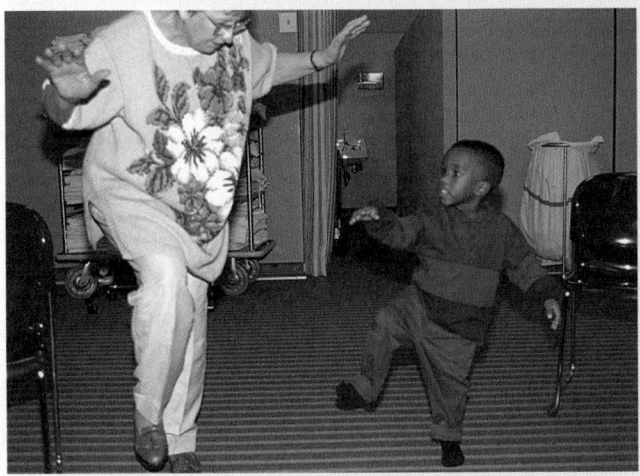

As the nurse shows T how to hop, he hops quickly in response. T's expression shows that he enjoys the gross motor part of the DDST-II.

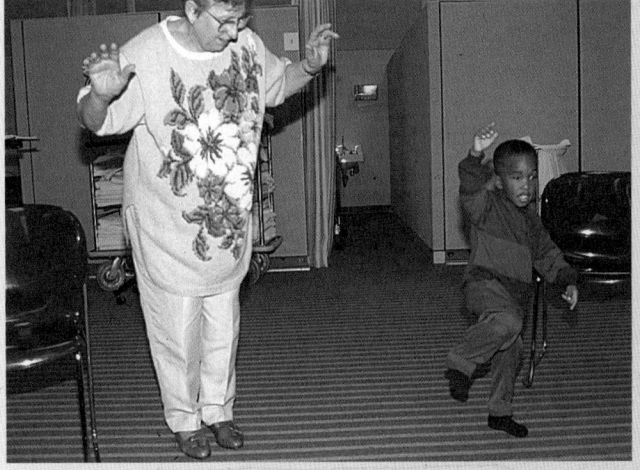

T shows the nurse that he can balance on each foot for 3 seconds. Note that he is effectively using his arms to help maintain his balance.

After completing the DDST-II, the nurse shares the results with T's mother. The screening indicates that T's development is appropriate for his age. The nurse recommends that TeVonte continue to have well-child screenings each year, including a DDST-II up to the age of 6 years.

adult observers, children's play may appear unorganized, meaningless, and even chaotic. Anyone who watches carefully, however, quickly discovers that play is a rich activity, intricately woven with meaning and purpose. In adulthood, work is any activity during which one uses time and energy to create a product or achieve a goal. Play in childhood is similar to adult work in that it is undertaken by the child to accomplish developmental tasks and master the environment.

Play is also an important part of the developmental process. Play is how children learn about shape, color, cause and effect, and themselves. In addition to cognitive thinking, play helps the child learn social interaction and psychomotor skills. It is a way of communicating joy, fear, sorrow, and anxiety.

Classifications of Play

Piaget (1962) described the following three types of play that relate to periods of sensorimotor, preoperational, and concrete operational functioning.

Practice play, which is also known as *functional* or *sensorimotor play*, involves repetitive muscle movements and the introduction of a deliberate complication into the way of doing something. Children who are running, gathering, dumping, and manipulating objects are displaying practice play (Ross, 1997).

Symbolic play, as its name suggests, uses games and interactions that represent an issue or concern to be addressed. Garvey (1979) identified three elements of symbolic play: one or more objects, a theme or plan, and roles. As children play, they incorporate some object (a syringe), use a theme (getting an injection), and then play the roles each player will have (child, nurse). Because there are no rules in symbolic play, the child can use this play not only to reinforce or learn the good things in life but also to alter those things that are painful.

Games include rules and usually are played by more than one person, although some games can be played by oneself. For example, the card game *solitaire* is played by one person, as are many video games. Games with rules rarely occur before age 4 years and are most common with the school-age child (Piaget, 1962). Games continue throughout life as adults play board games, cards, and sports.

Through games, children learn to play by the rules and to take turns. One common way children accomplish this is through board games. Young children often make up games with unique sets of rules, which may change each time the game is played. Older children have games with specific rules; younger children tend to change the rules.

Social Aspects of Play

As the child develops, more interaction with people occurs. Play becomes a vehicle for socialization with others through exploration of the social environment (Kritt, 2000). Certain types of play are associated with, but not limited to, specific age-groups.

Solitary Play. Solitary play is characterized by independent play (Fig. 4-2). The child plays alone with toys that are very different from those chosen by other children in the area. This type of play begins in infancy and is common in toddlers because of their limited social, cognitive, and physical skills. It is important for children in all age-groups, however, to have some time to play by themselves.

Parallel Play. Parallel play is usually associated with toddlers, although it can be found in any age-group. Children play side by side with similar toys, but there is a lack of interactive activity.

Associative Play. Associative play is characterized by group play without group goals. Children in this type of play do not set group rules, and although they may all be playing with the same types of toys and may even trade toys, there is a lack of formal organization. This type of play can begin during toddlerhood and continue into the preschool age.

Cooperative Play. Cooperative play begins in the late preschool years. This type of play is organized and has group goals. There is usually at least one leader, and children are definitely in or out of the group. following the leader

Onlooker Play. Onlooker play is present when the child observes others playing. Although the child may ask questions of the players, the child does not attempt to join the play (Fig. 4-2). Onlooker play is usually during the toddler years but can be observed at any age.

Types of Play

Dramatic Play. Dramatic play allows children to act out roles and experiences that may have happened to them, that they fear will happen, or that they have observed in others. This type of play can be spontaneous or guided, and it often includes medical or nursing equipment. It is especially valuable for children who have experienced or will experience multiple procedures or hospitalizations.

Hospitals and clinics with child life specialists on staff usually have a medical play area as part of the activity room. Nurses may provide opportunities for spontaneous as well as guided dramatic play. The nurse may choose to observe spontaneous play or be an active participant with the child. Occasionally nurses will want to structure the dramatic play to review a specific treatment or procedure. In guided play situations, the nurse directs the focus of the play. Specialized play kits may be developed for specific procedures, such as central line care, casting, bone marrow aspirations, lumbar punctures, and surgery, using supplies related to the hospital or clinic setting.

Familiarization Play. Familiarization play allows children to handle and explore health care materials in nonthreatening and fun ways (see Fig. 4-2). This type of play is especially helpful for but not limited to preparing children for procedures and the whole experience of hospitalization.

Examples of familiarization activities include using sponge mouth swabs as painting and gluing tools; making jewelry from Band-Aids, tape, gauze, and lid tops; creating mobiles and collages with health care supplies; making finger puppets using plaster casting material; filling a basin with water and using tubing, syringes, medicine cups, and bulb syringes for water play; decorating beds, wheelchairs, and intravenous (IV) poles with health care supplies; and using syringes for painting activities.

Functions of Play

Play enhances the child's growth and development. Play contributes to physical, cognitive, emotional, and social development.

Physical Development. Play aids in the development of both fine and gross motor activity. Children repeat certain body movements purely for pleasure, and these movements in turn aid in the development of body control. For example, an infant will first hit at a rattle, then will attempt to grasp it, and eventually will be able to pick up that same rattle. Next the infant will shake the rattle or perhaps bring it to the mouth.

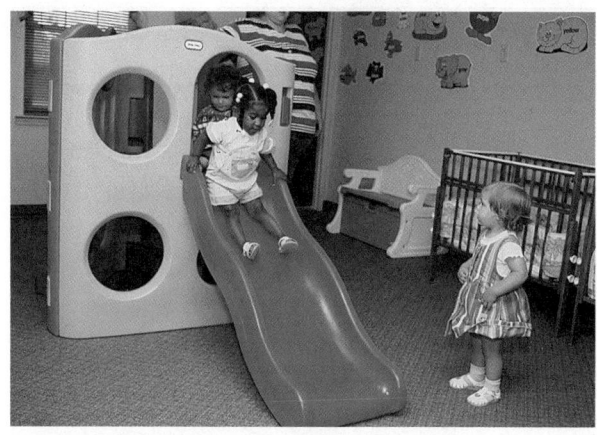

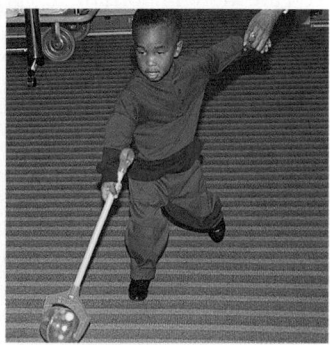

When engaging in solitary play, the child is playing apart from other children and with different types of toys. (Courtesy The University of Texas at Arlington School of Nursing.)

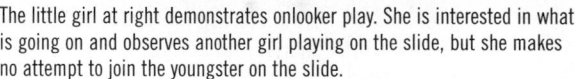

The little girl at right demonstrates onlooker play. She is interested in what is going on and observes another girl playing on the slide, but she makes no attempt to join the youngster on the slide.

Playing safely with medical equipment (familiarization play) lessens its unfamiliarity to the child and can allay fears. A less fearful child is likely to be more cooperative and less traumatized by necessary care. (Courtesy The University of Texas at Arlington School of Nursing.)

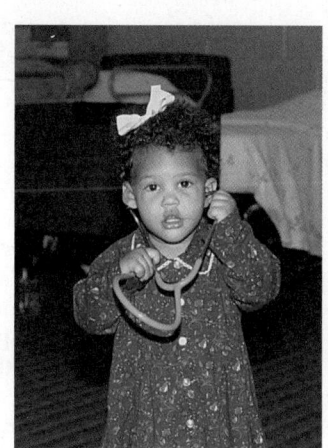

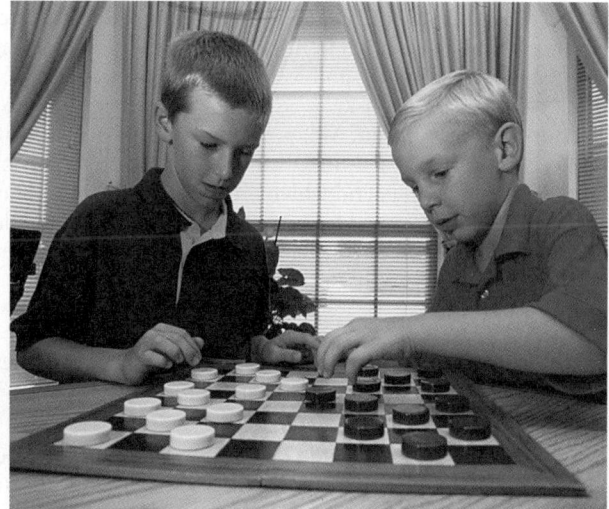

Games with rules, such as board games, help children learn boundaries, teamwork, taking turns, and competition. (Courtesy Cook Children's Medical Center, Fort Worth, TX.)

Figure 4-2 Types of play.

The parent and child may make a game of repeating sounds such as "ma ma" or "da da," which increases the child's language ability. Repeating rhymes and songs can be a fun way for children to increase their vocabulary. Children love to color on a paper with a crayon and will scribble before being able to draw pictures and to color. This assists the child with eventually learning how to write letters and numerals.

Cognitive Development. Play is a key element in the cognitive development of children. Once a child has learned a general concept, further experiences with that concept expand from that beginning knowledge. Piaget gave the example of an infant learning to swing an object and then subsequently swinging other objects (Piaget, 1962). This could apply, for example, to things to be eaten, read, or ridden. Progression takes place as the child begins to have certain experiences, test beliefs, and understand the surrounding world.

Children can increase their problem-solving abilities through games and puzzles. Pretend play can stimulate several types of learning. Language abilities are strengthened as the child models significant others in role-playing. The child must organize thoughts and be able to communicate with others involved in the play scenario. Children who play "house" create elaborate details of what the characters do and say.

Children also increase their understanding of size, shape, and texture through play. They begin to understand relationships as they attempt to put a square peg into a round hole, for example. Books and videos increase a child's vocabulary while increasing understanding of the world.

Emotional Development. Children who are experiencing an anxiety-producing situation are often helped by role playing. Play can be a way of coping with emotional conflict. Play can be a way to determine what is real and what is not. Children may escape through play into a world of fantasy and make-believe to make sense out of a sometimes senseless world. Play can also increase a child's self-awareness as an event or situation is explored through role playing or symbolic play.

As significant others in children's lives respond to their initiation of play, children begin to learn that they are important and cared for. Whether the child initiates the play or the adult does, when a significant person plays a board game with a child, shares a bike ride, plays baseball, or reads a story, the child gets the message, "You are more important than anything else at this time." This increases the child's self-esteem.

Social Development. The newborn cannot distinguish self from others and therefore is narcissistic. As the infant begins to play with others and things, a realization of self and others begins to develop. The infant begins to experience the joy of interacting with others and soon initiates behavior that involves others. Infants discover that when they coo, their mothers coo back. Children will soon expect this response and make a game of playing with their mothers.

Playing make-believe allows the child to try on different roles. When children play "restaurant" or "hospital," they experiment with rules that govern these settings.

Of course, most games, from board games to sports, involve interaction with others. The child learns boundaries, taking turns, teamwork, and competition. Children also learn how to negotiate with different personalities and the feelings associated with winning and losing. They learn to share and to take turns (see Fig. 4-2).

Moral Development. When children engage in play with their peers and their families, they begin to learn which behaviors are acceptable and which are not. Quickly they learn that taking turns is rewarded and cheating is not. Group play assists the child in recognizing the importance of teamwork, sharing, and being aware of the feelings of others.

HEALTH PROMOTION

Immunizations

Immunizations are effective in decreasing and, in some cases, eliminating childhood infectious diseases. Naturally occurring smallpox has been virtually eliminated, and the incidence of diphtheria, pertussis, tetanus, measles, mumps, rubella, and poliomyelitis has greatly declined in the United States. The incidence of diseases caused by *Haemophilus influenzae* type b (Hib) has been reduced by 95% since the 1980s. This pathogen was responsible for serious bacterial infections in infants and children (Centers for Disease Control and Prevention [CDC], 2002). In 2000, the American Academy of Pediatrics issued a policy regarding the administration of pneumococcal conjugate vaccine to prevent pneumococcal infections in children younger than 2 years. This vaccine is presently administered in a four-dose schedule (at 2, 4, and 6 months and between 12 and 15 months) (AAP, 2000b).

The threat of bioterrorism has generated interest in reintroducing smallpox vaccine. In 2002 the AAP issued a policy statement regarding routine administration of smallpox vaccine to children (AAP, 2002). Because children have a higher risk for adverse effects from the existing smallpox vaccine, the AAP supports the CDC recommendation for "ring" vaccination. This includes isolation of infected individuals and vaccinating contacts and contacts of contacts to contain the spread of disease (AAP, 2002).

Obstacles to Immunizations

Major reasons identified for low immunization rates during health care visits are presented in Box 4-3. In the 1980s the safety of the pertussis portion of the diphtheria-tetanus-pertussis (DPT) vaccine was questioned. Some parents

---

> **BOX 4-3**
> *Barriers to Immunization*
>
> - *Complexity of the health care system,* which may lead to a delay in vaccinating children when parents become confused or frustrated with the health care system; special barriers include:
>   —Appointment-only clinics
>   —Excessively long waiting periods
>   —Inconvenient scheduling
>   —Inaccessible clinic sites
>   —The need for formal referral from a primary health care provider
>   —Language and cultural barriers
> - *Expense* of immunization services
> - *Parental misconceptions* about disease severity, vaccine efficiency and safety, complications, and contraindications
> - *Inaccurate record keeping* by parents and health care workers
> - *Reluctance of the health care worker* to give more than two vaccines during the same visit
> - *Lack of public awareness* of the need for immunizations

---

elected not to immunize their children, which resulted in an increase in pertussis cases. Medical concern has led to the use in the United States of the acellular pertussis vaccine, which has fewer side effects.

The media play an important part in the immunization status of children. News programs that highlight the side effects of vaccines, rather than their individual and collective protective effect, create fear and misunderstanding in the public. Health care providers need to address this issue when recommending various immunizations to parents. It is important for nurses to be aware of vaccine controversies and know how to access appropriate, research-based information. The National Network for Immunization Information, an initiative of the Infectious Diseases Society of America, the Pediatric Infectious Diseases Society, the American Academy of Pediatrics, and the American Nurses Association, provides up-to-date information about immunization research. It can be accessed online at www.immunizationinfo.org.

Informed Consent

The National Childhood Vaccine Injury Act of 1986 requires that the benefits and risks associated with immunizations be discussed with parents before immunizations. The act also requires that families receive vaccine information statements (VISs) before immunization.

All health care providers who administer immunizations are required by federal law to provide general information about immunizations to the child and parents, preferably in the family's native language. This information describes why the vaccine is being given, the benefits and risks, and common side effects. Before providers administer a vaccine, parents should read the federally required information about that vaccine and have the opportunity to ask questions. The providers must use either VISs or a handout that provides all required information (American Academy of Pediatrics Committee on Infectious Diseases [APCID], 2003). It is necessary that the parents feel comfortable with the information, as well as with the answers to any questions. It has been shown that VISs do increase the parent's knowledge level and are beneficial. Providing the information before scheduled vaccinations allows parents the time to read all the information. Providers are encouraged to obtain written informed consent for each vaccine administered. If signatures are not obtained, the client's medical record should document that the vaccine information was reviewed.

Immunization Schedule

Each January, recommendations regarding vaccinations in the United States are made by the Advisory Committee on Immunization Practices (ACIP) of the Centers for Disease Control and Prevention (CDC), the American Academy of Pediatrics (AAP) Committee on Infectious Diseases, and the American Academy of Family Physicians (AAFP). All states require immunizations for children enrolled in licensed childcare programs and school. Some states further require immunizations in the upper grades and at the time of college entrance. One group who may be overlooked includes children who receive home schooling. It is of utmost importance therefore that immunization records be traced and that vaccinations be given over the course of the fewest visits possible. State requirements can be obtained from each state health department. Appendix D outlines the current recommendations for immunization of healthy children in the United States.

Children With an Uncertain History of Immunization

When a lapse in immunization occurs, the entire series does not have to be restarted. Children's charts should be flagged to remind health care providers of these children's immunization status. For children of unknown or uncertain immunization status, appropriate immunization should be administered. Readministration of measles, mumps, and rubella (MMR) vaccine, Hib vaccine, inactivated poliovirus vaccine (IPV), or hepatitis B vaccine to someone who is immune has no harmful effects. For children older than 7 years, the tetanus-diphtheria (Td) vaccine rather than the diphtheria-tetanus-acellular pertussis (DTaP) vaccine should be administered (CDC, 2003).

International adoptees, refugees, and exchange students should be immunized according to recommended schedules for healthy infants and children. If written records of prior immunization are not available, the child begins the schedule for children not immunized during infancy. Table 4-2 presents recommendations for immunizing children who were not immunized during infancy.

When taking an immunization history, the nurse should avoid asking the question, "Are your child's immunizations up-to-date?" This question will frequently be answered with a "yes," but that does not give the nurse sufficient information. The nurse may gain more information by asking, "Can you tell me when and what was the last immunization your child had?"

Administration of Vaccines

The manufacturer's packaging insert for each vaccine includes recommendations for handling, storage, administration site, dosage, and route. Nurses responsible for handling vaccines should be familiar with storage requirements to minimize the risk of vaccine failures. When multidose vials are

---

! **CRITICAL** **TO REMEMBER**

Special Considerations Related to Immunizations

- The gluteal site is not recommended at any age for the administration of the hepatitis B vaccine. This is because there is diminished immunogenicity in the gluteal site. (AAPCID, 2003).
- When giving DTaP, Hib, and hepatitis B vaccines simultaneously, it is advisable to administer the most reactive vaccine (DTaP) in one leg and to inject the others, which cause less reaction, into the other leg.
- Siblings and household contacts of immunocompromised children should not receive the oral poliovirus vaccine but may be given the inactivated poliovirus vaccine.
- Live measles vaccine is produced by chick embryo cell culture, so there is a remote possibility of anaphylactic hypersensitivity in children with egg allergies. Most reactions from the MMR are reactions to other components of the vaccine, so MMR is not usually contraindicated for children with egg hypersensitivity (AAPCID, 2003).
- Any immunization may cause an anaphylactic reaction. All offices and clinics must have epinephrine 1:1000 available.

DTaP, Diphtheria, tetanus, acellular pertussis; *Hib*, *Haemophilus influenzae* type B; *MMR*, measles, mumps, rubella.

---

used, sterile technique should be used to prevent contamination. To ensure safe administration, the vaccines should be given by the recommended route. In children whose gluteal muscle has not yet developed (those younger than 2 years), the preferred site for intramuscular (IM) injections is the anterolateral aspect of the thigh. The deltoid muscle can be used in children 18 months and older. The ventrogluteal site may be used in older children (see Chapter 38). Vaccines given intramuscularly need to be injected deep into the muscle mass to avoid irritation and possible necrosis.

More than one immunization may be administered at the same age or time. Some vaccines are given as a combined vaccine. When more than one injection is to be given, vaccines should be administered using separate syringes, not mixed into one. They should be given at different sites (preferably in different thighs), and the site used for each vaccine should be recorded to identify possible reactions. The nurse should also record the lot number for each vaccine given. Box 4-4 lists nursing responsibilities associated with administering vaccines. *expiration date*

Precautions and Contraindications

The main purpose of vaccination is to achieve immunity with the fewest possible side effects (Box 4-5). Most vaccines have no side effects; when side effects do occur, they are usually mild. Fever and local irritation are not uncommon after administration of DTaP vaccine, and fever and rash can occur 1 to 2 weeks after administration of live-virus measles vaccine.

Some severe side effects have been reported, however. These events are usually not predictable. Because cases have been reported of healthy children developing paralytic polio after administration of oral polio vaccine (OPV), the AAP and the CDC now recommend a full schedule of IPV. Reactions to the MMR vaccine have in-

TABLE 4-2 Catch-up Immunization Schedules for Children and Adolescents Who Start Late or Who Are More Than 1 Month Behind*

4 Months to 6 Years of Age: Minimum Interval Between Doses

Dose 1 (Minimum Age)	Dose 1 to Dose 2	Dose 2 to Dose 3	Dose 3 to Dose 4	Dose 4 to Dose 5
DTaP (6 wk)	4 wk	4 wk	6 mo	6 mo[1]
IPV (6 wk)	4 wk	4 wk	4 wk[2]	
HepB[3] (birth)	4 wk	3 wk (and 16 wk after first dose)		
MMR (12 mo)	4 wk[4]			
Varicella (12 mo)				
Hib[5] (6 wk)	4 wk: if first dose given at younger than 12 mo of age 8 wk (as final dose): if first dose given at 12 to 14 mo of age No further doses needed: if first dose given at 15 mo of age or older	4 wk[6]: if current age younger than 12 mo 8 wk (as final dose)[6]: if current age 12 mo or older and second dose given at younger than 15 mo of age No further doses needed: if previous dose given at 15 mo of age or older	8 wk (as final dose): this dose only necessary for children 12 mo to 5 yr of age who received 3 doses before 12 mo of age	
PCV[7]: (6wk)	4 wk: if first dose given at younger than 12 mo of age and current age younger than 24 mo 8 wk (as final dose): if first dose given at 12 mo of age or older or current age 24 to 59 mo No further doses needed: for healthy children if previous dose given at 24 mo of age or older	4 wk: if current age younger than 12 mo 8 wk (as final dose): if current age 12 mo or older No further doses needed: for healthy children if previous dose given at 24 mo of age or older	8 wk (as final dose): this dose only necessary for children 12 mo to 5 yr of age who received 3 doses before 12 mo of age	

7 to 18 Years of Age: Minimum Interval Between Doses

Dose 1 to Dose 2	Dose 2 to Dose 3	Dose 3 to Booster Dose
Td: 4 wk	Td: 6 mo	Td[8]: 6 mo: if first dose given at younger than 12 mo of age and current age younger than 11 yr 5 y: if first dose given at 12 mo of age or older and third dose given at younger than 7 yr of age and current age 11 yr or older 10 yr: if third dose given at 7 yr of age or older
IPV[9]: 4 wk	IPV[9]: 4 wk	IPV[2,9]
HepB: 4 wk	HepB: 8 wk (and 16 wk after first dose)	
MMR: 4 wk		
Varicella[10]: 4 wk		

From American Academy of Pediatrics Committee on Infectious Diseases. (2003). *2003 Red book: Report of the Committee on Infectious Diseases,* (26th ed.). Elk Grove, IL: American Academy of Pediatrics. Reprinted with permission.

*Catch-up schedules and minimum intervals between doses for children who have delayed immunizations. There is no need to restart a vaccine series regardless of the time that has elapsed between doses. Use the chart appropriate for the child's age. For additional information about vaccines, including precautions and contraindications for immunization and vaccine shortages, please visit the National Immunization Program Web site at www.cdc.gov/nip or call the National Immunization Information Hotline at 800-232-2522 (English) or 800-232-0233 (Spanish). Report adverse reactions to vaccines through the federal Vaccine Adverse Event Reporting System. For information on reporting reactions following vaccines, please visit www.vaers.org or call the 24-hour national toll-free information line at 800-822-7967. Report suspected cases of vaccine-preventable diseases to your state or the local health department.

[1] Diphtheria and tetanus toxoids and acellular pertussis (DTaP) vaccine: The fifth dose is not necessary if the fourth dose was given after the fourth birthday.

[2] Inactivated poliovirus (IPV) vaccine: For children who received an all-IPV or all-OPV series, a fourth dose is not necessary if third dose was given at 4 years of age or older. If both OPV and IPV were given as part of a series, a total of 4 doses should be given, regardless of the child's current age.

[3] Hepatitis B (HepB) vaccine: All children and adolescents who have not been immunized against hepatitis B should begin the hepatitis B immunization series during any visit. Providers should make special efforts to immunize children who were born in, or whose parents were born in, areas of the world where hepatitis B virus infection is moderately or highly endemic.

[4] Measles-mumps-rubella (MMR) vaccine: The second dose of MMR is recommended routinely at 4 to 6 years of age but may be given earlier if desired.

[5] *Haemophilus influenzae* type b (Hib) vaccine: Vaccine generally is not recommended for children 5 years of age or older.

[6] Hib: If current age younger than 12 months and the first 2 doses were PRP-OMP (PedvaxHIB or ComVax [Merck Vaccine Division, West Point, PA]), the third (and final) dose should be given at 12 to 15 months of age and at least 8 weeks after the second dose.

[7] Pneumococcal conjugate vaccine (PCV): Vaccine generally is not recommended for children 5 years of age or older.

[8] Tetanus and diphtheria toxoids (Td) vaccine: For children 7 to 10 years of age, the interval between the third and booster dose is determined by the age when the first dose was given. For adolescents 11 to 18 years of age, the interval is determined by the age when the third dose was given.

[9] IPV: Vaccine generally is not recommended for people 18 years of age or older.

[10] Varicella: Give 2-dose series to all susceptible adolescents 13 years of age or older.

BOX 4-4
Nursing Responsibility in Administering Vaccines

- Know the recommended immunization schedule and the recommended alternative schedule for those with lapsed immunizations or unknown immunization history.
- Acquire up-to-date information because recommendations are revised frequently.
- Assess the family's beliefs and values to assist in the education of the family as to the rationale for immunizations, the risks and side effects, and the risks of nonimmunization.
- Take a careful history to determine possible contraindications or precautions, and report any pertinent information to the practitioner. Educate the family as to the rationale for any contraindications.
- "Gloves are not required when administering vaccinations unless the persons who administer the vaccine will come in contact with potentially infectious body fluids or have open lesions" (AAPCID, 2003).
- Some vaccines come mixed in one syringe (e.g., DTaP-Hib). Other vaccines should not be mixed. Check manufacturer's recommendations.
- Administer vaccines according to the manufacturer's recommended sites.
- Aspirate to make sure that the needle has not been placed in a blood vessel.
- Wash hands before vaccine administration and between children.
- Review with the parents common side effects and the signs of potentially severe reactions that warrant contacting the practitioner.
- Instruct the parents that they may administer age-appropriate doses of acetaminophen every 4 to 6 hours for 24 hours if the child experiences discomfort related to vaccine administration.
- For painful or red injection sites, advise the parents to apply cold compresses for the first 24 hours; then use warm or cold compresses as long as needed.
- Give multiple administrations in different sites, and record those sites in the medical record.
- Document parental consent in the medical record. Documentation should also include the type of vaccine, date of administration, manufacturer and lot number, expiration date, administration site, any data pertinent to risks and side effects, and the signature and title of the person administering the immunization.

---

cluded anaphylactic reactions, both in children with and in those without a history of egg allergy. This has prompted consideration of other possible causative agents. For instance, the MMR vaccine contains neomycin, which may be the cause of the sensitivity.

Before a second dose of any vaccine is given, the nurse needs to ascertain and record whether any side effects or possible reactions occurred after the previous dose of that vaccine. The National Childhood Vaccine Injury Act of 1986 requires health care providers who administer vaccines to maintain permanent vaccination records and to report occurrences of certain adverse events stipulated in the act. Anaphylaxis or anaphylactic shock and encephalopathy are examples of two reportable events associated with the tetanus and pertussis vaccines. Providers administering immunizations must be aware of reportable events and comply with the provisions of the act.

Immunocompromised Children

In general, children who are immunologically compromised should not receive live bacterial or viral vaccines (e.g., MMR, varicella vaccine). There are some exceptions related to children with human immunodeficiency virus (HIV) and in some specific instances of children in remission from cancer. Children with HIV who are not severely compromised should receive MMR; varicella vaccine can be given, depending on the CD4 count (see Chapter 41).

Education

Immunization is a critical component of a child's health care. Knowledge of immunization schedules and an awareness of potential delays will aid the health care provider in identifying children who have not been fully immunized. Health care providers must provide parents with accurate information re-

BOX 4-5
Common Misconceptions About Administration and Safety of Vaccines

The following conditions or circumstances are *not* contraindications to the administration of vaccines:
- Mild acute illness with low-grade fever or mild diarrhea in an otherwise healthy child
- A reaction to a previous dose of DTaP vaccine with only soreness, redness, or swelling in the immediate vicinity of the injection site

DTaP, Diphtheria, tetanus, acellular pertussis.

garding immunizations, because immunizations are the primary and safest means of managing preventable infectious diseases. All children in the United States should have access to appropriate immunization. The State Children's Health Insurance Program (see Chapter 1) and the Vaccines for Children program ensure that there are no financial barriers. Nevertheless, health providers need to be aware that, although immunization rates are increasing through efforts of the federal and state governments, disparities in immunization access for the poor and certain racial or ethnic minorities still exist (United States Department of Health and Human Services [USDHHS], 2000).

Nutrition and Activity

To provide care for infants and children, the nurse must understand the nutritional needs of the body. The body is nourished by food. Carbohydrates, fats, proteins, water, vitamins,

---

BOX 4-6
Common Sources of Nutrients

Carbohydrates		**Proteins**	
Breads	Vegetables	Meat	Cheese
Cereals	Rice	Poultry	Eggs
Pasta	Fruits	Fish	Legumes
Dried peas and legumes		Milk	

Fats	
Butter	Cream
Margarine	Cheeses
Shortening	Nuts
Oils	Meats

BOX 4-7
ABC Dietary Guidelines for Americans Older Than 2 Years

- Aim for fitness
  —Aim for a healthy weight
  —Be physically active each day
- Build a healthy base
  —Let the pyramid guide food choices
  —Eat a variety of grains daily, especially whole grains
  —Eat a variety of fruits and vegetables daily
  —Keep food safe to eat
- Choose sensibly
  —Choose a diet low in saturated fat and cholesterol and moderate in total fat
  —Choose beverages and foods that limit your intake of sugars
  —Choose and prepare foods with less salt

From United States Department of Agriculture (USDA). (2001). *Dietary guidelines for Americans, 2000* (5th ed.). Available on-line: www.usda.gov/cnpp.

---

and minerals (Box 4-6) are the basic *nutrients* in food. Carbohydrates, fats, and proteins provide energy, which is required by the cells of the body to transport all substances across the cell membrane, to synthesize substances within the cell, and to dispose of waste products.

Carbohydrates

Complex carbohydrates should be the major dietary source of energy. Most complex carbohydrates are found in starch from cereal grains, roots, vegetables, and legumes. Foods that are good sources of complex carbohydrates are relatively inexpensive and easily obtained. Insufficient calorie intake causes the body to break down protein and fat for energy and glucose production. There is no recommended dietary allowance for carbohydrates. The more mature the vegetable, the higher the starch content. The U.S. Department of Agriculture (USDA) recommends that complex carbohydrates be the foundation of any diet; eaten in variety, they provide a healthy eating pattern (USDA, 2001).

Fats

Fats serve as the secondary source of energy by providing 30% or less of daily calorie intake. Of this amount, 10% or less should be saturated and the remaining 20% should be monounsaturated (olive, canola, and peanut oils) and polyunsaturated (corn and fish oils). Dietary fat allows the absorption of the fat-soluble vitamins (A, D, E, K) and adds flavor to foods. The layer of fat beneath the skin plays a role in regulating body temperature. Fat is a component of cell membranes and acts as a protective padding for the internal organs. When excess calories are consumed, dietary fats are stored as excess body fat. The monounsaturated and polyunsaturated fats can raise high-density lipoproteins and decrease low-density lipoproteins. For this reason, emphasis should be placed on replacing saturated fats with these fats whenever possible.

Proteins

Dietary *protein* is necessary for building and maintaining body tissues. Proteins are involved in homeostasis by working with other elements in the blood to maintain fluid balance. Many vitamins and minerals are bound to protein carriers for trans-

port. Proteins, as antibodies, aid in the regulation of the body's immune system.

Water

Water is essential for life. It transports nutrients to cells and waste products away from cells. It assists in the regulation of body temperature and in chemical reactions. Water lubricates joints and provides form and structure to the cells and the medium for body fluids. Water is found in most foods, including solids. Water requirements can be estimated by a variety of methods. The child's activity level and ambient temperature influence the amount of water needed.

Vitamins and Minerals

Vitamins and *minerals* are necessary in the regulation of metabolic processes. They are present in a wide variety of foods. Vitamins and minerals are added to processed formulas and to other foods such as cereals. It is generally not necessary for children to receive supplementation after infancy unless they are at nutritional risk (e.g., have anorexia or a chronic disease).

Dietary Guidelines

New guidelines for a healthful diet for Americans age 2 years or older were published by the USDA in 2001 (Box 4-7). The guidelines recommend that a variety of foods be eaten to get the energy, proteins, vitamins, minerals, and fiber needed for good health. The diet should be low in fat, saturated fat, and cholesterol. Vegetables, fruits, and grain products should be ample to provide needed vitamins, minerals, fiber, and complex carbohydrates. Sugars, salt, and sodium should be used in moderation.

The Food Guide Pyramid was developed by the USDA to show what should be eaten each day. Recent research on adults suggests that some changes are needed in the food pyramid, especially in regard to fat and carbohydrate intake (Harvard School of Public Health, 2003). The Food Guide Pyramid for Young Children (Fig. 4-3), however, illustrates

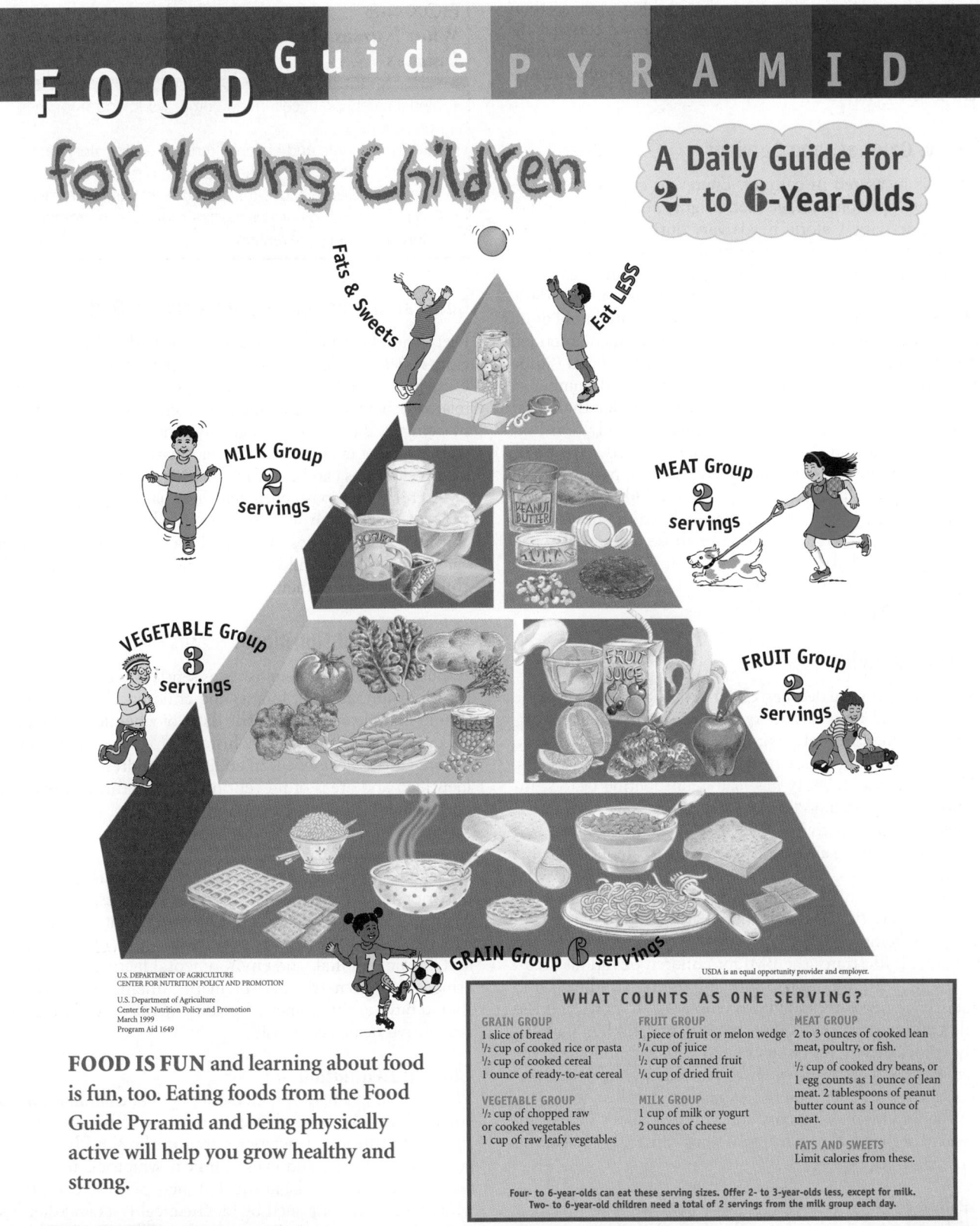

FOOD IS FUN and learning about food is fun, too. Eating foods from the Food Guide Pyramid and being physically active will help you grow healthy and strong.

WHAT COUNTS AS ONE SERVING?

GRAIN GROUP
1 slice of bread
½ cup of cooked rice or pasta
½ cup of cooked cereal
1 ounce of ready-to-eat cereal

VEGETABLE GROUP
½ cup of chopped raw or cooked vegetables
1 cup of raw leafy vegetables

FRUIT GROUP
1 piece of fruit or melon wedge
¾ cup of juice
½ cup of canned fruit
¼ cup of dried fruit

MILK GROUP
1 cup of milk or yogurt
2 ounces of cheese

MEAT GROUP
2 to 3 ounces of cooked lean meat, poultry, or fish.

½ cup of cooked dry beans, or 1 egg counts as 1 ounce of lean meat. 2 tablespoons of peanut butter count as 1 ounce of meat.

FATS AND SWEETS
Limit calories from these.

Four- to 6-year-olds can eat these serving sizes. Offer 2- to 3-year-olds less, except for milk.
Two- to 6-year-old children need a total of 2 servings from the milk group each day.

Figure 4-3 Food Guide Pyramid for Young Children. (From U.S. Department of Agriculture, Center for Nutrition Policy and Promotion.)

the Food Guide Pyramid in a way that children younger than 6 years can understand. The Pyramid focuses on eating a variety of foods to get the required nutrients and adequate energy. The importance of grains, fruits, and vegetables is evident in the Pyramid.

Energy, Calories, and Servings

Energy is measured in calories. Energy or calorie needs depend on the person's age, gender, height, weight, and level of physical activity. Calorie needs vary during childhood. Infants need sufficient calories to support rapid growth; therefore fat is not restricted in children younger than 2 years. After 2 years, fats should comprise no more than 30% of daily calories. Children can obtain the appropriate number of calories by eating the minimum number of recommended daily servings from all the food groups on the Food Guide Pyramid. Toddlers should consume the required number of servings, but the serving size should be smaller than that recommended for a preschooler (Center for Nutrition Policy and Promotion, 2001). Adolescents need to eat the maximum number of recommended servings, particularly if they are physically active. Very active children and those going through rapid growth spurts have higher energy needs than more sedate children or those who are in periods when growth is slower. Milk servings are particularly important, especially for adolescents, to avoid osteoporosis later in life.

Physical Activity

Over the past several decades, children of all ages have become less active and more sedentary. Obesity has become an epidemic in American children; in fact, approximately 20% to 27% of American children are considered obese (Roberts, 2000). Childhood obesity has many contributing factors: increased calorie consumption, low levels of physical activity, increased sedentary activities such as watching television and playing computer games, and overweight parents (Roberts, 2000).

A person's body mass index (BMI) provides an indication of relative obesity, and this number (a function of weight and height) is being used more frequently to assess for obesity. Appendix E illustrates the BMI for children of various ages.

Any health promotion counseling during childhood and adolescence needs to include an emphasis on increasing the child's and parents' daily physical activity. Children particularly enjoy activity if it is associated with fun and group involvement and are more likely to participate in physical exercise if they see their parents exercising as well.

When counseling parents and children about increasing physical activity, the nurse can emphasize the following (Story, Holt, & Sofka, 2002):

- Plan regular activities the family can do together.
- Schedule time for regular, daily physical activity.
- Encourage activity that is fun and meets the child's interests (e.g., dancing, ball games, karate, biking, water sports).
- Mix competitive with noncompetitive sports participation.
- Encourage the community to provide safe play and recreation areas for spontaneous games and activities.

BOX 4-8
What Nurses Can Do to Prevent Childhood Injuries

- Model safety practices in the home, work, and community.
- Educate parents and children through anticipatory safety guidance to help reduce needless injuries.
- Support legislative efforts that advocate prevention measures.
- Collaborate with other health care providers to promote safety and injury prevention.

Cultural and Religious Influences on Diet

Dietary intake is profoundly affected by both cultural and religious beliefs. An understanding of these patterns will assist the nurse in both the assessment and implementation of nutrition-related behaviors. Hospitalized children who become stressed by being in a new and strange environment do not need the added stress of unfamiliar foods. Information regarding a child's food preferences can be obtained during a dietary history.

A child's religious beliefs may also have an impact on the types of foods eaten and the way in which they are served. Within religious groups there may be a variety of dietary observances. The nurse should assist and encourage the child and the child's family in communicating specific dietary needs.

Assessment of Nutritional Status

A nutritional assessment is an essential component of the health examination of infants and children. This assessment should include anthropometric data, biochemical data, clinical examination, and dietary history. From these data, a plan of care can be developed. In addition, children at risk can be identified and areas of prevention pursued through teaching and further evaluation and follow-up.

Anthropometric Data
Height and head circumference reflect past nutrition or chronic nutritional problems. Weight, skinfold thickness, midarm circumference, and BMI better reflect present nutritional status. The nurse should always be aware of the roles of birth weight and ethnic, familial, and environmental factors when evaluating anthropometric measurements. Infants and children should have anthropometric measurements done during each preventive health care visit.

Clinical Evaluation
The clinical evaluation includes a physical examination and complete history. Special attention is paid to the areas where signs of nutritional deficiencies appear: the skin, hair, teeth, gums, lips, tongue, and eyes. Clinical symptoms usually are not by themselves diagnostic but may suggest conditions, which are then confirmed by biochemical tests and diet histories. More than one deficiency may be present. (See also the section "Failure to Thrive" in Chapter 53.)

Dietary History
Obtaining an accurate history of dietary intake is difficult. The knowledge that what the child is eating is being recorded can influence what the parent feeds the child or what the child eats.

CRITICAL TO REMEMBER

Relationship Between Safety and Childhood Development

Developmentally, children are vulnerable to injury, for the following reasons:

- Children are naturally curious and enjoy exploring their surroundings.
- Children are driven to test and master new skills.
- Children frequently attempt activities before they have developed the cognitive and physical skills required to accomplish the task safely.
- Children often assert themselves and challenge rules.
- Children develop a strong desire for peer approval as they grow older.

Children often cannot remember what they have eaten. If the child or parent is not committed to the process, incomplete information may be obtained. It is still a useful assessment process, however, and should be used. Client teaching includes an understanding of the importance of recording the child's dietary intake and the need for accuracy. Common methods of assessing dietary intake include 24-hour recall, a food frequency questionnaire, or a food diary.

Twenty-Four-Hour Recall. With the 24-hour recall method, the child or parent is asked to recall everything the child has eaten in the past 24 hours. A questionnaire may be used, or the nurse may conduct an interview asking the pertinent questions.

The child or parent may have difficulty remembering the kinds and amounts of food eaten, or the family may have had an atypical day on the previous day or may not feel comfortable relating what was eaten the day being evaluated. How the child or parents see the nurse may influence the response; they may say what they think the interviewer wants to hear. Asking for information in relation to meals eaten as opposed to food groups may increase the accuracy of the assessment.

Food Frequency Questionnaire. The food frequency questionnaire elicits information on the intake of particular foods or food groups on a daily, weekly, or monthly basis. This tool can be used to validate the 24-hour recall data. As for all methods of assessment, this requires the interviewer to be nonjudgmental and objective. Putting the information into a questionnaire may be less threatening to the child and family and will save time.

Food Diary. When keeping a food diary, the child or parent records everything consumed during a specified period. Various sources recommend different lengths of time for keeping the diary; 3-day to 7-day records may be used. As in all nursing care, the nurse must evaluate what is a reasonable time to expect the family or child to keep the records. The time, place, and people present when the food was eaten may also be recorded. This provides the nurse with additional information, which may identify trends and other information related to the child's eating behaviors.

Safety

Unintentional injury is the most significant but underrecognized public health threat facing children today. Unintentional injury is the leading cause of death in children.

Across age-groups, motor vehicle traffic injuries and firearm injuries are the two major causes of injury (Scheidt, Overpeck, Trifiletti, & Cheng, 2000). (See Chapter 34 for a more detailed discussion of the causes of injury in childhood.)

The number of childhood deaths is staggering, but it is only a fraction of the number of children who are hospitalized and require emergency treatment and who suffer permanent disability as a result of injury. The economic burden to society is equally astounding, reaching billions of dollars yearly. What cannot be quantified are the emotional loss, suffering, and pain the child and family must endure once an injury has occurred.

All children are at risk for injury because of their normal curiosity, impulsiveness, and impatience. Everywhere they venture, they are exposed to potentially hazardous situations.

Injury Prevention

Injury prevention is a relatively new focus of health promotion. The term *accident*, with its implied meaning of random chance or lack of responsibility, is being replaced with *injury*, with its implication that injuries have causes that can be modified to prevent or lessen their frequency and severity. Safety education is a critical component of injury prevention. It increases awareness, attempts to modify human behavior, and reinforces changes implemented through legal mandates (e.g., seat belt laws) or product modification (e.g., crib design, air bags).

Nurses need to become proactive in childhood injury prevention by increasing children's and adults' awareness of safety issues (Box 4-8). Nurses who care for children are acutely aware of the devastating effects and complex problems injuries cause. From their experiences, they become well-informed advocates for childhood safety.

Anticipatory Guidance

To be most effective in providing anticipatory safety guidance, nurses must gear educational strategies to the child's level of growth and development. Knowledge of growth and development also helps the nurse understand the risks associated with each age-group and choose the educational strategy appropriate to a child's developmental level.

Early in their parenting experience, parents need to know how to provide a safe environment for their children as well as what behaviors they can expect at various developmental levels. Anticipatory guidance builds on the safety principles of the previous stage. Awareness of a child's changing capabilities allows the parent to be more alert and reactive to safety hazards that the child is likely to encounter. This awareness is especially important for first-time parents.

Simply telling parents to "watch your children" or to "child-proof" the home or telling a child to "be careful" has little educational impact. Educational efforts are much more likely to be effective if they focus on specific problems with specific solutions rather than providing broad or vague advice.

Teaching Strategies

Teaching can be formal or informal, simple or elaborate, as long as it provides relevant safety information and coincides with the child's or parent's cognitive abilities. For children younger than 5 or 6 years, it is advisable to incorporate the parent into the teaching process so that the parents can assist with reinforcement or questions the child later has about the safety issue. With younger children, who are easily distracted, the information should be presented in short sessions.

Many local and national organizations have safety information available for distribution. This information can be used to supplement the teaching process. Prepared materials range from pamphlets, booklets, posters, and audiovisual materials to entire teaching programs that can assist in providing injury prevention education to all age-groups. Some programs offer the materials free of cost. Internet information, such as that obtained at www.kidsafe.com can be extremely helpful to parents. Appendix I gives a partial listing of organizations that provide safety information.

KEY CONCEPTS

- Growth, development, maturation, and learning are complex, interrelated processes that produce complicated series of changes in individuals from conception to death.
- Growth and development proceed from simple to complex, proximal to distal, and head to lower extremities.
- As children grow and develop, wide variations within normal limits occur.
- Weight, height, and head circumference, common parameters used to monitor growth, should be measured and evaluated at regular intervals.
- The earlier that delays and deviations from normal are treated, the less severe the effect will be on growth and developmental outcomes.
- Numerous factors, including genetics, environment, culture, nutrition, health status, and family structure, affect how children grow and develop.
- Piaget's theory of cognitive development describes how children learn to deal with their environment through thinking and reasoning. Progress in learning during various periods is based on the child's ability to create patterns of understanding and behavior.
- Freud's psychosexual theory attempts to explain how humans struggle in both conscious and unconscious ways to become individual

beings. During each stage of sexual development in children, a different area of the body is the focus of attention and pleasure.
- Erikson's theory of psychosocial development describes a series of crises emerging at specific times and in a particular order. These stages occur throughout life, and each must be resolved for an individual to progress emotionally.
- Kohlberg discusses moral development as a complex process involving progressive acceptance of the values and rules of society in a way that determines behavior. A maturing individual becomes less concerned with avoiding punishment and more interested in human rights and universal justice.
- Language development, a complex process involving extensive neuromuscular maturation, begins as undifferentiated crying at birth and proceeds throughout life to provide a vehicle for communication, thought, and creativity.
- A variety of prescreening and screening tools, such as the DDST-II, are used by nurses to gain an overall picture of a child's developmental progress and to alert the nurse to potential developmental delays.
- To provide high-quality, developmentally appropriate care to children and parents, nurses must be aware of normal patterns of growth and development.

- Piaget described three types of play, related to periods of sensorimotor, preoperational, and concrete operational functioning: practice play, symbolic play, and games.
- Play enhances the child's growth and development through physical, cognitive, emotional, social, and moral development.
- Personnel who administer and handle vaccines must be aware of recommendations for handling, storing, and administering the vaccines. Special attention should be given to the site of administration, dosage, and route.
- When a lapse in immunization occurs, the entire series does not have to be restarted.
- Children who are immunologically compromised should not receive live bacterial or viral vaccines.
- The six basic nutrients are carbohydrates, protein, fat, vitamins, minerals, and water.
- Components of a nutritional assessment are anthropometric data, biochemical data, clinical examination, and dietary history.
- Many childhood injuries and deaths are predictable and preventable.
- Understanding the developmental milestones of each age-group is important for promoting safety awareness for parents, caregivers, and children.

REFERENCES and READINGS

American Academy of Pediatrics [AAP]. (2000a). *Common household environmental dangers.* Available on-line: www.medem.com/MedLB.

American Academy of Pediatrics. (2000b). Policy statement: Recommendations for the prevention of pneumococcal infections, including the use of pneumococcal conjugate vaccine (Prevnar), pneumococcal polysaccharide vaccine, and antibiotic prophylaxis. *Pediatrics, 106*(2), 362-366.

American Academy of Pediatrics. (2001). Developmental surveillance and screening of infants and young children. *Pediatrics, 108*(1), 192-196.

American Academy of Pediatrics. (2002). Smallpox vaccine (Electronic version). *Pediatrics, 110*(3).

American Academy of Pediatrics Committee on Infectious Diseases. (2003). *2003 Red book: Report of the Committee on Infectious Diseases* (26th ed.). Elk Grove Village, IL: Author.

American Academy of Pediatrics Committee on Nutrition. (1998). *Pediatric nutrition handbook.* Elk Grove Village, IL: Author.

Bear, G.G., Richards, H.C., & Gibbs, J.C. (1997). Sociomoral reasoning and behavior. In G.C. Bear, K.M. Minke, & A. Thomas (Eds.), *Children's needs II: Development, problems and alternatives.* Bethesda, MD: National Association of School Psychologists.

Bowen, A., & Dammeyer, M. (1999). Reducing children's immunization distress in a primary care setting. *Journal of Pediatric Nursing, 14*(5), 296-302.

Brazelton, T.B. (1992). *Touchpoints.* Menlo Park, CA: Addison-Wesley.

Bricker, D., & Squires, J. (1999). *Ages & stages questionnaires: A parent-completed, child-monitoring system* (2nd ed.). Baltimore, MD: Brookes.

Calamaro, C. (2000). Infant nutrition in the first year of life: Tradition or science? *Pediatric Nursing, 26*(2), 211-214.

Carey, W. (2002). Rapid, competent, and inexpensive developmental-behavioral screening is possible. *Pediatrics, 109*(2), 316-318.

Center for Nutrition Policy and Promotion. (2001). *Food Guide Pyramid for young children.*

U.S. Department of Agriculture. Available on-line: www.usda.gov/cnpp.

Centers for Disease Control and Prevention [CDC]. (1999). Achievements in public health, 1900-1999 impact of vaccines universally recommended for children—United States, 1990-1998. *MMWR: Morbidity and Mortality Weekly Report, 48*(12), 243-248.

Centers for Disease Control and Prevention. (2002). *Haemophilus influenzae serotype b (HIB) disease.* Retrieved August 18, 2003, from www.cdc.gov.

Centers for Disease Control and Prevention. (2003). *Recommended childhood and adolescent immunization schedule—United States, 2003.* Retrieved August 18, 2003, from www.cdc.gov.

Colby, A., Kohlberg, L., & Kauffman, K. (1987). Theoretical introduction to the measurement of moral judgement. In A. Colby & L. Kohlberg (Eds.), *The measurement of moral judgment* (Vol. 1). Cambridge, England: Cambridge University Press.

Crawley-Coha, T. (2001). Childhood injury: A status report. *Journal of Pediatric Nursing, 16*(5), 371-374.

Crawley-Coha, T. (2002). Childhood injury: A status report, part 2. *Journal of Pediatric Nursing, 17*(2), 133-136.

Elkind, D. (1970). *Children and adolescents: Interpretive essays on Jean Piaget.* New York: Oxford University Press.

Emde, R.N. (1998). Early emotional development: New modes of thinking for research and intervention. *Pediatrics, 102*(5), 1236-1243.

Erikson, E.H. (1963). *Childhood and society* (2nd ed.). New York: Norton.

Feldman, R.S. (1998). *Child development.* Upper Saddle River, NJ: Prentice-Hall.

Flavell, J. (1963). *The developmental psychology of Jean Piaget.* Princeton, NJ: Van Nostrand.

Ford, C.A., & Coleman, W.L. (1999). Adolescent development and behavior: Implications for the primary care physician. In M.D. Levine, W.B. Carey, & A.C. Crocker (Eds.), *Developmental behavioral pediatrics.* Philadelphia: Saunders.

Frankenburg, W.K. (2002). Developmental surveillance and screening of infants and young children. *Pediatrics, 109*(1), 144-145.

Frankenburg, W.K., & Dodds, J.B. (1992). *Denver II screening manual.* Denver: Developmental Materials.

Freud, A. (1974). *Introduction to psychoanalysis.* New York: International Universities Press.

Freud, S. (1960). *The ego and the id* (J. Riviere, Trans.). New York: Norton. (Original work published 1923.)

Garvey, C. (1979). What is play? In P. Chance (Ed.). *Learning through play.* New York, NY: Gardner Press.

Glascoe, F.P. (1999). Using parents' concerns to detect and address developmental and behavioral problems. *Journal of Society of Pediatric Nurses, 4*(1), 24-35.

Glascoe, F.P., & Shapiro, H.L. (2003). *Developmental screening.* Retrieved on August 12, 2003, from www.dbpeds.org.

Harvard School of Public Health. (2003). *Fats and cholesterol.* Retrieved August 19, 2003, from www.hsph.harvard.edu/nutritionsource/fats.html.

Institute for Clinical Systems Improvement. (2001). Preventive services for children. *Journal of Child and Family Nursing, 4*(2), 156-158.

Kelly, D.P., & Sally, J.I. (1999). Disorders of speech and language. In M.D. Levine, W.B. Carey, & A.C. Crocker (Eds.), *Developmental behavioral pediatrics.* Philadelphia: Saunders.

Kohlberg, L. (1964). Development of moral character. In M. Hoffman & L. Hoffman (Eds.), *Review of child development research* (Vol. 1). New York: Russell Sage Foundation.

Kohlberg, L. (1984). *The psychology of moral development.* San Francisco: Harper & Row.

Kritt, D. (2000). Young children's play offers insight into developmental transitions. *The Brown University Child and Adolescent Behavior Letter, 16*(4), 1.

Litt, I. F., & Martin, J.A. (1999). Development of sexuality and its problems. In M.D. Levine, W.B. Carey, & A.C. Crocker (Eds.), *Developmental behavioral pediatrics.* Philadelphia: Saunders.

Melmed, M.E. (1998). Talking with parents about emotional development. *Pediatrics, 102*(5), 1317-1326.

Monsen, R. (2002). Children playing. *Journal of Pediatric Nursing, 17*(2), 137-138.

Offit, P., Quarles, J., Gerber, M., Hackett, C., Marcuse, E., Kollman, T., Gellin, B., & Landry, S. (2002). Addressing parents' concerns: Do multiple vaccines overwhelm or weaken the infant's immune system? *Pediatrics, 109*(1), 124-129.

Piaget, J. (1962). *Play, dreams and imitation childhood.* New York: Norton.

Piaget, J. (1967). *Six psychological studies.* New York: Random House.

Rice, M., & Howell, C. (2000). Measurement of physical activity, exercise, and physical fitness in children: Issues and concerns. *Journal of Pediatric Nursing, 15*(3), 148-155.

Richmond, P.G. (1971). *An introduction to Piaget.* New York: Basic Books.

Roberts, S. (2000). The role of physical activity in the prevention and treatment of childhood obesity. *Pediatric Nursing, 26*(1), 33-41.

Ross, R.P. (1997). Play. In G.G. Bear, K.M. Minke, & A. Thomas (Eds.), *Children's needs II: Development, problems and alternatives.* Bethesda, MD: National Association of School Psychologists.

Scheidt, P., Overpeck, M., Trifiletti, L., & Cheng, T. (2000). Child and adolescent injury research in 1998: A summary of abstracts submitted to the Ambulatory Pediatrics Association and the American Public Health Association. *Archives of Pediatrics and Adolescent Medicine, 154*(5), 442-445.

Story, M., Holt, K., & Sofka, D. (2002). *Bright futures in practice: Nutrition* (2nd ed.). Arlington, VA: National Center for Education in Maternal and Child Health.

Udovic, S.L., Lieu, T.A., Black, S.B., Ray, P.M., Ray, G.T., & Shinefield, H.R. (1998). Parent reports on willingness to accept childhood immunizations during urgent care visits. *Pediatrics, 102*(4), e47.

United States Department of Agriculture (USDA). (2001). *Dietary guidelines for Americans, 2000* (5th ed.). Available on-line: www.usda.gov/cripp.

United States Department of Health and Human Services [USDHHS]. (2000). *Healthy People 2010* (Conference edition, in 2 volumes). Washington, DC: Author.

Wilson, C. (1999). Parental preparation of children for routine physical examinations. *Journal of Pediatric Nursing, 14*(5), 329-334.

Woods, C. & Abramson, J. (2002). Immunization practices. In F.D. Burg, J.R. Ingelfinger, R.A. Polin, & A.A. Gershon (Eds.), *Gellis & Kagan's current pediatric therapy* (17th ed.). Philadelphia: Saunders.

5

Health Promotion for the Infant

◆ LEARNING OBJECTIVES

After studying this chapter, you should be able to:
- Describe the physiologic changes that occur during infancy.
- Describe the motor, psychosocial, language, and cognitive development of the infant.
- Discuss common problems of infancy, such as separation anxiety, sleep, irritability, and colic.
- Discuss the importance of immunizations and recommended immunization schedules for infants.
- Provide parents with anticipatory guidance for common concerns during infancy, such as immunizations, nutrition, elimination, dental care, sleep, hygiene, safety, and play.

◆ DEFINITIONS

asphyxiation A state of suffocation that severely compromises oxygen delivery to the body.

critical milestones Developmental milestones that, if not reached appropriately, would initiate a full developmental assessment. Critical milestones are based on the DDST-II milestones (see Chapter 4) and appear in the Growth and Development boxes throughout the chapter.

developmental milestones Benchmarks of development that indicate whether the infant is developing normally; not achieving milestones within a certain time frame might be cause for concern.

egocentrism Complete absorption with self; an inability to understand that others have a different point of view.

mistrust The negative resolution of the first developmental task, according to Erikson's theory; results in acute emotional tension and behavioral signs of unmet needs.

object permanence The realization that objects continue to exist even though they are out of sight.

parent-infant attachment A sense of belonging to or connection between a parent and infant.

pincer grasp The use of index finger and thumb to grip objects.

sensorimotor stage Piaget's first stage of cognitive development, in which infants and young toddlers use mainly senses and movement to begin to understand and control their environment.

stranger anxiety The infant's ability to distinguish between caregivers and others, to prefer parents to other caregivers, and to become distressed when separation occurs.

trust The basic emotion established during infancy as a result of satisfying interactions between child and caregiver; provides the foundation on which a healthy personality is built.

During no time after birth does a human being grow and change as dramatically as during infancy. Between the ages of 1 month and 1 year, the infancy period, a child grows and develops from a tiny bundle of physiologic needs to a dynamo, capable of locomotion and language and ready to embark on the adventures of the toddler years.

GROWTH AND DEVELOPMENT OF THE INFANT

Even though historically adults considered infants unable to do much more than eat and sleep, it is now well documented that even young infants can organize their experiences in meaningful ways and adapt to changes in the environment. Evidence shows that infants form strong bonds with their caregivers, communicate their needs and wants, and interact socially. By the end of the first year of life, infants can move about on their own, elicit responses from adults, communicate through the use of rudimentary language, and solve simple problems.

Infancy is characterized by the need to establish harmony between the self and the world. To achieve this harmony, the infant needs food, warmth, comfort, oral satisfaction, environmental stimulation, and opportunities for self-exploration and self-expression. Competent caregivers satisfy the needs of helpless infants, providing a warm, nurturing relationship so that the children experience a sense of trust in the world and in themselves. These challenges make infancy an exciting yet demanding period for both child and parents.

Nurses play an important role in promoting and maintaining health in infants. Although the infant mortality rate in the United States has declined markedly over the past 30 years (see Chapter 1), there are still many infant deaths before their first birthday. The leading cause of death in infants older than

1 month is sudden infant death syndrome (U.S. Department of Health and Human Services, 2000). Unintentional injuries contribute to mortality as well as morbidity in the infant population. Nurses provide anticipatory guidance for families with infants to reduce morbidity and mortality. Providing parents with information about immunization, feeding, sleep, hygiene, safety, and other common concerns is an important nursing responsibility. Appropriate anticipatory guidance can assist with achieving some of the goals and objectives determined by the U.S. government to be important in improving the overall health of infants (Box 5-1). Nurses are in a good position to offer anticipatory guidance based on the infant's growth and achievement of developmental milestones. Table 5-1 summarizes growth and development during infancy.

Physical Growth and Development

Growth is an excellent indicator of overall health during infancy. Although growth rates are variable, infants usually double their birth weight by 6 months and triple it by 1 year of age. During the first 5 to 6 months, the average weight gain is 1½ lb (0.68 kg) per month. Throughout the next 6 months, weight increase is approximately 1 lb (0.45 kg) per month. Weight gain in formula-fed infants is slightly greater than in breast-fed infants.

BOX 5-1
Healthy People 2010 Objectives for Infants

1-12	Establish a single toll-free telephone number for access to poison control centers on a 24-hour basis throughout the United States.
8-11	Eliminate elevated blood lead levels in children.
14-1	Reduce or eliminate indigenous cases of vaccine-preventable disease.
14-5	Reduce invasive pneumococcal infections.
15-7,8	Reduce nonfatal and fatal poisonings.
15-9	Reduce deaths caused by suffocation.
15-13	Reduce deaths caused by unintentional injuries.
15-20	Increase use of child restraints.
15-33	Reduce maltreatment and maltreatment fatalities of children.
28-11	Increase the proportion of newborns who are screened for hearing loss by age 1 month, who have audiologic evaluation by age 3 months, and who are enrolled in appropriate intervention services by age 6 months.

Modified from U.S. Department of Health and Human Services. (2000). *Healthy People 2010* (Conference edition, in 2 volumes). Washington, DC: Author.

TABLE 5-1 Summary of Growth and Development: The Infant

Physical	Motor	Psychosocial	Sensory/Cognitive	Language/ Communication
1-2 MO				
Fast growth; weight gain of 1½ lb (0.68 kg) per mo and height gain of 1 in (2.54 cm) per mo during first 6 mo. Upper limbs and head grow faster. Primitive reflexes present; strong suck and gag reflex. Obligate nose breather. Posterior fontanel closes by 2-3 mo.	**Gross** May lift head when held against shoulder. Head lag. **Fine** Palmar grasp. *1 mo:* Immediately drops object placed in hand. Fist usually clenched (grasp reflex). *2 mo:* Holds objects momentarily. Hands often open (grasp reflex fading).	Erikson's stage of trust vs. mistrust. Infant learns that world is good and "I am good." This stage is the foundation for other stages. Child is entirely dependent on parents and other caregivers. Needs should be met in a timely fashion. Touch is important.	Piaget's sensorimotor phase. *1 mo:* Notes bright objects if in line of vision. Vision 20/100. Reflexes dominate behavior. *2 mo:* Begins to follow objects.	Strong cry. Throaty sounds. Responds to human faces. *6-8 wk:* Begins to smile in response to stimuli.
3 MO				
Primitive reflexes fading.	**Gross** Can get hand to mouth. Can lift head off bed when in prone position. Head lag still present but decreasing. **Fine** Holds objects placed in hands. Grasp reflex absent.	Smiles in response to others. Uses sucking to soothe self.	Follows an object with eyes. Plays with fingers.	Babbles, coos. Enjoys making sounds. Responds to voices, watches speaker.

Continued

TABLE 5-1 Summary of Growth and Development: The Infant—cont'd

Physical	Motor	Psychosocial	Sensory/Cognitive	Language/ Communication
4-5 MO				
Can breathe when nose is obstructed. Growth rate declines. Drooling begins in preparation for teething. Moro, tonic neck, and rooting reflexes have disappeared.	**Gross** Plays with feet; puts foot in mouth. Bears weight when held in a standing position. Turns from abdomen to back. **Fine** Begins reaching and grasping with palm. Hits at object, misses.	Mouth is a sensory organ used to explore the environment. Attachment is an ongoing process throughout infancy. Has increased interest in parent, shows trust, knows parent. Shows emotions of fear and anger.	*4 mo:* Brings hands together at midline. Vision 20/80. Begins to play with objects. Recognizes familiar faces. Turns head to locate sounds. Shows anticipation and excitement. Memory span is 5-7 min. Plays with favorite toys.	Crying becomes differentiated. Babbling is common. Begins consonant sounds: *H, N, G, K, P, B* (4 mo). Makes vowel sounds: *ee, ah, ooh* (5 mo).
6-7 MO				
Weight gain slows to 1 lb (0.45 kg) per mo. Length gain of $\frac{1}{2}$ in (1.27 cm) per mo. Birth weight doubles; tooth eruption begins; chewing and biting occur. Maternal iron stores are depleted.	**Gross** Sits, leaning forward on both hands; when supine, lifts head off table. Turns from back to abdomen. **Fine** Transfers objects from one hand to another. Picks up object well with the whole hand.	Smiles at self in mirror. Plays peek-a-boo. Begins to show stranger anxiety.	Can fixate on small objects. Adjusts posture to see. Responds to name. Exhibits beginning sense of object permanence. Recognizes parent in other clothes, places. Is alert for $1\frac{1}{2}$-2 hr.	Produces vowel sounds and chained syllables. Begins to imitate sounds. Belly laughs. Babbles (one syllable) with pleasure. Calls for help. "Talks" to toys and image in mirror.
8-9 MO				
Continues to gain weight, length. Patterns of bladder and bowel elimination begin to become more regular.	**Gross** Sits steadily unsupported. Can crawl and pull up. **Fine** Pincer grasp develops. Reaches for toys. Rakes for objects and releases objects.	Stranger anxiety is at its height. Separation anxiety is increasing. Follows parent around the house.	Beginning development of depth perception. Object permanence continues to develop. Uses hands to learn concepts of in and out.	Stringing together of vowels and consonants begins. First few words begin to have meaning (Mama, Daddy, bye-bye, baby). Begins to understand and obey simple commands, such as, "Wave bye-bye." Responds to "No!" Shouts for attention.
10-12 MO				
Birth weight triples; birth length increases by 50% *(12 mo)*. Head and chest circumference equal. Babinski reflex disappears.	**Gross** Can stand alone. Can walk with one hand held but crawls to get places quickly. **Fine** Releases hold on cup. Finger-feeds self *(10 mo)*. Feeds self with spoon *(12 mo)*. Holds crayon to mark on paper. Pincer grasp is complete *(12 mo)*.	Has mood changes. Quiets self. Is quieted by music. Tenderly cuddles toy.	Vision 20/40. Searches for hidden toy. Explores boxes, inserts objects in container. Symbol recognition is developing (enjoys books).	Can say two or more words. Says "Mama" or "Dada" specifically. Waves bye-bye. Begins to differentiate between words. Enjoys jabbering. Vocalization decreases when walking. Knows own name.

During the first 6 months, infants increase their birth length by approximately 1 inch (2.54 cm) per month, slowing to $\frac{1}{2}$ inch (1.27 cm) per month over the next 6 months. By 1 year of age, most infants have increased their birth length by 50%.

The head circumference growth rate during the first year is approximately $\frac{4}{10}$ inch (1 cm) per month. Usually the posterior fontanel closes by 2 to 3 months of age, whereas the larger anterior fontanel may remain open until 18 months. Head circumference and fontanel measurements indicate brain growth and are obtained, along with height and weight, at each well-baby visit. Chapter 33 discusses growth rate monitoring throughout infancy.

Maturation of Body Systems

In addition to height and weight, organ systems grow and mature rapidly in the infant. Even though body systems are developing rapidly, the infant's organs differ from those of older children and adults in both structure and function. These differences place the infant at risk for problems that might not be expected in older individuals. Knowledge of these differences provides the nurse with important rationales on which to base anticipatory guidance and specific nursing interventions.

Neurologic System. Brain growth and differentiation occur rapidly during the first year of life and depend on nutrition and the function of the other organ systems. At birth, the brain accounts for approximately 10% to 12% of body weight. By 1 year of age, the brain has doubled its weight, with a major growth spurt occurring between 15 and 20 weeks of age and another between 30 weeks and 1 year of age. Increases in the number of synapses and expanded myelination of nerves contribute to maturation of the neurologic system during infancy. Primitive reflexes disappear as the cerebral cortex thickens and motor areas of the brain continue to develop, proceeding in a cephalocaudal pattern: arms first, then legs.

Respiratory System. In the first year of life, the lungs increase to three times their weight and six times their volume at birth. In the newborn, alveoli number approximately 20 million, increasing to the adult number of 300 million by age 8 years. During infancy, the trachea remains small, supported only by soft cartilage.

The diameter and length of the trachea, bronchi, and bronchioles increase with age. These tiny, collapsible air passages, however, leave infants vulnerable to respiratory difficulties caused by infection or foreign bodies. The eustachian tube is short and relatively horizontal, increasing the risk for middle-ear infections.

Cardiovascular System. The cardiovascular system undergoes dramatic changes in the transition from fetal to extrauterine circulation. Fetal shunts close, and pulmonary circulation increases drastically (see Chapter 46). During infancy, the heart doubles in size and weight, the heart rate gradually slows, and blood pressure increases.

Immune System. Transplacental transfer of maternal antibodies supplements the infant's weak response to infection until approximately 3 to 4 months of age. Although the infant begins to produce immunoglobulins (Ig) soon after birth, by 1 year of age, the infant has only approximately 60% of the adult IgG level, 75% of the adult IgM level, and 20% of the adult IgA level. Breast milk transmits additional IgA protection. The activity of T lymphocytes also increases after birth. Even though the immune system matures during infancy, maximum protection against infection is not achieved until early childhood. This immaturity places the infant at risk for infection.

Gastrointestinal System. The stomach capacity of a newborn is approximately 90 ml, but with feedings, the capacity increases rapidly to approximately 200 ml at 1 year of age. In the gastrointestinal system, enzymes needed for the digestion and absorption of proteins, fats, and carbohydrates mature and increase in concentration. Although the newborn's gastrointestinal system is capable of digesting protein and lactase, the ability to digest and absorb fat does not reach adult levels until approximately 6 to 9 months of age.

Renal System. Kidney mass increases threefold during the first year of life. Although the glomeruli enlarge considerably during the first few months, the glomerular filtration rate remains low. Thus the kidney is not effective as a filtration organ or efficient in concentrating urine until after the first year of life. Because of the functional immaturity of the renal system, the infant is at great risk for fluid and electrolyte imbalance.

Motor Development

During the first few months after birth, muscle growth and weight gain allow for increased control of reflexes and more purposeful movement. At 1 month, movement occurs in a random fashion, with the fists tightly clenched. Because the neck musculature is weak and the head is large, infants can lift their heads only briefly. By 2 to 3 months, infants can lift their heads 90 degrees from a prone position and can hold them steadily erect in a sitting position. During this time, active grasping gradually replaces reflexive grasping and increases in frequency as eye-hand coordination improves (see Table 5-1).

The Moro, tonic neck, and rooting reflexes disappear at approximately 3 to 4 months. These primitive reflexes, which are controlled by the midbrain, probably disappear because they are suppressed by growing cortical layers. Head control steadily increases during the 3rd month. By the 4th month, the head remains in a straight line with the body when the infant is pulled to a sitting position. Most infants play with their feet by 4 to 5 months, drawing them up to suck on their toes. Parents need anticipatory guidance about ways to prevent accidents by "baby-proofing" their homes before each motor development milestone is reached.

The nurse might, for instance, explain, "Infants grow and mature very rapidly, and you will be very busy with a new baby. Now is the time to 'baby-proof' your home before Mary turns over and begins crawling and reaching for objects. By doing this now, you can prevent later injuries and worries."

During the 5th and 6th months, motor development accelerates rapidly. Infants of this age readily reach for and

> ! **CRITICAL TO REMEMBER**
>
> **Risks Caused by the Infant's Immature Body Systems**
>
> - An immature respiratory system places the infant at risk for respiratory infection.
> - An immature immune system places the infant at risk for infection.
> - An immature renal system places the infant at risk for fluid and electrolyte imbalances.

PARENTS
Want to Know

How to "Baby-Proof" the Home

By the time babies reach 6 months of age, they begin to become much more active, curious, and mobile. Even though your baby might not be creeping or crawling yet, it is difficult to predict when that will happen. For this reason, you need to be prepared by making sure your house and the toys with which the baby plays are safe. Babies learn through exploring and participating in many different types of experiences. By keeping the baby's environment safe, you can encourage these experiences for your baby.

Be sure to check the following:

- All small or sharp objects or dangerous substances should be out of the baby's reach. Get down to the baby's eye level to be sure. This includes plants and paint chips, which can be poisonous. Be sure to check that any bedside table near the baby's crib is kept clear of ointments, creams, pins, or any other small objects. Be sure to check that small pieces from older siblings' toys are put away. Keep money put away.
- Put plastic fillers in all electrical outlets, and put cabinet and drawer locks on all cabinets and drawers. Doorknob covers are also available that prevent the infant from opening the door.
- Remove front knobs from the stove. Be sure to keep all pot and pan handles turned away from the edge of the stove.
- Remove from lower cabinets and lock away all dangerous or poisonous substances, including such items as pet food, household cleaning agents, cosmetic aids, pesticides, plant fertilizers, paints, matches, medicines, and plastic bags. Be sure to store these products in their original containers. Never give a small child a latex balloon.
- Place a gate on the top and bottom of stairways. Be sure the gate does not have openings that can trap the baby's head, hands, or fingers.
- Remove heavy containers from table tops covered with a tablecloth. Do not hold the baby on your lap while drinking or eating any kind of hot foods.
- Pad furniture that has sharp edges. Be sure all windows have screens.
- Keep household hot water temperature at less than 120° F; always test water temperature before bathing the baby. **Never leave a baby unattended near water** (toilet, bathtub, swimming pool). Keep water containers or tubs empty when not in use. Be sure there is no direct entrance to a back yard swimming pool through the house.
- Shorten all hanging cords (appliance, window cords, telephone) so they are out of the baby's reach. Be sure pull toy cords are shorter than 12 inches.
- Have your house tested for sources of lead.
- Never leave your baby unattended or in the care of a young sibling.

! CRITICAL TO REMEMBER

Possible Signs of Developmental Delays

- Lack of eye muscle control after 4 to 6 months suggests vision impairments and the need for further evaluation.
- Lack of a social smile by 8 to 12 weeks requires further evaluation and close follow-up.

---

grasp objects. They can bear weight when held in a standing position and can turn from abdomen to back. By 5 months, some infants rock back and forth as a precursor to crawling.

Six-month-old infants can sit alone, leaning forward on their hands. This ability provides them with a wider view of the world and creates new ways to play. Infants of this age can roll from back to abdomen and can raise their heads from the table when supine. At 6 to 7 months, they transfer objects from one hand to another. In addition, they can grab small objects with the whole hand and insert them into their mouths with lightning speed.

At 6 to 9 months, infants begin to explore the world by crawling. By 9 months, most infants have enough muscle strength and coordination to pull themselves up and cruise around furniture. These new methods of mobility enable the infant to follow a parent or caregiver around the house.

By 6 to 7 months, infants become increasingly adept at pointing to make their demands known. Six-month-olds grasp objects with all their fingers in a raking motion, but 9-month-olds use their thumbs and forefingers in a fine motor skill called the *pincer grasp*. This grasp provides infants with a useful yet potentially dangerous ability to grab, hold, and insert tiny objects into their mouths.

Nine-month-old infants can wave bye-bye and clap their hands together. They can pick up objects but have difficulty releasing them on request. By 1 year of age, they can extend an object and release it into an offered hand. Most 1-year-old children can balance well enough to walk when holding another person's hand. They often resort to crawling, however, as a more rapid and efficient way to move about.

An increased ability to move about, reach objects, and explore their world places infants at great risk for accidents and injury. Nurses provide information to parents about how quickly infant motor skills develop.

Cognitive Development

Many factors contribute to the way in which infants learn about their world. Besides innate intellectual aptitude and motivation, infants' sensory capabilities, neuromuscular control, and perceptual skills all affect how their cognitive processes unfold during infancy and throughout life. In addition, variables such as the quality and quantity of parental interaction and environmental stimulation contribute to cognitive development.

Cognitive development during the first 2 years of life begins with a profound state of egocentrism. Egocentrism is the child's complete self-absorption and the inability to view the world from anyone else's vantage point. As infants' cognitive capacities expand, they become increasingly aware of the outside world and their separateness from it. Gradually, with maturation and experience, they become capable of differentiating themselves from others and their surroundings.

According to Piaget's theory, cognitive development occurs in stages or periods (see Chapter 4). Infancy is included in the *sensorimotor stage* (birth to 2 years), during which infants experience the world through their senses and their attempts to control the environment. Learning activities progress from simple reflex behavior to trial-and-error experiments.

During the first month of life, infants are in the first substage, *reflex activity*, of the sensorimotor period. In this substage, behavior such as grasping, sucking, or looking is dominated by reflexes. Piaget believed that infants organize their activity, survive, and adapt to their world with the use of reflexes.

Primary circular reactions dominate the second substage, occurring from age 1 to 4 months. During this substage, reflexes become more organized and new schemata are acquired, usually centering on the infant's body. Sensual activities such as sucking and kicking become less reflexive and more controlled and are repeated because of the stimulation they provide. The baby also begins to recognize objects, especially those that bring pleasure, such as the breast or bottle.

During the third substage, or the stage of *secondary circular reactions*, infants perform actions that are more oriented toward the world outside their own bodies. The 4- to 8-month-old infant in this substage begins to play with objects in the external environment, such as a rattle or stuffed toy. The infant's actions are labeled *secondary* because they are intentional (repeated because of the response that is elicited). For example, a baby in this substage intentionally shakes a rattle to hear the sound.

By age 8 to 12 months, infants in the fourth substage, *coordination of secondary schemata*, begin to relate to objects as if they realize that the objects exist even when they are out of sight. This awareness is referred to as *object permanence* and is illustrated by a 9-month-old infant seeking a toy after it is hidden under a pillow. In contrast, 6-month-olds can follow the path of a toy that is dropped in front of them; however, they will not look for the dropped toy or protest its disappearance until they are older and have developed the concept of object permanence.

Infants in the fourth substage solve problems differently from how they solve problems in earlier substages. Rather than randomly selecting approaches to problems, they choose actions that were successful in the past. This tendency suggests that they remember and can perform some mental processing. They seem to be able to identify simple causal relationships, and they show definite intentionality. For example, when an 11-month-old child sees a toy that is beyond reach, the child uses the blanket that it is resting on to pull it closer (Flavell, 1964; Piaget, 1952).

Cognitive development in the infant parallels motor development. It appears that motor activity is necessary for cognitive development and that cognitive development is based on interaction with the environment, not simply maturation. Infancy is the period when the child lays the foundation for later cognitive functioning. Nurses can promote the cognitive development of infants by encouraging parents to interact with their infants and provide them with novel, interesting stimuli.

At the same time, parents should maintain familiar, routine experiences through which their infants can develop a sense of security about the world. Within this type of environment, infants will thrive and learn.

Sensory Development

Vision

The size of the eye at birth is approximately one-half to three-quarters the size of the adult eye. Growth of the eye, including its internal structures, is rapid during the first year. As infants grow and become more interested in the environment, their eyes remain open for longer periods. They show a preference for familiar faces and are increasingly able to fixate on objects. Visual acuity is estimated at approximately 20/100 to 20/150 at birth but improves rapidly during infancy and toddlerhood. Infants show a preference for high-contrast colors, such as black and white and primary colors. Pastel colors are not easily distinguished until about 6 months of age.

Young infants may lack coordination of eye movements and extraocular muscle alignment but should achieve proper coordination by age 4 to 6 months. Persistent lack of eye muscle control beyond the age of 4 to 6 months needs further evaluation. Depth perception appears to begin at approximately 7 to 9 months and contributes to the infant's new ability to move about independently.

Hearing

Hearing seems to be relatively acute, even at birth, as shown by reflexive generalized reactions to noise. With myelination of the auditory nerve tracts during the first year, responses to sound become increasingly more specialized. By 4 months, infants should turn their eyes and heads toward a sound coming from behind, and by 10 months, infants should respond to the sound of their names. The National Institutes of Health and the American Academy of Pediatrics have recommended that all newborns be screened for hearing impairment either as newborns or before 1 month of age and that infants who fail newborn screening have audiologic examination to verify hearing loss before age 3 months (American Academy of Pediatrics [AAP], 2000b). Because some children manifest hearing loss later in infancy and childhood, periodic, objective, and age-appropriate hearing screening should be performed throughout childhood (Cunningham & Cox, 2003).

Language Development

The acquisition of language has its roots in infancy as the child becomes increasingly intrigued with sound, begins to realize that words have meaning, and eventually uses simple sounds to communicate (Box 5-2). Although young infants probably understand tones and inflections of voice rather than words themselves, it is not long before repetition and practice of sounds enable them to understand and communicate with words. Infants can understand more than they can express.

The social smile develops early in the infant, usually by 3 to 5 weeks of age (Fig. 5-1). This powerful communication tool helps to foster attachment and demonstrates that the infant can differentiate between people and objects within the environment. The infant who does not display a social smile by the age of 8 to 12 weeks needs further evaluation and close follow-up because of the possibility of developmental delay.

The First Year: Growth and Development Milestones

During the first year after birth, the infant's development is dramatic as the child grows toward independence. Knowledge of developmental milestones helps caregivers determine whether the baby is growing and maturing as expected. One should remember that these markers are averages and that healthy infants often vary. Some infants reach each milestone later than most. Knowledge of normal growth and development helps the nurse promote the safety of children. Parents should be taught to prepare for the child's safety before the child reaches each milestone.

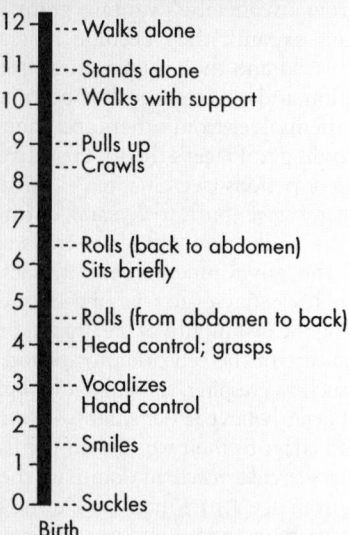

12	Walks alone
11	Stands alone
10	Walks with support
9	Pulls up
8	Crawls
7	
6	Rolls (back to abdomen) Sits briefly
5	Rolls (from abdomen to back)
4	Head control; grasps
3	Vocalizes Hand control
2	
1	Smiles
0	Suckles

Birth

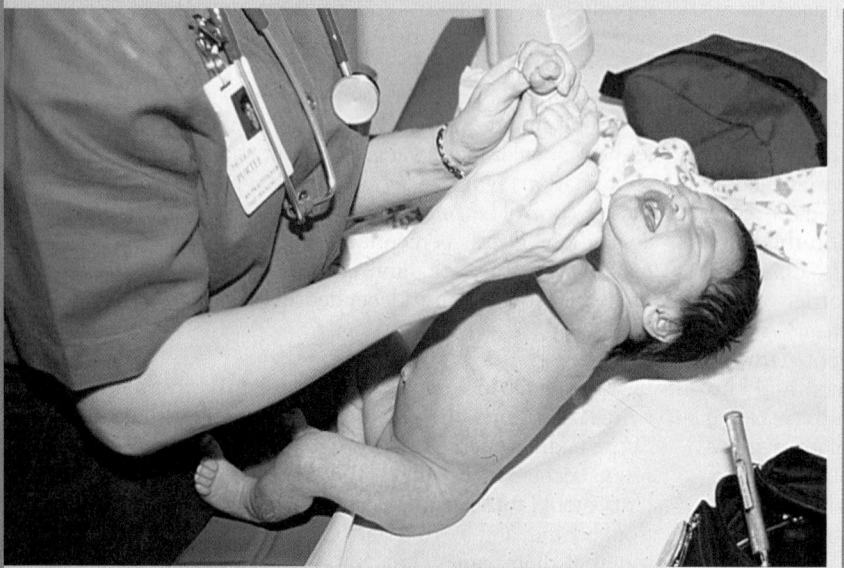

This 18-day-old infant demonstrates substantial head lag as the nurse lifts her trunk from the examining table. Weak neck muscles, combined with a large head, limit her ability to keep her head aligned with her spine as she is pulled toward a sitting position.

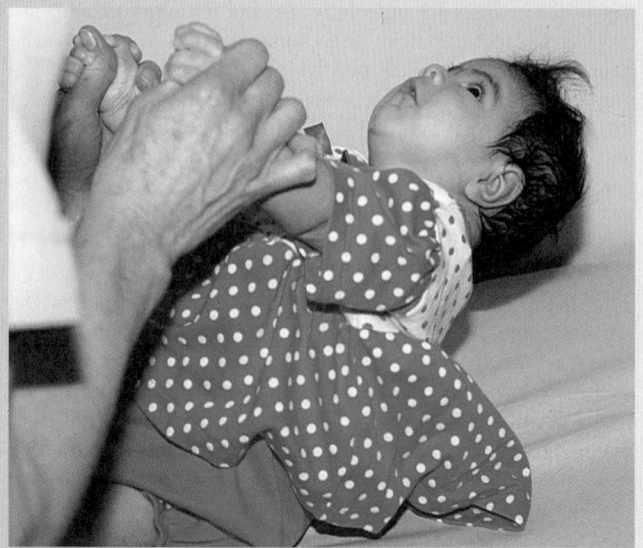

By 2 months, this infant has much less head lag as her neck muscles become stronger and better able to support her head.

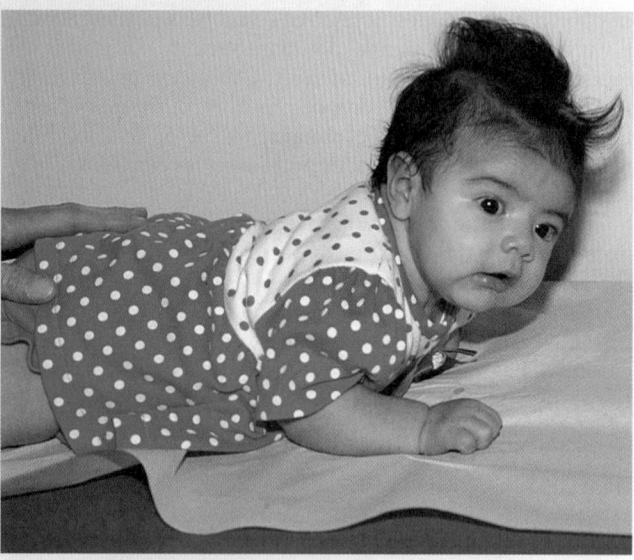

This 2-month-old infant can lift her head from the prone position and briefly hold it erect.

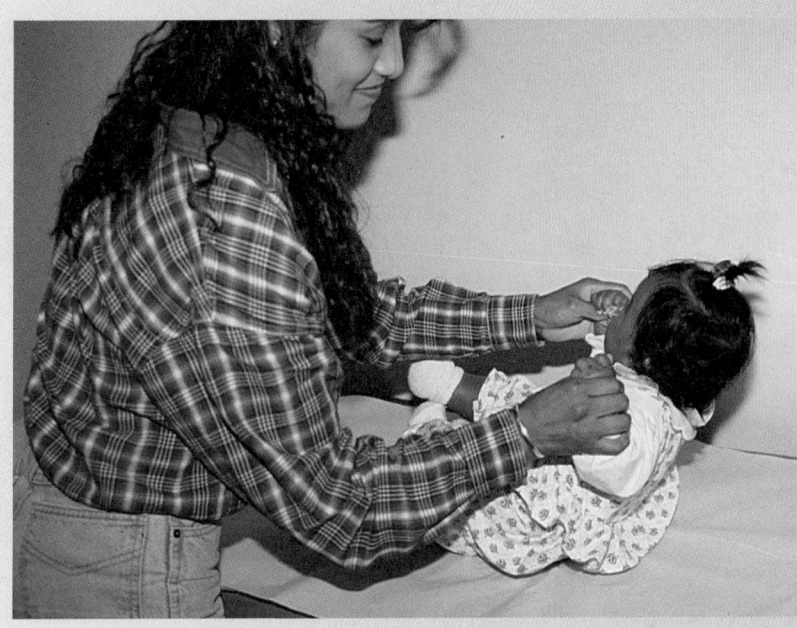

Head control steadily increases so that by 4 months, this infant keeps her head in a straight line as her mother pulls her to a sitting position.

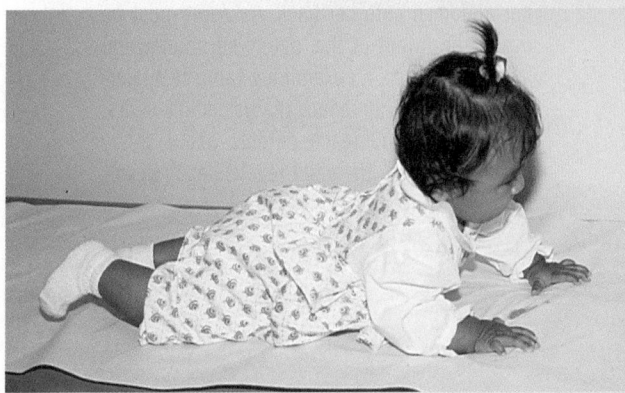

This 4-month-old infant can easily lift her head from a prone postition and hold it steadily erect.

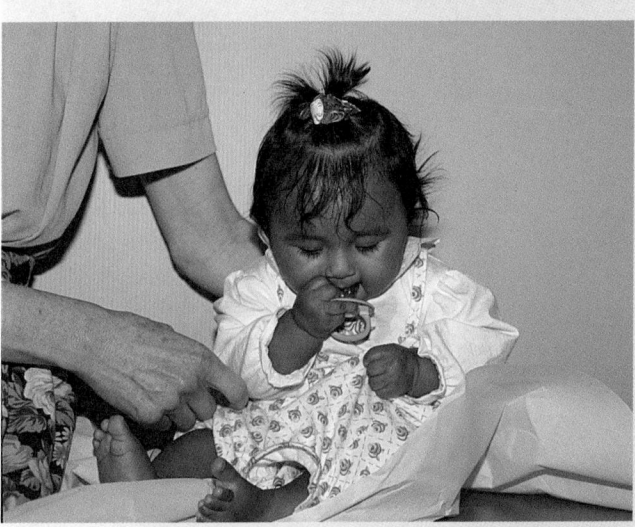

By 4 months, the infant can purposefully grasp objects with the palms of her hands.

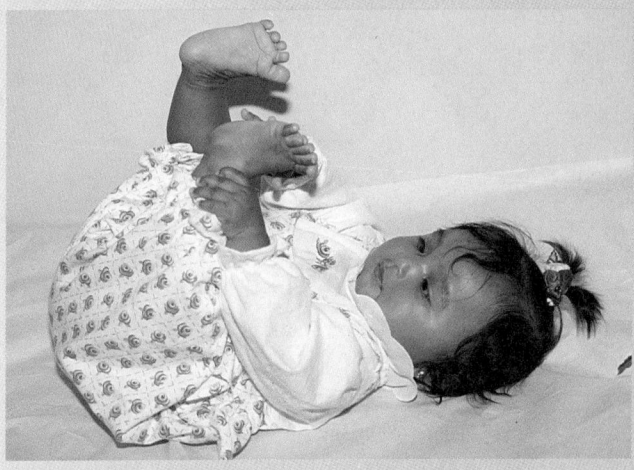

This 4-month-old infant takes pleasure in exploring her own body. She begins playing with her feet and often puts her toes in her mouth.

Continued

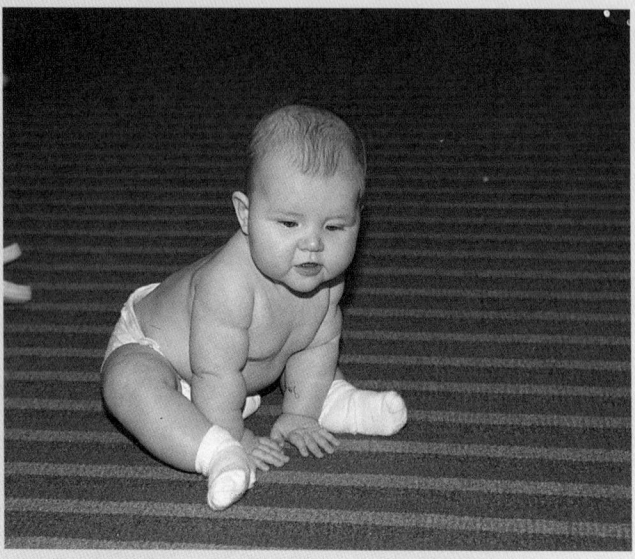

At 6 months, this infant can sit briefly if she leans forward on both hands for support. This position is called the *tripod sitting position*.

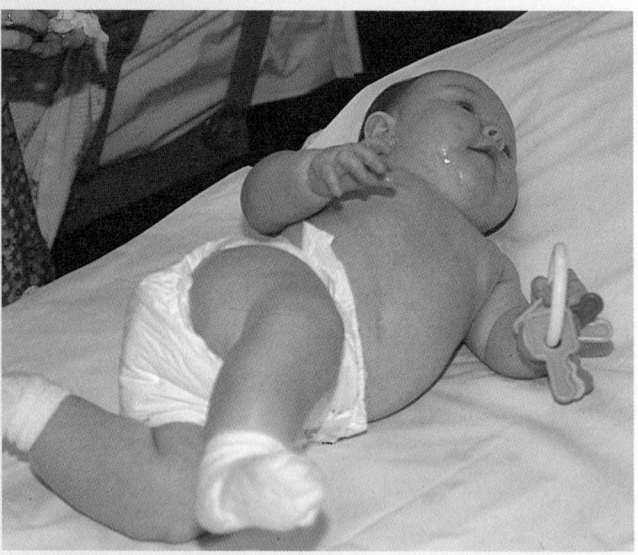

This 6-month-old infant can easily turn from her abdomen onto her back. An adult must be near if an infant of this age is on an elevated surface, such as an examining table or diaper-changing table. To reduce the risk of accidents, the nurse should teach parents about safety measures before the child reaches each developmental milestone.

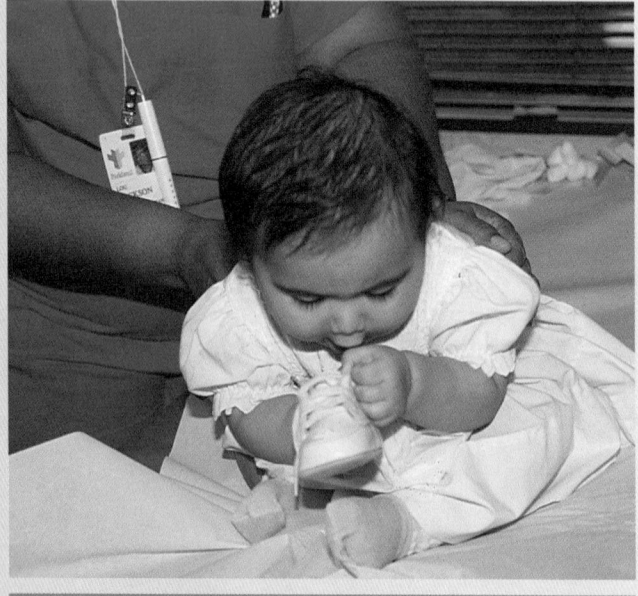

This 7-month-old infant can sit unsupported and hold her shoe. Note also that she explores it with her mouth. The nurse should teach parents that everything infants of this age can hold in their hands will go into their mouths. Parents must put dangerous materials, such as medications, cleaning solutions, and items small enough to swallow, well out of reach.

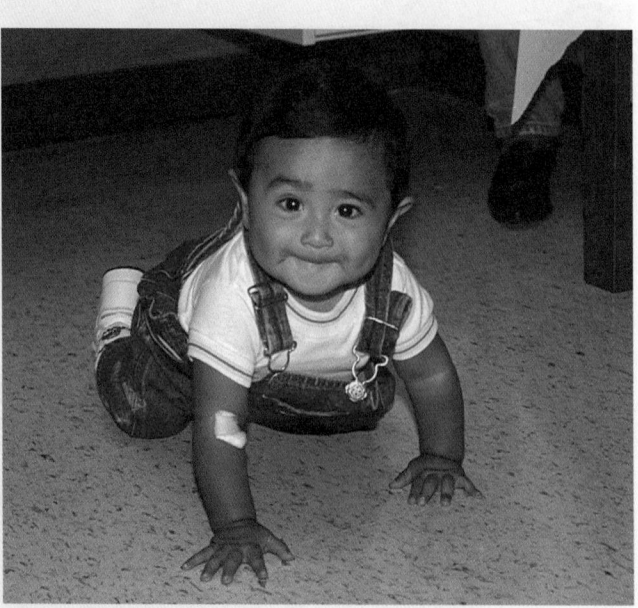

This 9-month-old infant crawls quickly, keeping his belly off the floor.

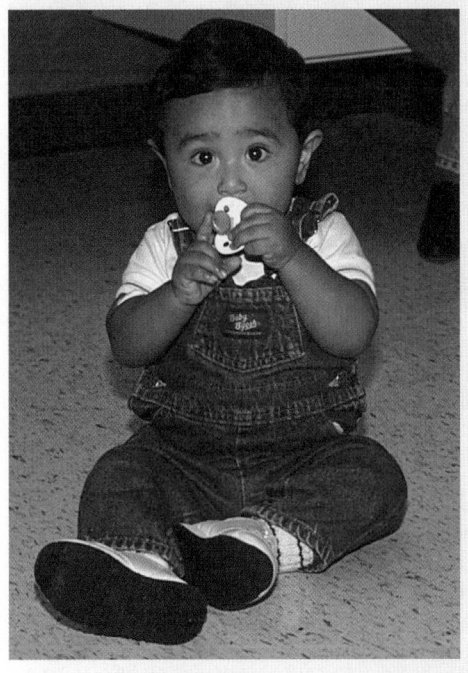

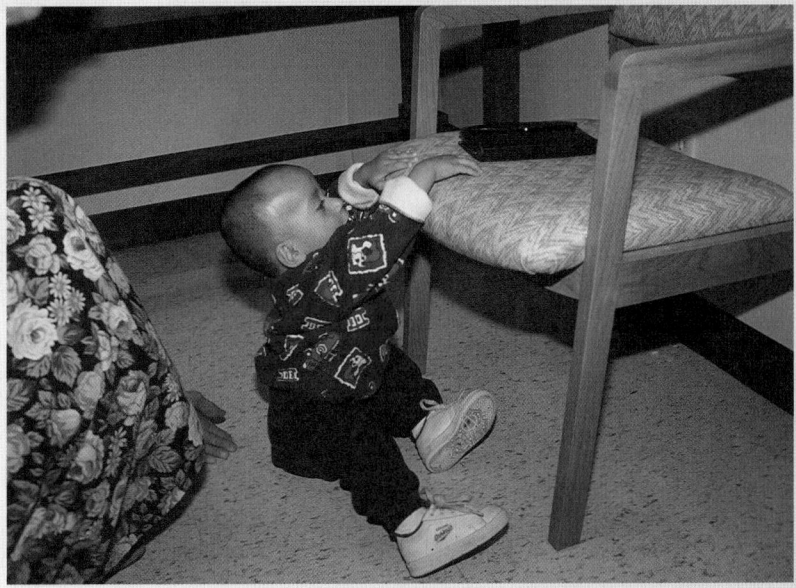

At 1 year, this infant can pull to a standing position. On a slick, hard floor such as this, an adult should be near to catch him if he slips backward while trying to pull up.

At 9 months, this infant can move easily from a crawling to a sitting position and can sit steadily with no support. He also begins grasping objects with the finer pincer grasp rather than the palmar grasp. If a parent tries to hide something, such as a pacifier, he will not forget the object and will search for it.

After pulling himself to a standing position, this 1-year-old can stand alone.

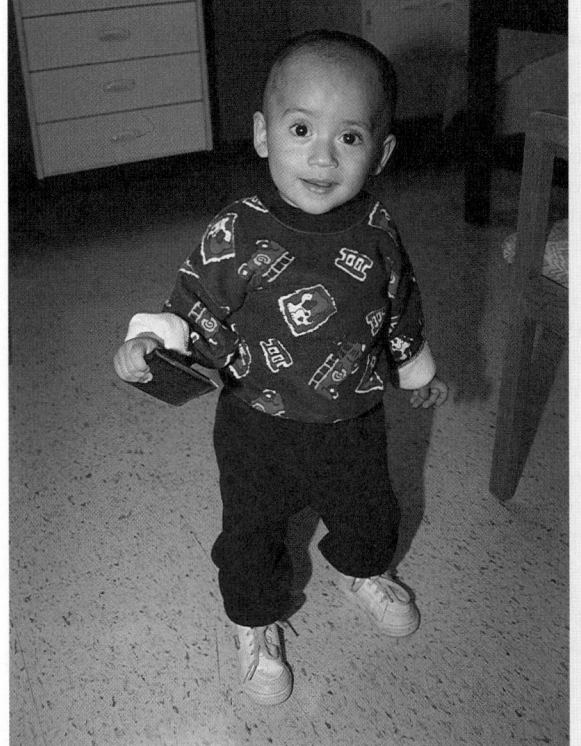

After the first year, motor development is less dramatic. Nevertheless, to promote the child's safety and normal development, nurses must continue to prepare parents for new milestones.

Photos courtesy Parkland Health and Hospital Systems Community Oriented Primary Care Clinic, Dallas; and The University of Texas at Arlington School of Nursing.

BOX 5-2
Language and Development: Developmental Milestones in Infancy

1 to 3 Months
Reflexive smile at first, and then smile becomes more voluntary; sets up a reciprocal smiling cycle with parent. Cooing.

3 to 4 Months
Crying becomes more differentiated. Babbling is common.

4 to 6 Months
Plays with sound, repeating sounds to self. Can identify mother's voice. May squeal in excitement.

6 to 8 Months
Single consonant babbling occurs. Increasing interest in sound.

8 to 9 Months
Stringing of vowels and consonants together begins. First few words begin to have meaning (Mama, Daddy, bye-bye, baby). Begins to understand and obey simple commands such as "Wave bye-bye."

9 to 12 Months
Vocabulary of two or three words. Gestures are used to communicate. Speech development may slow temporarily when walking begins.

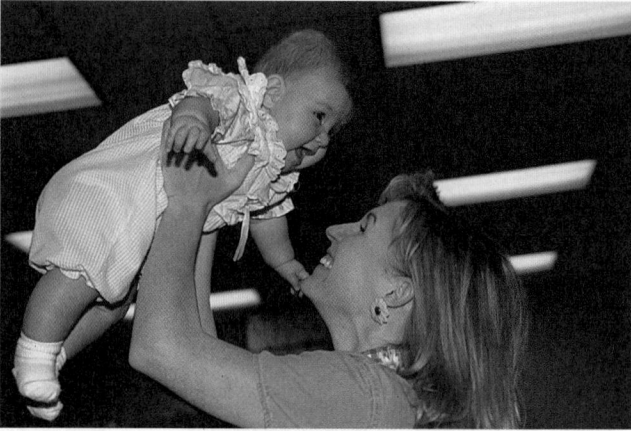

Figure 5-1 This 6-month-old infant responds delightedly to her mother with a true social smile. Such interactive responses between parent and child promote communication and emotional development.

During infancy, connections form within the central nervous system, providing fine motor control of the numerous muscles required for speech. Maturation of the mouth, jaw, and larynx; bone growth; and development of the face help prepare the infant to speak.

Vocalization does not appear to be reflexive but rather is a relatively high-level activity similar to conversation. Parents usually elicit vocalization in infants better than other adults can. Infants' brains process speech and language in the environment, using cues, structure, and distributional patterns to construct their native tongue (Karmiloff-Smith, 1995).

Although there is great variability, most children begin to make nonmeaningful sounds, such as "ma," "da," or "ah," by 4 to 6 months. The sounds become more meaningful and specific by 9 to 15 months, and by age 1 year, the child usually has a vocabulary of several words, such as "mama," "dada," and "bye-bye." Infants who have older siblings or who are raised in verbally rich environments sometimes meet these developmental milestones earlier than other infants.

Psychosocial Development

Most experts agree that infancy is a crucial period during which children develop the foundation of their personalities and their sense of self. According to Erikson's theory of psychosocial development (1963), infants struggle to establish a sense of basic *trust* rather than a sense of basic *mistrust* in their world, their caregivers, and themselves. If provided with consistent, satisfying experiences delivered in a timely manner, infants come to rely on the fact that their needs will be met and that, in turn, they will be able to tolerate some degree of frustration and discomfort until those needs are met. This sense of confidence is an early form of trust and provides the foundation for a healthy personality.

On the other hand, if infants' needs are ignored or met in a consistently haphazard, inadequate manner, they have no reason to believe that their needs will be met or that their environment is a safe, secure place. According to Erikson, without consistent satisfaction of needs, the individual develops a basic sense of suspicion or mistrust.

Parallel to this viewpoint is Freudian theory, which regards infancy as the oral stage. The mouth is the major focus of this stage. Observation of infants for a few minutes shows that most of their behavior centers on their mouths. Sensory stimulation and pleasure as well as nourishment are experienced through their mouths. Sucking is an adaptive behavior that provides comfort and satisfaction while enabling infants to experience and explore their world. Later in infancy, as teething progresses, the mouth becomes an effective tool for aggressive behavior (see Chapter 6).

Parent-Infant Attachment
One of the most important aspects of infant psychosocial development is parent-infant attachment. Attachment is a sense of belonging to or connection with each other. This significant bond between infant and parent is critical to normal development and even survival. Initiated immediately after birth, attachment is strengthened by many mutually satisfying interactions between the parents and the infant throughout the first months of life.

For example, noisy distress in infants signals a need, such as hunger. Parents respond by providing food. In turn, infants respond by quieting and accepting nourishment. The infants derive pleasure from having their hunger satiated and the parents from successfully caring for their children. A basic reciprocal cycle is set in motion in which parents learn to regulate infant feeding, sleep, and activity through a series of interactions. These interactions include rocking, touching, talking, smiling, and singing. The infants respond by quieting, eating, watching, smiling, or sleeping.

Conversely, chronic inability or unwillingness of parents to meet the dependency needs of their infants fosters insecurity and dissatisfaction in the infants. A cycle of dissatisfaction is established in which parents become frustrated as caregivers and have further difficulty providing for the infant's needs.

If parents can adapt to their infant, meet the infant's needs, and provide nurturance, attachment is secure. Psychosocial development can proceed based on a strong foundation of attachment. On the other hand, if parents' personalities and abilities to cope with infant care do not match their infant's needs, the relationship is considered at risk.

Although the establishment of trust depends heavily on the quality of the parental interaction, the infant also needs consistent, satisfying social interactions within a family structure. Family routines can help to provide this consistency. Touch is an important tool that can be used by all family members to convey a sense of caring.

Stranger Anxiety

Another important aspect of psychosocial development is stranger anxiety or separation anxiety. By 6 to 7 months, expanding cognitive capacities and strong feelings of attachment enable infants to differentiate between caregivers and strangers and to be wary of the latter. Infants display an obvious preference for parents over other caregivers and other unfamiliar people. Anxiety, demonstrated by crying, clinging, and turning away from the stranger, is manifested when separation occurs. This behavior peaks at approximately 7 to 9 months and again during toddlerhood, when separation may be difficult (see Chapter 6).

Although stressful for parents, stranger anxiety is a normal sign of healthy attachment and occurs because of cognitive development (object permanence). Nurses can reassure parents that although their infants seem distressed, leaving the infant for short periods does no harm. Separations should be accomplished swiftly, yet with care, love, and emphasis on the parents' return.

HEALTH PROMOTION FOR THE INFANT AND FAMILY

Parents, particularly new parents, often need guidance in caring for their infant. Nurses can provide valuable information about health promotion of the infant. Specific guidance about everyday concerns, such as sleep, crying, and feeding, can be offered, as well as anticipatory guidance about injury prevention. An important nursing responsibility is to provide parents with information about immunizations and dental care. Nurses can offer support to new parents by identifying strategies for coping with the first few months with an infant. The schedule of well visits corresponds with the schedule recommended by the American Academy of Pediatrics (see Appendix C). At each well visit the nurse assesses development, administers appropriate immunizations, and provides anticipatory guidance. The nurse asks the parent a series of general assessment questions and then focuses the assessment on the individual infant.

Immunization

The importance of childhood immunization against disease cannot be overemphasized. Infants are especially vulnerable to infectious disease because their immune systems are immature. Term newborns are protected from certain infections by transplacental passive immunity from their mothers. Breast-fed infants receive additional immunoglobulins against many types

---

> **Critical Thinking** EXERCISE 5-1
>
> Mary Brown and her 4-week-old daughter, Tonja, are being seen for a well-baby checkup. Tonja is Mrs. Brown's first child. Mrs. Brown looks very tired and begins to cry when you ask her how she is doing.
> 1. What are some of the possible causes the nurse should explore?
> 2. How can you explore these possible causes?
> 3. What are some of the appropriate nursing measures?

of viruses and bacteria. Transplacental immunity is effective only for approximately 3 months, however, and for a variety of reasons, many mothers choose not to breast-feed. In any case, this passive immunity does not cover all diseases, and infection in the infant can be devastating. Immunization offers protection that all infants need.

Nurses play an important role in health promotion and disease prevention related to immunization. Nursing responsibilities include assessing current immunization status, removing barriers to receiving immunizations, tracking immunization records, providing parent education, and recognizing contraindications to the receipt of vaccines. Chapter 4 provides detailed information regarding immunizations and their schedule.

Feeding and Nutrition

Because infancy is a period of rapid growth, nutritional needs are of special significance. During infancy, eating progresses from a principally reflex activity to relatively sophisticated, yet messy, attempts at self-feeding. Because the infant's gastrointestinal system continues to mature throughout the first year, changes in diet, the introduction of new foods, and even upsets in routines can result in feeding problems.

Parents often have many questions and concerns about nutrition. They are influenced by a variety of sources, including relatives and friends who may not be aware of current scientific practices regarding infant feeding. To provide anticipatory guidance, the nurse must have a clear understanding of gastrointestinal maturation and knowledge about breast-feeding and various infant formulas and foods. Families and cultures vary widely in food preferences and infant feeding practices. The nurse must remain cognizant of these differences when providing anticipatory guidance related to infant nutrition.

Breast-Feeding

The American Academy of Pediatrics (AAP) strongly recommends breast-feeding for all infants, including premature and sick newborns, with rare exceptions (AAP, 1997). Mothers

---

> ### ! CRITICAL TO REMEMBER
> **Essential Information for Infant Nutrition**
> - Breast milk or commercially prepared iron-fortified formula provides optimal nutrition throughout infancy.
> - Formula must be prepared according to instructions, and leftover formula should be stored according to the manufacturer's directions.
> - Some health care providers discourage the use of powdered formula until the infant is older than 6 weeks.

Health Promotion

The 2-Month-Old Infant

FOCUSED ASSESSMENT

How have things been going in the family?
Are you getting enough opportunities to continue relationships and activities away from the baby?
Will you describe the baby's personality?
Did the baby have any reaction to the last immunizations? If so, what happened?

DEVELOPMENTAL MILESTONES

Personal/social: smiles spontaneously; enjoys interacting with others
Fine motor: follows past midline; reflexes disappear
Language/cognitive: vocalizes "ooh" and "ah" sounds; attends to voices
Gross motor: beginning head control when upright; lifts head 45 degrees onto forearms

CRITICAL MILESTONES*

Personal/social: smiles responsively; looks at faces
Fine motor: follows to midline
Language/cognitive: vocalizes making cooing or short vowel sounds; responds to a bell
Gross motor: lifts head; equal movements

HEALTH MAINTENANCE

Physical Measurements
  Measure length, weight, and head circumference, and plot on growth charts
Immunizations
  Diphtheria, tetanus, acellular pertussis (DTaP) #1; inactivated poliovirus (IPV) #1; *Haemophilus influenzae* type b (Hib) #1; pneumococcal #1
  Discuss potential effects
Health Screening
  Hearing screen if not done at birth
  Check eyes for strabismus
  Assess ability to follow past midline

ANTICIPATORY GUIDANCE

Nutrition
  Breast-feed on demand with increasing intervals
  Formula, 4 to 6 oz six times per day
Elimination
  Six wet diapers
  Stools related to feeding method; may decrease in number

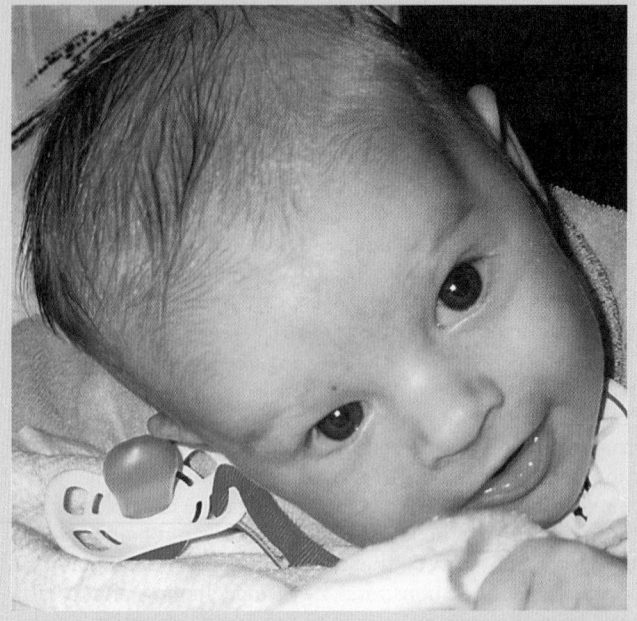

Photo courtesy Lisa Newton.

Dental
  Continue prenatal vitamins and calcium if breast-feeding
  Do not prop baby's bottle
Sleep
  Place on back to sleep
  Move to separate room
  Begin to establish nighttime routine
  Play with baby when awake
Hygiene
  Bathe several times per week
  Watch for diaper rash and seborrheic dermatitis
Safety
  Review house and environmental safety and conditions for calling the doctor; posting of emergency numbers near the telephone, car safety, and violence
  Discuss preventing falls; burns from hot liquids
Play
  Imitate vocalizations and smile
  Sing
  Change infant's environment
  Encourage rolling over

*Guided by DDST II

---

who breast-feed need instruction and support as they begin. They are more likely to succeed if they are given practical information. Many facilities provide lactation consultants or home visits, or they may call to assess the mother's needs. Significant others are included in teaching to provide a support system for the mother. An in-depth discussion of breast-feeding can be found in Chapter 24.

Bottle Feeding

Formula. Infant formula does not have the immunologic properties and digestibility of human milk, but it does meet the energy and nutrient requirements of infants. If bottle-feeding is chosen as the preferred feeding method, the formula should be iron-fortified. The Infant Formula Act of 1980, which was revised in 1986, establishes the standards for infant formulas. It also requires that the label show the quantity of each nutrient contained in the formula. Special formulas are available for low-birth-weight infants and for infants allergic to cow's milk–based formulas.

Mothers choose to use formula for many reasons. Some mothers simply do not want to breast-feed. Others may use formula to supplement an omitted breast-feeding, rather than pump their breasts. Infants with galactosemia or whose mothers use illegal drugs, are taking certain prescribed

Health Promotion

The 4-Month-Old Infant

FOCUSED ASSESSMENT
What new activities is the baby doing?
Is the baby able to settle down to sleep without needing to be consoled?
Are both parents included in the baby's care?
Is the mother considering going back to work in the near future?

DEVELOPMENTAL MILESTONES
Personal/social: loves moving faces; knows parents' voices
Fine motor: follows an object 180 degrees; binocular vision; bats objects; begins to hold own bottle
Language/cognitive: initiates conversation by cooing; turns head to locate sounds
Gross motor: supports weight on feet when standing; pulls to sit without head lag; begins to roll prone to supine

CRITICAL MILESTONES*
Personal/social: smiles responsively; smiles spontaneously; stares at own hand
Fine motor: grasps a rattle; follows past midline; brings hands to middle of body
Language/cognitive: laughs and squeals out loud; vocalizes; makes "ooh" sounds
Gross motor: lifts head and chest 45 and 90 degrees when prone; head steady when sitting

HEALTH MAINTENANCE
Physical Measurements
    Continue to measure and plot length, weight, and head circumference
    Posterior fontanel closed
Immunizations
    Diphtheria, tetanus, acellular pertussis (DTaP) #2; inactivated poliovirus (IPV) #2; *Haemophilus influenzae* type b (Hib) #2; pneumococcal #2
    Review side effects, and ask about previous reactions
Health Screening
    Assess for strabismus
    No additional screening required

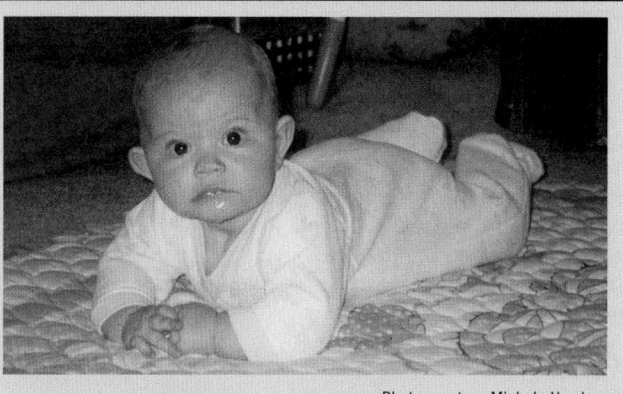

Photo courtesy Michele Hayden.

ANTICIPATORY GUIDANCE
Nutrition
    Maintain breast-feeding schedule
    Formula, 5 to 6 oz five or six times per day
    Bottle supplement if breast-feeding mother has returned to work
Elimination
    Similar to 2-month-old
Dental
    May begin drooling in preparation for tooth eruption
Sleep
    Place on back to sleep
    Total sleep: 15 to16 hours
    Encourage self-consoling techniques
Hygiene
    Continue daily routine of cleanliness
Safety
    Review car safety and violence
    Discuss choking hazards and management of choking; avoidance of walkers; playpen and swing safety; begin child-proofing
Play
    Talk with the baby frequently and from different locations
    Respond verbally and smile as infant does; cuddle
    Sing; expose to different environmental sounds
    Supervised water play
    Provide bright rattles, tactile toys, mirror

*Guided by DDST II

---

drugs, have untreated active tuberculosis, or are infected with the human immunodeficiency virus (HIV) should not be breast-fed. In countries where there is an increased risk for other infectious diseases and nutritional deficiencies resulting in infant death, the risk associated with not breast-feeding may outweigh the possible risk of the infant acquiring HIV infection (AAP, 1997). Whatever the family's choice of infant feeding method, the nurse should be helpful and supportive. For additional information about formula- and bottle-feeding, refer to Chapter 24.

Cow's Milk. Cow's milk (whole, skim, 1%, 2%) is not recommended in the first 12 months. Cow's milk contains too little iron, and its high renal solute load and unmodified derivatives can put small infants at risk for dehydration. The tough, hard curd is difficult for infants to digest. In addition, skim milk and reduced-fat milk deprive the infant of needed calories and essential fatty acids. The incidences of allergy and iron deficiency anemia are higher in infants who are given cow's milk than in those who receive breast milk or formula.

Juices. Once the infant takes fluids from a cup, the parent can introduce small amounts (no more than 5 oz/day) of fruit juice. Too much fruit juice can interfere with adequate amounts of calcium intake from milk and can cause a variety of gastrointestinal symptoms (Calamaro, 2000). Citrus fruits and juices should be avoided initially to reduce the chance of allergies. White grape juice is considered to be a better alternative to apple or pear juice for young infants because it is lower in sugar content (Calamaro, 2000). In infants with a family history of allergies, orange and tomato juice should be delayed until age 1 year. Some prepared foods and dinners contain orange juice and tomato juice. Parents should be taught to read labels. Juice is not warmed because heating destroys vitamin C. Juices should be kept in a covered container in the refrigerator to prevent the loss of the vitamin. Juices should not be given in the bottle at night to avoid the development of nursing-bottle caries.

Water. Sufficient water is provided in breast milk and in prepared formula during the nursing period. When solid foods are introduced, it may be necessary to add water because some foods (e.g., strained meats, high-meat dinners) have a high renal solute load. Infants should be offered water as part of a feeding or during the day. Additional water is necessary when intake is low or the infant is experiencing fluid loss because of illness (fever, respiratory disease). Young infants do not need fluoridated water.

Weaning

Weaning is the replacement of breast- or bottle-feedings with drinking from a cup. Infants usually have a decreasing interest in the breast or bottle starting between ages 6 and 12 months. This varies from infant to infant, but if solids and a cup have been introduced, the infant will probably begin to indicate a readiness for the cup. Even young infants can be weaned to a regular plastic cup, although they will not be ready to hold the cup themselves until later. Some parents choose to use a sippy cup—a cup with a tight cover that prevents contents from spilling when dropped. When weaning is begun after age 18 months, the infant may resist because of increased attachment to the breast or bottle.

Behaviors that might indicate a readiness to begin weaning include:

- Throwing the bottle down
- Chewing on the nipple
- Taking only a few ounces of formula
- Refusing the breast or dawdling

Weaning should not take place during times of change or stress (e.g., illness, starting child care, the arrival of a new baby). Weaning is a gradual process and should start with the replacement of one bottle- or breast-feeding at a time. If breast-feeding must be terminated before age 6 months, it should be replaced with bottle feedings to meet the infant's sucking needs. The older infant who has learned to use a cup may not need to use a bottle.

The first bottle- or breast-feeding eliminated should be the one in which the infant is least interested. Initially the infant may accept the cup only after drinking some formula from the bottle or milk from the breast. The infant is next offered the cup before the feeding. In approximately 1 week, another feeding can be eliminated if the infant is not resisting the change. The bedtime feeding is usually the last feeding to be eliminated.

During weaning, the child is giving up time that had been spent being held in the parent's arms. The parent needs to respond to the infant's continued need to be held and cuddled. Infants should not be allowed to carry bottles or sippy cups around as toys, to take them to bed, or to use them as pacifiers. Infants who indicate sucking needs should be given pacifiers.

Solid Foods

The early introduction of solid food is associated with a higher incidence of food allergy. In addition, the solids the infant eats cannot be adequately digested and the nutrients

---

> **BOX 5-3**
> *Readiness for Introduction of Solids*
>
> - Infant can sit.
> - Birth weight has doubled, and infant weighs at least 13 lb.
> - Infant can reach for an object and maintain balance.
> - Infant reaches for objects and brings to mouth.
> - Infant indicates a desire for food by opening mouth and leaning forward.
> - Extrusion reflex has disappeared (4 to 5 months).
> - Infant moves food to back of mouth and swallows during spoon feedings.

in breast or formula milk will not be taken in because the infant's appetite has been satisfied. In contrast, failure to offer solids by age 6 months may result in difficulty accepting solid feedings at a later time (AAP, 1998).

The feeding of semisolid foods should be delayed until the infant's consumption of foods is no longer a reflexive process and the infant has the fine and gross motor skills needed to consume them (usually between 4 and 6 months of age) (Story, Holt, & Sofka, 2002). The infant goes through a so-called *transitional period*, during which prepared foods are introduced and given together with human milk or formula. The growth and development of each infant vary, and milestones indicate the infant's readiness for solid foods (Box 5-3).

Solids should be introduced one at a time in small amounts (1 teaspoon to 2 tablespoons) for several days before introducing a new food. This is done to avoid confusion should a food intolerance be present. The order of introduction is not critical, but iron-fortified rice cereal is most often recommended as a first food because it is high in iron, is easily digested, and has a low allergenic probability. Other commercially available infant cereals include oatmeal, barley, mixed grain, and cereals with added fruit. When foods are first being introduced, mixed grains and cereals with added fruit should be avoided. Foods should not be mixed with formula and fed through a nipple with a large hole. This deprives the child of the chewing experience and changes the texture and taste of the food. There may be medical conditions (e.g., gastroesophageal reflux) in which an exception to this rule is made.

Several commercially prepared fruits and vegetables are available. In addition, fruits and vegetables can easily be steamed or boiled and then pureed in a blender or food processor at home. It is usually necessary to add a small amount of water during the blending process. The parent should not give an infant home-prepared orange or dark leafy vegetables before age 6 months because of the elevated nitrate levels, which can cause methemoglobinemia (Story, Holt, & Sofka, 2002). As with cereals, mixed fruits should be avoided until the infant is older and has tolerated individual foods.

Although most sources indicate that the order of introduction of foods is arbitrary, the introduction of meat usually follows cereal, fruit, and vegetables after age 6 months. The infant may be given ground liver, lean beef, or a variety of commercially prepared meats. The parent should avoid giving the infant mixed meats and vegetables; these baby foods may not contain enough meat.

Salt and sugar should not be added to commercial or home-prepared foods. Parents should avoid using canned foods or home-prepared foods that contain large amounts of sugar and salt. Feeding honey to infants under age 12 months has been associated with botulism and should therefore be avoided.

Finger Foods

Between age 8 and 10 months the infant can be introduced to finger foods. At this time the pincer grasp is developing and the infant can pick up foods. The infant will have a palmar grasp before this time and soft foods can be given, but the infant will mainly "play" with the food. This can be a positive experience that enables the infant to feel different textures and increase fine motor skills.

Finger foods should be bite-size pieces of soft food. Arrowroot biscuits, cheese sticks, slices of canned peaches or pears, cut pieces of bananas, and breads can be offered. As children's fine motor skills increase, they may enjoy eating some of the dry cereals, such as Cheerios. Be sure pieces of finger foods are not round and are small enough that they will not block the infant's airway, causing a choking hazard. Encourage parents to remain with an infant who is eating finger foods.

Snacks

When the infant is on a three-meals-a-day schedule, small snacks are an appropriate addition to the nutritional intake. Because infants have small stomachs, they may not be content to wait until the next meal before eating. Snacks should be nutritious, and parents should resist the urge to give infants a bottle to satisfy their hunger. Some of the finger foods just listed are good nutritious snacks. If the infant is not hungry at mealtime, the snack should be given in a smaller portion or eliminated.

Food Allergies

Food allergies can occur at any age, but the incidence for development of certain food allergies is increased before age 1 year. Some of the more common food allergies are allergies to milk, egg, soy products, peanuts, chocolate, corn, and wheat. Cow's milk protein intolerance is the most common food allergy during infancy, but this usually does not last past age 3 or 4 years.

Some of the common clinical manifestations of food allergies are abdominal pain, diarrhea, nasal congestion, cough, wheezing, vomiting, and rashes. Many children will outgrow their allergic response to certain foods; for example, 70% to 80% of infants with a milk allergy will tolerate milk by age 4 years. Children who develop food allergies after age 3 years tend not to outgrow them.

Dental Care

Eruption of the infant's first teeth is a developmental milestone that has great significance for many parents. Deciduous, or "baby," teeth usually erupt between 5 and 9 months of age. The first to appear are the lower central incisors, followed by the upper central incisors, and then the upper lateral incisors. The next teeth to erupt are usually the lower lateral incisors, first primary molars, canines, and the second primary molars. The average child has six to eight teeth by the first birthday.

Teething

Although sometimes asymptomatic, teething is often signaled by behavior such as night wakening, daytime restlessness, an increase in nonnutritive sucking, excess drooling, and temporary loss of appetite. Some degree of discomfort is normal, but a health care professional should further investigate elevated temperature, irritability, ear tugging, or diarrhea.

To help parents cope with teething, nurses can suggest that they provide cool liquids and hard foods (e.g., dry toast, Popsicles, frozen bagels) for chewing. Hard, cold teethers and ice wrapped in cloth may also provide comfort for inflamed gums. Nurses should explain to parents that over-the-counter topical medications for gum pain relief should be used only as directed. Home remedies, such as rubbing the gums with whiskey or aspirin, should be discouraged, but acetaminophen administered as directed for the child's age can relieve discomfort. Although these interventions can be helpful, parents should understand that absolute relief comes only with tooth eruption.

Assessment of Dental Risk

The American Academy of Pediatrics and the American Dental Association have issued recommendations about prevention and treatment of dental caries in infants and young children (AAP, 2003b). The risk of tooth decay begins in infancy and is higher in families with a history of dental caries. Viewed as an infectious process, mothers with dental caries can transmit bacteria that cause caries to their infants through sharing of eating utensils, toothbrushes, or a pacifier given to an infant after having been in the mother's mouth (AAP, 2003b). Taking a dental history from a mother can provide information about an infant's risk, and this should occur as early as the infant's teeth begin to erupt. Infants with observable dental caries should be referred to a dentist as soon as these are observed by the health care provider (AAP, 2003b).

Cleaning Teeth

Because the primary teeth are used for chewing until the permanent teeth erupt and because decay of the primary teeth often results in decay of the permanent teeth, dental care must begin in infancy. The parent can use cotton swabs or a soft washcloth and water to clean the teeth with the infant positioned in the parent's lap or on a changing table. The teeth should be cleaned at least twice a day, and juice should be limited to no more than one cup a day given at meals (AAP, 2003b). Toothpaste is not recommended because infants tend to swallow it, possibly ingesting excessive amounts of fluoride. Too much fluoride can cause fluorosis, which results in staining of the teeth (AAP, 2000a).

Appropriate amounts of fluoride, however, are necessary for the development of healthy teeth. Infants receive fluoride when formula and cereal are mixed with water from fluoridated water supplies. Fluoride supplementation usually begins at the 6-month visit.

Bottle-Mouth Caries

Bottle-mouth caries, or nursing-bottle caries, is a well-described form of tooth decay that can develop in infants and children. The decay pattern usually involves the incisors initially and then spreads to other teeth. Decay may be so serious that tooth loss occurs prematurely. When the infant is allowed to fall asleep with a bottle containing milk or juice, the carbohydrate-rich solution bathes the teeth for a long period and may cause dental caries.

Nurses should discourage parents from giving bedtime bottles of milk or juice to infants. If a nighttime bottle is necessary, plain water is an acceptable substitute for carbohydrate-rich liquids. A pacifier is an acceptable alternative to a nighttime bottle, although the practice of dipping the pacifier in corn syrup or honey to encourage acceptance poses the same problem. An additional danger of the use of honey in infancy is botulism.

Sleep, Rest, and Crying

Newborns may sleep as much as 17 to 20 hours per day. Sleep patterns vary widely, with some infants sleeping only 2 to 3 hours at a time. At approximately 3 to 4 months of age, most infants begin to sleep for longer periods during the night, although some children do not sleep through the night consistently until the 2nd year.

Often one of the most difficult tasks for new parents is the regulation of their infants' sleep-wake cycles. Parents need anticipatory guidance about what to expect regarding sleep, rest, and crying. It is important to remember that rocking an infant to sleep provides warmth and security for the infant; however, to initiate good sleep habits, the parent should put the infant in the crib while the infant is drowsy and before the infant falls completely asleep.

Patterns of Crying

Nurses can suggest that parents console their infants when they cry by holding them, talking softly, or humming. Gently stroking an infant's head, back, and arms may also be soothing. Infant massage techniques and simply "centering" are easily accomplished by positioning the infant's arms and legs toward the midline of the body. Swaddling a new infant is a consoling technique that assists the infant to center. Some infants respond readily to attempts to comfort them, sleep a great deal, and fit easily into their family's life-style.

On the other hand, some infants cry more readily and for longer periods and spend more time in a fretful, restless state than others. These infants often experience more colic symptoms and sleep problems. This irritability may be caused by health problems, such as feeding difficulties, infection, or allergies, but often no clear cause emerges. In some cases, infant temperament or the combination of a sensitive, irritable infant and parents who have not yet learned to respond to the infant's needs correctly may be the cause (Thiedke, 2001).

Strategies for Soothing Infants

Specific strategies to diminish infant irritability include activities such as taking the baby for a car ride, carrying the infant in a front pack close to the parent's chest, or swinging the baby in an infant swing. Vertical positioning and constant motion, such as that obtained when walking with the baby carried over the shoulder, are sometimes helpful. The football-carry position, with gentle patting on the back, can also be tried. Sometimes irritable infants need to be left alone to cry for brief periods. If parents choose this strategy, they must be cautioned to limit the crying time and to check the baby frequently.

Few interventions are consistently successful because infant responses may vary. Providing parents with strategies, however, helps decrease their anxiety and increase their feelings of control and competence. As infants grow and develop, they are better able to regulate their sleep-wake cycles.

Generally, during the 3rd or 4th month of life, sleep problems and irritability improve.

The Infant With Colic

Colic usually refers to unexplained crying or fussing in infants, which may be characterized by infants pulling up their arms and legs. Periods of crying tend to occur at the same time of day, often in the late afternoon or evening. Colic occurs in approximately 10% of infants younger than 3 months (Story, Holt, & Sofka, 2002). To be diagnosed with colic, an infant must experience the symptoms several times daily for several days a week. Most infants outgrow symptoms of colic by 3 months of age.

Etiology

The cause of colic is unknown, but several theories have been researched. The possibilities include but are not limited to allergy, cow's milk intolerance, maternal anxiety, familial stress, and too rapid feeding or overfeeding. It is highly likely that more than one factor may be involved. Colic is more common in infants with sensitive temperaments, who seem to need increased attention.

Management

The physician must determine whether, in fact, the infant is crying because of colic and not because of an acute condition such as intussusception, otitis media, or a fracture. Symptoms of milk allergy other than crying should be present before formula changes are made. Anticholinergics, motility-enhancing agents, barbiturates, and antiflatulents might be prescribed. Many practitioners avoid using these drugs because of their limited success, lack of scientific data, and possible side effects. Chamomile tea has a calming and sedating effect and is effective in some infants (Garrison & Christakis, 2000). It has been used for thousands of years and is readily available in most grocery stores, and allergic reactions are rare. If parents are using herbs such as chamomile, be sure they know the appropriate dose, are aware of possible allergic reactions, and do not use so much as to interfere with adequate breast milk or formula intake.

Nursing Considerations

Because the etiology of colic and the care of an infant with colic are so individualized, it is very important that the nurse obtain a thorough history. Provide a concerned and caring atmosphere during the assessment, and reassure the parents that colic is not related to bad parenting. Determine whether any other symptoms are associated with the crying. Discuss the infant's eating habits, including whether the infant is breast-fed or bottle-fed. Ask the parents if commonalities are associated with the crying (time of day, associated activities, family members present). Ask what has been tried, what works, and what does not work. If the parents are unsure, suggest they keep a diary for 48 to 72 hours to determine patterns. Assess the parents' stress level and support system.

Educate the parents regarding the normal growth and development needs of infants related to sleep and awake times, feeding, soothing, and holding. Listen to the parents with an empathic ear. Encourage parents to soothe their infant by rocking and cuddling. Some infants will quiet when given a massage, pacifier, or warm bath. If the parent is busy, a swing may provide a soothing, rhythmic effect. Some of the same

Health Promotion

The 6-Month-Old Infant

FOCUSED ASSESSMENT
What kind of new activities is the baby doing?
Have you begun to give the baby solid foods?
How is any childcare working out?
Have you done anything about child-proofing your home?

DEVELOPMENTAL MILESTONES
Personal/social: interacts readily and noisily with parents and
familiar people; may be cautious with strangers
Fine motor: rakes objects with the whole hand; begins to
transfer; mouths; can hold an object in each hand
Language/cognitive: begins to imitate sounds (raspberries,
clucking, kissing); babbles; says single sounds; beginning
object permanence; awareness of time sequence
Gross motor: tripod sitting unsupported; gets on hands and
knees; bears full weight on legs; "swims" when prone

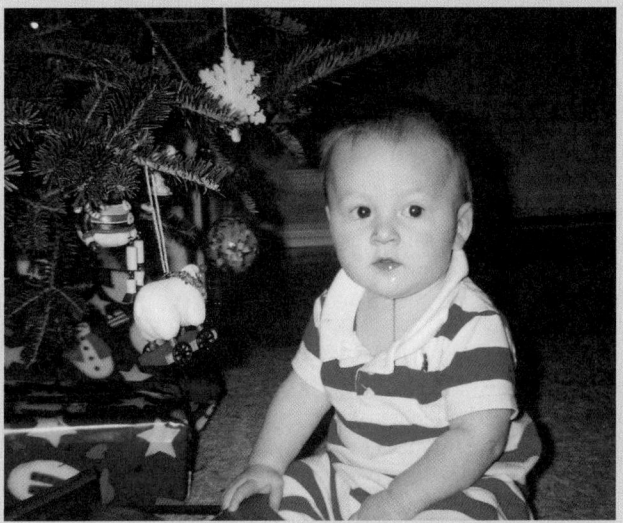

CRITICAL MILESTONES*
Personal/social: reaches for toy out of reach; looks at hand;
smiles spontaneously
Fine motor: looks at raisin placed on contrasting surface;
reaches out; follows completely side to side
Language/cognitive: turns to rattle sound made out of vision
on each side; squeals; laughs
Gross motor: rolls over both directions; no head lag; lifts head
and chest completely

HEALTH MAINTENANCE
Physical Measurements
  Birth weight doubles
  Continue to measure and plot length, weight, and head
    circumference
Immunizations
  Diphtheria, tetanus, acellular pertussis (DTaP) #3;
    Haemophilus influenzae type b (Hib) #3; pneumococcal
    #3; inactivated poliovirus (IPV) #3 may be given between
    now and 18 months
  Ask about previous reactions
  Review side effects
Health Screening
  Initial lead screening risk assessment (see Box 5-4)

ANTICIPATORY GUIDANCE
Nutrition
  Begin introducing solid foods one at a time by spoon; use
    iron-fortified cereals
  Avoid citrus and egg white; read labels
  Hold or place in infant seat for feeding
  Begin using a cup

Elimination
  Stools darken and become more formed as solids are
    increased
Dental
  Tooth eruption begins with lower incisors
  May have some pain and low-grade fever (<101° F)
  May be fussy
  Begin fluoride supplements as recommended
  Clean teeth and gums with wet cloth
  Do not put to sleep with a bottle
Sleep
  Place on back to sleep (infant may roll over to prone position)
  12 to 16 hours each day
  Sleeps all night; two or three naps
  Maintain or establish sleep routine
Hygiene
  Continue daily routine of cleanliness
  Clean toys frequently
Safety
  Review choking, walkers, violence
  Discuss child-proofing, drowning prevention, poison
    prevention (see Chapter 34)
Play
  Expose to different sounds and sights
  Begin social games (pat-a-cake, peek-a-boo)
  Provide bath toys, rattles, mirror, large ball, soft stuffed animals
  Encourage to sit unsupported
  Encourage to rock on hands and knees

*Guided by DDST II

---

strategies for soothing infants may also be effective in quieting infants with colic.

Some infants seem most distressed during high-activity times when the family may be busy preparing meals, doing chores, gathering at the end of the day, and so forth. By assisting parents to see such trends, the nurse can help them establish alternative routines to decrease the infant's stimuli. The parent may choose to feed the infant away from all the

activity or to have a later dinner. Each family will be unique, and the nurse's role is to facilitate problem solving.

If, after 30 minutes, none of the interventions are effective, the infant should be placed in the crib. If crying continues for more than 15 to 20 minutes, pick the infant up again and try to soothe.

All families need extra support after the birth of an infant. If the infant has colic, the need increases. During the first few months after the addition of a new baby, demanding work schedules, lack of recovery time from childbirth, the needs of other family members, physical exhaustion, and sleep deprivation can combine with the presence of a fretful infant to create stressful situations for the entire family. Sometimes infant temperament and parental coping styles are not compatible.

The nurse might, for example, explain to new parents, "Parenting is very much a challenge even when parents care about their baby as much as you do. It is difficult at first even to discern what Avery is telling you when she cries. But you will feel more and more comfortable, even see that she has a different cry when she is hungry and when she is tired."

In validating the parents' feelings, the nurse recognizes that the infant's irritability or colic is real, not imagined, and that the infant is a challenge to handle. The nurse can reassure the parents that the infant is healthy, normal, and gaining weight and that the parents are competent in their nurturing role.

The emotional reserves of the parents can be restored through rest and pleasurable activities. Parents may need brief periods of relief from infant care responsibilities. Grandparents or other family members may be able to provide the parents with an evening out or a night of uninterrupted sleep. This direct support can help restore the parents' energy to cope with daily activities and feel more relaxed and confident in their parenting.

Safety

The rapidly growing infant becomes mobile seemingly overnight. With newfound mobility comes the potential for unintentional injury. As the infant's musculature strengthens and coordination improves, the infant has an insatiable desire to explore. Without the cognitive skills needed to differentiate danger from safety, the rolling, crawling, toddling infant is at great risk for accidents.

Infants are totally dependent on others for safety and protection. They are especially vulnerable to serious injury because of their relatively large head size. Motor development progresses to the point where infants quickly master new skills to learn more about their environment. They begin impulsively to reach out and move toward interesting objects around them.

Because of an infant's dependence, parents and caregivers are the primary recipients of anticipatory safety guidance. From the first day of life, safety must be considered and incorporated into the infant's world. Providing a safe environment for a rapidly growing infant is challenging. Potential safety hazards multiply as the baby learns to creep, crawl, climb, and explore. Some parents may not have a complete awareness of the safety issues that must be addressed to protect the infant from injury.

Motor Vehicle Safety

Injuries associated with automobile accidents constitute the single greatest threat to an infant's life and health. Restraining seats are the only practical means of reducing this risk. The crushing forces of a crash or sudden stop, even at low speed, can cause serious injury to the infant. Without a car safety seat, an infant involved in a collision or sudden stop becomes an unguided missile, colliding with the interior of the car or, worse, being ejected from the vehicle. In a collision, infants are usually thrust headfirst, placing them at greater risk for head,

facial, or spinal injuries because of the weight of the head combined with poor neck muscle support (Kamerling, 2002).

Infant safety in motor vehicles depends entirely on adults. Parents must be informed that they cannot protect their child from injury in a crash by cradling or holding the infant in their laps. Adults are neither strong enough nor quick enough to prevent the sudden forward motions or to overcome the inertial forces (external forces of motion caused by impact) exerted in a crash. An unrestrained adult is propelled forward, trapping and crushing the infant between the adult's body and the hard surfaces inside the car on impact. The only way to prevent injuries and death to an infant in a car is to use a car safety seat for each trip, no matter how short.

A lifelong practice begins with the newborn's first ride home. Getting a child accustomed to using a safety seat at a young age establishes a safety habit and may reduce resistance later (Fig. 5-2). All car safety seats should be placed in the rear seat of the vehicle, preferably in the middle, away from the possibility of injury from a side crash. Newborns and infants should be in a rear-facing seat with a three- or five-point harness until they are 1 year of age and 20 pounds (AAP, 2003a). Front-facing seats (Fig. 5-3) should be tethered to the tether anchor (available in cars made after 2000). LATCH (Lower Anchors and Tethers for Children) systems, which secure the seat without need for the seat belt, keep the seat tightly anchored to the car. Both car (those made after 2002) and seat must have the LATCH system for it to work without the seatbelt (AAP, 2003a). Children should remain in an approved car safety seat or booster seat until they are approximately 4' 9" tall (between 8 and 12 years) (AAP, 2003a).

Some injuries and deaths have been associated with the deployment of air bags. Infants and children younger than 12 years should not be restrained in the front seat of cars equipped with passenger-side air bags. When deployed, the air bag can severely jolt the car safety seat and harm the infant. The National Highway Traffic Safety Administration recommends placing all children 12 years and younger in the rear seat with the appropriate restraint (Kamerling, 2002). Young children also can be severely injured in a side-impact crash from the deployment of side airbags; placing the child in the middle rear seat is advisable.

Providing a Safe Home Environment

During infancy and early childhood, when children are typically limited to the home environment, safety in and around the home is a top priority. With the exception of injuries and deaths related to motor vehicle crashes, most childhood injuries occur in the home. Parents must also consider safety as a factor when selecting daycare facilities for their child.

Burn Safety

Infants are especially vulnerable to inflicted burns, particularly scald burns, and scald burns are a leading cause of emergency admissions in infants and young children (Titus, Baxter, & Starling, 2003). Infants' limited mobility makes it impossible for them to escape from immersion in hot water. Parents should be instructed to decrease the setting on hot water heaters to 120° F to prevent accidental scalds. Infant skin is thin, causing burns to occur faster at lower temperatures than in adults. With water temperature settings of 140° F, it takes only 3 seconds for the child to suffer serious burns. Lowering the temperature by 20° F causes the same degree of burn injury

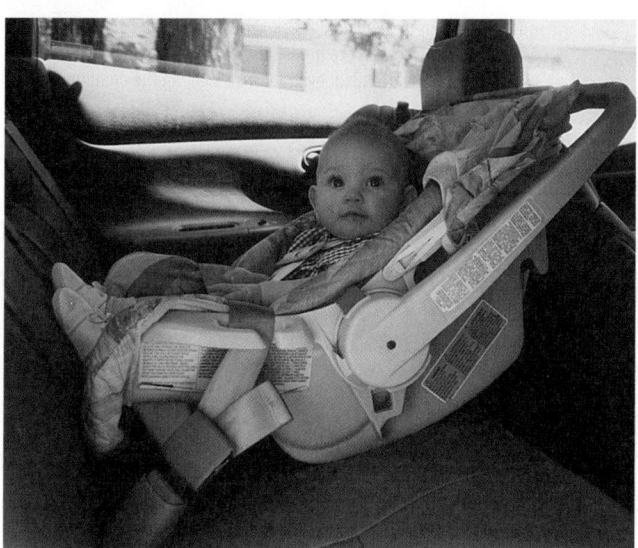

Figure 5-2 The infant rides facing the rear of the vehicle, ideally in the middle of the back seat. The infant seat is secured to the vehicle with the seat belts, and straps on the car seat adjust to accommodate the growing baby. The smaller infant will need a rolled blanket to prevent excess head movement.

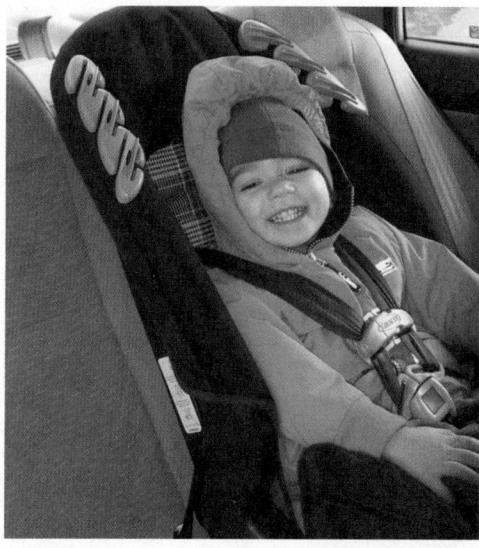

Figure 5-3 When the child reaches one year of age and 20 pounds, the car safety seat can be adjusted to a forward-facing, upright position. This seat is appropriate for the toddler until the child reaches about 40 lb. The safety straps should be adjusted to provide a snug fit, and the seat should be placed in the back seat of the car, ideally in the middle.

in 8 to 10 minutes of submersion. An adult should test the water temperature before the infant is submerged to decrease the risk of accidental scald injuries.

Burn injuries in infants can also be caused by a variety of other sources. Exposure to sunlight can result in serious sunburn to their delicate skin. Parents should be encouraged to apply sun blocks and sunscreens (minimum sun protection factor [SPF] 15) liberally to older infants and to protect the face and head with a hat when exposing the infant or toddler to sunlight, even for brief periods and on cloudy days. Young infants should not be exposed to strong sunlight, and sunscreen should not be used on infants younger than 6 months (AAP, 2003c).

Advise parents to avoid smoking, drinking hot liquids, or cooking while holding an infant. As infants begin to crawl around on the floor, open electrical sockets should be covered with appropriate socket protectors. Open stoves or fireplaces are especially intriguing to an exploring infant and should be outfitted with a guard or grid. Cool mist vaporizers should be used rather than steam vaporizers to prevent scald injuries to a curious infant.

Safe Baby Furnishings

Baby furniture, although seemingly benign, can present lethal hazards to a growing infant. Parents should be aware of safety considerations when planning or decorating the infant's room. Parents need to be aware that older furniture that has been handed down may not meet current safety regulations. In older cribs, the gaps between slats may be large enough that infants could entrap their heads, or the paint may contain lead.

Hanging toys or mobiles placed over the crib should be positioned well out of the infant's reach to prevent entanglement and strangulation. Encourage the parent to avoid placing large toys in the crib because an older infant may use them as steps to climb over the side, resulting in a serious fall. Cribs should be positioned away from curtains or blinds to prevent accidental entanglement in dangling cords.

PARENTS
Want to Know

Crib Safety

- The distance between slats must be no more than 2³/₈ inches wide to prevent entrapment of the infant's head or body. Mesh-sided cribs should have mesh openings smaller than ¹/₄ inch (6 mm).
- The interior of the crib must snugly accommodate a standard-size mattress so that the gap is minimal, less than the width of two adult fingers. Excessive space could allow the infant to become wedged, potentially suffocating.
- Decorative enhancements on the crib are not recommended because they can break apart and be aspirated by the infant. Design cutouts can trap an infant's arm or neck, causing death or serious injury.
- Corner posts or finials that rise above the end panels can snag garments and inadvertently strangle infants.
- The drop side must be impossible for an infant to release. Activating the drop side must take either a strong force (at least 10 lb) or a distinct action at each locking device. Never leave the drop side down when an infant is in the crib.
- Wood surfaces should be free of splinters, cracks, and lead-based paint.

Preventing Falls

Infants are often placed on surfaces at heights that are convenient for the adult, such as on changing tables, counters, or furniture. These surfaces often have no restraining barriers. Infants begin to roll over as early as 2 months, and as they begin to scoot or crawl, fall injuries from these elevations are common. There must be constant adult supervision when infants are placed at such heights (Fig. 5-4). If the par-

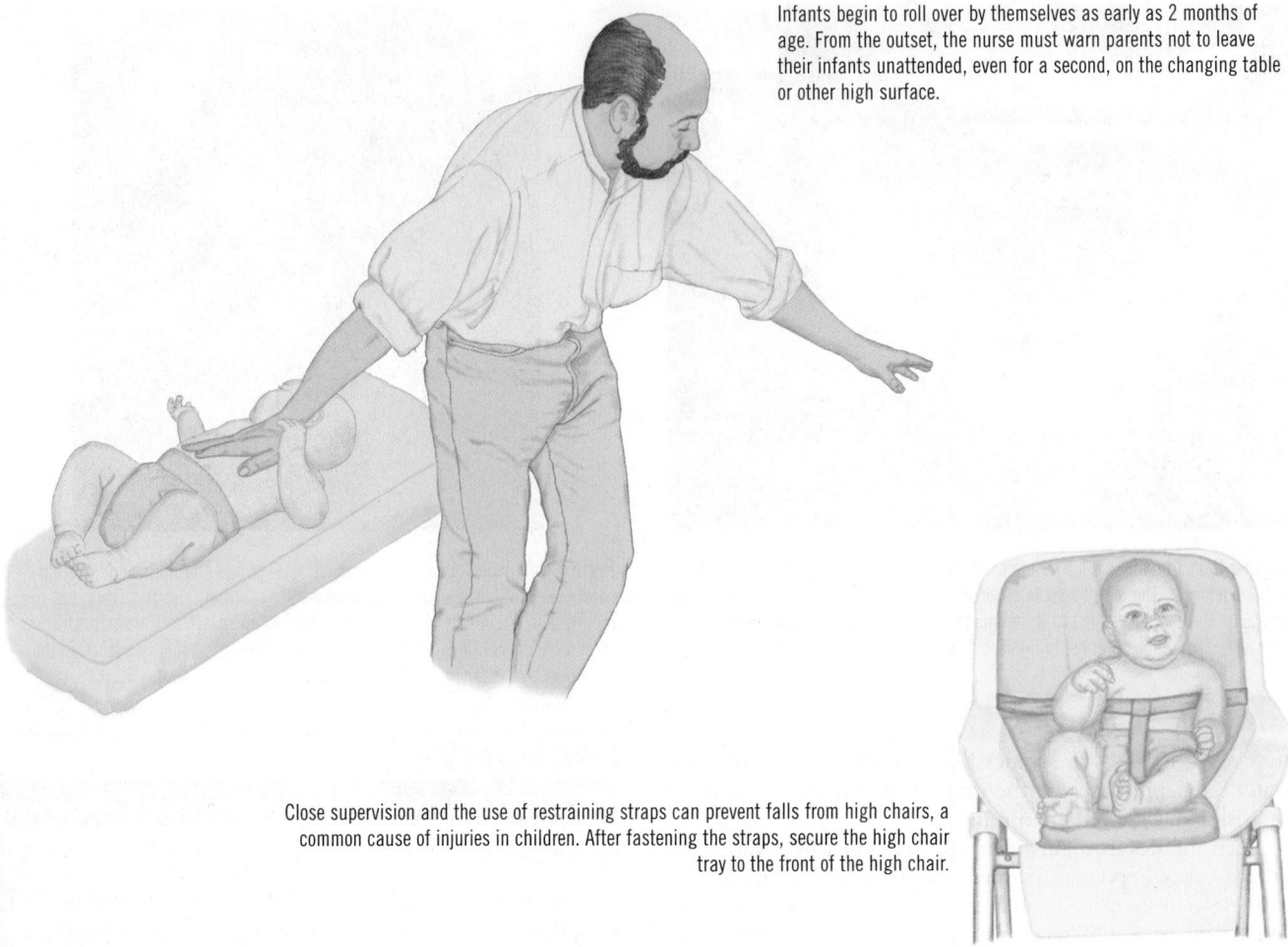

Infants begin to roll over by themselves as early as 2 months of age. From the outset, the nurse must warn parents not to leave their infants unattended, even for a second, on the changing table or other high surface.

Close supervision and the use of restraining straps can prevent falls from high chairs, a common cause of injuries in children. After fastening the straps, secure the high chair tray to the front of the high chair.

Figure 5-4 Safety education for parents of infants should emphasize the need for constant supervision and the use of restraining devices to prevent falls.

ent or nurse must move away from the infant, the adult should either take the infant or, if supplies are close, place a hand on the infant while reaching. At home, parents may choose to place their child on the floor for changing diapers or providing other care.

Falls from infant seats or out of highchairs are common, and falls from infant strollers have resulted in significant injury to young children improperly restrained in the stroller (Powell, Jovtis, & Tanz, 2002). Injuries can be prevented with supervision and the use of safety restraining straps to limit the mobility of the infant (see Fig. 5-4).

As infants begin to crawl, using gates at the top and bottom of stairs can prevent falls. Infant walkers are dangerous and are not recommended. They allow infants mobility and the freedom to explore surroundings before they have developed the ability to interpret heights or protect themselves from falls.

Preventing Asphyxiation

Asphyxiation (suffocation) occurs when air cannot get into or out of the lungs and oxygen supplies are consequently depleted. Carbon dioxide levels then increase, causing life-threatening disruption of cardiac and cerebral functioning. Choking occurs when substances or objects are *aspirated* into the airway or into the branches of the lower airways, causing partial or complete obstruction of the lungs. Strangulation is typically thought of as a constriction of the neck, but it also includes blockage of the nose and mouth by airtight materi-

als, such as plastic. This blockage prevents air exchange. Store all plastic bags or covers out of the infant's reach. Choking is a major concern in the first few months of an infant's life, when aspiration of feedings or vomit can occur easily because of the immature swallowing mechanism. Parents should be taught to position infants on their sides after feedings and to avoid placing small infants in bed with a bottle propped in their mouths.

As infants grow, they begin to explore the world around them by placing anything and everything in their mouths. Size, shape, and consistency are major determinants of whether a food or object is likely to be aspirated by an infant. Food that is round or similar to the size of the airway is especially dangerous. Dangerous foods include sliced hot dogs, hard candy, peanuts, grapes, raisins, and chewing gum. These foods should be avoided until the child is able to chew thoroughly before swallowing. Food should be cut into small pieces, and the child should be supervised while eating. Advise parents to strongly discourage infants and young children from playing, singing, or other activities while eating, to avoid choking. Infants are equally endangered by rattles, pieces of toys, ribbons from stuffed animals, and common household objects such as coins, buttons, pins, or beads found on the floor or within their reach. Balloons should not be given to infants or young children or used where an infant or young child plays.

Anticipatory guidance for parents includes performing a thorough inspection of the infant's surroundings to remove all

Health Promotion

The 9-Month-Old Infant

FOCUSED ASSESSMENT
What kind of new things is your baby doing?
How has the baby reacted to solid foods?
Do you live in a house built before 1978?
Do you live near sources of environmental lead?
Do you regularly come in contact with someone who uses lead?
Do you have a family member who has had lead poisoning?

DEVELOPMENTAL MILESTONES
Personal/social: stranger wariness; waves bye-bye; plays social
   games; begins to indicate wants
Fine motor: beginning pincer grasp; actively searches for out-
   of-sight objects; bangs toys together
Language/cognitive: uses consonant sounds and several vowel
   sounds; beginning to attach meaning to words; understands
   some symbolic language (blow a kiss); knows own name;
   says Mama and Dada specifically
Gross motor: gets to a sitting position; pulls up to stand;
   creeps and crawls; walks holding on to furniture; may briefly
   stand alone

CRITICAL MILESTONES*
Personal/social: feeds self finger foods; tries to get toys; looks
   at hands
Fine motor: transfers; rakes a raisin or Cheerio; picks up and
   holds a small object in each hand
Language/cognitive: imitates sounds; says single syllables; begins to put syllables together
Gross motor: no head lag; sits without support; stands holding
   on to furniture

HEALTH MAINTENANCE
Physical Measurements
   Continue to measure and plot length, weight, and head
      circumference
Immunizations
   Hepatitis B #3 (can give between 6 and 12 months)
   Provide information about upcoming measles, mumps,
      rubella (MMR) and varicella vaccines
Health Screening
   Lead risk assessment (routine lead screen at 9 or
      12 months, usually in conjunction with hemoglobin and
      hematocrit)
   Hemoglobin or hematocrit (screen at 9 or 12 months)

ANTICIPATORY GUIDANCE
Nutrition
   Continue to breast-feed on established schedule
   Formula, 16 to 32 oz/day
   Continue iron-fortified cereal
   Begin to introduce soft, mashed table foods
   Encourage cup, rather than bottle
   Avoid giving large pieces of food

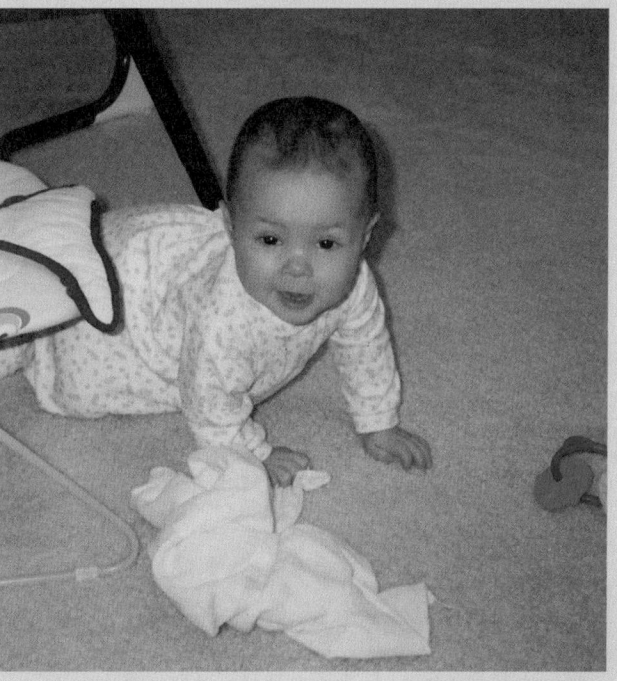

Photo courtesy Cindi Anderson.

Elimination
   Urinary and bowel patterns consistent
   Appearance of undigested food in stools
Dental
   Four teeth
   Brush erupted teeth with soft toothbrush and water
   Continue fluoride supplementation as recommended
Sleep
   Night waking diminishes if managed appropriately
Hygiene
   More vigilant cleanliness of diaper area as bladder volume
      increases
   Wash infant's hands and face frequently
   Keep toys clean
Safety
   Review child-proofing, violence
   Discuss lowering crib mattress, household and plant poi-
      sons, burn prevention, sunscreen use, avoiding sources
      of lead
Play
   Social games
   Provide cloth, cardboard, or plastic books
   Cuddle, rock, hug
   Ball rolling
   Pots and pans with wooden spoons
   Plastic stacking or nesting containers
   Hide-and-seek games with toys

*Guided by DDST II

potential items that infants could grasp, place in their mouths, and choke on. Parents can be encouraged to crawl through the home to gain a better perspective of the infant's environment. Parents can then substitute safe objects for exploration.

Ornaments or toys with detachable parts are not recommended for infants because of the aspiration risk. In 1979 the Consumer Product Safety Commission established a toy standard to prevent choking hazards in nonfood products targeted for children younger than 3 years. Parents should take extra care to note the presence of small detachable parts on toys before allowing the infant to play with the items. Although the government regulates the size of parts on infants'

Health Promotion

The 12-Month-Old Infant

FOCUSED ASSESSMENT

Have parents discussed and agreed on approaches to discipline?

Is the baby able to follow directions and carry out requests?

Have the parents assessed the home and environment for sources of lead?

DEVELOPMENTAL MILESTONES

Personal/social: rolls or throws a ball with another person; explores; drinks from a cup; indicates wants without crying

Fine motor: actively looks for hidden objects; puts blocks in containers; uses simple toys appropriately

Language/cognitive: names the appropriate parent; begins to say one to three single words; understands simple requests

Gross motor: stands alone for increasing lengths of time; stoops and recovers; walks holding onto a hand; may begin to walk alone and climb stairs (on knees)

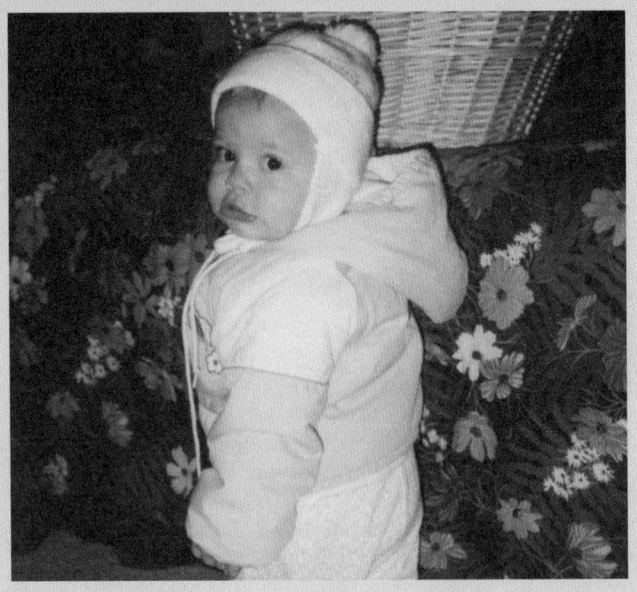

Photo courtesy Michele Hayden.

CRITICAL MILESTONES*

Personal/social: plays pat-a-cake; feeds self; works to get a toy

Fine motor: developed pincer grasp; bangs objects together; picks up two cubes

Language/cognitive: jabbers; combines syllables; mama/dada is nonspecific

Gross motor: stands briefly without support; gets to sitting position; pulls to stand

HEALTH MAINTENANCE

Physical Measurements

Continue to measure and plot length, weight, and head circumference

Weight is usually triple birth weight

Length is 50% over birth length

Immunizations

Hepatitis B #3 (if not given at 9 months); measles, mumps, rubella (MMR) #1; varicella vaccine; pneumococcal booster (if not scheduled to be given at 15 months)

Health Screening

Hemoglobin/hematocrit if not done earlier

Lead screen if not done earlier

Tuberculosis (TB) if at risk

ANTICIPATORY GUIDANCE

Nutrition

May begin whole milk (2 or 3 cups daily)

Offer a variety of table foods from different food groups

Begins to use table utensils

Usually eats three meals and snacks

Avoid giving foods high in salt and sugar

Discuss highchair safety

Elimination

Remains dry for longer periods

Bowel movements decrease in number and become more regular

Dental

Eight teeth

Continue fluoride as recommended and brushing

Sleep

Sleeps through the night and has one or two naps

Hygiene

Continue as previously

Safety

Review poisons, burns, violence

Discuss changing to front-facing car seat (if 20 lb) placed in rear seat, falls, water safety, toy and toy box safety, bike passenger helmet

Play

Beginning parallel play

Push-pull toys

Various-size balls

Picture books

Dolls and stuffed animals

"Busy" box

Sandbox

*Guided by DDST II

---

toys, older children's toys are not regulated by the same standard. As the infant explores an older sibling's or a playmate's territory, adult supervision is important.

To prevent strangulation injuries, caution parents not to place a pacifier on a string or cord around the infant's neck, not to put an infant to sleep with a bib in place, and not to position a crib near blinds or curtain cords. Crib slats should comply with the 2⅜-inch width requirement to prevent head entrapment.

In addition to inspecting and providing a safe environment for the infant, instruct parents in the appropriate action to take if the infant chokes (see Chapter 34 for a discussion of emergency procedures).

BOX 5-4
Lead Exposure Risk Assessment

- Do you live in, or is your child exposed to, housing that was built before 1950 that has peeling paint or plaster, or before 1978 that is being renovated?
- Do you live near any sources of environmental lead, such as smelters, or places that use leaded gasoline?
- Does your child regularly come in contact with a household member who works with lead or lead solder (e.g., plumber, construction worker, stained glass artisan)?
- Does your child have a sibling who has or has had lead poisoning, or has any other household member had lead poisoning?
- In addition, ask the parent if the infant or child has been exposed to any other sources of lead: vinyl mini-blinds, ceramics or toys imported from abroad, old baby furniture, leaded crystal. If the infant has any risk factors, do a capillary test for lead. Otherwise, wait until the 9-month or 1-year visit to do a routine capillary lead screening.

Modified from Rhode Island Department of Health. (2003). Lead screening and referral guidelines. Retrieved Feb. 27, 2004 from www.health.state.ri.us.

BOX 5-5
Age-Related Activities and Toys for Infants

General Activities
The infant enjoys watching other members of the family, being rocked, being taken for a walk in a stroller, time spent in a swing, supervised time on a blanket on the floor, crawling, walking, and being sung and read to.
Play is narcissistic; it is difficult, if not impossible, to direct play. Human interaction is the most important component of play.

Toys and Specific Types of Play
Oral movements (playing with the nipple of the bottle, lip movements unrelated to sucking); peek-a-boo; playing with the caretaker's fingers, hair, and face and the infant's own body parts; and playing in water.
Soft stuffed animals, crib mobiles, squeeze toys, rattles, busy boxes, mirrors, musical toys, water toys during the bath, blocks, safe kitchen utensils, push toys (after infant begins to walk).
Contrasting colors for young infants (black-and-white mobiles).
Large picture books.

Preventing Lead Exposure

Although lead poisoning in the United States has decreased markedly since the elimination of lead paint and solder used in homes and leaded gasoline, lead poisoning remains a significant risk, especially in cities where old housing predominates. In addition, paint from old homes can enter the soil and get on children's hands when they are playing. Children inhale lead dust as homes are being renovated. The lead risk assessment begins as the infant begins to be mobile (6 months of age). Risk should be assessed at every well visit beginning at the 6-month visit and education or treatment initiated as appropriate (see Box 5-4 and Chapter 34).

Play

One sign of infants' cognitive development is the beginning evidence of play. Early signs of play are related to infants' motor and cognitive development. They mouth, shake, inspect, and reach for objects. Infants observe and engage other members of the family. In fact, human involvement is the most important component of play. A familiar game that we all have played is peek-a-boo. Not only is this game fun, but also it is associated with the development of object permanence. Box 5-5 outlines appropriate play activities and toys for the infant. See Chapter 4 for more information related to play.

KEY CONCEPTS

- During the first year of life, the infant's organs grow and mature at a rapid rate, yet organ systems of infants remain very different from those of older children and adults.
- Weight gain and muscle growth during infancy allow the infant to have increased control of reflexes and increasingly coordinated movement.
- Sensory capabilities, neuromuscular control, perceptual skills, the quality and quantity of parental interaction, and environmental stimulation all affect cognitive development during infancy.
- Infants develop language first by listening to sounds of caregivers, then by realizing that certain sounds have special meaning, and eventually by using simple words to communicate.
- Infancy is the period during which children develop the foundation of their personalities, struggling to establish a sense of basic trust rather than mistrust.
- One of the most important features of psychosocial development during infancy is parent-

infant attachment, or the sense of belonging with one another.
- Common problems during infancy, such as separation anxiety, sleep disorders, and fretfulness, cause parents concern and distress. Nurses should be available with information and support to provide anticipatory guidance.
- Nurses play an important role in health promotion and disease prevention related to immunizations.
- Because infancy is a period of very rapid growth and development, nutritional needs are of special significance. Parents frequently have many questions and concerns about nutrition.
- Breast milk or commercially prepared formulas provide the foundation of nutrition throughout infancy.
- Solid foods are usually introduced between 4 and 6 months of age in small amounts, one food at a time, based on the infant's growth and development.
- Weaning usually begins between ages 6 and 12 months. It should never take place dur-

ing stress, and the infant should receive breast milk or formula in the cup until age 12 months.
- Teething usually begins between 5 and 9 months of age. Some degree of discomfort is normal, and parents often need suggestions for coping with teething.
- Bottle-mouth caries or nursing-bottle syndrome is a form of tooth decay that can develop in infants and children as a result of prolonged breast-feeding or bottle-feeding, especially at night.
- Colic can be very stressful for parents. The cause of colic is unknown, and care of the infant must be individualized. Support of the parents is very important.
- Improved motor development coupled with a keen desire to explore the environment places the infant at great risk for unintentional injury.
- Play enhances the infant's growth and development.

ANSWERS to Critical Thinking Exercise 5-1

1. Because this is Mrs. Brown's first child, she might be insecure about caring for Tonja. She might not be aware of normal growth and developmental milestones for this age. Tonja may be awake for long periods at night or she may have colic, depriving Mrs. Brown of sleep. Mr. Brown may travel or need to be away from home with his job and may not be available to help with Tonja. Mrs. Brown may not have an extended family to help her with the care of the infant. Mrs. Brown may be experiencing postpartum depression.

2. Trust must be established, and this can be accomplished by supporting Mrs. Brown and encouraging her to verbalize her concerns. Mothers of newborns often need reassurance that they are doing a good job, and they need to be given permission to ask any question, no matter how insignificant they or the nurse might think the question is. The nurse can validate Mrs. Brown's feelings of being overwhelmed.

3. The nurse must determine if Mrs. Brown has a support system and, if not, problem solve with her to provide the support she needs. If Tonja is colicky, Mrs. Brown will need added support and the various interventions will need to be discussed. The nurse ends the visit by giving Mrs. Brown permission to contact her as questions and problems arise. The nurse also makes a note to contact Mrs. Brown by phone in a couple of days to see how she is doing.

REFERENCES and READINGS

American Academy of Pediatrics. (2000a). *A guide to children's dental health.* Retrieved August 20, 2003, from www.medem.com.

American Academy of Pediatrics. (2000b). Year 2000 position statement: Principles and guidelines for early hearing detection and intervention programs. *Pediatrics, 106*(4), 798-817.

American Academy of Pediatrics. (2001). *Establishing good sleep habits.* Retrieved March 23, 2001, from www.medem.com.

American Academy of Pediatrics. (2003a). *Car safety seats: A guide for families.* Retrieved June 10, 2003, from www.aap.org/family/carseatguide.htm.

American Academy of Pediatrics. (2003b). Oral health risk assessment timing and establishment of the dental home. *Pediatrics, 111*(5), 1113-1116.

American Academy of Pediatrics. (2003c). *Summer safety tips.* Retrieved June 10, 2003, from www.aap.org.

American Academy of Pediatrics Committee on Nutrition. (1998). *Pediatric nutrition handbook.* Elk Grove Village, IL: American Academy of Pediatrics.

American Academy of Pediatrics Work Group on Breastfeeding. (1997). Breastfeeding and the use of human milk. *Pediatrics, 100*(6), 1035-1039.

Agran, P., Anderson, C., Winn, D., Trent, R., Walton-Haynes, L., & Thayer, S. (2003). Rates of pediatric injuries by 3-month intervals for children 0 to 3 years of age. *Pediatrics, 111*(6), e683-e692.

Calamaro, C. (2000). Infant nutrition in the first year of life: Tradition or science? *Pediatric Nursing, 26*(2), 211-214.

Carey, W. (1998). Let's give temperament its due. *Contemporary Pediatrics, 15*(5), 91-113.

Cunningham, M., & Cox, E. (2003). Hearing assessment in infants and children: Recommendations beyond neonatal screening. *Pediatrics, 111*(2), 436-441.

Erikson, E.H. (1963). *Childhood and society* (2nd ed.). New York: Norton.

Flavell, J.H. (1964). *The developmental psychology of Jean Piaget.* New York: Van Nostrand.

Garrison, M., & Christakis, D. (2000). A systematic review of treatments for infant colic. *Pediatrics, 106*(1), 184-190.

Graham, J., Goldie, S., Segui-Gomez, M., Thompson, K., Nelson, T., Glass, R., Simpson, A., & Woerner, L. (1998). Reducing risks to children in vehicles with passenger airbags. *Pediatrics, 102*(1), e3.

Green, M., & Palfrey, J.S. (2000). *Bright futures: Guidelines for health supervision of infants, children, and adolescents* (2nd ed.). Arlington, VA: National Center for Education in Maternal and Child Health.

Huff, G., Bagwell, S., & Bachman, D. (1998). Airbag injuries in infants and children: A case report and review of the literature. *Pediatrics, 102*(1), e2.

Huffman, G. (2001). Are there any effective treatments for infant colic? *American Family Physician, 63*(2), 369.

Iglowstien, I., Jenni, O., Molinari, L., & Largo, R. (2003). Sleep duration from infancy to adolescence: Reference values and generational trends. *Pediatrics, 111*(2), 302-307.

Kamerling, S.N. (2002). Airbags & children: Making correct choices in child passenger restraints. *MCN, The American Journal of Maternal/Child Nursing, 27*(5), 264-273.

Karmiloff-Smith, A. (1995). The extraordinary cognitive journey from foetus through infancy. *Journal of Child Psychology and Psychiatry, 36*(8), 1293-1313.

Levine, M., Carey, W., & Crocker, A. (1999). *Developmental-behavioral pediatrics* (3rd ed.). Philadelphia: Saunders.

Mack, R. (1998). "Something wicked this way comes": Herbs even witches should avoid. *Contemporary Pediatrics, 15*(6), 49-64.

Moore, M.L., & Krowchuk, H. (1997). Parent line: Nurse telephone intervention for parents and caregivers of children from birth through age 5. *Journal of the Society of Pediatric Nursing, 2*(4), 179-184.

Olsen, R., Barbaresi, W., & Olsen, G. (1998). Development in the first year of life. *Contemporary Pediatrics, 15*(7), 81-115.

Piaget, J. (1952). *The origins of intelligence in children.* New York: International Universities Press.

Powell, E., Jovtis, E., & Tanz, R. (2002). Incidence and description of stroller-related injuries to children. *Pediatrics, 110*(5), e62.

Roberts, M., Keels, M., Sharp, M., & Lewis, J. (1998). Fluoride supplement prescribing and dental referral patterns among academic pediatricians. *Pediatrics, 101*(1), e6.

Schmitt, B. (1999). Instructions for pediatric patients. Philadelphia: Saunders.

Story, M., Holt, K., & Sofka, D. (2002). *Bright futures in practice: Nutrition* (2nd ed.). Arlington, VA: National Center for Education in Maternal and Child Health.

Thiedke, C.C. (2001). Sleep disorders and sleep problems in childhood. *American Family Physician, 63*(2), 277-284.

Titus, M.O., Baxter, A., & Starling, S. (2003). Accidental scald burns in sinks. *Pediatrics, 111*(2), e191-e194.

U.S. Department of Health and Human Services. (2000). *Healthy People 2010* (Conference edition, in 2 volumes). Washington, DC: Author.

Velsor-Friedrich, B. (2002). The silent epidemic: Lead poisoning. *Journal of Pediatric Nursing, 17*(1), 59-61.

White, B.L. (1975). *The first three years of life.* Englewood Cliffs, NJ: Prentice-Hall.

Wright, A., Bauer, M., Naylor, A., Sutcliffe, E., & Clark, L. (1998). Increasing breastfeeding rates to reduce infant illness at the community level. *Pediatrics, 101*(5), 837-844.

6

Health Promotion During Early Childhood

◆ LEARNING OBJECTIVES

After studying this chapter, you should be able to:
- Describe the physiologic changes and the motor, cognitive, language, and psychosocial development of the toddler and preschooler.
- Provide parents with anticipatory guidance related to the toddler and preschooler.
- Discuss the causes of and identify interventions for common toddler behaviors—temper tantrums, negativism, and ritualism.
- Identify strategies to alleviate a preschool child's fears and sleep problems.
- Discuss strategies for disciplining a toddler and a preschooler.
- Describe signs of a toddler's readiness for toilet training, and offer guidelines to parents.
- Offer parents suggestions for promoting school readiness in the preschool child.

◆ DEFINITIONS

associative play Group play without group goals.
autonomy The ability to function independently without the control of others.
caries Tooth decay.
cooperative play Organized play with group goals.
dysfluency Disorders in the rhythm of speech in which individuals know precisely what they wish to say but are unable to do so because of an involuntary, repetitive prolongation or cessation of sound.
irreversibility The inability to understand a process in reverse or mentally to undo an action that has been performed.
negativism The attitude of opposing or resisting the directions of others.

parallel play Playing alongside but not with other children.
physiologic anorexia Decreased appetite because of relatively decreased caloric need.
regression The return to a behavior characteristic of an earlier stage of development.
ritualism The need to maintain sameness and reliability.
symbolic play The use of games and interactions that represent an issue or concern to be addressed.
symbolic thought The ability to allow a mental image (word or object) to represent something that is not present.
transductive reasoning Reasoning from the particular to the particular rather than from the general to the particular.

The developmental changes that mark the transition from infancy to early childhood are dramatic. During the toddler years, ages 12 through 36 months, the child begins to venture out independently from a secure base of trust established during the first year. The preschool period, ages 3 through 5 years, is a time of relative tranquility after the tumultuous toddler period.

GROWTH AND DEVELOPMENT DURING EARLY CHILDHOOD

The toddler years are characterized by a struggle for autonomy as the child develops a sense of self separate from the parent. Boundless energy and insatiable curiosity drive the toddler to explore the environment and master new skills (Fig. 6-1). The combination of increased motor skills, immaturity, and lack of experience places the toddler at risk for un-

intentional injury. Toddlers' egocentric and demanding behaviors, often marked by temper tantrums and negativism, have given this age the label "the terrible twos."

The preschooler becomes increasingly independent, mastering many self-care and motor skills and developing greater social and emotional maturity (Fig. 6-2). The preschooler is imaginative, creative, and curious. Many parents describe this period as their favorite age as they watch the dramatic transformation of a chubby toddler into an agile, articulate child who is ready to enter the world of peers and school.

The nurse's roles as health care provider, family counselor, and child advocate continues during the toddler and preschool years. Well-child checkups provide the nurse with opportunities for anticipatory guidance related to growth and development, safety, nutrition, and some of the common age-related concerns of parents (Box 6-1).

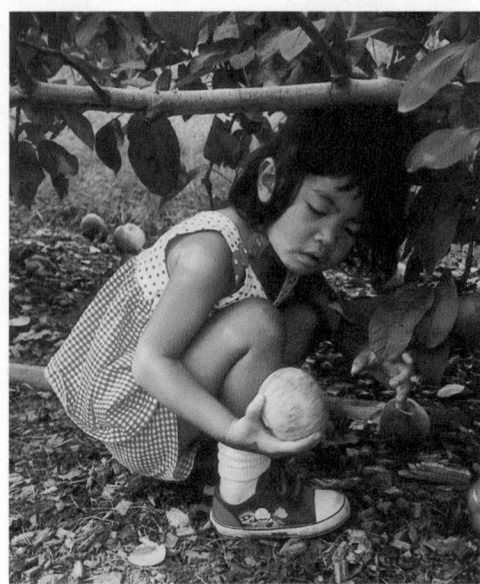

The toddler is enchanted by a world filled with discovery. Curiosity provides resources for the tremendous cognitive growth that occurs during this period.

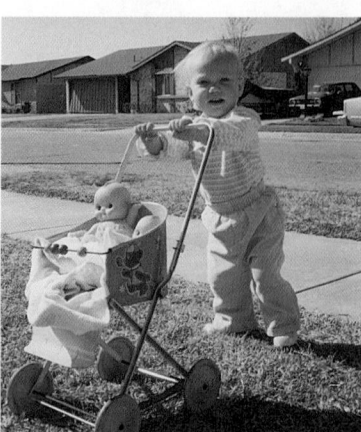

Toddlers enjoy push-pull toys. Toys should be strong and sturdy; wheeled toys should not tip over easily.

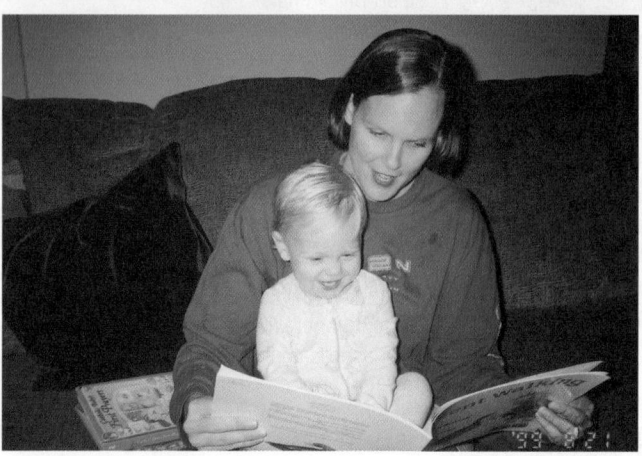

Reading simple stories provides quiet, enjoyable times for toddlers and parents and enhances speech and language development.

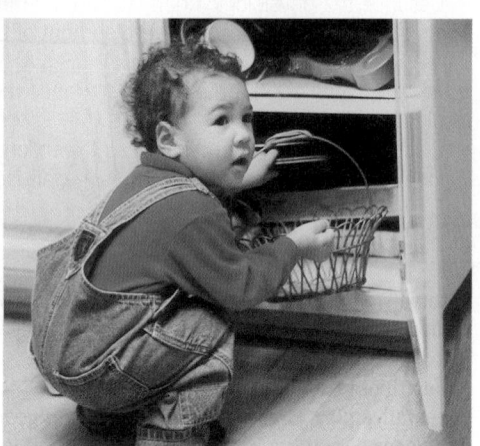

Pots and pans are popular toys for inquisitive toddlers. However, exploring cupboards can be a dangerous activity for toddlers. Toxic cleaning substances and other dangerous objects must be kept behind locked doors or otherwise out of reach.

Figure 6-1 Growth and development of the toddler.

BOX 6-1
Healthy People 2010 Objectives for Toddlers and Preschoolers

14-4	Reduce bacterial meningitis in young children.
14-24	Increase the proportion of young children who receive all vaccines that have been recommended for universal administration for at least 5 years.
15-3	Reduce firearm-related deaths.
	Reduce deaths caused by unintentional injuries.
15-29	Reduce drownings.
19-4	Reduce growth retardation among low-income children under age 5 years.
21-2	Reduce the proportion of children, adolescents, and adults with untreated dental decay.
27-9	Reduce the proportion of children who are regularly exposed to tobacco smoke at home.

Modified from U.S. Department of Health and Human Services. (2000). *Healthy People 2010* (Conference edition, in 2 volumes). Washington, DC: Author.

Physical Growth and Development

The Toddler

Physical growth slows during the toddler years. The average weight gain is 2.25 kg (5 lb) per year. A child's birth weight has quadrupled by age 2 to 3 years. The rate of increase in height also slows, with the average toddler growing approximately 7.5 cm (3 inches) per year.

The brain grows at a slower rate during this period than during infancy. Head circumference reflects this growth, increasing approximately 3.7 cm (1½ inches) during the toddler years, compared with the growth of 12 cm (4⁸/₁₀ inches) in the first 12 months. By the age of 2 years, the head circumference has reached 90% of its adult size.

Immature abdominal musculature gives the toddler a pot-bellied appearance, with an exaggerated lumbar curve. The child's short legs may appear slightly bowed, and the feet seem flat because of a plantar fat pad that disappears around the age of 2 years. During the toddler years, muscle tissue gradually replaces much of the adipose tissue (baby fat) pres-

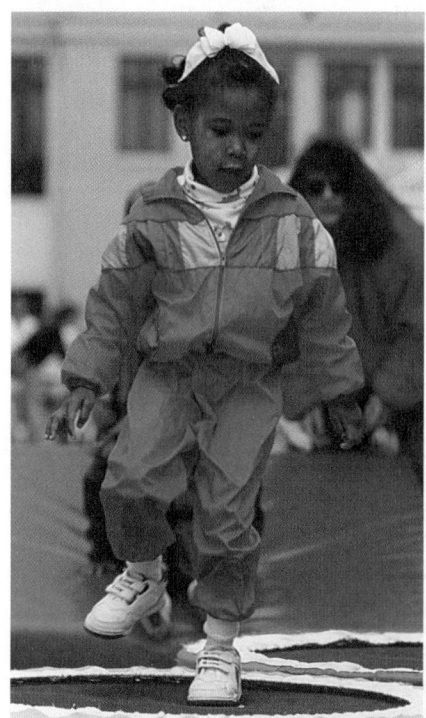

As the brain matures, the preschool child's motor development matures. Opportunities for practice contribute to the development of motor skills. (Courtesy Cook Children's Medical Center, Fort Worth, TX.)

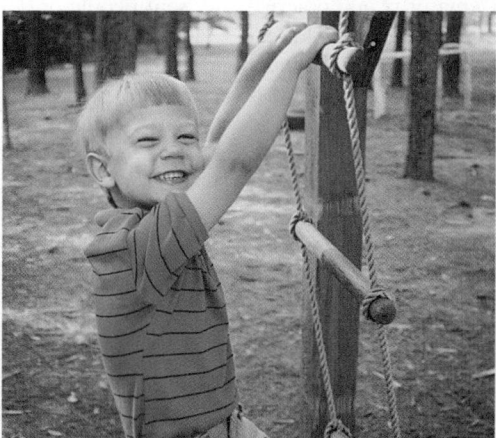

This 4-year-old's motor development has increased to the point that he can jump and climb well. The 4-year-old can also throw a ball overhand and cut on a curved line with scissors.

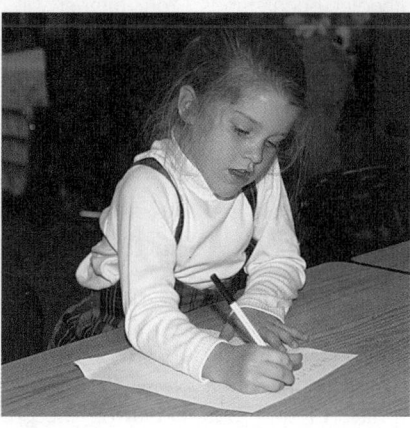

This 5-year-old is printing her name in readable letters. Children of this age can usually skip and can both throw and catch a ball. (Courtesy The University of Texas at Arlington School of Nursing.)

Figure 6-2 Growth and development of the preschooler.

ent during infancy. As the musculoskeletal system matures and the child walks and runs more, the cherubic toddler disappears and the child grows into a taller, leaner preschooler.

The Preschooler

The growth of the preschool child is slow and steady. Height and weight gains are minimal during this period. The average weight gain is about 2.25 kg (5 lb) per year, and the height gain averages 5 to 7.5 cm (2 to 3 inches) per year. Children attain half their adult height between the ages of 2 and 3 years. During this time, growth occurs more rapidly in the legs than in the trunk, accumulation of adipose tissue declines, and the child's appetite decreases. As a result, the preschooler loses the potbellied appearance of the toddler, becoming slimmer and more agile. Muscles grow faster than bones during the preschool period. Muscle strength is influenced by nutrition, genetic makeup, and the opportunity to exercise and use the muscles. Knock-knees (see Chapter 50) are common in 3-year-olds and are often associated with occasional stumbling and falling. Maturation of the knee and hip joints usually corrects this problem by age 4 or 5 years.

As the lungs grow, the vital capacity increases and the respiratory rate slows. Respirations remain primarily diaphragmatic until age 5 or 6 years. The heart rate decreases and the blood pressure increases as the heart increases in size (see Chapter 33 for vital sign ranges). Cardiovascular maturation enables the preschooler to engage in more sustained and strenuous activity.

All 20 deciduous teeth are present by age 3 years. Deciduous teeth may begin to fall out at the end of the preschool period. The first permanent teeth to erupt, the back molars, usually appear in the early school-age years.

Motor Development

The Toddler

Learning to walk well is the crowning achievement of the toddler period. The child is in perpetual motion, seemingly compelled to pull up, take a few steps, fall, and repeat the process over and over, oblivious to bumps and bruises. The toddler will repeat this performance hundreds of times, until the skill of walking has been perfected.

The age at which children learn to walk varies widely. Most children can walk alone by 15 months. By 18 months of age, toddlers walk well and try to run but fall often. At approximately 15 months of age, many toddlers become avid climbers. Chairs, tables, and bookcases all present irresistible challenges and risks for injury. Parents may have difficulty keeping the toddler in a crib and may decide it is time to move the child to a regular bed.

Toddlers are also engaged in perfecting fine motor skills. Hand-eye coordination improves with maturity and practice. Mealtimes are still messy. Although most 18-month-olds can hold a cup with both hands and drink from it without much spilling, eating with a spoon is difficult. Most of the food conveyed in a spoon is spilled. Children need a great deal of practice with a spoon before they can feed themselves without spilling. Most toddlers can feed themselves with a spoon by their 2nd birthday if they have been allowed to practice.

At 18 months of age, the toddler enjoys removing clothing. By 24 months, the toddler can put on simple items of clothing but cannot differentiate front from back. Children at this age also can zip large zippers, put on shoes, and wash and dry their hands. Two-year-olds brush their teeth but need help in adequately removing plaque.

The toddler's increasing motor skills allow more independence in all areas of daily life. Feeding, dressing, and play provide opportunities for the child to develop autonomy. Motor development in this age-group is far ahead of development of judgment and perception. This different timing of the development of different skills increases the risk for injury.

The Preschooler

Coordination and muscle strength increase rapidly between the ages of 3 and 5 years. Increases in brain size and nerve myelinization enable the child to perfect fine and gross motor skills.

Motor abilities vary widely among children. Although motor skill is less influenced by environment than other areas of development, such as language, opportunities to practice may contribute to better motor skills. For example, a 4-year-old who often plays catch with a sibling or parent generally finds playing Little League baseball as a 7-year-old easier than a child without a similar experience.

Handedness begins to emerge at about 3 years and is usually clearly established by 4 years. The nurse should encourage parents to provide left-handed children with appropriate tools, particularly left-handed scissors. Left-handed children should not be forced to use their right hand, because coordination is usually better when they use the dominant side. Eye-hand coordination is usually good enough by age 5 years for a child to hit a nail on the head with a hammer. Increased coordination allows the child to perform many self-care skills and to become more independent.

By age 4 or 5 years, the child is independent and can dress, eat, and go to the bathroom without help. Unlike the toddler, who must be restrained to avoid injury, the older preschooler can usually be trusted to heed verbal warnings of danger.

Cognitive and Sensory Development

The Toddler

Toddlers are consumed with curiosity. Their boundless energy and insatiable inquisitiveness provide them with resources for the tremendous cognitive growth that occurs during this period.

Toddlers between the ages of 12 and 18 months are in Piaget's sensorimotor period (see Chapter 4). Learning in this stage occurs mainly by trial and error. Toddlers spend most of a busy day experimenting to see what will happen as they dump, fill, empty, and explore every accessible area of their environment. Between 19 and 24 months, the child enters the final stage of the sensorimotor period. Object permanence is firmly established by this age. The child has a beginning ability to use symbols and words when referring to absent people or objects and begins to solve problems mentally rather than by repeating an action over and over. A toddler at this stage is often seen imitating the parent of the same gender performing household tasks (termed *domestic mimicry*). Late in this stage, the child displays *deferred imitation* (e.g., imitating the parent putting on makeup or shaving hours after that parent has left for work). The 18-month-old has a beginning ability to wait, as evidenced by the toddler responding appropriately to a parent or caregiver who says, "just a minute." The child's concept of time is still immature, however, and "a minute" may seem like an hour to the toddler.

Toddlers think in terms of the predictable routines of their daily schedule. When talking with the toddler, the nurse should use time orientation in relation to familiar activities. For example, a toddler understands "Your mother will be here after your nap" better than "Your mother will be here at 2 o'clock."

Many hours each day are spent putting objects into holes and smaller objects into each other as the child experiments with sizes, shapes, and spatial relations. Toddlers enjoy opening drawers and doors, exploring the contents of cabinets and closets, and generally wreaking havoc throughout the house as well as exposing themselves to potential danger.

According to Piaget, the preoperational stage of cognitive development characterizes the second half of early childhood (see Chapter 4). This stage is divided into two phases: the preconceptual phase (2 to 4 years) and the intuitive phase (4 to 7 years). During the preconceptual phase, the child is beginning to use symbolic thought—the ability to allow a mental image (words or ideas) to represent objects or ideas. Mental symbols allow the child to remember the past and to describe events that happened in the past. At around 24 months, children enter the preconceptual phase, which ends at age 4 years. Children begin to think and reason at a primitive level. Two-year-olds have a beginning ability to retain mental images. This ability allows them to internalize what they see and experience. Symbols in the form of words can be used to represent ideas. Increasing amounts of play time are spent pretending. A box may become a spaceship or a hat; pebbles may be money or popcorn. The child's rapidly increasing vocabulary enhances symbolic play. The toddler begins to think about alternative solutions to a problem and can even consider the consequences of an action without carrying it out (touching a hot stove, running too fast on a slippery sidewalk).

The toddler's thinking is immature, limited in its logic, and bound to the present. Egocentrism, animism, irreversibility, magical thinking, and centration characterize the preoperational thought of the toddler (Table 6-1). The predominant words in the toddler's language repertoire are "me," "I," and "mine."

Health Promotion

The 15- to 18-Month-Old Child

FOCUSED ASSESSMENT

What new activities is your child doing?

Can the child say single words? Put words together? Understand most of what you say? Communicate needs and wants?

What kinds of foods does your child eat and how often? Does the child have a problem with eating nonfood items? Is your child able to eat independently?

How does your child move from one area in the house to another?

How does your child behave when frustrated? How do you and your partner handle this?

What kinds of activities do you enjoy doing with your child?

DEVELOPMENTAL MILESTONES

Personal/social: may exhibit negativism, ritualism, and increasing tolerance of separation from parents; undresses; beginning temper tantrums when frustrated; may have a transition object; beginning understanding of gender differences

Fine motor: turns book pages; begins to imitate vertical and circular strokes; vision 20/50 by 18 months; drinks from a cup holding the cup with two hands

Language/cognitive: increasing receptive language; begins to understand and say "no"; may begin to put two words together; can point to familiar objects; beginning memory and understanding of spatial and temporal relationships; increased object permanence; has a basic moral understanding (reward and punishment); understands simple directions; by 18 months has a vocabulary of approximately 30 words; holographic speech (uses single words with gestures to express whole ideas)

Gross motor: walks with increasing confidence and begins to run; climbs stairs first by creeping, then walking with hand held; jumps in place; begins to throw a ball overhand without falling

CRITICAL MILESTONES*

Personal/social: begins to imitate; helps in the house; feeds self with increasing skill (still rotates the spoon, if used) and holds a cup

Fine motor: builds a tower with increasing number of blocks; scribbles; able to put a block in a cup

Language/cognitive: says 3 to 10 single words; can point to several body parts

Gross motor: walks well forward and backward; stoops and recovers

HEALTH MAINTENANCE

Physical Measurements

Continue to measure and plot length, weight, and head circumference

Anterior fontanel closed by 18 months

Immunizations

15 months: *Haemophilus influenzae* type b (Hib) #4; measles, mumps, rubella (MMR) #1 (if not given at 1 year); varicella (if not given at 1 year); pneumococcal (if not given at 1 year); hepatitis B #3 (if not given earlier)

18 months: diphtheria, tetanus, acellular pertussis (DTaP) #4; inactivated poliovirus (IPV) #3 (if not given earlier); hepatitis B #3 (if not given earlier); varicella (if not given earlier)

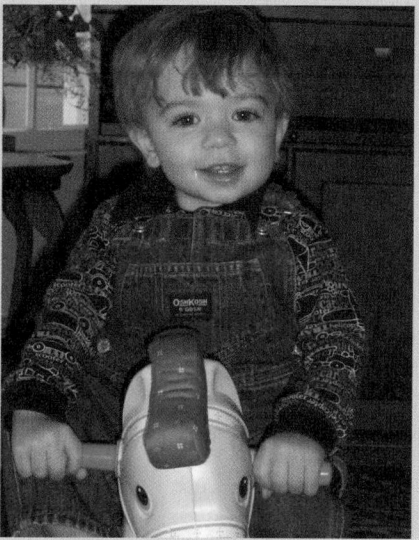

ANTICIPATORY GUIDANCE

Nutrition

Calorie, protein, and fluid requirements decrease slightly; offer a variety of foods every 2 to 3 hours

Give 2 or 3 cups of whole milk daily for calcium

Make mealtimes pleasant: use appropriate-size utensils, colorful dinnerware

Child may have fussy eating habits (physiologic anorexia)

Resist giving food as a comfort measure

Do not allow child to walk or play with food in the mouth

Elimination

Sphincters become physiologically under voluntary control, but child is usually not ready for toilet training; advise parents to wait, but discuss signs of readiness

Dental

Continue to brush with a soft toothbrush twice daily

Give fluoride if water is not fluoridated

Maintain a diet low in sugar

Do not put the child to sleep with a bottle

Sleep

Sleep cycles decrease, and the child has longer awake periods

Still naps one or two times per day

May resist going to bed; likes a bedtime routine

Hygiene

Begins to participate in self-care (washes face and hands with assistance)

Safety

Review car safety, violence, falls, water safety, toy and toy-box safety, bike passenger helmet, poisons

Discuss choking, toy safety, firearm access, burn prevention, sun protection

Play

Provide push-pull toys with short strings

Noise-making toys

Dolls and stuffed animals (watch for small parts)

Musical toys

Art supplies: large crayons, finger paints, clay

Large blocks and balls

* Guided by DDST II

TABLE 6-1 Characteristics of Preoperational Thinking

Characteristic	Example
Egocentrism: Views everything in relation to self; is unable to consider another's point of view.	Toddler takes a toy away from another child and cannot understand that the other child wants (or has a right to) the toy, too.
Animism: Believes that inert objects are alive and have wills of their own.	Toddler trips over a toy and scolds the toy for hurting her. She believes that the toy hurt her on purpose.
Irreversibility: Cannot see a process in reverse order. Cannot follow a line of reasoning back to its beginning. Cannot hold on to two or more sequential thoughts simultaneously.	If the child takes a toy apart, the child cannot remember the sequence for putting it back together. If a child is taken on a walk, the child cannot retrace steps and find the way home.
Magical thought: Believes that magical thought is the cause of events, and that wishing something will make it so.	Toddlers often feel extremely powerful and believe that their thoughts cause events to happen. May believe that parents are all-powerful and can read minds or have magical powers.
Centration: Tends to focus on only one aspect of an experience, ignoring other possible alternatives. Focuses on the dominant characteristic of an object, excluding other characteristics.	May have difficulty putting together a puzzle, concentrating on only one detail of a piece (e.g., shape) and ignoring other qualities (e.g., color, detail). Cannot follow more than one direction at a time.

The Preschooler

By age 3 years, the brain has reached two thirds of its adult size. Maturation of the central nervous system contributes to the child's increasing cognitive abilities.

The 3-year-old can retain a mental image of a loved one and can periodically "refuel" by thinking about that person. A photograph can help some children cope with separation by bridging the gap between physical presence and mental image. Preschoolers' ability to remember their parents and to recognize that their needs can be met even though their parents are not present increases their ability to tolerate separation.

Because preschoolers still engage in animism, they often endow inanimate objects with lifelike qualities during play. A doll may become a crying baby, or a teddy bear may become a friend who listens sympathetically. Symbolic play is important for emotional development because it allows the child to work through distressing feelings. For this reason, it is therapeutic to allow a child to play with medical equipment after a painful procedure. Four-year-olds who have received injections may be found working out their feelings by giving their dolls "lots of shots."

During the preconceptual phase, reality may be distorted by transductive reasoning. The preschool child reasons from particular to particular, rather than from particular to general and vice versa, as adults do. The child cannot understand that relationships exist and cannot view the whole in relation to its parts. The preschool child has difficulty focusing on the important aspects of a situation. To a child, everything is important and interdependent. This type of thinking is called *field dependency*. For example, the preschooler may have difficulty falling asleep at night because the parent did not follow the usual bedtime routine. Objects, routine, and sameness are important to the preschool child. Rituals provide the preschool child with a feeling of control.

The second phase of Piaget's preoperational stage, the intuitive phase, is characterized by centration and lack of reversibility. *Centration* is the tendency to center or focus on one part of a situation and ignore the other parts. The child cannot understand logical relationships and is unable to fo-

cus on more than one aspect of a situation at a time. For example, the child may not be able to follow a sequence of directions but will perform well if the directions are given one at a time.

The 4- or 5-year-old shows *irreversibility* in thought. Children this age cannot reverse a process or the order of events. They may be able to take a complex puzzle apart but have difficulty putting it back together. The 4- or 5-year old also lacks reversibility for mathematical processes. The child may be able to add 3 and 1 and get 4, but reversing the problem ($4 - 1 = 3$) would be too difficult.

The preschool years are a period of rapid learning. The preschool child is curious and wants to know how things work. Preschoolers' thinking is still magical and egocentric (self-centered). Children at this age tend to understand events only as these events affect them, believing that everyone else has had the same experience. Children seeing their mother in distress may bring her a doll, assuming that it would comfort the mother as it does the child.

Preschool children often think that their thoughts are powerful enough to cause things to happen. They may frighten themselves with some of their ideas, believing that they may become what they imagine they will be. Preschoolers may feel overwhelmed by guilt when a sibling is hospitalized because they believe that their hostile feelings caused the sibling's illness. Likewise, a child of this age may say, "I got sick because I was bad."

Language Development

The Toddler

The acquisition of language is one of the most dramatic developments of early childhood. Although the age at which children begin to talk varies widely, most can communicate verbally by their second birthday. The rate of language development depends on physical maturity and the amount of reinforcement that the child has received. Between 15 and 24 months of age, language ability develops rapidly. Toddlers understand many more words than they can say because receptive language (what the child understands) develops sooner and more quickly than speech. Sometime after 18 months, many children experience a sudden spurt in speech production and comprehension, resulting in a vocabulary of 300 or more words at 24 months. By 2 years of age, roughly 60% to 70% of toddlers' speech should be understandable. Because children of 24 to 30 months are less egocentric and better able to consider another's point of view, they engage in more conversation with others and less monologue.

If language development is not progressing normally, parents should be advised to pursue follow-up care. Children of bilingual families, children who are twins, and children other than firstborns may have slower language development. Because language development depends on adequate hearing, delayed language can be seen in children who have had repeated ear infections or who have undiagnosed hearing loss (see Chapter 55).

Parents can promote language development by talking to their child and incorporating teaching into daily routines. Feeding, bathing, dressing, and going on outings to both new and familiar places offer opportunities for verbal interaction and the practice of growing language skills. The child should be encouraged to express needs rather than the parent anticipating and providing what the child wants before the child asks for it. Reading simple, entertaining stories with colorful pictures provides quiet, enjoyable times for toddlers and parents and enhances speech and language development.

The Preschooler

A dramatic increase in language skill in the preschool period promotes self-control and increases the child's ability to direct and be directed by others. Children at this age may be heard talking to themselves about things they have heard or been taught.

The preschooler's vocabulary increases rapidly, from 300 words at 2 years of age to more than 2100 words at 5 years. In less than 3 years, the child grows from a toddler who knows only a few words into a child who skillfully uses an extensive vocabulary to describe events, share feelings, and ask questions. Three-year-olds speak in short, telegraphic sentences. They may talk to themselves or to imaginary friends. A delightful characteristic of young preschoolers is the tendency to engage in lengthy monologues, regardless of whether anyone is listening or even present. Such self-talk provides the child with opportunities to practice speech and is often accompanied by symbolic play.

By 4 years old, children talk incessantly and tend to boast and exaggerate. They enjoy rhymes and silly ways to use similar words. Four-year-olds expect more detailed answers to their questions. They may use speech aggressively and may use profanity to gain attention. "Bad" language should be ignored, thus depriving the child of reinforcement of the behavior. When children feel that they gain power over their parents by using bad language, these verbalizations will continue.

Five-year-olds speak in sentences of adult length and use all parts of speech. They usually are proficient storytellers who produce elaborate tales for anyone who will listen. Their tendency to mix fantasy with reality may be perceived by adults as lying. The child of 5 years usually can recite the days of the week and can name the seasons.

Nurses can teach parents strategies to promote their child's language development. It is important for parents to talk with the child and respond to the child's attempts at communication. Reading to the child and making reading materials available can help build vocabulary and promote a lifelong love of reading. Watching educational television programs with their child may augment parents' communication skills with their child. Preschoolers spend a lot of time asking "how" and "why" questions, often taxing parents' patience. Short, simple, honest answers encourage vocabulary building and boost self-esteem.

Psychosocial Development

The Toddler

The toddler is developing a sense of autonomy, giving up the comfort of dependence enjoyed during infancy. If a basic sense of trust was established during the first year, the toddler can venture forward and separate from parents for short periods to explore and experience the world.

According to Erikson (1963), the toddler is struggling with the developmental task of acquiring a sense of autonomy while overcoming a sense of shame and doubt. Toddlers discover that they have wills of their own and that they can control others. Asserting their wills and insisting on their own way, however, often lead to conflict with those they love, whereas submissive behavior is rewarded with affection and approval. Toddlers experience conflict because they want to assert their own will but do not want to risk losing the approval of loved ones. If the child continues to practice dependent behavior, doubt related to abilities develops. Toddlers may feel shame for independent impulses, particularly if frequent punishment is associated with their actions.

The toddler learns which behaviors gain approval and which result in censure and punishment. Two-year-olds do not have a conscience but avoid punishment by controlling their behavior. Right and wrong are determined by the consequences of actions.

At around 15 months, toddlers begin to demonstrate their developing autonomy with two almost universal behaviors: negativism and ritualism.

Negativism. Negativism, one of the most dramatic expressions of independence, is shown in a variety of ways. The toddler's favorite word seems to be "no." Unable to distinguish between requests and directives, the toddler seems to feel that saying "yes" would mean giving up free will. The child often seems to delight in this test of wills between parent and child. Negativism may result in screaming, kicking, hitting, biting, or breath holding. Parents often interpret the child's negative behavior as being bad or stubborn. Nurses can help parents understand their toddler's behavior as an important sign of the child's progress from dependence to autonomy and independence. The nurse should give support and encourage the parent to deal with the toddler's trying behavior with patience and a sense of humor. Although general permissiveness is not recommended, too much pressure and forceful methods of control often lead to defiance, tantrums, and prolonged negative behavior.

Ritualism and the Importance of Routine. Ritualism helps the child venture out and away from the safety of the parents by ensuring uniformity and security. Ritualism allows the toddler to have a sense of control. The child feels more confident with a secure home base. The toddler insists on sameness. Milk may have to be poured into the same cup,

Health Promotion

The 2-Year-Old Child

FOCUSED ASSESSMENT

How are you handling any discipline problems your child may be having?

Do you have any concerns about any daycare arrangements you have?

Does your child use a bottle or a cup?

How do you deal with temper tantrums?

How does your child communicate with others?

What, if anything, have you done to begin toilet training your child?

What activities do you enjoy doing together?

DEVELOPMENTAL MILESTONES

Personal/social: imitates household activities and begins to do helpful tasks; uses table utensils without much spilling; drinks from a lidless cup; removes a difficult article of clothing; begins developing sexual identity; stubborn and negativistic: wants own way in everything; brushes teeth with help; learning to walk; understands "soon"

Fine motor: puts blocks into a cup after demonstration; builds tower of four to six blocks; able to imitate a horizontal and circular stroke with a crayon; opens a doorknob; turns book pages one at a time; can unzip and unbutton

Language/cognition: has an approximately 300-word vocabulary, two-word sentences; points to six body parts and pictures of several familiar objects (e.g., bird, man, dog, horse); understands cause and effect, object permanence, sense of time; follows two-step directions; uses egocentric language (I, me, mine)

Gross motor: stoops and recovers well; walks forward and backward; climbs stairs holding the railing; runs, jumps, kicks a ball

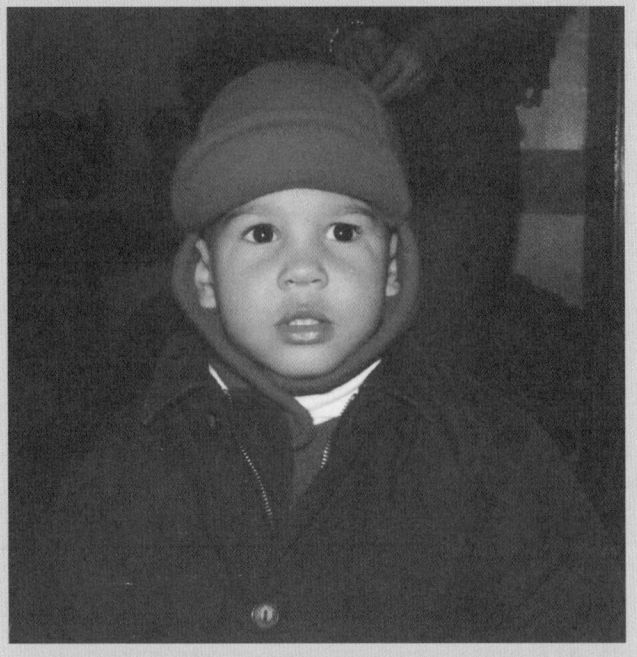

CRITICAL MILESTONES*

Personal/social: removes one article of clothing; feeds a doll; uses a spoon or fork

Fine motor: holds a pencil and scribbles spontaneously; dumps a raisin out of a bottle on command after demonstration; builds a two-block tower

Language/cognitive: points to two pictures; says three to six words

Gross motor: runs; walks up steps; kicks a ball forward

---

parents may have to sit in the same chairs at dinnertime, and a specified routine may have to be followed countless times throughout the day. The child may be unable to go to sleep unless a bedtime ritual is followed exactly (e.g., a drink of water, two stories, prayers, and a teddy bear). The child may experience distress if this routine is not followed exactly the next night. Failure to recognize the importance of such rituals may increase stress and insecurity.

Events such as hospitalization, where continuity of routine cannot be ensured, are difficult for the toddler. The nurse can decrease the stress of hospitalization by incorporating the child's usual rituals and routines from home into nursing care activities. Keeping hospital routines as similar to those of home as possible and recognizing ritualistic needs give the toddler some sense of control and security and decrease feelings of helplessness and fear. See Chapter 35 for further discussion of the hospitalized child.

Separation Anxiety. Separation anxiety peaks again in the toddler period. Although the concept of object permanence is fully developed in the toddler, children at this stage have difficulty differentiating their own feelings from those of their parents. Although the children experience a strong desire to be independent and leave their mothers, they fear that

their mothers also want to leave them. A toddler may strike out independently across the room, only to rush back in tears to the mother, as if the child were frightened and angry with the mother for leaving. For a brief period, the parent may find it almost impossible to talk on the telephone without interruption or even to go into the bathroom without being followed. Leave-taking and brief separations are acceptable to a toddler if they are the toddler's idea, but the parent's departure may cause desperate clinging and crying. Games such as hide-and-seek help the child master fears of separation. By repeating separation under conditions the child can control, the toddler is helped to overcome the anxiety associated with separation. The child learns from experience that loved ones will return after separation.

Being left with a stranger can be stressful. Toddlers should be told honestly and clearly about a separation shortly before it occurs. The parent or nurse should reassure the child that the parent is coming back. When a parent returns, the toddler often shows anger at being left by ignoring the parent or by pretending to be more interested in play than in going home. Parents of hospitalized toddlers are frequently distressed by such behavior when they visit their child (see Chapter 35).

Health Promotion—cont'd

The 2-Year-Old Child—cont'd

HEALTH MAINTENANCE

Physical Measurements
  Gains approximately 5 lb (2.25 kg) per yr
  Length is approximately half eventual adult height
  Grows approximately 3 inches (7.5 cm) per yr
Immunizations
  None needed unless making up for a delay
Health Screening
  Hemoglobin and lead screen
  Baseline cholesterol (if at risk)
  Tuberculosis (TB) screening (if at risk)

ANTICIPATORY GUIDANCE

Nutrition
  May begin low-fat milk
  Daily diet: 2 or 3 cups milk, two servings of protein, three
    small servings of vegetables, two servings of fruit, and six
    servings of bread
  Modify diet for children with elevated cholesterol (<300 mg/day,
    no more than 30% calories from fat and 10% from satu-
    rated fat): egg substitute, low-fat cheeses and meats
  Decrease added fat and high-calorie, high-fat desserts;
    increase fruits, vegetables, and carbohydrates
Elimination
  Bowel movements decrease in number and become more
    regular
  Child remains dry for several hours
  Begin to think about a positive approach to toilet training
Dental
  Sixteen teeth; may use pea-sized amount of fluoridated
    toothpaste, encourage not to swallow
  Increase fluoride dosage to 0.5 mg/day as recommended
  Schedule first dental visit

Sleep
  12 to 14 hr/day
  Usually a long afternoon nap
  Limit television viewing to no more than 1 hour daily
Hygiene
  Girls are prone to vaginal irritation; advise to wipe from front
    to back; adding 1/4 cup vinegar to bath water can relieve
    irritation
  Boys' foreskin begins to retract; retract gently to clean;
    never force
Safety
  Review toy safety, firearm safety, burn prevention, and other
    previously discussed subjects
  Discuss choking on food, street safety, water safety, outside
    poisons, playground safety, sun protection
Self-Esteem and Competence
  Model appropriate social behavior
  Encourage your child to learn to make choices
  Help your child to appropriately express emotions
  Spend individual time with your child daily
  Provide consistent and loving limits to help your child learn
    self-discipline
  Begin toilet training only when your child is ready (dry for
    2 hours, able to pull pants down, can use appropriate
    toileting words, can indicate the need to use the toilet)
Play
  Parallel play; play begins to become imitative and imaginative
  Choose toys that are safe and durable: balls, picture
    books, puzzles with large pieces, sandbox toys, trucks,
    riding toys, household toys (e.g., broom, mop, carpet
    sweeper)

*Guided by DDST II

Tolerating brief separations from parents is an important developmental task of the toddler. Transition objects, such as a favorite blanket or toy, provide comfort to the toddler in stressful situations, such as separation, illness, or even bedtime. Such objects help children make the transition from dependency to autonomy. Toddlers may become so attached to an object that they can hardly bear to part with it, even for a brief time while it is being laundered.

The nurse can offer support by explaining that the behavior is a normal growth and development milestone and telling the parents that plenty of affection and attention are needed to help the toddler cope with the stress of separation. The nurse counsels parents to leave a toddler only briefly at first and, if possible, to delay extended separations until the toddler can handle them better. The nurse who helps parents understand normal toddler behavior in response to separation helps parents cope with the frustrations of this transition.

Play. Toddlers spend most of their time at play. Play is serious business to the toddler—it is the child's work. Many hours are spent each day in play, perfecting fine and gross motor skills, learning to control inner urges, and gaining self-esteem. Play during this period reflects the developmental level of the egocentric toddler. The toddler engages in parallel play, in which children play alongside but not with other children (Fig. 6-3). Little regard is given to the feelings of others. Children engaged in this type of play frequently grab toys away from other children or may hit or fight to obtain a wanted toy. Because toddlers are egocentric, they do not realize that they are hurting the other child and feel no shame for aggressive actions.

Imitation or acting out of scenes of everyday life is common as the toddler begins to try out roles and identify with adults. Active, large-muscle play helps the toddler vent frustrations and dissipate excess energy. The nurse can help parents understand how play enhances the toddler's development. The nurse should encourage parents to play with their toddler and to provide opportunities for the toddler to play with other children. The nurse teaches parents about childproofing the house on a daily basis. Toys must be strong, safe, and too large to swallow or place in the ear or nose. Toddlers need supervision at all times. A variety of play materials, which need not be expensive, and a safe play environment enhance the toddler's development (Box 6-2).

Psychosexual Development. At around 18 months, toddlers enter Freud's anal stage. Freud theorized that as children focus on mastery of bowel and bladder functions, their

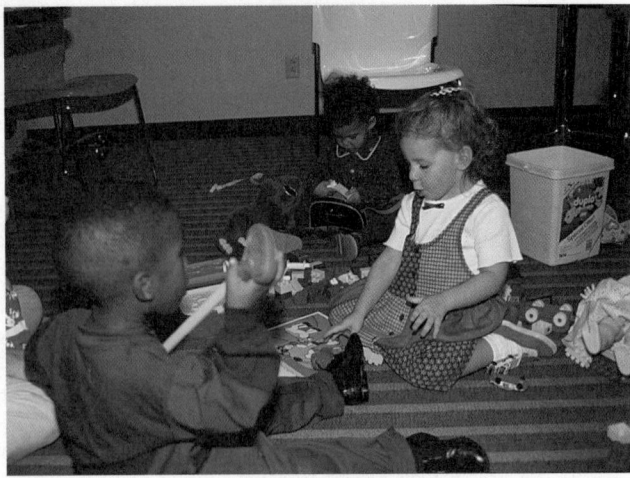

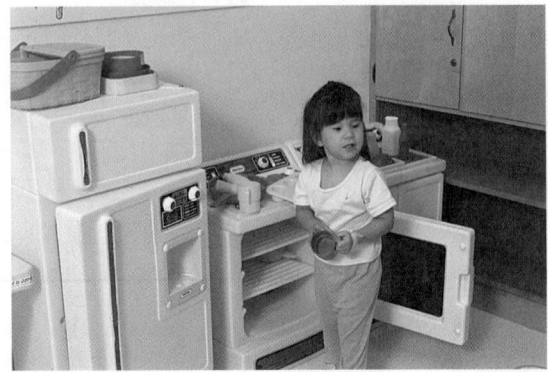

Parallel play occurs when children play side by side with similar toys but there is no organized group activity. The children play *beside* each other but not *with* each other. (Courtesy The University of Texas at Arlington School of Nursing.)

Symbolic play consists of activities that children use to express their perception of reality. This little girl is acting out a familiar adult scenario as she manipulates child-size toys that represent kitchen equipment.

Figure 6-3 Types of play.

attention is also directed to the genital area. Even before the age of 2 years, children are aware of their own gender and begin to develop a sense of gender identity. By 2½ or 3 years, toddlers can correctly identify anatomic pictures of boys and girls. It is not until 5 years of age that gender identity is fully established and the child understands gender as permanent (e.g., that gender does not change with the addition of a wig or a dress) (Kohlberg, 1966).

Children begin to be aware of expected gender role behaviors at an early age. By 3 years old, most toddlers show an awareness of gender role stereotypes and tend to imitate the same-gender parent during play. Gender role identification continues throughout the toddler and preschool years as the child incorporates the attitudes, roles, and values of the same-gender parent. Although gender role stereotypes have relaxed somewhat in recent years, children behave according to adult expectations. Children learn behavior by reinforcement and punishment as well as by imitation. If a boy repeatedly hears that boys do not play with dolls, he will spurn such "girls' toys" and will play with toys that his parents consider masculine to gain their praise and approval. Nurses should be aware of their own biases about gender-typed behaviors and should support the parents in their choice of toys and activities for their child. The nurse can be most helpful by encouraging parents to make traditionally gender-typed toys available to both boys and girls if this approach is consistent with the parents' beliefs. Parents' expectations of appropriate gender role behavior differ according to their cultural backgrounds. In most cultures, boys and girls are treated differently and thus are taught "male" and "female" behaviors.

Parents are often concerned about their toddler's interest in and curiosity about gender differences. Sex play and masturbation are common among toddlers. Nurses can reassure parents that self-exploration or exploration of another toddler's body is normal behavior during early childhood. Par-

ents should respect the child's curiosity as normal without judging the child as "bad." The child should be told that touching private parts is something that is done only in private. When parents discover children involved in sex play, casually telling them to dress and directing them to another activity can limit sex play without producing feelings of shame or anxiety. The nurse should explain to parents that positive attitudes toward sexuality are learned from parents who are comfortable with their own sexuality. As young children learn about their bodies and explore anatomic differences, they frequently ask questions about where babies come from or why "Brian looks different from Emily." Honest, straightforward answers using the correct terminology satisfy the toddler's curiosity and lay the foundation for healthy sexual attitudes.

The Preschooler

The preschool years are a critical period for the development of socialization. Children need opportunities to play with others to learn communication and social skills. They also need appropriate guidance to learn acceptable behavior.

According to Erikson, the developmental task of the preschooler is to achieve a sense of initiative. The preschooler is busy learning how to do things and takes great pride in new accomplishments. If the child acts inappropriately or is repeatedly criticized or punished for attempts to explore and learn, feelings of guilt, anxiety, shame, and fear may result. For example, an adult's comment, "That's nice, but it would look better if you did it this way," may cause the child to feel inferior. Such subtle criticism can make the child reluctant to try new activities. A feeling of inferiority also may develop if adults are always doing things for the child rather than encouraging independence. The child who does not achieve a sense of initiative will feel defeated, angry, and afraid of people and new situations. Nurses can promote the healthy psychosocial development of preschoolers and help them gain a sense of initiative by teaching parents the importance of providing the child with opportunities to explore in a safe, stimulating environment. Adults should encourage the preschooler's imagination and creativity and should praise appropriate behavior.

Play. Learning to relate to age mates is another developmental task that is significant during the preschool period. Preschoolers need experience playing with other children to learn how to relate to other people. Three-year-olds are capable of sharing and are more likely to do so than toddlers. Four-year-olds tend to be more argumentative and less generous with playmates. Although this behavior may appear to be a step backward to parents, it is actually a sign of growth because 4-year-olds feel more secure in a group and are testing their roles and communication skills. The 5-year-old enjoys playing with other children and generally can play with another child for longer periods before arguments develop.

Children between the ages of 3 and 5 years enjoy parallel and associative play. Children learn to share and cooperate as they play in small groups. During play, preschoolers learn simple games and rules, language concepts, and social roles. Play is often imitative, dramatic, and creative. Various roles are explored through play as children imitate significant adults. Preschoolers enjoy dress-up clothes, housekeeping toys, doll houses, and other toys that encourage pretending (see Fig. 6-3). Tricycles and climbing toys help to develop muscles and coordination. Preschoolers also enjoy materials for cutting, pasting, and painting. Such manipulative and creative materials stimulate imagination and fine motor development (see Box 6-2).

Imaginary friends are common about 3 years of age. Boundaries between reality and fantasy are blurred at this age, and "pretend" can seem real, especially during play. Imaginary friends serve many purposes. They may take the blame when the child misbehaves, allowing the child to save face when feeling guilty about a certain behavior. Imaginary friends may be companions during lonely times. They may accomplish a task with which the child is struggling or allow the child to practice roles. For example, the child may scold an imaginary friend and administer punishment, just as a parent would. Imaginary friends seem to be more common in highly imaginative and intelligent children.

Psychosexual Development. Sexual identity and body image are developing. Sexual curiosity and explorations are normal. Preschoolers are curious about anatomic differences and seek to investigate them. Preschoolers show interest in the differences between the genders and often compare their bodies with those of others. Playing doctor and hiding with a friend to investigate anatomic differences are common activities during the preschool period. The nurse can reassure parents that the child is simply learning about his or her body and that the parents can direct the child to another activity. Preschoolers are interested in where they came from and how babies are made. Parents should be encouraged to assess what the child already knows about the subject and to determine why the child is asking the question. The parent should answer questions simply, honestly, and matter-of-factly. The child usually neither wants nor understands detailed explanations.

Parents greatly influence their children's sexual development. Positive signs of physical and emotional intimacy between parents send a positive signal to the child. A warm, accepting, matter-of-fact attitude toward sexual matters

---

BOX 6-2
Age-Related Activities and Toys for Toddlers and Preschoolers

General Activities
Toddler
The toddler fills and empties containers, begins dramatic play, has increased use of motor skills, enjoys feeling different textures, explores the home environment, imitates orders, likes to be read to and to look at books and television that are age-appropriate.
Toys should meet the child's need for activity and inquisitiveness.
The child also enjoys manipulating small objects such as toy people, cars, and animals.

Preschooler
Dramatic play is prominent.
The child likes to run, jump, hop, and, in general, increase motor skills.
The child likes to build and create things, whether it is sand castles or mud pies.
Play is simple and imaginative.
Simple collections begin.

Toys and Specific Types of Play
Toddler
Continued exploring of the body parts of self and others; mechanical toys; objects of different textures such as clay, sand, finger paints, and bubbles; push-pull toys; large ball; sand and water play; blocks; painting; coloring with large crayons; nesting toys; large puzzles; trucks; dolls.
Therapeutic play can begin at this age.

Preschooler
Riding toys, building materials such as sand and blocks, dolls, drawing materials, crayons, cars, puzzles, books, appropriate television and videos, nonsense rhymes, singing games, pretending to be something or somebody, dressing up, finger paints, clay, cutting, pasting, simple board and card games.

---

promotes a positive, healthy perspective in children. Parents can create an atmosphere of acceptance in the early preschool years when the first questions arise. A parental attitude of "You can ask me anything" can set the stage for healthy interaction from early childhood on into adolescence, when parental guidance is so important.

Masturbation is common and may increase in frequency when the child is under stress. Parents often express concern about such behavior. The nurse can help parents handle these situations by explaining that such self-comforting behaviors are normal for this age. If the parent discovers the child masturbating, it is best to simply redirect the child's attention without punishing, shaming, or reprimanding. Children should be taught that touching their genitals is not appropriate in public.

At this age, a sense of rivalry with the same-gender parent develops. It is common for a preschool boy to compete with his father for the attention of his mother. A girl likewise may become "Daddy's girl," often cuddling and flirting with her father

---

❗ CRITICAL TO REMEMBER

Important Tasks of the Toddler Period

- Recognition of self as a separate person, with own will
- Control of impulses and acquisition of socially acceptable ways to communicate wants and needs
- Control of elimination
- Toleration of separation from the parent

BOX 6-3
Nutritious Snacks

- Fresh fruit
- Celery sticks with cheese spread
- Yogurt
- Bagels
- Carrot sticks
- Graham crackers
- Pretzels
- Puddings

---

while excluding her mother from the relationship. This rivalry is usually resolved early in the school-age period as the child identifies strongly with the same-gender parent and same-gender peers. According to Freudian theory, the oedipal stage is resolved when the child strongly identifies with the parent of the same gender. By the end of the preschool period, the child identifies with and imitates the same-gender parent. In single-parent homes, if the parent and child are not of the same gender it is important for the child to have a friendly, stable relationship with an adult relative or friend of the same gender who can serve as a role model. By age 3 years, children know gender differences. They imitate masculine and feminine behaviors in play, and gender identity is well established by 6 years.

Spiritual and Moral Development. Learning the difference between right and wrong (the development of a conscience) is another important task of the preschool period. According to Kohlberg (1964), children between the ages of 4 and 7 years are in the second stage of the preconventional level of moral development. In this stage, children obey rules out of self-interest. They tend to believe that if the consequences of an action are personally advantageous, the action is right. An "eye-for-an-eye" orientation guides their behavior.

The preschooler begins to use self-control to resist temptation and tries to "be good" to avoid feelings of guilt. Preschoolers determine right from wrong by the consequences of disobeying their parents' rules. At this age, children have little understanding of the reason for a rule. For example, when asked why it is wrong to hit another child, the preschooler might reply, "Because my mother says so." Preschoolers adhere to parents' rules dogmatically, deciding whether to break a rule based on the resulting punishment.

Preschoolers often have difficulty applying rules in different situations. The child may know that it is wrong to hit a sibling but may not understand that it is also wrong to hit another child at daycare. Because the preschooler is egocentric, understanding another's viewpoint is difficult. The child begins to develop a conscience as a result of consistent rewards for good behavior and punishment for bad behavior.

The preschool child's concept of God is concrete. The family's religious beliefs and customs, such as bedtime prayers, mealtime grace, and Bible stories, are important to preschoolers. Such rituals, practiced in an atmosphere of love, can be deeply meaningful and comforting to children of this age.

HEALTH PROMOTION FOR THE TODDLER OR PRESCHOOLER AND FAMILY

Nutrition

The rate of growth slows during the toddler and preschool period and so does the child's appetite. This is sometimes referred to as *physiologic anorexia*. The child's food experiences during this period can have a lasting effect on how food and meals are viewed. The family is the primary influence at this time, although television plays an important role. Children should be discouraged from eating while watching television, and family mealtimes should be encouraged.

Nutritional Requirements

The U.S. Department of Agriculture, Center for Nutrition Policy and Promotion has a Food Guide Pyramid specifically directed toward children ages 2 to 6 years (see Fig. 4-5 and Box 4-8). The serving recommendations associated with the Pyramid reflect the dietary guidelines for Americans, which include aiming for a healthy weight, daily physical activity, eating a variety of healthy foods, and limiting fats, sugars, and salt (U.S. Department of Agriculture, 2001). Fat and cholesterol intake, however, should not be restricted in children younger than 2 years (American Academy of Pediatrics [AAP] Committee on Nutrition, 1998a).

Many similarities exist in the nutritional needs of the toddler and the preschooler. Children this age who eat well-balanced diets should not experience iron deficiency. If milk remains the primary food, however, it will replace foods rich in iron, vitamins, and minerals, such as dark-green leafy vegetables, meats, and legumes. Three or four servings from the milk group each day are more than adequate for this age child. (See Chapter 47 for a discussion of iron deficiency anemia.) The child who is healthy does not need vitamin supplementation. However, giving a daily children's multivitamin containing 100% of the recommended daily allowance (RDA) is not harmful.

After 2 years of age, low-fat (2%) milk may be given. Milk intake should be limited to 2 or 3 cups per day. Yogurt and cheese are other milk-group sources. Poultry, fish, and lean meat are good sources of iron. Low-sugar breakfast cereals are sources of iron and vitamins. Snacks of fruits and vegetables assist in meeting the child's nutritional requirements (Box 6-3).

Solid Foods

Children at this age are increasing their proficiency in using a spoon and cup. By age 2 years, children can hold a cup in one hand and use a spoon well (Fig. 6-4). By age 12 months, most children are eating the same foods as the rest of the family. The child should be offered three meals and two snacks each day.

By age 3 to 4 years, the child begins to use a fork. The child continues to develop fine motor skills and by the end of the preschool period should begin to use a rounded knife for cutting.

One method to determine serving size for children is 1 tablespoon of solid food per year of age. Children may be more

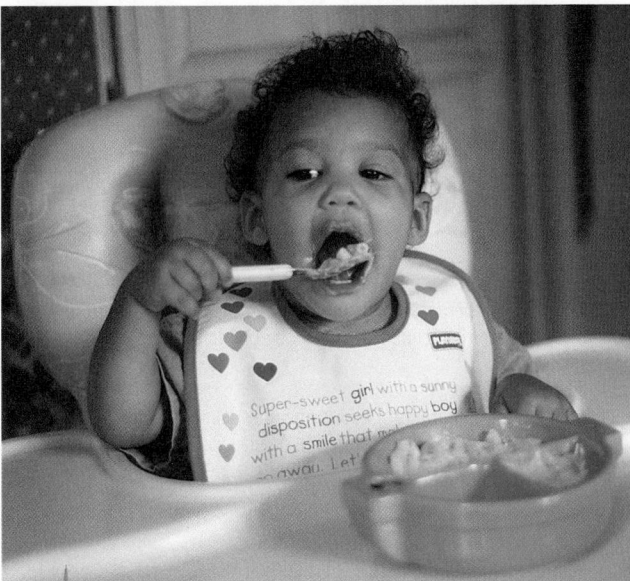

Figure 6-4 By age 1 year, most children are eating the same foods as the rest of the family. Toddlers should be offered three meals and two healthy snacks each day. Most 2-year-olds can drink from a cup and use a spoon well if given the opportunity to practice.

likely to try new foods and eat nutritious meals if smaller portions are served. Foods of different textures, colors, consistencies, tastes, and temperatures should be offered. The child should sit in a chair that allows easy access to the food; the dishes should be small, nonbreakable, and, when possible, steady enough to prevent spilling. Thick, short-handled spoons and forks and shallow bowls increase the toddler's ability to eat successfully.

Foods that could be aspirated should continue to be avoided during the toddler period. Soft drinks and candy need to be discouraged. Sugar is a source of calories and is naturally present in breast milk as lactose, in fruits as fructose, and in grain products as maltose. A diet with too much sugar, however, can replace other more nutritious foods and increase tooth decay. Artificial sweeteners and foods that contain artificial sweeteners are not recommended for children younger than 2 years.

Age-Related Nutritional Challenges

Food Jags. The volume of food the child eats may vary from day to day. The child may want the same food at every meal for several days and then suddenly reject the food completely. Children this age may refuse foods because of odor and temperature. They may not like mixing foods and therefore may not eat casseroles. This dislike does not seem to apply to foods such as pizza, spaghetti, and macaroni and cheese. Many children prefer juices to milk and water. Too much milk is not good, but neither is too much juice, because it can replace other foods and their nutrients. Juices should be limited to no more than one cup a day. Parents and older siblings can affect how a child views a food and should be careful about making negative comments about a certain food. Children should be assisted in developing tastes for new foods through role modeling and making the foods available.

Physiologic Anorexia. It is important for the nurse to teach parents appropriate ways to approach the child who is

---

BOX 6-4
Increasing Nutritional Intake

- Limit to two nutritious snacks per day, and give only at toddler's request.
- Limit to 6 oz of juice per day.
- Introduce to finger foods at age 8 to 10 months, and continue to make these types of food available.
- Limit to 16 to 24 oz of milk per day.
- Keep mealtimes pleasant.
- Do not force feed.
- Do not feed children who can feed themselves.

experiencing physiologic anorexia. Advise parents not to allow their child to fill up with snacks, milk, and juices. Small portions should be offered so that the child does not feel overwhelmed by the amount of food. Mealtimes should be pleasant and not times to discuss discipline problems or even the child's poor appetite. Children should not be made to sit at the table after the rest of the family has left. This will only create a negative association with mealtime. Parents need to maintain a balance between ignoring their child's nutritional intake and making it the focus of their parenting.

The nurse can encourage parents to focus more on their child's weekly nutritional intake, rather than on one day's intake. Frequently, children are the best judge of what they need, and they may eat primarily fruit one day and peanut butter the next. Nutritional consumption tends to balance out over a week. Box 6-4 illustrates ways parents can increase their child's nutritional intake.

Dental Care

Most toddlers have a complete set of 20 deciduous teeth by the time they are 30 months old. Although the exact time of eruption of teeth varies, an approximate rule of thumb to assess the number of teeth is the age of the toddler in months minus 6. Usually, one tooth erupts for each month of age past 6 months up to 30 months of age.

Permanent teeth are calcifying during the toddler period, long before they are visible. Proper care of the deciduous teeth is crucial for the toddler's general health and for the health and alignment of the permanent teeth. Deciduous teeth play an important role in the growth and development of the jaws and face and in speech development. Premature loss of the deciduous teeth complicates eruption of the permanent teeth, often leading to malocclusion. Nurses need to be aware that some parents do not understand the value of preserving primary teeth.

Because toddlers do not have the manual dexterity to remove plaque adequately, parents must be responsible for cleaning their teeth (Fig. 6-5). Children can be encouraged to brush their teeth after the teeth have been thoroughly cleaned by a parent. Because toddlers like to imitate, watching parents brush their teeth can be motivating. A small, soft, nylon bristle brush works best. Optimal access and visibility are provided if the parent sits on the floor or bed with the child's head in the parent's lap and the child's body perpendicular to the parent's. This position also gives the parent some control of the child's head movement. Toothpaste is not recommended for young children because they often do not

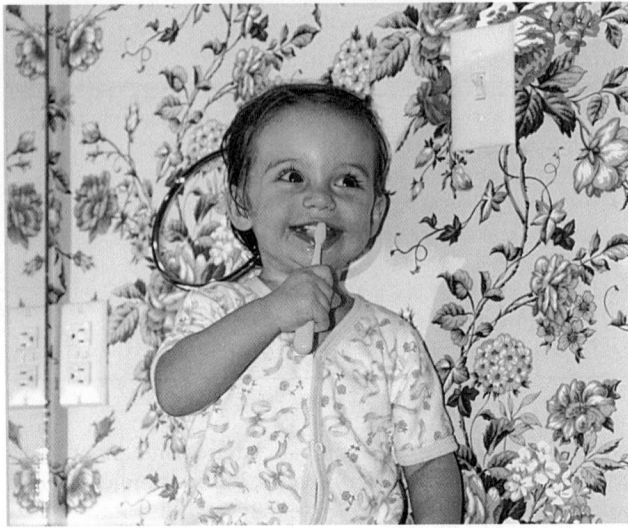

Figure 6-5 Care of the deciduous teeth promotes healthy development of the permanent teeth. Because 2-year-olds lack the manual dexterity to remove plaque adequately, parents must assume responsibility for cleaning the toddler's teeth.

TABLE **6-2** Fluoride Supplementation Schedule for Infants and Children (Revised 1994)		
	Fluoride in Home Water (PPM)		
Age of Child	<0.3 milligrams	0.3-0.6	>0.6
Birth to 6 mo	0	0	0
6 mo to 3 yr	0.25	0	0
3-6 yr	0.5	0.25	0
6-16 yr	1.0	0.5	0

Reprinted with the permission of the American Dental Association, copyright owner. Reproduction or republication strictly prohibited without prior written permission.
ppm, Parts per million.
NOTE: Numbers are milligrams of fluoride per day. Jointly endorsed by the American Academy of Pediatrics, the American Academy of Pediatric Dentistry, and the American Dental Association.

like the taste or, if they do, tend to swallow it. If the child receives fluoride from other sources, such as water or supplements, excess amounts of fluoride may be ingested if fluoride toothpaste is swallowed. Ingestion of excessive amounts of fluoride may lead to *fluorosis,* which produces white speckles or brown discoloration of the enamel. Ideally, teeth should be brushed after every meal and especially at bedtime. Flossing between teeth helps remove plaque and should be done daily by the parent after the toddler's teeth are brushed.

Fluoride makes tooth enamel resistant to acid attack, preventing decay. Fluoride supplementation is no longer recommended from birth, and doses during the first 6 years of life have been decreased (Roberts, Keels, Sharp, and Lewis, 1998). Supplements are recommended for children in some age-groups living in areas with less-than-optimal fluoride in the drinking water supply (Table 6-2).

A diet that is low in sweets and high in nutritious food promotes dental health. Sweets are most likely to cause caries if they are sticky or if they are eaten between meals rather than with meals. Encourage the parent to offer nutritious snacks, such as fresh fruit, yogurt, or cheese, instead of candy, soda, or cookies.

The child should first see the dentist 6 months after the first primary tooth erupts and no later than age 30 months. The first appointment should precede any needed dental work so that the visit is enjoyable and free from discomfort. This visit provides an opportunity for early assessment of the child's dental health as well as for teaching parents good preventive dental health practices.

Because the enamel on primary teeth is thinner than on permanent teeth, preschoolers' teeth are prone to destruction from decay. The distance from the tooth surface to the pulp is shorter also, so tooth abscesses from caries can occur rapidly. Untreated caries can lead to pain, abscess formation, and poor digestion because of ineffective chewing. Many parents do not realize that the deciduous teeth are important to protect the dental arch. If deciduous teeth are lost early (e.g., because of decay), the remaining teeth may drift out of posi-

tion, block proper eruption of the permanent teeth, and lead to malocclusion.

Nurses play an important role in the promotion of dental health by teaching proper tooth cleaning, including the removal of plaque and the importance of adequate fluoride ingestion; encouraging a balanced diet, limited in sweets; and recommending twice-yearly visits to the dentist. Preschoolers can usually brush their own teeth. Short back-and-forth or up-and-down strokes are easiest for the child to manage. Parents should monitor the child's tooth brushing and inspect the child's teeth to be sure that all plaque has been removed. Parents must help with flossing because it requires more manual dexterity than preschoolers have.

Sleep and Rest

During the 2nd year, children require approximately 12 to 14 hours of sleep each day. Most 2-year-olds take one nap each day until the end of the 2nd or 3rd year, when many children give up the habit. Toddlers often resist going to bed, using dawdling or even temper tantrums to postpone separation from loved ones and the exciting events of the day. Firm, consistent limits are needed when toddlers try stalling tactics, such as asking for one more drink of water.

Warning the child a few minutes before it is time for bed may reduce bedtime protests. Winding down with a quiet activity for 30 minutes before bedtime also helps toddlers prepare for sleep. Bedtime offers an opportunity for some snuggle time, when the parent and toddler can read a story and share the events of the day. Children of this age often have trouble relaxing and falling asleep. A warm bath before bedtime promotes relaxation. Bedtime rituals are important and should be followed consistently. Transition objects, such as a favorite blanket or stuffed animal, are often an important part of the child's bedtime routine.

Because preschoolers expend so much energy growing and learning, they need adequate rest. The preschooler needs an average of 10 to 12 hours of sleep in a 24-hour period. Some preschoolers do well without a nap during the day, but others still need a nap. Resistance to naps is common at this age. The child usually does not want to leave family or playmates, toys, and exciting activities to go into a darkened room to lie down and rest. A quiet time spent listening to music or looking at a favorite book may help the child relax and get some rest. Insufficient rest during the day may lead to irritability, decreased resistance to infection, and difficulty sleeping at night.

Sleep problems are more common during the preschool years than in any other period of childhood. Because of their active imaginations and immaturity, preschoolers often have nightmares and have trouble falling asleep at night. Because the boundaries between reality and fantasy are not well defined for children of this age, monsters and scary creatures that lurk in the preschooler's imagination become real to the child after the light is turned off. Patient and repeated reassurance from a caring parent may be needed. Nightmares—frightening dreams that awaken the child from sleep—are common among preschoolers. A familiar environment and comforting with a hug and verbal reassurance from a parent usually enable the child to return to sleep. Night terrors differ from nightmares. Night terrors occur during deep sleep, and the child remains asleep even though the eyes may be open. The child does not awaken but moans, screams, or cries and does not recognize parents. Efforts to comfort the child may lead to agitation. The child does not remember the episode in the morning, even if awakened during the night terror. Parents should be instructed not to attempt to comfort or awaken the child during a night terror but should allow the child to sleep.

The nurse should assess sleep patterns during well-child visits and address parental concerns. The nurse can reassure parents that resistance to going to bed, fears, and nightmares are normal for children of this age. The nurse should assess the frequency of sleep problems and parents' reactions to them. If sleep problems occur often and are disruptive to the family, further investigation and intervention may be indicated.

Ritualistic techniques and transition objects that helped decrease bedtime resistance in the toddler are continued during the preschool period. Avoiding high-carbohydrate snacks and excitement before bedtime promotes relaxation. Children should not be forced to face their fears alone by sleeping in a completely dark room or with the door shut. Parents can search the room to reassure the preschooler that the room is safe. Progressive head-to-toe relaxation is an effective technique for helping preschoolers fall asleep. A set bedtime promotes security and healthy sleep habits.

A child who has slept for a long time at the baby-sitter's or at daycare may not be ready to sleep again. Communication with the child's daytime caretaker is important to determine whether the child is maintaining a balance of activity, rest, and sleep.

Discipline

Effective discipline strategies should include a comprehensive approach that includes consideration of the parent-child relationship, reinforcement of desired behaviors, and consequences for negative behaviors (AAP Committee on Psychosocial Aspects of Child and Family Health, 1998; Banks, 2002). One goal of discipline and limit setting is to teach self-control. Eventually the child internalizes controls established by parental limits and begins to develop a conscience.

Toddlers need and want discipline to feel secure. They have little control over their behavior and need limits to learn how to behave and how to follow the rules and expectations of society. Toddlers' negativism, intense emotions, and curiosity place them at risk for injury. Because they are

---

Critical Thinking EXERCISE 6-1

Mr. and Mrs. Thomas have brought 2-year-old Todd to the clinic for his annual physical examination. The parents report that bedtime is a major production almost every night. They state that he cries, comes out of his room, and displays various other behaviors that delay sleep. They wonder if he has a sleep disorder. They relate that, other than an occasional temper tantrum, they do not have any other concerns.
1. What information do you need from the parents to assess the problem?
2. After you have the above information, what advice should you give the Thomases?

---

usually unaware of the consequences of their actions, vigilance and limits are needed for safety. Toddlers are frightened by a lack of limits and will deliberately test their parents until they are shown how far they can go. Firm discipline promotes the development of autonomy by giving the child a feeling of freedom within bounds.

Toddlers often repeat parental prohibitions to themselves while engaging in a forbidden activity. For example, a toddler may walk over to an electrical outlet, knowing that it is out of bounds, and mumble, "No, no, hurt!" while playing with the outlet. Although remembering the prohibition, the toddler lacks sufficient self-control to prevent the behavior.

Effective discipline techniques for children of this age include a time-out (1 minute per year of age), diversion, and positive reinforcement. Teaching parents how to discipline their child helps avoid problems related to the incorrect use of discipline. It is very important that the parent be consistent. Physical punishment, such as spanking, is one of the least effective discipline techniques (see Chapter 3).

Preschoolers are struggling to gain control over their strong inner impulses. To achieve this control, they need limits set on their behavior. When limits are set, the child feels more secure and can explore the environment and try out new roles in an atmosphere of freedom and safety. Appropriate limit setting helps the child learn self-confidence, self-control, and moral values. The child must be consistently disciplined for acts that are destructive, socially unacceptable, or morally wrong. Limits must be clearly defined and consistently enforced to be effective. To prevent confusion and anxiety, the consequences of misbehavior should be spelled out in advance and carried out immediately after misbehavior occurs. When the child is disciplined for misbehavior, a simple, truthful explanation of why the behavior was unacceptable should be given.

The focus of the explanation should be on the behavior rather than on the child. For example, "I don't like to see you throwing toys" is a better response than "I don't want to be around you when you act like that" or "You're a bad girl for doing that."

Discipline techniques that are effective with preschoolers include:

- Time-out (removing the child from a situation for a short period and offering an explanation for the punishment).
- Time-in (frequent, brief, nonverbal, physical contact when the child is acting appropriately). For example, the mother periodically strokes the child's hair or rubs his back

PARENTS
Want to Know

Guidelines for Disciplining a Toddler

- Discipline must be consistent. Inconsistency is confusing and counterproductive. It is important to follow through every time.
- Discipline must be immediate. Consequences of behavior should occur as soon as possible after the behavior occurs. Threats such as "Just wait until your father gets home!" are confusing and ineffective for a child of this age.
- Discipline must be realistic and age-appropriate. Toddlers should not be expected to act like "little ladies" or "little gentlemen."
- Discipline must be related to the incident. Consequences that are logical results of a behavior are most effective.
- Limits must be clearly explained to the child.
- Toddlers must be given time to respond to instructions.
- Withdrawal of love should never be used as punishment. Comforting the child after discipline promotes positive feelings. Love is the key to effective discipline.
- Arguments and extensive explanations should be avoided.
- Praise for good behavior should be used to build self-confidence and self-esteem.
- The toddler must be separated from the behavior: "I love you very much. Hitting your sister needs to stop."

! CRITICAL TO REMEMBER

Car Safety

Toddlers should be restrained in an upright, forward-facing position in a car safety seat until they outgrow the manufacturer's weight or height recommendations (usually 40 lb [18.14 kg] and at 3 to 5 years of age).

Car doors should be locked while the car is in motion to prevent a curious toddler from opening the door.

Until passenger vehicles are equipped with air bags that are safe and effective for children, children younger than 13 years should not ride in a front passenger seat that is equipped with an air bag.

A booster seat with lap and shoulder belt is recommended for a preschooler who weighs more than 40 lb. It raises the child to a level that accommodates the car's seat belt system. Children usually use a booster seat until they are tall enough to properly wear the seat/shoulder belt (height >4' 9")(AAP, 2003a).

when he is quietly playing on the floor near his mother while she talks on the telephone. The child who receives this type of reinforcement is more likely to continue what he is doing and much less likely to interrupt the mother.

- Offering restricted choices (e.g., "You may drink your juice in the kitchen or you may go into the living room without your juice.").
- Diversion (e.g., "You must stop marking on the wall with crayons. Here, mark on this paper instead.").

Consistent positive reinforcement for desired behavior is a powerful tool. If the parent does not care or is too busy to enforce rules consistently, the child will not internalize rules and will not feel guilty about breaking them. The child will be unruly and will be unable to follow the rules set by society.

Spending enjoyable time with their children is another way parents can model positive behaviors. Having good times with children increases the children's self-esteem and reinforces good behavior. Chapter 3 present additional discussions of discipline.

Toddler Safety

Understanding the developmental changes a toddler undergoes helps the nurse and parent appreciate why children are more injury-prone in this stage of development than at any other time. Constant supervision is challenging for parents but is the most important factor in preventing injuries in this energetic age-group.

Car Safety

Motor vehicle injuries are a significant threat to the toddler. Although toddlers begin to develop more independent behaviors, they are still wholly reliant on an adult for protection while traveling in a car. Once a toddler is able to sit up alone, car safety seats can be adjusted to face forward in an upright position. Safety straps should be adjusted to provide a snug fit.

Because children begin to imitate their parents at an early age, the nurse encourages parents to model safe behavior by consistently wearing their seat belts. As the toddler's cognitive and fine motor skills develop, some children wiggle free of the restraining system, despite releases that are designed to be difficult for a child to operate. Parents must insist on compliance in spite of temper tantrums.

Because of the toddler's short physical stature, adults should visually inspect the area surrounding the automobile before placing it in gear. A toddler near the car may not be visible and can sustain serious crushing injuries if run over by the car or trapped between the car and a stationary object. There is always the potential for a toddler to dart out on foot into oncoming traffic. Parents need to closely supervise play activities and remain physically close to the toddler to prevent these types of injuries.

Toddlers or infants should never be left unattended in a car, even for a moment. Exposure to extreme heat or cold is dangerous in this age-group. Injuries have occurred when parents have left cars running for various reasons and curious toddlers have disengaged the gears, causing the car to roll and collide with other objects.

Airplane Safety

There is ongoing concern regarding the lack of regulations to ensure that children younger than 2 years are restrained properly during airplane flights. Encourage parents to use a forward-facing restraint for children weighing more than 20 lb (9.07 kg) and older than 1 year, until they are able to sit properly in a standard aircraft seat with the seat belt fastened securely and low across their laps (AAP, 1998).

Fire and Burn Safety

Toddlers, with their increased mobility and developing fine motor skills, can reach hot water, open fires, or hot objects placed on counters and stoves above their eye level. They may pull objects off stoves, pull down cords attached to small appliances, open oven doors, and place electric cords or frayed wires into their mouths. They may drink liquids that are dangerously hot. The nurse emphasizes to parents to remain in the kitchen when preparing a meal, to use the back burners on the stove, and to turn pot handles inward and toward the middle of the stove to reduce the toddler's risk of burn injuries. Dangling cords from irons or other small appliances should not be accessible to toddlers. Open fires and heaters are also inviting. Sturdy guards fixed to the wall prevent young children from getting too close to these burn hazards. In addition, the curious toddler is fascinated with matches and lighters; therefore they must be kept out of reach.

Toddlers depend on adults for their protection in the event of a house fire. Anticipatory guidance emphasizes the importance of smoke detectors and escape plans.

Preventing Falls

Toddlers move quickly and climb everywhere. Toddlers can fall from playground equipment, off tricycles, and out of windows. Falls from above the first floor of a building can result in serious injury. A chair next to a kitchen counter or table allows the toddler easy access to dangerously high places. Because climbing and exploration are normal aspects of the developmental process, safety education for the parent emphasizes constant supervision and some anticipatory planning, such as moving furniture, installing screen guards, or restricting access to potential climbing hazards.

Water Safety

Toddlers love to play in water. Most drownings occur when a child is left alone in a bathtub or falls into a residential pool. Even when a child survives a submersion injury, the risk of permanent brain and lung damage is great. Parents should not leave a child alone in or near a bathtub, pail of water, wading or swimming pool, or any other body of water, even for a moment. A toddler can drown in as little as 1 inch of water. Toilet lids need to remain closed. Toddlers can inadvertently fall headfirst into a toilet or bucket, and they lack the upper-body strength and coordination to remove themselves from submersion. Fencing on all four sides with a locked entry should surround in-ground swimming pools. Preventing drowning requires constant parental supervision of the toddler.

Preventing Poisoning

Children younger than 5 years are the most common victims of poisoning, and children ages 1 to 3 years are at the highest risk. The home is the site of exposure in most cases, with poisoning from medication ingestion being the major cause (Agran et al., 2003). With exploration, everything eventually finds its way to the child's mouth, even if it does not smell or taste good. Small children who are thirsty or hungry will ingest poisons that look or smell inviting.

The nurse can help parents poison-proof the home (see Parents Want to Know box) and teach them the appropriate actions to take if an ingestion occurs: immediately contacting a poison control center or a physician. The American Academy of Pediatrics no longer recommends keeping syrup of ipecac in the home (AAP, 2003c). In case of an ingestion, the parent should immediately call the local poison control center. If the child is unconscious, having a seizure, or not breathing, the parent should immediately call 911 or the local emergency number (AAP, 2003b)

Medicine should never be called candy, and because young children often mimic their parents, adults should be

---

PARENTS
Want to Know

Childhood Poison Prevention

- Keep all poisons, medicines, cleaners, and toxic substances out of the reach of children. Never discard poisons in a wastebasket.
- Parents should be familiar with poisons commonly found in or near the home, including detergents, drain cleaner, dishwashing soap, furniture polish, cleaning agents, window cleaners, all medicines, vitamins, children's medications, sprays, powders, cosmetics, fingernail preparations, hair care products, sachets, mothballs, rodent poisons, fertilizers, gasoline, antifreeze, paints, glues, insecticides, cigarette butts, plants, and shrubs.
- Poisons should be stored in areas that are secured with locks or protected by child-resistant safety latches.
- Medicines and all harmful substances should be purchased in child-resistant packages.
- Alcoholic beverages should be kept out of the reach of children or locked in a separate cabinet. Parents should be discouraged from giving sips of alcohol to children, because small amounts can be toxic to young children.
- Children should not be allowed to chew on plants or shrubs.
- Ashtrays should be kept empty and out of the reach of small children.
- Handbags and overnight luggage of guests in the home often contain medicines or other toxic substances and should be kept out of a child's reach.
- Poisons or harmful substances should always be stored in the original container. Parents should be discouraged from placing toxic substances in food or beverage containers for storage.
- Children should be taught to ask an adult before they touch a nonfood substance.
- Parents should poison-proof all areas of the home, especially the following areas: kitchen, bathroom, pantry, bedroom, garage, basement, and work areas. Grandparents and other caregivers should be encouraged to do the same.
- The telephone number of the local poison control center should be posted for immediate access in the event of a poisoning. The National Poison Help Line number 1-800-222-1222 will connect to the local poison control number, which is staffed 24 hours a day, seven days a week. Parents should be instructed, when contacting the poison control center, to have on hand the substance with the label for prompt identification of toxic ingredients. Additionally, parents should not administer anything to the child without contacting the poison control center first.

---

discouraged from taking medicine in the child's presence. The nurse needs to advise parents to take the same precautions when small children go to a grandparent's home to visit. Childproof caps slow the child but are not an absolute barrier. Labeling poisons with characteristic symbols, such as the skull and crossbones or "Mr. Yuk," helps provide visual cues to young children; however, labels are not absolute deterrents for a determined child. The best way to prevent toxic ingestions is by carefully storing all potential poisons in a place that is inaccessible to children.

Health Promotion

The 3-Year-Old Child

FOCUSED ASSESSMENT

How are you handling any discipline problems your child may be having?

Have you been able to encourage your child to be independent and express ideas that may be different from yours?

Is your child in preschool or daycare? How many hours or days?

How does your child get along with other children the same age?

How well does your child communicate with others?

How well is your child doing with toilet training?

What activities do you enjoy doing together?

DEVELOPMENTAL MILESTONES

Personal/social: puts on articles of clothing; brushes teeth with help; washes and dries hands using soap and water; notices gender differences and identifies with children of own gender; exhibits sexual curiosity, may begin to masturbate; knows own name and names one or more friends; increasing independence, may start preschool; ritualistic; understands taking turns and sharing but may not be ready to do so; beginning fears (dark, shadows, animals)

Fine motor: vision approaches 20/20; builds a tower of at least eight blocks; begins purposeful drawing, can imitate a circle and a cross and draw a person with three parts; feeds self well

Language/cognition: increasing vocabulary with intelligible speech, although stuttering is common (thinks faster than can talk); names four familiar objects and begins to describe qualities or actions of objects; knows meaning of common adjectives (sleepy, hungry, hot); begins color identification; uses symbolic language; still egocentric; increased concept of time, space, causality; constantly asks "how" and "why" questions; can count to 3; can tell full name, age, and gender

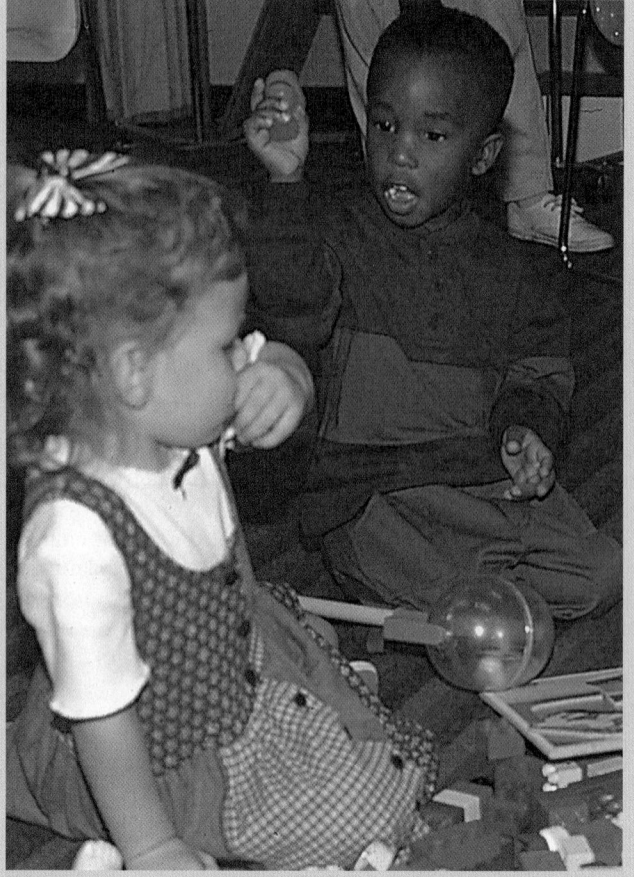

Gross motor: jumps with both feet up and down and over a short distance; throws a ball overhand; catches a large ball with both hands; balances on each foot for at least 2 seconds; begins to ride a tricycle

Preschooler Safety

Preschoolers are active and inquisitive. They have greater self-control, but their understanding of danger is not fully developed. Safety becomes even more challenging for the parent because preschoolers are no longer content with their own back yards. Preschoolers are mesmerized by cartoons that depict make-believe situations. They see cartoon characters engaging in daring endeavors and walking away unharmed. Because of their magical thinking, preschoolers may believe that these feats are possible and may attempt them.

Safety education can now be directed toward the child as well as the parent. Children of this age have a strong sense of rhythm, and songs and rhymes about safety can enhance the learning process. Instruction should be simple, with one concept introduced at a time. Short stories, puppet shows, songs, coloring activities, and role-playing games are all suitable learning activities that help preschoolers learn safety-conscious behaviors.

Car Safety

Preschoolers need to remain in a car safety seat until they weigh 40 lb (18.14 kg) or are too tall for the safety seat according to manufacturer's recommendations. Once a child has outgrown the child car safety seat, an approved booster seat, positioned high enough to safely use the lap/shoulder belt, is strongly recommended (Fig. 6-6). Although preferable to no restraints at all, standard seat belts alone can contribute to injury because they fit poorly over the small frame of the preschooler. The standard shoulder harness often crosses the child's face or neck, and the lap belt is positioned across the mid-abdomen rather than across the bony structure of the pelvis. Booster seats are designed to raise the child high enough so that the restraining straps are correctly positioned over the child's smaller body frame.

Parents continue to have primary responsibility for ensuring that a child is safely restrained before the vehicle is started and in motion. Parents must insist that children remain restrained at all times and that seat belts be used cor-

Health Promotion—cont'd

The 3-Year-Old Child—cont'd

CRITICAL MILESTONES*

Personal/social: brushes teeth with help, puts on clothing, feeds a doll

Fine motor: builds a tower of at least four to six cubes

Language/cognition: points to and names four familiar pictures (cat, horse, bird, dog, man); speech understandable 50% of the time

Gross motor: throws a ball overhand; jumps; kicks a ball forward

HEALTH MAINTENANCE

Physical Measurements
  Continue to plot height and weight
  Change to height growth chart if child able to stand while being measured
  Growth rate is similar to that of a 2-year-old
Immunizations
  Administer any immunizations not given previously according to the recommended schedule
Health Screening
  Objective vision screening using an appropriate chart
  Objective hearing screening using age-appropriate audiometry equipment
  Blood pressure measurement
  Hemoglobin, hematocrit, and lead screening
  Tuberculosis (TB) screening if at risk
  Cholesterol screening if at risk

ANTICIPATORY GUIDANCE

Nutrition
  Similar to that of a 2-year-old
Elimination
  Usually is toilet trained but not at night

Dental
  Continue to have the child brush with toothpaste and take recommended fluoride
  Child should see the dentist every 6 months
Sleep
  Similar to that of a 2-year-old
  May relinquish the nap
  Consider changing to a full bed if climbing out of the crib
  May begin to experience night terrors
Hygiene
  Similar to that of a 2-year-old
  Remind the child about good handwashing, especially after toileting and before meals
Safety
  Review choking on food, street safety, water safety, sun protection, outside poisons, playground safety
  Discuss bike and tricycle safety, fire safety, car seats (change to a forward-facing approved booster seat when the child reaches 40 lb)
Self-Esteem and Competence
  Model appropriate social behavior
  Encourage your child to learn to make choices
  Help your child to appropriately express emotions
  Spend individual time with your child daily, and encourage your child to talk about the day's events
  Provide consistent and loving limits to help your child learn self-discipline
Play
  Similar to that of a 2-year-old
  Likes imitative toys, large Legos, musical toys, blocks, and riding toys such as large trucks

* Guided by DDST II

---

rectly. Although it may seem fun and relatively harmless, riding in the open bed of a pickup truck or in the cargo area of a van or station wagon can be deadly in the event of a crash. It is outlawed in some states.

Fire and Burn Safety

Preschoolers imitate adults in all types of daily routines and activities. They may attempt these activities before they are able to manage an appliance safely (e.g., stove, iron, oven), increasing the risk of burn injuries. Matches and lighters continue to fascinate preschoolers. With their increased fine motor skills, preschoolers may be able to ignite a flame. Teaching a preschooler that lighters and matches are adult tools and instructing them to tell an adult immediately if they find these items can prevent burn injuries.

Children younger than 5 years are at the greatest risk for burn deaths in a house fire. They often panic and hide in closets or under beds rather than escaping safely. Parents need to practice fire drills with their children to teach them what to do in the event of a house fire. Preschoolers should become fa-

miliar with the sounds emitted by smoke alarms and be taught to crawl under smoke and to check doors for heat.

Preschoolers are at an ideal age to learn what to do if their clothing ignites in flames. Instruct preschoolers to stop immediately if their clothes catch on fire and to cover their face and mouth with their hands. They should then drop to the ground and roll to smother the flames. This simple command (stop, drop, roll) can help prevent severe burn injuries. Teaching specific behaviors educates children to remain calm and not panic.

Firearm Safety

Many guns are kept in the home loaded and readily accessible to young children. Parents should be encouraged to evaluate critically their need for a firearm in the home. Do the potentially devastating risks outweigh any benefits of keeping a weapon in the home? The nurse needs to talk to all parents about gun safety at every well visit because, even though parents may not keep a gun in the house, children may visit friends whose parents do. Parents who choose to

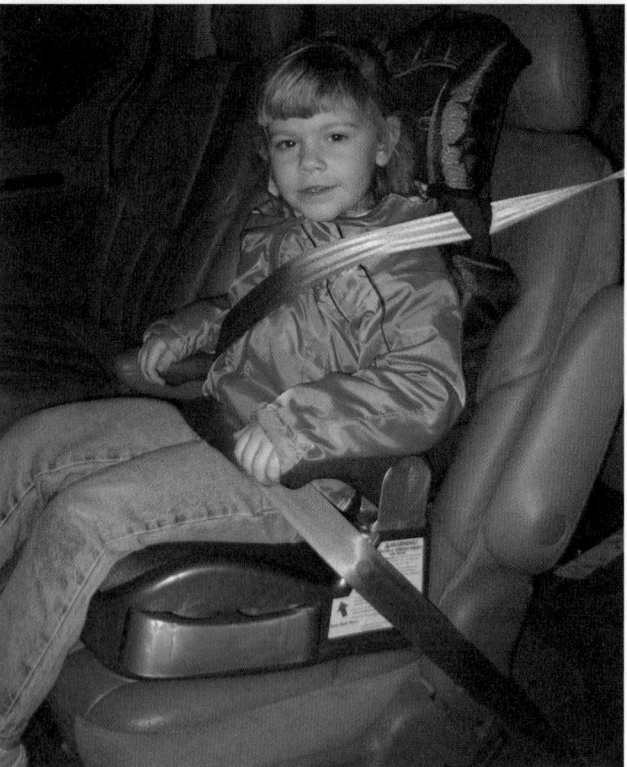

Figure 6-6 A high-back booster seat designed to properly hold a car lap and shoulder belt is strongly recommended for children who have outgrown a child safety seat. Booster seats raise the young child high enough to allow the car seatbelts to be correctly positioned over the child's chest and pelvis. Photo courtesy M. Hayden.

keep a gun in the home should receive anticipatory guidance about injury prevention. Guns kept in the home should always be unloaded, stored with trigger guards in place, securely locked in metal vaults, and inaccessible to all children.

Personal Safety

Preschoolers have an interest in establishing relationships with others as they expand the boundaries of their world. With the child's increasing assertion of independence, parents are less able to provide the constant protection they once did.

Teaching children about personal safety encourages them to develop skills to detect danger and teaches appropriate ways to handle threatening situations. Strangers are often portrayed as evil characters, when in reality their appearance and approach may be nonthreatening and friendly. Distinguishing a stranger from a well-intentioned person is challenging and often difficult for the preschooler. Basic guidelines that a child needs to know about personal safety include saying no, getting away, and telling an adult.

Children need to know how to access emergency help if they need it. Parents should help their children learn to identify safety officials and how to dial 911 or other locally appropriate emergency numbers. Children need to respond to emergency operators with their full name, address, parent's name, and other appropriate information and should remain on the phone until help arrives. Parents can practice this safety skill with their children to ensure proper reactions in

an emergency and to help the child understand what constitutes an emergency situation.

Sexual Abuse

Sexual abuse is another threat to personal safety. Preventing sexual abuse begins with teaching children the normal, healthy boundaries of their bodies and what constitutes inappropriate behavior. Often the perpetrators are known and trusted by the child. Abusers frequently intimidate the child into silence with threats of personal harm or suggestions that the child initiated the behavior. Children need to know that no matter how great the threat, if someone is touching their body in an inappropriate way, they should always tell an adult. If that adult cannot help them, they should tell as many adults as necessary until the inappropriate behavior is stopped (see Chapter 53).

Selected Issues Related to the Toddler

Toilet Training

Control of elimination is one of the major tasks of toddlerhood. Successful toilet training depends on both the child's and parent's readiness. The parent must be willing to spend the necessary time and emotional energy to encourage the child on a daily basis.

Toilet training is one of the most frustrating and time-consuming tasks that parents face. It can be so frustrating for some that researchers have linked toilet training accidents with many cases of child abuse. Parents who do not understand normal growth and development patterns often have unrealistic expectations and can become frustrated to the point of rage.

The nurse can assist parents by explaining developmental milestones and encouraging parents not to begin training until the child shows signs of readiness. Toilet training proceeds at different times in different cultures. Helping the parent to recognize both signs of readiness (Box 6-5) and factors that interfere with toilet training, such as stress, can make the training easier. The parent may not have the necessary reserves of patience and energy for toilet training during stressful times, such as near the birth of another child or while moving to a new house. Training may be easier if it is postponed until routines return to normal.

The nurse can assist parents in toilet training the toddler by explaining the importance of maturation to successful toilet training. Parents need to know that both physical readiness and psychologic readiness are necessary for toilet training to be successful. Myelinization of the spinal cord, which usually occurs between 12 and 18 months, must be complete before the child can voluntarily control bowel and bladder sphincters. The nurse can offer anticipatory guidance to parents by teaching them the signs that the toddler is ready for toilet training. The average toddler is not ready for toilet training to begin until 18 to 24 months of age. Waiting until the child is 24 to 30 months old makes the task considerably easier because toddlers of this age are less negative and usually are more willing to control their sphincters to please their parents.

There are no set rules or timetables for toilet training (Fig. 6-7). The age at which toilet training is usually begun varies from culture to culture. If the child resists, it is helpful to stop training and wait 30 to 60 days and begin again. Bowel control is usually achieved before bladder control.

BOX 6-5
Signs of Readiness for Toilet Training

Physical Readiness
Child can remove own clothing.
Child is willing to let go of a toy when asked.
Child is able to sit, squat, and walk well.
Child has been walking for 1 year.

Psychologic Readiness
Child notices if diaper is wet.
Child may indicate that diaper needs to be changed by
   pulling on diaper, squatting, or repeating a word or phrase.
Child communicates need to go to the bathroom or can get
   there by self.
Child wants to please parent by staying dry.

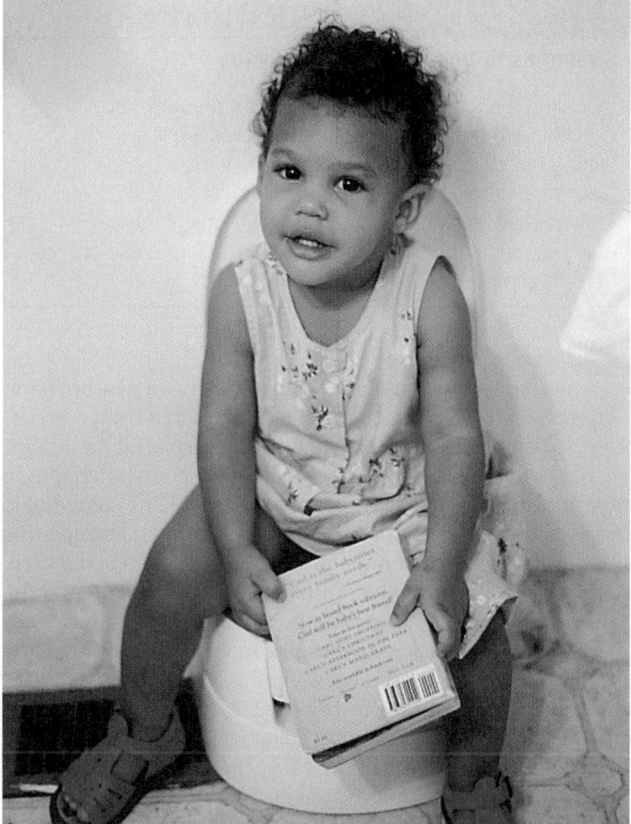

Figure 6-7 There are no set rules for toilet training. The nurse can help parents understand that both physical readiness and psychologic readiness are necessary for success.

Daytime bladder control occurs before nighttime bladder control. Some children do achieve daytime bladder control before bowel control. This phenomenon is referred to as *toileting refusal*, and it can be distressful to parents. Studies suggest that the earlier intensive toilet training begins, the longer it takes for the child to be trained. Optimal age for beginning toilet training is 27 months (Blum, Taubman & Nemeth, 2003).

A relaxed, child-centered approach is most successful, with plenty of praise for each success. Punishment and coercive techniques cause feelings of shame and lead to power struggles. The child should not be forced to sit on the potty for long periods. Successful toilet training is a gradual process, and relapses must be expected. Accidents often occur when children are too busy playing to notice a full bladder until it is too late. Many children cannot remain completely dry until the age of 3 years. Parents should respond to accidents with tolerance instead of scolding or shaming the child.

Temper Tantrums

Temper tantrums are a common toddler response to anger and frustration and often result from thwarted attempts at mastery and autonomy. Tantrums may also occur as an emotional release of tension after a long, tiring day. Unable to express anger in more productive ways because of limited language and reasoning abilities, toddlers may react by screaming, kicking, throwing things, or even biting themselves or banging their heads. Tantrums occur more often when toddlers are tired, hungry, bored, or excessively stimulated.

The nurse can help parents by identifying strategies to decrease the frequency of tantrums. Limiting situations that are too much for the child to handle is helpful. Anticipating periods of fatigue, having a snack ready before the child gets too hungry, and offering the toddler choices when possible can minimize temper tantrums. Parental practices such as inconsistency, permissiveness, excessive strictness, and overprotectiveness increase the probability of tantrums.

Toddlers need appropriate and consistent limits. Letting the child know that temper tantrums will not be tolerated gives the child a sense of security. The intensity of a tod-

dler's outburst almost seems to be a plea for someone to stop the behavior. Probably the most effective method for handling tantrums is to safely isolate and ignore the child. The child should learn that nothing is gained from a tantrum, not even attention. Giving in to the child's demands or scolding the child only increases the behavior. Toddlers stop using tantrums when they do not achieve their goals and as their verbal skills increase. Once the tantrum has subsided and the toddler has regained some self-control, the parent should comfort and let the child know that limits are necessary and that the child is loved. Acknowledging the child's angry feelings and rewarding more mature ways of expressing them assist the child to gain self-control.

Sibling Rivalry

Sharing parents' love and attention is difficult for most toddlers. Often toddlers have intense feelings of jealousy and envy toward a new infant sibling. Toddlers' egocentrism makes it difficult for them to understand that a parent can love more than one child at a time.

Because the infant needs a great deal of time and attention, the toddler's routine is disrupted. The toddler has limited resources to cope with such stress and may react by treating the baby roughly, damaging property, or harming pets. The toddler may seem to regress by asking for a bottle or pacifier or by using baby talk.

! CRITICAL TO REMEMBER

Strategies to Decrease Sibling Rivalry

Including the toddler in preparations for the new baby
Explaining to the toddler what new babies are like
Letting the child feel the fetus move
Reading picture books about new siblings
Talking about changes that the newborn might create
Acknowledging the older child's feelings about these changes
Referring to the baby as "ours"

Any changes, such as moving the toddler to a new bedroom or beginning daycare, should be made as far in advance as possible so that the toddler will not feel displaced by abrupt changes when the baby arrives. Many hospitals offer sibling preparation classes. When the mother and infant come home from the hospital, the mother's first concern should be greeting the older sibling. The father or another caregiver should carry the newborn, allowing the mother's arms to be free to hug the waiting toddler and to express how the child was missed. A toddler's jealous feelings can become intense when visitors lavish gifts and praise on the baby. Giving an inexpensive gift to the toddler each time the baby receives one can minimize these feelings. Visitors should be encouraged to pay attention to the older child as well as the baby. Parents should anticipate behavior changes, even if the toddler has been prepared for the arrival of a new baby. The parents should be present when the toddler is with the infant to prevent the toddler from inadvertently harming the newborn sibling.

It is important to help toddlers recognize and identify negative feelings toward a new sibling. Firm limits must be set, however, if the toddler tries to harm the baby. The child may be told "It's okay to feel jealous, but it's not okay to hurt the baby." Praise should be given for affectionate, cooperative behavior.

Planned, uninterrupted private time is important to maintain feelings of closeness between parent and toddler. Even 10 or 15 minutes each day while the baby is sleeping is valuable. Allowing the toddler to choose an activity for this time with the parent makes it even more special. This special time should be given to the child each day, regardless of the child's behavior.

Selected Issues Related to the Preschooler

Stuttering

Stuttering or stammering is a disturbance in the flow and time patterning of speech. During the preschool years, children often have experiences they want to share but have difficulty putting the words together. It is common for children at this age to repeat whole words or phrases and to interject "uh" and "um" in their speech. As the child's communication skills develop, most children grow out of their normal dysfluency. Dysfluency tends to be more common during times of excitement, when formulating long and complex sentences, when trying to think of a particular word, and during times of stress.

Reactions to stuttering can increase the dysfluency. No definite clinical signs clearly indicate the prognosis or need for referral of an individual child. Health care providers

PARENTS
Want to Know

How to Help the Child Who Stutters

- Listen closely when your child speaks.
- Speak slowly, and pause frequently. This provides a model for the child and gives the child more time to understand what is being said as well as to formulate thoughts.
- Provide opportunities for the child to talk without distractions or competition from other family members.
- Reduce pressure to communicate by limiting the number of questions asked that require an immediate answer.
- Limit time pressure. Do not ask a second question before the first question is answered.
- Observe situations that increase or decrease fluent behavior. Increase those times when the child is more fluent.
- Recognize that certain environmental factors may have a negative effect on fluency: competition to speak, excitement, time pressure, arguing, fatigue, new situations, unfamiliar listeners.
- Repeat or rephrase what your child says to verify that you have understood it.

Modified from American Speech-Language-Hearing Association. (1998). Stuttering: Do's & don'ts for parents. *Healthtouch On-line for Better Health.* Available on-line at www.healthtouch.com.

should intervene on the cautious side and refer the child to a fluency specialist if the child's speech is not understandable (older than 2 years) or only partially understandable (older than 3 or 4 years). Any of the following could also precipitate a referral (Schmidt, 2001):

- The child shows self-consciousness or fear of talking in reaction to the dysfluency.
- There is a physical struggle to get words out or the child displays grimacing or tics when trying to talk.
- The frequency of dysfluency is excessive.
- There is a family history of stuttering during adulthood or the parents are strongly concerned about possible stuttering. (Schmidt, 2001)

Parents can help their child by focusing on the ideas the child is expressing, not on the way the child is speaking. Parents should not complete their child's sentences or draw attention to their child's speech. They should not criticize or correct the child's speech.

Preschool and Daycare Programs

A quality daycare program provides an environment in which the child can expand social and play skills as well as manipulate play materials unavailable at home.

Working mothers often express guilt and concern about the effect of daycare on their child's emotional well-being and cognitive development. Some concerns about the effect of daycare on the child's development can be minimized by careful selection of the daycare facility.

The nurse is in an excellent position to advise parents about childcare. Parents need specific advice about options that are affordable but will not compromise the child's health and development. It is imperative that parents visit the daycare center to evaluate the quality of the program. They need to evaluate the attitude and qualifications of the caregivers as well as operating procedures, costs, childcare and disciplinary practices, meals, safety precautions, sanitary conditions, and the child/staff ratio.

The child needs preparation before beginning daycare and information about what to expect in simple, concrete terms. Emphasizing the exciting parts of the experience will help the child view the experience positively. The parent should also explain the reason for separation. It is not uncommon for imaginative preschoolers to believe that they are being "sent away" because of some misdeed.

When parents must take their child to a baby-sitter or daycare center, they should give the child an explanation for the separation. A statement such as "I have to work so I can buy food and clothes for the family and toys for you" is not adequate. In response to this explanation, one 3-year-old boy wailed, "But I have enough toys!" More effective would be to explain the separation by saying, "We both have work to do. My work is at my office, and your work is at school."

It is important for the parent to reassure the child ("I'm really going to miss you today, and I wish you could be with me.") and to let the child know that separation is painful for the parent as well but necessary. At the end of the day, when picking up the child, it is equally important to let the child know how happy the parent is to see the child. By responding to the child's feelings, parents can lessen the stress of separation.

Transition objects may help the child adjust to the new environment. Providing the staff with information about the child's interests, home routine, special terms, and names of pets and siblings helps the new caregiver make the child feel more comfortable. Parents should always assure the child that they will return to take the child home at the end of the day.

Preparing the Child for School

Preparation for school begins long before the preschool period. The earliest interactions between parent and infant lay the foundation for school readiness. Probably the most important factor in the development of academic competency is the relationship between parent and child. Parents who are attuned to their child and who structure the environment to provide challenges as well as security facilitate the child's cognitive growth. An interesting environment, combined with parental encouragement and support, maximizes the child's potential.

Parents are the child's first and most important teachers. They structure the child's environment and offer opportunities for learning. Visiting a zoo, fire station, or museum and talking about the experience increase the child's general knowledge and vocabulary. Cooking together, playing simple games, or putting together puzzles also fosters intellectual development. Playing with clay, paint, and scissors promotes fine motor skills and provides opportunity for self-expression. Reading to the child is one of the most valuable activities for promoting school readiness. Listening to stories and discussing them can promote reading readiness. Dramatic play encourages reading readiness by providing opportunities for symbolic thinking and problem solving.

Preschool and daycare programs can supplement the developmental opportunities provided by parents at home. Opportunities to play with other children and to learn how to share the attention of an adult are some benefits of a good preschool program. Head Start programs offer low-income children and their families opportunities for remedial and supportive activities. Kindergarten provides a transition between home and first grade through a structured learning environment. In kindergarten, children prepare for school by learning to cooperate with other children, developing listening skills, and forming a positive attitude toward school.

Nurses can provide parents with strategies designed to promote safety as part of preparation for school. Teaching children about street safety and dealing with strangers and ensuring that children know their telephone number and address are important aspects of preparation for school.

Not every 5-year-old is ready for kindergarten. Both chronologic age and developmental maturity should be considered when assessing a child's readiness for school (Box 6-6). At this age, boys tend to lag behind girls developmentally by about 6 months.

BOX 6-6
Checklist for School Readiness

- Child is physically healthy and strong enough to enjoy the challenge of going to school and to handle the increased stresses involved.
- Child attends to own toileting needs and washes hands independently.
- Child can separate from parent and spend several hours each day in an unfamiliar place with adults and children who are largely unknown at first.
- Child's attention span is long enough that child can sit for a fairly long period and concentrate on one thing at a time, gradually learning to enjoy the practicing and problem-solving activity involved.
- Child can listen to and follow two- or three-part instructions.

- Child can restrict talking to appropriate times.
- Child is able to tolerate the frustration of not receiving immediate attention from the teacher or others; can wait for and take turns.
- Child has some basic hand-eye skills necessary for learning to read and write.
- Child can hold a pencil properly and turn pages one at a time.
- Child knows the alphabet and can recognize some letters visually.
- Child counts to 10.
- Child recognizes the colors of the rainbow.

Health Promotion

The 4- and 5-Year-Old Child

FOCUSED ASSESSMENT

Have you been able to encourage your child to be independent and express ideas that may differ from yours?

Is your child in preschool or daycare? How many hours or days?

How does your child get along with other children the same age?

How well does your child communicate with others?

Has your child's play become more imaginative? Does your child describe any fears?

Has your child become independent in feeding, cleanliness, toileting, and dressing?

Do you give your child small responsibilities or chores to do around the house?

What activities do you enjoy doing together?

DEVELOPMENTAL MILESTONES

Personal/social: develops a sense of initiative; learns new skills and games; begins problem solving; develops a positive self-concept; develops a conscience: begins to learn right from wrong and good from bad (based on reward and punishment); learns to understand rules; identifies with parent of same gender, often closely imitating characteristics; aware of gender differences; independence in self-care; sociable and outgoing (might be aggressive or bossy); has an attention span of about 20 minutes

Fine motor: proficient holding a crayon or pencil, draws purposefully; copies circle, cross, square, diamond, and triangle; draws a person with several body parts; drawings resemble familiar objects or people; may begin to write name or numbers; can tie shoelaces

Language/cognitive: vocabulary of 1500 words; begins to understand concepts of size and time (related to familiar events such as meals and bedtime); understands two opposites (e.g., same/different, hot/cold, big/little); can follow several directions consecutively; four-word sentences using prepositions (e.g., on, under, behind); defines five words, counts to five, names four colors; begins to see others' viewpoints; uses magical thinking; very imaginative; can complete an 8- to 10-piece puzzle

Gross motor: hops on one foot or alternate feet; walks heel to toe (front and back); balances on each foot for longer time; begins to ride bike with training wheels; throws and catches a ball; walks downstairs using alternate feet

CRITICAL MILESTONES*

Personal/social: puts on a tee shirt; washes and dries hands; names a friend

Fine motor: imitates a vertical line; wiggles thumbs; builds a tower of eight cubes

Language/cognitive: knows two adjectives (e.g., tired, hungry, cold); identifies one color; knows the use of two objects (e.g., cup, chair, pencil)

Gross motor: balances on each foot for 1 second; jumps forward; throws a ball overhand

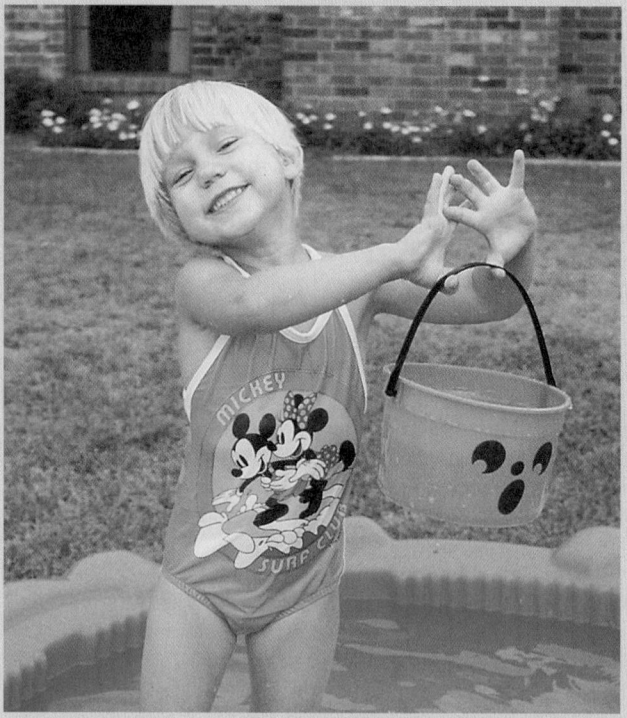

HEALTH MAINTENANCE

Physical Measurements
  Weight increases 5 lb (2.25 kg) per yr
  Height increases approximately 3 inches (7.5 cm) per yr
Immunizations
  Diphtheria, tetanus, acellular pertussis (DTaP) #5; inactivated poliovirus (IPV) #4; measles, mumps, rubella (MMR) #2
Health Screening
  Hemoglobin and lead screen
  Vision
  Audiometry
  Blood pressure
  Cholesterol if at risk
  Tuberculosis (TB) if at risk

ANTICIPATORY GUIDANCE

Provide information and health teaching to the child as well as the parent
Nutrition
  Continue as for a 3-year-old
  Provide nutritious snacks (child too often in a hurry to eat at mealtime)
  Begin to emphasize table manners
Elimination
  Bowel movements once or twice daily
  Urinary output 1000 ml/day
  Nighttime control achieved

Health Promotion

The 4- and 5-Year-Old Child—cont'd

Dental
- Dental examinations every 6 months
- Continue brushing and fluoride
- Child might begin to lose deciduous teeth

Sleep
- 10 to 12 hours, no nap *
- May experience night terrors or nightmares

Safety
- Review bicycle safety, playground safety, fire safety, poisoning (outside plants), pedestrian safety, automobile safety, sun protection
- Discuss gun safety, stranger awareness, good touch versus bad touch

Self-Esteem and Competence
- Model appropriate social behavior; begin to include participation in religious services
- Encourage your child to learn to make choices
- Help your child to appropriately express emotions
- Spend individual time with your child daily, and encourage your child to talk about the day's events

- Provide consistent and loving limits to help your child learn self-discipline
- Encourage curiosity, and provide formal learning experiences
- Establish opportunities for your child to do small household chores
- Assess your child's readiness for kindergarten entrance, and begin to prepare the child for the school experience

Play
- Peak of imaginative play: misbehavior projected onto inanimate object or "imaginary friend"; participate in imaginary play; encourage curiosity and creativity
- Teach songs and nursery rhymes
- Read to the child frequently
- Teach basic skills of sports and games
- Provide playground equipment, household and garden tools, dress-up clothes, building and construction toys, art supplies, more sophisticated books and puzzles

* Guided by DDST II

KEY CONCEPTS

- The slower physical growth rate of the toddler (in comparison with an infant) leads to a reduced demand for calories and decreased appetite (physiologic anorexia).
- The combination of increased motor skills, immaturity, and lack of experience places the toddler at risk for unintentional injury. Anticipatory guidance for the parents about childproofing the home is an essential nursing role.
- Children's coordination and muscle strength increase rapidly between the ages of 3 and 5 years. Increases in brain size and nerve myelinization enable the child to perfect fine and gross motor skills. The preschool child has the skills needed to engage in activities such as running, riding a tricycle, cutting with scissors, and drawing.
- Toddlers' behavior is characterized by negativism, ritualism, and egocentrism.
- The preschool years are a critical period for the development of socialization. Children need opportunities to play with others to learn communication skills and ways to get along with others. Preschool children learn to share and cooperate as they play in small groups. Their play is often imitative, dramatic, and creative.
- Preschoolers' thinking is still magical and egocentric. They tend to understand events only as those events affect them, believing that everyone else has the same experience. Preschool children may be overwhelmed by guilt feelings if a loved one is injured or becomes ill because they believe their thoughts are powerful enough to cause events to happen.

- Toddlerhood is characterized by the struggle for autonomy as the child develops a sense of self as separate from the parent. Erikson defines the toddler's task as centered on autonomy versus shame and doubt.
- According to Erikson, the developmental task of the preschooler is to gain a sense of initiative. The preschooler is busy learning how to do things and takes great pride in new accomplishments.
- Gender identity and body image are developing in the preschool period. Sexual curiosity, anatomic explorations, and masturbation are common. The nurse should encourage parents to answer the preschooler's questions simply and honestly. Children should not be shamed or punished for self-comforting behaviors or for investigating gender differences.
- Food jags and physiologic anorexia are common occurrences in the young child.
- Toddlers need approximately 12 to 14 hours of sleep per day.
- The preschooler needs an average of 10 to 12 hours of sleep in a 24-hour period. Because of the preschooler's active imagination and immaturity, sleep problems are common.
- Firm, consistent discipline helps toddlers learn self-control. Effective discipline techniques include time-outs, diversion, and positive reinforcements.
- Preschool children need consistent discipline to learn acceptable behavior. Appropriate limit setting helps the child learn self-confidence, self-control, and moral values. Discipline

techniques that are effective at this age include time-out, time-in, the use of restricted choices, and diversion.
- All 20 deciduous teeth are present by age 3 years. Proper care of deciduous teeth is crucial for the child's general health and for the health and alignment of permanent teeth. Nurses should teach parents the importance of good oral hygiene, adequate fluoride intake, good nutrition, and regular dental checkups.
- Nurses can help parents with toilet training by explaining the signs of physical and psychologic readiness. Readiness depends on myelinization of the nerve pathways that enable the child to control the bowel and bladder sphincters.
- Sibling rivalry can be minimized with techniques such as including the toddler in preparations for the new baby, acknowledging the toddler's negative feelings while setting appropriate limits, and affirming the toddler as special and loved.
- The nurse plays an important role in helping parents prepare their children for school and in assessing children's readiness for school. Parents can help their child succeed in school by providing a stimulating environment and encouragement and support.
- Health promotion for the preschool child includes ensuring adequate sleep, optimal nutrition, dental care, immunizations, and prevention of injuries.

ANSWERS to Critical Thinking Exercise 6-1

1. The nurse needs to know if there is a bedtime ritual. If a ritual exists, the nurse determines what it is and whether it is implemented consistently. Even though the parents volunteered that they did not have any other concerns, the nurse should ask about Todd's daily routine. Questions related to his play activities, eating habits, and daily routine might be helpful. The parents should be asked what discipline methods they use and if they are effective (i.e., what the parents do when Todd resists their instructions). This information will give the nurse a general idea of what the child's environment is

like. The nurse is trying to determine whether the parents are supporting this child's need for structure while allowing him to venture out. The nurse is looking for balance and gathering information to determine whether consistent limits are set within the family.

2. Two-year-old children need limits set to feel secure. They do not have the maturity to control their behavior. They must be taught the rules. It is not unusual for toddlers to delay going to bed. The parents should be told that this behavior is part of normal growth and development. By providing a bedtime ritual,

which may include quiet time, a snack, a story, and perhaps a prayer, parents help children find security in a routine that is repeated night after night. Children begin to know that their parents expect them to stay in bed and that they cannot manipulate their parents. Children who "wear their parents down" are confused and are not given the sense of control that they need to explore and become autonomous. Parents should be assured that by creating a consistent environment, they will not only help their child but also save themselves a good deal of frustration.

REFERENCES and READINGS

Agran, P., Anderson, C., Winn, D., Trent, R., Walton-Haynes, L., & Thayer, S. (2003). Rates of pediatric injuries by 3-month intervals for children 0 to 3 years of age. *Pediatrics, 111*(6), e683-e692.

American Academy of Pediatrics. (1998). Airline seats for infants. *AAP News, 14*(8), 5.

American Academy of Pediatrics. (1999). *Choosing child care.* Retrieved March 23, 2001, from www.medem.com.

American Academy of Pediatrics. (2000). *Age 2 to 3 years: Sleeping.* Retrieved March 23, 2001, from www.medem.com.

American Academy of Pediatrics. (2003a). *Car safety seats: A guide for families 2003.* Retrieved June 10, 2003, from www.aap.org/family/carseatguide.htm.

American Academy of Pediatrics. (2003b). Handling a poison emergency. Retrieved November 20, 2003, from www.aap.org.

American Academy of Pediatrics. (2003c). Poison treatment in the home. Retrieved November 20, 2003, from www.aap.org.

American Academy of Pediatrics Committee on Nutrition. (1998a). Cholesterol in childhood. *Pediatrics, 101*(1), 141-147.

American Academy of Pediatrics Committee on Nutrition. (1998b). *Pediatric nutrition handbook* (4th ed.). Elk Grove Village, IL: American Academy of Pediatrics.

American Academy of Pediatrics Committee on Psychosocial Aspects of Child and Family Health. (1998). Guidance for effective discipline. *Pediatrics, 101*(4), 723-728.

Ateah, C. (2003). Disciplinary practices with children: Parental sources of information, attitudes, and educational needs. *Issues in Comprehensive Pediatric Nursing, 26*, 89-101.

Banks, J.B. (2002). Childhood discipline: Challenges for clinicians and parents. *American Family Physician, 66*(8), 1447-1452.

Berry, B., Simons, B., Siatkowski, R., Schiffman, J., Flynn, J., & Duthie, M. (2001). Preschool vision screening using the MTI-Photoscreener™. *Pediatric Nursing, 27*(1), 27-34.

Bloom, L. (1998). Language development and emotional expression. *Pediatrics, 102*(5), 1272-1277.

Blum, N., Taubman, B., & Nemeth, N. (2003). Relationship between age at initiation of toilet training and duration of training: A prospective study. *Pediatrics, 111*(4), 810-814.

Center for Nutrition Policy and Promotion. (2001). *Food guide pyramid for young children.* U.S. Department of Agriculture. Available online: www.usda.gov/cnpp.

Dennison, B., Erb, T., & Jenkins, P. (2002). Television viewing and television in bedroom associated with overweight risk among low-income preschool children. *Pediatrics, 109*(6), 1028-1035.

Duncan, P., Dixon, R., & Carlson, J. (2003). Childhood and adolescent sexuality. *Pediatric Clinics of North America, 50*(4), 741-764.

Emude, R.N. (1998). Early emotional development: New modes of thinking for research and intervention. *Pediatrics, 102*(5), 1236-1243.

Erikson, E.H. (1963). *Childhood and society* (2nd ed.). New York: Norton.

Fox, N.A. (1998). Temperament and regulation of emotion in the first years of life. *Pediatrics, 102*(5), 1230-1235.

Green, M., & Palfrey, J.S. (Eds.). (2000). *Bright futures: Guidelines for health supervision of infants, children, and adolescents* (2nd ed.). Arlington, VA: National Center for Education in Maternal and Child Health.

Kamerling, S.N. (2002). Airbags & children: Making correct choices in child passenger restraints. *MCN: The American Journal of Maternal/Child Nursing, 27*(5), 264-273.

Kennedy, C.M., & Lipsitt, L.P. (1998). Risk-taking in preschool children. *Journal of Pediatric Nursing, 13*(2), 77-84.

Kinservik, M., & Friedhoff, M. (2000). Control issues in toilet training. *Pediatric Nursing, 26*(3), 267-272.

Kohlberg, L. (1964). Development of moral character. In M. Hoffman & L. Hoffman (Eds.), *Review of child development research* (Vol. 1). New York: Russell Sage Foundation.

Kohlberg, L. (1966). A cognitive developmental analysis of children's sex-role concepts and attitudes. In E.E. Maccoby (Ed.), *The development of sex differences.* Stanford, CA: Stanford University Press.

Litt, I., & Martin, J. (1999). Development of sexuality and its problems. In M. Levine, W. Carey, & A. Crocker (Eds.). *Developmental-behavioral pediatrics* (pp.457-470). Philadelphia: Saunders.

Roberts, M.W., Keels, M.A., Sharp, M.C., & Lewis, J.L. (1998). Fluoride supplement prescribing and dental referral patterns among academic pediatricians. *Pediatrics, 101*(1), e6.

Rodgers, G.B. (1998). Let's welcome a new generation of child-resistant packaging. *Contemporary Pediatrics, 15*(3), 57-72.

Schmidt, B. (2001). Stuttering and normal dysfluency. *Clinical Reference Systems, Annual 2001,* 1864.

Stein, M.T. (1998). Preparing families for the toddler and preschool years. *Contemporary Pediatrics, 15*(1), 88-110.

Stevenson, M., Rimajova, M., Edgecombe, D., & Vickery, K. (2003). Childhood drowning: Barriers surrounding private swimming pools. *Pediatrics, 111*(2), e115-e119.

Story, M., Holt, K., & Sofka, D. (Eds.). (2002). *Bright futures in practice: Nutrition.* Arlington, VA: National Center for Education in Maternal and Child Health.

Thiedke, C. (2001). Sleep disorders and sleep problems in childhood. *American Family Physician, 63*(2), 277-284.

U.S. Department of Agriculture. (2001). *Dietary guidelines for Americans, 2000* (5th ed.). Available on-line: www.usda.gov/cnpp.

Yoshinaga-Itano, C., Sedey, A.L., Coulter, D.K., & Mehl, A.L. (1998). Language of early- and later-identified children with hearing loss. *Pediatrics, 102*(5), 1161-1171.

Zurbrugg, E.B. (1998). When time-out fails, try plan B. *Contemporary Pediatrics, 15*(1), 79-84.

Health Promotion for the School-Age Child

◆ LEARNING OBJECTIVES

After studying this chapter, you should be able to:
◎ Describe the school-age child's normal growth and development, and assess the child for normal developmental milestones.
◎ Describe the maturational changes that take place during the school-age period, and discuss implications for health care.
◎ Identify the stages of moral development in the school-age child, and discuss implications for effective parenting strategies.
◎ Discuss the effect school has on the child's development and implications for teachers and parents.
◎ Discuss anticipatory guidance related to various health and safety issues seen in the school-age child.
◎ Describe anticipatory guidance that the nurse can offer to decrease children's stress.

◆ DEFINITIONS

caries Decay of the teeth.
conservation Ability to understand that certain properties of objects do not change simply because their order, form, or appearance has changed.
malocclusion Misalignment of the teeth or dental arches; teeth may be crowded, crooked, or out of alignment.

menarche Onset of menstruation.
self-care children Children who care for themselves at home after school; formerly called latch-key children.

iddle childhood, ages 6 to 12 years, is probably one of the healthiest periods of life. Slow, steady physical growth and rapid cognitive and social development characterize this time. During these 6 years, the child's world expands from the tight circle of the family to include children and adults at school, at church or synagogue, and in the community. The child becomes increasingly independent. Peers become important as the child starts school and gradually moves away from the security of home. This period is a time for best friends, sharing, and exploring.

The school years also are a time that can be stressful for a child, and this stress can impede the child's successful achievement of developmental tasks. The *Healthy People 2010* objectives (Box 7-1) that relate to school-age children include such goals as reducing stress and obesity, improving access to dental care, and preventing high-risk behaviors.

GROWTH AND DEVELOPMENT OF THE SCHOOL-AGE CHILD

The school-age child develops a sense of industry and learns the basic skills needed to function in society. The child develops an appreciation of rules and a conscience. Cognitively, the child grows from the egocentrism of early childhood to more mature thinking. The ability to solve problems and make independent judgments based on reason characterizes this new maturity. The child is invested in the task of middle childhood: learning to do things and do them well. Competence and self-esteem increase with each academic, social, and athletic achievement. The relative stability and security of the school-age period prepare the child to enter the storm of adolescence.

Physical Growth and Development

The school-age years are characterized by slow and steady growth. The physical changes that occur during this period are gradual and subtle. Although growth rates vary among children (Fig. 7-1), average weight gain is 2.5 kg (5½ lb) per year and the average increase in height is approximately 5.5 cm (2 in) per year. During the early school-age period, boys are approximately 1 inch taller and 2 lb heavier than girls. At around age 10 or 12 years, girls begin to catch up in size as they experience the preadolescent growth spurt. By age 12 years, girls are 1 inch taller than boys and 2 lb heavier. This growth spurt, which signals the onset of puberty, occurs usually between ages 12 and 14 years and occurs 2 years later in boys than in girls.

BOX 7-1
Healthy People 2010 Objectives for School-Age Children

6-2	Reduce the proportion of children and adolescents with disabilities who are reported to be sad, unhappy, or depressed.
6-9	Increase the proportion of children and youth with disabilities who spend at least 80% of their time in regular education programs.
15-23	Increase the use of helmets by bicyclists.
18-7	Increase the proportion of children with mental health problems who receive treatment.
19-3	Reduce the proportion of children and adolescents who are overweight or obese.
19-5, 6, 7	Increase the proportion of persons aged 2 years and older who consume at least two daily servings of fruit; three daily servings of vegetables, with at least one-third being dark-green or deep-yellow vegetables; and six daily servings of grain products, with at least three being whole grain.
19-8, 9	Increase the proportion of persons aged 2 years and older who consume less than 10% of calories from saturated fat; and who consume no more than 30% of calories from fat.
19-15	Increase the proportion of children and adolescents aged 6 to 19 years whose intake of meals and snacks at schools contributes proportionally to good overall dietary quality.
20-1	Reduce the proportion of children and adolescents who have dental caries experience in their primary or permanent teeth.
21-8	Increase the proportion of children who have received dental sealants to their molar teeth.
22-11	Increase the proportion of children and adolescents who view television 2 or fewer hours per day.
27-3	Reduce initiation of tobacco use among children and adolescents.

Modified from U.S. Department of Health and Human Services. (2000). *Healthy People 2010* (Conference edition, in 2 volumes). Washington, DC: Author.

Body Systems

School-age children appear thinner and more graceful than preschoolers do. Musculoskeletal growth leads to greater coordination and strength. The muscles are still immature, however, and can be injured from overuse. Growth of the facial bones changes facial proportions. As the facial bones grow, the eustachian tube assumes a more downward and inward position, resulting in fewer ear infections than in the preschool years. Lymphatic tissues continue to grow until about age 9 years; immunoglobulin A and G (IgA, IgG) levels reach adult value at approximately 10 years. Enlarged tonsils and adenoids are common during these years and are not always an indication of illness. Frontal sinuses develop at age 7 years. Brain growth is complete by 10 years. The respiratory system also continues to mature. During the school-age years, the lungs and alveoli develop fully and fewer respiratory infections occur.

Dentition

During the school-age years, all 20 primary (deciduous) teeth are lost and are replaced by 28 of the 32 permanent teeth. All permanent teeth, except the third molars, erupt during the school-age period. The order of eruption of permanent teeth and loss of primary teeth is shown in Figure 33-7. The first teeth to be lost are usually the lower central incisors, at around age 6 years. Most first-graders are characterized by a snaggle-tooth appearance (see Fig. 7-1), and visits from the "tooth fairy" are important signs of growing up.

Sexual Development

Puberty is a time of dramatic physical change. It includes the growth spurt, development of primary and secondary sexual characteristics, and maturation of the sexual organs. The age at onset of puberty varies widely, and puberty is occurring at an earlier age than previously thought. Onset of puberty is no longer unusual in girls who are 9 or 10 years old. On the average, African-American girls begin puberty 1 year earlier than white girls (Russell et al., 2001). The reason for the earlier development among African-American girls is not known. Puberty begins about 1½ to 2 years later in boys. Menarche, the onset of menstruation, occurs, on the average, during the 12th year. Females who are significantly overweight tend to have earlier onset of puberty and menarche. Because puberty is occurring increasingly earlier, many 10- and 11-year-old girls have already experienced menarche. Wide variations in maturity at this age are a common cause of embarrassment because the school-age child does not want to appear different from peers. Children who mature either early or late may struggle with feelings of self-consciousness and inferiority. Table 8-1 describes the usual sequence of appearance of secondary sex characteristics during the school-age and adolescent periods.

Because of earlier onset of puberty, sex education programs should be introduced in elementary school. Nurses are in an excellent position to serve as resource persons for parents and teachers who are responsible for sex education. Children's questions about sexuality and related issues should be answered honestly and matter-of-factly. If sex education is presented within the context of learning about the human body, with its wonders and mysteries, children are less likely to feel embarrassed and anxious. Regardless of whether sex education is a part of a formal school curriculum, children need accurate information. Basic anatomy and physiology, information about body functions, and the expected changes of puberty should be introduced to children before the onset of puberty. Older school-age children need information about menstruation, nocturnal emissions, and reproduction. Sex education programs must also include information about responsible sexuality and related issues, such as teenage pregnancy, human immunodeficiency virus (HIV), and sexually transmissible diseases.

Motor Development

Development of Gross Motor Skills

During the school years, coordination improves. A developed sense of balance and rhythm allows children to ride a two-wheeled bicycle, dance, skip, jump rope, and participate in a variety of sports. As puberty approaches in the late school-age period, children may become more awkward, as their bodies grow faster than their ability to compensate.

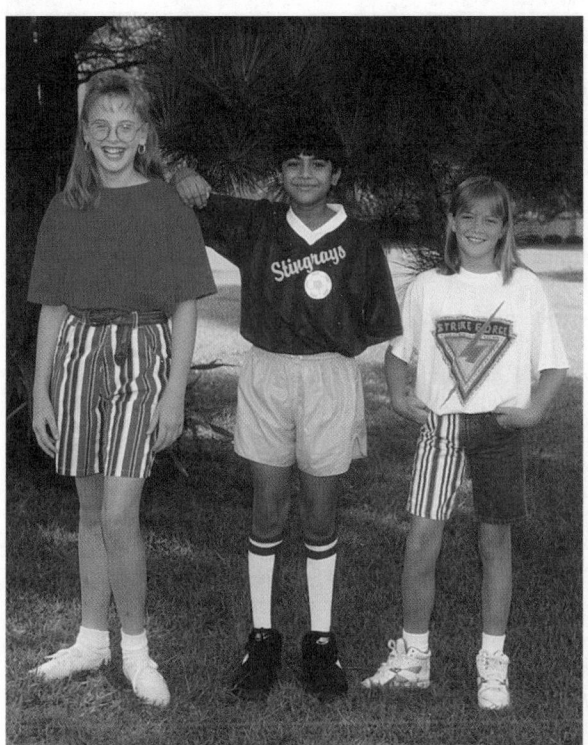

Children of the same age can vary significantly in height and physical development.

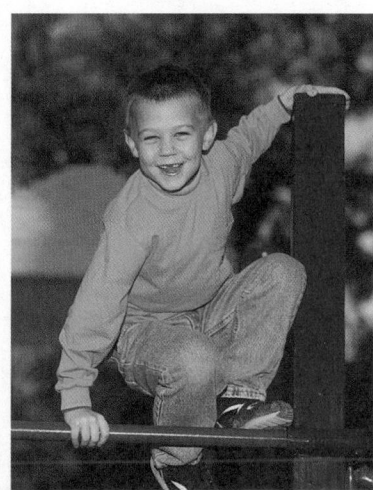

School-age children often have a snaggle-tooth appearance while they are losing their primary teeth.

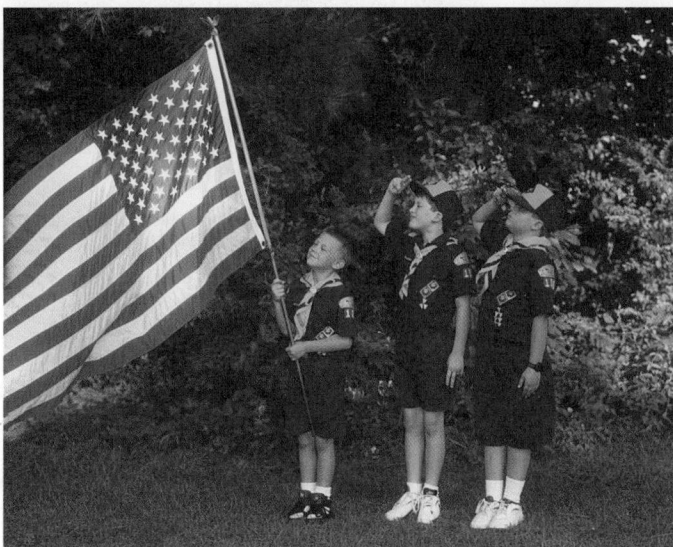

Organizations such as Boy Scouts help foster self-esteem and competence.

Figure 7-1 Growth and development of the school-age child.

Importance of Active Play

School-age children spend much of their time in active play, practicing and refining motor skills. They seem to be constantly in motion. Children of this age enjoy active sports and games as well as crafts and fine motor activities (Box 7-2). Activities requiring balance and strength, such as bicycle riding, tree climbing, and skating, are exciting and fun for the school-age child. Coordination and motor skills improve as the child is given an opportunity to practice.

Children should be encouraged to engage in physical activities. During the school-age years, children learn physical fitness skills that contribute to their health for the rest of their

---

! CRITICAL TO REMEMBER

Components of Sex Education

- Basic anatomy and physiology
- Body functions
- Expected changes related to puberty
- Menstruation, nocturnal emissions
- Reproduction
- Teenage pregnancy
- Human immunodeficiency virus (HIV) infection prevention
- Sexually transmissible diseases

BOX 7-2
*Age-Related Activities and Toys for the
School-Age Child*

General Activities
Play becomes organized with more direction.
Early school-age child continues dramatic play with increased
    creativity but loses some spontaneity.
Child is aware of rules when playing games.
Child begins to compete in sports.

Toys and Specific Types of Play
Collections, drawing, construction, dolls, pets, guessing
    games, complicated puzzles, board games, riddles, physi-
    cal games, competitive play, reading, bike riding, hobbies,
    sewing, listening to the radio, watching television and
    videos, cooking.

PARENTS
Want to Know

*Assessing an Organized Recreational
Sports Program*

Whenever your child begins playing in an organized recreational sports program, you need to consider the following:
- *Coaches' training:* Coaches not only need to understand
  how to play a sport and to teach it to young children but also
  should have undergone a training program in injury prevention and first aid. Check to see that the training emphasizes preventing overuse injuries.
- *Coaches' attitude:* Coaches should have a positive, encouraging manner with children—not critical and demeaning.
  Check whether the coach emphasizes skill development
  and plays all the children, whether required to or not. Be
  sure the coach is a good role model on the field and is cour-
  teous to referees, other coaches, and the children. Avoid
  coaches who have a "win at all costs" philosophy.
- *Safety:* Check to see that protective and athletic equipment
  is used correctly by all children participating in the sport.
  Facilities and equipment should be well maintained and
  safe. Children should be divided into teams according to
  size and maturation level, rather than by age. Many sports
  programs require a preseason physical examination.
- *Enjoyment:* Sports programs can do wonderful things for
  your child's skill development, confidence, sense of cooperation, and self-esteem. Remember that it is your child
  playing the sport and not you. Be encouraging and positive,
  help the child when asked, and cheer the team on in an appropriate manner.

---

lives. Cardiovascular fitness, strength, and flexibility are improved by physical activity. Popular games such as tag, jump
rope, and hide-and-seek provide a release of emotional tension
and enhance the development of leader and follower skills.

Team sports, such as soccer and baseball, provide opportunities not only for exercise and refinement of motor skills but
also for the development of sportsmanship and teamwork.
Nurses should advise parents on ways to prevent sports injuries and how to assess a recreational sports program (Parents Want to Know box). Sports activities should be well supervised, and protective gear (e.g., helmets for T-ball, shin
guards for soccer) should be mandatory.

Obesity is the most common cause of abnormal growth acceleration in childhood in the United States (Kaplowitz, Slora,
Wasserman, Pedlow, & Herman-Giddens, 2001). Time spent
watching television or playing computer games often diminishes a child's interest in active play outside. Nurses can help
reverse this trend by advising parents to limit their children's
television-watching time to 2 hours or less per day and to encourage them to engage in more active play. Parents should
provide adequate space for children to run, jump, and scuffle.
Children should have enough free time to exercise and play.
Parents need to role model both good nutrition and exercise.

Preventing Fatigue and Dehydration
Because children enjoy active play and are so full of energy,
they often do not recognize fatigue. Six-year-olds in particular will not stop an activity to rest. Parents must learn to recognize signs of fatigue or irritability and enforce rest periods
before the child becomes exhausted. Because the child's
metabolic rate is higher than an adult's and sweating ability
is limited, extremes in temperature while exercising can be
dangerous. Dehydration and overheating can pose threats to
the child's health. Frequent rest periods and adequate hydration are essential for the child during physical exercise.

Development of Fine Motor Skills
Increased myelinization of the central nervous system is
shown by refinement of fine motor skills. Balance and hand-
eye coordination improve with maturity and practice.
School-age children take pride in activities that require dex-

terity and fine motor skill, such as model building, playing a
musical instrument, and drawing.

Cognitive Development

Thought processes undergo dramatic changes as the child
moves from the intuitive thinking of the preschool years to the
logical operations of the school-age years. The school-age child
gains new knowledge and develops more efficient problem-
solving ability and greater flexibility of thinking. The 6-year-
old and 7-year-old remain in the intuitive thought stage
(Piaget, 1962) characteristic of the older preschool child. By
age 8 years, the child moves into the stage of concrete operations, followed by the stage of formal operations at around
12 years. See Chapter 4 for a discussion of formal operations; see
Chapter 54 for a discussion of the child with cognitive deficits,
including mental retardation and developmental disabilities.

Intuitive Thought Stage
In the intuitive thought stage (6 to 7 years), thinking is based
on immediate perceptions of the environment and the child's
own viewpoint. Thinking is still characterized by egocentrism,
animism, and centration (see Chapter 6). At 6 and 7 years
old, children cannot understand another's viewpoint, form
hypotheses, or deal with abstract concepts. The child in the
intuitive thought stage has difficulty forming categories and
often solves problems by random guessing.

Concrete Operations Stage

By age 7 or 8 years, the child enters the stage of concrete operations. Children learn that their point of view is not the only one as they encounter different interpretations of reality and begin to differentiate their own viewpoints from those of peers and adults (Piaget, 1962). This newly developed freedom from egocentrism enables children to think more flexibly and to learn about the environment more accurately. Problem solving becomes more efficient and reliable as the child learns how to form hypotheses. The use of symbolism becomes more sophisticated, and children now can manipulate symbols for things in the way that they once manipulated the things themselves. The child learns the alphabet and how to read. Attention span increases as the child grows older, facilitating classroom learning.

Reversibility. Children in the concrete operations stage grasp the concept of *reversibility*. They can mentally retrace a process, a skill necessary for understanding mathematical problems ($5 + 3 = 8$ and $8 - 3 = 5$). The child can take a toy apart and put it back together or walk to school and find the way back home without getting lost. Reversibility also enables a child to anticipate the results of actions—a valuable tool for problem solving.

The understanding of time gradually develops during the early school-age years. Children can understand and use clock time at around age 8 years. Although 8- or 9-year-olds understand calendar time and memorize dates, they do not master historical time until later.

Conservation. Gradually, the school-age child masters the concept of *conservation*. The child learns that certain properties of objects do not change simply because their order, form, or appearance has changed. For example, the child who has mastered conservation of mass recognizes that a lump of clay that has been pounded flat is still the same amount of clay as when it was rolled into a ball. The child understands conservation of weight when able to correctly answer the classic nonsense question, "Which weighs more, a pound of feathers or a pound of rocks?" The concept of conservation does not develop all at once. The simpler conservations, such as number and mass, are understood first, and more complex conservations are mastered later. An understanding of conservation of weight develops at 9 or 10 years old, and an understanding of volume is present at 11 or 12 years.

Classification and Logic. Older school-age children are able to classify objects according to characteristics they share, to place things in a logical order, and to recall similarities and differences. This ability is reflected in the school-age child's interest in collections. Children love to collect and classify stamps, stickers, sports cards, shells, dolls, rocks, or anything imaginable. School-age children understand relationships such as larger and smaller, lighter and darker. They can comprehend class inclusion—the concept that objects can belong to more than one classification. For example, a man can be a brother, father, and son at the same time.

School-age children move away from magical thinking as they discover that there are logical, physical explanations for most phenomena. The older school-age child is a skeptic, no longer believing in Santa Claus or the Easter Bunny.

Humor. Children in the concrete operations stage have a delightful sense of humor. Around the age of 8 years, increased mastery of language and the beginning of logic enable children to appreciate a play on words. They laugh at incongruities and love silly jokes, riddles, and puns ("How do you keep a mad elephant from charging? You take away its credit cards!"). Riddle and joke books make ideal gifts for young school-age children. Research suggests that children who have a good sense of humor use it as a positive coping mechanism for stress associated with maturational and situational life events (Dowling & Fain, 1999).

Sensory Development

Vision

The eyes are fully developed by age 6 years. Visual acuity, ocular muscle control, peripheral vision, and color discrimination are fully developed by age 7 years. Just before puberty, some children's eyes experience a growth spurt, resulting in myopia. Children with poor visual acuity usually do not complain of vision problems because the changes occur so gradually that they are difficult to notice. Usual behaviors that parents notice include squinting, moving closer to the television, or complaints of frequent headaches. The young child may never have had 20/20 vision and has nothing with which to compare the imperfect vision. For these reasons, yearly vision screening is important for school-age children.

Hearing

With maturation and growth of the eustachian tube, middle-ear infections occur less frequently than in younger children. However, chronic middle-ear infections are a problem for a few children, resulting in hearing loss. Annual audiometric screening tests are important to detect hearing loss before unrecognized deficits lead to learning problems (see Chapter 55).

Language Development

Language development continues at a rapid pace during the school-age years. Vocabulary expands, and sentence structure becomes more complex. By age 6 years, the child's vocabulary is approximately 8,000 to 14,000 words. There is an increase in the use of culturally specific words at this age. Bilingual children may speak English at school and a different language at home.

Reading effectively improves language skills. Regular trips to the library, where the child can check out books of special interest, can promote a love of reading and enhance school performance. School-age children enjoy being read to as well as reading on their own. Older children enjoy horror stories, mysteries, romances, and adventure stories.

School-age children often go through a period in which they experiment with profanity and dirty jokes. Children may imitate parents who use such words as part of their vocabulary.

Psychosocial Development

Development of a Sense of Industry

According to Erikson (1963), the central task of the school-age years is the development of a sense of industry. Ideally, the child is prepared for this task with a secure sense of self as separate from loved ones in the family. The child should have learned to trust others and should have developed a sense of autonomy and initiative during the preceding years. The school-age child replaces fantasy play with "work" at school, crafts, chores, hobbies, and athletics. The child is rewarded with a sense of satisfaction from achieving a skill as well as with external rewards, such as good grades, trophies, or an allowance. School-age children enjoy undertaking new tasks and carrying them through to completion. Whether it is baking a cake, hitting a home run, or scoring 100 on a math test, purposeful activity leads to a sense of worth and competence. Successful resolution of the task of industry depends on learning to do things and do them well. School-age children learn skills that they will need later to compete in the adult world. A person's fundamental attitude toward work is established during the school-age years.

Fostering Self-Esteem

The negative component of this developmental stage is a sense of inferiority. If a child cannot separate psychologically from the parent or if expectations are set too high for the child to achieve, the child develops feelings of inferiority. If a child believes that success is unattainable, confidence is lost and the child will not take pleasure in attempting new experiences. Children who have this experience will then have a pervasive feeling of inferiority and incompetence that will affect all aspects of their lives. The child who lacks a sense of industry has a poor foundation for mastering the tasks of adolescence. The reality is that no one can master everything. Every child will feel deficient or inferior at something. The task of the caring parent or teacher is to identify areas in which a child is competent and to build on successful experiences to foster feelings of mastery and success. Nurses can suggest ways in which parents and teachers can promote a sense of self-esteem and competence in school-age children (Parents Want to Know box).

At this age, the approval and esteem of those outside the family, especially peers, become important. Children learn that their parents are not infallible. As they begin to test parents' authority and knowledge, the influence of teachers and other adults is felt more and more. The peer group becomes the school-age child's major socializing influence. Although parents' love, praise, and support are needed, even craved during stressful times, the child begins to prefer activities with friends to activities with the family. As the child becomes more independent, increasing time is spent with friends and away from the family.

The concept of friendship changes as the child matures. At 6 and 7 years old, children form friendships merely on the basis of who lives nearby or who has toys that they enjoy. By the time children are 9 or 10 years old, friendships are based more on emotional bonds, warm feelings, and trust-building experiences. Children learn that friendship is more than just being together. Children at 11 and 12 years are loyal to their friends, often sharing problems and giving emotional support. School-age children tend to form friendships with peers of the same gender. Developing friendships and succeeding in social interactions lead to a sense of industry. Friendships are important for the emotional well-being of school-age children. Friends teach children skills they will use in future relationships.

Children learn a body of rules, sayings, and superstitions as they enter the culture of childhood. Rules are important to children because they provide predictability and offer security. Learning the sayings, jokes, and riddles is an important part of social interaction among peers. Sayings such as "Step on a crack and you'll break your mother's back" or "Finders, keepers; losers, weepers" have been part of the lore of childhood for generations.

PARENTS Want to Know

How to Promote Self-Esteem in School-Age Children

- Give your children household responsibilities according to their developmental level and capabilities. Set reasonable rules, and expect the child to follow them.
- Allow your child to solve problems and make responsible choices.
- Give praise for what is praiseworthy. Do not be afraid to encourage your child to do better. Refrain from being critical, but gently point out areas that could be improved.
- Allow your children to make mistakes, and encourage them to take responsibility for the consequences of the mistakes.
- Emphasize your child's strengths, and help improve weaknesses.
- Do not do your children's homework for them because this will make them think you do not trust them to do a good job; provide assistance and suggestions when asked, and praise their best efforts.
- Model appropriate behavior toward others.
- Provide consistent and demonstrative love.

Children become sensitive to the norms and values of the peer group because pressure to conform is great. Children often find that it is painful to be different. Peer approval is a strong motivating force and allows the child to risk disapproval from parents.

The school-age years are a time of formal and informal clubs. Informal clubs among 6-, 7-, and 8-year-olds are loosely organized, with fluid membership. Membership changes frequently and is based on mutual interests, such as playing ball, riding bikes, or playing with dolls. Children learn interpersonal skills, such as sharing, cooperation, and tolerance, in these groups.

Clubs among older school-age children tend to be more structured, often characterized by secret codes, rituals, and rigid rules. A club may be formed for the purpose of exclusion, in which children snub another child for some reason. Formal organizations, such as Boy Scouts, Girl Scouts, Campfire Boys and Girls, and 4-H, organized by adults, also foster self-esteem and competence as children earn ranks and merit badges. Transmission of societal values, such as service to others, duty to God, and good citizenship, is an important goal of these organizations.

Spiritual and Moral Development

Middle childhood years are pivotal in the development of a conscience and the internalization of values. Tremendous strides are made in moral development during these 6 years. Several theorists have described the dramatic growth that occurs during this stage.

Piaget

Piaget asserted that young school-age children obey rules because powerful, all-knowing adults hand them down. During this stage, children know the rules but not the reasons behind them. Rules are interpreted in a literal way, and the child is unable to adjust rules to fit differing circumstances. The perception of guilt changes as the child matures. Piaget stated that up to about age 8 years, children judge degrees of guilt by the amount of damage done. No distinction is made between accidental and intentional wrongdoing. For example, the child believes that a child who broke five china cups by accident is guiltier than a child who broke one cup on purpose. By age 10 years, children are able to consider the intent of the action. Older school-age children are more flexible in their decisions and can take into account extenuating circumstances.

Kohlberg

Kohlberg described moral development in terms of three levels containing six stages (see Chapter 4). According to Kohlberg's theory, children 4 to 7 years old are in stage 2 of the preconventional level, in which right and wrong are determined by physical consequences. The child obeys because of fear of punishment. If the child is not caught or punished for an act, the child does not consider the act wrong. At this stage, children conform to rules out of self-interest or in terms of what others can do in return ("I'll do this for you if you'll do that for me."). Behavior is guided by an eye-for-an-eye philosophy.

Kohlberg describes children between the ages of 7 and 12 years as being in stage 3 of the conventional level. A good-boy or good-girl orientation characterizes this stage, in which the child conforms to rules to please others and avoid disapproval. This stage parallels the concrete operations stage of cognitive development. Around the age of 12 years, children enter stage 4 of the conventional level. There is an orientation toward respecting authority, obeying rules, and maintaining social order. Most religions place the age of accountability at approximately 12 years.

Family Influence

Children manifest antisocial behaviors during middle childhood. Behaviors such as cheating, lying, and stealing are not uncommon. Often, children lie or cheat to get out of an embarrassing situation or to make themselves look more important to their peers. In most cases, these behaviors are minor; however, if they are severe or persistent, the child may need referral for counseling.

Parents and teachers profoundly influence moral development. Parents can teach children the difference between right and wrong most effectively by living according to their values. A father who lectures his child about the importance of honesty gives a mixed message when he brags about fooling his boss or cheating on his income tax return. The moral atmosphere in the home is a critical factor in the child's personality development.

Children learn self-discipline and internalization of values through obedience to external rules. School-age children are legalistic, and they feel loved and secure when they know that firm limits are set on their behavior. They want and expect discipline for wrongdoings. For moral teaching to be effective, parents must be consistent in their expectations of their children as well as in administering rewards and punishment.

Spirituality and Religion

Spiritually, school-age children become acquainted with the basic content of their faith. Children reared within a religious tradition feel a part of their religion. Although their thinking is still concrete, children begin to use abstract concepts to describe God and are able to comprehend God as a power greater than themselves or their parents. Because school-age children think literally, spiritual concepts take on materialistic and physical expression. Heaven and hell fascinate them. Concern for rules and a maturing conscience may cause a nagging sense of guilt and fear of going to hell. Younger school-age children still tend to associate accidents and illness with punishment for real or imagined wrongdoing. One 6-year-old child hospitalized for an appendectomy said, "God saw all the bad things I did, and He punished me." Reassurance that God does not punish children by making them sick reduces anxiety.

HEALTH PROMOTION FOR THE SCHOOL-AGE CHILD AND FAMILY

It is recommended that during middle childhood, children should visit the health care provider every 2 years. Many school districts require documentation of a routine physical examination at least once during the elementary school years after the kindergarten visit.

Nutrition During Middle Childhood

Nutritional Requirements

Growth continues at a slow, regular pace, but the school-age child begins to have an increased appetite. Energy needs increase during the later school-age years. Children in this age-group tend to have few eating idiosyncrasies and generally enjoy eating to satisfy appetite and as a social function. Children who developed dislikes for certain foods during earlier periods may continue to refuse those foods. School-age children are influenced by family patterns and the limitations their activities put on them. They may rush through a meal to go out to play or watch a favorite program on television.

Children should choose culturally appropriate foods and snacks daily according to the Food Guide Pyramid: 6 to 11 servings of grains, 3 to 5 servings of vegetables, 2 to 4 servings of fruit, 2 or 3 servings of protein, and 2 or 3 servings of milk or dairy products. They need to limit saturated fat intake and processed sugars. Caloric and protein requirements begin to increase at about age 11 years because of the preadolescent growth spurt. The requirements for boys and girls also begin to vary at this age. A gradual increase of food intake will also take place. The nurse should ask children to describe specifically what they eat at meals and for snacks to develop a more comprehensive picture of their eating habits.

When assessing children's nutritional status, it is important to also assess any body image concerns; be sure to ask children how they feel about the way they look. Eating disorders, although thought to be a problem of adolescence, can begin in the late elementary school years.

Age-Related Nutritional Challenges

During the school years, the child's schedule changes and more time is spent away from home. Most children eat lunch at school, and they usually have a choice of foods. Even if the parent packs a lunch for the child to take to school, there are no guarantees that the child will eat the lunch. Children sometimes trade foods with other children or may not eat a particular item. It is also during this period that the child becomes more active in clubs, sports, and other activities that interrupt the normal meal schedule.

The federal government funds the School Lunch Program, which provides lunches for low-income children for free or at a reduced cost. The School Lunch Program includes approximately one third of the recommended daily dietary allowances

Health Promotion

The 6- to 8-Year-Old Child

FOCUSED ASSESSMENT

Ask the child the following:

- Can you tell me how often and what foods you like to eat? How often do you eat at fast-food restaurants? How do you feel about how much you weigh? Do you think you need to gain or lose any weight?
- What types of physical activities do you like to do? How often do you do them? Do you have any quiet hobbies that interest you? How many hours each day do you watch television? What is your favorite television program?
- How often do you brush your teeth, floss, and see the dentist? Do you take fluoride?
- What time do you go to bed at night? What time do you get up in the morning? Do you have any trouble falling asleep, or do you wake up in the middle of the night?
- How often do you have a bowel movement? Are there any problems with urination? (Use the child's familiar terminology if known.) Do you wet the bed? If so, how often?
- What grade in school are you? Are you doing well in school or having any problems? Do you feel safe at school? Do you participate in any before-school or after-school programs?
- Tell me about your friends. Do they like to do the same things you like to do?
- How do you get along with other members of your family? Is there a special family member you could talk to if you are having a problem? If so, who?
- Do you do any or all of the following: use a seatbelt every time you get in a car; wear a helmet every time you ride a bike; wear a helmet and protective pads every time you skate or use a scooter; use sunscreen; swim with a buddy and only when an adult is present; always look both ways before crossing the street; use the right equipment when you play sports; know to avoid strangers and how to call for help if needed?
- Has anyone ever physically harmed you or touched you in a way that made you uncomfortable?

Ask the parent the following:

- Are there any concerns related to the child's nutrition, body image, physical activity, oral health, sleep, elimination,

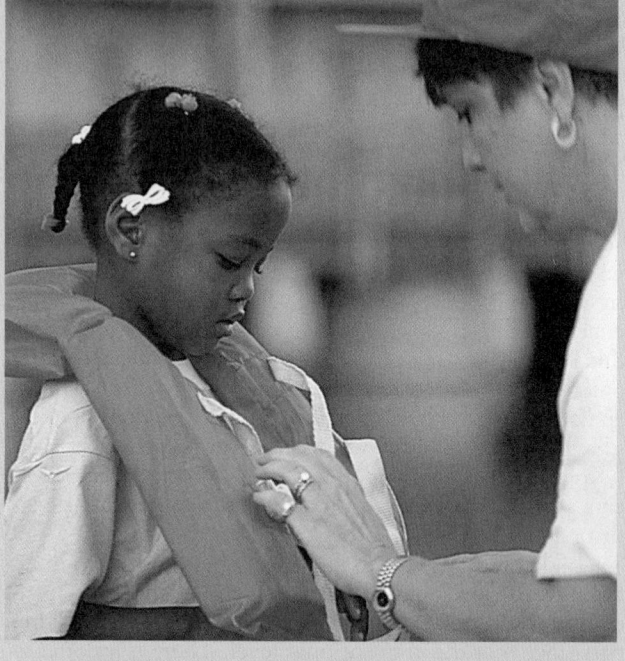

school, family interactions, self-esteem, and ability to practice safety precautions?
- Is there a gun in the home? If so, is it locked away and the ammunition stored in a separate place?
- Do you have a swimming pool? If so, is it fenced on all four sides and not directly accessible from the house?
- Do you have a fire escape plan that you practice regularly?

DEVELOPMENTAL MILESTONES

Personal/social: develops a positive self-esteem through skill acquisition and task completion; peer group becoming the primary socializing force; outgoing and boisterous, "know-it-all," but becomes more reflective and quiet by age 8 years; loves new ideas and places; has a good sense of humor, may tell crude jokes; may be argumentative and use tension-releasing behaviors such as nail biting, hair twisting, wriggling; likes to

for a child. School lunch programs usually follow the Food Guide Pyramid to meet recommended nutritional requirements; however, many school lunches are somewhat high in fat. Some schools also offer breakfast and milk programs. Many schools offer low-nutrient, high-calorie snacks as an add-on to the school lunch or in snack machines available in various locations throughout the school. In some cases, children use their lunch money to buy snacks. Advise parents to communicate with their children about appropriate lunch and snacks in school and to know what is being offered in the school cafeteria.

School-age children usually request a snack after school and in the evening. Parents should be encouraged to provide their child with healthy choices for snacks. By not buying foods high in calories and low in nutrients the parent can remove the temptation for the child to choose the less healthy foods.

Unpredictable schedules, advertising, easy access to fast food, and peer pressure all have an effect on the foods a child chooses. The child may begin to prefer "junk foods," which do not have much nutritional value. Most of these foods are high in fat and sugar. In addition, school-age children often skip breakfast. The family plays an important role in modeling good eating habits for the child. Schools also have a responsibility to provide nutritious meals for children.

Dental Care

Although the incidence of dental caries (tooth decay) has declined in recent years, tooth decay remains a significant health problem among school-age children. Unfortunately, many parents and school-age children consider dental hygiene to be of minor importance. Many parents erroneously believe that dental care, even brushing, is not important for primary teeth because they will all fall out anyway. However, premature loss of these deciduous teeth can complicate eruption of permanent teeth and lead to malocclusion.

Health Promotion

The 6- to 8-Year-Old Child—cont'd

make things but often does not finish projects; loves family members but worries about them; has a strong sense of fairness and justice—uses rules to define cooperative relationships with others (sees rules as being imposed by others)

Fine motor: ties shoelaces, buttons and zips clothes, dresses and undresses without help; can print, draw, color well, model clay, and cut with scissors; visual acuity is fully developed

Language/cognitive: vocabulary expands; understands the different properties of language: play on words, puns, mnemonics, jokes; adapts well to changing physical properties of objects (e.g., conservation, reversibility, identity); improved long-term memory; organizes concepts and classifies in several ways; uses various memory strategies to improve school work

Gross motor: improved muscle mass and coordination allow for participation in a variety of sports and games

HEALTH MAINTENANCE

Physical Measurements
Average weight gain is 2.5 kg (5½ lb) per year
Average increase in height is approximately 5.5 cm (2 in) per year
Continue to plot height and weight
Plot body mass index (see Appendix E)
Note any breast budding or signs of other secondary sex characteristics

Immunizations
If not given earlier, administer measles, mumps, rubella (MMR) #2; diphtheria, tetanus, acellular pertussis (DTaP) #5; and inactivated poliovirus (IPV) #4
Administer other immunizations if not up-to-date

Health Screening
Objective hearing and vision screening
Speech assessment for fluency
Hemoglobin or hematocrit
Urine for sugar and protein
Blood pressure
Lipid screen if at risk
Tuberculosis screening if at risk (see Chapter 45)

ANTICIPATORY GUIDANCE

Provide health teaching to the child as well as the parent.
Nutrition
Follow recommended servings according to the Food Guide Pyramid; teach the child how to keep track of servings and to give input into meal preparation
Advise to avoid fast foods and to eat a nutritious breakfast
Watch calcium and iron intake

Elimination
Regular bowel movements according to the child's pattern; treat constipation by increasing water intake and intake of fresh fruits and vegetables
Occasional bed-wetting is within the norm; refer for more serious problems (see Chapter 44)

Dental
Provide regular dental care every 6 months
Continue regular brushing with fluoride toothpaste and flossing (may need assistance with this)
Continue fluoride supplements if water is not fluoridated
May need dental sealants as permanent molars erupt

Sleep
Facilitate an individually appropriate sleep pattern; school-age children usually go to bed by 9 PM and are up by 7 AM
If the child is not tired, advise the parent to allow a quiet reading time in bed

Safety
Review gun safety; bicycle, skating, and scooter safety; playground safety; fire safety; automobile and pedestrian safety; water safety; sun protection; good touch versus bad touch, stranger awareness
Discuss exposure to contact allergens (poison ivy, oak, sumac), tick checks, sports safety, use of reflective clothing if out at night

Play
Encourage developing collections, playing complicated board and card games, crafts, electronic and science-related games
Advise limiting television watching to no more than 2 hours a day

Self-Esteem and Competence
See "Parents Want to Know" box, p. 134

School-age children are able to assume responsibility for their own dental hygiene. Good oral health habits tend to be carried into the adult years, reducing cavity formation for a lifetime. Thorough brushing with fluoride toothpaste followed by flossing between the teeth should be done after meals and especially before bedtime. Proper brushing and flossing and a well-balanced diet promote healthy gums as well as prevent cavities. Sugary or sticky between-meal snacks should be limited. Candy that dissolves quickly, such as chocolate, is less cariogenic than sticky candy, which stays in contact with teeth longer. Information related to fluoride supplementation is given in Chapter 6.

Malocclusion

Good *occlusion*, or alignment, of the teeth is important for tooth formation, speech development, and physical appearance. Many school-age children need orthodontic braces to correct malocclusion, a condition in which the teeth are crowded, crooked, or out of alignment. Factors such as heredity, cleft palate, premature loss of primary teeth, and mouth breathing lead to malocclusion. Thumb sucking is not believed to cause malocclusion unless it persists past the age of 5 or 6 years. Malocclusion becomes particularly noticeable between the ages of 6 and 12 years, when the permanent teeth are erupting.

Children with braces are at increased risk for dental caries and must be scrupulous about their dental hygiene. School nurses can encourage children who wear braces to brush after every meal and snack, eat a nutritious diet, and visit the dentist at least once every 6 months. Use of a water pick keeps gums healthy and helps remove food particles from around wires and bands.

Braces cause many children to feel self-conscious and may be difficult for a school-age child to accept. However, for some children, orthodontic appliances may be a status symbol. Parental support and encouragement are important to help the child adjust to orthodontic treatment.

Preventing Dental Injuries

During the school-age years, injuries to the teeth can occur easily. Many injuries can be avoided by using mouth protectors. These resilient shields protect against injuries by cushioning blows that might otherwise damage teeth or lead to jaw fractures (American Dental Association, 1998). Children should wear a mouth protector when participating in contact sports, bike riding, or in-line skating. Custom-made mouth protectors constructed by the dentist are more expensive than stock mouth protectors purchased in stores, but their better fit makes them more comfortable and less likely to interfere with speech and breathing.

Dental Health Education

Health education curricula need to be designed to foster attitudes and behaviors among children that promote good personal oral hygiene practices and awareness of the risks of dental disease. The school nurse is in an excellent position to educate children about dental health as well as to detect problems such as untreated caries, inflamed gums, or malocclusion. The nurse should look for signs of smokeless tobacco use (irritation of the gums at the tobacco placement site, gum recession, stained teeth) and should take this opportunity to explain to the child the risks of using tobacco. The use of snuff and chewing tobacco carries multiple dangers, including a greatly increased risk of oral cancer and heart disease.

Sleep and Rest

The number of hours spent sleeping decreases as the child grows older. Children ages 6 and 7 years need about 12 hours of sleep per night. Some children also continue to need an afternoon quiet time or nap to restore energy levels. The 12-year-old needs about 9 to 10 hours of sleep at night. More sleep is needed when the child enters the preadolescent growth spurt. Adequate sleep is important for school performance and physical growth. Inadequate sleep can cause irritability, inability to concentrate, and poor school performance.

To promote rest and sleep, a period of quiet activity just before bedtime is helpful. A leisurely bedtime routine, with adequate time for the child to read, listen to the radio or compact discs (CDs), or just daydream, promotes relaxation. Children who do not obtain adequate rest often have difficulty getting up in the morning, creating a family disturbance as they rush to get ready for school, perhaps skipping breakfast or leaving the house in the heat of frustration. A set bedtime and waking time, consistently enforced, promote security and healthful sleep habits. Bedtime offers an ideal opportunity for parent and child to share important events of the day or give a kiss and a hug, unthinkable in front of peers earlier in the day.

Occasionally, school-age children experience sleep problems, most commonly sleepwalking and sleep terrors (night terrors). Both conditions occur during deep sleep. Children with night terrors scream and appear excessively frightened; they may be difficult to console during the episode, but the episode is self-limiting, usually lasting less than 30 minutes. Children who walk in their sleep do not respond to their environment and are in danger of injuring themselves. Episodes of both sleep terrors and sleepwalking are frightening to parents, but the child is unlikely to remember the episode on awakening. The nurse can advise a parent to quietly soothe the child during an episode and protect the child from harm. Episodes may increase when the child is experiencing stress.

Discipline

Because school-age children possess a strong sense of justice and believe in the importance of rules, they want and expect limits to be set on their behavior. Firm, consistent limits increase children's sense of security and reinforce the message that an adult cares about them. Realistic expectations, clearly defined rules, and logical consequences help children develop self-discipline and increased self-esteem. Some families have meetings where they discuss how responsibilities in the family will be shared. The child is made to feel more a part of the solution rather than the problem.

Responsibility can be developed in children through the use of natural and logical consequences related to actions. Children become accountable for their actions. If a child leaves a toy outside and it is damaged, the parent is empathetic but does not replace the toy. The parent does not get in a power struggle, nor does the parent verbally attack the child. The child begins to understand that there are consequences to actions. This type of discipline, correctly used, will allow the parent to separate the deed from the doer; not pass moral judgment; focus on the present, not the past; and show respect and firm kindness. In addition, the child will be given choices and the consequence will relate to the logic of the situation.

Teachers' disciplinary efforts are often thwarted when parents do not support them or show no concern about their children's misbehavior in school. Teamwork between parents and teachers is essential for effective discipline. Regular parent-teacher conferences help make discipline effective.

Safety

Unintentional injury is the leading cause of death in children of every age-group. Although the death rate from unintentional injury is lower in children ages 5 to 9 years than it is during early childhood, with the exception of injury from falls, the annual incidence of nonfatal unintentional injury is higher (Rivara & Grossman, 2004).

Approaches to safety education vary as the child grows older. Physically, middle childhood is a period of great activity, with the child moving back and forth between the home environment and the community. The school-age child experiences less fear when playing and frequently imitates

---

Critical Thinking EXERCISE 7-1

Mrs. George states that Megan, 11 years old, has recently started to leave her belongings throughout the house and that her room is always a mess. Mrs. George states that she is frustrated and feels as if she is constantly asking Megan to pick her things up and to clean her room.

1. What assumptions might a nurse make, based on Mrs. George's report about her daughter's behavior?
2. What other data does the nurse need to clarify to best help Mrs. George and Megan in this situation?
3. What are some possible approaches the nurse might suggest to Mrs. George?

adults by using tools and household items. Children in this age-group enjoy helping with adult routines and chores around the home. Anticipatory guidance related to safety is very important as children develop and try new projects that require use of more dangerous or sophisticated equipment.

Safety education is best accomplished by simply stating safety rules and providing reinforcement through short projects and immediate rewards. Role-playing activities and error-detection picture games are excellent ways to reinforce safety lessons. Children in this age-group are inquisitive and will frequently ask questions. The answers to their questions should contain concrete rationales. Group projects with safety topics help foster independent thinking while promoting interactions with the child's peer group.

Car Safety

If the child has attained a height of 4' 9" and is between the ages of 8 and 12 years, the child may be large enough to use the vehicle's three-point restraining system. Compliance often is determined by family values, with use or nonuse reflecting parental practices. For the younger, smaller child, correct positioning of the seatbelt is important. Parents should help adjust the belts so that the lap belt fits snugly over the bony pelvis and the shoulder harness is positioned across the chest. Children should sit in a rear seat away from car passenger safety airbags.

Fire and Burn Safety

Parents should continue to reinforce safety procedures associated with fire safety. Routine fire drills should be practiced in the home. Repetition of family drills helps ensure that the child will respond correctly and automatically to smoke alarms. Children of this age can better comprehend cause-and-effect relationships, so they can understand why they should not play with potentially flammable substances.

School-age children are eager to help parents with daily chores such as cooking or ironing. Parents need to invest the time to teach their children how to use tools and appliances properly and must establish guidelines to avoid burn injuries as a result of the child's inexperience.

Fireworks create another burn hazard for children. Each summer, many children are seriously burned or permanently scarred by fireworks. To prevent serious burn injuries, the federal government, under the federal Hazardous Substance Act, prohibits the sale of the more dangerous fireworks to the general public. However, a degree of risk always is associated with any fireworks. There are no absolutely safe fireworks for children or adults. Fireworks are best left to the experts and viewed from a safe distance. En-

courage families to enjoy the many community-sponsored fireworks displays.

Bicycle, In-Line Skate, Scooter, and Skateboard Safety

Mastering the ability to ride a bicycle is a milestone in a child's life, leading to independence. The bicycle is typically considered a toy but is actually a vehicle that is capable of speedy transportation. It is also a major cause of death and serious head trauma in children (National Center for Injury Prevention and Control, 2000). For this reason, the public health community supports the mandatory use of bicycle helmets. Research has demonstrated that the use of a helmet can reduce the incidence of head injury by as much as 85% when fitted properly (Logan et al., 1998).

Bicycle safety practices actually begin when the child is a passenger in a bicycle seat on the back of a parent's bike. They continue as the child learns to ride a tricycle and progressively build as the child becomes more skilled and begins to ride a bicycle. A helmet and other safety accessories are essential for protection, but they are only an adjunct to the child's skill level and knowledge of the rules of the road. A young cyclist is unpredictable and may be preoccupied with managing the bicycle itself. For this reason, parents should set limits on where, when, and how far the child may ride until the child can competently maneuver the bicycle. When parents on bicycles accompany children, it is essential that the parents wear helmets and follow the rules of the road to role model appropriate safety and emphasize the importance of the helmet and the rules.

In-line skating and skateboarding are recreational activities that are popular with school-age children. Balancing, stopping, and turning are challenging and require motor skills similar to those required for bicycling. As the child begins to learn these skills, falls are frequent and protective gear is essential. Helmets and protective pads covering the knees and elbows help protect the most vulnerable areas of the child's body from serious injury. Key educational points and an overview of safety principles are described in the Parents Want to Know box.

Unpowered scooters are very lightweight, small versions of an older, more stable type of scooter used by children in the 1950s. They are propelled by one foot and have a very narrow base and small wheels. Because of their portability, both adults and children use them, many times on crowded city sidewalks. Since the introduction of unpowered scooters in the late 1990s, scooter-related injuries have markedly increased and approximately 85% of the visits to emergency rooms for scooter-related injuries were for children (Centers for Disease Control and Prevention [CDC], 2000b). Recommendations for safe operation of scooters are similar to those for in-line skating, with the exception of wrist pad use.

Pedestrian Safety

Children between the ages of 5 and 9 years are at the greatest risk for auto-pedestrian injuries. The tremendous forces of impact and the lack of protection for the pedestrian can lead to severe injury. Children are commonly struck when they dart into traffic, especially where parked cars obscure the driver's view of the child (e.g., crossing the street in front of a school bus, playing near cars in driveways or yards). Several

---

! CRITICAL TO REMEMBER

Fire Safety Rules

- Know two specific escape routes from each area in the home.
- Know how to access 911.
- Know how to crawl under the smoke to leave a burning house.
- Have a predetermined meeting area outside the house.
- Never return to a burning house.
- Practice fire drills.

PARENTS
Want to Know

Bicycle, In-Line Skating, Scooter, and Skateboard Safety

- Children should always wear a helmet when bike riding, in-line skating, or skateboarding. This safety practice should begin when the child begins to learn these activities.
- Helmets should fit properly and snugly on the head. Helmets need to be lightweight and ventilated and have reflective trim.
- Children should be taught not to ride at dusk or in the dark. They should always call home for a ride if it is after dark.
- Children should not ride two on a bicycle.
- Riding barefoot, in thongs, or in slippers is dangerous. Children need to avoid using audio headsets while riding a bicycle because they can diminish hearing capabilities.
- Encourage children to stay on sidewalks, paths, or driveways until they have mastered advanced biking skills and know the rules of the road.
- While riding or in-line skating, children should avoid uneven road surfaces, gravel, potholes, or bumps.
- Bicycles should be equipped with reflectors and lights. With their parents' help, encourage children to routinely inspect their own bicycles to ensure that they are functioning properly (e.g., brakes, tires, lights).
- Proper sizing is important when purchasing a bicycle for a child. Oversized bicycles are responsible for many injuries. The child should be able to place the balls of both feet on the ground when sitting on the seat with the hands on the handlebars.
- The child should be able to straddle the center bar with both feet flat on the ground. There should be about 1 inch of clearance between the crotch and the bar.
- The handlebars should be within easy reach for the child.

Rules of the Road
- Children younger than 8 years should ride only with adult supervision and not in the street. Limit in-line skating or skateboarding to areas where there is no car traffic.
- Children should not ride bicycles on roads with heavy traffic.
- A bicycle should be ridden on the right side of the road, with the traffic. Bike riders must obey all traffic laws, traffic signs, and lights.
- Children need to learn the appropriate hand signals and use them every time before turning.
- Bicycles should be walked across busy intersections, not ridden.
- Children need to learn to stop, look left, look right, and look left again before entering a street or leaving a driveway, alley, or parking lot.
- Children should stop at all intersections, marked and unmarked.
- Children riding bicycles should obey all stop signs and red lights.
- Children should look back and yield to traffic coming from behind before turning left at intersections.
- Basic bicycle safety rules apply to in-line skating and skateboarding.

factors predispose this age-group to such injuries. Their smaller physical stature limits their visibility to drivers until too late. In addition, children in this age-group have the misconception that if they can see the car, the driver must be able to see them and will be able to stop instantly. Focused on play activities, they often impulsively dart into the street, oblivious to boundaries and potential traffic dangers.

Children learn traffic safety by watching and doing. Exposure to traffic increases as the child begins to walk to and from school and friends' houses. Parents have the responsibility of practicing pedestrian safety hundreds of times before the child is allowed to venture across streets alone.

Water Safety
School-age children learn to swim well enough to keep their heads above water for a short time at about 8 years old. The length of time they can keep their heads above water and their swimming ability increase with age and experience. The incidence of drowning decreases in this age-group; however, adult supervision is still needed to prevent a water-related injury. School-age children often overestimate their swimming capabilities and endurance. As their swimming abilities improve, anticipatory guidance can include general swimming safety. Children should be taught to stay away from canals and the fast-moving waters of creeks and rivers. Advise parents to teach children to wade into shallow water or to jump

feet first into water of unknown depth to prevent neck injuries. Safety near the water includes never running, pushing, or jumping on others who are in the water.

Selected Issues Related to the School-Age Child

Adjustment to School
Most children are eager to start school, particularly if they have older siblings. They even look forward to bringing home their books and doing "real" homework. This enthusiasm usually fades quickly, however. Most children adjust well to first grade, enjoying the opportunities it provides for peer interaction and stimulating experiences. First grade may be the child's first experience of being away from home. For these children, starting school may be a frightening experience. Even children who have attended preschool have some anxiety about beginning first grade. Adjustment to school depends on a variety of factors, including the child's physical and emotional maturity, the child's experiences, and the parents' ability to support the child and accept the separation (see Chapter 6).

Peer Influence. School is often the first experience a child has with a large number of children of the same age. From peers children learn how to cooperate, compete, bargain, and follow rules. Peer approval is of major importance as children look to their friends for recognition and support. The influence of peers becomes stronger as the child grows older.

Influence of Teachers. Teachers have a significant influence on the social and intellectual development of children. An effective teacher makes learning fun and capitalizes on the child's interests and talents. Teachers guide the child's learning by rewarding success and helping the child learn from and deal with failures. The teacher plays an important role in preventing feelings of inferiority in the child. By structuring the learning environment so that the child experiences success, the teacher bolsters feelings of industry.

The student-teacher relationship is a key factor in school success. Effective teachers motivate students by being warm and understanding, showing interest, and communicating at the child's level. Children value the opinion of such teachers and will work to gain their approval. Favorite teachers serve as role models and are often objects of hero worship by their students.

Even excellent teachers cannot do an effective job alone. They need the support of parents and school administrators to maximize children's learning potential.

Parents' Role. Parents play a key role in their children's academic success. By taking an active interest in children's progress and encouraging them to do their best, parents can foster learning. Positive reinforcement should be given for honest efforts, not just good grades. Parents should enforce rules that encourage self-discipline and good study habits (e.g., no television until homework is finished). The child must create and adhere to a schedule for completing large assignments to prevent last-minute panic. If the child does not have a desk or another private place for homework, the kitchen table or another quiet, well-lighted area should be made available during study time. The television should be turned off during study time and distractions kept to a minimum. Adequate sleep is important for school performance. Parents may need to enforce bedtime rules to meet the child's needs. Rewarding children for meeting deadlines and for being organized encourages them to take responsibility for their learning and fosters skills that are important for success in jobs as adults.

Parents need to communicate with teachers and stay informed about their children's progress. Visiting the classroom and attending parent-teacher conferences and school activities are important. Showing respect and support for the teacher facilitates learning.

School Refusal. *School refusal* is a descriptive term for behavior that may indicate the presence of a specific phobia, separation anxiety, truancy, or social phobia (Ruggiero, 1999). In the past, the term was used interchangeably with *school phobia* and *school avoidance*. There is much discussion over the diagnosis and treatment of children who refuse to attend school and the appropriate label for these children. School phobia can be distinguished from a separation anxiety disorder in that with school phobia, the child does not experience distressing symptoms anywhere else but in school. Children with separation anxiety disorder experience distress any time they are separated from their parents, including at school (Varley & Smith, 2003).

School refusal has been defined as frequent absences from school, academic disengagement or disruption, or dropping out (Ruggiero, 1999). Some school-refusing children show specific fears of school or school-related situations (tests, bullies, teacher reprimands, undressing for gym). Because some children with school refusal behaviors have intense emotional distress related to school attendance, they are labeled *phobic*. The confusion over the use of these terms can make assessment and treatment of these children difficult. For an additional discussion of separation anxiety, see Chapter 53.

Children may go to school unwillingly or may refuse and have temper tantrums if the parents insist on taking the child to school. Younger children may complain of stomachaches, headaches, nausea, and vomiting. Older children may complain of palpitations and feeling faint. These symptoms typically resolve when the child returns home.

Helping a Child Overcome School Refusal. In uncomplicated cases, the parent needs to return the child to school as soon as possible. If symptoms are severe, a limited period of part-time or modified school attendance may be necessary. For example, part of the day may be spent in the counselor's or school nurse's office, with assignments obtained from the teacher. The child should be gently questioned about factors at school that cause worry or fear. Specific causes, such as a bully or an overly critical teacher, should be dealt with immediately. Parents must support each other because the child may play one parent against the other to avoid school. Parents should be empathetic yet firm and consistent in their insistence that the child attend school. Parents should not pick the child up at school once the child is there. Positive reinforcement for school attendance is essential. Encouraging and maintaining peer contacts and emphasizing the positive aspects of school are helpful. The principal and teacher should be told about the situation so that they can cooperate with the treatment plan.

Self-Care Children

The number of children who let themselves into their homes after school and are left alone continues to grow as the number of dual-income and single-parent families increases. These children are called *self-care children*, previously referred to as *latch-key children*. Approximately 12% of all children ages 5 to 12 years in the United States care for themselves at least once per week, and 1% are preschool-age children (Kerrebrock & Lewit, 1999).

Parents often feel guilty about leaving children alone and may feel concern for their children's safety. Potential positive outcomes of this experience are learning to be independent and responsible. Because of time spent unsupervised at home, the risk of children engaging in problem behaviors (smoking, alcohol use, inappropriate eating) increases. The quality of the parent-child relationship and parents who are emotionally supportive and establish firm rules play a role in moderating adverse effects on the child in self-care.

Nurses can help families by offering support and education to parents and children to reduce the risks for self-care children. Parents need to know how to prepare their children for self-care, teaching them specific strategies for staying safe at home alone. Nurses can serve as child advocates by working to develop expanded after-school childcare programs in the community. A number of communities have established after-school telephone help lines to provide information, support, and assistance to self-care children. Nurses should also know the laws relating to self-care in their state of practice. Some state and local regulations

Health Promotion

The 9- to 11-Year-Old Child

FOCUSED ASSESSMENT

Ask the child the following:

- Can you tell me how often and what foods you like to eat? How often do you eat at fast-food restaurants? How do you feel about how much you weigh? Do you think you need to gain or lose any weight?
- What types of physical activities do you like to do? How often do you do them? Do you have any quiet hobbies that interest you? How many hours each day do you watch television? What is your favorite television program?
- How often do you brush your teeth, floss, and see the dentist? Do you take fluoride?
- What time do you go to bed at night? What time do you get up in the morning? Do you have any trouble falling asleep, or do you wake up in the middle of the night?
- How often do you have a bowel movement? Are there any problems with urination? (Use the child's familiar terminology if known.) Do you wet the bed? If so, how often?
- What grade in school are you? Are you doing well in school or having any problems? Do you feel safe at school? In what before- or after-school programs do you participate?
- Tell me about your friends. Do they like to do the same things you like to do? Do they pressure you to do things you would rather not do? Do you or your friends smoke or take any substances (alcohol, drugs)?
- How do you get along with other members of your family? Is there a special family member you could talk to if you are having a problem? If so, who?
- Do you do any or all of the following: use a seatbelt every time you get in a car; wear a helmet every time you ride a bike; wear a helmet and protective pads every time you skate or use a scooter; use sunscreen; swim with a buddy and only when an adult is present; always look both ways before crossing the street; use the right equipment when you play sports; know to avoid strangers and how to call for help if needed?
- Has anyone ever physically harmed you or touched you in a way that made you uncomfortable? Have you ever thought about harming yourself?

Ask the parent the following:

- Are there any concerns related to the child's nutrition, body image, physical activity, oral health, sleep, elimination, school, family interactions, self-esteem, and ability to practice safety precautions?

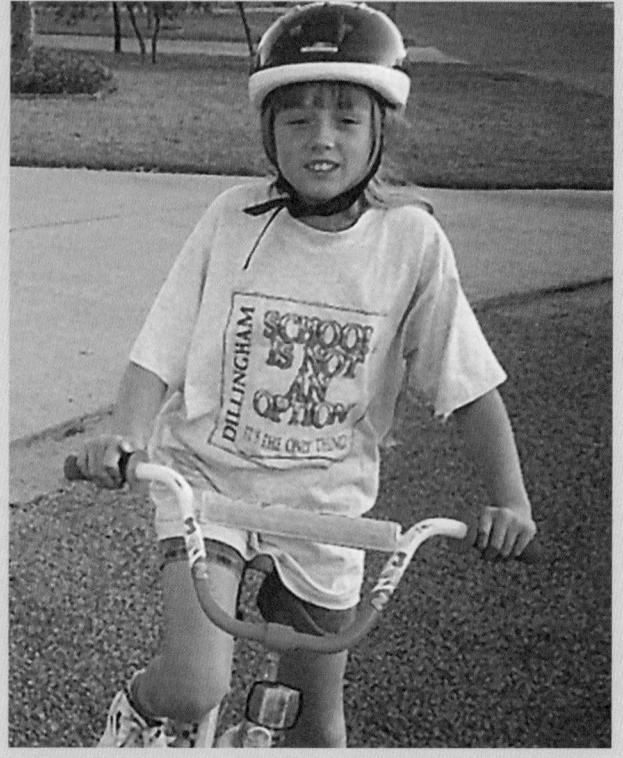

- Is there a gun in the home? If so, is it locked away and the ammunition stored in a separate place?
- Do you have a fire escape plan that you practice regularly?
- What types of information have you given to your child about puberty and sexual activity?
- Do you feel uncomfortable talking with your child about sensitive issues?

DEVELOPMENTAL MILESTONES

Personal/social: peers' opinions become more important than parents'; clubs, with secret codes and rituals, are at a peak; hero worship; fairly responsible, dependable, and polite to adults; boys tease girls, and girls may become "boy crazy"; may become angry but is learning to control it; critical of own work; rebelliousness may begin; ready for away-from-home experiences, such as camp

---

prohibit self-care in children younger than 6 to 11 years of age (Kerrebrock & Lewit, 1999).

Obesity

When intake of food exceeds expenditure, the excess is stored as fat. Obesity is an excessive accumulation of fat in the body. There is an increase of weight beyond that considered desirable with regard to age, height, and bone structure.

Obesity can be a precursor of hyperlipidemia, sleep apnea, cholelithiasis (gallstones), orthopedic problems, hyperten-

sion, and diabetes. In addition, children who are obese can have psychosocial difficulties, eating disorders, and inappropriate expectations because their greater growth makes them appear older than they are (Dietz, 1998; Hodges, 2003). Because the obese child develops increased numbers of fat cells, which are carried into adulthood, preventing obesity in childhood can reduce the risk of obesity in adulthood and plays a role in preventing disease.

Cultural, genetic, environmental, and socioeconomic factors have been linked to childhood obesity. Children with

Health Promotion

The 9- to 11-Year-Old Child—cont'd

Fine motor: hand-eye coordination fully developed; fine motor control approximates adults'

Language/cognitive: reads more and enjoys comics and newspapers; understands fractions, conservation of volume and weight; likes to talk on the telephone; interested in how things work

Gross motor: may begin to be more awkward as growth spurt begins; may drop out of team sports to avoid embarrassment

HEALTH MAINTENANCE

Physical Measurements

Girls are 2.54 cm (1 in) taller and 0.9 kg (2 lb) heavier on average than boys

About 90% of facial growth has been attained

Boys have greater physical strength

Girls may experience rapid growth spurt and menarche

Immunizations

Review immunization records

Administer immunizations if not up to date; some children may need measles, mumps, rubella (MMR) #2; varicella; hepatitis B series; tetanus and diphtheria (Td) if more than 5 years since last dose

Health Screening

Objective hearing and vision screening (may become myopic as growth spurt begins)

Hemoglobin or hematocrit

Urine for sugar and protein

Blood pressure

Baseline lipid screen

Tuberculosis screening if at risk (see Chapter 45)

Scoliosis screening

ANTICIPATORY GUIDANCE

Provide health teaching to the child as well as the parent.

Nutrition

Follow recommended servings according to the Food Guide Pyramid; teach the child how to keep track of servings and to give input into meal preparation

Advise to avoid fast foods and to eat a nutritious breakfast

Watch calcium and iron intake

Assess adequacy of diet and snacks

Elimination

Regular bowel movements according to the child's pattern

Dental

Provide regular dental care every 6 months

Continue regular brushing with fluoride toothpaste and flossing

Continue fluoride supplements if water is not fluoridated

May need dental sealants as permanent molars erupt

May need referral to orthodontist for malocclusion

Sleep

Facilitate an individually appropriate sleep pattern; school-age children usually go to bed by 9 PM and are up by 7 AM

If the child is not tired, advise the parent to allow a quiet reading time in bed

Hygiene

May resist baths and showers, may wear the same clothes every day, bedroom is usually messy

Early reluctance to keep clean may be followed by a period of overcleanliness (multiple showers daily, new outfit after each shower)

Safety

Review gun safety; bicycle, skating, and scooter safety; playground safety; fire safety; automobile and pedestrian safety; water safety; sun protection; exposure to outside allergens and ticks; sports safety; use of reflective clothing if out at night

Continue to have child belted in the back seat of the car away from airbags

Discuss not allowing others into the home if parent is not there; how to contact emergency services; not to open doors to strangers; avoiding listening to loud music through earphones

Play

Encourage reading age-appropriate fiction, developing collections, playing complicated board and card games, crafts, electronic and science-related games

Advise limiting television watching to no more than 2 hours a day

Self-Esteem and Competence

See "Parents Want to Know" box, p. 134

---

low metabolic rates and an increased number of fat cells tend to gain more weight. Children with one or both parents overweight are at increased risk for obesity (Strauss & Dietz, 1999). It is often very difficult to separate out factors contributing to obesity in a family in which the parents are obese. When a parent lacks nutritional knowledge, it is reflected in the meals and snacks provided in the home. The child is at risk for developing the same habits. Obesity is more prevalent among children raised in urban communities and in smaller families. In addition, obesity varies among different ethnic groups, geographic regions, and socioeconomic classes (Cowell & Agruss, 2000).

Unstructured meals, "meals on the run," and meals at fast-food restaurants can lack proper nutrition and be high in calories. Lack of exercise also contributes to obesity. Recent studies have shown that as school-age children get older, they are less likely to be involved in regular physical education classes (CDC, 2002; Cowell & Agruss, 2000). The child who is given food for reward or punishment attaches more to eating than gaining nutrition. Some people

PARENTS
Want to Know

How to Prevent and Manage Obesity

You can help prevent and manage obesity in your child by doing the following:
- Do not use food as a reward.
- Establish consistent times for meals and snacks, and do not allow in-between eating.
- Offer only healthy food options (ask the child to choose between an apple or popcorn, not an apple or a cookie). Avoid keeping unhealthy food in the house, and minimize trips to fast-food restaurants.
- Be a role model by improving your own eating habits and levels of activity.
- Encourage the child to do fun, physical activities with the family.
- Praise the child for making appropriate food choices and for increasing physical activity levels.

BOX 7-3
Manifestations of Stress in Children

How children perceive stress influences its effects. It is not just the stress but how the child perceives and responds to the stress that determines whether the child experiences symptoms of stress.

Intervention is needed when a child shows the following signs of stress:
- Unhappiness, moodiness
- Irritability, increased aggressive behavior
- Fatigue, inability to concentrate
- Hyperactivity
- Changes in eating or sleeping habits
- Physical complaints (nausea, headaches, stomachaches)
- Bed-wetting
- Substance abuse
- Diminished school performance
- Suicidal behavior

---

still think that a fat baby is a healthy baby. This type of thinking leads to overfeeding.

Although the child may experience an initial weight loss, the long-term success rate for the elimination of obesity is poor. Positive outcomes are increased when the child has a support system and understands the importance of diet and exercise.

Assessing the Scope of the Problem. There is no generally accepted definition of obesity. The child who is obese looks overweight. In addition, a body mass index (BMI) greater than the 95th percentile for age or a triceps skinfold measurement above the 95th percentile indicates obesity (Story, Holt, & Sofka, 2002).

Generally, obesity is caused by increased calorie intake combined with decreased physical activity. The amount of time spent watching television, at a computer, and playing video games takes away from time the child could be participating in active exercise. The possibility of disease as a contributing factor must be evaluated. Increased weight gain has been associated with central nervous system tumors, hypothyroidism, Cushing syndrome, and Turner syndrome.

Prevention. Early identification of risk factors can target the child who needs special attention and support. All children should be taught healthy eating habits and the importance of exercise. Three critical periods appear to exist for the development of childhood obesity: early infancy (1 year or younger), middle childhood (4 to 7 years), and puberty (Strauss & Dietz, 1999). Special attention should be given during these periods so that early intervention can take place.

Interventions and Anticipatory Guidance. Take a dietary history, and evaluate the child's eating habits and patterns. The child or parents (or both) should keep a food diary for 1 week. The diary should include the time, place, and type and amount of food eaten and the reason for eating. The general dietary habits of the family should also be assessed.

One of the key elements of successful weight reduction in the child or adolescent is ownership by the child of whatever plan is proposed. Care should be taken to avoid a power struggle between the parent and child. Obviously the young child will need more parental involvement than the older child or adolescent. The family should be willing to support the child but should not take on the role of watchdog (Parents Want to Know box).

Caloric requirements vary depending on the age and gender of the child. By changing the obese child's life-style to include exercise and nutritional foods in smaller servings, the possibility of success is increased. Teach the family and child how to select and prepare foods that are tasteful and how to restrict serving size. The child's favorite foods should be identified and incorporated whenever possible. Because snacks are an important aspect in childhood nutrition, nutritious snacks should be identified. Involvement of the whole family will create family behaviors that support the child's new eating and activity behaviors.

The parent needs to limit television and computer game time. Children should be involved in regular physical exercise at school and at home. Children can be encouraged to ride their bicycles or to walk rather than ride in a car to a friend's house to play. Planned physical activities should be part of the child's after-school and weekend routine.

Some older children and adolescents may find success in a support group, such as Weight Watchers or Overeaters Anonymous. Some centers have a special group for children. Other support groups may be associated with schools, summer camps, and children's hospitals in the community.

A team approach is often necessary for successful weight reduction. Psychologic support may be essential for the child and family to be successful. A registered dietitian can provide expertise in the identification and planning of foods not only that are nutritional but also that the child likes.

Stress. Today's children are subjected to stress as no generation has been before. Alarming increases in drug abuse, childhood suicide, child abduction and murder, and school failure attest to the overwhelming stress that children experience. Rapid, bewildering social change and ever-increasing demands for achievement often pressure children to grow up too quickly.

Stressed children may not show serious symptoms during childhood but may develop patterns of emotional response that can lead to serious illness as adults (Box 7-3).

Sources of Stress in Children. Growing up is stressful, even for well-adjusted children with loving, supportive families. Children experience stress from societal change, school, competitive athletics, rushed schedules, and the media.

Middle-class children in particular are pressured to grow up quickly. Achievement-oriented parents, focused on success and financial gain, often view children as extensions of themselves and unwittingly expect too much of their children. Pressure on children to succeed, to win, and to be the best and brightest is great, especially when parents value academic achievement. Children are often pressured into a frenzied schedule of music, dance, sport, and art lessons and may have little time for family meals or playing with friends. Self-esteem and peer relationships often suffer.

Economically deprived children must cope with an even greater burden of stress. Faced with the dangers of violence, drug and alcohol addiction, and gangs, these children must fight daily for survival. Children from lower-income families travel dangerous streets to and from school and suffer from the insecurity and uncertainty of poverty. Children who are homeless—as is increasingly common—have the added stress of living on the street or in shelters and having decreased access to appropriate nutritional, health, and educational resources. Both homeless and low-income children experience significant adversity in their lives, with homeless children having increased stress (Culbertson, Newman, & Willis, 2003).

School Pressures. School can be a source of stress for children. Some children are unable to cope with the competitive, test-regulated curricula of school. They find it difficult to keep up with the unrelenting academic pressure. School imposes long-term stress on these children, and they tend to dislike school and stay home whenever they can. They are often tardy and may abuse alcohol and drugs. Eventually, they may drop out of school. These children rarely return to complete their education.

Other children, particularly those who are academically gifted, find school stressful because it is tedious. Boredom can be stressful. Meaningless, repetitive schoolwork can cause bright, talented children to become chronically fatigued, inattentive, and careless.

Physical Threats. Children also face other types of stress at school. Violence and theft in schools are national problems. School-age children commonly voice fears of being beaten up or held up. The child who leaves a bike unlocked or a watch or jacket unattended quickly learns the hazards of such carelessness. Students who abuse drugs or participate in gang activity create a pervasive attitude of wariness and fear and are a real source of stress for children.

Competitive Sports. Participation in competitive sports is stressful for some children. Fear of failure, especially in front of a cheering crowd, can be overwhelming. Some parents contribute to competitive stress by overemphasizing the importance of winning. Because of their own needs or interests, some parents push their children to participate in organized sports at an early age (Fig. 7-2).

> **! CRITICAL TO REMEMBER**
>
> **Sources of Stress for School-Age Children**
>
> - Societal change
> - School
> - Competitive sports
> - Tight schedules
> - Family pressures
> - Influence of the media
> - Fear of violence
> - Chaotic living conditions

Tight Schedules and Adaptation Overload. As the number of single parents and working mothers increases, so does the stress on children who must adapt to parents' work schedules. Many children are rushed from home to school to carpool to daycare or a baby-sitter. Children must draw on their energy reserves to exercise self-control in these varying situations and may not be able to cope. Fatigue and exhaustion from such demands often result in behavioral problems and regression.

Family Pressures. In today's mobile society it is not unusual for families to move and for children to have to leave other family members and friends. Attending a new school, making new friends, and losing former support systems can be very stressful for children. This happens at a time when one or both parents are also making major adjustments in their lives, and they may not have the time and energy to meet all of the child's needs.

Overhearing parents quarrel produces anxiety and fear in children and erodes a child's sense of security. Some parents, although physically present, may be emotionally unavailable to children because of their own stresses. Divorce and separation are especially painful. Changes frequently caused by divorce, such as moving to a new house, attending a new school, and, usually the most stressful of all, separation from one of the parents, can cause great stress for children.

Media Influence. The media are a common source of stress for today's children. Sexual and violent material portraying loss of control may frighten children because it suggests that they may not be able to master their own sexual and aggressive impulses. Television exposes children to vivid portrayals of the problems of today's society for many hours of their day. It also tends to isolate children from their parents and peers. Hours spent watching television can limit children's participation in more creative play as well as contact and interaction with others.

Interventions and Anticipatory Guidance. The nurse is in an ideal position to help parents and children identify factors that produce stress and to suggest ways to cope with its effects. Parents can meet basic psychologic needs, influence self-esteem, shape values, control exposure to stressful events, and provide support. Parents may need guidance about realistic expectations from their children. Parents should watch for behavior changes in their children that may indicate signs of stress and offer appropriate reassurance. If significant tension is in the home, parents can try to resolve conflicts by negotiating rather than continuing to build an emotionally charged atmosphere. Parents should examine

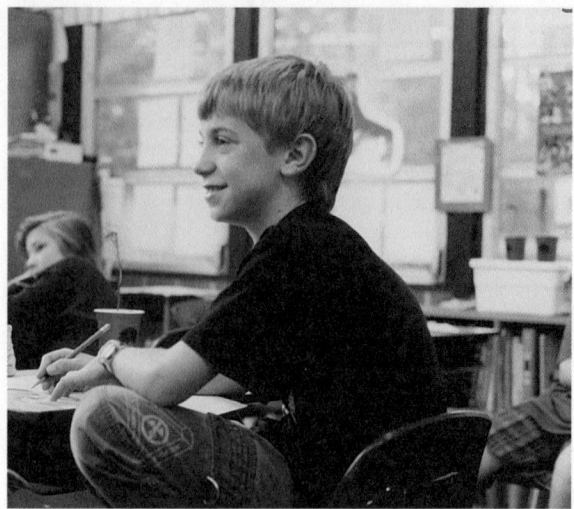

Attention span increases during the school-age years, facilitating classroom learning.

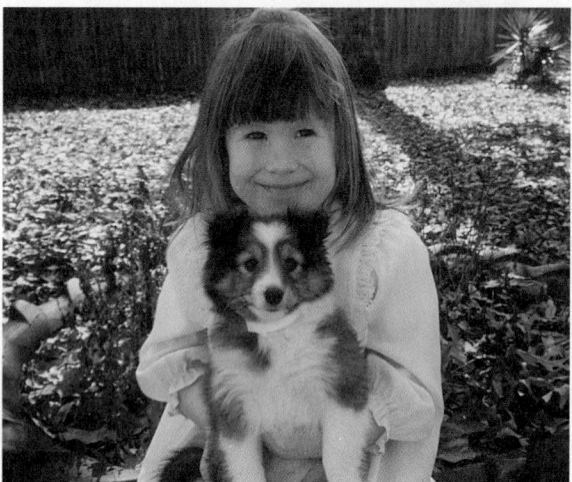

Spending time playing with and caring for pets can be fun and relaxing. Children who are given time and encouragement to play are better able to deal with the stresses of life.

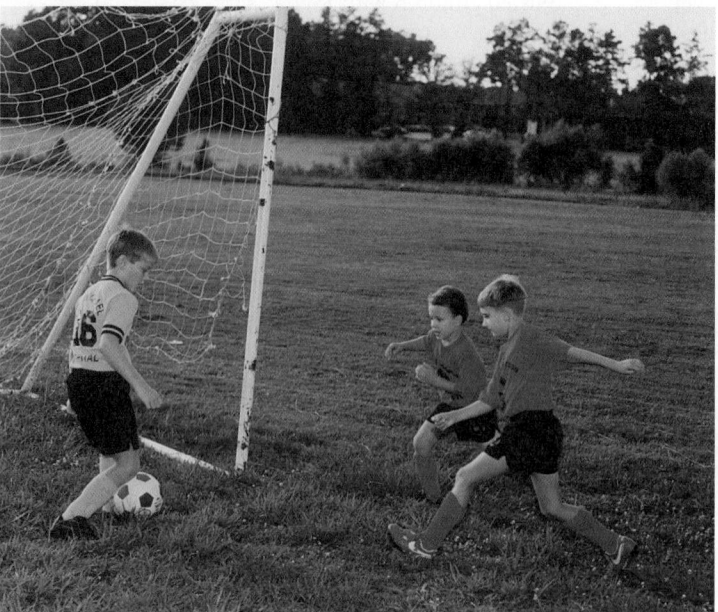

The nurse is in an excellent position to help parents and children identify factors that produce stress and to suggest ways to cope with its effects. Participation in competitive sports is stressful for some children, especially if parents push their child to play organized sports at an early age or overemphasize the importance of winning. Focusing on having fun and on the excitement of the game decreases competitive stress.

Figure 7-2 Health promotion for the school-age child and family.

the child's schedule to make sure the child is not overburdened with school and extracurricular activities.

Close communication with teachers is important to prevent and deal with school-related stress. Becoming interested in and involved with the child's schoolwork conveys support and caring. Parents need to become active in parent-teacher associations and other community organizations to find solutions to the problems of violence and crime in the schools.

Children should be allowed to decide whether to participate in competitive athletics. It is important for parents to talk to coaches to determine what is expected of their children. Corrective instruction rather than punishment should be given for errors. Parents should serve as role models for good sportsmanship.

Limiting the number of hours that children watch television and helping them select appropriate programs can decrease its negative effects. Watching television with children and discussing the content of programs are also helpful.

Children need to have time just to play. Parents should recognize that play is the child's work. Whether it is shooting baskets in the driveway, working on a collection, or building a model, play reduces stress for children. Toys and games that provide the greatest opportunity to use imagination are the best stress relievers. Most children love animals. Spending time playing with and caring for pets can be relaxing and fun. Children who are given the time and encouragement to play are better able to deal with the stresses of life (see Chapter 4).

One of the most effective antidotes for childhood stress is a loving, attentive parent who takes the time to listen. A sympathetic adult who understands the stresses of childhood can offer valuable support. Discussion and modeling of ways to deal with the inevitable stresses of life can teach the child valuable lessons for living in today's society.

KEY CONCEPTS

- Slow, steady physical growth and rapid social and cognitive development characterize the school-age period, from 6 to 12 years. Average weight gain in the school-age child is 2.5 kg (5½ lb) per year, and the increase in height is approximately 5.5 cm (2 in) per year. During the early school-age period, boys are approximately 2.54 cm (1 in) taller and 0.9 kg (2 lb) heavier than girls.

- During the school-age years, children gradually move away from home and parents as a primary source of support and they enter the wider world of peers and school.

- Physical changes include increased height and weight, increased muscle mass, maturation of body systems, and increased antibody production. During the school-age period, all 20 primary teeth are lost and are replaced by 28 of the 32 permanent teeth.

- The age at onset of puberty varies widely, but puberty is occurring at an earlier age than in the past. On average, African-American girls enter puberty approximately 1 year earlier than white girls.

- School-age children enjoy a variety of activities. Cooperative play and team sports are typical of this age-group.

- According to Erikson, the developmental task of this period is the development of a sense of industry.

- The child develops a conscience and internalizes cultural and social values. The child is able to understand and obey rules.

- Thinking becomes less egocentric as children learn to consider viewpoints different from their own. School-age children can solve problems, form hypotheses, and make judgments based on reason.

- School-age children experience an increase in appetite, and older school-age children have increased energy needs as they approach puberty.

- Sources of stress for school-age children include societal change, school, competitive athletics, rushed schedules, fear of violence from gangs or bullies, chaotic living conditions if homeless, and the media. Teaching children coping strategies can reduce the effects of stress.

- Dental care is increasingly important as the primary teeth are replaced by permanent teeth.

- Safety issues are related to the child moving more from the home environment to the community, less fear when playing, and the increased use of tools and household items.

ANSWERS to Critical Thinking Exercise 7-1

1. The nurse might assume that Mrs. George is inconsistent in her expectations. Consequences may not be associated with Megan's behavior. Mrs. George is engaging in a power struggle with Megan. Mrs. George's expectations of a clean room may differ from Megan's.

2. The nurse can begin to gather data by asking Mrs. George to describe a typical day when she feels upset with Megan's behavior. The nurse can further ask, "What is your response to her behavior?" Based on Mrs.

George's response, the nurse can determine how the mother is reacting to Megan's behavior and begin to develop strategies. The nurse can determine if Mrs. George has an emotional response to the situation and reacts or if she remains focused and has a plan of action.

3. Some children respond to family meetings where they are involved in the decision making related to the goals of the household. After the family agrees on a solution, there

must be consequences to not following the plan. The family might discuss putting items left in a public area into a holding box for a time. Or, if Megan does not pick up her room and dirty clothes do not make it to the hamper, her clothes will not be washed. Consistency and consequences are the foundation for making such a plan work. This is one way to develop a responsible child.

REFERENCES and READINGS

American Academy of Pediatrics. (2000a). *A guide to children's dental health*. Retrieved March 23, 2001, from www.medem.com.

American Academy of Pediatrics. (2000b). *Establishing good sleep habits*. Retrieved March 23, 2001, from www.medem.com.

American Academy of Pediatrics. (2003). *Car safety seats: A guide for families 2003*. Retrieved June 10, 2003, from www.aap.org/family/carseatguide.htm.

American Academy of Pediatrics Committee on Injury and Poison Prevention and Committee on Sports Medicine and Fitness. (1998). In-line skating injuries in children and adolescents. *Pediatrics, 101*(4), 720-722.

American Academy of Pediatrics Committee on Psychosocial Aspects of Child and Family Health. (1998). American Academy of Pediatrics: Guidance for effective discipline. *Pediatrics, 101*(4), 723-728.

American Dental Association. (1998, February). *Teeth and gums change rapidly as kids go through the wonder years*. Chicago: Author. News release.

Behrman, R. (Ed.). (1999). When school is out. *The Future of Children, 9*(2), 1-95.

Centers for Disease Control and Prevention. (2000a). Motor-vehicle occupant fatalities and restraint use among children aged 4-8 years—United States, 1994-1998. *MMWR: Morbidity and Mortality Weekly Report, 49*(07), 135-137.

Centers for Disease Control and Prevention. (2000b). Unpowered scooter-related injuries—United States, 1998-2000. *MMWR: Morbidity and Mortality Weekly Report, 49*(49), 1108-1110.

Centers for Disease Control and Prevention. (2001a). *Facts about violence among youth and violence in schools*. Available on-line: www.cdc.gov/ncipc/factsheets/schoolvi.htm.

Centers for Disease Control and Prevention. (2001b). *School health programs: An investment in our nation's future, at a glance, 2001*. Available online: www.cdc.gov/nccdphp/dash/ataglance.htm.

Centers for Disease Control and Prevention. (2001c). Surveillance for fatal and nonfatal firearm-related injuries—United States, 1993-1998. *MMWR: Morbidity and Mortality Weekly Report, 50*(SS02), 1-32.

Centers for Disease Control and Prevention. (2002). Youth risk behavior surveillance—United States, 2001. *MMWR: Morbidity and Mortality Weekly Report, 51*(SS04).

Cowell, J., & Agruss, J. (2000). Cardiovascular risk among middle school children: Implications for primary care. *Nurse Practitioner Forum, 11*(2), 141-148.

Culbertson, J., Newman, J., & Willis, D. (2003). Childhood and adolescent psychologic development. *Pediatric Clinics of North America, 50*(4), 741-764.

Dietz, W.H. (1998). Health consequences of obesity in youth: Childhood predictors of adult disease. *Pediatrics, 101*(3), 518-525.

Dowling, J., & Fain, J. (1999). A multidimensional sense of humor scale for school-aged children: Issues of reliability and validity. *Journal of Pediatric Nursing,14*(1), 38-41.

Edwards, C. (2001). Worlds of experience after school. *Human Development, 44*(1), 59.

Erikson, E. (1963). *Childhood and society* (2nd ed.). New York, NY: Norton.

Feldman, R.S. (1998). *Child development*. Upper Saddle River, NJ: Prentice-Hall.

Green, M., & Palfrey, J. (Eds.). (2000). *Bright futures: Guidelines for health supervision of infants, children, and adolescents* (2nd ed.). Arlington, VA: National Center for Education in Maternal and Child Health.

REFERENCES and READINGS

Gresham, L., Zirkle, D., Tolchin, S., Jones, C., Maroufi, A., & Miranda, J. (2001). Partnering for injury prevention: Evaluation of a curriculum based intervention program among elementary school children. *Journal of Pediatric Nursing, 16*(2), 79-87.

Guilleminault, C., Palombini, L., & Chervin, R. (2003). Sleepwalking and sleep terrors in prepubertal children: What triggers them? *Pediatrics, 111*(1), e17-e25.

Hernandez, B., Uphold, C.R., Graham, M.V., & Singer, L. (1998). Prevalence and correlates of obesity in preschool children. *Journal of Pediatric Nursing, 13*(2), 68-76.

Hodges, E. (2003). A primer on early childhood obesity and parental influence. *Pediatric Nursing, 29*(1), 13-17.

Kaplan, D.W., Brindis, C., Naylor, K.E., Phibbs, S.L., Ahlstrand, K.R., & Melinkovich, P. (1998). Elementary school-based health center use. *Pediatrics, 101*(6), 12.

Kaplowitz, P., Slora, E., Wasserman, R., Pedlow, S., & Herman-Giddens, M. (2001). Earlier onset of puberty in girls: Relation to increased body mass index and race. *Pediatrics, 108*(2), 347-353.

Kennedy, C. (2000). Examining television as an influence on children's health behaviors. *Journal of Pediatric Nursing, 15*(5), 272-280.

Kerrebrock, N., & Lewit, E. (1999). Children in self-care. In R. Behrman (Ed.), *The future of children*. Los Altos, CA: David and Lucille Packard Foundation.

Larsen, M., & Tentis, E. (2003). The art and science of disciplining children. *Pediatric Clinics of North America, 50*(4), 817-840.

Logan, P., Leadbetter, S., Gibson, R.E., Schieber, R., Branche, C., Bender, P., Zane, D., Humphreys, J., & Anderson, S. (1998). Evaluation of a bicycle helmet giveaway program—Texas, 1995. *Pediatrics, 101*(4), 578-582.

Lytle, L. Seifert, S., Greenstein, J., & McGovern, P. (2000). How do children's eating patterns and food choices change over time? Results from a cohort study. *American Journal of Health Promotion, 14*(4), 222-228.

Muscari, M.E., Catalino, C., & Faherty, J. (1998). Little women: Early menarche in rural girls. *Pediatric Nursing, 24*(1), 11-15.

National Center for Injury Prevention and Control. (2000). *Bicycle-related injuries.* Available on-line: www.cdc.gov/ncipc/pub-res/FactBook/fkbike.htm.

Piaget, J. (1962). *Play, dreams, and imitation in childhood* (C. Gattegno & F.M. Hodgson, Trans.). New York, NY: Norton.

Pratt, H., Patel, D., & Greydanus, D. (2003). Behavioral aspects of children's sports. *Pediatric Clinics of North America, 50*(4), 879-899.

Rivara, F., & Grossman, D. (2004). Injury control. In R. Behrman, R. Kliegman, & H. Jenson (Eds.). *Nelson textbook of pediatrics* (17th ed.; pp. 256-263). Philadelphia, PA: Saunders.

Robinson, T., & Killen, J. (2001). Obesity prevention for children and adolescents. In J. Thomplson & L. Smola (Eds.), *Image, eating disorders and obesity in youth* (pp. 261-292). Washington, DC: American Psychological Association.

Ruggiero, M. (1999). Maladaptation to school. In M. Levine, W. Carey, & A. Crocker (Eds.), *Developmental-behavioral pediatrics* (pp. 542-550). Philadelphia: Saunders.

Russell, D., Keil, M., Bonat, S., Uwaifo, G., Nicholson, J., McDuffie, J., Hill, S.C., & Yanovski, J. (2001). The relation between skeletal maturation and adiposity in African American and Caucasian children. *The Journal of Pediatrics, 139*(6), 844-848.

Stevenson, M., Rimajova, M., Edgecombe, D., & Vickery, K. (2003). Childhood drowning: Barriers surrounding private swimming pools. *Pediatrics, 111*(2), e115-e119.

Story, M., Holt, K., & Sofka, D. (Eds.). (2002). *Bright futures in practice: Nutrition.* Arlington, VA: National Center for Education in Maternal and Child Health.

Strauss, R.S., & Dietz, W.H. (1999). Obesity. In F.D. Burg, E.R. Wald, J.R. Ingelfinger, & R.A. Polin (Eds.), *Gellis and Kagan's current pediatric therapy* (pp. 8-10). Philadelphia: Saunders.

Thiedke, C. (2001). Sleep disorders and sleep problems in childhood. *American Family Physician, 63*(2), 277-284.

United States Department of Agriculture [USDA]. *National school lunch program.* Retrieved April, 26, 2003, from www.fns.usda.gov/cnd/Lunch/AboutLunch/AboutNLSP.htm.

Varley, C., & Smith, C. (2003). Anxiety disorders in the child and teen. *Pediatric Clinics of North America, 50*(5), 1107-1138.

Velsor-Friedrich, B. (2001). Guns killing our children: A status report. *Journal of Pediatric Nursing, 16*(2), 127-129.

Weinreb, L., Goldberg, R., Bassuk, E., & Perloff, J. (1998). Determinants of health and service use patterns of homeless and low-income housed children. *Pediatrics, 102*(3), 554-562.

Wilson, D., Nicholson, S., & Krishnamoorthy, J. (1997). *The role of diet in minority adolescent health promotion.* Washington, DC: American Psychological Association.

8

Health Promotion for the Adolescent

◆ LEARNING OBJECTIVES

After studying this chapter, you should be able to:

◎ Describe the adolescent's normal growth and development.

◎ Identify the sexual maturity rating and Tanner stages, and recognize deviations from normal.

◎ Describe the developmental tasks of adolescence.

◎ Describe the concept of identity formation in relation to adolescent psychosocial development.

◎ Describe appropriate health-promoting behaviors for adolescents and young adults.

◎ Provide anticipatory guidance for adolescents and their families with respect to risk-taking behaviors, nutrition, and safety.

◎ Discuss the prevalence of adolescent violence and strategies to deal with aggressive behavior.

◎ Discuss adolescent sexuality and related health risks.

◆ DEFINITIONS

adolescence Period between the onset of puberty and the cessation of physical growth; the passage from childhood to adulthood.

autonomy Independent will and the capacity to be self-governing.

egocentrism Concern with oneself; the lack of differentiation between one's own views and those of others.

identity formation The acquisition of psychosocial, sexual, and vocational identity.

primary sexual characteristics Internal and external reproductive organs in males and females (i.e., uterus, fallopian tubes, ovaries, vagina, vulva, penis, testes, spermatic cord).

puberty Period of time during which adolescents experience a growth spurt, develop secondary sexual characteristics, and achieve reproductive maturity.

pubescence Period of time before sexual maturity, characterized by the development of breast tissue and pubic hair in girls and genital growth and pubic hair in boys.

reproductive maturity The establishment of menstruation and ovulation in females and the development of spermatogenesis in males.

risk-taking behaviors Behaviors that predispose the adolescent to physical or psychosocial harm.

secondary sexual characteristics Physical characteristics of males and females influenced by reproductive hormones but having no direct role in reproduction (i.e., voice, body shape, pubic hair distribution, breasts).

sexual maturity rating (SMR) Stages of sexual maturation based on pubic hair and breast development in girls and pubic hair and genital development in boys.

A dolescence spans ages 11 to 21 years although the developmental tasks of early adolescence, as well as the beginning stages of sexual maturation, may overlap with the school-age years. Adolescence is a time of change for teenagers and their families, a transition from childhood to adulthood. During this transition period, dramatic physical, cognitive, psychosocial, and psychosexual changes take place that are exciting and, at the same time, frightening.

Healthy People 2010 (U.S. Department of Health and Human Services [USDHHS], 2000) objectives address many areas of adolescent health (Box 8-1). These areas include access to comprehensive health care and education about and practice of appropriate reproductive health, violence reduction, and decrease in risk factors.

ADOLESCENT GROWTH AND DEVELOPMENT

The adolescent tries out many new roles during this time as part of the important developmental task of identity formation. The peer group is of the utmost importance as adolescents experiment with new roles outside the confines of the family unit. When identity formation is complete, the young adult is emancipated from the family and establishes independence.

The rapid rate of physical growth during adolescence is second only to that of infancy. Adolescents come in many shapes and sizes, and the changes that take place during the teen years are obvious and dramatic. With physical changes come the development of secondary sexual characteristics and an intense interest in romantic relationships. In general,

BOX 8-1
Healthy People 2010 Objectives for Adolescents

3-9a	Increase the proportion of adolescents in grades 9 through 12 who follow protective measures that may reduce the risk of skin cancer.
7-1	Increase high school completion.
7-2	Increase the proportion of middle, junior high, and senior high schools that provide comprehensive school health education to prevent health problems in the following areas: unintentional injury; violence; suicide; tobacco use and addiction; alcohol or other drug use; unintended pregnancy; human immunodeficiency virus/acquired immunodeficiency syndrome (HIV/AIDS) and sexually transmitted disease (STD) infection; unhealthy dietary patterns; inadequate physical activity; and environmental health.
9-7	Reduce pregnancies among adolescent females.
9-8	Increase the proportion of adolescents who have never engaged in sexual intercourse before age 15 years.
9-9	Increase the proportion of adolescents who have never engaged in sexual intercourse.
9-10	Increase the proportion of sexually active, unmarried adolescents age 15 to 17 years who use contraception that both effectively prevents pregnancy and provides barrier protection against disease.
9-11	Increase the proportion of young adults who have received formal instruction before turning age 18 years on reproductive health issues, including all of the following topics: birth control methods, safer sex to prevent HIV, prevention of STDs, and abstinence.
13-1, 5	Reduce AIDS and the number of HIV infections among adolescents and adults.
14-27	Increase routine vaccination coverage levels of adolescents.
15-32	Reduce homicides.
15-38	Reduce physical fighting among adolescents.
15-39	Reduce weapon carrying by adolescents on school property.
18-2	Reduce the rate of suicide attempts by adolescents.
19-12	Reduce iron deficiency among young children and females of childbearing age.
22-6, 7	Increase the proportion of adolescents who engage in moderate physical activity for at least 30 minutes on 5 or more of the previous 7 days and vigorous physical activity that promotes cardiorespiratory fitness 3 or more days per week for 20 or more minutes per occasion.
25-1	Reduce the proportion of adolescents and young adults with *Chlamydia trachomatis* infections.
26-6	Reduce the proportion of adolescents who report that they rode, during the previous 30 days, with a driver who had been drinking alcohol.
26-9	Increase the age and proportion of adolescents who remain alcohol- and drug-free.
26-14	Reduce steroid use among adolescents.
26-15	Reduce the proportion of adolescents who use inhalants.
26-16	Increase the proportion of adolescents who disapprove of substance abuse.
27-2	Reduce tobacco use by adolescents.
27-17	Increase adolescents' disapproval of smoking.

Modified from U.S. Department of Health and Human Services. (2000). *Healthy People 2010* (Conference edition, in 2 volumes). Washington, DC: Author.

adolescents move from the same-gender friendships of childhood to the capacity for intimate, long-lasting relationships as young adults. Sexual orientation and gender identity are often recognized during adolescence as the teenager engages in exploration and self-discovery.

Parents as well as adolescents need the nurse's support and guidance in understanding and facilitating health-promoting behaviors. Nurses can assist adolescents and their families in the areas of health promotion, disease prevention, and management of common problems by using effective communication strategies, knowledge of normal growth and development, anticipatory guidance, and early identification of potential problems.

Physical Growth and Development

Physical development during the adolescent years is characterized by dramatic changes in size and appearance. Girls experience budding of the breasts followed by the appearance of pubic hair. About 1 year after breast development, height increases rapidly. Growth in height in girls typically ceases 2 to 2½ years after menarche.

Boys also experience physical changes, but those changes are not as obvious as in girls. Boys first experience testicular enlargement, followed in about 1 year by penile enlargement. Pubic hair usually precedes the growth of the penis. The growth spurt in boys occurs later than it does in girls, beginning between ages 10½ and 16 years and ending between 13½ and 17½ years. Growth does continue at a much slower pace for several years after the spurt but usually ceases between 18 and 20 years of age.

Muscle mass increases in boys, and fat deposits increase in girls. Because of greater muscle mass, fully developed adolescent boys tend to be larger and stronger than adolescent girls.

Psychosexual Development, Hormonal Changes, and Sexual Maturation

The physical development, hormonal changes, and sexual maturation that occur during adolescence correspond to Freud's final stage of psychosexual development, the genital stage (see Chapter 4 for a discussion of Freud's stages of psychosexual development). The genital stage begins with the production of sex hormones and maturation of the reproductive system. Sexual tension and energy are manifested in the development of sexual relationships with others, and sexual gratification is sought. Freud's theory suggests that personality development is closely related to psychosexual development, with an emphasis on aggressive and sexual impulses as determining factors of personality. Freud's theories about male dominance, sexual repression, and the Oedipus and Electra complexes make the psychosexual theory of development highly controversial even today.

Girls generally reach physical maturation before boys with the onset and establishment of menstruation (menarche). Menarche usually occurs between the ages of 9 and 15 years (average 12.43 years) (Chumlea et al., 2003). African-American girls experience menarche slightly earlier (approximately 1 year) than whites (Kaplowitz, Slora, Wasserman, Pedlow, & Herman-Giddens, 2001). Over the past 25 years in the United States, the age of menarche has decreased, while general body mass index has increased; population weight gain appears to significantly affect maturity in girls (Anderson, Dallal, & Must, 2003). Most young women achieve reproductive maturity 2 to 5 years after the start of menstruation. During the 2 to 5 years before reproductive maturity, the female sex hormones gradually increase, ovulation occurs more frequently, and menstrual periods become more regular.

Ultimately, diet, exercise, and hereditary factors influence the height, weight, and body build of adolescents. Over the past 3 decades, adolescents have become taller and heavier than their ancestors and the age of puberty has fallen. The earlier onset of puberty has implications for the timing of sex education programs and anticipatory guidance.

The physical growth of boys and girls is directly related to sexual maturation and occurs in a relatively predictable sequence. The secretion of sex hormones—estrogen in girls and testosterone in boys—stimulates the development of breast tissue, pubic hair, and genitalia. Hormonal secretion at the time of puberty is the result of a complex regulatory process among the environment, the central nervous system, the hypothalamus, the pituitary gland, the gonads, and the adrenal glands. Puberty is a biologic process that brings about the period of peak height velocity (PHV), or the "growth spurt," the changes in body composition, and the development of primary and secondary sexual characteristics in both genders. Although variable in both genders, the PHV occurs at approximately age 12 years in girls and age 13½ years in boys. Table 8-1 describes five distinct stages in a *sexual maturity rating* (SMR) based on breast and pubic hair development in girls and genital and pubic hair development in boys and includes approximate age ranges for early, middle, and late puberty (Tanner, 1962). The beginning Tanner stages frequently occur in the school-age child, and Tanner stages 3 to 5 occur in adolescence.

In boys, puberty is considered delayed if there is a lack of testicular enlargement or pubic hair development by the age of 14 years. Absence of breast budding or pubic hair development in girls by 13 years or lack of menses by 15 years requires referral (Misra & Park-Bennett, 2002). Some of the more common causes of delayed puberty are chronic illnesses, malnutrition, extreme exercise, and hypothyroidism.

Female Sexual Maturation

Sexual maturation in girls begins with the appearance of breast buds (*thelarche*), which is the first sign of ovarian function. Thelarche occurs at approximately age 9 to 11 years and is fol-

---

> **！ CRITICAL TO REMEMBER**
>
> **Understanding Tanner Staging**
>
> Knowledge of Tanner staging is essential for nurses to assess normal growth and development and to provide adolescents and their parents with anticipatory guidance regarding sexual development. Nurses must remember, however, that sexual maturation and physical development are *highly variable* and that Tanner stages may overlap one another. A description of the adolescent's sexual maturity rating provides greater information about the child's physical development than does chronologic age (age in years).

lowed by the growth of pubic hair. The PHV is reached during thelarche, usually in Tanner stage 2 or 3. Linear growth slows, and menarche begins approximately 1 year after the PHV. As pubic hair increases in amount and becomes dark, coarse, and curly, axillary hair develops and the apocrine sweat glands reach secretory capacity in Tanner stage 3 or 4. Frequent showers and deodorants become important to the adolescent. With increasing hormonal activity, girls develop a more adult body contour by age 14 to 15 years. As breasts mature, the nipples project more and the pubic hair extends to the medial thighs; the young female is estimated to be at Tanner stage 5. Ovulation may be established, and conception can occur.

Male Sexual Maturation

The first sign of pubertal changes in boys is testicular enlargement in response to testosterone secretion, which usually occurs in Tanner stage 2. There are also some slight pubic hair and some alteration in the smooth skin texture of the scrotum. As testosterone secretion increases, the penis as well as the testes and scrotum enlarge. The PHV usually occurs during Tanner stages 3 and 4, and the voice deepens and "cracks" as the cartilage in the larynx enlarges. Axillary hair develops, and the eccrine and apocrine sweat glands respond to stressful or emotional stimuli. Skin surface bacteria metabolize secretions from the apocrine glands, and body odor develops. Gynecomastia (male breast enlargement) occurs in about 69% of young males during early adolescence and may be unilateral or bilateral (Wolfsdorf, 2002). This phenomenon is often disturbing to boys, and they need considerable reassurance that the breast tissue will decrease over time. During Tanner stages 4 and 5, increasing levels of testosterone cause sebaceous glands to enlarge and excessive sebum may result in acne. The voice continues to deepen, facial hair appears at the corners of the upper lip and chin, and ejaculation may occur. Nurses need to provide anticipatory guidance to adolescent boys regarding involuntary nocturnal emissions of seminal fluid ("wet dreams") and assure them that this occurrence is normal. By Tanner stage 5, genital maturation is complete, spermatogenesis is well established, facial hair is present on the sides of the face, and the male physique is adultlike in appearance. Gynecomastia significantly decreases or disappears, much to the adolescent male's relief.

Motor Development

Adolescents often engage in various forms of motor activity, from aerobic exercise to football. Motor activities, such as sports and dancing, provide an outlet for the adolescent's en-

TABLE 8–1 Sexual Maturity Rating (SMR): Tanner Stages of Adolescent Sexual Development

BOYS

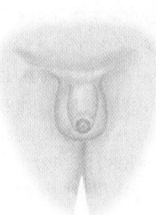 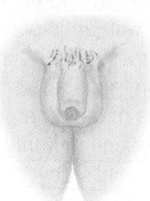 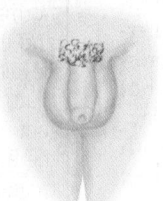 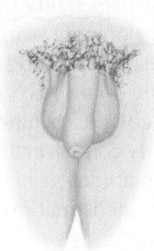 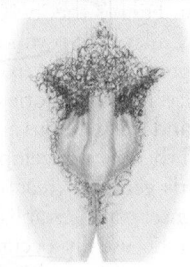

Stage 1
Pubic hair: None
Penis: Preadolescent
Testes: Preadolescent

Stage 2
Pubic hair: Slight, long, straight, slightly pigmented at the base of the penis
Penis: Slight enlargement
Testes: Enlarged scrotum, pink, slight alteration in texture

Stage 3
Pubic hair: Darker in color, starts to curl, small amount
Penis: Longer
Testes: Larger

Stage 4
Pubic hair: Coarse, curly, similar to adult but less quantity
Penis: Larger, glans and breadth increase in size
Testes: Larger, scrotum darker

Stage 5
Pubic hair: Adult distribution spread to inner thighs
Penis: Adult in size and shape
Testes: Adult

Early puberty: Testes, $9\frac{1}{2}$-$13\frac{1}{2}$ yr; penis, $10\frac{1}{2}$-$14\frac{1}{2}$ yr; pubic hair, 12-$12\frac{1}{2}$ yr

Middle puberty: Testes, $13\frac{1}{2}$-$14\frac{1}{2}$ yr; penis, $13\frac{1}{2}$-15 yr; pubic hair, $12\frac{1}{2}$-$14\frac{1}{2}$ yr

Late puberty: Testes, $13\frac{1}{2}$-17 yr; penis, $13\frac{1}{2}$-16 yr; pubic hair, $13\frac{1}{2}$-$16\frac{1}{2}$ yr

BREAST DEVELOPMENT IN GIRLS*

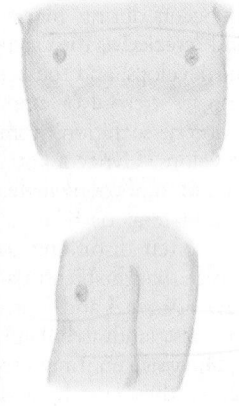 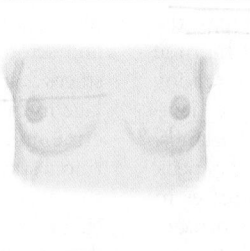 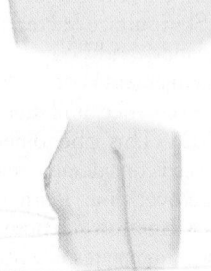 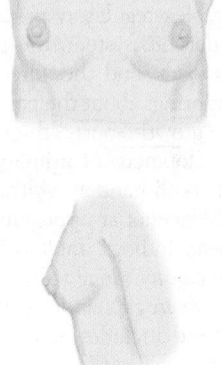 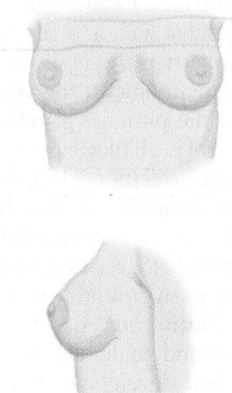

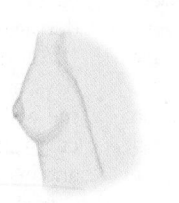

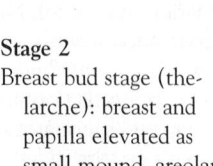

Stage 1
Preadolescent

Stage 2
Breast bud stage (thelarche): breast and papilla elevated as small mound, areolar diameter increased

Stage 3
Breast and areola enlarged, no contour separation

Stage 4
Areola and papilla form secondary mound

Stage 5
Mature, nipple projects, areola part of general breast contour

Early puberty: 9-13 yr

Middle puberty: 12-13 yr

Late puberty: 14-17 yr*

Modified from Tanner, J.M. (1962). *Growth at adolescence* (2nd ed.). Oxford: Blackwell Scientific Publications; Marshall, W.A., & Tanner, J. (1969). Variations in pattern of pubertal changes in girls. *Archives of Disease in Childhood, 44*(235), 291-303. Modified with permission from Blackwell Scientific Publications and The BMJ Publishing Group.
*Breast and pubic hair development may continue into late adolescence and increase with pregnancy.

Continued

TABLE 8-1 Sexual Maturity Rating (SMR): Tanner Stages of Adolescent Sexual Development—cont'd

PUBIC HAIR DEVELOPMENT IN GIRLS

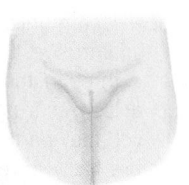 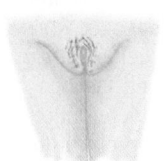 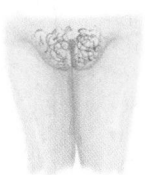 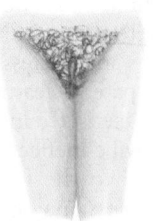 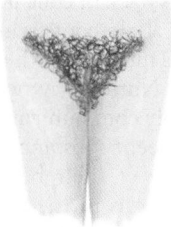

Stage 1	**Stage 2**	**Stage 3**	**Stage 4**	**Stage 5**
Preadolescent (none)	Sparse, lightly pigmented, straight medial border of labia	Darker, coarser, beginning to curl, increased over pubis	Coarse, curly, less in amount than adult, typical female triangle	Adult female triangle, adult quantity spread to medial surface of thighs

Early puberty: 10-11½ yr

Middle puberty: 11½-13 yr

Late puberty: 14½-16½ yr

BOX 8-2
Nursing Goals for Preparticipation Sports Physical Examination

- Assess the adolescent athlete's general health.
- Identify conditions that could limit participation or predispose to injury.
- Assess the adolescent athlete's physical and psychosocial maturity.
- Determine the athlete's fitness relative to performance requirements.
- Assess legal insurance requirements for participation.
- Provide wellness counseling and anticipatory guidance.

⚠ CRITICAL TO REMEMBER

The Adolescent Who Is Involved in Athletics

Adolescents participating in athletics need:
- Adequate equipment
- Appropriate training schedules
- Frequent rest periods
- Adequate fluids to prevent injury, dehydration, and exhaustion

---

ergy as well as an opportunity for competition, teamwork, and social relationships. Large muscle mass increases in adolescents, and coordination of gross and fine muscle groups improves. With practice, adolescents become more adept at athletics and also at art, music, sewing, and other activities using fine motor skills. The bones are not completely calcified until after puberty and are still fairly resistant to breaks in the young adolescent. Participants in sports activities should be grouped according to their size and their sexual maturity rating rather than their chronologic age. A small, thin, late-maturing boy is less capable of competing with an early-maturing, muscular classmate, and injuries are more likely to occur.

Nurses, particularly school nurses, may be helpful in assessing the growth and development of adolescents and counseling them about sports activities in which they can succeed, rather than those in which they will meet with physical and psychologic failure. It is important that adolescents have a yearly physical examination if participating in high school athletics (Box 8-2); the school nurse keeps documentation of this. Because it is generally superficial, the school sports examination should not substitute for the recommended complete adolescent physical examination with counseling.

The development of the cardiovascular pump plays an essential role in the adolescent's participation in gross motor activities. Cardiopulmonary capacity increases during adolescence and is relatively mature in the late adolescent. The cardiovascular pump is not as efficient in young adolescents, whose lungs are smaller. Adolescents generally cannot run as fast or as long as young adults. The athlete's aerobic power, body composition, joint flexibility, and strength of skeletal muscles determine physical fitness.

Cognitive Development

Cognitive development influences every aspect of adolescent psychosocial development. Cognition moves from concrete to abstract thinking during the three phases of adolescent development. According to Piaget, formal operations, or abstract thinking, characterize the last stage of cognitive development. Early abstract thinking encompasses inductive and deductive reasoning, the ability to connect separate events, and the ability to understand later consequences. Abstract thinking in late adolescence is increasingly logical, and young adults are capable of scientific reasoning, understanding complex concepts, and using analytic methods. Because of logical reasoning, adolescents are able to differentiate between others' perceptions and their own and to view social situations from a societal perspective.

For example, sex education for ninth graders is very different from that for college freshmen or adolescents with their first full-time jobs. The college freshman should be able to appreciate the later consequences of sexual behavior, whereas the young adolescent is focused on the here and now. Ask the ninth grader and the college freshman how an unwanted baby will affect their lives, and compare their answers.

For a variety of reasons (including poor comprehension ability, lack of education, and chronic substance abuse), some older adolescents remain concrete thinkers. Nurses and educators must know their audiences and address them appropriately. Nurses may need to help parents learn how to appropriately communicate with their teens. Counseling a group of adolescent substance abusers may be ineffective if the consequence of their behavior is tied to the future when their thinking is in the present. A professional approach to communicating with teens includes the following:

- Enjoy them.
- Be patient and flexible.
- Know adolescent development; consider how the teen will look to peers.
- Be open to their ideas and opinions and willing to negotiate choices.
- Listen nonjudgmentally, keeping criticism to a minimum.
- Encourage problem solving and mutual decision making.
- Maintain confidentiality.
- Be an advocate, but do not take sides against a parent.
- Explore feelings about health care choices, and allow for questions and analysis of health care options.

Sensory Development

Adolescents' eyes and ears are fully developed, and with the exception of refractive errors and occasional minor infections of the eyes, ears, and sinuses, the sensory system remains quite healthy. Myopia occurs in early adolescence, between ages 11 and 13 years, often requiring frequent changes in corrective lenses.

Because of increased participation in competitive sports and outdoor activities, eye injuries are common in adolescence. Boys are more prone to eye injuries than girls. Adolescents should always be required to wear safety or protective equipment when competing in sports or participating in any activity that may compromise eye safety.

Language Development

With the acquisition of formal operational thought and adequate intellectual capacity, adolescents are able to understand abstract concepts, process complex thoughts, and express themselves verbally. Adolescents who read extensively are generally more articulate and have a larger vocabulary than those who do not. Social development and self-confidence play a significant role in how well adolescents express themselves verbally to others. Shy, introverted adolescents may have difficulty speaking to a group or to members of the opposite sex but may write expressively. Conversely, extroverted, social adolescents who have no trouble with verbal expression may lack the reading and writing skills for effective written communication.

Computer technology has added to the adolescent's avenues for creative expression. Adolescents are capable of expressing ideas in symbols and abstract concepts, and many enjoy interpreting or even developing complex computer programs. Computers have a symbolic language of their own that some adolescents find fascinating. Teens may become

---

PARENTS
Want to Know

Communicating With Adolescents

Parents need encouragement to maintain open communication with their teenager while not appearing too intrusive. Inundating adolescents with questions or going through their belongings causes feelings of invasion and a lack of trust. Adolescents get more out of discussions in which they participate than they do out of lectures and are more likely to respond positively to adults who listen and appear interested in what they have to say.

---

more proficient with computer technology than their parents. As well as teaching teens basic computer literacy, many high schools have computer clubs where students who excel in computer languages share ideas and knowledge of computer information systems. Because of safety concerns with young adolescents using the Internet, parents need to monitor computer use, as well as investigate whether parental controls available through some Internet access companies are appropriate for their child.

Communicating with adolescents sometimes presents a challenge to parents and other adults. Although adolescents are capable of verbal expression, they are also intensely private and may not wish to divulge their thoughts and feelings to others. Developmentally, the verbally expressive 12-year-old may turn into a relatively uncommunicative 14-year-old. Conflict with parents increases tension in communication.

Nurses who work with adolescents must develop communication skills that include assuring confidentiality, making no assumptions, remaining nonjudgmental, and posing open-ended questions. Questions such as "Tell me about your plans for the future" will glean more information than "Do you plan to go to college?" The question "Do you live with your parents?" makes an assumption about the living situation that could make the adolescent feel uncomfortable. "Describe where you live and who lives with you" gives the adolescent an opportunity to discuss the living situation.

Confidentiality is often an issue when adolescents are seen in the health care setting. Nurses should encourage adolescents to involve their parents (Parents Want to Know box), but it is not unusual for adolescents to ask that communication be kept confidential. The adolescent must understand that the nurse will respect this confidentiality unless the information shared suggests a potentially life-threatening danger either to the adolescent or to others.

Screening tools are used in some settings to target areas of concern. Two of the more popular tools are HEADSS, which includes assessment of home, education, activities, drugs, sex, and suicide; and Guidelines for Adolescent Preventive Services (GAPS), which includes parenting, development, drugs, sex, learning problems, depression, abuse, safety, and diet and fitness. GAPS is a comprehensive packet of services that includes not only screening but also preventive services. The West Virginia University Adolescent Risk Score (WVUARS) includes the areas in the tools just listed but adds some other features, such as nutrition, exercise, friends and recreation, and self-perception. This particular tool assesses and also focuses on intervention and prevention (Perkins et al., 1997). Facility staff must identify which tool best suits their philosophy of care.

Some clinics send a questionnaire before the visit so that the adolescent can complete it at home and return it during the visit. Some settings display their policy on confidentiality, always underlining the need to share information only if someone is in danger. The following four critical areas need to be assessed (Prazer & Friedman, 1997):

1 • The adolescent's strengths and difficulties, as the family sees them
2 • The adolescent's functioning at home
3 • The adolescent's functioning at school
4 • Peer relationships

Depending on the issues identified, it may be decided to set a time to meet with the adolescent alone. Issues related to the time it takes to do an adequate interview may arise in the present managed care environment. Nurses should be knowledgeable about communicating with adolescents and aware of when referral is warranted.

CRITICAL THINKING EXERCISE 8-1

The nurse is caring for a 15-year-old girl, Heidi, who has been admitted to the hospital with dehydration. She is very quiet and answers questions with a simple "yes" or "no." On the day Heidi is to be discharged, she says, "I'll tell you something, but you can't tell anyone else."
1. What factors does the nurse have to consider in this situation?
2. What would be the nurse's best response?

Psychosocial Development

Identity formation is the major developmental task of adolescence; other tasks include the formation of a sexual and vocational identity and the ability to emancipate oneself from the family or to become independent (Fig. 8-1). Energy is focused within the self, and the adolescent is described as egocentric or self-absorbed. Frustrated parents often describe teenagers during this phase as self-centered, lazy, or irresponsible. In fact, they just need time to think, concentrate on themselves, and

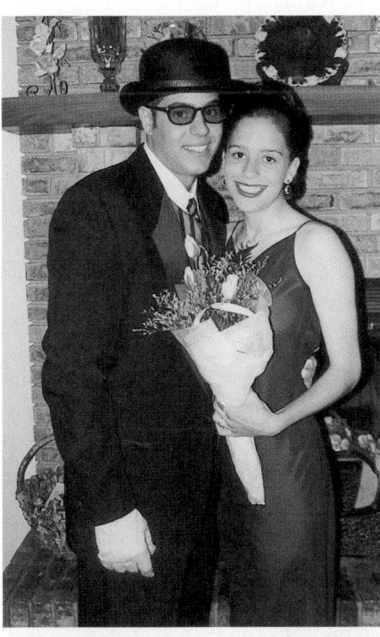

Relationships with the opposite sex are more mature by late adolescence. Late adolescents have more realistic expectations of both themselves and those who are important to them. They devote many hours and much anxious thought toward making events such as prom night memorable for a lifetime. Some adolescents may be left out because they are unpopular or shy or do not have the financial resources to participate in these special events.

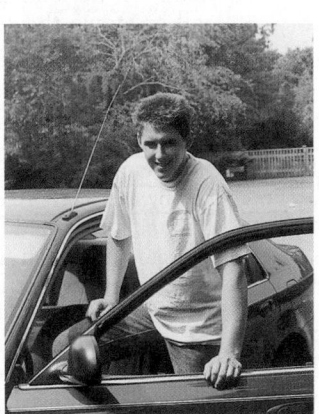

With the freedom driving brings to the adolescent comes responsibility. The adolescent's inexperience and risk-taking behaviors can be a lethal combination.

Computers in school and in many homes provide the adolescent with opportunities for learning, creative expression, communication, and entertainment. Adolescents often enjoy "surfing" the Internet, which can provide them with information not readily available locally. Parents must monitor their computer connections, however, for these networks sometimes allow access to people and activities that conflict with family values.

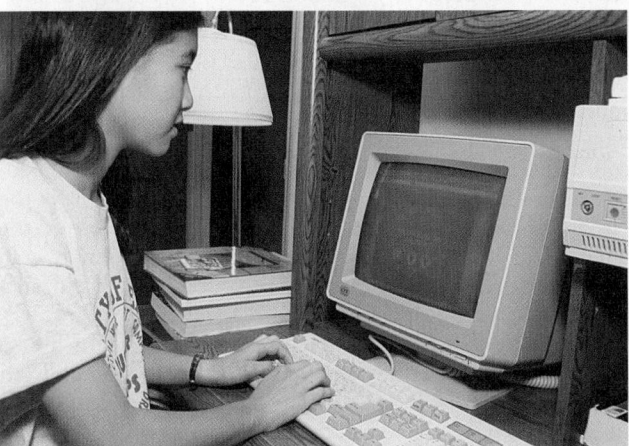

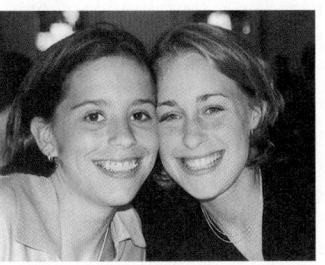

Although teens often have friends of both sexes, they are more comfortable sharing their hopes, dreams, secrets, and even embarrassing incidents with friends of the same sex.

Figure 8-1 Adolescent growth and development.

BOX 8-3
Age-Related Activities and Games for Adolescents

General Activities
Games and athletics are the most common forms of play.
Strict rules are in place.
Competition is important.

Games and Special Types of Play
Sports, videos, movies, reading, parties, hobbies, listening to favorite music on video or compact disc, experimenting with makeup and hairstyles, talking on the telephone.

⚠ CRITICAL TO REMEMBER
The Adolescent and Erikson

- Identity formation and establishment of autonomy
- Acquisition of abstract reasoning leading to:
  Analytic thinking
  Problem solving
  Planning for the future

---

determine who they are going to be. Erikson (1968) described the conflict of this phase of psychosocial development as identity formation versus role confusion; this phase corresponds to Freud's genital stage of psychosexual development (see Chapter 4 for information on developmental theories).

In the transition period from childhood to adulthood, adolescents try on new roles and experiment with the environment until they find a role that fits. The phase of experimentation has been termed the *moratorium*, meaning a period of delay granted to someone not yet ready to make more than a tentative commitment (Erikson, 1968). The adolescent's changing interests from year to year illustrate the lack of commitment. Parents may invest in expensive sports equipment or a musical instrument only to find it abandoned after a short time.

The peer group plays an essential role in adolescent identity formation. Teenagers take their cues on appearance, social behavior, and language from the peer group. The peer group serves as a safe haven as adolescents emotionally move away from the family and struggle to determine who they are. The peer group validates acceptable behavior, and teenagers feel secure in trying on new roles with peer group approval. It is not unusual for teens to spend all day with friends in school and all evening rehashing the day's events over the phone (Box 8-3). Changes in the adolescent's body image, psychosocial development, and peer group acceptance are closely related. Early and middle adolescents are particularly audience-conscious and feel that they are the focus of everyone's attention. A bad hair day or a blemish may throw the adolescent into despair. Clothing, hairstyles, and material possessions that are accepted by the group become the most important. Nurses should counsel parents to negotiate choices with teens but always to consider how peers will judge the child.

Early adolescence and middle adolescence are the periods when teens are prone to gang formation and activities. Peer modeling and peer acceptance, being of the utmost importance, lead some adolescents to form gangs that provide a collective identity and give them a sense of belonging. Peer pressure, companionship, and protection are the most frequently reported reasons for joining gangs, particularly those associated with violent or criminal acts.

There are marked developmental differences between early and late adolescence. Each age-group has unique reactions to the developmental tasks, which are influenced by the adolescent's cognitive thinking. According to Swiss psychologist Jean Piaget (1969), adolescent cognition is characterized by the transition from concrete operational thought to formal operational thought, the ability to think logically and use deductive and abstract reasoning (see Chapters 4 through 7 for further information on Piaget's theory of cognition). The acquisition of formal operational thinking allows the adolescent to draw on past experience and apply knowledge to the future by drawing on logical consequences from a set of observations. Adolescents are capable of using abstract symbols such as those derived from higher-order mathematics, making and testing hypotheses, and considering and arguing philosophic issues. Problem-solving and decision-making skills become more highly developed, although adolescents may still be conflicted about idealism versus reality.

Early Adolescence
The early adolescent (11 to 14 years) has intense feelings about body image and the many physical changes taking place. Less confident with members of the opposite sex, early adolescents tend to group together and have best friends of the same gender. One has only to visit the local mall or movie theater to see groups of young teens of the same gender, observing but rarely speaking to groups of the opposite sex.

The early adolescent is very egocentric and may go from obedience to rebellion with respect to parental authority. Parents are often shocked by the sudden turn of events and are hurt by the teen's rejection. Providing parents with anticipatory guidance regarding age-specific developmental changes is a primary nursing function. For example, the happy-go-lucky 11-year-old may turn into the shy, self-absorbed 12-year-old who seems comfortable only in the presence of friends. Young teens, who are developmentally egocentric, fail to differentiate between how others see them and their own mental preoccupations, thinking everyone is as obsessed with them as they are with themselves. Elkind (1993) describes this phenomenon as a reaction to the imaginary audience. The belief in the imaginary audience is probably why young teens are so self-conscious—they believe everyone is critical of them, and indeed teens are very critical of each other, especially of one who is different. Self-conscious behavior may also be the result of the physical and emotional transition to middle adolescence. The early adolescent is losing the familiar role of the child but does not yet feel comfortable with the role of the adult. Ambivalence toward independence is common, and the teen who feels too grown up for a good-night kiss from a parent still falls asleep with a favorite teddy bear.

Elkind (1993) believes that because young teens are so audience-conscious, they see themselves as unique and tell themselves a "personal fable" that supports feelings of invulnerability. They believe bad things will happen to others but not to them. Adolescent suicide attempts serve as a dramatic message to others, but young teens often do not realize the very final consequences of their actions.

Middle Adolescence

Middle adolescence (15 to 17 years) is often described by parents as the most frustrating period of adolescent development. The real audience gradually replaces the imaginary audience, and teens become even more introspective and narcissistic. Conformity to peer group norms becomes even more important, and conflicts between teenagers and parents often escalate. Testing of limits, sulky withdrawal, and overt rebellion may occur over conflicts with regard to curfews, friends, activities, appearance, cars, and money. The adolescent may feel more secure by associating with or becoming a member of a gang (Box 8-4). It is important for nurses to counsel parents to negotiate choices where possible and to set limits that are perceived as reasonable by the adolescent. Consistent discipline and structure actually make adolescents feel more secure and assist them with decision making. With parental guidance, adolescents are able to make decisions that will result in desirable outcomes. Adults must keep in mind that middle adolescents are impulsive and impatient, however. Parental concern may be seen as interference rather than guidance and may be met with resistance and resentment.

Feelings about self-image and social relationships are intense. Middle adolescence is generally a time of transition from same-sex friendships to an extreme interest in the opposite sex; it is also a time when adolescents may acknowledge homosexual feelings. The proportion of teens who are sexually experienced and sexually active has declined slightly, as has the teen pregnancy rate (Duncan, Dixon, & Carlson, 2003). Explanations for this slight decrease generally fall into two schools: one school points to abstinence education; the other cites sex education that promotes more widespread and effective contraceptive use (Duncan, Dixon, & Carlson, 2003). Nurses and other health care providers cannot become complacent in response to this change in trends. The United States still has one of the highest adolescent pregnancy rates, and in a recent survey by the Centers for Disease Control and Prevention (CDC) (2002), 6.6% of adolescents had initiated sexual intercourse before age 13 years, and 46% of the 9th- through 12th-graders surveyed had had sexual intercourse at least once.

Sexual activity is often related to peer pressure and self-esteem issues. Adolescents with low self-esteem are more vulnerable and are apt to engage in negative risk-taking activities associated with sexuality. Decisions about sexual activity are often impulsive and made with little regard to later consequences or prior preparation. In fact, according to the recent Youth Risk Behavior Surveillance (CDC, 2002), 42% of teenagers who are sexually active did not use a condom at last intercourse. Nurses may help by providing accurate information to assist adolescents in making appropriate sexual choices. Parents need encouragement to maintain open communication and guide teenagers in sexual decision making. Providing parental guidance about sexual behavior is not easy during middle adolescence, when privacy is of extreme importance and communication with parents tends to decrease. In addition, some parents may find sexual behavior a difficult topic to discuss and often avoid talking with teens regarding sexual issues altogether.

In the initial stages of establishing a vocational identity, adolescents are more likely to experience role confusion and

BOX 8-4
Signs of Gang Involvement

- Associating with new friends while ignoring old friends. The child usually will not talk about the new friends or what they do together.
- A change in hairstyle or clothing and associating with other youths with the same style. Usually some of the clothing, such as a hat or jacket, has the gang's initials or "street" name on it. Parents may note tattoos on the body.
- Unexplained source of money or possessions (stereos, jewelry, cars).
- Indications of drug, alcohol, or inhalant abuse (e.g., paint or correction fluid on the clothes, the smell of chemicals on the breath or clothes).
- Change in attitude toward activities such as sports, Scouts, or church. Discipline problems at school, in public, or at home. Youth no longer accepts parents' authority and challenges it frequently.
- Problems at school, such as failing classes, skipping school, or causing problems in class.
- Fear of the police.
- Unexplained signs of fighting, such as bruises, cuts, or complaints of pain.
- Graffiti on or around residence or possessions.
- Threats from rival gang members. Sometimes a family member is a victim of a drive-by shooting before the family realizes the youth is involved in a gang.

have unrealistic expectations of themselves. Some adolescents will identify a role that holds their interest, whereas others will experiment with many roles, moving quickly from one role to another. Overidentification with glamorous roles takes precedence over reality and is enriched by daydreams and fantasy. It is not unusual for a 15-year-old girl to spend time with her friends describing her future as a popular media star, while failing to fold the laundry or do the dishes.

During middle adolescence, some teens acquire part-time jobs and identify various skills and interests. Part-time jobs are often a source of income for material possessions and activities not provided by parents. Such experiences help adolescents set realistic expectations about work, become more independent, and develop their self-esteem. Those who are successful in the working world demonstrate a sense of responsibility and tend to have more positive social interactions. However, some adolescents may allow work to interfere with educational activity and have difficulty setting priorities. School nurses, in collaboration with parents and teachers, are in an excellent position to identify working students and to assist them in setting realistic guidelines for work and education.

Late Adolescence (18 to 21 Years)

Late adolescence is characterized by the ability to think abstractly, conceptualize verbally, and express one's thoughts and feelings about various aspects of life. Late adolescents tend to be idealistic about love, social issues, ethics, and lifestyles until their experiences modify their beliefs. Conformity becomes less important as teens progress through late adolescence. With the development of a unique identity, self-esteem increases and adolescents are able to resist group pressure if it is not in their best interest. Interactions with parents are less turbulent unless values clash, and relationships with both friends and family are maintained.

Emancipation (leaving home) is a major issue; late adolescents prepare themselves to meet this task through education or vocational training. Identifying realistic career goals is important, but many adolescents are not quite ready to make life-long commitments. Changing career goals is not uncommon, but the nurse should watch for those adolescents who have set no career goals, who demonstrate apathy about the future, and who appear committed only to the present. Boredom and apathy are often symptoms of a greater problem—depression.

Social relationships are more mature, although partner selection often continues to fluctuate. Friendships developed in late adolescence may last a lifetime, and expectations of friends and lovers become more realistic and less self-serving. The ability to consider others' needs increases, and recognition of societal needs is more apparent as the adolescent moves from adolescence to adulthood.

Failure to achieve identity formation may leave adolescents in role confusion and impede the successful mastery of the tasks of young adulthood. A positive ego identity depends on the adolescent's ability to accept the past, learn from experience, and become engaged in the future. Most adolescents move through the identity versus role confusion stage of development with minimal difficulty.

Moral and Spiritual Development

Children develop moral reasoning in a sequential manner, as described by American psychologist Lawrence Kohlberg (1984). As adolescents move from concrete to analytic thinking, they advance to Kohlberg's stage 4 conventional level or Kohlberg's stage 5 postconventional level of moral development. Adolescents who remain concrete thinkers may never advance beyond Kohlberg's stage 3 of moral reasoning: conformity to please others and avoid punishment. The teenager's sense of justice is developed through interpersonal relationships with peers, family, and other adult role models. Behaviors that are modeled and rewarded, such as helping the less fortunate and showing loyalty to friends, contribute to the development of a conscience, which operates as a moral guide for subsequent behavior. The middle to late teenager can appreciate that stealing from others is wrong regardless of whether one is caught and punished.

Adolescents and young adults develop a respect for law and order and a society-maintaining orientation (Kohlberg's

stage 4). Young adults may even advance to the societal-perspective stage (Kohlberg's stage 5), which honors the moral rules of right and wrong, contractual agreements, majority opinion, and overall utility or the greatest good for the greatest number. (See Chapter 4 for all stages of Kohlberg's theory of moral development.)

Older adolescents and young adults question the values of family and society and challenge existing moral codes before integrating their experiences and beliefs into a personal moral framework. Once the moral framework is developed, interpersonal relationships tend to be with those whose values and beliefs are similar.

Young adolescents in the stage of concrete operational thought are able to think logically. In this stage, children deal well with the observable but also begin to see other points of view and to examine what they have learned. The young adolescent will accept religious teaching and examine how religious concepts relate to everyday life. Young adolescents are especially inclined to look to God for guidance when troubled.

Middle to late adolescents are capable of analytic thought and may begin to question the religious affiliation of the family, much as they question other family values. Older adolescents may explore different kinds of religion and share religious activities with the peer group.

HEALTH PROMOTION FOR THE ADOLESCENT AND FAMILY

Adolescence is generally a period of wellness. Young people may seek health care for school or sports physicals, skin conditions (acne, contact dermatitis), acute minor illnesses (colds, flu), conditions related to sexuality (birth control, pregnancy, sexually transmissible diseases [STDs]), and the management of chronic illness (diabetes, epilepsy). Health promotion and disease prevention are achieved through adequate nutrition, rest, balanced exercise, and proper immunization against disease.

Nutrition During Adolescence

The accelerated growth (in linear height, weight, and muscle mass) and sexual maturation during adolescence increase teenagers' nutritional needs, including needs for protein, calories, zinc, calcium, and iron. Periods of intense growth require increased caloric intake, and the adolescent appears constantly hungry. Snacks and regular meals must contain adequate nutrients to meet the body's anabolic needs. Adolescents are generally interested in nutrition and the effect food has on their bodies. Teenagers tend to be concerned about their weight, complexion, sexual development, and acceptance by their peers. These issues, together with the adolescent's increasing independence, can have nutritional implications.

Age-Related Nutritional Challenges

The adolescent's food habits are influenced by many factors (Box 8-5). Unfortunately, this happens at a time when the body has increased nutritional needs. Boys tend to have fewer nutritional deficiencies than girls have because they take in more food and are less likely to be dieting. Milk is frequently replaced by soft drinks. Fast foods and "junk foods" sometimes become the mainstay of the adolescent's diet. The social aspect of food consumption gains impor-

---

BOX 8-5
Factors Influencing the Adolescent's Diet

- Busy schedule (sports, activities, jobs)
- Body image concerns, which can lead to undereating
- Skipping breakfast
- Eating away from home
- Eating fast food frequently
- Beginning to buy and prepare own food
- Peer pressure
- Psychologic and emotional problems

PARENTS
Want to Know

Caring for a Child With an Avulsed Tooth

A tooth that has been completely knocked out of the mouth (avulsed) can sometimes be reimplanted. The sooner the reimplantation occurs, the greater is the likelihood of success. If the tooth can be recovered, it should be rinsed in lukewarm tap water and placed in the tooth socket. The tooth should not be scrubbed, and cleaning agents and disinfectants should be avoided. If the tooth cannot be repositioned, it should be placed in a container of milk or water and the child should proceed to the dentist immediately. The prognosis is best if the injury is treated within 30 minutes.

---

tance, and adolescents may prefer to eat meals with peers at social gatherings and restaurants of their choice. Parental supervision of meals declines as the adolescent spends more time away from home and engages in extracurricular activities with peers.

Nutritional Guidance for the Adolescent

The nurse must understand growth and development to be successful in counseling adolescents and their parents about nutrition. Adolescents' increasing need to be independent and to make their own choices should guide the nurse in teaching nutrition. The adolescent should always be involved in the planning.

The nurse should assess the adolescent's present diet and determine habits and eating patterns. The assessment should elicit how often the adolescent eats food from the different food groups and what foods the adolescent does not eat. Based on this information, nutritious foods for meals can be identified and a plan developed.

The nurse can also assist the adolescent by pointing out nutritious fast foods and snacks. An awareness of nutritious fast foods can also aid the adolescent in meal selection. Many fast-food chains have salads with nonfat or low-fat dressings, grilled chicken sandwiches, pasta, and nonfat yogurt. Fat and salt contents have been reduced, and vegetable fats have replaced animal fats at some restaurants. Adolescents should be guided to mix an occasional hamburger and fries with a regular selection of more nutritious foods. Permission should be given to eat foods that may be untraditional at a particular meal, such as pizza for breakfast.

Body image is of particular importance to adolescents. The media reinforce the belief that "thin is in." Adolescents hold themselves to standards set by the entertainment and advertising worlds, which emphasize fitness, glamour, and sexuality. Products that promise a quick weight loss or enhanced muscle mass with a lean physique are appealing to adolescents. Weight management techniques may include fasting, diet pills and laxatives, self-induced vomiting, and fad diets instead of low-fat, low-calorie, nutritionally sound diets and more aerobic exercise. Adolescents may not realize that unsound nutritional habits often follow them for a lifetime or that growth and development may be delayed or permanently impaired. School nurses are in an excellent position to identify adolescents who have nutritional problems and to provide counseling or referral for adolescents and their families (see Chapter 53 for information on eating disorders).

Hygiene

Adolescents in general are meticulous about personal hygiene. A major concern, however, is acne. Acne contributes to adolescent self-consciousness and, if severe, to decreased self-image. Nursing interventions to address acne are discussed in detail in Chapter 49.

Dental Care

The incidence of dental caries decreases in adolescence, but dental hygiene remains very important. Most permanent teeth have erupted with the possible exception of the third molars (wisdom teeth), which erupt by late adolescence or remain impacted and might be removed surgically. Several dental conditions are prevalent during the adolescent years: gingivitis, malocclusion, and dental trauma. Gingivitis is the inflammation and breakdown of the gingival epithelium; the gums appear pale and swollen and bleed easily. Increased hormonal activity at the time of puberty, diets high in sugar and simple carbohydrates, and the use of dental braces and appliances that make cleaning less effective are thought to contribute to the development of gingivitis.

Malocclusion (improper contact) occurs in approximately 50% of adolescents because of facial and mandibular bone growth and dental crowding. Treatment varies but generally entails dental devices such as braces to correct tooth position and redirect facial growth. Adolescents may be self-conscious if their peers are no longer in braces and may need reassurance that the condition is temporary. For economic reasons, some adolescents are unable to correct malocclusions and suffer the consequences indefinitely. Nurses can help by referring adolescents with no dental care to free clinics or agencies providing dental care at low cost. People with uncorrected malocclusions are at greater risk for dental trauma.

A tooth that has been completely knocked out of the mouth (avulsed) can sometimes be reimplanted. The sooner the reimplantation occurs, the greater is the likelihood of success. The prognosis is best if the injury is treated within 30 minutes. School and clinic nurses may be the first health professionals to see a child with a complete tooth avulsion

Health Promotion

The Adolescent

FOCUSED ASSESSMENT

Ask the adolescent the following:

- Can you tell me how often and what foods you like to eat? How often do you eat at fast-food restaurants? How do you feel about how much you weigh? Do you think you need to gain or lose any weight? Do you ever make yourself vomit or take laxatives to control your weight?
- In what types of physical activities or organized sports do you participate? How often do you do them?
- How often do you brush your teeth, floss, and see the dentist? Do you take fluoride?
- What time do you go to bed at night? What time do you get up in the morning? Do you have any trouble falling asleep, or do you wake up in the middle of the night?
- How often do you have a bowel movement? Are there any problems with urination?
- What grade in school are you? How well do you think you are doing in school? Are there any circumstances at school where you feel unsafe or threatened?
- Tell me about your friends. What types of activities do you do with them for fun? Do your friends pressure you to do things you would rather not do? Do you or your friends smoke cigarettes or take any substances (alcohol, drugs)?
- How do you get along with other members of your family? Is there a special family member you could talk to if you are having a problem? If so, whom?
- Do you do any or all of the following: use a seatbelt every time you get in a car; avoid getting into a car if the driver has been drinking; wear a helmet every time you ride a bike or motorcycle; wear a helmet and protective pads every time you skate; use sunscreen; swim with a buddy?
- Has anyone ever physically harmed you or touched you in a way that made you uncomfortable? Have you ever thought about harming yourself? Do you or does anyone you know own a gun?

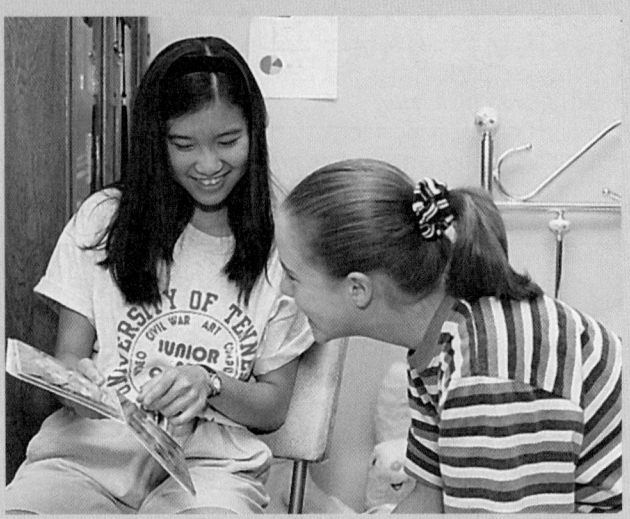

- Have you begun dating? Have you been or are you sexually active (if sexually active, ask about condom use and birth control methods and any incidence of sexually transmissible diseases [STDs])? Do you have any questions or concerns about your sexual development (ask girls about the pattern and frequency of menstruation)?
- What kind of job do you have, if any? How many hours per week do you work?
- What kind of things do you do to stay healthy? Do you take any medications or dietary supplements regularly? Do you do regular breast or testicular self-examinations? Do you have any concerns about any aspect of your health?

Ask the parent the following:

- Are there any concerns related to the adolescent's nutrition, body image, physical activity, oral health, sleep, elimination, school, family interactions, self-esteem, and ability to practice safety precautions?
- Do you continue to stay involved in your child's life?
- What types of family rules do you consistently enforce?

---

and should be aware of the proper procedure (see Chapter 34). Parents should also know how to care for their child if such an incident occurs (Parents Want to Know box).

Sleep and Rest

Along with increasingly independent activities, adolescents show a propensity for staying up late (particularly if working on a school project or attending a weekend party) and having difficulty waking up in the morning. Setting one's own bedtime and sleeping late on weekends are behaviors associated with gaining independence. Hours of sleep may vary from 6 to 8 hours during the week to 12 hours on the weekends, but an overall average of 8 hours per night is recommended for adolescents and young adults.

Rapid physical growth and increased activities contribute to the adolescent's fatigue, and frustrated parents may complain that their teenager has energy for everything but household and family chores. Nurses can educate teens and their parents to set realistic schedules that allow time for adequate rest and relaxation. Some teens may find themselves so overscheduled that they develop sleep disturbances from excess fatigue and anxiety. Adult sleep cycles are formed during adolescence, and sleep disturbances continue into the adult years. Persistent difficulty in falling asleep, wakefulness during the night, or early waking may be signs of emotional problems associated with tension, anxiety, or depression and may warrant referral.

Exercise and Activity

Although adolescents are often involved in many activities, these activities do not always promote physical fitness. A recent study found that only 32.2% of the students were enrolled in a daily physical education (PE) class and that the

Health Promotion—cont'd

The Adolescent—cont'd

DEVELOPMENTAL MILESTONES

Personal/social: emotional and social turmoil associated with rapid changes in development and altered body image; interested in opposite-sex relationships (some lead to a level of intimacy for which the adolescent is not ready); assumes varying roles to integrate social skills with new aspirations and to gain a sense of self; clarifies values and career directions; more stable emotional control in later adolescence; may exhibit imaginary audience ("everyone is staring at me") or personal fable ("it will never happen to me")

Fine motor: adult fine motor control

Language/cognitive: becomes future-oriented; views the world in broad perspective; hypothesizes several alternatives to a problem; thinks and reasons abstractly; develops moral reasoning

Gross motor: early growth-related awkwardness develops into coordinated muscle control

HEALTH MAINTENANCE

Physical Measurements

  Girls achieve peak height velocity (PHV) approximately 2 years before boys

  Average weight gain during growth spurt is 50% of adult weight, largely from body fat in girls and muscle mass in boys

  Average height gain is 20% to 25% of adult height over 2 to 3 years (girls 8.3 cm/yr, boys 9.4 cm/yr)

  Achieve Tanner stage 5 (see Table 8-1)

Immunizations

  Review immunization records; administer immunizations if not up-to-date

  Consider immunizing college-bound students with meningococcal vaccine

Health Screening

  Objective hearing and vision screening (may become myopic as growth spurt begins)

  Hemoglobin or hematocrit

  Urinalysis by dip stick

  Blood pressure

  Lipid screen if at risk

  Tuberculosis screening if at risk (see Chapter 45)

  Pap smear for sexually active girls

  STD screening if applicable

  Emotional and stress screening

ANTICIPATORY GUIDANCE

Nutrition

  Follow recommended servings according to the Food Guide Pyramid; teach the adolescent how to keep track of servings and to give input into meal preparation

  Advise to avoid fast foods and to eat a nutritious breakfast; watch calcium and iron intake; assess adequacy of diet and snacks; folic acid supplementation for adolescent girls

  Teach principles of a vegetarian diet if applicable

Elimination

  Regular bowel movements according to individual pattern

Dental

  Provide regular dental care every 6 months

  Continue regular brushing with fluoride toothpaste and flossing

  Discuss emergency care for fractured or avulsed teeth (see Chapter 34)

Sleep

  Facilitate an individually appropriate sleep pattern; usually needs 8 hours

Safety

  Review gun safety; automobile and motorized vehicle driver and passenger safety; water safety; sun protection; fire safety; avoiding listening to loud music through earphones

  Discuss techniques to combat violence, particularly dating violence; wearing protective equipment in the workplace; no drinking and driving; learning cardiopulmonary resuscitation (CPR)

Emotional Health

  Tell another if concerned about a friend

  Take every threat of suicide as real

  Learn stress reduction techniques

  Seek help if depressed or angry

---

older the adolescents, the less likely they were to be enrolled in a PE class (CDC, 2002). Regular exercise enhances physical and emotional development and promotes healthy sleep patterns. Healthy diet and exercise habits formed during adolescence can follow into adulthood and significantly reduce the risk of cardiovascular disease.

Adolescence is an ideal time to initiate an exercise program, either as a team sport or as an individual activity. Exercise need not always involve an athletic activity but should provide for a program that gradually increases exercise over a 1- to 3-week period with a goal of vigorous exercise of at least 20 minutes three or more times per week to enhance cardiovascular fitness (USDHHS, 2000). Nurses can assist adolescents in designing an exercise program that allows for gradual fitness and provides for warm-up and cool-down sessions. Exercise programs are highly personal and should be structured for enjoyment, with consideration of physical capabilities and limitations.

Safety

Injuries claim more lives during adolescence than all other causes of death combined. The predominance of injuries during adolescence results from a combination of factors: physical growth, psychomotor function, insufficient physical coordination for the task, energy, impulsivity, peer pressure, and inexperience. Impulsivity, inexperience, and peer pressure may place adolescents in unsafe situations. Feelings of invulnerability ("it can't happen to me") persist, and little thought may be given to the negative consequences of certain behaviors. Alcohol and other drugs that impair judgment are known to contribute to fatal injuries among adolescents, especially those involving firearms and motor vehicles (see Chapter 53 for a complete discussion of alcohol and substance abuse). The sad fact is that most serious or fatal injuries involving adolescents are preventable.

Nurses need to educate adolescents and their families about safety issues and injury prevention. Nurses in school and community action programs are focusing more on preventing firearm and traumatic head injuries. Factual information with supportive explanations should be provided. Expressing a genuine interest in adolescents as individuals and listening in a nonjudgmental way are also important steps to gain confidence and trust. Helping the adolescent recognize that there are choices when faced with difficult or potentially dangerous situations is an important component of safety promotion with this age-group.

The adolescent period is also a frightening time for parents because they are aware of the risks predisposing the adolescent to injury or death. Parents may request guidance from health care professionals in setting appropriate limits and establishing methods of effective enforcement. Parents should be encouraged to model the safe behaviors that they expect from the adolescent.

Car Safety

Obtaining a driver's license signifies a passage into adulthood and provides the adolescent with the means to explore and experience the world more freely. Driving is a complex activity, and proficiency requires skill, judgment, and experience. The adolescent's lack of judgment, opposition to authority, and need to express independence often result in a disregard for sound defensive driving practices. Risk-taking behaviors appear to play a major role in the high incidence of car-related injuries and deaths among teenagers. The young, inexperienced driver tends to drive faster and take more chances while operating a car than older drivers do. The Youth Risk Behavior Surveillance Survey of high school students found that 14.1% had rarely or never worn a seatbelt. In addition, during the 30 days preceding the survey, 30.7% had ridden with a driver who had been drinking alcohol (CDC, 2002).

There is an alarming association between the use of alcohol and motor vehicle crashes in adolescents. Despite legal drinking age laws, alcohol is easily accessible to adolescents. The greater social activity of the teenager, combined with the availability of alcohol, increases the incidence of impaired driving.

Nurses can promote car safety by supporting driver education programs for teenagers and the use of seatbelts. In addition, many schools and community organizations have developed prevention programs that are helpful in presenting the facts about drinking and driving to adolescents. Nurses should encourage teens and their parents to set up a ride-home agreement to discourage any driving after drinking alcohol. Adolescents need to know that they have an option available to them if they find themselves in a situation where the driver has been drinking. Dealing with the inconveniences of finding another ride home is much better than dealing with the injuries and damages of motor vehicle crashes.

Water Safety

Drowning is a needless cause of death in teenagers. Most drowning deaths occur in lakes, rivers, and ponds, with the rest occurring in public or private swimming pools. Risk-taking behaviors contribute greatly to deaths from drowning and to the incidence of spinal cord injuries. Adolescents are able to travel to areas that are free of adult supervision. Frequently, alcohol and drugs are contributing factors. Given the combination of freedom and alcohol, adolescents may inadvertently place themselves at risk for injury by exceeding the limits for safe swimming and diving.

Safety promotion includes encouraging swimming lessons, water safety classes, and the completion of a course in cardiopulmonary resuscitation. Adolescents need to know how alcohol and drugs impair their ability to perform activities at which they are usually competent.

Suicide

Suicide is the third leading cause of death for teenagers 15 to 19 years (CDC, 2003). Between 1980 and 1990, suicide rates increased by 30% but have gradually decreased since. In the year 2001, the rate of suicide in the 15- to 19-year-old population was 7.9/100,000—a decrease of 7% from 1990 (National Center for Health Statistics, 2003). In a survey of adolescents, 19% seriously considered committing suicide during the previous 12 months (CDC, 2002). The identification of adolescents at risk for suicide is a priority. Depression is a common finding among suicidal youths; other risk factors include declining mental health, poor impulse control, poor school performance, family disorganization, conduct disorders, substance abuse, homosexuality, and recent stress. Nurses must be involved in identifying high-risk adolescents through the scientific study of these phenomena. Adolescents identified as at risk for suicide and their families should be targeted for supportive guidance and counseling before a crisis situation. Nurses should counsel parents that *all* adolescent suicidal gestures should be taken very seriously. Many adolescents do not know what type of drug ingestion or action will actually harm them. The suicidal gestures may appear minor to adults, but the actions may have serious intent. (See Chapter 53 for more in-depth information on suicide and nursing interventions.)

Violence Toward Others

Violence continues to threaten the health and well-being of adolescents and society as a whole (see Chapter 1). Homicide is the fourth leading cause of death in children ages 10 to 14 years, and for teens ages 15 to 19 years it is the second leading cause of death after unintentional injury. The homicide rate increased dramatically during the 1990s but has decreased since then to 9.4/100,000 (National Center for Health Statistics, 2003). Factors contributing to violence are multiple and complex (Box 8-6). Contributing factors related to behavior provide the greatest opportunity for interventions initiated by health care professionals.

Nurses working with children, adolescents, and their families have the opportunity to include violence prevention as a component of anticipatory guidance. Ideally, prevention should begin when the child is young. Violence is a learned behavior. It is often reinforced by the actions of those closest to the child and by ever-increasing exposure to violence in the media. Assessing how a family deals with anger and resolves conflict provides insight into the way the child will be likely to react in similar situations. A family with violent tendencies should be referred to a counselor. Learning to react to anger or stress with nonviolent actions through conflict resolution is the goal for the youth. Unfortunately, intervention cannot be a one-time educational session. Efforts must be reinforced in multiple facets of the adolescent's life, such as in school, youth organizations, religious organizations, and home.

Parents need to be aware of the amount and type of violence to which their children are exposed in the media. Growing evidence suggests that exposure to media violence does lead to aggressive behavior by the children who watch the programs (Strasburger & Donnerstein, 1999). It is unrealistic to expect parents to isolate their children from all media violence, but they can be encouraged to monitor and limit their children's television viewing and to co-view and discuss with their children the implications of violence.

The availability of firearms is related to violent acts. In a survey of students in grades 9 through 12 conducted by the U.S. Centers for Disease Control and Prevention, it was found that 17% had carried a weapon within the 30 days preceding the survey (CDC, 2002). Carrying a weapon can establish a feeling of control or power, or it may be a response to fear of those with power. Regardless of the reasons, firearms in the hands of adolescents are impulsively used, before the ramifications of such actions can be logically considered.

As society urgently seeks a solution to the growing problem of violence, health care professionals must become advocates of violence prevention. Opportunities for adolescents to discover and use less violent means to express themselves or resolve day-to-day issues should be taught and promoted. Peer mediation programs in schools have been successful in preventing violent behavior among teens. Given the tragic effects of violence on the safety and health of American children, nurses should participate in efforts to resolve the complex issues of violence in our society. A product-oriented focus on firearms that incorporates several strategies, including legislation, education, regulation, litigation, and firearm modification, may be an effective approach to this problem (Freed, Vernick, & Hargarten, 1998).

Selected Issues Related to the Adolescent

Body Piercing

Ear piercing has been popular with teens for many years. Today the tongue, lip, eyebrow, nose, navel, and nipple are also common sites. Generally, body piercing is harmless, but nurses should caution teens about performing these procedures under unsterile conditions and should educate teens about complications, such as bleeding, infection, keloid formation, and allergies to metal. Qualified personnel using sterile needles

should perform piercing procedures. The area needs to be cleaned twice each day (more often for a tongue piercing).

Tattoos

Tattoos are increasingly popular among mainstream adolescents and are not usually a mark of gang membership (Carroll, Riffenburgh, Roberts, & Myhre, 2002). Like clothing and hairstyles, tattoos serve to define one's identity. Unfortunately, tattoos are often the result of an impulsive decision by the adolescent and are performed by amateurs who are not qualified to do the procedure. Recent studies of a large sample of adolescents suggest an increase in behavioral risk factors (eating disorders, drug and alcohol use, increased sexual activity and risk for suicide) among adolescents who have body piercings or tattoos (Carroll et al., 2002; Roberts & Ryan, 2002). Because of the invasiveness of the tattoo procedure, it should be considered a health-risk situation. Little regulation exists in the tattoo industry, and nurses should educate adolescents about the risks of bloodborne infections, skin infections, and allergic reactions to dyes used in the tattoo process. In addition, nurses need to be informed about tattoo removal to provide correct information to adolescents and their families (Adolescents Want to Know box). Impulsive decisions to tattoo are often regretted, and teens or their parents may want the tattoo removed. Laser therapy is available for tattoo removal but is costly and not usually covered by insurance. Amateur tattoos are removed quite easily, but studio tattoos made with red and green dyes are quite difficult to remove. Tattoo removal requires several visits, and adolescents have to tolerate the tattoo's appearance during the removal process. Nurses need to caution adolescents with tattoos to notify health professionals of the tattoo if magnetic resonance imaging (MRI) is to be performed. The iron oxide in the tattooing dye can contribute to injury during MRI (Selekman, 2003).

Suntanning

There is no such thing as a "good" tan. It is difficult, however, to convince adolescents that tanning not only is harmful to their skin but also is a risk factor for developing skin cancer

---

BOX 8-6
Factors Contributing to Adolescent Violence

- Low socioeconomic status
- Crowded urban housing
- Single-parent family or limited parental supervision
- History of family violence or child abuse
- Access to guns
- Peer pressure or gang involvement
- Limited education
- Racism
- Drug or alcohol use or abuse
- Low self-esteem and hopelessness about the future
- Aggression

ADOLESCENTS
Want to Know

Tattooing

- Talk with other tattooed people to get their ideas about tattooing.
- Avoid getting a tattoo during a stressful period.
- Check the artist's technique, equipment sterilization, gloving, and skin care instructions.
- Understand the dangers of bloodborne diseases, such as hepatitis B and HIV, and be alert for skin reactions.
- Assess the cost of future tattoo removal, because it is expensive and not easy to obtain.

Modified from Armstrong, M.L. (1995). Adolescent tattoos: Educating vs. pontificating. *Pediatric Nursing, 21*(6), 561-564.
HIV, Human immunodeficiency virus.

later in life. The media (advertising, movies, television) promote the image of beach glamour: young, well-built, and tanned. Although most companies that manufacture tanning products promote the sun protection factor (SPF) in their products, the advertised image remains a bronzed, attractive, young person. Most exposure to ultraviolet radiation occurs during childhood and adolescence, and skin cancers could be prevented with the appropriate and consistent use of sunscreens and sun blocks.

A recent study of the prevalence of indoor tanning salon use among adolescents suggests that approximately 10% of adolescents in the United States obtain a tan in a tanning salon (Cokkinides, Weinstock, O'Connell, & Thun, 2002). Very problematic in this piece of research is the fact that a percentage of the adolescents who use tanning salons do not use sun protection (either in the salon or when under natural sunlight). Adolescents most likely to use tanning salons are girls whose parent(s) also report tanning salon use (Cokkinides et al., 2002). It is essential for nurses who are doing anticipatory guidance with teens to address this issue along with the risks of tanning in natural sunlight.

Nurses need to educate teens about the benefits and side effects of different sun protection products and encourage use not only for water sports but also for all activities that involve sun exposure. Teens involved in athletic activities are often exposed to the sun for long periods without protection. Teenagers may be cognizant of body exposure at a beach but may forget about the exposure of body parts during a long tennis match or a baseball game, especially on a cloudy day, when up to 80% of the sun's radiation reaches the ground. Nurses should caution teens receiving any type of medication about the side effects related to sun exposure. Some medications may potentiate the sun's ultraviolet rays, resulting in quicker burning. The side effects of sunscreen products include itching, burning, and redness immediately or up to 24 hours after the product is applied. Some people are allergic or sensitive to the sunscreen agent (e.g., para-aminobenzoic acid [PABA], PABA esters, cinnamates, anthranilates, benzophenones) or to other ingredients used, such as fragrances or preservatives. Sunscreen use should be discontinued if an allergic dermatitis is noted, and the teen should try another type of sunscreen. Numerous products are on the market with various ingredients that have sun-screening capabilities. Sun damage can be prevented, and simple measures can minimize the effects of ultraviolet radiation on the skin.

Sexual Activity

Adolescent Sexuality. Adolescent sexuality refers to the thoughts, feelings, and behaviors related to the adolescent's sexual identity. Middle adolescence typically marks the initial period of dating and experimentation with heterosexual and homosexual behaviors, although in some cultures sexual experimentation occurs much earlier. Initially, group dating may be popular, but this is quickly replaced by dating in couples, who may be sexual partners. Intimate relationships in middle adolescence are usually short-lived as adolescents experiment with their sexual identity. Of greatest concern to parents during the adolescent's stage of sexual experimentation are unwanted pregnancies, STDs, and the teen's feelings

of despair over failed relationships. Adolescents themselves are often impervious to the possibility of negative consequences of their sexual experimentation and believe that "it can't happen to me."

Homosexual behavior in adolescence does not necessarily indicate that the adolescent will maintain a homosexual orientation. Gay and lesbian adolescents face many challenges growing up in a society that is often unaccepting. Those adolescents who self-identify their sexual preference as homosexual during high school are at increased risk for a variety of health risks and problem behaviors, including suicide, victimization, risky sexual behaviors, and multiple substance abuse (Duncan et al., 2003; Garofalo, Wolf, Kessel, Palfrey, & DuRant, 1998).

Most very young teens have not had intercourse. The likelihood of teenagers having intercourse increases with age, however. The Youth Risk Behavior Surveillance System showed that more than 6% of the group had sexual intercourse before age 13 years and that 46% of all adolescents had been involved in sexual activity (CDC, 2002). Adolescence is a period of risk taking, and many adolescents choose not only to be sexually active but also to do so unprotected. In addition, sexual activity in adolescents is greatly correlated with other risk behaviors, especially alcohol and other substance use, so nurses must approach the issue from multiple perspectives.

Some underlying themes influence whether an adolescent delays engaging in sexual activity. Adolescents who demonstrate high levels of self-esteem are more likely to delay intercourse. If adolescents value personal health and see sexual activity as dangerous, involving the risk of pregnancy or human immunodeficiency virus (HIV) or other STDs, they are more likely to recognize that intercourse should be postponed (Johnson, Rozmus, & Edmisson, 1999).

The adolescent's limited cognitive abilities or lack of abstract thinking may influence contraceptive practices. Adolescents who feel invulnerable to pregnancy often cannot assimilate and apply to themselves information about sexual behavior, conception, and birth control. Lack of self-esteem and peer pressure also play a role in determining adolescents' sexual behavior. Teens may use sex to feel loved or desired, and they may fear abandonment by a partner if sex is refused. Some teens lack correct reproductive information and do not plan ahead for sexual encounters. Sexual activity is often impulsive, erratic, and unplanned, because the relationships are relatively short-term.

Nurses in schools and community clinics are in a position to identify teens at risk for pregnancy and to provide guidance with appropriate information and referral in a confidential atmosphere. Nurses should strongly encourage adolescents to discuss sexuality, sexual behavior, and contraception with their parents whenever possible but must guarantee confidentiality of communication.

School sex education programs have had varying success. Many are either abstinence-based or protection-based. A combination of providing information about protection methods while emphasizing the benefits of abstinence may be more successful than either emphasis alone (American Academy of Pediatrics Committee on Adolescence, 1999; USDHHS, 2000).

The nurse's professional role is to ensure that adolescents have the knowledge, skills, and opportunities that enable them to make responsible decisions regarding sexual behavior. Education regarding sexuality and contraception should be oriented to the developmental level of the individual or group. The nurse uses primary preventive intervention by assisting adolescents to develop coping strategies to meet their needs in ways other than through sexual behavior.

Contraception. Complete protection from pregnancy and STDs is achievable only through sexual abstinence. Because approximately half of adolescents between ages 15 and 19 years are sexually active, however, nurses need to feel comfortable with managing health concerns related to sexuality. Comprehensive health care includes providing services for sexually active adolescents. Health care providers should provide screening for and management of STDs, contraceptive services, and psychosocial counseling.

In the United States, nearly 1 million teens unintentionally become pregnant annually, and of these pregnancies, nearly 50% end in abortion (USDHHS, 2000). The average age for girls to initiate sexual activity is between 15 and 17 years and is slightly earlier in black girls (American Academy of Pediatrics Committee on Adolescence, 1999). Most teens do not seek contraceptive information for 1 year after first intercourse; many (20%) become pregnant within the first month (American Academy of Pediatrics Committee on Adolescence, 1999).

When educating adolescents about birth control methods, it is ideal to see partners together. Open communication between partners is essential, and decisions about contraception should be mutual. Both male and female adolescents

need to assume responsibility for sexual behavior. Regardless of the method of birth control selected, all adolescents need frequent follow-up to maintain consistent contraception behaviors. Counseling teens about sexuality and contraception requires nurses who are open, forthright, and respectful of the decisions teens make about sexual activity (see Chapter 31 for information on STDs and Chapter 10 for information relating to contraception).

! CRITICAL TO REMEMBER

Factors to Consider in Selecting Adolescent Contraception

- Cognitive development (concrete versus abstract thinking)
- Understanding and acceptance of attitudes and values
- Sexual maturity rating
- Communication between partners
- Opportunity to counsel both partners
- Use of more than one method
- Frequency of intercourse
- Appropriate information (three messages per visit)
- Problem-solving abilities (appeal to logic and feelings of power over body)
- Communication with parents or other adults
- Physical and mental health
- Motivation of both partners
- Concrete, graphic instruction in all methods
- Number and gender of partners
- Encouragement that abstinence is alright

KEY CONCEPTS

- Adolescence is a period of transition from childhood to adulthood that is marked by important biologic and psychologic changes.
- Biologic development during adolescence is variable. Primary and secondary sexual characteristics are acquired through the influence of reproductive hormones in males and females.
- Sexual maturity ratings (SMR; Tanner stages) are somewhat variable but predictable stages of sexual maturation that are based on pubic hair and breast development in girls and pubic hair and genital development in boys.
- According to Erikson, the major developmental task in adolescence is the development of an identity and self-perception. Other developmental tasks include the development of a sexual identity, avocational/ educational identity, and independence and autonomy.
- Early and middle adolescents are egocentric and concerned with themselves.
- Cognitive thinking during adolescence moves from concrete to abstract reasoning.
- According to Kohlberg, adolescents and young adults develop a respect for law and order and a society-maintaining orientation.
- Adolescents question the values of family and society before integrating their experiences and beliefs into a personal moral framework.
- Adolescents may be emotionally labile, with extreme highs and extreme lows.
- The pace of physical growth during adolescence is second only to the pace of growth during infancy.
- Poor eating habits and lack of aerobic exercise contribute to obesity and decreased overall physical fitness.
- Suntanning, body piercing, and tattooing are behaviors associated with identity formation.
- Risk-taking behavior is considered part of normal growth and development.
- Safety issues related to sports activity, sexual activity, firearms, and the use of motor vehicles should be emphasized.
- Sexual maturation precipitates sexual activity; teen pregnancy and sexually transmissible diseases are related issues.

ANSWERS to Critical Thinking Exercise 8-1

1. The main issues will be confidentiality and trust. To establish trust, the nurse must be honest with Heidi. The nurse must be clear about the boundaries before the conversation continues. Depending on what Heidi tells the nurse, she may want to encourage Heidi to share the information with her parents. Finally, there should be no question that if the information has the potential to cause harm to either Heidi or others, it cannot be kept confidential.

2. A therapeutic response would be, "Heidi, I want you to feel comfortable talking with me. I will keep what you tell me confidential unless it is something that might be harmful to you or others."

REFERENCES and READINGS

Akinbami, L., Gandhi, H., & Cheng, T. (2003). Availability of adolescent health services and confidentiality in primary care practices. *Pediatrics, 111*(2), 394-401.

American Academy of Pediatrics Committee on Adolescence. (1999). Contraception and adolescents. *Pediatrics, 101*(5), 1161-1166.

American Academy of Pediatrics Committee on Nutrition. (1998). *Pediatric nutrition handbook.* Elk Grove Village, IL: American Academy of Pediatrics.

Anderson, S., Dallal, G., & Must, A. (2003). Relative weight and race influence average at menarche: Results from two nationally representative surveys of U.S. girls studied 25 years apart. *Pediatrics, 111*(4), 844-850.

Beall, S. (2000). Talking with teens: Successfully screening for high-risk behavior. *Journal of Society of Pediatric Nurses, 5*(3), 139-141.

Carroll, R., Riffenburgh, R., Roberts, T., & Myhre, E. (2002). Tattoos and body piercings as indicators of adolescent risk-taking behaviors. *Pediatrics, 109*(6), 1021-1028.

Centers for Disease Control and Prevention. (2002). Youth risk behavior surveillance—United States, 2001. *MMWR: Morbidity and Mortality Weekly Report, 51*(SS04), 1-68.

Centers for Disease Control and Prevention. (2003). Deaths: Leading causes for 2001 [Electronic version]. *National Vital Statistics Reports, 52*(9), 13. Retrieved December 8, 2003 from www.cdc.gov/nchs/.

Chumlea, W.C., Schubert, C.M., Roche, A.F., Kulin, H.E., Lee, P.A., Himes, J.H., & Sun, S.S. (2003). Age at menarche and racial comparisons in U.S. girls. *Pediatrics, 111*(1), 110-113.

Cohen, D., Farley, T., Taylor, S., Martin, D., & Schuster, M. (2002). When and where do youths have sex? The potential role of adult supervision. *Pediatrics, 110*(6), e66.

Cokkinides, V., Weinstock, M., O'Connell, M., & Thun, M. (2002). Use of indoor tanning sunlamps by U.S. youth ages 11-18 years and by their parent or guardian caregivers: Prevalence and correlates. *Pediatrics, 109*(6), 1124-1131.

Davis, K., Cokkinides, V., Weinstock, M., & Wingo, P. (2002). Summer sunburn and sun exposure among U.S. youths ages 11 to 18: National prevalence and associated factors. *Pediatrics, 110*(1), 27-35.

Duncan, P., Dixon, R., & Carlson, J. (2003). Childhood and adolescent sexuality. *Pediatric Clinics of North America, 50*(4), 765-780.

Elfenbein, D., & Felice, M. (2003). Adolescent pregnancy. *Pediatric Clinics of North America, 50*(4), 781-800.

Elkind, D. (1993). *Parenting your teenager.* New York: Ballantine Books.

Erikson, E. (1968). *Identity: Youth and crisis.* New York: Norton.

Federal Interagency Forum on Child and Family Statistics. (2000). *America's children: Key national indicators of well being.* Vienna, VA: National Maternal and Child Health Clearinghouse.

Feroli, K. (2003). Adolescent sexually transmitted diseases: New recommendations for diagnosis, treatment, and prevention. *MCN: The American Journal of Maternal/Child Nursing, 28*(2), 113-118.

Fletcher, J., & Slap, G. (1999). Menstrual disorders. *Pediatric Clinics of North America, 46*(3), 505-518.

Ford, C.A., & Coleman, W.L. (1999). Adolescent development and behavior: Implications for the primary care physician. In M.D. Levine, W.B. Carey, & A.C. Crocker (Eds.), *Developmental-behavioral pediatrics* (3rd ed., pp. 69-79). Philadelphia: Saunders.

Freed, L.H., Vernick, J.S., & Hargarten, S.W. (1998). Prevention of firearm-related injuries and deaths among youth. *Pediatric Clinics of North America, 45*(2), 427-438.

Frenn, M., & Porter, C. (1999). Exercise and nutrition: What adolescents think is important. *Applied Nursing Research, 12*(4), 179-183.

Garofalo, R., Wolf, R.C., Kessel, S., Palfrey, J., & DuRant, R.H. (1998). The association between health risk behaviors and sexual orientation among a school-based sample of adolescents. *Pediatrics, 101*(5), 895-902.

Gidwani, P., Sobol, A., DeJong, W., Perrin, J., & Gortmaker, S. (2002). Television viewing and initiation of smoking among youth. *Pediatrics, 110*(3), 505-508.

Green, M., & Palfrey, J. (Eds.). (2000). *Bright futures: Guidelines for health supervision of infants, children, and adolescents* (2nd ed.). Arlington, VA: National Center for Education in Maternal Child Health.

Hern, M.J., Marine, S., & Morris, T. (1999). Nursing's role in NetWellness: A children and adolescent health information resource via the web. *Journal of Pediatric Nursing, 14*(4), 222-230.

Hollen, P.J., & Brickle, B.B. (1998). Quality parental decision making and distress. *Journal of Pediatric Nursing, 13*(3), 140-150.

Honig, J. (2002). Perceived health status in urban minority young adolescents. *MCN: The American Journal of Maternal/Child Nursing, 27*(4), 233-237.

Johnson, L., Rozmus, C., & Edmisson, K. (1999). Adolescent sexuality and sexually transmitted diseases: Attitudes, beliefs, knowledge, and values. *Journal of Pediatric Nursing, 14*(3), 177-184.

Kaplowitz, P., & Oberfield, S. (1999). Reexamination of the age limit for defining when puberty is precocious in girls in the United States: Implications for evaluation and treatment. *Pediatrics, 104*(4), 936.

Kaplowitz, P., Slora, E., Wasserman, R., Pedlow, S., & Herman-Giddens, M. (2001). Earlier onset of puberty in girls: Relation to increased body mass index and race. *Pediatrics, 108*(2), 347-353.

Kohl, H.W., & Hobbs, K.E. (1998). Development of physical activity behaviors among children and adolescents. *Pediatrics, 101*(3), 549-554.

Kohlberg, L. (1984). *Essays on moral development.* San Francisco: Harper & Row.

Litt, I.F., & Martin, J.A. (1999). Development of sexuality and its problems. In M.D. Levine, W.B. Carey, & A.C. Crocker (Eds.), *Developmental-behavioral pediatrics* (3rd ed., pp. 457-470). Philadelphia: Saunders.

Longo, H. (1999). Meningococcal disease increasing in subgroups of college students. *Infectious Diseases in Children, 12*(7), 11.

Marshall, W.A., & Tanner, J. (1969). Variations in pattern of pubertal changes in girls. *Archives of Disease in Childhood, 44*(235), 291-303.

McCaleb, A., & Cull, V. (2000). Sociocultural influences and self-care practices of middle adolescents. *Journal of Pediatric Nursing, 15*(1), 30-35.

Misra, M., & Park-Bennett, S. (2002). Disorders of puberty. In F. Burg, J. Ingelfinger, R. Polin, & A.

Gershon (Eds.), *Gellis & Kagan's current pediatric therapy* (17th ed., pp. 706-710). Philadelphia: Saunders.

National Center for Health Statistics. (2003). *Health, United States, 2003.* Retrieved November 1, 2003, from www.cdc.gov/nchs.

Perkins, K., Ferrari, N., Rosas, A., Bessette, R., Williams, A., & Hatim, O. (1997). You won't know unless you ask: The biopsychosocial interview for adolescents. *Clinical Pediatrics, 36*(2), 79-86.

Piaget, J. (1969). *The theory of stages in cognitive development.* New York: McGraw-Hill.

Prazer, G.E., & Friedman, S.B. (1997). An office-based approach to adolescent psychosocial issues. *Contemporary Pediatrics, 14*(5), 59-76.

Riesch, S., Bush, L., Nelson, C., Ohm, B., Portz, P., Abell, B., Wightman, M., & Jenkins, P. (2000). Topics of conflict between parents and young adolescents. *Journal of Society of Pediatric Nursing, 5*(1), 27-38.

Roberts, T., & Ryan, S. (2002). Tattooing and high-risk behavior in adolescents. *Pediatrics, 110*(6), 1058-1064.

Russell, D., Keil, M., Bonat, S., Uwaifo, G., Nicholson, J., McDuffie, J., Hill, S., & Yanovski, J. (2001). The relation between skeletal maturation and adiposity in African American and Caucasian children. *The Journal of Pediatrics, 139*(6), 844-848.

Selekman, J. (2003). A new era of body decoration: What are kids doing to their bodies? *Pediatric Nursing, 29*(1), 77-80.

Steger, S. (2000). Killed in school. *RN, 63*(4), 36-38.

Steinberg, L. (2000). The family at adolescence: Transition and transformation. *Journal of Adolescent Health, 27*(3), 170-178.

Steom, K.F., Roeser, R., & Markus, H.R. (1998). Self-schemas and possible selves as predictors and outcomes of risky behaviors in adolescents. *Nursing Research, 47*(2), 96-106.

Strasburger, V.C., & Donnerstein, E. (1999). Children, adolescents, and the media: Issues and solutions. *Pediatrics, 103*(1), 129-139.

Tanner, J. (1962). *Growth at adolescence* (2nd ed.). Oxford: Blackwell Scientific Publications.

Trickett, P.K., & Schellenbach, C.J. (1998). *Violence against children in the family and community.* Washington, DC: American Psychological Association.

U.S. Department of Health and Human Services. (1998). *America's adolescents: Are they healthy?* San Francisco: National Adolescent Health Information Center.

U.S. Department of Health and Human Services. (2000). *Healthy People 2010* (Conference edition, in 2 volumes). Washington, DC: Author.

Wang, Y. (2002). Is obesity associated with early sexual maturation? A comparison of the association in American boys versus girls. *Pediatrics, 110*(5), 903-911.

Wolfsdorf, J. (2002). Gynecomastia. In F. Burg, J. Ingelfinger, R. Polin, & A. Gershon (Eds.), *Gellis & Kagan's current pediatric therapy* (17th ed., pp. 704-705). Philadelphia: Saunders.

Xiaoming, L., Stanton, B., & Feigelman, S. (2000). Impact of perceived parental monitoring on adolescent risk behavior over 4 years. *Journal of Adolescent Health, 27*(1), 49-56.

9

Hereditary and Environmental Influences on Development

 ## LEARNING OBJECTIVES

After studying this chapter, you should be able to:

◎ Describe the structure and function of normal human genes and chromosomes.
◎ Give examples of ways genes and chromosomes are studied.
◎ Describe the transmission of single gene traits from parent to child.
◎ Relate chromosomal abnormalities to spontaneous abortion and to birth defects in the infant.

◎ Explain characteristics of multifactorial birth defects.
◎ Identify environmental factors that can interfere with prenatal development, and explain how their effects can be avoided or reduced.
◎ Describe the process of genetic counseling.
◎ Explain the role of the nurse in caring for individuals or families with concerns about birth defects.

DEFINITIONS

allele An alternate form of a gene.

autosome Any of the 22 pairs of chromosomes other than the sex chromosomes.

birth defect An abnormality of structure, function, or body metabolism present at birth that results in physical or mental disability, or is fatal (according to the March of Dimes Birth Defects Foundation).

congenital Present at birth.

cytogenetics The study of chromosomes and chromosome abnormalities.

diploid Having a pair of chromosomes (46, or 23 pairs, in humans) that represents one copy of every chromosome from each parent; the number of chromosomes normally present in body cells other than gametes.

familial Presence of a trait or condition in a family more often than would be expected by chance alone.

gamete Reproductive cell; in the female an ovum and in the male a spermatozoon.

genetic Pertaining to the genes or the chromosomes.

genogram A graphic representation of a family's medical and hereditary history and the relationships among the family members; often called a pedigree.

genotype Genetic makeup of an individual.

haploid Having one copy of a chromosome from each pair (23 in humans, or half the diploid number). Gametes normally have a haploid number of chromosomes.

heterozygous Having two different alleles for a genetic trait.

homozygous Having two identical alleles for a genetic trait.

karyotype A picture of a cell's chromosomes, arranged from largest to smallest pairs.

monosomy Presence of only one of a chromosome pair in every body cell.

mutation Change in a gene that usually affects its function. Mutations may be in either the gametes or the somatic cells.

phenotype The outward expression of one's genetic makeup.

polymorphism A gene having two or more alternate forms (alleles), each of which occurs in more than 1% of the population.

polyploidy Having additional full sets of chromosomes.

sex chromosome The X or Y chromosome. Females have two X chromosomes; males have one X and one Y chromosome.

somatic cells Body cells other than the gametes, or germ cells.

teratogen An agent that can cause defects in a developing baby during pregnancy.

translocation Attachment of all or part of a chromosome to another chromosome.

trisomy Presence of three copies of a chromosome in each body cell.

Hereditary and environmental forces influence one's development from before conception until death. The nurse needs a basic knowledge of these forces to understand disorders evident at birth and those that develop later in life.

HEREDITARY INFLUENCES

Hereditary influences on development result from the directions for cellular functions provided by genes that make up the 46 chromosomes in every somatic cell. Abnormal struc-

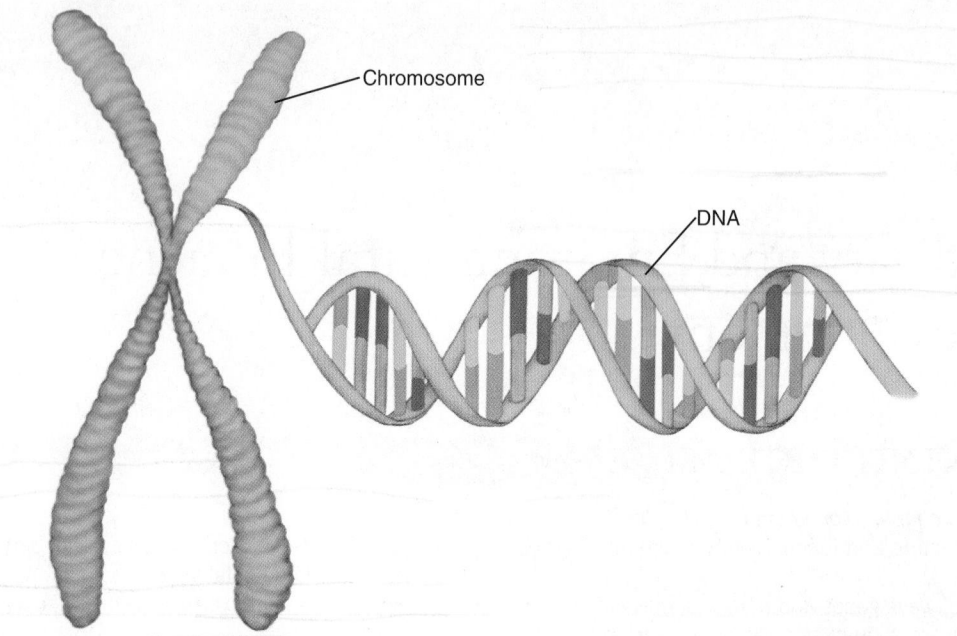

Figure 9-1 Diagrammatic representation of the deoxyribonucleic acid (DNA) helix, which is the building block of genes and chromosomes.

ture or function results if too much or too little genetic material is present in the cells or if an abnormal gene provides incorrect directions. The disorders that result may be merely annoying, or they may be devastating.

Structure of Genes and Chromosomes

A review of the structure of genes and chromosomes aids in understanding how disorders occur. Chromosomes are composed of genes that in turn are composed of deoxyribonucleic acid (DNA) (Fig. 9-1).

DNA

DNA is the basic building block of genes and chromosomes. It has three units: (1) a sugar (deoxyribose), (2) a phosphate group, and (3) one of four nitrogen bases (adenine, thymine, guanine, and cytosine).

DNA resembles a spiral ladder, with a sugar and a phosphate group forming each side of the ladder and a pair of nitrogen bases forming each rung. The four bases of the DNA molecule pair with one another in a fixed way, allowing accurate duplication of the DNA during each cell division.

- Adenine pairs with thymine.
- Guanine pairs with cytosine.

The sequence of base pairs within the DNA determines which amino acids are assembled to form a protein and the order in which they are assembled. Some of these proteins form the structure of body cells; others are enzymes that control metabolic processes within the cell. If the sequence of nitrogen bases in the DNA is incorrect or if some bases are missing or added, a defect in body structure or function may result.

Genes

A gene is a segment of DNA that directs the production of a specific product needed for body structure or function. Humans probably have between 30,000 and 40,000 genes, fewer

than previous estimates that ranged from 50,000 to 140,000 (Guyton & Hall, 2000; National Human Genome Research Institute, 2003).

Genes that code for the same trait often have two or more alternate forms (alleles). Many alleles are normal, such as those that code for a person's blood type. Normal alleles that are common in the population, or polymorphisms, provide genetic variation and sometimes a biologic advantage. However, mutations often involve change in a gene that harms function, such as those that cause the production of abnormal hemoglobin in sickle cell disease or cause cells to grow in an uncontrolled way, causing cancer.

Genes are too small to be seen under a microscope, but many can be studied by tissue analysis:

- By measuring the products that the genes direct cells to produce, such as an enzyme or other substance
- By studying the gene's DNA directly
- By analyzing the gene's close association (linkage) with another gene that can be studied in one of the previous two ways.

The Human Genome Project is an international effort begun in 1990 to identify all genes contained in the 46 human chromosomes. The full sequence of human genes was completed in April, 2003 (National Human Genome Research Institute, 2003). Information gained from this project may allow advances such as:

- Genetic testing to determine the risk for a disorder or the actual or probable presence of the disorder
- Basing reproductive decisions on more accurate and specific information than has previously been available
- Identifying genetic susceptibility to a disorder so that interventions to reduce risk can be instituted
- Using gene therapy to modify a defective gene
- Modifying therapy such as medication based on an individual's genetic code or the genetic makeup of tumor cells

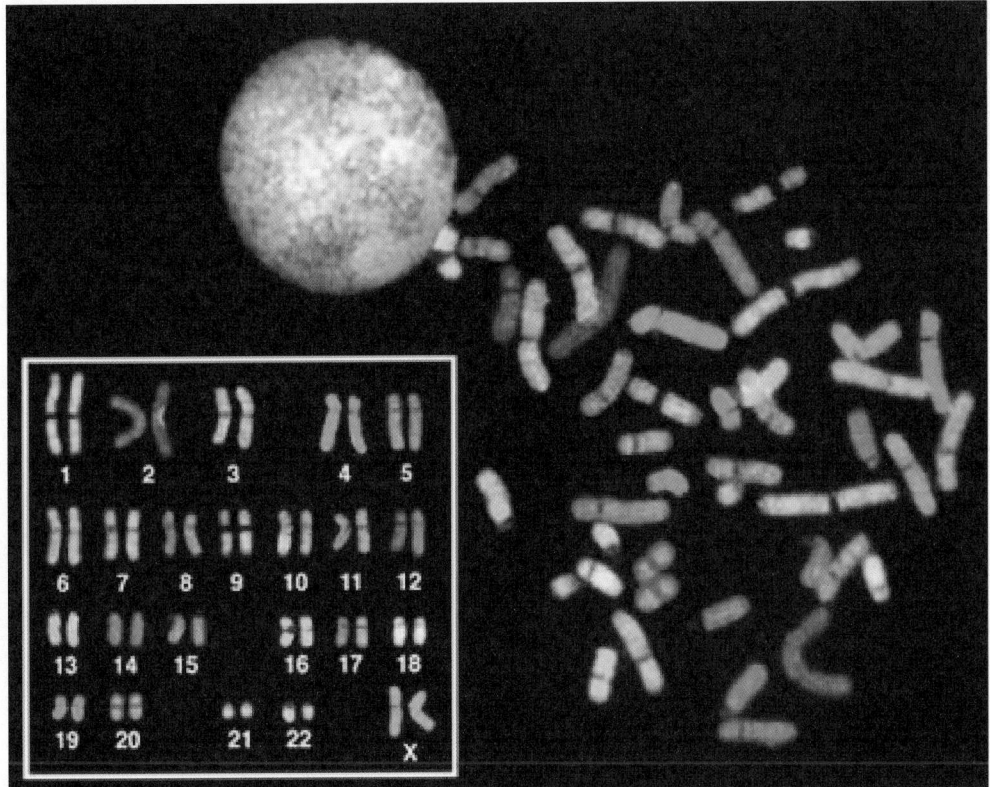

Figure 9-2 When viewed before karyotyping, chromosomes appear jumbled. This photo is a spectral karyotype from a normal female. (From National Human Genome Research Institute. [2002]. Retrieved July 19, 2003, from www.genome.gov/10000208.)

The explosion of knowledge about the genetic basis for many diseases raises many legal and ethical issues for which we do not yet have answers. As our knowledge base grows, new issues are likely to emerge:

- Genetic information has implications for others in the person's family, raising privacy issues.
- Identification of genetic problems could lead to poor self-esteem, guilt, and excessive caution, or, conversely, a reckless lifestyle.
- Presymptomatic identification of genetically influenced illness would be a source of long-term anxiety.
- Genetic knowledge could affect one's choice of a partner.
- Discrimination may occur, such as the imposition of high insurance rates, the denial of insurance coverage, or an employer's decision not to hire a qualified person who has a greater chance of genetically influenced illness.

Chromosomes

Genes are organized into 46 paired chromosomes in the nucleus of most somatic cells. Twenty-two chromosome pairs are autosomes, and the 23rd pair makes up the sex chromosomes. Added or missing chromosomes or structurally abnormal chromosomes are usually harmful.

Mature gametes have half the chromosomes (23) of other body cells. One chromosome from each pair is distributed randomly in the gametes, allowing variation of genetic traits among people. When the ovum and sperm unite at conception, the total is restored to 46 paired chromosomes.

Cells for chromosomal analysis must have a nucleus and must be living. Chromosomes can be studied using any of several types of cells: white blood cells, skin fibroblasts, bone marrow cells, and fetal cells from the chorionic villi (future placenta) or those suspended in amniotic fluid.

Unlike genes, chromosomes can be seen under the microscope, but only during division of live cells. Specimens must be obtained and preserved carefully to provide enough living cells for chromosomal analysis. Temperature extremes, clotting of blood, or adding improper preservatives can kill the cells and render them useless for analysis.

Chromosomes look jumbled when viewed under a microscope (Fig. 9-2). Photographing or using computer imaging allows the chromosomes to be displayed from largest to smallest pairs into a karyotype (Fig. 9-3). The karyotype is then analyzed.

Finer analysis of chromosomes is possible using fluorescent in-situ hybridization and spectral karyotyping. Fluorescent in-situ hybridization (FISH) uses fluorescent-labeled DNA probes that attach to specific chromosomes and permits testing for added, missing, or rearranged chromosome material that otherwise may not be visible. FISH analysis does not require living cells, unlike other chromosome analyses. Spectral karyotyping (SKY) colors, or "paints," each chromosome differently to identify small rearrangements, losses, or gains of chromosome material (Jorde, Carey, Bamshad, & White, 1999; National Human Genome Research Institute, 2003).

Transmission of Traits by Single Genes

Inherited characteristics are passed from parent to child by the genes in each chromosome. These traits are classified according to whether they are dominant (strong) or recessive (weak) and

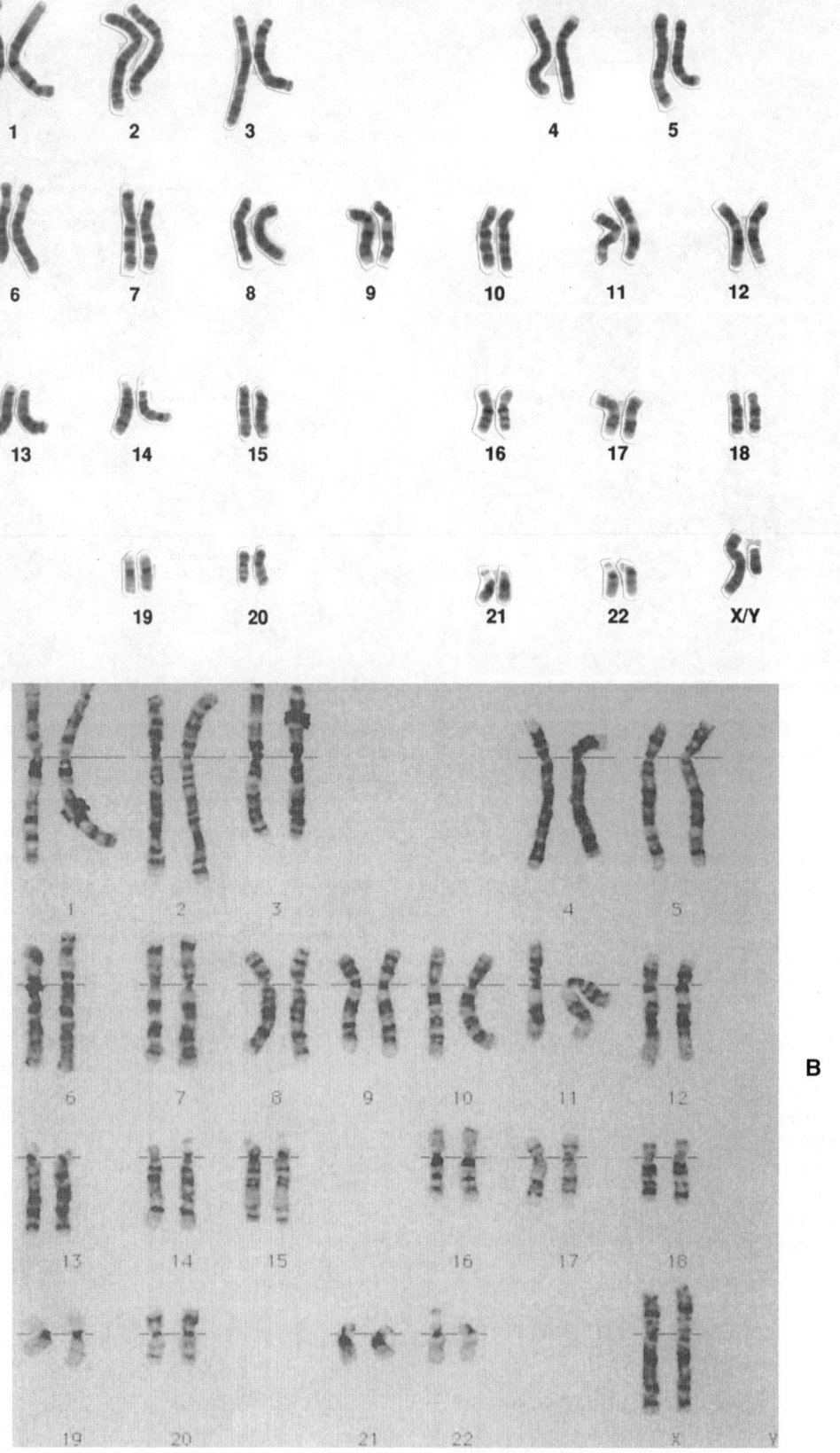

Figure 9-3 Karyotypes of chromosomes that were stained, creating bands to distinguish each chromosome and identify missing or duplicated chromosome material. *A,* Normal male karyotype: 46,XY. *B,* Normal female karyotype: 46,XX. (*A* from National Human Genome Research Institute. [2002]. *Fact sheet: Karyotype.* Retrieved July 19, 2003, from www.genome.gov; *B* from Jorde, L.B., Carey, J.C., Bamshad, M.J., & White, R.L. [2003]. *Medical genetics* [3rd ed., p. 108]. St. Louis, Mosby.)

whether the gene is located on one of the autosome pairs or on the sex chromosomes. Both normal and abnormal hereditary characteristics are transmitted by these mechanisms.

Alleles

Because humans have a pair of matched chromosomes (except the sex chromosomes in the male), they have one allele for a gene at the same location on each member of the chromosome pair. The paired alleles may be identical (homozygous) or different (heterozygous).

Some alleles, both normal and abnormal, occur more frequently in certain groups than they do in the population as a whole. For example, the gene that causes Tay-Sachs disease is carried by about 1 of every 27 Ashkenazi Jews, whose families have their roots in Eastern Europe. Some non-Jewish French-Canadians and Cajun people from Louisiana also have a higher incidence of the disorder. However, an estimated 1 of every 250 people outside this group, including non-Ashkenazi Jews, carries the gene (National Tay-Sachs and Allied Diseases Association, Inc., 2003). Other disorders that are prevalent in certain ethnic groups are cystic fibrosis (primarily whites of northern European descent) and sickle cell disease (primarily people of African, Mediterranean, Indian, or Middle Eastern descent).

A new trait (harmful, neutral, or sometimes beneficial) may emerge because of a change in the gene within the gamete. The DNA in the gamete is then different from that in the person's somatic cells. The offspring who receives the new version of the gene will have it in all somatic cells and can transmit it to future generations.

Dominance

Dominance describes how one's genetic composition is translated into the phenotype, or observable characteristics. In the case of a dominant gene, one copy is enough to cause the trait to be expressed. For example, in the ABO blood system, genes for type A and type B are dominant. Therefore a single copy of either of these genes is enough to be expressed in the person's blood type.

Two identical copies of a recessive gene are required for the trait to be expressed. The gene for blood group O is recessive. Only if a person receives a gene for blood group O from both parents will laboratory testing identify his or her blood group as O. If the person receives a gene for group O from one parent and group A from the other parent, group A will be expressed in laboratory blood typing.

Other alleles are equally dominant. The person who receives a gene for blood group A from one parent and group B from the other will have type AB blood because both alleles are equally dominant and both are expressed in blood typing.

Dominance and recessiveness are not absolute for all genes. Some people with a single copy of an abnormal recessive gene (carriers) may have a slightly abnormal level of the gene product (e.g., an enzyme) that can be detected by laboratory methods. These people usually do not have the disease because the normal copy of the gene directs production of enough of the required product to allow normal or near-normal function.

Chromosome Location

Genes located on autosomes are either autosomal dominant or autosomal recessive, depending on the number of identical copies of the gene needed to produce the trait. However, genes located on the X chromosome are paired only in fe-

males because males have one X and one Y chromosome.

A female with an abnormal recessive gene on one of her X chromosomes usually has a normal gene on the other X chromosome that compensates and maintains relatively normal function. However, the male is at a disadvantage if his only X chromosome has an abnormal gene. The male has no compensating normal gene because his other sex chromosome is a Y. The abnormal gene will be expressed in the male because it is unopposed by a normal gene.

Patterns of Single-Gene Inheritance

Three important patterns of single-gene inheritance are (1) autosomal dominant, (2) autosomal recessive, and (3) X-linked. Table 9-1 summarizes characteristics and transmission of each pattern. The inheritance patterns are graphically illustrated with a genogram, or pedigree, to represent a family's history and the relationships among family members.

The nurse may need to interpret the genogram for the client. For example, when taking a genetic family history, the nurse might say, "I'm going to use several symbols to depict your family tree and its members' health histories. This diagram is often called a *genogram* or a *pedigree*."

Single-gene traits have mathematically predictable and fixed rates of occurrence. For example, if a couple has a child with an autosomal recessive disorder, the risk that future children from the same couple will have the disorder is one in four (25%) at every conception. The *risk* for the disorder is the same at every conception, regardless of how many of the couple's children are or are not affected.

Autosomal Dominant Traits

An autosomal dominant trait is produced by a dominant gene on a non-sex chromosome. The expression of abnormal autosomal dominant genes may result in multiple and seemingly unrelated effects in the person. The gene's effects may vary substantially in severity, leading a family to think that a trait skips a generation. A careful physical examination may reveal subtle evidence of the trait in each generation. Some people may carry the dominant gene but may have no apparent expression of it in their physical makeup.

! CRITICAL TO REMEMBER

Single-Gene Abnormalities

- A person affected with an autosomal dominant disorder has a 50% chance of transmitting the disorder to each of his or her children.
- Two healthy parents who carry the same abnormal autosomal recessive gene have a 25% chance of having a child affected with the disorder caused by this gene.
- Parental consanguinity increases the risk for having a child with an autosomal recessive disorder.
- One copy of an abnormal X-linked recessive gene is enough to produce the disorder in a male.
- Abnormal genes can arise as new mutations that are then transmitted to future generations.

TABLE 9-1 Single-Gene Traits

GENOGRAM (PEDIGREE) SYMBOLS

A genogram symbolically represents a family's medical history and the relationships of its members to one another. It helps identify patterns of inheritance that may help distinguish one type of disorder from another.

☐ Male

○ Female

◇ Sex not specified
(number indicates the number of persons represented by the symbol)

■ ● Affected

◧ ◑ Carriers (heterozygous) for an autosomal recessive trait

⊙ Female carrier of an X-linked recessive trait

⊘ Deceased

☐—○ Mating/marriage

☐═○ Consanguineous mating/marriage

I   Roman numerals indicate generations

AUTOSOMAL RECESSIVE

Characteristics

Two autosomal recessive genes are required to produce the trait.
Males and females are equally likely to have the trait.
There is often no prior family history of the disorder before the first affected child.
If more than one family member is affected, they are usually full siblings.
Consanguinity (close blood relationship) of the parents increases the risk for the disorder.
Disorders are more likely to occur in groups isolated by geography, culture, religion, or other factors.
Some autosomal recessive disorders are more common in specific ethnic groups.

Transmission of Trait from Parent to Child

Unaffected parents are carriers of the abnormal autosomal recessive trait.
Children of carriers have a 25% (1 in 4) chance for receiving both copies of the defective gene and thus having the disorder.
Children of carriers have a 50% (1 in 2) chance of receiving one copy of the gene and being carriers like the parents.
Children of carriers have a 25% (1 in 4) chance of receiving both copies of the normal gene. They are neither carriers nor affected.

Examples

Normal traits: Blood group O; Rh-negative blood factor.
Abnormal traits: Tay-Sachs disease; sickle cell disease; cystic fibrosis.

Genogram

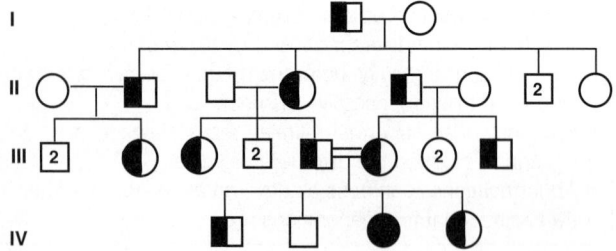

AUTOSOMAL DOMINANT

Characteristics

A single copy of the gene is enough to produce the trait.
Males and females are equally likely to have the trait.
Often appears in every generation of a family, although family members having the trait may have widely varying manifestations of it.
May have multiple and seemingly unrelated effects on body structure and function.

Transmission of Trait from Parent to Child

A parent with the trait has a 50% (1 in 2) chance of passing the trait to the child.
The trait may arise as a new mutation from an unaffected parent. The child who receives the mutated gene can then transmit it to future generations.

Examples

Normal traits: Blood groups A and B; Rh-positive blood factor.
Abnormal traits: Huntington's disease; neurofibromatosis.

Genogram

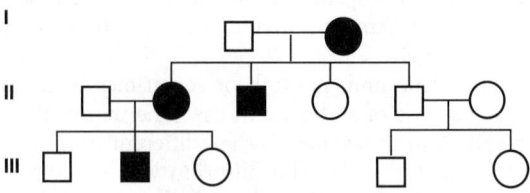

X-LINKED RECESSIVE

Characteristics

Although recessive, only one copy of the gene is needed to cause the disorder in the male, who does not have a compensating X without the trait.
Males are affected, with rare exceptions.
Females are carriers of the trait but not usually adversely affected.
Affected males are related to one another through carrier females.
Affected males do not transmit the trait to their sons.

Transmission of Trait from Parent to Child

Males who have the disorder transmit the gene to 100% of their daughters and none of their sons.
Sons of carrier females have a 50% (1 in 2) chance of being affected. They also have a 50% chance of being unaffected.
Daughters of carrier females have a 50% (1 in 2) chance of being carriers like their mothers. They also have a 50% chance of being neither affected nor carriers.
A new X-linked recessive gene also may arise by mutation.

Examples

Colorblindness; Duchene muscular dystrophy; hemophilia A.

Genogram

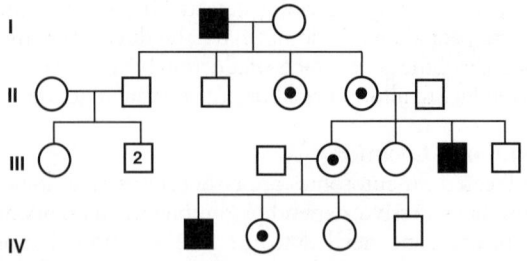

In some autosomal dominant disorders, such as Huntington's disease, the person having the gene will always have the disease if he or she lives long enough. In other disorders, only a portion of those carrying the gene will ever exhibit the disease.

New mutations often account for the introduction of autosomal dominant traits into a family that has no prior history. Men who father children in their fifth decade or later are more likely to have offspring with a new autosomal dominant mutation.

The person who is affected with an autosomal dominant disorder is usually heterozygous for the gene—that is, the person has a normal gene on one chromosome and an abnormal gene on the other chromosome of the pair that overrides the influence of the normal gene. Occasionally, a person receives two copies of the same abnormal autosomal dominant gene. Such an individual is usually much more severely affected than someone with only one copy.

Autosomal Recessive Traits

An autosomal recessive trait occurs when a person receives two copies of a recessive gene carried on an autosome. Most people carry a few abnormal autosomal recessive genes without problems because a compensating normal gene produces enough of the gene's product for normal function. Because the probability that two unrelated people will share even one of the same abnormal genes is low, the incidence of autosomal recessive diseases is relatively low in the general population.

Situations that increase the likelihood that two parents will share the same abnormal autosomal recessive gene are:

- Consanguinity (blood relationship of the parents)
- Membership in groups that are isolated by culture, geography, religion, or other factors

Many autosomal recessive disorders are severe, and affected persons may not live long enough to reproduce. Two exceptions are phenylketonuria and cystic fibrosis. Improved care of people with these disorders has allowed them to live into their reproductive years. If one member of the couple has the autosomal recessive disorder, all of their children will be carriers. Their risk for having similarly affected children is higher as well, depending on the prevalence of the abnormal gene in the general population.

X-Linked Traits

X-linked Recessive Disorders. X-linked recessive traits are more common than X-linked dominant ones. Sex differences in the occurrence of X-linked recessive traits and the relationship of affected males to one another distinguish these disorders from autosomal dominant or recessive disorders. Males usually show full effects of an X-linked recessive disorder because their only X chromosome has the abnormal gene on it. Females can show the full disorder in two uncommon circumstances:

- When a female has a single X chromosome (Turner's syndrome, p. 174)
- When a female child is born to an affected father and a carrier mother.

X-linked recessive disorders can be relatively mild, such as colorblindness, or they may be severe, such as hemophilia. Also, those having the disorder may be affected with varying degrees of severity.

Chromosomal Abnormalities

Chromosomal abnormalities can be numerical or structural. They are quite common (50% or more) in the embryo or fetus that is spontaneously aborted. Chromosomal abnormalities often cause major defects because they involve many added or missing genes.

Numerical Abnormalities

Numerical chromosomal abnormalities are those involving added or missing single chromosomes and those with multiple sets of chromosomes. Trisomy and monosomy are numerical abnormalities of single chromosomes. *Polyploidy* describes abnormalities involving entire sets of chromosomes.

Trisomy. A trisomy exists when each body cell contains an extra copy of one chromosome, bringing the total number to 47 (Fig. 9-4). Each chromosome is normal, but there is an extra one in every cell. The most common trisomy is *Down syndrome,* or trisomy 21. In Down syndrome, each body cell has three copies of chromosome 21. Trisomies of chromosomes 13 and 18 are less common and have more severe effects. The incidence of trisomies increases with maternal age, so that most women who are 35 years old or older at conception are offered prenatal diagnosis to determine whether the fetus has Down syndrome or another trisomy (see Chapter 16).

Infants with Down syndrome have characteristic features that are apparent shortly after birth. Chromosomal analysis is done during the neonatal period if the trisomy was not expected to confirm the diagnosis and to determine whether Down syndrome is caused by trisomy 21 or a rarer chromosomal anomaly that involves a structural rather than a numerical addition of chromosome 21 material.

Monosomy. A monosomy occurs when each body cell has a missing chromosome, with a total number of 45. The only monosomy that is compatible with extended postnatal life is *Turner's syndrome,* or monosomy X (Fig. 9-5). People with Turner's syndrome have a single X chromosome and are female.

Liveborn infants with Turner's syndrome have excess skin around the neck and edema that is most noticeable in the hands and feet. If Turner's syndrome is not identified and treated during infancy or childhood, an affected girl will remain very short and will not have menstrual periods or develop secondary sex characteristics. Heart and aortic defects are common. Severe defects are surgically repaired. Children with Turner's syndrome usually have normal intelligence,

---

⚠ CRITICAL TO REMEMBER

Chromosome Abnormalities
Chromosome abnormalities are either numerical or structural.

Numerical
- Entire single chromosome added (trisomy)
- Entire single chromosome missing (monosomy)
- One or more added sets of chromosomes (polyploidy)

Structural
- Part of a chromosome missing or added
- Rearrangements of material within chromosome(s)
- Two chromosomes that adhere to each other
- Fragility of a specific site on the X chromosome

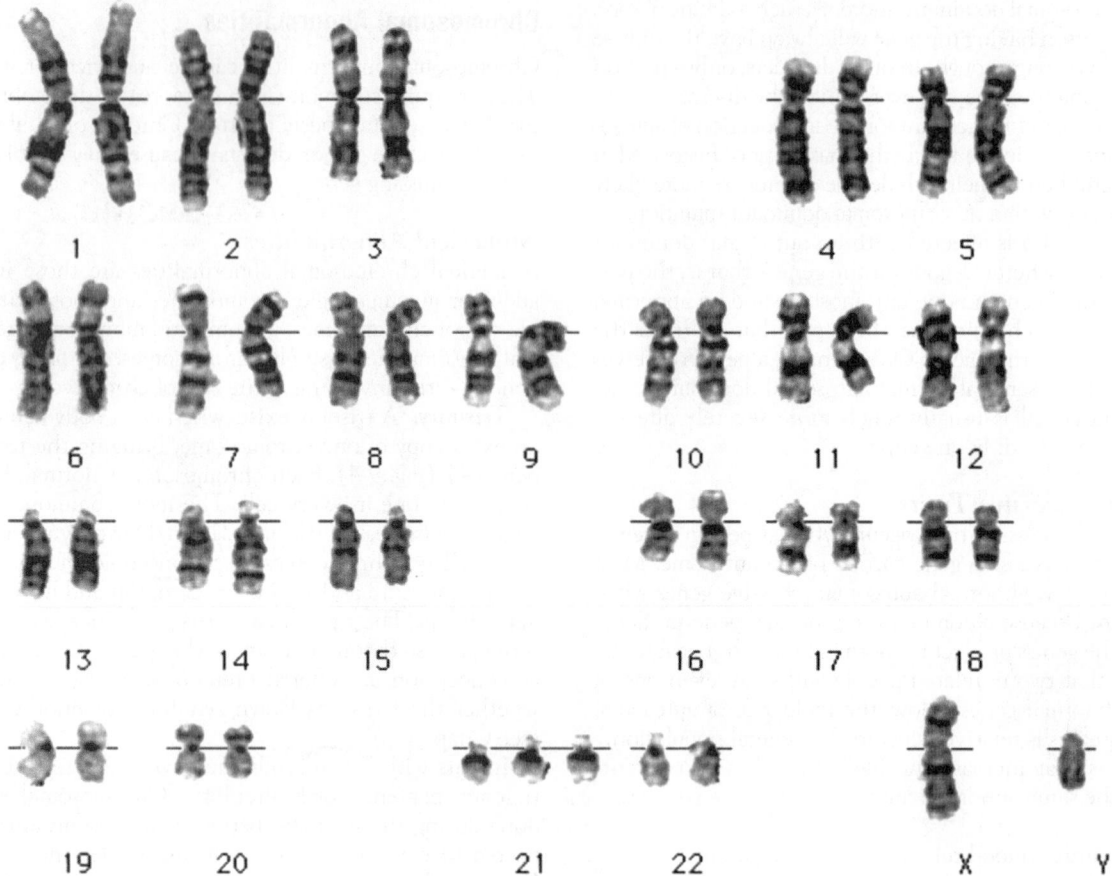

Figure 9-4 Karyotype of a male with trisomy 21 (Down syndrome: 47,XY, +21). (From Jorde, L.B., Carey, J.C., Bamshad, M.J., & White, R.L. [2003]. *Medical genetics* [3rd ed., p. 114]. St. Louis, Mosby.)

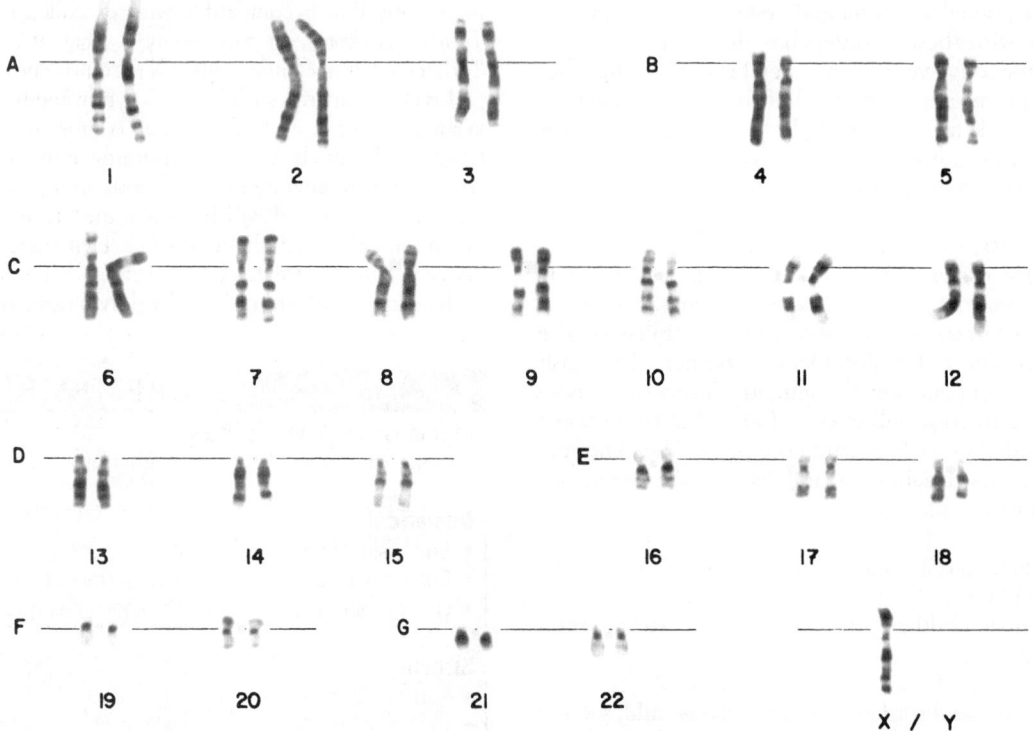

Figure 9-5 Karyotype of a female with monosomy X (Turner's syndrome: 45,X). (Courtesy Dr. Mary Jo Harrod, University of Texas Southwestern Medical Center.)

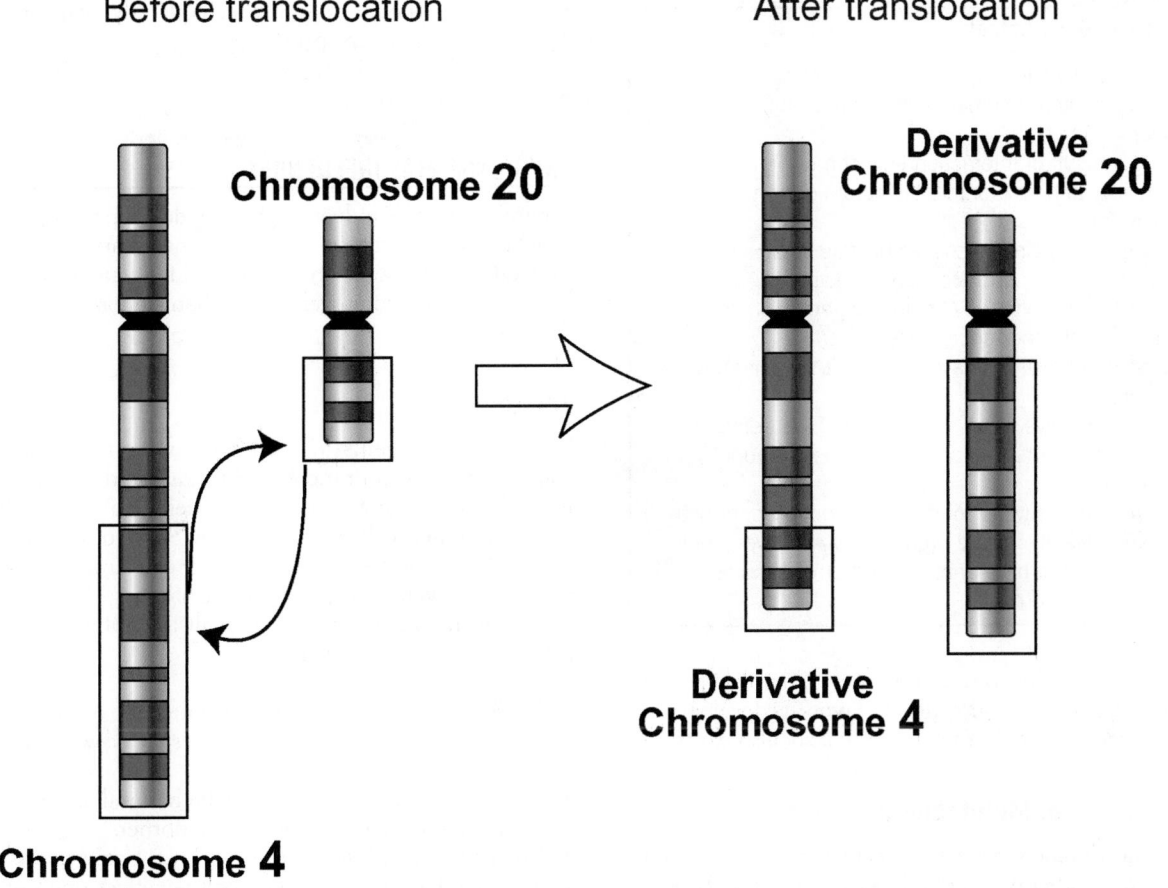

Figure 9-6 Illustration of a translocation of chromosome material between chromosomes 4 and 20. (From National Human Genome Research Institute. [2003]. *Fact sheet: Translocation.* Retrieved July 19, 2003, from www.genome.gov/glossary).

although they may have difficulty with spatial relationships or solving visual problems, such as reading a map.

Polyploidy. Polyploidy occurs when gametes do not halve their chromosome number during meiosis and retain both members of the pair or when two sperm fertilize an ovum simultaneously. The result is an embryo with one or more extra sets of chromosomes. The total number of chromosomes is a multiple of the haploid number of 23 (69 or 92 total chromosomes). Polyploidy usually results in an early spontaneous abortion but is occasionally seen in a liveborn infant.

Structural Abnormalities

The structure of one or more chromosomes may be abnormal. Part of a chromosome may be missing or added, or DNA within the chromosome may be rearranged. Some of these rearrangements are harmless polymorphisms. Others are harmful, however, because important genetic material is lost or duplicated in the structural abnormality or the position of the genes in relation to other genes is altered so that normal function is not possible.

Another structural abnormality occurs when all or part of a chromosome is attached to another (translocation). Many people with a translocation chromosomal abnormality are clinically normal because the total of their genetic material is normal, or balanced (Fig. 9-6). If a parent has a balanced translocation, the offspring may have normal chromosomes or may have a balanced translocation like the parent. However, the offspring may receive too much or too little chromosomal material at conception and may be spontaneously aborted or may have birth defects. Either balanced or unbalanced chromosomal translocations may occur spontaneously in the child of parents who have no translocation.

Fragile X syndrome is a structural chromosome abnormality that often causes mental retardation among males. With this abnormality, a site on the X chromosome is more fragile than normal. Although females can also be affected with fragile X syndrome, males are more severely affected because the female has a second X chromosome that is usually normal. The fragile X syndrome is inherited in an X-linked dominant pattern, with males being most severely affected (Jorde, Carey, Bamshad, & White, 2003).

MULTIFACTORIAL DISORDERS

Multifactorial disorders result from an interaction of genetic and environmental factors. The genetic tendency toward the disorder is modified by the environment. These interactions may influence prenatal and postnatal development either positively or negatively. For example, two embryos may have an equal genetic susceptibility for the development of a disorder

> **⚠ CRITICAL TO REMEMBER**
>
> **Multifactorial Birth Defects**
>
> - Multifactorial defects are some of the most common birth defects encountered in maternity and pediatric nursing practice.
> - They are a result of interaction between one's genetic susceptibility and environmental factors during prenatal development.
> - These are usually single, isolated defects, although the primary defect may cause secondary defects.
> - Some occur more often in certain geographic areas.
> - A greater risk of occurrence exists if
>   Several close relatives have the defect, whether mild or severe.
>   One close relative has a severe form of the defect.
>   The defect occurs in a child of the less frequently affected sex.
> - Infants who have several major or minor defects, or both, that are not directly related probably *do not* have a multifactorial defect but have another syndrome, such as a chromosomal abnormality.

such as spina bifida (open spine). However, the disorder will not occur unless an environment that favors its development, such as deficient maternal intake of folic acid, also exists.

Characteristics of Multifactorial Disorders

Multifactorial disorders have two characteristics that distinguish them from other types of birth defects. They are typically (1) present and detectable at birth and (2) isolated defects rather than ones that occur with other unrelated abnormalities.

A multifactorial defect may *cause* a secondary defect, however. For example, infants with spina bifida often have hydrocephalus because abnormal development of the spine and spinal cord disrupts spinal fluid circulation, allowing it to build up within the brain's ventricular system.

The infant who has spina bifida plus one or more defects that are not associated with disrupted central nervous system development probably does *not* have a multifactorial disorder. In this case, the spina bifida is more likely to be part of a syndrome that may pose a much different risk for recurrence in the parents' future children.

Multifactorial disorders represent some of the most common birth defects that a maternal-child nurse encounters. Examples include:

- Many heart defects
- Neural tube defects such as anencephaly (absence of most of the brain and skull) and spina bifida
- Cleft lip and cleft palate
- Pyloric stenosis

Risk for Occurrence

Unlike single-gene traits, multifactorial disorders are not associated with a fixed risk of occurrence or recurrence in a family. The risks are an average rather than a constant percentage. Factors that may affect the degree of risk are:

- Number of affected close relatives
- Severity of the disorder in affected family members
- Sex of affected person(s)
- Geographic location
- Seasonal variations

ENVIRONMENTAL INFLUENCES

Environment may influence prenatal development positively, as when good nutrition supplies all necessary raw materials for fetal growth. Some environmental influences are harmful, however, such as teratogens or mechanical forces that disrupt development.

Teratogens

Teratogens are agents in the fetal environment that either cause a birth defect or increase the likelihood that a birth defect will occur. People often ask whether a certain drug or other substance will harm the baby. Some drugs have been definitely established as either safe or harmful. For most agents, however, their potential for harming the fetus is not clear. Several factors make it difficult to establish the teratogenic potential of an agent:

- *Retrospective study.* Investigators must rely on the mother's memory about substances she ingested or was exposed to during pregnancy.
- *Timing of exposure.* Agents may be harmful at one stage of prenatal development but not at another.
- *Different susceptibility of organ systems.* Some agents affect only one fetal organ system, or they affect one system at one stage of prenatal development and another system if exposure occurs at a different stage of development.
- *Noncontrolled fetal exposure.* Exposures cannot be controlled to eliminate extraneous agents or to ensure a consistent dose.
- *Placental transfer.* Agents vary in their ability to cross the placenta.
- *Individual variations.* Fetuses show varying susceptibility to harmful agents.
- *Nontransferability of animal studies.* Results of animal studies cannot always be applied to humans.
- *Risk for damage from an uncontrolled maternal disorder.* Some maternal disorders, such as epilepsy or hypertension, may themselves cause fetal damage if not controlled, raising a question about whether the medication or the disorder caused the damage.

Teratogens typically cause more than one defect, which distinguishes teratogenic defects from multifactorial disorders. Children affected by single-gene and chromosome defects, however, are also likely to have multiple defects, often making diagnosis difficult.

Hundreds of individual agents are either known or suspected teratogens. Types of teratogens include:

- Maternal infectious agents (viruses or bacteria) that cross the placenta and damage the embryo or fetus
- Drugs and other substances used by the woman (therapeutic agents, illicit drugs, botanical preparations, tobacco, alcohol)

- Pollutants, chemicals, or other substances to which the mother is exposed in her daily life
- Ionizing radiation
- Maternal hyperthermia
- Effects of maternal disorders, such as diabetes mellitus or phenylketonuria

It is theoretically possible to eliminate all or some of the risk to the developing fetus by avoiding exposure to the agent or changing the fetal environment in some way.

Avoiding Fetal Exposure

Ideally, avoiding exposure to harmful influences begins before conception because major organ systems develop early in pregnancy, often before a woman realizes she is pregnant. To avoid some agents, such as alcohol or illicit drugs, pregnant women must be committed to make substantial lifestyle changes (Box 9-1).

Infections. Rubella immunization at least 3 months before pregnancy virtually eliminates the risk that the mother will contract this infection, which can damage the fetus severely. For infections that cannot be prevented by immunization, the nurse can counsel the woman to avoid situations in which acquiring the disease is more likely.

Drugs and Other Substances. The U.S. Food and Drug Administration has established pregnancy categories for therapeutic drugs based on their potential to harm the fetus. The categories range from A through D, and X. Class A drugs have no demonstrated fetal risk in well-controlled studies. At the opposite end, pregnancy category X drugs are well established as being harmful. For about 80% of therapeutic drugs, it is unknown whether they are definitely safe or definitely unsafe. (See Appendix B for a list of common drugs and other substances that may affect the fetus adversely.) In deciding whether to prescribe a drug, the physician must often balance the woman's need for the drug's therapeutic effects against the fetal need to avoid exposure to it. In addition, stopping a therapeutic drug may result in the mother's disease being uncontrolled, such as reappearance of seizures or hypertension, which adversely affects the fetus.

It is especially difficult to establish whether an illicit drug can cause prenatal damage, because women who abuse substances often have other problems that complicate analysis of fetal effects. For example, these women may use multiple drugs and often have poor nutrition, untreated diseases, inadequate prenatal care, and a stressful life. In addition, illicit drugs are unlikely to be pure, and the substances used to dilute them may themselves be harmful.

The best action is for the woman to eliminate use of nontherapeutic drugs and substances such as alcohol. If she takes therapeutic drugs, the physician may be able to prescribe an alternative drug with a lower risk to the fetus or may temporarily eliminate some therapeutic drugs when possible.

Ionizing Radiation. Nonurgent radiologic procedures may be done during the first 2 weeks after the menstrual period begins. This is usually before ovulation and thus before conception is possible. For urgent procedures, the lower abdomen should be shielded with a lead apron, if possible. The radiation dose is kept as low as possible to reduce fetal exposure.

BOX 9-1
Selected Environmental Substances Known or Thought to Harm the Fetus

- Alcohol
- Aminoglycosides
- Antineoplastic agents
- Antithyroid drugs
- Cocaine
- Diethylstilbestrol
- Diphenylhydantoin (phenytoin)
- Folic acid antagonists
- Infections
  Cytomegalovirus
  Herpes simplex virus
  Human immunodeficiency virus
  Rubella
  Syphilis
  Toxoplasmosis
  Varicella
- Lithium
- Mercury
- Retinoic acid
- Tetracycline
- Tobacco
- Trimethadione
- Valproic acid
- Warfarin

Maternal Hyperthermia. The mother's temperature may rise unavoidably during illness. However, pregnant women should be cautioned to avoid or limit exposure to heat such as saunas or hot tubs.

Manipulating the Fetal Environment

Appropriate medical therapy can help a woman avoid fetal damage that could result from her illness. For example, a woman who has diabetes should try to keep her blood glucose levels normal and stable before and during pregnancy for the best possible fetal outcomes. A woman with phenylketonuria should closely adhere to a low-phenylalanine diet before conception to avoid buildup of toxic metabolic products in her body that may damage the fetus.

Occasionally, a pregnant woman is given a drug for fetal therapy—for example, digoxin or propranolol for fetal cardiac dysrhythmias. In these cases, it is the fetus who has the disorder, not the mother. The mother is the conduit for medicating the fetus to allow normal development and function.

Mechanical Disruptions to Fetal Development

Mechanical forces that interfere with normal prenatal development include oligohydramnios and fibrous amniotic bands.

Oligohydramnios, an abnormally small volume of amniotic fluid, reduces the cushion surrounding the fetus and may result in deformations such as clubfoot. Prolonged oligohydramnios interferes with fetal lung development because it does not allow normal development of the alveoli. Oligohydramnios may not be the primary fetal problem but rather may be related to other fetal anomalies.

Fibrous amniotic bands may result from tears in the inner sac (amnion) of the fetal membranes and can result in fetal deformations or intrauterine limb amputation. Fibrous bands are usually sporadic and unlikely to recur. Because these bands can cause multiple defects, they may be confused with birth defects from other causes such as chromosome or single-gene abnormalities.

GENETIC COUNSELING

Genetic counseling provides services to help people understand the disorder about which they are concerned and the risk that it will occur in their family.

Availability

Genetic counseling is often available through facilities that provide maternal-fetal medicine services. State departments of mental health and mental retardation or rehabilitation services also may provide counseling services. Local chapters of the March of Dimes are an important source of information about birth defects and counseling sites. Fact sheets and other information about birth defects and their prevention are available on-line from the March of Dimes (www.modimes.org). Organizations that focus on specific birth defects provide

valuable support and assistance in obtaining needed services for individuals and families affected by that disorder.

Focus on the Family

Genetic counseling focuses on the family rather than on an individual. One family member may have a birth defect, but study of the entire family is often needed for accurate counseling. This may involve obtaining medical records or performing physical examinations or laboratory studies on numerous family members. Counseling is impaired if family members are unwilling to provide their medical records or agree to examinations or laboratory studies. Moreover, those who seek counseling may be unwilling to request cooperation from other family members or to share genetic information they acquire.

Process of Genetic Counseling

Genetic counseling is often a slow process that is not always straightforward. Several visits spread over months may be needed. In addition, some tests may be performed at only one or a few laboratories in the world, and several weeks may be needed to complete them. Despite a comprehensive evaluation, a diagnosis may never be established. An accurate diagnosis is crucial to provide families with the best information about the risks for a specific birth defect, the prognosis for one affected, and options available to avoid or manage the disorder. Advances in knowledge about birth defects may allow a definite diagnosis later, and families are encouraged to contact the center for updates. Box 9-2 lists examples of procedures that may be used before conception, prenatally, and after birth to establish an accurate diagnosis related to birth defects.

A genetic evaluation may include many factors, such as:

- A complete medical history, including prenatal and perinatal history
- The medical history of other family members
- Laboratory, imaging, or other diagnostic studies
- Physical assessment of a child with the birth defect and other family members as needed
- Examination of photographs, particularly for family members who are deceased or unavailable
- Construction of a genogram, or pedigree, to identify relationships among family members and their relevant medical history

If a diagnosis is established, genetic counseling educates the family about:

- What is known about the cause of the disorder
- The natural course of the disorder
- Options for care of an affected person
- The likelihood that the disorder will occur or recur
- The availability of prenatal diagnosis for the disorder
- How a couple may be able to avoid having an affected child
- The availability of treatment and services for the person with the disorder

Genetic counseling is nondirective; that is, the counselor does not tell the individual or parents what decision to make but educates them about options for dealing with the disor-

---

BOX 9-2
Diagnostic Methods That May Be Used in Genetic Counseling

Preconception Screening
Family history to identify hereditary patterns of disease or birth defects
Examination of family photographs
Physical examination for obvious or subtle signs of birth defects
Carrier testing
Persons from ethnic groups with a higher incidence of some disorders
Persons with a family history suggesting that they may carry a gene for a specific disorder
Chromosomal analysis
Deoxyribonucleic acid (DNA) analysis

Prenatal Diagnosis for Fetal Abnormalities
Maternal tests to screen for abnormalities
Chorionic villus sampling
Amniocentesis
Ultrasonography
Percutaneous umbilical blood sampling

Postnatal Diagnosis for an Infant With a Birth Defect
Physical examination and measurements
Imaging procedures (ultrasonography, radiography, echocardiography)
Chromosomal analysis
DNA analysis
Tests for metabolic disorders (phenylketonuria, cystic fibrosis)
Hemoglobin analysis for disorders such as sickle cell disease
Immunologic testing for infections
Autopsy

der. Families often interpret the counseling subjectively, however. Some parents may regard a 50% risk of occurrence or recurrence as low, whereas others may think that a 1% risk is unacceptably high. The family's values and beliefs also influence whether they seek counseling and what they do with the information that is provided.

Supplemental Services

Comprehensive genetic counseling includes services of professionals from many disciplines, such as biology, medicine, nursing, social work, and education. These professionals provide added support for families; they may offer referral to parent support groups, grief counseling, and intervention for problems that accompany the birth of a child with a birth defect, such as socioeconomic or family dysfunction.

NURSING CARE OF FAMILIES CONCERNED ABOUT BIRTH DEFECTS

Nurses have an important role in helping families who are concerned about birth defects. Some nurses work directly with family members who are undergoing genetic counseling. Many more nurses are generalists who bring their knowledge about birth defects and their prevention to those they encounter in everyday practice.

Nurses as Part of a Genetic Counseling Team

Genetic nursing may include:

- Providing counseling (after having additional education)
- Guiding a woman or couple through prenatal diagnosis
- Supporting parents as they make decisions after receiving abnormal prenatal diagnostic results
- Helping the family deal with the emotional impact of a birth defect
- Assisting parents who have had a child with a birth defect locate needed services and support
- Coordinating services of other professionals, such as social workers, physical and occupational therapists, psychologists, and dietitians
- Helping families find appropriate support groups to help them cope with the daily stresses associated with a child who has a birth defect

Nurses in General Practice

Nurses who work in women's health care and those who work in antepartum, intrapartum, newborn, or pediatric settings often encounter families who are concerned about birth defects. These families may include a member who has a birth defect. Other families may believe that they have an increased risk for having a child with a birth defect. Generalist

---

PARENTS
Want to Know

About Birth Defects

How can this birth defect be genetic? No one else in our family has ever had anything like it.
Autosomal recessive disorders are carried by parents who themselves are unaffected. The abnormal gene may have been passed down through many generations, but there is no risk for an affected child until *two* carrier *parents* mate.

Isn't there only a one-in-a-million chance that this birth defect will happen to another of our children?
Autosomal recessive disorders have a 25% (1 in 4) chance of recurring in children of the same parents. Autosomal dominant disorders may pose a 50% risk for recurrence unless they resulted from a new mutation in the egg or sperm that created the baby.

Isn't this birth defect very likely to recur? We'd better not have any more children.
Some birth defects are associated with a relatively high risk of recurrence; others have a relatively low risk. How high a risk is perceived also varies among people. Prenatal diagnosis may offer parents a way to avoid having an affected child, or some disorders may be treated before birth.

Since we've already had a child with this birth defect (an autosomal recessive one), will the next three be normal?
If both parents are carriers for an autosomal recessive disorder, there is a 25% (1 in 4) risk for the birth defect to occur that is constant with *each* child conceived. The chance is the same (1 in 4) that each child will not receive the gene from either parent and will be neither affected nor a carrier for the gene.

If I have an amniocentesis or other prenatal diagnostic test, can the test detect all birth defects?
Although many disorders can be prenatally diagnosed, not all can be diagnosed in the same fetus. Testing is offered for one or more specific disorders after a careful family history is taken to determine appropriate tests.

If the prenatal test is normal, will my baby be normal?
Normal results from prenatal testing exclude those disorders that were specifically tested for with varying accuracy. Every healthy couple has about a 5% risk of having a child with a birth defect, some of which are not obvious at birth. This baseline risk remains even if all prenatal test results are normal.

Will I have to have an abortion if my prenatal tests show that my baby is abnormal?
Abortion may be an option for parents whose fetus is affected with a birth defect, but most parents are reassured by normal test results. If results are abnormal, some parents appreciate the time to prepare for a child with special needs. Better medical management can be planned for a newborn who is expected to have problems. Prenatal diagnosis gives many parents the confidence to have children despite their increased risk for having a child with a birth defect.

BOX 9-3
Reasons for Referral to a Genetic Counselor

- Pregnant women who will be 35 years of age or older when the infant is born
- Men who father children after age 40
- Members of a group with an increased incidence of a specific disorder
- Carriers of autosomal recessive disorders
- Women who are carriers of X-linked disorders
- Couples closely related by blood (consanguineous relationship)
- Family history of birth defect or mental retardation
- Family history of unexplained stillbirth
- Women who experience multiple spontaneous abortions
- Pregnant women exposed to known or suspected teratogens or other harmful agents, either before or during pregnancy
- Pregnant women with abnormal prenatal screening results, such as triple screen or suspicious ultrasound findings

---

BOX 9-4
Problems Encountered in Genetic Counseling and Prenatal Diagnosis

- Inadequate medical records
  - Family members' refusal to share information
  - Records that are incomplete, vague, or uninformative
- Inconclusive testing
  - Too few family members available when family studies are needed
  - Inadequate number of live fetal cells obtained during amniocentesis or chorionic villus sampling
  - Failure of cells for chromosome analysis to grow in culture
  - Ambiguous prenatal test results that are neither clearly normal nor clearly abnormal
- Unexpected results from prenatal diagnosis
  - Finding an abnormality other than the one tested for
  - Nonpaternity revealed
- Inability to determine the severity of a prenatally diagnosed disorder
- Inability to rule out all birth defects

---

nurses provide care and support that complements those of nurses who work on a genetic counseling team.

Women's Health Nurses

The ideal time to provide counseling is before conception so the childbearing couple has more options if problems are identified. As in antepartum care, the primary nursing role is to identify families who might benefit from counseling before conception. Personal and family histories are commonly taken at primary health care visits, and the nurse may identify a history that could affect a future child that the couple might conceive.

Antepartum Nurses

During the initial antepartum interview, the nurse may identify the pregnant woman or family who may benefit from genetic counseling. The antepartum nurse also assists families with decision making, teaching, and emotional support.

Identifying Families for Referral. Nurses in antepartum settings often identify a woman or family who is appropriately referred for genetic counseling. The personal and family history of the woman and her partner may reveal factors that increase their risks for having a child with a birth defect. In addition to the usual medical history about disorders such as hypertension or diabetes, the woman should be questioned about a family history of birth defects, diseases that seem to "run in the family," mental retardation, or developmental delay.

Some people are reluctant to disclose that they have a family member with mental retardation or a birth defect. The nurse can gently probe for sensitive information by asking questions about whether there are family members who have learning problems or who are "slow." Using words that are lay-oriented often elicits more information than using clinical terms that may seem harsh.

Helping the Family Decide About Genetic Counseling.
If genetic counseling is appropriate, the physician usually discusses it with the woman and offers to refer her and her part-

ner to an appropriate center. The final decision, however, rests with the couple. The nurse can help the family decide whether they want genetic counseling at all and weigh issues that are important to them.

Genetic counseling can raise issues that are uncomfortable, such as whether to undergo prenatal diagnosis, what to do if a condition cannot be prenatally diagnosed, and what options are acceptable if prenatal diagnosis shows abnormal results. Counseling may open family conflicts if information from other family members is needed or if family values differ on issues such as abortion of an abnormal fetus. In addition, the tests can show unexpected results (Boxes 9-3 and 9-4). The nurse must be careful not to allow personal values to influence the family's decision. It is the family members who must live with the decision they make.

Teaching About Lifestyle. Nurses can teach a pregnant woman about harmful factors in her lifestyle that can be modified to reduce the risk of defects to her offspring. The nurse can support the woman in making lifestyle changes that may be difficult, such as stopping alcohol consumption, reducing or eliminating smoking, or improving her diet. Liberal praise can motivate a woman to continue her efforts to promote an optimal outcome. A negative attitude from nurses or other professionals may make her feel like a failure, and she may abandon her efforts to create a healthier lifestyle.

Providing Emotional Support. The time between prenatal testing and results sometimes spans several difficult weeks. In the meantime, the pregnancy is becoming more obvious and the woman may begin to feel fetal movement. Many women delay telling friends or family about their pregnancy until they know that prenatal test results are normal. They often delay investing emotionally in their pregnancy because it seems so tentative until test results are known. When results are abnormal, women face more difficult decisions about whether to terminate or continue the pregnancy.

Helping the Family Deal With Abnormal Results. Because prenatal diagnostic tests are performed to detect disorders involving serious physical and often mental effects, the woman or couple whose test results are abnormal must confront painful decisions. For many of these disorders, no effective prenatal or postnatal treatment exists. In many cases, there are only two choices: continue the pregnancy, or terminate it. In addition, the decision to terminate a pregnancy must be made in a short time. Arriving at "no decision" is effectively a decision to continue the pregnancy. Although the physician or genetic counselor is the one who discusses abnormal results and available options, the nurse reinforces the information given to these anxious families.

When test results are abnormal, nurses can expect the couple to grieve. Even if a pregnancy was unplanned, the woman who reaches the time of prenatal diagnosis has already made the initial decision to continue the pregnancy. If results are abnormal, she must decide all over again about terminating the pregnancy. Women who continue their pregnancies grieve over the expected normal infant.

Intrapartum and Neonatal Nurses

Nurses working in intrapartum and neonatal settings encounter families who have given birth to an infant with a birth defect that often was unexpected. Stillborn infants sometimes have birth defects that contributed to their intrauterine death. Besides the loss of their baby, these parents face added pain because of the associated abnormality. An autopsy documents all anomalies and helps establish the most accurate diagnosis of the birth defect for counseling. Nursing care for families experiencing a perinatal loss, whether a result of the infant's death or the loss of the expected normal infant, is addressed in Chapter 25.

Nurses who care for these families in the intrapartum and neonatal settings will find the parents anxious, depressed, and sometimes hostile because of the unexpected event. The family's usual coping mechanisms may be inadequate for the situation. Various diagnostic studies are often recommended soon after the birth of an abnormal infant to establish a diagnosis and to give parents accurate information about the disorder and their options. However, a high anxiety level reduces their ability to understand the often massive amount of information received. The nurse is in the best position to evaluate the family's perception of the problem, help them understand the diagnostic tests, reinforce correct information, and correct misunderstandings. Moreover, the nurse is often most therapeutic by just being an available, active listener, helping to ease the family's pain over the event.

Nurses should encourage families to contact lay support groups. These groups are a significant source of support because they understand fully the daily problems encountered when caring for a child with a birth defect. They can help the parents deal with the stress and chronic grief associated with prolonged care of these children. Support groups can also help the parents see the positive aspects and victories when caring for their special-needs child.

Pediatric Nurses

Children with birth defects typically have numerous recurrent medical problems. They usually are hospitalized more often and for longer periods than children without birth defects. They may have to travel to specialized hospitals for care, adding to the family's stress. Their families often have large expenses for medical care and equipment that are not covered by insurance or public assistance programs. There may be lost income because one parent, usually the mother, stops working to care for the child.

Family dysfunction is common, and the strain of having a child with a serious birth defect may lead to divorce. Siblings of the child often feel left out of their parents' attention because the needs of the sick child demand so much of the parents' time.

The pediatric nurse can reduce the family's stress by helping them locate appropriate support services. The nurse can contact social services departments to help the family find financial and other resources needed to care for the child. If parents have not connected with a lay support group, the pediatric nurse can encourage them to do so.

KEY CONCEPTS

- The 46 human chromosomes are long strands of DNA, each containing up to several thousand individual genes.
- With the exception of those genes located on the X and Y chromosomes in males, genes are inherited in pairs that may be identical or different. Some genes are dominant, and some are recessive.
- Many genes can be analyzed by the products they produce, their DNA, or their close association with another gene that is more easily analyzed.
- Cells for chromosome analysis must be living. Specimens must be handled carefully to preserve their viability.

- Chromosome abnormalities are either numerical, with the addition or deletion of an entire chromosome or chromosomes, or structural, with deletion, addition, rearrangement, or fragility of the chromosome material.
- Single-gene disorders are associated with a fixed risk of occurrence or recurrence. The type of single-gene abnormality (autosomal dominant, autosomal recessive, or X-linked) determines the level of risk.
- Multifactorial disorders occur because of a genetic predisposition combined with environmental factors.

- Relatively few agents that can enter the fetal environment are known to be either definitely teratogenic or definitely safe.
- The purpose of genetic counseling is to educate individuals or families, providing them with accurate information so they can make informed decisions about reproduction and appropriate care for affected members.
- The nurse cares for people with concerns about birth defects by identifying those needing referral, by teaching, by coordinating services, and by offering emotional support.

REFERENCES and READINGS

American Academy of Pediatrics and American College of Obstetricians and Gynecologists. (2002). *Guidelines for perinatal care* (5th ed.). Elk Grove Village, IL, and Washington, DC: Author.

Blackburn, S.T. (2003). *Maternal, fetal, and neonatal physiology: A clinical perspective.* Philadelphia: Saunders.

Guyton, A.C., & Hall, J.E. (2000). *Textbook of medical physiology* (10th ed.). Philadelphia: Saunders.

Hall, J.G. (2004a). Chromosomal clinical abnormalities. In R.E. Behrman, R.M. Kliegman, & H.B. Jenson (Eds.), *Nelson textbook of pediatrics* (17th ed., pp. 382-391). Philadelphia: Saunders.

Hall, J.G. (2004b). Genetic counseling. In R.E. Behrman, R.M. Kliegman, & H.B. Jenson (Eds.), *Nelson textbook of pediatrics* (17th ed., pp. 395-396). Philadelphia: Saunders.

Hasenau, S.M. (2002). Neural tube defects. *MCN: American Journal of Maternal-Child Nursing, 27*(2), 87-91.

Hoyme, H.E. (2004a). Molecular diagnosis of genetic diseases. In R.E. Behrman, R.M. Kliegman, & H.B. Jenson (Eds.), *Nelson's textbook of pediatrics* (17th ed., pp. 371-376). Philadelphia: Saunders.

Hoyme, H.E. (2004b). Patterns of inheritance. In R.E. Behrman, R.M. Kliegman, & H.B. Jenson (Eds.), *Nelson's textbook of pediatrics* (17th ed., pp. 376-382). Philadelphia: Saunders.

Hoyme, H.E. (2004c). The molecular basis of genetic disorders. In R.E. Behrman, R.M. Kliegman, & H.B. Jenson (Eds.), *Nelson's textbook of pediatrics* (17th ed., pp. 367-371). Philadelphia: Saunders.

Jenkins, T.M., & Wapner, R.J. (2003). Prenatal genetic diagnosis. In R.K. Creasy, R. Resnik & J.D. Iams (Eds.), *Maternal-fetal medicine* (5th ed., pp. 235-280). Philadelphia: Saunders.

Jones, S.L. (2000). Reproductive genetic technologies: Exploring ethical and policy implications. *AWHONN Lifelines 4*(5), 33-36.

Jones, S.L., & Fallon, L.A. (2002). Reproductive options for individuals at risk for transmission of a genetic disorder. *Journal of Obstetric, Gynecologic, and Neonatal Nursing, 31*(2), 193-199.

Jorde, L.B., Carey, J.C., Bamshad, M.J., & White, R.L. (2003). *Medical genetics.* St. Louis: Mosby.

Kay, M.A. (2004). Gene therapy. In R.E. Behrman, R.M. Kliegman, & H.B. Jenson (Eds.), *Nelson's textbook of pediatrics* (17th ed., pp. 391-395). Philadelphia: Saunders.

Kenner, C., Hilse, M.A., & Hetteberg, C. (2003). Human genetics and implications for nursing care. In C. Kenner, J.W. Lott, & A.A. Flandermeyer (Eds.), *Comprehensive neonatal nursing: A physiologic perspective* (3rd ed., pp. 132-150). Philadelphia: Saunders.

Lea, D.H., & Williams, J.K. (2002). Genetic testing and screening. *American Journal of Nursing, 102*(7), 36-43.

Lewis, J.A. (2001). Understanding genetics. *AWHONN Lifelines 5*(2), 50-56.

Lewis, J.A. (2002). Genetics in perinatal nursing: Clinical applications and policy considerations. *Journal of Obstetric, Gynecologic, and Neonatal Nursing, 31*(2), 188-192.

March of Dimes. (2003). *Professionals and researchers: Quick reference and fact sheets.* Retrieved July 16, 2003, from www.marchofdimes.com/professionals/681_1206.asp.

Moore, K.L., & Persaud, T.V.M. (2003). *Before we are born: Essentials of embryology and birth defects* (6th ed.). Philadelphia: Saunders.

National Human Genome Research Institute. (2003). *About the Human Genome Project.* Retrieved July 6, 2003, from www.genome.gov/10001772.

National Tay-Sachs and Allied Diseases Association, Inc. (2003). *Tay-Sachs disease: Classic infantile form.* Retrieved July 7, 2003, from www.ntsad.org/pages/t-sachs.htm.

Shapiro, L.J. (2000a). The molecular basis of genetic disorders. In R.E. Behrman, R.M. Kliegman, & H.B. Jenson (Eds.), *Nelson textbook of pediatrics* (16th ed., pp. 313-317). Philadelphia: Saunders.

Shapiro, L.J. (2000b). Molecular diagnosis. In R.E. Behrman, R.M. Kliegman, & H.B. Jenson (Eds.), *Nelson textbook of pediatrics* (16th ed., pp. 317-321). Philadelphia: Saunders.

Shapiro, L.J. (2000c). Patterns of inheritance. In R.E. Behrman, R.M. Kliegman, & H.B. Jenson (Eds.), *Nelson textbook of pediatrics* (16th ed., pp. 321-325). Philadelphia: Saunders.

Spahis, J. (2002). Human genetics: Constructing a family pedigree. *American Journal of Nursing, 102*(7), 44-49.

Tinkle, M., & Cheek, D.J. (2002). Human genomics: Challenges and opportunities. *Journal of Obstetric, Gynecologic, and Neonatal Nursing, 31*(2), 178-187.

10

Management of Fertility and Infertility

After studying this chapter, you should be able to:

◎ Describe the role of the nurse in helping couples choose contraceptive methods.

◎ Compare and contrast contraceptive methods in terms of safety, effectiveness, convenience, education needed to use, interference with spontaneity, availability, expense, and preference.

◎ Explain why informed consent is important for contraception.

◎ Compare and contrast contraceptive needs of adolescent and perimenopausal women.

◎ Explain the mechanism of action for each method of family planning available: sterilization, hormonal contraceptives,

intrauterine contraceptives, barrier, and natural family planning.

◎ Explain factors that can impair a couple's ability to conceive.

◎ Describe factors that can cause repeated pregnancy losses.

◎ Specify evaluations that may be performed when a couple seeks help for infertility.

◎ Explain the use of procedures and treatments that may aid a couple's ability to conceive and carry the fetus to viability.

◎ Discuss the nurse's role for families needing care related to fertility or infertility.

◆ DEFINITIONS

azoospermia Absence of sperm in semen.

assisted reproductive techniques (ART) Use of medical, surgical, laboratory, and/or micromanipulation techniques to handle the ovum and sperm to improve chances of conception.

basal body temperature Body temperature at rest.

cervical cap A small cuplike device placed over the cervix to prevent sperm from entering, thus preventing pregnancy.

climacteric Endocrine, body, and psychic changes occurring at the end of a woman's reproductive period. Also informally called menopause.

coitus Sexual union between a male and a female.

coitus interruptus Withdrawal of the penis from the vagina before ejaculation.

condom Latex, polyurethane, or natural membrane shield covering the penis or lining the vagina to prevent sperm from entering the cervix and to prevent infection.

contraception Prevention of pregnancy.

contraceptive vaginal ring Flexible ring releasing small amounts of estrogen and progestin to prevent pregnancy over the 3 weeks it is in place.

diaphragm A contraceptive device consisting of a latex dome that covers the cervix and prevents entrance of sperm; must be used with a spermicide to be effective.

endometriosis Presence of endometrial tissue (uterine lining) outside the uterine cavity.

ferning (or fern test) Microscopic fernlike appearance of dried cervical mucus that is most apparent at the time of ovulation.

gametogenesis Development and maturation of the sperm and ova.

gestational surrogate A woman who carries the embryo of an infertile couple and relinquishes the child after birth.

hormone implant Small capsules of progestin inserted subcutaneously to provide contraception.

impotence Inability of a man to achieve or maintain an erection of the penis that is sufficiently rigid to permit successful sexual intercourse.

incompetent cervix Inability of the cervix to remain closed long enough during pregnancy for the fetus to survive.

infertility Inability of a couple to conceive after 1 year of regular intercourse (two or three times weekly) without using contraception; also the involuntary inability to conceive and produce viable offspring when the couple chooses. Primary infertility occurs in a couple who have never conceived; secondary infertility occurs in a couple who have conceived at least once before.

intrauterine device (IUD) A mechanical device inserted into the uterus to prevent pregnancy.

libido Sexual desire.

mittelschmerz Low abdominal pain that occurs at ovulation.

natural family planning Method of predicting ovulation based on normal changes in a woman's body.

oligospermia A decreased number of sperm in semen, usually considered to be fewer than 20 million per milliliter.

oral contraceptive Drug that inhibits ovulation; contains progestins alone or in combination with estrogen.

◆ DEFINITIONS

progestin Any natural or synthetic form of progesterone.

retrograde ejaculation Discharge of semen into the bladder rather than from the end of the penis.

semen Spermatozoa with their nourishing and protective fluid, discharged at ejaculation.

sexually transmissible (or transmitted) disease (STD) A disease passed to others primarily through sexual contact. Also called sexually transmissible (or transmitted) infections (STI).

spermicide A chemical that kills sperm.

spinnbarkeit Clear, slippery, stretchy quality of cervical mucus during ovulation.

sterility Total inability to conceive.

surrogate mother A fertile woman inseminated with the purpose of conceiving and relinquishing a child to an infertile couple.

transdermal contraceptive patch Adhesive patch containing estrogen and progestin, which are absorbed through the skin to prevent pregnancy.

tubal ligation Cutting or otherwise occluding the fallopian tubes to prevent passage of ova or sperm, thus preventing pregnancy.

varicocele Abnormal dilation or varicosity of veins in the spermatic cord.

vasectomy Occluding the vas deferens to prevent passage of sperm, thus preventing pregnancy.

Family planning involves choosing the time to have children. It includes contraception—the prevention of pregnancy—as well as methods to achieve pregnancy. If both partners are fertile, approximately 90% of women will conceive within 1 year if they do not use contraception (Cunningham et al., 2001). Therefore those who wish to control the timing of pregnancies cannot leave contraception to chance.

A *Healthy People 2010* goal is to increase the number of pregnancies that are intended to 70% (U.S. Department of Health and Human Services [USDHHS], 2000). At this time approximately half of all pregnancies are unintended. Unintended pregnancies are those that are unwanted or mistimed. Mistimed pregnancies are those that occur in women who want to become pregnant at some time in the future but not at the time the pregnancy occurs (Moos, 2003). Unintended pregnancies may result in economic hardship, interference with educational or career plans, health problems, and other disruptions in the lives of women and their families. About half of the unintended pregnancies occur in women who are using a contraceptive method but use it incorrectly or have a contraceptive failure.

ROLE OF THE NURSE IN CONTRACEPTION

The nurse's role in family planning is that of counselor and educator. To fulfill this role, nurses need current, correct information about contraceptive methods. Nurses must also feel comfortable discussing contraception and be sensitive to the woman's concerns and feelings. Nurses must be careful not to introduce their own biases toward or against specific methods. The nurse's personal experiences and choices regarding contraception are not pertinent. The needs and feelings of the woman and her partner must be the focus of counseling, and their preferences take precedence (Fig. 10-1).

Many women who do not wish to become pregnant do not use any contraception during the month before they become pregnant (Peterson, Gazmararian, Clark, & Green, 2001). Women are more likely to use contraception if they have received counseling that is directed to their own needs instead of general information about contraception (Weisman, Maccannon, Henderson, Shortridge, & Orso, 2002). Therefore the nurse must provide individualized family planning information to women in every situation where it would be appropriate.

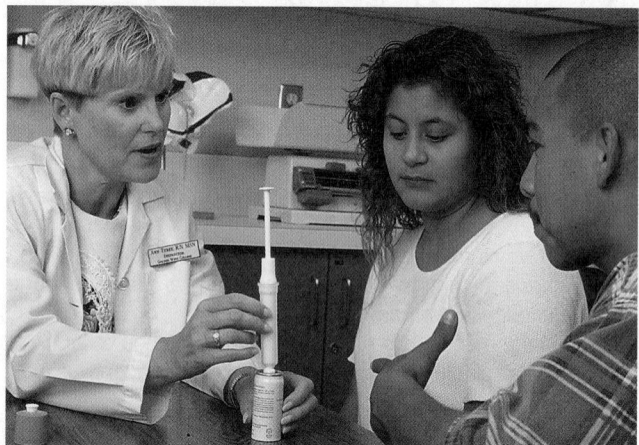

Figure 10-1 Success of contraception is more likely when both the woman and her partner are involved in discussions. The nurse demonstrates filling a foam applicator.

INFORMED CONSENT

Because some methods have potentially dangerous side effects, it is necessary for the woman to sign an informed consent form to show that she received and understands information about risks and benefits. For example, written consent may be obtained from women choosing surgical sterilization, oral contraceptives (OCs), hormone injections, and intrauterine devices (IUDs). Of course, whether or not a consent form is used, every woman should receive information about the chosen contraceptive method and its proper use, risks and benefits, and alternative methods available.

CONSIDERATIONS WHEN CHOOSING A CONTRACEPTIVE METHOD

No contraceptive method is perfect. Each has advantages and disadvantages (Table 10-1). Women change contraceptive methods as circumstances in their lives change and in response to dissatisfaction with side effects or other traits of their contraceptive. Thirty percent of married women and 61% of unmarried women switch contraceptive methods within 2 years (Grady, Billy, & Kepinger, 2002). Some women have an inter-

TABLE 10-1 Advantages and Disadvantages of Most Common Contraceptive Methods

Method	Advantages	Disadvantages
Sterilization (tubal ligation and vasectomy)	Ends concern about contraception. Tubal ligation can be performed in the hospital right after childbirth or as an outpatient at another time. Vasectomy may be performed in the physician's office under local anesthesia. Although expensive initially, long-term cost is low.	Does not protect against STDs. Reversal is difficult, expensive, and may be unsuccessful. Requires surgery with potential complications of all surgeries. Vasectomy requires another contraceptive method until semen is free of sperm.
Progestin injections (Depo-Provera)	Unrelated to coitus. Requires use only every 12 weeks. May cause eventual amenorrhea, which some women see as advantage. Taken at time unrelated to coitus.	Does not protect against STDs. Must remember to repeat every 12 weeks. Side effects similar to other progestin contraceptives.
Oral contraceptives	See Box 10-2 (Potential Benefits and Risks of Oral Contraceptives).	Does not protect against STDs. Must be taken every day at near same time. May cause side effects and complications. See Box 10-2.
Transdermal contraceptive patch	Requires only weekly application. Regulates menstrual cycles.	Does not protect against STDs. Must remember to apply on the right day. Less effective for women over 90 kg (198 lbs). May have skin irritation. Other side effects similar to OCs.
Vaginal contraceptive ring	In place for 3 weeks at a time. No fitting required.	Does not protect against STDs. Requires prescription. Must remember when to remove and when to insert. Side effects include expulsion, vaginitis, vaginal discomfort, and others similar to OCs.
Intrauterine devices or intrauterine system	In place at all times. Low long-term cost.	Does not protect against STDs. High initial cost. Can be expelled without the woman's knowledge—must check for strings. Potential side effects or complications: menorrhagia, infection, ectopic pregnancy, abortion, perforation.
BARRIER		
All methods	Avoid use of systemic hormones. Offer some protection against STDs.	Most coitus-related (must be used just before coitus). May interfere with sensation. Some people are sensitive to components of spermicide or latex.
Chemical (spermicides)	Quick and easy. No prescription needed. Inexpensive per single use.	Films and suppositories must melt to be effective. Usually effective for only 1 hr. May be messy. New application needed for subsequent intercourse.
Condoms	Quick and easy. No prescription needed. Best protection available for STDs. Inexpensive per single use. Can be carried discreetly. Vaginal condoms increase women's control over contraceptive use and protection from STDs.	Must be checked for expiration date and holes. Can break or slip off. Can be used only once. Vaginal condom may seem unattractive.
Diaphragm	Can be inserted several hours before coitus.	Initially expensive. Requires nurse practitioner, certified nurse-midwife, or physician to fit. Requires education on proper use. Some women have difficulty with correct insertion or removal. Added spermicide necessary for repeat coitus. Possibility of toxic shock or bladder infection. Should be checked for fit annually and after birth, abortion, or weight change of 10 or more lbs.
Cervical cap	Smaller than a diaphragm and may fit women who cannot wear a diaphragm. Requires less spermicide and no additional spermicide for repeated intercourse. No pressure against bladder. Less noticeable than diaphragm. Can remain in place 48 hr.	Sizes are limited. Initially expensive. Requires health care provider to fit. Requires education on proper use. Somewhat more difficult to insert than diaphragm. Can be dislodged during intercourse. Possibility of toxic shock. Must be refitted each year and after birth, abortion, or surgery.
NATURAL FAMILY PLANNING		
All methods	Inexpensive. No drugs or hormones. Help woman learn about her body. Can combine with barrier methods to increase effectiveness. Acceptable to most religions. May be used to help achieve pregnancy.	Does not protect against STDs. Requires high level of motivation and extensive education. Requires abstinence for large part of each cycle. High risk of pregnancy from error. Many factors may change ovulation time.

STD, Sexually transmissible disease; *OC*, oral contraceptive.

BOX 10-1
Comparison of Effectiveness of Common Types of Contraception

METHOD	EFFECTIVENESS RATE: ACTUAL OR TYPICAL USE (%)
Sterilization:	
Tubal ligation	99.50
Vasectomy	99.85
Injectable hormones	99.70
Intrauterine devices:	
Copper	99.20
LNG-IUS (Mirena)	99.9
Transdermal contraceptive patch	99.2
Vaginal contraceptive ring	98.8
Oral contraceptives	95.00
Condoms:	
Male	86.00
Female	79.00
Diaphragm with spermicide	80.00
Cervical cap:	
Nulliparous women	80.00
Parous women	60.00
Spermicides, gel, foam, films, suppositories (used alone)	74.00
Natural family planning (all types)	75.00
Coitus interruptus (withdrawal)	81.00
No contraceptive use	15.00

Percent of women remaining free of unintended pregnancy during first year of use. Data from Trussell, J., & Vaughan, B. (1999). Contraceptive failure, method-related discontinuation and resumption of use: Results from the 1995 national survey of family growth. *Family Planning Perspectives, 31*(2), 64-72, 93; Speroff, L., & Darney, P.D. (2001). *A clinical guide for contraception* (3rd ed.). Philadelphia: Lippincott Williams & Wilkins; Zieman, M., Guillebaud, J., Weisberg, E., Shangold, G.A., Fisher A.C., & Creasy, G.W. (2002). Contraceptive efficacy and cycle control with the Ortho Evra/Evra transdermal system: The analysis of pooled data. *Fertility and Sterility, 77*(2 Suppl. 2), S13-S18; & Organon website, retrieved Aug. 14, 2003, www.nuvaring.com/hcp.

val of using no contraception before beginning a new method, even though they do not wish to become pregnant. Careful consideration of all factors can help women choose methods that best meet their needs and that they will continue to use.

Safety

The safety of the method is a primary consideration. Medical conditions may make some methods unsafe for certain women. For example, OCs should not be used by women who have had thrombophlebitis or strokes because the hormones used may cause these conditions to recur.

Protection From Sexually Transmissible Diseases

No contraceptive (other than abstinence) is 100% effective in preventing sexually transmissible diseases (STDs). The risk of exposure to STDs should be considered in counseling women about contraceptive choices. The male condom offers the best protection available. It should be used whenever there is a risk that one partner may have an STD, even when another form of contraception is practiced.

Effectiveness

The importance of avoiding pregnancy must be considered when choosing a contraceptive method. Effectiveness is determined by how often the method prevents pregnancy. Effectiveness rates reflect two different types of contraceptive failure. The ideal, perfect, or theoretic effectiveness rate refers to perfect use of the method with every act of intercourse. The typical, actual, or user effectiveness rate is most useful because it refers to the occurrence of pregnancy in real people using the method (Box 10-1).

Effectiveness drops greatly when the user does not understand how to use the method. The failure rate commonly decreases after the first year of use because experience with the method leads to more accurate use. Combining two less reliable methods, such as a condom with a spermicide, increases effectiveness.

Acceptability

The effectiveness of a method must be balanced against the acceptability of the method to the couple. Sterilization is the most effective method but would not be chosen by those who want more children. Side effects of some methods may cause some women to choose less-effective methods.

A contraceptive such as spermicide that seems "messy" may be considered unacceptable. It may drip from the vagina and decrease satisfaction for the couple. Teenagers may not be comfortable with their bodies and are unlikely to be accepting of methods that require insertion of a device into the vagina.

Convenience

Convenience is another important factor in choosing a contraceptive method. If the woman perceives her contraceptive as difficult to use, time-consuming, or too much "bother," she is unlikely to use it consistently. Methods that can be used monthly or weekly instead of daily or with each intercourse are more convenient and likely to lead to better compliance. Spotting or bleeding between periods, common side effects with some methods, may be viewed as very inconvenient by many women.

Education Needed

Women may fail to use contraception because they do not understand their risk of pregnancy. They may not be familiar with the various methods available or the risks and benefits involved in the different types of contraception. Some methods of contraception, such as condoms, involve very little education, whereas others are more complicated. Women using natural family-planning methods need extensive education to practice these methods successfully. Women knowledgeable about a contraceptive technique are less likely to feel that the contraceptive is difficult to use.

Side Effects

Many methods of contraception have bothersome side effects that should be discussed. When women know what to expect, they are often more willing to tolerate side effects, especially if they know they do not indicate a health risk

Benefits

Some methods have special benefits that should be pointed out to the woman. Oral contraceptives have many beneficial side effects such as improvement of acne and decreased bleeding with periods. Natural family-planning methods offer freedom from exposure to hormones.

Interference With Spontaneity

Coitus-related contraceptive methods, such as spermicides and barrier methods, must be used just before sexual intercourse. They interrupt love making, increasing the chance that the method will not be used. Some couples remedy this problem by making placement of the contraceptive device a part of foreplay.

Availability

Condoms and spermicides are readily available without prescriptions. They can be purchased anonymously at any time. Their availability may be important to an adolescent who wants to hide her sexual activity or to women who are embarrassed to discuss contraception with a health care provider.

Expense

The cost of family-planning methods is important. Less-effective contraceptives are often chosen by some couples to save money. These methods may be less expensive but may result in pregnancy, which costs more than the yearly expense of any contraceptive method. Publicly funded clinics may provide free or low-cost contraceptives but may require a long wait to see a different health care provider each visit. Although family planning is covered by Medicaid, women with other insurance may or may not have coverage for contraceptives. Some states require that insurance companies pay for contraceptives, but just what is covered varies widely among states and insurance companies.

Cost of a contraceptive per use can be compared with long-term expense. The price of condoms and spermicides is relatively low, but frequent use makes them expensive over a period of years. Methods that depend on periodic visits to a health care provider are more costly than over-the-counter methods. However, these visits provide an opportunity for the provider to teach the woman about the contraceptive and to discuss other health concerns as well. Although they require a health practitioner visit, the IUD and injectable contraceptives are very cost-effective over a 5-year period because they are so effective in preventing pregnancy.

Preference

The woman usually makes the final decision about her contraceptive method. Consistent use of any method depends on whether it meets the needs of the woman and her partner. If a chosen method fails to live up to her expectations or the woman feels pressured to choose a certain method, use is likely to be inconsistent. The opinion of the woman's partner and her friends may also influence what method she decides is best for her.

Religious and Personal Beliefs

Religious or other personal beliefs also affect the choice of contraceptives. Roman Catholics may not believe in the use of any contraceptives other than natural family planning.

Culture

Culture may also influence the method chosen. Some cultures place a high value on large families and especially on sons. A woman may have more pregnancies in an effort to have sons. Asian and Hispanic women are often very modest and do not talk about sexuality with others. They need to feel very comfortable with the nurse before talking about sexual matters. Taking time to establish rapport before discussing intimate subjects is important.

Although there is much diversity within each group, many Hispanic adolescents may engage in risk-taking behavior such as beginning to have sex at an earlier age, having multiple partners, and having unprotected intercourse (Villarruel & Rodriguez, 2003). First generation Mexican-American women have different values from many women born in the United States and engage in less risky sexual behavior (Kelly & Morgan-Kidd, 2001). For Hispanic women, emphasizing the importance of her health to her family may be an effective way to encourage family planning and well-woman care because of the high importance of the family to this culture.

Some women may cling to less-effective methods even though others are available. For example, although 45% of Turkish women in one study used modern methods of contraception, more than a third of the women used coitus interruptus (withdrawal), a much less effective method (Aytekin, Pala, Irgil, & Aytekin, 2001). Use of contraception in a group may vary because of special needs. African-American women are more likely than other groups to use condoms (Upchurch, Kusunoki, Simon, & Doty, 2003). This may be true because they are more aware of the high incidence of STDs than other women.

ADOLESCENTS

Fifty percent of high school students report that they are sexually active (MacKay, Fingerhut, & Duran, 2000). Although the rate of adolescent pregnancies has diminished in recent years, adolescent pregnancy is still a major problem. More than 900,000 teenage girls become pregnant each year (USDHHS, 2000). Because of the severe impact of pregnancy on the teenager, finding methods to enhance contraception use among adolescents is extremely important. (See Chapter 25 for information about adolescent pregnancy.)

Because of this concern, the United States *Healthy People 2010* goals include:

- Increasing the number of sexually active, unmarried adolescents ages 15 to 17 years who use contraceptives that are effective against pregnancy and STDs

- Increasing condom use at first intercourse to 75% of females from a baseline of 68% and for males to 83% from a baseline of 72%
- Reducing pregnancies in women ages 15 to 17 years to no more than 46 per 1000 adolescents from the 1995 baseline of 72 per 1000 in this age-group (USDHHS, 2000)
- Increasing the use of contraceptives at last intercourse for females ages 15 to 17 years to 41% from a baseline of 38% and for males ages 15 to 17 years to 72% from a baseline of 70% (USDHHS, 2000)

Adolescent Knowledge

Many adolescents have little knowledge about their own anatomy and physiology, including how and when conception occurs. They are likely to learn about contraception from other teenagers, who often pass on incorrect information. Even adolescents who have been pregnant do not understand contraceptive techniques, and they may become pregnant again because of lack of information about family planning. In addition, adolescent mothers are more likely to use non-hormonal, less-effective methods like condoms and to use them less consistently than sexually active adolescents who have never been pregnant (Paukku, Quan, Darney, & Raine, 2003).

Misinformation

Misinformation and erroneous beliefs cause adolescents to use ineffective methods of contraception or no method at all. Some teenagers think they cannot become pregnant the first time they have intercourse. Others think they must have an orgasm or must have been menstruating a certain length of time. Pregnancy, however, can result from any intercourse near ovulation. Although many adolescents have anovulatory menstrual cycles during the early months after menarche, they cannot depend on anovulation to prevent pregnancy because some will ovulate before their first menses.

Teenagers and older women may douche (insert a solution into the vagina) after intercourse to prevent pregnancy. Douching, however, is ineffective because sperm may enter the cervix soon after ejaculation. Coitus interruptus (withdrawal) is another unreliable method used by teenagers. It requires more control over timing of ejaculation than most adolescent boys have. In addition, semen and preejaculatory fluid spilled near the vagina can enter and cause pregnancy even without penetration by the penis.

Risk-Taking Behavior

Adolescents are more likely than adults to take risks in sexual activity because they believe that their chances of becoming pregnant are small. They often do not plan intercourse and are not prepared with contraceptives. They are more likely to engage in risk-taking behavior than older women, and this may lead to STDs and pregnancy.

CRITICAL THINKING EXERCISE 10-1

A 15-year-old girl approaches the nurse with questions about contraception. She says she does not want to become pregnant, but her boyfriend does not want to use condoms and she is too embarrassed to go to see a physician for other contraceptive methods. How should the nurse handle the situation?

Counseling Adolescents

Nurses who counsel adolescents about sexuality must be sensitive to the feelings, concerns, and needs of the teenager (Fig. 10-2). They must be prepared to be accepting of the teenager regardless of personal feelings about adolescent sexuality. The teenager may not ask about contraception because she does not want anyone to know that she is sexually active. Her need for secrecy may cause her to miss appointments for family planning. The nurse must provide reassurance that her visits are confidential and will not be shared with others.

Visits to a health care provider for reasons other than contraception or after a teenager comes for a pregnancy test can provide unplanned opportunities for the nurse or other health care provider and adolescent to discuss contraception. School nurses may supply information about abstinence as well as contraception. Family planning clinics that are open after school and in the evenings may be a source of contraception education and supplies. Some health care providers put off the pelvic examination until a later visit because so many young women are fearful of it.

Because of her youth and possible lack of knowledge about anatomy and physiology, the adolescent often needs more extensive teaching than the older woman. Liberal use of audiovisual materials, such as pictures, anatomic models, and samples of various methods, helps the teenager understand the information more easily. Giving her a patch, vaginal ring, or condom to manipulate or showing her the packet of pills she will be using may be an important aid.

Using understandable terminology is especially important when teaching adolescents. The nurse must know street terms for body parts and sexual intercourse; they may be the only words with which the teenager is familiar.

Adolescents have higher failure rates with all methods of contraception (Speroff & Darney, 2001). They are most successful when they choose contraceptive methods that are easy to use and that seem unrelated to coitus. Many teenagers choose oral or injectable contraceptives. These methods are safe, seem unrelated to sex, and are not difficult or messy. In

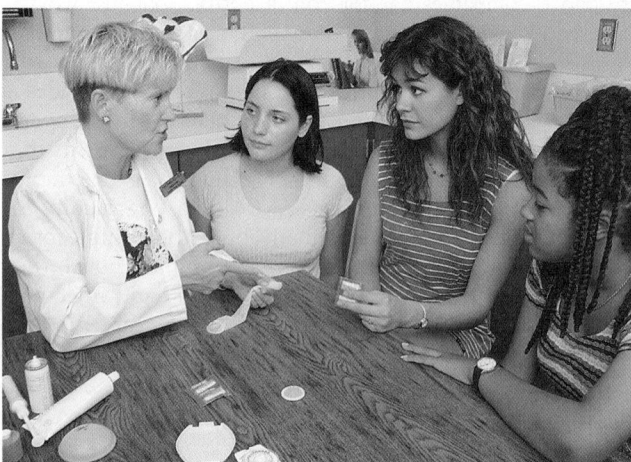

Figure 10-2 Although many adolescents choose oral contraceptives, the nurse emphasizes the need to use condoms for protection against sexually transmissible diseases. Demonstrating with actual contraceptives increases understanding.

addition, OCs increase bone density and can be used to decrease acne (Cunningham et al., 2001).

Adolescents may be inconsistent in taking pills every day, however. They are more likely to discontinue any method for minor side effects, such as nausea or spotting. Their concerns should be taken seriously, and attempts should be made to alleviate side effects or they are likely to stop using the method, with pregnancy as a possible result.

Adolescents may use condoms alone to prevent pregnancy and STDs, especially at the beginning of a relationship or with casual partners. With long-term partners, they may switch from condoms to hormonal methods if they are concerned about pregnancy prevention. Increased use of hormonal methods is associated with decreased use of condoms for many adolescents. Some use condoms, with or without hormonal methods, only if they also have casual partners or if they are very concerned about both pregnancy and STDs (Ott, Adler, Millstein, Tschann, & Ellen, 2002). Many young women are uneasy about asking a partner to use a condom. Discussions about how to negotiate condom use with a partner are helpful.

PERIMENOPAUSAL WOMEN

Perimenopausal women may continue to ovulate as long as they have regular menstrual periods, and some ovulate even when indications of menopause are present. Women older than 40 years are less likely to receive counseling about contraception even though they are more likely to have an unintended pregnancy than women in their 30s (Weisman et al., 2002). Therefore the nurse must offer these women contraceptive counseling whenever possible.

Pregnancy is rare after age 50, and contraception can be discontinued sooner if menstruation has ceased for at least 2 years (Cunningham et al., 2001). Low-dose OCs may be used in nonsmokers to provide contraception and help regulate the irregular bleeding that often occurs during the perimenopause. The mature woman who does not smoke and has no other contraindications can use any method of contraception.

METHODS OF CONTRACEPTION

Sterilization

Sterilization is a very popular method of contraception for couples who have completed their families. Although it is expensive at the time of surgery, sterilization ends all further contraceptive costs. It should always be considered a permanent end to fertility because reversal surgery is difficult, expensive, not always successful, and often not covered by insurance.

Couples considering sterilization need counseling to ensure that they understand all aspects of the procedure. When surgery is planned for immediately after childbirth, the decision should be made well before labor begins. Future marriage, divorce, or death of a child may cause couples to regret their decision. Although pregnancy is rare after sterilization, the risk of failure should be discussed. Pregnancies that occur after tubal ligation are more likely to be ectopic.

Tubal Ligation
Female sterilization is the most widely used contraceptive method in the world (Grimes, 2000). The effectiveness rate is 99.5%. The fallopian tubes may be cut or occluded so that fertilization cannot occur. The surgery is easiest during ce-

sarean birth or the first 48 hours after vaginal birth, when the fundus is located near the umbilicus and the fallopian tubes are just below the abdominal wall. At other times, the procedure is often performed in an outpatient surgery department. General anesthesia is common, but regional or local anesthesia may also be used.

There are various procedures for tubal ligation. A minilaparotomy incision is made near the umbilicus in the postpartum period or just above the symphysis pubis at other times. The surgeon brings the tubes through the incision, where a piece is removed and the ends are tied or cauterized or both. Surgery can also be performed through a laparoscope inserted through a small incision. The surgeon identifies the fallopian tubes and blocks them with clips or rings or destroys a portion of the tubes with electrocoagulation. Tubal ligation may also be performed during other surgery, generally a cesarean birth, when a woman is sure that she wants the procedure regardless of the outcome of the birth.

A nonsurgical method of sterilization is the insertion of a small coil into each fallopian tube. The tubes become permanently blocked during the next 3 months as tissue grows into the inserts. During this time the woman uses another contraceptive method. A hysterosalpingogram is performed at the end of 3 months to ensure the tubes are completely blocked.

Vasectomy
Vasectomy, the male sterilization procedure, is 99.85% effective. It involves making a small puncture or incision in the scrotum and cutting the vas deferens, which carries sperm from the testes to the penis. Cautery may also be used. After vasectomy, semen no longer contains sperm.

Vasectomy involves lower morbidity rates than tubal ligation, and because it can be performed in a physician's office under local anesthesia, it is less expensive. After surgery, the man applies ice to the area and watches for excessive swelling or bleeding.

The couple should understand that complete sterilization does not occur until all sperm have left the system, a process that may take a month or more. The man should submit semen specimens for analysis until two specimens show no sperm present.

Hormonal Contraceptives

Hormonal contraceptives alter the normal hormone fluctuations of the menstrual cycle. They may be given by injection, patch, vaginal ring, or orally.

Hormone Implant
The progestin implant (Norplant), six flexible capsules inserted subcutaneously into the upper inner arm, is currently unavailable in the United States. A single rod implant containing progestin may be available in the United States in the near future. Other implants are currently under study and may be available later.

Hormone Injections
Depo-Provera (medroxyprogesterone acetate or DMPA) is an injectable progestin. It is 99.7% effective, convenient, free of estrogen, and prevents ovulation for 12 weeks. Action and side effects are similar to those of other progestin contraceptives. Menstrual irregularities are the major reason for discontinuation. Although spotting and breakthrough bleeding

BOX 10-2
Potential Benefits and Risks of Oral Contraceptives

BENEFITS	RISKS*
Highly effective contraception.	No protection against STDs.
Reduces ovarian and endometrial cancer by as much as 50%. Protection continues for years after use.	May affect carbohydrate metabolism and may affect diabetics.
Regulates menstrual cycles and reduces cramping, menstrual blood loss, and associated anemia.	May slightly increase risk of breast and cervical cancer.
	Increased incidence of:
	Deep and superficial vein thrombosis
Decreased incidence of:	Pulmonary embolism
Benign breast disease	Myocardial infarction
Ovarian cysts	Stroke
Pelvic inflammatory disease	Hypertension
Ectopic pregnancy	Migraines
Rheumatoid arthritis	Chlamydial infection
	Benign liver tumors
Improves:	Gallbladder disease
Acne	Depression
Endometriosis	
Premenstrual syndrome (for some)	
Dysmenorrhea	
Fibroids (leiomyomas)	
Bone mass (combined OCs only)	

*Incidence of many risks is significantly reduced with low-dose oral contraceptives presently used. Avoiding oral contraceptive use in women who smoke or have other risk factors significantly lowers risk for cardiovascular disease. *STD,* Sexually transmissible disease; *OC,* oral contraceptive.

are common, amenorrhea occurs in 50% of women at 1 year. Weight gain averages about 4 pounds per year. Other side effects include headaches, depression, hair loss, and decreased bone density with long-term use. The bone density loss is reversible after the method is discontinued. Women who should not use other hormone contraceptives generally should avoid Depo-Provera as well.

Depo-Provera is given by deep intramuscular injection. The site should not be massaged after injection, because massage accelerates absorption and decreases the period of effectiveness. The injection is best given within 5 days of the menstrual period. If given later in the cycle, an additional form of contraception should be used for the first week.

Women can use Depo-Provera at any age if they are in good health. For breastfeeding women, it is often started 6 weeks after delivery, when lactation is well established. There are no adverse effects on production of breast milk. Fertility returns in approximately 10 to 18 months (Kaunitz, 2001).

Oral Contraceptives

Oral contraceptives (OCs) are a widely used reversible contraceptive method. They are available as combination OCs containing both estrogen and progestin or as "minipills" that contain only progestin. Both types contain much lower hormone levels than the original OCs, thus decreasing the risk of long-term side effects. Oral contraceptives have an overall typical effectiveness rate of 95%. The rate is higher for women who always take their OCs perfectly.

Combination. Estrogen and progestin combinations are the most common OCs and have an action similar to pregnancy in preventing ovulation. The elevated level of estrogen and progestin prevents the release of follicle-stimulating and luteinizing hormones from the pituitary. This process inhibits maturation of the follicle and ovulation. In addition, movement of sperm is impaired by thick cervical mucus and the endometrium becomes less hospitable to implantation.

Combination OCs are available in packets of 21 or 28 tablets. With 21-tablet packets, the woman takes one pill daily for 3 weeks and then stops for a week, during which menses occurs. Packets of 28 tablets include 21 active tablets and 7 tablets made of an inert substance that the woman takes during the fourth week. These extra pills avoid disrupting the everyday routine of taking pills. The OC is also available in a form in which the woman takes active pills for 12 weeks at a time and then takes 7 inactive pills, during which she has a period.

Monophasic or multiphasic dosages are available. Monophasic pills have an estrogen and progestin content that remains constant throughout the cycle. With multiphasic pills, the estrogen and progestin levels vary at different times during the cycle. The changes in hormone levels help reduce side effects. Because there may be two or three phases of dosage changes, women must take the pills in the proper order.

Progestin Only. Oral contraceptives containing progestin without estrogen are called *minipills* and are useful for women who cannot take estrogen. They are less effective at inhibiting ovulation but cause thickening of the cervical mucus, which helps prevent penetration by sperm and makes the endometrial lining unfavorable for implantation. These pills avoid the side effects and risk factors associated with estrogen. If the woman misses any pills or does not take them at the same time each day, however, chances of pregnancy increase. Breakthrough bleeding and higher risk of pregnancy have made these OCs less popular than the combination OCs.

Benefits, Risks, and Cautions. When choosing OCs, the balance between the benefits and risks must be weighed for each individual (Box 10-2). Women often believe the risks of OCs are higher than they are and do not realize the many benefits OCs offer in addition to safe, reliable contraception. Some formulations may reduce symptoms of premenstrual syndrome, reduce acne, and improve bone density. OCs provide cycle control so that women can have regular periods and minimal bleeding.

Although OCs were once thought unsafe for older women, studies show that women in good health who do not smoke can continue to take low-dose OCs until menopause (Siebert, Barbouche, & Fagan, 2003; Speroff & Darney, 2001). Smoking significantly increases the incidence of complications for women of all ages. Other risk factors include hypertension, high cholesterol levels, obesity, and diabetes. Diabetics younger than 35 years and in good health otherwise may use OCs with adequate supervision of their condition.

Although there are risks in using OCs, it is important for women to know that the chances of complications and death during pregnancy and childbirth are greater except in women who are heavy smokers (Cunningham et al., 2001). Oral contraceptives provide no protection against STDs and may increase susceptibility to chlamydia. A woman should be advised to use a condom and spermicide if her partner may be infected.

Side Effects. A large number of women who do not wish to become pregnant discontinue OCs within a year, usually because of side effects. Most side effects are minor and often decrease after the first few months of use. They are less frequent in low-dose OCs. Decreasing the amount of estrogen helps relieve nausea, headaches, or breast tenderness. Increasing the estrogen content prevents breakthrough bleeding. Other side effects include weight gain or loss, fluid retention, amenorrhea, and chloasma (brownish pigmentation of the face).

Teaching. Education about proper use of OCs greatly increases their effectiveness. Many unintended pregnancies result from failure to follow instructions correctly. Because the instructions can be complicated, they should be written clearly and simply in the woman's own language, if she can read.

The nurse should listen carefully to women's concerns about side effects and help them find methods to relieve them. Teaching about side effects that are temporary may help the woman endure them until they are no longer present. When women discontinue OCs because they are unhappy with the side effects, they may not use another contraceptive or may use one that is less effective and become pregnant as a result. Women should be instructed that they need a back-up contraceptive method readily available should they decide to stop taking their OCs.

Blood Hormone Levels. Because maintaining a constant blood hormone level is important for effectiveness, the woman must take the pills at the same time each day. Many women make them a part of their bedtime routine, whereas others take them with a meal to avoid nausea. Illness may affect the blood hormone levels. A woman who experiences vomiting or diarrhea should use a back-up method of contraception for 7 days because the hormones may not have been properly absorbed (Speroff & Darney, 2001).

The woman can begin the first cycle of pills during the first 5 days of the menstrual cycle or during the first 3 weeks after giving birth. If she starts the pills at any other time, she should use another contraceptive method during the first week of the first cycle until the blood hormone levels are established (Cunningham et al., 2001). Some women begin their OC on the first day of their menses. Many women use a Sunday start schedule (i.e., they begin a package on the first Sunday after the start of the menstrual period). This makes it easy to remember when to begin a new pack and often avoids having a period on the weekend.

Some health care providers give information about postponing a menstrual period for special occasions. Women are instructed to omit nonactive pills following the 21 active pills and to begin a new package at that time. The hormone levels remain high, and the menstrual period is delayed until the next month (Speroff & Darney, 2001).

Missed Doses. The woman should follow instructions from her provider if she misses one or more doses of her OC. Instructions may vary according to the type of OC she uses, the number of doses missed, and the time in the cycle the OC is missed. Missing one tablet usually does not require use of another contraceptive method, but a woman who misses more

---

> **⚠ CRITICAL TO REMEMBER**
>
> **Cautions in Using Oral Contraceptives**
>
> Oral contraceptives should not be used by women with a history of any of the following:
> - Thrombophlebitis and thromboembolic disorders
> - Cerebrovascular or cardiovascular diseases
> - Any estrogen-dependent cancer or breast cancer
> - Benign or malignant liver tumors
> - Hypertension (unless well controlled by medication)
>
> Oral contraceptives should not be used by women who currently have any of the following:
> - Any of the above conditions
> - Impaired liver function
> - Suspected or known pregnancy
> - Undiagnosed vaginal bleeding
> - Heavy cigarette smoking (or any cigarette smoking in women older than 35). Any use of cigarettes is discouraged and should be evaluated individually.

---

than one tablet should use another form of contraception to avoid pregnancy.

Instructions for missed OCs commonly include (Speroff & Darney, 2001):

- One missed dose: Take the pill as soon as remembered. Take the next dose at the usual time. No back-up contraception is necessary.
- Two missed doses in the first 2 weeks: Take two pills for 2 days, and then take one tablet each day. Use back-up contraception for the next 7 days.
- Two missed doses in the 3rd week or more than two pills missed at any time: If using the Sunday start schedule, take one active pill each day until Sunday. On Sunday start a new package. If on a different schedule, start a new package immediately. Use another form of contraception for 7 days.

Missed doses of inactive tablets are of no concern. The tablet can be discarded so the woman remains on schedule. If a woman misses a period and thinks she may be pregnant because she missed one or more doses, she should stop taking the pills and get a sensitive pregnancy test immediately. It is essential that she use another contraceptive method during this time. Although there is no established association with significant fetal anomalies, continued use of OCs during pregnancy is not advisable.

Nutrition. Low-estrogen OCs now used do not interfere with nutritional status. Women do not need to take vitamin supplements just because they are taking OCs (Haken, 2000).

Postpartum and Lactation. Women have an increased risk of thrombosis after giving birth. They are usually advised to wait 2 to 3 weeks to begin OCs (Bowes & Katz, 2002). Combination OCs reduce milk production in lactating women, and small amounts may be transferred to the milk. Progestin-only contraceptives may be a better choice because they do not affect milk production. They are often started at 6 weeks' postpartum.

Other Medications. Oral contraceptives may interact with other medications, and the effectiveness of each may be

BOX 10-3
"ACHES"* Warning Signs of Oral Contraceptive Complications

	Warning Sign	Possible Complication
A	Abdominal pain (severe)	Benign liver tumor, gall-bladder disease
C	Chest pain, dyspnea, hemoptysis	Pulmonary embolism or myocardial infarction
H	Severe headache, weakness or numbness of extremities	Stroke
E	Eye problems (visual changes such as blurred or double vision or visual loss), speech disturbance	Stroke
S	Severe leg pain or swelling (calf or thigh)	Deep vein thrombosis

Data from Hatcher, R.A., & Guillebaud, J. (1998). The pill: Combined oral contraceptives. In R.A. Hatcher, J. Trussell, F. Stewart, W. Cates, G.K. Stewart, F. Guest, & D. Kowal. *Contraceptive technology* (17th ed., pp. 405-466). New York: Ardent Media.

*The acronym ACHES can be used to help women remember warning signs that may indicate complications when using oral contraceptives. Other signs include jaundice, a breast lump, and depression. The woman should contact her health care provider if any of these signs develop.

changed. For example, some antibiotics and some anticonvulsants may decrease the effectiveness of OCs. Therefore the woman should always tell any health care provider prescribing medications for her about other drugs she is taking.

Follow-Up. The woman who takes OCs should have a yearly pelvic examination and a Papanicolaou (Pap) smear, breast examination, and blood pressure measurement. She should report any signs of adverse reaction immediately. Use of the acronym ACHES may help the woman remember signs that may indicate complications (Box 10-3). The woman's ability to remember to take a pill every day should be evaluated and other methods should be discussed if this is a problem. Return of fertility usually occurs within 2 to 3 months after the pills are discontinued for women who wish to become pregnant.

Transdermal Contraceptive Patch
The contraceptive patch (Evra) releases small amounts of estrogen and progestin to suppress ovulation and make cervical mucus thick. It also regulates menstrual cycles. The patch is applied to the abdomen, buttock, upper torso (but not on the breasts), or upper outer arm. It should not be placed in areas such as the waistline where it would be creased by bending or stretching. A new patch is applied each week for 3 weeks and worn continuously for 7 days. Then the woman goes without a patch for 1 week. During the patch-free week, she has a period. After 7 patch-free days, the woman applies a new patch and begins the cycle again.

The contraceptive patch is more than 99% effective, if used perfectly. A non-hormonal contraceptive should be used during the first week of use unless the patch is started on the first day of the menstrual period. The patch adheres to the skin even in the shower or when exercising or swimming. The patch should not be cut or altered, and no more than one patch should be worn at a time. Side effects include breakthrough bleeding, especially during the first few cycles, breast tenderness, headaches, and skin reactions. Other side effects and risks are similar to combination oral contraceptives. The patch may be less effective in women who weigh more than 90 kg (198 lb).

Contraceptive Vaginal Ring
Women using the contraceptive vaginal ring (NuvaRing) insert a soft, flexible ring into the vagina and leave it in place for 3 weeks. The ring releases small amounts of progestin and estrogen continuously to prevent ovulation. The woman removes the ring at the end of the 3rd week, and bleeding occurs. A new ring is inserted to begin the next cycle a week after the old ring was removed. Although a prescription is required, no fitting or particular placement in the vagina is necessary. A back-up contraceptive should be used during the first 7 days of the first cycle of use.

Some women experience side effects such as expulsion, vaginal discharge, headache, upper respiratory infection, vaginitis, or vaginal discomfort because they feel the ring in the vagina. The ring can be removed for short periods of time, but if more than 3 hours elapse, a back-up method of contraception is needed until the ring has been used continuously for the next 7 days. Other side effects and risks are similar to combination oral contraceptives.

Postcoital Emergency Contraception
Postcoital contraception (often called *emergency contraception* [EC] or the "morning-after pill") is a method to prevent pregnancy after unprotected intercourse. This method may be used after contraceptive failure, such as a condom breaking during intercourse. It may also be used after rape or in situations when contraceptives were used incorrectly or not at all.

Many women are unaware of the availability of EC. Information about it and how to obtain it should be included any time education about contraception is offered to women, in case they might later wish to use it. Women who require EC should receive counseling about their regular contraceptive method. They may not understand how to use their method correctly or may wish information about other, more effective options.

The most common method for emergency contraception involves taking a larger-than-usual dose of estrogen and progestin as soon as possible within 72 hours after unprotected intercourse. A second dose is taken 12 hours after the first. Regular OCs can be used for this purpose, but the dose varies with the brand and may require taking a large number of tablets. Two OCs are available by prescription specifically for emergency contraception. They are Plan B, which requires two progestin-only tablets and Preven, a kit with four combination estrogen/progestin tablets and a pregnancy test.

Treatment reduces the risk of pregnancy by 75%. The high hormone levels prevent or delay ovulation, thicken cervical mucus, and alter sperm transport to prevent fertilization and affect endometrial development. The treatment is ineffective if implantation has already occurred, and it does not harm a developing fetus. Antiemetics may be prescribed to treat the side effects of nausea and vomiting, which are more severe with combination tablets.

Progestin-only contraceptives are very effective and may be preferable for women who cannot take estrogen or wish to decrease the nausea. Insertion of the copper IUD within 5 days of intercourse may also be used and is 99% effective. An IUD inserted at this time would alter the endometrium to prevent implantation.

Mifepristone (RU 486) may also be used for emergency contraception. The drug inhibits ovulation and prevents endometrial development. Unlike the other drugs used for postcoital contraception, mifepristone will disrupt an existing pregnancy. Because it is also used for medically induced abortion, some women will prefer to use another method.

Intrauterine Devices

Intrauterine devices are inserted into the uterus to provide continuous pregnancy prevention. The copper-T 380A (ParaGard) (Fig. 10-3) and the levonorgestrel intrauterine system (LNG-IUS or Mirena) are both shaped like the letter T. Although there was a concern about safety with early models, IUDs are considered very safe at this time. They are often inserted at the 6-week postpartum checkup and are safe during lactation.

Action
The exact mechanism of action is unknown, but current belief is that IUDs cause a sterile inflammatory response resulting in a spermicidal intrauterine environment (Speroff & Darney, 2001). Very few sperm reach the fallopian tubes. The uterine environment would also prevent implantation if fertilization did occur. The ParaGard IUD has copper wire wound around it and remains effective for 10 years. Progestin is continuously released from the LNG-IUS, Mirena, which must be replaced in 5 years.

Once they are inserted, IUDs provide long-term, continuous contraception without the need to take pills, get injections, or perform other tasks before or during intercourse. They are appropriate for many women who cannot use other hormonal contraception and can be inserted at any time the woman is not pregnant. Fertility returns when the device is removed.

Side Effects
Side effects include cramping and bleeding with insertion. Menorrhagia (increased bleeding during menstruation) and dysmenorrhea (painful menstruation) are common reasons for removal. They are more common with the copper device. Spotting may occur during the early months with the LNG-IUS but may be followed by less bleeding with periods or amenorrhea. Ibuprofen may relieve cramping, and some women need iron for anemia.

Complications include expulsion of the IUD and perforation of the uterus. Women who become pregnant using the IUD are more likely to have ectopic pregnancies or spontaneous abortions. Nulliparous women and those with recent or recurrent pelvic infections, a history of ectopic pregnancy, bleeding disorders, or abnormalities of the uterus should choose another contraceptive method. Pelvic infections may occur in the first few weeks after insertion or may be caused by STDs. Therefore only women in mutually monogamous relationships and at low risk for STDs should use IUDs.

Teaching
Teaching the woman about side effects and about checking for the presence of the plastic strings, or "tail," extending from the IUD into the vagina is important. The woman

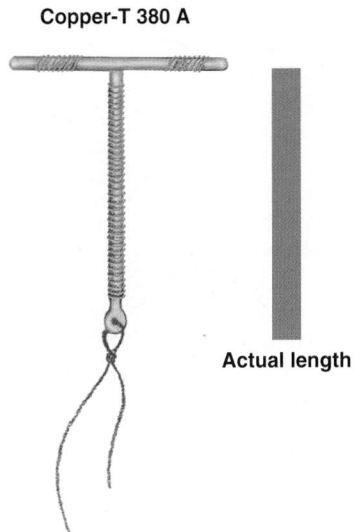

Copper-T 380 A

Actual length

Figure 10-3   The copper-T 380A (ParaGard) intrauterine device (IUD). Currently, IUDs are considered a very safe method for preventing pregnancy.

should feel for the strings once a week during the first 4 weeks, then monthly after menses, and if she has signs of expulsion (cramping or unexpected bleeding). If the strings are longer or shorter than they were previously, she should see her health care provider. Signs of infection, such as unusual vaginal discharge, pain or itching, low pelvic pain, and fever, should prompt a call to the health care provider. Any signs of pregnancy should be reported to rule out ectopic pregnancy and remove the device if pregnancy has occurred. The woman should return yearly for a Pap smear and to check for anemia if menses are heavy.

Barrier Methods

The barrier methods of contraception involve chemicals or devices that prevent sperm from entering the cervix. All of the barrier methods are coitus-related and may interfere with spontaneity. They avoid use of systemic hormones, however, and provide some protection from STDs.

Chemical Barriers
Chemicals that kill sperm are called *spermicides* and come in many forms. Creams and gels are generally used with mechanical barriers such as the diaphragm or cervical cap. Foams, foaming tablets, suppositories, and vaginal film are used alone. They are inserted deep into the vagina so they are in contact with the cervix. They should be used just before sexual intercourse and are effective for about 1 hour. Vaginal films and suppositories must melt before they become effective. This process takes approximately 15 minutes. Another application is necessary before repeated intercourse.

Spermicides are readily available without a prescription, are inexpensive per use, and are easy to use. Spermicides should be used with condoms to increase lubrication, decreasing the risk of condom breakage. They may be helpful during lactation or in the menopausal woman when vaginal secretions are decreased.

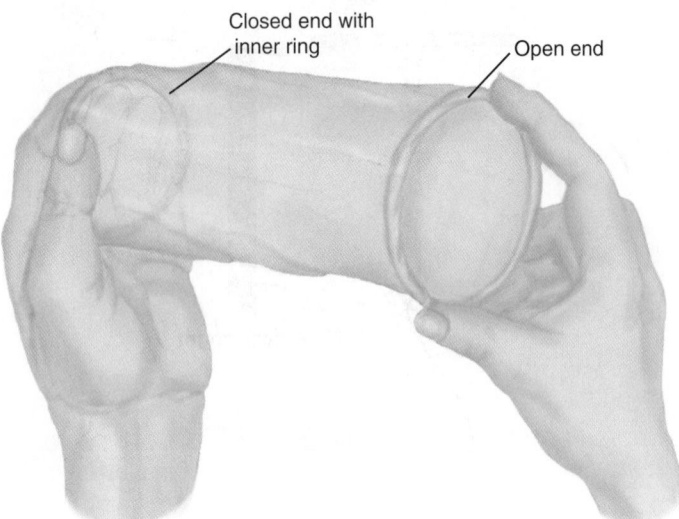

Figure 10-4   The female condom. A woman can protect herself from sexually transmissible diseases without relying on use of the male condom.

Women should avoid douching for at least 6 hours after intercourse and should add more spermicide if coitus is repeated. Frequent use or sensitivity to the products may cause genital irritation, which could increase susceptibility to infection. Some women and their partners think that spermicides are messy and interfere with sensation during intercourse. When used alone, spermicides are 74% effective. Effectiveness is increased when spermicides are used with a mechanical barrier method.

Mechanical Barriers

Mechanical barriers are devices placed over the penis or cervix to prevent sperm from entering the uterus. They include the condom, diaphragm, and cervical cap.

Male Condom. Condoms, one of the most popular contraceptive methods in the United States, cover the penis to prevent sperm from entering the vagina. They are most often made of latex and may be coated with spermicide. Couples who have an allergy to latex may use condoms made from polyurethane, other synthetic materials, or natural membrane. Polyurethane condoms are thinner than latex but may require lubrication to avoid breakage. Natural membrane condoms do not prevent passage of viruses and do not provide protection from STDs caused by viruses. Latex condoms provide the best protection available (other than abstinence) against STDs. Condoms should be used during any possible exposure to an STD, even if another contraceptive technique is practiced or if the woman is pregnant.

Condoms are readily available, are inexpensive, and can be carried inconspicuously by the man or the woman. The typical failure rate of 14% can be decreased greatly by combining condom use with another method, such as a vaginal spermicide. Reservoir tips and water-based lubricants help prevent breakage. Some couples reject condoms because they interfere with spontaneity or sensation. People allergic to latex should avoid the use of latex condoms because severe reactions are possible. Condoms may be affected by vaginal medications and should not be used concurrently.

Female Condom. The female condom (also called a *vaginal pouch*) is a polyurethane sheath inserted into the vagina.

COUPLES
Want to Know

What Is the Proper Way to Use Condoms?

Although condoms are easy to use, proper use increases their effectiveness.

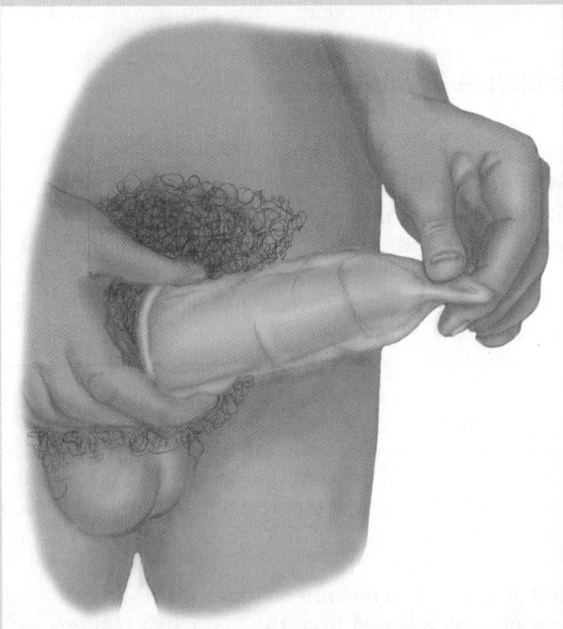

Condoms are available in a variety of colors, textures, and materials, but those made of latex are most effective. Others may help protect against pregnancy but may not protect against sexually transmissible diseases (STDs).

Check the expiration dates on packages because condoms may deteriorate after 5 years. Also check the condom to see that it is not damaged before using it.

Lubrication may increase comfort for the woman and reduce the risk of breakage. Use a water-soluble lubricant or a spermicide because oil-based products (such as petroleum jelly or baby oil) cause deterioration.

Because sperm may be present in pre-ejaculatory fluid, always apply the condom before there is any contact of the penis with the vagina.

Squeeze the air out of the tip of the condom, and leave ½ inch of space at the tip as the condom is rolled onto the erect penis. This space allows a place for sperm to collect and helps prevent breakage.

Withdraw the penis from the vagina before it becomes soft, and hold the condom in place so it does not slip off and no semen spills into the vagina.

Use a new condom each time intercourse is repeated.

A flexible ring fits over the cervix like a diaphragm, and another ring extends outside the vagina to cover the perineum partially (Fig. 10-4).

The female condom is the first contraceptive device that allows a woman some protection from STDs without relying on the male condom. It is less effective in preventing pregnancy, however, and many women object to it on aesthetic grounds. It has a typical failure rate of approximately 21%. Use of the condom is more likely if the

WOMEN
Want to Know

How to Use a Diaphragm

Follow instructions carefully when using your diaphragm. Skill at insertion and removal increases with practice.

Plan to insert the diaphragm during lovemaking or before you begin. Empty your bladder before insertion.

Spread about a teaspoon of spermicidal cream or gel inside the dome and around the rim.

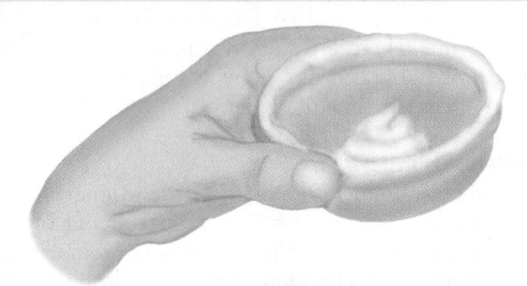

Insert it into the vagina with the spermicide toward the cervix. A squatting position or placing one foot on a chair makes insertion and removal easier.

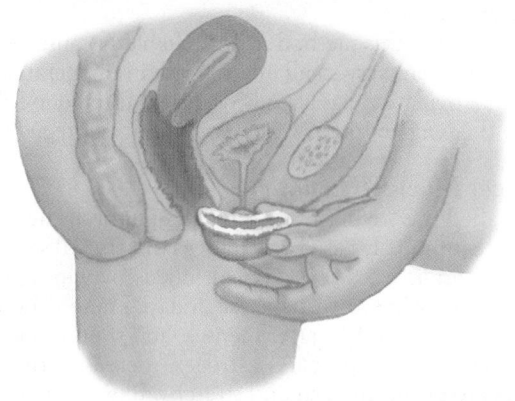

Be sure that the front rim fits behind your pubic bone and that you can feel the cervix through the center of the diaphragm.

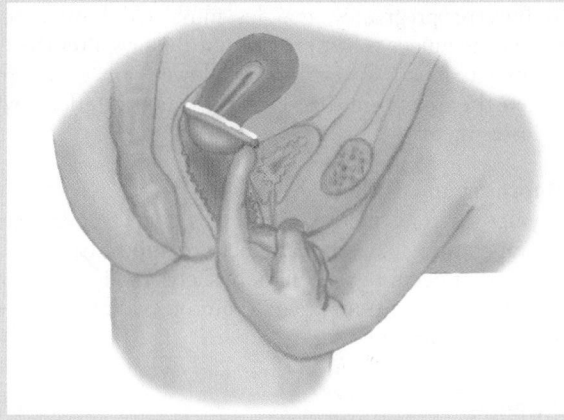

If more than 2 hours elapse between insertion and intercourse or if you have intercourse again, insert more spermicide into the vagina without removing the diaphragm.

Leave the diaphragm in place for at least 6 hours after the last intercourse. To reduce risk of infection, leave it in place for no more than a total of 24 hours.

Douching with the diaphragm in place is unnecessary and will lessen the effectiveness.

To remove the diaphragm, assume a squatting position and bear down. Hook a finger around the front rim to break the suction, and pull down.

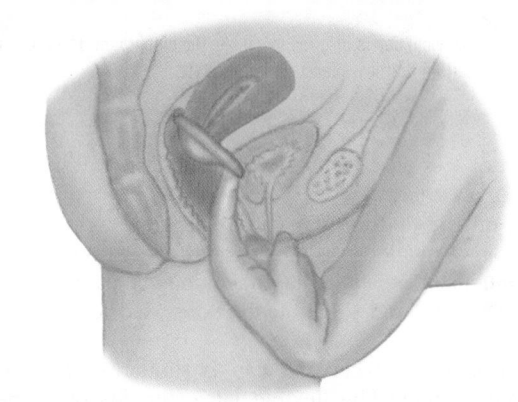

Wash the diaphragm with mild soap and dry well after each use. Inspect it for holes by holding it up to a light or filling it with water. If you find a hole, use another contraceptive method and go to your health care provider for a new diaphragm.

woman has training in how to use it and can practice on a pelvic model (Van Devanter et al., 2002).

Diaphragm. The diaphragm is a latex dome surrounded by a spring or coil. The woman places spermicidal cream or gel into the dome and around the rim and then inserts it over the cervix by hand or with a plastic introducer. The diaphragm prevents passage of sperm into the cervix while holding spermicide in place for additional protection. It must be fitted by a nurse practitioner, nurse-midwife, or physician. The woman should be checked for size changes yearly, after a

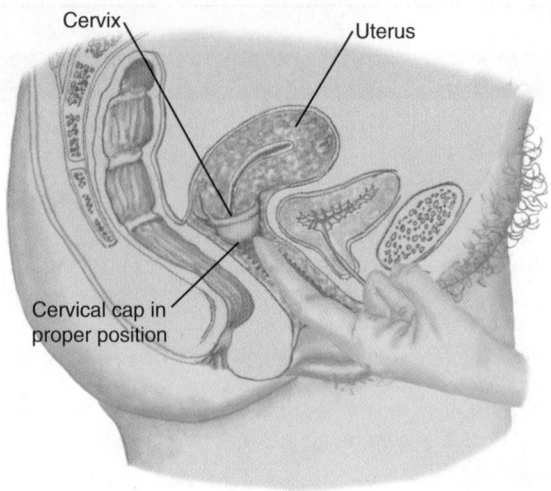

Figure 10-5 The cervical cap is inserted much like the diaphragm. The woman should check to be certain that it is placed over the cervix.

weight gain or loss of more than 10 pounds, and after each pregnancy or abortion.

Pressure on the urethra may cause irritation and urinary tract infections. An allergy to latex or a history of toxic shock syndrome precludes use. The diaphragm may be damaged by oil-based lubricants and some medications used for vaginal infections.

Cervical Cap. The cervical cap is similar to the diaphragm but smaller. The flexible latex cup fits over the cervix and remains in place by suction (Fig. 10-5). Women with cervical abnormalities may not be able to use it. It is 80% effective for nulliparous women but only 60% effective for women who have already given birth.

Because it is smaller than the diaphragm, the cervical cap is less noticeable and causes no pressure on the bladder. It can remain in place for 48 hours, and more spermicide is not needed if intercourse is repeated. It should not be removed for 6 hours after the last intercourse. The nurse should teach the woman to feel her cervix to check placement before and after intercourse, because the cap can be dislodged. It should not be used during menses or in women with a history of toxic shock syndrome (see Chapter 31). The fit should be checked yearly; after abortion, childbirth, or surgery; or if it dislodges frequently.

Natural Family-Planning Methods

Natural family-planning methods, also called *fertility awareness* or *periodic abstinence* methods, use physiologic cues to predict ovulation and avoid coitus when conditions are favorable for fertilization. They can also help women who wish to become pregnant. The methods are based on knowledge that the ovum may be fertilized for approximately 24 hours, and some sperm may live up to 5 days in the female genital tract (Guyton & Hall, 2000).

Natural family planning helps women learn about how their bodies change throughout the menstrual cycle. It is acceptable to most religious groups and avoids the use of drugs, chemicals, and devices. Couples must be highly motivated, however, because they must abstain from intercourse during as much as half the menstrual cycle. Natural

family-planning methods may be very effective if used perfectly. The methods are unforgiving, however, and errors in predicting ovulation or intercourse during the fertile times carry a high risk of pregnancy. Some women use the methods to determine when they are fertile and use a barrier contraceptive at that time.

Calendar

The calendar method is based on the timing of ovulation, approximately 14 days before the onset of menses. To determine the range in cycle length, the woman keeps track of the length of her cycles for 6 months. She subtracts 18 to 20 days from the shortest cycle and 10 days from the longest cycle to predict the time when fertilization is possible. The calendar method is unreliable because many factors, such as illness or stress, can affect the time of ovulation.

Basal Body Temperature

In the basal body temperature method, the woman charts her oral temperature each morning before getting out of bed or increasing her activity, which would cause her temperature to rise (Procedure 10-1). Her temperature may drop slightly before ovulation and then rise approximately 0.2° to 0.4° C (0.4° to 0.8° F) with ovulation. The temperature remains higher throughout the second half of the cycle. The woman is no longer fertile on the night of the third day after the rise in temperature.

Used alone, this method is not reliable because temperature changes are very small and the rise in temperature indicates that ovulation has already occurred. Intercourse the day before the temperature rise may well result in pregnancy.

Cervical Mucus (Ovulation)

Also called the "ovulation" or *Billings* method, the cervical mucus technique is based on changes in cervical secretions. The woman assesses the cervical mucus by wiping it from the vaginal orifice with tissue each day. There is no mucus for the first 3 to 4 days after menses, and then thick, sticky mucus begins to appear. As estrogen increases, the mucus changes to clear, slippery, and stretchy, like egg white. This condition is called *spinnbarkeit* (see Procedure 10-1). After ovulation, mucus decreases in amount and becomes thick and sticky again.

To prevent pregnancy, couples must avoid intercourse from the time mucus is first present until 4 days after the end of the slippery mucus. Intercourse is allowed only every other day when there is no mucus, because semen interferes with mucus assessment.

Symptothermal Method

The symptothermal method combines the calendar, basal body temperature, and cervical mucus methods. In addition, symptoms that occur near ovulation, such as weight gain, abdominal bloating, mittelschmerz (pain on ovulation), or increased libido, are noted.

Abstinence

Abstinence involves avoidance of sexual intercourse and any activity that may allow sperm to enter the vagina. Although it is the only completely effective method of preventing pregnancy and STDs, abstinence requires perfect use to be effective. Depending on the time within the menstrual cycle it oc-

Procedure 10-1

Teaching Women Fertility Awareness

PURPOSES To identify whether ovulation occurs and the probable time of ovulation.

To monitor therapeutic effects of drugs given to induce ovulation.

Basal Body Temperature

The basal body temperature (BBT) is designed to detect the slight elevation in temperature that accompanies increased progesterone secretion in response to the luteinizing hormone (LH) surge and ovulation.

1. Teach the woman the relationship between her BBT and ovulation:
   a. The BBT is the lowest, or resting, temperature of the body.
   b. During the first half of the woman's menstrual cycle, her temperature is lower than during the second half of the cycle.
   c. The basal temperature often drops slightly just before ovulation. Not all women experience this fall in basal temperature.
   d. Progesterone is secreted during the second half of the cycle, rising just after ovulation. The BBT rises after the slight drop near ovulation and remains higher during the second half of the cycle.
   e. The BBT remains higher if conception occurs and falls about 2 to 4 days before menstruation if conception does not occur.

This method of fertility awareness requires careful assessment and record keeping by the woman. She is more likely to have an accurate record if she understands the relationship between her basal temperature and ovulation.

2. Explain the occurrences that can interfere with the accuracy of her BBT. Examples include illness, restless or inadequate sleep (fewer than 6 hours), waking later than usual, traveling across time zones (jet lag), alcohol intake the evening before, sleeping under an electric blanket or on a heated waterbed, or performing any activity before taking the temperature. *Temperature changes are very slight at ovulation; these factors can cause the temperature to rise even if ovulation has not occurred.*

3. Teach the woman how to take her basal temperature:
   a. Show the woman an electronic thermometer that digitally displays tenths of a degree. Determine if she knows how to use it, and answer any questions.
   b. Explain that she should place the thermometer under her tongue as soon as she awakens each morning and before any activity. It should remain in place until the electronic signal sounds.

The temperature rise is slight (about 0.2°-0.4° C or 0.4°-0.8° F higher than during the first half of the cycle). Understanding thermometer use increases the accuracy of the assessment.

4. Show the woman the chart for recording her BBT and the symbols for marking relevant events, such as menstrual periods, intercourse, illness, or other occurrences that may

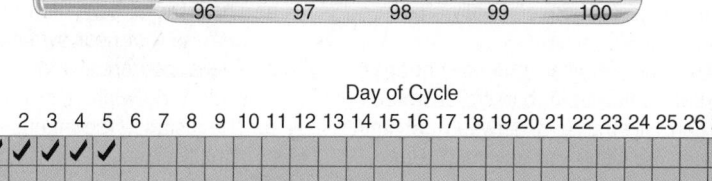

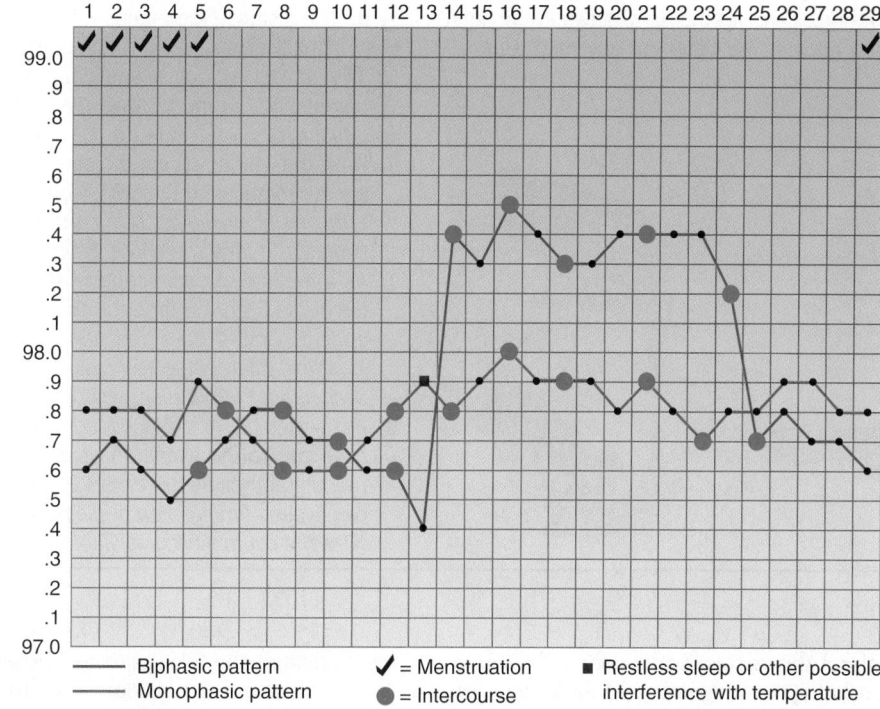

| Biphasic pattern | ✔ = Menstruation | ■ Restless sleep or other possible |
| Monophasic pattern | ● = Intercourse | interference with temperature |

Continued

Procedure 10-1—cont'd

alter her BBT. The chart allows a more accurate interpretation of temperature fluctuations.

5. Encourage the woman to demonstrate taking her temperature and recording the result. Ask her to list events other than ovulation that can alter the BBT. *Discussion verifies that she has correctly understood the teaching and allows correction of misunderstandings.*

6. As a method to avoid pregnancy: Explain that for the greatest effectiveness, a woman should avoid intercourse from the onset of the menstrual period until the night of the third day of elevated temperature. *The most conservative approach requires a long period of abstinence because the rise in temperature shows that ovulation has already occurred. Also, sperm can remain viable in the woman's reproductive tract up to 5 days. To reduce the time of abstinence, couples usually combine methods, such as BBT and the cervical mucus assessment or use a barrier method during the fertile period.*

7. To enhance the chances of conception, this method has limited value because the rise in temperature indicates that ovulation has already occurred. It is helpful as a screening method to identify whether the woman is likely to be ovulating and if progesterone is secreted to prepare the endometrium for implantation. *The woman receiving infertility therapy should understand limitations of the BBT technique.*

Cervical Mucus Assessment

To facilitate survival of the sperm and promote their passage into the woman's uterus, the cervical mucus normally changes just before ovulation.

1. Teach the woman how her cervical mucus changes throughout the menstrual cycle. Spinnbarkeit describes how much the mucus can be stretched between her fingers or between a microscope slide and coverslip. Before

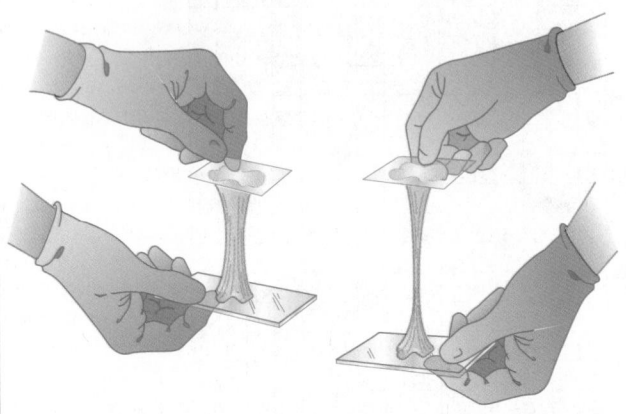

and after ovulation, the cervical mucus is scant, thick, sticky, and opaque. It stretches less than 6 cm (2.3 inches). Just before and for 2 to 3 days after ovulation, the cervical mucus is thin, slippery, and clear and is similar to raw egg white. It stretches 6 cm or more. When this ovulatory mucus is present, the woman has probably ovulated and could become pregnant. *This method requires careful assessment and record keeping by the woman. She is more likely to perform the assessment and record changes in her cervical mucus accurately if she understands how the changes relate to fertility.*

2. Explain common causes of changes in the mucus. It may be thicker if she takes antihistamines. Vaginal infections, contraceptive foams or jellies, sexual arousal, and semen can make the mucus thinner even if ovulation has not occurred. Tell her to record these factors. *The woman should understand that these factors can interfere with the accuracy of her assessment.*

3. Suggest that the woman simulate stretching mucus using raw egg white at home. *Visual and tactile experiences enhance learning.*

4. Teach the woman to wash her hands before and after assessing her mucus. *Handwashing reduces the chance of introducing infection into the reproductive tract and of transferring infectious organisms from the vagina to other areas.*

5. Teach the woman to use a tissue to obtain a small sample of mucus several times a day from just inside her vagina and to note the following:
   a. The general sensation of wetness (around ovulation) or dryness (not near ovulation) on her labia
   b. The appearance and consistency of the mucus: thick, sticky, and whitish; or thin, slippery, and clear or watery
   c. The distance the mucus will stretch between her fingers, usually at least 6 cm (2.3 inches) at the time of ovulation.
   This measurement allows the woman to identify cyclic changes in her mucus over the entire duration of her menstrual cycle.

6. Have the woman record the day's mucus characteristics (often combined with the BBT recording). *Recording provides a means of evaluating signs and symptoms associated with ovulation during the entire cycle.*

7. As a method of contraception, the woman should avoid intercourse from the time the thin, stretchy ovulatory mucus appears until 4 days after the end of the slippery mucus. *Avoiding intercourse reduces the chance that sperm are available for fertilization while the ovum is viable.*

8. As a method to enhance conception, the couple should have intercourse every 2 days during the period of ovulatory mucus (approximately days 12 to 16 if the woman has a 28-day cycle). *Timing intercourse makes sperm available to fertilize the ovum while it is viable.*

curs, intercourse without the use of a contraceptive has up to an 85% chance of resulting in pregnancy. Most women are not abstinent all of their reproductive lives but many practice abstinence at various intervals. Some women practice absti-

nence part of the time but have other methods available to use if they decide to become sexually active. Periodic abstinence is also practiced by women using the natural family-planning methods.

Least Reliable Methods of Contraception

The following methods of contraception are not considered reliable but are used by women who lack information about their risks and other options or who will not use other methods for medical or personal reasons. To help women understand the risks involved, the nurse needs to be familiar with these methods.

Breastfeeding

Breastfeeding inhibits ovulation because suckling and prolactin interfere with secretion of gonadotropin-releasing hormone and luteinizing hormone. The frequency, intensity, and duration of suckling are very important in inhibiting ovulation.

Women who breastfeed completely (at least 10 times in 24 hours with no supplementary feedings) may avoid ovulation and resumption of menstrual cycles. Use of formula or solid foods decreases breastfeeding frequency and may lead to ovulation. The menstrual cycle generally resumes by 6 months. Another method of contraception should be used by this time.

Coitus Interruptus

Also called *withdrawal*, coitus interruptus is the removal of the penis from the vagina before ejaculation. Although it has an effectiveness rate of 81%, coitus interruptus requires great control by the man and may be unsatisfying for both partners. Fluid that escapes from the penis before ejaculation is not felt by the man or woman and may contain sperm. Sperm spilled on the vulva may enter the vagina and cause pregnancy.

■ NURSING CARE
Choosing a Contraceptive Method

Assessment

Perform the assessment in a quiet area where interruptions are unlikely. Assure the woman that her confidentiality will be maintained.

Introducing the Subject

In the postpartum setting, introduce the subject by asking the woman if she plans to have more children. Most women indicate a desire to wait a period of time before the next pregnancy. Introduce the subject during well-woman checks by asking what contraceptive, if any, the woman is currently using. This will help identify problems and questions that the woman may have about contraception.

Determining the Woman's Understanding

Determine the woman's understanding of her contraceptive technique. For example, ask where she places her patch or what time of day she takes her OC. The woman should know how to use her technique effectively and what to do in special circumstances, such as missing an OC dose. Explore any misinformation, concerns, or problems that she may have in regard to effectiveness, technique, or common side effects of the method.

Assessing the Woman's Satisfaction

Assess the woman's satisfaction with her contraceptive. Women may be unsure about their method in the early months until they gain comfort from repetitive use. Side effects also affect satisfaction. They may be severe enough to cause the woman to consider another method, or they may be relieved by simple techniques.

Discussing Available Choices

If the woman is considering a change in contraceptive method, assess for factors that would help determine the best method for her. Include history of medical conditions, childbearing history, cultural and religious beliefs, and intensity of desire to prevent pregnancy. The woman's ability to understand and follow complicated directions is important as well.

The relationship of the couple is important. If the relationship is mutually monogamous, there is no risk of STDs if neither partner is infected. If either of the couple has more than one partner, protection against STDs with a barrier method is essential, even if the woman uses another contraceptive method.

Nursing Diagnosis and Planning

Lack of knowledge about family planning is common. A nursing diagnosis that addresses this problem is:

■ Risk for Ineffective Health Maintenance related to lack of understanding about contraceptive methods chosen and available.

Expected Outcomes: By the end of the visit the woman will correctly describe how to use her contraceptive method, including solving common problems, and will describe common side effects, indications of complications, and correct follow-up. The woman will report that she and her partner are satisfied with their contraceptive method or will explore choosing another method.

Interventions

Increasing Understanding of the Chosen Method

Fill in gaps in the woman's knowledge about how her contraceptive method works, its effectiveness, advantages and disadvantages, common side effects and complications, and when to seek help. Use demonstrations and return demonstrations for using the method. Give suggestions for managing side effects and common problems.

Teaching About Other Methods

Provide information about other forms of contraceptives, if the woman wishes. Discuss characteristics of other methods that are most important to the woman and her lifestyle. Include benefits, disadvantages, and risks of each method. If a prescription or fitting is needed, discuss what may happen during the visit.

Protecting Against Sexually Transmissible Diseases

Address defense against STDs, particularly if the woman is using a method that does not provide protection. This is a delicate subject. A way to approach it might be to say, "The method you are using is very effective against pregnancy but does not protect you against diseases, like HIV, you might catch from a partner. If there is any chance that you or your partner might have sex with more than one person or that your partner might have an infection, you should protect yourself by using condoms with your regular contraceptive."

Including the Woman's Partner

Invite the woman to include her partner in discussions, if possible. If the partner understands the proper method of use, he may be more cooperative and willing to help ensure contraceptive success.

Evaluation

- Can the woman explain the proper use of her contraceptive technique?
- Can she describe side effects, complications, and how to solve common problems?
- Do she and her partner report satisfaction with their chosen method?
- Has she discussed other methods if she is unhappy with her present contraceptive?

ROLE OF THE NURSE IN INFERTILITY CARE

Although infertility care is a specialty, many general-practice nurses meet persons who are seeking help for infertility or who have had infertility treatment in varied settings, such as perioperative and maternity settings. In addition, parenthood after infertility is not always easy, and nurses who work in pediatric or psychosocial settings may counsel families needing help with parenting and changes in their personal relationships. Friends and family members often see the nurse as one who can answer questions and refer them to appropriate resources when they have problems conceiving.

Extent of Infertility

The extent of infertility depends on how the problem is defined. Infertility is not an absolute condition but instead is a reduced ability to conceive. Infertility is strictly defined as the inability to conceive after 1 year of unprotected regular sexual intercourse. A more workable definition does not specify a time limit but recognizes that infertility is any involuntary inability to conceive at the time desired. The definition is commonly expanded to include couples who conceive but repeatedly lose a pregnancy (*pregnancy wastage*) before the fetus is old enough to survive. Couples with primary infertility have never conceived. Couples with secondary infertility may have conceived before but are unable to conceive again.

From 10% to 20% of U.S. couples cannot have a baby when they desire (American Society for Reproductive Medicine, 2000-2003a; Carcio, 1998). Although the rate of infertility has not increased, more couples are seeking help for impaired conception. Some couples delay childbearing until their middle to late 30s, when a natural decline in fertility begins. As improved diagnostic and treatment options become available, couples who might have accepted childlessness may enter infertility therapy or resume therapy they had abandoned. In addition, women who want to have a child without a male partner may be served by infertility services.

Factors Contributing to Infertility

The ability to conceive depends not only on normal reproductive function in each partner but also on a sensitive interaction between the partners. For some couples, identification and treatment of infertility are simple; for other couples, complex evaluation and treatment are required. Because some factors contributing to infertility remain unknown, treatment of an identified problem does not always lead to a successful pregnancy.

Factors in the Man

The test of a man's fertility is his ability to initiate pregnancy in a fertile woman. Few absolute criteria distinguish normal from abnormal male fertility, although an adequate number of sperm having normal structure and function must be deposited near the woman's cervix. Problems may occur with the sperm, with erection or ejaculation, or with the seminal fluid that carries the sperm into the woman's reproductive tract.

Abnormalities of the Sperm. Many factors can impair the number, structure, or function of sperm. Some conditions, such as an acute illness, are temporary; other conditions, such as a genetic disorder, are permanent. A single finding or several findings may be abnormal. Further complicating evaluation of a man's fertility are the normal daily variations in semen.

Evaluation of the semen may reveal that the man has azoospermia or oligospermia. The average number of sperm released at ejaculation is 40 to 250 million (Blackburn, 2003). Twenty million sperm per milliliter of semen is considered the minimum number adequate for unassisted fertilization.

A sufficient number of normal sperm must move in a purposeful direction to reach the ovum in the fallopian tube. Abnormal sperm structure or movement may reduce fertility, regardless of the actual number of sperm. Inflammatory processes in the man's reproductive organs may cause the sperm to clump, inhibiting their motility and fertilizing ability. Other sperm may look normal but may be unable to penetrate the ovum.

Many factors can impair the number and function of the sperm, such as:

- Abnormal hormonal stimulation of sperm production
- Acute or chronic illness such as mumps, cirrhosis, or renal failure
- Infections of the genital tract
- Anatomic abnormalities, such as a varicocele or obstruction of the ducts that carry sperm to the penis
- Exposure to toxins, such as lead, pesticides, or other chemicals
- Therapeutic treatments, such as antineoplastic drugs or radiation for cancer
- Excessive alcohol intake
- Use of illicit drugs, such as marijuana or cocaine
- An elevated scrotal temperature resulting from febrile illness, repeated use of saunas or hot tubs, or sitting for prolonged periods
- Immunologic factors produced by the man against his own sperm (autoantibodies) or by the woman, causing the sperm to clump or be unable to penetrate the ovum

Abnormal Erections. Abnormal erections reduce the man's ability to deposit sperm-bearing seminal fluid in the woman's upper vagina near her cervix. Erections are influenced by both physical and psychologic factors. Central nervous system dysfunction, which may be caused by drugs, psychiatric disturbance, or chronic illness, can interfere with erections. Spinal cord disorders and disorders or surgery affecting the autonomic nervous system may also disrupt normal erections. Peripheral vascular disease reduces the amount of blood entering the penis and thus reduces the ability to maintain an erection. Drugs, such as antihypertensives, may reduce the erection or shorten its duration.

Abnormal Ejaculation. Abnormal ejaculation prevents deposition of the sperm in the ideal place to achieve pregnancy. Retrograde ejaculation may occur in the man who has diabetes or neurologic disorders, has had surgery that impairs function of the sympathetic nerves, or takes drugs such as antihypertensives and psychotropics. Men who have suffered spinal cord injury may retain the ability to ejaculate, depending on the level of cord damage.

Anatomic abnormalities, such as hypospadias (urethral opening on the underside of the penis), may cause deposition of semen near the vaginal outlet rather than near the cervix.

Excessive alcohol intake or use of illicit drugs can adversely affect ejaculation as well as sperm number and function. Ejaculation may be slow, absent, or retrograde if a man takes drugs that affect the neurologic coordination of this event. Premature ejaculation is usually related to psychologic disorders, such as performance anxiety or unresolved conflicts.

Abnormalities of Seminal Fluid. The seminal fluid nourishes, protects, and carries sperm into the vagina until they enter the cervix. Only sperm enter the uterus. Most seminal fluid remains in the vagina because it contains prostaglandins that would cause intense uterine contractions if large amounts entered the uterus. Semen coagulates immediately after ejaculation but liquefies within 30 minutes or less, permitting forward movement of sperm. Seminal fluid that remains thick traps the sperm, impeding their movement into the cervix. The pH of seminal fluid is slightly alkaline to protect the sperm from the acidic secretions of the vagina. Adequate fructose, citric acid, and other nutrients must be present to provide energy for the sperm to move forward in the woman's reproductive tract. Seminal fluid that is abnormal in amount, consistency, or chemical composition suggests obstruction, inflammation, or infection. The presence of large numbers of leukocytes suggests infection.

Factors in the Woman

A woman's fertility depends on:

- Regular production of normal ova
- An open path from her cervix to the fallopian tube to permit fertilization and movement of the embryo into the uterus for implantation
- A uterine endometrium that supports the pregnancy after implantation

Disorders of Ovulation. Normal ovulation depends on delicately timed and balanced secretions from the hypothalamus and pituitary and an ovarian response to mature and release an ovum. The hypothalamus secretes gonadotropin-releasing hormone (GnRH) beginning at puberty. This hormone, in turn, causes the pituitary to release follicle-stimulating hormone (FSH) and luteinizing hormone (LH). FSH stimulates maturation of several follicles in the ovary. As the follicles mature, the ovary secretes estrogen to thicken the endometrium. About 24 to 36 hours before ovulation, there is a marked surge of LH, which stimulates final maturation and release of one ovum from its follicle. The collapsed follicle from which the ovum was released, now called a *corpus luteum,* produces progesterone and estrogen, which further prepare the endometrium for implantation and nourishment of the fertilized ovum.

Ovulation can be disrupted by:

- Dysfunction in the hypothalamus or pituitary gland that alters the secretion of GnRH, FSH, and LH
- Failure of the ovaries to respond to FSH and LH stimulation, preventing maturation and release of the ovum

Disruption of hormone secretion or of the ovarian or endometrial responses to hormone secretion can be caused by many factors, such as cranial tumors, stress, obesity, anorexia, systemic disease, and abnormalities in the ovaries or other endocrine glands. A few women have premature ovarian failure, also known as *early menopause*.

As a woman approaches the end of her reproductive life, she ovulates and menstruates more erratically as her pool of ova diminishes and fewer are available for fertilization. Oocytes are produced only during prenatal life and are vulnerable to cumulative toxic effects of therapeutic drugs, abused substances, and environmental agents. In addition to normal aging of oocytes, factors that may impair normal ovulation include cancer chemotherapeutic agents, excessive alcohol intake, and cigarette smoking.

Women with ovulation disorders often have abnormal menses because hormone levels do not permit normal development and shedding of the endometrium. Some women have absent, scant, or heavy menstrual periods, but others have no menstrual disorders. Inability to conceive may be a woman's only complaint.

Abnormalities of the Fallopian Tubes. At least one open fallopian tube is needed for normal conception and implantation. Tubal obstruction may occur because of scarring and adhesions following reproductive tract infections. STDs, such as chlamydia and gonorrhea, are responsible for many cases of infertility from tubal obstruction.

Endometriosis may cause tubal adhesions, painful menstrual periods, and painful intercourse. Small lesions are unlikely to affect tubal function, but large lesions can distort tubal anatomy and lead to infertility.

Tubal obstruction also may occur if adhesions develop after pelvic surgery, ruptured appendix, peritonitis, or ovarian cysts. In addition, the fallopian tubes and other reproductive organs may have congenital anomalies that disrupt normal function.

The conditions that cause obstruction also may interfere with normal motility within the fallopian tube. Poor movement of the fimbriated (distal) end of the tube may prevent the pickup of the ovum from the ovarian surface after ovulation. Abnormal action of the cilia within the tube prevents normal transport of the ovum toward the uterine cavity.

Depending on the extent and location of the blockage, fallopian tube obstructions can prevent fertilization of the ovum or lead to an ectopic pregnancy. Complete tubal occlusion prevents fertilizing sperm from reaching the ovum, and the woman will be sterile without the use of advanced techniques, such as *in vitro fertilization* (IVF). Because sperm can reach the ovum to fertilize it but the embryo cannot reach the uterine cavity to implant, partial obstruction may result in a tubal pregnancy.

Abnormalities of the Cervix. Estrogen levels from the ovary peak twice during the menstrual cycle—once before ovulation and again about 1 week after ovulation. The first peak occurs about 2 days before ovulation and causes the woman's cervix to dilate slightly and produce the clear, thin, slippery mucus described on p. 198. This mucus facilitates passage of sperm into the uterus and capacitation to prepare them for fertilization. Low estrogen levels prevent development of this mucus and are usually associated with anovulation.

Polyps or scarring from past surgical procedures, such as cauterization or conization, may obstruct the woman's cervix. Abnormal cervical mucus caused by estrogen deficiency, surgical destruction of the mucus-secreting glands, and cervical damage

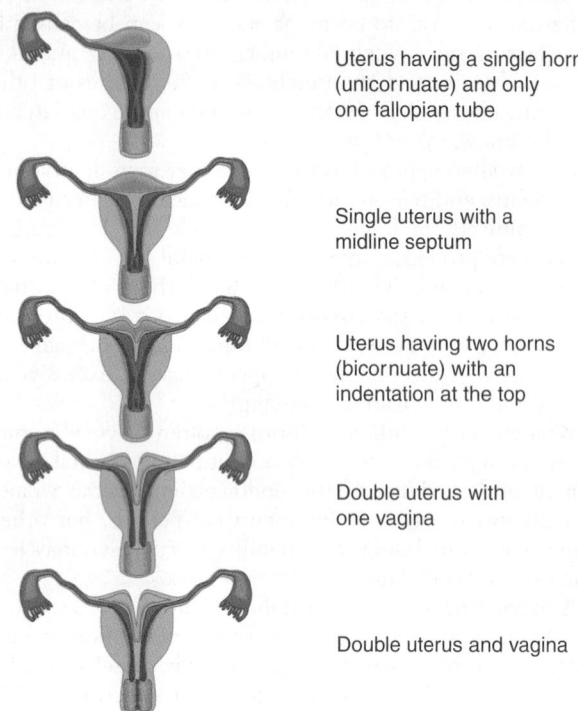

Uterus having a single horn (unicornuate) and only one fallopian tube

Single uterus with a midline septum

Uterus having two horns (bicornuate) with an indentation at the top

Double uterus with one vagina

Double uterus and vagina

Figure 10-6 Types of uterine malformations that may cause infertility or repeated pregnancy loss.

secondary to infection or other factors prevent normal capacitation and movement of the sperm into the uterus and fallopian tubes for fertilization.

Repeated Pregnancy Loss

Couples who repeatedly lose pregnancies have the same result as those unable to conceive: no living child. Repeated losses may result from abnormalities in the fetus or placenta or from maternal factors.

Abnormalities of the Fetal Chromosomes

Errors in the fetal chromosomes may result in spontaneous abortion, usually in the first trimester. Chromosomal abnormalities often disrupt development severely, and the embryo or fetus cannot survive to live birth. Maternal age–associated chromosome abnormalities in the ova increase spontaneous abortions and decrease live births in older women who conceive.

Abnormalities of the Cervix or Uterus

Stenosis or congenital malformations of the cervix or uterine cavity may cause repeated loss of a normal embryo or fetus (Fig. 10-6). These malformations may prevent normal implantation of the fertilized ovum or may prevent normal prenatal growth of the placenta or fetus.

Women who were exposed prenatally to diethylstilbestrol (DES), prescribed to pregnant women as recently as the early 1970s to prevent several pregnancy complications, are more likely to have uterine malformations or an incompetent cervix. Cervical or uterine abnormalities and possibly hysterectomy also may occur after surgery or trauma from a previous birth. Painless and premature cervical dilation, often

early in the second trimester, is characteristic in women with an incompetent cervix.

Uterine myomas, or fibroids (benign tumors of the uterine muscle), and adhesions inside the uterine cavity may cause repeated fetal losses. These problems can alter the blood supply to the developing fetus or cause uterine irritability that leads to preterm labor and birth.

Endocrine Abnormalities

Inadequate progesterone secretion by the corpus luteum (luteal phase defect) prevents normal implantation and establishment of the placenta. The embryo may not implant, or it may implant poorly. In other cases, the corpus luteum may develop and function properly but the woman's endometrium may not respond to its progesterone secretion.

Hypothyroidism and hyperthyroidism may be associated with the inability to conceive and with recurrent pregnancy loss. Because of its effects on maternal blood glucose levels and the vascular system, poorly controlled diabetes can result in repeated pregnancy loss as well as many other complications of pregnancy.

Immunologic Factors

Immunologic factors are implicated in some cases of recurrent pregnancy loss, although not all are established conclusively. The embryo has antigens different from those of the mother and ordinarily would be rejected as any other foreign tissue would be rejected. The mother's body, however, normally blocks this rejection response and tolerates the developing baby. Some women's bodies respond inappropriately to the embryo, rejecting it. These women often have recurrent spontaneous abortions.

Women with autoimmune disease, such as systemic lupus erythematosus (SLE), are more likely to experience spontaneous abortion. Pregnancy loss in these women appears related to thrombosis or other damage in placental blood vessels. Women with SLE may have other complications during pregnancy, such as exacerbation of their symptoms, fetal heart block, fetal distress, and stillbirth (also see Chapter 26).

Environmental Agents

Some environmental agents have a well-established relationship to impairment of fertility and pregnancy loss. In addition to DES, other common toxic agents are ionizing radiation, alcohol, and isotretinoin (Accutane). Suspected toxins are numerous; among them are cigarette smoke, anesthetic gas, chemicals such as organic solvents or pesticides, and lead and mercury. These agents may be directly toxic to the embryo or fetus, causing its death, or they may interfere with normal placental function necessary to sustain the pregnancy.

Infections

Infections of the reproductive tract are associated with poor pregnancy outcomes in general, and they may be related to early pregnancy losses as well (see Chapter 26). These infections are often asymptomatic, making their link to pregnancy loss difficult to establish.

EVALUATION OF INFERTILITY

Devine (2003) has likened the infertility evaluation to opening a mystery novel, moving from the simpler evaluations to the more complex ones. Couples are often in a hurry for de-

INFERTILE COUPLES
Want to Know

What Is Infertility Treatment Like?

General

Both members of the couple are evaluated systematically to identify the most time- and cost-effective therapy.

Simpler evaluations and therapies are done before more complex efforts are undertaken.

A complete medical history and physical examination are done for each partner.

The ages of the partners, particularly the woman's, are considered. Evaluations and therapy proceed more quickly if the woman is in her mid-30s or older.

Costs may be partially covered by insurance; check to see what your insurance covers.

Difficult decisions may be required at different times during evaluation and treatment. Decisions might include whether to proceed to more complex and expensive tests and therapies, whether to take a break from treatment, or whether to abandon treatment altogether.

Infertility treatment can be stressful, can occupy many hours per week, and requires a substantial commitment to self-care.

Infertility remains unexplained in as many as 20% of couples.

Internet resources for infertility include the Centers for Disease Control and Prevention (www.cdc.gov) and American Society of Reproductive Medicine (www.asrm.org).

Men

Semen analysis is usually the first test. Several semen specimens are obtained over a period of several weeks to obtain the best evaluation.

Depending on your medical history, physical examination, and semen analysis, other diagnostic tests may be done (hormone assay, an ultrasound of your reproductive organs, a biopsy of your testicles, and specialized tests of sperm function).

Corrective measures may include medications, surgery, and methods to reduce the scrotal temperature.

Women

The first evaluation is usually to determine whether you are ovulating each month. An ovulation predictor kit is most often used for this purpose. Self-assessment of your basal body temperature and cervical mucus may also be taught. These assessments are often done at the same time as other tests.

Other common evaluations include an ultrasound examination of your reproductive organs, a laparoscopy or hysteroscopy, and a hysterosalpingogram (x-ray of your uterus and tubes).

For some tests and therapies, an operative procedure is required (e.g., hysteroscopy, laparoscopy, laser surgery, microsurgery).

Typically, infertility evaluations and treatments require more of the woman's time, energy, physical discomfort, and risk than the man's.

Corrective measures depend on the problem identified. Examples include medications, surgery, and advanced reproductive techniques, such as in vitro fertilization.

---

finitive therapy, but a thorough assessment of their problem is essential for effective and financially sound treatment. Some tests, such as semen evaluation, must be repeated sequentially for an accurate picture. The prolonged evaluation process is frustrating to many couples, especially those who are anxious for a child before the end of the woman's reproductive years. In addition, the usefulness and well-accepted normal values are not yet established for some tests and other diagnostic tests are investigational. Despite many examinations and tests, infertility remains unexplained in 10% to 20% of couples who seek care (American Society for Reproductive Medicine, 2000-2003a; Angard, 1999; Devine, 2003).

Numerous professionals may be involved in evaluation and care of infertile couples: nurses, physicians specializing in reproductive medicine, gynecologists, urologists, microsurgeons, biologists, embryologists, laboratory technical workers, and ultrasonographers. In addition, general and specialized laboratory facilities may provide diagnostic services to enhance treatment. Nurses working in infertility clinics often coordinate communication among the many providers and help the couple negotiate the maze of evaluation and treatment.

Preconception Counseling

Couples may be offered preconception counseling to help them evaluate their risk for birth defects and perhaps reduce their risk for bearing a child with a serious birth de-

fect. Many women seeking infertility care are older than 35, an age at which having an infant with a chromosome defect increases (see Chapter 9). A thorough history and physical examination of both members of the couple, including their family histories, may identify increased risk for having a child with a single-gene defect. Counseling can help the woman understand *before conception* the importance of an adequate diet and avoidance of teratogens that can harm the developing fetus before she knows she is pregnant.

History and Physical Examination

A thorough history and physical examination of each partner can help identify the appropriate diagnostic tests and therapy and identify risks for birth defects in the couple's offspring.

History

The partners' general health history is reviewed to determine problems that affect their general health as well as their fertility. An extensive reproductive history is also taken. It includes:

- The woman's age at menarche and menstrual characteristics (frequency, regularity, duration, amount of flow, presence of pain)
- Pattern of intercourse in relation to the woman's menstrual cycles

BOX 10-4
Selected Diagnostic Tests in Infertility

Test/Purpose	Nursing Implications
Male	
Semen Analysis	
Evaluates structure and function of sperm and composition of seminal fluid. Semen volume: 2.0-6.0 ml pH: 7.2-7.8 Sperm concentration: 20 million/ml or more Motility: 50% or more with normal forms Morphology: 60% or more with normal forms Viability: 50% or more live Liquefaction: within 30 min Leukocytes (white blood cells): fewer than 1 million/ml Fructose: 150-600 mg/dl	Explain purpose of semen analysis: three or more specimens are usually collected over several weeks' time for accurate analysis. Explain to the man that he should collect the specimen by masturbation after a 2- to 3-day abstinence; semen may be collected in a condom if masturbation is unacceptable. Teach the man to note the time the specimen was obtained so the laboratory can evaluate liquefaction of the semen. To maintain warmth, the specimen should be transported near the body and should arrive in the laboratory within 1 hr.
Endocrine Tests	
Evaluate function of hypothalamus, pituitary gland, and the response of the testicles. Assays are made to determine testosterone, estradiol, luteinizing hormone (LH), and follicle-stimulating hormone (FSH) levels. Additional tests may be done based on history and physical findings.	Teach the man about the relationship between hypothalamic and pituitary function and sperm formation; LH stimulates testosterone production by Leydig cells of the testes, and FSH stimulates Sertoli cells of the testes to produce sperm.
Ultrasonography	
Evaluates structure of prostate gland, seminal vesicles, and ejaculatory ducts by use of a transrectal probe.	Teach the man that ultrasonography uses sound waves to evaluate these structures; no radiation is involved.
Testicular Biopsy	
An invasive test for obtaining a sample of testicular tissue; identifies pathology and obstructions.	Explain the purpose of the test; a local anesthetic is used, and there should be little discomfort.
Sperm Penetration Assay	
Evaluates fertilizing ability of sperm; assesses ability of sperm to undergo changes that allow penetration of a hamster ovum from which the zona pellucida has been removed.	Explain the purpose of the test; abnormal penetration does not necessarily mean that the sperm cannot fertilize a human ovum.
Female	
Ovulation Prediction	
Identifies the surge of LH, which precedes ovulation by 24 to 36 hr; improves ability to time intercourse to coincide with ovulation, and identifies the absence of ovulation. Common prediction methods include commercial ovulation predictor kits, basal body temperature, and cervical mucus assessment (see Procedure 10-1).	Explain the purpose of the assessments. Teach the woman to follow the instructions on commercial ovulation predictor. Teach her how to do the basal body temperature and cervical mucus assessment if that is used.

- Contraceptive history
- Previous pregnancies and their outcomes
- Previous surgeries, infections (including childhood infections), serious illness, injuries
- Previous fertility of the man and woman with other partners
- Length of time the couple has had unprotected intercourse
- Exposure to potential toxins, prescribed medications
- Family history of multiple pregnancy losses, birth defects, mental retardation
- Any home tests the couple has used, such as over-the-counter ovulation predictor kits or basal body temperature

The medical history, including childhood illnesses and surgery and any exposure to toxins, provides clues to the possible cause of infertility. Determination of toxin exposure may identify adverse influences on conception and successful pregnancy outcomes. Intercourse not timed to coincide with ovulation impairs conception.

Physical Examination

Couples who seek help for infertility are usually healthy. A thorough physical examination of each partner, however, may identify endocrine disturbances, cranial tumors, or undiagnosed chronic disease. Examination of the reproductive organs may reveal structural defects, infection, cysts,

BOX 10-4—cont'd
Selected Diagnostic Tests in Infertility

Test/Purpose	Nursing Implications
Ultrasonography Evaluates structure of pelvic organs. Identifies ovarian follicles and release of ova at ovulation. Evaluates for presence of ectopic or multifetal pregnancy.	Teach the woman that ultrasonography uses sound waves to evaluate these structures; no radiation is involved. Explain preparations needed for specific evaluations.
Postcoital Test Evaluates characteristics of cervical mucus and sperm function within that mucus at time of ovulation. Ultrasonography ensures proper timing for test.	Explain that the test is performed 6 to 12 hours after intercourse; the woman may have to rearrange her personal or work commitments each time this test is done. Use is becoming less frequent but remains a valid diagnostic tool.
Endocrine Tests Evaluates functions of hypothalamus, pituitary gland, and ovary. Assays are made to determine LH, FSH, estrogen, and progesterone levels. Additional hormone evaluations may be done on the basis of the history and physical findings.	Explain the purpose of each test: FSH and LH stimulate ovulation; estrogen and progesterone prepare uterine endometrium for implantation of a fertilized ovum. Explain the importance of timing within the cycle to provide best information.
Hysterosalpingogram X-ray that uses contrast medium to evaluate the structure and patency of the uterus and fallopian tubes.	The test is performed after the menstrual period during the first half of the cycle to avoid flushing menstrual debris through the tubes into the pelvic cavity and to avoid disrupting a pregnancy that might be in place. Explain the purpose of the test. Contrast medium is injected through the cervix, and x-ray films are taken at the same time.
Endometrial Biopsy (Endometrial Sampling) An invasive test for obtaining a small sample of endometrial tissue; determines whether endometrium is responding properly to estrogen and progesterone stimulation from ovary.	Explain the purpose of the test. The test is done 2 to 3 days before the woman expects her menstrual period; some cramping may occur, but it should be relieved with mild analgesics, such as ibuprofen.
Hysteroscopy and Laparoscopy Examines uterine interior and pelvic organs with an endoscope; general anesthesia is used. Identifies abnormalities (polyps, endometrial adhesions). Some surgical procedures may be done via the endoscope.	Explain the purpose of the test and any procedures that will be done at the same time. The woman takes nothing by mouth and should urinate before the procedure. Carbon dioxide gas, used to separate pelvic organs for better visibility, may cause temporary shoulder pain.

or other abnormalities. Chromosomal analysis may be performed for couples experiencing repeated pregnancy loss that is not explained by other factors.

Diagnostic Tests

Each couple's evaluation is individualized, but testing generally proceeds from the simple and less expensive to the more complex and expensive diagnostics. Simple evaluations are done simultaneously, but more complex tests are delayed until the need for them is established. Two methods of identifying ovulation, basal body temperature and as-sessment of cervical mucus, can be used as contraceptive measures in addition to their use in infertility care (see Procedure 10-1).

Several basic tests are common in early infertility evaluation, and others may be used as indicated:

- Basal body temperature (see Procedure 10-1) or, more commonly, ovulation predictor kits
- Hormone evaluations such as estrogen, progesterone, LH, FSH, thyroid function
- Ultrasound
- Hysterosalpingogram
- Endometrial biopsy
- Semen analysis

Box 10-4 describes selected diagnostic tests that may be offered to the infertile couple and the nursing care associated with each.

THERAPIES TO FACILITATE PREGNANCY

Evaluation of the couple identifies whether therapy might improve their chances to conceive and complete a pregnancy. A variety of procedures may be used, depending on the couple's initial and ongoing evaluations and on their personal choices. Some therapy, like timing intercourse to better coincide with ovulation, is simple; other procedures may involve considerable expense, discomfort, or unpleasant side effects. Many couples need a combination of treatments to improve their chances of conception.

Identification of appropriate infertility therapy is not always straightforward. Many factors must be considered, including the couple's history, their medical evaluations, financial resources, age and other time constraints, and religious and cultural values. Generally, simpler treatments are indicated before more complex ones, but the needs of each couple are considered individually.

Medications

Medications may be used to improve semen quality, reduce endometriosis, induce ovulation, prepare the uterine endometrium, or support the pregnancy once it is established. Box 10-5 summarizes medications that may be used in infertility therapy.

Ovulation Induction

Medications to induce ovulation may be prescribed for the woman who does not ovulate or who ovulates erratically. Medications may also be given to provide multiple ova if a woman plans to have intrauterine insemination, in vitro fertilization, gamete intrafallopian transfer, or tubal embryo transfer. Clomiphene citrate (Clomid) is a drug often used to stimulate follicle development. Human chorionic gonadotropin (hCG) can then be given to induce release of several ova.

Ovulation induction, also known as *superovulation*, increases the risk of multiple births because several ova may be released and fertilized. Another serious complication is *ovarian hyperstimulation syndrome*, which involves marked ovarian enlargement with exudation of fluid into the woman's peritoneal and pleural cavities. Careful adjustment of medication dosage and serial ultrasound examinations prevent most cases of high-order multifetal pregnancy (triplets or more) and ovarian hyperstimulation syndrome.

Surgical Procedures

Endoscopic procedures may be used to correct obstructions, with minimal invasiveness in either the man or the woman. The woman may need a laparotomy to relieve pelvic adhesions and obstructions caused by endometriosis, infection, or previous surgical procedures if these cannot be corrected via laparoscopy. Laser surgical techniques may be used to reduce adhesions because they are minimally invasive, precise, and less likely to cause formation of new adhesions. Correction of a varicocele by ligating or embolizing the dilated vein may improve sperm quality and quantity, although there is not a consensus on its usefulness. Microsurgical techniques may be attempted for correction of obstructions in the fallopian tubes or male tubal structures.

Transcervical balloon tuboplasty is a minimally invasive method to unblock the fallopian tubes. A thin catheter is threaded through the cervix and uterus into the fallopian tube. The balloon is then inflated to clear the blockage.

Therapeutic Insemination

The technique of therapeutic insemination (once called *artificial insemination*) may use either the partner's semen or that of a donor to overcome a low sperm count. Donor insemination also may be used if the man carries a genetic defect or if a woman wants a biologic child without having a relationship with a male partner. Intrauterine insemination (IUI) is a variation that allows the sperm to bypass cervical mucus and reduces immunologic incompatibilities by injecting prepared sperm directly into the uterus.

Sperm for therapeutic insemination or IUI are obtained from semen collected by masturbation. The sperm are washed in a series of solutions in the laboratory and then concentrated before they are used for inseminations. This process also removes many of the antibodies that interfere with sperm motility and ability to penetrate the ovum.

Men who donate semen for insemination are screened to reduce the risk of transmitting diseases or genetic defects. They are questioned about their personal and family health history, including genetic disorders or birth defects. Questions about their social habits and personality can disclose high-risk behaviors and also give recipient parents information about traits their child might have. Physical and laboratory examinations are performed to evaluate the man's general health, determine his blood type and Rh factor, and screen for infections such as STDs or human immunodeficiency virus (HIV). Carrier testing for specific genetic defects, such as sickle cell and Tay-Sachs diseases, reduces the risk of passing on these disorders. To reduce the risk of transmitting diseases that may not be apparent at the initial screening, donor semen is frozen and held for 6 months before use. The man is retested for diseases such as HIV several times during the 6 months.

Inadvertent consanguinity (blood relationship) can occur because half-siblings from two families may not know they were conceived with donor gametes. They could later conceive a child who shares a larger number of genes, both normal and abnormal, than the general population. For this reason, the number of donations from a single donor may be limited.

Egg Donation

Use of donor eggs (oocytes) may be an option for some women who do not produce ova because of premature ovarian failure, who do not respond to ovarian stimulation, or whose ova are not successfully fertilized despite apparently normal sperm. It is less successful if used for women who have a birth defect such as Turner's syndrome, in which the ova regress early in life, or for women who have had radiation therapy to the pelvis (Balen & Jacobs, 2003).

As in use of donor semen, egg donation carries with it the risk for infecting the recipient, the fetus, and possibly the male partner of the recipient. Inadvertent consanguinity is a risk with multiple donations as it is in use of donor semen. In addition to these risks, the procedure carries risks for the

BOX 10-5
Selected Medications for Infertility Therapy

Drug	Primary Use
Bromocriptine (Parlodel)	Corrects excess prolactin secretion by anterior pituitary, improving gonadotropin-releasing hormone (GnRH) secretion, in turn normalizing follicle-stimulating hormone (FSH) and luteinizing hormone (LH) release. These drug actions increase ovulation and support early pregnancy by stimulating progesterone secretion by the corpus luteum.
Chorionic gonadotropin, human (hCG; Pregnyl); recombinant deoxyribonucleic acid (DNA) origin (r-hCG; Ovidrel)	Used in conjunction with gonadotropins to stimulate ovulation in the female or sperm formation in the male. Stimulates progesterone production by corpus luteum.
Clomiphene citrate (Clomid)	Induction of ovulation in women who have specific types of ovulatory dysfunction. The drug increases frequency of GnRH secretion from the hypothalamus, thus increasing FSH and LH release and maturing the ovarian follicle and release of the ovum.
FSH, recombinant DNA origin (follitropin [Gonal-F])	Stimulation of ovarian follicle growth; ovulation-induction gonadotropin.
GnRH antagonists (e.g., cetrorelix [Cetrotide], ganirelix [Antagon]	Reduces endometriosis; adjunct to drugs given to stimulate ovulation by suppressing LH and FSH. Depending on drug, doses may be given intranasally, subcutaneously, or intramuscularly.
GnRH agonists (gonadarelin); gosarelin [Zoladex], leuprolide [Lupron], nafarelin [Synarel])	Stimulates release of FSH and LH from the pituitary gland in men and women who have deficient GnRH secretion by their hypothalamus. FSH and LH, in turn, stimulate ovulation in the female and stimulate testosterone production and spermatogenesis in the male. The drug is given with an automated pump at 75- to 90-minute intervals or by twice-daily nasal puff (Synarel).*
Gonadotropins, human (urofollitropin [Bravelle; Fertinex]; menotropin [Humegon, Pergonal, Repronex])	Induction of ovulation with human-derived FSH and LH; brands may differ in the proportions of FSH to LH; recombinant DNA preparations are becoming more common because of their greater purity
Luteinizing hormone, recombinant DNA origin	Replacement of luteinizing hormone; promotes ability of mature ovarian follicle to rupture and luteinize when hCG is secreted; usefulness of drug requires more study.†
Progesterone (intramuscular or vaginal preparations)	Luteal phase support; prepares uterine lining and promotes implantation of embryo.
Erectile agents (sildenafil [Viagra], vardenafil [Levitra])	Increase blood flow to the penis, improving erectile function.

*Daly, D.C. (2000). Induction of ovulation. In E.J. Quilligan & F.P. Zuspan (Eds.). *Current therapy in obstetrics and gynecology* (5th ed., pp. 80-83). Philadelphia: Saunders.
Leibowitz, D., & Hoffman, J. (2000). Fertility drug therapies: Past, present, and future. *Journal of Obstetric, Gynecologic, and Neonatal Nursing, 29*(2), 201-210.
Richard-Davis, G. (2002). Ovulation induction for in vitro fertilization: The role of gonadotropin-releasing hormone antagonists. *Infertility and Reproductive Medicine Clinics of North America, 13*(3), 437-444.
†Thornton, K.L. (2002). Recombinant gonadotropins and IVF. *Infertility and Reproductive Medicine Clinics of North America, 13*(3), 445-458.

donor because she will need medications to stimulate ovulation and an ova retrieval procedure as is done in IVF. Because of the complexity of egg donation, donors are fewer than for sperm donation (American Society for Reproductive Medicine, 2000; Balen & Jacobs, 2003; Penzias, 2002).

Surrogate Parenting

A surrogate mother may enter the picture if the woman is infertile because she does not have a uterus or if she cannot carry a fetus to live birth even though no problems with the baby, such as chromosome defects, are identified. Surrogacy is different from therapeutic insemination or egg donation because it is not anonymous. In addition, the woman who carries the child inevitably forms bonds with the fetus during the months of pregnancy. For these and many other reasons, extensive interview and counseling of both the infertile couple and the surrogate mother are required.

Custody issues are clearer when the birth mother is a gestational surrogate than when she also donates her ovum to the child. Courts have more often recognized the genetic parents as the legal parents and upheld the contracts between them and the gestational surrogate.

Advanced Reproductive Techniques

Several advanced reproductive technologies (ART) procedures are available to bypass natural obstacles to conception by placing gametes together to promote fertilization. One class includes in vitro fertilization (IVF), gamete intrafallopian transfer (GIFT), and zygote intrafallopian transfer (ZIFT). Each procedure begins with ovulation induction to permit retrieval of several ova, thus improving the likelihood of a successful pregnancy. Sperm are prepared and concentrated as they are for therapeutic insemination.

Couples who have concerns about a specific genetic defect in the family may be offered preimplantation genetic testing of their fertilized ova. As in other types of prenatal screening, preimplantation genetic testing cannot rule out every potential abnormality in the offspring. Rather, the testing allows

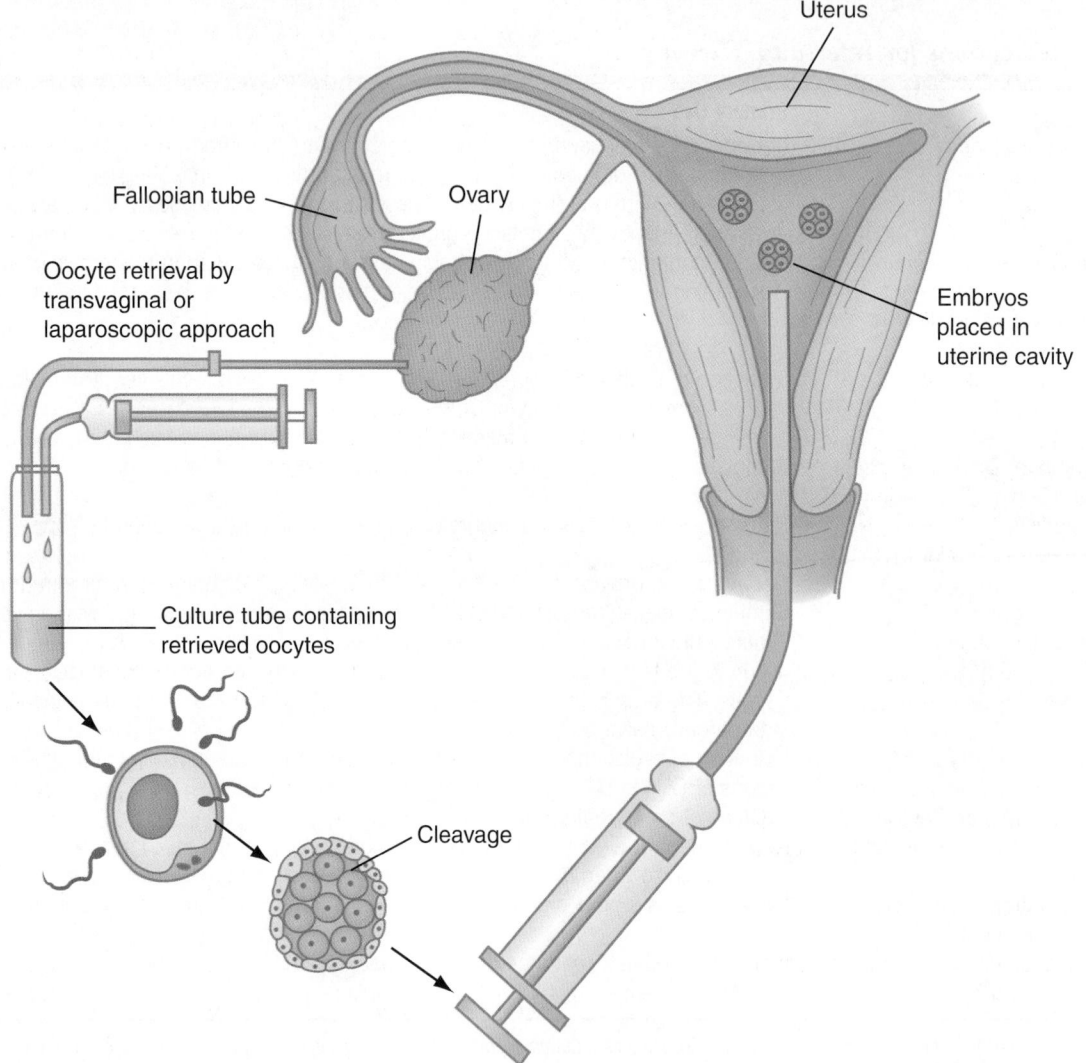

Uterus

Fallopian tube   Ovary

Oocyte retrieval by
transvaginal or
laparoscopic approach

Embryos
placed in
uterine cavity

Culture tube containing
retrieved oocytes

Cleavage

Figure 10-7 In vitro fertilization (IVF). Multiple oocytes are obtained by using a transvaginal or laparoscopic approach. The retrieved oocytes are mixed with prepared sperm and incubated 1 to 2 days. Embryos are then transferred to the uterine cavity to allow implantation and continued development.

parents to make informed decisions about whether to implant the fertilized ova into the uterus.

The success rates for ART therapy in carefully selected couples now average 25% to 30% (American Society for Reproductive Medicine, 2000-2003a; Centers for Disease Control and Prevention [CDC], 2002). Clinics that provide therapy for couples with poorer prognoses for pregnancy may have a lower overall success rate because they may be a "last resort" option for these couples.

In Vitro Fertilization
The technique of IVF involves bypassing blocked or absent fallopian tubes (Figure 10-7). The physician removes the ova by ultrasound-guided transvaginal retrieval or occasionally laparoscopy and mixes them with prepared sperm from the woman's partner or a donor. Fertilized ova are returned to the uterus 1 to 2 days after conception. The number of fertilized ova returned is individualized but is approximately 3 or 4. Older women usually have more ova transferred than younger women to improve their chances of pregnancy

without greatly increasing the risk of having a triplet or higher pregnancy. Supplemental progesterone is given to the woman to promote implantation and support the early pregnancy (luteal phase support). Because of the supplemental progesterone, the woman will not have a menstrual period even if she is not pregnant. Four weeks after implantation, transvaginal ultrasound is used to detect whether one or more gestational sacs are present and to identify if a tubal pregnancy occurred (see Chapter 26).

Gamete Intrafallopian Transfer
The woman must have at least one patent fallopian tube for GIFT to be an option. The procedure begins in a manner similar to that of IVF, with retrieval of multiple ova and washed sperm. The retrieved ova are drawn into a catheter that also carries prepared sperm. Sperm and up to two ova per tube are injected into each fallopian tube through a laparoscope. Additional prepared sperm may be injected into the uterus through the cervix to improve the chance of successful fertilization. Progesterone is given as it is in IVF.

Zygote Intrafallopian Transfer

Zygote intrafallopian transfer (ZIFT) is a hybrid of IVF and GIFT. The woman's ova are fertilized outside her body as in IVF, but the resulting fertilized ova are placed in the distal fallopian tube and enter the uterus naturally for implantation. The woman must have at least one patent fallopian tube.

Comparison of In Vitro Fertilization, Gamete Intrafallopian Transfer, and Tubal Embryo Transfer

One advantage of GIFT and ZIFT is that some people or religious groups may find these procedures more natural and thus more acceptable than IVF. With IVF or ZIFT, there is evidence of fertilization before placement in the uterus or tubes. GIFT and ZIFT have minimally higher success rates than IVF in some clinics, although the success rate for IVF rises with the number of cycles attempted. The GIFT and ZIFT procedures are more invasive, requiring a laparoscopy to place the gametes or fertilized ova in the distal fallopian tube. Tubal pregnancy may result if embryos cannot reach the uterine cavity to implant. For these reasons, IVF is used about 98% of the time if a couple requires assisted reproductive technology (American Society for Reproductive Medicine, 2000-2003a; CDC, 2003).

These reproductive techniques can result in multifetal pregnancy, sometimes high multiples. Pregnancies with more than twins carry a substantially higher risk to both mother and infants because of preterm labor and birth, placental insufficiency, and a high demand on maternal body systems. Selective reduction in the number of fetuses may give those remaining a better chance to progress to a live birth. Such a procedure is, of course, heavily laden with emotional and ethical concerns.

Intracytoplasmic Sperm Injection. Intracytoplasmic sperm injection (ICSI) is a method in which a single prepared sperm is injected into an ovum. Several ova are injected and then incubated for 48 to 72 hours. Up to three fertilized ova are returned to the uterus as in IVF or sometimes returned to the fallopian tube. Excess fertilized ova are frozen for future transfers or may be donated to another infertile couple.

Men who have obstructions to or absence of their epididymis may be able to father children with the use of percutaneous or microsurgical sperm aspiration. The sperm are retrieved from the epididymis by percutaneous aspiration with a small-gauge butterfly needle. Alternately, a microsurgical incision may be made to aspirate the sperm if the percutaneous approach cannot be used. The sperm obtained are then used to fertilize ova by ICSI.

RESPONSES TO INFERTILITY

The desire for children is strong in many couples. If a couple does not achieve pregnancy or produce a living child as expected, the man and woman often experience psychologic distress and a threat to their self-images. Either or both partners may feel like failures. Their marital and family relationships may be stressed, and they may withdraw from relationships with others that they previously found satisfying.

Assumption of Fertility

Many couples use contraception for a few years before they decide to have a baby. When they want a child, they discontinue contraception and assume that pregnancy will occur within a few months at most.

Either or both partners may experiment with the role of parent as they anticipate pregnancy. They develop a heightened awareness of children and parenting. Being with others who are expecting or who already have children is exciting because they plan to join their ranks shortly. They may discuss issues such as full-time parenting by one partner, child care, and future lifestyle changes. They may begin acquiring toys and furnishings a child will need and perhaps move to a larger home. Both partners may develop a fantasy child or a concept of what their baby will be like.

Growing Awareness of a Problem

As the months pass, the couple gradually becomes concerned about the inability to conceive. If the woman is older, they feel the urgency of the limited time before her reproductive years end.

The couple begins to feel uneasy with child-related activities. Now they are not so sure when they will be parents. Events such as baby showers or christenings may become melancholy rather than joyful occasions. Family members and friends who are having children may feel guilty at their good fortune when they are around the couple that cannot conceive.

The potential grandparents may feel that their children are waiting too long to start a family or even that they are selfish. If they are aware that the couple is trying to conceive, they become even more worried as the months pass without the longed-for announcement of a pregnancy. They are twice saddened by the lack of a grandchild and by the hurt their adult children are enduring.

Seeking Help for Infertility

Eventually, couples must decide whether to seek help to conceive. They may reach this point after only a few menstrual cycles or, at the opposite extreme, may never seek help. Many factors enter into their decision. These include their ages (especially the woman's), how long they have been unable to conceive, how much they want a biologic child, how they regard adoption, and how they feel about a child-free life.

Identifying the Importance of Having a Baby

Each partner may place a different priority on having a baby. Conflicts may arise when one partner wants help to conceive sooner than the other. In addition, cultural or religious beliefs influence how each feels about procreation and whether options such as assisted reproductive procedures or adoption are acceptable. How the couple resolves these differences is crucial to the stability of the relationship.

Men and women often differ in their reactions to infertility. Women may want to talk about their feelings and frustrations, but men often internalize their feelings or feel that they must be strong for their partner. The woman may interpret her partner's reluctance to express his feelings and his stoicism as disinterest or lack of concern and care for her.

Sharing Intimate Information

Although the infertility specialist will limit questions to those necessary, evaluation and treatment for infertility require that both partners reveal intimate information about their sexual relationship, such as the frequency and timing of intercourse. In addition, infertile couples may feel that the evaluation calls their sexual adequacy into question.

Considering Financial Resources

Financial concerns enter into the couple's decision about whether to seek treatment and how far to carry it. Techniques such as ovulation predictor kits or basal body temperature assessment are fairly inexpensive but have limited usefulness in achieving a pregnancy when there are complex problems. Advanced techniques, such as IVF, are expensive and have a very low likelihood of success for some couples. Health insurance may not cover infertility treatment at all or may not cover all procedures because the problem does not directly threaten the health of either partner. Also, investigational treatments are often not covered. The drugs that must be taken to achieve pregnancy are often quite expensive. Expense and restricted coverage limit treatment choices for many low-income or middle-income couples.

Ethical Issues

Ethical issues enter infertility care as well (see also Chapter 1). Those who seek and pursue infertility treatment usually have greater financial resources than those who do not, creating a disparity in availability to pursue parenthood. Money paid to a woman who donates ova or a surrogate mother may raise issues of baby selling. Participation by professionals in arranging surrogacy even may be illegal in some states. Could a poor but fertile woman feel compelled to provide her body for a more well-to-do couple? Yet not compensating a woman for the real physical and emotional risks of this undertaking can be construed as exploitative as well. Not implanting live embryos that have a genetic defect or reducing the number of fetuses in a high multiple pregnancy may be viewed as abortion by many people.

Committing to Involvement in Care

Infertility evaluation and treatment require commitment of the couple's time, energy, and money. Couples participate on a day-to-day basis as they do home assessments, take medications, and keep detailed records. For infertility diagnosis and therapy to be most effective, couples must consider their ability and desire to be directly involved in the process over what may be a long time.

Reactions During Evaluation and Treatment

Couples undergoing infertility evaluation and treatment have different reactions to the process. In addition, their reactions may change as infertility care progresses.

Influences on Decision Making

If their evaluation shows that a treatment or procedure may enable them to conceive, the couple must then decide whether to proceed. The decision-making process begins early and must be repeated during therapy if pregnancy does not occur. A complex array of factors enters into their decisions about beginning and continuing treatment or whether to end their pursuit of pregnancy. These factors interact dynamically as the couple makes each decision. As part of an interdisciplinary team, the nurse helps both partners examine each factor and arrive at a decision that is best for them.

Social, Cultural, and Religious Values. Some medically appropriate options may not be acceptable to every couple. Surrogate parenting, IVF, and therapeutic insemination (especially with donor sperm) are inconsistent with the personal or religious beliefs of many people. If a procedure offers the partners hope for a child but is incompatible with their beliefs, their choices are two: use the technology despite their beliefs, or accept childlessness. Adoption may be a third alternative for some couples if the desire for a biologic child is not absolute. As in other decisions, couples must work out conflicting personal values about what therapy is acceptable.

Difficulty of Treatment. The couple must consider how difficult, risky, and uncomfortable therapy will be. The level of difficulty involves physical, psychologic, geographic, and time factors. Employment constraints often affect treatment decisions as well.

Several infertility treatments involve invasive procedures or surgery. The person who undergoes the procedure must be the one who ultimately decides whether to do it. That person alone can decide whether the hope of a child is worth the risks and discomfort of the procedure.

Infertility treatment is stressful. Often partners feel or are willing to tolerate different levels of stress. To reduce the stress, they may abandon treatment completely or may take a vacation for a few months from the constant preoccupation with conceiving. Women nearing or in their 40s often feel that they do not have the luxury of skipping a treatment cycle.

Some couples encounter geographic difficulties if they must travel a long distance for therapy. Time stresses are substantial. The partners, particularly the woman, feel that achieving pregnancy is their new career. One or both partners may spend many hours every week in pursuit of pregnancy.

Employment constraints may be a barrier to infertility therapy because of the time required for treatment. The impact of time is usually greatest on the woman. Time away from work may burden the employer or co-workers. Stopping work may not be an option because the family needs the money and often needs the insurance coverage that comes with employment.

Probability of Success. Couples often have a biased interpretation of their statistical probability of success, especially when they begin treatment with a new procedure. For example, if a procedure has a 20% likelihood of success in any given cycle, they may expect that they will be in the successful group rather than in the 80% who do not conceive. As time goes by, however, they must weigh the likelihood of success of any therapy against financial concerns and their own willingness to accept the discomfort and difficulty associated with it. The fact that a couple with no infertility problems will conceive in any given month is also about 20% is little comfort to those investing so much time, money, and effort.

Financial Concerns. Some couples, particularly those with ample resources and a strong desire for a biologic child, pursue expensive treatments and pursue them longer than others of more limited means. They may do so despite a low probability of success. Couples with financial limitations find that they must abandon treatment sooner than they want. Other couples go heavily into debt, adding financial strain to the other stresses of treatment in their quest for a biologic child.

Psychologic Reactions

A couple's initial reaction to infertility is often one of shock because the partners are usually healthy and do not expect to have problems conceiving. Their reactions vary according to how easily their infertility is alleviated, their personalities and self-images, and the strength of their relationship.

Guilt. A partner having the only identified problem might feel that he or she is depriving the other of children. This feeling may be compounded if the "normal" partner has children from another relationship. It may be difficult for this person to understand that not all factors affecting fertility can be detected and that what seems like the one partner's problem is often the couple's problem.

Either partner may feel guilty about past choices that now affect fertility. A woman with adhesions resulting from a sexually acquired infection may regret her past choices. The man who wanted to delay pregnancy longer than the woman may feel guilty if her age is now limiting the time she has for conceiving.

Isolation. Infertile couples often feel different from friends and relatives who do not have difficulty conceiving. To insulate themselves from painful reminders of their infertility, they may withdraw from these relationships. Some couples develop supportive relationships with others who are also infertile, which somewhat diminishes their sense of isolation.

Depression. One or both partners may experience depression as their sense of competence and control over their bodies is challenged, especially if therapy is not successful quickly. They often feel as if they are on a roller coaster of hope alternating with despair when the woman has her menstrual period each month. In an attempt to insulate themselves from disappointment, couples with long-term infertility try not to expect too much with each cycle.

The couple may feel envious of those who conceive easily. They may become judgmental and angry when they see those who seem to "have no business having a baby," such as an adolescent, a woman who abuses drugs, or a woman who cannot support an added child.

Stress on the Relationship. Because infertility can challenge one's identity and self-esteem, the partners may find less satisfaction in their relationship. They may feel unlovable or unappealing to their mates.

The man may find it difficult to perform on demand for examinations that require him to ejaculate, feeling that others will judge his sexual function. The fact that semen samples are best obtained by masturbation is unacceptable to some men. Both partners are stressed when intercourse must be scheduled to coincide with specific evaluations or with ovulation. Intercourse can become a chore or a medical procedure more than an expression of love. It may come to be associated with failure rather than fulfillment.

If sperm from an anonymous donor is used for therapeutic insemination or other techniques, the man may feel that his masculinity is further threatened. He may have difficulty distinguishing fatherhood as a biologic achievement from fatherhood as a relationship.

The partners find their relationship strained if they disagree on which treatments are appropriate and how long they should be pursued. One partner may want to keep trying "one more month," and the other may want to abandon treatment. If they are considering adoption, their relationship may be strained if they differ on whether to adopt and what kind of child they are willing to accept.

Outcomes After Infertility Therapy

After infertility therapy, three outcomes are possible. Pregnancy may be achieved and then lost, causing mixed emotions of grief and optimism. The couple may become parents, either biologically or through adoption. The couple also may decide to remain childless after unsuccessful infertility therapy.

Pregnancy Loss After Infertility Therapy

Couples who suffer pregnancy loss after infertility therapy may interpret the experience with mixed feelings of loss and gain. Couples undergoing infertility evaluation and treatment are often aware of a pregnancy much earlier than fertile couples. They want to hope yet expect to be disappointed again. If a miscarriage or birth before fetal viability occurs, they may grieve profoundly for what they achieved and then lost.

Yet despite their grief about the pregnancy loss, the partners may be encouraged because they have proved that they can achieve a pregnancy. They may feel that if they succeeded once, they can do it again.

Parenthood After Infertility Therapy

Couples who conceive experience varied emotions. Pregnancy after infertility therapy is emotionally tentative for many infertile couples, especially those who have been trying to conceive for a long time or those who have lost a pregnancy. They may distance themselves from the pregnancy until late in gestation, emotionally "holding their breath" until the baby is born. The woman has grown accustomed to sensing and reporting every symptom and may interpret normal physiologic changes and discomforts of pregnancy as threatening.

The previously infertile couple may find little sympathy from those who do not understand why they are tentative about the pregnancy. Friends or family may be annoyed because they expect the couple to be overjoyed at a successful and apparently normal pregnancy. Outsiders may feel that the partners are self-centered and cannot decide what they want. Other infertile couples, who were previously a source of mutual support, may withdraw from the expectant couple.

The parents' anxiety may be heightened during labor. They are afraid that something will go wrong at the last moment. Even after the birth of a healthy infant, some parents have difficulty relaxing and enjoying their baby.

These new parents often need much nursing support as they gain experience with their child. Infertile couples who eventually have biologic or adopted children may have unrealistic expectations about parenting. After investing so much financial, physical, and emotional resources into having a child, they may be reluctant to express any unhappiness or frustration over the realities of childrearing.

Choosing to Adopt

Couples who consider adoption must confront their personal preferences, limitations, and biases. As much as they want a child, couples may not be willing to adopt *any* child. Most couples prefer to adopt a newborn or an infant of their race. Some prefer an infant but are also willing to adopt an older child, one with special needs, one of a mixed or different race, or a group of siblings. Other couples, for a variety of reasons, will not consider adopting these children. Couples, particularly older ones, may turn to foreign adoption because they are considered too old to be adoptive parents by most U.S. agencies.

Some couples fear adopting a child because the woman might become pregnant. Although pregnancy has been the goal for a long time, they may worry that they would love their adopted child differently from their biologic child.

Couples who decide to adopt face further scrutiny of their personal lives. Agencies investigate their home, financial means (which may be drained), and fitness as parents. Once again, they may feel that their personal competence is questioned. Their age also may limit their options.

The couple that decides on adoption may have emotions similar to those who achieve a pregnancy. They may be slow to invest in the process emotionally because they expect disappointment. In addition, the adopted child often comes to them suddenly and unexpectedly. Although they may have been waiting months for this happy event, they have little time to adjust to the reality that they are becoming parents.

■ NURSING CARE
The Infertile Couple

Nursing care of the infertile couple is challenging but can be most satisfying. Regardless of the clinical setting where the nurse encounters infertile couples, meeting the emotional needs associated with infertility evaluation, treatment, and outcomes of therapy is an important part of their care.

Assessment

Most infertile couples have previously had a positive self-image and feelings of competence about themselves. The diagnosis of infertility shakes their positive view. The nurse should be aware that these feelings may underlie their physical concerns.

Determine at what point the couple is in their infertility treatment. Couples who have just discovered that they may have difficulty conceiving may be shocked yet optimistic that therapy will result in a baby for them. Couples with long-standing infertility may have a deeper sense of failure and a pessimistic outlook. Listen for remarks that are negative, expressing guilt or helplessness.

Evaluate how infertility has affected the partners' relationships with each other. Are there conflicts or differences in their values? Observing their body language, such as eye contact, may provide clues about how similarly or differently they are committed to diagnosis and treatment. Ask them how their relationship has changed. Are they more or less satisfied with their marital relationship than they were before they had problems conceiving?

Ask about support systems. Couples suffering from infertility often withdraw from old relationships but do not form new supportive ones. Do others who are significant in the partners' lives know that they are trying to conceive? Are family members and friends nearby, and are they supportive? Have they encountered others' assumptions that infertility is the "fault" of one partner or the other? Are they subjected to questions that invade their privacy, such as, "When are you two going to have a baby of your own?"

Elicit information about how the couple's culture, religion, or personal values view infertility and the impact of these values on treatment. Are any therapies unacceptable to one or both partners?

Determine how the couple is coping with the stresses of treatment. How much has infertility cost them in time, money, and discomfort? Identify the successes and failures they have experienced. Their ages, especially the woman's, add another stressor that they cannot avoid.

If the woman is pregnant or has given birth recently or if the couple has adopted a child recently, observe for high levels of anxiety in either or both parents. Assess them for negative behaviors and comments, such as reluctance to feel joy or a sense that they will "fail" again.

Nursing Diagnosis and Planning

A nursing diagnosis commonly encountered is:

■ Situational Low Self-Esteem related to perception of reproductive inadequacy.

Expected Outcomes: The person(s) will express feelings about infertility and its evaluation and treatment, will explore ways to increase control within the situation of infertility, and will identify aspects of self that are positive. Expected outcomes may apply to the man, the woman, or both partners.

Interventions

Assisting Communication

Use a variety of communication techniques, such as active listening and exploration, to encourage the partners to express their feelings honestly, both as a couple and individually. Provide privacy and acceptance of their feelings.

Encourage the partners to accept their feelings, both positive and negative. For example, the couple that has finally achieved pregnancy may be living a lie to some extent. The partners may act elated because they believe they should feel happy yet inside feel cautious and hesitant to become attached to their baby. Explain that feelings are neither right nor wrong. It may be helpful to open the subject of negative feelings (fear of attachment) within a successful situation (pregnancy or birth) to reinforce the normality of their mixed emotions. This technique gives them the opportunity to talk about emotional reactions that they or others feel are inappropriate and might otherwise be reluctant to discuss.

Discuss possible differences in ways the man and the woman communicate. For example, explain that the woman may feel more comfortable than the man in talking about their problem and concerns about treatment. Explain that these differences in communication style can cause misunderstandings because one partner believes that the other does not care as much about their problem. Encourage them to be open with each other for the best mutual support.

Increasing the Couple's Sense of Control

Explore how the couple has dealt with stressors in the past and how these techniques might be used to cope with the present crisis. Reinforce positive coping skills, such as learning more about infertility and the proposed therapy for it.

Couples who experience undue stress may benefit from relaxation techniques, such as visualization and moderate exercise. Frequent strenuous exercise may reduce the woman's ability to ovulate. Although a hot tub is relaxing for many people, it should be avoided because the high temperatures may inhibit spermatogenesis. The woman also could become pregnant with any cycle, and high body temperature in early pregnancy has been associated with fetal anomalies.

Discuss behaviors that enhance the ability to handle stress and that provide a good environment for a pregnancy that might occur. Reinforce healthy choices, such as good nutrition and balance between exercise and rest. Teach the couple ways to enhance general health if deficiencies are identified.

Explain any procedures and their purpose in language that the couple can understand. Reinforce any medical explanations they have been given. Clarify information they may have obtained from outside sources such as the Internet. Encourage questions so that the couple is fully informed. Have the partners review teaching to reduce misunderstandings.

Help the couple explore options at each decision point. No one else can decide the best course of action, but the nurse can help identify pros and cons of each choice so that the partners can arrive at a decision appropriate for them. Be nondirective so that the choices are theirs and do not reflect the biases of the nurse or other caregivers.

Reducing Isolation

Because couples often distance themselves from friends and family relationships that they find painful, they may have few social supports. Refer them to available support groups to provide emotional outlets, a sense of belonging, and a source of information. Help them to identify ways they can improve communication with family and friends. Remind them that they have undergone significant shifts in self-image that have also affected those around them.

Promoting a Positive Self-Image

Explore with them areas of competence and activities that make them feel good about themselves. Reinforce positive attitudes and self-evaluations. Encourage them to maintain activities such as hobbies, sports, or volunteer work. The career of either partner may be a source of stress that needs relief, or it may be an avenue that fosters a positive self-perception.

Evaluation

- Did the partners express their feelings about their situation over a period of time?
- Did the partners explore ways to increase personal control over their lives and express feelings of reduced helplessness and dependence?
- Did the partners identify one or more aspects of self perceived as positive and identify areas of competence?

KEY CONCEPTS

- The nurse plays an important role in educating women about contraceptive techniques available and their correct use.
- In choosing the best contraceptive method for an individual woman, important issues include safety, protection from STDs, effectiveness, convenience, education needed, side effects, interference with spontaneity, availability, expense, preference, religious beliefs, and culture.
- Because some methods have potentially serious complications, written informed consent specific to the method may be necessary.
- Adolescents often have erroneous beliefs and incorrect information about contraception that increase their risk of pregnancy and STDs.
- Adolescents feel more comfortable talking about contraception with a nurse who has an accepting attitude, provides extra time for education, and uses understandable terms and audiovisual materials.
- Contraception is necessary to prevent pregnancy until menstruation has ceased for 2 years. The healthy perimenopausal woman who does not smoke or have contraindications can use any method of contraception safely.
- Sterilization offers permanent contraception. A tubal ligation can be performed soon after childbirth or at any time. Vasectomy is less expensive and can be performed in a physician's

office with the client under local anesthesia. Although surgery to reverse sterilization is possible, it is expensive and not always successful.
- Hormonal contraceptives include OCs, or the hormone injection, patches, or vaginal rings. Hormonal contraceptives inhibit ovulation and make the cervical mucus unreceptive to sperm. Side effects and complications make these unsuitable for some women.
- Intrauterine devices are very effective and safe in women with no risk of STDs. Women must learn how to check for the device's strings and when to seek medical treatment.
- Barrier methods may be chemical or mechanical. They kill sperm or prevent sperm from entering the cervix and provide some protection against STDs.
- Natural family-planning methods involve avoidance of coitus when physiologic cues suggest that ovulation is likely. They are acceptable to most religions but involve extensive education and high motivation and have a high risk of pregnancy should error occur.
- Up to 20% of infertile couples have no identified problem explained by current evaluation techniques.
- Because of the many unknown factors in reproduction, identification and correction of problems in one or both partners do not necessarily resolve their infertility.

- A variety of structural and functional abnormalities may contribute to a couple's infertility. The man may have abnormalities of the sperm or of the seminal fluid or with ejaculation. The woman may have ovulation disorders, anatomic problems such as fallopian tube occlusion, or physiologic disorders such as hormone imbalances.
- A systematic evaluation of both partners, proceeding from simple to complex, identifies therapy most likely to be successful and cost effective. The couple may decide to stop evaluation or therapy at any point.
- Infertility is a crisis for the couple and often for the extended family. Either or both partners may feel that the inability to conceive represents a personal failure.
- Infertile couples must make choices at many points before and during evaluation and therapy. Some major factors that enter into their decisions involve social, cultural, and religious values; difficulty of treatment; probability of success; financial resources; and age, particularly the woman's.
- The possible outcomes after infertility therapy may present new challenges to the partners and their families: unsuccessful therapy and the choice of whether to pursue adoption, pregnancy loss after infertility, and parenthood after infertility.

ANSWER to Critical Thinking Exercise 10-1

Find a private place to talk without interruption. Use therapeutic communication to explore this girl's feelings further. Help her think through the ways a pregnancy might change her life and how she would feel about those changes. Discuss what happens when a woman is examined during a visit for contraceptive counseling. Explore what she feels would be most embarrassing about seeing a health care provider. Would a female care provider be more acceptable? Some providers will prescribe contraceptives for a healthy woman without requiring a pelvic examination on the first visit. Discuss common contraceptive methods, and determine her understanding and concerns about them. Also discuss negotiation skills for condom use, because condoms are important for prevention of STDs as well as pregnancy. Try role-playing, with the adolescent acting the role of her partner and the nurse taking the role of the adolescent.

REFERENCES and READINGS

Alper, M.M. (2002). Improving and facilitating the delivery of care to patients undergoing in vitro fertilization. *Infertility and Reproductive Medicine Clinics, 13*(3), 431-436.

American Society for Reproductive Medicine. (2000). *Practice committee report: Optimal evaluation of the infertile female.* Retrieved July 27, 2003, from www.asrm.org/Media/Practice/eval_infertile_female.pdf.

American Society for Reproductive Medicine. (2000). *Practice committee report: Repetitive oocyte donation.* Retrieved August 19, 2003, from www.asrm.org/Media/Practice/oocyte_donation.pdf.

American Society for Reproductive Medicine. (2001a). *Patient's fact sheet: Diagnostic testing for male factor infertility.* Retrieved August 2, 2003, from www.asrm.org/Patients/FactSheets/Testing_Male-Fact.pdf.

American Society for Reproductive Medicine. (2001b). *Patient's fact sheet: Intracytoplasmic sperm injection (ICSI).* Retrieved August 2, 2003, from www.asrm.org/Patients/FactSheets/ICSI-Fact.pdf.

American Society for Reproductive Medicine. (2001c). *Practice committee report: Preimplantation genetic diagnosis.* Retrieved August 1, 2003, from www.asrm.org/Media/Practice/preimplantation.pdf.

American Society for Reproductive Medicine. (2002). *Practice committee report: Aging and infertility in women.* Retrieved July 27, 2003, from www.asrm.org/Media/Practice/ageandinfertility.pdf.

American Society for Reproductive Medicine. (2000-2003a). *Frequently-asked questions about infertility.* Retrieved July 27, 2003, from www.asrm.org?patients/faqs.html.

American Society for Reproductive Medicine. (2000-2003b). *Fact sheet: In vitro fertilization (IVF).* Retrieved August 2, 2003, from www.asrm.org/Patients/FactSheets/invitro.html.

Angard, N.T. (1999). Diagnosis: Infertility. *AWHONN Lifelines, 3*(3), 22-29.

Aytekin, N.T., Pala, K., Irgil, E., & Aytekin, H. (2001). Family planning choices and some characteristics of coitus interruptus users in Gemlik, Turkey. *Women's Health Issues, 11*(5), 442-447.

Balen, A.H., & Jacobs, H.S. (2003). *Infertility in practice* (2nd ed.). Edinburgh: Churchill-Livingstone.

Blackburn, S.T. (2003). *Maternal, fetal, & neonatal physiology: A clinical perspective.* Philadelphia: Saunders.

Borenstein, J., Yu, H., Wade, S., Chiou, C., & Rapkin, A. (2003). Effect of an oral contraceptive containing ethinyl estradiol and drospirenone on premenstrual symptomatology and health-related quality of life. *Journal of Reproductive Medicine, 48*(2), 79-85.

Bowes, W.A., & Katz, V.L. (2002). Postpartum care. In Gabbe, S.G., Niebyl, J.R., & Simpson, J.L. (Eds.). *Obstetrics: normal and problem pregnancies* (4th ed., pp 701-726). New York: Churchill Livingstone.

Carcio, H.A. (1998). *Management of the infertile woman.* Philadelphia: Lippincott.

Centers for Disease Control and Prevention. (2002). *Assisted reproductive technology reports: 2000 assisted reproductive technology success rates.* Retrieved August 2, 2003, from www.cdc.gov/nccdphp/drh/ART00/index.htm.

Chantilis, S.J., & Carr, B.R. (2000). Infertility. In E.J. Quilligan &F.P. Zuspan (Eds.). *Current therapy in obstetrics and gynecology* (5th ed., pp. 83-90). Philadelphia: Saunders.

Creasy, G.W., Fisher, A.C., Hall, N, & Shangold, G.A. (2003). Transdermal contraceptive patch delivering norelgestromin and ethinyl estradiol effects on the lipid profile. *Journal of Reproductive Medicine, 48*(3), 179-186.

Cunningham, F.G., Gant, N.F., Leveno, K.J., Gilstrap, L.C., Hauth, J.C., & Wenstrom, K.D. (2001). *Williams obstetrics* (21st ed.). New York: McGraw-Hill.

Daly, D.C. (2000). Induction of ovulation. In E.J. Quilligan & F.P. Zuspan (Eds.). *Current therapy in obstetrics and gynecology* (5th ed., pp. 80-83). Philadelphia: Saunders.

Dardano, K., & Burkman, R.T. (2002). The contraceptive and noncontraceptive health benefits of oral contraceptives: An update. In S.B. Ransom, M.P. Donbrowski, M.I. Evans, & K.A. Ginsburg (Eds.). *Contemporary therapy in obstetrics and gynecology* (pp. 349-353). Philadelphia: Saunders.

Devine, K.S. (2003). Caring for the infertile woman. *MCN: American Journal of Maternal-Child Nursing, 28*(2), 100-105.

Dieben, T.O.M., Roumen, F.J.M.E., & Apter, D. (2002). Efficacy, cycle control, and user acceptability of a novel combined contraceptive vaginal ring. *Obstetrics & Gynecology, 100*(3), 585-593.

Flynn, D.M., Clark, J.B., & Hume, R.F. (2002). Unintended pregnancy. In S.B. Ransom, M.P. Donbrowski, M.I. Evans, & K.A. Ginsburg (Eds.). *Contemporary therapy in obstetrics and gynecology* (pp. 157-163). Philadelphia: Saunders.

Garcia, F.A.R,. & Huggins, G.R. (2002). Emergent postcoital contraception. In S.B. Ransom, M.P. Donbrowski, M.I. Evans, & K.A. Ginsburg (Eds.). *Contemporary therapy in obstetrics and gynecology* (pp. 359-361). Philadelphia: Saunders.

Gold, C., Nardontonia, T., & Condon, M.C. (2004). Gynecological wellness and illness. In M.C. Condon. *Women's health: Body, mind, spirit* (pp. 319-364). Upper Saddle River, NJ: Prentice Hall.

Grady, W.R., Billy, J.O.G., & Kepinger, D.H. (2002). Contraceptive method switching in the United States. *Perspectives on Sexual and Reproductive Health, 34*(3), 135-145.

Grimes, D.A. (2000). Updates in contraception from the XVI World Congress of the International Federation of Gynecology and Obstetrics, Washington DC. *Medscape Women's Health, 5*(5).

Gutman, J.N., & Braverman, A.M. (2002). What's in a name? The evolution of gestational surrogacy. *Infertility and Reproductive Medicine Clinics of North America, 13*(3), 595-613.

Guyton, A.C., & Hall, J.E. (2000). *Textbook of medical physiology* (10th ed.). Philadelphia: Saunders.

Haken, V. (2000). Interactions between drugs and nutrients. In L.K. Mahan & S. Escott-Stump. *Krause's food, nutrition, and diet therapy* (10th ed.). Philadelphia: Saunders.

Hatcher, R.A., & Guillebaud, J. (1998). The pill: Combined oral contraceptives. In R.A. Hatcher, J. Trussell, F. Stewart, W. Cates, G.K. Stewart, F. Guest, & D. Kowal. *Contraceptive technology* (17th ed., pp. 405-466). New York: Ardent Media.

Hatcher, R.A., Trussell, J., Stewart, F., Cates, W., Stewart, G.K., Guest, F., & Kowal, D. (1998). *Contraceptive technology* (17th ed.). New York: Ardent Media.

Holt, V.L., Cushing-Haugen, K.L., & Daling, J.R. (2002). Body weight and risk of oral contraceptive failure. *Obstetrics & Gynecology, 99*(5), 820-827.

Hutti, M.H. (2003). New and emerging contraceptive methods. *AWHONN Lifelines, 7*(1), 34-39.

Johnson, Julia. (2003). Infertility. In J.R. Scott, R.S. Gibbs, B.Y. Karlan, and A.F. Haney (Eds.), *Danforth's obstetrics and gynecology* (9th ed., pp. 685-695). Philadelphia: Lippincott.

Jones, G.S. (2000). Luteal phase defect. In E.J. Quilligan & F.P. Zuspan (Eds.). *Current therapy in obstetrics and gynecology* (5th ed., pp. 101-104). Philadelphia: Saunders.

Jones, M.E., Bond, M.L., Garnner, S.H., & Hernandez, M.C. (2002). A call to action: Acculturation level and family-planning patterns of Hispanic immigrant women. *MCN: American Journal of Maternal-Child Nursing, 27*(1), 26-32.

Katz, A. (2002). "Where I come from, we don't talk about that." *AWHONN Lifelines, 6*(6), 533-536.

Kaunitz, A.M. (2001). Choosing an injectable contraceptive. *Contemporary OB/GYN, 46*(6), 29-46.

Kelly, P.J., & Morgan-Kidd, J. (2001). Social influences on the sexual behaviors of adolescent girls in at-risk circumstances. *Journal of Obstetric, Gynecologic, and Neonatal Nursing, 30*(5), 481-489.

Leibowitz, D. & Hoffman, J. (2000). Fertility drug therapies: Past, present, and future. *Journal of Obstetric, Gynecologic, and Neonatal Nursing, (29)*2, 201-210.

Lindberg, C.E. (2003). Emergency contraception for prevention of adolescent pregnancy. *MCN: American Journal of Maternal-Child Nursing, 28*(3), 199-204.

MacKay, A.P., Fingerhut, L.A., & Duran, C.R. (2000). *Adolescent health chartbook, Health, United States, 2000.* Hyattsville, MD: National Center for Health Statistics.

Maifeld, M., Hahn, S., Titler, M.G., and Mullen, M. (2003). Decision making regarding multifetal reduction. *Journal of Obstetric, Gynecologic, and Neonatal Nursing, 32*(3), 357-369.

March of Dimes Birth Defects Foundation. (2003). *Perinatal profiles, 2003: United States.* Retrieved April 13, 2003, from the World Wide Web: http://peristats.modimes.org/ataglance/us.pdf.

Marions, L., Hultenby, K. Lindell, I., Sun, X., Stabi, B., & Danielsson, K.G. (2002). Emergency contraception with mifepristone and levonorgestrel: Mechanism of action. *Obstetrics & Gynecology, 100*(1), 65-71.

Moos, M.K. (2003). Unintended pregnancies: A call for nursing action. *MCN: American Journal of Maternal-Child Nursing, 28*(1), 24-30.

Murphy, P.A. (2003). New methods of hormonal contraception. *Nurse Practitioner, 28*(2), 11-21.

Ott, M.A., Adler, N.E., Millstein, S.G., Tschann, J.M., & Ellen, J.M. (2002). The trade-off between hormonal contraceptives and condoms among adolescents, *Perspectives on Sexual and Reproductive Health, 34*(1), 6-14.

Patrizio, P. (2000). Male infertility: Intrauterine insemination. In E.J. Quilligan & F.P. Zuspan (Eds.). *Current therapy in obstetrics and gynecology* (5th ed., pp. 104-107). Philadelphia: Saunders.

Patrizio, P. (2000). Microsurgical and percutaneous epididymal sperm aspiration. In E.J. Quilligan & F.P. Zuspan (Eds.). *Current therapy in obstetrics and gynecology* (5th ed., pp. 113-115). Philadelphia: Saunders.

Patrizio, P., & Khorram, O. (2000). GIFT procedure. In E.J. Quilligan & F.P. Zuspan (Eds.). *Current therapy in obstetrics and gynecology* (5th ed., pp. 64-66). Philadelphia: Saunders.

Paukku, M., Quan, J., Darney, P., & Raine, T. (2003). Adolescents' contraceptive use and pregnancy history. Is there a pattern? *Obstetrics & Gynecology, 101*(3), 534-538.

Penzias, A.S. (2002). Oocyte donation, 2002. *Infertility and Reproductive Medicine Clinics of North America, 13*(3), 587-594.

Peterson, R., Gazmararian, J.A., Clark, K.A., & Green, D.C. (2001). How contraceptive use patterns differ by pregnancy intention: Implications for counseling. *Women's Health Issues, 11*(5), 427-435.

Postlethwaite, D. (2003). Preconception health counseling for women exposed to teratogens: The role of the nurse. *Journal of Obstetric, Gynecologic, and Neonatal Nursing, (32)*4, 523-532.

Richard-Davis, G. (2002). Ovulation induction for in vitro fertilization: The role of gonadotropin-releasing hormone antagonists. *Infertility and Reproductive Medicine Clinics of North America, 13*(3), 437-444.

Richlin, S.S., Shanti, A., & Murphy, A.A. (2003). Assisted reproductive technology. In J.R. Scott, R.S. Gibbs, B.Y. Karlan, & A.F. Haney (Eds.). *Danforth's obstetrics and gynecology* (9th ed., pp. 697-712). Philadelphia: Lippincott.

Schnare, S.M. (2002). Progestin contraceptives. *Journal of Midwifery & Women's Health, 47*(3), 157-166.

Siebert, C., Barbouche, E., & Fagan, J. (2003). Prescribing oral contraceptives for women older than 35 years of age (Electronic version). *Annals of Internal Medicine, 138*(1), 54-64.

Speroff, L., & Darney, P.D. (2001). *A clinical guide for contraception* (3rd ed.). Philadelphia: Lippincott Williams & Wilkins.

Thornton, K.L. (2002). Recombinant gonadotropins and IVF. *Infertility and Reproductive Medicine Clinics of North America, 13*(3), 445-458.

Tinkle, M., Reifsnider, E., & Ransom, S.P. (December 2001/January 2002). A quality assurance problem: Why women quit using Depo-Provera. *AWHONN Lifelines, 5*(6), 36-41.

Trussell, J., & Vaughan, B. (1999). Contraceptive failure, method-related discontinuation and resumption of use: Results from the 1995 national survey of family growth. *Family Planning Perspectives, 31*(2), 64-72, 93.

Upchurch, D.M., Kusunoki, Y., Simon, P., & Doty, M.M. (2003). Sexual behavior and condom practices among Los Angeles women. *Women's Health Issues, 13*(1), 8-15.

U.S. Department of Health and Human Services. (2000). *Healthy people 2010: Healthy People 2010* (Conference edition, in 2 volumes). Washington, DC.

U.S. Food and Drug Administration. (2003). FDA talk paper T03-63: *FDA approves new drug for treatment of erectile dysfunction in men.* Retrieved August 22, 2003, from www.fda.gov/bbs/topics/ANSWERS/2003/ANS01249.html.

Van Devanter, N., Gonzales, V., Merzel, C., Parikh, N., Celantano, D., & Greenberg, J. (2002). Effect of an STD-HIV behavioral intervention on women's use of the female condom. *American Journal of Public Health, 92*(1), 109-115.

Villarruel, A.M., & Rodriguez, D. (2003). Beyond stereotypes: Promoting safer sex behaviors among Latino adolescents. *Journal of Obstetric, Gynecologic, and Neonatal Nursing, 32*(2), 258-263.

Weisman, C.S., Maccannon, D.S., Henderson, J.T., Shortridge, E., & Orso, C.L. (2002). Contraceptive counseling in managed care: Preventing unintended pregnancy in adults. *Women's Health Issues, 12*(2), 79-95.

11

Reproductive Anatomy and Physiology

◆ LEARNING OBJECTIVES

After studying this chapter, you should be able to:

◎ Explain female and male sexual development from prenatal life through sexual maturity.

◎ Describe normal anatomy of the female and male reproductive systems.

◎ Explain normal function of the female and male reproductive systems.

◎ Explain normal structure and function of the female breast.

◆ DEFINITIONS

amenorrhea Absence of menstruation. Primary amenorrhea is a delay of the first menstruation. Secondary amenorrhea is cessation of menstruation after its initiation.

cilia Hairlike processes on the surface of a cell. Cilia beat rhythmically to move the cell or to move fluid or other substances over the cell surface.

climacteric Physical and emotional changes occurring at the end of a woman's reproductive period. Also informally called menopause although this term does not encompass all changes.

coitus Sexual union between a male and a female.

fornix (pl. fornices) An arch or pouchlike structure at the upper end of the vagina. Also called a cul-de-sac.

gamete Reproductive cell: in the female an ovum, and in the male a spermatozoon.

genetic sex Sex determined at conception by union of two X chromosomes (female) or an X and a Y chromosome (male). Also called chromosomal sex.

gonad Reproductive (sex) gland that produces gametes and sex hormones. The female gonads are ovaries; the male gonads are testes.

gonadotropic hormones Secretions of the anterior pituitary gland that stimulate the gonads, specifically follicle-stimulating hormone and luteinizing hormone. Chorionic gonadotropin is secreted by the placenta during pregnancy.

graafian follicle A small sac within the ovary that contains the maturing ovum.

menarche Onset of menstruation.

menopause Permanent cessation of menstruation during the climacteric.

puberty Period of sexual maturation accompanied by the development of secondary sex characteristics and the capacity to reproduce.

ruga (pl. rugae) Ridge or fold of tissue, as on the male's scrotum and in the female's vagina.

secondary sex characteristics Physical differences between mature males and females that are not directly related to reproduction.

somatic sex Gender assignment as male or female on the basis of form and structure of the external genitalia.

spermatogenesis Formation of male gametes (sperm) in the testes.

spinnbarkeit Clear, slippery, stretchy quality of cervical mucus during ovulation.

This chapter reviews basic prenatal development, sexual maturation, and structure and function of both female and male reproductive systems.

SEXUAL DEVELOPMENT

Sexual development begins at conception, when the genetic sex is determined by union of an ovum and a sperm. During childhood, the sex organs are quiet.

Prenatal Development

The mother's ovum carries a single X chromosome. Each of the father's spermatozoa carries either an X chromosome or a Y chromosome. If an X-bearing spermatozoon fertilizes the ovum, the offspring's genetic sex is female. If a Y-bearing spermatozoon fertilizes the ovum, a male offspring results.

Although genetic sex is determined at conception, the reproductive system of both males and females is similar, or sexually undifferentiated, for the first 6 weeks of prenatal life. During the seventh week, differences between males and females appear in the internal structures. The external genitalia look similar until the ninth week, when these outer structures begin to change. Differentiation of the external sexual organs is complete at about 12 weeks.

During fetal life, both ovaries and testes secrete their primary hormones, estrogen and testosterone, respectively. Testosterone causes development of male sex organs and external genitalia, and its absence results in development of female sex characteristics. Although estrogen is secreted by the fetal ovary, this hormone is not required to initiate development of female sex structures. The trend for prenatal sexual development is to have female structures unless a Y chromosome is present.

Childhood

The sex glands of both girls and boys are inactive during infancy and childhood. At sexual maturity, the hypothalamus stimulates the anterior pituitary gland to produce hormones that will stimulate sex hormone production by the gonads.

Sexual Maturation

Puberty refers to the time during which the reproductive organs become fully functional. Puberty is not a single event but a series of changes occurring over several years during late childhood and early adolescence.

Initiation of Sexual Maturation

Some factors that initiate sexual maturation remain unknown. Secretions of the hypothalamus, the anterior pituitary, and the gonads all play a part. The hypothalamus is capable of secreting gonadotropin-releasing hormone (GnRH) to initiate puberty during infancy and early childhood, but it does not do so in significant amounts until late childhood. Production of even tiny quantities of sex hormones by the young child's ovaries or testes inhibits secretions of the hypothalamus, avoiding premature onset of puberty. Maturation of another unknown brain area probably triggers the hypothalamus to initiate puberty (Guyton & Hall, 2000).

The maturing child's hypothalamus gradually increases production of GnRH beginning at 9 to 12 years of age (Blackburn, 2003; Guyton & Hall, 2000). The level of GnRH increases slowly until it is adequate to stimulate the anterior pituitary to increase its production of follicle-stimulating hormone (FSH) and luteinizing hormone (LH). The ovaries and testes increase production of sex hormones and begin maturing gametes in response to higher levels of FSH and LH. The sex hormones also induce development of secondary sex characteristics. Table 11-1 presents the major hormones that play a role in reproduction.

There is individual variation in the age at which the changes of puberty begin and in the time required to complete these changes. Nutritional state can influence the start of puberty, with the well-nourished child having an earlier onset. Girls are about 6 months to 1 year younger than boys when hormonal changes of puberty begin, although the girl's growth spurt early in puberty makes it seem that she begins puberty about 2 years before boys of the same age. Changes of puberty occur in an orderly sequence in both sexes. Increases in height and weight are dramatic during puberty but slow after puberty until the mature height and weight are attained. Box 11-1 lists secondary sex

characteristics of males and females. (See Chapter 8 for detailed information about the changes of puberty.)

Female Puberty Changes

As the girl matures, the anterior pituitary gland secretes increasing amounts of FSH and LH in response to the hypothalamic secretion of GnRH. These pituitary secretions stimulate secretion of estrogens and progesterone by the ovary, resulting in maturation of the reproductive organs and breasts and in development of secondary sex characteristics such as axillary and pubic hair. The first noticeable changes of puberty begin at about 8 to 13 years in girls, with the development of breast buds. The first menstrual period occurs 2 to $2^1/_2$ years later, with an average range from 9 to 16 years (Needlman, 2000).

Breast Changes. The earliest outward changes of puberty occur in the breasts. First, the nipple enlarges and protrudes. The areola surrounding the nipple enlarges and becomes somewhat protuberant, although less so than the nipple. These changes are followed by growth of the glandular and ductal tissue. Fat is deposited in the breasts. During puberty, a girl's breasts may develop at different rates, resulting in a lopsided appearance.

Body Contours. The pelvis widens and assumes a rounded, basinlike shape that is favorable for passage of the fetus during childbirth. Fat is deposited selectively in the hips, giving them a rounder appearance than those of the male.

Body Hair. Pubic hair appears downy at first but becomes thicker as puberty progresses. Axillary hair appears near the time of menarche. The texture and quantity of pubic and axillary hair vary among women and in different ethnic groups. Women of African descent usually have body hair that is coarser and curlier than that of white women. Asian women often have sparser body hair than women of other racial groups.

Skeletal Growth. In response to estrogen stimulation, the girl grows taller for several years during early puberty. The growth spurt begins about 1 year after initial breast development. Estrogen's other powerful effect on the skeleton is to cause the epiphyses (growth areas of the bone) to unite with the shaft of the bones; this development eventually stops growth in height.

Reproductive Organs. The girl's external genitalia enlarge as fat is deposited in the mons pubis, labia majora, and labia minora. The vagina, uterus, fallopian tubes, and ovaries grow larger. Vaginal mucosa changes, becoming more resistant to trauma and infection in preparation for sexual activity. Cyclic changes in the reproductive organs occur during each female reproductive cycle.

Menarche. Early menstrual periods are often irregular and scant. Early menstrual cycles are not usually fertile because ovulation occurs inconsistently. Fertile reproductive cycles require preparation of the uterine lining precisely timed with ovulation. Ovulation may occur during any female reproductive cycle, however, including the first. The sexually active girl can conceive even before her first menstrual period.

Delayed onset of menstruation is called *primary amenorrhea* if the girl's periods have not begun by the age of 16 years. It may also be considered if the girl is more than 1 year older than her mother or sisters were when their menarche occurred. *Secondary amenorrhea* describes absence of menstruation for at least three cycles after regular cycles have been es-

TABLE 11-1 Major Hormones in Reproduction

Produced by	Target Organs	Action in Female	Action in Male
GONADOTROPIN-RELEASING HORMONE (GNRH)			
Hypothalamus	Anterior pituitary	Stimulates release of FSH and LH, initiating puberty and sustaining female reproductive cycles; release is pulsatile	Stimulates release of FSH and LH, initiating puberty; release is pulsatile
FOLLICLE-STIMULATING HORMONE (FSH)			
Anterior pituitary	Ovaries (female) Testes (male)	1. Stimulates final maturation of follicle 2. Stimulates growth and maturation of graafian follicles before ovulation	Stimulates Leydig cells of testes to secrete testosterone
LUTEINIZING HORMONE (LH)			
Anterior pituitary	Ovaries (female) Testes (male)	1. Stimulates final maturation of follicle 2. Surge of LH about 14 days before next menstrual period causes ovulation 3. Stimulates transformation of graafian follicle into corpus luteum, which continues secretion of estrogens and progesterone for about 12 days if ovum is not fertilized. If fertilization occurs, placenta gradually assumes this function	Stimulates Leydig cells of testes to secrete testosterone
ESTROGENS			
1. Ovaries and corpus luteum (female) 2. Placenta (pregnancy) 3. Formed in small quantities from testosterone in Sertoli cells of testes (male); other tissues, especially the liver, produce estrogen in the male	Internal and external reproductive organs; Breasts (female) Testes (male)	1. Reproductive organs a. Maturation at puberty b. Stimulation of endometrium before ovulation 2. Breasts: induce growth of glandular and ductal tissue; initiate deposition of fat at puberty 3. Stimulate growth of long bones but cause closure of epiphyses, limiting mature height 4. Pregnancy: stimulate growth of uterus, breast tissue; inhibit active milk production; relax pelvic ligaments	Necessary for normal sperm formation

---

BOX 11-1
Comparison of Secondary Sex Characteristics in Females and Males

Females	Males
Development of glandular and ductal systems in the breast; deposition of fat selectively in the breast, buttocks, and thighs	Muscle mass 50% greater
Wide, round pelvis	Narrow, upright, and heavier pelvis
Pubic and axillary hair	Pubic and axillary hair; facial and chest hair; increased amount of hair on upper back in some males; male-pattern baldness, beginning on top of head
Soft, smooth skin texture	Coarser skin
Higher-pitched voice	Deeper voice

tablished. Both primary and secondary amenorrhea are more common in females who are thin because they may have too little fat to produce enough sex hormones to stimulate ovulation and menstruation. Pregnancy is a common cause of secondary amenorrhea as well.

Male Puberty Changes

Secretion of GnRH by the hypothalamus begins increasing as the boy enters puberty, stimulating secretion of LH and FSH from the anterior pituitary. LH and FSH then stimulate secretion of testosterone and eventually spermatogenesis. Testosterone stimulates development of a boy's reproductive organs and secondary sex characteristics.

Growth of the Testes and Penis. The first outward evidence of male sexual maturation is growth of the testes between about 9½ and 17 years. Growth in circumference and lengthening of the penis follow about a year after testicular growth begins. The skin of the scrotum thins and darkens.

Nocturnal Emissions. Often called "wet dreams," nocturnal emissions are common during adolescence. The boy experiences a spontaneous ejaculation of seminal fluid during

TABLE **11-1** Major Hormones in Reproduction—cont'd

Produced by	Target Organs	Action in Female	Action in Male
PROGESTERONE			
Ovary, corpus luteum, placenta	Uterus, female breasts	1. Stimulates secretion of endometrial glands; causes endometrial vessels to become dilated and tortuous in preparation for possible embryo implantation 2. Pregnancy: induces growth of cells of fallopian tubes and uterine lining to nourish embryo; decreases contractions of uterus; prepares breasts for lactation but inhibits prolactin secretion	Not applicable
PROLACTIN			
Anterior pituitary	Female breasts	Stimulates secretion of milk (lactogenesis); estrogen and progesterone from placenta have an inhibiting effect on milk production until after placenta is expelled at birth; sucking of newborn stimulates prolactin secretion to maintain milk production	Not applicable
OXYTOCIN			
Posterior pituitary	Uterus, female breasts	1. Uterus; stimulates contractions during birth and stimulates postpartum contractions to compress uterine vessels and control bleeding 2. Stimulates let-down, or milk-ejection reflex during breastfeeding	Not applicable
TESTOSTERONE			
Adrenal glands (female) Ovaries (female)	Sexual organs (male) Male body conformation after puberty	Small quantities of androgenic (masculinizing) hormones from adrenal glands cause growth of pubic and axillary hair at puberty Most androgens, such as testosterone, are converted to estrogen	1. Induces development of male sex organs in fetus 2. Induces growth and division of the cells that mature sperm 3. Induces development of male secondary sex characteristics

sleep, often accompanied by dreams with sexual content. Boys should be prepared for this normal occurrence so that they do not feel abnormal or ashamed.

Body Hair. Pubic hair growth begins at the base of the penis. Gradually the hair coarsens and spreads upward and in the midline of the abdomen. About 2 years later, axillary hair appears. Facial hair begins as a fine, downy mustache and progresses to the characteristic beard of the adult male. In most boys, chest hair develops, and some have hair on their upper backs. The amount and character of body hair vary among men of different racial groups, with Asian and Native American men often having less than white or African men.

Body Composition. Testosterone causes the male to develop a greater muscle mass than the female. At maturity, the man's muscle mass exceeds the woman's by 50%.

Skeletal Growth. Testosterone causes boys to undergo a rapid growth spurt, especially in height. A boy's linear growth begins about a year later than a girl's and lasts for a longer time, resulting in the male's greater average height at maturity. Testosterone causes union of the epiphysis with the shaft of long bones, as does estrogen. The height-limiting effect of testosterone in the male is not as strong as that of estrogen in the female, so boys grow in stature for several years more than girls.

A boy's shoulders broaden as his height increases. His pelvis assumes an upright shape, with a narrower diameter and heavier structure than the female's.

Voice Changes. Hypertrophy of the laryngeal mucosa and enlargement of the larynx cause the male's voice to deepen. Before reaching the lower-pitched voice at maturity, many boys experience "cracking" or "squeaking" of their voices when they speak.

Decline in Fertility

A woman's ability to reproduce decreases over a period of years, called the *climacteric*. In most women, the climacteric occurs between the ages of 45 and 50. At this time, maturation of ova and production of ovarian hormones decline. The external and internal reproductive organs atrophy somewhat as well. *Menopause* is the term used to describe the final menstrual period. Menopause and climacteric, however, are often

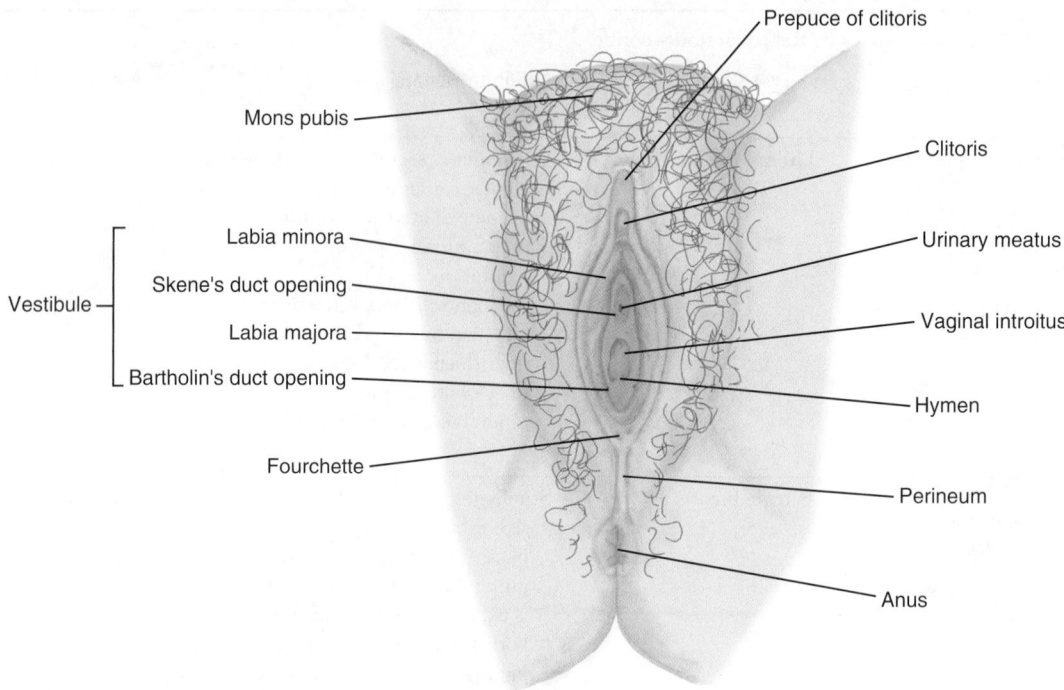

Figure 11-1 External female reproductive structures.

used interchangeably to describe the entire gradual process of change. *Perimenopause* is the time from onset of symptoms associated with the climacteric until at least 1 year after the last menstrual period.

Males do not experience a marker event like menopause. Their production of testosterone and sperm gradually declines, but men in their 50s, 60s, and beyond may still be able to father children.

FEMALE REPRODUCTIVE ANATOMY

External Female Reproductive Organs

Collectively, the external female reproductive organs are called the *vulva* (Fig. 11-1).

Mons Pubis
The mons pubis is the rounded, fleshy prominence over the symphysis pubis that forms the anterior border of the external reproductive organs. It is covered with varying amounts of pubic hair.

Labia Majora and Labia Minora
The labia majora are two rounded, fleshy folds of tissue that extend from the mons pubis to the perineum. They have a slightly deeper pigmentation than surrounding skin and are covered with pubic hair. The labia majora protect the more fragile tissues of the external genitalia.

The labia minora run parallel to and within the labia majora. The labia minora extend from the clitoris anteriorly and merge posteriorly to form the fourchette, or posterior rim of the vaginal introitus. The labia minora do not have pubic hair. They are highly vascular and respond to stimulation by becoming engorged with blood.

Clitoris
The clitoris is a small projection at the anterior junction of the labia minora. The clitoris is composed of highly sensitive erectile tissue that is similar to tissue of the penis. The labia majora merge to form a prepuce over the clitoris.

Vestibule
The vestibule refers to structures enclosed by the labia minora. The urinary meatus, vaginal introitus, and ducts of Skene and Bartholin glands lie within the vestibule. Skene, or periurethral, glands provide lubrication for the urethra. Bartholin glands provide lubrication for the vaginal introitus, particularly during sexual arousal. The vaginal introitus is surrounded by erectile tissue. During sexual stimulation, blood flows into the erectile tissue, allowing the introitus to tighten around the penis. This process adds a massaging feeling that heightens the male's sexual sensations, encouraging release of semen.

The hymen is a thin fold of mucosa partially separating the vagina from the vestibule. The hymen may be broken with injury, with the use of tampons, during intercourse, or during childbirth. The intactness, or lack thereof, of the hymen is not a criterion of virginity.

Perineum
The perineum is the most posterior part of the external female reproductive organs. It extends from the fourchette anteriorly to the anus posteriorly and is composed of fibrous and muscular tissues that support pelvic structures.

Internal Female Reproductive Organs

The internal reproductive structures are the vagina, uterus, fallopian tubes, and ovaries (Figs. 11-2 and 11-3).

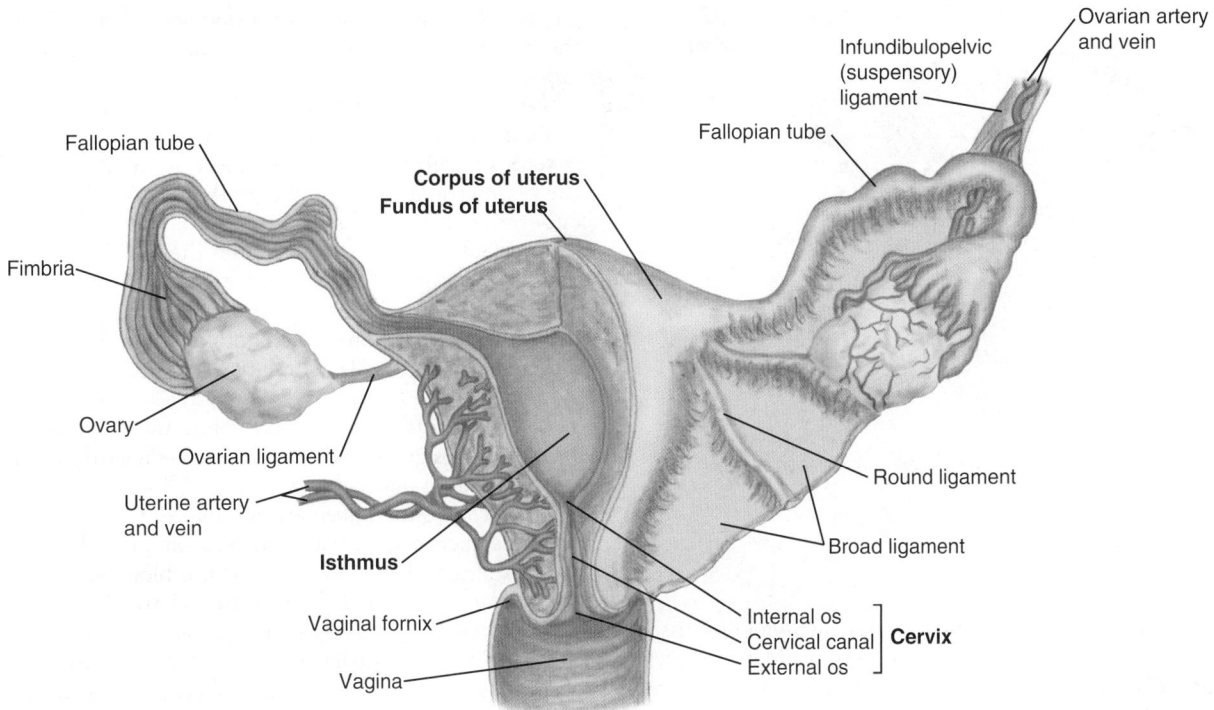

Figure 11-2 Internal female reproductive structures, *anterior view.*

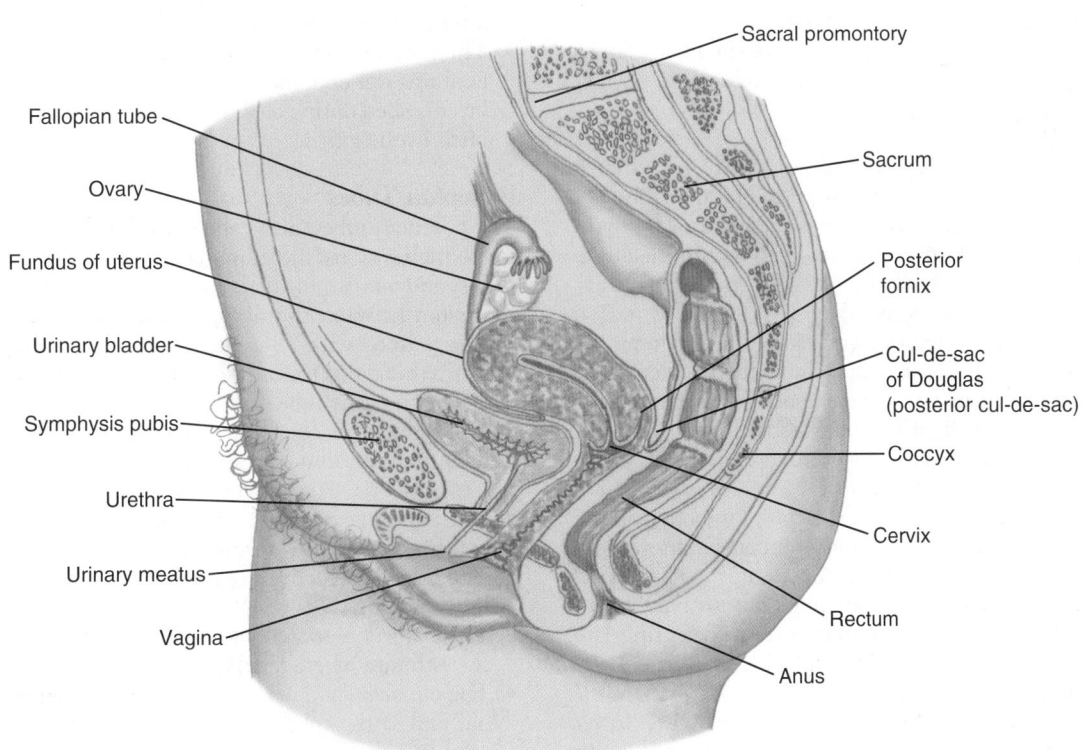

Figure 11-3 Internal female reproductive structures, *midsagittal view.*

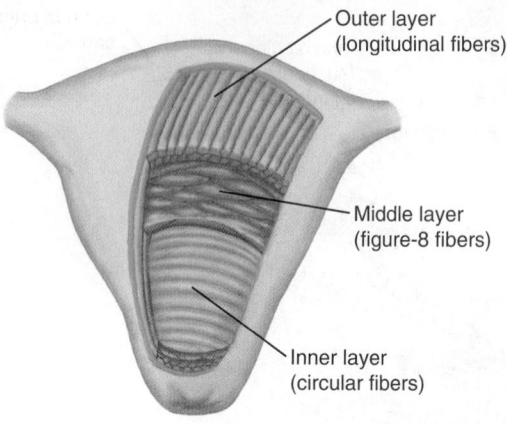

Figure 11-4 Layers of the myometrium, showing the three types of smooth muscle fiber.

Vagina

The vagina is a tube of muscular and membranous tissue about 8 to 10 cm long, lying between the bladder anteriorly and the rectum posteriorly. The vagina connects the uterus above with the vestibule below. The vaginal lining has multiple folds, or rugae, and a muscular layer that are capable of marked distention during childbirth. The vagina is lubricated by secretions of the cervix, the lowermost part of the uterus, and by the Bartholin glands.

The vagina does not end abruptly at the uterine opening but arches to form the vaginal fornix. Each fornix is described by its location: anterior, posterior, or lateral.

The three major functions of the vagina are:

- To allow discharge of the menstrual flow
- As the female organ of coitus, to receive the male penis
- To allow passage of the fetus from the uterus

Uterus

The uterus is a hollow, thick-walled, muscular organ that is shaped like a flattened upside-down pear. The uterus houses and nourishes the fetus until birth and then contracts rhythmically during labor to expel the fetus. Each month the uterus is prepared for a pregnancy, whether or not conception occurs.

The uterus measures about 7.5 × 5 × 2.5 cm (3 × 2 × 1 inch) and is larger in a woman who has borne children than in one who has not. It is suspended above the bladder and is anterior to the rectum. Its normal position is anteverted (rotated forward) and slightly anteflexed (flexed forward).

Divisions of the Uterus. The uterus is divided into three parts.

Corpus. The upper part is the corpus, or body, of the uterus. The *fundus* of the uterus is the part of the corpus above the area where the fallopian tubes enter the uterus.

Isthmus. A narrower transition zone, the isthmus, is between the corpus of the uterus and the cervix. During late pregnancy, the isthmus elongates and is known as the lower uterine segment.

Cervix. The cervix is the tubular "neck" of the lower uterus and is about 2 to 3 cm long. The os is the opening in the cervix that runs between the uterus and the vagina. The upper part of the cervix is marked by the internal os, and the lower cervix is marked by the external os. The external os of a childless woman is round and smooth. After vaginal birth, the external os has an irregular, slitlike shape and may have tags of scar tissue.

Layers of the Uterus. The uterus has three layers.

Perimetrium. The perimetrium is the outer peritoneal layer of serous membrane that covers most of the uterus. Laterally, the perimetrium is continuous with the broad ligaments on either side of the uterus.

Myometrium. The myometrium is the middle layer of thick muscle. Most of the muscle fibers are concentrated in the upper uterus, and their number diminishes progressively toward the cervix. The myometrium contains three types of smooth muscle fiber (Fig. 11-4). These types are:

- *Longitudinal fibers*, which are found mostly in the fundus and are designed to expel the fetus efficiently toward the pelvic outlet during birth.
- *Interlacing figure-8 fibers*, which make up the middle layer. These fibers contract after birth to compress the blood vessels that pass between them to limit blood loss.
- *Circular fibers*, which form constrictions where the fallopian tubes enter the uterus and surround the internal cervical os. Circular fibers prevent reflux of menstrual blood and tissue into the fallopian tubes, promote normal implantation of the fertilized ovum by controlling its entry into the uterus, and retain the fetus until the appropriate time of birth.

Endometrium. The endometrium is the inner layer of the uterus. It is responsive to the cyclic variations of estrogen and progesterone during the female reproductive cycle (see p. 226). The two layers of the endometrium are:

- The *basal layer*, which is nearest the myometrium. This layer regenerates the functional layer of the endometrium after each menstrual period and after childbirth.
- The *functional layer*, which lies above the basal layer and contains the endometrial arteries, veins, and glands. This layer is shed during each menstrual period and after childbirth in the *lochia*.

Fallopian Tubes

The fallopian tubes, also called *oviducts*, are 8 to 14 cm (3.2 to 5.6 inches) long and quite narrow (2 to 3 mm at their narrowest and 5 to 8 mm at their widest). They are a pathway for the ovum between the ovary and the uterus. The fallopian tubes are lined with folded epithelium containing cilia that beat rhythmically toward the uterine cavity to propel the ovum through the tube. Each fallopian tube enters the upper uterus at the *cornu*, or horn, of the uterus.

The four divisions of the tubes are:

- The *interstitial* portion, which runs into the uterine cavity and lies within the uterine wall.
- The *isthmus*, which is the narrow part of the tube adjacent to the uterus.
- The *ampulla*, which is the wider area of the tube lateral to the isthmus, where fertilization occurs.
- The *infundibulum*, which is the wide, funnel-shaped terminal end of the tube. *Fimbriae* are fingerlike processes surrounding the infundibulum.

The fallopian tubes are not directly connected to the ovary. At ovulation, the ovum is expelled into the abdominal

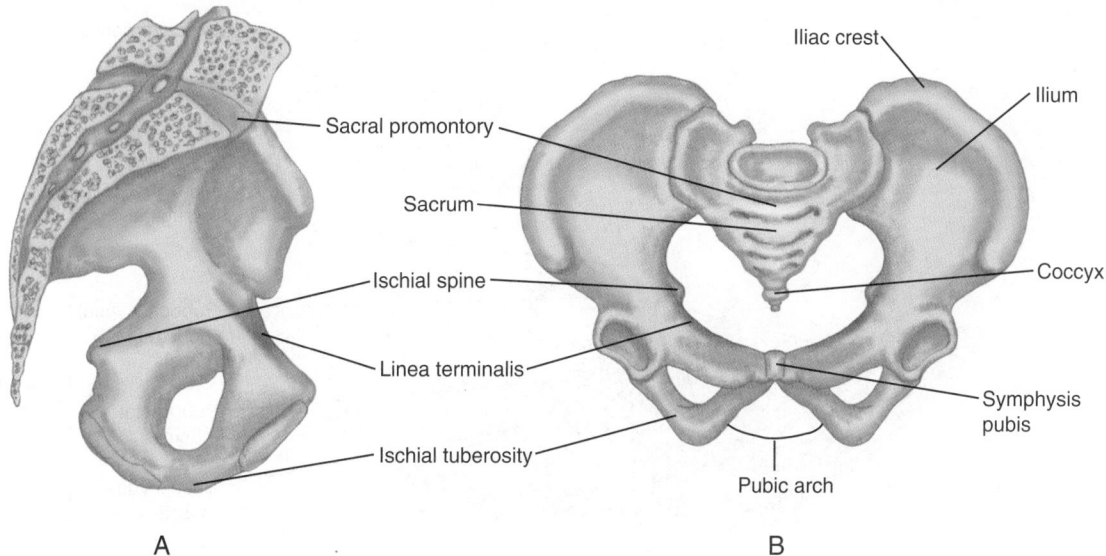

Figure 11-5 Structures of the bony pelvis, shown in lateral, **A,** and anterior, **B,** views.

cavity. Wavelike motions of the fimbriae, which are very near the ovary, draw the ovum into the tube. The tubal isthmus, however, remains contracted until 3 days after conception to allow the fertilized ovum to develop within the tube. Initial growth of the fertilized ovum within the fallopian tube promotes its normal implantation in the fundal portion of the uterine corpus.

Ovaries

The ovaries have two functions: to produce sex hormones and to develop an ovum to maturity during each reproductive cycle.

The ovaries secrete estrogen and progesterone in varying amounts during a woman's reproductive cycle to prepare the uterine lining for pregnancy. Ovarian hormone secretion gradually declines to very low levels during the climacteric.

At birth, the ovary contains all the ova that it will ever have. About 2 million immature ova are present at birth. Many of these degenerate until fewer than 300,000 remain at puberty. Many ova begin the maturation process during each reproductive cycle but most never reach maturity. During the course of a woman's reproductive life, only about 400 of the ova ever mature enough to be released and fertilized. By the time a woman reaches the climacteric, almost all of her ova have been released during ovulation or have regressed. The few remaining ova are unresponsive to stimulating hormones and do not mature (Blackburn, 2003; Moore & Persaud, 2003).

Support Structures

The bony pelvis supports and protects the lower abdominal and internal reproductive organs. Muscles and ligaments provide added support for the internal organs of the pelvis against the downward force of gravity and the increases in intraabdominal pressure.

Pelvis

The bony pelvis is a basin-shaped structure at the lower end of the spine. Its posterior wall is formed by the sacrum. The side and anterior pelvic walls are composed of three fused

bones: the *ilium*, the *ischium*, and the *pubis*. Figure 11-5 illustrates important anatomic landmarks on the pelvis.

The *linea terminalis*, also called the *pelvic brim* or *iliopectineal line*, is an imaginary line that divides the upper, or false, pelvis from the lower, or true, pelvis. The false pelvis provides support for the internal organs and the upper part of the body. The true pelvis is most important during childbirth, and its divisions and measurements are discussed in Chapter 17.

Muscles

Paired muscles enclose the lower pelvis and provide support for internal reproductive, urinary, and bowel structures (Fig. 11-6). A fibromuscular sheet, the *pelvic fascia*, also supports the pelvic organs. Vaginal and urethral openings are in the pelvic fascia.

The levator ani is a collection of three pairs of muscles: the *pubococcygeus*, which is also called the *pubovaginal muscle* in the female; the *puborectal*; and the *iliococcygeus*. These muscles support internal pelvic structures and resist increases in the intraabdominal pressure.

The *ischiocavernosus muscle* extends from the clitoris to the ischial tuberosities on each side of the lower bony pelvis. The two *transverse perineal muscles* extend from fibrous tissue of the perineum to the two ischial tuberosities, stabilizing the center of the perineum.

Ligaments

Seven pairs of ligaments maintain the internal reproductive organs, with their nerve and blood supplies, in their proper positions within the pelvis (see Fig. 11-2).

Lateral Support. Paired ligaments stabilize the uterus and ovaries laterally and keep them in the midline of the pelvis. The *broad ligament* is a sheet of tissue extending from each side of the uterus to the lateral pelvic wall. The *round ligament* and fallopian tube mark the upper border of the broad ligament; the lower edge is bounded by the uterine blood vessels. Within the two broad ligaments are the ovarian ligaments, blood vessels, and lymphatics.

The right and left *cardinal ligaments* provide support to the lower uterus and vagina. They extend from the lateral walls of the cervix and vagina to the side walls of the pelvis.

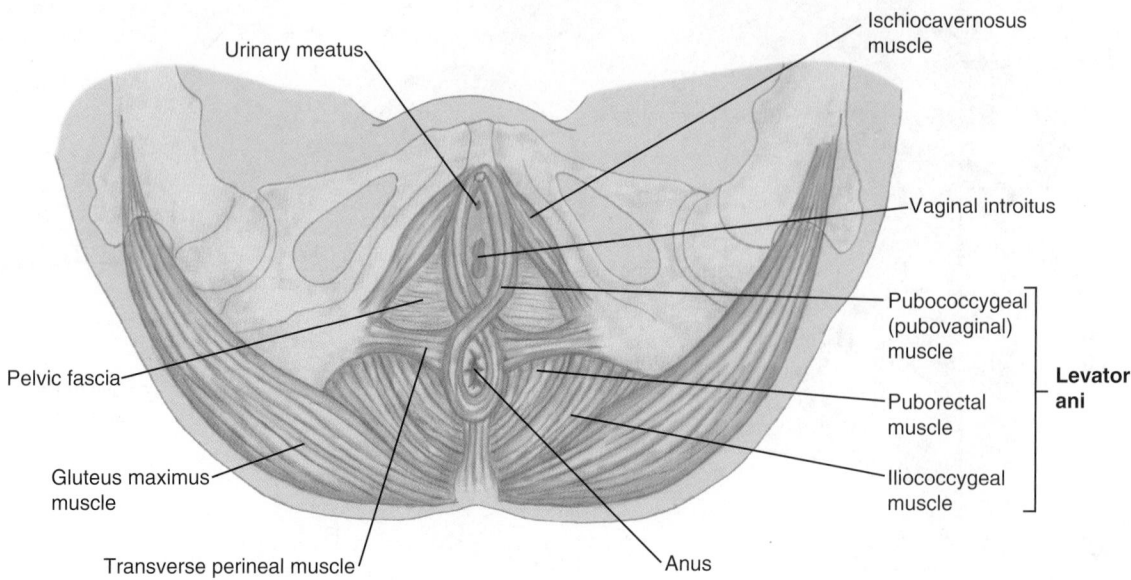

Figure 11-6 Muscles of the female pelvic floor.

The two *ovarian ligaments* connect the ovaries to the lateral uterine walls. The *infundibulopelvic*, or *suspensory*, *ligaments* connect the lateral ovary and distal fallopian tubes to the pelvic side walls. The infundibulopelvic ligament also carries the blood vessel and nerve supply for the ovary.

Anterior Support. Two pairs of ligaments provide anterior support for the internal reproductive organs. The *round ligaments* connect the upper uterus to the connective tissue of the labia majora. These ligaments maintain the uterus in its normal anteflexed position and help guide the fetal presenting part against the cervix during labor.

The *pubocervical ligaments* support the cervix anteriorly. They connect the cervix to the interior surface of the symphysis pubis.

Posterior Support. The *uterosacral ligaments* provide posterior support, extending from the lower posterior uterus to the sacrum. These ligaments also contain sympathetic and parasympathetic nerves of the autonomic nervous system.

Blood Supply

The uterine blood supply is carried by the *uterine arteries*, which are branches of the internal iliac artery. These vessels enter the uterus at the lower border of the broad ligament, near the isthmus of the uterus. The vessels branch downward to supply the cervix and vagina and upward to supply the uterus. The upper branch also supplies the ovaries and fallopian tubes. The vessels are coiled to allow for elongation as the uterus expands during pregnancy. Blood drains into the *uterine veins* and from there into the internal iliac veins.

Additional ovarian and tubal blood supply is carried by the *ovarian artery*, which arises from the abdominal aorta. The ovarian blood supply drains into the two *ovarian veins*.

Nerve Supply

Most functions of the reproductive system are under involuntary, or unconscious, control. Nerves of the autonomic nervous system from the uterovaginal plexus and inferior hypogastric plexus control automatic functions of the reproductive system. Sensory and motor nerves that innervate the reproductive organs enter the spinal cord at the T12 through L2 levels. These nerves are important during childbearing for pain management.

FEMALE REPRODUCTIVE CYCLE

The female reproductive cycle describes the regular and recurrent changes in the anterior pituitary secretions, ovaries, and uterine endometrium that are designed to prepare the body for pregnancy (Fig. 11-7). The female reproductive cycle is often called the *menstrual cycle* because menstruation provides a marker for each cycle's beginning and end if pregnancy does not occur.

The duration of the cycle is about 28 days, although it may range from 20 to 45 days (Guyton & Hall, 2000). Significant deviations from the 28-day cycle are associated with reduced fertility. The first day of the menstrual period is counted as day 1 of the woman's cycle. The female reproductive cycle is further divided into two cycles that reflect changes in the ovaries and uterine endometrium.

Ovarian Cycle

In response to GnRH from the woman's hypothalamus, the anterior pituitary secretes FSH and LH. The FSH and LH stimulate the ovaries to mature an ovum, release it, and secrete other hormones that will prepare the endometrium for implantation of a fertilized ovum. The ovarian cycle consists of three phases: the follicular phase, the ovulatory phase, and the luteal phase.

Follicular Phase

The follicular phase is the period during which an ovum matures. It begins with the first day of menstruation and ends about 14 days later in a 28-day cycle. The length of this phase varies more among different women than do the lengths of

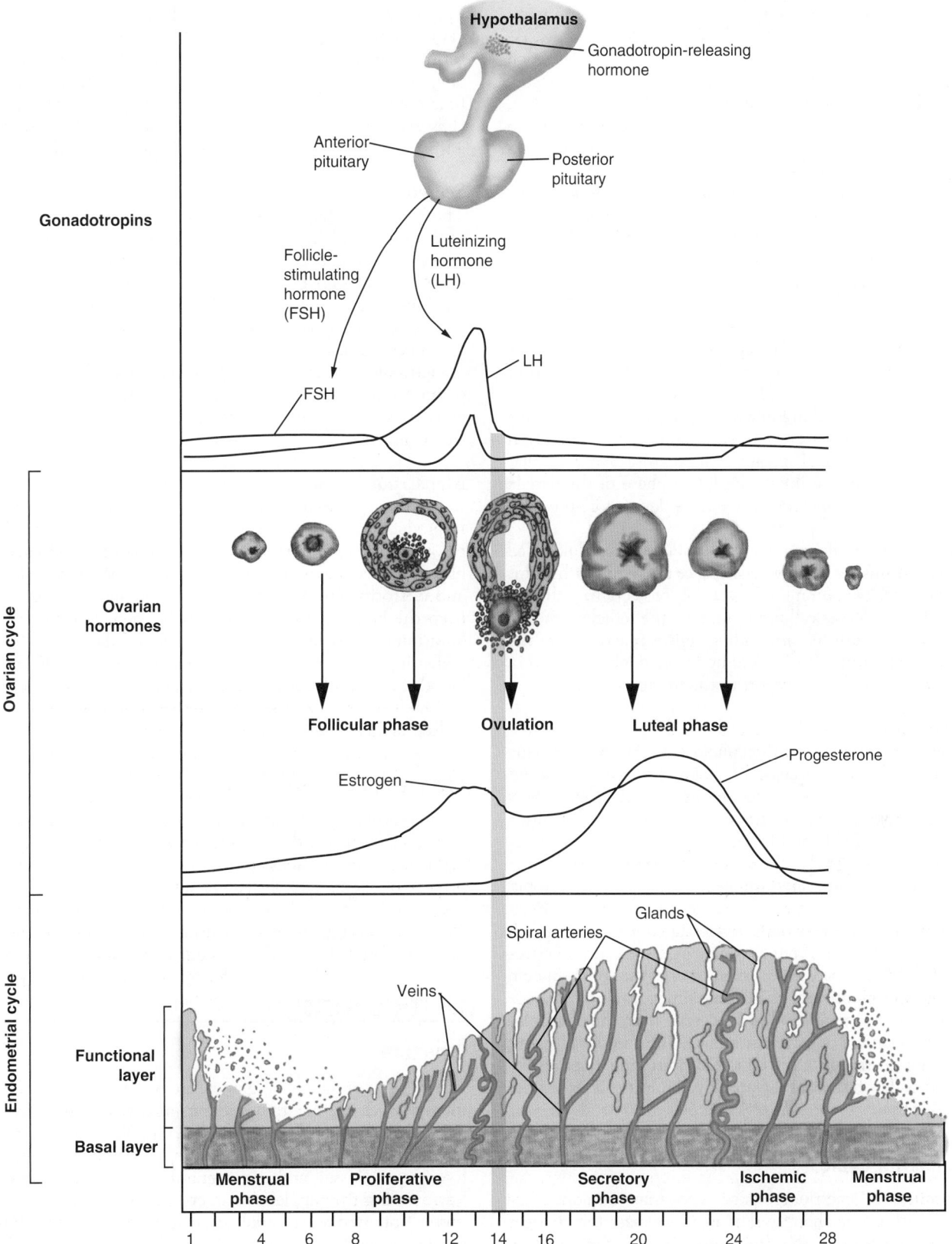

Figure 11-7 The female reproductive cycle, showing the changes in hormone secretion from the anterior pituitary and interrelated changes in the ovary and uterine endometrium.

the other two phases. The decrease in estrogen and progesterone secretion by the ovary just before menstruation stimulates secretion of FSH and LH by the anterior pituitary. As the FSH and LH levels rise, 6 to 12 graafian follicles, each containing an oocyte (immature ovum), start growing faster. Each follicle secretes fluid containing high levels of estrogen, which accelerates maturation by making the follicle more sensitive to the effects of FSH. Eventually, one follicle matures before the others. The mature follicle secretes large amounts of estrogen, which depresses FSH secretion. The brief dip in FSH secretion just before ovulation blocks further maturation of the less-developed follicles. Occasionally, more than one follicle matures and releases its ovum; this condition can lead to a multifetal pregnancy.

Ovulatory Phase

Near the middle of a 28-day reproductive cycle, about 2 days before ovulation, LH secretion rises markedly. Secretion of FSH also rises, but less than LH does. These surges in LH and FSH cause a slight fall in follicular estrogen production and a rise in progesterone secretion, stimulating final maturation of a single follicle and release of its mature ovum. Ovulation marks the beginning of the luteal phase of the female reproductive cycle and occurs about 14 days before the next menstrual period.

The mature follicle is a mass of cells with a fluid-filled chamber. A smaller mass of cells houses the ovum within this chamber. At ovulation, a blisterlike projection, called a *stigma*, forms on the wall of the follicle, the follicle ruptures, and the ovum with its surrounding cells is released from the surface of the ovary. It is picked up by the fimbriated end of the fallopian tube for transport to the uterus.

Luteal Phase

After ovulation and under the influence of LH, the remaining cells of the old follicle persist for about 12 days as a *corpus luteum*. The corpus luteum secretes estrogen and large amounts of progesterone to prepare the endometrium for a fertilized ovum. Levels of FSH and LH decrease during this phase in response to higher levels of estrogen and progesterone. If the ovum is fertilized, it secretes human chorionic gonadotropin (hCG) that causes the corpus luteum to persist to maintain an early pregnancy. If the ovum is not fertilized, FSH and LH fall to low levels and the corpus luteum regresses. Decline of estrogen and progesterone with the regression of the corpus luteum results in menstruation as the uterine lining breaks down.

The loss of estrogen and progesterone from the corpus luteum at the end of one cycle stimulates the anterior pituitary to increase secretion of FSH and LH, initiating a new cycle. The old corpus luteum is replaced by fibrous tissue called the *corpus albicans*.

Endometrial Cycle

The uterine endometrium responds to ovarian hormone stimulation with cyclic changes. Three phases mark the changes in the endometrium: the proliferative phase, the secretory phase, and the menstrual phase.

Proliferative Phase

The proliferative phase takes place as the ovum matures and is released during the first half of the ovarian cycle. After completion of a menstrual period, the endometrium is very thin, with only the basal layer of cells remaining. These cells multiply to form new endometrial epithelium and endometrial glands under the stimulation of estrogen secreted by the maturing ovarian follicles. Endometrial spiral arteries and endometrial veins elongate to accompany thickening of the functional endometrial layer and to nourish the proliferating cells. As ovulation approaches, the endometrial glands secrete a thin, stringy mucus that aids entry of sperm into the uterus.

Secretory Phase

The secretory phase occurs during the second half of the ovarian cycle as the uterus is prepared to receive a fertilized ovum. The endometrium continues to thicken under the influence of estrogen and progesterone from the corpus luteum, reaching its maximum thickness of 5 to 6 mm. The blood vessels and endometrial glands become twisted and dilated.

Progesterone from the corpus luteum causes the thick endometrium to secrete substances that nourish a fertilized ovum. Large quantities of glycogen, proteins, lipids, and minerals are stored within the endometrium, awaiting arrival of the ovum.

Menstrual Phase

If fertilization does not occur, the corpus luteum regresses and its production of estrogen and progesterone falls. About 2 days before the onset of the menses, vasospasm of the endometrial blood vessels causes the endometrium to become ischemic and necrotic. The necrotic areas of endometrium separate from the basal layers, resulting in the menstrual flow. The duration of the menstrual phase is about 5 days.

During a menstrual period, women lose about 40 ml of blood. Because of the recurrent loss of blood, many women are mildly anemic during their reproductive years, especially if their diets are low in iron.

Changes in Cervical Mucus

During most of the female reproductive cycle, the mucus of the cervix is scant, thick, and sticky. Just before ovulation, cervical mucus becomes thin, clear, and elastic to promote passage of sperm into the uterus and fallopian tube, where they can fertilize the ovum. *Spinnbarkeit* refers to the elasticity of cervical mucus. A woman may assess the elasticity of her cervical mucus either to avoid or to promote conception.

THE FEMALE BREAST

Structure

The breasts, or mammary glands, are not directly functional in reproduction, but they secrete milk after childbirth to nourish the infant. The small, raised nipple is at the center of each breast (Fig. 11-8). The nipple is composed of sensitive erectile tissue and can respond to sexual stimulation. Surrounding the nipple is a larger circular areola. Both the nipple and areola are darker than surrounding skin. Montgomery tubercles are sebaceous glands in the areola. They are inactive and not obvious except during pregnancy and lactation, when they enlarge and secrete a substance that keeps the nipple soft.

Within each breast are lobes of glandular tissue that secrete milk. These lobes are arranged like spokes of a wheel around the hub. Fifteen to 20 of these lobes are arranged

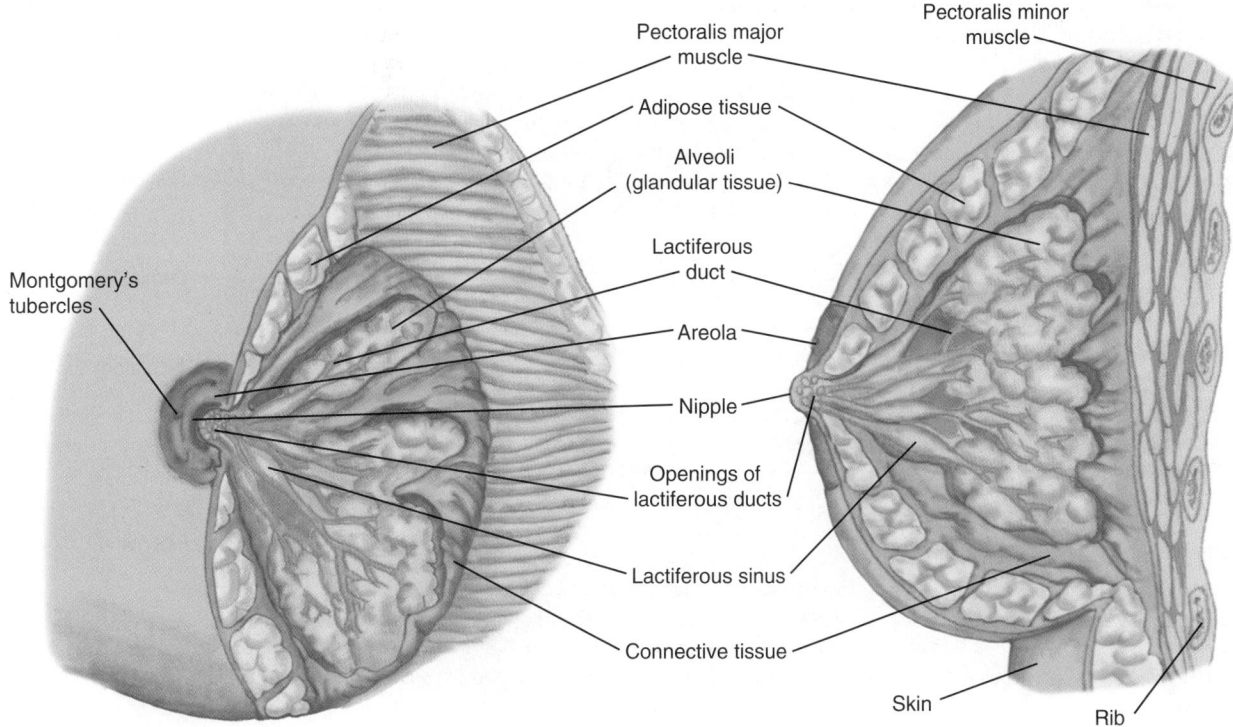

Pectoralis major muscle

Pectoralis minor muscle

Adipose tissue

Alveoli (glandular tissue)

Lactiferous duct

Montgomery's tubercles

Areola

Nipple

Openings of lactiferous ducts

Lactiferous sinus

Connective tissue

Skin

Rib

Figure 11-8 Structures of the female breast.

around and behind the nipple and areola. Fibrous tissue and fat in the breast support the glandular tissue, blood vessels, lymphatics, and nerves.

Alveoli are small sacs that contain milk-secreting cells called *acini*. Acini extract substances needed from the mammary blood supply to manufacture milk when the breasts are properly stimulated by the anterior pituitary gland. Myoepithelial cells surround the alveoli to contract and eject the milk into the ductal system when signaled by secretion of the hormone *oxytocin* from the posterior pituitary gland.

The alveoli drain into lactiferous ducts, which join to drain milk from all areas of the breast. The lactiferous ducts become wider under the areola and are called *lactiferous sinuses* in this area. The lactiferous sinuses narrow again as they open to the outside in the nipple.

Function

The breasts are inactive until puberty, when rising estrogen levels stimulate growth of the glandular tissue. Fat is deposited in the breasts, resulting in the mature female contour. The amount of fat is the major determinant of breast size; the amount of glandular tissue is similar for all mature women. Breast size is therefore unrelated to the amount of milk a woman can produce during lactation.

During pregnancy, high levels of estrogen and progesterone, produced by the placenta, stimulate growth of the alveoli and ductal system to prepare them for lactation. Prolactin secreted by the anterior pituitary gland stimulates milk production during pregnancy, but this effect is inhibited by estrogen and progesterone produced by the placenta. Inhibit-

ing effects of estrogen and progesterone stop when the placenta is expelled after birth, and active milk production occurs in response to the infant's nursing.

MALE REPRODUCTIVE ANATOMY AND PHYSIOLOGY

External Male Reproductive Organs

The male has two external organs of reproduction: the penis and the scrotum (Fig. 11-9).

Penis

The penis has two functions. As part of the urinary tract, it carries urine from the bladder to the exterior during urination. As a reproductive organ, the penis carries semen into the female vagina during coitus.

The penis is composed mostly of erectile tissue, which is spongy tissue with many small spaces inside. There are three areas of erectile tissue: the corpus spongiosum, which surrounds the urethra; and two columns of the corpus cavernosum, one on each side of the penis.

The penis is flaccid most of the time because small spaces within the erectile tissue are collapsed. During sexual stimulation, arteries within the penis dilate and veins are partly occluded, trapping blood in the spongy tissue. Entrapment of blood within the penis causes erection and enables the man to penetrate the vagina during sexual intercourse.

The glans is the distal end of the penis. The urinary meatus is centered in the end of the glans. Covering the glans is the loose skin of the prepuce, or foreskin. The prepuce may be removed during *circumcision*.

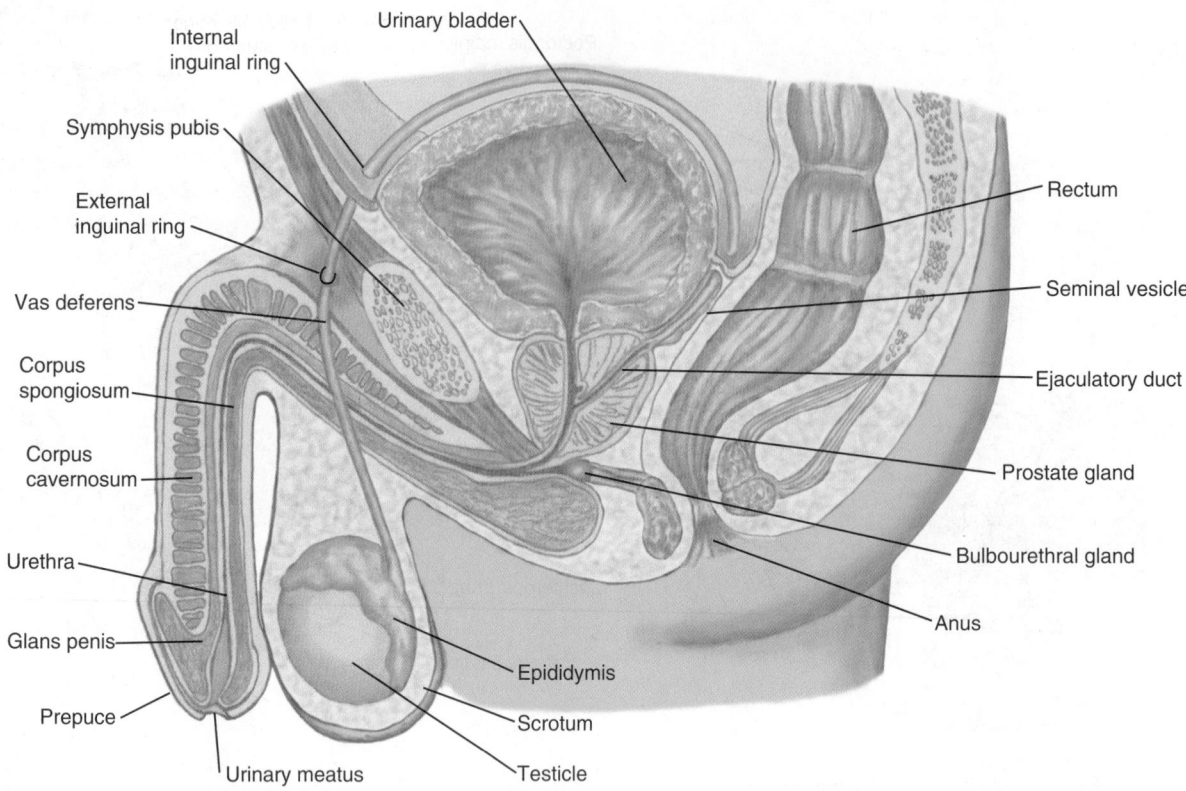

Figure 11-9 Structures of the male reproductive system, *midsagittal view.*

Scrotum

The scrotum is a pouch of thin skin and muscle suspended behind the penis. The skin of the scrotum is darker than the surrounding skin and is covered with rugae. The scrotum is divided internally by a septum. One testicle is contained within each pocket of the scrotum.

The scrotum's main function is to keep the testes cooler than the core body temperature. Formation of normal sperm requires that the testes not be too warm. A cremaster muscle is attached to each testicle. This muscle can tighten, drawing the testes closer to the body and warming them, or it can relax, allowing the testes to fall away from the body and become cooler.

Internal Male Reproductive Organs

Testes

The male gonads, or testes, have two functions: they serve as endocrine glands; and they produce male gametes, or sperm, also called *spermatozoa*. Androgens, which are the male sex hormones, are the primary endocrine secretions of the testes. Androgens are produced by Leydig cells of the testes. The primary androgen produced by the testes is testosterone.

Unlike the female, who experiences a cyclic pattern of hormone secretion, the male secretes testosterone in a relatively even pattern. A small amount of testosterone is converted to estrogen in the male and is necessary for sperm formation.

Spermatogenesis occurs within tiny coiled tubes, called the *seminiferous tubules*, of the testes (Fig. 11-10). Leydig cells are interstitial cells that support the seminiferous tubules and secrete testosterone, a hormone necessary for

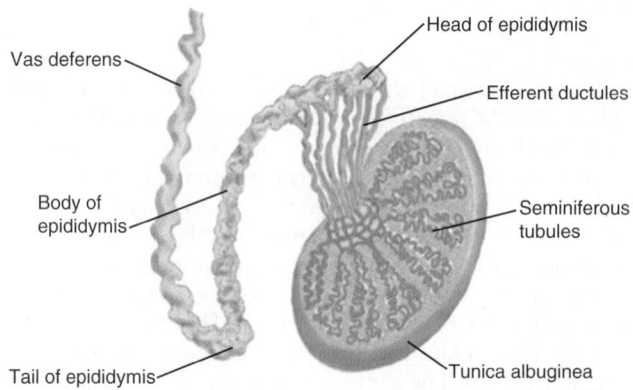

Figure 11-10 Internal structures of the testis. Production of sperm begins within the tiny, coiled seminiferous tubules. Immature sperm pass from the seminiferous tubules to the epididymis and then to the vas deferens. During their passage through these structures, the sperm mature and acquire the ability to propel themselves.

forming new cells that will mature into sperm. Sertoli cells within the seminiferous tubules respond to FSH secretion by nourishing and supporting sperm as they mature. Unlike the female, who has a lifetime supply of ova in her gonads at birth, the male does not begin producing sperm until puberty. The normal male produces new sperm throughout life, although production declines with age.

At ejaculation, 40 to 250 million sperm are deposited in the vagina (Blackburn, 2003). This large number is needed for normal fertility, although a single sperm fertilizes the ovum. Only a few sperm ever reach the fallopian tube, where an ovum may be available for fertilization.

Accessory Ducts and Glands

From the seminiferous tubules, sperm pass into the epididymis within the scrotum for storage and final maturation. In the epididymis, sperm develop the ability to be motile. Secretions within the epididymis, however, inhibit actual motility until ejaculation occurs.

The epididymis empties into the vas deferens, where larger numbers of sperm are stored. The vas deferens then leads upward into the pelvis and then back down toward the penis through the internal and external inguinal rings. Within the pelvis, the vas deferens joins the ejaculatory duct before connecting to the urethra.

Three glands—the *seminal vesicles*, the *prostate*, and the *bulbourethral glands*—secrete seminal fluids that carry sperm into the vagina during intercourse. The seminal fluid (1) nourishes the sperm, (2) protects the sperm from the acidic environment of the vagina, (3) enhances the motility of the sperm, and (4) washes the sperm out of the urethra so that the maximum number are deposited in the vagina.

KEY CONCEPTS

- Initial prenatal development of the reproductive organs is similar for both males and females. If a critical part of the Y chromosome is not present at conception, female reproductive structures will develop.
- Puberty is the time when the reproductive organs become fully functional and secondary sex characteristics develop.
- Puberty begins about 6 months to 1 year earlier in girls than in boys, although the girl's early growth spurt makes it seem that she begins puberty much earlier than the boy.
- Females are generally shorter than males because they begin their growth spurt at an earlier age and complete it more quickly than boys.
- Girls often do not ovulate in early menstrual cycles, although it is possible for them to ovulate even before the first one. A sexually active girl can become pregnant before her first menstrual period.
- The onset of puberty is more subtle in boys than in girls and begins with growth of the testes and penis.
- Nocturnal emission of seminal fluids may be distressing to boys unless they are prepared for this normal event.
- At birth, a woman has all the ova she will ever have. New ova are not formed after birth; almost all are depleted when she reaches the climacteric.
- The female reproductive cycle is often called the menstrual cycle. It includes changes in the anterior pituitary gland, ovaries, and uterine endometrium to prepare for a fertilized ovum. The character of cervical mucus also changes to encourage fertilization.
- Breast size is unrelated to glandular tissue or to the quantity or quality of milk a woman can produce for her infant after childbirth. Breast size is primarily related to the amount of fat present.
- For normal sperm to form, a man's testes must be cooler than his core body temperature.
- Seminal fluids secreted by the seminal vesicles, prostate, and bulbourethral glands nourish and protect the sperm, enhance their motility, and ensure that most sperm are deposited in the vagina during sexual intercourse.

REFERENCES and READINGS

Blackburn, S.T. (2003). *Maternal, fetal, and neonatal physiology: A clinical perspective*. Philadelphia: Saunders.

Cunningham, F.G., Gant, N.F., Leveno, K.J., Gilstrap, L.C., Hauth, J.C., & Wenstrom, K. (2001). *Williams obstetrics* (21st ed.). Norwalk, CT: Appleton & Lange.

Garibaldi, L. (2004). Physiology of puberty. In W.E. Nelson, R.E. Behrman, R.M. Kliegman, & A.M. Arvin (Eds.). *Nelson textbook of pediatrics* (14th ed., p. 1862). Philadelphia: Saunders.

Georges, J M. (2000). Female genital and reproductive function. In L.C. Copstead & J.L. Banasik (Eds.). *Pathophysiology: Biological and behavioral perspectives* (2nd ed., pp. 742-760). Philadelphia: Saunders.

Guyton, A.C, & Hall, J.C. (2000). *Textbook of medical physiology* (10th ed.). Philadelphia: Saunders.

Mikkelson, D., & Cagle, C.S. (2000). Male genital and reproductive function. In L.C. Copstead & J.L. Banasik (Eds.). *Pathophysiology: Biological and behavioral perspectives* (2nd ed., pp. 708-725). Philadelphia: Saunders.

Moore, K.L., & Persaud, T.V.N. (1998). *The developing human: Clinically oriented embryology* (6th ed.). Philadelphia: Saunders.

Moore, K.L., & Persaud, T.V.N. (2003). *Before we are born* (6th ed.). Philadelphia: Saunders.

Needlman, R.D. (2004). Growth and development: Adolescence. In W.E. Nelson, R.E. Behrman, R.M. Kliegman, & A.M. Arvin (Eds.). *Nelson textbook of pediatrics* (17th ed., pp. 53-58). Philadelphia: Saunders.

12

Conception and Prenatal Development

◆ LEARNING OBJECTIVES

After studying this chapter, you should be able to:

◉ Describe formation of the female and male gametes.
◉ Relate ovulation and ejaculation to the process of human conception.
◉ Explain implantation and nourishment of the embryo before development of the placenta.
◉ Describe normal prenatal development from conception through birth.

◉ Explain structure and function of the placenta, umbilical cord, and fetal membranes.
◉ Describe how common deviations from usual conception and prenatal development occur.
◉ Describe prenatal circulation and the circulatory changes after birth.
◉ Explain how multifetal pregnancies can occur.

◆ DEFINITIONS

autosome Any of the 22 pairs of chromosomes other than the sex chromosomes.

conceptus Cells and membranes resulting from fertilization of the ovum at any stage of prenatal development.

corpus luteum Graafian follicle cells remaining after ovulation. These cells produce estrogen and progesterone.

diploid Having a pair of chromosomes (46 in humans) that represents one copy of every chromosome from each parent. The number of chromosomes normally present in body cells other than gametes.

ejaculation Expulsion of semen from the penis.

embryo The developing baby from the beginning of the 3rd week through the 8th week after conception.

endometrium Lining of the uterus.

fertilization age Prenatal age of the developing baby, calculated from the date of conception. Also called postconceptional age.

fetus The developing baby from 9 weeks after conception until birth. In everyday practice, this term is often used to describe a developing baby during pregnancy, regardless of age.

gamete Reproductive cell: in the female an ovum, and in the male a spermatozoon.

gestational age Prenatal age of the developing baby (measured in weeks) calculated from the first day of the woman's last menstrual period. Also called menstrual age, about 2 weeks longer than the fertilization age.

graafian follicle A small sac within the ovary. The graafian follicle contains the maturing ovum.

haploid Having one copy of a chromosome from each pair (23 in humans, or half the diploid number). Gametes normally have a haploid number of chromosomes.

meiosis Reduction cell division in gametes that halves the number of chromosomes in each cell.

mitosis Cell division in body cells other than the gametes.

nidation Implantation of the fertilized ovum (zygote) in the uterine endometrium.

oogenesis Formation of gametes (ova) in the female.

ovulation Release of the mature ovum from the ovary.

placenta Fetal structure that provides nourishment to and removes wastes from the developing baby and secretes hormones necessary for the pregnancy to continue.

sex chromosome The X and Y chromosomes. Females have two X chromosomes; males have one X and one Y chromosome.

somatic cells Body cells other than the gametes, or germ cells.

spermatogenesis Formation of male gametes (sperm) in the testes.

teratogen An agent that can cause defects in a developing baby during pregnancy.

zygote Cell formed by union of an ovum and sperm.

basic understanding of conception and prenatal development helps the nurse provide care to parents during normal childbearing and better understand problems such as infertility and birth defects. This chapter addresses formation of the gametes, the process of conception, prenatal development, and important auxiliary structures that support prenatal development. A short discussion of multifetal pregnancy is included.

TABLE **12-1** Comparison of Female and Male Gametogenesis

	Oogenesis	Spermatogenesis
Time during which primary germ cells are produced	Fetal life. No others develop after about 30 weeks of gestation.	Continuously after puberty.
Hormones controlling process	GnRH. FSH. LH. Estrogen.	GnRH. FSH. LH. Testosterone. Estrogen (small amounts converted from testosterone). Growth hormone.
Number of mature germ cells that develop from each primary cell	One.	Four.
Quantity	One during each reproductive cycle of about 28 days.	40-250 million are released with each ejaculation.
Size	Large. Visible to naked eye. Abundant cytoplasm to nourish embryo until implantation.	Tiny compared with ovum. Little cytoplasm. Head is almost all nuclear material (chromosomes).
Motility	Relatively nonmotile. Carried along by action of cilia and currents within fallopian tubes.	Independently motile by means of whiplike tail. Mitochondria in middle piece provide energy for motility.
Chromosome complement	23 total: 22 autosomes plus one X sex chromosome.	23 total: 22 autosomes, plus either an X or a Y sex chromosome.

GnRH, Gonadotropin-releasing hormone; *FSH*, follicle-stimulating hormone; *LH*, luteinizing hormone.

GAMETOGENESIS

To develop ova in females and spermatozoa in males, gametogenesis requires a special reduction division called *meiosis*. Unlike *mitosis*, in which the diploid number of chromosomes (46) is retained in each new cell, meiosis halves the number of chromosomes (haploid number). Only one of each chromosome pair is directed to the gamete, 22 autosomes and 1 sex chromosome.

When the sperm and ovum unite at conception, the "halves" form a new cell and restore the chromosome number to 46. Table 12-1 summarizes human gametogenesis in males and females.

Oogenesis

Oogenesis begins during prenatal life, when primitive ova (oogonia) multiply by mitosis, like other cells in the body. Each oogonium contains 46 chromosomes (22 pairs of autosomes and a pair of X chromosomes), as do other body cells. Before birth, the oogonia enlarge to form primary oocytes with a layer of follicular cells surrounding each one (Fig. 12-1, A). These are called *primary follicles*. The primary oocyte begins its first meiotic division during fetal life but does not complete the process until puberty. The primary oocytes (still containing 46 chromosomes) remain dormant throughout childhood.

By the 30th week of gestation, the female fetus has all the ova she will ever have. Many of these ova regress during childhood until fewer than 300,000 remain at puberty (Blackburn, 2003). When a girl's reproductive cycles begin at puberty, some of the primary follicles present at birth begin maturing. The cyclical process of gamete maturation continues throughout her reproductive years until the climacteric, or "change of life."

When the oocyte matures, two meiotic divisions reduce the chromosome number from 46 paired to 23 unpaired chromosomes: 22 autosomes and an X chromosome. Shortly before ovulation, the primary oocyte completes its first meiotic division, which began during fetal life. A secondary oocyte, now containing 23 unpaired chromosomes, results. The cytoplasm in the primary oocyte is divided unequally with this division, with most retained by the secondary oocyte. The remainder of cytoplasm, plus the other 23 chromosomes, goes into a tiny, nonfunctional polar body that soon degenerates.

At ovulation, the secondary oocyte begins dividing again (second meiotic division) to form a mature ovum. The 23 chromosomes duplicate themselves in the second meiotic division, but half of the duplicated chromosomes will be discarded if fertilization occurs. The second meiotic division is prolonged, and the mature ovum remains suspended in metaphase, the middle part of cell division. If fertilization occurs, the second meiotic division is completed, resulting in a mature ovum containing 23 chromosomes and a second tiny polar body containing the 23 discarded chromosomes that degenerates. If the ovum is not fertilized, it does not complete the second meiotic division and degenerates. In oogenesis, one primary oocyte results in a single mature ovum.

When released from the ovary, the mature ovum is surrounded by two layers—the zona pellucida and the cells of the corona radiata. These layers protect the ovum and prevent fertilization by more than one sperm. For fertilization to occur, the sperm must penetrate these two layers to reach the ovum's cell nucleus.

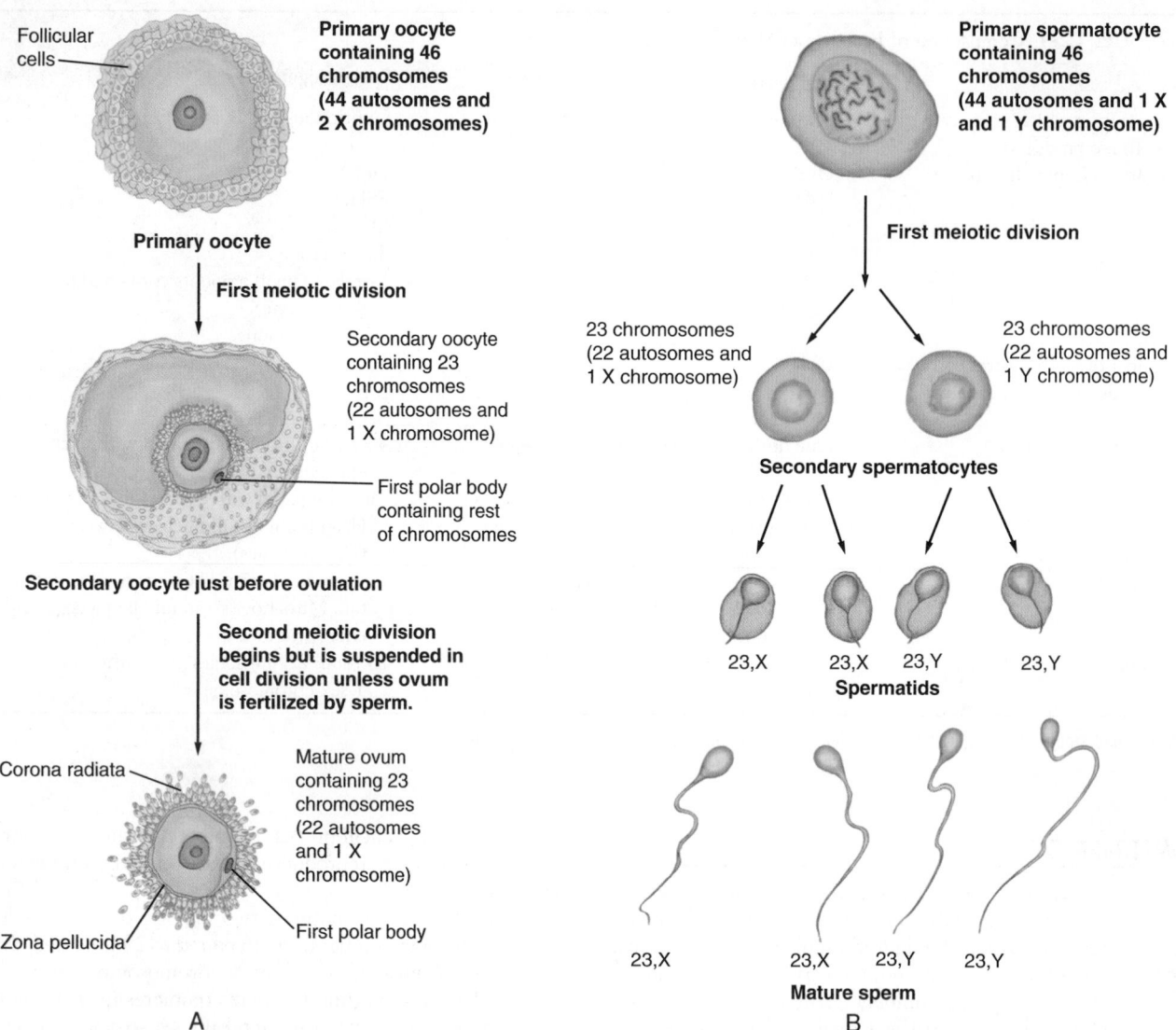

Figure 12-1 Gametogenesis. **A,** Formation of the mature ovum. **B,** Formation of mature sperm.

Spermatogenesis

Spermatogenesis (see Fig. 12-1, *B*) begins during puberty in the male. Primitive sperm cells (*spermatogonia*) develop during fetal life and begin multiplying by mitosis during puberty. Unlike the female, the male produces new spermatogonia that can mature into sperm throughout his lifetime. Although male fertility gradually declines with age, men can father children in their 50s, 60s, and beyond.

Each spermatogonium contains 46 paired chromosomes, like other body cells. In the mature male, a spermatogonium enlarges to become a primary spermatocyte, still containing all 46 chromosomes. The first meiotic division forms two secondary spermatocytes and reduces the number to 23 unpaired chromosomes: 22 autosomes and 1 sex chromosome, either an X or a Y. Each secondary spermatocyte divides again in the second meiotic division to form two spermatids. Therefore half of the four spermatids that result from the two meiotic divisions of the spermatogonium carry an X chromosome and half carry a Y. The spermatids gradually mature into sperm.

The gamete from a male determines the sex of the new baby. If an X-bearing spermatozoon fertilizes the ovum, the baby is a girl. If a Y-bearing spermatozoon fertilizes the ovum, the baby is a boy.

The mature sperm has three sections: a head, a middle portion, and a tail (Fig. 12-2). The head is almost entirely the cell nucleus. The head contains the male chromosomes that join the chromosomes of the ovum. The middle portion supplies energy for the tail's whiplike action. The movement of the tail propels the sperm toward the ovum.

CONCEPTION

Conception requires correct timing between release of a mature ovum at ovulation and ejaculation of enough healthy, mature, motile sperm into the vagina. The ovum may have the capacity to be fertilized no longer than 24 hours after ovulation, although the exact duration of its viability is unknown. Most sperm survive no more than 1 to 2 days although a few may remain fertile in the woman's reproductive tract as long as 5 days (Guyton & Hall, 2000).

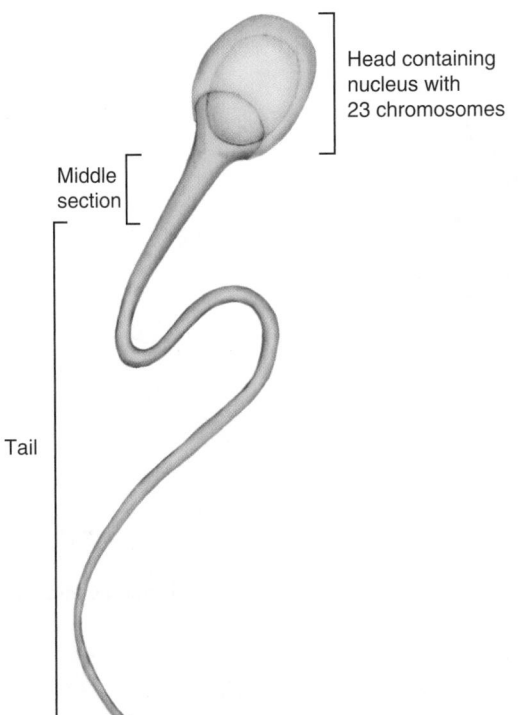

Head containing
nucleus with
23 chromosomes

Middle
section

Tail

Figure 12-2 Mature sperm.

Preparation for Conception in the Male

The male preparation for fertilizing the ovum consists of ejaculation, movement of the sperm in the female reproductive tract, and preparation of the sperm for actual fertilization.

Ejaculation

When a male ejaculates during sexual intercourse, 40 to 250 million sperm are deposited in the upper vagina and over the cervix (Blackburn, 2003). The sperm are suspended in seminal fluid, which nourishes and protects them from the acidic vaginal environment. To hold the semen deeply in the vagina, the seminal fluid coagulates somewhat after ejaculation. The sperm are relatively immobile for about 15 to 30 minutes until other seminal enzymes dissolve the coagulated fluid and allow the sperm to begin moving upward through the cervix.

Transport of Sperm in the Female Reproductive Tract

Whiplike movement of the tails of spermatozoa propels them through the cervix, uterus, and fallopian tubes. Uterine contractions induced by prostaglandins in the seminal fluid enhance movement of the sperm toward the ovum. Only sperm cells enter the cervix. The seminal fluid remains in the vagina.

Many sperm are lost along the way. Some are digested by vaginal enzymes and phagocytes in the female reproductive tract, whereas others move into the wrong tube or past the ovum and out into the peritoneal cavity. Only a few hundred reach the fallopian tube where the ovum waits.

Preparation of Sperm for Fertilization

Sperm are not immediately ready to fertilize the ovum when they are ejaculated. While making the trip to the ovum, the sperm undergo changes (*capacitation*) that enable one to penetrate the protective layers surrounding the ovum. During capacitation, a glycoprotein coat and seminal proteins are removed from the acrosome (tip of the sperm head). After capacitation, the sperm look the same but are more active and can better penetrate the corona radiata and zona pellucida that surround the ovum.

The sperm that reach the ovum release an enzyme (hyaluronidase) to digest a pathway through the corona radiata and zona pellucida. Their tails beat harder to propel them toward the center of the ovum. Eventually, one spermatozoon penetrates the ovum.

Fertilization

Fertilization occurs when one spermatozoon enters the ovum and the two nuclei containing the parents' chromosomes merge (Fig. 12-3).

Entry of One Spermatozoon Into the Ovum

Entry of a spermatozoon into the ovum has two results:

- Changes in the zona pellucida surrounding the ovum prevent other sperm from entering.
- The ovum, which has been suspended in the middle of its second meiotic division, completes meiosis.

Preparation for Conception in the Female

Before ovulation, several oocytes begin to mature under the influence of follicle-stimulating hormone (FSH) and luteinizing hormone (LH) from the woman's anterior pituitary gland. The maturing oocytes are contained in a sac called the *graafian follicle*, which produces estrogen and progesterone to prepare the endometrium for a possible pregnancy. Eventually, one follicle outgrows the others. The less mature oocytes permanently regress.

Release of the Ovum

Ovulation occurs about 14 days before a woman's next menstrual period would begin. The follicle develops a thin spot on the surface of the ovary and ruptures, releasing the mature ovum with its surrounding cells on the surface of the ovary. There the collapsed follicle becomes the corpus luteum, which maintains the high estrogen and progesterone secretion necessary to make final preparation of the uterine lining for a fertilized ovum.

Ovum Transport

Released on the surface of the ovary, the mature ovum is picked up by the fimbriated (fringed) ends of the fallopian tube near the surface of the ovary. The ovum is transported through the tube by muscular action of the tube and movement of cilia within the tube. Fertilization normally occurs in the distal third of the fallopian tube, near the ovary. The ovum, fertilized or not, enters the uterus about 3 days after its release from the ovary.

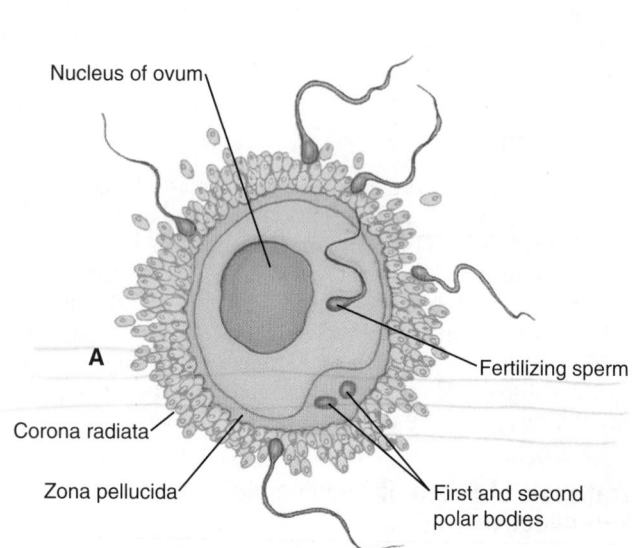

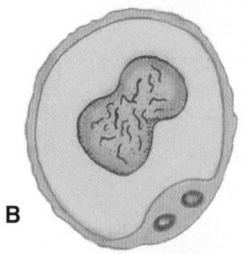

**Mixing of cell nuclei and
chromosomes of ovum and sperm**

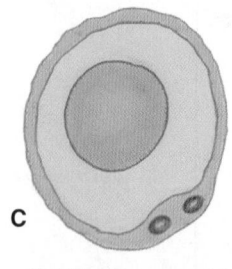

Fertilization complete

Figure 12-3 Process of fertilization. **A,** A sperm enters the ovum. **B,** The 23 chromosomes from the sperm mingle with the 23 chromosomes from the ovum, restoring the diploid number to 46. **C,** The fertilized ovum, now called a *zygote,* is ready for the first mitotic cell division.

The results are a nucleus with 23 chromosomes and expulsion of a second nonfunctional polar body. The mature ovum now contains 23 unpaired chromosomes, 22 autosomes, and 1 X chromosome, in its nucleus.

Fusion of the Nuclei of Sperm and Ovum

Fusion of the nuclei of the sperm and ovum begins when the sperm enters the ovum. The sperm head enlarges, and the tail degenerates. The nuclei of the gametes move toward the center of the ovum, where the membranes surrounding their nuclei touch and dissolve. The 23 chromosomes from the sperm mingle with the 23 from the ovum, restoring the diploid number to 46. Fertilization is complete, and cell division can begin when the nuclei of the sperm and ovum unite.

PRE-EMBRYONIC PERIOD

The pre-embryonic period is the first 2 weeks after conception. Figure 12-4 illustrates the period from fertilization through implantation.

Initiation of Cell Division

The zygote divides into 2 cells, then 4, then 8 cells while in the fallopian tube. Up to the 16-cell stage, the cells become smaller with each division, so they occupy about the same amount of space as the original ovum. When the conceptus is a solid ball of 12 to 16 cells, it is called a *morula* because it resembles a mulberry.

The outer cells of the morula secrete fluid, creating a sac of cells (the *blastocyst*) that has an inner cell mass placed off-center within the sac. The inner cell mass of the blastocyst develops into the fetus. Part of the outer layer of blastocyst cells develops into the placenta and fetal membranes.

Entry of the Zygote Into the Uterus

The conceptus enters the uterus about 3 to 4 days after conception, when it contains about 100 cells. It lingers in the uterus another 2 to 4 days before beginning implantation. The endometrium, now called the *decidua,* is in the secretory phase of the reproductive cycle, 1½ weeks before the woman would begin her menstrual period. The endometrial glands are secreting at their maximum, providing rich fluids to nourish the conceptus before placental circulation is established. The endometrial spiral arteries are well developed in the secretory phase, providing easy access for developing the placental blood supply.

Implantation in the Decidua

The conceptus carries a small supply of nutrients for early cell division, but implantation (*nidation*) at the proper time and location in the uterus is crucial for continued development. Complete implantation is a gradual process that occurs between the 6th and 10th days. Embryonic structures continue developing during implantation.

Maintaining the Decidua

Implantation and survival of the conceptus are critically dependent on a continuing supply of estrogen and progesterone to maintain the decidua in the secretory phase. The zygote secretes human chorionic gonadotropin (hCG) to signal that a pregnancy has begun. With continued hCG production by the conceptus, the corpus luteum continues to secrete estrogen and progesterone rather than regressing.

Location of Implantation

The conceptus must be in the right place at the right time for normal implantation to occur. The site of implantation is important because that is the place that the placenta develops.

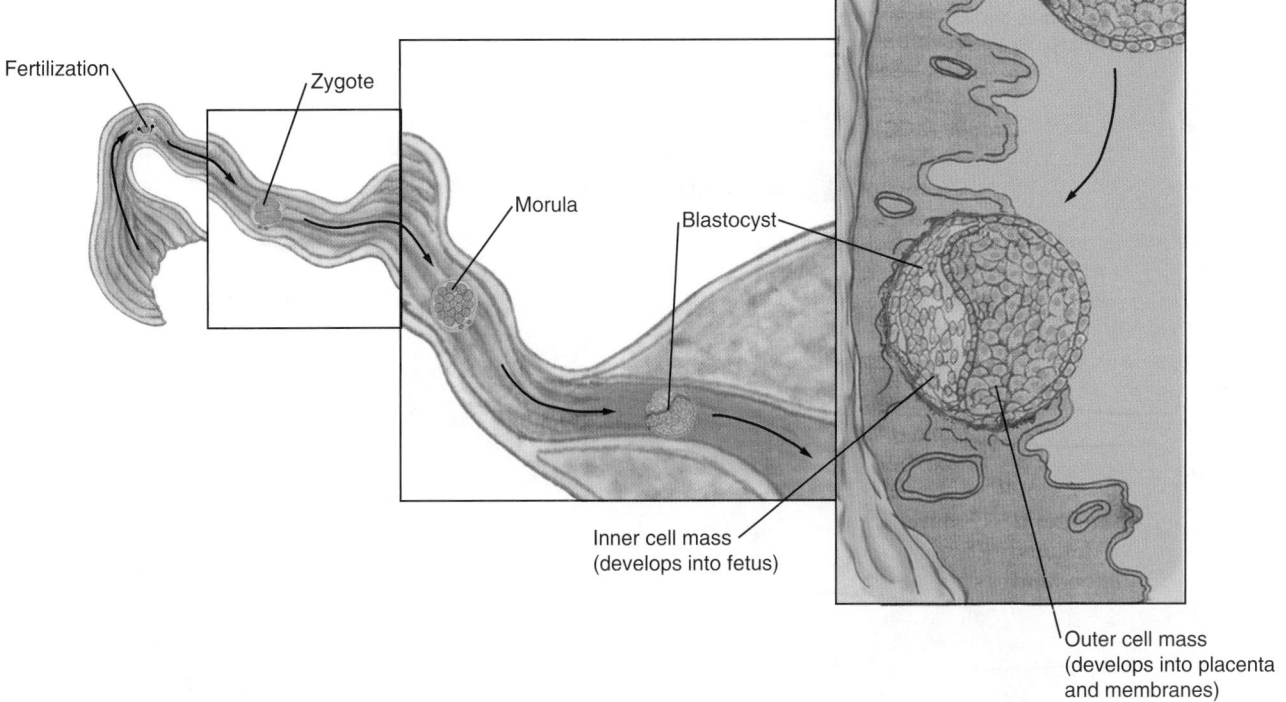

Figure 12-4 Prenatal development from fertilization through implantation of the blastocyst. Implantation gradually occurs from the 6th through the 10th day. Implantation is complete by the 10th day.

Normal implantation occurs in the upper uterus (fundus). The upper uterus is the best area for implantation and placental development for three reasons:

- The upper uterus is richly supplied with blood for optimal fetal gas exchange and nutrition.
- The uterine lining is thick in the upper uterus, preventing the placenta from attaching so deeply that it does not easily detach after birth.
- Implantation in the upper uterus limits blood loss after birth because strong interlacing muscle fibers in this area compress open vessels after the placenta detaches.

Mechanism of Implantation

Enzymes produced by the conceptus erode the decidua, tapping maternal sources of nutrition. Primary chorionic villi are tiny projections on the surface of the conceptus. They extend into the decidua basalis that lies between the conceptus and the wall of the uterus. The chorionic villi eventually form the fetal side of the placenta; the decidua basalis forms the maternal side of the placenta (see Figure 17-14).

At this early stage, nutritive fluid passes to the embryo by *diffusion* (passive movement across a cell membrane from an area of higher concentration to one of lower concentration) because no circulatory system is yet established. By 10 days, the conceptus is fully embedded within the mother's uterine decidua.

As the conceptus implants, usually near the time of the next expected menstrual period, a small amount of bleeding may occur at the site. The woman may think implantation bleeding is a normal menstrual period.

EMBRYONIC PERIOD

The embryonic period of development extends from the beginning of the 3rd week through the 8th week after conception. Basic structures of all major body organs are completed during the embryonic period. Table 12-2 presents major developments in body systems during prenatal life. Figure 12-5 illustrates the external appearance of the embryo from the 3rd through the 8th week after conception.

Differentiation of Cells

The embryo progresses from having cells with identical functions (undifferentiated) to differentiated, or specialized, body cells. By the end of the 8th week, all major organ systems are in place, and many are functioning in a simple way.

Development of the specialized structures is controlled by three factors: (1) the genetic information in the chromosomes received from the parents, (2) interaction between adjacent tissues, and (3) timing. Although basic instructions are carried within the chromosomes, one tissue may induce change toward greater specialization in another but only if a signal between the two tissues occurs at a specific time during development. In this way, structures develop with appropriate size and relationships to each other.

During the embryonic period, organs are especially vulnerable to structural damage from teratogens because they are developing rapidly. Normal development of one structure often requires normal and properly timed development of another. Unfortunately, a woman may not realize she is pregnant at this sensitive time. For this reason, the possibility of pregnancy should be explored with her before potentially

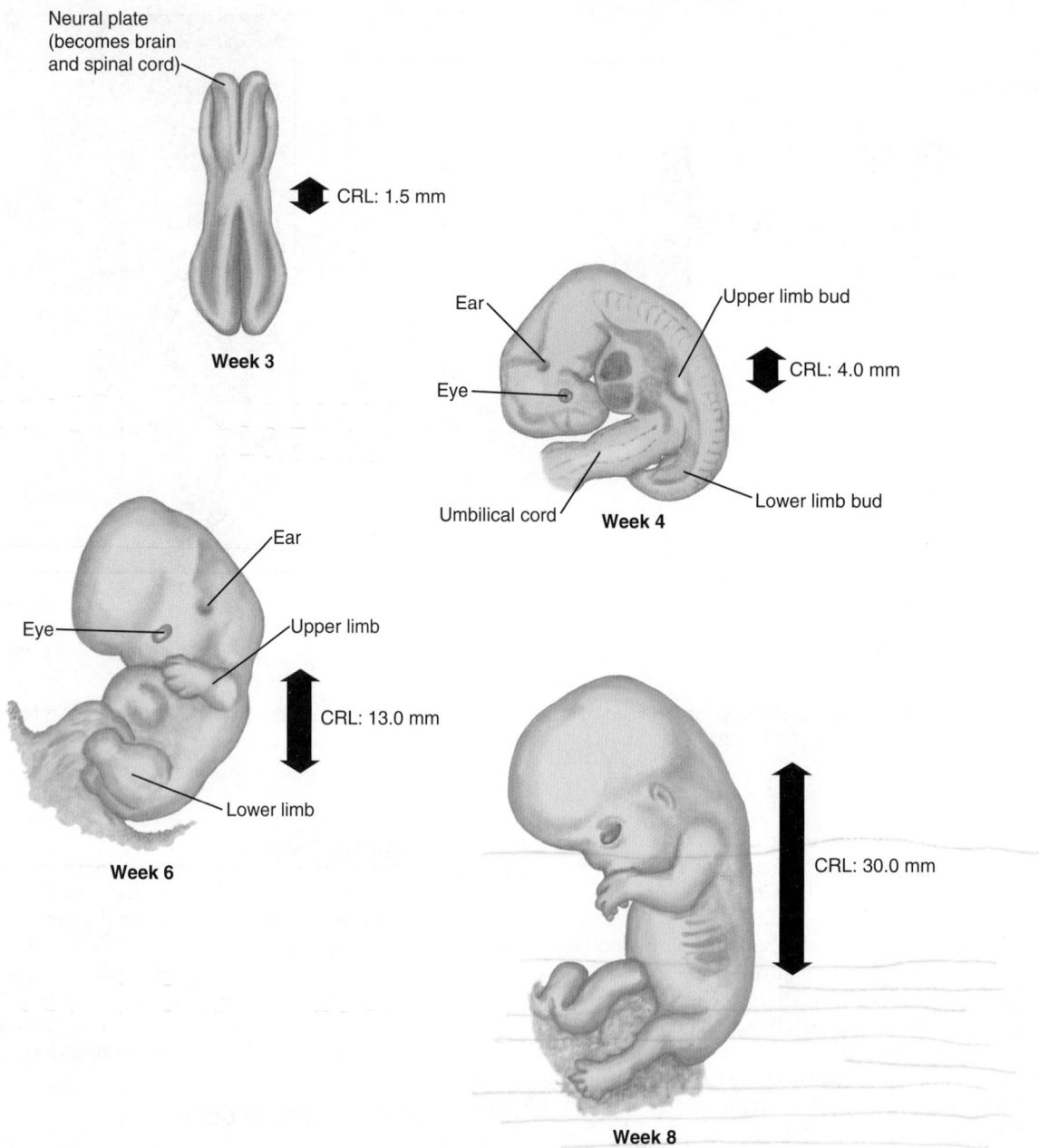

Figure 12-5 Embryonic development from 3 weeks through the 8th week after fertilization. *CRL,* Crown-rump length.

harmful drugs or diagnostic procedures are prescribed. Some agents may be damaging at one time during pregnancy but not at another. Others may be damaging at any time during pregnancy. Appendix B contains information about substances that may cause prenatal damage.

Other teratogenic effects may cause fetal damage because a beneficial substance is not taken in by the mother, either before or during pregnancy. One prominent example of causing teratogenic damage is maternal intake of an inadequate amount of folic acid, a substance that can reduce neural tube defects. Some mothers need standard amounts of folic acid, while a mother having a higher risk for an infant with the neural tube defect often needs several times the most frequently advised

Prenatal growth and development proceed in patterns that continue after birth:

Cephalocaudal (head-to-toe)
Central-to-peripheral direction (from center outward)
Simple-to-complex (early cells may become any cell of the body before they become specialized into specific structures with specific functions)
General-to-specific (upper extremities begin as limb buds before detailed development of bones, joints, muscles, ligaments, and fingers)

See p. 56.

TABLE 12-2 Timetable of Prenatal Development Based on Fertilization Age*

Nervous/Sensory System	Cardiorespiratory System	Digestive System	Genitourinary System	Musculoskeletal System	Integumentary System
3 WEEKS: 1.5 MM CRL					
Flat neural plate begins closing to form neural tube. Neural tube still open at each end.	Heart consists of two parallel tubes that fuse into a single tube. Contractions of heart tube begin. Chorionic villi of early placenta connect with heart.	Endoderm (inner germ layer) will become digestive tract.		Paired, cube-shaped swellings (somites) appear and will form most of the head and trunk skeleton. Muscle, bone, and cartilage develop from mesoderm.	Epidermis (outer skin layer) will develop from ectoderm (outer germ layer). Dermis (deep skin layer) and connective tissue will develop from mesoderm (middle germ layer).
4 WEEKS: 4.0 MM CRL					
Neural tube closed at each end. Cranial end of neural tube will form brain; caudal end will form spinal cord. Eye development begins as an outgrowth of forebrain. Nose development begins as two pits. Inner ear begins developing from hind brain.	Heart begins partitioning into four chambers and begins beating. Blood circulating through embryonic vessels and chorionic villi. Tracheal development begins as a bud on the upper gut and branches into two bronchial buds.	Development of primitive gut as embryo folds laterally. Stomach begins as a widening of the tube-shaped primitive gut. Liver, gallbladder, and biliary ducts begin as a bud from primitive gut.	Primordial germ (reproductive) cells are present on embryonic yolk sac.	Upper limb buds are present and look like flippers. Lower limb buds appear.	Mammary ridges that will develop into mammary glands appear.
6 WEEKS: 13 MM CRL					
Development of pituitary gland and cranial nerves. Head sharply flexed because of rapid brain growth. Eyelid development beginning. External ear development begins in neck region as six swellings.	Blood formation primarily in liver. Three right and two left lung lobes develop as out-growths of the right and left bronchi.	Most intestines are contained within the umbilical cord because the liver and kidneys occupy most of the abdominal cavity. Stomach nearing final form. Development of upper and lower jaws.	Kidneys are near bladder in the pelvis. Kidneys occupy much of the abdominal cavity. Primordial germ cells incorporated into developing gonads. Male and female gonads are identical in appearance.	Arms paddle-shaped, fingers webbed. Feet and toes develop similarly, but a few days later than arms and hands. Bones cartilaginous, but ossification of skull begins.	Mammary glands begin development. Tooth buds for primary (deciduous) teeth begin developing.
8 WEEKS: 30 MM CRL					
Spinal cord stops at end of vertebral column. Taste buds begin developing. Eyelids fuse. Ears have final form but are low-set.	Heart partitioned into four chambers. Heart beat detectable with ultrasound. Additional branching of bronchi.	Stomach has reached final form. Lips are fused. Intestines remain in umbilical cord.	Testes begin developing under influence of Y chromosome. Ovaries will develop if a Y chromosome is not present. External genitalia begin to differentiate but still appear quite similar.	Fingers and toes still webbed, but distinct by end of 8th week. Bones begin to ossify. Joints resemble those of adults.	Auricles of ear low-set but beginning to assume final shape.

*Fertilization age is about 2 weeks less than gestational age.
*Fertilization age is about 2 weeks less than gestational age.
CRL, Crown-rump length.

Continued

TABLE 12-2 Timetable of Prenatal Development Based on Fertilization Age—cont'd

Nervous/Sensory System	Cardiorespiratory System	Digestive System	Genitourinary System	Musculoskeletal System	Integumentary System
10 WEEKS: 61 MM CRL; WEIGHT, 14 G					
Head flexion still present, but straighter. Eyelids closed and fused. Top of external ear slightly below eye level.	May be possible to detect heartbeat with Doppler transducer. Blood produced in spleen and lymphatic tissue.	Intestines contained within abdominal cavity as growth of this cavity catches up with digestive system development. Digestive tract patent from mouth to anus.	Kidneys in their adult position. Male and female external genitalia have different appearance but are still easily confused.	Toes distinct; soles face each other.	Fingernails begin developing. Tooth buds for permanent teeth begin developing below those for primary teeth.
12 WEEKS: 87 MM CRL; WEIGHT, 45 G					
Surface of brain is smooth, without sulci (grooves) or gyri (convolutions). Nasal septum and palate complete development.	Heart beat should be detected with Doppler transducer.	Sucking reflex present. Bile formed by liver.	Kidneys begin producing urine. Male and female external genitalia can be distinguished by appearance.	Limbs are long and thin. Involuntary muscles of viscera develop.	Downy lanugo begins developing at end of this week.
16 WEEKS: 140 MM CRL; WEIGHT, 200 G					
Face is human-looking because eyes face forward rather than to side.	Pulmonary vascular system developing rapidly.	Fetus swallows amniotic fluid and produces meconium (bowel contents).	Urine excreted into amniotic fluid.	Lower limbs reach final relative length, longer than upper limbs. A woman who has been pregnant before may begin to feel fetal movements.	External ears have enough cartilage to stand away from head somewhat. Blood vessels easily visible through the delicate skin. Fingerprints developing.
20 WEEKS: 160 MM CRL; WEIGHT, 460 G					
Myelination of nerves begins and continues through first year of postnatal life.	Heartbeat should be detectable with regular fetoscope.	Peristalsis well developed.	Over 40% of nephrons are mature and functioning. Testes contained in abdomen but begin descent toward scrotum. Primordial follicles of ovary reach peak of 5 to 7 million and then gradually decline.	Fetal movements felt by mother and may be palpable by an experienced examiner.	Skin is thin and covered with vermix caseosa. Brown fat production complete. Nipples begin development.

24 WEEKS: 230 MM CRL; WEIGHT, 820 G				
Spinal cord ends at level of first sacral vertebra because of more rapid growth of vertebral canal.	Primitive thin-walled alveoli (air sacs) have developed and are surrounded by capillary network. Surfactant production begins in lungs. Respiration possible, but most fetuses die if born at this time.	Testes descending toward inguinal rings.	Fetus is active. Fetal movements become progressively more noticeable to both mother and examiner.	Body appearance lean. Skin wrinkled and red. Fingerprints and footprints developed. Fingernails present. Eyebrows and lashes present.

28 WEEKS: 270 MM CRL; WEIGHT, 1300 G				
Major sulci and gyri are present. Eyelids no longer fused after 26 weeks. Responds to bitter substances on tongue.	Erythrocyte formation completely in bone marrow. Sufficient alveoli, surfactant, and capillary network to allow respiratory function, although respiratory distress syndrome is common. Many infants born at this time survive with intensive care.	Testes descended through inguinal canal into scrotum by end of 26th week.		Skin slightly wrinkled but smoothing out as subcutaneous fat is deposited under it.

32 WEEKS: 300 MM CRL; WEIGHT, 2100 G				
Maturation of parasympathetic nears that of sympathetic nervous system, resulting in fetal heart rate variability on electronic fetal monitor tracing.	Surfactant production nears mature levels. Respiratory distress still possible if born at 32 weeks.			Skin smooth and pigmented. Large vessels visible beneath skin. Fingernails reach fingertips. Lanugo disappearing.

38 WEEKS: 360 MM CRL; WEIGHT, 3400 G				
Sulci and gyri developed. Visual acuity about 20/600 at birth.	Newborn infant has about one-eighth to one-sixth the number of alveoli of an adult. Well-developed ability to exchange gas.	Both testes usually palpable in scrotum at birth. The newborn girl's ovaries contain about 1 million follicles. No new ones are formed after birth; their numbers continue to decline after birth.		Fetus plump, and skin smooth. Vernix caseosa present in major body creases. Lanugo present on shoulders and upper back only. Fingernails extend beyond the fingertips. Ear cartilage firm.

TABLE 12-3 Derivatives of the Three Germ Layers: Developing Structures

Ectoderm	Mesoderm	Endoderm
Brain and spinal cord	Cartilage	Lining of gastrointestinal and respiratory tracts
Peripheral nervous system	Bone	
	Connective tissue	
Pituitary gland	Muscle tissue	
Sensory epithelium of the eye, ear, and nose	Heart	Tonsils
	Blood vessels	Thyroid
	Blood cells	Parathyroid
Epidermis	Lymphatic system	Thymus
Hair	Spleen	Liver
Nails	Kidneys	Pancreas
Subcutaneous glands	Adrenal cortex	Lining of urinary bladder and urethra
	Ovaries	
	Testes	
Mammary glands	Reproductive system	Lining of ear canal
Tooth enamel	Lining membranes (pericardial, pleural, peritoneal)	

Second Week

Implantation is complete by the end of the 2nd week. The most growth occurs in the outer cells (*trophoblast*), which eventually become the fetal part of the placenta. The inner cell mass that will develop into the baby becomes flattened into the *embryonic disk*. Cells that eventually form part of the fetal membranes develop.

Third Week

Many women miss their first menstrual period during the 3rd week of pregnancy. The embryonic disk develops three layers (*germ layers*) that, in turn, give rise to the major organ systems of the body. The three germ layers are the ectoderm, the mesoderm, and the endoderm. Table 12-3 lists structures that develop from each germ layer.

The central nervous system begins developing during the 3rd week. A thickened flat neural plate appears, extending toward the end of the embryonic disk that will become the head. The neural plate develops a longitudinal groove that folds to form the neural tube. At the end of the 3rd week, the neural tube is fused in the middle but is still open at each end.

Early heart development consists of a pair of parallel tubes that run longitudinally and join. The early heart begins beating at 21 to 22 days. Vessels developing in the chorionic villi and membranes join the heart tubes. Primitive blood cells arise from the endoderm lining the distal blood vessels.

Fourth Week

The shape of the embryo changes. It folds at the head and tail end and laterally. The embryo resembles a **C**-shaped cylinder by the end of the 4th week. A "tail" is apparent during the embryonic period because the brain and spinal cord develop more rapidly than other systems.

The neural tube completes closure during the 4th week. If the neural tube does not close, defects such as anencephaly and spina bifida result.

Formation of the face and upper respiratory tract begins. Beginnings of the internal ear and the eye are apparent. The upper extremities appear as buds on the lateral body walls.

Because the embryo is sharply flexed anteriorly, the heart is near the embryo's mouth. Partitioning of the heart into four chambers begins during the 4th week and is completed by the end of the 6th week.

The lower respiratory tract begins growth as a branch of the upper digestive tract, which is tubular at this time. Gradually, the esophagus and trachea separate completely. The trachea branches to form the right and left bronchi. These bronchi in turn branch to form the three lobes of the right lung and two lobes of the left lung. Continued branching of the bronchi eventually forms the terminal air sacs (*alveoli*). The alveoli proliferate and become surrounded by a rich capillary network that allows oxygen and carbon dioxide exchange at birth.

Fifth Week

The head is very large because the brain grows rapidly during the 5th week. The heart is beating and developing four chambers. Upper limb buds are paddle-shaped, with notches between the fingers. Lower limbs are also paddle-shaped, but the area between the toes is less defined as the division between the fingers.

Sixth Week

The head is prominent because of rapid development and is bent over the chest. The heart reaches its final four-chambered form. Upper and lower extremities continue to become more defined.

The eye continues to develop, and the beginning of the external ear is apparent as six small bumps near each side of the neck. Facial development begins with eyes, ears, and nasal pits widely separated, aligned with the body walls. Gradually, the embryo grows so that the face comes together at the midline.

Seventh Week

Growth and refinement of all systems occur. The face is now human-looking. The eyelids begin to grow, and the extremities become longer and better defined. The trunk elongates and straightens, although a **C**-shaped spinal curve remains at birth.

During the embryonic period, the intestines grow faster than the abdominal cavity. The relatively large liver and kidneys also occupy much of the abdominal cavity. Therefore most of the intestines are contained within the umbilical cord while the abdominal cavity grows to accommodate them. By 10 weeks, the abdomen is large enough to contain all its normal contents.

Eighth Week

The embryo has a definite human form, and refinements to all systems continue. The ears are low-set but are approaching their final location. The eyes are pigmented but not fully covered by eyelids. Fingers and toes are stubby but well defined. The external genitalia begin to differentiate, but male and female characteristics are not distinct until after the 10th week.

FETAL PERIOD

The fetal period begins 9 weeks after conception and ends with birth. Dramatic growth and refinement in the structure and function of all organ systems occur during the fetal period. Teratogens may damage already formed structures but are less likely to cause major structural alterations. The central nervous system is vulnerable to damaging agents through the entire pregnancy. Figure 12-6 illustrates growth and development during the fetal period.

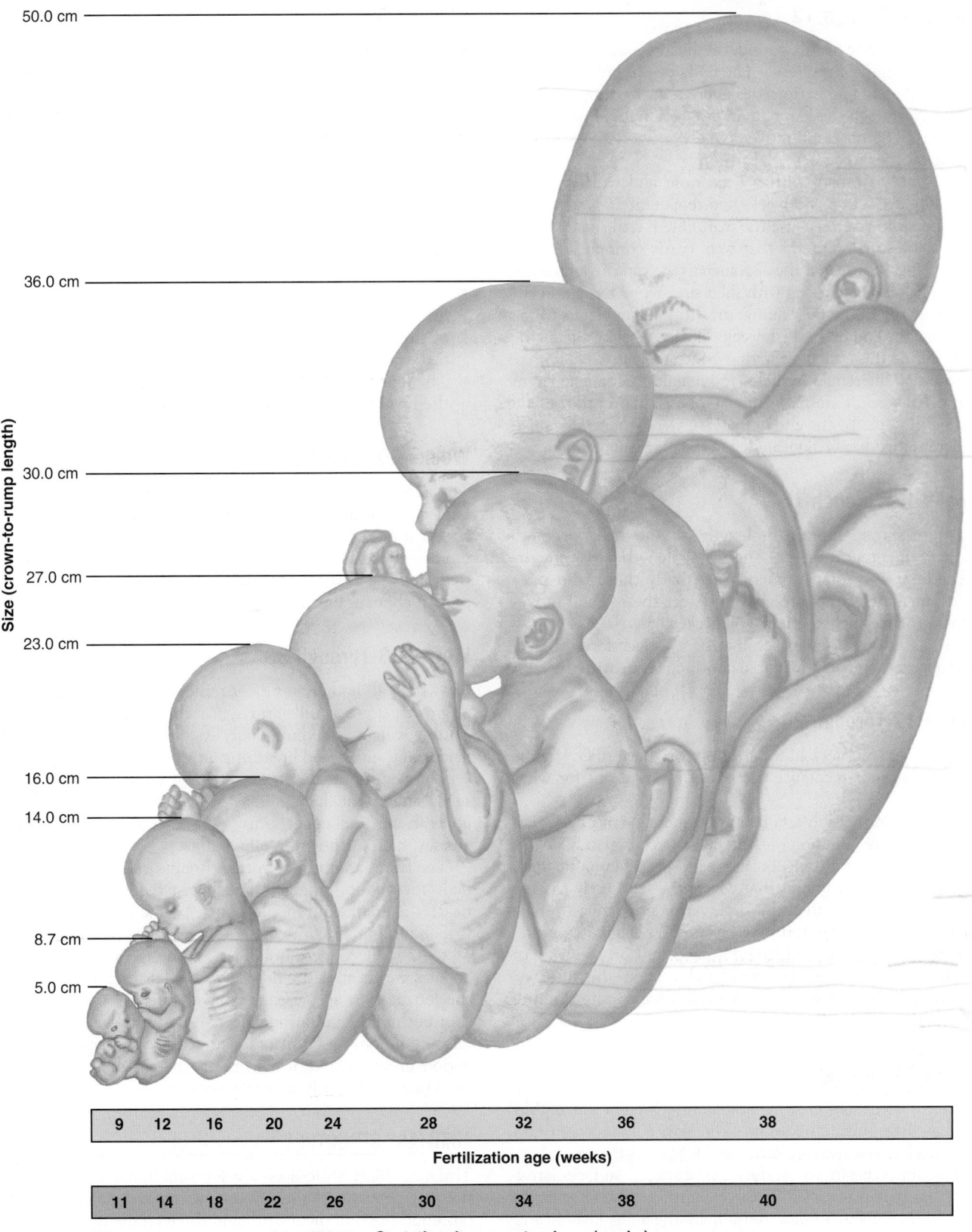

Figure 12-6 Fetal development from 9 weeks of fertilization age through 38 weeks of fertilization age. Gestational age, measured from the first day of the last menstrual period, is about 2 weeks longer than the fertilization age.

Weeks 9 Through 12

At the beginning of this period, the head is large, about half the total length of the fetus. The body begins growing faster than the head. The extremities approach their final relative lengths, although the legs remain proportionally shorter than the arms. The first fetal movements begin but are too slight for the mother to detect.

The face is broad, with a wide nose and widely spaced eyes. The eyes close at 9 weeks and reopen at 26 weeks. The ears appear low-set because the mandible is still small.

The intestinal contents that were partly contained within the umbilical cord enter the abdomen as the capacity of the abdominal cavity catches up with their size. Blood formation occurs primarily in the liver during the 9th week but shifts to the spleen by the end of the 12th week. The fetus begins producing urine during this period, excreting it into the amniotic fluid.

Internal differences in males and females become apparent in the 7th week. External genitalia look similar until the end of the 9th week. By the end of the 12th week, the fetal sex can be determined by the appearance of the external genitalia.

Weeks 13 Through 16

The fetus grows rapidly in length, so the head becomes smaller in proportion to the total length. Movements strengthen, and some women, particularly those who have been pregnant before, are able to detect them. Fetal movements produce the experience of *quickening*.

The face looks human because the eyes face forward. The external ears approach their final position, in line with the eyes.

Weeks 17 Through 20

Fetal movements feel like fluttering, or "butterflies." Some women may not recognize these subtle sensations for what they are.

Changes in the skin and hair are evident. *Vernix caseosa*, a fatty, cheeselike secretion of the fetal sebaceous glands, covers the skin to protect it from constant exposure to amniotic fluid. *Lanugo* is fine, downy hair that covers the fetal body to help the vernix adhere to the skin. Both vernix and lanugo diminish as the fetus reaches term. Eyebrows and head hair appear.

Brown fat is heat-producing fat deposited on the back of the neck, behind the sternum, and around the kidneys. Brown fat helps the neonate maintain temperature stability after birth.

Weeks 21 Through 24

The fetus continues growing and gaining weight but is thin and has little subcutaneous fat. The skin is translucent and looks red because the capillaries are close to its fragile surface.

The lungs begin to produce *surfactant*, a surface-active lipid that makes it easier for the baby to breathe after birth. Surfactant reduces surface tension in the lung alveoli and keeps them from collapsing with each breath.

The capillary network surrounding the alveoli is increasing but is still very immature, although some gas exchange is possible. If born at the end of this period, the baby may survive. However, multiple complications related to immaturity of all systems are likely and the survivor has a high risk for permanent disability.

Weeks 25 Through 28

With maturation of the lungs, pulmonary capillaries, and central nervous system, the fetus is more likely to survive if born after 24 weeks. The fetus becomes plumper and smoother-skinned as subcutaneous fat is deposited under the skin. The skin becomes less red. The eyes, closed since 9 weeks, reopen. Head hair is abundant. Blood formation shifts from the spleen to the bone marrow.

During early pregnancy, the fetus floats freely within the amniotic sac. The fetus usually assumes a head-down position during this time, however, for two reasons:

- The uterus is shaped like an inverted egg. The shape of the fetus in flexion is similar, with the head as the small pole of the egg shape, and with the buttocks, flexed legs, and feet as the larger pole.
- The fetal head is heavier than the feet, and gravity causes the head to drift downward in the pool of amniotic fluid.

Weeks 29 Through 32

The skin is pigmented according to race and is smooth. Larger vessels are visible over the abdomen, but small capillaries cannot be seen. Toenails are present, and fingernails extend to the fingertips. The fetus has more subcutaneous fat, rounding the body contours. If the fetus is born during this period, chances of survival are good.

Weeks 33 Through 38

Growth of all body systems continues until birth, but the rate of growth slows as full term approaches. The fetus is mainly gaining weight. The pulmonary system matures to enable efficient and unlabored breathing after birth.

The well-nourished term fetus is rotund, with abundant subcutaneous fat. Lanugo may be present over the forehead, upper back, and upper arms. Vernix may remain in major creases, such as the groin and axillae.

The testes are in the scrotum. Breasts of both male and female infants are enlarged, and breast tissue is palpable beneath the areola and nipple.

Full term ranges from 36 to 40 weeks of fertilization age, or 38 to 42 weeks of gestational age. Because conception occurs about 2 weeks after the first day of the last menstrual period, the fertilization age, used in this chapter, is about 2 weeks shorter than the gestational age. Gestational age, however, is most commonly used in practice because the last menstrual period provides a known marker, whereas most women do not know exactly when they conceived.

AUXILIARY STRUCTURES

Three auxiliary structures develop simultaneously to sustain the pregnancy and permit normal prenatal development: the placenta, the umbilical cord, and the fetal membranes.

Placenta

The placenta is a thick, disk-shaped organ (Fig. 12-7). Its major functions are (1) metabolic, (2) transfer of substances between mother and fetus, and (3) endocrine. The fetal side is smooth, with branching vessels covering the membrane-

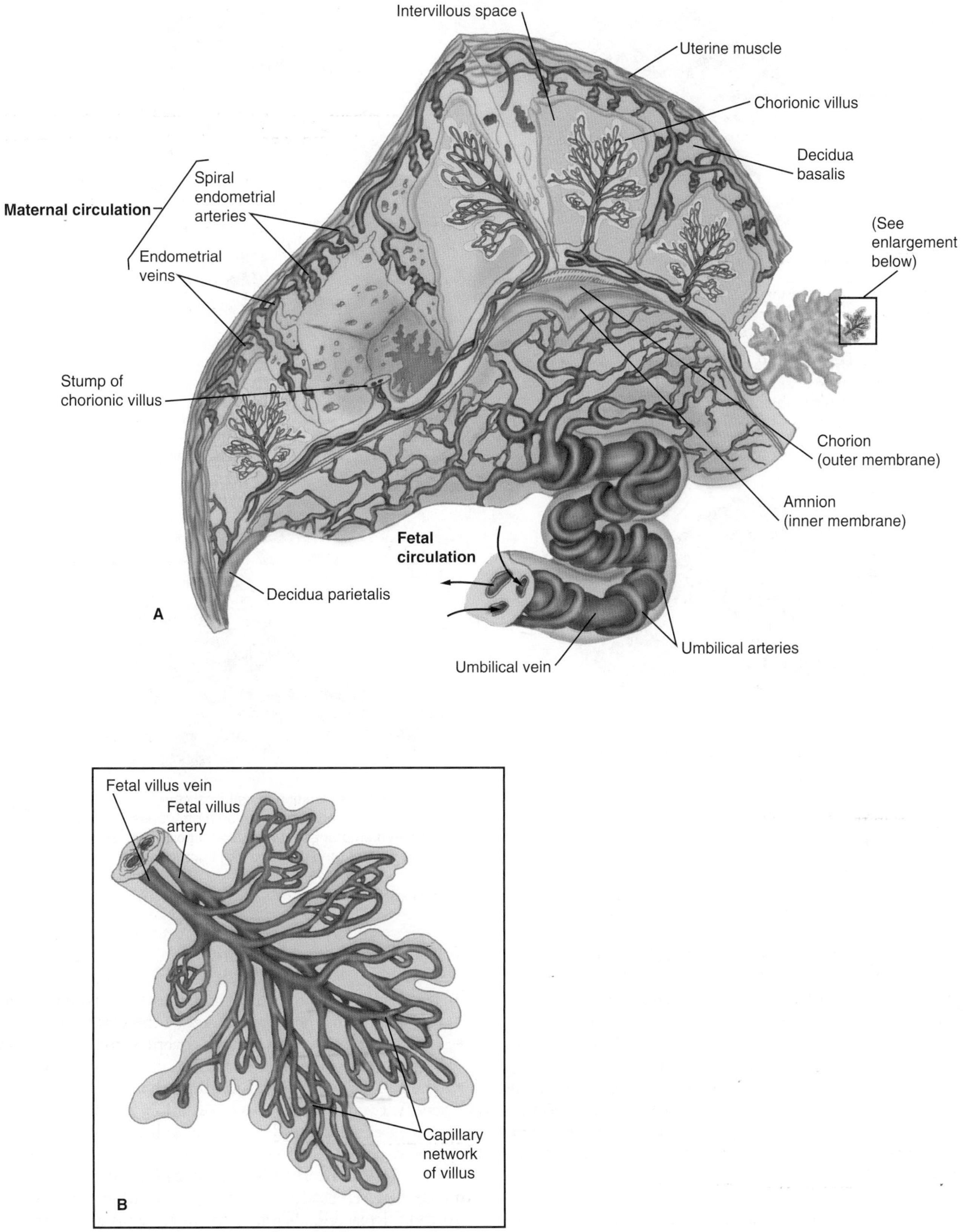

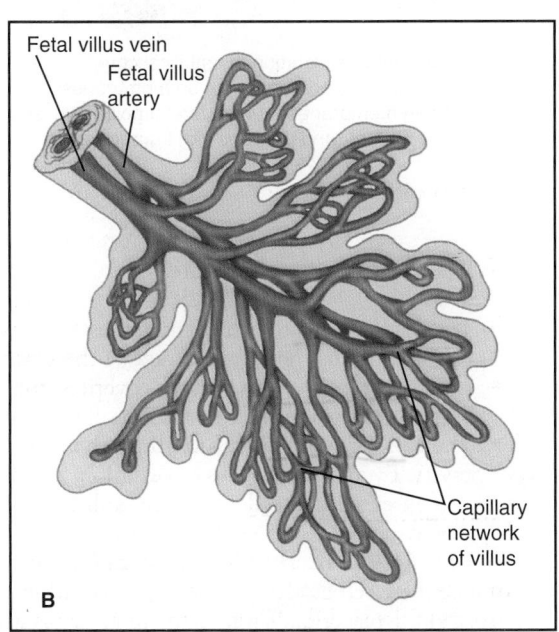

Intervillous space

Uterine muscle

Chorionic villus

Decidua basalis

Maternal circulation

Spiral endometrial arteries

Endometrial veins

(See enlargement below)

Stump of chorionic villus

Chorion (outer membrane)

Amnion (inner membrane)

Fetal circulation

Decidua parietalis

Umbilical arteries

Umbilical vein

A

Fetal villus vein

Fetal villus artery

Capillary network of villus

B

Figure 12-7 **A,** Placental structure, showing relationship of placenta, fetal membranes, and uterus. *Arrows* indicate the direction of blood flow between the fetus and placenta through the umbilical arteries and vein. Blood from the woman bathes the fetal chorionic villi within the intervillous spaces to allow exchange of oxygen, nutrients, and waste products without gross mixing of maternal and fetal blood. **B,** Structure of a chorionic villus, showing its fetal capillary network.

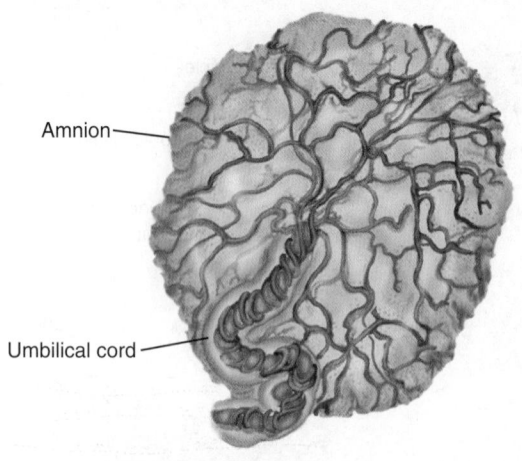

Amnion

Umbilical cord

Normal placenta, with insertion of umbilical
cord near center and branching of fetal umbilical
vessels over the surface

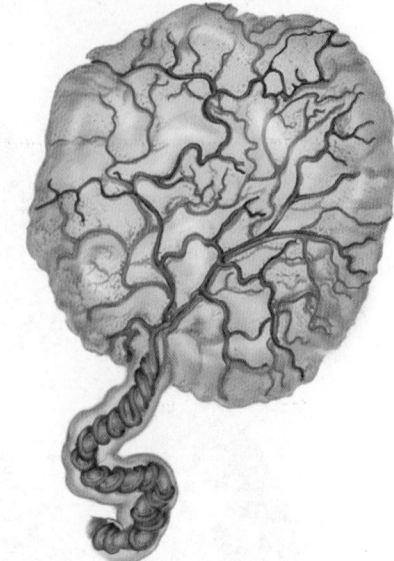

Placenta with cord inserted near margin
of placenta

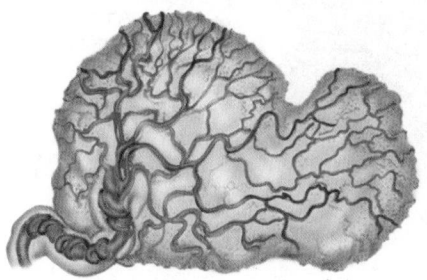

Placenta with a small accessory lobe

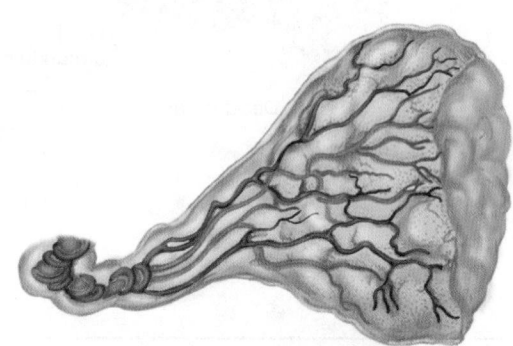

Velamentous insertion of umbilical cord.
Cord vessels branch far out on membranes.
When membranes rupture, fetal umbilical vessels
may be torn, and the fetus can hemorrhage.

Figure 12-8 Placental variations.

covered surface. The maternal side is rough where it attaches
to the uterus (see Fig. 17-14).

The umbilical cord is normally inserted on the fetal side of
the placenta, near the center. It may insert off-center or even
out on the fetal membranes, however. Figure 12-8 illustrates
the normal insertion and variations from normal.

During early pregnancy, the placenta is larger than the
embryo or fetus. The fetus grows faster than the placenta,
however, so that the placenta is about one-sixth the weight
of the fetus at the end of a term pregnancy.

Maternal Component

Development. When conception occurs, cells of the decidua undergo changes that promote early nutrition of the
embryo and enable most of the uterine lining to be shed after
birth. These changes convert endometrial cells into the *decidua*. In addition to providing nourishment for the embryo,
the decidua may protect the mother from uncontrolled invasion of fetal placental tissue into the uterine wall.

The three decidual layers are:

- The *decidua basalis*, which underlies the developing embryo and forms the maternal side of the placenta.
- The *decidua capsularis*, which overlies the embryo and
  bulges into the uterine cavity as the embryo and fetus grow.
- The *decidua parietalis*, which lines the rest of the uterine
  cavity. By about 22 weeks of gestation, the decidua capsularis fuses with the decidua parietalis, filling the uterine
  cavity.

Circulation in the Maternal Side. Exchange of substances between mother and fetus occurs within the *intervillous
space* of the placenta. While in the intervillous space, maternal
blood is briefly outside her circulatory system. About 150 ml of
maternal blood is contained within the intervillous space, and
it is changed about three to four times per minute.

Maternal blood enters the intervillous spaces through 80
to 100 spiral arteries in the decidua. After the oxygenated
and nutrient-bearing maternal blood washes over the chori-

TABLE 12-4 Mechanisms of Placental Transfer

Mechanism	Description	Examples of Substances Transferred
Simple diffusion	Passive movement of substances across a cell membrane from an area of higher concentration to one of lower concentration	Oxygen and carbon dioxide Carbon monoxide Water Urea and uric acid Most drugs and their metabolites
Facilitated diffusion	Passage of substances across a cell membrane by binding with carrier proteins that assist transfer	Glucose
Active transport	Transfer of substances across a cell membrane against a pressure or electrical gradient, or from an area of lower concentration to one of higher concentration	Amino acids Water-soluble vitamins Minerals: Calcium, iron, iodine
Pinocytosis	Movement of large molecules by ingestion within cells	Maternal IgG class antibodies Some passage of maternal IgA antibodies

IgG, Immunoglobulin G; *IgA,* immunoglobulin A.

onic villi containing fetal capillaries, it returns to the maternal circulation through the endometrial veins for elimination of fetal waste products.

Fetal Component

Development. The fetal side of the placenta develops from the outer cell layer (trophoblast) of the blastocyst at the same time that the inner cell mass develops into the embryo and fetus. The primary chorionic villi are the initial structures that eventually form the fetal side of the placenta.

Circulation in the Fetal Side. Blood is circulated to and from the fetal side of the placenta by the fetal heart. The umbilical cord contains two umbilical arteries that spiral around one vein to transport blood between the fetus and placenta. The chorionic villi are bathed by oxygen-rich and nutrient-rich maternal blood in the maternal intervillous spaces. Each chorionic villus is supplied by a tiny fetal artery carrying deoxygenated blood and waste products from the fetus. The vein of the chorionic villus returns oxygenated blood and nutrients to the fetus.

Fetal capillaries in the chorionic villi are separated from actual contact with the mother's blood by the membranes of each villus. This arrangement allows contact close enough for exchange and avoids mixing of fetal and maternal blood, which may not be compatible.

Metabolic Functions

The placenta produces some nutrients needed for the embryo and for its own functions. Substances synthesized include glycogen, cholesterol, and fatty acids (Moore & Persaud, 2003).

Transfer Functions

Exchange of oxygen, nutrients, and waste products across the chorionic villi occurs by several methods. Table 12-4 presents examples of substances transferred between the mother and the developing fetus.

Placental transfer of harmful substances also may occur. Most substances that enter the mother's bloodstream can enter the fetal circulation, and many agents enter it almost immediately.

Gas Exchange. A key function of the placenta is respiration. Oxygen and carbon dioxide pass through the placental membrane by simple diffusion. The average oxygen partial pressure (PO_2) of maternal blood in the intervillous space is 50 mm Hg. The average blood PO_2 in the umbilical vein (af-

ter oxygenation) is about 30 mm Hg (Guyton & Hall, 2000). The fetus can thrive in this low-oxygen environment for three reasons:

- Fetal hemoglobin can carry 20% to 50% more oxygen than adult hemoglobin.
- The fetus has a higher oxygen-carrying capacity because of a higher average hemoglobin (14.5 to 22.5 g/dl) and hematocrit value (about 48% to 69%).
- Hemoglobin can carry more oxygen at low carbon dioxide partial pressure (PCO_2) levels than it can at high ones (Bohr effect). Blood entering the placenta from the fetus has a high PCO_2, but carbon dioxide diffuses quickly to the mother's blood, where the PCO_2 is lower, reversing the levels of carbon dioxide in maternal and fetal blood supplies. Therefore the fetal blood becomes more alkaline and the maternal blood becomes more acidic. This difference allows the mother's blood to give up oxygen and the fetal blood to combine with oxygen readily.

Nutrient Transfer. The growing fetus requires a constant supply of nutrients from the pregnant woman. Glucose, fatty acids, electrolytes, and vitamins pass readily across the placenta.

Waste Removal. In addition to carbon dioxide, urea, uric acid, and bilirubin are readily transferred from the fetus to the mother for disposal.

Antibody Transfer. The immunoglobulin G (IgG) class of maternal antibodies are the primary ones transferred to the fetus by the placenta. Transfer of IgG antibodies to the fetus may provide temporary (passive) immunity against diseases such as rubella or tetanus if the mother is immune. The preterm or small-for-gestational-age infant has little disease protection because many maternal antibodies are not transferred until late pregnancy and are poorly transferred if placental function is inadequate.

Passage of antibodies from expectant mother to fetus may be harmful. If maternal and fetal blood types are not compatible, the mother either may already have or may produce antibodies against fetal erythrocytes. The mother's antibodies may then destroy the fetal erythrocytes, causing fetal anemia or even fetal death.

Transfer of Maternal Hormones. Most maternal protein hormones do not reach the fetus in amounts sufficient to cause abnormalities.

Endocrine Functions

The placenta produces many hormones necessary for normal pregnancy. Human chorionic gonadotropin (hCG) causes the corpus luteum to persist and secrete estrogens and progesterone for the first 6 to 8 weeks. The placenta gradually takes over production of estrogens and progesterone, and the corpus luteum regresses after 20 weeks. When a Y chromosome is present in the male fetus, hCG also causes the fetal testes to secrete testosterone necessary for normal development of male reproductive structures.

Human placental lactogen, also called *human chorionic somatomammotropin*, promotes normal nutrition and growth of the fetus and maternal breast development for lactation. The hormone decreases maternal insulin sensitivity and utilization of glucose, making more glucose available for fetal growth.

Steroid hormones secreted by the placenta include estrogens and progesterone. Estrogens cause enlargement of the woman's uterus, enlargement of the breasts, growth of the ductal system of the breasts, and enlargement of the external genitalia. Estrogens enhance uterine activity, particularly as term approaches, playing a role as labor begins.

Progesterone causes the endometrium to change into the decidua, providing nourishment for the early conceptus. Progesterone reduces uterine contractions and suppresses maternal reactions to fetal antigens to prevent spontaneous abortion. Progesterone acts with estrogens and other hormones to cause growth of the breasts, budding of the alveoli that will secrete milk, and development of secretory characteristics in the alveolar cells.

Other hormones produced by the placenta include human chorionic thyrotropin and human chorionic adrenocorticotropin as well as many growth factors.

Fetal Membranes and Amniotic Fluid

The two fetal membranes are the *amnion* (inner membrane) and the *chorion* (outer membrane). The two membranes are so close as to be one, although they can be separated. Together, they are often called the *bag of waters*. If they rupture in labor, amnion and chorion usually rupture together, releasing the amniotic fluid within the sac.

The amnion is continuous with the surface of the umbilical cord, joining the epithelium of the fetus's abdominal skin. Chorionic villi proliferate over the entire surface of the gestational sac for the first 8 weeks after conception. A conceptus observed at this time looks like a shaggy sphere with the embryo suspended inside. As the embryo grows, it bulges into the uterine cavity. The villi on the outer surface gradually atrophy and form the smooth-surfaced chorion. The remaining villi continue to branch and enlarge to form the fetal side of the placenta.

Amniotic fluid protects the growing fetus and promotes normal prenatal development. Amniotic fluid protects the fetus by:

- Cushioning against an impact to the maternal abdomen
- Providing a stable temperature

Amniotic fluid promotes normal prenatal development by:

- Allowing symmetric development of the fetus
- Keeping the membranes from adhering to developing fetal parts

- Providing room and buoyancy for fetal movement
- Maintaining constant intrauterine temperature
- Providing a cushion to distribute pressure within the uterus

Amniotic fluid is derived from two sources: fetal urine and fluid transported from the maternal blood across the amnion. Cast-off fetal epithelial cells and vernix are suspended in the amniotic fluid. The water of the amniotic fluid changes by absorption across the amnion, returning to the mother. Some fluid is absorbed by the fetal lungs with breathing movements. Additional amniotic fluid is swallowed and absorbed by the fetal digestive tract.

The volume of amniotic fluid increases during pregnancy, until it is about 500 to 1000 ml at term (Guyton & Hall, 2000). An abnormally small quantity of fluid (less than 50% of the amount expected for gestation, or less than 500 ml at term) is called *oligohydramnios* and is associated with poor fetal lung development and malformations that result from compression of fetal parts. Oligohydramnios may occur because the kidneys fail to develop, urine excretion is blocked, or placental blood flow is inadequate. *Hydramnios* (also called *polyhydramnios*) is the opposite situation, in which the quantity may exceed 2000 ml. Hydramnios may occur when the fetus has a severe malformation of the central nervous system or gastrointestinal tract that prevents normal ingestion of amniotic fluid.

Fetal Circulation

The course of fetal blood circulation is from the fetal heart, to the placenta for exchange of oxygen and waste products, and back to the fetus for delivery to fetal tissues (Fig. 12-9, A).

Umbilical Cord

The umbilical cord has two arteries that carry blood that is high in carbon dioxide and other waste products away from the fetus to the placenta, where these substances are transferred to the mother's circulation for elimination. The umbilical vein carries freshly oxygenated and nutrient-rich blood from the placenta back to the fetus. The umbilical arteries and vein are coiled within the cord to allow them to stretch and prevent obstruction of blood flow through them. The entire cord is cushioned by a soft substance called *Wharton's jelly* to prevent obstruction caused by pressure.

Fetal Circulatory Circuit

Because the fetus does not breathe air or metabolize substances in the liver, several alterations of the postbirth circulatory route are needed. Three shunts—the ductus venosus, the foramen ovale, and the ductus arteriosus—divert most circulating blood away from the lungs and liver.

Oxygenated blood from the placenta enters the fetal body through the umbilical vein. About half the blood goes through the liver, and the rest bypasses the liver and enters the inferior vena cava through the first shunt, the *ductus venosus*. The blood then enters the right atrium. Most of the blood passes directly into the left atrium through the second shunt, the *foramen ovale*, where it mixes with the small amount of blood returning from the lungs. Blood is pumped from the left ventricle into the aorta to nourish the body. A small amount of blood from the right ventricle is circulated to the lungs to nourish the lung tissue. The rest of the blood from the right ventricle joins oxygenated blood in the aorta

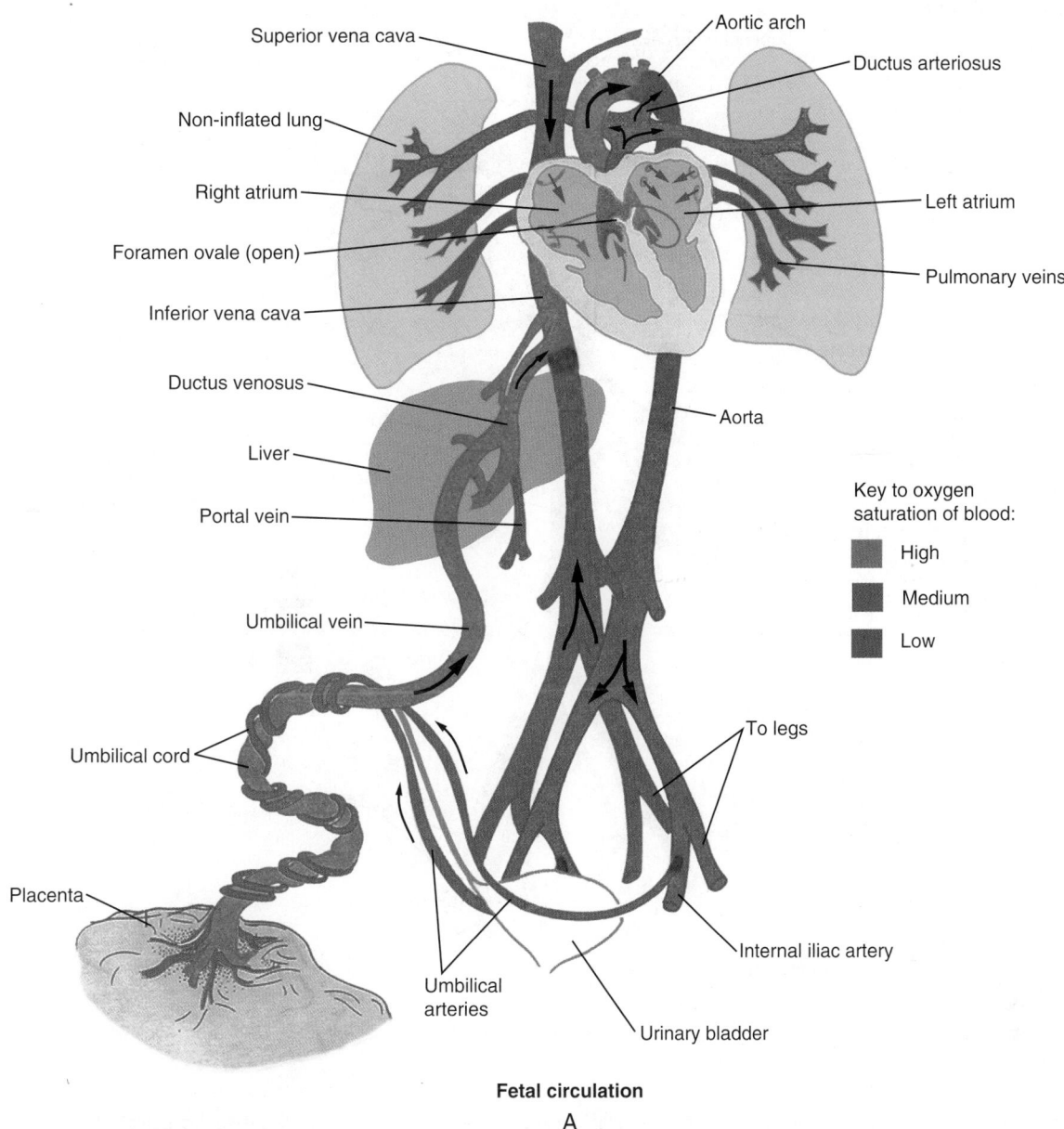

Figure 12-9 A, Fetal circulation. Three shunts—the ductus venosus, the ductus arteriosus, and the foramen ovale—allow most blood from the placenta to bypass the fetal lungs and liver.

Continued

through the third shunt, the *ductus arteriosus*. The head and upper body receive the greatest amount of oxygenated blood.

Resistance to blood flow through the uninflated lungs is high, causing the right ventricle to work harder and have a thicker wall than the left. After breathing is established, resistance to pulmonary blood flow falls and systemic resistance rises, causing the right ventricular wall to become thinner while the left becomes thicker.

Changes in Blood Circulation After Birth

Fetal circulatory shunts are not needed after birth because the infant oxygenates blood in the lungs, metabolizes substances in the liver, and stops circulating blood to the pla-

centa (see Fig. 12-9, B). As the infant breathes, blood flow to the lungs increases, pressure in the right heart falls, and the foramen ovale closes. Pressure in the aorta rises as pressure in the pulmonary artery falls, causing the direction of blood flow through the ductus arteriosus to reverse, from the aorta into the pulmonary artery. The ductus arteriosus constricts as the arterial oxygen level rises. The ductus venosus constricts when blood flow from the umbilical cord stops.

The foramen ovale and ductus venosus permanently close as tissue proliferates in these structures. The ductus venosus and ductus arteriosus become ligaments, as do the umbilical vein and arteries.

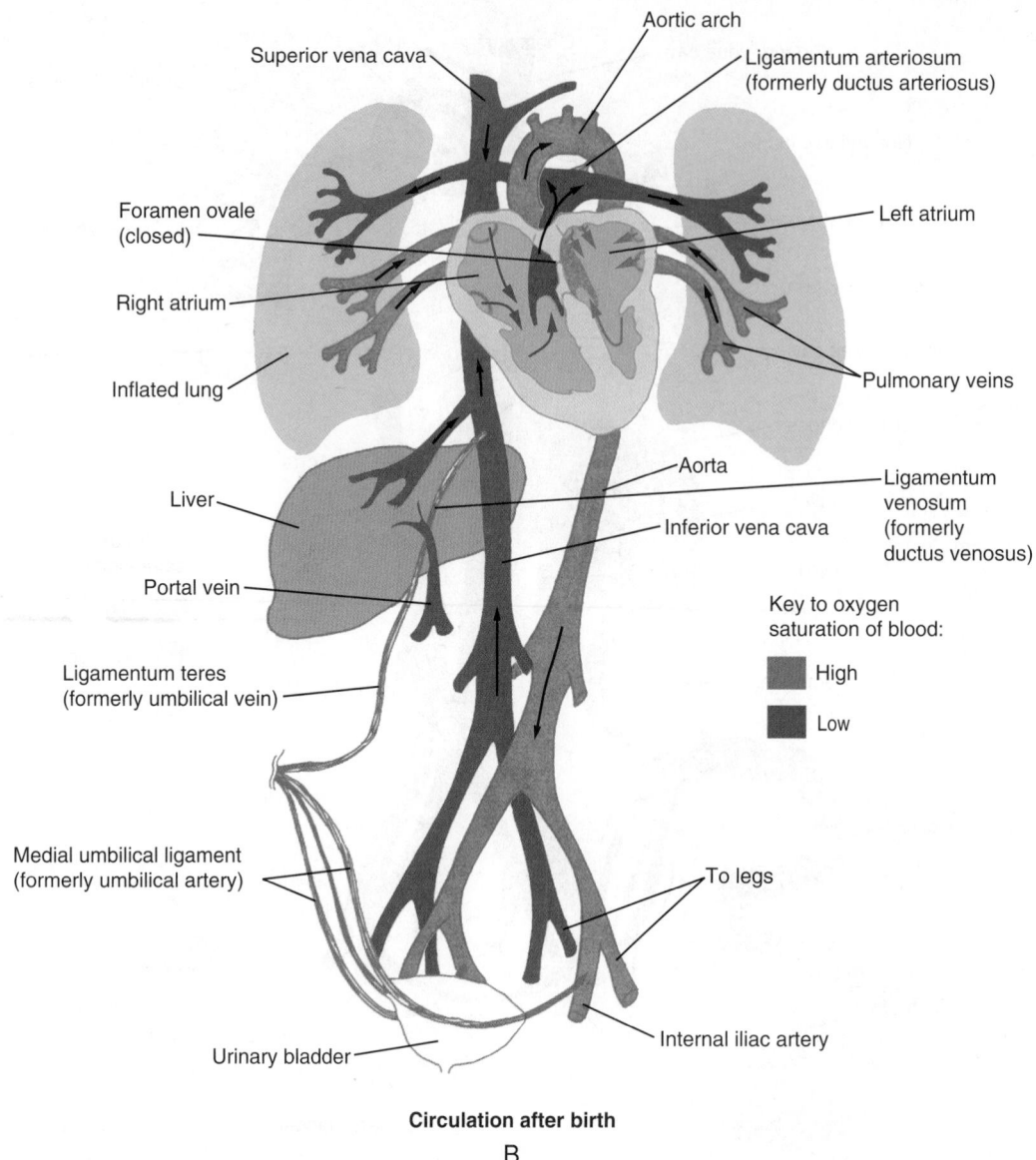

Figure 12-9, cont'd **B**, Circulation after birth. Note that the fetal shunts have closed. The umbilical vessels, the ductus venosus, and the ductus arteriosus have been converted to ligaments.

MULTIFETAL PREGNANCY

Multifetal pregnancy is a deviation from the usual course of gestation. Twins occur *spontaneously* about once in 85 pregnancies, triplets about once in 8100 pregnancies, quadruplets once in 729,000 pregnancies, and quintuplets only once in more than 65 million pregnancies (Moore & Persaud, 2003). The number of twin births has increased in recent years to 31.1 per 1000 births in 2002. Rates of high-order multiples (triplets or more) declined after 1998 but are now increasing.

Twinning is the most common form of multifetal pregnancy. Processes that cause a twin pregnancy also may cause other multiple gestations. Twins are most accurately described by their genetic origin or by the number of ova and sperm involved. The two types of twins are monozygotic and dizygotic. Figure 12-10 illustrates these two mechanisms of twinning.

Monozygotic Twinning

Monozygotic twins are conceived by the union of a single ovum and spermatozoon, with later division of the conceptus into two. Monozygotic twins have identical genetic complements and are of the same sex and are often called "identical" by laypeople. They may not always look identical at birth because one twin may be larger than the other or one may have a birth defect, such as a cleft lip. Monozygotic twinning occurs at random and is unrelated to the use of assisted reproductive techniques (Atlanta Maternal-Fetal Medicine, 1994; Blackburn, 2003; Moore & Persaud, 2003).

In monozygotic twinning, a single conceptus divides early in gestation. In most cases of monozygotic twins (65%), the formed *blastocyst* has two inner cell masses instead of one. With two inner cell masses, the fetuses have

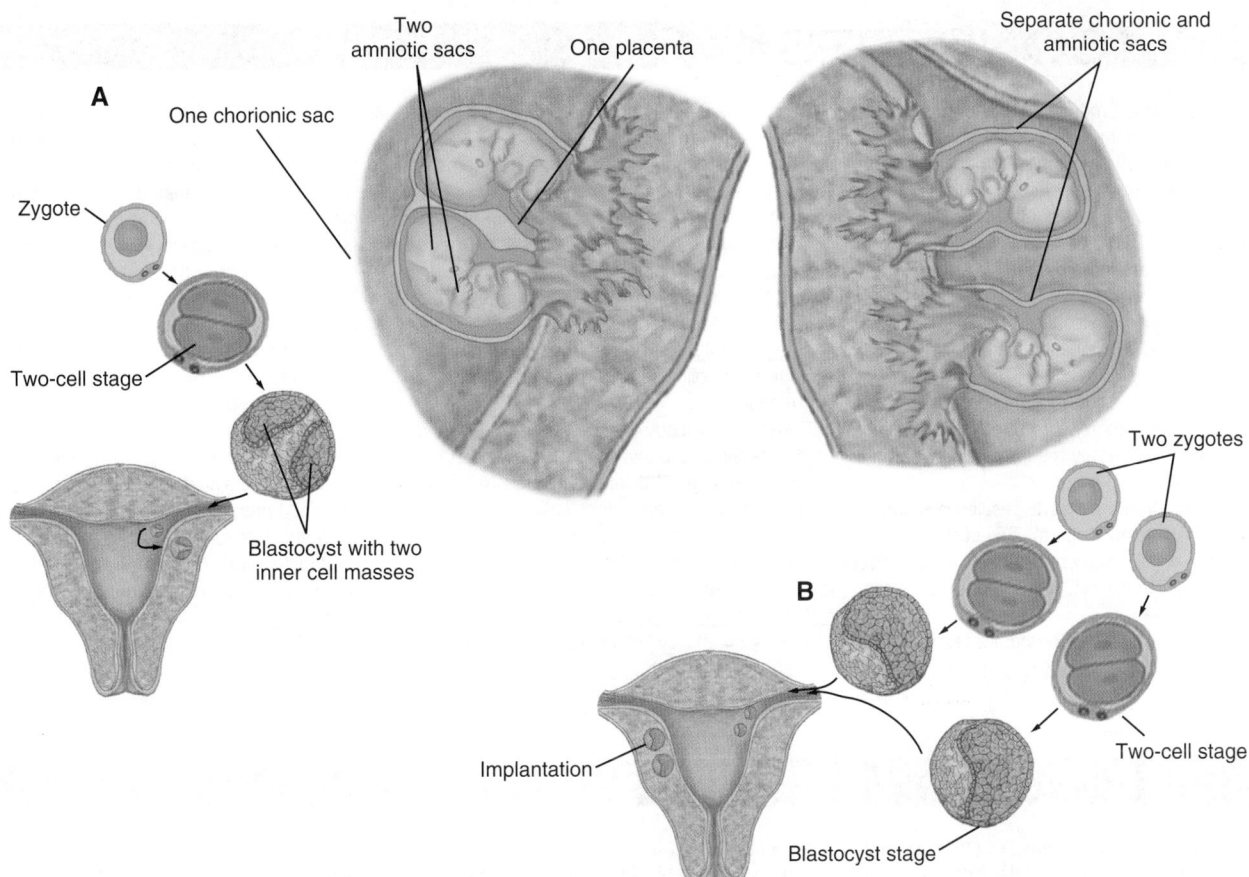

Figure 12-10 A, Monozygotic twinning. The single inner cell mass divides into two inner cell masses during the blastocyst stage. These twins have a single placenta and chorion, but each twin develops in its own amnion. **B,** Dizygotic twinning. Two ova are released during ovulation, and each is fertilized by a separate spermatozoon. The ova may implant near each other in the uterus, or they may be far apart.

two amnions (inner membranes) but a single chorion (outer membrane).

If the conceptus divides earlier, two separate but identical morulas (and then blastocysts) develop and implant separately. These monozygotic twins have two amnions and two chorions. Although their placentas develop separately, they may fuse and appear as one at birth. Their chorions also may fuse during prenatal development. Therefore examining the placenta and membranes after birth cannot always establish whether twins are monozygotic or dizygotic.

Late separation of the inner cell mass may result in twins with a single amnion and a single chorion. These twins often die because their umbilical cords become entangled. Incomplete separation of the inner cell mass may result in conjoined twins.

Dizygotic Twinning

Dizygotic twins arise from two ova that are fertilized by different sperm. Because dizygotic twins are no more alike than siblings, laypeople often refer to them as "fraternal." Dizygotic twins may be the same or different sex, and they may or may not have similar physical traits. Dizygotic twins are associated with the use of assisted reproductive techniques because these therapies involve induction of multiple ovulation and implantation of multiple fertilized ova. Advancing ma-

ternal age is also associated with an increased incidence of dizygotic twin births.

Dizygotic twinning may be hereditary in some families, presumably because of an inherited tendency of the women to release more than one ovum per cycle. Women of some races are more likely to have dizygotic twins as well (Moore & Persaud, 2003):

- African: 1 in 20 births
- White: 1 in 125 births
- Asian: 1 in 500 births

The membranes and placentas of dizygotic twins are separate because they arise from two separate zygotes. The membranes, placentas, or both may fuse during development if they implant closely. Dizygotic twins are not conjoined because they do not involve division of a single cell mass into two.

Other Multifetal Gestations

Pregnancies resulting in more offspring than twins may arise from a single zygote or a combination of a single and multiple zygotes, or each may arise from a separate zygote. High-multiple pregnancies pose greater hazards to both the expectant mother and fetuses. The incidence of long-term handicaps is higher as the number of fetuses increases.

KEY CONCEPTS

- Gametogenesis produces ova and sperm that have half the full number of chromosomes, or 23 unpaired chromosomes. When an ovum and a sperm unite at conception, the number is restored to 46 paired chromosomes as in other body cells.
- No new ova are formed after 30 weeks of prenatal gestation.
- One primary oocyte results in one mature ovum that contains 23 unpaired chromosomes (22 autosomes and an X chromosome).
- A male can continuously produce new sperm from puberty through the rest of his life, although fertility declines somewhat after age 40.
- One primary spermatocyte results in production of four mature sperm. Two of the mature sperm have 22 autosomes and an X sex chromosome. Two have 22 autosomes and a Y sex chromosome.
- The male determines the baby's sex because sperm carry either an X or a Y sex chromosome. The female contributes only an X chromosome to the baby.
- The basic structure of all organ systems is established during the first 8 weeks of pregnancy. Teratogens during this period may cause major structural and functional damage to the developing organs.
- The fetal period is one of growth and refinement of established organ systems.
- The placenta is an embryonic or fetal organ with metabolic, respiratory, and endocrine functions.
- Transfer of substances between mother and her developing baby occurs by four mechanisms: simple diffusion, facilitated diffusion, active transport, and pinocytosis.
- Most substances in the maternal blood can be transferred to the fetus.
- The fetal membranes contain the amniotic fluid, which cushions the fetus, allows normal prenatal development, and maintains a stable temperature.
- Two umbilical arteries carry deoxygenated blood and waste products to the placenta for transfer to the mother's blood. One umbilical vein carries oxygenated and nutrient-rich blood to the fetus. Coiling of the vessels and enclosure in Wharton's jelly reduce compression and torsion of the umbilical vessels.
- Three fetal circulatory shunts partially bypass the fetal liver and lungs: the ductus venosus, the foramen ovale, and the ductus arteriosus. These structures close functionally after birth but are not closed permanently until several weeks or months later.
- Multifetal pregnancy may be monozygotic or dizygotic. Twins are the most common form of multifetal pregnancy.
- Dizygotic twins are more likely to occur in certain families and racial groups, in older mothers, and in women who undergo fertility therapy.

REFERENCES and READINGS

Atlanta Maternal-Fetal Medicine, PC. (1994). *Clinical discussions: Twin pregnancy, 2*(4), April 19, 1994. Retrieved June 13, 2003, from www.atlanta-mfm.com/clindisc/vol2no4.html.

Benirschke, K. (2004a). Multiple gestation: Incidence, etiology and inheritance. In R.K. Creasy, R. Resnik, & J.D. Iams (Eds.). *Maternal-fetal medicine: Principles and practice* (5th ed., pp. 55-67). Philadelphia: Saunders.

Benirschke, K. (2004b). Normal development. In R.K. Creasy, R. Resnik, & J.D. Iams (Eds.). *Maternal-fetal medicine: Principles and practice* (5th ed., pp. 37-44). Philadelphia: Saunders.

Blackburn, S.T. (2003). *Maternal, fetal, and neonatal physiology: A clinical perspective*. Philadelphia: Saunders.

Guyton, A.C., & Hall, J.E. (2000). *Textbook of medical physiology* (10th ed.). Philadelphia: Saunders.

Martin, J.A., Hamilton, B.E., Sutton, P.D., Ventura, S.J., Menacker, F., & Munson, M.L. (2003). Births: Final data for 2002. *National Vital Statistics Reports* (vol 52, no. 10). Hyattsville, MD: National Center for Health Statistics. Retrieved January 28, 2004, from www.cdc.gov/nchs/data/nvsr/nvsr52/nvsr52_10.pdf

Moore, K.L., & Persaud, T.V.N. (2003). *Before we are born: Essentials of embryology and birth defects* (6th ed.). Philadelphia: Saunders.

13

Physiologic Adaptations to Pregnancy

◆ LEARNING OBJECTIVES

After studying this chapter, you should be able to:

◎ Describe the physiologic changes that occur during pregnancy.
◎ Differentiate presumptive, probable, and positive signs of pregnancy.
◎ Compute gravida, para, and estimated date of delivery (birth) based on the woman's last menstrual period.
◎ Describe initial antepartum assessments in terms of history, physical examination, and risk assessment.

◎ Identify subsequent antepartum assessments.
◎ Discuss maternal adaptations to multifetal pregnancy.
◎ Describe the common discomforts of pregnancy in terms of causes, and describe measures that prevent or relieve them.
◎ Use nursing process and critical thinking skills to develop a plan of nursing care for the most common problems and discomforts of pregnancy.

◆ DEFINITIONS

abortion In the United States, a spontaneous or elective termination of pregnancy before the 20th week of gestation, based on the date of the last menstrual period. Spontaneous abortion is frequently called "miscarriage" by the lay public.

amenorrhea Absence of menstruation.

Braxton Hicks contractions Irregular, mild uterine contractions that occur throughout pregnancy and become stronger in the last trimester.

Chadwick's sign Bluish purple discoloration of the cervix, vagina, and labia during pregnancy as a result of increased vascular congestion.

chloasma Brownish pigmentation of the face during pregnancy, also called melasma or "mask of pregnancy."

colostrum Breast fluid secreted during pregnancy and the first 2 to 3 days after childbirth.

diastasis recti Separation of the longitudinal muscles of the abdomen (rectus abdominis) during pregnancy.

Goodell's sign Softening of the cervix, uterus, and vagina during pregnancy.

gravida A woman who is or has been pregnant, regardless of the duration or the outcome of the pregnancy.

hyperemia Excess of blood in a part of the body.

multigravida A woman who has been pregnant more than once.

multipara A woman who has given birth two or more times at 20 or more weeks of gestation.

nullipara A woman who has never completed a pregnancy beyond a spontaneous or elective abortion.

para Number of pregnancies that have progressed to 20 or more weeks at delivery, whether the fetus was born alive or was stillborn; refers to the number of pregnancies, not the number of fetuses.

physiologic anemia of pregnancy Decrease in hemoglobin and hematocrit values caused by dilution of erythrocytes by expanded plasma volume rather than by an actual decrease in erythrocytes or hemoglobin.

postterm birth A birth that occurs after 42 weeks of gestation.

preterm birth A birth that occurs after the 20th week and before the start of the 38th week of gestation.

primigravida A woman who is pregnant for the first time.

primipara A woman who has given birth once after a pregnancy of at least 20 weeks of gestation.

quickening The first movements of the fetus in the uterus felt by the mother.

striae gravidarum Irregular reddish streaks on the abdomen, breasts, or thighs resulting from tears in connective tissue.

term birth A birth that occurs between the 38th and 42nd week of gestation.

trimester A division of pregnancy into three equal parts of 13 weeks each.

From the moment of conception, important changes occur in the pregnant woman's body. These changes are necessary to support and nourish the fetus and to prepare the woman for childbirth and lactation. Nurses must understand not only the physiologic changes but also the ways these changes affect the daily lives of expectant mothers.

CHANGES IN BODY SYSTEMS

Pregnancy challenges each body system to adapt to the increasing demands of the fetus.

Reproductive System

Uterus

Growth. Before conception the uterus is a small, pear-shaped organ entirely contained in the pelvic cavity. It weighs approximately 50 to 70 g (1.8 to 2.5 oz) and has a capacity of about 10 ml (one third of an ounce). At the end of pregnancy, the uterus extends to the level of the xiphoid process, weighs approximately 1000 g (2.2 lb), and has a capacity of about 5000 ml.

Uterine growth occurs as the result of both hyperplasia and hypertrophy. During the first trimester, growth is due mainly to hyperplasia resulting from stimulation of the myometrium by estrogen and growth factors. During the second and third trimesters, uterine growth is due to hyperplasia and hypertrophy as the muscle fibers stretch to accommodate the growing fetus (Blackburn, 2003). Fibrous tissue accumulates in the outer muscle layer of the uterus, and the amount of elastic tissue increases. These changes greatly increase the strength of the muscle wall.

Muscle fibers in the myometrium increase in both length and width. As a result, by the third trimester the uterine muscles are thin and the fetus can be easily palpated through the abdominal wall. As the uterus expands into the abdominal cavity, it gradually displaces the intestines upward and laterally as it rotates to the right. The rotation is probably the result of pressure of the rectosigmoid colon on the left side of the pelvis.

Pattern of Uterine Growth. The uterus grows in a predictable pattern that provides information about fetal growth and helps to confirm the expected date of delivery (EDD), sometimes called the *expected date of birth (EDB)* (Fig. 13-1). By 12 weeks of gestation, the uterus can be palpated above the symphysis pubis. At 16 weeks, the fundus reaches midway between the symphysis pubis and the umbilicus. It is located at the umbilicus by 20 weeks.

The fundus reaches its highest level at the xiphoid process at 36 weeks. Because it pushes against the diaphragm, many expectant mothers experience shortness of breath. By 40 weeks, the fetal head descends into the pelvic cavity and the uterus sinks to a lower level. This descent of the fetal head is called *lightening* because it reduces pressure on the diaphragm and makes breathing easier.

Contractility. Throughout pregnancy, the uterus undergoes irregular, painless contractions called *Braxton Hicks contractions*. During the first two trimesters, the contractions are infrequent. During the third trimester, the contractions occur more frequently and they may cause some discomfort. They are called *false labor* when they are mistaken for the onset of early labor.

Uterine Blood Flow. As the uterus increases in size, blood flow increases dramatically. In early pregnancy, when the uterus and placenta are relatively small, most of the blood

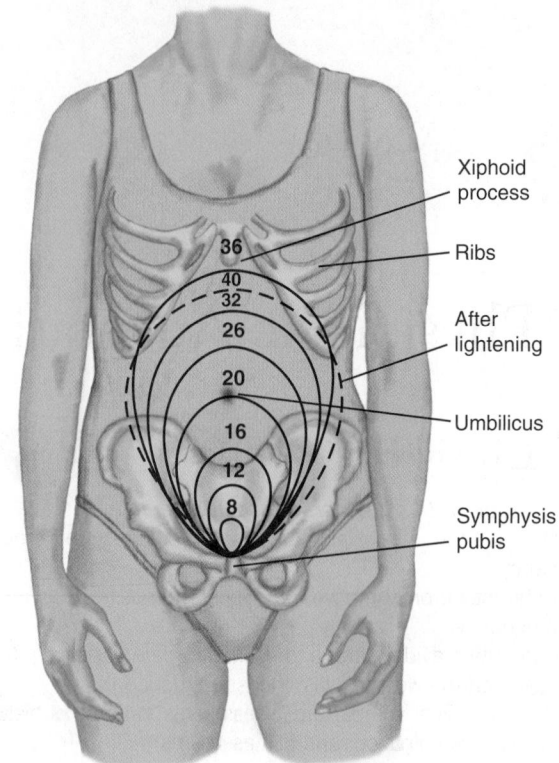

Figure 13-1 Uterine growth pattern during pregnancy.

flow is to the myometrium and endometrium. During late pregnancy, blood flow to the uterus and placenta reaches 450 to 650 ml/min (Cunningham et al., 2001). Adequate perfusion of the placental intervillous spaces is necessary for the delivery of most substances needed for fetal growth and the removal of metabolic wastes.

Cervix

The most obvious cervical changes occur in color and consistency. Estrogen causes the cervix to becomes congested with blood (i.e., hyperemic), resulting in the characteristic bluish purple color that extends to include the vagina and labia. This discoloration, referred to as *Chadwick's sign*, is one of the earliest signs of pregnancy.

Collagen fibers in the connective tissue of the cervix decrease, causing the cervix to soften. Before pregnancy, the cervix has a consistency similar to that of the tip of the nose. After conception, the cervix feels more like the lobe of the ear. The cervical softening is referred to as *Goodell's sign*.

The cervical glands proliferate during pregnancy, and the endocervical tissue resembles a honeycomb that fills with mucus. The mucus forms a plug in the cervical canal and blocks the ascent of bacteria from the vagina into the uterus during pregnancy (Fig. 13-2). One of the earliest signs of labor may be "bloody show," which consists of the mucous plug plus a small amount of blood produced by disruption of the cervical capillaries as the mucous plug is dislodged when the cervix begins to thin and dilate.

Vagina and Vulva

Increased vascularity of the vagina causes the vaginal walls, as well as the cervix, to appear bluish. Softening of the abundant connective tissue allows the vagina to distend during

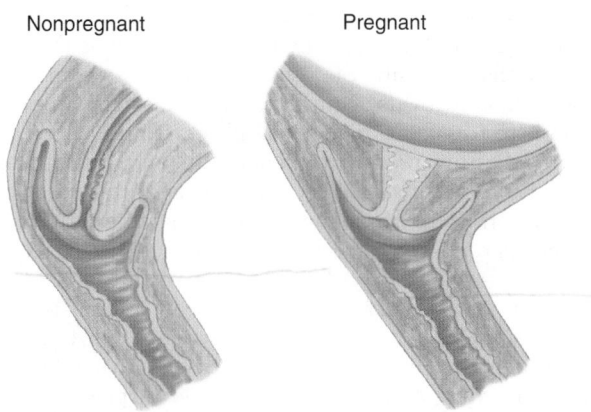

Nonpregnant   Pregnant

Figure 13-2 Cervical changes that occur during pregnancy. Note enlargement of spaces in cervical mucosa, which are filled with a thick mucous plug.

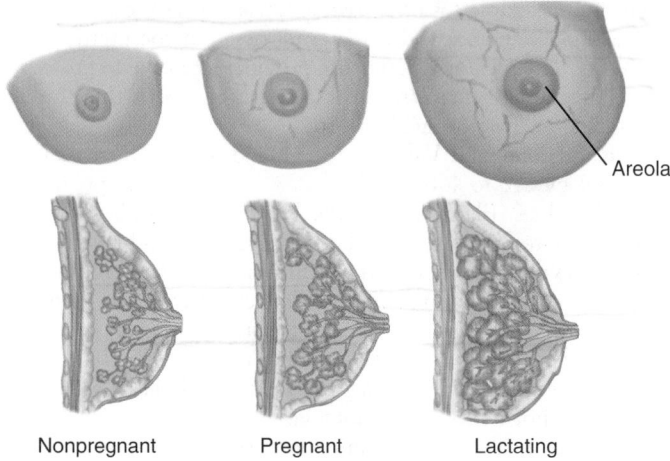

Areola

Nonpregnant   Pregnant   Lactating

Figure 13-3 Breast changes that occur during pregnancy. The breasts increase in size and become more vascular, the areolae become darker, and the nipples become more erect.

childbirth. The vaginal mucosa thickens, and vaginal rugae (folds) become very prominent.

Vaginal cells contain increasing amounts of glycogen, which causes rapid sloughing and increased vaginal discharge. The pH of the vaginal discharge is acidic because of the increased production of lactic acid that results from the action of *Lactobacillus acidophilus* on glycogen in the vaginal epithelium (Cunningham et al., 2001). The acidic condition works to prevent growth of harmful bacteria found in the vagina. The glycogen-rich environment, however, favors the growth of *Candida albicans*, so that persistent yeast infections (candidiasis) are common during pregnancy.

Increased vascularity, edema, and connective tissue changes make the tissues of the vulva and perineum more pliable. Pelvic congestion during pregnancy can lead to heightened sexual interest and increased orgasmic experiences.

Ovaries

After conception, the major function of the ovaries is to secrete progesterone for the first 6 to 7 weeks of the pregnancy. Progesterone is called the *hormone of pregnancy*, and if the pregnancy is to be maintained, adequate progesterone must be available from the earliest stages. The corpus luteum secretes progesterone until the placenta is developed. Once developed, the placenta secretes progesterone throughout pregnancy.

Ovulation ceases during pregnancy because the circulating levels of estrogen and progesterone are high, inhibiting the release of follicle-stimulating hormone (FSH) and luteinizing hormone (LH) from the pituitary, which are necessary for ovulation.

Breasts

During pregnancy, the breasts change in size and appearance because of the effects of estrogen and progesterone (Fig. 13-3). Estrogen stimulates the growth of mammary ductal tissue, and progesterone promotes the growth of lobes, lobules, and alveoli. The breasts become highly vascular, and a delicate network of veins is often visible. If the increase in breast size is extensive, striations ("stretch marks") may develop.

Characteristic changes in the nipples and areolae occur during pregnancy. The nipples increase in size and become more erect, and the areolae become larger and more pigmented. Women with very light complexions exhibit less change in

pigmentation than those who have darker skin. Sebaceous glands, called *tubercles of Montgomery*, become more prominent during pregnancy and secrete a substance that lubricates the nipples. In addition, a thin, yellowish breast fluid (*colostrum*) is present in varying amounts throughout pregnancy and can readily be expressed by the third trimester.

Cardiovascular System

Heart

Heart Size and Position. Cardiac changes are slight, and they reverse soon after childbirth. The muscles of the heart (myocardium) enlarge slightly because of an increased workload during pregnancy. The heart is pushed upward and toward the left as the uterus elevates the diaphragm during the third trimester. As a result of the change in position, the locations for auscultating heart sounds may be shifted upward and laterally in late pregnancy.

Heart Sounds. During pregnancy, some heart sounds may be altered to the extent that they would be considered abnormal in a nonpregnant state. The changes are first heard between 12 and 20 weeks and continue for 2 to 4 weeks after childbirth. The most common variations in heart sounds include splitting of the first heart sound and a systolic murmur that is found in 90% of pregnant women (Cunningham et al., 2001). Although the second heart sound remains normal, many women have a third heart sound because of rapid filling during diastole.

Blood Volume

Plasma Volume. Total blood volume is a combination of plasma and other components, such as red blood cells (erythrocytes), white blood cells (leukocytes), and platelets (thrombocytes). Plasma volume increases progressively from 6 to 8 weeks' gestation to approximately 5000 ml at 32 weeks. This is an increase of 50% (about 1200 to 1300 ml or more) above nonpregnant values (Gordon, 2002). Increases may be higher in multifetal pregnancies. The increase may be related to estrogen stimulation of the renin-angiotensin-aldosterone system, which stimulates sodium and water retention.

The increased volume is needed for two reasons: (1) to transport nutrients and oxygen to the placenta, where they become available for the growing fetus; and (2) to meet the demands of the expanded maternal tissue in the uterus and breasts. The greater volume also provides a reserve to protect the pregnant woman from the adverse effects of the blood loss that occurs during childbirth.

Red Blood Cell Volume. Red blood cell (RBC) mass increases by 250 to 450 ml, about 25% to 33% above prepregnancy values (Blackburn, 2003). The increase in plasma volume is more pronounced and occurs earlier than the increase in RBC volume. The resulting dilution of RBC mass causes a decline in maternal hematocrit. This condition is frequently called *physiologic anemia* or *pseudoanemia of pregnancy* because it reflects the dilution of RBCs rather than an actual decline in the number of RBCs in a greatly expanded plasma volume and does not indicate true anemia.

Frequent laboratory examinations may be needed to distinguish physiologic anemia from true anemia. Generally, iron deficiency anemia occurs when the hemoglobin is less than 11 g/dl in the first and third trimesters or less than 10.5 g/dl in the second trimester (Cunningham et al., 2001). Iron supplementation is often prescribed for all pregnant women by the second trimester to prevent anemia.

Dilution of red blood cells by plasma may also have a protective function. By decreasing blood viscosity, dilution may counter the tendency to form clots (thrombi) that can obstruct blood vessels and cause serious complications (see Chapter 28).

Cardiac Output

The expanded vascular volume of pregnancy causes an increase in cardiac output—the amount of blood discharged from the heart each minute. It is based on stroke volume (the amount of blood pumped from the heart with each contraction) and heart rate (the number of times the heart beats each minute). Cardiac output rises rapidly during the first trimester and remains elevated throughout pregnancy. During pregnancy, the increase in cardiac output is caused primarily by a gain in stroke volume, but the heart rate also rises about 10 to 20 beats per minute (bpm) (Blackburn, 2003).

Peripheral Vascular Resistance

Peripheral vascular resistance falls during pregnancy. This change is likely the result of (1) smooth muscle relaxation in vessel walls caused by the effects of progesterone; (2) the addition of the uteroplacental unit, which provides a greater area for circulation; (3) fetal heat production, which may cause vasodilation; and (4) an increased synthesis of prostaglandins that cause resistance to circulating vasoconstrictors, such as angiotensin II and norepinephrine.

Blood Pressure

As a result of decreased peripheral vascular resistance, blood pressure remains stable during pregnancy despite the increase in blood volume. Systolic pressure remains largely unchanged or decreases slightly and diastolic pressure may decrease (by about 10-15 mm Hg) during the first and second trimesters (Blackburn, 2003). By the end of the third trimester, blood pressure returns to nonpregnant levels.

Effect of Position on Blood Pressure. Arterial blood pressure is affected by position during pregnancy. Pressure is lowest when the pregnant woman is in a lateral recumbent position. Pressures are higher when she is standing than when she is sitting. Moreover, an increase in both systolic and diastolic pressures occurs when the arm is held in a dependent position.

Each agency needs to standardize the way blood pressure is taken and to document the position as well as the pressure so that the site of assessment remains consistent. Moreover, controversy continues over whether Korotkoff's fifth phase (disappearance of sound) correlates better with the true diastolic pressure than does the fourth phase (muffling). Facilities should select which phase is to be used and remain consistent throughout the prenatal, intrapartum, and postpartum periods. Blood pressures of 140/90 require additional assessment.

Mean Arterial Pressure. The mean arterial pressure (MAP) is the average pressure within an artery over a complete cycle of one heartbeat. The MAP is estimated by computing one third of the pulse pressure (systolic pressure minus diastolic pressure) and adding that figure to the diastolic pressure. According to some researchers, an elevated MAP (above 85 mm Hg) is predictive of hypertension.

Supine Hypotension. When the pregnant woman is in the supine position, particularly during the second half of pregnancy, the weight of the *gravid* (pregnant) uterus partially occludes the vena cava and the descending aorta (Fig. 13-4). The occlusion impedes return of blood from the lower extremities and, as a consequence, reduces cardiac return, cardiac output, and blood pressure. Collateral circulation developed in pregnancy generally allows blood flow from the legs and pelvis to return to the heart when the woman is in a supine position (Blackburn, 2003). Some women develop supine hypotensive syndrome.

Symptoms include faintness, lightheadedness, dizziness, and agitation. Some may experience syncope, a brief lapse in consciousness. Blood flow through the placenta also decreases if the woman remains in the supine position for a prolonged period, and decreased blood flow could result in fetal hypoxia.

Turning to a lateral recumbent position alleviates the pressure on the blood vessels and quickly corrects supine hypotension. Women should be advised to rest in a side-lying position to prevent supine hypotension. If they must assume a supine position for fetal surveillance testing, a wedge or pillow under the right hip is effective in decreasing supine hypotension.

Blood Flow

Four major changes in blood flow occur during pregnancy:

- Blood flow is altered to include the uteroplacental unit. Approximately 500 ml/min is required to perfuse the placenta adequately.
- Approximately 30% more blood must circulate through the maternal kidneys to remove the increased metabolic wastes generated by the mother and fetus.
- The woman's skin requires increased circulation to dissipate the heat generated by increased metabolism during pregnancy.
- The weight of the expanding uterus on the inferior vena cava and iliac veins partially obstructs blood return from veins in the legs, causing stasis of blood and venous distension. Prolonged engorgement of the veins of the lower legs may result in varicose veins of the legs, vulva, or rectum (hemorrhoids).

Blood Components

During pregnancy, erythrocytes increase by 25% to 33%. The rise reflects accelerated production of erythrocytes rather than prolonged red cell life. The gain in erythrocytes greatly

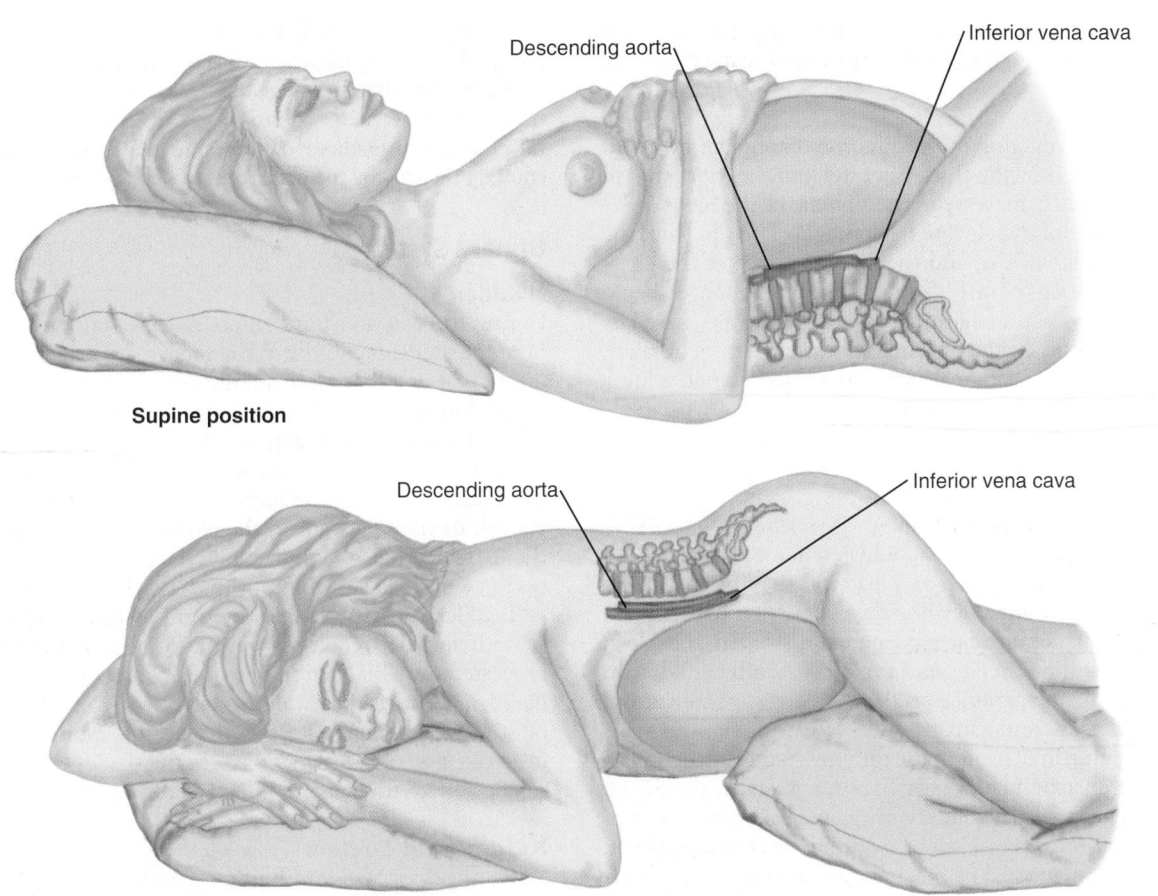

Figure 13-4 Supine hypotensive syndrome. When the woman is supine, the weight of the gravid uterus partially occludes the vena cava and the descending aorta. A lateral recumbent position corrects supine hypotension.

increases the maternal demand for iron, which is necessary for hemoglobin formation.

Although iron absorption and iron-binding power are increased during pregnancy, sufficient iron is not always supplied by diet. Iron supplementation is needed to promote hemoglobin synthesis and ensure that erythrocyte production is sufficient to prevent iron deficiency anemia (see Chapter 26).

Leukocytes increase during pregnancy, ranging from 5,000 cells/mm^3 to 12,000 cells/mm^3. Leukocytes increase further during labor and the early postpartum period, reaching as high as 25,000 cells/mm^3 (Cunningham et al., 2001).

During pregnancy, plasma fibrinogen (factor I) rises by about 50%. Elevated fibrinogen levels increase the ability to form clots. This offers some protection from hemorrhage during childbirth, but it also increases the risk of thrombus formation in the legs and the development of thrombophlebitis. The risk is a particular concern if the woman must stand or sit for prolonged periods, with stasis of blood in the veins of the legs. (See Appendix A for additional changes in blood components.)

Respiratory System

Oxygen Consumption

Oxygen consumption increases by about 15% to 20% in pregnancy. Half the oxygen is used by the fetus and placenta. The rest is consumed by the uterus, the breast tissue, and the increased respiratory and cardiac demands. To compensate for the increased need for oxygen, the woman breathes more deeply, although her respiratory rate remains unchanged. As a result, the tidal volume (the volume of gas moved into or out of the respiratory tract with each breath) as well as the respiratory minute volume (the volume of air inspired or expired in 1 minute) increase by about 40%. As a consequence of the elevated minute volume, the partial pressure of carbon dioxide (P_{CO_2}) is lowered. Renal excretion of bicarbonate partially compensates for the resulting respiratory alkalosis. Decreased partial pressure of P_{CO_2} also promotes the transfer of carbon dioxide from fetal to maternal circulation.

Hormonal Factors

Progesterone. Progesterone and prostaglandins play a role in decreasing airway resistance by relaxing the smooth muscle in the respiratory tract. Progesterone is also believed to raise the sensitivity of the respiratory center (medulla oblongata) to carbon dioxide, thus stimulating the increase in minute ventilation and lowering the P_{CO_2}. These two factors are responsible for the heightened awareness of the need to breathe experienced by many women during pregnancy.

Estrogen. Estrogen causes increased vascularity of the mucous membranes of the upper respiratory tract. As the capillaries become engorged, edema and hyperemia develop within the nose, pharynx, larynx, and trachea. This congestion may result in nasal and sinus stuffiness, epistaxis (nosebleeds), and changes in the voice. Increased vascularity also causes edema of the eardrum and eustachian tubes, which may result in a sense of fullness in the ears or earaches.

Physical Changes

Although the enlarging uterus lifts the diaphragm by about 4 cm (1.6 inches) by the third trimester, movement of the diaphragm is slightly increased. The volume of the lungs is decreased because of the elevated diaphragm. The ribs flare, the substernal angle widens, and the circumference of the chest expands by about 6 cm (2.5 inches). These changes begin when the uterus is just beginning to enlarge and are caused by relaxation of the ligaments around the ribs from relaxin. Breathing becomes thoracic rather than abdominal, adding to the dyspnea many women experience.

Gastrointestinal System

Mouth

Elevated levels of estrogen cause hyperemia of the tissues of the mouth and gums, which may lead to gingivitis and bleeding gums. Some women develop severe vascular hypertrophy of the gums, which appear reddened and swollen and bleed easily. The condition regresses spontaneously after childbirth.

Some women experience *ptyalism*, or excessive salivation, that is unpleasant and embarrassing. The cause of ptyalism is unknown, but stimulation of the salivary glands by the ingestion of starch may play a part (Cunningham et al., 2001). Small, frequent meals, gum chewing, and oral lozenges offer limited relief for some women. Contrary to common belief, the teeth are unaffected by pregnancy and do not lose minerals to the fetus.

Esophagus

The lower esophageal sphincter tone decreases during pregnancy, primarily because of the effect of progesterone on the smooth muscles. The reduced tone allows reflux of acidic stomach contents into the esophagus and produces heartburn (*pyrosis*).

Stomach and Small Intestine

Elevated levels of progesterone relax all smooth muscle, decreasing gastrointestinal tone and motility. The stomach and small intestine take longer to empty, allowing additional time for nutrients to be absorbed. This slowed process benefits the growing fetus, but it may contribute to the nausea many expectant mothers experience. Calcium, iron, and some other nutrients are better absorbed during pregnancy, but absorption of some of the B vitamins is reduced.

Large Intestine

Decreased motility in the large intestine allows time for more water to be reabsorbed from bowel contents, which may lead to constipation. Hemorrhoids may be caused or exacerbated by constipation if the expectant mother must strain to have bowel movements.

Liver and Gallbladder

Progesterone causes functional changes of the liver and gallbladder. The gallbladder becomes hypotonic and emptying time is prolonged, resulting in thicker bile, which can predispose to the development of gallstones. Reduced gallbladder tone also leads to a tendency to retain bile salts, which can lead to itching (pruritus).

During the last trimester, the liver is pushed upward and backward by the enlarging uterus and liver function is also altered. Serum alkaline phosphatase rises 2 to 4 times that of nonpregnant women, whereas levels of serum albumin and total protein fall gradually (Gordon, 2000). These changes are caused primarily by the effect of estrogen and by hemodilution.

Urinary System

Bladder

During the first and third trimesters, pressure on the bladder from the uterus causes the woman to experience frequency and urgency of urination. The uterus extends into the abdominal cavity during the second trimester, so pressure on the bladder is relieved and frequency may lessen. Nocturia is also common. Although uterine expansion within the pelvis is one cause of these urinary changes, frequency begins before the uterus is big enough to exert pressure on the bladder. Hormonal influences, the increased blood volume, and changes in glomerular filtration rate may play a significant role (Blackburn, 2003).

Bladder capacity doubles by term as the bladder, like all smooth muscle, relaxes in response to increasing levels of progesterone. Bladder mucosa becomes congested with blood, and the bladder walls become hypertrophied as a result of stimulation from estrogen. Decreased drainage of blood from the base of the bladder makes the tissues edematous and susceptible to trauma and infection during childbirth.

Kidneys and Ureters

Changes in Size and Shape. During pregnancy, the kidneys change in both size and shape because dilation of the renal pelves, calyces, and ureters occurs above the pelvic brim. The dilation is caused by (1) the effect of progesterone, which causes the ureters to become elongated and more distensible, and (2) compression of the ureters between the enlarging uterus and the bony pelvic brim. As the flow of urine through the ureters is obstructed, particularly on the right side, the ureters and renal pelvis dilate. The resulting stasis of urine allows time for bacteria to multiply and increases the risk of urinary tract infection during pregnancy.

Functional Changes. Renal plasma flow, the total amount of plasma to flow through the kidneys, increases by 35% to 60%. The rise is the result of increases in plasma volume and cardiac output. The glomerular filtration rate, the rate at which water and dissolved substances are filtered in the glomerulus, increases by as much as 50%. This increase is the result of the increase in renal plasma flow and of decreased colloid osmotic pressure caused by a reduction in the concentration of plasma proteins.

The increases in renal plasma flow and glomerular filtration rate are necessary to excrete additional metabolic waste from the mother and fetus, but they also affect the excretion of glucose. As the glomerular filtration rate increases, the filtered load of glucose exceeds the ability of the renal tubules to reabsorb it, and glucose spills into the urine. Therefore glycosuria is common during pregnancy, particularly after the consumption of foods such as candy or cookies that are high in simple sugars. Furthermore, small quantities of amino acids and water-soluble vitamins are excreted. Bacteria thrive in urine that is rich in nutrients, so glycosuria is one more reason why the incidence of urinary tract infections increases during pregnancy.

Mild proteinuria is common and does not mean there is abnormal kidney function or preeclampsia (Blackburn, 2003).

Protein levels are monitored throughout pregnancy to identify increases that would indicate a problem. Tests of renal function may be misleading during pregnancy. As a result of increased glomerular filtration rate, plasma concentrations of both creatinine and urea normally decline.

Integumentary System

Skin

Circulation to the skin increases during pregnancy and encourages activity of the sweat and sebaceous glands. Pregnant women feel warmer and perspire more, particularly during the last trimester. Accelerated activity of the sebaceous glands fosters the development of facial blemishes. Additional changes include hyperpigmentation and vascular changes in the skin.

Hyperpigmentation. Increased pigmentation may begin as early as the 2nd month, when levels of melanocyte-stimulating hormone (MSH) become elevated because of the effects of estrogen and progesterone. Brunettes and dark-skinned women exhibit more hyperpigmentation than women with very light skin. Areas of pigmentation include brownish patches, called *chloasma, melasma*, or the *mask of pregnancy*, over the forehead, cheeks, and bridge of the nose. Chloasma increases with exposure to sunlight, but use of sunscreen may reduce the severity. A dark line of pigmentation (*linea nigra*) may extend up the center of the abdomen from the symphysis pubis as high as the top of the fundus. Preexisting moles become darker, and the areolae become darker as pregnancy progresses. Hyperpigmentation usually disappears after childbirth, when the levels of estrogen and progesterone decline, although chloasma may persist in some women.

Cutaneous Vascular Changes. Blood vessels dilate and proliferate during pregnancy. This change is thought to be caused largely by the effect of estrogen. Changes in surface blood vessels are obvious during pregnancy, especially in white women. These include angiomas that appear as tiny red elevations that branch in all directions. Commonly called *vascular spider nevi*, they appear most often on the face, neck, upper chest, and arms. Redness of the palms or soles of the feet, known as *palmar erythema*, also occurs in many white women and in some African-American women. Although vascular changes may be emotionally distressing for the expectant mother, they are clinically insignificant and usually disappear shortly after childbirth.

Connective Tissue

Linear tears may occur in the connective tissue, most often on the abdomen, breasts, and buttocks, appearing as slightly depressed, pink to purple streaks called *striae gravidarum* or "stretch marks" (Fig. 13-5). Women are concerned about striae because they fade to silvery lines but do not disappear after childbirth. Laser therapy is sometimes used after childbirth to reduce or eliminate severe striae. Many women believe that striae can be prevented by massage with oil or vitamin E, but the effectiveness of this treatment has not been documented. Antipruritic ointments may be effective in controlling the itching that accompanies severe striae.

Hair and Nails

Because fewer follicles are in the resting phase, hair grows more rapidly and less hair falls out during pregnancy. After childbirth, hair follicles return to normal activity. Many women become concerned about the rate of hair loss that be-

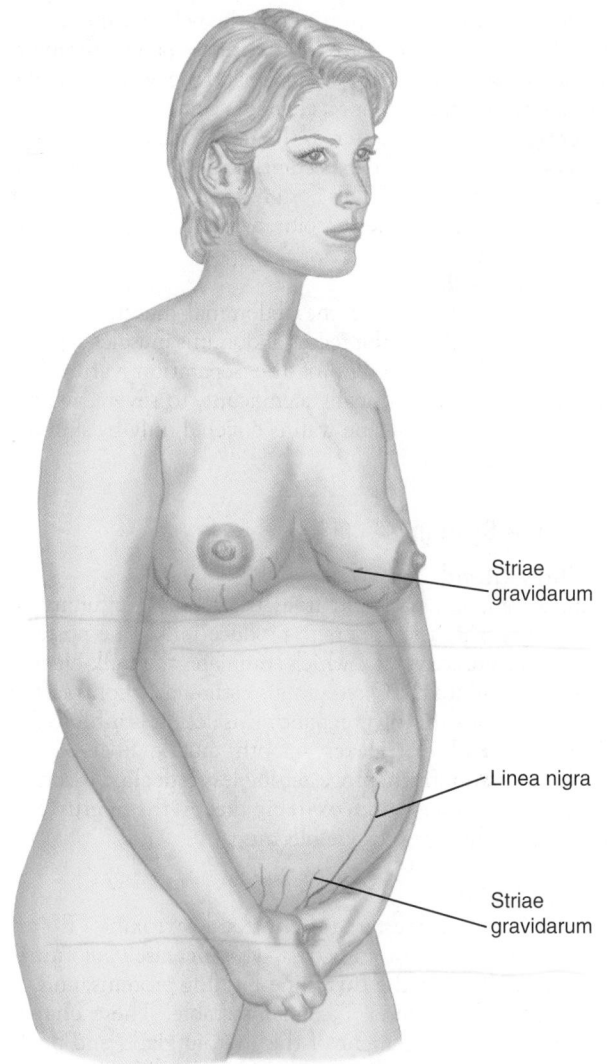

Figure 13-5 Striae gravidarum are linear tears that may occur in the connective tissue. Linea nigra, a dark line of pigmentation from the umbilicus to the symphysis pubis, may also appear.

Striae gravidarum

Linea nigra

Striae gravidarum

gins 1 to 4 months postpartum. They need reassurance that more follicles have returned to the normal resting phase and that excessive hair loss will not continue.

Nail growth increases during pregnancy. Many women notice thinning and softening of the nails as pregnancy progresses, although the reasons for this change are unclear.

Musculoskeletal System

Calcium Storage

During pregnancy, fetal demands for calcium increase, especially in the third trimester. Absorption of calcium from the intestine is increased from the first trimester, and calcium is stored to meet the later needs of the fetus. There is no loss of maternal bone density to supply fetal needs.

Postural Changes

Musculoskeletal changes are progressive. They begin in the second trimester, when the hormones *relaxin* and *progesterone* initiate increased mobility of the pelvic ligaments and joints. This facilitates passage of the fetus through the pelvis at the time of birth. Relaxation of the pelvic joints creates pelvic instability, and the woman assumes a wide stance and the waddling gait of pregnancy to compensate for a changing center of gravity.

During the third trimester, as the uterus increases in size, it becomes necessary for the expectant mother to lean backward to maintain her balance. This posture creates a progressive *lordosis*, or curvature of the lower spine, and may lead to backache.

Abdominal Wall

During the third trimester the abdominal muscles may become so stretched that the rectus abdominis muscles separate (*diastasis recti*). The extent of the separation varies from slight, which is not clinically significant, to severe, when a large portion of the uterine wall is covered only by skin and fascia (see Figure 21-5).

Endocrine System

Pituitary Gland

During pregnancy, prolactin from the anterior pituitary increases to prepare the breasts to produce milk. The posterior pituitary secretes oxytocin, which stimulates the milk-ejection reflex after childbirth. Oxytocin also stimulates contractions of the uterus, but during pregnancy this action is inhibited by progesterone, which relaxes smooth muscle fibers of the uterus. After childbirth, progesterone levels decline when the placenta is removed and oxytocin keeps the uterus contracted, preventing excessive bleeding.

Thyroid Gland

Early in the first trimester, a rise in total thyroxine (T_4) and thyroxine-binding protein occurs. The increased amounts of T_4 bind readily with the thyroxine-binding proteins, and the serum level of unbound T_4 remains stable. These changes produce slight enlargement of the thyroid gland and an increase in basal metabolic rate (BMR). The BMR increases during pregnancy, causing greater cardiac output, pulse rate, and heat intolerance. The BMR returns to normal within a few weeks after childbirth.

Parathyroid Glands

Parathyroid hormone is slightly decreased during the first trimester and normal during the rest of pregnancy. Although it was once thought that parathyroid hormone was involved in protecting the mother's bones from the loss of calcium to the fetus, this is no longer considered accurate (Gordon, 2002).

Pancreas

Significant changes in the pancreas during pregnancy are caused by alterations in maternal blood glucose concentrations and consequent fluctuations in insulin production. During the first trimester, the increasing glucose demand by the fetus causes a fall in maternal blood glucose. As a result, the islets of Langerhans produce less insulin.

During the second trimester, maternal tissue sensitivity to insulin begins to decline, mainly because of the effects of human placental lactogen, prolactin, progesterone, estrogen, and cortisol. The resulting higher blood glucose level makes more glucose available for fetal energy needs and stimulates the pancreas of a healthy woman to produce additional insulin. Inadequate insulin production results in gestational diabetes, described in Chapter 26.

Adrenal Glands

During pregnancy, there is a significant change in two adrenal hormones: cortisol and aldosterone. Although production of cortisol does not increase during pregnancy, the unbound level of cortisol is elevated because of a decreased metabolic clearance rate. Cortisol regulates carbohydrate and protein metabolism. It stimulates gluconeogenesis (formation of glycogen from non-carbohydrate sources such as amino or fatty acids) whenever the supply of glucose is inadequate to meet the body's needs for energy.

Aldosterone regulates the absorption of sodium from the distal tubules of the kidneys. It increases during pregnancy to overcome the salt-wasting effects of progesterone to maintain the necessary level of sodium in the greatly expanded blood volume and to meet the needs of the fetus. Aldosterone is closely related to water metabolism.

Changes Caused by Placental Hormones

Human Chorionic Gonadotropin. In early pregnancy, human chorionic gonadotropin (hCG) is produced by the trophoblastic cells that surround the developing embryo. This hormone stimulates the corpus luteum to produce progesterone and estrogen until the placenta is sufficiently developed to assume that function. It also causes a positive pregnancy test.

Estrogen. After the 6th or 7th week of pregnancy, estrogen is produced primarily by the placenta. Estrogen has numerous functions during pregnancy: (1) it stimulates uterine growth and increases blood supply to uterine vessels; (2) it aids in developing the ductal system in the breasts in preparation for lactation; and (3) it is associated with hyperpigmentation, vascular changes in the skin, increased activity of the salivary glands, and hyperemia of the gums and nasal mucous membranes.

Progesterone. Progesterone is produced first by the corpus luteum and then by the fully developed placenta. Progesterone is the most important hormone of pregnancy. The major functions include:

- Maintaining the endometrial layer for implantation of the fertilized ovum
- Preventing spontaneous abortion by relaxing smooth muscles of the uterus
- Stimulating the development of the lobes and lobules in the breast in preparation for lactation
- Facilitating the deposit of maternal fat stores, which provide a reserve of energy for pregnancy and lactation

Progesterone relaxes not only the smooth muscle of the uterus but also all other smooth muscle. As a consequence, progesterone is associated with decreased motility of the bowel, dilation of the ureters, and increased bladder capacity. Progesterone raises the respiratory sensitivity to carbon dioxide and thus stimulates increased ventilation.

Human Placental Lactogen. Also called *human chorionic somatomammotropin (hCS)*, human placental lactogen (hPL) increases the availability of glucose for the fetus, who needs a constant supply. Human placental lactogen does this by decreasing the sensitivity of maternal cells to insulin, which decreases maternal metabolism of glucose, thereby freeing glucose for transport to the fetus. In addition, hPL causes free fatty acids to be quickly metabolized to provide energy for the pregnant woman.

Relaxin. Relaxin is produced by the corpus luteum and by the placenta. Relaxin inhibits uterine activity, softens connective tissue in the cervix, and relaxes pelvic joints.

Changes in Metabolism

Weight Gain. As a result of the correlation between infant mortality and low birth weights, women are encouraged to gain an adequate amount of weight during pregnancy. (See Table 15-1 for the recommended weight gain for women of normal weight and those with special needs.)

The normal distribution of weight gain is illustrated in Figure 15-1. The fetus, placenta, and amniotic fluid make up less than half the recommended weight gain. The remainder is found in the increased size of the uterus and breasts, increased blood volume, increased interstitial fluid, and maternal stores of subcutaneous fat.

Water Metabolism. The requirements for water increase during pregnancy, and the kidneys must compensate for the many factors that influence the balance of fluid at this time. An increased glomerular filtration rate, decreased concentration of plasma proteins, and increased progesterone level all result in an increase in sodium excretion. However, increased concentrations of estrogen, cortisol, prolactin, and aldosterone all tend to promote the reabsorption of sodium. The net effect of the combined hormonal action is that sodium balance is maintained.

Dependent Edema. Because of hemodilution, a slight decrease occurs in colloid osmotic pressure, which favors the development of edema during pregnancy. Edema is further increased toward term, when the weight of the uterus compresses the veins of the pelvis. This process delays venous return, causing the veins of the legs to become distended, and increases venous pressure, resulting in additional fluid shifts from the vascular compartment to interstitial spaces.

Even women without edema accumulate water during pregnancy to allow for the added fluid needs of the fetus as well as those of the woman. About 1.5 to 5 L of fluid is retained during pregnancy (Blackburn, 2003).

Edema of the feet and ankles is obvious at the end of the day, particularly if a pregnant woman stands for prolonged periods. Dependent edema is clinically insignificant. If edema of the face or hands is noted, however, further assessment for hypertension or proteinuria is essential to determine whether preeclampsia is developing.

Carpal Tunnel Syndrome. Fluid retention is also associated with carpal tunnel syndrome, believed to result when edema compresses the median nerve at the point where it goes through the carpal tunnel of the wrist. Symptoms include pain, burning, numbness, or tingling of the hand and wrist. Splinting of the wrist during the night may be necessary. The condition usually resolves when the pregnancy ends.

Carbohydrate Metabolism. Carbohydrate metabolism changes markedly during pregnancy because more insulin is required as pregnancy progresses. As hormones such as progesterone and hPL cause maternal tissue to be resistant to insulin, insulinase, an enzyme produced by the placenta, speeds the breakdown of insulin.

Decreasing the mother's ability to use insulin is a protective mechanism to supply glucose for the fetus. The mother's pancreas produces more insulin so that she can metabolize enough glucose to meet her energy needs and to prevent hyperglycemia. In some women, however, insulin production cannot be increased, and these women experience periodic hyperglycemia. This pregnancy-induced glucose intolerance is called *gestational diabetes* (see Chapter 26).

CONFIRMATION OF PREGNANCY

Although many women have an early ultrasound that proves they are pregnant, the diagnosis of pregnancy has traditionally been based on symptoms experienced by the woman as well as on signs observed by a health care provider. Figure 13-6 summarizes fetal and maternal changes that occur throughout pregnancy. These signs and symptoms are grouped into three classifications: presumptive, probable, and positive indications of

Gestational age 1–4 weeks

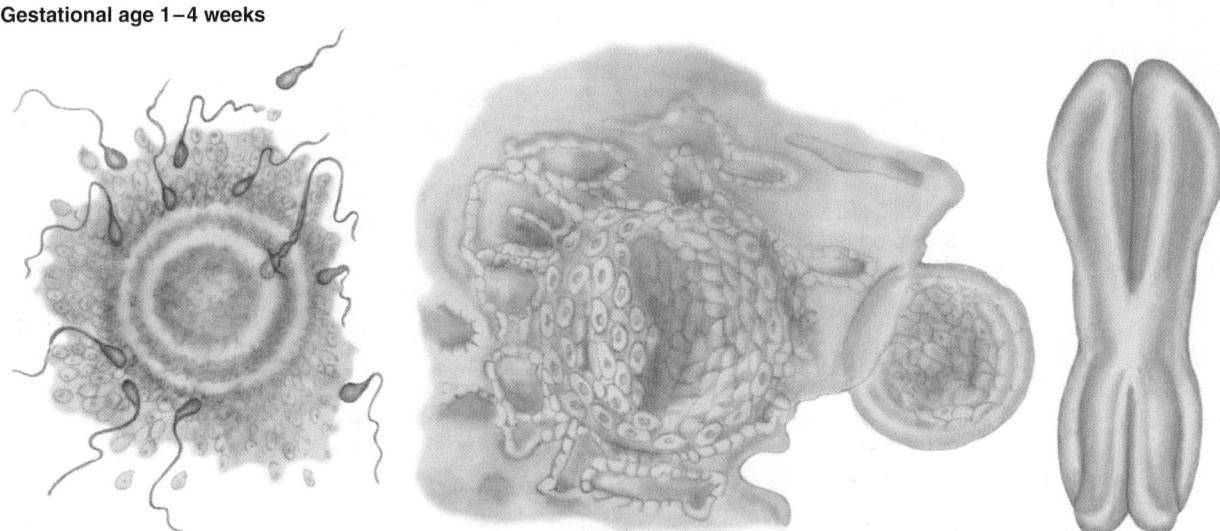

Fertilization, implantation. Woman's basal body temperature and hCG become elevated, pregnancy tests positive. Pre-embryonic stage. Crown-rump length reaches 4 mm.

Figure 13-6 Fetal growth and development and maternal responses based on the date of the last menstrual period.

Continued

Gestational age 5–8 weeks

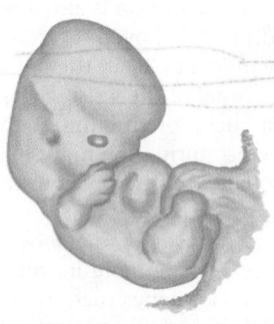

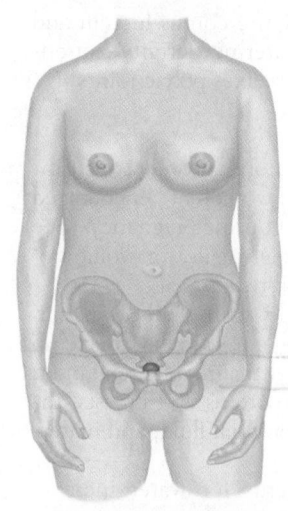

Crown-rump length 13 mm. Embryonic stage. Heart developed, beginning to pump. Arm and leg buds present. Head large, with facial features beginning to form.

Woman misses menstrual period. Nausea; fatigue. Tingling of breasts. Uterus is size of a lemon; positive Chadwick's, Goodell's and Hegar's sign. Urinary frequency as enlarging uterus presses on the bladder; increased vaginal discharge.

Gestational age 9–12 weeks

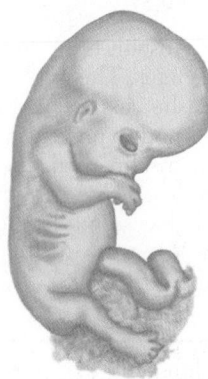

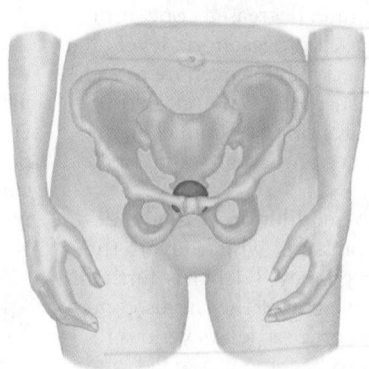

Crown-rump length 6–7 cm (2.4-2.8 in). Fetal stage begins at 10 weeks after last menstrual period. Extremities developed; fingers and toes differentiated; external genitalia show signs of male or female sex. Weight 14 g (0.5 oz).

Nausea usually decreases after 12 weeks. Uterus is size of an orange; palpable above symphysis pubis. Vulvar varicosities may appear.

Gestational age 13–16 weeks

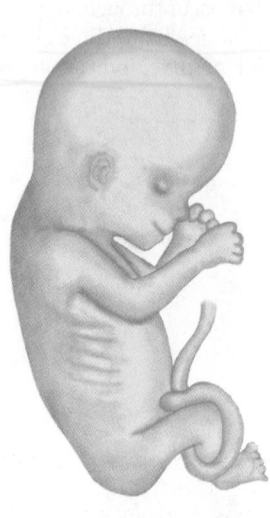

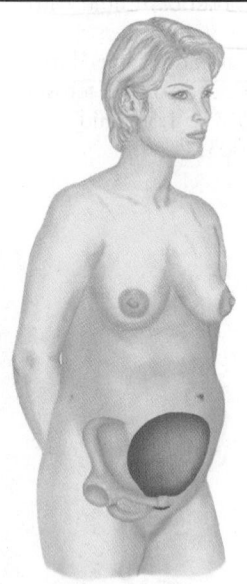

Crown-rump length 12 cm (4.7 in). Weight 110 g (4 oz). Fetus begins to move. Head and thorax can be identified by ultrasound; sexual organs formed. Urine formation begins.

Fetal movements may be felt at about 16 weeks. Uterus has risen into the abdomen; fundus midway between symphysis pubis and umbilicus. Urinary frequency decreases; blood volume increases; uterine souffle heard.

Figure 13-6, cont'd

Gestational age 17–20 weeks

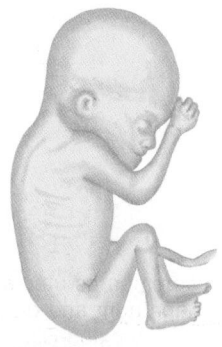

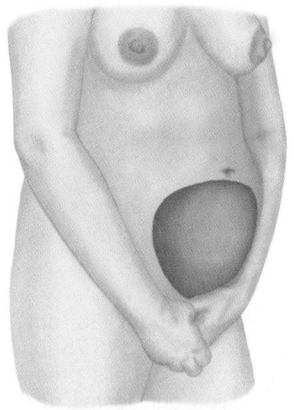

Crown-rump length 16 cm (6.3 in). Weight 320 g (11 oz). Heart beat can be heard with fetoscope or electronic device. Meconium begins collecting in bowel. Period of very rapid growth.

Fetal movements felt. Skin pigmentation increases: areolae darken; chloasma and linea nigra may be obvious. Colostrum may be expressed. Braxton Hicks contractions palpable. Fundus at level of umbilicus at about 20 weeks.

Gestational age 21–24 weeks

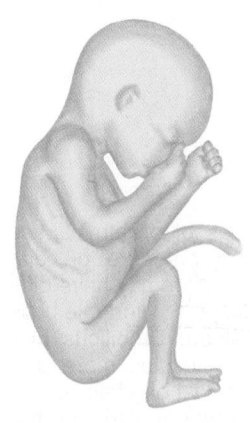

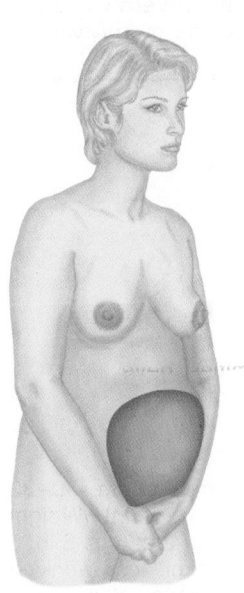

Crown-rump length 21 cm (8 in). Weight 630 g (1 lb, 6 oz). Skin wrinkled and red; vernix present; head and body covered with lanugo.

Relaxation of smooth muscles of veins and bladder increases the chance of varicose veins and urinary tract infections. Woman is more aware of fetal movements.

Gestational age 25–28 weeks

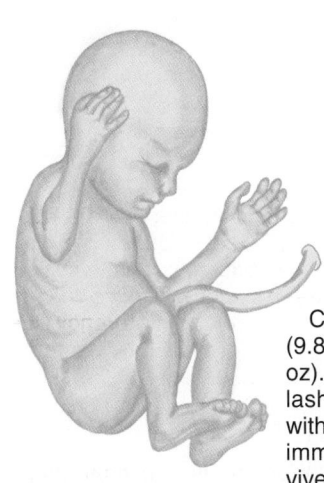

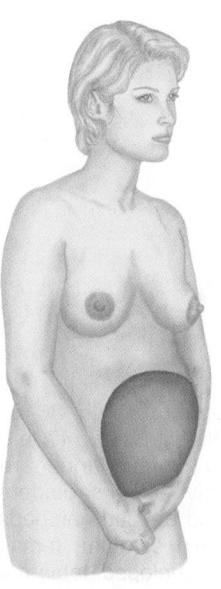

Crown-rump length 25 cm (9.8 in). Weight 1000 g (2 lb, 3 oz). Eyes partially open; eyelashes present. Skin covered with vernix. Respiratory system immature, but fetus may survive if born.

Period of greatest weight gain and lowest hemoglobin level begins. Fundal height is 3 to 4 fingerbreadths above umbilicus. Lordosis may cause backache.

Figure 13-6, cont'd

Continued

Gestational age 29–32 weeks

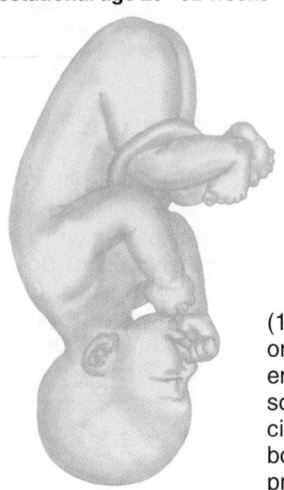

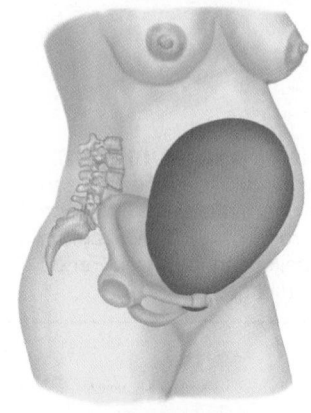

Crown-rump length 28 cm (11 in). Weight 1700 g (3.75 lb, or 3 lb, 12 oz). Toenails present. Body filling out, testes descending. Iron, nitrogen, calcium stored. Vernix covers body. Chances of survival improving.

Heartburn common as uterus presses on diaphragm and displaces stomach. Braxton-Hicks contractions more noticeable. Lordosis increases; waddling gait develops due to increased mobility of pelvic joints.

Gestational age 33–36 weeks

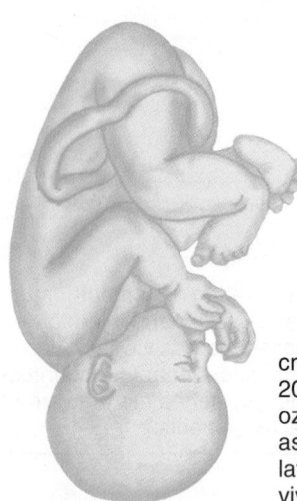

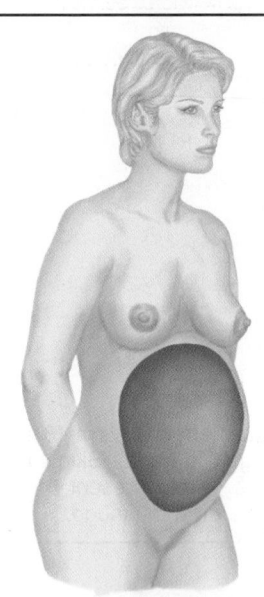

Crown-rump length 30–32 cm (11.8 to 12.6 in). Weight 2000–2500 g (4 lb, 6 oz-5 lb, 8 oz). Skin thicker, less wrinkled as subcutaneous fat accumulates. Excellent chance for survival.

Shortness of breath caused by upward pressure on diaphragm; woman may have difficulty finding a comfortable position for sleep. Umbilicus protrudes. Varicosities more pronounced; pedal or ankle edema may be present. Urinary frequency noted following lightening when presenting part settles into pelvic cavity.

Gestational age 37–40 weeks

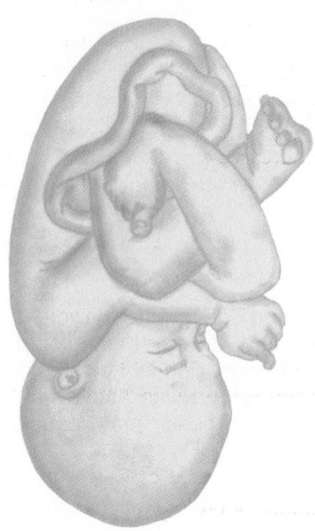

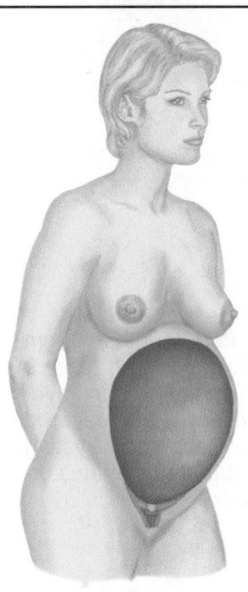

Crown-rump length 36 cm (14 in). Weight 3400 g (7 lb, 8 oz). Body plump; lanugo remains only over shoulders; nails extend beyond nail beds; testes within scrotum; female labia well developed; labia majora cover labia minora.

Woman is uncomfortable; looking forward to birth of baby. Cervix softens, begins to efface; mucus plug is often lost.

Figure 13-6, cont'd

BOX 13-1
Indications of Pregnancy and Other Possible Causes

SIGN	OTHER POSSIBLE CAUSES
Presumptive Indications	
Amenorrhea	Emotional stress, strenuous physical exercise, endocrine problems, chronic disease, early menopause
Nausea and vomiting	Gastrointestinal virus, food poisoning, emotional stress
Fatigue	Illness, stress, sudden changes in lifestyle
Urinary frequency	Urinary tract infections
Breast and skin changes	Premenstrual changes, use of oral contraceptives
Vaginal and cervical color changes	Infection or hormonal imbalance
Quickening	Abdominal gas, peristalsis, or pseudocyesis (false pregnancy)
Probable Indications	
Abdominal enlargement	Abdominal or uterine tumors
Cervical softening	Infection or hormonal imbalance
Ballottement	Uterine or cervical polyps
Braxton Hicks contractions	Soft uterine fibroids (leiomyomas)
Palpation of fetal outline	Large leiomyoma (may feel like the fetal head); small, soft leiomyoma (may simulate small parts of the fetus)
Pregnancy tests	Certain medications, premature menopause, blood in urine, or malignant tumors that produce human chorionic gonadotropin may result in false-positive findings
Positive Indications	
Auscultation of fetal heart sounds	
Fetal movements felt by examiner	
Visualization of embryo or fetus	

pregnancy. A diagnosis of pregnancy cannot be made solely on the presumptive or probable signs. Box 13-1 lists other possible causes for these signs. A definitive diagnosis of pregnancy can be based only on positive signs.

Presumptive Indications of Pregnancy

Presumptive indications are mainly subjective changes that the woman experiences and reports. These changes are the least reliable indicators of pregnancy because they can be caused by conditions other than pregnancy.

Amenorrhea

Absence of menstruation in a sexually active woman who regularly menstruates strongly suggests that conception has occurred. Menses cease after conception because progesterone and estrogen, secreted from the corpus luteum, maintain the endometrial lining in preparation for implantation of the fertilized ovum.

Nausea and Vomiting

Many women experience nausea and vomiting, which generally begin about 6 weeks after the start of the last menstrual period. Symptoms generally disappear by about 14 weeks (Cunningham et al., 2001). Nausea and vomiting are believed to be caused by the increased levels of hormones (hCG, estrogen) and decreased gastric motility (an effect of progesterone).

Fatigue

Fatigue and drowsiness during the first trimester are very common. The direct cause is unknown, but it may be related to progesterone and other hormone changes.

Urinary Frequency

Urinary frequency begins in the first few weeks of pregnancy from hormonal changes and continues later when pressure is exerted on the bladder by the expanding uterus. This symptom may be decreased during the second trimester, when the uterus expands into the abdominal cavity. Late in the third trimester, the fetus settles into the pelvic cavity and the woman experiences frequency and urgency of urination because the uterus presses against the bladder.

Breast and Skin Changes

Breast changes occur at about the 6th week of pregnancy. Breast tenderness, tingling, feelings of fullness, and increased size and pigmentation of the areolae are present. These changes are caused by the influence of estrogen and progesterone. Many women observe increased pigmentation of the skin (chloasma, linea nigra, darkening of the areolae of the breasts) during pregnancy.

Vaginal and Cervical Color Changes

The vagina changes from pink to a dark bluish purple. The color change, called Chadwick's sign, extends to the cervix and labia as well. The bluish purple color is caused by increased vascularity of the pelvic organs and is one of the earliest signs of pregnancy.

Fetal Movement

Unlike other presumptive indications of pregnancy, fetal movement is not perceived until the second trimester. Although some women feel movement sooner, most expectant mothers first notice subtle fetal movements (quickening) between 16 and 20 weeks. These movements gradually increase in intensity.

Probable Indications of Pregnancy

Probable indications of pregnancy are objective findings that can be documented by an examiner. They are related primarily to physical changes in the reproductive organs. Although these signs are stronger indicators of pregnancy, a positive diagnosis of pregnancy cannot be based on these findings because they may be caused by other conditions.

Abdominal Enlargement

Enlargement of the abdomen during the childbearing years is a fairly reliable indication of pregnancy, particularly if it corresponds to a slow, gradual increase in uterine growth. Evidence of pregnancy is even more reliable when uterine growth is accompanied by amenorrhea.

Cervical Softening

Softening of the cervix (Goodell's sign) is noted by the examiner during pelvic examination. At about the 6th week of pregnancy, the lower uterine segment is so soft that it can be compressed to the thinness of paper. This is called Hegar's sign (Fig. 13-7). Because of the softening, the uterus can be easily flexed against the cervix.

Changes in the Uterus

Ballottement. Near midpregnancy, a sudden tap on the cervix during vaginal examination may cause the fetus to rise in the amniotic fluid and then rebound to its original position (Fig. 13-8). Ballottement is a strong indication of pregnancy, but the same sensation may be caused by other factors such as uterine or cervical polyps.

Braxton Hicks Contractions. Irregular, painless contractions occur throughout pregnancy, although many expectant mothers do not notice them until the third trimester. As the woman nears the end of pregnancy, the contractions become stronger and more frequent.

Palpation of the Fetal Outline. An experienced practitioner is able to palpate the outlines of the fetal body by the second half of pregnancy. Palpating the fetal outline becomes easier as the pregnancy progresses and the uterine walls thin to accommodate the growing fetus.

Uterine Souffle. A soft, blowing sound may be auscultated over the uterus. This sound is caused by blood circulating through the placenta, and it corresponds to the maternal pulse. Therefore, to identify uterine souffle, the rate of the maternal pulse must be checked simultaneously. Uterine souffle differs from *funic souffle*, the soft, purring sound heard over the umbilical cord and corresponding to the fetal heart rate.

Pregnancy Tests

Pregnancy tests detect hCG or the beta subunit of hCG, which is secreted by the placenta and present in maternal blood or urine shortly after conception. There are many different kinds of tests, but only the most common tests are discussed here.

Radioimmunoassay. Because radioimmunoassays use radioactively labeled markers to detect antibodies against beta-subunit hCG in blood or urine, they must be performed in a laboratory. They are the most sensitive pregnancy tests available and are accurate as early as 1 week after ovulation.

Enzyme-Linked Immunosorbent Assay (ELISA). The ELISA uses antibodies to detect hCG in blood or urine. The test is quick and ideal for early diagnosis of pregnancy. It

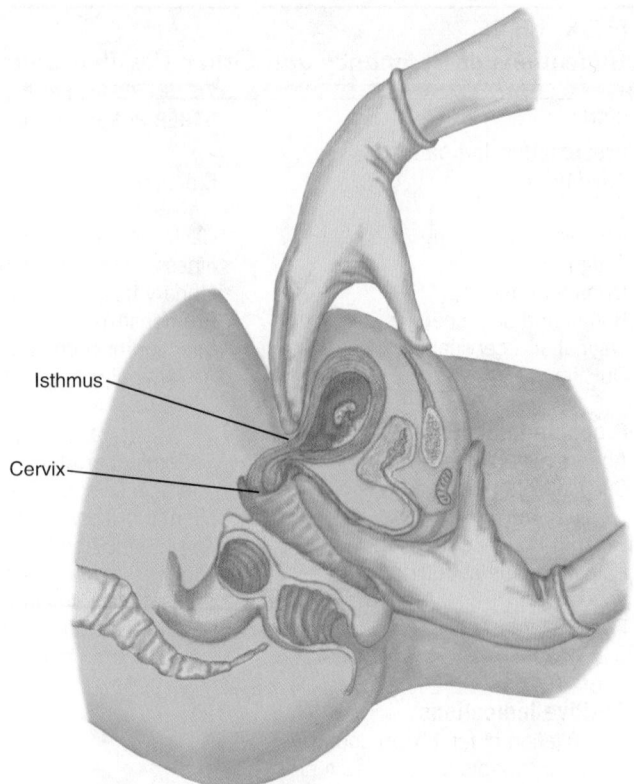

Figure 13-7 Hegar's sign—compressibility of the lower uterus—reflects softening of the isthmus of the cervix.

can detect hCG in serum at very low concentrations and is positive as early as 5 days before the woman misses a period (Buster & Carson, 2002).

Home Pregnancy Tests. Home pregnancy test kits, often based on ELISA, are available for purchase over the counter and are uncomplicated and convenient. The woman places urine on a strip or wick and watches for a color change. Although the first morning void is most concentrated, samples from any time of day can be used for most kits.

When pregnancy test results are reported as negative and the woman is in fact pregnant, the results are called *false negative*. False-negative results may occur when the instructions are not followed properly, it is too early in the pregnancy, the urine is too dilute, or the woman has an ectopic pregnancy or impending spontaneous abortion. Certain drugs may affect the accuracy of the test. The woman should check with the manufacturer's instructions or her health care provider if she is taking drugs.

Positive Indications of Pregnancy

Positive signs of pregnancy are those caused only by pregnancy.

Auscultation of Fetal Heart Sounds

Fetal heart sounds can be heard with a fetoscope by 18 to 20 weeks of gestation. The electronic Doppler detects heart motion and makes a sound that is audible by 10 weeks.

It is necessary to distinguish the fetal heartbeat from the maternal pulse. The fetal heart rate ranges between 110 and

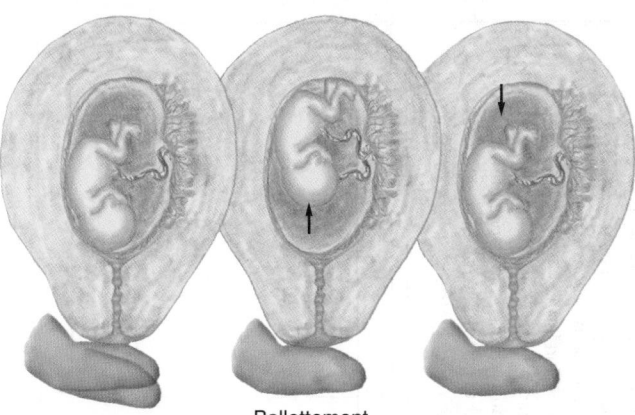

Ballottement

Figure 13-8 When the cervix is tapped, the fetus floats upward in the amniotic fluid. A rebound is felt by the examiner when the fetus falls back.

160 bpm during the third trimester. It should be auscultated while the radial pulse of the expectant mother is being palpated. The fetal heart rate is muffled by amniotic fluid, and the location changes because the fetus moves freely in the amniotic fluid.

Fetal Movements Felt by Examiner
Fetal movements are considered a positive sign of pregnancy when felt by an experienced examiner who is not likely to be deceived by similar sensations produced by peristalsis in the large intestine.

Visualization of the Fetus
Confirmation of pregnancy has become much simpler since the development of ultrasonography, which makes it possible to view the fetal outline and observe the fetal heartbeat very early in pregnancy. Positive confirmation of pregnancy is possible by transvaginal ultrasonography as early as 4 weeks after the last menstrual period (Buster & Carson, 2002). The gestational sac and movements of the fetal heart are readily identifiable in the maternal pelvis.

ANTEPARTUM ASSESSMENT AND CARE

Prenatal care includes assessment to identify potential problems as well as health education, counseling, and social support. Approximately 83% of American women begin antepartum care in the first trimester. The *Healthy People 2010* goal is for at least 90% of American women to begin antepartum care in the first trimester (U.S. Department of Health and Human Services, 2000).

Antepartum care is considered adequate when it begins in the first trimester and continues on a regular basis thereafter. Inadequate antepartum care is associated with low birth weight and an increased incidence of prematurity in neonates. A strong correlation has been found between these two complications and increased infant mortality.

Figure 13-9 is an example of a clinical pathway for prenatal care. Such pathways provide guidelines and a time sequence for specific assessments and interventions. Note that the most common family problems and risk factors are listed at the top of the page and alert the team that additional assessments or care may be needed.

Preconception Visit
Ideally, the first visit takes place before conception with a complete history and physical examination. Health problems or social situations that might be detrimental in pregnancy can be discussed at this time. If not immune to rubella, the woman can be immunized and instructed to wait at least 1 month before conceiving. Vaccines for varicella and hepatitis may be offered at the same time. The woman is advised to consume 0.4 mg of folic acid daily before becoming pregnant and 0.6 mg daily throughout pregnancy to decrease the risk of neural tube defects. Avoidance of common teratogens or other harmful substances is also discussed. Referral to smoking cessation programs may be indicated.

Initial Visit
If the woman had a preconception visit, many of the initial prenatal assessments will have been completed. If not, the initial visit is a time to establish rapport with the family and to perform a thorough assessment of the physiologic and psychosocial needs of the family. The health care provider must complete a thorough history and physical examination.

History
Obstetric History. The obstetric history provides essential information about prior pregnancies that may alert the health care provider to possible problems in the present pregnancy. Components of the obstetric history include:

- Gravida, para, abortions, and living children
- Weight of infants at birth, length of gestation
- Labor experience, type of delivery, location of birth, name of caregiver
- Type of anesthesia and any difficulties with anesthesia during childbirth or previous surgeries
- Maternal complications, such as hypertension, diabetes, infection, bleeding
- Complications with the infant
- Method of infant feeding planned (breast or formula)
- Special concerns

Gravida refers to the number of pregnancies, regardless of the duration of the pregnancy. *Para* refers to the number of pregnancies that end at 20 or more weeks. The number of fetuses in a pregnancy does not change the para. Thus a woman pregnant with twins will be a gravida 1, para 1 if birth occurs at 20 or more weeks of pregnancy.

Use of the TPAL acronym allows a more complete description of pregnancy outcomes than use of gravida and para alone. *TPAL* stands for term (*T*), preterm (*P*), abortions (*A*), and live (*L*) births. The TPAL method obtains complete information. A G for gravida is sometimes added (GTPAL) (Box 13-2).

Nurses must exercise caution when discussing obstetric history with the expectant mother in the presence of her family or significant other. Although the antepartum record may indicate a previous pregnancy or childbirth, she may not have shared this information with her family, and her right to privacy could be jeopardized by probing questions. The confidentiality of the pregnant woman must always be protected.

YORK HEALTH SYSTEM
YORK, PENNSYLVANIA
PRENATAL CARE
CLINICAL PATHWAY

DEMOGRAPHIC LABEL

EDC _____

PRETERM LABOR RISK
1. ☐ Substance abuse
2. ☐ Prior preterm delivery
3. ☐ >2 abortions
4. ☐ <90 lb prepregnancy weight
5. ☐ Placental anomaly
6. ☐ STD current pregnancy
7. ☐ Multiple gestation
8. ☐ Persistent bleeding
9. ☐ Incompetent cervix

DOCUMENTATION CODES
Initialed box = Meets standard   ★ = Exception on pathway identified   N = Not applicable

CONSULTS/PROBLEM MANAGEMENT
FOR PATIENTS INCLUDE:
- Social Service prn
- Perinatologist prn
- Genetic Counseling prn
- Nutritionist prn
- WIC prn
- Pastoral Care prn
- Lactation Consultant prn (3rd trimester)

STANDARD OF CARE FOR PRENATAL
PATIENTS INCLUDES:
- Activity ad lib
- Diet to meet needs of pregnancy
- Prenatal vitamins
- FeSO$_4$, if needed

Clinical Path Visits	Expected Patient/ Family Outcomes	Multidisciplinary Assessment (Refer to STD-0011)	Tests	Education & DC Planning (Refer to STD-0011)
Nurse Interview Date _____ RN Name _____	☐ Referrals made as indicated following prenatal standard of care ☐ Verbalizes understanding of normal vs. abnormal signs and symptoms of pregnancy ☐ Verbalizes agreement to complete labs, obtain prenatal vitamins and keep scheduled appointments ☐ Verbalizes signs and symptoms of preterm labor ☐ No risk factors PTL identified ☐	• Refer to Standard 0011-Nurse interview • Weight, height • Physical, psych/social, behavioral, nutritional risk factors • Knowledge of normal vs. abnormal signs and symptoms of pregnancy • Premature labor risk assessment	• CCMS-UA, for nitr/leuk/ glucose, C and S if applicable • Prenatal group _____ • HIV • Sickle cell if applicable • Dating ultrasound scheduled	☐ Childbirth ed., baby care and postpartum classes. Exercise during pregnancy. Effects of risk factors on pregnancy. Sexuality during pregnancy. Nutrition education. Normal effects of pregnancy on the body. Fetal growth/development. S and S of complications/preterm labor. Preadmission form. Contraceptives/STD Prevention/HIV counseling. Schedule return-to-clinic appointment. Orient to clinic hours/physical setup, emergency protocol.
1st OB Exam RN Name _____	☐ Prenatal group tests within normal limits ☐ Demonstrates measures to relieve normal complaints of pregnancy ☐ No change in preterm labor risk factors ☐	• Signs and symptoms of normal physical changes, complications • Behavioral risks • BP, weight • Urine dipstick for sugar/ ketone/protein • Fetal heart sounds • Fundal height • Pelvimetry	• Pap • GC • Chlamydia (if indicated) • Wet smear bacterial/ trich./vaginosis, vaginal ph and Whiff Test	

(1-14 Weeks)

Date _____

Outcomes:
- ☐ Demonstrates measures to relieve the normal complaints of pregnancy during 1st trimester.
- ☐ Established exercise routine
- ☐ Exhibits minimum weight loss/gain
- ☐ 1st trimester test results within normal limits
- ☐ Avoids or demonstrates decrease in risk associated behavior (ie. smoking)
- ☐ No change in preterm labor risk factors
- ☐ Takes prenatal vitamins
- ☐ _____

Assessments:
- Signs and symptoms of normal physical changes, complications
- Behavioral risks
- BP, weight
- Urine dipstick for sugar, ketone, protein
- Fetal heart sounds
- Fundal height

Interventions/Consultations:
- ☐ Reinforce (STD-0011) (Prenatal Standard of Care)
  Importance of compliance
  _____

RN Name _____

(15-28 Weeks)

Outcomes:
- ☐ Demonstrates measures to relieve the normal complaints of pregnancy during 2nd trimester.
- ☐ Exhibits normal weight gain.
- ☐ 2nd trimester test results within normal limits.
- ☐ Continues exercise routine.
- ☐ Avoids risk-associated behavior.
- ☐ Demonstrates self-palpation technique and verbalizes signs and symptoms of preterm labor.
- ☐ No change in preterm labor risk factors.
- ☐ _____

Assessments:
- Signs and symptoms of normal physical changes, complications including:
- Behavioral risks
- BP, weight
- Urine dipstick for sugar/ketone/protein
- Fetal heart sounds, fundal height
- Fundal movement at 16-20 weeks
- Premature labor

Tests:
- Triple Screen (16 to 19 weeks)
- Ultrasound, as needed
- Fibronectin (24 to 26 weeks)
  ORDER AT 26 WEEKS:
- Trutol
- Antibody screen (Rh Neg)
- Repeat WCBC
- RhoGAM at 28 weeks, if indicated

Interventions/Consultations:
- ☐ Fetal growth/development for 2nd tri.
  Encourage childbirth, baby care and postpartum classes
  Reinforce (STD-0011) (Prenatal Standard of Care)
  Review S and S of preterm labor at 24 week appointment
  Importance of compliance
  Home visit

RN Name _____

(29-42 Weeks)

Outcomes:
- ☐ Demonstrates measures to relieve the normal complaints of pregnancy during 3rd trimester.
- ☐ Exhibits normal weight gain.
- ☐ Continues exercise routine.
- ☐ Normal physical changes of pregnancy w/o complications.
- ☐ Avoids risk-associated behaviors.
- ☐ Attends childbirth, baby care and postpartum classes
- ☐ Responds appropriately to signs and symptoms of preterm labor or other complications when indicated.
- ☐ Performing nipple preparation, if needed.
- ☐ No change in preterm labor risk factors.
- ☐ _____

Assessments:
- Signs and symptoms of normal physical changes, complications including:
- Behavioral risks
- BP, weight
- Urine dipstick for sugar/ketone/protein
- Fetal heart sounds, fundal height
- Fetal movement
- Planned method of infant feeding
- Nipple exam, if planning to breast feed
- Premature labor

Tests:
- Ultrasound as needed
  ORDER AT 36 WEEKS:
- Recto vaginal cultures for GBS
- Order at 41 Weeks:
- NST and AFI Biweekly (amniotic fluid index)

Interventions/Consultations:
- ☐ Fetal growth/development for 3rd trimester
  Review signs and symptoms and admission procedures for normal labor at 36 weeks.
  Reinforce (STD-0011) (Prenatal Standard of Care)
  Review S and S of preterm labor
  Importance of compliance
  Update perinatal risk assessment
  Childbirth education, babycare and postpartum classes
  Tubal forms, if indicated by 34 weeks
  Treatment for inverted nipples if indicated
  Home visit

RN Name _____

Figure 13-9 Prenatal clinical pathway that identifies outcomes, assessments, interventions, and consultations performed during pregnancy. (Courtesy Women and Children Services of the York Health System, York, PA. Reprinted with modifications.)

BOX 13-2
Calculation of Gravida and Para

A useful method for calculating gravida and para is to use the acronym *TPAL* to divide pregnancy outcome into the number of term births (*T*), preterm pregnancies (*P*), abortions (*A*), and living children (*L*).

To illustrate: Sally Lam is pregnant for the fifth time. She underwent one spontaneous abortion and one elective abortion in the first trimester. She has a son who was born at 40 weeks' gestation and a daughter who was born at 36 weeks' gestation. She is gravida 5, para 2. T = 1 (the son born at 40 weeks); P = 1 (the daughter born at 36 weeks); A = 2; L = 2. The two abortions are counted in the gravida but are not included in the para because they occurred before 20 weeks.

CRITICAL THINKING EXERCISE 13-1

Wilma Turner gave birth to twin girls at 38 weeks of gestation 3 years ago. She had a spontaneous abortion last year at 12 weeks of gestation and thinks she may be pregnant now because she has missed a menstrual period and is experiencing morning sickness. Wilma's last normal menstrual period began June 22.
1. If Wilma is pregnant now, what would be the gravida and para?
2. Explain to Wilma why amenorrhea and morning sickness are not positive indications of pregnancy.
3. Use Nägele's rule to compute the expected date of delivery (EDD).

EDD - Estimated delivery date

Menstrual History. A complete menstrual history is necessary to establish the EDD (or EDB). It is common practice to estimate the EDD on the basis of the first day of the last normal menstrual cycle, although ovulation and conception occur approximately 2 weeks after the beginning of menstruation in a regular 28-day cycle. The average duration of pregnancy from the first day of the last normal menstrual period is 40 weeks, or 280 days. Nägele's rule is often used to establish EDD. To use this method, subtract 3 months, add 7 days to the first day of the last normal menstrual period (LNMP), and correct the year, if appropriate.

> *For example:* LNMP June 30, 2005
>
> Subtract 3 months = March 30, 2005
>
> Add 7 days and change the year = April 6, 2006

Many health care providers also use a gestational calculator or wheel to calculate EDD quickly, although some wheels are prone to error. A sonogram is often used to confirm the date.

Contraceptive History. A detailed history of contraceptive methods is important. Use of oral contraceptives during early unrecognized pregnancy is a concern because of the effect of estrogens and some synthetic progestins on the fetus. Intrauterine devices can cause complications if pregnancy occurs with an intrauterine device in place. Risks include abortion, premature delivery, and puncture of the uterus.

Medical and Surgical History. Chronic conditions, such as diabetes mellitus, hypertension, and renal disease, can affect the outcome of the pregnancy and must be investigated. Infections such as hepatitis or pyelonephritis, as well as surgical procedures and trauma that may complicate the pregnancy or childbirth, must be documented. The history includes:

- Age, race, ethnic background (risk for specific genetic problems, such as sickle cell disease, thalassemia, and Tay-Sachs disease)
- Childhood diseases and immunizations
- Chronic illnesses, such as asthma and heart disease
- Previous illnesses, surgical procedures, injuries
- Previous infections: hepatitis, sexually transmissible diseases, and tuberculosis

- History of anemia
- Bladder, bowel function (problems or changes)
- Amount of caffeine and alcohol consumed each day
- Tobacco use (number of years and number of packs per day)
- Prescription or other drugs
- Complementary or alternative therapies
- General nutrition, history of eating disorders
- Contact with pets, particularly cats (increased risk of infections such as toxoplasmosis)
- Allergies and drug sensitivities
- Occupation and related risk factors

Family Health History. A family history for the woman and her partner provides valuable information about the general health of the family, including chronic diseases such as diabetes and heart disease, and infections such as tuberculosis and hepatitis. Moreover, information about patterns of genetic or congenital anomalies may be revealed.

The use of drugs such as cocaine or alcohol may affect the family's ability to cope with pregnancy and childbirth. Tobacco use by the father poses a risk to both the mother and infant for upper respiratory tract complications as a result of passive smoking. In addition, the father's blood type and Rh factor are important if the mother is Rh negative because there is a possibility of a blood incompatibility between the mother and the fetus.

Psychosocial History. The psychosocial history, which should be completed at the same time, is discussed in Chapter 14.

Physical Examination

Many women have not had a recent physical examination before becoming pregnant. A thorough evaluation of all body systems is necessary to detect previously undiagnosed physical problems that may affect the pregnancy outcome. It also allows the examiner to establish baseline levels that will guide the treatment of the expectant mother and fetus throughout pregnancy.

Vital Signs

Blood Pressure. Position affects blood pressure in the pregnant woman. Blood pressure should be obtained with the woman seated and her arm supported in a horizontal position at the level of the heart. Documentation should include the position, the arm used, and the pressures obtained.

Pulse. The normal adult pulse rate is 60 to 90 bpm. Tachycardia is associated with anxiety, hyperthyroidism, and infection and should be investigated. The apical pulse should be assessed for at least 1 minute to determine the amplitude and regularity of the heartbeat. Presence of murmurs should be noted. Pedal pulses should be strong, equal, and regular.

Respiratory Effort. Respiratory rate during pregnancy is in the range of 16 to 24 breaths per minute. Tachypnea may indicate respiratory infection or cardiac disease. Breath sounds should be equal bilaterally, chest expansion should be symmetric, and lung fields should be free of all abnormal breath sounds.

Temperature. Normal temperature during pregnancy is 36.6° to 37.6° C (97.8° to 99.6° F). Increased temperature suggests infection that may require medical management.

Cardiovascular System

Venous Congestion. Additional assessment of the cardiovascular system includes observation for venous congestion, which can develop into varicosities. Venous congestion is most commonly noted in the legs, vulva, or rectum.

Edema. Edema of the legs may be a benign condition that reflects pooling of blood in the extremities, which results in a shift of intravascular fluid into interstitial spaces. When pressure exerted by a finger or thumb leaves a persistent depression, the condition is termed *pitting edema*. Edema of the hands or face may be a sign of preeclampsia.

Musculoskeletal System

Posture and Gait. Body mechanics, as well as changes in posture and gait, should be addressed. Body mechanics during pregnancy may place strain on the muscles of the lower back and legs.

Height and Weight. An initial weight is needed to establish a baseline for weight gain throughout pregnancy. Weight should be compared with the ideal-weight-for-height charts. A preconception weight of less than 45 kg (100 lb) or height under 150 cm (60 inches) is associated with preterm labor and low-birth-weight infants. A preconception weight more than 91 kg (200 lb) is associated with an increased incidence of gestational diabetes and hypertension.

Pelvic Measurements. Early in pregnancy, the bony pelvis is evaluated to determine whether the diameters are adequate to permit vaginal delivery (see Chapter 12).

Abdomen. The contour, size, and muscle tone of the abdomen should be assessed. Fundal height should be measured if the fundus is palpable above the symphysis pubis. The woman lies on her back with her knees slightly flexed after emptying her bladder to avoid elevation of the uterus by a full bladder. The top of the fundus is palpated, and a tape is stretched from the top of the symphysis pubis, over the abdominal curve, to the top of the fundus (Fig. 13-10).

From 16 to 38 weeks, the fundal height, measured in centimeters, is equal to the gestational age of the fetus in weeks, within 3 cm (Johnson & Niebyl, 2002). If there is a discrepancy between fundal height and weeks of gestation, additional assessment is necessary. The EDD may be incorrect and the pregnancy more or less advanced than thought. The number of fetuses present and fetal growth should also be evaluated.

Fetal heart rate should be counted and recorded if the pregnancy is advanced enough so that it is audible.

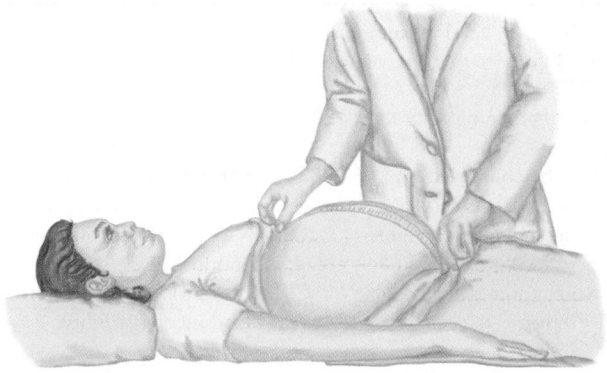

Figure 13-10 Measuring the uterus entails measuring from the upper border of the symphysis pubis to the top of the fundus.

Neurologic System. A complete neurologic assessment is not necessary for women who are free of signs or symptoms that indicate a problem. Deep tendon reflexes should be assessed, however, because hyperreflexia is associated with complications of pregnancy. (See Procedure 26-1 for assessment of deep tendon reflexes.)

Integumentary System. Skin color should be consistent with racial background. Pallor may indicate anemia. Jaundice may indicate hepatic disease. Lesions, bruising, or areas of hyperpigmentation (chloasma, linea nigra) related to pregnancy, as well as stretch marks (striae), should be noted. Nail beds should be pink, with instant capillary return.

Endocrine System. The thyroid enlarges slightly during the second trimester. Gross enlargement or tenderness, however, may indicate hyperthyroidism and requires further medical evaluation.

Gastrointestinal System

Mouth. Mucous membranes should be pink, smooth, glistening, and uniform. The lips should be free of ulcerations. The gums may be red, tender, and edematous as a result of increased estrogen, which produces hyperplasia. The woman should be referred for regular dental care because periodontal disease may result in infections that precipitate preterm labor.

Intestine. Bowel sounds may be diminished because of the effects of progesterone on smooth muscle. Bowel sounds are often increased if a meal is overdue or if diarrhea is present. Constipation can be discussed at this time.

Urinary System. Urine collected for testing should be a clean-catch midstream sample. Urine is tested to detect signs of urinary tract infection and substances that may indicate a problem.

Protein. Although a small amount of protein may be present in the urine, the amount should not increase. Its presence may indicate contamination by vaginal secretions, kidney disease, or preeclampsia.

Glucose. Small amounts of glucose may indicate physiologic "spilling" that occurs during normal pregnancy. Larger amounts require glucose screening of the blood.

Ketones. Ketones may be found in the urine after heavy exercise or as a result of inadequate intake of food and fluid.

Bacteria. Increased bacteria in the urine is associated with urinary tract infection, which is common during pregnancy.

TABLE 13-1 Common Laboratory Tests

Test	Purpose	Significance
Blood grouping	To determine blood type and Rh.	Identifies possible causes of incompatibility with the blood of the fetus that may cause jaundice.
Hemoglobin (Hgb) or hematocrit (Hct)	To detect anemia. Often checked several times during pregnancy.	Hgb <11 g/dl or Hct <33% may indicate a need for iron supplementation.
Complete blood count (CBC)	To detect infection, anemia, or cell abnormalities.	12,000/mm³ or more white blood cells or decreased platelets require followup.
Rh factor and antibody screen	To screen for possible maternal-fetal blood incompatibility.	If mother is Rh-negative and father is Rh-positive or antibodies present, additional testing and treatment required. If negative, RhoGAM will be given at 26-28 weeks.
Venereal Disease Research Laboratory (VDRL) or rapid plasma reagin (RPR)	To screen for syphilis.	Treat if positive. Retest at 36 weeks.
Rubella titer	To determine immunity.	If titer is 1:8 or less, mother is not immune. Immunize postpartum if not immune.
Tuberculin skin test	To screen for tuberculosis.	If positive, refer for additional testing or therapy.
Hemoglobin electrophoresis	To screen for sickle cell trait if client is African-American.	If mother is positive, check partner. Infant is at risk only if both parents are positive.
Hepatitis B	To detect presence of antigens in maternal blood.	If present, infants should be given hepatitis immune globulin and vaccine soon after birth.
Human immunodeficiency virus (HIV) screen	Voluntary test encouraged at first visit to detect HIV antibodies.	Positive results require retesting, counseling, and treatment to lower infant infection.
Urinalysis	To detect renal disease or infection.	Requires further assessment if positive for more than trace protein (renal damage, preeclampsia, or normal), glucose (diabetes or normal), ketones (fasting or dehydration), or bacteria (infection).
Papanicolaou (Pap) test	To screen for cervical neoplasia.	Treat and refer if abnormal cells are present.
Cervical culture	To detect group B streptococci and sexually transmissible diseases.	Treat and retest as necessary, treat group B streptococci during labor.
Triple screen: Maternal serum alpha-fetoprotein, human chorionic gonadotropin, and estriol	To screen for fetal anomalies.	Abnormal results may indicate Down syndrome or neural tube defects.
Maternal blood glucose	To screen for gestational diabetes.	If elevated, a 3-hour glucose tolerance test is recommended.

Reproductive System

Breasts. Breast size and symmetry, the condition of the nipples, and the presence of colostrum should be noted. Any lumps, dimpling of the skin, or asymmetry of the nipples requires further evaluation.

External Reproductive Organs. The skin and mucous membranes of the perineum, vulva, and anus are inspected for excoriations, growths, ulcerations, lesions, varicosities, warts, chancres, and perineal scars. Enlargement, tenderness, redness, or discharge from Bartholin's glands or Skene's glands may indicate gonorrheal or chlamydial infection. The examiner should obtain a specimen for culture of any discharge from lesions or inflamed glands to determine the causative organisms and to provide effective care.

Internal Reproductive Organs. A speculum inserted into the vagina permits the examiner to see the walls of the vagina and the cervix. Chadwick's sign and Goodell's sign are seen during pregnancy. The external cervical os is closed in primigravidas, but one fingertip may be admitted in multiparas. Routine cervical cultures for gonorrhea and chlamydial infection are standard practice during the initial pregnancy examination at most agencies. The examiner also collects a specimen for a Papanicolaou (Pap) smear, a screening test for cervical cancer.

A bimanual examination involves using both hands, one on the abdomen and the other in the vagina, to palpate the internal genitalia. The examiner palpates the uterus for size, contour, tenderness, and position. The uterus should be movable between the two examining hands and should feel smooth. The ovaries, if palpable, should be about the shape and size of almonds and should not be tender.

Laboratory Data

Table 13-1 lists laboratory examinations that are commonly performed during pregnancy. The table briefly describes their purpose and the significance of each test.

Risk Assessment

Risk assessment begins at the initial visit, when the health care team identifies factors that put the expectant mother or the fetus at risk for complications and thus in need of specialized care. Many women identified as high risk give birth to healthy term infants. Furthermore, risk factors change as pregnancy progresses, and risk assessment must be updated throughout pregnancy. Box 13-3 lists the major risk factors and identifies maternal and fetal-neonatal implications.

BOX 13–3
Summary of High-Risk Factors in Pregnancy

FACTORS	IMPLICATIONS
Demographic Factors	
<16 years or >35 years	Increased risk for preterm labor, preeclampsia, congenital anomalies
Low socioeconomic status or dependent on public assistance	Increased risk for preterm labor, low-birth-weight infants
Nonwhite race	Incidence of infant and maternal death often higher than that of whites
Multiparity: >4 pregnancies	Increasing parity increases risk for pregnancy loss, antepartum or postpartum hemorrhage, cesarean birth
Social-Personal Factors	
Weight <45 kg (100 pounds)	Associated with low-birth-weight infant
Weight >91 kg (200 pounds)	Increased risk for preeclampsia, difficult labor, large-for-gestational-age infant, and cesarean birth
Height <152 cm (5 feet)	Increased incidence of cesarean birth because of cephalopelvic disproportion
Smoking	Associated with low-birth-weight infant, preterm birth
Use of alcohol or unprescribed drugs	Increased risk for congenital anomalies, neonatal withdrawal syndrome, fetal alcohol syndrome
Obstetric Factors	
Birth of previous infant >4000 g (8.8 pounds)	Increased need for cesarean birth; increased risk for infant birth injury, neonatal hypoglycemia, maternal gestational diabetes
Previous fetal or neonatal death	Maternal psychologic distress
Rh sensitization	Fetal anemia, erythroblastosis fetalis, kernicterus
Existing Medical Conditions	
Diabetes mellitus	Increased risk for preeclampsia, cesarean birth, infant either small or large for gestational age, neonatal hypoglycemia, fetal or neonatal death, congenital anomalies
Thyroid disorder:	
Hypothyroidism	Increased incidence of spontaneous abortion, congenital anomalies, congenital hypothyroidism
Hyperthyroidism	Maternal risk for preeclampsia, thyroid storm, or postpartum hemorrhage; neonatal risk for thyrotoxicosis
Cardiac disease	Maternal risk for cardiac decompensation and increased death rate; increased risk for fetal and neonatal death
Renal disease	Maternal risk for renal failure and preterm delivery; fetal risk for intrauterine growth restriction
Concurrent Infections	
	Severe fetal implications (heart disease, blindness, deafness, bone lesions) if maternal disease occurred in the first trimester
	Increased incidence of spontaneous abortion or congenital anomalies are associated with some infections

Subsequent Assessments

Ongoing antepartum care is important to the successful outcome of pregnancy. Although the recommended number of visits can be reduced for women with no complications, the usual schedule for prenatal assessment in a normal pregnancy is:

Conception to 28 weeks: every 4 weeks

29 to 36 weeks: every 2 to 3 weeks

37 weeks to birth: weekly

Vital Signs

To be accurate, the blood pressure must be measured in the same arm with the mother in the same position each time. Deviations from baseline values in blood pressure, pulse, or respiratory rate indicate the need for further assessment. The temperature should remain within normal limits.

Weight

Weight should be plotted to document that the expected pattern of weight gain is occurring. A gain of 11.5 to 16 kg (25-35 lb) is recommended for the average woman (see Chapter 15). Inadequate weight gain may signify that the pregnancy is not as advanced as first thought or that the fetus is not growing as expected. A sudden, rapid weight gain may indicate fluid retention, and further assessment for preeclampsia is indicated.

Urinalysis

Urine is tested at each visit for protein, glucose, and ketones. A screen for bacteria may be repeated later in the pregnancy if the woman has a history of previous urinary tract infections.

The urine may be checked for nitrates with a dipstick. A positive result indicates infection may be present, and a urine culture may be performed.

Fundal Height

Measuring fundal height is an inexpensive and noninvasive method for evaluating fetal growth and confirming gestational age.

Leopold Maneuvers

Leopold maneuvers provide a systematic method for palpating the fetus through the abdominal wall during the later part of pregnancy. These maneuvers provide valuable information about the location and presentation of the fetus (see Chapter 17).

Fetal Heart Rate

The fetal heart rate may be heard in early pregnancy with a Doppler transducer or, in later pregnancy, with a fetoscope. The location of the fetal heart sounds provides information that may help determine the position in which the fetus is entering the pelvis. For instance, a fetal heart rate heard in an upper quadrant of the abdomen suggests that the fetus is in a breech presentation.

Fetal Activity

Usually first noticed by the expectant mother at 16 to 20 weeks of gestation, fetal movements (quickening) gradually increase in both frequency and strength. In the last trimester, the woman may be asked to count fetal body movements. These are commonly called "kick counts." In general, fetal activity indicates that the fetus is physically healthy.

Ultrasound Screen

Although an ultrasound examination is not necessary for all women, the test may be performed at 12 to 20 weeks of gestation. Ultrasound helps determine gestational age and may show some fetal anomalies and determine the sex (see Chapter 16).

Glucose Screen

Blood glucose is often screened between 24 and 28 weeks, and additional testing is indicated if the result is elevated (see Chapter 26). Glucose testing may not be necessary in women younger than 25 years and at low risk for developing gestational diabetes (Cunningham et al., 2001).

Isoimmunization

Antibody tests may be repeated at 26 to 28 weeks in women who are Rh negative when the father of the baby is Rh positive. If unsensitized, the woman should receive anti-D immune globulin (RhoGAM) prophylactically at this time (see Chapter 26).

Pelvic Examination

During the last month of pregnancy the health care provider may perform a pelvic examination to determine cervical changes. The descent of the fetus and the presenting part can also be assessed at this time.

Signs of Labor

The woman should be asked about signs of labor at each visit. A discussion of contractions, bleeding, and rupture of membranes will help the woman know how to identify preterm labor.

Multifetal Pregnancy

A multifetal pregnancy is a pregnancy in which two or more embryos or fetuses exist simultaneously (see Chapter 12).

Diagnosis

Women with multifetal pregnancies are larger than expected for the weeks of gestation, have more fetal movements, and gain more weight. The fundal height is often 4 cm larger than expected on the basis of gestational age computed from the last menstrual period.

The maternal history may be of some help in making the diagnosis. A maternal family history that includes fraternal twins slightly increases the chance of twins. Recent administration of fertility drugs greatly increases the chance of multifetal pregnancy. When more than one fetus seems likely, the diagnosis should be confirmed by sonography. Separate gestational sacs may be seen as early as 6 weeks of gestation.

Maternal Adaptation to Multifetal Pregnancy

Maternal physiologic change is greater with multiple fetuses than with a single fetus. There is a 500-ml increase in blood volume over that needed for a single fetus. This increases the workload of the heart and may contribute to fatigue and activity intolerance. The uterus may achieve a volume of 10 liters or more and weigh more than 20 lb (Cunningham et al., 2001). Respiratory difficulty increases because the overdistended uterus causes greater elevation of the diaphragm.

The uterus may also cause more compression of the large vessels, resulting in more pronounced and earlier supine hypotension. Greater compression of the ureters can occur, and maternal edema and proteinuria are common. Compression of the bowel makes constipation a persistent problem.

Antepartum Care in Multifetal Pregnancy

Many health care providers increase the number of times women with a multifetal pregnancy are seen during the antepartum period. More frequent visits permit extra vigilance in the detection of common complications such as anemia, hypertension, premature labor, and congenital anomalies.

Education about the need for increased rest, signs of preterm labor and diet is important. The need for calories, iron, vitamins, and folic acid increases. Women carrying twins are advised to gain 16 to 20.5 kg (35 to 45 lb).

Common Discomforts of Pregnancy

Many women experience discomforts of pregnancy that are not serious in themselves but detract from the woman's feeling of comfort and well-being.

(See Women Want to Know: How to Overcome the Common Discomforts of Pregnancy.)

Nausea and Vomiting

Nausea and vomiting of pregnancy are frequently called *morning sickness* because these symptoms are more acute on arising. They may, however, occur at any time of the day. Women need reassurance that nausea and vomiting, however distressing, are common and that the condition is temporary. Morning sickness must be distinguished from hyperemesis gravidarum—severe vomiting accompanied by weight loss, dehydration, electrolyte imbalance, and ketosis (see Chapter 26).

Although the cause of nausea and vomiting is unknown, these symptoms are believed to be related to increased levels of hCG and estrogen, as well as periodic hypoglycemia. Symptoms may be aggravated by cooking odors, fatigue, and emotional stress.

Heartburn

Heartburn is described as an acute burning sensation in the epigastric and sternal regions. It occurs when reverse peristaltic waves cause regurgitation of acidic stomach contents into the esophagus. The underlying causes are diminished gastric motility, displacement of the stomach by the enlarging uterus, and relaxation of the lower esophageal sphincter. Improper diet and nervous tension may be precipitating factors.

Backache

Backache is a common complaint during the third trimester. A primary focus is to prevent backache by teaching correct posture (Fig. 13-11) and body mechanics (Fig. 13-12). Figure 13-13 suggests exercises that relax the shoulders and thighs and help prevent backache.

Round Ligament Pain

Round ligament pain is a sharp pain in the side or inguinal area, usually on the right side. It is caused by softening and stretching of the ligament from hormones and uterine growth. Because the uterus turns slightly to the right during pregnancy, the right round ligament is stretched more than the left.

Urinary Frequency

Although urinary frequency is a common complaint of women, especially during the first trimester and near term, the condition is temporary and is managed by most women without undue distress. Kegel exercises are sometimes recommended to help maintain bladder control.

Varicosities

Varicosities occur in 40% of pregnancies because the weight of the uterus partially compresses the veins that return blood from the legs and estrogen causes elastic tissue to become more fragile (Blackburn, 2003). This process causes the vessels to dilate, and they may become engorged, inflamed, and

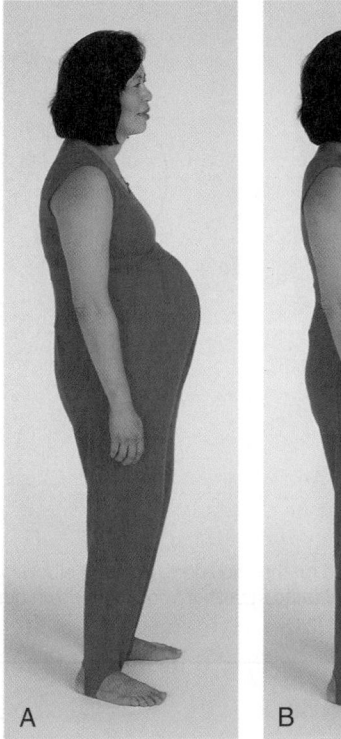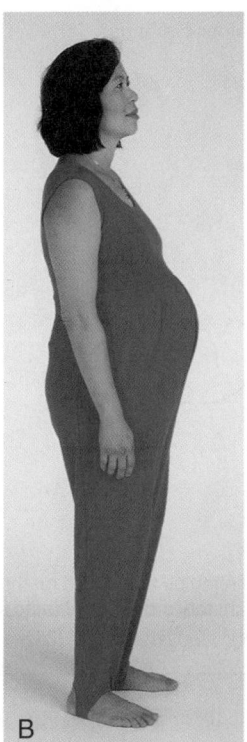

Figure 13-11 Posture during pregnancy may cause or alleviate backache. *A,* Incorrect posture. The neck is jutting forward, the shoulders are slumping, and the back is sharply curved, creating back pain and discomfort. *B,* Correct posture. The neck and shoulders are straight, the back is flattened, and the pelvis is tucked under and slightly upward.

painful. The condition is usually confined to the legs but may involve the veins of the vulva or rectum (hemorrhoids).

Varicosities occur most often in women with a family history of varicose veins and are more likely to be a problem in women who are obese or who are multiparas. The problem is exacerbated by prolonged standing, when the force of gravity makes blood return more difficult. There may be minimal discomfort at the end of each day or large, tortuous veins that produce severe discomfort with any activity.

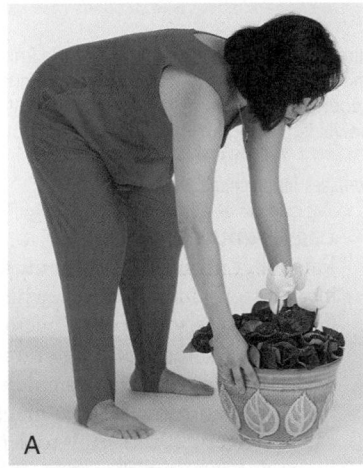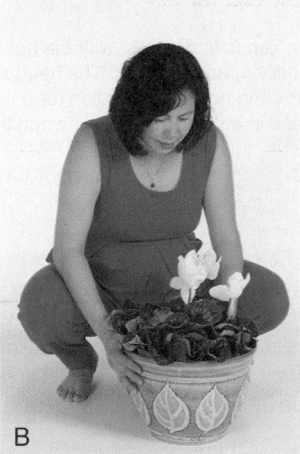

Figure 13-12 Techniques for lifting. Squatting places less strain on the back. *A,* Incorrect technique. Stooping or bending places a great deal of strain on muscles of the lower back. *B,* Correct technique. Squatting and moving the object close permits the stronger muscles of the legs to do the lifting.

Shoulder circling

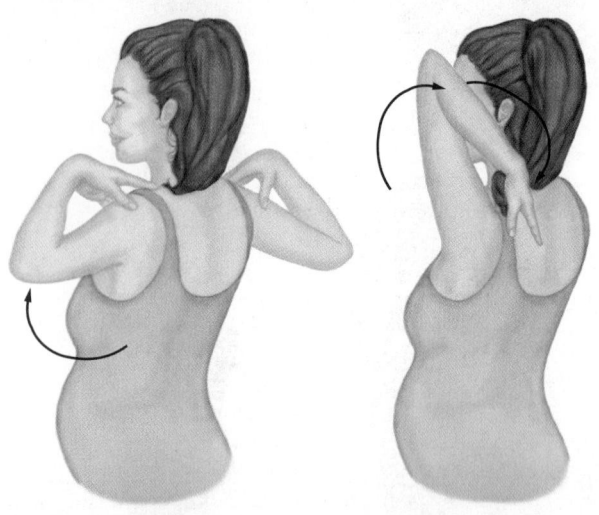

The fingertips are placed on the shoulders, then the elbows are brought forward and up during inhalation, back and down during exhalation. Repeat five times.

Tailor sitting

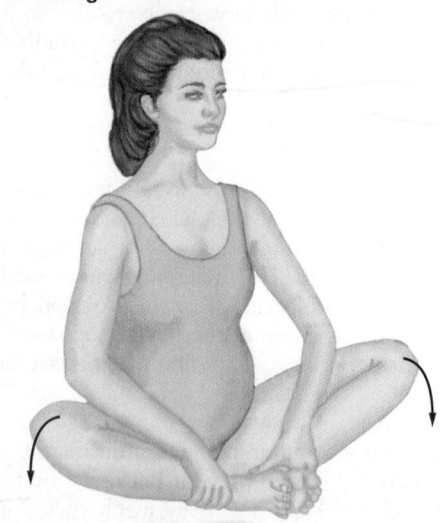

The woman uses her thigh muscles to press her knees to the floor. Keeping her back straight, she should remain in the position for 5 to 15 minutes.

Pelvic tilt or pelvic rocking

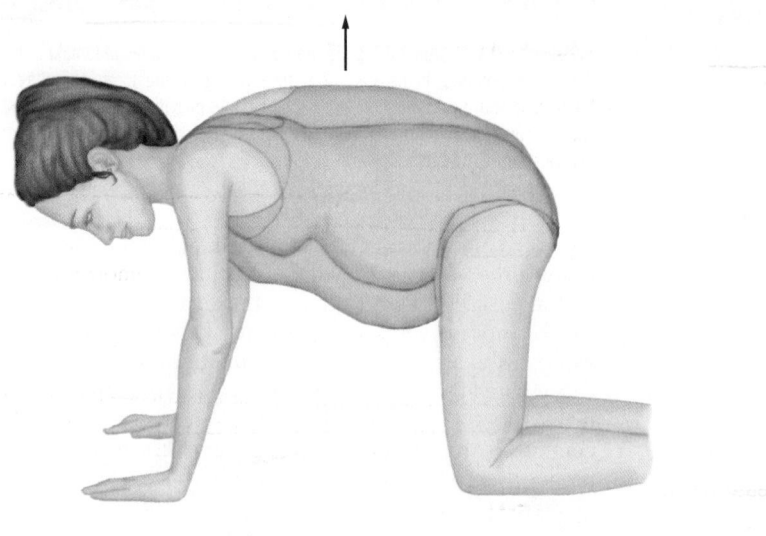

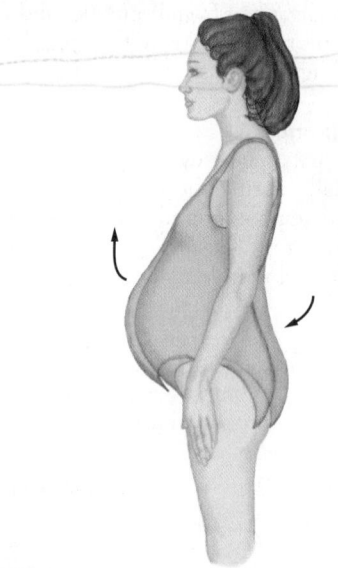

This exercise can be performed on hands and knees, with the hands directly under the shoulders and the knees under the hips. The back should be in a neutral position, not hollowed. The head and neck should be aligned with the straight back. The woman then presses up with the lower back and holds this position for a few seconds, then relaxes to a neutral position. Repeat 5 times. The exercise may also be performed in a standing position when the pelvis is rotated forward to flatten the lower back.

Figure 13-13 Exercises for pregnancy.

Hemorrhoids

Hemorrhoids are varicosities of the rectum that may be external (outside the anal sphincter) or internal (above the sphincter). Common causes include vascular engorgement of the pelvis, constipation, straining at stool, and prolonged sitting or standing. Pushing during the second stage of labor exacerbates the problem, which may continue into the postpartum period.

Constipation

Intestinal motility is reduced during pregnancy as a result of progesterone. This change may cause hard, dry stools and decreased frequency of bowel movements. Iron supplementation also causes constipation in some women.

Leg Cramps

Painful contraction of the muscles of the lower legs occurs most often during sleep, when the muscles are relaxed. Cramps are also likely to occur when the woman stretches and extends her foot. Leg cramps are believed to be caused by an imbalance of serum calcium and phosphorus, but this has not been proven. Low magnesium levels may also be a cause (Fagen, 2000). A 1-to-1 ratio of calcium to phosphorus is desired, but this ratio is difficult to achieve in pregnancy, when many women consume large amounts of dairy products high in calcium and phosphorus. Venous congestion in the legs during the third trimester also contributes to leg cramps.

▪NURSING CARE

Family Responses to Physical Changes of Pregnancy

The nursing process focuses on identifying each family's unique responses to the physiologic changes of pregnancy, determining factors that might interfere with the ability to adapt to changes that occur, and finding solutions to identified problems.

Assessment

Assess the family's responses to the physiologic processes of pregnancy and the family's preparation for the birth. Include structured interviews, planned teaching-learning sessions, and informal discussions. Review the history and physical examination findings. Gather information from the expectant mother as well as from the partner and other significant family members, if appropriate.

Nursing Diagnosis and Planning

Most families express an intense desire to protect the health of the unborn child and the well-being of the mother. Perhaps the most encompassing nursing diagnosis for the prenatal period is:

■ Health-Seeking Behaviors: prenatal care and health practices that provide optimum benefit to the fetus and mother.

Expected Outcomes: The family will explain practices that promote the safety and well-being of the mother and fetus throughout pregnancy and will describe measures that provide relief from the common discomforts of pregnancy. The family will describe a realistic plan during the first trimester to modify behaviors or habits that do not promote the health of the mother and fetus.

Interventions

After the initial assessment, the woman is usually not seen by the health care provider for 4 weeks. Instruct her and her family about signs and symptoms that indicate a serious danger and should be reported immediately.

Teaching Health Behaviors

Bathing Bathing protects pregnant women from potential infection and promotes comfort by dissipating heat produced by increased metabolism. During the last trimester, when balance is altered by a changing center of gravity, caution the woman to use nonskid pads in the tub or shower.

WOMEN
Want to Know

How to Overcome the Common Discomforts of Pregnancy

Nausea and Vomiting
- Eat dry crackers or toast before arising in the morning; then get out of bed slowly.
- Eat small amounts of carbohydrate foods frequently during the day and 5 to 6 small meals.
- Drink fluids separately from meals.
- Avoid fried, greasy, or spicy foods or those with strong odors.
- Try peppermint or combining salty and tart foods like potato chips and lemonade at the same time.
- Vitamin B$_6$ (pyridoxine) may also be helpful. Check with primary caregiver for the dosage.
- Eat a protein snack before bedtime.
- Use an acupressure band that applies pressure over a point approximately 3 finger-widths above the wrist crease on the inner arm.

Heartburn
- Eat several small meals daily, and avoid fatty or spicy foods.
- Curtail smoking and coffee drinking, which stimulate acid formation in the stomach.
- Sit upright for at least 1 hour after meals to reduce reflux and relieve symptoms.
- Do not eat or drink just before bedtime, and sleep with an extra pillow.
- Sip water to help relieve the burning sensation.
- Use antacids but avoid those that are high in sodium (Alka-Seltzer, baking soda), which cause fluid retention. Antacids high in calcium (Tums, Alka-Mints) provide relief but may cause rebound hyperacidity. Liquid antacids may be more effective.

Backache
- Maintain correct posture: head up, shoulders back.
- Avoid high-heeled shoes to improve posture.

- To pick up objects, squat rather than bend at the waist.
- When sitting, use foot supports, arm rests, and pillows behind the back.
- Exercise using tailor sitting, shoulder circling, and pelvic rocking strengthens the back and prepares for labor.

Round Ligament Pain
- Use good body mechanics, and avoid very strenuous exercise.
- Avoid stretching and twisting at the same time. When getting out of bed, turn to the side first and then get up slowly.
- Bend toward the pain, squat, or bring the knees up to the chest to relieve pain by relaxing the ligament.
- Apply heat and lie on the right side to relieve the pain.

Urinary Frequency
- Performing Kegel exercises helps maintain bladder control:
  Identify the muscles to be exercised by stopping the flow of urine midstream. Do not, however, perform the exercise while urinating because urinary retention increases the risk of urinary tract infection.
  Slowly contract the muscles around the vagina, and hold for 10 seconds. Relax at least 10 seconds.
  Repeat the contraction-relaxation cycle 30 times per day.

Varicosities
- Avoid constricting clothing and crossing the legs at the knees, which impedes blood return from the legs.
- Rest frequently with the legs elevated above the level of the hips.
- Wear support hose or elastic stockings that reach above the varicosities. Apply them before getting out of bed each morning.
- If working in one position for prolonged periods, walk around for a few minutes at least every 2 hours.

Continued

WOMEN
Want to Know

How to Overcome the Common Discomforts of Pregnancy—cont'd

Hemorrhoids
- To prevent hemorrhoids, establish a regular pattern of bowel elimination that does not require straining. Drink plenty of water, eat foods rich in fiber, and exercise regularly.
- To relieve existing hemorrhoids, take frequent, tepid baths. Apply cool witch hazel compresses or anesthetic ointments. Lie (on the side) with the hips elevated on a pillow.
- Gently push the hemorrhoids back into the rectum. To do so, put on a glove and lubricate the index finger. Maintain pressure for 1 to 2 minutes.
- If pain persists or bleeding occurs, call your health care provider.

Constipation
- Self-care measures generally are as effective as using laxatives, but they do not interfere with absorption of nutrients or lead to laxative dependency.
- Drink at least eight glasses of water each day. These should not include coffee, tea, or carbonated drinks because of their diuretic effect. After drinking one of these beverages, add a glass of water.
- Add foods high in fiber such as unpeeled fresh fruits and vegetables, whole-grain cereals, bran muffins, oatmeal, baked potatoes with skins, and fruit juices. Four pieces of fruit plus a large salad provide enough fiber for 1 day.
- Restrict cheese consumption, which causes constipation.
- Curtail intake of sweets, which increase bacterial growth in the intestine and can lead to flatulence.
- Do not discontinue taking iron supplements if they have been prescribed. If constipation persists, consult your health care provider for advice about stool softeners.
- A brisk walk of at least 1 mile per day stimulates peristalsis and improves muscle tone. Swimming and riding a stationary bicycle are also helpful.

- Establish a regular pattern by allowing a consistent time each day for elimination. One hour after meals is ideal to take advantage of the gastrocolic reflex (the peristaltic wave in the colon that is induced by taking food into the fasting stomach). Using a footrest during elimination provides comfort and decreases straining.

Leg Cramps

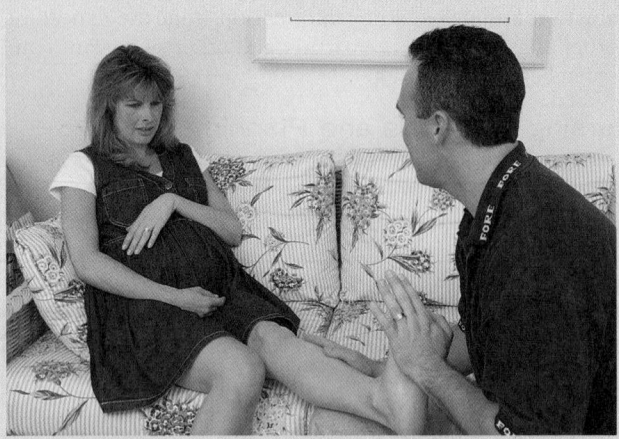

- To prevent cramps, elevate the legs often during the day to improve circulation.
- To relieve cramps, extend the affected leg, keeping the knee straight. Bend the foot toward the body, or ask someone to assist. If alone, stand and apply pressure on the affected leg.
- Avoid excessive foods high in phosphorus. Additional calcium or magnesium may be helpful but should be taken only with the advice of the health care provider.

! CRITICAL TO REMEMBER
Danger Signs During Pregnancy
- Vaginal bleeding, with or without discomfort
- Rupture of membranes (escape of fluid from the vagina)
- Swelling of the fingers (rings become tight) or puffiness of the face or around the eyes
- Continuous, pounding headache
- Visual disturbances (blurred vision, dimness, spots before the eyes)
- Persistent or severe abdominal pain
- Chills or fever
- Painful urination
- Persistent vomiting
- Change in frequency or strength of fetal movements

Hot Tubs and Saunas Instruct the woman to avoid activities that may cause maternal hyperthermia. Maternal hyperthermia, particularly during the first trimester, may be associated with fetal anomalies. A pregnant woman

should not stay in a sauna for more than 15 minutes or a hot tub for more than 10 minutes and should keep her head and chest out of the water (American Academy of Pediatrics and American College of Obstetricians and Gynecologists, 2002).

Douching Despite increased vaginal discharge in pregnancy, there is no need for douching during pregnancy or at any other time. Some women douche because they believe it increases cleanliness and prevents infection. However, douching is associated with infections, preterm labor, and low birth weight (Cottrell, 2003). Discuss women's reasons for douching, and explain the detrimental effects.

Breast Care Instruct the expectant mother to avoid soap on her nipples because it removes the natural lubricant that forms there. A supportive bra helps prevent loss of muscle tone as the breasts become heavier during pregnancy. Wide bra straps distribute the weight evenly across the shoulders and provide greater comfort. Breast stimulation, which increases oxytocin secretion and thus initiates uterine contractions, is unsafe if there has been a history of preterm labor or if signs of preterm labor are present.

Nursing Care Plan

Discomfort During Early Pregnancy

ASSESSMENT

Maria Gomez, a thin, 21-year-old primigravida 8 weeks' pregnant, states that she is experiencing nausea with occasional vomiting throughout the day. She reports that the nausea is intensified by the odor of cooking food and that she has little appetite. Although she is always thirsty, she restricts fluids because "they make me sicker." She has no signs of dehydration.

Nursing Diagnosis

Risk for Imbalanced Nutrition: Less Than Body Requirements related to nausea, vomiting, and anorexia.

Goals/Expected Outcomes

Maria will

- Maintain adequate intake of calories and nutrients to meet her needs, as evidenced by a weight gain of 10 lb by 20 weeks.
- Report less nausea and a decrease in the episodes of vomiting within 2 weeks.
- Demonstrate no signs or symptoms of dehydration.

INTERVENTION	RATIONALE
1. Recommend that Maria eat two dry crackers half an hour before arising in the morning and that she get out of bed slowly.	1. Food counteracts the hypoglycemia resulting from nightlong fasting and prevents an initial episode of nausea that may become difficult to control.
2. Suggest that Maria consume a high-protein bedtime snack, such as cottage cheese or half a turkey sandwich.	2. Proteins are metabolized at a slower rate, which helps prevent morning hypoglycemia.
3. Instruct Maria to eat small, dry meals five to six times a day rather than three large meals.	3. Frequent, dry meals prevent the stomach from becoming empty, which increases the feeling of nausea.
4. Suggest that fluids be taken separately from meals.	4. Fluids stretch the stomach and may cause vomiting.
5. Suggest that Maria avoid fried or greasy foods, foods that are highly seasoned, and foods that have strong odors. Suggest salty and tart combinations.	5. Odors and greasy textures are associated with nausea and increased episodes of vomiting. Various food combinations may be helpful.
6. Teach Maria to keep a record of daily intake of food and fluids, episodes of vomiting, and measures that reduce nausea.	6. A record is essential to determine whether adequate nutrients and fluids are being retained and to identify the most helpful measures to control nausea.
7. Recommend that Maria eat dry crackers, unbuttered popcorn, or dry toast every 2 hours.	7. Nausea is more intense when the stomach is empty.
8. Recommend frequent, small amounts of ice chips, water, and clear liquids like Jell-O or popsicles. Suggest that Maria avoid coffee and tea.	8. Clear fluids may be tolerated better during periods of nausea. Coffee and tea act as diuretics.
9. Suggest that Maria try ice cream, pudding, watermelon, soups, and vegetable drinks.	9. These foods have more nutrients and are often tolerated well when taken separately.
10. Reassure Maria that nausea and vomiting usually disappear by the second trimester and do not indicate a problem with the pregnancy.	10. Reassurance reduces anxiety, so that the woman knows the condition is self-limiting and does not threaten the fetus.
11. Assess Maria's weight at each prenatal visit, and compare her weight gain with that expected for the weeks of gestation.	11. If weight gain is adequate, the focus remains on relieving the discomfort of nausea and vomiting. If weight gain is less than adequate or if signs of dehydration are present, she can be referred for medical management.
12. Tell Maria to call if she is unable to retain recommended amounts of fluid or has signs of dehydration such as dry, cracked lips; elevated pulse; fever; and concentrated urine.	12. Dehydration should be treated promptly.

Evaluation

Periodic nausea and vomiting continued throughout the first trimester but gradually decreased during the second trimester. Maria did not become dehydrated and gained 4 kg (9 lb) by 20 weeks.

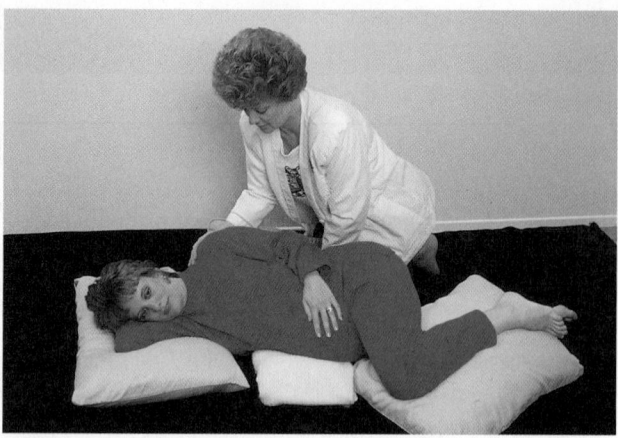

Figure 13-14 During the third trimester, pillows supporting the abdomen and back provide a comfortable position for rest.

Clothing Clothing should be comfortable and nonconstricting. Tight jeans or pantyhose that may constrict venous circulation should be worn only for short periods. Explain that low heels do not interfere with balance, but high heels increase the curvature of the lower spine (lordosis) that is prevalent during the last trimester.

Exercise Teach women who have no medical or obstetric complications to exercise in moderation each day for 30 minutes or more during pregnancy (American Academy of Pediatrics and American College of Obstetricians and Gynecologists, 2002). Recreational sports can generally be continued if there is no risk for falling or abdominal trauma. Exercise that requires balance or may cause injury and exercise in the supine position are not safe.

Walking is an ideal exercise because it stimulates muscular activity of the entire body, gently increases respiratory and cardiovascular effort, and does not result in fatigue or strain. Swimming is also an excellent exercise because the buoyancy of the water helps prevent injuries.

Instruct the women not to *begin* strenuous exercise programs or intensify training during pregnancy. Women who have been exercising strenuously should consult the health care provider but may be able to continue much of their usual routine. As pregnancy progresses, it may be necessary to reduce the level of exercise to prevent physiologic stress. The woman can take her pulse every 10 to 15 minutes and should not exceed a heart rate that has been determined in consultation with her health care provider.

Pregnant women must avoid becoming overheated because heat is transmitted to the fetus. They should allow a cool-down period of mild activity after exercising. It is important to take liquids frequently while exercising to prevent dehydration. The woman should stop exercising and seek medical advice if she has chest pain, dizziness, headache, decreased fetal movement, or signs of labor while exercising.

Sleep and Rest Finding a comfortable position for rest becomes a problem in the third trimester. Suggest she use pillows to support the abdomen and back and to provide the best opportunity for sleep (Fig. 13-14).

Nutrition A discussion of nutrition should be part of each visit. The woman's use of prenatal vitamins is assessed, and any questions she has are answered (see Chapter 15).

Sexual Activity Sexual activity is generally safe for healthy pregnant women (see Chapter 14).

Employment Most women of childbearing age in the United States are employed outside the home, and most continue to work during pregnancy.

Maternal Safety Work should not lead to undue fatigue. Frequent rest periods are essential. For jobs that require constant standing or sitting, suggest that the woman change positions frequently or walk briefly to stimulate circulation and reduce fatigue. Tasks that require balance may be hazardous because the uterus enlarges and the center of gravity shifts. Heavy lifting should be avoided.

Exposure to Teratogens Intrauterine exposure to toxic substances is of particular concern during the first trimester, the period of organogenesis. Advise women to investigate their own occupational hazards. For example, hairdressers are exposed to toxic substances in hair dyes and aerosol sprays; nurses and hospital personnel may be exposed to radiation and anesthetic gases; and laundry and dry cleaning workers may be exposed to fetotoxic compounds. In addition, passive smoking is harmful to both mother and fetus.

Travel Although travel by car is generally safe for uncomplicated pregnancy, suggest frequent stops to allow the expectant mother to empty her bladder and walk around. She must fasten the seat belt snugly, with the lap belt under the abdomen. This position is uncomfortable for some women, and it causes concern about internal injuries should a collision occur. It is much safer to wear the belt, however, than to leave it off and risk being ejected from the car during an accident.

Travel by plane is generally safe up to 36 weeks. If travel is necessary, advise the women to walk frequently to maintain adequate peripheral circulation and avoid thromboembolism. The woman should not travel to remote areas where medical care is unavailable.

Immunizations In general, immunizations that use live virus vaccines are contraindicated during pregnancy because of teratogenic effects on the fetus. These vaccines include measles, mumps, rubella, and oral polio vaccines. Use of inactivated vaccines such as those for tetanus, hepatitis A and hepatitis B, and influenza, should be safe and can be used in women who have a risk for developing these diseases (Jones, 2002).

Teaching Necessary Lifestyle Changes

Many expectant parents are willing to make lifestyle changes to avoid adversely affecting the fetus.

Prescription and Over-the-Counter Drugs Advise the pregnant woman to consult with her health care provider before taking any drugs. This precaution is important for over-the-counter drugs as well as for prescription drugs. Nonprescription drugs such as acetaminophen are considered safe, but nonsteroidal antiinflammatory drugs such as aspirin are generally to be avoided because they may increase bleeding. When prescription drugs are necessary, consideration must be given to the risks and benefits during pregnancy. In general, the health care provider must weigh the risks against the benefits and decide if a drug can safely be used or if changes are necessary.

Complementary and Alternative Therapies Some complementary and alternative therapies are very safe and helpful during pregnancy. Some, however, can be harmful. For example, herbs such as black or blue cohosh and goldenseal may cause contractions if used in pregnancy (Kuhn & Winston, 2000). Ask about any of these therapies that are used, and advise the woman to discuss them with her health care provider.

Tobacco Identify women who smoke, and explain the effects of smoking during pregnancy. It is well documented that pregnant women who smoke have smaller infants and a higher rate of perinatal mortality and preterm births than women who do not smoke. Moreover, developmental problems, such as short attention span and lower cognitive skills, are also more common in children when the mother continues to smoke during pregnancy.

Make every effort to motivate the expectant mother to stop smoking and to avoid contact with others who smoke. Discuss methods that will help the woman stop smoking, and make referrals as necessary. Generally the use of nicotine replacement products is discouraged because their effect during pregnancy is unknown.

Alcohol Alcohol is a known teratogen, and maternal alcohol use is a leading cause of mental retardation in the United States. Alcohol produces a characteristic cluster of developmental anomalies known as *fetal alcohol syndrome* (see Chapter 25). There is no known safe amount of alcohol that can be consumed during pregnancy. Therefore women who are pregnant or who plan to become pregnant should abstain from all alcohol use.

Illegal Drugs Use of so-called *street drugs*, such as cocaine, heroin, and methamphetamines, is harmful to the fetus. Advise the pregnant woman to seek help to discontinue all illicit drug use (see Chapter 25).

Evaluation

- Does the woman perform self-care practices as she was taught?
- Can she discuss ways to obtain relief from the common discomforts of pregnancy?
- Does she develop a plan early in pregnancy to modify habits that do not promote health?

KEY CONCEPTS

- Pregnancy causes a predictable pattern of uterine growth. In general, the uterus can be palpated at the level of the umbilicus at 20 weeks of gestation and at the xiphoid process by 36 weeks.
- Thick mucus fills the cervical canal and protects the fetus from infection caused by bacteria ascending from the vagina.
- The plasma volume expands faster and to a greater extent than red blood cell volume, resulting in a dilution of hemoglobin concentration called physiologic (pseudo) anemia.
- Although blood volume increases, blood pressure is not elevated during normal pregnancy.
- The gravid uterus partially occludes the vena cava and the descending aorta when the mother is supine. The occlusion causes supine hypotensive syndrome, which can be prevented or corrected by assuming a lateral position.
- During the last trimester, the uterus pushes the diaphragm upward, decreasing lung capacity.

- The ribs flare, the substernal angle widens, and the circumference of the chest increases.
- Increased renal plasma flow results in an increased glomerular filtration rate, which often results in "spilling" of glucose and other nutrients into the urine.
- Increased blood flow to the skin helps reduce the heat generated by the fetus and by the increased maternal metabolic rate.
- Increased hCG and estrogen levels may cause nausea in early pregnancy.
- Increased progesterone causes relaxation of all smooth muscles, resulting in stasis of urine and the risk of urinary tract infections and constipation.
- Alterations in hormones are also responsible for cutaneous changes, such as hyperpigmentation.
- The expanding uterus plus the hormone relaxin result in progressive changes that can lead to muscle strain and backache during the last trimester.

- Progesterone maintains the uterine lining, prevents uterine contractions, and helps prepare the breasts for lactation.
- Presumptive and probable signs of pregnancy may be caused by conditions other than pregnancy and thus cannot be considered positive or diagnostic signs. Positive signs can have no other cause.
- A complete history and physical examination are necessary at the initial antepartum visit to determine the potential risks to the mother and fetus and to obtain baseline data so that a plan of care can be developed.
- Multifetal pregnancies impose greater physiologic changes than a single-fetus pregnancy and require extra vigilance to detect possible complications.
- Families need information on self-care and health promotion during pregnancy as well as information on ways to deal with the common discomforts of pregnancy that do not need or respond to medical management.

ANSWERS to Critical Thinking Exercise 13-1

1. If pregnant now, Wilma is gravida 3, para 1 (the twin birth counts as one parous experience). If the acronym GTPAL is used, G = 3; T = 1; P = 0 (no preterm infants); A = 1 (one pregnancy ended before 20 weeks' gestation); L = 2 (living twins).

2. Amenorrhea and nausea and vomiting are only presumptive (subjective) indications of pregnancy because they can be caused by conditions other than pregnancy.

3. Count back 3 months to March 22, and add 7 days. This brings the date to March 29.

Wilma's EDD is March 29. Add 1 to the current year.

REFERENCES and READINGS

American Academy of Pediatrics and American College of Obstetricians and Gynecologists. (2002). *Guidelines for perinatal care* (5th ed.). Elk Grove Village, IL. and Washington, DC: Author.

Association of Women's Health, Obstetric, and Neonatal Nurses. (2003). *Standards and guidelines for professional nursing practice in the care of women and newborns* (6th ed.). Washington, DC: Author.

Barron, M.L. (2001). Antenatal care. In K.R. Simpson & P.A. Creehan. *AWHONN perinatal nursing* (2nd ed., pp.125-160). Philadelphia: Lippincott.

Blackburn, S.T. (2003). *Maternal, fetal, and neonatal physiology* (2nd ed.). Philadelphia: Saunders.

Bond, L. (2000). Physiology of pregnancy. In S. Mattson & J.E. Smith (Eds.). *Core curriculum for maternal-newborn nursing* (2nd ed., pp 85-100). Philadelphia: Saunders.

Buster, J.E., & Carson, S.A. (2002). Endocrinology and diagnosis of pregnancy. In S.G. Gabbe, J.R. Niebyl, & J.L. Simpson (Eds.). *Obstetrics, normal and problem pregnancies* (4th ed., pp. 3-36). New York: Churchill Livingstone.

Cottrell, B.H. (2003). Vaginal douching. *Journal of Obstetric, Gynecologic, and Neonatal Nursing, 32*(1), 12-18.

REFERENCES and READINGS

Cunningham, F.G., Gant, N.F., Leveno, K.J., Gilstrap, L.C., Hauth, J.C., & Wenstrom, K.D. (2001). *Williams obstetrics* (21st ed.). New York: McGraw-Hill.

Driscoll, J.W. (2001). Psychosocial adaptation to pregnancy and postpartum. In K.R. Simpson & P.A. Creehan. *AWHONN perinatal nursing* (2nd ed., pp.115-124). Philadelphia: Lippincott.

Fagen, C. (2000). Nutrition during pregnancy and lactation. In L.K. Mahan & S. Escott-Stump. *Krause's food, nutrition, and diet therapy* (10th ed., pp. 167-195). Philadelphia: Saunders.

Georges, J.M. (2000). Female genital and reproductive function. In L.C. Copstead & J.L. Banasik. *Pathophysiology: Biological and behavioral perspectives* (2nd ed., pp. 742-760). Philadelphia: Saunders.

Glover, D.D., Amonkar, M., Rybeck, B.F., & Tracy, T.S. (2003). Prescription, over-the-counter, and herbal medicine use in a rural, obstetric population. *American Journal of Obstetrics & Gynecology, 188*(4), 1039-1045.

Gordon, M.C. (2002). Maternal physiology in pregnancy. In S.G. Gabbe, J.R. Niebyl, & J.L. Simpson (Eds.). *Obstetrics, normal and problem pregnancies* (4th ed., pp. 63-91). New York: Churchill Livingstone.

Johnson, T.R.B., & Niebyl, J.B. (2002). Preconception care and prenatal care: part of the continuum. In S.G. Gabbe, J.R. Niebyl, & J.L. Simpson (Eds.). *Obstetrics, normal and problem pregnancies.* (4th ed., pp. 139-159). New York: Churchill Livingstone.

Jones, T.B. (2002). Vaccines in pregnancy. In S.B. Ransom, M.P. Dombrowski, M.I. Evans, & K.A. Ginsburg (Ed.). *Contemporary therapy in obstetrics and gynecology* (pp. 57-64). Philadelphia: Saunders.

Kronenberg, F., Murphy, P.A., & Wade, C. (2003). Select populations: Women. In J.W. Spencer & J.J. Jacobs. *Complementary and alternative medicine: An evidence-based approach* (2nd ed., pp. 458-481). St. Louis: Mosby.

Kuhn, M.A., & Winston, D. (2000). *Herbal therapy and supplements.* Philadelphia: Lippincott Williams & Wilkins.

Luppi, C.J. (2001). Physiologic changes of pregnancy. In K.R. Simpson & P.A. Creehan. *AWHONN perinatal nursing* (2nd ed., pp. 96-114). Philadelphia: Lippincott.

Mills, L.W., & Moses, D.T. (2002). Oral health during pregnancy. MCN: *The American Journal of Maternal Child Nursing, 27*(5), 275-280.

Moos, M. (2003). *Preconception health promotion: A focus for women's wellness.* White Plains, NY: March of Dimes Birth Defects Foundation.

Repke, J.T. (2002). Medication use during pregnancy. In S.B. Ransom, M.P. Dombrowski, M.I. Evans, & K.A. Ginsburg (Ed.). *Contemporary therapy in obstetrics and gynecology* (pp. 137-141). Philadelphia: Saunders.

Steele, N.M., French, J., Gatherer-Boyles, J., Newman, S., & Leclaire, S. (2001). Effect of acupressure by Sea-Bands on nausea and vomiting of pregnancy. *Journal of Obstetric, Gynecologic, and Neonatal Nursing, 30*(1), 61-70.

Tillett, J., Kostich, J.M., & VandeVusse, L. (2003). Use of over-the-counter medications during pregnancy. *Journal of Perinatal Neonatal Nursing, 17*(1), 3-18.

Tiran, D. (2002). Nausea and vomiting in pregnancy: Safety and efficacy of self-administered complementary therapies. *Complementary Therapies in Nursing and Midwifery, 8*(4), 191-196.

U.S. Department of Health and Human Services. (2000). *Healthy People 2010* (Conference edition, in 2 volumes). Washington, DC: Author.

Watson-Blasioli, J. (2001). Doubletake—Defining the need for specialized prenatal care for women expecting twins: A Canadian perspective. *AWHONN Lifelines, 5*(2), 34-42.

Psychosocial Adaptations to Pregnancy

14

◆ LEARNING OBJECTIVES

After studying this chapter, you should be able to:

◎ Describe the psychological responses of the expectant mother to pregnancy.
◎ Identify the process of role transition.
◎ Explain the maternal tasks of pregnancy.
◎ Describe the developmental processes of the transition to the father role.
◎ Describe the responses of prospective grandparents and siblings to pregnancy.

◎ Discuss factors that influence psychosocial adaptation to pregnancy such as age, parity, social support, socioeconomic status, and absence of a partner.
◎ Describe cultural influences on pregnancy and cultural assessment and negotiation.
◎ Describe the various types of education for childbearing families.

◆ DEFINITIONS

ambivalence Simultaneous conflicting emotions, attitudes, ideas, or wishes.
attachment Development of strong affectional ties as a result of interaction between an infant and a significant other (mother, father, sibling, caretaker).
birth plan A plan describing a couple's preferences for their birth experience.
body image Subjective image of one's physical appearance and capabilities derived from own observations and from the evaluation of significant others.
bonding Development of a strong emotional tie of a parent to a newborn; also called claiming or binding in.
couvade Pregnancy-related ritual or a cluster of symptoms experienced by some prospective fathers during pregnancy and childbirth.

developmental task A step in growth and maturation that one must complete before additional growth and maturation are possible.
disturbance in body image Negative feelings about characteristics, functions, or limits of one's body.
fantasy Mental images formed to prepare for the birth of a child.
introversion Inward concentration on oneself and one's body.
mimicry Copying the behaviors of other pregnant women or mothers as a method of "trying on" the role of advanced pregnancy or motherhood.
narcissism Undue preoccupation with oneself.
role transition Changing from one pattern of behavior and one image of self to another.

lthough each couple adapts to pregnancy in a unique manner, the psychological responses of prospective parents change as the pregnancy progresses. By the time the infant is born, the woman and her partner have completed developmental tasks that make it possible for them to become parents in the true sense of the word. Both social and cultural factors influence the way the woman adjusts to pregnancy.

MATERNAL RESPONSES

A woman's psychological response to pregnancy changes over time. Initially she may be uncertain or ambivalent about the pregnancy and her primary focus is on herself. Gradually her focus shifts, and she becomes increasingly concerned about how she can protect and provide for the fetus she is carrying.

First Trimester

Uncertainty
During the early weeks, the woman is unsure whether she is pregnant and tries to confirm it. She observes her body carefully for changes indicating pregnancy. She may use an over-the-counter pregnancy test kit for validation.

Reaction to the uncertainty of pregnancy depends on the individual. A woman may be eager to find confirming signs, or she may dread the possibility. Usually, she seeks confirmation from a physician, certified nurse-midwife, or

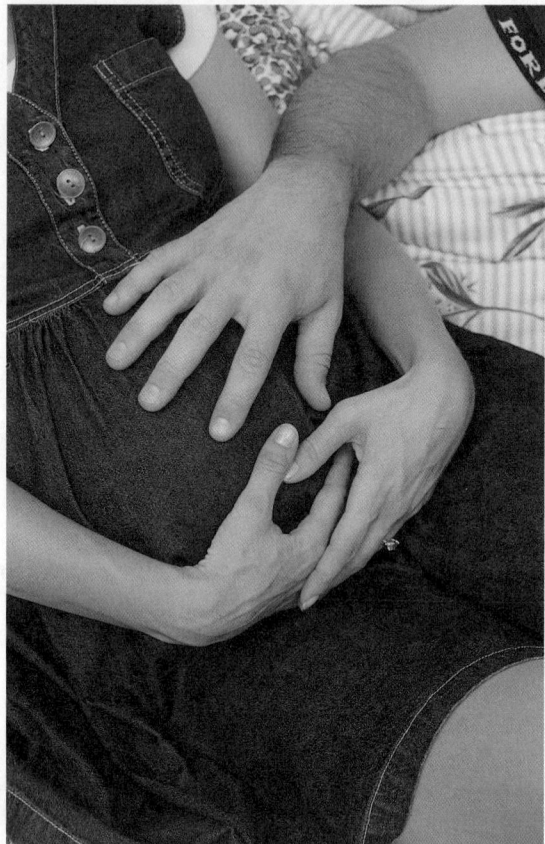

Figure 14-1 Fetal movement (*quickening*) confirms that a separate life is developing.

nurse practitioner within 12 weeks of the first missed menstrual period.

Ambivalence

Because almost half of pregnancies are unintended, pregnancy is often unexpected. Once the pregnancy is confirmed, most women have conflicting feelings, or ambivalence, about being pregnant. Some feel that this is not the right time, even if the pregnancy is wanted and planned. Women who had planned to become pregnant often say they thought it would take longer and that they feel unprepared for it. Many pregnancies are desired but unplanned, and these women may wish they had not become pregnant until some specific goals were met.

Pregnancy results in permanent life changes for the woman, and she begins to examine those changes and how she will cope with them. If it is a first pregnancy, the woman may worry about the added responsibility and feel unsure of her ability to be a good parent. She may be apprehensive about how this pregnancy will affect her relationship with other children or with the father.

The Self as Primary Focus

Throughout the first trimester, the woman's primary focus is on herself, not the fetus. Early physical responses to pregnancy confirm that something is happening to her, but the fetus remains vague and unreal.

Physical changes and increased hormone levels may cause emotional lability (unstable moods). Her mood can change quickly from contentment to irritation or from optimistic planning to an overwhelming need for sleep. These changes may be confusing to her partner, who is accustomed to a more stable relationship.

Nurses should concentrate on the mother's physical and psychological feelings during this period of maternal self-focus. Teaching should be aimed at the common early changes of pregnancy and their normality. Dealing with morning sickness and mood swings is an important subject to explore with the couple. They need to understand that these changes are normal and that they do not necessarily indicate problems.

Second Trimester

Physical Evidence of Pregnancy

During the second trimester, physical changes occur in the expectant mother and make the fetus "real." The uterus can be palpated in the abdomen, weight increases, and breast changes occur. Ultrasound examination allows her to see the fetus, and she may be given an ultrasound picture or video to share with her family. During this time she feels the fetus move (*quickening*). This experience is important because it confirms the presence of the fetus with each movement. As a result, she no longer thinks of the fetus as simply a part of her body but now perceives it as separate, although entirely dependent on her (Fig. 14-1).

The Fetus as Primary Focus

The woman's major focus during the second trimester becomes the fetus. Most pregnant women feel well because the discomforts of the first trimester have usually decreased. The woman is now concerned about how she can produce a healthy infant. She often seeks information about diet and about how the fetus grows and develops. She experiences a feeling of creative energy and satisfaction.

Narcissism and Introversion

During this time many women become increasingly concerned about their ability to protect and provide for the fetus. This concern is often manifested as narcissism and introversion. Selecting exactly the right foods to eat or the right clothes to wear may assume more importance than ever before. Some women may lose interest in their jobs because the work seems alien to the events taking place inside them. They may be less interested in current events as they focus on the pregnancy, or they may become fearful that world events threaten them and therefore present a danger to the fetus.

If she is a primigravida, the expectant mother wonders what the infant is like. She looks at baby pictures of herself and her mate and wants to hear stories about them as infants. Multiparas have concerns about how this child will be accepted by siblings and grandparents. Expectant mothers may also examine their relationships with others and how they will change after the birth.

Body Image

Rapid and profound changes take place in the body during the second trimester. Changes in body size and contour are noticeable, with obvious bulging of the abdomen, thickening of the waist, and enlargement of the breasts. The changes may be welcomed because they signify growth of the fetus, and this growth creates pride in the woman and her partner. For some women, however, the change in body size and shape, coupled with hyperpigmentation of the skin and striae gravidarum (stretch marks), may contribute to a negative body image. Moreover, changes in body function, such as altered balance, less physical endurance, and discomfort in the pelvis and lower back areas, may also contribute to a negative body image.

Changes in Sexuality

Sexual interest and activity of pregnant women and their partners are unpredictable: they may increase, decline, or remain unchanged. The culture of the couple is also important. Intercourse during pregnancy is allowed and encouraged in some cultures but strictly forbidden in others. Unless there are complications, intercourse is safe throughout pregnancy.

During the first trimester, freedom from worry about becoming pregnant or need for contraceptive use may enhance sexuality for both partners. For some women, however, nausea, fatigue, and breast tenderness interfere with erotic feelings. Fear of miscarriage may cause couples to avoid intercourse, particularly if the woman has previously lost a pregnancy. Nurses can help reassure the couple that there is no evidence that intercourse is related to pregnancy loss when no other complications are present.

As a result of pelvic vasocongestion, women experience increased sensitivity of the labia and clitoris and increased vaginal lubrication during the second trimester. Orgasm may occur more frequently and with greater intensity during pregnancy because of these changes. In addition, nausea is generally no longer a problem by this time. These changes, coupled with not having to worry about getting pregnant, may increase sexual responsiveness for many women.

During the third trimester, the "missionary position" (male on top) may cause discomfort from abdominal pressure. Heartburn, indigestion, and supine hypotensive syndrome may also occur in this position. The nurse can suggest alternate positions include side-lying, female-superior, and rear-entry. Fatigue, ligament pain, urinary frequency, and shortness of breath may also interfere with vaginal intercourse. Hugging, kissing, mutual massage, and cuddling are expressions of affection that do not always lead to intercourse.

As they become larger, some women believe that their bodies are ugly, and they may worry about how their partners react to their increased size. Sexual response varies widely among males. Some report heightened feelings of sexual interest, but some men perceive the woman's body in late pregnancy as unattractive. Moreover, for some men, fear of harming the fetus or causing discomfort interferes with sexual activity.

The expectant couple should be made aware of the normal changes in sexual desire that occur during pregnancy and the importance of communicating their feelings openly with each other. Despite the need for information, most women are reluctant to ask questions about sexual activity. Health professionals often do not initiate such discussions because of discomfort with introducing the topic or concern about the client's response.

It may be helpful to use a broad opening statement to initiate discussion about sexual activity. For example, "Sometimes couples are concerned about having sex during pregnancy." Such a statement provides a method of introducing the subject so that the woman feels comfortable to pursue it or to let it drop.

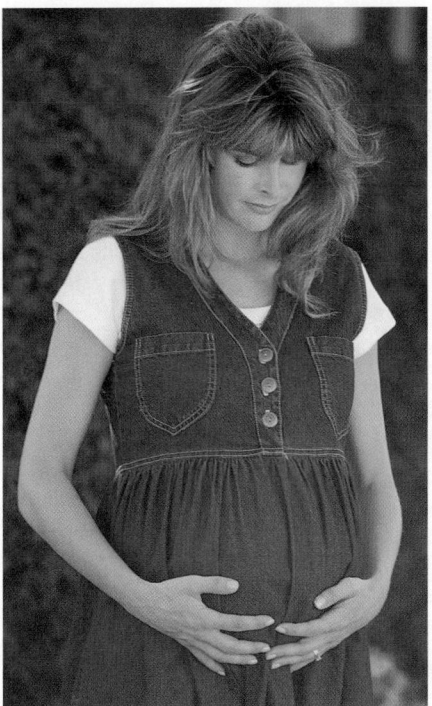

Figure 14-2 During the third trimester, the mother feels increasingly vulnerable. She cradles her fetus to signify her protectiveness.

The nurse should advise the couple to curtail all sexual activity if the client is at risk for preterm labor, because uterine contractions may be initiated by orgasm. Explaining that nipple stimulation, orgasm, and semen can cause uterine contractions helps them understand the reasons. Intercourse should also be avoided if bleeding or ruptured membranes occurs or if the cervix is incompetent. In addition, blowing into the vagina should be avoided because it may cause air embolus (Mullaly, 2000).

Third Trimester

Vulnerability

During the third trimester, pregnant women have increasing feelings of vulnerability. They often feel that the precious baby may be lost or harmed if not protected at all times (Fig. 14-2). Many mothers have fantasies or nightmares about harm coming to the infant and become very cautious as a result. They may avoid crowds because they feel unable to protect the infant from infectious diseases or physical dangers that may be present. They should be reassured that such dreams are not unusual in pregnancy (Ramer & Frank, 2001).

Increasing Dependence

The expectant mother often becomes increasingly dependent on her partner in the last weeks of pregnancy. She may insist that he be readily available at all times and may call his place of work several times during the day. She may rely on others more at this time and seek their help in making decisions. Her need for love and attention from her partner is even more pronounced in late pregnancy. When she is assured of his concern and willingness to provide assistance, she feels more secure and able to cope.

Nursing Care Plan

Body Image During Pregnancy

ASSESSMENT

Dolores White is a 34-year-old primigravida in the 26th week of pregnancy. Both she and her husband have been runners for several years. With her physician's permission, Dolores continued running until 6 weeks ago. She no longer runs because she finds it uncomfortable. She says she now walks "like other old ladies." She verbalizes concern about her increasing size and says she feels "fat, awkward, and ugly." She states, "I hate the way I look; I can't wait to get back into shape."

Nursing Diagnosis

Disturbed Body Image related to changes in body size, contour, and function secondary to pregnancy.

Goals/Expected Outcomes

By the end of her next prenatal visit, Dolores will
- Make statements that indicate acceptance of expected body changes during pregnancy.
- Express her feelings about body changes to her husband as well as to the health care team.
- Set realistic goals for weight loss and the resumption of a running program after childbirth.

INTERVENTION	RATIONALE
1. Acknowledge Dolores's feelings. "I can see you're disappointed at not being able to run, and I sense you are concerned about how your body has changed as a result of pregnancy."	1. Feelings must be acknowledged, reflected, and dealt with before the underlying cause can be addressed.
2. Clarify Dolores's concerns. "You've always been an athlete. You may be wondering how much permanent change will result from pregnancy."	2. An underlying, unvoiced concern may be that pregnancy and childbirth will change the woman from athlete to mother. This altered perception of herself causes fear and/or grief.
3. Suggest that Dolores share her feelings with her husband and seek his support.	3. Although one may assume that the partner observes and understands when negative feelings exist, this may not be true.
4. Describe the expected pattern of weight gain from 26 weeks to term gestation, and correlate this change with the growth and development of the fetus.	4. Knowledge that weight gain shows growth of the fetus may allay unexpressed fears of excessive weight gain.
5. Discuss types of low-impact, moderate exercise, such as walking or swimming, that would be beneficial for Dolores.	5. Moderate daily exercise is permissible and encouraged during uncomplicated pregnancy.
6. Help Dolores make realistic plans to lose weight and regain strength after childbirth: a. Discuss the expected pattern of weight loss after birth. Initial weight loss is 10 to 12 pounds. An additional 5½ pounds may be lost in the first few postpartum days. By the end of 6 months, many women have returned to their prepregnancy weight. b. Demonstrate graduated exercises that increase muscle tone and strength. c. Explain the purpose of adipose tissue gained during pregnancy. Discuss a diet that provides sufficient calories to meet needs during breastfeeding.	6. Adipose tissue provides a needed source of energy during birth and lactation. Many women are relieved to know that there is a purpose and that the added weight will be lost gradually. Breastfeeding requires at least 500 additional calories per day.

Evaluation

At the next prenatal visit, Dolores makes statements that show more acceptance of body changes during pregnancy. She reports she has discussed her feelings with her husband and that he is very supportive. She has explored other types of exercises and has found several she will use during the rest of her pregnancy. She also discusses her plans for diet and exercise after birth.

Additional Nursing Diagnoses to Consider

- Risk for Situational Low Self-Esteem
- Interrupted Family Processes

TABLE 14-1 Progressive Changes in Maternal Responses to Pregnancy

First Trimester	Second Trimester	Third Trimester
EMOTIONAL RESPONSE		
Uncertainty, ambivalence, focus on self	Wonder, increased narcissism, introversion, concern about changes in her body and sexuality	Vulnerability, increased dependence, acceptance that fetus is separate but totally dependent
PHYSICAL VALIDATION		
No obvious signs of fetal growth	Quickening	Obvious fetal growth, discomfort, decreased maternal activity
ROLE		
May begin to seek safe passage for self and fetus	Seeks acceptance of fetus and her role as mother	Prepares for birth

Although the woman may not be able to explain the increasing dependence, she expects her partner to understand the feeling and may become angry if he is not sympathetic. The nurse can encourage couples to discuss their fears and feelings openly so that misunderstandings can be avoided.

Some pregnant women have difficulty with tasks that require direct, sustained attention, particularly in the third trimester. Women may feel they have trouble concentrating or focusing on learning new material or skills at this time (Stark, 2000). Teaching should be clear and concise to help women learn most easily.

Preparation for Birth

Gradually the feelings of vulnerability decrease as the woman comes to terms with her situation. The fetus continues to grow, and fetal movements are no longer gentle. The woman's relationship with the fetus changes as she acknowledges that although she and the fetus are interrelated, the baby is not a part of herself. Although she may not consciously acknowledge the increasing feelings of separateness, she longs to *see* the baby and to become acquainted with her child.

Most pregnant women are concerned with their ability to determine when they are in labor. They review the signs of labor taught in childbirth education classes and question friends and family members who have given birth. Many couples worry that they will not get to the hospital or clinic in time for the birth, and they may be concerned about how they will cope with labor.

During the last several weeks, the woman becomes increasingly concerned with her expected date of delivery and with the experience of labor and delivery. Some women fear labor and dread the due date, whereas others are so uncomfortable that they look forward to that day, anticipating that it will be the exact day the birth will occur.

Women pregnant for the first time are more likely to fear childbirth than multiparas. Many women fear the pain of childbirth or that something will go wrong during labor (Melender, 2002). Multiparas who had a previous negative pregnancy or birth experience worry about having another problem with the present pregnancy. Women may seek help for their fears by talking to members of their support system or by seeking information from health professionals, books, or on the Internet.

During the third trimester, an expectant mother prepares for the infant, if that is appropriate for her culture. "Nest-ing" behavior includes obtaining clothing and arranging a place for the infant to sleep. Negotiation of how household tasks will be shared with her partner also often occurs at this time. In addition, many couples complete childbirth education classes.

Table 14-1 summarizes the progressive changes in maternal responses during pregnancy.

MATERNAL ROLE TRANSITION

The transition into mothering begins during pregnancy and increases with gestational age. Some aspects of this transition must be accomplished before moving on to the next part of the process. The woman must accept the pregnancy and the changes that will result. She must develop a relationship with the unborn child, first as part of herself and then as a separate individual. Near the end of pregnancy she must prepare herself for the birth and for parenting the new baby (Ramer & Frank, 2001).

Transitions Experienced Throughout Pregnancy

The woman undergoes transitions in relationships that continue throughout the pregnancy. She becomes more aware of herself and the changes occurring in her life. There are alterations in her relationship with the father as they both prepare for parenthood. Her relationship with her own mother is examined and may change as the expectant mother develops a view of herself as a mother and what that role entails. In addition, she must develop a relationship with this particular child (Ramer & Frank, 2001).

Steps in Maternal Role Taking

Rubin (1984) observed specific steps that provide a framework for understanding the process of maternal role taking: mimicry, role play, fantasy, looking for a role fit, and grief work.

Mimicry

Mimicry involves observing and copying the behavior of other women who are pregnant or already mothers. It is an attempt to discover what the role is like. Mimicry often begins early, when the woman may wear maternity clothes before they are needed to see how women in more advanced pregnancy feel and to see how people react to her.

Role Play

Role play consists of acting out some aspects of what mothers actually do. The pregnant woman searches for opportunities to hold or provide care for infants in the presence of another person. Role playing gives her an opportunity to practice the expected role and to receive validation from an observer that she has functioned well. She is particularly sensitive to the responses of her partner and her own mother.

Fantasy

Fantasies allow the woman to explore a variety of possibilities and to daydream or to "try on" a variety of behaviors. Fantasies often have to do with how the infant will look and what characteristics he or she will have. The woman may daydream about taking her daughter to the park or about holding the child and reading or playing music.

At times, fantasies are fearful. What happens if something is wrong with the infant? What if the baby cries and won't stop? Fearful fantasies often provoke a pregnant woman to respond by seeking information or reassurance.

Looking for a Role Fit

Looking for a role fit is a process that occurs once the woman has built a set of role expectations for herself and has internalized a view of a "good" mother's behavior. She then observes the behaviors of mothers and compares them with her own expectations of herself. She imagines herself acting in the same way and either rejects or accepts the behaviors, depending on how well they fit her sense of what is right. This process implies that the woman has explored the role of mother long enough to have developed a sense of herself in the role and to be able to select behaviors that reaffirm her sense of herself fulfilling the role.

Grief Work

Grief work may seem incongruous with maternal role taking, but women often experience a sense of sadness when they realize that they must permanently give up certain aspects of their previous selves. A new mother will never again be a carefree girl without a child. She must relinquish some of her old patterns of behavior so that she can move into the new identity of mother. Even simple things such as going shopping or going to the movies will require planning to include the infant or to find alternative care. Changes may be particularly difficult for the adolescent who is not used to planning ahead and who may have to give up or change school plans as well.

Maternal Tasks of Pregnancy

The psychological work of pregnancy has been grouped into four maternal tasks (Rubin, 1984):

1. Seeking safe passage for herself and the baby through pregnancy, labor, and childbirth
2. Securing acceptance of the baby and herself by her partner and family
3. Learning to give of herself
4. Developing attachment and interconnection with the unknown child

Seeking Safe Passage

Seeking safe passage for herself and her baby is the woman's priority task. If she cannot be assured of that safety, she cannot move on to the other tasks. Behaviors that ensure safe passage include seeking the care of a physician or certified nurse-midwife and following recommendations about diet, vitamins, rest, and subsequent visits to the office or clinic.

In addition to following the advice of health care professionals, the pregnant woman must adhere to cultural practices that ensure the safety of herself and the infant. For instance, a Hmong woman may avoid raising her arms above her head because she believes it may cause preterm labor. She does not cut her hair during pregnancy because it might harm the fetus (Moore & Moos, 2003).

Securing Acceptance

Securing acceptance is a process that continues throughout pregnancy. It involves reworking relationships so that the important persons in the family accept the woman in the role of mother and welcome the baby into the family. For example, she and the father of the baby must give up an exclusive relationship and make a place in their lives for a child. When the partner expresses pride and joy in the pregnancy, the woman feels valued and comforted. This feeling is so important that many women retain a memory of the partner's reaction to the announcement of pregnancy for many years. Women with supportive partners are more likely to report the pregnancy is wanted (Kroelinger & Oths, 2000).

Support and acceptance of the pregnancy from her own mother is also important. The pregnant woman gains energy and contentment when her mother freely offers acceptance and support. Many expectant mothers develop an increased closeness with their mothers during pregnancy.

Problems may occur if the family strongly desires a child with particular characteristics and the woman believes that the family may reject an infant who does not meet the criteria. For example, if family members wish for a boy, will they accept a girl?

Learning to Give of Self

Giving is one of the most idealized components of motherhood but one that is essential. Learning to give to the coming child begins in pregnancy when the woman allows her body to give space to the fetus. She tests her ability to derive pleasure from giving, often by providing food or care for her family. Their acceptance and enjoyment of the "gift" enhance her pleasure, so the role is strengthened. She may explore further by making and giving small gifts to friends, especially those who are pregnant.

Pregnant women also learn to give by receiving. Gifts received at baby showers are more than needed items—they also confirm continued interest and commitment from friends and family and enhance the woman's ability to give. Intangible gifts from others, such as companionship, attention, and support, help to increase her energy and affirm the importance of giving.

Committing Herself to the Unknown Child

Developing attachment to the unborn baby begins in early pregnancy when the woman accepts or "binds in" to the idea that she is pregnant, although the baby is not yet real to her.

During the second trimester, the baby becomes real and feelings of love and attachment surge. This is especially true after quickening or after an ultrasound late in pregnancy that shows recognizable parts of the baby. Mothers report feedback from their unborn infants during the third trimester and describe unique characteristics of the fetus with regard to sleep-wake cycles, temperament, and communication. Love of the infant becomes possessive and leads to feelings of vulnerability. The woman integrates the role of mother into her image of herself. She becomes comfortable with the idea of herself as mother and finds pleasure in contemplating the new role.

PATERNAL ADAPTATION

Expectant fathers must also make major psychosocial changes to adapt to their new role. Moreover, the changes may be more difficult because the male partner is often neglected by the health care team as well as by his peer group as attention is focused on the woman. His anxieties and concerns may remain unknown because of the lack of focus on him.

Variations in Paternal Adaptation

Wide variations exist in how men respond to pregnancy. Some are emotionally invested and explore every aspect of pregnancy, childbirth, and parenting. Others are more task-oriented and see themselves as managers. They may direct the woman's diet and act as coaches during childbirth but remain detached from the emotional aspects of the experience. Other men are more comfortable as observers and prefer not to participate. Some men are culturally conditioned to see pregnancy and childbirth as "women's work," and they may not be able to express their true feelings about pregnancy and fatherhood.

Readiness for fatherhood is more likely if there is a stable relationship between the partners, financial security, and a desire for parenthood. Additional factors include the man's relationship with his own father, his previous experience with children, and his confidence in his ability to care for the infant.

Unintended pregnancy is more likely than a planned pregnancy to cause distress for fathers-to-be. Distress is also more likely in younger fathers, those where the relationship with the mother has been less than 2 years' duration, and those without full-time employment (Buist, Morse, & Durkin 2003).

Fathers have many concerns during a pregnancy. These include anxiety about the health of the mother and the baby, financial concerns, and worry about his role during the birth and about the changes that will result from the birth of the baby. Financial concerns may be especially acute in a two-income family if the mother develops complications that prevent her from working as long as expected. A reduction in income coupled with an increase in expenses can result in added stress for both parents.

Developmental Processes

Jordan (1990) described the developmental processes that an expectant father must work through as he deals with the reality of pregnancy and the new child, works to be recognized as a parent, and makes an effort to be seen as relevant to childbearing.

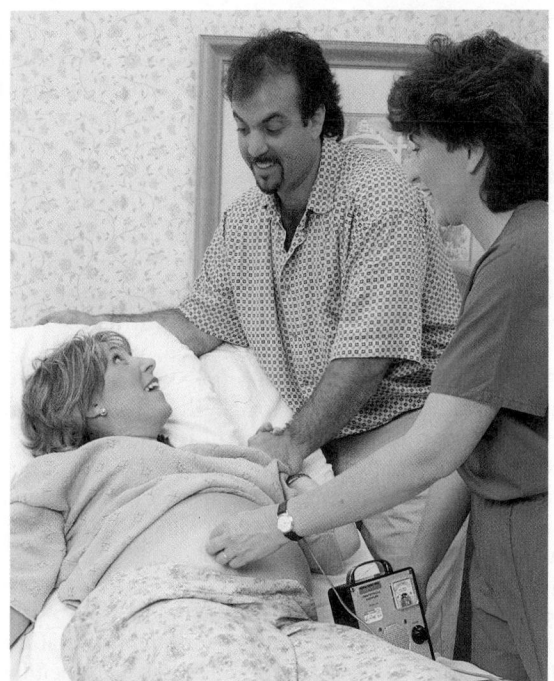

Figure 14-3 Reality booster: the existence of the fetus becomes real for the father when he hears sounds of the fetal heart through the transducer.

Grappling With the Reality of Pregnancy and the Child

The pregnancy and the child must become real before a man can take on the identity of father. Initially, early pregnancy changes, such as the woman's nausea and fatigue, are perceived as symptoms of illness that have little to do with having a baby.

A man's initial reaction to the announcement of pregnancy may be pride and joy, but he often experiences the same ambivalence that his partner does, particularly if he is unprepared for the added responsibility or commitment. Various experiences act as catalysts or "reality boosters" that make the child more real (Fig. 14-3). These include hearing sounds of the baby's heartbeat, feeling the infant move, and seeing the fetus on a sonogram.

Preparing the nursery and accumulating supplies for the new addition also reinforce the reality of the forthcoming child. These tasks often represent the first time that the expectant father has the opportunity to do something for the child directly. The birth itself is the most powerful "reality booster," and the infant becomes real to the father when he has an opportunity to see and hold the infant.

Support groups just for expectant fathers are sometimes available. These groups allow a father-to-be to talk with other men about changes resulting from the pregnancy. Knowing his experiences and feelings are shared by other men in the same situation is very helpful.

Struggling for Recognition as a Parent

Men are often perceived by others to be helpmates but not parents in their own right. Many men find it upsetting that there is often little validation of their feelings or recognition that they want to be considered a parent as well as a helper.

Expectant mothers play an important role in helping their partners gain recognition as parents. Women who openly share the physical sensations and emotions that they experience help the expectant father feel that he is part of the process. These women often refer to it as "our" pregnancy and insist that the man be included in all discussions and decisions.

Nurses must learn to view the mother, father, and child as the client and not focus exclusively on the mother and fetus. The nurse should encourage the man to ask questions about his partner's pregnancy. These men are entitled to as much advice and reassurance as expectant women.

The nurse can also guide the couple in looking at the role the father will play after the birth. Will he be involved in infant care from the start or wait until the baby is older? Will he change diapers and help with night-time care, or does he see those tasks as belonging to the mother? The couple must consider the views of both the woman and her partner to determine roles each will play.

Creating the Role of Involved Father

Men use various means to create a parenting role that is comfortable for them. They may seek closer ties with their fathers to reminisce about their own childhood. They also observe men who are already fathers and "try on" fathering behaviors to determine whether they are comfortable and fit their own concept of the father role. Some change their image of themselves and even change their appearance to fit their new image (Mullaly, 2000). Many men assertively seek information about infant care and growth and development so that they will be prepared.

Parenting Information. Fathers may not receive enough parenting information to prepare them for care of their infants. Although adequate information may have been given them, fathers may not be ready for the information at the time it is provided. As a result, they may be unprepared to care for their infants and have unrealistic expectations of the newborn. Nurses must review information about infant care and growth and development after the infant is born, when the information is immediately relevant.

Couvade. The term *couvade* refers to pregnancy-related symptoms and behavior in expectant fathers. In primitive cultures, couvade took the form of rituals involving special dress, confinement, limitations of physical work, avoidance of certain foods, sexual restraint, and in some instances performance of "mock labor."

In modern practice, expectant fathers sometimes experience a cluster of physical symptoms similar to those experienced by women during pregnancy: loss of appetite, nausea and vomiting, headache, fatigue, and weight gain. Couvade symptoms are more likely to occur in early pregnancy and diminish as the pregnancy progresses. Symptoms may be caused by stress, anxiety, or empathy for the pregnant partner. They are usually harmless but may persist and result in nervousness, insomnia, restlessness, and irritability. Although the symptoms are rarely observed by the health care team, anticipatory guidance is beneficial for both partners.

ADAPTATION OF GRANDPARENTS

The initial reaction of grandparents depends on a number of different factors.

Age

Age is a major factor in determining the emotional responses of prospective grandparents. Older grandparents have usually dealt with their feelings about aging and react with joy when they find that they are to become grandparents. Younger grandparents may feel conflict and must resolve their self-image with the stereotype of grandparents as old persons. They often have career responsibilities and may not be accessible because of the continuing demands of their own lives.

Number and Spacing of Other Grandchildren

The number and spacing of other grandchildren also determine how grandparents feel. A first grandchild may be an exciting event that creates great joy. If there are several other grandchildren, however, the birth of another may cause less excitement than with the first grandchild. The subdued reaction may be disappointing to the couple.

Perceptions of the Role of Grandparents

Many grandparents see their relationship with the grandchild as second in importance only to the parent-child relationship. They want to be involved in the pregnancy and look forward to being intimately involved in child care. They offer to care for older children while the mother gives birth, and they assist during the first weeks after childbirth.

In the past, grandparents were often looked to for advice about childbearing and child rearing. Health care personnel have now become the "experts," and many grandparents have difficulty adjusting to this change. Special classes are available for grandparents to bring them up to date with current childbearing practices and to help them deal with the changes in their role.

Some contemporary grandparents hold different beliefs about the role of grandparents and plan much less participation in pregnancy or child care. This expectation often results in conflict with the parents, who may feel hurt by such an attitude. Parents and grandparents may need to negotiate how the grandparents can be involved without feeling that they must assume care of the child.

ADAPTATION OF SIBLINGS

Toddlers

How siblings adapt to the birth of an infant depends largely on their age and developmental level. Children 2 years or younger are unaware of the maternal changes that occur during pregnancy and are unable to understand that a new brother or sister is going to be born. Because toddlers have little perception of time, many parents delay telling them that a baby is expected until shortly before the birth.

The nurse can make suggestions about helping prepare young children for the birth and what to expect from toddlers when the new baby comes home. Changes in sleeping arrangements should be made several weeks before the birth so that the child does not feel displaced by the new baby. Parents need to realize that toddlers may have feelings of jealousy and resentment when they must share attention with a baby. Frequent reassurances of parental love and affection are of primary importance.

Older Children

Children from 3 to 12 years are more aware of changes in the mother's body and may be aware that a baby is to be born. They enjoy listening to the heart beat and may have questions about how the fetus develops, how it started, and how it will get out of the abdomen. Younger children may expect that the infant will be a full-fledged playmate, however, and are shocked when the infant is small and helpless. They also need preparation for the fact that the mother will go away for several days.

School-age children benefit from being included in preparations for the new baby. They are interested in preparing space and supplies for the infant. These children should be encouraged to feel the fetus move, and many come close to the mother's abdomen and talk to the fetus. School-age children may wonder how the birth will affect their role in the family. Parents should address these concerns and reassure the children about their continued importance. Providing books about children's experiences after the birth of a sibling may be helpful.

Children as young as 3 years benefit from sibling classes. The classes also provide an opportunity for them to discuss what newborns are like and what changes the new baby will bring to the family.

In some settings, siblings are permitted to be with the mother during childbirth. When they are to be present, children should attend a class that prepares them for the event. A familiar person who has no other role than to provide support and care for a younger child should be present at the birth.

Adolescents

The response of adolescents also depends on their developmental level. Some may be embarrassed because the pregnancy confirms the continued sexuality of their parents. Others may be indifferent to the pregnancy unless it directly affects them or their activities. Some adolescents, on the other hand, become very involved and want to help with preparations for the baby.

FACTORS THAT INFLUENCE PSYCHOSOCIAL ADAPTATIONS

Age

Pregnancy presents a challenge for teenagers, who must cope with the conflicting developmental tasks of pregnancy and adolescence at the same time. The major developmental task of adolescence is to form and become comfortable with a sense of self. On the other hand, one of the major tasks of pregnancy involves learning to give of self, a process that includes sacrificing personal desires for the benefit of the fetus.

Nurses who work with pregnant teenagers should help them tune in to their changing body and the developing fetus. Adolescents also need prompting to follow a lifestyle that promotes the best outcomes for them and for their infants. Concerns relating to the pregnant adolescent and the woman older than 35 years are discussed further in Chapter 25.

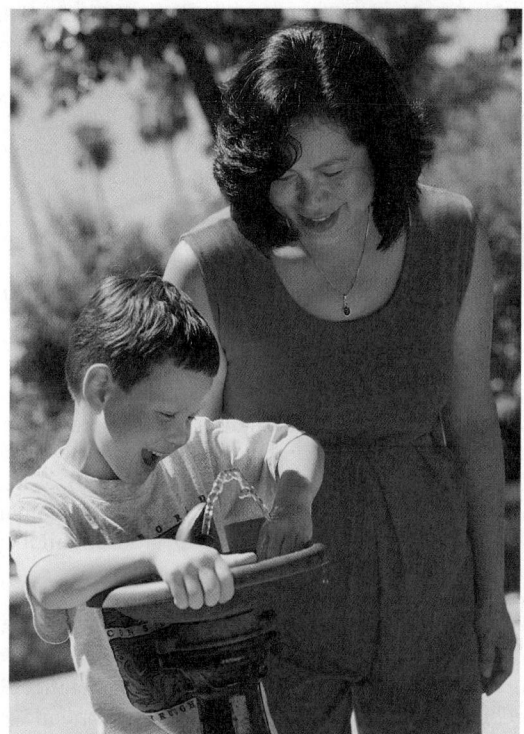

Figure 14-4 A pregnant multipara seeks to rework her relationship with other children.

Multiparity

Pregnancy tasks are much more complex for the multipara than for the primigravida (Mercer, 1990). The multipara does not have time to take special care of herself as she did during the first pregnancy. Multiparas report more fatigue, and significantly fewer report feeling very well or excellent. They report having serious worries about other children and about finding time and energy for additional responsibilities. When seeking acceptance of the new baby, the multipara may find family members less excited than they were for the first child.

The woman spends a great deal of time working out a new relationship with the first child, who often becomes demanding. This behavior may foster feelings of guilt as she tries to expand her love to include the second child. Developing attachment for the coming baby is hampered by feelings of loss between herself and the first child. She senses that the child is growing up and away from her, and she may grieve for the loss of their special relationship (Fig. 14-4).

Nurses must remember that multiparas may need information about labor, breastfeeding, and infant care. They also need special assistance in integrating an additional infant into the family structure.

Social Support

Social support includes that from the woman's partner, family, friends, and co-workers. Generally, support from the woman's partner and her mother are particularly important. Benefits of social support include improved coping, compliance with health care regimens, satisfaction with intimate relationships, and attachment to the infant. Reduced physical symptoms and increased breastfeeding are other effects (Logsdon, 2000).

Women who have little support during pregnancy are more likely to begin prenatal care late and to be depressed during and after pregnancy (Webster et al., 2000). When social support is inadequate, the nurse can help the woman explore potential sources such as support groups, childbearing education classes, church, work, or school.

Socioeconomic Status

One of the greatest influences on childbearing practices is the socioeconomic status of the family. Socioeconomic status refers to the resources that the family has to meet the needs for food, shelter, and health care. Socioeconomic status can be divided into the affluent, middle class, working poor, and new poor. Table 14-2 summarizes the impact of socioeconomic status on the family's response to pregnancy.

Absence of a Partner

Pregnant single women may have special concerns. Although some unmarried women have the financial and emotional support of a partner, many do not. These women often experience more stress about how to tell their family and friends about the pregnancy. They may have to enlist more social support to substitute for that of a partner. They may have legal concerns regarding the father's rights.

Single women without partners often live below the poverty level. They are more likely to delay prenatal care until the second or third trimester and are at increased risk for pregnancy complications and delivery of a low-birth-weight infant. Nurses must be prepared to offer special supportive care for single mothers. Needed social services may include Medicaid, WIC for food vouchers, and transportation to prenatal appointments.

Other Factors

Other factors influencing psychosocial adaptation during pregnancy include abnormal situations such as abuse (discussed in Chapter 25) and depression (discussed in Chapter 28). All women should be screened for both of these risk factors during pregnancy so that appropriate referrals for help can be given.

BARRIERS TO PRENATAL CARE

The value of prenatal care has been extensively documented. Women who receive inadequate prenatal care are likely to have poor pregnancy outcomes, including higher rates of low-birth-weight babies and increased infant mortality rates.

Women's access to prenatal care, however, is limited by financial, systemic, and attitudinal barriers.

Financial barriers are one of the most important factors that limit prenatal care. Many women have no insurance or not enough insurance to cover maternity care. Although Medicaid finances prenatal care for indigent women, the enrollment process is burdensome and lengthy. Some women may not know how to access this resource.

Systemic barriers include institutional practices that interfere with consistent care. For instance, women must often wait 6 to 8 weeks before being seen for their first visit. Prenatal visits are usually scheduled during daytime hours, when some working women cannot attend. Moreover, child care is rarely available, and some women are unable to find it. Lack of transportation and inability to take time off from work also prevent women from getting prenatal care.

An important barrier to health care results from the unsympathetic attitude of some health care workers toward those who are unable to pay for prenatal care. Poor families may experience long delays, hurried examinations, rudeness, and arrogance from members of the health care team who work in public clinics. Women may wait hours for an examination that lasts only a few minutes. Many never see the same health care provider more than once. Women often fail to keep clinic appointments because they do not see the importance of the hurried examinations.

Nurses must understand the importance of treating each family with respect and consideration, and they must insist that poor families who are unable to pay receive the same standard of care as that received by families who can pay. Scheduling prenatal visits in the evening or on weekends, having times set aside for walk-in prenatal visits, and offering other services such as Medicaid applications and WIC at the same time might increase use of prenatal services (Beckman, Buford, & Witt, 2000).

Some women may not obtain early prenatal care because they do not want the pregnancy confirmed, do not want anyone to know about the pregnancy, or are considering an abortion. One study found that only 17.5% of women who did not want to be pregnant began prenatal care during the first trimester. Poor housing and use of substances also decreased early prenatal care (Pagnini & Reichman, 2000). Many women believe prenatal care is unimportant if they are healthy and having no problems.

CULTURAL INFLUENCES ON CHILDBEARING

More distinct cultural groups live in the United States than anywhere else in the world. Each culture has its own health and healing belief system about major life events such as pregnancy and childbirth. The success of health care depends on how well it fits in with the beliefs of those being served. Therefore ignorance of culturally divergent beliefs may lead to failure in health care delivery.

Differences Within Cultures

Wide variations of beliefs and practices exist within each culture, and nurses must recognize that not everyone who shares a culture has identical beliefs. Those who have lived in Western societies for years or even for generations often do not exhibit behaviors prescribed by their culture of origin. Nurses must be careful not to stereotype families or to

TABLE 14-2 Impact of Socioeconomic Factors on Family's Response to Pregnancy

Affluent	Middle Class	Working Poor and Unemployed	New Poor
RESOURCES			
Is confident of ability, has financial reserves to protect from economic fluctuations, owns or rents home in a safe neighborhood, has health insurance or can pay for health care, able to provide enriched environment	Has relative security, but fewer reserves and more debt, owns or rents home in relatively safe neighborhood, depends on employment for health insurance	Lacks skills and bargaining power, is most vulnerable to economic fluctuations, struggles for basic needs	Was previously self-sufficient, but has lost prior resources, may have recently lost job and insurance, unused to public assistance
VALUE PLACED ON HEALTH CARE			
Values preventive care	Values health care but must rely on health insurance related to employment	May value health care but often does not see a way to improve situation	Values health care but may no longer have finances to access it
TIME ORIENTATION			
Seeks prenatal care early	Is future oriented and seeks early prenatal care, makes plans to provide best possible care and education for children	Priority is to meet needs of present, often seeks prenatal care late, uncertain future	Has middle-class time orientation but must meet present needs, may begin prenatal care late

expect a certain set of behaviors from every family in a particular cultural group. Individual differences are as important as cultural variations.

Cultural Differences That Can Cause Conflict

Cultural differences that cause conflict between health care workers and families during pregnancy are observed most often in the areas of health care beliefs, communication, and time orientation. When health professionals violate cultural norms, women are less likely to follow health education given (Ramer & Frank, 2001).

Health Beliefs

For many cultures, health is the balance of mind, body, and spirit. Health-promoting behaviors are the actions used in each of these dimensions to maintain health, prevent illness, or restore health (Spector, 2000).

Health Maintenance During Pregnancy. The predominant American culture treats pregnancy similar to an illness, with frequent visits to a physician, frequent laboratory tests, and hospitalization for delivery with various medical interventions. Many other cultures, however, see pregnancy as a natural condition that does not require medical care. Visits to a health care provider are often later in pregnancy than for American women.

Different cultures have various requirements for behaviors needed to maintain health during pregnancy. Such practices include wearing proper clothing, which is believed by some Hispanics to ensure a safe birth. Some American Indians may avoid tying knots during pregnancy to prevent complications of the umbilical cord (Cesario, 2001).

Avoidance of unclean things and strong emotions like anger is believed necessary by some groups to prevent harm to the fetus or a difficult childbirth. Concentration, silence, prayer, and meditation to maintain mental and spiritual health are practiced by some. In many cultures, women must avoid contact with illness and death and may not attend funerals during pregnancy. They also must surround themselves with beautiful things and positive people (Shilling, 2000).

Belief in Fate. Some cultures (Southeast Asian, Middle Eastern) promote a strong belief in fate. Women often believe that the only way they can affect the outcome of pregnancy is by eating correctly and observing the taboos of their culture. Because of this belief, it is sometimes difficult to convince women to seek early and regular prenatal care.

Preventing Illness. Practices that prevent illness include the use of protective religious objects or charms, such as amulets and talismans. Some women also believe that the type of food one eats can prevent illness or provide a good pregnancy outcome. For instance, those from many backgrounds eat raw garlic or onion or adhere to food taboos and prescribed combinations of foods. American Indians may believe that eating berries during pregnancy will cause a birthmark. Strict adherence to religious codes, morals, and practices is also believed to prevent illness.

Modesty. Fear, modesty, and a desire to avoid examination by men may keep some women from seeking health care during pregnancy. In many cultures (Muslim, Hindu, Hispanic), exposure of the genitals to men is considered demeaning. Nurses must remember that the reputations of women from these cultures depend on their demonstrated modesty. If necessary, female health care providers can perform examinations. If this is not possible, the woman should be carefully draped, with the legs completely covered. A female nurse needs to remain with the woman at all times. It may be necessary to obtain permission from the husband before any examination or treatment can be performed.

Female Genital Mutilation. Female genital mutilation is also called *female circumcision*. It involves removal of part or all of the clitoris, labia minora, and labia majora. The procedure is practiced in parts of Africa and some areas of Asia and the Middle East. The practice has been associated with premarital chastity and is a prerequisite for marriage in some cultures.

Women who have had the procedure and are now living in the United States need care from physicians and nurses who are knowledgeable about the custom and prepared for the appearance of the women's genitals. Pelvic examination is very painful because the introitus is so small and inelastic scar tissue makes the area especially sensitive.

Nurses must assist the woman in locating a health care provider with whom she is comfortable. Pelvic examinations should be made as comfortable as possible by maintaining utmost privacy and draping the woman to provide maximum coverage. The woman may not give any verbal or nonverbal sign of pain, but this lack of response does not indicate an absence of pain.

Restoring Health. Traditional ways to restore health include natural folk medicine such as herbs and plants. Charms, holy words, and holy actions as well as traditional healers are often used before other medical advice is sought. Hispanics, for instance, often consult *curanderas* (faith healers), who work with women to maintain balance and harmony, which has been lost during illness (Spector, 2000). Some (Africans, Haitians) rely on folk medicine that includes witchcraft, voodoo, and magic.

To be certain that all essential information about folk medicine is obtained, nurses should inquire whether the client is taking folk remedies. "What do pregnant women take to protect themselves and the baby?" "How often and how much of this do you take?" "Tell me about special foods and drinks that are important."

Communication Techniques

Language. Language is a major barrier to health care. The ideal is to have trained interpreters, preferably women. Sometimes others may be used, but considerations of confidentiality, use of medical jargon, and the possible need to discuss sensitive issues indicate the need for professional interpreters. Adults who came to the United States as children may speak English well and can interpret for their parents and grandparents. Other family members or friends, as well as coworkers in the clinic or hospital, may be helpful but not fluent. They can misunderstand instructions, particularly if medical jargon is used. Women may not want to discuss sensitive issues if the interpreter is a family member.

Communication Style. Styles in communication differ among cultures. For example, among Asians, nodding and smiling do not necessarily show agreement or even understanding but simply "Yes, I hear you." When presenting information, the nurse should validate how much the person understands by requesting that the listener repeat the information: "Tell me what you understood"; or "Show me what you learned."

Knowing the "rules" of communication helps the nurse avoid making errors. Hispanics are traditionally diplomatic and tactful. They frequently engage in small talk before bringing up questions they may have about their care. Nurses can use small talk to establish rapport and help accomplish the goals of care. Native Americans often converse in a low tone that may be difficult to hear in a noisy setting. They may consider note-taking taboo and expect the caregiver to remember what is said (Spector, 2000).

Eye Contact. Many Americans and African-Americans consider eye contact important to communication. Some American Indian groups avoid direct eye contact, which is like looking into the soul and endangers both people (Moore & Moos, 2003). Southeast Asians often believe eye contact shows disrespect. Some Hispanics believe eye contact is not appropriate with an authority figure, such as a physician or nurse (Mattson, 2003). Eye contact between unmarried men and women is considered seductive by those from Middle Eastern cultures.

Touch. Touch is also an important component of communication. In some cultures (Hindu, Muslim), touch by a woman other than the wife is offensive to men. Hispanics are from a "high touch" culture and are more likely to appreciate touch (Mattson, 2003). Nurses must remain sensitive to the response of the person being touched and should refrain from touching if the person indicates that touch is not welcomed.

Time Orientation

Time orientation varies among cultures. American Indian, Middle Eastern, Hispanic, and African-American women tend to emphasize the moment rather than the future. This attitude causes conflicts in a health care setting, where tests or appointments are scheduled at particular times. If a woman does not place the same importance on keeping appointments, she may encounter anger and frustration in the health care setting that leaves her bewildered and ashamed.

Culturally Competent Nursing Care

Culturally competent nursing care requires an awareness of, sensitivity to, and respect for the diversity of the clients served. It involves assessment of the family's culture and cultural negotiation when necessary.

Cultural Assessment

Although nurses should be aware of the important aspects of the predominant cultures seen in their practice, they cannot be expected to know all the specific aspects of every culture. Some questions to help the nurse understand the family's beliefs about appropriate care during pregnancy include:

- How will you and your family prepare for the baby?
- What concerns do you have about the pregnancy?
- What would provide the greatest assistance?
- Where do you obtain most health care information?
- What foods are encouraged? Curtailed?
- Who will be with you during labor and birth?
- Who will help you at home?

Cultural Negotiation

Cultural negotiation involves providing information while acknowledging that the family may hold different views. If the family indicates that the information would be helpful, it can be incorporated into the teaching plan.

If family members indicate that the information is not helpful or is harmful in their opinion, the conflict must be acknowledged openly and clarified. "I sense that you are unsure of this. Help me understand your reluctance to try it." After allowing the family to express their beliefs, the nurse explains why the recommendation was made and works with the family to find a compromise.

Cultural negotiation also involves being sensitive to specific concerns. For example, when caring for childbearing

Nursing Care Plan

Language Barrier During Pregnancy

ASSESSMENT

Diep Tran, a young Vietnamese primigravida of 16 weeks' gestation, speaks very little English. She listens quietly to the nurse's health care instructions, and although she appears confused, she asks no questions. Her husband, Bao Nguyen, has difficulty responding to questions about his wife's health, although he frequently nods and smiles.

Nursing Diagnosis

Impaired Verbal Communication related to foreign language barriers.

Goals/Expected Outcomes

The family will
- Keep scheduled appointments.
- Follow health care instructions.
- Verbalize basic needs and concerns at each prenatal visit.

INTERVENTION	RATIONALE
1. Assess the couple's ability to speak, read, and write in English, and determine the languages in which each is fluent.	1. Clients who are not fluent in speaking a language may be more adept at reading it.
2. Obtain the assistance of a fluent interpreter: a. Establish a list of bilingual staff members who are willing to interpret and be educated about the importance of confidentiality and exactness. b. Enlist adult family members or friends who can interpret for the client if a professional interpreter is not available. c. Use a translator to develop written material in Vietnamese about common teaching topics. Use cards with common questions and answers printed in Vietnamese.	2. A fluent interpreter is essential because Asians do not always reveal they do not understand instructions. Printed instructions reinforce information that was given verbally and may answer unasked questions. Communication cards convey interest in communicating and provide a means of eliciting basic information.
3. Talk to the client rather than the interpreter, using quiet tones. Use the same interpreter whenever possible.	3. Talking directly to the client shows respect and concern for the client. Soft speech protects the privacy and modesty of the patient. A natural response when people do not understand is to raise the voice. This may convey impatience or anger. A consistent interpreter enhances communication.
4. Consider nonverbal factors when communicating: a. Speak slowly, and smile when appropriate. b. Keep an open posture. Avoid crossing the arms over the chest or turning away from the family. c. Attend carefully to what the family says by nodding, leaning forward, or encouraging continued talk with frequent "uh-huhs." d. Avoid fidgeting or watching a clock. e. Determine Diep's response to light touch on the arm, and use or avoid touch depending on her response. f. Do not expect prolonged eye contact.	4. Even subtle body language can indicate interest and empathy or impatience, annoyance, or hurry. Touch and eye contact are sensitive cultural variables, and nurses must be aware that they are not always welcomed.
5. Locate prenatal classes in Vietnamese. Explain what is included in such classes, and encourage the couple to attend.	5. Information is more easily learned in one's own language. Appropriate cultural concerns are likely to be discussed in classes taught in Vietnamese.

Evaluation

Diep kept all prenatal appointments throughout her pregnancy, bringing an English-speaking family member with her. She followed recommendations and asked appropriate questions at each visit.

Additional Nursing Diagnoses to Consider
- Deficient Knowledge
- Risk for Ineffective Health Maintenance

TABLE 14-3 Psychosocial Assessment

Findings (Normal and Unusual)*	Sample Questions	Nursing Implications
PSYCHOLOGICAL RESPONSE		
First trimester: uncertainty, ambivalence, mood changes, self as primary focus Second trimester: wonder, joy, focus on fetus Third trimester: vulnerability, preparing for birth (fear, anger, apathy, ambivalence, lack of preparation)	"How do you and your partner feel about being pregnant?" "How will your lives change as a result of being pregnant?" "How do you feel about the changes in your body?" "What preparations have you made for the baby?"	Use active listening and reflection to establish a sense of trust. Reevaluate negative responses (fear, apathy, anger) in subsequent assessments.
AVAILABILITY OF RESOURCES		
Financial concerns (lack of funds or insurance) Availability of grandparents, friends, family (family geographically or emotionally unavailable)	"What are your plans for prenatal care and birth?" "How do your parents feel about being grandparents?" "Who else can you depend on besides the family?" "Who provides strength when there is a problem?"	Determine adequacy of financial means. Refer to resources such as a public clinic for care, WIC for food. Help the couple discover alternative resources if the family is unavailable. Identify family conflicts early to allow time for resolution.
CHANGES IN SEXUAL PRACTICES		
Mutual satisfaction with changes (excessive concern with comfort or safety, excessive conflict)	"How have sexual patterns or satisfaction changed?" "How do you cope with the changes?" "What concerns you most?"	Offer reassurance that intercourse is usually safe. Suggest alternative positions and open communication.
EDUCATIONAL NEEDS		
Many questions about pregnancy, childbirth, and infant care (no questions, absence of interest in educational programs)	"How do you feel about caring for an infant?" "What are your major concerns?" "Whom do you count on for information?"	Respond to priority needs that are expressed. Refer couple to appropriate child and parenting classes.
CULTURAL INFLUENCES		
Ability of either the woman or her family to speak English or availability of fluent interpreters, cultural influences support a healthy pregnancy and infant (harmful cultural beliefs or health practices)	"What foods are recommended during pregnancy?" "What practices are recommended?" "What is forbidden?" "What is most important to you in your care?" "How do your religious beliefs affect pregnancy?"	Locate fluent interpreters if needed. Avoid labeling beliefs as superstition. Reinforce beliefs that promote a good pregnancy outcome. Elicit help from accepted source of information to overcome harmful practices.

*Findings that require additional assessment or intervention are shown in parentheses.

Muslim women, nurses must be aware of Islamic laws that require the woman to keep her hair, body, arms to the wrist, and legs to the ankles covered at all times in the presence of a man. Moreover, a Muslim woman is not to be alone in the presence of a man other than a close relative. Female providers should be available to care for these women.

When talking to the woman's significant others, the nurse must call them by the right name. For example, a Vietnamese woman usually keeps her maiden name when she marries. Therefore the husband and wife will have different last names.

NURSING CARE

Psychosocial Concerns

Assessment

The purpose of a psychosocial assessment is to monitor the adaptation of the family to pregnancy, which has been called a maturational crisis that requires a major transition in role function and relationships. Some data required for a psychosocial assessment can be obtained from the physical assessment. For example, age, gravida, para, and general health status provide important information in both areas. Table 14-3 identifies areas for assessment, provides sample questions, and indicates nursing implications.

Nursing Diagnosis and Planning

Most families strive to maintain the health of the expectant mother and fetus and to complete developmental tasks needed for parenting. The most encompassing nursing diagnosis probably is:

■ Health-Seeking Behaviors: developmental tasks needed to prepare for parenthood.

Expected Outcomes: The family will verbalize emotional responses appropriate to each trimester and will verbalize methods that assist the expectant parents to complete the developmental processes of pregnancy. The family will identify cultural factors that may produce conflicts and collaborate to reduce those conflicts.

Interventions

Providing Information

Provide family members with information and anticipatory guidance about the emotional changes that occur during pregnancy, the developmental tasks of the mother and father, and role transition. Guidance is necessary to prepare prospective parents for the progressive changes that occur during pregnancy and to reassure them that their feelings and behaviors are normal. It also gives them an opportunity to ask questions and explore their feelings.

Discussing Resources

Help couples who have no financial resources or insurance coverage to find the most convenient location to obtain prenatal care and to determine where the woman will give birth. This concern is particularly important for the new poor, who have little idea of how to gain access to government-sponsored care.

Emotional resources include those that assist the new family to adjust to the demands of pregnancy and parenting. If family members who traditionally offer support in times of stress are unavailable, refer the prospective parents to community resources, such as childbirth education classes, support groups, and sibling classes, and later to breastfeeding and new parenting classes.

Helping the Family Prepare for the Birth

During the last trimester, discuss lifestyle changes that will occur when the infant is born. Unanticipated changes that accompany this dramatic life event may add stress and disrupt family processes. Help the prospective parents make practical plans for the infant, such as obtaining clothing and choosing the method of feeding. Siblings should be prepared several weeks or months before the birth, depending on their ages. Older children often benefit from participating in planning for the baby.

Suggest that parents consider how they will work out the division of household and parenting tasks, as well as child care if the mother must return to work after childbirth. If these issues are not addressed, the couple can experience frustration and anger as one parent, usually the mother, assumes total care of the infant and attempts to complete all household tasks. Moreover, exhaustion and frustration can overwhelm the joys of parenting when one parent must provide all care.

Modeling Communication Techniques

When disagreements are evident, it is often helpful to discuss and model therapeutic communication techniques that include all significant family members. Techniques that clarify, summarize, and reflect feelings can defuse negative feelings that might result in family disruption.

Identifying Cultural Factors That Could Cause Conflict

Explore possible areas of conflict related to cultural beliefs and health practices that affect pregnancy.

It is reassuring to expectant mothers when nurses support health beliefs that are beneficial before confronting them with health care beliefs that cause concern. For example, "It is so good for you and the baby when you eat so many vegetables, but I am worried because you missed your last appointment."

If there is conflict as a result of differences in time orientation, acknowledge the problem, convey understanding of the differences, and emphasize the importance of calling when appointments cannot be kept. Many families do not realize that when they miss their appointment, another family misses the opportunity for health care.

Evaluation

- Does the family verbalize concerns and emotions at each visit?
- Do the partner and significant family members appear interested and involved?
- Do the family members discuss compromises when cultural health practices are harmful?

PERINATAL EDUCATION

Perinatal education has become increasingly important in helping couples learn about pregnancy, birth, and parenting. Classes focus not only on preparing for childbirth but also include information formerly received during the birth facility stay.

The goals of perinatal education are to help parents become knowledgeable consumers, take an active role in maintaining health during pregnancy and birth, and learn coping techniques to deal with pregnancy, childbirth, and parenting. A national *Healthy People 2010* goal is to increase the proportion of women who attend a series of prepared childbirth classes (U.S. Department of Health and Human Services, 2000).

Providers of Education

Most perinatal education classes are taught by registered nurses, but some are taught by physical therapists or others with special preparation. Many instructors are certified by organizations such as the American Society for Psychoprophylaxis in Obstetrics (ASPO) or the International Childbirth Education Association (ICEA). Certification ensures that the instructors have received special preparation to provide sound education that adheres to the certifying organization's general philosophy. The Association of Women's Health, Obstetric, and Neonatal Nurses (2000) has published guidelines for educator competencies and class curricula.

Class Participants

Participants in classes about childbearing have traditionally been middle-income couples who are older and better educated than those who do not take classes. Low-income women may not have money or transportation to take classes. Although inexpensive or free classes are available in some areas, women with little or no prenatal care may not know about this form of education. Classes in languages other than English are often available in areas where they are needed.

People take classes for a variety of reasons. Many want to participate actively in all aspects of childbearing. Others are looking for coping strategies to deal with their fear of childbirth or pain. When women feel informed and believe that they have some control over what happens to them, they are more likely to expect birth to be satisfying and fulfilling and to experience it as such.

Choices for Childbearing

One purpose of any perinatal education program is to help parents learn about available options so that they can make appropriate choices. Parents learn that there are many ways

BOX 14-1
Birth Plan Considerations

- Use of intermittent (Doppler or fetoscope) or continuous (electronic) fetal monitoring
- Intravenous fluids: use, avoidance, saline lock
- Food and oral fluids allowed in labor
- Enemas
- Position and activity for labor, position for delivery
- Use of tubs, showers
- Episiotomy
- Methods of pain relief
- Support person(s) present during labor
- Breastfeeding only, formula only, combination feeding
- Participation of siblings during/after birth
- Mother/baby couplet care
- Time of discharge
- Follow-up care

of birthing and that no one "right" method exists. Knowledgeable parents can communicate assertively with their health care providers about their needs and desires.

Some women make a birth plan as they consider the various choices possible in childbirth. The plan may be very simple, such as the desire to keep the infant with the mother at all times, or it may be a list of very specific items to be included in the childbirth experience. Cultural preferences can be incorporated into the birth plan (see Box 14-1).

Setting

The woman and her partner must choose a birth setting and select a care provider who practices in that setting. Hospitals are the most common setting for birth in North America. They often have birthing suites that provide a homelike atmosphere. A freestanding birth center provides an atmosphere that is less institutional than that of the hospital. Home birth allows the woman to give birth in her own surroundings, with delivery managed by a midwife.

Support Person

During labor, the woman needs to have someone with her to help her through the experience. The support person is most often the father of her baby, but a relative or friend may also take this role (Fig. 14-5). Some women wish to share the birth experience with several relatives or close friends. Other women hire a doula to provide support during labor.

A doula is a trained labor support person who is employed by the mother to provide labor support. She gives physical support such as massage and helping with relaxation and provides emotional support and advocacy throughout labor. Some doulas also help during the postpartum period.

Education

Expectant mothers must also decide on prenatal education classes. Their decisions are based on the classes available in the area, the costs, and the kinds of information they need.

Some areas have a vast array of classes from which to choose. In others, the selection is limited to childbirth preparation classes only.

Types of Classes Available

Preconception Classes
Classes for couples who are thinking about having a baby are designed to help them have a healthy pregnancy from the beginning. Information about nutrition before conception, signs of pregnancy, healthy lifestyle, and choosing a caregiver is presented. Preconception classes emphasize early and regular prenatal care and ways to reduce risk factors for poor pregnancy outcome.

Early Pregnancy Classes
Early pregnancy classes focus on the first two trimesters. First-trimester classes are sometimes called "earlybird" or "right start" classes. They cover information on adapting to pregnancy, dealing with early discomforts such as morning sickness and fatigue, sexuality, and understanding what to expect in the months ahead. Emphasis is placed on obtaining prenatal care and avoiding hazards to the fetus.

Second-trimester classes focus on changes that occur during middle pregnancy, fetal development, and alterations in roles. Information on body mechanics, working during pregnancy, and what to expect during the third trimester is included. Teachers discuss childbirth choices and information to help students become more knowledgeable consumers.

In these classes, parents may begin to learn about the needs of the mother and infant after birth, or they may attend other classes to meet this need. This information is especially important because of the short birth-facility stay after birth.

Exercise Classes
Exercise classes help women keep fit and healthy during pregnancy. Exercises should be low impact and preceded by warm-up routines. To prevent diversion of blood away from the uterus, women should avoid excessive heart rate elevation. An added benefit of the classes is the opportunity for women to meet others with similar concerns.

Childbirth Preparation Classes
In childbirth preparation classes, women and their support persons learn self-help measures and what to expect during labor and birth. Couples learn coping methods that help them approach childbirth in a positive manner. Teachers do not promise prevention of all pain in labor. The increased confidence and the techniques learned in prepared childbirth classes may help decrease perception and increase tolerance of pain during labor.

Classes include information about labor, pharmacologic and nonpharmacologic methods of pain relief, and a tour of the birth setting. Practice of relaxation, breathing techniques, and coping strategies are part of "labor rehearsals" in every class (Fig. 14-6) (see Chapter 19). Films assist women to develop a realistic picture of the birth process.

Class series range from a 1-day class to four to nine meetings, depending on the content included. Women who have taken classes for a previous birth often take a refresher class for an update of current practices and review of techniques.

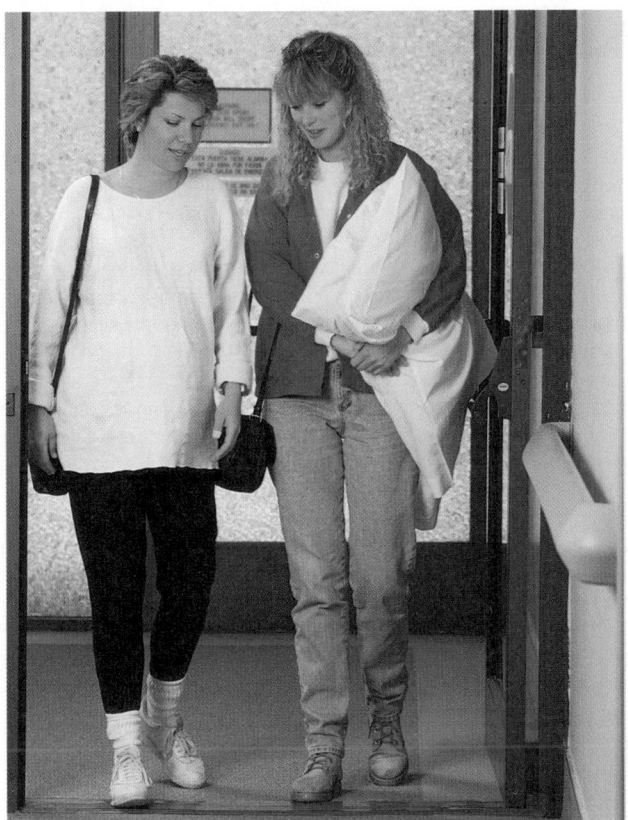

Figure 14-5 An expectant mother may ask a sister or close female friend to be her labor partner and to attend classes with her.

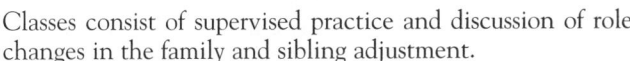

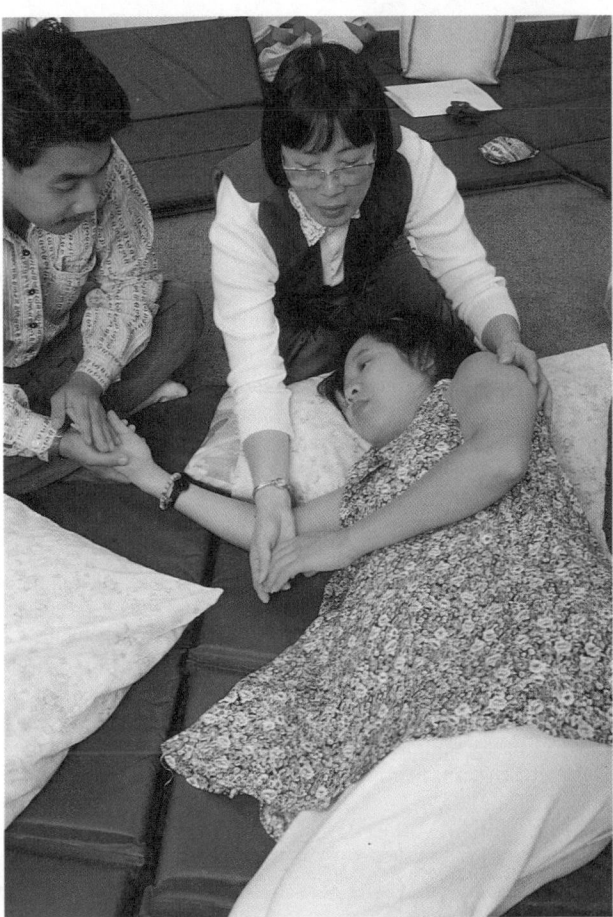

Figure 14-6 The nurse teaches the support person how to check for relaxation.

Classes consist of supervised practice and discussion of role changes in the family and sibling adjustment.

Prepared childbirth classes based in birth facilities include detailed information on what to expect in that particular setting but may not cover options that are unavailable at that agency. Hospital classes have sometimes been criticized for teaching clients to be "good," or compliant, patients. A woman may wish to talk to the instructor before taking a class to ask about class size and the teacher's philosophy, background, and teaching methods.

Cesarean Birth Preparation Classes

Although cesarean birth is discussed in general childbirth classes, women planning a cesarean birth may take a separate class. Topics include indications, options, surgical procedure, and postoperative course. For those who had a cesarean birth previously, the class offers an opportunity to share experiences and feelings and to clarify misconceptions. Class discussion helps couples feel that they have some control over what happens and provides a basis for discussion with caregivers.

Special classes are available for women who have previously had a cesarean birth but want to attempt a vaginal birth. Vaginal birth after cesarean (VBAC) is also called a *trial of labor after cesarean (TLAC)*. Class content includes explanations of when a VBAC is possible, what to expect during labor and birth, coping techniques, and possible problems that would necessitate another cesarean birth.

Breastfeeding Classes

Prenatal breastfeeding classes help increase a woman's confidence in her ability to breastfeed successfully and provide her with sources of help if she encounters difficulties. Breastfeeding classes include information on physiology of lactation, feeding techniques, establishing a milk supply, and dealing with common problems. Partners who attend learn methods of providing support during breastfeeding.

Parenting Classes

Instruction on parenting and newborn care may be included in prepared childbirth classes or provided separately. Content typically includes general care and common concerns, such as the crying infant and advantages and disadvantages of circumcision. Baby equipment, such as various types of infant car seats, is often displayed. Practice with dolls may also be included. Classes sometimes continue after the birth of the infant.

Postpartum Classes

Although the postpartum period is covered in childbirth preparation classes, the mother can also attend classes after birth. Content includes the physiologic and psychological changes of the postpartum period, role transition, sexuality, and nutrition. Some classes focus on exercise for the postpartum period.

KEY CONCEPTS

- Maternal psychological responses progress during pregnancy from uncertainty and ambivalence to feelings of vulnerability and preparation for the birth of the infant.
- As the fetus becomes real, usually in the second trimester, maternal focus shifts from self to the fetus, and the woman turns inward to concentrate on the processes going on in her body.
- Changes in the maternal body during pregnancy may result in a negative body image that affects sexual responses. This change may be especially troubling if the couple does not discuss emotions and concerns related to the changes in sexuality.
- It takes time for a woman to make the transition to the role of mother, and the process involves mimicking the behavior of other mothers, fantasizing about the baby, developing a sense of self as mother, and grieving for the loss of previous roles.
- To complete the maternal tasks of pregnancy, the woman must take steps to seek safe passage for herself and the infant, gain acceptance of significant persons, give of herself,

and form an attachment to the unknown child.
- Paternal responses change throughout pregnancy and depend on the ability to perceive the fetus as real, to gain recognition for the role of parent, and to create a role as involved father.
- The most powerful reality boosters for the expectant father during pregnancy are hearing the fetal heart beat, feeling the fetus move, and viewing the infant on a sonogram.
- In primitive cultures, couvade refers to pregnancy-related rituals performed by the man; in modern society, it often refers to a cluster of pregnancy-related signs and symptoms experienced by the man.
- The response of grandparents to the announcement of pregnancy depends on their age, the number and ages of other grandchildren, and their perception of the role of grandparents.
- The response of siblings to pregnancy depends on their ages and developmental levels. Toddlers may feel displaced in their parents' affection unless measures are taken to reassure them.

- It is more difficult for multiparas to complete the developmental tasks of pregnancy because they have less time, experience more fatigue, and must negotiate a new relationship with the older child or children.
- Socioeconomic status is a major factor in determining health practices during pregnancy. Poor families have competing priorities for food and shelter and seek prenatal care late in pregnancy.
- Cultural differences can create major conflicts between expectant families and health care workers. Language, time orientation, and health beliefs are the areas in which conflicts are most likely to occur.
- Education for childbearing helps couples become knowledgeable consumers and active participants in pregnancy and childbirth.
- Many classes are available for pregnant women and their support persons. Early pregnancy classes emphasize having a healthy pregnancy. Those conducted in later pregnancy focus on preparing for childbirth, breastfeeding, and early parenting.

ANSWERS to Critical Thinking Exercise 14-1

1. The tasks of pregnancy are more complex for the multipara than for a primigravida. Multiparas have less time and are more likely to be fatigued. They are often very concerned about the effect of the pregnancy on other children and about their ability to handle the added responsibilities of another child.

2. Respond by acknowledging her concerns and reflecting her feelings so that she can fully express how she feels. "You worry that your son will be upset when the new baby is born." Or "You feel guilty that your son will have to share your time and energy with the baby."

3. Suggest that Emma make any changes in sleeping arrangements now so that her son

will not feel displaced by the infant. Recommend that she plan ways to have time alone with the older child when the baby arrives, and review measures to reduce sibling rivalry. The mother can tell her 2-year-old how much she loves him; she can hug and cuddle him frequently. She can remind others to pay attention to her son as well as to the new baby.

REFERENCES and READINGS

American Academy of Pediatrics (AAP), Committee on Bioethics. (1998). Female genital mutilation. *Pediatrics, 102*(1), 153-156.

American College of Obstetricians & Gynecologists (ACOG). (1999). *ACOG Educational Bulletin No. 255: Psychosocial risk factors: Perinatal screening and intervention.* Washington, DC: Author.

Association of Women's Health, Obstetric, & Neonatal Nurses (AWHONN). (2000). *Nurse providers of perinatal education: Competencies and program guide.* Washington, DC: Author.

Beckmann, C.A., Buford, T.A., & Witt, J.B. (2000). Perceived barriers to prenatal care services. *MCN: The American Journal of Maternal/Child Nursing, 25*(1), 43-46.

Braveman, P., Marchi, K., Egerter, S., Pearl, M., & Neuhaus, J. (2000). Barriers to timely prenatal care among women with insurance: The impor-

tance of prepregnancy factors. *Obstetrics & Gynecology, 95*(1), 874-880.

Buist, A., Morse, C.A., & Durkin, S. (2003). Men's adjustment to fatherhood: Implications for obstetrical health care. *Journal of Obstetric, Gynecologic, and Neonatal Nursing, 32*(2), 172-180.

Callister, L.C. (2001). Integrating cultural beliefs and practices into the care of childbearing women. In K.R. Simpson & P.A. Creehan. *AWHONN perinatal nursing* (2nd ed., pp. 68-94). Philadelphia: Lippincott.

Cesario, S.K. (2001). Care of the Native American woman: Strategies for practice, education, and research. *Journal of Obstetric, Gynecologic, & Neonatal Nursing, 30*(1), 13-19.

Driscoll, J.W. (2001). Psychosocial adaptation to pregnancy and postpartum. In K.R. Simpson & P.A. Creehan. *AWHONN perinatal nursing* (2nd ed., pp.115-124). Philadelphia: Lippincott.

Gichia, J.E.U. (2000). Mothers and others: African-American women's preparation for motherhood. *MCN: The American Journal of Maternal/Child Nursing, 25*(2), 86-91.

Jimenez, S.L. (2000). Comfort and pain management. In F.H. Nichols & S.S. Humenick (Eds.). *Childbirth education: Practice, research, and theory* (2nd ed., pp. 157-177). Philadelphia: Saunders.

Jordan, P.L. (1990). Laboring for relevance: Expectant and new fatherhood. *Nursing Research, 39*(1), 11-16.

Keppler, A.B., & Simpson, K.R. (2001). Discharge planning. In K.R. Simpson & P.A. Creehan. *AWHONN perinatal nursing* (2nd ed., pp. 610-632). Philadelphia: Lippincott.

Kridli, S.A. (2002). Health beliefs and practices among Arab women. *MCN: The American Journal of Maternal Child Nursing, 27*(1), 178-182.

Kroelinger, C.D., & Oths, K.S. (2000). Partner support and pregnancy wantedness. *Birth, 27*(2), 112-119.

Logsdon, M.C. (2000). *Social support for pregnant and postpartum women.* Washington, DC: AWHONN.

Matteson, P.S. (2001). *Women's health during the childbearing years: A community-based approach.* St. Louis: Mosby.

Mattson, S. (2000). Ethnocultural considerations in the childbearing period. In S. Mattson & J.E. Smith (Eds.). *Core curriculum for maternal-newborn nursing* (2nd ed., pp. 70-84.). Philadelphia: Saunders.

Mattson, S. (2000). Providing culturally competent care: Strategies and approaches for perinatal clients. *AWHONN Lifelines, 4*(5), 39-41.

Mattson, S. (2003). Caring for Latino women. *AWHONN Lifelines, 7*(3), 258-260.

Melender, H. (2002). Experiences of fears associated with pregnancy and childbirth: A study of 329 pregnant women. *Birth, 29*(2), 101-111.

Melender, H. (2002). Fears and coping strategies associated with pregnancy and childbirth in Finland. *Journal of Midwifery & Women's Health, 47*(4), 256-263.

Mercer, R.T. (1990). *Parents at risk.* New York: Springer.

Mercer, R.T., & Ferketich, S.L. (1994). Maternal-infant attachment of experienced and inexperienced mothers during infancy. *Nursing Research, 43*(6), 344-351.

Midmer, D. (2000). Psychosocial support for childbearing families. In H. Nichols & S.S. Humenick. *Childbirth education: Practice, research, and theory* (2nd ed., pp. 476-500). Philadelphia: Saunders.

Moore, M.L., & Moos, M. (2003). *Cultural competence in the care of childbearing families.* White Plains, NY: March of Dimes.

Mullaly, L.M. (2000). Psychology of pregnancy. In S. Mattson & J.E. Smith (Eds.). *Core curriculum for maternal-newborn nursing* (2nd ed., pp. 101-114). Philadelphia: Saunders.

Pagnini, D.L., & Reichman, N.E. (2000). Psychosocial factors and the timing of prenatal care among women in New Jersey's HealthStart program. *Family Planning Perspectives, 32*(2), 56-64.

Ramer, L., & Frank, B. (2001). *Pregnancy: Psychosocial perspectives.* White Plains, NY: March of Dimes.

Redman, B.K. (2001). *The practice of patient education* (9th ed.). St. Louis: Mosby.

Rubin, R. (1975). Maternal tasks in pregnancy. *MCN: The American Journal of Maternal/Child Nursing, 4*(3), 143-153.

Rubin, R. (1984). *Maternal identity and the maternal experience.* New York: Springer.

Schneider, Z. (2001). An Australian study of women's experiences of their first pregnancy. *Midwifery, 18*(3), 238-249.

Shilling, T. (2000). Cultural perspectives on childbearing. In F.H. Nichols & S.S. Humenick.

Childbirth education: Practice, research, and theory (2nd ed., pp. 138-154). Philadelphia: Saunders.

Sleutel, M.R. (2003). Intrapartum nursing: Integrating Rubin's framework with social support theory. *Journal of Obstetric, Gynecologic, and Neonatal Nursing, 32*(1), 76-82.

Spector, R.E. (2000). *Cultural diversity in health and illness* (5th ed.). Norwalk, CT: Appleton & Lange.

Stark, M.A. (2000). Is it difficult to concentrate during the 3rd trimester and postpartum? *Journal of Obstetric, Gynecologic, and Neonatal Nursing, 29*(4), 378-389.

U.S. Department of Health and Human Services. (2000). *Healthy people 2010: Healthy People 2010* (Conference Edition, in Two Volumes). Washington, D.C.

Webster, J., Linnane, J.W.J., Dibley, L.M., Hinson, J.K., Starrenburg, S.E., & Roberts, J.A. (2000). Measuring social support in pregnancy: Can it be simple and meaningful? *Birth, 27*(2), 97-101.

Wilkerson, N.N., & Shrock, P. (2000). Sexuality in the perinatal period. In F.H. Nichols & S.S. Humenick. *Childbirth education: Practice, research, and theory* (2nd ed., pp. 48-65). Philadelphia: Saunders.

Zwelling, E. (2000). The pregnancy experience. In F.H. Nichols & S.S. Humenick. *Childbirth education: Practice, research, and theory* (2nd ed., pp. 35-47). Philadelphia: Saunders.

15

Nutrition for Childbearing

After studying this chapter, you should be able to:

- Explain the importance of adequate nutrition and weight gain during pregnancy.
- Compare the nutrient needs of pregnant and nonpregnant women.
- Describe common factors that influence a woman's nutritional status and choices.
- Describe how common nutritional risk factors affect nutritional requirements during pregnancy.
- Compare the nutritional needs of the postpartum woman who is breastfeeding with those of one who is not breastfeeding.
- Apply the nursing process to nutrition during pregnancy, the postpartum period, and lactation.

 DEFINITIONS

anorexia nervosa Refusal to eat because of a distorted body image and a feeling of obesity.

bulimia Eating disorder characterized by ingestion of large amounts of food, followed by purging behavior such as induced vomiting or laxative abuse.

complete protein food Food containing all the essential amino acids.

Dietary Reference Intakes A label for several terms that estimate nutrient needs; includes recommended dietary allowance, adequate intake, tolerable upper intake level, and estimated average requirement.

essential amino acids Amino acids that cannot be synthesized by the body and must be obtained from foods.

gynecologic age Number of years since menarche (first menstrual period).

heme iron Iron obtained from meat, poultry, or fish sources; the form most usable by the body.

incomplete protein food Food that does not contain all the essential amino acids.

kilocalorie A unit of heat used to show the energy value in foods, commonly called a calorie.

lacto-ovovegetarian A vegetarian whose diet includes milk products and eggs.

lactose intolerance Inability to digest most dairy products owing to a deficiency in the enzyme lactase.

lactovegetarian A vegetarian whose diet includes milk products.

nonheme iron Iron obtained from plants and fortified foods.

nutrient density Quantity and quality of protein, vitamins, and minerals per 100 calories in foods.

ovovegetarian A vegetarian whose diet includes eggs.

pica Ingestion of nonnutritive substances, such as laundry starch, dirt, or ice.

recommended dietary allowance Level of intake of a nutrient considered to meet the needs of healthy individuals.

vegan A complete vegetarian who does not eat any animal products.

vegetarian An individual whose diet consists wholly or mostly of plant foods and who avoids animal food sources.

At no time in a woman's life is nutrition as important as it is during pregnancy and lactation. The nurse has ongoing contact with women throughout this period and can provide education about nutritional needs on a continuing basis. This is especially important because studies often show that many women do not adequately understand the nutritional needs of pregnancy (Fowles, 2002; Hilton, 2002).

WEIGHT GAIN DURING PREGNANCY

Weight gain during pregnancy, especially after the first trimester, is an important determinant of fetal growth. Low birth weight (less than 2500 g or 5½ lb), preterm labor, and an increased risk of fetal and newborn mortality and morbidity have been associated with insufficient weight gain

TABLE **15-1**   Recommended Weight Gain During Pregnancy

Weight Before Pregnancy	Total Gain	Total Gain (First Trimester)	Weekly Gain (Second and Third Trimesters)
Normal weight (BMI 19.8-26.0)	11.5-16 kg (25-35 lb)	1.6 kg (3.5 lb)	0.44 kg (0.97 lb)
Underweight (BMI <19.8)	12.5-18 kg (28-40 lb)	2.3 kg (5 lb)	0.49 kg (1.07 lb)
Overweight (BMI >26, <29)	7-11.5 kg (15-25 lb)	0.9 kg (2 lb)	0.3 kg (0.67 lb)
Obese (BMI >29)	At least 6.8 kg (15 lb)	Individually determined	Individually determined
Twin pregnancies	16-20.5 kg (35-45 lb)	1.6 kg (3.5 lb)	0.75 kg (1.5 lb)

Data from National Academy of Sciences. (1990). *Nutrition during pregnancy, Part I: Weight gain.* Washington, DC: National Academy Press.
BMI: Body mass index.

during pregnancy. Poor maternal weight gain indicates not only lower caloric intake but also low intake of other important nutrients. Excessive weight gain is another problem. It is associated with increased birth weight, prolonged labor, birth trauma, asphyxia, and cesarean birth. An infant birth weight of 3 to 4 kg ($6\frac{1}{2}$ to $8\frac{4}{5}$ lb) is associated with the lowest rates of infant mortality (Mitchell, 2003; Strychar et al., 2000).

Recommendations for Total Weight Gain

Recommendations for weight gain in pregnancy are based on the woman's prepregnancy weight for her height or her body mass index (BMI). BMI is calculated by dividing the weight in kilograms by the height in meters squared. Another method is to divide the weight in pounds by the height in inches squared and multiplying the result by 704.5. Tables are available that show the BMI for various weights and heights.

The recommended weight gain during pregnancy is 11.5 to 16 kg (25 to 35 lb) for women who begin pregnancy at normal weight for height or a BMI of 19.8 to 26. This amount of weight gain is believed to reduce intrauterine growth restriction caused by inadequate maternal intake.

Suggested gains vary according to the woman's BMI before pregnancy (Table 15-1). Prepregnancy weight below 45 kg (100 lb) is associated with preterm labor and low-birth-weight infants. Women with BMIs less than 19.8 should gain more during pregnancy to meet the needs of pregnancy as well as their own need to gain weight.

Prepregnancy weight above 90 kg (200 lb) is associated with increased incidence of gestational diabetes, pregnancy-induced hypertension, neural tube defects, cesarean birth, and postpartum infection (Morin, 1998). The recommended gain for overweight women (BMI above 26 to 29) is 7 to 11.5 kg (15 to 25 lb). This provides sufficient nutrients for the fetus. The weight gain for the obese woman (BMI above 29) is at least 6.8 kg (15 lb), which is equivalent to the weight of the products of conception (e.g., fetus, placenta).

Women who are shorter than 157 cm (62 inches) may not need to gain as much as taller women and should gain only to the lower limits of the recommended range. Young adolescents need to gain to the upper end of the range to provide for their own growth during pregnancy as well as growth of the fetus. Infants of a multifetal pregnancy are often born be-

fore term and tend to weigh less than infants born of single pregnancies. A greater weight gain in the mother may help prevent low birth weight.

Pattern of Weight Gain

The pattern of weight gain is as important as the total increase. The general recommendation is for an increment of about 1.6 kg ($3\frac{1}{2}$ lb) during the first trimester, when the mother may be nauseated and the fetus needs fewer nutrients for growth. During the rest of the pregnancy, the expected weight gain is 0.44 kg (almost 1 lb) a week.

Maternal and Fetal Distribution

Women often wonder why they should gain so much weight when the fetus weighs only 3.2 to 3.6 kg (7 to 8 lb). Explaining the distribution of weight helps them understand this need (Fig. 15-1).

Factors That Influence Weight Gain

Knowing about factors that may negatively influence nutrient intake and weight gain helps the nurse devise plans for improving nutrition. Women at risk for inadequate weight gain include those who are young, unmarried, low income, poorly educated, in poor general health, or receiving insufficient prenatal care. African-American, Southeast Asian, and Hispanic women are more at risk for low weight gain during pregnancy than are white women.

Adequate weight gain is especially important for African-Americans and teenagers, who tend to have smaller infants even when they gain weight in the same amount as whites or older mothers. The reasons for this difference are not fully understood. Multiparas are at higher risk for low weight gain than women in their first pregnancy. Smoking or substance abuse may interfere with food intake and weight gain.

NUTRITIONAL REQUIREMENTS DURING PREGNANCY

Nutrient needs during pregnancy increase to meet the demands of the mother and fetus. Usually the increases are not large and are relatively easy to obtain through the diet.

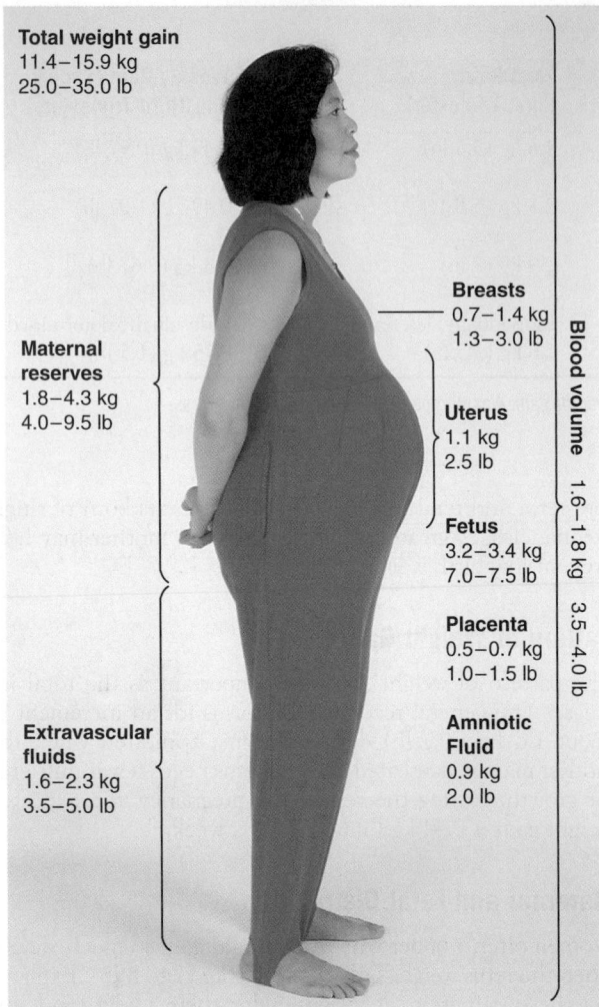

Total weight gain
11.4–15.9 kg
25.0–35.0 lb

Maternal reserves
1.8–4.3 kg
4.0–9.5 lb

Extravascular fluids
1.6–2.3 kg
3.5–5.0 lb

Breasts
0.7–1.4 kg
1.3–3.0 lb

Uterus
1.1 kg
2.5 lb

Fetus
3.2–3.4 kg
7.0–7.5 lb

Placenta
0.5–0.7 kg
1.0–1.5 lb

Amniotic Fluid
0.9 kg
2.0 lb

Blood volume 1.6–1.8 kg 3.5–4.0 lb

Figure 15-1 Distribution of weight gain in pregnancy. The numbers represent a general distribution because there is a great deal of variation among women. The component with the greatest fluctuation is the amount of weight increase attributed to extravascular fluids (edema) and maternal reserves of fat.

Dietary Reference Intakes

In the United States, Dietary Reference Intakes (DRIs) are used to estimate nutrient needs. DRIs include four categories:

Recommended Dietary Allowance (RDA), the amount of a nutrient that meets the needs of almost all (97%-98%) healthy people in an age-group. The actual needs of individuals (particularly for calories and protein) may vary according to body size, previous nutritional status, and usual activity level.
- Adequate Intake (AI), the nutrient intake assumed to be adequate when an RDA cannot be determined. The AI is chosen because it appears to sustain nutritional status.
- Tolerable Upper Intake Level, the highest amount of a nutrient that can be taken without probable adverse health effects by most people.
- Estimated Average Requirement (EAR), the amount of a nutrient estimated to meet the needs of half the healthy people in an age-group.

Table 15-2 shows the current recommendations for DRIs.

Energy

The energy provided by foods for body processes is calculated in kilocalories. Kilocalories (often used interchangeably with the term *calories*) are obtained from carbohydrates and proteins, which provide 4 calories in each gram, and fats, which provide 9 calories in each gram.

Carbohydrates

Carbohydrates may be simple or complex. Simple carbohydrates include sucrose (table sugar) and those found in fruits and vegetables. Complex carbohydrates are present in starches, such as cereals, and supply vitamins, minerals, and fiber. Because of their value in providing other nutrients, complex carbohydrates should be the major source of carbohydrates in the diet. Fiber, the nondigestible product of plant foods, is important because it produces bulk in the diet. Fiber absorbs water and stimulates peristalsis to help prevent constipation. It also slows gastric emptying, causing a sensation of fullness.

Fats

Fats provide energy as well as fat-soluble vitamins. When reduction of calories is necessary, it is important to reduce but not eliminate carbohydrates and fats. If carbohydrate and fat intake provides insufficient calories, the body uses protein to meet energy needs. This use decreases the amount of protein available for building and repairing tissue.

Fat intake is also important because it provides essential fatty acids such as DHA, an n-3 or omega-3 fatty acid, that help in formation of the placenta, fetal brain development, and visual function. It is also transferred to the infant after birth during breastfeeding. Sources for these fatty acids are fish and red meat (Brooks, Mitchell, & Steffenson, 2000).

Calories

Between 68,000 and 80,000 additional calories are needed during pregnancy (Grodner, Anderson, & DeYoung, 2000). These extra calories furnish energy for the production and maintenance of the fetus, placenta, added maternal tissues, and increased basal metabolic rate. The caloric RDA for women of childbearing age is approximately 2200 calories per day. Although there is little need for additional calories during the first trimester of pregnancy, daily caloric intake should increase by 300 calories after that time. A 300-calorie increase can be achieved relatively easily with a variety of foods. For example, a banana, a carrot, a piece of whole-wheat toast, and a glass of low-fat milk consumed over 1 day would provide the extra calories along with other important nutrients.

Nutrient density, the quantity and quality of the various nutrients in each 100 calories of food, is an important consideration. Foods of high nutrient density have large amounts of good-quality nutrients per serving. During pregnancy, the increased need for most nutrients may not be met unless calories are selected carefully. The term *empty calories* refers to foods that are high in calories but low in other nutrients. Many snack foods not only contain excessive calories and low nutrient density but also are high in fat and sodium (Box 15-1). Increased calories should be "spent" on foods that provide the nutrients needed in increased amounts during pregnancy.

TABLE **15-2** Recommended Energy and Protein Intakes

Nonpregnant Adult Female	Pregnancy	Lactation
ENERGY		
Varies greatly according to body size, age, and physical activity level	Age 14-50: *First trimester:* No change from nonpregnant need *Second and third trimesters:* 300 kcal above nonpregnant needs	500 kcal above nonpregnant needs
CARBOHYDRATE		
Age 14-50: 130 g RDA	Age 14-50: 175 g RDA	Age 14-50: 210 g RDA
PROTEIN		
Age 14-50: 46 g RDA	Age 14-50: 71 g RDA	Age 14-50: 71 g RDA

Data from Institute of Medicine, Food and Nutrition Board. (2002). *Dietary reference intakes for energy, carbohydrates, fiber, protein and amino acids (macronutrients)*. Washington, DC: National Academy Press; Kaiser, L.L., & Allen, L. (2002). Position of the American Dietetic Association: Nutrition and lifestyle for a healthy pregnancy outcome. *Journal of the American Dietetic Association, 102*(10), 1479-1490.
RDA, Recommended dietary allowance.

Protein

Protein is necessary for metabolism, tissue synthesis, and tissue repair. The RDA for adults is 0.80 g of protein per 1 kg of body weight daily. This RDA averages to a daily need of 46 g for females, depending on their age and size. During pregnancy and lactation, a protein intake of 1.1 g/kg or approximately 71 g each day is recommended to expand the blood volume and support the growth of maternal and fetal tissues (Institute of Medicine, 2002). This is an increase of 25 g of protein daily.

Protein is generally abundant in diets in most industrialized nations, but diets low in caloric intake may also be low in protein. If calories are low and protein is used to provide energy, fetal growth may be impaired.

The nurse should counsel women at risk for poor-protein diets about determining protein intake and ways to increase food sources of protein. When a woman needs to increase her protein intake, she should eat more high-protein foods rather than use high-protein powders or drinks. Protein substitutes increase protein but do not have the other nutrients provided by foods.

Vitamins

Although most people do not eat as much as they should of every vitamin each day, true deficiency states are uncommon in North America. Pregnant women, however, may not eat enough foods high in vitamins B_6, D, or E and folic acid to obtain the recommended levels (Table 15-3).

The fat-soluble vitamins (A, D, E, and K) are stored in the liver. Deficiency states are not likely to occur, but fat-soluble vitamins can be toxic in excessive amounts. For example, too much vitamin A can cause fetal defects.

Water-soluble vitamins (B_6, B_{12}, and C, and folic acid, thiamine, riboflavin, and niacin) are not stored in the body as well as fat-soluble vitamins. Therefore water-soluble vitamins should be included in the daily diet. Excess amounts are excreted in the urine, so there is less chance of toxicity from excessive intake.

BOX 15-1
High-Sodium Foods

- Products that contain the word "salt," "soda," or "sodium," such as table salt, seasoning salt, monosodium glutamate, bicarbonate of soda (baking soda)
- Foods that taste salty, including snack foods like popcorn, potato chips, pretzels, crackers
- Condiments and relishes, such as ketchup, horseradish, mustard, soy sauce, bouillon cubes, pickles, green and black olives
- Smoked, dried, or processed foods, such as ham, bacon, lunch meats, corned beef
- Canned soups, meats, and vegetables unless label states low in sodium
- Packaged mixes for sauces, gravies, cakes and other baked foods

During pregnancy, foods high in sodium should be consumed in moderation. Expectant mothers should be taught to read labels and to avoid products in which sodium is listed among the first ingredients.

These vitamins are easily transferred from food to water in cooking so foods should be steamed, microwaved, or prepared in only small amounts of water. The remaining water can be used in other dishes, such as soups.

Folic Acid

Folic acid (also called *folate*) can decrease the occurrence of neural tube defects in newborns. Adequate intake of folic acid is especially important in the month just before conception and during the first trimester after conception. Because many pregnancies are unplanned, all women of childbearing age should consume at least 400 micrograms (μg) (0.4 milligrams [mg]) of folic acid each day. However, women often do not realize the importance of folic acid in their diet before pregnancy begins and many do not meet the recommended

TABLE 15–3 Recommendations for Vitamins and Minerals

Adult Females: Nonpregnant	Pregnancy and Lactation	Sources	Purpose	Importance in Pregnancy
FAT-SOLUBLE VITAMINS				
Vitamin A Age 14-50: 700 μg	*Pregnancy:* Age 14-18: 750 μg Age 19-50: 770 μg *Lactation:* Age 14-18: 1200 μg Age 19-50: 1300 μg	Green leafy and dark-yellow vegetables, whole or fortified low-fat or nonfat milk, egg yolk, butter and fortified margarine.	Important for vision and cell reproduction, growth, and functioning of skin and mucous membranes.	Fetal growth and cell differentiation. Excessive intake causes spontaneous abortions or serious fetal defects. Isotretinoin (Accutane), a vitamin A derivative for acne, should not be taken during pregnancy because it causes fetal defects.
Vitamin D Age 14-50: 5 μg (AI)	*Pregnancy and Lactation:* Age 14-50: 5 μg (AI)	Fortified milk, margarine, and soy products, butter, egg yolks. Synthesized in skin exposed to sunlight. Vegans who are not exposed to sun and who do not eat fortified foods need supplements.	Necessary for metabolism of calcium and prevention of rickets.	Inadequate amounts may cause neonatal hypocalcemia, hypoplasia of tooth enamel, and maternal osteomalacia (softening of the bones). Excessive intake causes hypercalcemia and possible fetal deformities. Supplements should be taken cautiously.
Vitamin E Age 14-50: 15 mg (RDA)	*Pregnancy:* Age 14-50: 15 mg *Lactation:* Age 14-50: 19 mg (RDA)	Vegetable oils, whole grains, nuts, and green leafy vegetables.	Antioxidant, important for tissue growth and integrity of cells, particularly red blood cell membranes.	Rarely deficient in pregnant women but can cause anemia in mother and fetus.
Vitamin K Age 14-18: 75 μg Age 19-50: 90 μg (AI)	*Pregnancy and Lactation:* Age: 14-18: 75 μg Age 19-50: 90 μg (AI)	Green leafy vegetables. Also produced by normal bacterial flora in small intestine.	Necessary for blood clotting.	Newborns are temporarily deficient and receive one dose by injection at birth to prevent hemorrhage.
WATER-SOLUBLE VITAMINS				
Vitamin B$_6$ (Pyridoxine) Age 14-18: 1.2 mg Age 19-50: 1.3 mg (RDA)	*Pregnancy:* Age 14-50: 1.9 mg *Lactation:* Age 14-50: 2.0 mg (RDA)	Chicken, fish, pork, eggs, peanuts, whole grains.	Important in amino acid metabolism and in blood, hormone, and immune function.	Increased metabolism of amino acids during pregnancy.

Data from Food & Nutrition Board (FNB), National Academy of Sciences. (1989.) *Recommended dietary allowances* (10th ed.), Washington, DC: National Academy Press; Institute of Medicine (IOM), FNB. (1998). *Dietary reference intakes for thiamin, riboflavin, niacin, vitamin B$_6$, folate, vitamin B$_{12}$, pantothenic acid, biotin, and choline.* Washington, DC: National Academy Press; IOM, FNB. (1997). *Dietary reference intakes for calcium, phosphorus, magnesium, vitamin D, and fluoride.* Washington, DC: National Academy Press; IOM, FNB. (2000). *Dietary reference intakes for vitamin C, vitamin E, selenium, and carotenoids.* Washington, DC: National Academy Press; IOM, FNB. (2002). *Dietary reference intakes for vitamin A, vitamin K, arsenic, boron, chromium, copper, iodine, iron, manganese, molybdenum, nickel, silicon, vanadium, and zinc.* Washington, DC: National Academy Press.
RDA, Recommended dietary allowances; *AI*, adequate intake; μg, microgram or mcg; *mg*, milligram; *DNA*, deoxyribonucleic acid; *RNA*, ribonucleic acid.

TABLE **15–3** Recommendations for Vitamins and Minerals—cont'd

Adult Females: Nonpregnant	Pregnancy and Lactation	Sources	Purpose	Importance in Pregnancy
WATER-SOLUBLE VITAMINS—cont'd				
Vitamin B₁₂ Age 14-18: 2.4 μg (RDA)	*Pregnancy:* Age 14-50: 2.6 μg *Lactation:* Age 14-50: 2.8 μg (RDA)	Meat, fish, eggs, milk, fortified soy and cereal products.	Cell division and protein synthesis. Prevents megaloblastic anemia.	Increased formation of red blood cells and protein synthesis.
Folic Acid Age 14-18: 400 μg (RDA)	*Pregnancy:* Age 14-50: 600 μg *Lactation:* Age 14-50: 500 μg (RDA)	Beans, peanuts, orange juice, asparagus, spinach, and fortified cereal and pasta. May be lost in cooking.	Important for cell replication and metabolism and for prevention of megaloblastic anemia.	Expanded blood volume and tissue growth. Deficiency in first 6 weeks of pregnancy may cause spontaneous abortion and neural tube defects.
Thiamine Age 14-18: 1.0 mg Age 19-50: 1.1 mg (RDA)	*Pregnancy and Lactation:* Age 14-50: 1.4 mg (RDA)	Pork, whole or enriched grain products, milk, legumes, organ meats, corn, seeds, nuts.	Forms coenzymes necessary to release energy.	Increased because of intake of calories.
Riboflavin Age 14-18: 1.0 mg Age 19-50: 1.1 mg (RDA)	*Pregnancy:* Age 14-50: 1.4 mg *Lactation:* Age 14-50: 1.6 mg (RDA)	Milk, pork, beef, enriched grain products, and deep-green vegetables.	Forms coenzymes necessary to release energy.	Increased because of greater intake of calories.
Niacin Age 14-50: 14 mg (RDA)	*Pregnancy:* Age 14-50: 18 mg *Lactation:* Age 14-50: 17 mg (RDA)	Meats, legumes, fish, poultry, enriched grains.	Forms coenzymes necessary to release energy.	Increased because of greater intake of calories.
Vitamin C Age 14-18: 65 mg Age 19-50: 75 mg (RDA)	*Pregnancy:* Age 14-18: 80 mg Age 19-50: 85 mg *Lactation:* Age 14-18: 115 mg Age 19-50: 120 mg (RDA)	Citrus fruit, peppers, strawberries, cantaloupe, green leafy vegetables, tomatoes, potatoes. Destroyed by heat and oxidation.	Important in collagen formation, tissue integrity, healing, immune response, and metabolism. Severe deficiency causes scurvy.	Necessary for formation of fetal tissue. Need increased with smoking, drug or alcohol abuse, or aspirin use.
MINERALS				
Iron Age 14-18: 15 mg Age 19-50: 18 mg (RDA)	*Pregnancy:* Age 14-50: 27 mg *Lactation:* Age 14-18: 10 mg Age 19-50: 9 mg (RDA)	Meats, green leafy vegetables, eggs, grain products, tofu, legumes, nuts, blackstrap molasses.	Formation of hemoglobin and enzymes for metabolism.	Expanded maternal blood volume, formation of fetal red blood cells, and storage in the fetal liver for use after birth.

Continued

TABLE **15–3** Recommendations for Vitamins and Minerals—cont'd

Adult Females: Nonpregnant	Pregnancy and Lactation	Sources	Purpose	Importance in Pregnancy
MINERALS—cont'd				
Calcium Age 14-18: 1300 mg Age 19-50: 1000 mg (AI)	*Pregnancy and Lactation:* Age 14-18: 1300 mg Age 19-50: 1000 mg (AI)	Dairy products, salmon or sardines with bones, legumes, nuts, dried fruits, dark-green leafy vegetables, tofu, broccoli.	Needed in bone formation, cell membrane permeability, coagulation, and neuromuscular function.	Mineralization of fetal bones and teeth.
Phosphorus Age 14-18: 1250 mg Age 19-50: 700 mg (RDA)	*Pregnancy and Lactation:* Age 14-18: 1250 mg Age 19-50: 700 mg (RDA)	Dairy products, lean meat. High in processed foods, snacks, carbonated drinks.	Needed with calcium for bone formation and cell metabolism.	Mineralization of fetal bones and teeth. Excessive intake causes binding of calcium in intestines and prevents calcium absorption.
Zinc Age 14-18: 9 mg Age 19-50: 8 mg (RDA)	*Pregnancy:* Age 14-18: 13 mg Age 19-50: 11 mg *Lactation:* Age 14-18: 14 mg Age 19-50: 12 mg (RDA)	Meat, poultry, seafood, eggs, nuts, seeds, legumes, wheat germ, whole grains, yogurt.	Used in cell differentiation and reproduction, DNA and RNA synthesis, metabolism, acid-base balance.	Fetal and maternal tissue growth.
Magnesium Age14-18: 360 mg Age 19-30: 310 mg Age 31-50: 320 mg (RDA)	*Pregnancy:* Age 14-18: 400 mg Age 19-30: 350 mg Age 31-50: 360 mg *Lactation:* Age 14-18: 360 mg Age 19-30: 310 mg Age 31-50: 320 mg (RDA)	Whole grains, nuts, legumes, dark-green vegetables, small amounts in many foods.	Important in cell growth and neuromuscular function; activates enzymes for metabolism of protein and energy.	Same as for nonpregnant. Excessive intake may interfere with absorption of iron.
Iodine Age 14-50: 150 μg (RDA)	*Pregnancy:* Age 14-50: 220 μg *Lactation:* Age 14-50: 290 μg (RDA)	Seafood, iodized salt.	Important in thyroid function.	Deficiency may cause abortion, stillbirth, congenital hypothyroidism, neurologic conditions.

level, in spite of a national campaign to make the public more aware of this problem.

Women who have given birth to an infant with a neural tube defect should take higher doses of folic acid. This practice can decrease the risk of recurrence of neural tube defects by 70% (American Academy of Pediatrics [AAP] and American College of Obstetricians and Gynecologists [ACOG], 2002). *Healthy People 2010* goals are to increase the adequate intake of folic acid in childbearing women to 80% and to cut the incidence of neural tube defects in half by the year 2010 (U.S. Department of Health and Human Services [USDHHS], 2000).

Minerals

Although most minerals (see Table 15-3) are supplied in adequate amounts in normal diets, the intake of iron, calcium, zinc, and magnesium may drop below recommended levels for pregnancy (Giddens et al., 2000, Swensen, Harnack, & Ross, 2001).

Iron

A total of approximately 1000 mg of iron is needed during pregnancy. This provides for the 25% to 33% increase in maternal red blood cells and for transfer to the fetus for stor-

PREGNANT WOMEN
Want to Know

About Vitamins and Minerals

- Take only vitamin and mineral supplements prescribed by a physician, nurse practitioner, or certified nurse-midwife. Over-the-counter supplements may not be formulated to meet your individual needs and could be harmful to you and your baby.
- Take iron on an empty stomach, if possible. If you have nausea, heartburn, constipation, or diarrhea, try taking your iron at different times of the day, such as at bedtime or 1 to 2 hours after meals. Taking it with orange juice or another source of vitamin C may increase absorption. Do not take iron with calcium supplements, milk, tea, or coffee because these substances decrease absorption.
- Keep all vitamin and mineral supplements away from children because they can cause accidental poisoning.

BOX 15-2
Foods High in Iron Content

FOOD AND AMOUNT	AVERAGE AMOUNTS OF IRON SUPPLIED (MG)
Meats and Poultry (3 oz)	
Red meats (average)	2.5
Chicken	0.9
Turkey	1.4
Legumes (½ c)	
Kidney beans	2.3
Lentils	2.1
Peanuts	1.4
Sunflower seeds	7.6
Chickpeas (garbanzo beans)	2.4
Black-eyed peas	1.8
Lima beans, baby	1.7
Peas	1.3
Eggs	
Eggs (each)	1.0
Grains (1 c)	
Rice	1.8
Bran flakes	6.8
with raisins	9.0
Oatmeal	1.6
Bread (slice)	0.9
Fruits	
Raisins (⅓ c)	1.0
Prunes (4)	1.2
Dried apricots (½ c)	3.0
Vegetables (1 c)	
Asparagus (frozen)	1.2
Broccoli	1.8
Collards	1.9
Spinach	
Raw	1.5
Cooked (frozen)	2.9
Other	
Tofu (2½ × 2¾ × 1 inch)	2.3

The Recommended Daily Dietary Allowance for iron during pregnancy is 30 mg. Although many women do not eat enough iron-containing foods in their daily diet to meet this need and take supplements, iron in foods is often better absorbed. Therefore the nurse should suggest ways a woman can increase her dietary iron.
Data from Mahan, L.K., & Escott-Stump, S. (2000). *Krause's food, nutrition, and diet therapy* (10th ed.). Philadelphia: Saunders.

age and production of red blood cells (Blackburn, 2003; Mitchell, 2003). Infants use stored iron during the first 4 to 6 months, when their intake of iron is low. Iron is probably the only nutrient that cannot be supplied completely and easily from the diet during pregnancy. Box 15-2 lists common foods high in iron.

Iron is present in many foods, but in small amounts. The average American diet contains only about 6 mg of iron for each 1000 calories of food. Thus many adult women do not meet their daily nonpregnancy requirement for iron and begin pregnancy already anemic or with low iron stores. (See Chapter 26 for a discussion of anemia in pregnancy.)

Absorption of iron is affected by many other substances. Calcium and phosphorus in milk and tannin in tea decrease iron absorption from plant sources and fortified foods (called *nonheme iron*) if consumed during the same meal. Coffee binds iron, preventing it from being fully absorbed. Foods cooked in iron pans contain more iron. Foods containing ascorbic acid and meats eaten with other iron-containing foods increase absorption. Iron from animal sources (called *heme iron*) is more readily absorbed than nonheme iron and is less affected by other foods.

Because of the difficulty of obtaining enough iron in the diet, health care providers often prescribe iron supplements of 30 mg/day during pregnancy. Women who are anemic may need 60 to 120 mg/day. Supplementation should begin during the second trimester, when the need increases and morning sickness has usually ended.

Iron taken on an empty stomach is absorbed more completely, but many women find iron difficult to tolerate without food. Side effects occur more often with higher doses and include nausea, vomiting, heartburn, epigastric pain, constipation, diarrhea, and black stools. Taking iron at bedtime may make it easier to tolerate. For best absorption, it should be taken with water or orange juice but not with coffee, tea, or milk.

Women should be reminded to keep iron, like all other medicines, out of the reach of children. Accidental overdose with iron is a leading cause of childhood poisoning.

Calcium

Calcium is necessary for bone formation, maintenance of cell membrane permeability, coagulation, and neuromuscular function. It is transferred to the fetus, especially in the last trimester, and is important for mineralization of fetal bones and teeth. Calcium absorption increases during the

BOX 15-3
Calcium Sources Approximately Equivalent to 1 Cup of Milk

1 c yogurt
1½ oz hard cheese
2 c low-fat cottage cheese
1¾ c ice cream or ice milk
3 c sherbet
2¼ c peanuts
1 c almonds
9 oz sunflower seeds
2 c refried beans
3 pieces (2½ × 2¾ × 1 inch) tofu processed with calcium
1¾ c broccoli
1½ c cooked kale
1 c cooked collard greens
4 oz salmon with bones
2½ oz sardines with bones
7 corn tortillas
5 tsp blackstrap molasses

This list can be used to counsel women who are vegans or lactose-intolerant. Lactose-intolerant women can often tolerate yogurt and cheese without distress. Although the amounts of some foods listed are more than would be likely to be eaten within a day, they serve for comparison.
Data from Mahan, L.K., & Escott-Stump, S. (2000). *Krause's food, nutrition, and diet therapy* (10th ed.). Philadelphia: Saunders.

second trimester. Calcium from the mother's bones may be used to meet the needs of pregnancy, but changes are reversed after pregnancy. A common myth is that calcium is removed from the teeth during pregnancy, leading to excessive decay. Actually, calcium in the teeth is stable and is not affected by pregnancy.

The best source of calcium is dairy products. Whole, low-fat, and skim milk all contain the same amount of calcium and may be used interchangeably to increase or reduce calorie intake. However, women with lactose intolerance (lactase deficiency resulting in gastrointestinal problems when dairy products are consumed) need other sources of calcium (Box 15-3). Calcium is also present in legumes, nuts, dried fruits, dark-green leafy vegetables, and broccoli. Although spinach contains calcium, it also contains oxalates, which decrease calcium availability; thus spinach is not a good source of calcium.

Calcium needs are unchanged during pregnancy and lactation. Women who eat inadequate amounts of calcium-rich foods or avoid dairy products for cultural reasons, because of lactose intolerance, to avoid ingesting animal products, or for other reasons should take calcium and vitamin D supplements. Women with little or no exposure to the sun especially need vitamin D added because they may not have enough to ensure adequate metabolism of calcium. Women younger than 18 years need more calcium because their bone density is not complete. To ensure absorption of calcium, women should take supplements with meals, separately from the time they take iron supplements. Caffeine increases the excretion of calcium.

Nutritional Supplementation
Purpose
Food is the best source for nutrients. Although health care providers frequently prescribe prenatal vitamin-mineral supplements, women do not routinely need to take vitamin and mineral supplements during pregnancy unless there is reason to believe that the diet is inadequate. The exceptions are iron and folic acid, which may not be obtained in adequate amounts through normal food intake. Expectant mothers who are vegetarians or lactose intolerant or who have special problems in obtaining nutrients through diet alone may need supplements. Assessment of each woman's individual needs determines whether supplementation is appropriate.

Disadvantages and Dangers of Nutritional Supplementation
Because many people think supplements are a harmless way to improve their diets, some women take them without consulting a health care provider. There is no standardization or regulation of the amounts of ingredients contained in supplements. Some supplements may not have the amount of an ingredient that is listed on the label and may not fulfill the health claims made for it.

The use of supplements may increase the intake of some nutrients to doses much higher than the recommended amounts. Excessive amounts of some vitamins and minerals may be toxic to the fetus. Vitamin A can cause fetal anomalies of the bones, urinary tract, and central nervous system when more than 10,000 IU is taken per day. This is double the amount in most prenatal vitamins. No more than 5000 IU a day should be taken during pregnancy (AAP/ACOG, 2002). Large amounts of vitamin A are taken by women using the drug isotretinoin (Accutane) for acne. Other nutrients that may cause harm in excessive amounts include vitamins B_6, C, and D and the minerals iron, selenium, and zinc (Cunningham et al., 2001).

Water

Water is important during pregnancy for the expanded blood volume and as a part of the increased maternal and fetal tissues. Women should drink approximately eight to ten 8-ounce glasses of fluids each day, with water constituting most of the fluid intake. Fluids low in nutrients should be limited because they are filling and replace other more nutritional foods and drinks.

Food Guide Pyramid

The U.S. Department of Agriculture's (USDA) Food Guide Pyramid provides a guide for healthy eating for adults and children. It has been adapted to provide a guide for pregnancy in Figure 15-2.

Whole Grains
At the base of the Pyramid are breads, cereals, rice, and pastas. They provide complex carbohydrates and fiber as well as vitamins and minerals. Whole grains provide more nutrients than processed grain products. The USDA recommends 6 to 11 servings of this group for healthy adults older than 25 years. Pregnant women should have at least 7 servings.

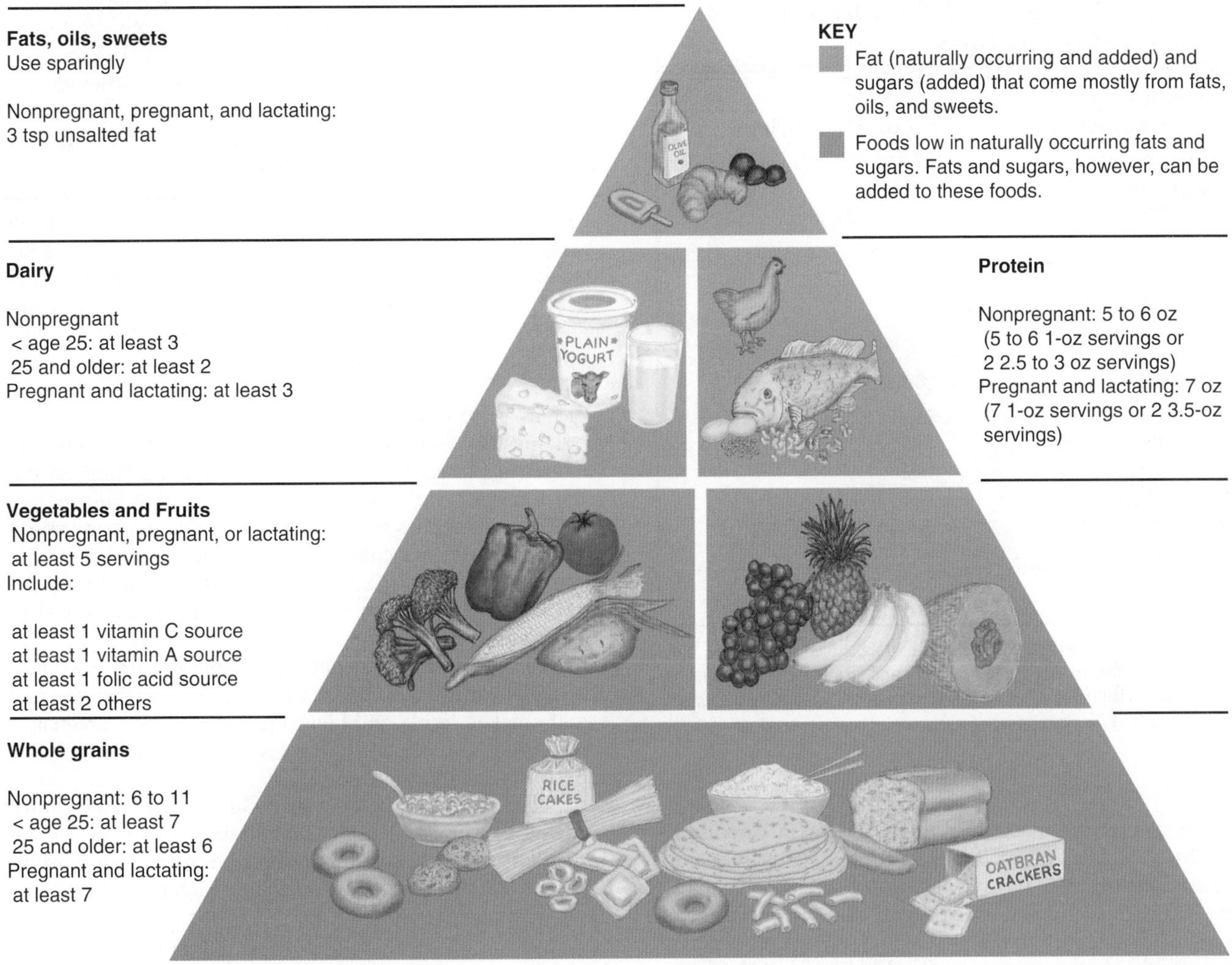

Fats, oils, sweets
Use sparingly

Nonpregnant, pregnant, and lactating:
3 tsp unsalted fat

KEY

▨ Fat (naturally occurring and added) and sugars (added) that come mostly from fats, oils, and sweets.

▨ Foods low in naturally occurring fats and sugars. Fats and sugars, however, can be added to these foods.

Dairy

Nonpregnant
< age 25: at least 3
25 and older: at least 2
Pregnant and lactating: at least 3

Protein

Nonpregnant: 5 to 6 oz
(5 to 6 1-oz servings or
2 2.5 to 3 oz servings)
Pregnant and lactating: 7 oz
(7 1-oz servings or 2 3.5-oz servings)

Vegetables and Fruits
Nonpregnant, pregnant, or lactating:
at least 5 servings
Include:

at least 1 vitamin C source
at least 1 vitamin A source
at least 1 folic acid source
at least 2 others

Whole grains

Nonpregnant: 6 to 11
< age 25: at least 7
25 and older: at least 6
Pregnant and lactating:
at least 7

Figure 15-2 Nutrient needs during pregnancy and lactation. Eating at least the number of servings listed meets the minimum nutrient need for pregnancy. Additional calories may be necessary to meet individual requirements. (Modified from California Department of Health Services, Maternal and Child Health. [1990]. *Nutrition during pregnancy and the postpartum period: A manual for health care professionals* [Summary]. Sacramento: Author; U.S. Department of Agriculture, 1992.)

Vegetables and Fruits

Vegetables and fruits form the next two groups of the Pyramid and are important sources of vitamins, minerals, and fiber. At least one food that provides vitamin C and one that provides vitamin A should be selected from the fruit and vegetable group each day. Healthy adults should have at least five servings of fruits and vegetables, with a range of three to five servings of vegetables and two to four servings of fruits. The pregnant or lactating woman needs the same amount.

Dairy Foods

Dairy foods include milk, yogurt, and cheese. They contain approximately the same nutrient values whether they are whole (4% fat), low fat (2% fat), or nonfat (skim), but the calories and fat are less in the latter two forms. Dairy products are especially good sources of calcium. Adults older than 25 years need two to three servings from this group each day. Younger women

and those who are pregnant or lactating need at least three servings.

In the past, calcium supplements and decreased milk intake were recommended to prevent leg cramps from an imbalance of calcium and phosphorus. However, the effectiveness of this treatment has not been proven (Fagen, 2000). Adding magnesium to the diet may offer some improvement, but more research is necessary.

Protein

Many adults think of meat, poultry, fish, and eggs as the only sources of protein, but legumes (beans, peas, lentils), nuts, and soybean products such as tofu are also good sources. Adults should consume 5 to 6 ounces of protein foods each day; pregnant or lactating women need 7 or more ounces. A typical serving of meat, fish, or poultry is approximately 3 ounces. Three ounces is about the size of a deck of playing cards.

BOX 15-4
Common "Hot" and "Cold" Foods: Southeast Asian and Hispanic Diets

Southeast Asian

"HOT" (YANG) FOODS	**"COLD" (YIN) FOODS**
Peppers, onions	Most fruits and juices
Meat and poultry	Flour
Fish and fish sauce	Cold fluids
Broth	Sour foods
Eggs	
Spices, sweets	

Hispanic

"HOT" FOODS	**"COLD" FOODS**
Potatoes, peas, onions, chili peppers	Most fruits and vegetables
Cheese, evaporated milk	Milk
Chicken, lamb	Fish
Flour tortillas	Corn tortillas
Chickpeas and kidney beans	Green and red beans

Although there are variations within cultural groups, foods considered "hot" are used for conditions thought to be "cold" and vice versa. This influences what women are willing to eat during pregnancy or illness, and these customs must be respected as part of nursing care.

Although fish are an excellent source of protein, certain precautions should be taken. Shark, swordfish, king mackerel, tuna, and tilefish often have high levels of mercury, which can damage the fetal central nervous system. Other types of fish may have smaller amounts of mercury. Women should restrict their intake of fish during pregnancy to 6 to 12 ounces a week (Evans, 2002). Raw fish should also be avoided (James, Mahomed, Stone, van Wijngaarden, & Hill, 2003).

Other Elements

The tip of the USDA's Food Guide Pyramid represents fats, oils, and concentrated sugars, which should be ingested sparingly. They provide calories for energy but few other nutrients. Three teaspoons of unsaturated fats per day are adequate for this group.

FACTORS THAT INFLUENCE NUTRITION

The nurse must consider cultural background, age, and knowledge about nutrition when counseling women about their diets.

Culture

Food may have special cultural meaning during pregnancy or childbirth. Nurses need knowledge about the habits of a variety of cultures so that they can provide culturally appropriate nutritional counseling. Before making assumptions about the influence of a woman's culture on her diet, the nurse must assess each woman individually. Not all women follow food practices considered typical for their culture.

The nurse should assess the woman's age, her length of time in North America, and whether she has adopted prevalent American eating habits. Some women who follow an American diet may return to some aspects of their culture's traditional diet during pregnancy to "be sure" they do not harm the fetus.

Nurses often use pamphlets as a part of teaching and may be able to obtain them in various languages.

The nurse should determine if the woman can read her own language before giving her written materials. People who cannot read may not readily admit it. In addition, the translation may be too complicated for the woman with little education to understand. Having an interpreter discuss the material with the woman helps discover whether she can read and aids in other teaching.

Many cultures believe that certain foods, conditions, and medicines are "hot" or "cold" and that they must maintain a balance to preserve health. Foods considered "hot" in one culture may not fit in that category in another culture, and the designation does not necessarily match the temperature of the food. In Asian cultures, this may be referred to as "yin" (cold) and "yang" (hot) and may influence what the mother eats during pregnancy and the postpartum period. Box 15-4 lists common "hot" and "cold" foods.

Food taboos also influence what some women eat during the childbearing period. For example, Korean women may avoid chicken, pork, and blemished fruits during pregnancy. These foods are thought to have a harmful effect on the infant's physical appearance.

Special foods may be customary during pregnancy or after birth. For example, a Korean family may bring the woman miyuk-kuk, a hot seaweed soup served to new mothers (Kim-Godwin, 2003). Hispanic women are encouraged to satisfy food cravings (Mattson, 2003).

Great variety exists in cultural preferences for foods. For instance, some African-Americans may follow a diet that is similar to that of people living in the southeastern United States. Common foods include okra, collards, mustard greens, ham hocks, black-eyed peas, and hominy or grits. The diets of other African-Americans, however, vary according to the geographic area in which they live.

Iron deficiency anemia occurs in 15% of African-American women of childbearing age, compared with 10% of white women (USDHHS, 2000). Lactose intolerance is common, resulting in lack of calcium if other sources are not present in the diet. Intake of high-sodium and fried foods may present health problems.

Some Jewish women follow a strictly kosher diet. This diet includes meat only from animals with cloven hooves (no pork) and processed to remove all blood. Milk and meat are not eaten in the same meal. Muslim women do not eat pork and may fast on certain days. The religion exempts pregnant and nursing women from obligatory fasting, but women may not always choose to omit fasting.

The diet of Native American women may contain corn, beans, and squash but lack fresh fruits and vegetables. Lactose intolerance is common, and milk is avoided. Fat, carbohydrate, sodium, and sugar intakes are often high. Low-income Native Americans living on reservations may receive foods such as white flour, corn meal, white rice, and processed meats from federal programs.

Food preferences for two cultures, Southeast Asian and Hispanic, are explored further here to show the influence of culture on diet. Immigrants and refugees from Southeast Asia are likely to continue following diets similar to those in their homelands. Hispanics are a large minority group in the United States, and nurses throughout the United States need information about Hispanic food preferences.

Southeast Asian Dietary Practices

Southeast Asians come from Cambodia, Laos, and Vietnam. Traditional cooking in these countries includes searing fresh vegetables quickly with a small portion of meat, poultry, or fish in a little oil over high heat. Meals cooked in this manner are low in fat and retain vitamins. Most meals are accompanied by rice, which increases the intake of complex carbohydrates. Soups are commonly served with meals. A salty fish sauce called *nuoc mam* and fresh vegetables are part of most meals.

Many Southeast Asians have added more American foods to their diets. The addition of more eggs, beef, pork, and bread has added nutrients but also fat to the diet. Coffee, candy, soft drinks, butter or margarine, and fast foods have been less favorable influences because they are low in nutrients but high in sugar or fat. Southeast Asians have decreased their intake of fish, a low-fat source of protein (Williams, 2003a).

Effect of Southeast Asian Culture on Diet During Childbearing. In Southeast Asian cultures, pregnancy, especially the third trimester, is considered "hot," and women eat "cold" foods to maintain a balance of hot and cold. Their diet includes sour foods, fruits, noodles, spinach, mung beans, and sweets and avoids fish, excessively salty or spicy foods, alcohol, and rice. The woman also avoids unfamiliar foods for fear that they may harm her or her fetus.

The postpartum period is considered "cold," partly because of the loss of blood, which is "hot." Mothers avoid losing more heat, which would have ill effects on their health. They stay warm physically and choose "hot" foods to eat, including rice with fish sauce, broth, salty meats, fish, chicken, and eggs. They may refuse cold drinks but welcome hot fluids, requesting tea or plain hot water. Families frequently bring food to the mother while she is in the hospital because hospital food may not meet her preferences.

The diet of Southeast Asians, especially those with low incomes, may be below recommended levels for energy, calcium, iron, zinc, magnesium, and vitamins B_6 and D, but high in sodium. These deficiencies may be of special concern during pregnancy. The woman can often increase her intake of needed nutrients without deviating greatly from her usual diet.

Increasing Nutrients With Traditional Foods. Milk products are not part of the traditional Southeast Asian diet, and lactose intolerance is common. Increasing the intake of commonly used dark-green leafy vegetables, such as mustard greens, bok choy, and broccoli, however, increases levels of calcium, iron, magnesium, and folic acid. Tofu contains good amounts of calcium and iron. A broth made from pork or chicken bones soaked in vinegar (which removes calcium from the bones) is frequently taken. If the mother avoids fortified milk, she may need vitamin D supplementation. Increasing the intake of meats or poultry elevates levels of vitamin B_6 and zinc.

Hispanic Dietary Practices

Spanish-speaking people, such as Mexican-Americans, Puerto Ricans, and Cuban-Americans, are often referred to as *Hispanics* or *Latinos*. Like Asians, Hispanics follow the theories of "hot" and "cold" foods and conditions. They also consider pregnancy to be "hot" and the postpartum period to be "cold" and adjust the diet accordingly.

Dried beans (especially pinto beans) are a staple of the Mexican-American diet and are part of most meals, either eaten alone, as refried beans, or mixed with other foods, such as rice. Corn or flour tortillas are eaten with most meals. Corn tortillas are a good source of calcium. Rice is also an important grain.

Although milk is not commonly drunk except by infants, cheese is part of many dishes. Chili peppers and tomatoes are the most common vegetables used. Green leafy and yellow vegetables are seldom included.

Hispanic foods are often hot and spicy and frequently fried. The diet is high in fiber and complex carbohydrates but also high in calories and fat. It may be low in iron, calcium, and vitamins A and D, which should be increased through foods or supplements during pregnancy.

Puerto Ricans and Cubans may add tropical fruits and vegetables from the homeland, when available. Viandas (starchy fruits and vegetables like plantain, green bananas, sweet potatoes, yams, and breadfruit) are common. They may be cooked with codfish and onion. Guava, papaya, mango, and eggplant are also used when available.

Age

Age is an important consideration. The adolescent who is not fully mature needs nutritional support for her own growth. Older women who are in good health, however, have the same nutritional requirements as younger pregnant women.

Nutritional Knowledge

Once pregnancy is confirmed, women often become interested in the relationship between what they eat and the effect on the fetus. Some lack basic understanding about nutrition and have misconceptions based on common food myths. They may seek out information from books, magazines, and the Internet. They benefit from help from nurses in learning about nutrition.

NUTRITIONAL RISK FACTORS

The nurse must identify risk factors that may interfere with a woman's ability to meet the nutritional needs of pregnancy.

Socioeconomic Status

Poverty

Low-income women may have deficient diets because of lack of financial resources and nutritional education. Carbohydrate foods are often less expensive than other foods. Therefore the diet may be high in calories but low in vitamins and minerals. A referral to Temporary Assistance for Needy Families (TANF) or the Special Supplemental Food Program for Women, Infants, and Children (WIC) may be helpful. Vitamin and mineral supplementation may be important for the woman, especially if her diet is inconsistent.

Food Supplement Programs

The WIC program is administered by the USDA to provide nutritional assessment, counseling, and education to low-income women and children up to age 5 years who are at nutritional risk. The program also provides food vouchers for foods such as milk, cheese, eggs, iron-fortified cereal, fruit juice, dried beans, peanut butter, and formula to qualified women and their children. Eligibility is based on an income below 185% of the federal poverty level. Women are eligible throughout pregnancy and for 6 months after birth if bottle-feeding or 1 year if breastfeeding.

Adolescence

Adolescent pregnancies are associated with higher risk for complications for both the expectant mother and the fetus (Chapter 25). Adolescents at greatest risk are the youngest in terms of gynecologic age (number of years since menarche) and those who are still growing. Growing adolescents continue to add fat to their own bodies in late pregnancy rather than use it for support of the fetus. As a result, they tend to have smaller infants even with good weight gains (Spear, 2000).

Weight gain for the young adolescent should be in the upper part of the range for her BMI.

Nutrient Needs

The DRIs for nutrients needed by pregnant adolescents are the same as those for older women for most nutrients. They need more calcium, magnesium, and phosphorus to meet their own growth needs. These amounts are adequate for most adolescents, but individualized assessment of gynecologic age, nutritional status, and daily diet may indicate the need for increases in some areas. More energy and iron may be needed for younger teens who are still growing.

Common Problems

The diets of teenagers may be low in vitamins C and A, folic acid, calcium, iron, and zinc (Schlenker, 2003). Supplements may be prescribed, but the adolescent may not take them regularly. This combination of poor intake and unreliable supplementation may further deplete nutrient stores and general nutrition.

Peer pressure is an important influence on nutritional status. Adolescents are often concerned about their body image. If weight is a major focus for a teenager and her peers, she may restrict calories to avoid weight gain during pregnancy. Teenagers tend to skip meals, especially breakfast. The fetus requires a steady supply of nutrients, and the expectant mother's stores may be used if intake is not sufficient to meet fetal needs.

Teenagers are often in a hurry, and they want foods that are fast and convenient. Meals may be irregular and often eaten away from home. Fast foods from restaurants or snack machines are a significant part of many teenagers' diets. These foods may be high in calories, fat, and sodium yet low in vitamins, minerals, and fiber. Iron, calcium, riboflavin, vitamins A and C and folic acid are likely to be low in fast foods (Spear, 2000). Choosing fast foods that do not make her appear different to her peers yet meet her added nutrient needs is important.

Teaching the Adolescent

Teaching the adolescent about nutrition can be a challenge for nurses. It is essential to establish an accepting, relaxed atmosphere and show willingness to listen to the teenager's

TABLE 15-4 Food Plan for Pregnant or Lactating Vegetarians

Food	Number of Servings for Pregnancy	Number of Servings for Lactation
Whole and enriched grains	6	6
Protein-rich foods: legumes, nuts, soy, meat substitutes, eggs, dairy	7	8
Vegetables	4	4
Fruits	2	2
Fats	2	2
Calcium-rich foods (included in the above food group servings)	8	8

A serving of a calcium-rich food is also counted as a serving of one of the other food groups. Adolescents need 6 servings of protein-rich foods and 10 servings of calcium-rich foods. Vitamin and mineral supplements may be necessary according to individual needs.
Data from Messina, V., Melina, V., & Mangels, A.R. (2003). A new food guide for North American vegetarians. *Journal of the American Dietetic Association,* *103*(6), 771-775.

concerns. Her lifestyle, pattern of eating, and food likes and dislikes should be explored.

In making suggestions, the nurse should focus on only those changes that are necessary. Suggestions should be kept to a minimum, and snacks should be included in the meal plan. Asking for the adolescent's input increases the likelihood that she will follow suggestions. When changes are necessary, the nurse should explain the reasons. A teenager, like other pregnant women, often makes changes for the sake of her unborn child that she would not consider for herself alone.

The need to be like her peers is of major importance to the adolescent, especially when she is going through the changes of pregnancy. With education about what foods to choose, she can eat fast foods with her friends and still maintain a nourishing diet. Giving her plenty of examples of alternatives from which she can choose should be very helpful.

Vegetarianism

Although the vegetarian may eat a very nutritional diet, she is at higher risk during pregnancy. If she is new to vegetarian food practices, uninformed about pregnancy needs, or careless with her diet, she could fail to meet her nutrient needs. Guidelines for vegetarian foods during pregnancy (see Table 15-4) are similar to the Food Guide Pyramid groups followed by nonvegetarians.

Vegetarianism occurs in a variety of forms. Vegans avoid all animal products and may have the most difficulty meeting their nutrient needs. Their diet may be lacking in adequate calcium, iron, zinc, and vitamins D and B_{12} (Grodner et al., 2000). It is easier for lactovegetarians, ovovegetarians, and lacto-ovovegetarians to meet their nutrient needs.

Meeting the Nutritional Requirements of the Pregnant Vegetarian

Energy. Vegetarian diets are low in calories and fat and may not meet the energy needs of pregnancy. The diets are high in fiber and may cause a feeling of fullness before enough

Nursing Care Plan

Nutrition for the Pregnant Adolescent

ASSESSMENT

Vicki, age 15, is 20 weeks pregnant and has gained 4.5 kg (10 lb). Her 24-hour diet history shows areas of deficiency and many food dislikes. Vicki skips breakfast and eats from snack machines and fast-food restaurants for lunch and after school. Vicki says she is disgusted with how heavy she is and wants to go on a diet to lose some weight. Her hemoglobin is 10.4 g/dl. She appears interested in nutrition, and her statements show concern about her baby's needs. Vicki's weight was normal before her pregnancy, and a weight gain of approximately 16 kg (35 lb) is appropriate for her. Her gynecologic age is 2½ years.

Nursing Diagnosis

Imbalanced Nutrition: Less Than Body Requirements related to concern about weight gain and diet choices inadequate to meet nutrient requirements of adolescent pregnancy.

Expected Outcomes

Vicki will
- Choose a diet that meets the recommended servings from each food group for adolescent pregnancy.
- Gain approximately 1 to 1¼ lb (0.44 to 0.57 kg) a week for the rest of her pregnancy.
- Maintain a hemoglobin level above 10.5 g/dl throughout her pregnancy.

INTERVENTION	RATIONALE
1. Praise Vicki for her interest in nutrition and her concern about gaining too much weight.	1. Praise helps foster rapport and may focus attention on learning.
2. Discuss the reasons for appropriate weight gain during pregnancy and its effect on the fetus.	2. Adolescents may not understand how diet affects the fetus and themselves during pregnancy.
3. Assist Vicki in comparing her food intake with the recommended servings from each food group. Point out areas of strength, and praise her for these.	3. Active involvement of the learner and positive reinforcement help increase motivation.
4. Ask Vicki what problems she sees in her diet. Point out areas she may have missed. Explain the effect that lack of specific nutrients may have on the fetus.	4. Adolescents learn best when they see how the material applies to them.
5. Discuss the high caloric intake of fast foods in relation to her present diet. Discuss "spending calories" to "buy" nutrients needed during pregnancy.	5. Relating information to concepts already understood increases understanding.
6. Determine, from Vicki's food preferences, low-calorie foods to meet her nutrient needs. Point out fruits and vegetables high in vitamins A and C yet low in calories.	6. Individualizing the recommended diet to meet the woman's likes and dislikes increases compliance.
7. Suggest nutritional foods that Vicki could choose at fast-food restaurants, and ask which ones are acceptable to her.	7. The adolescent needs to feel that she is part of her peer group. Including her input on what she likes to eat may increase her compliance.
8. Discuss the importance of breakfast during pregnancy. Explain that the fetus needs a steady supply of nutrients and needs food in the morning after the long fast during the night.	8. Prolonged periods without maternal food intake can lead to a state of ketosis that is hostile to the fetus.
9. Discuss breakfast foods and the nutrients found in whole-grain breads and cereals.	9. Whole grains are often part of a well-balanced breakfast.
10. Suggest that Vicki eat foods not usually considered breakfast foods if she prefers. For example, cold pizza provides calcium and protein.	10. Nontraditional methods of meeting the adolescent's nutritional needs may be very effective.
11. Suggest foods high in nutrient density that are available from snack dispensers. Ask which of these are acceptable to Vicki.	11. Adolescents are unlikely to give up foods that help them feel part of their peer group.

Continued

Nursing Care Plan

Nutrition for the Pregnant Adolescent—cont'd

INTERVENTION—cont'd	RATIONALE—cont'd
12. Ask Vicki if she is willing to eat more dairy products after explaining their importance to her and her baby. Ask her to help plan which ones she will eat to meet her needed intake.	12. Compliance is increased when clients maintain a feeling of control.
13. Reinforce the importance of consistent intake of vitamin-mineral supplements. Offer suggestions on how to deal with any problems she is having in this area.	13. Adolescents generally need supplements but may be inconsistent in taking them, especially if they experience side effects.
14. Ask Vicki to bring in another 24-hour diet history on her next visit.	14. Reassessment of dietary intake identifies new or continuing problems.
15. Ask Vicki to share ways she has found to meet her diet needs that you could tell other teenagers. Ask for feedback on the methods discussed.	15. It is important for the adolescent to feel that the nurse values her thoughts and ideas.

Evaluation

Vicki's 24-hour diet histories show that she is meeting the recommendations for each food group. She gains 1.8 to 2.7 kg (4 to 6 lb) a month throughout the rest of her pregnancy, for a total weight gain of 15 kg (33 lb). Her hemoglobin level rises to 11 g/dl. A healthy 3.4-kg (7½-lb) baby girl is born at term.

Additional Nursing Diagnoses to Consider

- Disturbed Body Image
- Situational Low Self-Esteem

---

calories are eaten. A pregnant woman can increase caloric intake by eating between-meal snacks or higher-calorie foods. If carbohydrate and fat intake are too low, her body may use protein for energy.

Protein. Protein intake may be a concern in vegetarian diets. "Complete" proteins contain all the essential amino acids the body cannot synthesize from other sources. Animal proteins are complete, but plant proteins lack one or more of the essential amino acids. Combining incomplete plant proteins with other plant foods that have complementary amino acids allows intake of all essential amino acids. Dishes that contain grains (wheat, rice, corn) and legumes (garbanzo, navy, kidney, pinto or soy beans; peas; peanuts) are combinations that provide complete proteins. Complementary proteins do not have to be eaten at the same meal if they are consumed in a single day. Tofu, made from soybeans, is often used by vegetarians to provide protein.

Incomplete proteins can also be combined with small amounts of complete protein foods like cheese to provide all amino acids. Therefore women who include even small amounts of animal products have less difficulty meeting their protein needs.

Calcium. Vegetarians who include milk products in their diet may meet their pregnancy needs for calcium. Vegans obtain calcium from vegetables, but their high-fiber diet may interfere with calcium absorption. Calcium-fortified soy products, such as soy milk or tofu, may meet the requirements, or calcium supplements may be necessary. Vitamin D supplementation is especially important if the woman drinks no milk and has little exposure to sunlight. Soy milks may be enriched with vitamin D.

Iron. Iron in the vegetarian diet is poorly absorbed because of the lack of heme iron (from meats), which improves absorption. Absorption is enhanced by eating a vitamin C source at the same meal as the nonheme iron. Iron supplementation may be important for vegetarian women during pregnancy.

Zinc. The best sources of zinc are meat and fish. Vegans may be deficient in this mineral and need supplements to meet their needs.

Vitamin B_{12}. Vitamin B_{12} is obtained only from animal products. Because vegetarian diets contain large amounts of folic acid, anemia caused by inadequate intake of vitamin B_{12} may not be apparent at first. Vegans may eat fortified foods such as cereal and soy products or take B_{12} supplements.

Vitamin A. Vitamin A is abundant in vegetarian diets. If the woman takes a daily multiple vitamin-mineral supplement, she may experience toxic effects, such as anorexia, irritability, hair loss, dry skin, and damage to the fetus from excessive intake of vitamin A. Supplementation should be individualized for each woman, based on her diet and her needs.

Lactose Intolerance

Intolerance of lactose is caused by deficiency of the small intestine enzyme *lactase*, necessary for absorption of the milk sugar *lactose*. Some degree of lactose intolerance is normal for most of the world's population after early childhood. Groups with a high incidence of lactose intolerance include many African-American, Hispanic, Asian, Native American, and Middle Eastern women. Although women with lactose intolerance may tolerate cultured or fermented milk products, such as aged cheese, buttermilk, and some brands of yogurt, symptoms may occur after drinking as little as a cup of milk. Symptoms include nausea, bloating, flatulence, diarrhea, and intestinal cramping.

Although the ability to tolerate lactose may increase during pregnancy, women who avoid dairy foods may not consume the recommended amounts of calcium. Most women tolerate small amounts ($\frac{1}{2}$ cup) of milk with meals, and they should increase their intake of other foods that provide calcium. Soy milk, low-lactose milk, and milk treated with lactase are available. The enzyme can be purchased to be added to milk or taken as a tablet. Calcium supplements may be necessary for some lactose-intolerant women.

Nausea and Vomiting of Pregnancy

Morning sickness usually ends with the first trimester, but some women experience nausea at other times of the day and for longer than 12 weeks. These women are often able to manage frequent, small meals better than three large meals. Protein and complex carbohydrates are tolerated best, but fatty foods increase nausea. Drinking liquids between meals instead of with meals often helps. At bedtime, a protein snack such as cheese helps maintain glucose levels through the night. Eating a carbohydrate food like dry toast or crackers before getting out of bed in the morning helps prevent nausea.

Anemia

Anemia is a common concern during pregnancy. Hemoglobin values drop during the second trimester of pregnancy as a result of the dilution of the blood caused by plasma increases. This is often called *physiologic anemia* because it is normal (see Chapter 13). During the third trimester, hemoglobin levels generally return to prepregnancy levels because of increased absorption of iron from the gastrointestinal tract, even though iron is transferred to the fetus primarily during this time. Fetal iron stores during the third trimester are sufficient to prevent anemia in the newborn for the first 4 to 6 months after birth.

Iron stores may be measured by determining the serum ferritin level in the blood. A ferritin level less than 10 micrograms per liter (μg/L) indicates that the anemia is caused by iron deficiency (Pagana & Pagana, 2001). Generally, a woman is considered anemic if her hemoglobin is less than 11 g/dl during the first and third trimesters or less than 10.5 during the second trimester (Cunningham et al., 2001). A *Healthy People 2010* goal is to reduce iron deficiency anemia in females of childbearing age from the baseline of 11% to 7% and to reduce anemia in low-income pregnant women in the third trimester from the baseline of 29% to 20% (USDHHS, 2000).

Anemic women need iron supplements and help in choosing foods high in iron (see Box 15-2). Iron supplements are better absorbed if taken between meals or at bedtime with a dietary source of vitamin C to increase absorption. Because high intakes of iron inhibit the body's use of zinc and copper, anemic women may need to take these minerals also.

Abnormal Prepregnancy Weight

In addition to teaching about dietary changes, the nurse should be alert for other problems associated with abnormal prepregnancy weight. The woman who is below normal weight may not have enough money for food or may have an eating disorder. An obese woman may have other health problems, such as hypertension or gestational diabetes, that may affect the nurse's nutritional counseling plan.

Eating Disorders

Eating disorders include anorexia nervosa (refusal to eat because of a distorted body image and feelings of obesity) and bulimia (overeating, sometimes followed by induced vomiting). Women with anorexia often have amenorrhea and do not become pregnant. Women with eating disorders are likely to have medical complications as well as complications of pregnancy and birth. Some women eat normally during pregnancy for the sake of the fetus, but others continue their previous eating patterns during pregnancy or in the early postpartum period when they do not lose weight immediately. They need a great deal of individual counseling to be sure that they meet the increased nutrient needs of pregnancy and understand normal postpartum weight loss.

Pica

The practice of eating nonnutritive substances not normally considered food is called *pica*. Ice, clay or dirt, and solid laundry starch are the most common materials involved, but other items, such as chalk, freezer frost, baking soda, burnt matches, or ashes, may be included. Pica is more common in the southeastern United States, in African-Americans, and in women who live in poverty and have poor nutrition. However, pica is not limited to any one socioeconomic group or geographic area.

The cause of pica is unknown, although cultural values may make pica a common practice. Pica may be related to beliefs about the effect of the material eaten on labor or the baby. Some women may fear that their eating habits are harmful but may be unable to ignore the cravings. They often keep their eating practices secret from caregivers who might disapprove.

The major concern with pica is that it decreases the intake of foods and, therefore, essential nutrients. Iron deficiency was once thought to be a cause of pica but is now considered a result. Clay and dirt in the gut may decrease the absorption of nutrients such as iron, be contaminated with organisms, and cause intestinal blockage (Grodner et al., 2000). It may also contain toxic substances such as lead.

CRITICAL THINKING EXERCISE 15-1

A pregnant woman very hesitantly confides that the reason she is not gaining much weight is that she eats large amounts of ice. She buys bags of crushed ice daily. "I know I should be gaining more weight, but I'm just not hungry for anything besides ice," she says.

1. How should the nurse handle this situation?

Multiparity

The number and spacing of pregnancies as well as the presence of more than one fetus influence nutritional requirements. The woman who has had more than five pregnancies may begin a pregnancy with a nutritional deficit. In addition, she may be too busy meeting the needs of her family to be attentive to her own nutritional needs.

Closely spaced pregnancies may not allow a woman to make up any nutritional deficits originating during a previous pregnancy. Thus she begins a new pregnancy with inadequate nutrient stores to maintain her own needs and fetal requirements. Morning sickness from a new pregnancy may further interfere with an expectant mother's ability to eat an adequate diet.

The woman with a multifetal pregnancy must provide enough nutrients to meet the needs of each fetus without depleting her own stores. The suggested weight gain for women pregnant with twins is 10 to 20 lb more than for women with single pregnancies. Supplementation with calcium, iron, and folic acid may also be necessary.

Substance Use and Abuse

Substance abuse often accompanies a lifestyle that is unlikely to promote good eating habits. The expense of supporting a substance abuse habit may decrease the amount of money available to purchase food. Therefore nutrition in pregnant women who abuse substances should be explored fully. Usually more than one substance is involved, and the effects on nutrition of various combinations of substances are not fully understood. The damaging effects of smoking, alcohol, and drug use on the fetus are discussed in Chapter 25.

Smoking

Cigarette smoking increases maternal metabolic rate and decreases appetite, which may result in a lower weight gain. Infant birth weight decreases in spite of adequate diet as the amount of smoking increases. Prematurity, spontaneous abortion, and other complications may also result. Smoking decreases the availability of some vitamins and minerals, and vitamin-mineral supplements are important during pregnancy. Counseling to help the woman stop smoking or at least decrease the number of cigarettes smoked during pregnancy is essential.

Caffeine

The effect of caffeine on nutrition during pregnancy is controversial. Most studies show no association between caffeine and preterm labor or congenital defects, but more research is needed. Caffeine changes calcium, zinc, and iron absorption or excretion. Until more is known about its effects on nutrition and the fetus, caffeine intake should be limited during pregnancy to 300 mg/day (equal to 2-3 cups of coffee, 6 cups of tea, or 5 carbonated beverages with caffeine). The nurse should discuss other sources of caffeine including chocolate and some medications.

Alcohol

Because of the association between drinking and fetal alcohol syndrome (see Chapter 25), women should avoid alcohol completely during pregnancy. Alcohol interferes with the absorption and use of protein, thiamine, folic acid, and zinc; impairs metabolism; and often takes the place of food in the diet. Vitamin-mineral supplementation may be necessary for women whose intake of alcohol before pregnancy was large, because their nutrient stores may be depleted.

Drugs

The use of drugs other than those prescribed during pregnancy increases danger to the fetus and may interfere with nutrition. Abusers often use a combination of various drugs. The interaction of various drugs with nutrients is not fully understood.

Marijuana increases appetite, but women may not satisfy their hunger with foods of good nutrient quality. Heroin interferes with insulin response to glucose and metabolism. Heroin may therefore cause the woman to be malnourished. Cocaine acts as an appetite suppressant, interfering with nutrient intake. Cocaine users tend to drink more beverages with alcohol or caffeine. Amphetamines depress appetite. Women who use amphetamines for dieting should be warned that the drugs should be discontinued during pregnancy.

Other Risk Factors

Women who follow food fads may not meet the nutritional requirements of pregnancy. Each diet must be carefully analyzed to determine its nutrient content. Women who have followed a severely restricted diet for a long period of time may have depleted nutrient stores. The nurse can help them understand nutrition and what diet changes they need to make during pregnancy.

Women with complications of pregnancy, such as diabetes, heart disease, and pregnancy-induced hypertension, may need dietary alterations. Those with other medical conditions, such as extreme obesity, cystic fibrosis, and celiac disease, may need nutritional counseling from a dietitian.

NUTRITION AFTER BIRTH

Nutritional requirements after birth depend on whether the mother breastfeeds her infant or gives formula. If the mother plans to breastfeed, the nurse should teach her how to adapt her diet to meet the needs of lactation. If the mother plans to use formula, the nurse can review the woman's nutritional knowledge as she returns to her prepregnancy diet.

Nutrition for the Lactating Mother

The DRIs for lactating women are higher than the needs of nonpregnant adult women for almost every nutrient (see Table 15-2). DRIs are lower for iron, niacin, folic acid, and magnesium. Lactating women with poor diets may have reduced milk levels of iodine and some of the B vitamins (Fagen, 2000). Milk volume is usually adequate for the infant even if a mother's diet is less than optimal.

Energy

The RDA for energy during the first 6 months of lactation is 500 calories each day above the normal needs for women according to age, weight, and height. Another 140 calories a day is drawn from maternal stores to produce breast milk for a total of 640 calories needed each day.

Protein

The RDA for protein is 71 grams each day during pregnancy and lactation. Although there is no change in protein needed, it is important for the woman to keep up her protein intake throughout the breastfeeding period.

Vitamins and Minerals

Lactating women who take in at least 1800 calories (which is well below the energy intake recommended) probably consume adequate amounts of other essential nutrients to meet the infant's and their own needs. The vitamin content of the milk may be decreased if the mother's diet is consistently low in vitamins. Mineral levels in the milk may remain constant because some minerals, such as calcium, are drawn from the mother's stores if her intake is poor. Routine vitamin-mineral supplements are not necessary unless there is concern that the diet is lacking in vitamins or minerals.

Specific Nutritional Concerns

Some women are unlikely to consume all the nutrients they require, and they need special counseling.

Dieting. Women who are concerned about losing weight after pregnancy need special consideration. After the initial losses in the first month, weight gradually decreases as maternal fat is used to meet a portion of the energy needs of lactation. Breastfeeding mothers tend to lose body fat even without dieting (Grodner et al., 2000). However, breastfeeding does not necessarily result in weight loss and 20% of women maintain or even gain weight during lactation (Matteson, 2001). This is more likely when weight gain during pregnancy was excessive.

Dieting should be postponed for at least 3 weeks after birth to allow the woman to recover fully from childbirth and establish her milk supply if she is breastfeeding. Gradual weight loss is preferable and should be accomplished by a combination of moderate exercise and a diet high in nutrients, with at least 1800 calories per day. Weight loss of 500 g weekly is safe and does not affect infant growth (Lovelady, Garner, Moreno, & Williams, 2000). Nursing mothers should avoid appetite suppressants, which may pass into the milk and harm the infant.

Adolescence. The problems of the adolescent diet continue to be of concern during lactation. The adolescent may be deficient in the same nutrients listed for other mothers during lactation, and she may also be lacking in iron. If she avoids fruits and vegetables, her intake of vitamin A may be inadequate.

Vegan Diet. The milk of the vegan mother may contain inadequate vitamin B_{12}, and she and her infant may need supplements. The amounts of vitamin D and calcium in the diet may also be low. Vegans can meet their need for other nutrients during lactation by diet alone with careful planning. Those who are not knowledgeable about nutrition should take supplements.

Avoidance of Dairy Products. The recommendation for calcium remains the same for pregnancy and lactation, and the calcium content of breast milk is not affected by maternal intake. Less calcium is excreted in the urine during lactation. Calcium is removed from the mother's bones during lactation but replaced when she is no longer breastfeeding (Witt & Mihok, 2003). Prolonged lactation with inadequate calcium intake, however, may cause excessive loss of calcium

from the mother's bones. Women who do not eat dairy products should obtain calcium from other sources or take a calcium supplement. Unless they consume foods fortified with vitamin D or have exposure to sunlight, they may also need to take vitamin D supplements.

Inadequate Diet. Women who have cultural or other food prohibitions may need help choosing a diet adequate for lactation. Those with inadequate income may need referral to social agencies and programs such as WIC. If the mother must take medications that interfere with absorption of certain nutrients, her diet should be high in foods containing those nutrients.

Alcohol. Although it was once thought that the relaxing effect of alcohol would be helpful to the nursing mother, the deleterious effects of alcohol are too important for this suggestion to be considered appropriate today. An occasional single alcoholic beverage may not be detrimental, but larger amounts may interfere with the milk-ejection reflex and be harmful to the infant.

Caffeine. Foods high in caffeine should also be limited. The mother should restrict her caffeine intake to two cups of coffee or the equivalent each day. Caffeine in excessive amounts may make the infant irritable and may decrease the iron content of the milk.

Fluids

Nursing mothers should drink fluids sufficient to relieve thirst, which often increases in the early breastfeeding period. Eight to ten glasses of fluids, other than those containing caffeine, is adequate.

Foods to Avoid

Lactating mothers are often concerned about whether they should avoid certain foods that might adversely affect the infant. Most mothers find that few foods affect the infant and that fussiness is related to other factors. If the family history places the infant at risk for developing allergies, the woman should avoid highly allergenic foods including cow's milk, eggs, fish, and nuts (AAP, 2000).

If an infant shows signs of reacting to something in the mother's diet (excessive irritability, crying as if in pain, passing gas, diarrhea, or rash), the mother should review what she ate during the previous 8 to 12 hours. Foods that may cause a problem for some infants include the cabbage family, onions, garlic, nuts, chocolate, large amounts of fresh fruits, and highly allergenic, spicy, or acidic (orange juice) foods. Eliminating the suspected food from the mother's diet and then trying it again can often pinpoint whether it was the cause of the problem.

Nutrition for the Nonlactating Mother

The postpartum woman who is not breastfeeding can return to her prepregnancy diet, provided that it meets the RDAs for the adult woman. Her diet should contain protein and vitamin C foods to promote healing. She may continue to take her prenatal vitamin-mineral supplements until her supply is finished. This supplementation ensures adequate intake during the early weeks and helps renew nutrient stores.

The nurse should assess the mother's understanding of the number of servings she needs from each food group. A review of important nutrient sources for calcium and iron may be relevant. If a woman was anemic during pregnancy, an iron supplement is important until the hemoglobin value returns to normal.

When her baby is born, a woman can expect to lose about 12 lb immediately. She loses approximately another 8 lb during the early weeks and probably all but about 2 lb by the end of the first year if she follows a well-balanced diet. To avoid retaining weight, she should take in 300 calories per day less than she did during pregnancy.

Some women are impatient with slow weight loss. Because they need energy to meet the demands of infant care, new mothers should wait at least 3 weeks to start dieting to lose weight. Suggestions for sensible calorie reduction combined with exercise are appropriate. Women who gain excess weight during pregnancy may have more difficulty losing it after birth and may need help from a dietitian in planning a weight loss program.

Mothers may snack instead of planning meals for themselves, especially during the early weeks. The nurse should remind them that snacking often involves high caloric intake without meeting nutritional needs. Meals and snacks should be high in nutrient content.

■NURSING CARE
Nutrition for Childbearing

Assessment

Interview
The interview provides an opportunity to develop rapport and to determine whether any specific problems are present that affect dietary intake.

Appetite Begin the interview by discussing the woman's appetite. Morning sickness may decrease food intake during the first trimester. Determine the severity and duration of nausea and vomiting. Hyperemesis gravidarum is the most serious form of this problem, often requiring intravenous correction of fluid and electrolyte imbalance (see Chapter 26).

Eating Habits Assess the usual pattern of meals to discover poor food habits, such as skipping breakfast or eating only snack foods for lunch. Determine who does the cooking for the family. If someone else does the cooking, discuss nutritional needs during pregnancy with that person.

Food Preferences Ask about the woman's food preferences and dislikes. During pregnancy, some women experience an aversion to certain foods, such as meats, that they do not have at other times. Determine whether she has food cravings or eats large amounts of any one particular food or group of foods. Discuss pica in a matter-of-fact way to avoid giving an impression of disapproval.

In assessing for pica, you might say, "Have you had cravings for special things to eat during your pregnancy?" This can be followed by "Women sometimes eat things like ice, clay, or starch during pregnancy. Have you tried these?" This provides an opening for a discussion of substitutes, such as nonfat dry milk powder for laundry starch, the woman may be willing to try.

Psychosocial Influences Identify factors that interfere with adequate nutrition. Women with low incomes may not know about sources of help. Question the vegetarian to

determine how long she has followed the practice and her awareness of changes necessary during pregnancy. A woman's smoking habits, alcohol intake, and substance abuse may become obvious during the interview. Determine whether she takes medications that interfere with nutrient absorption. Ask whether cultural or religious considerations affect the woman's diet. Provide an opportunity for the woman to ask about special diet concerns. This may bring out fears about weight gain, worry that specific foods could hurt the fetus, or other issues not yet addressed.

Diet History Diet histories provide information about a woman's usual intake of nutrients. They form a basis for counseling about any changes required to meet pregnancy needs.

Twenty-Four-Hour Diet History Ask the woman to recall what she ate at each meal and snack during the previous 24 hours. Use specific questions about the size of portions and ingredients used. Inquire about beverages as well as food snacks. Determine whether this sample is typical of her usual daily food intake; if not, ask which foods are more representative. Analyze the 24-hour diet history to determine whether the woman has met the recommendations for specific food groups, calories, and protein. Detailed analysis for individual nutrients is unnecessary.

Food Intake Records Food intake records are used to report foods eaten over one or more days. Ask the woman to list everything she eats throughout the day. The list is more accurate if she writes down each food immediately after eating.

Food-Frequency Questionnaires Use of food-frequency questionnaires provides information about diet over a longer period. Ask the woman how often she eats each of the common foods listed. Analyze the list to determine whether foods from each food group are eaten in adequate amounts to meet pregnancy needs.

Physical Assessment
Information about nutritional status includes measurement of weight and examination for signs of nutritional deficiency.

Weight at Initial Visit To get a baseline value for future comparison, weigh the woman at the first prenatal visit. Ask if this is her usual weight or if she has gained or lost weight. Measure her height without shoes. If her weight is low for height, nutritional reserves are marginal. If it is high, she may be overweight or obese.

Weight at Subsequent Visits Weigh the woman at each visit on the same scale with approximately the same amount of clothing. Record the weight on a weight grid at each visit throughout the pregnancy (Figure 15-3). This grid allows examination of the pattern as well as the total gain to date. It also helps show the weight gain between individual visits.

Be careful not to overemphasize weight gain. In some instances, a woman may be afraid that caregivers will be disapproving if she gains weight and consequently she may diet or fast a day or two before her prenatal visit.

Signs of Nutrient Deficiency Observe for indications of nutritional status or signs of deficiency. For example, bleeding gums may indicate inadequate intake of vitamin C. Actual deficiency states, however, are not likely to occur in women in most industrialized countries. The exception is iron defi-

Trimester

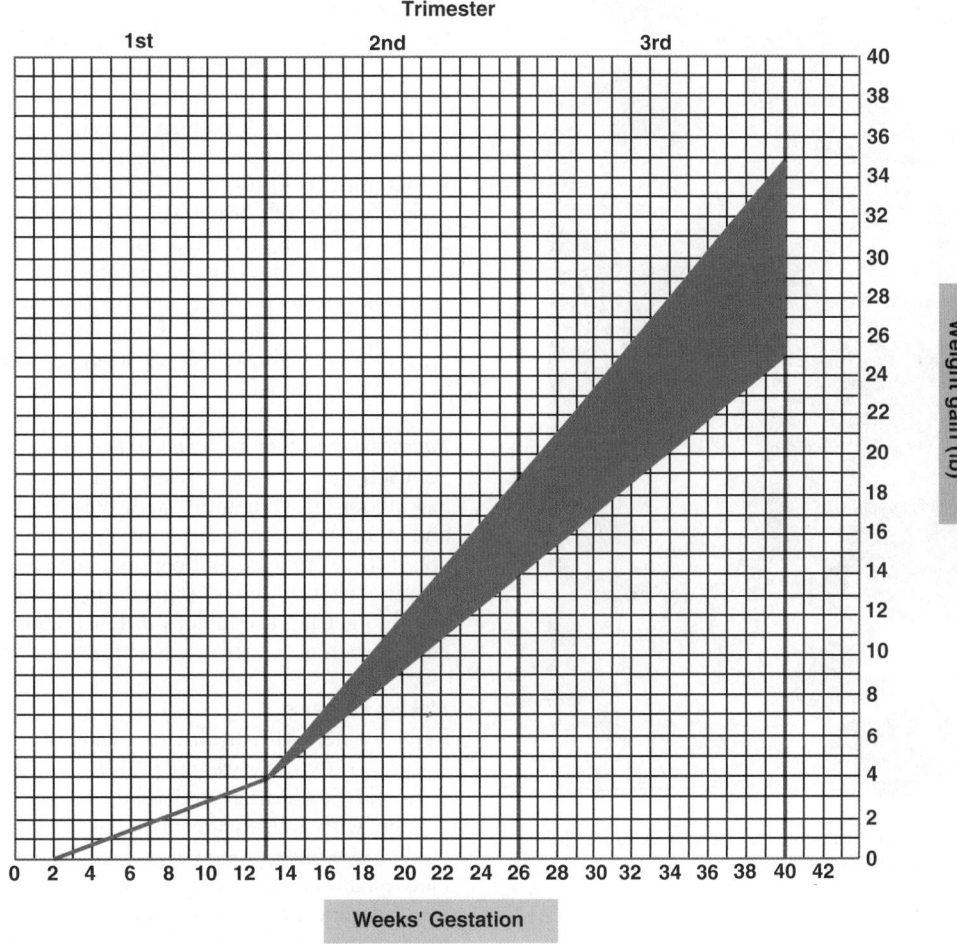

Figure 15-3 Weight-gain grid for pregnancy. The normal range for weight gain is 25 to 35 lb. Adolescents often need to gain in the higher end of the range. Women who are shorter than 62 inches should gain in the lower portion.

ciency anemia, which is common in a mild form. Signs and symptoms include pallor, low hemoglobin level, fatigue, and increased susceptibility to infection.

Laboratory Tests
Laboratory tests for in-depth analysis of nutrient intake are generally impractical. Hemoglobin, hematocrit, and in some cases serum ferritin levels may be measured to detect anemia, particularly iron deficiency anemia.

Nursing Diagnosis and Planning
Although some women consume more calories than they need during pregnancy, the most important nursing diagnosis concerning nutrition is:

■ Imbalanced Nutrition: Less Than Body Requirements related to lack of understanding about the nutrient needs of pregnancy.
   Expected Outcomes: The woman's diet will follow the recommended number of servings for each food group for pregnancy. The woman (with a normal BMI before pregnancy) will gain approximately 1.4 to 1.8 kg (3 to 4 lb) during the first trimester and 0.44 kg (1 lb) per week during the second and third trimesters, for a total gain of 11.5 to 16 kg (25 to 35 lb).

Interventions
Identifying Problems
Identify any obvious areas of potential deficiency. For example, the woman might eat little meat, avoid vegetables, be lactose intolerant, or follow a vegetarian diet. Also determine the woman's knowledge about nutritional needs during pregnancy.

Explaining Nutrient Needs
Use the woman's diet history as a basis to introduce information about nutrition during pregnancy. Help the woman analyze her own diet for the number of food group servings included so that she understands the process. Explain which important nutrients are provided in each food group and why they are necessary for her and for the fetus.

Make a rough estimate of calories, protein, iron, folic acid, and calcium in the diet. To help her determine whether she eats enough of these foods on a regular basis, compare the usual sources of these major nutrients with her diet history and favorite foods. Suggest ways she can increase her intake of nutrients that she is lacking by increasing servings of specific food groups.

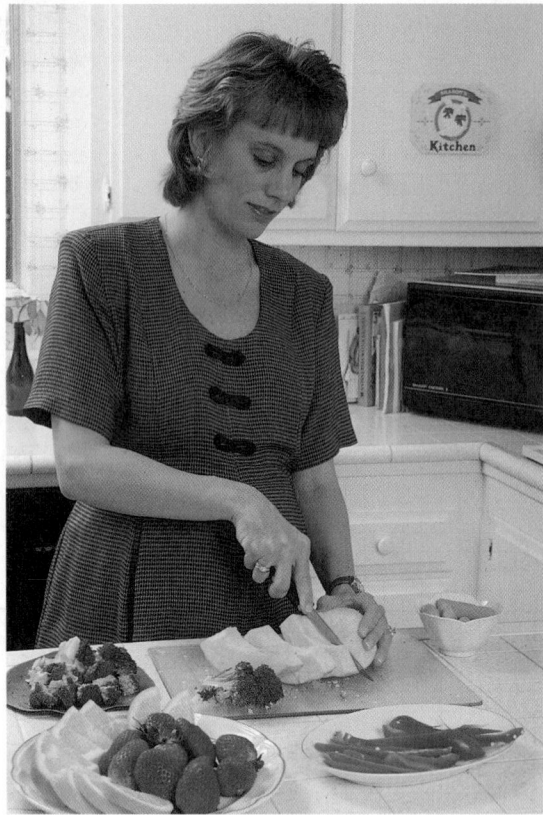

Figure 15-4 Women often make changes in their diets for the sake of their unborn child that they would not consider for themselves alone.

Providing Reinforcement

Give frequent positive reinforcement when the woman is eating appropriately. Assist her in evaluating where changes in her diet may be necessary, and plan ways to overcome weaknesses in her present diet (Fig. 15-4).

If the woman can read, give her written materials on nutrition during pregnancy and review them with her. A small pamphlet with pictures might be placed on the refrigerator to help her remember what foods she needs each day.

Evaluating Weight Gain

Compare the woman's weight with a weight-gain grid to ascertain whether she has gained the appropriate amount of weight for this point in her pregnancy. Discuss the importance and expected pattern of weight gain for her. Explain the concept of eating foods high in nutrient density when she is increasing calories.

For women of normal weight, a monthly gain of less than 2 lb (1 kg) should lead to a discussion of possible problems in food intake. A gain of more than 6½ lb (3 kg) per month may signify a serious problem such as pregnancy-induced hypertension (see Chapter 26). Errors in calculation of gestation may, however, also reflect a pattern of weight gain different from that expected.

Reassessing Nutritional Status at Each Visit

At each prenatal visit, reassess the woman's dietary status. Ask about any difficulties with her diet. Check weight gain and evaluate hemoglobin and hematocrit levels, if appropriate. If the woman is taking vitamin-mineral supplements, determine whether she is taking them regularly. Suggest ways to avoid forgetting the tablets, if that is a problem. Explain side effects, such as constipation with iron supplements.

Making Referrals

Refer women with health problems such as diabetes, celiac disease, or extreme weight problems for an initial consultation with a dietitian and follow-up with the nurse. Refer women with inadequate financial resources to buy food to public assistance programs such as Temporary Assistance to Needy Families (TANF) or the WIC program. At the next visit, determine whether the woman obtained the help needed and whether other assistance is necessary.

Evaluation

- Does the woman report eating the recommended food group servings each day?
- Does the woman gain 1.4 to 1.8 kg (3 to 4 lb) during the first trimester and 0.44 kg (1 lb) per week during the second and third trimesters?
- Is her total pregnancy weight gain between 11.5 and 16 kg (25 and 35 lb)?

KEY CONCEPTS

- Weight gain during pregnancy is an important determinant of fetal growth. Poor weight gain in pregnant women is associated with low birth weight in infants. Excessive weight gain may lead to macrosomia and labor complications.
- The recommended weight gain during pregnancy is 25 to 35 lb. The amount is greater for women who are underweight or who carry more than one fetus, and it is less for obese women.
- The pattern of weight gain is as important as the total increase in weight. The average should be 3 to 4 lb during the first trimester and 1 lb per week thereafter.
- The recommended increase in energy intake during pregnancy is 300 calories per day. Calorie increases should be attained by

choosing foods high in nutrient density to meet the other needs of pregnancy.
- Protein should be increased to 71 g/day during pregnancy, an increase of 25 g/day over nonpregnancy needs.
- Women may not eat enough foods high in vitamins B_6, D, and E and folic acid to meet recommendations.
- Fat-soluble vitamins (A, D, E, and K) are stored in the liver. Excess consumption may result in toxic effects.
- Daily intake of water-soluble vitamins (B and C) is necessary because excesses are not stored but excreted.
- Minerals most likely to be consumed in less-than-recommended amounts during pregnancy are iron, calcium, zinc, and magne-

sium. Iron and folic acid are often added as a supplement, whereas calcium is added for women with low intake. The nurse can suggest foods high in these nutrients.
- The routine use of vitamin-mineral supplements is unnecessary and may lead to excessive intake and toxic effects. Increased intake of some nutrients interferes with the use of others and may result in deficiencies.
- Pregnant women should drink eight to ten 8-ounce glasses of fluids each day. They should eat at least seven servings of whole grains, five servings of fruits and vegetables, three servings of dairy products, and 7 ounces of protein foods daily.
- Culture can influence diet during pregnancy. The nurse should learn whether a woman fol-

KEY CONCEPTS

- lows traditional dietary practices and whether her food practices are consistent with good nutrition.
- Southeast Asian and Hispanic dietary practices include balancing yin and yang or "cold" and "hot" foods. The nurse must know which foods are acceptable at what times.
- Low-income women may not have enough money or knowledge to meet the nutrient needs of pregnancy. The nurse should refer them for financial assistance and nutritional counseling.
- Adolescents may skip meals and eat snacks and fast foods of low nutrient density. They are subjected to peer pressure that may decrease their nutritional intake.

- Pregnant vegetarians may need help in choosing an adequate diet that includes non-animal sources of energy, protein, iron, calcium, vitamin B_{12}, and other nutrients. Vegetarians may need vitamin-mineral supplements during pregnancy.
- Lactose-intolerant women should increase calcium intake from foods other than milk, such as calcium-rich vegetables.
- Abnormal prepregnancy weight, anemia, eating disorders, pica, more than five pregnancies, substance abuse, closely spaced pregnancies, and multifetal pregnancies are all nutritional risk factors that warrant adaptations of diet during pregnancy.

- Lactating women need more of almost every nutrient than women who are not lactating. The increased calories needed for milk production can be met by an added daily intake of 500 calories, and the rest can come from maternal fat stores.
- During lactation, mothers should avoid alcohol, caffeine, and foods that seem to cause distress in the infant.
- The postpartum woman who does not breastfeed should decrease her daily calorie intake by 300 calories but should eat a well-balanced diet to enhance recovery from childbirth. Weight loss should be accomplished slowly and sensibly.

ANSWER to Critical Thinking Exercise 15-1

It is important to be accepting and nonjudgmental in responding to this woman. It is unlikely that she will discontinue her pica, and she may withdraw and continue to practice it in secret if she feels that the nurse is disapproving. Therapeutic communication techniques are important to explore the woman's feelings about her cravings. A discussion of her feelings can then lead to teaching about nutrition. The nurse should determine how much ice the woman eats each day and whether she has other cravings. A 24-hour diet history assists in identifying deficient areas in the diet. The nurse can work with the woman to find ways to modify the diet to include more of the food groups that are lacking. She should be referred to a dietitian for further counseling, but the nurse should also discuss the diet at each prenatal visit.

REFERENCES and READINGS

American Academy of Pediatrics (AAP) Committee on Nutrition. (2000). Hypoallergenic infant formulas. *Pediatrics, 106*(2), 346-349.

American Academy of Pediatrics & American College of Obstetricians and Gynecologists. (2002). *Guidelines for perinatal care* (5th ed.). Elk Grove Village, IL, and Washington, DC: Author.

American Dietetics Association & Dietitians of Canada. (2003). Position of the American Dietetic Association and Dietitians of Canada: Vegetarian diets. *Journal of the American Dietetic Association, 103*(6), 748-765.

Blackburn, S. T., (2003). Maternal, fetal, and neonatal physiology (2nd ed). Philadelphia: Saunders.

Brodeur, M.A. (2002). Understanding dietary supplement regulation. *AWHONN Lifelines, 6*(2), 106-109.

Bronner, Y.L., & Auerbach, K.G. (1999). Maternal nutrition during lactation. In J. Riordan & K.G. Auerbach (Eds.), *Breastfeeding and human lactation* (2nd ed., pp. 515-539). Sudbury, MA: Jones & Bartlett.

Brooks, S.L., Mitchell, A., & Steffenson, N. (2000). Mothers, infants, and DHA: Implications for nursing practice. *MCN: The American Journal of Maternal/Child Nursing, 25*(2), 71-75.

Cesario, S.K. (2003). Obesity in pregnancy: What every nurse needs to know. *AWHONN Lifelines, 7*(2), 118-125.

Corbett, R.W., Ryan, C., & Weinrich, S.P. (2003). Pica in pregnancy: Does it affect pregnancy outcomes? *Journal of Obstetric, Gynecologic, and Neonatal Nursing, 28*(3), 183-189.

Cunningham, F.G., Gant, N.F., Leveno, K.J., Gilstrap, L.C., Hauth, J.C., & Wenstrom, K.D. (2001). *Williams obstetrics* (21st ed.). New York: McGraw-Hill.

Evans, E.C. (2002). The FDA recommendations on fish intake during pregnancy. *Journal of Obstetric, Gynecologic, and Neonatal Nursing, 31*(6), 715-720.

Fagen, C. (2000). Nutrition during pregnancy and lactation. In L.K. Mahan & S. Escott-Stump, *Krause's food, nutrition, and diet therapy* (10th ed., pp. 167-195). Philadelphia: Saunders.

Fowles, E.R. (2002). Comparing pregnant women's nutritional knowledge to their actual dietary intake. *MCN: The American Journal of Maternal/Child Nursing, 27*(3), 171-177.

Giddens, J.B., Krug, S.K., Tsang, R., Guo, S., Miodovnik, M., & Prada, J.A. (2000). Pregnant adolescent and adult women have similarly low intakes of selected nutrients. *Journal of the American Dietetic Association, 100*(11), 1334-1340.

Grodner, M., Anderson, S.L., & DeYoung, S. (2000). *Nutrition, a nursing approach* (2nd ed.). St. Louis: Mosby.

Hassenau, S.M., & Covington, C. (2002). Neural tube defects: Prevention and folic acid. *MCN: The American Journal of Maternal/Child Nursing, 27*(1), 87-91.

Hilton, J.J. (2002). Folic acid intake of young women. *Journal of Obstetric, Gynecologic, and Neonatal Nursing, 31*(2), 172-177.

Institute of Medicine, Food and Nutrition Board. (1997). *Dietary reference intakes for calcium, phosphorus, magnesium, vitamin D, & fluoride.* Washington, DC: National Academy Press.

Institute of Medicine, Food and Nutrition Board. (1998). *Dietary reference intakes for thiamin, riboflavin, niacin, vitamin B_6, folate, vitamin B_{12}, pantothenic acid, biotin, & choline.* Washington, DC: National Academy Press.

Institute of Medicine, Food and Nutrition Board. (2000). *Dietary reference intakes for vitamin C, vitamin E, selenium, and carotenoids.* Washington, DC: National Academy Press.

Institute of Medicine, Food and Nutrition Board. (2002). *Dietary reference intakes for vitamin A, vitamin K, arsenic, boron, chromium, copper, iodine, iron, manganese, molybdenum, nickel, silicon, vanadium, and zinc.* Washington, DC: National Academy Press.

Institute of Medicine, National Academy of Sciences, Food and Nutrition Board. (1990). *Nutrition during pregnancy. Pt. I: Weight gain. Pt. II: Nutrient supplements.* Washington, DC: National Academy Press.

Institute of Medicine, National Academy of Sciences, Food and Nutrition Board. (1991). *Nutrition during lactation.* Washington, DC: National Academy Press.

Institute of Medicine, National Academy of Sciences, Subcommittee for a Clinical Application Guide. (1992). *Nutrition during pregnancy and lactation: An implementation guide.* Washington, DC: National Academy Press.

REFERENCES and READINGS

James, D.C. (2001). Eating disorders, fertility, and pregnancy: Relationships and complications. *Journal of Perinatal & Neonatal Nursing, 15*(2), 36-48.

James, D.K., Mahomed, K., Stone, S., van Wijngaarden, W., & Hill, L.M. (2003). *Evidence-based obstetrics.* Philadelphia: Saunders.

Kaiser, L.L., & Allen, L. (2002). Position of the American Dietetic Association: Nutrition and lifestyle for a healthy pregnancy outcome. *Journal of the American Dietetic Association, 102*(10), 1479-1490.

Kim-Godwin, Y.S. (2003). Postpartum beliefs and practices among non-western cultures. *MCN: The American Journal of Maternal/Child Nursing, 28*(2), 74-78.

Lawrence, R.A., & Lawrence, R.M. (1999). *Breastfeeding: A guide for the medical profession* (5th ed.). St. Louis: Mosby.

Lovelady, A.A., Garner, K.E., Moreno, K.L., & Willams, J.P. (2000). The effect of weight loss in overweight, lactating women on the growth of their infants. *New England Journal of Medicine, 342*(7), 449-453.

Matteson, P.S. (2001). *Women's health during the childbearing years: A community-based approach.* St. Louis: Mosby.

Mattson, S. (2003). Caring for Hispanic women. *AWHONN Lifelines, 7*(3), 258-260.

Messina, V., Melina, V., & Mangels, A.R. (2003). A new food guide for North American vegetarians. *Journal of the American Dietetic Association, 103*(6), 771-775.

Mitchell, M.K. (2003). *Nutrition across the life span* (9th ed.). Philadelphia: Saunders.

Mohrbacher, N., & Stock, J. (2003). *The breastfeeding answer book* (3rd ed.). Schaumburg, IL: La Leche League International.

Moore, M.L., & Moos, M. (2003). *Cultural competence in the care of childbearing families.* White Plains, NY: March of Dimes.

Morin, K.H. (1998). Perinatal outcomes of obese women: A review of the literature. *Journal of Obstetric, Gynecologic, and Neonatal Nursing, 27*(4), 431-440.

Pagana, K.D., & Pagana, T.J. (2001). *Mosby's diagnostic and laboratory test reference.* St. Louis: Mosby.

Peckenpaugh, N.J., & Poleman, C.M. (2003). *Nutrition essentials and diet therapy* (9th ed.). Philadelphia: Saunders.

Ramer, L., & Frank, B. (2001). *Pregnancy: Psychosocial perspectives.* White Plains, NY: March of Dimes.

Reifsnider, E., & Gill, S.L. (2000). Nutrition for the childbearing years. *Journal of Obstetric, Gynecologic, and Neonatal Nursing, 29*(1), 43-55.

Schlenker, E.D. (2003). Nutrition for growth and development. In S.R. Williams & E.D. Schlenker, *Essentials of nutrition and diet therapy* (8th ed., pp. 293-319). St. Louis: Mosby.

Spear, B.A. (2000). Nutrition in adolescence. In L.K. Mahan & S. Escott-Stump, *Krause's food, nutrition, and diet therapy* (10th ed., pp. 257-270). Philadelphia: Saunders.

Strychar, I.M., Chabot, C., Champagne, F., Ghadirian, P., Leduc, L., Lemonnier, M., &

Raynauld, P. (2000). Psychosocial & lifestyle factors associated with insufficient and excessive maternal weight gain during pregnancy. *Journal of the American Dietetic Association, 100*(3), 353-356.

Swensen, A.R., Harnack, L.J., & Ross, J.A. (2001). Nutritional assessment of pregnant women enrolled in the Special Supplemental Program for Women, Infants, and Children (WIC). *Journal of the American Dietetic Association, 101*(8), 903-908.

U.S. Department of Health and Human Services. (2000). *Healthy People 2010: Healthy People 2010* (Conference edition, in 2 volumes). Washington, DC.

Wilkerson, N.N. (2000). Nutrition. In F.H. Nichols & S.S. Humenick, *Childbirth education: Practice, research, & theory,* Philadelphia: Saunders.

Williams, S.R. (2003a). The food environment and food habits. In S.R. Williams & E.D. Schlenker, *Essentials of nutrition and diet therapy* (8th ed., pp. 219-245). St. Louis: Mosby.

Williams, S.R. (2003b). Nutrition during pregnancy and lactation. In S.R. Williams & E.D. Schlenker, *Essentials of nutrition and diet therapy* (8th ed., pp. 269-292). St. Louis: Mosby.

Witt, K.A., & Mihok, M.A. (2003). Lactation and breastfeeding. In M.K. Mitchell, *Nutrition across the life span* (9th ed., pp. 177-206). Philadelphia: Saunders.

16

Prenatal Diagnostic Tests

 LEARNING OBJECTIVES

After studying this chapter, you should be able to:
◎ Identify indications for fetal diagnostic procedures.
◎ Discuss the purpose, procedure, advantages, and risks of each diagnostic procedure presented in the chapter.

◎ Provide information in response to common questions parents have about procedures.

 DEFINITIONS

alpha-fetoprotein Plasma protein produced by the fetus.

amniocentesis Transabdominal puncture of the amniotic sac to obtain a sample of amniotic fluid that contains fetal cells and biochemical substances for laboratory examination.

biophysical profile Method for evaluating fetal status during the antepartum period based on five fetal variables: fetal heart rate variability, fetal breathing movements, gross movements, muscle tone, and amniotic fluid volume.

chorionic villus sampling Transcervical or transabdominal sampling of chorionic villi (projections on the outer fetal membrane) for analysis of fetal cells.

contraction stress test Method for evaluating fetal status during the antepartum period by observing the response of the fetal heart to intermittent stress of uterine contractions.

late deceleration Slowing of the fetal heart rate after the onset of a uterine contraction that persists after the contraction ends.

lecithin/sphingomyelin ratio (L/S ratio) Ratio of two phospholipids in amniotic fluid that is used to estimate fetal lung maturity.

neural tube defect A congenital defect in the closure of the bony encasement of the spinal cord or of the skull.

nonstress test A method for evaluating fetal status during the antepartum period by observing for accelerations of the fetal heart rate.

percutaneous umbilical blood sampling (cordocentesis) Procedure for obtaining fetal blood through ultrasound-guided puncture

of an umbilical cord vessel to detect fetal problems such as inherited blood disorders, acidosis, or infection.

phosphatidylglycerol A phospholipid component of surfactant; its presence in amniotic fluid indicates fetal lung maturity.

phosphatidylinositol A phospholipid component of surfactant that is produced and secreted in increasing amounts as the fetal lungs mature.

placenta previa Abnormal implantation of the placenta in the lower uterus, at or near the cervical os.

surfactant A mixture of lipoproteins produced by mature fetal lungs that reduces surface tension in the alveoli, thus promoting lung expansion after birth.

triple-marker screening Analysis of maternal serum for abnormal levels of alpha-fetoprotein, human chorionic gonadotropin, and estriols that may predict chromosomal abnormalities of the fetus.

ultrasonography Technique for visualizing deep structures of the body by recording the reflections (echoes) of sound waves directed into the tissue.

uteroplacental insufficiency Decreased ability of the placenta to exchange oxygen, carbon dioxide, nutrients, and waste products properly between the maternal and fetal circulations.

vibroacoustic stimulation Use of sound and vibration to elicit acceleration of the fetal heart rate.

Methods to detect physical abnormalities in the fetus and to monitor the fetal condition in a high-risk pregnancy with greater accuracy are becoming common as knowledge about their usefulness accumulates. Many pregnant women now expect to know the sex of their baby before birth because of routine use of technology such as ultrasonography.

The ability to predict fetal outcome offers reassurance for most parents but not all. If the fetus is free of anomalies and

is determined to be in good condition, the parents are relieved. However, testing may raise questions about fetal health rather than answer them, forcing parents to make decisions about having other tests or perhaps increasing their anxiety throughout the remainder of pregnancy. If fetal anomalies are identified, the parents must then decide whether to continue or terminate the pregnancy. This decision can create emotional conflict and raise ethical dilemmas that impose a great deal of stress on the family.

BOX 16-1
Indications for Fetal Diagnostic Procedures

Medical Conditions
Preexisting diabetes mellitus or gestational diabetes
Hypertension (chronic or pregnancy-induced)
Chronic infections (e.g., pyelonephritis)
Sexually transmissible diseases
Severe anemia
Parents carry or express a genetic disorder (e.g., sickle cell anemia, cystic fibrosis)

Demographic Factors
Maternal age <16 or >35 years
Poverty
Nonwhite (greater risk for prematurity or neonatal or infant death)
Inadequate prenatal care (initial visit after 20 weeks' gestation or fewer than five prenatal visits to physician or nurse-midwife)

Obstetric Factors
History of low-birth-weight (<2500 g) or preterm infant
Multifetal pregnancy
Malpresentation (breech, shoulder)

Previous fetal loss or birth of infant with congenital anomaly
Previous infant >4000 g at birth
Hydramnios (>2000 ml at term; amniotic fluid index >18-20)
Oligohydramnios (<500 ml at term; amniotic fluid index <5)
Decrease in or absence of fetal movements
Uncertainty about gestational age
Suspected intrauterine growth restriction
Discordant (unequal) fetal growth of twins
Postmaturity (>42 weeks)
Preterm labor (>20 weeks and <38 weeks gestation)
Grand multiparity (>5 pregnancies)

Concurrent Maternal Factors
Prepregnancy weight less than 45 kg (100 lb) or body mass index (BMI) less than 19.8
Prepregnancy weight more than 90 kg (200 pounds) or more than 20% above ideal weight for height at conception
Inadequate weight gain or poor pattern of weight gain
Excessive weight gain
Use of drugs, alcohol, tobacco

INDICATIONS FOR PRENATAL DIAGNOSTIC TESTS

In general, three reasons exist for performing fetal diagnostic and surveillance procedures: to detect congenital anomalies; to evaluate the condition of the fetus if the pregnancy is high risk and allow appropriate intervention; and to provide baseline information such as a more accurate gestational age. Procedures that were once done only if the pregnancy was high risk are now being done routinely. Tests such as ultrasonography or maternal serum screening are often offered to all pregnant women. Box 16-1 lists some risk factors for which prenatal diagnostic procedures are often recommended.

ULTRASONOGRAPHY

When high-frequency sound waves are aimed in a specific direction, they are deflected by objects in their path and return as echoes. The amount of energy returned as an echo depends on the density of the object that deflected the ultrasonic wave. In obstetrics, when ultrasonic waves are directed through the abdomen of a pregnant woman, they are deflected by tissues of the mother and fetus. The returning sound waves are converted to two- or three-dimensional images that show structures of different densities (Fig. 16-1).

Ultrasound procedures in obstetrics typically use real-time scanning in which a rapid sequence of fixed images is displayed on the screen, showing movement as it happens. This technique allows the observer to detect movement such as fetal heartbeat, fetal breathing activity, and fetal body movement.

Emotional Responses

Some expectant mothers are excited and pleased and report feelings of love and protectiveness when they view the fetus. Others, however, report increased feelings of vulnerability

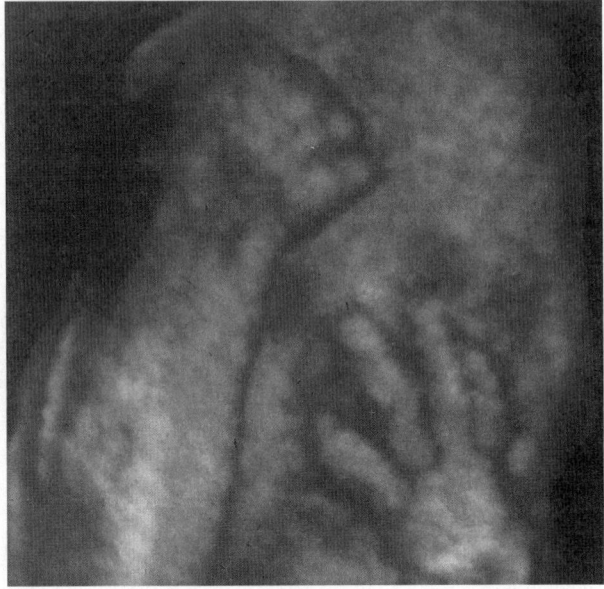

Figure 16-1 Three-dimensional sonogram showing normal fetal hands in front of the face. (From Pretorius, D.H., Nelson, T.R., & Lev-Toaff, A.S. [2000]. Three dimensional ultrasound in obstetrics and gynecology. In P.W. Callen [Ed.], *Ultrasonography in obstetrics and gynecology* [4th ed]. Philadelphia: Saunders.)

and anxiety about the fetus, fearing that something wrong will be found.

Expectant fathers are often fascinated by fetal movement and insist that the fetus "waved" at them or that they could see the facial expression as the fetus looked directly at them. Some couples wish to know the sex of the fetus, but others prefer to wait and "be surprised" even if the sex is obvious. Also, determining the fetal sex by ultrasound is sometimes not possible. Occasionally a couple is surprised at birth if the infant's sex is not what they expected.

Although ultrasonography is not yet a standard of care for all women, it is widely used because a great deal of information can be obtained with minimum risk to mother or fetus. Ultrasonography may be used during any trimester, but the procedure and the reasons for its use vary for each trimester.

First Trimester

Transvaginal ultrasonography is often used during the first trimester because the uterus, gestational sac, embryo, ovaries, and fallopian tubes are deep in the pelvis.

Procedure

The woman is placed in a lithotomy position for transvaginal ultrasonography. A transvaginal probe that is encased in a disposable cover and coated with a gel that provides lubrication and promotes sound wave conduction is inserted into the vagina. The woman may feel more comfortable if she inserts the probe herself. The procedure takes about 10 to 15 minutes.

Purposes

Common uses for ultrasonography during the first trimester include:

- Determining the presence and location (intrauterine or elsewhere) of pregnancy
- Detecting multifetal gestations
- Estimating gestational age
- Confirming fetal viability
- Identifying the need for follow-up testing
- Identifying ultrasound characteristics that suggest fetal abnormality, such as chromosome defects
- As an adjunct for transcervical or transabdominal chorionic villus sampling

During the first trimester, measurement of the crown-rump length of the embryo is the most reliable indicator of gestational age (Fig. 16-2). Fetal viability is confirmed by observation of the fetal heartbeat, which is visible as early as 38 days after the last normal menstrual period (Manning, 2004). Maternal structures and some abnormalities such as uterine fibroids, ovarian cysts, and a bicornuate uterus also can be seen.

Second and Third Trimesters

Transabdominal ultrasonography is common during the second and third trimesters because the uterus is out of the pelvis and accessible. Transvaginal ultrasound continues to be useful to evaluate the cervical and lower uterine areas.

Procedure

The expectant mother is positioned on her back with her head and knees supported by pillows. Her head should be elevated, and she should be turned slightly to one side with a wedge or rolled blanket under one hip to avoid supine hypotension (see p. 255). If she desires, the screen can be positioned so that she (and the father) can see the images. Transmission gel is spread over her abdomen, and the sonographer (nurse, physician, or ultrasound technician) moves a transducer over the abdomen to obtain a picture (Fig. 16-3).

The procedure takes 10 to 30 minutes. The sonographer can "freeze" a picture and copy it for permanent records or for the parents if they wish. Many ultrasound systems offer videotaping of the evaluation, and some facilities provide a section of videotape for the parents.

During the second trimester a full bladder may be needed to displace the intestines and elevate the uterus for better visibility. If indicated, the woman should be instructed to drink several glasses of clear fluid an hour before the time of the examination and not to urinate until the examination is completed.

Purposes

Ultrasonography is used during the second and third trimesters for many reasons, including to:

- Confirm fetal viability
- Evaluate fetal anatomy
- Estimate gestational age
- Assess progress of fetal growth over a series of scans
- Compare growth of fetuses in multifetal gestations
- Evaluate amniotic fluid volume (see also "Biophysical Profile," p. 333)
- Determine location and relation of the placenta and umbilical cord to each other and the insertion of the cord into the fetal abdomen
- Determine fetal presentation
- Guide needle placement for procedures such as amniocentesis or percutaneous umbilical blood sampling

Several body measurements are done to estimate gestational age during the last half of pregnancy, such as biparietal diameter, femur length, and abdominal circumference. Sequential assessments of multiple fetal measurements will help date the pregnancy more accurately than a single measurement. Estimating fetal age by ultrasonography after 32 weeks is subject to major error. At this time the fetus may be evaluated for other signs of maturity and for signs of excessive or reduced growth rate (Manning, 2004).

Knowing the true gestational age is needed when screening for maternal serum alpha-fetoprotein (MSAFP), which changes with fetal age. Accurate gestational age is also important if intrauterine growth restriction is suspected or the expected date of delivery is uncertain.

A comprehensive ultrasound in the second trimester is used to evaluate the fetus when risk factors are present or the basic examination shows abnormal findings. Examples include prior birth of an infant with anomalies or abnormal clinical findings such as hydramnios (excessive amniotic fluid), oligohydramnios (insufficient amniotic fluid), or abnormal levels of MSAFP. Fetal anatomy is systematically examined to identify major system and organ structures. Anomalies that can be detected with comprehensive ultrasonography include most neural tube defects such as myelomeningocele and anencephaly; abdominal wall defects such as gastroschisis and omphalocele; malformed kidneys; hydrocephalus; obstruction in fetal bowel and urinary systems; cleft lip and palate; and limb abnormalities.

Advantages

Ultrasonography allows clear visualization of the fetus and surrounding structures, and it is safe. Ultrasonography is noninvasive and relatively comfortable, and the results are immediately

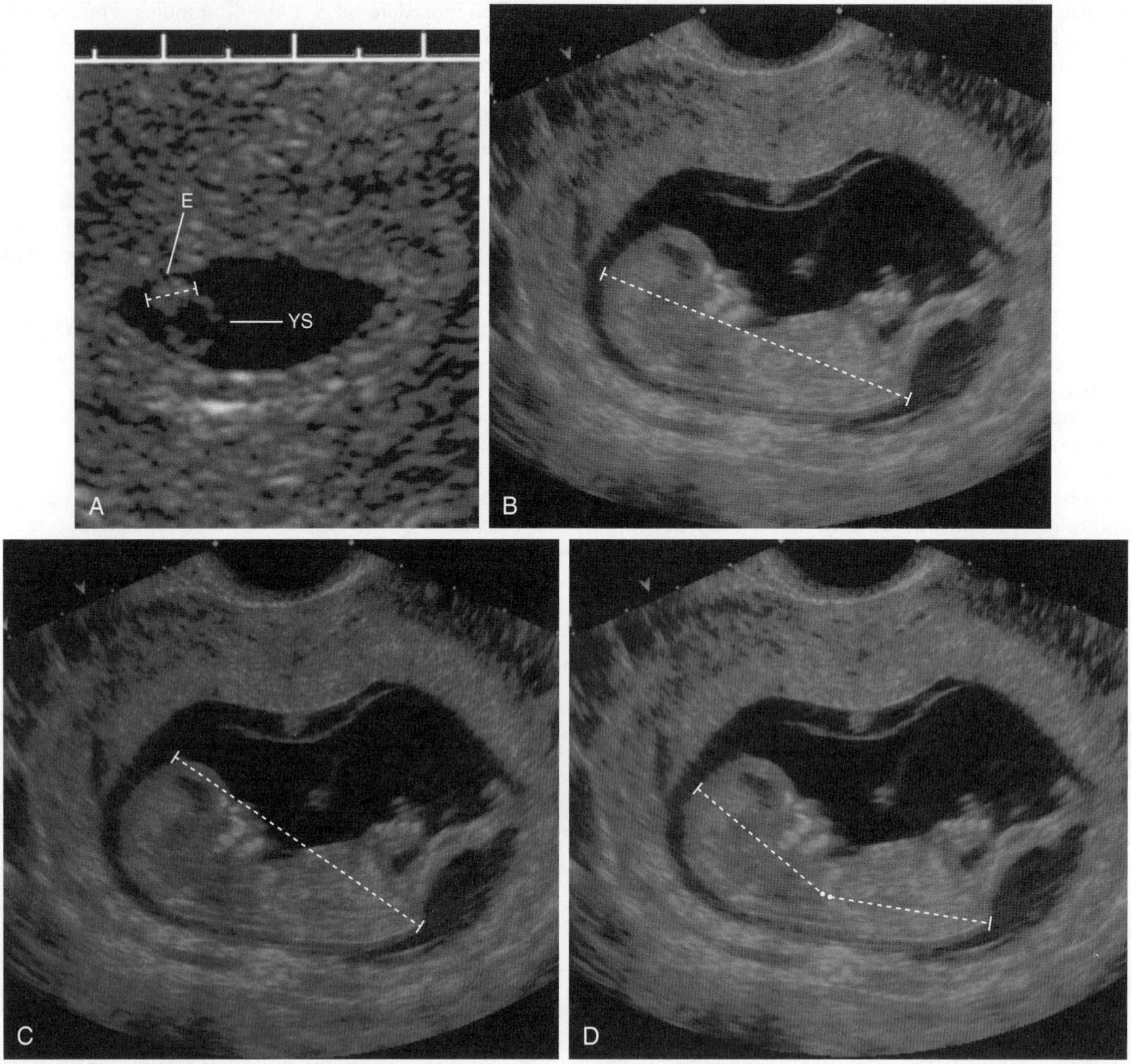

Figure 16-2 Measurement of the crown-rump length with ultrasound. (From Filly, R.A., & Hadlock, F.P. [2000]. In P.W. Callen [Ed.], *Ultrasonography in obstetrics and gynecology* [4th ed.]. Philadelphia: Saunders.)

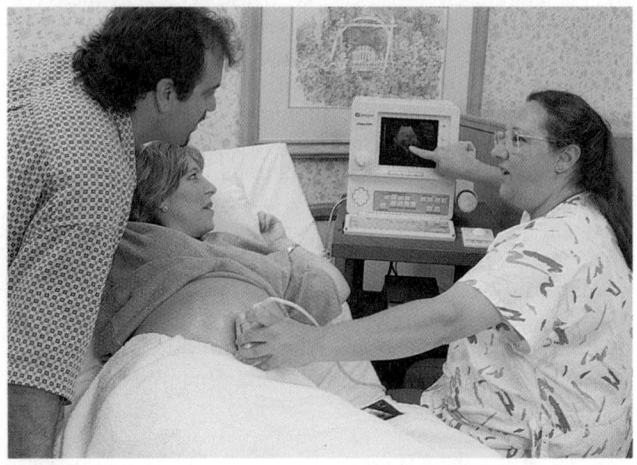

Figure 16-3 The nurse trained in obstetrical ultrasound provides information as she moves the transducer over the mother's abdomen to obtain an image.

available. Small portable scanners allow the machine to be moved easily for quick scans, such as in the case of a questionable fetal presentation in a laboring woman.

Disadvantages

Women who do not have prenatal care in the first trimester of pregnancy lose many benefits of ultrasound examinations, such as accurate dating of the pregnancy. In addition, ultrasonography and other prenatal diagnostic procedures cannot identify every fetal structural defect or defects that do not affect body structures, such as an inborn error of metabolism. Cost may be a problem if the woman has no insurance or if the cost of the procedure is not covered by insurance.

Ultrasound findings that are not normal but for which little is known about their implications may occur. The next step in the fetal diagnostic process may be unknown, causing greater parental anxiety.

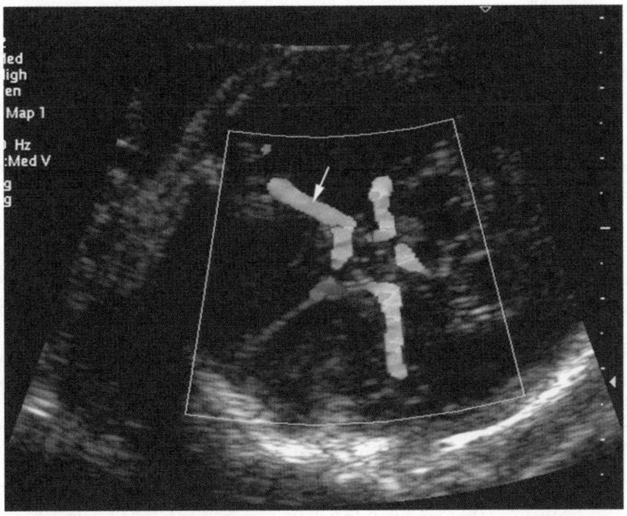

Figure 16-4 Color Doppler visualization of the circle of Willis in the fetal head. (From Tekay, A., & Campbell, S. [2000]. In P.W. Callen [Ed.], *Ultrasonography in obstetrics and gynecology* [4th ed.]. Philadelphia: Saunders.)

DOPPLER ULTRASOUND BLOOD FLOW ASSESSMENT

When an ultrasound wave is directed at an acute angle to a moving target, as with blood flowing through a vessel, the frequency of echoes changes as the cardiac cycle goes through systole and diastole. This change, referred to as the *Doppler shift*, indicates forward movement of blood within a vessel.

Purpose

Pregnancies complicated by hypertension or fetal growth restriction caused by placental insufficiency may have Doppler ultrasound assessment of blood flow through the umbilical artery to identify abnormalities in the diastolic flow. The most common measurement is the systolic/diastolic (S/D) ratio, which normally decreases throughout gestation. Normal S/D ratios for different gestations have not yet been established (Maulik, 2000). If fetal peripheral resistance rises, the diastolic flow falls, resulting in an increased S/D ratio. In severe cases of growth restriction caused by placental insufficiency, diastolic flow may be absent or even reversed (American Academy of Pediatrics [AAP] & American College of Obstetricians and Gynecologists [ACOG], 2002; Opipari & Johnson, 2000).

COLOR DOPPLER

Color Doppler imaging is useful to clarify the relationships of body structures to each other. Nondirectional color Doppler imaging uses a single color to identify structures such as the number of vessels in the umbilical cord. Directional color Doppler uses two or more colors to determine the direction and speed of blood flow and pulsations within cardiovascular structures (Fig. 16-4). It helps determine whether the heart has normal structure and whether major vessels have correct relationships to the heart chambers. Color Doppler imaging can determine blood flow and pulsations within umbilical cord vessels and other major vessels such as cranial vessels.

> **BOX 16-2**
> ### *Conditions Associated With Abnormal Maternal Serum Alpha-Fetoprotein (AFP) Levels*
>
> **Elevated Levels of AFP**
> Open neural tube defects (anencephaly, spina bifida)
> Esophageal obstruction
> Abdominal wall defects (omphalocele, gastroschisis)
> Increased amount leaked by fetal kidney (hydronephrosis)
> Threatened abortion
> Fetal demise
> Normal fetus in conjunction with one or more of the following:
>   Amniotic fluid contaminated with fetal blood during amniocentesis
>   Underestimation of fetal age
>   Multifetal gestation
>   Incorrect maternal weight (lower than true weight)
>   Maternal insulin-dependent diabetes
>
> **Low Levels of AFP**
> Chromosomal trisomies (e.g., Down syndrome)
> Gestational trophoblastic disease
> Normal fetuses in conjunction with the following:
>   Overestimation of gestational age
>   Incorrect maternal weight (higher than true weight)

ALPHA-FETOPROTEIN SCREENING

Alpha-fetoprotein (AFP) is the main protein in fetal plasma. It diffuses from fetal plasma into fetal urine and is excreted into the amniotic fluid. Some AFP crosses placental membranes into the maternal circulation. Therefore AFP can be measured both in maternal serum (MSAFP) and in amniotic fluid (AFAFP). Abnormal concentrations of AFP are associated with serious fetal anomalies, requiring additional testing to determine the reason for the abnormal concentration.

The AFP concentration increases with advancing gestational age of the fetus. It is higher in multifetal gestations because more than one fetus is producing the protein. Interpretation of MSAFP values must be corrected for maternal weight because AFP diffuses into a larger maternal compartment in heavier women. Other factors that influence interpretation of AFP levels include race and maternal diabetes.

Purpose

Low levels of MSAFP are associated with chromosomal anomalies, such as trisomy 21 (Down syndrome). The most common cause of elevated AFP is failure of the embryonic neural tube or anterior body wall to close properly. In these conditions, neural or abdominal cavity tissues are exposed or covered with only a very thin layer of tissue, allowing high concentrations of AFP to seep into amniotic fluid and then enter maternal serum.

The most common open neural tube defects are anencephaly, in which the cranial vault is absent and most of the brain is undeveloped, and spina bifida, which has a wide range of severity (see Chapter 52). See Box 16-2 for other conditions that are associated with abnormal MSAFP.

Procedure

Pregnant women should be offered MSAFP screening, ideally between 16 and 18 weeks of gestation (AAP & ACOG, 2002). The mother is informed that MSAFP is a screening test rather than a diagnostic test. Further tests will be indicated to investigate abnormal concentrations. If MSAFP levels are abnormal, ultrasonography is recommended initially to determine whether the abnormal concentration is caused by multifetal gestation, inaccurate gestational age, or fetal death.

If ultrasonography fails to explain the abnormal levels of AFP, amniocentesis is the next step offered. Amniotic fluid is analyzed for elevated levels of AFP and for acetylcholinesterase (AChE). Elevations of AChE may help distinguish neural tube defect from other body wall defects. Amniotic fluid can also be analyzed for chromosome makeup if MSAFP values are lower than expected.

Advantages

MSAFP evaluation has several advantages:

- It is a simple procedure that requires only a sample of maternal blood.
- It is the least invasive and most economic procedure to screen for an open body wall defect such as neural tube defect or for chromosome abnormality.
- Prenatal diagnosis allows parents time to examine their options or to prepare for the birth of an infant who will need special care.

Limitations

Limitations of MSAFP evaluation are:

- It is a screening test and must be viewed as the first step in a series of diagnostic procedures that are indicated if abnormal concentrations are found. Parents must decide about whether to proceed each time another diagnostic test is offered.
- Benign conditions, such as inaccurate estimation of gestational age, can result in apparently abnormal levels, causing the parents greater anxiety and expense if follow-up tests are indicated.
- Timing imposes limits on the usefulness of MSAFP. Evaluation is best performed between 16 and 18 weeks of pregnancy, but many women do not seek prenatal care until well after the 18th week, thus limiting their options.
- Because closed defects that are covered by skin do not produce elevated levels of AFP, normal levels of AFP do not guarantee that the baby will be free of structural anomalies.

TRIPLE-MARKER SCREENING

Two other markers, human chorionic gonadotropin (hCG) and unconjugated estriol, have been added to routine MSAFP evaluation to screen for chromosomal abnormalities. This triple-marker screening (also called *multiple-marker screening*) increases the detection of trisomy 18 and trisomy 21 (Gilbert & Harmon, 2003; Jorde, Carey, Bamshad, & White, 2003; Ward, 2003). Maternal serum samples are taken between 16 and 18 weeks' gestation, and the results are considered positive if MSAFP and estriol are low and if hCG is high. If testing is positive, the woman should be offered additional testing, such as amniocentesis for karyotyping or additional ultrasonography to look for physical characteristics associated with the chromosome defects.

A fourth marker, inhibin A, is being evaluated to determine if its use can increase the accuracy of multiple-marker screening for identifying trisomy 21. Inhibin A is elevated in the fetus with Down syndrome. Levels do not rise until the second trimester, limiting its usefulness as an early screening test.

CHORIONIC VILLUS SAMPLING

Chorionic villi are microscopic projections from the outer membrane (chorion) that develop and burrow into endometrial tissue as the placenta is formed. The villi are composed of rapidly dividing cells of fetal origin that reflect the chromosomal and genetic makeup of the fetus. Chorionic villus cells can be used for diagnosis of fetal chromosomal, metabolic, or DNA abnormalities between 10 and 12 weeks of gestation.

Purpose

Chorionic villus sampling (CVS) can be used to diagnose fetal chromosome or metabolic abnormalities. It cannot be used to diagnose anomalies for which amniotic fluid is essential, such as open neural tube defects, which require measuring AFP levels (AAP & ACOG, 2002; Beall, 2000).

Indications

CVS is recommended only for women who are at high risk for giving birth to an infant with genetic anomalies that can be diagnosed from the fetal cells. Women older than 35 years, those with a history of a previous fetus with anomalies that can be detected with fetal cells, or couples who are carriers or who exhibit genetic defects are at the greatest risk for giving birth to an infant with similar anomalies. CVS may be used to identify the Rh type of a fetus at risk for complications because of maternal isoimmunization, so that the best treatment can be planned (see Chapter 26).

Procedure

As with all diagnostic procedures, the woman should receive both counseling about the procedure itself and genetic counseling about the specific defect for which CVS is being performed. The benefits and limitations of the procedure should be carefully explained, and a signed informed consent is obtained.

CVS can be performed by a transcervical or transabdominal approach (AAP & ACOG, 2002; Beall, 2000). In the transcervical technique, a flexible catheter is inserted through the cervix and a sample of chorionic villi is aspirated (Fig. 16-5). In the transabdominal technique, a needle is inserted through the abdominal and uterine walls to collect chorionic tissue.

After the procedure, the woman is shown the fetal heart motion and maternal vital signs are assessed. Heavy bleeding or the passage of amniotic fluid, clots, or tissue suggests possible miscarriage and should be reported. The woman should rest at home for several hours after the procedure.

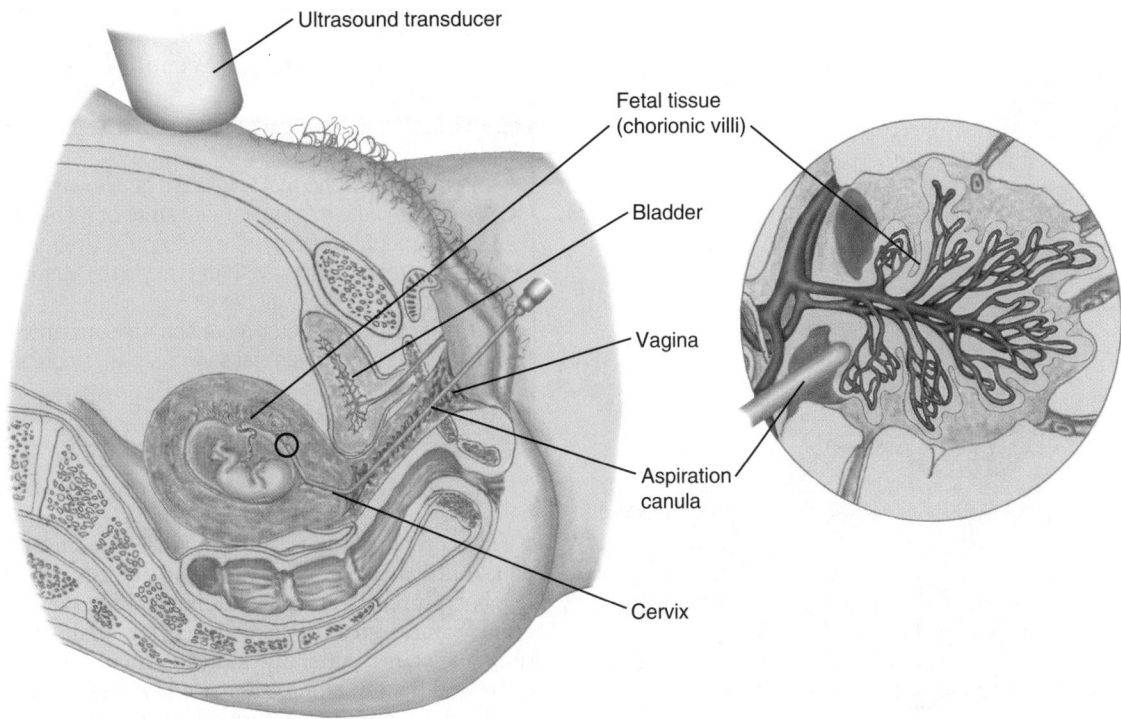

Figure 16-5 Transcervical chorionic villus sampling. Tissue is aspirated to identify some genetic defects in the fetus. Transabdominal aspiration is an alternative method.

Advantages

CVS is performed between 10 and 12 weeks of gestation, providing earlier results than amniocentesis to women who find later procedures unacceptable. Furthermore, if results are abnormal and the woman chooses abortion, she may consider the earlier abortion less physically and emotionally traumatic than a later procedure.

Limitations

Although chorionic villus sampling is now considered a safe and effective technique for first-trimester prenatal diagnosis, there are limitations:

- The pregnancy loss rate is 0.5%-1%—slightly higher than with amniocentesis. Factors that decrease the risk of pregnancy loss include an experienced team, an anterior placenta, and the ease with which the sample is obtained.
- Reports of a higher-than-expected rate of limb reduction defects has occurred in CVS performed before 10 weeks. Although CVS is now performed at 10 to 12 weeks, families should be given information about earlier CVS before they choose the procedure.
- The risk for uterine infection is low, but it occasionally occurs. Presence of cervical or vaginal infection is a contraindication for the transvaginal approach (Gilbert & Harmon, 2003).
- Rh sensitization may occur as a result of entry of fetal Rh-positive blood cells into the circulation of a Rh-negative mother. Rh$_o$ (D) immune globulin should be administered

to all unsensitized Rh-negative women following the procedure (see Chapter 26).
- CVS is labor intensive because maternal cells may be aspirated with the fetal cells. Maternal cells must be removed from the sample before culture, adding to the procedure's cost. Third-party payers may not pay for these added costs.

AMNIOCENTESIS

Amniocentesis is aspiration of amniotic fluid from the amniotic sac for examination (Fig. 16-6). Amniocentesis may be performed during the second or third trimester of pregnancy, depending on the purpose. Second-trimester amniocentesis for fetal genetic abnormalities is best performed between 15 and 20 weeks because amniotic fluid volume is adequate and there are many viable fetal cells in the fluid.

Early amniocentesis is possible between 11 and 14 weeks. Early amniocentesis is associated with a higher fetal loss rate than later amniocentesis (Cunningham et al., 2001). Fetal foot deformations are more likely to occur with removal of amniotic fluid and earlier gestations.

Purposes

Second-Trimester Amniocentesis

The primary purpose for midtrimester amniocentesis is to examine fetal cells present in amniotic fluid to identify chromosomal or biochemical abnormalities and detect high levels of AFP. Amniocentesis is also used to evaluate the fetal condition when the woman is sensitized to Rh-positive blood, to

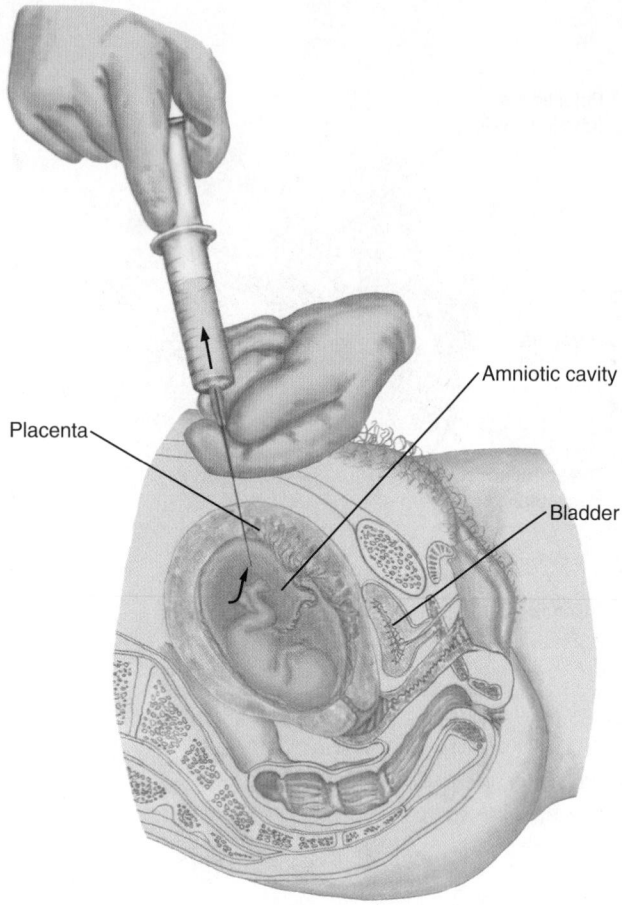

Placenta

Amniotic cavity

Bladder

Figure 16-6 In amniocentesis, a needle is inserted through the expectant mother's abdomen to aspirate fluid from the amniotic sac. The fluid can then be tested to detect chromosomal abnormalities in fetal cells or other problems and to determine fetal lung maturity.

diagnose amnionitis (intrauterine infection), and to test the amniotic fluid AFP when MSAFP is abnormal and a cause for the abnormal levels cannot be determined by noninvasive tests (Box 16-3).

Third-Trimester Amniocentesis

During the third trimester, amniocentesis is usually performed to determine fetal lung maturity or to diagnose fetal hemolytic disease that is often caused by Rh incompatibility. Reduction amniocentesis is a variation in which excess amniotic fluid is removed and discarded when hydramnios occurs. Samples of the fluid removed in a reduction amniocentesis may be evaluated for presence of infection or for substances that help evaluate fetal condition.

Tests to Determine Fetal Lung Maturity. A test for fetal lung maturity is recommended when delivery is contemplated before 38 weeks' gestation. The lecithin/sphingomyelin (L/S) ratio is the best-known test for estimating fetal lung maturity. Lecithin and sphingomyelin are lipoproteins that make up surfactant, which is present in the pulmonary alveoli in term infants. Surfactant keeps the alveoli open by reducing surface tension on their inner walls. The decreased surface tension prevents collapse of the alveoli when the infant exhales, reducing the effort of breathing.

The proportion of lecithin to sphingomyelin is about equal until about the 30th week of gestation. At this time the level of sphingomyelin plateaus but lecithin continues to rise. An L/S ratio greater than 2:1 (twice as much lecithin as sphingomyelin) generally indicates that surfactant is adequate and the fetal lungs are mature. An L/S ratio of 2:1 does not ensure fetal lung maturity, however, particularly for the fetus of a woman who has diabetes. Amniotic fluid is therefore also tested for the presence of phosphatidylglycerol (PG) and phosphatidylinositol (PI), which are other phospholipids that boost the properties of lecithin.

Test for Fetal Hemolytic Disease. Amniocentesis is used to obtain fluid for determination of fetal bilirubin concentration if the mother is Rh-negative and is sensitized (i.e., has been exposed to the Rh antigen and has developed antibodies against Rh-positive erythrocytes). The level of bilirubin in amniotic fluid reflects the amount of fetal red blood cell destruction that occurs when maternal antibodies destroy Rh-positive fetal red blood cells, leaving the fetus vulnerable to erythroblastosis fetalis and hydrops fetalis (see Chapter 30).

Procedure

The woman is placed in a supine position with a pillow or rolled towel under one buttock to shift the weight of the uterus off the major vessels. Maternal blood pressure and fetal heart tones are assessed to establish baseline levels.

Ultrasonography is used to locate the fetus and placenta, to identify the largest pockets of amniotic fluid that can safely be sampled, and to guide needle insertion. The skin is prepared with antiseptic solution. A small amount of local anesthetic is injected into the skin. This step causes the only pain the woman experiences, although she may experience the sensation of pressure as the needle is inserted and mild cramping as the needle enters the myometrium.

A 3- to 4-inch, 20- or 21-gauge needle is inserted into the pocket of fluid. The first 1 to 2 ml of fluid is discarded to avoid contamination of the fetal sample with maternal cells. Approximately 20 ml of fluid is removed for analysis. After fluid removal, the woman is shown the fetal heart beating and that fluid remains (Cunningham et al., 2001). Electronic fetal monitoring for 30 to 60 minutes is often done to identify continuing uterine contractions or nonreassuring fetal heart activity. She may resume normal activities after 24 hours. She should report persistent uterine contractions, vaginal bleeding, leakage of amniotic fluid, or fever.

As with chorionic villus sampling, Rh_o (D) immune globulin is administered to unsensitized Rh-negative women after amniocentesis to prevent sensitization.

Advantages

Amniocentesis has several advantages:

- It is a simple, relatively safe procedure that permits the diagnosis of many fetal anomalies and confirms fetal lung maturity.
- It is a brief and relatively painless procedure.
- It has been done for many years, with few reported complications. The fetal loss rate is less than 1% more than the baseline risk for miscarriage during midtrimester.

Disadvantages

The major disadvantage of midtrimester amniocentesis for genetic prenatal diagnosis is timing. It is done between 15 and 20 weeks of gestation, and some test results may take 2 or more weeks if they are uncommon tests. By this time, the pregnancy is obvious, the woman has felt fetal movement, and the woman may face an even more difficult decision about continuing the pregnancy if the results are abnormal.

Early amniocentesis avoids some of the timing disadvantages associated with later amniocentesis for prenatal diagnosis. Early amniocentesis does, however, carry a higher fetal loss rate after the procedure.

Risks

Amniocentesis is a relatively safe prenatal diagnostic procedure. The risk of injury to the fetus or umbilical cord is minimal when ultrasound is used to guide needle insertion. The risk of infection is also minimal, because aseptic technique is used throughout the procedure. The risk of spontaneous abortion associated with amniocentesis is 0.5% or less (Cunningham et al., 2001).

As with all fetal diagnostic procedures, amniocentesis cannot guarantee the birth of a perfect infant. Parents must be counseled that not all defects are detectable by amniocentesis.

ANTEPARTUM FETAL SURVEILLANCE

Antepartum fetal surveillance has three goals: to determine fetal health or compromise as accurately as possible, to guide intervention by the obstetric team, and to reduce perinatal morbidity and mortality. The three most common methods of fetal surveillance are the nonstress test, the contraction stress test, and the biophysical profile.

Nonstress Test

Purpose

One way to assess fetal well-being is to evaluate the ability of the fetal heart to accelerate, often in association with fetal movement. Accelerations of the fetal heart rate are associated with adequate oxygenation of the autonomic nervous system, a healthy neural pathway from the fetal central ner-

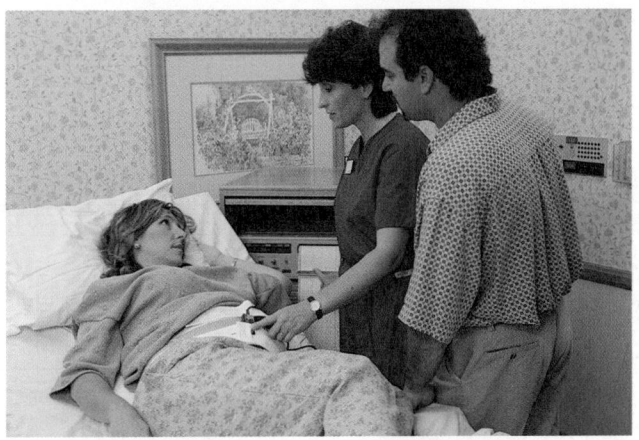

Figure 16-7 A nonstress test is a noninvasive test that measures the ability of the fetal heart to accelerate, often in response to fetal movements. Here the nurse reassures the parents by pointing to fetal heart rate accelerations detected by the external fetal monitor.

vous system to the fetal heart, and the ability of the fetal heart to respond to stimuli. If the fetal heart does not accelerate, an additional test, such as the contraction stress test or the biophysical profile, is necessary to better ascertain the metabolic condition of the fetus.

Procedure

The nonstress test (NST) is performed by a nurse with training in fetal monitoring. The nurse instructs the woman about the test and explains why it is recommended. The test is termed "nonstress" because it consists of monitoring only; the fetus is not challenged or stressed by stimulated uterine contractions to obtain the necessary data. A physician reviews and makes the final interpretation of the data.

The woman usually sits in a reclining chair or in bed in a semi-Fowler's position to prevent supine hypotension. If she is lying down, she should be side-lying or in a lateral tilt. If symptoms of maternal supine hypotension occur, such as faintness, dizziness, or pallor, her position is changed. One study found that a reactive, or reassuring, NST was more likely if the woman was in a sitting position, reducing testing time (Nathan, Haberman, Burgess, & Minkoff, 2000).

The nurse applies external electronic fetal monitoring equipment to the woman's abdomen to detect the fetal heart rate and any contractions or fetal movement (Fig. 16-7). The woman may also be given a remote event marker to press each time she senses movement. (See Chapter 18 for more information about fetal monitoring.)

Interpretation

Results are judged to be reactive (reassuring) or nonreactive (nonreassuring) (AAP & ACOG, 2002) if the following characteristics are present:

- *Reactive:* At least two fetal heart rate accelerations, with or without fetal movement, occurring within a 20-minute period and peaking at least 15 beats per minute (bpm) above the baseline and lasting 15 seconds ("15 by 15") from baseline to baseline (Fig. 16-8). Acoustic stimulation with a vibroacoustic stimulator of 1 second that elicits similar fetal heart rate accelerations is also reassuring. Extending

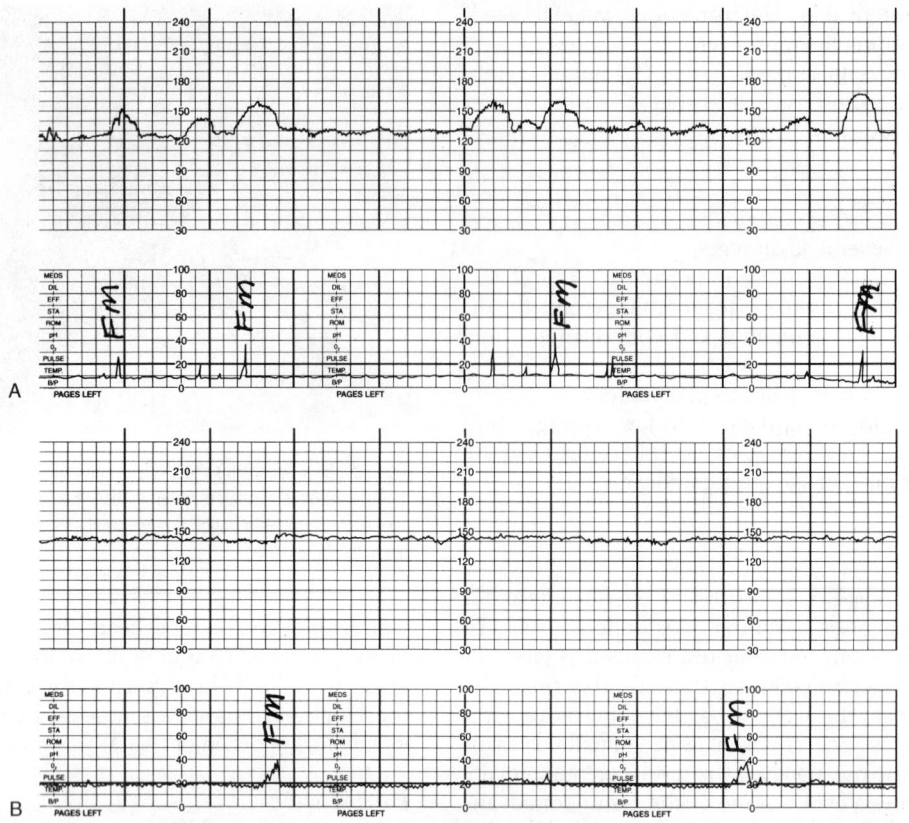

Figure 16-8 A, In this recording of a reactive nonstress test, the fetal heart rate acceleration peaks at least 15 beats per minute (bpm) and lasts for at least 15 seconds in response to fetal movement. Comparable accelerations without fetal movement are also reassuring. **B,** In this recording of a nonreactive nonstress test, accelerations are absent following fetal movement (FM). (Courtesy Graphic Controls, Buffalo, NY.)

the testing time for an additional 40 minutes or longer may be needed to allow for normal fetal sleep-wake cycles.

- *Nonreactive:* Tracing does not demonstrate the required characteristics of a reactive tracing within a 40-minute period.

Fetal heart reactivity occurs with maturation of the fetal autonomic nervous system. More than 15% of NSTs done before 32 weeks of gestation are likely to be nonreactive even with normal fetal oxygenation (AAP & ACOG, 2002). Different criteria for reassuring status on the preterm fetus younger than 32 weeks may be used although these are not definitively established. Suggested criteria for a reassuring NST in the fetus younger than 32 weeks include accelerations that peak 10 bpm above the baseline with a duration of 10 seconds ("10 by 10") within a 30-minute time window (Atterbury, Mikkelsen, & Santa-Donato, 2003).

Vibroacoustic, or acoustic, stimulation can reduce overall testing time and the incidence of false-positive nonreactive NSTs. A vibroacoustic stimulator is applied to the maternal abdomen in the area of the fetal head, and stimulation is given for up to 3 seconds. Acoustic stimulation can be repeated at 1-minute intervals for up to 3 times.

Advantages

The nonstress test is not invasive, is painless, and is believed to be without risk to mother or fetus. For these reasons it is the primary means of fetal surveillance in pregnancies that are at increased risk for uteroplacental insufficiency and consequent fetal hypoxia and acidosis. The nonstress test is easy to administer and may be repeated weekly or even daily if necessary. Results are available immediately.

Disadvantages

False-positive results often occur with nonstress testing. A common correctable reason for false-positive results is fetal sleep. Forty minutes gives most sleeping fetuses time to awaken, and acoustic stimulation reduces many other false-positive results.

Awaiting accelerations can prolong the nonstress test. Various methods have been used to stimulate the fetus to elicit accelerations in the fetal heart rate. Some of these methods include having the mother drink orange juice to raise her glucose level, manipulating the woman's abdomen, and fetal sound stimulation. Of these, only vibroacoustic stimulation of the fetus through the maternal abdomen has been shown by research to be both safe and effective.

Contraction Stress Test

Purpose

A contraction stress test (CST) may be suggested if nonstress test findings are nonreactive. The concern is that if fetal oxygenation is only marginally adequate when the uterus is at rest, it will be decreased further during uterine contractions. As the name implies, a contraction stress test involves recording the response of the fetal heart rate to stress that is induced by uterine contractions. Uterine contractions compress the arteries supplying the placenta with oxygenated maternal blood, causing a recurrent decrease in fetal oxygen levels.

The fetus with adequate oxygen reserves can tolerate the temporary hypoxia induced by uterine contractions, so the fetal heart rate pattern remains reassuring. If the fetus has inadequate reserves, however, and if hypoxia has led to anaerobic metabolism, fetal acidosis may result. This condition leads to myocardial depression that is evidenced by late decelerations in the fetal heart rate. If fetal heart rate variability is also decreased in the presence of persistent late decelerations, the correlation with fetal compromise is increased. Late decelerations begin after the contraction peaks and do not return to the baseline until after the contraction ends. (Chapter 18 reviews electronic fetal monitoring and nonreassuring patterns.)

Procedure

The nurse is responsible for administering the test and for protecting the safety of the mother and fetus throughout the testing period. The woman is positioned in a semi-Fowler's position or in a lateral or lateral tilt position if recumbent. External electronic fetal monitoring devices are applied to record both uterine activity and fetal heart rate. The fetal heart rate and patterns must be evaluated in relation to uterine contractions. Three contractions of at least 40 seconds each and occurring within a 10-minute period are required to interpret the contraction stress test. Two methods may be used to initiate uterine contractions if none are present:

1. *Nipple stimulation* causes the release of oxytocin from the posterior pituitary, which then causes uterine contractions. The woman brushes her palm across one nipple through her clothing for 2 minutes, stopping if a contraction begins. The nipple stimulation is repeated after a 5-minute rest period if no contractions occur.
2. If nipple stimulation does not result in adequate contractions, *intravenous infusion of low-dose oxytocin* is used to stimulate uterine contractions. The nurse conducting the test inserts a primary intravenous line plus a "piggyback" line to administer the oxytocin solution. Administration of oxytocin is similar to that for induction of labor (see Chapter 20).

Interpretation

Contraction stress test results are assigned one of five interpretations (AAP & ACOG, 2002):

- *Negative:* No late decelerations.
- *Positive:* Late decelerations follow 50% or more of contractions, even if fewer than three contractions occur in 10 minutes.
- *Equivocal-suspicious:* Intermittent late or significant variable decelerations.
- *Equivocal-hyperstimulation:* Fetal heart rate decelerations occur in the presence of excessive contractions (more frequent than every 2 minutes or lasting longer than 90 seconds).
- *Unsatisfactory:* Fewer than three contractions within 10 minutes or a tracing that cannot be interpreted.

See Figure 16-9 for a summary of contraction stress test interpretations.

Advantages

Contraction stress testing has a few advantages, although availability of other tests that are more diagnostic of fetal well-being and placenta function has reduced its original advantages.

- The test allows follow-up of a nonreactive NST result.
- A positive CST result allows the physician to analyze available options and to make plans for the birth of an infant who may be compromised because of decreased placental functioning before or during labor.

Disadvantages

Several significant disadvantages of the CST exist:

- A contraction stress test cannot be done if uterine contractions are contraindicated. Examples of these conditions include placenta previa (see Chapter 26), a previous classic cesarean incision (see Chapter 20), preterm rupture of the membranes, prematurity or high risk for premature delivery (ACOG, 1999).
- Uterine hyperstimulation may occur, possibly reducing uteroplacental perfusion. Hyperstimulation may result in late decelerations that would not occur with normal contractions, making test interpretation difficult.
- The test is time-consuming and thus more expensive, usually requiring about 2 hours.
- The contraction stress test is tedious, requiring either the participation of the woman in breast self-stimulation or controlled infusion of oxytocin to obtain an adequate contraction pattern without causing hyperstimulation of the uterus.
- Errors in interpretation are common. These may be caused by technical difficulties in obtaining tracings or problems in interpreting the data. For example, the fetal heart rate may accelerate with fetal movement, and late decelerations may occur with contractions (a reactive nonstress test but a positive contraction stress test). Such an interpretation requires further evaluation to confirm the well-being of the fetus.
- A contraction stress test is done in a hospital setting, where equipment and supplies, such as intravenous lines, oxytocin, and infusion pumps, are costly. The time spent by a nurse who is educated to administer the test must also be factored into the total cost.

Biophysical Profile

Predicting the condition of the fetus is more accurate if several parameters are evaluated. Unlike the nonstress test and contraction stress test, which assess only fetal heart activity, the biophysical profile (BPP) assesses five parameters of fetal well-being: the nonstress test, fetal breathing movements, gross fetal movements (large trunk movements), fetal tone (small or fine body movements such as limb or hand extension and flexion or sucking movements), and amniotic fluid volume. The last four parameters require ultrasound evaluation. If all four ultrasound components are reassuring, the nonstress test is not essential (AAP & ACOG, 2002).

Purpose

The individual components of the examination are a combination of both acute and chronic markers of fetal well-being to improve prognostic ability of the BPP. The acute markers

Negative   No late decelerations   Reassuring that the fetus can tolerate labor

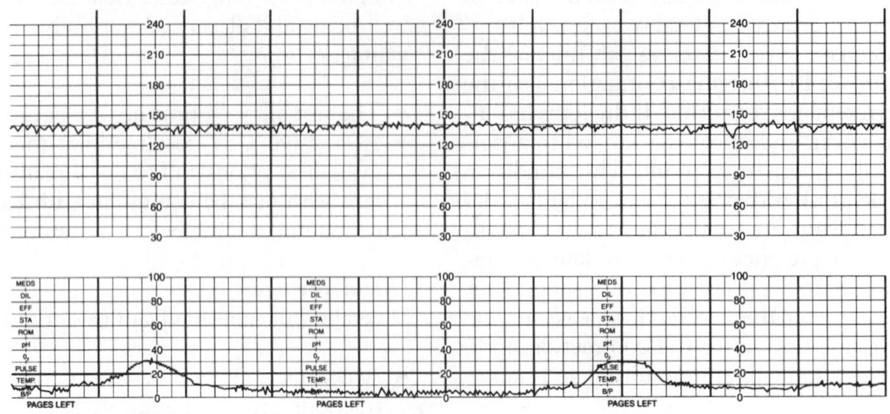

A

Positive   Consistent late decelerations in ≥ 50% of the con-   Indicates UPI and fetal compromise during con-
                                  tractions, even if contraction frequency is less   tractions
                                  than 3 in 10 minutes

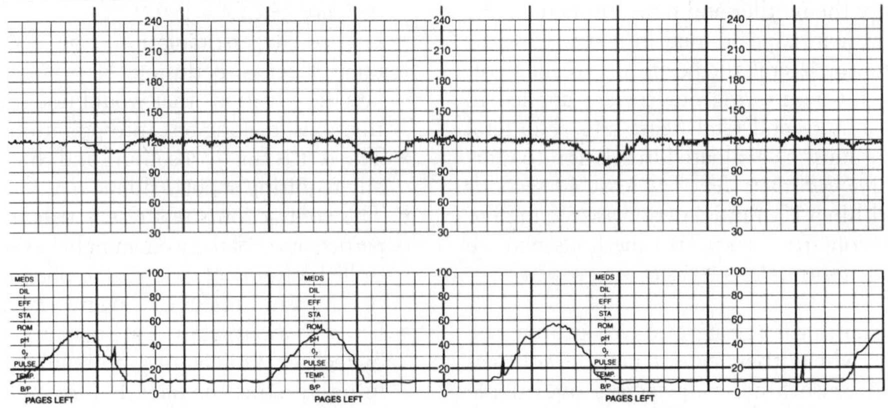

B

Equivocal-suspicious   Intermittent late or significant variable decelerations   A second CST should be repeated within 24 hours
Equivocal-Hyperstimulation   Late decelerations with excessive uterine activity   Repeat CST within 24 hours with careful monitor-
                                  (contractions closer than every 2 minutes or   ing of the situation
                                  lasting longer than 90 seconds)

Unsatisfactory   Test cannot be interpreted; either not enough data   Repeat CST with careful attention to maternal po-
                                  or unsatisfactory tracing; fewer than 3 contractions   sition, oxytocin infusion, and placement of toco-
                                  in 10 minutes   transducer

Figure 16-9 Interpretation of contraction stress test (CST). *UPI,* Uteroplacental insufficiency. (Courtesy Graphic Controls, Buffalo, NY.)

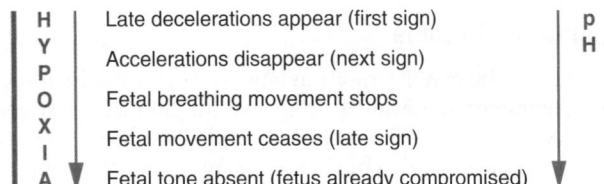

H Y P O X I A	Late decelerations appear (first sign)	p H
	Accelerations disappear (next sign)	
	Fetal breathing movement stops	
	Fetal movement ceases (late sign)	
	Fetal tone absent (fetus already compromised)	

Figure 16-10 Effects of gradual hypoxemia and worsening fetal acidosis.

are fetal heart rate reactivity and fetal breathing movements. Chronic markers include the volume of amniotic fluid, gross body movements, and fetal tone. Normal values for each suggest adequate neurologic function and oxygenation.

The fetal central and autonomic nervous systems that control some parameters of the biophysical profile react differently to hypoxemia. Late-developing control centers require higher oxygen levels than earlier-developing centers and are first to re-

act when oxygen levels fall. Fetal activities that develop earliest in gestation are the last to disappear when fetal oxygenation is compromised. Thus, as hypoxemia begins, fetal heart rate reactivity will be reduced, then absent. Fetal breathing movements will slow, then cease. As hypoxemia progresses, characteristics that developed earlier in gestation disappear, such as gross body movements and muscle tone, as the fetus conserves energy and oxygen. Figure 16-10 illustrates the effects of gradual hypoxemia on the central nervous system of the fetus.

The amount of amniotic fluid provides important information about long-term hypoxia. During periods of hypoxemia, the fetus shunts blood from areas that are not critical to fetal life, such as the kidneys and lungs, toward the vital organs (heart, brain, and placenta). If the hypoxemia is prolonged, blood flow to the fetal kidneys and lungs, which help produce amniotic fluid, may virtually cease. Therefore oligohydramnios indicates prolonged fetal hypoxia and strongly suggests fetal compromise.

TABLE **16-1** Scoring the Biophysical Profile for a Term Fetus

| | Points | |
Criterion	Present (2 points)	Absent (0 points)
Nonstress test (NST) (if used)	Reactive NST (≥2 fetal heart rate [FHR] accelerations peaking at least 15 beats per minute [bpm] above baseline for 15 sec within a 20-min period)	Nonreactive NST (absence of required characteristics for reactive test after 40 min of testing)
Fetal breathing movements (FBM)	≥1 episode of rhythmic FBM of 30 sec or more within 30 min	Absent FBM or none that meet criterion for "present"
Gross body movements	≥3 trunk movements in 30 min; limb and trunk movement is considered one movement	≤2 trunk movements in 30 min
Fetal tone	≥1 episode of fetal extremity extension with return to flexion; opening or closing of hand	Extension with return to partial flexion; absence of flexion
Amniotic fluid volume	At least one pocket of fluid that measures at least 2 cm in two planes perpendicular to each other	Amniotic fluid volume that does not meet this criterion

Interpretation: Normal (reassuring) = 8 to 10 points; equivocal = 6 points; abnormal = ≤4 points and delivery may be considered. If oligohydramnios is present, more frequent testing is warranted and delivery may be considered.
From American Academy of Pediatrics (AAP) & American College of Obstetricians and Gynecologists (ACOG). (2002). *Guidelines for perinatal care* (5th ed.). Elk Grove Village, IL, and Washington, DC: Author.

Procedure and Interpretation

Fetal heart rate reactivity is measured and interpreted from a nonstress test. The other four parameters are measured by real-time ultrasound scanning for a maximum of 30 minutes. A scoring technique is used to quantify the data, with each of the five parameters contributing either 2 or 0 points out of 10 total points, or 8 total points if the NST is not done (Table 16-1). A score of 10 (8 for BPPs that do not include the NST) is perfect; a score of 0 is the worst possible score. A total score of 8-10 out of 10 (expressed as "8/10" to "10/10") is reassuring; a score of 4 or less is nonreassuring. Oligohydramnios may indicate chronic fetal hypoxia and warrants more frequent biophysical profile testing or consideration of delivery (AAP & ACOG, 2002).

Amniotic Fluid Index

The amniotic fluid index (AFI) has become a popular measurement for the volume of amniotic fluid. Ultrasound is used to calculate the vertical depth of the largest pocket of amniotic fluid in each of four uterine quadrants, and the four numbers are added. Although standard guidelines for the AFI do not exist, values of more than 5 cm and less than 18 to 20 cm are usually recognized as normal (Callen, 2000a).

Modified Biophysical Profile

Some physicians assess the fetus only by ultrasonography and omit the nonstress test if all ultrasound parameters are normal. Another modification includes only two parameters: an amniotic fluid index and a nonstress test (AAP & ACOG, 2002).

Advantages

The BPP is noninvasive and is less costly than some tests because it can be done on an outpatient basis. Results are immediately available, and it may decrease the number of false-positive nonreactive nonstress test findings. Nurses educated in ultrasonography may perform the ultrasound part of the BPP. The evaluation allows conservative treatment of high-risk patients because delivery can be delayed if reassurance of fetal well-being exists.

Disadvantages

Additional research is needed to refine interpretation of the test. For example, each variable is given equal weight, although some variables may be more important. Oligohydramnios is an indicator for more frequent testing or for delivery, regardless of results from the other parameters (AAP & ACOG, 2002). At present, knowledge about the relationship of low BPP scores to long-term development of the child is not complete.

PERCUTANEOUS UMBILICAL BLOOD SAMPLING

Percutaneous umbilical blood sampling (PUBS), also called *cordocentesis*, involves the aspiration of fetal blood from the umbilical cord for prenatal diagnosis or therapy (Fig. 16-11). Major indications for PUBS include the diagnosis and intrauterine management of Rh disease, genetic studies, diagnosis of abnormal blood-clotting factors, severe fetal growth restriction, and acid-base status of the fetus.

Procedure

Ultrasonography is used to locate the fetus, placenta, and umbilical cord. A needle is inserted through the abdomen and into the uterine cavity. The puncture is made into the umbilical cord near the site at which the cord meets the placenta because the cord is more stable at this site. The umbilical vein is targeted more commonly than one of the umbilical arteries because it is larger and is less likely to constrict during the procedure. It is not important to know which vessel (vein or artery) was used when sampling fetal

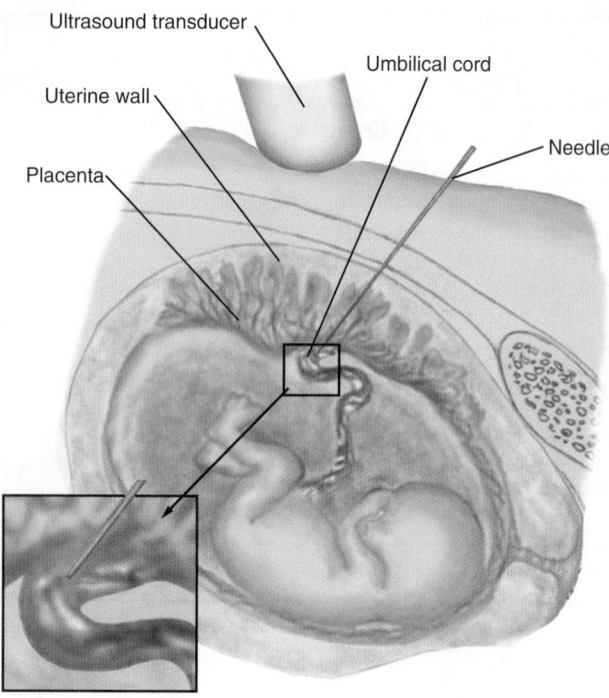

Figure 16-11 In percutaneous umbilical blood sampling, a needle is inserted through the expectant mother's abdomen and into an umbilical vessel (vein or artery) to withdraw a sample of fetal blood.

blood for genetic or coagulation studies, but it is very important to know which was used when testing fetal acid-base parameters. Blood from the umbilical vein contains oxygenated blood and has a lower carbon dioxide content (and thus a higher pH) than blood from an umbilical artery, which comes directly from the fetus after circulation throughout the body.

Risks

In addition to fetal loss, complications of PUBS include infection, fetal bradycardia, cord laceration, cord hematoma, thrombosis, thromboembolism, premature labor, and premature rupture of membranes. After needle withdrawal, the duration of bleeding from the umbilical cord is usually short and can be monitored by ultrasound examination. In addition, the fetal heart can be monitored electronically to identify reassuring or nonreassuring patterns.

MATERNAL ASSESSMENT OF FETAL MOVEMENT

Movements by the fetus, as assessed by the mother, are often called "kick counts." Fetal movement is associated with fetal condition, and daily evaluation of these movements provides a way of evaluating the fetus.

Procedure

Numerous protocols exist for assessing kick counts. Examples of kick count protocols include the following:

- Count fetal movements for 30 minutes three times per day (Fig. 16-12). Further evaluation is recommended for fewer than four movements in 30 minutes.

- Count fetal movements daily for 1 hour. If fewer than 10 movements are felt, continue counting for another hour. Fewer than 10 movements in a 2-hour period should be reported to the health care provider.
- The Cardiff count-to-10 method entails counting the first 10 movements and noting the amount of time required to reach the 10th movement. The health care provider should be notified if the 10th movement occurs progressively later or fewer than 10 movements occur in 12 hours.
- Count fetal movements for 30 minutes in the morning and evening to establish a baseline. If a 50% decrease or no fetal movement occurs, extend the counting period for 30 minutes. If no improvement occurs, the woman should report to the hospital or clinic (Devoe, 2000).

If another protocol for fetal movement evaluation is used, the physician may give slightly different guidelines for notification.

Advantages

Counting fetal movements is one of the oldest methods for evaluating the condition of the fetus. There are some obvious advantages:

- It is inexpensive.
- It is noninvasive.
- It is convenient for the client and encourages her participation in care.

Disadvantages

Many variables make interpretation of fetal movement counts difficult:

- Fetal resting state normally decreases movements.
- Maternal perception of fetal movement varies considerably, even in the same woman at different times.
- Time of day may affect fetal movement (less in the morning, greater in the evening).
- Maternal use of drugs (sedative drugs, methadone, heroin, cocaine, alcohol, tobacco) may affect fetal activity.

■NURSING CARE
The Client Who Has Diagnostic Testing

Assessment

Nurses collect information that is important to conducting the diagnostic tests or that is helpful to the physician interpreting the results. Necessary information includes:

- Gravida, para, living children, gestation.
- Maternal health problems (hypertension, diabetes, heart disease).
- Current obstetric problems (vaginal bleeding, decreased fetal movement, multifetal gestation, intrauterine growth restriction, malpresentation, hydramnios, oligohydramnios, preeclampsia).
- Prior obstetric problems (birth of stillborn infant or infant with congenital anomalies, birth of low-birth-weight infant or large-for-gestational-age infant).

Dates: 11/14/98 to 11/20/98							
Time of day	Sunday	Monday	Tuesday	Wednesday	Thursday	Friday	Saturday
Morning 8-9 a.m.	╫╫ ╫╫	╫╫ ‖	╫╫ ‖‖				
Afternoon 1-2 p.m.	╫╫		╫╫ ‖‖‖	╫╫				
Evening 9-10 p.m.	╫╫ ‖ ╫╫	╫╫ ‖‖‖‖					
Total	28	24					

Figure 16-12 Example of a fetal movement record. The mother counts the number of fetal movements, or "kicks," within a specified period several times a day and indicates each movement on a chart. She reports any abnormality to her health care provider.

- History of substance abuse, including alcohol and tobacco.
- Client knowledge of reasons for the test and the procedure to be performed. The nurse may ask, "What questions can I answer before we start the test?"
- Client knowledge of surveillance regimen if additional testing is necessary: "Will you tell me what you understand about the need to repeat the test every week?"
- The woman's emotional response to the tests: "What are your major concerns?" "What can we do to make the tests easier for you?"
- The woman's or couple's expectations of the diagnostic tests. The risks and limitations for testing should be discussed as well as the indications. It may also be necessary to remind the couple that results from one test may indicate that others are appropriate. They must decide at each step about whether to continue.

Nursing Diagnosis and Planning

The following nursing diagnosis is common when a woman requires fetal diagnostic testing:

■ Anxiety related to lack of knowledge of diagnostic procedures and the uncertain condition of the fetus.

Expected Outcomes: The woman and her support person will verbalize knowledge of how, when, and why she is to be tested before testing procedures are initiated. The woman and her family will verbalize concerns and seek knowledge about the fetus.

Interventions

Providing Information

Provide the woman and her family simple, clear explanations of what the test assesses and the purpose and frequency of any tests. Tell them how long the test takes, and describe the testing procedure to reduce anxiety caused by lack of knowledge. Some tests require teaching about follow-up care and events that should be reported to the health care team.

Providing Support

It is critical that the nurse identify and respond to feelings expressed by prospective parents when antepartum testing procedures are recommended or when fetal problems are con-

firmed. The woman often experiences frustration with the discomfort, limitations, and time-consuming demands of the pregnancy and the regimen of fetal testing. Skill in therapeutic communication is never more important than when counseling about fetal diagnostic tests.

- Active listening conveys interest and concern.
- Paraphrasing allows for interpretation because it expresses in different words what concerns the family.
- Reflecting what is expressed about feelings helps the family "hear" their feelings.
- Clarifying helps prospective parents "see" the issues and what options are available.
- Comforting measures such as touch convey empathic concern and are especially important during difficult procedures.

Although nurses offer caring concern and careful reflection of feelings, they do not offer advice. The decisions must be made by the woman and her family, but nurses frequently help clients contact persons to whom they turn in troubled times, such as a member of the clergy or a close relative.

Women benefit from knowing that compliance with the testing regimen is beneficial for the fetus. Each day in the uterus allows time for growth and development and increases the chance that the infant will be strong and healthy. The fetus has an improved chance of surviving as long as the test results remain reassuring.

Nurses must examine their own ethical beliefs before they become involved in fetal diagnostic testing. They must be prepared to support whatever decision a woman and her family make, even if it is not one they would make. For example, whether a woman decides to continue or terminate a pregnancy, she is entitled to compassionate care regardless of the nurse's personal views about the decision.

Evaluation

- Did the woman (and her family) verbalize knowledge of why tests are recommended and express an idea of how and when they will be performed?
- Does she actively seek information about the fetal condition to relieve her anxiety?

KEY CONCEPTS

- Ultrasonography is widely used during pregnancy to determine a variety of fetal and placental conditions and to aid in the performance of other tests, such as amniocentesis. Doppler ultrasound is a variation that allows estimation of blood flow and vascular resistance in fetal structures.
- Alpha-fetoprotein (AFP) assessment, a screening test performed on maternal serum or amniotic fluid, is used primarily to detect open neural tube defects and chromosomal abnormalities. Additional tests are required if AFP levels are abnormal. Two other markers, human chorionic gonadotropin and estriol, are assessed along with AFP to screen for chromosomal anomalies.
- Chorionic villus sampling can be performed as early as 10 weeks of gestation to provide parents with information about many chromosomal defects in the first trimester of pregnancy. The risk for pregnancy loss is somewhat higher than it is for amniocentesis.

- Amniocentesis is usually performed in the second trimester to identify fetal genetic anomalies or open defects such as neural tube defects. It is done during the third trimester to evaluate fetal lung maturity or Rh incompatibility problems. Early amniocentesis (11 to 14 weeks) may also be done but is associated with higher fetal loss.
- The nonstress test evaluates fetal heart rate (FHR) accelerations, with or without fetal movement. FHR reactivity with accelerations is a reassuring sign associated with adequate fetal oxygenation and intact neural pathway from the fetal brain to the heart. Reactivity may not develop until 32 weeks in many fetuses.
- A biophysical profile provides information on five parameters: the nonstress test, fetal breathing movements, gross fetal movements, fetal tone, and amniotic fluid volume.
- The amniotic fluid index is a method to quantify the amount of amniotic fluid. Values over

5 cm and less than 18 to 20 cm are presently considered normal.
- Contraction stress tests (CSTs) are used to determine how the fetal heart responds to uterine contractions that temporarily decrease placental blood flow. A positive test result suggests that the placental function has deteriorated. The CST cannot be done if stimulated uterine contractions are contraindicated.
- Percutaneous umbilical blood sampling involves aspirating blood from umbilical vessels to detect blood disorders, acid-base imbalance, infection, or fetal genetic disease.
- Maternal assessment of fetal movement ("kick counts") is an inexpensive and noninvasive method of evaluating the placental function.
- All perinatal nurses must be prepared to offer clear explanations of diagnostic procedures and to provide support for the family requiring fetal diagnostic tests.

REFERENCES and READINGS

Alteneder, R.R., Kenner, C., Greene, D., & Pohorecki, S. (1998). The lived experience of women who undergo prenatal diagnostic testing due to elevated maternal serum alpha-fetoprotein screening. *MCN: The American Journal of Maternal/Child Nursing, 23*(4), 180-186.

American Academy of Pediatrics (AAP), & American College of Obstetricians and Gynecologists (ACOG). (2002). *Guidelines for perinatal care* (5th ed.). Elk Grove Village, IL, and Washington, DC: Author.

American College of Obstetricians and Gynecologists (ACOG). (1999). *ACOG practice bulletin: Antepartum fetal surveillance.* Washington, DC: Author.

Association of Women's Health, Obstetric, & Neonatal Nurses. (1998). Clinical competencies and education guide: Antepartum and intrapartum fetal heart rate monitoring.

Atterbury, J.L., Mikkelsen, G.M., & Santa-Donato, A. (2003). Antenatal fetal assessment and testing. In N. Feinstein, K.L. Torgersen, & J. Atterbury (Eds.), *AWHONN's fetal heart monitoring principles and practices* (3rd ed., pp. 261-288). Dubuque, IA: Kendall/Hunt.

Beall, M.H. (2000). Chorionic villus sampling for prenatal diagnosis. In E.J. Quilligan & F.P. Zuspan (Eds.), *Current therapy in obstetrics and gynecology* (5th ed., pp. 253-256). Philadelphia: Saunders.

Callen, P.W. (2000a). Amniotic fluid: Its role in fetal health and disease. In P.W. Callen (Ed.), *Ultrasonography in obstetrics and gynecology* (4th ed., pp. 638-659). Philadelphia: Saunders.

Callen, P.W. (2000b). The obstetric ultrasound examination. In P.W. Callen (Ed.), *Ultrasonography in obstetrics and gynecology* (4th ed., pp. 1-17). Philadelphia: Saunders.

Cunningham, F.G., Gant, N.F., Leveno, K.J., Gilstrap, L.C., Hauth, J.C., & Wenstrom, K.D. (2001). *Williams obstetrics* (21st ed.). New York: McGraw-Hill.

Devoe, L.D. (2000). Antepartum fetal surveillance. In E.J. Quilligan & F.P. Zuspan (Eds.), *Current therapy in obstetrics and gynecology* (5th ed., pp. 372-376). Philadelphia: Saunders.

Farkouh, L.J., & Hobbins, J.C. (2000). Percutaneous umbilical blood sampling. In E.J. Quilligan & F.P. Zuspan (Eds.), *Current therapy in obstetrics and gynecology* (5th ed., pp. 427-429). Philadelphia: Saunders.

Filly, R.A. (2000a). Obstetrical sonography: The best way to terrify a pregnant woman. *Journal of Ultrasound in Medicine, 19*(1), 1-5.

Filly, R.A., & Hadlock, F.P. (2000). Sonographic determination of menstrual age. In P.W. Callen (Ed.), *Ultrasonography in obstetrics and gynecology* (4th ed., pp. 146-170). Philadelphia: Saunders.

Gilbert, E.S., & Harmon, J.S. (2003). *Manual of high-risk pregnancy and delivery* (3rd ed.). St. Louis: Mosby.

Harman, C.R. (2004). Assessment of fetal health. In R.K. Creasy, R. Resnik, & J. D. Iams (Eds.), *Maternal-fetal medicine* (5th ed., pp. 357-401). Philadelphia: Saunders.

Harris, R.D., & Alexander, R.D. (2000). Ultrasound of the placenta and umbilical cord. In P.W. Callen (Ed.), *Ultrasonography in obstetrics and gynecology* (4th ed., pp. 597-625). Philadelphia: Saunders.

Jenkins, T.M., & Wapner, R.J. (2004). Prenatal diagnosis of congenital disorders. In R.K. Creasy, R. Resnik, & J.D. Iams (Eds.), *Maternal-fetal medicine: principles and practice* (5th ed., pp. 235-280) Philadelphia: Saunders.

Johnson, D.D., & Vandorsten, J.P. (2000). In S.B. Ransom, M.P. Dombrowski, S.G. McNeeley, K.S. Moghissi, & A.R. Munkarah (Eds.), *Practi-*

cal strategies in obstetrics and gynecology (pp. 239-248). Philadelphia: Saunders.

Jorde, L.B., Carey, J.C., Bamshad, M.J., & White, R.L. (2003). *Medical genetics* (3rd ed.). St. Louis: Mosby.

Lettieri, L., Vintzileos, A.M., & Nochimson, D.J. (2000). Biophysical profile. In E.J. Quilligan & F.P. Zuspan (Eds.), *Current therapy in obstetrics and gynecology* (5th ed., pp. 376-380). Philadelphia: Saunders.

Manning, F.A. (2004). General principles and applications of ultrasonography. In R.K. Creasy R. Resnik, and J.D. Iams (Eds.), *Maternal-fetal medicine* (5th ed., pp. 315-355). Philadelphia: Saunders.

Maulik, D. (2000). Doppler velocimetry in fetal surveillance. In E.J. Quilligan & F.P. Zuspan (Eds.), *Current therapy in obstetrics and gynecology* (5th ed., pp. 388-393). Philadelphia: Saunders.

Nathan, E.B., Haberman, S., Burgess, T., & Minkoff, H. (2000). The relationship of maternal position to the results of brief nonstress tests: A randomized clinical trial. *American Journal of Obstetrics and Gynecology, 182*(5), 1070-1072.

Opipari, A.W., & Johnson, T.R.B. (2000). Fetal assessment. In S.B. Ransom, M.P. Dombrowski, S.G. McNeeley, K.S. Moghissi, & A.R. Munkarah (Eds.), *Practical strategies in obstetrics & gynecology* (pp. 224-233). Philadelphia: Saunders.

Pretorius, D.H., Nelson, T.R., & Lev-Toaff, A.S. (2000). Three-dimensional ultrasound in obstetrics and gynecology. In P.W. Callen (Ed.), *Ultrasonography in obstetrics and gynecology* (4th ed., pp. 747-762). Philadelphia: Saunders.

Richardson, B. S., & Gagnon, R. (1999). Fetal breathing and body movements. In R. K. Creasy & R. Resnik (Eds.), *Maternal-fetal medicine* (4th ed., pp. 231-247). Philadelphia: Saunders.

Stringer, M., Miesnik, S.R., Brown, L.P., Menei, L., & Macones, G.A. (2003). Limited obstetric ultrasound examinations: Competency and cost. *Journal of Obstetric, Gynecologic, & Neonatal Nursing, 32*(3): 307-312.

Tekay, A., & Campbell, S. (2000). Doppler ultrasonography in obstetrics. In P.W. Callen (Ed.), *Ultrasonography in obstetrics and gynecology* (4th ed., pp. 677-723). Philadelphia: Saunders.

Treadwell, M.C. (2000). First trimester ultrasonography. In S.B. Ransom, M.P. Dombrowski, S.G. McNeeley, K.S. Moghissi, & A.R. Munkarah (Eds.), *Practical strategies in obstetrics and gynecology* (pp. 234-238). Philadelphia: Saunders.

Treanor, C. (1998). Exploring nurses' roles in limited ultrasound. *AWHONN Lifelines, 2*(2), 13-14.

Yankowitz, J., & Williamson, R.A. (1999). Abnormalities of alpha-fetoprotein and other biochemical tests. In D.K. James, P.J. Steer, C.P. Weiner, & B. Gonik (Eds.), *High-risk pregnancy: Management options* (2nd ed., pp. 157-170). Philadelphia: Saunders.

Ward, K. (2003). Genetics and prenatal diagnosis. In J.R. Scott, R.S. Gibbs, B.Y. Karlan, & A.F. Haney (Eds.), *Danforth's obstetrics and gynecology* (9th ed., pp. 105-128). Philadelphia: Lippincott.

17

Giving Birth

◆ DEFINITIONS

abortion A pregnancy that ends before 20 weeks' gestation, either spontaneously or electively. *Miscarriage* is a lay term for a spontaneous abortion that is being more frequently used by professionals.

amniotomy Artificial rupture of the amniotic sac (fetal membranes).

attitude Relationship of fetal body parts to one another, such as flexion or extension.

bloody show Mixture of cervical mucus and blood from ruptured capillaries in the cervix. Bloody show often precedes labor and increases with cervical dilation.

Braxton Hicks contractions Irregular, mild uterine contractions that occur throughout pregnancy. These contractions become stronger in the last trimester.

caput succedaneum Area of edema over the presenting part of the fetus or newborn, resulting from pressure against the cervix. Usually called simply *caput*.

crowning Appearance of the fetal scalp or presenting part at the vaginal opening.

EDD Abbreviation for estimated date of delivery. This date may also be abbreviated EDB (estimated date of birth).

engagement Descent of the widest diameter of the fetal presenting part to at least a zero station (the level of the ischial spines in the maternal pelvis).

episiotomy Surgical incision of the perineum to enlarge the vaginal opening.

ferning (or fern test) Microscopic appearance of amniotic fluid that resembles fern leaves when the fluid dries on a microscope slide.

fontanel Space at the intersection of sutures connecting fetal or infant skull bones.

gravida A pregnant woman. Also refers to a woman's total number of pregnancies, including the one in progress, if applicable.

lie Relationship of the long axis of the fetus to the long axis of the mother.

lightening Descent of the fetus toward the pelvic inlet before labor.

lochia Vaginal drainage after birth.

molding Shaping of the fetal head during movement through the birth canal.

multipara A woman who has given birth after two or more pregnancies of at least 20 weeks' gestation. Also informally used to describe a pregnant woman before the birth of her second or later child.

nitrazine paper Paper to determine pH. Nitrazine paper helps determine whether the amniotic sac has ruptured.

nuchal cord Umbilical cord around the fetal neck.

nullipara A woman who has not completed a pregnancy to at least 20 weeks' gestation.

para A woman who has given birth after a pregnancy of at least 20 weeks' gestation. Para also designates the number of pregnancies that end after at least 20 weeks' gestation. (A multifetal gestation, such as twins, is considered one birth when calculating parity.)

position Relation of a fixed reference point on the fetus to the quadrants of the maternal pelvis.

presentation Fetal part that first enters the pelvic inlet; also, the presenting part.

primipara A woman who has given birth after a pregnancy of at least 20 weeks' gestation. The term is also used informally to describe a pregnant woman before the birth of her first child.

station Measurement of fetal descent in relation to the ischial spines of the maternal pelvis. See also *engagement*.

sutures Narrow areas of flexible tissue that connect the fetal skull bones, permitting slight movement during labor.

VBAC Abbreviation for vaginal birth after cesarean birth.

Care of the woman and her family during labor and birth is a rewarding field of nursing. The birth of a baby is more than a physical event; it has deep personal and social significance for the family. Family roles and relationships are forever altered by this event.

ISSUES FOR NEW NURSES

Common issues face new nurses and nursing students when caring for families during birth.

Pain Associated With Birth

Working with people in pain is difficult, and most nurses feel compelled to relieve pain promptly. Yet pain is an expected part of labor and cannot be eliminated for all of labor, even with the newest techniques. Helping the woman manage the pain of birth is a crucial part of nursing care.

Inexperience or Negative Experiences

The nurse who has never given birth may feel inadequate to care for laboring women, although she or he rarely feels it necessary to experience a fracture to care for someone with that problem. Nursing skills needed by the intrapartum nurse are basic: observation, critical thinking, problem solving, therapeutic communication, comfort promotion, empathy, and common sense.

Nurses also may be anxious because of their own difficult experiences during pregnancy or birth. They must be careful not to convey negative attitudes to the laboring woman and her partner.

Unpredictability

Labor is a natural process that follows its own timetable. Some occurrences simply are not easily predicted or explained. Some nurses find the uncertain nature of intrapartum care troubling, whereas others find it exciting. Some days are busy from the start, while others are uncannily quiet, only to erupt in adrenaline-charged action with no warning.

Intimacy

The intimate nature of intrapartum care and its sexual overtones also make some nurses uncomfortable. They may feel that they are intruding on a private time.

The male nurse often finds this aspect of intrapartum care most anxiety-provoking. Although he may have cared for other female clients, his care has not been this focused on the reproductive system. He often wonders how a woman's male partner will accept him as a care provider.

The best approach for both male and female nurses is to maintain professional conduct and take cues from the couple. If they want privacy, the nurse should intervene only as needed to assess the woman and fetus. In more advanced labor, both partners often welcome the presence of a competent, caring nurse of either sex.

PHYSIOLOGIC EFFECTS OF THE BIRTH PROCESS

Labor and birth affect the physiologic systems of both the pregnant woman and her fetus. These effects are most striking in the maternal reproductive system and in relation to fetal and neonatal oxygenation.

Maternal Response

Significant changes during labor occur in the woman's cardiovascular, respiratory, gastrointestinal, urinary, and hematopoietic systems as well as in her reproductive system.

Reproductive System

Characteristics of Contractions. Normal labor contractions are coordinated, involuntary, and intermittent.

Coordinated Contractions. The uterus can contract and relax in a coordinated way, as can other smooth muscles such as the heart. As the woman approaches full term, contractions become organized and gradually assume a regular pattern of increasing frequency, duration, and intensity during labor. Coordinated labor contractions begin in the uterine fundus and spread downward toward the cervix to propel the fetus through the pelvis.

Involuntary Contractions. Uterine contractions are not under conscious control, as are skeletal muscles. The mother cannot cause labor to start or stop by conscious effort. Walking or other activity may stimulate existing labor contractions. Anxiety and excessive stress can diminish them.

Intermittent Contractions. Labor contractions are intermittent rather than sustained, allowing relaxation of the uterine muscle and resumption of blood flow to and from the placenta to permit gas, nutrient, and waste exchange for the fetus.

Contraction Cycle. Each contraction consists of three phases (Fig. 17-1). The *increment* occurs as the contraction begins in the fundus and spreads throughout the uterus. The *peak*, or *acme*, is the period during which the contraction is most intense. The *decrement* is the period of decreasing intensity as the uterus relaxes.

The contraction cycle and the overall pattern of contractions are also described in terms of frequency, duration, and intensity. *Frequency* is the period from the beginning of one uterine contraction to the beginning of the next; it is usually expressed in minutes and fractions of minutes. For example, the nurse states, "Contractions are $3\frac{1}{2}$ to 4 minutes apart."

Duration is the length of each contraction from beginning to end; it is usually expressed in seconds. For example, the nurse might report, "Her contractions last 55 to 65 seconds."

Intensity is the strength of the contractions. The terms "mild," "moderate," and "strong" are used to describe contraction intensity as palpated by the nurse. Mild contractions are often described as feeling like the tip of the nose, moderate contractions like the chin, and firm contractions like the forehead. Different descriptions of intensity may apply when the electronic fetal monitor is used to record contractions (see Chapter 18).

The *interval* is the period between the end of one contraction and the beginning of the next. The interval is the time when most fetal exchange of oxygen, nutrients, and waste products occurs.

Uterine Body. Uterine activity during labor is characterized by opposing features. The upper two thirds of the uterus contracts actively to push the fetus down. The lower one third of the uterus remains less active, allowing downward passage of the fetus. The cervix is similar to the lower uterine segment in that it is also passive. The net effect of labor contractions is enhanced because the downward push from the upper uterus is accompanied by reduced resistance to fetal descent in the lower uterus.

Myometrial (uterine muscle) cells in the upper uterus remain shorter at the end of each contraction rather than returning to their original length. In contrast, myometrial cells in the lower uterus become longer with each contraction.

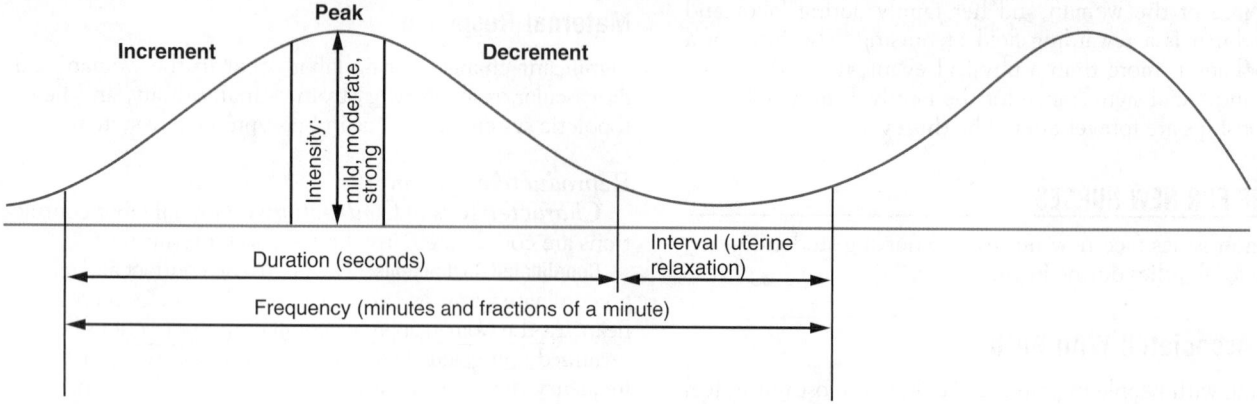

Figure 17-1 Contraction cycle.

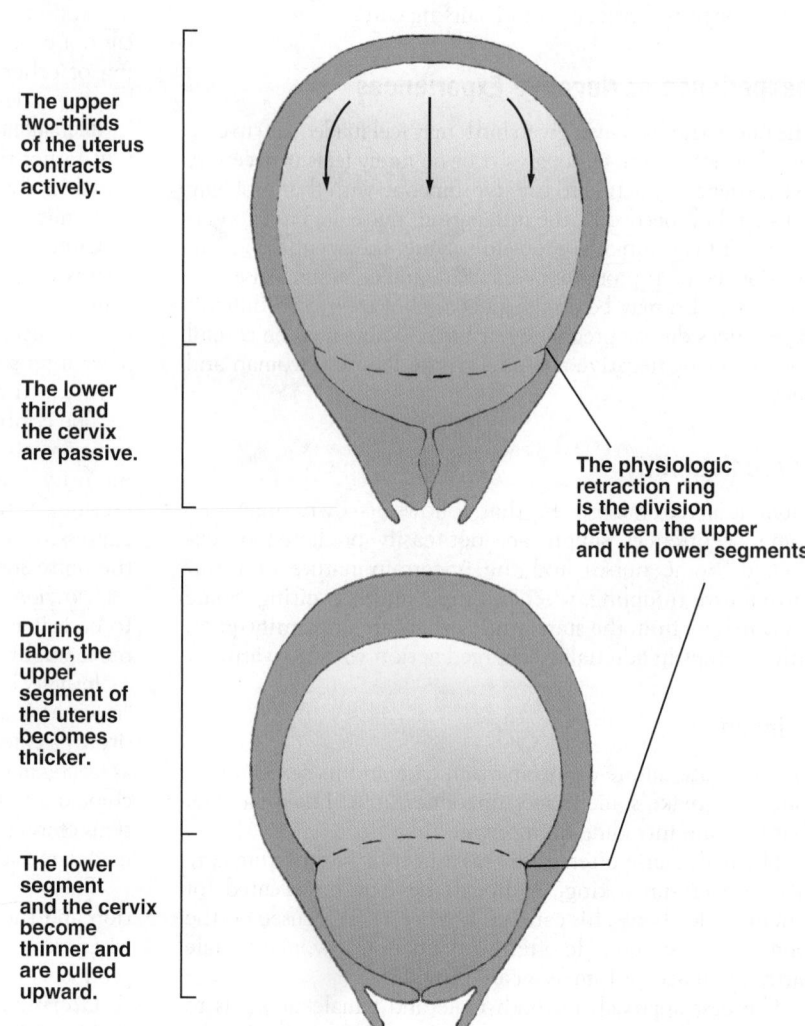

The upper two-thirds of the uterus contracts actively.

The lower third and the cervix are passive.

The physiologic retraction ring is the division between the upper and the lower segments.

During labor, the upper segment of the uterus becomes thicker.

The lower segment and the cervix become thinner and are pulled upward.

Figure 17-2 Opposing characteristics of uterine contraction in the upper and lower segments of the uterus.

These two characteristics enable the upper uterus to maintain tension between contractions to preserve the cervical changes and downward fetal progress made with each contraction.

The opposing characteristics of myometrial contraction in the upper and lower uterine segments cause changes in the thickness of the uterine wall during labor. The upper uterus becomes thicker while the lower uterus becomes thinner and pulled upward during labor. The physiologic retraction ring marks the division between the upper and lower segments of the uterus (Fig. 17-2).

The opposing characteristics of contractions in the upper and lower uterine segments change the shape of the uterine cavity, which becomes more elongated and narrower as labor progresses. This change in uterine shape straightens the fetal body and efficiently directs it downward in the pelvis.

Primigravida   **Multigravida**

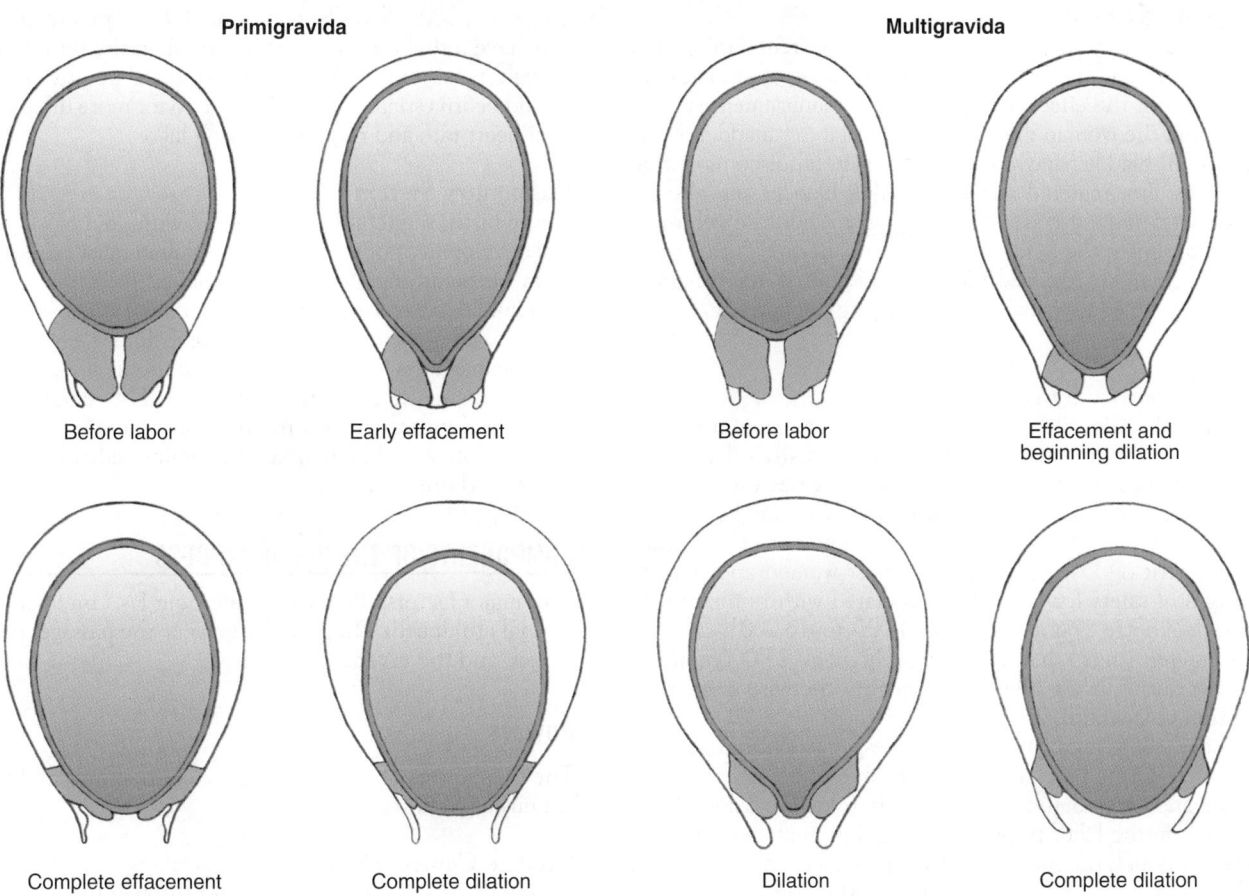

| Before labor | Early effacement | Before labor | Effacement and beginning dilation |

| Complete effacement | Complete dilation | Dilation | Complete dilation |

Figure 17-3 Cervical dilation and effacement. During labor, the multigravida's cervix remains thicker than the nullipara's.

Cervical Changes. *Effacement* (thinning and shortening) and *dilation* (opening) are the major cervical changes during labor. Effacement and dilation occur together during labor but at different rates. The nullipara completes most cervical effacement early in the process of cervical dilation. In contrast, the parous woman's cervix is usually thicker than a nullipara's cervix at any point during labor.

Effacement. Before labor, the cervix is a cylindric structure, about 2 cm long, at the lower end of the uterus. Labor contractions push the fetus downward against the cervix as they pull the cervix upward. The cervix becomes shorter and thinner as it is drawn over the fetus and amniotic sac (Fig. 17-3). The cervix merges with the thinning lower uterus rather than remaining a distinct cylindric structure. Effacement is estimated as a percentage of the amount the cervix has thinned, so that a fully thinned cervix is 100% effaced. Effacement also may be recorded as cervical length, estimated in centimeters during vaginal examination.

Dilation. As the cervix is pulled upward and the fetus is pushed downward, the cervix dilates. Dilation is expressed in centimeters, with approximately 10 cm being full dilation, large enough to allow passage of the average-size term fetus. The action during effacement and dilation can be likened to pushing a tennis ball out the cuff of a sock.

Cardiovascular System

During each uterine contraction, blood flow to the placenta gradually decreases, causing a relative increase in the woman's blood volume. This temporary change increases her blood pressure slightly and slows her pulse. Therefore the mother's vital signs are best assessed during the interval between contractions.

Although it is more likely to occur during the antepartum period, supine hypotension also may occur during labor if the mother lies on her back (see Fig. 13-4). *The mother should be encouraged to rest in positions other than the supine to promote blood return to her heart and therefore enhance blood flow to the placenta and promote fetal oxygenation.*

Respiratory System

The depth and rate of respirations increase, especially if the woman is anxious or in pain. A woman who breathes rapidly and deeply may experience symptoms of hyperventilation if she exhales too much carbon dioxide. She may also feel tingling in her hands and feet, numbness, and dizziness. Helping her to slow her breathing and to breathe into a paper bag or her cupped hands can restore normal blood levels of carbon dioxide and relieve these symptoms.

Gastrointestinal System

Gastric motility is reduced to varying degrees during labor. Most women are not hungry but are often thirsty and have a dry mouth. Food and large volumes of liquids are usually limited to reduce the risk of vomiting and aspiration if unexpected surgery is needed. Ice chips are commonly provided, as are small amounts of other clear liquids or juices, Popsicles, or hard candy. Large amounts of sugar are not desirable because they may cause rebound hypoglycemia in the newborn when the sugar supply abruptly ends at birth.

Urinary System

The most common change in the urinary system during labor is reduced sensation of a full bladder. Because of intense contractions or the effects of regional pain management such as epidural, the woman may be unaware that her bladder is full. Yet a full bladder may contribute to general discomfort that remains after regional analgesia. A full bladder can also inhibit fetal descent because it occupies space in the pelvis.

After birth, the fluid retention that is normal during pregnancy is quickly reversed and urine is excreted in large quantities. The bladder may fill rapidly during the first few days after birth.

Hematopoietic System

Most authorities recognize 500 ml as the maximum normal blood loss during vaginal birth. Women usually tolerate this loss well because the blood volume increases during pregnancy by 1 to 2 liters (Blackburn, 2003; Cunningham et al., 2001; Guyton & Hall, 2000). A hemoglobin of 11 g/dl and a hematocrit of 33% or higher give most women an adequate margin of safety for blood loss associated with normal birth. The leukocyte count averages 14,000 to 16,000 per cubic millimeter (mm^3) but may be as high as 25,000/mm^3 or higher during labor, a level that might otherwise suggest infection (Blackburn, 2003, Cunningham et al., 2001).

Levels of several clotting factors, especially fibrinogen, are elevated during pregnancy and continue to be higher during labor and after delivery. Fibrinolysis (clot breakdown) decreases during labor to promote coagulation at the placental site. Although the increase in clotting factors and decrease in fibrinolysis protect from hemorrhage, the combination also raises the mother's risk for venous thrombosis during pregnancy and after birth.

Fetal Response

Fetal responses are most notable in the placental circulation, the cardiovascular system, and the pulmonary system.

Placental Circulation

Exchange of oxygen, nutrients, and waste products between mother and fetus occurs in the intervillous spaces (see Chapter 12). During strong labor contractions, the maternal blood supply to the placenta stops intermittently as the spiral arteries supplying the intervillous spaces are compressed by the uterine muscle. Therefore most placental exchange occurs during the interval between contractions.

The placental circulation usually has enough reserve over fetal basal needs to tolerate the intermittent interruption of blood flow. The fetus has protective mechanisms, such as fetal hemoglobin (which more readily takes on oxygen and releases carbon dioxide), a high hematocrit, and a high cardiac output. The fetus may not tolerate labor contractions well in conditions associated with reduced placental function, such as maternal diabetes or hypertension, or in conditions associated with reduced fetal oxygen-carrying capacity, such as fetal anemia.

Cardiovascular System

The fetal cardiovascular system reacts quickly to events during labor. The fetal heart rate is rapid, ranging from 110 to 160 beats per minute (bpm) at term (Cypher, Adelsperger, &

Torgersen, 2003; King & Simpson, 1999). The preterm fetus may have a slightly higher heart rate than the term fetus, although persistent high fetal heart rates at any gestation should be investigated (see Chapter 18 for more discussion of fetal heart rate and responses during labor).

Pulmonary System

Before birth, the fetal lungs are filled with fluid to allow normal development of the airways. This fluid must be cleared to allow air breathing. As term approaches, production of fetal lung fluid decreases and its absorption increases. Labor intensifies the absorption of lung fluid. Some fluid is expelled from the upper airways as the fetal head and thorax are compressed during passage through the birth canal. The remaining fluid is absorbed into the newborn's pulmonary and lymphatic circulations after birth. Chapter 22 contains added information about newborn transition.

COMPONENTS OF THE BIRTH PROCESS

Four major factors, often called the "four P's," interact during normal childbirth. They are the powers, the passage, the passenger, and the psyche.

Powers

The two powers of labor are uterine contractions and maternal pushing efforts.

Uterine Contractions

During the first stage of labor (onset through full cervical dilation), uterine contractions are the primary force moving the fetus through the maternal pelvis.

Maternal Pushing Efforts

At some point during the second stage of labor (full cervical dilation through birth of the baby), the woman adds her voluntary pushing efforts to the force of uterine contractions to propel the fetus through the pelvis.

Passage

The passage for birth of the fetus consists of the maternal pelvis and its soft tissues. The bony pelvis is usually more important to the outcome of labor than the soft tissue because the bones and joints do not readily yield to the forces of labor. Softening of the cartilage linking the pelvic bones, however, occurs at term because of an increase in the hormone *relaxin*.

The bony pelvis is divided by the linea terminalis (or pelvic brim) into the false pelvis above and the true pelvis below (see Chapter 11). The true pelvis is most important in childbirth. The true pelvis has three subdivisions: (1) the inlet, or upper pelvic opening; (2) the midpelvis, or pelvic cavity; and (3) the outlet, or lower pelvic opening. The true pelvis is like a curved cylinder with different dimensions at different levels. Figure 17-4 illustrates important pelvic measurements.

Passenger

The passenger is the fetus plus the membranes and placenta.

Inlet

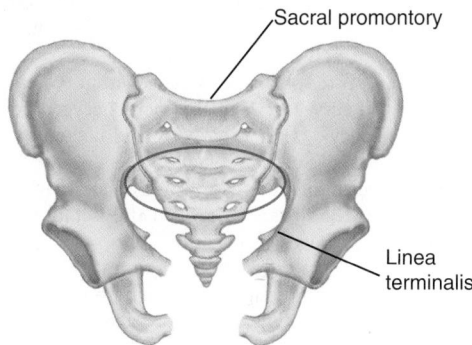

Frontal view, cutaway

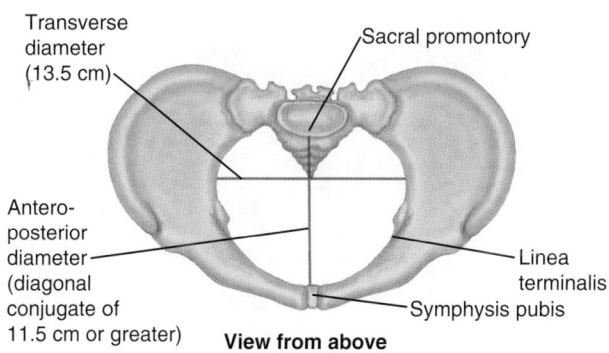

View from above

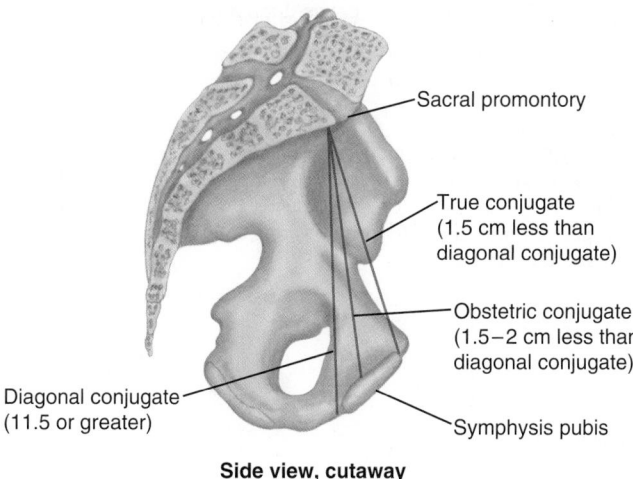

Side view, cutaway

The boundaries of the inlet are the symphysis pubis anteriorly, the sacral promontory posteriorly, and the linea terminalis on the sides. The inlet is slightly wider in its transverse diameter (13.5 cm) than in its anteroposterior (diagonal conjugate) diameter (11.5 cm or greater).

The diagonal conjugate is slightly larger than both the obstetric and true conjugates. The obstetric conjugate is the narrowest of the three conjugate diameters but cannot be measured directly. The obstetric conjugate is estimated by first measuring the diagonal conjugate and then subtracting 1.5 to 2 cm.

If the inlet is small, the fetal head may not be able to enter it. Because it is almost entirely surrounded by bone, except for cartilage at the sacroiliac joint and symphysis pubis, the inlet cannot enlarge much to accommodate the fetus. The bony measurements are essentially fixed.

Midpelvis

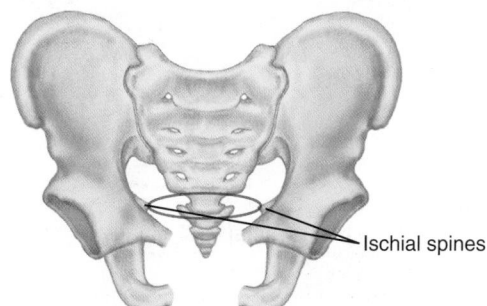

Frontal view, cutaway

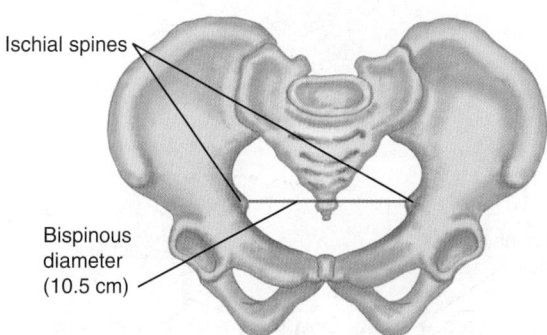

View from above, with pelvis tilted anteriorly

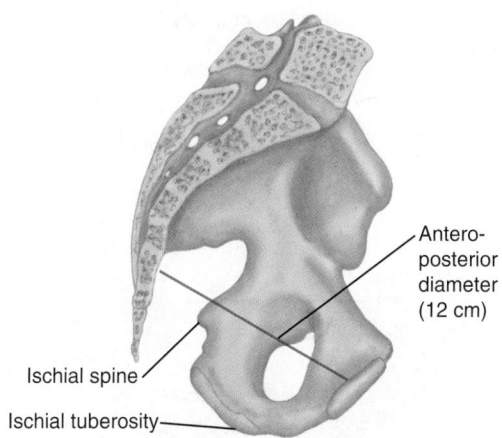

Side view, cutaway

The midpelvis, or pelvic cavity, is the narrowest part of the pelvis through which the fetus must pass during birth. Midpelvic diameters are measured at the level of the ischial spines. The anteroposterior diameter averages 12 cm.

The transverse diameter (bispinous or interspinous) averages 10.5 cm. Prominent ischial spines that project into the midpelvis can reduce the bispinous diameter.

Figure 17-4 Pelvic divisions and measurements.

Continued

Outlet

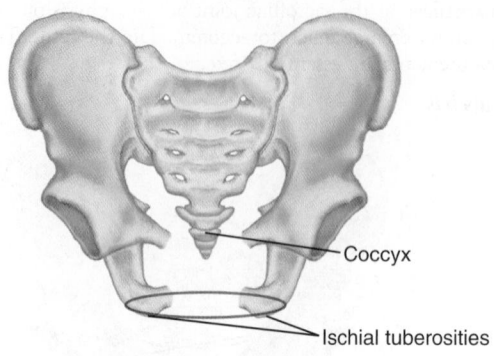

Frontal view, cutaway

Three important diameters of the pelvic outlet are (1) the anteroposterior, (2) the transverse (bi-ischial or intertuberous), and (3) the posterior sagittal. The angle of the pubic arch is also an important pelvic outlet measure.

The anteroposterior diameter ranges from 9.5 to 11.5 cm, varying with the curve between the sacrococcygeal joint and the tip of the coccyx. The anteroposterior diameter can increase if the coccyx is easily movable.

The transverse diameter is the bi-ischial, or intertuberous, diameter. This is the distance between the ischial tuberosities ("sit bones"). It averages 11 cm.

The posterior sagittal diameter is normally at least 7.5 cm. It is a measure of the posterior pelvis. The posterior sagittal diameter measures the distance from the sacrococcygeal joint to the middle of the transverse (bi-ischial) diameter.

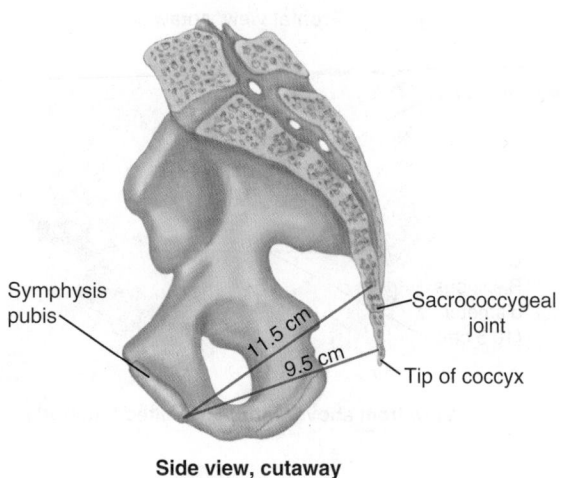

Side view, cutaway

Frontal view, with pelvis tilted anteriorly

The angle of the pubic arch is important because it must be wide enough for the fetus to pass under it. The angle of the pubic arch should be at least 90 degrees. A narrow pubic arch displaces the fetus posteriorly toward the coccyx as it tries to pass under the arch.

View from below (woman is in lithotomy position)

Figure 17-4, cont'd Pelvic divisions and measurements.

Fetal Head

The fetus enters the birth canal in the cephalic presentation 96% of the time. The fetal shoulders are important because of their width, but they usually flex and adapt to the pelvis.

Bones, Sutures, and Fontanels. The bones of the fetal head involved in birth are the two frontal bones on the forehead, the two parietal bones at the crown of the head,

and the occipital bone at the back of the head (Fig. 17-5). The five major bones are not fused but are connected by sutures composed of strong but flexible fibrous tissue. The fontanels are wider spaces at the intersections of the sutures.

The *anterior fontanel* is diamond shaped and formed by the intersection of four sutures: the two coronal, the frontal, and the sagittal, which connect the two frontal and

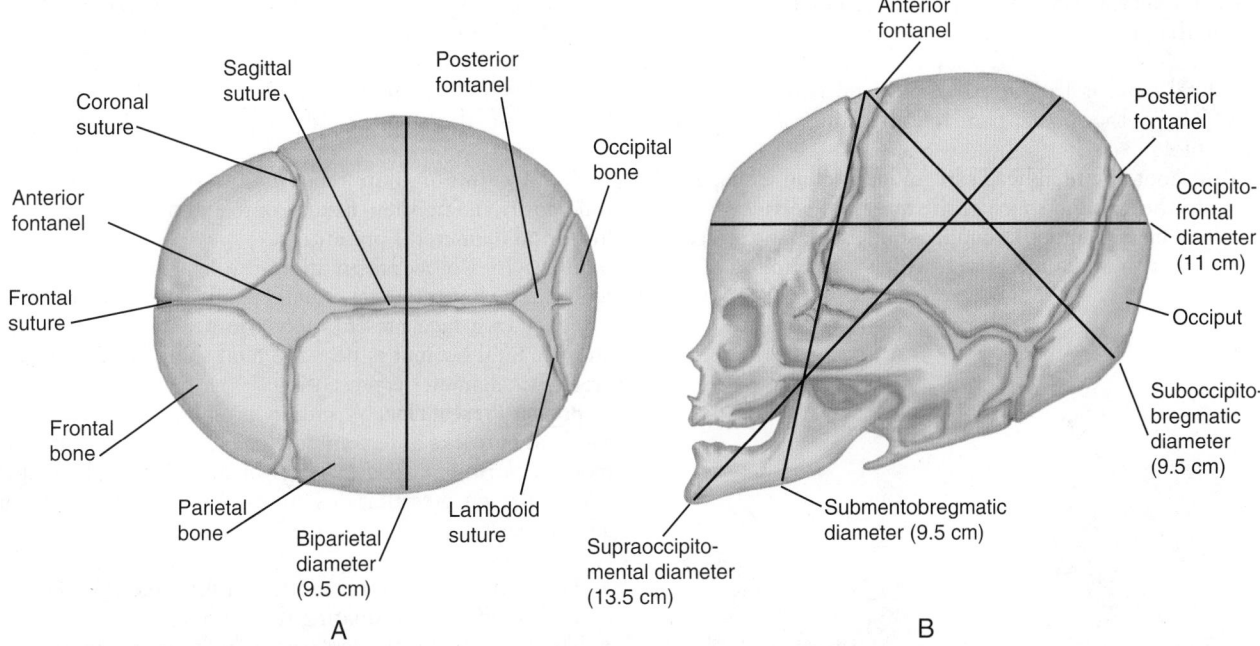

Figure 17-5 **A,** Bones, sutures, fontanels of the fetal head. Note that the anterior fontanel has a diamond shape, whereas the posterior fontanel is triangular. **B,** Lateral view of the fetal head. Anteroposterior diameters vary with the amount of flexion or extension.

the two parietal bones. The *posterior fontanel* has a triangular shape formed by the intersection of three sutures, one sagittal and two lambdoid, which connect the two parietal bones and the occipital bone. The posterior fontanel is very small, often more like a slight depression in the skull. The sutures and fontanels allow the bones to move slightly, changing the shape of the fetal head so that it can adapt to the size and shape of the pelvis by molding. The sutures and the different shapes of the fontanels provide landmarks to determine fetal position and head flexion during vaginal examination.

Fetal Head Diameters. Although most fetuses enter the pelvis in the cephalic presentation, several variations are possible. The major transverse diameter of the fetal head is the biparietal, measured between the two parietal bones. The biparietal diameter averages 9.5 cm in a term fetus.

The anteroposterior diameter of the head varies with the degree of flexion. In the most favorable situation, the head becomes fully flexed during labor and the anteroposterior diameter is the suboccipitobregmatic, averaging 9.5 cm. See Figure 17-5, *B*, for anteroposterior head diameters in different degrees of head flexion and extension.

Variations in the Passenger

Fetal Lie. The orientation of the long axis of the fetus to the long axis of the woman is the fetal lie (Fig. 17-6). In more than 99% of pregnancies, the lie is longitudinal, or parallel to the long axis of the woman. In the *longitudinal lie,* either the head or buttocks of the fetus enter the pelvis first. A *transverse lie* exists when the long axis of the fetus is at right angles to the woman's long axis; it occurs in fewer than 1% of pregnancies. An *oblique lie* is one at some angle between the longitudinal lie and the transverse lie.

Attitude. The attitude of the fetus is the relation of fetal body parts to each other (Fig. 17-7). The normal fetal at-

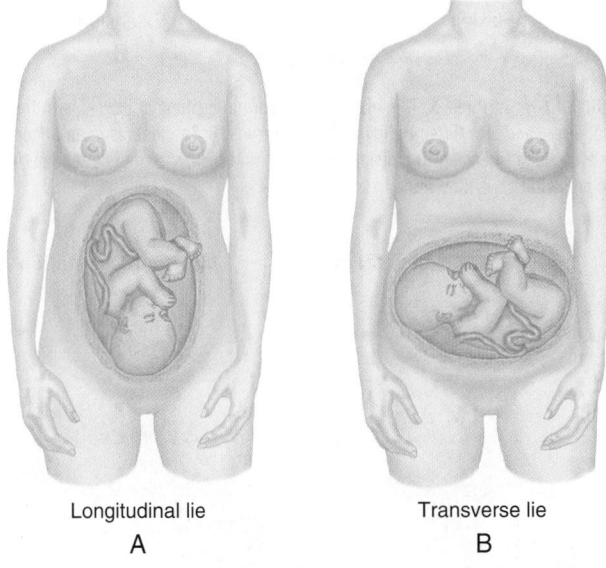

Longitudinal lie
A

Transverse lie
B

Figure 17-6 Lie. **A,** In a longitudinal lie, the long axis of the fetus is parallel to the long axis of the woman. **B,** In a transverse lie, the long axis of the fetus is at right angles to the long axis of the mother. The woman's abdomen has a wide, short appearance.

titude is one of flexion, with the head flexed toward the chest and the arms and legs flexed over the thorax. The back is curved in a convex **C** shape as labor starts.

Presentation. The fetal part that enters the pelvis first is the presenting part. Presentation falls into three categories: (1) cephalic, (2) breech, and (3) shoulder. The cephalic presentation with the fetal head flexed is the most common (Fig. 17-8). Other presentations are associated with prolonged labor or other problems and are more likely to require cesarean birth.

Cephalic Presentation. The cephalic presentation is more favorable than others, for several reasons:

- The fetal head is the largest single fetal part. After the head is born, the smaller parts follow easily as the extremities unfold.
- During labor, the fetal head can gradually change shape to adapt to the size and shape of the maternal pelvis.
- The fetal head is smooth, round, and hard, making it an effective part to dilate the cervix, which is also round.

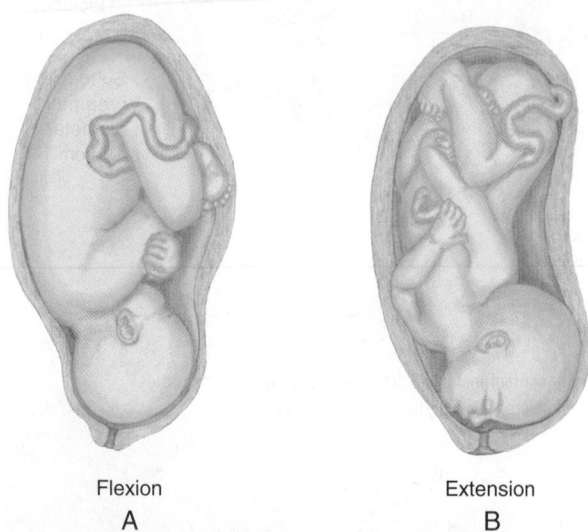

Flexion
A

Extension
B

Figure 17-7 Attitude. **A,** The fetus is in the normal attitude of flexion, with the head, arms, and legs flexed tightly against the trunk. **B,** The fetus is in an abnormal attitude of extension. The head is extended, and the right arm is extended. A face presentation is illustrated.

Cephalic presentation has four variations (see Fig. 17-8).

Vertex. The vertex presentation is the most common type of cephalic presentation. The fetal head is fully flexed. This presentation is the most favorable for normal progress of labor because the smallest suboccipitobregmatic diameter is presenting.

Military. In a military presentation, the head is in a neutral position, neither flexed nor extended. The occipitofrontal diameter is presenting.

Brow. In a brow presentation, the fetal head is partly extended. The longest supraoccipitomental diameter is presenting.

Face. In a face presentation, the head is fully extended and the fetal occiput is near the fetal spine. The submentobregmatic diameter is presenting.

Breech Presentation. A breech presentation occurs when the fetal buttocks or feet enter the pelvis first. They are common, occurring in about 3.5% of births (Cunningham et al., 2001). Breech presentations are associated with several disadvantages:

- The buttocks are not smooth and firm like the head and are less effective at dilating the cervix.
- The fetal head is the last part to be born. By the time the fetal head is deep in the pelvis, the umbilical cord is subject to compression between the baby's head and the maternal pelvis.
- Because the umbilical cord can be compressed after the fetal chest is born, the head must be delivered quickly to allow the infant to breathe. This necessary speed does not permit gradual molding of the fetal head as it passes through the pelvis.

The breech presentation has three variations, depending on the relationship of the legs to the body (Fig. 17-9).

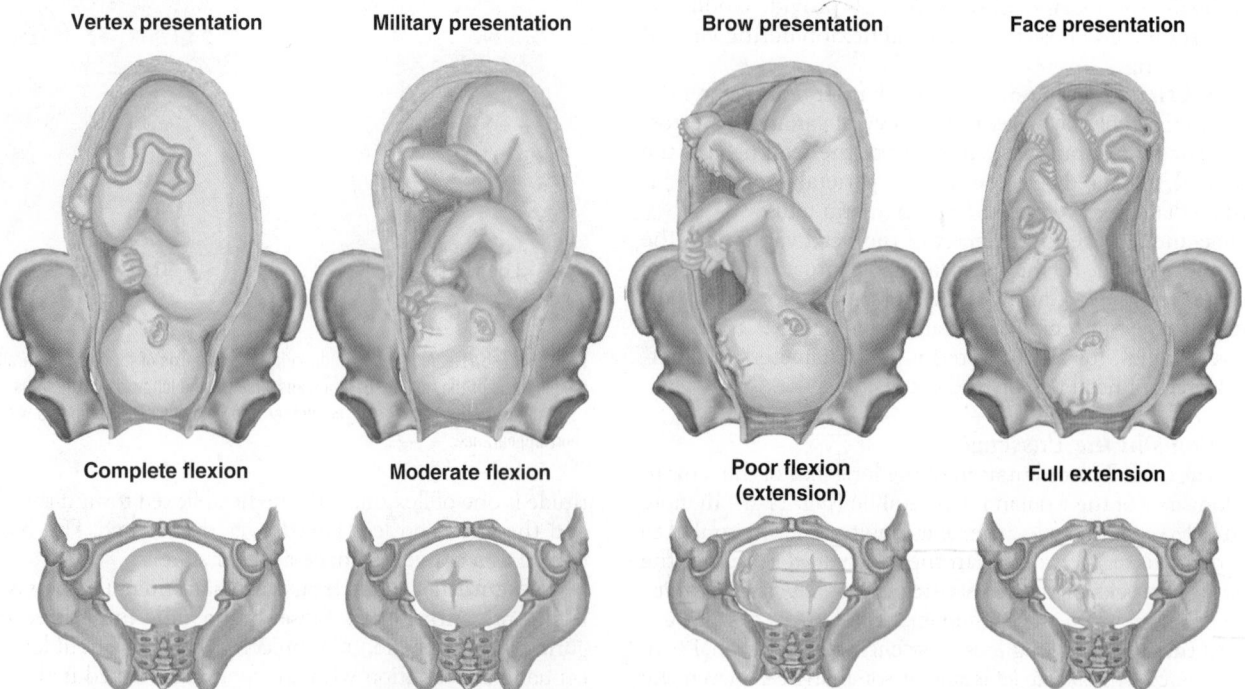

Vertex presentation   Military presentation   Brow presentation   Face presentation

Complete flexion   Moderate flexion   Poor flexion (extension)   Full extension

Figure 17-8 Four types of cephalic presentation. The vertex presentation is normal. Note postional changes of the anterior and posterior fontanels in relation to the maternal pelvis.

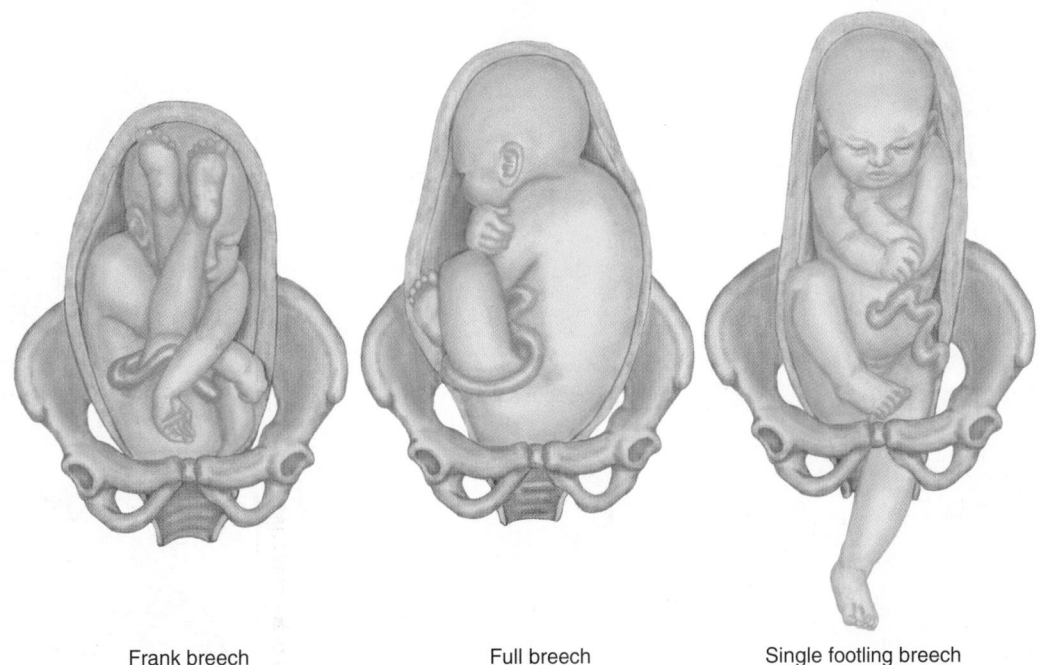

Frank breech   Full breech   Single footling breech

Figure 17-9 Three variations of a breech presentation. Frank breech is the most common variation. Footling breeches may be single or double.

Frank Breech. The frank breech is the most common variation. In a frank breech presentation the fetal legs are extended across the abdomen toward the shoulders.

Full (or Complete) Breech. The full breech is a reversal of the usual cephalic presentation. The head is flexed, and the knees and hips are also flexed, but the buttocks are presenting.

Footling Breech. The footling breech occurs when one or both feet are presenting.

Shoulder. The shoulder presentation is a transverse lie and accounts for only 0.4% of births (Cunningham et al., 2001). A cesarean birth is almost always necessary.

Position. Fetal position describes the location of a fixed reference point on the presenting part in relation to the four quadrants of the maternal pelvis (Fig. 17-10): right and left anterior and right and left posterior. The fetal position is not fixed but rather changes during labor as the fetus moves downward and adapts to the pelvic contours. Abbreviations indicate the relationship between the fetal presenting part and the maternal pelvis.

Right (R) or Left (L). The first letter of the abbreviation describes whether the fetal reference point is in the right or the left of the mother's pelvis. If the fetal point is neither to the right nor to the left of the pelvis, this letter is omitted.

Occiput (O), Mentum (M), or Sacrum (S). The second letter of the abbreviation refers to the fixed fetal reference point, which varies with the presentation. The occiput is used in a vertex presentation. The chin, or mentum, is the reference point in a face presentation. The sacrum is used for breech presentations. Letters may also designate the less common brow (F for fronto) and shoulder (Sc for scapula) presentations.

Anterior (A), Posterior (P), or Transverse (T). The third letter describes whether the fetal reference point is in the anterior or the posterior quadrant of the mother's pelvis. If the fetal reference point is in neither the anterior nor the posterior quadrant, it is described as transverse.

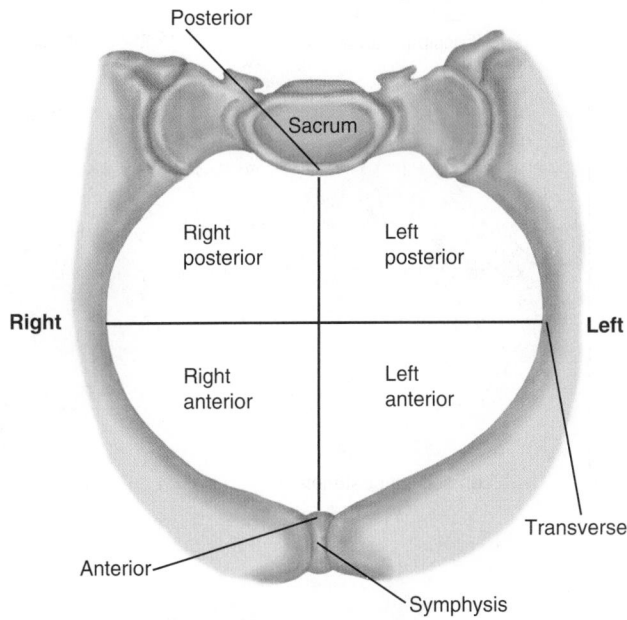

Figure 17-10 Four quadrants of the maternal pelvis, used to describe fetal position.

If the fetal occiput is located in the left anterior quadrant of the mother's pelvis, the position is described as left occiput anterior (LOA). If the occiput is in the mother's anterior pelvis, neither to the right nor to the left, it is described as occiput anterior (OA). If the fetal sacrum is located in the mother's right posterior pelvis, the description is R (right) S (sacrum) P (posterior). See Figure 17-11 for different fetal presentations and positions.

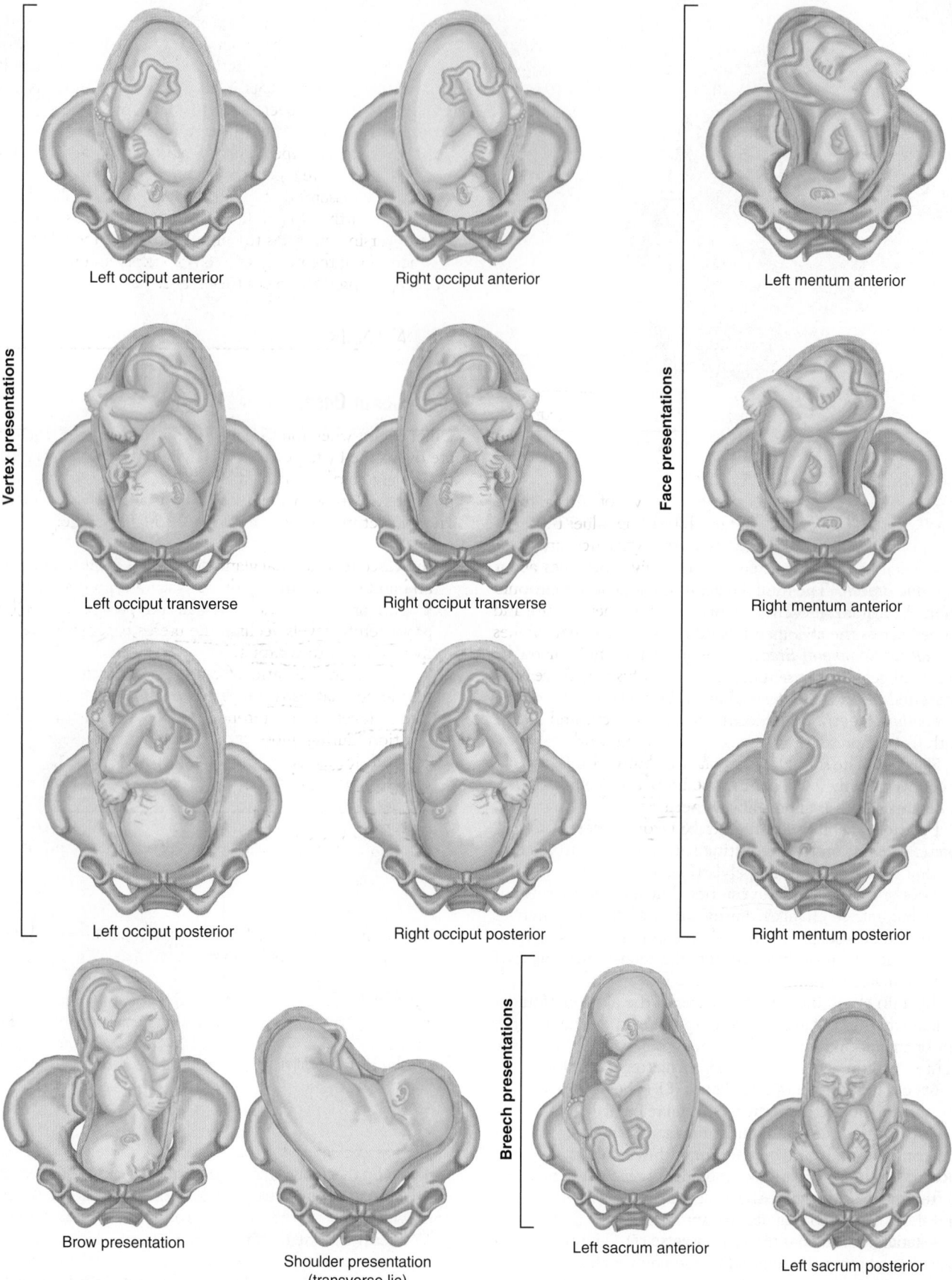

Vertex presentations

Left occiput anterior

Right occiput anterior

Left occiput transverse

Right occiput transverse

Left occiput posterior

Right occiput posterior

Face presentations

Left mentum anterior

Right mentum anterior

Right mentum posterior

Brow presentation

Shoulder presentation
(transverse lie)

Breech presentations

Left sacrum anterior

Left sacrum posterior

Figure 17-11 Fetal presentations and positions.

Psyche

The psyche is a crucial part of childbirth. Marked anxiety, fear, or fatigue decreases a woman's ability to cope with pain in labor. Maternal catecholamines secreted in response to anxiety or fear can inhibit uterine contractility and placental blood flow. Relaxation, however, augments the natural process of labor.

Interrelationships of the Components of Birth

The four P's—the powers, passage, passenger, and psyche—are an interrelated whole. For instance, a woman with a small pelvis (passage) and a large fetus (passenger) can have a normal labor and birth if the fetus is ideally positioned and the uterine contractions and maternal bearing-down efforts (powers) are vigorous. The nurse's supportive attitude strengthens positive psychologic elements (psyche) and enhances the processes of birth. The nurse can act as an advocate for the laboring woman and her family or partners to increase their sense of control and mastery of labor, often reducing anxiety and fear.

Individual and Cultural Values

A family's culture affects its members' views of birth and the practices that surround it. Culture shapes the values that people hold, their expectations of the birth experience, and their responses to birth. A woman's culture gives her cues about how she should behave and react to labor and how she should interact with her newborn. If the woman, her family, and caregivers have similar views, little conflict in their values and expectations is likely. If these individuals hold markedly different views, however, they may be confused because each expects something different of the other.

Knowledge of the values and practices of cultural groups that the nurse encounters provides a framework to assess and care for the woman and her family, but within a culture, people are individuals. The nurse must assess the personal expectations and birth-related values of each woman and her family within this general framework. Aspects of cultural assessment for the intrapartum period might include:

- How long has the family been in the area? Are they recent immigrants, or have their relatives and friends lived in the area for generations?
- What is the family's primary language? Are they comfortable communicating in the nurse's language if the two are different? If an interpreter is needed, are there people the family considers unacceptable (e.g., a male or a member of certain religious groups)?
- Who is the woman's primary support person for labor? What is that person's role? How extensively will that support person interact with the laboring woman?
- If the woman's primary support is to be the baby's father, how does the couple view his role? Will he actively support the woman (e.g., by coaching her breathing), or will he take a less active role?
- Is a caregiver of the same sex and cultural group essential?
- What are the woman's feelings about touch? Is she comfortable telling the nurse when she does or does not welcome touch?
- Are specific symbols, practices, or ceremonies used during the birth period? Who will conduct any ceremonies?

Birth as an Experience

Childbirth is a physical and emotional experience. It is also an irrevocable event that changes a woman and her family forever. Families describe the births of children as they describe other pivotal events in life: marriages, anniversaries, religious events, and even deaths. Women often have specific expectations about the experience of childbirth. The more realistic a woman's expectations about the birth are, the more likely she is to have a positive experience.

Nursing measures that increase a sense of control and mastery during birth help families perceive the birth as a positive event. Nursing measures to empower families include teaching them about their choices in childbirth in an unbiased way and supporting the choices they make.

NORMAL LABOR

Theories of Onset

Labor begins when forces favoring continuation of pregnancy are overcome by forces favoring its end. The body's preparation to give birth occurs gradually over the last few weeks of pregnancy. Although all reasons for initiation of labor are not known, factors that have a role in its onset include:

- Increased fetal adrenal gland production of glucocorticoids and androgens, which reduces placental progesterone secretion and increases prostaglandin production. When progesterone levels decline, the uterus becomes more easily stimulated to contract.
- A change in the ratio of maternal estrogen to progesterone so that estrogen levels are higher than progesterone levels. Progesterone promotes uterine muscle relaxation during most of pregnancy. Relatively higher estrogen levels enhance uterine sensitivity to substances that stimulate uterine contractions: prostaglandins from the fetal membranes and oxytocin from the maternal posterior pituitary gland.
- Stretching, pressure, or irritation of the uterus and cervix.

Premonitory Signs

Before spontaneous labor begins, women usually notice one or more premonitory, or warning, signs that labor is near:

- Braxton Hicks contractions, which occur throughout pregnancy, increase in frequency and are sometimes painful. They may become regular at times, only to decrease spontaneously.
- Lightening ("dropping") occurs as the fetus descends toward the pelvic inlet. Lightening is most noticeable in nulliparas, occurring about 2 to 3 weeks before the onset of labor.
- Increased clear and nonirritating vaginal secretions occur as fetal pressure causes congestion of the vaginal mucosa.
- "Bloody show," a mixture of thick mucus and pink or dark brown blood, may occur as the cervix begins to soften, dilate, and efface slightly ("ripening").
- An energy spurt ("nesting").
- A small weight loss of up to 3 lb may occur because changing levels of estrogen and progesterone cause excretion of some of the extra fluid that accumulates during pregnancy.

True Labor and False Labor

False labor, also called *prodromal labor*, is common because the time of spontaneous labor's onset is rarely known and the onset is usually gradual. False labor often causes women to be disappointed when their symptoms are not "the real thing." The term *false labor* may discourage a woman, because she does not realize that these "false" contractions are simply preparation for the main event of true labor, rather than true labor itself.

Several characteristics distinguish true labor from false labor: contractions, discomfort, and cervical change. The best distinction between the two is that the contractions of true labor cause *progressive changes in the cervix*. Effacement and dilation occur with true labor contractions.

Mechanisms of Labor

The mechanisms (cardinal movements) of labor occur as the fetus is moved through the pelvis during birth. The fetus undergoes several positional changes to adapt to the size and shape of the mother's pelvis at different levels (Fig. 17-12). Although the mechanisms of labor are described separately in Figure 17-12, some occur concurrently. In a vertex presentation, the mechanisms are:

- *Descent* of the fetal presenting part through the true pelvis.
- *Engagement* of the fetal presenting part as its widest diameter reaches the level of the ischial spines of the mother's pelvis.
- *Flexion* of the fetal head so that the smallest head diameters pass through the pelvis.
- *Internal rotation* to allow the largest fetal head diameters to match the largest maternal pelvic diameters.
- *Extension* of the fetal head as it passes beneath the mother's symphysis pubis.
- *External rotation* of the fetal head to allow the shoulders to rotate internally to fit the mother's pelvis.

- *Expulsion* of the fetal shoulders and fetal body.

The mechanisms of labor are different in presentations other than the vertex, but the reason is the same: effective use of available space in the maternal pelvis.

✳ Stages and Phases of Labor

Each stage and phase of labor has qualities that set it apart from the others. Individual women vary in their labor patterns and responses to labor. Table 17-1 provides details of the characteristics of each stage of labor. Use of regional anesthetics, such as the epidural block, is likely to modify the typical maternal behaviors. Also, labor that is induced or augmented often differs from spontaneous labor.

First Stage of Labor

Cervical effacement and dilation occur in the first stage of labor, or *stage of dilation*. It begins with the onset of true labor contractions and ends with complete dilation (10 cm) and effacement (100%) of the cervix. The first stage of labor is the longest for both nulliparous and parous women. Labor progress may be plotted on a graph, often called a *Friedman curve* (Fig. 17-13, p. 356).

First-stage labor differs from the other stages because it has three phases: latent (early), active, and transition. Each phase is characterized by typical maternal behaviors. These behaviors vary with the woman's preparation, use of coping skills, and analgesia.

Latent Phase. The latent, or early, phase lasts from the beginning of labor until about 3 cm of cervical dilation. Its length varies among women. Despite being called *latent*, cervical effacement and subtle fetal position change occur during this phase, preparing for more rapid changes during active labor. The woman is usually sociable and excited during this early phase of labor.

Active Phase. The cervix dilates from 4 to 7 cm and dilates more rapidly than in the latent phase. Effacement of the cervix is completed. The fetus descends in the pelvis,

---

WOMEN
Want to Know

How to Know Whether Labor Is "Real"

True labor differs from false labor in three categories.

FALSE LABOR	TRUE LABOR
Contractions	
Inconsistent in frequency, duration, and intensity.	A consistent pattern of increasing frequency, duration, and intensity usually develops.
A change in activity, such as walking, does not alter contractions, or activity may decrease them.	Walking tends to increase contractions.
Discomfort	
Felt in the abdomen and groin.	Begins in lower back and gradually sweeps around to the lower abdomen like a girdle.
May be more annoying than truly painful.	Back pain may persist in some women. Early labor often feels like menstrual cramps.
Cervix	
No significant change in effacement or dilation of the cervix.	Effacement and/or dilation of cervix occurs. Progressive effacement and dilation of cervix are most important characteristics.

Descent, Engagement, and Flexion

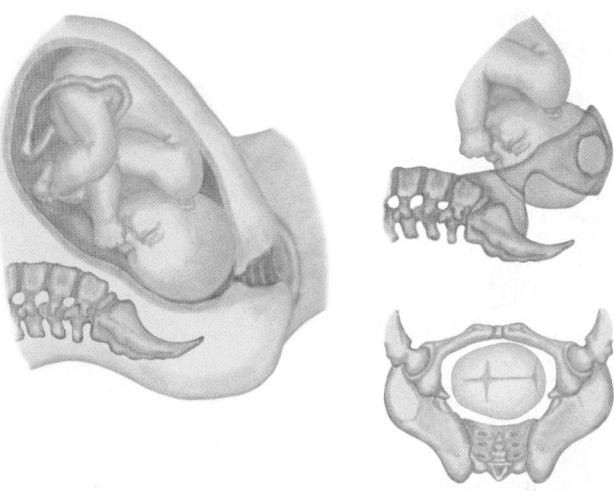

Descent of the fetus is a mechanism of labor that accompanies all the others. Without descent, none of the mechanisms will occur.

Station

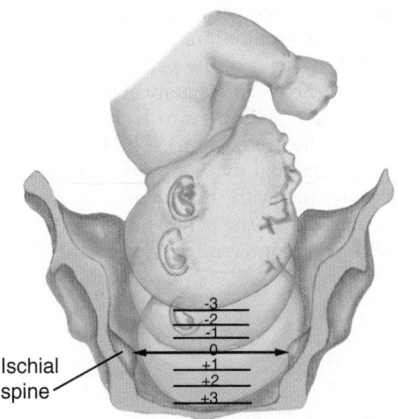

Ischial spine

Station describes the descent of the fetal presenting part in relation to the level of the ischial spines. The level of the ischial spines is a zero station. Other stations are described with numbers representing the approximate number of centimeters above (negative numbers) or below (positive numbers) the ischial spines. As the fetus descends through the pelvis, the station changes from higher negative numbers (−3, −2, −1) to zero to higher positive numbers (+1, +2, +3, etc.). Sometimes the terms *floating* or *ballottable* may describe a fetal presenting part that is so high that it is easily displaced upward during abdominal or vaginal examination, similar to tossing a ball upward.

Engagement

Engagement occurs when the largest diameter of the fetal presenting part (normally the head) has passed the pelvic inlet and entered the pelvic cavity. Engagement is presumed to have occurred when the station of the presenting part is zero or lower. Engagement often takes place before onset of labor in nulliparous women. In many parous women and in some nulliparas, it does not occur until after labor begins.

Flexion

As the fetus descends, the fetal head is flexed further as it meets resistance from the soft tissues of the pelvis. Head flexion presents the smallest anteroposterior diameter (suboccipitobregmatic) to the pelvis.

Internal Rotation

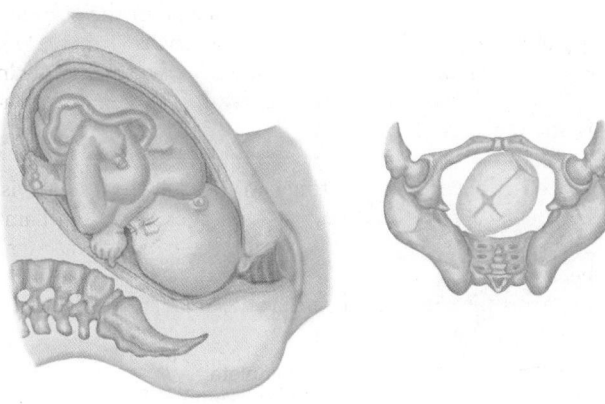

The fetus enters the pelvic inlet with the sagittal suture in a transverse or oblique orientation to the maternal pelvis because that is the widest inlet diameter. Internal rotation allows the longest fetal head diameter (the anteroposterior) to conform to the longest diameter of the maternal pelvis.

The longest pelvic outlet diameter is the anteroposterior. As the head descends to the level of the ischial spines, it gradually turns so that the fetal occiput is in the anterior of the pelvis (OA position, directly under the maternal symphysis pubis). When internal rotation is complete, the sagittal suture is oriented in the anteroposterior pelvic diameter (OA). Less commonly, the head may turn posteriorly so that the occiput is directed toward the mother's sacrum (OP).

Figure 17-12 Mechanisms (cardinal movements) of labor.   *Continued*

Extension

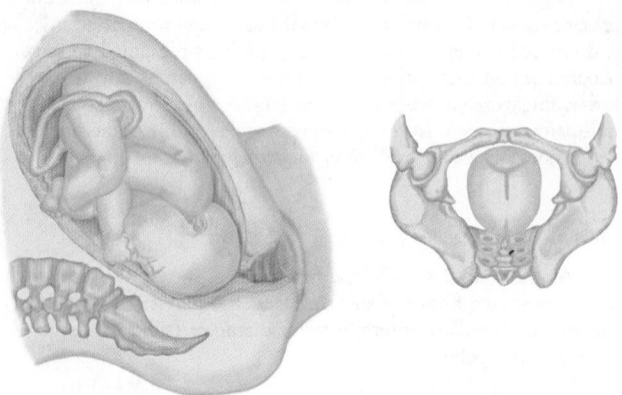

Extension beginning (internal rotation complete)

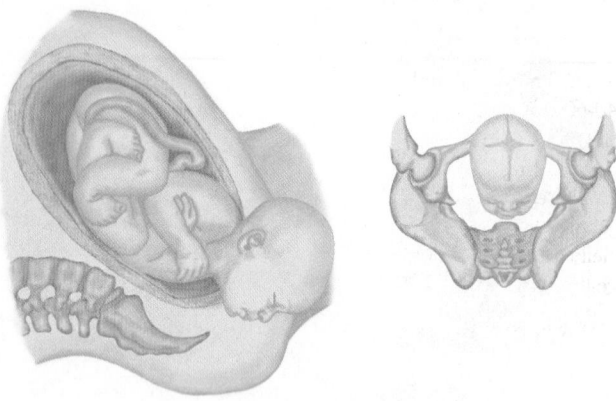

Extension complete

Because the true pelvis is shaped like a curved cylinder, the fetal head is directed posteriorly toward the rectum as it begins its descent. To negotiate the curve of the pelvis, the fetal head must change from an attitude of flexion to one of extension.

While still in flexion, the fetal head meets resistance from the tissues of the pelvic floor. At the same time, the fetal neck stops under the symphysis, which acts as a pivot. The combination of resistance from the pelvic floor and the pivoting action of the symphysis causes the fetal head to swing anteriorly, or extend, with each maternal pushing effort. The head is born in extension, with the occiput sliding under the symphysis and the face directed toward the rectum. The fetal brow, nose, and chin slide over the perineum as the head is born.

External Rotation

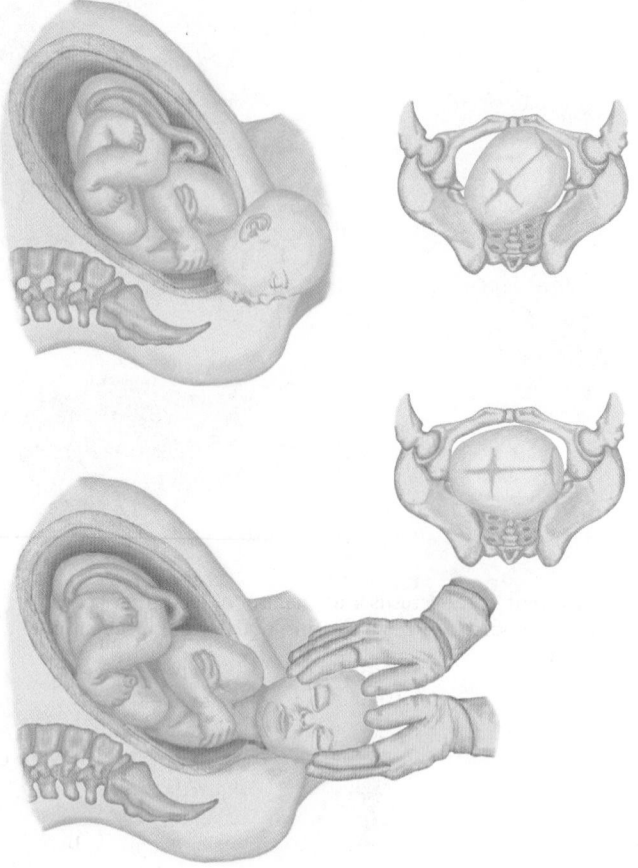

When the head is born with the occiput directed anteriorly, the shoulders must rotate internally so that they align with the anteroposterior diameter of the pelvis.

After the head is born, it spontaneously turns to the same side as it was in utero as it realigns with the shoulders and back (through a process called restitution). The head then turns further to that side in external rotation as the shoulders internally rotate and are positioned with their transverse diameter in the anteroposterior diameter of the pelvic outlet. External rotation of the head accompanies internal rotation of the shoulders.

Expulsion

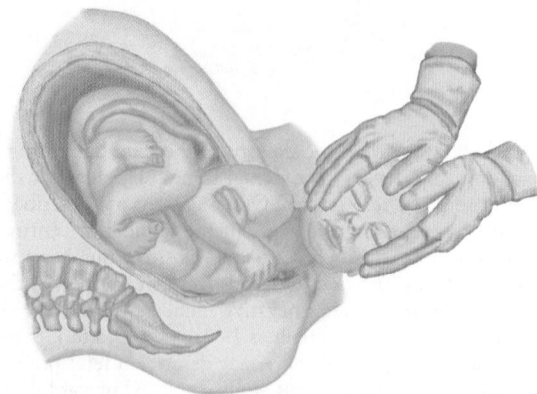

Expulsion occurs first as the anterior, then the posterior, shoulder passes under the symphysis. After the shoulders are born, the rest of the body follows.

Figure 17-12, cont'd Mechanisms (cardinal movements) of labor.

TABLE **17-1** Characteristics of Normal Labor

	First Stage	Second Stage	Third Stage	Fourth Stage
Work accomplished	Effacement and dilation of cervix	Expulsion of fetus	Separation of placenta	Physical recovery and bonding with newborn
Forces	Uterine contractions	Uterine contractions and voluntary bearing-down efforts	Uterine contractions	Uterine contraction to control bleeding from placental site
Average duration:				
• Nullipara	8-10 hr after reaching active phase; dilation averages 1 cm/hr	Average 50 min (range, 30 min-3 hr)	5-10 min; up to 30 min is normal for unassisted placental separation	1-4 hr after birth
• Multipara	6-7 hr (range, 2-10 hr) after reaching active phase; dilation averages 1.2 cm/hr	Average 20 min (range, 5-30 min)	Same as for nullipara	Same as for nullipara
Cervical dilation	*Latent phase:* 0-3 cm *Active phase:* 4-7 cm *Transition phase:* 8-10 cm	10 cm (complete dilation)	Not applicable	Not applicable
Uterine contractions	*Latent phase:* Initially mild and infrequent; progress to moderate strength, every 5 min with a regular pattern; duration increases to 30-40 sec by end of latent phase *Active phase:* Increase in frequency, duration, and intensity until every 2-5 min, 40-60 sec, and moderate to strong intensity *Transition phase:* Strong, every 1½-2 min, 60 sec	Strong, every 2-3 min, lasting 40-60 sec; may be slightly less intense than during transition phase of first stage; may pause briefly as second stage begins	Firmly contracted	Firmly contracted
Discomfort*	Often begins with a low backache and sensations similar to those of menstrual cramps; back discomfort gradually sweeps to the lower abdomen in a girdlelike fashion, discomfort intensifies as labor progresses	Urge to push or bear down with contractions, which becomes stronger as fetus descends; distention of vagina and vulva may cause a stretching or splitting sensation	Little discomfort; sometimes slight cramp is felt as placenta is passed	Discomfort varies; some women have afterpains, more common in multigravidas or those who have had a large baby; as anesthesia wears off, perineal discomfort may become noticeable
Maternal behaviors*	Sociable, excited, and somewhat anxious during early labor; becomes more inwardly focused as labor intensifies; may lose control during transition	Intense concentration on pushing with contractions; often oblivious to surroundings and appears to doze between contractions	Excited and relieved after baby's birth; usually very tired; often cries	Tired, but may find it difficult to rest because of excitement; eager to become acquainted with her newborn

*Maternal discomfort and behaviors often vary with pain-relief method chosen.

and internal rotation begins. Discomfort usually increases as the pace of labor picks up.

The woman becomes more anxious and may feel helpless as the contractions intensify. The sociability of early labor is gone, replaced with a serious, inward focus.

Transition Phase. The cervix dilates from 8 to 10 cm, and the fetus descends further into the pelvis. Bloody show often increases with completion of cervical dilation. Transition is a short but intense phase, with very strong contractions. The woman may have an urge to push down during

contractions as the fetal presenting part reaches her pelvic floor. Leg tremors, nausea, and vomiting are common.

The woman may be irritable and lose control. Her partner may be confused because actions that were helpful just a short time before now bother her.

Second Stage of Labor

The second stage (*expulsion*) begins with complete (10 cm) dilation and full (100%) effacement of the cervix and ends with the birth of the baby. As the fetus descends, pressure of

Composite Normal Dilation Curves

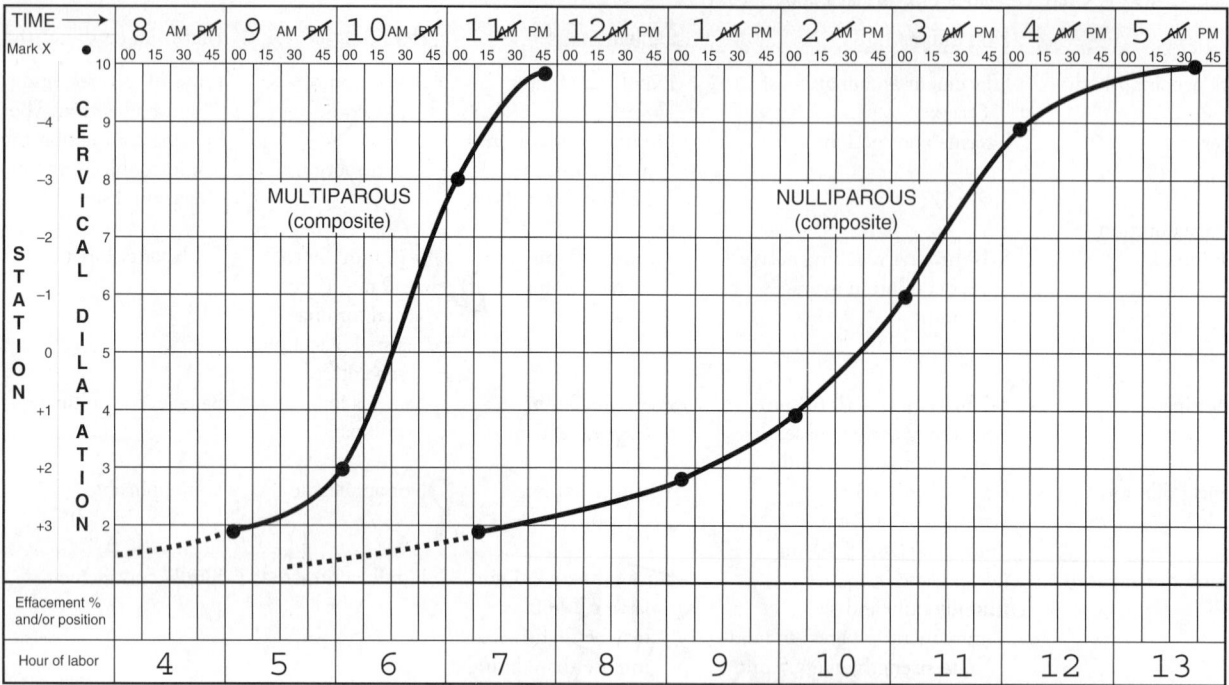

Figure 17-13 A labor curve, often called a *Friedman curve*, may be used to identify whether a woman's cervical dilation is progressing at the expected rate. Typical labor curves for a multiparous and a nulliparous woman are illustrated for comparison of patterns.

the presenting part on the rectum and the pelvic floor causes the mother to have an involuntary pushing response. She may say that she needs to have a bowel movement or "The baby's coming" or "I have to push." Her voluntary pushing efforts augment involuntary uterine contractions. As the fetus descends low in the pelvis and the vulva distends with crowning of the fetal head, she may feel a sensation of stretching or splitting even if no trauma occurs.

Contractions are strong, but the woman may feel more in control because she is actively completing the process by pushing with them. "Labor" describes the second stage well. The woman exerts intense effort to push her baby out. Between contractions, she may be oblivious to her surroundings and may appear asleep. She feels tremendous relief and excitement as the second stage ends with the birth of the baby.

Third Stage of Labor

The third (*placental*) stage begins with the birth of the baby and ends with the expulsion of the placenta (Fig. 17-14). When the infant is born, the uterine cavity becomes much smaller. The reduced size decreases the size of the placental site, causing the placenta to separate from the uterine wall. Four signs suggest placenta separation:

- The uterus has a spherical shape.
- The uterus rises upward in the abdomen as the placenta descends into the vagina and pushes the fundus upward.
- The cord descends further from the vagina.
- A gush of blood appears as blood trapped behind the placenta is released.

The placenta may be expelled in one of two ways. In the more common *Schultze* mechanism, the placenta is expelled

with the shiny, fetal side first (see Fig. 17-14, B). The *Duncan* mechanism is less common, with the rough maternal side presenting (see Fig. 17-14, A).

The uterus must contract firmly and remain contracted after the placenta is expelled to compress open vessels at the implantation site. Inadequate uterine contraction after birth may result in hemorrhage.

Pain during the third stage of labor results from uterine contractions and brief stretching of the cervix as the placenta passes through it.

Fourth Stage of Labor

The fourth stage of labor is the *stage of physical recovery* for the mother and infant. It lasts from the delivery of the placenta through the first 1 to 4 hours after birth.

Immediately after birth, the firmly contracted uterus can be palpated through the abdominal wall as a firm, rounded mass about 10 to 15 cm (4 to 6 in) in diameter at or below the level of the umbilicus. The uterus is larger when the infant is large or the mother is a multipara.

The vaginal drainage during the fourth stage is *lochia rubra*, which consists mostly of blood. Small clots may also be present. See Chapter 21 for more information about lochia.

Many women have a chill after birth. The chill lasts for about 20 minutes and subsides spontaneously. A warm blanket, hot drink, or soup may help shorten the chill and make the woman more comfortable.

Discomfort during the fourth stage usually results from birth trauma or afterpains. Ice packs on the perineum limit discomfort and hematoma formation.

Afterpains are uterine contractions similar to menstrual cramps that occur after birth as the uterus begins its return to the prepregnancy state. The discomfort is similar to that

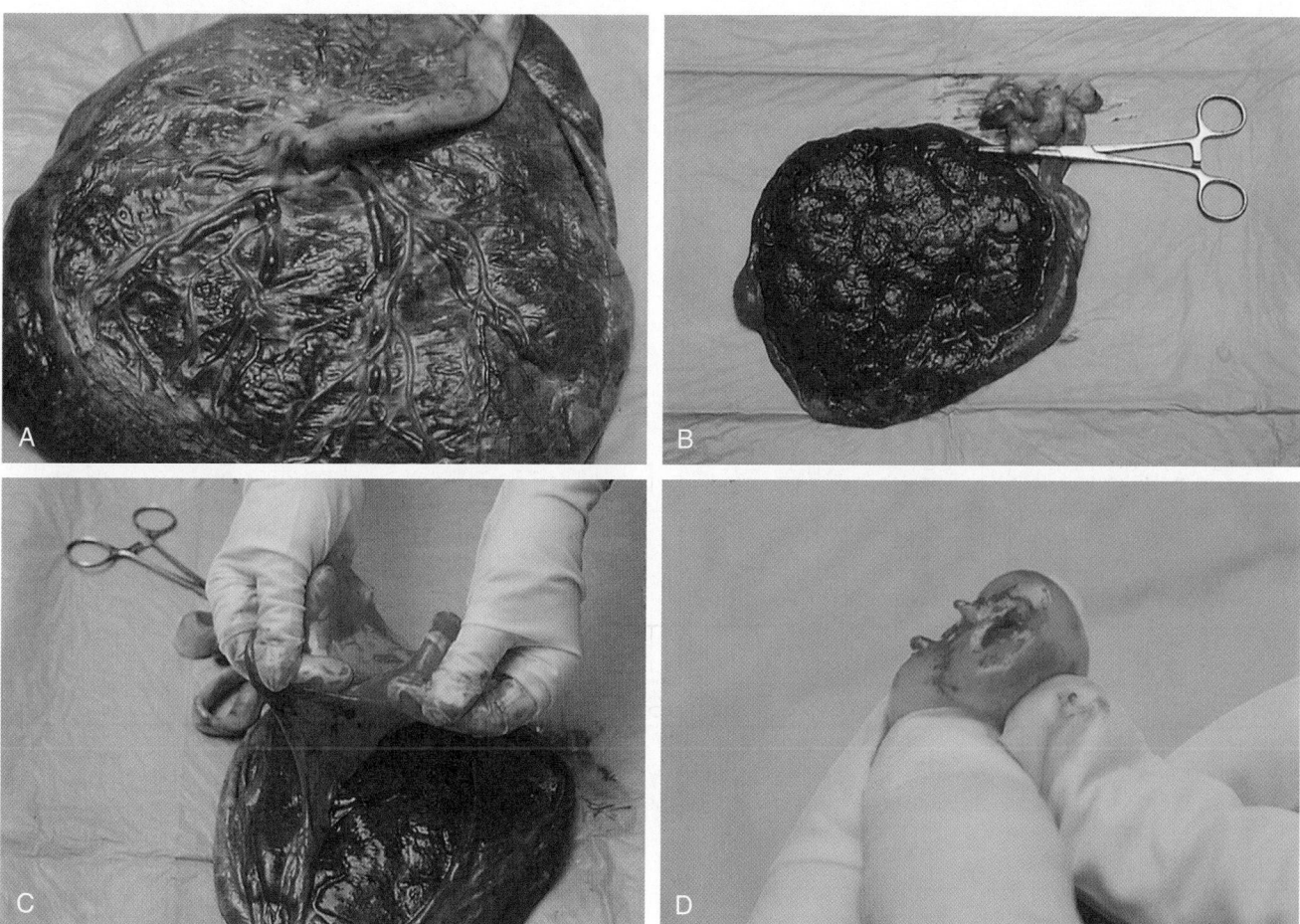

Figure 17-14 **A,** Fetal side of the placenta. **B,** Maternal side of the placenta. **C,** Separating membranes. **D,** Umbilical cord vessels—two arteries and one vein.

of menstrual cramps. Afterpains are more intense in multiparas, in women who breastfeed, in women who have large babies or other causes of uterine overdistention during pregnancy, or when something interferes with uterine contraction, such as a full bladder or a blood clot that remains in the uterus.

The mother is simultaneously excited and tired after birth. She may be exhausted but too full of nervous energy to rest. The fourth stage of labor is an ideal time for bonding of the new family because the interest of both parents and newborn is high. It is also the best time to start breastfeeding if no maternal or infant problems are present. The baby is alert and seeks to make eye contact with the new parents, giving powerful reinforcement for the parents' attachment to their newborn.

Duration of Labor

The total duration of labor is different for women who have never given birth and for those who have previously given birth vaginally. The parous woman usually delivers more quickly than does the nulliparous woman. Women, however, are individuals. Some nulliparas progress through labor quickly, whereas labor for some parous women resembles that of women who have never given birth. A woman who experienced a long labor with her first child may not have a long labor with every baby. If she has a history of rapid labor, however, later births are often rapid as well.

NURSING CARE DURING LABOR AND BIRTH

Admission to the Birth Center

During the last trimester, the woman needs to know when she should go to the hospital or birth center. Nurses teach women differences between false labor and true labor and offer guidelines for going to the birth center. Not everyone has a typical labor, so a woman should be encouraged to go to the birth center if she is uncertain or has other concerns.

Nursing Responsibilities During Admission

The nurse has two priorities when the woman arrives at the birth center: (1) assessing the condition of the mother and fetus and (2) establishing a therapeutic relationship.

Establishing a Therapeutic Relationship
Making the Family Feel Welcome. A family's first impression influences how family members feel about the quality of the birth experience. Even if the unit is busy, the nurse should communicate interest, friendliness, caring, and competence. Families understand if the nurse is busy;

WOMEN
Want to Know

When to Go to the Hospital or Birth Center

These are guidelines for providing individualized instruction to women about when to enter the hospital or birth center.

Contractions

A pattern of increasing regularity, frequency, duration, and intensity:

    Nullipara: Regular contractions, 5 minutes apart, for 1 hour.

    Multipara: Regular contractions, 10 minutes apart, for 1 hour.

Ruptured Membranes

A gush or trickle of fluid from the vagina should be evaluated, whether or not you have contractions, to determine if your membranes have ruptured (if your "water has broken").

Bleeding

Bright red bleeding that is not mixed with mucus should be evaluated promptly. Normal bloody show is thicker, pink or dark red, and mixed with mucus.

Decreased Fetal Movement

If you notice a decrease in the baby's movement, notify your physician or nurse-midwife or come to the labor unit.

Other Concerns

These guidelines cannot cover all situations. Therefore go to the hospital for evaluation of any concerns or feelings that something may be wrong.

CRITICAL THINKING EXERCISE 17-1

Alan Lindsey phones you as you are working in the birth unit of your hospital one night. He says, "My wife's baby is almost due. She's been having some contractions off and on all day, and they are keeping her awake now. Should we come to the hospital?"

1. Do you need any other information? If so, what information do you need?

You next speak to Heather Lindsey about her symptoms. You find out that her first baby is due the following week and that she has had no leaking of fluid from her vagina. She says, "My contractions are coming every 2 to 10 minutes, and most of them last about 30 seconds. They didn't bother me much until I tried to go to sleep, but now they are keeping me awake. I'm so tired of all this!"

2. What should you tell Heather about her symptoms? What advice should you give her?

---

they do not understand rudeness or insensitivity to their needs.

When caring for the woman who has not had prenatal care or childbirth classes, behaviors most nurses value, the nurse should avoid being judgmental in either words or actions. The woman's priorities and values may not be the same as those of the nurse, but she deserves the same respect, support, and care as the woman who made every preparation for her baby's birth.

Nurses often encounter women who speak a language other than English. Arranging for a culturally acceptable interpreter who is fluent in the woman's language makes the woman and family feel more welcome and promotes safety because it enhances understanding among the woman, her family, and the nurse.

Determining Family Expectations About Birth. Regardless of how many children they have, women and their partners have expectations about the birth experience. The partners have often studied their options extensively and have planned a birth that best fits their ideals. Some may have a written birth plan filed with their prenatal records. Those who have not made specific plans also have expectations shaped by contact with relatives and friends or by previous birth experiences.

Conveying Confidence. From the first encounter, the nurse should convey confidence in the woman's ability to give birth and her partner's ability to support her. Contractions and discomfort intensify as labor progresses. A woman having her first baby may find the power of normal labor contractions overwhelming. The nurse can reassure the woman

that intense contractions are normal in active labor while helping her deal with them and watching for problems.

Consider the different perspective implied by the phrases "give birth" and "be delivered." The woman who gives birth is an active and able participant; she is the principal action figure. When her baby is "delivered," however, the language implies that she is passive. The nurse might ask, "Who will attend you as you give birth?" or "Who is your doctor (or midwife)?" rather than, "Who will deliver your baby?"

Assigning a Primary Nurse. Birth, even if induced, does not fit neatly into nursing schedules. Thus having one nurse give care during all of labor is unrealistic. The number of different caregivers should, however, be limited as much as possible. The woman should know who each caregiver is and what to expect from each.

Using Touch for Comfort. Touch can communicate acceptance and reassurance and can provide physical and emotional comfort to many laboring women. Women who do not usually welcome touch may appreciate it during labor. Cultural norms and personal history influence whether a woman is comfortable with touch from a stranger such as a nurse. One should not assume that the woman desires touch but should ask her if she wants it or benefits from it. As labor progresses, her desire for touch may change; during late labor, it may become an irritant rather than a comfort measure.

Respecting Cultural Values. Cultural beliefs and practices give structure and meaning to the birth experience. The nurse should incorporate a family's cultural practices into care as much as possible.

Assessments at the Time of Admission

A record of prenatal care is sent to the center where the woman plans to give birth a few weeks before her due date. Her record of prenatal care is added to her chart when she is admitted. The information can be verified or updated as needed on admission. Women who have not had prenatal care need a more extensive assessment by the nurse and physician. Table 17-2 lists intrapartum assessments, usual findings, significant findings, and appropriate nursing actions.

TABLE 17-2 Intrapartum Assessment Guide
Women who have had prenatal care have much of this information available on their prenatal record. The nurse need only verify it or update it as needed.

Assessment, Method (Selected Rationales)	Common Findings	Significant Findings, Nursing Action
INTERVIEW		
Purpose: To obtain information about the woman's pregnancy, labor, and conditions that may affect her care. The interview is curtailed if she seems to be in late labor.		
Introduction: Introduce yourself, and ask the woman how she wants to be addressed. Ask her if she wants her partner and/or family to remain during the interview and assessment. (Shows respect for the woman and gives her control over those she wants to remain with her.)	Many women prefer to be addressed by their first names during labor.	The surname (family name) precedes the given name in some cultures. Clarify which name is used to properly address the woman and to properly identify both mother and newborn
Culture/language: If she is from another culture, ask what her preferred language is and what language(s) she speaks, reads, or verbally understands. (Identifies the need for an interpreter and enables the most accurate data collection.)	Common non-English languages of women in the United States are Spanish and some Asian dialects. The most common non-English language varies with location.	Try to secure an interpreter fluent in the woman's primary language. Ask her if there are people who are not acceptable to her as interpreters (e.g., males or one from a group in conflict with her culture). Family members may not be the best interpreters because they may interpret selectively, adding or subtracting information as they see fit. Telephone interpreters are available in many facilities. Hearing-impaired women may read lips well, or they may need sign-language interpreters or other assistance.
Communication: Ask the woman to tell you when she has a contraction, and pause during the interview and physical assessment. (Shows sensitivity to her comfort and allows her to concentrate more fully on the information the nurse requests.)	Women in active labor have difficulty answering questions or cooperating with a physical examination while they are having a contraction.	If contractions are very frequent, assess the woman's labor status promptly rather than continuing the interview. Ask only the most critical questions.
Nonverbal cues: Observe the woman's behaviors and interactions with her family and the nurse. (Permits estimation of her level of anxiety. Identifies behaviors indicating that she should have a vaginal examination to determine whether birth is imminent.)	*Latent phase:* Sociable and mildly anxious. *Active phase:* Concentrating intently with contractions; often uses prepared childbirth techniques.	The unprepared or extremely anxious woman may breathe deeply and rapidly, displaying a tense facial and body posture during and between contractions. These behaviors suggest that birth is imminent: 1. Her statement that the baby is coming. 2. Grunting sounds (low-pitched, guttural sounds). 3. Bearing down with abdominal muscles. 4. Sitting on one buttock. Euphoria, combativeness, or sedation suggests recent illicit drug ingestion.
Reason for admission: "What brings you to the hospital/birth center today?" (Open-ended question promotes more complete answer.)	Labor contractions at term, induction of labor, or observation for false labor are common reasons for admission.	Bleeding, preterm labor, pain other than labor contractions. Report these findings to the physician or nurse-midwife promptly.
Prenatal care: "Did you see a doctor or nurse-midwife during your pregnancy?" "Who is your doctor or nurse-midwife?" "How far along were you in your pregnancy when you saw the physician or nurse-midwife?" "Have you ever been admitted here before during this pregnancy?" (Enables location of prenatal record and prior visit records.)	Early and regular prenatal care promotes maternal and fetal health.	No prenatal care or care that was irregular or begun in late pregnancy means that complications may not have been identified.

Continued

TABLE **17-2** Intrapartum Assessment Guide—*cont'd*

Assessment, Method (Selected Rationales)	Common Findings	Significant Findings, Nursing Action
Estimated date of delivery (EDD): "When is your baby due?" (Determines if gestation is term.) "When did your last menstrual period begin?" (For estimation of EDD if woman did not have prenatal care.)	*Term gestation:* 38-42 wk. The woman's gestation may have been confirmed or adjusted during pregnancy with an ultrasound or other clinical examination.	Gestations earlier than the beginning of the 38th wk (preterm) or later than the end of the 42nd wk (postterm) are associated with more fetal or neonatal problems. The physician may try to stop labor that occurs earlier than 36 weeks.
Gravidity, parity, abortions: "How many times have you been pregnant?" "How many babies have you had? Were they full-term or premature?" "How many children are now living?" "Have you had any miscarriages or abortions?" "Were there any problems with your babies after they were born?" (Helps estimate probable speed of labor and anticipate neonatal problems.)	Labor may be faster for the woman who has given birth before than for the nullipara. Miscarriage is used to describe a spontaneous abortion because many lay people associate the term "abortion" with only induced abortions.	Parity of 5 or more (grand multiparity) is associated with placenta previa (see Chapter 26) and postpartum hemorrhage (see Chapter 28). Women who have had several spontaneous abortions or who have given birth to infants with abnormalities may face a higher risk for an infant with a birth defect.
Pregnancy history (Identifies problems that may affect this birth.) Present pregnancy: "Have you had any problems during this pregnancy, such as high blood pressure, diabetes, infections, or bleeding?"	Complications are not expected.	Women who have diabetes or hypertension may have poor placental blood flow, possibly resulting in fetal compromise. Some complications of past pregnancies, such as diabetes, may recur in another pregnancy. The woman who plans a VBAC may need more support and reassurance to give birth vaginally.
Past pregnancies: "Were there any problems with your other pregnancy(ies)?" "Were your other babies born vaginally or by cesarean birth?"	Women who had previous cesarean birth(s) may have a trial of labor and vaginal birth (VBAC). A woman who previously had a difficult labor or a cesarean birth may be more anxious than one who had an uncomplicated labor and birth.	
Other: "Is there anything else you think we should know so that we can better care for you?"	This open-ended question gives the woman a chance to share information that may not be elicited by other questions.	
Labor status: "When did your contractions become regular?" "What time did you begin to think you might really be in labor?" (Facilitates a more accurate estimation of the time labor began.)	Varies among women. Many women go to the birth facility when contractions first begin. Others wait until they are reasonably sure that they are really in labor.	Women who say they have been "in labor" for an unusual length of time (e.g., "for 2 days") have probably had false labor. These women may be very tired from the annoying, nonproductive contractions.
Contractions: "How often are your contractions coming?" "How long do they last?" "Are they getting stronger?" "Tell me if you have a contraction while we are talking." (Obtains the woman's subjective evaluation of her contractions. Alerts the nurse to palpate contractions that occur during the interview.)	Varies according to her stage and phase of labor. Labor contractions are usually regular and show a pattern of increasing frequency, duration, and intensity.	Irregular contractions or those that do not increase in frequency, duration, or intensity are more likely to represent false labor. Contractions that are too frequent or too long can reduce placental blood flow. Incomplete uterine relaxation between contractions also can reduce placental blood flow (see Chapter 18).
Membrane status: "Has your water broken?" "What time did it break?" "What did the fluid look like?" "About how much fluid did you lose—was it a big gush or a trickle?" (Alerts the nurse of the need to verify whether the membranes have ruptured if it is not obvious. Identifies possible prolonged rupture of membranes or preterm rupture.)	Most women go to the birth facility for evaluation soon after their membranes rupture. If a woman is not already in labor, contractions usually begin within a few hours after the membranes rupture at term.	If the woman's membranes have ruptured and she is not in labor or if she is not at term, a vaginal examination is often deferred. Labor may be induced if she is at term with ruptured membranes.

VBAC, Vaginal birth after cesarean.

TABLE **17-2** Intrapartum Assessment Guide—*cont'd*

Assessment, Method (Selected Rationales)	Common Findings	Significant Findings, Nursing Action
Allergies: "Are you allergic to any foods, medicines, or other substances?" "Do you have allergy to latex?" "What kind of reaction do you have?" "Have you ever had a problem with anesthesia when you had dental work?" (Determines possible sensitivity to drugs that may be used.)	Record any known allergies to food, medication, or other substances. As needed, describe how they affected the woman.	Allergy to seafood, iodized salt, or x-ray contrast media may indicate iodine allergy. Because iodine is used in many prep solutions, alternative ones should be used. Allergy to latex is becoming more common. Allergy to dental anesthetics may indicate possible allergy to the drugs used for local or regional anesthetics. These drugs usually end in the suffix *-caine.*
Food intake: "When was the last time you had something to eat or drink?" "What did you have?" (Provides information needed to most safely administer general anesthesia if required. Identifies possible fluid or energy deficit.)	Record the time of the woman's last food intake and what she ate. Include both liquids and solids.	If the woman says she has not had any intake for an unusual length of time, question her more closely: "Is there any food you may have forgotten, such as a snack or a drink of water?"
Recent illness: "Have you been ill recently?" "What was the problem?" "What did you do for it?" "Have you been around anyone with a contagious illness recently?"	Most pregnant women are healthy. An occasional woman may have had a minor illness such as an upper respiratory tract infection.	Urinary tract infections are associated with preterm labor. The woman who has had contact with someone having a communicable disease may become ill and possibly infect others in the facility.
Medications: "What drugs do you take that your doctor or nurse-midwife has prescribed?" "Are there any over-the-counter drugs that you use?" "I know this may be uncomfortable to discuss, but we need to know about any illegal substances that you use, to more safely care for you and your baby." (Permits evaluation of the woman's drug intake and encourages her to disclose nonprescribed use.)	Prenatal vitamins and iron are commonly prescribed. Record all drugs the woman takes, including time and amount of last ingestion. Women who use illegal substances often conceal or diminish the extent of their use because they fear reprisals.	Drugs may interact with other medications given during labor, especially analgesics and anesthetics. Substance abuse is associated with complications for the mother and infant (see Chapter 25). If the woman discloses that she uses illegal drugs, ask her what kind and the last time she ingested them (often referred to as a "hit"). A nonjudgmental approach is more likely to result in honest information.
Tobacco or alcohol: "Do you smoke or use tobacco in any other form? About how many cigarettes a day?" "Do you use alcohol? About how many drinks do you have each day (or week)?" (Evaluates use of these legal substances.)	As in substance abuse, women may underreport the extent of their use of tobacco or alcohol.	Infants of heavy smokers are often smaller and may have reduced placental blood flow during labor. Infants of women who use alcohol may show fetal alcohol effects (see Chapter 30).
Birth plans (Shows respect for the woman and her family as individuals and promotes achievement of their expectations. Enables more culturally appropriate care): Coach or primary support person: "Who is the main person you want to be with you during labor?" Ask that person how he or she wants to be addressed, such as "Mr. Ramos," or "Carlos."	This is usually the woman's husband or the baby's father, but it may be her mother, sister, or a friend, especially if she is single.	The woman who has little or no support from significant others probably needs more intense nursing support during labor and after the birth. These clients are more likely to have problems with parent-infant attachment.
Other support: "Is there anyone else you would like to be present during labor?"	Women often want another support person present.	
Preparation for childbirth: "Did you attend prepared childbirth classes?" "Did someone go with you?"	Ideally, the woman and a partner have had some preparation in classes or self-study. Women who attended classes during previous pregnancies do not always repeat the classes during subsequent pregnancies.	The unprepared woman may need more support with simple relaxation and breathing techniques during labor. Her partner may need to learn techniques to assist her.

Continued

TABLE 17-2 Intrapartum Assessment Guide—*cont'd*

Assessment, Method (Selected Rationales)	Common Findings	Significant Findings, Nursing Action
Preferences: "Are there any special plans you have for this birth?" "Is there anything you want to avoid?" "Did you plan to record the birth with pictures or video?" *Cultural needs:* "Are there any special cultural practices that you plan when you have your baby?" "How can we best help you to fulfill these practices?"	Some women or couples have strong feelings regarding certain interventions. Common ones are: (1) analgesia or anesthesia; (2) intravenous lines; (3) fetal monitoring; (4) use of episiotomy or forceps. Women from Asian and Hispanic cultures may subscribe to the "hot/cold" theory of illness and want specific foods after birth, such as soft-boiled eggs. They may not want their water or other fluids iced.	Conflict may arise if the woman has not previously discussed her preferences with her physician or nurse-midwife or if she is unaware of what services are available where she gives birth. Try to incorporate all positive or neutral cultural practices. If a practice is harmful, explain why and try to find a way to work around it if the family does not want to give it up.

FETAL EVALUATION

Purpose: To determine if the fetus seems to be healthy and tolerating labor well. Fetal heart rate (FHR): Assess by intermittent auscultation, or apply an external fetal monitor if that is the facility's policy (most common in the United States). Document fetal heart rate according to the risk status and stage of labor (see Chapter 18).	Average rate at term is 110-160 bpm. Rate usually increases when the fetus moves and is reassuring.	These signs may indicate fetal stress and should be reported to the physician or nurse-midwife: 1. Rate outside the normal limits 2. Slowing of the rate that persists after the contraction ends 3. No increase in rate when the fetus moves 4. Irregular rhythm More frequent assessments should be made of the fetal heart rate and contractions if any finding is questionable.

LABOR STATUS

Purpose: To identify whether the woman is in labor and if birth is imminent. If she displays signs of imminent birth, this assessment is done as soon as she is admitted. Contractions (Yields objective information about labor status): In addition to asking the woman about her contraction pattern, assess the contractions by palpation with the fingertips of one hand. Contractions should be assessed each time the fetal heart rate is assessed.	See interview section earlier in table.	See interview section earlier in table. Women who have intense contractions or who are making rapid progress should be assessed more frequently.
Vaginal examination (Determines cervical dilation and effacement; fetal presentation, position, and station; bloody show; and status of the membranes.)	Varies according to the stage and phase of labor. It may not be possible to determine the fetal position by vaginal examination when membranes are intact and bulging over the presenting part.	A vaginal examination is not performed if the woman reports or has evidence of active bleeding (not bloody show) and may not be done if her gestation is 36 weeks or younger and she does not seem to be in active labor. Report reasons for omitting a vaginal examination to the physician or nurse-midwife.

bpm, beats per minute.

TABLE **17-2** Intrapartum Assessment Guide—*cont'd*

Assessment, Method (Selected Rationales)	Common Findings	Significant Findings, Nursing Action
Status of membranes: During a vaginal examination a flow of fluid suggests ruptured membranes. A nitrazine test and/or fern test may be done, often using a sterile speculum exam. (Test not needed if it is obvious that the membranes have ruptured.)	Amniotic fluid should be clear, possibly containing flecks of white vernix. Its odor is distinctive but not offensive. The nitrazine test with a color change of blue-green to dark blue (pH >6.5) suggests true rupture of the membranes but is not conclusive. The fern test is more diagnostic of true rupture of membranes because it is less likely to be affected by vaginal infections, recent intercourse, or other factors.	A greenish color indicates meconium staining, which may be associated with fetal compromise or postterm gestation. Thick meconium with heavy particulate matter ("pea soup") is most significant (see Chapter 30). Thick green-black meconium may be passed by the fetus in a breech presentation and is not necessarily associated with fetal compromise. Cloudy, yellowish, strong-, or foul-smelling fluid suggests infection. Bloody fluid may indicate partial placental separation (see Chapter 27).
Leopold's maneuvers: Often done before assessing the fetal heart rate to locate the best place to assess the fetal heart rate. (Identifies fetal presentation and position. Most accurate when combined with information from vaginal examination.)	A cephalic presentation with the head well flexed (vertex) is normal. The fetal head is often easily displaced upward ("floating") if the woman is not in labor. When the head is engaged, it cannot be displaced upward with Leopold's maneuvers.	A hard, round, freely movable object in the fundus suggests a fetal head, meaning the fetus is in a breech presentation. Less commonly, the fetus may be crosswise in the uterus: a transverse lie.
Pain: Note discomfort during and between contractions. Note tenderness when palpating contractions. (Distinguishes between normal labor pain and abnormal pain that may be associated with a complication.)	There may be verbal or nonverbal evidence of pain with contractions, but the woman should be relatively comfortable between contractions. The skin around the umbilicus is often sensitive.	Constant pain or a tender, rigid uterus suggests a complication, such as abruptio placentae (separated placenta) (see Chapter 26) or, less commonly, uterine rupture (see Chapter 27).

PHYSICAL EXAMINATION

Purpose: To evaluate the woman's general health and identify conditions that may affect her intrapartum and postpartum care.		
General appearance: Observe skin color and texture, nutritional state, and appearance of rest or fatigue. Examine the woman's face, fingers, and lower extremities for edema.	Women are often fatigued if their sleep has been interrupted by Braxton Hicks contractions, fetal activity, or frequent urination. Ask her if she can take her rings off and on. Mild edema of the lower extremities is common in late pregnancy.	Pallor suggests anemia. Substantial edema of the face and fingers or extreme (pitting) edema of the lower extremities is associated with pregnancy-induced hypertension (see Chapter 26).
Vital signs: Take the woman's temperature, pulse, respirations, and blood pressure. Reassess the temperature every 4 hr (every 2 hr after membranes rupture or if elevated); repeat blood pressure, pulse, and respirations every hour.	*Temperature:* 35.8°-37.3° C (96.4°-99.1° F). *Pulse:* 60-100/min. *Respirations:* 12-20/min, even and unlabored. Blood pressure near baseline levels established during pregnancy. Transient elevations of blood pressure are common when the woman is first admitted, but they return to baseline levels within	Report abnormalities to physician or nurse-midwife. Temperature of 38° C (100.4° F) or higher suggests infection. Pulse and respirations may also be elevated. Pulse and blood pressure may be elevated if the woman is extremely anxious or in pain. A blood pressure of 140/90 mm Hg or higher is considered hypertensive. For women who did not have prenatal care, there is no baseline to compare.

Continued

TABLE 17-2 Intrapartum Assessment Guide—*cont'd*

Assessment, Method (Selected Rationales)	Common Findings	Significant Findings, Nursing Action
Heart and lung sounds: Auscultate all areas with a stethoscope.	about ¹/₂ hr. Heart sounds should be clear with a distinct S₁ and S₂. A physiologic murmur is common because of the increased blood volume and cardiac output. Breath sounds should be clear, with respirations even and unlabored.	The woman who is breathing rapidly and deeply may have symptoms of hyperventilation: tingling and spasm of the fingers, numbness around the lips.
Breasts: Palpate for a dominant mass.	Breasts are full and nodular. Areola is darker, especially in dark-skinned women. Breasts may leak colostrum (clear, sticky, straw-colored fluid) during labor.	Report a dominant mass to the physician or nurse-midwife.
Abdomen: Observe for scars at the same time Leopold's maneuvers and the fetal heart rate are assessed. It is usually sufficient to assess the fundal height by observing its relation to the xiphoid process.	Striae (stretch marks) are common. If scars are noted, ask the woman what surgery she had and when. The fundus at term is usually slightly below the xiphoid process.	Report a previous cesarean birth to the physician or nurse-midwife. Transverse uterine scars are least likely to rupture if the woman is in labor (see Chapter 27). Measure the fundal height (see p. 269) if the fetus seems small or if the gestation is questionable.
Deep tendon reflexes: Assess patellar reflex (see Chapter 26). Upper extremity deep tendon reflexes should be used if epidural block analgesia is planned because they are normally not as strong as the patellar reflex.	A brisk jerk without spasm or sustained muscle contraction is normal. Some women normally have hypoactive reflexes but at least a slight twitch is expected. Obese women may appear to have diminished reflexes because of the fat tissue over the tendon.	Report absent (uncommon unless the woman is receiving magnesium sulfate) or hyperactive reflexes. Hyperactive reflexes and clonus (repeated tapping when the foot is dorsiflexed) are associated with pregnancy-induced hypertension and often precede a seizure (see Chapter 26).
Midstream urine specimen: Assess protein and glucose levels with a dipstick. Follow instructions on the package for waiting times. Check for ketones if the woman has not eaten for a prolonged period or has been vomiting. Send for urinalysis if ordered.	Negative or trace of protein; negative glucose and ketones.	Proteinuria is associated with preeclampsia but may also be associated with urinary tract infections or a specimen that is contaminated with vaginal secretions. Glucosuria is associated with diabetes. Ketonuria is common in poorly-controlled diabetes or if the woman does not eat adequate carbohydrates to meet her energy needs.
Laboratory tests: Women who have had prenatal care may not need as many admission tests. Common tests include: 1. Complete blood cell count (or hematocrit done on unit). 2. Blood type and Rh factor. 3. Serologic tests for syphilis.	1. Hemoglobin at least 11 g/dl; hematocrit at least 33%. 2. The woman who is Rh-negative receives Rh immune globulin at 28 weeks' gestation to prevent formation of anti-Rh antibodies if she has regular prenatal care. 3. Negative.	1. Values lower than these reduce maternal reserve for normal blood loss at birth. 2. Rh-negative mothers need Rh immune globulin after birth if their infant is Rh-positive. 3. A positive test indicates that the baby could be infected and needs treatment after birth. The mother should be treated if she has not been treated already.

Focused Assessment. In the intrapartum unit, an initial focused assessment is done before the broader database assessment—opposite of the usual order. Assessment priorities are to determine the condition of the mother and fetus and whether birth is imminent.

Fetal Assessment. Leopold's maneuvers (Procedure 17-1) help identify the best place to assess the fetal heart rate (FHR). The rate, rhythm, and other characteristics should be assessed on admission and at intervals appropriate to the woman's risk status and labor. Fetal movement should be noted. If the membranes are ruptured, assess the color, odor, and clarity of leaking fluid. Chapter 18 provides detailed information about intrapartum fetal surveillance.

Maternal Vital Signs. Assess maternal vital signs primarily for signs of hypertension or infection. Hypertension during pregnancy is defined as a sustained blood pressure increase to 140 mm Hg systolic or 90 mm Hg diastolic (ACOG, 2002). A temperature of 38° C (100.4° F) or higher suggests infection.

Impending Birth. Occasionally a woman enters the intrapartum unit almost ready to give birth. Grunting sounds, bearing down, sitting on one buttock, or saying urgently something like "The baby's coming" suggests imminent birth. The nurse abbreviates the initial assessment and collects other information after birth.

Vital information to obtain if birth is imminent includes:

- Mother's name
- Support person's name
- Whether the woman had prenatal care
- Physician's or nurse-midwife's name
- Number of pregnancies and prior births, including whether vaginal or cesarean birth
- Status of membranes
- Expected date of birth
- Any problems during this pregnancy
- Allergies
- Time and type of last oral intake
- Maternal vital signs and fetal heart rate
- Pain: location, intensity, intensifying or relieving factors, duration, whether it is constant or intermittent, acceptability to the woman

If focused assessments of mother and fetus are normal and birth is not imminent, complete the admission assessment. If the initial assessments are not normal or birth is near, notify the physician or nurse-midwife promptly.

Database Assessment. In addition to the focused assessment, assess the mother and fetus and available maternal support.

Basic Information. Most intrapartum admission forms guide the nurse to ask for essential information. Typical information includes:

- The woman's reason for coming to the hospital or birth center (e.g., contractions, rupture of membranes)
- Prenatal care
- Estimated date of birth
- Number of pregnancies, births, and abortions
- Allergies (medications, food, substances such as latex)
- Food intake: what food and when it was eaten
- Medical, surgical, and pregnancy history

- Recent illness, including treatment
- Medications, including prescription and over-the-counter drugs, tobacco, alcohol, and substances of abuse
- Her subjective evaluation of her labor
- Birth plans, including expected pain management methods
- Support persons: who they are and the role of each
- Screening for domestic abuse (see Chapter 25)

Be careful when discussing prior pregnancies and births when a woman's family is present. She may have had an abortion or relinquished a baby for adoption, and her family may not know about it. Even if her partner knows about previous pregnancies, other family and friends may not.

Fetal Assessments. Assess the fetal presentation and position and the fetal heart rate. Note the color of the amniotic fluid and the time of rupture if the membranes have ruptured.

Labor Status. Determine the woman's labor status by:

- Assessing her contraction pattern
- Determining cervical dilation and effacement; and fetal station, presentation, and position
- Determining if her membranes have ruptured

Physical Examination. If birth is not imminent, perform a brief physical examination to evaluate the woman's overall health. Important general observations that relate to birth include the presence and location of edema, abdominal scars, and the height of the fundus.

Admission Procedures

Notifying the Physician or Midwife. After assessment, contact the woman's birth attendant to report on her status and obtain orders. Include the following data in the report:

- Gravidity, parity, and abortions
- Estimated date of delivery
- Contraction pattern
- Fetal presentation and position
- Cervical dilation and effacement, station of the presenting part
- Fetal heart rate and pattern
- Maternal vital signs
- Any identified abnormalities or concerns about the maternal or fetal condition
- Pain, anxiety, or other reactions to labor

If the woman is admitted, any of several procedures may be done.

Consent Forms. The woman signs consent for care during labor, anesthesia, vaginal birth, cesarean birth, and often blood transfusion. Consent for newborn care is often completed as

Procedure 17-1

Leopold's Maneuvers

PURPOSES

To determine the presentation and position of the fetus.
To aid in locating the best place to check the fetal heart rate. Leopold's maneuvers are less likely to yield useful information if the woman has a thick abdominal fat pad, excessive amniotic fluid, or a very preterm fetus.

1. Explain the procedure to the woman, the rationale for each step, and what is found at each step to teach her and reassure her when the assessment findings are normal.
2. Ask the woman to empty her bladder if she has not done so recently to reduce discomfort during palpation and make fetal parts easier to feel. Have her lie on her back with her knees flexed slightly or head slightly elevated to help her relax her abdominal muscles. Place a small pillow or folded towel under one hip to prevent supine hypotension.
3. Wash your hands with warm water to prevent transmission of microorganisms and to make your hands warmer when touching the woman. Wear gloves to avoid contact with the woman's secretions as indicated.
4. Stand beside the woman, facing her head, with your dominant hand nearest her, because the first three maneuvers are most easily performed in this position.

FIRST MANEUVER

5. Palpate the uterine fundus to distinguish between a cephalic and breech presentation. The breech (buttocks) is softer and more irregular in shape than the head. Moving the breech also moves the fetal trunk. The head is harder, with a round, uniform shape. The head can move without the entire fetal trunk moving.

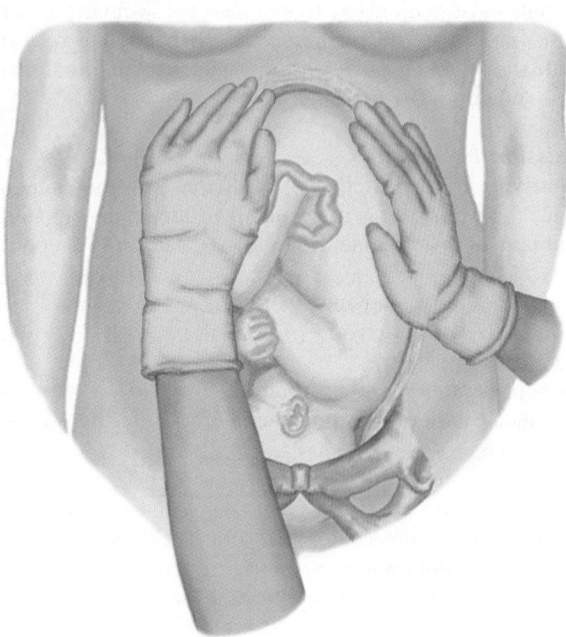

SECOND MANEUVER

6. Hold your left hand steady on one side of the uterus while palpating the opposite side of the uterus with your right hand to determine which side the fetal back is on and which side the arms and legs ("small parts") are on. Then hold your right hand steady while palpating the opposite side of the uterus with your left hand. The fetal back is a smooth, convex surface. The fetal arms and legs feel nodular, and the fetus often moves them during palpation.

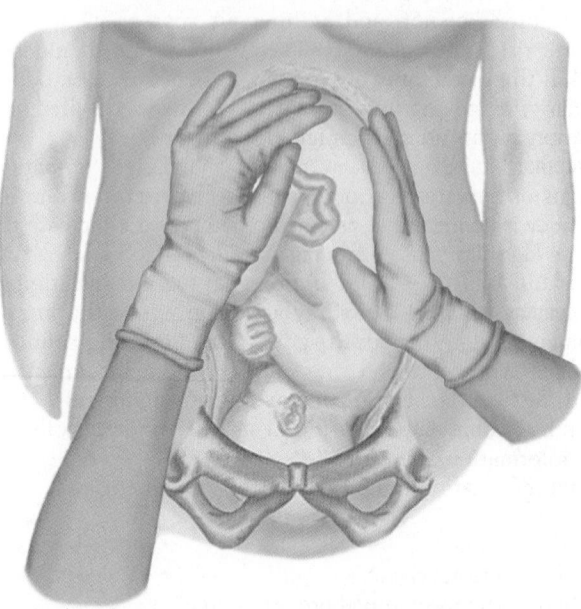

THIRD MANEUVER

7. Palpate the suprapubic area to confirm the presentation felt in the first maneuver and to determine if the presenting part is engaged. If a breech was palpated in the fundus, expect a hard, rounded head in this area. Grasp the presenting part gently between the thumb and fingers. If the presenting part is not engaged, grasping with the fingers moves it upward in the uterus.

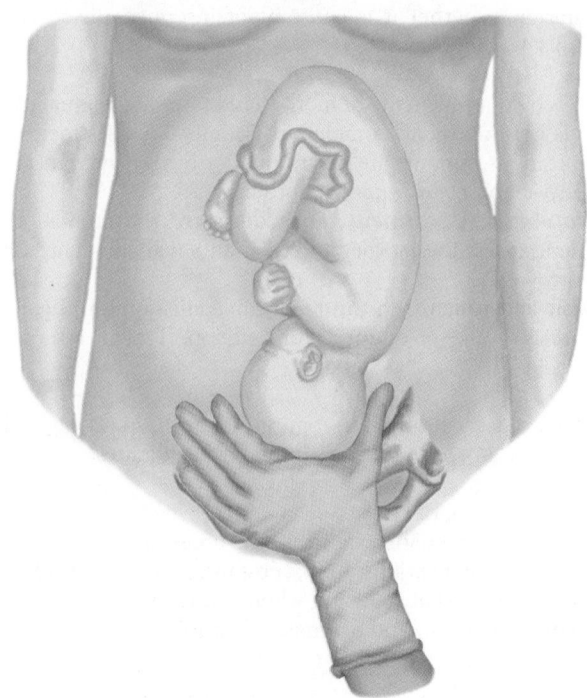

Procedure 17-1

Leopold's Maneuvers—cont'd

8. Omit the fourth maneuver if the fetus is in a breech presentation, because this maneuver is done only in cephalic presentations to determine if the fetal head is flexed.

FOURTH MANEUVER

9. To perform this maneuver most easily, turn so that you face the woman's feet.
10. Place your hands on each side of the uterus with your fingers pointed toward the pelvic inlet to determine whether the head is flexed (vertex) or extended (face). Slide your hands downward on each side of the uterus. On one side, your fingers easily slide to the upper edge of the symphysis. On the other side, your fingers meet an obstruction, the cephalic prominence. If the head is flexed, the cephalic prominence (the forehead in this case) is felt on the opposite side from the fetal back. If the head is extended, the cephalic prominence (the occiput in this case) is felt on the same side as the fetal back.

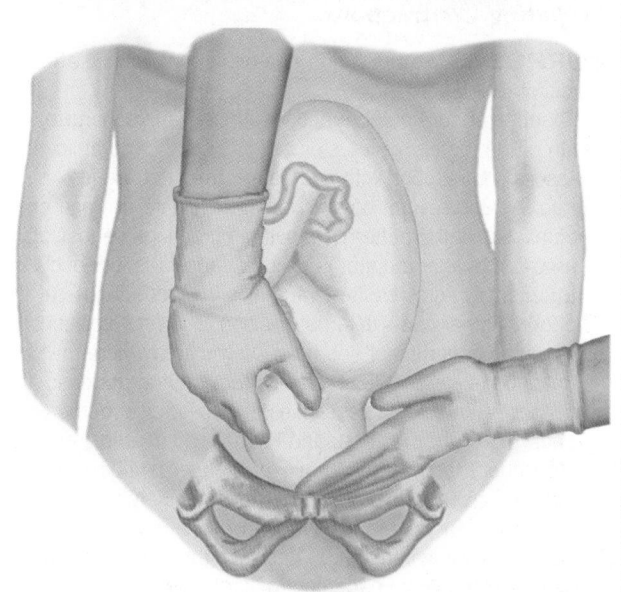

well. A separate consent for tubal ligation must be signed for women desiring permanent sterilization at delivery.

Laboratory Tests. A woman usually has routine admission laboratory tests plus other tests if indicated by her history and physical examination. If her prenatal record is available, some tests may be omitted, such as blood type and Rh. Simple tests may be done on the unit, such as:

- Hematocrit
- Blood glucose levels
- Midstream urine specimen for dipstick evaluation of protein, glucose, and ketone levels. Leukocytes may be assessed, but a catheterized specimen is best to diagnose possible urinary tract infection.

Other common routine tests done for every admitted perinatal patient include:

- Complete blood count
- Blood type and Rh factor
- Rapid plasma reagin (RPR) or other test for syphilis
- Hepatitis B surface antigen
- Human immunodeficiency virus (HIV) testing, if the woman consents

Intravenous Access. If used, intravenous access is started with at least an 18-gauge catheter. A saline lock may be used, or the woman may receive continuous infusion of fluids. The lock facilitates walking during early labor and is less associated with illness, but it provides quick access if fluids or drugs are needed. Continuous fluid infusion helps prevent or relieve dehydration and is needed if epidural block analgesia is used. Isotonic electrolyte solutions, such as lactated Ringer's solution, are common. Glucose-containing fluids are avoided during labor except for specific indications because they may cause neonatal hypoglycemia.

Assessments After Admission

After the admission assessment, the woman and her fetus need regular assessments based on their risk status and on whether interventions such as epidural analgesia are needed. General guidelines for continuing assessments are listed here.

The woman is usually observed if it is unclear after the initial assessment whether she is in true labor. After 1 or 2 hours, progressive cervical changes (effacement, dilation, or both) suggest true labor. Assess the woman and fetus during the observation period as if she were in labor.

Fetal Assessments. Fetal assessments continue to identify signs of well-being and signs that suggest compromise. The principal fetal assessments include the fetal heart rate and patterns and the character of the amniotic fluid. Abnormalities revealed in these assessments may be associated with impaired fetal gas exchange or infection.

Fetal Heart Rate. The fetal heart rate is usually assessed using electronic fetal monitoring. However, intermittent auscultation may be done with a Doppler transducer or a fetoscope (see Chapter 18).

Amniotic Fluid. The membranes may rupture spontaneously (spontaneous rupture of membranes [SROM]), or amniotomy (artificial rupture of membranes [AROM]) may be done. Assess the fetal heart rate for at least 1 minute after the membranes rupture. The umbilical cord could be displaced in a large fluid gush, resulting in compression and interruption of blood flow through it. Charting related to membrane rupture includes the time, fetal heart rate (which may appear on an electronic fetal monitor strip), and character of the fluid.

Amniotic fluid should be clear and may include bits of vernix, the creamy fetal skin lubricant. Cloudy, yellow, or foul-smelling amniotic fluid suggests infection. Green fluid indicates that the fetus has passed meconium before birth. Meconium passage may have been a response to transient hypoxia, although the cause may remain unknown. Meconium-stained fluid is rarely noted in the preterm fetus.

Procedure 17-2

Palpating Contractions

PURPOSES: To determine whether a contraction pattern is typical of true labor.

To identify abnormal contractions that may jeopardize the health of the mother or fetus or indicate another complication.

1. Assess contractions with each assessment of the fetal heart rate. Assess several contractions to evaluate average characteristics of the pattern. Palpate contractions periodically if an external fetal monitor is used because it is less accurate for intensity as a result of variations in the thickness of the abdominal fat pad, maternal position, and fetal position.
2. Place the fingertips of one hand on the area where the contractions are best felt, usually the uterine fundus. The mother usually feels sensations in her lower abdomen and back. Use light pressure, and keep your fingertips relatively still rather than moving them over the uterus, because moving your hand over the uterus may stimulate contractions and give an inaccurate view of their true pattern. The fingertips are more sensitive to the first tightening of the uterus.
3. Note the time when each contraction begins and ends:
   a. Determine the frequency by noting the average time that elapses from the beginning of one contraction to the beginning of the next one.

   b. Determine the duration of contractions by noting the average time in seconds from beginning to end of each contraction.
   c. Determine the interval between contractions by noting the average time between the end of one contraction and the beginning of the next one.
4. Estimate the average intensity of contractions by noting how easily the uterus can be indented during the peak of the contraction:
   a. Mild contractions are easily indented with the fingertips. They feel similar to the tip of the nose.
   b. Moderate contractions can be indented with more difficulty. They feel similar to the chin.
   c. Firm contractions feel "woody" and cannot be readily indented. They feel similar to the forehead.
5. Report excessive contractions that can reduce placental blood flow. Note incomplete relaxation of the uterus. See Chapter 18 for details and interventions.

Describe quantity in approximate terms. At term, a "large" amount is more than 1000 ml; a "moderate" amount is about 500 to 1000 ml; and "scant" amniotic fluid is only a trickle, barely enough to detect. If the fetus is well down into the pelvis when the membranes rupture, a small amount of fluid in front of the fetal head may be discharged (forewaters), with the rest lost at birth.

Maternal Assessments. Several maternal assessments, such as vital signs and contractions, also relate to the health of the fetus.

Vital Signs. Guidelines for maternal vital signs assessment are listed in Table 17-2. Hypotension, hypertension, elevated pulse and respiratory rates, and elevated temperature should be reported, and repeat assessments should be done more frequently.

Contractions. Contractions can be assessed by palpation (Procedure 17-2) or with the electronic fetal monitor, using the guidelines in Table 18-1. With external monitoring, a combination of techniques is often used.

Progress of Labor. Periodic vaginal examinations determine cervical dilation and effacement and fetal descent. The frequency of vaginal examinations depends on the woman's parity, the status of her membranes, and the overall speed of her labor. Vaginal examinations are limited to avoid introducing microorganisms from the perineal area into the uterus.

Intake and Output. Oral and intravenous intakes are recorded. Each voiding is recorded. Labor or regional anesthesia reduces a woman's urge to void, so check her suprapubic area every 2 hours to identify bladder distention. Check more frequently if she has received large amounts of intravenous fluid.

Pressure of the fetal head on the rectum in late labor makes many women feel the need to defecate, even if they had epidural analgesia. Look at the woman's perineum for crowning of the fetal head if she abruptly expresses a need to defecate or says "something feels different down there" or a comparable remark.

Response to Labor. The woman's behavioral responses change as labor intensifies. She withdraws from interactions but needs more nursing presence and reassurance. She may become more anxious because of pain and fear of bodily injury, unknown outcome, loss of control, unresolved psychologic issues that influence her readiness to give birth (e.g., sexual abuse, previous birth experiences), or unexpected occurrences during labor.

Women vary in the way they handle the pain of labor. The nurse must constantly assess whether added pain control measures are needed, because laboring women are often uncertain about when they are ready for added relief measures. Behaviors that suggest the woman needs help with pain management include:

- Expressing that nonpharmacologic measures are ineffective.
- Tensing her muscles or arching her back during contractions.
- Persistence of muscle tension between contractions.
- A tense facial expression; rolling in the bed.
- Expressions such as "I can't take it anymore."
- Specific requests for medication or other pain control.

The Support Person's Response. Labor is stressful for the woman's support person, often the baby's father. He may become anxious, fearful, or tired. He feels a responsibility to protect and support the woman but may have limited resources for doing so. It is difficult for him to watch the woman he loves in pain, even if the pain is normal and she declines medication. He may respond to stress in many ways: by becoming quiet, suffering silently, pacing, expressing anger, or even vomiting. Some fathers respond by leaving the room frequently or for long periods, whereas others resist taking even short breaks.

Nurses encourage and value the father's presence during labor and birth. This attitude, however, may conflict with a couple's cultural norms, which may dictate that birth is a strictly female activity. The father may be pulled in two directions, wanting to be included but hesitant because it is not customary in his culture to be part of the birth. The nurse should respect the values of each couple and their wishes about the father's involvement.

The support person also may be a parent or other relative, a friend of either sex, or a homosexual partner. The nurse must remember that anyone who assists the woman during labor may feel anxious or helpless at times. Reassurance and care for the labor partner strengthen that person's ability to support the woman and increase the likelihood that both will view the birth experience as positive.

▪NURSING CARE
The Woman With False or Early Labor

Assessment
After assessment, it may be apparent that the woman is not in true labor. If findings are normal and her membranes are intact, she is usually discharged home. The woman who is in very early labor may be discharged to await active labor, especially if she is a nullipara and lives nearby.

Nursing Diagnosis and Planning
The woman may be frustrated because she cannot tell whether labor is real. She may resist returning to the birth center, possibly delaying care needlessly. A nursing diagnosis that applies to many women with false labor contractions is:

■ Deficient Knowledge
   Expected Outcome: The woman and her support person will describe reasons for returning to the birth center for evaluation.

Interventions
Providing Reassurance
A woman sent home after observation often feels foolish and frustrated. Reassure her that even professionals cannot always identify true labor and that false labor and early true labor have similar characteristics. Tell her that important preparation occurs during late pregnancy, such as softening of her cervix, even if objective progress like cervical dilation has not yet occurred.

Teaching
Review guidelines for returning to the birth center with her: regular contractions, leaking of amniotic fluid, active bleeding (more than bloody show and often not mixed with mucus), and decreased fetal movement. Explain that these are only guidelines and that she should call or return if she has

any concerns. It is better for her to return with another false alarm than to arrive at the birth center in advanced labor or to develop complications at home.

Evaluation
• Can the woman and her support person describe guidelines for returning to the birth center?

▪NURSING CARE
The Woman in True Labor

The admission assessment may confirm that the woman is in true labor, or true labor may be evident after observation. Nursing diagnoses and collaborative problems change during labor because the intrapartum period is an evolving process. Those covered in this chapter relate to fetal oxygenation, maternal discomfort, and maternal injury.

Nursing diagnoses are often interrelated during labor. For example, anxiety or fear can affect pain relief measures. A fluid volume deficit can alter fetal oxygenation because less blood is available to circulate to the placenta.

FETAL OXYGENATION
Assessment
Refer to assessments listed in Table 17-2 for intrapartum assessments. The main assessments related to fetal well-being are:

• Fetal heart rate
• Contractions: frequency, duration, intensity, resting tone, interval
• Character of amniotic fluid and time of rupture
• Maternal vital signs

Chapter 18 contains detailed information about fetal heart rate and related observations.

Nursing Diagnosis and Planning
A collaborative problem is appropriate for nursing care related to fetal well-being during labor. Most fetuses tolerate labor well, but conditions such as maternal hypotension or hypertension, maternal fever, excessive (tetanic) contractions, or compression of the umbilical cord can compromise fetal oxygenation. Client-centered goals are not made for collaborative problems as they are for nursing diagnoses. Planning includes nursing responsibilities to (1) promote normal placental function and (2) observe for and report problems to the physician or nurse-midwife.

Interventions
Promoting Placental Function
Maternal positioning is the most common measure to promote placental function during normal labor. The woman can choose any position other than the supine to avoid aortocaval compression that would reduce blood flow to the placenta. If she must be in the supine position for a procedure such as catheterization, a small pillow or rolled towel or blanket wedged under one hip shifts her uterus to one side to maintain good placental blood flow.

! CRITICAL TO REMEMBER

Conditions Associated With Fetal Compromise

- A fetal heart rate outside the normal range of 110-160 beats per minute (bpm) for a term fetus.
- Meconium-stained (greenish) amniotic fluid.
- Cloudy, yellowish, or foul odor to the amniotic fluid (suggests infection).
- Excessive frequency or duration of contractions.
- Incomplete uterine relaxation.
- Maternal hypotension (may divert blood flow away from the placenta to ensure adequate perfusion of the maternal brain and heart).
- Maternal hypertension (may be associated with vasospasm in spiral arteries, which supply the intervillous spaces of the placenta).
- Maternal fever (38° C [100.4° F] or higher).

NOTE: Chapter 18 provides detailed fetal assessments and interpretation of data.

Observing for Conditions Associated With Fetal Compromise

Determine whether any conditions associated with fetal compromise exist. If any are identified, assess the fetus more frequently and notify the birth attendant.

Evaluation

Evaluation of client goals or expected outcomes does not apply to a collaborative problem. Throughout labor, the nurse compares actual data with the norms for the mother and fetus. See Chapter 18 for integration of fetal assessments into intrapartum care planning.

DISCOMFORT

Assessment

See Table 17-2 for continuing assessments of the laboring woman.

Nursing Diagnosis and Planning

Labor is painful. Women vary in their responses to pain and in the pain management methods they choose. Providing choices for pain management and supporting the woman's choice increase her sense of control over her birth experience. The woman who successfully masters the pain and other physical demands of labor is more likely to view her experience as positive. Her support person is likely to feel more satisfaction with the experience as well.

Pain and Anxiety are related nursing diagnoses. Excess anxiety intensifies pain perception, and pain worsens anxiety. The nurse clusters assessment data and considers both pain and anxiety when determining the best approach to pain relief. Several cues may suggest that anxiety is a major contributor to labor pain that the woman might otherwise easily manage: a previous poor experience during birth or expressions of worry and concern. The nursing diagnosis is therefore:

■ Pain related to effects of uterine contractions.

Expected Outcomes: The woman will state that she is able to tolerate the pain satisfactorily and will use breathing and relaxation techniques. The woman's partner will express satisfaction with his or her ability to support her.

Interventions

Providing Comfort Measures

Ordinary measures reduce irritating surroundings that impair a woman's ability to relax and use coping skills. Nurses must be creative when providing comfort to the laboring woman.

Lighting Soft, indirect lighting is soothing, whereas a bright overhead light is an irritant. Bright lights imply a hospital ("sick") atmosphere rather than the normal life event that birth is. Use the overhead light only when needed. A small flashlight is handy if the woman wants her room truly dark.

Temperature Labor is work. Women in labor are often hot and perspiring. Cool, damp washcloths on the woman's face and neck promote comfort. Keep an ample supply of damp washcloths available, and change them often to keep them cool. An electric fan circulates air in the labor room and directs a breeze on the woman. Be sure that the fan does not blow on the infant after birth, because cool air might cause hypothermia.

Have the woman wear socks if her feet are cold. She may shake, sometimes intensely, although her temperature is normal and she denies being cold.

Cleanliness Bloody show and amniotic fluid leak from the woman's vagina during labor. Change the sheets and gown as needed to keep her dry and comfortable. Let her preferences be the guide, because she may not want to be disturbed during late labor. Change the underpad regularly to reduce microorganisms that may ascend into the vagina. A folded towel absorbs larger quantities of amniotic fluid than the pad alone. If using pillows near where fluid will leak, protect them with underpads.

Mouth Care Ice chips, Popsicles, or hard candy on a stick reduces the discomfort of a dry mouth. Avoid excess sugar intake that might contribute to neonatal hypoglycemia after birth. If oral intake is contraindicated, brushing the teeth (without swallowing water) or simply rinsing the mouth helps. Many women appreciate a moist washcloth applied to their lips.

Bladder A full bladder intensifies pain during labor and can delay fetal descent. Remind the woman to empty her bladder at least every 2 hours. Catheterization is often needed.

Positioning Occasionally, a specific maternal position reduces discomfort or assists the labor process. Otherwise, encourage the woman to assume any position that she finds comfortable, avoiding the supine position with no side tilt. Frequent changes reduce discomfort from constant pressure, help the fetus adapt to the pelvic contours, and promote fetal descent. Figure 17-15 illustrates various maternal positions for labor.

The woman often has "back labor" if her fetus is in the occiput posterior position, because the fetal occiput presses on the mother's sacral promontory with each contraction. Positions that encourage the fetus to fall away from the sacral promontory, such as those in which the mother leans forward or uses the hands-and-knees position, promote her comfort and enhance internal rotation to an occiput anterior position.

Water Water in the form of a shower, tub, or whirlpool is relaxing and helps many women tolerate contractions. Nipple stimulation by water currents causes release of oxytocin by the posterior pituitary gland, which increases contractions and promotes labor progress. If contractions become too strong, she simply removes her breasts from the water stream.

Teaching

Teaching the woman in labor is a constant and changing task.

First Stage of Labor Many women become discouraged because several hours are needed to reach 4 or 5 cm of cervical dilation. They believe that the last 5 cm will take as long as the first 5 cm. It may help them to know that 5 cm is more like two thirds of the way to full dilation rather than half the way because the rate of dilation increases during the active phase.

The urge to push usually occurs when the woman's cervix is fully dilated and effaced and when the fetus descends deep into the pelvis and internally rotates. As she nears the second stage, however, her baby may descend enough to give her an urge to push before full cervical dilation. If her cervix, which is usually 8 or 9 cm dilated at this time, yields easily to downward pressure, pushing in response to her spontaneous urge rarely causes problems. Either of two problems may occur if she pushes

Standing

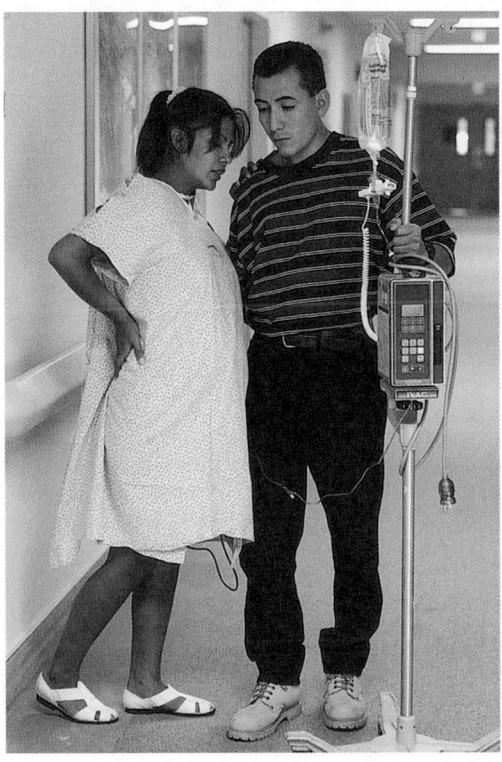

Advantages

Adds gravity to force of contractions to promote fetal descent.
Contractions are less uncomfortable and more efficient.
Variation: Standing, leaning forward with support reduces back pain because fetus falls forward, away from the sacral promontory.

Disadvantages

Tiring over long periods.
Continuous electronic fetal monitoring is not possible without telemetry if woman is walking in the hall.

Nursing Implications

If the woman has intravenous fluid running, give her a rolling pole. Encourage her to alternate walking with other positions whenever she tires or desires to do so.
Remind the woman and her partner when she should return to the labor area for evaluation of the fetal heart rate and her labor status.

Sitting Upright

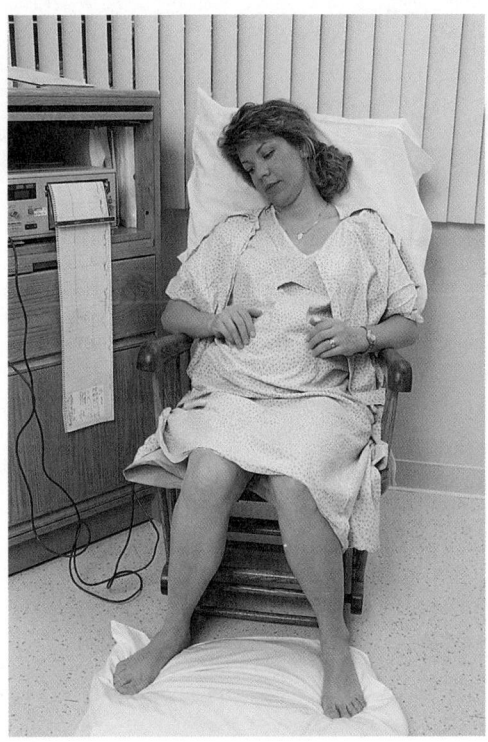

Advantages

Uses gravity to aid fetal descent.
Can be done when sitting on side of bed, in a chair, or on the toilet.
Can be used with continuous fetal monitoring.
Avoids supine hypotension.

Disadvantages

May increase suprapubic discomfort.
Contractions are the most efficient when the woman alternates sitting with other positions.

Nursing Implications

A rocking chair is soothing.
Place a pillow on a chair with a disposable underpad over the pillow to absorb secretions.
Use pillows or a footstool to keep the short woman's legs from dangling.
Encourage the woman to alternate positions periodically; for example, she can alternate walking with sitting or sitting with side-lying.

Figure 17-15 Maternal positions for labor. *Continued*

Sitting, Leaning Forward with Support

Semi-sitting

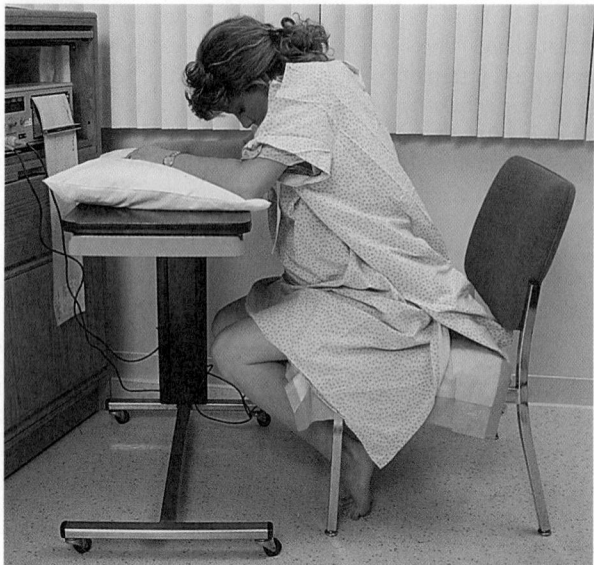

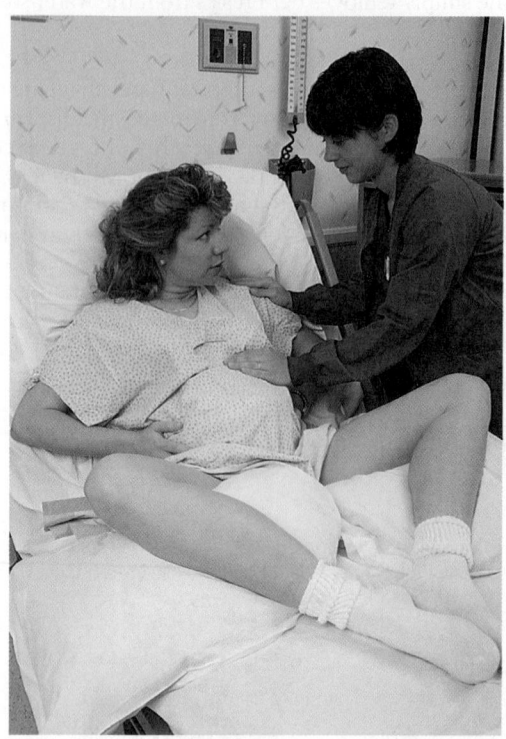

Advantages

Same as for sitting.
Reduces back pain because fetus falls forward, away from sacral promontory.
Partner or nurse can rub back or provide sacral pressure to relieve back pain.

Disadvantages

Same as for sitting.

Nursing Implications

Same as for sitting.

Advantages

Same as for sitting.
Aligns long axis of uterus with pelvic inlet, which applies contraction force in the most efficient direction through pelvis.

Disadvantages

Same as for sitting.
Does not reduce pain as well as the forward-leaning positions.

Nursing Implications

Same as for sitting.
Raise bed to about a 30- to 45-degree angle.
Encourage the woman to use sitting (leaning forward) or side-lying position if she has back pain so that the caregiver can rub her back or apply sacral pressure.

Figure 17-15, cont'd Maternal positions for labor.

against a cervix that does not easily open as the fetus applies pressure:

- The cervix may become edematous, which can block progress.
- The cervix may be lacerated.

Teach the woman to blow out in short breaths if she should not yet push.

Second Stage of Labor The woman may need help to push most effectively during second-stage labor.

Laboring Down Two hours was once considered the upper limit for the duration of the second stage. It is now recognized that a second stage longer than 2 hours is safe if the mother and fetus show no signs of compromise.

Women push most effectively when they feel the reflex urge to do so. Many women do not immediately feel the urge to push when the cervix is fully dilated, especially if

they received epidural analgesia. Repeated prolonged episodes of breath-holding while bearing down (the Valsalva maneuver) can reduce fetal oxygenation. Pushing vigorously before the urge is present contributes to birth canal injury, because vaginal tissues are stretched more forcefully and rapidly than they would be if she pushed spontaneously and in response to her body's signals. In addition, early pushing adds to maternal fatigue, with instrumental delivery (e.g., vacuum extractor) being a common result.

The weight of evidence does not support the validity of having a woman push just because her cervix is fully dilated. Also, studies have shown that a second stage longer than 2 hours is not harmful if progress continues. If maternal and fetal assessments are reassuring, the woman does not need to push before she feels the urge. For these reasons, many nurses practice a second stage technique that goes by any of several names, such as "laboring down" or "rest and descend."

Side-Lying

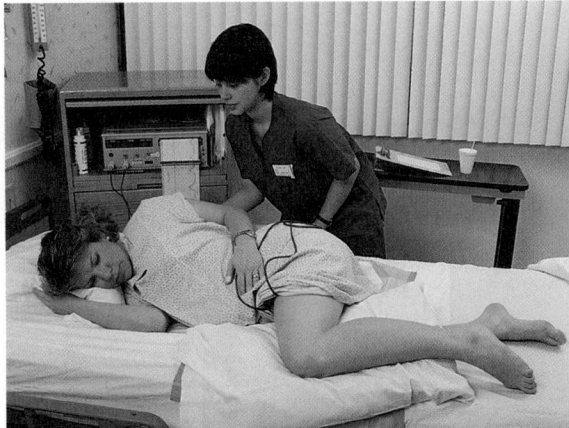

Kneeling, Leaning Forward with Support

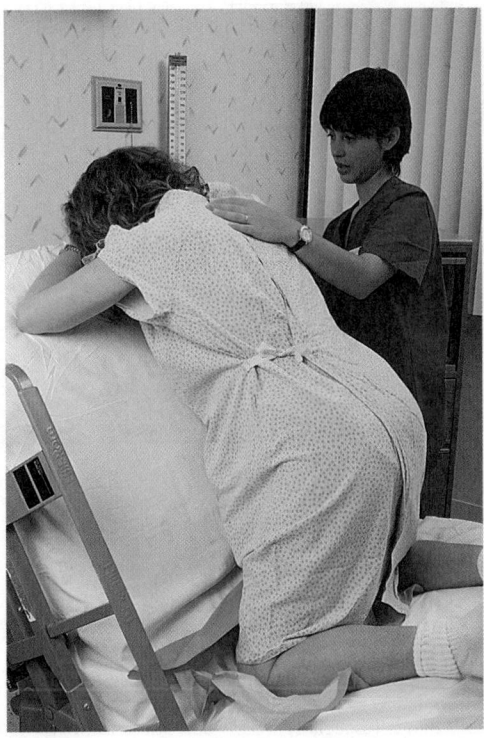

Advantages

Is a restful position.
Prevents supine hypotension and promotes placental blood flow.
Promotes efficient contractions, although they may be less frequent than with other positions.
Can be used with continuous fetal monitoring.

Disadvantages

Does not use gravity to aid fetal descent.

Nursing Implications

Teach the woman and her partner that although the contractions are less frequent, they are more effective.
This position offers a break from more tiring positions.
Use pillows for support and to prevent pressure: at her back, under her superior arm, and between her knees.
Use disposable underpads to protect the pillow between the woman's knees from secretions.
Some women like to put their superior leg on the bed rail. If the woman wants this variation, pad the bed rail with a blanket to prevent pressure.
If she wants to remain recumbent, she should use this position to promote placental blood flow.

Advantages

Reduces back pain because fetus falls forward, away from sacral promontory.
Adds gravity to force of contractions to promote fetal descent.
Can be used with continuous fetal monitoring.
Caregivers can rub her back or apply sacral pressure.
Promotes normal mechanisms of birth.

Disadvantages

Knees may become tired or uncomfortable.
Tiring if used for long periods.

Nursing Implications

Raise the head of the bed, and have the woman face the head of the bed while she is on her knees.
Another method is for the partner to sit in a chair, with the woman kneeling in front, facing her partner, and leaning forward on him or her for support.
Use pillow under the knees and in front of the woman's chest, as needed, for comfort.
Encourage her to change positions if she becomes tired.

Figure 17-15, cont'd Maternal positions for labor. *Continued*

Simply put, laboring down means allowing uterine contractions to cause most fetal internal rotation and descent after full cervical dilation. The woman rests before actively pushing her baby out. When the woman senses rectal pressure or an urge to push, she is then supported to push in response to her natural urge. Nursing and medical research continue about the effectiveness of laboring down and whether any time limit should be applied (Mayberry, Hammer, Kelly, True-Driver, & De, 2000b; Minato, 2000/2001).

Positions The mother can push in any position she prefers if her lower body is not affected by an epidural block. Position changes promote her natural pushing ef-

forts. Many women prefer semi-sitting and side-lying positions. Squatting enlarges the pelvic outlet slightly and adds the force of gravity to the mother's efforts; this is an advantage if she has a small pelvis or the fetus is large. Some women push most effectively while sitting on the toilet because that is where they are accustomed to giving in to that sensation. The woman can also turn backward while sitting on the toilet, letting the tank (with a pillow on top) support her upper body.

When the mother pushes, teach her to curve her body around her uterus in a **C** shape with her chin on her chest. For most effectiveness, teach her to pull on her knees, hand-holds,

Hands and Knees

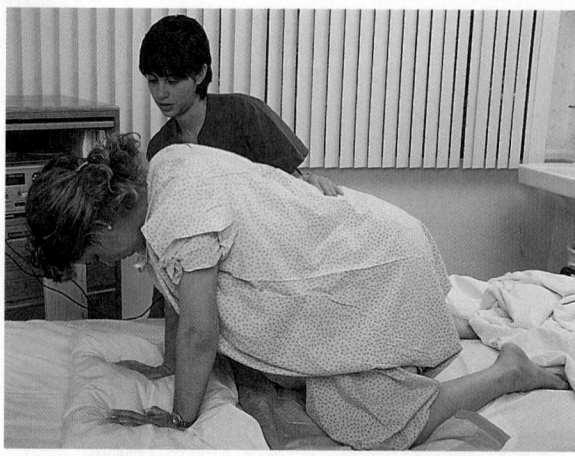

Squatting

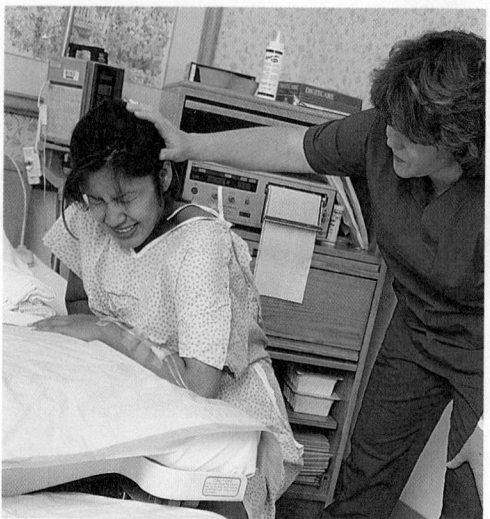

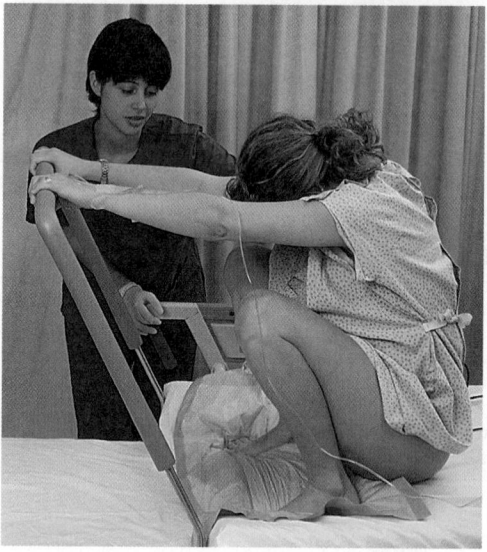

Advantages

Reduces back pain because the fetus falls forward, away from the sacral promontory.

Promotes normal mechanisms of birth.

The woman can use pelvic rocking to decrease back pain.

Caregivers can rub the woman's back or apply sacral pressure easily.

Disadvantages

The woman's hands (especially wrists) and knees can become uncomfortable.

Tiring when used for a long time.

Some women are embarrassed to use this position.

Nursing Implications

Encourage the woman to change to less tiring positions occasionally.

Ensure privacy when encouraging the reluctant woman to try this position if she has back pain.

A second hospital gown with the opening in front covers her back and hips but may be too warm.

Positions for Pushing in Second Stage

Standing

This position may be tiring, and access to the woman's perineum is difficult. Because the infant could fall to the ground if birth occurs rapidly, provide padding under the mother's feet. Gravity aids fetal descent.

Hands and Knees

Advantages and disadvantages are similar to those during first-stage labor. In addition, caregivers must reorient themselves because the landmarks are upside down from their usual perspective.

A variation is for the mother to kneel and lean forward against a beanbag or the side of the bed. This variation reduces some of the strain on her wrists and hands.

Advantages

Adds gravity to force of contractions to promote fetal descent.

Straightens the pelvic curve slightly for more direct fetal descent.

Increases dimensions of pelvis slightly.

Promotes effective pushing efforts in the second stage.

Caregivers can rub back or provide sacral pressure.

Disadvantages

Knees and hips may become uncomfortable because of prolonged flexion.

Tiring over a long time.

Nursing Implications

Provide support with a squat bar attached to the bed or by two people standing on each side of the woman.

If she becomes tired, or between contractions, she can lean back into the sitting position.

Variation: Have the woman squat beside the bed as she pushes.

Figure 17-15, cont'd Maternal positions for labor.

Semi-sitting

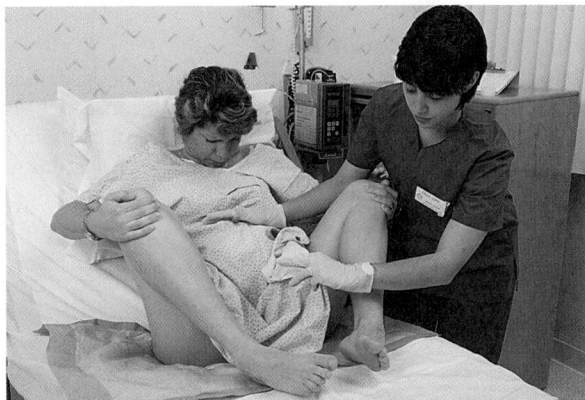

Many women prefer this because they have the security of a back rest; it is also familiar to caregivers and allows easy observation of the perineum. Elevate the woman's back at least 30 to 45 degrees so that gravity aids fetal descent. The woman pulls on her flexed knees (behind or in front of them) as she pushes. She should keep her head flexed and her sacrum flat on the bed to straighten the pelvic curve.

Side-Lying

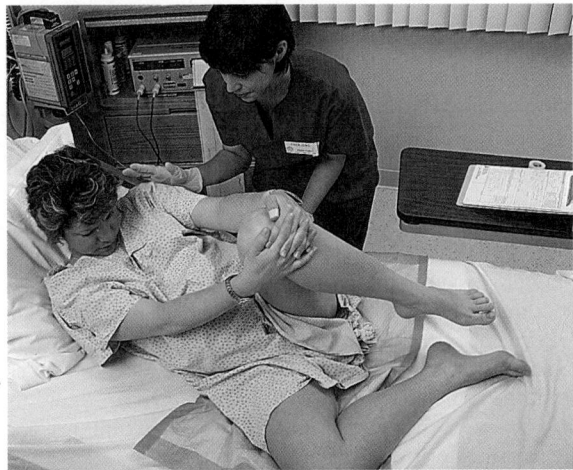

The woman flexes her chin on her chest and curls around her uterus as she pushes. She pulls on her flexed knees or the knee of the superior leg as she pushes.

Figure 17-15, cont'd Maternal positions for labor.

or a squatting bar while pushing. Women often find that pulling on something from above is efficient.

Method and Breathing Pattern If she is pushing effectively and safely, do not interfere, but support the woman's spontaneous techniques. Prolonged breath-holding (more than 6-8 sec per push) or pushing more than 4 times per contraction is discouraged. A deep breath helps her relax at the end of the contraction. The woman may grunt or groan when pushing and should be reassured that this is normal.

A woman who is modest or fears losing control may inhibit her best pushing efforts if she is instructed to push as if she were having a bowel movement, particularly if she is in a bed or chair. A more anatomically correct image is to teach the woman to push down and out under her symphysis ("pubic bone"), following the pelvic curve. Seeing a diagram of the pelvis helps her to visualize the curve.

Providing Encouragement Success breeds success. Tell the woman when her labor is progressing. If she can see that her efforts are effective, she has more courage to continue. Help her touch or see the baby's head with a mirror as crowning occurs.

Praise the woman and her labor partner when they use breathing or other coping techniques effectively. This encouragement reinforces their actions, gives them a sense of control, and conveys the respect and support of the nurse. If one technique is not helpful after a reasonable trial (three to five contractions), encourage them to try other techniques.

Giving of Self The nurse's caring presence is a crucial element in labor support. Even women who are very independent may become dependent during labor and need human contact. Many times the woman simply needs reassurance that all is going well and that the nurse is there for her. The nurse's presence helps allay her fears of abandonment and conveys safety, acceptance, support, and comfort.

Although the woman and her support person may have prepared for childbirth, they often welcome suggestions and affirmation from the nurse. The nurse who is familiar with the techniques they are using can better support them and avoid contradicting what they have learned and practiced. The nurse's presence, gentle coaching, and encouragement help the laboring woman have confidence in her own body and her fitness to give birth. See Chapter 19 for nonpharmacologic support and pain-relief measures.

Offering Pharmacologic Measures Some women do not need pharmacologic pain relief during labor. Birth is usually a normal process, and the prepared woman and labor partner can deliver their infant without medication. Most, however, do choose to have pharmacologic pain management. Inform the woman about medications available to her without pressuring her to take them. See Chapter 19 for additional information about pharmacologic measures.

A few women have a firm goal of avoiding all pain medication during labor. These women may then feel let down or guilty if they need medication. Other women may plan to use a specific pain-relief method, such as epidural analgesia. If something prevents use of their chosen method, they may be upset about this unexpected development in their birth experience. In either case, allow the woman to ventilate her feelings about her experience. Although this development may not be what she wanted, expressing her feelings helps her put it into perspective.

Caring for the Birth Partner The woman's support person is an integral part of her labor care. Her labor partner can provide care and comfort, which support the woman's ability to give birth. Do not expect too much of the partner or make assumptions about the desired type and amount of involvement.

Some partners are coaches in the true sense of the word, actively assisting the woman through labor. Others want the woman and nurse to lead them and tell them how to help.

They are eager to do what they can but expect instructions about how and when to do it. Many couples see the partner's role as one of encouragement, moral support, and just being there for the woman.

To impose unrealistic expectations of leadership, care, and comfort on the partner makes the birth experience unnecessarily stressful. To ensure a positive experience for both people, accept whatever pattern of support the partner is able and willing to provide and whatever the couple finds comfortable. Without taking over or diminishing this role, provide support that the partner cannot.

Encourage the partner to conserve physical strength. The partner may have missed sleep during the hours of early labor or may need a break. The nurse may need to encourage the partner to eat or bring a snack. Remind the partner that support will be more effective if the partner's own needs are met. Support persons who do not eat for a long time are more likely to faint during the birth.

Evaluation

- Is the woman satisfied with her pain control, whether it is nonpharmacologic or pharmacologic?
- Does the woman use the breathing and relaxation techniques that she was taught or that she creates for herself?
- Does her partner express satisfaction with his or her labor support?

As a nursing diagnosis, Pain and related goals for pain management are constantly re-evaluated during labor.

PREVENTING INJURY
Assessment

Nursing assessments of the mother and fetus continue as the woman nears birth. During the second stage of labor, observe the woman's perineum to determine when to make final birth preparations.

The exact time for final birth preparations varies according to the woman's parity, the overall speed of labor, the fetal station, and the distance of the physician or nurse-midwife from the labor and delivery unit. Final preparations are usually completed when crowning in the nullipara reaches a diameter of about 3 to 4 cm. The multipara is prepared sooner, when her cervix is fully dilated and the fetal head is well down in the pelvis but before much crowning has occurred.

Nursing Diagnosis and Planning

The woman is vulnerable to injury immediately before and after birth for several reasons: (1) altered physical sensations, such as responses to intense pressure or medication; (2) positional changes for birth; and (3) unexpectedly rapid progress. The nursing diagnosis selected for the laboring woman near the time of birth is therefore:

■ Risk for Injury (maternal) related to altered sensations and positional or physical changes.

   Expected Outcome: The woman does not have an avoidable injury, such as muscle strains, thrombosis, or lacerations, during birth.

Interventions

Transferring the woman to the delivery site or positioning her in the birthing bed is the first step in the sequence of events that culminates in birth of the baby. During the period surrounding birth, the nurse reduces factors that contribute to maternal injuries.

Transfer to a Delivery Room
Most vaginal births occur in a combination labor, delivery, and recovery room. With some client conditions, such as a twin birth, the woman is transferred to a separate room for birth. Transfer her early enough to avoid rushed, last-minute preparations, which are stressful for all.

Positioning for Birth
To promote effective pushing and take advantage of gravity, raise the woman's back, shoulders, and head. Experimenting with the level of head elevation will probably be needed.

Padded stirrups or footrests support the woman's legs and feet and make her perineum more accessible. To reduce strain on muscles and ligaments, raise and lower her legs together (if regional block limits her movement) and do not separate them too widely for her leg length. Surfaces that contact the popliteal space behind the knee should be padded to reduce pressure that can lead to thrombus formation. Do not leave her legs in stirrups for a prolonged time.

Observing the Perineum
The exact time at which a woman is ready to give birth is an educated guess. A woman who has been having a slow labor may suddenly make rapid progress. Birth is near when the fetal head swings anteriorly in extension as the occiput slips under the symphysis pubis. Observe the woman's perineum, especially during late second-stage labor.

A classic sign of imminent birth is the mother's urgent cry, "The baby's coming!" Look at her perineum, and if the baby will be born before the physician or nurse-midwife arrives, remain calm and support the infant's head and body with gloved hands as it emerges (Box 17-1).

Evaluation

- During the postpartum period, does the woman show evidence of muscle strains or thrombus formation?

NURSING CARE DURING THE LATE INTRAPARTUM PERIOD

Responsibilities During Birth

The nurse has added responsibilities during the birth. These may include:

- Preparation of a table with sterile gowns, gloves, drapes, solutions, and instruments (Fig. 17-16)
- Perineal cleansing preparation
- Initial care and assessment of the newborn
- Administration of medications such as oxytocin to contract the uterus and control blood loss (see Chapter 20)

Staff from the newborn or special care nursery and often a pediatrician, neonatologist, or neonatal nurse practitioner are usually present if the newborn is at risk for problems (e.g., aspiration of amniotic fluid containing meconium) or has shown nonreassuring signs during labor. Nursery staff may routinely attend deliveries in some facilities (Fig. 17-17, pp. 378-379).

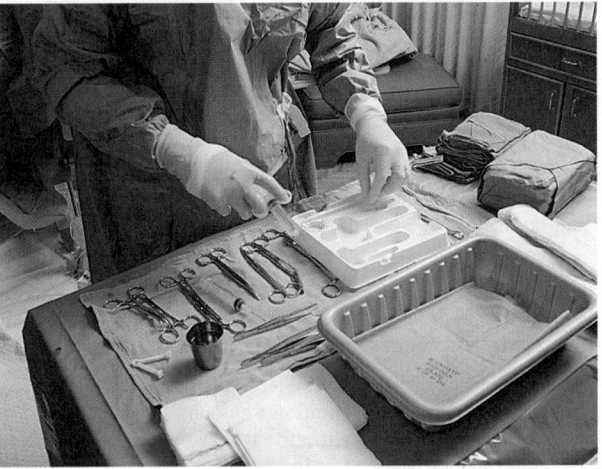

Figure 17-16 The physician arranges instruments in final preparation for birth. Although the vagina is not sterile, a sterile table is prepared to limit introduction of outside organisms into the birth canal. Included on the sterile table are infant care materials (e.g., a cord clamp, cord blood tube), instruments for repair of maternal injury or episiotomy, and anesthesia materials (if needed).

Standard Precautions protect personnel from potentially infectious substances from mother or baby. At birth, the newborn is covered with blood, amniotic fluid, vernix, and other body substances (Fig. 17-18, pp. 380-381). To avoid contact with potentially infectious secretions, personnel involved in infant contact should wear gloves and other protective equipment until after the first bath. (The Nursing Care Plan: Normal Labor and Birth illustrates a normal labor and birth experience.)

Responsibilities After Birth

Intrapartum nursing care extends through the fourth stage of labor and includes care of the infant, the mother, and the family unit. See Chapters 21 through 24 for discussion of later postpartum care of the mother and infant.

Care of the Infant
Immediate nursing care of the newborn includes supporting cardiopulmonary and thermoregulatory function and placing identifying bands on the infant. In addition, the nurse assesses the infant for approximate gestational age and whether large or small for gestational age. Additional assessment of the blood glucose level is common for infants who are large or small for gestation. Assessment for obvious anomalies or birth injuries and number of cord vessels (see

Figure 17-14, *D*) should also be done. If the newborn stays with parents longer than 1 hour after birth, a full assessment and admission procedures are often done in the birthing room.

Maintaining Cardiopulmonary Function. Maintaining the infant's cardiopulmonary function begins before birth by ensuring that equipment needed for neonatal resuscitation, such as suction equipment, oxygen, an appropriate-size Ambu bag and mask, and intubation equipment, is ready. Most infants need only gentle stimulation such as drying, but a few need more vigorous resuscitation measures.

Assess the infant's Apgar score (Table 17-3, p. 385) at 1 and 5 minutes after birth for evaluation of early cardiopulmonary adaptation. If the Apgar score is 8 or higher, no intervention is needed other than supporting normal respiratory efforts. If the infant is obviously in distress (i.e., no or low heart rate and/or respirations, limp muscle tone, lack of response to stimulation, blue or pale color), interventions to correct the problem are instituted immediately rather than awaiting the 1-minute Apgar score.

Suction secretions from the infant's mouth and nose with a bulb syringe as needed. If deeper suction is needed for large amounts of fluid, use a neonatal suction apparatus with a mucus trap that is connected to regulated wall suction. Teach parents how to use the bulb syringe (see Procedure 23-1). Avoid keeping the infant in a head-dependent position without a specific indication, because the position limits diaphragm movement by upward pressure from the intestines.

Supporting Thermoregulation. To reduce evaporative heat loss, dry the infant. Dry the head well, because substantial heat loss can occur from the head, which is about one fourth of the neonate's body surface area. Discard damp linens.

Place the infant in a prewarmed radiant warmer to limit heat loss while giving initial care. Skin-to-skin contact with a parent has the same effect and also promotes bonding. Avoid coming between the infant and the heat source. Wrap the infant in warm blankets when he or she is not in the warmer or making skin-to-skin contact. A stockinette cap

Transfer and Positioning for Birth

Action: When the woman is almost ready to give birth, transfer her to the delivery room or position the birthing bed. The exact time varies with several factors (such as overall speed of labor and rate of fetal descent). *Rationale:* Rushed, last-moment preparations are anxiety-producing for the woman, her partner, and the nurse. Remaining in the birth position for a long time can be tiring.

Action: Continue observing her perineum while making final preparations for birth. *Rationale:* Birth may occur unexpectedly, and the nurse should be prepared to "catch" the infant if the attendant (physician or nurse-midwife) is not in the room.

Action: Continue observing the fetal heart rate (FHR) with continuous monitoring or intermittent auscultation. *Rationale:* Detects changes in fetal condition that may require interventions by the attendant to speed birth.

Action: Elevate the woman's back, shoulders, and head with a wedge (on a delivery table) or by raising the head of the birthing bed. *Rationale:* Allows more effective maternal pushing and uses gravity to aid fetal descent.

Action: Stirrups or foot rests to support the woman's legs and feet may be used on a birthing bed. Pad the surface. *Rationale:* Padding reduces pressure, preventing venous stasis and possible thrombus formation.

Action: When placing the woman's legs in stirrups, elevate them and remove them simultaneously. Do not separate her legs widely. *Rationale:* Reduces strain on muscles and ligaments.

Prepping and Draping

Action: After the woman is in position, cleanse the perineal area with a sterile iodophor and water preparation unless she is allergic. Use warm water to dilute the iodophor scrub. *Rationale:* Removes secretions and feces from perineal area.

Action: After hand washing, apply sterile gloves for the prep procedure. Take a fresh sponge to begin each new area, and do not return to a clean area with a used sponge. Six sponges are needed. The proper order and motions are as follows:

1. Use a zig-zag motion from clitoris to lower abdomen just above the pubic hairline.

2, 3. Use a zig-zag motion on the inner thigh from the labia majora to about halfway between the hip and knee. Repeat for the other inner thigh.

4, 5. Apply a single stroke on one side from clitoris over labia, perineum, and anus. Repeat for the other side.

6. Use a single stroke in the middle from the clitoris over the vulva and perineum.

Rationale: Prevents cross-contamination or recontamination of an area that is already clean.

Action: The attendant may apply sterile drapes if desired. *Rationale:* A vaginal birth is a clean procedure rather than a sterile one because the vagina is not sterile. Sterile drapes are unnecessary, but some attendants may prefer to use them.

Birth of the Head

Action: If an episiotomy is needed, the attendant will perform it when the head is well crowned (see Chapter 20). *Rationale:* Minimizes blood loss from the episiotomy.

Action: As the vaginal orifice encircles the fetal head, the attendant applies gentle pressure to the woman's perineum with one hand while applying counterpressure to the fetal head with the other hand (Ritgen's maneuver). The attendant may ask the mother to blow so that she avoids pushing, or to push gently. *Rationale:* Controls the exit of the fetal head so that it is born gradually rather than popping out; this minimizes trauma to the maternal tissues.

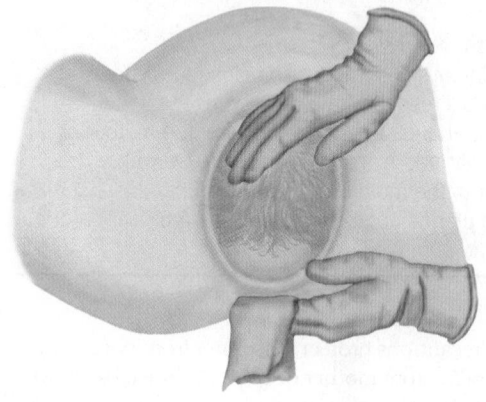

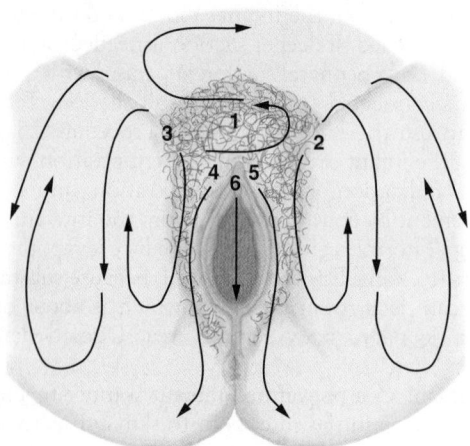

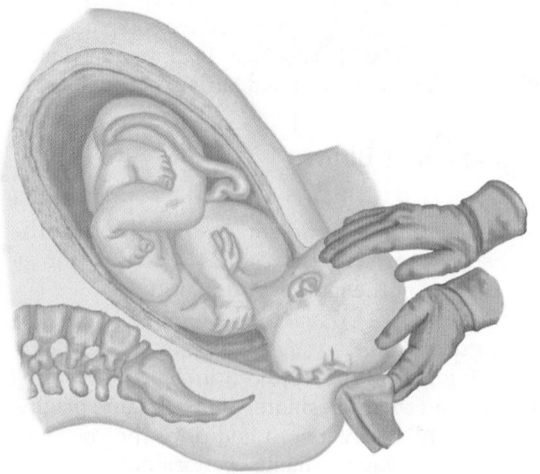

Figure 17-17 Sequence of delivery.

Action: The attendant wipes secretions from the infant's face and suctions the nose and mouth with a bulb syringe. *Rationale:* Removes blood and secretions, preventing the infant from aspirating them with the first breaths.

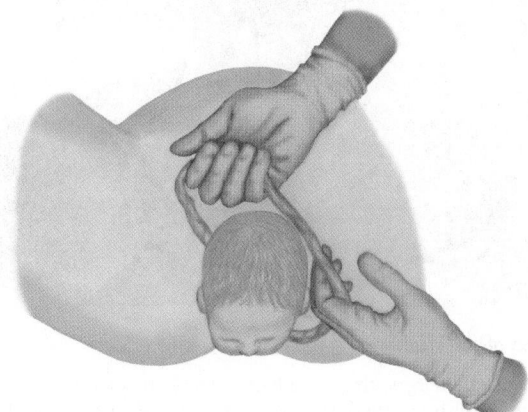

Action: The attendant feels for a cord around the fetal neck (nuchal cord). If it is loose, it is slipped over the head. If tight, it is clamped and cut between two clamps before the rest of the baby is born. *Rationale:* Allows the rest of the birth to occur and prevents stretching or tearing the cord.

Birth of the Shoulders

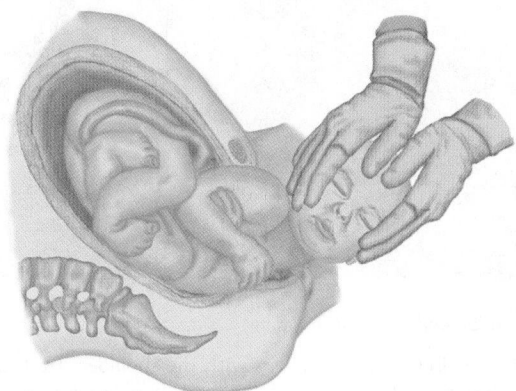

Action: After external rotation, the attendant applies gentle traction on the fetal head in the direction of the mother's perineum. *Rationale:* External rotation allows the shoulders to rotate internally and aligns their transverse diameter with the anteroposterior diameter of the mother's pelvic outlet. Traction on the head in the direction of her perineum allows the anterior fetal shoulder to slip under the symphysis pubis.
—

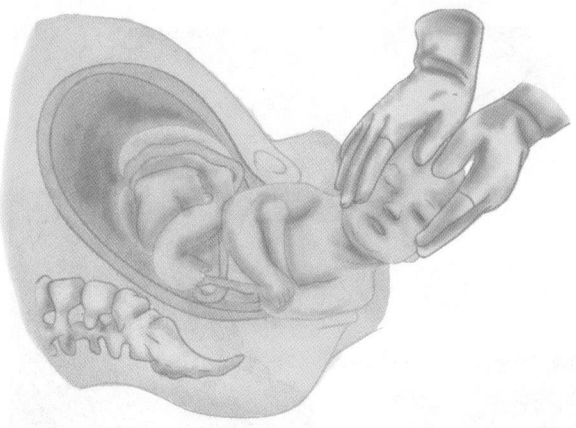

Action: The attendant then lifts the head toward the mother's symphysis pubis. *Rationale:* Permits the posterior fetal shoulder to be eased over the perineum, minimizing trauma to the maternal tissues.

Clearing the Infant's Airway and Cutting the Cord

Action: The rest of the infant's body is born quickly after the shoulders are born. The attendant maintains the infant in a slightly head-dependent position while suctioning excess secretions with a bulb syringe. The infant is often placed on the mother's abdomen. *Rationale:* Gravity aids spontaneous drainage of secretions and prevents aspiration of oral mucus and secretions.

Action: The attendant clamps the cord. Either the father or the attendant cuts the cord above the clamp. *Rationale:* Allows parents to interact more freely with their infant. Prevents flow of blood between placenta and infant, which might result in anemia (if infant is higher than placenta) or polycythemia (if infant is below the placenta).

Delivery of the Placenta

Action: After the placenta separates, it can usually be delivered if the mother bears down. The attendant may pull gently on the cord. *Rationale:* Excess traction on the cord may cause it to break, making the placenta harder to deliver.

Action: The attendant inspects both sides of the placenta. *Rationale:* Ensures that no fragments remain inside the uterus that might cause hemorrhage and infection.

After the infant and placenta are born, the attendant inspects the birth canal for injuries. If needed, any injuries and the episiotomy (if one was done) are repaired.

Figure 17-17, cont'd Sequence of delivery.

further reduces heat loss if placed on the baby's *dry* head. A cap is not worn in the radiant warmer because the cap slows transfer of heat to the baby.

Identifying the Infant. Bands with matching imprinted numbers and identifying information are the primary means to ensure that the baby goes to the right mother after any separation (Fig. 17-19, p. 386). Apply two bands on the infant, one on an arm and another on an ankle or one on each ankle to prevent facial scratching. Infant bands are applied more snugly than they would be if worn by an adult: leave about one slender adult fingerwidth of slack in the bands. Apply the larger band to the mother's wrist, similar to adult identification for any patient. A fourth band is provided to the father or other primary support person. Check that imprinted numbers and names are identical on each set of bands. A set is needed for each baby in a multiple birth.

A photograph of the infant's face may be taken at birth for added identification. Digital cameras have the advantage of electronic data storage.

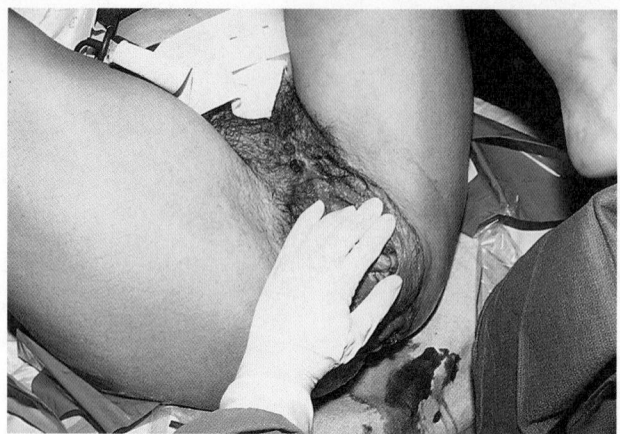

A. Crowning

The fetal head distends the labial and perineal tissues. The anus is stretched wide, and it is not unusual to see the woman's anterior rectal wall at this time. Any feces expelled are wiped posteriorly to avoid contaminating the vulva. The attendant (physician or nurse-midwife) is not holding the fetal head back but rather controlling its exit by using gentle pressure on the fetal occiput.

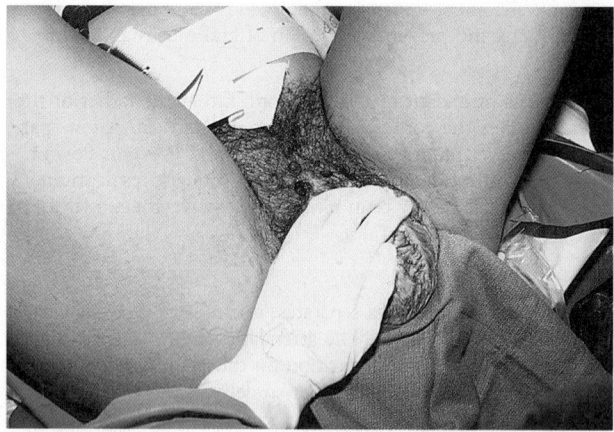

B. Ritgen Maneuver

Pressure is applied to the fetal chin through the perineum at the same time pressure is applied to the occiput of the fetal head. This action aids the mechanism of extension as the fetal head comes under the symphysis.

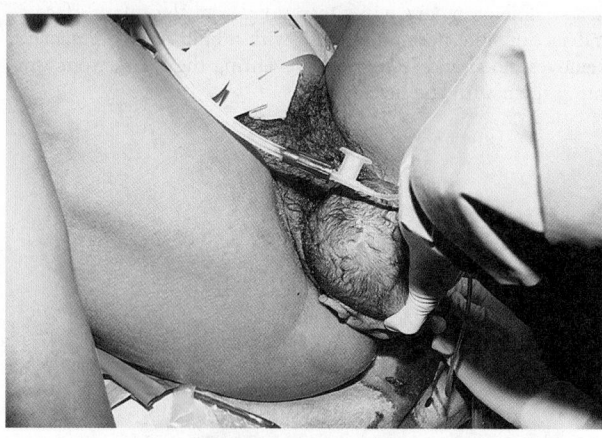

C. Birth of the Head

As the head emerges, the attendant prepares to suction the nose and mouth to avoid aspiration of secretions when the infant takes the first breath.

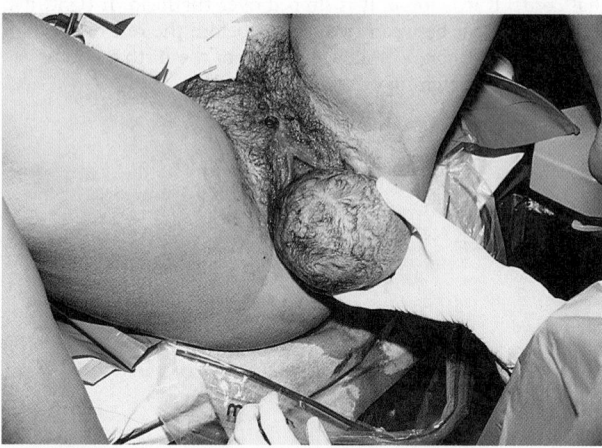

D. Restitution and External Rotation

After the head emerges, it realigns with the shoulders (restitution). External rotation occurs as the fetal shoulders internally rotate, aligning their transverse diameter with the anteroposterior diameter of the pelvic outlet.

Figure 17-18 Vaginal birth.

Care of the Mother

Nursing care of the mother during the fourth stage of labor focuses on observing for hemorrhage and relieving discomfort. Table 17-4 summarizes possible problems during the fourth stage of labor.

Observing for Hemorrhage. Important assessments related to hemorrhage are the woman's vital signs, uterine fundus, bladder, and lochia. For detailed information about these assessments, see Chapter 21.

Vital Signs. Assess the woman's temperature when recovery care begins and before transfer to a postpartum room. Added temperature checks will be needed for the woman who requires an extended recovery period. Assess her blood pressure, pulse, and respirations every 15 minutes during the first hour and every 30 minutes to 1 hour after the first hour,

or as indicated by her condition. A rising pulse is an early sign of excessive blood loss, because the heart contracts faster to compensate for reduced blood volume. The blood pressure may fall much later as the blood volume is severely reduced. A rising pulse rate also accompanies an elevated temperature.

If an indwelling catheter is in place, observe the urine output for adequacy. A low urine output (≤25-30 ml/hr) identifies water conservation by the kidneys in response to falling blood volume from any of several causes (e.g., dehydration, excess bleeding).

Fundus. The most common reason for excessive postpartum bleeding is that the uterus does not firmly contract and compress open vessels at the placental site. Assess the firmness, height, and positioning of the uterine fundus with each vital sign assessment. The fundus should be firm, in the midline, and

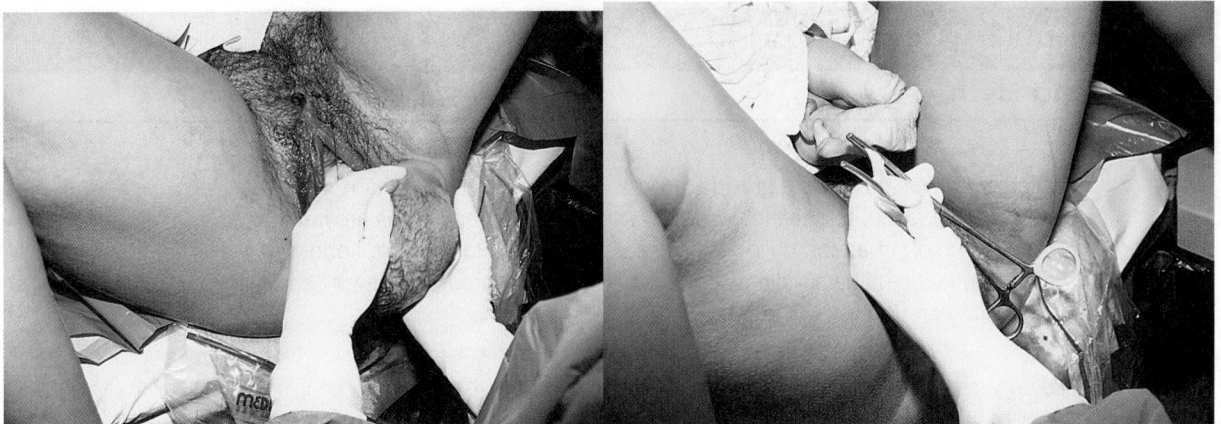

E. Birth of the Anterior Shoulder

The attendant gently pushes the fetal head toward the woman's perineum to allow the anterior shoulder to slip under her symphysis. The bluish skin color of the fetus is normal at this point; it becomes pink as the infant begins air breathing.

H. Cord Clamping

While the infant is in skin-to-skin contact on the mother's abdomen, the attendant doubly clamps the umbilical cord. The cord is then cut between the two clamps. Samples of cord blood are collected after it is cut.

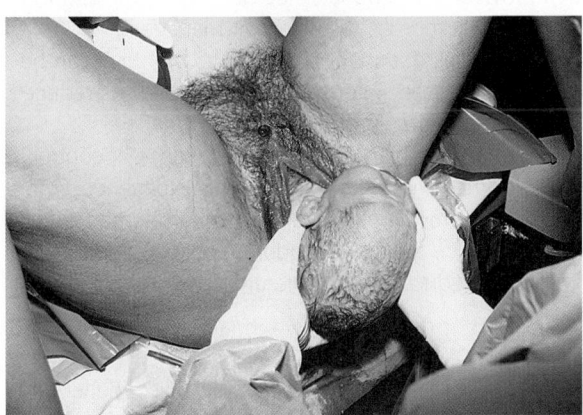

F. Birth of the Posterior Shoulder

The attendant now pushes the fetal head upward toward the woman's symphysis to allow the posterior shoulder to slip over her perineum.

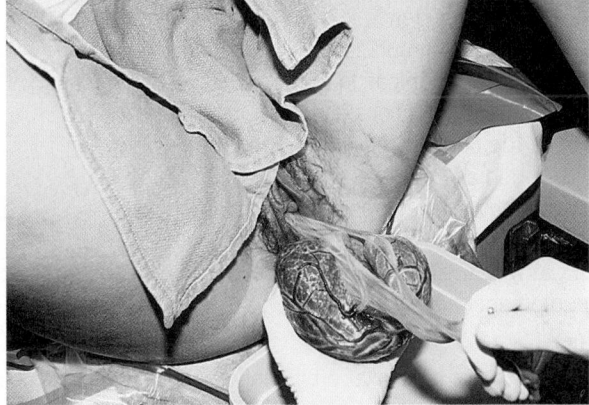

I. Birth of the Placenta

The attendant applies gentle traction on the cord to aid expulsion of the placenta. This placenta is expelled in the more common Schultze mechanism, with the shiny fetal surface and membranes emerging. Note the fetal membranes that surrounded the fetus and amniotic fluid during pregnancy. The chorionic vessels that branch from the umbilical cord are readily visible on the fetal surface of the placenta.

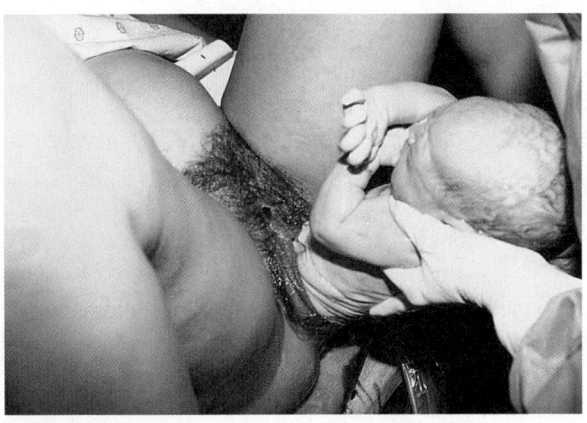

G. Completion of the Birth

The attendant supports the fetus during expulsion. Note that the fetus has excellent muscle tone, as evidenced by facial grimacing and flexion of the arms and hands.

Figure 17-18, cont'd Vaginal birth.

Nursing Care Plan

Normal Labor and Birth

ASSESSMENT

Cathy Taggart, 17 years old, is a gravida 1, para 0, who is admitted in early labor. Her cervix is 3 cm dilated and completely effaced, and the fetus is at a 0 station. Her membranes are intact. Cathy's husband, Tim, is with her. They did not attend childbirth classes. Cathy is holding Tim's hand tightly and breathing rapidly with each contraction. She says in a shaky voice, "I'm so scared. I've never been in a hospital before. I just don't know if I can do this."

Nursing Diagnosis

Anxiety related to unfamiliar environment and lack of birth preparation.

Goals/Expected Outcomes

Cathy will:
- Express being less anxious after admission procedures are completed.
- Have a relaxed facial expression and body posture between contractions.

INTERVENTION	RATIONALE
1. Maintain a calm and confident manner when caring for Cathy. Express confidence in her ability to give birth.	1. Calm provides reassurance that labor is normal and that she has the resources within her to manage it.
2. Use therapeutic communication when talking with Cathy. Adapt communication to the situation; simplifying explanations and directions as labor intensifies.	2. Clarity identifies dominant concerns so that they can be properly addressed. Intense physical sensations reduce the ability to comprehend complex information.
3. Determine the couple's plans for birth, and work within them as much as possible.	3. Determining their plan enhances their sense of control and helps them have a satisfying birth experience.
4. Stay with Cathy as much as possible during labor.	4. A nurse can provide reassurance through human contact and reduce fears of abandonment.
5. Orient Cathy to the labor room, and explain procedures and equipment she will encounter.	5. Information reduces fear of the unknown.

Evaluation

Cathy relaxes a bit after talking with the nurse and slows her breathing. Cathy says, "I feel a little better now. I hope I can have my baby before you go home."

ASSESSMENT

Cathy's admission vital signs are all normal: temperature, 37.1°C (98.8° F); pulse, 88; respirations, 20; and blood pressure, 112/70 mm Hg. The fetal heart rate averages 140 to 150 beats per minute (bpm). Her contractions occur every 4 minutes, last 50 seconds, and are of moderate intensity.

Potential Complication

Fetal compromise.

Goals/Expected Outcomes

Goals are not formulated for a potential complication because the nurse cannot independently manage fetal compromise. The nurse will:
- Take actions to promote normal placental function.
- Observe for and report signs associated with fetal compromise.

INTERVENTION	RATIONALE
1. Encourage Cathy to use any position she desires except the supine. If she lies flat, a wedge should be placed under one hip to displace her uterus to one side.	1. The supine position can cause aortocaval compression, reducing blood flow to the placenta.
2. Assess and document the fetal heart rate using the guidelines in Table 18-1. Report rates or patterns that are not reassuring. Assess the fetal heart rate more frequently if deviations from normal are identified. (Refer to Chapter 18 for detailed information.)	2. Observation allows prompt identification of changes in the rate or of abnormal rates. Fetal heart rate assessments that are outside expected limits need corrective action and should be reported for possible medical intervention.

Nursing Care Plan

Normal Labor and Birth—*cont'd*

INTERVENTION	RATIONALE
3. When the membranes rupture, observe the color, odor, and approximate amount of fluid, and note the time of rupture. Note the fetal heart rate after rupture.	3. Meconium-stained fluid may be associated with fetal compromise and should be reported. Cloudy, yellow, or foul-smelling fluid suggests infection. Prolonged rupture of membranes increases the risk of infection. A low fetal heart rate suggests significant cord compression.
4. Assess contractions when the fetal heart rate is assessed. Report incomplete uterine relaxation between contractions or excessively strong or long contractions (longer than 90-120 sec or having <30 sec of full relaxation). Keep in mind that the fetus with risk factors may not tolerate even less-than-normal labor contractions.	4. Most placental exchange occurs during the interval between contractions. Contractions that are too long or have an inadequate interval between them decrease the time available for the intervillous spaces of the placenta to eliminate wastes and refill with oxygenated blood and nutrients.
5. Assess Cathy's blood pressure, pulse, and respirations every hour. Assess her temperature every 4 hr until her membranes rupture, then every 2 hr. If elevated, assess temperature every 2 hr or more frequently.	5. Maternal hypotension or hypertension can decrease blood flow to the placenta. Maternal fever increases the fetal temperature and metabolic rate, possibly raising fetal demand for oxygen beyond the mother's ability to supply it. A rising maternal pulse or fetal heart rate may precede the temperature elevation.
6. See the nursing care plan in Chapter 18, p. 408, for additional interventions if signs of fetal compromise occur.	6. This nursing care plan addresses basic actions to promote fetal oxygenation and identify possible problems.

Evaluation

Because no client goal is established for a potential complication, goal evaluation is not done. The fetal heart rate remains approximately the same, and there are no signs of fetal compromise. Cathy finds that sitting in a rocking chair is most comfortable.

ASSESSMENT

In 1½ hours, Cathy's cervical dilation progresses to 5 cm and the fetus descends to a +1 station. Her contractions occur every 3 minutes, last 60 seconds, and are of strong intensity. The fetal heart rate remains near its admission level. Cathy is having difficulty relaxing between contractions and is complaining of back pain. She is relieved that her labor is progressing normally.

Nursing Diagnosis

Pain related to effects of uterine contractions.

Goal/Expected Outcome

Cathy will express assurance that she can manage labor pain satisfactorily.

INTERVENTION	RATIONALE
1. Encourage Cathy to try positions such as standing/sitting and leaning forward, side-lying, leaning over the back of the bed, or on her hands and knees. Remind her to change positions about every half hour or when she feels the need for a change.	1. These positions shift the weight of the fetus away from the sacral promontory, reducing back pain. Alternating positions relieves strain and constant pressure and also helps the fetus adapt to the pelvis.
2. Teach Tim to rub or apply firm pressure to Cathy's back. Ask her where the best place is and how hard to press. Apply powder to the area rubbed.	2. Back rubs or firm pressure counteract some of the back pain. Powder decreases friction and promotes skin comfort.

3. Offer thermal pain management options:
  a. A warm blanket or warm pack applied to her back.
  b. Cold packs applied to her back.
  c. Alternating warm and cold packs, or use of them for 20 minutes on and 20 minutes off.
  d. Warm water in a shower or whirlpool.
	3. Thermal stimulation interferes with transmission of pain impulses. Changing the thermal stimulation prevents habituation. Nipple stimulation in a shower or whirlpool causes release of oxytocin from the posterior pituitary and enhances contractions.

Continued

Nursing Care Plan

Normal Labor and Birth—cont'd

INTERVENTION	RATIONALE
4. Teach Cathy simple breathing and relaxation techniques (see Chapter 19).	4. Breathing techniques provide distraction from pain and give her a sense of control. Relaxation enhances a woman's ability to manage pain and enhances normal labor processes.
5. Observe Cathy's suprapubic area and palpate for a full bladder at least every 2 hours. Remind her to void if she has not done so recently.	5. A full bladder contributes to discomfort and can prolong labor by obstructing fetal descent.
6. Tell Cathy about her progress in labor. Explain that she will probably begin to dilate faster now that she has entered active labor.	6. Encouragement and the knowledge that her efforts are having the desired results increase a woman's willingness to continue.
7. Tell Cathy what pharmacologic pain relief measures are available to her.	7. Knowing available options gives the woman a sense of control because she can choose whether she wants these measures. (This action may be done during early labor to give a woman more time to consider her options.)

Evaluation

Cathy continues to have back pain that is 6 on a 0-to-10 scale but says that she is more comfortable sitting on the side of the bed with her head on a pillow on the overbed table. Tim rubs her back during contractions. She says she is able to manage the pain and does not want medication yet.

ASSESSMENT

After another 2 hours, Cathy is quite uncomfortable and requests pain medication. She is occasionally feeling an urge to push. Cathy cries and says she is "losing it" and "can't take it anymore." Tim asks anxiously, "What's wrong? Is Cathy OK? Why is she acting this way?" The fetal heart rate remains near the admission range and shows no signs suggesting fetal compromise. Contractions occur every 2 minutes, last 70 seconds, and are strong.

Cathy's cervix is now 8 cm dilated and the station is +1. She asks for pain relief but does not want an epidural. Butorphanol (Stadol), 1 mg slow IV push, helps her regain control and work with her contractions. She avoids pushing by blowing out at the peak of each contraction.

Cathy is fully dilated in 45 minutes, and the fetal station is +2. She pushes spontaneously several times with each contraction but tends to stiffen her back and push on the bed with her arms with each push. She pushes for about 10 to 15 seconds at a time, holding her breath each time. She prefers a semi-sitting position.

Nursing Diagnosis

Deficient Knowledge: effective pushing techniques.

Goal/Expected Outcome

After instruction in more effective pushing techniques, Cathy will use the techniques until the birth occurs.

INTERVENTION	RATIONALE
1. Observe Cathy's perineum for fetal crowning with each push.	1. A woman having her first baby can still give birth rapidly. Observation permits the nurse to maintain her safety and that of the baby should rapid birth occur.
2. Encourage Cathy to exhale as she pushes strongly for about 4-6 sec at a time.	2. Prolonged pushing against a closed glottis reduces blood return to the heart and maternal oxygen saturation and decreases placental blood flow, especially if it is done with every contraction.
3. Teach Cathy techniques to make each push more effective: a. Instruct her to flex her head with each push.	3. a. Flexing her head directs each push downward into the pelvic cavity.
b. Instruct her to pull against her flexed knees (or handholds on the bed) as she pushes, curving her body around her uterus. Encourage upright positions, including squatting.	b. Pulling provides leverage to gain a more effective push from the abdominal muscles. Upright positions take advantage of gravity, and squatting enlarges the pelvic outlet slightly.

Nursing Care Plan

Normal Labor and Birth—cont'd

INTERVENTION	RATIONALE
c. Have her push toward the vaginal outlet.	c. The vagina is the anatomically correct direction.
d. Help her relax her perineum as she pushes down.	d. Relaxation reduces soft tissue resistance to fetal descent.
e. Keep her sacrum flattened against the bed when she pushes in a semi-sitting position.	e. A flat sacrum straightens the pelvic curve somewhat (and is similar to squatting).
4. Do not talk to Cathy unnecessarily between contractions.	4. Silence allows her to conserve her energy for pushing efforts.

Evaluation

Cathy pushes more effectively with the nurse coaching her during each contraction. In another hour she gives birth to a 7-lb, 6-oz (3346-g) boy. The baby's Apgar scores are 9 at both 1 and 5 minutes. Cathy has a small first-degree laceration that is sutured with a local anesthetic. The new family gets acquainted during the recovery period.

TABLE **17-3** Apgar Score*

Assessment	Points		
	0	**1**	**2**
Heart rate	Absent	Below 100/min	100/min or higher
Respiratory effort	No spontaneous respirations	Slow respirations or weak cry	Spontaneous respirations with a strong, lusty cry
Muscle tone	Limp	Minimal flexion of extremities; sluggish movement	Flexed body posture; spontaneous and vigorous movement
Reflex response	No response to suction or gentle slap on soles	Minimal response (grimace) to suction or gentle slap on soles	Responds promptly to suction or a gentle slap to the sole with cry or active movement
Color	Pallor or cyanosis	Bluish hands and feet only	Pink (light-skinned) or absence of cyanosis (dark-skinned); pink mucus membranes

* The Apgar score is a method for rapid evaluation of the infant's cardiorespiratory adaptation after birth. The nurse scores the infant at 1 minute and 5 minutes in each of five areas. The assessments are arranged from most important (heart rate) to least important (color). The infant is assigned a score of 0 to 2 in each of the five areas and the scores are totaled. Resuscitation should not be delayed until the 1-minute score is obtained. However, general guidelines for the infant's care are based on three ranges of 1-minute scores:

0	1	2	3	4	5	6	7	8	9	10

Infant needs resuscitation.	Gently stimulate by rubbing the infant's back while administering oxygen. Determine whether mother received narcotics, which may have depressed infant's respirations. Have naloxone (Narcan) available for administration.	Provide no action other than support of the infant's spontaneous efforts and continued observation.

---

at or below the umbilicus; it is about the size of a large grapefruit. If the fundus is firm, no massage is needed; if it is soft (boggy), massage it until it is firm. Nipple stimulation from the infant's suckling releases natural oxytocin from the mother's posterior pituitary to maintain firm uterine contraction. Oxytocin in the intravenous solution or given intramuscularly has the same effect.

Bladder. A full bladder interferes with contraction of the uterus and may lead to hemorrhage. Suspect a full bladder if the fundus is above the umbilicus or is displaced to one side, usually the right. If there is no contraindication, such as altered sensation, the mother can walk to the bathroom (with assistance the first few times). Often, the first two voidings are measured until it is evident that the woman voids with-

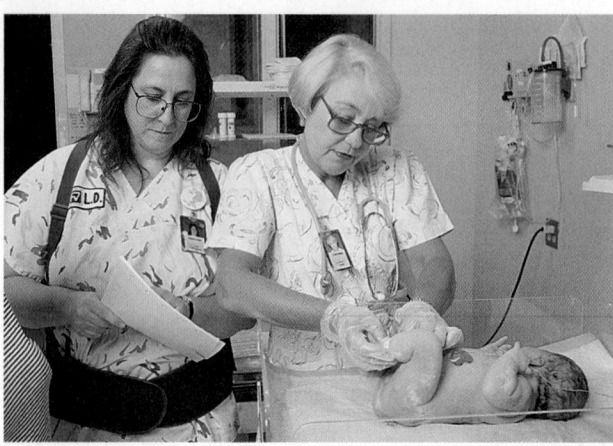

Figure 17-19 When the birthing room nurse turns care of the newborn over to the nursery nurse, both check the identification bands and record for the same information.

out difficulty and empties her bladder completely. Each voiding is usually at least 300 to 400 ml if she is emptying her bladder.

Lochia. Assess lochia with each vital sign and fundal assessment. The amount of lochia seems large to the inexperienced nurse and the new mother. Perineal pads vary in their absorbency, but *saturation* of one pad within the first hour is a guideline for the maximum normal lochia flow. Observe for lochia that pools under the mother's buttocks and back. Small clots are often present, but the presence of large clots is not normal, and the physician or nurse-midwife should be notified. A continuous trickle of bright red blood when the fundus is firm suggests a laceration in the birth canal. A hematoma causes bleeding into the tissues, but excess visible bleeding is unusual.

Relieving Discomfort. Uterine contractions (afterpains) and perineal trauma are common causes of pain after birth. A postpartum chill is often annoying. Pain is usually mild and readily relieved by simple measures. Pain that is intense or does not respond to common relief measures requires investigation, and the birth attendant should be notified.

Ice Packs. To reduce edema and limit hematoma formation, apply an ice pack to the perineum promptly after vaginal birth. Small hematomas are common, but a rapidly enlarging hematoma causes significant concealed blood loss and pain. Some perineal pads containing chemical cold packs vary in the amount of lochia they can absorb, which should be considered when estimating pad saturation. Many facilities use a glove filled with ice and wrapped in a washcloth because it is economical and often colder than the pads with cold packs.

Analgesics. Afterpains and perineal pain respond well to mild oral analgesics such as ibuprofen. Regular urination re-

---

TABLE 17-4 Maternal Problems During the Fourth Stage of Labor

Sign	Potential Problem	Immediate Nursing Action
Rising maternal pulse rate and/or falling blood pressure; possibly accompanied by low or no urine output	An early sign of hypovolemia caused by excessive blood loss (visible or concealed).	Identify the probable cause of the blood loss, usually a poorly contracted uterus. Take steps to correct it (see below). Indwelling catheter may be inserted to observe urine output.
Soft (boggy) uterus	A poorly contracted uterus does not adequately compress large open vessels at the placental site, resulting in hemorrhage.	With one hand securing the uterus just above the symphysis and the other on the fundus, massage the uterus until firm. Push downward on the firm uterus to expel any clots. Empty the woman's bladder (by voiding or catheterization) if that is contributing to the uterine atony.
High uterine fundus, often displaced to one side	Suggests a full bladder, which can interfere with uterine contraction and result in hemorrhage.	Massage the uterus if it is not firm. Help the woman urinate in the bathroom or on the bedpan. If she cannot void, catheterize her (usually a routine postpartum order).
Lochia exceeding 1 saturated perineal pad per hour during the fourth stage	Suggests hemorrhage; however, perineal pads vary in their absorbency, and this must be considered.	Identify cause of hemorrhage, usually uterine atony, which is manifested by a soft uterus. Correct the cause. If lacerations are the suspected cause (excess bleeding with a firm fundus), notify the birth attendant. Keep the woman NPO until the birth attendant evaluates her.
Intense perineal or vaginal pain, poorly relieved with analgesics	Hematoma, usually of vaginal wall or perineum; signs of hypovolemia may occur with substantial blood loss into tissues.	If the hematoma is visible, apply cold packs to the area to slow bleeding into tissues. Notify the birth attendant, and anticipate possible surgical drainage. Keep the woman NPO.

duces the severity of afterpains because the uterus contracts most effectively.

Warmth. A warm blanket is soothing and shortens the chill that is common after birth. A portable radiant warmer provides warmth to both the mother and infant. The mother may enjoy warm drinks or prefer cool ones.

Promoting Early Family Attachment

The first hour after birth is an ideal time for parent-infant attachment because the healthy neonate is alert and responsive. Provide privacy while unobtrusively observing the parents and infant. The infant can remain in the parent's arms while vital signs, minor suctioning of secretions, and many initial assessments are completed.

Assist the mother to breastfeed during the recovery period, if she desires. The infant is usually attentive and nurses briefly. Early nipple stimulation helps initiate milk production.

When the parents are ready, allow siblings, other family members, and friends to visit. Help siblings to see and touch their new brother or sister by putting a stool at the bedside or letting them sit on the bed.

Observe for signs of early parent-infant attachment. Parent behaviors are tentative at first, progressing from fingertip touch to palm touch to enfolding of the infant. Expect parents to make eye contact with the infant and talk to a baby in higher-pitched, affectionate tones.

Cultural variations should be considered when assessing early attachment. The nurse should be knowledgeable about the typical practices of the populations commonly served. In some cultures, great attention to the newborn is considered unlucky (sometimes because of an "evil eye").

KEY CONCEPTS

- Labor contractions are intermittent, allowing placental blood flow and exchange of oxygen, nutrients, and waste products between maternal and fetal circulations during the interval.
- The upper uterus contracts actively during labor, maintaining tension to pull the more passive lower uterus and cervix over the fetal presenting part. These actions bring about cervical effacement and dilation.
- Fetal lung fluid production decreases and its absorption into lung tissue increases during late pregnancy and labor. Thoracic compression during labor aids in expulsion of additional fluid.
- Four interrelated components affecting the process of birth are the powers, the passage, the passenger, and the psyche. Presentation and position further describe the relation of the fetus (passenger) to the maternal pelvis.
- The mechanisms of labor favor the most efficient passage of the fetus through the mother's pelvis.
- As labor approaches, the woman may notice one or more premonitory signs that precede its onset: an increase in the frequency and intensity of Braxton Hicks contractions, lightening, increased vaginal secretions, bloody show, a spurt of energy, and weight loss.

- The conclusive difference between true labor and false labor is progressive effacement and dilation of the cervix.
- Some women do not have symptoms typical of true labor. They should enter the birth center for evaluation if they are uncertain or have concerns other than those listed in the guidelines.
- The four stages and phases of labor are characterized by different physiologic events and maternal behaviors. In the first stage, these are cervical dilation and effacement; in the second stage, expulsion of the fetus; in the third stage, expulsion of the placenta; in the fourth stage, maternal physiologic stabilization and parent-infant bonding.
- Normal labor is characterized by consistent progression of uterine contractions, cervical dilation and effacement, and fetal descent.
- The initial intrapartum assessments are assessments of maternal and fetal health and labor status.
- Because of complete dependence on the mother's physiologic systems, the fetus is the more vulnerable of the maternal-fetal pair.
- The normal fetal heart rate at term averages 110 to 160 bpm. Other reassuring findings include the presence of variability in the electronically monitored term fetus, accelerations that peak at least 15 bpm above existing

baseline with a total duration for the acceleration of at least 15 seconds, and absence of decelerations following contractions.
- Persistent contractions lasting longer than 90 to 120 seconds or having rest intervals of less than 30 seconds may reduce placental blood flow and fetal oxygen, nutrient, and waste exchange. The fetus with low reserves may be unable to cope with normal contractions.
- A maternal supine position can reduce placental blood flow because the uterus compresses the aorta and inferior vena cava.
- General comfort measures promote the woman's ability to relax and cope with labor.
- Regular changes in position during labor promote maternal comfort and help the fetus adapt to the pelvis.
- The nurse must be alert for signs of impending birth. The woman may urgently state, "The baby's coming," or she may make grunting sounds or bear down.
- The priority nursing care of the newborn immediately after birth is to promote normal respirations, maintain normal body temperature, and promote attachment.
- The priority nursing care of the mother after birth is to assess for hemorrhage, promote firm uterine contraction, and promote parent-infant attachment.

ANSWERS to Critical Thinking Exercise 17-1

1. First, you need to speak directly to the woman who is having the contractions. You need some additional information as well: Which baby is this for her? What is her due date? Have her membranes ruptured? What are the characteristics of her contractions (frequency, duration, intensity, effect of activity)?

2. Heather's symptoms sound like those typical of false labor: irregular contractions that are mild, fairly short, and more annoying than painful. Although not harmful, these frequent contractions in late pregnancy interrupt the woman's rest. You should tell Heather that these contractions do not sound like true labor; then you should review with her the typical signs and symptoms of true labor. Advise her to come to the hospital if she believes she is in labor, if the contractions intensify and become more consistent, if her "water breaks," if the baby seems to move much less, or if she has bleeding. And because it is impossible to diagnose labor over the phone, tell her to come to the hospital for assessment if she has any continuing concern.

ANSWERS to Critical Thinking Exercise 17-2

1. The woman's behavior may have changed for any of several reasons, so the nurse must not make assumptions. For example, she may have been offended that the nurse asked her questions about illicit drug use, not realizing that this is part of routine assessment questions. Or she may use other drugs (licit or illicit) but prefers not to admit it. She may, however, simply have been surprised by the question about drug use. Women often want their family to remain during the admission assessment but may not admit substance or domestic abuse in their presence. Nonverbal cues, such as a too-quick denial, avoidance of eye contact, or vague responses, are clues that the woman may not be answering these questions truthfully.

2. The nurse should follow up on maternal behaviors privately to clarify the facts that underlie them.

REFERENCES and READINGS

American Academy of Pediatrics (AAP), & American College of Obstetricians and Gynecologists (ACOG). (2002). *Guidelines for perinatal care* (5th ed.). Elk Grove Village, IL, and Washington, DC: Authors.

Association of Women's Health, Obstetric, & Neonatal Nurses (AWHONN). (2003). *Standards for professional nursing practice in the care of women and newborns* (6th ed.). Washington, DC: Author.

Blackburn, S.T. (2003). *Maternal, fetal, and neonatal physiology: A clinical perspective* (2nd ed.). Philadelphia: Saunders.

Bowers, B.B. (2002). Mother's experiences of labor support: Exploration of qualitative research. *Journal of Obstetric, Gynecologic, and Neonatal Nursing, 31*(6), 742-752.

Challis, J.R.G., & Lye, S.J. (2004). Characteristics of parturition. In R. Creasy, R. Resnik, & J.D. Iams (Eds.), *Maternal-fetal medicine: Principles and practice* (5th ed., pp. 79-87). Philadelphia: Saunders.

Chalmers, B., Mangiaterra, V., & Porter, R. (2001). WHO principles of perinatal care: The essential antenatal, perinatal, and postpartum care course. *Birth, 28*(3), 202-207.

Chen, C.H., Wang, S.Y., & Chang, M.Y. (2001). Women's perceptions of helpful and unhelpful nursing behaviors during labor: A study in Taiwan. *Birth, 28*(3), 180-185.

Copeland, D.B., & Douglas, D. (1999). Communication strategies for the intrapartum nurse. *Journal of Obstetric, Gynecologic, and Neonatal Nursing, 28*(6), 579-586.

Creehan, P.A. (2001). Pain relief and comfort measures during labor. In K.R. Rice & P.A. Creehan (Eds.), *Perinatal nursing* (2nd ed., pp. 417-444). Philadelphia: Lippincott.

Cunningham, F.G., Gant, N.F., Leveno, K.J., Gilstrap, L.C., Hauth, J.C., & Wenstrom, K.D. (2001). *Williams obstetrics* (21st ed.). New York: McGraw-Hill.

Cypher, R.L., Adelsperger, D., & Torgersen, K.L. (2003). Interpretation of fetal heart rate patterns. In N. Feinstein, K.L. Torgersen, & J. Atterbury (Eds.), *AWHONN's fetal heart monitoring principles and practices* (3rd ed., pp. 113-158). Philadelphia: Lippincott Williams & Wilkins.

Enkin, M.W., Marc, J.N.C., Neilson, J.P., Crowther, C., Duley, L., Hodnett, E., & Hofmeyr, G.J. (2000). Effective care in pregnancy and childbirth: A synopsis. *Birth, 28*(1), 41-51.

Feinstein, N.F., Sprague, A., & Trépanier, M.J. (2000). *Fetal heart rate auscultation*. Washington, DC: Association of Women's Health, Obstetric and Neonatal Nurses.

Gale, J., Fothergill-Bourbonnais, F., & Chamberlain, M. (2001). Measuring nursing support during childbirth. *MCN: The American Journal of Maternal/Child Nursing, 26*(5), 264-271.

Gilliland, A.L. (2002). Beyond holding hands: The modern role of the professional doula. *Journal of Obstetric, Gynecologic, and Neonatal Nursing, 31*(6), 762-769.

Greenhaigh, R., Slade, P., & Spiby, H. (2000). Fathers' coping style, antenatal preparation, and experiences of labor and the postpartum. *Birth, 27*(3), 177-184.

Guyton, A.C., & Hall, J.C. (2000). *Textbook of medical physiology* (10th ed.). Philadelphia: Saunders.

Haddad, G.G., & Pérez Fontán, J.J. (2004). Development of the respiratory system. In R.E. Behrman, R.M. Kliegman, & H.B. Jenson (Eds.), *Nelson textbook of pediatrics* (17th ed., pp. 1357-1359). Philadelphia: Saunders.

Hunter, L.P. (2002). Being with woman: A guiding concept for the care of laboring women. *Journal of Obstetric, Gynecologic, and Neonatal Nursing, 31*(6), 650-657.

Kendrick, J.M., & Simpson, K.R. (2001). Labor and birth. In K.R. Simpson & P.A. Creehan (Eds.), *AWHONN's perinatal nursing* (2nd ed., pp. 298-365). Philadelphia: Lippincott Williams & Wilkins.

King, T.L., & Simpson, K.R. (1999). Fetal assessment during labor. In K.R. Rice & P.A. Creehan (Eds.), *Perinatal nursing* (pp. 378-416). Philadelphia: Lippincott.

Manogin, T.W. (2000). Caring behaviors for nurses: Women's perceptions during childbirth. *Journal of Obstetric, Gynecologic, and Neonatal Nursing, 29*(1), 153-157.

Mayberry, L.J., Gennaro, S., Strange, L., & Williams, M. (1999a). Maternal fatigue: Implications of second stage labor nursing care. *Journal of Obstetric, Gynecologic, and Neonatal Nursing, 28*(2175-2181), 721-732.

Mayberry, L.J., Hammer, R., Kelly, C., True-Driver, B., & De, A. (1999b). Use of delayed pushing with epidural anesthesia: Findings from a randomized, controlled trial. *Journal of Perinatology, 19*(1), 26-30.

Mayberry, L.J., Wood, S.H., Strange, L.B., Lee, L., Heisler, D.R., & Nielsen-Smith, K. (2000a). Managing second-stage labor: Exploring the variables during the second stage. *AWHONN Lifelines, 3*(6), 28-34.

Mayberry, L.J., Wood, S.H., Strange, L.B., Lee, L., Heisler, D.R., & Nielsen-Smith, K. (2000b). *Second stage labor management: Promotion of evidence-based practice and a collaborative approach to patient care*. Washington, DC: Association of Women's Health, Obstetric and Neonatal Nurses.

Miltner, R.S. (2002). More than support: Nursing interventions provided to women in labor. *Journal of Obstetric, Gynecologic, and Neonatal Nursing, 31*(6), 753-761.

Minato, J.F. (2000/2001). Is it time to push? Examining rest in second-stage labor. *AWHONN Lifelines, 4*(6), 20-23.

Mozingo, J.N., Davis, M.W., Thomas, S.P., & Droppleman, P.G. (2002). I felt violated: Women's experience of childbirth-associated anger. *MCN: The American Journal of Maternal/Child Nursing, 27*(6), 342-347.

Righard, L. (2001). Making childbirth a normal process. *Birth, 28*(1), 1-4.

Roberts, J.E. (2003). A new understanding of the second stage of labor: Implications for nursing care. *Journal of Obstetric, Gynecologic, and Neonatal Nursing, 32*(6), 794-801.

Sauls, D.J. (2002). Effects of labor support on mothers, babies, and birth outcomes. *Journal of Obstetric, Gynecologic, and Neonatal Nursing, 31*(6), 721-732.

Simkin, P. (2002). Supportive care during labor: A guide for busy nurses. *Journal of Obstetric, Gynecologic, and Neonatal Nursing, 31*(6), 733-741.

Simkin, P. (2003). Maternal positions and pelves revisited. *Birth, 30*(2), 130-132.

Simpson, K.R. (1999). Routine care during labor and birth: Is this really how we want to practice perinatal nursing, or are we ready to advocate for childbearing women and insist on evidence-based care? *Mother-Baby Journal, 4*(4), 5-7.

Sleutel, M., & Golden, S.S. (1999). Fasting in labor: Relic or requirement. *Journal of Obstetric, Gynecologic, and Neonatal Nursing, 28*(5), 507-512.

Sleuthel, M.R. (2000). Intrapartum nursing care: A case study of supportive interventions and ethical conflicts. *Birth, 27*(1), 38-45.

Spiby, H. Slade, P., Escott, D., Henderson, B., & Fraser, R.B. (2003). Selected coping strategies in labor: An investigation of women's experiences. *Birth, 30*(3), 189-194.

Sprague, A., & Trépanier, M.J. (1999). Charting in record time. *AWHONN Lifelines, 3*(5), 25-30.

Tumblin, A., & Simkin, P. (2001). Pregnant women's perceptions of their nurse's role during labor and delivery. *Birth, 28*(1), 52-56.

Winslow, E.H., & Crenshaw, J. (2000). Managing labor: Does walking help or hurt? *American Journal of Nursing, 100*(3), 50-51.

Intrapartum Fetal Surveillance

After studying this chapter, you should be able to:
- Identify the purposes of fetal surveillance during labor.
- Explain the normal and pathologic mechanisms that influence fetal heart rate.
- Identify the advantages and limitations of each method of intrapartum fetal surveillance: auscultation and electronic monitoring.
- Explain the types of equipment used for electronic fetal monitoring during labor and the advantages and limitations of each.

- Describe the interpretation of electronic fetal monitoring data.
- Explain the methods that may be used in addition to electronic fetal monitoring to judge fetal well-being.
- Describe appropriate responses to nonreassuring fetal heart rate patterns.
- Use the nursing process to plan care for a woman having intrapartum electronic fetal monitoring.

acidosis A condition resulting from the accumulation of acid (hydrogen ions) or the depletion of base (bicarbonate) in the blood or body tissues. The pH measures acid-base balance.

amnioinfusion Infusion of a sterile isotonic solution into the uterine cavity during labor to reduce umbilical cord compression; also done to dilute meconium in amniotic fluid, reducing the risk that the infant will aspirate thick meconium at birth.

asphyxia Insufficient oxygen and excess carbon dioxide in the blood and tissues.

baroreceptors Cells that are sensitive to blood pressure changes.

chemoreceptors Cells that are sensitive to chemical changes in the blood, specifically changes in oxygen and carbon dioxide levels and in acid-base balance.

hypercapnia Excess carbon dioxide in the blood, evidenced by an elevated P_{CO_2}.

hypertonic contractions Uterine contractions that are too long or too frequent, have too short a resting interval, or have an inadequate relaxation period to allow optimal uteroplacental exchange.

hypoxemia Reduced oxygenation of the blood, evidenced by a low P_{O_2}.

hypoxia Reduced availability of oxygen to the body tissues.

intermittent monitoring A variation of electronic fetal monitoring in which an initial strip is obtained on admission. If patterns are reassuring, the woman is remonitored for periods of 15 minutes at regular intervals (about every 30 to 60 minutes).

Montevideo units A method to quantify intensity of labor contractions with internal uterine activity monitoring. The baseline intrauterine pressure for each contraction in a 10-minute period is subtracted from the peak pressure. The resulting net pressures (peak minus baseline) are added to calculate Montevideo units, or MVUs.

nadir Lowest point, such as the lowest pulse rate in a series.

nuchal cord Umbilical cord around the fetal neck.

telemetry Wireless transmission of electronic fetal monitoring data to a bedside or central monitor unit.

tocolytic A drug that inhibits uterine contractions.

transducer A device that translates one physical quantity into another, such as fetal heart motion into an electrical signal for rate calculation, generation of sound, or a written record.

uterine resting tone Degree of uterine muscle tension when the woman is not in labor or during the interval between labor contractions.

Intrapartum fetal surveillance uses any of several methods to identify signs associated with well-being or with compromise. Accurate assessment of these signs promotes appropriate and timely care to reduce hazards to the fetus. During labor there are two clients: the expectant mother and her fetus. The purposes of intrapartum fetal surveillance are to evaluate how the fetus tolerates labor and to identify possible hypoxic insult to the fetus during labor. Fetal surveillance cannot identify every compromised fetus.

Two basic approaches are taken to intrapartum fetal surveillance—low-technology approach and high-technology approach. Each has advantages and limitations. The low-technology approach uses auscultation of the fetal heart rate and palpation of uterine activity. Electronic fetal monitoring is the second approach to intrapartum fetal surveillance. Although electronic fetal monitoring is dominant in U.S. hospital births, its routine use remains controversial because its benefits to the fetus are not always clear. Other data, such as assessment for fetal movement (see Chapter 16), fetal pulse oximetry, or cord blood gases, may be added to fetal heart rate and contraction data to provide a balanced view of the fetal condition.

FETAL OXYGENATION

Adequate fetal oxygenation requires five related factors:

- Normal maternal blood flow and volume to the placenta
- Normal oxygen saturation in maternal blood
- Adequate exchange of oxygen and carbon dioxide in the placenta
- An open circulatory path between the placenta and the fetus through vessels in the umbilical cord
- Normal fetal circulatory and oxygen-carrying functions

Labor is stressful for a fetus, but several mechanisms exist to compensate for these stresses. One must understand the dynamics of uteroplacental exchange and fetal circulation to understand fetal responses to labor. (See also Chapter 12 for a discussion of fetal circulation and placental functions.)

Uteroplacental Exchange

Oxygen-rich and nutrient-rich blood from the mother enters the intervillous spaces of the placenta via the spiral arteries (see Fig. 12-7). Oxygen and nutrients in the maternal blood pass into the fetal blood that circulates in capillaries in the intervillous spaces. Carbon dioxide and other waste products pass from the fetal blood into the maternal blood at the same time. Maternal blood carrying fetal waste products drains from the intervillous spaces through endometrial veins and returns to the mother's circulation for elimination by her body. Substances pass back and forth between mother and fetus without mixing of maternal and fetal blood.

During labor, contractions gradually compress the spiral arteries, temporarily stopping maternal blood flow into the intervillous spaces. During contractions, the fetus depends on the oxygen supply already present in body cells, fetal erythrocytes, and the intervillous spaces. The oxygen supply in these areas is enough for about 1 to 2 minutes. As each contraction relaxes, freshly oxygenated maternal blood re-enters the intervillous spaces and waste-laden blood drains out.

Fetal Circulation

The fetal heart circulates oxygenated blood from the placenta throughout the body and returns deoxygenated blood to the placenta. The umbilical vein carries oxygenated blood to the fetus, and the two umbilical arteries carry deoxygenated blood from the fetus to the placenta (see Fig. 12-7).

Regulation of Fetal Heart Rate

Mechanisms that regulate the fetal heart rate are balanced to maintain cardiac output at a level that keeps the fetal heart and brain oxygenated. Fetal cardiac output increase is accomplished primarily by an increase in the heart rate. Conversely, a marked decrease in fetal heart rate decreases the cardiac output.

Five fetal factors interact to regulate the fetal heart rate:

1. The autonomic nervous system
2. The baroreceptors
3. The chemoreceptors
4. The adrenal glands
5. The central nervous system

The balance among forces that increase and those that slow the heart rate result in the characteristic fluctuations in fetal heart rate during the final trimester of pregnancy.

Autonomic Nervous System

The sympathetic and parasympathetic branches of the autonomic nervous system are balanced forces that regulate the fetal heart rate. Sympathetic stimulation increases the heart rate and strengthens myocardial contractions through release of epinephrine and norepinephrine. The net result of sympathetic stimulation is an increase in cardiac output.

The parasympathetic nervous system, through stimulation of the vagus nerve, reduces the fetal heart rate and maintains short-term variability. The parasympathetic branch gradually exerts greater influence as the fetus matures, beginning between 28 and 32 weeks of gestation. Therefore the average fetal heart rate in the term fetus is slightly lower than in the preterm fetus. However, variability of the fetal heart rate near full term is often more dramatic than a fetus just a few weeks younger than full term.

Baroreceptors

Cells in the carotid arch and major arteries respond to stretching when the fetal blood pressure increases. The baroreceptors stimulate the vagus nerve to slow the fetal heart rate and decrease the blood pressure, thus lowering cardiac output. As fetal blood pressure falls, the heart rate accelerates to maintain normal cardiac output.

Chemoreceptors

Cells that respond to changes in oxygen, carbon dioxide, and pH are found in the medulla oblongata and in the aortic and carotid bodies. Decreased oxygen content, increased carbon dioxide content, or a lower pH in the blood or cerebrospinal fluid triggers an increase in the heart rate. However, prolonged hypoxia, hypercapnia, and acidosis depress the fetal heart rate.

Adrenal Glands

The adrenal medulla secretes epinephrine and norepinephrine in response to stress, causing a response from the sympathetic nervous system that accelerates the fetal heart rate. The adrenal cortex responds to a fall in the fetal blood pressure with release of aldosterone and retention of sodium and water, resulting in an increase in the circulating fetal blood volume.

Central Nervous System

The fetal cerebral cortex causes the heart rate to increase during fetal movement and to decrease when the fetus sleeps. The hypothalamus coordinates the two branches of the autonomic nervous system. The medulla oblongata maintains the balance between stimuli that speed and stimuli that slow the heart rate.

Pathologic Influences on Fetal Oxygenation

Fetal oxygenation may be compromised by alterations in any of the placental or fetal factors or those of the pregnant woman.

Maternal Cardiopulmonary Alterations

Actual or relative reductions in the mother's circulating blood volume reduce perfusion of the intervillous spaces with oxygenated maternal blood. Hemorrhage causes an actual decrease in her blood volume. Relative reductions in maternal circulating volume result from altered distribution of the blood volume without blood loss. For example, epidural block analgesia may result in vasodilation, which increases the capacity of the maternal vascular bed. However, the amount of blood available to fill the vessels is unchanged. Hypotension can result, reducing placental blood flow.

Maternal hypertension may reduce blood flow to the placenta because of vasospasm and narrowing of the spiral arteries.

A lowered oxygen level in the mother's blood reduces the amount available to the fetus. Maternal acid-base alterations, which often accompany respiratory abnormalities or diabetic ketoacidosis, may also compromise exchange in the placenta. A lower maternal oxygen tension may result from respiratory disorders, such as asthma or acute pulmonary infections, or from smoking.

Uterine Activity

Hypertonic uterine activity can reduce the time available for exchange of oxygen and waste products in the placenta. Contractions may be too long (over 90-120 sec) or too frequent (closer than every 2 min) or have too short an interval (less than 30 sec of complete relaxation). Additional criteria may be specified when internal electronic fetal monitoring is used. The uterus may never fully relax between contractions, applying continuous compression to the spiral arteries and reducing maternal-fetal exchange in the intervillous spaces. Excess uterine activity may occur spontaneously or with prostaglandin or oxytocin administration. However, a fetus with good oxygen reserve may never show signs of compromise, even with excessive contractions. Likewise, the fetus with little reserve may show compromise, even with weak uterine activity.

Placental Disruptions

Conditions such as abruptio placentae (separation of the placenta before birth) and infarcts (necrosis of varying amounts of placental tissue) reduce the placental surface area available for exchange. The amount and location of placental disruption relate to the degree of impairment in uteroplacental exchange.

Interruptions in Umbilical Flow

The usual cause of interrupted blood flow through the umbilical cord is compression. Blood flow through the umbilical cord may be reduced by compression between the fetal presenting part and the pelvis, a nuchal cord or one that is wrapped around the fetal body, or a knot in the cord. It may occur with oligohydramnios, because the amount of amniotic fluid is inadequate to cushion the cord. The umbilical cord also may become entangled around fetal body parts.

The thin-walled umbilical vein is compressed initially, reducing flow of more highly oxygenated blood into the fetus. This results in initial hypoxia with hypotension. Barorecep-tors and chemoreceptors respond by accelerating the fetal heart rate. Flow from the fetus to the placenta through the firmer-walled umbilical arteries falls as cord compression continues, resulting in hypertension from increased fetal blood volume. Baroreceptors respond to hypertension by stimulating the vagus nerve, thus reducing blood pressure and slowing the fetal heart. The fetal heart rate again accelerates as pressure on the arteries is relieved, and then pressure on the vein.

Fetal Alterations

Fetal tissues may be hypoxic despite an adequate oxygen supply from the mother and adequate exchange within the placenta. A low circulating fetal blood volume, fetal hypotension, or fetal anemia reduces the ability of fetal erythrocytes to deliver oxygen to body cells. Central nervous system or cardiac abnormalities may cause an abnormal rate or rhythm. For example, a fetus with complete heart block may not respond to stimuli that would normally cause a rate increase.

Prolonged fetal bradycardia may be both a response to hypoxia and a contributing factor to hypoxia because fetal oxygenation is rate-dependent. Prolonged tachycardia can also decrease cardiac output because the ventricles have less time to fill with oxygenated blood during diastole.

Risk Factors for Fetal Compromise

When conditions associated with reduced fetal oxygenation exist (Box 18-1), surveillance by either intermittent auscultation and palpation or electronic fetal monitoring should be done more often. No difference in perinatal outcome has been demonstrated between properly performed intermittent auscultation and electronic fetal monitoring (American Academy of Pediatrics, & American College of Obstetricians and Gynecologists. [2002]. *Guidelines for perinatal care,* 5th ed. Elk Grove Village, IL, and Washington, DC: Author.)

AUSCULTATION AND PALPATION

The nurse may use intermittent auscultation of the fetal heart rate and palpation of uterine activity for intrapartum fetal surveillance (Procedure 18-1). Intermittent auscultation can be done using either the fetoscope or Doppler ultrasound (Fig. 18-1). Doppler auscultation is most common in actual practice because of its ease of use and the ability to adjust the volume. Many Doppler devices also have a digital display of the rate, and some may be used under water. The Doppler creates an electronic sound based on movements of the fetal heart and may be the only way to use auscultation if a woman has thick abdominal fat. However, the nonelectronic fetoscope is useful in cases of fetal cardiac dysrhythmias because its sound is that of actual opening and closing of heart valves, similar to the amplified sounds one hears with a stethoscope.

Advantages

Mobility is the primary advantage of auscultation and palpation for intrapartum fetal monitoring. The woman is free to change position and walk, which is especially helpful during early labor or with a fetal occiput posterior position (see Chapter 17). She can use water-based methods of pain management, such as whirlpool baths or showers. The atmosphere

Potential Maternal, Fetal, or Neonatal Risk Factors

ANTEPARTUM PERIOD
Maternal History

Prior stillbirth (unexplained or potentially recurrent cause)
Prior cesarean birth
Poor nutrition, low prepregnancy weight, poor weight gain
Chronic diseases, such as cardiac disease, anemia, hypertension, diabetes, asthma, and autoimmune diseases
Acute infections, such as urinary tract, pneumonia, gastrointestinal
Hematologic problems, such as anemia, deep vein thrombosis
Drug use (includes prescription, over-the-counter, herbal preparations, illegal)
Psychosocial stress, domestic violence

Problems Identified During Pregnancy

Intrauterine growth restriction
Gestation >42 weeks
Marked decrease in fetal movement
Multifetal gestation
Preeclampsia, eclampsia
Gestational diabetes
Placental abnormalities (placenta previa, abruptio placentae)
Maternal severe anemia
Maternal infection
Maternal trauma

INTRAPARTUM PERIOD
Maternal Problems

Hypotension or hypertension
Hypertonic uterine contractions
Abnormal labor: preterm or dysfunctional
Prolonged rupture of membranes
Chorioamnionitis
Fever

Fetal or Placental Problems

Fetal anemia
Abnormal fetal heart rate or pattern
Meconium-stained amniotic fluid
Abnormal presentation or position
Prolapsed cord
Abruptio placentae

---

is more natural than technologic, which is important to some families during their birth experience.

Limitations

One disadvantage of auscultation and palpation as the primary method of fetal assessment is that fetal heart rate and uterine activity are assessed for a small part of the total labor. Labor contractions place stress on the fetus because of the normal reduction of blood flow to the placenta at that time. Although the fetal heart rate is assessed during some contractions, it is not recorded during every contraction. Moreover, no continu-

ous printed record is available to show the fetal response throughout labor or to identify subtle trends in the response.

Some women find that interruptions for auscultation are distracting. The pressure of the instrument on the abdomen is uncomfortable for some, and it may require several moves to locate the best place for auscultation with each assessment.

Intermittent auscultation is more staff-intensive than electronic monitoring, primarily during first-stage labor. When the nurse-patient ratio is high, auscultation may not be a realistic option as the primary method of intrapartum fetal surveillance.

ELECTRONIC FETAL MONITORING

Electronic fetal monitoring may be continuous, starting shortly after the woman is admitted, or intermittent, with a short recording made at regular intervals during labor, similar to auscultation.

Subjectivity of interpretation and use of varying descriptive terminology have made outcomes of research difficult to evaluate. Between 1995 and late 1996, a series of workshops was held to clarify and standardize definitions for electronic fetal monitoring data (National Institute of Child Health and Human Development (NICHD) Research Planning Workshop, 1997). A major purpose was to develop standard definitions to improve data collection and evaluation. Many health care facilities have adopted these definitions in their policies. Guidelines from AWHONN's *Fetal Heart Rate Monitoring: Principles and Practices* (3rd ed.) (2003) and terminology from the NICHD workshops are used in a simplified form here.

Advantages

The electronic monitor supplies more data about the fetus than auscultation, and it prints a permanent record. Gradual trends in fetal heart rate and uterine activity are more apparent because the strip provides a graphic record for review. Continuous electronic fetal monitoring shows the fetal response before, during, and after every contraction while it is in use rather than providing a sampling of fetal responses to contractions.

Electronic fetal monitoring, done in 85.2% of live births, was the most prevalent obstetric procedure in the United States in 2002 (Martin, Hamilton, Sutton, Ventura, Menacker, & Munson, 2003). Most women in the United States expect electronic monitoring and may find the constant sound of the fetal heartbeat comforting. The coach can use the tracing of contractions on the monitor strip to help the woman anticipate the beginning and end of each contraction.

Electronic monitoring allows one nurse to observe two laboring women, primarily during uncomplicated early labor. A 1-to-1 nurse-patient ratio is needed during the second stage of labor or if high-risk conditions exist, regardless of the monitoring method used. Electronic monitoring can give the nurse more time for teaching and supporting the laboring woman with breathing and relaxation techniques if the nurse maintains the primary focus on the woman, not on the technology.

Limitations

Reduced mobility is a limitation of electronic fetal monitoring. Frequent maternal position changes or an active fetus may require constant adjustment of equipment. It is often dif-

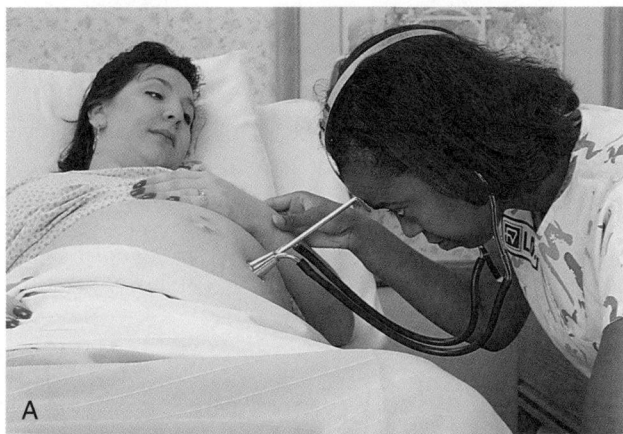
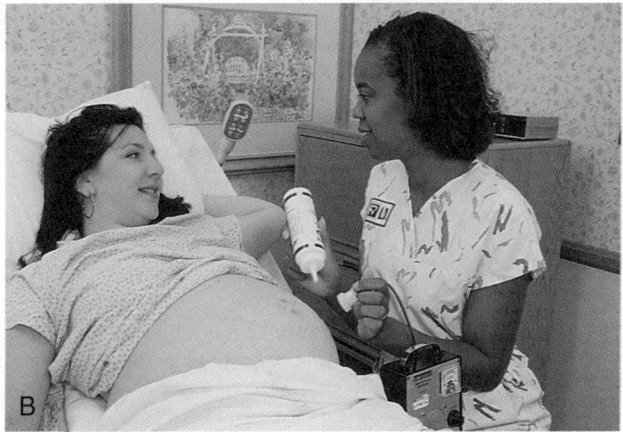
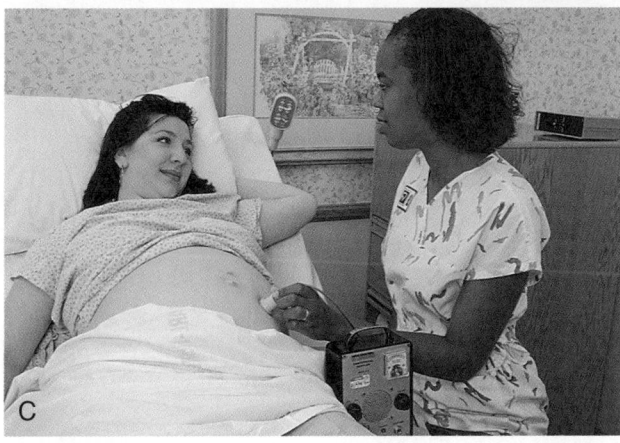

Figure 18-1 Low-intervention methods for evaluating the fetal heart rate during labor. **A,** Fetoscope, with head attachment to enhance conduction of faint fetal heart sounds. **B,** Transmission gel improves the clarity of the fetal heart movement sensed by the Doppler ultrasound transducer. **C,** The nurse moves the transducer until the fetal heart sounds are heard clearly. This location is usually over the fetus's back, which is most likely to be located in the woman's right or left lower abdomen.

ficult to obtain a clear tracing in overweight women. In addition, repositioning the equipment is necessary as the baby moves downward in the pelvis during labor. The belts or stockinette used to keep sensors positioned properly for external monitoring are uncomfortable for some women. A woman may concentrate on maintaining a good tracing rather than making herself comfortable or using a position to enhance fetal rotation and descent.

The electronic fetal monitor imparts a technical air to the surroundings and may be objectionable to a woman and her partner.

ELECTRONIC FETAL MONITORING EQUIPMENT

Electronic fetal monitoring equipment consists of the bedside monitor unit and sensors for fetal heart rate and uterine activity. Sensors for each function may be either internal or external. Computer interfaces allow addition of chart annotations and admission and delivery information and provide electronic storage of information. Telemetry-equipped models enable wireless transmission of data to the base for observation and storage, thus allowing ambulation while monitoring.

Fetal monitor clocks should be synchronized throughout the unit, often by connection to an atomic clock. Using the fetal monitor clock to determine the birth time allows the most accurate reconstruction of the events of labor. In legal proceedings, the amount of time required to accomplish corrective interventions can make a difference in the defense of a lawsuit.

Bedside Monitor Unit

The bedside fetal monitor unit uses the information from the fetal heart rate and uterine activity sensors to provide a visual output in the form of a numeric display and a graphic strip. The strip may be printed by the monitor itself, similar to an electrocardiogram (ECG) strip, or viewed on a computer screen. The strip can be printed if electronic storage is not available in facilities that use a computer interface with the bedside monitor. Simultaneous monitoring of twins is possible for most fetal monitors.

Paper Strip

Data about the fetal heart rate and uterine activity are displayed on two horizontal grids—one for the fetal heart rate and another for the uterine activity (Fig. 18-2). Each segment of paper between perforations is numbered for identification and reassembly of a multipart strip. Electronic strips do not have numbered segments because time and date markers provide sequencing.

The fetal heart rate is recorded on the upper strip. The range of recorded rates is from 30 to 240 beats per minute (bpm).

Uterine activity is recorded on the lower grid as bell-shaped curves with continuous smaller rises and falls that represent maternal breathing superimposed on the larger curve. Fetal movements, maternal coughing, vomiting, or position changes cause erratic curves or spikes on the uterine activity line. Contraction intensity and uterine resting tone (from 0 to 100 mm Hg) are recorded on the lower grid.

Procedure 18-1

Auscultating the Fetal Heart Rate

PURPOSE: To evaluate the fetal condition and tolerance of labor.

1. Explain the procedure to give information to the woman and her partner. Wash your hands with warm water to reduce the transmission of microorganisms and to make your hands more comfortable when touching the woman's abdomen.

2. Use Leopold's maneuvers to identify the fetal back (Procedure 17-1) because it usually is closest to the surface of the maternal abdomen, where fetal heart sounds are clearest. Illustrations show approximate locations of the fetal heart rate in different presentations and positions.

3. Assess the fetal heart rate with a fetoscope or Doppler transducer. The external fetal monitor may be used but is more often used for intermittent electronic fetal monitoring (short periods of electronic monitoring interspersed with periods with no fetal surveillance, such as maternal ambulation).

4. Fetoscope (see Fig. 18-1, *A*): Place the bell of the fetoscope over the fetal back with the head plate pressed against your forehead to add bone conduction to the sound coming through the earpieces. Move the fetoscope until you locate where the sound is loudest. Use your forehead to maintain pressure during auscultation to enhance the faint fetal heart sounds.

5. Doppler transducer (see Fig. 18-1, *B*): Review the manufacturer's instructions for operating the Doppler device. Place water-soluble conducting gel over the transducer to make an interface for clear signal transmission, and turn it on. Place the transducer over the fetal back and move it until you hear clear sounds that represent the fetal heart motion.

6. With one hand, palpate the mother's radial pulse to verify that the fetal heart rate is what is actually heard. If her pulse is synchronized with the sounds from the fetoscope or Doppler transducer, try another location for the fetal heart. Other sounds that may be represented by the Doppler are the funic souffle (blood flowing through the umbilical cord) or uterine souffle (blood flowing through the uterine vessels). The funic souffle is synchronized with the fetal heart and is the same rate; the uterine souffle is synchronized with the mother's pulse.

7. Count the baseline fetal heart rate for 30 to 60 seconds between contractions. Assessment during a contraction may clarify findings, but auscultation is difficult during contractions. Note accelerations or slowing of the rate.

8. Note reassuring signs that suggest the fetus is tolerating labor well:
   a. An average rate of 110 to 160 beats per minute
   b. Regular rhythm
   c. Accelerations from the baseline rate
   d. No decrease in rate from the baseline rate

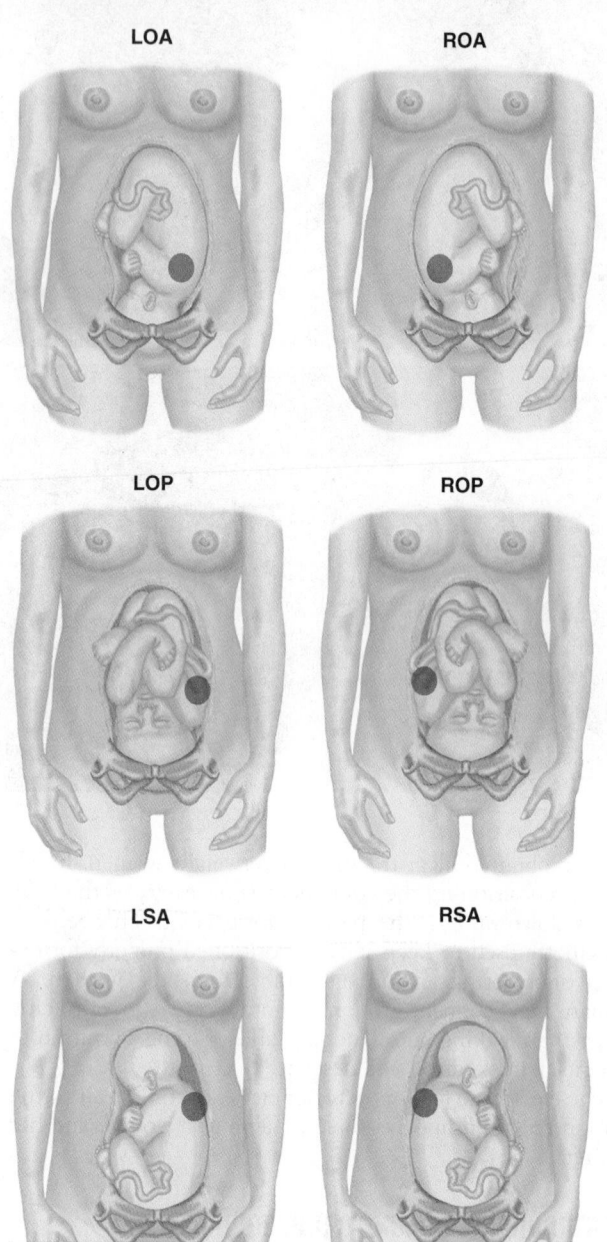

9. Note nonreassuring signs, and make more frequent assessments. Notify the physician or nurse-midwife for further evaluation.
   a. Heart rate outside normal limits. Unexplained tachycardia or bradycardia for 10 minutes or longer
   b. Irregular rhythm
   c. Gradual or abrupt decrease in rate

Modified from Feinstein, N.F., Torgersen, K.L., & Atterbury, J. (Eds.). (2003). *AWHONN's Fetal heart monitoring: Principles and practices* (3rd ed.). Dubuque, IA: Kendall/Hunt.

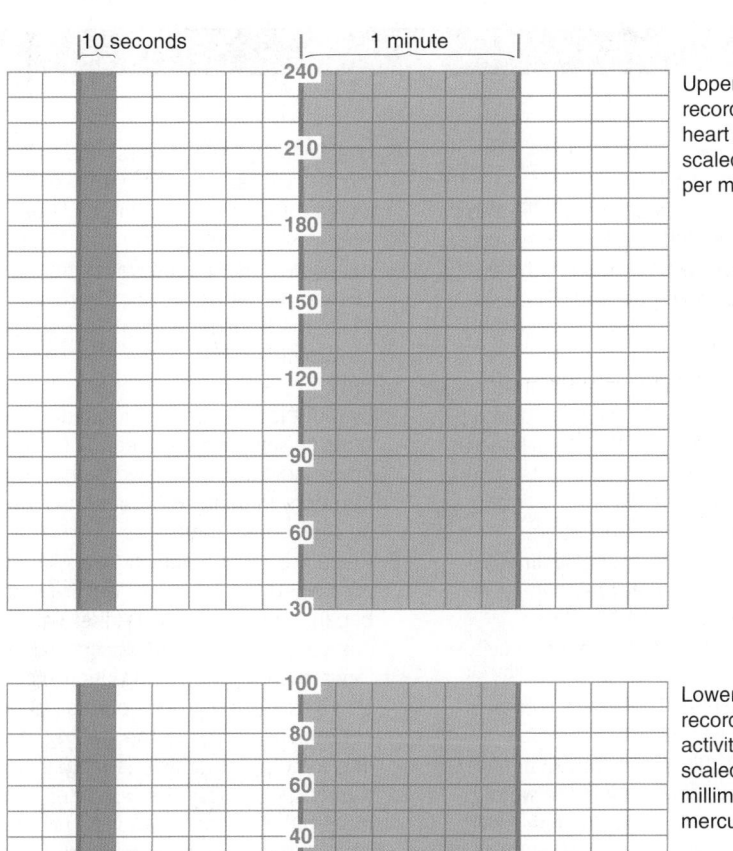

Figure 18-2 Paper strip for recording electronic fetal monitoring data. Each dark vertical line represents 1 minute, and each lighter vertical line represents 10 seconds. Paperless computerized displays that depict the fetal heart rate and uterine activity patterns have a similar appearance.

Vertical lines on both upper and lower grids are time divisions. At a paper speed of 3 cm per minute, dark vertical lines are 1 minute apart. Lighter lines subdivide the 1-minute divisions into six 10-second segments. The vertical lines are used to time the frequency and duration of contractions and to identify the fetal response to the contractions. The scroll speed of a screen display uses similar time divisions as a printed strip.

Remote Surveillance

Many facilities have a display for each patient at central locations to allow surveillance when the nurse is not at the bedside. These units display the tracing on a screen and have settings for audible and visual alerts, such as an abnormal fetal heart rate, or maternal blood pressure.

Devices for External Fetal Monitoring

Both the fetal heart rate and uterine activity can be monitored by external sensors, or transducers. External devices are secured on the mother's abdomen by elastic straps, a tube of wide stockinette, or an adhesive ring (Fig. 18-3). External devices are less accurate than internal ones but are noninvasive

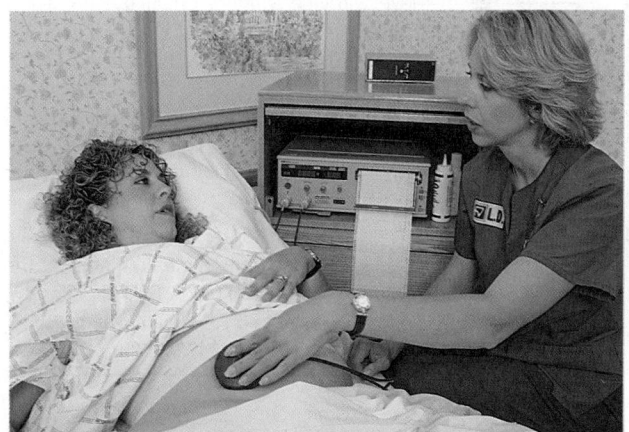

Figure 18-3 The nurse applies the uterine activity transducer to the woman's upper abdomen, in the fundal area. The Doppler transducer for sensing the fetal heart rate is usually placed on her lower abdomen when the fetus is in the cephalic presentation.

and are suitable for most women in labor. Procedure 18-2 contains instructions for using the external electronic fetal monitor.

Procedure 18-2

External Fetal Monitor

PURPOSES:

To apply the electronic fetal monitor properly.

To perform a basic evaluation of the fetal heart rate (FHR) and uterine activity patterns to identify data needing further assessment by the experienced nurse, physician, or nurse-midwife.

1. Read instruction manual for the equipment to become familiar with proper operation of the equipment and to be able to identify the equipment.
2. Verify that the date and time for the monitor are accurate.
3. Perform a function test, following the manufacturer's instructions, to ensure that the bedside monitor unit is calibrated properly to give accurate data. Each manufacturer sets standards for indicators of proper function. Press the TEST button, and observe for result. Common correct test results are:
   a. *Fetal heart rate:* The monitor prints a line or lines at 120, 150, 180, or 200 beats per minute, depending on the model.
   b. *Uterine activity:* The monitor adds 50 to uterine activity display.
   c. *Maternal electrocardiogram (ECG):* The monitor creates an artificial ECG waveform.
4. To decrease the woman's fear of the unknown, explain the basic procedure of electronic fetal monitoring to the woman and her partner or family. Teaching her that she can move with the monitor in place enhances her comfort and promotes normal labor. Vary instructions according to equipment used and hospital protocols. A sample is:
   a. Using the electronic fetal monitor does not mean that you or the baby has a problem. It is the usual way we assess the baby's response to labor contractions.
   b. Two belts go around your abdomen—one for the fetal heart rate sensor and one for contractions. (At least three belts are needed for most twin pregnancies.)
   c. Feel free to move with the monitor on. If the tracing is poor, we can adjust the sensors.
5. Apply belts, an adhesive ring, or other method to secure the sensors:
   a. Slide both belts under the woman's back without the sensors attached. To enhance comfort, keep the belts smooth under her back.
   b. An additional belt that is tied in a knot rather than attached to the ultrasound transducer may apply pressure against the sensor to better maintain ideal tilt against the maternal abdomen. A folded washcloth, roll of tape, or other simple techniques may be used similarly to maintain the best tracing.
6. Use Leopold's maneuvers (see Procedure 17-1) to locate the fetus's back because the fetal heart rate is best detected through the back of the fetus.
7. Apply ultrasound gel to the Doppler ultrasound transducer because gel improves transmission and reception of the ultrasound waves to provide more accurate data. Place the transducer on the woman's abdomen at the approximate location of the fetal back. Move the transducer until a clear signal is heard, tilting the sensor slightly (without losing contact) if needed for a clear signal. Most bedside units have a green light, flashing heart shape, or other indicator of a good signal. Continuously changing numbers indicate the fluctuations of the fetal heart rate on many machines.
8. Place the uterine activity sensor in the fundal area or the area where contractions feel the strongest when palpated because the external uterine activity monitor senses the change in the abdominal contour as the uterus rotates forward with each contraction. Contractions are usually strongest in the upper uterus. When the woman has a contraction, observe the tracing for the bell shape. The line for uterine activity is jagged because it also senses the rise and fall of the abdomen with breathing. Fetal or maternal movement causes a larger spike in the line. Observe through several contractions to verify correct placement, and improve placement if needed.
9. Observe the strip for baseline fetal heart rate, presence of variability, periodic changes, and uterine activity (contraction duration and frequency). Palpate contractions for intensity and relaxation between contractions to identify reassuring and nonreassuring fetal heart rate patterns (see Table 18-1). Contractions having a frequency greater than every 2 minutes, duration longer than 90 to 120 seconds, rest interval of under 30 seconds, or incomplete uterine relaxation between contractions may reduce maternal blood flow into the intervillous spaces and impair exchange of oxygen and waste products. The external uterine activity sensor is useful for assessing contraction frequency and duration. It is not accurate for determining actual intensity or uterine resting tone.
10. Take corrective actions for nonreassuring patterns (see p. 406). Notify the physician or nurse-midwife of nonreassuring patterns, corrective actions, and maternal and fetal responses. Document all calls, their content, and provider response.

Fetal Heart Rate Monitoring With an Ultrasound Transducer

A Doppler ultrasound transducer detects fetal heart movement for rate calculation. It is similar to the hand-held Doppler unit. The transducer sends high-frequency sound waves into the uterus. The sound waves are reflected, and the monitor's computer continuously calculates the fetal heart rate based on the movement sensed as the heart beats.

Fetal heart motion does not always correlate with electrical heart activity. Other movements, such as fetal or maternal activity or blood flow through the umbilical cord and the woman's aorta, can also be detected. Modern monitors ignore most of these extraneous sounds to provide a clean tracing.

The Doppler transducer produces a two-part sound with each heartbeat. Fetal or maternal activity produces a rough, erratic sound rather than the crisp, rhythmic sound characteristic of fetal heart motion. Fetal hiccups cause a "th-thump" sound at regular intervals that is superimposed on sounds created by heart activity. Volume can be adjusted or turned off.

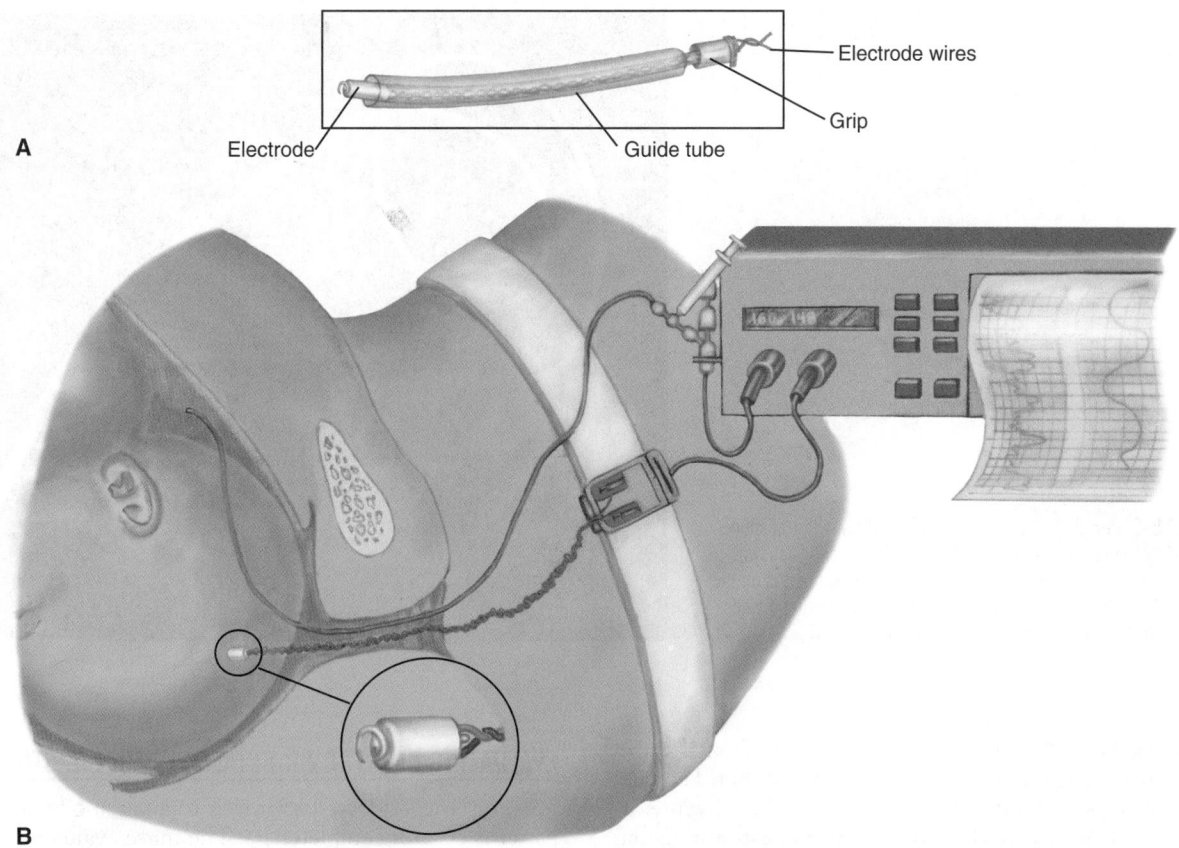

Figure 18-4 Fetal scalp electrode and intrauterine pressure catheter. **A,** Parts of the fetal scalp electrode before it is applied. **B,** Fetal scalp electrode and intrauterine pressure catheter in place and connected to the bedside monitor unit.

Uterine Activity Monitoring With a Tocotransducer

A tocotransducer ("toco") with a pressure-sensitive area detects changes in abdominal contour to measure uterine activity. The uterus pushes outward against the mother's anterior abdominal wall with each contraction. The monitor calculates changes in this signal and prints them as bell shapes on the lower grid of the strip.

Movement other than uterine activity also registers on the monitor. For example, maternal respirations superimpose a zigzag appearance on the uterine activity line. Other fetal or maternal movements appear as spikes on the uterine activity tracing.

Because uterine activity is sensed through the woman's abdomen, a tocotransducer is useful for observing the frequency and duration of contractions. It does not reliably measure internal contraction intensity and uterine resting tone. Factors that affect apparent intensity as printed on the strip include:

- *Fetal size.* A small fetus does not allow the uterus to push firmly against the abdominal wall with each contraction, making contractions appear less intense. In addition, an immature fetus floats in a relatively larger quantity of amniotic fluid than a term fetus.
- *Abdominal fat thickness.* A thick layer of abdominal fat absorbs energy from uterine contractions, reducing their apparent intensity on the printed strip. Conversely, a thin woman whose uterus rotates sharply forward with each contraction may appear to have intense contractions when they are actually mild.
- *Maternal position.* Different maternal positions may increase or decrease pressure against the transducer.
- *Location of the transducer.* Uterine activity is best detected where it is strongest and where the fetus lies close to the uterine wall. This location is usually over the upper uterus. Uterine contractions may not be detectable if the transducer is located elsewhere.

Devices for Internal Fetal Monitoring

Accuracy is the main advantage of using internal devices for electronic fetal monitoring, but they are invasive, slightly increasing the risk for infection. Their use requires ruptured membranes and about 2 cm of cervical dilation.

Fetal Heart Rate Monitoring With a Scalp Electrode

The fetal scalp electrode (FSE) detects electrical signals from the fetal heart (Fig. 18-4). Fetal or maternal movement interferes less with accuracy because the rate is calculated from electrical events in the fetal heart. The monitor unit generates a beeping sound with each fetal heartbeat; the volume of the sound can be adjusted.

Areas to avoid for electrode application are the fetal face, fontanels, and genitals. The wire from the electrode protrudes from the mother's vagina and is attached to a leg plate to provide electrical grounding.

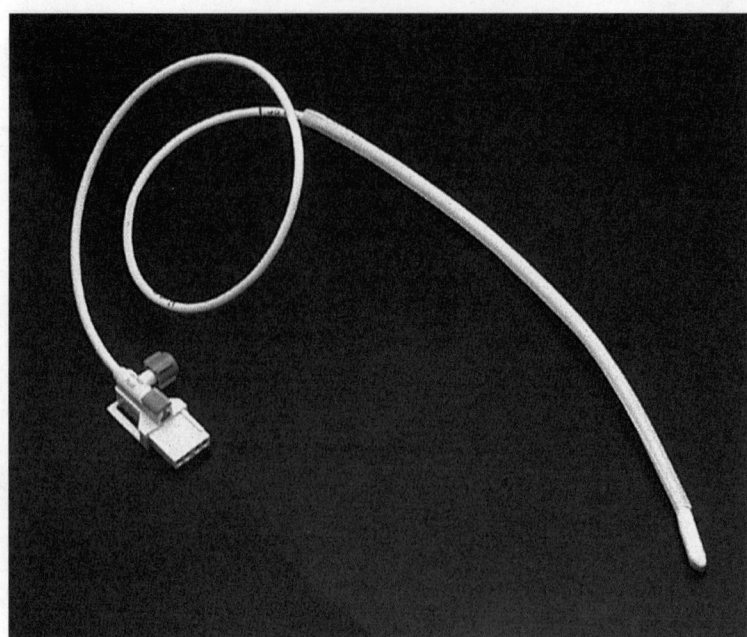

Figure 18-5 Intrauterine pressure catheter (IUPC) with transducer in its tip. This model has a lumen for amnioinfusion and is shown with its introducer over the catheter. The amnioinfusion port is on the side of the catheter connection and has a blue cap covering it when not in use. (Courtesy Utah Medical Products, Midvale, UT.)

Because it barely penetrates the fetal skin (about 1 mm), the electrode is easily displaced. The tracing then becomes erratic or stops if the electrode is fully detached. Secure attachment of the electrode is often difficult if the fetus has thick hair. The electrode is removed by turning it counterclockwise about one and one-half turns until it detaches.

Uterine Activity Monitoring With an Intrauterine Pressure Catheter

Two kinds of intrauterine pressure catheters can be used to measure uterine activity, including contraction intensity and resting tone. These are:

- A solid catheter with a pressure transducer in its tip (Fig. 18-5). This catheter usually has an additional lumen for amnioinfusion.
- A hollow, fluid-filled catheter that connects to a pressure transducer on the bedside monitor unit.

Both types sense intrauterine pressure and increases in intraabdominal pressure, such as with coughing or vomiting.

The solid catheter is not affected by height because its transducer is in the catheter. However, the sensor in its tip measures hydrostatic pressure from the amniotic fluid above the fetal presenting part as well as the pressure from uterine activity. Therefore recorded intrauterine pressures from the solid catheter are higher than those from the fluid-filled catheter, and the nurse must consider this fact when assessing whether uterine activity is normal or hypertonic.

The tip of the fluid-filled catheter in the uterus should be at the level of the transducer on the outside for best accuracy. If the tip is lower than the transducer, the recorded pressure is lower than the actual intrauterine pressure. If the tip is higher, the recorded pressure may be artificially high. Changes in the mother's position may alter the height of the catheter tip, requiring adjustment of the transducer's height. Because it is simpler to use, the solid catheter is more commonly used.

EVALUATING ELECTRONIC FETAL MONITORING STRIPS

A consistent, organized approach to analyzing fetal monitor patterns ensures completeness. The nurse evaluates the fetal heart rate tracing for baseline rate, variability, and any pattern of rate changes from the baseline. Uterine activity is evaluated by determining the frequency, duration, and intensity of contractions and by assessing uterine resting tone. Fetal heart rate and uterine activity patterns must be evaluated together when assessing whether the fetal status is reassuring.

Other data relevant to strip interpretation are maternal vital signs; maternal position; drug, anesthetic, or oxygen administration; character of the amniotic fluid; labor status; and procedures performed. These are recorded on the strip as well as in the labor record.

Terms such as *fetal distress* or *birth asphyxia* should be avoided because they do not yet have clear definitions with broad acceptance. In addition, fetal monitor strips that are diagnosed as nonreassuring result in the birth of a baby who neither is hypoxic nor has acidemia over 50% of the time (Cypher, Adelsperger, & Torgersen, 2003). Electronic fetal heart monitoring appears to be the most accurate in diagnosis of fetal oxygen and acid-base status at the extremes, either clearly reassuring or definitely nonreassuring. Strips for the large number of babies that fall between the two extremes may be evaluated quite differently by different experts, with major differences in interventions.

Baseline Fetal Heart Rate

The baseline is described by rate and variability, and the numbers are rounded to 5 bpm (Fig. 18-6). A baseline fetal heart rate assesses the average rate for at least 2 minutes within a 10-minute window. During this 2 or more minutes, the uterus must be at rest and episodes of significant increases or decreases in rate must not occur (see Fig. 18-6). The baseline also excludes temporary increases or decreases in rate that are (1) periodic (recurrent, associated with contrac-

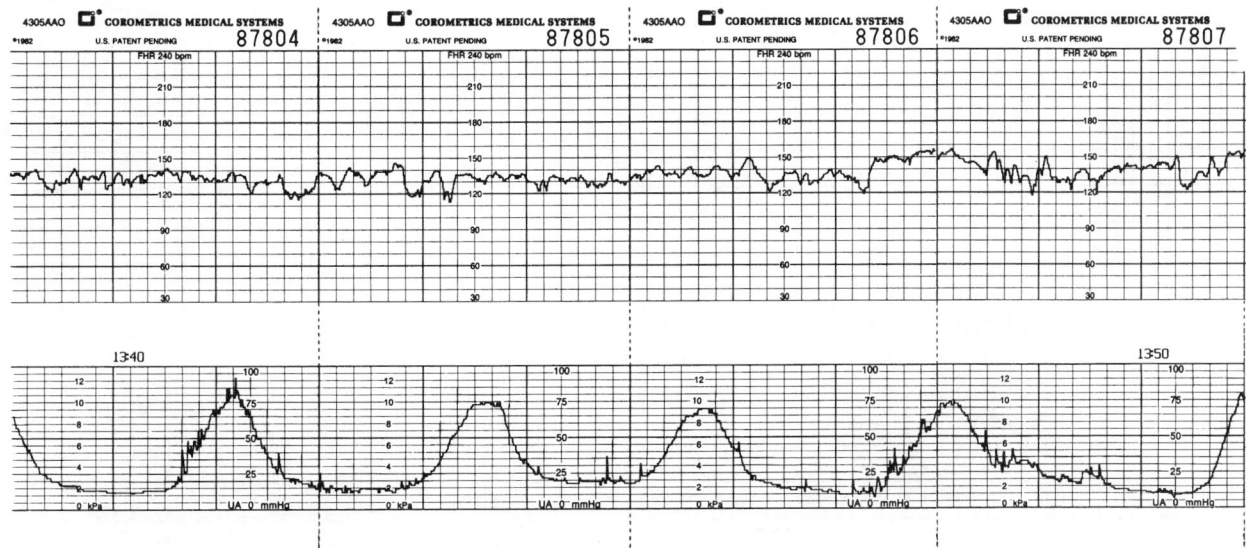

Figure 18-6 Electronic fetal monitor strip showing a reassuring pattern of fetal heart rate and uterine activity. The baseline fetal heart rate is 130 to 140 beats per minute (bpm), with a variability of about 10 bpm. There are no periodic changes in this strip. The contraction frequency is approximately every 2 to 3 minutes, duration is about 50 to 60 seconds, intensity is 75 to 90 mm Hg, and uterine resting tone is approximately 10 mm Hg. Fetal scalp electrode and intrauterine pressure catheter are being used. (Courtesy Corometrics Medical Systems, Inc., Wallingford, CT. Redrawn with permission.)

tions) or (2) nonperiodic (irregular). Segments of extreme fluctuations of rate (>25 bpm) that are not characteristic of the usual pattern are excluded when determining baseline.

The baseline rate is classified as follows (Cypher et al., 2003; NICHD, 1997):

- *Normal:* A rate that averages from 110 to 160 bpm. The preterm fetus at 26 to 28 weeks often averages a rate at the upper end of this range because the parasympathetic nervous system, which slows the rate, is immature. Some healthy full-term fetuses have a rate that averages 100 to 110 bpm.
- *Bradycardia:* Less than 110 bpm, persisting for at least 10 minutes.
- *Tachycardia:* More than 160 bpm, persisting for at least 10 minutes.

Baseline Fetal Heart Rate Variability

Variability describes the fluctuations in the baseline fetal heart rate that cause the printed line to have an irregular, wavelike appearance rather than a smooth, flat one (Fig. 18-7). Two types of variability exist together, but facilities that use the NICHD definitions do not distinguish between short- and long-term variability.

- Short-term variability (STV): changes in the fetal heart rate from one beat to the next (beat-to-beat). This variability is most accurately assessed with an internal spiral electrode because it detects cardiac electrical activity rather than heart motion. Presence of STV gives the line for the fetal heart rate a rough appearance, whereas the line is smooth if STV is absent.
- Long-term variability (LTV): broader fluctuations that are apparent over 1-minute intervals. About three to six of these broad rate changes occur each minute. LTV may be assessed with either external or internal placement.

Variability may be decreased by several nonpathologic and pathologic factors, such as:

- Fetal sleep (usually lasting 40 min or less at term, but may last up to 2 hr [Blackburn, 2003; Cunningham et al., 2001; Harmon, 2004])
- Narcotics or other sedative drugs, such as magnesium sulfate, given to the woman
- Alcohol, illicit drugs
- Fetal tachycardia
- Gestation younger than 28 weeks
- Fetal anomalies that affect central nervous system regulation of the heart rate, such as anencephaly
- Hypoxia that is severe enough to affect the central nervous system
- Abnormalities of the central nervous system, heart, or both
- Maternal acidemia or hypoxemia

Both kinds of variability occur because multiple factors constantly speed and slow the fetal heart in a push-and-pull manner. Evaluation of variability helps clarify how a fetus is tolerating the stress of labor, including factors that cause hypoxia. Variability is a significant component of the fetal heart rate tracing on the electronic monitor, for two reasons:

- Adequate oxygenation promotes normal function of the autonomic nervous system and helps the fetus adapt to the stress of labor.
- Variability evaluates the function of the fetal autonomic nervous system, especially the parasympathetic branch.

No consensus exists on terms to describe variability. Some sources describe short-term and long-term variability separately, whereas others describe the two as a unit. The NICHD Research Planning Workshop (1997) recommended that no distinction be made between short-term and long-term variability because the two are evaluated visually

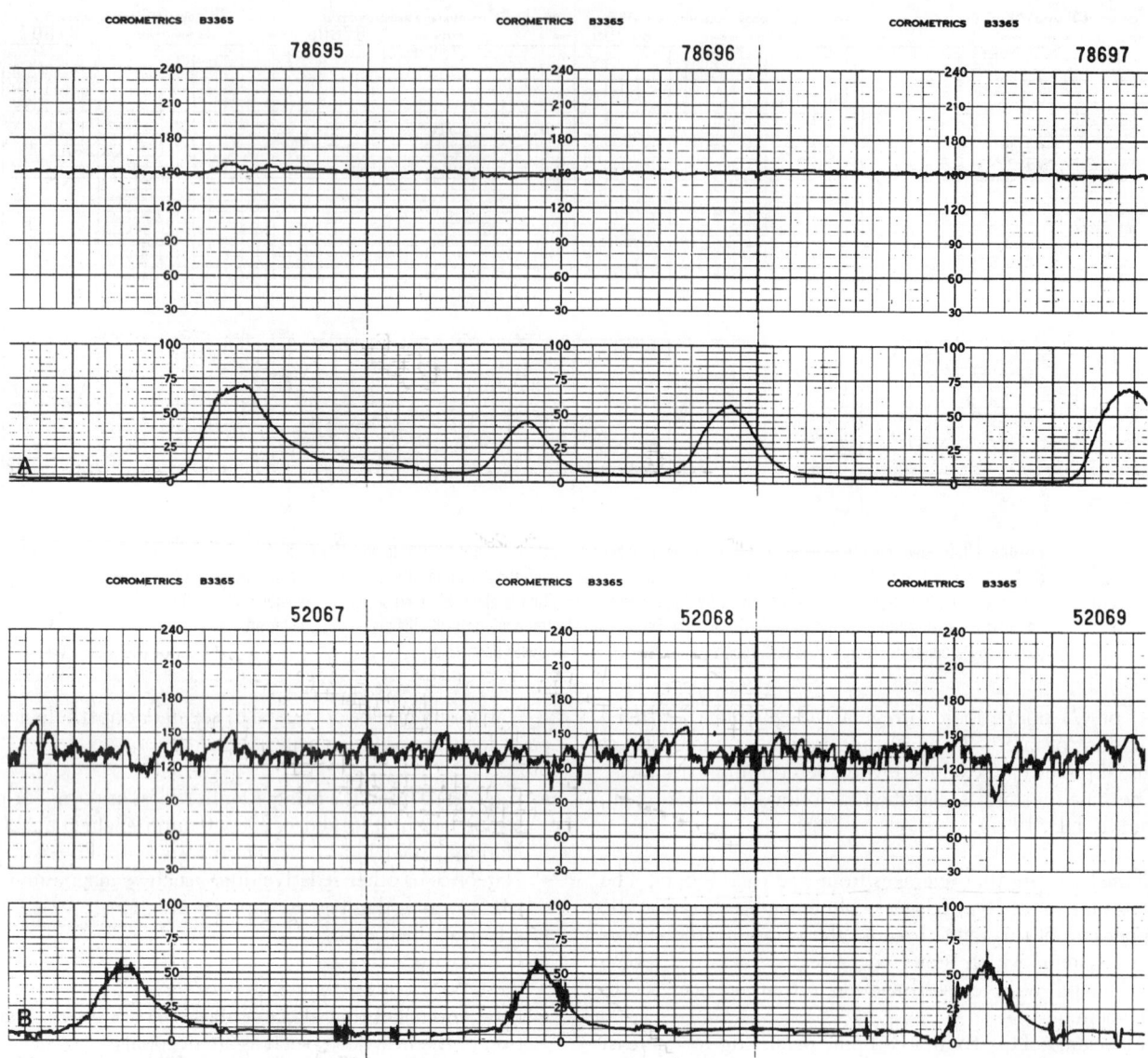

Figure 18-7 Contrasts in fetal heart rate variability. A fetal scalp electrode is being used. **A,** Minimal variability (less than 5 beats per minute). Note the smooth, flat line in the upper graph for the fetal heart rate. **B,** Moderate variability (average 20 bpm variability). Note the zigzag appearance of the fetal heart rate line compared with the flat appearance in **A.** (Courtesy Corometrics Medical Systems, Inc., Wallingford, CT. Redrawn with permission.)

as a unit. Although the usefulness and validity of the recommendations of the NICHD group is not fully tested, many hospitals have adopted the workshop's proposed terminology. Because of its wide use, the NICHD terminology will be used to describe variability in this text.

NICHD (1997) developed four categories of variability. Moderate variability is 6 to 25 bpm, meaning that the rate changes over time fall within the 6- to 25-bpm range. Variability is *absent* if it cannot be detected, *minimal* if it is detectable at 5 or fewer bpm, and *marked* if over 25 bpm. Moderate variability of 6 to 25 bpm is accepted by most authorities as reassuring.

Periodic Patterns in the Fetal Heart Rate

Periodic patterns are temporary, recurrent changes from the baseline rate that are associated with uterine contractions. They include accelerations and decelerations. Periodic patterns are evaluated with baseline characteristics (rate and variability).

Accelerations

An acceleration is a temporary increase in the FHR that peaks at least 15 bpm above the baseline and lasts at least 15 seconds (Fig. 18-8). Accelerations often occur with fetal movement. They may occur with vaginal examinations, uterine contractions, and mild cord compression and when the fetus is in a breech presentation. They may be nonperiodic (having no relation to contractions) as well as periodic. Accelerations are usually a reassuring sign, reflecting a fetus that has a responsive central nervous system and is not in acidosis.

The healthy preterm fetus may have shorter FHR accelerations less than 15 bpm. Before 32 weeks of gestation, an increase in the FHR that peaks at least 10 bpm above the baseline and lasts at least 10 seconds is considered an acceleration.

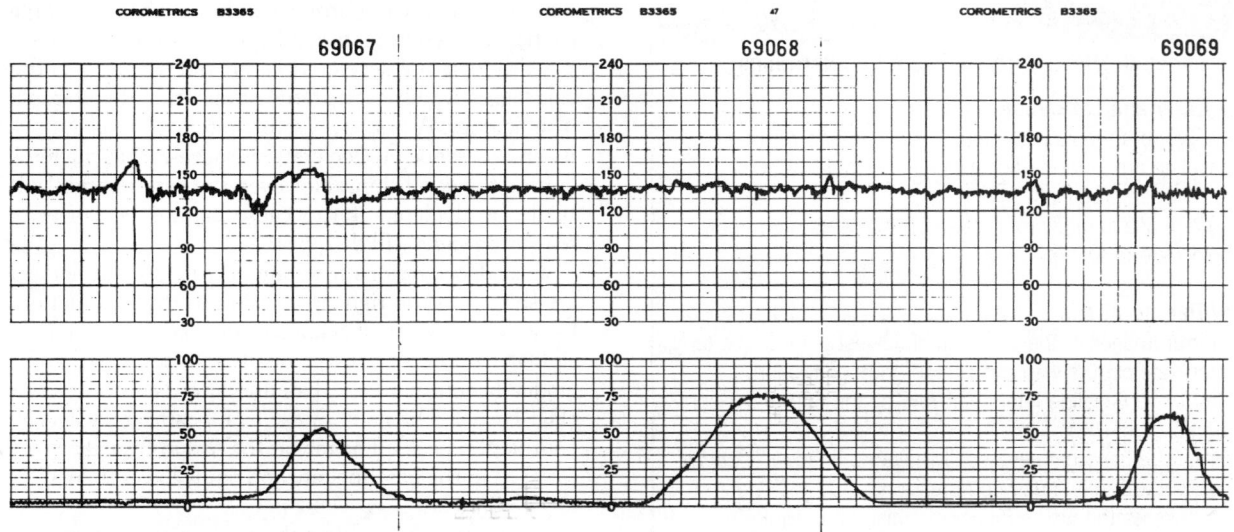

Figure 18-8 Accelerations in the fetal heart rate. (Courtesy Corometrics Medical Systems, Inc., Wallingford, CT. Redrawn with permission.)

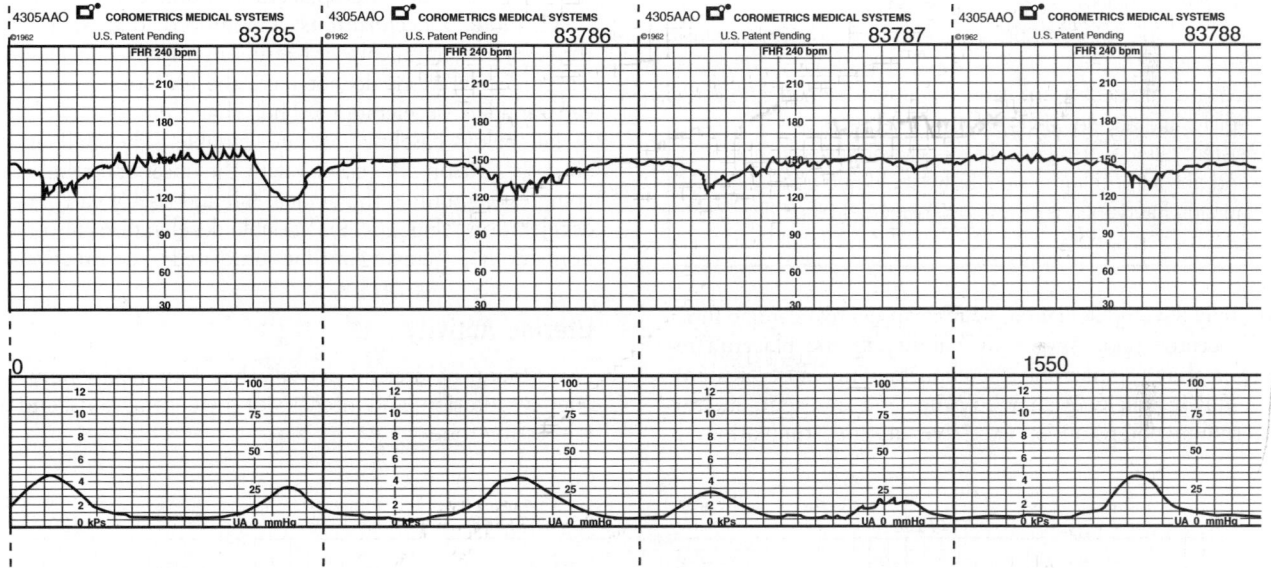

Figure 18-9 Early decelerations. The slowing of the fetal heart rate is gradual, and the nadir of the deceleration occurs at the peak of the contraction. It returns to the baseline by the end of the contraction. Cause: fetal head compression. (Courtesy Corometrics Medical Systems, Inc., Wallingford, CT. Redrawn with permission.)

Accelerations lasting longer than 2 minutes but less than 10 minutes are prolonged accelerations. Accelerations that last longer than 10 minutes are a change in the baseline rate or they may reflect a merging of several accelerations that later return to the previous baseline.

Decelerations
Periodic decelerations are classified into three types, based on their shape and relationship to uterine contractions.

Early Decelerations. Fetal head compression for any reason increases intracranial pressure, causing the vagus nerve to slow the heart rate. Early decelerations are not associated with fetal compromise and require no intervention. They oc-

cur *during* contractions as the fetal head is pressed against the woman's pelvis or soft tissues, such as the cervix.

Early decelerations are consistent in appearance; they are uniform in that one early deceleration looks similar to others. They mirror the contraction, gradually falling from the baseline and gradually returning to the baseline by the end of the contraction (Fig. 18-9). The nadir (low point) of the fetal heart rate occurs at the same time the contraction peaks. The rate at the nadir is usually no lower than 30 to 40 bpm from the baseline.

Late Decelerations. Impaired exchange of oxygen and waste products in the placenta (uteroplacental insufficiency) may result in a pattern of late (delayed) decelerations. The

! CRITICAL TO REMEMBER

Differences Between Early and Late Decelerations

Both Early and Late Decelerations

Decrease from the baseline fetal heart rate and return to baseline are gradual (onset to nadir of at least 30 sec).

Occur with contractions.

Rate decrease is rarely more than 30-40 beats per minute below the baseline.

Early Decelerations

Are mirror images of the contraction (lowest point in the fetal heart rate occurs with the peak of the contraction).

Return to the baseline fetal heart rate by the end of the contraction.

Maternal position changes usually have no effect on pattern.

Associated with fetal head compression.

Are not associated with fetal compromise and require no added interventions.

Late Decelerations

Look similar to early decelerations but begin after the contraction begins (often near the peak).

Nadir occurs after the peak of the contraction.

Reflect possible impaired placental exchange (uteroplacental insufficiency).

Occasional late decelerations accompanied by moderate variability, and accelerations are not ominous.

Persistent late decelerations, especially with no accelerations and absent or minimal variability, should be addressed by nursing interventions to improve placental blood flow and fetal oxygen supply.

fetus may develop acidemia, which can depress cardiac function, because poor oxygen availability in the placenta requires a shift to anaerobic metabolism. The cause of uteroplacental insufficiency may be acute and transient, such as maternal hypotension or excessive uterine stimulation. It may also occur with chronic conditions that impair placental exchange, such as maternal hypertension or diabetes.

Although late decelerations are not reassuring, other signs can suggest whether the fetus is tolerating the uteroplacental insufficiency. A normal baseline rate with moderate variability and presence of accelerations suggests that the fetus is tolerating the conditions. However, the fetal reserves will eventually be depleted if the cause cannot be corrected, and reassuring signs will disappear.

Late decelerations look similar to early decelerations but are shifted to the right in relation to the contraction. They have a consistent appearance; one late deceleration looks similar to others. They gradually fall from the baseline and gradually return to the baseline after the contraction ends (Fig. 18-10). The nadir of the fetal heart rate occurs after the contraction peaks. The rate at the nadir is usually 5 to 30 bpm lower than the baseline rate and rarely lower than 40 bpm below baseline.

They often begin after the peak of the contraction. The rate returns to baseline *after* the contraction ends. They have a consistent appearance. The fetal heart rate may remain in the normal range and may not fall much below its baseline level. The amount of rate decrease from the baseline does not indicate how much uteroplacental insufficiency exists.

Variable Decelerations. Conditions that reduce flow through the umbilical cord result in variable decelerations. These decelerations do not have the uniform appearance of early and late decelerations. Their shape, duration, and degree of fall below baseline rate are variable. They fall and rise abruptly (within 30 seconds) with the onset and relief of cord compression, unlike the gradual fall and rise of early and late decelerations (Fig. 18-11). Variable decelerations also may be nonperiodic, occurring at times unrelated to contractions.

Uterine Activity

Assessment of uterine activity has four components: frequency, duration, and intensity of the contractions; and uterine resting tone.

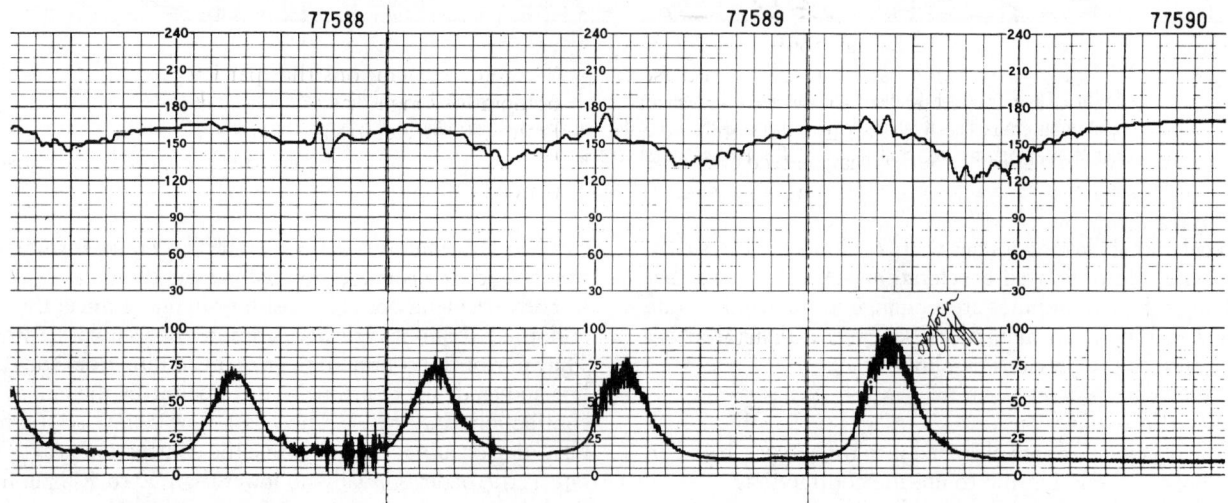

Figure 18-10 Late decelerations. Note that the decelerations look similar to early decelerations but are offset to the right. They begin at about the peak of the contraction, and the nadir occurs well after the peak of the contraction, often during the interval. Cause: uteroplacental insufficiency. (Courtesy Corometrics Medical Systems, Inc., Wallingford, CT. Redrawn with permission.)

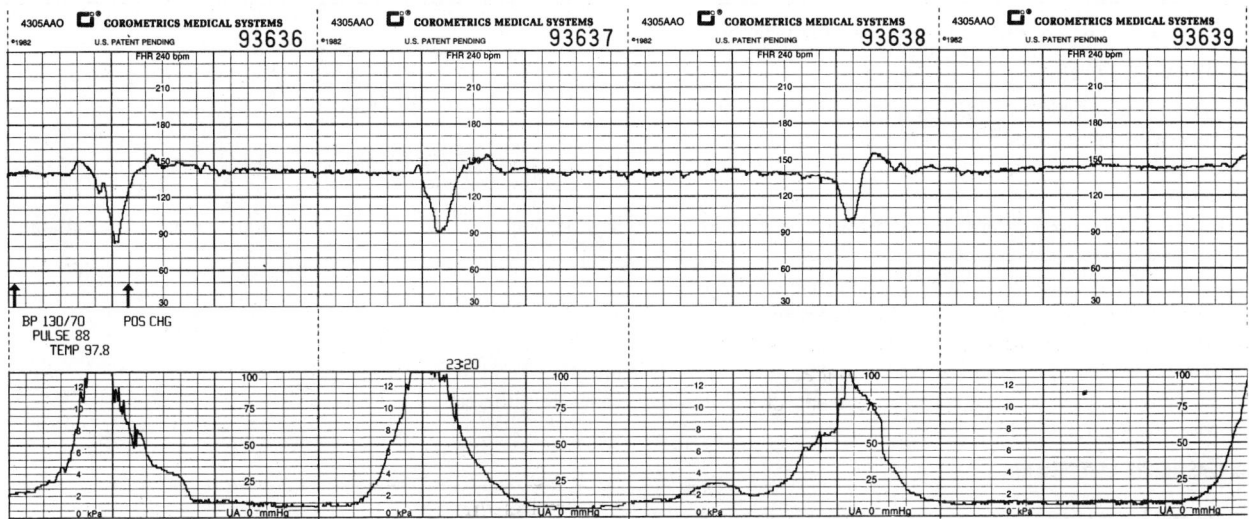

Figure 18-11 Variable decelerations. The decelerations are sharp in onset and offset. Note slight rate accelerations (shoulders) after each variable deceleration. These variable decelerations are periodic, in that they occur during contractions. Cause: umbilical cord compression. (Courtesy Corometrics Medical Systems, Inc., Wallingford, CT. Redrawn with permission.)

Palpation is used to estimate contraction intensity and uterine resting tone when an external uterine activity monitor is used (see Procedure 17-2). Contraction intensity is described as *mild*, *moderate*, or *strong*. The uterus should relax between contractions for at least 30 seconds.

With the intrauterine pressure catheter, the scale on the paper is used to describe intensity and resting tone. Intensity increases as labor progresses. Uterine contraction intensity changes as labor progresses. When measured internally, intrauterine pressure is about 20 to 30 mm Hg above resting values during early labor. Intrauterine pressure increases to about 75 to 80 mm Hg in the active phase and may reach 100 to 150 during second stage as the mother pushes vigorously. Average resting tone is 5 to 15 mm Hg (Blackburn, 2003; Cypher et al., 2003).

SIGNIFICANCE OF FETAL HEART RATE PATTERNS

Fetal heart rate patterns on the electronic monitor are classified as either "reassuring" or "nonreassuring." Between these two classifications are patterns that are "equivocal"—neither clearly reassuring nor clearly nonreassuring. For equivocal (ambiguous) patterns, several methods may be used to further evaluate the fetal condition. Table 18-1 summarizes reassuring and nonreassuring patterns.

Reassuring Patterns

Reassuring patterns, such as accelerations with fetal movement, are associated with fetal well-being. The nurse need only support optimal oxygenation because the patterns suggest that the fetus is tolerating intrapartum stressors.

Nonreassuring Patterns

Nonreassuring patterns are those in which favorable signs are absent or signs that are associated with fetal hypoxia or acidosis are present. ***Nonreassuring patterns do not necessarily***

indicate that fetal hypoxia or acidosis has occurred. Electronic fetal monitoring best identifies the well-oxygenated fetus; it less reliably identifies the compromised fetus. Thus electronic fetal monitoring is a screening rather than a diagnostic tool.

Nonreassuring patterns are more significant if they occur together and are persistent. For example, bradycardia with short-term variability of less than 5 bpm and late decelerations suggests greater physiologic stress than bradycardia with normal variability of the heart rate. The healthy fetus may demonstrate an occasional late deceleration, but a persistent pattern of late decelerations is more likely to represent compromise in a fetus. Nonreassuring patterns include but are not limited to:

- Tachycardia
- Bradycardia
- Absent or minimal variability
- Late decelerations
- Variable decelerations that persistently fall to less than 60 bpm for longer than 60 seconds
- Prolonged decelerations
- Hypertonic uterine activity, whether spontaneous or stimulated by drugs

Nonreassuring patterns do not always indicate that labor should end immediately. Several interventions may be used to clarify the fetal condition and to determine the best course of action. Other interventions may increase fetal oxygenation, allowing the fetal heart patterns to return to normal.

Clarification of Data
Any of four methods may clarify data to better understand the fetal condition. Four methods are used during the intrapartum period: fetal scalp stimulation, vibroacoustic stimulation, fetal oxygen saturation monitoring, and fetal scalp blood sampling. A fifth method, analysis of umbilical cord blood gases and pH, is used immediately after birth.

TABLE **18-1** Reassuring and Nonreassuring Fetal Surveillance Assessments

REASSURING ASSESSMENTS

- Baseline FHR: Stable, rate 110-160 beats per minute (bpm)
- Moderate variability (6-25 bpm)
- Accelerations: Peaking at least 15 bpm above the baseline with a duration of 15 sec or more (10 bpm and 10 sec if gestation 32 weeks or less)
- Variable decelerations of less than 60 sec with rapid return to baseline, accompanied by normal baseline rate and moderate variability
- Uterine activity:
  Contraction frequency: no more frequent than every 2 min
  Contraction duration: no longer than 90-120 sec
  Interval between contractions: at least 30 sec
  Uterine resting tone: uterus relaxed between contractions (by palpation when intermittent auscultation or external fetal monitoring is used); uterine resting tone <20 mm Hg (with intrauterine pressure catheter)
  Montevideo units: <400

NONREASSURING ASSESSMENTS

Pattern and Description	Possible Cause or Causes
Tachycardia Baseline FHR >160 bpm for at least 10 min	Maternal fever (fetal tachycardia may precede fever or other signs of infection) Maternal dehydration Maternal or fetal hypoxia Fetal acidosis Maternal or fetal hypovolemia Fetal cardiac dysrhythmias Maternal severe anemia Maternal hyperthyroidism Drugs administered to mother (e.g., terbutaline, bronchodilators, decongestants, stimulant drugs)
Bradycardia Baseline FHR <110 bpm for at least 10 min Baseline rates between 100 and 110 bpm are usually not associated with fetal compromise if there are no nonreassuring patterns	Fetal head compression Fetal hypoxia Fetal acidosis Fetal heart block Umbilical cord compression Late second-stage labor with maternal pushing

Decreased or Absent Variability
FHR baseline has a smooth, flat appearance
	Fetal sleep episodes (usually 40 min or less; occasionally as long as 2 hr)
	Fetal hypoxia with acidosis
	Drug effects:
	  CNS depressants
	  Local anesthetic agents

Late Decelerations
Gradual decelerations having a uniform appearance and a consistent relation to the contraction
Onset to nadir of 30 sec or longer
Nadir occurs after the peak of the contraction
	Uteroplacental insufficiency, which may be secondary to:
	  Maternal hypotension or hypertension
	  Excess uterine activity, spontaneous or stimulated
	  Placental interruption, such as abruptio placentae or placenta previa
	  Maternal diabetes
	  Maternal severe anemia
	  Maternal cardiac disease

Variable Decelerations
Sharp in onset and offset
May occur as a periodic or nonperiodic (random) pattern
Nonreassuring if:
  Fall to less than 60 bpm for more than 60 sec
  Return to baseline prolonged
  Overshoots (exceeding baseline after deceleration) are present
  Accompanied by tachycardia and/or loss of variability
	Umbilical cord compression, which may be secondary to:
	  Prolapsed cord
	  Nuchal cord (around fetal neck)
	  Cord around fetal body parts
	  Oligohydramnios (abnormally small amount of amniotic fluid)
	  Cord between fetus and mother's uterus or pelvis, without obvious prolapse
	  Knot in cord

FHR, Fetal heart rate; *bpm*, beats per minute; *CNS*, central nervous system.

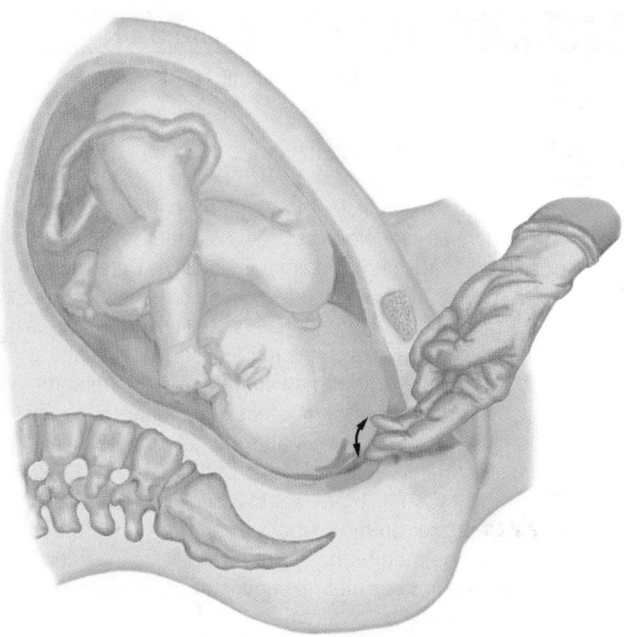

Figure 18-12 Fetal scalp stimulation identifies fetal response to gentle massage. An acceleration in the fetal heart rate of 15 beats per minute for 15 seconds suggests that the fetus is in normal oxygen and acid-base balance. Accelerations often occur with vaginal examination unrelated to nonreassuring fetal heart rate patterns.

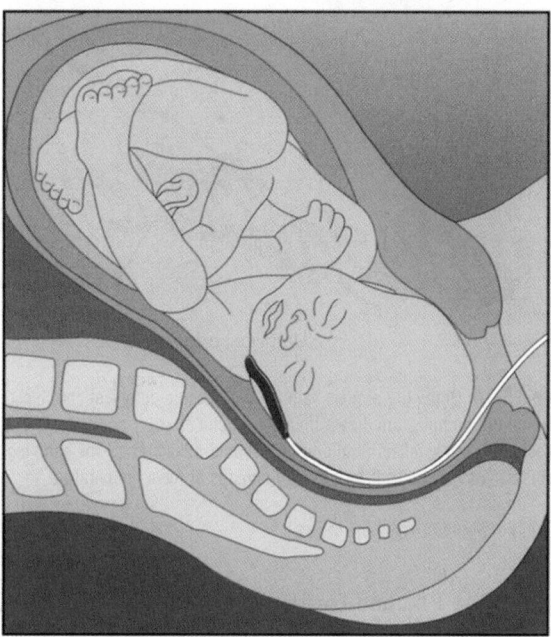

Figure 18-13 Fetal pulse oximeter.

Fetal Scalp Stimulation. Scalp stimulation evaluates the fetus's response to tactile stimulation during labor (Fig. 18-12). This procedure may be performed by the nurse, physician, or nurse-midwife. The examiner applies pressure to the scalp (or other presenting part) with a gloved finger or fingers and sweeps the fingers in a circular motion. An acceleration in the fetal heart rate of 15 bpm for at least 15 seconds is a reassuring response, suggesting a fetus in normal oxygen and acid-base balance. The acceleration may be delayed rather than immediate.

Fetal scalp stimulation is not done in some cases. These situations are similar to those in which vaginal examination would be restricted:

- Preterm fetus (may cause contractions)
- Prolonged rupture of membranes (higher risk of infection)
- Chorioamnionitis (intrauterine infection)
- Placenta previa (may cause hemorrhage)
- Maternal fever of unknown origin (possibility of introducing microorganisms into the uterus)

Vibroacoustic Stimulation. Acoustic, or vibroacoustic, stimulation (VAS) may be used by the nurse, physician, or nurse-midwife to supplement fetal scalp stimulation or if scalp stimulation is contraindicated. Because of its simplicity and noninvasive nature, vibroacoustic stimulation is common.

A stimulator that uses a combination of sound and vibration or an electronic larynx is applied to the mother's lower abdomen, and it is turned on for up to 3 seconds. The reassuring response is the same as with fetal scalp stimulation: an acceleration in the fetal heart rate of 15 bpm for 15 seconds or more. An absent response, however, does not necessarily mean that the fetus is hypoxic or in acidosis.

Fetal Oxygen Saturation Monitor. This fetal surveillance method, also called *fetal pulse oximetry*, ideally will help caregivers make better judgments about whether a nonreassuring fetal heart rate pattern is one that requires immediate operative intervention (cesarean or forceps birth) or if labor can safely continue (Cypher & Adelsperger, 2003; Seelbach-Göbel, Heupel, Kühnert, & Butterwegge, 1999; Simpson, 1998 & 2003).

A special sensor is placed alongside the fetal cheek or temple area to pick up the fetal pulse for estimation of oxygen saturation (Fig. 18-13). An oxygen saturation of 30% to 65% is considered a normal range for fetuses because of their high hemoglobin and hematocrit (compared with a normal of 95% to 100% oxygen saturation for the mother). The low value of 30% is considered the *critical threshold* because values above this saturation are unlikely to be associated hypoxia sufficient to lead to metabolic acidosis (Cypher & Adelsperger, 2003). Technical difficulties include fetal pulses that are normally faint, vernix and other debris interfering with the sensor, and sensor displacement.

Fetal Scalp Blood Sampling. Occasionally, the physician may obtain a sample of fetal scalp blood to evaluate the pH. This procedure is more complex than other intrapartum techniques already described. It requires rupture of membranes. Normal scalp pH is 7.25 to 7.35. Acidosis is present if the pH is less than 7.20, and the clinician may hasten the birth by using forceps or cesarean delivery. The scalp sample may be repeated for a borderline pH of 7.20 to 7.24.

Although fetal scalp blood sampling directly measures fetal acid-base status, it is the most invasive of methods now available. In addition, scalp sampling reflects acid-base status in the recent past rather than providing dynamic information during birth.

Cord Blood Gases and pH. Umbilical cord blood analysis is used to assess the infant's status immediately after birth for oxygenation and acid-base balance. The samples are analyzed

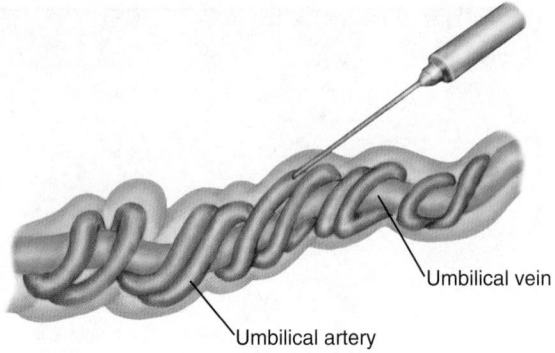

Figure 18-14 Obtaining a blood sample to determine umbilical cord blood gas values and pH. Samples are drawn from the umbilical artery and vein. Arterial samples most closely reflect fetal oxygen and acid-base status. The samples in capped syringes may be kept for up to 60 minutes at room temperature.

for pH, P_{CO_2}, P_{O_2}, and bicarbonate and for base deficit. This information helps identify whether acidosis exists and whether it is respiratory (short-term), metabolic (prolonged), or mixed. Normal cord blood gases and pH can confirm that the fetus was adjusting normally to the stresses of labor, although the fetal monitoring pattern may have been nonreassuring or the Apgar score may have been low (see p. 385).

Within 20 to 30 seconds **after** birth, the cord is double-clamped and cut to isolate a 10- to 30-cm (4- to 12-in) segment. Arterial cord blood best reflects fetal oxygenation and acid-base status because this blood is leaving the fetus on its way to the placenta. Blood is drawn into heparinized syringes to prevent coagulation, air is expelled, and the syringes are capped to avoid altering values by exposure to room air (Fig. 18-14). Samples should be carefully labeled as containing arterial or venous cord blood. Samples kept at room temperature are reliable for 30 to 60 minutes; they should be kept in ice if there is a delay beyond this time (American Academy of Pediatrics [AAP] & American College of Obstetricians and Gynecologists [ACOG], 2002; Cypher & Adelsperger, 2003).

Interventions for Nonreassuring Patterns

Any of several nursing or medical interventions, or both, may be indicated if a nonreassuring fetal heart rate pattern is present. All are directed toward identifying the cause of the nonreassuring pattern and improving fetal oxygenation.

Identifying the Cause of a Nonreassuring Pattern. Careful examination of the strip may suggest a cause for the nonreassuring fetal heart rate pattern and direct interventions most likely to correct the presumed problem. For example, a pattern of late decelerations suggests uteroplacental insufficiency. Uteroplacental insufficiency, however, may be secondary to a variety of causes, such as maternal hypotension and excessive uterine activity. Different causes require different corrective interventions. Checking the mother's vital signs may disclose hypotension, hypertension, or fever. Maternal sedative medications may alter variability in a well-oxygenated fetus.

A vaginal examination may reveal a prolapsed cord, which may cause variable decelerations, bradycardia, or both, as it is compressed. A vaginal examination also evaluates the

---

! CRITICAL TO REMEMBER

Nursing Responses to Nonreassuring Fetal Heart Rate Patterns

1. Identify the nonreassuring pattern to plan appropriate interventions:
   - Evaluate characteristics of the pattern that are nonreassuring (late or variable decelerations, bradycardia or tachycardia, absent or minimal variability). Determine if combinations of nonreassuring characteristics exist (i.e., late decelerations with minimal variability).
   - Evaluate maternal vital signs to identify hypotension, hypertension, or fever that may contribute to the fetal response associated with a nonreassuring pattern.
   - If indicated, perform a vaginal examination to identify a prolapsed umbilical cord. Do not perform a vaginal examination if there is active vaginal bleeding, diagnosed placenta previa, preterm labor or preterm premature rupture of the membranes, or a high risk for infection.
2. Stop oxytocin or other uterine stimulants. A tocolytic such as terbutaline may be ordered.
3. Reposition the woman, avoiding the supine position, for patterns associated with cord compression. Repositioning often improves other nonreassuring patterns as well.
4. Increase the rate of infusion of a nonadditive intravenous fluid to expand the mother's blood volume and improve placental perfusion.
5. Administer oxygen by facemask at 8 to 10 L/min to increase maternal blood oxygen saturation, making more oxygen available to the fetus. Maternal pulse oximetry, available on many fetal monitors, allows ongoing assessment of maternal oxygen saturation and documentation on the strip if the information is crucial.
6. Consider starting continuous electronic fetal monitoring with internal devices if no contraindication exists.
7. Notify the physician or nurse-midwife as soon as possible, or ask another nurse to notify. Report and document the following:
   - The pattern that was identified.
   - Nursing interventions taken in response to the pattern.
   - The fetal response after nursing interventions.
   - The response of the physician or nurse-midwife (orders, other response).
8. If the nonreassuring pattern is severe, other staff members should be alerted to the possibility of immediate delivery (usually cesarean birth, unless operative vaginal birth is possible).

---

woman's labor status, which helps the birth attendant decide if labor should continue or be ended with a cesarean birth.

Increasing Placental Perfusion. The woman is positioned on her side to eliminate aortocaval compression, which reduces placental blood flow. Giving a bolus of isotonic intravenous fluid such as lactated Ringer's solution increases the maternal blood volume, which in turn improves perfusion of the placenta if hypotension develops secondary to regional block (see "Epidural Block," p. 425, in Chapter 19).

Uterine activity reduces blood flow into the intervillous spaces, and a fetus with little reserve for stress may be unable

---

CRITICAL THINKING EXERCISE 18-1

Nancy Joe is having her labor induced with oxytocin and is having internal electronic fetal monitoring. Her contractions occur every 2 minutes, are 110 seconds in duration, and reach 75 mm Hg using an intrauterine pressure catheter. Uterine resting tone between contractions is 20 mm Hg. The baseline fetal heart rate is 135 to 145 beats per minute (bpm) with about 15 bpm variability.

Her nurse, Jackie Brown, notes a pattern of uniform decelerations that begin at the peak of each contraction. The rate falls to 125 bpm before returning to the previous baseline about 30 seconds after the contraction ends.
1. What pattern do these findings describe? What is the probable cause?
2. What is the most appropriate nursing response? Why? If needed, are corrective actions urgent?

CRITICAL THINKING EXERCISE 18-2

LaShonda Blair is in active labor and is having external electronic fetal monitoring for fetal assessment. LaShonda has not had medication, and her labor has been normal so far. Her membranes ruptured about 1 hour ago, and the amniotic fluid was clear. Contractions occur every 3 minutes, are 60 seconds in duration, and are moderately intense. Her uterus fully relaxes between each contraction.

The nursing student who is helping to care for LaShonda notes abrupt slowing of the fetal heart rate to 90 beats per minute during the next two contractions, each time lasting about 30 seconds.
1. What pattern do these findings describe? What is the probable cause?
2. Are any nursing actions needed? Why? If nursing actions are needed, what are they? In what order should they be done?

---

to tolerate even normal contractions. Persistent hypertonic uterine activity may compromise a fetus with normal reserves. If a woman is receiving oxytocin, it is discontinued so that uterine activity is not stimulated. A tocolytic drug such as terbutaline (0.125 to 0.25 mg intravenously or 0.25 mg subcutaneously) may be given to reduce uterine activity.

Increasing Maternal Blood Oxygen Saturation. Administration of 100% oxygen at 8 to 10 L/min through a snug facemask makes more oxygen available for transfer to the fetus.

Reducing Cord Compression. If cord compression is suspected, the woman is repositioned. She may be turned from side to side, or her hips may be elevated to shift the fetal presenting part toward her diaphragm. Several position changes may be required before the pattern improves or resolves. The fetal presenting part may be pushed upward slightly. See also Chapter 27 for information about prolapsed umbilical cord, an intrapartum emergency.

Amnioinfusion increases the fluid around the fetus and cushions the cord. Lactated Ringer's solution or normal saline is infused into the uterus through an intrauterine pressure catheter. The underpads must be changed as the fluid leaks out. Possible complications include overdistention of the uterus and increased uterine resting tone. These complications are relieved by withdrawing some of the fluid or by disconnecting the amnioinfusion and allowing excess fluid to drain through that port. Amnioinfusion also may be used to wash out and dilute fluid that is stained with thick meconium so that the infant does not aspirate it at birth (see "Meconium Aspiration Syndrome," Chapter 30).

■ NURSING CARE
The Woman Having Intrapartum Fetal Monitoring

Either fetal heart auscultation with palpation or electronic monitoring is acceptable for both low- and high-risk women, although the frequency of assessments changes with risk status. The nurse may identify any of several problems if a woman has electronic fetal monitoring. The woman or couple who prefer a nontechnical environment for birth may en-

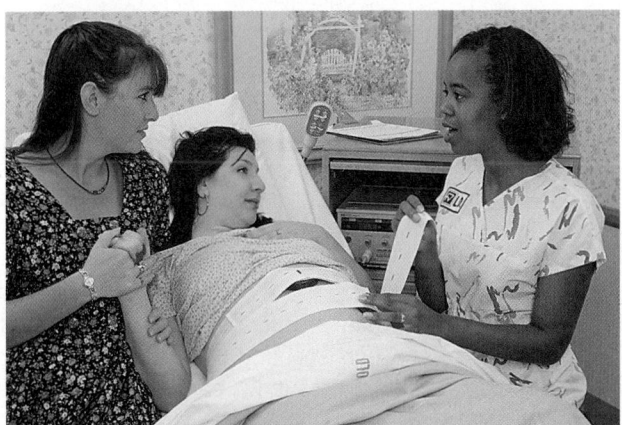

Figure 18-15 The nurse teaches the woman and her partner about electronic fetal monitoring to reduce anxiety and promote the woman's comfort during labor. Electronic fetal monitoring is only one method used to evaluate fetal well-being during labor.

counter a decision conflict because electronic fetal monitoring may be routine or recommended for a problem. Anxiety is likely if the woman does not understand the electronic monitor or if complications develop. Pain may be increased if mobility is restricted during labor.

Two nursing care needs related to intrapartum fetal monitoring are the woman's (or couple's) learning needs and an expansion of nursing care related to fetal oxygenation. Care related to fetal monitoring by either electronic means or auscultation should be combined with that for normal or complicated intrapartum nursing as needed.

LEARNING NEEDS
Assessment

Determine what the woman and her partner already know about fetal surveillance during labor. Does she believe that use of the electronic monitor (Fig. 18-15) indicates the development of a complication, or does she expect its use? Is the woman comfortable with intermittent auscultation with palpation of contractions for fetal assessment?

Nursing Care Plan

Intrapartum Fetal Compromise

ASSESSMENT

Glenda Brown is a 30-year-old African-American woman who is accompanied by her husband Paul. She is a gravida 4, para 1, who has had two spontaneous abortions. Glenda has had type 1 diabetes for 15 years. Her insulin dose required periodic increases as pregnancy progressed. Labor is being induced with oxytocin (Pitocin) at 39 weeks' gestation because she had a blood pressure elevation at today's antepartum care appointment. Her blood pressure was 146/94 mm Hg on admission, and repeat assessments have shown little change. A random urine sample shows 1+ protein. Glenda will have electronic fetal monitoring during labor.

Nursing Diagnosis

Deficient Knowledge: electronic fetal monitoring.

Goals/Expected Outcomes

Glenda and Paul will:
- State that they understand the reason for electronic monitoring, related equipment and procedures, and the data that are expected.

INTERVENTION	RATIONALE
1. Evaluate the parents' present knowledge about electronic fetal monitoring.	1. This evaluation allows the nurse to build on existing accurate knowledge and to correct misunderstandings about the technology's uses, benefits, and limitations.
2. Provide information about the monitor to Glenda and Paul.	2. Reassure Glenda and Paul that use of the electronic fetal monitor or making care changes based on its data does not mean that something is wrong with Glenda or the baby.
a. *Purposes:* To provide an audible and written record of the fetal response to labor and help caregivers choose appropriate interventions if nonreassuring patterns are identified.	a. Information tells the parents how the monitor is used. The fetal scalp electrode (if used) penetrates the outer layer of skin no more than a dime's thickness. The intrauterine pressure catheter or fetal pulse oximeter lies between the baby and the wall of the uterus.
b. *Safety:* The monitoring sensors are electrically isolated from the wall current.	b. Information explains common safety concerns of parents.
c. *Misleading data:* Encourage Glenda to call for assistance if she cannot hear the fetal heartbeat or if she notices that her contractions do not seem to be evident on the strip.	c. Sensors, especially external devices, can easily be displaced and stop picking up data. Preparing Glenda and Paul for this common occurrence reduces their fears if they should stop hearing the fetal heartbeat.
d. Encourage Glenda to move about freely. Tell her that a nurse will readjust her monitor if it stops recording properly. Explain that she should urinate at least every 2 hours and that the nurse can help her roll the monitor to the bathroom door or temporarily disconnect the sensor cables.	d. Maternal movement and regular urination enhance normal labor processes. A woman is likely to become anxious and uncomfortable if she concentrates more on maintaining data from the monitor than on coping with labor.

Evaluation

Glenda and Paul say that they expected electronic fetal monitoring during labor. Glenda is familiar with the external monitor because it was used for several biophysical profiles. She agrees to have internal monitoring if advised by her physician, saying that she understands that greater accuracy may be desirable because diabetes and hypertension are added risk factors for her baby.

Nursing Care Plan

Intrapartum Fetal Compromise—cont'd

ASSESSMENT

The nurse applies the external fetal monitor because Glenda's membranes are intact. She is having irregular spontaneous contractions. The fetal heart rate baseline averages 125 to 135 beats per minute (bpm) and accelerates when the fetus moves. The nurse begins an oxytocin infusion to induce labor. Glenda's blood pressure is 154/94.

Potential Complication

Fetal compromise.

Goals/Expected Outcomes

Client goals for the fetus are inappropriate because nurses cannot independently manage fetal compromise. Planning for Glenda should reflect the need to:

- Compare fetal heart rate and uterine activity data with baseline levels before oxytocin induction.
- Promote normal fetal oxygenation.
- Take corrective actions for nonreassuring patterns.
- Notify Glenda's physician if nonreassuring patterns develop.

INTERVENTION	RATIONALE
1. Identify relevant risk factors for fetal compromise.	1. Women who have risk factors that could reduce fetal oxygenation should have fetal surveillance by either electronic fetal monitor or intermittent auscultation done more frequently.
2. Encourage Glenda to assume any comfortable position other than the supine position.	2. Compression of the aorta reduces blood return to the heart and reduces cardiac output and placental perfusion.
3. Evaluate the strip, signing the printed strip each time if annotations are not automatically printed. Summarize the evaluation on the labor record as required by the facility policy. Guidelines for evaluation include:	3. Documentation creates a record that assessment was done. Documenting on both strip and the labor record allows each to stand alone.
a. Every 15 min during the first stage and every 5 min during the second stage.	a. Regular documentation provides a framework for regular assessment of the fetal response to labor in the high-risk pregnancy.
b. Before and after procedures such as amniotomy, medications or changes in medication rates, and start of epidural anesthesia.	b. Documenting a "paper (or electronic) trail" of the fetal status before and after procedures that may alter fetal heart rate patterns demonstrates that the standard of care was met. Documentation shows not only that changes in rate were recorded but also that a trained professional observed and interpreted data and took action appropriately.
c. With changes of activity, such as urination and repositioning.	c. Changes in activity or position could alter the uterine or umbilical cord blood flow. External sensors often need adjustment.
4. Use a four-step approach to evaluate the strip:	4. The four-step approach provides a systematic framework to evaluate the fetal response to labor.
a. Baseline fetal heart rate, rounded to 5 and expressed as a range (i.e., 130-140 bpm)	a. Tachycardia may be an early response to hypoxia or maternal fever. Bradycardia may occur in response to vagal stimulation or prolonged hypoxia.
b. Variability. If short-term variability is evaluated separately at the facility, a fetal scalp electrode provides the most accurate data. Consider effects of medication or preterm gestation and fetal sleep when evaluating variability.	b. Moderate variability (6 to 25 bpm) provides reassurance that the fetal central nervous system (CNS) is currently well oxygenated and that the fetal heart is responsive to CNS signals. Nonhypoxic causes that may reduce variability include fetal sleep, maternal sedative medications, prematurity, or fetal CNS anomalies (e.g., anencephaly).

Continued

Nursing Care Plan

Intrapartum Fetal Compromise—cont'd

INTERVENTION	RATIONALE
c. Periodic changes: Accelerations, decelerations. Note relationship of periodic changes to fetal movement, contractions, and the woman's status and activity. Note nonperiodic (random) accelerations or variable decelerations.	c. Accelerations are a reassuring sign. Early decelerations are a normal response to head compression, but care must be taken to distinguish them from late decelerations. Late (uteroplacental insufficiency) and variable (umbilical cord compression) decelerations are nonreassuring.
d. Uterine activity: Evaluate frequency and duration using either external or internal devices. Estimate their intensity with an external device by palpating three or more contractions. Note whether the uterus relaxes between contractions for at least 30 sec. If an intrauterine pressure catheter is used, read the contraction intensity and uterine resting tone from a scale on the strip.	d. Contractions that are too long (over 90-120 sec) or too frequent (closer than every 2 min), a resting interval of less than 30 sec, or intrauterine resting pressure of more than 20 mm Hg (average normal is 5-15 mm Hg) can reduce placental exchange.
5. If nonreassuring patterns develop, take appropriate corrective actions such as discontinuing the oxytocin, increasing the rate of the nonadditive intravenous solution, positioning Glenda on her side, and administering oxygen. Notify the birth attendant of nonreassuring patterns, corrective actions taken, and the fetal response. Document the birth attendant's response and any orders.	5. The first priority is to identify the cause of the nonreassuring pattern and improve fetal oxygenation. The physician should be updated on the maternal-fetal status for needed medical orders or interventions.

Evaluation

Goals are not established for collaborative problems. The nurse should continuously compare current data from the fetal monitor and other sources, such as maternal blood pressures, with baseline assessment and fetal monitoring data before starting oxytocin induction and during labor.

For the first 4 hours of the oxytocin induction, the fetal heart rate continued near its baseline of 125 to 135 bpm, with variability averaging 10 bpm. Fetal heart rate accelerations continued. No nonreassuring patterns were noted.

ASSESSMENT

The physician ruptures Glenda's membranes and inserts internal devices for assessing the fetal heart rate and uterine activity. Glenda's blood pressure remains near 145/90, and her oxytocin infusion continues. A pattern of repeated late decelerations with baseline variability less than 5 bpm develops 1 hour after the membranes are ruptured. The nurse stops the oxytocin infusion and increases the rate of nonadditive intravenous fluid, positions Glenda on her left side, and administers oxygen at 10 L/min by facemask. Maternal pulse oximeter readings range from 97%-100%. The physician is notified. Glenda is holding Paul's hand tightly and breathing rapidly. Her vital signs are now: blood pressure, 145/90; pulse, 98; and respirations, 32. Uterine activity is normal (contractions, every 3-4 min; duration, 45-60 sec; intensity, 50 mm Hg; resting tone, 15 mm Hg).

Lack of knowledge contributes to anxiety. Note the anxiety level of the woman and her partner when the electronic monitor is used. For example, is the woman afraid to move because the fetal heart sounds and tracing skip at that time? Does she place the monitor's data above her own comfort? Note questions about the monitor and its data. Reassess after teaching to identify information that is still unclear or causing anxiety.

Nursing Diagnosis and Planning

Many women expect to have continuous electronic fetal monitoring during labor, and they have often been introduced to it during prepared childbirth classes. Most women have additional questions, however, and some women know little about this mode of fetal surveillance. The nursing diagnosis selected is

■ Deficient Knowledge: fetal monitoring.
Expected Outcome: After being taught about intrapartum fetal surveillance, the woman and her partner will express understanding of the equipment, procedures, limitations, and expected data.

Interventions

Explaining Fetal Heart Rate Auscultation With Uterine Palpation

Many women are surprised to know that auscultation and palpation are accepted modes of fetal surveillance during labor because they do not know of anyone who had this "low-tech" approach. Explain that the frequency of assessment by either method varies with risk status and stage of labor. Also explain that the physician or midwife may recommend electronic fetal monitoring for several reasons and that this does not necessarily indicate a complication.

Nursing Care Plan

Intrapartum Fetal Compromise—cont'd

Nursing Diagnosis

Anxiety related to unexpected development of complications.

Goals/Expected Outcomes

Glenda will:

- Have a reduced respiratory rate (14 to 22 breaths per minute) after interventions.
- Have a more relaxed face and body posture after interventions.

INTERVENTION	RATIONALE
1. Maintain calm behavior while performing corrective actions and notifying the physician.	1. Calm behavior communicates to Glenda and Paul that mother and fetus are receiving competent care. Anxious or dramatic behavior on the part of caregivers will increase the parents' anxiety.
2. Use simple, concise language for all explanations.	2. High anxiety or intense physical sensations impair one's ability to comprehend explanations.
3. Explain the following to Glenda and Paul: a. The problem that was identified b. The usual cause or causes of the problem c. Reasons for corrective actions d. Expected results e. That Glenda can talk with the oxygen mask on	3. If Glenda and Paul understand what is happening and why the corrective actions are taken, they are more likely to comply with the care. Knowledge decreases fear of the unknown. Assuring Glenda that she can talk with the oxygen mask on allows her to ask questions and ventilate feelings to reduce anxiety and fear.
4. Inform Glenda and Paul if the pattern improves or resolves.	4. Knowledge that the nonreassuring pattern has improved or resolved reassures parents about the fetus's condition.

Evaluation

Over the next hour, the fetal heart rate pattern gradually improves. Glenda gradually relaxes her grip on Paul's hand, and her body relaxes. Her respiratory rate slows to 22 breaths per minute. Oxygen is continued because of her risk status, but no further nonreassuring patterns occur.

Explaining the Electronic Fetal Monitor

Teaching is continuous as circumstances change. Explain the purposes of the monitor and the equipment to be used. A simple explanation entails telling the parents that the monitor is a tool to assess how the fetus reacts to labor, especially during contractions. If true, assure the woman that its use does not mean that something is wrong with her baby. Explain the reason for changes in the monitoring mode (external to internal). It may be helpful to explain that the physician or nurse-midwife evaluates many factors during labor and that the monitor strip is only one of those factors.

Addressing Parents' Safety Concerns

Parents are often concerned about attachment of the scalp electrode to the fetal presenting part. Show them that the electrode is a very fine wire that penetrates the outer layer of skin only (about 1 mm, or the thickness of a dime). If she is concerned about the intrauterine pressure catheter or fetal pulse oximeter, tell her that it lies beside the fetus, next to the inner wall of the uterus.

Coping With Misleading Data

Teach the woman that the monitor data sometime suggest a problem when none exists. For example, the fetal heart rate may suddenly fall to zero and the audible tone stop if the sensor (external or scalp electrode) is displaced. Tell her to call the nurse for adjustment or replacement of the sensor. Explain that normal labor progress and fetal movement may alter the best location for assessing the fetal heart rate externally by either auscultation or electronic monitor.

The woman may be discouraged because the curves representing contractions on the electronic monitor do not look as

PARENTS
Want to Know

About Electronic Fetal Monitoring

When women have electronic fetal monitoring during labor, they often have questions that the nurse may answer. Here are some commonly asked questions and answers the nurse might use.

Can I move around with the monitor?
You can move freely with the monitor. If you notice that the machine isn't picking up the fetal heart sounds or contractions as well, call me and I'll readjust it. Make yourself comfortable; then we'll adjust the machine if necessary.

What if I need to go to the bathroom?
If you need to go to the bathroom, we'll unplug the cords from the machine and you can walk in there or we can roll the monitor to the door of the bathroom. There may be some circumstances in which ambulation or discontinuation of the monitor is not recommended.

Will the monitor shock me? I don't know if I want to be hooked to an electrical outlet, especially since my water has broken.
Any monitor parts that are attached to you and your baby only transmit information into the machine for processing. The sensors on your body are isolated from electrical parts in the monitor.

Why is the baby's heart beating so fast?
A baby's heart normally beats faster than an adult's, both before and after birth. The normal rate is about 110 to 160 beats per minute. A higher or lower rate does not necessarily mean that the baby has a problem, but we do look at the monitor strip closely to see how the baby is doing.

Why do those numbers for the baby's heart rate change all the time?
The heart rate of a healthy baby who is awake changes constantly. When the baby moves, the heart often speeds up, just as yours does. If the baby sleeps, the heart rate may change less.

What do those numbers for contractions on the machine (external monitor) **mean? They change all the time.**
The numbers reflect a change in the pressure that the monitor senses. The monitor senses many changes in pressure other than those from contractions, such as changes from breathing, coughing, or movement of you or the baby.

My contractions don't look very strong, but they sure seem strong to me! (External uterine activity monitor is being used.)
The external monitor senses contractions indirectly rather than sensing the actual pressure inside the uterus. Their appearance on the tracing varies because of many factors, such as your position, the position of the sensor on your abdomen, and the thickness of your abdominal wall.

Will the internal monitor hurt my baby?
The spiral electrode attaches only to the outer layer of skin on the baby's head. We avoid sensitive areas on the head, such as the fontanels (soft spots) or the face. The uterine catheter or fetal pulse oximeter slides up beside the baby.

---

strong on the strip as they feel to her. This situation is more likely if an external transducer is used. Explain the many factors that may cause the contraction curves to appear stronger or weaker than they really are. When an external tocotransducer is used, tell her that the strip is used mainly to assess the timing of contractions and the fetus's reaction. Explain that an intrauterine pressure catheter may be recommended if knowledge of intrauterine pressure is crucial. Explain also that data from the catheter may become inaccurate because of obstruction by amniotic fluid debris or pressure between the fetal head and pelvic structures during late labor.

Reassure the woman that her perception of her contractions and discomfort is important. Value the woman-generated data as well as the machine-generated data. Palpate contractions at intervals as well as evaluating their appearance on the monitor strip.

It is natural for the nurse's attention to be drawn to the electronic fetal monitor when entering the room. Stay focused on the woman and her family rather than devoting excessive attention to the monitoring equipment. The woman is having the baby, not the monitor.

Including the Labor Partner
Tell the partner how to identify the onset and peak of contractions. During active labor, some women discover that contractions become intense before they can prepare for them. If this is the case, have the coach tell the woman when

each contraction begins. The coach also can tell her when the peak has passed, to encourage her.

Enhancing Comfort
Auscultation and palpation allow intermittent fetal surveillance with minimal interruption of the woman's comfort measures for labor. However, the reassuring sounds generated by the electronic fetal monitor may also enhance emotional comfort.

Some women are reluctant to make themselves more comfortable when an electronic monitor is used. Nursing care involves finding ways to make the mother comfortable and the monitor as nonintrusive as possible. Teach her ways to improve comfort while still obtaining an adequate tracing.

Explain that staying in one position is uncomfortable and does not promote normal labor. The woman may assume any position other than supine unless a specific position is needed. Encourage her to find the position in which she is most comfortable; then adjust the external devices to best detect contractions and the fetal heartbeat. Internal devices may be an option if external devices cannot be adjusted to provide useful data.

If the woman finds the sound produced by the electronic fetal monitor distracting or inconsistent with the atmosphere she desires, lower the sound or turn it off. Remember that the auditory cues for rate accelerations and decelerations are absent.

If no other contraindications to walking exist, the woman may go to the bathroom to urinate or defecate when an electronic fetal monitor is used. Unplug the sensors at the machine and let her walk to the bathroom. Reconnect and adjust them when she returns. Alternatively, you may roll the machine to the door of the bathroom, keeping the cables connected. Sensors will need adjustment when she returns to bed, even if they were not disconnected. Document ambulation interruptions in monitoring on the strip. If the fetus has a persistent nonreassuring pattern or internal sensors, it may be best not to interrupt the recording.

Evaluation

The evaluation of parental knowledge is continuous because most parents think of questions after initial explanations and as conditions change. Do the partners indicate their understanding after each explanation? Their understanding may be accompanied by a decrease in anxiety as well.

FETAL OXYGENATION

Assessment

Use a systematic approach to evaluate data from intermittent auscultation with palpation or a fetal monitoring strip. Assess the fetal heart rate for baseline and for variability and periodic changes if using the electronic fetal monitor. Assess uterine activity for frequency, duration, and intensity of contractions and for uterine resting tone. Calculate Montevideo units for intrauterine pressure catheter data if that is unit policy. Intervals for assessment and documentation are the same as those recommended for intermittent auscultation:

- Women without risk factors: every 30 minutes during active first-stage labor and every 15 minutes during the second stage
- Women with risk factors: every 15 minutes during active first-stage labor and every 5 minutes during the second stage

See Table 18-2 for additional guidelines for evaluating and documenting the fetal heart rate.

Take the woman's temperature every 4 hours and then every 2 hours after the membranes rupture. Maternal fever increases the fetal temperature and fetal oxygen requirements. Assess the woman's pulse, respirations, and blood pressure at least hourly or with fetal assessments. Hypotension or hypertension may reduce maternal blood flow to the intervillous spaces.

Assessment of mother and fetus is continuous during the dynamic process of labor. Compare data about fetal heart rate patterns, uterine activity, and maternal vital signs with baseline data and normal ranges. Observe for subtle trends in the data. Distinguish between patterns having similar appearances, such as early and late decelerations.

Vaginal examination (see Chapter 17) may be performed to evaluate specific fetal heart rate patterns—for example, to check for a prolapsed cord if a pattern of variable decelerations occurs.

Nursing Diagnosis and Planning

The collaborative problem potential complication: fetal compromise is selected for nursing care related to fetal oxygenation when electronic fetal monitoring is used.

TABLE 18-2 Guidelines for Assessment and Documentation of Fetal Heart Rate Using Auscultation

Women Without Risk Factors	Women With Risk Factors Present on Admission or That Develop During Labor
ACTIVE FIRST-STAGE LABOR	
At least every 30 min, just after a contraction	At least every 15 min, just after a contraction
SECOND-STAGE LABOR	
At least every 15 min	At least every 5 min

Other Times to Document Fetal Heart Rate
- Before artificial rupture of the membranes; after rupture of the membranes, either artificially or spontaneously.
- Before and after ambulation.
- If contractions become too frequent or last too long or if there is an inadequate interval between them.
- Before administration of oxytocin and when evaluating the dose for increase, maintenance, or decrease.
- Before administration of sedative medications or central nervous system depressants and at time of peak action.
- Before epidural analgesia is started and every 15 min for 1 hr after it is started.

Because the nurse cannot manage every instance of fetal distress independently, client (fetal) goals are not made. The nurse's responsibility includes planning to:

- Promote adequate fetal oxygenation.
- Take corrective actions to increase fetal oxygenation if nonreassuring patterns are identified.
- Report nonreassuring patterns to the physician or nurse-midwife.
- Support the woman and her partner if a complication develops.
- Document assessments and care.

Interventions

Measures to promote fetal oxygenation are discussed with the care of the woman in normal labor (see Chapter 17) and of the woman having an epidural or subarachnoid block (see Chapter 19).

Taking Corrective Actions

If a nonreassuring pattern is noted, take actions to identify its cause and improve fetal oxygenation. Birth facilities have protocols for interventions if nonreassuring patterns develop. Nursing interventions may include both independent and delegated actions.

Reassuring Parents

Parents understandably become anxious when a nonreassuring fetal assessment occurs. Remain at the bedside and use a calm manner to avoid increasing their anxiety. Use the call bell to summon other nurses if needed to help with corrective actions and to notify the physician or nurse-midwife.

Explain the problem that was identified and the reason for corrective actions in simple, concise language. Severe anxiety

---

BOX 18-2
Documenting Electronic Fetal Monitoring

Documentation When Monitoring is Inititated
Monitor Strip
Woman's name and hospital or other permanent identifying number
Physician's or nurse-midwife's name
Date and time of admission
Date and time monitoring begins (verify accuracy of electronic monitor date and time)
Gravidity, parity, abortions, living children
Gestation in weeks
Presence of identified risk factors
Character of amniotic fluid (when membranes rupture)
Function test of monitor accuracy
Initial mode of monitoring (external or internal devices)

Labor Record
Patient and healthcare provider identifying information
Date and time of admission, mode of admission (ambulatory, wheelchair, stretcher)
Date, time, and monitor mode (external or internal)
Prenatal record if available
Admission database and assessment
Signs and symptoms displayed by woman (e.g., bloody show, pain, nonlabor problems)
Admission procedures such as laboratory work or intravenous access
First panel number when strip begins (paper strips)

Continuing Documentation
Monitor Strip
Maternal vital signs at appropriate intervals for stage of labor, membrane status, and interventions such as labor stimulation or pain management measures
Notations of strip review at intervals appropriate for risk factors and labor status (see Table 18-2)
Vaginal examinations, including cervical dilation and effacement and fetal station
Rupture of membranes (spontaneously or artificially)
Color, quantity, and character (e.g., foul odor, cloudiness) of amniotic fluid
Maternal position changes
Maternal or fetal movement that affects tracing
Maternal vomiting, coughing, or other movement that affects tracing
Summaries while pushing in second stage
Equipment adjustments, problems maintaining continuous tracing (e.g., an active fetus)
Medication and anesthetic, including related interventions
Changes of equipment mode such as external to internal device
Interventions for nonreassuring patterns and maternal-fetal response
Interruptions or discontinuation of electronic monitoring

Labor Record
Notations of vital signs, procedures or interventions and maternal responses, pain level and control measures, support of labor partner, teaching and patient understanding
Periodic summary of maternal vital signs, baseline fetal heart rate, variability, periodic changes, and uterine activity (frequency, duration, and intensity of contractions and uterine resting tone) at intervals specified by the facility
Nonreassuring maternal or fetal assessments, interventions, responses, provider notification, and provider response

---

NOTE: The term "strip" refers to an onscreen display of the electronic fetal monitor strip as well as a paper strip. Some annotations listed may be automatically entered by the monitor according to settings chosen by the nurse. Information documented in a labor record is often entered on several different chart forms or flowsheets.

reduces the parents' ability to understand information. Inform them if the fetal heart rate returns to a reassuring pattern. Some corrective actions, such as oxygen administration and positioning, may continue after a reassuring pattern returns. Tell the woman that she may talk with the oxygen mask on.

Reporting Nonreassuring Patterns
Notify the birth attendant of nonreassuring patterns as soon as possible after taking corrective actions. The priority of nursing care is to improve fetal oxygenation. Document the time and content of all consultations with the physician or

nurse-midwife about the mother or fetus and document the birth attendant's response.

Documenting Assessments and Care

Data related to fetal well-being in both the labor record and on the monitor strip are permanent records and should be complete. Box 18-2 shows guidelines for documentation on the monitor strip and labor record. Documentation can demonstrate good nursing care and show that the standard of care has been met.

Label a paper strip with the woman's name, the date, and the time when electronic fetal monitoring begins. If a break in the strip occurs, such as to change paper, label the new strip with the woman's name, the date, and the time. Label each section of a multi-part strip so that the entire paper record can be reassembled sequentially. Electronic "strips" include time for automatic and typed notations. Late entries can also be made as on a paper chart. Some units do not print all parts of strips if they are stored electronically. Printing may be required if electronic storage is not functional at the time or if a printed view of a specific section of the strip is desired.

Continue documenting the heart rate and maternal observations until vaginal birth occurs. If a cesarean birth is needed, a minimum of one fetal heart rate assessment is done after arrival in the operating room, with additional assessments done if surgery is delayed. Remove internal devices before securing the woman's legs to the operating table. Document the time of arrival in the operating room, all fetal heart rate and contraction assessments, the time of abdominal incision, and the time of birth. The unit should have a consistent method to document times, often by the electronic fetal monitor clock.

Evaluation

Client-centered goals are not formulated for a collaborative problem. The nurse compares data with established standards to determine whether they are within normal limits. If nonreassuring patterns are identified, the nurse:

- Takes measures to increase fetal oxygenation
- Notifies the physician or nurse-midwife
- Documents all relevant data

KEY CONCEPTS

- The purpose of intrapartum fetal surveillance is to identify fetal well-being and to identify the fetus who may be having hypoxic stress beyond the ability to compensate for it.
- The two approaches to intrapartum fetal monitoring are intermittent auscultation with palpation of uterine activity and electronic fetal monitoring. Each type has distinct advantages and limitations. Electronic fetal monitoring has not been shown to be superior to auscultation with palpation.
- Fetal oxygenation depends on a normal flow of oxygenated maternal blood into the placenta, normal exchange within the placenta,

patent umbilical cord vessels, and normal fetal circulatory and oxygen-carrying function.
- Stimulation of the sympathetic nervous system increases the fetal heart rate and strengthens the heart contraction. Stimulation of the parasympathetic nervous system slows the heart rate. The push-pull action of speeding and slowing the heart rate is evidenced by the wavy appearance of the baseline in the fetus who is monitored electronically.
- Intermittent auscultation and palpation allow the greatest amount of maternal movement but also require a 1-to-1 nurse-patient ratio for proper surveillance.

- External electronic fetal monitoring is less accurate for fetal heart rate and uterine activity patterns than internal monitoring, but it is noninvasive and does not require ruptured membranes.
- Greater accuracy is the main advantage of internal electronic fetal monitoring devices, but these are invasive and require ruptured membranes.
- Nursing responsibilities related to intrapartum fetal surveillance by any mode include promoting fetal oxygenation, identifying and reporting nonreassuring findings, supporting parents, communicating with the physician or nurse-midwife, and documenting all care.

ANSWERS to Critical Thinking Exercise 18-1

1. The pattern described is one of late decelerations, probably caused by excess uterine activity secondary to the use of oxytocin. Presence of moderate variability in the fetal heart rate suggests that the fetus is currently tolerating the uterine hyperstimulation.
2. Although the fetus seems to be tolerating the hyperstimulation, continued excess contractions may exceed fetal reserves, so corrective actions should be taken promptly, but

not urgently. Jackie's initial action should be to stop the oxytocin infusion to reduce stimulation of uterine activity and increase the rate of Nancy's nonadditive intravenous fluid. Oxygen should be given through a snug facemask at 8 to 10 L/min. Nancy should be placed on her side, if she is not already in this position, to increase placental blood flow. Turning to the opposite side may be helpful if she is already on her side. After

the immediate corrective actions are completed, Jackie should contact Nancy's physician or nurse-midwife, documenting interventions and patient/fetal response, the content of the call, and the healthcare provider's response.

ANSWERS to Critical Thinking Exercise 18-2

1. The pattern described is one of variable decelerations, usually associated with cord compression. The student should use the call bell to summon a more experienced nurse. At the same time, LaShonda should be asked to change her position. If she is on her left side, she should turn to the right.

Changing position may relieve pressure on the cord. The experienced nurse will further evaluate LaShonda and her baby and may perform other interventions.
2. The physician should be contacted, but attempting to correct the cause of the variable decelerations is the priority. Document all

corrective actions and the patient/fetal response, any contact with the physician, and physician responses.

REFERENCES and READINGS

Adelsperger, D., & Waymire, V.J. (2003). Physiological interventions for fetal heart rate patterns. In N. Feinstein, K.L. Torgersen, & J. Atterbury (Eds.), *Association of Women's Health, Obstetric, and Neonatal Nurses' Fetal heart monitoring: Principles and practices* (3rd ed., pp. 159-175). Dubuque, IA: Kendall/Hunt.

American Academy of Pediatrics, & American College of Obstetricians and Gynecologists. (2002). *Guidelines for perinatal care* (5th ed.). Elk Grove Village, IL, and Washington, DC: Author.

American College of Obstetricians and Gynecologists. (1995). *Fetal heart rate patterns: Monitoring, interpretation, and management* (ACOG Technical Bulletin No. 207). Washington, DC: Author.

Association of Women's Health, Obstetric, and Neonatal Nurses (AWHONN). (1998). *Clinical competencies and education guide: Antepartum and intrapartum fetal heart rate monitoring.* Washington, DC: Author.

Blackburn, S.T. (2003). *Maternal, fetal, and neonatal physiology: A clinical perspective* (2nd ed.). Philadelphia: Saunders.

Cunningham, F.G., Gant, N.F., Leveno, K.J., Gilstrap, L.C., Hauth, J.C., & Wenstrom, K.D. (2001). *Williams obstetrics* (21st ed.). New York: McGraw-Hill.

Cypher, R.L., & Adelsperger, D. (2003). Assessment of fetal oxygenation and acid-base status. In N. Feinstein, K.L. Torgersen, & J. Atterbury (Eds.), *Association of Women's Health, Obstetric, and Neonatal Nurses' Fetal heart monitoring: Principles and practices* (3rd ed., pp. 177-198). Dubuque, IA: Kendall/Hunt.

Cypher, R.L., Adelsperger, D., & Torgersen, K.L. (2003). Interpretation of fetal heart rate patterns. In N. Feinstein, K.L. Torgersen, & J. Atterbury (Eds.), Association of Women's Health, Obstetric, & Neonatal Nurses. *Fetal Heart Monitoring Principles and Practices* (3rd ed., pp. 113-158). ADubuque, IA: Kendall/Hunt.

Feinstein, N.F., Sprague, A., & Trépanier, M.J. (2000). *Fetal heart rate auscultation.* Washington, DC: Association of Women's Health, Obstetric, and Neonatal Nurses.

Gilstrap, L.C. (2004). Fetal acid-base balance. In R. Creasy, R. Resnik, & J.D. Iams (Eds.), *Maternal-fetal medicine: Principles and practice* (5th ed., pp. 429-439). Philadelphia: Saunders.

Glantz, J.C., & Woods, J.R. (2004). Significance of amniotic fluid meconium. In R. Creasy, R. Resnik, & J.D. Iams (Eds.), *Maternal-fetal medicine: Principles and practice* (5th ed., pp. 441-450). Philadelphia: Saunders.

Guyton, A.C., & Hall, J.E. (2000). *Textbook of medical physiology* (10th ed.). Philadelphia: Saunders.

Harman, C.R. (2004). Assessment of fetal health. In R.K. Creasy, R. Resnik, & J.D. Iams (Eds.), *Maternal-fetal medicine: Principles and practice,* (5th ed., pp. 357-401). Philadelphia: Saunders.

King, T.L., & Simpson, K.R. (1999). Fetal assessment during labor. In K.R. Simpson & P.A. Creehan (Eds.), *AWHONN perinatal nursing* (pp. 378-416). Philadelphia: Lippincott.

Mahoney, K., Torgersen, K.L., & Feinstein, N. (2003). Maternal-fetal assessment. In N. Feinstein, K.L. Torgersen, & J. Atterbury (Eds.), *Association of Women's Health, Obstetric, and Neonatal Nurses' Fetal heart monitoring: Principles and practices* (3rd ed., pp. 61-76). Dubuque, IA: Kendall/Hunt.

Martin, J.A., Hamilton, B.E., Sutton, P.D., Ventura, S.J., Menacker, F., & Park, M.M. (2003). Births: Final data for 2002. *National Vital Statistics Reports, 52*(10). Hyattsville, MD: National Center for Health Statistics.

National Institute of Child Health and Human Development (NICHD) Research Planning Workshop. (1997). Electronic fetal heart rate monitoring: Research guidelines for interpretation. *Journal of Obstetric, Gynecologic, and Neonatal Nursing, 26*(6), 635-640.

Parer, J.T., & King, T. (2000). Fetal heart rate monitoring: Is it salvageable? *American Journal of Obstetrics and Gynecology, 182*(4), 982-987.

Parer, J., & Nageotte, M.P. (2004). Intrapartum fetal surveillance. In R. Creasy, R. Resnik, & J.D. Iams (Eds.), *Maternal-fetal medicine: Principles and practice* (5th ed., pp. 403-427). Philadelphia: Saunders.

Seelbach-Göbel, B., Heupel, M., Kühnert, M., & Butterwegge, M. (1999). The prediction of fetal acidosis by means of intrapartum fetal pulse oximetry. *American Journal of Obstetrics and Gynecology, 180*(1 Pt. 1), 73-81.

Simpson, K.R. (1998). Fetal oxygen saturation monitoring during labor. *Journal of Perinatal and Neonatal Nursing, 12*(3), 26-37.

Simpson, K.R. (2003). Fetal pulse oximetry update. *AWHONN Lifelines, 7*(5), 411-412.

Tucker, S.M. (2000). *Mosby's fetal monitoring and assessment* (4th ed.). St. Louis: Mosby.

Williams, K.P., & Galerneau, F. (2003). Intrapartum fetal heart rate patterns in the prediction of neonatal acidemia. *American Journal of Obstetrics and Gynecology, 188*(3), 820-823.

Wood, S.H. (2003). Should women be given a choice about fetal assessment in labor? *MCN: The American Journal of Maternal/Child Nursing, 28*(5), 292-298.

19

Pain Management for Childbirth

LEARNING OBJECTIVES

After studying this chapter, you should be able to:

◎ Compare childbirth pain with other types of pain.
◎ Describe how excessive pain can affect the laboring woman and her fetus.
◎ Examine how physical and psychologic forces interact in the laboring woman's pain experience.
◎ Describe the use of nonpharmacologic pain management techniques in labor.

◎ Describe how medications may affect a pregnant woman and the fetus or neonate.
◎ Identify the benefits and risks of specific pharmacologic pain-control methods.
◎ Explain nursing care related to different types of intrapartum pain management.

DEFINITIONS

agonist A substance that causes a physiologic effect.

analgesic A systemic agent that relieves pain without loss of consciousness.

anesthesia Loss of sensation, especially pain sensation, with or without loss of consciousness.

anesthesiologist A physician who specializes in the administration of anesthesia.

antagonist A drug that blocks the action of another drug or of body secretions.

aspiration pneumonitis A chemical injury to the lungs that may occur with regurgitation and aspiration of acidic gastric secretions.

cleansing breath A deep breath taken at the beginning and end of each labor contraction.

effleurage Massage of the abdomen or other body part performed during labor contractions.

endorphins Morphine-like substances that occur naturally in the central nervous system and modify pain sensations.

epidural space The area outside the dura, between the dura mater and the vertebral canal.

general anesthesia Systemic loss of sensation with loss of consciousness.

motor block Loss of voluntary movement caused by regional anesthesia.

nurse anesthetist A registered nurse who has advanced education and certification in administration of anesthetics. Also called a *certified registered nurse anesthetist (CRNA)*.

pain threshold (or pain perception) The lowest level of stimulus one perceives as painful. Pain threshold is relatively constant under different conditions.

pain tolerance Maximum pain one is willing to endure. Pain tolerance may increase or decrease under different conditions.

regional anesthesia Anesthesia that blocks pain impulses in a localized area without loss of consciousness.

sensory block Loss of sensation caused by regional anesthesia.

subarachnoid space Space between the arachnoid mater and the pia mater that contains the cerebrospinal fluid.

Each woman has unique expectations about birth, including expectations about pain and her ability to manage it. The woman who successfully handles the pain of labor is more likely to view her experience as a positive life event. A woman's experience with labor pain varies with several physical and psychologic elements, and each woman responds differently. Nonpharmacologic and pharmacologic methods give the nurse and laboring woman a selection of pain management techniques to choose from.

UNIQUE NATURE OF PAIN DURING BIRTH

Pain involves two components:

• A physiologic component, which includes reception by sensory nerves and transmission to the central nervous system.
• A psychologic component, which involves recognizing the sensation, interpreting it as painful, and reacting to the interpretation.

Pain is subjective and personal; no one can feel another's pain. One must simply believe what another person says about his or her pain experience.

Childbirth pain, however, differs from other pain in several important respects:

- Childbirth pain is part of a normal process, whereas other types of pain usually indicate an injury or illness. Pain may encourage the unmedicated woman to assume different positions in labor, favoring rotation and descent of the fetus.
- The pregnant woman has several months to prepare for birth, including acquiring skills to help manage pain. Realistic preparation and knowledge about the birth process help her develop skills to cope with labor pain.
- Labor pain has a foreseeable end. A woman can expect her labor to end in hours, rather than days, weeks, or months. Other kinds of pain may also be brief, but the baby's birth brings a rapid decrease in pain.
- Labor pain is not constant but intermittent. A woman may describe little discomfort with contractions during early labor. Even during late labor, she may be relatively comfortable during the short rest periods between contractions.
- Labor ends with the birth of a baby. The emotional significance of her child's birth cannot be ignored when trying to understand a woman's response to pain. Concern about her fetus often motivates a woman to tolerate more pain during labor than she otherwise might be willing to endure.

ADVERSE EFFECTS OF EXCESSIVE PAIN

Although expected during labor, pain that exceeds a woman's tolerance can have harmful effects on her and the fetus.

Physiologic Effects

Labor increases a woman's metabolic rate and her demand for oxygen. Pain and anxiety escalate her already high metabolic rate by increasing production of catecholamines (epinephrine and norepinephrine), cortisol, and glucagon. She breathes fast to obtain more oxygen, exhaling too much carbon dioxide in the process, and having less oxygen to share with her fetus. Significant changes, more than those expected during labor, can occur in the woman's PaO_2 and $PaCO_2$ and in her arterial pH. These maternal respiratory and metabolic changes alter placental exchange of oxygen and waste products, even in the presence of normal placental circulation. The fetus has less oxygen available for uptake and is less able to unload carbon dioxide to the mother. The net result is that the fetus shifts to anaerobic metabolism, with the buildup of hydrogen ions (metabolic acidosis).

Excessive catecholamine secretion inhibits uterine response to oxytocin secretion of the posterior pituitary. Contractions become shorter, less frequent, and less effective, slowing labor progress.

High catecholamine levels reduce blood flow to the uterus and placenta. The fetus is more likely to become hypoxic and eventually shift to anaerobic metabolism if good placental blood flow is not restored. In addition, contractions become irritable and poorly effective, possibly resulting in dystocia and inhibiting labor progress (see Chapter 27).

Psychologic Effects

Poorly relieved pain lessens the pleasure of this extraordinary life event for both partners. The mother may find it difficult to interact with her infant because she is depleted from a painful, exhausting labor. Unpleasant memories of the birth may affect her response to sexual activity or another labor. Her partner may feel inadequate as a support person during birth.

VARIABLES IN CHILDBIRTH PAIN

Physical and psychosocial factors contribute to a woman's response to the pain of labor.

Physical Factors

Childbirth pain is of two types—visceral and somatic. Visceral pain is a slow, deep pain that is poorly localized. It is often described as dull or aching. Visceral pain dominates during first-stage labor as the uterus contracts and the cervix dilates.

Somatic pain is a faster, sharp pain. It can be precisely localized. Somatic pain is most prominent during late first-stage labor and during second-stage labor as the descending fetus puts direct pressure on maternal tissues.

Sources of Pain

Four potential sources of labor pain exist in most labors. Other physical factors may modify labor pain, increasing or decreasing it.

Tissue Ischemia. The blood supply to the uterus decreases during contractions, leading to tissue hypoxia and anaerobic metabolism. Ischemic uterine pain has been likened to ischemic heart pain.

Cervical Dilation. Dilation and stretching of the cervix and lower uterus are a major source of pain. Pain stimuli from cervical dilation travel through the hypogastric plexus, entering the spinal cord at the T10, T11, T12, and L1 levels (Fig. 19-1).

Pressure and Pulling on Pelvic Structures. Some pain results from pressure and pulling on pelvic structures such as ligaments, fallopian tubes, ovaries, bladder, and peritoneum. The pain is a visceral pain; a woman may feel it as referred pain in her back and legs.

Distention of the Vagina and Perineum. Marked distention of the vagina and perineum occurs with fetal descent, especially during the second stage. The woman may describe a sensation of burning, tearing, or splitting (somatic pain). Pain from vaginal and perineal distention and pressure and pulling on adjacent structures enters the spinal cord at the S2, S3, and S4 levels (see Fig. 19-1).

Factors Influencing the Perception or Tolerance of Pain

Although physiologic processes cause labor pain, a woman's tolerance of pain may be affected by other physical influences.

Intensity of Labor. The woman who has a short, intense labor often complains of severe pain because each contraction does so much work (effacement, dilation, and fetal descent). A rapid labor may limit her options for pharmacologic pain relief as well.

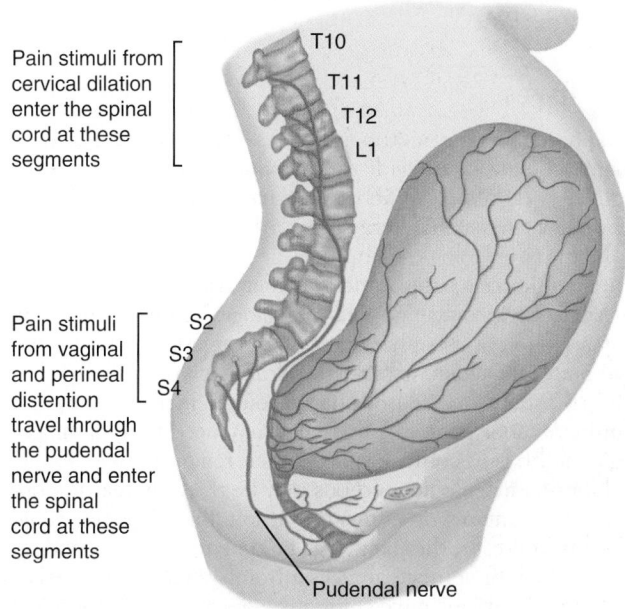

Pain stimuli from cervical dilation enter the spinal cord at these segments

T10
T11
T12
L1

Pain stimuli from vaginal and perineal distention travel through the pudendal nerve and enter the spinal cord at these segments

S2
S3
S4

Pudendal nerve

Figure 19-1 Pathways of pain transmission during labor.

Cervical Readiness. If prelabor cervical changes (softening, with some dilation and effacement) are incomplete, the cervix does not open as easily. More contractions are needed to achieve dilation and effacement, resulting in a longer labor and greater fatigue in the laboring woman.

Fetal Position. Labor is likely to be longer and more uncomfortable when the fetus is in an unfavorable position. An occiput posterior fetal position is a common variant seen in otherwise normal labors. In this position, each contraction pushes the fetal occiput against the woman's sacrum. She experiences intense back discomfort (*back labor*) that persists between contractions. Often a woman cannot deliver her infant in the occiput posterior position. The fetal head must therefore rotate in a wider arc before the mechanisms of extension and expulsion occur, so labor is often longer (see Chapter 17). Back pain may decrease dramatically when a fetus rotates into the more favorable occiput anterior position. The rate of labor progress usually increases as well.

Characteristics of the Pelvis. The size and shape of a woman's pelvis influence the course and length of her labor. Abnormalities may cause a difficult and longer labor and may contribute to fetal malpresentation or malposition.

Fatigue. Fatigue reduces a woman's ability to tolerate pain and to use coping skills she has learned. She may be unable to focus on relaxation and breathing techniques that would otherwise help her tolerate labor.

Many women sleep poorly during the last weeks of pregnancy. Shortness of breath when lying down, frequent urination, and fetal activity interrupt sleep so that a woman often begins labor with a sleep deficit. If labor begins late in the evening, she may have been awake well over 24 hours by the time she gives birth. Even if a woman begins labor well rested, slow progress may exhaust her. Women who have scheduled labor induction may have as much fatigue as those who have spontaneous labor.

Prolonged, intense pushing during the second stage is exhausting as well. For this reason, promoting a physiologic second stage in which the woman delays pushing until she feels an urge to do so ("laboring down") is preferred (see Chapter 17).

Intervention of Caregivers. Although they may be appropriate for the well-being of a woman and fetus, some interventions add discomfort to the natural pain of labor. Intravenous lines cause pain when they are inserted and remain noticeable to many women during labor. Fetal monitoring equipment and the frequent need to adjust the sensors is uncomfortable to some women. Both may hamper a woman's mobility, which she might use to assume a more comfortable position.

A woman whose labor is induced or augmented often reports more pain and increased difficulty coping with it because contractions reach peak intensity quickly. Vaginal examinations and amniotomy are uncomfortable because of vaginal and cervical stretching.

Psychosocial Factors

Several psychosocial variables influence a woman's experience of pain.

Culture

A woman's sociocultural roots influence how she perceives, interprets, and responds to pain during childbirth. Some cultures encourage loud and vigorous expression of pain, whereas others value self-control. Women are individuals within their cultural groups, however. The experience of pain is personal, and one should not make assumptions about how a woman from a specific cultural or ethnic group will behave during labor.

Women should be encouraged to express themselves in any way they find comforting, and the diversity of their expressions must be respected. Accepting a woman's individual response to labor and pain promotes a therapeutic relationship.

The nurse should avoid praising some behaviors (e.g., stoicism) while belittling others (e.g., noisy expression). This restraint is difficult because noisy women are challenging to work with and may disturb others.

The unique nature of childbirth pain and women's diverse responses to it make nursing management complex. The nurse can miss important cues if the woman is either stoic, having little outward expression of pain, or expresses herself loudly and constantly. With either extreme, the nurse may not readily identify critical information such as impending birth or the symptoms of a complication.

Anxiety and Fear

Extreme anxiety and fear magnify sensitivity to pain and impair a woman's ability to tolerate it. They consume energy she needs to cope with the birth process, including its painful aspects.

Anxiety and fear increase muscle tension, diverting oxygenated blood to the brain and skeletal muscles. Tension in pelvic muscles counters the expulsive forces of uterine contractions and the laboring woman's pushing efforts during the second stage. Prolonged tension results in general fatigue, increased pain perception, and reduced ability to use skills to cope with pain.

Previous Experiences With Pain

Early in life a child learns that pain is a symptom of bodily injury. Consequently, fear and withdrawal are a woman's natural reactions to pain during labor. Learning about the normal sensations of labor, including pain, helps a woman suppress her natural reactions of fear and withdrawal, allowing her body to do the work of birth.

A woman who has given birth previously has a different perspective. If she has had a vaginal delivery, she is probably aware of normal labor sensations and is less likely to associate them with injury or abnormality. Also, time has a way of blunting the memory of painful experiences.

A woman who had a child by cesarean birth and has never experienced labor may be particularly anxious. The experience of cesarean birth is known to her, whereas labor is unknown. A repeat cesarean birth may seem like the quicker and less painful option. She may have difficulty yielding to the normal forces of birth.

A woman who has previously had a long and difficult labor is more likely to be anxious about the outcome of the present one. If she had a cesarean birth following the difficult labor, she may doubt her ability to give birth vaginally. Her anxiety often intensifies when she reaches the point at which her prior labor ended with the cesarean birth.

Previous experiences do not always adversely affect a woman's ability to deal with pain. She may have learned ways to cope with pain during other episodes of pain or during other births and may use these skills adaptively during labor.

Preparation for Childbirth

Preparation for childbirth does not ensure a pain-free labor. A woman should be prepared for pain realistically, including reasonable expectations about analgesia and anesthesia. She may feel that her entire preparation is invalid if what she expects does not happen when she is in labor.

Preparation reduces anxiety and fear of the unknown. It allows a woman to rehearse for labor and learn a variety of skills to master pain as labor progresses. She and her partner learn about expected behavioral changes during labor, and their knowledge decreases their anxiety when those changes occur.

Support System

An anxious partner is less able to provide the support and reassurance that the woman needs during labor. In addition, anxiety in others can be contagious and an anxious partner can increase her anxiety. She may assume that if others are worried, something is probably wrong.

The birth experiences of a woman's family and friends cannot be ignored. Those individuals can be an important source of support if they convey realistic information about labor pain and its control. If they describe labor as intolerable, however, she may have needless distress. It is equally detrimental for a woman to hear that labor is painless. No two labors are alike, even for the same woman.

NONPHARMACOLOGIC PAIN MANAGEMENT

The nurse who cares for women in labor and birth can offer nonpharmacologic and pharmacologic pain management methods. Education about nonpharmacologic pain management is the foundation of prepared childbirth classes. To be most helpful to women and their labor partners, the intrapartum nurse should know methods that are taught in local childbirth classes.

Advantages

Nonpharmacologic methods have several advantages over pharmacologic methods if they produce adequate pain control. They do not slow labor and have no side effects, nor do they carry the risk of allergy or sedation.

Nonpharmacologic techniques are both an alternative to and an adjunct to drugs. Most women use a combination of pharmacologic and nonpharmacologic techniques. The woman who chooses pharmacologic analgesia needs alternative pain management until the drug is given, usually after labor is established. Also, pharmacologic methods may not eliminate labor pain and a woman may need nonpharmacologic methods to control the pain that remains.

Nonpharmacologic methods may be the only realistic option for a woman who enters the hospital in advanced, rapid labor. In this case, there may not be time to obtain a good regional block or achieve analgesia from systemic drugs. Also, the newborn might have respiratory depression if a systemic opioid narcotic reaches its peak action near the time of birth.

Limitations

Nonpharmacologic methods of pain control have limitations, especially if they are used as the sole method of pain control. Women do not always achieve their desired level of pain control using these methods alone. Because of the many variables in labor, even a well-prepared and highly motivated woman may have a difficult labor and need pharmacologic analgesia or anesthesia.

Preparation for Pain Management

The ideal time to learn nonpharmacologic pain control is before labor. During the last few weeks of pregnancy, the woman learns about labor, including its painful aspects, in childbirth classes. She can prepare to confront the pain, learning a variety of skills to use during labor. Her support person learns specific methods to encourage and support her. After admission, the nurse can review and reinforce what the partners learned in class.

The nurse can teach the unprepared woman and her support person nonpharmacologic techniques. The latent phase of labor is the best time for intrapartum teaching because the woman is usually anxious enough to be attentive and interested, yet comfortable enough to understand.

Many methods may become less effective after prolonged use, a process called *habituation*. Changing techniques counters habituation. The nurse who knows a variety of methods can select those that are most helpful to an individual woman.

Application of Nonpharmacologic Techniques

Four categories can be applied to intrapartum care: relaxation, cutaneous stimulation, mental stimulation, and breathing.

Relaxation

Promoting relaxation provides a base for all other methods, both nonpharmacologic and pharmacologic, because it does the following:

- Promotes uterine blood flow, thus improving fetal oxygenation
- Promotes efficient uterine contractions
- Reduces tension that increases pain perception and decreases pain tolerance
- Reduces tension that can inhibit fetal descent

Environmental Comfort. Comfortable surroundings support relaxation. The nurse can reduce irritants such as bright lights and can adjust the room temperature.

Music masks outside noise and provides a background for use of imagery and breathing techniques. It is a distraction that shifts the woman's attention from bodily sensations. Television may have the same effect for some women.

General Comfort. Promoting the woman's personal comfort helps her focus on pain management techniques during labor (Fig. 19-2). This includes actions to increase comfort and reduce the effect of irritants, such as a hot environment or wet bedding.

Reducing Anxiety and Fear. The nurse may reduce a woman's anxiety and increase her self-control by providing accurate information and focusing on the normality of birth. Hospitals are typically associated with illness or injury, situations that are anxiety provoking. Yet hospitals are the most common site for the normal event of birth in the United States.

Simple nursing actions keep the focus on the normality of childbirth, regardless of the setting. For example, referring to a woman as a *patient* reinforces the atmosphere of illness associated with being in a hospital, whereas calling her by name helps her to see birth as a normal process. Empowerment of the woman and her partner by giving them choices whenever possible helps them see themselves as competent people who can accomplish the task of giving birth.

Implementing Specific Relaxation Techniques. Relaxation techniques work best if they are learned and practiced before labor. During practice sessions at home, cou-

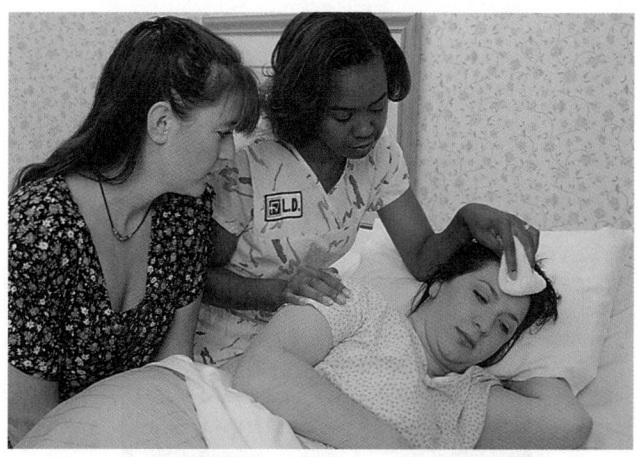

Figure 19-2 General comfort measures such as the nurse's reassuring presence or a cool, damp cloth applied to the face supplement other methods of nonpharmacologic and pharmacologic pain control.

ples may practice *progressive relaxation,* in which the woman contracts and then releases specific muscle groups until all muscles are relaxed. *Neuromuscular dissociation* helps the woman learn to relax all muscles except those that are working (the uterus or the abdominal muscles when pushing). The woman can learn *touch relaxation* in response to her partner's touch, and *relaxation against pain* as the partner deliberately causes mild pain and the woman learns to relax despite the pain.

Even if the woman did not practice these relaxation techniques at home, the nurse can teach her how to consciously relax as labor goes by. The partner can learn to watch for signs of tension, touch that area, and direct the woman to relax.

Water therapy (Box 19-1) can supplement any relaxation technique. The buoyancy afforded by immersion supports the

---

BOX 19-1
Use of Water Therapy During Labor

Use of water therapy has accompanied trends toward a low-intervention approach to intrapartum care. Water therapy can be delivered in several ways:
- Shower
- Standard tub
- Whirlpool

Benefits
- Associated with a more natural, homelike atmosphere.
- Gives a woman greater control over her labor.
- Upright position facilitates progress of labor.
- Faster labor progress if contractions are frequent when woman enters the tub.
- Buoyancy relieves tired muscles and reduces pressure.
- Facilitates fetal rotation from occiput posterior or transverse positions to the occiput anterior position. The woman can also assume different positions to aid rotation.
- Many women report a perception of less pain.
- Reduction in the mean arterial pressure, edema, and increased diuresis. This is especially helpful if the woman has pregnancy-induced hypertension.

Disadvantages
- May reduce frequency of contractions and dilation during the latent phase of labor.
- Fetus must be assessed with intermittent auscultation rather than electronic fetal monitoring.

Contraindications and Precautions
- No specific contraindications if the woman can safely be out of bed.
- Thick meconium in the amniotic fluid is an indication for continuous electronic fetal monitoring in most birth facilities and would preclude use of water therapy.
- Bleeding.
- Oxytocin induction or augmentation. The use of both oxytocin and water therapy could cause excess uterine activity.

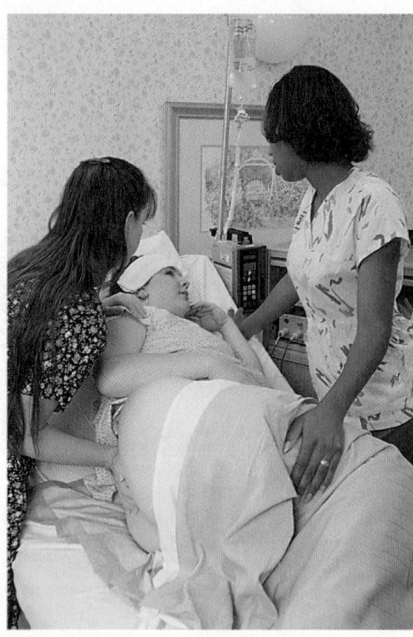

Figure 19-3 The coach applies sacral pressure to counter the back pain that is common during labor.

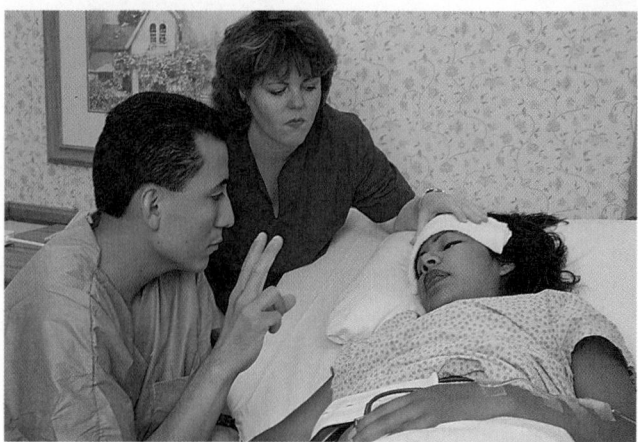

Figure 19-4 A woman and her partner who are prepared for labor have learned a variety of skills to master pain as labor progresses. The coach uses hand signals to tell the woman how to change her pattern of paced breathing.

body, equalizes pressure on the body, and aids muscle relaxation. In addition, fluid shifts from the extravascular space to the intravascular space, reducing edema as the excess fluid is excreted by the kidneys.

Cutaneous Stimulation

Cutaneous stimulation has several variations that are often combined with each other or with other techniques.

Self-Massage. The woman may rub her abdomen, legs, or back in a self-massage called *effleurage* to counteract discomfort. Some women find abdominal touch irritating, especially near the umbilicus. Women in labor may find firm stroking more helpful than very light stroking. They can trace figure-8s or circles on the bed if touch irritates them.

Some women benefit from firm palm or sole stimulation during labor. They may like to have their palms rubbed vigorously by another, rub their hands or feet together, or bang their palms on, or grip, a cool surface. They may hold another person's hand tightly during a contraction. The nurse should determine if these actions indicate excess pain or if they are a woman's way of countering pain and therefore useful.

Massage by Others. The partner or the nurse can rub the woman's back, shoulders, legs, or any area where she finds massage helpful. Sacral pressure is a variation that may help when the woman has back pain, which is usually most intense when the fetus is in an occiput posterior position. Sacral pressure may be applied using the palm of the hand, the fist or fists, or a firm object such as two tennis balls in a sock (Fig. 19-3).

Nonclinical touch by the nurse is a powerful tool if the woman does not object to it. Holding her hand, stroking her hair, or similar actions convey caring, comfort, affirmation, and reassurance at this vulnerable time.

Thermal Stimulation. Many women like to have warmth applied to their back, abdomen, or perineum during labor. A warm shower, tub bath, or whirlpool bath is relaxing and provides thermal stimulation. A sock filled with dry rice and microwaved provides gentle warmth and can be used to apply pressure to the sacral area.

Cool, damp washcloths may be comforting, especially if a woman is hot. She may put them on her head, throat, abdomen, or any place she wants. She also may want to put them in or over her mouth to relieve dryness.

Acupressure. Acupressure is a directed form of massage in which the support person applies pressure to specific pressure points using hands, rollers, balls, or other equipment. It is related to its invasive counterpart, acupuncture, in which tiny needles are inserted into similar points. Acupuncture and acupressure have data to support effectiveness to relieve nausea and vomiting, including "morning sickness" of pregnancy. Few controlled studies exist on its usefulness during birth. For updated objective information on acupressure and other complementary and alternative medicine (CAM) techniques, visit the website for the National Center for Complementary and Alternative Medicine, one of the institutes of the National Institutes of Health (www.nncam.nih.gov).

Mental Stimulation

Mental techniques occupy the woman's mind and compete with pain stimuli. They also aid relaxation by providing a tranquil imaginary atmosphere.

Imagery. If the woman has not practiced a specific imagery technique, the nurse can help her create a relaxing mental scene. Most women find images of warmth, softness, security, and total relaxation most comforting.

Imagery can help the woman dissociate herself from the painful aspects of labor. For example, the nurse can help her visualize the work of labor: the cervix opening with each contraction or the fetus moving down toward the outlet each time she pushes. This technique is like visualizing success or movement toward a goal with each contraction.

Focal Point. When using nonpharmacologic techniques, a woman may prefer to close her eyes or may want to concentrate on an external focal point. Classes emphasize that keeping the eyes open on a focal point helps her concentrate on something outside her body and thus away from the pain from contractions. She may bring a picture of a relaxing scene or an object to use as a focal point and to aid in the use of imagery. She can use any point in the room as a focal point.

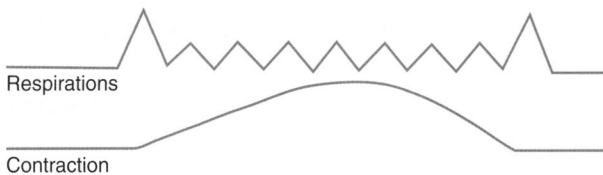

Figure 19-5 Slow-paced breathing. Although a specific rate may or may not be taught, slow-paced breathing should be *no slower than half* the woman's usual respiratory rate to ensure adequate oxygenation. This pace is generally about six to nine breaths per minute.

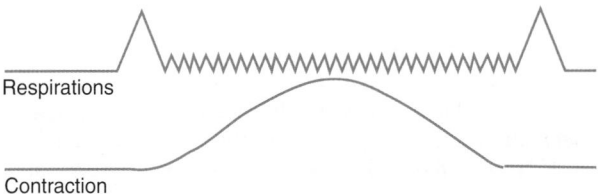

Figure 19-6 Modified-paced breathing. The pattern for modified-paced breathing should be comfortable to the woman and *no faster than twice* her normal respiratory rate to prevent hyperventilation or interference with relaxation.

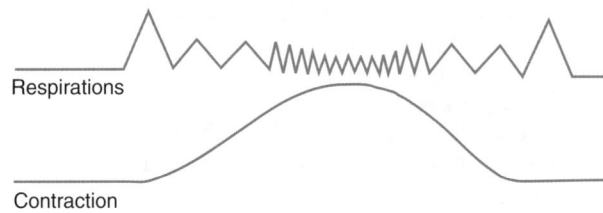

Figure 19-7 Combining breathing techniques during a contraction. Slow- and modified-paced breathing can be combined by using the slower breathing at the beginning and end of the contraction and the more rapid breathing over the peak of the contraction.

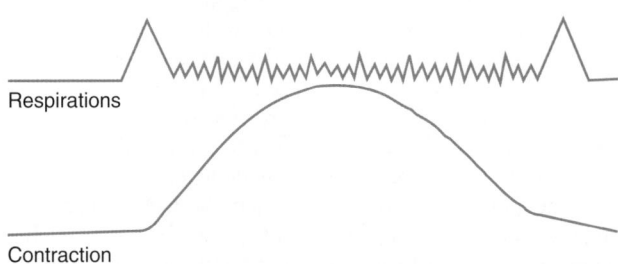

Figure 19-8 Pattern-paced breathing. Pattern-paced breathing adds a slight emphasis or "blow" on the exhalation in a pattern. The diagram shows the emphasis after every third inhalation.

Breathing

Breathing techniques provide a different focus during contractions, interfering with pain sensory transmission (Fig. 19-4). Breathing techniques begin with simple patterns and progress to more complex ones as needed. There is no single right time to begin using breathing techniques or to change patterns during labor. Prolonged use of complex breathing techniques can be tiring, however.

First-Stage Breathing. Breathing in the first stage of labor consists of a cleansing breath and various breathing techniques known as *paced breathing*. The method begins with a very simple technique that is used as long as possible. When it is no longer effective, breathing that requires more concentration is added.

Cleansing Breath. Each contraction begins and ends with a deep inspiration and expiration known as the *cleansing breath*. Like a sigh, a cleansing breath helps the woman release tension. It provides oxygen to help prevent myometrial hypoxia, one cause of pain in labor. The cleansing breath also helps the woman clear her mind to focus on relaxing and signals her labor partner that the contraction is beginning or ending. The woman may inhale through the nose and exhale through the mouth or take her cleansing breath in any way comfortable for her.

Slow-Paced Breathing. The first breathing is slow-paced breathing, a slow, deep breathing that increases relaxation (Fig. 19-5). The woman should concentrate on relaxing her body rather than on regulating the rate of her breathing. Relaxation naturally brings about slower breathing, similar to that which occurs during sleep. She can use nose, mouth, or combination breathing, depending on which is most comfortable.

The woman uses slow-paced breathing as long as possible during labor because it promotes relaxation and sufficient oxygenation. Slow-paced breathing is easy for the unprepared woman to learn between contractions and, with the support of the nurse, helps even a frightened woman become calm and able to work with her contractions.

Modified-Paced Breathing. When the woman finds that slow-paced breathing is no longer effective, she begins modified-paced breathing (Fig. 19-6). This chest breathing at a faster rate matches the natural tendency to use more rapid breathing during stress or physical work, such as labor. Although modified-paced breathing is more shallow than slow-paced breathing, the faster rate allows oxygen intake to remain about the same. As with slow-paced breathing, the focus is on release of tension rather than on the actual number of breaths taken.

Women can combine slow- and modified-paced breathing during the course of a contraction (Fig. 19-7). They begin slowly and use shallow, faster breathing at the peak of the contraction. Breathing should not interfere with relaxation but enhance it.

Pattern-Paced Breathing. Pattern-paced breathing (sometimes called "pant blow," "hee hoo," or "hee blow" breathing) involves focusing on a rhythmic pattern of breathing (Fig. 19-8). It is similar to modified-paced breathing. It differs in that after a certain number of breaths, the woman exhales with a slight emphasis or blow and then begins the modified-paced breathing again. The addition of a blow causes her to focus more on her breathing and reduces habituation. Some educators teach women to make a sound such as "hee" during this breathing and to blow through pursed lips with a "hoo" sound. Others avoid special sounds, which tighten the vocal cords and may decrease relaxation.

The number of breaths before the blow may remain constant (usually between two and six) or may change in a pattern. Variations include a set pattern such as 3-1 or a stairstep pattern such as 6-1, 5-1, 4-1, 3-1. Some couples use a random pattern determined by the coach, who uses hand signals to show the number of breaths the woman should take before each blow.

Controlling the Urge to Push. If a woman pushes strenuously before the cervix is completely dilated, she risks injury to the cervix and the fetal head. Blowing prevents closure of the glottis and breath holding, which are a part of strenuous pushing. The woman blows repeatedly using short puffs when the urge to push is strong. The support person may learn to blow along with her to help the woman concentrate. Some women vary the blowing by using one short breath and one blow.

Common Problems. Hyperventilation and mouth dryness may occur during breathing techniques. Hyperventilation is the result of rapid deep breathing that causes excessive loss of carbon dioxide, eventually resulting in respiratory alkalosis. The woman may feel dizzy or lightheaded and have impaired thinking. Vasoconstriction leads to tingling and numbness in fingers and lips. If hyperventilation continues, tetany caused by decreased calcium in tissues and blood may result in stiffness of the face and lips and carpopedal spasm.

The woman can blow into a paper bag or her own cupped hands if she feels dizzy. Containment of exhaled air in this way increases her blood carbon dioxide levels.

Dryness of the mouth occurs when the woman uses prolonged mouth breathing. To avoid dryness, she can place her tongue gently against the roof of her mouth to moisturize entering air. The support person can offer ice, mouthwash, or liquids or encourage her to brush her teeth.

Second-Stage Breathing. Care in the second stage of labor encourages a physiologic completion of labor, assisting the mother to respond to her urge to push rather than directing her to push as soon as her cervix is completely dilated even if she does not feel the urge. Lengthy pushing in second stage has been shown to result in greater maternal fatigue, more operative births, and nonreassuring fetal heart rate patterns and does not significantly shorten second stage (Mayberry et al., 2000).

With newer techniques of epidural block, women who choose this method of labor pain control often feel the urge to push, although not as strongly as unmedicated women. Using their natural urge to push, even if reduced, helps them push with contractions most effectively. Delaying pushing for up to 1 to 2 hours after complete dilation has shown benefits similar to those of women who do not have epidural analgesia.

Prolonged breath-holding while pushing (more than 6-8 sec) with a closed glottis involves use of the Valsalva maneuver. Closed-glottis pushing causes recurrent increases in intrathoracic pressure with a resulting fall in cardiac output and blood pressure. The woman's lower blood pressure then causes less blood to be delivered to the placenta, resulting in fetal hypoxia that is reflected in nonreassuring fetal heart patterns. Repeating this pushing technique more than 4 times per contraction increases the adverse effects more.

Promoting a physiologic second stage involves several variations of breathing rather than a specified technique. The woman may grunt, groan, sigh, or moan as she pushes, and the nurse should validate that these sounds are normal. Either open-glottis pushing or limiting breath-holding to 6 to 8 seconds promotes best fetal oxygenation.

PHARMACOLOGIC PAIN MANAGEMENT

Pharmacologic methods for pain management include systemic drugs, regional pain management techniques, and general anesthesia.

Special Considerations When Medicating a Pregnant Woman

Medicating a woman when she is pregnant is not straightforward for several reasons:

- Any drug taken by the woman may affect her fetus.
- Drugs may have unusual effects in pregnancy.
- Drugs can affect the course and length of labor.
- Complications may limit the choice of pharmacologic pain management methods.
- Women who need other therapeutic drugs or who practice substance abuse may have fewer safe choices for pain relief.

Effects on the Fetus

The effects on the fetus of drugs given to the mother may be direct or indirect. Direct effects result from passage of the drug or its metabolites across the placenta to the fetus. An example of a direct effect on the fetus is decreased fetal heart rate variability after administration of an analgesic to the woman. Indirect effects are secondary to drug effects on the mother. For example, a drug that causes maternal hypotension may reduce blood flow to the placenta. Fetal hypoxia and acidosis may result from major reductions in placental perfusion.

Maternal Physiologic Alterations

Normal pregnancy changes in four body systems have the greatest implications for pharmacologic pain management methods.

Cardiovascular Changes. Compression of the aorta and inferior vena cava (aortocaval compression) by the uterus can occur when a woman lies in the supine position. If placing a regional block or other procedure requires that the woman lie on her back, the uterus must be displaced to one side with the hands or with a small wedge placed under one hip. Operating room tables can often be tilted slightly to one side during a cesarean birth to provide a comparable safety measure.

Respiratory Changes. A pregnant woman's full uterus reduces her respiratory capacity. To compensate, she breathes more rapidly and deeply. As a result, she is more vulnerable to reduced arterial oxygenation during induction of general anesthesia and is more sensitive to inhalational anesthetic agents.

Gastrointestinal Changes. A pregnant woman's stomach is displaced upward by her large uterus; the stomach's interior also has a higher pressure. Progesterone slows peristalsis and reduces the tone of the sphincter at the junction of the stomach and esophagus. These changes make a pregnant woman more vulnerable to regurgitation and aspiration of acidic gastric contents during general anesthesia.

Nervous System Changes. During pregnancy and labor, circulating levels of endorphins are high. Endorphins modify pain perception and reduce requirements for analgesia and anesthesia.

The epidural and subarachnoid spaces are smaller during pregnancy, enhancing the spread of anesthetic agents used for epidural or subarachnoid blocks. Cerebrospinal fluid pressure is higher, reaching a peak during the second stage of labor. Nerve fibers are more sensitive to local anesthetic agents, probably because of acid-base or hormonal alterations. High intraabdominal pressure causes engorgement of the epidural veins, increasing the risk for intravascular injection of anesthetic agents. The net result of these changes is that a smaller volume of local anesthetic is needed to achieve satisfactory epidural or subarachnoid block.

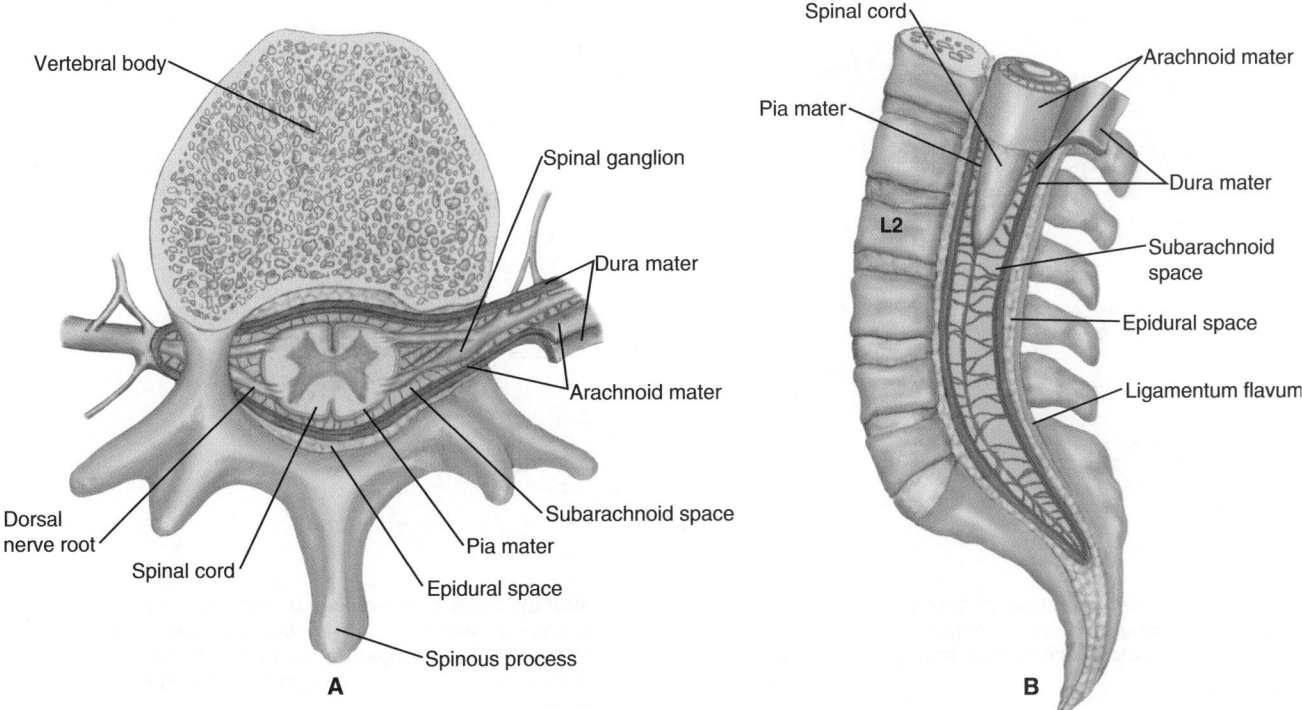

Figure 19-9 A, Cross section of spinal cord, meninges, and protective vertebra. The dura and arachnoid lie close together. The pia mater is the innermost of the meninges and covers the brain and spinal cord. The subarachnoid space is between the arachnoid and pia mater. **B,** Sagittal section of spinal cord, meninges, and vertebrae. The epidural and subarachnoid spaces are illustrated. Note that the spinal cord ends at the L2 vertebra.

Effects on the Course of Labor

Most analgesics are not given until labor is well established, because they may slow progress if given too early. Caregivers, however, must consider the adverse effects of excessive pain on labor's progress when helping a woman choose methods of pain relief. Regional anesthetics, primarily the epidural block, can slow progress during the second stage if they impair the laboring woman's natural urge to push.

Effects of Complications

Complications during pregnancy may limit the choices of analgesia or anesthesia. For example, large volumes of intravenous fluids may be infused to prevent hypotension with regional anesthesia. If a pregnant woman has heart disease, this fluid load could be detrimental. Yet without it, she is vulnerable to hypotension.

Interactions With Other Substances

A woman who ingests drugs (therapeutic, over-the-counter, or illicit) or other substances may have fewer options that are also safe for the fetus because of interactions between these substances and analgesics or anesthetics.

Regional Pain Management Techniques

Regional pain-control methods may be used for intrapartum analgesia, anesthesia, or both. These methods provide pain relief without loss of consciousness.

Epidural block analgesia or anesthesia provides pain control during much of labor and for the birth itself. Intrathecal opioids are used for pain control during labor; additional measures are needed during late labor and for the birth. Regional anesthetics that are used only during the birth include the local, pudendal, and subarachnoid blocks.

The major advantage of regional pain management methods is that the woman can participate in birth yet still have good pain control. The woman usually feels some pressure and discomfort, although these sensations are greatly reduced. She can interact with her infant and partner and does not lose her protective airway reflexes, as can happen with general anesthesia. The disadvantages of regional pain control techniques depend on the specific technique used. The effects on the fetus depend on how the woman responds rather than on direct drug effects.

Epidural Block

The epidural block is a popular and versatile regional block for relief of pain in labor and birth. It is useful for both vaginal and cesarean births.

The epidural space is outside the dura mater, between the dura and the spinal canal. It is loosely filled with fat, connective tissue, and epidural veins that are dilated during pregnancy (Fig. 19-9).

The epidural block is done by injecting local anesthetic into the tiny epidural space. It provides substantial relief of pain from contractions and birth canal distention. The level of the epidural block can be extended upward to provide anesthesia for a cesarean birth or tubal ligation after birth. The woman usually retains some motor function and sensation when low concentrations of anesthetic are used. Higher concentrations of the anesthetic agent that are used for abdominal surgery result in loss of both motor and sensory functions.

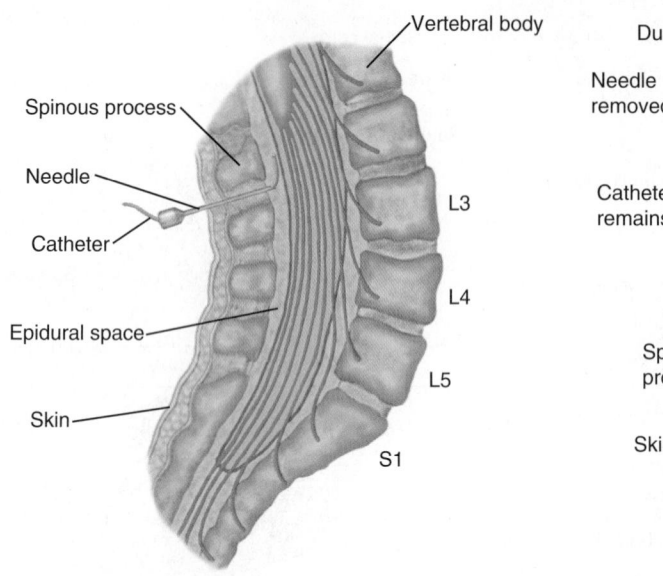

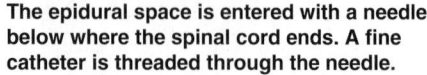

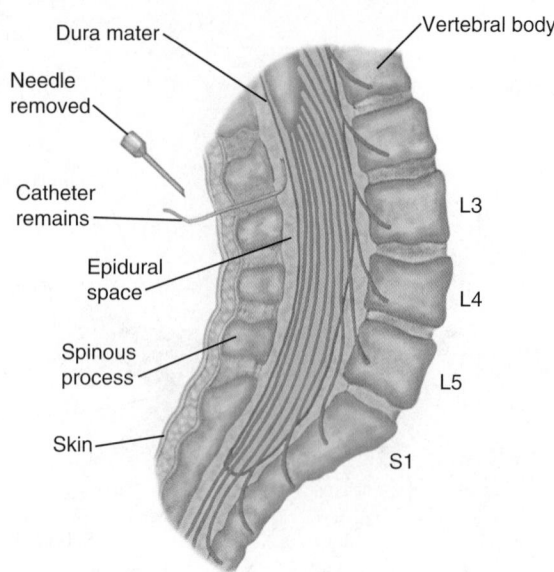

The epidural space is entered with a needle below where the spinal cord ends. A fine catheter is threaded through the needle.

After the catheter is threaded into the epidural space, the needle is removed. Medication can then be injected into the epidural space intermittently or by continuous infusion for pain relief during labor and birth.

Figure 19-10 Technique for epidural block.

Technique. The epidural block is started after labor is established or just before a scheduled cesarean birth. The epidural space is entered at about the L3-L4 interspace (below the end of the spinal cord), and a catheter is passed through the needle into the epidural space (Fig. 19-10). The catheter allows continuous infusion or intermittent injection of medication to maintain pain relief during labor and vaginal or cesarean birth.

A small (3-ml) test dose of local anesthetic may be injected before the full dose is given and before subsequent intermittent doses. Alternatively, the anesthesia provider may inject the total initial dose of the drug in small increments. A small dose of anesthetic may also be injected into the subarachnoid (spinal) space with an injection of an epidural dose that immediately follows. If a large dose of anesthetic is injected into the subarachnoid space instead of the epidural space, the woman may experience rapid, intense motor and sensory block. The test dose also can detect accidental intravascular injection. The woman has numbness of the tongue and lips, lightheadedness, dizziness, and tinnitus with intravascular injection. Epinephrine in the test dose produces tachycardia if injected intravascularly, helping distinguish tachycardia caused by labor pain from that caused by intravascular injection.

Local anesthetic drugs are usually combined with a very small dose of an opioid analgesic such as fentanyl (Sublimaze), sufentanil (Sufenta), or morphine (Duramorph). All drugs injected into the epidural or subarachnoid spaces are preservative-free. The drug combination provides rapid onset of relief and permits a lower total dose of local anesthetic with less motor block. Epidural analgesics also are given after cesarean birth to provide long-acting pain relief with a low dose. The mother is comfortable enough to interact with her infant and family. Oral analgesics are often sufficient for added pain relief.

Dural Puncture. Because the tough dura and the fragile weblike arachnoid membranes lie close together, dural puncture also punctures the arachnoid. If the dura is unintentionally punctured with the needle used to introduce the catheter, substantial leakage of cerebrospinal fluid can occur, which may result in a spinal headache. Dural puncture and spinal headache also can occur without obvious cerebrospinal fluid leakage.

Contraindications and Precautions. An epidural block is not suitable for all laboring women. Contraindications include the woman's refusal, coagulation defects, uncorrected hypovolemia, an infection in the area of insertion or a severe systemic infection, allergy, or a fetal condition that demands birth sooner than the block can become effective. Women who have had spinal surgery, such as for scoliosis (spinal curvature), are evaluated individually.

Adverse Effects of Epidural Block. An epidural block can have adverse effects.

Maternal Hypotension. Sympathetic nerves are blocked along with pain nerves, which may result in vasodilation and hypotension. Maternal hypotension with possible reduction in placental perfusion is most likely to occur within the first 15 minutes of an epidural's initiation or injection of intermittent bolus doses to maintain pain relief. However, a significant percentage of women may have hypotension that occurs within 1 hour of initiation or repeat bolus doses (Association of Women's Health, Obstetric, and Neonatal Nurses [AWHONN], 2001). In addition, the fetus is more likely to have nonreassuring signs on an electronic fetal monitor strip, such as a rising baseline, tachycardia, or late decelerations, if the mother has hypotension (see Chapter 18). Nonreassuring fetal signs may also have other etiologies, however.

Rapid infusion of intravenous (IV) solution, which is often warmed, such as lactated Ringer's solution, before initiation of the block offsets vasodilation by filling the vascular system. Preload IV quantities are at least 500 to 1000 ml infused rapidly (Creehan, 1999). If hypotension occurs, IV ephedrine in 5- to 10-mg increments promotes vasoconstriction to raise the blood pressure. Additional non-dextrose IV fluid is given rapidly, accompanied by maternal oxygen administration and uterine displacement as needed (see Chapter 18 for added information about care for nonreassuring fetal signs).

Bladder Distention. A woman's bladder fills quickly because of the large quantity of IV solution, yet her sensation to void is reduced. Bladder distention may cause pain that remains after initiation of the block.

Prolonged Second Stage. The urge to push is often less intense than if a woman does not have an epidural block. Forceps- or vacuum extractor–assisted births are more likely because of the reduced urge to push.

Migration of the Epidural Catheter. The catheter may move after accurate placement. A woman may then have symptoms of intravascular injection, an intense block or one that is too high, absence of anesthesia, or a unilateral block.

Fever. Fever with no apparent relation to infection may occur in a woman who has epidural analgesia, and its cause is not clear. The neonate's temperature may be elevated as well, possibly leading to unnecessary treatment for neonatal sepsis. Several possible explanations for epidural-associated fever in the absence of infection have been proposed (AWHONN, 2001; Lieberman, et al, 2000; Rolbin & Morningstar, 2000; Segal, Carp, & Chestnut, 1999):

Explanations for causes of epidural-associated fevers include the following list of possibilities:

1. Decreased hyperventilation, sweating, and activity after onset of pain relief reduce heat production.
2. Vasodilation redistributes heat from the core to the periphery of the body, where it is lost to the environment. The lower core temperature then signals the hypothalamus to increase heat production.
3. Shivering often occurs with sympathetic blockade accompanied by a dissociation between warm and cold sensations. In effect, the body believes that the temperature is lower than the true temperature and raises the "thermostat" to produce heat by shivering, thus increasing the core temperature.

Adverse Effects of Epidural Opioids. Adverse maternal effects associated with epidural opioids may include nausea and vomiting, pruritus, and delayed respiratory depression.

Nausea and Vomiting. As when opioids are given by other routes, nausea and vomiting may occur. Adjunctive drugs such as promethazine (Phenergan) reduce nausea and vomiting.

Pruritus. Itching of the face and neck is a harmless but annoying side effect of epidural opioids. Although she may not specifically complain of itching, a woman may rub or scratch her face and neck frequently. Diphenhydramine (Benadryl) or very small doses of naloxone (Narcan), nalbuphine (Nubain), or naltrexone (Trexan) may relieve bothersome pruritus (Sinatra, Ayoub, & Sevarino, 2000) (Table 19-1).

Delayed Respiratory Depression. The possibility of late respiratory depression in the mother persists for up to 24 hours after the administration of an epidural opioid for cesarean pain relief, depending on the drug used.

Nursing Care. The nurse should record baseline maternal vital signs and fetal heart rate and patterns for comparison with prenatal levels and those after the block. Intravenous access is ensured, and the prescribed preload of fluid is given. The nurse supports the woman in the correct position and tells the anesthesia provider when the woman is having a contraction. The woman may feel a brief "electric shock" sensation as the catheter is passed. The nurse should assist her in remaining still while the block is completed. After the medication is injected, the nurse observes for signs of subarachnoid puncture or intravascular injection.

Newest evidence-based practice guidelines from the Association of Obstetric, Gynecologic, and Neonatal Nurses (AWHONN) state that insufficient evidence exists to set firm guidelines for frequency of maternal blood pressure and fetal heart monitoring with an epidural block. However, based on a literature review, the committee suggests assessing the blood pressure and fetal heart rate every 5 minutes during the first 15 minutes after initiation of the epidural or any additional bolus doses. Until further research is available to identify the optimal time for assessment, facilities are free to use this recommendation or to develop their own protocols.

The woman's bladder must be assessed frequently because of the large IV fluid load and her reduced sensation to void. Intermittent or indwelling catheterization is usual.

The nurse should observe for signs associated with catheter migration from the epidural space and for adverse effects from epidural opioids, such as nausea and vomiting and pruritus. Reassurance about the harmless and temporary nature of pruritus is often sufficient.

Intrathecal (Subarachnoid) Opioid Analgesics

Intrathecal injection of an opioid analgesic provides labor pain management without sedation. The drug binds to opiate receptors in the subarachnoid space, allowing much smaller doses than systemic opioids. The woman can feel her contractions but not the pain.

The advantages of intrathecal analgesics include:

- Rapid onset of pain relief without sedation
- No motor block, enabling the woman to ambulate during labor (unless she receives a concurrent epidural block)
- No sympathetic block, with its hypotensive effects

The disadvantages include:

- Limited duration of action, possibly requiring another procedure for continued pain relief
- Inadequate pain relief for late labor and the birth itself, requiring added measures to manage pain at that time

A hybrid technique is the combined spinal-epidural (CSE), in which the woman receives the intrathecal opioid for rapid pain control at the time an epidural catheter is placed. Epidural drugs are then given to provide a long-acting block for labor.

TABLE **19-1** **Drugs Commonly Used for Intrapartum Pain Management**

Drug/Dose	Comments
OPIOID ANALGESICS	
Meperidine (Demerol) 12.5-50 mg every 2-4 hr IV; may be given by PCA	Respiratory depression (primarily in the neonate) is the main side effect.
Fentanyl (Sublimaze) 50-100 mcg; may be repeated every hour; may be given by PCA Adjunct to epidural analgesia during labor (dose individualized)	Onset is quick (5 min for IV administration), but duration of action is short. Less nausea, vomiting, and respiratory depression occurs than with meperidine. Epidural use may cause pruritus.
Butorphanol (Stadol) 1 mg every 3-4 hr; range 0.5-2 mg IV; may be given by PCA	Has some narcotic antagonist effects; should not be given to the opiate-dependent woman (may precipitate withdrawal) or after other narcotics such as meperidine (may reverse their analgesic effects); also a respiratory depressant.
Nalbuphine (Nubain) 10 mg every 3-6 hr IV; may be given by PCA	Same as butorphanol. 5-10 mg may be given to relieve pruritus associated with epidural narcotics.
ADJUNCTIVE DRUGS	
Promethazine (Phenergan) 12.5-25 mg every 4-6 hr IV	Given for nausea and vomiting in labor. Duration of action is longer than most narcotics; may enhance respiratory depressant effects of narcotics.
Diphenhydramine (Benadryl) 10-50 mg every 4-6 hr IV	Given to relieve pruritus from epidural narcotics.
Hydroxyzine (Atarax, Vistaril) 25-100 mg IM Z-track only	See promethazine.
NARCOTIC ANTAGONISTS	
Naloxone (Narcan) Adult: To reduce respiratory depression induced by opioids: 0.4-2 mg IV To reverse pruritus from epidural opioids: 0.04-0.2 mg IV or IV infusion 5-10 mcg/kg/hr Neonatal resuscitation: 0.1 mg/kg IV (umbilical vein) or intratracheal	Action shorter than most narcotics it reverses; must observe for recurrent respiratory depression and be prepared to give additional doses. Small doses (0.04-0.08 mg) may be given to reduce pruritus from epidural opioids. Neonatal resuscitation dose (see Chapter 30).
Naltrexone (Trexan) 3-6 mg PO × 1 dose	Long-acting drug to relieve pruritus from epidural narcotics. May reduce some analgesic effect when given for pruritus.

IV, Intravenously; *PCA*, patient-controlled analgesia; *IM*, intramuscularly; *PO*, orally.

Technique. The subarachnoid space is entered with a spinal needle, as in the subarachnoid block. A preservative-free opioid analgesic is then injected.

The drug chosen depends on the expected duration of labor at the time it is given. Drugs that may be used by this route include fentanyl, sufentanil, and morphine.

One technique of performing the CSE is to insert the epidural needle into the epidural space. The much thinner spinal needle is then inserted through the larger epidural needle to reach the subarachnoid space for injection of the intrathecal opioid. The smaller needle is then withdrawn and an epidural catheter placed for injection of epidural medication.

Adverse Effects of Intrathecal Opioids. As with epidural opioids, nausea, vomiting, and pruritus may occur. Delayed respiratory depression may occur, depending on the drug used.

Nursing Care. Vital signs and fetal heart rate are taken at the usual intervals for the woman's stage of labor. Side ef-

fects, such as nausea and vomiting or pruritus, are reported and managed similarly to those occurring with the epidural block. Reduced effectiveness suggests that the drug's duration of action is ending or that the woman is in late labor. Other pain management methods may be needed for the remainder of labor and for birth.

Care of the woman having a CSE is the same as that for a non-combined block.

Subarachnoid (Spinal) Block
A subarachnoid block (SAB) may be done when a quick cesarean birth is necessary and an epidural catheter is not in place. The typical subarachnoid block provides no pain relief during most of labor. Because of the popularity of epidurals for labor and the ability to give epidural opioids for long-lasting postoperative analgesia, the subarachnoid block is less common.

The anesthesia provider injects local anesthetic, often combined with an opioid such as fentanyl, into the sub-

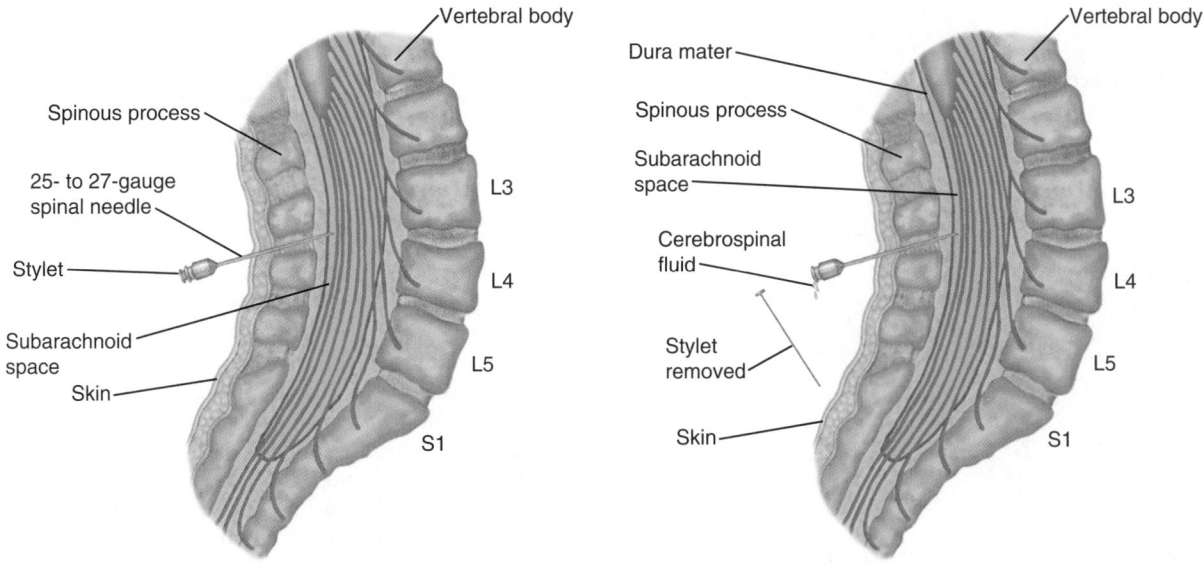

A 25- to 27-gauge spinal needle with a stylet occluding its lumen is passed into the subarachnoid space below where the spinal cord ends.

The stylet is removed, and one or more drops of clear cerebrospinal fluid at needle hub confirm correct needle placement. Medication is then injected, and the needle is removed.

Figure 19-11 Technique for subarachnoid block.

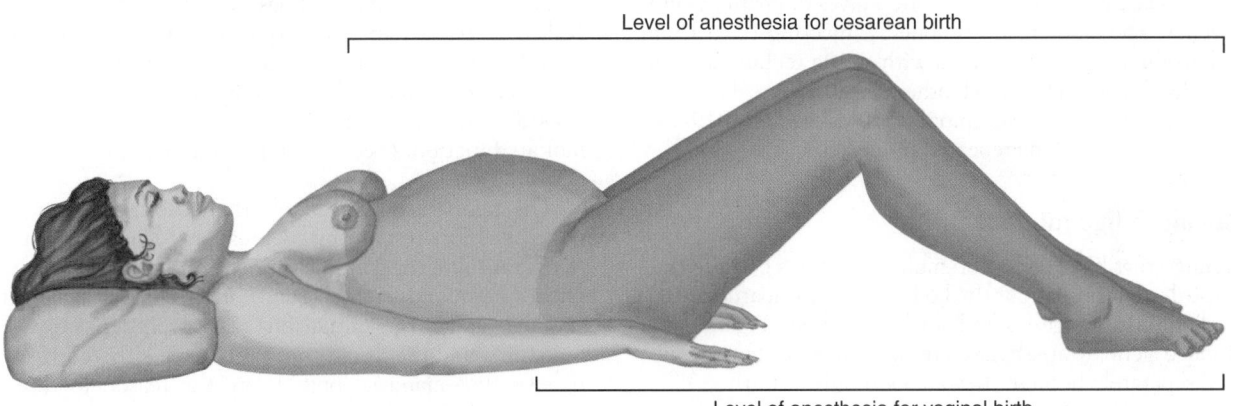

Figure 19-12 Levels of anesthesia for epidural and subarachnoid blocks. A level of T10 through S5 is adequate for vaginal birth. A higher level, to T4-T6, is needed for cesarean birth.

arachnoid space in a single dose. The woman loses both sensory and motor function below the level of the subarachnoid block, with complete relief of pain from contractions. A much lower dose of anesthetic agent is required because less absorption into surrounding tissues occurs than with the epidural block.

Technique. A spinal needle is placed in the subarachnoid space. Appearance of cerebrospinal fluid at the needle hub assures correct placement, and the local anesthetic combination is injected (Fig. 19-11).

The level of anesthesia for both epidural and subarachnoid blocks is determined by the volume, concentration, and density of the drug (Fig. 19-12).

Contraindications and Precautions. Contraindications and precautions are similar to those for epidural block: the woman's refusal, coagulation defects, uncorrected hypovolemia, infection in the area of insertion, systemic infection, and allergy.

Adverse Effects of a Subarachnoid Block. Three adverse effects of a subarachnoid block are maternal hypotension, bladder distention, and spinal headache. Hypotension occurs because of sympathetic blockade as in epidural block but can be more severe. Treatment is the same, but a larger preload of IV fluid is common.

Postspinal headache may occur after subarachnoid block in some women because of cerebrospinal fluid leakage at the

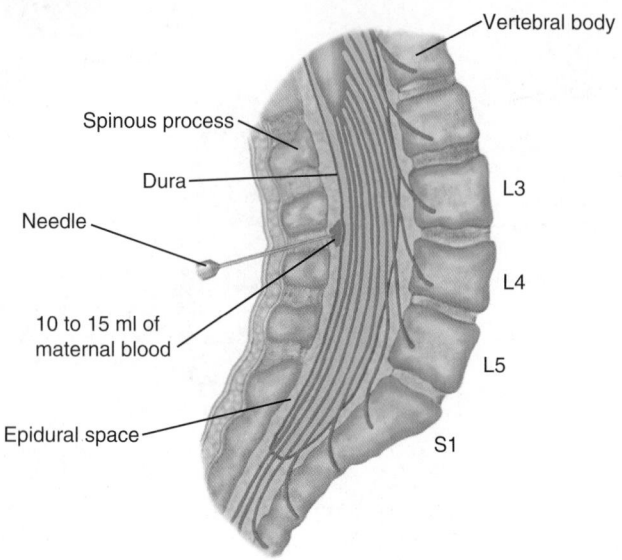

Figure 19-13 Blood patch for relief of spinal headache. Ten to 15 ml of the woman's blood is injected into the epidural space to seal a dural puncture.

site of dural puncture. A spinal headache is postural; it is worse when a woman is upright and may disappear when she is lying flat. The incidence of spinal headache is lower if a small-gauge needle is used.

Bed rest with oral or IV hydration helps relieve the post-spinal headache. A blood patch often gives dramatic, defini-tive relief. The blood patch is done by injecting 10 to 15 ml of the woman's blood (obtained with sterile technique) into the epidural space. The blood forms a gelatinous seal over the hole in the dura, stopping spinal fluid leakage (Fig. 19-13). The blood patch can be repeated if needed.

Systemic Drugs for Labor

Systemic drugs have effects on multiple systems because they are distributed throughout the body. These intrapartum drugs include opioid analgesics and adjunctive drugs. Agents used to induce general anesthesia are also systemic but are dis-cussed separately because they are used only at birth.

Opioid Analgesics
Opioid analgesics reduce the perception of pain without loss of consciousness. Injectable opioid analgesics are the sys-temic drugs of choice in labor. Analgesics that may be used in labor are meperidine (Demerol), fentanyl (Sublimaze), bu-torphanol (Stadol), and nalbuphine (Nubain). Table 19-1 summarizes common drugs used for intrapartum pain relief.

Although often prescribed for labor analgesia, meperidine often produces a dysphoric, rather than an analgesic, effect in the woman. She may be restless or irritable and have twitch-ing, jerking, shaking, tremors, or even delirium. Of more con-cern is that meperidine produces a long-lasting active metabo-lite, normeperidine, which has a half-life of 3 to 6 hours in the woman but 15 to 23 hours in the newborn (Bricker & Lavender, 2002; Britt & Pasero, 1999).

Meperidine is a pure opioid agonist, but butorphanol and nalbuphine have mixed opioid agonist and antagonist effects. These agonist-antagonist drugs should not be given to a woman who is opiate dependent (on a drug such as heroin) to avoid withdrawal effects. These drugs also should not be given if she has already received a pure opioid agonist such as meperidine, because some analgesic effect of the first drug will be reversed. Respiratory depression is limited with the mixed agonist-antagonist opioids, but pain relief also reaches a ceiling, making them poorly suited for intense pain as labor progresses.

Opioid analgesics can cause respiratory depression, which is more likely to occur in the newborn than in the mother. An infant born at the peak of the drug's action is more likely to have respiratory depression than if born earlier or later. Prolonged action of active metabolites of drugs such as meperidine must also be considered.

During labor, opioid analgesics are usually given intra-venously in small, frequent doses to provide a rapid onset of analgesia and a predictable duration of action. A woman ben-efits from rapid pain control, and there is less likelihood of neonatal respiratory depression. Starting the injection at the beginning of the contraction, when blood flow to the pla-centa is normally reduced, limits transfer to the fetus. When placental blood flow resumes, much of the drug is in maternal tissues.

Opioid Antagonists
Naloxone (Narcan) reverses opioid-induced respiratory de-pression. Small doses may be given to the woman to reduce pruritus from epidural opioids. Naloxone does not reverse res-piratory depression from other causes, such as barbiturates, anesthetics, non-opioid drugs, or pathologic conditions. Naloxone has a shorter duration of action than most of the opioids it reverses. In an opiate-dependent woman or new-born, naloxone may induce withdrawal symptoms. Naloxone is used with other measures as needed to support cardiopul-monary function. (See Chapter 30 for discussion of neonatal resuscitation.)

The neonate is more likely than the mother to receive naloxone for respiratory depression. The recommended neonatal route for administration is intravenous or intratra-cheal for the most reliable absorption. Airway management (i.e., bag and mask ventilation) takes precedence over use of naloxone, and the drug is not given unless there is reason to believe that maternal opioids are the reason for the new-born's respiratory depression.

Adjunctive Drugs
Adjunctive drugs during the intrapartum period include those with antiemetic and tranquilizing effects and sedatives. These drugs are given to reduce nausea and anxiety and to promote rest (see Table 19-1). They have no analgesic effects and do not potentiate analgesic drugs.

Promethazine (Phenergan) relieves the nausea and vomit-ing that may occur when opioid drugs are given. Promethazine is usually given intravenously but may be given by the intra-muscular route.

Sedatives
Sedatives such as barbiturates are not routinely given because they have prolonged depressant effects on the neonate. How-ever, a small dose of a short-acting barbiturate may be given to promote rest if a woman is fatigued from false labor or a prolonged latent phase.

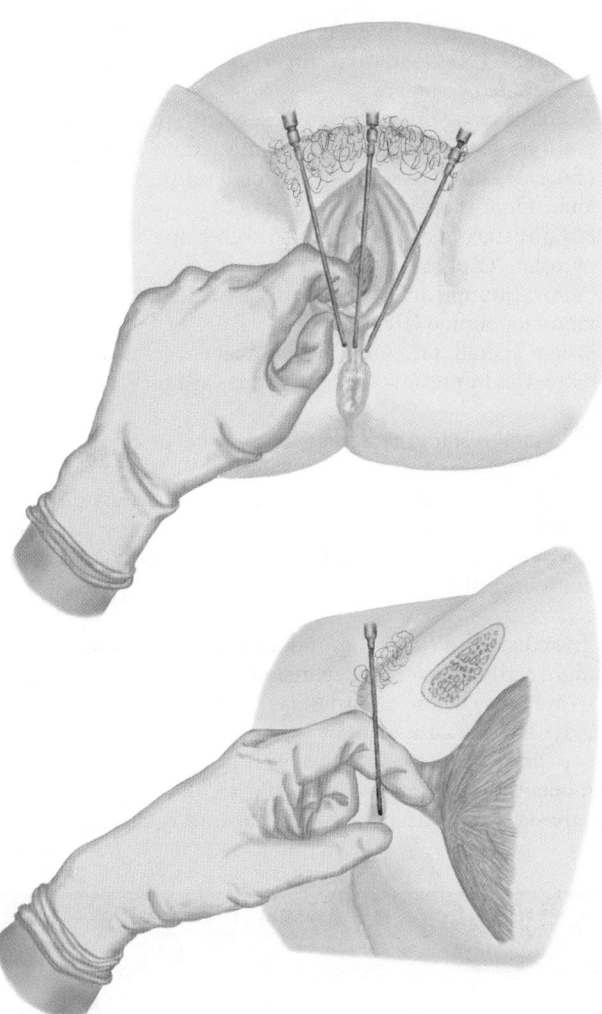

Figure 19-14 Local infiltration anesthesia numbs the perineum just before birth for an episiotomy or after birth for suturing of a laceration. The birth attendant protects the fetal head by placing a finger inside the vagina while injecting the perineum in a fanlike pattern or as needed.

Vaginal Birth Anesthesia

Local Infiltration Anesthesia

Infiltration of the perineum with a local anesthetic is done by the physician or nurse-midwife just before performing an episiotomy or suturing a laceration (Fig. 19-14). Local infiltration does not alter pain from uterine contractions or distention of the vagina. The local agent provides anesthesia in the immediate area of the episiotomy or laceration. There is a short delay between anesthetic injection and the onset of numbness, and the drug burns before its anesthetic action begins. Local infiltration rarely has adverse effects on either mother or infant.

Pudendal Block

A pudendal block anesthetizes the lower vagina and part of the perineum to provide anesthesia for an episiotomy and vaginal birth, using low forceps if needed. A pudendal block does not block pain from uterine contractions, and the mother feels pressure.

The physician or nurse-midwife injects the pudendal nerves near each ischial spine with local anesthetic (Fig. 19-15). The perineum is infiltrated with local anesthetic because the pudendal block does not fully anesthetize this area. As in local infiltration, a delay occurs between injection and the onset of numbness. Possible maternal complications include a toxic reaction to the anesthetic, rectal puncture, hematoma, and sciatic nerve block. If maternal toxicity is avoided, the fetus is usually not affected.

General Anesthesia

General anesthesia is a systemic pain control that involves loss of consciousness. It is rarely used for vaginal births, but it still has a place in cesarean birth. Some women either refuse or are not good candidates for epidural or subarachnoid block but require surgery. Occasionally, a planned epidural or subarachnoid block proves inadequate for surgical anesthesia. Or, it may be necessary to perform a cesarean birth so quickly

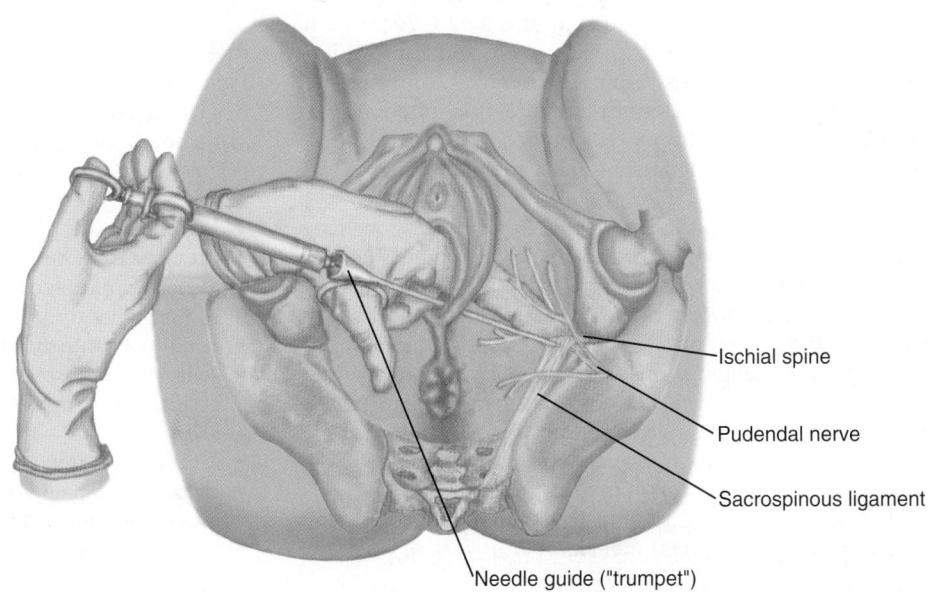

Figure 19-15 Pudendal block provides anesthesia for an episiotomy and the use of low forceps. A needle guide ("trumpet") protects the maternal and fetal tissues from the long needle needed to reach the pudendal nerve. Only about 1.25 cm (¹/₂ in) of the long needle protrudes from the guide.

Ischial spine

Pudendal nerve

Sacrospinous ligament

Needle guide ("trumpet")

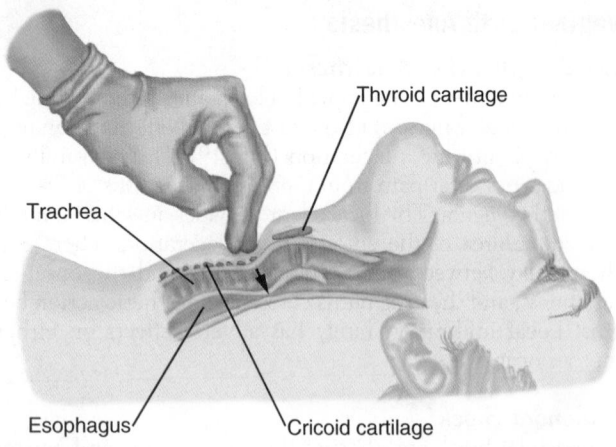

Figure 19-16 Sellick maneuver to prevent vomitus from entering the woman's trachea while she is being intubated for general anesthesia. An assistant applies pressure to the cricoid cartilage to obstruct the esophagus. Once the woman is successfully intubated with a cuffed endotracheal tube, gastric secretions cannot enter the trachea.

that no time is available to establish either type of regional block. General anesthesia may be required for emergency procedures at any stage of pregnancy, such as to repair injury that might result from an accident or domestic violence.

Technique

Before induction of anesthesia, a woman breathes oxygen for 3 to 5 minutes, or 4 deep breaths, to increase her oxygen stores and those of her fetus for the short period of apnea during anesthesia induction. A wedge is placed under the woman's right side (or the operating table is tilted toward her left side) to displace the uterus from the aorta and inferior vena cava, promoting placental blood flow.

Adverse Effects of General Anesthesia

Major adverse effects are possible with the use of general anesthesia.

Maternal Aspiration of Gastric Contents. Regurgitation with aspiration of acidic gastric contents is a potentially fatal complication of general anesthesia. Aspiration of food particles may result in airway obstruction. Aspiration of acidic secretions results in chemical injury to the airways (aspiration pneumonitis). Infection often occurs after the initial lung injury. For purposes of general anesthesia, anesthesia providers assume a pregnant woman has a full stomach.

Respiratory Depression. Respiratory depression may occur in either the mother or the infant but is more likely in the baby if delivery after starting anesthesia is delayed.

Uterine Relaxation. Some inhalational anesthetics may cause uterine relaxation. This characteristic is desirable for treating some complications, such as replacing an inverted uterus (see Chapter 27). However, postpartum hemorrhage may occur if the uterus relaxes after birth.

Methods to Minimize Adverse Effects

Measures to reduce the risk of maternal aspiration (or of lung injury, if aspiration occurs) include:

- Restricting intake to clear fluids or maintaining nothing-by-mouth (NPO) status if surgery is expected, such as with a scheduled cesarean.
- Administering drugs to raise the gastric pH and make secretions less acidic, such as sodium citrate and citric acid (Bicitra), ranitidine (Zantac), cimetidine (Tagamet), or famotidine (Pepcid).
- Administering drugs to reduce secretions, such as glycopyrrolate (Robinul).
- Administering drugs to speed gastric emptying, such as metoclopramide (Reglan).
- Using cricoid pressure (Sellick maneuver) to block the esophagus by pressing the rigid trachea against it (Fig. 19-16).

Neonatal respiratory depression may be averted by:

- Reducing the time from induction of anesthesia until the umbilical cord is clamped.
- Keeping use of sedating drugs and anesthetics to a minimum until the cord is clamped.

To reduce the time from induction of anesthesia to cord clamping, the woman is prepared and draped and the physicians are ready before anesthesia is begun. Before cord clamping, the anesthesia is so light that the woman may move on the operating table as the incision is made, but she rarely remembers the experience or does not recall it as painful. The anesthesia level is deepened after the cord is clamped.

■ NURSING CARE
Pain Management

The nurse assists laboring women with both nonpharmacologic and pharmacologic methods of pain control as needed (see Nursing Care Plan: Intrapartum Pain Management). Nursing care related to pain management should be combined with that for normal labor and any complications that arise. Two problems that commonly affect the woman are pain and her potential for respiratory compromise if she needs general anesthesia.

PAIN
Assessment

Pain assessment begins at admission and continues throughout labor. The assessments discussed in Table 17-1 guide the nurse in obtaining data related to pain management. Pain-related assessments include:

- Preferences for pain management
- Previous surgeries, type of anesthesia, and any anesthesia-associated problems
- Maternal vital signs
- Fetal heart rate and monitor patterns
- Allergies, focusing especially on allergy to opioid analgesics, dental anesthetics, and iodine (used in most prep solutions)
- Oral intake time and type of intake
- Evidence of pain: verbal evidence—verbal statement, requests for pain-relief measures, crying, moaning; and nonverbal evidence—tense, guarded posture or facial expression

Nursing Care Plan

Intrapartum Pain Management

ASSESSMENT

Beth Anderson is a 28-year-old gravida 1, para 0, who was admitted 1 hour ago. Beth's cervix is 3 cm dilated and 100% effaced, the station is –2, and her membranes are intact. Contractions occur every 3 minutes, last 40 to 50 seconds, and are of moderate intensity. The fetal heart rate averages 135 to 145 beats per minute (bpm) and has no nonreassuring patterns. Beth says that back pain is most troubling. Beth and her husband Sam attended prepared childbirth classes and are using breathing techniques they learned.

Nursing Diagnosis

Pain related to effects of uterine contractions and pressure on pelvic structures.

Goals/Expected Outcomes

During labor, Beth will
- Continue to use techniques she learned in prepared childbirth classes.
- Have a relaxed facial and body posture between contractions.

INTERVENTION	RATIONALE
1. Adjust the environment for comfort: a. Adjust room thermostat. b. Add warm blankets and socks for warmth. c. Offer small electric fan or hand fan if Beth is hot.	1. A comfortable environment is conducive to relaxation. Relaxation underlies all other interventions because it increases a woman's ability to use her coping skills to tolerate discomfort.
2. Reduce distractions: a. Close door to reduce outside noise. b. Play music of Beth's choice to mask external noise. c. Do not stand in front of her focal point. d. Try to delay assessments or questions until after a contraction is over.	2. Distractions interfere with use of the skills for pain management taught in prepared childbirth classes.
3. Reduce irritating stimulants: a. Keep sheets and underpads dry. b. Dim the lights as Beth desires. Use bright lights only when necessary. c. Do all procedures and nursing interventions as gently as possible. d. Avoid bumping the bed. e. Limit visitors as the couple wishes.	3. Irritating stimulants are distractions that decrease the woman's ability to use learned childbirth skills and add to her discomfort.
4. Encourage Beth to assume the most comfortable positions and to change positions regularly (about every 30-60 min). If there is no contraindication, she may walk around or sit in a chair or on a birth ball at the bedside. A rolled pillow or blanket provides a wedge in a side-tilt position.	4. Frequent position changes favor fetal descent by encouraging the fetal head to adapt to the pelvic diameters most efficiently. Position changes also reduce muscle tension and unrelieved pressure: a. Upright positions enhance descent with gravity. b. If lying down, a side-lying or side-tilt position is more comfortable and reduces aortocaval compression with decreased placental perfusion.
5. Check for bladder distention hourly or more often if she has had large quantities of intravenous (IV) or oral fluid. Encourage voiding at least every 2 hours. With an order, catheterize her if her bladder is full and she cannot void.	5. The sensation to void may be decreased during labor. A full bladder contributes to overall discomfort and may impede fetal descent and prolong labor.
6. Give Beth small amounts of clear fluids such as ice chips. If oral intake is prohibited or she does not want fluids, moisten her mouth with a damp washcloth or have her rinse her mouth with water.	6. Women often use rapid mouth breathing during labor, resulting in a dry mouth. These methods may relieve some of the discomfort associated with a dry mouth. Clear liquids limit the risk of aspiration if general anesthesia is needed.

Continued

Nursing Care Plan

Intrapartum Pain Management—cont'd

7. Offer a back rub or firm, constant sacral pressure. Ask Beth where and how firm pressure should be applied. Use baby powder when rubbing her back. Have her tell caregivers if this technique becomes uncomfortable or if the location on her back needs to be changed. If Sam is rubbing her back, offer to relieve him occasionally and encourage him to take a break.
8. Keep Beth and Sam informed about the progress of labor and their baby's condition.

7. Back rubs may somewhat reduce discomfort associated with back labor by stimulating large-diameter fibers and interfering with transmission of the pain impulse to the brain. As labor continues, back rubs may become less effective or even uncomfortable. Powder reduces friction, which could be another source of discomfort. The partner needs a break to conserve energy and better help the woman in later labor.
8. Information reduces anxiety and fear of the unknown. Anxiety and fear increase pain perception and reduce pain tolerance.

Evaluation

Beth concentrates on her breathing techniques with each contraction but has a relaxed body posture between them. She continues to use learned skills effectively for about 2 hours, when she begins to have more difficulty coping with her contractions.

ASSESSMENT

Three hours after admission, Beth's cervix is 4 cm dilated and 100% effaced, and the fetal station is –1. Membranes have ruptured, and the amniotic fluid is clear. Contractions occur every 2 to 3 minutes, last 50 seconds, and are firm. Fetal heart rate and monitor patterns are reassuring. Back discomfort persists, and she is having difficulty relaxing between contractions and is discouraged that labor is not progressing as quickly as she expected. She is no longer able to use prepared childbirth techniques effectively and rates her labor pain as "8" on a 0-10 scale. Beth reluctantly requests an epidural block, which will be given by continuous infusion.

The nurse gives Beth 500 ml or more of ordered IV solution before the block begins, which offsets its hypotensive effects. Fetal monitoring, usually by continuous electronic means, helps identify nonreassuring patterns that may occur.

Nursing Diagnosis

Risk for Injury related to altered sensation in her lower extremities.

Goals/Expected Outcomes

- Beth will not fall or suffer other injury while experiencing the effects of epidural block.
- The fetus will not be born in an uncontrolled manner.

Labor status

In addition to these routine assessments, ask the woman if she needs help with pain management. A stoic woman may give little outward evidence of pain yet may say she wants medication or other pain control if asked.

When assessing pain, clarify the words a woman uses. When asked if she has "pain," the woman may deny it. Changing the word used to "discomfort," "aching," "pulling," "pressure," or other words that may describe labor pain may bring a different response. Do not assume that everyone uses the same words to describe their pain. Just as pain is an individual experience, so also is the expression of pain, including verbal expression.

Asking a woman to rate her pain on a scale of 0 to 10 or a similar scale helps clarify her pain's intensity. Zero represents no pain, whereas 10 is the worst possible pain. (Other scales that use drawings that range from smiling faces to crying are readily available.) Ask the woman to rate her pain on this scale before and after pain-relief mea-

sures to evaluate their effectiveness. A surprising number of women have difficulty using a pain scale because they have little experience with pain. They may want to allow for an increase in the number later in labor, possibly underrating current pain. Or, they may say that they have no idea what the "worst pain imaginable" is and thus cannot guess what pain rated as 10 feels like. A scale does, however, provide one measure of how pain feels before and after relief measures.

The woman who remains tense between contractions may be having difficulty coping with pain. Moaning, crying, thrashing, and an inability to use nonpharmacologic techniques suggest that she needs pharmacologic pain relief.

Assess the woman's labor status to help her choose the most appropriate method of pain control. If she has reached a point in labor at which she needs to decide for or against a specific pharmacologic method, inform her. This point does not occur at an exact time or with an exact amount of cervical dilation but is estimated according to when she is

Nursing Care Plan

Intrapartum Pain Management—cont'd

INTERVENTIONS	RATIONALE
1. Assist Beth to change positions regularly. Ambulation after birth should be delayed until movement and strength return, and assistance should be available until her legs have normal strength.	1. Changing positions reduces constant pressure on one area and helps prevent muscle strain. The epidural block causes a varying degree of motor block and weakness. An assistant helps prevent falls when first ambulating.
2. Observe for signs of labor progress: a. Contractions increasing in frequency, duration, and intensity. b. Fetal heart rate changes such as early or variable decelerations that reflect head or cord compression. c. Increase in bloody show. d. Statement reflecting urge to push (not always present).	2. Rectal pressure associated with fetal descent may be reduced. To prevent the fetus from being born unattended, the nurse must observe for other signs that birth is near.
3. Support Beth's pushing efforts. Teach her to avoid holding her breath while pushing and to push no longer than 6-8 seconds at a time. Explain to Beth and Sam that she may make grunting, moaning, or other sounds when pushing to avoid excessive breath-holding.	3. The urge to push may not be as strong but it is usually felt when the fetus descends low in the pelvis. Prolonged breath-holding or multiple long pushing efforts (see also Chapter 17) can cause fetal hypoxia and non-reassuring fetal heart rate patterns. Women may make a variety of sounds when they push.

Evaluation

Beth is satisfied with her pain relief after the epidural block, rating her pain as "0 out of 10." She has little motor block. Her blood pressure and the fetal heart rate remain within expected limits. Cervical dilation progresses to 10 cm (complete) without injury to Beth or her fetus. However, despite her vigorous pushing efforts, the fetal station remains at 0. Beth has a cesarean birth, delivering an 8-lb, 10-oz girl (3912 g).

Additional Nursing Diagnoses and Collaborative Problems to Consider

- Anxiety
- Risk for Aspiration
- Powerlessness
- Situational Low Self-Esteem
- Urinary Retention
- Potential complication: Fetal compromise

---

likely to give birth, the time needed to establish a specific method, and the pharmacology of the drug or drugs.

Avoid making assumptions about the amount of pain a woman is having on the basis of her rate of labor progress, cervical dilation, or apparent intensity of contractions. It is tempting to assume that a woman whose cervix is 2 cm dilated has little pain and that a woman whose cervix is dilated 8 cm has intense pain. An obese woman's contractions may be strong, but they may seem mild if they are assessed by palpation or an external monitor because of her thick abdominal fat pad. *Labor progress or contraction intensity cannot be equated with a woman's pain perception or tolerance.*

A woman's need for pain relief should not be based on her outward expression alone. A quiet woman may need medication but may be reluctant to ask, whereas an expressive woman may be satisfied with nonpharmacologic measures. Because women who do not speak the prevailing language may not know what is available, seek an interpreter to communicate accurately.

CRITICAL THINKING EXERCISE 19-1

Truc Pham is a Vietnamese-American in labor with her first baby. Her cervix is dilated 6 cm, effacement is 100%, and the fetus is at a +1 station. Truc's contractions occur every 3 minutes, last 50 to 60 seconds, and are of strong intensity. She smiles at the nurse each time the nurse talks to her but talks little. Truc stiffens her body during contractions and interacts little with her husband or the nurse at those times.
1. How should the nurse interpret these data?
2. Does the nurse need additional data?
3. What nursing actions are appropriate?

Observe for pain that is not typical of labor. Although labor pain is often intense, it should not be constant but should come and go with each contraction. The uterus should not be tender or board-like between contractions. Report atypical pain to the physician or nurse-midwife.

Nursing Diagnosis and Planning

Because pain is an expected part of normal childbirth, a common nursing diagnosis is:

■ Pain related to effects of uterine contractions and fetal descent.

Expected Outcomes: The woman will describe the pain-relief measures as satisfactory during labor and will use learned breathing and relaxation techniques during labor. These two goals are realistic for the unique pain of labor.

Interventions

Nursing care for intrapartum pain management is to reduce factors that hinder the woman's pain control and to enhance those that benefit it. Refer to Chapter 17 for nursing measures that should be included in the care of all laboring women, such as positioning, teaching, encouragement, and care of the partner.

Promoting Relaxation

Simple attention to details helps the woman relax. Adjust her environment so that it is more comfortable. If noise is a problem, suggest music or television to mask it.

A warm blanket or a cool cloth provides tangible comfort and conveys the nurse's caring attitude. Change the linens or underpads as needed to keep the woman reasonably clean and dry.

Offer the woman a warm shower or bath, especially if she is tense and if no contraindications exist (see Box 19-1). In general, walking is good during early labor, and water therapy is better during active labor. The mild nipple stimulation that occurs in a whirlpool or shower may intensify contractions in a woman whose labor has slowed, because it causes her posterior pituitary gland to secrete oxytocin.

Reduce intrusions as much as possible. For example, wait until a contraction is over before asking questions or doing a procedure. Longer assessments and procedures may span several contractions, but try to stop during each contraction.

Reducing Outside Sources of Discomfort

If inserting the intravenous line is expected to be difficult or the woman is very anxious, anesthetize the site with 0.1 ml of 1% lidocaine (Xylocaine) before insertion if the woman is not allergic and if facility policy permits. Remind her to change position regularly to reduce tension and discomfort from constant pressure. Support her with pillows or folded blankets.

Observe the woman's bladder for distention hourly, and encourage her to void every 2 hours or more often if she has received a large quantity of IV fluids. Catheterization is needed if she cannot void and her bladder is full.

Reducing Anxiety and Fear

Accurate information reduces the negative psychologic impact of the unknown. Tell the woman about her labor and its progress. It is impossible to predict when she will give birth, but tell her if her labor progress is or is not on course. Sometimes she needs only the reassurance from an experienced nurse that her intense contractions are indeed normal. The woman may be willing to endure more discomfort than she otherwise would if she is making progress.

Be honest if problems do occur. A woman usually knows if there is a problem and is more anxious if she does not know what it is. Explain all measures taken to correct the problem, and keep her informed about the results.

Helping the Woman Use Nonpharmacologic Techniques

If the nonpharmacologic method is safe for the woman and fetus and if it is effective, do not interfere with its use. Try not to distract the woman from whatever technique she is using.

Massage Fetal monitor belts hinder abdominal effleurage. Encourage the woman to do effleurage on uncovered areas of her abdomen or to stroke her thighs. Consider using intermittent fetal monitoring if this method is appropriate.

During massage, baby powder reduces friction and skin irritation. The woman needs to tell the person who is providing sacral pressure or other massage how much pressure helps and the best location for it. Because this information may change during labor or massage may become uncomfortable rather than helpful, seek the woman's feedback regularly.

Mental Stimulation Use a low, soothing voice when helping a woman use imagery. It is often helpful to speak close to her ear when trying to create a tranquil imaginary scene or to calm her. Music can enhance mental stimulation techniques.

Breathing Women learn a variety of breathing techniques in prepared childbirth classes and often modify them or invent some of their own during labor. Encourage the woman to change techniques when she needs to, avoiding the complex ones during early labor. If she has trouble maintaining her concentration, the nurse or her partner can make eye contact (if culturally appropriate) and breathe the pattern with her.

Symptoms of hyperventilation (dizziness, tingling and numbness of the fingers and lips, carpopedal spasm) are likely if a woman breathes fast and deep, whether or not she is using patterned breathing techniques. Breathing into her cupped hands, a paper bag, or a washcloth placed over her nose and mouth promotes rebreathing exhaled carbon dioxide to lessen the symptoms.

Teach breathing techniques to the unprepared woman when she is admitted. Review them when she seems to need a different method. Many women make up their own breathing techniques.

When teaching nonpharmacologic pain management techniques to the woman who is in advanced labor, follow these guidelines:

- Teach one method at a time.
- Demonstrate the method between contractions.
- Use breathing techniques with the woman while maintaining eye contact.
- Allow her control over her labor: who is present, what technique she will use, and the like.

Incorporating Pharmacologic Methods

All pharmacologic methods require collaboration with medical personnel for orders. Tell the woman soon after admission what medication is available if she needs it. This is not done to undermine her self-confidence but so that she can better understand when she needs to make a choice about medication. Also, analgesia is most effective if it is given before pain is severe.

Tell her that her preferences about pain-relief methods will be honored if possible, but it is impossible to predict the course of her labor. Assure her that no pharmacologic method will be given without her understanding and consent.

If a woman finds some nonpharmacologic methods inadequate, try other nonpharmacologic methods or offer her available medication. When contacting the birth attendant for medication orders, report the fetal and maternal status and vital signs, labor status, and the woman's request for medication, including her pain rating on a scale. If she has a continuous epidural block, contact the person who inserted it if problems occur or added relief is needed. Observe special nursing considerations associated with the method used (Table 19-2).

Evaluation

- Is the woman satisfied with her ability to manage her pain?
- Is she using coping skills somewhat consistently during labor?
- How did her pain scale rating change before and after the method (either nonpharmacologic or pharmacologic) was used? Is she satisfied with its relief?

RESPIRATORY COMPROMISE

Assessment

General anesthesia may be needed any time during birth, most often for cesarean birth. Document the type (solids or liquids) and time of the woman's last food intake. Question her closely if she reports an unusually long interval since her last oral intake. Anesthesia providers can anticipate and prevent problems better if they know the actual oral intake.

Nursing Diagnosis and Planning

Nursing care of laboring women includes monitoring for the short-term risk for aspiration, because it is impossible to predict every woman who will require general anesthesia. The nursing diagnosis is:

- Risk for Aspiration related to impaired protective laryngeal reflexes.

    Expected Outcome: The woman will not aspirate gastric contents during the perioperative period.

Interventions

Nursing interventions relate to identifying factors that increase a woman's risk for aspiration, and collaborative and nursing measures to reduce the risk of aspiration or lung injury.

Identifying Risk Factors

Report oral intake both before and after admission to the anesthesia provider. Oral intake during labor is often restricted to medications, clear liquids, ice chips, Popsicles, or hard candies.

Vomiting is a common discomfort during normal labor, regardless of the mother's oral intake. If vomiting occurs, chart the time, quantity, and character (amount, color, presence of undigested food).

Reducing Risk for Aspiration or Lung Injury

Nursing and medical personnel collaborate to reduce a woman's risk for pulmonary complications.

Perioperative Care Restrict oral intake as ordered if surgery is expected. Give ordered medications such as sodium citrate and citric acid (Bicitra). Either the nurse or anesthesia provider may give parenteral drugs, such as glycopyrrolate (Robinul), depending on when they are administered.

An experienced nurse or a trained anesthesia assistant provides cricoid pressure (Sellick maneuver) to block the

---

PARENTS
Want to Know

How Will This Medicine Affect Our Baby?

Women and their partners often ask whether pain medication or anesthesia will harm their baby. The nurse can help parents choose wisely from available options by providing honest information:

- Pain that you cannot tolerate is not good for you or your baby, and it reduces the joy of this special event.
- Some risk is associated with every type of pain medication or anesthesia, but careful selection and the use of preventive measures minimize this risk. If complications occur, corrective measures can reduce the risk to you and your baby.
- Some pain relievers can cause your baby to be slow to breathe at birth, but carefully controlling the timing and dose of the medication reduces the likelihood that this will occur. We can use another medication to reverse this effect if needed.
- Epidural or spinal anesthesia can cause your blood pressure to fall, which can reduce the blood flow to your baby. However, we give you lots of intravenous fluids to reduce this effect. We have other medications to increase your blood pressure if the fluids are not enough.
- General anesthesia can cause your baby to be slow to breathe at birth. To reduce this risk, the anesthesia will not be started until everything is ready for the surgery, and the doctors will clamp the baby's umbilical cord as quickly as possible.

---

esophagus until the woman is intubated and the cuff of the endotracheal tube is inflated. Successful intubation with the cuffed endotracheal tube blocks passage of any gastric contents into the trachea.

Postoperative Care Birth facility protocols guide postoperative care, including pre- and post-extubation care for the woman who had general anesthesia. The woman is extubated when her protective laryngeal reflexes have returned. Suction equipment and an Ambu bag with appropriate-size mask should be immediately available. Administer oxygen by mask or face tent for 2 to 5 minutes until the woman is awake and alert, because the agents used for general anesthesia are respiratory depressants. Monitor oxygen saturation with a pulse oximeter. If her oxygen saturation falls below 95%, have her take several deep breaths. Deep breathing also helps her eliminate inhalational anesthetics and reduces stasis of pulmonary secretions.

Assess the woman's pulse, respiration, and blood pressure every 15 minutes for 1 hour or until stable; then continue according to policy. Observe her color for pallor or cyanosis, which suggests shock or hypoventilation.

Evaluation

Interventions for this nursing diagnosis are preventive and short-term because it is a temporary high-risk situation. The goal is met if the woman does not aspirate gastric contents during the perioperative period.

TABLE 19-2 Pharmacologic Methods of Intrapartum Pain Management

Method and Uses	Nursing Considerations
OPIOID ANALGESICS	
Systemic analgesia during labor and for postoperative pain after cesarean birth. May be combined with an adjunctive drug such as promethazine to reduce the nausea and vomiting that sometimes occur with narcotic use and after surgery. Often delivered by PCA pump in postoperative period.	1. Assess the woman for drug use at admission. Women who are opiate-dependent should not receive analgesics having mixed agonist and antagonist actions (butorphanol and nalbuphine). 2. Observe neonate for respiratory depression, especially if the mother had opioid narcotics within 4 hr of birth or at time of the drug's peak action or if the mother received multiple opioid doses during labor: • Delay in initiating or sustaining normal depth and rate of respirations • Respiratory rate <30/min • Poor muscle tone: limp, floppy 3. The use of adjunctive drugs for nausea, such as promethazine, enhances respiratory depressant effects. 4. Have naloxone available for infants exposed to opioids during labor. Respiratory and cardiac support precede drug administration in neonatal resuscitation. Observe for recurrent respiratory depression after administration of naloxone.
EPIDURAL OPIOIDS	
Labor: Mixed with a local anesthetic agent to give better pain relief with less motor block. *Postoperatively:* Gives long-acting analgesia without sedation, allowing the mother and infant to interact more easily.	1. Observe same nursing implications as with epidural block. 2. Do not give additional opioids or other CNS depressants except as ordered by the anesthesia provider. Nonsteroidal antiinflammatory drugs or oral analgesics are often prescribed in routine orders. 3. Maternal respiratory depression may be delayed for up to 24 hr and varies with drug given. Observe respiratory rate, depth, oxygen saturation, and arousability hourly for 24 hr. Notify anesthesia provider for rate of <12/min, persistent oxygen saturation of <95% on pulse oximetry, reduced respiratory effort, difficulty arousing, or as ordered by the provider. Cyanosis is a late sign of respiratory depression. 4. Have naloxone, 0.4 mg, an oral airway, and an Ambu bag and mask immediately available, such as on a "crash cart." 5. Observe for pruritus or rubbing of the face and neck. Routine postoperative orders to relieve pruritus are usually provided. Notify anesthesia provider if these are insufficient. 6. Urinary retention may occur after indwelling catheter removal. Observe for adequacy of voiding, as in all postpartum women. 7. Notify anesthesia provider for relief of nausea or vomiting. 8. Assess sensation and mobility before allowing ambulation.
INTRATHECAL OPIOID ANALGESICS	
Provides analgesia for most of first-stage labor without maternal sedation. A very small dose of the drug is needed because it is injected very near the spinal cord where sensory fibers enter. Usually not adequate for late labor or the birth itself. Often combined with epidural block for the combined spinal-epidural (CSE) technique for labor.	1. Observe for the common side effects of nausea, vomiting, and pruritus. Notify the anesthesia provider if these effects occur, and have an antagonist such as naloxone or naltrexone available. 2. Observe for delayed respiratory depression, depending on the drug given. Use a pulse oximeter as indicated. 3. Observe for nonreassuring fetal heart rate patterns that may be associated with reduced maternal oxygenation.
LOCAL INFILTRATION ANESTHESIA	
Numbs perineum for episiotomy or repair of laceration at vaginal birth. No relief of labor pain. Not adequate for forceps-assisted birth.	1. Assess for drug allergies, especially to dental anesthetics because they are related to those used in maternity care. 2. Apply ice to perineum after birth to reduce edema and hematoma formation and to increase comfort.

PCA, Patient-controlled analgesia; *CNS,* central nervous system; *BP,* blood pressure; *IV,* intravenous.

TABLE **19-2** Pharmacologic Methods of Intrapartum Pain Management—cont'd

Method and Uses	Nursing Considerations
PUDENDAL BLOCK	
Numbs the lower vagina and perineum for vaginal birth. No relief of labor pain because it is done just before birth. Provides adequate anesthesia for many forceps-assisted births.	1. Use the same interventions as for local infiltration. A woman or her partner may be alarmed if she notices the long needle (about 6 inches [15 cm]). Teach her that it must be long to reach the pudendal nerve through the vagina and that it will be inserted only about 1/2 inch (1.25 cm) near the location of the nerve. Tell her that a guide ("trumpet") will be used to avoid injuring her vaginal tissue or that of her baby.
EPIDURAL BLOCK	
Labor: Insertion of catheter provides pain relief for labor and vaginal birth (T10-S5 levels). *Cesarean birth:* If epidural was used during labor, level of block can be extended upward (T4-T6 level). Also used for cesarean birth.	1. Prehydrate the woman with warmed nonglucose crystalloid solution such as Ringer's lactate solution. Common minimum amounts: 500-1000 ml for labor and vaginal birth; 1500-2000 ml for planned cesarean birth and postbirth tubal ligation. 2. Displace uterus to left manually or with a wedge placed under the woman's right side to enhance placental perfusion. 3. Assess for hypotension at least every 5 min for 15 min after block is begun and with each new dose until vital signs are stable. Report to anesthesia provider: systolic BP of <110 mm Hg or a fall of 20% or more from baseline levels, pallor, or diaphoresis. Facility procedures give further guidance. 4. Assess fetal heart rate for signs of impaired placental perfusion, and report to anesthesia provider and nurse-midwife: tachycardia (>160/min for 10 min) or bradycardia (<110/min for 10 min), late decelerations (see Table 18-1). 5. If hypotension or signs of impaired placental perfusion occur, increase the rate of infusion of nonadditive IV fluid, reposition the woman to her side, and administer oxygen by face mask (8-10 L/min). Have ephedrine available (usually included in epidural tray). 6. Observe for a full bladder, and catheterize as ordered. 7. Leg movement and strength vary after an epidural block. Transfer with help to avoid muscle strains to nurse or woman. 8. Ambulate only after sensation and movement have returned. Have another person's assistance with the first ambulation.
SUBARACHNOID BLOCK	
Cesarean birth: Can be established slightly faster than epidural block. May rarely be used for complicated vaginal birth. Does not provide pain relief for labor because it is done just before birth. May be combined with an epidural block in a combined spinal-epidural (CSE). See "Intrathecal Opioid Analgesics" for more information.	1. See "Epidural Block" for these interventions: • IV prehydration • Uterine displacement • Observation of blood pressure and fetal heart rate • Care for hypotension or signs of impaired placental perfusion • Observation and intervention for bladder distention • Transfer and ambulation precautions 2. Observe for postspinal headache: a headache that is worse when the woman is upright and that may disappear when she is lying flat. Notify anesthesia provider if it occurs (a blood patch may be done). 3. Nursing interventions for postspinal headache: encourage bed rest, increase oral fluids if not contraindicated, give oral caffeine, and give analgesics as ordered.
GENERAL ANESTHESIA	
Cesarean birth if epidural or spinal block is not possible or if the woman refuses regional anesthesia. May be required for emergency procedures such as replacement of inverted uterus.	1. Determine type and time of last food intake on admission. 2. Restrict oral intake to clear liquids or as ordered. Consult with physician or nurse-midwife if surgical intervention is likely. 3. Report to anesthesia provider: oral intake before and during labor, vomiting.

Continued

TABLE 19-2 Pharmacologic Methods of Intrapartum Pain Management—cont'd

Method and Uses	Nursing Considerations
GENERAL ANESTHESIA—cont'd	
	4. Displace uterus (see "Epidural Block"). 5. Give ordered drugs such as sodium citrate and citric acid (Bicitra). 6. Maintain cricoid pressure (Sellick maneuver) during intubation. 7. The woman will remain intubated until protective (gag) reflexes have returned. Have oral airway and suction immediately available. Oxygen by face tent or face mask should be given after extubation. 8. Interventions for postoperative respiratory depression: give positive-pressure oxygen by face mask; observe oxygen saturation with pulse oximetry until woman is awake and alert; have woman take several deep breaths if oxygen saturation falls below 95%. Notify anesthesia provider.

KEY CONCEPTS

- Childbirth pain is unique because it is normal and self-limiting, can be prepared for, and ends with a baby's birth.
- Excess or poorly relieved pain can be harmful to the mother and fetus.
- Pain is a complex physical and psychologic experience. It is subjective and personal.
- Four sources of pain are present in most labors, but other physical and psychologic factors may increase or decrease the pain felt from these sources. These sources are cervical dilation, uterine ischemia, pressure and pulling on pelvic structures, and distention of the vagina and perineum.
- Relaxation enhances other pain management techniques.
- Any drug that the expectant mother takes, whether therapeutic or abused, also may affect the fetus. Fetal effects may be direct or indirect.
- Cutaneous and mental stimulation techniques reduce pain perception. Techniques should be varied to prevent habituation.
- The purpose of breathing techniques is to increase relaxation. Lamaze breathing should be no slower than half the woman's normal respiratory rate and no faster than twice her normal rate.
- The physiologic alterations of pregnancy may affect a woman's response to medications.
- The major advantages of regional pain management methods are that the woman can participate in the birth and that she retains her protective airway reflexes.
- The nurse should observe for and take actions to prevent maternal hypotension with an epidural or subarachnoid block.
- The nurse should observe for fetal heart rate changes associated with impaired placental perfusion if the woman is at risk for hypotension, such as with epidural or subarachnoid blocks.
- The main nursing observations for the woman who receives epidural or intrathecal opioids are for nausea and vomiting, pruritus, and delayed respiratory depression.
- The nurse should observe for respiratory depression, primarily in the newborn, when the mother has received opioid analgesics during labor.
- Regurgitation with aspiration of acidic gastric contents is the greatest risk for a woman who receives general anesthesia.

ANSWERS to Critical Thinking Exercise 19-1

1. Truc's labor progress and pattern of contractions plus her tension suggest that she may need medication. However, the nurse should not assume that she needs or wants medication. Breathing techniques or other nonpharmacologic measures may be adequate for Truc.

   The nurse must not assume that Truc does not need pain relief because she smiles and has not requested pain medica-

tion. Asian women often value stoicism and are concerned with harmonious relationships. Truc may be smiling to please the nurse rather than because she is comfortable. In addition, Truc may not fully understand what the nurse says about pain relief if she is not comfortable speaking and understanding the nurse's language.

2. The nurse needs additional data about Truc's needs and plans for pain relief.

3. The nurse can share observations about Truc's body posture during contractions. If Truc does not speak English well, an interpreter may improve assessment of her need for pain relief. The nurse can demonstrate nonpharmacologic actions, such as breathing techniques, for Truc to use with or without medication.

REFERENCES and READINGS

American Academy of Pediatrics (AAP), & American College of Obstetricians and Gynecologists (ACOG). (2002). *Guidelines for perinatal care* (5th ed.). Elk Grove Village, IL, and Washington, DC: Authors.

Association of Women's Health, Obstetric, and Neonatal Nurses (AWHONN). (2001). *Evidence-based clinical practice guideline: Nursing care of the woman receiving regional analgesia/anesthesia in labor*. Washington, DC: Author.

Blackburn, S.T. (2003). *Maternal, fetal, and neonatal physiology: A clinical perspective* (2nd ed.). Philadelphia: Saunders.

Bricker, L., & Lavender, T. (2002). Parenteral opioids for labor pain relief: A systematic review.

American Journal of Obstetrics and Gynecology, 186(5), S94-S109.

Britt, R., & Pasero, C. (1999). Pregnancy, childbirth, postpartum, and breastfeeding: Use of analgesics. In M. McCaffery & C. Pasero, *Pain: Clinical manual* (2nd ed., pp. 608-625). St. Louis: Mosby.

Browning, C. (2000). Using music during childbirth. *Birth,* 27(4), 272-276.

Caton, D., Frölich, M.A., & Euliano, T.Y. (2002). Anesthesia for childbirth: Controversy and change. *American Journal of Obstetrics and Gynecology,* 186(5), S25-S30.

Chapman, L.L. (2000). Expectant fathers and labor epidurals. *MCN: The American Journal of Maternal/Child Nursing,* 25(3), 133-138.

Crafter, H. (2000). Psychology of pain in normal labour. In M. Yerby, *Pain in childbearing: Key issues in management* (pp. 43-60). Edinburgh: Balliére-Tindall.

Creehan, P.A. (2001). Pain relief and comfort measures during labor. In K.R. Simpson & P.A. Creehan (Eds.), *AWHONN's perinatal nursing* (2nd ed., pp. 417-444). Philadelphia: Lippincott.

Cunningham, F.G., Gant, N.F., Leveno, K.J., Gilstrap, L.C., Hauth, J.C., & Wenstrom, K.D. (2001). *Williams obstetrics* (21st ed.). New York: McGraw-Hill.

Eckert, K., Turnbull, D., & MacLennan, A. (2001). Immersion in water in the first stage of labor: A randomized controlled trial. *Birth,* 28(2), 84-93.

Faucher, M.A., & Brucker, M.C. (2000). Intrapartum pain: Pharmacologic management. *Journal of Obstetric, Gynecologic, and Neonatal Nurses,* 29(2), 169-180.

Fehder, W.P., & Gennaro, S. (1998). Immune alterations associated with epidural analgesia for labor and delivery. *MCN: The American Journal of Maternal/Child Nursing,* 23(6), 292-299.

Gilder, K., Mayberry, L.J., Gennaro, S., & Clemmens, D. (2002). Maternal positioning in labor with epidural analgesia. *AWHONN Lifelines,* 6(1), 40-45.

Goldberg, A.B., Cohen, A., & Lieberman, E. (1999). Nulliparas' preferences for epidural analgesia: Their effects on actual use in labor. *Birth,* 26(3), 139-143.

Hodnett, E.D. (2002). Pain and women's satisfaction with the experience of childbirth. *American Journal of Obstetrics and Gynecology,* 186(5), S160-S172.

Kabler, J. (2000). Water immersion during labor and birth. In F.N. Nichols & S.S. Humenick (Eds.), *Childbirth education: Practice, research, and theory* (2nd ed., pp. 284-294). Philadelphia: Saunders.

Klein, M.C., Grzybowski, S., Harris, S., Liston, R., Spence, A., Le, G., Brummendorf, D., Kim, S., & Kaczorowski, J. (2001). Epidural analgesia use as a marker for physician approach to birth: Implications for maternal and neonatal outcomes. *Birth,* 28(4), 243-248.

Koehn, M.L. (2000). Acupuncture and acupressure. In F.N. Nichols & S.S. Humenick (Eds.), *Childbirth education: Practice, research, and theory* (2nd ed., pp. 295-306). Philadelphia: Saunders.

Leighton, B.L., & Halpern, S.H. (2002). The effects of epidural analgesia on labor, maternal, and neonatal outcomes: A systematic review. *American Journal of Obstetrics and Gynecology,* 186(5), S69-S77.

Lieberman, E., Lang, J., Richardson, D.K., Frigoletto, F.D., Heffner, L.J., & Cohen, A. (2000). Intrapartum maternal fever and neonatal outcome. *Pediatrics,* 105(1), 8-13.

Lieberman, E., & O'Donoghue, C. (2002). Unintended effects of epidural analgesia during labor: A systematic review. *American Journal of Obstetrics and Gynecology,* 186(5), S31-S68.

Lowe, N.K. (2002). The nature of labor pain. *American Journal of Obstetrics and Gynecology,* 186(5), S16-S24.

Mayberry, L.J., Clemmens, D., & De, A. (2002). Epidural analgesia side effects, co-interventions, and care of women during childbirth: A systematic review. *American Journal of Obstetrics and Gynecology,* 186(5), S81-S93.

Mayberry, L.J., Strange, L.B., Suplee, P.D., & Gennaro, S. (2003). Use of upright positioning with epidural analgesia: Findings from an observational study. *MCN: The American Journal of Maternal/Child Nursing,* 28(3), 152-159.

Mayberry, L.J., Wood, S.H., Strange, L.B., Lee, L., Heisler, D.R., & Nielsen-Smith, K. (2000). *Second-stage labor management: Promotion of evidence-based practice and a collaborative approach to patient care.* Washington, DC: Association of Women's Health, Obstetric, and Neonatal Nurses.

Newton, E.R. (2000). Commentary: Epidural analgesia, intrapartum fever, and neonatal outcomes. *Birth,* 27(3), 206-208.

Nichols, F.H. (2000). Paced breathing techniques. In F.N. Nichols & S.S. Humenick (Eds.), *Childbirth education: Practice, research, and theory* (2nd ed, pp. 509-520). Philadelphia: Saunders.

Parker, R. (1999). Postoperative analgesia: Systemic techniques. In D.H. Chestnut, *Obstetric anesthesia: Principles and practice* (2nd ed., pp. 711-724). St. Louis: Mosby.

Pasero, C. L., & Britt, R. (1998). Managing pain during childbirth. *American Journal of Nursing,* 98(8), 10-11.

Paull, J. (2000). Epidural analgesia for labor. In D.J. Birnbach, S.P. Gatt, & S. Datta (Eds.), *Textbook of obstetric anesthesia* (pp. 145-156). New York: Churchill Livingstone.

Ransjö-Arvidson, A.B., Matthiesen, A.S., Lilja, G., Nissen, E., Widström, A.M., & Uvnäs-Moberg, K. (2001). Maternal analgesia during labor disturbs newborn behavior: Effects on breastfeeding, temperature, and crying. *Birth,* 28(1), 5-12.

Rolbin, S.H., & Morningstar, B.A. (2000). The febrile parturient. In D.J. Birnbach, S.P. Gatt, & S. Datta, (Eds.), *Textbook of obstetric anesthesia* (pp. 375-391). New York: Churchill Livingstone.

Segal, S., Carp, H., & Chestnut, D.H. (1999). Fever and infection. In D.H. Chestnut, *Obstetric anesthesia: Principles and practice* (2nd ed., pp. 711-724). St. Louis: Mosby.

Simkin, P. (2002). Nonpharmacologic relief of pain during labor: Systematic reviews of five methods. *American Journal of Obstetrics and Gynecology,* 186(5), S131-S159.

Sinatra, R.S., & Ayoub, C.M. (1999). Postoperative analgesia: Epidural and spinal techniques. In D.H. Chestnut, *Obstetric anesthesia: Principles and practice* (2nd ed., pp. 521-555). St. Louis: Mosby.

Sinatra, R.S., Ayoub, C.M., & Sevarino, F.B. (2000). Postcesarean analgesia: Patient-controlled analgesia and neuraxial techniques. In D.J. Birnbach, S.P. Gatt, & S. Datta (Eds.), *Textbook of obstetric anesthesia* (pp. 320-341). New York: Churchill Livingstone.

Walker, N.C., & O'Brien, B. (1999). The relationship between method of pain management during labor and birth outcomes. *Clinical Nursing Research,* 8(2), 119-134.

Yancy, M.K., Zhang, J., Schweitzer, D.L., Schwarz, J., & Klebanoff, M.A. (2001). Epidural analgesia and fetal head malposition at vaginal delivery. *Obstetrics & Gynecology,* 97(4), 608-612.

Yerby, M. (2000). Physiology of labour pain. In M. Yerby, *Pain in childbearing: Key issues in management* (pp. 29-42). Edinburgh: Balliére-Tindall.

20

Nursing Care During Obstetric Procedures

LEARNING OBJECTIVES

After studying this chapter, you should be able to:

◎ Identify clinical situations in which specific obstetric procedures are appropriate.

◎ Explain risks, precautions, and contraindications for each procedure.

◎ Identify nursing considerations for each procedure.

◎ Identify methods to provide effective emotional support to the woman having an obstetric procedure.

◎ Apply the nursing process to plan care for the woman having a cesarean birth.

DEFINITIONS

abruptio placentae Premature separation of a normally implanted placenta.

amniotomy Artificial rupture of the amniotic sac (fetal membranes).

augmentation of labor Artificial stimulation of uterine contractions that have become ineffective.

cephalopelvic disproportion Fetal head size that is too large to fit through the maternal pelvis at birth. Also called *fetopelvic disproportion.*

cesarean birth Surgical birth of the fetus through an incision in the abdominal wall and uterus.

chignon Newborn scalp edema created by a vacuum extractor.

chorioamnionitis Inflammation of the amniotic sac (fetal membranes), usually caused by bacterial or viral infections. Also called *amnionitis.*

dystocia Difficult or prolonged labor, often associated with abnormal uterine activity and cephalopelvic disproportion.

episiotomy Surgical incision of the perineum to enlarge the vaginal opening.

hydramnios Excessive volume of amniotic fluid (more than 2000 ml at term). Also called *polyhydramnios.*

iatrogenic An adverse condition resulting from treatment.

induction of labor Artificial initiation of labor.

nuchal cord Umbilical cord around the fetal neck.

oligohydramnios Abnormally small quantity of amniotic fluid (less than 500 ml at term).

placenta previa Abnormal implantation of the placenta in the lower uterus.

premature rupture of the membranes Spontaneous rupture of the membranes before the onset of labor. The gestation may be term, preterm, or postterm.

version Turning the fetus from one presentation to another before birth, usually from breech to cephalic.

Although labor is a normal process, special procedures are sometimes needed to help the mother or fetus. A physician or nurse-midwife performs these procedures; nursing considerations for each are addressed.

AMNIOTOMY

Indications

Almost 1 million women had an amniotomy in 2000 (National Center for Health Statistics, 2003). Amniotomy is done to induce or stimulate labor or to permit internal electronic fetal monitoring (Chapter 18). Although amniotomy is often used for induction or stimulation of labor, its actual effectiveness and benefits for these purposes are not well established (Bricker & Luckas, 2001; Cunningham et al., 2001).

Risks

Amniotomy is seen by many professionals and expectant mothers as harmless, but the nurse must observe for three major associated risks and assist in emergency procedures.

Prolapse of the Umbilical Cord

An immediate and continuing risk is that the umbilical cord will slip down in the gush of fluid. The cord can be compressed between the fetal presenting part and the woman's pelvis, obstructing blood flow to and from the placenta and reducing fetal gas exchange.

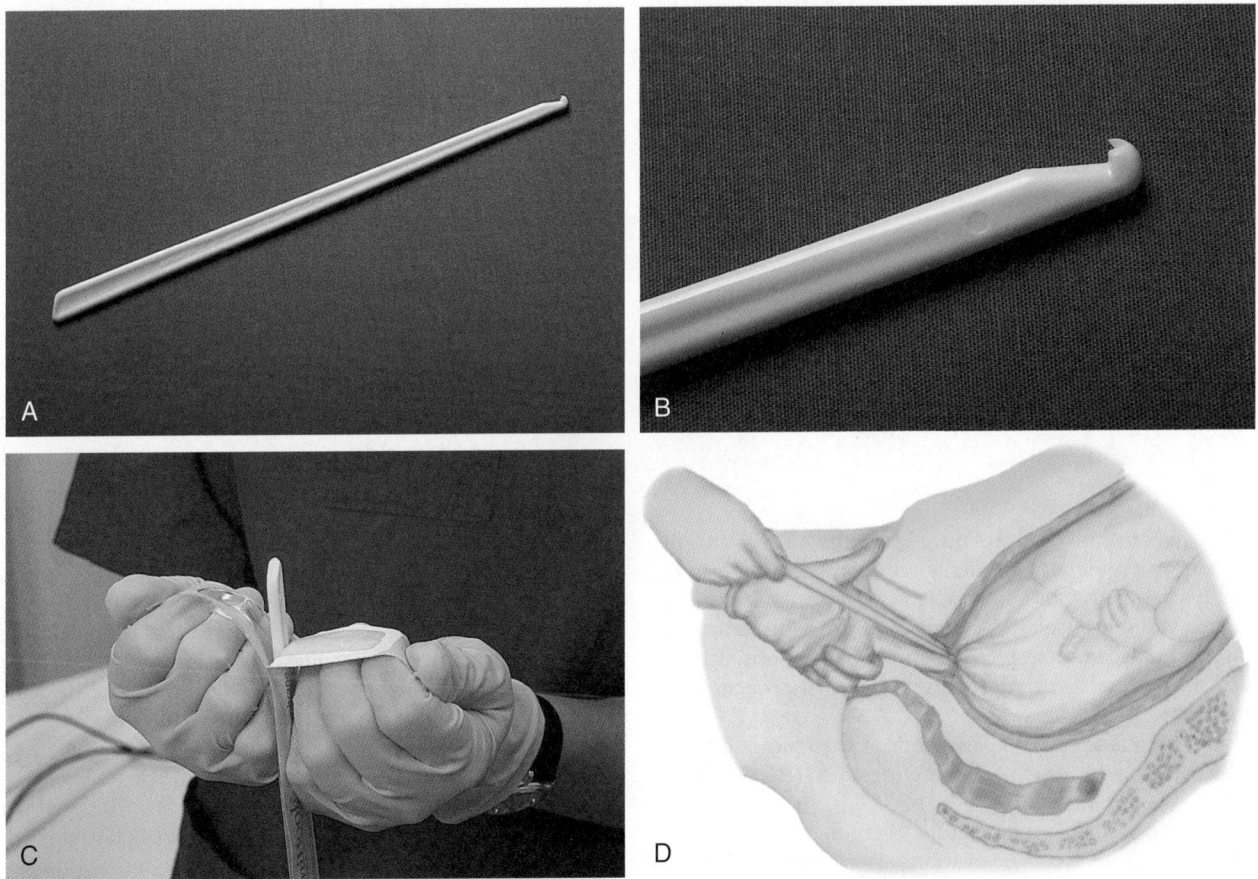

Figure 20-1 **A,** Disposable plastic membrane perforator (Amnihook). **B,** Hook end of plastic membrane perforator. **C,** Correct method of opening the package. **D,** Technique for artificial rupture of membranes.

Infection

With interruption of the membrane barrier, vaginal organisms have free access to the uterine cavity and may cause chorioamnionitis. The risk is low at first but increases as the interval between membrane rupture and birth increases. Birth within 24 hours of amniotomy is desirable although there is no absolute time when infection occurs.

Abruptio Placentae

Abruptio placentae may occur if the uterus is distended when the membranes rupture. The risk is greater if there is excessive amniotic fluid in the uterus (hydramnios), because of greater uterine distention. The area of placental attachment shrinks as the uterus collapses with discharge of the amniotic fluid. The placenta then no longer fits its implantation site and partially separates. A large area of placental disruption reduces fetal oxygenation, nutrition, and waste disposal.

Technique

A disposable plastic hook (Amnihook) is commonly used to perforate the amniotic sac (Fig. 20-1). The physician or nurse-midwife does a vaginal examination to determine cervical dilation and effacement, fetal station, and fetal presenting part. Amniotomy is deferred if the fetal presenting part is high or if the presentation is not cephalic. The risk for a prolapsed cord is greater in these situations because more room is available for the cord to slip down. In addition, a cesarean birth is usually performed for a non-cephalic presentation.

The hook is passed through the cervix, and the membranes are snagged. The hole is enlarged with the finger, allowing fluid to drain.

Nursing Considerations

Obtaining Baseline Information

The fetal heart rate is assessed with auscultation or electronic monitoring to identify a reassuring rate and pattern before amniotomy is done. A minimum of 20 to 30 minutes is needed for adequate baseline fetal evaluation and can be obtained while obtaining other admission information.

Assisting With Amniotomy

Before amniotomy, place underpads under the woman's buttocks to absorb the fluid. One or more folded bath towels under the buttocks absorb amniotic fluid well. Other supplies needed are a disposable plastic hook, a sterile glove or pair of gloves, and a packet of sterile lubricant.

Providing Care After Amniotomy

Nursing care after amniotomy is the same as that after spontaneous membrane rupture.

Identifying Complications. Assess the fetal heart rate for at least 1 full minute after amniotomy. Nonreassuring rate or other electronic fetal monitor patterns or significant changes from previous assessments are reported promptly to the birth attendant. Cord compression is suspected if deep or prolonged variable decelerations occur during contractions or persistent bradycardia is present after contractions. Other nonreassuring fetal heart rate patterns may also occur (see Chapter 18).

Chart the quantity, color, and odor of the amniotic fluid. Refer to Chapter 17 for expected findings and signs of abnormality in the amniotic fluid.

Assess the woman's temperature every 2 hours after the membranes rupture. Report elevations above 38° C (100.4° F). Fetal tachycardia (sustained rate above 160 beats per minute [bpm]) often precedes maternal fever.

Promoting Comfort. Amniotic fluid leaks from the woman's vagina after membranes rupture. Change the underpads regularly for comfort and to reduce the moist environment that favors bacterial growth.

INDUCTION AND AUGMENTATION OF LABOR

Induction and augmentation of labor use artificial methods to stimulate uterine contractions. Techniques and nursing care are similar for both induction and augmentation. The U.S. prevalence of labor induction is 19.9%, more than twice the 1989 rate of 9%. Augmentation rates have also increased from 10.9% in 1989 to 20.6% in 2002 (Martin, Hamilton, Ventura, Menacker, & Munson, 2003). Few women who have regular prenatal care expect to deliver more than a few days past their due date.

Indications

Induction of labor is considered when ending the pregnancy benefits the woman or fetus and when labor and vaginal birth are considered safe. Labor induction is not done if the fetus must be delivered more quickly than the process permits; a cesarean birth would be performed instead. Examples of specific conditions that are indications for induction include (American College of Obstetricians and Gynecologists [ACOG], 1999b):

- Conditions in which the intrauterine environment is hostile to fetal well-being (e.g., intrauterine fetal growth restriction, maternal-fetal blood incompatibility)

- Spontaneous rupture of the membranes at or near term without onset of labor
- Postterm pregnancy
- Chorioamnionitis (inflammation of the amniotic sac)
- Hypertension associated with pregnancy or chronic hypertension, both of which are associated with reduced placental blood flow
- Abruptio placentae (large abruptions require immediate delivery, see Chapter 26)
- Maternal medical conditions that are worsening with continuation of the pregnancy (e.g., diabetes, renal disease, pulmonary disease, chronic hypertension)
- Fetal death

Factors such as a history of rapid labors or living a long distance from the hospital are valid reasons to induce labor, because of the real possibility that the baby would otherwise be born in uncontrolled circumstances. Psychosocial indications such as availability of the infant's father or other family to help after birth may be considered *if term gestation and/or fetal lung maturity have been confirmed.* Convenience for the medical provider or woman is not included on the list of indications.

Prenatal testing sometimes reveals a fetal anomaly for which specialized neonatal care at a distant facility will be needed. The mother may be transported to that facility for labor induction or cesarean birth, with the necessary equipment and specialists assembled to care for the newborn.

Augmentation of labor with oxytocin is considered when labor has begun spontaneously but progress has slowed or stopped because of poor contractions. The medical provider may use augmentation if progress is slower than expected, even if contractions seem to be adequate.

Contraindications

Any contraindication to labor and vaginal birth is a contraindication to induction or augmentation of labor. These conditions may include:

- Placenta previa, which may result in hemorrhage during labor
- Vasa previa, in which fetal umbilical cord vessels branch over the amniotic sac rather than inserting into the placenta; fetal hemorrhage is a possibility if the membranes rupture
- Transverse fetal lie, in which the fetus is lying crosswise in the uterus
- Umbilical cord prolapse, because immediate birth by cesarean is indicated
- Some uterine surgery, such as classic cesarean (see p. 456 and Fig. 20-9) or extensive surgery for uterine fibroids

Other maternal or fetal conditions are not contraindications to induction but require individual evaluation:

- One or more previous low transverse cesarean births (see Fig. 20-9)
- Breech presentation (vaginal birth may be more hazardous; also, the fetus may turn to a normal position by the time spontaneous labor occurs)
- Maternal heart disease, which varies in severity
- Severe maternal hypertension
- Multifetal pregnancy (high-multiple gestations, such as triplets, are rarely induced because of the uterine distention)

TABLE 20-1 Bishop Scoring System to Evaluate the Cervix

Factor	Score			
	0	1	2	3
Dilation	0 cm	1-2 cm	3-4 cm	5-6 cm
Effacement	0%-30%	40%-50%	60%-70%	>80%
Fetal Station	−3	−2	−1 or 0	+1 or +2
Cervical consistency	Firm	Medium	Soft	
Cervical position	Posterior	Middle	Anterior	

NOTE: This system is used to estimate how easily a woman's labor can be induced. Higher scores are associated with a greater likelihood of successful induction because her cervix has undergone prelabor changes, often called *ripening*. A woman who has given birth before usually has a successful induction when her Bishop score is 5 or higher. Delivery in a woman who is having her first baby is most successfully induced if her score is 7 or higher.
Modified from Bishop, E. H. (1964). Pelvic scoring for elective induction. *Obstetrics & Gynecology, 24*(2), 266-268.

- Hydramnios, which results in uterine distention
- Fetal presenting part above the pelvic inlet, which may be associated with cephalopelvic disproportion or a preterm fetus
- Nonreassuring fetal heart rate patterns that do not yet mandate emergency delivery

Risks

Induction and augmentation of labor are associated with risks, as is spontaneous labor. These risks include:

- Uterine hyperstimulation, which can reduce placental perfusion and fetal oxygenation caused by excessive frequency, duration, or intensity of contractions, or from poor uterine relaxation between contractions. The hyperstimulation may or may not be accompanied by nonreassuring fetal heart rate patterns.
- Uterine rupture, more likely to occur with overdistention.
- Maternal water intoxication caused by oxytocin's antidiuretic effects; more likely if hypotonic solutions are used to dilute the oxytocin and infusion rates exceed 20 mU/min (ACOG, 1999b ; Cunningham et al., 2001).
- Greater risk for cesarean birth (see p. 455).

Technique

Surgical, medical, or mechanical methods may be used for labor induction or augmentation. Amniotomy is the method of surgical induction and augmentation, because rupturing membranes stimulates uterine contractions if the cervix is favorable. Medical methods for induction or augmentation use drugs such as prostaglandins or intravenous (IV) oxytocin (Pitocin), or both, to stimulate contractions. Mechanical methods of induction use a variety of intracervical inserts to gradually stretch and soften the cervix.

Determining Whether Induction Is Indicated

The birth attendant evaluates whether labor and birth are safer for the woman or fetus than continuing the pregnancy. Labor is not induced if term gestation and/or fetal lung maturity are not established unless there is a compelling reason. Induction is more likely to be successful at term because prelabor cervical changes favor dilation.

The Bishop scoring system (Table 20-1) uses five factors to estimate cervical readiness for labor: cervical dilation, effacement, consistency, position, and fetal station. The Bishop score remains popular because of its ability to predict probable success of induction. The likelihood of vaginal birth is similar to that of spontaneous labor if the score is greater than 8 (ACOG, 1999b).

Cervical Ripening

Procedures to ripen (soften) the cervix and make it more likely to dilate with the forces of labor are a common adjunct to induction. Cervical ripening may be done the morning of induction or possibly the day before.

Medical Methods. Preparations containing prostaglandin E_2 (PGE$_2$, or dinoprostone) may be used to facilitate cervical ripening. Prostaglandin may be given as an intravaginal or intracervical gel or a timed-release vaginal insert (Table 20-2). It is administered in a setting in which fetal monitoring and emergency care, including immediate cesarean birth, are readily available.

Prostaglandin should be given cautiously to women who have asthma, glaucoma, ischemic heart disease, or pulmonary, hepatic, or renal disease. The major adverse reaction to prostaglandin for induction is hyperstimulation of uterine contractions, which can reduce placental blood flow and fetal oxygen exchange. The fetal heart rate and uterine activity should be monitored before prostaglandin insertion for a baseline and at least 30 minutes afterward for nonreassuring fetal heart rate patterns or excessive contractions.

Misoprostol (Cytotec) is popular for preinduction cervical ripening and labor induction because of its low cost, stability, and ease of use (see Table 20-2). Misoprostol is a synthetic prostaglandin tablet that is used for prevention of gastric ulcers. Use for cervical ripening or labor induction is currently an unlabeled one, and its manufacturer does not plan to seek approval from the U.S. Food and Drug Administration for this use.

Mechanical Methods. Although other mechanical methods for cervical ripening exist, a common method involves placement of hydrophilic (moisture-attracting) inserts into the cervical canal, where they absorb water and expand, gradually dilating the cervix. Examples of these dilators are:

- Dilapan—a synthetic material
- Lamicel—a synthetic sponge containing 450 mg of magnesium sulfate
- Laminaria tents—sterile, cone-shaped preparations of dried seaweed; more than one can be placed

TABLE 20-2 Prostaglandin Preparations for Cervical Ripening at Term

Prostaglandin Gel (dinoprostone, or Prepidil)	Vaginal Insert (dinoprostone, or Cervidil)	Misoprostol (Cytotec)
DOSAGE		
0.5 mg applied to cervix. May be repeated 6-12 hr later. 2.5 mg vaginally.	10 mg in a time-release vaginal insert.	One-quarter of 100-mcg tablet vaginally (approximately 25 mcg; see cautions below). Also used for labor induction by repeating 25-mcg dose every 3-6 hr. A 50-mcg dose is associated with hypertonic contractions.
ACTIONS FOR HYPERTONIC CONTRACTIONS, WITH OR WITHOUT NONREASSURING FETAL HEART RATE PATTERN		
Place woman in side-lying position. Provide oxygen by face mask at 8-10 L/min. Administer tocolytic drug such as terbutaline or magnesium sulfate. Typically begins 1 hr after gel application. Higher incidence with vaginal application.	Same as for dinoprostone gel. Remove insert. Hypertonic uterine activity may occur up to $9\frac{1}{2}$ hr after insert placement. Greater incidence than with lower-dose intracervical dinoprostone gel.	Same as for dinoprostone gel. Higher doses or more frequent administration is more likely to cause excessive contractions, which may or may not be accompanied by a nonreassuring fetal heart rate pattern.
WHEN OXYTOCIN INDUCTION MAY BEGIN		
Safe interval has not been established. Delaying oxytocin administration for 6-12 hr after total intracervical dose of 1.5-mg or 2.5-mg vaginal dose recommended.	30-60 min after removal of insert.	At least 4 hr after last dose.
PRECAUTIONS AND COMMENTS		
Limit dinoprostone gel to maximum of 1.5 mg dinoprostone gel in 24 hr. Woman should remain recumbent with lateral uterine displacement for 15-30 min after application. Has increased effect if combined with other oxytocics such as oxytocin (Pitocin). Increases hypertensive effect of the herb ephedra. Use caution in women with asthma, hypertension, glaucoma, or severe renal or hepatic dysfunction, ischemic heart disease.	Removed after 12 hr or when active labor begins. Adverse effects can be reduced within 15 min of removal. Most expensive of the prostaglandin options.	Misoprostol is currently FDA-approved only for treatment of peptic ulcers but is widely used for cervical ripening and induction of labor. Manufacturer does not intend to seek approval, but American College of Obstetricians and Gynecologists supports its use for these purposes. 100-mcg tablet is not scored. Hospital pharmacy should prepare the 25-mcg dose for greater accuracy. Cost is about 1%-2% that of other prostaglandin preparations. Contraindicated in the woman with a previous cesarean or other uterine surgery.

NOTE: Doses may be higher in cases of fetal death.
From American College of Obstetricians and Gynecologists (ACOG). (1999). *Induction of labor* (ACOG Practice Bulletin No. 10). Washington, DC: Author.

Oxytocin induction of labor begins the following morning.

Oxytocin Administration

Oxytocin is a powerful drug, and it is impossible to predict a woman's response to it. Several precautions reduce the chance of adverse reactions in the mother and fetus:

- Oxytocin is diluted in an isotonic solution and given as a secondary (piggyback) infusion so that it can be stopped quickly if complications develop (Fig. 20-2).
- The oxytocin line is inserted into the primary (nonadditive, or maintenance) intravenous line as close as possible to the venipuncture site (the proximal port) to limit the amount of drug infused after changing to the nonadditive fluid.

- Oxytocin is started slowly, increased gradually, and regulated with an infusion pump. The primary line may also be regulated with a pump.
- Uterine activity and fetal heart rate and patterns are monitored before induction, when oxytocin is started, and throughout labor.

The woman's uterus becomes more sensitive to oxytocin as labor progresses. Oxytocin administration is therefore titrated to uterine and fetal response. The rate of oxytocin infusion may be gradually reduced when she is in the active phase of labor, about 5 to 6 cm of cervical dilation. It may be stopped or reduced after her membranes rupture. When labor is augmented with oxytocin, a lower total dose is usually needed to achieve adequate contractions.

Drug Guide

Oxytocin (Pitocin)

Classification: Oxytocic.

Action: Synthetic compound identical to the natural hormone from the posterior pituitary. Stimulates uterine smooth muscle, resulting in increased strength, duration, and frequency of uterine contractions. Uterine sensitivity to oxytocin increases gradually during gestation. Oxytocin has vasoactive and antidiuretic properties.

Indications: Induction or augmentation of labor at or near term. Maintenance of firm uterine contraction after birth to control postpartum bleeding. Management of inevitable or incomplete abortion.

Dosage and Route

Induction or Augmentation of Labor

1. *Intravenous infusion* via a secondary (piggyback) line. Oxytocin infusion is controlled with a pump. Various dilutions of oxytocin and balanced electrolyte solution may be used. Mixtures having 60 mU/ml are convenient because the ml/hr setting on the infusion pump is the same number as the milliunits/min infused, reducing the chance for errors. Common mixtures that provide 60 mU/ml of oxytocin include (1) 15 units of oxytocin (1.5 ml) plus 250 ml of solution; (2) 30 units (3 ml) of oxytocin plus 500 ml solution; (3) 60 units oxytocin plus 1000 ml solution. Lower concentrations, such as 10-20 units of oxytocin plus 1000 ml of solution may also be used. The drug may be given in 10-minute pulsed infusions rather than continuously.

2. Guidelines for oxytocin administration from the American College of Obstetricians and Gynecologists* provide examples of low- and high-dose oxytocin labor induction protocols. Depending on the protocol followed, the following recommendations are provided: (1) starting dosages of 0.5 to 6 mU/min, and (2) increasing dosage by 1 to 2 mU/min—increments every 15 to 40 minutes. High-dose protocols may increase the dose in increments of up to 6 mU/min. The actual oxytocin dose is based on uterine response and absence of adverse effects. Higher starting doses, higher dose increases, and shorter intervals between dose increases are most likely to result in uterine hyperstimulation. A lower starting dose and lower rate increase increments are usually required to augment labor.

3. After an adequate contraction pattern is established and the cervix is dilated 5 to 6 cm, the oxytocin may be reduced by similar increments.

Control of Postpartum Bleeding

Intravenous infusion: Dilute 10 to 40 units in 1000 ml of intravenous solution. The rate of infusion must control uterine atony. Begin at a rate of 20 to 40 mU/min, increasing or decreasing the rate according to uterine response and the rate of postpartum bleeding. Correcting any identifiable cause of the hemorrhage should also be done. *Intramuscular injection:* Inject 10 units after delivery of the placenta.

Inevitable or Incomplete Abortion

Dilute 10 units in 500 ml of intravenous solution and infuse at a rate of 10 to 20 mU/min. Other dilutions are acceptable.

Absorption: Intravenous, immediate; intramuscular, 3 to 5 minutes.

Excretion: Liver and urine.

Contraindications and Precautions: Include, but are not limited to, placenta previa, vasa previa, nonreassuring fetal heart rate patterns, abnormal fetal presentation, prolapsed umbilical cord, presenting part above the pelvic inlet, previous classic or other fundal uterine incision, active genital herpes infection, pelvic structural deformities, invasive cervical carcinoma.

Adverse Reactions: Most result from hypersensitivity to drug or excessive dosage. Adverse reactions include hypertonic uterine activity, impaired uterine blood flow, uterine rupture, and abruptio placentae. Uterine hypertonicity may result in fetal bradycardia, tachycardia, reduced fetal heart rate variability, and late decelerations. Fetal asphyxia may occur with diminished uterine blood flow. Fetal or maternal trauma, or both, may occur from rapid birth. Prolonged administration may cause maternal fluid retention, leading to water intoxication. Hypotension (seen with rapid intravenous injection), tachycardia, cardiac dysrhythmias, and subarachnoid hemorrhage are rare adverse reactions.

Drug interactions include vasopressors and the herb ephedra, causing hypertension.

NURSING CONSIDERATIONS

Intrapartum: Assess the fetal heart rate for at least 20 minutes before induction to identify reassuring or nonreassuring patterns. Perform Leopold's maneuvers, a vaginal examination, or both to verify a cephalic fetal presentation. If nonreassuring fetal heart rate patterns are identified or if fetal presentation is other than cephalic, notify the physician and do not begin induction until an ultrasound is done to ascertain fetal presentation.

Observe uterine activity for establishment of effective labor pattern: contraction frequency every 2 to 3 minutes, duration of 40 to 90 seconds, intensity of 50 to 80 mm Hg (measured with an intrauterine pressure catheter). Observe for hypertonic uterine activity: contractions less than 2 minutes apart, rest interval shorter than 30 seconds, duration longer than 90-120 seconds, or an elevated resting tone greater than 20 mm Hg (measured with an intrauterine pressure catheter).

Observe fetal heart rate for nonreassuring patterns such as tachycardia, bradycardia, decreased variability, and late decelerations.

If uterine hypertonicity or a nonreassuring fetal heart rate pattern occurs, intervene to reduce uterine activity and increase fetal oxygenation: stop the oxytocin infusion; increase the rate of nonadditive solution; position the woman in a side-lying position; and administer oxygen by snug facemask at 8 to 10 L/min. Notify the physician of adverse reactions, nursing interventions, and response to interventions. Record the maternal blood pressure, pulse, and respirations every 30 to 60 minutes and with each dosage increase. Record intake and output.

Postpartum: Observe uterus for firmness, height, and deviation. Massage until firm if uterus is soft ("boggy"). Observe lochia for color, quantity, and presence of clots. Notify birth attendant if uterus fails to remain contracted or if lochia is bright red or contains large clots. Assess for cramping. Assess vital signs every 15 minutes or according to protocol. Monitor intake and output and breath sounds to identify fluid retention or bladder distention.

Inevitable or Incomplete Abortion: Observe for cramping, vaginal bleeding, clots, and passage of products of conception. Observe maternal vital signs, intake, and output as noted under postpartum nursing implications.

---

*American College of Obstetricians and Gynecologists. (1999). *Induction of labor* (ACOG Practice Bulletin No. 10). Washington, DC: Author; American College of Obstetricians and Gynecologists. (2003). *Dystocia and augmentation of labor* (ACOG Practice Bulletin No. 49). Washington, DC: Author.

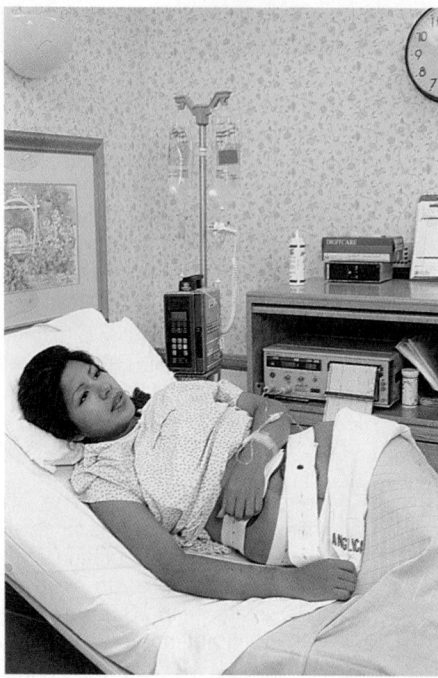

Figure 20-2 Intravenous oxytocin setup for induction or augmentation of labor. The primary line (nonadditive, or maintenance line) on the left side of the pole contains no medication. The secondary line with the orange "medication added" label contains oxytocin. The secondary oxytocin line should be regulated by the infusion pump and is inserted into the lowest port in the primary fluid line. An external fetal monitor is used to assess the fetal and uterine response to oxytocin-stimulated contractions. The woman lies on her side to promote uterine blood flow.

Nursing Considerations

In addition to basic intrapartum care, the nurse observes the woman and fetus for complications and takes corrective actions if abnormalities are noted. Nursing care is similar for the woman who has cervical ripening.

The nurse has a great responsibility when administering oxytocin or other uterine stimulants to a pregnant woman. The nurse must decide, within the facility's protocols and medical orders, when to start, change, or stop the oxytocin infusion. This responsibility requires additional education and refinement of the nurse's critical thinking skills.

Observing the Fetal Response

Oxytocin stimulates uterine contractions, and they may become too strong (hypertonic). Hypertonic contractions can reduce placental blood flow and therefore reduce exchange of fetal oxygen and waste products. Before induction or augmentation of labor, the nurse determines whether the fetal heart rate and patterns are reassuring. The fetal heart rate is charted in the labor record at least every 15 minutes during first-stage labor and every 5 minutes during the second stage (King & Simpson, 2001).

The nurse remains alert for fetal heart rate patterns that suggest reduced placental exchange secondary to hypertonic contractions. Examples of these patterns are fetal bradycardia (rate less than 110 bpm at term), tachycardia (persistent rate more than 160 bpm at term), late decelerations (slowing after the peak of the contraction), and decreased fetal heart rate variability (reduced rate fluctuations) that is not explained by

CRITICAL THINKING EXERCISE 20-2

A woman is having labor induced with oxytocin following earlier cervical ripening with prostaglandin. Her cervix is 4 cm dilated and fully effaced, and the fetal head is at station 0. The nurse notes that the fetal heart rate (internal monitor) is near its baseline of 120 to 130 bpm, with variability of 10 bpm. Contractions are firm (100 mm Hg with intrauterine pressure catheter), occur every 1½ to 2 minutes, with a duration of 95 to 100 seconds. The baseline intrauterine pressure is 25 to 30 mm Hg.
1. What is the correct interpretation of these assessments?
2. What are appropriate nursing actions in this situation, and why are they done?

medications or fetal sleep. Reduced placental exchange also may have causes other than excess uterine activity, such as maternal hypotension or maternal diabetes. The nurse must assess the woman and fetus carefully to identify the most likely cause of the problem and the indicated corrective actions.

If nonreassuring patterns occur or if contractions are hypertonic, the nurse takes steps to reduce uterine activity and increase fetal oxygenation. These steps include:

1. Reducing or stopping the oxytocin infusion and increasing the rate of the primary nonadditive infusion.
2. Keeping the woman on her side to prevent aortocaval compression and increase placental blood flow.
3. Giving 100% oxygen by snug facemask at a rate of 8 to 10 L/min to increase the woman's oxygen saturation, making more oxygen available for the fetus.

The physician may order a drug to reduce uterine activity, such as terbutaline (Brethine) or magnesium sulfate. Terbutaline, 0.25 mg subcutaneously, can be given quickly to stop the uterine hyperstimulation.

Observing the Mother's Response

Uterine activity must be assessed for hypertonus, which can reduce fetal oxygenation and contribute to uterine rupture. Contractions are assessed for frequency, duration, and intensity, and uterine resting tone is assessed for relaxation of at least 30 seconds between contractions. Uterine activity observations are charted at the same intervals as the fetal heart rate patterns. Corrective actions for hypertonic uterine activity are the same as those listed in the discussion of the fetal response. In addition, a tocolytic drug such as terbutaline may be given.

The woman's blood pressure and pulse are taken every 30 minutes or with each increase in the oxytocin dose to identify changes from her baseline. Her temperature is checked every 4 hours (every 2 hours after membrane rupture) to identify infection.

Recording intake and output identifies fluid retention, which precedes water intoxication. Signs and symptoms of water intoxication include headache, blurred vision, behavioral changes, increased blood pressure and respirations, decreased pulse, rales, wheezing, and coughing.

After birth, observe for postpartum hemorrhage caused by uterine relaxation. Postpartum uterine atony is more likely if the woman has received oxytocin for a long time, because the uterine muscle becomes fatigued and does not contract effec-

! CRITICAL TO REMEMBER

Signs of Hypertonic Uterine Activity

- Contraction duration longer than 90-120 seconds.
- Contractions occurring less than 2 minutes apart or relaxation of less than 30 seconds between contractions.
- Uterine resting tone above 20 mm Hg or peak pressure higher than 80 mm Hg during first-stage labor (with intrauterine pressure catheter).
- Montevideo units greater than 400.
- A fetal heart rate pattern of late decelerations may accompany hypertonic uterine activity.

Nursing Actions for Hypertonic Uterine Activity

- Reduce or stop the oxytocin infusion.
- Increase the rate of the primary nonadditive infusion.
- Keep the laboring woman in a lateral position.
- Give oxygen by snug facemask, 8 to 10 L/min.
- Notify the physician or nurse-midwife.

tively to compress vessels at the placental site. It is manifested by a soft uterine fundus and excess amounts of lochia, usually with large clots. Hypovolemic shock may occur with hemorrhage.

VERSION

Either of two methods may be used to change fetal presentation: external version or internal version. Each has different indications and a different technique. External version is much more common.

Indications

External Cephalic Version

The fetus may be changed from a breech, shoulder (transverse lie), or oblique presentation to a cephalic presentation using external cephalic version (ECV). Successful version may allow the woman to avoid a cesarean birth. ECV can change the fetal presentation from breech to cephalic an average of 58% of the time. In current studies (ACOG, 2000b) birth outcomes after ECV have shown mixed results. Some studies have found that the cesarean rate is still higher than average after successful ECV, whereas others have not demonstrated a difference (ACOG, 2000b; Laros, Flanagan, & Kilpatrick, 1995; Regalia et al., 2000). Even if ECV does not reduce the cesarean rate to the same level as for women who had a cephalic presentation in late pregnancy, it is a procedure that greatly increases a woman's chance for vaginal birth.

Internal Version

Malpresentation in twin gestations is usually managed by cesarean birth, but internal version is sometimes used for the vaginal birth of the second twin.

Contraindications

Version is not done if a woman cannot or is unlikely to deliver vaginally. Maternal conditions that may contraindicate external version or reduce its success include:

- Uterine malformations that limit the room available to perform the version and may contribute to the abnormal fetal presentation.
- Previous cesarean birth with a vertical uterine incision. Manipulation of the fetus within the uterus may strain and rupture the old incision, and a vertical incision is most likely to rupture.
- Disproportion between fetal size and maternal pelvic size.

Fetal conditions also may contraindicate the use of version:

- Placenta previa. Manipulation of the fetus within the uterus may cause hemorrhage, endangering both mother and fetus. Placenta previa other than marginal is an indication itself for cesarean birth.
- Multifetal gestation, which reduces available room to turn the fetus or fetuses. External version may be done after the first twin is born.
- Oligohydramnios, ruptured membranes, or a cord around the fetal body or neck (nuchal cord). These conditions limit the room in which to turn the fetus and may lead to cord compression and fetal hypoxia.
- Uteroplacental insufficiency. Uterine contractions occurring during the version or during labor may worsen the insufficiency and cause fetal compromise.
- Engagement of the fetal presenting part into the pelvis.

Risks

There are few risks to the woman, and serious adverse effects on the fetus are few. Fetal heart rate changes are common during the procedure but usually return to normal after the procedure. The fetus may become entangled in or compress the umbilical cord, possibly resulting in transient or prolonged hypoxia. Abruptio placentae may occur if fetal manipulation disrupts the placental site. Mixing of fetal and maternal blood within small breaks in placental vessels may result in maternal sensitization to the fetal blood type. Cesarean birth may be needed for fetal compromise at the time of version or later if the fetus returns to an abnormal presentation.

Technique

External Version

A nonstress test or biophysical profile (see Chapter 16) is done before external version to evaluate fetal health and placental function. If the test is nonreactive or other nonreassuring signs are present, the procedure is not done. Version adds stress to the fetus already functioning with reduced physiologic reserve. An ultrasound examination confirms fetal gestational age and fetal presentation and demonstrates adequacy of amniotic fluid (an amniotic fluid index [AFI] >5).

External version is usually attempted after 37 weeks of gestation but before the woman is in labor, for the following reasons:

- As term nears, the fetus may spontaneously turn to a cephalic presentation.
- The fetus is more likely to return to an abnormal presentation if version is attempted before 37 weeks.
- If fetal compromise or onset of labor occurs, the fetus will be at or near term at birth.

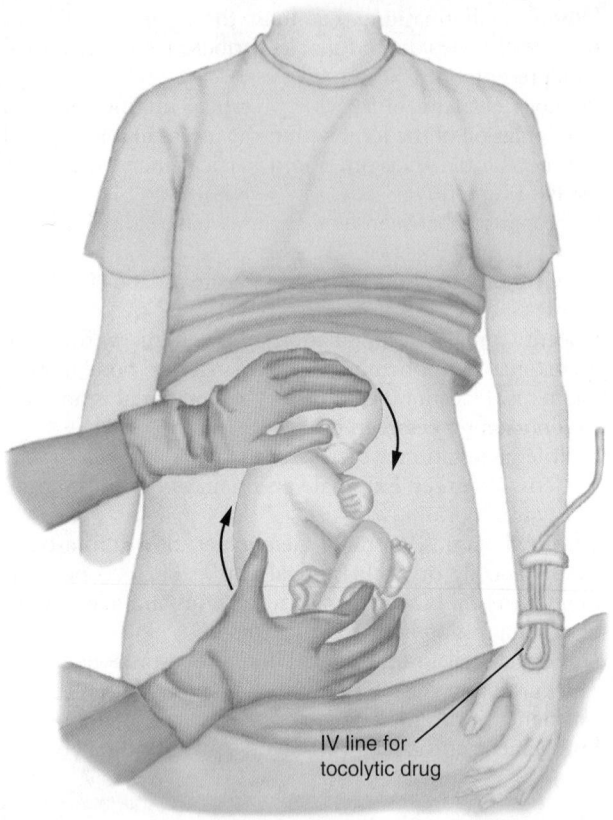

Figure 20-3 External version. IV access is established in case of emergency or for some tocolytic drugs. If terbutaline is the tocolytic drug, it is given by subcutaneous injection.

The woman is usually given a tocolytic drug, such as terbutaline 0.25 mg subcutaneously, to relax the uterus while the version is performed.

An epidural block or other analgesic may be given to increase maternal comfort and relaxation.

Ultrasonography guides fetal manipulations during external version and helps monitor the fetal heart rate. The physician gently pushes the breech out of the pelvis in a forward or backward roll (Fig. 20-3).

If indicated, Rh immune globulin is given to the Rh-negative woman after external version to prevent Rh sensitization.

Labor induction may be done immediately after a successful version, or the woman may await spontaneous labor or a later induction.

Internal Version

Internal version is an unexpected and urgent procedure. The physician reaches into the uterus with one hand and, with the other hand on the maternal abdomen, maneuvers the fetus into a longitudinal lie (cephalic or breech) to allow delivery.

Nursing Considerations

When caring for the woman having external version, the nurse provides information, assesses the woman and fetus, and helps reduce her anxiety.

Providing Information

The physician explains the indications and risks for external version to the woman before she signs an informed consent form. The nurse verifies the woman's understanding of the purposes, risks, and limitations of version. Consent for cesarean birth is usually obtained as well.

The purposes and side effects of any tocolytic drug are reviewed. Tachycardia, flushing, headache, and tremors are common side effects of tocolytics such as terbutaline.

Promoting Maternal and Fetal Health

Admission information is collected as if the woman were in labor or having a cesarean birth, because the need for operative intervention may arise suddenly.

Maternal vital signs are assessed for baseline value, and the initial nonstress test is done. Abnormalities or nonreassuring fetal heart rate patterns should be reported promptly.

An IV line is established for possible drug administration or fluid resuscitation if the fetal heart rate is nonreassuring.

The nurse administers the tocolytic drug. Terbutaline onset of action is 6 to 15 minutes after subcutaneous injection.

Real-time ultrasonography is used to guide the version and check the fetal heart rate periodically.

After the version, the mother and fetus are observed for at least 1 hour. Reassuring fetal signs are a heart rate near the same range as baseline, resolution of bradycardia, and the presence of rate accelerations with fetal movement.

Maternal tachycardia, flushing, or headache may be present for up to 4 hours if terbutaline was given to relax the uterus.

Maternal vital signs are measured every 15 to 30 minutes until they return to near their baseline level. Maternal pulse should be no higher than 120 bpm.

The presence of regular contractions suggests the onset of labor. Spontaneous rupture of membranes sometimes occurs.

Rh immune globulin is given to the Rh-negative woman.

The woman usually has some discomfort during the version, but it should diminish quickly afterward. Persistent or continuous pain suggests a complication such as abruptio placentae.

Because the woman undergoing external version is near term, the nurse should review the signs of true labor or membrane rupture with her and explain guidelines for returning to the hospital if she is not having induction immediately after the procedure (see Chapter 17).

Reducing Anxiety

The woman may be anxious before version because its success is not certain and complications may require rapid cesarean delivery. After version, she may still be anxious because the fetus can return to its previous position. Supporting her as she expresses her concerns and during the procedure helps reduce her anxiety somewhat.

Pointing out reassuring fetal monitor patterns, such as a normal heart rate and rate accelerations, can help reduce her anxiety about her baby. If problems such as bradycardia develop, the nurse should explain what has happened, what steps are being done to relieve it, and the result of these interventions. Explanations of tocolytic-associated side effects and when they should disappear should be provided.

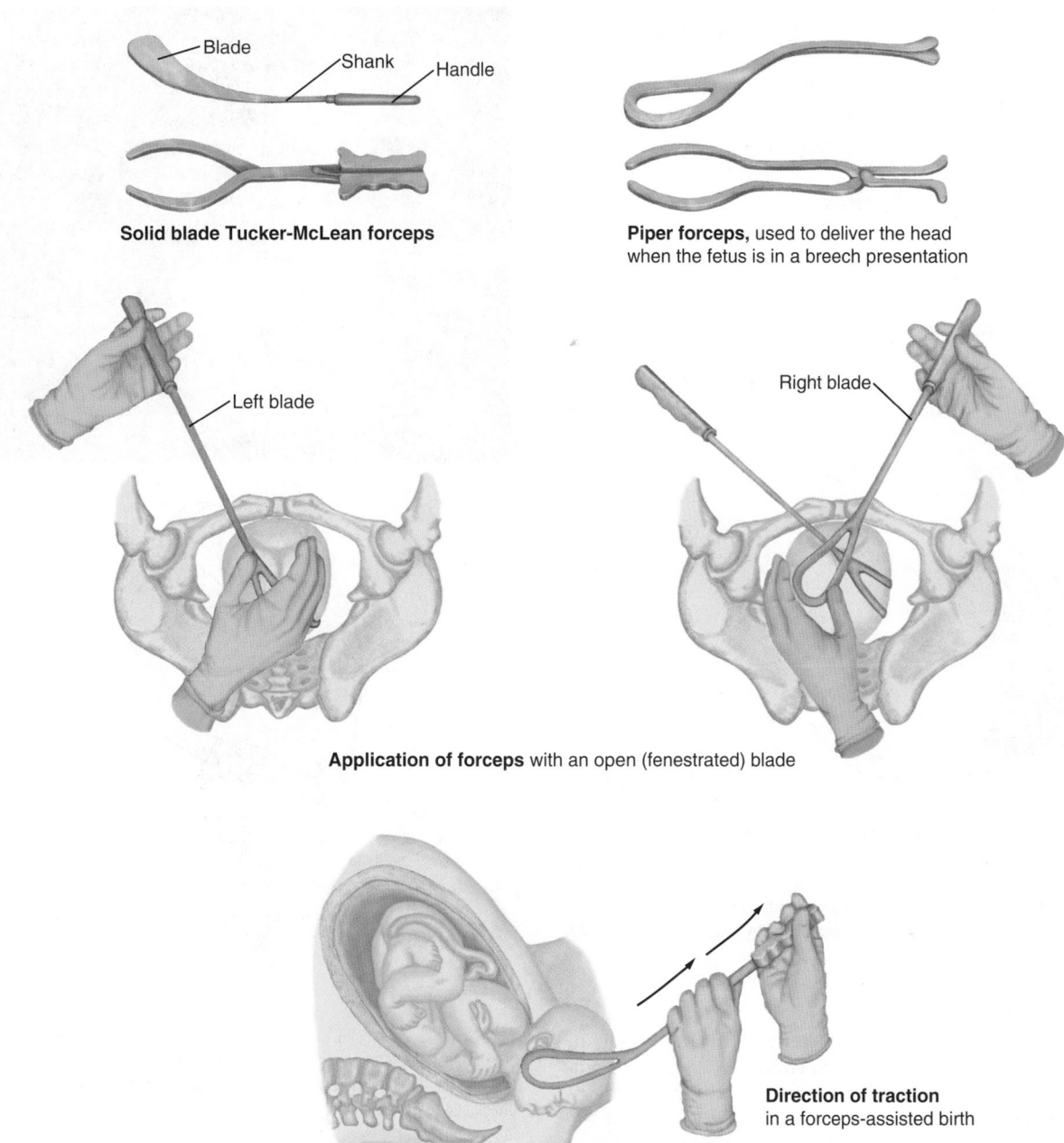

Solid blade Tucker-McLean forceps

Blade   Shank   Handle

Piper forceps, used to deliver the head when the fetus is in a breech presentation

Left blade

Right blade

Application of forceps with an open (fenestrated) blade

Direction of traction in a forceps-assisted birth

Figure 20-4 Obstetric forceps and their application.

OPERATIVE VAGINAL BIRTH

An operative vaginal birth is one in which the physician applies traction to the fetal head during birth with a vacuum extractor or forceps, to aid the woman's expulsive efforts. The use of forceps has fallen while use of vacuum extractors has risen. The rate of births assisted by vacuum extraction is now double the rate of forceps-assisted births (Kozak & Weeks, 2002). However, as the rate of cesarean births has risen, vaginal births assisted by either vacuum extractor or forceps have decreased since 1996 (Martin, Hamilton, Sutton, Ventura, Menacker, & Munson, 2003).

Forceps are metal instruments having two curved blades with rounded edges that can be locked in the center. Many styles are available for different needs. The blades may be closed or open as they partly surround the fetal head (Fig. 20-4). Disposable foam pads are available to cushion the fetal head. Piper forceps are a special type used to assist birth of the head as it is born last in a vaginal breech birth. Forceps or a vacuum extractor also may be used during a cesarean birth.

A vacuum extractor uses suction to grasp the fetal head as traction is applied (Figs. 20-5 and 20-6). It is not used to deliver the fetus in a nonvertex presentation, such as breech or face; otherwise, its use is similar to that for forceps.

Indications

Forceps or vacuum extraction is considered if the second stage should be shortened for the well-being of the woman, fetus, or both and if a vaginal birth can be accomplished

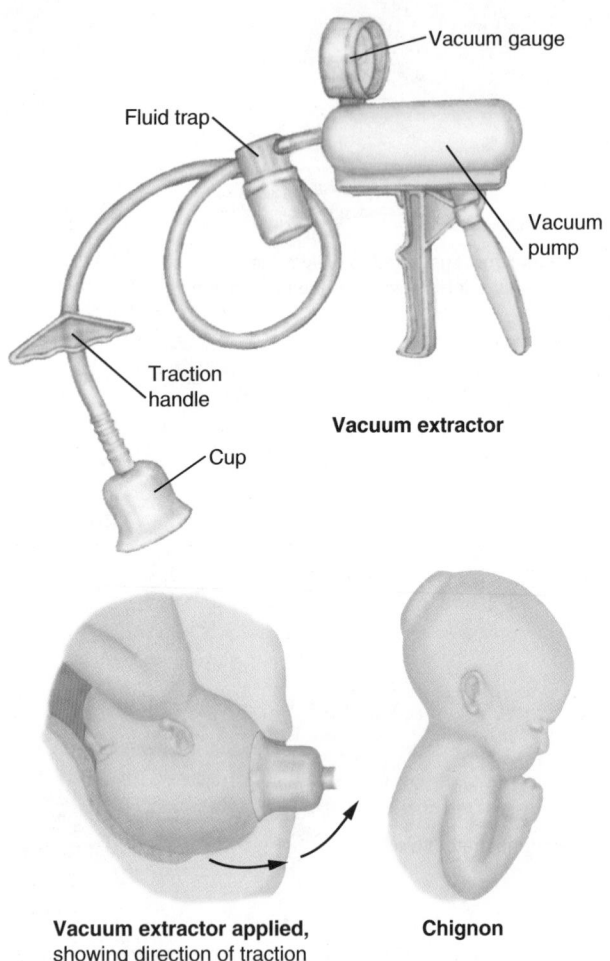

Vacuum gauge

Fluid trap

Vacuum pump

Traction handle

Vacuum extractor

Cup

Vacuum extractor applied,
showing direction of traction

Chignon

Figure 20-5 Birth assisted with a vacuum extractor. The chignon is scalp edema that often forms under the suction cup when the vacuum extractor is used.

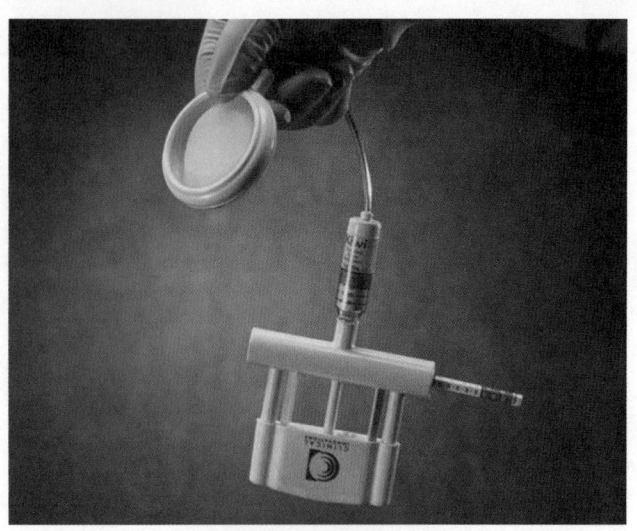

A

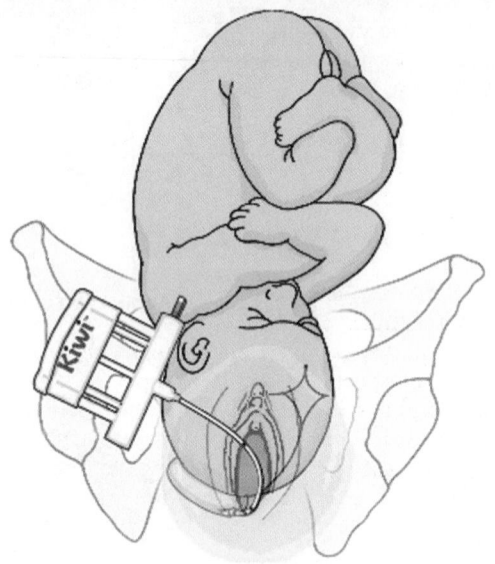

B

Figure 20-6 A, Vacuum extractor with a low-profile cup that can be used for occiput posterior fetal positions. Note the green band that denotes adequate suction and the red band that warns of excess suction. **B,** Application of the low-profile cup to the fetal head in an occiput posterior position. (Courtesy Clinical Innovations, Inc.)

quickly without undue trauma. Maternal indications may include exhaustion, inability to push effectively, cardiac or pulmonary disease, and intrapartum infection. Fetal indications may include cord compression, premature separation of the placenta, or nonreassuring fetal heart rate patterns.

Contraindications

A cesarean birth is preferable if the maternal or fetal condition mandates a more rapid birth than can be accomplished with forceps or a vacuum extractor or if the procedure would be too traumatic. Examples of these conditions are severe fetal compromise, acute maternal conditions such as congestive heart failure and pulmonary edema, a high fetal station, and disproportion between the size of the fetus and the maternal pelvis.

Risks

The main risk of forceps or vacuum extraction is trauma to maternal or fetal tissues. Because of the relative safety of cesarean birth, the attempt at an instrumental birth is usually abandoned if the fetal head does not descend easily.

Maternal risks include laceration or hematoma of the vagina, perineum, or periurethral area and a very large episiotomy. The infant may have ecchymoses, facial and scalp lacerations or abrasions, facial nerve injury, cephalhematoma, subgaleal hemorrhage, and other intracranial hemorrhage. A vacuum extractor creates circular scalp edema and redness or bruising called a *chignon* at the application area (see Fig. 20-5), which resolves quickly after birth.

Technique

Preparation for forceps or vacuum extraction is the same as for any vaginal birth. The woman's bladder should be empty to limit bladder trauma. Membranes must be ruptured and the cervix completely dilated for forceps or vacuum extraction birth. The woman needs adequate anesthesia, usually with a regional block such as an epidural or pudendal block.

Forceps- and vacuum extractor–assisted births are classified according to how far the fetal head has descended into the pelvis when these instruments are applied (American Academy of Pediatrics & American College of Obstetricians and Gynecologists [AAP & ACOG], 2002). The three classifications are outlet, low, and midpelvis (or midforceps):

- *Outlet operative vaginal delivery:* The fetal head is on the perineum, with the scalp visible at the vaginal opening without separating the labia. The position is occiput anterior or either right or left occiput anterior (ROA, LOA) or posterior (ROP, LOP).
- *Low operative vaginal delivery:* The leading edge of the fetal skull is at station +2 (about 4 cm below the level of the mother's ischial spines) or lower. Low operative vaginal birth is subdivided according to the amount of rotation of the fetal head needed. Births requiring 45° or less of fetal head rotation are simpler.
- *Midpelvis operative vaginal delivery:* The leading edge of the fetal skull is between a 0 (at the level of the ischial spines) and a +2 station.

The physician determines the presentation, position, and station of the fetal head and the amount of cervical dilation. With correct application, the long axis of the forceps blades lies over the fetal cheeks and parietal bones. After checking for proper application, the physician locks the two blades in the center and pulls gently as the woman pushes, following the curve of the pelvis. An episiotomy may be done as the fetal head distends the perineum. The physician may keep the forceps on until the head is born or may remove the blades just before expulsion. The rest of the fetus is born in the usual way.

A hand pump is used to create suction to hold the vacuum cup on the fetal head in the midline of the occiput. The physician applies traction intermittently, as in a forceps-assisted birth. A vacuum release allows removal of the cup. The vacuum should go no higher than the green zone, indicated on the vacuum pump. Hospital policies often limit to three the number of times the vacuum cup can be applied.

Nursing Considerations

The woman's bladder should be empty, usually by catheterization, before attempting an operative vaginal birth. The physician specifies the type of forceps or vacuum cup. The fetal heart rate should be assessed, and any rate lower than 100 bpm should be reported.

After birth, the mother and infant are observed for trauma. The mother may have vaginal wall lacerations or hematoma (see Chapter 28). Cold applications for the first 12 hours reduce pain by numbing the area and limit bruising and edema of the tissues. Intermittent applications after 12 hours aid resolution of the edema and bruising. The fundus is usually firm unless uterine atony is also present.

The infant often has reddening and mild bruising of the skin where the forceps were applied. Observe for skin breaks that allow entry of microorganisms; keep skin breaks clean.

Facial asymmetry, most obvious when the infant cries, suggests facial nerve injury that is usually temporary. Neurologic abnormalities such as seizures suggest that the newborn has had an intracranial hemorrhage. Seizures may also occur with neonatal hypoglycemia or sepsis, however.

After a forceps-assisted birth, a parent may ask why the baby's cheeks are reddened or bruised. A response is to explain that the pressure of the forceps on the baby's delicate skin may cause minor bruising that usually resolves without treatment. Parents of an infant born with assistance of a vacuum extractor may likewise be concerned about the edema on their baby's head. Reassure them that this edema will soon resolve. Point out improvement in the baby's cheeks or scalp during the postpartum stay.

EPISIOTOMY

Performance of an episiotomy remains controversial, despite research disputing its usefulness. It may be done based on tradition and personal beliefs rather than based on research. Episiotomy was performed in 64% of vaginal births in 1980. By 2000, the rate had fallen to 32.7%. Repair of perineal or other genital tract lacerations during vaginal birth rose in the same period, from 11.1% to 39.2% (Kozak & Weeks, 2002). The decision about whether an episiotomy is needed must be made just before birth, however, and indications are not always clear.

Indications

Few indications exist for routine episiotomy, based on a large body of research. However, the following conditions justify the use of selective, rather than routine, episiotomy (Cunningham et al., 2001):

- Fetal shoulder dystocia, in which the shoulder of a fetus becomes lodged under the mother's symphysis during birth
- Vaginal breech birth, in which the fetal head must be quickly delivered after the body is born
- Forceps- or vacuum extractor–assisted births
- Birth with the fetus in an occiput posterior (face up) position
- If an obvious risk for serious tears of the soft tissues of the genital tract exists

Risks

Infection is a risk of episiotomy, as it is in any disruption of skin or mucus membrane integrity. Perineal pain occurs with both episiotomy and spontaneous tears. However, perineal pain may last longer with episiotomy, because the incision often extends into deeper lacerations. Episiotomy increases blood loss and is associated with poor sexual satisfaction and comfort 3 months after birth as compared with birth over an intact perineum (Eason & Feldman, 2000; Kendrick, 2001). Research has not supported the presumption that episiotomy reduces damage to the pelvic floor that causes later dysfunction such as urinary incontinence.

Also there is no guarantee the woman will not tear in addition to the episiotomy.

Median or Midline

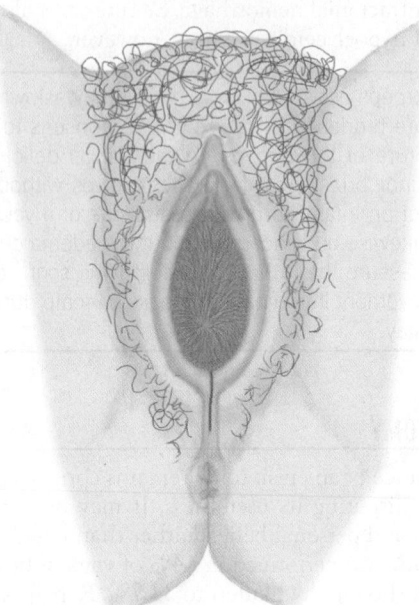

Mediolateral

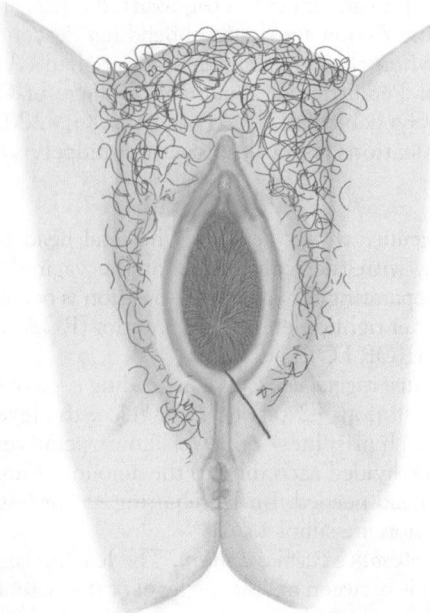

Advantages
Minimal blood loss
Neat healing with little scarring
Less postpartum pain than the
   mediolateral episiotomy

Disadvantages
An added laceration may extend the median episiotomy
   into the anal sphincter
Limited enlargement of the vaginal opening because perineal length is limited by the
   anal sphincter

Advantages
More enlargement of the vaginal opening
Little risk that the episiotomy
   will extend into the anus

Disadvantages
More blood loss
Increased postpartum pain
More scarring and irregularity
   in the healed scar
Prolonged dyspareunia (pain-
   ful intercourse)

Figure 20-7 Types of episiotomies.

Technique

An episiotomy is done when the fetal presenting part has crowned to a diameter of about 3 to 4 cm. The two types of episiotomies have different advantages and disadvantages: *median* or *midline*; and *mediolateral* (Fig. 20-7).

Nursing Considerations

Gradual stretching of the perineum is the key to reducing the risk for episiotomy. An upright position while pushing promotes gradual stretching of the woman's perineum. Laboring down, or delaying pushing until the urge is felt, also gradually distends the soft tissues of the pelvic floor. When the woman pushes, use of an open-glottis technique rather than prolonged breath-holding when pushing also promotes gradual perineal stretching.

Daily perineal massage and stretching by the woman from 34 to 35 weeks' gestation until birth has been shown to reduce the risk for perineal trauma during birth for women having their first birth (Eason, Labrecque, Wells, & Feldman, 2000; Labrecque et al., 1999).

Nursing interventions during the recovery and postpartum periods are similar for episiotomy and perineal laceration. Observe the perineum for hematoma and edema. As with forceps use, perineal cold applications are done for the first 12 hours, followed by intermittent perineal heat applications after at least 12 hours if needed.

CESAREAN BIRTH

More than 1 million births in the United States during 2002 were by cesarean, the highest ever recorded (Martin, Hamilton, Ventura, Menacker, & Munson, 2003). At one time, cesarean births made up only 5% to 6% of births, and then the number gradually rose to 22.8% of births in 1989. Efforts to curb the rapid rise reduced the cesarean birth rate to just under 21% in 1995 before the rate again rose to the 2002 level of 26.1%. The primary (first) cesarean rate was 18% during 2002.

Several factors contribute to the high U.S. cesarean birth rate (Cunningham et al., 2001; Martin, Hamilton, Ventura, Menacker, & Munson, 2003):

- More women are having their first baby, and these women are more likely to have a cesarean than a woman who has had one or more births vaginally.
- The high primary cesarean rate adds to the overall rate because more women will have repeat cesareans rather than attempting vaginal birth for their next children.
- Women are having children later, and cesareans are more common in the older pregnant woman.
- Electronic fetal monitoring often prompts concerns about fetal oxygen and acid-base status or progress of labor.
- Preference for cesarean birth if the baby remains in a breech presentation may be chosen.

- A high threat of litigation if birth outcomes are not good causes physicians to opt for surgery quickly if the maternal or fetal condition or both seem to be at risk.

Evidence is accumulating that links labor induction to increased risk for cesarean birth. Studies have demonstrated that women who have their labor induced are 2 to 3 times more likely to have a surgical birth. Women having a Bishop score of less than 5 at the time of induction, indicating a cervix that is not favorable, had a greater risk for cesarean than women who had a score of 5 or more. Approximately 25% of inductions had no clearly documented medical or obstetric indication but were elective. The risk for cesarean following failed induction was similar whether women had medical or elective inductions (Johnson, Davis, & Brown, 2003; Martin, Hamilton, Ventura, Menacker, & Munson, 2003; Seyb, Berka, Socol, & Dooley, 1999; Yeast, Jones, & Poskin, 1999).

Healthy People 2010 goals related to reducing cesarean birth rates are to reduce the primary (first) cesarean rate to 15% and the repeat cesarean rate to no more than 63% for women at low risk for complications. Promotion of vaginal birth after cesarean in women for whom it is appropriate is a major way to accomplish the goal. Other possibilities include more careful evaluation of dystocia of labor as a reason for cesarean and careful selection of women who are appropriate candidates for vaginal breech birth. External cephalic version (p. 449) is an option to attempt changing the presentation of a near-fetus in a cephalic presentation.

The American Academy of Pediatrics and American College of Obstetricians and Gynecologists (2002 and 1999c) have affirmed their support for vaginal birth after cesarean birth (VBAC) (Box 20-1) but have urged caution in approaching a trial of labor because VBAC is associated with a small but significant risk of uterine rupture. The risks and benefits of VBAC for each woman must be considered by her and her physician. For example, the risk of uterine rupture increases as the number of prior uterine incisions increases, and a woman who has had two prior cesarean deliveries might be reluctant to attempt VBAC for her third birth because of this added risk. In addition, the woman who tries VBAC and still needs a repeat cesarean birth incurs more costs because she has both labor and surgical expenses. She and her infant are more likely to have infections that further complicate their recovery and add to costs. The hospital also incurs greater costs for personnel and supplies.

Experience with electronic fetal monitoring has improved knowledge of normal fetal responses to labor, promoting interventions for fetal benefit that may avoid cesarean delivery. Nurses and birth attendants increasingly recognize that simple interventions, such as walking or squatting during the second stage, may promote normal labor progress. Interventions, both nursing and medical, that reduce the primary cesarean birth rate will also reduce the need for repeat (secondary) cesareans.

Indications

Cesarean birth is performed when awaiting a vaginal birth would compromise the mother, the fetus, or both. Possible indications for cesarean birth include but are not limited to:

- Dystocia
- Cephalopelvic (fetopelvic) disproportion
- Hypertension, if prompt delivery is necessary

BOX 20-1
Vaginal Birth After Cesarean Birth

Approximately 60% to 80% of women with one low transverse uterine incision from a previous cesarean birth have successful vaginal births.

Women who had their previous cesarean for a nonrecurring reason, such as breech presentation, are more likely to have a successful vaginal birth after cesarean birth (VBAC) than women who had their previous cesarean for dystocia.

Women who have had a vaginal birth before or since the prior cesarean birth are more likely to have successful VBAC.

Candidates for VBAC include:
- A woman who has one or two previous low transverse uterine incisions.
- No other uterine scars (e.g., removal of fibroid tumors) or a previous uterine rupture.
- A pelvis that is clinically adequate for the estimated fetal size.
- Immediate availability of a physician during active labor if a an emergency cesarean is needed.
- Availability of anesthesia and personnel to perform an emergency cesarean.

Management of women who plan VBAC:
- External cephalic version may be as successful for women having a previous cesarean as for women with an unscarred uterus.
- Epidural analgesia and anesthesia may be used.
- Induction and augmentation of labor with oxytocin may be done. Use of prostaglandin gel appears to be safe. Misoprostol (Cytotec) is currently contraindicated.
- Most authorities recommend electronic fetal monitoring.

Data from American College of Obstetricians and Gynecologists (1999). *Vaginal birth after previous cesarean delivery* (ACOG Practice Bulletin No. 5). Washington, DC: Author.

- Maternal diseases such as diabetes, heart disease, or cervical cancer, if labor is not advisable
- Active genital herpes at the time of birth
- Some previous uterine surgical procedures, such as a classic cesarean incision
- Persistent nonreassuring fetal heart rate patterns
- A prolapsed umbilical cord
- Fetal malpresentations, such as breech or transverse lie
- Hemorrhagic conditions, such as abruptio placentae or placenta previa

A prior cesarean birth alone is not an indication for another cesarean birth for most women. Many women will choose repeat cesarean rather than a trial of labor even if they are appropriate candidates for VBAC, because of the small, but real, added risk for uterine rupture. In other cases they choose elective (scheduled) repeat cesarean to avoid another unsuccessful experience or the pain of labor. For other women, trying to deliver their next baby vaginally—whether successful or not—is important.

Contraindications

There are few absolute contraindications to cesarean birth, but there are conditions in which it is not desirable because the risks to the woman are too great when compared with the potential benefit to mother or fetus. These conditions include fetal death, a fetus that is too immature to survive, and maternal coagulation defects.

Risks

Cesarean birth is one of the safest major surgical procedures; however, it poses greater risk for the mother than does vaginal birth. The risk for complications is much higher if the woman is obese (Cunningham et al., 2001). Maternal risks include the following, many of which are associated with any major surgery:

- Infection
- Hemorrhage
- Urinary tract trauma or infection
- Thrombophlebitis, thromboembolism
- Paralytic ileus
- Atelectasis
- Anesthesia complications

Cesarean delivery poses added risks for the infant, which may include:

- Inadvertent preterm birth
- Transient tachypnea of the newborn caused by delayed absorption of lung fluid (see Chapter 30)
- Persistent pulmonary hypertension of the newborn (see Chapter 30)
- Injury, such as laceration, bruising, fractures, or other trauma

Validation of fetal maturity is essential when a cesarean birth is planned. Gestational age of at least 39 weeks can be confirmed by (AAP & ACOG, 2002):

- Documentation of fetal heart sounds for 20 weeks by non-electronic means or for 30 weeks by Doppler ultrasound
- An interval of 36 weeks since positive results for a serum or urine pregnancy test performed by a reliable laboratory
- An ultrasound examination between 6 and 11 weeks of pregnancy that supports a gestational age of 39 weeks or more
- Clinical history and later ultrasound examinations support a gestational age of 39 weeks or more

For women with questionable due dates, amniocentesis (see Chapter 16) may be done to establish fetal maturity if the cesarean is elective. Another alternative is to await spontaneous onset of labor to do the cesarean.

Technique

Preparation

Routine laboratory studies vary with the mother's condition and type of anesthesia but may include a complete blood count, clotting studies such as prothrombin and partial thromboplastin times, and blood typing and screening. The physician may order one or more units of blood to be typed and crossmatched to have available for transfusion if the woman's hemoglobin and hematocrit values are low or she has a high risk for hemorrhage, such as grand multiparity (five or more births).

Regional anesthesia, such as epidural block, is typical for cesarean birth. General anesthesia may be required for either known or unexpected reasons. For emergency cesarean with no epidural block in place, a general anesthetic may be needed because it can be established the most quickly. A drug such as famotidine (Pepcid) or sodium citrate with citric acid (Bicitra) is given to reduce gastric acidity before surgery. The woman does not have routine premedication other than drugs to control gastric and respiratory secretions.

Fetal surveillance continues until just before the sterile abdominal skin prep (intermittent auscultation or external monitor) or just after the prep (internal monitor) (AAP & ACOG, 2002). A wedge placed under one hip prevents aortocaval compression and promotes placental blood flow.

A single intravenous dose of a prophylactic antibiotic such as ampicillin or a cephalosporin is often ordered. Additional antibiotic doses are given to a woman who has an increased risk for infection, such as one who has had prolonged rupture of membranes.

If a Pfannenstiel (transverse or "bikini") skin incision is planned, the woman's abdomen is shaved from about 3 inches above the pubic hairline to the mons pubis, about where her legs come together. The fronts of the upper thighs are also shaved. For a vertical skin incision, the upper border of the shave is near the umbilicus. Cordless electric clippers with disposable heads are available to reduce skin nicks that provide an entry point for microorganisms.

An indwelling catheter inserted after the regional block is established but before the surgery keeps the bladder away from the operative area, reducing the risk for injury. The catheter may also be placed before the epidural. The catheter allows accurate observation of urine output during and after surgery, which helps evaluate circulatory status. The catheter also allows delay of ambulation to the restroom for urination until the woman can safely ambulate.

A grounding pad for the electrocautery (Bovie) is applied to an area with no bony prominences, usually the thigh. After application of the pad, the woman's legs are secured to the operating table with a wide, padded strap.

A sterile abdominal skin prep is done just before sterile draping. As in other surgical skin preparations, the direction of the scrub is generally circular, from the center of the operative area outward and from the pubic area downward on each upper thigh. It may be necessary to use wide tape to hold excess abdominal fat (the pannus, or "apron") upward, pulling it away from the skin incision area.

Preoperative preparations are completed before a general anesthetic is begun to reduce neonatal exposure to anesthesia. The team scrubs, dons gowns and gloves, and drapes the woman before general anesthesia is induced.

Incisions

Two incisions are made: one in the abdominal wall (skin incision) and the other in the uterine wall. Either of two skin incisions is used: a midline vertical incision between the umbilicus and the symphysis or a Pfannenstiel incision just above the symphysis (Fig. 20-8).

Three types of uterine incisions are possible (Fig. 20-9): (1) low transverse; (2) low vertical; and (3) classic, a vertical incision into the upper uterus. The low transverse uterine incision is preferred unless a very large fetus or placenta previa in the lower uterus prevents its use. The uterine incision does not always match the skin incision. For example, a woman may have a vertical skin incision and a low transverse uterine incision, particularly if she is very obese.

Vertical

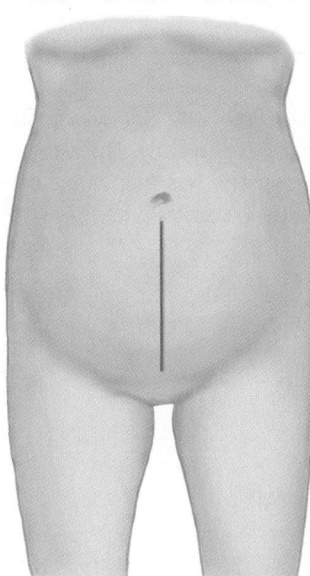

Advantages
Quicker to perform
Better visualization of the
  uterus
Can quickly extend upward
  for greater visualization if
  needed
Often more appropriate for
  obese women

Disadvantages
Easily visible when healed
Greater chance of dehis-
  cence and hernia formation

Pfannenstiel

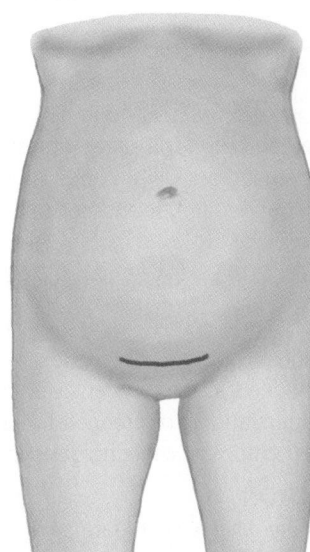

Advantages
Less visibility when healed
  and the pubic hair grows
  back
Less chance of dehiscence or
  formation of a hernia

Disadvantages
Less visualization of the
  uterus
Cannot be done as quickly,
  which may be important in
  an emergency cesarean
  birth
Cannot easily be extended to
  give greater operative exposure
Re-entry at a subsequent cesarean birth may require
  more time

Figure 20-8 Skin (abdominal wall) incisions for cesarean birth.

Low Transverse

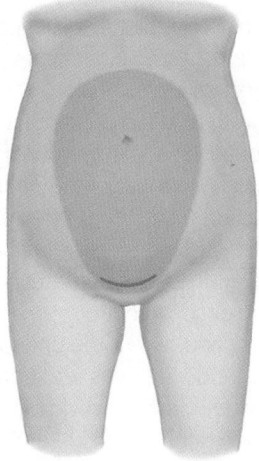

Low Vertical

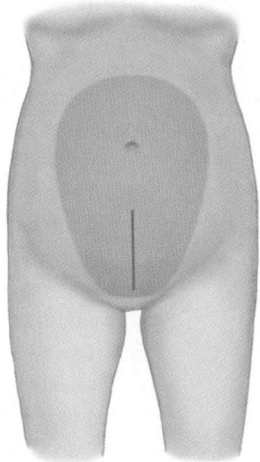

Classic

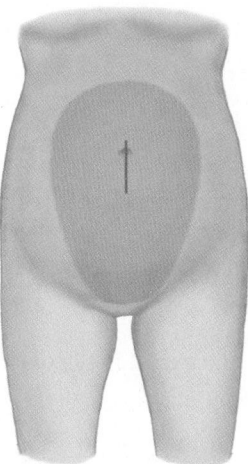

Advantages
Unlikely to rupture during a subsequent
  birth
Makes VBAC possible for subsequent
  pregnancy
Less blood loss
Easier to repair
Less adhesion formation

Advantage
Can be extended upward to make a larger
  incision if needed

Advantage
May be the only choice in these situations:

  Implantation of a placenta previa on the
    lower anterior uterine wall
  Presence of dense adhesions from
    previous surgery
  Transverse lie of a large fetus with the
    shoulder impacted in the mother's
    pelvis

Disadvantage
Limited ability to extend laterally to enlarge the incision

Disadvantages
Slightly more likely to rupture during a
  subsequent birth
A tear may extend the incision downward
  into the cervix

Disadvantages
Most likely of the uterine incisions to rupture during a subsequent birth
Eliminates VBAC as an option for birth of
  a subsequent infant

Figure 20-9 Uterine incisions for cesarean birth. The abdominal and uterine incisions do not always match. *VBAC,* Vaginal birth after cesarean.

Nursing Care Plan

Cesarean Birth

ASSESSMENT

Christina Cole is 22 years old and in early labor at 37 weeks' gestation with her first baby. She was scheduled for a cesarean birth for a breech presentation the following week, but labor began early. The baby remains breech, so surgery will be done as soon as possible. Christina is anxious and has many questions about what will happen to her and her baby. Christina's mother and husband Bruce are with her.

Nursing Diagnosis

Anxiety related to unfamiliarity with the setting and procedures for cesarean birth.

Goals/Expected Outcomes

After interventions, Christina will
- State that she feels less apprehensive.
- Verbalize understanding of preoperative and postoperative care.
- Demonstrate postoperative techniques for coughing and deep breathing.

INTERVENTION	RATIONALE
1. Assess Christina's level of anxiety. Mild to moderate anxiety is expected.	1. Assessment enables the nurse to approach preoperative care of the woman in the most appropriate manner. Mild to moderate anxiety facilitates learning, but high levels impair learning.
2. Remain with Christina as much as possible while completing preoperative procedures. Allow her to express her fears. Encourage her mother and Bruce to remain with her.	2. The presence of significant others and a caring nurse provides support. Expression of her fears enables the nurse to answer the woman's concerns specifically.
3. Elicit Christina's feelings about surgery by using broad leads, such as, "What were your thoughts when you found out you might have your baby by cesarean?"	3. Identification of expectations of the birth experience allows actions to be taken to make it a positive one. If a woman's expected and actual experience closely match, she is likely to be more satisfied with it. Misunderstandings and possible feelings of inadequacy or anger are identified.
4. Explain preoperative preparations using simple language, verifying Christina's understanding and giving her the opportunity to ask questions.	4. Knowledge decreases anxiety and fear of the unknown. Simple language facilitates understanding when a woman's attention is narrowed from anxiety. Explanations and the chance to ask questions show respect and give the woman a greater sense of control.
5. Explain what to expect postoperatively, demonstrating as needed.	5. Knowledge reduces anxiety and fear of the unknown. The explanation promotes understanding and acceptance of care that will be painful while providing reassurance of pain control. Return demonstration verifies learning and identifies the need for additional teaching.
6. Reduce unnecessary stimulation. Work efficiently, but calmly.	6. Unnecessary stimulation can add to the woman's anxiety. Its reduction emphasizes that a cesarean delivery is a birth, not just a surgical procedure.

Evaluation

Christina agrees that a cesarean birth is best for her baby. She asks a few other questions and then states that she understands preoperative and postoperative care but that she is still "a little nervous." She demonstrates effective coughing and deep-breathing techniques.

Nursing Care Plan

Cesarean Birth—cont'd

ASSESSMENT

Christina will have epidural anesthesia for her birth. Her vital signs are: temperature, 37.2° C (99° F); pulse, 90 bpm; respirations, 22 breaths per minute; and blood pressure, 122/70 mm Hg. The fetal heart rate is 130 to 140 bpm and accelerates with fetal movement.

Christina walks to the operating room, and epidural anesthesia is begun.

Nursing Diagnosis

Risk for Injury related to altered sensation from epidural anesthesia and the use of electrical equipment during surgery.

Goals/Expected Outcomes

Christina will not have injury, such as pressure areas, muscle strains, and electrical injury, during the perioperative period.

INTERVENTION	RATIONALE
1. Pad bony prominences. Avoid obstructing her popliteal area. Place a wedge under her hip to slightly tilt her uterus to one side.	1. Padding reduces potential for tissue damage caused by pressure. An unobstructed popliteal area reduces venous stasis and possible thrombus formation. Padding includes a uterine displacement wedge to avoid aortocaval compression.
2. Transfer Christina from the operating table carefully after surgery, using enough staff members to keep her body in alignment. Brake the bed and operating table to keep them from separating. Be certain that the indwelling catheter tubing and IV line are free during the transfer.	2. Having adequate staff reduces the risk for a fall or muscle strains in both Christina and the staff.
3. After anesthesia is begun, position Christina on the operating table and secure her legs with a safety strap.	3. The safety strap prevents falls or displacement of the woman's legs, which have lost sensation.
4. Apply a grounding pad if electrocautery is to be used.	4. A grounding pad prevents electrical shock or burn.

Evaluation

During surgery, Christina's body was secured in proper alignment, with proper padding of all her bony prominences. The grounding pad ensured electrical safety when the electrocautery was used. She gave birth to an appropriate-for-gestational-age baby, 3318 g (7 lb, 5 oz). Christina was transferred to the recovery room without incident. During recovery and postpartum she showed no signs of pressure, electrical, or musculoskeletal injury.

Additional Nursing Diagnoses to Consider

- Risk for Aspiration (general anesthesia)
- Pain
- Risk for Impaired Spontaneous Ventilation
- Hypothermia
- Readiness for Enhanced Family Coping

NOTE: Only nursing diagnoses related to the preoperative and intraoperative care of the woman are discussed here. See Chapter 18 for nursing care related to fetal oxygenation. See Chapter 19 for care related to anesthesia. See Chapters 17 and 21 for nursing care of the mother during the recovery and postpartum periods.

BOX 20-2
Nursing Care for a Woman Having Cesarean Birth

Before the Cesarean Birth
1. Assess the time of last oral intake and what was eaten.
2. Assess for allergies. Include drug, food, and substance (e.g., latex) allergies.
3. Determine medications taken and last dose. Include herbal preparations.
4. Have the woman sign informed consents for surgery, anesthesia, and usually blood transfusion.
5. Obtain ordered laboratory work.
6. Do preoperative teaching: what the woman can expect in the operating and recovery rooms, infant care, and who will be present.
7. Start ordered intravenous infusion and begin bolus dose for regional anesthetic at appropriate time (see "Epidural Block" in Chapter 19).
8. Do abdominal shave (or use electric clipper).
9. Administer ordered medication to control gastric secretions if not done by anesthesiologist.
10. Insert a urinary indwelling catheter (or insert in operating room after regional block).
11. Assist woman to operating table, positioning her with a wedge under her hip to displace the uterus.
12. Apply grounding pad for electrocautery.
13. Do sterile prep of abdomen.
14. Call infant care team if it is routine in the facility or for anticipated newborn complications.

During the Recovery Period
1. Begin anesthesia-related interventions: pulse oximeter, oxygen administration, cardiac monitor.
   a. Assess for return of sensation and movement if regional anesthesia was used.
   b. Assess level of consciousness if general anesthesia was used.
2. Do routine assessments every 15 minutes for the first hour, every 30 minutes during the second hour, and hourly thereafter until the woman is transferred to the postpartum unit. Assess:
   a. Vital signs; oxygen saturation.
   b. ECG pattern.
   c. Uterine fundus for firmness, height, and deviation (massage if poorly contracted).
   d. Lochia for color, quantity, and presence of large clots.
   e. Urine output for color, quantity, and patency of the catheter and tubing.
   f. Abdominal dressing for drainage.
3. Assess need for analgesia, and administer as ordered.
4. Change position hourly if no contraindication exists. Have her breathe deeply and cough at each routine assessment time. Provide a small pillow to support her incision when coughing or turning if sensation is present.

Nursing Considerations

Nursing care for a woman who has a cesarean birth varies according to the situation (see Nursing Care Plan: Cesarean Birth). She may be planning a cesarean birth, or a surgical birth may be unexpected. A planned cesarean may be her first, or she may have had a cesarean birth before. Her previous cesarean may have been planned or an emergency, and her feelings about the prior cesarean birth may be positive or negative.

Nursing care for all women having cesarean childbirth is similar, but the approach in each situation is different. For example, although preoperative teaching is important, it must be abbreviated or even omitted in a true emergency.

Providing Emotional Support
Emotional support begins well before the birth and extends well after it. A mother who has had a previous cesarean birth may harbor unresolved feelings of grief, guilt, or inadequacy because she perceives that she somehow failed in her expected birth experience.

The nurse in the prenatal setting can open the subject of a woman's previous cesarean or vaginal birth with a broad lead, such as "Tell me about when you had your other baby."

The staff's behavior can either reduce or increase the woman's anxiety. A calm and confident manner helps her feel that she is being cared for by competent professionals. A quiet, controlled voice is calming to the patient, her family, and the nurse and other staff.

The nurse and the woman's significant others are important sources of emotional support. Therapeutic communication with a caring nurse helps clarify her concerns, so explanations to reduce her fear of the unknown can be most effective.

The father or other support person should be encouraged to remain with her during surgery if she has regional anesthesia. In many hospitals, the support person also may come into the operating room after the woman is intubated for general anesthesia to foster attachment with the infant and help the mother integrate her birth experience.

Nurses also support a woman's partner and significant others during the cesarean birth. The partner may be as anxious as the woman but may be afraid to express it because the woman needs so much support. The partner may be physically exhausted after hours of labor coaching. The staff should not expect more support from the partner than he or she can provide.

Although cesarean births are routine in the intrapartum unit, they are not routine to women who undergo them or to their families. Avoid belittling their fears by telling women and their families not to worry or that everything will be all right, especially if an emergency occurs.

Talking with the mother and her family after birth allows the nurse to answer questions about the surgery and fill in any gaps in their understanding. This helps them understand the experience and promotes a positive perception of the birth.

Teaching

Knowledge helps reduce fear of the unknown and increases a woman's sense of control over her infant's birth. The nurse cannot assume that a woman who had a previous cesarean birth already knows what will happen and why. If her previous surgery was done after a long labor or in an emergency, she may recall only part of it and may not understand what she does remember. Teaching should be done in simple language and should include her partner.

The nurse explains preoperative procedures and their purposes, such as the abdominal shave, indwelling catheter, intravenous lines, and dressings. The catheter and intravenous lines usually remain in place no longer than 24 hours after birth. The nurse may need to reinforce anesthetic information provided by the anesthesia clinician.

Women who have regional anesthesia, such as an epidural or subarachnoid block, often fear that they will feel pain during surgery. They do feel pressure and pulling, but these sensations do not mean that the anesthesia is wearing off. The nurse reassures her that her anesthesia clinician will regularly assess her needs for pain management.

If a woman is having general anesthesia, the nurse explains why operative preparations are completed before the woman is anesthetized. She should be reassured that her surgery will not begin until she is asleep and that she will not wake up during the procedure.

The nurse describes the operating room and everyone who will be present to make it less intimidating to her. The operating room may seem cool, and the surgery table is narrow. Her labor nurse is often the circulating nurse during surgery, reassuring her with a familiar face and voice.

The support person should be told when he or she can expect to come into the operating room. If it is not already in place, an epidural block is often established after the woman goes to the operating room. Bringing the partner in may be delayed until the regional block and other preparations, such as placement of the indwelling catheter, are complete. These preparations may take up to 30 to 45 minutes for a scheduled cesarean birth, varying with facility and provider practices. Assure the support person that he or she will not be forgotten. Estimating wait time helps reassure the partner that no problem has occurred during the preparation phase.

The nurse explains the recovery room and any equipment that will be used, such as a pulse oximeter, electrocardiogram (ECG) monitor, and automatic blood pressure cuff. The need for routine assessments and interventions such as fundus and lochia checks, coughing, and deep breathing are explained. The woman is taught simple exercises to promote normal circulation in her legs when movement returns. The nurse reassures her that every effort will be made to promote her comfort with medication, positioning, and other interventions. She should be encouraged to ask for pain relief early, before it is severe, for best results.

Promoting Safety

Although the need for general anesthesia during pregnancy occurs infrequently, the nurse must assume that it may be needed. The woman's food intake is assessed for type and time on admission. Oral intake and emesis during labor are recorded and reported to the anesthesia clinician. Usually the woman is on NPO status or only ice is given if a cesarean birth is expected. Anesthesia-related drugs to control gastric and respiratory secretions are administered as ordered.

The woman is transferred and positioned carefully to prevent injury, especially if she has received regional anesthesia that reduces motor control and sensation. Her bony prominences are well padded. A safety strap placed across her thighs secures her on the narrow operating table. A wedge placed under one hip or tilting the operating table avoids aortocaval compression and reduced placental blood flow. During positioning, the drain tube of the indwelling catheter should be routed under her leg to promote drainage and keep the tube away from the operative area. The catheter bag is placed near the head of the table so that the anesthesia clinician can monitor urine output.

The nurse verifies proper function of machines such as suction devices, monitors, and electrocautery. Leads for the cardiac monitor and pulse oximeter are placed to observe heart and respiratory functions. A grounding pad permits safe use of the electrocautery. Infant care equipment should be readied for immediate use.

After the surgery, the incision area is cleansed with sterile water and a sterile dressing is applied. Blood and amniotic fluid are cleaned from the woman's abdomen, buttocks, and back before she is transferred to a bed. Smooth transfers done by an adequate number of personnel reduce pain and hypotension.

Providing Postoperative Care

Postoperative care for the mother who has had a cesarean birth is similar to that for one who has had a vaginal birth, with added interventions. Her temperature is assessed on admission to the post anesthesia care unit (PACU) and according to protocol thereafter. If her condition is stable, other assessments are done on admission and every 15 minutes during the first 1 to 2 hours, progressing to every 30 minutes to 1 hour until transfer to her postpartum room. In addition to temperature, routine postoperative assessments include:

- Vital signs and character of respirations; oxygen saturation; ECG pattern (usually normal sinus rhythm)
- Return of motion and sensation (if a regional block was given)
- Level of consciousness (particularly if general anesthetic or sedating drugs were given)
- Abdominal dressing
- Uterine firmness and position (midline or deviated)
- Lochia (color, quantity, presence and size of any clots)

- Urine output (quantity, color, other characteristics)
- Intravenous infusion
- Pain-relief needs

The nurse observes for return of motion and sensation if the woman had epidural or subarachnoid block anesthesia. The level of consciousness and respiratory status (skin or mucous membrane color; rate and quality of respirations; oxygen saturation) are important observations if she had general anesthesia. Detailed respiratory observations are essential for a longer period if the woman received epidural opioid narcotics, which can cause delayed respiratory depression. Have naloxone (Narcan) available to reverse opioid-induced respiratory depression. (See Chapter 19 for more information about anesthesia and analgesia for cesarean birth.)

The pulse, respirations, and blood pressure provide important clues to the woman's circulatory and respiratory status. If oxygen saturation falls below 95%, having her take several deep breaths usually raises it. Supplemental oxygen by nasal cannula, face tent, or mask is occasionally needed. A respiratory rate of less than 12 breaths per minute suggests respiratory depression. Deep breathing and coughing move secretions out of the lungs and promote full expansion. A small pillow to support her incision reduces pain when she coughs. Position changes every 2 hours improve ventilation and decrease discomfort from constant pressure.

As with a vaginal birth, the fundus is assessed for height, firmness, and position. To relax abdominal muscles, thus reducing pain from fundus checks if sensation has returned, she should flex her knees and take slow, deep breaths. The nurse gently "walks" his or her fingers toward the woman's fundus to determine uterine firmness. The woman who has a Pfannenstiel skin incision usually has less pain with fundus checks than the woman with a vertical skin incision. A firm fundus does not need massage. The dressing is checked for drainage with each fundus check.

The nurse assesses the lochia and urine output with other assessments. Lochia may pool under the mother's buttocks and lower back. Urine may be bloody temporarily if the cesarean delivery was done after a long labor or an attempted forceps delivery. The urine drainage tube should be observed for gradual clearing of the blood. Urine should drain freely to prevent bladder distention, which worsens pain and increases the risk for postpartum hemorrhage. The nurse must remember that a falling urine output is an early sign of hypovolemia, occurring well before the fall in blood pressure.

The woman's needs for pain relief should be assessed with her vital signs. The woman who received an epidural analgesic may not need other analgesia during the early postpartum period. If she needs added pain relief while the epidural analgesic is still in effect, an oral analgesic often suffices. One to 2 doses of a nonsteroidal antiinflammatory (NSAID) drug such as rofecoxib (Vioxx) provide long-acting analgesia to supplement the epidural drug. Parenteral analgesic is usually given by a patient-controlled analgesia pump or occasionally intermittent injections. Oral analgesics usually replace parenteral ones the day after surgery.

Presenting Vaginal Birth After Cesarean

Teaching the woman about VBAC presents a challenge to nurses. Women have often heard the outdated saying, "once a cesarean, always a cesarean," and are anxious about attempting vaginal birth in a later pregnancy. Scheduling a repeat cesarean often seems safer, simpler, and predictable. The prospect of laboring and perhaps still needing a cesarean birth is unattractive as well. Also, the nurse cannot promise the woman that she will not ultimately need a cesarean birth after hours of labor.

If the woman at low risk for uterine rupture is planning VBAC, the nurse should reinforce the appropriateness of attempting it and the advantages of a successful vaginal birth, such as fewer overall complications. Vaginal birth after cesarean should be presented in a positive way, at the same time acknowledging that a cesarean delivery may be needed. The nurse should also acknowledge the slightly increased risk for uterine rupture if she attempts VBAC and support her decision if she opts for a repeat cesarean birth.

KEY CONCEPTS

- Prolapse and compression of the umbilical cord are the primary risks of amniotomy. As the fluid gushes out, the cord can become compressed between the fetal presenting part and the expectant woman's pelvis.
- The risk for infection is greater the longer membranes have been ruptured, especially if over 24 hours has elapsed.
- Labor may be induced if continuing the pregnancy is more hazardous to the maternal or fetal health than is the induction. Induction is not done if a maternal or fetal contraindication exists to labor or vaginal birth.
- Oxytocin- or prostaglandin-stimulated uterine contractions may be hypertonic, decreasing placental perfusion.

- External version promotes vaginal birth by changing the fetal presentation from a breech or transverse lie to a cephalic lie. Internal version is occasionally used to change the presentation of the second twin after the birth of the first twin.
- Giving birth over an intact perineum results in less blood loss, less pain, and earlier resumption of comfortable intercourse postpartum. Therefore episiotomy should be done selectively rather than routinely, to every woman.
- Trauma to maternal and fetal tissue is the primary risk associated with use of forceps or a vacuum extractor. Possible trauma to the mother includes vaginal wall laceration and

hematoma. Trauma to the infant may include ecchymoses, lacerations, abrasions, facial nerve injury, and intracranial hemorrhage.
- The preferred uterine incision for cesarean birth is the low transverse incision because it is least likely to rupture in a subsequent pregnancy. The skin incision does not always match the uterine incision and is unrelated to the risk of later uterine rupture.
- Some women have feelings of guilt or inadequacy if they have a cesarean birth. Therapeutic communication and sensitive, family-centered care are essential to help them achieve a positive perception of their birth experience.

ANSWERS to Critical Thinking Exercise 20-1

1. The amount of amniotic fluid is normal, but the pale yellow color and strong odor suggest chorioamnionitis, or infection of the amniotic sac. The risk for chorioamnionitis increases as the duration of ruptured membranes increases, but it can be apparent at any time, including at initial rupture. The fetal heart rate is slightly elevated from the normal maximum rate at term of 160 bpm. Accelerations with fetal movement are a reassuring sign.

The maternal temperature, pulse, and respirations are slightly elevated. It is difficult to accurately interpret these values because the baseline values are not stated. These contractions are typical for a woman entering the active phase of first-stage labor.

2. The nurse should continue to assess the fetus for tachycardia, which often precedes maternal fever. Assess the woman's temperature at least every 2 hours for a temperature of 38° C (100.4° F) or higher. Report abnormalities to the physician. Observe also for fetal tachycardia and signs of fetal compromise that may occur with maternal infection.

ANSWERS to Critical Thinking Exercise 20-2

1. The woman is having hypertonic uterine activity because the rest interval is often under 30 seconds. Also, her peak intrauterine pressure during contractions is 10 mm Hg higher than expected for first-stage labor and the baseline intrauterine pressure is high. Oxytocin stimulation is the probable cause of the excessive contractions. The reassuring fetal heart rate suggests that the fetus is now tolerating the excessive contractions.

2. Fetal oxygenation may be compromised if the excessive contractions continue. Reduce or stop the oxytocin infusion to decrease uterine stimulation. Increase the primary (nonadditive) intravenous infusion as needed to maintain adequate circulating volume and ensure maximum uterine blood flow. Keep the woman in a lateral position to reduce aortocaval compression and increase placental blood flow. Oxygen given at 10 L/min with a snug facemask increases her blood oxygen saturation, making more available to the fetus. (See Chapter 18 for further information about fetal responses to reduced placental perfusion.)

REFERENCES and READINGS

Alexander, J.M., McIntire, D.D., & Leveno, K.J. (2001). Prolonged pregnancy: Induction of labor and cesarean births. *Obstetrics & Gynecology, 97*(6), 911-915.

American Academy of Pediatrics, & American College of Obstetricians and Gynecologists. (2002). *Guidelines for perinatal care* (5th ed.). Elk Grove Village, IL, and Washington, DC: Author.

American College of Obstetricians and Gynecologists (ACOG). (2003). *Dystocia and the augmentation of labor* (ACOG Practice Bulletin No. 49). Washington, DC: Author.

American College of Obstetricians and Gynecologists. (1999a). *Induction of labor* (ACOG Practice Bulletin No. 10). Washington, DC: Author.

American College of Obstetricians and Gynecologists. (1999b). *Vaginal birth after previous cesarean delivery* (ACOG Practice Bulletin No. 5). Washington, DC: Author.

American College of Obstetricians and Gynecologists (ACOG). (2000a). *ACOG news release: ACOG writes FDA on safety of misoprostol*. Retrieved Oct. 1, 2003, from www.acog.org/from_home/publications/press_releases/nr10-27-00.cfm.

American College of Obstetricians and Gynecologists (ACOG). (2000b). *External cephalic version* (ACOG Practice Bulletin No. 13). Washington, DC: Author.

American College of Obstetricians and Gynecologists (ACOG). (2000c). *Operative vaginal delivery* (ACOG Practice Bulletin No. 17). Washington, DC: Author.

American College of Obstetricians and Gynecologists (ACOG). (1999, reaffirmed 2001). *Induction of labor with misoprostol* (ACOG Committee Opinion No. 228). Washington, DC: Author.

Belfort, M.A. (2003). Operative vaginal delivery. In J.R. Scott, R.S. Gibbs, B.Y. Karlan, & A.F. Haney, *Danforth's obstetrics and gynecology* (9th ed., pp. 419-447). Philadelphia: Lippincott.

Bishop, E.H. (1964). Pelvic scoring. *Obstetrics & Gynecology, 24*(2), 266-268.

Bowes, W.A., & Thorpe, J.M. (2004). Clinical aspects of normal and abnormal labor. In R. K. Creasy, R. Resnik, & J.D. Iams (Eds.), *Maternal-fetal medicine: Principles and practice* (5th ed., pp. 671-705). Philadelphia: Saunders.

Bricker, L, & Luckas, M. (2001). Selected Cochrane systematic reviews: Amniotomy alone for induction of labour. *Birth, 28*(2), 138-139.

Clayworth, S. (2000). The nurse's role during oxytocin administration. *MCN: The American Journal of Maternal/Child Nursing, 25*(5), 80-84.

Crenshaw, J.T., & Winslow, E.H. (2002). Preoperative fasting: Old habits die hard. *American Journal of Nursing, 102*(5), 36-44.

Cunningham, F.G., Gant, N.F., Leveno, K.J., Gilstrap, L.C., Hauth, J.C., & Wenstrom, K.D. (2001). *Williams obstetrics* (21st ed.). New York: McGraw-Hill.

Depp, R. (2002). Cesarean delivery. In S.G. Gabbe, J.R. Niebyl, & J.L. Simpson (Eds.), *Obstetrics: Normal and problem pregnancies* (4th ed., pp. 539-606). New York: Churchill Livingstone.

Eason, E., & Feldman, P. (2000). Clinical commentary: Much ado about a little cut: Is episiotomy worthwhile? *Obstetrics & Gynecology, 95*(4), 616-617.

Eason, E., Labrecque, M., Wells, G., & Feldman, P. (2000). Preventing perineal trauma during childbirth: A systematic review. *Obstetrics & Gynecology, 95*(3), 464-471.

Flamm, B.L. (2000). Cesarean section: A worldwide epidemic? *Birth, 27*(2), 139-140.

Flamm, B.L., Berwick, D.M., & Kabcenell, A. (1998). Reducing cesarean section rates safely: Lessons from a "breakthrough series" collaborative. *Birth, 25*(2), 117-124.

Gamble, J.A., Health, M., & Creedy, D.K. (2000). Women's request for a cesarean section: A critique of the literature. *Birth, 27*(4), 256-263.

Gifford, D.S., Morton, S.C., Fiske, M., Keesey, J., Keeler, E., & Kahn, K.L. (2000). Lack of progress in labor as a reason for cesarean. *Obstetrics & Gynecology, 95*(4), 589-595.

Goer, H. (2003). "Spin doctoring" the research. *Birth, 30*(2), 124-129.

Goetzl, L., Shipp, T.D., Cohen, A., Zelop, C.M., Repke, J.T., & Lieberman, E. (2001). Oxytocin dose and the risk of uterine rupture in trial of labor after cesarean. *Obstetrics & Gynecology, 97*(3), 381-384.

Goldberg, J., Holtz, D., Hyslop, T., & Tolosa, J.E. (2002). Has the use of routine episiotomy decreased? Examination of episiotomy rates from 1983 to 2000. *Obstetrics & Gynecology, 99*(3), 395-400.

Greene, M.F. (2001). Vaginal delivery after cesarean section—Is the risk acceptable? *New England Journal of Medicine, 345*(1), 54-55.

Hall, M.J., & Owings, M.F. (2002). 2000 National hospital discharge survey. Advance data from *Vital & Health Statistics*; number 329. Hyattsville, MD: National Center for Health Statistics, 2003. Retrieved Jan. 24, 2004, from www.cdc.gov/nchs/data/ad/ad329.pdf.

Hall, R.S., Duarte-Gardea, M., & Harlass, F. (2002). Oral versus vaginal misoprostol for labor induction. *Obstetrics & Gynecology, 99*(6), 1044-1048.

Hall, S.P. (2002). Amniotomy: Necessary intervention or bad habit? *AWHONN Lifelines, 5*(6), 10-13.

REFERENCES and READINGS

Johnson, D.P., Davis, N.R., & Brown, A.J. (2003). Risk of cesarean delivery after induction at term in nulliparous women with an unfavorable cervix. *American Journal of Obstetrics and Gynecology, 188*(6), 1565-1672.

Kaczorowski, J., Levitt, C., Hanvey, L., Avard, D., & Chance, G. (1998). A national survey of use of obstetric procedures and technologies in Canadian hospitals: Routine or based on existing evidence? *Birth, 25*(1), 11-18.

Kendrick, J.M. (2001). Labor and birth. In K.R. Simpson & P.A. Creehan (Eds.), *AWHONN's perinatal nursing* (2nd ed., pp. 298-365). Philadelphia: Lippincott.

King, T.L., & Simpson, K.R. (2001). Fetal assessment during labor. In K.R. Simpson & P.A. Creehan (Eds.), *AWHONN's perinatal nursing* (2nd ed., pp. 378-416). Philadelphia: Lippincott.

Kozak, L.J., & Weeks, J.D. (2002). U.S. trends in obstetric procedures, 1990-2000. *Birth, 29*(3), 157-161.

Labrecque, M., Eason, E., Marcoux, S, Lemieu, F., Pinault, J.J., Feldman, P., & Laperrière, L. (1999). Randomized controlled trial of prevention of perineal trauma by perineal massage during pregnancy. *American Journal of Obstetrics & Gynecology, 180*(3 Pt. 1), 593-600.

Landon, M.B. (2000). Cesarean section. In S.B. Ransom, M.P. Dombrowski, S.G. McNeeley, K.S. Moghissi, & A.R. Munkarah (Eds.), *Practical strategies in obstetrics and gynecology* (pp. 299-310). Philadelphia: Saunders.

Laros, R.K., Flanagan, T.A., & Kilpatrick, S.J. (1995). Management of term breech presentation: A protocol of external cephalic version and selective trial of labor. *American Journal of Obstetrics and Gynecology, 172*(6), 1916-1925.

Lowe, N.K. (2003). Amazed or appalled, apathy or action? *Journal of Obstetric, Gynecologic, and Neonatal Nursing, 32*(3), 281-282.

Mancuso, K.M., Yancey, M.K., Murphy, J.A., & Markenson, G.R. (2000). Epidural analgesia for cephalic version: A randomized trial. *Obstetrics & Gynecology, 95*(5 Pt. 1), 648-651.

Martin, J.H., Hamilton, B.E., Ventura, S.J., Menacker, F., & Munson, M.L. (2003). Births: Final data for 2002. *National Vital Statistics Reports, 52*(10). Hyattsville, MD: National Center for

Health Statistics. Retrieved Jan. 24, 2004, from www.cdc.gov/nchs/data/nvsr52/nvsr5_10.pdf.

Maslow, A.S., & Sweeny, A.L. (2000). Elective induction of labor as a risk factor for cesarean delivery among low-risk women at term. *Obstetrics & Gynecology, 95*(6 Pt. 1), 917-922.

Nager, C.W., & Helliwell, J.P. (2001). Episiotomy increases perineal laceration length in primiparous women. *American Journal of Obstetrics & Gynecology, 185*, 444-450.

Norwitz, E.R., Robinson, J. N., & Repke, J.T. (2002). Labor and delivery. In S.G. Gabbe, J.R. Niebyl, & J.L. Simpson (Eds.), *Obstetrics: Normal and problem pregnancies* (4th ed., pp. 353-394). New York: Churchill Livingstone.

Porter, T.F., & Scott, J.R. (2003). Cesarean delivery. In J.R. Scott, R.S. Gibbs, B.Y. Karlan, & A.F. Haney, *Danforth's obstetrics and gynecology* (9th ed., pp. 449-460). Philadelphia: Lippincott Williams & Wilkins.

Puder, K.S., & Dombrowski, M.P. (2000). Vaginal delivery, operative and breech. In S.B. Ransom, M.P. Dombrowski, S.G. McNeeley, K.S. Moghissi, & A.R. Munkarah (Eds.), *Practical strategies in obstetrics and gynecology* (pp. 291-298). Philadelphia: Saunders.

Rayburn, W.F., & Zhang, J. (2002). Rising rates of labor induction: Present concerns and future strategies. *Obstetrics & Gynecology, 100*(1), 164-167.

Regalia, A.L., Curiel, P., Natale, N., Galluzzi, A., Spinelli, G., Ghezzi, G.V.L. Tampieri, A., & Terzian, E. (2000). Routine use of external cephalic version in three hospitals. *Birth 27*(1), 19-24.

Rice-Simpson, K., & Poole, J.H. (1998). *Cervical ripening and induction and augmentation of labor.* Washington, DC: Association of Women's Health, Obstetric, and Neonatal Nurses.

Ridley, R.T., Davis, P.A., Bright, J.H., & Sinclair, D. (2002). What influences a woman to choose vaginal birth after cesarean? *Journal of Obstetric, Gynecologic, and Neonatal Nursing, 31*(6), 665-672.

Robinson, J.N., Norwitz, E. R., Cohen, A.P., & Lieberman, E. (2000). Predictors of episiotomy use at first spontaneous vaginal delivery. *American Journal of Obstetrics & Gynecology, 96*(2), 214-218.

Ruchala, P.L., Metheny, N., Essenpreis, H., & Borcherding, K. (2002). Current practice in oxytocin dilution and fluid administration for induction of labor. *Journal of Obstetric, Gynecologic, and Neonatal Nursing, 31*(5), 545-550.

Sanchez-Ramos, L., Oliver, F., Delke, I., & Kaunitz, A.M. (2003). Labor induction versus expectant management for postterm pregnancies: A systematic review with meta-analysis. *Obstetrics & Gynecology, 101*(6), 1312-1318.

Searing, K.A. (2001). Induction vs. post-date pregnancies: Exploring the controversy of who's really at risk. *AWHONN Lifelines, 5*(2), 44-48.

Seyb, S.T., Berka, R.J., Socol, M.L., & Dooley, S.L. (1999). Risk of cesarean delivery with elective induction of labor at term in nulliparous women. *Obstetrics & Gynecology, 94*(4), 600-607.

Siddiqui, D., Stiller, R.J., Collins, J., & Laifer, S.A. (1999). Pregnancy outcome after successful external cephalic version. *American Journal of Obstetrics and Gynecology, 181*(5 Pt. 1), 1092-1095.

Signorello, L.B., Harlow, B.L., Chekos, A.K., & Repke, J.T. (2001). Postpartum sexual functioning and its relationship to perineal trauma: A retrospective cohort study of primiparous women. *American Journal of Obstetrics & Gynecology, 185*(5), 881-890.

Simpson, K.R., & Poole, J.H. (1998). *Cervical ripening and induction and augmentation of labor.* Washington, DC: Association of Women's Health, Obstetric, and Gynecologic Nurses (AWHONN).

U.S. Department of Health and Human Services. (2003.). *Healthy People 2010.* Retrieved Sept. 16, 2003, from www.healthypeople.gov/document/html/objectives/16-09.htm.

Webb, D.A., & Culhane, J. (2002). Hospital variation in episiotomy use and the risk of perineal trauma during childbirth. *Birth, 29*(2), 132-136.

Wing, D.A., Park, M.R., & Paul, R.H. (2000). A randomized comparison of oral and intravaginal misoprostol for labor induction. *Obstetrics & Gynecology, 95*(6 Pt. 1), 905-908.

Yeast, J.D., Jones, A., & Poskin, M. (1999). Induction of labor and the relationship to cesarean delivery. *American Journal of Obstetrics and Gynecology, 180*(3 Pt. 1), 626-633.

21

Postpartum Adaptations

After studying this chapter, you should be able to:

◎ Explain the physiologic changes that occur during the postpartum period.
◎ Describe nursing assessments and nursing care during the postpartum period.
◎ Discuss the role of the nurse in health education and identify important areas of teaching.
◎ Describe postpartum home care in terms of criteria for discharge, common problems, and available health care services.
◎ Compare nursing assessments and care for women who have undergone cesarean birth and vaginal birth.
◎ Explain the process of bonding and attachment, including the role of maternal touch and verbal interactions.

◎ Describe the progressive phases of maternal adaptation to childbirth and the stages of maternal role attainment.
◎ Identify maternal concerns and how they change over time.
◎ Discuss the cause, manifestations, and interventions related to postpartum blues.
◎ Describe the processes of family adaptation to the birth of a baby.
◎ Discuss factors that affect family adaptation.
◎ Discuss cultural influences on family adaptation.
◎ Describe assessments and interventions related to postpartum psychosocial adaptations.
◎ Explain the need for additional care after discharge of the mother and infant from the birth facility.

◆ DEFINITIONS

afterpain Cramping pain after childbirth, caused by alternating relaxation and contraction of uterine muscles.

atony Absence or lack of usual muscle tone.

attachment Development of strong affectional ties as a result of interaction between an infant and a significant other (mother, father, sibling, caretaker).

bonding Development of a strong emotional tie of a parent to a newborn. Also called *claiming* or *binding in.*

catabolism A destructive process that converts living cells into simpler compounds. Process involved in involution (normal changes) of the uterus after childbirth.

deciduas The endometrium during pregnancy. All except the deepest layer is shed after childbirth.

diastasis recti Separation of the longitudinal muscles of the abdomen (rectus abdominis) during pregnancy.

dyspareunia Difficult or painful coitus in women.

en face Position that allows eye-to-eye contact between the newborn and a parent. Optimal distance is 20 to 22 cm (8-9 in).

engorgement Swelling of the breasts resulting from increased blood flow and the presence of milk.

engrossment Intense fascination and close face-to-face observation between father and newborn.

entrainment Newborn movement in rhythm with adult speech, particularly high-pitched tones, which are more easily heard.

episiotomy Surgical incision of the perineum to enlarge the vaginal opening.

fingertipping First tactile (touch) experience between mother and newborn. The mother explores the infant's body with her fingertips only.

fourth trimester First 12 weeks after birth, a time of transition for parents and siblings.

fundus Part of the uterus that is farthest from the cervix, above the openings of the fallopian tubes.

involution Retrogressive changes that return the reproductive organs, particularly the uterus, to their nonpregnant size and condition.

Kegel exercises Alternate contracting and relaxing of the pelvic muscles. These movements strengthen the pubococcygeal muscle, which surrounds the urinary meatus and vagina.

lactation Secretion of milk from the breasts. Also describes the period of time of breastfeeding.

letting go A phase of maternal adaptation that involves relinquishing previous roles and assuming a new role as a parent.

lochia alba White, cream-colored, or light-yellow vaginal discharge that follows lochia serosa. Occurs when the amount of blood is decreased and the number of leukocytes is increased.

lochia rubra Red vaginal discharge that occurs immediately after childbirth; composed mostly of blood.

lochia serosa Pinkish or brown-tinged vaginal discharge that follows lochia rubra; composed largely of serous exudate, blood, and leukocytes.

milk-ejection reflex Release of milk from the alveoli into the ducts. Also known as the *letdown reflex.*

oxytocin Posterior pituitary hormone that stimulates uterine contractions and the milk-ejection reflex. Also prepared synthetically.

postpartum blues Temporary, self-limiting period of weepiness experienced by many new mothers within the first few days after childbirth.

prolactin Anterior pituitary hormone that promotes growth of breast tissue and stimulates production of milk.

puerperium Period from the end of childbirth until involution of the uterus is complete, approximately 6 weeks.

reciprocal bonding behaviors Repertoire of infant behaviors that promotes attachment between parent and newborn.

REEDA Acronym for redness, ecchymosis, edema, discharge, and approximation. Useful for assessing wound healing or the presence of inflammation or infection.

sibling rivalry Feelings of jealousy and fear of replacement when a young child must share parental attention with a newborn infant.

subinvolution Delayed return of the uterus to its nonpregnant size and consistency.

taking hold Second phase of maternal adaptation, during which the mother assumes control of her own care and initiates care of the infant.

taking in First phase of maternal adaptation, during which the mother passively accepts care and comfort and details about the newborn.

The first 6 weeks after the birth of an infant is known as the *postpartum period,* or *puerperium.* During this time, mothers experience numerous physiologic and psychosocial changes. Many postpartum physiologic changes are retrogressive—that is, changes that occurred in body systems during pregnancy are reversed as the body returns to the nonpregnant state. Progressive changes also occur. Most obvious are the return of normal menstrual cycles and the initiation of lactation.

REPRODUCTIVE SYSTEM

Involution of the Uterus

Involution refers to the changes that the reproductive organs, particularly the uterus, undergo after childbirth as they return to their nonpregnant size and condition. Uterine involution entails three processes: (1) contraction of muscle fibers, (2) catabolism, and (3) regeneration of uterine epithelium. Uterine involution begins immediately after delivery of the placenta, when uterine muscle fibers contract firmly around maternal blood vessels at the area where the placenta was attached. This contraction controls bleeding from the area left denuded when the placenta separated. The uterus becomes smaller as the muscle fibers, which have been stretched for many months, contract and gradually regain their former contour and size.

The enlarged uterine muscle cells are affected by catabolic changes in protein cytoplasm, which cause a reduction in individual cell size. The products of this catabolic process are absorbed by the bloodstream and excreted in the urine as nitrogenous waste.

Regeneration of the uterine epithelial lining begins soon after childbirth. The outer portion of the endometrial layer is expelled with the placenta. Within 2 to 3 days, the remaining decidua separates into two layers. The first layer is superficial and is shed in lochia. The basal layer remains to provide the source of new endometrium. Regeneration of the endometrium, except at the site of placental attachment, occurs by 2 to 3 weeks.

The placental site, which is about 7 cm ($2^{7}/_{10}$ in) in diameter, heals by a process of exfoliation (scaling off of dead tissue). New endometrium is generated at the site from glands and tissue that remain in the lower layer of the decidua after separation of the placenta (Cunningham et al., 2001). This process leaves the uterine lining free of scar tissue, which would interfere with implantation of future pregnancies. Healing at the placental site takes approximately 6 to 7 weeks.

Descent of the Uterine Fundus

The location of the uterine fundus helps determine whether involution is progressing normally. Immediately after delivery, the uterus is about the size of a large grapefruit and weighs approximately 1000 g (2.2 lb). The fundus can be palpated midway between the symphysis pubis and umbilicus (James, 2001). Within a few hours, the fundus rises to the level of the umbilicus and should remain at this level for about 24 hours.

After 24 hours, the fundus begins to descend by approximately 1 cm, or one fingerbreadth, per day, so that by the 10th to 14th day it is in the pelvic cavity and cannot be palpated abdominally. The fundus may be slightly higher in multiparas or in women who delivered a large infant or more than one infant. Descent is documented in relation to the umbilicus. For instance, U – 1 indicates that the fundus is palpable one fingerbreadth below the umbilicus. Within a week, the weight of the uterus decreases to about 500 g (1 lb); at 6 weeks, the uterus weighs 60 g (2 oz), which is roughly the prepregnancy weight. Figure 21-1 illustrates normal descent of the uterine fundus as involution occurs.

Afterpains

Etiology. Intermittent contractions, known as *afterpains,* are a source of discomfort for many women. The discomfort is more acute for multiparas because repeated stretching of muscle fibers leads to loss of the muscle tone that enables alternate contraction and relaxation of the uterus. The uterus of a primipara tends to remain contracted, but she may also experience severe afterpains if the uterus has been overdistended by twins, a large infant, hydramnios (excess of amniotic fluid), or retained blood clots. Oxytocin released from the posterior pituitary during breastfeeding may also cause strong contractions of the uterine muscles.

Nursing Considerations. Analgesics are frequently used to lessen the discomfort of afterpains. If the mother is breastfeeding, she achieves maximum relief by taking the medication at least 30 minutes before nursing the infant. There is general agreement that analgesics may be used for short-term pain relief without harm to the infant. The benefits of pain

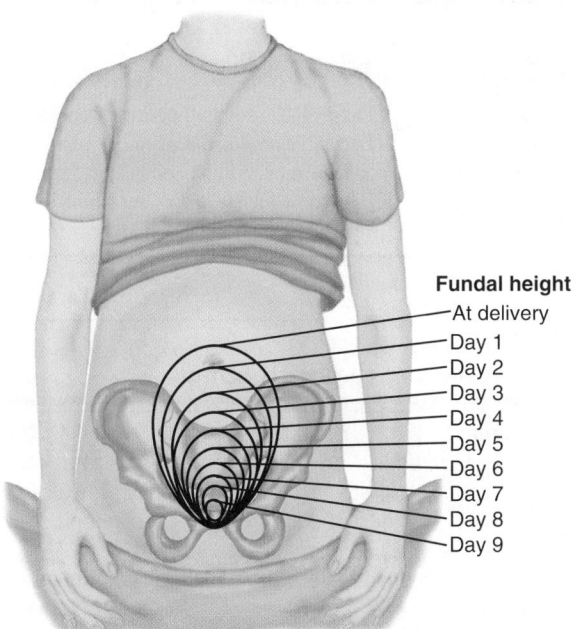

Fundal height
At delivery
Day 1
Day 2
Day 3
Day 4
Day 5
Day 6
Day 7
Day 8
Day 9

Figure 21-1 Involution of the uterus. Height of the uterine fundus decreases by approximately 1 cm/day.

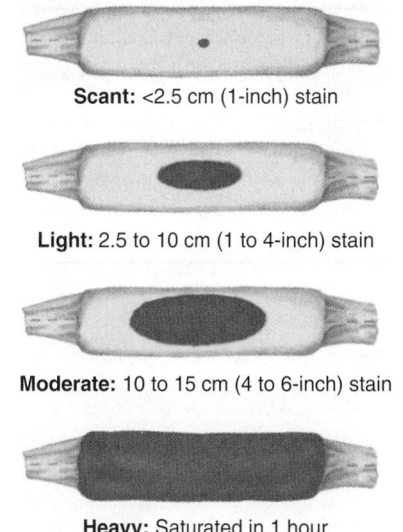

Scant: <2.5 cm (1-inch) stain

Light: 2.5 to 10 cm (1 to 4-inch) stain

Moderate: 10 to 15 cm (4 to 6-inch) stain

Heavy: Saturated in 1 hour

Figure 21-2 Guidelines for assessing the volume of lochia based on the amount of stain on the perineal pad.

relief, such as comfort and relaxation, which facilitate the milk-ejection reflex, usually outweigh the negligible effects of the medication on the infant.

Some mothers also find that lying in a prone position with a small pillow or folded blanket under the abdomen helps keep the uterus contracted and provides relief. Afterpains are self-limiting and decrease rapidly after 48 hours.

Lochia — vaginal discharge

Changes in the color and amount of lochia also provide information about whether involution is progressing normally.

Changes in Color. For the first 3 days after childbirth, lochia consists almost entirely of blood, with small particles of decidua and mucus. Because of its red color, it is termed *lochia rubra*. The amount of blood decreases by about the 4th day. The color of lochia then changes from red to pink or pinkish brown (*lochia serosa*). Lochia serosa is composed of serous exudate, erythrocytes, leukocytes, and cervical mucus. By about the 11th day, the erythrocyte component decreases. The discharge becomes white, cream-colored, or light-yellow (*lochia alba*). Lochia alba contains leukocytes, decidual cells, epithelial cells, fat, cervical mucus, and bacteria. It is present in most women until the 3rd week after childbirth but may persist for 6 weeks.

Amount. Because estimating the amount of lochia is difficult, nurses frequently record lochia in terms that are difficult to quantify, such as "scant," "moderate," and "heavy." One method for estimating the amount of lochia in 1 hour uses the following labels (Scoggin, 2000):

Scant: Less than a 2.5-cm (1-in) stain on the perineal pad ("peripad")
Light: 2.5- to 10-cm (1- to 4-in) stain
Moderate: 10- to 15-cm (4- to 6-in) stain

Large: Saturated peripad in 1 hour
Excessive: Saturated peripad in 15 minutes.

Determining the time the peripad has been in place is important in assessing lochia. What appears to be a light flow may be heavier if the peripad has been in use less than an hour (Figure 21-2). Lochia is often heavier when the new mother first gets out of bed, because gravity allows blood that has pooled in the vagina during the hours of rest to flow freely when she stands. Table 21-1 summarizes the characteristics of normal and abnormal lochia.

Cervix

Immediately after childbirth, the cervix is formless, flabby, and open wide. Small tears or lacerations may be present, and the cervix is often edematous. Healing occurs rapidly, and by the end of the first week the cervix feels firm and the external os is the width of a pencil. The internal os closes as before pregnancy, but the shape of the external os is permanently changed. It remains slightly open and appears slit-like rather than round, as in the nulliparous woman (Fig. 21-3).

Vagina

Soon after childbirth, the vaginal walls appear edematous and multiple small lacerations may be present. Very few vaginal rugae (folds) are present. The hymen is permanently torn and heals with small, irregular tags of tissue visible at the vaginal introitus.

Although the vaginal mucosa heals and rugae are regained by 3 weeks, it takes the entire postpartum period (6 weeks) for the vagina to complete involution and to gain approximately the same size and contour it had before pregnancy. The vagina does not, however, entirely regain the nulliparous size.

During the postpartum period, vaginal mucosa becomes atrophic, and vaginal walls do not regain their thickness until estrogen production by the ovaries is re-established. Be-

TABLE 21-1 Characteristics of Lochia

Time and Type	Normal Discharge	Abnormal Discharge
Days 1-3: lochia rubra	Bloody; small clots; fleshy, earthy odor	Large clots; saturated perineal pads; foul odor
Days 4-10: lochia serosa	Decreased amount; serosanguineous; pink or brown	Excessive amount; foul smell; continued or recurrent reddish color
Days 11-21: lochia alba	White, cream-colored, or light-yellow; decreasing amounts	Persistent lochia serosa; return to lochia rubra, foul odor; discharge continuing

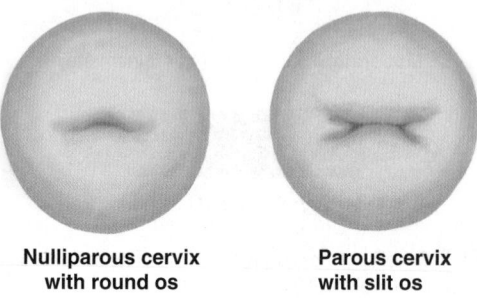

Nulliparous cervix with round os   **Parous cervix with slit os**

Figure 21-3 A permanent change occurs in the external cervical os after childbirth.

cause ovarian function, and therefore estrogen production, is not well established during lactation, breastfeeding mothers are likely to experience vaginal dryness and may experience dyspareunia, or discomfort during intercourse.

Perineum

Because of pressure from the fetal head, the muscles of the pelvic floor stretch and thin greatly during the second stage of labor. After childbirth, the perineum may be edematous and bruised. In the United States, many women who give birth also have a surgical incision (episiotomy) of the perineal area. The episiotomy site may take 4 to 6 months to heal completely (Blackburn, 2003).

Lacerations of the perineum may also occur during delivery. Lacerations and episiotomies are classified according to tissue involved (Box 21-1). (See discussion of episiotomy in Chapter 20.)

Discomfort

Although the episiotomy is relatively small, the muscles of the perineum are involved in many activities (walking, sitting, stooping, squatting, bending, defecating, urinating). An incision in this area can cause a great deal of discomfort. In addition, many pregnant women are affected by hemorrhoids (distended rectal veins), which are pushed out of the rectum during the second stage of labor.

Nursing Considerations

Hemorrhoids, as well as perineal trauma, episiotomy, or lacerations, can make physical activity or bowel elimination difficult during the postpartum period. Relief of perineal discomfort is a nursing priority and includes teaching self-care measures, such as sitz baths, perineal care, and the use of topical anesthetics.

BOX 21-1
Lacerations of the Birth Canal

Perineum
Perineal lacerations are classified in degrees to describe the amount of tissue involved. Some physicians or nurse-midwives also describe the extent of median episiotomies by degree of tissue involvement:
- *First-degree:* Involves the superficial vaginal mucosa or perineal skin.
- *Second-degree:* Involves the vaginal mucosa, perineal skin, and deeper tissues, which may include muscles of the perineum.
- *Third-degree:* Same as second-degree laceration but involves the anal sphincter.
- *Fourth-degree:* Extends through the anal sphincter into the rectal mucosa.

Periurethral Area
A laceration in the area of the urethra that may cause women to have difficulty urinating after birth. An indwelling catheter may be necessary for a day or two.

Vaginal Wall
A laceration involving the mucosa of the vaginal wall.

Cervix
Tears in the cervix may be a source of significant bleeding after birth.

CARDIOVASCULAR SYSTEM

Hypervolemia, which produces a 50% increase in blood volume at term, allows the woman to tolerate a substantial blood loss during childbirth without ill effect. On the average, 500 ml of blood is lost in vaginal deliveries and 1000 ml is lost in cesarean births (Blackburn, 2003).

Cardiac Output

Despite the blood loss, a transient increase in maternal cardiac output occurs after childbirth. This increase is caused by (1) an increased flow of blood back to the heart when blood from the uteroplacental unit returns to the central circulation and (2) the mobilization of excess extracellular fluid into the vascular compartment. The rise in cardiac output, which persists for about 48 hours after childbirth, is probably caused by an increase in stroke volume because bradycardia is often noted during the postpartum period.

Bradycardia is defined as a pulse rate of 50 to 60 beats per minute. Gradually, cardiac output decreases and returns to normal levels by 12 weeks after childbirth (Blackburn, 2003).

Plasma Volume

The body rids itself of excess plasma volume by diuresis and diaphoresis:

- Diuresis (increased excretion of urine) is facilitated by a decline in the adrenal hormone aldosterone, which increases during pregnancy to counteract the salt-wasting effect of progesterone. As aldosterone production decreases, sodium retention declines and fluid excretion accelerates. A decrease in oxytocin, which promotes reabsorption of fluid, also contributes to diuresis. A urinary output of 3000 ml/day is not uncommon, especially on days 2 to 5 of the postpartum period (Blackburn, 2003).
- Diaphoresis (profuse perspiration) also rids the body of excess fluid. Although it is not clinically significant, diaphoresis can be uncomfortable and unsettling for the mother who is not prepared for it. Explanations of the cause and provision of comfort measures, such as showers and dry clothing, are generally sufficient.

Blood Values

Several components of the blood change during the postpartum period. Marked leukocytosis occurs, with the white blood cell count (WBC) increasing to as high as 30,000/mm^3 (Cunningham et al., 2001). The average range is 14,000/mm^3 to 16,000/mm^3 (Scoggin, 2000). The WBC falls to normal values by 4 to 7 days after birth (Blackburn, 2003). Neutrophils, which increase in response to inflammation, pain, and stress, account for the major increase in white blood cells.

Maternal hemoglobin and hematocrit values are difficult to interpret during the first few days after birth because of the remobilization and rapid excretion of excess body fluid. The hematocrit is low when plasma (the liquid part of blood) increases and dilutes the concentration of blood cells and other substances carried by the plasma. As excess fluid is excreted, the dilution is gradually reduced. The hematocrit returns to normal values within 4 to 6 weeks (Blackburn, 2003).

Coagulation

During pregnancy, plasma fibrinogen and other factors necessary for coagulation increase. As a result, the mother's body has a greater ability to form clots and thus prevent excessive bleeding. Fibrinolytic activity (to break down clots) is decreased during pregnancy. Although fibrinolysis increases shortly after delivery, elevations in clotting factors continue for several days or longer, causing a continued risk of thrombus formation. It takes 3 to 4 weeks before the hemostasis returns to normal prepregnant levels (Blackburn, 2003).

Although the incidence of thrombophlebitis has declined greatly in recent years, probably as a result of early postpartum ambulation, new mothers are still at increased risk. Women who have varicose veins, a history of thrombophlebitis, or a cesarean birth are at further risk, and the lower extremities should be monitored closely. Antiembolism hosiery or sequential compression devices are often applied when the woman has a cesarean birth or if the mother is at particular risk because of a history of previous phlebitis or the presence of varicosities (see Chapter 28).

GASTROINTESTINAL SYSTEM

Soon after childbirth, digestion begins to be active and the new mother is usually hungry because of the energy expended in labor. She is also thirsty because of the long period of fluid restriction during labor, fluid loss from exertion, and early diaphoresis. Nurses anticipate the mother's needs and provide food and fluids soon after childbirth.

Constipation is a common problem during the postpartum period, for a variety of reasons. First, bowel tone, which was diminished during pregnancy as a result of progesterone, remains sluggish for several days. Second, restricted food and fluid intake during labor often results in small, hard stools. Third, perineal trauma, episiotomy, and hemorrhoids cause discomfort and interfere with effective bowel elimination. In addition, many women anticipate pain when they attempt to defecate and are unwilling to exert pressure on the perineum.

Temporary constipation is not harmful, although it can cause a feeling of abdominal fullness and flatulence. Stool softeners and laxatives are frequently prescribed to prevent or treat constipation. The first stool usually occurs within 2 to 3 days postpartum. Normal patterns of bowel elimination usually resume by 8 to 14 days after birth (Blackburn, 2003).

URINARY SYSTEM

Physical Changes

As a result of many changes that occur during pregnancy, the bladder of the postpartum woman has an increased capacity and has lost some of its muscle tone. During childbirth, the urethra, bladder, and tissue around the urinary meatus may become edematous and traumatized as the fetal head passes beneath the bladder. This condition often results in diminished sensitivity to fluid pressure, and many new mothers have no sensation of needing to void even when the bladder is distended.

The bladder fills rapidly because of the diuresis that follows childbirth. As a consequence, the mother is at risk for overdistention of the bladder, incomplete emptying of the bladder, and retention of residual urine. Women who have received regional anesthesia are at particular risk for bladder distention and for difficulty voiding until feeling returns.

Urinary retention and overdistention of the bladder may cause urinary tract infection and postpartum hemorrhage. Urinary tract infection occurs when urinary stasis allows time for bacteria to multiply. Risk of postpartum hemorrhage increases because uterine ligaments, which were stretched during pregnancy, allow the uterus to be displaced upward and laterally by the full bladder. The displacement results in an inability of the uterine muscles to contract (uterine atony), a primary cause of excessive bleeding (Fig. 21-4).

Chemical Changes

Both protein and acetone may be present in the urine in the first few postpartum days. Acetone suggests dehydration, which often occurs during the exertion of labor. Mild pro-

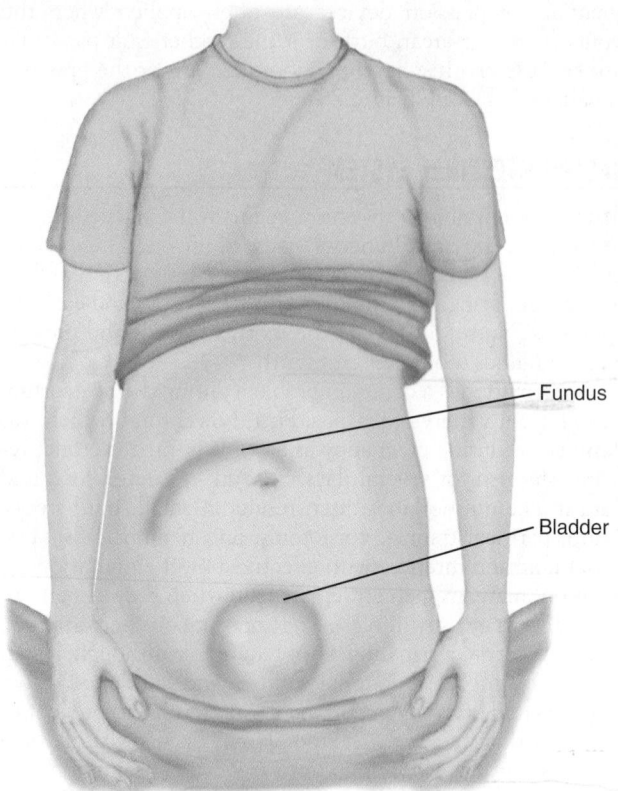

Figure 21-4 A full bladder displaces and prevents contraction of the uterus.

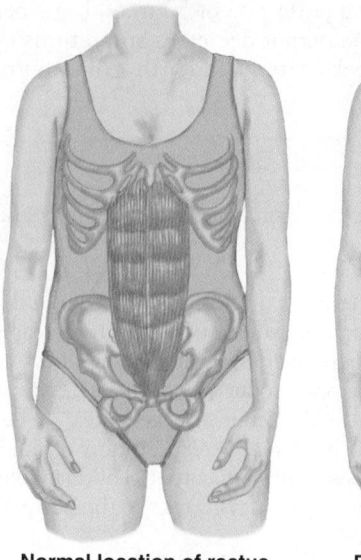
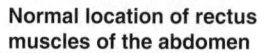
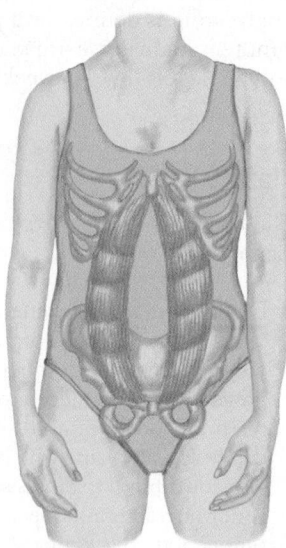

Normal location of rectus muscles of the abdomen

Diastasis recti: separation of the rectus muscles

Figure 21-5 Diastasis recti occurs when the longitudinal muscles of the abdomen separate during pregnancy.

teinuria is usually the result of the catabolic processes involved in uterine involution.

MUSCULOSKELETAL SYSTEM

Muscles and Joints

In the first 1 to 2 days after childbirth, many women experience muscle fatigue and aches, particularly of the shoulders, neck, and arms, because of exertion during labor. Warmth and gentle massage increase circulation to the area and provide comfort and relaxation.

During the first few days, levels of the hormone relaxin gradually subside and the ligaments and cartilage of the pelvis begin to return to their prepregnancy position. These changes can cause hip or joint pain that interferes with ambulation and exercise. It is helpful if the mother understands that the discomfort is temporary and does not indicate a medical problem. Good body mechanics and correct posture are extremely important during this time and should prevent low back pain and injury to the joints. (See Figures 13-11 and 13-12 for correct and incorrect posture and body mechanics.)

Abdominal Wall

During pregnancy, the abdominal walls stretch to accommodate the growing fetus and muscle tone is diminished. Many women, expecting that the abdominal muscles will return to the prepregnancy condition immediately after childbirth, are dismayed to find the abdominal muscles weak, soft, and flabby.

The longitudinal muscles of the abdomen may also separate (diastasis recti) during pregnancy (Fig. 21-5). The separation may be minimal or severe. The mother may benefit from special exercises to strengthen the abdominal wall. Figure 21-6 illustrates exercises that help to correct diastasis recti.

INTEGUMENTARY SYSTEM

Many skin changes that occur during pregnancy are caused by an increase in hormones. When the hormone levels decline after childbirth, the skin gradually reverts to the prepregnancy state. For example, melanocyte-stimulating hormone, which caused hyperpigmentation during pregnancy, decreases rapidly after childbirth and pigmentation begins to recede. This change is particularly noticeable when the "mask of pregnancy" (chloasma) and linea nigra disappear.

Striae gravidarum (stretch marks), which develop during pregnancy when connective tissue in the abdomen and breasts is stretched, gradually fade to silvery lines but do not disappear.

NEUROLOGIC SYSTEM

Many women experience discomfort and fatigue after childbirth. Afterpains, discomfort from episiotomy or incisions, muscle aches, and breast engorgement may contribute to a woman's discomfort and inability to sleep. Anesthesia or analgesia may produce temporary neurologic changes such as lack of feeling in the legs and dizziness. During this time, the priority is prevention of injury that could occur as a result of falling.

Complaints of headache need careful assessment. Although they are uncommon, postpuncture headaches after regional anesthesia may occur. They may be most severe when the woman is in an upright position and are relieved by a supine position. They should be reported to the appropriate health care provider, usually an anesthesiologist. Headache,

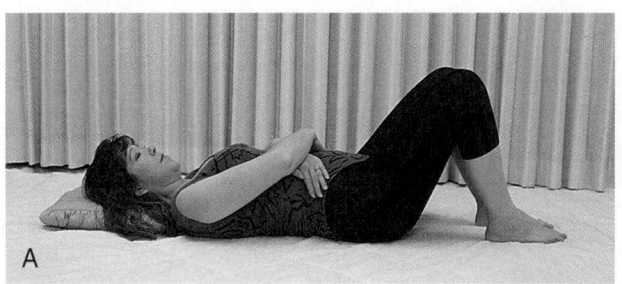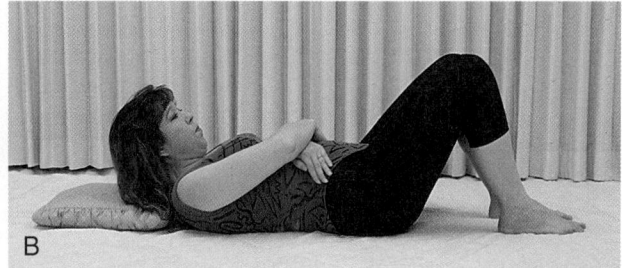

Figure 21-6 Abdominal exercises for diastasis recti. **A,** The woman inhales and supports the abdominal wall firmly with her hands. **B,** Exhaling, the woman raises her head as she pulls the abdominal muscles together.

along with blurred vision, photophobia, abdominal pain, and proteinuria, may also indicate development or worsening of preeclampsia (see Chapter 26).

ENDOCRINE SYSTEM

After expulsion of the placenta, a fairly rapid decline occurs in placental hormones such as estrogen, progesterone, and human placental lactogen. Human chorionic gonadotropin may remain several weeks. Adrenal hormones, such as aldosterone, return to prepregnancy levels. If the mother is not breastfeeding, the pituitary hormone prolactin, which stimulates milk secretion, returns to nonpregnant levels in about 2 weeks.

Resumption of Ovulation and Menstruation

Most non-nursing mothers resume menstruation within 7 to 9 weeks after childbirth, although times vary widely (Blackburn, 2003). Menses while lactating may resume as early as 12 weeks or as late as 18 months (Scoggin, 2000). Frequent feedings with no supplements are more likely to delay menses. Although the first few cycles for both lactating and non-lactating women are often anovulatory, ovulation may occur before the first menses. Therefore contraceptive measures are important considerations when sexual relations are resumed for both lactating and non-lactating women.

Lactation

During pregnancy, estrogen and progesterone prepare the breasts for lactation. Although prolactin also rises during pregnancy, lactation is inhibited at this time by the high level of estrogen and progesterone. After expulsion of the placenta, estrogen and progesterone decline rapidly, and prolactin initiates milk production within 2 to 3 days after childbirth. Once milk production is established, it continues because of frequent removal of milk from the breast.

Oxytocin is necessary for milk ejection, or "let down." A hormone secreted by the posterior pituitary gland, oxytocin, causes milk to be expressed from the alveoli into the lactiferous ducts during suckling (see Chapter 24).

Weight Loss

Approximately 5.5 kg (12 lb) is lost during childbirth. This includes the weight of the fetus, placenta, and amniotic fluid and blood lost during the birth. An additional 2.3 to 3.6 kg (5 to 8.8 lb) is lost by diuresis and involution (Scoggin, 2000). Adipose (fatty) tissue that was gained during pregnancy to meet the energy requirements of labor and breastfeeding is not lost initially, and the usual rate of loss is quite slow.

Most women approach their prepregnancy weight about 6 months after childbirth, but a year may elapse before almost all weight is lost. This period may be frustrating for mothers who desire an immediate return to prepregnancy weight. Nurses can provide information about diet and exercise that will produce an acceptable weight loss but does not deplete energy or impair the mother's health (see Chapter 15).

POSTPARTUM ASSESSMENTS

Providing essential, cost-effective postpartum care to new families is a challenge for maternity nurses. Legislation allows women with an uncomplicated vaginal birth to stay in the birth facility for 48 hours. Those who gave birth by cesarean section may remain in the facility for 96 hours. Many choose to go home earlier, however.

Although the length of stay is short, the family's need for care and information remains the same. This need causes nurses a great deal of concern for families who are discharged without adequate preparation or support. Nurses are actively involved in developing ways to provide continuing care in the home.

Clinical Pathways

Many institutions use clinical pathways (also called *critical pathways, care paths, care maps,* or *multidisciplinary action plans*) to provide necessary care while reducing the length of stay. Clinical pathways identify expected outcomes and establish time frames for specific assessments and interventions that prepare the mother and infant for discharge. The clinical pathway is a guideline and documentation tool. Figure 21-7 shows an example of a clinical pathway for normal spontaneous vaginal birth.

Initial Assessments

When caring for postpartum patients, the nurse faces a high risk for contact with body fluids (colostrum, breast milk, amniotic fluid, and lochia from the mother as well as urine, stool, and blood from the infant). Therefore the recommendations of the Centers for Disease Control and Prevention (CDC) for standard blood and body fluid precautions must be followed diligently.

YORK HEALTH SYSTEM

YORK, PENNSYLVANIA

CLINICAL PATHWAY

VAGINAL DELIVERY

CLINICAL PATH DAY		EXPECTED PATIENT/ FAMILY OUTCOMES	INTERDISCIPLINARY ASSESSMENT	TESTS	CONSULT
Pre-Natal	DATE	☐ Prenatal test results available [4] ☐ 8 or more prenatal visits complete [4] ☐ Attended baby care and post-partum classes [3] ☐ Risk assessment complete and referral(s) to appropriate agency made as needed.[5] ☐ Low risk pregnancy or monitored high risk pregnancy [4] ☐ _____ ☐ _____	Each visit-maternal weight; BP; urine dipstick-sugar, protein ketones; FHT S/S of pregnancy complication Perinatal risk assessment Social support Knowledge of self and newborn care Knowledge of warning signs of complications Knowledge of signs of labor	Type and Rh Antibody Screen H and H Sickle cell Rubella RPR HBSAG Trutol or 3h GTT GC, Chlamydia Triple Screen Group B Strep	☐ Perinatologist ☐ Diabetic Educator ☐ Behavioral Health ☐ Social Service ☐ _____ ☐ _____ ☐ _____
Admission		☐ Demonstrates knowledge of pain management options [1, 2, 3] ☐ Support person present [2] ☐ Referral made for identified risk factors ☐ Admission procedures completed [4] ☐ _____	Admission assessment Patient needs/desires for pain relief in labor Support system _____	WCBC Type and Rh prn Tube to hold US scan prn _____	☐ Perinatologist ☐ Behavioral Health ☐ Social Service ☐ Neonatology ☐ _____
Labor First Stage		☐☐ Achieves desired level of pain relief [1, 2, 3] ☐☐ Support person present [2] ☐☐ Referral made for identified maternal/fetal risk during labor ☐☐ Mother demonstrates normal physiologic parameters [4] ☐☐ Fetus demonstrates normal physiologic parameters [4] ☐☐ _____	FHR q 30 min UC q 30-60 min P, R, BP q 2h T q 4° (q2 if ROM) Support system Progress of labor Level of comfort _____	_____ _____	☐ Neonatology ☐ _____
Labor Second Stage		☐ Pushing effectively [4] ☐ Support person present {2} ☐ Referral made for identified maternal/fetal risk during labor [4] ☐ Mother demonstrates normal physiological parameters [4] ☐ Fetus demonstrates normal physiological parameters [4] ☐ _____	FHR q 5 min BP q 30 min Vaginal exam prn _____	_____ _____	☐ Neonatology ☐ _____

NAME	INITIALS		NAME	INITIALS

Figure 21-7 Clinical pathway for uncomplicated vaginal birth. (Courtesy Women and Children's Services of the York Health System, York, PA.)

DOCUMENTATION CODES
Initial=Meets Standard
★=Exception on pathway identified
C=Chronic problems
N=Not applicable

PARENT/FAMILY PROBLEMS
1. Pain r/t childbirth
2. Anxiety r/t childbirth and/or parenting
3. Knowledge deficit r/t childbirth and/or parenting
4. Potential alteration maternal/fetal homeostasis

5. Potential for ineffective parenting
6. _____
7. _____

INTERVENTIONS/ACTIVITIES	MEDS	NUTRITION	EDUCATION AND DC PLANNING
_____ _____	Prenatal vitamin, Fe as per order _____ _____	Regular diet _____ _____	Childbirth preparation class Baby care class Breastfeeding class when appropriate Prenatal education
Bed rest with fetal monitor x 30 minutes _____	IV/mini cath _____	NPO with ice chips _____	☐ Orient pt/SO/family to L and D area ☐ Reinforce breathing and relaxation techniques ☐ _____
Insertion of scalp electrode and IUPC as appropriate Warm/cold compress, massage, position change, ambulates and warm showers prn Encourage to void q 1-2° EFM as ordered Vaginal exam prn Catheterize prn _____	IV as ordered Analgesia prn as ordered Epidural as ordered Induction/augmentation of labor as ordered _____ _____	NPO with ice chips _____	☐☐☐ Reinforce breathing and relaxation technique ☐☐☐ Review options for pain management ☐☐☐ Encourage support person involvement ☐☐☐ Provide explanation of labor progress prn
Position for comfort Catheterize prn Warm/cold compress, massage, position change and void prn _____	IV as ordered Continue epidural as ordered Augmentation of labor as ordered _____ _____	NPO with ice chips _____	☐ Assist with pushing ☐ Encourage support person involvement ☐ _____ ☐ _____

NAME	INITIALS	NAME	INITIALS

Figure 21-7, cont'd

Continued

CLINICAL PATH DAY		EXPECTED PATIENT/ FAMILY OUTCOMES	INTERDISCIPLINARY ASSESSMENT	TESTS	CONSULT
Delivery	DATE ___ TIME ___	☐ Deliver live newborn vaginally [4] ☐ Support person present [2] ☐ Mother demonstrates normal physiologic parameters ☐ _____	Fundus, bleeding _____ _____	Cord blood Rh studies when indicated Placenta to pathology as ordered	_____
Early Recovery	DATE ___	☐ Postpartum parameters stable [4] ☐ Achieves desired level of pain relief [1] ☐ _____ ☐ _____	Temp X 1 P, R, BP, fundus, lochia, bladder, episiotomy q 15 min x 4, and q 30 min x 2 Level of comfort	_____ _____	_____
2-24 Hours	DATE ___	☐☐☐ Achieves desired level of pain relief [1] ☐☐☐ Cares for self and infant [3] ☐☐☐ Postpartum parameters stable ☐☐☐ Voiding qs [4] ☐☐☐ Adequate home support system identified [5] ☐☐ _____ ☐☐ _____	T, P, R, BP, Breasts, fundus, lochia, bladder, episiotomy q 4h Readiness to learn Knowledge of self and newborn care Level of comfort Home support system	_____ _____	_____
24-48 Hours	DATE ___	☐☐☐ Achieves desired level of pain relief [1] ☐☐☐ Postpartum parameters stable [4] ☐☐☐ Referral made for potential or identified risk (physical/psychosocial) ☐ Cares for self and infant [3] ☐☐ _____	T, P, R, BP, bid Breasts, fundus, lochia, bladder, episiotomy q shift WA Level of comfort Readiness to learn Knowledge of self and newborn care _____	WCBC _____ _____	_____
Day of Discharge	DATE ___	☐☐☐ Achieves desired level of pain relief [1] ☐☐☐ Postpartum physiological parameters within D/C guidelines [4] ☐ Patient/SO/family verbalization of D/C instructions [3] ☐ Postpartum Home Visit not needed based on Interqual Criteria ☐ Discharge within 2 days after delivery ☐ _____ ☐ _____	T, P, R, BP, bid Breasts, fundus, lochia, bladder, episiotomy bid Level of comfort Readiness to learn Pt/SO/family knowledge of self and newborn care _____ _____	_____ _____	_____ _____

NAME	INITIALS		NAME	INITIALS

NOTE: EACH PATIENT REQUIRES AN INDIVIDUAL ASSESSMENT AND TREATMENT PLAN. THIS CLINICAL PATH IS A RECOMMENDATION FOR THE AVERAGE PATIENT WHICH REQUIRES MODIFICATION WHEN NECESSARY BY THE PROFESSIONAL STAFF.

Figure 21-7, cont'd

INTERVENTIONS/ACTIVITIES	MEDS	NUTRITION	EDUCATION AND DC PLANNING
Catheterize prn Continue IV Continue epidural or local anesthetic _____ _____	Oxytocin after placenta delivered as ordered ☐ _____ ☐ _____	NPO _____ _____	☐ Support parent/infant bonding ☐ _____ ☐ _____
OOB with assist first time Perineal ice pack q 30 min prn Cath prn Shower _____ _____	Analgesia prn Continue epidural if PPTL Continue IV oxytocin as ordered D/C IV or cap IV ☐ _____ ☐ _____	Reg diet as tolerated _____ _____	☐ Support parent/infant bonding ☐ Teach pericare ☐ _____ ☐ _____
OOB with assist first time, then OOB ad lib Catheterize per protocol Epifoam, Tucks prn Ice pack prn Sitz bath 12° after delivery prn _____ _____	Analgesia prn _____ _____	Adv to reg diet as tolerated _____ _____	☐☐☐ Initiate and continue maternal/newborn education record, D/C instructions ☐☐☐ _____ _____ ☐☐☐ _____
OOB ad lib Epifoam, Tucks prn Sitz bath prn _____ _____	Analgesia prn _____ _____	Regular diet _____ _____	☐☐☐ Continue maternal newborn education record ☐☐☐ _____ ☐☐☐ _____

OOB ad lib
Epifoam, Tucks prn
Sitz bath prn
_____
_____
	Analgesia prn
	☐ RhoGAM, when indicated
	☐ Rubella, when indicated
	_____
		Regular diet
		_____
		_____
			☐ Completion of maternal newborn education record
			☐ Physician discharge instructions
			☐ Support services in community:
			  ☐ Breastfeeding Support Services
			  ☐ Perinatal Coaching
			  ☐ City/State Health
			  ☐ Other
			☐ D/C after Pt./family review instructions

DISCHARGE DATE	DISCHARGE TIME	DISCHARGED TO	ACCOMPANIED BY ☐ W/C ☐ AMBULATE

Figure 21-7, cont'd

Drug Guide

Rubella Vaccine

Classification: Attenuated live virus vaccine.

Action: Produces a modified rubella infection that is not communicable, causing the formation of antibodies against rubella virus.

Indications: Administered after childbirth or abortion to women whose antibody screen shows they are not immune to rubella (German measles). This vaccine prevents rubella infection and possible severe congenital defects in the fetus during a subsequent pregnancy.

Dosage and Route: The entire reconstituted volume of a single-dose vial or 0.5 ml from a multiple-dose vial. Inject subcutaneously into the upper outer aspect of the arm.

Absorption: Well absorbed.

Contraindications and Precautions: The vaccine is contraindicated in women who have a respiratory or febrile infection, active untreated tuberculosis, or conditions that affect the bone marrow or lymphatic systems or are immunosuppressed, pregnant, or sensitive to neomycin or eggs. The attenuated virus may appear in breast milk but is not a contraindication to vaccination of lactating women. It should be deferred for 3 months in clients receiving immune serum globulin or blood transfusions.

Adverse Reactions: Lymphadenopathy, rash, urticaria, fever, malaise, sore throat, headache, dizziness, nausea, vomiting, arthralgia, arthritis.

Nursing Implications: In the past, the mother and her partner were warned to avoid pregnancy for at least 3 months after vaccination because of the possibility that a fetus might be affected by the live virus in the vaccine. This time period was shortened to 28 days by the Centers for Disease Control and Prevention (2001).

Vials should be refrigerated. Reconstitute only with diluent supplied with the vial. Use immediately after reconstitution, and discard if not used within 8 hours. Protect from light. Do not give at the same time as immune globulin.

Postpartum assessments begin during the fourth stage of labor (the first 1 to 2 hours after childbirth). During this time the mother is examined to determine whether she is physically stable. Initial assessments include:

- Vital signs
- Skin color
- Location and firmness of the fundus
- Amount and color of lochia
- Perineum (edema, episiotomy, lacerations, hematoma)
- Presence and location of pain
- Intravenous infusions (type of fluid, rate, added medications, patency, site for redness, pain, edema)
- Urinary output (time and amount of last voiding or catheterization or presence of catheter, color and character of urine)
- Abdominal incision, if present
- Level of feeling and ability to move if regional anesthesia was administered

Chart Review

When the initial assessments confirm that the mother's physical condition is stable, nurses should review the chart to obtain pertinent information and to determine whether there are factors that increase the risk of complications during the postpartum period. Relevant information includes:

- Gravida, parity
- Time and type of delivery (use of forceps, vacuum extractor)
- Degree of episiotomy or laceration, if present
- Anesthesia or medications administered during labor
- Significant medical and surgical history, such as diabetes, hypertension, or heart disease
- Medications routinely taken and reasons why they are needed
- Food and drug allergies

- Chosen method of infant feeding
- Condition of the baby

Laboratory data are also examined. Of particular interest are the prenatal hemoglobin and hematocrit values, the blood type and Rh factor, hepatitis B surface antigen, rubella immune status, syphilis screen, and group B streptococcus status (see Chapter 28).

Need for Rh$_o$ (D) Immune Globulin

Prenatal and neonatal records are checked to determine whether Rh$_o$ (D) immune globulin should be administered. Rh$_o$ (D) immune globulin may be necessary if the mother is Rh-negative and the newborn is Rh-positive. To prevent the development of maternal antibodies that would affect subsequent pregnancies, Rh$_o$ (D) immune globulin should be administered within 72 hours after childbirth (see Chapter 26).

Need For Rubella Vaccine

A prenatal rubella antibody screen is performed on each pregnant woman to determine if she is immune to rubella. If she is not immune, rubella vaccine is offered after childbirth to prevent her from acquiring rubella during subsequent pregnancies, when it can cause serious fetal anomalies. Rubella vaccine is a live virus that can produce serious consequences for the fetus if the mother becomes pregnant soon after it is administered. Before administration, some agencies require that she sign a statement indicating that she understands the risks of becoming pregnant again too soon after the injection (see Drug Guide). If this statement is not required, the nurse should record in the chart that the risk has been explained and the parents have verbalized their understanding.

Risk Factors for Hemorrhage and Infection

Nurses must be aware of conditions that increase the risk of hemorrhage and infection, the two most common complications of the puerperium.

Focused Assessments After Vaginal Birth

Nurses perform postpartum assessments according to facility protocol. For example, a protocol might require assessment every 15 minutes for the first hour, every half hour for the next hour, every 4 hours for the first 24 hours, and every 8 hours thereafter. Of course, assessments are performed more frequently if findings are abnormal.

Although assessments vary according to particular problems presented, a focused assessment for a vaginal delivery generally includes the vital signs, fundus, lochia, perineum, bladder elimination, breasts, and lower extremities. The assessment for postcesarean mothers is more complete (see p. 483).

Vital Signs

Blood Pressure. Blood pressure varies with position. To obtain accurate results, it should be measured with the mother in the same position each time. Therefore nurses must record both the mother's position when taking blood pressure and the pressure obtained. Postpartum blood pressure should be compared with that of the predelivery period so that deviations from the parameters that are normal for the mother can be quickly identified. An increase from the baseline suggests preeclampsia. A decrease may indicate dehydration or hypovolemia resulting from excessive bleeding.

Orthostatic Hypotension. After birth, a rapid decrease in intraabdominal pressure results in dilation of blood vessels supplying the viscera. The resulting engorgement of abdominal blood vessels contributes to a rapid fall in blood pressure of 15 to 20 mm Hg when the woman moves from a recumbent to a sitting position. This change causes mothers to feel dizzy or lightheaded or to faint when they stand. The nursing diagnosis *Risk for Injury* applies to women with orthostatic hypotension. (For application of this nursing diagnosis, see Nursing Care Plan: Postpartum Hypotension, Fatigue, and Pain.)

Hypotension may also indicate hypovolemia. Careful assessments for hemorrhage (location and firmness of the fundus, amount of lochia, pulse rate for tachycardia) should be made if the postpartum blood pressure is significantly less than the prenatal baseline blood pressure.

Pulse. The average pulse rate is 60 to 90 beats per minute (bpm), although a pulse of 50 to 60 may occur. The lower pulse rate reflects the large amount of blood that returns to the central circulation after delivery of the placenta. The increase in central circulation results in increased stroke volume and allows a slower heart rate to provide adequate maternal circulation.

Tachycardia may indicate excitement, fatigue, pain, dehydration, hypovolemia, anemia, or infection. If tachycardia is noted, additional assessments should include blood pressure, location and firmness of the uterus, amount of lochia, estimated blood loss at delivery, and hemoglobin and hematocrit values. The objective of the additional assessments is to rule out excessive bleeding and to intervene at once if hemorrhage is suspected.

Respirations. A normal respiratory rate of 12 to 20 breaths per minute should be maintained. It is not necessary to assess breath sounds if the mother has had a normal vaginal delivery, is ambulatory, and is without signs of respiratory distress. Breath sounds should always be auscultated for mothers who have a cesarean birth, are smokers, have a history of frequent or recent upper respiratory infections, those receiving mag-

nesium sulfate (see Chapter 26), and women with a history of asthma.

Temperature. A temperature of up to 38° C (100.4° F) is common during the first 24 hours after childbirth and may be caused by dehydration or normal postpartum leukocytosis. If the elevated temperature persists for longer than 24 hours or if it exceeds 38° C, infection should be suspected and the fever reported to the physician or nurse-midwife.

Pain. Pain, the fifth vital sign, should be assessed to determine the type, location, and severity on a pain scale. Nurses must remain alert to signs of afterpains, perineal discomfort, and breast tenderness. Nonspecific signs of discomfort include an inability to relax or sleep, a change in vital signs, restlessness, irritability, and facial grimaces. The effectiveness of pain-relief measures should also be assessed.

Fundus

The fundus should be assessed for consistency and location. It should be firmly contracted and at or near the level of the umbilicus. If the uterus is above the expected level or is shifted from the midline position (usually to the right), the bladder may be distended. The location of the fundus should be rechecked after the woman has emptied her bladder. Procedure 21-1 illustrates how to locate and palpate the fundus. If the fundus is difficult to locate or is soft or "boggy," the nurse stimulates the uterine muscle to contract by gently massaging the uterus.

The nondominant hand must support and anchor the lower uterine segment if it is necessary to massage an uncontracted uterus. Uterine massage is not necessary if the uterus is firmly contracted.

The uterus can contract only if it is free of intrauterine clots. To expel clots, the nurse must support the lower uterine segment, as illustrated in Procedure 21-1. This support pre-

Nursing Care Plan

Postpartum Hypotension, Fatigue, and Pain

ASSESSMENT

Four hours after giving birth, Jacqueline Tilden became weak and dizzy when she attempted to ambulate the first time. Her gait was unsteady, and the nurse had to lower her back to bed to prevent her fainting. Her color was pale, and her pulse was rapid. Jacqueline's hemoglobin at the end of pregnancy was 10.8 g/dl.

Nursing Diagnosis

Risk for Injury related to physiologic effects of orthostatic hypotension.

Goal/Expected Outcome

Jacqueline will:
- Remain free of injury caused by fainting and falling during the postpartum period.

INTERVENTION	RATIONALE
1. Obtain the assistance of a second staff person the next time ambulation is attempted and at other times if Jacqueline becomes faint with subsequent ambulation attempts.	1. A second person is necessary to help prevent injury to the client and the staff members if Jacqueline should start to fall.
2. Check the mother's blood pressure while she is in a supine position and in a sitting position before attempting to get her out of bed again. Use the same arm each time the blood pressure is taken.	2. A decrease of 20 mm Hg in systolic pressure in the upright position indicates orthostatic hypotension. Measuring from the same arm provides more accurate information because the reading may differ slightly in each arm.
3. Assist the mother to elevate the head of the bed for a few minutes and then to sit on the side of the bed for several minutes before standing. Help her to stand slowly.	3. Sitting and dangling the legs allows time for blood pressure to stabilize before she is fully upright, thus maintaining circulation to the brain.
4. Instruct the mother to move her feet constantly when she first stands.	4. Moving the feet increases venous return from the lower extremities, which maintains cardiac output and increases cerebral circulation.
5. Suggest that Jacqueline take brief, tepid (not hot) showers and that she bend her knees and "march" during the shower.	5. Hot water dilates peripheral blood vessels, allowing additional blood to remain in the vessels of the legs. Moving the feet and legs increases blood return from the legs and increases blood to the brain.
6. Initiate measures to prevent injuries that could be sustained if Jacqueline were to faint: a. Stay with her when she ambulates, and be prepared to assist her in sitting down or to lower her gently to the floor if she becomes faint. b. Call for additional assistance, if needed, before attempting to return her to bed. c. Remind her to call for assistance before trying to ambulate. Check to see that the call light is conveniently located.	6. Gravity increases blood flow to the brain when the head is lowered and thus prevents fainting. Adequate assistance prevents falling and possible injury during a fainting episode.

Evaluation

Jacqueline has participated in self-care and has sustained no injury during her hospital stay.

ASSESSMENT

On the 2nd day after delivery, Jacqueline expresses concern about her third-degree episiotomy and asks what she can do to prevent the pain she experienced during intercourse for several months after the birth of her first child, who is now 18 months old.

Nursing Diagnosis

Risk For Ineffective Sexuality Pattern related to fatigue and pain.

Goals/Expected Outcomes

The couple will:
- Verbalize measures to promote comfort during sexual activity by discharge.
- Verbalize a plan to reduce fatigue, which interferes with interest in and energy for sexual activity by discharge.

Nursing Care Plan

Postpartum Hypotension, Fatigue, and Pain—cont'd

INTERVENTION	RATIONALE
1. Recommend that the parents postpone vaginal intercourse until the perineum is well healed, usually about 3 weeks. Suggest that the mother continue perineal care, sitz baths, and the use of topical agents until the perineum is healed.	1. These measures promote rapid healing and reduce pain or fear of pain when sexual activity is resumed.
2. Suggest that the infant be breastfed just before the parents initiate sexual activity.	2. Breastfeeding reduces the chance of leaking milk, which interferes with sexual pleasure for some couples. Feeding the infant may also allow uninterrupted time while the infant sleeps.
3. Suggest the use of a water-soluble vaginal lubricant (Lubrin, Replens, KY Jelly) if the mother is planning to breastfeed for longer than 6 weeks.	3. Breastfeeding delays the return of ovarian hormones to nonpregnant levels, including estrogen, which may result in vaginal dryness that is most noticeable after 6 weeks of breastfeeding.
4. Before vaginal intercourse, as part of foreplay, suggest that one finger be inserted into the vaginal introitus to determine areas of tenderness or pain.	4. A finger locates areas of discomfort and stretches the perineal scar gently.
5. Remind parents that sexual arousal may be slower because of decreased hormone levels and fatigue. More stimulation may be necessary before the mother is sexually aroused.	5. Knowledge of postpartum physiologic changes reduces the anxiety and tension that occur if the parents are unprepared for them.
6. Suggest that the woman assume the superior position during intercourse.	6. In this position the woman controls the depth and location of penetration, which can help reduce her discomfort.
7. Remind the mother to perform Kegel exercises until she can comfortably do 30 each day.	7. Kegel exercises strengthen the muscles around the vagina and promote increased sexual satisfaction.
8. Suggest measures that may lessen fatigue: a. Recommend that each partner nap for 30 minutes sometime during the day or evening. b. Suggest that sexual activity occur in the morning or afternoon rather than at the end of a tiring day. c. Suggest that parents rest when the infant has long periods of sleep and that they postpone additional home projects that will increase fatigue until the infant is older and is sleeping through the night.	8. Fatigue is a major cause of decreased interest in sexual activity after childbirth for both mothers and fathers.
9. Discuss the need for frank communication between partners about measures that reduce discomfort, as well as specific concerns and needs.	9. Communication facilitates understanding and fosters a feeling of closeness that can enhance sexual interest.

Evaluation

The couple expresses interest in trying various measures to reduce fatigue and discomfort. They verbalize a plan to use the instructions provided.

Additional Nursing Diagnoses to Consider

Interrupted Family Processes
Ineffective Health Maintenance
Impaired Parenting
Health-Seeking Behaviors
Sleep Deprivation

Procedure 21-1

Assessing the Uterine Fundus

PURPOSE: To determine the location and firmness of the uterus.

1. To reduce anxiety and elicit cooperation, explain the procedure and rationale before beginning the procedure.
2. Ask the mother to empty her bladder if she has not voided recently, because a distended bladder lifts and displaces the uterus.
3. Place the mother in a supine position with her knees slightly flexed to relax the abdominal muscles and to permit accurate location of the fundus.
4. Put on clean gloves, because there may be contact with body fluids. Lower the perineal pads to observe lochia as the fundus is palpated.
5. Place your nondominant hand above the woman's symphysis pubis to support and anchor the lower uterine segment during palpation or massage of the fundus.
6. Use the flat part of your fingers (not the fingertips) for palpation (see illustration), because the larger surface provides more comfort.
7. Begin palpation at the umbilicus, and palpate gently until the fundus is located. Notice how the hand "cups" the uterus to determine firmness and location of the fundus. The fundus should be firm, in the midline, and approximately at the level of the umbilicus.
8. If the fundus is difficult to locate or is "boggy" (soft), keep your nondominant hand above the woman's symphysis pubis and massage the fundus with your dominant hand until the fundus is firm. The nondominant hand anchors the lower segment of the uterus and prevents trauma while the uterus is massaged. The uterus contracts in response to tactile stimulation.
9. After massaging a boggy fundus until it is firm, press firmly to expel clots. Keep one hand pressed firmly just above the symphysis (over the lower uterine segment) during the entire time. Removing clots allows the uterus to contract properly. Providing pressure over the lower uterine segment prevents uterine inversion.

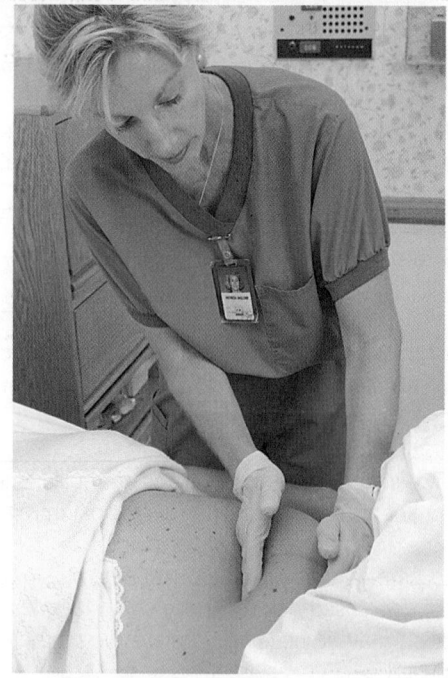

10. If the fundus is above or below the umbilicus, use your fingers to determine the number of fingerbreadths between the fundus and the umbilicus. Using the fingers to measure allows an approximation of the number of centimeters.
11. Document the consistency and location of the fundus to promote accurate communication and identify deviations from expected findings. Record consistency as "fundus firm," "firm with massage," or "boggy." Record fundal height in fingerbreadths above or below the umbilicus. For example, "fundus firm, midline, U – 2" (two fingerbreadths below umbilicus) or "fundus firm with light massage, U + 2, displaced to right."

---

vents inversion of the uterus (turning inside out) when the nurse applies firm pressure downward toward the vagina to express clots that have collected in the uterus. Nurses should observe the perineum for the number and size of clots expelled. Table 21-2 describes normal and abnormal findings of the uterine fundus and includes follow-up nursing actions for abnormal findings.

Drugs are sometimes needed to maintain contraction of the uterus and thus to prevent postpartum hemorrhage. The most commonly used drug is oxytocin (Pitocin). A drug Guide for oxytocin is presented on p. 447.

Lochia

Important assessments include the amount, color, and odor of lochia. Nurses observe the amount and color of lochia on perineal pads and while checking the perineum (see Table 21-1 and Figure 21-2). They also watch vaginal discharge while palpating or massaging the fundus so that the amount of lochia as well as the number and size of any clots expressed during these procedures can be observed. The nurse should note these important guidelines:

- A constant trickle of lochia indicates excessive bleeding and requires immediate attention.
- Excessive lochia in the presence of a contracted uterus suggests lacerations of the birth canal, and the health care provider must be notified so that the laceration can be located and repaired.

The odor of lochia is usually described as "fleshy," "earthy," or "musty." A foul odor suggests endometrial infection, and assessments should be made for additional signs of infection.

TABLE **21–2** Observations of the Uterine Fundus Requiring Nursing Actions

Normal Findings	Abnormal Findings	Nursing Actions
Fundus is firmly contracted.	Fundus is soft, "boggy," uncontracted, or difficult to locate.	Support lower uterine segment, and massage until firm.
Fundus remains contracted when massage is discontinued.	Fundus becomes soft and uncontracted when massage is stopped.	Continue to support lower uterine segment; massage until firm and apply pressure to fundus to express clots that may be accumulating in uterus. Notify health care provider and begin oxytocin administration, as prescribed, to maintain a firm fundus.
Fundus is located at level of umbilicus and midline.	Fundus is above umbilicus and/or displaced from midline.	Assess bladder elimination. Assist mother in urinating or catheterize, if necessary, to empty bladder.

Procedure 21-2

Assessing the Perineum

PURPOSE: To observe perineal trauma and the state of healing.

1. Provide privacy, and explain the purpose of the procedure to elicit cooperation and reduce anxiety.
2. Put on clean gloves to implement Standard Precautions.
3. Ask the mother to assume a Sims position and flex her upper leg. Lower the perineal pads and lift her superior buttocks to provide an unobstructed view of the perineum. If necessary, use a flashlight for better visibility during inspection of the perineal area.
4. Note the extent and location of edema or bruising. Extensive bruising or asymmetric edema may indicate formation of a hematoma.
5. Examine the episiotomy or laceration for redness, ecchymosis, edema, discharge, and approximation (REEDA), which may indicate infection or problems with healing.
6. Note the number and size of hemorrhoids. Swollen hemorrhoids interfere with activity and bowel elimination.

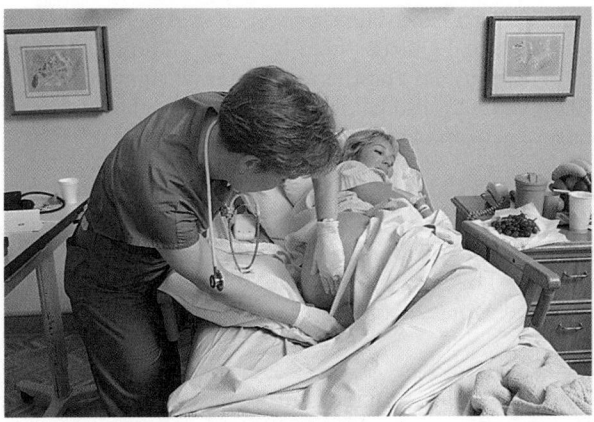

These signs include maternal fever, tachycardia, and uterine tenderness and pain.

Absence of lochia, like the presence of a foul odor, may also indicate infection. If the birth was cesarean, lochia may be scant because the cavity of the uterus was wiped by

! CRITICAL TO REMEMBER

Signs of a Distended Bladder

- Location of fundus above baseline level, which is determined when the bladder is empty
- Fundus displaced from midline
- Excessive lochia
- Bladder discomfort
- Bulge of bladder above symphysis
- Frequent voidings of less than 150 ml of urine, which indicates urinary retention with overflow

sponges, removing some of the endometrial lining. Lochia should not, however, be entirely absent.

Perineum

The acronym REEDA is used as a reminder that the site of an episiotomy or a perineal laceration should be assessed for five signs: redness (R), edema (E), ecchymosis (bruising) (E), discharge (D), and approximation (A) (the edges of the wound should be close, as though stuck or glued together).

Redness of the wound may indicate the usual inflammatory response to injury. If accompanied by excessive pain or tenderness, however, it may indicate the beginning of localized infection. Ecchymosis or edema indicates soft tissue damage that can delay healing. There should be no discharge from the wound. Rapid healing necessitates that the edges of the wound be closely approximated. Procedure 21-2 describes the perineal examination.

Bladder Elimination

Because the mother may not experience the urge to void even if the bladder is full, nurses must rely on physical assessment to determine whether the bladder is distended. Bladder distention often produces an obvious or palpable bulge that feels like a soft, movable mass above the symphysis pubis. Other signs include an upward and lateral displacement of the uterine fundus and increased lochia. Frequent voidings of less than 150 ml suggest urinary retention with overflow. Signs of an empty bladder include a firm fundus in the midline and a nonpalpable bladder.

Some facilities measure the first two voidings to determine whether normal bladder function has returned. When the mother can void at least 300 to 400 ml, the bladder is usually empty. Regardless of the amount voided, however, the fundus must be assessed after the woman voids to confirm that the bladder is empty. Subjective symptoms of urgency, frequency, or dysuria suggest urinary tract infection and should be reported to the health care provider.

Breasts

For the first day or two after delivery, the breasts should be soft and nontender. After that, breast changes depend largely on whether the mother is breastfeeding or is taking measures to prevent lactation. The breasts should be examined even if she chooses formula feeding, because engorgement may occur despite preventive measures. The size, symmetry, and shape of the breasts should be observed. The skin should be inspected for dimpling or thickening, which, although rare, can indicate a breast tumor.

The areola and nipple should be carefully examined for potential problems such as flat or retracted nipples; these problems sometimes make breastfeeding more difficult. Signs of nipple trauma (redness, blisters, fissures) are often noted during the first days of breastfeeding, especially if the mother needs assistance in positioning the infant correctly (see Chapter 24).

The breasts should be palpated for firmness and tenderness, which indicate increased vascular and lymphatic circulation that may precede milk production. The breasts may feel "lumpy" as various lobes begin to produce milk.

The breast assessment is an excellent opportunity to provide information or reassurance about breast care and breastfeeding techniques.

Lower Extremities

The legs are examined for signs or symptoms of thrombophlebitis. These indications include localized areas of redness, heat, edema, and tenderness. Pedal pulses may be obstructed by thrombophlebitis and should be palpated with each assessment.

Homans Sign

Discomfort in the calf with sharp dorsiflexion of the foot may indicate deep vein thrombosis. A negative Homans sign is indicated by absence of discomfort. A positive Homans sign is indicated by the presence of discomfort and should be reported to the health care provider, along with redness, tenderness, or warmth of the leg. Assessment of Homans sign can be confusing because a deep venous thrombosis may not produce pain with dorsiflexion. In addition, the woman may report pain that is caused by strained muscles from positioning and pushing during delivery.

Edema and Deep Tendon Reflexes

Pedal or pretibial edema may be present for the first few days, until excess interstitial fluid is remobilized and excreted. Diuresis is highest between the 2nd and 5th days after birth and should be complete by 21 days (Blackburn, 2003).

Deep tendon reflexes should be 1+ to 2+. Report brisker-than-average and hyperactive reflexes (3+ to 4+), which suggest preeclampsia. (See Procedure 26-1 For an explanation of assessing deep tendon reflexes.)

CARE IN THE IMMEDIATE POSTPARTUM PERIOD

The postpartum period is often divided into three periods. The first 24 hours is called the *immediate postpartum period*; the 1st week is referred to as the *early postpartum period*; and the 2nd week to the 6th week is the *late postpartum period*. Care of the mother during the immediate postpartum period focuses on:

- Maintaining the mother's physiologic safety through frequent assessments
- Providing comfort measures
- Establishing bladder elimination
- Providing health education

Providing Comfort Measures

Ice Packs

Both cold and warmth are used to alleviate perineal pain after childbirth. Ice causes vasoconstriction and is most effective if applied soon after the birth to prevent edema and to numb the area. Some perineal pads have cold packs incorporated into them. Chemical ice packs, non-latex gloves filled with ice and tied at the cuff, or reclosable plastic bags are also used during the first 12 to 24 hours after a vaginal birth. The ice pack is wrapped in a washcloth or paper before it is applied to the perineum. It should be left in place until the ice melts or about 20 minutes. It is then removed for 10 minutes before a fresh pack is applied. Condensation from ice may dilute lochia and make it appear to be heavier than it actually is.

20 min on   20 min off

Perineal Care

Perineal care consists of squirting warm water over the perineum after each voiding or bowel movement. Perineal care cleanses, provides comfort, and prevents infection. The perineum is gently patted rather than wiped dry.

Topical Medications

Anesthetic sprays decrease surface discomfort and allow more comfortable ambulation. The mother is instructed to hold the nozzle of a benzocaine spray, such as Americaine or Dermoplast, 6 to 12 inches from her body and direct it toward the perineum. An anesthetic and steroid combination such as Epifoam may also be used. The spray should be used after perineal care and before clean pads are applied.

Sitting

The mother should be advised to squeeze her buttocks together before sitting and to lower her weight slowly onto her buttocks. This measure prevents stretching of the perineal tissue and avoids sharp impact on the traumatized area.

Sitz Baths

Sitz baths, which provide continuous circulation of water, cleanse and comfort the traumatized perineum. Cool water reduces pain caused by edema and may be most effective within the first 24 hours. Warm water increases circulation and promotes healing and may be most effective after 24 hours. Nurses must be sure that the emergency bell is within easy reach in case the mother feels faint during the sitz bath.

Analgesics

Mothers should be encouraged to take prescribed medications for afterpains and perineal discomfort. Analgesics, such as acetaminophen (Tylenol, Panadol), and nonsteroidal antiinflammatory drugs (NSAIDs), such as ibuprofen (Motrin, Advil) or rofecoxib (Vioxx), are frequently prescribed for relief of mild to moderate discomfort. Percocet, Lortab, Vicodin, or Tylenol No. 3 is often prescribed for more severe discomfort. NSAIDs such as ketorolac (Toradol) may be given intravenously for several doses to help relieve cesarean incisional pain. Because a side effect of ketorolac is prolonged bleeding, the nurse should monitor lochia carefully.

In some agencies, women receive a self-administered medication kit for use during their postpartum stay. The kit may include routine stool softeners, gas-relieving drugs, and non-narcotic or a limited supply of certain narcotic pain medications. Women are instructed on how to take their medications and given a log to record each dose. This allows them to receive pain medication quickly because they do not have to wait for a nurse to bring it to them (Werrbach & Wroblewski, 2003).

Promoting Bladder Elimination

Many new mothers have difficulty voiding because of edema and trauma of the perineum as well as diminished sensitivity to fluid pressure in the bladder. As soon as they are able to ambulate safely, mothers should be assisted to the bathroom. It is important to provide privacy and to allow adequate time for the first voiding. Some common measures to promote relaxation of the perineal muscles and to stimulate the sensation of needing to void include:

- Medicating the woman for perineal pain
- Running water, placing the mother's hands in water, and pouring water over the vulva
- Encouraging urination in the shower or sitz bath
- Providing hot tea or fluids of choice
- Asking the mother to blow bubbles through a straw

A distended bladder lifts and displaces the uterus, making it difficult for the uterus to remain contracted. Thus urinary retention is a major cause of uterine atony (loss of tone), which permits excessive bleeding. Moreover, stasis of urine in the bladder predisposes the woman to urinary tract infection. Therefore the mother must be catheterized if:

- She is unable to void.
- The amount voided is less than 150 ml.
- The fundus is elevated or displaced from the midline.

Repeated catheterizations increase the chance of urinary tract infection because bacteria may be pushed into the bladder despite scrupulous aseptic technique. To decrease the risk of infection, an indwelling catheter is usually inserted for 24 hours if catheterization is necessary more than once or twice.

Providing Fluids and Food

Adequate fluids help restore the balance altered by fluid loss during labor and the birth process. Women should be encouraged to drink approximately 2500 ml of fluids each day. Offering ice water or cold drinks may be culturally inappropriate for some mothers. They may prefer hot or room-temperature water instead.

New mothers generally have a hearty appetite, and nurses should encourage healthy food choices, with respect for ethnic background. Meals and snacks should be available at all times.

Preventing Thrombophlebitis

The mother should be assisted to ambulate early after childbirth to prevent the development of thrombi. Frequent trips to the bathroom will help accomplish this.

NURSING CARE AFTER CESAREAN BIRTH

The usual length of stay for mothers after a cesarean birth is 72 to 96 hours after surgery. Many facilities have developed clinical pathways or care maps that are similar to those used for uncomplicated vaginal births. The clinical pathway identifies outcomes and establishes a time frame for assessments and interventions for postcesarean mothers and their infants. Clinical pathways, however, are guidelines only. If a problem arises, sometimes called a *variance*, additional assessments and interventions are necessary.

Assessment

In addition to the usual postpartum assessments, the postcesarean mother must be assessed as any other postoperative patient.

Pain Relief

Assessment of pain level and the effectiveness of pain medication is important for postcesarean clients. Pain relief may be provided in various ways. Patient-controlled analgesia (PCA) is administered by continuous intravenous infusion of a low-concentration narcotic solution using a pump specifically designed for that purpose. If the analgesia is insufficient, the woman can self-administer intermittent small doses of narcotic from the infusion pump. The machine limits the total amount of narcotic available.

A single dose of narcotic (often morphine) may be injected into the epidural or subarachnoid space immediately after the surgery to provide 18 to 24 hours of postcesarean

---

CRITICAL THINKING EXERCISE 21-1

Linda Welker, a 22-year-old multipara, was admitted from the labor, delivery, and recovery unit 2 hours after the birth of an 8-lb (3600-g) baby boy. An hour later her fundus is firm, located three fingerbreadths above the umbilicus, and displaced to the right. Her perineal pads, which were changed just before transfer, are saturated.

1. What do these data suggest? Why?
2. What nursing action should be taken first? What follow-up assessments are necessary?
3. Why is it necessary to remind Linda to void?

analgesia. If the woman has pain, oral analgesics usually suffice. Itching is a major side effect, with an incidence as high as 84% (Zuspan, 2000). Side effects of both patient-controlled analgesia and epidural narcotics include respiratory depression, itching (pruritus), nausea and vomiting, and urine retention.

Pain relief can also be provided by local anesthetic delivered into the incision site through a catheter attached to a pump. This allows the woman to move about more freely than with a PCA and avoids the side effects of narcotics. Occasionally, intramuscular analgesics are given for one or two doses.

Respirations

When mothers receive epidural narcotics for postoperative pain relief, respirations must be assessed frequently because narcotics depress the respiratory center. In some facilities, a pulse oximeter or an apnea monitor is used for 18 to 24 hours to detect a decreased respiratory rate. If these devices are not used, the respiratory rate and depth should be checked according to hospital policy, such as every 15 minutes for the first hour, every 30 minutes for 3 to 6 hours, and every 30 minutes to 1 hour for the remainder of the first 24 hours.

If the respiratory rate begins to decline or if the respiratory rate is less than 12 breaths per minute, the nurse should:

- Notify the anesthesiologist immediately.
- Elevate the head of the bed to facilitate lung expansion.
- Administer oxygen, and apply a pulse oximeter to measure oxygen saturation.
- Follow facility protocol to administer narcotic antagonists, such as naloxone hydrochloride (Narcan).
- Observe for recurrence of respiratory depression, because the effect of naloxone lasts only approximately 30 minutes.
- Recognize that naloxone reduces the level of pain relief.

In addition to observing respiratory rate and depth, the mother's breath sounds should be auscultated, because depressed respirations as well as a longer period of immobility allow secretions to pool in the bronchioles.

Abdomen

Nurses assess gastrointestinal function by auscultating for bowel sounds until normal peristalsis is noted in all abdominal quadrants. Although paralytic ileus (lack of movement in the bowel) is rare after cesarean birth, nurses must be aware of the signs, which include abdominal distention, absent or decreased bowel sounds, and no passage of flatus or stool.

The surgical dressing should be observed for intactness and discharge. When the dressing is removed, nurses observe the incision, which should be approximated, and use the acronym REEDA to assess for signs of infection, such as redness and edema.

The fundus must be palpated gently because of increased discomfort caused by the uterine incision.

Intake and Output

The intravenous infusion should be monitored for the rate of flow and the condition of the intravenous site. Any signs of infiltration, such as edema or coolness at the site, as well as signs of infection, such as edema, redness, and pain, should be reported. Ice chips and fluids are usually allowed soon after cesarean birth. The amount as well as the color and clarity of urine should be monitored.

Interventions

The First 24 Hours

Nursing care for the mother who gave birth by cesarean section is similar to that for other postoperative clients.

Providing Pain Relief. The nurse should offer pain relief on a regular basis. If the woman has a PCA, the nurse should check how often she is using it. The effectiveness of any type of medication must be observed. Pain relief aids ambulation, helps prevent thrombophlebitis, and promotes healing.

Overcoming the Effects of Immobility. The new mother is on bed rest for the first 8 to 12 hours. To counteract this risk, the mother must be assisted to turn, cough, and expand the lungs by breathing deeply. Splinting the abdomen with a small pillow reduces incisional discomfort when she coughs. An incentive spirometer may also be used to help expand the lungs.

Antiembolism stockings or sequential compression devices may be used to prevent the pooling of blood in the lower extremities while the woman is on bed rest. She should be encouraged to flex her legs and to move her feet and legs frequently to improve peripheral circulation and prevent thrombi.

Activity will be gradually increased. The woman needs assistance to sit and dangle her feet for the first few times before she gets out of bed. She will need help ambulating with the IV and catheter still in place at first.

Providing Comfort. Placing a pillow behind her back and one between her knees when the mother is in a side-lying position prevents strain and discomfort. Excellent physical care (oral hygiene, perineal care, a sponge bath, clean linen) comforts and refreshes her.

After 24 Hours

Resuming Normal Activities. After 24 hours, several normal functions return as postcesarean women are able to participate more actively in their own care:

- The indwelling catheter and intravenous infusion are usually discontinued.
- The dressing is usually removed, and often staples or clamps are removed on the 2nd or 3rd day. Steri-Strips (small strips of adhesive), a small, nonadherent dressing, or a peripad may be placed over the incision.
- Mothers are usually helped to ambulate by the 1st postpartum day and are comfortable sitting in a chair for brief periods.
- Clear liquids are changed to a soft or regular diet once bowel sounds are audible. In some agencies solids are given earlier.

Nurses must encourage the mother to increase her activity and ambulation each postpartum day. By the 2nd day, she is usually allowed to shower.

Assisting the Mother With Infant Feeding. It is important to help the mother find a comfortable position for holding and feeding her infant. A side-lying position or football hold may be most comfortable because these positions avoid pressure on the incision. Some mothers prefer sitting with a pillow on the lap to protect the incisional area (see Chapter 24).

Preventing Abdominal Distention. Abdominal distention is a major source of discomfort, and measures should be taken to prevent or minimize it. Early, frequent ambulation is perhaps the best method. Additional measures include:

- Pelvic lifts. Lying supine with her knees bent, the woman lifts her pelvis from the bed. These exercises may be repeated up to 10 times, several times each day.
- Tightening and relaxing the abdominal muscles.
- Avoiding carbonated beverages and the use of straws, which increase the accumulation of intestinal gas.
- Simethicone to help disperse upper gastrointestinal flatulence.
- Rectal suppositories to stimulate peristalsis and the passage of flatus.

■NURSING CARE
Teaching After Birth

Assessment

Nurses are responsible for providing health education before the family is discharged from the birth facility. This is difficult because so much must be taught during a short time and women have not fully recovered from the birth process. Some women feel they have difficulty concentrating during the first week of postpartum although studies show they function better than they did during the last trimester of pregnancy (Stark, 2000).

Before beginning teaching, determine the learning needs and the major concerns of the family. For example, multiparas may remember some aspects of self-care but would benefit from a review. On the other hand, primiparas may be anxious about self-care measures and all aspects of infant care. They may need more thorough teaching and more practice. Identify the most common barriers to learning: age and developmental level, cultural factors, and difficulty understanding the language.

Nursing Diagnosis and Planning

In general, mothers adapt to the physiologic changes after childbirth, and most nursing care is wellness-oriented. Some new mothers, however, lack knowledge of self-care and need education to prevent later problems. A nursing diagnosis that applies to these women is

- Health-Seeking Behaviors: knowledge of self-care, signs of complications, and preventive measures.

  Expected Outcomes: The mother will verbalize or demonstrate understanding of self-care instructions by discharge and verbalize understanding of practices that promote maternal health by a specified date. By the day of discharge, the mother will describe plans for follow-up care and the signs and symptoms that should be reported to the health care provider.

Additional diagnoses include Risk for Injury and Ineffective Sexuality Pattern. These are discussed in Nursing Care Plan: Postpartum Hypotension, Fatigue, and Pain, p. 478.

Interventions

Teaching the Process of Involution

Provide the mother with basic information about involution, including how to assess lochia and how to locate and palpate the fundus. This information allows her to recognize abnormal signs, such as prolonged lochia or uterine tenderness, which should be reported to the health care provider. If the mother is a young teenager, another family member may also need to be given the information.

Teaching Self-Care

Handwashing Emphasize the importance of thorough handwashing before touching the breasts, after diaper changes, after bladder and bowel elimination, and always before handling the infant.

Breast Care for Lactating Mothers Instruct the breast-feeding mother to avoid using soap on her nipples because it will remove the natural lubrication secreted by Montgomery's glands. Keeping the nipples dry between feedings helps prevent tissue damage, and wearing a good bra provides necessary support as breast size increases.

Measures to Suppress Lactation If the mother chooses not to breastfeed, initiate measures to suppress lactation. The safest method is to prevent breast distention either by having the mother wear a well-fitting support bra or by binding the breasts with an elastic bandage 24 hours a day until the breasts become soft. A support bra may be more comfortable and leaking may be less with a support bra (Swift & Janke, 2003).

Discomfort can usually be managed by applying ice, which reduces vasocongestion, and with analgesics. Advise the woman to refrain from stimulating milk production (i.e., she should not allow warm water to fall directly on the breasts during showers and should not pump or massage the breasts).

Care of the Cesarean Incision If the birth was by cesarean, the woman may have concerns about care of the incision. If strips of adhesive have been applied over the incision, teach the woman that she can shower with these in place and that they will gradually detach. Explain that the incision is closed and is unlikely to come apart. There should be little or no drainage from the incision. Instruct her to call her provider if the incision separates or drainage increases or has a foul smell.

Perineal Care Nurses are responsible for teaching perineal cleansing as soon as possible after childbirth. The most common method is to fill a squeeze bottle with warm water and spray the perineal area from the front toward the back. Remind the new mother not to separate the labia during this procedure so that water does not enter the vagina. If a commercial product that includes a nozzle attached to the faucet is used, teach the mother that the nozzle should not touch the perineum during use.

Moist antiseptic towelettes or toilet paper is used in a patting motion to dry the perineum. Teach the mother to dry from front to back to prevent fecal contamination from the anal area to the vaginal introitus. She should perform perineal cleansing and change peripads after each voiding or defecation.

Many women do not use peripads for menstrual protection and must be taught how to use them correctly. Mesh panties and adhering pads are used in most facilities. Careful handling of the pads is important to prevent localized perineal infection:

- Thorough handwashing is a must before and after changing the pads.
- Unused pads should be stored inside their package.
- Pads should be applied without touching the side that comes into contact with the perineum.
- The pads should be applied and removed in a front-to-back direction to prevent contamination of the vagina and perineum.
- Used pads must be disposed of properly.

Kegel Exercises All mothers should become familiar with Kegel exercises. These movements strengthen the pubococcygeal muscle, which surrounds the vagina and urinary meatus. This exercise helps prevent the loss of muscle tone that can occur after childbirth.

The Kegel exercise involves contracting muscles around the vagina (as though stopping the flow of urine), holding tightly for 10 seconds, and then relaxing for 10 seconds. The woman should work up to 30 contraction-relaxation cycles each day.

Promoting Rest and Sleep

Postpartum fatigue is common during the early days after birth and often continues for weeks or months (Troy, 2003). The extreme fatigue that mothers experience in the puerperium has several causes. Women are tired when they begin the postpartum period because they often did not sleep well during the third trimester and are exhausted by the exertion of labor. New mothers commonly experience feelings of excitement and euphoria for some time after childbirth and are unable to rest. Numerous visitors interfere with periods of rest. Hospital routines and noise, an unfamiliar environment, and physical discomfort also make it difficult for the new mother to rest.

Most mothers go home with a tremendous deficit in sleep and energy. Yet new parents may be unprepared for the conflict between their need for sleep and the infant's need for care and attention. The joys of parenting can easily be overshadowed by the exhaustion and frustration that result.

Rest at the Birth Facility Hospital routines often make uninterrupted rest difficult and increase the probability that the mother is fatigued when she is discharged. Group assessments and care to minimize interruptions, and plan with the mother for a time for napping. Suggest that she restrict phone calls and visitors during these times. Encourage the use of the side-lying position for breastfeeding to allow her to rest during feedings.

Rest at Home Help the mother understand the impact that her physical discomfort and the demands of the newborn will have on her energy when she returns home. If she understands that fatigue is normal and will continue for some time, she can plan ahead of time ways to obtain extra help and conserve her energy. Start with the following suggestions:

• Maintain a flexible routine that focuses on care of the mother and infant.
• Nap whenever the infant sleeps, if possible.
• Plan simple meals and flexible mealtimes.
• Accept assistance with food shopping, meal preparation, and housework.
• Postpone major household projects.
• Involve friends and family to provide care for other children.

Explain to the mother that she should delay her return to employment, if possible, until the infant sleeps through the night (usually by 4 months) or later. It takes time to recover from childbearing as well as adjust to the changes of parenting. Advise the mother to restrict coffee, tea, colas, and chocolate (which all contain the stimulant caffeine) or to use decaffeinated versions for the first few weeks.

Relaxation Exercises Total relaxation exercises (lying quietly, alternately tightening and relaxing the muscles of the neck, shoulders, arms, legs, and feet) are helpful when a nap is not possible. Emphasize to the mother the importance of asking for help when she begins to feel exhausted or overwhelmed. Encourage her to share these feelings with family, friends, and other new mothers.

Providing Nutrition Counseling

Food Supply Families of low socioeconomic status may benefit from referral to government-sponsored programs, such as food stamps or the Special Supplemental Food Program for Women, Infants, and Children (WIC) to help them obtain adequate food. It may also be necessary to determine what facilities are available for cooking and storing food. Sometimes the new family must be referred to a social worker for solutions for their unique problems.

Diet Although many women are unsatisfied with slow weight loss, they should avoid severe restriction of caloric intake. Explain the need to select foods that provide adequate calories to meet energy needs, taking into account the time and energy needed to care for a newborn. Strict dieting can leave the mother feeling tired, lower her immunity, and interfere with the lactating mother's ability to synthesize milk (Lawrence & Lawrence, 1999).

One study found that women often lost weight by decreasing carbohydrate consumption. However, their fat intake increased slightly, partly as a result of skipping meals and eating high-fat snacks or fast foods (Gennaro & Fehder, 2000). A balanced, low-fat diet with adequate protein, complex carbohydrates, fruits, and vegetables provides the nutrients needed (see Chapter 15).

Promoting Regular Bowel Elimination

Explain the role of progressive exercise, adequate fluid, and dietary fiber in preventing constipation. Walking is perhaps the best exercise, and the distance can be increased as strength and endurance increase. Drinking at least eight glasses of water daily will help maintain normal bowel elimination. Dietary fiber is present in fruits and vegetables, particularly when they are unpeeled. Prunes act as a natural laxative. Additional fiber is found in whole-grain cereals, bread, and pasta.

A regular schedule of bowel elimination is also important in overcoming constipation. For instance, bowel elimination after breakfast allows the mother to take advantage of the gastrocolic reflex (stimulation of peristalsis induced in the colon when food is consumed on an empty stomach). Measures that reduce perineal and hemorrhoidal pain, such as sitz baths, prepackaged witch hazel astringent compresses, and hydrocortisone ointments, also facilitate bowel elimination.

Promoting Good Body Mechanics

Exercise Teach exercises in the early postpartum period to strengthen the abdominal muscles and firm the waist. The exercises can be started soon after childbirth and repeated up to five times twice a day, at first (Figure 21-8). The number of exercises is gradually increased as the mother gains strength.

ABDOMINAL BREATHING

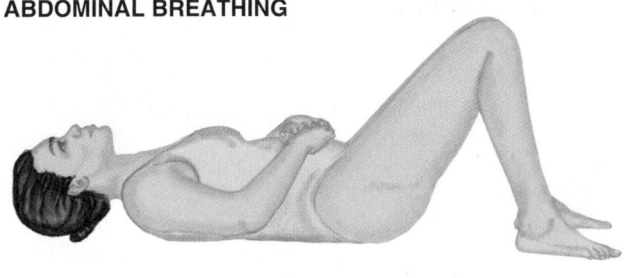

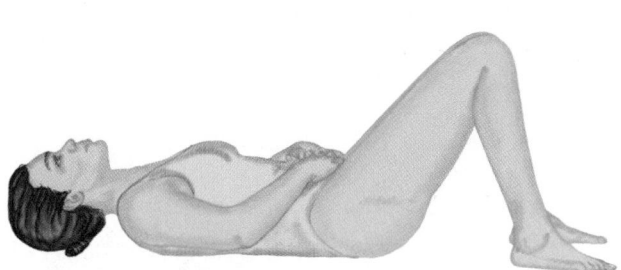

This is one of the simplest exercises and can be started on the first postpartum day. The woman assumes a supine position with knees bent. She inhales through the nose, keeps the rib cage as stationary as possible, and allows the abdomen to expand. She then contracts the abdominal muscles as she exhales slowly through the mouth.

HEAD LIFT

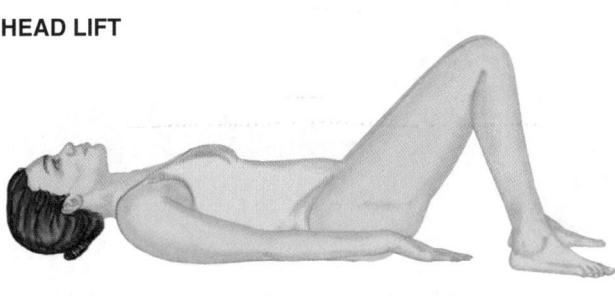

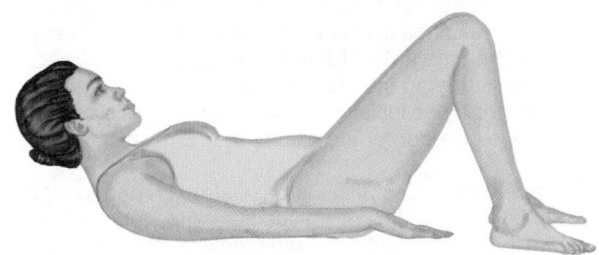

This exercise can be started within a few days after child-birth. The mother is supine with knees bent and arms out-stretched at her side. She inhales deeply to begin, then exhales while lifting the head slowly; she holds the position for a few seconds and relaxes.

MODIFIED SIT-UPS

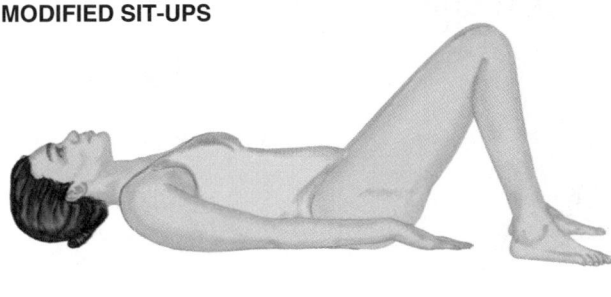

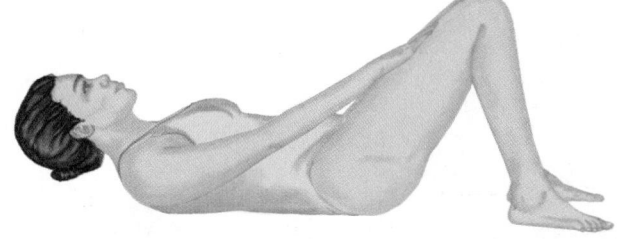

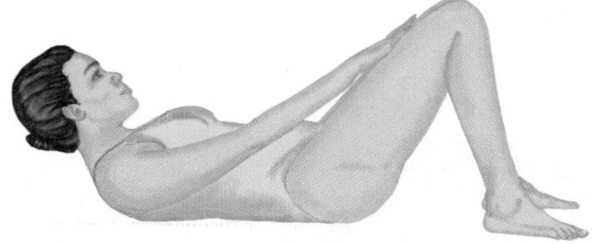

Head lifts may progress to modified sit-ups with the approval of the health care provider; the mother should follow the advice of the health care provider about the number of repetitions.

The exercise begins with the mother supine with arms outstretched and the knees bent. She raises her head and shoulders as her hands reach for her knees. She raises the shoulders only as far as the back will bend; her waist remains on the floor.

Continued

Figure 21-8 Postpartum exercises.

KNEE AND LEG ROLLS   **CHEST EXERCISES**

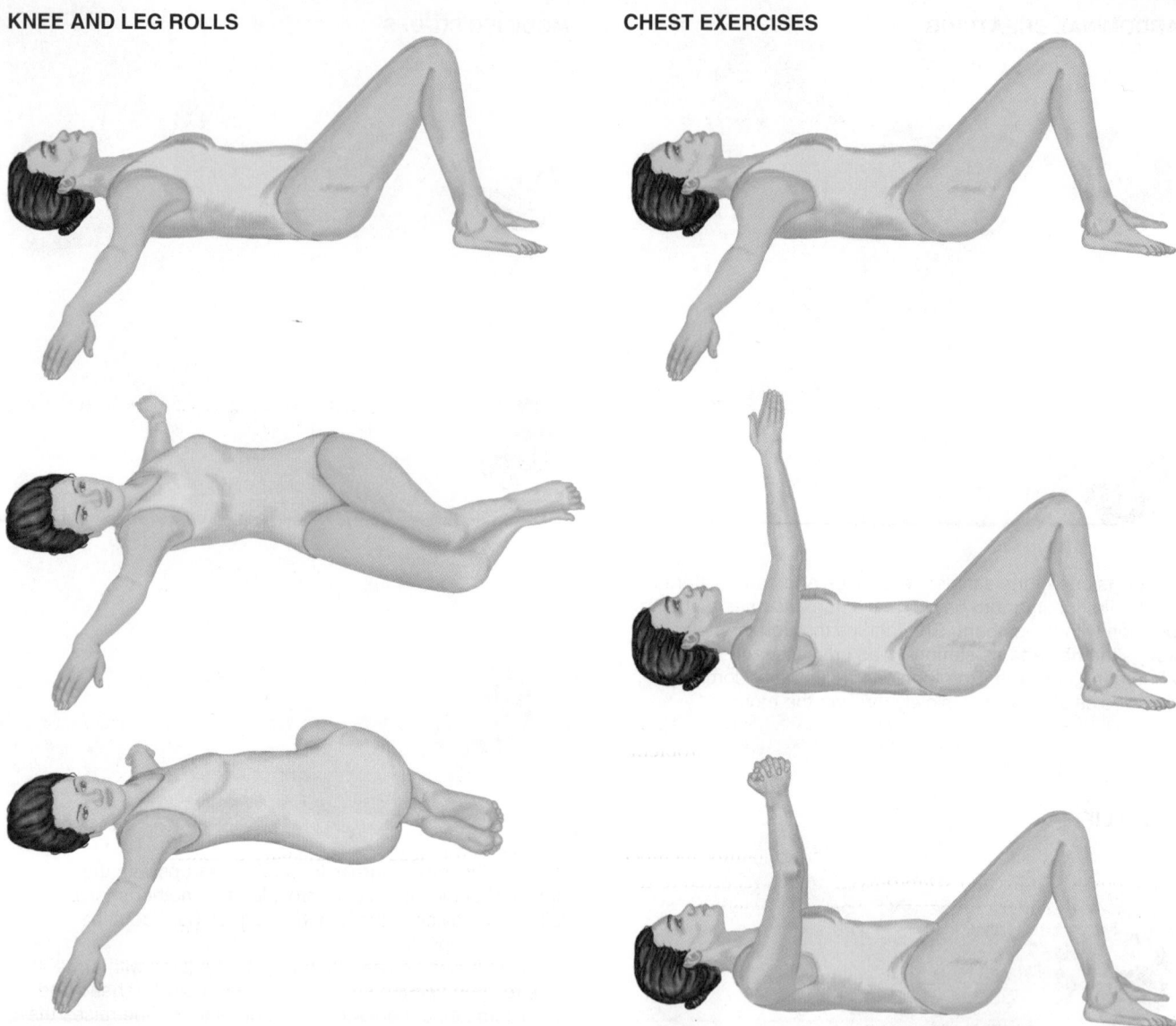

This is an excellent exercise to begin firming the waist. The mother lies flat on her back with knees bent and feet flat on the floor or bed; she keeps the shoulders and feet stationary and rolls the knees to touch first one side of the bed, then the other. She maintains a smooth motion as the exercise is repeated five times. Later, as flexibility increases, the exercise can be varied by the rolling of one knee only. The mother rolls her left knee to touch the right side of the bed, returns to center, and rolls the right knee to touch the left side of the bed.

This is an excellent exercise to strengthen the chest muscles. The mother lies flat with arms extended straight out to the side; she brings the hands together above the chest while keeping the arms straight; she holds for a few seconds and returns to the starting position. She repeats the exercise five times initially and follows the advice of the health care provider for increasing the number of repetitions.

Isometric exercises also increase strength and tone; the mother bends her elbows, clasps her hands together above her chest, and presses her hands together for a few seconds. This is repeated at least five times.

Figure 21-8, cont'd Postpartum exercises.

Instruct postcesarean mothers to follow the instructions of their health care provider. Generally they should not begin a strenuous exercise program for 4 to 6 weeks. Less-vigorous exercise, like walking, is more appropriate at first.

Preventing Back Strain Back strain often can be prevented if the mother and father find a location for infant care, such as a kitchen table or bathroom counter, that does not require bending or leaning forward. For lifting objects,

teach parents to hold the back straight as they squat and use the legs rather than bending at the waist (see Fig. 13-12).

Counseling About Sexual Activity

The couple may have concerns about resuming sexual intercourse and contraceptive choices. Fatigue, fear of pain, and concerns about the baby may interfere with a woman's sexual desire. Women who have a 2nd-degree or more extensive laceration or episiotomy may report pain and interference with sexual activities at 6 months postpartum (Signorello, Harlow, Chekos, & Repke, 2001).

Many new parents are reluctant to ask about when to resume sexual activity and about potential alterations in sexuality resulting from pregnancy and childbirth. If couples do not indicate such concerns, introduce the topic in a general, nonspecific manner, such as by saying, "You have an episiotomy, which may cause some discomfort with intercourse until it has completely healed," or "Sometimes couples are not aware that some vaginal dryness occurs as a result of breastfeeding." Such broad opening statements permit the family to pursue the topic as they desire.

The nursing diagnosis "Risk for Ineffective Sexuality Pattern" is appropriate for many postpartum women. The Nursing Care Plan: Postpartum Hypotension, Fatigue, and Pain, p. 478, explores this diagnosis.

Cultural or religious convictions may restrict the choice of contraceptive methods for some couples, whereas the availability of health care or limited finances may dictate the choice for others. Discuss previous experience with contraceptives and the satisfaction with those methods.

Instructing About Follow-up Appointments
The new mother generally returns to her physician or nurse-midwife for postpartum examination between 2 weeks and 6 weeks after childbirth. Explain that examination at that time allows early identification and treatment of problems that may develop.

Teaching About Signs and Symptoms That Should Be Reported
Teach new mothers and at least one other family member which physical signs and symptoms should be reported to the health care provider immediately. These signs and symptoms include:

- Fever
- Localized area of redness, swelling, or pain in either breast that is not relieved by support or analgesics
- Persistent abdominal tenderness
- Feelings of pelvic fullness or pelvic pressure
- Persistent perineal pain
- Frequency, urgency, or burning on urination
- Change in character of lochia (increased amount, resumption of bright red color, passage of clots, foul odor)
- Localized tenderness, redness, or warmth of the legs
- Separation of or foul drainage from the cesarean incision

Ensuring That All Elements Have Been Taught
Streamline and organize information so that it can be presented in the time available. Group instruction and hospital classes, such as those that demonstrate infant care and provide breastfeeding instructions, are an efficient use of time for teaching. Individual teaching is necessary, in addition, to meet individual needs.

Documentation is an important aspect of teaching, just as it is for other aspects of nursing care. Documentation that discharge teaching was performed and that the client indicates comprehension of teaching is required by accrediting agencies. To prevent omissions, many hospitals use teaching "check-off" sheets listing the areas that must be covered.

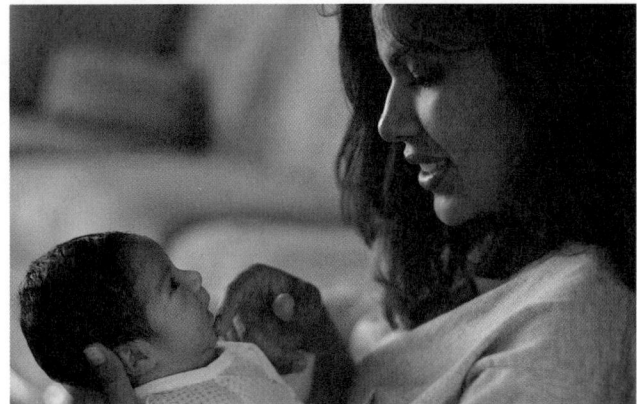

Figure 21-9 The infant is quiet and alert during the initial sensitive period. The newborn gazes at the mother and responds to her voice and touch.

Although there are many subjects that must be discussed in parent teaching, avoid covering too much information at a time. Interspersing small segments of teaching throughout the day will help keep the woman from being overwhelmed and help her remember information better.

Evaluation
- Does the mother demonstrate correct breast and perineal hygiene?
- Can the mother verbalize her plan to manage diet, rest, and exercise after discharge?
- Can she describe her plan for follow-up care and signs that indicate the need for immediate treatment?

THE PROCESS OF BECOMING ACQUAINTED
Perhaps no other event requires such rapid change in family structure and function as the birth of a baby. The addition of a new baby requires that all family members adjust their roles. The role of maternity nurses includes not only the care of the mother-infant dyad but the well-being of the entire family, as well. Nurses are concerned about the family's adjustment to childbearing during the hospital stay and the early weeks at home as new parents make the transition to parenthood.

A great deal of information has appeared in nursing literature that describes how parents and newborns become acquainted and progress to develop feelings of love, concern, and deep devotion that last throughout life. The terms *bonding* and *attachment* are commonly used to describe the initial steps. Although the terms are sometimes used interchangeably, their meanings differ.

Bonding
Bonding describes the initial attraction felt by parents. It is unidirectional, from parent to child, and is enhanced when parent and infant are permitted to touch and interact during a so-called *sensitive period* that extends through the first 30 to 60 minutes after birth. During this time the infant is in a quiet, alert stage. The eyes are open, and the infant seems to gaze directly at the parents (Fig. 21-9). Nurses frequently de-

lay procedures such as instillation of prophylactic eye medications that can interfere with this time between parents and newborns. Bonding can also occur later if parent-infant interaction does not occur immediately after birth.

Attachment

Attachment is the process by which an enduring bond to a child is developed through pleasurable, satisfying parent-child interaction. The process begins in pregnancy and extends for many months after childbirth. The infant receives warmth, food, and security from the parent. The parent (usually the mother) places the child's needs above her own for years to come. In return, she receives enjoyment and establishes her identity as a mother. Both benefit from the formation of irreplaceable links that continue long after the child ceases to be dependent.

Attachment follows a progressive course that changes over time. It is rarely instantaneous. Attachment behaviors of inexperienced or first-time mothers do not differ significantly from those of experienced mothers (Mercer & Ferketich, 1994). Attachment occurs through mutually satisfying experiences. Therefore if the new mother is in severe pain or is exhausted, she needs pain relief and assistance for her to enjoy the early experiences with the baby.

Unlike bonding, attachment is reciprocal—that is, it goes in both directions between parent and infant. Attachment is facilitated by positive feedback, either real or perceived. For example, an infant's grasp reflex around a parent's finger means "I love you" to the parent. Alert infants have a whole repertoire of responses called *reciprocal attachment behaviors*. They are the infant's part in the process of early attachment that progresses to lifelong mutual devotion.

Maternal Touch

Maternal behavior, particularly maternal touch, changes rapidly as the mother progresses through a discovery phase with her infant. Initially the mother may not reach for the infant, but if the infant is placed in her arms, she holds the baby in an *en face* position, with the infant's face in the same vertical plane as her own. When the infant is awake, the two engage in prolonged mutual gazing (see Fig. 21-9).

Fingertipping is common during the early minutes as the mother gets acquainted with the tiny stranger. She may gently explore the infant's face, fingers, and toes with her fingertips only (Fig. 21-10). She then begins to stroke the baby's

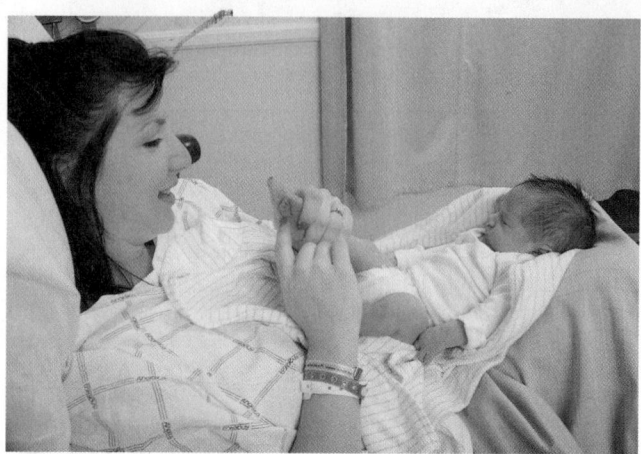

Figure 21-10 The mother's initial touch includes fingertipping, whereby she becomes acquainted with her infant by touching only with her fingertips.

chest and legs with her palm. Next, the mother uses her entire hand to enfold the infant and to bring the child close to her body. She strokes the baby's hair, presses her cheek against the infant's cheek, and finally feels comfortable enough to engage in a full range of consoling behaviors (Fig. 21-11).

The mother next begins to identify specific features of the newborn. "Look at his little pink mouth." Then she begins to relate features to family members. "He has his father's chin and nose (Fig. 21-12). This identification process has been called *claiming* or *binding in* (Rubin, 1977).

Verbal Behaviors

Verbal behaviors are also important indicators of maternal attachment. Most mothers speak to the infant in a high-pitched voice and progress from calling the baby "it" to "he" or "she" and then to using the given name. Verbal behaviors may provide clues to a mother's early psychologic relationship with her infant. Nurses observe the interactions of mothers and their infants and, if necessary, teach and model interactions that foster early attachment between them.

THE PROCESS OF MATERNAL ROLE ADAPTATION

Puerperal Phases

In the early 1960s, Rubin identified restorative phases that the mother must go through to replenish the energy lost during labor and to attain comfort in the role of mother. The puerperal phases are called *taking in*, *taking hold*, and *letting go*. They provide one method of observing change in maternal behavior that can be helpful in anticipating maternal needs and in intervening to meet those needs.

Taking-In Phase

During the taking-in phase, the mother is focused primarily on her own need for fluid, food, and sleep. Inexperienced nurses may be puzzled by the mother's passive behavior as she takes in or receives attention and physical care. She also

---

> ⚠ **CRITICAL TO REMEMBER**
>
> **Reciprocal Attachment Behaviors**
>
> Newborn infants have the ability to:
> - Make eye contact and engage in prolonged, intense, mutual gazing
> - Move their eyes and attempt to "track" the parent's face
> - Grasp the parent's finger and hold on
> - Move synchronously in response to rhythms and patterns of the parent's voice. This is called *entrainment*
> - Root, latch on to the breast, and suckle
> - Be comforted by the parent's voice or touch

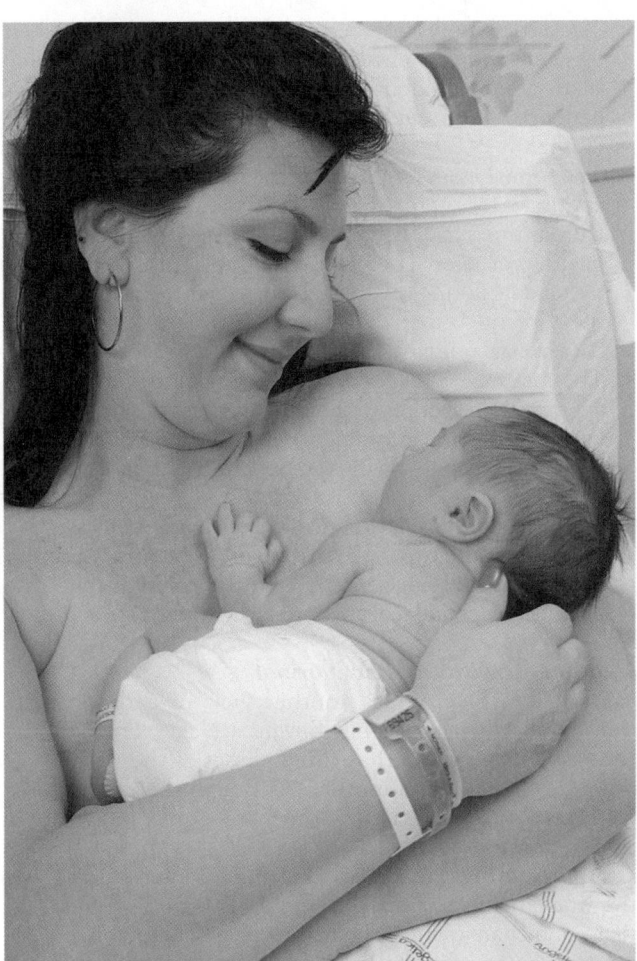
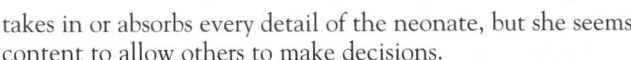

Figure 21-11 Mothers progress from exploratory touching to enfolding the infant. Their pleasure is enhanced by skin-to-skin contact.

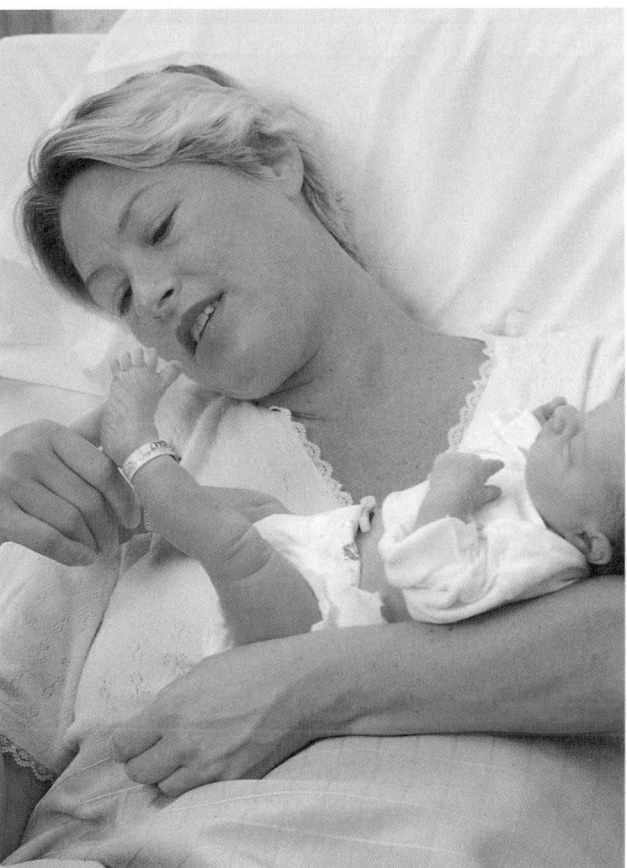

Figure 21-12 The binding-in, or claiming, process includes the mother's identification of her baby's specific features, relating them to other family members. This mother states, "His long toes are exactly like mine."

takes in or absorbs every detail of the neonate, but she seems content to allow others to make decisions.

A major task for the mother during this time is to integrate her birth experience into reality. To do this she discusses her labor and delivery in detail with visitors or on the telephone. This process helps the mother realize that the pregnancy is over and the infant is an individual separate from her.

Although Rubin believed that the taking-in phase lasted for approximately 2 days, it probably lasts a day or less today. The phase may be prolonged when a cesarean birth, especially in an emergency, has been necessary. These women may have difficulty assimilating the unfamiliar and intrusive procedures that occurred very rapidly, and they may express negative perceptions of the birth experience.

Taking-Hold Phase

The mother becomes more independent in the taking-hold phase. She exhibits concern about managing her own body functions and assumes responsibility for her own self-care. When she feels more comfortable and in control of her body, she shifts her attention to the performance of the infant. She welcomes information about the wide variety of behaviors exhibited by newborns.

During the taking-hold phase, the mother may verbalize anxiety about her competence as a mother. She may compare her caretaking skills unfavorably with those of the nurse.

Nurses must be careful not to assume the mothering role but to allow the mother to perform as much of the caretaking as possible and to praise each attempt, even if the mother's early care is awkward.

The taking-hold phase, which extends over several days, has been called the "teachable, reachable, referable moment." Nurses who provide home or clinic care can take advantage of this ideal time to review previously taught material and to provide additional instructions and demonstrations.

Letting-Go Phase

The letting-go phase is a time of relinquishment for the mother and often for the father. If this is a first child, the couple must give up their previous role as a childless couple and acknowledge the loss of a more carefree lifestyle. Many mothers must also give up idealized expectations of the birth experience. For example, they may have planned to have a vaginal birth with minimal or no anesthesia, but instead they required a cesarean birth.

CRITICAL THINKING EXERCISE 21-2

Ju-An, a 35-year-old primipara, had a cesarean birth after failure to progress in labor. She is very tired, although she is relatively comfortable. Her husband is excited about being a father but expresses concern because neither he nor Ju-An has experience with infants and his job requires almost constant travel.

The day of delivery, Ju-An readily accepts attention and assistance with hygiene. She recounts the details of her labor to friends on the telephone. She examines her baby girl closely and touches the infant's face and hands gently with her fingertips. She remarks that she plans to breastfeed and is surprised that the infant sleeps so much.
1. What are Ju-An's priority needs at this time?
2. What phase of recovery is she manifesting? Why does she "fingertip" the infant?

On the first postoperative day, Ju-An's indwelling catheter is removed and intravenous fluids are discontinued. She ambulates with minimal assistance and is pleased that she is able to urinate without difficulty. She asks about bowel function and requests the prescribed stool softener. She spends a great deal of time getting the baby to breastfeed. She is very frustrated that the infant does not breastfeed well and asks for assistance from the lactation educator.
3. What are Ju-An's priority needs now?
4. How have her behaviors changed?

Before discharge, Ju-An is breastfeeding well. The infant latches on and nurses for 10 to 15 minutes on each side, and Ju-An's nipples are free of tenderness or signs of trauma. Ju-An has no relatives in the area, and her husband is home for the weekend only. She states that she will just have to get along by herself after that.
5. What anticipatory guidance should Ju-An receive about her own care? About the infant's care?
6. What further nursing interventions would be most helpful to her and the baby?

In addition, some mothers (and fathers) are disappointed by the size, sex, or characteristics of the infant who does not "match up" with the fantasy baby of pregnancy. They must relinquish the infant of their fantasies and accept the real infant. These losses often provoke feelings of grief that may be so subtle that they are unexamined or unacknowledged. Both parents may benefit, however, if given the opportunity to verbalize unexpected feelings and to realize that these feelings are common. If the mother is very young or the pregnancy was unplanned, the feelings of loss and grief may be acute.

Maternal Role Attainment

Role attainment is a process in which the mother achieves confidence in her ability to care for her infant and becomes comfortable with her identity as a mother. The process begins during pregnancy and continues for several months after childbirth. The transition to the maternal or paternal role follows four stages (Mercer, 1995b):

1. The anticipatory stage begins during the pregnancy when pregnant women choose a physician or nurse-midwife. Many attend childbirth classes to prepare for the birth experience. They seek out role models to learn the role of mother.
2. The formal stage begins with the birth of the infant and continues for approximately 4 to 6 weeks (Mercer, 1995a). During this stage, behaviors are guided largely by others: health professionals, close friends, or parents. A major task for parents during this stage is to become acquainted with their infant so that they can mesh their caregiving with cues from the infant.
3. The informal stage begins once the parents have learned appropriate responses to their infant's cues or signals. They begin to respond according to the unique needs of the infant rather than following textbook or health professionals' directives.
4. The personal stage is attained when parents feel a sense of harmony in their role, see the infant as a central person in their lives, and have internalized the parental role. The parents accept and feel comfortable with the role of parent.

Heading Toward a New Normal
Martell (2003) provides another view of early postpartum changes with *Heading Toward a New Normal* as the theme. This view also has three phases as the woman reorganizes her life as a mother. Although the phases have distinctive characteristics, they are continuous rather than separate.

Appreciating the Body. This phase centers on the way the woman feels physically as she deals with discomfort, fatigue, and changes in her body. The phase also involves dealing with emotional lability and changes in the way women think and retain information.

Settling In. During settling in, mothers become more secure with their infants. They gradually gain in competence and in confidence about their abilities to care for their infants without help from others. They accommodate their needs and activities to meet the needs of the infant. Some find ways to integrate the infant into their usual activities with minor changes.

Becoming a New Family. As women work toward becoming a new family, they modify relationships with their partners and other family members. They develop new routines to include the infant and enjoy spending time alone with the newly developed family.

Redefining Roles
The mother is particularly concerned about redefining roles and focuses on maintaining a strong, adaptive relationship with her partner. She observes him carefully for any change in behavior and is acutely sensitive to his interaction with the infant. From the father's perspective, anxieties about succeeding in his new role put added pressure on the family. Conflicting demands between work and home, feelings of exclusion, and concerns about his relationship with his partner present additional challenges.

It may be essential for the new parents to agree on a division of tasks and responsibilities that was not necessary before the birth of the infant. This process is accomplished quickly and with very little discord in some families. Role assignment in other families is much less flexible, and any change can be a source of tension and frustration.

Although nurses are not actively involved in redefining family roles, they can use their skills in communication to assist the family in expressing their feelings and concerns so that the changes can be accomplished with minimal stress.

Role Conflict

Role conflict occurs when one's perception of role responsibilities differs significantly from reality. For example, if the mother perceives that her responsibility is to provide most of the care and comfort for the infant but reality dictates that she must return to full-time employment, role conflict may occur. In the United States over 50% of mothers with children younger than 1 year are employed (United States Department of Labor Bureau of Labor Statistics, 2003).

Primiparas often do not realize how strong their attachment to the infant will be or how difficult it will be for them to leave the infant to return to work (Nelson, 2003). Many women report feelings of guilt for leaving the infant and experience intense "separation grief" when they first leave the infant with a caregiver. Some report feeling jealous of the caregiver and fear that the caregiver will supplant the mother in the infant's affection.

Acknowledging these feelings and reassuring the mother that her emotions are normal may be helpful. The mother also needs time to reestablish feelings of closeness when she comes home from work, and she needs to develop a schedule that allows maximum time with the infant when she is at home. She may have to negotiate with another family member to take over some of the household tasks until she feels more comfortable with the situation. (See Nursing Care Plan: Adaptation of the Working Mother).

Nursing Care Plan

Adaptation of the Working Mother

ASSESSMENT

Rebecca Sanders, a 30-year-old single mother, gave birth to a baby boy by cesarean delivery 4 days ago. She cares for herself with minimal assistance and demonstrates confidence in breastfeeding. Rebecca must return to work in 6 weeks. She states that she does not want to leave the baby with someone else while she works: "I've always wanted to stay home for at least 6 months when I had a baby, but it is just impossible. How can I be a mother and work full time?"

Nursing Diagnosis

Anticipatory Grieving related to inability to perform the role of mother as she wishes secondary to the need to return to full-time employment.

Goals/Expected Outcomes

Rebecca will:
- Describe her concerns and feelings about leaving her infant with a caregiver by (specific date).
- Verbalize plans to achieve maximum satisfaction in her role as mother by the time she returns to work.

INTERVENTION	RATIONALE
1. Allow Rebecca to describe her perception of her role as mother and to express concerns about how employment will interfere with her ability to fulfill this role.	1. Role conflict, stress, and grief can result when a mother must leave the infant with another caregiver and return to her job.
2. Recommend free expression of feelings to significant others and to the care provider who is selected.	2. Candid expression of feelings helps to resolve them and opens the way for a discussion of measures that will help to overcome feelings of conflict.
3. Acknowledge the feelings Rebecca expresses, and reassure her that the feelings are common.	3. Knowledge that the feelings are not trivial and that they are common reinforces their validity and importance.
4. Help Rebecca develop a schedule that allows her maximum time with the infant:	4. Feelings of frustration and stress can be alleviated if the mother has a plan that allows her long periods of uninterrupted time with the infant.
a. Make a list of errands and supplies needed, to avoid frequent stops that delay getting home from work.	
b. Double the recipe when cooking, and freeze half for future use.	
c. Pick up nutritious take-out meals to avoid cooking each evening.	
d. Work out plans that include the baby in daily walks, exercise, or social visits.	

Continued

Nursing Care Plan

Adaptation of the Working Mother—cont'd

5. Recommend that Rebecca allow 30 to 45 minutes to hold the infant when she first gets home. Delay all other activities until this need is met.
6. Suggest that Rebecca delay her return to employment, if possible, until the infant is at least 16 weeks old.

7. Recommend that Rebecca investigate several day care providers. She should check references, make unannounced visits, insist on seeing required licenses and certification, discuss the number and ages of children cared for, request a schedule of planned care, determine the provider's philosophy of infant care, determine whether the care provider is trained in emergency measures, and know what plans are in place if a fire or disaster occurs.
8. Suggest that Rebecca leave the infant with the chosen day care provider for 2 or 3 days before resuming full-time employment.
9. Recommend that Rebecca pump her breasts and feed the infant by bottle at least once a day before returning to work.

5. Time is needed to reestablish feelings of closeness, comfort, and attachment.
6. By 16 weeks most infants are able to sleep through the night. This development reduces the chance that sleep deprivation will add to other stressors.
7. A great deal of stress is eliminated if parents feel confident that a competent and nurturing day care provider has been found.

8. Allowing both mother and infant to "practice separating" while there is still some flexibility in their schedules makes the first day back at work less traumatic.
9. Becoming proficient at pumping the breasts and introducing the infant to bottle feeding prepares both the mother and infant for all-day separation.

Evaluation

Rebecca freely expresses her feelings of guilt, anxiety, and concern about leaving her infant. She has organized a plan to investigate day care in her area and verbalized plans to reorganize her work and social schedule so that she can spend as much time as possible with her son.

Additional Nursing Diagnoses to Consider

Deficient Diversional Activity
Parental Role Conflict
Ineffective Role Performance

Postpartum Blues

Mild depression, also known as *postpartum blues* or *maternity blues*, is a frequently expressed concern. This transient condition affects more than 70% of American women who have given birth (American Academy of Pediatrics [AAP] & American College of Obstetricians and Gynecologists [ACOG], 2002). The condition begins in the 1st week and usually lasts no longer than 2 weeks. It is characterized by insomnia, irritability, fatigue, tearfulness, mood instability, and anxiety. The symptoms are usually unrelated to events, and the condition does not seriously affect the mother's ability to care for the infant.

Although the direct cause is unknown, it may be caused by the letdown that occurs after birth, postpartum discomforts, fatigue, anxiety about the mother's ability to care for the infant, and concern about her attractiveness (Cunningham et al., 2001). Hormonal fluctuations have been implicated in the past, but they have not been proven to be a cause. Although postpartum blues is self-limiting, mothers benefit greatly when empathy and support are freely given by the family and the health care team.

Postpartum blues must be distinguished from postpartum depression and postpartum psychosis, which are disabling conditions and require therapeutic management for full recovery (see Chapter 28). Nurses should teach women to call their provider if their depression becomes severe or lasts longer than expected.

THE PROCESS OF FAMILY ADAPTATION

The birth of an infant requires that roles and relationships within the family be reorganized. Each family member is affected.

Fathers

The father's developing bond to his newborn is called *engrossment*. It is characterized by intense interest in how the infant looks and responds and a desire to touch and hold the baby. Many fathers comment on the baby's distinctive features. They experience strong attraction to the infant and elation after the baby's birth. The father's attachment behaviors increase when the infant is awake, makes eye contact, and responds to the father's voice (Fig. 21-13).

Many fathers eagerly look forward to co-parenting with their mate. They may, however, lack confidence in providing infant care and are sensitive to being left out of instructions and demonstrations of infant care. They may feel that others expect them only to provide support to the mother. The nurse can assist the new father by involving him in child care activities soon after birth to help him feel more confident and competent (Matteson, 2001).

Siblings

Sibling response to the birth of a new brother or sister depends on age and developmental level. Toddlers are usually not completely aware of the impending birth. They may view the infant as competition or fear that they will be replaced in the parents' affection. Negative behaviors such as sleep problems, an increase in attention-seeking efforts, and more infantile behaviors like renewed bed-wetting may surface. Some may exhibit hostile behaviors toward the mother, particularly when she holds or feeds the newborn. Parents must find opportunities to affirm their continued love and affection for the very vulnerable sibling.

Preschool siblings engage in more looking than touching. Most spend at least some time in proximity to the infant and talk to the mother about the infant (Fig. 21-14). A relaxed, natural setting, without time constraints, may make it easier for young children to interact with the infant. Special care must be taken by the parents, visitors, and nurses to pay as much attention to the sibling as to the new baby.

Grandparents

The involvement of grandparents with grandchildren depends on many factors. One of the most important factors is proximity. Grandparents who live near the child frequently develop strong attachment. This evolves into unconditional love and a special relationship that brings joy to the grandparents and an added sense of security to the grandchildren (Fig. 21-15). Grandparents who live many miles from grandchildren must try to devise ways to foster a relationship with grandchildren they seldom see.

Expectations of the role of grandparents are also a factor in how the grandparents adapt to the birth of a grandchild. Many grandparents strive to be fully involved in the care and upbringing of the child. Others desire less involvement.

Grandparents are often a major part of the support system that new parents need. Grandmothers in particular provide assistance with household tasks and infant care, which allows the mother to recover from childbirth and make the transition to parenthood.

Factors Affecting Family Adaptation

Numerous factors influence the family's adjustment. Some, such as discomfort and fatigue, can be anticipated because they are so common. Unanticipated events, such as cesarean birth, birth of a preterm or ill infant, or the birth of more than one infant, also affect the ease and speed with which the family adjusts.

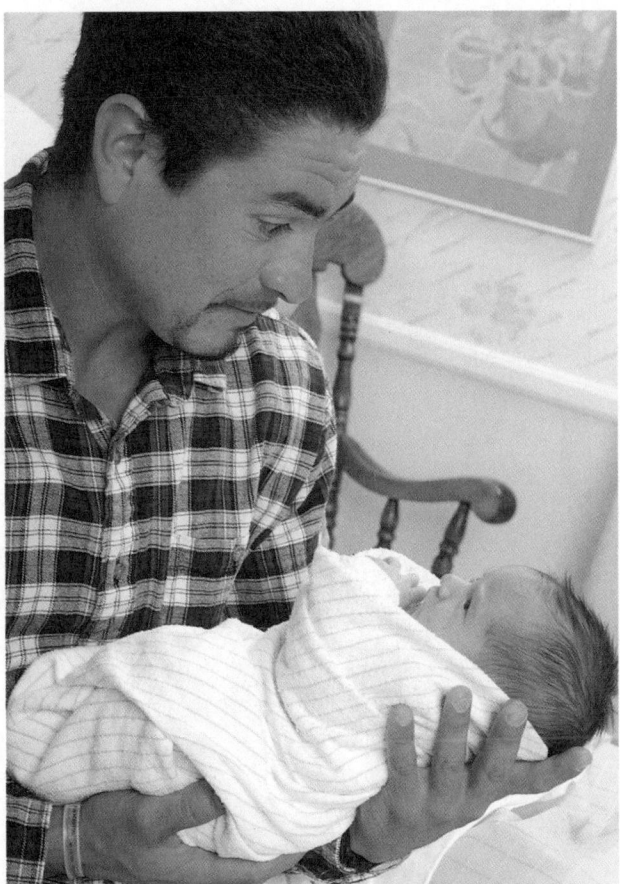

Figure 21-13 Fathers' behaviors at initial contact with their infants often correspond to maternal behaviors. The intense fascination that fathers exhibit is called *engrossment*. Note the eye-to-eye contact between father and infant.

Discomfort and Fatigue

Normally, discomfort associated with childbirth resolves within the first days after birth. Discomfort may make it difficult to focus on the needs of the newborn. Fatigue often continues during the first few weeks or even months, when the infant's schedule is erratic and uninterrupted sleep is minimal. When the infant begins to sleep through the night (at about 16 weeks), fatigue becomes less of a factor.

Knowledge of Infant Needs

First-time parents are often unsure of how to care for the newborn and become very anxious if they are unable to console a crying infant. Moreover, many are concerned about specific procedures, such as care of the umbilical cord or the circumcision. They want to know if the infant is receiving adequate nutrition. Breastfeeding benefits both mother and infant. It may, however, add to the stress that parents experience initially when they lack knowledge about it.

Some parents have concerns about spoiling the infant. They may believe that responding each time the infant cries causes the infant to cry to get his or her way. It may be necessary to remind parents that infants cry to indicate a need and to reassure the parents that responding to crying does not spoil the child. Suggesting a variety of methods to cope with crying may be helpful.

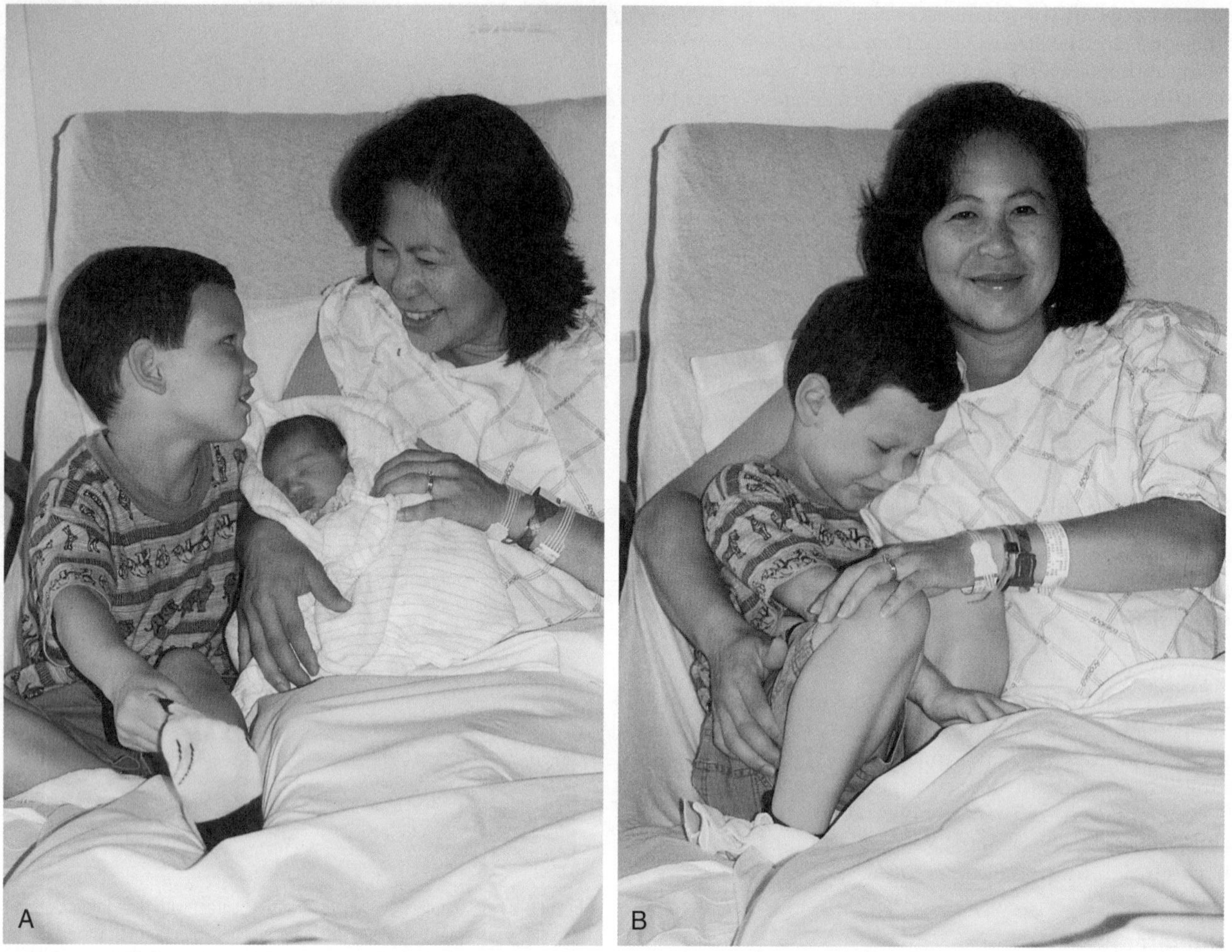

Figure 21-14 A, Although they may hesitate to touch the infant, children often want to be close. **B,** This boy's relief and joy are obvious as he reclaims a favorite spot.

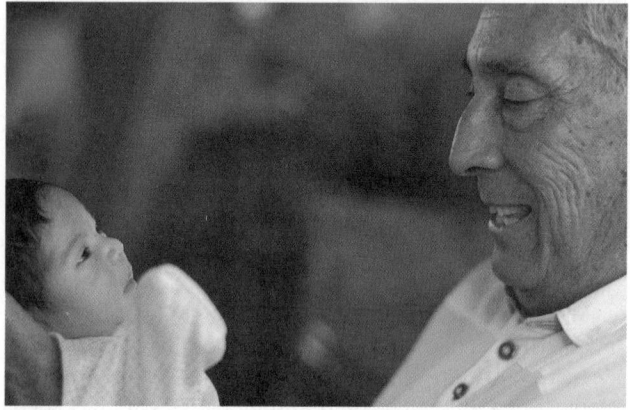

Figure 21-15 Grandparents may develop strong bonds with grandchildren.

Previous Experience

Previous experience with newborns may also affect family adjustment. Multiparas are more comfortable with infants and exhibit attachment behaviors earlier than do primiparas, who may spend many more hours in the early discovery phase of attachment. Mothers who have previously given birth to infants with anomalies or to infants who did not survive may need more time to feel comfortable with this infant.

Expectations of the Newborn

Unrealistic expectations of the infant may also influence adjustment. Many parents have very little experience with newborns and are disappointed at the way a newborn looks. Mothers often report that it took them 3 to 6 months to feel they really knew their infants (Nelson, 2003).

Nurses must be prepared to teach normal growth and development and to assist the parents in working through their misconceptions. For instance, the capacity of an infant's stomach is small and the infant must be fed frequently. Also, infants are neurologically unable to sleep through the night for several months. Increasing the time the mother spends with the infant during the postpartum stay increases opportunities for her to care for the infant when a nurse is available to help her.

Some parents may be very disappointed in the sex of the child, or they may sense that their partners are disappointed. These feelings must be acknowledged and dealt with before attachment can take place.

Maternal Age

Adjustment to parenthood is a challenge for teenagers who have not achieved a strong sense of their own identity. In general, adolescents tend to talk less, respond less, appear more passive, and sometimes appear less affectionate with their children than do adult parents. They need special assistance to develop necessary parenting skills that promote optimal development of the infant.

Maternal Temperament

Maternal personality traits are a major influence on attachment. Mothers who are calm and secure in their ability to learn adjust more easily to the demands of motherhood. Conversely, mothers who are excitable, insecure, and anxious have more difficulty.

Temperament of the Infant

The infant also affects maternal adjustment. Infants who are calm, easily consoled, and enjoy cuddling increase parental confidence and feelings of competence. In contrast, irritable infants who are difficult to console and who do not respond to cuddling interfere with attachment.

Availability of a Strong Support System

A strong, consistent support system is a major factor in the adjustment of the new mother. Friends and relatives who are parents can provide role modeling that is particularly important to first-time mothers. They also provide encouragement, praise, and reassurance that she is a good mother. In addition, the woman needs practical assistance with household tasks such as meal preparation, laundry, and shopping.

Other Factors

Cesarean Birth. A cesarean birth, especially one that is not anticipated, may make parental adjustment more difficult. The surgical birth may result in financial strain, a longer recovery time for the mother, additional discomfort, and increased stress for the family. The mother's needs for both recovery and attachment with her infant must be considered in nursing care.

Preterm or Ill Infant. Birth of a preterm or ill infant results in additional concern about the condition of the infant. Prolonged separation of parents and child may be necessary. Although attachment can occur in these situations, the separation may delay the process of attachment and create stress on the normally functioning family (see Chapter 29).

Birth of Multiple Infants. The birth of more than one infant may present problems of attachment. It is believed the process of attachment is structured so that the parents become attached to only one infant at a time. Therefore parents should be encouraged to interact with each child individually, especially in the early getting-acquainted period. Nurses must help the parents relate to each infant as an individual rather than as part of a unit by pointing out the individual responses and uniqueness of each infant. Early, frequent contacts or rooming-in helps the parents gain confidence in caretaking and facilitates the attachment process. Mothers are sometimes overwhelmed at the prospect of breastfeeding more than one infant. They need reassurance that they will produce an ample supply of milk for each infant because supply increases with demand. Some mothers choose to combine breastfeeding with formula feeding.

CULTURAL INFLUENCES ON ADAPTATION

A major goal of nursing practice in the postpartum period is to provide culturally specific nursing care that fits the health beliefs, values, and practices of each client. This effort can be difficult because of the wide ethnic diversity in the United States and Canada. A major challenge for nurses is to be aware of cultural beliefs and to acknowledge their importance in family adaptation. Postpartum is often thought to be a time of vulnerability for the woman and the infant (Mattson, 2000b). Many cultural factors relevant to the postpartum period can be grouped into communication, dietary practices, and health beliefs.

Communication

Verbal communication may be difficult because of the numerous dialects and languages spoken. An interpreter should be fluent in the language, of the same religion, and of the same country of origin if possible. This compatibility is particularly important for Middle Eastern families, whose religious orientation may vary widely and who come from countries with long histories of social and religious conflict.

Respecting the privacy and modesty of all people is important, but modesty is especially important to Hispanic and Middle Eastern and Asian women. Laws of modesty require that Muslim women keep their hair, body, arms to the wrist, and legs to the ankles covered.

Health care workers must remember that tactfulness and warmth are important. Direct communication can be distressing, particularly for Hispanics and Native Americans, who approach a subject only after exchanging polite and gracious comments.

When the nurse and the family speak different primary languages, it is important to verify that the family has understood what is being said. Nodding or saying "Yes" may be a sign of courtesy rather than of understanding or agreement. To be certain the message has been received, the nurse should ask family members to repeat in their own words what they have been told.

Health Beliefs

Cultural beliefs and practices provide a sense of security for new mothers. Provision of care of the mother and baby by relatives is a common thread among cultures. Women from

BOX 21-2
Assessing Maternal Adaptation

Assessments	Nursing Considerations
Progression Through Puerperal Phases	
Taking in (passive, dependent)	Consider the mother's need for rest, her need to recount the details of her labor
Taking hold (autonomous, seeks information)	and childbirth, and her readiness to learn infant care and assume control of her
Letting go (relinquishes fantasy baby, begins to see self as mother)	own care.
Maternal Mood	
Mood and energy level, eye contact, posture, comfort	Tense body posture, crying, or anxiety may indicate discomfort, fatigue, or the beginning of postpartum blues.
Factors That Affect Maternal Adaptation	
Age of mother	May need additional support if younger than 18 years.
Previous experience	Primiparas often progress through puerperal phases at a slower pace and may need additional assistance. Multiparas have more experience with infant care. Previous birth of a child with anomalies or death of an infant may delay adaptation.
Maternal/infant temperament	Mothers who are calm, secure in their ability to learn, and free from anxiety need less assistance.
Other factors	Cesarean birth may result in increased discomfort and longer recovery. The birth of a preterm or ill infant or more than one infant can create problems with attachment.
Interaction With Infant	
Maternal touch	Mother progresses from "fingertipping" to enfolding and a variety of comforting behaviors.
Verbal interaction	Mother may call infant "it" initially but progresses quickly to using given name and identifying specific characteristics.
Response to infant cues or signals	Prompt, gentle, consistent response indicates progressive adaptation to parenting role.
Preparation for Parenting	
Classes in breastfeeding, parenting, or infant care	Many mothers feel more prepared after completing classes and participate in care sooner.

Japan practice *satogaeri bunben,* in which the women stay in their parents' home from near the end of pregnancy until 1 to 2 months after birth (Moore & Moos, 2003). Women from parts of India also return to the parents' home and stay for 16 weeks postpartum, where the new mother is cared for by her mother (Bowes & Katz, 2002). In Native American families, decisions are often made by the women in the family. Therefore the matriarch of the family should be included in teaching (Cesario, 2001).

For many Southeast Asians, the postpartum period is important to ensure health in later years. New mothers are expected to rest for 1 to 3 months while the grandmother or other female relatives take over the mother's usual responsibilities and care for her and her baby. Lack of adequate rest or the proper diet during this period is believed to cause varicose veins, early aging, problems with eyesight and digestion, and head and back pain (Davis, 2001). Korean women believe new mothers must keep warm to protect their loose bones and to prevent bone pain in later years (Kim-Godwin, 2003).

Southeast Asians and Hispanics believe that the mother should be kept warm to avoid upsetting the balance of hot and cold. Southeast Asian women drink hot water or other beverages to keep warm. Some women do not wish to take baths or wash their hair during the postpartum period. This practice is upsetting for nurses who are concerned about hygiene. Tact and sensitivity are needed to find a compromise.

Dietary Practices

Some dietary practices that must be considered center on the hot-cold theory of health and diet. This theory refers to the intrinsic properties and effects of certain foods rather than the temperature. For example, Southeast Asians (Cambodians, Vietnamese, Hmong, and Laotians) believe that after childbirth the woman should eat only foods that are considered hot in effect on the body. Examples are chicken, pork, and rice.

Some Chinese believe that a combination of yin and yang maintains balance. Yin foods include bean sprouts, broccoli, carrots, and cauliflower. Yang foods include broiled meat, chicken, soup, and eggs.

NURSING CARE
Maternal Adaptation

Assessment

Factors such as how the mother progresses through the puerperal phases, her mood, and interaction with the infant affect maternal adaptation to the birth. Box 21-2 summarizes the psychosocial assessment of the mother and nursing considerations related to each assessment.

Nursing Diagnosis and Planning

Parenting involves the parents' ability to create an environment that nurtures the growth and development of the infant. Parenting may be difficult when factors such as maternal discomfort, fatigue, and lack of knowledge or confidence in infant care come into play. Therefore a common nursing diagnosis is

■ Risk for Impaired Parenting related to multiple factors, such as fatigue, discomfort, and lack of knowledge of infant care.

Expected Outcomes: The mother will verbalize feelings of comfort and support as she progresses through the phases of recovery and will demonstrate progressive attachment behaviors by (specific date) and participate in care of the newborn by (date).

Interventions

Assisting the Mother Through Recovery Phases

"Mother" the Mother The early taking-in phase is a time to mother the mother so that she can move on to more complex tasks of maternal adjustment. During the first few hours after childbirth, she has a great need for physical care and comfort. Provide ample fluids and favorite foods. Keep linens dry, tuck warm blankets around her until chilling has stopped, and use warm water for perineal care.

Monitor and Protect The new mother depends on nurses to monitor and protect her. Remind her of the need to void, and assist her to ambulate. Offer pain medication before discomfort is severe, at which time the analgesic is less effective. At the first signs of fatigue, encourage the mother to sleep.

Listen to the Birth Experience Be prepared to listen to details of the birth experience and to offer sincere praise for her efforts during labor.

Many mothers spend so much time on the telephone that it is difficult to complete assessments and care. It is often helpful to offer a choice. "Excuse me for a moment. I need to check you soon. I can do it now or come back in 5 minutes."

Fostering Independence

As the mother becomes more independent, allow her to schedule her care as much as possible. Collaborate with her to plan when procedures, such as sitz baths, will be done. Encourage her to assume responsibility for self-care, and emphasize that the nurse's role at this point is to assist and to teach.

Promoting Bonding and Attachment

Early, unlimited contact between parents and infants is of primary importance to facilitate the attachment process (Fig. 21-16). In many hospitals and birth centers, infants remain in the room with the parents unless complications intervene. This arrangement may be called *mother-baby care*, *couplet care*, or *dyad care*. One nurse cares for both the mother and the baby and provides teaching and help with bonding as a part of ongoing nursing care.

Prolonged contact between mothers and infants leads to more touching and caring for the infant, which enhances bonding. Specific nursing measures to promote bonding and attachment include:

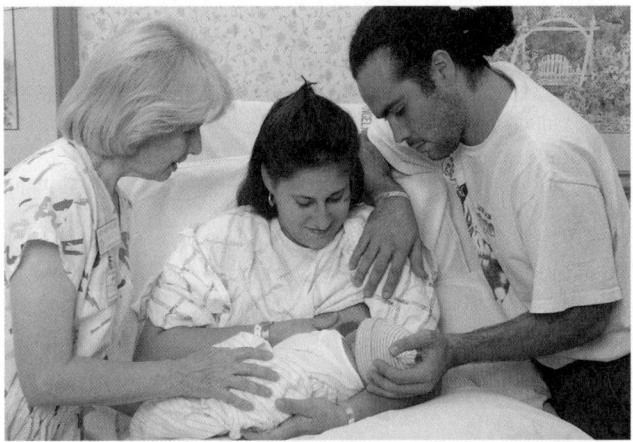

Figure 21-16 By teaching about the newborn and family, the nurse helps parents develop confidence in their ability to provide care for the infant.

- Assist the parents in unwrapping the baby to inspect the toes, fingers, and body. This process allows the parents to become acquainted with the "real" baby that must replace the fantasy baby that many parents imagined during the pregnancy.
- Position the infant in an *en face* position because eye-to-eye contact is a first step in establishing mutual interaction between the infant and the parent.
- Point out the reciprocal bonding activities of the infant: "Look how she holds your finger"; "He has not taken his eyes off you."
- Encourage the parents to spend time with the infant so they can progress at their own speed through the discovery or getting-acquainted phase.
- Assist the mother in feeding the infant, and answer her questions about feeding.
- Model behaviors by holding the infant close and speaking in high-pitched, soothing tones.
- Refer to the infant's characteristics positively: "She has the tiniest pink ears and such a lot of dark hair."

Involving Parents in Infant Care

Providing care for the infant fosters feelings of responsibility and nurturing and is an important component of attachment. In addition, it allows parents to develop confidence in their ability to care for an infant before they go home.

Help the parents take over the care of the infant gradually while providing assistance to enhance their self-confidence in their abilities. Although teaching begins during pregnancy, review information and repeat demonstrations if time allows. It is important for the entire staff to agree on how basic care is to be taught. Mothers seek confirmation of information, and they become confused and lose faith in the credibility of the staff if information varies.

Offer parents repeated praise and encouragement, because they become easily discouraged if they think they have failed at some attempt to care for their infants.

Suggestions for care must be tactfully phrased to avoid the implication that the parents are inept: "You burped that baby like a professional. There are a couple of little hints I can share about diapering."

BOX 21-3
Assessing Family Adaptation

Assessments	Nursing Considerations
Characteristics of Infant That May Affect Family Adaptation	
Sex and size of infant	Disappointment in the sex or concern about the small size may interfere with bonding.
Unexpected characteristics (cephalhematoma, jaundice, cranial molding, newborn rash)	Explain unexpected appearance or behavior in words parents can comprehend.
Infant behavior (irritable, easily consoled, cuddles)	An easily consoled, cuddly infant increases bonding and attachment.
Paternal Adaptation	
Response to mother and to infant	The father often provides the most important support for the mother, and his involvement with the infant indicates his acceptance of his parenting role.
Knowledge of infant care	Useful in planning teaching that includes the father.
Response to infant cues or signals (crying, fussing)	Many fathers feel awkward handling the infant but want to become proficient in infant care.
Ages and Developmental Levels of Siblings	
Reaction of siblings	Young children often fear that the newborn will replace them in the affection of parents. Parents may need anticipatory guidance about sibling rivalry.
Support System	
Interest and availability of family or friends to assist during early weeks	Family may need assistance in identifying available support.
Plans for first few days at home	Review plans for care, support, and rest. Provide resources.
Follow-up plans	Appointments should be scheduled for follow-up with clinic or health care provider.
Cultural Factors	
Cultural beliefs and practices that may affect nursing care	Culture-specific care can be planned for hygiene, dietary preferences, usual care of infants, and role of mate and family.
Expectations of the health care team	

Evaluation

- Does the mother verbalize feelings of comfort as she cares for her infant?
- Does she demonstrate attachment behaviors such as enfolding the infant, using the infant's name, and responding gently when the infant cries?
- Does she participate in infant care (diapering, feeding, and care of the umbilical cord and circumcision)?

■ NURSING CARE
Family Adaptation

Assessment

Fathers

The father's emotional status and interaction with the infant are particularly important because he usually serves as the mother's primary support person. The nurse should assess the father's interaction with the mother and the infant and his knowledge about infants. Unrealistic expectations of the infant may lead to problems. Moreover, if the father expects the mother to recover her energy and libido rapidly, he may become resentful if her recovery takes longer than anticipated.

Siblings

Note the ages of siblings and how they react to the newborn. Also assess the parents' reaction to sibling behaviors.

Support System

Family members often provide a powerful support system, and their involvement is important to the adaptation of the family. Ask about who will assist the mother when she returns home.

Nonverbal Behavior

Nonverbal behavior is equally important. Are the parents' words congruent with what they do? For example, does the mother verbalize satisfaction with her infant's characteristics but respond slowly to infant signals? Box 21-3 summarizes the family assessment and briefly indicates nursing considerations.

Nursing Diagnosis and Planning

Sometimes a family who usually functions effectively is unable to cope because of a specific event, such as the birth of a baby. A common nursing diagnosis is

■ Risk for Interrupted Family Processes related to lack of knowledge of infant needs and behaviors, stress during the early weeks at home, and sibling rivalry.
Expected Outcomes: The family will verbalize understanding of infant needs and behaviors and identify methods for reducing stress during the early weeks at home. The family will describe measures to reduce sibling rivalry and identify external resources and support system.

Expected outcomes often cannot be evaluated before discharge from the birth facility and overlap with home care. The expected outcome should therefore specify a date.

Interventions

Teaching the Family About the Newborn

Infant Needs Some new parents have unrealistic expectations of the newborn, and nurses are in the best position to explain what the infant is capable of doing and what the infant needs to thrive. Provide them with information about the infant's capabilities as well as the emotional and physical needs.

Infant Signals Discuss the importance of responding promptly and gently to cues such as crying or fussing. Reassure parents that responding to cues does not "spoil" their child but helps the infant learn to trust that the world is a safe, secure place.

Help parents recognize signals that indicate when their infant has had enough and wants to avoid further stimulation. The so-called *avoidance cues*, such as looking away, splaying the fingers, arching the back, and fussiness, indicate that the infant needs a quiet time.

Helping the Family Adapt

Providing Anticipatory Guidance About Stress Reduction Help the family plan for the first weeks at home, when the family must adjust to the demands of a newborn. This is a time when the need for rest is great but the opportunity for uninterrupted sleep is minimal. As a result, fatigue is a common problem.

Emphasize that the priority during the first 4 to 6 weeks should be caring for the mother and baby. The mother should sleep when the infant sleeps and delay visits and phone calls until she is rested. She can reduce family tension by establishing a relaxed home atmosphere and a flexible meal schedule. Enlisting the aid of grandparents, other relatives, and friends to help with meal preparation, shopping, and care of the other children will provide the mother more time for rest.

Teach mothers breathing exercises and progressive relaxation techniques to reduce stress and to energize, especially when a nap is not possible. To help them cope with stress, encourage parents to discuss their feelings openly. Remind them of the need for healthy nutrition and for favorite recreation. It is easy for fatigue and tension to overwhelm the anticipated joys of parenting if no respite is available from constant care.

Providing Ways to Reduce Sibling Rivalry Suggest that parents plan time alone with the older child and that they offer frequent expressions of love and affection. It is also helpful if visitors and family do not focus exclusively on the infant but also include the older child in their gift giving and exclamations about the newborn.

Emphasize the importance of responding calmly and with understanding when the child regresses to more infantile behaviors or expresses hostility toward the infant. Acknowledging the child's feelings and offering prompt reassurance of continued love are most valuable.

Identifying Resources In many homes, women assume the major responsibilities of day-to-day homemaking. With the birth of an infant, this task becomes more difficult. A division of labor must be negotiated to prevent undue stress and fatigue. This division of labor is particularly important if there are other children whose needs for time, attention, and comfort must also be met.

The mother's primary support is often the father of the baby. Members of the extended family, particularly grandmothers and sisters, or friends also provide valuable support. Community resources such as day care centers, parenting classes, and breastfeeding support groups are available in many areas. Remind the mother that resources are available when she begins to feel isolated and exhausted.

Evaluation

- Do the parents respond to the infant's crying promptly and gently?
- Do the parents have a plan to reduce family stress and sibling anxiety?
- Are they able to describe resources for support?

POSTPARTUM HOME COMMUNITY CARE

Criteria for Discharge

Most women leave the hospital when they are just beginning to recover from giving birth and beginning to learn how to care for themselves and their infants. The following criteria for discharge of mothers were developed by the American Academy of Pediatrics and the American College of Obstetricians and Gynecologists (2002):

- The mother has no complications, and assessments are normal (including vital signs, lochia, fundus, urinary output, incisions, ambulation, ability to eat and drink, and emotional status).
- Pertinent laboratory data including hemoglobin or hematocrit have been reviewed, and immune globulin has been administered, if necessary.
- The mother has received instructions on self-care, deviations from normal, and the proper response to danger signs and symptoms.
- The mother demonstrates readiness to care for herself and her baby.
- The mother has received instructions on postpartum activity, exercises, and relief measures for common postpartum discomforts.
- Arrangements have been made for postpartum care.
- Family members or other support persons are available to the mother for the first few days after discharge.

Home Care Services

New parents must be made aware of the services offered for home care. These services include information lines, follow-up telephone calls, home visits, and nurse-managed postpartum outpatient clinics. In addition, some facilities offer breastfeeding and parenting classes, "baby and me" walks or exercise sessions, and postpartum support groups.

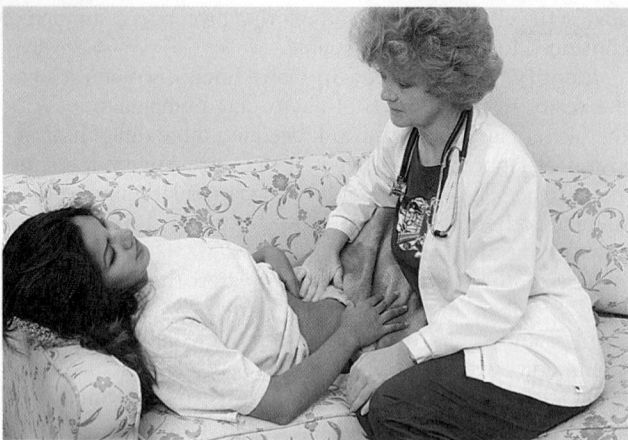

Figure 21-17 Postpartum home visits include assessments and health education. Here the nurse evaluates involution while teaching the mother how to palpate her fundus.

Information Lines

Ideally, information lines should be open 24 hours a day, 7 days a week. They should be staffed by qualified nurses who use agency protocols to respond to the family's questions. Moreover, these nurses must be prepared to triage. That is, they must be skilled at soliciting information to identify problems and at determining the priority of the problems identified.

Legal liability is a concern for all agencies and personnel who identify problems, set priorities, and provide information by telephone. Not only must the staff be educated and evaluated for the task, but protocols must also be devised, a documentation system developed, and adequate consultation or "backup" support made available.

A major disadvantage of information lines is that they rely on families to initiate a request for assistance. Not all families recognize a problem as it begins to develop and, as a result, may delay seeking information.

Telephone Calls

Some facilities initiate telephone interviews to assess new families and to provide information to families at home. The calls are usually made 1 to 3 days after discharge. As with information lines, a qualified nurse, following the facility protocol, conducts a systematic assessment of the mother and infant. The nurse solicits questions and reinforces important information. Telephone calls are relatively inexpensive. Their major disadvantage, however, is that the nurse cannot confirm the data but must rely on observations made by the family.

Home Visits

Home visits allow physical examination of the mother and infant and assessment of family adaptation and the home environment. Maternal assessment should include the breasts, fundus, lochia, perineum, and psychosocial status (Fig. 21-17). Postpartum visits can provide opportunities for further teaching. If possible, nurses should allow time to observe breastfeeding and to provide encouragement and reassurance that is badly needed during the first days before lactation is well established.

The newborn's weight, color, and elimination pattern are important parts of the home visit. Time should be allowed to reinforce previous learning, to answer questions, and to introduce new topics. Although home visits are expensive, they provide the most comprehensive nursing care.

Outpatient Clinics

Nurse-managed outpatient clinics offer another option for postpartum care. Although transportation is a problem for some families, clinic visits are less costly for the agency than home visits. Like home care, clinic visits include an examination of the mother and infant. There should be time to answer questions about maternal self-care, to provide assistance with infant feeding, and to deal with special concerns, such as care of the umbilical cord or circumcision and postpartum blues.

KEY CONCEPTS

- After childbirth, the uterus returns to its nonpregnant size and condition by involution, which involves contraction of muscle fibers, catabolic processes, and regeneration of uterine epithelium.
- The site of placental attachment heals by a process of exfoliation, which leaves the endometrium smooth and without scars.
- Involution can be evaluated by measuring the descent of the fundus (about 1 cm/day). By the 10th day after childbirth, the fundus should no longer be palpable abdominally.
- Afterpains, or intermittent uterine contractions, cause discomfort for many women, particularly multiparas who breastfeed.
- Vaginal discharge (lochia) progresses from lochia rubra, to lochia serosa, to lochia alba in a predictable time frame. Lochia should be assessed for volume, type, and odor. Foul odor suggests endometrial infection.

- Although vaginal mucosa heals within 3 weeks, it takes 6 weeks for the vagina to regain the same size and contour.
- Perineal trauma and hemorrhoids cause discomfort and can interfere with bladder and bowel elimination.
- As blood from the uteroplacental unit returns to central circulation and extracellular fluid is mobilized into the vascular compartment, the cardiac output increases and excess fluid is excreted by diuresis and diaphoresis.
- Increased clotting factors predispose the postpartum woman to clot formation. Early ambulation helps prevent thrombophlebitis.
- Constipation may occur from decreased food and fluid intake during labor, diminished bowel tone, or fear of pain during defecation.
- Increased bladder capacity and decreased sensitivity to fluid pressure may result in urinary retention. Stasis of urine allows time for

bacteria to grow and can lead to urinary tract infection.
- A distended bladder lifts and displaces the uterus. This condition can interfere with uterine contraction and result in excessive bleeding.
- Exercises to strengthen the abdominal muscles as well as good posture and body mechanics may reduce musculoskeletal discomfort.
- As hormone levels decline, the skin gradually returns to its prepregnancy state.
- Breastfeeding may delay the return of ovulation and menstruation, but it is not a reliable method of contraception. All mothers need information about family planning.
- Breastfeeding mothers are more likely to experience dyspareunia as a result of vaginal dryness that results from inadequate estrogen.
- Lactation may be suppressed by wearing a snug bra, by binding the breasts, and by avoiding stimulation of the breasts.

KEY CONCEPTS

- The postpartum woman should be afebrile. Because of exertion, dehydration, and leukocytosis, however, her temperature may be higher during the first 24 hours after delivery.
- Bradycardia is expected. Tachycardia may be caused by excitement, dehydration, hypovolemia, or infection. Additional assessments are required to determine if excessive bleeding is the cause.
- Orthostatic hypotension occurs when the mother goes from a supine to a standing position quickly.
- The common practice of early discharge challenges nurses to develop a plan for teaching self-care and infant care in a short period.
- The postcesarean woman requires postoperative as well as postpartum assessments and care. She is at increased risk for problems associated with immobility and discomfort.
- Bonding and attachment are gradual processes that begin before childbirth and

progress to feelings of love and deep devotion that last throughout life.
- Nurses foster bonding and attachment by providing early, unlimited contact between the parents and infant and by modeling attachment behaviors.
- Maternal touch changes over time as many mothers progress from exploratory "fingertipping" to enfolding and finally to demonstrating a full range of comforting behaviors.
- Verbal behaviors are important indicators of maternal attachment. Nurses often model how to speak to the infant and point out the infant's response to verbal stimulation.
- Maternal adjustment to parenthood is a gradual process that involves restorative phases. Nurses play a valuable role in the process by "mothering the mother" and fostering her independence.
- Postpartum blues, a temporary, self-limiting period of weepiness, is often ignored by the health care team. Explanations and support

can assist the mother through this distressing episode.
- Parents usually progress through four stages of role attainment (anticipatory, formal, informal, and personal) as they learn to structure their parenting behaviors to mesh with the infant's needs.
- Many women experience role conflict when they must leave the infant with a caregiver and return to work. Nurses can offer anticipatory guidance that makes the conflict less difficult.
- The birth of a baby necessitates reorganization of family structure and renegotiation of family responsibilities. Nurses can assist the father in co-parenting the infant and help the new parents identify family resources.
- Siblings feel jealousy and fear that they will be replaced by the newborn in the affection of the parents. Nurses can help by providing information about how to reduce sibling rivalry.

ANSWERS to Critical Thinking Exercise 21-1

1. The birth of a large infant increases the risk of postpartum hemorrhage. Saturation of pads in a short time suggests excessive bleeding. The location of the fundus above the umbilicus and displaced to the side indicates that the cause of excessive bleeding might be a distended bladder.

2. Assisting the mother to void is the most appropriate nursing action. If, after voiding, the

fundus is located at the level of the umbilicus and firmly contracted, the cause of the bleeding was probably a distended bladder, which made it difficult for the uterus to contract firmly. The location and consistency of the uterus, amount of lochia, blood pressure, and pulse should be assessed frequently so that further excessive bleeding can be identified and controlled.

3. Linda does not experience the urge to void because the bladder has not regained the muscle tone lost during pregnancy and the sensitivity to pressure is decreased.

ANSWERS to Critical Thinking Exercise 21-2

1. Ju-An's priority needs are for physical care and comfort. She also needs to make the experience of childbirth part of her reality by recounting the details of her birth experience to anyone who will listen and by trying to fill in the missing pieces about the cesarean birth.

2. Ju-An is in the taking-in phase. She is getting acquainted with her "real" baby by exploring with her fingertips. This is usually the first maternal touch observed.

3. Ju-An's priorities are to assume control of her own body functions and to manage her

care so that she can "take hold" and assume care of the baby.

4. Ju-An has become more independent and demonstrates readiness to learn by requesting the assistance of the lactation educator.

5. Anticipatory guidance should focus on how Ju-An can manage the care of the infant while still getting adequate rest and nutrition. A flexible schedule, resting while the infant sleeps, and preparing simple meals are some of the most important items to emphasize.

6. It would be helpful to assist her in identifying a friend or neighbor who could provide some support while her husband is away. She should have telephone numbers for community resources, such as the hospital "baby line." A follow-up telephone call or a home visit by a perinatal nurse should be scheduled, if possible. The nurse could assess both the mother and the infant, reinforce teaching, and provide encouragement.

REFERENCES and READINGS

American Academy of Pediatrics, & American College of Obstetricians and Gynecologists. (2002). *Guidelines for perinatal care* (5th ed.). Elk Grove Village, IL, and Washington, DC: Author.

American College of Obstetricians and Gynecologists. (2002). Exercise during pregnancy and the postpartum period. *Obstetrics & Gynecology*, 99(1), 171-173.

Association of Women's Health, Obstetric and Neonatal Nurses. (2003). *Standards for professional nursing practice in the care of women and newborns* (6th ed.). Washington, DC: Author.

Blackburn, S.T. (2003). *Maternal, fetal, and neonatal physiology* (2nd ed.). Philadelphia: Saunders.

Bowes, W.A., & Katz, V.L. (2002). Postpartum care. In S.G. Gabbe, J.R. Niebyl, & J.L. Simpson (Eds.), *Obstetrics, normal and problem pregnancies*

(4th ed., pp. 701-725). New York: Churchill Livingstone.

Buist, A., Morse, C.A., & Durkin, S. (2003). Men's adjustment to fatherhood: Implications for obstetrical health care. *Journal of Obstetric, Gynecologic, and Neonatal Nursing, 32*(2), 172-180.

Callister, L.C. (2001). Integrating cultural beliefs and practices into the care of childbearing women. In K.R. Simpson & P.A. Creehan,

REFERENCES and READINGS

AWHONN perinatal nursing (2nd ed., pp. 68-94). Philadelphia: Lippincott.

Centers for Disease Control and Prevention. (2001). Notice to readers: Revised ACIP recommendation for avoiding pregnancy after receiving a rubella-containing vaccine. *Morbidity and Mortality Weekly Report, 50*(49), 1117, Dec. 14, 2001.

Cesario, S.K. (2001). Care of the Native American woman: Strategies for practice, education, and research. *Journal of Obstetric, Gynecologic, & Neonatal Nursing, 30*(1), 13-19.

Cunningham, F.G., Gant, N.F., Leveno, K.J., Gilstrap, L.C., Hauth, J.C., & Wenstrom, K.D. (2001). *Williams obstetrics* (21st ed.). New York: McGraw-Hill.

Davis, R.E. (2001). The postpartum experience for Southeast Asian women in the United States. *MCN: The American Journal of Maternal/Child Nursing, 26*(4), 208-213.

Driscoll, J.W. (2001). Psychosocial adaptation to pregnancy and postpartum. In K.R. Simpson & P.A. Creehan, *AWHONN perinatal nursing* (2nd ed., pp.115-124). Philadelphia: Lippincott.

Ewy-Edwards, D. (2000). Transition to parenthood. In F.H. Nichols & S.S. Humenick, *Childbirth education: Practice, research, and theory* (2nd ed., pp. 84-113). Philadelphia: Saunders.

Gennaro, S., & Fehder, W. (2000). Health behaviors in postpartum women. *Family & Community Health, 22*(4), 16-26.

Hayashi, R.H., & Zettelmaier, M.A. (2000). Postpartum management. In S.B. Ransom, M.P. Dombrowski, S.G. McNeeley, K.S. Moghissi, & A.R. Munkarah (Eds.), *Practical strategies in obstetrics and gynecology* (pp. 321-325). Philadelphia: Saunders.

James, D.C. (2001). Postpartum care. In K.R. Simpson & P.A. Creehan, *AWHONN perinatal nursing* (2nd ed., pp. 446-472). Philadelphia: Lippincott.

Kim-Godwin, Y.S. (2003). Postpartum beliefs and practices among non-Western cultures. *MCN: The American Journal of Maternal/Child Nursing, 28*(2), 74-78.

Klaus, M., & Kennell, J. (1982). *Maternal-infant bonding.* St. Louis: Mosby.

Lawrence, R., & Lawrence, R.M. (1999). *Breastfeeding: A guide for the medical profession* (5th ed.). St. Louis: Mosby.

Logsdon, M.C. (2000). *Social support for pregnant and postpartum women.* Washington, DC: AWHONN.

Martell, L.K. (2000). Heading toward the new normal: A contemporary postpartum experience. *Journal of Obstetric, Gynecologic, and Neonatal Nursing, 30*(5), 496-506.

Martell, L.K. (2003). Postpartum women's perceptions of the hospital environment. *Journal of Obstetric, Gynecologic, and Neonatal Nursing, 32*(4), 478-485.

Matteson, P.S. (2001). *Women's health during the childbearing years: A community-based approach.* St. Louis: Mosby.

Mattson, S. (2000a). Providing culturally competent care: Strategies and approaches for perinatal clients. *AWHONN Lifelines, 4*(5), 39-41.

Mattson, S. (2000b). Ethnocultural considerations in the childbearing period. In S. Mattson & J.E. Smith (Eds.), *Core curriculum for maternal-newborn nursing* (2nd ed., pp. 70-84.). Philadelphia: Saunders.

Mattson, S. (2003). Caring for Latino women. *AWHONN Lifelines, 7*(3), 258-260.

Mercer, R.T. (1985). The process of maternal role attainment. *Nursing Research, 34*(4), 198-204.

Mercer, R.T. (1990). *Parents at risk.* New York: Springer.

Mercer, R.T. (1995a). *Becoming a mother: Research on maternal identity from Rubin to the present.* New York: Springer.

Mercer, R.T. (1995b). Predictors of maternal role attainment. *Nursing Research, 34*(4), 198-204.

Mercer, R.T., & Ferketich, S.L. (1994). Maternal-infant attachment of experienced and inexperienced mothers during infancy. *Nursing Research, 43*(6), 344-351.

Moore, M.L., & Moos, M. (2003). *Cultural competence in the care of childbearing families.* White Plains, NY: March of Dimes.

Nelson, A.M. (2003). Transition to motherhood. *Journal of Obstetric, Gynecologic, and Neonatal Nursing, 32*(4), 465-477.

Resnik, R. (1999). The puerperium. In R.K. Creasy & R. Resnik (Eds.), *Maternal-fetal medicine: Principles and practice* (4th ed., pp. 102-105). Philadelphia: Saunders.

Rubin, R. (1961). Puerperal change. *Nursing Outlook, 9*(12), 743-755.

Rubin, R. (1977). Binding-in in the postpartum period. *Maternal-Child Nursing Journal, 6*(1), 65-75.

Rubin, R. (1984). *Maternal identity and the maternal experience.* New York: Springer.

Ruchala, P.L. (2000). Teaching new mothers: Priorities of nurses and postpartum women. *Journal of Obstetric, Gynecologic, and Neonatal Nursing, 29*(3), 265-273.

Scoggin, J. (2000). Physical and psychological changes. In S. Mattson & J.E. Smith (Eds.), *Core curriculum for maternal-newborn nursing* (2nd ed., pp. 302-316). Philadelphia: Saunders.

Signorello, L.B., Harlow, B.L., Chekos, A.K., & Repke, J.T. (2001). Postpartum sexual functioning and its relationship to perineal trauma: A retrospective cohort study of primiparous women. *American Journal of Obstetrics & Gynecology, 184*(5), 881-890.

Stark, M.A. (2000). Is it difficult to concentrate during the 3rd trimester and postpartum? *Journal of Obstetric, Gynecologic, and Neonatal Nursing, 29*(4), 378-389.

Swift, K. & Janke, J. (2003). Breast binding…is it all that it's wrapped up to be? *Journal of Obstetric, Gynecologic, & Neonatal Nursing, 32*(3), 332-339.

Troy, N.W. (2003). Is the significance of postpartum fatigue being overlooked in the lives of women? *MCN: The American Journal of Maternal/Child Nursing, 28*(4), 252-257.

United States Department of Labor, Bureau of Labor Statistics. *Employment status of mothers with own children under 3 years old by single year of age of youngest child, and marital status, 2001-02 annual averages.* Retrieved August 11, 2003, from stats.bls.gov/news.release/famee.t06.htm.

Werrbach, K., & Wroblewski, M. (2003). Self-administered pain medications: A practical approach in an OB/GYN setting. *AWHONN Lifelines, 7*(2), 132-138.

Wilkerson, N.N., & Shrock, P. (2000). Sexuality in the perinatal period. In F.H. Nichols & S.S. Humenick, *Childbirth education: Practice, research, and theory* (2nd ed., pp. 48-65.) Philadelphia: Saunders.

Zuspan, K. (2000). Control of postpartum pain. In F.P. Zuspan & E.J. Quilligan (Eds.), *Current therapy in obstetrics and gynecology* (5th ed., pp. 261-263). Philadelphia: Saunders.

22

The Normal Newborn: Adaptation and Assessment

◆ LEARNING OBJECTIVES

After studying this chapter, you should be able to:

◎ Explain the physiologic changes that occur in the respiratory and cardiovascular systems during the transition from fetal to neonatal life.

◎ Describe thermoregulation in the newborn.

◎ Compare gastrointestinal functioning in the newborn and adult.

◎ Explain the causes and effects of hypoglycemia.

◎ Describe the steps in normal bilirubin excretion and the development of physiologic, pathologic, and breast milk jaundice.

◎ Describe kidney functioning in the newborn.

◎ Explain the functioning of the newborn's immune system.

◎ Describe the periods of reactivity and behavioral states of the newborn.

◎ Describe nursing assessments of the newborn.

◎ Explain the importance and the components of gestational-age assessment.

◆ DEFINITIONS

acrocyanosis Bluish discoloration of the hands and feet caused by reduced peripheral circulation.

asphyxia Insufficient oxygen and excess carbon dioxide in the blood and tissues.

bilirubin Unusable component of hemolyzed (broken down) erythrocytes.

brown fat (or brown adipose tissue) Highly vascular specialized fat found in the newborn that provides more heat than other fat when metabolized.

café au lait spots Light brown birthmarks.

caput succedaneum Area of edema over the presenting part of the fetus or newborn, resulting from pressure against the cervix. Often called simply "caput."

cephalhematoma Bleeding between the periosteum and skull from pressure during birth; does not cross suture lines.

choanal atresia Abnormality of the nasal septum that obstructs one or both nasal passages.

craniosynostosis Premature closure of the sutures of the infant's head.

cryptorchidism Failure of one or both testes to descend into the scrotum.

epispadias Abnormal placement of the urinary meatus on the dorsal side of the penis.

erythema toxicum Benign rash of unknown cause in newborns, with blotchy red areas that may have white or yellow papules or vesicles in the center.

fetal lung fluid Fluid that fills the fetal lungs, expanding the alveoli and promoting lung development.

first period of reactivity Period beginning at birth in which newborns are active and alert. It ends when the infant first falls asleep.

hyperbilirubinemia Excessive amount of bilirubin in the blood.

hypospadias Abnormal placement of the urinary meatus on the ventral side of the penis.

jaundice Yellow discoloration of the skin and sclera caused by excessive bilirubin in the blood.

lanugo Fine, soft hair covering the fetus.

milia White cysts, 1 to 2 mm in size, from distended sebaceous glands.

molding Shaping of the fetal head during movement through the birth canal.

mongolian spots Bruiselike marks that occur mostly in newborns with dark skin tones.

neutral thermal environment Environment in which body temperature is maintained without an increase in metabolic rate or oxygen use.

nevus flammeus Permanent purple birthmark; also called *port-wine stain*.

nevus vasculosus Rough, red collection of capillaries with a raised surface that disappears with time. Also called *strawberry hemangioma*.

nonshivering thermogenesis Process of heat production, without shivering, by oxidation of brown fat.

periodic breathing Cessation of breathing lasting 5 to 10 seconds without changes in color or heart rate.

point of maximum impulse Area of the chest in which the heart sounds are loudest when auscultated.

polycythemia Abnormally high number of erythrocytes.

polydactyly More than 10 digits on the hands or feet.

pseudomenstruation Vaginal bleeding in the newborn, resulting from withdrawal of placental hormones.

second period of reactivity Period after the first sleep following birth when the newborn may have an elevated pulse and respiratory rate and excessive mucus.

strabismus A turning inward ("crossing") or outward of the eyes caused by poor tone in the muscles that control eye movement.

surfactant Combination of lipoproteins produced by the lungs of the mature fetus to reduce surface tension in the alveoli, thus promoting lung expansion after birth.

syndactyly Webbing between fingers or toes.

tachypnea Respiratory rate above 60 breaths per minute in the newborn after the first hour of life.

telangiectatic nevi (stork bites, salmon patch, nevus simplex) Flat, pink areas on the nape of the neck or midforehead or over the eyelids resulting from dilation of the capillaries.

thermogenesis Heat production.

thermoregulation Maintenance of body temperature.

vernix caseosa Thick, white substance that protects the skin of the fetus.

At birth, neonates make profound physiologic changes to adapt to extrauterine life to meet their own respiratory, digestive, and regulatory needs. During nursing assessments, nurses must be aware of those changes so that they can identify behaviors signifying problems or abnormalities.

INITIATION OF RESPIRATIONS

The first vital task in newborn adaptation is the initiation of respirations. Forces occurring throughout pregnancy and during birth bring about this change.

Development of the Lungs

During fetal life, the respiratory tract produces fetal lung fluid that expands the alveoli. As the fetus nears term, production of lung fluid decreases. During labor, the fluid begins to move into the interstitial spaces, where it is absorbed. Absorption is accelerated by the process of labor and may be delayed after cesarean birth that occurs without labor. This continues throughout labor and during the early hours after birth (Blackburn, 2003).

As the lungs mature, they begin to produce surfactant—a slippery, detergent-like lipoprotein that reduces surface tension within the alveoli. Without surfactant, the alveoli collapse as the infant exhales. They must be reexpanded with each breath, greatly increasing the work of breathing. Sufficient surfactant is usually produced beginning at 34 to 36 weeks of gestation.

Causes of Respirations

Because the alveoli are collapsed, the infant's first breath requires a much larger negative pressure (suction) than subsequent breathing. Breathing is initiated by chemical, mechanical, and thermal factors that stimulate the respiratory center in the medulla of the brain and trigger respirations (Fig. 22-1).

Chemical Factors

Chemoreceptors in the carotid arteries and the aorta respond to changes in blood chemistry brought about by the hypoxia that occurs with normal birth. The decrease in blood oxygen level (PO_2) and pH and increase in blood carbon dioxide level (PCO_2) cause stimulation of the respiratory center in the medulla. A forceful contraction of the diaphragm results, causing air to enter the lungs.

Mechanical Factors

During a vaginal birth, the fetal chest is compressed by the narrow birth canal. A small amount of the fetal lung fluid is forced out of the lungs into the upper air passages and expelled during birth. When the pressure against the chest is released at birth, recoil of the chest draws a small amount of air into the lungs. This reduces the amount of negative pressure needed for the first breath after birth. Tactile stimuli and the stimulation of the sounds and lights at delivery may also aid in initiating respirations.

Thermal Factors

The temperature change that occurs with birth also stimulates the initiation of respirations. Sensors in the skin respond to this sudden change in temperature by sending impulses that stimulate the respiratory center and breathing.

Continuation of Respirations

As the alveoli expand, surfactant allows them to remain partially open between respirations. Approximately half of the air from the first breath remains in the lungs to become the functional residual capacity.

With the first cry, the pressure within the lungs increases, causing fetal lung fluid to move into the interstitial spaces, where it is absorbed by the circulatory and lymphatic systems. Although most fluid is absorbed within a few hours, complete absorption may take as long as 24 hours. Therefore the lungs may sound moist when first auscultated but become clear a short time later.

CARDIOVASCULAR ADAPTATION: TRANSITION FROM FETAL TO NEONATAL CIRCULATION

During fetal life, the *ductus arteriosus, foramen ovale,* and *ductus venosus* shunt most of the blood away from the lungs and some of the blood away from the liver. High pressures within the collapsed, fluid-filled lungs permit only a small amount of blood flow into the narrow pulmonary vessels (see Chapter 12).

At birth, the shunts close and the pulmonary vessels dilate. These changes occur in response to increases in blood oxygen, shifts in pressure within the heart and pulmonary and systemic circulations, and clamping of the umbilical cord. The changes necessary for transition from fetal to neonatal circulation occur simultaneously within the first few minutes after birth.

Ductus Arteriosus

In the fetus, the ductus arteriosus connects the pulmonary artery and the aorta. Most of the blood that enters the pulmonary artery passes into the aorta and bypasses the nonfunctioning lungs. A small amount travels to the lungs to perfuse the tissues there.

As the newborn takes the first breaths of air at birth, the rise in oxygen causes the ductus arteriosus to constrict. At the

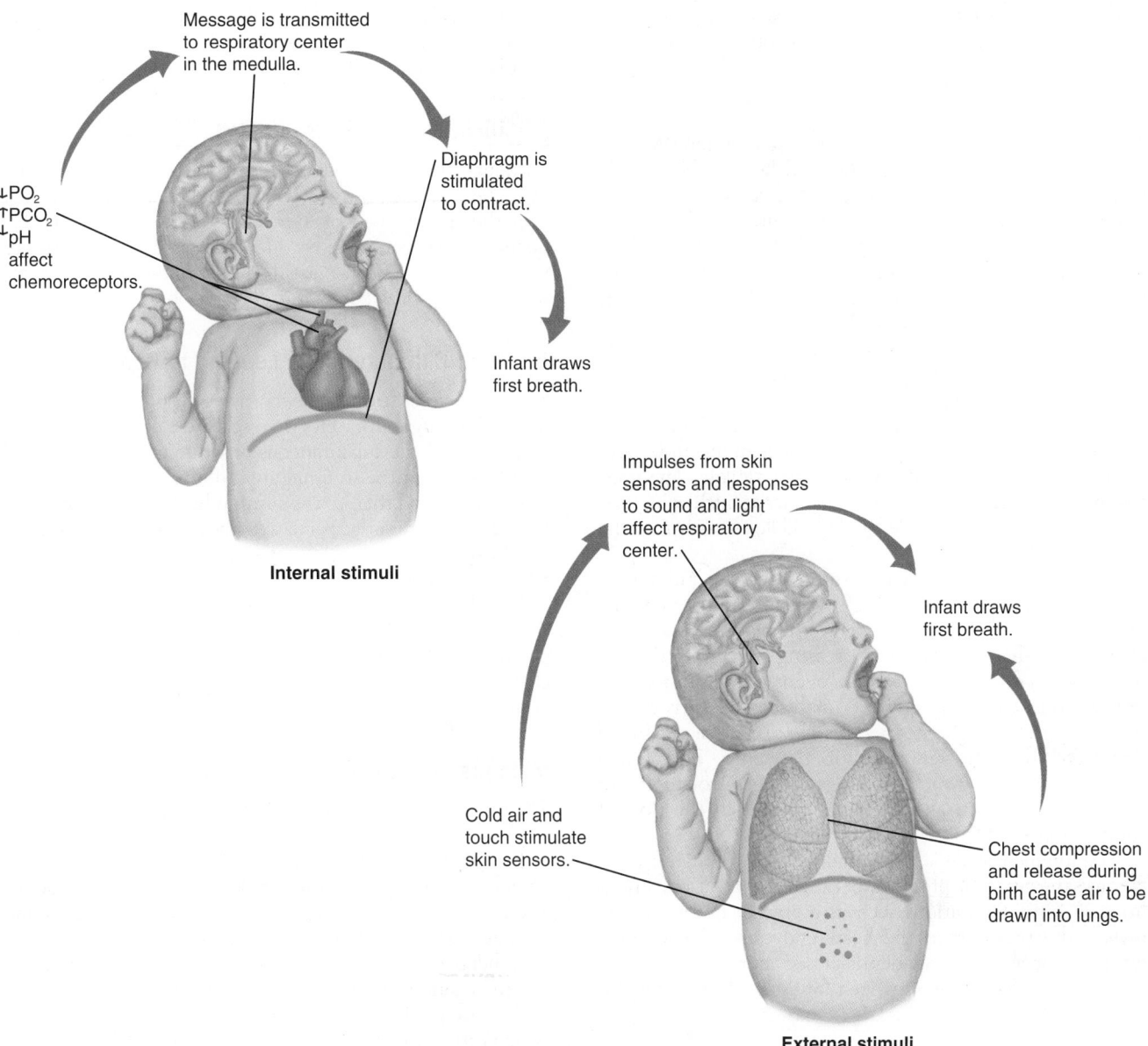

Message is transmitted
to respiratory center
in the medulla.

Diaphragm is
stimulated
to contract.

↓PO$_2$
↑PCO$_2$
↓pH
affect
chemoreceptors.

Infant draws
first breath.

Internal stimuli

Impulses from skin
sensors and responses
to sound and light
affect respiratory
center.

Infant draws
first breath.

Cold air and
touch stimulate
skin sensors.

Chest compression
and release during
birth cause air to be
drawn into lungs.

External stimuli

Figure 22-1 Internal causes of the initiation of respirations are the chemical changes that take place at birth. External causes of respirations include thermal and mechanical factors.

same time, resistance in the pulmonary circulation decreases and resistance throughout the systemic circulation increases. These responses cause blood to flow from the pulmonary artery into the lungs for oxygenation.

The ductus arteriosus closes gradually as oxygenation improves and prostaglandins from the placenta, which help keep it open, are metabolized. Functional closure occurs for most term infants within 15 to 24 hours (Lott, 2003).

Until closure is complete, the blood that does flow through the vessel reverses, moving from the aorta to the pulmonary artery and increasing blood flow to the lungs. This sequence occurs because pressure in the aorta is now higher than that in the pulmonary artery. A murmur may be heard as a result of blood flow through the partially open vessel.

The ductus arteriosus closes permanently by 3 to 4 weeks and is then called the *ligamentum arteriosum* (Lott, 2003).

Until permanent closure occurs, low levels of oxygen in the blood may cause the ductus arteriosus to dilate and the pulmonary vessels to constrict. These processes may cause a return to fetal blood flow patterns—a serious complication. A patent ductus arteriosus may occur in the infant who experiences asphyxia at birth, becomes hypoxic, or is preterm (see Chapter 46).

Pulmonary Blood Vessels

Although the ductus arteriosus constricts in response to the increased oxygenation that occurs at birth, the pulmonary blood vessels dilate. At the same time, fetal lung fluid shifts into the interstitial spaces and is removed by the blood and lymph system. These changes allow more room for dilation of the pulmonary blood vessels and decrease pulmonary vascular resistance. As a result, the vessels can expand to hold the suddenly increased blood flow from the pulmonary artery.

Foramen Ovale

The foramen ovale is a flap in the septum between the right atrium and the left atrium of the fetal heart. About 50 to 60 percent of the fairly well oxygenated blood from the inferior vena cava moves through the foramen ovale from the right atrium to the left atrium (Blackburn, 2003). Little mixing occurs with the less oxygenated blood that enters the right atrium from the superior vena cava and continues to the right ventricle. Thus most of the better oxygenated blood travels away from the nonfunctioning fetal lungs to the aorta and the vessels of the heart and the head.

The foramen ovale opens only from right to left. The higher pressure in the right side of the heart from the restricted flow of blood to the lungs during fetal life allows this right-to-left shunting through the foramen ovale. The pressure in the right side of the heart decreases at birth, when the umbilical vessels are occluded and blood flows easily into the pulmonary circulation.

As blood enters the left atrium from the pulmonary veins, pressure in the left side of the heart builds. Systemic resistance increases as blood flow to the placenta ends with clamping of the cord, further increasing pressure in the left heart. Because the foramen ovale opens only from right to left, it closes when the pressure in the left heart is higher than that in the right heart. This change increases blood flow from the right ventricle into the lungs. Thus blood flow through the heart and lungs changes from fetal to neonatal circulation and is similar to that in the normal adult (see Fig. 12-9).

The foramen ovale is functionally closed soon after birth because the unequal pressures between the atria prevent it from opening. Conditions such as asphyxia, however, may reverse the pressures in the heart and cause the foramen ovale to reopen. It is permanently closed after several months in most infants but may stay open for 9 months or longer in some infants (Blackburn, 2003).

Ductus Venosus

During fetal life, it is not necessary for the liver to filter the blood. The ductus venosus directs about a third of the blood flow from the umbilical vein away from the liver and directly to the inferior vena cava. Near the end of pregnancy, the liver needs more perfusion and 70% to 80% of the oxygenated blood goes to the liver instead of the ductus venosus (Blackburn 2003). It then enters the inferior vena cava and mixes with blood from the lower part of the fetal body to travel to the heart.

After birth, very little blood enters the ductus venosus and the vessel constricts. Fibrosis of the ductus venosus occurs by 7 to 14 days after birth (Lott, 2003).

NEUROLOGIC ADAPTATION: THERMOREGULATION

Although the fetus produces heat in utero, the consistently warm temperature of the amniotic fluid makes thermoregulation, the maintenance of body temperature, unnecessary. The neonate, however, must produce and maintain heat to prevent the serious effects of cold stress when it moves from the warm uterus to the cooler outside environment.

Newborn Characteristics Leading to Heat Loss

Some characteristics of newborns predispose them to lose heat. The skin is thin, blood vessels are close to the surface, and there is little subcutaneous or white fat. Heat is readily transferred from the internal areas of the body to the cooler skin surfaces and then to the surrounding air. Newborns have three times more surface area to body mass than the adult and lose heat at a rate four times greater than adults do (Stoll & Kliegman, 2004b).

The flexed position of the healthy, full-term infant reduces the amount of skin surface exposed to the surrounding temperatures and decreases heat loss. Because of decreased muscle tone, the sick or preterm infant does not maintain a flexed position.

Methods of Heat Loss

The four methods of heat loss in the neonate are (Fig. 22-2):

- *Evaporation:* Air-drying of the skin that results in cooling. Insensible water loss from the skin and respiratory tract increases heat loss by evaporation. Drying the infant immediately when wet helps prevent loss of heat.
- *Conduction:* Movement of heat away from the body occurs when newborns come in direct contact with objects that are cooler than their skin. Contact with warm objects increases body heat by conduction. Warming objects that will touch the infant or placing the unclothed infant against the mother's skin prevents conductive heat loss.
- *Convection:* Transfer of heat to the air surrounding the infant. Providing a warm, draft-free environment avoids convective heat loss.
- *Radiation:* Heat transfer to cooler objects that are not in direct contact with the infant. Placing cribs away from outside windows helps avoid this type of heat loss. Using a radiant heater transfers warmth from the heater to the cooler infant.

Nonshivering Thermogenesis

When newborns become cold they get restless, which increases flexion and activity to help maintain heat. Vasoconstriction occurs to decrease heat loss, and body metabolism increases. Acrocyanosis may result. Shivering, however, is not an effective method of heat production for newborns. Instead, nonshivering thermogenesis is used when the infant becomes cold.

CRITICAL THINKING EXERCISE 22-1

Understanding the changes that occur during the transition from fetal to neonatal circulation helps in predicting the effect on blood flow of various defects in the heart. What would be the effect on blood flow of an opening in the septum of the atria of the heart?

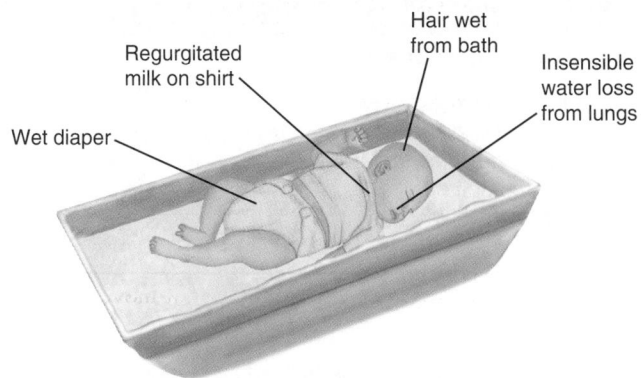

Evaporation can occur during birth or bathing from moisture on skin, as a result of wet linens or clothes, and from insensible loss.

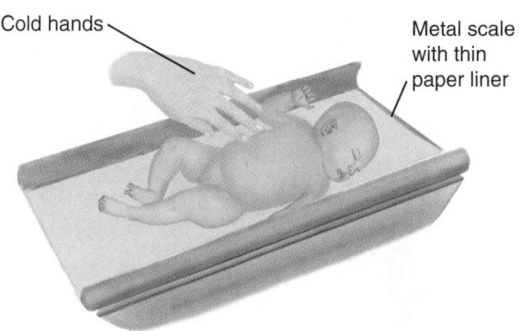

Conduction occurs when the infant comes in contact with cold objects or surfaces such as a scale, a circumcision restraint board, cold hands, or a stethoscope.

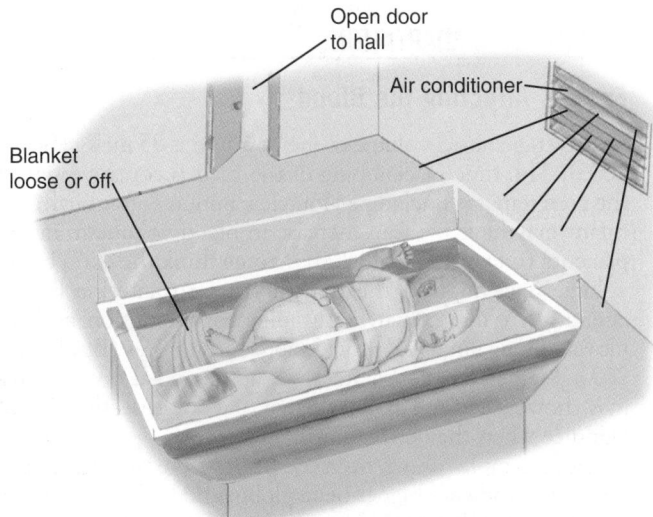

Convection occurs when drafts come from open doors, air conditioning, or even air currents created by people moving about.

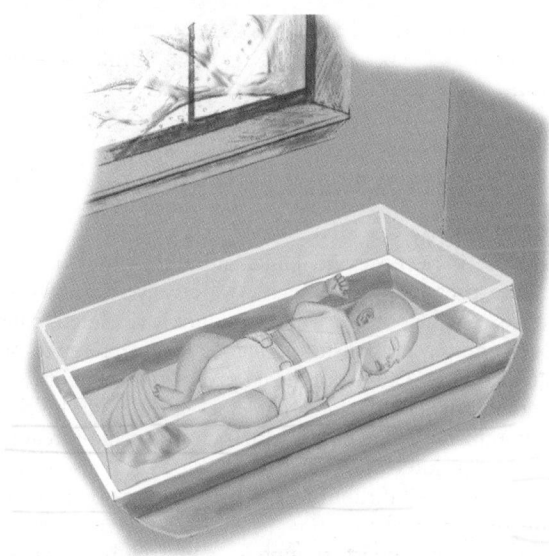

Heat is lost by radiation when the infant is near cold surfaces. Thus, heat is lost from the infant's body to the sides of the crib or incubator and to the outside walls and windows.

Figure 22-2 Methods of heat loss.

Nonshivering thermogenesis is the oxidation of brown fat (also called *brown adipose tissue*) to produce heat. This highly vascular fat is located primarily around the back of the neck; in the axillae; around the kidneys, adrenals, and sternum; between the scapula; and along the abdominal aorta (Fig. 22-3). As brown fat is metabolized, it generates more heat than white subcutaneous fat. Blood passing through brown fat is warmed and carries heat to the rest of the body.

Nonshivering thermogenesis begins when thermal receptors in the skin detect a drop in skin temperature. Thermal receptor stimulation causes release of norepinephrine, which initiates metabolism of brown fat. The process goes into effect even before a change occurs in core or interior body temperature, as measured with a rectal thermometer. Therefore nonshivering thermogenesis may begin in an infant when skin temperature is cool, even though a temperature taken rectally shows a normal reading. A decreased core tempera-ture will not occur until nonshivering thermogenesis is no longer effective.

Preterm infants and those with intrauterine growth restriction may have inadequate brown fat stores. These infants are not able to raise their body temperature if they are subjected to cold stress and may have serious complications. Hypoxia, hypoglycemia, and acidosis may interfere with the infant's ability to generate heat.

Effects of Cold Stress

Cold stress causes many body changes (Fig. 22-4). An increase in metabolic rate can lead to a significant rise in the need for oxygen. If an infant is having even mild respiratory distress, the problem may be increased as oxygen is used for heat production. Cold stress also causes diminished production of surfactant, impeding lung expansion and leading to more respiratory distress.

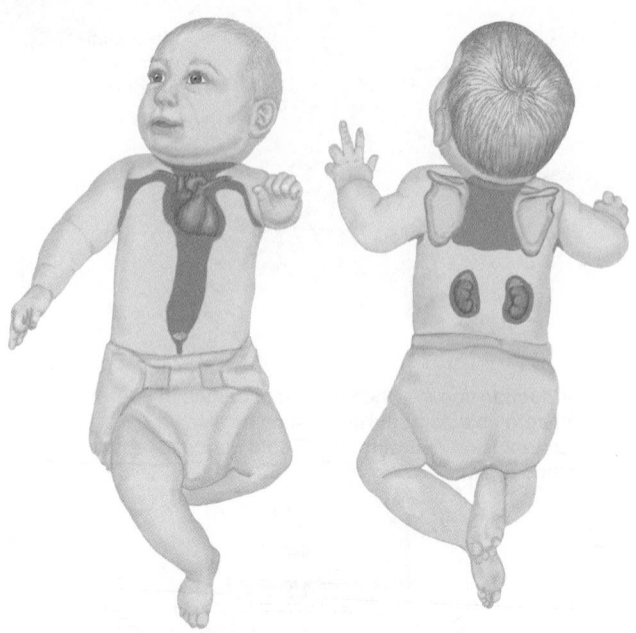

Figure 22-3 Sites of brown fat in the neonate.

Glucose is necessary in larger amounts when the metabolic rate rises to produce heat. When glycogen stores are converted to glucose, they may be quickly depleted, causing hypoglycemia. Metabolism of glucose in the presence of insufficient oxygen causes increased production of acids.

Metabolism of brown fat also releases fatty acids. This release can cause metabolic acidosis, which can be a life-threatening condition. Elevated fatty acids in the blood can also interfere with transport of bilirubin to the liver, increasing the risk of jaundice.

As the infant's body attempts to conserve heat, vasoconstriction of the peripheral blood vessels occurs to reduce heat loss from the skin's surface. Decreased oxygen levels in the blood, however, may also cause vasoconstriction of the pulmonary vessels. This may result in a shunting of blood from the left to the right side of the heart, further increasing respiratory distress.

Neutral Thermal Environment

A neutral thermal environment is one in which the infant can maintain a stable body temperature without an increase in oxygen consumption or metabolic rate. The range of environmental temperature that allows this maintenance is called the *thermoneutral zone.* In healthy full-term newborns, an environmental temperature of 32° to 33.5° C (89.6° to 92.3° F) provides a thermoneutral zone (Blackburn, 2003).

Hyperthermia

Infants also respond poorly to hyperthermia. With an elevated temperature, the metabolic rate rises, causing an increased need for oxygen and glucose. In addition, vasodilation leads to increased insensible fluid losses. Sweating may occur but is often delayed because sweat glands are immature.

Newborns may be overheated by poorly regulated equipment designed to keep them warm. When infants are under

---

> **! CRITICAL TO REMEMBER**
>
> **Hazards of Cold Stress**
>
> - Increased oxygen need
> - Respiratory distress
> - Decreased surfactant production
> - Hypoglycemia
> - Metabolic acidosis
> - Jaundice

radiant warmers, warming lights, or in warmed incubators, the temperature mechanism must be set to vary the heat according to the infant's skin temperature and thus prevent heat that is too high or too low. Alarms to signal that the infant's temperature is too high or too low should be functioning properly.

HEMATOLOGIC ADAPTATION

Factors Affecting the Blood

The average blood volume of the newborn is 85 ml/kg (Shaw, 2003). The time of clamping of the cord is controversial. If the cord remains unclamped for a few minutes after birth, the infant may have a 75-ml increase in blood volume from the placenta (Guyton & Hall, 2001). Some think the extra blood volume may improve the transition to extrauterine life by opening the lungs, increasing pulmonary perfusion and removal of lung fluid, and provide added iron stores (Blackburn, 2003; Mercer & Skovgaard, 2002). The added erythrocytes may, however, cause polycythemia and increase the risk of jaundice when they break down.

Blood samples drawn from the heel, where the circulation is sluggish, indicate higher hemoglobin and hematocrit levels than samples taken from central areas. Venous blood samples are more accurate and are taken when precise measurement is essential. (Newborn laboratory values for common tests are listed in Appendix A.)

Blood Values

Erythrocytes and Hemoglobin

At birth, the infant has comparatively more erythrocytes (red blood cells) and higher hemoglobin and hematocrit levels than the adult. This difference is necessary because the partial pressure of oxygen of fetal blood is much lower than the normal adult level. The large number of erythrocytes and higher hemoglobin level enable the fetal cells to receive enough oxygen. Adequate oxygenation to the cells is also possible because fetal hemoglobin (hemoglobin F) carries 20% to 50% more oxygen than adult hemoglobin (Guyton & Hall, 2001).

Erythrocytes in the newborn have a shorter life span than those of the adult. Excess bilirubin caused by the breakdown of large numbers of red blood cells may lead to jaundice.

Hematocrit

The hematocrit level in the normal infant is 48% to 69% from peripheral sites (Nicholson & Pesce, 2004). A level above 65% from a central site indicates polycythemia—an

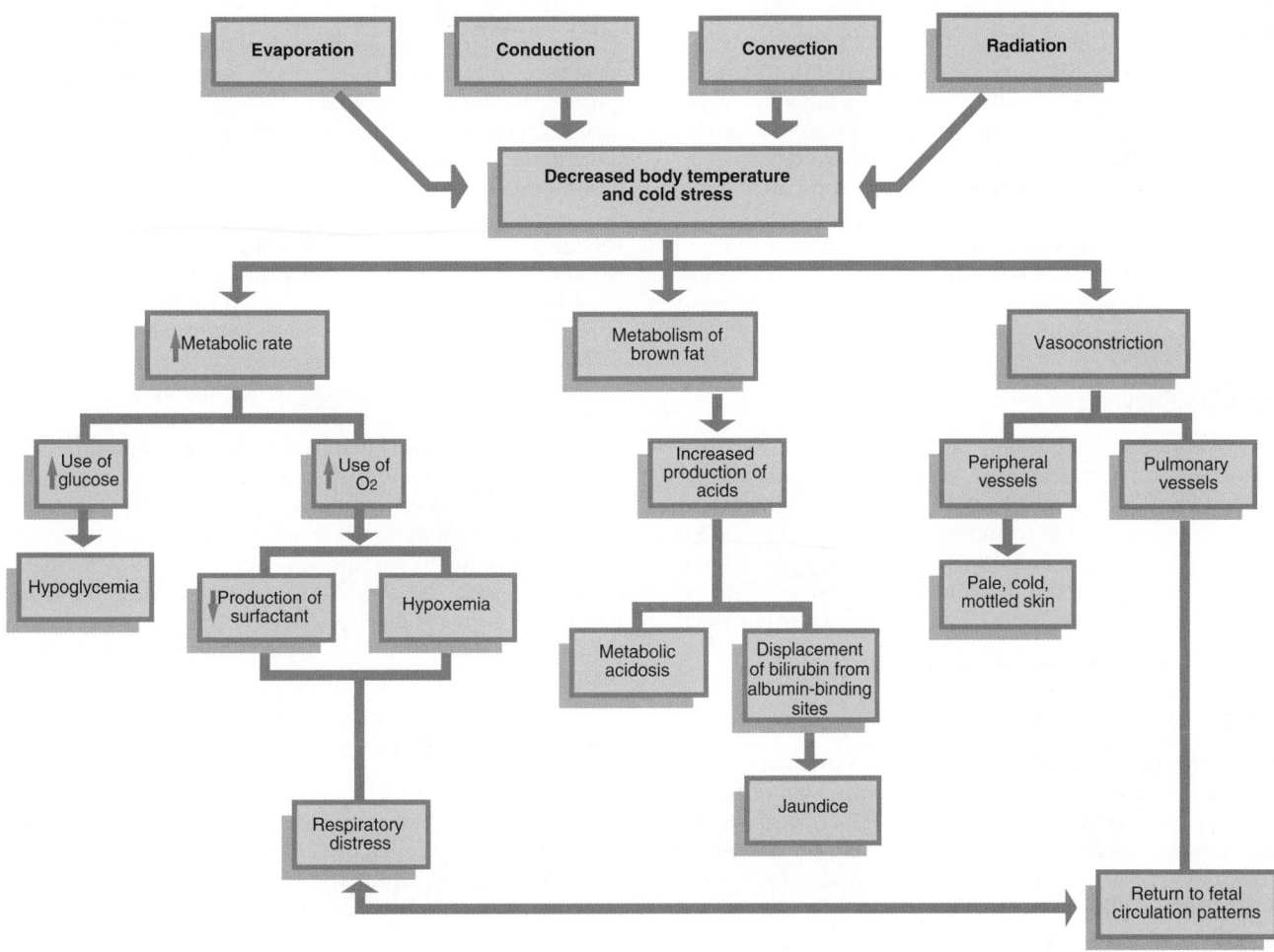

Figure 22-4 Effects of cold stress.

abnormally high erythrocyte count. Polycythemia increases the risk of jaundice and damage to the brain and other organs as a result of blood stasis. Respiratory distress and hypoglycemia are more common in these infants. Hematocrit testing is not necessary unless the infant has risk factors or signs of polycythemia or anemia (American Academy of Pediatricians [AAP] & American College of Obstetricians and Gynecologists [ACOG], 2002).

Leukocytes

In newborns, an elevated white blood cell (leukocyte) count does not necessarily indicate infection. In fact, the white blood cell count may decrease in infections. The leukocytes normally rise during the first 12 hours and then decline slowly (Shaw, 2003). Increased numbers of immature leukocytes are a sign of infection or sepsis. Platelets (thrombocytes) may also decrease as a result of infections.

Risk of Clotting Deficiency

Although platelet counts in term newborns are near adult levels, platelet response to stimuli is decreased during the first few days of life. Newborns lack vitamin K, which is necessary to activate several of the clotting factors (factors II [prothrombin], VII, IX, and X). Vitamin K is synthesized in the intestines, but food and normal intestinal flora are necessary for this process. To decrease the risk of hemorrhagic disease of the newborn, vitamin K is administered intramuscularly to most newborns. Drugs such as phenytoin (Dilantin), phenobarbital, and aspirin taken by the mother during pregnancy interfere with clotting ability in the infant after birth.

GASTROINTESTINAL SYSTEM

Stomach

The newborn's stomach capacity is approximately 6 ml/kg at birth (Blackburn, 2003) but expands to approximately 90 ml within the first week. Gastric emptying may be delayed at first. It is more rapid after ingestion of human milk and slower if the infant has swallowed mucus. The gastrocolic reflex is stimulated when the stomach fills, causing increased intestinal peristalsis. Infants frequently pass a stool during or after a feeding. The cardiac sphincter between the esophagus and the stomach is relaxed, which explains the newborn's tendency to regurgitate feedings easily.

Intestines

The newborn's intestines are long in proportion to the infant's size and compared with those of the adult. The added length allows more surface area for absorption, but it also makes infants more prone to water loss should diarrhea develop. Air enters the gastrointestinal tract soon after birth, and bowel sounds are present within the first hour.

The digestive tract is sterile at birth. Once the infant is exposed to the external environment and begins to take in fluids, however, bacteria enter the gastrointestinal tract. Normal intestinal flora is established within the first few days of life.

Digestive Enzymes

The newborn can digest simple carbohydrates but is deficient in pancreatic amylase and lipase. Amylase is needed to digest complex carbohydrates such as those in cereal. Sufficient amylase is present at 3 to 6 months of age. Lipase, needed for fat digestion, is present in breast milk and may make it more digestible for the newborn than formula. Protein and lactose, the major carbohydrate in the infant's milk diet, are both well digested.

Stools

Meconium is the first stool excreted by the newborn. It consists of particles from amniotic fluid such as vernix, skin cells, and hair, along with cells shed from the intestinal tract, bile, and other intestinal secretions. Meconium is greenish black with a thick, sticky, tar-like consistency. The first meconium stool is usually passed within 12 hours of birth, and 99% of newborns have the first stool within 48 hours (Stoll & Kliegman, 2000b). If meconium is not passed within that time, obstruction is suspected.

Meconium stools are followed by transitional stools, which are greenish brown and of a looser consistency than meconium. They are followed by milk stools that are characteristic of the type of feeding that the infant receives.

The stools of infants fed with breast milk are seedy and have the color and consistency of mustard with a sweet-sour smell. The breastfed infant in general has more frequent stools than the infant who is formula-fed. Breastfed newborns excrete as many as 10 small stools each day, although some older infants pass only one stool every 2 to 3 days. The normal breastfed newborn should have at least three or more stools daily after the first few days.

The formula-fed infant excretes pale-yellow to light-brown stools. They are firmer in consistency than those of the breastfed infant. The infant may excrete several stools daily, or only one or two. The stools have the characteristic odor of feces.

HEPATIC SYSTEM

Liver functions include maintenance of blood glucose levels, conjugation of bilirubin, production of factors necessary for blood coagulation, storage of iron, and metabolism of drugs.

Blood Glucose Maintenance

During the last 4 to 8 weeks of pregnancy, glucose is stored in the fetal liver as glycogen for use after birth. Glucose is used rapidly in the newborn for energy during the stress of delivery and for breathing, heat production, movement against gravity, and activation of all the functions that the neonate must take on at birth. The brain requires a constant supply of glucose, or damage may result.

Until newborn feedings are adequate to meet energy requirements, stored glycogen is converted by the liver to glucose for use. In the term infant, blood glucose levels should be 40 to 60 mg/dl on the first day and 50 to 90 mg/dl thereafter (Nicholson & Pesce, 2004). There is no general consensus for the level of blood glucose that defines hypoglycemia, but a level below 40 to 45 mg/dl in the term infant is often used (Blackburn, 2003; McGowan, Hagedorn, & Hay, 2002).

Many newborns are at increased risk for hypoglycemia. In the preterm and small-for-gestational-age infant, adequate stores of glycogen may not have accumulated. Stores may be used up before birth in the post-term infant because of poor intrauterine nourishment from a deteriorating placenta. Large-for-gestational-age infants and those with diabetic mothers may produce excessive insulin that consumes available glucose quickly (see Chapter 30). Infants exposed to such stressors as asphyxia or infection may exhaust their stores of glycogen. Newborns who are cold may deplete glycogen to increase metabolism and raise body temperature.

Conjugation of Bilirubin

A major function of the liver is the conjugation of bilirubin (Fig. 22-5). The newborn's liver may not be mature enough to prevent the development of jaundice during the first week of life. Jaundice occurs in 60% of term newborns and 80% of preterm infants (Stoll & Kliegman, 2004a).

Source and Effect of Bilirubin

The principal source of bilirubin is the hemolysis of erythrocytes. This is a normal occurrence after birth, when fewer erythrocytes are needed than during fetal life. Bilirubin is toxic to the body and must be excreted.

Bilirubin is released in an unconjugated form. Unconjugated bilirubin, also called *indirect bilirubin*, is not soluble in water. Before excretion can occur, the liver must change it to a water-soluble form by a process called *conjugation*. The bilirubin is then known as *conjugated* or *direct bilirubin*.

Because unconjugated bilirubin is fat-soluble, it may be absorbed by the subcutaneous fat, causing the yellowish discoloration of the skin called *jaundice*. If enough unconjugated bilirubin accumulates in the blood, staining of the tissues in the brain may occur. This condition, known as *kernicterus*, may result in bilirubin encephalopathy, which may cause severe brain damage.

Normal Conjugation

When unconjugated bilirubin is released into the bloodstream, it attaches to binding sites on albumin in the plasma and is carried to the liver. There, the enzyme *glucuronyl transferase* changes the bilirubin to the conjugated form. Conjugated bilirubin is excreted into the bile and then into the duodenum. In the intestines, the normal flora acts on bilirubin to reduce it to urobilinogen and stercobilin, which are excreted in the stool. A small amount of urobilinogen is excreted by the kidneys.

A small percentage of conjugated bilirubin may be converted back to the unconjugated state by the intestinal en-

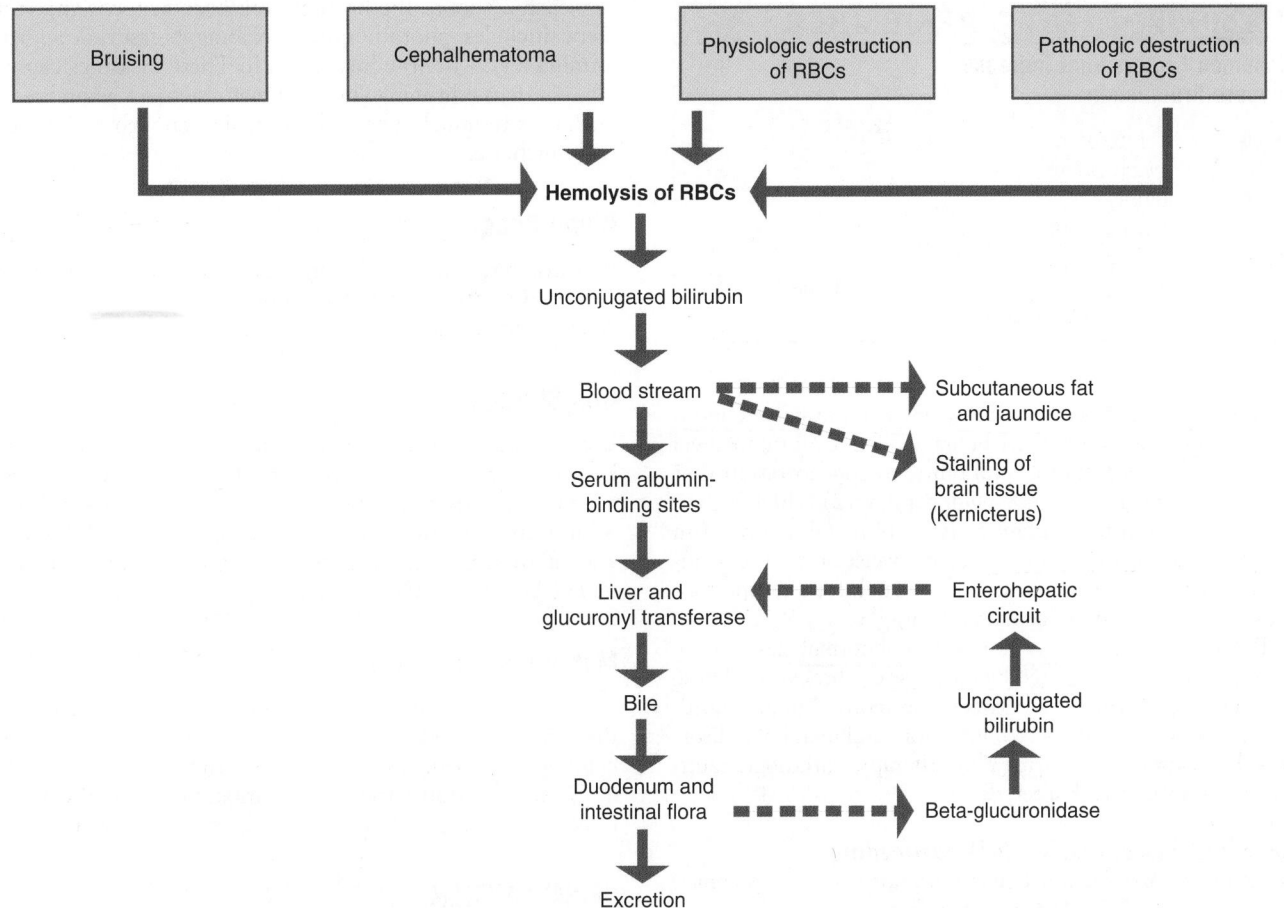

Figure 22-5 Sources of bilirubin and how it is removed from the body.

zyme *beta-glucuronidase*. The deconjugated bilirubin is absorbed into the bloodstream and carried back to the liver, where it once again undergoes the conjugation process. This recirculation of bilirubin is called the *enterohepatic circuit*.

Factors in Increased Bilirubin

Factors that result in an increased incidence of jaundice in the first week of life include:

- *Excess production:* Bilirubin is produced in infants during the first 2 weeks of life at a rate 2½ times that of adults (Maisels, 2001).
- *Red blood cell life:* Fetal red blood cells break down more quickly than do adult erythrocytes.
- *Liver immaturity:* The newborn's immature liver may not produce adequate amounts of glucuronyl transferase and other substances during the first few days of life. This limits the amount of bilirubin that can be conjugated.
- *Intestinal factors:* Conjugated bilirubin cannot be reduced to urobilinogen or stercobilin for excretion until intestinal flora is established. Large amounts of the enzyme *beta-glucuronidase* change bilirubin back to the unconjugated state.
- *Delayed feeding:* When feedings are delayed or taken poorly, normal intestinal flora is not established, and passage of meconium, which is high in bilirubin, is delayed. Delayed feedings may therefore allow more time in the intestine for conjugated bilirubin to be deconjugated by beta glucuronidase.

- *Trauma:* Trauma during birth (bruising, cephalhematoma) causes increased hemolysis of red blood cells.
- *Fatty acids:* Fatty acids have a greater affinity than bilirubin for the binding sites on albumin and bind to albumin in place of bilirubin. Cold stress or asphyxia may increase circulating fatty acids.

Hyperbilirubinemia

Physiologic Jaundice

Physiologic jaundice is also called *nonpathologic* or *developmental jaundice*. It is caused by transient hyperbilirubinemia and is considered normal. It is not present during the first 24 hours of life but appears on the 2nd or 3rd day after birth. Jaundice becomes visible when the serum bilirubin reaches 5 to 7 mg/dl. In physiologic jaundice, the serum bilirubin peaks at 5 to 6 mg/dl between the 2nd and 4th day of life. The bilirubin then begins to fall, declining to adult levels of 1 mg/dl by 10 to 14 days of age (Stoll & Kliegman, 2004a). Bilirubin normally rises higher and falls more slowly in Asian infants.

Pathologic Jaundice

Physiologic jaundice must be differentiated from pathologic jaundice, which is abnormal and requires further investigation. One of the most important differences is the time at which the jaundice appears. Pathologic jaundice may occur

! CRITICAL TO REMEMBER

Common Factors That Increase Hyperbilirubinemia

- Hemolysis of excessive erythrocytes
- Short red blood cell life
- Liver immaturity
- Lack of intestinal flora
- Delayed feeding
- Trauma resulting in bruising or cephalhematoma
- Fatty acids from cold stress or asphyxia

during the first 24 hours after birth, whereas physiologic jaundice begins after the first 24 hours. A direct bilirubin level that is above 2 mg/dl or a total bilirubin concentration that (1) increases by more than 5 mg/dl per day, (2) is higher than 12 mg/dl in a full-term infant or 10 to 14 mg/dl in a preterm infant, or (3) persists after the second week of life is considered pathologic and should lead to a search for a nonphysiologic cause (Stoll &, Kliegman, 2004a).

Pathologic jaundice is the result of abnormalities causing excessive destruction of red blood cells (erythrocytes). These include incompatibilities between the mother's and infant's blood types (see Chapter 26), infection, and metabolic disorders. It is often treated with phototherapy. Pathologic jaundice is discussed in Chapter 30.

Jaundice Associated With Breastfeeding

More than 50% of breastfed infants develop jaundice (Halamek & Stevenson, 2002). Jaundice may begin early or late after birth.

Early-Onset Breast Milk Jaundice. Bilirubin levels above 12 mg/dl develop in 13% of breastfed infants by 1 week of age (Stoll & Kliegman, 2004a). The most common cause of jaundice in breastfed infants is insufficient intake, often called *early-onset jaundice* or *breastfeeding jaundice*. Jaundice begins within the first week of life, and serum bilirubin may rise above 12 mg/dl and reach dangerous levels if intake is not increased.

Infants who are sleepy, have a poor suck, or nurse infrequently may not receive enough colostrum, the substance that precedes true breast milk, to take advantage of its normal laxative effect in eliminating bilirubin-rich meconium. Lack of adequate suckling depresses production of breast milk and increases the problem further. Helping the mother with breastfeeding to increase intake and stimulate milk production is the most important treatment. If this is not possible, temporary supplementing with formula is necessary. Glucose water will not reduce bilirubin levels and should be avoided.

True Breast Milk Jaundice. True breast milk jaundice, also called *late-onset breast milk jaundice*, occurs after the first 3 to 5 days of life. The serum bilirubin usually peaks at 5 to 10 mg/dl at approximately 2 weeks, but some infants (fewer than 1%) reach levels over 20 mg/dl. Serum bilirubin falls gradually over several months (Halamek & Stevenson, 2002). The exact cause of breast milk jaundice is unknown. Substances in the breast milk may increase absorption of bilirubin from the intestine, but the exact cause is unknown. This may be a form of physiologic jaundice in breastfed infants.

Treatment of breast milk jaundice includes close monitoring of serum bilirubin in the blood and at least 8 to 10 feedings each 24 hours. If bilirubin levels become too high, treatment includes phototherapy, replacing breastfeeding with formula for 24 to 48 hours, or both. These measures cause a rapid drop in bilirubin. The level may rise again when breastfeeding is resumed but usually not high enough to interfere with further breastfeeding.

Blood Coagulation

Prothrombin and coagulation factors II, VII, IX, and X are produced by the liver and activated by vitamin K, which is deficient in the newborn (see p. 511).

Iron Storage

Iron is stored in the liver during the last weeks of pregnancy. Full-term infants who are breastfeeding usually do not need added iron until 6 months of age. At that time, they should begin iron-containing foods or iron supplements. All infants who are not breastfeeding should be given iron-fortified formula (AAP & ACOG, 2002).

Metabolism of Drugs

The liver metabolizes drugs inefficiently in the newborn. Breastfeeding mothers should alert their primary caregiver before taking medications, because harmful amounts of some drugs may be transferred to the infant through the breast milk.

URINARY SYSTEM

Kidney Development

The kidneys are completely developed at 35 weeks of gestation. Full kidney function, however, does not occur until after birth. Blood flow to the kidneys increases after birth because of decreased resistance in the renal vessels. The improved perfusion results in a steady improvement in kidney function during the first few days of life.

Kidney Function

The newborn's kidney function is immature compared with that of the adult. The ability of the glomeruli to filter and the renal tubules to reabsorb is considerably less than in adults. The glomerular filtration rate doubles during the first weeks of life but does not reach adult levels until 1 to 2 years of age (Swinford, Bonilla-Felix, Cerda, & Portman, 2002). Therefore infants have a decreased ability to remove waste products from the blood.

Small amounts of substances such as glucose and protein may escape into the urine of the neonate. They disappear within the first few days of life as kidney function improves. Urate crystals may give a pink color to the urine that is sometimes mistaken for blood.

Voiding occurs by 12 to 24 hours of birth in most newborns (Stoll & Kliegman, 2004b). Absence of kidneys or anomalies that interfere with excretion of urine are usually discovered before birth because they cause low amniotic fluid volume. Only one or two voidings may occur during the first 2 days of life. The infant voids at least 6 times a day by the 4th day.

! CRITICAL TO REMEMBER

Intake and Output in the Newborn

First 2 Days of Life

Intake: 40 to 60 ml/kg (18-27 ml/lb) a day
Output: At least 1 to 2 voids

After the First 2 Days

Intake: 100 to 150 ml/kg (45-68 ml/lb) a day
Output: At least 6 voids by the 4th day

Fluid Balance

Newborns have a lower tolerance for changes in total volume of body fluid than do older infants. In addition, the fluid turnover rate is greater than that in adults. To maintain fluid balance, full-term infants need 40 to 60 ml/kg (18-27 ml/lb) daily during the first 2 days of life and then 100 to 150 ml/kg (45-68 ml/lb) a day (Tsang, DeMarini, & Rath, 2003). For example, an infant who weighs 3.4 kg (7^1/$_2$ lb) on the 3rd day of life needs 340 to 510 ml of fluid each day.

Water Distribution

Seventy-eight percent of the newborn's body is composed of water, which is distributed differently from the distribution in the adult. The percentage of extracellular water in newborns is more than twice as high as in adults. Because infants have more fluid for their size than adults and because a larger proportion of it is located outside the cells, total body water is easily depleted. Conditions such as vomiting and diarrhea can quickly result in life-threatening dehydration.

Insensible Water Loss

Water lost from the skin and respiratory tract contributes to insensible water loss. The newborn's large body surface area and rapid respiratory rate cause increased insensible water loss. Fluid losses increase greatly when infants are placed under radiant heaters, which accelerate evaporation from the skin. An elevated respiratory rate or low humidity in the air surrounding the infant raises insensible water losses even further.

Urine Dilution and Concentration

The ability of a newborn's kidneys to dilute urine is similar to that of adults, to a specific gravity of 1.001 to 1.005 (Swinford et al., 2002). A newborn's kidneys, however, cannot handle large increases in fluids, which result in fluid overload. This is most likely to happen if infants receive too much intravenous fluid. Normal urine output is 1 to 3 ml/kg/hr (Brodsky & Martin, 2003).

Because they have only half the adult's ability to excrete concentrated urine, newborns have more difficulty preventing loss of fluid in the urine than do adults (Blackburn, 2003; Guyton & Hall, 2001). Neonates can concentrate urine only to a specific gravity of 1.015 to 1.020 (Swinford et al, 2002), compared with the adult level of 1.040. The newborn's limited ability to conserve water may result in dehydration more quickly than in the older infant or child.

Acid-Base and Electrolyte Balance

The maintenance of acid-base and electrolyte balance is a primary function of the kidneys and may be precarious in neonates. Newborns tend to lose bicarbonate at lower levels than adults, increasing their risk for acidosis. The excretion of solutes is less efficient in newborns as well. Although newborns conserve needed sodium well, they are less able to excrete sodium efficiently if they receive excessive amounts.

IMMUNE SYSTEM

The neonate is less effective in fighting off infection than the older infant or child. Leukocytes are delayed in moving to the site of invasion and are not efficient in destroying the invader. The infant's decreased ability to localize infection leads to a tendency toward generalized sepsis. Fever and leukocytosis, which occur during infection of the older child, are often not present in the newborn with infection. This lack of response is the result of immaturity of the hypothalamus and the inflammatory response.

Because of their immature immune system, infants are susceptible to pathogens such as Group B streptococci and *Escherichia coli* that do not usually affect older children. Full-term newborns received antibodies from the mother during the last trimester of pregnancy. If the mother breastfeeds, the infant continues to receive antibodies in breast milk that provide passive immunity to the infant. Immunoglobulins (serum globulins with antibody activity) help protect the newborn from infection. The major immunoglobulins are IgG, IgM, and IgA.

IgG

IgG crosses the placenta readily and provides the fetus with passive temporary immunity to bacteria, bacterial toxins, and viruses to which the mother has immunity. It is the only immunoglobulin that crosses the placenta. Preterm infants have less IgG because transfer is greatest during the third trimester. The full term infant has IgG levels near those of the mother.

Although the fetus begins to make IgG at 20 weeks of gestation, production at significant levels is delayed until after 6 months of age (Blackburn, 2003). The passive immunity from the mother gradually disappears over the first 6 to 8 months of life (Buckley, 2004).

IgM

IgM helps protect against gram-negative bacteria. Production increases rapidly a few days after birth and reaches adult levels at 1 year of age (Buckley, 2004). IgM is not actively transported across the placenta because the molecules are too large. If IgM is found in larger-than-normal amounts in the neonate, exposure to infection in utero is probable.

IgA

IgA does not cross the placenta and must be produced by the infant. Because IgA is important in protection of the gastrointestinal and respiratory systems, newborns are particularly susceptible to infections of those systems. A form of IgA is included in colostrum and breast milk. Therefore breastfed infants receive protection that formula-fed infants do not.

PSYCHOSOCIAL ADAPTATION

Periods of Reactivity

In the early hours after birth, the infant goes through changes called *periods of reactivity*. There are two periods of reactivity, separated by a period of sleep.

First Period of Reactivity

The first period of reactivity begins at birth. Infants are wide awake and alert and appear interested in their surroundings. Parents enjoy this phase, as the infant gazes directly at them when held in the *en face* (face-to-face) position. Infants move their arms and legs energetically, root, and appear hungry. If allowed to nurse, many infants latch on to the nipple and suck well.

Respirations during the first period of reactivity may be as high as 80 breaths per minute. The heart rate may be elevated to 180 beats per minute (bpm). There may be crackles, retractions, nasal flaring, and increased mucous secretions. The pulse and respirations gradually slow, and the infant becomes sleepy after approximately 30 minutes to 2 hours.

Period of Sleep

After the first period of reactivity, infants fall into a deep sleep, which may last several hours. During this time, the pulse and respirations drop to the normal range but the temperature may be low.

Second Period of Reactivity

When infants waken, they enter the second period of reactivity. They become interested in feeding and may pass meconium. The pulse and respiratory rates may increase, and some infants become cyanotic or have periods of apnea. Mucous secretions increase, and infants may gag or regurgitate. The second period of reactivity occurs 4 to 6 hours after birth and lasts a very short time or several hours. Many infants pass through all stages within 8 hours.

Behavioral States

Six gradations in the infant's behavioral state, ranging from deep sleep to crying, have been identified.

Quiet Sleep State

In the quiet sleep state, the infant is in a deep sleep with no eye movements. Respirations are quiet, regular, and slower than in the other states. Although startles occur at intervals, the infant's body is quiet. Little or no response to noise or stimuli occurs, and the infant returns to deep sleep quickly if not disturbed.

Active Sleep State

Sleep is lighter in the active sleep state, and infants move their extremities, stretch, change facial expressions, and fuss briefly. During this period, respirations tend to be more rapid and irregular and rapid eye movements (REM) occur. Infants are more likely to startle from noise or disturbances and may return to sleep or move to an awake state.

Drowsy State

The drowsy state is a transitional period between sleep and waking. The eyes may remain closed or, if open, appear glazed and unfocused. Infants startle and move their extremities slowly. They may go back to sleep or, with gentle stimulation, gradually awaken.

Quiet Alert State

The quiet alert state should be pointed out to parents because it is an excellent time to increase bonding. Infants focus on objects or people and seem bright and interested in their surroundings. Body movements are minimal as infants seem to concentrate on the environment.

Active Alert State

In the active alert state, infants are often fussy. They seem restless, have faster and more irregular respirations, and seem more aware of feelings of discomfort from hunger or cold. Although their eyes are open, infants seem less focused on visual stimuli than during the quiet alert state.

Crying State

The crying state may quickly follow the active alert state if no intervention occurs to comfort the infant. The cries are continuous and lusty, and the infant does not respond positively to stimulation. It may take a period of comforting to move the infant to a state in which feeding or other activities can be accomplished.

EARLY ASSESSMENTS

Assessment of the newborn is important to identify abnormalities or problems in adapting to life outside the uterus. Table 22-1 summarizes newborn assessments.

Assessing for Anomalies

Immediately after birth, the infant is examined quickly for respiratory problems and obvious anomalies. The nurse determines whether resuscitation (see Chapter 30) or other immediate intervention is necessary. When the infant is stable and oxygenating well, a more thorough assessment can be performed.

It is important for the nurse to wear gloves when handling newborns until they are bathed and all blood is removed from their skin and hair. This precaution helps protect the nurse from blood-borne infections.

Head

The newborn's head and neck constitute one fourth of the body surface (Gardner, Johnson, & Lubchenco, 2002). The head is palpated to assess the shape and to identify abnormalities. The degree of molding, size of the fontanels, and presence of caput succedaneum or later development of a cephalhematoma are noted.

The hair should be fine with a consistent hair pattern. Abnormal hair growth patterns may indicate genetic abnormalities. The nurse separates the hair, if necessary, to display bruises, rashes, or other marks on the scalp. A small red mark is present if a fetal monitor electrode was inserted into the skin of the scalp.

TABLE **22-1** Summary of Newborn Assessment

Normal	Abnormal (Possible Causes)	Nursing Considerations
INITIAL ASSESSMENT		
Assess for obvious problems first. If infant is stable and has no problems that require immediate attention, continue with complete assessment.		
VITAL SIGNS		
Temperature 36.5°-37.5° C (97.7°-99.5° F) axillary. 36.5°-37.6° C (97.7°-99.7° F) rectal. Axilla is preferred site.	Decreased (cold environment, hypoglycemia, infection, CNS problem). Increased (infection, environment too warm).	Decreased: Institute warming measures and check in 30 min. Check blood glucose. Increased: Remove excessive clothing. Check for dehydration. Decreased or increased: Look for signs of infection. Check radiant warmer or incubator temperature setting. Check thermometer for accuracy if skin is warm or cool to touch. Report abnormal temperatures to physician.
Respirations Rate 30-60 (average 40) per min. Respirations irregular, shallow, unlabored. Chest movements symmetric. Breath sounds present and clear bilaterally.	Tachypnea, especially after the first hour. Slow respirations (maternal medications). Nasal flaring. Grunting (respiratory distress syndrome). Gasping (respiratory depression). Periods of apnea more than 20 sec or with change in heart rate or color (respiratory depression, sepsis, cold stress). Asymmetry or decreased chest expansion (pneumothorax). Intercostal, xiphoid, or supraclavicular retractions or seesaw respirations (respiratory distress). Moist, coarse breath sounds (crackles, rhonchi) (fluid in lungs). Bowel sounds in chest (diaphragmatic hernia).	Mild variations require continued monitoring and usually clear in early hours after birth. If persistent or more than mild, suction, give oxygen, call physician, and initiate more intensive care.
Pulses Heart rate 120-160 bpm (100 sleeping, 180 crying). Rhythm regular. PMI at third to fourth intercostal space, slightly to left of midclavicular line. Brachial, femoral, and pedal pulses present and equal bilaterally.	Tachycardia (respiratory problems, anemia, infection, cardiac conditions). Bradycardia (asphyxia, increased intracranial pressure). PMI to right (dextrocardia, pneumothorax). Murmurs (functional or congenital heart defects). Dysrhythmias. Absent or unequal pulses (coarctation of the aorta).	Note location of murmurs. Refer abnormal rates, rhythms and sounds, pulses.
Blood Pressure See Appendix G. Varies with activity and gestational age and size.	Hypotension (hypovolemia, shock, sepsis). Blood pressure 15 mm Hg or more higher in arms than legs (coarctation of the aorta).	Refer abnormal blood pressures. Prepare for intensive care if very low.
MEASUREMENTS		
Weight Weight 2500-4000 g (5 lb, 8 oz to 8 lb, 13 oz). Weight loss up to 10% in early days.	High (LGA, maternal diabetes). Low (SGA, preterm, multifetal pregnancy, medical conditions in mother that affect fetal growth). Weight loss above 10% (dehydration, feeding problems).	Determine cause. Monitor for complications common to cause.

Continued

TABLE 22-1 Summary of Newborn Assessment—cont'd

Normal	Abnormal (Possible Causes)	Nursing Considerations
MEASUREMENTS—cont'd		
Length 48-53 cm (19-21 in).	Below normal (SGA, congenital dwarfism). Above normal (LGA, maternal diabetes).	Determine cause. Monitor for complications common to cause.
Head Circumference 33-35.5 cm (13-14 in). Head approximately one fourth of infant's length.	Small (SGA, microcephaly, anencephaly). Large (LGA, hydrocephalus, increased intracranial pressure).	Determine cause. Monitor for complications common to cause.
Chest Circumference 30.5-33 cm (12-13 in). Is 2-3 cm less than head circumference.	Large (LGA). Small (SGA).	Determine cause. Monitor for complications common to cause.
POSTURE		
Flexed extremities resist extension, return quickly to flexed state. Hands usually clenched. Movements symmetric. Slight tremors on crying. Breech: extended, stiff legs. "Molds" body to caretaker's body when held, responds by quieting when needs met.	Limp, flaccid, "floppy," or rigid extremities (preterm, hypoxia, medications, CNS trauma). Hypertonic (neonatal abstinence syndrome, CNS damage). Jitteriness or tremors (low glucose or calcium level). Opisthotonus, seizures, stiff when held (CNS damage).	Seek cause, refer abnormalities.
CRY		
Lusty, strong.	High-pitched (increased intracranial pressure). Weak, absent, irritable, cat-like "mewing" (neurologic problems). Hoarse or crowing (laryngeal irritation).	Observe for changes, report abnormalities.
SKIN		
Color pink or tan with acrocyanosis. Vernix caseosa in creases. Small amounts of lanugo over shoulders, sides of face, forehead, upper back. Skin turgor good with quick recoil. Some cracking and peeling of skin. **Normal variations:** Milia. Erythema toxicum ("flea bite" rash). Puncture on scalp (from electrode). Mongolian spots.	**Color:** Cyanosis of mouth and central areas (hypoxia). Facial bruising (nuchal cord). Pallor (anemia, hypoxia). Gray (hypoxia, hypotension). Red, sticky, transparent skin (very preterm). Ruddy (polycythemia). Greenish brown discoloration of skin, nails, cord (possible fetal compromise, post-term). Harlequin color (normal or cardiac problems, sepsis). Mottling (normal or cold stress, hypovolemia, sepsis). Yellow vernix (blood incompatibilities). Jaundice (pathologic if first 24 hr). Thick vernix (preterm). **Delivery marks:** Bruises on body (pressure), scalp (vacuum extractor), or face (cord around neck). Petechiae (pressure, low platelet count, infection). Forceps marks. **Birthmarks:** Mongolian spots. Telangiectatic nevi (nevus simplex, salmon patch, or "stork bites"). Nevus flammeus (port-wine stain). Nevus vasculosus (strawberry hemangioma). Café au lait spots (6 or more or >0.5 cm in size, neurofibromatosis). **Other:** Excessive lanugo (preterm). Excessive peeling, cracking (post-term). Skin tags. Milia. Erythema toxicum. Pustules or other rashes (infection). "Tenting" of skin (dehydration).	Differentiate facial bruising from cyanosis. Central cyanosis requires suction, oxygen, and further treatment. Refer jaundice that appears in first 24 hr. Watch for respiratory problems in infants with meconium staining. Look for other signs and complications of preterm or post-term birth. Record location, size, shape, color, type of rashes and marks. Differentiate mongolian spots from bruises. Check for facial movement with forceps marks. Watch for jaundice with bruising. Point out and explain normal skin variations to parents.

TABLE **22-1** Summary of Newborn Assessment—cont'd

Normal	Abnormal (Possible Causes)	Nursing Considerations
HEAD		
Sutures palpable with small separation between each. Anterior fontanel diamond-shaped, 2-4 cm, soft, and flat. May bulge slightly with crying. Posterior fontanel triangular, 0.5-1 cm. Hair silky and soft with individual hair strands. **Normal variations:** Overriding sutures (molding). Caput succedaneum or cephalhematoma (pressure during birth).	Head large (hydrocephalus, increased intracranial pressure) or small (microcephaly). Widely separated sutures (hydrocephalus) or hard, ridged area at sutures (craniosynostosis). Anterior fontanel depressed (dehydration, molding), full or bulging at rest (increased intracranial pressure). Woolly, bunchy hair (preterm). Unusual hair growth (genetic abnormalities).	Seek cause of variations. Observe for signs of dehydration with depressed fontanel, increased intracranial pressure with bulging of fontanel and wide separation of sutures. Refer for treatment. Differentiate caput succedaneum from cephalhematoma, and reassure parents of normal outcome. Observe for jaundice with cephalhematoma.
EARS		
Ears well formed and complete. Area where upper ear meets head even with imaginary line drawn from outer canthus of eye. Startle response to loud noises. Alerts to high-pitched voices.	Low-set ears (chromosomal disorders). Skin tags, preauricular sinuses, dimples (kidney or other anomalies). No response to sound (deafness).	Check voiding if ears abnormal. Look for signs of chromosomal abnormality if position abnormal. Refer for evaluation if no response to sound.
FACE		
Symmetric in appearance and movement. Parts proportional and appropriately placed.	Asymmetry (pressure and position in utero). Drooping of mouth or one side of face, "one-sided cry" (facial nerve damage). Abnormal appearance (chromosomal abnormalities).	Seek cause of variations. Check delivery history for possible cause of damage to facial nerve.
EYES		
Symmetric. Eyes clear. Transient strabismus. Scant or absent tears. Pupils equal, react to light. Alerts to interesting sights. Follows objects across midline. Doll's-eye sign, red reflex present. May have subconjunctival hemorrhage or edema of eyelids from pressure during birth.	Inflammation or drainage (chemical or infectious conjunctivitis). Constant tearing (plugged lacrimal duct). Unequal pupils. Failure to follow objects (blindness). White areas over pupils (cataracts). Setting-sun sign (hydrocephalus). Yellow sclera (jaundice). Blue sclera (osteogenesis imperfecta).	Clean and monitor any drainage; seek cause. Reassure parents that subconjunctival hemorrhage and edema will clear. Refer other abnormalities.
NOSE		
Both nostrils open to air flow. May have slight flattening from pressure during birth.	Blockage of one or both nasal passages (choanal atresia). Malformations (congenital conditions). Flaring, mucus (respiratory distress).	Observe for respiratory distress. Report malformations.
MOUTH		
Mouth, gums, tongue pink. Tongue normal in size and movement. Lips and palate intact. Sucking pads. Sucking, rooting, swallowing, gag reflexes present. **Normal variations:** Precocious teeth, Epstein's pearls.	Cyanosis (hypoxia). White patches on cheeks or tongue (candidiasis). Protruding tongue (Down syndrome). Diminished movement of tongue, drooping mouth (facial nerve paralysis). Cleft lip or palate, or both. Absent or weak reflexes (preterm, neurologic problem). Excessive drooling (tracheoesophageal fistula, esophageal atresia).	Oxygen for cyanosis. Expect loose teeth to be removed. Obtain order for nystatin medication for candidiasis. Check mother for vaginal or breast infection. Refer anomalies.
FEEDING		
Good suck/swallow coordination. Retains feedings.	Poorly coordinated suck and swallow. Duskiness or cyanosis during feeding (cardiac defects). Choking, gagging, excessive drooling (tracheoesophageal fistula, esophageal atresia).	Feed slowly. Stop frequently if difficulty occurs. Suction and stimulate if necessary. Refer infants with continued difficulty.

Continued

TABLE 22-1 Summary of Newborn Assessment—cont'd

Normal	Abnormal (Possible Causes)	Nursing Considerations
NECK/CLAVICLES		
Short neck turns head easily side to side. Infant raises head when prone. Clavicles intact.	Weakness, contractures, or rigidity (muscle abnormalities). Webbing of neck, large fat pad at back of neck (chromosomal disorders). Crepitus, lump, or crying when clavicle palpated, diminished or absent arm movement (fractured clavicle).	Fracture of clavicle occurs especially in large infants with shoulder dystocia at birth. Immobilize arm. Look for other injuries. Refer abnormalities.
CHEST		
Cylinder shape. Xiphoid process may be prominent. Symmetric. Nipples present and located properly. May have engorgement, white nipple discharge (maternal hormone withdrawal).	Asymmetry (diaphragmatic hernia, pneumothorax). Supernumerary nipples. Redness (infection).	Report abnormalities.
ABDOMEN		
Rounded, soft. Bowel sounds present soon after birth. Liver palpable 1-3 cm below costal margin. Skin intact. Three vessels in cord. Clamp tight and cord drying. Meconium passed within 12-48 hr. Urine passed within 12-24 hr. **Normal variation:** "Brick dust" staining of diaper (urate crystals).	Sunken abdomen (diaphragmatic hernia). Distended abdomen or loops of bowel visible (obstruction, infection, enlarged organs). Absent bowel sounds after first hour (paralytic ileus). Masses palpated (kidney tumors, distended bladder). Enlarged liver (infection, heart failure, hemolytic disease). Abdominal wall defects (umbilical or inguinal hernia, omphalocele, gastroschisis, extrophy of bladder). Two vessels in cord (other anomalies). Bleeding (loose clamp). Redness, drainage from cord (infection). No passage of meconium (imperforate anus, obstruction). Lack of urinary output (kidney anomalies) or inadequate amounts (dehydration).	Refer abnormalities. Look for other anomalies if only two vessels in cord. Tighten or replace loose cord clamp. If stool and urine output abnormal, check to see none was unrecorded, increase feedings, report.
GENITALS		
Female Labia majora dark, cover clitoris and labia minora. Small amount of white mucous vaginal discharge. Urinary meatus and vagina present. **Normal variations:** Vaginal bleeding (pseudomenstruation). Hymenal tags.	Clitoris and labia minora larger than labia majora (preterm). Large clitoris (ambiguous genitalia). Edematous labia (breech birth).	Check gestational age for immature genitalia. Refer anomalies.
Male Testes within scrotal sac, rugae on scrotum, prepuce nonretractable. Meatus at tip of penis.	Testes in inguinal canal or abdomen (preterm, cryptorchidism). Lack of rugae on scrotum (preterm). Edema of scrotum (pressure in breech birth). Enlarged scrotal sac (hydrocele). Small penis, scrotum (preterm, ambiguous genitalia). Urinary meatus located on upper side of penis (epispadias), underside of penis (hypospadias), or perineum.	Check gestational age for immature genitalia. Refer anomalies. Explain to parents why no circumcision can be performed with abnormal placement of meatus.

TABLE **22-1** Summary of Newborn Assessment—cont'd

Normal	Abnormal (Possible Causes)	Nursing Considerations
EXTREMITIES		
Upper and Lower Extremities		
Equal and bilateral movement of extremities. Correct number and formation of fingers and toes. Nails to ends of digits or slightly beyond. Flexion, good muscle tone.	Crepitus, redness, lumps, swelling (fracture). Diminished or absent movement, especially during Moro reflex (fracture, nerve damage, paralysis). Polydactyly (extra digits). Syndactyly (webbing). Fused or absent digits. Poor muscle tone (preterm, neurologic damage, hypoglycemia, hypoxia).	Refer all anomalies, look for others.
Upper Extremities		
Two transverse palm creases.	Simian crease (Down syndrome). Diminished movement of arm with extension and forearm prone (Erb-Duchenne paralysis).	Refer all anomalies, look for others.
Lower Extremities		
Legs equal in length, abduct equally, gluteal and thigh creases and knee height equal, no hip "clunk." Normal position of feet.	Ortolani and Barlow tests abnormal, unequal leg length, unequal thigh or gluteal creases (developmental dysplasia of the hip). Malposition of feet (position in utero, talipes equinovarus).	Refer all anomalies, look for others. Check malpositioned feet to see if they can be manipulated back to normal position.
BACK		
No openings observed or felt in vertebral column. Anus patent. Sphincter tightly closed.	Failure of vertebra to close (spina bifida), with or without sac with spinal fluid and meninges (meningocele) or cord (myelomeningocele) enclosed. Tuft of hair over spina bifida occulta. Pilonidal dimple or sinus. Imperforate anus.	Refer abnormalities. Observe for movement below level of defect. If sac, cover with sterile dressing wet with sterile saline. Protect from injury.
REFLEXES		
Moro, palmar and plantar grasp, rooting sucking, swallowing, tonic neck, Babinski, Gallant, and stepping reflexes present (see Table 22-2).	Absent, asymmetric, or weak reflexes.	Observe for signs of fractures, nerve damage, or injury to CNS.

CNS, Central nervous system; *bpm*, beats per minute; *PMI*, point of maximum impulse; *LGA*, large for gestational age; *SGA*, small for gestational age.

Suture Lines. All suture lines should be palpated. Separation of more than 1 cm may indicate increased intracranial pressure. Overriding of the cranial bones at the sutures is the result of molding—changes in the shape of the head that allow it to pass through the birth canal. The condition usually resolves within a few days to a week after birth. A hard, ridged area may be caused by premature closure of the sutures, called *craniosynostosis*. This condition may impair brain growth and the shape of the head and necessitates surgery.

Fontanels. The nurse palpates the fontanels—the areas where the sutures of the head meet (Fig. 22-6). The infant's head is elevated during palpation for accurate assessment. The anterior fontanel is a diamond-shaped area where the frontal and parietal bones meet (see Fig. 17-5). It measures 2 to 4 cm, although this varies greatly because of molding and individual differences (Howard-Glenn, 2000). The fontanel closes by 12 to 18 months of age.

The anterior fontanel should be soft and even with the surrounding bones or only slightly depressed. Vigorous crying may cause the fontanel to bulge. Fullness or bulging of the anterior fontanel of a quiet infant may indicate increased intracranial pressure. After molding resolves, a depressed fontanel may be a sign of dehydration. Abnormal signs are reported to the primary care provider.

The posterior fontanel is a triangular area where the occipital and parietal bones meet. It is much smaller than the anterior fontanel, measuring 0.5 to 1 cm (Howard-Glenn, 2000). This fontanel closes by the time the infant is 2 to 3 months of age.

Caput Succedaneum. A caput succedaneum often appears over the vertex of the newborn's head as a result of pressure against the mother's cervix during labor (Fig. 22-7). The edematous area crosses suture lines, is soft, and varies in size. It resolves quickly and disappears within 12 hours to several

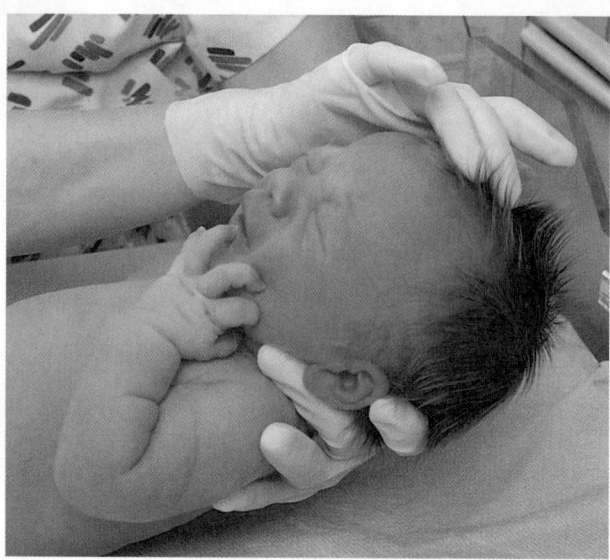

Figure 22-6 Palpation of the anterior fontanel. Note elevation of the head.

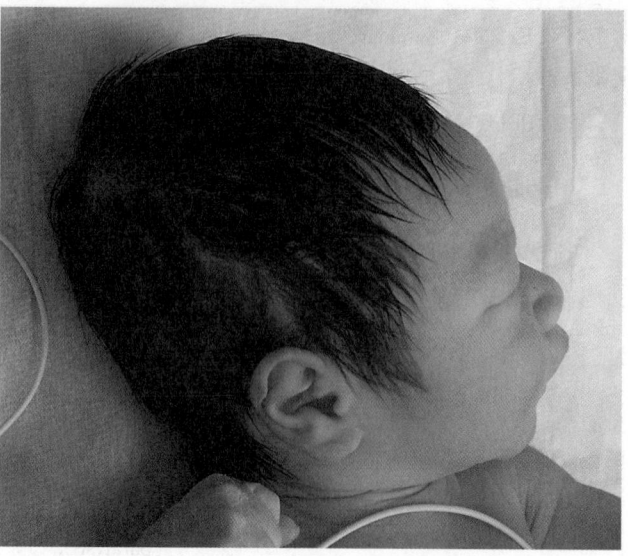

Figure 22-7 Caput succedaneum is an edematous area on the head from pressure against the cervix. It may cross suture lines.

days after birth. Caput may also occur when a vacuum extractor is used to hasten birth and corresponds to the area where the extractor was placed on the skull. The amount of edema and presence of bruising are assessed.

Cephalhematoma. A cephalhematoma results when there is bleeding between the periosteum and the skull from pressure during birth (Fig. 22-8). It occurs on one or both sides of the head, usually over the parietal bones. The firm swelling is usually not present at birth but develops within the first 24 to 48 hours.

A cephalhematoma has clear edges that end at the suture lines. It does not cross the suture lines like a caput succedaneum because the bleeding is held between the bone and its covering, the periosteum. A cephalhematoma reabsorbs slowly and may take weeks to months before it is completely resolved. Because of the breakdown of the red blood cells within the hematoma, affected infants are at greater risk for jaundice.

Both caput succedaneum and cephalhematoma may be frightening to parents. They need information, even if they do not ask, about the causes and how long it takes for the areas to resolve.

Facies. The face is examined for symmetry, positioning of the facial features, and movement and expression. A transient asymmetry from intrauterine pressure may be present, which lasts a few weeks or months. Irregularities of the facial features should be reported.

Neck and Clavicles
The nurse assesses the infant's neck and notes the infant's ability to turn the head from side to side. The neck is very short. Webbing or an unusually large fat pad between the occiput and the shoulders may indicate a chromosomal anomaly. There should be no masses.

Fractures of the clavicle are more likely to occur in large infants. A lump, swelling, or crepitus (grating of the bone) may be palpated if a fracture is present. The site may be tender. Decreased movement of the affected arm is especially noticeable when the Moro reflex is elicited. Damage to the brachial plexus may cause paralysis of the arm on the side of

the fracture. Treatment of a fractured clavicle includes immobilization of the affected arm.

Cord
The umbilical cord should contain three vessels. The two arteries are small and may stand up at the cut end. The single vein is larger than the arteries and resembles a slit because its walls are more easily compressed. A two-vessel cord is associated with chromosomal and renal defects. The amount of Wharton's jelly in the cord is noted. If the cord appears thin, the infant may have been poorly nourished in utero. A yellow-brown or green tinge to the cord indicates that meconium was released before birth, perhaps as a result of fetal compromise.

Extremities
The infant should actively move the extremities equally in a random manner. The limbs of a term infant should remain sharply flexed and resist extension during examination. Poor muscle tone results in a limp or "floppy" infant. This finding may be the result of inadequate oxygen during birth but should resolve within a few minutes as oxygen intake increases. Continued poor muscle tone may be caused by prematurity or neurologic damage. Infants with previously good muscle tone may show decreased flexion if they become hypoglycemic or experience respiratory difficulty.

All extremities are examined for signs of fractures such as crepitus, redness, lumps, or swelling. Lack of movement of an extremity may indicate nerve damage. Injury to the brachial nerve plexus may result in Erb's palsy (Erb-Duchenne paralysis)—paralysis of the shoulder and arm muscles. The affected arm is extended at the infant's side with the forearm prone, and movement is diminished.

Hands and Feet. The fingers and toes are examined for extra digits (polydactyly) or webbing between digits (syndactyly). Extra digits are often small and may not have a bone. Tying the extra digits with sutures causes them to atrophy and fall off. Presence of a bone in the extra digit requires surgical removal. Webbed fingers or toes may be corrected by surgery. Nails in a term infant should extend to the end of the fingers or slightly beyond.

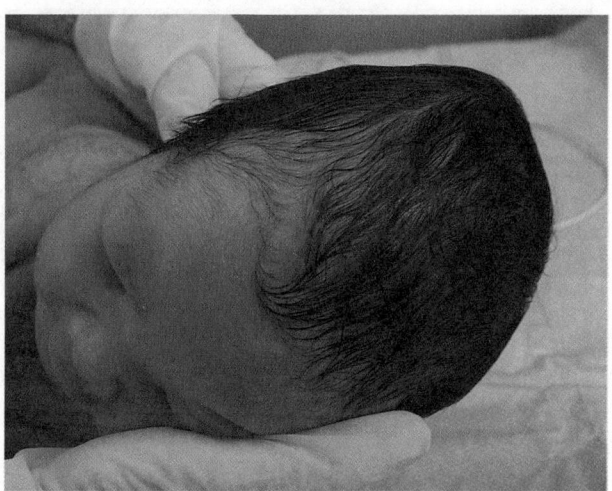

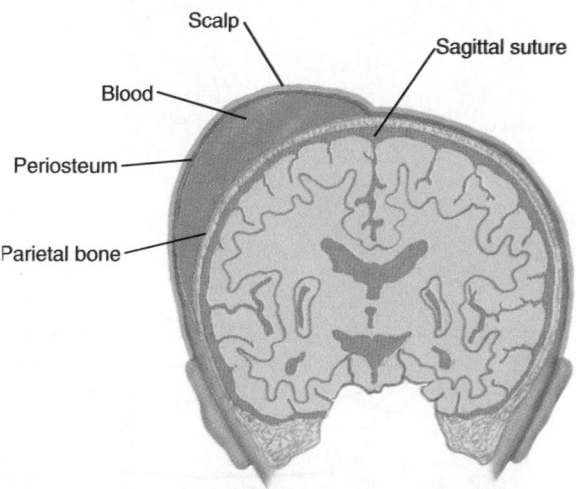

Scalp

Sagittal suture

Blood

Periosteum

Parietal bone

Figure 22-8 A cephalhematoma is characterized by bleeding between the bone and its covering, the periosteum. It may occur on one or both sides and does not cross suture lines.

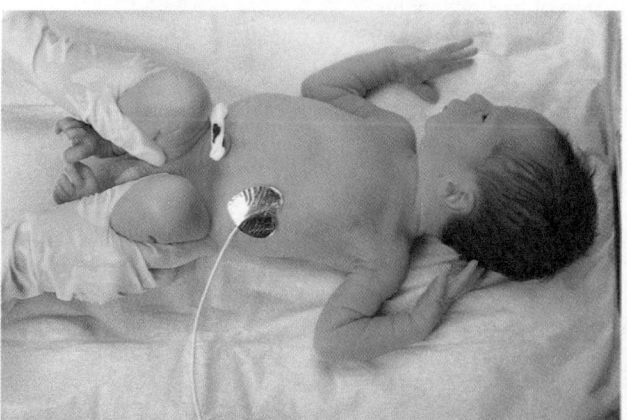

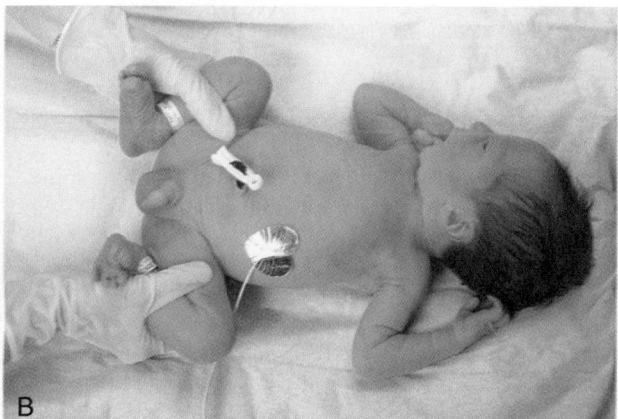

B

Figure 22-9 Assessment of the hips. Place the fingers over the infant's greater trochanter and thumbs over the femur. Bend the knees and hips at a 90-degree angle. **A,** Barlow test: adduct the hips, and apply gentle pressure down and back with the thumbs. In hip dysplasia, the examiner can feel the femoral head move out of the acetabulum. **B,** Ortolani test: abduct the thighs, and apply gentle pressure forward over the greater trochanter. A "clunking" sensation indicates a dislocated femoral head moving into the acetabulum. A hip click may be felt or heard but is usually normal.

Normally, two long transverse creases extend most of the way across the palm. The hands are examined for a simian crease, or line. This is a single crease parallel with the base of the fingers that crosses the palm without a break. It may be seen with incurving of the little finger in Down syndrome. The simian line alone is not diagnostic of Down syndrome, however, and may occur in normal infants.

The feet are assessed for talipes equinovarus, or clubfoot, a common malformation of the feet (see Chapter 50). If a foot looks abnormal, it should be gently manipulated. If it moves to a normal position, the abnormality is probably temporary, resulting from the position of the infant in the uterus. In true clubfoot, the foot turns inward and cannot be moved to a midline position.

Hips. The hips are examined for developmental dysplasia (see Chapter 50). This is an incomplete development of the acetabulum, which may allow the head of the femur to slip out of the acetabulum and become dislocated.

Barlow and Ortolani tests are methods of assessing for hip instability in the newborn period (Fig 22-9). Both legs should abduct equally when the test is performed. It may be more

difficult to abduct the affected hip. A hip click may be felt or heard but is usually normal and is different from the "clunk" of hip dysplasia (Thompson, 2004).

The legs are extended to determine if they are equal in length and if thigh and gluteal creases are symmetric (Fig. 22-10). If the hip is dislocated, the leg on the affected side is shorter and the creases are asymmetric. When the infant's legs are bent, the knee on the affected side is lower if the hip is dislocated. Because the hip may be unstable but not yet dislocated, these signs are not always present at birth. Treatment of developmental dysplasia of the hip involves immobilizing the leg in a flexed, abducted position, usually with a harness.

Vertebral Column

The nurse palpates the newborn's vertebral column to discover any defects in the vertebrae (see Chapter 52). An indentation, especially with a tuft of hair over it, is a sign of spina bifida occulta—failure of a vertebra to close. Other, more obvious neural tube defects include a meningocele or myelomeningocele. These are protrusions of spinal fluid and meninges or the spinal cord, or both, through the defect in

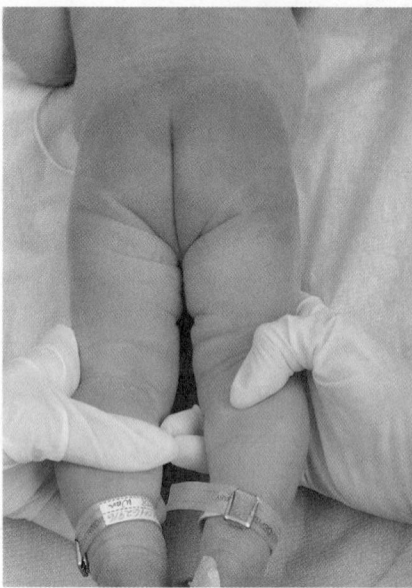

Figure 22-10 Note the symmetry of gluteal and thigh creases.

the vertebrae. They appear as a sac on the back and may be covered by skin or only the meninges.

A pilonidal dimple may be present at the base of the spine. It should be examined for a sinus and the depth noted.

Measurements

Measurements provide information about the infant's growth in utero. The weight, length, and head and chest circumferences are compared with the norms for the infant's gestational age.

Weight
The newborn's weight ranges between 2500 and 4000 g (5 lb, 8 oz and 8 lb, 13 oz) (Howard-Glenn, 2000). The average weight of a full-term newborn is 3400 g (7½ lb). Factors affecting weight include gestational age, placental functioning, genetic factors, and maternal diabetes, substance abuse, or hypertension.

Infants are weighed each day they are in the birth facility and at follow-up visits. They can be expected to lose 5% to 10% of their birth weight during the first few days of life (Bell & Oh, 1999). This weight loss is caused by excretion of meconium from the bowel, normal loss of extracellular fluid, and inadequate intake of calories in the early days after birth. Infants normally regain birth weight by 10 to 14 days of life. Thereafter, they gain approximately 25 to 30 g/day during the early months (Walker & Creehan, 2001).

Length
The infant's length is measured from the top of the head to the heel of the outstretched leg (Fig. 22-11). The average length of a full-term newborn is 48 to 53 cm (19 to 21 in) (Howard-Glenn, 2000).

Head and Chest Circumference
The diameter of the head is measured around the occiput, just above the eyebrows. The average head circumference of the term newborn is 33 to 35.5 cm (13 to 14 in) (Howard-Glenn, 2000). The measurement may be affected by molding

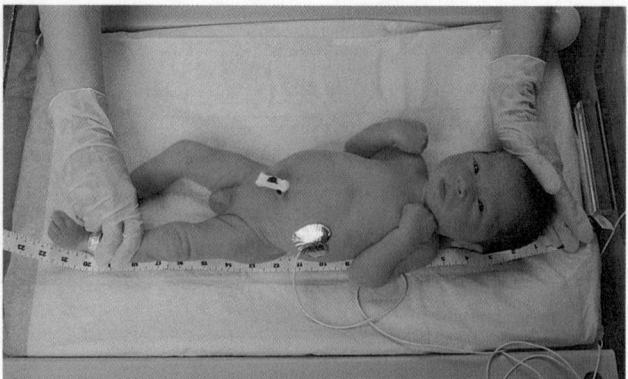

Figure 22-11 Measuring length.

of the skull during the birth process. If a large amount of molding occurred, the head is remeasured when it regains its normal shape. An abnormally small head may indicate poor brain growth and microcephaly. A very large head may be a sign of hydrocephalus.

The chest is measured at the level of the nipples. It is usually 2 to 3 cm smaller than the head. The average circumference of the chest is 30.5 to 33 cm (12 to 13 in) (Howard-Glenn, 2000). If molding of the head is present, the head and chest measurement may be equal at birth.

ASSESSMENT OF CARDIORESPIRATORY STATUS

Assessments of respiratory and cardiovascular status are performed together because transitional changes take place in both systems at birth.

History

Information about the pregnancy, labor, and delivery is important in assessing the infant's cardiovascular and respiratory status and the likelihood of problems at birth.

Airway

During birth, some fetal lung fluid is forced into the upper airway. Excessive fluid or mucus in the infant's respiratory passages may cause respiratory difficulty for several hours after birth.

Respiratory Rate
The nurse assesses respirations at least once every 30 minutes until the infant has been stable for 2 hours after birth (AAP & ACOG, 2002). If abnormalities are noted, respirations are assessed more often. The normal respiratory rate is 30 to 60 breaths per minute. The infant may breathe faster immediately after birth, during crying, and during the first and second periods of reactivity. Respirations should not be labored, and

---

! CRITICAL TO REMEMBER

Normal Vital Signs in the Newborn

- Temperature: 36.5° to 37.5° C (97.7° to 99.5° F) axillary; 36.5° to 37.6° C (97.7° to 99.7° F) rectal
- Apical pulse: 120 to 160 beats/min (100 sleeping; 180 crying)
- Respirations: 30 to 60 breaths/min

Procedure 22-1

Assessing Vital Signs in the Newborn

PURPOSE: To obtain an accurate measurement of newborn vital signs.

RESPIRATIONS

1. Assess respirations when the infant is quiet or sleeping, if possible, so that lung sounds can be heard more clearly. Count the respirations (and apical pulse) before disturbing the infant for other assessments.
2. Observe, palpate, or auscultate the chest and abdomen. Using more than one method increases accuracy and helps differentiate rapid, irregular respirations from other movements.
3. Lift the infant's blanket and shirt to see the chest and abdomen. Observation of the pattern of respirations before beginning to count makes it easier to count the rate.
4. If desired, place a hand lightly to the side of the infant's chest or abdomen to feel the movement and palpate the rate. Avoid covering the chest completely so the chest excursions can be watched as well as palpated.
5. To auscultate respirations, place a stethoscope on the right side of the infant's chest to decrease the sounds of the heart. Then listen to breath sounds in all areas.
6. Count for a full minute to increase accuracy, because respirations are normally irregular in the newborn.
7. A crying infant may become quiet if allowed to suck on a pacifier or gloved finger. If the infant continues to cry, count the respirations but make a note in the chart, because the rate may be faster than when the infant is quiet. Recheck later when the infant is calm.
8. Expect the respiratory rate to be 30 to 60 breaths/min when the infant is at rest. Report signs of respiratory distress (tachypnea, retractions, flaring, cyanosis, grunting, seesawing, apneic periods, and asymmetry of chest movements) to ensure follow-up care.

PULSE

1. If possible, listen to the apical pulse on a quiet or sleeping infant so the sounds can be heard more clearly.
2. Use a stethoscope with a pediatric head to listen, if available. A pediatric head allows better contact between the stethoscope and the chest wall and eliminates some of the sounds from the lungs and intestines.
3. If the infant is crying, insert a pacifier or a gloved finger into the mouth to quiet the infant.

4. If the infant cannot be quieted, increase concentration and time spent listening. This increase helps separate the sounds heard and helps focus in on the heartbeat.
5. Listen briefly before beginning to count. Tapping a finger in rhythm with the beat may be helpful. Count for a full minute to allow time to identify abnormalities. Expect the heart rate to be 120 to 160 beats/min at rest.
6. Move the stethoscope to listen over the entire heart area to increase the chance of hearing abnormal sounds. Refer any abnormal sounds (dysrhythmias, murmurs) for follow-up.

TEMPERATURE

Axillary

1. Place the thermometer vertically along the chest wall in the center of the axillary space with the infant's arm firmly over it to keep the thermometer positioned properly and avoid injury to the infant. If the thermometer is held horizontally, it may protrude behind the axilla and give an inaccurate reading.
2. Read the thermometer at the proper time. *Electronic:* when the indicator sounds; *other types:* according to manufacturer's directions. Normal range: 36.5° to 37.5° C (97.7° to 99.5° F).

Rectal

NOTE: Taking rectal temperatures is not recommended because of possible injury.

1. Place the infant in a supine position, and hold the ankles firmly in one hand. Bend the infant's knees against the abdomen and raise the legs to expose the anus, or place the infant prone or on the side and separate the buttocks. This provides visibility and prevents excessive movement that might cause injury.
2. Lubricate the tip of the thermometer with water-soluble lubricant to ease insertion. Insert the thermometer carefully and gently without force into the rectum. The rectum turns to the right 3 cm (1.2 in) from the sphincter.
3. To maintain control and avoid injury to the infant, hold the thermometer securely throughout the time it remains in the rectum.
4. Read the thermometer at the proper time: *Electronic:* when indicator sounds; *other types:* according to manufacturer's directions. Normal range: 36.5° to 37.6° C (97.7° to 99.7° F).

---

the chest movements should be symmetric. Because the pattern and depth of respirations are irregular, they must be counted for a full minute for accuracy (Procedure 22-1).

Periodic breathing, pauses in breathing lasting up to 10 seconds without other changes, may occur in some full-term infants during the first few days but is more common in preterm infants. Apnea lasting longer than 20 seconds, or accompanied by cyanosis, heart rate changes, or other signs of difficult breathing, is abnormal.

Breath Sounds

The anterior and posterior lung fields are auscultated for breath sounds, which should be present equally throughout. Breath sounds should be clear over most areas. It is not unusual, however, to hear sounds of moisture in the lungs during the first hour or two after birth because fetal lung fluid has not been completely absorbed. Abnormal or diminished sounds should always be reported to the primary care provider if they continue.

Choanal Atresia

Assessment for choanal atresia is important because newborns are preferential nose breathers for approximately the first 3 weeks of life. Therefore they breathe mostly through the nose, except when crying. In choanal atresia, one or both nasal passages are blocked by an abnormality of the septum.

The nurse can assess for choanal atresia by closing the infant's mouth and occluding one nostril at a time. The infant

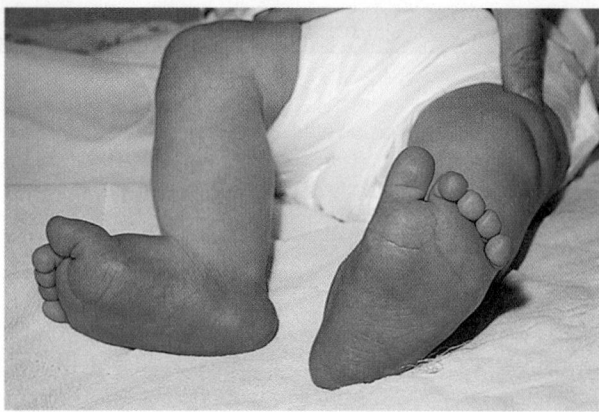

Figure 22-12 Acrocyanosis. (From Eichenfeld LF, Frieden IJ, Esterly NB. [2001.] *Textbook of Neonatal Dermatology*. St. Louis, Saunders.)

is observed for breathing, and breath sounds are auscultated while each nostril is occluded. Another method of assessment is to pass a catheter (5 to 8 French [Fr]) through each nostril to check for patency. Infants with choanal atresia may become cyanotic when quiet but pink when crying.

Bilateral choanal atresia causes severe respiratory distress and requires surgery. Blockage of one side puts the infant at risk for respiratory distress if the other side becomes occluded by mucus or edema.

Signs of Respiratory Distress

The nurse must be alert for signs of respiratory distress, which may be present at birth or develop later.

Tachypnea. Tachypnea, a respiratory rate above 60 breaths per minute, is the most common sign of respiratory distress. It is not unusual during the first hour after birth and during the second period of reactivity. Continued tachypnea, however, is abnormal.

Retractions. Retractions result when the soft tissue around the bones of the chest is drawn in with the effort of pulling air into the lungs. Substernal (xiphoid) retractions occur when the area under the sternum retracts each time the infant inhales. When the muscles between the ribs are pulled in so that each rib is outlined, intercostal retractions are present. The muscles above the sternum and around the clavicles may also be used to aid in respirations (supraclavicular retractions). Occasional mild retractions are common immediately after birth but should not continue after the first hour.

Flaring of the Nares. A reflex widening of the nostrils occurs when the infant is receiving insufficient oxygen. Flaring of the nares helps to decrease airway resistance and increase the amount of air entering the lungs. Intermittent flaring may occur in the first hour after birth. Continued flaring indicates a more serious respiratory problem.

Cyanosis. Cyanosis is a purplish blue discoloration that indicates the infant is not getting enough oxygen. It may be preceded by a dusky or gray hue to the skin. Central cyanosis involves the lips, tongue, mucus membranes, and trunk and shows true hypoxia. It indicates that not enough oxygen is reaching the vital organs and requires immediate attention. To differentiate cyanosis from bruising, apply pressure to the area. A cyanotic area will blanch, but a bruised area remains blue.

Acrocyanosis, which involves just the extremities, is normal during the first day or if the infant becomes cold. It is caused by poor perfusion of blood to the periphery of the body (Fig. 22-12).

Grunting. Grunting describes a noise made on expiration when pressure is increased within the alveoli to keep them open and allow more oxygen to be absorbed. Grunting may be very mild and heard only with a stethoscope, or it may be loud enough to hear unaided in an infant having severe respiratory difficulty. Grunting is a common sign of respiratory distress syndrome and necessitates expanded assessment and referral for treatment.

Seesaw Respirations. If the infant's chest falls when the abdomen rises and the chest rises when the abdomen falls during respirations, seesaw respirations are present. These respirations are a sign of respiratory difficulty.

Asymmetry. Chest expansion should be equal on both sides. Asymmetry, or decreased movement on one side, may indicate the collapse of a lung (pneumothorax).

Color

In addition to cyanosis, the nurse assesses for pallor and ruddiness.

Pallor

Pallor can indicate that the infant is slightly hypoxic or anemic. A laboratory examination of hemoglobin and hematocrit or a complete blood count may be ordered by the physician.

Ruddy Color

A ruddy or reddish skin color may indicate polycythemia—an excessive number of red blood cells. A hematocrit determination confirms polycythemia. Infants with elevated hematocrit levels are at increased risk for jaundice from the normal destruction of excessive red blood cells that occurs after birth. Jaundice may occur in infants with hematocrit levels above 65%.

Heart Sounds

The heart is auscultated for rate, rhythm, and the presence of murmurs or abnormal sounds. The nurse should count the apical pulse for a full minute for accuracy and listen for abnormalities. The rate should range between 120 and 160 bpm with normal activity. It may elevate to 180 bpm when infants are crying or drop as low as 100 bpm when they are in a deep sleep.

If no problems are present at birth, the heart rate should be recorded at least once every 30 minutes until the infant has been stable for 2 hours after birth (AAP & ACOG, 2002). Monitoring is more frequent if there are abnormalities. Once stable, the heart rate is checked once every 8 hours unless a reason develops to assess it more frequently.

Position

The apex of the heart is located at the point of maximum impulse, where the pulse is most easily felt and the sound is loudest. This is at the third or fourth intercostal space, slightly left of the midclavicular line (a line drawn from the middle of the left clavicle). Conditions that affect the position of the heart include pneumothorax and dextrocardia (in which the heart position is reversed from normal).

Rhythm and Murmurs

The rhythm of the heart should be regular, and the first and second sounds should be heard clearly. Abnormalities in rhythm or sounds such as murmurs should be noted. Murmurs are sounds of abnormal blood flow through the heart and may indicate openings in the septum of the heart or problems with blood flow through the valves. Most murmurs in the newborn are normal functional murmurs caused by incomplete transition from fetal to neonatal circulation. A murmur is not uncommon until the ductus arteriosus is functionally closed. Any abnormal sounds of the heart are investigated further because they may be signs of cardiac defects.

Brachial and Femoral Pulses

The brachial and femoral pulses should be present and equal bilaterally. The brachial pulse is located over the antecubital space, and the femoral pulse is located at the groin. Pulses should be equal bilaterally, and the brachial and femoral pulses should be the same. Femoral pulses that are weaker than the brachial pulses may indicate impaired blood flow such as in coarctation of the aorta—a congenital heart defect (see Chapter 46).

Blood Pressure

Measurement of blood pressure is not a necessary part of a routine assessment of the newborn (AAP & ACOG, 2002). The blood pressure is taken on all extremities, however, if the infant has unequal pulses or murmurs. Doppler ultrasonography or other electronic measurement is used. To ensure accurate measurement, the infant should be quiet when the blood pressure is taken, because crying elevates it. The width of the blood pressure cuff should cover the upper arm or leg without encroaching on the joints (Swinford et al., 2002).

Blood pressure varies according the infant's age, weight, and gestational age. (See Appendix G for normal blood pressure readings.) Hypotension may occur in the sick infant. The blood pressure of the lower extremities should be the same as or slightly higher than that of the upper extremities. A blood pressure in the upper extremities that is over 15 mm Hg higher than that in the lower extremities may indicate coarctation of the aorta (Montoya & Washington, 2002).

Capillary Refill

Capillary refill is assessed to help determine if perfusion is adequate. It is checked by depressing the skin over the abdomen or an extremity until the area blanches. The color should return in less than 3 seconds (Sansoucie & Cavaliere, 2003).

ASSESSMENT OF THERMOREGULATION

The neonate's temperature is taken soon after birth while the infant is being held by the mother or is in a radiant warmer with a skin probe attached to the abdomen. The probe allows the warmer to measure and display the infant's skin temperature continuously. It should not be attached over bony prominences. The temperature control is set to regulate the amount of heat produced according to the infant's skin temperature. The temperature should be assessed at least once every 30 minutes until it has been stable for 2 hours after

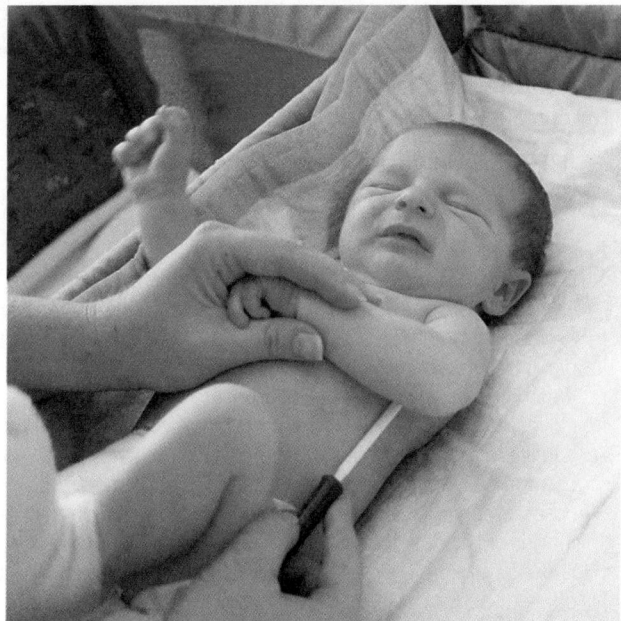

Figure 22-13 The infant is held securely to prevent injury and obtain an accurate reading when taking the temperature.

birth (AAP & ACOG, 2002). It is often checked again at 4 hours and then once every 8 hours as long as it remains stable (see Procedure 22-1; Fig. 22-13).

The normal range for axillary temperature is 36.5° to 37.5° C (97.7° to 99.5° F) (Blake & Murray, 2002). Axillary temperatures provide a reading close to rectal measurements. Taking axillary temperatures is safer than taking rectal temperatures because it avoids the possibility of irritation or damage to the rectum, which turns at a right angle approximately 3 cm (1.2 in) from the anal sphincter. If a rectal temperature is necessary, the nurse should use great care, because inserting the thermometer farther might result in potentially fatal perforation of the intestinal wall. A thermometer should never be forced into the rectum, because there could be an imperforate (closed) anus.

Temperatures are usually measured with an electronic thermometer. Use of glass thermometers with mercury is discouraged because of possible injury or contamination with mercury if the thermometer breaks. Tympanic thermometers, used in some facilities, have moderate correlation with skin and rectal measurements, but there may be variation in the measurement when used with newborns. These thermometers are not as accurate in infants with fevers or in radiant warmers (Blackburn, 2003).

ASSESSMENT OF HEPATIC FUNCTION

The major early assessments of the hepatic system are related to blood glucose and bilirubin conjugation.

Blood Glucose

Observing for signs of hypoglycemia is necessary throughout routine assessment and care. The American Academy of Pediatrics (AAP) and American College of Obstetricians and

Procedure 22-2

Obtaining Blood Samples From the Newborn by Heel Puncture

PURPOSE: To obtain blood by heel puncture for various laboratory testing. (Instructions are given here for measuring the infant's blood glucose using a glucometer or reagent strips, but the same method applies to other testing.)

1. Bathe the infant or wash the area (if the infant has not received a bath since birth) before puncturing the skin, to avoid contamination of the puncture site with maternal blood on the infant's skin.
2. Wash hands and gather appropriate supplies needed: gloves, alcohol wipe, 2 × 2–inch gauze, microlancet or commercial lancing device, adhesive bandage, cloth or commercial warming pack to warm heel, glucometer or glucose screening reagent strips, blotting paper for phenylketonuria (PKU) tests, capillary tubes. A cotton ball or a pipette is used with some systems. Having all supplies ready allows efficient performance of the procedure.
3. If using a glucometer, calibrate or program it and use quality-control measures according to manufacturer's guidelines to ensure proper functioning of the machine.
4. Warm the infant's foot if it is cold or if blood is needed for several tests. Dampen a cloth with warm water and wrap it over the heel, or use a heel-warming pack according to directions. Use caution to avoid burning the infant's foot. Warming causes vasodilation and allows blood to flow more easily.
5. Provide comforting measures such as swaddling, providing a pacifier, allowing the mother to hold, or giving oral sucrose (according to hospital policy) to help decrease the infant's pain.
6. Apply gloves to prevent contamination of the hands with blood.
7. Locate the site. Palpate the bone of the heel to avoid puncturing the calcaneus bone, which could result in infection. Place the thumb or finger over the walking surface to avoid damage to area nerves and arteries. Choose a puncture site on the lateral heel that has not been used before, to avoid infection or scarring.

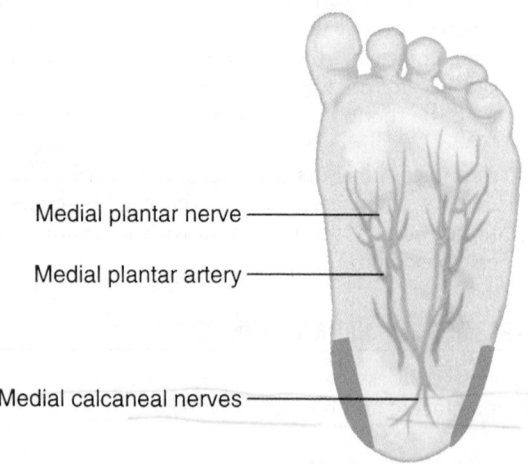

Medial plantar nerve

Medial plantar artery

Medial calcaneal nerves

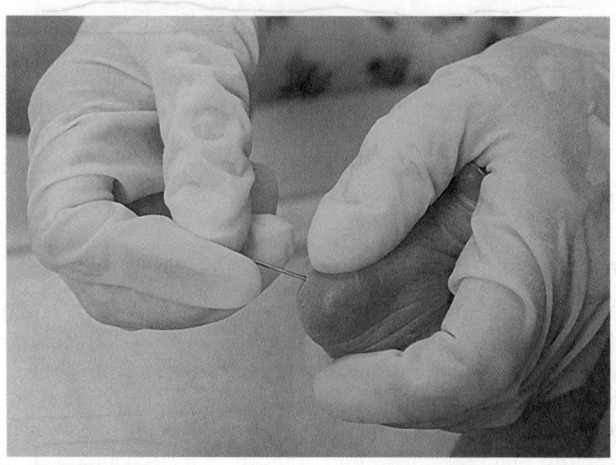

8. Clean the area with alcohol and dry with sterile gauze, or allow to air-dry to prevent diluting the specimen with alcohol.
9. Puncture the side of the heel with a lancet to a depth of less than 2 mm to avoid piercing the bone. Place the lancet in a sharps container to prevent injury to the infant and injury or unnecessary exposure of others to the infant's blood.
10. If an automatic puncture device is used, place it over the site and activate according to manufacturer's directions.
11. Wipe away the first drop of blood with gauze to avoid dilution with fluid from the area of the puncture (if directed by manufacturer).
12. Collect a large drop of blood at the puncture site. Avoid excessive squeezing of the foot because it dilutes the sample with tissue fluid. If using reagent strips, place the drop of blood on the treated area of the strip. To ensure accuracy, cover the entire treated area of the strip and do not smear it. Some glucometers require that blood be drawn into a pipette and then placed on the reagent strip that has been positioned in the glucometer.
13. If using a strip without a glucometer, remove the blood from the strip at the exact time and by the method recommended by manufacturer. More or less time affects accuracy of reading.
14. Obtain results. If using a glucometer, read the results when the machine indicates they are ready. For strips used without a glucometer, compare the strip with the color chart on the bottle.
15. Apply a bandage to prevent bleeding. Remove it as soon as the bleeding has stopped.
16. Record the results. Have the laboratory draw blood for verification of abnormal results according to agency policy. To provide calories needed for metabolism and prevent further decrease in glucose levels, feed the infant according to agency policy or for readings below 40 to 45 mg/dl.

<table>
<tr><td>

! CRITICAL TO REMEMBER

Risk Factors for Hypoglycemia

- Prematurity
- Postmaturity
- Intrauterine growth restriction
- Asphyxia
- Cold stress
- Large for gestational age
- Small for gestational age
- Maternal diabetes
- Maternal intake of terbutaline

</td></tr>
</table>

Gynecologists (ACOG) (2002) state that screening for the blood glucose level is necessary only for infants in risk categories. Normal blood glucose during the first day of life is 40 to 60 mg/dl, and it is 50 to 90 mg/dl after that (Nicholson & Pesce, 2004). Capillary blood is used in screening tests, and these tests are less accurate than laboratory tests using venous blood. Therefore a laboratory analysis (per agency policy) is often used to verify low readings.

It is important to avoid injuring the infant's foot when taking blood from the heel. If the lancet goes into the calcaneus bone, osteomyelitis may result. To avoid piercing the bone, the skin should be punctured to a depth of less than 2 mm (Meehan, 1998). The site chosen must avoid the major nerves and arteries in the area (Procedure 22-2).

Bilirubin

The nurse identifies infants at increased risk for hyperbilirubinemia. Jaundice is identified by pressing the infant's skin over a firm surface, such as the end of the nose or the sternum. Because jaundice begins at the head and moves down the body, the nurse can make a rough estimate of the severity. Jaundice of the face occurs when the bilirubin level reaches 5 mg/dl; jaundice of the midabdomen at about 15 mg/dl; and jaundice of the soles of the feet at about 20 mg/dl (Stoll & Kliegman, 2004a).

Jaundice becomes visible when serum bilirubin reaches 5 to 7 mg/dl. If it appears before the 2nd day of life, the bilirubin level may not be physiologic. The physician or nurse practitioner may order laboratory determinations of the bilirubin level on the basis of the nurse's assessment.

<table>
<tr><td>

! CRITICAL TO REMEMBER

Common Risk Factors for Hyperbilirubinemia

- Prematurity
- Cephalhematoma
- Bruising
- Delayed or poor intake
- Cold stress
- Asphyxia
- Rh incompatibility
- ABO incompatibility
- Sepsis
- Sibling with jaundice
- Breastfeeding

</td></tr>
</table>

<table>
<tr><td>

! CRITICAL TO REMEMBER

Signs of Hypoglycemia

- Jitteriness
- Poor muscle tone
- Sweating
- Tachypnea
- Dyspnea
- Apnea
- Cyanosis
- Low temperature
- Poor suck
- High-pitched cry
- Lethargy
- Irritability
- Seizures, coma

</td></tr>
</table>

NOTE: Some infants may be asymptomatic.

ASSESSMENT OF BODY SYSTEMS

Neurologic System

Reflexes

The nurse notes the presence and strength of the reflexes and whether both sides of the body respond symmetrically (Fig. 22-14). A diminished overall response occurs in preterm or ill infants. Absence of reflexes may indicate a serious neurologic problem. Asymmetric responses may indicate that trauma during birth caused nerve damage, paralysis, or fracture. Some of the newborn reflexes gradually weaken and disappear over a period of months (Table 22-2).

Sensory Assessment

Ears. The ears are assessed for placement, overall appearance, and maturity. An imaginary horizontal line drawn from the outer canthus of the eye should be even with the area where the upper ear joins the head (Fig. 22-15). Low-set ears may indicate chromosomal abnormalities. The nurse examines the ears for skin tags and preauricular sinuses or dimples. If abnormalities of the ear are present, the newborn may have chromosomal abnormalities, mental retardation, or kidney defects. The stiffness of the cartilage and the degree of incurving of the pinna are checked as part of the gestational-age assessment.

Hearing is assessed by noting the infant's reaction to sudden loud noises, which should cause a startle response. The

<table>
<tr><td>

CRITICAL THINKING EXERCISE 22-2

What might be the effect on normal development if reflexes are retained beyond the age when they should disappear?

</td></tr>
</table>

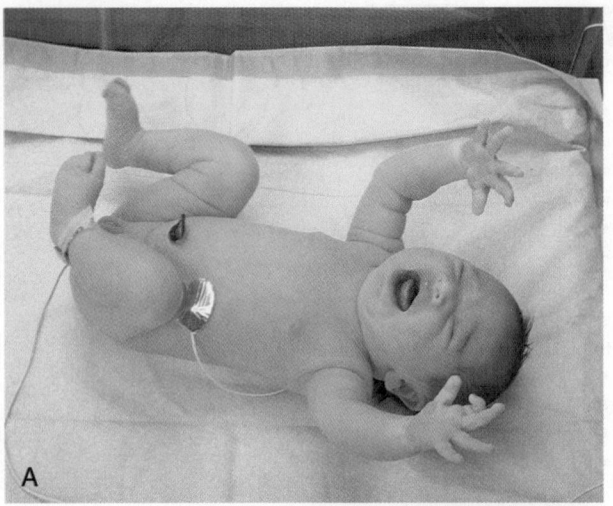

A. **Moro Reflex.**
The Moro reflex is the most dramatic reflex. It occurs when the infant's head and trunk are allowed to drop back 30 degrees when the infant is in a slightly raised position. The infant's arms and legs extend and abduct, with the fingers fanning open and thumbs and forefingers forming a C position. The arms then return to their normally flexed state with an embracing motion. The legs may also extend and then flex.

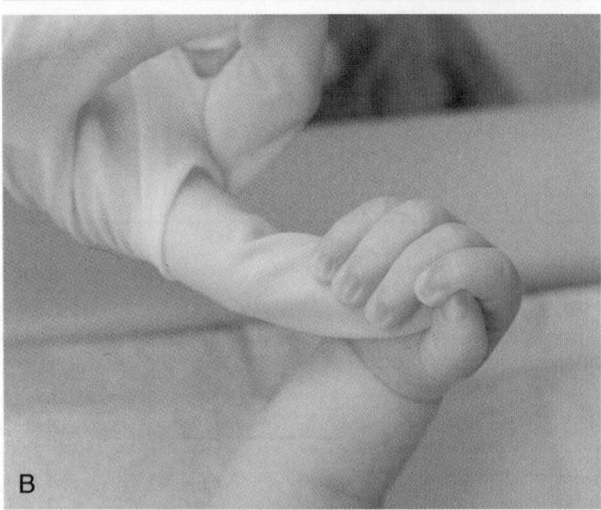

B. **Palmar grasp reflex.**
The palmar grasp reflex occurs when the infant's palm is touched near the base of the fingers. The hand closes into a tight fist. The grasp reflex may be weak or absent if the infant has damage to the nerves of the arms.

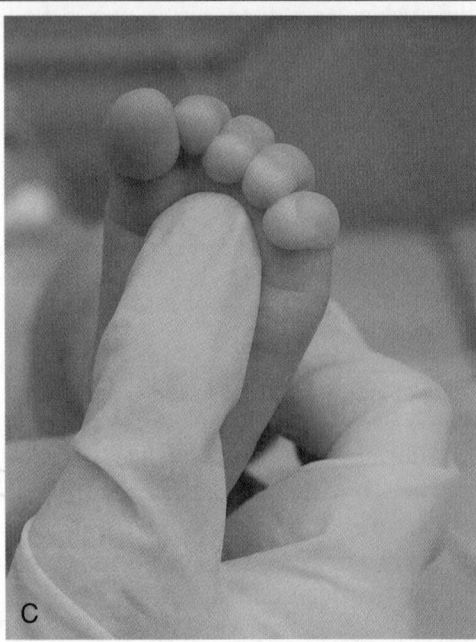

C. **Plantar grasp reflex.**
The plantar grasp reflex is similar to the palmar grasp reflex. When the area below the toes is touched, the infant's toes curl over the nurse's finger.

Figure 22-14 Reflexes.

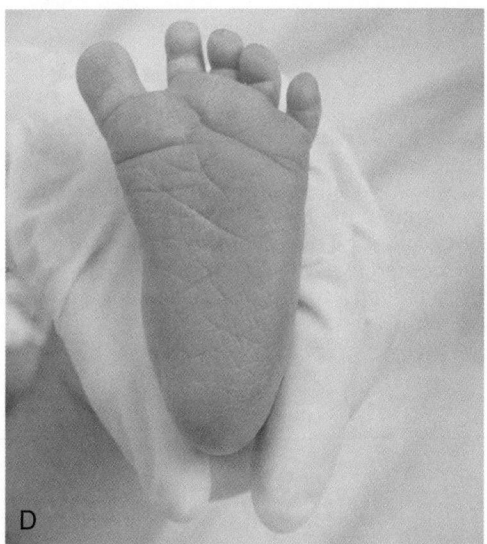

D. **Babinski reflex.**
The Babinski reflex is elicited by stroking the lateral sole of the infant's foot from the heel forward and across the ball of the foot. This causes the toes to flare outward and the big toe to dorsiflex.

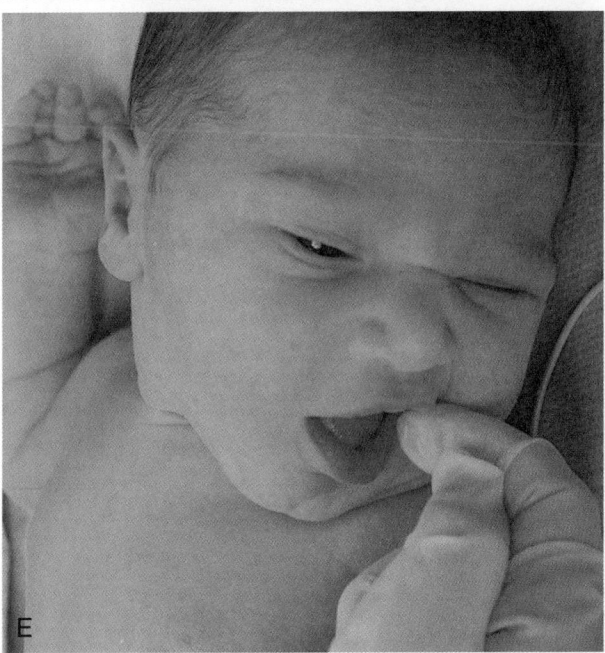

E. **Rooting reflex.**
The rooting reflex is important in feeding and is most often demonstrated when the infant is hungry. When the infant's cheek is touched near the mouth, the head turns toward the side that has been stroked. This response helps the infant find the nipple for feeding. The reflex occurs when either side of the mouth is touched. Touching the cheeks on both sides at the same time confuses the infant.

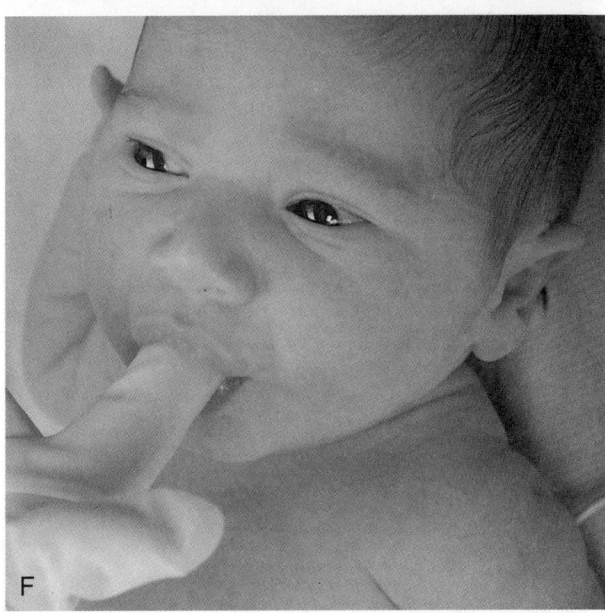

F. **Sucking reflex.**
The sucking reflex is essential to normal life. When the mouth or palate is touched by the nipple or a finger, the infant begins to suck. The sucking reflex is assessed for its presence and strength. Feeding difficulties may be related to problems in the infant's ability to suck and to coordinate sucking with swallowing.

Figure 22-14, cont'd Reflexes.   *Continued*

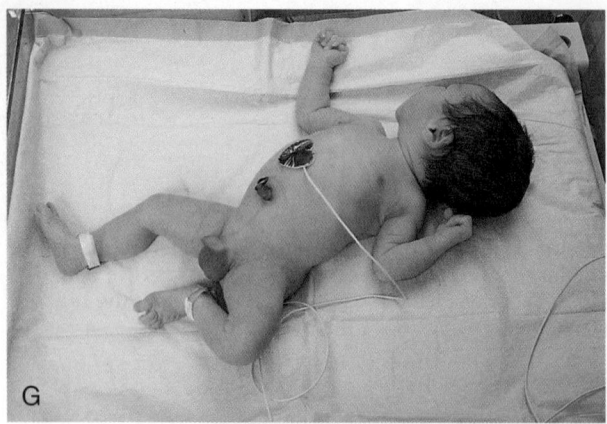

G. **Tonic neck reflex.**
The tonic neck reflex refers to the posture assumed by new-borns when in a supine position. The infant extends the arm and leg on the side to which the head is turned and flexes the extremities on the other side. This response is some-times referred to as the "fencing reflex" because the infant's position is similar to that of a person engaged in a fencing match.

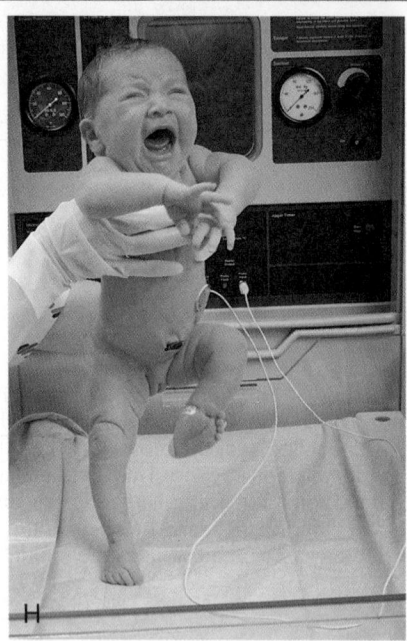

H. **Stepping reflex.**
The stepping reflex occurs when infants are held upright with their feet touching a solid surface. They lift one foot and then the other, giving the appearance that they are trying to walk.

Figure 22-14, cont'd Reflexes.

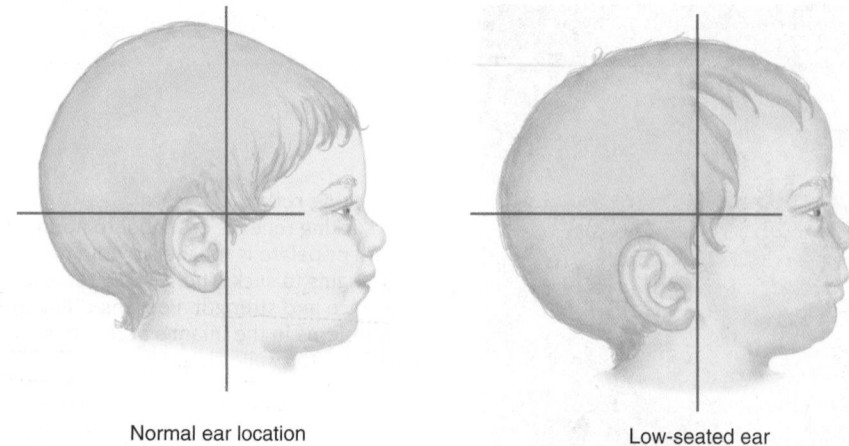

Normal ear location   Low-seated ear

Figure 22-15 An imaginary line is drawn from the outer canthus of the eye and then to the ear. The line should intersect with the area where the upper ear joins the head.

TABLE 22-2 Summary of Neonatal Reflexes

Reflex	Method of Testing	Expected Response	Abnormal Response/ Possible Cause	Time Reflex Disappears
Babinski	Stroke lateral sole of foot from heel to across base of toes.	Toes flare with dorsiflexion of the big toe.	No response. Bilateral: CNS deficit. Unilateral: local nerve damage.	12 mo.
Gallant (trunk incurvation)	Lightly stroke the back lateral to the vertebral column.	Entire trunk flexes toward side stimulated.	No response: CNS deficit.	1 mo.
Grasp reflex (palmar and plantar)	Press finger against base of fingers or toes.	Fingers curl tightly; toes curl forward.	Weak or absent: neurologic deficit or muscle damage.	Palmar grasp lessens by 3 mo. Plantar grasp lessens by 8 mo.
Moro	Let infant's head drop back approximately 30 degrees.	Sharp extension and abduction of arms with thumbs and forefingers in "C" position. Followed by flexion and adduction to "embrace" position. Legs follow similar pattern.	Absent: CNS dysfunction. Asymmetry: brachial plexus injury, paralysis, or fractured bone of extremity. Exaggerated: maternal drug use.	6 mo.
Rooting	Touch or stroke from side of mouth toward cheek.	Infant turns to side touched. Difficult to elicit if infant sleeping or just fed.	Weak or absent: prematurity, neurologic deficit, depression from maternal drug use.	3-4 mo.
Startle	Make a loud noise.	Similar to Moro, but hands remain clenched.	Weak or absent: neurologic damage, deafness.	4 mo.
Stepping	Hold infant so feet touch solid surface.	Infant lifts alternate feet as if walking.	Asymmetry: fracture of extremity, neurologic deficit.	4-7 mo.
Sucking	Place nipple or finger in mouth, rub against palate.	Infant begins to suck Weak if recently fed.	Weak or absent: prematurity, neurologic deficit, maternal drug use.	By 1 yr.
Swallowing	Place fluid on the back of the tongue.	Infant swallows fluid. Should be coordinated with sucking.	Coughing, gagging, choking, cyanosis: tracheoesophageal fistula, esophageal atresia, neurological deficit.	Present throughout life.
Tonic neck reflex	Gently turn head to one side while infant is supine.	Extension of extremities on side to which head turned, with flexion on opposite side.	Prolonged period in position: neurologic deficit.	May be weak at birth. Disappears by 4 mo.

CNS, Central nervous system.

infant should respond to the sound of voices, particularly if it is high-pitched or the mother's voice. Auditory testing is performed in many birth facilities before the infant is discharged. The goal of universal hearing testing is discussed in Chapter 23.

Eyes. The eyes should be symmetric and equal in size. The usual slate gray–blue color of the eyes of infants with light skin tones gradually changes to the true color by 3 to 12 months of age. Infants with dark skin may have dark brown eyes. The eyes are examined for abnormalities and signs of inflammation. A slant of the epicanthal fold in a non-Asian infant may indicate Down syndrome. Edema of

the eyelids or subconjunctival hemorrhages (reddened areas of the sclera) result from pressure on the head during birth.

The sclera should be white or bluish white. A yellow color indicates jaundice. A blue color occurs in osteogenesis imperfecta—a congenital bone condition.

Conjunctivitis may result from infection or a chemical reaction to medications. *Staphylococcus, Chlamydia,* and *Neisseria gonorrhoeae* are common organisms that cause infection. Maternal gonorrhea can infect the infant's eyes (ophthalmia neonatorum) and lead to blindness. All infants are treated prophylactically with antibiotics to the eyes to prevent this condition. Any discharge from the eyes is reported for possible culture and treatment.

Transient strabismus ("crossed eyes") is common for the first 3 to 4 months after birth, because infants have poor control of their eye muscles. The doll's-eye sign is a normal finding in the newborn: when the head is turned quickly to one side, the eyes move toward the other side. The setting-sun sign (the iris appears low in the eye, and part of the sclera can be seen above the iris) may be an indication of hydrocephalus.

The pupils should be equal in size and react equally to light. Cataracts (opacities of the lens) appear as white areas over the pupils. They may develop in infants of mothers who had rubella or other infections during the pregnancy. When a light is directed into the eyes, the normal red reflex may not be seen if large cataracts are present. Tears are scant or absent for the first 2 to 4 weeks of life. Excessive tearing may indicate a plugged lacrimal duct, which is treated with massage or surgery.

Although visual acuity is not well developed and the eyes cannot accommodate for distance, newborns should show a visual response to the environment. They should make eye contact when held in a cradle position during a period of alertness and focus on objects that are 20 to 30 cm (8-12 in) away. Newborns can follow interesting objects horizontally across midline. They should respond well to human faces and geometric patterns of black and white or medium-bright colors, but they show little interest in pastel colors.

Newborns should blink or close their eyes in response to bright lights. Any infant who does not respond to visual stimuli should be reported to the physician or nurse practitioner for further investigation.

Other Neurologic Signs

The newborn is assessed for jitteriness or tremors, usually caused by hypoglycemia, low calcium levels, or prenatal exposure to drugs. Tremors increase each time the infant is touched or moved but stop briefly if the extremity is flexed and held firmly.

Seizures indicate central nervous system abnormality. To differentiate jitteriness from seizures, the infant's extremities are held in a flexed position. This position causes tremors to stop, but a seizure continues. Seizure activity may also include abnormal movements of the eyes or mouth and other subtle signs. Any infant thought to be having seizures is referred for further assessment and treatment (see Chapter 52).

The pitch of the cry is important. A shrill or high-pitched cry, a cat-like "mewing," or a hoarse cry is abnormal. These cries may indicate a neurologic disorder or other problem.

Normal infants respond to holding and appear content when their needs are met. Rocking motions are often effective in quieting an irritable infant. Most infants "mold" their bodies to that of the people holding them, making them easy to hold and cuddle. The neonate who stiffens the body, pulls away from contact, or arches the back when held is showing signs of central nervous system damage. Infants should react to painful stimuli with crying and an increase in vital signs. Excessive irritability may also be a sign of damage to the nervous system. All such abnormal signs are reported for further neurologic assessment.

Gastrointestinal System

The initial assessment of the gastrointestinal tract occurs during the first hours after birth, as the nurse observes the parts that can be seen and the infant takes the initial feeding.

Mouth

The mouth is inspected visually and by palpation. Some infants are born with precocious teeth, usually incisors. If the teeth are loose, the physician usually removes them to prevent aspiration. Epstein's pearls are small, white, hard cysts on the hard palate that disappear without treatment.

The nurse examines the tongue for size and movement. A large, protruding tongue is present in hypothyroidism and chromosomal disorders such as Down syndrome. Paralysis of the facial nerve causes drooping of the mouth and affects the movement of the tongue.

Although candidiasis (thrush) is not apparent in the mouth immediately after birth, it may appear a day or two later. The lesions resemble milk curds on the tongue and cheeks that bleed if attempts are made to wipe them away. Newborns may become infected with *Candida albicans* during passage through the birth canal if the mother has a candida vaginal infection. The infant is treated with nystatin suspension.

A cleft lip or palate results if the lip or palate fails to close (see Chapter 43). Cleft palate may involve the hard or the soft palate or both, and the condition may appear alone or with a cleft lip. The palate is inspected when the infant cries. A gloved finger is inserted into the mouth to palpate both the hard and the soft palate. A very small cleft of the soft palate may be missed if only a visual examination is done.

Suck

The normal full-term infant should have a strong suck reflex, which is elicited when the lips or palate is stimulated. The reflex is weaker in the neonate who is preterm or ill or has just been fed. The newborn's cheeks have well-developed muscles and sucking pads that enhance the ability to suck.

Abdomen

The abdomen should be rounded and protrude slightly but should not be distended. A distended abdomen with stretched, shiny skin may indicate obstruction. Loops of bowel should not be visible through the abdominal wall. Visible bowel could indicate that air and meconium are not passing through the intestines normally.

A sunken or scaphoid appearance of the abdomen occurs in diaphragmatic hernia, in which the intestines are located in the chest cavity instead of the abdomen (see Chapter 43). The nurse listens over the abdomen for bowel sounds, which usually appear within the first hour after birth. Bowel sounds heard in the chest may indicate diaphragmatic hernia.

An umbilical hernia occurs when the intestinal muscles fail to close around the umbilicus, allowing the intestines to protrude through the weak area. The condition is more common in African-American infants. It often disappears when the infant is walking well, although some hernias require surgical repair.

Palpating the abdomen is easiest when the infant is relaxed and quiet. The abdomen should feel soft because the muscles are not yet well developed. Masses may indicate tumors of the kidneys. Palpation of the liver is usually not part of the routine nursing assessment of the abdomen; it is performed by the primary provider instead. When palpated, the liver is normally felt 1 to 2 cm below the right costal margin. If the organ seems large, it should be reported to the physician or nurse practitioner because it may be a sign of congestive heart failure or congenital infection.

Initial Feeding

The initial feeding is an opportunity to assess the newborn further. The nurse observes for choking, coughing, and cyanosis, indicating a connection between the trachea and the esophagus, such as tracheoesophageal fistula. If the mother is breastfeeding, the nurse can observe the infant's response unobtrusively while assisting the mother to position the infant. To decrease regurgitation from overdistention of the stomach, a formula feeding should be no more than 1 ounce.

The infant's ability to suck, swallow, and breathe in a coordinated manner is evaluated. Some newborns choke or gag during the first feeding. Others may become dusky or cyanotic because they become apneic while they are feeding. In either case, the nurse should stop the feeding immediately, suction if necessary, and stimulate the infant to cry by rubbing the back.

Most infants learn to coordinate sucking, swallowing, and breathing by the time the first feeding is finished. Neonates who continue to have difficulty may have a cardiac anomaly (see Chapter 46), tracheoesophageal fistula, or esophageal atresia (see Chapter 43). Infants with tracheoesophageal fistula or esophageal atresia may also have excessive secretions. Further assessment and referral are necessary.

Stools

Stools should be assessed for type, color, and consistency. There should never be a "water ring" around the solid part of any stool. This indicates diarrhea, with the watery part absorbed into the diaper.

The nurse should be aware of the time that the infant's last stool occurred and whether any stools have been passed since birth. Newborns often pass the first meconium stool within 12 hours of birth and most within 48 hours.

Genitourinary System

Kidney Palpation

Palpation of the kidneys is not usually part of the routine nursing assessment of the newborn. The kidneys may be felt, however, just above the level of the umbilicus on each side of the abdomen during the first hours after birth. Abdominal masses may indicate enlargement or tumors of the kidneys. Anomalies of the kidney may accompany other defects because an insult early in fetal development often affects other organs being formed at that time. For example, an infant with only one umbilical artery or defects involving the ears may have renal anomalies. The nurse should observe carefully for urinary output in these infants to determine if the kidneys are functioning.

Urine

Most newborns void within 24 hours of birth, and almost all void by 48 hours. Because absence of urine output during this time may indicate anomalies, the first void should be carefully noted on the chart. The newborn's bladder empties as few as one to two times during the first 2 days, and the first void may be missed. Sometimes it occurs in the delivery room but goes unnoticed because attention is focused on the infant's overall condition. If there is no void in the expected time, the physician or nurse practitioner is alerted.

Each void is recorded in the infant's chart, including diapers the mother changes. The total number is correlated with what is appropriate for the age of the infant. Mothers should be taught that at least six wet diapers, after the first 3 days, indicate the infant is taking adequate fluid.

The newborn's urine may contain urate crystals that cause a reddish or pink stain on the diaper. This is known as "brick dust staining" and may be frightening to parents, who may think the infant is bleeding. It does not continue beyond the first few days as the kidneys mature.

Genitalia

Female. In the full-term female infant, the labia majora should be large and completely cover the clitoris and labia minora. The labia may be darker than the surrounding skin from exposure to the mother's hormones before birth. Edema of the labia and white mucous vaginal discharge are normal. A small amount of vaginal bleeding, known as *pseudomenstruation*, may occur from the sudden withdrawal of the mother's hormones at birth. Hymenal or vaginal tags are small pieces of tissue at the vaginal orifice. These are normal and disappear in a few weeks. The urinary meatus and vagina should be present.

Male. The scrotum should be pendulous at term and may be dark brown from maternal hormones. Pressure during a breech delivery may cause it to be edematous. Rugae (creases in the scrotum) are deep and cover the entire scrotum in the full-term infant. Enlargement of one or both sides of the scrotum may be caused by a hydrocele—a collection of fluid around the testes, which usually resolves without treatment.

Palpation of the scrotum determines if the testes have descended (Fig. 22-16). Testes feel like small, round, movable objects that "slip" between the fingers. If the testes are not present in the scrotal sac, they may be felt in the inguinal canal. Undescended testis (cryptorchidism) occurs on one or both sides. An empty scrotal sac appears smaller than one with testes (see Chapter 44).

The meatus should be at the tip of the glans penis. It may be abnormally located on the underside of the penis (hypospadias), on the upper side (epispadias), or on the perineum. The prepuce, or foreskin, of the penis covers the glans and is adherent to it. Attempts to retract it in the newborn are unnecessary and can cause damage. Abnormal placement of the meatus may not be visible because it is covered by the prepuce, but often the prepuce in these infants is incompletely formed. Hypospadias may be accompanied by chordee, a condition in which fibrotic tissue causes the penis to curve downward (see Chapter 44).

Parents are very concerned about any abnormalities of the genitalia. If the meatus is abnormally positioned, parents

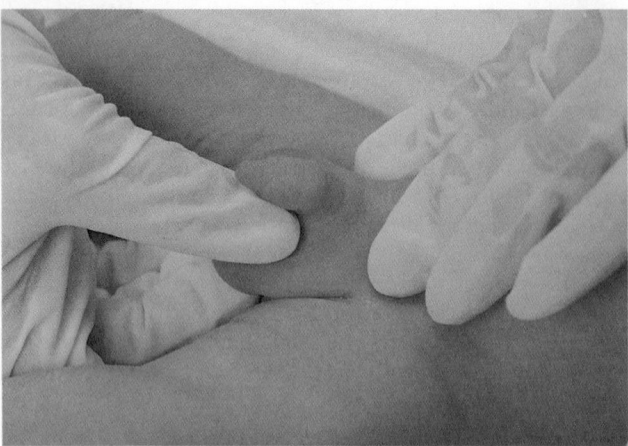

Figure 22-16 The testes are palpated from front to back with the thumb and forefinger. Placing a finger over the inguinal canal holds the testes in place for palpation.

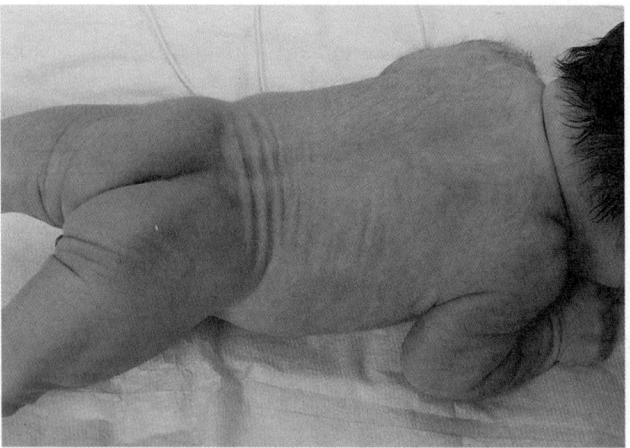

Figure 22-17 Lanugo is abundant on this slightly preterm infant. Preterm infants and those with dark coloring have more lanugo than full-term infants and those with fair skin.

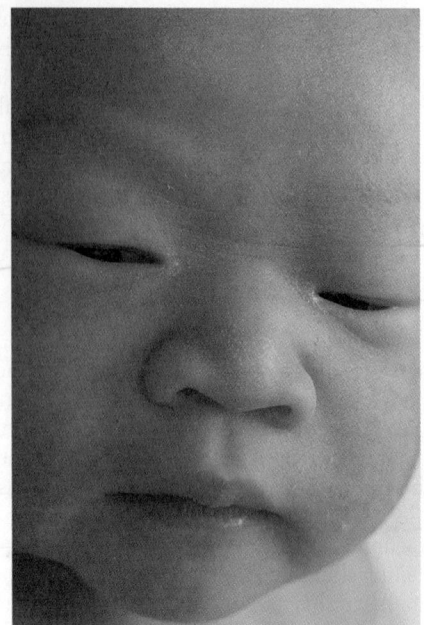

Figure 22-18 Milia.

need an explanation of the condition and why the infant should not be circumcised. The foreskin may be needed for later plastic surgery to repair the defect.

Integumentary System

Skin

The skin of the newborn is fragile, and reddened areas or rashes may develop during the early days of life. The nurse must examine every inch of skin surface carefully during the initial assessment and at the beginning of each shift.

Color. The newborn's skin should be pink or tan. Red, thin skin occurs in preterm infants. Redness (ruddy color) in the full-term infant may indicate polycythemia. Acrocyanosis is common during the first day as a result of poor peripheral circulation. The infant's mouth and central body areas should not be cyanotic at any time. Blanching the skin over the nose or chest shows the presence of jaundice.

Jaundice is abnormal during the first day of life but common during the first week.

A greenish brown discoloration of the skin, nails, and cord results if meconium was passed before birth. This discoloration may indicate that the infant was compromised at some time before birth, and it is more common in the postterm infant. These infants must be watched for other complications, such as respiratory difficulty.

Vernix Caseosa. Vernix, a thick, white substance, resembles cream cheese and provides a protective covering for the fetal skin in utero. The full-term infant has little vernix left on the body except small amounts in the creases. A thick covering of vernix may indicate a preterm infant. Yellow-tinged vernix may indicate elevated bilirubin levels in utero, and green-tinged vernix is caused by meconium staining.

Lanugo. Lanugo is fine hair that covers the fetus during intrauterine life (Fig. 22-17). It is assessed with the gestational-age assessment.

Milia. Milia are white cysts, 1 to 2 mm in size, caused by distention of sebaceous glands (oil glands) that are not yet functioning properly. They occur on the face over the forehead, nose, and chin and disappear within 2 months without treatment (Fig. 22-18).

Erythema Toxicum. The nurse notes the presence of erythema toxicum—red, blotchy areas that may have white or yellow papules in the center (Fig. 22-19). It is commonly called "flea bite" rash or *newborn rash* and resembles small bites or acne. The rash appears during the first 24 to 48 hours after birth, although occasionally not until 1 to 2 weeks. It is most common over the back, shoulders, and chest. The cause of erythema toxicum is unknown, and it disappears within hours or up to 10 days.

Birthmarks. The size, location, color, elevation, and texture of all birthmarks should be carefully documented. Marks should be explained to parents, who are often concerned.

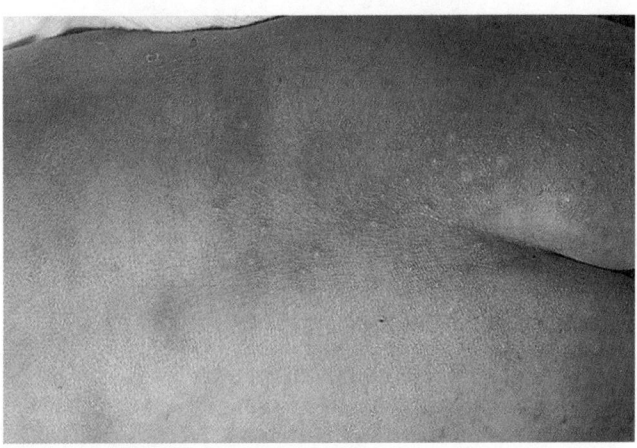

Figure 22-19 Erythema toxicum. (From Hurwitz, S. [1993]. *Clinical pediatric dermatology* [2nd ed., p. 13]. Philadelphia: Saunders.)

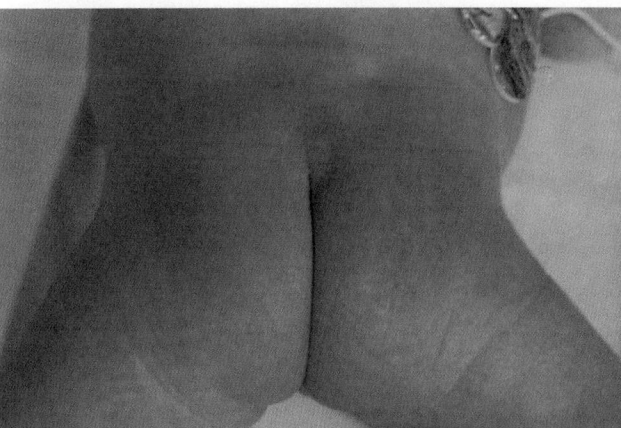

Figure 22-20 Mongolian spots.

- Mongolian spots are bluish black marks that resemble bruises on the sacrum, buttocks, arms, shoulders, or other areas (Fig. 22-20). They occur most frequently in newborns with dark skin and usually disappear after the first few years of life. Some continue into adulthood.
- A telangiectatic nevus is also called *nevus simplex, salmon patch,* or "stork bite" (Fig. 22-21). It is a flat, pink or reddish discoloration from dilated capillaries that occurs on the eyelids, middle of the forehead, or nape of the neck. The color blanches when pressed and is more prominent during crying. Stork bites disappear by age 2 years, although those at the nape of the neck may persist.
- Nevus flammeus (port-wine stain) is a permanent, flat, dark reddish purple mark (Fig. 22-22). It varies in size and location and does not blanch with pressure. It can be removed by laser surgery.
- Nevus vasculosus (strawberry hemangioma) consists of enlarged capillaries in the outer layers of skin. It is dark red and raised with a rough surface, giving a strawberry-like appearance. The hemangioma is usually located on the head. It may grow larger for 5 to 6 months but usually disappears by the early school years. No treatment is necessary.
- Café au lait spots are permanent, light brown areas that may occur anywhere on the body. Although they are harmless, the number and size are important. Six or more spots or spots larger than 0.5 cm are associated with neurofibromatosis, a genetic condition of neural tissue.

Marks From Delivery. The nurse inspects the infant for marks that may have occurred from injury or pressure during labor or delivery.

- Bruises may occur on any part of the body where there was pressure during delivery. Bruising of the face may be present if the cord was wrapped around the neck during birth. Bruising on the head may occur from use of a vacuum extractor.

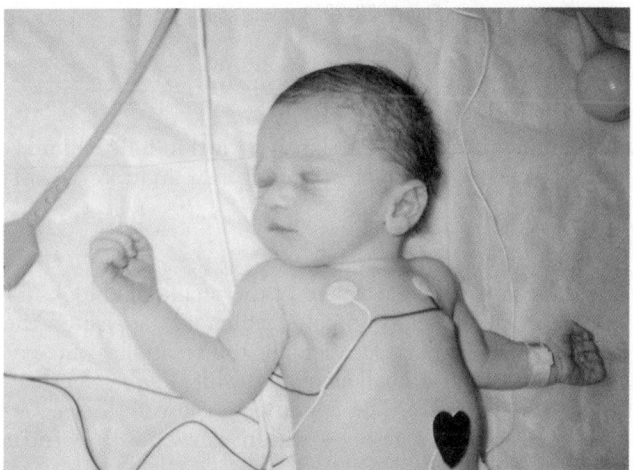

Figure 22-21 Stork bite or salmon patch.

- Petechiae, pinpoint bruises that resemble a rash, may appear on the back or face or in the groin. They are caused by pressure during the birth process. Widespread petechiae or continued formation of petechiae may indicate infection or a low platelet count.
- A small puncture mark is present on the newborn's head if a fetal monitor scalp electrode was attached. The area should scab and heal normally but should be observed for signs of infection.
- Forceps marks occur over the cheeks and ears where the instruments were applied. They are carefully documented as to size, color, and location. Lack of movement or symmetry of the face may indicate damage to the facial nerve.

Other Aspects of Skin Assessment. The nurse notes other aspects of the skin that may indicate abnormalities. Localized edema may be caused by trauma of delivery. Generalized edema indicates more serious conditions, such as

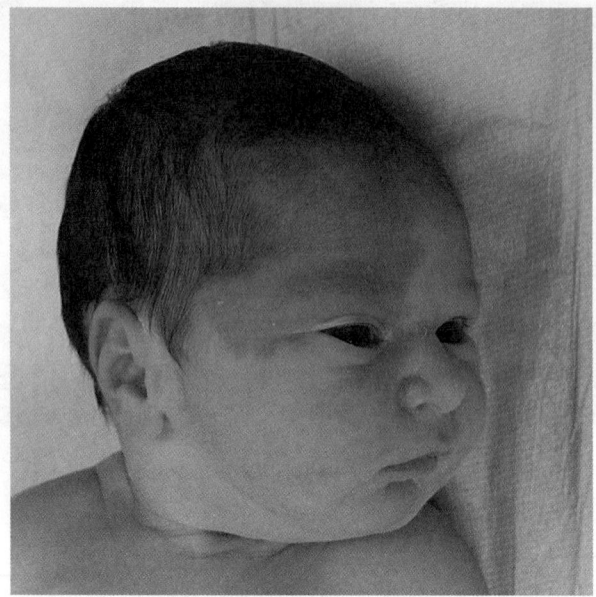

Figure 22-22 Port-wine stain.

heart failure. Peeling of the skin is normal in full-term newborns. Excessive amounts of peeling may indicate a post-term infant.

Breasts

The nurse notes the placement of the nipples and looks for extra (or supernumerary) nipples, which may appear on the chest or in the axilla. Occasionally, the breasts become engorged and secrete a small amount of white fluid (sometimes called "witch's milk"). This condition is caused by hormones from the mother. It resolves within a few weeks without treatment.

Hair and Nails

The hair on the full-term infant should be silky and soft, whereas that on the preterm infant is woolly or fuzzy. The nails come to the end of the fingers or beyond. Very long nails may indicate a post-term infant.

ASSESSMENT OF GESTATIONAL AGE

The gestational-age assessment is an examination of the newborn to determine the number of weeks from conception to birth. The determination is based on physical and neurologic characteristics. It is important because neonates born before or after term and those whose size is not appropriate for gestational age are at increased risk for complications.

Assessment Tools

The New Ballard Score (Fig. 22-23) is frequently used to determine gestational age based on neuromuscular and physical characteristics. A score is given to each assessment,

and the total score is used to determine the gestational age of the infant.

Neuromuscular Characteristics

Posture

The posture and degree of flexion of the extremities are scored before disturbing the quiet infant to perform the remainder of the examination (Fig. 22-24). Preterm neonates with immature flexor muscles have extended, limp arms and legs. The limbs of full-term infants are sharply flexed. The legs should be flexed at the hips, knees, and ankles. Infants who were in a frank breech position may have legs that are less flexed and do not resist extension, even when they are full term.

Square Window

The "square window" sign is elicited by bending the hand at the wrist until the palm is as flat against the forearm as possible with gentle pressure (Fig. 22-25). The angle between the palm and the forearm is measured. The more mature the neonate, the smaller the angle, until the palm folds flat against the forearm at term.

Arm Recoil

To test for arm recoil, the nurse holds the neonate's arms fully flexed at the elbows for 5 seconds and then pulls the hands straight down to the sides (Fig. 22-26). The hands are quickly released, and the degree of flexion is measured as the arms return to their normally flexed position. Preterm infants may not move the arms at all, whereas the full-term infant has a quick return to flexion.

Popliteal Angle

To measure the popliteal angle, the newborn's lower leg is folded against the thigh, with the thigh on the abdomen (Fig. 22-27). Then the lower leg is straightened just until resistance is met. Continued pressure causes the infant to extend the leg further and results in an inaccurate score. The angle at the popliteal space is scored when resistance is first felt. A frank breech position in utero may cause the legs to extend with less resistance.

Scarf Sign

For the scarf sign, the nurse grasps the infant's hand and brings the arm across the body to the opposite side, keeping the shoulder flat on the bed and the head in the middle of the body (Fig. 22-28). The position of the elbow in relation to the midline of the infant's body is noted.

Heel to Ear

For the heel-to-ear assessment, the nurse grasps the infant's foot and pulls it straight up toward the ears while the hips remain flat on the surface of the bed (Fig. 22-29). When resistance is first felt, the position of the foot in relation to the head and the amount of flexion of the leg are compared with the diagrams. The more resistance and flexion, the more mature the infant. This assessment is also affected when the baby was in a frank breech position before birth.

NEWBORN MATURITY RATING & CLASSIFICATION

ESTIMATION OF GESTATIONAL AGE BY MATURITY RATING
Symbols: X - 1st Exam   O - 2nd Exam

Gestation by Dates_____wks

Birth Date_____Hour_____ am pm

APGAR_____1 min_____5 min

NEUROMUSCULAR MATURITY

	-1	0	1	2	3	4	5
Posture							
Square Window (wrist)	>90°	90°	60°	45°	30°	0°	
Arm Recoil		180°	140°-180°	110°-140°	90-110°	<90°	
Popliteal Angle	180°	160°	140°	120°	100°	90°	<90°
Scarf Sign							
Heel to Ear							

PHYSICAL MATURITY

Skin	sticky friable transparent	gelatinous red, translucent	smooth pink, visible veins	superficial peeling &/or rash, few veins	cracking pale areas rare veins	parchment deep cracking no vessels	leathery cracked wrinkled
Lanugo	none	sparse	abundant	thinning	bald areas	mostly bald	
Plantar Surface	heel-toe 40-50mm:-1 <40mm:-2	>50mm no crease	faint red marks	anterior transverse crease only	creases ant. 2/3	creases over entire sole	
Breast	imperceptible	barely perceptible	flat areola no bud	stippled areola 1-2mm bud	raised areola 3-4mm bud	full areola 5-10mm bud	
Eye/Ear	lids fused loosely:-1 tightly:-2	lids open pinna flat stays folded	sl. curved pinna; soft; slow recoil	well-curved pinna; soft but ready recoil	formed &firm instant recoil	thick cartilage ear stiff	
Genitals male	scrotum flat, smooth	scrotum empty faint rugae	testes in upper canal rare rugae	testes descending few rugae	testes down good rugae	testes pendulous deep rugae	
Genitals female	clitoris prominent labia flat	prominent clitoris small labia minora	prominent clitoris enlarging minora	majora & minora equally prominent	majora large minora small	majora cover clitoris & minora	

MATURITY RATING

score	weeks
-10	20
-5	22
0	24
5	26
10	28
15	30
20	32
25	34
30	36
35	38
40	40
45	42
50	44

SCORING SECTION

	1st Exam=X	2nd Exam=O
Estimating Gest Age by Maturity Rating	_____Weeks	_____Weeks
Time of Exam	Date_____ Hour_____am pm	Date_____ Hour_____am pm
Age at Exam	_____Hours	_____Hours
Signature of Examiner	_____ M.D.	_____ M.D.

Figure 22-23 New Ballard Score. (Courtesy Bristol-Myers Company, Evansville, IN. From Ballard, J.L., Khoury, J.C., Wedig, K., Wang, L., Eilers-Walsman, B.L., & Lipp, R. [1991]. New Ballard Score, expanded to include extremely premature infants. *Journal of Pediatrics, 19* [3], 417-423.)

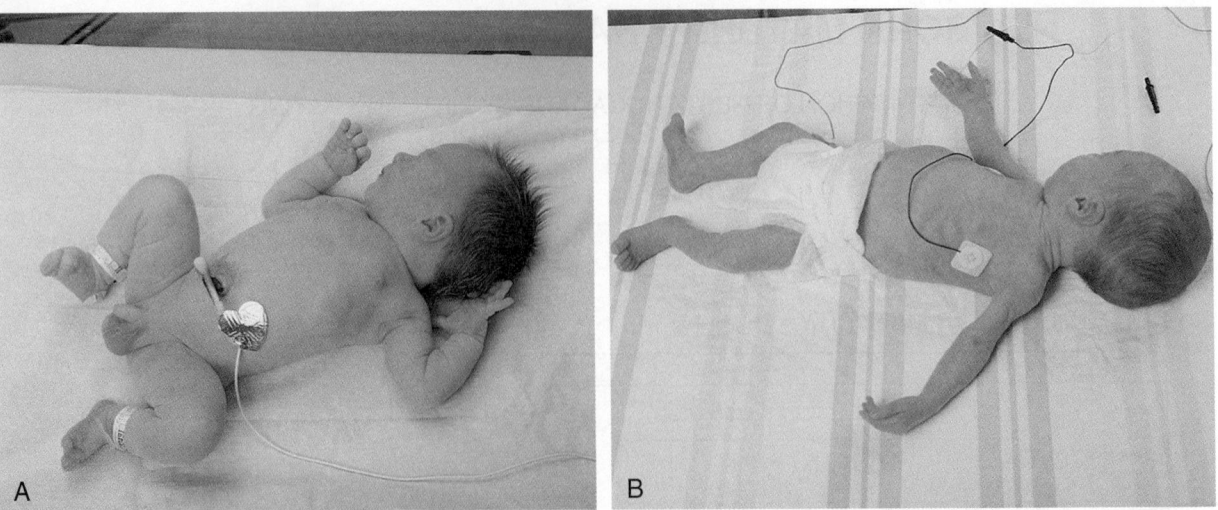

Figure 22-24 Posture in newborns. **A,** The healthy, full-term infant remains in a strongly flexed position. **B,** The preterm infant's extremities are extended.

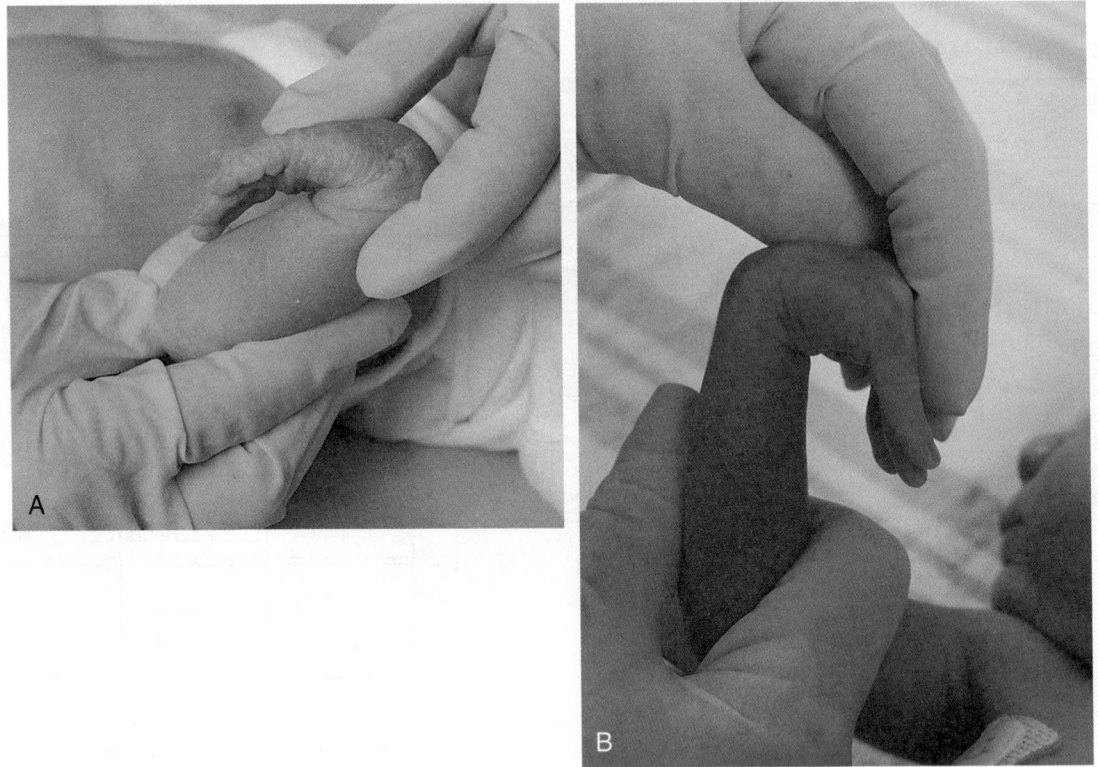

Figure 22-25 The square window sign is performed on the arm without the identification bracelet. The nurse bends the wrist and measures the angle. **A,** Infant near full term. **B,** Preterm infant.

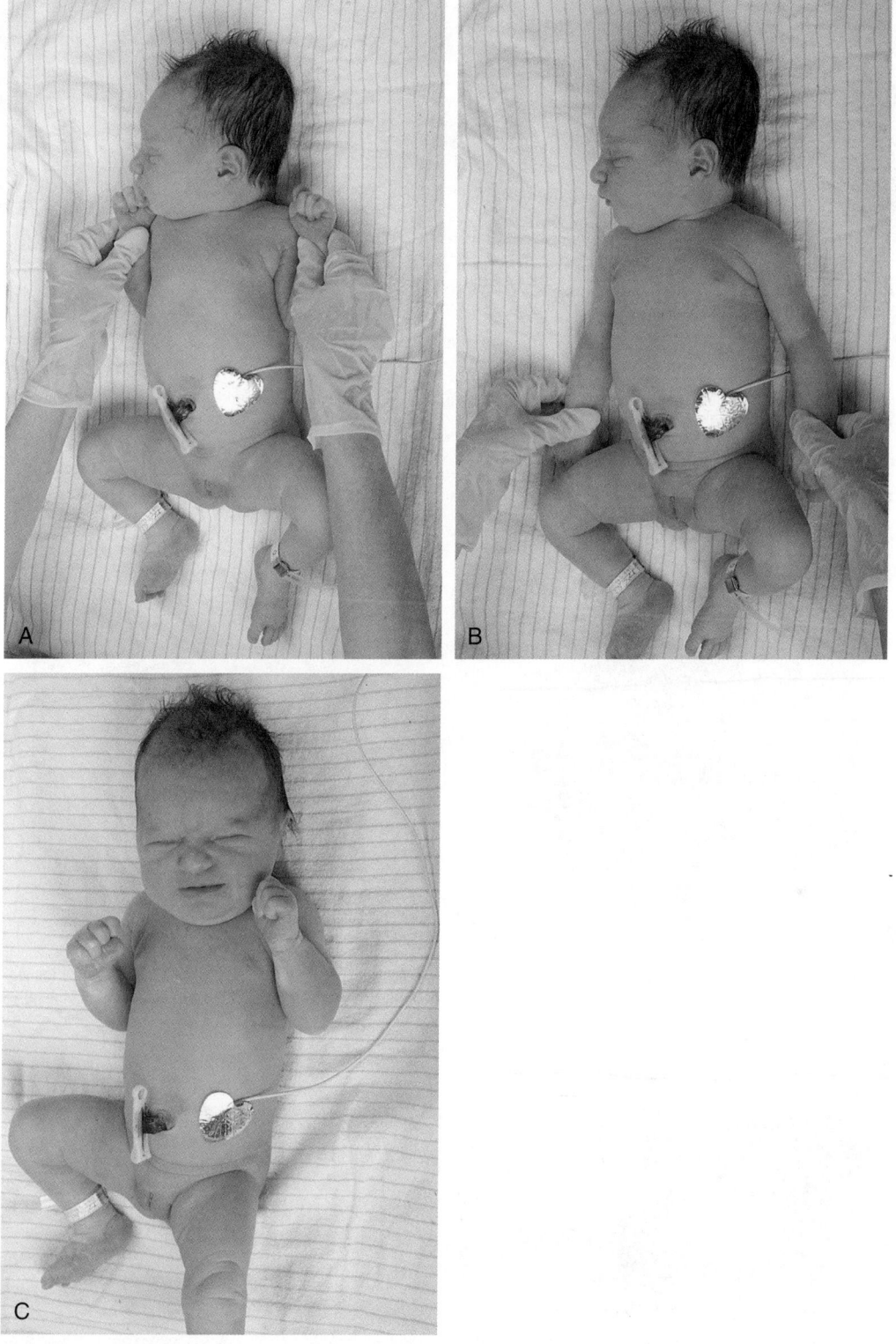

Figure 22-26 Arm recoil. **A,** Arms flexed. **B,** Arms extended. **C,** Recoil for the full-term infant.

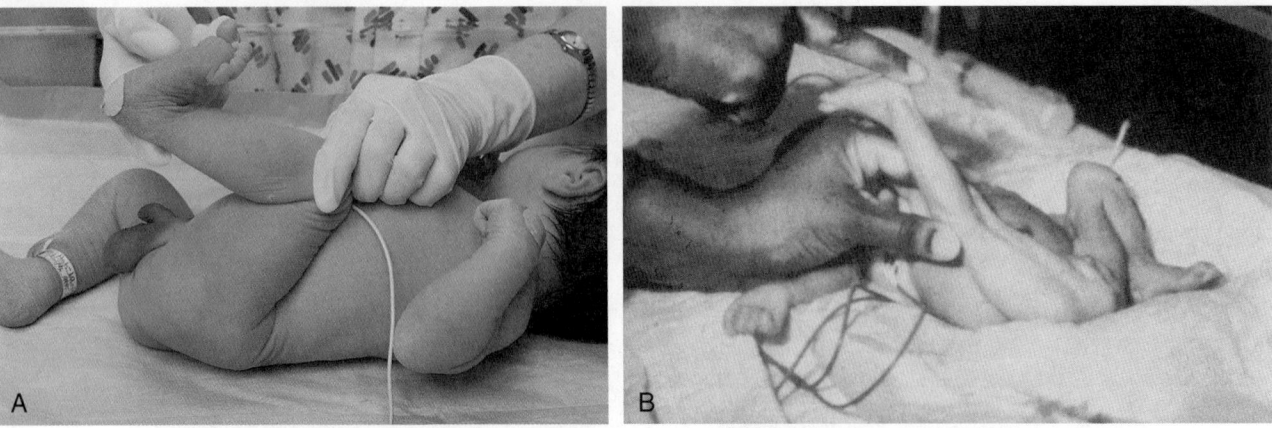

Figure 22-27 The popliteal angle is measured by flexing the thigh against the abdomen and extending the lower leg to the point of resistance. **A,** Full-term infant. **B,** Preterm infant.

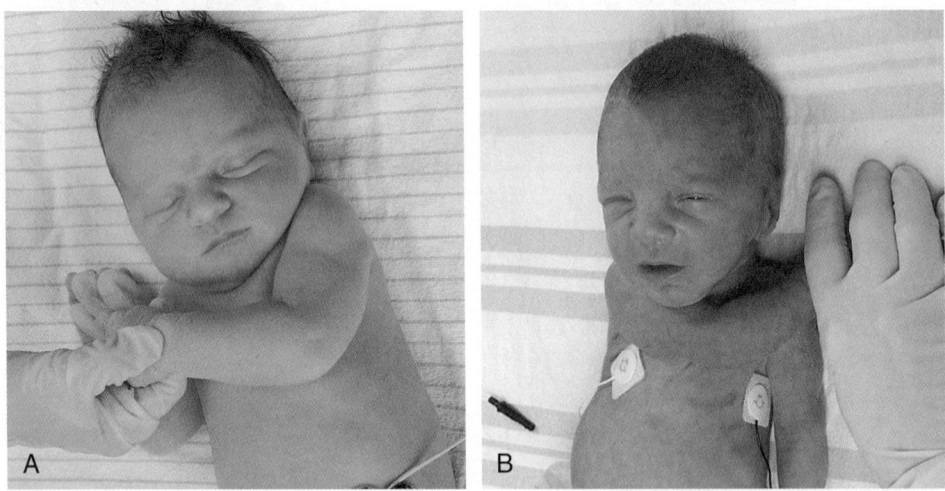

Figure 22-28 Scarf sign. The nurse determines how far the arm will move across the chest and observes the position of the elbow when resistance is felt. **A,** Full-term infant. **B,** Preterm infant. (Note the many visible veins in the preterm infant and the absence of visible veins in the full-term infant.)

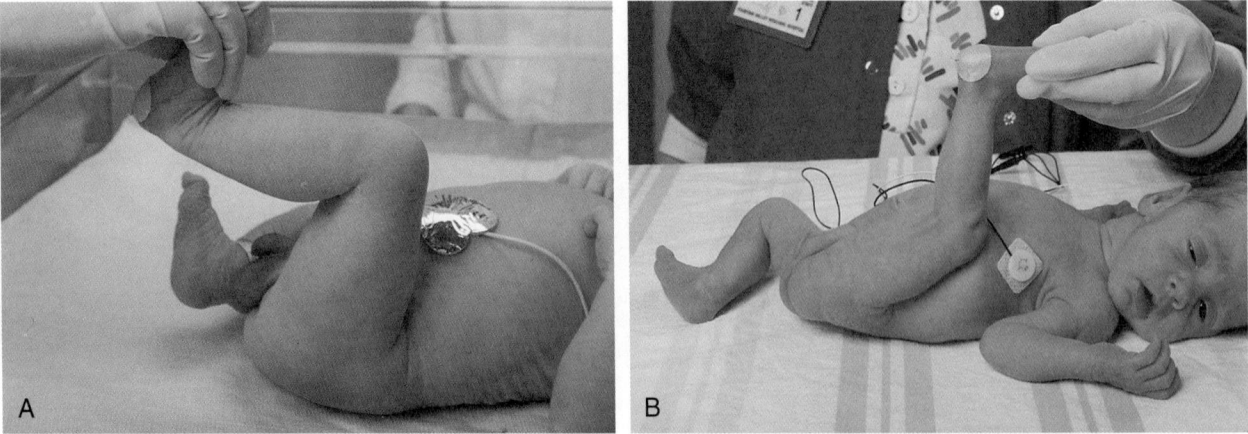

Figure 22-29 Heel to ear. The nurse grasps the foot and brings it up toward the ear, keeping the hips flat. The score is recorded when resistance is felt. **A,** Full-term infant. **B,** Preterm infant.

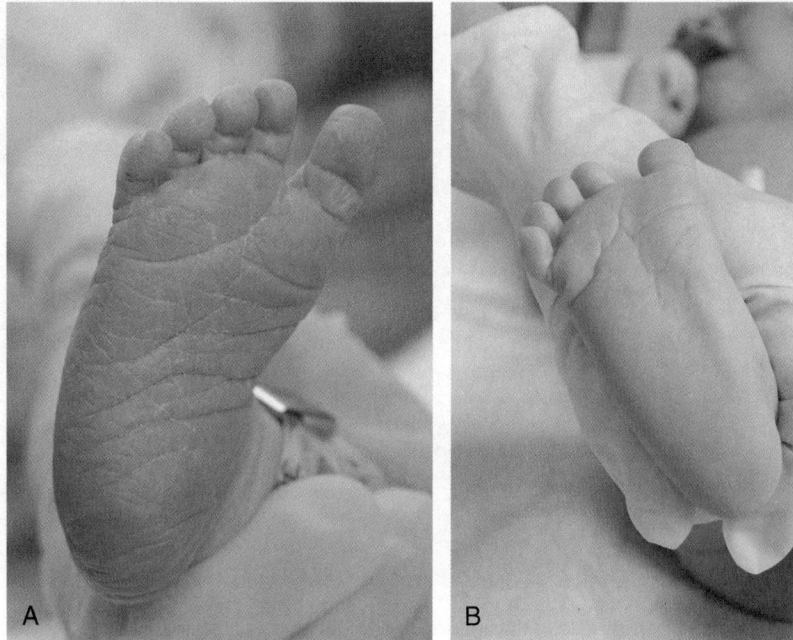

Figure 22-30 Plantar creases begin to develop at the base of the toes and extend to the heel. **A,** The post-term infant has deep creases. **B,** The preterm infant has few creases on the entire foot.

Physical Characteristics

Skin

The skin is assessed for color, visibility of veins, and peeling and cracking. The very preterm infant's skin is red, sticky, and fragile, with veins that are easily visible. In the mature newborn, the skin color is paler; few veins are visible; and there is peeling and cracking. Peeling becomes even more apparent in the post-term infant and during the hours after birth as the skin loses moisture.

Lanugo

Lanugo appears at 20 weeks of gestation and increases in amount until 28 weeks (see Fig. 22-17), when it begins to disappear. At term, a small amount may remain over the upper back and shoulders, over the ears, or on the sides of the forehead. Infants with dark coloring have more lanugo (which is dark and more easily noticed) than infants with fair skin and very light hair, even though they are the same gestational age. The infant receives a score based on the amount of lanugo present on the back.

Plantar Surface

Plantar creases begin to appear at 32 weeks of gestation and gradually spread down toward the heel and become deeper (Fig. 22-30). The plantar creases must be assessed during the early hours after birth because, as the infant's skin begins to dry, the creases appear more prominent.

Breasts

The formation of the nipples and areolae and size of the breast buds are assessed and scored. To determine the size of the breast buds, the nurse places a finger on each side and measures the diameter (Fig. 22-31). Use of the thumb and

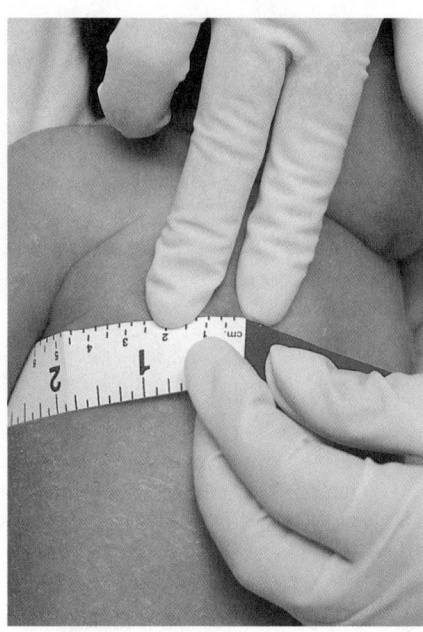

Figure 22-31 The nurse places a finger on either side of the breast bud tissue and measures the size. In the full-term infant, the areola is raised and the nipple is easily distinguished from surrounding skin. (Note the peeling skin.)

forefinger may cause excess tissue to be drawn together, resulting in an inaccurate score.

Eyes and Ears

The eyelids are fused until 26 to 28 weeks. The incurving of the upper pinnae begins at the top and continues around the ear. In assessing the ear, the incurving and thickness of each

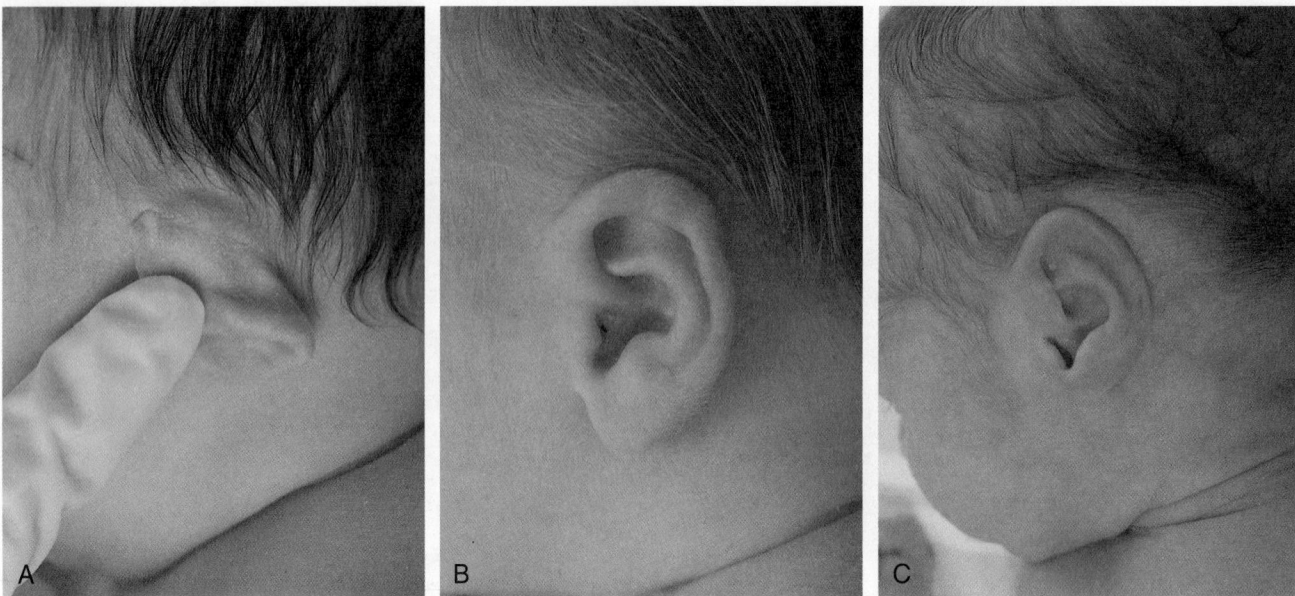

Figure 22-32 Ear maturation. **A,** The nurse folds the ears and notes how quickly they return to position. **B,** Ears in the full-term infant are well formed and have instant recoil. **C,** In the preterm infant, ears show less curving of the pinna and recoil slowly or not at all.

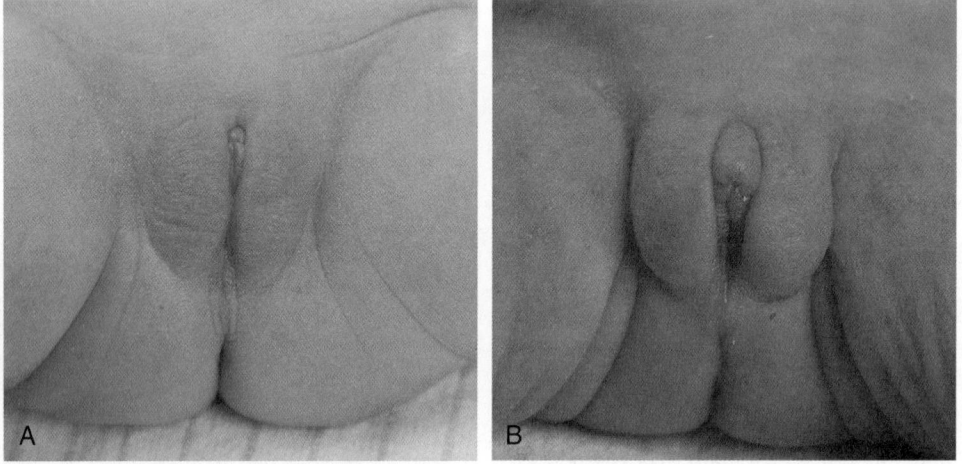

Figure 22-33 Female genitals. As the female fetus matures, the labia majora cover the labia minora and clitoris completely; in the preterm infant, these structures are not covered. **A,** Near-term infant. **B,** Preterm infant.

pinna are rated (Fig. 22-32). The ear is folded to assess the resistance and how fast the ear returns to its original state. In infants younger than 32 weeks of gestational age, the ear has little cartilage to keep it stiff. In the term neonate, the ear springs back to its original position immediately.

Genitals

In the female infant, the relationship in size of the clitoris, labia minora, and labia majora is noted (Fig. 22-33). As the infant nears term, the labia majora enlarge until the clitoris and labia minora are completely covered.

In the male infant, the location of the testes and the rugae on the scrotum are assessed (Fig. 22-34). The testes originate in the abdominal cavity but have moved through

the inguinal canal into the scrotum by term. Rugae forming on the surface of the scrotum are more obvious by 36 weeks and cover the sac by 40 weeks. Once the testes are completely down into the scrotum, it appears large and pendulous.

Scoring

As each part of the assessment is performed, the infant's response is matched with the diagrams and descriptions on the assessment tool (Fig. 22-23). The total score is compared with the corresponding gestational age. It is important to understand that the total score of *all* assessed characteristics determines the gestational age. One or two characteristics alone are not enough to assign a gestational age.

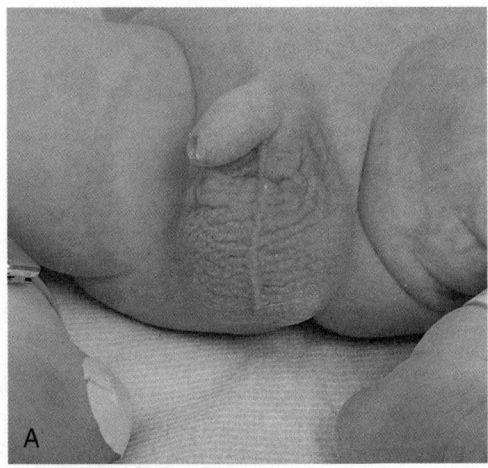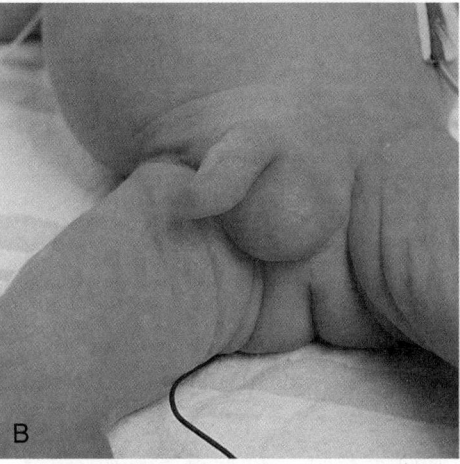

Figure 22-34 Male genitals. **A,** The full-term infant has a pendulous scrotum with deep rugae. **B,** In the preterm infant, the testes may not be descended and rugae are few.

Gestational Age and Infant Size

The appropriateness of the neonate's size for gestational age is determined by plotting the gestational age, weight, length, and head circumference on a graph of intrauterine development (see Fig. 22-35). This score determines how well the infant has grown for the amount of time spent in the uterus. The infant who is appropriate for gestational age falls between the 10th and 90th percentiles on the graph. The large-for-gestational-age (LGA) infant is above the 90th percentile, whereas the small-for-gestational-age (SGA) infant is below the 10th percentile.

When an infant's gestational age or measurements fall outside the range expected, the nurse monitors for complications specific to the preterm, post-term, SGA, and LGA infant (see Chapter 29).

ASSESSMENT OF BEHAVIOR

Assessment of the infant's behavior helps determine intactness of the central nervous system and provides information about ability to respond to caretaking activities.

Periods of Reactivity

During the first and second periods of reactivity, newborns may have elevated pulse and respiratory rates, low temperatures, and excessive respiratory secretions. It is important to observe infants carefully during this time. During the sleep period between the first and second periods of reactivity, newborns cannot be awakened easily and are not interested in feeding.

Behavioral Changes

Nurses assess the infant's behavior and alert the physician to abnormalities. Assessment includes the six different behavioral states: deep sleep, active sleep, drowsy, quiet alert, active alert, and crying. Movement between states should be smooth and not abrupt. The Brazelton Neonatal Behavioral Assessment Scale is often used when detailed knowledge about the infant is needed. In addition to assessing behavioral states, the scale analyzes other aspects of the newborn's behavior, such as orientation, habituation, self-consoling behaviors, and social behaviors.

Orientation

The nurse notes the infant's orientation (ability to pay attention) to interesting visual or auditory stimuli. It is most prominent during the quiet alert state. Infants focus their eyes and turn their heads toward a stimulus in an attempt to prolong contact with it.

Habituation

The infant's response to a visual, auditory, or tactile stimulus is assessed. Usually, the first response of a healthy newborn to an interesting stimulus, such as a brightly colored object or a bell, is a period of alertness. If the stimulus is disturbing, like a bright light flashed in the eyes, the infant startles and attempts to escape by averting the eyes.

Infants gradually stop responding to continued noxious stimuli. This gradual habituation allows them to ignore the stimuli and save energy for physiologic needs. Newborns may go into a dull, drowsy state or fall into a deep sleep. Those who seem unresponsive in a bright, noisy nursery may be in a state of habituation. The preterm infant or one with damage to the central nervous system may not be able to habituate.

Self-Consoling Activities

Normal newborns are able to console themselves for short periods. Self-consoling activities include attempting to bring their hands to the mouth and sucking on their fists. Infants who are ill, preterm, or exposed to drugs prenatally have less ability to console themselves.

Parents' Response

The parents' growing ability to respond to the infant's behavioral cues should be noted. To facilitate bonding and help the parents learn how to interpret the infant's cues, the nurse can point out the infant's behavioral changes.

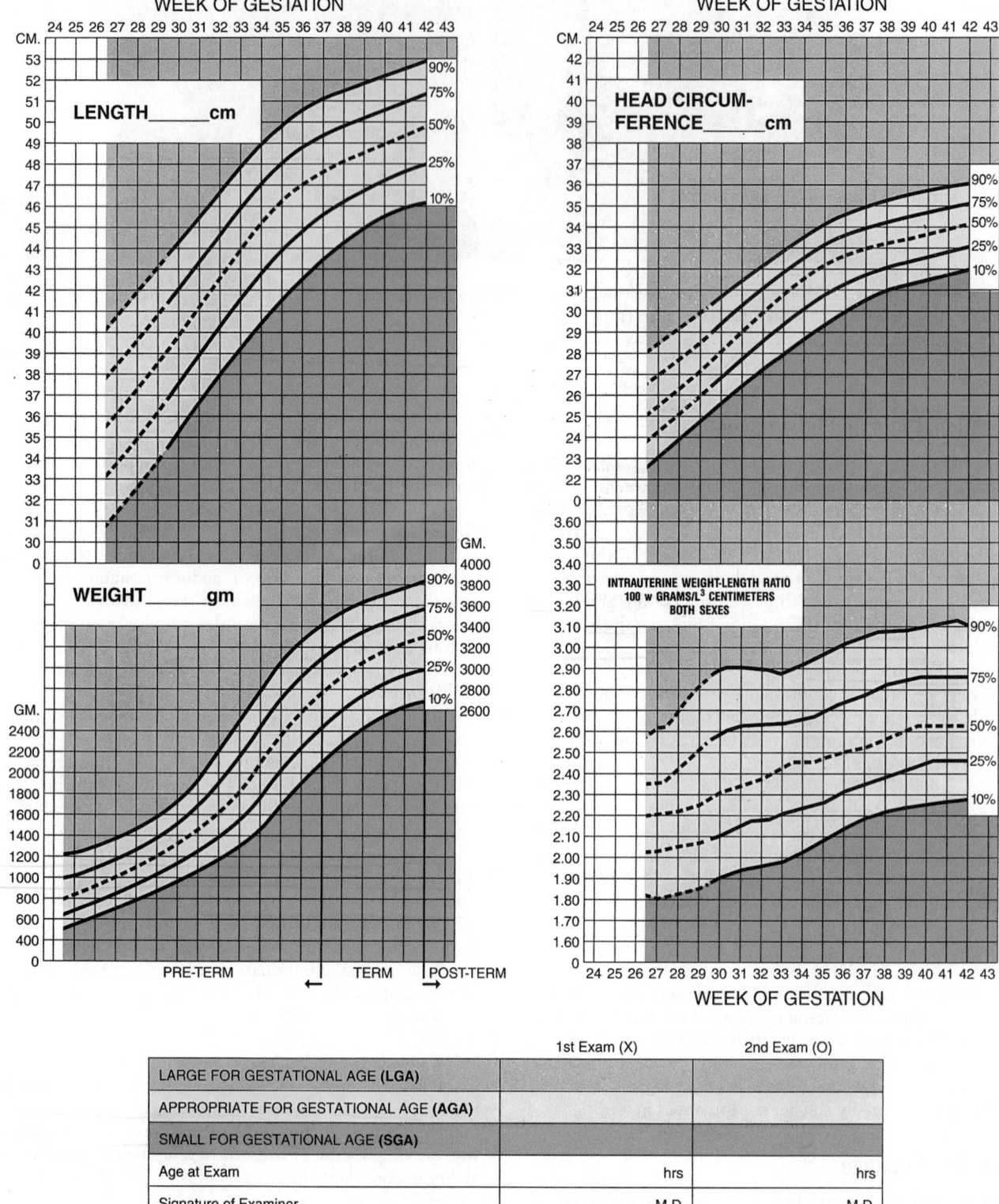

Figure 22-35 Intrauterine growth grids. (Courtesy Bristol-Myers Company, Evansville, IN. Modified from Lubchenko, L.C., Hansman, C., & Boyd, E. [1966]. *Pediatrics, 37,* 403. Modified by permission of *Pediatrics,* Vol. 37, p. 403, 1966; and from Battaglia, F.C., & Lubchenko, L.C. [1967]. *Journal of Pediatrics, 71,* 159.)

KEY CONCEPTS

- Chemical, thermal, and mechanical factors combine to stimulate the respiratory center in the brain and initiate respirations at birth.
- Surfactant lines the alveoli and reduces surface tension to keep the alveoli open. Fetal lung fluid moves into the interstitial spaces before, during, and after birth and is absorbed by the lymphatic and vascular systems.
- Increases in blood oxygen levels, shifts in pressure in the heart and lungs, and closing of the umbilical vessels cause closure of the ductus arteriosus, foramen ovale, and ductus venosus at birth.
- Infants are predisposed to heat loss because they have thin skin with little subcutaneous (white) fat, blood vessels close to the surface, and a large skin surface area. They lose heat by evaporation, conduction, convection, and radiation.
- Heat is produced in newborns by nonshivering thermogenesis, vasoconstriction, and an increase in metabolism. These factors increase oxygen and glucose consumption and may cause respiratory distress, hypoglycemia, acidosis, and jaundice.
- Laboratory values for erythrocytes, hemoglobin, and hematocrit are higher for newborns than for adults because less oxygen was available in fetal life than after birth.
- The stools progress from thick, greenish black meconium to loose, greenish brown transitional stools to milk stools. Stools of breastfed infants are frequent, soft, seedy, and mustard-colored, whereas those of formula-fed infants are pale yellow to light brown, firmer, and less frequent.
- The brain needs a constant supply of glucose and may be damaged without it.
- Physiologic jaundice occurs in normal newborns after the first 24 hours of life as a result of hemolysis of red blood cells and immaturity of the liver. Pathologic jaundice is abnormal, may begin within the first 24 hours, and often requires treatment with phototherapy. Breast milk jaundice begins later than physiologic jaundice and may be caused by substances in the milk.
- The ability of the newborn's kidneys to filter, reabsorb, and maintain fluid and electrolyte balance is less than that of the adult's kidneys. The newborn's body is composed of a greater percentage of water, and fluid is more easily lost.
- Newborns receive passive immunity when IgG crosses the placenta in utero. After birth, IgM and IgA are produced to protect against infection.
- During the first and second periods of reactivity, newborns are active and alert and may be interested in feeding. They may have a low temperature, elevated pulse and respirations, and excessive respiratory secretions. Between these periods, the infant is in a deep sleep with relaxed muscle tone.
- Newborns progress through six behavioral states: quiet sleep, active sleep, drowsy, quiet alert, active alert, and crying.
- Nurses assess newborns immediately after birth to detect serious abnormalities. If no problems are detected with a quick assessment, a more comprehensive examination is performed.
- Molding of the head is normal during birth and may cause the head to appear misshapen. Caput succedaneum or a cephalhematoma may be present.
- Measurements are an important way to learn about growth before birth. Abnormal measurements alert the nurse that complications may occur.
- Assessment of cardiorespiratory status includes history, airway, color, heart sounds, pulses, and blood pressure.
- Axillary temperatures are preferred over rectal temperatures because they are safer and provide accurate measurement.
- Hypoglycemia can cause damage to the brain. Early signs of hypoglycemia include jitteriness, poor muscle tone, respiratory distress, sweating, low temperature, and poor suck.
- In performing heel sticks for blood glucose, the nurse must choose the site carefully to avoid damage to the bone, nerves, or blood vessels of the heel.
- Reflexes are an indication of the health of the central nervous system. Asymmetry or retention of reflexes beyond the time when they should disappear is abnormal.
- The initial feeding provides information about the neonate's ability to coordinate sucking, swallowing, breathing, and tolerance to feeding.
- Newborns usually pass the first stool within 12 hours of birth. Absence of stool for 48 hours may signify an obstruction.
- The newborn's first void occurs within 24 to 48 hours. Only 1 or 2 voids a day may occur during the first 2 days. By the 4th day, the infant voids at least 6 times a day.
- Marks on the skin should be documented, including location, size, and a general description. Explain marks to parents, and offer emotional support if they are upset.
- The gestational-age assessment provides an estimate of the infant's age from conception. It alerts the nurse to possible complications of age and development.

ANSWER to Critical Thinking Exercise 22-1

If there were an opening between the right atrium and left atrium after birth, blood would flow from the left atrium, where pressures are high, into the right atrium, where pressures are low. This process is the reverse of blood flow through the foramen ovale during fetal life. The blood would then flow to the right ventricle, the pulmonary artery, and the lungs. This sequence would cause an increased workload on the lungs and could lead to serious complications.

ANSWER to Critical Thinking Exercise 22-2

Failure of the reflexes to fade on schedule may interfere with normal development. For example, the palmar grasp reflex must disappear so that the infant can learn to grasp voluntarily and later to release objects at will. Persistence of the plantar reflex would interfere with walking. Retention of reflexes beyond the age when they should disappear indicates a pathologic process and should prompt further investigation.

REFERENCES and READINGS

American Academy of Pediatrics, & American College of Obstetricians and Gynecologists. (2002). *Guidelines for perinatal care* (5th ed.). Elk Grove Village, IL, and Washington, DC: Author.

Askin, D.F. (2001). Newborn adaptation to extrauterine life. In K.R. Simpson & P.A. Creehan (Eds.), *Perinatal nursing* (2nd ed., pp. 307-335). Philadelphia: Lippincott.

Askin, D.F. (2002). Complications in the transition from fetal to neonatal life. *Journal of Obstetric, Gynecologic, and Neonatal Nursing, 31*(3), 318-327.

Ballard, J.L., Khoury, J.C., Wedig, K., Wang, L., Eilers-Walsman, B.L., & Lipp, R. (1991). New Ballard Score, expanded to include extremely premature infants. *Journal of Pediatrics, 19*(3), 417-423.

Bell, E.F., & Oh, W. (1999). Fluid and electrolyte management. In G.B. Avery, M.A. Fletcher, & M.G. MacDonald (Eds.), *Neonatology: pathophysiology and management of the newborn* (5th ed., pp. 345-361). Philadelphia: Lippincott.

Blackburn, S.T. (2003). *Maternal, fetal, and neonatal physiology* (2nd ed.). Philadelphia: Saunders.

Blake, W.W., & Murray, J.A. (2002). Heat balance. In G.B. Merenstein & S.L. Gardner (Eds.), *Handbook of neonatal intensive care* (5th ed., pp. 100-115). St. Louis: Mosby.

Brazelton, T.B. (1999). Behavioral competence. In G.B. Avery, M.A. Fletcher, & M.G. MacDonald (Eds.), *Neonatology: pathophysiology and management of the newborn* (5th ed., pp. 321-332). Philadelphia: Lippincott.

Brodsky, D., & Martin, C. (2003). *Neonatology review*. Philadelphia: Hanley & Belfus.

Buckley, R.H. (2004). The T lymphocytes, B lymphocytes, and natural killer cells. In R.E. Behrman, R.M. Kliegman, & A.M. Arvin (Eds.), *Nelson textbook of pediatrics* (17th ed., pp. 683-689). Philadelphia: Saunders.

Buschbach, D., & Bordeaux, M.S. (2002). *Newborn physiological and developmental transitions: Integrating key components of perinatal and neonatal assessment*. Washington DC: Association of Women's Health, Obstetric, and Neonatal Nurses (AWHONN).

Creehan, P.A. (2001). Newborn physical assessment. In K.R. Simpson & P.A. Creehan (Eds.), *Perinatal nursing* (2nd ed., pp. 513-542). Philadelphia: Lippincott.

D'Harlingue, A.E., & Duran, D.J. (2001). Recognition, stabilization, and transport of the high-risk newborn. In M.H. Klaus & A.A. Fanaroff, *Care of the high-risk neonate* (5th ed., pp. 65-99). Philadelphia: Saunders.

Frank, C.G., Cooper, S.C., & Merenstein, G.B. (2002). Jaundice. In G.B. Merenstein & S.L. Gardner (Eds.), *Handbook of neonatal intensive care* (5th ed., pp. 443-461). St. Louis: Mosby.

Gardner, S.L., Johnson, J.L., & Lubchenco, L.O. (2002). Initial nursery care. In G.B. Merenstein & S.L. Gardner (Eds.), *Handbook of neonatal intensive care* (5th ed., pp. 70-99). St. Louis: Mosby.

Guyton, A.C., & Hall, J.E. (2001). *Textbook of medical physiology* (10th ed.). Philadelphia: Saunders.

Hackman, P.S. (2001). Recognizing and understanding the cold-stressed term infant. *Neonatal Network, 20*(8), 35-41.

Hagedorn, M.I., Gardner, S.L., & Abman, S.H. (2002). Respiratory diseases. In G.B. Merenstein & S.L. Gardner (Eds.), *Handbook of neonatal intensive care* (5th ed., pp. 485-575). St. Louis: Mosby.

Halamek, L.P., & Stevenson, D.K. (2002). Neonatal jaundice and liver disease. In A.A. Fanaroff & R.J. Martin (Eds.), *Neonatal-perinatal medicine* (Vol. 2, 7th ed., pp. 1309-1350). St. Louis: Mosby.

Howard-Glenn, L.H. (2000). Newborn biological/behavioral characteristics and psychosocial adaptations. In S. Mattson & J.E. Smith (Eds.), *Core curriculum for maternal-newborn nursing* (pp. 360-373). Philadelphia: Saunders.

Jobe, A.H. (2002). Lung development and maturation. In A.A. Fanaroff & R.J. Martin (Eds.), *Neonatal-perinatal medicine* (Vol. 2, 7th ed.). St. Louis: Mosby.

Kenner, C. (2003). Resuscitation and stabilization of the newborn. In C. Kenner & J.W. Lott (Eds.), *Comprehensive neonatal nursing: A physiologic perspective* (3rd ed., pp. 210-227). Philadelphia: Saunders.

Lissauer, T., & Izatt, S.D. (2002). Physical examination and care of the newborn. In A.A. Fanaroff & R.J. Martin (Eds.), *Neonatal-perinatal medicine* (Vols. 1 and 2, 7th ed., pp. 441-459). St. Louis: Mosby.

Lott, J.W. (2003). Assessment and management of the cardiovascular system. In C. Kenner & J.W. Lott (Eds.), *Comprehensive neonatal nursing: A physiologic perspective* (2nd ed., pp. 376-408). Philadelphia: Saunders.

Maisels, M.J. (2001). Neonatal hyperbilirubinemia. In M.H. Klaus & A.A. Fanaroff, *Care of the high-risk neonate* (5th ed, pp. 324-362). Philadelphia: Saunders.

Matteson, P.S. (2001). *Women's health during the childbearing years: A community-based approach*. St. Louis: Mosby.

McGowan, J.E., Hagedorn, M.I.E., & Hay, W.W. (2002). Glucose homeostasis. In G.B. Merenstein & S.L. Gardner (Eds.), *Handbook of neonatal intensive care* (5th ed., pp. 298-313). St. Louis: Mosby.

Meehan, R.M. (1998). Heelsticks in neonates for capillary blood sampling. *Neonatal Network, 17*(1), 17-24.

Mercer, J.S., & Skovgaard, R.L. (2002). Neonatal transitional physiology: A new paradigm. *Journal of Perinatal & Neonatal Nursing, 15*(4), 56-75.

Montoya, K.D., & Washington, R.L. (2002). Cardiovascular diseases and surgical interventions. In G.B. Merenstein & S.L. Gardner (Eds.), *Handbook of neonatal intensive care* (5th ed., pp. 576-608). St. Louis: Mosby.

Nelson, N. (1999). The onset of respirations. In G.B. Avery, M.A. Fletcher, & M.G. MacDonald (Eds.), *Neonatology: Pathophysiology and management of the newborn* (5th ed., pp. 257-278). Philadelphia: Lippincott.

Nicholson, J.F., & Pesce, M.A. (2004). Reference ranges for laboratory tests and procedures. In

R.E. Behrman, R.M. Kliegman, & A.M. Arvin (Eds.), *Nelson textbook of pediatrics* (17th ed., pp. 2396-2421). Philadelphia: Saunders.

Reiser, D.J. (2001). *Hyperbilirubinemia: Identification and management in healthy term and near term newborns*. White Plains, NY: March of Dimes.

Sansoucie, D.A., & Cavaliere, T.A. (2003). Newborn and infant assessment. In C. Kenner & J.W. Lott (Eds.), *Comprehensive neonatal nursing: A physiologic perspective* (3rd ed., pp. 308-347). Philadelphia: Saunders.

Savaser, S. (2001). Coming to arms: Calming newborns during heel stick procedures: A Turkish perspective. *Lifelines, 5*(4), 42-46.

Shaw, N.M. (2003). Assessment and management of the hematologic system. In C. Kenner & J.W. Lott (Eds.), *Comprehensive neonatal nursing: A physiologic perspective* (3rd ed., pp. 580-623). Philadelphia: Saunders.

Sifuentes, M. (2000). Neonatal examination and nursery visit. In C.D. Berkowitz (Ed.), *Pediatrics: A primary care approach* (2nd ed., pp. 20-23). Philadelphia: Saunders.

Smith, J.E. (2000). Hyperbilirubinemia. In S. Mattson & J.E. Smith (Eds.), *Core curriculum for maternal-newborn nursing* (2nd ed., pp. 705-715). Philadelphia: Saunders.

Southgate, W.M. & Pittard, W.B. (2001). Classification and physical examination of the newborn infant. In M.H. Klaus & A.A. Fanaroff, *Care of the high-risk neonate* (5th ed., pp. 100-129). Philadelphia: Saunders.

Stoll, B.J., & Kliegman, R.M. (2004a). Digestive system disorders. In R.E. Behrman, R.M. Kliegman, & H.B. Jenson (Eds.). *Nelson textbook of pediatrics* (17th ed., pp. 588-599). Philadelphia: Saunders.

Stoll, B.J., & Kliegman, R.M. (2004b). The newborn infant. In R.E. Behrman, R.M. Kliegman, & H.B. Jenson (Eds.), *Nelson textbook of pediatrics* (17th ed., pp. 523-531). Philadelphia: Saunders.

Swinford, R.D., Bonilla-Felix, M., Cerda, R.D., & Portman, R.J. (2002). Neonatal nephrology. In G.B. Merenstein & S.L. Gardner (Eds.), *Handbook of neonatal intensive care* (5th ed., pp. 609-643). St. Louis: Mosby.

Thompson, G.H. (2004). The hip. In R.E. Behrman, R.M. Kliegman, & H.B. Jenson (Eds.), *Nelson textbook of pediatrics* (17th ed., pp. 2273-2280). Philadelphia: Saunders.

Tsang, R.C., DeMarini, S., & Rath, L.L. (2003). Fluids, electrolytes, vitamins, and trace minerals. In C. Kenner & J.W. Lott (Eds.), *Comprehensive neonatal nursing: A physiologic perspective* (3rd ed., pp. 409-424). Philadelphia: Saunders.

Walker, M. & Creehan, P. (2001). Newborn nutrition. In K. R. Simpson & P. A. Creehan (Eds.), *Perinatal nursing* (2nd ed., pp. 550-574). Philadelphia: Lippincott

23

The Normal Newborn: Nursing Care

LEARNING OBJECTIVES

After studying this chapter, you should be able to:

- Describe the purpose and use of routine prophylactic medications for the normal newborn.
- Explain the nurse's responsibility in cardiorespiratory and thermoregulatory assessments and care.
- Describe collaborative interventions for hypoglycemia.
- Discuss prevention and parent teaching for jaundice.
- Explain the risks and benefits of circumcision.
- Describe the care of circumcised and uncircumcised male infants.

- Describe ongoing nursing assessments and care of the newborn.
- Describe methods to protect newborns by proper identification.
- Explain how nurses can help prevent infant abductions.
- Describe methods to prevent infections in newborns.
- Discuss important considerations in parent teaching.
- Explain the importance of newborn screening tests.
- Describe postdischarge nursing care included in home visits, clinic visits, and telephone follow-up.

DEFINITIONS

hyperbilirubinemia Excessive amount of bilirubin in the blood.
jaundice Yellow discoloration of the skin and sclera caused by excessive bilirubin in the blood.
ophthalmia neonatorum Severe conjunctivitis in the newborn often caused by gonorrhea or chlamydia infection in the mother. May cause blindness.

prepuce Fold of skin covering the glans penis; foreskin; may be removed by circumcision.
thermoregulation Maintenance of body temperature.

The nurse's role in ongoing assessments and care of the newborn is to identify changes in the newborn's condition as the infant adapts to life outside the uterus. Nurses also intervene to keep infants safe and teach parents to provide care.

CLINICAL PATHWAYS

Birth facilities use clinical pathways (also called *care paths, care maps, multidisciplinary action plans*) to see that all the necessary tasks involved in helping infants and mothers prepare for discharge are accomplished in the time available. Clinical pathways are also used to see that mothers and infants meet the criteria for discharge. Figure 23-1 provides one example of a clinical pathway for newborns. Pathways are individualized by each institution and based on protocols to meet the needs of their clients.

EARLY CARE

Early care after birth involves the assignment of Apgar scores, assessment, and stabilization of the infant as necessary. Immediate care is discussed in Chapter 17, and infant resuscita-

tion is discussed in Chapter 30. Assessment is discussed in Chapter 22. Once the infant is stable, prophylactic medications are given.

Administering Vitamin K

A parenteral dose of vitamin K should be given to the neonate to prevent vitamin K deficiency bleeding (formerly known as *hemorrhagic disease of the newborn*) (American Academy of Pediatrics [AAP], 2003). Because infants cannot synthesize vitamin K in the intestines without bacterial flora, they are deficient in clotting factors. One dose of vitamin K, given intramuscularly within the first hour after birth, prevents bleeding problems until the infant is able to produce the vitamin independently. (See Chapter 38 for administration of injections to infants.)

Providing Eye Treatment

Infants also receive prophylactic eye treatment to prevent ophthalmia neonatorum in case the mother is infected with gonorrhea. Erythromycin (0.5%) or tetracycline (1%) ophthalmic ointment (Fig. 23-2) or povidone-iodine oph-

YORK HOSPITAL
YORK, PENNSYLVANIA
CLINICAL PATHWAY

NEWBORN

CLINICAL PATH DAY		EXPECTED PATIENT/ FAMILY OUTCOMES	MULTIDISCIPLINARY ASSESSMENT	TESTS	CONSULT
Immediate Newborn Care	Date & Time	☐ Apgar score >7 at 5 min. [4] ☐ Maintains axillary temp of 36.5C to 37.2C while in radiant warmer or in double blankets [1] ☐ Physiologic parameters WNL [4} ☐ Demonstrates proper latch when breastfeeding [2]	☐ Apgar score 1 & 5 min. ☐ Transitional newborn assessment q 30 min. ☐ Suck reflex	☐ Hypoglycemia protocol when indicated	☐ _____
Newborn Admission	Date & Time	☐ Maintains axillary temp of 36.5C to 37.2C while in radiant warmer or in double blankets [1] ☐ Physiologic parameters WNL [4] ☐ Tolerates initial feeding [2] ☐ _____	☐ Weight ☐ V/S q 30 min x 4 ☐ Multisystem admission assessment ☐ Suck reflex ☐ _____	☐ Hypoglycemia protocol when indicated ☐ _____	☐ _____ ☐ _____
Day of Birth	Date	N D E ☐☐☐ Maintains axillary temp of 36.5C to 37.2C independent of external heat source [1] ☐☐☐ Parents/family verbalize understanding of safety & security measures [6] ☐☐☐ Physiologic parameters WNL [4] ☐☐☐ Parent(s)/family & infant demonstrate attachment behaviors [3] ☐☐☐ Feeding [2] ☐☐☐ Latch score is 7 or greater for breastfed newborn [2] ☐☐☐ No jaundice [4] ☐☐☐ Infant seen by physician within 12 hours [6]	N D E ☐☐☐ Temp, apical pulse, neuro, cardiac, resp., GI, GU, integ. q shift ☐☐☐ Parent/infant attachment ☐☐☐ Positioning and LATCH score of breastfed newborn ☐☐☐ Freq. and amount of bottlefeeding ☐☐☐ _____	N D E ☐☐☐ Hypoglycemia protocol when indicated ☐☐☐ _____	N D E ☐☐☐ _____ ☐ Social service consult if indicated

NAME	INITIALS		NAME	INITIALS

8035 (4/96)

Figure 23-1 An example of a clinical pathway for the newborn from birth through the 2nd day and discharge. This form is printed on both sides and is used by all caregivers to plan and document care. (Courtesy Women and Children Services of the York Health System, York, PA. Modified with permission.)

DOCUMENTATION CODES
Initial = Meets Standard
★ = Exception on pathway identified
C = Chronic problems
N/A = Not applicable

PATIENT/FAMILY PROBLEMS
1. Thermoregulation
2. Nutrition
3. Parent-Infant attachment
4. Potential alteration in newborn metabolism
5. Risk for infection
6. Infant safety
7. _____
8. _____

TREATMENTS	MEDS	NUTR.	EDUC & DC PLANNING
☐ Clamp cord ☐ Dry newborn ☐ Radiant warmer or double blanket while being held until temp stable ☐ ID bands	☐ Neonatal eye prophylaxis & Aquamephyton ☐ HBIG if indicated	☐ Determine if bottlefeeding or breastfeeding ☐ Assist with initial breastfeeding	☐ Initiate safety & security measures with parents/family ☐ Teach breastfeeding mother proper latch
☐ Cord care ☐ Admission bath	☐ _____	Initial feeding: ☐ _____	
N D E ☐☐☐ Cord care ☐☐☐ _____	N D E ☐☐☐ _____	N D E ☐☐☐ Breast/bottle feed on demand (breast: q 2–3 hrs, bottle: q 3–4 hrs)	N D E ☐☐☐ Reinforce safety and security measures w/ parents/family ☐☐☐ Observe & reinforce proper latch and instruct breastfeeding mother/family in alternative positioning ☐☐☐ Give and review new pamphlets: -Message to mothers -Newborn screening -Car seat -Health insurance for newborns -Preparing formula -Breastfeeding, A Guide for Success

NAME	INITIALS	NAME	INITIALS

Figure 23-1, cont'd

Continued

CLINICAL PATH DAY	EXPECTED PATIENT/ FAMILY OUTCOMES	MULTIDISCIPLINARY ASSESSMENT	TESTS	CONSULT
Day 1 Date	N D E ☐ Maintains axillary temp of 36.5C to 37.2C independent of external heat source [1] ☐ Parent(s)/family & newborn demonstrate attachment behaviors [3] ☐ Physiologic parameters WNL [4] ☐ Feeding [2] ☐ LATCH score 7 or greater for breastfed newborn [2] ☐ No jaundice [4] ☐ No signs of infection [5] ☐ _____	N D E ☐ Temp, apical pulse, cardiac, resp., neuro, GI, GU, integ. q 8 hr. N/A N/A N/A Weight ☐ Parent(s)/family & infant attachment behaviors ☐ LATCH score of breastfed newborn ☐ Frequency & amt. of bottle feeding ☐ _____	N D E ☐ _____	N D E ☐ Referral made to lactation consultant for LATCH score <7 ☐ _____
Day 2 Date	☐ Maintains axillary temp of 36.5C to 37.2C independent of external heat source [1] ☐ Parent(s)/family & newborn demonstrate attachment behaviors [3] ☐ Physiologic parameters WNL [4] ☐ Feeding [2] ☐ LATCH score 7 or greater for breastfed newborn [2] ☐ No jaundice [4] ☐ No signs of infection [5] ☐ _____	☐ Temp, apical pulse, cardiac, resp., neuro, GI, GU, integ. q 8 hr. N/A N/A N/A Weight ☐ Parent(s)/family & infant attachment behaviors ☐ LATCH score of breastfed newborn ☐ Frequency & amt. of bottle feeding ☐ _____	☐ _____	☐ Referral made to lactation consultant for LATCH score <7 ☐ _____
Discharge Date	☐ Maintains axillary temp of 36.5C to 37.2C independent of external heat source [1] ☐ Parent(s)/family & newborn demonstrate attachment behaviors and appropriate care of newborn [3] ☐ Physiologic parameters WNL [4] ☐ Circumcision w/o bleeding [5] ☐ Voided at least x 1 [4] ☐ Stooled at least x 1 [4] ☐ Feeding [2] ☐ LATCH score 7 or greater for breastfed newborn [2] ☐ Parent(s)/family verbalize newborn D/C instruction [6] ☐ No jaundice [4] ☐ Physician aware of Coombs results ☐ Discharge Day 2 ☐ No signs of infection	☐ Temp, apical pulse, cardiac, resp., neuro, GI, GU, integ. q 8 hr. ☐ Discharge weight ☐ Parent(s)/family & infant attachment behaviors ☐ LATCH score of breastfed newborn ☐ Frequency & amt. of bottle feeding ☐ _____	☐ Newborn screening tests prior to D/C ☐ _____	☐ Referral made to lactation consultant for LATCH score <7 ☐ _____

NAME	INITIALS	NAME	INITIALS

NOTE: EACH PATIENT REQUIRES AN INDIVIDUAL ASSESSMENT & TREATMENT PLAN. THIS CLINICAL PATH IS A RECOMMENDATION FOR THE AVERAGE PATIENT WHICH REQUIRES MODIFICATION WHEN NECESSARY BY THE PROFESSIONAL STAFF.

Figure 23-1, cont'd

TREATMENTS	MEDS	NUTR.	EDUC & DC PLANNING
N D E □N/A □ □N/A Cord care □ □ □ _____	N D E □ □ □ _____	N D E □ □ □ Breast/bottle feed on demand (breast: q 2–3 hrs, bottle: q 3–4 hrs)	N D E □ □ □ Observe return demonst. of breast-feeding mother's use of alternative positioning □ □ □ Observe parent(s) providing appropriate newborn care; reinforce. □ □ □ _____
□N/A □ □N/A Cord care □ □ □ _____	□ □ □ _____	□ □ □ Breast/bottle feed on demand (breast: q 2–3 hrs, bottle: q 3–4 hrs)	□ □ □ Observe return demonst. of breast-feeding mother's use of alternative positioning □ □ □ Observe parent(s) providing appropriate newborn care; reinforce. □ □ □ _____
□ Cord care □ Circumcision care when indicated □ Cord clamp removed prior to D/C □ _____	□ Hepatitis B vaccine per order □ _____	□ NPO for circumcision when indicated □ Breast/bottle feed on demand (breast: q 2–3 hrs, bottle: q 3–4 hrs)	□ Review D/C instructions with parent(s)/family □ Discuss plan for follow-up care □ D/C to mother's care

NAME	INITIALS	NAME	INITIALS

Figure 23-1, cont'd

Drug Guide

Vitamin K₁ (Phytonadione)

Other Names: AquaMEPHYTON, Konakion.

Classification: Fat-soluble vitamin, antihemorrhagic.

Action: Promotes the formation of factors II (prothrombin), VII, IX, and X by the liver for clotting. Provides vitamin K, which is not synthesized in the intestines for the first 5 to 8 days after birth because the newborn lacks intestinal flora necessary for vitamin K production.

Indication: Prevention or treatment of vitamin K deficiency bleeding (hemorrhagic disease of the newborn).

Neonatal Dosage and Route: 0.5 to 1 mg (0.25 to 0.5 ml of solution containing 1 mg/2 ml) given once intramuscularly within 1 hour of birth for prophylaxis. (The lower dose may be used for small infants weighing less than 2500 g.) May be repeated or higher doses used if the mother took anticonvulsants during pregnancy. May be repeated if the infant shows bleeding tendencies.

Absorption: Readily absorbed after intramuscular injection. Effective within 1 to 2 hours.

Adverse Reactions: Pain and edema at site of administration. Hemolysis or hyperbilirubinemia, especially in a preterm infant or when large doses are used.

Nursing Considerations: Protect the drug from light until just before administration because it decomposes and loses potency on exposure to light. Incompatible with other drugs. Observe all infants for signs of vitamin K deficiency: ecchymoses or bleeding from any site.

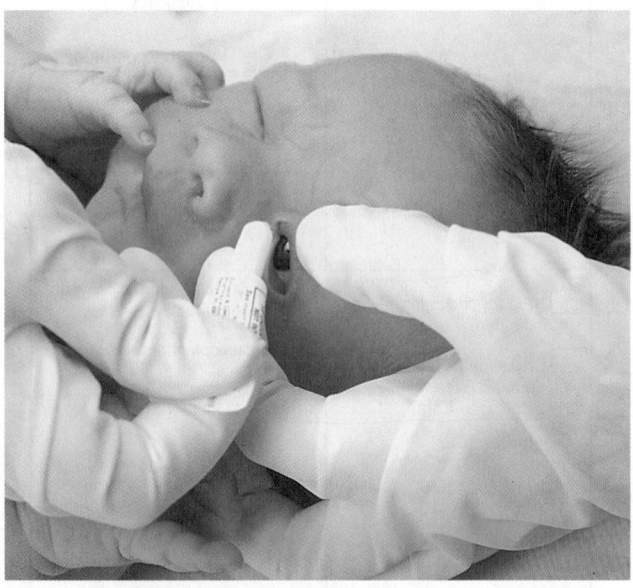

Figure 23-2 Administration of ophthalmic ointment. The nurse gently cleans the blood or vernix from around the eyes. Then, placing a finger and thumb near the edge of each lid, the nurse gently presses against the periorbital ridges to open the eyes, avoiding pressing on the eye itself. A ribbon of ointment is squeezed into each conjunctival sac.

thalmic solution (2.5%) may be used (American Academy of Pediatrics [AAP] & American College of Obstetricians & Gynecologists [ACOG], 2002). Because the ointment may temporarily blur the infant's vision, the treatment may be given near the end of the first hour to allow for bonding with the parents.

In some infants, a mild inflammation develops a few hours after prophylactic treatment. Any discharge from the eyes, however, especially if it is purulent, should alert the nurse to the possibility of infection. Drainage should be removed with sterile saline and cotton. If the mother is infected, the infant needs additional antibiotics because routine prophylactic treatment may not completely prevent infection.

▪ NURSING CARE

Cardiorespiratory Status

In the early newborn period, problems of transition may include temporary problems in cardiorespiratory status.

Assessment

Assess the infant for signs of difficult transition to newborn life. Note the rate and character of the heart rate, pulses, respirations, and breath sounds. Look for signs of respiratory distress, including tachypnea, retractions, flaring of the nares, pallor or cyanosis, grunting, seesaw respirations, and asymmetry.

Nursing Diagnosis and Planning

Fluid from the lungs must be removed by absorption or drainage from the respiratory passages after birth. This does not happen immediately and may cause a temporary problem during the early hours after birth. One of the most common nursing diagnoses for the newborn is

■ Ineffective Airway Clearance related to excessive secretions in the respiratory passages.

   Expected Outcomes: The newborn will maintain a patent airway as evidenced by a respiratory rate within the normal range of 30 to 60 breaths per minute and no signs of respiratory distress.

Interventions

Suctioning Secretions

Position the infant on the back with the head in a neutral position or to the side. Use the bulb syringe frequently to suction secretions as they drain into the infant's mouth or nose (Procedure 23-1). Suction the mouth first, because the infant may gasp and aspirate fluids in the mouth if the nose is suctioned first. Suction the nose gently and only if necessary, because suctioning is traumatic to the tissues of the nose.

Keep the bulb syringe in the crib near the infant's head, where it is available if needed quickly. Teach both parents how to use the bulb syringe correctly. Send the syringe home with the infant so that the parents can use it if the infant experiences a problem.

Drug Guide

Erythromycin Ophthalmic Ointment

Other Name: Ilotycin ophthalmic ointment.

Classification: Antibiotic.

Action: Inhibits protein synthesis in bacteria, bacteriostatic or bacteriocidal (depending on organism).

Indications: Prophylaxis against the organisms *Neisseria gonorrhoeae* and *Chlamydia trachomatis*. Prevents ophthalmia neonatorum in infants of mothers with gonorrhea and prevents conjunctivitis in infants of mothers with chlamydial infection. Prophylaxis against gonorrhea is required by law for all infants, regardless of whether the mother is known to be infected.

Neonatal Dosage and Route: A "ribbon" of 0.5% erythromycin ointment, 1 to 2 cm (0.4 to 0.8) long, is applied to the lower conjunctival sac of each eye within 1 hour after birth.

Adverse Reactions: Irritation may result in chemical conjunctivitis, lasting 24 to 48 hours. Ointment may cause temporary blurred vision.

Nursing Considerations: Cleanse the infant's eyes before application, as needed. Hold the tube in a horizontal rather than a vertical position to prevent injury to the eye from sudden movement. Administer from the inner canthus to the outer canthus. Do not touch the tip of the tube to any part of the eye because this may spread infectious material from one eye to the other. Do not rinse. Excess ointment may be wiped away after 1 minute. Observe for irritation. Use a new tube for each infant to prevent spread of infection. Other medications used for prevention of gonorrhea include tetracycline and povidone-iodine ophthalmic solution.

If mechanical suctioning is necessary to remove deeper secretions, choose a small catheter to avoid damaging the tissues of the respiratory tract. Suction for no more than 5 seconds at a time using minimal negative pressure to avoid trauma, laryngospasm, and bradycardia.

Providing Continuing Care

Continue monitoring the infant for problems throughout the birth facility stay. By the time of the second period of reactivity, the infant may be alone with the mother without constant attendance by the nurse. Although nurses know that regurgitation, gagging, and brief episodes of cyanosis are normal during the second periods of reactivity, these may be very frightening to the mother. Check frequently with her to see if the infant is having difficulty.

Evaluation

- Is the respiratory rate between 30 and 60 breaths per minute?
- Is the infant free of signs of respiratory distress?

NURSING CARE

Thermoregulation

Because any neonate may have difficulty with thermoregulation, the nurse must identify problems and intervene to prevent complications.

Assessment

Assess the newborn's temperature every half hour until it has been stable for 2 hours. Thereafter, the temperature is often checked again at 4 hours and then every 8 hours. Assess the newborn more often if the temperature is abnormal.

Nursing Diagnosis and Planning

A common diagnosis is

- Risk for Ineffective Thermoregulation related to immature compensation for changes in environmental temperature.
  Expected Outcome: The infant will maintain an axillary temperature within the normal range of 36.5° to 37.5° C (97.7° to 99.5° F).

Procedure 23-1

Using a Bulb Syringe

PURPOSE: To maintain an open airway by removing secretions or regurgitated feeding from the infant's mouth and nose.

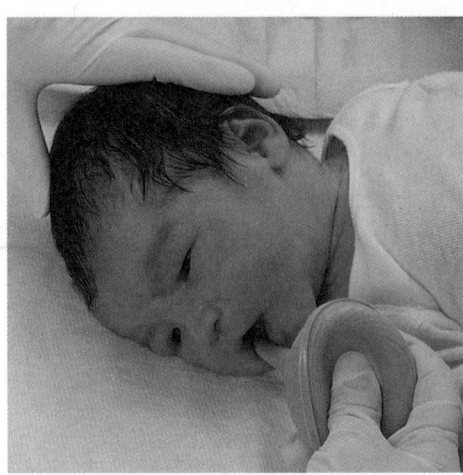

1. To allow drainage from the mouth, position the infant's head to the side.
2. Compress the bulb before inserting it into the mouth. Do not compress the bulb while it is in the infant's mouth or secretions in the bulb will be expelled back into the mouth.
3. Insert the syringe into the side of the infant's mouth. Avoid inserting it straight to the back of the throat, which (a) could stimulate the gag reflex, causing more regurgitation, and (b) could stimulate a vagal response, resulting in bradycardia or even apnea.
4. Release the bulb slowly to draw in the secretions from the mouth. Remove and empty bulb by compressing several times before using again.
5. Suction the nose, only if necessary, after the mouth is suctioned. Infants often gasp when the nose is suctioned and might aspirate secretions in the mouth if it is not cleared first.
6. Suction the nose gently because trauma could cause edema and obstruction of nasal passages.

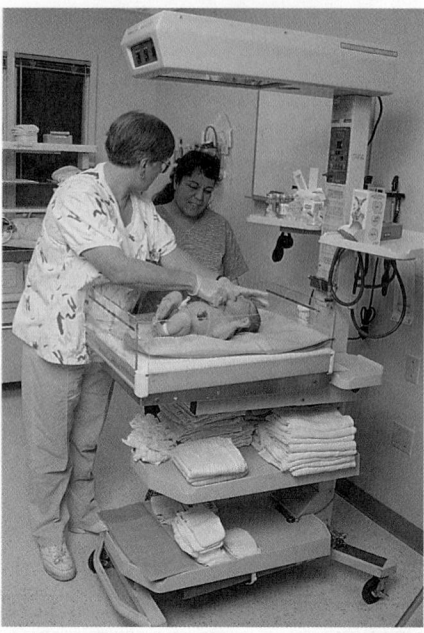

Figure 23-3 Radiant warmers allow easy access to the infant without increasing heat loss caused by exposure. The nurse should be careful not to come between the infant and the overhead source of heat when giving care.

Interventions

Preventing Heat Loss

Preparing the Environment Before Birth Before the birth, prepare a neutral thermal environment with a radiant warmer to use during initial assessments (Fig. 23-3). Check the radiant warmer to be sure it is functioning properly before the delivery. Turn it on early enough to warm the bed before the birth. Set the servocontrol between 36.0° and 36.5° C (96.8° and 97.7° F). This setting regulates the amount of heat produced by the warmer to maintain the infant's skin temperature at the normal level.

Providing Immediate Care Immediately after birth, place the infant on the mother's abdomen or under the radiant warmer to counteract the cool temperature of the delivery room. Dry the wet infant quickly with warm towels to prevent heat loss by evaporation. Dry the hair well because the head is a large surface area and hair that remains damp increases heat loss. Remove towels or blankets as soon as they become wet, and replace them with dry, warmed linens. Cover the infant's head with a cap when the infant is not under a radiant warmer. Use of a hat when the infant is under the warmer prevents transfer of heat to the infant's head.

Providing Ongoing Prevention To avoid conduction of heat away from the body, warm anything that comes in contact with the infant. Pad cool surfaces such as scales before placing infants on them. Warm stethoscopes and clothing before using them. Before touching the infant, run warm water over your hands if they are cold.

To prevent heat loss by radiation, in cold weather position the newborn's crib or incubator away from walls or windows that are part of the outside of the building. When the objects and air around the infant seem warm, it is easy to overlook the fact that infants lose heat to objects not in close contact with them. Keep this possibility in mind when positioning cribs in mothers' rooms, which are often short of space. Place the crib at the end of the mother's bed or between the beds (in a two-bed room) rather than next to the windows. Avoid areas with drafts. Keep traffic low around radiant warmers, because movement increases air currents.

When assessing or caring for newborns, avoid exposing more of their bodies than necessary. Remove clothing and blankets only from the areas being assessed. Keep the upper part of the infant covered when changing diapers. Wrap infants in blankets, and use a stockinette or insulated hat to prevent heat loss from the large surface area of the head.

Restoring Thermoregulation

If an infant with a previously normal temperature develops a low temperature, institute nursing measures to assist thermoregulation immediately. If the axillary temperature is low, some nurses check the rectal temperature to determine core temperature. However, the process of nonshivering thermogenesis begins before the core temperature becomes abnormal. Core temperature changes indicate that the infant's thermoregulatory resources are exhausted. Nurses must intervene before this happens.

Correct obvious causes first. The infant may be unwrapped or wearing wet clothing. The mother's room may be cold, or the crib may be placed near the air conditioner.

A slight drop in temperature may require only the addition of extra clothing. Put a shirt on the infant upside down by placing the infant's legs in the sleeves for added warmth. Use two blankets, each wrapped separately around the infant, to increase insulation of heat by trapping air between the layers. Place another blanket over the infant in the crib, and be sure that a hat is on the infant's head. Place linens in a warmer before use if added warmth is desired.

A greater drop in temperature requires additional measures. Place the infant under a radiant warmer for a short time. For an infant with a markedly decreased temperature, set the temperature control on the warmer to warm the infant slowly. Too-rapid warming can cause complications, including apnea.

Performing Expanded Assessments

Expanded assessments are necessary whenever temperature is decreased in a newborn. Observe for signs of respiratory distress brought on by the additional oxygen requirement of nonshivering thermogenesis.

Because the cold infant uses more glucose to produce heat, test the blood glucose level when the temperature is abnormal. If the glucose is low, have the mother breastfeed or use heated formula. Warm milk helps warm the infant.

Notify the physician or nurse practitioner if the infant does not respond to these measures. Place the infant in an incubator for close observation until the temperature stabilizes. Because low temperature is a common sign of infection, observe for signs of infection.

CRITICAL THINKING EXERCISE 23-1

You are caring for Nancy Belinsky and her son, Andy, who have both been doing well since Andy was born early this morning. As you enter the room after lunch, Nancy says, "Andy's hands and feet are so cold! And his hands are so shaky. Is he all right?"

1. What are the nursing priorities in this situation?
2. What expanded assessments are necessary?
3. What interventions are necessary?
4. How will you respond to Nancy?

Evaluation

- Is the temperature within normal range?
- Are there signs of complications from cold stress?

■ NURSING CARE

Hepatic Function

The major early assessments and care of the hepatic system are related to blood glucose levels and bilirubin conjugation.

BLOOD GLUCOSE

Assessment

Assess all infants for risk factors and signs of hypoglycemia (see Chapter 22). Perform screening tests for blood glucose according to signs exhibited and agency policy.

Nursing Diagnosis and Planning

For infants who have glucose levels below 40 to 45 mg/dl (or value used by the agency), the *collaborative problem potential complication: hypoglycemia* is appropriate. Client-centered goals for hypoglycemia are not made because this problem requires collaboration between the nurse and the physician. Planning revolves around the nurse's role in:

- Assessing for signs of hypoglycemia
- Notifying the physician about signs of hypoglycemia, or following routine orders left by the physician for infants with hypoglycemia
- Intervening to minimize hypoglycemia

Interventions

Maintaining Safe Glucose Levels

If glucose is not constantly available to the brain, permanent damage may occur. To prevent this, follow agency policy and physician orders regarding feeding infants with low glucose levels. The infant may be fed a small amount of glucose water immediately followed with breast milk or formula. Glucose water is not recommended alone for newborns because the rise in glucose results in increased insulin production, causing further drop in blood glucose. The other nutrients included in milk provide a longer-lasting supply of glucose.

Assist the breastfeeding mother with the first feeding. If she is unable to nurse the infant immediately (because of pain or exhaustion from delivery), feed the infant formula and help her breastfeed at the next feeding. Assist formula-feeding mothers to give the bottle.

Repeating Glucose Tests

Until glucose levels are stable, closely observe newborns who have shown signs of hypoglycemia. Repeat glucose screenings may be performed. Keep the physician or nurse practitioner aware of the newborn's status. If the blood glucose does not remain at an adequate level, other causative factors are investigated. The infant may be transferred to a nursery for more intensive treatment, including intravenous feedings, until blood glucose is regulated with oral feedings.

Providing Other Care

Watch for signs of other complications. Infants who do not have enough glucose may experience a drop in temperature that could lead to respiratory distress as oxygen is used for nonshivering thermogenesis. Explain the situation to par-

ents. They will be distressed over the multiple heel sticks their infant must endure. Explain the importance of maintaining adequate blood glucose levels and why the tests and frequent feedings are necessary. Encourage parents to feed the newborn as instructed so that enough glucose is available to meet the infant's needs.

Evaluation

Evaluate the collaborative interventions for hypoglycemia by noting the infant's response to interventions and the presence or absence of continued signs of hypoglycemia.

BILIRUBIN

Elevated bilirubin levels are common in newborns. Infants who need treatment for hyperbilirubinemia are discussed in Chapter 30. Prevention, however, is an important aspect of care.

Assessment

Assess for jaundice by blanching the infant's skin on the nose or sternum. Determine how far down the body the jaundice extends. When serum bilirubin tests are ordered, compare the results with what is expected for the infant's age and with previous results.

Nursing Diagnosis and Planning

Hyperbilirubinemia may not occur until after infants are at home, especially if discharge is early. A nursing diagnosis to address this situation is

- Risk for Injury related to lack of parental knowledge about hyperbilirubinemia.
  Expected Outcomes: Infants with jaundice will be identified early in the birth facility or at home. Parents will identify methods of preventing or reducing jaundice when at home.

Interventions

Determine which infants are at increased risk for hyperbilirubinemia (see Chapter 22). By using extra vigilance in caring for infants at higher risk, nurses can detect jaundice earlier and take measures to decrease it.

Explain the significance of jaundice to parents, and show them how to assess the color changes in the skin. Answer parents' questions about blood testing and care.

Discuss the importance of adequate feedings to stimulate passage of stools and help prevent high levels of bilirubin in the infant. When a newborn is feeding poorly, determine the reasons and intervene appropriately. Help mothers wake sleepy infants to feed, and encourage them to spend extra time with an infant with a poor suck. Instruct breastfeeding mothers to nurse every 2 to 3 hours. Avoid giving water to jaundiced infants, because water does not stimulate stool excretion.

Before discharge, instruct parents to contact their care provider if they see an increase in jaundice or if the infant is not eating every 3 to 4 hours, is not voiding at least six times a day by the 4th day, and is not producing stools appropriately (at least once daily for formula-fed infants; at least three stools daily for breastfed infants).

Continue to check the infant for jaundice during the early home or clinic visits. A device to measure transcutaneous bilirubin or end-tidal carbon monoxide may also be used to determine the degree of jaundice. Reinforce teaching about identification of jaundice and importance of feedings and stooling. Answer questions that have occurred to parents since discharge from the birth facility.

If an infant develops true breast milk jaundice, explain it to the parents. The mother who must discontinue breastfeeding for a day or two will be very concerned. Reassure her that her milk is adequate and not harmful to the infant. Help her maintain her milk supply by using a breast pump during the time the infant is taking formula.

Evaluation

- Can parents describe what they will look for regarding jaundice?
- Are parents able to verbalize methods to prevent or reduce jaundice?

ONGOING ASSESSMENTS AND CARE

A complete assessment is necessary every 8 hours or according to the birth facility's routine, but the nurse must always watch for signs of change in the newborn's condition (see Nursing Care Plan: Normal Newborn). Vital signs are assessed once every 8 hours or more often if they are abnormal. The infant is weighed once daily, and weight loss or gain noted.

Providing Skin Care

The skin is checked for new marks or changes in old ones. To assess skin turgor, the nurse pinches up a small area of skin over the chest or abdomen and notes how quickly it returns to its normal position. The return should be immediate in the normal newborn, with no "tenting." Skin that remains tented is an indication of dehydration.

Bathing

The infant receives a bath to remove blood, amniotic fluid, and excessive vernix as soon after birth as the temperature is stable. It is not necessary to remove all vernix. Early bathing decreases exposure to maternal blood and possible bloodborne organisms on the infant's skin. The nurse wears gloves during all contact with the infant until the bath is completed, because of the blood on the infant's skin from birth. After the bath, gloves are necessary only when contact with body fluids or stools will occur. If latex gloves are used, early bathing also decreases exposure to the allergen *latex* in the gloves.

Studies have shown that infants with stable temperatures and no complications can be bathed within 1 hour of birth with no significant drop in temperature when compared with infants bathed 2 to 6 hours after birth (Behring, Vezeau, & Fink, 2003; Penny-MacGillivray, 1996; Varda & Behnke, 2000). Giving the bath under a radiant warmer helps maintain the infant's temperature.

While shampooing the hair, the nurse combs through it to remove dried blood. After the bath, the infant is thoroughly dried to prevent heat loss by evaporation. Combing the hair hastens drying.

After the initial bath, the infant may not receive another full bath during the birth facility stay. The skin, however, is cleansed at diaper changes and to remove regurgitated milk. Clear water or a mild soap solution is used according to agency policy.

Bathing the infant in the presence of the parents allows the nurse to point out infant characteristics in addition to demonstrating the bath procedure. This may be helpful in promoting bonding in the parents (Amy, 2001).

Providing Cord Care

The cord should be checked for bleeding or oozing during the early hours after birth. The cord clamp must be securely fastened with no skin caught in it. Purulent drainage or redness or edema at the base indicates infection. The cord becomes brownish black within 2 to 3 days and falls off within approximately 10 to 14 days.

Care of the cord varies in different agencies. It may be treated with a bactericidal substance such as triple-dye solution, antibiotic ointment, or alcohol 3 times a day or allowed to dry naturally. Evidence-based practice guidelines state that none of the treatments commonly used are superior to keeping the cord clean and dry. When soiled, the cord should be cleaned with water. This natural treatment of cords may shorten the time to cord separation and does not lead to increased infections (Association of Women's Health, Obstetric and Neonatal Nurses [AWHONN], 2001). The diaper is folded below the cord to keep it dry and free from contamination by urine.

The cord clamp is removed about 24 hours after birth if the end of the cord is dry (Fig. 23-4). Although the base of the cord is still moist, there is no danger of bleeding if the end is dry and crisp.

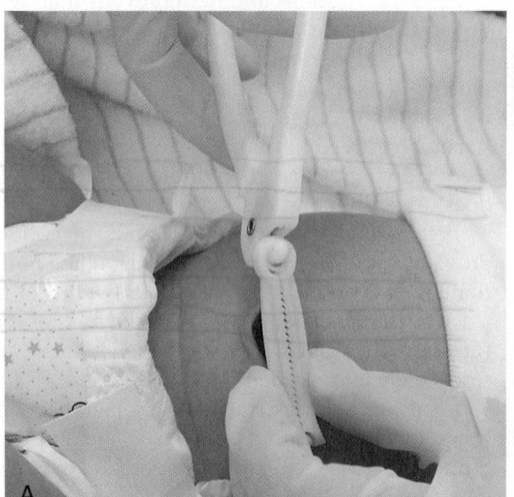
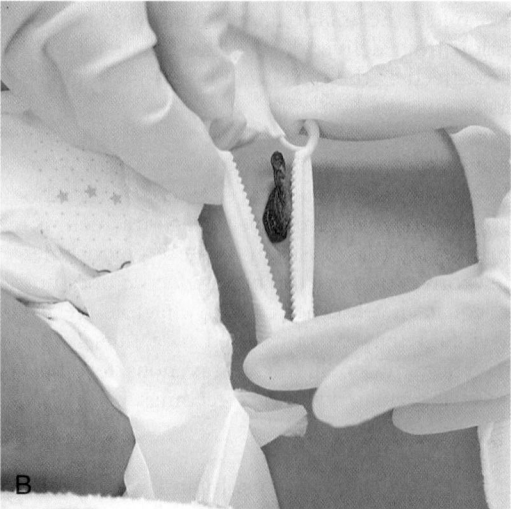

Figure 23-4 The cord clamp is removed when the end of the cord is dry and crisp. The clamp is cut (**A**) and separated (**B**).

Nursing Care Plan

Normal Newborn

ASSESSMENT

Nicholas, a full-term newborn, weighs 3402 grams (7 lb, 8 oz), and is 50 cm (20 in) long. He is the first baby for his mother, Vicki. Nicholas receives Apgar scores of 8 at 1 minute and 9 at 5 minutes. During the initial assessment, he has an excessive amount of mucus. His respiratory rate is 62, apical pulse is 156, and breath sounds are slightly moist. He has mild substernal retractions. His color is pink with acrocyanosis.

Nursing Diagnosis

Ineffective Airway Clearance related to excessive secretions in airways.

Goal/Expected Outcome

Nicholas will:

- Maintain a patent airway and have no signs of respiratory distress throughout the birth facility stay as demonstrated by respiratory rate of 30 to 60 breaths per minute, clear breath sounds, and no cyanosis, retractions, flaring, or grunting.

INTERVENTION	RATIONALE
1. Suction Nicholas as needed with a bulb syringe. If the nose also requires suctioning, suction it gently after suctioning the mouth.	1. Suctioning the mouth first prevents aspiration of oral secretions should Nicholas gasp when his nose is suctioned. Suctioning the nose can be traumatic to nasal tissues.
2. Change the infant's position frequently.	2. Position changes promote expansion and drainage of all parts of the lungs.
3. Provide reassurance for Vicki, who may be concerned.	3. The mother may be worried that something is wrong.
4. Explain use of the bulb syringe, and show Vicki how to use it. Make suggestions as needed when Vicki uses the bulb syringe.	4. Demonstration and return demonstration help ensure that parents learn correct techniques.
5. Continue to observe Nicholas for signs of respiratory distress. Count pulse and respirations every 30 minutes until they have been stable for 2 hours. Assess more often if there is any sign of abnormality. Continue to watch for other signs of ineffective airway clearance and respiratory difficulty, such as cyanosis, retractions, flaring, and grunting.	5. Monitoring should be based on history of excessive mucus, ability to cope with mucus, and other signs of respiratory difficulty and changes in the infant's condition.

Evaluation

Nicholas has clear breath sounds within 3 hours of birth, and his respiratory rate stays within normal limits. He has no further signs of respiratory difficulty. Vicki uses the bulb syringe to suction Nicholas appropriately.

ASSESSMENT

Nicholas's temperature is stable during the initial assessments, but later the axillary temperature is 36.2° C (97.2° F). His mother frequently removes his blankets to admire him and has him unwrapped while changing his diaper.

Nursing Diagnosis

Risk for Ineffective Thermoregulation related to parental lack of knowledge of newborn thermoregulation abilities and needs.

Goals/Expected Outcomes

Nicholas will:

- Maintain a temperature within the normal range of 36.5° to 37.5° C (97.7° to 99.5° F) axillary throughout his birth facility stay.

Vicki will:

- Verbalize and practice methods of preventing heat loss by the end of the first day.

Continued

Nursing Care Plan

Normal Newborn—cont'd

INTERVENTION	RATIONALE
1. Explain to Vicki the reasons newborns have problems with thermoregulation.	1. When parents understand the reasons behind precautions given them, they are more likely to practice them.
2. Teach Vicki to keep Nicholas wrapped as much as possible. Show her how to look at him and change his diaper while exposing only small areas of his body at a time.	2. Exposing the skin to the surrounding air increases heat loss by convection and radiation.
3. Teach Vicki to dry Nicholas promptly whenever he is wet, such as during bathing and when changing wet diapers or clothing.	3. Heat loss from evaporation occurs when the infant's skin is wet.
4. Instruct Vicki to keep Nicholas's crib away from cold walls, windows, or drafts from air conditioners and open doors or windows.	4. Heat loss by radiation and convection occurs from exposure to cold objects or air drafts.
5. Point out common objects that may be cold when they touch Nicholas. Explain the effect of this contact, and suggest methods to warm them before use.	5. Heat can be gained or lost by conduction.
6. Assess the infant's axillary temperature every 30 minutes until it is once again stable for 2 hours.	6. Continued assessment shows response to interventions.
7. If Nicholas becomes jittery or lethargic, check blood sugar according to birth facility routine. If the blood sugar is low, help Vicki breastfeed him or use formula if she prefers.	7. Nonshivering thermogenesis may cause hypoglycemia. Feeding provides calories for heat production. The contact with the mother's skin during breastfeeding will also help warm the infant by conduction.
8. Monitor for tachypnea or other signs of respiratory distress. Suction and apply oxygen if needed.	8. Nonshivering thermogenesis requires use of large amounts of oxygen, increases the work of the respiratory system, and may lead to hypoxia.
9. If Nicholas is slow to warm or has repeated episodes of low temperature, place him under a radiant warmer. Alert the physician or nurse practitioner.	9. Radiant heat warms infants and can be adjusted according to their needs. Temperature instability is one sign of infection in newborns.
10. When Nicholas is ready to go into an open crib, dress him in warmed clothes and blankets. Apply a stockinette or insulated hat to his head.	10. Warming clothing and blankets warms infants by conduction. Covering the head decreases heat loss.
11. Remove extra blankets according to the infant's temperature.	11. Overheating increases oxygen and glucose consumption.
12. After transfer to an open crib, monitor the infant's temperature every 30 to 60 minutes until it is stable.	12. Continued monitoring provides prompt identification of problems that develop.
13. Teach Vicki how to take her son's axillary temperature at home.	13. Teaching increases parents' competence in infant care.

Evaluation

Nicholas's axillary temperature rises to 37° C (98.6° F) and remains stable during his birth facility stay. Vicki is conscientious in using correct measures to keep Nicholas warm.

Additional Nursing Diagnoses to Consider

- Risk for Impaired Parenting.
- Risk for Infection.
- Health-Seeking Behaviors.

Cleansing the Diaper Area

Because contact with body fluids is likely while changing diapers, it is important to wear gloves. Meconium is very thick and sticky and can be difficult to remove from the skin. Plain water or mild soap solutions may be used for cleaning the diaper area. Commercial diaper wipes should be avoided because they may affect skin pH (AWHONN, 2001).

Assisting with Feedings

The nurse must ensure that infants are eating well and that parents understand their chosen feeding method. This is particularly important for breastfeeding infants (see Chapter 24). A short period of observation at the start of feedings followed by checking back during the feedings can help the nurse identify any problems.

Positioning the Infant

Teaching parents how to position infants properly is important. Placing infants in the prone position for sleep is associated with an increased risk of sudden infant death syndrome (SIDS). The American Academy of Pediatricians recommends that mothers be taught to place infants on the back for sleep because this position has the lowest rate of SIDS. The side position also reduces the risk, although not as much as the back position (AAP & ACOG, 2002). Parents should also be taught to avoid loose or soft bedding that might interfere with breathing (see Chapter 45).

Protecting the Infant

Safeguarding the infant is a major role of the nurse. Primary ways nurses protect newborns are by (1) ensuring that infants always go to the correct parents, (2) taking precautions to prevent infant abductions, and (3) preventing or recognizing early signs of infection.

Identifying the Infant

Identification bands are placed on the mother, the infant, and the father or other support person at the infant's birth to ensure that an infant is never given to the wrong person. This type of mistake could result in interference with bonding, exposure to infection, lack of confidence in the staff, and lawsuits.

Information on each band is identical and includes a number imprinted on the plastic band. The imprinted number is used to identify the mother and the infant every time the infant is brought to the mother (or significant other) after a period of separation, however brief (Fig. 23-5).

Other methods to identify infants include taking footprints of the infant and a fingerprint of the mother or photographs of the infant. A notation of birthmarks or other distinguishing features is made on the nurses' notes. Cord blood may be used for deoxyribonucleic acid (DNA) analysis if there is a later need for identification.

Preventing Infant Abduction

An unfortunate but essential role of the nurse is protection of the infant from abduction (kidnapping). Precautions include teaching parents how to recognize the picture identification badge worn by birth facility personnel. There may be other identifying measures such as color-coded badges for maternity staff. Parents receive written and oral information, including a picture of special identification badges worn by staff. Parents must be cautioned never to give their infant to anyone who does not have proper identification.

Staff members who are working temporarily on the unit are assigned special identification badges that are carefully monitored so that none can be removed from the premises without alerting the staff. In some agencies, an electronic sensor is attached to each infant by a bracelet or tag. The sensor activates an alarm if it goes near an exit or if it is cut or removed from the infant. With some systems, all exits lock automatically if an alarm is activated.

Entrances to the maternity unit should be in areas where staff can watch people entering and leaving. Unit doors may be locked at all times. Entrance requires knocking, pressing a call signal, or using a card-key or a code on the lock (Fig. 23-6). Visitors to maternity units may be required to check in with security guards or other staff members and wear special visitor identification tags.

Remote exits are locked and often equipped with video cameras and alarms. Staff must respond quickly whenever a door alarm sounds. Although alarms are usually triggered accidentally, it is always possible that a kidnapper is using a remote exit for a quick getaway.

Newborns are usually abducted by women who are familiar with the birth facility and its routines. They are of childbearing age, usually overweight, and may live near the birth facility. They usually visit several times to learn the routines so that they can impersonate birth facility staff to gain access to a newborn. They often know the layout of the facility and the locations of exits well. The woman may have had a previous pregnancy loss or has been unable to have a child of her own. She may want an infant to solidify a relationship with her husband or boyfriend. Although the woman plans the kidnapping, she waits for an appropriate opportunity to take any infant (Box 23-1).

Preventing Infection

Many nursing actions help prevent infection. Nurses wash their hands and arms at the beginning of their shift and before and after touching any infant. It is essential not to handle one neonate and then go to another without again washing one's hands. An infection that develops in one infant could quickly spread to others without these precautions. A special disinfectant for cleansing the hands may be used in place of handwashing when the hands are not visibly soiled. Dispensers may be placed in each mother's room and at other locations throughout the unit.

The nurse should instruct parents and visitors to wash their hands before handling infants. Parents should be instructed to discourage visitors with colds or other infections from coming in contact with the mother or newborn at the birth facility or during the early weeks at home.

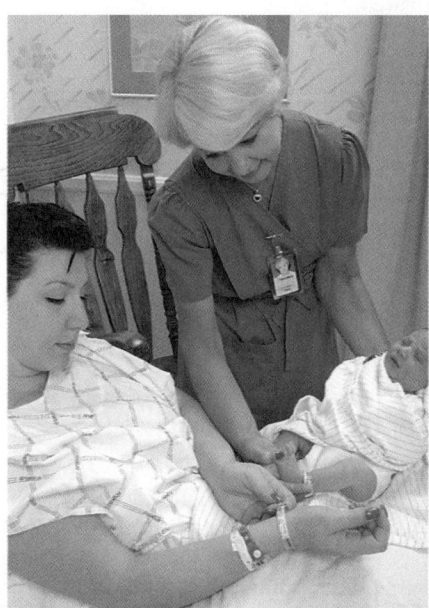

Figure 23-5 The nurse unwraps the infant to compare the infant's identification band with the mother's band. The mother may be asked to read the identification number on her band as the nurse checks the infant's band.

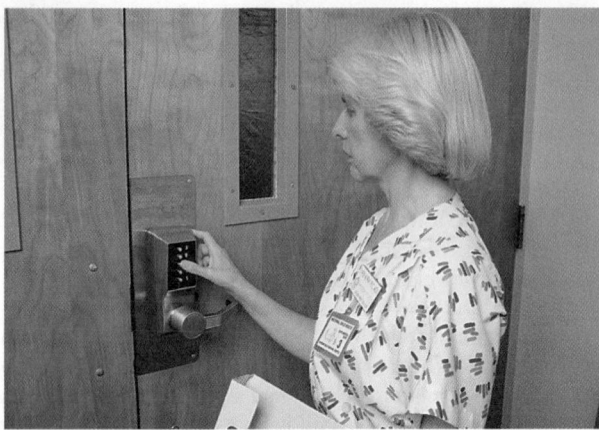

Figure 23-6 The nurse uses a code to open the door to the nursery.

To avoid cross-contamination, each infant's supplies should be kept separate from those used for other infants. Supplies in drawers or cupboards of each crib unit should be used only for that infant. Using them for another neonate could result in the transfer of infectious organisms.

When the mother has an infection, the health care provider decides whether it is safe for the newborn to remain with her. Although mothers and infants may well share the same organisms, the infant of a mother who is acutely ill may need to stay in the nursery until the mother is no longer contagious and feels able to perform infant care. Often the degree of the mother's fever is one of the determining factors. Nurses must be vigilant for signs of infection during assessment and care of the infant (see Chapter 30). Instead of a fever, there may be a decrease in temperature. The infant may feed poorly, be lethargic, or have periods of apnea. Any change in behavior that is unexplained should be recorded and investigated.

CIRCUMCISION

Circumcision is the most common surgical procedure of the neonate (Stoll & Kliegman, 2004). It is the removal of the prepuce (foreskin), a fold of skin that covers the glans penis. Although it can be retracted easily for cleaning in the older child, the prepuce is not usually fully retractable until age 3 years or older. The prepuce should never be forcibly retracted in any infant, because trauma and adhesions can result. Circumcision is a controversial procedure, and parents may have questions about whether to choose to have it performed.

Reasons for Choosing Circumcision

The American Academy of Pediatrics (AAP) states that although there are potential benefits of the procedure, data are not sufficient to recommend routine neonatal circumcision (AAP & ACOG, 2002). Circumcision may reduce urinary tract infections, some sexually transmitted infections, inflammation of the glans or prepuce, and cancer of the penis. Other factors may be causative factors in these conditions as well.

Some parents choose circumcision for religious, cultural, or social reasons. Jewish parents may have their infants circum-

BOX 23-1
Precautions to Prevent Infant Abductions

1. All personnel must wear appropriate identification *that is easily visible* at all times. No one without appropriate identification should handle or transport infants.
2. Enlist parents' help in preventing kidnapping. Teach them to allow only hospital staff with proper identification to take their infants from them.
3. Teach parents and staff to transport infants only in their cribs and never by carrying them. Question anyone walking in the hallway carrying an infant.
4. Investigate anyone with a newborn near an exit or in an unusual part of the facility.
5. Be suspicious of anyone who does not seem to be visiting a specific mother or who asks detailed questions about nursery or discharge routines.
6. Be suspicious of unknown people carrying large bags or packages that could contain an infant.
7. Respond immediately when an alarm sounds signaling that a remote exit has been opened or an infant has been taken into an unauthorized area.
8. Never leave infants unattended at any time. Teach parents that infants must be observed at all times. If there are no family members present, infants can be taken into the bathroom with mothers, if necessary. Infants can be sent back to the nursery if the mother is napping and no family members are present.
9. Take infants to mothers one at a time. Never leave an infant in the hall unsupervised.
10. When infants are left in mothers' rooms, place the cribs away from the doorways.
11. If entrances to the maternity unit or nurseries are equipped with locks that open to codes or card keys, protect them from others.
12. When a parent or family member comes to the nursery to take an infant, always match the infant and adult identification bracelet numbers. Never give an infant to anyone without the correct identification bracelet or other proper identification.
13. Alert hospital security immediately of any suspicious activity.
14. Suggest that parents do not place announcements in the paper or signs in their yard that might alert an abductor that a new baby is in the home.

cised on the 8th day after birth as part of a special ceremony. Muslim culture also includes circumcision. Some parents want their son to look like his circumcised father or peers. Others feel circumcision is an expected part of newborn care, and some do not realize that they have a choice in the matter.

Parents may be concerned that when older, the child might acquire phimosis, a tightening of the prepuce that prevents its retraction and requires circumcision. Although the number of such cases is small, surgery after the newborn period involves hospitalization and anesthesia and can be psychologically disturbing to the young child.

Lack of knowledge about the care of the prepuce leads to some circumcisions. Poor hygiene may increase the risk of in-

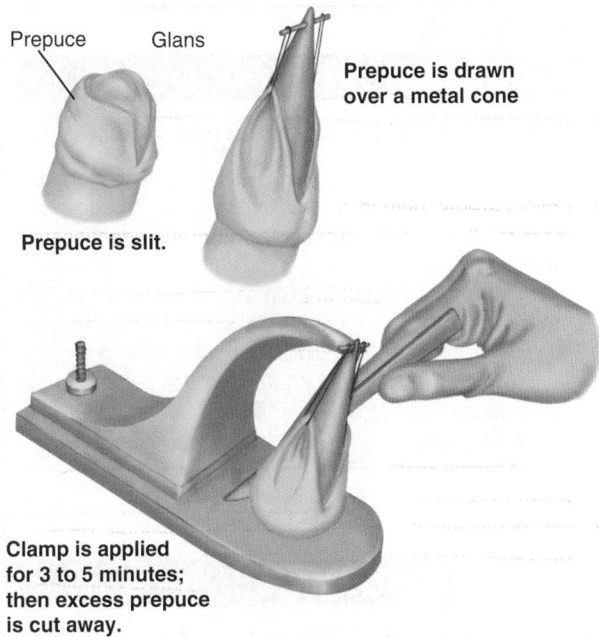

Prepuce Glans

Prepuce is drawn over a metal cone

Prepuce is slit.

Clamp is applied for 3 to 5 minutes; then excess prepuce is cut away.

Figure 23-7 Circumcision using the Gomco (Yellen) clamp. The physician pulls the prepuce over a cone-shaped device that rests against the glans. A clamp is placed around the cone and prepuce and is tightened to provide enough pressure to crush the blood vessels. This procedure prevents bleeding when the prepuce is removed after 3 to 5 minutes.

fections and other problems. Teaching the parents and child the proper care of the uncircumcised penis can prevent surgery and complications related to inadequate cleanliness.

Reasons for Rejecting Circumcision

Reasons parents decide against circumcision are varied. Some parents believe that the incidence of conditions more common in uncircumcised males is still too uncommon to warrant surgery. Others believe that having the infant circumcised to look like the father or peers is cosmetic surgery and therefore unnecessary. These parents especially object to subjecting their sons to pain during and after surgery. Circumcision is uncommon in many countries and less frequent among families from Asian, Latino, and Native American cultures.

Parents may be concerned about removing the prepuce, which serves to protect the glans. The glans is more prone to irritation from constant exposure to urine and rubbing against diapers when unprotected by the prepuce. Many believe that circumcision decreases sexual pleasure later in life because the glans becomes less sensitive.

Complications are unusual but most often include hemorrhage and infection. Other complications include the removal of too much or too little of the prepuce, stenosis or fistulas of the urethra, adhesions, necrosis, or other damage to the glans penis.

Only healthy newborns should undergo circumcision. The preterm or sick infant should not be circumcised until he is healthy enough to tolerate the procedure. Infants with blood dyscrasias may have excessive bleeding if circumcised. For the repair of anatomic abnormalities of the penis, such as hypospadias or epispadias, an intact prepuce may be needed for use in plastic surgery.

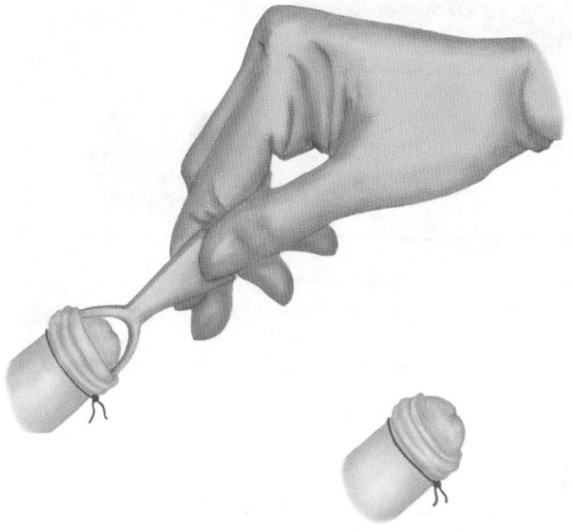

Figure 23-8 Circumcision using the Plastibell. The physician places the Plastibell, a plastic ring, over the glans, draws the prepuce over it, and ties a suture around the prepuce and Plastibell. This procedure prevents bleeding when the excess prepuce is removed. The handle is removed, leaving only the ring in place over the glans. The Plastibell falls off in 5 to 8 days.

Pain Relief

Some circumcisions are performed without anesthesia. Although it was once commonly thought that newborns do not feel pain, it is now known that pain stimuli pass along myelinated pathways by the third trimester (Agarwal, Hagedorn, & Gardner, 2002). During circumcision, newborns show changes in vital signs, oxygen saturation levels, and responses by the adrenals, indicating that they feel pain. Infants may show irritability, altered sleep-wake states, and abnormal feeding patterns for up to 22 hours after being circumcised without pain medication (Agarwal et al., 2002).

Injection of the dorsal penile nerves or the base of the penis with an anesthetic such as lidocaine is a safe method to eliminate pain during circumcision. Complications are uncommon but include hematomas, local skin necrosis, and absorption of the medication into the bloodstream. Eutectic mixture of local anesthetic (EMLA) is a cream that may be applied to anesthetize the skin before the procedure, but it is less effective than anesthetic injection and requires a longer waiting period before it is effective.

Acetaminophen may be given just before the procedure or throughout the first day for postprocedure pain. Infants receiving acetaminophen are more likely to be alert and responsive during postprocedure feedings and have improved mother/infant interaction during this time (Macke, 2001).

Nonpharmacologic pain-relief methods include pacifiers, oral sucrose, soothing music, recordings of intrauterine sounds, decreased lights, and talking softly to the infant. They are especially helpful at decreasing the stress of the procedure when combined with regional anesthesia (Geyer et al., 2002).

Methods

The Gomco (Yellen) clamp (Fig. 23-7) and the Plastibell (Fig. 23-8) are two commonly used devices for performing circumcisions. In each method, the prepuce is first separated

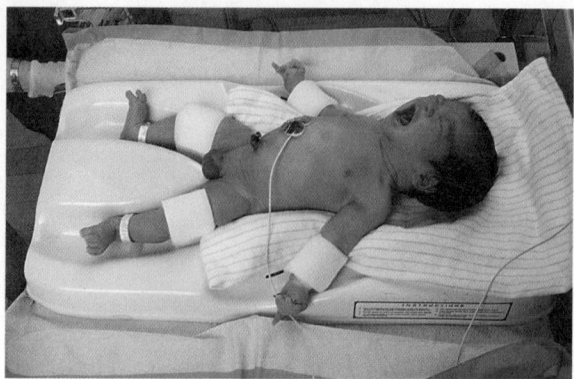

Figure 23-9 The infant is placed on the circumcision board just before the procedure is begun.

from the glans with a probe and incised to expose the glans. A Mogen clamp may also be used for circumcisions, especially for ritual circumcisions for Jewish infants.

Nursing Considerations

Assisting in Decision Making

Ideally, parents decide about circumcision early in pregnancy on the basis of careful consideration of the risks and benefits. This ideal, however, is not always the case. Nurses may be called on to answer parents' questions or clarify misconceptions.

Nurses must be certain that their own biases about circumcision do not interfere with their ability to give objective information to parents. Once the parents come to a decision, the nurse should support it.

Preparing for the Procedure and Providing Care During Circumcision

As with any surgical procedure, informed consent is necessary from the parents before a circumcision is performed. The nurse sees that the consent has been signed and that the infant has received vitamin K and informs the physician of problems that might impair the infant's ability to withstand circumcision. The infant should be at least 12 hours old and stable.

The nurse gathers equipment and supplies before the procedure. To prevent regurgitation and possible aspiration while the infant is restrained in a supine position, feedings may be withheld for 2 to 4 hours before the procedure. A bulb syringe should be placed nearby in case suction is necessary.

When the physician and equipment are ready, the infant is placed on a circumcision board and restrained (Fig. 23-9). A blanket is placed under the infant, and a drape provides warmth and maintains sterility. A heat lamp or radiant warmer helps prevent cold stress. During the procedure, the nurse provides comfort measures.

Providing Postprocedure Care

The infant should be removed from the restraints immediately after the circumcision is completed. If a Gomco clamp was used, the nurse uses petrolatum gauze strips or squeezes petroleum jelly ointment over the circumcision site and covers it with gauze to prevent the diaper from sticking to it. Petroleum jelly should not be used with a Plastibell because it might make the Plastibell slip off too soon. The diaper is attached loosely to prevent pressure. The infant should be comforted and returned to his mother, who may be anxious about her son.

PARENTS Want to Know

How to Care for the Uncircumcised Penis

Wash your son's penis daily and when soiled diapers are changed. Do not retract the foreskin, because it is does not separate from the glans or end of the penis for 3 or more years after birth.

Occasionally, gently pull back on the foreskin to see how much separation has occurred. *Never,* however, force the foreskin to retract, because it would be painful and might cause bleeding, infection, and adhesions. As your son gets older and takes over his own care, teach him to wash under the foreskin by gently pulling it back as far as it retracts each day.

PARENTS Want to Know

How to Care for the Circumcision Site

Observe the circumcision site at each diaper change. Call the physician if there are more than a few drops of blood with diaper changes during the first day or any bleeding thereafter. Continue to apply petroleum jelly to the penis with each diaper change for the first 24 hours. If a Plastibell was used, petroleum jelly should not be applied.

Squeeze warm water from a clean washcloth over the penis to wash it. Fasten the diaper loosely to prevent rubbing or pressure on the incision site.

A yellow crust over the area is normal and should not be removed. Watch for signs of infection such as fever or drainage that smells bad or has pus in it. *Call your physician if you suspect any abnormalities.* The area should be fully healed in approximately 10 days. If a Plastibell was used, the plastic rim will fall off in 5 to 8 days. If it does not fall off by that time, notify your physician.

The nurse watches carefully for signs of complications after the circumcision. The wound is checked frequently for bleeding during the first few hours after the procedure. If the infant is to be discharged after the circumcision, he should be observed for 1 to 2 hours before release.

If excessive bleeding occurs, pressure is applied to the site and the physician is notified. A small amount of blood loss may be significant in an infant, who has a small total blood volume. The physician may apply Gelfoam or epinephrine or may suture the site.

Noting the first urination after circumcision is important because edema could cause an obstruction. If the infant goes home before voiding, the mother is instructed to call the physician if there is no urinary output within 6 to 8 hours.

Teaching Parents

Each time the site is checked for bleeding, the nurse should show the parents the amount of blood on the diaper to help them understand how much to expect. The normal yellowish exudate that forms over the site should be described and differentiated from purulent drainage. Signs of complications should be discussed fully.

! CRITICAL TO REMEMBER

Signs of Complications After Circumcision

- Bleeding more than a few drops with first diaper changes
- Failure to urinate
- Signs of infection: fever or low temperature, purulent or foul-smelling drainage
- Displacement of the Plastibell

Although nurses usually teach parents of circumcised infants how to care for the penis, they may not think about providing teaching for parents who decide against circumcision. They should include care of the intact penis in the teaching plan for these parents.

NURSING CARE
Parents' Knowledge of Newborn Care

The nurse must use every contact with the parents as an opportunity for further teaching.

Assessment

Assess parents' changing learning needs throughout the birth facility stay. Consider the mother's and infant's physical conditions and any special concerns that the mother may have.

Determine learning needs for experienced mothers. They may be unaware of information that has changed since the birth of the last infant. Some examples are current recommendations about positioning infants for sleep and immunization against hepatitis B. Experienced mothers may also be concerned about helping their other children adjust to the newborn.

Also assess the father's learning needs and his plans for involvement with infant care. Determine if there are cultural dictates about the father's involvement with the infant.

Nursing Diagnosis and Planning

A common nursing diagnosis for the family with learning needs is

- Health-Seeking Behaviors: desire for information about infant care.

    Expected Outcomes: The parents will seek assistance from nurses to meet their information needs, will correctly demonstrate infant care before discharge, and will express confidence in their ability to meet their infant's needs.

Interventions
Determining Who Teaches

Because several different nurses care for mothers and infants during each 24-hour period, coordinate the teaching so that all concerns are addressed. Many facilities use a checklist to ensure that all important topics are covered with every parent.

Setting Priorities

With only a short time available for teaching, it is important to set priorities in determining what to teach. Make a teaching plan with the parents. Use a topic list to help them point out major concerns regarding infant care to ensure effective use of time. Begin by discussing their most pressing concerns to decrease anxiety. Then, as time allows, go on to other subjects.

Using Various Teaching Methods

Use a variety of teaching methods to increase effectiveness. Use verbal and written methods, as well as demonstrations. Parents often learn best by seeing skills performed correctly and then practicing them while the nurse gives suggestions. To increase the likelihood that parents will follow the nurse's instructions, explain the rationale for each point made during teaching sessions.

Discuss information with the mother alone or with her family members, roommate, or a group of mothers. Group teaching is a more efficient use of nursing time, but some mothers learn better with 1-to-1 teaching. Use audiovisual materials, including pamphlets, magazines, videos, and television programs. Highlight the most important areas and clarify information as necessary to reinforce learning.

Modeling Behavior

Modeling by the nurse is an important teaching tool. Mothers watch closely when nurses handle infants. The nurse demonstrates mothering behavior by the way the infant is held and care is given and by talking to the infant. This guidance is particularly important for the mother with no experience in infant care.

Teaching Intermittently

Plan teaching in small segments that are interspersed with infant care. Check the parents' understanding often. Encourage them to take over until they are performing all of the infant's routine care.

Including the Father

Identify fathers who would like to participate in care of their infants but hesitate. Offer them the same teaching given the inexperienced mother. Give praise liberally when mothers and fathers practice their new infant care skills. Praise increases their confidence and skill.

Documenting Teaching

Document all teaching performed and the parents' abilities to carry out infant care. This information helps other nurses know what teaching is still needed. It also provides legal proof that teaching was completed before discharge.

Providing for Follow-up Care

Provide information about unmet learning needs to the home or clinic nurse who will see the mother and infant, especially if they are discharged early. Reinforcement can then be provided during outpatient care.

Give as much information as possible in written form. The parents can then refer to areas where they have concerns. Also provide telephone numbers that they can call for further help. Offer written information in the parents' primary language, if possible. Even if they speak English, parents may prefer to read in their own language.

Incorporating Cultural Considerations

When teaching, consider the family's cultural beliefs about childcare. For example, some Southeast Asian and Latino women are hesitant to breastfeed in the birth facility and wish to wait until the milk comes in when they are home. Asian parents may be uneasy when caregivers are too complimentary about the baby or casually touch the infant's head. Latino parents, however, may prefer that a person who compliments the infant touch the infant to ward off *mal ojo,* or the "evil eye."

Teaching should include family members who will be caring for the infant. The people involved may vary according to the culture and the availability of the traditional caregiver. The woman's mother is often a major support person. In the Korean culture, however, the husband's mother is the primary caregiver for the infant and the mother in the early weeks. If the new mother will not be the primary infant caregiver, she may appear uninterested in the nurse's teachings. Asking the parents who will be helping them care for the infant helps determine family members to be included in the teaching.

Elicit questions during the discussions. However, be aware that women from some cultures will not ask questions. For many Native Americans, asking questions is considered rude (Cesario, 2001). Other women may be too shy. When questions are not asked, discuss topics often brought up by other parents.

Evaluation

- Do the parents ask questions about the infant's care?
- Can they demonstrate correct infant care?
- Do they verbalize growing confidence in their caregiving abilities?

IMMUNIZATION

Hepatitis B is a growing problem in the United States. Immunization for this disease is now included with other routine childhood vaccinations (see Appendix D). Newborns of mothers with acute or chronic hepatitis B infection (hepatitis B surface antigen [HbsAg] positive) may become infected from exposure to the mother's blood at birth. They have a very high chance for development of a chronic infection, which may cause later cancer or other serious liver damage.

These infants should receive both the vaccine and hepatitis B immune globulin (HBIG). The immune globulin provides passive immunity to hepatitis to protect infants until they develop their own antibodies and should be given within 12 hours of birth. The vaccine promotes antibody formation to protect infants from further exposure to the disease.

NEWBORN SCREENING TESTS

Blood Tests

In the United States, all states require newborn screening for phenylketonuria (PKU) (see Chapter 30) and hypothyroidism (see Chapter 51). Each state also requires testing for certain other conditions in which early treatment may prevent or lessen serious consequences such as mental retardation. Although conditions tested vary by state, other conditions often tested for are galactosemia (absence of the enzyme necessary to use the milk sugar *galactose*), and hemoglobinopathies such as sickle cell disease and thalassemia (see Chapter 47). Screening may also be performed for adrenal congenital hyperplasia, maple syrup urine disease, biotinidase deficiency, homocystinuria, and other conditions. The tests are easy and inexpensive. Further testing is necessary to confirm any abnormal test results.

Hearing Tests

Hearing loss in infants is estimated to be approximately 1 per 1000 in newborns without other complications (AAP & ACOG, 2002). Because early identification and treatment can prevent developmental delays and help the child communicate better, auditory screening of all newborns is recommended by the American Academy of Pediatrics. A goal of *Healthy People 2010* is to increase the proportion of newborns who are screened for hearing loss by age 1 month, have audiologic evaluation by age 3 months, and caregivers enroll infant in appropriate intervention services by age 6 months (U.S. Department of Health and Human Services, 2000). More than 37 states and the District of Columbia require hearing screening of all newborns (Marlowe, 2003).

To accomplish this goal, a screening test is given infants before discharge from the birth facility and referrals are made for further testing if the infant shows signs of hearing problems. Auditory brainstem response and otoacoustic emissions testing are used for screening. The nurse ensures that infants receive screening and explains the testing to the parents. Parents of infants referred for further testing will need more explanation and emotional support (see Chapter 55).

DISCHARGE AND NEWBORN FOLLOW-UP CARE

Discharge

Although state and federal legislation allow women and infants to stay in the birth facility for 48 hours after vaginal birth and 96 hours after cesarean birth, some women choose to go home earlier. The time of discharge varies according to the mother's and newborn's needs, the mother's wishes, and the primary caregivers' assessment of their conditions.

Discharge is allowed for term newborns who are appropriate for gestational age and have normal physical examination results. Infants should have normal vital signs, have fed successfully at least twice, passed urine and stool, have no excessive bleeding from the circumcision site for at least 2 hours, show no significant jaundice in the first 24 hours of life, and show that they are making the transition from fetal to neonatal life without difficulty. The mother should demonstrate knowledge, ability, and confidence to provide adequate care of the newborn. The family should have an adequate support system (AAP & ACOG, 2002).

Follow-up Care

Care after discharge from the birth facility is very important. The AAP recommends that follow-up by a health care professional be provided to all newborns who go home from the birth facility less than 48 hours after birth. This should occur within 48 hours of discharge and can be provided in the home, clinic, or office (AAP & ACOG, 2002).

Nursing follow-up care can be provided in a number of ways. These include home visits, clinic visits, and telephone counseling.

Home Visits

The home visit is ideally scheduled during the first 24 to 72 hours after discharge. This timing allows early assessment and intervention for problems in nutrition, jaundice, newborn adaptation, and maternal-infant interaction. Visits usually

PARENTS
Want to Know

Techniques for Infant Care

This guide is written in language that the nurse might use when teaching parents about infant care. Adapt the subjects to meet the needs of individual parents.

Handling the Infant
Head Support
An infant cannot support the heavy head when held in an upright position for the first few months of life. To help support the head, place a hand behind the head whenever you hold the baby.

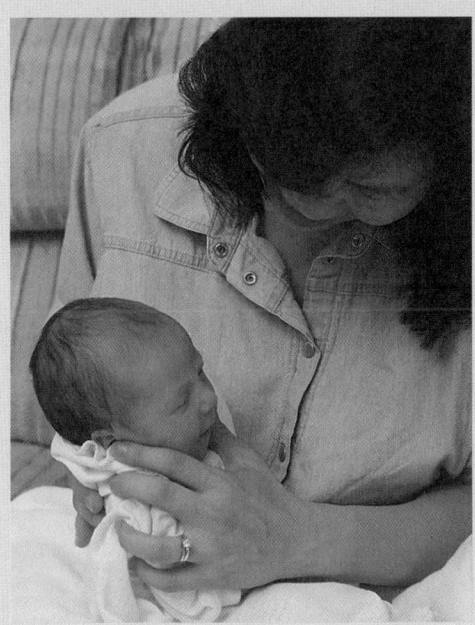

Positions
Most mothers hold the infant in the cradle position. For the "football" position, support the baby's head in the palm of your hand with the body along your arm, supported against your side. This position allows one hand to be free when washing the baby's hair or breastfeeding.

The shoulder hold is good for burping the baby. You can also set the baby on your lap and support the head and chest with one hand while gently patting or rubbing the infant's back with the other hand. This position allows you to see the baby's face in case of "spit ups."

Always place your baby on the back for sleep, unless your care provider tells you otherwise. This position is recommended by the American Academy of Pediatrics because it helps prevent sudden infant death syndrome (SIDS), the sudden, unexplained death of an infant. The baby should sleep on a firm mattress.

Wrapping
Young infants feel secure when wrapped firmly in a blanket. To swaddle the infant, turn down one corner of a blanket and position the baby's head over the edge. Fold one side of the blanket over the body and arm. Bring the lower corner up, and fold it over the chest. Then bring the other side around the infant and tuck it underneath.

Normal Body Processes
Breathing
Newborns normally breathe about 30 to 60 times a minute. Their breathing is irregular and may vary from loud to very soft. Sneezing is usually a normal response to lint from new baby clothes rather than a sign of a cold.

Using a Bulb Syringe
Use the bulb syringe when the infant has excessive mucus in the mouth or nose or spits up milk. Be very gentle, and use the bulb only if necessary. Squeeze the bulb before you insert the tip into the mouth and aim it to the side of the mouth rather than to the back. Extra mucus is common in the first days of life but is usually not a problem unless a cold develops. Clean the bulb with soap and water and dry well before using again. Call your physician if the baby's skin becomes blue or if the baby stops breathing for more than 15 seconds, has difficulty breathing, or has yellow or green drainage from the nose.

Temperature
When newborns become cold, they need more calories and oxygen than when they are warm, which can be dangerous to them. Dress your baby as you would like to be dressed. Add a light receiving blanket, except in very hot weather.

Using a Thermometer
Check your baby's temperature under the arm during illness. Hold the arm firmly over the thermometer, and be sure the bulb does not protrude behind the arm. Read it according to the manufacturer's directions. A digital thermometer is quick and is easy to read. Call your physician if the baby has a temperature higher than 100° F or lower than 97.7° F (37.8 and 36.5 if a Celsius thermometer is used at home).

Urine Output
Your baby will have at least one or two wet diapers a day during the first day or two and at least six wet diapers a day by the 4th day. Counting the number of wet diapers helps you know if the baby is getting enough milk. *Call your baby's doctor if the baby has no wet diapers for more than 12 hours.*

Stool Output
Breastfed infants pass at least three very soft, seedy stools that have a sweet-sour odor and are mustard-yellow. Formula-fed infants pass one to several stools each day. Stools are pale yellow to light brown and formed. Babies are not constipated when they turn red when passing a stool. Constipated infants pass small, hard stools. There are often fewer stools per day than usual.

Diarrhea
Babies with diarrhea pass more frequent stools that are greener and more liquid than usual. There may be a water ring—an area in the diaper where the liquid has absorbed, sometimes around an area of more solid stool. Call your physician if your baby has more than two diarrhea stools.

Continued

PARENTS
Want to Know

Techniques for Infant Care—cont'd

Skin Care

A number of normal marks occur on the newborn's skin. The normal newborn rash resembles small insect bites. Small whiteheads disappear without treatment. Do not squeeze them or they may become infected. Newborns have very dry, peeling skin that will be soft after peeling. It is not necessary to use lotions or creams because they may cause irritation.

Cord

If you have been instructed to let the cord dry naturally, do not put anything on it. Clean it with water it if it becomes soiled, and keep it dry. If you have been instructed to use alcohol, apply it to the cord three times a day. Follow the directions of your health care provider regarding use of other substances on the cord. *Notify your physician if you see bleeding or signs of infection, such as redness, drainage, or a foul odor.*

Fold the diaper below the cord so that it is not wet by urine. The cord usually falls off in about 10 to 14 days. Do not start tub baths until the cord is off and the area is well healed.

Diaper Area

Clean the diaper area with each diaper change. For girls, separate the labia (folds) and remove all stool. For boys, wash under the scrotum to help prevent rashes. Changing the diaper frequently, avoiding commercial diaper wipes, and using absorbent diapers may help prevent diaper rash. If the diaper area becomes red, change the diaper more often. Leaving the diaper off to expose the area to air is also helpful. If an ointment is needed, petroleum jelly or a barrier-type zinc oxide ointment may be used. *If redness persists, ask your baby's doctor for suggestions.*

Bathing

Give your baby a sponge bath until the cord and circumcision areas are healed. Then begin tub baths. Because infants are washed as needed after regurgitation and with diaper changes, it is not necessary to give them a bath every day.

Sponge Baths

Before the bath, gather all the supplies. You need a container or sink for the warm water, washcloth, towel, baby shampoo, alcohol, cotton-tipped swabs, and clean clothes. Soap is not necessary for the young infant, but if it is used, it should be gentle and non-alkaline.

Give the bath in a room that is warm and free of drafts. Bathe the baby on a surface that is comfortable and safe. If you use a counter, pad it with blankets or towels.

Never leave the infant alone on an unprotected surface, even for a minute. Keep one hand on the infant at all times to prevent falls. Taking the phone off the hook during the bath prevents distractions. If you must leave the room, take the baby along or place the baby in the crib.

Keep the baby warm by uncovering only the area you are washing. Wash the face with clear water. Use a separate clean area of the washcloth to wipe across the eyelids and around each eye. Clean in and around the ears, where regurgitated milk may accumulate. Do not use cotton-tipped swabs in the infant's ears or nose because injury may occur.

To clean the neck folds, put one hand under the baby's shoulders and lift slightly. This maneuver causes the head to drop back enough that the creases in the neck can be washed.

Clean the diaper area last. For baby girls, wipe the diaper area from front to back. Wiping back and forth may move stool into the vagina or urethra, causing infection.

Shampoo the head while holding the baby in a football position. The fontanel, or "soft spot," is covered with a tough membrane and is not injured by washing. Pulse movements in the fontanel are normal. Dry the hair well to prevent heat loss.

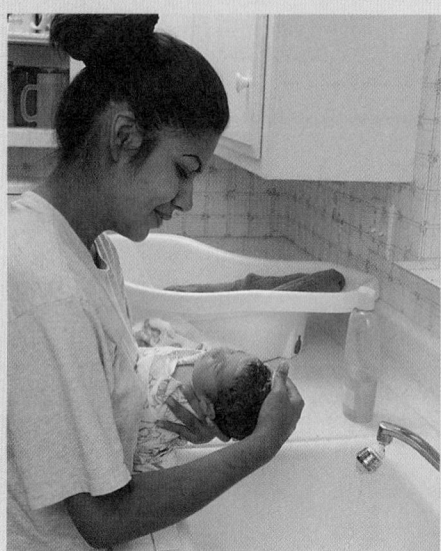

Tub Bath

For a tub bath, use a small plastic tub or a clean sink. Pad the bottom with a towel or foam pad. Place about 3 inches of warm water in the tub. Wash the face and hair before placing the baby in the tub. Keeping the baby dressed until after the hair is washed helps prevent chilling.

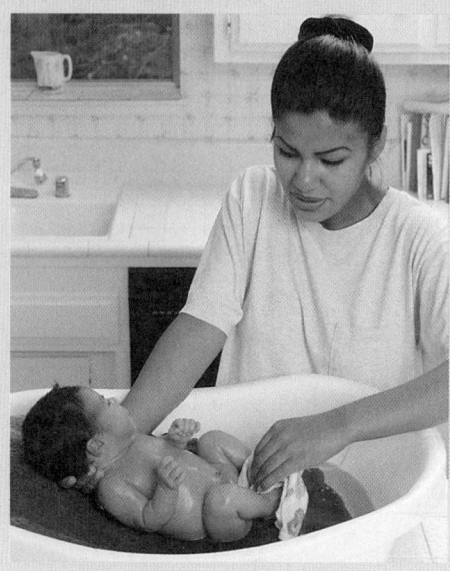

PARENTS
Want to Know

Techniques for Infant Care—cont'd

It may be easier, at first, to lather the infant's body and then immerse the baby in the tub for rinsing. It is not unusual for young infants to be frightened when they are first put in water. To help the baby adjust, talk softly and calmly while holding your baby securely.

Behavior

Knowing infants' different behavioral states helps you learn about your baby's individual characteristics.

Sleep Phases

During quiet sleep, the infant sleeps soundly with quiet breathing and little movement. Your baby will not be disturbed by noises from appliances or other children at this time. In active sleep, the baby moves or fusses while still asleep. During the drowsy state, the baby is beginning to wake but may go back to sleep if not disturbed. If it is time for feeding or other activities, however, talk softly to help the baby awaken.

Awake Phases

The quiet alert state is a good time for infant stimulation because the infant seems interested in objects and people. In the active alert, or "fussy," phase, infants signal hunger or discomfort. If you do not intervene, the baby soon moves to the crying state. The baby who cries too long may not respond at first to care activities. A few minutes of rocking and holding close may be necessary before the infant settles down.

Socialization

Infants enjoy contact with people. Use an infant seat or an infant carrier to keep the baby near you and the rest of the family. Talking and holding the baby close provide social stimulation. Infants enjoy music that is not too loud. Because they focus their eyes best at a distance of 7 to 12 inches, items such as mobiles should be placed within this range. Infants especially like black-and-white geometric figures. Babies respond best to gentle stimulation during the quiet alert state. Too much stimulation can cause the baby to be irritable and have difficulty going to sleep.

---

are 60 to 90 minutes to allow enough time for assessment and teaching (Fig. 23-10). When mothers and infants are seen within 2 days of discharge, there is an increase in maternal satisfaction with care and a reduction in infant morbidity (Lieu et al., 2000).

Content of the Home Visit. During the home visit, the nurse performs a physical examination of the mother and infant. Family adaptation to the addition of a new member and the adequacy of the mother's support system are assessed. The nurse reinforces and continues the teaching about self-care and infant care that was begun at the birth facility, and parents have an opportunity to ask questions. A feeding session should be assessed, especially if the mother is breastfeeding. Blood may be obtained for metabolic screening if the infant went home too early for reliable testing in the birth facility (Fig. 23-11).

Home visits provide reassurance for parents and may increase a woman's confidence and competence in caring for herself and her infant. Early return to her own environment, coupled with the knowledge that she can receive needed assistance from nurses, helps the woman feel more in control of her experience.

Identification of Jaundice. Home visits are especially valuable in recognizing jaundice and intervening before bilirubin levels become dangerously high (Fig. 23-12). When jaundice is found, the nurse can discuss the implications and draw blood for testing bilirubin levels. Appropriate care is discussed, as necessary, including hydration and phototherapy (see Chapter 30).

Feeding Concerns. Feeding is a subject about which mothers often have questions, especially when they are breastfeeding. When the nurse observes a feeding and helps a woman deal with

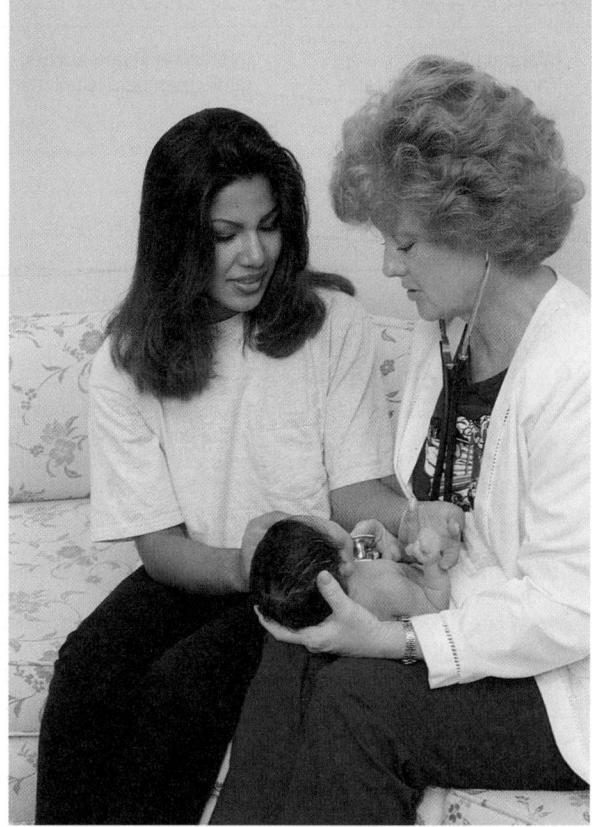

Figure 23-10 During the home visit, the nurse performs a complete assessment of the infant. Here a nurse is checking the apical pulse and listening to breath sounds.

EXPECTED NEWBORN/FAMILY OUTCOMES	ASSESSMENTS	INTERVENTIONS	RESPONSE
Physical assessment: The newborn assessment is within normal limits.	Vital signs, weight Respiratory status (color, retractions, etc.) Skin (rash, jaundice, cord, circumcision) Fontaneles Activity, sleep, behavior, crying Elimination (number of voids and stools in 24 hours)	Complete systematic assessment.	Outcomes met. Outcome not met (requires further documentation).
Nutrition: Infant's intake is adequate. LATCH score is over 7 if infant breastfed.	Infant's and mother's behaviors during a feeding	Discuss frequency, length of feedings, and amount (in oz. or time at breast). Discuss breastfeeding or other problems. Provide written educational materials.	Outcome met. Outcome not met (requires further documentation). Referral made
Caregiving: Parents correctly describe infant characteristics and needs and demonstrate care.	Parent's knowledge and performance of infant care	Teach and clarify as necessary. Provide written educational materials.	Outcome met. Outcome not met (requires further documentation).
Infant/family relationships: The family demonstrates attachment behaviors.	Interaction of parents and family members with infant	Discuss emotional adjustment of all family members, sibling rivalry, postpartum blues. Provide written educational materials.	Outcome met. Outcome not met (requires further documentation).
Support system: Parents have an adequate support system.	Interaction of family members, sources of support within and outside the immediate family	Discuss availability and need for support, resources. Provide written educational materials.	Outcome met. Outcome not met (requires further documentation). Referral made.
Environment: The home is safe and has adequate facilities and baby equipment and supplies are safe.	Safety and potential hazards in the home; availability of heat, electricity, telephone, sanitation, sleeping arrangements	Provide written educational materials.	Outcome met. Outcome not met (requires further documentation).
Need for care: The parents understand need for well baby care. They recognize signs of infant illness and how to get help.	Knowledge about well baby checkups and immunizations, signs of illness, how to take a temperature, where to get care	Discuss areas in which there is need; demonstrate temperature taking. Provide written educational materials.	Outcome met. Outcome not met (requires further documentation).

Figure 23-11 An example of a clinical pathway for a home visit by a nurse to the family of a normal newborn.

EXPECTED NEWBORN/FAMILY OUTCOMES	ASSESSMENTS	INTERVENTIONS	RESPONSE
Other care: Metabolic screening or other care is received, as ordered.	Need for specimen collection or other care	Collect blood specimens for newborn metabolic screening; give other care (phototherapy, etc.) as ordered. Provide written educational materials.	Outcome met. Outcome not met (requires further documentation).
Referrals: Parents receive necessary referrals.	Need for referrals	Refer to physician, lactation consultant, WIC, community resources, etc. Provide written educational materials.	Outcome met (document to whom referral made). Outcome not met (requires further documentation).

Figure 23-11, cont'd

problems, the infant's intake may increase. Increased intake helps prevent dehydration and possible hospital readmission. It also leads to increased excretion of bilirubin, which may prevent a need for phototherapy at home or in the hospital.

General Considerations in Home Visits. The nurse making a home visit is a guest of the family and must adapt nursing care usually given in the birth facility to the home setting. The needs of other family members may make care in the home quite different from care given in the hospital. For example, the examination of the infant may need to wait for a short time while the mother attends to her other small children.

Careful planning before the visit is essential to make the most of the limited time available. A telephone call allows the nurse to schedule the visit at a time convenient for the family and obtain directions to the home. It is important to set priorities very carefully based on the needs identified by the nurse and the family, especially when only one visit is planned. After the home visit, the nurse may schedule additional visits or provide the family with a telephone number where they may receive further help if needed.

Communication skills are particularly important when the setting is the home and the client is the family. The nurse must develop rapport with family members quickly and work with them to meet shared goals for the visit. A brief social interaction may be beneficial at the beginning of the visit to develop a trusting relationship. The purpose of the visit should be explained and the family's expectations and desires discussed. Open-ended questions and therapeutic communication techniques help the nurse identify and address the family's needs. It is important to make suggestions in a positive manner.

The nurse should be aware of any cultural practices affecting the family's view of care. For example, many Asians find direct eye contact, pointing a finger, or showing the bottom of the shoe offensive. In patriarchal cultures, the father is the head of the family and teaching should be performed through him. The elder members of the family may also play a large role in determining what health care is essential. In some cultures, the mother-in-law is a very important influence in the care of the mother and infant.

Documentation of the visit is essential. The results of the assessments, teaching, nursing care, referrals, and plans for

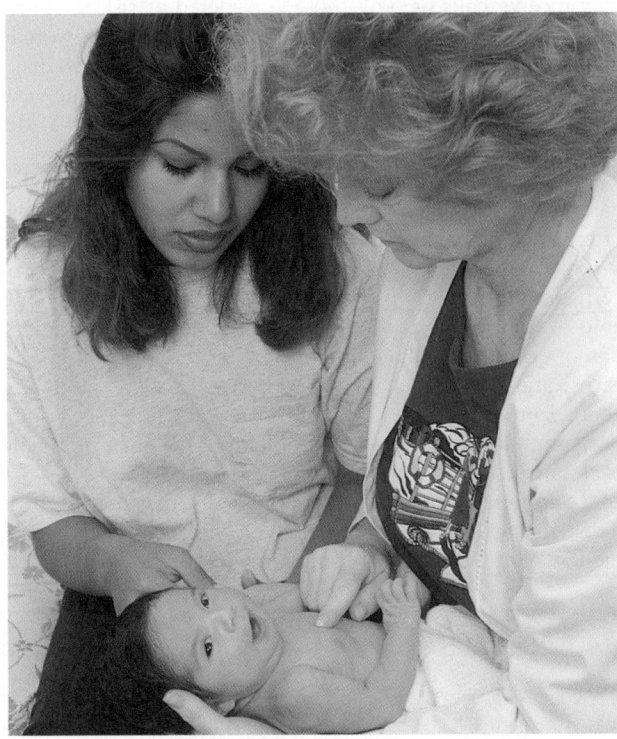

Figure 23-12 Jaundice is of particular concern when infants are discharged early after birth. The nurse shows the mother how to blanch the skin to check for jaundice and discusses what the mother should do if she sees it.

follow-up should be recorded. Copies of the record are usually sent to the primary caregiver.

Outpatient Visits

Outpatient visits may be provided by the pediatrician or by the birth facility in clinics managed by nurses. In nurse-managed clinics, mothers and infants are seen by a nurse within the first 48 to 72 hours after discharge. The charge is often included in the maternity care package. Assessment and care are essentially the same as those provided for home visits. The advantage of outpatient visits is that the nurse does not have to travel to the home and can see more clients each day, thereby reducing the cost of the service. The disadvantage is that the nurse does not have the opportunity to assess the home setting and the family interaction there. Clinic visits usually last 30 to 45 minutes. Clinic appointments may be made during the discharge procedure from the birth facility.

Telephone Counseling

Telephone counseling can occur during follow-up calls to discharged clients or when parents call "warm lines" for help with problems or questions. Telephone calls have the advantage of being much less expensive than home or clinic visits. The major disadvantage is that the nurse cannot perform an in-person assessment of the mother, infant, or home environment and must rely on the caller to present an accurate picture of the situation.

Follow-up Calls. Follow-up calls are placed by nurses in the first few days after discharge. The nurse asks a series of questions to assess the physical condition of the mother and infant and to identify any needs or problems. All mothers may receive calls or only those considered at risk for problems. In some facilities, the nurse who cared for the woman makes the calls. In others, certain nurses are assigned to make all calls. The nurse may schedule another call or a home visit, if available, or refer the woman to her primary care provider if problems are discovered.

Warm Lines. Warm lines, also called *help lines*, provide parents with an opportunity to ask a nurse the questions that often arise after they have faced the reality of parenting. Warm lines are used for situations that cause parents concern but are not emergencies. The service should be available 24 hours each day to best meet the needs of the callers. Parents often call about infant feeding, breastfeeding concerns, and basic care of the mother and infant. Calls last about 15 to 20 minutes. The nurse answers the caller's questions and assesses for other problems. The nurse may call back later to see if the situation has resolved.

Telephone Techniques. It is important that nurses caring for clients by telephone understand telephone counseling techniques. They need special training in telephone communication and triage. Open-ended questions such as "How have you been getting along since you left the hospital?" or "Have there been situations where you weren't sure what to do?" help the mother describe any problems in her own terms.

Telephone triage involves determining whether a serious problem exists and what needs to be done about it. The nurse should help the mother (or caller) describe the major concerns, which may not be those discussed first. "What worries you most?" may help focus on the most important problems. Although most problems discussed are concerns about normal infants, the nurse must be alert for serious situations needing immediate referral.

The nurse should determine if the parents know where and when to obtain more care if the problem is not resolved. They should be told approximately how long it is appropriate to wait before calling the primary care provider or telephone warm line if the situation does not improve. Nurses often call parents back to check on the progress of the problem.

Guidelines and Documentation. When nurses are giving care by telephone, it is important that they have written protocols and policies that provide guidelines for care. This procedure helps ensure that all who perform this service provide clients with similar information. A list of common questions can be compiled to help nurses obtain appropriate information when parents call about a problem.

Parents should always be told when and how to seek more care if problems are not resolved. If the infant appears ill, referral to the pediatrician or hospital emergency department is most appropriate. The nurse's judgment, based on education, expertise, and experience, is the most important factor in how helpful the service is to clients.

All calls should be documented so that accurate legal records are available for future reference. The nurse may use a check-off form or a simple written description of the call. Documentation should include identifying information for the caller, including address and phone number. The reason for the call, problems described, advice given, and any referrals should also be recorded. In some agencies, all calls are audiotaped. A copy of the information is sent to the primary caregiver to provide continuity of care.

KEY CONCEPTS

- Prophylaxis against vitamin K–deficiency bleeding (hemorrhagic disease of the newborn) and ophthalmia neonatorum is necessary shortly after birth. It is provided by an injection of vitamin K and use of erythromycin ophthalmic ointment.
- Newborns may need help in clearing the airway. Positioning, suction, and close observation may be necessary.
- Nurses can prevent heat loss in newborns by keeping them dry and covered, avoiding contact between them and cold objects or surfaces, and keeping them away from drafts and outside windows and walls.
- The nurse must identify actual or potential hypoglycemia and intervene appropriately.
- Important interventions for jaundice are to monitor for its occurrence, to be sure that the infant is feeding well, and to explain the condition to the parents.

- Reasons parents choose circumcision include decreased incidence of urinary tract infections and inflammation of the glans, prepuce, or meatus; religious dictates; parent preference; and lack of knowledge about care of the foreskin.
- Risks of circumcision include hemorrhage, infection, over-removal, urethral stenosis or fistula, adhesions, damage to the glans, and pain during and after the surgery.
- Parents may reject circumcision because of cultural practices, the belief that surgery is unnecessary, and concern about pain.
- Parents with uncircumcised sons should be taught not to retract the foreskin until it becomes separate from the glans later in childhood.
- Parents of circumcised infants should be taught signs of complications and how to care for the area.

- The nurse must prevent mistaken identification of infants by checking the mother and infant identification bands whenever they have been separated.
- Parents and nurses must work together to prevent infant abductions. Parents must know how to identify hospital staff. Nurses should be alert for suspect behavior.
- Infection can best be prevented by scrupulous handwashing by staff and all who come in contact with newborns.
- Every nursing contact with parents should be used as an opportunity to teach.
- Screening tests are commonly performed to rule out phenylketonuria, hypothyroidism, galactosemia, and hemoglobinopathies. Other tests may also be included.

ANSWERS to Critical Thinking Exercise 23-1

1. Determine whether Andy is showing signs of inadequate thermoregulation, hypoglycemia, or both. Reassure and teach Nancy about her son's condition.

2. While taking the infant's temperature, assess for skin temperature, jitteriness, and general behavior. Check the blood glucose level if indicated.

3. If Andy's temperature is slightly low, change any wet linens, double-wrap him, and apply a hat. Have Nancy feed him if it is near feeding time. Recheck the temperature in 30 minutes, and place Andy in a radiant warmer if necessary. Notify the physician if the problem continues. (See Nursing Care Plan 23-1 for other interventions.)

4. Praise Nancy for being so observant of her son. Explain that peripheral circulation is sluggish in newborns and causes cool hands and feet. If "shakiness" is the Moro reflex or normal newborn behavior, discuss this. Explain all interventions.

REFERENCES and READINGS

Agarwal, R., Hagedorn, M.I.E., & Gardner, S.L. (2002). Pain and pain relief. In G.B. Merenstein & S.L. Gardner (Eds.), *Handbook of neonatal intensive care* (5th ed., pp. 191-218). St. Louis: Mosby.

American Academy of Pediatrics. (2003). Policy statement: Controversies concerning vitamin K and the newborn. *Pediatrics, 112*(1), 191-192.

American Academy of Pediatrics, & American College of Obstetricians and Gynecologists (AAP & ACOG). (2002). *Guidelines for perinatal care* (5th ed.). Elk Grove Village, IL, and Washington, DC: Author.

Amy, E. (2001). Reflections on the interactive newborn bath demonstration. *MCN: The American Journal of Maternal/Child Nursing, 26*(6), 320-322.

Association of Women's Health, Obstetric, and Neonatal Nurses (AWHONN). (2001). *Evidence-based clinical practice guideline: Neonatal skin care*. Washington, DC: Author.

Association of Women's Health, Obstetric, and Neonatal Nurses (AWHONN). (2003). *Standards for professional nursing practice in the care of women and newborns* (6th ed.). Washington, DC: Author.

Behring, A., Vezeau, T.M., & Fink, R. (2003). Timing of the newborn first bath: A replication. *Neonatal Network, 22*(1), 39-46.

Berkowitz, C.D. (2000). Circumcision. In C.D. Berkowitz (Ed.), *Pediatrics: A primary care approach* (2nd ed., pp. 30-33). Philadelphia: Saunders.

Burns, A.L. (2003). Protecting infants in healthcare facilities from abduction. *Journal of Perinatal and Neonatal Nursing, 17*(2), 139-147.

Buschbach, D., & Bordeaux, M.S. (2002). *Newborn physiological and developmental transitions: Integrating key components of perinatal and neonatal assessment*. Washington DC: Association of Women's Health, Obstetric, and Neonatal Nurses (AWHONN).

Cesario, S.K. (2001). Care of the Native American woman: Strategies for practice, education, and research. *Journal of Obstetric, Gynecologic, & Neonatal Nursing, 30*(1), 13-19.

Chagnon, L. (2002). Newborn hearing screening. *AWHONN Lifelines, 6*(5), 398-400.

Dana, S.N., & Wambach, K.A. (2003). Patient satisfaction with an early discharge home visit program. *Journal of Obstetric, Gynecologic, and Neonatal Nursing, 32*(2), 190-198.

Ewy-Edwards, D. (2000). Transition to parenthood. In F.H. Nichols & S.S. Humenick, *Childbirth education: Practice, research, and theory* (2nd ed., pp. 84-113). Philadelphia: Saunders.

Geyer, J., Ellsbury, D., Kleiber, C., Litwiller, D., Hinton, A., & Yankowitz, J. (2002). An evidence-based multidisciplinary protocol for neonatal circumcision pain management. *Journal of Obstetric, Gynecologic, and Neonatal Nursing, 31*(4), 403-410.

Hale, K., & Incao, D. (2002). Infant security education: A multidisciplinary approach. *AWHONN Lifelines, 6*(3), 235-239.

Howard-Glen, L. (2000). Adaptation to extrauterine life and immediate nursing care. In S. Mattson & J.E. Smith (Eds.), *Core curriculum for maternal-newborn nursing* (2nd ed., pp. 346-359). Philadelphia: Saunders.

Howard-Glenn, L.H. (2000). Newborn biological/behavioral characteristics and psychosocial adaptations. In S. Mattson & J.E. Smith (Eds.), *Core curriculum for maternal-newborn nursing* (pp. 360-373). Philadelphia: Saunders.

Kaufman, M.W., Clark, J.Y., & Castro, C.L. (2001). Neonatal circumcision: Benefits, risks, and family teaching. *MCN: The American Journal of Maternal/Child Nursing, 26*(4), 197-201.

Kepler, A.B., & Simpson, K.R. (2001). Discharge planning. In K.R. Simpson & P.A. Creehan (Eds.), *Perinatal nursing* (pp. 610-632). Philadelphia: Lippincott.

Kim-Godwin, Y.S. (2003). Postpartum beliefs and practices among non-Western cultures. *MCN: The American Journal of Maternal/Child Nursing, 28*(2), 74-78.

Knott, C. (2001). Universal newborn hearing screening coming soon: "Hear's" why. *Neonatal Network, 20*(8), 25-33.

Lashley, F.R. (2002). Newborn screening: New opportunities and new challenges. *Newborn and Infant Nursing Reviews, 2*(4), 228-242.

Lieu, T.A., Braveman, P.A., Escobar, G.J., Fischer, A.F., Jensvold, N.G., & Capra, A.M. (2000). A randomized comparison of home and clinic follow-up visits after early postpartum hospital discharge. *Pediatrics, 105*(5), 1058-1065.

Lloyd-Puryear, M.A., & Forsman, I. (2002). Newborn screening and genetic testing. *Journal of Obstetric, Gynecologic, and Neonatal Nursing, 31*(2), 200-207.

Macke, J.K. (2001). Analgesia for circumcision: Effects on newborn behavior and mother/infant interaction. *Journal of Obstetric, Gynecologic, and Neonatal Nursing, 30*(5), 507-514.

Malnory, M., Johnson, T.S., & Kirby, R.S. (2003). Newborn behavioral and physiological responses to circumcision. *MCN: The American Journal of Maternal/Child Nursing, 28*(5), 313-317.

Marlowe, J.A. (2003). *Newborn hearing screening: Testing, follow-up and communication with families*. Washington, DC: AWHONN.

Matteson, P.S. (2001). *Women's health during the childbearing years: A community-based approach*. St. Louis: Mosby.

Mattson, S. (2003). Caring for Latino women. *AWHONN Lifelines, 7*(3), 258-260.

McGregor, L.A. (1996). Short, shorter, shortest: Continuing to improve the hospital stay for mothers and newborns. *MCN: The American Journal of Maternal/Child Nursing, 21*(4), 191-196.

Penny-MacGillivray, T. (1996). A newborn's first bath: When? *Journal of Obstetric, Gynecologic, and Neonatal Nursing, 25*(6), 481-487.

Rabun, J.B. (2003). *For healthcare professionals: Guidelines on prevention of and response to infant abductions* (7th ed.). Alexandria, VA: National Center for Missing & Exploited Children.

Shogan, M.G. (2002). Emergency management plan for newborn abduction. *Journal of Obstetric, Gynecologic, and Neonatal Nursing, 31*(3), 340-346.

Sifuentes, M. (2000). Screening in newborns. In C.D. Berkowitz (Ed.), *Pediatrics: A primary care approach* (2nd ed., pp. 24-26). Philadelphia: Saunders.

Stoll, B.J., & Kliegman, R.M. (2004). Genitourinary system. In R.E. Behrman, R.M. Kliegman, & H.B. Jenson (Eds.), *Nelson textbook of pediatrics* (17th ed., p. 608). Philadelphia: Saunders.

U.S. Department of Health and Human Services. (2000). *Healthy People 2010* (Conference edition, in 2 volumes). Washington, DC.

Varda, K.E., & Behnke, R.S. (2000). The effect of timing of initial bath on newborn's temperature. *Journal of Obstetric, Gynecologic, and Neonatal Nursing, 29*(1), 24-32.

24

Newborn Feeding

◆ LEARNING OBJECTIVES

After studying this chapter, you should be able to:

◎ Identify the nutritional and fluid needs of the infant.
◎ Compare the composition of breast milk with that of formula.
◎ Explain important factors in choosing a method of infant feeding.
◎ Explain the physiology of lactation.
◎ Describe nursing management of initial and continued breastfeeding.

◎ Describe nursing assessments and interventions for common problems in breastfeeding.
◎ Describe nursing assessments and interventions in formula feeding.

◆ DEFINITIONS

colostrum Breast fluid secreted during pregnancy and the first week after childbirth.

engorgement Swelling of the breasts resulting from enlarged lymph glands, increased blood flow, and accumulation of milk when milk begins to be produced.

foremilk First breast milk received in a feeding.

hindmilk Breast milk received near the end of a feeding; contains higher fat content than foremilk.

latch-on Attachment of the infant to the breast.

let-down reflex See *milk-ejection reflex.*

mastitis Inflammation of the breast, usually caused by stasis of milk in the ducts or by infection.

mature milk Breast milk that appears after the first 2 weeks of lactation.

milk-ejection reflex Release of milk from the alveoli into the ducts; also known as the *let-down reflex.*

nonnutritive sucking Sucking during which no milk flow is obtained.

nutritive suckling or **sucking** Steady, rhythmic suckling at the breast or sucking at a bottle to obtain milk.

oxytocin Hormone produced by the posterior pituitary gland that stimulates uterine contractions and the milk-ejection reflex; also prepared synthetically.

prolactin Anterior pituitary hormone that promotes growth of breast tissue and stimulates production of milk.

suckling Giving or taking nourishment from the breast. Sometimes used interchangeably with *sucking,* which refers to drawing into the mouth with a partial vacuum, as with a bottle or pacifier.

transitional milk Breast milk that appears between secretion of colostrum and mature milk.

Helping women choose a feeding method and become comfortable using it are important nursing contributions that require knowledge of the infant's nutritional needs and the techniques to meet those needs.

NUTRITIONAL NEEDS OF THE NEWBORN

Calories

The full-term newborn needs 110 to 120 kcal/kg (50-55 kcal/lb) of body weight each day. Breast milk and formulas used for the normal newborn contain 20 kcal/oz. The average newborn weighing 3.4 kg (7½ lb) requires approximately 570 to 630 ml (19-21 oz) of breast milk or formula each day to meet caloric requirements.

During the early days after birth, many infants lose 5% to 10% of their birth weight. This loss is the result of normal loss of extracellular water and the consumption of fewer calories than needed. Newborns may fall asleep before feeding adequately and have a small stomach capacity at birth. Capacity increases rapidly so that many infants take 60 to 90 ml (2-3 oz) by the end of the first week. Infants usually regain the lost weight by age 10 to 14 days. This information should be explained to parents.

> **! CRITICAL TO REMEMBER**
>
> ### Daily Calorie and Fluid Needs of the Newborn
>
> - *Calories:* 110 to 120 kcal/kg (50-55 kcal/lb).
> - *Fluid:* 40 to 60 ml/kg (18-36 ml/lb) for the first 2 days of life; 100 to 150 ml/kg (45-68 ml/lb) after the first 2 days of life.

Other Nutrients

The calories needed by the newborn are provided by carbohydrates, proteins, and fat in breast milk or formula. Full-term neonates digest simple carbohydrates and proteins well. Fats are less well digested because of the lack of pancreatic lipase in the newborn. Vitamins and minerals are provided by both breast milk and formula.

Water

Because newborns lose water easily from the skin, kidneys, and intestines, they must have adequate fluid intake each day. The normal newborn needs approximately 40 to 60 ml/kg (18-36 ml/lb) during the first 2 days of life and 100 to 150 ml/kg (45-68 ml/lb) a day by the end of the first week (Tsang, DeMarini, & Rath, 2003). Breast milk or formula supplies the infant's fluid needs. Additional water is unnecessary.

BREAST MILK AND FORMULA COMPOSITION

Breast Milk

Breast milk is species-specific for human infants and offers many advantages over formula. The nutrients in breast milk are proportioned appropriately for the neonate and change to meet the newborn's changing needs. Breast milk provides protection against infection and is easily digested.

Changes in Composition

The composition of breast milk changes in three phases: colostrum, transitional milk, and mature milk.

Colostrum. The major secretion of the breasts during the first week of lactation is colostrum—a thick, yellow substance. Colostrum is higher in protein, fat-soluble vitamins, and minerals than mature milk but lower in calories, fat, and lactose. It is rich in immunoglobulins, especially secretory IgA, which helps protect the infant's gastrointestinal tract from infection. Colostrum helps establish the normal flora in the intestines, and its laxative effect speeds the passage of meconium.

Transitional Milk. Transitional milk appears as the milk changes from colostrum to mature milk. Immunoglobulins and proteins decrease while lactose, fat, and calories increase. The vitamin content is approximately the same as that of mature milk.

Mature Milk. After the first 2 weeks of lactation, mature milk replaces transitional milk. Because breast milk is bluish and not as thick as colostrum, some mothers think their milk is not "rich" enough for the infant. Nurses should explain the normal appearance of breast milk. Mature milk contains approximately 20 kcal/oz and nutrients sufficient to meet the infant's needs. Discussions of breast milk and its contents refer to mature milk unless otherwise stated.

Nutrients

Protein. The concentrations of amino acids in breast milk are suited to the infant's needs and ability to metabolize them. Breast milk is high in taurine, which is important for bile conjugation and brain development. Breast milk is low in tyrosine and phenylalanine, corresponding to the infant's low levels of enzymes to digest them. The proteins produce a low solute load for the infant's immature kidneys.

Casein and whey are the proteins in milk. Casein forms a large, insoluble curd that is harder to digest than the curd from whey, which is very soft. Breast milk is easily digested because it has a high ratio of whey to casein. Commercial formulas must be adapted to increase the amount of whey so that the curd is more digestible.

The protein in cow's milk causes allergies in many infants fed cow's milk formulas. Because breast milk is made for the human infant, it is unlikely to cause allergies. Although breast milk does not cause allergies, allergenic foods the mother has eaten may pass to her milk. If the infant reacts to the mother's diet, the offending food should be identified and eliminated. When there is a high family incidence of allergies, a mother can reduce the risk by restricting highly allergenic foods such as cow's milk, eggs, fish, peanuts, and tree nuts (American Academy of Pediatrics [AAP], 2000).

Carbohydrate. Lactose is the carbohydrate in breast milk. Its higher level in breast milk may improve absorption of calcium, phosphorus, and magnesium (Biancuzzo, 2003; Lawrence & Lawrence, 1999). Lactose also promotes growth of the normal bacterial flora in the intestines.

Fat. Fat provides 30% to 55% of the calories in breast milk. Triglycerides form the majority of fat content. Cholesterol and essential fatty acids such as long-chain polyunsaturated fatty acids, docosahexaenoic acid (DHA) and arachidonic acid (ARA), which are important for growth of the brain and other parts of central nervous system, are also present. These fatty acids must be added to formulas. The fat in breast milk is more easily digested by the newborn than that in cow's milk.

The amount of fat in breast milk varies during the feeding and according to the time of day. More fat is present in the hindmilk—the milk produced at the end of the feeding.

Vitamins. Vitamin C must be added to commercial formulas to match the levels in human milk, which meet the infant's needs if the mother has an adequate intake. The vitamin D content of breast milk is low, and supplementation is often given. Infants who are not exposed to the sun and those with dark skin are particularly at risk for insufficient vitamin D. The infant of a vegan mother may need supplementation with vitamin B_{12}.

Minerals. The casein protein in cow's milk interferes with iron absorption. Although iron in breast milk is lower than in formula, approximately 49% is absorbed, compared with only 4% of that in iron-fortified formula (Lawrence & Lawrence, 1999). The full-term infant who is breastfed exclusively maintains iron stores for the first 6 months of life. Generally iron is added at 4 to 6 months. Preterm infants need iron supplements earlier. All formula-fed infants should receive formula fortified with iron (American Academy of Pediatrics [AAP] & American College of Obstetricians and Gynecologists [ACOG], 2002).

Sodium, calcium, and phosphorus are higher in cow's milk than in human milk. This difference could cause an excessively high renal solute load if formula is not diluted properly.

Enzymes

Breast milk contains enzymes that aid in digestion. Pancreatic amylase, necessary to digest carbohydrates, is low in the newborn, but the enzyme is present in breast milk. Breast milk also contains lipase to increase fat digestion.

Infection-Preventing Components

Substances in breast milk such as *bifidus factor, lysozymes,* and *lactoferrin* help to prevent infection in the infant. *Immunoglobulins* are present in highest amounts in colostrum but are present throughout lactation. Lymphocytes in the milk produce secretory IgA, which helps prevent intestinal and respiratory infections. Infants who are breastfed, even partially, have a decreased incidence not only of respiratory and gastrointestinal infections but also of ear infections and sudden infant death syndrome (Newton, 2002).

Effect of Maternal Diet

Although the fatty acid content of breast milk is influenced by the mother's diet, malnourished mothers have about the same proportions of protein, carbohydrates, and most minerals as those who are well nourished. Levels of vitamins in breast milk, however, are affected by the mother's intake and stores. It is important that breastfeeding women eat a well-balanced diet to maintain their own health and energy levels. (See "Nutrition for the Lactating Mother" in Chapter 15.)

Formulas

Commercial formulas are produced to replace or supplement breast milk. Manufacturers adapt commercial formulas to correspond to the components in breast milk as much as possible, although an exact match is impossible. A variety of formulas that differ in price and ingredients are available.

Cow's Milk

Unmodified cow's milk (whole milk, low-fat milk, or fat-free milk) is not recommended for infants younger than 12 months because it contains too much protein, potassium, and sodium, lacks enough iron and linoleic acid, and may cause gastrointestinal bleeding and anemia (Heird, 2004; Trahms, 2000). Modified cow's milk is the source of most commercial formulas. Manufacturers specifically formulate it for infants by reducing protein to decrease renal solute load. Saturated fat is removed and replaced with vegetable fats. Vitamins and other nutrients are added to simulate the contents of breast milk. Examples of formulas are Similac, Enfamil, and Good Start.

Formulas for Infants With Special Needs

Infants with galactosemia or lactase deficiency or those whose families are vegetarians may be given soy formula. Many infants with cow's milk allergy are also allergic to soy formulas. Casein hydrolysate formulas are more universally tolerated by infants with allergies. The protein in these formulas is less allergenic than other formulas. The formulas are also used for infants with fat malabsorption.

The preterm infant may require a more concentrated formula with more calories in less liquid. Human milk fortifiers can be added to human milk to adapt it to the needs of preterm infants. Lactose-free formula uses primarily glucose instead of lactose for infants who do not tolerate lactose. Low-phenylalanine formulas are needed for infants with phenylketonuria, a deficiency in the enzyme to digest phenylalanine found in standard formulas.

CONSIDERATIONS IN CHOOSING A FEEDING METHOD

Many women decide on a feeding method well ahead of birth, but some wait until late in their pregnancy. Nurses can help mothers decide on a method and gain confidence in feeding their infants. Nurses should explain the many benefits to the mother and the infant of breastfeeding when the woman is undecided. However, it is very important for nurses to be sensitive to mothers' feelings about feeding. Although nurses should encourage breastfeeding as the best method of feeding in most circumstances, they should be supportive of the mother's chosen method once the decision is made.

Breastfeeding

Mothers choose breastfeeding because it offers many advantages for the mother and the infant (Table 24-1). Both the American Academy of Pediatrics (AAP) and the U.S. Surgeon General recommend breastfeeding. The AAP and American Dietetics Association recommend that only breast milk be given for the first 6 months after birth and that breastfeeding continue after the addition of solids until the infant is at least 12 months old (AAP, 1997; AAP, 2002; Dobson & Murtaugh, 2001).

A goal set by the U.S. Department of Health and Human Services (USDHHS) for the year 2010 is for 75% of all new mothers to breastfeed at the time of birth facility discharge, for at least 50% to be breastfeeding at 6 months, and 25% at 1 year (USDHHS, 2000). In 2000, 68.4% of mothers began to breastfeed their newborns. At 6 months, 31.4% of mothers were breastfeeding. At 12 months, the rate was 17.6% breastfeeding. These statistics show a gradual but steady increase since 1991 (Ross Products Division, 2003), but continued improvement is needed.

In an effort to promote breastfeeding, the United Nations Children's Fund (UNICEF) and the World Health Organization (WHO) advocate that birth facilities become certified as "baby-friendly" hospitals, where policies are initiated to encourage breastfeeding actively. Guidelines to becoming certified as a baby-friendly hospital emphasize education of staff and parents about breastfeeding, early initiation of breastfeeding, demand feedings, avoidance of formula and pacifiers, and rooming-in.

Formula Feeding

Mothers choose formula feeding for many reasons. Some women are embarrassed by breastfeeding, seeing the breasts only in a sexual context. Many mothers have little experience with family or friends who have had breastfeeding experiences. The woman's partner or mother may not be supportive of breastfeeding.

Occasionally a woman requires medications that would harm the infant. A frequent reason that mothers choose formula feeding instead of breastfeeding is a lack of adequate understanding about the two methods.

TABLE **24-1** Benefits of Breastfeeding

FOR THE INFANT	FOR THE MOTHER
Allergies are less likely to develop.	Oxytocin release enhances involution of uterus.
Immunologic properties help prevent infections. May have fewer respiratory, ear, and gastrointestinal infections and less risk for sudden infant death syndrome (SIDS).	Mother loses less blood because of delayed return of menses.
Composition meets infant's specific nutritional needs.	Mother more likely to rest while feeding.
Nutritional and immunologic properties change according to infant's needs.	Mother likely to eat balanced diet that improves healing.
Breast milk easily digested.	Frequent, close contact may enhance bonding.
Protein, fat, and carbohydrate in most suitable proportions.	Convenient: always available, no bottles to prepare, no formula to buy or heat.
No possibility of improper (and potentially dangerous) dilution.	Economical: eliminates cost of formula and bottles.
Breast milk unlikely to be contaminated; not affected by water supply.	Traveling easier: no bottles to prepare, carry, refrigerate, or warm.
Less likely to result in overfeeding.	May reduce the risk of some cancers.
Infant unlikely to have constipation.	

Combination Feeding

Some parents prefer a combination of breastfeeding and bottle feeding. Giving breastfeeding infants formula leads to a decrease in breastfeeding frequency and milk production, making successful breastfeeding less likely (AAP & ACOG, 2002). Women who use a combination of breast milk and formula are likely to breastfeed for shorter durations than women who breastfeed exclusively (Chezem, Friesen, & Boettcher, 2003).

Unless medically indicated, it is best to delay giving formula until lactation has been well established. However, if the mother chooses to feed both breast milk and formula, the nurse should support her so that the infant receives the benefits of breast milk at least part of the time.

Some mothers choose to give a bottle daily or only occasionally, such as when a babysitter is with the infant. This allows the mother to be away from the infant for longer periods of time yet allows the closeness with the infant that many mothers enjoy, as well as the physical advantages of breastfeeding, to continue. Mothers may choose to use breast milk or formula for occasional bottle feedings.

Factors Influencing Choice

Many factors influence a woman's choice of feeding method. These factors must be considered when educating women about their choices.

Support From Others

The influence of family members is often an important determinant of whether mothers breastfeed. The mother with little support or with active discouragement from her family will probably have a difficult time nursing. Educating family members about the advantages of breastfeeding and how to deal with problems may lead to their encouragement of the breastfeeding mother. Some women choose not to breastfeed because their partner objects. However, one study of men from African-American, Hispanic, and other cultures found that 81% wanted their infants to be breastfed (Pollock, Bustamante-Forest, & Giarratano, 2002).

Encouragement from the woman's health care provider may increase the chance that she will breastfeed. One study found that women were more likely to still be breastfeeding at 12 weeks if they had received encouragement from their provider (Taveras et al., 2003). The support the mother receives from the nursing staff plays a significant part in whether she feels comfortable with the feeding method she chooses. Those who do not feel confident in their ability to breastfeed before they leave the birth facility are less likely to continue breastfeeding if they encounter difficulties at home.

Culture

Cultural influences may dictate decisions about how a mother feeds her infant. For example, many Mormon women believe that breastfeeding is an important part of motherhood. Muslim women often breastfeed for the first 2 years. Immigrants from countries where breastfeeding is the norm may breastfeed for shorter durations or not at all because they lack the support system they had in their own country. In addition, formula feeding may be seen as a symbol of the new way of life.

Nurses should be particularly watchful for ways to help mothers from other cultures who might wish to breastfeed but fail to do so because of lack of support. Canadian Mohawk mothers were more likely to breastfeed when a woman from their community worked with them and the grandmother in promoting the value of breastfeeding (Banks, 2003).

Some Asian and Latino mothers give their infants formula while in the birth facility and do not begin to breastfeed until at home. This practice may be because of modesty about nursing in front of others in the birth facility, as well as lack of understanding about the value of colostrum. Some Korean women believe they should not breastfeed for the first 3 days after birth (Windsor, 2003). Women in some cultures believe that colostrum may be "spoiled" because it has been in the breasts for a long time. They may express colostrum and discard it before they begin to breastfeed the infant.

Certain foods are used to increase milk production in some cultures. Examples include broth from blue cornmeal for Navajo Indians, chocolate for women from Guatemala, and anise or sesame seed for Hispanic women (Biancuzzo, 2003).

Employment

Returning to work or school is a major cause of discontinuation of breastfeeding by 10 to 12 weeks (Taveras et al., 2003). The mother may choose formula from the begin-

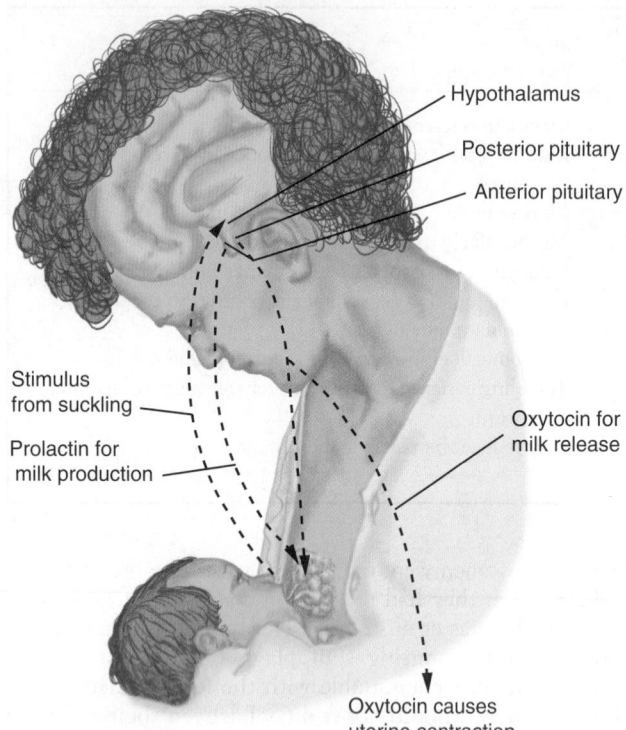

Figure 24-1 Effect of prolactin and oxytocin on milk production. When the infant begins to suckle at the breast, nerve impulses travel to the hypothalamus, which causes the anterior pituitary to secrete prolactin to increase milk production. Suckling also causes the posterior pituitary to secrete oxytocin, producing the let-down reflex, which releases milk from the breast. Oxytocin also causes the uterus to contract, which aids in involution.

ning, plan a short period of breastfeeding before weaning the infant to formula, or use a combination of breastfeeding and bottle feeding with breast milk or formula. Nurses who provide practical information about breastfeeding and working may help a mother continue breastfeeding for a longer period.

Women who will be using a breast pump at work should have a place to pump once or twice during her breaks or lunch time. The place should be clean and private. If she pumps a couple of times a day for a week or two before returning to work, she will be adept at using the pump and will have a supply of breast milk for the caregiver to use while she is at work. Frequent breastfeeding during the evening and weekends will help her maintain her milk supply.

Other Factors

Other factors may also influence a woman's decision. Her knowledge and past experience with infant feeding are important. Women who are most likely to breastfeed are older than 35 years, are white, have a college education, and live in the western part of the United States. Those with the lowest breastfeeding rates are African American, have a grade-school education, are employed full-time, are younger than 20 years, and live in the southern United States (Ross Products Division, 2003). Although African-American women still have the lowest rates of breastfeeding, they have shown a greater increase in breastfeeding than other groups in recent years (USDHHS, 2000).

NORMAL BREASTFEEDING

Breast Changes During Pregnancy

Breast changes begin early in pregnancy (see Chapters 11 and 13 and Figures 11-8 and 13-3). The ducts, lobules, and alveoli develop in response to estrogen, progesterone, placental lactogen, prolactin, and chorionic gonadotropin. Prolactin levels are high but milk production is prevented by estrogen, progesterone, and placental lactogen, which inhibit breast response to prolactin. Changes such as increase in breast size indicate that the breasts are responding adequately to hormonal stimulation to prepare for lactation.

Milk Production

Milk is produced in the alveoli of the breasts through a complex process by which materials are removed from the mother's bloodstream and reformulated into breast milk. Most milk is synthesized when the infant is suckling.

The milk is ejected from the secretory cells of the alveoli into the alveolar lumen by contraction of the myoepithelial cells. It travels through the lactiferous ducts to the lactiferous sinuses (or ampullae), which the infant compresses during nursing to eject a stream of milk through pores in the nipple.

Hormonal Changes at Birth

Prolactin

At birth, loss of progesterone, estrogen, and placental lactogen from the placenta results in increasing levels and effectiveness of prolactin and causes milk production. Suckling and the removal of colostrum or milk cause continued increased levels of prolactin. Levels are high during the early months and then gradually decrease until weaning.

Oxytocin

Oxytocin increases in response to nipple stimulation and causes the milk-ejection reflex, commonly known as the *let-down reflex*. During a feeding, the milk-ejection reflex occurs a number of times. When mothers see, hear, or think about their infants, they often have an increase in oxytocin level, bringing about a let-down of milk. Pain or lack of relaxation can inhibit oxytocin release. Oxytocin also causes the uterine contractions mothers may feel at the beginning of nursing sessions (Fig. 24-1).

Continued Milk Production

The amount of milk produced depends primarily on adequate stimulation of the breast and removal of the milk. This "supply-and-demand" effect continues throughout lactation—that is, increased demand with more frequent and longer nursing results in more milk available for the infant. If milk (or colostrum) is not removed from the breasts, the milk in the ducts is eventually absorbed, the alveoli become smaller, the secretory cells return to a resting state, and milk production ends.

Preparation of Breasts for Breastfeeding

Little preparation is needed during pregnancy for breastfeeding. The mother should avoid soap on her nipples to prevent removal of the natural protective oils from the Montgomery tubercles of the breasts. The use of creams, nipple rolling, pulling, and rubbing to "toughen" nipples is unnecessary and may cause irritation or uterine contractions from release of oxytocin.

The breasts should be assessed during pregnancy to identify flat or inverted nipples (Fig. 24-2). Normal nipples protrude. Flat nipples appear soft, like the areola, and do not stand erect unless stimulated by rolling them between the fingers. Inverted nipples are drawn into the breast tissue. Both conditions make it difficult for infants to draw the nipples into the mouth. Some nipples appear normal but draw inward when the areola is compressed in the infant's mouth. Compressing the areola between the thumb and the forefinger determines whether the nipple projects normally or becomes inverted.

Women with flat or inverted nipples may find breast shells useful (Biancuzzo, 2003). The dome-shaped devices are worn during the last weeks of pregnancy and between feedings after birth. The shells are placed in the bra with the opening over the nipple. They exert slight pressure against the areola to help the nipples protrude. A breast pump may be used just before feedings to help bring the nipples out.

■NURSING CARE
Breastfeeding

Assessment

Assess the mother and the infant during the breastfeeding process. The LATCH breastfeeding assessment tool may be helpful to score the infant's ability to latch onto the breast and swallow as well as the mother's nipples, comfort and ability to hold and position the infant correctly. A score of 0 to 2 is given for each area. An infant who does not have a sustained latch receives a 0, the need for repeated attempts is scored 1, and a latch with the mouth positioned correctly and rhythmic sucking is scored 2. Scores of 0, 1, or 2 are given for no audible swallowing, a few swallows, or spontaneous swallows. The mother's nipples are scored 0 to 2 for inverted, flat, or everted nipples. Engorged breasts with cracks, bleeding or blisters of the nipples are scored 0. Redness or small blisters with some discomfort receives as score of 1. Soft, nontender breasts receive a score of 3. A score of 0 is given if the mother requires the staff to position the infant at the breast, a score of 1 if some assistance is needed, and a score of 2 if no assistance is needed for correct positioning (Jensen, Wallace, & Kelsay, 1994). A score of 7 or less indicates the mother needs more assistance in feeding.

Maternal Assessment

Assess the condition of the breasts and nipples and the mother's knowledge about breastfeeding to determine her needs for assistance.

Breasts and Nipples

Examine the breasts and nipples during late pregnancy, if possible, to identify problems that might interfere with feeding. After birth, palpate the breasts with each postpartum assessment to see if they are soft, filling, or engorged. Soft breasts feel like a cheek. If milk is beginning to come in, the breasts may be slightly firmer, which is charted as "filling." Engorged breasts are hard and tender, with taut, shiny skin.

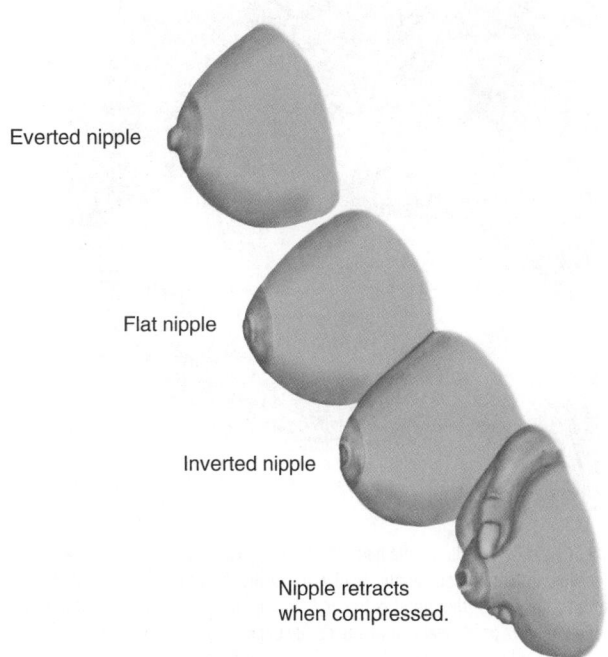

Figure 24-2 Normal everted nipple and other types of nipples that may cause the infant difficulty in latching-on. Nipples shown after stimulation.

Everted nipple

Flat nipple

Inverted nipple

Nipple retracts when compressed.

Redness, tenderness, or lumps within the breasts are also noted. The nipples may be red, bruised, blistered, fissured, bleeding, or tender.

Knowledge

The mother breastfeeding for the first time may have many questions and may need substantial guidance during her first attempts. If she has nursed before, she may have a better understanding of breastfeeding but may have questions or have forgotten some aspects.

Assessment of Infant Feeding Behaviors

Before initiating a breastfeeding session, assess the infant's readiness for feeding. The infant should be awake and hungry. Sucking on the hands, rooting when the cheek or side of the mouth is touched, smacking of the lips, and slight fussiness are common hunger cues. Crying is a late sign of hunger. Continue to assess for signs of infant problems throughout the feeding.

Nursing Diagnosis and Planning

Women with and without experience often need information to have a successful breastfeeding experience. Breastfeeding problems and lack of confidence during the first 1 to 2 days are good predictors of discontinuation of breastfeeding within the first 2 weeks (Taveras et al., 2003). Nurses can help prevent early weaning by using the nursing diagnosis

■ Risk for Ineffective Breastfeeding related to lack of understanding of breastfeeding techniques.

Expected Outcomes: The infant will breastfeed using nutritive suckling for 15 minutes or more for most feedings before discharge. The mother will demonstrate breastfeeding techniques as taught before discharge and will verbalize satisfaction and confidence with the breastfeeding process before discharge.

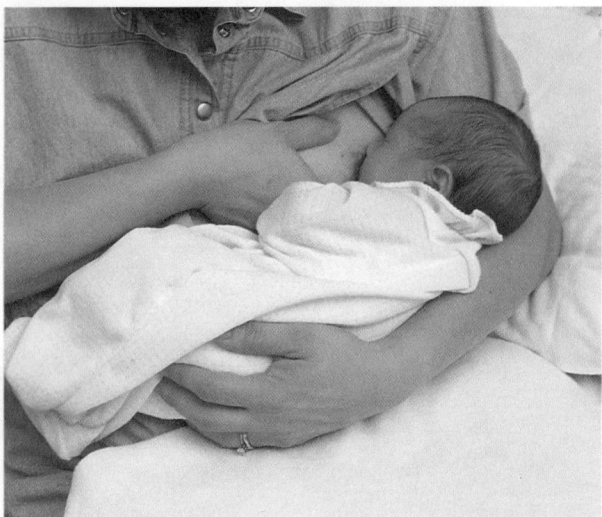

Figure 24-3 For the cradle hold, the mother positions the infant's head at or near the antecubital space and level with her nipple, with her arm supporting the infant's body. Her other hand is free to hold the breast. Once the infant is positioned, pillows or blankets can be used to support the mother's arm, which may tire from holding the baby.

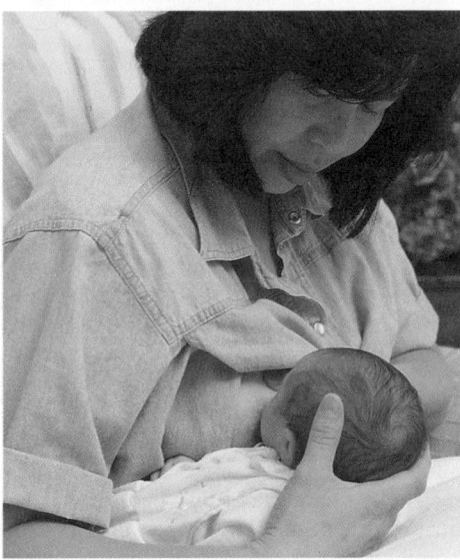

Figure 24-4 For the football hold, the mother supports the infant's head in her hand, with the infant's body resting on pillows alongside her hip. This method allows the mother to see the position of the infant's mouth on the breast, helps her control the infant's head, and is especially helpful for mothers with heavy breasts. This hold also avoids pressure against an abdominal incision.

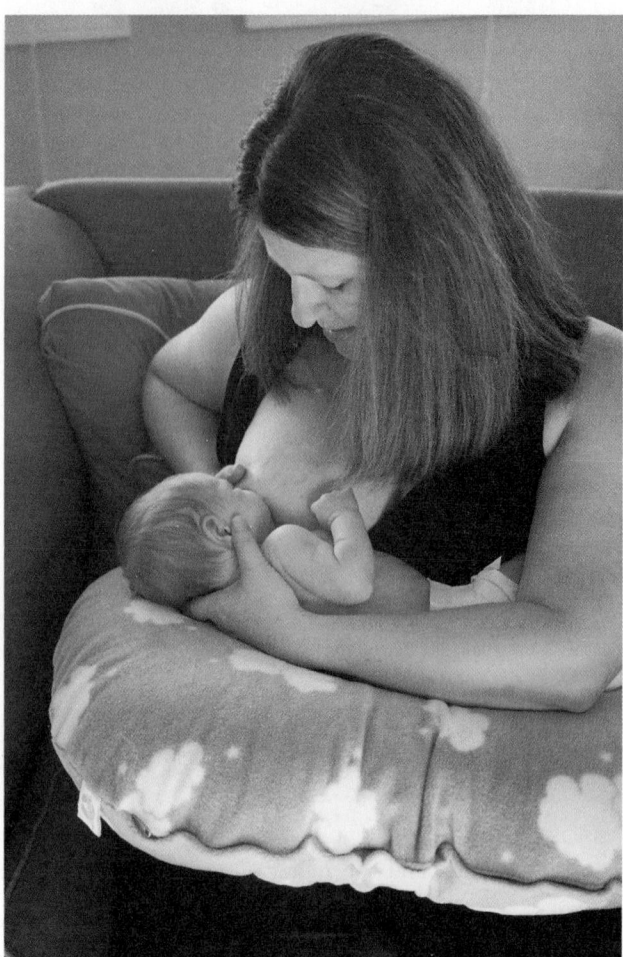

Figure 24-5 The cross-cradle or modified cradle hold is helpful for infants who are preterm or have a fractured clavicle. The mother holds the infant's head in the hand opposite from the side on which the infant will feed, with the arm supporting the body across the mother's lap. The other hand holds the breast. The mother can guide the infant's head to the breast and see the mouth on the breast during the feeding.

Interventions

Interventions are centered on teaching that nurses should provide to all inexperienced breastfeeding mothers. These techniques should be adapted as appropriate for mothers who have some knowledge of breastfeeding but need review or clarification.

Assisting With the First Feeding

The first feeding should take place within the first hour after birth if both mother and infant are stable. Early breastfeeding provides stimulation of milk production and improved suck-

ling and may increase the duration of breastfeeding (Biancuzzo, 2003). The mother may need assistance in positioning herself and the infant and a demonstration of how to hold the breast. Nurses should stay with the mother during the first few feedings and then check back frequently to answer questions.

Teaching Feeding Techniques

Position of the Mother and Infant Breastfeeding mothers most often use the cradle, football, and cross-cradle holds and the side-lying position (Figs. 24-3 through 24-6). To increase her comfort, position pillows behind the mother's back or over an abdominal incision. Her shoulders should be relaxed, and she should not be hunched over. Use pillows to elevate the infant to the level of the nipple and prevent pulling and tension on the nipple. The infant's head and body should directly face the breast, with the infant's nose, cheeks, and chin lightly touching the breast. If the infant must turn the head to reach the breast, swallowing is difficult. The infant's body should be aligned so that the ear, shoulder, and hips are in a straight line.

Position of the Mother's Hands The mother's hand position is also important. In the palmar or **C** hand position, the mother holds her breast with her thumb on top and the fin-

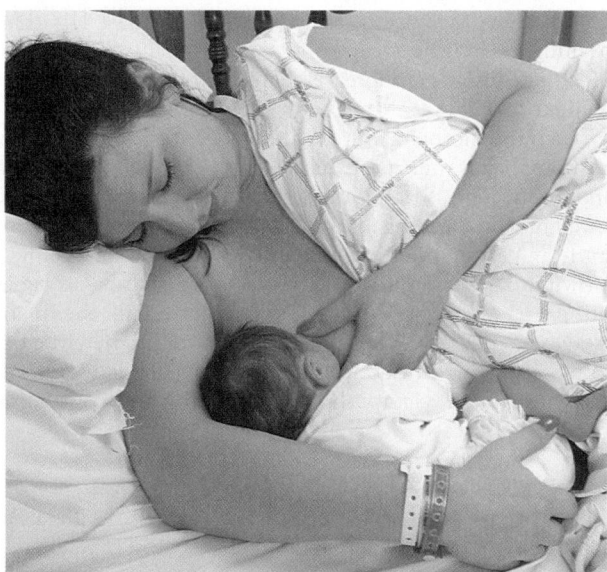

Figure 24-6 The side-lying position avoids pressure on episiotomy or abdominal incisions and allows the mother to rest while feeding. She lies on her side, with her lower arm supporting her head or placed around the infant. A pillow behind her back and between her legs provides comfort. Her upper hand and arm are used to position the infant on the side at nipple level and hold the breast. When the infant's mouth opens to nurse, the mother draws the infant to her to insert the nipple into the mouth.

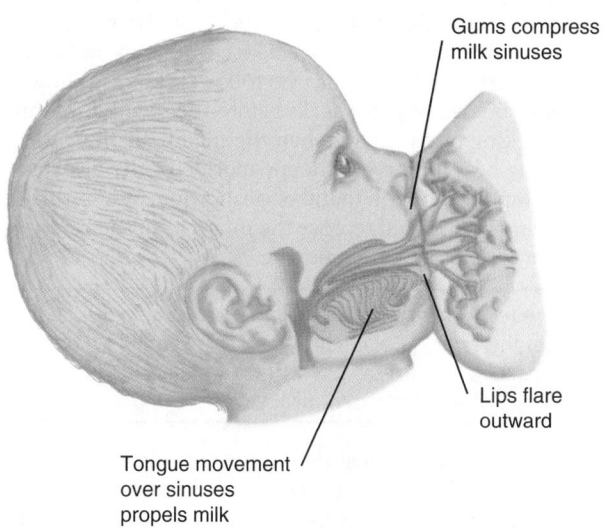

Figure 24-8 Position of infant's mouth while suckling. When the nipple and areola are properly positioned in the infant's mouth, the gums compress the milk sinuses behind the areola. The tongue is between the lower gum and the breast. The tongue moves over the sinuses like a peristaltic wave to bring the milk forward into the infant's mouth. The infant's lips are flared outward.

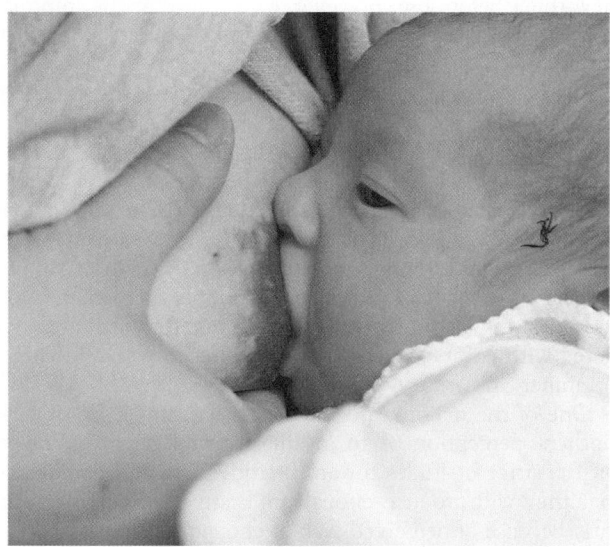

Figure 24-7 C position of hand on breast. The hand is positioned so the thumb is on top of the breast while the fingers support the breast from below. Note the flaring of the infant's lips.

gers against the chest wall and supporting the underside of the breast (Fig. 24-7). Her fingers should be behind the areola and her thumb should not press on the breast enough to make the nipple tip upward, or the infant will suck improperly and the nipple may become sore.

In the "scissors" or V hold, the woman uses her forefinger and middle finger to support the breast. The fingers must be well behind the areola, or they may slip down the wet areola and interfere with the placement of the infant's mouth.

The mother should support her breast in place for the first few weeks if the weight of it makes it difficult for the infant to hold it in the mouth. As the infant becomes more adept at breastfeeding, the mother will not need to hold the breast.

Although mothers worry about the infant's ability to breathe while nursing, it is unnecessary to indent the breast tissue near the infant's nostrils. This might cause improper positioning of the nipple in the infant's mouth, interfere with the grasp of the nipple, or impede milk flow.

Latch-On Techniques Teach the mother techniques to help the infant latch on to the breast.

Eliciting Latch-On. After positioning the awake and hungry infant to face the breast, instruct the mother to hold her breast so that the nipple brushes against the center of the infant's lips. The infant will respond by opening the mouth, although up to a minute of stroking may be necessary. The breast should not be inserted until the infant's mouth is opened wide, or the infant will compress the end of the nipple, causing pain and little milk flow. When the mouth opens wide, the mother should quickly bring the infant close to her so that the infant can latch on to the areola.

Position of the Mouth. The position of the infant's mouth on the breast is important (Fig. 24-8). As much of the areola as possible should be in the infant's mouth to allow the nipple to be drawn toward the back of the mouth. This position prevents the infant from sucking on the nipple only, which leads to sore nipples and insufficient milk production. The infant's lips should be about 1 to $1^1/_2$ inches from the base of the nipple and curled outward (Lawrence & Lawrence, 1999). This places the gums over the milk sinuses behind the areola so that milk is released into the infant's mouth as the gums compress the sinuses.

Suckling Pattern Teach the mother about the infant's suckling pattern. During nutritive suckling, the infant sucks with smooth, continuous movements with only occasional pauses to rest. Each suck may be followed by a swallow, or there may be two or three sucks before the swallow. Nonnutritive sucking often occurs when the infant is falling asleep. There may be a fluttery or choppy motion of the jaw that is not accompanied by the sound of swallowing. When this occurs, the mother should remove the infant from the breast because her nipples may become sore.

Mothers often wonder whether their infants are actually receiving milk from the breast. Point out to them the sound of swallowing when it occurs. A soft "ka" or "ah" sound indicates that the infant is swallowing colostrum or milk.

Short pauses are normal during nursing. Caution mothers not to jiggle the breast in the infant's mouth in an effort to start the suckling again. This process may cause the infant to lose the grasp on the nipple and areola, resulting in "chewing" on the nipple and soreness. If necessary, she should take the infant off the breast to awaken the baby and then start again.

Removal from the Breast Demonstrate how to avoid trauma to the breast when removing the infant. To break the suction, the mother inserts her finger into the corner of the infant's mouth between the gums. She then removes the breast quickly before the infant begins to suck again.

Frequency of Feedings Because breast milk moves through the stomach within 1½ to 2 hours, infants usually feed every 2 to 3 hours. Frequent feedings are especially important in the early days after birth, while lactation is being established and stomach capacity is small. Explaining that the hormone *prolactin*, which is responsible for milk production, is released in increased amounts while the infant is suckling helps mothers understand the relationship of frequent feeding to milk supply.

During the early weeks of life, infants should be gently awakened, if possible, every 3 hours for feeding to stimulate milk production (Association of Women's Health, Obstetric, & Neonatal Nurses [AWHONN], 2000b). Infants should feed about every 4 hours during the night (Meek, 2002). Long periods between feedings increase the likelihood of breast engorgement. A total of 8 to 12 feedings should be given in each 24-hour period. However, strict scheduling of infant feedings is unnecessary and leads to frustration for both mother and infant. A mother should take her cues from her infant.

Length of Feedings Although early feedings were once limited to only a few minutes per breast to prevent sore nipples, improper positioning, rather than time at breast, is the usual cause of nipple trauma. When feedings are too short, the infant receives little or no colostrum or milk. It may take as long as 5 minutes for the milk-ejection (let-down) reflex to occur at first.

Generally, mothers can let infants determine the amount of time spent at each feeding. However, mothers who are uneasy without a specific length of time for feedings can be instructed to start with feedings lasting approximately 10 to 15 minutes on each side, or longer if the infant continues to nurse vigorously (AAP & ACOG, 2002). After burping, the feeding continues on the second breast until the infant falls asleep or begins nonnutritive suckling. Although variations in the length of feedings occur, early feedings that last less than 15 minutes may not be enough (Auerbach & Riordan, 1999). Feeding time increases as needed by the infant over the next few days.

Teach the mother about the differences between foremilk, the watery first milk that quenches the infant's thirst, and hindmilk, which is richer in fat, is more satisfying, and leads to weight gain. Feeding for too short a period prevents the infant from getting the hindmilk and decreases weight gain.

Switching back and forth between breasts several times during a feeding increases the amount of foremilk the infant receives but decreases the amount of hindmilk. Therefore the mother should continue feeding on the first side as long as the infant nurses vigorously before burping and continuing on the other breast.

Preventing Problems

Women who intend to breastfeed but encounter difficulties that cause them to switch to formula feeding may express guilt and disappointment for months after the experience (Mozingo, Davis, Droppleman, & Merideth, 2000). Nurses can help prevent early problems in several ways.

Check frequently on the woman as she feeds her infant so she can get her questions answered as she thinks of them. Intensive teaching during the short stay in the birth facility helps prevent problems after discharge. Include suggestions about common problems and their solutions, as well as how to improve positioning and techniques. Pamphlets and videos provide another means of providing education. Review them before use, however, to ensure that the information is correct and that they contain no advertisements for formula.

Although there is lack of agreement about the effects of formula gift packs given to mothers at discharge, it is likely that having formula available sets up an expectation, at least for some mothers, that formula may be necessary. This is contrary to the message nurses should give to parents about breastfeeding.

Avoid use of formula supplementation in the hospital unless there are medical indications. Formula supplementation and initiating feedings after the first hour after birth are associated with early termination of breastfeeding (DiGirolamo, Grummer-Strawn, & Fein, 2001).

One of the major reasons for early weaning to formula is mothers' perception of an insufficient milk supply. Women with positive attitudes toward breastfeeding and confidence that they will produce enough milk are less likely to wean early because of perceived lack of enough milk. Explanation of the normal course of breastfeeding and methods of handling problems can help mothers feel more confident in their abilities.

Teach the mother how to assess whether the infant is receiving enough milk. Infants should have at least three wet diapers and three stools a day by the 3rd day. Intake can also be gauged when the physician or nurse practitioner weighs the infant at well-baby checkups. After the initial weight loss after birth, infants generally gain approximately 15 to 30 g (½-1 oz) each day during the early months of life (Walker & Creehan, 2001). Weight gain generally begins by the 5th day of life.

Common causes of decreased milk supply include formula use, inadequate rest or diet, smoking by the mother or others in the home, and use of caffeine, alcohol, or some medica-

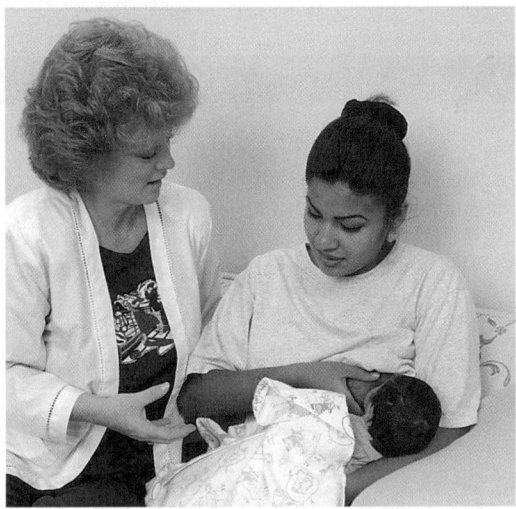

Figure 24-9 The nurse offers suggestions on hand position during the home visit.

tions. Intervene appropriately if any common causes are found. Because the breasts are soft during the first few days and the mother doesn't see large amounts of milk, she may believe that none is present. This may lead her to give the infant formula before or after the feeding, decreasing milk production. Teach mothers who need to increase milk supply to feed more often and use a breast pump after feedings. If problems persist, refer the mother to a lactation consultant.

Evaluation
- Does the infant nurse for 15 minutes or more per feeding, with good latch-on and nutritive suckling?
- Does the mother use correct techniques for latch-on and positioning?
- Does the mother say she feels confident about the process?

BREASTFEEDING CONCERNS

Because mothers may be discharged from the birth facility before problems arise, nurses should teach them how to prevent and treat common problems.

When the mother seeks help for problems that have developed, the nurse should ask the mother what has been done to try to solve the problem. It is important to ask about any complementary or alternative therapies the mother may have tried. The safety of any therapy should be determined. The mother may have tried teas from fennel, fenugreek, dill, or aniseed to help in milk production, hot parsley compresses for engorgement, and olive oil or washing the nipples with marigolds for sore nipples. Because there has not been adequate research on the use of these therapies, the mother should be referred to the health care provider before using any of these substances (Skidmore-Roth, 2004). Cabbage leaves have been used for engorgement, but most research does not show they are effective. Poultices of grated potato or carrot have also been suggested.

After discharge, guidance for breastfeeding problems can be continued at home by referring the mother to lactation specialists or organizations such as La Leche League—a support group that gives ongoing assistance to breastfeeding mothers. Some facilities provide home visits (Fig. 24-9), telephone follow-up,

---

MOTHERS
Want to Know

Is My Baby Getting Enough Milk?

Your baby is probably getting enough milk if:
- You hear the baby swallow frequently during feedings. It sounds like a soft "ka" or "ah" sound.
- You see nutritive suckling—a smooth series of sucking and swallowing with occasional rest periods. This pattern is different from short, choppy sucks that occur when the baby is falling asleep and not getting milk. After the first few days, you may feel a tingling of your nipples as a new let-down reflex occurs. This sensation is followed by more nutritive suckling as the infant swallows the increased milk available.
- Your breast is getting softer during the feeding. (However, your breasts do not have to be hard [engorged] for you to have enough milk.)
- You can see milk in the baby's mouth or dripping from your breast occasionally.
- You feed your baby 8 to 12 times every 24 hours. When you nurse often, you produce more milk.
- Your baby has at least three wet diapers a day by the 3rd day. If you are unsure if the diaper is wet, place a tissue or cotton ball inside it to show small amounts of urine. Urine should be light, not dark, yellow.
- By the 3rd day, your baby passes at least three bowel movements—and often more—every day during the 1st month. The bowel movements are yellow by the 4th day.
- Your baby seems satisfied after feedings. Babies remain quietly awake or go to sleep for at least an hour after most feedings. (An occasional fussy time is not unusual and does not mean that the baby is not getting enough to eat.)
- Your baby has gained weight at the first well-baby checkup.

---

or outpatient clinics. Women with more serious breastfeeding problems need referral to a lactation consultant—a professional educated to deal with more complex situations.

Infant Problems

Infant problems require prompt attention to ensure successful breastfeeding. See p. 584 for prevention and treatment of these problems.

! CRITICAL TO REMEMBER
Infant Signs of Breastfeeding Problems

- Falling asleep after feeding less than 5 minutes
- Refusal to breastfeed
- Tongue thrusting
- Smacking or clicking sounds
- Dimpling of cheeks
- Failure to open mouth wide at latch-on
- Lower lip turned in
- Short, choppy motions of jaw
- No audible swallowing
- Use of formula

MOTHERS
Want to Know

Solutions to Common Breastfeeding Problems

Problem
Infant is sleepy at feeding time or falls asleep shortly after beginning feeding.

Prevention
- Gently awaken your baby at feeding time. Talk, gently move the infant's arms and legs, and play with the infant for a short time before beginning the feeding.
- Unwrap the baby's blankets, and change the diaper. Leave the blanket off as you begin the feeding. Your body and a blanket added later will provide adequate warmth.

Solutions
If your baby goes to sleep during the feeding and has fed less than 5 minutes, try the following:
- Rub the baby's hair or cheeks gently, stroke around the infant's mouth, or shift the baby's position slightly to see if the infant will wake up.
- Remove the baby from the breast. Rub the infant's back to bring up bubbles of air and help awaken the baby.
- Express a few drops of colostrum onto the nipple. The baby tastes the colostrum when the nipple is offered and often begins renewed suckling.
- Wash the baby's face with a lukewarm washcloth to help the infant wake up.
- If your baby cannot be aroused with a few of the above gentle techniques, a longer sleep period may be needed. Let the infant sleep another half hour and then begin again.

Problem
Infant who has taken bottles pushes the nipple out of the mouth and sucks poorly during breastfeeding. Infant is using sucking movements used for bottle feeding.

Prevention
- Avoid all bottles and pacifiers unless necessary. If they are necessary, stop as soon as possible.
- Do not give the baby formula during the night.

- Avoid giving formula at the end of a breastfeeding session, because it is unnecessary for healthy newborns. Adding formula may cause the infant's stomach to become distended, resulting in more "spitting up." If the infant waits longer before nursing again, milk production will decrease.

Solution
Stop all bottle feeding and pacifier use so that the baby gets used to suckling from the breast instead of the bottle. Nurse more often to stimulate milk production and help the baby learn what to do.

Problem
Infant sucks on the end of the nipple or fails to open the mouth widely enough.

Prevention
- Be sure that the baby has the nipple at the back of the mouth and 1 to $1^{1}/_{2}$ inches of the areola in the mouth.
- Do not insert the breast into the infant's mouth until the infant opens the mouth wide. Then bring the baby to the breast.
- Pull down gently on the infant's chin to help the infant open the mouth wider if necessary.

Solution
Stop the feeding and start again if the infant is sucking on the end of the nipple or you see dimples in the infant's cheeks or hear "smacking" or clicking sounds.

Problem
Breasts are hard and tender from engorgement.

Prevention
- Breastfeed the infant every 2 to 3 hours day and night.
- Do not give a bottle during the night, because it increases the risk of engorgement.

Solutions
- To reduce edema and pain, apply cold packs to the breasts between feedings. Make inexpensive cold packs from clean

Sleepy Infant
During the first few days after birth, infants often sleep longer than expected or fall asleep at the breast after feeding for only a short time. The nurse should show mothers how to arouse sleepy infants for breastfeeding. When infants fall asleep during feedings, the nurse should evaluate whether the infant has fed adequately, should be awakened to feed longer, or should be fed again sooner than usual. Irritating stimuli should not be used to awaken infants, because feedings should be associated with pleasurable feelings. Infants who continue to be excessively sleepy or to nurse poorly need further evaluation. Poor feeding may be an early sign of a complication such as sepsis (see Chapter 30).

Nipple Confusion
Nipple confusion (or nipple preference) may occur when an infant who has received bottle feedings confuses the tongue movements necessary for bottle feeding with the suckling of

breastfeeding. The infant may refuse to breastfeed or may use tongue movements that push the breast out of the mouth. Some infants develop a preference for the bottle, from which milk flows freely without effort.

Movement of the mouth and tongue are different in breastfeeding and bottle feeding. In bottle feeding, infants must push their tongue over the latex nipple of a bottle to slow the flow of milk and prevent choking. If the infant uses the same thrusting tongue motion while nursing, the breast may be pushed out of the mouth. During breastfeeding, the tongue cups around the nipple and areola and presses against the breast like a peristaltic wave to bring milk from the sinuses into the infant's mouth.

Nurses should discourage use of formula in normal breastfeeding infants. It reduces breastfeeding time and decreases production of prolactin and, therefore, milk supply. Formula takes longer to digest, and the infant is not hungry again for about 4 hours. Formula feeding further limits

MOTHERS
Want to Know

Solutions to Common Breastfeeding Problems—cont'd

disposable gloves or plastic bags filled with crushed ice, a bag of frozen vegetables, or frozen washcloths. Cover with a washcloth before applying to the skin. A disposable diaper with ice placed between the layers may also be used.

- Before feedings, apply heat with compresses or a shower to stimulate milk flow. Use warm, wet disposable diapers applied over each breast. Fasten the tabs to keep the diapers in place and prevent dripping.
- To stimulate the let-down reflex so that the baby can nurse more easily, massage the breasts before and during feedings.
- For areolar engorgement where the breasts are so hard that your baby cannot latch on, express a little milk by hand or with a breast pump.
- Feed more often—every 1½ to 2 hours.
- Wear a well-fitting bra for support day and night.
- To help you feel more comfortable, take prescribed pain medication just before feedings.

Problem

Nipples are sore, cracked, blistered, or bleeding.

Prevention

- Position the baby at the breast with enough of the areola in the mouth that the nipple is not compressed between the baby's gums during nursing.
- Avoid engorgement by nursing frequently. Express enough milk to soften the areola if it becomes too hard for the infant to grasp.
- Do not use soap on the nipples because it removes the protective oils and causes drying.
- If you use breast pads for leaking milk, remove them when they become wet to prevent irritation of the skin. Avoid pads with plastic linings that retain moisture.
- Breast creams may cause sensitivity and irritation. If you choose to use lanolin, use only the purified form to protect against allergens and pesticides. Creams that must be removed before each feeding may increase soreness.

Solutions

- To start the let-down reflex, begin each feeding with the less-sore side first. This causes milk to flow more quickly on the second breast. Using warm compresses or massage will also help the milk flow more quickly.
- Do not use nipple shields (latex nipples that fit over your own nipples) without help from a lactation consultant. They decrease milk flow so that the baby receives less milk and milk production is decreased.
- Vary the position of the infant during nursing. The area of the nipple directly in line with the infant's nose and chin is most stressed during the feeding.
- Apply colostrum or breast milk to the nipples after feedings, because it has healing properties. Or try warm water or warm, wet tea bag compresses to the nipples.
- Hydrogel dressings may help relieve pain and promote healing. Use according to directions
- If you have burning, itching, or stabbing pain throughout your breast, look in the baby's mouth for the white patches of thrush—a yeast infection that can infect the nipples. Call the health care provider for medication to treat both you and your baby.

Problem

Flat or inverted nipples that the baby has difficulty drawing into the mouth.

Prevention

None.

Solutions

- Wear breast shells in your bra to help make the nipples protrude.
- Just before beginning breastfeeding, roll the nipple between your thumb and forefinger to help it protrude (see Fig. 24-11).
- To draw out inverted nipples, use a breast pump just before feedings. Put the baby to your breast immediately after the pump causes the nipple to become erect. The normal suckling process usually causes the nipple to stay erect.

---

breast stimulation and milk supply and may lead to engorgement.

Pacifiers are controversial. Although parents often find them helpful, their use may be associated with suckling problems and an earlier weaning of infants from the breast (Biancuzzo, 2003). Some infants can use a pacifier without ensuing problems with breastfeeding, but their use should be discouraged at least until the infant is breastfeeding successfully (AWHONN, 2000b).

Suckling Problems

Suckling problems may occur when the nipple is poorly positioned in the mouth. Dimpling of the cheeks and smacking or clicking sounds may indicate that the infant is sucking on the nipple only. Some infants do not open their mouths widely and suck on the end of the nipple.

Inserting a gloved finger into the infant's mouth helps assess suckling. The peristaltic motion of the tongue should be felt as the infant sucks. The infant who is thrusting the tongue may have become confused by the use of artificial nipples, which should be avoided until the problem is resolved. The tongue should be cupped under the breast and covering the lower gum. Helping the infant open the mouth widely may improve suckling. More complicated suckling problems may require assistance from a lactation consultant.

Infant Complications

Infant complications may be minor and cause minimal interference with breastfeeding. The very preterm or ill infant, however, may be unable to breastfeed for a long period (see Nursing Care Plan: Breastfeeding an Infant Who Has Complications).

Jaundice

Jaundice (hyperbilirubinemia) need not interfere with breastfeeding. Even when infants receive phototherapy, they can usually be removed from the lights for feedings. Concern over

Nursing Care Plan

Breastfeeding an Infant Who Has Complications

ASSESSMENT

Ruth James's son David develops respiratory complications at birth and is admitted to the neonatal intensive care unit. The infant will probably not be able to feed at the breast for a few days. Ruth is disappointed and worried about whether she will be able to breastfeed at all.

Nursing Diagnosis

Interrupted Breastfeeding related to separation from infant secondary to illness.

Goals/Expected Outcomes

Within 2 days, Ruth will
- Verbalize the importance of breastfeeding her infant and her desire to maintain lactation.
- Pump her breasts as taught.
- Breastfeed David successfully (when it becomes possible).

INTERVENTION	RATIONALE
1. Explore Ruth's perception of the problem and her understanding of the cause for separation and the effect on breastfeeding.	1. Discussion of the problem identifies misconceptions and determines the type of teaching and support required.
2. Use therapeutic communication to help Ruth express her feelings of disappointment with the unexpected change in plans.	2. Helping the mother express her feelings and accepting them helps her cope with the situation.
3. Explain to Ruth how valuable breast milk is for her infant and that she can use a breast pump to maintain lactation until David can breastfeed.	3. Reinforcing the value of breastfeeding and offering encouragement increase the chance of success.
4. Teach Ruth to use a breast pump and store her milk. Instruct her to pump her breasts for approximately 15 to 20 minutes every 3 hours during the day and at least once at night.	4. Frequent use of a breast pump helps establish lactation by causing release of prolactin and oxytocin so that milk is produced and released from the breasts.
5. Explain prevention and treatment of engorgement.	5. Frequent pumping should prevent engorgement. If it does not, the mother will need assistance in treating it.
6. Feed David breast milk if possible, whether by bottle or gavage. Teach Ruth how to store her milk and how to prepare it for use for her infant.	6. Breast milk has properties that are especially valuable for the sick infant.
7. Arrange for Ruth to spend as much time with David as possible. To answer her questions and provide support, accompany her during the early visits and when she begins to breastfeed.	7. Bonding occurs more easily if a mother can be with her baby. Accompanying a mother during visits allows the nurse an opportunity to offer support as needed.
8. When Ruth begins to breastfeed, offer the same teaching that mothers of well infants receive. In addition, provide continued support if she has concerns.	8. Women who must delay breastfeeding may be more anxious about the process.
9. Offer praise and realistic encouragement frequently.	9. A mother needs reinforcement of her abilities to increase self-esteem as a mother. Encouragement must be suited to actual circumstances.
10. If Ruth must go home before David is ready for discharge, provide her with information about purchase or rental of breast pumps. Give her containers to bring her milk into the nursery.	10. The mother who must pump her breasts for a longer period may find that an electric pump is more efficient.

Evaluation

Ruth verbalizes her determination to provide breast milk for David. She maintains lactation and brings breast milk at each visit. At 5 days of age, David is ready to begin breastfeeding. Ruth is very patient in helping David learn to breastfeed with the nurses' help. David is able to nurse well at each feeding by discharge.

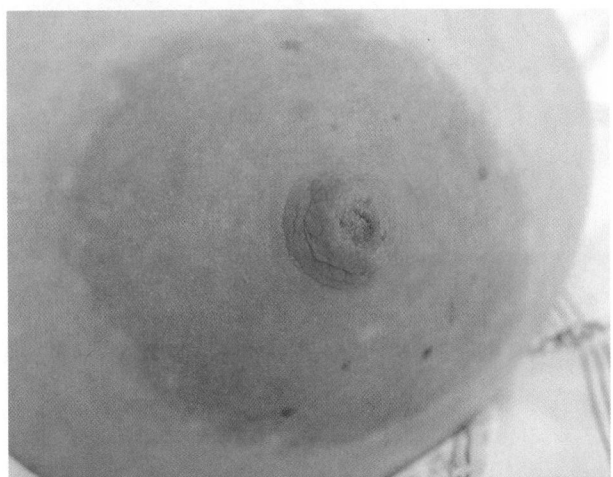

Figure 24-10 Note the cracked area on this nipple.

adequate intake may be more prevalent in caring for the infant with jaundice. Infants receiving phototherapy should not be given extra water, because it may decrease the intake of breast milk. Frequent breastfeeding is necessary to provide adequate intake of protein and fluid and stimulate production of milk. In addition, breastfeeding increases the number of stools and aids in excretion of bilirubin. Jaundice is discussed in Chapters 22, 23, and 30.

Prematurity

If the preterm infant cannot breastfeed immediately after birth, the mother needs encouragement and instruction on how to use a breast pump to establish and maintain her milk supply. Breast milk offers immunologic and nutritional benefits and is adapted to preterm needs. It may help prevent or minimize the severity of necrotizing enterocolitis, a serious complication of preterm infants. It also helps the mother feel she is providing care for her infant even if she cannot take the infant home with her. The woman can pump her milk and take it to the nursery for the infant's feedings. The nurse should provide sterile containers for the woman to take home and instruct her in special nursery requirements (see Chapter 29).

Illness and Congenital Defects

Illness in the infant and congenital defects such as a cleft palate may cause breastfeeding problems. Parents of these infants need the same type of assistance as parents with preterm infants. The focus is on helping the mother maintain lactation until she is able to nurse the infant. Referral to support groups can be particularly helpful.

! CRITICAL TO REMEMBER

Maternal Signs of Breastfeeding Problems

- Hard, tender breasts
- Painful, red, cracked, blistered, or bleeding nipples
- Flat or inverted nipples
- Localized edema or pain in either breast
- Fever, generalized aching, or malaise

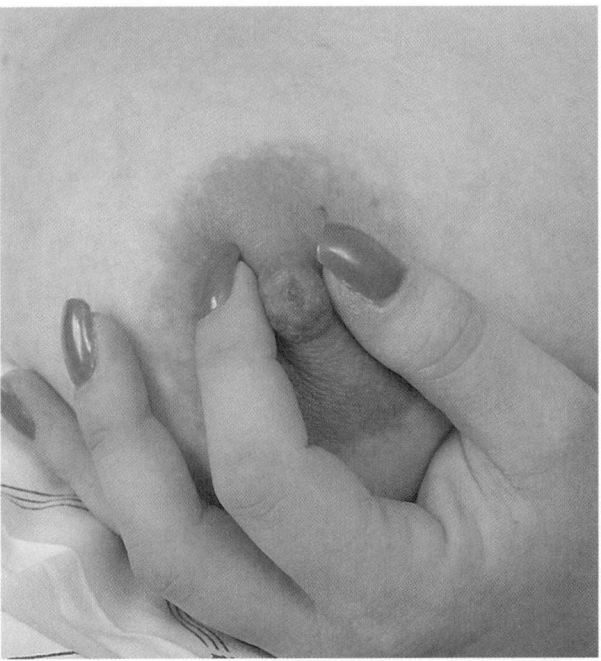

Figure 24-11 Rolling helps flat nipples become erect in preparation for latch-on.

Maternal Concerns

Common Breast Problems

Early nursing intervention can help the mother overcome common breast problems. See p. 584-585 for prevention and treatment of these problems.

Engorgement. Many women have a temporary swelling or fullness of the breasts on the 2nd or 3rd day after birth when the milk begins to "come in" or change from colostrum to transitional breast milk. This normal, temporary engorgement is caused by accumulation of milk, enlarged lymph glands, and increased blood flow and should not interfere with breastfeeding.

Engorgement may become a problem if feedings are delayed, too short, or not frequent enough. The breasts become edematous, hard, and tender, making feeding or even movement painful. The areola may become hard and the nipples flat, making it difficult for the infant to nurse. The condition may lead to nipple trauma, mastitis, and even the discontinuation of breastfeeding.

Nipple Trauma. Nipple pain lasting a minute or less at the beginning of feedings may occur during early breastfeeding as the infant stretches the tissue. Traumatized nipples appear red, cracked, blistered, or bleeding (Fig. 24-10). Minor nipple trauma can be treated by independent nursing interventions. Redness of breast tissue, purulent drainage, and fever indicate mastitis or breast abscess and require antibiotic treatment (see Chapter 28).

Flat and Inverted Nipples. Nipple abnormalities should be treated during pregnancy, if possible, but interventions can begin after birth. Use of breast shells can be taught at this time. Nipple rolling just before feeding helps flat nipples become more erect so that the infant can grasp them more readily (Fig. 24-11). A breast pump used for a few minutes just before feedings may help draw out inverted nipples.

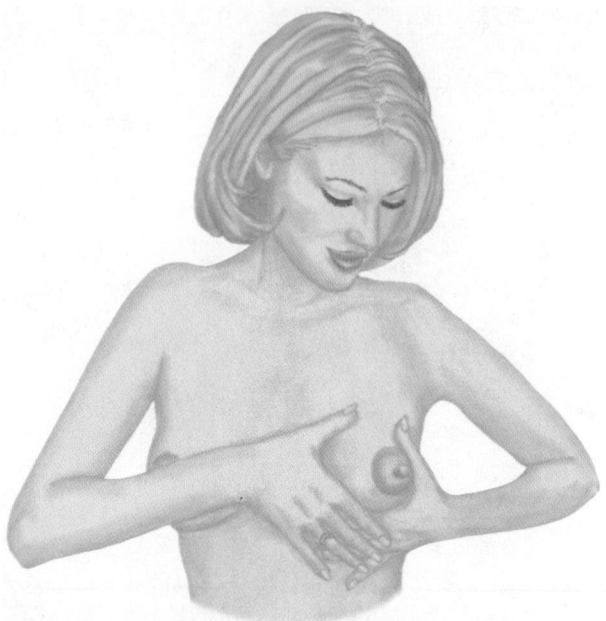

Figure 24-12 To massage the breasts, the mother places her hands against the chest wall with her fingers encircling the breasts. She gently slides her hands forward until the fingers overlap. The position of the hands is rotated to cover all breast tissue. Massaging with the fingertips in a circular motion over all areas of the breast is also helpful.

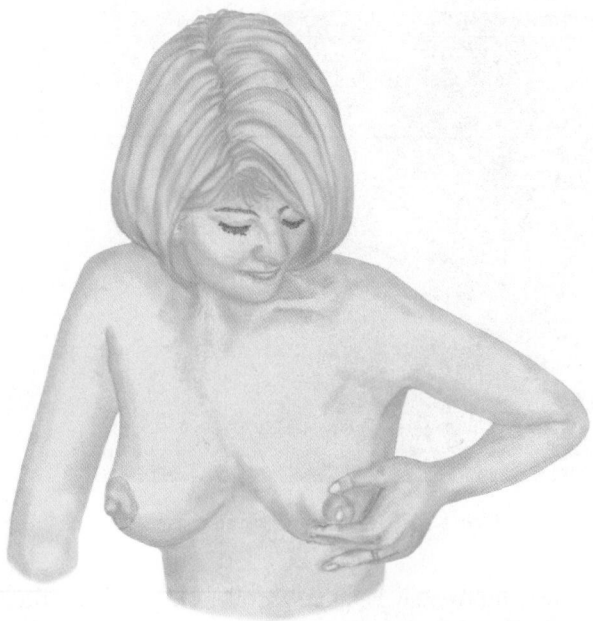

Figure 24-13 To express milk from the breast, the mother places her hand just behind the areola, with the thumb on top and the fingers supporting the breast. The tissue is pressed back against the chest wall; then the fingers and thumb are brought together and toward the nipple. This procedure compresses the milk sinuses and causes milk to flow. The action is repeated to simulate the suckling of the infant. Moving the hands around the areola allows compression of all sinuses and complete removal of milk from the breast. Compression should be gentle to avoid trauma.

Plugged Ducts. Although the exact cause of occlusion of a lactiferous duct is unknown, engorgement, missed feedings, or a constricting bra may be involved. Localized edema and tenderness are present, and a hard area may be palpated. A tiny white area may be on the nipple. Massage of the area (Fig. 24-12) followed by heat and continued breastfeeding using varied positions cause the duct to open. A plugged duct may progress to mastitis if not treated promptly. Mastitis involves localized pain accompanied by fever, generalized aching, and malaise (see Chapter 28).

Illness in the Mother
When the mother is ill, breastfeeding may have to be postponed temporarily because of the mother's condition or the drugs she receives. Abrupt weaning, however, may lead to mastitis as well as maternal depression from decreased prolactin, which has been associated with feelings of well-being (Lawrence & Lawrence, 1999). The nurse should assist the mother in using a breast pump until she resumes breastfeeding.

Drug Transfer to Breast Milk. Most medications taken by the mother cross into the breast milk to some degree, but many pass in small amounts and are safe during lactation. Some drugs interfere with milk production. Use of both prescription and over-the-counter drugs should be approved by a physician. Another drug can often be substituted for one that affects the infant. If a mother must take a drug that will be harmful to her infant, she should pump her breasts while she is taking the medication. Once the drug clears her bloodstream, she may resume breastfeeding. Some drugs may not reach the infant in harmful amounts if taken after a feeding or at night when there is a longer time between feedings. (See Appendix B for information about drug effects during breastfeeding.)

Conditions in Which Breastfeeding Should Be Avoided. In some situations, breastfeeding is contraindi-

cated. Examples are untreated active tuberculosis, human immunodeficiency virus (HIV) infection, galactosemia, and maternal drug abuse. Mothers with hepatitis A, B, or C may breastfeed. Infants of mothers with hepatitis B should receive hepatitis B immune globulin before breastfeeding. Mothers with herpes simplex may breastfeed if no lesion is on the breast and she performs good handwashing. (AAP & ACOG, 2002; Biancuzzo, 2003).

Previous Breast Surgery
Women who have had surgery for breast reduction or augmentation may have difficulty with lactation. The type of surgical technique used and the amount of tissue involved determine breastfeeding ability. Surgery may cause disruption of neural pathways, ducts, and blood supply. Some women can breastfeed without problem, and others may be able to do so using a supplementation device to help build up milk supply if milk production is low.

Employment
Although some mothers remain at home for 6 weeks or more after birth, others must return to work earlier. Working and breastfeeding can be combined very well with some planning. A week or two before she returns to work, the mother can begin using a breast pump once or twice a day to practice pumping her breasts and to build up a small supply of frozen breast milk.

Most working mothers use a battery-operated or electric pump once or twice a day during lunch or coffee breaks. The milk should be refrigerated or placed in an insulated container with ice to be used for later feedings.

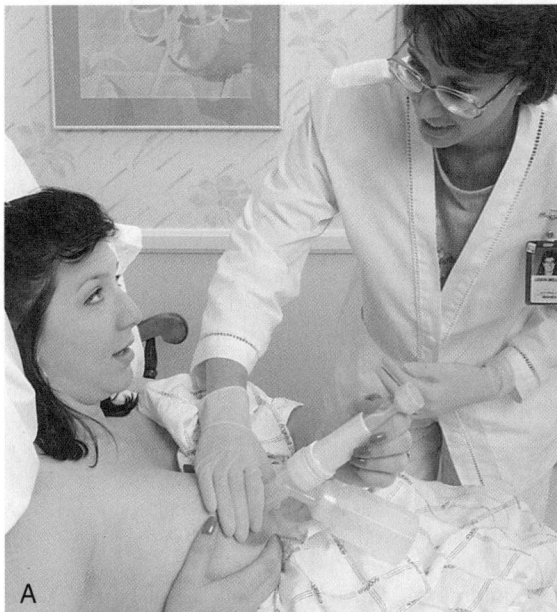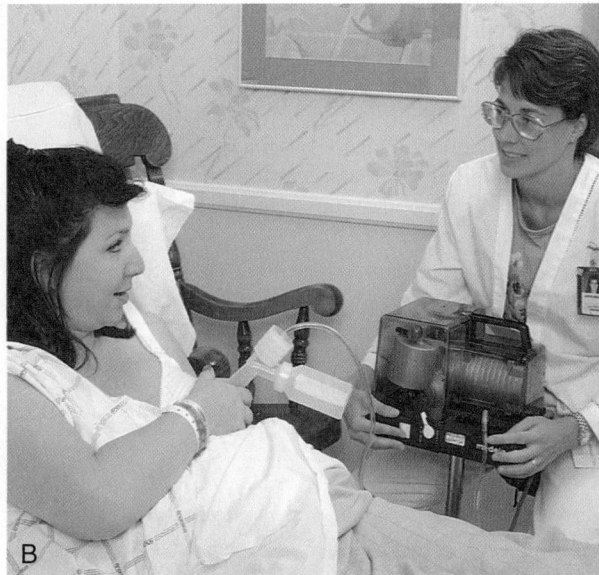

Figure 24-14 The nurse demonstrates methods of pumping breast milk. **A,** Manual breast pump. **B,** Electric breast pump.

Milk Expression and Storage

Hand Expression. When there is a need for milk expression, the nurse helps the mother use hand expression (Fig. 24-13) or a breast pump (Fig. 24-14). Hand expression can be done without other equipment but is not as effective as a breast pump. Hand expression or manual pumps are useful for the mother who wants to save breast milk for another feeding or whose areola is so engorged that the infant cannot grasp it.

Use of a Breast Pump. The mother who needs to pump her milk for a prolonged period may prefer using a battery-operated or electric breast pump. Battery-operated pumps are small, portable, and relatively inexpensive. Large electric pumps can often be rented for home use. They are more efficient than hand or battery pumps and are indicated when the mother must pump to maintain her milk supply for a long period. A double pump allows the mother to pump both breasts at one time, saving time and increasing milk production.

Use of the breast pump should begin within the first 24 hours after birth for the woman who cannot breastfeed her infant. She should pump her breasts approximately as often as her baby would nurse—about every 3 hours during the day and at least once at night. Sessions should last approximately 15 to 20 minutes. A total of at least 8 to 10 sessions in each 24 hours is best to maintain milk supply (Mohrbacher & Stock, 2003).

Use of massage and heat before pumping helps initiate the flow of milk. Massage during pumping may increase the volume of milk obtained at each session. The amount of suction should be set at a low level in the beginning and gradually increased, if necessary. Too much negative pressure traumatizes the breast. If the woman needs to increase her milk supply, pumping more often rather than for longer periods is more effective.

Milk Storage. Milk should be stored in glass or plastic containers with a tight cap. A nipple should not be used to cap the milk during storage because the hole allows passage of organisms. Rigid plastic containers are easier to use than plastic bottle liners, which may spill or be punctured.

Breast milk can be kept in a refrigerator for 48 hours, if colder than 4° C (39° F). It can be kept in a freezer that is in a separate compartment of a refrigerator at −20° C (−4° F) (approximately the temperature that keeps ice cream hard) for 3 months. It can be kept in a deep freeze for 6 months (Biancuzzo, 2003). Leukocytes are destroyed by freezing, but most of the other immunologic properties are preserved.

Breast milk should be thawed in a refrigerator or by holding the container under running lukewarm water or in a bowl of cool or lukewarm water rather than by heating it. It should not be refrozen or heated in a microwave. Milk that has been refrigerated rather than frozen should be used as much as possible so that the leukocytes are available for the infant.

Breastfeeding After Multiple Births

To be successful, mothers who have more than one newborn need help and support from nurses and family members. It is important for these mothers to nurse every 2 to 3 hours to build up the milk supply. If the infants cannot breastfeed, the woman will need to be taught how to use a breast pump.

If the woman decides to feed two infants simultaneously, she will need help positioning them using the football hold, cradle hold, or a combination of both. She should be encouraged to eat well, get enough rest, and ask for help from family and friends.

Weaning

There is no one "right" time to wean the infant. Mothers choose to wean their infants for a variety of reasons. The nurse should provide information so that the mother can make an informed decision about weaning and should support the woman once her decision is made. Explaining that even a short period of breastfeeding offers her infant many advantages is reassuring. Mothers may need help in planning a gradual weaning process to help avoid engorgement and allow the infant to get used to a bottle or cup slowly. Omitting one breastfeeding session a day and waiting several days or a week before omitting another will allow the mother and infant to adjust to the change more easily.

Home Care

Many infants have not breastfed well by the time of discharge from the birth facility, placing them at risk for failure to gain weight, dehydration, and hyperbilirubinemia. Problems with engorgement and sore nipples are more likely to occur after discharge. The nurse can refer mothers to lactation specialists or organizations such as La Leche League. La Leche League chapters are available in most communities and are listed in the telephone book. Support groups may also be provided by the birth facility.

FORMULA FEEDING

Although formula feeding may require less knowledge and skill than breastfeeding, the inexperienced mother often has many questions and may need assistance in learning to use formula correctly.

■ NURSING CARE
Formula Feeding

Assessment

To identify areas that need teaching, the nurse assesses the mother's method of positioning the infant and bottle and burping during the initial and subsequent feedings. The mother's knowledge about how to prepare formula should also be assessed.

Nursing Diagnosis and Planning

Because improper formula preparation and feeding techniques could harm the infant, an appropriate nursing diagnosis for the mother using formula feeding is

■ Risk for Ineffective Health Maintenance related to lack of understanding of formula preparation and feeding techniques.

  Expected Outcomes: The mother will demonstrate correct techniques in holding the infant and bottle during feedings and will describe how to prepare formula and the frequency of feedings.

Interventions
Teaching About Formula

Teach the mother how to prepare formula correctly. Infection may occur if the milk or water used for preparation is contaminated. Emphasize the importance of following directions in mixing the formula. Improper dilution of the formula may cause undernutrition or imbalances of sodium, which can be dangerous to the infant.

! CRITICAL TO REMEMBER

Formula Dilution

Formulas must be properly diluted to prevent serious illness and to promote weight gain and growth in the infant.
• *Ready-to-use preparations:* use as is without dilution.
• *Concentrated formulas:* dilute with equal parts of water.
• *Powdered formulas:* mix 1 scoop of powder with 2 ounces of water.

Types of Formula Formula may be purchased in three different forms.

Ready-to-Use Preparations. Ready-to-use formula is available in bottles to which a nipple is added or in cans to be poured directly into a bottle. It should not be diluted. Although expensive, it is practical when there is difficulty mixing the formula or the water supply is in question. An open can should be refrigerated and used within 48 hours.

Concentrated Liquid. Explain to the mother how to dilute concentrated liquid formula. Equal parts of formula and water are mixed together in a bottle to provide the amount desired for each feeding. Opened cans should be stored in the refrigerator and used within 24 hours.

Powdered Formula. Powdered formula is more economical and is particularly useful when a breastfeeding mother plans to give an occasional bottle of formula. Usually one scoop of powder is added to each 2 ounces of warm water in a bottle. Single-portion packets of powder are available for travel. Formula should be well mixed to dissolve the powder and make the solution uniform.

Equipment Many different types of bottles and nipples are available. Mothers may use glass or plastic bottles or a plastic liner that fits into a rigid container. Some nipples are designed to simulate the human nipple to promote jaw development. Selection of the type of bottles and nipples depends on individual preference.

Preparation The mother can prepare a single bottle or a 24-hour supply. If the water supply is safe, sterilization is not necessary. Bottles and nipples can be washed in hot, sudsy water using a brush to clean well and then rinsed and allowed to air-dry. Bottles may be washed in a dishwasher, but nipples tend to deteriorate quickly unless washed by hand. Instruct the mother to wash her hands, as well as the top of the can and the can opener. The formula and water are poured into the bottles, which are then capped. Emphasize that the proportion of water and liquid or powdered formula must be adhered to exactly to prevent illness in the infant.

Explain that if safety of the water supply is questionable, sterilization, by aseptic or terminal method, is required. In both methods, all equipment is washed and rinsed well before beginning.

In the aseptic method, equipment needed for the procedure is boiled for 5 minutes in a sterilizer or deep pan. Water for diluting the formula is boiled separately. The bottles are then assembled, using sterilized tongs to avoid contamination by the hands. The formula and boiled water are added, and the bottles are capped and refrigerated until needed.

In the terminal sterilization method, the formula is placed in clean, loosely capped bottles. The bottles are then placed in the sterilizer or pan of water and boiled for 25 minutes. After the bottles cool, the caps are tightened and the bottles refrigerated.

Explaining Feeding Techniques

Positioning Show the mother how to position the infant in a semi-upright position such as the cradle hold. This position allows the mother to hold the infant close with face-to-face contact. The bottle is held so that the nipple is kept full of formula to prevent excessive swallowing of air (Fig. 24-15). Place the infant in the opposite arm for each feeding to provide varied visual stimulation during feedings.

Burping Burping or "bubbling" the infant after every $1/2$ ounce is important for the first few days. The infant gradually can take more milk before burping and should be burped halfway through feedings. Show the mother how to place the infant over her shoulder or in a sitting position with the head supported while she pats and rubs the infant's back.

Frequency and Amount Tell the mother to feed the infant every 3 to 4 hours. The infant takes only ¹/₂ to 1 ounce per feeding during the 1st day of life but increases to 2 to 3 ounces per feeding by the 3rd day. Both the frequency and amount, however, should be adapted to the infant's needs. An infant who is satisfied often goes to sleep.

Cautions Formula should not be heated in a microwave oven because the heating is uneven and may result in some parts of the liquid being very hot, even when the outside of the bottle feels only warm. Formula can be heated by placing it in a container of hot water until it is warm. Suggest that the mother test the formula temperature by allowing a few drops from the bottle to fall on her inner arm.

Caution mothers not to prop the bottle. Propping increases the likelihood of choking if regurgitation occurs and eliminates the holding and cuddling that should accompany feeding. Infants who go to sleep with a bottle propped are at risk for aspiration. Pooled milk in the mouth leads to cavities once the teeth are in. Otitis media is more common in infants who sleep with a bottle or have a propped bottle.

The mother should not try to coax the infant to finish the bottle at each feeding. This action could result in regurgitation and excessive weight gain. Discarding unused formula within an hour prevents feeding the infant formula contaminated by rapidly growing bacteria.

Infant Variations Although formula is usually given at room temperature, some infants take heated or cold formula better. The mother of a sleepy infant needs to use the same wake-up techniques discussed for the breastfeeding mother.

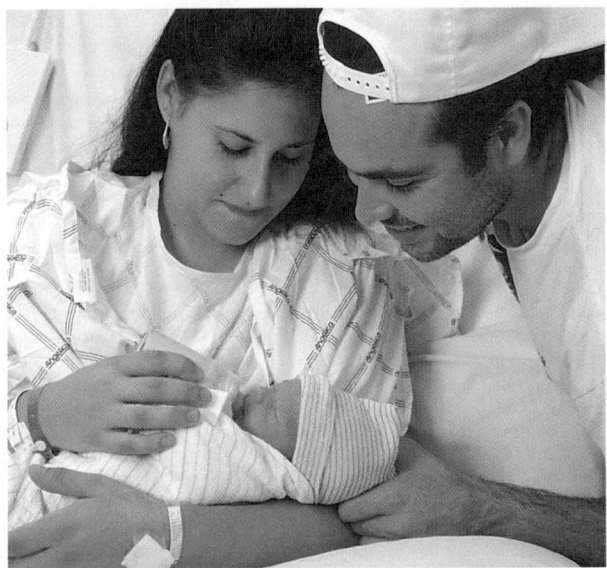

Figure 24-15 This mother holds her infant close during bottle feeding. The bottle is positioned so the nipple is filled with milk at all times. The father offers encouragement.

Angling the tip of the nipple so that it rubs the palate triggers the suck reflex in most infants.

Evaluation

- Does the mother position the infant and the bottle correctly?
- Does she feed the infant the right amount of formula?
- Can she explain how to prepare formula properly?

KEY CONCEPTS

- Full-term infants need 110 to 120 kcal/kg (50-55 kcal/lb) daily. They may lose weight in the first few days after birth as a result of insufficient intake and normal loss of extracellular fluid.
- Colostrum is rich in protein, vitamins, minerals, and immunoglobulins. Transitional milk appears between colostrum and mature milk. Mature milk is present after the first 2 weeks of lactation.
- Breast milk has nutrients in proportions that the newborn requires and in an easily digested form. Most commercial formulas are cow's milk adapted to simulate human milk.
- Breast milk contains factors that help establish the normal intestinal flora and prevent infection. These include *bifidus* factor, leukocytes, lysozymes, lactoferrin, and immunoglobulins.
- A variety of commercial formulas are available. They include modified cow's milk formula, soy-based or protein hydrolysate formulas, and formulas for preterm infants or those with special problems.
- Factors that influence the mother's choice of feeding method include knowledge about each method, support from family and friends, cultural influences, and employment.

- Suckling at the breast causes the mother's posterior pituitary to release oxytocin, which triggers the let-down reflex. It also causes the anterior pituitary to release prolactin, which increases milk production.
- The principle of "supply and demand" applies to breastfeeding. Milk production increases when the infant feeds frequently. When breastfeeding ceases, prolactin is decreased and eventually the alveoli of the breasts atrophy and stop producing milk.
- Flat and inverted nipples should be identified during pregnancy. Creams and methods to toughen the nipples are not necessary.
- The nurse can help the mother establish breastfeeding by initiating early feeding, assisting her to position the infant at the breast, and showing her how to position her hands. The nurse should teach the mother how to help the infant latch on to the breast, assess the position of the mouth on the breast, and remove the infant from the breast.
- The mother should feed the infant 8 to 12 times each day for an average of 15 minutes or more per feeding, nursing until the infant is satisfied at the second breast.
- Wake-up techniques for sleepy infants include unwrapping the blankets, talking to the

infant, changing the diaper, rubbing the infant's back, and expressing colostrum onto the breast.
- When infants suck from a bottle, they must push the tongue against the nipple to slow the flow of milk. When they suckle at the breast, they position the nipple far into the mouth so that the gums compress the areola as the tongue moves over the milk sinuses in a wavelike motion.
- The nurse can help the woman with engorged breasts by encouraging her to nurse frequently, apply heat and cold, and massage and express milk to soften the areola if necessary.
- The nurse should help the mother with sore nipples to check the positioning of the infant at the breast. The mother should vary the position of the infant at the breast and apply breast milk, warm-water compresses, or warm, wet tea bags to the nipples. She should also expose the nipples to air.
- Teaching for the mother who plans to work and breastfeed includes expression of breast milk by hand or pump and proper storage of the milk.
- Mothers who use formula need information about the types of formula available, preparing them correctly, and feeding techniques.

REFERENCES and READINGS

Adams, C., Berger, R., Conning, P., Cruikshank, L., & Dore, K. (2001). Breastfeeding trends at a community breastfeeding center: An evaluative survey. *Journal of Obstetric, Gynecologic, and Neonatal Nursing, 30*(4), 392-400.

American Academy of Pediatrics Committee on Nutrition. (2000). Hypoallergenic infant formula. *Pediatrics, 106*(2), 346-349.

American Academy of Pediatrics Work Group on Breastfeeding. (1997). Breastfeeding and the use of human milk. *Pediatrics, 100*(6), 1035-1039.

American Academy of Pediatrics, & American College of Obstetricians and Gynecologists (AAP & ACOG). (2002). *Guidelines for perinatal care* (5th ed.). Elk Grove Village, IL, and Washington, DC: Author.

Association of Women's Health, Obstetric, and Neonatal Nurses (AWHONN). (2000a). *Evidence-based clinical practice guideline: Breastfeeding support: Prenatal care through the first year* (Monograph). Washington, DC: Author.

Association of Women's Health, Obstetric, and Neonatal Nurses (AWHONN). (2000b). *Evidence-based clinical practice guideline: Breastfeeding support: Prenatal care through the first year* (Practice guidelines). Washington, DC: Author.

Association of Women's Health, Obstetric, and Neonatal Nurses (AWHONN). (2003). *Standards and guidelines for professional nursing practice in the care of women and newborns* (6th ed.). Washington, DC: Author.

Auerbach, K.D. (1999). Maternal employment and breastfeeding. In J. Riordan & K.C. Auerbach (Eds.), *Breastfeeding and human lactation* (2nd ed., pp. 577-636). Boston: Jones & Bartlett.

Auerbach, K D., & Riordan, J. (1999). The breastfeeding process: The perinatal and intrapartum period. In J. Riordan & K.C. Auerbach (Eds.), *Breastfeeding and human lactation* (2nd ed., pp. 279-309). Boston: Jones & Bartlett.

Banks, J.W. (2003). Ka'nistenhsera Teiakotihsnie's: A Native community rekindles the tradition of breastfeeding. *AWHONN Lifelines, 7*(4), 340-347.

Barton, S.J. (2001). Infant feeding practices of low-income rural mothers. *MCN: The American Journal of Maternal/Child Nursing, 26*(2), 93-97.

Biancuzzo, M. (2003). *Breastfeeding the newborn: Clinical strategies for nurses* (2nd ed.). St. Louis: Mosby.

Bronner, Y L., & Auerbach, K.G. (1999). Maternal nutrition during lactation. In J. Riordan & K.G. Auerbach (Eds.), *Breastfeeding and human lactation* (2nd ed., pp. 515-539). Boston: Jones & Bartlett.

Brooks, S.L., Mitchell, A., & Steffenson, N. (2000). Mothers, infants, and DHA: Implications for nursing practice. *MCN: The American Journal of Maternal/Child Nursing, 25*(2), 71-75.

Chezem, J., Friesen, C., & Boettcher, J. (2003). Breastfeeding knowledge, breastfeeding confidence, and infant feeding plans: Effects on actual feeding practices. *Journal of Obstetric, Gynecologic, and Neonatal Nursing, 32*(1), 40-47.

Cobb, M.A.B. (2003). Promoting breastfeeding. *AWHONN Lifelines, 5*(6), 418-423.

Dennis, C.L. (2002). Breastfeeding initiation and duration: A 1990-2000 literature review. *Journal of Obstetric, Gynecologic, and Neonatal Nursing, 31*(1), 12-32.

DiGirolamo, A. M., Grummer-Strawn, L.M., & Fein, S. (2001). Maternity care practices: Implications for breastfeeding. *Birth, 28*(2), 94-100.

Dobson, B., & Murtaugh, M.A. (2001). Position of the American Dietetic Association: Breaking the barriers to breastfeeding. *Journal of the American Dietetic Association, 101*(10), 1213-1220.

Dodd, V., & Chalmers, C. (2003). Comparing the use of hydrogel dressings to lanolin ointment with lactating mothers. *Journal of Obstetric, Gynecologic, and Neonatal Nursing, 32*(4), 486-494.

Gomez, L.T. (2000). Breastfeeding: Increasing primary adjustment milk supply. *International Journal of Childbirth Education, 15*(1), 29-35.

Groer, M.W., Davis, M.W., & Hemphil, J. (2002). Postpartum stress: Current concepts and the possible protective role of breastfeeding. *Journal of Obstetric, Gynecologic, and Neonatal Nursing, 31*(4), 411-417.

Grover, G. (2000). Nutritional needs. In C.D. Berkowitz (Ed.), *Pediatrics: A primary care approach* (2nd ed., pp. 34-39). Philadelphia: Saunders.

Hamelin, K., & McLennan, J. (2000). Examination of the use of an in-hospital breastfeeding tool. *Mother Baby Journal, 5*(3), 29-37.

Hauck, C.L. (2000). Breastfeeding and the workplace: A review of the literature. *Mother Baby Journal, 5*(2), 45-51.

Heird, W.C. (2004). The feeding of infants and children. In R.E. Behrman, R.M. Kliegman, & H.B. Jenson (Eds.), *Nelson textbook of pediatrics* (17th ed., pp. 157-167). Philadelphia: Saunders.

Hill, P.D. (2000). Update on breastfeeding: Health People 2010 objectives. *MCN: The American Journal of Maternal/Child Nursing, 25*(5), 248-251.

Hong, T.M., Callister, L.C., & Schwartz, R. (2003). First-time mothers' views of breastfeeding support from nurses. *MCN: The American Journal of Maternal/Child Nursing, 28*(1), 10-15.

Hornell, A., Hofvander, Y., & Kylberg, E. (2001). Solids and formula: Association with pattern and duration of breastfeeding. *Pediatrics, 107*(3), e38.

Humenick, S.S. (2000). Prenatal preparation for breastfeeding. In F.H. Nichols & S.S. Humenick, *Childbirth education: Practice, research, and theory* (2nd ed., pp. 114-137). Philadelphia: Saunders.

Lawrence, R.A., & Lawrence, R.M. (1999). *Breastfeeding: A guide for the medical profession* (5th ed.). St. Louis: Mosby.

MacMullen, N.J., & Dulski, L.A. (2000). Factors related to sucking ability in healthy newborns. *Journal of Obstetric, Gynecologic, and Neonatal Nursing, 29*(4), 390-396.

Meek, J.Y. (Ed.). (2002). *American Academy of Pediatrics new mother's guide to breastfeeding.* New York: Bantam.

Mohrbacher, N., & Stock, J. (2003). *The breastfeeding answer book* (3rd ed.). Schaumburg, IL: La Leche League International.

Moore, M.L., & Moos, M. (2003). *Cultural competence in the care of childbearing families.* White Plains, NY: March of Dimes.

Mozingo, J.N., Davis, M.W., Droppleman, P.G., & Merideth, A. (2000). "It wasn't working": Women's experiences with short-term breastfeeding. *MCN: The American Journal of Maternal/Child Nursing, 25*(3), 120-126.

Newton, E.R. (2002). Physiology of lactation and breastfeeding. In S.G. Gabbe, J.R. Niebyl, & J.L. Simpson (Eds.), *Obstetrics, normal and problem pregnancies,* (4th ed., pp. 105-136). New York: Churchill Livingstone.

Novotny, R., Hla, M.M., Kieffer, E.C., Park, C., Mor, J., & Thiele, M. (2000). Breastfeeding duration in a multiethnic population in Hawaii. *Birth, 27*(2), 91-96.

Orr, S.S. (2000). Breastfeeding. In S. Mattson & J.E. Smith (Eds.), *Core curriculum for maternal*

newborn nursing (2nd ed., pp. 317-344). Philadelphia: Saunders.

Pollock, C.A., Bustamante-Forest, R., & Giarratano, G. (2002). Men of diverse cultures: Knowledge and attitudes about breastfeeding. *Journal of Obstetric, Gynecologic, and Neonatal Nursing, 31*(6), 673-679.

Riordan, J. (1999a). The biologic specificity of breastmilk. In J. Riordan & K.C. Auerbach (Eds.), *Breastfeeding and human lactation* (2nd ed., pp. 121-161). Boston: Jones & Bartlett.

Riordan, J. (1999b). The cultural context of breastfeeding. In J. Riordan & K.C. Auerbach (Eds.), *Breastfeeding and human lactation* (2nd ed., pp. 29-52). Boston: Jones & Bartlett.

Riordan, J., & Gill-Hopple, K. (2001). Breastfeeding care in multicultural populations. *Journal of Obstetric, Gynecologic, and Neonatal Nursing, 30*(2), 216-223.

Robinson, L.B. (2003). Olive oil: A natural treatment for sore nipples? *AWHONN Lifelines, 6*(2), 110-112.

Ross Products Division. (2003). *Breastfeeding trends through 2000. Mothers' survey.* Columbus, OH: Ross Products Division, Abbott Laboratories, Inc. Retrieved Oct. 27, 2003, from www.ross.com/aboutross/survey.

Santa-Donato, A. (2001). Promoting breastfeeding. *AWHONN Lifelines, 5*(2), 10-12.

Skidmore-Roth, L. (2004). *Mosby's handbook of herbs & natural supplements* (2nd ed.). St. Louis: Mosby.

Spicer, K. (2001). What every nurse needs to know about breast pumping: instructing and supporting mothers of premature infants in the NICU. *Neonatal Network, 20*(4), 35-41.

Taveras, E.M., Capra, A.M., Braveman, P.A., Jensvold, N.G., Escobar, G.J., & Lieu, T.A. (2003). Clinician support and psychosocial risk factors associated with breastfeeding discontinuation. *Pediatrics, 112*(1), 108-115.

Tiedje, L.B., Schiffman, R., Omar, M., Wright, J., Buzzitta, C., McCann, A., & Metzger, S. (2002). An ecological approach to breastfeeding. *MCN: The American Journal of Maternal/Child Nursing, 27*(3), 154-162.

Tiran, D., & Mack, S. (Eds.). (2000). *Complementary therapies for pregnancy and childbirth.* Edinburgh: Bailliere Tindall.

Trahms, C.M. (2000). Nutrition in infancy. In L K. Mahan & S. Escott-Stump (Eds.), *Krause's food, nutrition, and diet therapy* (10th ed., pp. 196-213). Philadelphia: Saunders.

Tsang, R.C., DeMarini, S., & Rath, L.L. (2003). Fluids, electrolytes, vitamins, and trace minerals. In C. Kenner & J.W. Lott (Eds.), *Comprehensive neonatal nursing: A physiologic perspective* (3rd ed., pp. 409-424). Philadelphia: Saunders.

U.S. Department of Health and Human Services. (2000). *Healthy People 2010,* (Conference edition, in 2 volumes). Washington, DC: Author.

Walker, M., & Creehan, P. (2001). Newborn nutrition. In K.R. Simpson & P.A. Creehan (Eds.), *Perinatal nursing* (pp. 550-574). Philadelphia: Lippincott.

Williams, S.R. (2003b). Nutrition during pregnancy and lactation. In S.R. Williams & E.D. Schlenker, *Essentials of nutrition and diet therapy* (8th ed., pp. 269-292). St. Louis: Mosby.

Windsor, J.E. (2003). Korean women & breastfeeding. *AWHONN Lifelines, 7*(1), 61-64.

Witt, K.A., & Mihok, M.A. (2003). Lactation and breastfeeding. In M.K. Mitchell, *Nutrition across the life span* (2nd ed., pp. 177-206). Philadelphia: Saunders.

The Childbearing Family with Special Needs

After studying this chapter, you should be able to:

- Discuss the incidence of and identify the factors that contribute to teenage pregnancy.
- Identify the effects of pregnancy on the adolescent mother, her infant, and the family.
- Describe the role of the nurse in the prevention and management of teenage pregnancy.
- Relate the major implications of delayed childbearing to maternal and fetal health.
- Describe the effects of substance abuse on the mother and the infant.
- Identify nursing interventions to reduce or minimize the effects of substance abuse in the antepartum, intrapartum, and postpartum periods.

- Discuss parental responses when an infant is born with congenital anomalies, and identify nursing interventions to assist the parents.
- Describe parental responses to pregnancy loss, and identify nursing interventions to assist parents through the grieving process.
- Examine the role of the nurse when the mother relinquishes the infant for adoption.
- Identify the factors that promote violence against women, and describe the role of the nurse in assessment, prevention, and interventions.

abstinence syndrome A group of symptoms that occurs when a person who is addicted to a specific drug withdraws or abstains from taking that drug.

addiction Physical or psychologic dependence on a substance such as alcohol, tobacco, or drugs, either legal or illicit.

alcoholism A chronic, progressive, and potentially fatal disease characterized by tolerance for and physical dependency on alcohol or by pathologic organ changes resulting from alcohol abuse or both.

amphetamines Central nervous system stimulants that create a perception of pleasure unrelated to external stimuli.

crack A highly addictive form of cocaine that has been processed to be smoked.

egocentrism Interest centered on the self rather than on the needs of others.

fetal alcohol syndrome A group of physical and mental disorders of the offspring associated with maternal use of alcohol during pregnancy.

methadone A synthetic compound with opiate properties. Used as an oral substitute for heroin and morphine in the opiate-addicted person.

neonatal abstinence syndrome A cluster of physical signs exhibited by the newborn exposed in utero to maternal use of substances such as heroin. See also *abstinence syndrome*.

opiate Any narcotic containing opium or a derivative of opium.

withdrawal syndrome See *abstinence syndrome*.

All families must make major changes as they adapt to pregnancy and childbirth. For some families, however, the changes are particularly difficult. Those families have special needs related to the parents' age, substance abuse, the birth of an infant with congenital abnormalities, loss of a pregnancy, or family violence. Perinatal nurses can make a difference in the lives of these families.

ADOLESCENT PREGNANCY

Incidence of Teenage Pregnancy

Since 1991 there has been a trend toward fewer births to teenagers in the United States. The incidence has decreased to 43 births/1000 women ages 15 to 19 years in 2002 (Martin, et

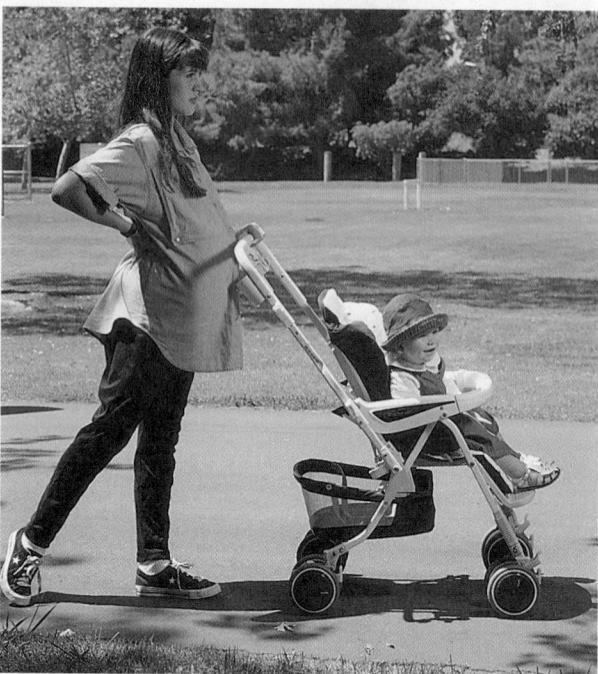

Figure 25-1 Pregnant adolescent. Of teenage girls who become pregnant, 30% to 50% will be pregnant again within 24 months.

al., 2004). This exceeds the *Healthy People 2010* goal of not more than 46 pregnancies per 1000 adolescent girls (U.S. Department of Health & Human Services [USDHHS], 2000).

Adolescent pregnancy remains a problem, however. In 2002, 425,493 teenage girls gave birth (Martin, et al., 2004). Of these, 30% to 50% have another pregnancy within 2 years (Hancock, Calhoun, & Hume, 2002) (Fig. 25-1).

Factors Associated With Teenage Pregnancy

The high level of sexual activity and lack of or inconsistent contraceptive use among adolescents are directly related to the incidence of teenage pregnancies in the United States. Fifty percent of high school students report that they are sexually active (MacKay, Fingerhut, & Duran, 2000). Approximately 75% of teen pregnancies are unintended (Davis, 2003).

Pregnancy occurs because many adolescents fail to recognize their vulnerability as a result of their sexual activity and believe that pregnancy cannot happen to them. Some risk pregnancy and parenthood as a means of gaining a love relationship. They often see themselves as lacking power in their relationships and defer to their partner's wishes (Kelly & Morgan-Kidd, 2001). Other teens see pregnancy as a means to gain independence.

When compared with other developed countries, the pregnancy and birth rate for teenagers in the United States is one of the highest (Singh & Darroch, 2000). Adolescents who give birth are more likely to be low income, which may mean they have less access to contraception and abortion. These teenagers may not believe finishing their education and obtaining good jobs are possibilities for them and may see little reason to postpone pregnancy (Breedlove & Schorfheide, 2001).

BOX 25-1
Factors Contributing to Teenage Pregnancy

- Lack of accurate information about how to use contraceptives
- Limited access to contraceptive devices
- Fear of reporting sexual activity to parents
- Ambivalence toward sexuality; intercourse not "planned"
- Feelings of invulnerability
- Peer pressure to begin sexual activity
- Low self-esteem and consequent inability to set limits on sexual activity
- Desire to attain love or to escape present situation
- Lack of appropriate role models
- Low level of education correlated with incorrect use of contraceptives

Sex Education

Sex education for teenagers should focus on helping them understand how to set limits on sexual activity and instruction in effective measures to prevent pregnancy and sexually transmissible diseases (STDs).

Learning how to set limits on sexual behavior is particularly important for younger teenagers, who may be pressured to become sexually active before they have developed the maturity to deal responsibly with intercourse, contraception, or unplanned pregnancy. They need advice about how to handle pressure so they can postpone sexual intercourse until they are emotionally and physically ready.

When providing sex education, nurses must keep in mind that adolescent males and females mature at different rates and may be more comfortable learning in separate groups. In talking with teenagers, nurses should use simple but correct language such as uterus, testicles, penis, and vagina (see "Methods of Contraception," Chapter 10; see Box 25-1).

Options When Pregnancy Occurs

An adolescent who becomes pregnant must choose one of three options: (1) to terminate the pregnancy, (2) to place the infant for adoption, or (3) to keep the infant. Although many pregnant teens choose abortion, this is not an acceptable option for some. Teenagers who might consider termination may not acknowledge the pregnancy until it is too late for abortion.

Few teenagers choose to place the infant for adoption. Those who do may have complicated feelings of grief, relief that a "bad" experience is over, and anger at parents who were unwilling to provide assistance and thus made adoption the only realistic option. The autonomous decision to relinquish the child "for the child's good," however, may be an important step toward maturity.

Adolescents who choose abortion or adoption receive less assistance in dealing with their experience than those who keep their infants. They need help in coping with their feelings about their decision (see "Relinquishment by Adoption," p. 610).

Socioeconomic Implications of Teenage Pregnancy

The financial cost of teenage pregnancy in the United States is estimated to be between $7 billion and $15 billion per year (USDHHS, 2000). Costs include funds for Temporary Assistance for Needy Families (TANF), Medicaid, food stamps, direct payment to care providers, and administrative costs. Teenage mothers are more likely than older mothers to be nonwhite, poor, less educated, and unmarried. Adolescents are more likely to have larger families at an earlier age, resulting in more children to feed and clothe on an already inadequate income.

Although the financial cost of teenage pregnancy is enormous, the cost in human terms is often tragic. The developmental tasks of adolescence, such as achieving independence from parents and establishing a lifestyle that is personally satisfying, may be interrupted. Instead of becoming independent, they often become more dependent on parents or a boyfriend as a result of pregnancy. Educational goals are curtailed for some young mothers, limiting employment opportunities and resulting in reliance on the welfare system.

For some adolescents, however, pregnancy motivates a desire to do well in school so they can provide for their infants (Rentschler, 2003). Pregnancy and birth may have a stabilizing effect in adolescents who change past poor lifestyle choices and become more goal-directed than they had previously been (Clemmens, 2003).

Children born into this situation do not escape unscathed. They show a higher incidence of impaired intellectual functioning and poor school adjustment. The negative cycle is often repeated: a large percentage of teenage parents were children of teenage parents. As a result, children of adolescent parents are often among the poorest people in the United States.

Implications of Teenage Pregnancy for Maternal Health

Pregnancy presents significant problems for the health of adolescent females. They are at increased risk for preeclampsia, anemia, gaining too much or not enough weight, urinary tract infections, and depression (Breedlove & Schorfheide, (2001). However, these risks may be lowered in adolescents with adequate prenatal care and elimination of other risk factors (Koniak-Griffin & Turner-Pluta, 2001).

Adolescents are often in abusive relationships and should be screened to identify violence so the nurse can help them access available resources. The high incidence of STDs among pregnant teenagers is another concern. Gonorrhea and chlamydial infection are particularly prevalent during these years, and these diseases can be transmitted to the infant, affecting the eyes and lungs.

The reason for the incidence of complications among teenagers is unclear. It may be caused by delayed prenatal care and economic problems rather than by age. Pregnant adolescents tend to see a health care provider to start prenatal care later than older women and may delay until the pregnancy is advanced. Early prenatal care that includes counseling about nutritional needs and close observation for complications is important.

Implications of Teenage Pregnancy for Fetal-Neonatal Health

The pregnant adolescent is more likely to smoke cigarettes, increasing the risk that her infant will be preterm or low birth weight (less than 2500 g) (Martin, et al., 2004). The cause of low birth weight may be intrauterine growth restriction, which means that the fetus does not grow as expected. This condition may result from a variety of causes, such as poor placental perfusion, which occurs during preeclampsia, or the underdeveloped vasculature of the uterus in young primigravidas. Prematurity is also a major cause of low-birth-weight infants. When the infant is born before 38 weeks' gestation, the baby is more likely to weigh less than 2500 g and has the added risks associated with immature organs. Even infants born at 37 weeks' gestation or more and healthy are more likely to die during the first year of life if they are born to teenage mothers when compared with those whose mothers are in their 20s (Phipps, Blume, & DeMonner, 2002).

The Teenage Expectant Father

Approximately 64% of adolescent mothers have partners within 2 years of their age, but 7% have partners 6 or more years older (Alan Guttmacher Institute, 2003). These men may accept responsibility for the child, or they may become "phantom fathers," who are absent or rarely involved in raising the child.

Almost all adolescent expectant fathers indicate that they are not ready for fatherhood. Many are depressed as they grapple with the conflicting roles of adolescence and fatherhood. Although some express interest in learning about childbirth and child care, those who do not want to be fathers are less likely to be supportive. Some do not wish to interact with the infant, leaving the pregnant girl to seek support elsewhere. Others are involved in some degree during the pregnancy and early years of the child's life but become less involved over time (Breedlove & Schorfheide, 2001).

A disproportionate number of teenage expectant fathers are from environments of poverty and lack job skills or educational preparation. Many need job training before they can earn enough money to contribute to the support of their children.

Impact of Teenage Pregnancy on Parenting

Adolescent mothers are at risk for becoming nonnurturing parents. Whether this risk results from adolescence per se, the higher incidence of premature births, the lower socioeconomic status, or the particular home environment is difficult to determine. Teenage mothers do tend to be less sensitive to infant cues. They display fewer instances of mutual gazing, verbal interaction, and touching than do older mothers (American Academy of Pediatrics [AAP], 2001).

Adolescent parents are likely to be surprised and dismayed at how difficult and time-consuming parenting can be. They may have little understanding of the expected growth and development of infants and may expect too much too soon from their children. For instance, they may expect that the infant will sleep through the night, smile, or be toilet-trained before it is possible for infants to do these things.

Preparing for parenthood is important. Although pregnant adolescents may want to be good mothers, they often do not actively seek information about infant care and development (Rentschler, 2003). The mother's relationship with the father of the baby may affect her parenting abilities. A close and satisfying relationship with the baby's father may increase attachment behaviors in the mother. Thus the father should be included, when appropriate, in care of the mother and baby. However, many adolescent mothers do not have a good relationship with the father of their baby and will need support in coping (Clemmens, 2003; Rentschler, 2003).

The ability to deal with stress plays an important part in mothering skills. Young adolescents have immature coping mechanisms, and they may be unable to separate the stress of other life events from the stress that occurs when the infant cries and cannot be consoled. They may respond with immature or punitive measures toward the infant when the source of stress is another factor, such as social isolation or inadequate financial resources.

NURSING CARE
The Pregnant Teenager

Assessment

Physical Assessment

Assessment of pregnant teenagers is similar to that of older women in many respects. At the initial visit, obtain a thorough health and family history to determine whether conditions such as diabetes or infectious diseases increase the risk for the mother and fetus. Monitor closely for signs of iron deficiency anemia, preeclampsia, or STDs. Attempt to identify behavioral risk factors, such as smoking, alcohol or drug use, or unprotected sex, that could harm the mother or fetus. Screen for physical or sexual abuse, which is elevated in pregnant teenagers (Hancock, Calhoun, & Hume, 2002). (See intimate partner violence, p. 610.)

Structure the interview so that questions can be interspersed in a more general conversation that explores the teenager's likes and concerns. This approach helps establish rapport and gain a better understanding of the teenager.

Knowledge of Infant Needs

Assess knowledge of infant needs and parenting skills. How does the teenager plan to feed the infant? What will she do when the infant cries? How will she know when the infant is ill and should be taken to a pediatrician? Does she know how much the infant should sleep? What plans have been made to provide for the hygiene and safety needs of the infant?

Cognitive Development

Determine the teenager's cognitive development and ability to absorb health counseling. The three most important areas of cognitive development are:

1. *Egocentrism*, which involves the ability to defer personal satisfaction to respond to the needs of the infant: "What would you do if the baby were sick?" "How would you make the baby better?"

2. *Present-future orientation*, which involves the ability to make long-term plans: "What are your plans for finishing high school?"

3. *Abstract thinking*, which involves identifying cause and effect: "Why is it important to keep clinic appointments?" "Why should condoms be used even though you are pregnant?"

Family Assessment

Begin assessment of the family unit by determining the degree of participation by the infant's father. Fathers may plan to marry the expectant mother, participate in the pregnancy and rearing of the child without marriage, or be totally uninvolved.

It is important to assess the adolescent without the presence of her parents, but it is also crucial to determine the availability and amount of family support. Families respond in a variety of ways. A family member (usually the adolescent's mother) may take over the mothering role, or all infant care may be performed by the teenager. In other families, care and responsibilities are shared. This arrangement allows the adolescent to complete the developmental tasks of adolescence as well as learning the mother role.

The pregnant teenager's mother is particularly important when assessing the family. She may feel that she has "failed" as a mother, or she may resent the new cycle of child care in which the pregnancy involves her. If the family is unable or unwilling to provide care for an adolescent with an infant, what other social support can be located?

Nursing Diagnosis and Planning

Many adolescents wait until the second or third trimester to seek prenatal care because they either do not realize that they are pregnant or continue to deny that they are pregnant. They may not know where to go for care and may fear the results of the pregnancy on their lives and relationships. Teenagers often have little information about physiologic demands, such as an increased need for nutrients, that pregnancy imposes on their bodies. As a result, they may have a pattern of sporadic prenatal care and missed appointments (see Nursing Care Plan: Adolescents' Responses to Pregnancy and Birth). One of the most relevant nursing diagnoses is

■ Risk for Ineffective Health Maintenance related to lack of knowledge of measures to promote health during pregnancy and increased family stress.

Expected Outcomes: The expectant mother will keep scheduled prenatal appointments and follow instructions that promote her health and the health of the fetus throughout pregnancy. She will participate in learning about infant needs by the end of the third trimester. The family will verbalize emotions and concerns and maintain functional support of the expectant mother and her infant.

Interventions

Eliminating Barriers to Health Care

Two major barriers to health care are scheduling conflicts and negative attitudes of health care workers. Help the adolescent locate the clinic closest to her that has appointments available when the girl (and her partner, if he wishes) is not in school. Provide information about public transportation to that location.

Nursing Care Plan

Adolescents' Responses to Pregnancy and Birth

ASSESSMENT

Ann Killian, a 16-year-old white female, presented at the prenatal clinic during the 20th week of her pregnancy. She lives with her mother and father, who both work, and a younger sister. She sees her boyfriend sporadically but is unsure if he will be involved with the baby. Ann remains in school but verbalizes concern about how she looks and feels: "How much bigger am I going to get?" "Why is my face so blotchy?"

Nursing Diagnosis

Disturbed Body Image related to perceived negative effects of pregnancy, as evidenced by verbalized concern about appearance.

Goals/Expected Outcomes

Ann will:

- Verbalize her feelings about pregnancy and her perception of herself during each antepartum visit.
- Make two positive statements about herself during the next antepartum visit.

INTERVENTION	RATIONALE
1. Allow time at each prenatal visit for Ann to express concerns about weight gain and other physiologic changes of pregnancy, such as hyperpigmentation and stretch marks.	1. The adolescent is often ashamed and uncomfortable with her pregnant body. She feels more comfortable if she is allowed to share these feelings and be reassured that they are a normal part of pregnancy.
2. Initiate interaction about body changes by asking open-ended questions such as "How do you feel about needing to wear maternity clothes?"	2. Adolescents are often intimidated by health care professionals and may think that their own feelings are not important enough to discuss.
3. Provide anticipatory guidance about normal changes, such as the pattern of weight gain during pregnancy and weight loss after childbirth.	3. Most adolescents do not know what to expect during pregnancy. Anticipatory guidance reduces fear and provides information about expected changes.
4. Explain the reason for changes that are most troublesome at each prenatal visit (weight gain, hyperpigmentation, stretch marks, breast changes).	4. It is helpful for the adolescent to know that some changes are temporary and that increasing weight indicates that the fetus is growing and developing. This often becomes a source of pride for the young teenager as well as for the older woman.
5. Promote positive self-image by praising grooming, posture, and responsible behavior such as keeping prenatal appointments and following recommendations: "You have never missed an appointment, and your baby is growing so well."	5. Positive reinforcement is particularly important to help the adolescent meet the developmental tasks of developing a sense of identity and self-worth.

Evaluation

Ann discusses her concerns about how she looks and feels about herself. She begins to make positive statements about herself at each prenatal visit.

ASSESSMENT

Ann reveals that her father has said that she has "shamed the family," and she is worried that her friends will reject her when they learn that she is pregnant. Ann states that she will have to "drop out of everything." She confides, in a trembling voice, that she feels guilty for "putting my family through this."

Nursing Diagnosis

Situational Low Self-esteem related to feelings of rejection by family and friends, as manifested by statements indicating guilt and uncertainty about future support for self and infant.

Goals/Expected Outcomes

Ann will:

- Identify at least two new measures to cope with anxiety by the end of the current antepartum visit.
- Demonstrate ability to implement these measures during subsequent antepartum visits.

Continued

Nursing Care Plan

Adolescents' Responses to Pregnancy and Birth—cont'd

INTERVENTION	RATIONALE
1. Help Ann identify what she can do to overcome anxiety about rejection from her family and friends before the next prenatal appointment.	1. Planning how to approach family and friends reduces anxiety.
a. Role-play how Ann can initiate a conversation with her friends to discuss activities that they can continue to share.	a. Acceptance by the peer group and participation in group activities are major concerns of adolescents. A change of status within the group is a threat to self-concept that precipitates acute anxiety.
b. Suggest that she talk to family members about her feelings (guilty for the unhappiness she is causing them and fearful they will not assist her through the pregnancy and birth).	b. Although adolescents strive for independence, family values continue to be a significant influence. Rejection by the family at this time would leave her vulnerable to great stress.
c. Recommend that she share her feelings with the father of the infant if she continues to see him.	c. Expectant fathers may be a source of emotional and financial support.
2. Encourage Ann to discuss her economic needs as well as her plans for continuing school when the infant is born.	2. Planning provides some sense of control and increases feelings of competency.
3. Assist Ann in locating and joining the school-age mothers' program if available through her school district.	3. Teenagers who are mothers or expectant mothers often replace the pregnant teenager's previous peer group. The programs allow for continuing high school classes, and the shared concerns and activities provide an opportunity for growth.
4. Point out and praise any positive actions Ann takes, such as keeping prenatal appointments or eating a nutritious diet.	4. Sincere praise helps reinforce a positive self-image.

Evaluation

Ann talks with her family and reports relationships are somewhat improved. She enters a school-age mothers' program and is very pleased.

ASSESSMENT

Ann has given birth to a 6-lb, 3-oz girl at 38 weeks' gestation. She does not want to breastfeed because she feels uncomfortable with it and plans to go back to school as soon as possible. Ann will live at home, and her mother has agreed to pay for child care for the infant while Ann is in school. Ann is very concerned about caring for the newborn. She seems unsure how to respond when the infant cries and handles her only during feedings.

Nursing Diagnosis

Risk for Impaired Parenting related to knowledge deficit of infant needs and lack of confidence in her ability to care for the infant, as evidenced by uncertain responses to the infant.

Pregnant women of all ages state that the negative attitude of some health care workers can discourage them from obtaining prenatal care. Nurses can be instrumental in finding ways to overcome these negative attitudes, thus encouraging pregnant women, including teenagers, to return for needed follow-up care.

Applying Teaching/Learning Principles

Adolescents often feel isolated from peers who may not understand the responsibilities of parenthood (Clemmens, 2003). They may no longer be able to participate in activities with their peers because of child care obligations. Arrange for the pregnant teenager to participate in small groups with common concerns. Specific needs that might be addressed are the benefits of prenatal care or help in eliminating unhealthful habits such as smoking, drug use, or alcohol consumption. Near the end of pregnancy, preparations for labor and delivery and infant care become the priorities.

Repetition is an important method of teaching and clarifying misinformation. Allow ample time for questions and discussions. Although teenagers do not read or benefit from printed materials to the same degree that older parents do, many learn well from audiovisual aids. Written materials prepared especially for adolescents may be helpful for some.

It is particularly important that the nurse does not sound like a parent when working with adolescents. Avoid using the word "should" or "ought" or making decisions for the teenagers.

Nursing Care Plan

Adolescents' Responses to Pregnancy and Birth—cont'd

Goals/Expected Outcomes

Ann will:
- Demonstrate basic infant care (cord care, bathing, burping, feeding, swaddling) by discharge.
- Verbalize infant needs for gentle, prompt response to crying on the first postpartum day.
- Demonstrate attachment behaviors (eye contact, gazing, holding, verbal stimulation, positive comments about the infant) before discharge.

INTERVENTION	RATIONALE
1. Demonstrate infant care on the first postpartum day, and obtain a return demonstration on the second postpartum day. (See Chapter 23.)	1. Confidence is increased by returning the demonstration of infant care.
2. Role-play for Ann the way to respond when the infant cries, and emphasize the importance of promptness and gentleness.	2. Observing nurses respond to the infant increases the likelihood that adolescents will respond in the same manner. Prompt response helps the infant develop trust.
3. Emphasize the importance of touch and verbal stimulation, and point out the reciprocal bonding behaviors, such as the infant following the mother with the eyes.	3. Many teenage parents do not provide adequate tactile and verbal stimulation for their infants, which may decrease the infant's ability to learn and respond to the environment. The infant has many behaviors that stimulate attachment between parent and child.
4. Include the grandparents and the father of the infant in as many demonstrations as possible.	4. When all primary caregivers are included, family cohesiveness and consistency of care are enhanced.
5. Instruct Ann in early growth and development of the infant (how often infants need to eat, how much they sleep, what to do when they cry).	5. Anticipatory guidance helps parents have realistic perceptions of the infant.
6. Encourage Ann to continue in the school-age mothers' program and to attend parenting classes along with other teenagers.	6. Learning along with her peers will help her increase her parenting skills and provides a continuing peer support group.

Evaluation

Ann shows a prompt and gentle response when her infant cries. She gives basic care as taught and discusses what to expect in early growth and development of her baby. She makes frequent positive comments about her daughter.

Additional Nursing Diagnoses to Consider

- Ineffective Coping.
- Interrupted Family Processes.
- Disabled Family Coping.
- Risk for Ineffective Health Maintenance.
- Risk for Delayed Growth and Development.

Counseling

Allow time to counsel teenagers about their specific problems, such as nutrition, stress reduction, and infant care.

Nutrition Nutrition counseling is one means of reducing the incidence of low-birth-weight infants. Determine the adolescent's general nutritional status, and assess for eating disorders that would reduce caloric intake and possibly affect fetal growth. Emphasize that the adolescent's nutrition must be adequate for her own growth needs as well as that of the fetus. Discuss nutrition during lactation, pointing out the advantages for both mother and baby. Tailor information to the individual adolescent's likes and peer group habits. Nutrition education must be socially and culturally appropriate. (See Chapter 15 for suggestions on nutrition for adolescents.)

Make referrals to food stamp providers, the Special Supplemental Food Program for Women, Infants, and Children (WIC), surplus food distributors, food banks, and food preparation equipment if necessary. Many teenagers have limited access to food and lack the ability to store or prepare food.

Self-care Provide the same teaching about self-care that would be given to an older woman (see Chapter 13). In addition, emphasize prevention of STDs by using a condom even though she is pregnant. Counsel the adolescent about lifestyle changes, such as smoking or substance abuse cessation, that will benefit mother and fetus, and refer her to resources to help her with these problems.

Stress Reduction Determine the stressors in the adolescent's life. Stress may be related to basic needs such as food, shelter, and health care. Fear of labor and delivery and fear of being single, alone, and unsupported all create stress. Meeting the developmental tasks of adolescence while working on the developmental tasks of pregnancy (overcoming ambivalence, attaining the role of parent) is another stressor.

A variety of measures may be used to reduce stress, depending on the teenager's age, situation, and available support. Refer adolescents with chronic life stress to a social worker to achieve stabilization. If the girl is very young or if the pregnancy occurred as a result of rape or incest, social service and law enforcement agencies must become involved to provide protection and assistance.

The pregnant teenager often experiences stress because she has not told her parents or the father of the infant about the pregnancy. Role-play the encounter with her to help her work out a plan for breaking the news. Although there is strain on the relationship when the teen first tells her parents, over time her relationship with her parents may become better than it was before the pregnancy if her parents are supportive (Clemmens, 2003).

Infant Care Explain and demonstrate basic infant care and infant cues (using behaviors of the infants in videos or in the group as examples). Emphasize that eye contact, holding, cuddling, and verbal stimulation are important for the child's development.

Because adolescents tend to have a more rigid and punitive approach to child care, explain that infants develop a sense of trust when their needs are met promptly and gently. Moreover, their future development depends on attaining a sense of trust during infancy. Emphasize that crying does not indicate that the infant is spoiled but simply that the infant has a need for food, warmth, or comfort and love.

If a support person will be involved in helping care for the infant, include that person in teaching, especially if the support person has little experience with babies. Having a support person learn with her may help the teenager remember the information better.

Promoting Family Support

The pregnant teenager needs encouragement to include her family in her decision making and problem solving. Discuss topics such as who will care for the infant, whether the teenager will return to school, and what financial assistance is available from the family and from the infant's father. Adolescent mothers who have adequate emotional support are more likely to learn appropriate parenting techniques.

If, however, the family has multiple problems that include substance abuse or domestic violence, involving family members may be inappropriate. The teenager should be encouraged instead to communicate with a family friend or other trusted adult.

Providing Referrals

Make referrals to conveniently located national and community resources for pregnant adolescents. These include well-baby clinics, programs for school-age mothers offered by many school districts, TANF, and WIC. Church and community organizations may also provide needed assistance. Home visit services, if available, would be helpful throughout the pregnancy and postpartum to help the mother cope with difficulties that occur during the early months. Home visits during pregnancy and the first year help decrease hospitalization of infants and repeat pregnancies (Koniak-Griffin et al., 2003).

Evaluation

- Does the pregnant adolescent keep prenatal appointments?
- Does she ask questions and follow the recommended plan of care?
- Can she explain basic needs and care of the infant?
- Is the family supportive, or have appropriate referrals been made?

DELAYED PREGNANCY

An increasing number of women become pregnant relatively late in their reproductive life. Advances in contraception and improved infertility treatment allow women more options in childbearing.

Maternal and Fetal Implications of Delayed Pregnancy

When the mature woman decides to conceive, she may experience a delay in becoming pregnant, particularly after the age of 35 years. This is because of the normal aging of the ovaries and the increased incidence of reproductive tract disorders. (See Chapter 10 for a discussion of infertility.)

Once she conceives, the mature woman is at increased risk for complications associated with pregnancy. The risks may be genetic, a result of preexisting medical conditions, or from obstetric complications. The increased risk for fetal chromosomal abnormalities with advancing maternal age is well documented. Trisomy 21 (Down syndrome) is the most common example. Genetic abnormalities also increase when the father is older than 40 years (Neumann & Graf, 2003).

The most common examples of preexisting diseases that can cause maternal or fetal jeopardy are hypertension and diabetes mellitus. Uterine myomas (fibroids) occur with greater frequency in women older than 35 years and may be associated with postpartum hemorrhage. The older primigravida is also at increased risk for obstetric complications, such as vaginal bleeding, preeclampsia, multiple gestation, preterm labor, gestational diabetes, dysfunctional labor, and cesarean birth.

However, women who are without medical problems have much lower risks for problems than previously thought (Cunningham et al., 2001). Those who do have some complications can often have a successful pregnancy with good medical and nursing care.

Advantages of Delayed Childbirth

Mature primigravidas come to the parenting role with a range of personal resources: psychosocial maturity, self-confidence, and a sense of control over their lives. In addition, they are capable of solving complex problems and are often adept at maintaining interpersonal relationships. Because they are more likely to be financially secure, these women can afford good care for their infants. They are experienced at setting priorities and developing plans. They are usually able to manage stress and will seek support and assistance when needed (Fig. 25-2).

Disadvantages of Delayed Childbirth

Mature primiparas need more time to recover from childbirth, and they have less energy than their younger counterparts. They may find child care an exhausting experience for the first few weeks, particularly if they had a cesarean birth or other complications of pregnancy.

Peer support may be less available for mature primigravidas. Many of their friends have teenage children and do not relate to the concerns of a new mother. Younger mothers have some of the same concerns, but they often do not share the perspective of older mothers.

Family support may also be lacking for the older woman. Her parents are usually in their 60s or 70s and may not be able to assist with child care to the extent that younger grandparents can.

Nursing Considerations

Reinforcing and Clarifying Information

Because the fetus of a mature woman is at increased risk for chromosomal anomalies, the woman will be informed about diagnostic tests that are available (see Chapter 16). The tests most often recommended are triple marker screening, chorionic villus sampling, amniocentesis, and ultrasonography. The family's beliefs and attitudes about abortion often determine whether to have the recommended tests. The woman who would not consider abortion regardless of the condition of the fetus may refuse diagnostic studies or have them to help prepare for the problems that will occur at birth. Nurses must respect the decision and acknowledge that it may have been a difficult one to make.

Facilitating Expression of Emotions

Several days or weeks may pass between the time when the diagnostic studies are performed and when the results of the tests are known. This is a particularly difficult time for many expectant parents, and nurses often assist the couple to express their concerns and emotions.

A broad statement such as "Many couples find it difficult to wait for the results" will often elicit free expression of their feelings. Follow-up questions such as "What concerns you most?" may reveal worry about the procedure itself or about the possible effects of the procedure on the fetus. Simply acknowledging that it is a stressful time helps the couple cope with their emotions.

Mature gravidas also worry about complications that may affect the fetus or their own health. They are aware that they may not have another opportunity for pregnancy because of their age. They may be concerned about their ability to balance their careers with increased family responsibilities.

Providing Parenting Information

Nurses often help the mature primipara prepare for effective parenting. Anticipatory guidance about measures that will help conserve energy after childbirth is very useful. Such measures include meal planning and setting realistic housekeeping goals. In addition, many older mothers need to mobilize all available support so that they can reserve their energy for infant care. During the first weeks after childbirth, the mother may experience feelings of social isolation, particularly if her friends have children who are a great deal

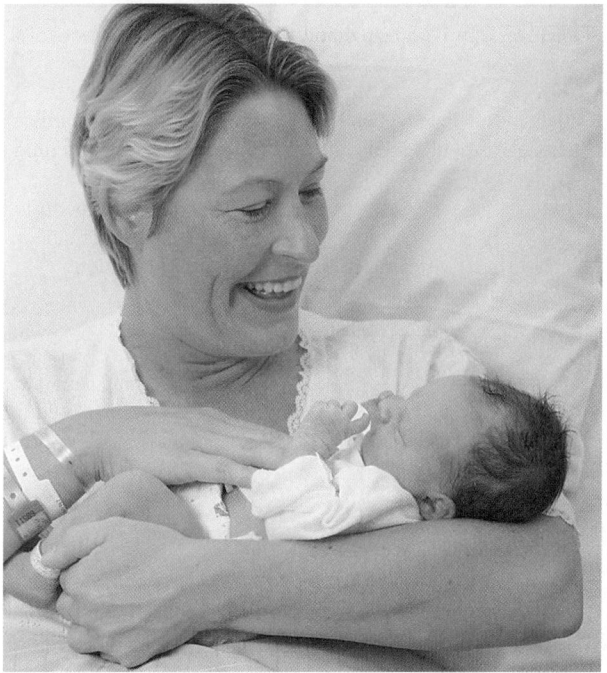

Figure 25-2   Older primigravidas bring maturity and problem-solving skills to the maternal role, but they are at somewhat increased risk for physiologic problems related to pregnancy and birth.

older. If she is accustomed to much mental stimulation, she may miss this while staying at home. If she elects to return to work, she is likely to experience guilt and grief because she must leave her infant.

First-time mothers older than 35 years are especially receptive to prenatal classes. Older gravidas are more likely to seek out information they need from a variety of sources. They often adopt health-promoting activities such as improving nutrition and eliminating harmful substances (Viau, Padula, & Eddy, 2002). They are interested in printed materials that can be used to reinforce teaching.

SUBSTANCE ABUSE

The use of legal substances, such as alcohol and tobacco, as well as illicit drugs, such as cocaine and marijuana, increases the risk for medical complications in the mother and poor birth outcomes in the infant.

Incidence of Substance Abuse

Approximately 1 in 10 infants is exposed to one or more mood-altering drugs during pregnancy (American Academy of Pediatrics [AAP] and American College of Obstetricians and Gynecologists [ACOG], 2002). Although tobacco, alcohol, and marijuana are the most commonly abused drugs, the use of cocaine and heroin has had a major impact on health care for pregnant women and their offspring.

Maternal and Fetal Effects of Substance Abuse

When the pregnant woman takes a substance, the fetus experiences the same systemic effects as the expectant mother but often more severely. For instance, cocaine raises the

TABLE **25-1** Maternal and Fetal or Neonatal Effects of Commonly Abused Substances

Substance	Maternal Effects	Fetal or Neonatal Effects
Caffeine (coffee, tea, cola, chocolate, cold remedies, analgesics)	Stimulates CNS and cardiac function, causes vasoconstriction and mild diuresis; half-life triples during pregnancy	Crosses placental barrier and stimulates fetus; teratogenic effects are undocumented
Tobacco	Decreased placental perfusion, anemia, PROM, preterm labor, spontaneous abortion	Prematurity, LBW, fetal demise, developmental delays, increased incidence of SIDS, pneumonia
Alcohol (beer, wine, mixed drinks, after-dinner drinks)	Spontaneous abortion	Fetal demise, IUGR, FAS (facial and cranial anomalies, developmental delay, mental retardation, short attention span), fetal alcohol effects (milder form of FAS)
Cocaine ("crack")	Hyperarousal state, generalized vasoconstriction, hypertension, increased incidence of spontaneous abortion, abruptio placentae, preterm labor, cardiovascular complications (stroke, heart attack), seizures, increased STDs	Tachycardia, stillbirth, prematurity, LBW, tremors, IUGR, irritability, decreased ability to interact with environmental stimuli, poor feeding reflexes, nausea, vomiting, diarrhea, decreased intellectual development; distended, flabby, creased abdomen (prune-belly syndrome) caused by absence of abdominal muscles
Narcotics (heroin, methadone, morphine)	Spontaneous abortion, PROM, preterm labor, increased incidence of STDs, HIV exposure, hepatitis, malnutrition	IUGR, perinatal asphyxia, intellectual impairment, neonatal abstinence syndrome, neonatal infections, fetal or neonatal death (SIDS, child abuse and neglect)
Sedatives (barbiturates, tranquilizers)	Lethargy, drowsiness, CNS depression	Neonatal abstinence syndrome, seizures, delayed lung maturity, possible teratogenic effects
Amphetamines ("speed," "crystal," or "ice" when processed in crystals to smoke)	Malnutrition, tachycardia, withdrawal symptoms (lethargy, depression)	Increased risk for IUGR, prematurity, cardiac anomalies, cleft palate, placental abruption, hypoglycemia, sweating, poor visual tracking, "glassy-eyed" look, lethargy, feeding problems
Marijuana ("pot" or "grass")	Often used with other drugs: alcohol, cocaine, tobacco; increased incidence of anemia and inadequate weight gain	Unclear, more study needed, believed related to prematurity, IUGR, tremors, sensitivity to light

CNS, Central nervous system; *PROM,* premature rupture of membranes; *LBW,* low birth weight; *SIDS,* sudden infant death syndrome; *IUGR,* intrauterine growth restriction; *FAS,* fetal alcohol syndrome; *STDs,* sexually transmissible diseases; *HIV,* human immunodeficiency virus.

blood pressure of the woman and the fetus and puts both at risk for intracranial bleeding. A drug that causes intoxication in the woman causes it for prolonged periods in the fetus. This prolonged effect occurs because the fetus cannot metabolize drugs efficiently and will experience the effects long after they have abated in the woman. Maternal, fetal, and neonatal effects of commonly abused substances are summarized in Table 25-1.

Tobacco

Exposure to maternal smoking occurs in 20% to 30% of pregnancies (Greene & Goodman, 2003). The active ingredients of cigarette smoke are nicotine, tar, and harmful gases, such as carbon monoxide and cyanide. Nicotine causes vasoconstriction and reduces placental blood circulation. Carbon monoxide inactivates fetal and maternal hemoglobin. Together these substances reduce the amount of oxygen delivered to the fetus. Indirect effects of cigarette smoking include decreased maternal appetite, which results in inadequate intake of calories as well as decreased absorption of some nutrients.

Neonatal consequences of smoking tobacco during pregnancy are prematurity and low birth weight. Infants are symmetrically smaller in all areas, including head circumference. Smoking during pregnancy is also associated with delayed neurologic and intellectual development of children. Problems include hyperactivity, shorter attention span, and lower reading and spelling scores during the primary grades. Sudden infant death syndrome is twice as frequent in children of smokers (Moran, 2000).

Alcohol

Approximately 1 in 30 women reports drinking seven or more drinks per week or binge drinking (five or more drinks on any one occasion) during pregnancy (Centers for Disease Control and Prevention, 2003). Alcohol is a teratogen, and its use during pregnancy may result in fetal alcohol syndrome (FAS), the leading cause of mental retardation and the only cause that is preventable (Botham, 2000). Alcohol passes easily across the placenta.

The amount and timing of alcohol intake influence the specific effects on the fetus. During the first trimester, it is believed to affect cell membranes and alter the organization of tissue. Throughout pregnancy, alcohol interferes with the metabolism of nutrients and thus retards cell growth and division. Binge drinking is especially harmful, but drinking in any amount and at any time may cause adverse fetal effects.

The teratogenic effects of alcohol include FAS, which is characterized by three clinical features: prenatal and postnatal growth restriction, central nervous system impairment, and a recognizable combination of facial features.

Growth restriction is noted in length, weight, and head circumference. Central nervous system impairment includes mental retardation, learning disabilities, high activity level, short attention span, and poor short-term memory. Common facial anomalies associated with FAS include short palpebral fissures (the openings between the eyelids), epicanthal folds, flat midface with a low nasal bridge, indistinct philtrum (median groove on the external surface of the upper lip), and a thin upper lip (Fig. 25-3).

Alcohol-related birth defects (or *fetal alcohol effects*) and *alcohol-related neurobehavioral defects* are terms used to describe infants who exhibit mild or partial manifestations of FAS, such as low birth weight, developmental delay that may not be obvious for 1 to 2 years, and hyperactivity. Not all fetuses exposed to alcohol in utero develop FAS, but no safe level of alcohol consumption during pregnancy has been established. It is therefore recommended that women abstain from drinking alcohol throughout their pregnancies.

Cocaine

Actions of Cocaine. Cocaine is a powerful, short-acting stimulant of the central nervous system. Cocaine blocks the presynaptic reuptake of the neurotransmitters *norepinephrine* and *dopamine*, producing a hyperarousal state that results in euphoria, physical excitement, reduced fatigue, and a heightened sense of well-being and power. Anorexia, hyperglycemia, hyperthermia, and tachypnea are among the side effects of cocaine use.

When the initial euphoria wears off, a period of irritability, fatigue, lethargy, depression, and impatience occurs. This state elicits a strong desire for additional cocaine so that the initial feelings can be recaptured.

Physical effects of cocaine use are related to cardiovascular stimulation and vasoconstriction. The heart rate, systolic blood pressure, and need for oxygen increase. Complications of generalized vasoconstriction include heart attacks, strokes, and pulmonary, renal, and gastrointestinal problems.

Maternal and Fetal Effects of Cocaine. Because many women who use cocaine also use additional drugs, such as alcohol or marijuana, to "come down" from the superarousal state that cocaine produces, it is difficult to define the precise effects of cocaine use on the fetus. In addition, women who abuse cocaine are less likely to seek prenatal care or to eat a diet that contains adequate nutrition. Sex is often exchanged for drugs, so the woman is at increased risk for STDs.

Cocaine stimulates uterine contractions, and premature delivery is common. Because of the vasoconstriction of placental vessels, the incidence of spontaneous abortion and abruptio placentae increases. Additional complications include premature rupture of membranes, precipitous delivery, and stillbirth.

Clearance of the drug takes a prolonged period in the fetus. Fetal effects include tachycardia, decreased beat-to-beat variability of the fetal heart rate baseline, fetal overactivity, and intrauterine growth restriction.

Neonatal Effects of Cocaine. Clinical symptoms observed in neonates exposed to cocaine in utero include low birth weight, tremors, tachycardia, marked irritability, muscular rigidity, hypertension, and exaggerated startle reflex. Infants are difficult to console and respond poorly to voices or

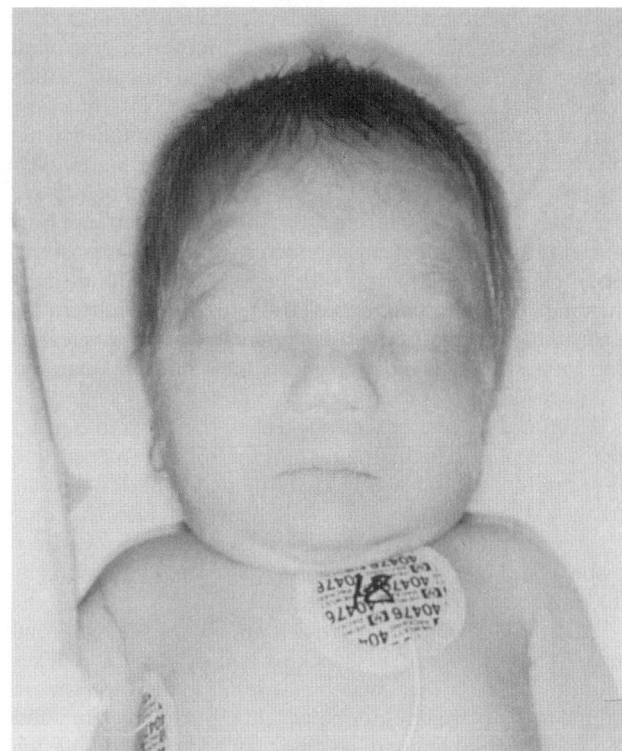

Figure 25-3 Infant with fetal alcohol syndrome. Subtle indicators are flat midface, indistinct philtrum, and low-set ears. (Courtesy Trish Beachy, M.S., R.N., Perinatal Program Coordinator. University of Colorado Health Sciences, Denver.)

environmental stimuli. They are often poor feeders and have frequent episodes of diarrhea.

Infants may continue to be irritable and have limited interaction with people and objects in their environment. There may be lifelong disabilities, such as learning problems, slower intellectual development, and delayed language and motor development.

Marijuana

The active constituent of marijuana is delta-9-tetrahydrocannabinol (THC), which crosses the placenta and accumulates in the fetus. Because marijuana is often paired with other drugs such as cocaine and alcohol, its precise effects are difficult to determine.

Repeated use of marijuana appears to increase the incidence of maternal anemia and inadequate maternal weight gain. The neonate may exhibit low birth weight, hyperirritability, tremors, and unusual sensitivity to light. Long-term effects of marijuana on the development of the child are unknown.

Heroin

Heroin, an illegal opiate derived from morphine, produces severe physical addiction. Like all opiates, heroin is a central nervous system depressant. It produces a feeling of mental dullness, drowsiness, and finally stupor. Addiction is present when discontinuing the drug causes withdrawal symptoms (abstinence syndrome) that are quickly relieved by a dose of heroin.

Women who abuse heroin have poor general health with multiple medical problems associated with their drug abuse and addicted lifestyle. Heroin is an appetite suppressant that also interferes with the absorption of nutrients, and many women start pregnancy malnourished and anemic. Additional problems include a high incidence of STDs. Infections such as hepatitis and exposure to human immunodeficiency virus (HIV) occur frequently as a result of sharing unclean needles.

Fetal Effects of Heroin. Because the street supply of heroin is usually not steady, the fetus suffers episodes of maternal overdose alternating with periods of withdrawal from the drug. These episodes expose the fetus to intermittent hypoxia, which increases the risk of prematurity, growth restriction, and stillbirth. Indirect effects are caused by maternal malnutrition and fetal exposure to STDs.

Neonatal Effects of Heroin. Infants born to mothers addicted to opiates, including heroin, methadone, meperidine, or morphine, exhibit neonatal abstinence (withdrawal) syndrome. This syndrome affects all body systems. The most consistent symptoms are neurologic: tremors, jitteriness, restlessness, and on occasion, seizures. Other manifestations include hypertonicity and irritability.

Additional symptoms of newborn abstinence syndrome include poorly coordinated sucking and swallowing reflexes, vomiting, and diarrhea, which may result in dehydration and failure to gain weight normally. Long-term developmental and learning problems are common. In addition, the lifestyle of parents who are substance abusers is strongly associated with child neglect and abuse. (See Chapter 30 for a discussion of management of the infant.)

Diagnosis and Management of Substance Abuse

In addition to toxicology screening, the pregnant woman who uses illicit drugs must be assessed throughout pregnancy for STDs, hepatitis, and exposure to HIV. Fetal diagnostic tests such as nonstress tests are used to identify problems with the fetus. Nurses monitor weight and provide guidance in nutrition to prevent maternal anemia and inadequate weight gain.

Therapeutic management depends on the type of drug used. In the case of opiates, such as heroin, withdrawal during pregnancy has been associated with significant fetal stress, fetal seizures, and even fetal death resulting from the effects of abstinence syndrome. One approach to treatment of the pregnant woman who uses heroin is to place her on an alternative drug such as methadone. Methadone can be taken orally once daily and is long-acting, providing consistent blood levels to decrease the adverse fetal effects of wide swings in blood level found with heroin use. The newborn, however, must withdraw from methadone after birth. In addition, women using methadone may use other illicit drugs such as cocaine or marijuana.

Treatment is aimed at establishing abstinence and preventing relapse. Outpatient or residential treatment may be used to provide education, individual and group therapy sessions, and peer support groups (Narcotics Anonymous, Alcoholics Anonymous, or Cocaine Anonymous). Written contracts that focus on abstinence for one day at a time are often used to help the client who has relapsed and experiences feelings of guilt and self-blame.

■ NURSING CARE
Maternal Substance Abuse

ANTEPARTUM PERIOD
Assessment

Polydrug abuse appears to be the most common substance abuse problem among women, and all women must be screened at the first prenatal visit for nicotine, alcohol, and other drugs. *Because substance abuse occurs in all populations, the nurse must not make assumptions based on class, race, or economic status.*

Certain behaviors are strongly associated with substance abuse: seeking prenatal care late in the pregnancy, failing to keep appointments, and following recommended regimens inconsistently. Poor grooming, inadequate weight gain, or a poor pattern of weight gain may be signs of a lifestyle that includes substance abuse.

Defensive or hostile behaviors may be overt signs of substance abuse. Women who use drugs have low self-esteem. They must deal with conflicting issues: the physical or psychologic need for the substance and the guilt that they may be responsible for harming the fetus. Fear of prosecution for use of illegal drugs may keep the woman from seeking prenatal care, increasing the risk of complications for the woman and the fetus.

Many women with substance abuse problems face discrimination and resentment from health care professionals who direct their frustration at the woman rather than at the problem. The nurse taking the health history must exhibit patience, empathy, and tolerance and must use a blend of approaches that reinforce concern for the woman and her infant.

Medical and Obstetric History
Determine whether the woman has medical conditions such as hepatitis, STDs, depression, cellulitis, or hypertension that are more common among women who use drugs. Evaluate for past and current complications of pregnancy. Spontaneous abortions, premature deliveries, abruptio placentae, and stillbirths are associated with substance abuse. Current complications may include an STD, vaginal bleeding, an inactive or hyperactive fetus, or intrauterine growth restriction.

Investigate emotional responses, such as anger or apathy, regarding the pregnancy. These feelings are particularly significant during the latter half of the pregnancy, when normal feelings of ambivalence are usually resolved. Negative feelings toward the pregnancy may interfere with prenatal compliance with recommended care.

History of Substance Abuse
Obtaining an accurate history of substance abuse is difficult and depends in large part on the way the health care worker approaches the woman. A sincere, nonjudgmental, empathic approach promotes an open exchange of information.

> **! CRITICAL TO REMEMBER**
>
> **Behaviors Associated With Substance Abuse**
>
> • Seeking prenatal care late in pregnancy
> • Failure to keep prenatal appointments
> • Inconsistent follow-through with recommended care
> • Poor grooming, inadequate weight gain
> • Needle punctures, thrombosed veins, cellulitis
> • Defensive or hostile reactions
> • Anger or apathy regarding pregnancy

Investigate all forms of drug use, including cigarettes, over-the-counter drugs, prescribed medications, alcohol, and illicit drugs such as amphetamines, cocaine, marijuana, and heroin. Examine patterns of drug use, which can range from occasional recreational use to weekly binges to daily dependence on a particular drug or group of drugs.

Nursing Diagnosis and Planning

Some women do not realize the adverse effects of the drugs they are using, and others are aware of the risks but are unable to stop using the substances. A nursing diagnosis that addresses both these factors is

- Ineffective Health Maintenance related to lack of knowledge of the effects of substance abuse on self and fetus and inability to manage stress without the use of drugs.

  Expected Outcomes: The woman will identify harmful effects of substances on herself and her infant, will verbalize feelings related to continued use of harmful substances, and will identify personal strengths and accept support offered by the health care delivery system to stop using drugs.

Interventions

Effective interventions for substance abuse require that nurses realize that progress is slow and frustrating. The major priority is to protect the fetus and the expectant mother from the harmful effects of drugs.

Examining Attitudes

When working with substance-abusing pregnant women, nurses must identify and acknowledge their own knowledge level, feelings, and prejudices. They may have limited knowledge about perinatal substance abuse and may have negative attitudes toward mothers who abuse substances. Maintaining feelings of empathy or concern without becoming judgmental or even unknowingly punitive to the pregnant woman may be difficult. Nurses may feel angry, helpless, and discouraged when the pregnant woman continues to abuse drugs despite the best efforts of the health care team. In-service education, professional consultation, and peer support are all helpful when working with pregnant women who abuse drugs.

Communicating With the Woman

Ask the woman about stressors in her life that may be contributing to the pattern of substance abuse. Additional stressors may include inadequate housing, economic predicaments, intimate partner violence, and emotional or physical illness.

Be honest at all times while displaying a patient, nonjudgmental attitude as well as genuine interest and concern. This approach is especially important when the woman relapses into substance-abusing patterns. Allow her to express guilt, and reassure her that abstinence is possible and that she must simply begin again.

Helping the Woman Identify Strengths

Because she generally has a poor self-image, assist the substance-abusing pregnant woman in identifying personal strengths. Acknowledge her actions when she abstains from drugs or alcohol for even a short time. Praise for maintaining an adequate weight gain and attending prenatal classes may increase self-esteem and compliance with the recommended regimen of care.

Providing Ongoing Care

At each antepartum visit, consider the current status of substance use, social service needs, education needs, and compliance with treatment referrals. In particular, address current drug use, because women may change their pattern of drug use during pregnancy. For instance, they may stop using cocaine but increase their use of marijuana or alcohol.

Verify compliance with recommended treatment regimens, such as antepartum clinics and chemical-dependence referral programs. Coordinate care among various service providers such as group therapy and prenatal classes.

Provide continuing prenatal education classes that include the anatomy and physiology of pregnancy and consequences of prenatal substance abuse. Describe how the newborn benefits when the mother abstains from drugs, including tobacco and alcohol. Praise any attempts at abstinence, and encourage the expectant mother to try again if she relapses.

Assess maternal attachment to the fetus as it may help her reduce or eliminate her substance use. Fetal movement often increases the woman's awareness of the fetus and may lead to a discussion about her plans for the infant and changes in her life that have and will occur.

Evaluation

- Can the expectant mother identify the effects of substance abuse on herself and her infant?
- Does she discuss her feelings about continued substance abuse?
- Does she identify her own strengths and work with the health care team to stop using drugs?

INTRAPARTUM PERIOD
Assessment

Nurses who work in labor and delivery units must become skilled at identifying drug-induced signs and symptoms.

Cocaine

Behaviors associated with frequent or recent use of crack cocaine include profuse sweating, hypertension, and irregular respirations, combined with a lethargic response to labor and lack of interest in the necessary interventions. Additional signs include dilated pupils, increased body temperature, and sudden onset of severely painful contractions. Fetal signs often include tachycardia and excessive activity.

Emotional signs of recent cocaine use may include angry, caustic, or abusive reactions to those attempting to provide care. Emotional lability and paranoia are signs of cocaine intoxication.

! CRITICAL TO REMEMBER

Signs and Symptoms of Recent Cocaine Use

- Diaphoresis, high blood pressure, irregular respirations
- Dilated pupils, increased body temperature
- Sudden onset of severely painful contractions
- Fetal tachycardia, excessive fetal activity
- Angry, caustic, abusive reactions and paranoia

Heroin

Typically, the pregnant woman addicted to heroin comes to the labor and delivery unit intoxicated from a recent drug administration. When the effects of the drug begin to wear off, withdrawal symptoms may be observed. These include yawning, diaphoresis, rhinorrhea, restlessness, and excessive tearing of the eyes.

Nursing Diagnosis and Planning

One of the most relevant nursing diagnoses during the intrapartal period is

- Risk for Injury related to physiologic and psychologic effects of recent drug use.

  Expected Outcome: The woman and the fetus will remain free from injury during labor and childbirth.

Interventions

Preventing Injury

When a laboring woman has recently used a substance such as cocaine, her life and the life of the fetus depend heavily on the nurse, who must intervene to meet the needs for safety, oxygen, and comfort.

Admitting Procedure Two nurses may be needed to admit the woman into the labor unit. One nurse helps the woman assume a safe position, initiates electronic fetal monitoring, and begins administration of oxygen, as needed. The other nurse acts as communicator.

Because the woman who has recently used a drug often has difficulty following directions, only one nurse should tell her what to do. This nurse states firmly what is happening and exactly what the woman must do: "This helps us watch how the baby is doing." "This gives you more oxygen." "Lie on your left side." Maintain eye contact with the woman while giving her instructions.

Setting Limits It is essential to set limits to protect the safety of the mother and the fetus. For instance, the mother cannot smoke when oxygen is in use. If she must remain in bed, she may become agitated. The nurse may say, "I know it's hard to stay in bed, but we can't take good care of the baby when you walk." If it is safe for the woman to walk, the nurse must set limits about where she can walk.

Initiating Seizure Precautions The laboring woman who recently used cocaine is at risk for hypertensive crisis. Take seizure precautions to protect her from injury in case of seizures. Keep the bed in a low, locked position. Pad the side rails and keep them up at all times. To prevent aspiration, make sure suction equipment functions properly. Reduce environmental stimuli (lights, noise) as much as possible.

Maintaining Effective Communication

Establishing a therapeutic pattern of communication is essential. Avoid confrontation; instead, acknowledge feelings: "I know you hurt and you are frightened. I'll do everything I can to make you comfortable." When the woman is abusive, be careful not to take the abuse personally or react in a nontherapeutic manner.

Examine your own feelings when women are abusive, and acknowledge when anger is getting in the way of providing care. To allow some relief from unrelenting abusive comments, another nurse may need to assume care of the woman for a time.

Providing Pain Control

Pain control for women who are substance abusers poses a difficult problem because it is often impossible to determine the type or combination of drugs that were used before admission. If pain medication can be administered safely, do not withhold it under the false assumption that the woman does not need it or medication will contribute to her addiction. Comfort measures should include nonpharmacologic nursing interventions, such as sacral pressure, back rubs, a cool cloth on the head, and continual support and encouragement.

Preventing Heroin Withdrawal

To prevent or stabilize heroin withdrawal during labor, administer methadone intramuscularly as ordered if the woman is nauseated or vomiting. Give oral methadone to the woman who usually takes methadone at chemical-dependence centers if she did not receive her daily dose. Avoid narcotic agonists-antagonists, such as butorphanol (Stadol), because they may cause acute withdrawal symptoms in the woman and the fetus.

Evaluation

- Are the woman and her fetus free of injury during labor and childbirth?

POSTPARTUM PERIOD

During the postpartum period, nursing care is focused on helping the mother with bonding, infant care, and planning to provide for the care of herself and the infant after discharge (see Chapter 30). Encourage the woman to continue her efforts to stop taking substances. Women who stop or reduce use during pregnancy may return to using at previous levels after pregnancy and need support to continue abstinence.

BIRTH OF AN INFANT WITH CONGENITAL ANOMALIES

Even when everything goes according to plan, childbirth is a time of stress for parents. When the infant is born with anomalies, the parents are often overwhelmed with shock and grief. Because nurses are with the parents more than other members of the perinatal team are, they have an opportunity to help the family adjust and cope with their feelings.

Factors Influencing Emotional Responses of Parents

Timing and Manner of Being Told

It was common practice at one time to remove the infant from the delivery area before parents could see a congenital anomaly. This practice changed, however, when it was realized that parents experienced less stress if they were told at once and were permitted to hold the newborn if the physical status of the infant allowed (Fig. 25-4). Physicians and nurses also became aware of the importance of helping the parents accept and bond with the newborn.

Prior Knowledge of the Defect

Although ultrasound does not identify all fetal anomalies, many parents become aware of fetal anomalies during ultrasound examinations performed during pregnancy. These parents may not experience the shock and disbelief at the birth seen in unprepared parents. Their reactions, however, should

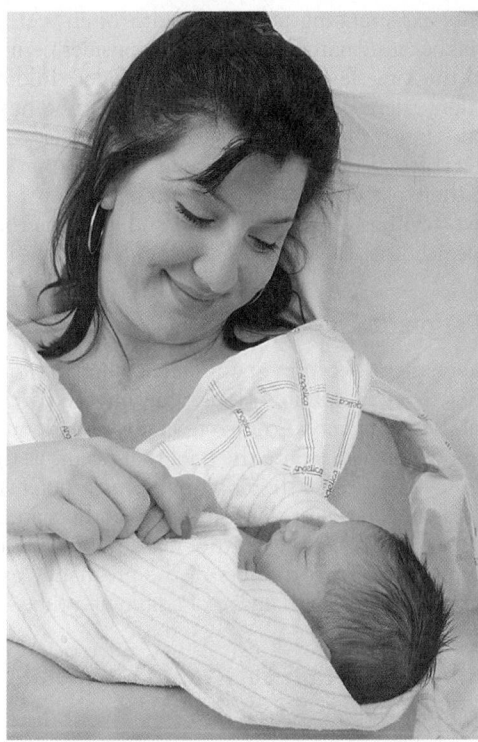

Figure 25-4 Touching and cuddling between parents and the infant with a congenital anomaly foster attachment and help resolve the grieving process.

not be interpreted to mean that they do not experience grief. Instead, they have completed some of the early stages of grieving before the birth. Their grief is real, even though it is expressed differently.

Type of Defect
Although any defect in a newborn produces extreme concern and anxiety, certain defects are associated with long-term parenting problems. It is particularly difficult for the family and the community to accept an infant with facial or genital anomalies. The face is visible to everyone, and parents are fearful about whether the child will be accepted. If the defect is cleft lip and palate, the parents are extremely concerned about surgical repair. Parents are often anxious about how grandparents and siblings will accept the child.

Gender is at the core of a person's identity, and any defect of the genitals arouses deep concern in both parents. Some anomalies, such as hypospadias (opening of the urethra on the underside of the penis), are repaired in early childhood. Other genital anomalies, such as ambiguous genitalia, when assignment of gender is in doubt, cause extreme concern in the family and affect such basic issues as what to name the infant, how to dress the infant, and how to respond to questions about the infant's sex.

Irreparable Defect
Although the initial impact of any defect is profound disappointment and concern, when the defect is irreparable, the parents must grapple with the knowledge that the infant will have a lifelong disability. Examples of irreparable defects include Down syndrome, microcephaly, and amelia (absence of an entire extremity).

Grief and Mourning

Grief describes the emotional response to loss. *Mourning* is the process of going through the phases of grief until the loss can be accepted and resolved. Birth of an infant with an anomaly evokes a grief response, and the family must mourn the loss of the perfect infant they fantasized about during pregnancy. Early emotions include denial, anger, and guilt.

Denial and disbelief are the initial reactions of most parents to the birth of an infant with a congenital defect. Anger is often a pervasive response, and it may take the form of fault-finding or resentment. Anger may be directed toward the family, the medical personnel, or the self, but it is seldom directed toward the infant. Guilt may be expressed as a question of responsibility for the defect: "I shouldn't have worked so much while I was pregnant."

Other emotions include fear, which may be expressed as concern about what must be done in the immediate or distant future (surgical procedures, complicated health care, the infant's potential for a normal life). Sadness and depression, manifested by crying, withdrawal from relationships, lack of energy, inability to sleep, and decreased appetite, may precede acceptance and resolution. Gradually, often after a prolonged period, feelings of sadness abate and the family can accept and resolve grief.

Nursing Considerations

Assisting With the Grieving Process
Parents must grieve for the loss of the perfect infant that they expected before they can form an attachment with this newborn. It is helpful if nurses remain with the parents through the initial phase of shock and disbelief and maintain an atmosphere that encourages them to express their feelings.

Nurses must recognize that grief responses vary with individuals. Moreover, cultural and religious beliefs affect the expression of grief. Some groups express grief openly by crying, becoming angry, or seeking comfort from a support group. Other cultures (e.g., Chinese, Japanese, Native Americans) do not. They may appear stoic and may not reveal the depths of their grief. In some cultures (such as Latino), it is acceptable for women, but not for men, to grieve publicly.

Promoting Bonding and Attachment
A priority nursing intervention is to promote bonding and attachment, which may be disrupted when parents who expected a perfect infant give birth to an infant with an abnormality. The process often begins when the nurse communicates acceptance of the infant.

To do this, the nurse handles the newborn gently and presents the infant as something precious. Parents are particularly sensitive to facial expressions of shock or distress. Many nurses emphasize the normal aspects of the infant's body: "She's so alert, and she has beautiful eyes." Perhaps it is most important to help the parents hold their infant as soon as possible. Touching and cuddling are essential to caring.

Providing Accurate Information

Nurses who work in perinatal settings are responsible for becoming informed about follow-up treatment and timing of surgical procedures so that they can clarify and reinforce information provided by the physician. This process involves discussing the plan of care with the physician as well as researching the nursing care that will be required. Parents develop trust in the health care team when consistent information is presented clearly and explained fully.

One primary nurse or team should work with the family throughout the hospital stay. Nurses should expect to repeat information frequently because it may be difficult for the grieving parents to retain it.

Facilitating Communication

Nurses are sometimes fearful of being asked questions that they cannot answer, or they fear that they will say the wrong thing.

The most helpful course of action is to answer questions as honestly as possible. If unsure of information, say so: "I'm not sure about that, but I'll find out about it for you." In addition to answers, parents need kindness, support, and genuine concern.

It is crucial that family members communicate with one another as well as with the health professionals. Fathers should be included in all discussions, demonstrations, and care of the infant. Information and empathy should be offered consistently to both parents. Without this attention, the father cannot be expected to support his partner, explain the infant's condition to relatives and friends, or begin to deal with his own shock and sadness.

Planning for Discharge

Teach parents the special feeding, holding, and positioning techniques that their infant needs. Early participation in infant care fosters feelings of attachment and responsibility for the infant.

Providing other anticipatory guidance may help prevent problems when the infant is discharged. The reaction and behavior of siblings depend on their age and ability to understand the needs of the infant. Young children, who are often jealous of the attention and care that the infant requires, may regress to infantile behaviors, such as bed-wetting or thumb-sucking. Remind parents that this response indicates a need for attention rather than naughtiness.

Although grandparents can be a great source of strength and support, they may also have difficulty adjusting to the infant with an abnormality. When appropriate, include grandparents when teaching special care the infant will need.

Providing Referrals

Initiate referrals to national and community resources, if appropriate. Besides a referral to the social worker in the hospital, parents may also benefit from information about the National Easter Seal Society for Crippled Children, the March of Dimes Birth Defects Foundation, or the disabled children's services of the public health department. In addition, organizations such as the Shriners provide funds for the care of children.

PREGNANCY LOSS

Perinatal death can occur at any time. Early spontaneous abortion, fetal demise during the latter half of pregnancy, stillbirth, or neonatal death when the infant survives for a few days or weeks can be equally devastating for the parents.

Parents experiencing perinatal death often feel alone in their grief because many people do not consider perinatal loss to be on the same level as the loss of an older child or adult. In addition, friends and family members may be hesitant to discuss the loss for fear of saying the wrong thing.

Fathers often feel a need to appear strong so that they can support their partners. As a result, fathers often hold back their own feelings of grief and pain and are sometimes perceived as needing less support than the mother.

Early Pregnancy Loss

Early pregnancy loss from spontaneous abortion or ectopic pregnancy may precipitate intense grief by the parents. The pregnancy may not yet be known to family and friends. Those who do know may minimize the grief that occurs at this time. Comments such as "You shouldn't have any problems getting pregnant again" discount the feelings of mothers and fathers. When ectopic pregnancy is the reason for the loss, the woman must deal with the loss of the pregnancy as well as with the possible loss or damage of a fallopian tube.

Concurrent Death and Survival in Multifetal Pregnancy

Parents experience conflicting and complex feelings of joy and grief when one or more infants in a multifetal pregnancy live and one or more infants in the same gestation die. Contrary to common belief, parents do not grieve less for the dead infant because of the joy that they experience in the surviving infant.

For parents experiencing both survival and death of an infant, the grieving process may be complicated. They may have fears about the health of the surviving infant, especially if the infant is preterm or ill. They may be unable to grieve for the dead child because of their concerns for the surviving child. They may also have problems with attachment to the surviving infant because of grieving. In addition, they may receive less support than parents who have lost the only child in a single gestation.

Previous Pregnancy Loss

Women who have experienced previous pregnancy losses may have higher levels of anxiety and lower levels of attachment during subsequent pregnancies, especially until they pass the point where the loss occurred or deliver a normal baby (Van & Meleis, 2003). They are also at risk for having a preterm or low-birth-weight infant in later pregnancies (Heinonen & Kirkinen, 2000). Therefore they should be counseled about obtaining early prenatal care and will need extra emotional support if they become pregnant again.

▪NURSING CARE
Pregnancy Loss

Assessment

Nursing assessment of the family that has experienced the loss of a fetus or infant requires a great deal of sensitivity. In the case of infant death, collect as much information as possible before meeting the woman and her family for the first time so that hurtful mistakes can be avoided. Knowing the child's sex, weight, length, gestational age, and whether any abnormalities were noted will help in communicating effectively.

Many perinatal units design a symbol to place on the door, chart, and Kardex so that all staff who come in contact with the family, including auxiliary, housekeeping, laboratory, and radiology personnel, will be alerted that the infant has not survived. Designs include a fallen leaf, a teardrop, or a rainbow. This visual symbol diminishes the chance that an uninformed person will make inadvertent comments that cause the family pain.

Nurses are often unsure how to interact with a family who has experienced the loss of an infant. It is helpful to acknowledge the situation and to clarify the nurse's role at once: "I am Claire Turner, and I'll be your nurse today. I'm so sorry for your loss. Let me know if there is any way I can be of help." This is not an appropriate time for self-disclosure or for false reassurance. Keep the focus on the family's response and their ability to support one another.

Nurses who provide home care or who make follow-up telephone calls must be aware of subtle cues of grief, such as sighing, excessive sleeping, apathy, poor hygiene, or loss of appetite. These are especially important when assessing members of cultural groups who do not display grief publicly.

Evaluate also the availability of a support system that includes family members or clergy. It may be necessary to ask whether a spiritual adviser would help the family cope with grief. Include the father in assessment, because he may not receive the support he needs.

Nursing Diagnosis and Planning

A common nursing diagnosis for families who experience perinatal death is

■ Interrupted Family Processes related to grief over newborn (or fetal) death.

Expected Outcomes: The parents will express the meaning of the loss and will share their grief with significant others.

Interventions

Acknowledging the Infant

It was once believed that, when an infant was stillborn or died shortly after birth, the parents would grieve less if the newborn were quickly taken away before the parents saw the infant. Relatives often disposed of the clothes and the crib of the expected infant before the mother returned home, and the parents were left with very few memories of the infant's birth.

The response to perinatal death changed as nurses discovered that the most helpful interventions for grieving parents were those that acknowledged the rights of the baby. These include the right to (Primeau & Lamb, 1995):

Be recognized as a person who was born and died
Be named
Be seen, touched, and held by the family
Have life-ending acknowledged
Be put to rest with dignity

Presenting the Infant to the Parents The infant's presentation to the parents is extremely important because these are the memories that they will retain. If necessary, wash the infant and apply baby lotion or powder. Wrap the infant in a soft, warm blanket. If possible, bring parents and infant together while the infant is still warm and soft. It may be necessary to keep the infant in a warmed incubator if some time elapses before the parents have contact with the infant. If this is not possible, tell the parents that the skin may feel cool. Allow parents to keep the infant as long as they wish, and allow them to unwrap the infant if they wish.

When the stillborn infant has severe deformities, explain the defect briefly and gently. Wrap the infant to expose the most normal aspect. Use diapers to cover genital defects, and use booties and mittens to cover abnormalities of the hands and feet. It is not advisable, however, to try to hide the defects completely. Allow parents to progress at their own speed in inspecting the infant. Parents may look at the abnormality or choose to leave the infant wrapped.

Allow as much privacy and time as the parents and other family members need to be together. Remain sensitive to cues that members of the family want to talk or prefer not to. A sympathetic smile and a promise to return in a specific time and then returning at that time are equally important. It is all right to ask, "Do you want to talk?" Then, listening quietly and reflecting the mother's or father's feelings are all that is required.

Preparing a Memory Packet Mourning requires memories. Nurses have explored measures that help the family create memories of the infant so that the existence of the child is confirmed and the parents can complete the grieving process.

Prepare a memory packet that includes a photograph; footprints or handprints; the crib card with the infant's name, weight, and length; identification bracelet; blanket used for the baby; and, if possible, a lock of hair. Give the parents pictures of the infant to help them remember the baby's features and assist them through the grieving process. Some parents and grandparents want pictures taken of themselves with the infant. The memory packet should be kept on file if the parents do not wish to take it home, because they may change their minds later.

Assisting With Other Needs

Help the parents plan how to tell other children about the death of the newborn. Provide the parents with written information about children's responses to death for later use. Offer to call clergy, if the parents wish, and discuss the funeral or memorial service. Discuss the normal grieving process with parents. Explain the steps of grieving and that a considerable amount of time may be involved. Describe common reactions that family members and friends may have and that grandparents will also go through grief because of the loss as well as the pain their children must endure.

Providing Referrals

Parents may find that friends and relatives expect them to recover quickly from perinatal loss and cannot understand their continued grief. The greatest help often comes from contact with persons who have experienced a similar loss, and a variety of support groups have been formed. Refer parents to Resolve Through Sharing; Aiding a Mother Experiencing Neonatal Death (AMEND); Source of Help in Airing and Resolving Experiences (SHARE); or Helping After Neonatal Death (HAND). Many hospitals have bereavement programs to offer ongoing help to parents.

Evaluation

- Have the parents acknowledged their grief and the meaning of the loss?
- Have they shared their grief with significant others?

RELINQUISHMENT FOR ADOPTION

Some women carry the pregnancy to term and then relinquish the newborn to the care of another family for adoption. The decision to place the infant for adoption is a painful one that can produce long-lasting feelings of ambivalence and chronic sorrow. On the one hand, the expectant mother may be satisfied that the infant is going into a stable home where a child is wanted and will receive excellent care. On the other hand, the social pressures against giving up one's child are often intense.

The relationship between the birth mother and the adoptive parents varies greatly. The adoptive parents may be unknown to the birth mother, or she may have chosen them. Some adoptive mothers participate in the birth. The birth mother may never see the infant again or may keep in contact with and participate in the child's life.

Nurses are sometimes unsure of how to communicate with the woman who is relinquishing her infant. First, the nursing staff who come into contact with the woman must be informed of her decision to place the infant for adoption. Information prevents inadvertent comments that could cause distress. Second, nurses must remember that adoption is *an act of love, not one of abandonment*, as the woman relinquishes the newborn to a family who is better able to provide financial and emotional support.

Nurses must also be prepared to respect any special wishes that the mother may have about the birth. For instance, most birth mothers want to know all about the infant. They may want to see and hold the newborn and give it a name. Many take photographs or save the crib card. Such actions provide memories of the infant and help the mother through the grieving process that may accompany relinquishment of the child.

The nurse should try to establish rapport and a trusting relationship with the mother. It is helpful to acknowledge the situation at the initial contact with the woman: "Hello, my name is Claire, and I'll be your nurse today. I understand the adoptive family is coming this morning. What can I do to help you get ready?" This communication is more helpful than providing care without reference to an event that is of utmost concern to the mother. It also provides an opening for her to express feelings that may include attachment to the infant, ambivalence about her decision, and profound sadness.

Nurses also teach adoptive families how to care for the newborn and what to expect in growth and development. Teaching requires adequate time and a private place. This family benefits from all the teaching provided to other new parents. They may be anxious, and demonstrations as well as return demonstrations are appropriate.

INTIMATE PARTNER VIOLENCE

Approximately 1.9 million American women are physically assaulted by an intimate partner each year (Tjaden & Thoennes, 2000). Intimate partner violence (IPV) may start or increase in frequency and severity during pregnancy and the postpartum period (Toohey, 2000). The incidence during pregnancy varies between 1% and 20% (AAP & ACOG, 2002) and as many as 324,000 pregnant women are affected

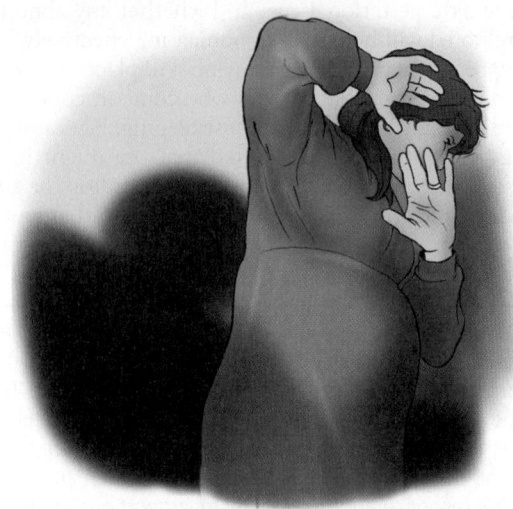

Figure 25-5   The woman who is abused by her partner lives with an ever-present risk of violence. Because they may not seek help, all women should be asked about abuse whenever they receive health care.

yearly (Gazmararian et al., 2000). IPV is recurrent, with 60% of abused women reporting two or more episodes of violence.

Physical abuse may involve threats, slapping, or pushing. It may also escalate to punching, kicking, and beating that result in internal injury or to wounds from weapons (Fig. 25-5). It may end in death. Sexual abuse, including rape, is often part of physical abuse, with almost half the abused women reporting being forced into sex by their male partner. Substance abuse by both the woman and her partner is often associated with IPV (El-Bassel et al., 2003).

Physical violence occurs within the context of continuous mental abuse, threats, and coercion. Women often feel shame, loss of self-respect, and powerlessness. They are more likely to experience depression and lower self-esteem and have a greater need for health and community services than other woman (Peterson, Gazmararian, & Clark, 2001).

Abuse of the mother may be an indication of what life holds for the unborn child. In over 50 percent of homes where there is domestic violence, the children are also injured (Toohey, 2000). Most men who batter women also batter their children, and some women who are victims abuse their children. Children who witness abuse of their mother often react with sleep problems, regression, aggression, or other behavioral disturbances (Lemmey, McFarlane, Wilson, & Malecha, 2001).

Factors That Promote Violence

Family violence occurs in cultures in which male and female roles are based on gender and little value is placed on the woman's role. Men hold power, and women are viewed as less worthy of respect than men.

Women earn less than men in the job market, and they are often victimized by marriage. For example, women who hold full-time jobs still carry the major responsibilities for housekeeping and child care. They may remain in unhealthy relationships because they are financially dependent on men. If they divorce, women often become single parents

TABLE 25-2 Myths and Realities of Violence Against Women

Myths	Realities
The battered woman syndrome affects only a small percentage of the population.	Battering is the single major cause of injury to women; approximately 1.9 million women suffer each year from intimate partner violence.
Violence against women occurs only in lower socioeconomic classes and in minority groups.	Violence occurs in families from all social, economic, educational, racial, and religious backgrounds.
The problem is really "partner abuse," couples who assault each other.	Approximately 95% of serious assaults are male against female; violence against women is about control and power.
Alcohol and drugs cause abusive behavior.	Substance abuse and violence against women are two separate problems. Substance abuse is a disease; violence is a learned behavior that can be unlearned.
The abuser is "out of control."	He is not out of control; he is making a decision, because he chooses who, when, and where he abuses.
The woman "got what she deserved."	No one deserves to be beaten. No one has the right to beat another person. Violent behavior is the responsibility of the violent person.
Women "like" it or they would leave.	Women are threatened with severe punishment or death if they attempt to leave; many have no resources and are isolated, and they and their children depend on the abuser.
Couples counseling is a good recommendation for abusive relationships.	Couples counseling is ineffective for the couple. It can also be dangerous for the abused woman.

with a standard of living much lower than that of their former husbands.

Stereotyping males as powerful and females as weak and without value has a profound effect on the self-esteem of women. Many women internalize the messages and come to believe that they are less worthy than their partners and that they are the cause of their own punishment. They accept the message from society that when women are battered or raped, "they got what they deserved."

Although alcohol is often stated as a cause of violence against women, chemical dependence and intimate partner violence are two separate problems. However, violence may become more severe or bizarre when alcohol or drugs are involved. See Table 25-2 for a summary of the myths and realities of violence against women.

Characteristics of the Abuser

Physical abuse concerns power, and it is only one of many tactics that abusive men use to control their partners. Other tactics include isolation, intimidation, and threats. Extreme jealousy and possessiveness are typical of the abuser. An abusive man often attempts to control all aspects of the woman's life, such as where she goes and what she wears. He controls access to money and transportation and may force the woman to account for every moment spent away from him.

The abusive man often has a low tolerance for frustration and poor impulse control. He does not perceive his violent behavior as a problem and often blames the woman. Most abusive men come from homes where they witnessed the abuse of their mothers or were themselves abused as children.

Cycle of Violence

Although IPV may be random, there is often a pattern. The violence occurs in a cycle that consists of three phases: a tension-building phase, a battering incident, and a "honeymoon phase." Being aware of the behaviors that accompany each phase will enable the nurse to counsel the woman. Figure 25-6 depicts these behaviors.

Effects of Intimate Partner Abuse During Pregnancy

Abuse during pregnancy is correlated with health problems for the mother and infant. These women are likely to have multiple injury sites, particularly of the abdomen as well as the face and breasts. They are twice as likely as nonabused women to start prenatal care in the third trimester (McFarlane, Parker, & Cross, 2001) and to have health problems such as STDs (Winn, Records, & Rice, 2003). Low weight gain, anemia, and use of alcohol and illicit drugs are more likely in women experiencing IPV. Infants born to women with IPV have an increased risk of prematurity, low birth weight, and neonatal death (Lipsky, Holt, Easterling, & Critchlow, 2003).

Nurses' Role in Prevention of Abuse

Nurses can do a great deal to prevent physical abuse. First, they must examine their beliefs to determine whether they accept the prevailing attitude that blames the victim: "Why does she stay with him?"

Second, nurses can consciously practice in ways that empower women. They should make it clear that the woman owns her body and has the right to decide how it should be treated. Nurses must use language that indicates that the woman is an active partner in her care: "You understand your body; what do you think?"

During examinations, nurses can introduce aspects of care that increase the woman's control over the situation. For example, make sure that the woman meets the physician or nurse practitioner who is to examine her while she is seated and clothed rather than while she is unclothed and in a lithotomy position.

School nurses are in an excellent position to influence how teenagers define gender roles: "Real men don't beat up women." "Girls don't have to put up with verbal or physical abuse from anyone."

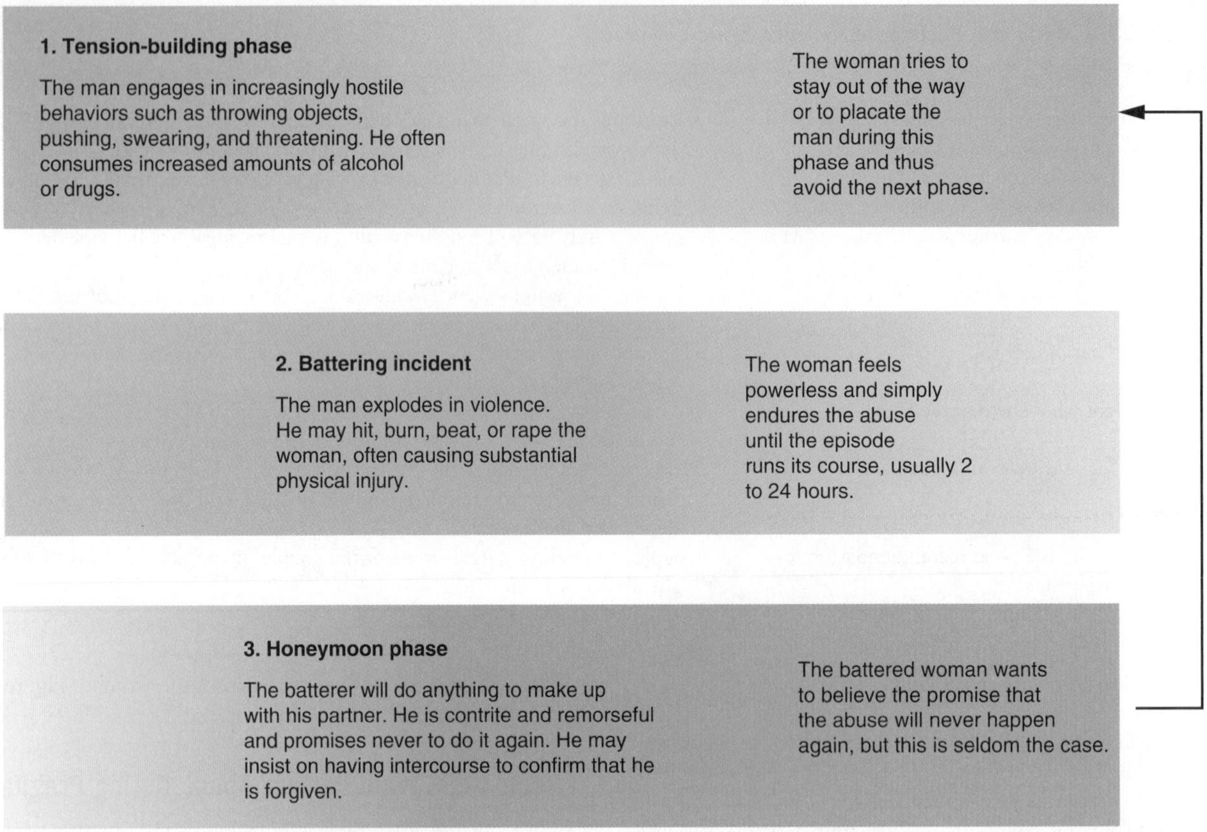

1. Tension-building phase

The man engages in increasingly hostile behaviors such as throwing objects, pushing, swearing, and threatening. He often consumes increased amounts of alcohol or drugs.

The woman tries to stay out of the way or to placate the man during this phase and thus avoid the next phase.

2. Battering incident

The man explodes in violence. He may hit, burn, beat, or rape the woman, often causing substantial physical injury.

The woman feels powerless and simply endures the abuse until the episode runs its course, usually 2 to 24 hours.

3. Honeymoon phase

The batterer will do anything to make up with his partner. He is contrite and remorseful and promises never to do it again. He may insist on having intercourse to confirm that he is forgiven.

The battered woman wants to believe the promise that the abuse will never happen again, but this is seldom the case.

Figure 25-6 Types of behaviors evident in each step of the cycle of violence.

CRITICAL THINKING EXERCISE 25-1

Joan Piszarek, a 28-year-old primigravida, is admitted to the labor, delivery, and recovery unit in active labor. The right side of her face is swollen, evidence of old bruises that look like fingerprints are present on her upper arms, and a large bruised area is evident on her abdomen. She is accompanied by her husband, who is very solicitous. He verbalizes concern about her labor status and remains close beside her at all times. Joan appears lethargic and avoids eye contact with the nurse who is admitting her. She states that she fainted at home and hurt herself when she fell against the bathtub. The nurse accepts the explanation and asks no further questions.
1. What assumptions has the nurse made?
2. What should make the nurse examine her conclusion that the injuries resulted from falling?
When the relief nurse arrives, she waits for time alone with Joan and asks, "Did you get these injuries from being hit?" Joan appears extremely anxious and says, "Don't say anything! He got so mad when I was late getting home from shopping. It was my fault."
3. Why did the nurse wait for time alone before asking questions?
4. How should the nurse respond? What bias must she guard against?
5. How can Joan be protected?

■NURSING CARE

The Battered Woman

Assessment

Because of the prevalence of IPV during pregnancy, it is recommended that all women be screened for physical abuse at each contact. When they are first approached, women may deny that abuse has occurred. Asking, and especially asking more than once, may lead the woman to seek help at a later time. Leaving written information in women's restrooms also implies that discussion of violence with the nurse is encouraged and safe.

Nurses are often unsure how to approach the issue of suspected abuse. Women often seek care and are assessed in the "honeymoon phase" of the violence cycle. It is during this phase that the man is often overly solicitous ("hovering husband syndrome") and eager to explain any injuries that the woman exhibits. *Introducing the subject of violence in the presence of the man who may be responsible for it places the woman in danger. It is essential to separate the woman from the man for the interview.*

When a private, secure place has been found, reassure the woman that her privacy will be protected and that confidentiality will be absolute. Ask questions directly, and let her know that the questions about abuse are standard for all clients. Commonly used questions to screen for violence are whether the woman has been hit, slapped, kicked, or otherwise physically hurt or forced to have sexual relations by anyone during the past year and during the pregnancy and if she is afraid of anyone. A "yes" answer to these questions requires further assessment into the situation.

If there is trauma, appropriate questions are "Did someone hurt you?" "Did you receive these injuries from being hit?" The abused woman often appears hesitant, embarrassed, or evasive. She may be unable to look the nurse in the eye and appears guilty, ashamed, jumpy, or frightened.

Evaluate and document all signs of injury, both past and present. This includes areas of welts, bruising, swelling, lacerations, burns, and scars. Injuries are most commonly noted on the face, breasts, abdomen, and genitalia. Many women have new or old fractures of the face, nose, ribs, or arms. A photograph or a drawing may be used to show areas of injury. If there has been sexual abuse, a gynecologic examination is necessary because there is often trauma to the labia, vagina, cervix, or anus. Record direct quotes of what the woman says about her experience.

Be particularly alert for nonverbal cues that indicate that abuse has occurred. Facial grimacing or a slow, unsteady gait may indicate pain. Vomiting or abdominal tenderness may indicate internal injury. A flat affect (absence of facial response) is indicative of women who mentally withdraw from the situation to protect themselves from the horror and humiliation they experience. Keep in mind that the woman may fear for her life because abusive episodes tend to escalate.

Nursing Diagnosis and Planning

Nursing diagnosis depends on the data collected during the assessment. The most meaningful diagnosis for perinatal nurses to make may be

- Fear related to possibility of severe injury to self and/or children during an unpredictable cycle of violence.

  Expected Outcomes: The woman will acknowledge the physical assaults, will develop a specific plan for when the abusive cycle begins, and will identify community resources that provide protection for herself and her children.

The abused woman is often unwilling to leave the abusive situation, and nurses frequently must work with the woman to plan realistic short-term goals that will protect her from injury.

Interventions

Developing a Personal Safety Plan

Help the woman make concrete plans to protect the safety of herself and her children. For example, describe the cycle of behavior that culminates in physical abuse and instruct her in factors such as use of alcohol or other drugs that precipi-

---

> **! CRITICAL TO REMEMBER**
>
> **Cues Indicating Violence Against Women**
>
> - *Nonverbal:* Facial grimacing, slow and unsteady gait, vomiting, abdominal tenderness, absence of facial response
> - *Injuries:* Welts, bruises, swelling, lacerations, burns, vaginal or rectal bleeding; evidence of old or new fractures of the nose, face, ribs, or arms
> - *Vague somatic complaints:* Anxiety, depression, panic attacks, sleeplessness, anorexia
> - *Discrepancy between history and type of injuries:* Wounds that do not match the woman's story, multiple bruises in various stages of healing, bruising on the arms (which she may have raised to protect herself), old, untreated wounds

---

tate a violent episode. Discuss behaviors that indicate that the level of frustration and anger is increasing to the point where the danger is escalating. Assist her to:

- Locate the nearest shelter or safe house and make specific plans to go there once the cycle of violence begins.
- Identify the safest, quickest routes out of the home.
- Hide extra keys to the car and house, money, personal information (social security numbers, birth certificate, drivers license, bank account numbers), and some clothes and personal necessities.
- Devise a code word, and prearrange with someone to call the police when the word is used.
- Memorize the telephone number of the shelter or hotline, because time is often a crucial element in the decision to leave. An easy number to remember is for the National Domestic Violence Hotline (1-800-799-SAFE), which provides immediate crisis assistance in the caller's community.
- Review the safety plan frequently, because leaving the partner is one of the most dangerous times.

Affirming She Is Not to Blame

The abused woman often believes that she is responsible for the abuse. Let her know that no one deserves to be hit for any reason. The one who hit her is the person responsible. She did not provoke it or cause it and could not have prevented it. Nurses are often responsible for teaching her that violence is not normal and it is usually repeated and usually escalates. She needs help to understand that battered women have alternatives.

She also needs nonjudgmental acceptance and recognition of the difficulties involved in making changes in her situation. Praise her for any actions she takes, even if they are only minor steps toward making her life safer. Reassure her that she is doing the right thing for herself and her children when she seeks help and makes plans for escape.

Providing Referrals

Refer the family to community agencies such as the police department, legal services, community shelters, and social service agencies as needed. Include mental health referrals, if necessary, for depression or counseling. Document that referrals were made and whether the woman accepts them.

It is essential to accept the decisions of the battered woman and acknowledge that she is on her own timetable. She may not take any actions at the time that they are recommended. Therefore listening to her and providing information about resources may be the only help the nurse can provide until the battered woman is ready to do more.

Do not become negative or pass judgment on the partner of an abused woman. She is often tied to the man by both economic and emotional bonds and may become defensive if her partner is criticized. Tell her that resources are available for her partner but that it is necessary for him to admit abuse and seek assistance before help can be offered. Initiating referrals for the partner before he asks for help will increase the danger to the woman if he feels that he has been betrayed.

Evaluation

- Does the woman acknowledge the violence?
- Has she made concrete plans to protect herself and her children from future injury?
- Does she use the community resources available to her?

KEY CONCEPTS

- Teenage pregnancy is a major health problem in the United States. Adolescents need to receive accurate information not only about contraceptives but also about setting limits on sexual behavior.

- Pregnancy poses serious physiologic risks for the adolescent and the fetus. These result in a higher incidence of preeclampsia, anemia, nutritional deficiencies, urinary tract infections, and depression for the expectant mother as well as prematurity and low birth weight for the infant.

- Teenage pregnancy interrupts the developmental tasks of adolescence and may result in childbirth before the parents are capable of providing a nurturing home for the infant without a great deal of assistance.

- The mature primigravida often has financial and emotional resources that younger women do not have. She may experience anxiety about recommended antepartum testing, however, and about her ability to be an effective parent.

- Polydrug abuse is a widespread problem that can have devastating fetal and neonatal effects. These may become long-term developmental problems for the child.

- The lifestyle associated with illicit drug abuse includes inadequate nutrition, inadequate prenatal care, and an increased incidence of STDs. It necessitates interdisciplinary interventions to prevent injury to the expectant mother and to the fetus.

- The birth of an infant with congenital anomalies produces strong emotions of shock and grief in the family. It calls for a sensitive response from the health care team to help the family grieve for the loss of the perfect or "fantasy" infant and to form an attachment to the newborn.

- Pregnancy loss at any stage of pregnancy produces grief that must be acknowledged and expressed before it can be resolved. Nurses realize that mourning requires memories, and they intervene to arrange unlimited contact between the family and the stillborn infant and to prepare a packet of mementos for the family.

- Nursing care for the mother who is placing her infant for adoption is based on the knowledge that relinquishment (adoption) is an act of love, not abandonment.

- Multiple factors are associated with intimate partner violence. It is deliberate, severe, and generally repeated in a predictable cycle that often causes severe physical harm (or death) to the woman.

- All perinatal nurses come into contact with abused women who require assistance to protect themselves and their children from serious injury.

ANSWERS to Critical Thinking Exercise 25-1

1. The nurse assumed that the husband's behavior showed concern for his wife. Instead, it may have been a "hovering husband syndrome" that occurs in the honeymoon phase of the cycle of violence.

2. Facial injury, signs of previous bruising that resemble "grab marks," and abdominal bruising. Joan's story of falling and hurting herself is not congruent with the location of abdominal injury and injuries on her arms. Joan's lethargy and avoidance of eye contact also suggest that she is afraid.

3. The nurse should not question Joan's explanation of the injury in her husband's presence because this action increases the danger of escalating violence when the mother and infant are discharged.

4. The nurse should respond, "No one deserves to be hurt. It's not your fault. There are resources to help you." Nurses must examine their own thinking to be certain that they do not accept a common bias that physical abuse is deserved by the victim.

5. Joan needs information about protecting herself and the coming infant from future harm. This is not, however, the appropriate time to give her this information. The nurse must inform the physician and the postpartum staff of the problem and must make the necessary referrals to the hospital's social service department for follow-up.

REFERENCES and READINGS

Alan Guttmacher Institute. (2003). *Teenagers' sexual and reproductive health*. Retrieved November 15, 2003, from http://agi-usa.org/pubs/fb_teens.html.

Alexander, K.V. (2001). "The one thing you can never take away:" Perinatal bereavement photographs. MCN: *The American Journal of Maternal/Child Nursing, 26*(3), 123-127.

American Academy of Pediatrics (AAP). (2001). Care of adolescent parents and their children. *Pediatrics, 107*(2), 429-434.

American Academy of Pediatrics (AAP), & American College of Obstetricians and Gynecologists (ACOG). (2002). *Guidelines for perinatal care* (5th ed.). Elk Grove Village, IL, and Washington, DC: Author.

Anderson, C. (2002). Battered and pregnant: A nursing challenge. MCN: *The American Journal of Maternal/Child Nursing, 6*(2), 95-99.

Askin, D.F., & Diel-Jones, B. (2001). Cocaine: Effects of in utero exposure on the fetus and neonate. *Journal of Perinatal and Neonatal Nursing, 14*(4), 83-102.

Botham, S. (2000). Perinatal substance abuse. In J. Deacon & P. O'Neill (Eds.), *Core curriculum for neonatal intensive care nursing* (2nd ed., pp. 618-634). Philadelphia: Saunders.

Breedlove, G.K., & Schorfheide, A.M. (2001). *Adolescent pregnancy* (2nd ed.). White Plains, NY: March of Dimes.

Campbell, J.C. (2002). Health consequences of intimate partner violence. *The Lancet, 359*, 1331-1336.

Cambell, S. (2003). Prenatal cocaine exposure and neonatal/infant outcomes. *Neonatal Network, 22*(1), 19-21.

Carolan, M. (2003). The graying of the obstetric population: Implications for the older mother. *Journal of Obstetric, Gynecologic, and Neonatal Nursing, 32*(1), 10-27.

Centers for Disease Control and Prevention. (2003). *Alcohol use and pregnancy*. Retrieved November 24, 2003, from www.cdc.gov/ncbddd/factsheets/alcoholuse.pdf.

Clemmens, D. (2001). The relationship between social support and adolescent mothers' interactions with their infants: A meta-analysis. *Journal of Obstetric, Gynecologic, and Neonatal Nursing, 30*(4), 410-420.

Clemmens, D. (2003). Adolescent motherhood: A metasynthesis of qualitive studies. MCN: *The American Journal of Maternal/Child Nursing, 28*(2), 93-99.

Cote-Arsenault, D. (2003). The influence of perinatal loss on anxiety in multigravidas. *Journal of Obstetric, Gynecologic, and Neonatal Nursing, 32*(5), 623-629.

Cunningham, F.G., Gant, N.F., Leveno, K J., Gilstrap, L.C., Hauth, J.C., & Wenstrom, K.D. (2001). *Williams obstetrics* (21st ed.). New York: McGraw-Hill.

Davis, A.H. (2003). Pediatric and adolescent gynecology. In J.R. Scott, R.S. Gibbs, B.Y. Karlan, & A.F. Haney (Eds.), *Danforth's obstetrics and gynecology* (9th ed., pp 529-540). Philadelphia: Lippincott.

Deitch, K.V. (2000). Age-related concerns. In S. Mattson & J.E. Smith (Eds.), *Core curriculum for maternal-newborn nursing* (2nd ed., pp. 116-123.). Philadelphia: Saunders.

Delaney-Black, V., Covington, C.Y., Dhar, S., & Sokol, R.J. (2000). Illicit substance abuse during pregnancy. In S.B. Ransom, M.P. Dombrowski,

S.G. McNeeley, K.S. Moghissi, & A.R. Munkarah (Eds.), *Practical strategies in obstetrics and gynecology* (pp. 390-402). Philadelphia: Saunders.

deLisser, R., & Trimmer, T. (2001). Teen talk: An intervention for pregnant and parenting adolescents. *AWHONN Lifelines, 5*(4), 36-41.

De Mendoza, V.B. (2001). Culturally appropriate care for pregnant Latina women who are victims of domestic violence. *Journal of Obstetric, Gynecology, and Neonatal Nursing, 30*(6), 579-588.

Dienemann, J., Campbell, J., Wiederhorn, N., Laughon, K., & Jordan, E. (2003). A critical pathway for intimate partner violence across the continuum of care. *Journal of Obstetric, Gynecologic, and Neonatal Nursing, 32*(5), 594-603.

El-Bassel, N., Gilbert, L., Witte, S., Wu, E., Gaeta, T., Schilling, R., & Wada, T. (2003). Intimate partner violence and substance abuse among minority women receiving care from an inner-city emergency department. *Women's Health Issues, 13*(1), 16-22.

Eustace, L.W., Kang, D., & Coombs, D. (2003). Fetal alcohol syndrome: A growing concern for health care professionals. *Journal of Obstetric, Gynecologic, and Neonatal Nursing, 32*(2), 215-221.

Fike, D.L. (2003). Assessment and management of the substance-exposed newborn and infant. In C. Kenner & J.W. Lott (Eds.), *Comprehensive neonatal nursing: A physiologic perspective* (3rd ed., pp. 773-802). Philadelphia: Saunders.

Foley, E.M. (2002). Drug screening and criminal prosecution of pregnant women. *Journal of Obstetric, Gynecologic, and Neonatal Nursing, 31*(2), 133-137.

Gazmararian, J.A., Petersen, R., Spitz, A.M., Goodwin, M.M., Salzman, L.E., & Marks, J.S. (2000). Violence and reproductive health: Current knowledge and future research. *Maternal and Child Health Journal, 4*(2), 79-84.

Gemma, P.B., & Arnold, J. (2002). *Loss and grieving in pregnancy and the first year of life: A caring resource for nurses.* White Plains, NY: March of Dimes.

Greene, C.M., & Goodman, M.H. (2003). Neonatal abstinence syndrome: Strategies for care of the drug-exposed infant. *Neonatal Network, 22*(4), 15-25.

Haggerty, L.A., & Goodman, L.A. (2003). Stages of change-based nursing interventions for victims of interpersonal violence. *Journal of Obstetric, Gynecologic, and Neonatal Nursing, 32*(1), 68-75.

Hancock, E.G., Calhoun, B.C., & Hume, R.F. (2002). Adolescent pregnancy: Improving outcomes through focused multidisciplinary obstetric care. In S.B. Ransom, M.P. Dombrowski, M.I. Evans, & K.A. Ginsburg (Eds.), *Contemporary therapy in obstetrics and gynecology* (pp. 152-155). Philadelphia: Saunders.

Heinonen, S., & Kirkinen, P. (2000). Pregnancy outcome after previous stillbirth resulting from causes other than maternal conditions and fetal abnormalities. *Birth, 27*(1), 33-37.

Jansen, J.L. (2003). A bereavement model for the intensive care nursery. *Neonatal Network, 22*(3), 17-23.

Kavanaugh, K., & Wheeler, S.R. (2003). When a baby dies: Caring for bereaved families. In C. Kenner, J.W. Lott, & A.A. Flandermeyer (Eds.), *Comprehensive neonatal nursing: A physiologic perspective* (3rd ed., pp. 108-126). Philadelphia: Saunders.

Kelly, P.J., & Morgan-Kidd, J. (2001). Social influences on the sexual behaviors of adolescent girls in at-risk circumstances. *Journal of Obstetric, Gynecology, and Neonatal Nursing, 30*(5), 481-489.

Koniak-Griffin. (2001). Health risks and psychosocial outcomes of early childbearing: A review of the literature. *Journal of Perinatal and Neonatal Nursing, 15*(2), 1-17.

Koniak-Griffin, D., Verzemnieks, I.L., Anderson, N.L.R., Brecht, M., Lesser, J., Kim, S., & Turner-Pluta, C. (2003). Nurse visitation for adolescent mothers. *Nursing Research, 52*(2), 127-136.

Kowalski, K. (2001). Perinatal loss and bereavement. In K.R. Simpson & P.A. Creehan (Eds.), *Perinatal nursing* (pp. 476-491). Philadelphia: Lippincott.

Lemmey, D., McFarlane, J., Wilson, P., & Malecha, A. (2001). Intimate partner violence: Mothers' perspectives of effects on their children. *MCN: The American Journal of Maternal/Child Nursing, 26*(2), 98-103.

Lipsky, S., Holt, V.L., Easterling, T.R., & Critchlow, C.W. (2003). Impact of police-reported intimate partner violence during pregnancy on birth outcomes. *Obstetrics & Gynecology, 102*(3), 557-564.

MacKay, A.P., Fingerhut, L.A., & Duran, C.R. (2000). *Adolescent health chartbook. Health, United States, 2000.* Hyattsville, MD: National Center for Health Statistics.

Maier, S.E., & West, J.E. (2001). Drinking pattern and alcohol-related birth defects. *Alcohol Research and Health, 25*(3), 168-174.

Marcellus, L. (2002). Care of substance-exposed infants: The current state of practice in Canadian hospitals. *Journal of Perinatal and Neonatal Nursing, 16*(3), 51-68.

Martin, J.A., Hamilton, B.E., Sutton, P.D., Ventura, S.J., Menacker, F., & Munson, M.L. (2003). Births: Final data for 2002. *National Vital Statistics Reports* (vol 52, no. 10). Hyattsville, MD: National Center for Health Statistics. Retrieved February 14, 2004, from www.cdc.gov/nchs/data/nvsr/nvsr52/nvsr52_10.pdf

Matteson, P.S. (2001). *Women's health during the childbearing years: A community-based approach.* St. Louis: Mosby.

McComish, F.F., Greenberg, R., & Shewmaker, K. (2002). Contemporary options in substance abuse treatment for women. In S.B. Ransom, M.P. Dombrowski, M.I. Evans, & K.A. Ginsburg (Eds.), *Contemporary therapy in obstetrics and gynecology* (pp. 387-395). Philadelphia: Saunders.

McFarlane, J., Parker, B., & Cross, B. (2001). *Abuse during pregnancy: A protocol for prevention and interventions* (2nd ed.). White Plains, NY: March of Dimes.

Montgomery, K.S. (2003a). Health promotion for pregnant adolescents. *MCN: The American Journal of Maternal/Child Nursing, 7*(5), 432-444.

Montgomery, K.S. (2003b). Nursing care for pregnant adolescents. *Journal of Obstetric, Gynecologic, and Neonatal Nursing, 32*(2), 249-257.

Moran, B.A. (2000). Substance abuse in pregnancy. In S. Mattson & J.E. Smith (Eds.), *Core curriculum for maternal-newborn nursing* (2nd ed., pp. 545-563). Philadelphia: Saunders.

Neumann, M., & Graf, C. (2003). Pregnant after age 35: Are these women at high risk? *AWHONN Lifelines, 7*(5), 422-430.

Peterson, R., Gazmararian, J., & Clark, K.A. (2001). Partner violence: Implications for health and community settings. *Women's Health Issues, 11*(2), 116-125.

Phipps, M.G., Blume, J.D., & DeMonner, S.M. (2002). Young maternal age associated with increased risk of neonatal death. *Obstetrics & Gynecology, 100*(3), 481-486.

Plichta, S.B., & Falik, M. (2001). Prevalence of violence and implications for women's health. *Women's Health Issues, 11*(3), 244-258.

Primeau, M.R., & Lamb, J.M. (1995). When a baby dies: Rights of the baby and parents. *Journal of Obstetric, Gynecologic, and Neonatal Nursing, 24*(3), 206-208.

Renker, P.R. (2002). "Keep a blank face. I need to tell you what has been happening to me." *MCN: The American Journal of Maternal/Child Nursing, 27*(2), 109-116.

Renker, P.R. (2003). Keeping safe: Teenagers' strategies for dealing with perinatal violence. *Journal of Obstetric, Gynecologic, and Neonatal Nursing, 32*(1), 58-67.

Rentschler, D.D. (2003). Pregnant adolescents' perspectives of pregnancy. *MCN: The American Journal of Maternal/Child Nursing, 28*(6), 377-383.

Rillstone, P., & Hutchinson, S.A. (2001). Managing the reemergence of anguish: Pregnancy after a loss due to anomalies. *Journal of Obstetric, Gynecologic, and Neonatal Nursing, 30*(3), 291-298.

Samuelsson, M., Radestad, I., & Segesten, K. (2001). A waste of life: Fathers' experience of losing a child before birth. *Birth, 28*(2), 124-130.

Savage, C., Wray, J., Ritchey, P.N., Sommers, M., Dyehouse, J., & Fulmer, M. (2003). Current screening instruments related to alcohol consumption in pregnancy and a proposed alternative method. *Journal of Obstetric, Gynecologic, and Neonatal Nursing, 32*(4), 437-446.

Shieh, C., & Kravitz, M. (2002). Maternal-fetal attachment in pregnant women who use illicit drugs. *Journal of Obstetric, Gynecologic, and Neonatal Nursing, 31*(2), 156-164.

Singh, S., & Darroch, J.E. (2000). Adolescent pregnancy and childbearing: Levels and trends in developed countries. *Family Planning Perspectives, 32*(1), 14-23.

Tillett, J., & Osborne, K. (2001). Substance abuse by pregnant women: Legal and ethical concerns. *Journal of Perinatal and Neonatal Nursing, 14*(4), 1-11.

Tjaden, P., & Thoennes, N. (2000). *Full report of the prevalence, incidence, and consequences of intimate partner violence against women: Findings from the National Violence Against Women survey.* Washington, DC: National Institute of Justice.

Toohey, J.S. (2000). Battered women. In E.J. Quilligan & F.P. Zuspan, *Current therapy in obstetrics and gynecology* (5th ed., pp. 453-456). Philadelphia: Saunders.

U.S. Department of Health and Human Services. (2000). *Healthy People 2010: Healthy People 2010* (Conference edition, in 2 volumes). Washington, DC.

Van, P., & Meleis, A.I. (2003). Coping after grief after involuntary pregnancy loss: Perspectives of African American women. *Journal of Obstetric, Gynecologic, and Neonatal Nursing, 32*(1), 28-39.

Viau, P.A., Padula, C.A., & Eddy, B. (2002). An exploration of health concerns & health-promotion behaviors in pregnant women over age 35. *MCN: The American Journal of Maternal/Child Nursing, 27*(6), 328-334.

Winn, N., Records, K., & Rice, M. (2003). The relationship between abuse, sexually transmitted diseases, & group B streptococcus. *MCN: The American Journal of Maternal/Child Nursing, 28*(2), 106-110.

26

The Pregnant Woman with Complications

⬥ LEARNING OBJECTIVES

After studying this chapter, you should be able to:
- Describe the hemorrhagic conditions of early pregnancy, including spontaneous abortion, ectopic pregnancy, and hydatidiform mole.
- Explain disorders of the placenta, such as placenta previa and abruptio placentae, that may result in hemorrhage during late pregnancy.
- Discuss the effects and management of hyperemesis gravidarum.
- Describe the development and management of hypertensive disorders of pregnancy.
- Compare Rh and ABO incompatibility in terms of etiology, fetal and neonatal complications, and management.
- Describe the effects of pregnancy on glucose metabolism.
- Discuss the effects and management of preexisting diabetes mellitus during pregnancy.

- Explain the effects and management of gestational diabetes mellitus.
- Describe management of the pregnant and postpartum woman who has heart disease.
- Explain the maternal and fetal effects of specific hematologic disorders and the required management during pregnancy.
- Identify the effects, management, and nursing considerations of specific preexisting conditions discussed in this chapter.
- Identify the major causes of trauma during pregnancy, and describe therapeutic management.
- Discuss the maternal, fetal, and neonatal effects of the most common infections that may occur during pregnancy.

⬥ DEFINITIONS

abortion Spontaneous or elective ending of a pregnancy before the pregnancy reaches a state's legal limit. Fetal death (later than abortion) occurs at 20 weeks or more by National Center for Health Statistics criteria but varies by state laws. *Miscarriage* is a lay term for a spontaneous abortion.

antiphospholipid antibodies Autoimmune antibodies directed against phospholipids in cell membranes, associated with recurrent spontaneous abortion, fetal loss, and severe pregnancy-induced hypertension.

bicornuate (bicornate) uterus Malformed uterus having two horns.

caudal regression syndrome Malformation that results when the sacrum, lumbar spine, and lower extremities fail to develop.

cerclage Encircling of the cervix with suture to prevent recurrent spontaneous abortion caused by early cervical dilation.

congestive heart failure Condition resulting from failure of the heart to maintain adequate circulation, characterized by weakness, dyspnea, and edema in body parts lower than the heart.

culdocentesis Needle puncture through the upper posterior vaginal wall (cul-de-sac of Douglas) to aspirate blood or fluid from the pelvic cavity.

diabetogenic Producing the effects of diabetes mellitus. Diabetogenic conditions include pregnancy.

dilation and curettage (D&C) Stretching the cervical os to permit suctioning or scraping of the walls of the uterus. The

procedure is performed in abortion, to obtain samples of uterine lining tissue for laboratory examination, and during the postpartum period to remove retained fragments of placenta.

dystocia Difficult or prolonged labor, often associated with abnormal uterine activity and cephalopelvic disproportion.

erythroblastosis fetalis Agglutination and hemolysis of fetal erythrocytes caused by incompatibility between maternal and fetal blood. In most cases the fetus is Rh-positive and the mother is Rh-negative. Other maternal-fetal blood incompatibilities can produce similar effects.

euglycemia Normal blood glucose level.

gestational trophoblastic disease A spectrum of diseases that includes benign hydatidiform mole and gestational trophoblastic tumors, such as invasive moles and choriocarcinoma.

gluconeogenesis Formation of glycogen by the liver from noncarbohydrate sources, such as amino acids or fatty acids.

hydramnios Excess volume of amniotic fluid (more than 2000 ml at term). Also called *polyhydramnios.*

hypovolemic shock Acute peripheral circulatory failure caused by loss of circulating blood volume.

kernicterus Staining of brain tissue caused by accumulation of unconjugated bilirubin in the brain. Also called *bilirubin encephalopathy.*

ketosis Accumulation of ketone bodies (metabolic products) in the blood; frequently associated with acidosis.

laparoscopy Insertion of an illuminated tube (laparoscope) into the abdominal cavity to observe contents, locate bleeding, and perform surgical procedures.

lipogenic substance Substance, such as insulin, that stimulates the production of fat.

maceration Discoloration and softening of tissues and eventual disintegration of a fetus retained in the uterus after its death.

Marfan syndrome A hereditary condition that involves weakness in connective tissue, bones, and muscles. The vascular system is affected, particularly the aorta.

osmotic diuresis Secretion and passage of large amounts of urine as a result of increased osmotic pressure that can result from hyperglycemia.

perinatologist A physician who specializes in the care of the mother, fetus, and infant during the perinatal period (from the 20th week of pregnancy to 4 weeks after childbirth).

seroconversion Change in a blood test result from negative to positive, indicating the development of antibodies in response to infection or immunization.

vacuum curettage (vacuum aspiration) Removal of the uterine contents by application of a vacuum through a hollow curette or cannula introduced into the uterus.

vasoconstriction Narrowing of the lumen of blood vessels.

Complications during pregnancy sometimes threaten the well-being of the expectant mother, her fetus, or both. These complications fall into two broad categories: complications of pregnancy, when problems develop in the normal processes; and complications related to other disorders that adversely affect the pregnancy or are adversely affected by the pregnancy.

PREGNANCY-RELATED COMPLICATIONS

The most common pregnancy-related complications are hemorrhagic conditions that occur in early pregnancy, hemorrhagic complications of the placenta in late pregnancy, hyperemesis gravidarum, hypertensive disorders of pregnancy, and blood incompatibilities between the mother and fetus.

HEMORRHAGIC CONDITIONS OF EARLY PREGNANCY

The three most common causes of hemorrhage during the first half of pregnancy are abortion, ectopic pregnancy, and hydatidiform mole.

Spontaneous Abortion

Abortion is the loss of pregnancy before the fetus is viable, that is, before it is capable of living outside the uterus. The medical consensus today is that a fetus of less than 20 weeks' gestation or one weighing less than 500 g is not viable. Abortion may be either spontaneous or induced. *Miscarriage* is a term used by lay people to denote an abortion that has occurred spontaneously as opposed to one that has been induced, and the term is becoming accepted by professionals as well. Induced abortion is described in Chapter 31. Spontaneous abortion denotes termination of a pregnancy without action taken by the woman or any other person.

Determining the exact incidence of spontaneous abortion is difficult because many unrecognized losses occur in early pregnancy. The incidence of spontaneous abortion increases with parental age. The incidence is 12% for women younger than 20 years, rising to 26% for women older than 40 years. Paternal age younger than 20 years is associated with a spontaneous abortion rate of 12%, rising to 20% for fathers older than 40 years. Most spontaneous abortions occur in the first 12 weeks of pregnancy, with the rate declining rapidly thereafter (Cunningham et al., 2001).

The most common cause of spontaneous abortion is severe congenital abnormalities that are often incompatible with life. Chromosomal abnormalities account for about 50% to 60% of early spontaneous abortions. Additional causes include maternal infections such as syphilis, listeriosis, toxoplasmosis, brucellosis, rubella, and cytomegalic inclusion disease. Intraabdominal infections also increase the risk. Maternal endocrine disorders such as hypothyroidism and abnormalities of the reproductive organs have also been implicated. Still other women who have repeated early pregnancy losses appear to have immunologic factors that play a role in their higher-than-expected spontaneous abortion incidence. Anatomic defects of the uterus or cervix may contribute to pregnancy loss at any gestation (Branch & Scott, 2003; Coulam, 2000; Cunningham et al., 2001).

Spontaneous abortion is divided into six subgroups: threatened, inevitable, incomplete, complete, missed, and recurrent. Figure 26-1 illustrates threatened, inevitable, and incomplete abortion.

Threatened Abortion

Manifestations. The first sign of threatened abortion is vaginal bleeding. Up to 25% of all women experience "spotting," or light bleeding, in early pregnancy, and about half of these pregnancies will not survive. Vaginal bleeding, which may be brief or last for weeks, may be followed by uterine cramping, persistent backache, or feelings of pelvic pressure. These added symptoms of pain and pressure are more likely to be associated with progression to loss of the pregnancy. When examined using a speculum, the cervix is closed. Laboratory tests show rising levels of beta–human chorionic gonadotropin (β-hCG), and the uterine size increases with embryonic growth if the pregnancy remains viable (Branch & Scott, 2003; Cunningham et al., 2001).

Therapeutic Management. Bleeding in the first half of pregnancy must be considered a threatened abortion, and women should be advised to notify their physician or nurse-midwife if they note vaginal bleeding. The nurse obtains a detailed history that includes length of gestation or time of last menstrual period and the onset, duration, and amount of vaginal bleeding. Accompanying discomfort, such as cramping, backache, abdominal pain, or pelvic pressure, is also evaluated. Fever or uterine tenderness suggests infection.

Ultrasound examination is often performed to determine whether the fetus is present and, if so, whether it is alive.

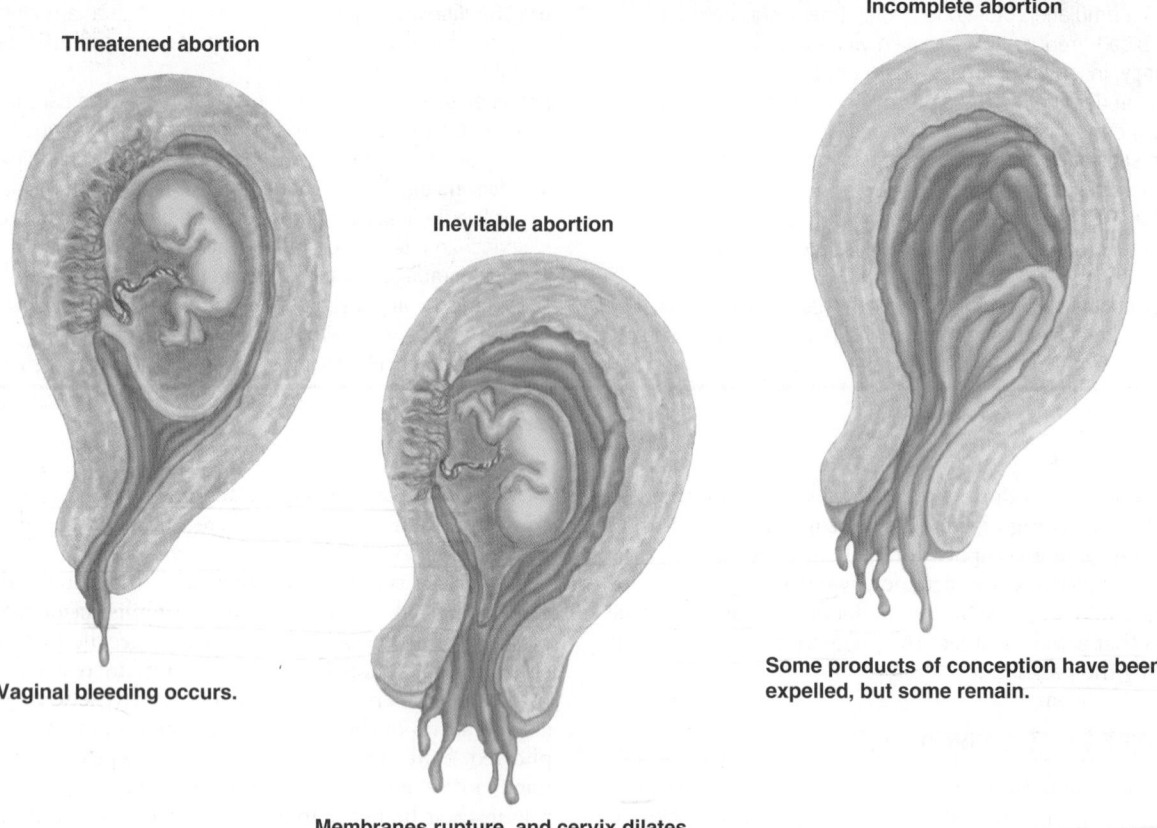

Threatened abortion

Vaginal bleeding occurs.

Inevitable abortion

Membranes rupture, and cervix dilates.

Incomplete abortion

Some products of conception have been expelled, but some remain.

Figure 26-1 Three types of spontaneous abortion.

Levels of β-hCG may be done to determine if they are appropriate for the gestation and if they are rising as the fetus grows.

The woman may be advised to curtail sexual activity until bleeding has ceased and for at least 2 weeks after the last evidence of bleeding. Bed rest has not been demonstrated to be effective in treatment of threatened abortion. Reduced activity is often recommended. The woman is instructed to count the number of perineal pads (peripads) used and to note the quantity and color of blood on the pads. She should also look for tissue passage. A drainage that has a foul odor suggests infection.

The woman often wonders whether her actions may have contributed to the situation and is anxious about her own condition and that of the fetus. The nurse should offer accurate information and avoid false reassurance, because the woman may lose the fetus despite every precaution. In addition, later complications, such as preterm birth or low birth weight may occur, even if the pregnancy progresses.

Inevitable Abortion

Manifestations. Abortion is usually inevitable (i.e., it cannot be stopped) when the membranes rupture and the cervix dilates. Active bleeding that is heavier than that of threatened abortion is common.

Therapeutic Management. Natural expulsion of the uterine contents is common, and no further treatment may be needed. If tissue remains or if bleeding is excessive, the physician performs a dilation and vacuum curettage (D&C) while the woman is under anesthesia.

Incomplete Abortion

Manifestations. Incomplete abortion occurs when some but not all of the products of conception are expelled from the uterus. The major manifestations are active uterine bleeding and severe abdominal cramping. The cervix is open, and fetal and placental tissue is passed. The products of conception may have been expelled from the uterus but remain in the vagina because of their small size, often no larger than a ping-pong ball if the gestation is very early.

Therapeutic Management. The retained tissue prevents the uterus from contracting firmly, thus allowing profuse bleeding from uterine blood vessels. Initial treatment should focus on ensuring the woman's cardiovascular stabilization. Blood is drawn for crossmatching and blood typing, and an intravenous (IV) line is inserted for fluid replacement and drug administration. Curettage is usually performed to remove remaining tissue. This procedure may be followed by IV administration of oxytocin (Pitocin) or intramuscular (IM) administration of methylergonovine (Methergine) to contract the uterus and control bleeding.

Because of the danger of excessive bleeding, curettage may not be performed if the pregnancy has advanced beyond 14 weeks. In this case, oxytocin or prostaglandin is administered to stimulate uterine contractions until all products of conception (fetus, membranes, placenta, amniotic fluid) are expelled.

Complete Abortion

Manifestations. Complete abortion occurs when all products of conception are expelled from the uterus. Uterine contractions and bleeding abate, and the cervix closes after all products of conception are passed.

Therapeutic Management. Once complete abortion is confirmed, no additional intervention is required unless excessive bleeding or infection develops. The woman should be advised to rest and watch for further bleeding, pain, or fever. She should abstain from intercourse until after a follow-up visit with her health care provider. Contraception will be discussed at this visit if she wishes to avoid pregnancy.

Missed Abortion

Manifestations. Missed abortion occurs when the fetus dies during the first half of pregnancy but is retained in the uterus. When the fetus dies, the early symptoms of pregnancy (nausea, breast tenderness, urinary frequency) disappear. The uterus stops growing and often decreases in size, reflecting the absorption of amniotic fluid and maceration of the fetus.

Therapeutic Management. In most cases, the pregnancy ends spontaneously after fetal death (Cunningham et al., 2001). If the fetus is not expelled, fetal death is confirmed by ultrasound examination. When fetal death is confirmed, the uterus may be evacuated by D&C. Prostaglandin compounds may be necessary to induce contractions and empty the uterus during the second trimester.

Two major complications of missed abortion are infection and disseminated intravascular coagulation (DIC). If there are signs of uterine infection, such as an elevated temperature, vaginal discharge with a foul odor, or abdominal pain, evacuation of the uterus is delayed until antibiotic therapy is initiated.

Disseminated Intravascular Coagulation (Consumptive Coagulopathy). DIC is a defect in coagulation that may occur if the fetus is retained for a prolonged period. Coagulation defects do not usually occur unless fetal death occurs after the first trimester. DIC is also associated with abruptio placentae and with pregnancy-induced hypertension.

With DIC, anticoagulation and procoagulation factors are activated simultaneously. DIC develops when the clotting factor *thromboplastin* is released into the maternal bloodstream as a result of placental bleeding and consequent clot formation. The circulating thromboplastin activates widespread clotting in small vessels throughout the body. This process consumes, or "uses up," other clotting factors such as fibrinogen and platelets. The condition is further complicated by activation of the fibrinolytic system to lyse, or destroy, clots. The result is a simultaneous decrease in clotting factors and increase in circulating anticoagulants, which leaves the circulating blood unable to clot. This situation allows bleeding to occur from any area, such as intravenous sites, incisions, or the gums or nose, as well as from expected sites such as the site of placental attachment during the postpartum period.

In DIC, fibrinogen and platelets are usually decreased, prothrombin and partial thromboplastin times may be prolonged, and fibrin degradation products, the most sensitive measurement, are increased. The D-dimer serum assay, which is normally negative, is a specific measurement of fibrin degradation activity.

The priority in treating DIC is delivery of the fetus and placenta to stop the production of thromboplastin, which is fueling the process. In addition, blood replacement products, such as whole blood, packed red blood cells, and cryoprecipitate, are administered to maintain the circulating volume and to transport oxygen to body cells.

Recurrent Spontaneous Abortion

Manifestations. Recurrent spontaneous abortion is sometimes referred to as *habitual abortion*; the current definition is three or more consecutive spontaneous abortions. The primary causes of recurrent abortion are believed to be genetic or chromosomal abnormalities and anomalies of the woman's reproductive tract, such as bicornuate uterus or incompetent cervix.

Additional causes include an inadequate luteal phase with insufficient secretion of progesterone and immunologic factors that involve increased sharing of human leukocyte antigens by the sperm and ovum of the man and woman who conceived. The theory is that, because of this sharing, the woman's immunologic system is not stimulated to produce blocking antibodies that protect the embryo from maternal immune cells or other damaging antibodies. Systemic diseases such as lupus erythematosus and diabetes mellitus have been implicated in recurrent abortions. Reproductive infections and some sexually transmitted diseases are also associated with recurrent abortions.

Therapeutic Management. The first step in managing recurrent spontaneous abortion is a thorough examination of the woman's reproductive organs to determine whether anatomic defects are the cause. If her reproductive organs are normal, the woman is usually referred for genetic screening to identify genetic factors that would increase the possibility of recurrent abortions. Additional therapeutic management of recurrent pregnancy loss depends on the cause. For example, antimicrobials are prescribed for the woman with infection or hormone-related drugs may be prescribed if imbalance preventing normal fetal implantation and support is found.

Recurrent spontaneous abortion may be caused by cervical incompetence, an anatomic defect that results in painless dilation of the cervix in the second trimester. In this instance, the cervix may be sutured to keep it from opening (i.e., cerclage). Sutures may be removed near term if vaginal delivery is expected, or they may be left in place if a cesarean birth is planned. Prophylactic antibiotics may be necessary if the woman is judged to be at high risk for infection. Preterm labor may still occur but, it is hoped, after the fetus is viable.

Nursing Considerations

Spontaneous abortion may be accompanied by various amounts of bleeding. Prevention or identification and treatment of hypovolemic shock are the nursing priorities when a woman is bleeding heavily. The nurse should observe for tachycardia (often the earliest sign), a falling blood pressure, pale skin and mucous membranes, confusion, restlessness, and cool and clammy skin. The nurse manages fluid and blood replacement as ordered.

Vaginal bleeding of any amount during pregnancy is frightening, and waiting and watching are difficult, although often the only reasonable treatment. Moreover, many families feel an acute sense of loss and grief with spontaneous abortion. Grief often includes feelings of guilt, which may be expressed as wondering if the woman could have done something to prevent the loss. Nurses can help by emphasizing that most spontaneous abortions occur because of factors or abnormalities that could not be avoided.

Anger, disappointment, and sadness are commonly experienced emotions, although the intensity of the feelings may vary. For many couples, the fetus has not yet taken on specific physical characteristics but they grieve for their fantasies of

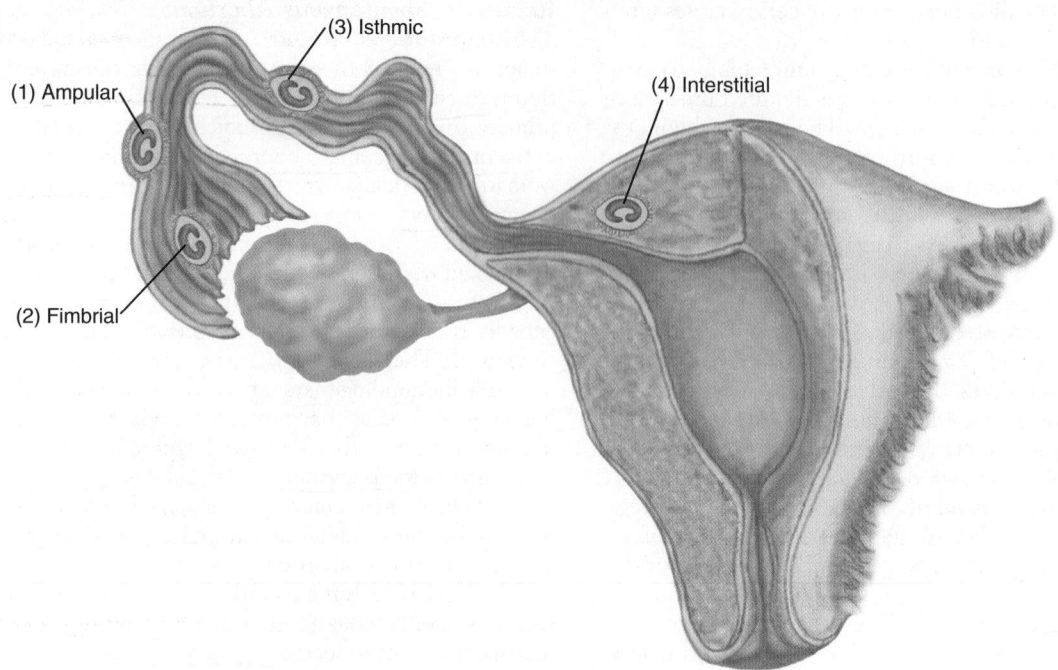

Figure 26-2 Sites of ectopic pregnancy. Numbers indicate the order of prevalence.

BOX 26-1
Risk Factors for Ectopic Pregnancy

- History of sexually transmitted diseases (gonorrhea, chlamydial infection)
- History of pelvic inflammatory disease
- History of previous ectopic pregnancies
- Failed tubal ligation
- Intrauterine device
- Multiple induced abortions
- Maternal age older than 35 years

---

the lost child. The couple may want to express their sadness but may feel that family, friends, and often health personnel are uncomfortable or diminish their loss.

To recognize the meaning of the loss to each family, nurses must listen carefully to what the couple say and observe how the partners behave. Nurses must attempt to convey unconditional acceptance of the feelings expressed or demonstrated. The couple should be permitted to remain together as much as possible. Providing information and simple, brief explanations of what has occurred and what will be done facilitates the family's ability to grieve.

It is helpful for the family to realize that grief may last from 6 months to a year, or even longer. Family support, knowledge of the grief process, spiritual counselors, and the support of other bereaved couples may provide needed assistance during this time.

Ectopic Pregnancy

Ectopic pregnancy refers to implantation of a fertilized ovum in an area outside the uterine cavity. More than 95% of ectopic pregnancies are in the fallopian tube, usually the am-

pulla, or middle part of the tube. Figure 26-2 shows common sites of tubal implantation. Anything that slows the transport of the fertilized ovum through the tube or causes it to implant too early increases the risk that implantation will occur in the tube rather than the uterus.

Incidence and Etiology

The incidence of ectopic pregnancy has increased dramatically throughout the world in the past 20 years. Ectopic pregnancy rates are higher in nonwhite women and older women. The highest rate is seen in nonwhite women older than 35 years (Cunningham et al., 2001). The rapid increase in incidence is attributed to the growing number of women of childbearing age who experience scarring of the fallopian tubes caused by pelvic infection, inflammation, or surgery. Pelvic infection or inflammation (pelvic inflammatory disease [PID]) is often the result of sexually transmitted infections such as *Chlamydia* or *Neisseria gonorrhoeae*. Pelvic infection may also occur after induced abortion or childbirth. Women who require assisted reproductive techniques to conceive also have a greater risk, probably the result of the underlying pathology that caused infertility (Box 26-1).

Additional risk factors for ectopic pregnancy include:

- Use of the intrauterine device (IUD) for contraception
- Anatomic or functional defects in the fallopian tubes
- Cigarette smoking
- Vaginal douching

Manifestations

Early signs and symptoms of ectopic pregnancy are:

- Missed menstrual period
- Abdominal and pelvic pain
- Vaginal "spotting" or light bleeding

More subtle signs and symptoms depend on the site of implantation. If implantation occurs in the distal end of the fallopian tube, which can accommodate the growing embryo longer, the woman may at first exhibit the usual early signs of pregnancy. Several weeks into the pregnancy, intermittent abdominal pain and small amounts of vaginal bleeding occur. These early manifestations are easily mistaken for those of threatened abortion. An embryo implanted in the tube may also die early and be reabsorbed by the body.

If implantation has occurred in the proximal end of the fallopian tube, rupture of the tube may occur within 2 to 3 weeks of the missed period. Symptoms include sudden, severe pain in one of the lower quadrants of the abdomen as the tube tears open and the embryo is expelled into the pelvic cavity. Pain is often accompanied by intraabdominal hemorrhage. Irritation of the diaphragm, manifested by shoulder or neck pain that is worse on inspiration, occurs in about half of women (Cunningham et al., 2001). Signs of hypovolemic shock (rapid pulse, lightheadedness, syncope, falling blood pressure) may develop with no or minimal external bleeding.

Diagnostic Evaluation

Ectopic pregnancy can usually be diagnosed before rupture occurs. Transvaginal ultrasound can confirm or rule out an intrauterine pregnancy reliably by 28 days after conception. Serum tests for β-hCG and progesterone provide added screening for a viable or nonviable pregnancy. Using multiple diagnostic tests, the physician can make a judgment about whether the pregnancy is intrauterine or ectopic and whether the conceptus is living (Cunningham, 2001; Lipscomb & Ling, 2000; Stovall, 2000).

Serum β-hCG normally rises during early gestation to cause the corpus luteum to persist and secrete progesterone. β-hCG then decreases at about 50 to 70 days' gestation as the placenta takes over production of progesterone to maintain the pregnancy. Lower-than-normal levels of β-hCG suggest an abnormal pregnancy. Progesterone should also be elevated in normal pregnancy because of β-hCG stimulation of the corpus luteum. If progesterone is very low, the pregnancy is unlikely to be viable.

The use of sensitive pregnancy tests and high-resolution ultrasound has largely eliminated invasive tests for ectopic pregnancy. Minimally invasive examinations, such as culdocentesis or laparoscopy, may be required. Aspiration of blood from the vaginal cul-de-sac in a culdocentesis suggests bleeding into the peritoneal cavity from rupture of a fallopian tube. Laparoscopy allows direct visualization of the abdominal cavity to identify the source of the problem.

Therapeutic Management

The management of tubal pregnancy depends on whether the tube is intact or ruptured. Medical management may allow preservation of the tube, thus improving the chance of future fertility. Medical management is most successful if the tube is intact, the pregnancy is early, the size of the pregnancy is less than 3.5 cm, and the fetus is not living. The cytotoxic drug methotrexate (a folic acid antagonist that interferes with cell reproduction) inhibits cell division in the embryo. Retreatment or surgical treatment may be needed if the initial treatment fails (Cunningham et al., 2001).

Surgical management of a tubal pregnancy that is unruptured may involve a *linear salpingostomy* to salvage the tube for future pregnancies. The tube is opened with a fine linear incision, the products of conception are removed, and to reduce scarring, the tubal incision is left to heal without suturing. Linear salpingostomy also may be attempted if the fallopian tube is minimally ruptured and a slightly greater tubal opening is needed for removal of tubal pregnancy material.

When ectopic pregnancy results in rupture of the fallopian tube, the goal of therapeutic management is to control the bleeding and prevent hypovolemic shock. When the woman's cardiovascular status is stable, a salpingectomy is performed to remove the affected tube and ligate bleeding vessels. Future pregnancies can still occur when only one tube is present, although the likelihood of fertility decreases. In addition, the same conditions that caused the ectopic pregnancy in the tube that was removed may exist in the other tube.

Nursing Considerations

Nursing care focuses on preventing or identifying hypovolemic shock, controlling pain, and providing psychologic support for the woman who experiences an ectopic pregnancy. If methotrexate is used, the nurse must explain temporary side effects (e.g., nausea and vomiting) and the importance of communicating to the health care team bothersome drug effects or worsening symptoms that suggest rupture (e.g., pelvic, shoulder, or neck pain; dizziness or faintness; increased vaginal bleeding). The woman must be instructed to refrain from drinking alcohol or ingesting vitamins that contain folic acid, which would decrease the drug's effectiveness. She should not have sexual intercourse until β-hCG levels are undetectable. If the treatment is successful, this hormone disappears from plasma within 2 to 3 weeks (Cunningham et al., 2001). The importance of keeping follow-up appointments should be emphasized because medical treatment is not always successful and surgical intervention may be needed.

The woman and her family often need emotional support to resolve emotions, which may include anger, grief, guilt, and self-blame. The woman may also be anxious about her ability to become pregnant in the future. Although the pregnancy is unsuccessful very early, the nurse should be aware that these women may feel an acute sense of loss similar to that of women suffering miscarriage. Nurses may need to clarify the physician's explanation and to use therapeutic communication techniques that assist the woman to deal with her anxiety and grief.

Gestational Trophoblastic Disease (Hydatidiform Mole)

Hydatidiform mole is a form of gestational trophoblastic disease that occurs when the trophoblasts (peripheral cells that attach the fertilized ovum to the uterine wall) develop abnormally. As a result of the abnormal growth, the placenta, but not the fetus, develops. The condition is characterized by proliferation and edema of the chorionic villi. The fluid-filled villi form grapelike vesicles that may grow large enough to fill the uterus to the size of an advanced pregnancy if not diagnosed and treated (Fig. 26-3). The mole may be *complete*, with no fetus present, or *partial*, in which fetal tissue or membranes are present. Malignant change and proliferation of residual trophoblastic tissue (gestational trophoblastic neoplasm, or choriocarcinoma) is a life-threatening complication that follows 15% to 20% of hydatidiform moles (Li &

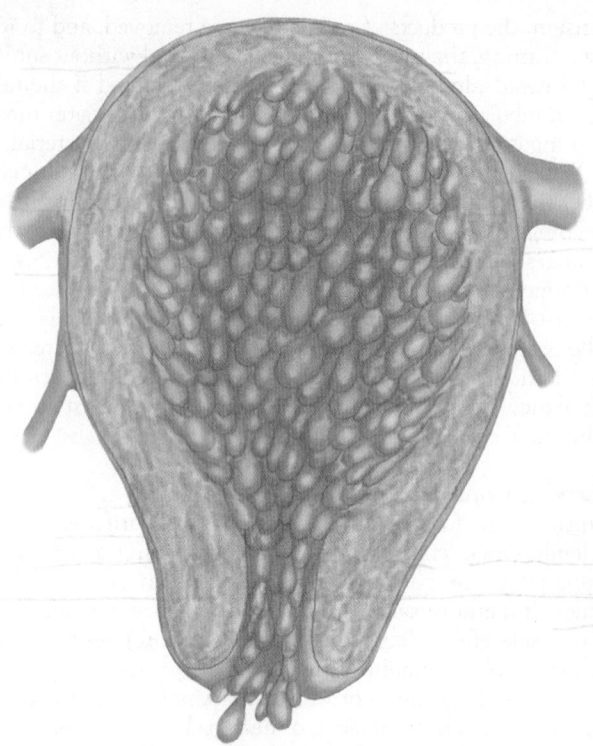

Figure 26-3 Hydatidiform mole.

Karlan, 2003). Acute respiratory distress may occur if vesicles of the hydatidiform mole enter the woman's circulation and embolize to her lungs.

Incidence and Etiology

In the United States and Europe, the incidence of hydatidiform mole is 1 in every 1500 to 2000 pregnancies (Li & Karlan, 2003). Hydatidiform mole is more likely to occur in older mothers. Women who have had one molar pregnancy are at slightly greater risk for having another.

A *complete mole* is believed to occur when the ovum is fertilized by a sperm that duplicates its own chromosomes while the chromosomes of the ovum are inactivated. In a *partial mole*, the maternal contribution is usually present but the paternal contribution is double, and thus the karyotype is triploid (69,XXY or 69,XYY). Anomalies are usually present if a fetus is present.

Manifestations

Most molar pregnancies can be diagnosed early by ultrasonography that reveals the vesicles and no fetal gestational sac or cardiac action. Levels of β-hCG are also high because of the rapidly proliferating abnormal villi. Other signs and symptoms of a complete molar pregnancy vary with gestation, but may include:

- Vaginal bleeding, which varies from dark brown spotting to profuse hemorrhage
- A uterus larger than expected for the duration of the pregnancy
- Excessive nausea and vomiting, which may be related to excessive β-hCG from the proliferating trophoblasts
- Early development (before 24 weeks) of preeclampsia or eclampsia (see p. 631)

Diagnostic Evaluation

Ultrasound examination allows a differential diagnosis to be made between two types of molar pregnancies. A complete mole shows multiple small cystic structures but no fetus. Current diagnostic techniques allow early identification and treatment of a molar pregnancy rather than later, when it ends spontaneously and is more likely to be accompanied by hemorrhage.

Therapeutic Management

Management includes (1) evacuation of the mole and (2) follow-up to detect any malignant changes in the remaining trophoblastic tissue. Before evacuation, chest radiography, metabolic and blood chemistry tests, and a baseline serum β-hCG level are done. A complete blood count, laboratory assessment of clotting factors, and blood typing and cross-matching are done in case a transfusion is needed. Treatment for hypertension or hyperemesis may be needed if these added complications have occurred (Cunningham et al., 2001; Li & Karlan, 2003).

Vacuum aspiration is usually used to extract the mole. After tissue has been removed, intravenous oxytocin is used to contract the uterus. It is important to avoid uterine stimulation with oxytocin before evacuation. Uterine contractions can cause trophoblastic tissue to be drawn into the venous circulation, resulting in embolization of the vesicles. Curettage with a sharp curette follows the evacuation to remove all remaining molar tissue, and the tissue obtained is sent for laboratory evaluation to identify malignant changes.

Follow-up is critical to detect choriocarcinoma. The follow-up protocol involves evaluation of serum β-hCG levels every 1 to 2 weeks until normal prepregnancy levels are attained. The test is repeated every 1 to 2 months for up to a year and following any subsequent pregnancies (Cunningham et al., 2001; Goldstein & Berkowitz, 2000b; Li & Karlan, 2003). Pregnancy, which normally raises β-hCG levels, must be avoided during follow-up because it would obscure the evidence of choriocarcinoma.

Malignant transformation of any remaining tissue is suspected if the β-hCG levels do not fall or if they rise after an initial fall. Computed tomography (CT) of the brain, chest, abdomen, and pelvis helps identify metastases of the cancer. Chemotherapy is the primary treatment for gestational trophoblastic neoplasm (choriocarcinoma) and has a high cure rate.

Nursing Considerations

Women who have had a hydatidiform mole experience many of the same emotions as those who have had any other type of pregnancy loss. In addition, they may be anxious about the possibility of malignancy and the need to delay pregnancy.

■ NURSING CARE

The Woman With a Hemorrhagic Condition of Early Pregnancy

Nurses play a vital role in the management of early pregnancy bleeding, regardless of its cause. Nurses monitor the condition of the pregnant woman and collaborate with the physician to provide treatment.

Assessment

Confirmation of pregnancy and length of gestation is an important initial step. Physical assessment priorities are to determine the amount and character of bleeding and the description, location, and severity of pain. Estimate the amount of vaginal bleeding by examining linen and peripads. If necessary, make a more accurate estimation by weighing the linen and peripads (1 g weight equals 1 ml volume). When asking a woman how much blood she lost at home, ask her to compare the amount lost with a common measure, such as a tablespoon or a cup. Ask how long the bleeding episode lasted and what she has done to control the bleeding.

Bleeding may be accompanied by pain. Uterine cramping usually accompanies spontaneous abortion; deep, severe pelvic pain is associated with ectopic pregnancy. Remember that in ruptured ectopic pregnancy, bleeding may be concealed within the abdomen and pain is the only symptom.

Assess the woman's vital signs to determine her cardiovascular status. Check laboratory values for hemoglobin and hematocrit, and report abnormal values to the physician. Determine the Rh factor so that all women who are Rh-negative can receive $Rh_o(D)$ immune globulin (see p. 644).

Moreover, because any spontaneous abortion may be associated with infections, assess the woman for fever, malaise, and prolonged or malodorous vaginal discharge.

Determine the family's knowledge of needed follow-up care and how to prevent complications such as infection.

Nursing Diagnosis and Planning

The potential complications *prenatal bleeding* and *Infection* are collaborative problems and nursing diagnosis that should be considered in the woman who has a bleeding complication in early pregnancy. Because current diagnostic techniques allow early diagnosis before hemorrhage, a nursing diagnosis that is more commonly encountered that would apply to early bleeding disorders is

■ Deficient Knowledge: diagnostic and therapeutic procedures, signs and symptoms of additional complications, dietary measures to prevent infection, and recommended follow-up care.

Expected Outcomes: The woman will verbalize understanding of diagnostic and therapeutic procedures, signs and symptoms of additional complications, and measures to reduce the risk for infection. The woman will develop a plan for obtaining follow-up care, including signs or symptoms that should be reported.

Interventions

Providing Information About Tests and Procedures

Women and their families experience less anxiety if they understand what is happening. Explain necessary diagnostic procedures, such as transvaginal or abdominal ultrasonography. Include the purpose of the tests, their duration, and whether the procedures cause discomfort. If surgical intervention is necessary, reinforce the explanations of the physicians who will perform the surgery and administer anesthetic. Briefly describe the reasons for blood tests, such as those for determining β-hCG, hemoglobin, or hematocrit values. Explain that diagnostic and therapeutic measures are performed quickly at times to prevent excessive bleeding.

Teaching Measures to Prevent Infection

The risk for infection is greatest during the first 72 hours after spontaneous abortion or operative procedures, but most women are discharged within a few hours of uterine evacuation. To prevent infection, perineal pads should be used instead of tampons until bleeding has stopped. Teach the woman to wash her hands before and after changing perineal pads. She should consult with the physician before resuming sexual intercourse.

Providing Dietary Information

Nutrition and adequate fluid intake help maintain the body's defense against infection and help correct anemia. The woman needs foods high in iron to increase hemoglobin and hematocrit values. These foods include liver, red meat, spinach, egg yolks, carrots, and raisins. In addition, she needs foods high in vitamin C, which may increase the utilization of iron (Fagen, 2000). These foods include citrus fruits, broccoli, strawberries, cantaloupe, cabbage, and green peppers.

Iron supplements may be prescribed. Gastric upset is less severe when iron is taken with meals, and a diet that is high in fiber and fluid (2500 ml/day) helps reduce the constipation experienced by many women who take iron supplements.

Teaching Signs of Infection to Report

Teach the woman where she can buy a thermometer if she does not have one, and instruct her to take her temperature every 8 hours for the first 3 days at home. Tell her to seek medical help if her temperature goes above 37.8° C (100° F) or as instructed by her physician. She should also report to the physician additional signs of infection, such as vaginal discharge with foul odor, pelvic tenderness, or general malaise.

Emphasizing the Importance of Follow-up Care

A variety of follow-up procedures such as repeat ultrasonic examinations or repeated determinations of serum β-hCG levels may be necessary, depending on the pregnancy disorder. The couple who experiences recurrent abortions may become involved in complex investigations of immunologic or genetic abnormalities.

The nurse should help couples who experience a pregnancy loss by answering questions about the cause of the pregnancy loss. The nurse should acknowledge the couple's grief, which often manifests as anger. Many women have guilt feelings that must be recognized. They often need repeated reassurance that the loss was not caused by anything they did or by anything they neglected. Older mothers are often more concerned about pregnancy loss or the need to delay pregnancy after hydatidiform mole, because their age imposes limits for successful subsequent pregnancy. Many women will be anxious about the possible development of choriocarcinoma as well.

Evaluation

- Did the woman verbalize comprehension of diagnostic and therapeutic procedures, signs and symptoms of additional complications, and hygienic and dietary measures to support the body's healing and reduce the risk for infection?
- Did the woman develop and follow the plan of care suggested for her complication?

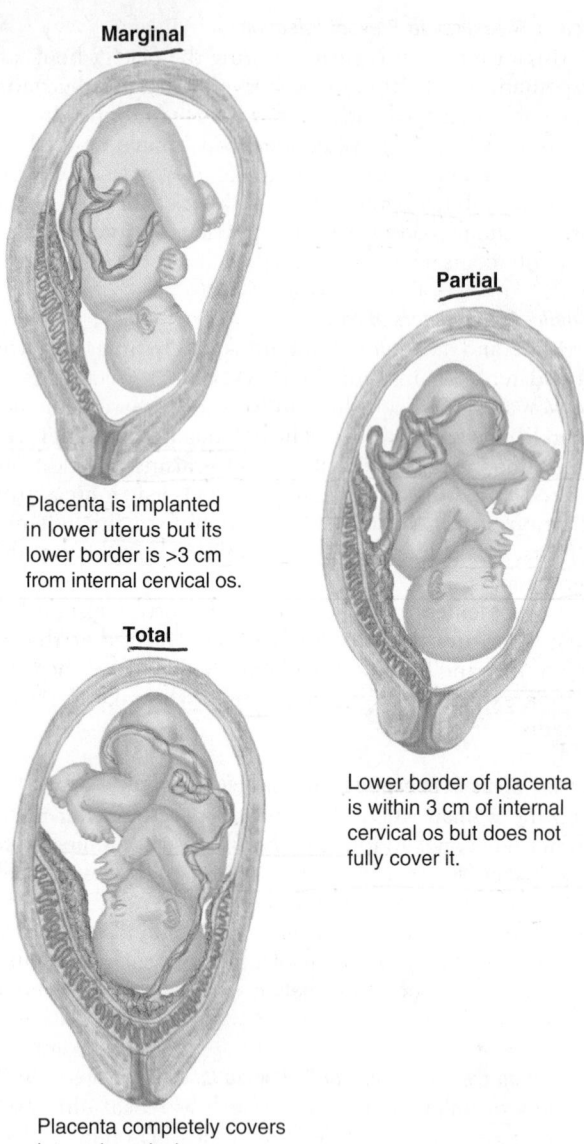

Marginal

Placenta is implanted in lower uterus but its lower border is >3 cm from internal cervical os.

Partial

Lower border of placenta is within 3 cm of internal cervical os but does not fully cover it.

Total

Placenta completely covers internal cervical os.

Figure 26-4 The three classifications of placenta previa.

HEMORRHAGIC CONDITIONS OF LATE PREGNANCY

After 20 weeks of pregnancy, the two major causes of hemorrhage are disorders of the placenta called *placenta previa* and *abruptio placentae*. Abruptio placentae may be further complicated by DIC.

Placenta Previa

Placenta previa is an implantation of the placenta in the lower uterus, near the fetal presenting part. Use of both abdominal and transvaginal ultrasound allows measurement of the distance between the internal cervical os and the lower border of the placenta to classify placenta previa (Figure 26-4):

- *Marginal* (sometimes called *low-lying*): Placenta is implanted in the lower uterus but its lower border is more than 3 cm from the internal cervical os.

- *Partial*: Lower border of the placenta is within 3 cm of the internal cervical os but does not completely cover the os.
- *Total*: Placenta completely covers internal cervical os.

Marginal placenta previa is common in early ultrasound examinations and often appears to "move" upward and away from the internal cervical os. The placenta does not move, however, but is drawn upward as the myometrium beneath it develops with pregnancy progression.

Incidence and Etiology

Placenta previa occurs in about 1 in 200 pregnancies in the United States. It is more common in older women, multiparas, women who have had cesarean births, and women who have had prior suction curettage for induced or spontaneous abortion. It is also more likely to recur if a woman had a previous placenta previa. Women of Asian or African ethnicity have an increased risk. Smoking and cocaine use are also associated with placenta previa. Placenta previa is also more likely to occur if the fetus is male (Clark, 2003).

Manifestations

The classic sign of placenta previa is the sudden onset of painless uterine bleeding in the latter half of pregnancy. Many cases of placenta previa, however, are diagnosed by ultrasound examination before the onset of bleeding. Bleeding occurs when the placental villi are torn from the uterine wall, resulting in hemorrhage from the uterine vessels. Bleeding is typically painless because it does not occur in a closed cavity and therefore does not cause pressure on adjacent tissue. Bleeding may be scanty or profuse, and it may cease spontaneously, only to recur later.

Bleeding may not occur until labor starts, when cervical changes disrupt placental attachment. The admitting nurse may be unsure whether the bleeding represents heavy "bloody show" or is a sign of a placenta previa. Also, the woman may have pain associated with the bleeding because of active labor contractions.

Digital examination of the cervical os when placenta previa is present can cause additional placental separation or can tear the placenta itself, causing severe maternal and fetal bleeding. *Until the location and position of the placenta are verified by ultrasound to determine the cause of excessive vaginal bleeding, manual examinations and administration of oxytocin to stimulate labor should be avoided. Manual vaginal examination or contraction stimulation can interrupt connections between maternal and placental vessels if the placenta is attached low in the uterus.*

Therapeutic Management

When the diagnosis of placenta previa is confirmed, medical interventions are based on the condition of the mother and fetus. The woman is evaluated carefully to determine the amount of hemorrhage, and external electronic fetal monitoring is initiated to determine if the patterns are reassuring (see Chapter 18). A third consideration is the fetal gestational age.

Options for management include conservative management if the mother's cardiovascular status is stable and the fetus is immature and has a reassuring status by monitoring and ultrasound examination. Delaying birth may increase birth weight and maturity and allow administration of corticosteroids to the mother to speed maturation of the fetal lungs.

Conservative management may take place in the home or hospital.

Home Care. Criteria for outpatient management include (Clark, 2003):

- The woman is clinically stable, with no evidence of active bleeding.
- The woman can remain on bed rest at home.
- Home is within a reasonable distance from the hospital.
- Emergency transportation is available 24 hours a day.

Nurses should help the family develop a plan of care that includes bed rest, the presence of a responsible adult at all times, and ready transportation to the hospital. Nurses must teach the mother and the family what to monitor and emphasize the importance of (1) assessing vaginal discharge or bleeding after each urination or bowel movement, or more often as needed, (2) counting fetal movements daily (see Chapter 16), (3) assessing uterine activity daily, and (4) omitting sexual intercourse to prevent disruption of the placenta. Spontaneous membrane rupture can occur at any time and with varying amounts of fluid loss, so the woman and her family should be taught to return to the hospital for evaluation. Home care nurses may provide assessments of uterine activity (cramping, regular or sporadic contractions), bleeding, fetal activity, and adherence to the prescribed treatment plan. In addition, nurses can make regular home visits for comprehensive maternal-fetal assessments with portable equipment, including nonstress tests. The family is instructed to report decreased fetal movements, uterine contractions, or increased vaginal bleeding at once.

Nurses should also provide specific, accurate information about the condition of the fetus. For example, parents are reassured when they hear that the fetal heart rate is within the expected range and daily "kick counts" are reassuring of fetal well-being. Moreover, it may be necessary for nurses to help the family understand the physician's plan of care, such as a cesarean delivery with possible blood transfusion.

Inpatient Care. Hospitalization is needed if the woman does not meet the criteria for home care. Nursing assessments in the hospital are similar to those done at home and are focused on observing the presence and character of bleeding and looking for signs of preterm labor. Periodic nonstress tests and biophysical profiles provide added information about the fetal condition. A significant change in fetal heart activity, an episode of increased vaginal bleeding, or signs of preterm labor should be reported immediately to the physician. Rupture of membranes should be reported, whether on home care or in the hospital.

At times, conservative management is not an option. For example, delivery by cesarean birth is scheduled if the fetus is 36 weeks' gestation and the lungs are mature. Immediate delivery of an immature fetus may be necessary if bleeding is excessive and does not stop, the woman's cardiovascular status is unstable, or there are signs of fetal compromise.

Nurses prepare the woman for surgery whenever cesarean birth becomes necessary (see Chapter 20). Signed consents for cesarean birth, blood transfusion, and anesthesia may be kept current for women with late pregnancy bleeding, because surgery may be required suddenly. Intravenous access is established if a woman has late pregnancy bleeding, and crossmatched blood may be kept on hold. A woman who must be hospitalized for several weeks during preterm pregnancy for ex-

cessive bleeding that is not severe enough to require immediate birth may continue intravenous access, often with a saline lock. When many emergency preparations occur at once, the nurse should constantly provide appropriate reassurance to reduce the woman's anxiety and that of her family.

Abruptio Placentae

Separation of a normally implanted placenta before the fetus is born (called *abruptio placentae*, *placental abruption*, or *premature separation of the placenta*) occurs when there is bleeding and formation of a hematoma on the maternal side of the placenta. As the clot expands, further separation occurs. The severity of the complication depends on the amount of bleeding and the size of the hematoma. The hematoma can expand and thus obliterate intervillous spaces where fetal gas and nutrient exchange occurs. Moreover, fetal vessels will be disrupted as placental separation occurs, resulting in fetal as well as maternal bleeding. Small abruptions may, however, be self-limiting.

The major danger for the woman is hemorrhage and consequent hypovolemic shock and clotting abnormalities such as DIC (see p. 619). The major dangers for the fetus are related to anoxia, blood loss, and preterm birth.

Incidence and Etiology

The incidence of abruptio placentae varies but is about 0.5% to 1% of pregnancies. However, abruptio placentae accounts for 10% to 15% of perinatal deaths. Some populations have a rising incidence because of the prevalence of cocaine use, a strong risk factor (Cunningham et al., 2001; Kay, 2003).

The cause of abruptio placentae is unknown, but several factors that increase the risk have been identified. The risk factors include maternal hypertension, maternal cigarette smoking, multigravida status, short umbilical cord, abdominal trauma, and a history of a previous premature separation of the placenta. Maternal use of cocaine, which causes vasoconstriction in the endometrial arteries, is a leading cause of abruptio placentae.

Recently identified factors that are associated with abruptio placentae can be grouped under the classification of autoimmune antibodies that result in various coagulopathies. This group includes anticardiolipin antibodies and lupus anticoagulant. Other coagulopathies may be caused by genetic factors, such as a factor V Leiden mutation. Women who have these coagulopathies have a tendency to form clots in the placenta. Hypertension, a frequent companion of abruptio placentae, occurs more frequently in women with some autoimmune disorders as well.

Manifestations

Five classic signs and symptoms of abruptio placentae are:

- Vaginal bleeding, which may not reflect the true amount of blood loss
- Abdominal and low back pain that may be described as aching or dull
- Uterine irritability with frequent low intensity contractions
- High uterine resting tone identified by use of an intrauterine pressure catheter
- Uterine tenderness that may be localized to the site of the abruption

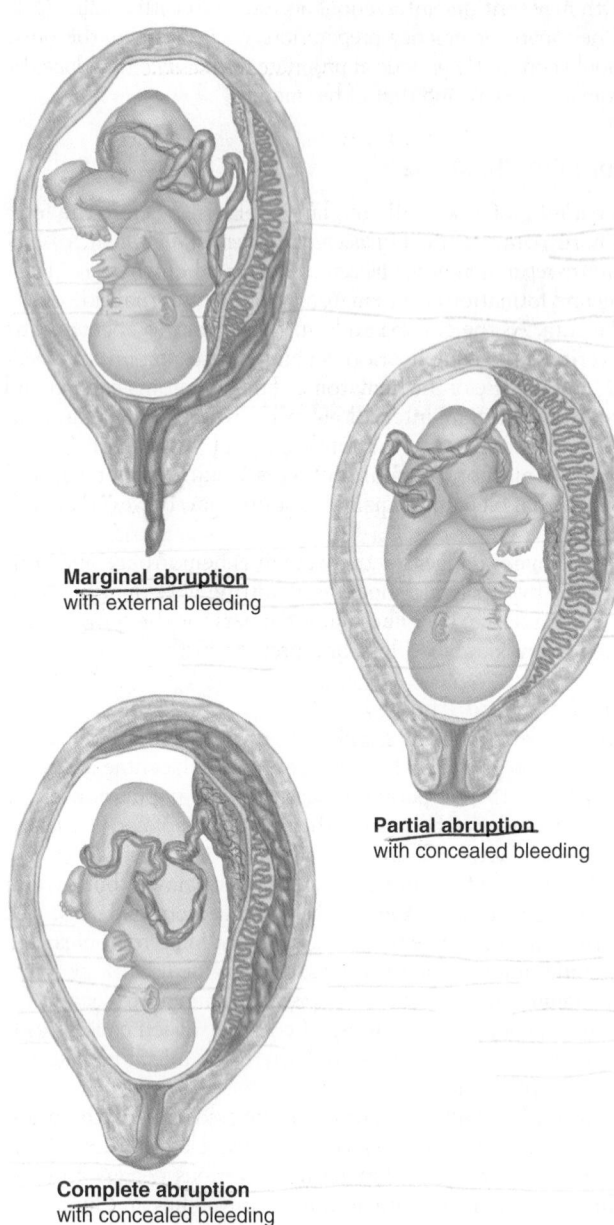

Marginal abruption
with external bleeding

Partial abruption
with concealed bleeding

Complete abruption
with concealed bleeding

Figure 26-5 Types of abruptio placentae.

Additional signs include back pain, nonreassuring fetal heart rate patterns, signs of hypovolemic shock, and fetal death.

Hemorrhage from abruptio placentae may be concealed or apparent. In either type, the placental abruption may be complete or partial. Concealed hemorrhage is bleeding that occurs behind the placenta while the margins remain intact. The hemorrhage is apparent when bleeding separates or dissects the membranes from the endometrium and blood flows out through the vagina. The amniotic fluid often has a classic "port-wine" color. Figure 26-5 illustrates variations of abruptio placentae with external and concealed bleeding. The actual amount of blood lost may be greater than the visible bleeding. Signs of maternal hypovolemia may be present when there is little or no external bleeding.

Abdominal pain is also related to the type of separation. It may be sudden and severe when there is bleeding into the myometrium (uterine muscle) or intermittent and difficult to distinguish from labor contractions. The abdomen may become exceedingly firm (boardlike) and tender, making palpation of the fetus difficult. Ultrasound examination is helpful to rule out placenta previa as the cause of bleeding, but it cannot be used to diagnose abruptio placentae because the separation and bleeding may not be obvious on ultrasonography.

Therapeutic Management

A woman who exhibits signs of abruptio placentae should be hospitalized and evaluated at once. Evaluation focuses on the condition of the fetus and the cardiovascular status of the mother. If the abruption is mild and the fetus is immature and shows no signs of distress, conservative management may be initiated. Measures include bed rest and may include administration of tocolytic medications to decrease uterine activity (Clark, 2003). Serial Kleihauer-Betke (K-B) tests determine if fetal bleeding is worsening.

Women may be observed for 24 hours after significant abdominal trauma such as a motor vehicle collision or domestic violence, because it may take this long for an abruptio placentae to develop. If they are not having contractions after the trauma and the fetal heart rate pattern is reassuring, monitoring for 4 to 6 hours may be sufficient (Clark, 2003).

If signs of fetal compromise are present or if the expectant mother or fetus exhibits signs of excessive bleeding, either obvious or concealed, immediate delivery of the fetus is necessary. Intensive monitoring of both the woman and the fetus is essential, because rapid deterioration of either can occur. One or more large-gauge intravenous lines should be placed for replacement of fluid and blood.

Nursing Considerations

If immediate cesarean delivery is necessary, the woman may feel powerless as the health care team hurriedly prepares her for surgery. If at all possible, nurses should explain anticipated procedures to the woman and her family to reduce their feelings of fear and anxiety.

! CRITICAL TO REMEMBER

Signs and Symptoms Suggesting Concealed Hemorrhage in Abruptio Placentae

- Increase in fundal height
- Hard, boardlike abdomen
- High uterine baseline tone on electronic monitoring strip
- Persistent abdominal pain
- Systemic signs of early hemorrhage (tachycardia [maternal and fetal], falling blood pressure, restlessness)
- Persistent late deceleration in fetal heart rate or decreasing baseline variability
- Vaginal bleeding that may be slight or absent

CRITICAL THINKING EXERCISE 26-1

All women who have experienced prenatal bleeding and invasive procedures are at increased risk for infection.

What common assumptions do nurses make about those who are at risk for developing infections?

Excessive bleeding and fetal hypoxia are always major concerns with abruptio placentae, and nurses are responsible for continuous monitoring of both the expectant mother and the fetus so that problems can be detected early, before the condition of the woman or the fetus deteriorates.

◾NURSING CARE

The Woman With a Hemorrhagic Condition of Late Pregnancy

Assessment

For hemorrhagic conditions of late pregnancy, medical and nursing assessments are concurrent. Some assessments are delayed if the maternal or fetal condition is not reassuring. The priority assessments are:

- *Amount and nature of bleeding*: Time of onset, estimated blood loss before admission to hospital, and description of tissue or clots passed. Peripads and underpads should be saved so that blood loss can be estimated accurately.
- *Pain:* Type (constant, intermittent, sharp, dull, severe), onset (sudden, gradual), and location (generalized over abdomen, localized). Is the uterus tender or irritable when palpated gently?
- *Maternal vital signs:* To identify hypertension or hypotension and tachycardia that occur with hypovolemia. A normal blood pressure can be misleading in a woman with abruptio placentae because she may have been hypertensive before the blood loss caused her blood pressure to fall to normal or hypotensive levels.
- *Condition of the fetus:* Application of an electronic monitor to identify trends and patterns in fetal heart rate, baseline variability, and fetal response to uterine activity (late decelerations or loss of baseline variability are of particular concern).
- *Uterine contractions:* If the membranes are ruptured, placement of an intrauterine pressure catheter allows more precise evaluation of baseline pressure and contraction intensity. Inadequate uterine relaxation, uterine irritability, and high baseline pressures (above 20 mm Hg) are common.
- *Obstetric history:* Gravida, para, previous abortions, preterm infants, previous pregnancy outcomes. History of abruptio placenta.
- *Length of gestation:* Date of last menstrual period, fundal height, correlation of fundal height with estimated gestation, results of ultrasound examinations performed during pregnancy. With bleeding into the myometrium, the fundus enlarges rapidly as bleeding progresses. A piece of tape can be used to mark the top of the fundus at a given time and then to observe and report increasing fundal size, which indicates that bleeding into uterine muscles is occurring.
- *Laboratory data:* Laboratory studies include a complete blood count and blood typing and screening. Blood crossmatching is done if transfusion is likely. Type and Rh factor identify possible need for $Rh_o(D)$ immune globulin (RhoGAM). Other tests may be done serially to identify whether the abruptio is stable or worsening. The K-B test identifies fetal blood cells in the maternal circulation. Coagulation studies include fibrinogen, fibrin split products (FSP), prothrombin and partial thromboplastin times (PT/PTT), and D dimer (a fibrin degradation fragment from fibrinolysis). A drug screen is done if illegal drug use is suspected.

Despite the emphasis on physical assessment, the emotional response of the expectant mother and her partner must also be addressed (Nursing Care Plan: Antepartum Bleeding). They will most likely be anxious, fearful, confused, and overwhelmed by the activity. They may have very little knowledge of expected medical management and may not realize that the fetus must be delivered as quickly as possible and that a surgical procedure is necessary. Moreover, they may fear for the life of the woman and the fetus. Also, the baby may be dead when the mother is admitted, adding shock and grief to their anxiety.

Nursing Diagnosis and Planning

The most dangerous potential complication is *hypovolemia*, which jeopardizes the life of the mother as well as the fetus. The nurse cannot independently manage this collaborative problem but must confer with physicians for medical orders for treatment. Planning should therefore reflect the nurse's responsibility to:

- Monitor for signs of hypovolemic shock.
- Consult the physician if signs of hypovolemic shock are observed.
- Perform actions to minimize the effects of hypovolemic shock.

Interventions

Monitoring for Signs of Hypovolemic Shock

Observe for any sign of developing hypovolemic shock. The body attempts to compensate for decreased blood volume and to maintain oxygenation of essential organs by increasing the rate and effort of the heart and lungs and by shunting blood from less essential organs. This compensatory mechanism results in the early signs and symptoms of hypovolemic shock before birth:

- Fetal tachycardia (often the first sign of either maternal or fetal hypovolemia)
- Maternal tachycardia, weak peripheral pulses
- Normal or slightly decreased blood pressure
- Increased respiratory rate
- Cool, pale skin and mucous membranes

The compensatory mechanism fails if hypovolemic shock progresses and blood volume is insufficient to perfuse the

---

❗ CRITICAL TO REMEMBER

Signs and Symptoms of Impending Hypovolemic Shock Caused by Blood Loss

- Increased pulse rate, falling blood pressure, increased respiratory rate
- Weak, diminished, or "thready" peripheral pulses
- Cool, moist skin, pallor, or cyanosis (late sign)
- Decreased urinary output (<30-ml/hr)
- Decreased hemoglobin, hematocrit levels
- Change in mental status (restlessness, agitation, difficulty concentrating)

Nursing Care Plan

Antepartum Bleeding

ASSESSMENT

Beth Dixon, a 28-year-old gravida 2, para 1, is admitted at 34 weeks' gestation after an episode of vaginal bleeding caused by total placenta previa. Vital signs are stable, and the fetal heart rate is 140-150 beats per minute with no nonreassuring signs. Beth and her husband, Bob, appear anxious about the condition of the fetus and the plan of care. Beth is particularly worried about her 5-year-old son, who is at home with a neighbor.

Nursing Diagnosis

Anxiety related to unknown effects of bleeding and lack of knowledge of predicted course of management.

Goals/Expected Outcomes

The couple will:
- Verbalize expected routines and projected management by the end of the first day after admission.
- Express less anxiety after teaching.

INTERVENTION	RATIONALE
1. Remain with the couple, and acknowledge the emotions that they exhibit: "I know this is unexpected, and you must have many questions. Perhaps I can answer some of them."	1. The nurse's presence and empathic understanding prepare the family to cope with the unexpected situation.
2. Determine the couple's level of understanding of the situation and the projected management: "Tell me what you've been told to expect."	2. Assessing understanding allows the nurse to reinforce the physician's explanations and to notify the physician if additional explanations are necessary.

3. Provide the couple with factual information about projected management. Examples of teaching may include these topics:
  a. Hospitalization, which may be necessary so that Beth's condition and the condition of the fetus can be watched closely.
  b. The necessity for a cesarean birth this time even though Beth delivered vaginally before.
  c. Information about hospital routines (meals, visiting hours) and monitoring techniques that will be used (electronic fetal monitoring, nonstress tests).
	3. Client education has proved effective in preventing and reducing anxiety.

4. Allow Beth and her family to participate in the routine as much as possible. Family involvement may mean scheduling procedures around times when Tom and their son can visit.	4. Reduces the sense of powerlessness that women often feel when they are confined to bed and a course of treatment is prescribed without consultation.

Evaluation

The interventions are judged to be successful if the couple demonstrates knowledge of the projected management, the reasons it is necessary, and how they may reduce their anxiety.

ASSESSMENT

Although Beth has no more episodes of vaginal bleeding, she cries frequently. She tells the nurse, "I miss my son so much. He just started kindergarten, and he is so shy. I feel useless, and he really needs me now. It's hard on Bob too; he has to do everything."

Nursing Diagnosis

Situational Low Self-Esteem related to temporary inability to provide care for family.

Goals/Expected Outcomes

Beth will:
- Identify positive aspects of self during hospitalization.
- Identify ways of providing comfort and affection for her son during the hospital stay.

Nursing Care Plan

Antepartum Bleeding—cont'd

INTERVENTION	RATIONALE
1. Encourage Beth to express her concerns about the need for hospitalization: "What bothers you most about being away from home?"	1. Major concerns may not be identified or may be misunderstood unless the woman clarifies them.
2. After acknowledging Beth's feelings, encourage examination of the need for hospitalization and its consequences: it provides time for the fetus to mature.	2. Careful consideration identifies positive aspects of Beth's important role in maturing her fetus.
3. Explore reality of Beth's self-appraisal ("I feel useless") by assisting her to investigate ways to provide nurturing care for her son while she is hospitalized: a. Keep in close touch by telephone (wake-up, good-night, and after-school calls). b. Make small handmade items such as bookmarks. c. Explain to him in simple, nonfrightening terms why she must stay in the hospital. d. Offer reassurances of continued love.	3. Daily involvement in the life of the older child helps reduce feelings of isolation and inability to meet needs of her family.
4. Assist Beth to involve her son in plans for the newborn. He might benefit from sibling classes or play time with his mother that involves caring for dolls.	4. Involving siblings provides goals for combined family interaction that increase feeling of self-worth. Young boys often benefit from understanding that they also can be beneficial to their new sibling's life.

Evaluation

Beth is able to make positive comments about the importance of bed rest to the health of the fetus, and she initiates numerous activities that permit her to continue close, comforting contact with her child during the period of hospitalization.

Additional Nursing Diagnoses to Consider

Interrupted Family Processes
Deficient Diversional Activity
Fear

---

brain, heart, and kidneys. Later signs of hypovolemic shock include:

- Falling blood pressure
- Pallor of skin and mucous membranes; cold, clammy skin
- Urine output less than 30 ml/hr
- Restlessness, agitation, decreased mentation

Monitoring the Fetus

Initiate continuous electronic fetal monitoring to identify nonreassuring signs that can occur as the placental surface area for gas exchange is disrupted, such as decreasing baseline variability or late decelerations (see Chapter 18). Notify the physician if nonreassuring patterns are noted, because these may occur before maternal signs of hypovolemia are obvious. The physician should be given a report on new laboratory data that suggest increasing abruptio, such as rising K-B levels.

Promoting Tissue Oxygenation

To promote oxygenation of tissues:

- Place the woman in a lateral position, with the head of the bed flat to increase cardiac return and thus to increase circulation and oxygenation of the placenta and other vital organs.

- Restrict maternal movements and activity to decrease the tissue demand for oxygen.
- Provide simple explanations, reassurance, and emotional support to the woman to help reduce anxiety, which increases the metabolic demand for oxygen.

Collaborating With the Physician for Fluid Replacement

To maintain circulating maternal blood volume:

- Insert intravenous lines, often two large-gauge catheters, to allow rapid blood replacement.
- Obtain an order for blood typing and screening (or cross-matching) so that blood is available for replacement if necessary.
- Administer fluids for replacement as directed by the physician to maintain a urinary output of at least 30 ml/hr.

Providing Emotional Support

Explain to the woman what is causing her discomfort, and reassure her that pain relief measures will be initiated as soon as possible without causing harm to the fetus. Although it is unwise to offer false reassurance about the condition of the fetus, provide accurate and timely information to the woman and her family.

Care Related to Surgery

It may be necessary to prepare the woman quickly for cesarean birth. (Care for the woman having a cesarean birth is discussed fully in Chapter 20.) Remain with the woman and her family as much as possible to provide information.

After birth, assess bleeding from the vagina as well as from any surgical sites or puncture wounds (epidural, intravenous sites). Report uncontrolled bleeding or bleeding from unexpected sites, which may indicate DIC. Perform all routine postpartum assessments as well as those related to surgery and to the hemorrhagic complication.

Evaluation

Although client-centered goals are not developed for collaborative problems, the nurse collects and compares data with established norms and judges whether the data are within normal limits. The desired outcome is that the maternal vital signs remain within normal limits and the fetal heart rate demonstrates no signs of compromise, such as late decelerations or decreasing baseline variability.

HYPEREMESIS GRAVIDARUM

Hyperemesis gravidarum is persistent, uncontrollable vomiting that begins in the first weeks of pregnancy and may continue throughout pregnancy. Hyperemesis is associated with weight loss, dehydration, acidosis from starvation, elevated blood and urine ketones, alkalosis from loss of hydrochloric acid in the gastric fluids, and hypokalemia. Short-term hepatic dysfunction with elevated liver enzymes may occur. Deficiency of vitamin K may cause coagulation disorders, and deficiency of thiamine can cause encephalopathy.

Etiology

The cause of hyperemesis gravidarum is not known, but the condition is more common among unmarried white women, during first pregnancies, and in multifetal pregnancies. Other possible causes include possible allergy to fetal proteins. Elevated levels of pregnancy-related hormones, such as estrogen and β-hCG, are considered a possible cause, as is maternal thyroid dysfunction. More recently, an association with the organism that causes peptic ulcer disease, *Helicobacter pylori* (*H. pylori*), has been associated with hyperemesis. Psychologic factors may interact with the nausea and vomiting that occurs during early pregnancy to worsen it (Buckwalter & Simpson, 2002; Cunningham et al., 2001; Gilbert & Harmon, 2003; Scott & Abu-Hamda, 2004; Weyerman et al., 2003).

Therapeutic Management

The physician will exclude other causes for persistent nausea and vomiting, such as cholecystitis or peptic ulcer disease, before diagnosing and treating hyperemesis. Laboratory studies include determining the hemoglobin and hematocrit, which may be elevated as a result of dehydration, which results in hemoconcentration. Electrolyte studies may reveal reduced sodium, potassium, and chloride. Elevated creatinine levels indicate renal dysfunction.

Treatment often occurs in the home, where the woman attempts to control the nausea by methods used for morning sickness (see Chapter 13). In addition, some physicians prescribe vitamins, such as pyridoxine (vitamin B_6), although its benefits have not been substantiated. Antiemetics, such as promethazine (Phenergan), provide some short-term relief. Drugs that act on the central nervous system, such as ondansetron (Zofran) or metoclopramide (Reglan), may be used. Ondansetron has not proven superior to promethazine, however. The steroid *methylprednisolone* has recently been found to reduce the nausea and vomiting (Magee, Mazzotta, & Koren, 2002; Modigliani, 2000).

If methods to relieve nausea and vomiting are unsuccessful and weight loss or electrolyte imbalance persists, intravenous fluid and electrolyte replacement or total parenteral nutrition may be necessary. Enteral nutrition via a feeding tube has also been used successfully (Cunningham et al., 2001).

Nursing Considerations

Physical assessment begins with determining the woman's intake and output. Intake includes intravenous fluids and parenteral nutrition as well as oral fluids and nutrition, which is allowed once vomiting is controlled. A description of the output includes the amount and character of emesis and urinary output. As a rule of thumb, the normal urinary output is about 1 ml/kg (2.2 lb)/hr. A record of bowel elimination also provides significant information about oral nutrition because bowel movements will be decreased and hard with dehydration. Findings associated with dehydration include decreased fluid intake (<2000 ml/day), decreased urinary output, increased urine specific gravity (>1.025), dry skin or dry mucous membranes, and nonelastic skin turgor.

The woman should be weighed daily during acute illness and her urine tested for ketones. Weight loss and the presence of ketones in the urine suggest that fat stores and protein are being metabolized to meet energy needs. Consultation with a dietitian is indicated.

Nursing interventions focus on reducing nausea and vomiting, maintaining nutrition and fluid balance, and providing emotional support.

Reducing Nausea and Vomiting

Food portions should be small so that the amount does not appear overwhelming. Present foods attractively, and eliminate foods with strong odors because nausea is often associated with food smells. Low-fat foods and easily digested carbohydrates, such as fruit, breads, cereals, rice, and pasta, provide important nutrients and help prevent low blood sugar, which can cause nausea. Soups and other liquids should be taken between meals so as not to overly distend the stomach and trigger vomiting. Sitting upright after meals reduces the frequency of gastric reflux.

Maintaining Nutrition and Fluid Balance

Intravenous fluids and total parenteral nutrition are administered as directed by the physician. Small oral feedings of clear liquids are started when nausea and vomiting begin to subside. When oral fluids are tolerated, parenteral fluids and nutrition are gradually discontinued. Any inability to tolerate oral feedings or continued episodes of vomiting should be reported to the physician so that continued parenteral fluids and nutrition can be prescribed.

Women with nausea and vomiting should eat every 2 to 3 hours. Salting food helps replace chloride lost when hy-

TABLE **26-1** Classifications of Hypertension in Pregnancy

Classification	Comments
Preeclampsia	Systolic blood pressure ≥140 mm Hg or diastolic blood pressure ≥90 mm Hg that develops after 20 weeks of pregnancy and is accompanied by proteinuria >0.3 g in a 24-hr urine collection (random urine dipstick is usually ≥1+).
Eclampsia	Progression of preeclampsia to generalized seizures that cannot be attributed to other causes.
Gestational hypertension	Systolic blood pressure ≥140 mm Hg or diastolic blood pressure ≥90 mm Hg that develops after 20 weeks of pregnancy, but without significant proteinuria (negative or trace on a random urine dipstick).
Chronic hypertension	Systolic blood pressure ≥140 mm Hg or diastolic blood pressure ≥90 mm Hg that was known to exist before pregnancy or develops before 20 weeks of gestation. Also diagnosed if the hypertension does not resolve during the postpartum period.
Preeclampsia superimposed on chronic hypertension	Development of new-onset proteinuria >0.3 g in a 24-hr collection in a woman who has chronic hypertension. In women who had proteinuria before 20 weeks, preeclampsia should be suspected if the woman has a sudden increase in proteinuria from her baseline levels, a sudden increase in blood pressure when it had been previously well controlled, development of thrombocytopenia (platelets <100,000/mm³), or abnormal elevations of liver enzymes (AST or ALT).

AST, Aspartate aminotransferase (formerly SGOT); *ALT,* alanine aminotransferase (formerly SGPT).

drochloric acid is vomited. Potassium- and magnesium-rich foods should be encouraged because these nutrients are likely to be depleted and magnesium deficiency can exacerbate nausea.

Providing Emotional Support

The woman with hyperemesis gravidarum needs the opportunity to express how it feels to be pregnant and to live with everpresent nausea, but these women often experience a curious lack of sympathy and support. This attitude may stem from reports that the cause of hyperemesis gravidarum is always psychologic. In addition, observation of the woman and her family may provide clues about family dynamics that may be contributing to her response to nausea of pregnancy. Observation may identify whether anticipation of nausea is a trigger. Whatever the cause, nurses must use critical thinking to examine their own beliefs and biases so that they can provide comfort and support. Case conferences and educational programs help nurses overcome preset beliefs and meet the woman's needs.

HYPERTENSION DURING PREGNANCY

The terminology used to describe hypertension in pregnancy is often nonuniform and confusing. In an effort to standardize classifications of hypertension occurring during pregnancy and to identify the best management, the National Heart, Lung, and Blood Institute assembled a working group to update older recommendations (Table 26-1).

Four categories of hypertensive disorders occurring during pregnancy were identified by a group working within the National Heart, Lung, & Blood Institute of the National Institutes of Health for the United States (2001):

- *Preeclampsia:* A systolic blood pressure of ≥140 mm Hg or diastolic blood pressure of ≥90 mm Hg occurring after 20 weeks of pregnancy that is accompanied by significant proteinuria (>0.3 g in a 24-hr urine collection, which usually correlates with a random urine dipstick evaluation of ≥1+). Edema, although common in preeclampsia, is now

considered to be nonspecific because it occurs in many pregnancies not complicated by hypertension.
- *Eclampsia:* Progression of preeclampsia to generalized seizures that cannot be attributed to other causes. Seizures may occur postpartum.
- *Gestational hypertension:* Blood pressure elevation after 20 weeks of pregnancy that is not accompanied by proteinuria. Gestational hypertension must be considered a working diagnosis because it may progress to preeclampsia. If gestational hypertension persists after birth, chronic hypertension is diagnosed.
- *Chronic hypertension:* The elevated blood pressure was known to exist before pregnancy. Unrecognized chronic hypertension may not be diagnosed until well after the end of pregnancy.

Preeclampsia

Preeclampsia affects about 5% to 8% of women in the United States each year, although its incidence varies. It is a major cause of perinatal death and is often associated with intrauterine fetal growth restriction (IUGR).

Risk Factors

Although the cause of preeclampsia is unknown, several factors increase a woman's risk that the condition will develop. Many risk factors are interrelated, such as overweight and prepregnancy diabetes.

Preeclampsia is most likely to occur in a first pregnancy, in women older than 35 years, in African-Americans, in those with a positive family history, and in those with chronic hypertension or renal disease. Overweight increases a woman's risk as it does for chronic hypertension. Women with diabetes or multifetal gestations are also more likely to have preeclampsia. Presence of immunologic disorders, such as lupus or antiphospholipid antibody syndrome, adds to the risk for preeclampsia that is often severe.

The father's contribution also appears to play a role in development of preeclampsia. Women who had prior pregnancies without hypertension are more likely to have preeclampsia if a new partner has previously fathered a pregnancy in another woman that was complicated by the disorder.

Pathophysiology

Preeclampsia is the result of generalized vasospasm. The underlying cause of the vasospasm remains a mystery, but some of the physiologic processes are known. In a normal pregnancy, vascular volume is significantly increased and cardiac output is increased. Despite these factors, blood pressure does not rise in a normal pregnancy, probably because pregnant women develop resistance to the effects of vasoconstrictors such as angiotensin II. Moreover, a decrease in peripheral vascular resistance occurs from the effects of certain vasodilators, such as prostacyclin (PGI$_2$), prostaglandin E (PGE), and endothelium-derived relaxing factor (EDRF).

In preeclampsia, however, peripheral vascular resistance increases because of the sensitivity of some women to angiotensin II and a decrease in vasodilators. For instance, there is an increase in the ratio of thromboxane A$_2$ to prostacyclin. Thromboxane, produced by kidney and trophoblastic tissue, causes vasoconstriction and platelet aggregation (clumping). Prostacyclin, produced by placental tissue and endothelial cells, causes vasodilation and inhibits platelet aggregation.

Vasoconstriction decreases the diameter of blood vessels, which results in endothelial cell damage and decreased EDRF. Vasoconstriction also results in impeded blood flow and elevated blood pressure. As a result, circulation to all body organs, including the kidneys, liver, brain, and placenta, is decreased. The following changes are most significant:

- Decreased renal perfusion reduces the glomerular filtration rate. Consequently, blood urea nitrogen, creatinine, and uric acid levels rise.
- Glomerular damage secondary to reduced renal blood flow allows protein to leak across the glomerular membrane.
- Loss of protein from the kidneys reduces colloid osmotic pressure and allows fluid to shift to interstitial spaces. This fluid shift may result in relative hypovolemia, which causes increased viscosity of the blood and a rise in hematocrit. Generalized edema often occurs.
- In response to hypovolemia, additional angiotensin II and aldosterone are secreted to trigger the retention of both sodium and water. The pathologic processes spiral: additional angiotensin II results in further vasospasm and hypertension; aldosterone increases fluid retention, and edema is worsened.
- Decreased circulation to the liver impairs liver function and leads to hepatic edema and subcapsular hemorrhage, which can result in hemorrhagic necrosis. This process is manifested by elevated liver enzyme levels in maternal serum. Epigastric pain is a common symptom.
- Vasoconstriction of cerebral vessels leads to pressure-induced rupture of thin-walled capillaries, resulting in small cerebral hemorrhages. Signs and symptoms of arterial vasospasm include headache and visual disturbances, such as blurred vision and "spots" before the eyes, as well as hyperreflexia.
- Decreased colloid oncotic pressure can lead to pulmonary capillary leaks that result in pulmonary edema. Dyspnea is the primary symptom.
- Decreased placental circulation results in infarctions that increase the risk for abruptio placentae and DIC. In addition, the fetus may experience IUGR and persistent fetal hypoxemia.

Preventive Measures

Although it does not prevent preeclampsia, early and regular prenatal care with attention to the pattern of weight gain as well as careful monitoring of blood pressure and urinary protein may minimize maternal and fetal morbidity and mortality.

Past attempts at prevention have included low-dose aspirin, calcium and magnesium supplements, and fish oil supplements. These measures have not proven to be beneficial for the general population, however.

More recent research assessed the benefits of antioxidant therapy with 1000 mg of vitamin C and 400 IU of vitamin E starting at 22 weeks. Although the results were promising, safety and effectiveness of antioxidant supplementation for the general population requires further study (National Heart, Lung, and Blood Institute, 2001).

Manifestations

Classic Signs. The first indication of preeclampsia is usually hypertension. Blood pressure measurements vary with the woman's position, so the blood pressure should be measured uniformly at each office visit. Blood pressure should be measured with the woman seated and her arm supported, and the cuff size should be appropriate for the size of her arm. The diastolic pressure should be recorded at Korotkoff phase V, disappearance of sound (National High Blood Pressure Education Program Working Group on High Blood Pressure in Pregnancy, 2000). Hospitalizing the woman for serial observations of her blood pressure may identify true elevations from those induced by anxiety.

Proteinuria can be identified by using a clean-catch specimen to prevent contamination of the specimen by vaginal secretions or blood. Women with a urinary tract infection often have erythrocytes and leukocytes in the urine, which would elevate urine protein in the absence of preeclampsia.

Additional Signs. When the retina is examined, vascular constriction and narrowing of the small arteries are obvious in most women with preeclampsia. The vasoconstriction that can be seen in the retina is occurring throughout the body. Deep tendon reflexes may be very brisk (hyperreflexia), suggesting cerebral irritability secondary to decreased circulation and edema.

Laboratory studies may identify liver, renal, and hepatic dysfunction if preeclampsia is severe. Coagulation may be impaired as evidenced by a fall in platelets, which are often in the high normal range in a woman without preeclampsia. See also disseminated intravascular coagulation, p. 619.

Although it is a nonspecific sign that may have many causes, generalized edema often occurs with preeclampsia and it may be severe. Edema may first present as a rapid weight gain caused by fluid retention. Edema may be present in the lower legs, which is common in pregnancy, and in the hands and face (Fig. 26-6). Edema may be so massive that the woman's appearance is distorted. Edema may not, however, be present in all women who develop preeclampsia, and it may be severe in women who do not have the disorder. Pulmonary edema is also more common in women with massive edema from any cause, including drug therapy such as that given to stop preterm labor.

Symptoms. Preeclampsia is dangerous for the expectant mother and fetus for two reasons: (1) it can develop and progress rapidly; and (2) the early symptoms are not often noticed by the woman or may be attributed to other causes. By the time she experiences symptoms, the disease has often progressed to an advanced state and valuable treatment time has been lost.

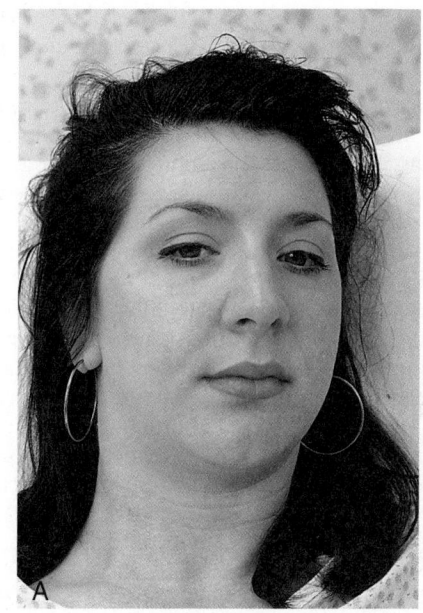
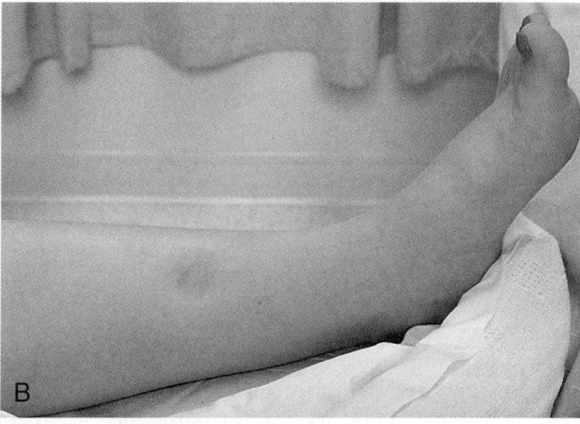

Figure 26-6 Generalized edema is a possible sign identified with preeclampsia although it may occur in both normal pregnancy or in a pregnancy complicated by another disorder. **A,** Facial edema may be subtle. **B,** Pitting edema of the lower leg.

Certain symptoms, such as continuous headache, drowsiness, or mental confusion, indicate poor cerebral perfusion and may be precursors of convulsions. Visual disturbances, such as blurred or double vision or spots before the eyes, indicate arterial spasms and edema in the retina. Some symptoms, such as epigastric pain or "upset stomach," are particularly ominous because they indicate distention of the hepatic capsule and often warn that a convulsion is imminent. Decreased urinary output indicates poor perfusion of the kidneys and may precede acute renal failure.

Therapeutic Management

Preeclampsia may be categorized as either mild or severe, depending on the frequency and intensity of presenting signs and symptoms (Table 26-2). Because the disease may progress rapidly, however, an apparently mild condition can become severe in a very short time or it may progress to eclampsia from mild disease.

Delivery is the only definitive treatment but may not be practical if preeclampsia is mild and the fetus is immature.

TABLE **26-2** Mild Versus Severe Preeclampsia

Parameter Evaluated	Mild	Severe
Systolic blood pressure	≥140 but <160 mm Hg	≥160 mm Hg (2 readings, 6 hours apart, while on bed rest)
Diastolic blood pressure	≥90 but <110 mm Hg	≥110 mm Hg
Proteinuria (24-hr specimen is preferred to eliminate hour-to-hour variations)	≥0.3 g but <2 g in 24-hr specimen (1+ on random dipstick)	≥5 g in 24-hr specimen (3+ or higher on random dipstick sample)
Creatinine, serum (renal function)	Normal	Elevated (>1.2 mg/dl)
Platelets	Normal	Decreased (<100,000 cells/mm³)
Liver enzymes (alanine aminotransferase [ALT] or aspartate aminotransferase [AST])	Normal or minimal increase in levels	Elevated levels
Urine output	Normal	Oliguria common, often <500 ml/day
Severe, unrelenting headache not attributable to other cause; mental confusion (cerebral edema)	Absent	Often present
Persistent right upper quadrant or epigastric pain or pain penetrating to the back (distention of the liver capsule); nausea and vomiting	Absent	May be present and often precedes seizure
Visual disturbances (spots or "sparkles"; temporary blindness; photophobia)	Absent to minimal	Common
Pulmonary edema; heart failure; cyanosis	Absent	May be present
Fetal growth restriction	Normal growth	Growth restriction; reduced amniotic fluid volume

From American Academy of Pediatrics, & American College of Obstetricians and Gynecologists. (2002). *Guidelines for perinatal care* (5th ed.). Elk Grove, IL: Author; National High Blood Pressure Education Program Working Group on High Blood Pressure in Pregnancy. (2000). Report of the national high blood pressure education program working group on high blood pressure in pregnancy. *American Journal of Obstetrics and Gynecology,* 183(1), S1-S22.

If the fetus is less than 34 weeks of gestation, steroids to accelerate fetal lung maturity will be given and an attempt made to delay birth for 48 hours. However, if the maternal or fetal condition deteriorates, the woman will be delivered, regardless of fetal age or administration of steroids. Vaginal birth is preferred because of the multisystem impairments.

Home Care for Mild Preeclampsia. Initial evaluation of the severity of preeclampsia will be done in the hospital. Home management is possible if preeclampsia is mild, if the woman and fetus are in stable condition, and if she can adhere to the treatment plan and follow-up visits every 3 to 4 days. The woman on home care should be taught blood pressure assessment and the signs of worsening preeclampsia, such as visual disturbance, severe headache, or epigastric pain. She must also be taught signs that suggest nonreassuring fetal status, such as diminished movements (see Chapter 16), and signs and symptoms that suggest onset of labor (see Chapter 17). If any of these occur, she should return to the hospital or clinic.

Activity Restrictions. Activity is usually restricted, although full bed rest is not required. The woman will most likely need to stop working for the duration of home management. Lying down for at least $1^1/_2$ hours per day in a side-lying position maximizes placental blood flow.

Fetal Activity. The woman often keeps a record of fetal movements, also called a "kick count" (see Chapter 16). She should report a significant decrease in movements or if no movement is felt during a 4-hour period.

Blood Pressure. The family must be taught to use electronic blood pressure equipment, readily available in drug, grocery, and discount stores. Blood pressure should be checked two to four times per day in the same arm and with the woman in the same position. For accuracy, a large cuff should be used for the woman with a large upper arm.

Weight. The woman should weigh herself each morning, preferably on the same scale and in clothing of similar weight.

Urinalysis. A urine dipstick test for protein, using the first voided midstream specimen, should be performed daily. The physician may request that she test at other times also.

Diet. A regular diet without salt or fluid restriction is usually prescribed. Women who also have chronic hypertension or diabetes should have diet management appropriate to these disorders.

Fetal Assessment. Fetal surveillance includes sonography for fetal growth and quantity of amniotic fluid or as part of a biophysical profile (BPP). A diminishing amount of amniotic fluid suggests placental impairment. If the pregnancy is less than 34 completed weeks and delivery is being considered, amniocentesis is often done to evaluate fetal lung maturity.

Inpatient Management for Severe Preeclampsia. Preeclampsia is severe if the systolic blood pressure is ≥160 mm Hg or the diastolic blood pressure is ≥110 mm Hg or if evidence of multisystem involvement is present (see Table 26-2). Delivery is usually necessary, even if the gestation is less than 34 weeks, because of disease severity.

Antepartum Management. The woman will be hospitalized for assessment and management. The goals of management are to prevent convulsions and to maintain the pregnancy until it is safe to deliver the fetus.

Bed Rest. The hospitalized woman is kept on bed rest, and her environment is kept quiet. External stimuli (lights, noise) that might precipitate a convulsion should be reduced.

Anticonvulsant Medications. Magnesium sulfate ($MgSO_4$) is the drug most commonly used to prevent convulsion. Magnesium acts as a central nervous system (CNS) depressant by blocking neuromuscular transmission and decreasing the amount of acetylcholine liberated. Magnesium is not an antihypertensive medication, but it relaxes smooth muscle, in-

---

Drug Guide

Magnesium Sulfate

Classification: Miscellaneous anticonvulsant.

Action: Decreases acetylcholine released by motor nerve impulses, thereby blocking neuromuscular transmission. Depresses the central nervous system (CNS) to act as an anticonvulsant; also decreases frequency and intensity of uterine contractions. Produces flushing and sweating due to decreased peripheral blood pressure.

Indications: Prevention and control of seizures in severe preeclampsia. Prevention of uterine contractions in preterm labor.

Dosage and Route: A common intravenous (IV) administration protocol for preeclampsia includes a loading dose and a continuous infusion. The loading dose is 4 to 6 g magnesium sulfate administered in 100 ml IV fluid over 15-20 minutes. The continuing infusion to maintain control is 2 g/hr. Doses are individualized for some women. Deep intramuscular (IM) injection is acceptable but is painful.

Magnesium sulfate may also be administered in a similar dose profile to stop preterm labor contractions.

Absorption: Immediate onset following IV administration.

Excretion: Excreted by the kidneys.

Contraindications and Precautions: Contraindicated in persons with myocardial damage, heart block, myasthenia gravis, or impaired renal function. Magnesium toxicity, possibly related to incomplete renal drug excretion, may be evidenced by thirst, mental confusion, or decrease in reflexes.

Adverse Reactions: Result from magnesium overdose and include flushing, sweating, hypotension, depressed deep tendon reflexes, and CNS depression, including respiratory depression.

Nursing Implications: Monitor blood pressure closely during administration. Assess client for respiratory rate of at least 12 breaths per minute, presence of deep tendon reflexes, and urinary output greater than 30 ml/hr before administering magnesium. Place resuscitation equipment (suction, oxygen) in the room. Keep calcium gluconate, which acts as an antidote to magnesium, in the room along with syringes and needles.

cluding the uterus, and thus reduces vasoconstriction, possibly resulting in modest blood pressure reduction. Decreased vasoconstriction promotes circulation to the vital organs of the expectant mother and increases placental circulation. Increased circulation to the maternal kidneys leads to diuresis, as interstitial fluid is shifted into the vascular compartment and excreted.

Magnesium is usually administered by intravenous infusion, which allows for immediate onset of action and does not cause the discomfort associated with intramuscular administration. Intravenous magnesium is administered via a secondary ("piggyback") line so that the medication can be discontinued at any time while the primary line remains functional.

Although magnesium sulfate is not risk-free, the major advantage of magnesium is its long record of safety for mother and baby while preventing maternal convulsions (Roberts, 2004). Fetal magnesium levels are nearly identical with those of the expectant mother. As a result, the fetal monitor tracing may show decreased fetal heart rate variability. No cumulative effect occurs, however, because the fetal kidneys excrete magnesium effectively.

The therapeutic serum level for magnesium is 4 to 8 mg/dl. Adverse reactions to magnesium sulfate usually occur if the serum level becomes too high. The most important is CNS depression, including depression of the respiratory center. Magnesium is excreted solely by the kidneys, and the reduced urine output that often occurs in preeclampsia allows magnesium to accumulate to toxic levels in the woman. Frequent assessment of serum levels, deep tendon reflexes (Procedure 26-1), and respiratory rate and oxygen saturation can identify CNS depression before it progresses to respiratory depression or cardiac dysfunction. Monitoring urine output identifies oliguria that could allow magnesium to accumulate and reach excessive levels.

Antihypertensive Medications. If the woman's systolic blood pressure is ≥160 mm Hg or her diastolic blood pressure is ≥110 mm Hg, the risk for stroke or congestive heart failure is higher. Hydralazine (Apresoline) is commonly used because of its record of safety. Hydralazine's major advantage over other antihypertensives is that it is a vasodilator that increases cardiac output and blood flow to the placenta. Other antihypertensive medications such as nifedipine (a calcium channel blocker) or labetalol (a beta-adrenergic blocker) may be used.

Intrapartum Management. Most seizures occur during labor and the postpartum period. During labor, the woman must be monitored continuously to detect signs of imminent convulsions. She should be kept in a lateral position to promote circulation through the placenta, and pain that may cause agitation and precipitate seizures should be controlled. Narcotic analgesics or epidural analgesia may be administered to reduce pain that could precipitate a convulsion.

Induction of labor by intravenous oxytocin is done if the maternal or fetal condition deteriorates. Vaginal birth is usually the first choice because depression of coagulation factors and other multisystem involvement adds to the surgical risk for cesarean birth. Oxytocin to stimulate uterine contractions and magnesium sulfate to prevent convulsions are often administered simultaneously during labor. The woman will have two secondary infusions in addition to her primary infusion: one for oxytocin and one for magnesium.

Continuous electronic fetal monitoring identifies fetal heart rate patterns that suggest compromise. If nonreassuring patterns occur, the corrective actions depend on the pattern identified (see Chapter 18). Late decelerations, associated with reduced placental perfusion, or decreased variability, associated with reduced placental perfusion or magnesium use, is more likely to occur, but any other nonreassuring pattern may occur as well.

A pediatrician, neonatologist, or neonatal nurse practitioner must be available to care for the newborn at birth.

Postpartum Management. After birth, careful assessment of the mother's blood loss and signs of shock is essential because the hypovolemia caused by preeclampsia may be aggravated by blood loss during the delivery. Assessments for signs and symptoms of preeclampsia must be continued for at least 48 hours, and magnesium may be continued to prevent seizures.

Signs that the woman is recovering from preeclampsia are:

- Urinary output of 4 to 6 L/day, which causes a rapid reduction in edema and rapid weight loss
- Decreased protein in the urine
- Return of blood pressure to normal, usually within 2 weeks

Management of Eclampsia. Eclampsia is a potentially preventable extension of severe preeclampsia marked by onset of one or more generalized seizures. Early identification of preeclampsia in a pregnant woman allows intervention before the condition reaches the seizure stage in most cases. Generalized seizures usually start with facial twitching, followed by rigidity of the body. Tonic-clonic movements then begin and last for about 1 minute. Breathing stops during a seizure but resumes with a long, noisy inhalation. The woman is temporarily in a coma and is unlikely to remember the seizure when she resumes consciousness. Transient fetal heart rate patterns may be nonreassuring, such as bradycardia, loss of variability, or late decelerations. Fetal tachycardia may occur as the fetus compensates for the period of maternal apnea during the seizures. Eclampsia may occur during pregnancy or in the intrapartum or postpartum period.

Magnesium is the drug of choice to control eclamptic seizures. Other anticonvulsants or sedatives are not routinely given.

The woman's blood volume is usually severely contracted in eclampsia, increasing the risk for poor placental perfusion. Fluid shifts from her intravascular space to the interstitial space, including the lungs, causing pulmonary edema and possibly heart failure as forward blood flow is impeded. Renal blood flow is severely reduced, with oliguria (<30 ml/hr urine output) and possible renal failure. Cerebral hemorrhage may accompany eclampsia because of the high blood pressure and coagulation deficits. The woman's lungs should be auscultated at regular intervals, usually hourly. A pulse oximeter provides continuous readings of oxygen saturation. Furosemide (Lasix) may be administered if pulmonary edema develops. Oxygen by facemask at 8 to 10 L/min improves maternal and fetal oxygenation. Digitalis may be needed to strengthen contraction of the heart if circulatory failure results. Urine output should be assessed hourly; if output drops below 30 ml/hr, renal failure should be suspected.

Because eclampsia stimulates uterine irritability, the woman should be monitored carefully for ruptured membranes, signs of labor, or abruptio placentae. While the

Procedure 26-1

Assessing Deep Tendon Reflexes

PURPOSE: To identify exaggerated reflexes (hyperreflexia) or diminished reflexes (hyporeflexia).

1. You will need a reflex hammer to best assess both the brachial and the patellar reflex.
2. Support the woman's arm and instruct her to let it go limp while it is being held so that the arm is totally relaxed and slightly flexed as you assess the brachial reflex. If you have difficulty identifying the correct tendon to tap, have the woman flex and extend her arm until you can feel it moving beneath your thumb. Have her fully relax her arm after you identify the tendon.
3. Place your thumb over the woman's tendon, as illustrated, to allow you to feel as well as see the tendon response when it is tapped. Strike the thumb with the small end of the reflex hammer. The normal response is slight flexion of the forearm.

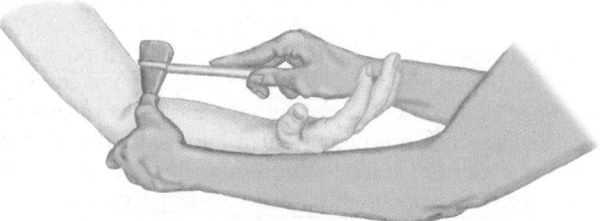

4. The patellar, or "knee-jerk," reflex can be assessed with the woman in two positions, sitting or lying. When the woman is sitting, allow her lower legs to dangle freely to flex the knee and stretch the tendons. If her patellar tendon is difficult to identify, have her flex and extend her lower legs slightly until you palpate the tendon. Strike the tendon directly with the reflex hammer just below the patella. The patellar reflex is less reliable if the woman has had epidural analgesia, and upper extremity reflexes should be assessed.

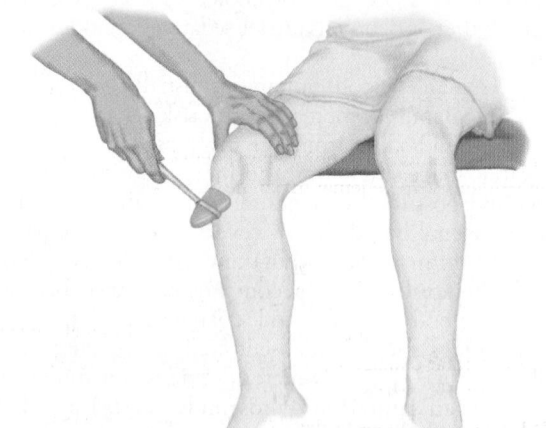

5. When the woman is supine, the weight of her leg must be supported to flex the knee and stretch the tendons. An accurate response requires that the limb be relaxed and the tendon partially stretched. Strike the partially stretched tendons just below the patella. Slight extension of the leg or a brief twitch of the quadriceps muscle of the thigh is the expected response.

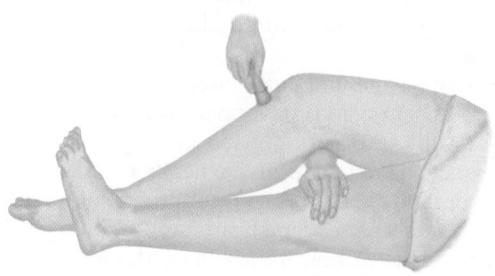

6. To assess clonus, the woman's lower leg should be supported, as illustrated, and the foot well dorsiflexed to stretch the tendon. Hold the flexion. If no clonus is present, no movement will be felt. When clonus (indicating hyperreflexia) is present, rapid rhythmic tapping motions of the foot are present.

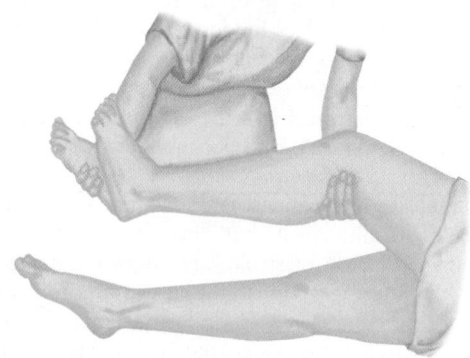

Deep Tendon Reflex Rating Scale

0:	Reflex absent
+1:	Reflex present, hypoactive
+2:	Normal reflex
+3:	Brisker than average reflex
+4:	Hyperactive reflex; clonus may also be present

NOTE: The rating scales of some facilities may omit the plus signs

woman is unresponsive, she should be kept on her side to prevent aspiration and to improve placental circulation. The side rails should be padded and raised to prevent an injury from a fall. When vital signs have stabilized, delivery of the fetus should be considered.

Aspiration of gastric contents is a leading cause of maternal morbidity after an eclamptic seizure. After initial stabilization, the nurse should anticipate orders for chest radiography and arterial blood gas determination to identify aspiration.

▪Nursing Care

The Woman With Preeclampsia

Assessment

The frequency of assessments will vary according to the severity of the woman's preeclampsia. Weigh her on admission and then daily. Check vital signs every 4 hours, and auscultate the chest for moist breath sounds that suggest pulmonary edema. Assess the location and severity of edema at least every 4 hours. Table 26-3 describes a useful method for describing edema if it is present. Measure urine output hourly. An indwelling catheter is often ordered. Check the urine for protein every 4 hours. Apply an electronic fetal monitor to identify changes in fetal heart rate or variability, which suggest poor placental perfusion or other problems.

Check brachial, radial, and patellar reflexes for hyperreflexia, which indicates cerebral irritability. Clonus (rapidly alternating muscle contraction and relaxation) may be present when reflexes are hyperactive. Procedure 26-1 details how to assess and rate deep tendon reflexes.

Question the woman carefully about symptoms she may be experiencing, such as headache, visual disturbances, epigastric pain, nausea or vomiting, or a sudden increase in edema.

An open-ended question such as "How do you feel?" may not be adequate. Ask targeted questions, such as "Do you have a headache? Describe it for me." "Do you have any pain in the abdomen? Show me where it is, and describe it." "Have you had an upset stomach or vomiting?" "Do you see spots before your eyes? Flashes of light? Double vision?" "Is your vision blurred?" "Does light bother your eyes?" "Have you had an increase in swelling? Where is it located? When did you notice it?"

Assessments for Magnesium Toxicity

Obstetrical units have protocols that address routine assessments when magnesium is being administered and their frequency. Hypotonic or absent reflexes indicate CNS depression that precedes respiratory depression. Determining the respiratory rate and oxygen saturations by pulse oximetry identifies the adequacy of maternal respirations. Checking urine output identifies oliguria (<30 ml/hr) that may result in magnesium toxicity as the drug accumulates. Assess the woman's level of consciousness (alert, drowsy [expected], confused, oriented). Table 26-4 summarizes nursing assessments and their implications

Psychosocial Assessment

The development of preeclampsia places a great deal of stress on the childbearing family. The woman may be on bed rest at home or hospitalized for some time. This situation creates

---

TABLE 26-3 Assessment of Edema

Characteristics	Grade
Minimal edema of lower extremities	+1
Marked edema of lower extremities	+2
Edema of lower extremities, face, hands, and sacral area	+3
Generalized massive edema that includes ascites (accumulation of fluid in peritoneal cavity)	+4

TABLE 26-4 Nursing Assessments for Preeclampsia and Magnesium Toxicity

Assessment	Implications
Daily weight	Provides estimate of fluid retention.
Blood pressure	To determine worsening condition, response to treatment, or both.
Respiratory rate, pulse oximeter readings	Drug therapy (MgSO$_4$) causes respiratory depression, and drug should be withheld and the physician notified if respiratory rate is <12/min or as specified by hospital policy. Pulse oximeter readings 95% or greater.
Breath sounds	To identify sounds of excess moisture in lungs associated with pulmonary edema
Deep tendon reflexes	Hyperreflexia indicates increased cerebral irritability and edema; hyporeflexia is associated with magnesium excess.
Edema	For estimation of interstitial fluid.
Urinary output	Output of at least 30 ml/hr indicates adequate perfusion of the kidneys. (25 ml/hr is used by some authorities.) Toxic magnesium levels may occur if urinary output is inadequate.
Urine protein	Normal protein in a random dipstick urine sample is negative or trace. Higher protein levels suggest greater leaking of protein secondary to glomerular damage with worsening preeclampsia. A 24-hour urine sample is most accurate for quantitative urine protein level.
Level of consciousness	Drowsiness or dulled sensorium indicates therapeutic effects of magnesium; no responsive behavior or muscle weakness is associated with magnesium excess.
Headache, epigastric pain, visual problems	These symptoms indicate increasing severity of the condition caused by cerebral edema, vasospasm of cerebral vessels, and liver edema. Eclampsia may develop quickly.
Fetal heart rate and baseline variability	Rate should be between 110 and 160 BPM in a term fetus. Decreasing baseline variability may be caused by therapeutic magnesium level or by inadequate placental perfusion.
Laboratory data	Elevated serum creatinine, elevated liver enzymes, or decreased platelets (thrombocytopenia) are significant signs of increasing severity of disease. Serum magnesium levels should be in the therapeutic range designated by the physician.

anxiety about the condition of the fetus as well as that of the expectant mother. Moreover, many families do not understand the seriousness of the disease; after all, the woman feels well initially.

Investigate how the family will function while the expectant mother is hospitalized or on bed rest at home. Determine how the woman is adapting to the "sick role" and the necessity of depending on others instead of functioning in her primary role. Ask how much support is available and who is willing to participate. Finally, determine the major concerns of the family.

Nursing Diagnosis and Planning

Analysis of the data collected can lead to both nursing diagnoses (Nursing Care Plan: Preeclampsia) and collaborative problems or potential complications. Potential complications require nurses to monitor for the onset of new problems or changes in status. Both physician-prescribed and nurse-prescribed interventions are used to minimize the complication. Potential complications for the woman with preeclampsia are *eclamptic seizures* and *magnesium toxicity*.

Client-centered goals are inappropriate for the potential complications of eclamptic seizures and magnesium toxicity because the nurse cannot independently manage these conditions but must confer with physicians and use established protocols for treatment. For seizures, planning should reflect the nurse's responsibility to:

- Perform actions that will minimize the risk for seizures occurring and prevent maternal or fetal injury if seizures do occur.
- Monitor for signs of impending seizures.
- Support the family of the woman with eclampsia.

For magnesium toxicity, planning should reflect these nursing responsibilities:

- Monitor for signs of magnesium toxicity.
- Consult with the physician if signs of magnesium toxicity are observed.
- Perform actions that will minimize the possibility of magnesium toxicity.

Interventions

Interventions for Seizures

Initiating Preventive Measures In the presence of cerebral irritability, seizures may be precipitated by excessive visual or auditory stimuli. Nurses should reduce external stimuli by:

- Limiting excessive stimulation by admitting the woman to a room in the quietest section of the unit and keeping the door to the room closed. The need for intense nursing observation and care exists regardless of the specific room location that is available.
- Reducing noise when the door must be opened and closed.
- Keeping lights low and noise to a minimum; this may include blocking incoming telephone calls or visitors.
- Grouping nursing assessments and care to allow the woman periods of undisturbed quiet.
- Moving carefully and calmly around the room, and avoiding bumping into the bed or startling the woman.
- Collaborating with the woman and her family to restrict visitors.

Monitoring for Signs of Impending Seizures Maternal findings that may precede seizures include:

- Hyperreflexia, the presence of clonus, or both
- Increasing signs of cerebral irritability (headache, visual disturbances)
- Epigastric or right upper quadrant pain, nausea, or vomiting

None of these signs is a predictor of imminent seizure in any woman. Nurses must be alert for subtle changes and be prepared for seizures in all women with preeclampsia.

Preventing Seizure-Related Injury Hard side rails should be padded and the bed kept in the lowest position with the wheels locked to prevent trauma during a convulsion.

Oxygen and suction equipment should be assembled and ready to use to remove secretions and to provide oxygen if it is not already being administered. Check equipment and connections at the beginning of each shift because there will not be time to set up equipment if convulsions occur.

Supplies specific for care in preeclampsia should be immediately available, often in a separate box or tray. Common supplies include a medium plastic airway, an Ambu bag with mask, endotracheal tubes in assorted sizes, an ophthalmoscope, a tourniquet, a reflex hammer, syringes, and needles. Medications that should be on hand include magnesium sulfate, sodium bicarbonate, heparin sodium, epinephrine, phenytoin, and calcium gluconate.

Protecting the Woman and Fetus During a Convulsion The nurse's primary responsibilities to protect the woman and the fetus during a convulsion are:

- Remain with the woman and press the emergency bell for assistance.
- If not on her side already, attempt to turn the woman on her side when the tonic phase begins. A side-lying position permits greater circulation through the placenta, and it may also help prevent aspiration.
- Note the time and sequence of the convulsion.
- Insert an airway after the convulsion, and suction the woman's mouth and nose to clear secretions and prevent aspiration. Provide oxygen by mask at 8 to 10 L/min to increase oxygenation of the placenta and all maternal body organs.
- Observe fetal monitor patterns for nonreassuring signs, such as bradycardia, tachycardia, or decreased variability. These usually resolve within a few minutes as maternal oxygenation is restored.
- Notify, or have another nurse notify, the physician that a convulsion has occurred. Administer medications and prepare for additional medical interventions as directed by the physician.

Providing Information and Support for the Family Explain to the family what has happened without minimizing the seriousness of the situation. A convulsion is frightening for anyone who witnesses it, and the family is often reassured when the nurse explains that the convulsion lasts only a few minutes and that the woman will probably not be conscious for some time afterward. Acknowledge that the convulsion indicates worsening of the condition and that it will be necessary for the physician to determine future management, which may include delivery of the infant as soon as possible. Vaginal birth is preferred if the maternal and fetal conditions

Nursing Care Plan

Preeclampsia

ASSESSMENT

Julie Frost, a 16-year-old primigravida, is seen in the prenatal clinic at 30 weeks of gestation. Her blood pressure is 136/90, and there is some edema of the lower legs and trace proteinuria. She is given instructions about home care for pregnancy-induced hypertension. The regimen includes bed rest; frequent monitoring of blood pressure, weight, and urine; and doing fetal "kick counts." Julie is told she must return to the clinic in a week. She states that she feels fine and doesn't want to miss school. She says that she doesn't see the reason for bed rest.

Nursing Diagnosis

Impaired Adjustment related to lack of knowledge of health status and the need for a change in lifestyle.

Goals/Expected Outcomes

Julie will:
- Verbalize the benefits of the recommended regimen by the end of the first prenatal appointment.
- Comply with the recommended care for the next week.
- Keep prenatal appointments.

INTERVENTION	RATIONALE
1. Allow Julie to verbalize her feelings about the recommended regimen: "What concerns you most about missing school?" Acknowledge her feelings as important: "It must be difficult to think of falling behind in your schoolwork. It isn't any fun to miss all the after-school activities."	1. When feelings are identified and acknowledged as important, anxiety decreases and teaching and learning can begin.
2. Identify family support that will permit compliance with the recommended regimen of bed rest and home care.	2. Compliance with the regimen is impossible without family assistance, which includes assistance with activities of daily living and necessary assessments.
3. Describe in general terms the pathophysiologic processes that affect Julie and her fetus.	3. Expectant mothers are usually motivated to comply with a therapeutic management that will benefit the fetus.
4. Explain that Julie may feel well even when the condition worsens and that she must be observed for signs and symptoms at home and at the clinic.	4. The expectant mother does not notice hypertension and proteinuria. Although edema is not always present in hypertensive complications during pregnancy, clients may not be aware that it may also be associated with other disorders.
5. Instruct Julie to call the clinic if she notices headache, double vision, or spots before her eyes.	5. These signs indicate rapid progression of the disease and that additional management is promptly needed.
6. Collaborate with Julie to arrange for contact with her boyfriend or selected friends and to arrange for ongoing home-bound classes.	6. Such an agreement will allow a schedule to provide peer support but allow for prolonged periods of quiet. Home-bound classes alleviate the concern that she is falling behind with schoolwork.

Evaluation

Despite maintaining the recommended regimen of bed rest with the help of her mother and sister and keeping prenatal appointments, Julie's condition worsened. She developed a rise in blood pressure and a rapid gain in weight, indicating generalized edema at 32 weeks.

ASSESSMENT

Julie is admitted to the hospital at 32 weeks of gestation with a blood pressure of 160/110, heart rate of 92, and respiratory rate of 22 per minute. There is 2+ proteinuria and marked edema of the hands and face as well as her lower extremities. Fetal heart rate is 136 with average variability. An intravenous infusion of magnesium sulfate ($MgSO_4$) is started, seizure precautions are initiated, and environmental stimuli are carefully reduced. Julie is agitated and verbalizes concern that the procedures are going to hurt her or the fetus. She frequently asks, "How sick am I?" "Is the baby going to be okay?" Her hands are perspiring, and they shake when she reaches for a tissue.

Continued

Nursing Care Plan

Preeclampsia—cont'd

Nursing Diagnosis

Anxiety related to hospitalization and concern about her health and the health of the fetus.

Goals/Expected Outcomes

Julie will:

- Verbalize her concerns and describe the benefits of the treatment while her family is present.
- Manifest less anxiety (agitation, physiologic signs such as tremors, tachycardia, and perspiration).

INTERVENTION	RATIONALE
1. Initiate measures to reduce anxiety:	1. Anxiety is an ominous feeling of tension resulting from a physical or emotional threat to the self. It is a global, often unnamed sense of doom, a feeling of helplessness, isolation, and insecurity. Anxiety needs to be ventilated and then addressed by conveying that the person is not alone and will be protected.
a. Provide positive reassurance that a solution to anxiety can be found: "I can see you are really worried, and I will try to answer all your questions."	
b. Allow Julie to cry, get angry, or express any feeling that is present.	
c. Encourage a discussion of feelings: "Tell me more about how you feel."	
d. Reflect observations: "I see you wringing your hands; do you want to talk about it?"	
e. Convey empathy and positive regard; use nonverbal behavior, including touch, when appropriate.	
2. Provide information about hospital routines and procedures when Julie's anxiety has diminished enough for learning to take place:	2. Knowledge of procedures to be performed and the purpose of these procedures provides a sense of control that reduces anxiety. Perception is somewhat narrowed when anxiety is high; therefore short, brief instructions are easier for the anxious person to understand than long explanations.
a. Be very specific about procedures, such as fetal monitoring, assessment of deep tendon reflexes, and vital signs. Explain the reasons for these procedures, who will do them, and how long they will be maintained.	
b. Focus on Julie's present concerns; she is not able to be future-oriented at this time.	
c. Speak slowly and calmly, give very short directions, and do not ask Julie to make decisions: "Turn on your side." "Breathe slowly."	
d. Allow a friend or family member to remain with Julie, and instruct the person on the need for a low-stimulus environment.	

Evaluation

Julie discusses her feelings with the nurse and with her sister. She feels in control of anxiety, as manifested by fewer signs of agitation and fewer physiologic signs (tachycardia, tachypnea) and by the ability to use relaxation techniques.

Potential Complications to Consider

Magnesium toxicity
Seizures

---

permit because of the abnormalities in the coagulation and other body systems.

Interventions for Magnesium Toxicity

Monitoring for Signs of Magnesium Toxicity Magnesium excess depresses the entire central nervous system, including the brainstem, which controls respirations and cardiac function, and the cerebrum, which controls memory, mental processes, and speech. Carbon dioxide accumulates if

the respiratory rate or depth is inadequate, leading to respiratory acidosis and further CNS depression, which could end in respiratory arrest.

Signs of magnesium toxicity may include:

- Respiratory rate less than 12 breaths per minute. (Hospitals may specify a respiratory rate of less than 14 breaths per minute as an alternative.)
- Maternal pulse oximeter reading lower than 95%.

- Absence of deep tendon reflexes.
- Sweating, flushing.
- Altered sensorium (confusion, lethargy, slurring of speech, drowsiness, disorientation).
- Hypotension.
- A serum magnesium concentration above the therapeutic range of 4 to 8 mg/dl.

Responding to Signs of Magnesium Toxicity Discontinue magnesium if the respiratory rate is less than 12 breaths per minute, a low pulse oximeter level (<95%) persists, or if deep tendon reflexes are absent. Notify the physician. Magnesium is excreted by the kidneys, and if the urinary output falls below 30 ml/hr, the physician should be notified.

Calcium opposes the effects of magnesium at the neuromuscular junction. Magnesium toxicity can be reversed by slow intravenous administration of 1 g (10 ml of 10%) calcium gluconate at 1 ml/min.

Evaluation

Collect and compare data with established norms and then judge whether the data are within normal limits. For seizures, interventions are judged to be successful if:

- Deep tendon reflexes remain within normal limits (+1 to +3).
- The woman is free of visual disturbances, severe headache, and epigastric or right upper quadrant pain.
- The woman remains free of seizures or free of preventable injury if a seizure occurs.

For magnesium toxicity, determine whether respiratory rates remain at least 12 breaths per minute, deep tendon reflexes are present, and maternal serum levels of magnesium do not exceed the therapeutic range.

HEMOLYSIS, ELEVATED LIVER ENZYMES, AND LOW PLATELETS SYNDROME

The acronym HELLP (Hemolysis, Elevated Liver enzymes, Low Platelets) describes a life-threatening occurrence that complicates about 10% of pregnancies. Half of the women affected with HELLP will also have severe preeclampsia, although hypertension may be absent. As in preeclampsia, HELLP syndrome may occur during the postpartum period (Abramovici, Mattar, & Sibai, 2000; Moldenhauer & Sibai, 2003).

Hemolysis is believed to occur as a result of the fragmentation and distortion of erythrocytes during passage through small damaged blood vessels. Liver enzyme levels increase when hepatic blood flow is obstructed by fibrin deposits. Hyperbilirubinemia and jaundice may occur as a result of liver impairment. Low platelet levels are caused by vascular damage resulting from vasospasm; platelets aggregate at sites of damage, resulting in systemic thrombocytopenia.

The prominent symptom of the HELLP syndrome is pain in the right upper quadrant, the lower chest, or epigastric area. There may also be tenderness because of liver distention. Additional signs and symptoms include nausea, vomiting, and severe edema (Moldenhauer & Sibai, 2003; Riely & Fallon, 1999). It is important to avoid traumatizing the liver by abdominal palpation and to use care in transporting the woman. A sudden increase in intraabdominal pressure, including a seizure, could lead to rupture of a subcapsular hematoma, resulting in internal bleeding and hypovolemic shock.

Women with the HELLP syndrome should be managed in a setting with full intensive care facilities available. Their treatment includes that which is appropriate for preeclampsia or eclampsia. After delivery, most women begin recovering within 72 hours.

CHRONIC HYPERTENSION

A diagnosis of chronic hypertension is made whenever evidence suggests that hypertension preceded the pregnancy or when a woman is hypertensive before 20 weeks' gestation. Chronic hypertension is seen most often in older women, in those who are obese, and in those with diabetes. Heredity, including race, plays a role in the development of chronic hypertension, which is more common in African-Americans at any age than in other races (Freid, Prager, MacKay, & Xia, 2003). Late childbearing and rising obesity rates will no doubt fuel an increase in hypertension. Chronic hypertension is usually essential, or primary. However, it may be secondary to another problem, such as renal disease or an autoimmune disorder.

The most common maternal hazard is the development of preeclampsia, which occurs in 20% of pregnant women with chronic hypertension. New-onset proteinuria or a significant rise in preexisting proteinuria identifies the development of superimposed preeclampsia. The rise in blood pressure with preeclampsia is likely to be greater in these women (Cunningham et al., 2001; National High Blood Pressure Education Program Working Group on High Blood Pressure in Pregnancy, 2000; Roberts, 2004).

A dietitian should be consulted about the appropriate diet and weight gain, because many of these women are obese and they frequently have diabetes. Adequate intake of protein helps counteract the protein lost in urine. A reduced salt intake may be advised, unlike for the woman with preeclampsia alone. More frequent prenatal visits will be needed. Regular fetal surveillance by biophysical profile and kick counts (see Chapter 16) are usual to identify poor growth patterns or signs that are nonreassuring, such as a falling amount of amniotic fluid.

Antihypertensive medications must be chosen carefully because they may reduce placental blood flow. Antihypertensive medication should be initiated if the diastolic pressure is consistently higher than 100 mm Hg in early pregnancy (Roberts, 2004). Methyldopa (Aldomet) is the drug of choice because of its record of safety and effectiveness in pregnancy. Beta blockers and calcium channel blockers may also be used if methyldopa is not effective, but their record of safety in pregnancy is less well established. Angiotensin-converting enzyme (ACE) inhibitors are contraindicated in pregnancy but may be used in the postpartum period. Hydralazine is a vasodilator reserved for hypertensive crisis. Diuretics are avoided if possible because they may shrink the blood volume, which may already be reduced if preeclampsia exists with the chronic hypertension.

INCOMPATIBILITY BETWEEN MATERNAL AND FETAL BLOOD

Rh Incompatibility

Rhesus (Rh) factor incompatibility during pregnancy is possible only when two specific circumstances coexist: (1) the expectant mother is Rh-negative; and (2) the fetus is Rh-positive. For such a circumstance to occur, the father of the

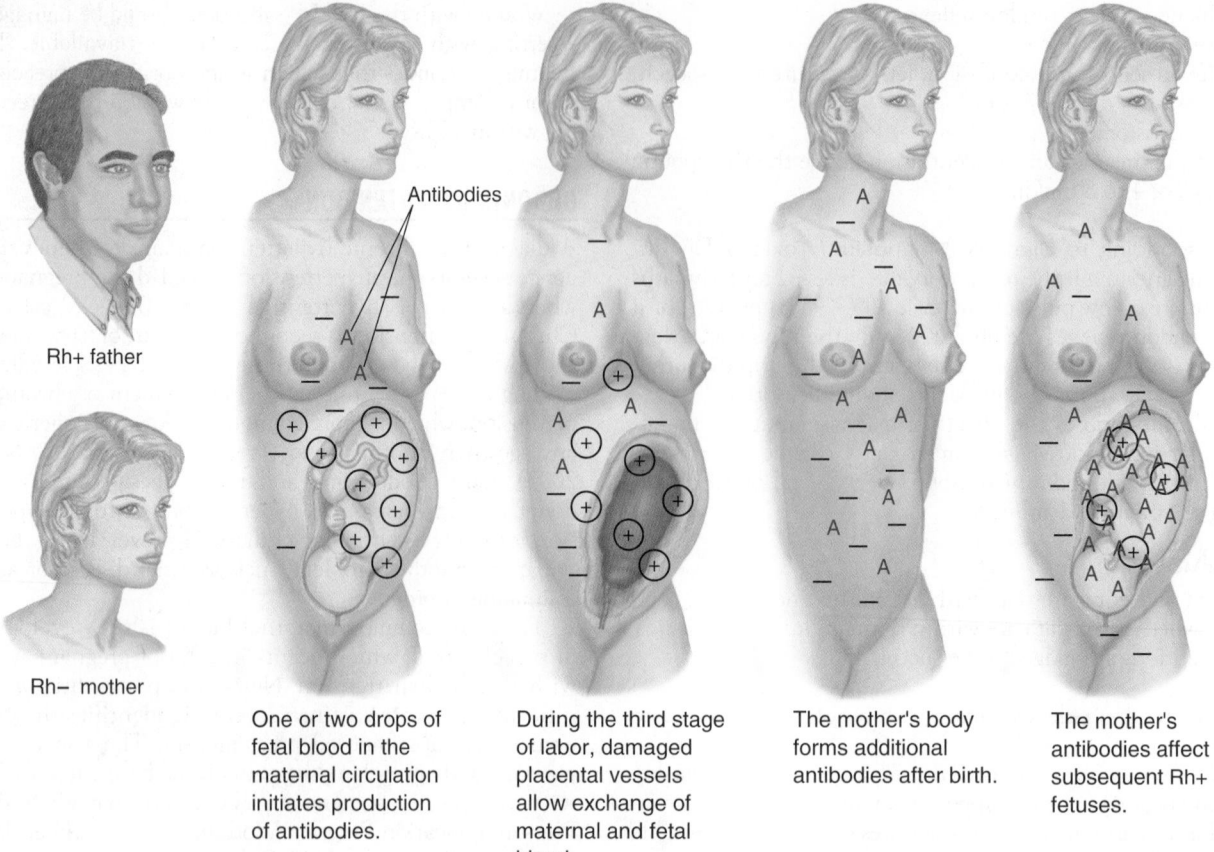

Antibodies

Rh+ father

Rh− mother

One or two drops of fetal blood in the maternal circulation initiates production of antibodies.

During the third stage of labor, damaged placental vessels allow exchange of maternal and fetal blood.

The mother's body forms additional antibodies after birth.

The mother's antibodies affect subsequent Rh+ fetuses.

Figure 26-7 The process of maternal sensitization to the Rh factor.

fetus must have an Rh-positive blood type. Rh incompatibility is a problem that affects the fetus; it causes no harm to the expectant mother during pregnancy.

Rh-negative blood is a recessive trait; therefore a person must inherit the same gene from both parents to be Rh-negative. Approximately 15% of the white population in the United States is Rh-negative. The incidence is lower in African-Americans and Asians.

Pathophysiology
People who are Rh-positive have the Rh antigen on their red blood cells, whereas people who are Rh-negative do not have the antigen. When blood from a person who is Rh-positive enters the bloodstream of a person who is Rh-negative, the body reacts as it would to any foreign substance: it develops antibodies to destroy the invading antigen. To destroy the Rh antigen, which exists as part of the red blood cell, the entire red blood cell must be destroyed.

Theoretically, no mixing of fetal and maternal blood occurs during pregnancy. In reality, however, small placental accidents may allow a drop or two of fetal blood to enter the maternal circulation and initiate the production of antibodies to destroy the Rh-positive blood (isoimmunization). Sensitization can also occur during a spontaneous or elective abortion or during antepartal procedures such as amniocentesis and chorionic villus sampling. Figure 26-7 illustrates the process of maternal sensitization.

Most exposure of maternal blood to fetal blood occurs during the third stage of labor, when active exchange of fetal and maternal blood can occur as the placenta separates. The woman's first child is usually unaffected because antibodies are formed after the birth of the infant. Subsequent Rh-positive fetuses may be affected, however, unless the mother receives $Rh_o(D)$ immune globulin (RhoGAM) to prevent antibody formation after the birth of each Rh-positive infant. Use of RhoGAM has greatly reduced the fetal and neonatal complications of Rh incompatibility. The complication does still occur, however, and may be fatal to the fetus.

Fetal and Neonatal Implications
If antibodies to the Rh factor are present in the expectant mother's blood, they cross the placental barrier and destroy fetal red blood cells. The fetus becomes deficient in red blood cells, which are needed to transport oxygen to fetal tissue. As fetal red blood cells are destroyed, fetal bilirubin levels increase (*icterus gravis*), which can lead to severe neurologic disease (*bilirubin encephalopathy*). This hemolytic process results in rapid production of erythroblasts (immature red blood cells), which cannot carry oxygen. The entire syndrome is termed *erythroblastosis fetalis*. The fetus may become so anemic that generalized fetal edema (*hydrops fetalis*) results and can end in fetal congestive heart failure. Management of the infant born with erythroblastosis fetalis is discussed in Chapter 30.

Prenatal Assessment and Management

All pregnant women should have a blood test to determine blood type and Rh factor at the initial prenatal visit. Rh-negative women should have an antibody titer (indirect Coombs test) to determine whether they are sensitized (have developed antibodies) as a result of previous exposure to Rh-positive blood. If the indirect Coombs test is negative, it is repeated at 28 weeks of gestation to identify cases of later sensitization. A negative indirect Coombs test result accurately identifies the fetus as not at risk for hemolytic disease of the newborn.

As a preventive measure, an $Rh_o(D)$ immune globulin (such as RhoGAM) is administered to the unsensitized, Rh-negative woman at 28 weeks of gestation. RhoGAM is a commercial preparation of passive antibodies against Rh factor. It effectively prevents the formation of active antibodies if a small amount of fetal Rh-positive blood enters the circulation of an Rh-negative mother during the remainder of the pregnancy. RhoGAM is repeated after birth if the woman delivers an Rh-positive infant.

A positive indirect Coombs test result indicates maternal sensitization and the presence of antibodies against Rh-positive erythrocytes. The indirect Coombs test is repeated at frequent intervals throughout the pregnancy to determine whether the antibody titer is rising, which indicates that the process is continuing. The fetus will be in jeopardy because fetal erythrocytes are being attacked by maternal anti-Rh antibodies.

Amniocentesis may be performed to evaluate change in the optical density (ΔOD 450) of amniotic fluid. This measure reflects the amount of bilirubin (residue of red blood cell destruction) present in the amniotic fluid. If the fluid optical density remains low, it may indicate that the fetus is Rh-negative and in no jeopardy or that the fetus is Rh-positive. If the optical density is elevated, the fetus is in jeopardy.

Ultrasound examination is used to noninvasively evaluate the condition of the fetus. Doppler studies allow evaluation of cardiac function and blood flow in fetal vessels. Generalized fetal edema, ascites, an enlarged heart, or hydramnios occur when the fetus is very anemic. Percutaneous umbilical blood sampling (PUBS), or cordocentesis (see Chapter 16), allows invasive sampling of fetal blood from cord vessels to determine the degree of erythrocyte destruction. Because it is invasive, PUBS is reserved for the fetus thought to be significantly affected.

Intrauterine transfusion is the direct infusion of O-negative erythrocytes into the umbilical cord by percutaneous umbilical blood transfusion (see Chapter 16). The transfused erythrocytes must be compatible with maternal blood to avoid destruction by her antibodies. Whole blood is usually used to replace fetal serum proteins. Erythrocytes may also be transfused into the fetal abdominal cavity where they are gradually absorbed into the circulation.

Postpartum Management

If the mother is Rh-negative, umbilical cord blood is taken at delivery to determine blood type, Rh factor, and antibody titer (direct Coombs test) of the newborn. Rh-negative, unsensitized mothers who give birth to Rh-positive infants are given an intramuscular injection of RhoGAM within 72 hours after delivery. If RhoGAM is given to the mother in the first 72 hours after delivery of an Rh-positive infant, fetal Rh antigens present in her circulation are destroyed and she does not form natural, permanent antibodies.

If the infant is Rh-negative, there is no possibility of antibody formation and RhoGAM is not necessary. RhoGAM is also administered after abortion, chorionic villus sampling, and amniocentesis, when fetal-to-maternal transfusion is possible, and at 28 weeks of gestation if the mother is Rh-negative and unsensitized. The drug may also be given after trauma if fetal-to-maternal hemorrhage is detected. More than the single 300 mcg dose may be needed for large fetal hemorrhages.

Families are often very concerned about the fetus. Nurses must be sensitive to cues and signals that indicate that the family is anxious, and must be able to offer honest reassurance. This is especially important if the expectant mother is sensitized and fetal testing is necessary throughout pregnancy.

At birth, the physician or nurse should collect cord blood to determine the blood type and Rh factor of the newborn. During the postpartum period, nurses are responsible for follow-up to determine whether RhoGAM is necessary and to administer the injection within the prescribed time.

ABO Incompatibility

ABO incompatibility occurs when the expectant mother is blood type O and the fetus is blood type A, B, or AB. Blood types A, B, and AB contain a protein component (antigen) that is not present in type O blood.

Drug Guide

Rh₀(D) Immune Globulin (RhoGAM, HypRho-D, Gamulin Rh)

Classification: Concentrated immunoglobulins directed toward the red blood cell antigen Rh₀(D).

Action: Prevents production of anti-Rh₀(D) antibodies in Rh-negative women who have been exposed to Rh-positive blood by suppressing the immune reaction of the Rh-negative woman to the antigen in Rh-positive blood. Prevents antibody response and subsequently prevents hemolytic disease of the newborn in future pregnancies of women who have conceived an Rh-positive fetus.

Indications: Administered to Rh-negative women who have been exposed to Rh-positive blood by:

- Delivering an Rh-positive infant
- Aborting an Rh-positive fetus
- Having chorionic villus sampling, amniocentesis, or intraabdominal trauma while carrying an Rh-positive fetus

- Accidental transfusion of Rh-positive blood to an Rh-negative woman

Dosage and Route: One *standard dose* administered intramuscularly:

- At 28 weeks of pregnancy and within 72 hours of delivery
- Within 72 hours following the termination of a pregnancy of 13 weeks or more of gestation

One *microdose* within 72 hours following the termination of a pregnancy of less than 13 weeks of gestation.

After accidental transfusion, dosage is calculated based on the volume of blood erroneously administered.

Absorption: Well absorbed from intramuscular sites.

Excretion: Metabolism and excretion unknown.

Contraindications and Precautions: Women who are Rh-positive or women previously sensitized to Rh₀(D) should not receive Rh₀(D) immune globulin. Used cautiously for women with previous hypersensitivity reactions to immune globulins.

Adverse Reactions: Local pain at intramuscular site, fever, or both.

Nursing Implications: Type and crossmatch of mother's blood and cord blood of the newborn must be performed to determine the need for the medication. The mother must be Rh-negative and negative for Rh antibodies; the newborn must be Rh-positive. If there is doubt regarding the fetus's blood type following termination of pregnancy, the medication should be administered. The drug is administered to the mother, not the infant. The deltoid muscle is recommended for intramuscular administration.

People with type O blood develop anti-A or anti-B antibodies naturally as a result of exposure to antigens in the foods that they eat or to infection by gram-negative bacteria. As a result, some women with type O blood have developed high serum anti-A and anti-B antibody titers before pregnancy. The antibodies may be either IgG or IgM. When the woman becomes pregnant, the IgG antibodies cross the placental barrier and cause hemolysis of fetal red blood cells. Although the first fetus can be affected, ABO incompatibility is less severe than Rh incompatibility because the primary antibodies of the ABO system are IgM, which do not cross the placenta.

No specific prenatal care is needed, but the nurse must be aware of the possibility of ABO incompatibility. At birth, cord blood is taken to determine the blood type of the newborn and the antibody titer (direct Coombs test). The newborn is carefully screened for jaundice, which indicates hyperbilirubinemia. See Chapter 30 for medical and nursing management of hyperbilirubinemia in newborns.

Other Blood Group Incompatibility

Although less common, maternal sensitization to several other erythrocyte antibodies, such as Kell, Duffy, and Kidd antibodies, may also cause isoimmunization. Management during pregnancy is similar to that of the Rh-sensitized mother.

CONCURRENT DISORDERS DURING PREGNANCY

Pregnancy may alter the course of a concurrent disease, or a disease and its treatment may have unwanted effects on the pregnancy. As a result, the usual antepartum care must be adapted to include increased surveillance of the mother and the fetus. Moreover, some disorders that are mild or even subclinical in the pregnant woman can cause massive damage to a fetus.

DIABETES MELLITUS

Pathophysiology

Etiology

Diabetes mellitus is a complex disorder of carbohydrate metabolism caused primarily by a partial or complete lack of insulin secretion by the beta cells of the pancreas. Some cells, such as those in skeletal and cardiac muscles and in adipose tissue, require insulin to carry glucose across the cell membranes. Without insulin, glucose accumulates in the blood, resulting in hyperglycemia. The body attempts to dilute the glucose load by any means possible. The first strategy is to increase thirst (*polydipsia*), one of the classic symptoms of diabetes mellitus. Next, fluid from the intracellular spaces is drawn into the vascular bed, resulting in dehydration at the cellular level but fluid volume excess in the vascular compartment. The kidneys attempt to excrete large volumes of this fluid plus the heavy solute load of glucose (osmotic diuresis). This excretion produces the second sign of diabetes, *polyuria*, as well as *glycosuria* (glucose in the urine). Without glucose, the cells starve, so weight loss occurs even though the person ingests large amounts of food (*polyphagia*).

Because the body is unable to metabolize glucose, it begins to metabolize protein and fat to meet energy needs. Metabolism of protein produces a negative nitrogen balance, and the metabolism of fat results in the buildup of ketone bodies (e.g., acetone, acetoacetic acid, or beta-hydroxybutyric acid) or ketosis (accumulation of acids in the body).

If the disease is not well controlled, serious complications may occur. Hypoglycemia or hyperglycemia can result if the amount of insulin does not match the diet. Moreover, fluctuating periods of hyperglycemia and hypoglycemia damage small blood vessels throughout the body. This damage can cause serious impairment, especially in the kidneys, eyes, and heart.

Effect Of Pregnancy On Fuel Metabolism

To comprehend the relationship of diabetes mellitus and pregnancy, it is necessary to understand how pregnancy and diabetes alter the metabolism of food.

Early Pregnancy. Metabolic changes can be divided into those that occur early in pregnancy (from 1 to 20 weeks) and those that occur late in pregnancy (from the end of 20 weeks until birth). During early pregnancy, maternal metabolic rates and energy needs change little. During this time, however, insulin release in response to serum glucose levels increases. As a result, significant hypoglycemia may occur, particularly in women who experience the nausea, vomiting, and anorexia that often occur during the first weeks of pregnancy.

In an uncomplicated pregnancy, the availability of glucose and insulin favors the development and storage of fat during the first half of pregnancy. Accumulation of fat prepares the mother for the rise in energy use by the growing fetus during the second half of pregnancy.

Late Pregnancy. During the second half of pregnancy, when fetal growth accelerates, levels of placental hormones rise sharply. These hormones, particularly estrogen, progesterone, and human placental lactogen, create resistance to insulin in maternal cells to provide an abundant supply of glucose for the fetus. The hormones have a diabetogenic effect, however, in that they may leave the woman with insufficient insulin and episodes of hyperglycemia.

For most women, insulin resistance is not a problem. The pancreas responds by simply increasing the production of insulin. If the pancreas is unable to respond, however, the woman will experience periods of hyperglycemia.

During late pregnancy, the fetus continuously withdraws nutrients, such as glucose and amino acids, from maternal blood. The result is an earlier-than-normal switch from carbohydrate metabolism to gluconeogenesis (formation of glycogen from noncarbohydrate sources such as proteins and fat). Because the fetus uses many of the amino acids, the process becomes predominantly one of fat utilization. This process produces high levels of free fatty acids that further inhibit the uptake and oxidation of glucose and thus preserve glucose for use by the central nervous system and the fetus. These metabolic changes are similar to those that occur during "accelerated starvation," when fat is metabolized to meet the body's energy needs.

Classification

Diabetes is classified as type 1 (insulin-dependent) or type 2 (non-insulin-dependent) according to the pathology underlying the condition. Type 1 diabetes, previously called *insulin-dependent diabetes mellitus (IDDM)*, occurs when pancreatic beta cells that produce insulin are destroyed by the body's immune cells. Type 1 diabetes can occur at any age but usually occurs in children through young adults. Insulin by intermittent injection or pump is required to sustain life.

The root cause for type 2 diabetes, previously called *non-insulin-dependent diabetes mellitus (NIDDM)*, is insulin resistance, in which body cells do not use glucose properly. The need for insulin rises, and the pancreas gradually loses the ability to supply enough of the hormone needed to metabolize glucose. Type 2 diabetes is associated with advancing age and obesity, among other factors, but is frequently being diagnosed in children and adolescents. Race plays a role, with African-Americans, Hispanics, Native Americans, and Pacific Islanders having a higher incidence than whites (Centers for Disease Control and Prevention [CDC], 2003a). Type 2 diabetes may be controlled by diet, exercise, and weight reduction, or it may require oral agents or insulin to control high glucose levels.

Gestational diabetes is the onset of glucose intolerance during pregnancy. Gestational diabetes accounts for 90% of the cases of diabetes during pregnancy, affecting 2% to 5% of all pregnancies. Of this number, 5% to 10% will be diagnosed with type 2 diabetes shortly after delivery, with up to 50% of them developing type 2 diabetes sometime within 20 years of birth. Gestational diabetes is more likely to recur in subsequent pregnancy. Women of African, Hispanic, American Indian, South or East Indian, and Pacific Islands ancestry are more frequently affected with gestational diabetes. Family history of diabetes, advancing age, and obesity are added risk factors for its development. Gestational diabetes is also more likely to occur in multifetal gestations (American College of Obstetricians & Gynecologists [ACOG], 2001b; CDC, 2003a; Cunningham et al., 2001) (Nursing Care Plan: Pregnancy and Diabetes Mellitus and Box 26-2).

Preexisting Diabetes Mellitus

Maternal Effects

Preeclampsia occurs more often in the woman with diabetes than in the unaffected population (ACOG, 2001b; Cunningham et al., 2001). The development of ketoacidosis is a threat to women who require insulin to properly control their diabetes. Ketoacidosis is often precipitated by infection

---

BOX 26-2
Classification of Diabetes Mellitus

- *Type 1, Insulin-Dependent:* Onset in childhood or young adulthood. Involves autoimmune destruction of pancreatic beta cells. Prone to ketosis.
- *Type 2, Non-Insulin-Dependent:* Usual onset after 40 years. Associated with obesity. Increasing insulin resistance. Ketosis less likely to occur than in type 1 diabetes mellitus.
- *Gestational:* Onset of glucose intolerance first diagnosed during pregnancy. Exogenous insulin may or may not be needed.

Data from American Diabetes Association. (2003). Position statement: Gestational diabetes mellitus. *Diabetes Care, 26*(Suppl. 1), S103-S105. Retrieved Nov. 25, 2003, from http://care.diabetesjournals.org/cgi/reprint/26/suppl_1/s103.pdf; American Diabetes Association. (2003). Position statement: Preconception care of women with diabetes. *Diabetes Care, 26*(Suppl. 1), S91-S93. Retrieved Nov. 25, 2003, from http://care.diabetesjournals.org/cgi/reprint/26/suppl_1/s103.pdf.

Nursing Care Plan

Pregnancy and Diabetes Mellitus

ASSESSMENT

Kathy Ringold is a 24-year-old primigravida at 9 weeks' gestation. She was diagnosed with type 1 diabetes mellitus 6 years ago. She has been on a daily regimen of insulin and is comfortable with insulin administration and blood glucose monitoring. She is experiencing daily nausea and vomiting. Kathy states that she is concerned because she is not eating as much as before becoming pregnant. She also reveals that she had sometimes "binged" on food before becoming pregnant and didn't always monitor blood glucose as often as directed. She does not see why her blood glucose has to be watched so carefully.

Nursing Diagnosis

Risk for Ineffective Health Maintenance related to knowledge deficit of the effects of pregnancy on diabetes control.

Goals/Expected Outcomes

Kathy will:
- Describe predicted changes in insulin needs throughout pregnancy.
- Follow prescribed schedule of blood glucose monitoring, insulin administration, diet, and exercise.
- Describe the importance of frequent fetal surveillance and follow the prescribed schedule.

INTERVENTION	RATIONALE
1. Reduce barriers to learning: a. Allow Kathy to express emotions and concerns before teaching. b. Examine her beliefs and past experiences related to diabetes. c. Assess readiness to learn, based on interest, attention, and participation in scheduled learning sessions.	1. Motivation and readiness to learn are essential for permanent learning to occur. Kathy will learn only if she sees the value of the information.
2. Instruct Kathy about the predicted changes in diabetes management during pregnancy: a. Explain the importance of blood glucose testing; Kathy will need less insulin because of the nausea and vomiting occurring in the first trimester. b. Emphasize that she will probably need more insulin as the second and third trimesters progress because of the effects of the placental hormones. Insulin requirements usually fall immediately after birth but will achieve ideal longer-term levels after the immediate postdelivery period. c. Describe the importance of following the prescribed diet and exercise regimen to maintain normal blood glucose levels.	2. Behaviors change when learning occurs. Understanding how insulin needs change throughout pregnancy, labor, and the postpartum period increases the likelihood that Kathy will follow the recommended regimen.
3. Inform Kathy about specific fetal surveillance techniques recommended during pregnancy (serial nonstress tests, contraction stress tests, biophysical profiles), and explain the importance of the tests.	3. Some frequently ordered tests are time-consuming and expensive. The woman is more likely to comply if she understands the importance of monitoring the fetal condition at frequent intervals.
4. Allow time for Kathy to focus on her feelings and concerns at each teaching session; offer praise and encouragement for her adherence to the prescribed regimen.	4. Motivation to comply with the regimen is strengthened by praise and the awareness that the woman's feelings are important.
5. Explain in simple, positive terms the advantages to the fetus of maintaining a normal maternal blood glucose level. These advantages include an optimal pattern of growth, the increased likelihood that the baby will be born near term, and fewer complications associated with prematurity.	5. Understanding that the fetus benefits when maternal glucose levels are normal reduces anxiety and increases the likelihood that the mother will comply with recommended treatment.

Nursing Care Plan

Pregnancy and Diabetes Mellitus—cont'd

6. Review the recommended plan for diet and exercise during pregnancy, and determine whether Kathy knows the importance of these factors in her care.

6. Maintenance of normal blood glucose depends on coordinating the amount of food, insulin, and exercise. If any of these factors is altered, the others must also be altered to prevent hypoglycemia or hyperglycemia.

Evaluation

Kathy verbalizes her understanding of changing insulin needs and the importance of glucose monitoring. She states that she feels in better control of the diabetes and plans to comply with the recommended schedule of fetal surveillance, diet, and exercise.

ASSESSMENT

At 32 weeks' gestation, Kathy's blood glucose is consistently above the desired level and twice-weekly nonstress tests are prescribed. The tests are reactive, indicating no present fetal compromise. Kathy, however, verbalizes anxiety about the condition of the fetus and asks when it will be safe for the baby to be born.

Nursing Diagnosis

Anxiety related to perceived threat to the health of the fetus, including his expected gestation when born.

Goals/Expected Outcomes

Kathy will:

- Relate her perception of the condition of the fetus and the significance of the reactive nonstress test as the tests are performed.
- Describe her concerns about the timing of the delivery at the conclusion of the next nonstress test.

INTERVENTION

1. Ask Kathy to describe her concern about the fetus and to clarify her feelings.
2. Explain that a reactive nonstress test indicates that the fetal heart rate accelerates whenever the fetus moves; this is a good sign that the fetus is not in immediate jeopardy. Frequency of the nonstress test will be changed if a need is identified.
3. Ask Kathy how she feels about the labor and delivery; determine whether she is taking childbirth education classes and whether she has selected her coach.

4. Assist Kathy in investigating a childbirth education class if she has not done so previously, and suggest that she and her coach begin classes.
5. Acknowledge that the prospect of labor and delivery causes many women some anxiety, even when the condition of the infant is not at risk.

RATIONALE

1. Kathy's concerns must be identified and clarified so that misconceptions do not occur.
2. Reassurance that the fetus is not in jeopardy and that the tests will detect early signs if a problem develops reduces anxiety about the fetal condition.

3. It is normal for women to become concerned about the birth process and how they will cope with labor during the last few weeks of pregnancy. Medical professionals should not neglect the need for normal pregnancy care for women with high-risk pregnancies.
4. Knowledge learned at childbirth classes may reduce the anxiety about the birth processes.

5. Knowledge that her feelings are common to most women may provide some relief from anxiety.

Evaluation

Kathy says she is reassured by explanations regarding the reactive nonstress test but is concerned about how she will do in labor. She initiates plans to attend a childbirth education class with her sister as the coach.

Additional Nursing Diagnoses to Consider

Readiness for enhanced family coping
Risk for Injury

or missed insulin doses, particularly in the woman with type 1 diabetes. Moreover, ketoacidosis may develop during pregnancy at lower thresholds of hyperglycemia than when the woman is not pregnant. Untreated ketoacidosis can progress to fetal and maternal death.

Urinary tract infections are more common, possibly because glucose-rich urine provides a good medium for bacterial growth. Other effects include hydramnios, which may result from fetal hyperglycemia and consequent fetal diuresis, and premature rupture of membranes, which may be caused by overdistention of the uterus by hydramnios or a large fetus. A difficult labor, shoulder dystocia (delayed or difficult birth of fetal shoulders after the head is born), and injury to the birth canal are more likely if the fetus is large. Large fetal size also increases the likelihood that a cesarean birth will be necessary and increases the risk for postpartum hemorrhage.

Production of excess amniotic fluid (hydramnios) may occur if maternal insulin control is not optimal. The excess fluid distends the uterus, possibly leading to early rupture of membranes, prolapsed cord (see Chapter 27), and abnormal labor and postpartum hemorrhage caused by failure of the uterus to contract effectively.

Fetal Effects

Fetal and neonatal effects of preexisting diabetes depend on the timing and severity of maternal hyperglycemia and the degree of maternal vascular impairment. During the first trimester, when major fetal organ development is occurring, the effects of the abnormal metabolic environment, such as hypoglycemia, hyperglycemia, and ketosis, may lead to an increased incidence of spontaneous abortion or major fetal malformations.

Congenital Malformation. The most common major congenital malformations associated with preexisting diabetes are neural tube defects, caudal regression syndrome, and cardiac defects. Women who are hyperglycemic during the first trimester have a risk that is 4 to 8 times higher than for women with normal serum glucose of having an infant with a structural anomaly. Fewer malformations occur in women with good glycemic control during formation of major body structures (Moore, 2004).

The occurrence of maternal and fetal-neonatal complications can be greatly diminished if the mother maintains normal and stable blood glucose levels before and throughout pregnancy. The objective of the team providing treatment is to devise a plan that allows the woman to maintain a blood glucose level as close to normal as possible (see Nursing Care Plan: Pregnancy and Diabetes Mellitus).

Variations in Fetal Size. Fetal growth is related to maternal vascular integrity. In women without vascular impairment, glucose and oxygen are easily transported to the fetus; if the woman is hyperglycemic, so is the fetus. Although maternal insulin does not cross the placental barrier, the fetus produces insulin by the 10th week of gestation. Fetal macrosomia results when elevated levels of blood glucose stimulate excessive production of fetal insulin, which acts as a powerful growth hormone.

Conversely, placental perfusion may be decreased with vascular impairment. Vascular impairment may be caused by complications of the diabetes or by vasoconstriction that occurs in preeclampsia, a common added complication for all women with diabetes. When placental perfusion is impaired, the supply of glucose as well as oxygen will be decreased. If placental perfusion is impaired for a prolonged period, the infant is likely to be small for gestational age (intrauterine fetal growth restriction, or IUGR).

Neonatal Effects

The four major complications of maternal diabetes for the newborn are hypoglycemia, hypocalcemia, hyperbilirubinemia, and respiratory distress syndrome. All can be minimized by stabilizing and maintaining maternal glucose levels near normal, particularly in the last weeks of pregnancy and during labor.

Cardiac Dysfunction. In addition to birth injuries, exceptionally large newborns, often weighing well over 4500 g (about 9 lb), may have cardiac problems. Congestive cardiomyopathy is characterized by thickening of the myocardium and the septum between chambers and may result in congestive heart failure. Treatment may include digoxin, diuretics, or both (Moore, 2004).

Hypoglycemia. The neonate is at higher risk for hypoglycemia because fetal insulin production was accelerated during pregnancy to metabolize excessive glucose received from the expectant mother. The constant stimulation of hyperglycemia leads to hyperplasia and hypertrophy of the islets of Langerhans in the pancreas. At birth, when the maternal glucose supply is withdrawn, the level of neonatal insulin exceeds the available glucose and hypoglycemia develops rapidly.

Hypocalcemia. Hypocalcemia, defined as a calcium concentration of under 7 mg/dl, usually occurs within 72 hours of birth. The risk for hypocalcemia is less if the maternal glucose level is controlled (Moore, 2004).

Hyperbilirubinemia. The fetus who experiences recurrent hypoxia caused by maternal vascular impairment compensates by producing additional erythrocytes to carry oxygen supplied by the mother, resulting in polycythemia. After birth, the excess in erythrocytes is broken down, releasing large amounts of bilirubin into the neonate's circulation.

Respiratory Distress Syndrome. Fetal hyperinsulinemia retards cortisol production, which is necessary for synthesis of surfactant that increases the risk that the newborn will experience respiratory distress syndrome. Reduced lung fluid clearance and delayed thinning of lung connective tissue may also play a part, although other authorities believe that gestational age is the primary determinant of whether an infant will have respiratory distress syndrome (Cunningham, 2001; Roberts, 2004). (See Chapters 29 and 30 for additional information about neonatal complications.)

Maternal Assessment

The initial prenatal assessment for the woman with preexisting diabetes includes a history, physical examination, and laboratory tests.

History. A detailed history should include the onset and management of the diabetic condition. How long has she had the disease? How does she maintain normal blood glucose levels? Can she monitor her blood glucose level and self-administer insulin? The degree of glycemic control before pregnancy is of particular interest. Effective management depends on her adherence to a plan of care. Therefore her knowledge of how diabetes and pregnancy interact must be determined. Her support person's knowledge also must be assessed, and specific learning needs should be identified. In addition, the woman's emotional status should be assessed to determine how she is coping with pregnancy superimposed on preexisting diabetes.

All women with diabetes should be seen by a qualified nurse educator for an individualized assessment to ensure that they can monitor blood glucose accurately. Accurate readings depend on performing the test correctly and as often as recommended by the health care team. Most women who need a hypoglycemic agent take insulin rather than an oral agent, although an occasional woman refuses to take injectable medication for blood glucose control. The nurse must observe the woman's skill in mixing and administering insulin, using a sliding scale for added insulin, or in using an insulin pump if the drug will be given that way.

Physical Examination. In addition to routine prenatal examination (see Chapter 13), specific efforts should be made to assess the effects of diabetes. A baseline electrocardiogram (ECG) determines cardiovascular status. Evaluation for retinopathy should be performed, with referral to an ophthalmologist if necessary. The woman's weight and blood pressure must be monitored carefully because of the increased risk for the development of preeclampsia. Fundal height should be measured, noting any abnormal increase in size that may indicate macrosomia or hydramnios. Reduced growth in fundal height suggests intrauterine growth restriction associated with maternal vascular impairment. Ultrasonography is indicated to determine true gestational age and to identify any abnormal fetal growth.

Laboratory Tests. In addition to routine prenatal laboratory examinations, baseline renal function should be assessed with a 24-hour urine collection for total protein excretion and creatinine clearance. A random midstream urine sample should be checked at each prenatal visit for possible urinary tract infections and for the presence of protein, glucose, and ketones. Thyroid function tests should be performed because of the risk for coexisting thyroid disease.

Glycemic control should be evaluated on the basis of *glycosylated hemoglobin,* or HbA_{1c}. Prolonged hyperglycemia causes some of the hemoglobin in erythrocytes to remain saturated with glucose for the life of the red blood cell. Unlike other tests, which reflect the amount of glucose in the plasma at that moment, the HbA_{1c} assay result is not affected by recent intake or restriction of food.

Fetal Surveillance

Because of the increased risk for congenital anomalies or fetal death, surveillance should begin early for women with preexisting diabetes. Testing for anomalies includes triple marker screening to identify possible neural tube or other open defects and for possible chromosome abnormalities. Testing also includes performing ultrasonography and fetal echocardiography at 20 to 22 weeks to determine the integrity of the fetal body and cardiac structure (ACOG, 2001b; Cunningham et al., 2001; Moore, 2004).

During the third trimester, the goal of fetal surveillance is to identify markers that suggest a worsening intrauterine environment with a higher probability of fetal death. Surveillance may include maternal assessment of fetal movement ("kick counts"), biophysical profiles, nonstress tests, and contraction stress tests. Ultrasonography is also used to document fetal growth rates. Doppler velocimetry may be recommended if vascular complications exist or if hypertension develops. See Chapter 16 for a description of fetal surveillance methods.

Therapeutic Management

The goals of therapeutic management for a pregnant woman with diabetes are (1) to normalize and maintain maternal blood glucose levels as near normal as possible, (2) to increase the likelihood that the baby will be born healthy, and (3) to avoid accelerated impairment of maternal blood vessels and other major organs. Pregnant women with diabetes are cared for by a team, which may include a diabetologist, who assists in regulation of maternal blood glucose; a perinatologist, who monitors the mother and fetus and determines the optimal time for birth; a dietitian, who provides a balanced meal plan that considers the woman's individual needs; and a nurse, who provides ongoing education and support. The team is completed by a neonatologist, who will care for the newborn, and by the family physician and the pediatrician, who will provide ongoing care for the infant and mother after birth.

Preconception Care. Ideally, care should begin before conception. Both prospective parents should participate in care sessions to learn more about the following issues:

- Establishing the optimal time to undertake pregnancy, based on maintenance of normal maternal blood glucose levels, to reduce the risk for major fetal malformations
- Evaluating the degree of maternal vascular complications and end organ damage
- Understanding the importance of maintaining normal blood glucose levels throughout the pregnancy
- Correctly performing home glucose monitoring techniques

Diet. Diet recommendations are individualized during a diabetic pregnancy. The average recommended caloric intake for the pregnant diabetic woman of normal weight is 30 kcal/kg/day. Approximately 40% to 45% of the calories should be from carbohydrates, 12% to 20% from protein (about 60 g), and up to 40% from fat. Caloric intake should be distributed among three meals and two or more snacks. The bedtime snack should include a complex carbohydrate and protein. Women who are overweight or underweight usually have lower or higher caloric goals.

Self-Monitoring of Blood Glucose. The best frequency for self-monitoring of glucose of capillary blood has not yet been established. One common testing regimen requires obtaining fasting and 2-hour postprandial levels. Another includes testing six times per day: a fasting capillary glucose, 1 to 2 hours after breakfast, before and after lunch, before dinner, and at bedtime. One study found that the postprandial levels were most effective at predicting fetal macrosomia and other adverse outcomes (ACOG, 2001b; Moore, 2004). In addition to regular monitoring, the woman should also perform a glucose test whenever she experiences symptoms of hypoglycemia. The woman should record all test results on a log sheet for review by the health care provider at each visit. Instruments for self-monitoring of blood glucose usually have a memory to provide accurate recall of times and glucose levels.

Insulin Therapy. The need to maintain rigorous control of maternal metabolism during pregnancy requires more frequent doses of insulin than usual. Most treatment regimens rely on three daily injections, with a combination of short-acting (regular) insulin and intermediate-acting (NPH) insulin given before breakfast, regular insulin before dinner, and NPH insulin at bedtime. Lispro and aspart (Humalog and Novolog respectively) insulins act rapidly and should be injected just before a meal. The rapid-acting insulins have been shown to control postprandial hyperglycemia with less between-meals hypoglycemia (Moore, 2004). Because placental hormones cause insulin needs to change throughout pregnancy, insulin coverage will need to be adjusted as pregnancy progresses.

First Trimester. Insulin needs generally decline during the first trimester because the secretion of placental hormones that are antagonistic to insulin remains low during this time. The woman may also experience nausea, vomiting, and anorexia, resulting in decreased intake of food, and thus may need less insulin. Moreover, the fetus receives its share of glucose, which reduces maternal plasma glucose levels and decreases the need for maternal insulin.

Second and Third Trimesters. Insulin needs increase markedly during the second and third trimesters, when placental hormones, which initiate maternal resistance to the effects of insulin, reach their peak. The nausea of early pregnancy usually resolves, and the woman needs additional calories per day to meet the increased metabolic demands of pregnancy.

During Labor. Maintenance of tight maternal glucose control during birth is desirable to reduce neonatal hypoglycemia. Continuous infusion of a regular or lispro insulin solution combined with a separate intravenous solution containing glucose, such as 5% dextrose in Ringer's lactate, allows titration to maintain blood glucose levels between 80 and 110 mg/dl. The insulin solution is raised, lowered, or discontinued to maintain euglycemia based on hourly capillary blood glucose levels. If blood glucose levels remain too high, the insulin infusion is adjusted and the primary intravenous infusion is changed to one without glucose.

Women with type 2 or gestational diabetes that has been controlled by diet during pregnancy can usually maintain normal glucose levels during labor if glucose-bearing intravenous solutions are avoided (Cunningham et al., 2001; Moore, 2004).

Postpartum. Insulin needs should decline rapidly after delivery of the placenta and the abrupt cessation of placental hormones. Blood glucose levels should be monitored at least four times daily, however, so that the insulin dose can be adjusted to meet individual needs.

Timing of Delivery. If possible, the pregnancy should be allowed to progress to 38 weeks to allow fetal lungs to mature, reducing the risk for neonatal respiratory distress syndrome. With evidence of fetal compromise, such as nonreassuring biophysical profile or reduced amniotic fluid, delivery may be required. If delivery before 38 weeks is contemplated for non-emergency causes, amniocentesis to determine fetal lung maturity is often done, since lung maturation may be slower than in non-diabetic pregnancies.

Gestational Diabetes Mellitus

Risk Factors

Gestational diabetes mellitus (GDM) is a carbohydrate intolerance of variable severity that develops or is first recognized during pregnancy. Some maternity women diagnosed with gestational diabetes may actually have unrecognized type 2 diabetes. Factors associated with a higher risk for gestational diabetes are similar to those for type 2 diabetes (ACOG, 2001b; American Diabetes Association, 2003a).

- Obesity (body mass index [BMI] >25)
- Maternal age older than 25 years
- Previous birth outcome often associated with GDM (neonatal macrosomia, maternal hypertension, infant with unexplained congenital anomalies, previous fetal death)
- Gestational diabetes in previous pregnancy
- History of abnormal glucose tolerance
- History of diabetes in a close (first degree) relative
- Member of a high-risk ethnic group (Hispanic, African, Native American, South or East Asian, or Pacific Islands ancestry)

Identifying Gestational Diabetes Mellitus

All pregnant women should be screened by identification of a history or risk factors that are consistent for GDM or by blood glucose testing. A common screening test is the glucose challenge test administered between 24 and 28 weeks. An oral glucose tolerance test may be used as the initial test if a woman is at high risk for GDM but is more likely to be used as a diagnostic test when abnormally high glucose challenge test results occur. Women with a fasting glucose level >126 mg/dl or a nonfasting level of >200 mg/dl meet the criteria for GDM, and no added testing is needed (ACOG, 2001b; American Diabetes Association, 2003a).

Glucose Challenge Test. Fasting is not necessary for a glucose challenge test, and the woman is not required to follow any pretest dietary instructions. The woman should ingest 50 g of oral glucose solution; 1 hour later a blood sample is taken. If the blood glucose concentration is 140 mg/dl or greater, a 3-hour oral glucose tolerance test (OGTT) is recommended. Some practitioners use a lower cutoff of 130 or 135 mg/dl to identify more women at risk (ACOG, 2001b; American Diabetes Association, 2003a; Moore, 2004).

Oral Glucose Tolerance Test. The OGTT is the gold standard for diagnosing diabetes, but it is a more complicated test. The woman must ingest a high-carbohydrate diet for 3 days before the scheduled test and must fast from midnight before the day of the test. After a fasting plasma glucose level is determined, the woman should ingest 100 g of oral glucose solution. Plasma glucose levels are then determined at 1, 2, and 3 hours. Gestational diabetes is the diagnosis if the fasting blood glucose level is abnormal or if two or more of the following values occur on the OGTT (ACOG, 2001b; American Diabetes Association, 2003a):

- Fasting, greater than 95 mg/dl
- 1 hour, greater than 180 mg/dl
- 2 hours, greater than 155 mg/dl
- 3 hours, greater than 140 mg/dl

Maternal, Fetal, and Neonatal Effects

With a few important exceptions, the effects of gestational diabetes are similar to those associated with preexisting type 2 diabetes. Because gestational diabetes develops after the first trimester, which is the critical period of major fetal organ development (organogenesis), it is not usually associated with an increase in the incidence of major congenital malformations. Nevertheless, poorly-controlled gestational diabetes, with maternal hyperglycemia during the third trimester, is associated with macrosomia and neonatal hypoglycemia.

TABLE **26-5** Major Effects of Diabetes Mellitus on Pregnancy

Increased Maternal Risks	Probable Cause
Pregnancy-induced hypertension	Unknown but increased even without renal or vascular impairment
Urinary tract infections	Increased bacterial growth in nutrient-rich urine
Ketoacidosis (risk for mother and fetus)	Uncontrolled hyperglycemia or infection; most common in woman with type 1 diabetes
Labor dystocia; cesarean birth; uterine atony with hemorrhage after birth	Hydramnios secondary to fetal osmotic diuresis caused by hyperglycemia; uterus is overstretched
Birth injury to maternal tissues (hematoma, lacerations)	Fetal macrosomia causing difficult birth

Increased Fetal and Neonatal Risks	Probable Cause
Congenital anomalies	Maternal hyperglycemia during organ formation in first trimester
Perinatal death	Poor placental perfusion because of maternal vascular impairment, primarily in woman with type 1 diabetes
Macrosomia (>4000 g)	Fetal hyperglycemia stimulating production of insulin to metabolize carbohydrates; excess nutrients transported to fetus
Intrauterine fetal growth restriction	Maternal vascular impairment
Preterm labor; premature rupture of membranes; preterm birth	Overdistention of uterus caused by hydramnios and large fetal size at preterm gestation
Birth injury	Large fetal size; shoulder dystocia or other difficult delivery
Hypoglycemia	Neonatal hyperinsulinemia after birth when maternal glucose is no longer available (but insulin production remains high)
Polycythemia	Fetal hypoxemia stimulating erythrocyte production
Hyperbilirubinemia	Breakdown of excessive red blood cells after birth
Hypocalcemia	Transfer of calcium abruptly stopped at birth, reduced fetal parathyroid function
Respiratory distress syndrome	Delayed maturation of fetal lungs; inadequate production of pulmonary surfactant; slowed absorption of fetal lung fluid

Hypocalcemia, hyperbilirubinemia, and respiratory distress may also occur. Table 26-5 summarizes maternal, fetal, and neonatal effects of diabetes mellitus and their probable causes.

Therapeutic Management

Diet. Ideally a registered dietitian or diabetes educator determines the dietary needs for the woman with GDM. The diet should provide the calories and nutrients needed for maternal and fetal health, result in euglycemia, avoid ketosis, and promote appropriate weight gain. Calories should be distributed in a way similar to that for preexisting diabetes. Simple sugars found in concentrated sweets should be eliminated from the diet. The obese woman may be prescribed a diet with a smaller percentage of carbohydrates than the woman of normal weight. Carbohydrates should be adequate to prevent ketosis in all women. Calories should be divided among three meals and at least three snacks (ACOG, 2001b; Moore, 2004).

Exercise. Exercise plays a significant role in managing blood glucose levels in women who develop gestational diabetes and in women with type 2 diabetes who become pregnant. The exercise regimen should be recommended by a physician who takes into account each woman's risk factors and risks to the fetus. Regular exercise improves glucose metabolism, offers cardiorespiratory benefits, and aids in weight control (ACOG, 2001b; American Diabetes Association, 2003b).

Glucose Level Monitoring. As in care of the woman with preexisting diabetes, self-monitoring of blood glucose levels helps guide diet and insulin therapy (see p. 653). Optimum frequency and timing of glucose monitoring also has not been established for GDM.

Fetal Surveillance. Fetal surveillance methods (see Chapter 16) for the woman with GDM are similar to those for the woman with preexisting diabetes. Ultrasound is used to identify macrosomia and abnormal amniotic fluid volume and is used to guide amniocentesis for fetal lung maturity if labor induction or cesarean is planned.

Nursing Considerations

The care of a pregnant woman with diabetes mellitus focuses primarily on helping her maintain normal blood glucose levels and optimum fetal condition. Some women respond calmly to the intense medical supervision; others respond with anxiety, fear, denial, or anger and feel inadequate or unable to control the diabetes to the degree expected by the health care team. Still others fear for their own or their baby's health, especially when the diagnosis is a new one.

Increasing Effective Communication. Nurses must ask specifically about the feelings and concerns the woman and her family have about the pregnancy.

Broad opening questions, such as "What are your major concerns?" and "How do you feel about the plan of care?" help identify the woman's greatest concerns. These should be followed with more specific questions, such as "How do you feel about the fetal testing?" and "What would you like to change about your diet?"

The nurse must be an active listener and allow time for the woman and her family to express concerns and feelings. The nurse must convey acceptance of feelings that are expressed, whether they are negative or positive. Sharing of emotions will help the woman avoid unnecessary guilt, anxiety, or frustration and thus promote her active participation in her plan of care.

Most women benefit from praise when diabetic control is well maintained. They feel competent and trusted by the health care team and are motivated to continue their efforts.

Providing Opportunities for Control. Providing ways for the woman to make decisions increases her sense of control. For instance, she can select foods from the exchange list that provide the necessary nutrients but still allow her some choice. She may also develop a regular schedule of exercise and sleep that helps keep the blood glucose level under control. Nurses should allow as much flexibility as possible when scheduling stressful events, such as fetal monitoring tests and amniocentesis.

Providing Normal Pregnancy Care. The nurse caring for a woman with diabetes should provide education and counseling regarding normal pregnancy changes and discomforts. Also, because women with diabetes are concerned about how they will manage during labor and delivery, nurses should offer childbirth preparation classes and discuss with them the experiences common to all pregnant women.

NURSING CARE
The Pregnant Woman With Diabetes Mellitus

Assessment

Determine how well the woman understands the prescribed management and how she plans to carry out the recommended regimen. She may be newly diagnosed and may have no experience in the necessary skills and procedures. On the other hand, she may be skilled in monitoring glucose levels and administering insulin but may have no knowledge of the effects of diabetes on pregnancy or the effects of pregnancy on diabetes management.

To determine whether her techniques are accurate, ask the expectant mother to demonstrate how she monitors her blood glucose level and observe how she mixes and injects insulins. Verify that she and her family are aware of the need to select appropriate sites and injection techniques.

Although diet is often prescribed by a dietitian or a diabetes educator, it is necessary to assess how well the family understands the diet. Diet recommendations include a target number of calories, plus targets for grams of carbohydrate, protein, and fat to meet calorie needs. Any of several methods to count and exchange foods may be used. One method uses exchange lists, in which the listed foods all have about the same grams of carbohydrate, protein, and fat. Thus one food from the list may be substituted, or exchanged, for another in the same list. Another method uses carbohydrate counting, in which foods on the starch, fruit, or milk list supply about 15 g of carbohydrate, or one carbohydrate choice. The diet plan would prescribe the number of carbohydrate choices for each meal and snack. Insulin is often adjusted according to the carbohydrate count for each meal or snack.

Identify special needs related to food preferences, culturally prescribed foods, or the availability of recommended foods. It may be necessary to review the exchange list and ask the woman how she plans to substitute and exchange foods to obtain the prescribed number of foods from each list.

Identify the woman's knowledge of potential complications, such as hypoglycemia and hyperglycemia, so that she and her family can be provided with pertinent information to avoid and treat it.

Determine her knowledge of fetal surveillance techniques and her response to the need for frequent tests. Some women are highly motivated to continue the treatment regimen when test results indicate the fetus is thriving. Other women find the frequent testing stressful and inconvenient.

Nursing Diagnosis and Planning

One of the most common nursing diagnoses is either

■ Risk for or actual Ineffective Health Maintenance related to knowledge deficit of specific measures to maintain normal blood glucose levels; signs, symptoms, and management of hypoglycemia and hyperglycemia; and recommended fetal surveillance procedures.

Goals/Expected Outcomes: The woman and her family will demonstrate competence in home glucose monitoring and administration of insulin before home management is initiated; describe a plan for meeting dietary recommendations that fits their lifestyle and food preferences; identify signs and symptoms of hypoglycemia and hyperglycemia and the management required for each; and verbalize knowledge of fetal surveillance procedures and keep scheduled appointments for testing.

Interventions

Although management of diabetes mellitus during pregnancy is a team effort, the nurse's major responsibility is to provide accurate information about the recommended therapeutic regimen and to offer consistent support for the woman's efforts to comply with the recommendations. It may be necessary to demonstrate specific skills that the woman and her family must master and to review and reinforce information that comes from other members of the health care team.

Teaching Self-Care Skills

Demonstration and return demonstration are effective ways to teach and evaluate psychomotor skills. The woman (and her family) must learn to use a meter and obtain a small sample of blood to test for glucose determination and to mix and inject insulin. Both procedures are invasive and cause mild discomfort, which may make the woman reluctant to start. Mixing insulins accurately or using a sliding scale may be intimidating at first. Using food exchanges is often unfamiliar to the woman who is newly diagnosed, but it is critical to glucose control. Acknowledge these feelings before teaching begins.

Self-Monitoring of Blood Glucose Spring-loaded lancets make home blood glucose monitoring easier. The side of the fingertip is less sensitive than the pad and may be less uncomfortable. Teach her to cleanse the area with warm water before obtaining a sample, to prevent infection. The first drop of blood is wiped away, and the second drop is used to place blood on the meter's strip. Each home monitoring kit contains specific instructions for use of the meter. Teach her how to record glucose values in a handwritten log.

Insulin Administration The woman is usually prescribed a combination of short- and intermediate-acting insulins. Teach the expectant mother the difference in onset, peak, and duration of action of each type of insulin. She also needs to learn how to mix the two insulins in the same syringe. If she will use a sliding scale to keep glucose levels closer to normal, she will need teaching about how to determine the dose of insulin in addition to scheduled injections if she has never used sliding scale insulin administration.

The use of programmable insulin infusion pumps allows tailoring of insulin administration to the woman's individual lifestyle and may result in more stable glucose levels within the target range. The woman will need instruction on programming, loading and changing syringes, and changing injection sites. Assistance should be available 24 hours a day to provide emergency counseling.

Insulin is administered subcutaneously. Common sites include the upper thighs, abdomen, and upper arms. Because the pregnant woman is injecting insulin frequently, emphasize these precautions:

- To prevent hypoglycemia, a meal should be taken 30 minutes after regular insulin is injected. Because of its 10-minute onset of action, lispro insulin is injected just before eating.
- Unless the woman is very thin, insulin should be injected with the short needle inserted at a 90-degree angle so that the tip of the needle reaches the fatty tissue layer.
- The needle should be inserted quickly to minimize discomfort.
- The tissue pinch, if used, is released after inserting the needle and before injecting insulin because pressure from the pinch can promote insulin leakage from the subcutaneous tissue.
- It is not necessary to aspirate to ensure the needle has not been placed in a blood vessel when injecting insulin into subcutaneous tissue.

- Insulin is injected slowly (over 2 to 4 seconds) to allow tissue expansion and to minimize pressure, which can cause insulin leakage.
- The needle is withdrawn quickly to minimize the formation of a track, which might permit insulin to leak out.

Emphasize the importance of administering the correct dosage at the correct time. Teach the woman and her family the function of insulin and the importance of following the directions of her physician in regard to coordinating meals with the administration of insulin.

Teaching Dietary Management

Although a dietitian prescribes the recommended diet, the nurse must be aware of the general requirements and must be sensitive to the expectant mother's dietary habits and preferences. There is often a need to review and clarify how the exchange lists are used to plan meals and snacks. Teach the woman to avoid simple sugars (candy, cake, cookies, juice), which raise the blood glucose levels quickly but may result in wide swings between high and low.

It may be necessary to help the woman select foods high in nutrients but low in cost or to meet cultural or religious constraints. Animal protein is especially expensive, and alternative sources of protein (beans, peas, corn, grains) can be substituted to meet some of the protein needs as well as provide high-quality carbohydrate and fiber.

Recognizing and Correcting Hypoglycemia and Hyperglycemia

Every woman and her family must be aware of the signs and symptoms that indicate abnormal blood glucose levels. If they are not identified and corrected quickly, hypoglycemia and hyperglycemia pose a threat to mother and fetus.

Hypoglycemia Treat hypoglycemia at once to prevent damage to the brain, which depends on glucose. If the woman is able to swallow, have her drink 8 ounces of milk and eat two crackers. Repeat the snack in 15 minutes if symptoms persist or her blood glucose level is between 40 and 80 mg/dl. Glucose tablets are often recommended to treat hypoglycemia because of their consistent glucose content.

Teach family members how to inject glucagon in the event that the woman cannot swallow or retain food. Notify the physician at once. Intravenous glucose will be administered if she is hospitalized. If untreated, hypoglycemia can progress to convulsions and death.

To prevent episodes of hypoglycemia, instruct the woman to have meals at a fixed time each day and to plan snacks at the recommended times. Suggest that she carry glucose tablets or a container of milk and some dry crackers whenever possible.

! CRITICAL TO REMEMBER

Signs and Symptoms of Maternal Hypoglycemia

- Shakiness (tremors)
- Sweating
- Pallor; cold, clammy skin
- Disorientation, irritability
- Headache
- Hunger
- Blurred vision

! CRITICAL TO REMEMBER

Signs and Symptoms of Maternal Hyperglycemia

- Fatigue
- Flushed, hot skin
- Dry mouth, excessive thirst
- Frequent urination
- Rapid, deep respirations; odor of acetone on the breath
- Drowsiness, headache
- Depressed reflexes

Hyperglycemia Because infection is the most common cause of hyperglycemia in a woman with preexisting diabetes, pregnant women must be instructed to notify the physician whenever they have an infection of any type.

If untreated, hyperglycemia can lead to ketoacidosis, coma, and maternal and fetal death. If signs and symptoms occur, notify the physician at once so that treatment can be initiated. Hospitalization is often necessary for monitoring blood glucose levels and intravenous administration of insulin.

Explaining Procedures, Tests, and Plan of Care

Explain the schedule and the reasons for frequent checkups and tests. Encourage the woman and her family to ask questions if any part of the schedule is confusing. Pregnant women and their families need to know why frequent non-stress tests or other tests are necessary. They need to know that their diabetic care will take more time and effort than it did before pregnancy but that this care greatly improves the likelihood that they will have healthy infants.

Evaluation

After the procedures, tests, and plan of care have been explained, the family should be evaluated:

- Can the expectant mother and one family member demonstrate competence in blood glucose monitoring and administration of insulin?
- Can the family describe a plan for meeting dietary requirements?
- Can the woman and her family list the signs and symptoms of hypoglycemia and hyperglycemia?
- Can the woman and her family describe the initial management of these conditions?
- Can the woman verbalize knowledge of the reason for fetal surveillance procedures and keep appointments for tests?

CARDIAC DISEASE

Cardiovascular function changes during pregnancy to meet additional maternal metabolic demands and the needs of the fetus. Plasma volume, venous return, and cardiac output all increase. Heart rate and stroke volume, the two components of cardiac output, increase during pregnancy. The heart rate gradually rises above baseline during the third trimester, but an increase in stroke volume is primarily responsible for the overall rise in cardiac output during early pregnancy.

A normal heart adapts to the changes so that the woman tolerates pregnancy and birth without difficulty. With underlying heart disease, however, the changes can impose an additional burden on an already compromised heart, and cardiac decompensation and congestive heart failure can result.

Incidence and Classification

Successful treatment of congenital cardiac anomalies or mitral stenosis resulting from rheumatic heart disease now allows many girls to reach childbearing age and bear children. Rheumatic heart disease, a complication of streptococcal infection, is not common in the United States but may be found in recent immigrants. Hypertensive heart disease, often a secondary effect of obesity, can be expected to affect more childbearing women because of the growing incidence in the general population (Cunningham et al., 2001; Freid et al., 2003). Cardiomyopathy is a disorder of the muscle structure of the heart that may have any of several causes. Congestive heart failure may be secondary to underlying heart disease or damage or may occur secondary to treatment for other conditions.

Rheumatic Heart Disease

Rheumatic heart disease is a complication that sometimes follows a streptococcal pharyngitis infection (strep throat). Even one bout of rheumatic fever may cause scarring of the heart valves, resulting in stenosis (narrowing) of the openings between the chambers of the heart. Early diagnosis and treatment of the streptococcal infection has resulted in a near-eradication of rheumatic fever in North America and Europe.

The mitral valve is the most common site of stenosis. Mitral stenosis obstructs free flow of blood from the left atrium to the left ventricle. The left atrium becomes dilated. As a result, pressure in the left atrium, the pulmonary veins, and pulmonary capillaries is chronically elevated. This elevation may lead to pulmonary hypertension, pulmonary edema, or congestive heart failure. The first warnings of heart failure include persistent rales at the base of the lungs, dyspnea on exertion, cough, and hemoptysis. Progressive edema and tachycardia are additional signs of heart failure.

Congenital Heart Disease

Congenital heart defects can be grouped into those that cause a left-to-right shunt and those that result in a right-to-left shunt. Those defects that produce left-to-right shunting include atrial and ventricular septal defects and patent ductus arteriosus. Right-to-left shunting occurs with a cyanotic heart defect, such as tetralogy of Fallot. Right-to-left shunting may also occur through a septal defect or a patent ductus arteriosus when pulmonary vascular resistance exceeds peripheral vascular resistance and pulmonary hypertension (Eisenmenger syndrome) occurs.

Left-to-Right Shunt

Atrial Septal Defect. Atrial septal defect is often first discovered in women of childbearing age because symptoms are absent or vague. This defect produces a left-to-right shunt because pressure in the left side of the heart is higher than it is in the right side. Pregnancy is well tolerated by patients with no complications. Bacterial endocarditis is rare, and prophylactic antibiotics are not required. Atrial septal defects are not associated with heart failure; therefore digitalis, diuretics, and extreme limitation of intravenous infusions are not warranted. Left-to-right shunting, however, may increase the chance of pulmonary hypertension because the additional blood that moves to the right side of the heart is transported to the lungs via the pulmonary artery (Blanchard & Shabetai, 2004; Caulin-Glaser & Setaro, 1999).

Ventricular Septal Defect. Although ventricular septal defects are more common at birth than atrial septal defects, ventricular septal defects are usually detected and corrected before girls reach childbearing age. Most women with these defects who become pregnant are asymptomatic, but occasionally fatigue or symptoms of pulmonary congestion occur.

How pregnancy is tolerated is directly related to the size of the defect. Small defects are unlikely to cause pulmonary hypertension and heart failure. If heart failure or dysrhythmias occur, they are managed as in nonpregnant patients. Bacterial endocarditis is common with unrepaired defects, and antibacterial prophylaxis is usual.

Patent Ductus Arteriosus. The communicating shunt between the pulmonary artery and aorta is usually discovered and treated in childhood. If untreated, the physiologic effects are related to size. If small, this lesion, like septal defects, may be well tolerated during pregnancy unless complicated by pulmonary hypertension. The patent ductus arteriosus tends to become infected, so antibiotic prophylaxis is recommended, particularly during labor.

Right-to-Left Shunt

Tetralogy of Fallot. The primary cause of right-to-left shunting is tetralogy of Fallot, a combination of four defects (ventricular septal defect, pulmonary valve stenosis, right ventricular hypertrophy, and displacement of the aorta so that it overrides part of the right ventricle). Untreated patients with tetralogy of Fallot have obvious symptoms of heart disease that include (1) cyanosis, (2) clubbing of the fingers, indicating proliferation of capillaries to transport blood to the extremities, and (3) inability to tolerate activity.

Women who have undergone repair and in whom cyanosis did not reappear may do well during pregnancy. With uncorrected tetralogy of Fallot, more common in women from undeveloped countries, maternal mortality approaches 10% (Blanchard & Shabetai, 2004; Cunningham et al., 2001).

Eisenmenger Syndrome. Eisenmenger syndrome is a cyanotic heart condition that develops when pulmonary resistance equals or exceeds systemic resistance to blood flow and a right-to-left shunt develops. Several underlying congenital defects may underlie the equalization of pressures within the ventricles, such as a large ventricular septal defect or a large patent ductus arteriosus (PDA). Operative closure of these defects must be done as soon as possible in defects that may cause Eisenmenger syndrome. A late surgical correction often results in the patient's death. If she survives delayed surgery, pregnancy may carry a 50% maternal mortality risk, usually from right ventricular failure (Blanchard & Shabetai, 2004).

Mitral Valve Prolapse

Mitral valve prolapse is one of the most common cardiac conditions among the general population. The incidence among otherwise healthy young women is 2% to 3%. Although the condition appears to be inherited, mitral valve prolapse is associated with a variety of other cardiac disorders, such as atrial septal defects and Marfan syndrome (Cunningham et al., 2001).

The leaflets of the mitral valve prolapse into the left atrium during ventricular contraction. Most women with mitral valve

---

BOX 26-3
New York Heart Association Functional Classification of Heart Disease

- *Class I:* Uncompromised. No limitation of physical activity. Asymptomatic with ordinary activity.
- *Class II:* Slightly compromised, requiring slight limitation of physical activity. Comfortable at rest, but ordinary physical activity causes fatigue, dyspnea, palpitations, or anginal pain.
- *Class III:* Marked limitation of physical activity. Comfortable at rest, but less than ordinary activity causes excessive fatigue, palpitation, dyspnea, or anginal pain. Markedly compromised.
- *Class IV:* Inability to perform any physical activity without discomfort. Symptoms of cardiac insufficiency even at rest.

In general, maternal and fetal risks with classes I and II disease are small but are greatly increased with classes III and IV.

---

prolapse are asymptomatic. Some women experience dysrhythmias or chest pain, but most women with mitral valve prolapse tolerate pregnancy well. The condition is considered by some to be a significant risk factor for bacterial endocarditis, and some physicians administer prophylactic antibiotics before and during labor and delivery. Beta blockers, such as atenolol or metoprolol, may be given for chest pain or dysrhythmias.

Diagnostic Evaluation of Cardiac Disease

Early recognition of underlying heart disease is essential, and careful assessment for specific signs and symptoms of heart disease is part of every initial prenatal visit. Signs and symptoms include dyspnea, syncope (fainting) with exertion, hemoptysis, paroxysmal nocturnal dyspnea, and chest pain with exertion. Additional signs that confirm the diagnosis are (1) diastolic, presystolic, or continuous heart murmur, (2) cardiac enlargement, (3) a loud, harsh systolic murmur associated with a thrill, or (4) serious dysrhythmias.

The diagnosis of heart disease may be made from clinical signs and symptoms and physical examination. It is confirmed by tests such as chest radiography, electrocardiography, or echocardiography.

Once the diagnosis is made, the severity of the disease can be determined by the woman's ability to endure physical activity. A clinical classification based on the effect of exercise on the heart has been developed by the New York Heart Association (Box 26-3).

Therapeutic Management

Class I and Class II Heart Disease

All pregnant women with heart disease should do the following (Blanchard & Shabetai, 2004; Caulin-Glaser & Setaro, 1999; Cunningham et al., 2001):

- Limit physical activity so that cardiac demand does not exceed the functional capacity of the heart. In other words, the woman should remain free of symptoms of cardiac stress, such as dyspnea, chest pain, or tachycardia.

- Avoid excessive weight gain, which places extra demands on the heart. A diet adequate in protein, calories, and sodium is necessary. A low-sodium diet may be advised to avoid congestive heart failure.
- Prevent anemia, which decreases the oxygen-carrying capacity of the blood and results in a compensatory increase in heart rate that a diseased heart may be unable to tolerate. Most anemia is prevented by administration of iron and folic acid.
- Prevent infection such as upper respiratory infections. Immunization for influenza and pneumonia are available. Prevention may include administration of prophylactic antibiotics.
- Undergo careful assessment for the development of congestive heart failure, pulmonary edema, or cardiac dysrhythmias. Characteristics of heart failure may include persistent basilar rales, often accompanied by a cough during the night as the woman tries to sleep, sudden inability to carry out usual activities, dyspnea, cough, hemoptysis, increasing edema, and tachycardia.

Class III and Class IV Heart Disease

The primary goal of management is to prevent cardiac decompensation and the development of congestive heart failure. Moreover, every effort is also made to protect the fetus from hypoxia and IUGR, which can occur if placental perfusion is inadequate. In addition to the precautions listed for classes I and II heart disease, the woman may require bed rest, especially during the last trimester because she has little reserve to tolerate rising metabolic demands. Reduced activity increases the risk for thrombus formation and will require prophylaxis such as elastic compression stockings or a serial or boot compression device. Prophylactic anticoagulation may be needed.

Drug Therapy

Anticoagulants. During pregnancy, clotting factors normally increase and thrombolytic activity decreases. These changes predispose the pregnant woman to thrombus formation. Superimposed cardiac problems, such as mitral valve stenosis, may require anticoagulant therapy during pregnancy because they add to the tendency to form thrombi. Warfarin (Coumadin) is associated with fetal malformations and should be restricted throughout pregnancy. Subcutaneous heparin, which does not cross the placental barrier, is an effective alternative anticoagulant for most women. Careful monitoring of the partial thromboplastin time, activated partial thromboplastin time, and platelet count is essential to achieve effective, safe anticoagulation. Enoxaparin (Lovenox) may be used instead of heparin because it requires less-frequent monitoring for bleeding complications. Enoxaparin and heparin are not interchangeable. Both are given subcutaneously.

Antidysrhythmics. Use of medications for heart disease during pregnancy must balance benefits to the mother against possible harm to the fetus. Another consideration is that maternal heart failure itself is harmful to the fetus. Digoxin, adenosine, and calcium channel blockers appear to be safe. Beta blockers have been associated with neonatal respiratory depression, sustained bradycardia, and hypoglycemia when administered late in pregnancy or just before delivery but may be needed in selected cases (Blanchard & Shabetai, 2004; Cunningham et al., 2001).

Antiinfectives. Antiinfective agents for endocarditis are chosen based on the infecting agent. Gram-positive staphylococcus infections are common in intravenous drug users, and the mortality is high. Maternal gonorrhea infection may cause acute, rapidly developing endocarditis. A woman with an increased risk for bacterial endocarditis may receive prophylactic antibiotics at delivery, such as amoxicillin, penicillin, ampicillin, and gentamicin. Ceftriaxone or vancomycin also may be given for acute endocarditis.

Drugs for Heart Failure. Diuretics may be needed when congestive heart failure is uncontrolled by restriction of activity and sodium intake. Careful monitoring of electrolytes and water balance is necessary to avoid excessively reducing maternal blood volume with resulting adverse effects on the fetus. Experience is greatest with furosemide and thiazide diuretics. Fetal growth restriction has been associated with furosemide, and neonatal jaundice, thrombocytopenia, anemia, and hypoglycemia have been associated with thiazide diuretics (Blanchard & Shabetai, 2004; Moore, 2004). Beta blockers, ACE inhibitors, or angiotensin receptor blockers, and digoxin also may be used if beneficial for treatment of pregnancy-associated heart failure.

Intrapartum Management

Every effort is made to minimize the effects of labor on the cardiovascular system. For example, with every contraction, 300 to 500 ml of blood is shifted from the uterus and placenta into the central circulation. This extra fluid causes a sharp rise in cardiac workload. Therefore careful management of intravenous fluid administration is essential to prevent fluid overload. The woman should be positioned on her side, with her head and shoulders elevated. Oxygen is administered to increase the blood oxygen saturation, which is monitored by pulse oximetry. Discomfort should be reduced to a minimum, but the use of epidural block is sometimes controversial because of its potential hemodynamic effects (see Chapter 19). The environment is kept as quiet and calm as possible to decrease anxiety, which can cause tachycardia.

The fetus is monitored electronically, and signs of fetal compromise as well as maternal signs of cardiac decompensation (tachycardia, rapid respirations, moist rales, exhaustion) should be reported immediately to the physician.

A vaginal delivery is recommended for a woman with heart disease unless there are specific indications for cesarean birth. Vacuum extraction or outlet forceps are often used to minimize the mother's use of the Valsalva maneuver when pushing during the second stage.

The fourth stage of labor is associated with special risks. After delivery of the placenta, about 500 ml of blood is added

---

! CRITICAL TO REMEMBER

Signs and Symptoms of Congestive Heart Failure

- Cough (frequent, productive, hemoptysis)
- Progressive dyspnea with exertion
- Orthopnea
- Pitting edema of legs and feet or generalized edema of face, hands, or sacral area
- Heart palpitations
- Progressive fatigue or syncope with exertion
- Moist rales in lower lobes, indicating pulmonary edema

to the intravascular volume. To minimize the risks of overloading the heart, abrupt positional changes should be avoided. Moreover, the uterus should not be massaged to expedite separation of the placenta. Careful assessment for signs of circulatory overload, such as a bounding pulse, distended neck and peripheral veins, and moist rales in the lungs, is performed throughout labor and the postpartum.

Postpartum Management

Women who have shown no evidence of cardiac distress during pregnancy, labor, or childbirth may still decompensate during the postpartum period. They must be observed closely for signs of infection, hemorrhage, or thromboembolism. These conditions can act together to precipitate postpartum heart failure in women with underlying heart disease.

Nursing Considerations

To plan care better, the nurse should determine what functional classification the physician has assigned the woman. Assess for changes in vital signs such as tachycardia. Note increasing fatigue or other signs of congestive heart failure at office visits. Review the chart to identify other factors that can increase the woman's cardiac workload, such as anemia, infections, anxiety, or inadequate support to manage the activities of daily living.

During pregnancy, nursing care focuses on helping the woman and her family understand factors that increase the workload of the heart and measures they can adopt to help the woman maintain any needed activity restrictions. Explain how gaining excessive weight during pregnancy or any other time increases the burden on the heart. Anemia causes the heart to pump faster to circulate available erythrocytes to the tissues. A well-balanced diet that yields approximately 2200 calories/day is recommended, with adequate high-quality protein. Emphasize the importance of taking iron and folic acid supplements to prevent anemia.

Identify modifications to allow the woman to live within her cardiac reserve. Explain how she can take rest periods during the day and for an hour after meals. Instruct her to sit rather than stand, if possible, when performing activities. If she performs an activity that increases her heart rate, teach her to rest every few minutes to allow the heart to recover. She should stop the activity if she experiences dyspnea, chest pain, or tachycardia. Chapter 27 contains suggestions for coping with bed rest if it is required.

The woman should avoid extremes of temperature when possible. Instruct her to dress for the cold in layers and to avoid exertion during hot and humid weather.

Emotional stress also increases cardiac demand. Discuss methods for stress management, such as meditation, progressive relaxation, and biofeedback. Teach that cigarette smoking and the use of illicit drugs, such as cocaine and amphetamines, greatly increase stress to her heart and are associated with hypertension.

The woman is vulnerable postpartum, as interstitial fluid is mobilized into the vascular space for elimination. Continue to observe for signs of congestive heart failure. Observe urine output because inadequate urine output may reflect the heart's inability to circulate blood adequately to the kidneys. If the mother cannot assume the care of her infant, nurses should make every effort to promote contact between the mother, her significant others, and the infant. Breastfeeding

imposes extra demands on the mother's heart, and whether it is advised is individualized.

The mother and new family may need help at home. Consult physicians and make any needed referrals for follow-up care, which may include home visits by a nurse or nursing assistant. Before the woman is discharged, review the signs and symptoms of cardiac complications and note the times when she should contact the physician.

ANEMIAS

Anemia is a condition in which a decline in circulating red blood cell mass reduces the capacity to carry oxygen to the vital organs of the mother or fetus. Significant maternal anemia is associated with preterm birth and low birth weight. A woman is usually considered anemic if her hemoglobin is less than 10.5 or 11 g/dl (Blackburn, 2003; Cunningham et al., 2001; Kilpatrick & Laros, 2004)

Anemia is one of the most common problems of pregnancy. The incidence varies according to geographic location and socioeconomic group. Anemia may be caused by a variety of factors, including nutrition, hemolysis, or blood loss. The most common types of anemia observed during pregnancy include iron deficiency anemia, folic acid deficiency anemia, the anemia associated with sickle cell disease, and thalassemia.

Iron Deficiency Anemia

It is difficult to meet pregnancy needs for iron through the diet alone, although iron is present in many foods. The primary sources of iron are meat, fish, chicken, and green leafy vegetables.

Maternal Effects

Signs and symptoms of iron deficiency anemia are often minimal but may include pallor, fatigue, lethargy, and headache. Clinical findings may also include inflammation of the lips and tongue. Pica (consuming nonfood substances such as clay, dirt, ice, or starch) is also a sign of iron deficiency anemia (Kilpatrick & Laros, 2004). Laboratory findings include red blood cells that are *microcytic* (small) and *hypochromic* (pale). The plasma iron and serum ferritin concentrations are low, whereas the total iron-binding capacity is higher than normal. Women who have multifetal pregnancies or bleeding complications are more likely to be anemic during pregnancy.

Fetal and Neonatal Effects

The effects of maternal iron deficiency anemia on the fetus and neonate are unclear. In general, even with significant maternal iron deficiency, the fetus will receive adequate stores at a cost to the mother. If the mother is severely anemic, the fetus may have reduced red cell volume, hemoglobin, and iron stores.

Therapeutic Management

Routine supplemental iron therapy rather than therapy based on an indication of anemia is controversial. Ferrous sulfate, 320 mg, one to three times per day is common. Many women experience less gastrointestinal discomfort if iron is taken with meals. Taking iron with 500 mg of vitamin C may enhance the iron absorption. Therapy is often continued for about 6 months after the anemia has been corrected. Parenteral therapy may be necessary for the woman who cannot or will not take oral iron and is significantly anemic (hemoglobin <8.5 g/dl) (Kilpatrick & Laros, 2004).

Folic Acid Deficiency (Megaloblastic) Anemia

Folic acid is essential for cell duplication and for fetal and placental growth. It is also an essential nutrient for the formation of red blood cells.

Maternal Effects

Maternal needs for folic acid double during pregnancy in response to the demand for greater production of erythrocytes and for fetal and placental growth. A deficiency in folic acid results in a reduction in the rate of deoxyribonucleic acid (DNA) synthesis and mitotic activity of individual cells, resulting in the presence of *large, immature erythrocytes (megaloblasts)*. Folate deficiency is the primary cause of megaloblastic anemia during pregnancy.

Nonnutritional factors that contribute to folic acid deficiency include hemolytic anemias with increased red blood cell turnover; some medications, such as phenytoin (Dilantin); and malabsorption entities. Folic acid deficiency is often present in association with iron deficiency anemia.

Fetal and Neonatal Effects

Folate deficiency is associated with an increased risk for spontaneous abortion, abruptio placentae, and fetal anomalies, especially neural tube defects such as spina bifida or anencephaly.

Therapeutic Management

The recommended daily allowance for folic acid doubles during pregnancy, and some women have difficulty ingesting the amount needed, even though folic acid occurs widely in foods. The best sources of folic acid are kidney beans, lima beans, and fresh, dark green leafy vegetables. As a result of the increased demands for this vitamin during pregnancy, supplementation with folic acid, 400 mcg (0.4 mg)/day, is recommended for all women of childbearing age. Women who have had a previous child with a neural tube defect should take 4 mg of folic acid for 1 month before and during the first trimester of pregnancy (AAP & ACOG, 2002; Blackburn, 2003).

Sickle Cell Anemia

Sickle cell disease is an autosomal recessive genetic disorder that causes anemia because an abnormal hemoglobin results in distortion and destruction of erythrocytes. It occurs when the gene for the production of hemoglobin S is inherited from both parents. The abnormal hemoglobin in the erythrocytes responds to hypoxia, acidosis, or dehydration by changing its shape to become a long, rigid rod. The change of hemoglobin S into rigid molecules distorts erythrocytes into a crescent, or sickle, shape. After erythrocytes lose their round, smooth, concave shape, they tend to clump together and occlude the smaller blood vessels.

The disease is characterized by chronic anemia, increased susceptibility to infection, and periodic crises when the abnormally shaped erythrocytes obstruct blood vessels. Sickle cell disease occurs most often in people who have ancestors

from sub-Saharan Africa, South America, Cuba, Central America, Saudi Arabia, India, and Mediterranean countries. About 1 in 500 African-American and 1 in 1000 to 1400 Hispanic births in the United States will result in an infant with sickle cell anemia. Sickle cell anemia affects 72,000 Americans. More than 2 million Americans are carriers of the sickle cell trait and may pass the gene on to their children even though they are not affected (Ashley-Koch, A., & Olney, R.S., 2000; National Institutes of Health: National Heart, Lung, and Blood Institute 1996; Sickle Cell Disease of America, Inc., 2004).

Maternal Effects

The physiologic anemia, increased coagulation factors, and venous stasis that are normal in pregnancy may bring on *sickle cell crisis*, sometimes for the first time. Any of several conditions may result, particularly temporary cessation of bone marrow function, hemolytic crisis with massive erythrocyte destruction resulting in jaundice, and severe pain caused by infarctions in the joints and all the major organs. In addition, expectant mothers with sickle cell disease are prone to pyelonephritis, bone infection, and heart disease. The incidence of preeclampsia in these women is about 15% (National Institutes of Health: National Heart, Lung, and Blood Institute, 2002).

Fetal and Neonatal Effects

In the absence of maternal sickle cell crisis, the fetus usually does well, although complications such as prematurity and intrauterine growth restriction are more common. The incidence of fetal death is high if sickle cell crisis occurs, because of placental infarctions with loss of exchange surface on the placenta (Blackburn, 2003; Kilpatrick & Laros, 2004).

Therapeutic Management

Most treatment of sickle cell anemia during pregnancy is symptomatic and directed toward avoiding sickle cell crisis. Evaluations of hemoglobin, complete blood count, serum iron, total iron-binding capacity, and serum folate determine the degree of anemia and iron and folic acid stores. Testing for infections, such as hepatitis, human immunodeficiency virus (HIV), tuberculosis, and sexually transmitted infections, is done. Hepatitis B vaccine may be given to the noninfected woman. Urinalysis identifies both clinical and subclinical infection that should be treated. Fetal surveillance studies (ultrasonography, nonstress tests, biophysical profiles) assess fetal growth and development and placental function. Exchange transfusions or prophylactic transfusions may be used to increase the amount of normal hemoglobin in the circulation and to reduce severe anemia (Cunningham et al., 2001; Kilpatrick & Laros, 2004; National Institutes of Health: National Heart, Lung, and Blood Institute, 2002).

The goal of nursing management is to help the pregnant woman maintain a healthy status and avoid hospitalization. Women must be encouraged to keep all prenatal care appointments, usually every other week. Topics in prenatal education include (1) the need to maintain adequate hydration to prevent sickling, (2) the need for adequate nutrition to meet metabolic needs, (3) the need for folic acid supplementation for erythrocyte production, (4) the need for rest periods throughout the day, (5) good hygiene practices and the avoidance of persons with infectious illnesses, and (6) the need for prompt treatment of fever or other signs of infection that could precipitate a crisis.

Nurses must be alert for signs of sickle cell crisis. The most common indications are pain in the abdomen, chest, vertebrae, joints, or extremities; pallor; and signs of cardiac failure. Nurses must also provide comfort measures, such as repositioning, good skin care, assisting with ambulation and movement in bed, and assisting the woman to splint the abdomen with a pillow when she must cough or breathe deeply.

Intrapartum care focuses on preventing the development of sickle cell crisis. Oxygen is administered continuously, and fluids should be administered to prevent dehydration because hypoxemia and dehydration as well as exertion, infection, and acidosis stimulate the sickling process. Packed red blood cells (PRBCs) may be administered to women who have a hematocrit lower than 20%.

Thalassemias

Like sickle cell disease, thalassemia is a genetic disorder that involves the abnormal synthesis of alpha or beta chains of hemoglobin. This leads to alterations in the red blood cell membrane and a decreased life span of red blood cells. Thalassemia is named and classified by the type of chain that is inadequately produced. Beta-thalassemia is most frequently encountered in the United States. Beta-thalassemia minor refers to the heterozygous form that results from the inheritance of one abnormal gene from either parent. Beta-thalassemia major refers to inheritance of the gene from both parents. Females with beta-thalassemia major (Cooley's anemia) usually die in young adulthood. Those who survive are often sterile (Cunningham et al., 2001; Kilpatrick & Laros, 2004). Beta-thalassemia is most often found in those of Mediterranean or Asian (particularly Chinese) origin.

Maternal Effects
Women with beta-thalassemia minor are often mildly anemic but healthy otherwise. Laboratory values normally associated with beta-thalassemia minor indicate a mild hypochromic and microcytic anemia. This can lead to the diagnosis of iron deficiency anemia and iron supplementation therapy. Large doses of iron are potentially dangerous because beta-thalassemia is associated with increased iron absorption and storage and a susceptibility to iron overload (Duffy, 1999).

Fetal and Neonatal Effects
Whether the disorders are associated with increased fetal or neonatal morbidity remains unresolved because of the many variants of thalassemia. There appears to be no increase in the rate of prematurity, low-birth-weight infants, or abnormal size for gestation. Fetal anemia may be serious if inadequate fetal hemoglobin is produced. The fetus may inherit the serious problem of beta-thalassemia major if both parents have beta-thalassemia minor.

Therapeutic Management
There is no specific therapy for beta-thalassemia minor during pregnancy. Most often the outcomes for the mother and fetus are satisfactory (Cunningham et al., 2001). Infections, which depress production of red blood cells and accelerate erythrocyte destruction, should be identified and treated promptly.

IMMUNE COMPLEX DISEASES

Systemic Lupus Erythematosus

Systemic lupus erythematosus (SLE) is a chronic, inflammatory, autoimmune disease that can affect any organ or system in the body. Although the cause is unknown, an imbalance appears to develop between immune response and tolerance of specific antigens, so that the body produces antibodies to its own cells and tissue. Signs and symptoms result from inflammation of multiple organ systems, especially the joints, skin, kidneys, and nervous system. The most common signs or symptoms are joint pain, photosensitivity, thrombocytopenia, and a "butterfly" rash on the face that is easily confused with normal pigmentation changes of pregnancy. Fatigue is one of the most common symptoms. Remissions occur periodically, during which no symptoms are present.

The disease tends to affect young women, but it may occur in any age-group. The exact incidence is unknown. It is more common in women of African, Hispanic, Asian, and Native American descent (Lupus Foundation of America, 2001).

SLE is associated with an increased incidence of abortion and fetal death during the first trimester. There is an increased risk for later pregnancy loss or premature birth because of hypertension, renal complications, and preterm rupture of membranes. Preeclampsia may be early and severe for the woman who has SLE.

The newborn may have a congenital heart block, which may be detected prenatally. Skin lesions resembling those of the adult with SLE may be present for most of the first year.

Because pregnancy can worsen SLE, the woman must be carefully observed for signs that the disease has progressed. Renal complications pose a special risk. Women with a history of kidney problems should be advised to seek the advice of a physician before becoming pregnant. Pregnancy is most likely to have a favorable outcome in the woman whose disease is under good control at the beginning and who does not have renal involvement.

Antiphospholipid Syndrome

Antiphospholipid syndrome (APS) is an autoimmune condition characterized by the production of antiphospholipid antibodies, combined with certain clinical features. The most specific clinical features include thrombosis, decreased platelets, and pregnancy loss. Stroke may occur as a consequence of arterial thrombosis. An unusually high rate of preeclampsia has been noted in women with APS. Preeclampsia and uteroplacental insufficiency contribute to the high rate of preterm births, intrauterine growth restriction, and fetal loss with APS.

Although the syndrome occurs most often in women with other underlying autoimmune diseases, such as SLE, it is also diagnosed in women with no other recognizable autoimmune disease.

Women with APS should be informed of the potential maternal and obstetric problems, ideally before conception. They should be assessed for evidence of anemia, thrombocytopenia, and underlying renal disease. Low-dose aspirin and prophylactic heparin are recommended for pregnant women with APS. Research for the best treatments continues (Lockwood & Silver, 2004).

Hashimoto's Thyroiditis

Hashimoto's thyroiditis, characterized by antithyroid antibodies, causes most cases of hypothyroidism in women. Maternal hypothyroidism during pregnancy can adversely affect the child's mental development. Thyroid-stimulating hormone should be tested before or in early pregnancy and hypothyroidism corrected.

SEIZURE DISORDERS: EPILEPSY

Convulsive seizures are the most common form of epilepsy, which is a recurrent disorder of cerebral function. Epilepsy occurs in 0.3% to 0.6% of pregnant women. Pregnancy may affect management of seizure disorders, and the seizure disorder may affect the course of pregnancy.

The effect of pregnancy on the course of epilepsy is variable and unpredictable. The frequency of seizures may increase, decrease, or remain the same. In general, the longer the woman has been seizure-free before pregnancy, the less likely she is to develop seizures during pregnancy. Those with partial (focal) seizures are more likely to have an increased frequency. Vomiting, reduced gastric motility, use of gastrointestinal medications, and weight gain affect the absorption and distribution of anticonvulsant drugs. Serum levels of anticonvulsants may rise, fall, or remain the same during pregnancy.

A major concern is the teratogenic effects of anticonvulsant drugs possibly related to folate deficiency. One specific syndrome is *fetal hydantoin syndrome*, which includes craniofacial abnormalities, limb reduction defects, growth restriction, mental retardation, and cardiac anomalies. Other anticonvulsants, such as trimethadione, paramethadione, and carbamazepine, are also associated with malformation syndromes. The teratogenic effects of phenobarbital are difficult to assess because it is usually combined with other drugs. Newer anticonvulsants, such as levetiracetam, have less data accumulated related to fetal effects.

Health professionals should recommend that the pregnant woman consult a neurologist before conception. The goals of treatment are to prevent generalized (grand mal) seizures and to reduce the adverse effects of anticonvulsant medications on the fetus. The woman and her family must be made aware of the risks involved of specific anticonvulsants that must continue during pregnancy. They also should realize that treatment cannot be stopped during pregnancy unless the woman has been free of seizures for a prolonged time. Generalized seizures result in fetal hypoxia and acidosis and thus pose a serious problem for the fetus (Aminoff, 2004).

TRAUMA IN PREGNANCY

Blunt Force Injuries

Automobile accidents cause most cases of blunt force injuries to the pregnant woman, followed by violent assault and suicide (Gonik, 2003). Maternal deaths are most often caused by head injury or intraabdominal hemorrhage, which may follow sudden premature separation of the placenta or rupture of the uterus. Pelvic fracture is a commonly reported injury in automobile accidents or as a result of falls.

During the first trimester, the fetus is protected from external forces by the bony pelvis, the amniotic fluid, and soft tissue surrounding the pelvis. As the uterus grows beyond the bony pelvis with progression, the fetus becomes more vulnerable to blunt force injury. Fetal injury may include skull fracture and intracranial hemorrhage. Moreover, disruption of uteroplacental blood flow caused by premature separation of the placenta can result in fetal anoxia. Traumatic uterine rupture is associated with a fetal mortality rate near 100% (Gonik & Foley, 2004).

The use of seatbelt restraints improves maternal and fetal outcomes in automobile accidents significantly. Current recommendations are that the pregnant woman wears three-point restraint seatbelts during automobile travel. The lower part of the belt should be over the lap and not placed over the protruding uterus.

Penetrating Injuries

Gunshot and knife wounds are the most common penetrating injuries and are associated with assaults or suicide attempts. Because the uterus acts as a shield for maternal abdominal structures, mortality rates from penetrating wounds in the pregnant woman are less than those in nonpregnant women. The fetus usually suffers high injury and mortality rates (Gonik & Foley, 2004).

Therapeutic Management

The initial management of trauma in pregnant women is similar to that in the nonpregnant person. Priority includes:

- Maintenance of maternal cardiopulmonary function
- Evaluation and stabilization of maternal injuries

The basic ABCs of resuscitation, Airway, Breathing, and Circulation, are the priority of care. To minimize compression of the large blood vessels by the heavy uterus, prolonged supine positioning should be avoided during resuscitation and other treatment. Lateral displacement of the uterus can be accomplished by placing a wedge along the right or left side of the woman. The need for large amounts of blood and fluid replacement should be anticipated; venous access is often by a central line. An arterial line is placed in critically ill patients to monitor hemodynamic status and oxygenation.

After resuscitation, evaluation continues for fractures, bleeding sites, and internal injuries. Exploratory abdominal surgery may be necessary to identify and control internal bleeding. The uterus and fetus must also be evaluated for injuries.

Electronic fetal monitoring may reflect the condition of the mother as well as that of the fetus. For example, although the mother is stable, electronic monitoring may detect signs of premature separation of the placenta, such as uterine contractions, fetal tachycardia, and late decelerations. Fetal tachycardia often precedes changes in maternal vital signs caused by hemorrhage. Fetal-to-maternal hemorrhage caused by disruption of the placenta is monitored by K-B testing. K-B tests that show a growing percentage of fetal erythrocytes in maternal blood suggest some disruption of the placenta, although the test alone is not diagnostic.

The necessity for a cesarean birth to deliver a live fetus depends on several factors, including the age of the fetus, the fetal condition, and the extent of uterine injury. Because placental abruption usually develops soon after severe trauma, electronic monitoring is begun as soon as the mother is stabilized. It is continued as long as there are signs of uterine contractions, vaginal bleeding, uterine tenderness, or ruptured membranes. Cesarean section may also be required to stabilize the mother by removing the fetus from her circulatory path.

INFECTIONS DURING PREGNANCY

Infections may harm the woman, the fetus, or both. A mild infection in the adult may have devastating effects on the developing fetus. Table 26-6 presents nursing considerations in relation to sexually transmitted diseases, vaginal, and urinary tract infections.

Viral Infections

Viral infections are often mild or even asymptomatic in adults, but they may have catastrophic fetal or neonatal consequences. Maternal infections with cytomegalovirus, rubella, varicella-zoster virus, herpes simplex, hepatitis B, and human immunodeficiency virus have the greatest potential for harming the fetus or neonate.

Cytomegalovirus

Cytomegalovirus (CMV), a member of the herpesvirus group, is widespread and eventually infects most humans. Although CMV is widespread, the most serious effects occur in the fetus and immunocompromised persons. CMV has been isolated from urine, saliva, blood, cervical mucus, semen, breast milk, and feces. Young children who have close contact with infected playmates are the most likely reservoirs for transmission to adults, including pregnant women. Many infections are asymptomatic or produce minimal symptoms, so they may not be suspected or diagnosed.

After primary (first) infection, the virus becomes latent, but like other herpesviruses, CMV may produce periodic reactivation and shedding of the virus. Primary CMV infection is the most dangerous to the fetus. The best way to establish the presence of CMV is by isolating the virus by culture or DNA study (Gibbs, Sweet, & Duff, 2004).

Fetal and Neonatal Effects. If a woman develops a primary CMV infection during pregnancy, her fetus has a 40% to 50% chance of being infected. Of infected fetuses, 5% to 18% are symptomatic at birth, having problems such as enlarged spleen and liver, CNS abnormalities, jaundice, chorioretinitis, hearing loss, and IUGR. Another 10% to 15% will develop manifestations within the first 2 years of life (Gibbs, Sweet, & Duff, 2004).

TABLE 26-6 Sexually Transmitted Diseases, Urinary Tract, and Vaginal Infections: Their Impact on Pregnancy

Maternal, Fetal, and Neonatal Effects	Nursing Considerations
SEXUALLY TRANSMITTED DISEASES	
Syphilis (Causative Organism: Spirochete Treponema pallidum*)*	
If untreated, the infection may cross the placenta to the fetus and result in spontaneous abortion, a stillborn infant, premature labor and birth, or congenital syphilis. Major signs of congenital syphilis are enlarged liver and spleen, skin lesions, rashes, osteitis, pneumonia, and hepatitis.	Penicillin is the primary treatment to cure the disease in both the woman and fetus. Women who are allergic are desensitized and then treated.*
Gonorrhea (Causative Organism: Bacterium Neisseria gonorrhoeae*)*	
Not transmitted via the placenta; vertical transmission from mother to newborn during birth may cause ophthalmia neonatorum. Endocervicitis and weakness of the fetal membranes increase the risk for premature rupture of membranes and preterm labor. *Chlamydia* infection is likely to accompany the gonorrhea infection.	Ceftriaxone or cefixime plus amoxicillin or azithromycin are now recommended for penicillin-resistant organisms because 20%-50% of women with gonorrhea will also have chlamydial infection.*† The partner must also be treated to prevent reinfection. Infants are treated with an ophthalmic antibiotic such as ceftriaxone at birth to prevent ophthalmia neonatorum.
Chlamydial Infection (Causative Organism: Bacterium Chlamydia trachomatis*)*	
Chlamydial infection is the most common sexually transmitted disease in the United States. The fetus may be infected during birth and suffer neonatal conjunctivitis or pneumonitis. Conjunctivitis is prevented by erythromycin ophthalmic ointment. *Chlamydia* may also be responsible for premature rupture of membranes, premature labor, and chorioamnionitis.	Education is particularly important because *Chlamydia* infection is the most common sexually transmitted disease in the United States and infection is usually asymptomatic. Both partners should be treated to prevent recurrent infection. As with all sexually transmitted diseases, the use of condoms decreases the risk for infection. Erythromycin or amoxicillin is the recommended treatment. Azithromycin is an alternate treatment.†
Trichomoniasis (Causative Organism: Protozoan Trichomonas vaginalis*)*	
Common cause of vaginitis in 10%-50% of pregnant women. Associated with premature rupture of membranes and postpartum endometritis.†	Metronidazole (Flagyl) may be given to the pregnant woman as a 2-g single oral dose. Consistent association between fetal abnormalities or injury and metronidazole use has not been upheld.†

Continued

TABLE 26-6 Sexually Transmitted Diseases, Urinary Tract, and Vaginal Infections: Their Impact on Pregnancy—cont'd

Maternal, Fetal, and Neonatal Effects	Nursing Considerations
Condyloma Acuminatum (Causative Organism: Human Papillomavirus) Transmission of condyloma acuminatum, also called *venereal* or *genital warts*, may occur during vaginal birth and is associated with the development of epithelial tumors of the mucous membranes of the larynx in children. Pregnancy can cause proliferation of lesions, which are associated with cervical dysplasia and cancer.	The common choices for nonpregnant therapy (podophyllin, podofilox, imiquimod) are not recommended during pregnancy. Excision of the maternal lesions by cryotherapy or cautery may be done.†

VAGINAL INFECTIONS

Maternal, Fetal, and Neonatal Effects	Nursing Considerations
Candidiasis (Causative Organism: Yeast Candida albicans) Oral candidiasis (thrush) may develop in newborns if infection is present at birth. Thrush is treated with application of nystatin (Mycostatin) over the surfaces of the oral cavity four times a day for several days. Characteristic "cottage cheese" vaginal discharge with vulvar pruritus, burning, and dyspareunia. Vulva may be red, tender, and edematous.	Candidiasis (sometimes called *Monilia vaginitis*) is a persistent problem for many women during pregnancy. Examples of maternal treatment choices include miconazole, clotrimazole, or fluconazole.†
Bacterial Vaginosis‡ (Causative Organism: Gardnerella vaginalis) No known fetal effects. May be associated with postpartum endometritis; has been associated with preterm birth. Marked by a major shift in vaginal flora from the normal predominance of lactobacilli to a predominance of anaerobic bacteria. Causes profuse, malodorous, "fishy" vaginal discharge, itching, and burning.	Metronidazole (oral therapy or intravaginal gel) or clindamycin intravaginal cream may be used in the pregnant woman.

URINARY TRACT INFECTIONS

Maternal, Fetal, and Neonatal Effects	Nursing Considerations
Asymptomatic Bacteriuria (Causative Organisms: Escherichia coli, Klebsiella, Proteus) Ascending bacterial infection can result in cystitis or pyelonephritis in later pregnancy if condition remains untreated.	Recovery of a urinary pathogen from a midstream, clean-catch urine specimen is defined as 100,000 colony-forming units (CFUs) per ml of urine. Rapid, less-expensive office tests to identify the infection may also be used. Treatment for aymptomatic bacteriuria may include treatment for pathogens that also cause symptomatic cystitis.
Cystitis (Causative Organisms: E. coli, Klebsiella, Proteus) Signs and symptoms include dysuria, frequency, urgency, and suprapubic tenderness. Ascending infection may lead to pyelonephritis.	Antibiotics used for both asymptomatic bacteriuria and cystitis may include amoxicillin, sulfisoxazole, trimethoprim-sulfamethoxazole, nitrofurantoin, or 3rd-generation cephalosporins such as cefixime or cefpodoxime. Emphasize importance of reporting signs of urinary tract infection. Stress the importance of taking all the medication prescribed even if the symptoms abate. Provide information about hygiene measures.
Acute Pyelonephritis (Causative Organisms: E. coli, Klebsiella, Proteus) Increased risk for preterm labor and premature delivery. Maternal complications include a high fever, septic shock and adult respiratory distress syndrome.	Inform women with asymptomatic bacteriuria or cystitis of signs and symptoms, such as sudden onset of fever (often higher than 39°(102.2°F), chills, flank pain or tenderness, nausea, and vomiting, so that treatment can begin promptly. Skin cooling equipment may be used to lower her temperature below 38° C (100.4°F) reducing possible compromise of fetal oxygen level. Woman may be hospitalized for intravenous administration of antibiotics. Common combinations include ampicillin or a cephalosporin plus an aminoglycoside. Serum levels of aminoglycosides are often done to ensure an adequate dose without its reaching a toxic level.

*Centers for Disease Control and Prevention. (2002b). Sexually transmitted diseases treatment guidelines, 2002. *Morbidity and Mortality Weekly Report, 51*(RR-6). Retrieved Dec. 11, 2003, from www.cdc.gov/STD/treatment/rr5106.pdf.
†Gibbs, R.S., Sweet, R.L., & Duff, W.P. (2004). Maternal and fetal infectious diseases. In R.K. Creasy, R. Resnik, & J.D. Iams (Eds.), *Maternal-fetal medicine: Principles and practice* (5th ed., pp. 741-801). Philadelphia: Saunders.
‡Formerly called *nonspecific vaginitis* or *Gardnerella vaginitis*.

Therapeutic Management. No effective therapy is currently available for the treatment of congenital infection. Ultrasound scanning may identify manifestations of the infection, such as cranial abnormalities or growth restriction. Antiviral agents, such as ganciclovir and foscarnet, may be used for severe infections, but these drugs are toxic and only temporarily suppress shedding of the virus. Primary prevention, such as emphasizing handwashing, especially to women who care for small children, warning of the risks imposed by having several sexual partners, and transfusing only CMV-free blood, is most effective (Gibbs, Sweet, & Duff, 2004).

Rubella

Rubella is caused by a virus that is transmitted by droplets or through direct contact with articles contaminated with nasopharyngeal secretions. Rubella is a mild disease; major symptoms are fever, general malaise, and a characteristic maculopapular rash that begins on the face and spreads over the body. Although the overall incidence has declined since rubella vaccine became available, many young adults remain at risk. Recent outbreaks of rubella have tended to occur where young adults congregate and in Latinos, who are more likely to remain unvaccinated (Gibbs, Sweet, & Duff, 2004).

Fetal and Neonatal Effects. Rubella remains a serious concern because the virus crosses the placental barrier and can infect the fetus. The greatest risk to the fetus occurs during the first trimester, when fetal organs are developing. If maternal infection occurs during this time, approximately one third of these cases will result in spontaneous abortions and the surviving fetuses may be seriously compromised. Deafness, mental retardation, cataracts, cardiac defects, IUGR, and microcephaly are the most common fetal complications. Moreover, infants born to mothers who had rubella during pregnancy shed the virus for many months and thus pose a threat to other infants as well as to susceptible adults who come in contact with them.

Therapeutic Management. Prevention is the only effective protection for the fetus. Because of widespread immunization against rubella, fewer than 50 cases of congenital rubella syndrome are identified each year. Women who are immune do not become infected, so it is critical to determine the immune status of all women of childbearing age. A rubella titer of 1:8 or greater provides evidence of immunity. Women who are not immune should be vaccinated before they become pregnant, and they should be advised not to become pregnant for 4 weeks after vaccination because the live-virus vaccine poses a possible risk to the fetus, although there is no evidence of fetal damage (CDC, 2003b). Many nonimmune women are vaccinated during the postpartum period so that they will be immune before becoming pregnant again (Gibbs, Sweet, & Duff, 2004).

Varicella-Zoster Virus

Varicella infection (chickenpox) is caused by varicella-zoster virus, a herpesvirus that is transmitted by direct contact or via the respiratory tract. The varicella virus can become latent in nerve ganglia. When the virus is reactivated, herpes zoster (shingles) results. Adults have usually acquired immunity by the time they reach childbearing age. Potential maternal complications of acute varicella infection include preterm labor, encephalitis, and varicella pneumonia, which can be fatal despite high doses of acyclovir, an antiviral drug (Gibbs, Sweet, & Duff, 2004).

Fetal and Neonatal Effects. Fetal and neonatal effects depend on the time of maternal infection. If the infection occurs during the first trimester, the fetus has a small risk for congenital varicella syndrome (0.4%-2%). The greatest risk for development of congenital varicella syndrome occurs from 13 to 20 weeks of pregnancy (2%). Clinical findings include limb hypoplasia, cutaneous scars, chorioretinitis, cataracts, microcephaly, and IUGR. In later pregnancy, transplacental passage of maternal antibodies usually protects the fetus. If the fetus is exposed to the virus in utero and is born before the development of maternal antibodies, however, the infant is at risk for the development of life-threatening neonatal varicella infection (CDC, 2001b; Gibbs, Sweet, & Duff, 2004).

Therapeutic Management. A live attenuated varicella vaccine (Varivax) is available, and the child or susceptible adult may receive the vaccine if they live in the same household as a susceptible pregnant woman. Varicella-zoster immune globulin (VZIG) should be administered within 96 hours to provide passive (temporary) immunity to women who have been exposed and are susceptible. A nonimmune postpartum woman should receive her first immunization before discharge and her second one at 6 weeks postpartum. Pregnancy should be avoided for 1 month (AAP & ACOG, 2002; CDC, 2001b).

Women should be instructed to report pulmonary symptoms, such as shortness of breath or cough, immediately. Hospitalization, fetal surveillance, full respiratory support, and hemodynamic monitoring should be available for women diagnosed with varicella pneumonia. Women and infants with varicella should be placed in airborne and contact isolation. Only staff members known to be immune to varicella should come in contact with these clients. Pregnant women with shingles should be in contact isolation.

The Centers for Disease Control and Prevention (CDC) (2001b) recommends administration of varicella-zoster immune globulin to infants born to mothers who develop varicella 5 days before birth or 2 days after birth for passive immunity. Preterm or low-birth-weight (<28 weeks or <1000 g) should also receive VZIG because they are born before maternal antibodies to the disease cross the placenta, even if their mother is immune.

Herpesvirus Serotypes 1 and 2

Genital herpes is one of the most common sexually transmitted diseases. It may be caused by herpesvirus serotype 1 or serotype 2, but 90% of episodes of genital herpes are caused by type 2. Infection occurs as a result of direct contact of the skin or mucous membrane with an active lesion. Lesions form at the site of contact and begin as a group of painful papules that progress rapidly to become vesicles, shallow ulcers, pustules, and crusts. The woman sheds the virus until the lesions are completely healed. The virus then migrates along the sensory nerves to reside in the sensory ganglion, and the disease enters a latent phase. It can be reactivated later as a recurrent infection.

Vertical transmission (from mother to infant) occurs in two ways: (1) after rupture of membranes, when the virus ascends from active lesions; and (2) during birth, when the fetus comes in contact with infectious genital secretions. The risk for neonatal infection is highest if the infant is exposed during the mother's primary (first) infection.

The diagnosis is usually based on clinical signs and symptoms. A definitive diagnosis, however, requires isolation of the virus from a lesion.

Fetal and Neonatal Effects. Complications during pregnancy from a recurrent maternal infection are rare. Neonatal herpes infection acquired during vaginal birth is the major perinatal problem, particularly if the maternal infection is primary. Evidence and severity of neonatal infection depend on the system or systems involved but may include skin lesions, cough, cyanosis, tachypnea, dyspnea, jaundice, seizures, or coagulation defects. Viral culture is the only reliable method of diagnosis.

Therapeutic Management. To reduce symptoms and shorten the duration of lesions, acyclovir may be given orally during pregnancy. Some specialists recommend acyclovir treatment during late pregnancy for women who have recurrent lesions, to reduce the likelihood of active lesions at term (CDC, 2002b).

For women with a history of genital herpes, vaginal delivery is allowed if there are no genital lesions at the time of labor. For women with active lesions, either recurrent or primary, at the time of labor, cesarean birth is recommended. Use of fetal scalp electrodes, which cause a break in the skin, should be limited in the woman with active lesions but is acceptable if there are no active lesions (American Academy of Pediatrics [AAP] & American College of Obstetricians & Gynecologists [ACOG], 2002).

After delivery, isolation of the mother from her infant is not necessary as long as direct contact with lesions is avoided and mothers use careful handwashing techniques. Mothers may breastfeed if there are no lesions on the breasts. The infant is observed carefully for signs of infection, including temperature instability, lethargy, poor sucking reflex, jaundice, seizures, and herpetic lesions. Acyclovir therapy is prescribed for neonatal infection.

Expectant mothers need information about effective ways to deal with the emotional as well as the physical effects of herpes. Many women are concerned about privacy and do not want family members to know why cesarean birth is necessary. Such women must be assured that their wishes will be respected. Many women need an opportunity to discuss their feelings of shame, anger, or anxiety about the disease.

Parvovirus B19

Erythema infectiosum, also called *fifth disease*, is caused by human parvovirus B19. It is an acute, communicable disease that is characterized by a distinctive rash. The rash starts on the face with a "slapped-cheeks" appearance, followed by a generalized maculopapular rash. Other symptoms include fever, malaise, and joint pain. Erythema infectiosum is more common among children and often occurs in community epidemics. The disease is most contagious the week before the rash appears. The prognosis is usually excellent. If the disease occurs in pregnancy, however, there are potential fetal and neonatal effects.

Fetal and Neonatal Effects. When infection occurs during pregnancy, fetal death can result, usually from failure of fetal red blood cell production, followed by severe fetal anemia, hydrops (generalized edema), and heart failure. Maternal serum alpha-fetoprotein (MSAFP) is sometimes elevated when fetal hydrops is present. Serial ultrasonography can also be performed to detect hydrops. Intrauterine transfusion is an option to treat severe fetal anemia if it does not spontaneously resolve. The risk to the fetus is greatest when the mother is infected in the first 20 weeks of pregnancy. The affected infant is examined for any defect, and the child is assessed regularly for several years to identify delayed complications.

Therapeutic Management. Infection with parvovirus B19 has no specific treatment. Starch baths may help reduce pruritus, and analgesics may be necessary to relieve mild joint pain.

Hepatitis B

Six types of hepatitis virus have currently been identified: A, B, C, D, E, and G. Hepatitis A accounts for about one third of cases in the United States. Hepatitis A is rarely transmitted perinatally, and supportive care is usually sufficient. Hepatitis B accounts for 40% to 45% of cases in the United States and can be transmitted perinatally and is thus of great interest to maternal-newborn caregivers. Hepatitis C may go undiagnosed until the woman develops chronic liver disease that often requires liver transplantation. The incidence of hepatitis C in pregnant women is 1% to 5% (Landon, 2004).

Hepatitis B is caused by a virus that is transmitted via blood, saliva, vaginal secretions, semen, or breast milk and readily crosses the placental barrier. The disease is prevalent in certain population groups, such as Africans, Asians, Southeast Asian immigrants, Native Americans, Eskimos, and intravenous drug users. Symptoms may include vomiting, abdominal pain, jaundice, fever, rash, and painful joints. Fortunately, most infected adolescents and adults recover within 6 months and acquire long-lasting immunity.

Fetal and Neonatal Effects. Hepatitis B infection in pregnancy is associated with an increased incidence of prematurity, low birth weight, and neonatal death. Infants born to mothers who had hepatitis B during pregnancy or who are chronic carriers of hepatitis B surface antigen (HBsAg) are at risk for the development of acute infection at birth. Newborns and children infected with hepatitis B virus before the age of 5 years are most likely to become chronic carriers of the virus, becoming reservoirs for continued infection in the population (CDC, 2002b).

Therapeutic Management. Hepatitis B infection is preventable. Simple hygiene measures such as safe sex and the use of Standard Precautions with body fluids provide primary prevention. Highly effective hepatitis B vaccines are available as a series of three intramuscular injections into the deltoid for adults, with the second and third doses given 1 and 6 months after the first. Vaccination is recommended for any population at risk, including nurses who frequently come in contact with infectious body fluids.

All pregnant women should be screened for HBsAg, and those having risk factors should be offered the vaccine. Household members and sexual contacts should be tested and offered vaccination if they are not immune. No specific treatment exists for acute hepatitis B. Recommended supportive treatment includes bed rest and a high-protein, low-fat diet.

Chronic infection of a newborn whose mother is known to be HBsAg-positive can usually be prevented by administration of hepatitis B immune globulin (HBIG, Hep-B-Gammagee), followed by hepatitis B vaccine (Recombivax-HB, Engerix-B) within 12 hours of birth. To prevent infection from contamination of the infant's skin with maternal blood, the newborn must be bathed before injections or heel sticks are done. The second and third doses should be given at 1 to 2 months and

6 months of age. The infant is tested 1 to 3 months after completing the hepatitis B immunization schedule to identify presence of chronic infection. Breastfeeding is considered safe as long as the newborn has been vaccinated (AAP & ACOG, 2002; CDC, 2002b).

Human Immunodeficiency Virus

Acquired immunodeficiency syndrome (AIDS) is caused by a retrovirus known as human immunodeficiency virus (HIV). HIV infection is most often transmitted to women or infants in three ways: (1) heterosexual transmission from an infected person, (2) parenteral exposure to infected blood or tissue, and (3) from an infected mother to an infant (vertical transmission) perinatally. Heterosexual transmission causes about two thirds of female infections, and infection by blood or tissue exposure occurs in about one fourth of the cases. Infection of the infant varies with the severity of maternal infection and the time and severity in which the retrovirus is transmitted to the infant. The continuing occurrence of HIV infections of infants demonstrates the importance of identifying and treating maternal infections during pregnancy to reduce the risks of infant infections (AAP & ACOG, 2002; CDC, 2001a; Minkoff, 2004).

The AIDS epidemic in women living in the United States is most pronounced in African-American and Hispanic women, who account for 78% of current cases. More female cases now occur in the southern United States. Infected women more often have heterosexual relationships rather than homosexual relationships that can cause their infection (Minkoff, 2004).

Pathophysiology. Like other retroviruses, HIV can integrate its viral genetic makeup into the genetic makeup of the cell when infecting it. This process produces a cell that cannot perform its functions properly. At the same time, this abnormal cell replicates and produces more viruses that invade more cells. The disease worsens as more and more cells cease to function, and at the same time, a greater number of viruses are produced. The principal mechanism whereby HIV leads to immunodeficiency is through its effect on helper (CD4) lymphocytes. These cells play a key role in organizing the body's immune response.

As the number of CD4 cells declines, the immune response becomes inadequate and opportunistic infections are able to overwhelm the person who is HIV-positive. A CD4 count of less than 200 cells/mm³ confirms the diagnosis of AIDS.

The clinical course of HIV infection follows four fairly predictable stages:

- An early, or acute, stage that occurs several weeks after HIV exposure. Flu-like symptoms may develop and last a few weeks. Antibodies to HIV (seroconversion) generally appear within a few months but may occasionally be delayed for more than a year.
- A middle, or asymptomatic, period of minor or no clinical problems. This period is characterized by continuous low-level viral replication and CD4 cell loss. The latent period from infection to AIDS is approximately 11 years but varies with whether the woman accepts treatment.
- A transitional period of symptomatic disease, characterized by immune dysfunction.
- A late, or crisis, period of symptomatic disease that may last months or years. This period is characterized by infec-

tions and cancers that occur principally in persons with immune system compromise.

During stages 1 and 2, the infected person is said to be HIV-positive; during stages 3 and 4, the immune system no longer offers adequate protection and opportunistic diseases occur. The person is then said to have AIDS.

Fetal and Neonatal Effects. Because of new antiretroviral drugs, the prognosis for HIV-infected women and their infants can improve. Low transmission (≤2% in 2000-2001) of the mother's HIV infection to the infant has occurred with the most current Public Health Service guidelines for viral prevention using zidovudine (ZDV) treatment. Additional actions to prevent infant infection may include cesarean birth before the onset of labor or membrane rupture. Mothers who receive no or minimal care may have higher rates of infected infants. Infant infection may occur during pregnancy, labor and birth, or after birth if the infant is breastfed (CDC, 2001a).

An infected newborn is typically asymptomatic at birth, but signs and symptoms may become obvious during the first year of life. Early signs may include enlargement of the liver and spleen, lymphadenopathy, failure to thrive, persistent thrush, and extensive seborrheic dermatitis (cradle cap). Infants frequently experience chronic bacterial infections, such as meningitis, pneumonia, osteomyelitis, septic arthritis, and septicemia. Infant tests for HIV infection diagnosis may include polymerase chain reaction (PCR) and viral culture in addition to standard antibody tests that can remain positive for up to 18 months after birth because of passive maternal antibodies.

Prompt treatment of the HIV-infected infant with appropriate antiretroviral medications and other prophylactic therapy may slow the infection's progress. See Chapter 41 for more information about HIV infection and its treatment in infants and children.

Prevention. Prevention remains the only way to avoid HIV infection. Sexual transmission can be avoided by several methods. Abstinence would render a person safe from all sexually transmitted diseases, including HIV, but for many people sexual expression adds to the quality of life, and many are not willing to practice total abstinence. Sexual transmission of HIV can also be prevented if infected persons do not have intercourse with susceptible persons.

Intravenous drug users who refuse rehabilitative treatment should be taught to wash the equipment with water, soap, and bleach before each use to prevent transmission of the virus from one person to another via a soiled needle.

Therapeutic Management. Drug therapy for HIV-infected women during pregnancies focuses on two goals: (1) improving maternal health as much as possible, and (2) reducing the rates of maternal-to-fetal infection as much as possible. Early maternal treatment with zidovudine (ZDV) can reduce transmission of the HIV infection to the fetus by 68% (AAP & ACOG, 2002; CDC, 2001a). Typical maternal treatment includes five daily doses of ZDV 100 mg beginning at 14 to 34 weeks of pregnancy. Intravenous ZDV is initiated during birth. The newborn's treatment begins within 8 to 12 hours after birth.

Other antiretroviral therapy may be considered for some pregnant women who are infected with HIV. Therapy may require combination drugs, added treatments for drug resistance, and treatment of opportunistic infections. Monitoring

---

BOX 26-4
Recommendations for Prevention of Perinatal HIV Infection of the Infant

- *Pregnancy:* Zidovudine, 100 mg orally 5 times per day initiated between 14 and 34 weeks of gestation.
- *Labor:* Intravenous zidovudine with a 1-hour loading dose of 2 mg/kg, followed by continuous infusion of 1 mg/kg/hr.
- *Newborn:* Oral zidovudine syrup, dose of 2 mg/kg every 6 hours for 6 weeks, beginning 8 to 12 hours after birth.

A cesarean at 38 weeks of pregnancy, before the onset of labor and rupture of membranes, is usual to reduce maternal transmission of HIV to the fetus. HIV-infected mothers are also advised not to breastfeed because of the presence of the virus in their milk.

Data from American Academy of Pediatrics, & American College of Obstetricians and Gynecologists. (2002). *Guidelines for perinatal care* (5th ed.). Elk Grove Village, IL, and Washington, DC: Author.

of the woman's HIV-related immune status may also be changed during pregnancy.

A cesarean at 38 weeks of pregnancy, before the onset of labor and rupture of membranes, is usual to reduce maternal transmission of HIV to the fetus. HIV-infected mothers are also advised not to breastfeed because of the presence of the virus in their milk (Box 26-4).

Nursing Considerations. Learning of HIV infection during pregnancy can have a devastating and immobilizing effect on the entire family. Even though appropriate antiretroviral drug treatment and birth interventions may reduce risk to both mother and infant, grief of the family is a real possibility. Anticipatory Grieving, a nursing diagnosis related to possible deaths of the mother and infant at some time during the future, should be considered. Crisis intervention may be necessary to help the family cope with a serious and unexpected diagnosis during pregnancy.

Nurses must frequently determine what the family perceives as the most pressing needs and worries. Some of the most common fears are loss of control, loss of support and love, social isolation, and loss of privacy. The nurse's response may involve finding ways for the woman to retain control while she is physically able and to assist her in selecting those in her family who will provide continued love and emotional support. Above all, it is necessary to reassure the woman that her right to privacy will not be violated.

Nurses can help the woman maintain the highest level of wellness possible. Adequate, high-quality nutrition decreases the risk for opportunistic infections and promotes vitality. A daily regimen should include sufficient rest and activity. It is important to avoid large crowds, travel to areas with poor sanitation, or exposure to infected individuals. Meticulous skin care is essential, especially during recurrent herpes infections.

The woman will need to know that breastfeeding is contraindicated but that she can provide all other care for her infant. She will almost certainly experience a great deal of anxiety about whether the infant will be HIV-positive. Nurses need to respond honestly that testing will be required but that many infants do not get the virus. Moreover, nurses must reinforce information about medications such as zidovudine that reduce the rate of vertical transmission.

Nonviral Infections

Toxoplasmosis

Toxoplasmosis is a protozoal infection caused by *Toxoplasma gondii*. Infection is transmitted through organisms in raw or undercooked meat, through contact with infected cat feces, or across the placental barrier to the fetus if the expectant mother acquires the infection during pregnancy.

Toxoplasmosis is often subclinical; the woman may experience a few days of fatigue, muscle pains, and swollen glands but may be unaware of the disease. If the infection is suspected, diagnosis can be confirmed by positive serologic test results, which include indirect fluorescent antibody tests for IgG and IgM.

Fetal and Neonatal Effects. The severity of fetal and neonatal effects secondary to toxoplasmosis vary with timing during pregnancy. Most severe infant effects result when acute infection occurs in the first trimester. Severe infant complications may include chorioretinitis, hydrocephaly, microcephaly, and calcifications within the cranium.

Therapeutic Management. Pregnant women should be advised to:

- Cook meat thoroughly, particularly pork, beef, and lamb.
- Avoid touching mucous membranes of the mouth or eyes while handling raw meat.
- Wash all kitchen surfaces that come in contact with uncooked meat.
- Wash the hands thoroughly after handling raw meat.
- Avoid uncooked eggs and unpasteurized milk.
- Wash fruits and vegetables before eating.
- Avoid contact with materials that are possibly contaminated with cat feces (cat litter boxes, sandboxes, garden soil).

Maternal treatment of toxoplasmosis during pregnancy is essential to reduce the risk for congenital infection. Sulfonamides can be used alone but are less effective than combination therapy. Spiramycin is successfully used in Europe for maternal toxoplasmosis and may be used under specific guidelines within the United States (Gibbs, Sweet, & Duff, 2004).

Group B Streptococcus Infection

Group B streptococcus (GBS) is a leading cause of life-threatening perinatal infections in the United States. The gram-positive bacterium colonizes the rectum, vagina, cervix, and urethra of pregnant and nonpregnant women. Approximately 10% to 30% of pregnant women are colonized with GBS in the vaginal or rectal area (AAP & ACOG, 2002; CDC, 2002a). Symptomatic maternal infections such as urinary tract infection, chorioamnionitis, and endometritis can occur in the mother. High fever within 12 hours of birth, tachycardia, abdominal distention, or fascitis or intraabdominal abscess may occur (Gibbs, Sweet, & Duff, 2004).

Fetal and Neonatal Effects. Early-onset GBS disease occurs within 7 days of birth and accounts for the majority of all GBS cases in newborns. In these newborns, the mortality rate ranges from 5% to 20%. Sepsis and pneumonia are the most common manifestations of early-onset disease, whereas late-onset GBS (after the first week of life) has a higher incidence of meningitis (AAP & ACOG, 2002; CDC, 2002a). See Chapter 30 for additional information about manifestations and recommended management of neonatal sepsis.

Therapeutic Management. Identifying women who are asymptomatic carriers of GBS is difficult because the duration of carrier status varies. Optimal identification of the GBS carrier status is obtained by vaginal and rectal culture between 35 and 37 weeks' gestation. Penicillin is the first-line agent for antibiotic treatment of the infected woman during birth. Ampicillin is an acceptable alternative. Patients who have clindamycin- and erythromycin-resistant GBS infections are more often observed than during the past.

Added guidelines based on CDC guidelines in 2002 include:

- Routine intrapartum antibiotic prophylaxis treatment for GBS infection is not required for the woman having a planned cesarean birth if labor or membrane rupture did not precede her planned cesarean birth.
- A woman whose GBS culture is not known at the time of birth is managed according to her risk. GBS infection risk is higher if the pregnancy is less than 37 weeks, membrane rupture has persisted 18 hours or more, or temperature is higher than 38° C (>100.4° F).
- A mother who previously gave birth to an infant with GBS disease or who had bacterial infection with GBS during pregnancy should receive antibiotic prophylaxis at birth.

Tuberculosis

Tuberculosis results from infection by *Mycobacterium tuberculosis*. It is transmitted by aerosolized droplets of liquid containing the bacterium, which are inhaled by a noninfected individual and taken into the lung. Initially, most individuals are asymptomatic. Women obtaining prenatal care should be screened for tuberculosis. This screening involves an intradermal injection of mycobacterial protein (purified protein derivative). If the reaction is positive, the woman's abdomen should be protected by a lead shield while a radiograph is taken of her chest. The diagnosis is confirmed by isolating and identifying the bacterium in the sputum.

Symptomatic persons have general malaise, fatigue, loss of appetite, weight loss, and fever. These symptoms occur in the late afternoon and evening and are accompanied by night sweats. As the disease progresses, a chronic cough develops and mucopurulent sputum is produced.

Tuberculosis is associated with poverty, malnutrition, and HIV infection. Worldwide, it is responsible for more deaths than any other communicable disease. Moreover, the incidence is increasing in inner-city areas and among homeless persons. It is also prevalent among immigrants from Southeast Asia and Central and South America.

Fetal and Neonatal Effects. Although perinatal infection is rare, it may be acquired as the fetus swallows infected amniotic fluid or is exposed through the umbilical vein. The diagnosis is made by finding the bacilli in a gastric aspirate of the neonate or in placental tissue. Signs of congenital tuberculosis include failure to thrive, lethargy, respiratory distress, fever, and enlargement of the spleen, liver, and lymph nodes. If the mother remains untreated, the newborn is at high risk for acquiring tuberculosis by inhalation of infectious respiratory droplets from the mother.

Therapeutic Management. Multidrug therapy is used to protect the woman and her fetus. Examples of drugs effective against tuberculosis include combinations such as isoniazid and rifampin, possibly supplemented with ethambutol. Pyrazinamide may be used in a multidrug regimen for 6 months, although safety data have not been well established (AAP & ACOG, 2002; Whitty & Dombrowski, 2004).

Management of the infant born to a mother with tuberculosis involves preventing the disease or treating early infection. Prevention focuses on teaching family members how the disease is transmitted so that they can protect the infant from airborne organisms. The infant should be skin tested at birth and may be started on preventive isoniazid therapy. Skin testing should be repeated at 3 to 4 months. Isoniazid is usually continued for at least 9 months. Infant tuberculosis medication may stop if the mother and family members are well treated and show no additional disease. If the skin test result converts to positive, a full course of drug therapy should be given.

KEY CONCEPTS

- Spontaneous abortion is a leading cause of pregnancy loss. Treatment focuses on preventing complications, such as hypovolemic shock and infection, and providing emotional support for grieving.
- The incidence of ectopic pregnancy in the United States is increasing as a result of pelvic inflammation associated with sexually transmitted diseases. The goals of therapeutic management are to prevent severe hemorrhage and to preserve the fallopian tube so that future fertility is retained.
- Management of hydatidiform mole involves two phases: (1) evacuation of the molar pregnancy, and (2) regular follow-up for 1 year to detect malignant changes.
- A woman with placenta previa typically presents with painless vaginal bleeding during the last half of pregnancy. Bleeding from abruptio placentae may be visible or concealed and is likely to be accompanied by pain, uterine tenderness, and uterine hyperactivity.
- Disseminated intravascular coagulation is a life-threatening complication of missed abortion, abruptio placentae, and preeclampsia, in which procoagulation and anticoagulation factors are simultaneously activated.
- The goals of management for hyperemesis gravidarum are to prevent dehydration, malnutrition, and electrolyte imbalance. Emotional support is a most important therapy and a responsibility of nurses.
- Generalized vasospasm, which occurs with pregnancy-induced hypertension, decreases circulation to all organs of the body, including the placenta. Major maternal organs affected include the liver, kidneys, and brain.
- The treatment of preeclampsia includes bed rest, reducing environmental stimuli, and administering anticonvulsants.
- Magnesium sulfate is used to prevent convulsions in pregnancy-induced hypertension. Its most serious adverse effect is central nervous system depression, which includes depression of the respiratory center. Hyporeflexia precedes respiratory depression.
- Nurses monitor the woman with preeclampsia to determine the effectiveness of medical therapy and to identify signs that the condition is worsening, such as increasing hyperreflexia. Nurses also control external stimuli and initiate measures to protect the woman in case of eclamptic seizures.
- Women who have chronic hypertension are at increased risk for preeclampsia and should be monitored closely for proteinuria and generalized edema. Antihypertensive medication should be continued or initiated if diastolic blood pressure is consistently higher than 100 mm Hg.

KEY CONCEPTS

- Rh incompatibility can occur when an Rh-negative woman conceives a child who is Rh-positive. As a result of exposure to the Rh-positive antigen, maternal antibodies may develop and cause hemolysis of fetal Rh-positive red blood cells in subsequent pregnancies. Administration of RhoGAM prevents production of anti-Rh antibodies, thus preventing destruction of Rh-positive red blood cells in subsequent pregnancies.
- ABO incompatibility usually occurs when the mother has type O blood and has naturally occurring anti-A and anti-B antibodies, which cause hemolysis if the fetal blood is not type O. ABO incompatibility may result in hyperbilirubinemia of the infant, but it usually is a mild condition.
- During early pregnancy, the release of insulin accelerates and may result in episodes of hypoglycemia. Placental hormones, which reach their peak during the second and third trimesters, create resistance to insulin in maternal cells and cause changes in insulin needs throughout pregnancy.
- Women with type 1 diabetes mellitus have a greater risk for pregnancy-induced hypertension, urinary tract infections, and ketosis.
- Because maternal hyperglycemia during the first trimester increases the risk for congenital anomalies in the fetus, a major goal of management is to establish normal blood glucose levels before pregnancy occurs.
- Fetal growth depends on the condition of maternal blood vessels and the blood glucose levels. With no vascular impairment and adequate placental perfusion, the infant is likely to be of normal size (if maternal glucose levels are normal) or large (i.e., having macrosomia). With high maternal glucose levels and vascular impairment, placental perfusion may be compromised and the fetus may be growth restricted.
- In addition to congenital anomalies, the infant of a diabetic mother is at increased risk for hypoglycemia, hypocalcemia, hyperbilirubinemia, and respiratory distress syndrome.
- The maternal effects of gestational diabetes include increased risks for urinary tract infections, hydramnios, premature rupture of membranes, and the development of pregnancy-induced hypertension.
- Gestational diabetes is responsible for two major complications for the fetus or neonate—fetal macrosomia and neonatal hypoglycemia.
- Gestational diabetes can usually be treated by diet and exercise. Insulin, however, may be administered if blood glucose remains high.
- Cardiovascular changes that occur in normal pregnancy impose an additional burden that may result in cardiac decompensation if the expectant mother has preexisting heart disease.
- The primary goal of management of the pregnant woman with heart disease is to prevent the development of congestive heart failure by restricting activity, limiting weight gain, and preventing anemia and infection, so that cardiac demand does not exceed cardiac reserves.
- Intrapartum and postpartum management of heart disease focuses on preventing fluid overload, which can cause a sharp rise in cardiac effort.
- Iron supplementation is needed during pregnancy because most women do not have sufficient iron stores to meet the demands of pregnancy.
- Folic acid deficiency is associated with an increased risk for spontaneous abortion, abruptio placentae, and fetal anomalies, such as neural tube defects. A folic acid supplement may be necessary to prevent maternal and fetal effects.
- Sickle cell disease is worsened by pregnancy, and a primary goal is to prevent sickle cell crisis during pregnancy.
- Laboratory values for thalassemia are similar to those of iron deficiency, but administration of iron is risky because increased iron absorption and storage make the woman susceptible to iron overload.
- Although women with systemic lupus erythematosus can have a normal pregnancy and give birth to a normal newborn, the preg-
- nancy must be treated as high risk because of the increased incidence of abortion, fetal death during the first trimester, and possible exacerbation of the disease.
- Antiphospholipid syndrome is a cluster of clinical entities and is associated with an increased risk for thrombosis, fetal loss, and decreased platelets. Preeclampsia has a higher incidence in the woman with antiphospholipid syndrome.
- The management of epilepsy is complicated by the teratogenic effects of anticonvulsant medications. Alterations in epilepsy therapy may be possible to reduce teratogenic effects on the fetus.
- Automobile accidents are the major cause of blunt force trauma that may result in premature separation of the placenta, hemorrhage, fractures, and internal injuries. Penetrating injuries caused by knives or bullets are particularly dangerous for the fetus.
- The treatment of trauma during pregnancy is similar to that in a nonpregnant person. Providing cardiopulmonary support and controlling bleeding are the priorities. Careful evaluation of the uterus and fetus is also essential.
- Viral infections that occur during pregnancy can be transmitted to the fetus in two ways: across the placenta or by exposure to organisms during birth. Although they are mild or even subclinical in the mother, viral infections can have serious effects for the fetus.
- Human immunodeficiency virus (HIV) is a retrovirus that gradually allows a fall in the effectiveness of the maternal immunity, often over many years in the treated woman. Maternal treatment with zidovudine (ZDV), sometimes with other antiretroviral medications, can substantially reduce infection of the fetus with HIV.
- Specific pregnancy and post-birth treatment of nonviral infections such as toxoplasmosis, group B streptococcus infection, and tuberculosis reduce long-term maternal and newborn complications.

ANSWER to Critical Thinking Exercise 26-1

Nurses often assume that clients know how to use a thermometer and that they know the signs of infection. Moreover, many nurses assume that clients recognize the connection between blood loss and the tendency to develop infection. As a result, nurses may not emphasize the need for a diet high in nutrients that increase hemoglobin and hematocrit.

ANSWERS to Critical Thinking Exercise 26-2

1. The team may have assumed that Marcia knew the maternal and fetal effects of gestational diabetes and the importance of following the plan of care.
2. The team could have explained the reasons for the recommended plan and allowed adequate time to answer all questions. It is particularly important to emphasize why it is necessary to monitor the condition of the fetus, because mothers are usually motivated to do whatever they can to ensure the health of the fetus.
3. The nurse should acknowledge Marcia's belief. "I realize that we haven't made our concerns clear to you. Let me explain why it is important for you and for your baby to be watched carefully during these last weeks." The nurse must then provide clear, simple explanations and allow time to answer questions.
4. The nurse must acknowledge that weekly tests are time-consuming but that they provide valuable information about the well-being of the baby. Usually the information is reassuring, but additional tests can be performed if there are questions.

REFERENCES and READINGS

Abramovici, D., Mattar, F., & Sibai, B. (2000). Hypertensive disorders in pregnancy. In S.B. Ransom, M.P. Dombrowski, S.G. McNeeley, K.S. Moghissi, & A.R. Munkarah (Eds.), *Practical strategies in obstetrics and gynecology* (pp. 380-389). Philadelphia: Saunders.

American Academy of Pediatrics (AAP), & American College of Obstetricians and Gynecologists (ACOG). (2002). *Guidelines for perinatal care* (5th ed.). Elk Grove Village, IL, and Washington, DC: Author.

American College of Obstetricians & Gynecologists (ACOG). (1999). *Management of herpes in pregnancy* (ACOG Practice Bulletin No. 8). Washington, DC: Author.

American College of Obstetricians & Gynecologists (ACOG). (2001a). *Chronic hypertension in pregnancy* (ACOG Practice Bulletin No. 29). Washington, DC: Author.

American College of Obstetricians & Gynecologists (ACOG). (2001b). *Gestational diabetes* (ACOG Practice Bulletin No. 30). Washington, DC: Author.

American College of Obstetricians & Gynecologists (ACOG). (2002). *Diagnosis and management of preeclampsia and eclampsia* (ACOG Practice Bulletin No. 33). Washington, DC: Author.

American Diabetes Association. (2003a). Position statement: Gestational diabetes mellitus. *Diabetes Care, 26*(Suppl.1), S103-S105. Retrieved Nov. 25, 2003, from http://care.diabetesjournals.org/cgi/reprint/26/suppl_1/s103.pdf.

American Diabetes Association. (2003b). Position statement: Preconception care of women with diabetes. *Diabetes Care, 26*(Suppl. 1), S91-S93. Retrieved Nov. 25, 2003, from http://care.diabetesjournals.org/cgi/reprint/26/suppl_1/s91.pdf.

Aminoff, M.J. (2004). Neurologic disorders. In R.K. Creasy, R. Resnik, & J.D. Iams (Eds.), *Maternal-fetal medicine: Principles and practice* (5th ed., pp. 1165-1191). Philadelphia: Saunders.

Ashley-Koch, A., Yang, Q., & Olney, R.S. (2000). Human genome epidemiology (HuGE) reviews. *American Journal of Epidemiology, 151*(9), 839-845.

August, P. (1999). Hypertensive disorders in pregnancy. In G.N. Burrow & T.P. Duffy (Eds.), *Medical complications during pregnancy* (5th ed., pp. 53-77). Philadelphia: Saunders.

Berman, M.L., DiSaia, P.J., & Tewari, K.S. (2004). Pelvic malignancies, gestational trophoblastic neoplasia, and nonpelvic malignancies. In R.K. Creasy, R. Resnik, & J.D. Iams (Eds.), *Maternal-fetal medicine: Principles and practice* (5th ed., pp. 1213-1242). Philadelphia: Saunders.

Birkhahn, R.H., Gaeta, T.J., Van Deusen, S.K., & Tlockowski, J. (2003). The ability of traditional vital signs and shock index to identify ruptured ectopic pregnancy. *American Journal of Obstetrics and Gynecology, 189*(5), 1293-1296.

Blackburn, S.T. (2003). *Maternal, fetal, & neonatal physiology: A clinical perspective.* Philadelphia: Saunders.

Blanchard, D.G., & Shabetai, R. (2004). Cardiac diseases. In R.K. Creasy, R. Resnik, & J.D. Iams (Eds.), *Maternal-fetal medicine: Principles and practice* (5th ed., pp. 815-843). Philadelphia: Saunders.

Branch, D.W., & Scott, J.R. (2003). Early pregnancy loss. In J.R. Scott, R.S. Gibbs, B.Y. Karlan, & A.F. Haney (Eds.), *Danforth's obstetrics and gynecology* (9th ed., pp. 75-87). Philadelphia: Lippincott Williams & Wilkins.

Buchbinder, A., Sibai, B.M., Caritis, S., MacPherson, C., Hauth, J., Lindheimer, M.D., Klebanoff, M., VanDorsten, P., Landon, M., Paul, R., Miodovnik, M., Meis, P., & Thurnau, G. (2002). Adverse perinatal outcomes are significantly higher in severe gestational hypertension than in mild preeclampsia. *American Journal of Obstetrics & Gynecology, 186*(1), 66-71.

Buckwalter, J.G., & Simpson, S.W. (2002). Psychological factors in the etiology and treatment of severe nausea and vomiting of pregnancy. *American Journal of Obstetrics and Gynecology, 186*(Suppl. 5), S210-S214.

Carolan, M. (2003). The graying of the obstetric population: Implications for the older mother. *Journal of Obstetric, Gynecologic, and Neonatal Nursing, 32*(1), 19-27.

Carpenito, L.J. (2004). *Handbook of nursing diagnosis* (10th ed.). Philadelphia: Lippincott.

Carson, S.A. (2000). Spontaneous abortion. In S.B. Ransom, M.P. Dombrowski, S.G. McNeeley, K.S. Moghissi, & A.R. Munkarah (Eds.), *Practical strategies in obstetrics and gynecology* (pp. 533-538). Philadelphia: Saunders.

Caulin-Glaser, T., & Setaro, J. (1999). Pregnancy and cardiovascular disease. In G.N. Burrow & T.P. Duffy (Eds.), *Medical complications during pregnancy* (5th ed., pp. 111-133). Philadelphia: Saunders.

Centers for Disease Control and Prevention. (2001a). Revised guidelines for HIV counseling, testing, and referral and revised recommendations for HIV screening of pregnant women. *Morbidity and Mortality Weekly Report: Recommendations and Research, 50*(RR-19), November 9, 2001. Retrieved Jan. 10, 2004, from www.cdc.gov/mmwr/pdf/rr/rr5019.pdf.

Centers for Disease Control and Prevention. (2001b). *Varicella vaccine: FAQs related to pregnancy.* Retrieved Dec. 9, 2003, from www.cdc.gov/nip/vaccine/varicella/faqs-clinic-vac-preg.htm.

Centers for Disease Control and Prevention. (2002a). Prevention of perinatal group B streptococcal disease: Revised guidelines from CDC. *Morbidity and Mortality Weekly Report, 45*(RR-11), 1-28. Retrieved Nov. 23, 2003, from www.cdc.gov/groupBstrep/docs/RR5111al.pdf.

Centers for Disease Control and Prevention. (2002b). Sexually transmitted diseases treatment guidelines, 2002. *Morbidity and Mortality Weekly Report, 51*(RR-6). Retrieved Dec. 11, 2003, from www.cdc.gov/STD/treatment/rr5106.pdf.

Centers for Disease Control and Prevention. (2003a). *National diabetes fact sheet: United States, November 2003.* Retrieved Nov. 23, 2003, from www.cdc.gov/diabetes/pubs/pdf/ndfs_2003.pdf.

Centers for Disease Control and Prevention. (2003b). *Rubella.* Retrieved Dec. 9, 2003, from www.cdc.gov/nip/publications/pink/rubella.pdf.

Centers for Disease Control and Prevention. (2003c). *Sexually transmitted diseases surveillance, 2002.* Atlanta, GA: U.S. Department of Health and Human Services, Centers for Disease Control and Prevention, September 2003. Retrieved Dec. 11, 2003, from www.cdc.gov/std/stats/copy&cite.htm.

Chames, M.C., Haddad, B., Barton, J.R., Livingston, J.C., & Sibai, B.M. (2003). Subsequent pregnancy outcome in women with a history of HELLP syndrome at ≤28 weeks of gestation. *American Journal of Obstetrics & Gynecology, 188*(6), 1504-1508.

Chames, M.C., Livingston, J.C., Ivester, T.S., Barton, J.R., & Sibai, B.M. (2002). Late postpartum eclampsia: A preventable disease? *American Journal of Obstetrics & Gynecology, 186*(6), 1174-1177.

Clark, S.H. (2003). Critical care obstetrics. In J.R. Scott, R.S. Gibbs, B.Y. Karlan, & A.F. Haney (Eds.), *Danforth's obstetrics and gynecology* (9th ed., pp. 461-475). Philadelphia: Lippincott Williams Wilkins.

Clark, S.H. (2004). Placenta previa and abruptio placentae. In R.K. Creasy, R. Resnik, & J.D. Iams (Eds.), *Maternal-fetal medicine: Principles and practice* (5th ed., pp. 707-722). Philadelphia: Saunders.

Classen, S.R., Paulson, P.R., & Zacharias, S.R. (1998). Systemic lupus erythematosus: Perinatal and neonatal implications. *Journal of Obstetric, Gynecologic, and Neonatal Nursing, 227*(5), 493-500.

Côté-Arsenault, D. (2003). The influence of perinatal loss on anxiety in multigravidas. *Journal of Obstetric, Gynecologic, and Neonatal Nursing, 32*(5), 623-629.

Coulam, C.B. (2000). Recurrent spontaneous abortion. In E.J. Quilligan & F.P. Zuspan (Eds.), *Current therapy in obstetrics and gynecology* (5th ed., pp. 349-354). Philadelphia: Saunders.

Cunningham, F.G., Gant, N.F., Leveno, K.J., Gilstrap, L.C., Hauth, J.C., & Wenstrom, K.D. (2001). *Williams obstetrics* (21st ed.). Norwalk, CT: Appleton & Lange.

Damato, E.G., & Winnen, C.W. (2002). Cytomegalovirus infection: Perinatal implications. *Journal of Obstetric, Gynecologic, and Neonatal Nursing, 31*(1), 86-92.

Donahue, D.B. (2002). Diagnosis and treatment of herpes simplex infection during pregnancy. *Journal of Obstetric, Gynecologic, and Neonatal Nursing, 31*(1), 99-106.

Duff, P. (1998). Hepatitis in pregnancy. *Seminars in Perinatology, 22*(4), 277-283.

Duffy, T.P. (1999). Hematologic aspects of pregnancy. In G.N. Burrow & T.P. Duffy (Eds.), *Medical complications during pregnancy* (5th ed., pp. 79-85). Philadelphia: Saunders.

Erlen, J.A., Sereika, S.M., Cook, R.L., & Hunt, S.C. (2002). Adherence to antiretroviral therapy among women with HIV infection. *Journal of Obstetric, Gynecologic, and Neonatal Nursing, 31*(4), 470-477.

Fagen, C. (2000). Nutrition during pregnancy and lactation. In L.K. Mahan & S. Escott-Stump (Eds.), *Krause's food, nutrition, & diet therapy,* (10th ed., pp. 167-195). Philadelphia: Mosby.

Farrell, M. (2003). Improving the care of women with gestational diabetes. *MCN: The American Journal of Maternal/Child Nursing, 28*(5), 301-305.

Flemming, D.R. (1999). Challenging traditional insulin injection practices. *American Journal of Nursing, 99*(2), 72-74.

Franz, M. (2000). Medical nutrition therapy for diabetes mellitus and hypoglycemia of nondiabetic origin. In L.K. Mahan & S. Escott-Stump (Eds.), *Krause's food, nutrition, and diet therapy* (10th ed., pp. 742-780). Philadelphia: Saunders.

Freid, F.M., Prager, K., MacKay, A.P., & Xia, H. (2003). *Health, United States, 2003, with chartbook on trends in the health of Americans.* National Center for Health Statistics (DHHS Publication No. 2003-1232): Hyattsville, MD.

Gabbe, S.G., & Landon, M.B. (2000). Diabetes mellitus in pregnancy. In E.J. Quilligan & F.P. Zuspan

REFERENCES and READINGS

(Eds.), *Current therapy in obstetrics & gynecology* (5th ed., pp. 263-268). Philadelphia: Saunders.

Gibbs, R.S., Sweet, R.L., & Duff, W.P. (2004). Maternal and fetal infectious diseases. In R.K. Creasy, R. Resnik, & J.D. Iams (Eds.), *Maternal-fetal medicine: Principles and practice* (5th ed., pp. 741-801). Philadelphia: Saunders.

Gilbert, E.S., & Harmon, J.S. (2003). *Manual of high risk pregnancy & delivery.* St. Louis: Mosby.

Goldstein, D.P., & Berkowitz, R.S. (2000a). Gestational trophoblastic disease. In E.J. Quilligan & F.P. Zuspan (Eds.), *Current therapy in obstetrics and gynecology* (5th ed., pp. 210-213). Philadelphia: Saunders.

Goldstein, D.P., & Berkowitz, R.S. (2000b). Gestational trophoblastic disease. In S.B. Ransom, M.P. Dombrowski, S.G. McNeeley, K.S. Moghissi, & A.R. Munkarah (Eds.), *Practical strategies in obstetrics and gynecology* (5th ed., pp. 511-518). Philadelphia: Saunders.

Goldstein, D.P., & Berkowitz, R.S. (2000c). Hydatidiform mole. In E.J. Quilligan & F.P. Zuspan (Eds.), *Current therapy in obstetrics and gynecology* (5th ed., pp. 213-217). Philadelphia: Saunders.

Gonik, B., & Foley, M.R. (2004). Intensive care monitoring of the critically ill pregnant patient. In R.K. Creasy, R. Resnik, & J.D. Iams (Eds.), *Maternal-fetal medicine: Principles and practice* (5th ed., pp. 975-1004). Philadelphia: Saunders.

Hankins, G.D.V., & Suarez, V.R. (2004). Rheumatologic and connective tissue disorders. In R.K. Creasy, R. Resnik, & J.D. Iams (Eds.), *Maternal-fetal medicine: Principles and practice* (5th ed., pp. 1147-1163). Philadelphia: Saunders.

Heard, M.J., & Buster, J.E. (2003). Ectopic pregnancy. In J.R. Scott, R.S. Gibbs, B.Y. Karlan, & A.F. Haney (Eds.), *Danforth's obstetrics and gynecology* (9th ed., pp. 89-103). Philadelphia: Lippincott Williams Wilkins.

Hill, J.A. (2004). Recurrent pregnancy loss. In R.K. Creasy, R. Resnik, & J.D. Iams (Eds.), *Maternal-fetal medicine* (5th ed., pp. 579-601). Philadelphia: Saunders.

Inzucchi, S.E. (1999). Diabetes in pregnancy. In G.N. Burrow & T.P. Duffy (Eds.), *Medical complications during pregnancy* (5th ed., pp. 25-51). Philadelphia: Saunders.

Jackson, D.J., Chopra, M., Witten, C., & Sengwana, M.J. (2003). HIV and infant feeding: Issues in developed and developing countries. *Journal of Obstetric, Gynecologic, and Neonatal Nursing, 32*(1), 117-127.

Katz, A. (2001). Waiting for something to happen: Hospitalization with placenta previa. *Birth, 28*(3), 186-191.

Katz, A. (2003). The evolving art of caring for pregnant women with HIV infection. *Journal of Obstetric, Gynecologic, and Neonatal Nursing, 32*(1), 102-108.

Katz, J.R., & Hirsch, A.M. (2003). When global health is local health: Infectious diseases travel easily. *American Journal of Nursing, 103*(12), 75-79.

Kay, H.H. (2003). Placenta previa and abruption. In J.R. Scott, R.S. Gibbs, B.Y. Karlan, & A.F. Haney (Eds.), *Danforth's obstetrics and gynecology* (9th ed., pp. 365-379). Philadelphia: Lippincott Williams & Wilkins.

Kendrick, J.M. (1999). Diabetes mellitus in pregnancy. In L.K. Mandeville & N.H. Troiano (Eds.), *AWHONN's high-risk and critical care intrapartum nursing* (2nd ed., pp. 224-255). Philadelphia: Lippincott.

Khanlian, S.A., Smith, H.O., & Cole, L.A. (2003). Persistent low levels of human chorionic gonadotropin: A premalignant gestational trophoblastic disease. *American Journal of Obstetrics & Gynecology, 188*(5), 1254-1259.

Kilpatrick, S.J., & Laros, R.K. (2004). Maternal hematologic disorders. In R.K. Creasy, R. Resnik, & J.D. Iams (Eds.), *Maternal-fetal medicine: Principles and practice* (5th ed., pp. 975-1004). Philadelphia: Saunders.

Lake, M.F. (2001). Tuberculosis in pregnancy: This old disease is presenting new challenges. *AWHONN Lifelines, 5*(5), 35-40.

Landon, M.B. (2004). Diseases of liver, biliary system, and pancreas. In R.K. Creasy, R. Resnik, & J.D. Iams (Eds.), *Maternal-fetal medicine: Principles and practice* (5th ed., pp. 1127-1145). Philadelphia: Saunders.

Landry, M.L. (1999). Viral infections. In G.N. Burrow & T.P. Duffy (Eds.), *Medical complications during pregnancy* (5th ed., pp. 337-362). Philadelphia: Saunders.

Larry, C.D., & Yeo, S. (2000). The circadian rhythm of blood pressure during pregnancy. *Journal of Obstetric, Gynecologic, and Neonatal Nursing, 29*(5), 500-508.

Larson, J.D., & Rayburn, W.F. (2000). Hyperemesis gravidarum. In E.J. Quilligan & F.P. Zuspan (Eds.), *Current therapy in obstetrics and gynecology* (5th ed., pp. 296-299). Philadelphia: Saunders.

Leicht, T.L., & Harvey, C.J. (1999). Hypertensive disorders in pregnancy. In L.K. Mandeville & N.H. Troiano (Eds.), *AWHONN's high-risk and critical care intrapartum nursing* (2nd ed., pp. 159-172). Philadelphia: Lippincott.

Li, A.J., & Karlan, B.Y. (2003). Gestational trophoblastic neoplasms. In J.R. Scott, R.S. Gibbs, B.Y. Karlan, & A.F. Haney (Eds.), *Danforth's obstetrics and gynecology* (9th ed., pp. 1019-1030). Philadelphia: Lippincott Williams & Wilkins.

Lipscomb, G.H., & Ling, F.W. (2000). Ectopic pregnancy. In E.J. Quilligan & F.P. Zuspan (Eds.), *Current therapy in obstetrics and gynecology* (5th ed., pp. 277-277). Philadelphia: Saunders.

Lipscomb, G.H., Meyer, N.L., Flynn, D.E., Peterson, M., & Ling, F.W. (2002). Oral methotrexate for treatment of ectopic pregnancy. *American Journal of Obstetrics and Gynecology, 186*(6), 1192-1195.

Lockwood, C.J., & Silver, R. (2004). Thrombophilias in pregnancy. In R.K. Creasy, R. Resnik, & J.D. Iams (Eds.), *Maternal-fetal medicine: Principles and practice* (5th ed., pp. 1005-1021). Philadelphia: Saunders.

Lucus, M.J., Sharma, S.K., McIntire, D.D., Wiley, J., Sidawi, J.E., Ramin, S.M., Leveno, K.J., & Cunningham, F.G. (2001). A randomized trial of labor analgesia in women with pregnancy-induced hypertension. *American Journal of Obstetrics & Gynecology, 185*(4), 970-975.

Lupus Foundation of America. (2001). *Lupus fact sheet.* Retrieved Dec. 5, 2003, from www.lupus.org/education/factsheet.htm.

MacKay, A.P., Berg, C.J., & Atrash, H.K. (2001). Pregnancy-related mortality from preeclampsia and eclampsia. *Obstetrics & Gynecology, 97*(4), 533-538.

Magee, L.A., Mazzotta, P., & Koren, G. (2002). Evidence-based view of safety and effectiveness of pharmacologic therapy for nausea and vomiting of pregnancy (NVP). *American Journal of Obstetrics and Gynecology, 186*(Suppl. 5), S256-S261.

Malee, M.P. (2003). Medical and surgical complications of pregnancy. In J.R. Scott, R.S. Gibbs, B.Y. Karlan, & A.F. Haney (Eds.), *Danforth's obstetrics and gynecology* (9th ed., pp. 273-311). Philadelphia: Lippincott Williams & Wilkins.

Martin, J.N., & Magann, E.F. (2000). HELLP syndrome. In E.J. Quilligan & F.P. Zuspan (Eds.), *Current therapy in obstetrics and gynecology* (5th ed., pp. 288-293). Philadelphia: Saunders.

Matteson, S., Roscoe, J., Hickok, J., & Morrow, G.R. (2002). The role of behavioral conditioning in the development of nausea. *American Journal of Obstetrics and Gynecology, 186*(Suppl. 5), S239-S243.

McCarter-Spaulding, D. (2002). Parvovirus B19 in pregnancy. *Journal of Obstetric, Gynecologic, and Neonatal Nursing, 31*(1), 107-112.

Minkoff, H.L. (2004). Human immunodeficiency virus. In R.K. Creasy, R. Resnik, & J.D. Iams (Eds.), *Maternal-fetal medicine: Principles and practice* (5th ed., pp. 803-814). Philadelphia: Saunders.

Modigliani, R.M. (2000). Gastrointestinal and pancreatic diseases. In W.M. Barron, M.D. Lindheimer, & J.M. Davison (Eds.), *Medical disorders during pregnancy* (3rd ed., pp. 257-271). St. Louis: Mosby.

Moise, K.J. (2004). Hemolytic disease of the fetus and newborn. In R.K. Creasy, R. Resnik, & J.D. Iams (Eds.), *Maternal-fetal medicine: Principles and practice* (5th ed., pp. 537-561). Philadelphia: Saunders.

Moldenhauer, J.S., & Sibai, B.M. (2003). Hypertensive disorders of pregnancy. In J.R. Scott, R.S. Gibbs, B.Y. Karlan, & A.F. Haney (Eds.), *Danforth's obstetrics and gynecology* (9th ed., pp. 273-311). Philadelphia: Lippincott Williams & Wilkins.

Moore, T.R. (2004). Diabetes in pregnancy. In R.K. Creasy, R. Resnik, & J.D. Iams (Eds.), *Maternal-fetal medicine: Principles and practice* (5th ed., pp. 1023-1061). Philadelphia: Saunders.

Nader, S. (2004). Thyroid disease in pregnancy. In R.K. Creasy, R. Resnik, & J.D. Iams (Eds.), *Maternal-fetal medicine: Principles and practice* (5th ed., pp.1063-1081). Philadelphia: Saunders.

National Center for Health Statistics. (2002). *Fetal death.* Retrieved Jan. 19, 2004, from www.cdc.gov/nchs/datawh/nchsdefs/fetaldeath.htm.

National Center for Health Statistics. (2003). *Abortion.* Retrieved Jan. 19, 2004, from www.cec.hchs/datawh/nchsdefs/abortion.htm.

National High Blood Pressure Education Program Working Group on High Blood Pressure in Pregnancy. (2000). Report of the national high blood pressure education program working group on high blood pressure in pregnancy. *American Journal of Obstetrics and Gynecology, 183*(1), S1-S22.

National Institutes of Health: National Heart, Lung, and Blood Institute. (1996). *Facts about sickle cell anemia* (NIH Publication No. 96-4057, November 1996). Retrieved Dec. 5, 2003, from www.nhlbi.nih.gov/health/public/blood/sickle/sca_fact.pdf.

National Institutes of Health: National Heart, Lung, and Blood Institute. (2001). *Report of the working group on research on hypertension during pregnancy.* Retrieved July 12, 2003, from www.nhlbi.nih.gov/resources/hyperten_preg/index.html.

National Institutes of Health: National Heart, Lung, and Blood Institute. (2002). *Management of sickle cell disease* (4th ed.) (NIH Publication No. 02-2114, June 2002). Retrieved Dec. 5, 2003, from www.nhlbi.nih.gov/health/prof/blood/sickle/sc_mngt.pdf.

National Institutes of Health: National Institute of Arthritis and Musculoskeletal and Skin Diseases. (May, 2001). *Lupus: A patient care guide for nurses and other health professionals.* Retrieved Dec. 5, 2003, from www.niams.nih.gov/ni/topics/lupus/lupusguide/chp4.htm.

Neuman, Mary, & Graf, C. (2003). Pregnancy after age 35: Are these women at high risk? *AWHONN Lifelines, 7*(5),422-430.

Nick, J.M. (2003). Deep tendon reflexes: The what, why, where, and how of tapping. *Journal of Obstetric, Gynecologic, and Neonatal Nursing (JOGNN), 32*(3), 297-306. See also Erratum Article printed in the 4th issue (*JOGNN, 32*[4]).

Olohan, K., & Zappitelli, D. (2003). The insulin pump: Making life with diabetes easier. *American Journal of Nursing, 103*(4), 48-56.

Porter, T.F., Peltier, M., & Branch, D.W. (2003). Immunologic disorders in pregnancy. In J.R. Scott, R.S. Gibbs, B.Y. Karlan, & A.F. Haney (Eds.), *Danforth's obstetrics and gynecology* (9th ed., pp. 313-338). Philadelphia: Lippincott Williams & Wilkins.

Potter, M.B., Lepine, L.A., & Jamieson, D.J. (2003). Predictors of success with methotrexate treatment of tubal ectopic pregnancy at Grady Memorial Hospital. *American Journal of Obstetrics and Gynecology, 188*(5), 1192-1194.

Public Health Service Task Force. (2003). *Recommendations for use of antiretroviral drugs in pregnant HIV-1-infected women for maternal health and interventions to reduce perinatal HIV-1 transmission in the United States.* Retrieved Nov. 17, 2003, from www.aidsinfo.nih.gov/guidelines/perinatal/PER_092203.pdf.

Reece, E.A., & Homko, C.J. (2003). Diabetes mellitus and pregnancy. In J.R. Scott, R.S. Gibbs, B.Y. Karlan, & A.F. Haney (Eds.), *Danforth's obstetrics and gynecology* (9th ed., pp. 247-256). Philadelphia: Lippincott Williams & Wilkins.

Riely, C.A., & Fallon, H.J. (1999). Liver diseases. In G.N. Burrow & T.P. Duffy (Eds.), *Medical complications during pregnancy* (5th ed., pp. 269-294). Philadelphia: Saunders.

Roberts, J.M. (2004). Pregnancy-related hypertension. In R.K. Creasy, R. Resnik, & J.D. Iams (Eds.), *Maternal-fetal medicine: Principles and practice* (5th ed., pp. 859-899). Philadelphia: Saunders.

Salmon, B, & Bruick-Sorge, C. (2003). Pneumonia in pregnant women: Exploring this high-risk complication & its links to preterm labor. *AWHONN Lifelines, 7*(5), 48-52.

Samuelsson, M., Rådestad, I., & Segesten, K. (2001). A waste of life: Fathers' experience of losing a child before birth. *Birth, 28*(2), 124-130.

Savoia, M.C. (1999). Bacterial, fungal, and parasitic disease. In G.N. Burrow & T.P. Duffy (Eds.), *Medical complications during pregnancy* (5th ed., pp. 295-335). Philadelphia: Saunders.

Scott, L.D., & Abu-Hamda, E. (2004). Gastrointestinal disease in pregnancy. In R.K. Creasy, R. Resnik, & J.D. Iams (Eds.), *Maternal-fetal medicine: Principles and practice* (5th ed., pp. 1109-1126). Philadelphia: Saunders.

Shames, K.H., & Youngkin, E.Q. (2002). The thyroid dance: New approaches to autoimmune low thyroid. *AWHONN Lifelines, 6*(1), 52-59.

Sibai, B.M. (2000). Chronic hypertension in pregnancy. In E.J. Quilligan & F.P. Zuspan (Eds.), *Current therapy in obstetrics and gynecology* (5th ed., pp. 256-261). Philadelphia: Saunders.

Sickle Cell Disease Association of America, Inc. (2004). *Break the sickle cycle.* Retrieved February 12, 2004, from www.sicklecelldisease.org/default.htm.

Sorokin, Y. (2000). Obstetric hemorrhage. In S.B. Ransom, M.P. Dombrowski, S.G. McNeeley, K.S. Moghissi, & A.R. Munkarah (Eds.), *Practical strategies in obstetrics and gynecology* (pp. 311-320). Philadelphia: Saunders.

Stovall, T.G. (2000). Ectopic pregnancy. In S.B. Ransom, M.P. Dombrowski, S.G. McNeeley, K.S. Moghissi, & A.R. Munkarah (Eds.), *Practical strategies in obstetrics and gynecology* (pp. 27-39). Philadelphia: Saunders.

Tiller, C.M. (2002). Chlamydia during pregnancy: Implications and impact on perinatal and neonatal outcomes. *Journal of Obstetric, Gynecologic, and Neonatal Nursing, 31*(1), 93-98.

Weinberger, S.E., & Weiss, S.T. (1999). Pulmonary disease. In G.N. Burrow & T.P. Duffy (Eds.), *Medical complications during pregnancy* (5th ed., pp. 363-400). Philadelphia: Saunders.

Weyermann, M., Brenner, H., Adler, G., Yasar, Z., Handke-Veseley, A., Grab, D., Kreineberg, R., & Rothenbacher, D. (2003). *Heliobacter pylori* infection and the occurrence and severity of gastrointestinal symptoms during pregnancy. *American Journal of Obstetrics and Gynecology, 189*(2), 526-531.

Wheeler, S.R., & Austin, J.K. (2001). The impact of early pregnancy loss on adolescents. *MCN: The American Journal of Maternal/Child Nursing, 26*(3), 154-159.

Whitty, J.E., & Dombrowski, M.P. (2004). Respiratory diseases in pregnancy. In R.K. Creasy, R. Resnik, & J.D. Iams (Eds.), *Maternal-fetal medicine: Principles and practice* (5th ed., pp. 953-974). Philadelphia: Saunders.

Zuspan, F.P. (2000). Preeclampsia. In E.J. Quilligan & F.P. Zuspan (Eds.), *Current therapy in obstetrics and gynecology* (5th ed., pp. 322-325). Philadelphia: Saunders.

27

The Woman with an Intrapartum Complication

 ## LEARNING OBJECTIVES

After studying this chapter, you should be able to:

◎ Explain abnormalities that may result in dysfunctional labor.
◎ Describe maternal and fetal risks associated with premature rupture of the membranes.
◎ Analyze factors that increase a woman's risk for preterm labor.
◎ Explain maternal and fetal problems that may occur if pregnancy persists beyond 42 weeks.

◎ Describe common intrapartum emergencies.
◎ Explain therapeutic management of each intrapartum complication.
◎ Apply the nursing process to care of women with intrapartum complications and to their families.

 ## DEFINITIONS

abruptio placentae Premature separation of a normally implanted placenta.

anaphylactoid syndrome A disorder in which amniotic fluid with its particulate matter enters the pregnant woman's circulation, lodging in her lungs. Previously called *amniotic fluid embolism.*

cephalopelvic disproportion (CPD) Fetal head size that is too large to fit through the maternal pelvis at birth. Also called *fetopelvic disproportion.*

chorioamnionitis Inflammation of the amniotic sac (fetal membranes); usually caused by bacterial or viral infection. Also called *amnionitis.*

dystocia Difficult or prolonged labor; often associated with abnormal uterine activity and cephalopelvic disproportion.

hydramnios Excessive volume of amniotic fluid (more than 2000 ml at term). Also called *polyhydramnios.*

hypertonic labor dysfunction Ineffective labor characterized by erratic and poorly coordinated contractions. Uterine resting tone is higher than normal.

hypotonic labor dysfunction Ineffective labor characterized by weak, infrequent, and brief but coordinated uterine contractions. Uterine resting tone is normal.

macrosomia Unusually large fetal size; infant birth weight more than 4000 g (8.8 lb).

multifetal pregnancy A pregnancy in which the woman is carrying two or more fetuses. Also called *multiple gestation.*

occult prolapse See *prolapsed cord.*

oligohydramnios Abnormally small volume of amniotic fluid (less than 500 ml at term).

placenta accreta A placenta that is abnormally adherent to the uterine muscle. If the condition is more advanced, it is called *placenta increta* (the placenta extends into the uterine muscle) or *placenta percreta* (the placenta extends through the uterine muscle).

placenta previa Abnormal implantation of the placenta in the lower uterus, at or very near the cervical os.

precipitate birth A birth that occurs without a trained attendant present.

precipitate labor An intense, unusually short labor (less than 3 hours).

preterm labor Onset of labor after 20 weeks and before the beginning of the 38th week of gestation.

prolapsed cord Displacement of the umbilical cord in front of or beside the fetal presenting part. An occult prolapse is one that is suspected on the basis of fetal heart rate patterns; the umbilical cord cannot be palpated or seen.

shoulder dystocia Delayed or difficult birth of the fetal shoulders after the head is born.

tocolytic A drug that inhibits uterine contractions.

uterine inversion Turning of the uterus inside out after birth of the fetus.

uterine resting tone Degree of uterine muscle tension when the woman is not in labor or during the interval between labor contractions.

uterine rupture A tear in the wall of the uterus.

Birth is usually free of major complications. Sometimes, however, complications make childbearing hazardous for the woman or her baby. The nurse's challenge is to identify and manage the complications promptly and to provide effective care for these mothers while supporting the entire family at this significant time in their lives.

DYSFUNCTIONAL LABOR

Normal labor is characterized by progress. Dysfunctional labor is one that does not result in normal progress of cervical effacement, dilation, and fetal descent. *Dystocia* is a general term that describes any difficult labor or birth. A dysfunctional labor may result from problems with the powers of labor, the passenger, the passage, the psyche, or a combination of these. Dysfunctional labor is often prolonged but may be unusually short and intense.

An operative birth (vacuum extractor– or forceps-assisted or cesarean) may be needed if dysfunctional labor does not resolve or if fetal or maternal compromise occurs. Signs that indicate the need for an operative birth include persistent non-reassuring fetal heart rate (FHR) patterns (see Chapter 18), fetal acidosis, and meconium passage. Maternal exhaustion or infection may occur, especially during long labors.

Problems of the Powers

The powers of labor may not be adequate to expel the fetus because of ineffective contractions or ineffective maternal pushing efforts.

Ineffective Contractions

Effective uterine activity is characterized by coordinated contractions that are strong and numerous enough to propel the fetus past the resistance of the woman's bony pelvis and soft tissues. It is not possible to say how frequent, long, or strong labor contractions must be. One woman's labor may progress with contractions that would be inadequate for another woman. Possible causes of ineffective contractions include:

- Maternal fatigue
- Maternal inactivity
- Fluid and electrolyte imbalance
- Hypoglycemia
- Excessive analgesia or anesthesia
- Maternal catecholamines secreted in response to stress or pain
- Disproportion between the maternal pelvis and the fetal presenting part
- Uterine overdistention, such as with multiple gestation or hydramnios

Two patterns of ineffective uterine contractions are hypotonic and hypertonic dysfunction (Table 27-1). Hypotonic dysfunction is more common than hypertonic. Characteristics and management of each are different, but the result—poor labor progress—is the same if they persist.

Hypotonic Dysfunction. Hypotonic contractions are coordinated but are too weak to be effective. They are infrequent and brief and can be easily indented with fingertip pressure at the peak.

Hypotonic dysfunction usually occurs during the active phase of labor, when progress normally quickens. Uterine overdistention is associated with hypotonic dysfunction because the stretched uterine muscle contracts poorly.

The woman may be fairly comfortable because her contractions are weak. Persistent hypotonic dysfunction is fatiguing and frustrating for the mother. Fetal hypoxia is not usually seen with hypotonic labor.

Management depends on the cause. Providing intravenous or oral fluids corrects maternal fluid and electrolyte imbalances or hypoglycemia. Maternal position changes, particularly upright positions, favor fetal descent and promote effective contractions. The woman who moves about actively typically has better labor progress and is more comfortable than one who remains in one position. Pain management techniques such as epidural block may have outcomes that reduce contraction effectiveness, requiring interventions specific to that factor.

The nurse should use therapeutic communication to help the woman identify anxieties or beliefs about labor and its progress. Helping her to get her anxieties in the open is the first step to managing them effectively so that the stress response does not slow her labor.

Some women need measures such as amniotomy or oxytocin infusion to promote labor progress. The birth attendant evaluates the woman's labor to confirm that she is having hypotonic active labor rather than a long latent phase (the first 3 cm of dilation) of labor. The maternal pelvis and fetal presentation and position are assessed to identify abnormalities.

Amniotomy or oxytocin augmentation (see Chapter 20) may be used to stimulate a labor that slows after it is established. Reduced placental perfusion caused by excessive uterine contractions is the most common risk of oxytocin labor augmentation.

Hypertonic Dysfunction. Hypertonic dysfunction of labor is less common than hypotonic. Contractions are uncoordinated and are erratic in their frequency, duration, and intensity. The contractions are painful but ineffective. Hypertonic dysfunction usually occurs during the latent phase of labor.

The uterine resting tone between contractions is high, reducing uterine blood flow. This ischemia decreases fetal oxygen supply and causes the woman to have almost constant cramping pain. Because high resting tone and constant pain are also seen in abruptio placentae, this complication should be considered as well.

The mother becomes very tired because of long yet non-productive discomfort. She may lose confidence in her ability to cope with labor and give birth. Frustration and anxiety further reduce her pain tolerance and interfere with normal processes of labor. The nurse should accept her frustration and discomfort. It is important not to equate cervical dilation with the amount of pain a woman "should" experience.

Management of hypertonic labor depends on the cause. Relief of pain is the primary intervention to promote a normal labor pattern. Warm showers or baths promote relaxation and rest, often allowing a normal labor pattern to ensue. Systemic analgesics or epidural analgesia may be required to achieve this purpose.

Oxytocin is not usually given because it can intensify the already high uterine resting tone. Very low doses of oxytocin, however, are sometimes given to promote coordinated uter-

TABLE 27-1 Patterns of Labor Dysfunction

Hypotonic Dysfunction	Hypertonic Dysfunction
CONTRACTIONS	
Coordinated but weak. Become less frequent and shorter in duration. Easily indented at peak. Woman may have minimal discomfort because the contractions are weak.	Uncoordinated, irregular. Short and poor intensity, but painful and cramp-like.
UTERINE RESTING TONE	
Not elevated.	Higher than normal. Important to distinguish from abruptio placentae, which has similar characteristics (see p. 625).
PHASE OF LABOR	
Active. Typically occurs after 4-cm dilation. More common than hypertonic dysfunction.	Latent. Usually occurs before 4-cm dilation. Less common than hypotonic dysfunction.
THERAPEUTIC MANAGEMENT	
Amniotomy (may increase the risk of infection). Oxytocin augmentation. Cesarean birth if no progress.	Correct cause if it can be identified. Light sedation to promote rest. Hydration. Tocolytics to reduce high uterine tone and promote placental perfusion.
NURSING CARE	
Interventions related to amniotomy and oxytocin augmentation. Encourage position changes. An abdominal binder may help direct the fetus toward the mother's pelvis if her abdominal wall is very lax. Ambulation if no contraindication and if acceptable to the woman. Emotional support: Allow her to ventilate feelings of discouragement. Explain measures taken to increase effectiveness of contractions. Include her partner/family in emotional support measures because they may have anxiety that will heighten the woman's anxiety.	Promote uterine blood flow: side-lying position. Promote rest, general comfort, and relaxation. Pain relief. Emotional support: Accept the reality of the woman's pain and frustration. Reassure her that she is not being childish. Explain reason for measures to break abnormal labor patterns and their goal/expected results. Allow her to ventilate her feelings during and after labor. Include partner/family (see hypotonic labor dysfunction).

ine contractions. Tocolytic drugs may be ordered to reduce uterine resting tone and improve placental blood flow.

Ineffective Maternal Pushing

A reflex urge to push with contractions usually occurs as the fetal presenting part reaches the pelvic floor during second-stage labor. Ineffective pushing may result from:

- Use of incorrect pushing techniques or inappropriate pushing positions
- Fear of injury because of pain and tearing sensations felt by the mother when she pushes
- Decreased or absent urge to push
- Maternal exhaustion
- Analgesia or anesthesia that suppresses the woman's urge to push
- Psychological unreadiness to "let go" of her baby

Management focuses on correcting the causes contributing to ineffective pushing. If maternal and fetal vital signs are normal, there is no maximum allowable duration for the second stage. Each woman is evaluated individually by her birth attendant to determine whether labor should be

ended with an operative delivery or can continue safely (see Chapter 17).

Nursing care to promote effective pushing helps the mother make each effort productive. Upright positions such as squatting add the force of gravity to her efforts. Semi-sitting, side-lying, and pushing while sitting on the toilet are other options. Regional analgesia methods may restrict possible maternal positions and may alter a woman's spontaneous urge to push. On the other hand, women who have regional pain management often feel an adequate urge to push that is not complicated by excessive painful sensation.

The woman who fears injury because of the sensations she feels when she pushes may respond to accurate information about the process of fetal descent. If she understands that sensations of tearing often accompany fetal descent but that her tissues can expand to accommodate the baby, she may be more willing to push with contractions.

The woman who is exhausted may push more effectively if she is encouraged to rest until she feels the urge. Encouraging her to push with intermittent contractions also allows her to maintain adequate pushing effort. Oral or intravenous fluids provide energy for the strenuous work of second-stage labor. Reassuring the woman if there is no ap-

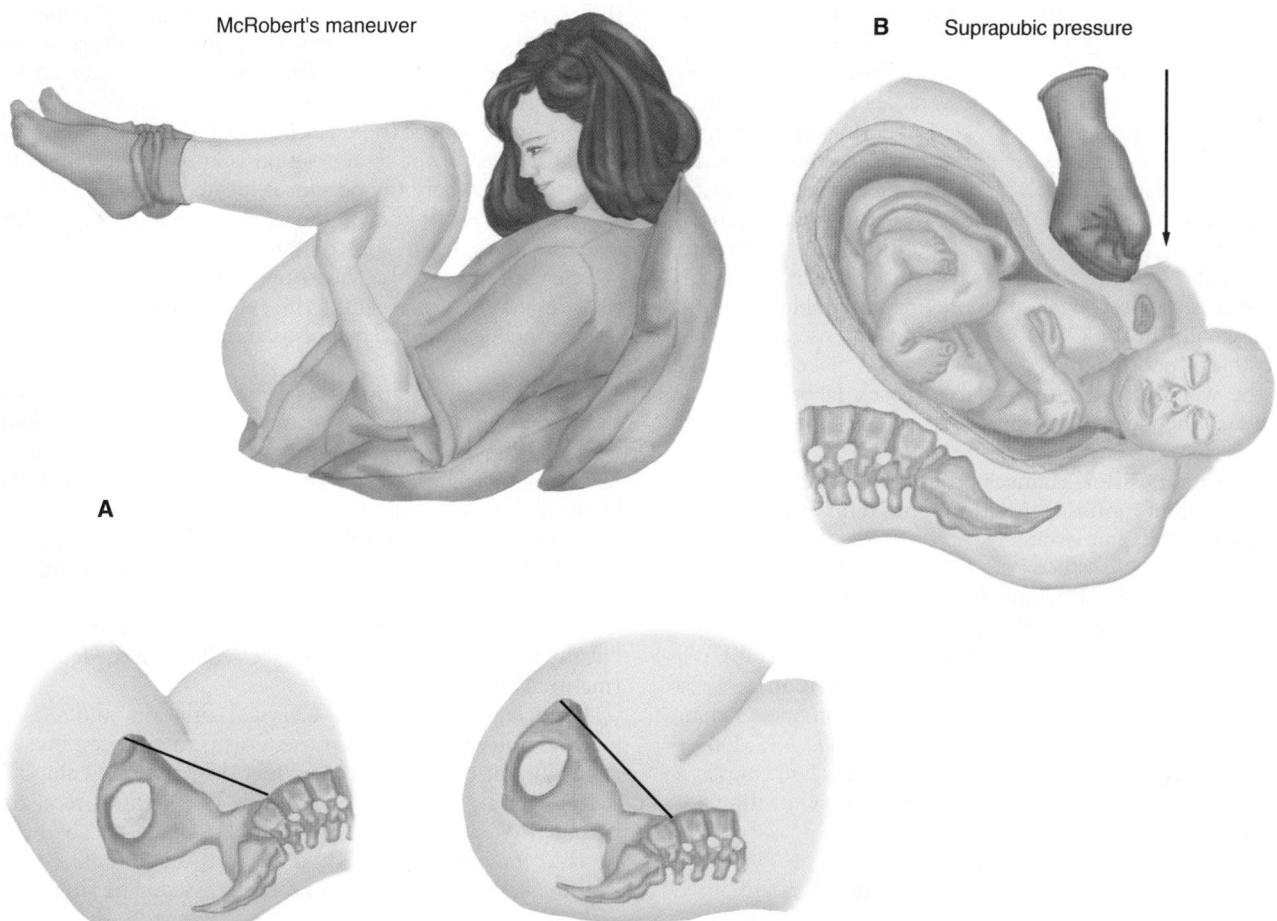

McRobert's maneuver

B   Suprapubic pressure

A

Figure 27-1 Methods that may be used to relieve shoulder dystocia. **A,** McRobert's maneuver. The woman flexes her thighs sharply against her abdomen, which straightens the pelvic curve. A supported squat has a similar effect and adds gravity to her pushing efforts. **B,** Suprapubic pressure by an assistant pushes the fetal anterior shoulder downward to displace it from above the mother's symphysis pubis. Fundal pressure should not be used, because it will push the anterior shoulder more firmly against the mother's symphysis.

parent fetal or maternal harm to a prolonged second stage may encourage her.

Problems With the Passenger

Fetal problems associated with dysfunctional labor are those related to:

- Fetal size
- Fetal presentation or position
- Multifetal pregnancy
- Fetal anomalies

These variations may cause mechanical problems and contribute to ineffective contractions.

Fetal Size

Macrosomia. The macrosomic infant weighs more than 4000 g (8.8 lb) at birth. The head or shoulders may not be able to adapt to the pelvis. In addition, distention of the uterus by the large fetus reduces the strength of contractions both during and after birth.

Size is relative, however. The woman with a small pelvis or one that is abnormally shaped may not be able to deliver an average-size or small infant. A woman with a large pelvis may easily give birth to a larger infant than the woman having a small or even average pelvic size. The actual fetal position as it descends through her pelvis also may alter the ease with which she completes the second stage of birth.

Shoulder Dystocia. Delayed or difficult birth of the shoulders may occur as they become impacted above the maternal symphysis pubis. As soon as the head is born, it retracts against the perineum, much like a turtle's head drawing into its shell (sometimes called the "turtle sign").

Shoulder dystocia requires urgent intervention because the umbilical cord is compressed but chest compression within the vagina prevents respirations. Any of several methods may be used to relieve the impacted fetal shoulders quickly (Fig. 27-1). The infant's clavicles should be checked for crepitus, deformity, or bruising, each of which suggests fracture.

Abnormal Fetal Presentation or Position

An unfavorable fetal presentation or position may interfere with cervical dilation or fetal descent.

Rotation Abnormalities. Persistence of the fetus in the occiput posterior (OP) or occiput transverse (OT) position can contribute to dysfunctional labor. These positions delay fetal descent and other mechanisms of labor (cardinal movements). Most fetuses in an OP position during early labor rotate spontaneously to an occiput anterior position while descending through the pelvis, promoting normal extension and expulsion of the head. Although many women cannot readily deliver their fetus in the OP position, the woman with a large pelvis relative to the fetal size may be able to do so.

Labor is usually longer and more uncomfortable when the fetus remains in the OP or OT position. Intense back or leg pain that is poorly relieved with analgesics makes it difficult for the woman to cope with labor. "Back labor" aptly describes the sensations a woman feels when her fetus is in an OP position.

Maternal position changes promote fetal head rotation to an occiput anterior position and fetal descent (see Chapter 17). Examples are:

- Hands and knees. Rocking the pelvis back and forth while on hands and knees encourages rotation.
- Side-lying (on her left side if the fetus is in a right OP position and on her right side for a left OP position).
- The lunge, in which the mother places one foot on a chair with her foot and knee pointed to that side. She lunges sideways repeatedly during a contraction for 5 seconds at a time. This action can also be performed in a kneeling position.
- Squatting (for second-stage labor).
- Sitting, kneeling, or standing while leaning forward.

Using a birthing ball—a large plastic ball capable of supporting an adult's weight—helps support the woman when in the hands-and-knees position. She can also sit on it, providing many of the benefits of squatting. In addition, the woman tends to move her hips back and forth, favoring fetal descent.

Upright maternal positions promote descent, which is usually accompanied by fetal head rotation. The hands-and-knees and the side-lying positions promote rotation because the mother's abdomen is dependent in relation to her spine. The convex surface of the fetal back tends to rotate toward the convex anterior uterus, similar to nesting two spoons together (Fig. 27-2). Moreover, these positions decrease the mother's discomfort by reducing fetal head pressure on her sacrum. A side-lying position has a similar effect.

The lunge widens the side of the pelvis toward which the woman lunges. If the fetal position is known, she lunges toward the side where the occiput is located (Fig. 27-3). If the fetal position is not known, the woman can lunge toward the side that gives her greater comfort.

All variations of the squatting position aid rotation and fetal descent by straightening the pelvic curve and by enlarging the pelvic outlet. They also add gravity to the force of maternal pushing.

If spontaneous rotation does not occur, the physician may assist rotation and descent of the head with forceps. Some types of vacuum extractors cannot be applied to the fetal head when it remains in an OP position. Cesarean birth may be needed if forceps use is not successful.

Deflexion Abnormalities. The poorly flexed fetal head presents a larger diameter to the pelvis than if flexed with the chin on the chest (see Fig. 17-8). In the *face presentation*, the head diameter is similar to that of the vertex presentation, but the maternal pelvis can be traversed only if the fetal chin (mentum) is anterior.

Breech Presentation. Cervical dilation and effacement are often slower when the fetus is in a breech presentation because the buttocks or feet do not form a smooth, round dilating wedge like the head. The greatest fetal risk is that the head—the largest fetal part—is last to be born. By the time the lower body is born, the umbilical cord is well into the pelvis and may be compressed. The shoulders,

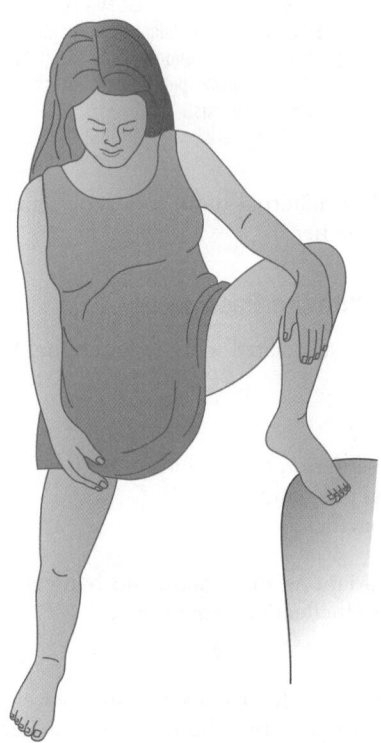

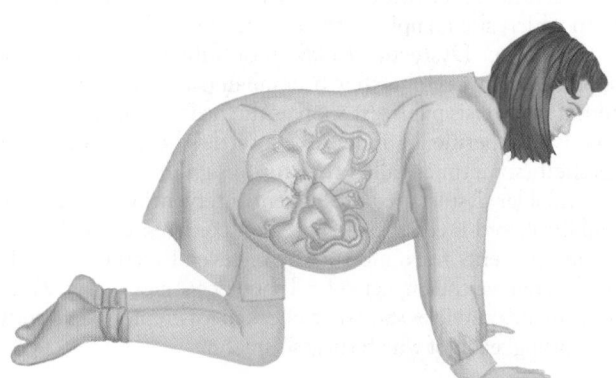

Figure 27-2 A "hands-and-knees" position helps the fetus rotate from a left occiput posterior (LOP) position to an occiput anterior position.

Figure 27-3 The "lunge" to one side promotes rotation of the fetal occiput from a posterior position to an anterior one.

arms, and head must be delivered quickly so that the infant can breathe.

A breech presentation is common well before term, but only 3% to 4% of term fetuses remain in this presentation. Adverse outcomes that are associated with breech birth may include:

- Fetal injury with a difficult vaginal birth
- Prolapsed umbilical cord
- Low birth weight as a result of preterm gestation, multifetal pregnancy, or intrauterine growth restriction
- Fetal anomalies contributing to the breech presentation, such as hydrocephalus
- Complications secondary to placenta previa or cesarean birth.

External cephalic version (ECV) may be attempted to change the fetus in a breech presentation or transverse lie to a cephalic presentation (see Chapter 20). If the fetus remains in the abnormal presentation, cesarean birth is recommended to avoid complications of a difficult vaginal birth if the woman is not in active labor. A woman who first enters the labor unit in advanced active labor may have a fetus remaining in a breech presentation and perhaps also a very immature fetus. In this case, ECV is not always possible and vaginal birth may be necessary simply because labor ends very quickly.

Multifetal Pregnancy

Multifetal pregnancy may result in dysfunctional labor because of uterine overdistention, which contributes to hypotonic dysfunction, and abnormal presentation of one or both fetuses (Fig. 27-4). In addition, the potential for fetal hypoxia during labor is greater. The risk for postpartum hemorrhage resulting from uterine atony because of uterine overdistention is greater.

Because of these problems, birth for a woman with a twin pregnancy is often cesarean, although it is also common for

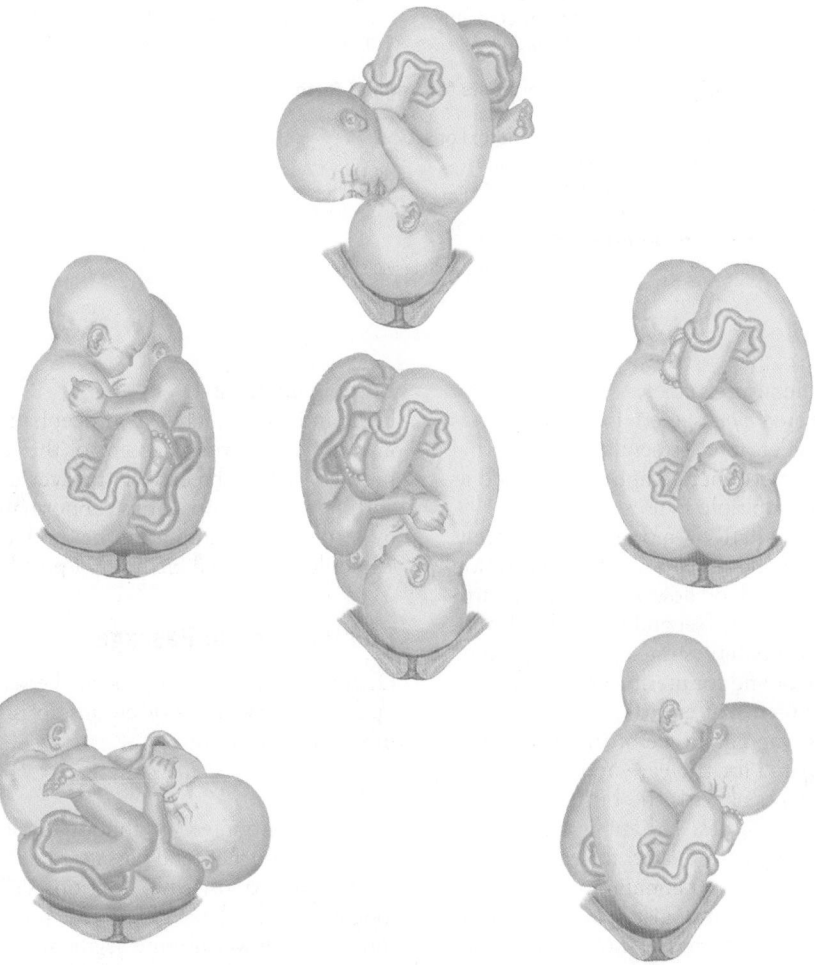

Figure 27-4 Twins can present in any combination of presentations and positions.

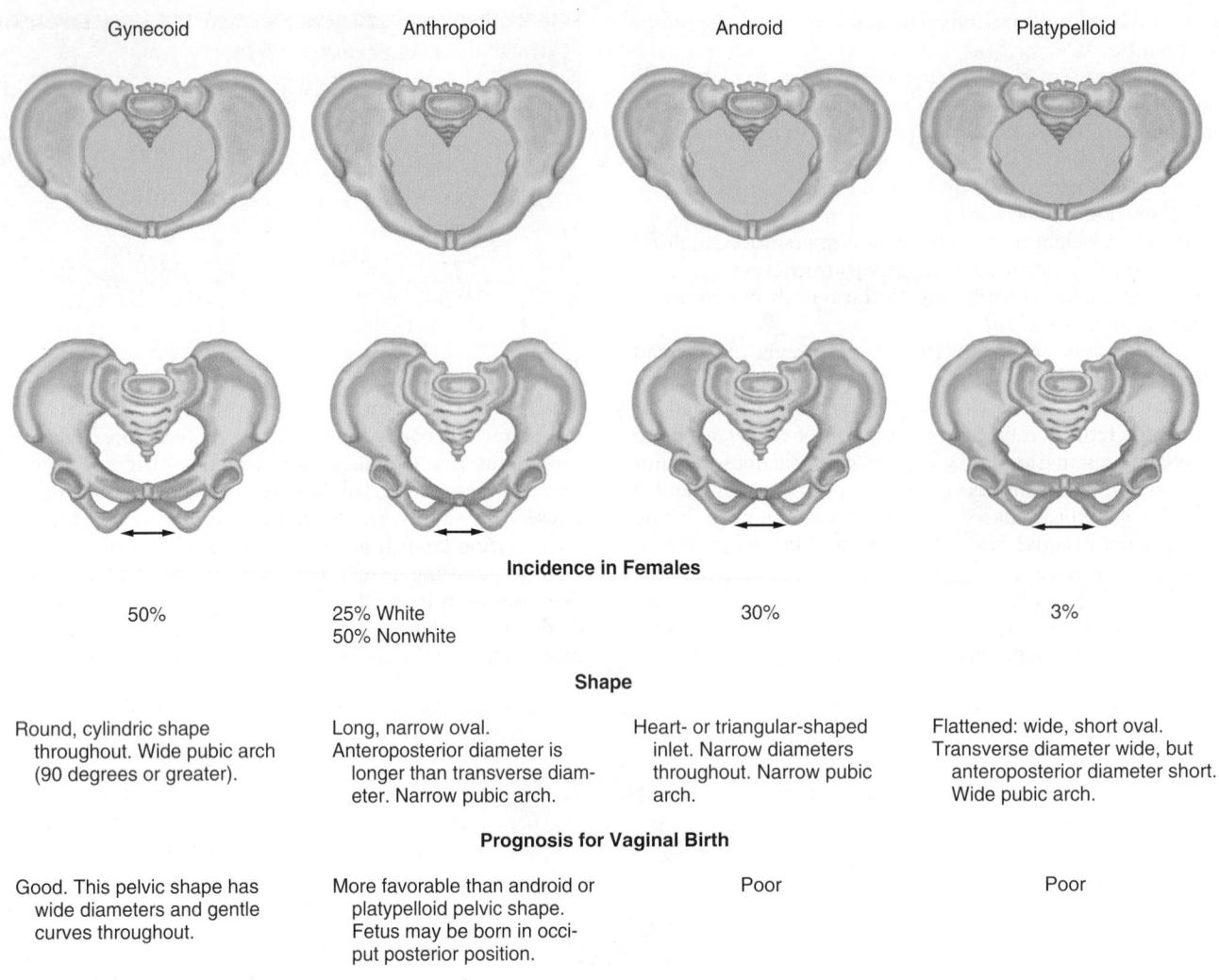

Gynecoid	Anthropoid	Android	Platypelloid
Incidence in Females			
50%	25% White 50% Nonwhite	30%	3%
Shape			
Round, cylindric shape throughout. Wide pubic arch (90 degrees or greater).	Long, narrow oval. Anteroposterior diameter is longer than transverse diameter. Narrow pubic arch.	Heart- or triangular-shaped inlet. Narrow diameters throughout. Narrow pubic arch.	Flattened: wide, short oval. Transverse diameter wide, but anteroposterior diameter short. Wide pubic arch.
Prognosis for Vaginal Birth			
Good. This pelvic shape has wide diameters and gentle curves throughout.	More favorable than android or platypelloid pelvic shape. Fetus may be born in occiput posterior position.	Poor	Poor

Figure 27-5 Pelvic shapes.

birth to be vaginal. Multifetal pregnancies with more than twins are most often delivered by cesarean if the gestation is viable. The physician considers fetal presentations, maternal pelvic size, and the presence of other complications, such as hypertension, as well as the multiple fetuses.

During labor, each twin's FHR is monitored separately. When in bed, the woman should remain in a lateral position to promote adequate placental blood flow. After vaginal birth of the first twin, assessment of the second twin's FHR continues until birth. The nurse observes for signs of hypotonic dysfunction throughout labor and for uterine atony, often related to the overdistended uterus, after birth.

Whether the birth is vaginal or cesarean, the intrapartum staff must be prepared for the care and possible resuscitation of multiple infants as with the birth of a single infant. Cord clamps, bulb syringes, radiant warmers, and resuscitation equipment must be prepared for each infant. One or more neonatal nurses, a neonatal nurse practitioner, a pediatrician, or a neonatologist should be available to care for each infant. One nurse should be free to care for the mother.

Fetal Anomalies

Fetal anomalies such as hydrocephalus or a large fetal tumor may prevent normal descent of the fetus. Abnormal presentations, such as breech or transverse lie, are also associated with fetal anomalies. These abnormalities may be discovered by ultrasound examination before labor. A cesarean birth is scheduled if vaginal birth is not possible or if it is inadvisable.

Problems of the Passage

Dysfunctional labor may occur because of variations in the maternal bony pelvis or because of soft tissue problems that inhibit fetal descent.

Pelvis

A small (contracted) or abnormally shaped pelvis may retard labor and obstruct fetal passage. The woman may experience poor contractions, slow dilation, slow fetal descent, and a long labor. The danger of uterine rupture is greater with thinning of the lower uterine segment, especially if contractions remain strong.

There are four basic pelvic shapes, each with different implications for labor and birth (Fig. 27-5). Most women have mixed characteristics from two or more types.

Maternal Soft Tissue Obstructions

During labor, a full bladder is a common soft tissue obstruction. Bladder distention reduces available space in the pelvis and intensifies maternal discomfort. The woman should be assessed for bladder distention regularly and encouraged to void every 1 to 2 hours. Catheterization may be needed if she cannot urinate or if she receives regional block analgesia such as an epidural (see Chapter 19).

Problems of the Psyche

A perceived threat caused by pain, fear, nonsupport, or one's personal situation can result in great maternal stress and interfere with normal labor progress. The woman's perception of stress more than the actual existence of a threat is important.

The body responds to stress, preparing itself for fight or flight. Responses to excessive or prolonged stress, however, interfere with labor in several ways:

- Increased glucose consumption reduces the energy supply available to the contracting uterus.
- Maternal catecholamines can impair labor by interfering with adequate uterine contractility. Maternal blood supply to the placenta may also be reduced.
- Labor contractions and maternal pushing efforts are less effective because these powers are working against the resistance of tense abdominal and pelvic muscles.
- Pain perception is increased and pain tolerance is decreased, which further increase maternal anxiety and stress.

Helping the woman relax helps her body work more effectively with the forces of labor and promotes normal progress. General nursing measures involve:

- Establishing a trusting relationship with the woman and her family
- Making the environment comfortable by adjusting temperature and light
- Promoting physical comfort, such as cleanliness
- Providing accurate information
- Implementing non-pharmacologic and pharmacologic pain management

Chapters 17 and 19 describe additional methods to encourage relaxation and promote comfort, including individual and family cultural values that are part of childbirth.

Abnormal Labor Duration

An unusually long or short labor may result in maternal, fetal, or neonatal problems.

Prolonged Labor

Prolonged labor is a type of dysfunctional labor that results from problems with any of the factors in the birth process. After the woman reaches the active phase of labor, cervical dilation should proceed at a minimum rate of 1.2 cm per hour in the nullipara and 1.5 cm per hour in the parous woman. Descent of the fetal presenting part is expected to occur at a minimum rate of 1.0 cm per hour in the nullipara and 2.0 cm per hour in the parous woman (Cunningham et al., 2001). If all previous births were by cesarean before much cervical dilation occurred, the criteria that apply to a nullipara may be applied to a multipara.

Potential maternal and fetal problems in prolonged labor include:

- Maternal infection, intrapartum or postpartum
- Neonatal infection, which may be severe or fatal
- Maternal exhaustion
- Higher levels of anxiety and fear during a subsequent labor

Maternal and neonatal infections are more likely if the membranes have been ruptured for a prolonged time, because organisms ascend from the vagina. The mother is more likely to have an intrapartum infection, a postpartum infection, or both. See also Chapter 19 for elevated maternal temperature that is often associated with epidural analgesia.

Nursing measures for the woman who has prolonged labor include promotion of comfort, conservation of energy, emotional support, position changes that favor normal progress, and assessments for infection. Nursing care for the fetus includes observation for signs of intrauterine infection and for compromised fetal oxygenation (see Chapter 18).

Precipitate Labor

Precipitate labor is a rapid birth that occurs within 3 hours of labor onset. There is often an abrupt onset of intense contractions rather than the more gradual increase in frequency, duration, and intensity that typifies most spontaneous labors. The mother or her fetus or newborn may be affected by several conditions that can be associated with the precipitate labor. These conditions may include abruptio placentae, fetal meconium, maternal cocaine use (also may be associated with abruptio placentae), postpartum hemorrhage, or low Apgar scores for the infant (Clark, 2003; Cunningham et al., 2001).

Precipitate labor is not the same as a precipitate birth. A precipitate birth occurs after a labor of any length, in or out of the hospital or birth center, when a trained attendant is not present to assist. A woman in precipitate labor may also have a precipitate birth. The nurse should simply wear gloves while supporting the baby as it emerges. The mother's legs should not be forced together or the fetal head held back to delay birth. Such actions can result in fetal hypoxia or other injury.

If the maternal pelvis is adequate and the soft tissues yield easily to fetal descent, little maternal injury is likely. However, trauma, such as uterine rupture, cervical lacerations, or hematoma, of the vagina or vulva may occur.

The fetus may suffer direct trauma, such as intracranial hemorrhage or nerve damage, during a precipitate labor. The fetus may become hypoxic because intense contractions with a short relaxation period reduce time available for gas exchange in the placenta.

Priority nursing care of the woman in precipitate labor includes promotion of fetal oxygenation and maternal comfort. The woman should remain in a side-lying position to enhance placental blood flow and reduce the effects of aortocaval compression. An added benefit of the side-lying position is to slow the rapid fetal descent and minimize perineal tears. Additional measures to enhance fetal oxygenation include administering oxygen to the mother and maintaining adequate blood volume with nonadditive intravenous fluids. If oxytocin is being used, it should be stopped. A tocolytic drug is often ordered.

Promoting comfort is difficult in a precipitate labor because intense contractions give the woman little time to prepare and to use coping skills, such as breathing techniques. Pharmacologic measures (opioid analgesia or regional block) may not be useful because rapid labor progression does not allow time for them to become effective. Also, possible newborn respiratory depression must be considered when opioids are given near birth. The nurse helps the woman focus on techniques to cope with pain one contraction at a time. The nurse must remain with her, both to provide support and to assist with an emergency birth if it occurs.

▶NURSING CARE
The Woman in Dysfunctional Labor

Several nursing diagnoses and collaborative problems may be appropriate in dysfunctional labor. The potential complication of fetal compromise should be part of all intrapartum management (see Chapter 18). If the woman had planned and practiced the use of coping skills while in labor, she may find that these skills are inadequate if labor is not normal. Anxiety or fear is often higher with abnormal labor, which also may reduce the effectiveness of pharmacologic or regional block (e.g., epidural block) pain control methods. Maternal or newborn injury sometimes becomes apparent after the birth.

In addition to these possible situations, nursing care in this section is directed toward two other concerns: possible intrauterine infection and maternal exhaustion.

INTRAUTERINE INFECTION
Assessment

Infection can occur with both normal and dysfunctional labors. Assess the FHR and maternal vital signs for evidence of infection:

- FHR: persistent fetal tachycardia (>160 beats per minute [bpm] for >10 min) is often an early sign of intrauterine infection.
- Maternal temperature: assess every 2 to 4 hours in normal labor and every 2 hours after membranes rupture; assess hourly if elevated (38° C, or 100.4° F) or if other signs of infection are present.
- Maternal pulse, respirations, and blood pressure: assess at least hourly to identify tachycardia or tachypnea, which often accompany temperature elevation. Maternal vital signs are usually added to the fetal monitor tracing.

Assess amniotic fluid for normal clear color and mild odor. Small flecks of white vernix are normal. Yellow or cloudy fluid or fluid with a foul or strong odor suggests infection and vernix may be stained by discolored fluid. The strong odor may be noted before birth or afterward on the infant's skin.

Nursing Diagnosis and Planning

For the woman without signs of infection but with risk factors, the nursing diagnosis selected is

- Risk for Infection related to presence of favorable conditions (specify) for development.
  Goals/Expected Outcomes: Maternal temperature will remain less than 38° C (100.4° F). The FHR pattern will remain 160 bpm or lower and near the baseline range. The amniotic fluid will remain clear and without a foul or strong odor.

Interventions
Reducing the Risk for Infection

Nurses should wash their hands before and after each contact with the woman and her infant to reduce transmission of organisms. Use gloves and other protective wear to prevent contact with potentially infectious secretions before and after birth (Standard Precautions).

Limit vaginal examinations to reduce transmission of vaginal organisms into the uterine cavity, and maintain aseptic technique during essential vaginal examinations. Keep underpads as dry as possible to reduce the moist, warm environment that favors bacterial growth. Periodically clean excessive secretions from the vaginal area in a front-to-back motion to limit fecal contamination and promote the mother's comfort.

Identifying Infection

Assess the woman and fetus for signs of infection. Increase the frequency of assessments if labor is prolonged. If signs of infection are noted, report them to the birth attendant for definitive treatment. Note the time at which the membranes ruptured to identify prolonged rupture, which adds to the risk for infection.

The birth attendant may collect specimens after birth from the uterine cavity or placenta for culture to identify infectious organisms and determine antibiotic sensitivity. Both aerobic and anaerobic culture specimens may be collected. Transport specimens to the laboratory promptly because living organisms are required for culture and sensitivity study.

Inform the newborn staff if maternal risk factors for infection exist and if signs of infection are noted. If available, specialized caregivers such as neonatal nurse practitioners should be notified of an increased risk for newborn infection and resuscitation requirements that also may be increased. Specimens of infants' secretions may be obtained for testing after birth. Prophylactic antibiotics to prevent neonatal sepsis are often given. See Chapter 30 for additional information about neonatal infection.

Evaluation

- Did the woman's temperature remain less than 38° C (100.4° F)?
- Did the amniotic fluid have normal characteristics?
- Did the FHR remain within the expected range and without tachycardia?

❗ CRITICAL TO REMEMBER

Signs Associated With Intrapartum Infection

- Fetal tachycardia (>160 beats per minute [bpm])
- Maternal fever (38° C, or 100.4° F)
- Foul- or strong-smelling amniotic fluid
- Cloudy or yellow amniotic fluid

The woman remains at higher risk for postpartum infection and should continue to be observed for signs and symptoms of infection.

MATERNAL EXHAUSTION
Assessment
Many women begin labor with a sleep deficit because of fetal movement, frequent urination, and shortness of breath associated with advanced pregnancy. As labor drags on, the mother's reserves are further depleted.

Assess the mother for signs and symptoms of exhaustion:

- Verbal expression of tiredness, fatigue, or exhaustion
- Verbal expression of frustration with a prolonged, unproductive labor ("I can't go on any longer. Why doesn't the doctor just take the baby?")
- Ineffectiveness of or inability to use coping techniques (e.g., patterned breathing) that she previously used effectively
- Changes in her pulse, respiration, and blood pressure (increased or decreased)

Nursing Diagnosis and Planning
The intense energy demands of a dysfunctional labor may exceed a woman's physical and psychological ability to meet them. For this reason, an appropriate nursing diagnosis is
- Activity Intolerance related to depletion of maternal energy reserves.
    Goals/Expected Outcomes: The woman will rest between contractions with her muscles relaxed. She will use coping skills, such as breathing and relaxation techniques.

Interventions
Conserving Maternal Energy
Reduce factors that interfere with the woman's ability to relax. Lower the light level, and turn off overhead lights. Reduce noise by closing the door or masking it with soft music or other comforting sounds. Maintain a comfortable maternal temperature with blankets or a fan. If there is no contraindication, a warm shower or bath is soothing.

Position the woman to encourage comfort, promote fetal descent, and enhance fetal oxygenation. Support her with pillows to reduce muscle strain and added fatigue. Help her change positions regularly (about every 30 min) to reduce muscle tension from constant pressure. Regular position changes also promote maternal comfort by maintaining an even distribution of regional analgesia such as an epidural block.

Even though an epidural block is a common pain relief for birth, a woman may become tense in the upper body areas that are not affected by epidural effects, such as the shoulders and upper or mid-back. Several pain management methods are options for women regardless of whether they choose any medical pain relief for labor. A soothing back rub may reduce muscle tension, which increases fatigue. Firm sacral pressure or assuming some of the positions that are helpful for fetal OP positions may reduce back pain. Using the birthing ball can relax and support her in some positions. Warmth to her back can reduce back pain. However, warm applications should be avoided if a regional block significantly lowers skin sensation and the mother's recognition of the higher temperature of the application is reduced compared to her sensation in areas unaffected by the block.

Maintain intravenous fluids at the rate ordered to provide fluid and electrolytes. Fluids containing glucose are sometimes given in this situation. Assess intake and output to identify dehydration, which may accompany prolonged labor. Dehydration may also cause maternal fever, which is usually preceded by fetal tachycardia. If there is no contraindication, provide juice, lollipops, Popsicles, or other clear liquids, as ordered by the physician or nurse-midwife, to moisten the woman's mouth and replenish her energy.

Promoting Coping Skills
When medical therapy or position changes are used to enhance labor, explain their purpose and expected benefits. Encourage the woman to visualize her baby passing downward smoothly through her pelvis as a result of her efforts. Provide her with mental images that allow her to "see" herself giving birth.

Generous praise and encouragement of the woman's use of skills, such as breathing techniques, motivate her to continue them even when she is discouraged. As with any laboring woman, tell her when she is making progress. Tell her that fetal heart rates and patterns are reassuring if this is true. Knowing that her efforts are having the desired results and that her fetus is doing well gives the woman courage to continue.

Evaluation
- Does the woman rest and relax between contractions? If she cannot relax, discuss analgesia options with her. Inability to relax between contractions is associated with pain beyond the woman's tolerance.
- Does the woman continue to demonstrate adequate use of learned skills to cope with labor?

PREMATURE RUPTURE OF THE MEMBRANES
Rupture of the amniotic sac before the onset of true labor, regardless of length of gestation, is called *premature rupture of the membranes* (PROM). A related term, *preterm premature rupture of the membranes* (PPROM, sometimes abbreviated pPROM), describes ruptured membranes earlier than the end of the 37th week of gestation, with or without contractions. PROM may be a normal occurrence that precedes term birth, even if labor induction is needed to initiate labor. However, PPROM is often associated with preterm labor, with the greatest risks from preterm birth occurring before completing 34 weeks' gestation (Garite, 2004). However, short delays of an inevitable preterm birth from PPROM may enable interventions to reduce these risks.

Etiology
Several conditions have been found when a woman's membranes rupture early, but the exact cause is not always identified, particularly if occurring before reaching a full term gestation. Possible causes are (ACOG, 2001; Garite, 2004):

- Infections of the vagina or cervix, such as chlamydia, gonorrhea, group B streptococcal infection, and *Gardnerella vaginalis* infection
- Amniotic sac with a weak structure
- Chorioamnionitis (intraamniotic infection) which may be associated with group B streptococci, *Neisseria gonorrhoeae*,

Listeria monocytogenes, or species such as *Mycoplasma*, *Bacteroides*, and *Ureaplasma* in the amniotic fluid
- Hydramnios
- Fetal abnormalities or malpresentation
- Incompetent cervix
- Overdistention of the uterus
- Maternal hormonal changes
- Recent sexual intercourse
- Maternal stress
- Maternal nutritional deficiencies

Complications

Both mother and newborn are at risk for infection during the intrapartum and postpartum periods. Chorioamnionitis, or intraamniotic infection, can be both a cause and a result of PROM. The mother is at higher risk for postpartum infection. The newborn is at greater risk for sepsis after birth, with the most immature preterm infants having the greatest risk for the systemic infection.

Chorioamnionitis, characterized by maternal fever and uterine tenderness, is most likely to precede preterm birth in the infant born before 34 weeks' gestation. Preterm infants with the lowest maturity, such as 24 weeks' gestation, have higher risk for the infection than a preterm infant who is even a few weeks more mature (Rao & Andersen, 2003). The exact time at which infection occurs cannot be predicted for either term or preterm infants. Frequently performing a digital examination of the cervix increases the risk for term or preterm infants.

Membranes ruptured before term may form a seal, stopping the fluid leak and allowing the amniotic fluid cushion to become reestablished. However, membranes may continue to leak, prolonging the loss of the amniotic fluid cushion (oligohydramnios) for the fetus. Umbilical cord compression, reduced lung volume, and deformities resulting from compression may occur, particularly in the fetus impacted at the earliest gestation.

Therapeutic Management

Management of PROM depends on the gestation and whether there is evidence of infection or other fetal or maternal compromise. If infection is present, further management also depends on the type of infection. For a woman at term, PROM may herald the imminent onset of true labor. Usually, the cervix is soft with some dilation and effacement and the fetal head is at or near zero station. Labor induction or cesarean birth is often reasonable if the fetus is 35 weeks' gestation or more because the impact of an active infection may be greater than a slightly preterm birth that occurs after the fetal lungs are basically mature.

If the woman is 34 weeks' gestation or earlier, therapeutic management is more complex. The risk for infection or preterm birth is weighed against the hazards of actively promoting birth, whether vaginally or by cesarean. An accurate gestational age is also important and something that may not be well defined in women who lack significant prenatal care.

Determining True Membrane Rupture
The first step is to determine whether the membranes are truly ruptured. Urinary incontinence, increased vaginal discharge, or loss of the mucus plug can cause a woman to believe her membranes have ruptured when they have not. A vaginal examination is avoided if possible, particularly if the gestation is preterm and there is no evidence of labor. Instead, the physician or nurse-midwife performs a sterile speculum examination to look for a pool of fluid near the cervix and to estimate cervical dilation and effacement. A nitrazine or fern test (see Chapter 17) may verify that the vaginal fluid is amniotic fluid. Tests to assess fetal lung maturity and identify infection may also be done, depending on the extent of the woman's prenatal care.

Gestation Near Term
If labor does not begin spontaneously, the woman's pregnancy is at or near term, and her cervix is favorable, labor induction may be done. If the cervix is not favorable and no infection is present, induction may be delayed 24 hours or longer to allow cervical softening and administration of drugs to combat infection associated with early membrane rupture. If induction is unsuccessful or if infection or other complications develop, a cesarean birth is most common. The nurse should remember, however, that cesarean birth also increases the risk for any mother's infection after birth.

Preterm Gestation
If the fetus is 34 or fewer weeks of gestation, the physician weighs the risks of infection against the infant's risk for complications of prematurity. Cesarean birth is more common if delivery at the earlier gestation is needed. The mother's physician considers factors such as gestational age, amount of amniotic fluid remaining, and fetal lung maturity in addition to possible infection of mother and infant.

Maternal Antibiotics

Maternal antibiotics are usually prescribed for premature membrane rupture because of the increased likelihood that an infection caused or further complicated the rupture for both mother and fetus or newborn. Antibiotics may stop the infection that caused or will occur with the rupture, thus delaying the onset of labor and allowing the fetus to mature. Drugs to stop infection if early membrane rupture occurs may include ampicillin, gentamicin, erythromycin, clindamycin, a cephalosporin antibiotic, and piperacillin. Group B streptococcus is also treated if indicated (see Chapter 26). Guidelines for drugs to correct infection associated with early membrane rupture vary with culture and sensitivity test results, other maternal laboratory results, or changes in the drugs most currently recommended for this purpose.

Additional therapeutic and nursing interventions that may be chosen for threatened preterm labor and birth are discussed in the "Preterm Labor" section, pp. 683-684.

Nursing Considerations

The woman may remain hospitalized until birth, or she may return home after a few days of hospital observation. If she is hospitalized, the nurse observes for signs of infection. Preparation for home management includes teaching the woman to:

- Avoid sexual intercourse, orgasm, or insertion of anything into the vagina, which increases the risk for infection, caused by ascending organisms, and can stimulate contractions.
- Avoid breast stimulation if the gestation is preterm because it may cause release of oxytocin from the posterior pituitary and thus stimulate contractions.

TABLE **27-2** Maternal Risk Factors for Preterm Labor

Medical History	Obstetric History	Present Pregnancy	Lifestyle and Demographics
Low weight for height	Previous preterm labor	Uterine distention (e.g., multifetal pregnancy, hydramnios)	Little or no prenatal care
Obesity	Previous preterm birth		Poor nutrition
Uterine or cervical anomalies, uterine fibroids	Previous first-trimester abortions (>2)	Abdominal surgery during pregnancy	Age <18 yr or >40 yr
History of cone biopsy	Previous second-trimester abortion	Uterine irritability	Low educational level
Diethylstilbestrol (DES) exposure as a fetus	History of previous pregnancy losses (2 or more)	Uterine bleeding	Low socioeconomic status
Chronic illness (e.g., cardiac, renal, diabetes, clotting disorders, anemia, hypertension)	Incompetent cervix	Dehydration	Smoking >10 cigarettes daily
Periodontal disease	Cervical length 25 mm (2.5 cm) or less at midtrimester of pregnancy	Infection	Nonwhite
	Number of embryos implanted (assisted reproductive techniques [AST])	Anemia	Employment with long hours and/or long standing
		Incompetent cervix	Chronic physical or psychological stress
		Preeclampsia	Intimate partner violence
		Preterm premature rupture of membranes (PPROM)	Substance abuse
		Fetal or placental abnormalities	

- Take her temperature at least four times a day, reporting any temperature of more than 37.8° C (100° F).
- Maintain any activity restrictions recommended.
- Note and report uterine contractions.

PRETERM LABOR

Preterm labor begins after the 20th week but before the end of the 37th week of pregnancy. The physical risks to the mother are no greater than labor at term unless complications, such as infection, hemorrhage, or the need for a cesarean delivery, also exist. Preterm labor, however, may result in the birth of an infant who is ill equipped for extrauterine life.

Associated Factors

Just as all of the causes of labor's onset at term are not known, the causes of preterm labor are not fully known either. Many factors are associated with preterm labor (Table 27-2):

- Maternal medical conditions such as infections of the urinary tract, reproductive organs, or systemic organs, dental disorder (periodontal disease), preexisting or gestational diabetes, connective tissue disorders, chronic hypertension, or drug abuse
- Conceptions assisted by assisted reproductive technology, including conceptions resulting in a single fetal gestation rather than a multifetal gestation
- Present and past obstetric conditions, such as unusually short cervical length, multifetal gestation, preterm membrane rupture, preeclampsia, or bleeding disorders that involve the woman, fetus, or placental implantation area
- Fetal conditions such as growth retardation, inadequate amniotic fluid volume, or chromosome or other birth defects
- Social and environmental factors such as inadequate or absent prenatal or dental care, maternal domestic violence episodes, maternal smoking, or housing deficiency such as homelessness
- Demographic factors such as race and age of the parents, financial stability, or the number and birth intervals of the woman's other children

However, about 50% or more women who have preterm labor and birth do not demonstrate known risk factors.

Manifestations

Signs and symptoms near the beginning of a preterm labor episode are more subtle than those of labor at term and often occur in normal pregnancies as well. The woman may be only vaguely aware that something seems different, or she may not detect that anything is amiss. Only when preterm labor reaches the active phase is it more typical of characteristics of labor at term. Signs and symptoms that a woman may experience when preterm labor begins include:

- Uterine contractions that may or may not be painful; the woman may not feel contractions at all.
- A sensation that the baby is frequently "balling up."
- Cramps similar to menstrual cramps.
- Constant low backache; intermittent or irregular mild low back pain
- Sensation of pelvic pressure or a feeling that the baby is pushing down.
- Pain, discomfort, or pressure in the vulva or thighs.
- Change or increase in vaginal discharge (increased, watery, bloody).
- Abdominal cramps with or without diarrhea.
- A sense of "just feeling bad" or "coming down with something."

Preventing Preterm Birth

Community Education

Preterm birth can impose substantial physical, emotional, and financial burdens on the child, family, and society. Ideally, nursing strategies to prevent preterm birth begin before conception, through community education. Programs often include teaching related to the:

- Role of early and regular prenatal care in preventing preterm birth
- Duration of normal pregnancy

- Conditions that increase a woman's risk for preterm birth
- Signs and symptoms that preterm labor may be occurring
- Consequences of preterm birth for mother and baby

Women who are aware of the consequences of preterm birth may be more likely to take action to prevent it. If they recognize that they have risk factors, they may seek prenatal care earlier in gestation than they otherwise might.

During Pregnancy

During pregnancy, measures to prevent preterm birth include:

- Reducing barriers and improving access to early and regular prenatal care for all women
- Assessing for risk factors to promote changes in those that can be reduced
- Promoting adequate nutrition and maternal smoking cessation
- Teaching women and their partners about often-subtle characteristics of early preterm labor and how these differ from normal pregnancy changes
- Empowering women and their partners to take an active approach in seeking care if they have signs and symptoms of preterm labor

Improving Access to Care. Improving access to prenatal care must consider the community setting. Difficult access is a serious problem for women who rely on public clinics for their care. Women who live in an area having a low population may find access difficult whether they seek public or private prenatal care. Long waits to see the provider for just a few minutes, fragmented care, language or cultural barriers, and insensitivity of caregivers may discourage women from obtaining any care. Expanding the number of caregivers by using nurses with advanced education, such as certified nurse-midwives and nurse practitioners, can reduce waits for care and enhance the communication process among professionals and the expectant woman and her family. Nurses can help coordinate various aspects of care to limit the number of appointments a woman needs to obtain complete care.

Identifying Risk Factors. Women who have risk factors for preterm birth can benefit from programs to reduce the risk and identify preterm labor early. These women benefit from care such as more frequent prenatal care appointments, reinforcement of the symptoms of preterm labor, telephone contacts, and assessments of fetal growth and health.

Some risk factors can be reduced or eliminated if the woman changes her lifestyle. Although it may have been difficult for them, many women have stopped smoking or using drugs to benefit their babies. A woman may need to rest more or to stop working, and this may be difficult or impossible for many. Nurses can work with the woman to help reduce her risks as much as possible by helping her identify sources of support.

Infections of the urinary and reproductive tracts are associated with PPROM and preterm labor. Screening for abnormal microorganisms in the urine, vagina, or cervix identifies women who may benefit from antibiotic therapy.

Promoting Adequate Nutrition. An adequate maternal diet contributes positively to the length of gestation and the infant's weight. Every pregnant woman should be offered culturally appropriate diet counseling that considers her means. The Women, Infants, and Children (WIC) program is available to supplement the diet of some low-income women. Anemia can be corrected with appropriate supplements. Women carrying more than one fetus need additional food intake.

Educating Women and Their Partners About Preterm Labor. *All pregnant women and their partners should be taught about symptoms of preterm labor, because most preterm births occur in women who have no identified risk factors.* Language barriers can be reduced by using fluent interpreters and printed materials in the woman's primary language. Diagrams should supplement the words of any language because some women have limited reading skills. Respecting cultural norms of the woman and her family is also an essential part of prenatal care.

The vague signs and symptoms of early preterm labor should be reinforced regularly as part of prenatal care. Women who often have uterine irritability may be given guidelines to observe at home before they must come to the hospital. Preterm labor often has vague sensations to the woman when the cervix has minimal dilation, so any home care guidelines are individualized according to the woman's risk for a preterm birth, the gestation and prenatal status, and the likelihood that specific interventions are beneficial to mother and baby. In addition, women are to enter the hospital for evaluation if they are not sure about the seriousness of their sensations. Examples of home care guidelines that may be given include:

- Drinking adequate amount of water to improve hydration or reduce bladder irritation that may accompany a urinary tract infection.
- Emptying the bladder frequently, because a full bladder may be associated with uterine irritability and contractions.
- Lying down in a side-lying position to promote uterine blood flow. Limiting physical activity also may increase diuresis, thus reducing hydration. Prolonged limitation of physical activity is not usually beneficial or safe for prevention of premature labor, although it may be required for serious maternal disorders, such as cardiac disease.
- Palpating contractions for 1 hour or as instructed because of the duration of any prior labor. However, the woman should notify her birth attendant or go directly to the labor unit for assessment if contractions increase in frequency, duration, or sensitivity.

The nurse should verify the woman's understanding by seeking feedback, such as having her restate the signs and symptoms of preterm labor and the appropriate responses to them.

Empowering Women and Their Partners. Delaying birth when preterm labor occurs depends on identifying it early. Women should be taught to report to the labor unit promptly for assessment if contractions or other discomfort intensifies. They should be encouraged to communicate their concerns when they arrive at the clinic or hospital; otherwise they may wait for hours to be seen in a public facility. It is equally important not to make the woman feel foolish if she reports signs and symptoms but is not in labor; otherwise she may not seek care for recurrent episodes when she truly is in labor, possibly losing the opportunity to stop the episodes.

The nurse might suggest that a woman who is seeking care for possible preterm labor say, "I'm not due for 8 more weeks, but I think I may be in labor. I need to be seen right away, or I might have a premature baby."

Therapeutic Management

Management focuses on identifying preterm labor early, delaying birth, and accelerating fetal lung maturity if preterm birth is likely.

Identifying Preterm Labor

The reason to identify preterm labor early is to delay birth, thus promoting further fetal maturation. These criteria are suggested for preterm labor (American Academy of Pediatrics [AAP] & American College of Obstetricians and Gynecologists [ACOG], 2002):

- Gestation from 20 weeks to before 37 weeks
- Persistent uterine contractions (four in 20 min or eight in 60 min), *and:*
  —Documented cervical change, *or*
  —Cervical effacement of 80% or greater, *or*
  —Cervical dilation of greater than 1 cm

Frequent Prenatal Visits. Women at risk for preterm labor have more frequent prenatal visits and are checked for signs and symptoms of preterm labor and their ability to follow therapy to prevent it. Gentle cervical examinations or ultrasound examinations identify the painless effacement or dilation that often precedes the onset of labor. Infections can be identified and treated promptly before they result in rupture of the membranes or labor.

Determining Preterm Labor. Methods to estimate how likely birth before 37 weeks is and determining probable causes of the pregnancy complication are essential to guide the best medical and nursing interventions. Clearly indicated diagnostic evaluation, such as physical assessment of the mother and baby by physicians, nurses, or other professionals, is common. Laboratory testing, such as a maternal urinalysis, is common. However, advantages of all professional assessments or diagnostic tests are not always clear because a woman's early signs and symptoms of preterm labor are not always apparent. Thus the nurse working with these women may find a variety of diagnostic and treatment options for the high-risk pregnancy.

Assessments to determine if the risk for preterm labor and birth is higher vary with signs and symptoms when a woman seeks treatment. A sterile speculum examination helps determine the status of cervical dilation and effacement, whether loss of amniotic fluid has occurred, or whether abnormal secretions are present in the vagina. The speculum examination can be used to obtain cervical or vaginal secretions such as those to verify membrane rupture (see "ferning" or "fern testing," Chapter 17) and to diagnose problems such as infection or mild blood loss. Recent sexual intercourse that may stimulate preterm labor symptoms in some women may be identified if semen is present.

Repeated digital vaginal examinations, common during active labor, are often minimized if the pregnancy is preterm and labor is not active. If the ideal goal of therapy is to increase gestation, repeated uninformative vaginal examinations may hasten birth by repeated introduction of organisms from the lower reproductive tract. The goal may be to add time to the gestational age to provide drugs to enhance fetal lung maturity. It may be much longer for the very immature fetus, however.

An ultrasound (see Chapter 16) may be performed to identify factors contributing to preterm labor. One example is diagnosis of a multifetal pregnancy that has not previously been determined. Another important example is that the transvaginal ultrasound examination may identify short cervical length that may accompany preterm contractions or infection in the area. For example, a woman whose cervix is no longer than 25 mm (2.5 cm) during the midtrimester has a substantially greater risk of giving birth before 35 weeks' gestation (Iams & Creasy, 2004).

Fetal fibronectin (fFN), a protein produced by fetal membranes, may improve diagnostic accuracy for preterm birth. Fetal fibronectin is found in vaginal secretions until 16 to 20 weeks' gestation and again at or near term. Fetal fibronectin is associated with maternal and fetal infections if found during the midtrimester of pregnancy when it is usually absent from vaginal secretions. Its most useful function is to improve the diagnosis of preterm labor and also to determine likelihood of preterm birth within 2 weeks (ACOG, 2001; Iams & Creasy, 2004; Maloni, 2000). A woman who has preterm contractions, cervical dilation greater than 3 cm, and a positive midtrimester fFN has the greatest risk for preterm birth within 2 weeks of the fFN test and is treated most aggressively.

Infections often increase the risk for preterm membrane rupture or birth, even if the woman does not initially have clinical signs or symptoms with the preterm labor. A urinary tract infection is common with preterm labor, so catheterized urine is often obtained for urinalysis and for culture and sensitivity testing. Tests for other infections associated with preterm birth risk include those that often are found if membranes rupture prematurely (see "Premature Rupture of the Membranes," p. 681).

Blood peak and trough levels of indicated antibiotics, such as gentamicin, ensure that the woman is receiving a therapeutic level (peak) of the drug. Determining if the drug blood level is excessive just before the next dose (a high trough level) is important to prevent possible damage to mother or baby with some drugs. Testing for peak and trough drug levels allows the dose to be adjusted appropriately for the drug.

A woman with an infection that is not always related to pregnancy may present for care. Relevant testing may relate to acute gastrointestinal or respiratory infections that affect pregnant women as well as other people of both sexes. More serious maternal infections may require cultures of maternal blood, respiratory, or other secretions to determine the ideal treatment. Maternal pneumonia, although rare during pregnancy, increases the risk for fetal or maternal death as well as increases the risk that a woman will give birth to a living preterm infant. Other poor health conditions during pregnancy, such as crowded living conditions or a chronic condition such as asthma, may increase a woman's risk for pneumonia as well.

Stopping Preterm Labor

Once the diagnosis of preterm labor is made, management focuses on stopping the uterine activity before it reaches the point of no return, usually after 3 cm dilation. If preterm delivery is inevitable, therapy is directed toward reducing the infant's risk for respiratory distress.

Initial Measures. Before attempting to halt preterm labor, the physician determines whether any maternal or fetal conditions contraindicate continuing the pregnancy. Examples of these conditions are:

- Preeclampsia or eclampsia; persistent hypertension from any cause
- Significant or prolonged maternal alterations, such as hypovolemia, hypoxemia, or acid-base imbalance
- Serious infection, including chorioamnionitis or maternal infection such as maternal pyelonephritis
- Fetal heart rate monitoring data showing inability to correct signs that are nonreassuring for the gestation of the fetus

Treating Infections. Infections associated with a more rapid preterm birth are likely if the membranes have ruptured. However, it may be unclear whether levels of various microorganisms found at diagnosis of preterm labor are significant if membranes remain intact.

The value of treating acute infections, such as pyelonephritis, is clear for improved maternal and fetal outcomes. Broad-spectrum antibiotics, such as ampicillin, penicillin, and an aminoglycoside, may be chosen for chorioamnionitis because multiple types of bacteria may be found in the infected amniotic fluid. Anaerobic organisms may also cause infection for a woman who requires a cesarean birth, and antibiotics such as clindamycin or metronidazole may be prescribed (AAP & ACOG, 2002; Iams & Creasy, 2004).

Restricting Activity. Activity restriction, usually by assuming a side-lying position, increases placental blood flow and reduces fetal pressure on the cervix. However, prolonged substantial activity restriction (e.g., complete bed rest) has not been shown to lengthen pregnancy significantly. As in other persons, activity restriction also is associated with serious maternal side effects, some of which develop within as few as 24 hours. Adverse effects of activity restriction during pregnancy may include:

- Muscle weakness, including aching; muscle atrophy and bone loss
- Diuresis as the body tries to reduce the normally higher fluid level of pregnancy
- Poor nutrition as a result of appetite loss, lower intake, and increased indigestion; weight loss or inadequate weight gain
- Orthostatic hypotension caused by the change in blood pressure regulation by baroreceptors
- Psychological effects, such as increased stress about separation from her family, anxiety about the pregnancy's outcome, depression; boredom from a decreased activity level and less contact with other people
- Sleep changes as depression increases or usual activities that direct her sleep-wake cycles are not present

Because of problems and lack of benefits for most women, limited and individualized activity reductions are now prescribed if preterm birth risk is higher. Changes may be relatively simple, such as a change in work hours or duties or finding ways to help the woman meet the needs for her other children, such as transportation to school or other activities. Several rest periods may be prescribed for home care when the woman's risk status is lower. Positions for rest may include semi-Fowler's position. If lying down for rest, a mother's frequent change of the side-lying position reduces discomfort from the pressure of remaining on one side for a prolonged time. Rest position changes are also beneficial to women who require hospitalization for their preterm labor.

Women hospitalized for care of preterm labor may have a greater activity restriction. Because of intravenous hydration and drug therapy, bed rest is common during initial care. Ambulating to the bathroom may be contraindicated because of maternal sedative effects from a drug that depresses uterine activity, such as magnesium sulfate (also given for preeclampsia; see Chapter 26). The woman usually has a Foley catheter for precise urine output assessment needed with administration of magnesium or other drugs. If stopping labor is successful, the woman may be able to walk to the restroom for voiding and bowel movements. Later, while on longer-term care, she may sit in a chair periodically or take occasional short trips to another area in a wheelchair that her family or friends pushes.

Hydrating the Woman. Hydration to stop preterm contractions has not been shown to be beneficial for all women. High-volume intravenous infusions may cause maternal respiratory distress if a drug such as magnesium sulfate to decrease uterine contractions is being administered because the drug may also reduce the respiratory rate, even if a woman has a normal blood pressure level.

However, dehydration may contribute to uterine irritability for some women. This is often the case in those who have had an infection such as an acute gastrointestinal infection in which loss of fluid through diarrhea may exceed the nauseated woman's ability to drink water or other fluids. Infections with maternal fever ($\geq$38° C, or 100.4° F) sometime reduce the woman's fluid ingestion. Intravenous fluids are ordered according to their expected benefit, such as magnesium sulfate drug therapy to stop preterm labor or initiation of an antibiotic.

Tocolytics. A tocolytic is most likely to be ordered if preterm labor occurs before the 34th week of gestation, because the infant's risk for respiratory and other complications of prematurity is high if born at that time. Tocolytic drugs usually delay preterm birth rather than prevent it. This delay may provide time to allow the use of corticosteroids to accelerate fetal lung maturity or to transfer the woman to a facility with a neonatal intensive care unit that is appropriate for the gestation of her fetus.

Most tocolytic drugs are used primarily for conditions other than preterm labor and therefore have effects on other body systems. Four types of drugs are used for tocolytic therapy: (1) magnesium sulfate, (2) beta-adrenergics, (3) prostaglandin synthesis inhibitors, and (4) calcium antagonists. Table 27-3 summarizes the doses and routes of administration for these drugs.

Magnesium Sulfate. Magnesium sulfate is used in the management of pregnancy-induced hypertension to prevent seizures (see Drug Guide: Magnesium Sulfate, p. 634, for nursing care related to the drug). Because of its added effect of quieting uterine activity also, it is often used to inhibit preterm labor.

Magnesium sulfate for tocolysis is given intravenously using a similar protocol to that for hypertension during pregnancy. The loading dose, given in 15 to 20 minutes, is 4 to 6 g. The maintenance dose of magnesium sulfate ranges from 1 to 4 g/hr

TABLE **27-3** Drugs Used in Preterm Labor

Drug/Purpose	Common Dose Regimens*	Side or Adverse Effects
Terbutaline (beta-adrenergic for tocolysis)	See Drug Guide: Terbutaline (p. 688). *Intravenous (IV):* Begin at 0.01-0.05 mg/min. Increase by 0.01 mg/min increments every 10-30 min until contraction frequency is 6 or fewer per hr or significant side effects develop. Maximum dose guideline 0.08 mg/min. When contraction frequency is no higher than 4-6 per hr, maintain the infusion for 1 hr; then reduce rate at 20-min intervals to reach the minimum maintenance dose, which may be continued for 12 hr after contractions stop or stabilize at acceptable maximum levels. *Subcutaneous (SC):* 0.25 mg q3-4h (maximum dose interval may be q6h, depending on client response). By SC infusion pump: continuous low dose baseline infusion plus intermittent bolus doses of 0.25 mg at times of greatest uterine activity. *Oral (PO):* 2.5 to 5 mg q2-4h. Hold for maternal pulse >120/min.	Cardiovascular: Maternal and fetal tachycardia, palpitations, cardiac dysrhythmias, chest pain, wide pulse pressure. Respiratory: Dyspnea, chest discomfort, pulmonary edema. Central nervous system: Tremors, restlessness, weakness, dizziness, headache. Metabolic: Hyperglycemia, hypokalemia. Gastrointestinal: Nausea, vomiting, reduced bowel motility. Skin: Flushing, diaphoresis. Infection at injection site for subcutaneous infusion pump.
Magnesium sulfate (use as tocolytic)	*IV:* Loading dose, 4-6 g in 15-20 min. Maintenance dose for tocolysis, 1-4 g/hr. When contraction frequency is no higher than 4-6 per hr, maintain infusion rate for 12-24 hr; then reduce rate. An oral drug may be ordered to continue tocolysis after magnesium sulfate is stopped for this purpose.	Side and adverse effects are dose-related, occurring at higher maternal serum levels. Depression of deep tendon reflexes, which should be present, although less active. Respiratory or cardiac depression if serum levels are high; greatest risk is in woman with poor urine elimination of drug. Less serious side effects: Lethargy, weakness, visual blurring, headache, sensation of heat, nausea, vomiting, constipation. Fetal-neonatal effects: Reduced fetal heart rate (FHR) variability, hypotonia
Indomethacin (Indocin); sulindac (Clinoril) (prostaglandin synthesis inhibitors)	Loading dose: up to 100 mg (rectal) or 50 mg (oral). Rectal preparation usually prepared by birth facility's pharmacy. Maintenance dose: 25-50 mg orally q6h. Ideal duration of treatment has not been established. Ultrasound examinations and fetal echocardiography help determine if maternal indomethacin has adverse effects on the fetus.	Epigastric pain, nausea, gastrointestinal bleeding. Asthma in aspirin-sensitive woman. Increased blood pressure in hypertensive woman. Fetus: Adverse fetal effects may include constriction of the ductus arteriosus, particularly if the mother receives indomethacin for more than 48-72 hr and the gestation is earlier than 32 weeks. Impairs fetal renal function, which may reduce the volume of amniotic fluid and result in cord compression.
Nifedipine (Procardia); nicardipine (Cardene) (calcium channel blockers for tocolysis)	Oral loading dose of 10-20 mg. Continued oral therapy: 10-20 mg q4-6h. Duration of calcium channel blocking drug for tocolysis has not been established.	Maternal flushing, dizziness, headache, nausea. Transient maternal tachycardia. Mild hypotension. Modest increases in blood glucose levels.

*Doses and frequency of administration are examples; actual protocols vary.
Data from American Academy of Pediatrics (AAP), & American College of Obstetricians and Gynecologists (ACOG). (2002). *Guidelines for perinatal care* (5th ed.). Elk Grove Village, IL, and Washington, DC: Author; Blackburn, S.T. (2003). *Maternal, fetal, & neonatal physiology: A clinical perspective.* Philadelphia: Saunders; Goldenberg, R.L. (2002). The management of preterm labor. *Obstetrics & Gynecology, 100*(5 Pt. 1), 1020-1037; Iams, J.D., & Creasy, R.K. (2004). Preterm labor and delivery. In R.K. Creasy & R. Resnik (Eds.), *Maternal-fetal medicine: Principles and practice* (5th ed., pp. 498-531). Philadelphia: Saunders.

to stop preterm labor, often a broader range than when the drug is used for preeclampsia. The magnesium sulfate infusion is continued for 12 to 24 hours, when uterine contractions are no more than 4 to 6 per hour. The magnesium sulfate infusion is then reduced. The woman is often changed to an oral medication to maintain tocolysis when the magnesium sulfate is discontinued.

Beta-Adrenergic Drugs. Ritodrine (Yutopar) is a beta-adrenergic currently approved by the U.S. Food and Drug Administration (FDA) to stop preterm contractions. Ritodrine is less-often used because of significant maternal side effects and minimal prolongation of pregnancy. Terbutaline (Brethine), considered investigational to treat preterm labor, is the more widely used drug in this class because it has a lower cost, longer duration of action between doses, and the ability to promptly administer a dose by the

subcutaneous rather than oral route if needed (AAP & ACOG, 2002).

The main side effects for beta-adrenergic drugs involve the cardiorespiratory system. Maternal and fetal tachycardia are common. Other maternal side effects may include decreased blood pressure, wide pulse pressure, dysrhythmias, myocardial ischemia, chest pain, and pulmonary edema. Metabolic changes include hyperglycemia and hypokalemia. Headaches, tremors, and restlessness are other side effects, with headaches often becoming less severe as the woman becomes accustomed to the drug. Propranolol, an agent that blocks beta-adrenergic drugs, should be available to reverse severe adverse effects.

A beta-adrenergic, such as terbutaline, may be given by the intravenous, subcutaneous, or oral route. Subcutaneous terbutaline may be given with a continuous, low-dose infu-

---

Drug Guide

Terbutaline

Classification: Beta-adrenergic agent.

Action: Stimulates beta-adrenergic receptors of the sympathetic nervous system. Action results primarily in bronchodilation and inhibition of uterine muscle activity. Increases pulse rate and widens pulse pressure.

Indications: Stop preterm labor. Reduce or stop hypertonic labor contractions, whether natural or stimulated. Tolerance and loss of tocolytic effect occur with prolonged use.

Dosage and Route:

1. *Intravenous (IV) infusion:* Begin at the ordered rate of approximately 0.01-0.05 mg/min. Increase rate if needed to stop contractions by 0.01 mg/min at 10- to 30-min intervals until contractions stop (maximum of 0.08 mg/min). The infusion rate is not increased or may be decreased if the maternal pulse rate remains over 120 beats per minute (bpm) or systolic blood pressure falls below 80-90 mm Hg. Maintain this dose for at least 1 hour; then reduce the rate at 20-min intervals to reach minimum maintenance dose. Continue maintenance dose for 12 hr after contractions stop.
2. *Subcutaneous (SC)* (most common parenteral route): Intermittent injections, 0.25 mg, q3-4h. A subcutaneous programmed infusion pump may be used for low-dose continuous (baseline) drug infusion plus intermittent bolus doses of approximately 0.25 mg at times of greatest uterine activity. The subcutaneous pump is

typically placed and its programming for continuous and bolus doses verified before removing the intermittent IV terbutaline line.
3. *Oral:* 2.5-5 mg q2-4h.

When changing from IV to oral therapy, give oral dose 30 min before discontinuing IV infusion.

Absorption:

1. *IV:* Prompt; duration about 2 hr
2. *SC:* 6-15 min; duration $1\frac{1}{2}$-4 hr
3. *Oral:* 1-2 hr; duration 4-8 hr

Excretion: Metabolized in the liver. Excreted in urine.

Contraindications: Hypersensitivity. Contraindicated before 20 weeks' gestation and if continuing the pregnancy is hazardous to the mother or fetus, as in fetal distress, hemorrhage, chorioamnionitis, and intrauterine fetal death. Contraindicated in conditions that may be adversely affected by beta-adrenergic agents (uncontrolled diabetes, hyperthyroidism, bronchial asthma treated with other beta-adrenergic agents or steroids, cardiac dysrhythmias, hypovolemia, uncontrolled hypertension).

Precautions: Terbutaline is not approved by the Food and Drug Administration (FDA) for inhibiting uterine activity, although it is widely used for this purpose. Research has been mixed regarding the drug effects of terbutaline for this purpose, but its lower risk for adverse side effects combined with some efficacy has maintained terbutaline's use as a tocolytic.

Adverse Reactions:

1. *Cardiovascular:* Maternal and fetal tachycardia, palpitations, cardiac dysrhythmias, chest pain, wide pulse pressure
2. *Respiratory:* Dyspnea, chest discomfort
3. *Central nervous system:* Tremors, restlessness, weakness, dizziness, headache
4. *Metabolic:* Hypokalemia, hyperglycemia
5. *Gastrointestinal:* Nausea, vomiting, reduced bowel motility
6. *Skin:* Flushing, diaphoresis

Nursing Considerations: Diagnostic studies that may be ordered related to terbutaline therapy: electrocardiogram, blood glucose, electrolytes, urinalysis. Explain common side effects that are usually well tolerated, such as palpitations, tremors, restlessness, weakness, headache. Assess fetal heart rate (FHR), usually with continuous electronic fetal monitoring when the drug is initiated, recording rate and patterns at recommended intervals and with IV dose increases. Assess maternal pulse, respirations, and blood pressure by same schedule as for FHR. Maintain adequate IV or oral hydration. Encourage the woman to empty her bladder every 2 hr. Notify the physician for significant or unacceptable side effects (maternal heart rate >120 bpm, respirations >24/min, dyspnea, pulmonary edema, systolic blood pressure <80-90 mm Hg, FHR >160 bpm, chest pain). Report continuing or recurrent uterine activity. Teach signs and symptoms of recurrent preterm labor and follow-up medical care after discharge.

sion pump. The subcutaneous pump for terbutaline allows the physician to order a baseline infusion rate plus greater doses at specific intervals for a bolus dose. Time intervals and doses for the bolus doses may be individualized to permit most efficient and safe reduction of contraction frequency.

Tolerance may develop when terbutaline is given, resulting in recurrent frequent contractions. Magnesium sulfate may be used to allow terbutaline to be eliminated from a woman's system while reducing contraction frequency. Terbutaline may be resumed or another tocolytic drug may be prescribed if indicated after contractions slow to acceptable frequency and intensity.

The nurse should assess a woman's apical heart rate and lung sounds before administering each intermittent dose of terbutaline for preterm labor. Addition of these maternal assessments to scheduled maternal vital signs and fetal heart rate is often adequate when a woman receives terbutaline by subcutaneous infusion pump. A maternal heart rate over 120 bpm or respiratory findings such as "wet" lung sounds or a more rapid rate, possibly accompanied by shortness of breath, suggest drug toxicity that may be a reason to discontinue terbutaline. Nonreassuring maternal and fetal assessments should be promptly reported to the physician.

Prostaglandin Synthesis Inhibitors. Because prostaglandins stimulate uterine contractions, drugs may be used to inhibit their synthesis. Indomethacin is the drug in this class that is most often used for tocolysis.

Constriction of the fetal ductus arteriosus may occur, particularly if the woman receives indomethacin for more than 48 to 72 hours and the gestation is earlier than 32 weeks. Indomethacin impairs fetal renal function, which reduces the volume of amniotic fluid, also making it a useful treatment for the fetus with excess volume (hydramnios). The amniotic fluid volume usually returns to its previous level when indomethacin treatment is discontinued. Regular ultrasound examinations and fetal echocardiography help determine if indomethacin is having adverse effects on the infant. Assessment of the infant after birth for other complications, such as pulmonary hypertension or intracranial hemorrhage, may be done related to the duration of maternal indomethacin intake, gestation, and the probability that delivery will occur less than 24 hours after the drug is discontinued (Iams & Creasy, 2004).

Maternal side effects are usually minimal because of the brief duration of indomethacin therapy. Bleeding times may be prolonged, becoming most important if birth, possibly by cesarean, occurs before the drug has been discontinued for 24 hours or more. Providing food when giving the drug can reduce gastrointestinal effects, such as heartburn, indigestion, or epigastric pain. Headache or dizziness is also a common side effect. Because indomethacin is an antiinflammatory drug, signs of infection may not be apparent.

Calcium Blockers. Nifedipine (Procardia) is a calcium channel blocker often given for problems such as chronic hypertension. Calcium is essential for muscle contraction in smooth muscles such as the uterus, so blocking calcium reduces the muscular contraction. Flushing of the skin, headache, and a transient increase in the maternal and fetal heart rates are common side effects. Because nifedipine is a vasodilator, postural hypotension may result in lightheadedness or dizziness with maternal position change (Iams & Creasy, 2004).

The nurse should observe for side effects of nifedipine, including an elevated maternal heart rate similar to that which may occur with terbutaline use. However, maternal and fetal tachycardia are usually of shorter duration if they occur. The woman should be assisted to a sitting or standing position gradually to reduce the effects of postural hypotension.

Accelerating Fetal Lung Maturity
Administration of corticosteroid therapy to the mother before preterm birth reduces the severity of complications associated with immature gestation. The incidence of neonatal respiratory distress syndrome (RDS) and intraventricular hemorrhage (IVH) can be lower if a woman receives corticosteroids, and the incidence of neonatal death is also lower. Betamethasone and dexamethasone are considered the best steroid drugs for accelerating maturation of the fetus likely to be born before 34 weeks. The mother of the fetus having a low lecithin/sphingomyelin (L/S) ratio may receive the corticosteroid drug through 37 weeks' gestation because her fetus may have less pulmonary maturity (AAP & ACOG, 2002; Iams & Creasy, 2004).

Corticosteroids are indicated if the woman is between 24 and 34 weeks' gestation because of the high incidence of problems such as RDS that affect an infant of this age. Delay of preterm birth for 24 hours after a woman begins corticosteroid therapy provides the greatest benefit in reducing critical problems associated with prematurity. Evidence also shows that a fetus born earlier than 24 hours after the mother begins taking the corticosteroid may have some maturation benefits of the drug. Thus one benefit of tocolytic drugs to the woman at risk for preterm birth is to prolong labor enough that her fetus may receive benefits of the corticosteroid drug given. Benefits of corticosteroids to the preterm infant are known to last for 7 days after the drug is initiated, although they may last longer. Any benefit for repeating the corticosteroid therapy 7 days after the prior dose is not now recommended but is being studied (AAP & ACOG, 2002; ACOG, 2001; Iams & Creasy, 2004; National Institutes of Health, 2000).

Current recommendations for the corticosteroids for threatened preterm birth are:

- Betamethasone 12 mg: two doses (intramuscular [IM]), 24 hours apart
- Dexamethasone 6 mg: four doses (IM), 12 hours apart

The woman may display a temporary increase in her leukocytes or glucose intolerance while she receives betamethasone or dexamethasone. An increase in the insulin dose may be required for both the woman with gestational diabetes and the woman whose diabetes is present when not pregnant.

■ NURSING CARE
The Woman in Preterm Labor

Nursing care for the woman with preterm labor may include interventions related to tocolytic, corticosteroid, or antibiotic drug therapy. If labor cannot be stopped, care is similar to that for other laboring women, with additional care to prepare for

Drug Guide

Betamethasone, Dexamethasone

Classification: Corticosteroids.

Indications: Acceleration of fetal lung maturity to reduce the incidence and severity of respiratory distress syndrome (RDS). Studies suggest that antenatal steroids can also reduce the incidence of intraventricular hemorrhage (IVH) and neonatal death in the preterm infant. Greatest benefits accrue if at least 24 hours elapse between the initial dose and birth of the preterm infant, but the drug is indicated if birth is not imminent.

Dosage and Route:

Betamethasone: 12 mg intramuscular (IM) for two doses, 24 hr apart.

Dexamethasone: 6 mg IM q12h for four doses.

Absorption: Rapid and complete after IM administration.

Excretion: Metabolized in the liver. Excreted in urine.

Contraindications: Active infection, such as chorioamnionitis, is a relative contraindication, although further study is needed. The National Institutes of Health recommend use of corticosteroids for the woman who has preterm rupture of the membranes (24-32 weeks' gestation), but the American College of Obstetrics and Gynecology has not yet endorsed this recommendation.

Precautions: Possible infection. Pregnancies complicated by diabetes.

Adverse Reactions: Few, owing to the short-term use of the drug. Pulmonary edema is possible secondary to sodium and fluid retention.

Nursing Considerations: Explain the potential benefits of corticosteroid administration to the preterm neonate. Explain that the drug cannot prevent or lessen the severity of all complications of prematurity. If the woman is diabetic, explain that more frequent blood glucose determinations are common because these levels are often elevated. Assess lung sounds. Report chest pain or heaviness or dyspnea.

---

a preterm infant's needs at birth. Support for anticipatory grieving may be needed if the infant is very immature and is expected to die.

Care for the family when an extremely preterm infant (about 20 through 24 weeks' gestation) is expected to be born can be heavily laden with ethical and legal issues. For example, what is the true accuracy of the gestational age? Have drugs that could accelerate fetal lung maturity been administered? If labor cannot be halted, is fetal monitoring beneficial? Nonreassuring fetal monitoring patterns in the very immature fetus can distress parents and caregivers alike. On the other hand, knowledge of the fetal response to labor helps the neonatologist make better decisions about how to treat the infant. In addition, ultrasound estimates of gestational age have considerable variation at this time. A fetus presumed to be 23 weeks of gestation before birth may be assessed to be 25 weeks or older after birth and suited to more intense treatment than planned, especially if the woman had no prenatal care before entering the hospital.

General nursing care for a woman having preterm labor often applies to women with other high-risk pregnancies. Women may need multiple hospitalizations, and these may occur in the middle of the night, disrupting sleep and family routines. These women often have some activity restriction and may have to stop working. Therefore this section focuses on the family's psychosocial concerns, management of home care, and the woman's boredom that may result from restrictions.

PSYCHOSOCIAL CONCERNS
Assessment

The entire family is affected by stressors associated with a complicated pregnancy. Assess how the woman and her family usually cope with crisis situations and how they are coping with this one. To set priorities for care, identify their greatest concerns.

The woman or her family may have physical, emotional, and cognitive impairments because of the unexpected problems. Physical signs of emotional distress, such as trembling,

palpitations, and restlessness, are also side effects of beta-adrenergic drugs such as terbutaline. The woman may express fear, helplessness, or disbelief. She may be irritable and tearful. Her ability to concentrate may be impaired at a time when she needs to absorb new information.

Her partner often feels at loose ends. He struggles to keep the household running if she must be inactive. Young children pick up on their parents' anxiety and may misbehave or regress.

The family may be under financial strain. The woman must often curtail or stop working. If she does not have sick time or other benefits, the family suffers an abrupt drop in income at a time when medical expenses are mounting. A woman may be admitted to a distant hospital having the better capacity to care for her and her preterm baby. A distant transfer to a higher-level maternity care facility removes the woman from familiar friends, family, or support groups.

Overlaid on the sudden change in lifestyle is the family's concern for fetal well-being. A woman may feel pulled in opposite directions by the needs of all her children—those already born and the fetus she is trying to mature. She may be concerned about the effects of drug therapy on the fetus and on her own body.

Nursing Diagnosis and Planning

The outcome of any pregnancy is never certain, and this is especially true when the pregnancy is a high-risk one for any reason. The unexpected development of complications during pregnancy can prevent a woman and her family from using their normal coping mechanisms. Goals focus on the family's ability to cope with the crisis of preterm labor. The nursing diagnosis is

- Anxiety related to uncertain outcome of the pregnancy, disruption of family relationships, and financial concerns.
  Goal/Expected Outcome: The woman and family will identify methods to cope with the temporary disruption in their lives.

Interventions

Providing Information

Knowledge decreases anxiety and fear related to the unknown. Include appropriate family members so that they are more likely to be supportive. Determine what the woman knows about preterm birth and about the specific therapy that is recommended. Determine what information the parents need about the problems that a preterm infant may face. Use this opportunity to correct misinformation and reinforce accurate information.

Initially, the woman for whom activity restriction is prescribed may be highly motivated to maintain the recommended level of activity. Because her contractions often diminish, even if for only a short time, she may become restless from minor restrictions. She may feel that there is now no need for a restriction, such as how far she can ambulate. Help her understand the purposes for activity restrictions as well as understand when these restrictions may diminish as the condition of her pregnancy stabilizes.

Promoting Expression of Concerns

Encourage the woman and her family to express their concerns. Begin by exploring common concerns of women with problem pregnancies. For example, say, "Most women are worried when they have to stop working. How has this affected your family?" An open question gives them a chance to ventilate their feelings so that they can take the next step: identifying constructive methods to cope with the situation. Collaboration with a social worker may identify financial or other community resources available. Offering to refer a chaplain to the woman may help her talk about her concerns associated with care related to her pregnancy, the pregnancy outcome, or her personal life.

Teaching What May Occur During a Preterm Birth

Because preterm birth may occur despite all interventions, a pregnant woman and her partner should be prepared for that possibility. If the hospital has a neonatal intensive care unit, a nurse often visits the parents to explain what might occur there if their baby is born early. One or both parents tour the unit to see the equipment and care infants receive there. A tour of the intensive care nursery may motivate the woman to maintain the recommended therapy to prevent preterm birth.

In hospitals with neonatal intensive care units, one or more neonatal nurses, a neonatal nurse practitioner, a neonatologist, or a combination of these professionals is present at birth to care for the infant. The woman who planned to give birth in a hospital that does not have a neonatal intensive care unit or has one of a lower level of critical care may be transferred before the birth to a facility with the appropriate unit to allow immediate care and stabilization of her newborn. The infant may also be transferred after birth if there is no time to transfer the woman before birth or if the infant has more problems than anticipated. Hospitalization of the mother, infant, or both at a distant location adds to the stress on the family. However, the pregnancy and fetal maturity also may progress after the early complications, allowing the woman to return to care in a familiar environment.

Evaluation

- Can the woman and her family identify constructive methods to deal with their anxiety?

If a high-risk pregnancy situation is prolonged or if the family has difficulty adapting constructively to the situation, a nursing diagnosis of Interrupted Family Processes may be more appropriate. (See Nursing Care Plan: Preterm Labor.)

MANAGEMENT OF HOME CARE
Assessment

Care of women with high-risk pregnancies, including a risk for preterm birth, often occurs in their homes if the gestation is sufficiently advanced and the signs and symptoms of preterm labor and birth have diminished significantly. Many daily household activities are managed by the woman, even if only by her directions to others. However, when preterm labor complication becomes greater, family roles are again disrupted because of the changed relationships among family members.

Clarify the level of activity prescribed by the physician, and identify the role of each family member. A good way to do this is to have the woman describe a usual day before any limitations were recommended. Determine the number and ages of children in the home.

Evaluate the home itself, either by visual inspection or by questioning the family. Does the home or apartment have more than one level? Determine if a telephone is available for emergency contact.

Evaluate the family's resources and their willingness to use them. Ask whether family members and friends in the area are available to help. Explore local support groups, such as churches or mother-to-mother networks, that the family might contact for assistance. Determine financial reimbursement that may be available through insurance coverage.

Nursing Diagnosis and Planning

The nursing diagnosis is

- Impaired Home Maintenance related to change in usual roles and responsibilities.

    Goals/Expected Outcomes: Two outcomes are often appropriate for the woman and family faced with a preterm birth that occurs at an unknown time:

- *Short-term:* The family will identify methods for managing daily household routines.
- *Long-term:* The woman will be able to maintain the prescribed level of activity and drug therapy.

Interventions

The pregnancy threatened by preterm labor or other complications is a self-limiting situation, making temporary adjustments somewhat easier. Needed changes in home routines may be brief but sometimes unexpectedly extend over several weeks.

Caring for Children

The woman who has children has different concerns than the woman who does not. Knowledge of growth and development helps the nurse identify the most appropriate way to ensure adequate care for the children and strengthen family relationships.

Toddlers and young preschoolers rarely understand why their mother does not play with them as usual. If they are already in day care, this may continue if the family can afford it. They may live with a relative or friend temporarily. Toddlers may feel that their parents have abandoned them if they

Nursing Care Plan

Preterm Labor

ASSESSMENT

Rhonda Ellis is a 28-year-old gravida 4, para 3. Her children were born at 40 weeks, 28 weeks, and 32 weeks of gestation. Her children are 7 and 4 years and 18 months old. She has mild cramping and pelvic pressure at 28 weeks and comes to the hospital right away. Her cervix is dilated 1 to 2 cm and is beginning to efface. She responds to intravenous (IV) magnesium sulfate to stop her contractions. The physician also orders betamethasone 12 mg intramuscular (IM) for two doses, 24 hours apart. After her contractions stop, Rhonda is started on oral terbutaline to maintain tocolysis and will be discharged home in 48 hours if no recurrent symptoms develop.

Nursing Diagnosis

Impaired Home Maintenance related to activity restrictions and family demands

Goal/Expected Outcome

By hospital discharge, Rhonda will:
- Relate ways that she can maintain prescribed activity restrictions.

INTERVENTION	RATIONALE
1. Assess what support systems are available and financially feasible to help Rhonda with child care and transportation, such as day care, "mother's day out" programs at churches, family, and friends.	1. Responsibilities for other children may impede a woman's ability to maintain activity limits. Coordination among several resources helps provide all day coverage for child care.
2. Encourage Rhonda to lower her standards for home management temporarily: a. Eat nourishing take-out or fast food. b. Set priorities regarding household tasks that must be done. c. Let her children do tasks that are within their abilities. d. Make lists of tasks for different people who ask to help her.	2. Many usual roles must be reallocated during this time. Having alternative arrangements increases the chance that the woman can maintain therapy.
3. Encourage Rhonda to accept help from others. Remind her that this situation is temporary and that she may be able to help someone else at another time.	3. If a woman feels that she can help others at another time, she may be more willing to accept help when she needs it.

Evaluation

Rhonda identifies three friends in addition to her mother-in-law who may be able to help with child care. She says she cannot afford to continue sending her children to their day care center if she is not working. She feels that if her children are cared for, her husband can handle the other home management needs.

---

are sent away, although this may be the only realistic solution if no one besides the mother is available to supervise them.

School-age children usually understand the situation better and are often quite helpful. They may assist with care of other children, but they should not be put into the role of an adult. They may resent responsibility that is excessive for their age. School-age children often enjoy learning new facts about their mother's pregnancy and tests the baby may need.

Adolescents may welcome the trust their parents have in them, but they also may resent the intrusion on independent activities with their peers. Teenagers who drive can be helpful in taking younger siblings to school and other activities. They may be enlisted for grocery shopping and meal prepara-

tion. If resentment flares, the parents and nurse can remind teenagers that the situation is temporary and that they are making valuable contributions to the health of the new baby.

Maintaining the Household

The first step to home maintenance during this time may be for the woman to lower her standards of housekeeping. Things may not be as clean or as organized as she would like. The partner may take over many household tasks, but these compete with his responsibilities outside the home.

Advise the woman to have a list of tasks ready when friends and family ask, "Can I do anything to help?" If they offer to bring a meal or do laundry, encourage her to accept.

Nursing Care Plan

Preterm Labor—cont'd

ASSESSMENT

At 31 weeks' gestation, Rhonda again experiences preterm labor and goes to the hospital. Her cervix is dilated 2 to 3 cm and is 75% effaced (about 0.5 cm long). Her contractions occur every 6 to 7 minutes, and last about 20 to 30 seconds each. The physician again orders a magnesium sulfate infusion and betamethasone injections. The physician explains that preterm birth may be delayed but will probably occur within the next 24 to 48 hours. Rhonda begins crying and says, "I did what I was supposed to do and now I'm still going to have another preemie! It will be weeks before I can be a real mother!"

Nursing Diagnosis

Anticipatory Grieving related to loss of expected birth experience.

Goal/Expected Outcome

Rhonda will:
- Express her feelings about the loss of her expected birth at term.

INTERVENTION	RATIONALE
1. Sit down and spend time with Rhonda. Use therapeutic communication to encourage her to express her feelings.	1. Unhurried time allows expression of feelings, which is the first step in dealing with the anticipated loss.
2. When she has expressed her frustration about this development in her pregnancy, explain that much remains unknown about why labor begins, whether at term, preterm, or postterm.	2. If a woman knows that professionals do not have all the answers but must make recommendations based on what is known or appears to work for an individual woman, she may be more accepting of the inevitability of preterm birth.
3. Explain that Rhonda's efforts have paid off because she has gained 3 valuable weeks of gestation for her baby. In addition, the drug betamethasone may reduce the chance that her preterm newborn will have the usual degree of common respiratory problems if born at that gestation.	3. Knowing that her self-care has benefits, although not the hoped-for term birth, reduces the sense of failure that she may feel.

Evaluation

Rhonda cries and expresses her frustration about the developments in her pregnancy. She says that she knew she was more likely to have another preterm infant but hoped that this time would be different. As the day goes by, Rhonda gradually begins expressing feelings that she did do something positive for this baby. She begins making specific plans to deal with the probable preterm birth.

Additional Nursing Diagnoses to Consider

Health-Seeking Behaviors
Family Coping, Readiness for Growth
Interrupted Family Processes
Ineffective Health Maintenance
Ineffective Individual Coping

Remind her that people who offer to help mean it and that she may be able to return the favor to someone else. Homemaker services may be an option to help the family deal with the woman's temporary disability.

Transportation of school-age children may be a concern. If no family or friends are available, the school nurse or parent-teacher association (PTA) may help find someone willing to take the children to school each day.

Evaluation

Goals/expected outcomes with a short term help the nurse and patient, often including the family, identify resolution of their immediate needs. Longer term outcomes may be evaluated over a series of days or weeks as the prescribed therapy for the complicated pregnancy changes.

- *Short-term:* Does the family identify how to manage minimal household care?
- *Long-term:* Can the woman maintain the prescribed therapy until birth?

BOREDOM
Assessment

If activity is to be restricted, determine what skills the woman has for coping with boredom. Although use of bed rest to prolong gestation is usually brief because of the questionable benefits and known problems, some reduction in activity is prescribed. The nurse should consider helping the woman choose appropriate activities, whether hospitalized or managing her care at home.

To identify activities that are still appropriate within the restrictions prescribed, ask about a usual day. Ask about hobbies, present and past. What type of leisure activities does the woman enjoy? Which activities are available or possible? Does she have more than one resting place to give her a change of scenery and surrounding activity?

Assess her personality. Is she calm and composed, taking whatever comes with serenity, or does she need to be busy most of the time? No matter how motivated, the woman who finds inactivity tiresome will find even limited activity restrictions difficult to maintain.

Nursing Diagnosis and Planning

A possible nursing diagnosis is

■ Deficient Diversional Activity related to lack of knowledge about appropriate activities for her pregnancy restrictions.
  Goal/Expected Outcome: The woman will pursue (with the help of others) appropriate activities to relieve boredom while maintaining recommended activity limits.

Interventions

Identifying Appropriate Activities

Determine the woman's understanding about needed activity restrictions to identify misunderstandings. The type and amount of ideal physical activities may vary with complications and the progression of pregnancy. Reinforce which usual activities are permitted and which ones should not be done and why. If she understands the rationale, she may be more willing to comply with restrictions.

Some women continue work activities, such as paperwork or phone calls, that can be accomplished with minimal physical exertion. Workplace deadlines can increase stress, even if she works at home. The feeling of usefulness gained by such activities, however, may be beneficial if it means she is willing to maintain activity restrictions. Moreover, work-related activities can reduce some of the family's financial concerns.

Suggest activities to help the woman keep busy and productive. These may include household activities that can be done at rest, volunteering for activities such as phone calls, and leisure activities such as puzzles, home movies, games, and needlework. Help her identify someone who can obtain the necessary supplies for her. This might be a good time to reactivate an old (quiet) hobby.

The woman can participate in many activities with her children while she rests. She can read to them and play board or card games. Encourage her to help the children with their homework and stimulate their development with thought-provoking discussions.

Changing the Physical Surroundings

Encourage the woman to identify at least two areas where she can maintain her prescribed rest periods. A change of location helps the woman be more willing to reduce her activities yet still feel like part of the family activities. Each area should include pillows, blankets, and a clipboard with writing materials. Small rolling carts made of plastic help keep small things organized and together. The carts may be used after the baby is born for any kind of household need. Ideally, the telephone is within reach and is cordless or she has effective use of a cell phone. Either programming or writing important phone numbers, such as family and friends, physicians, and emergency numbers, helps assure the family that phone contacts are easily available for emergency as well as social needs.

Evaluation

• Does the woman accurately identify appropriate and inappropriate activities that she pursues?

PROLONGED PREGNANCY

A prolonged pregnancy is one that lasts longer than 42 weeks. Many apparent cases of prolonged pregnancy are only miscalculation of the estimated date of delivery (EDD) because the woman has had irregular menstrual periods or has forgotten the date of her last normal one. Late prenatal care limits the use of clinical methods such as ultrasonography, which are most useful for pinpointing her EDD and reducing some potential problems associated with a prolonged gestation.

Complications

The main physical risk in prolonged pregnancy is to the fetus or newborn. Insufficiency of the placental function secondary to aging and infarctions of small areas reduces transfer of oxygen and nutrients to the fetus and removal of carbon dioxide and other wastes. Because the fetus with placental insufficiency has less reserve to tolerate uterine contractions, signs of fetal compromise, such as late decelerations and decreased variability, may develop during labor. In addition, the reduced amniotic fluid volume (oligohydramnios) that often accompanies placental insufficiency can result in umbilical cord compression. Meconium in the amniotic fluid may cause respiratory distress in the newborn if it is aspirated before or during birth. The infant may have growth restriction and may appear to have lost weight.

Many postterm fetuses do not suffer from placental insufficiency and may continue growing. The woman and fetus then may have complications related to dysfunctional labor, injury if the birth is traumatic, and the woman's postpartum uterine contraction may be inadequate to control bleeding. However, some women and their postterm fetus also may have an uneventful labor and birth.

Psychologically, the woman often feels as if her pregnancy will never end. She may fear induction of labor, a possible cesarean birth, and problems with her baby. The added fatigue imposed by prolonged pregnancy diminishes her resources for tolerating the added stress and anxiety.

Therapeutic Management

Therapeutic management begins with determination of the most accurate gestational age. If a woman did not have early prenatal care, several markers used to pinpoint gestation, such as ultrasonography, fundal height measurements, and dates of quickening and first auscultation of the fetal heart tones with a nonamplified fetoscope, may be lost. Also, the

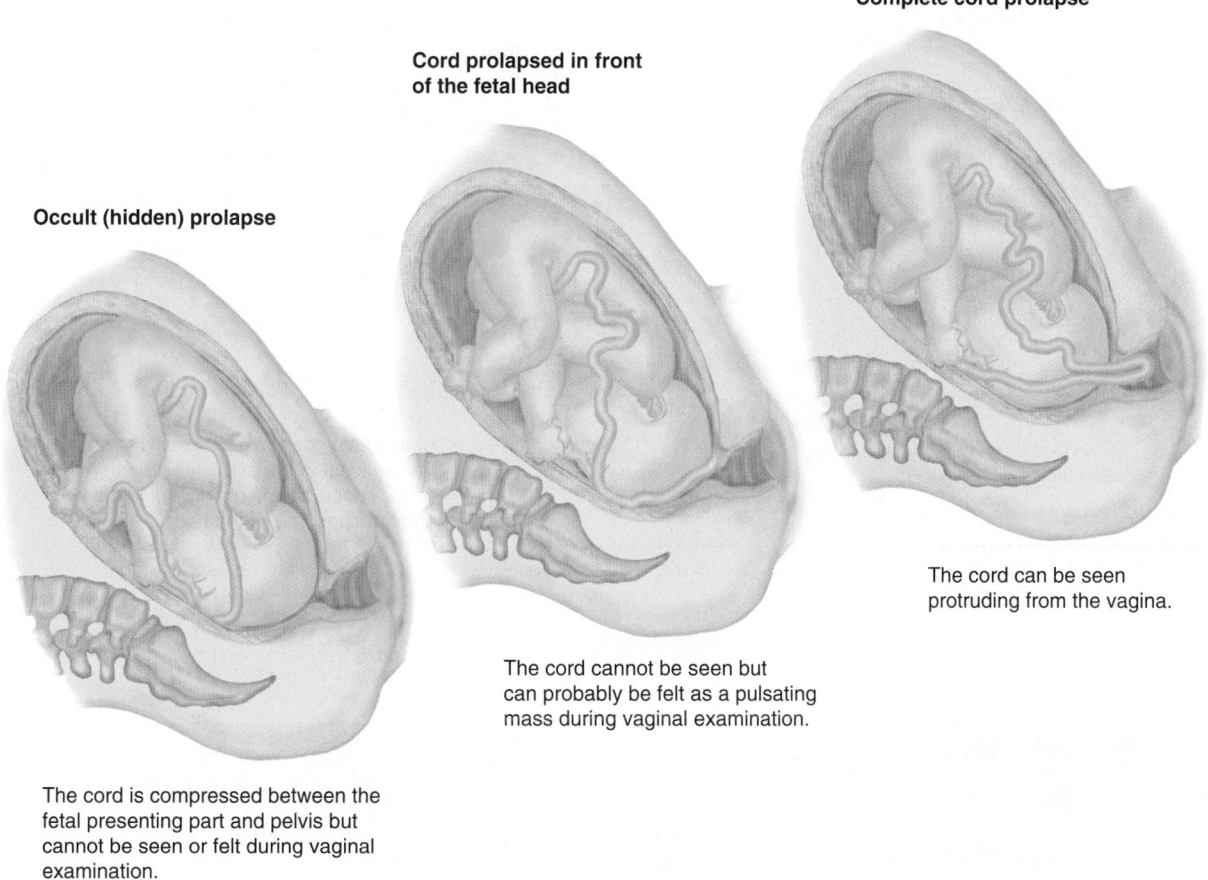

Complete cord prolapse

Cord prolapsed in front of the fetal head

Occult (hidden) prolapse

The cord can be seen protruding from the vagina.

The cord cannot be seen but can probably be felt as a pulsating mass during vaginal examination.

The cord is compressed between the fetal presenting part and pelvis but cannot be seen or felt during vaginal examination.

Figure 27-6 Variations of prolapsed umbilical cord.

woman may have forgotten the date of her last menstrual period or have irregular periods.

Another factor in management decisions is the fetal condition. If antepartum tests such as a biophysical profile (BPP) indicate that the fetus is doing well but other tests do not yet verify a term gestation, the birth attendant often takes a more conservative approach than if the fetus is suffering from reduced placental function.

If the gestation appears to be truly postterm and there is no fetal urgency to deliver quickly, management depends on whether the cervix is favorable for induction of labor. If the cervix is favorable, induction is often started. If the cervix is not favorable, the physician may take a "wait-and-see" approach, repeating fetal surveillance tests as needed. The woman often has a cervical ripening procedure (see Chapter 20) to make the cervix more favorable for induction.

Nursing Considerations

Nursing care for the woman with a prolonged pregnancy is tied to the management chosen. The nurse's role may include:

- Teaching about procedures, such as antepartum testing or induction of labor
- Support for the woman's psychological and physical fatigue

- Nursing care related to specific procedures, such as induction of labor

INTRAPARTUM EMERGENCIES

Placental Abnormalities

Women with placental abnormalities (see Chapter 26) may experience hemorrhage during the antepartum or intrapartum period. Placenta previa is sometimes associated with an abnormally adherent placenta (placenta accreta). Placenta accreta may cause immediate or delayed hemorrhage immediately after birth because the placenta does not separate cleanly, often leaving small fragments that prevent full uterine contraction. More extreme degrees of abnormal adherence occur when the placenta penetrates the uterine muscle itself (placenta increta) or even all the way through the uterus (placenta percreta). All or only part of the placenta may be involved. A hysterectomy is often required if a large portion of the placenta is abnormally adherent.

Prolapsed Umbilical Cord

A prolapsed umbilical cord slips down after the membranes rupture, subjecting it to compression between the fetus and pelvis (Fig. 27-6). It may slip down immediately with the

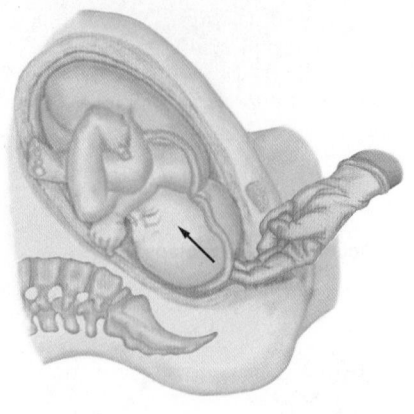

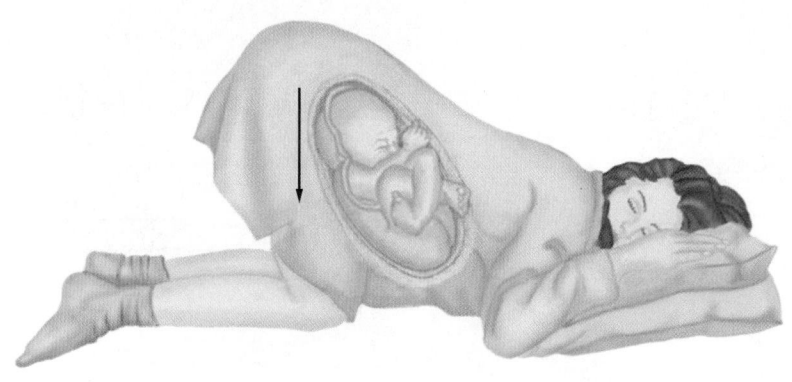

A gloved hand in the vagina pushes the fetus upward and off the cord.

Knee-chest position uses gravity to shift the fetus out of the pelvis. The woman's thighs should be at right angles to the bed and her chest flat on the bed.

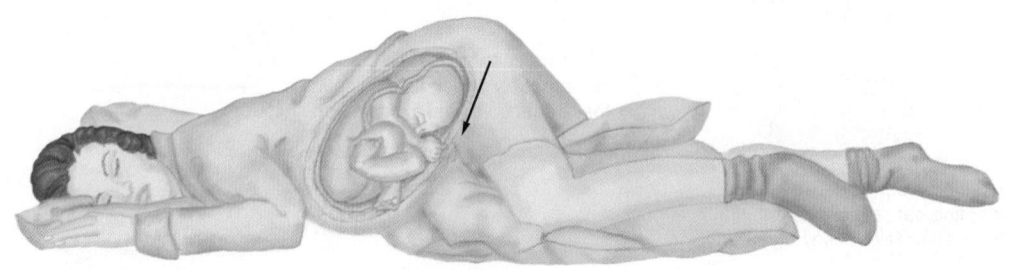

The woman's hips are elevated with two pillows; this is often combined with the Trendelenburg (head down) position.

Figure 27-7 Measures that may be used to relieve pressure on a prolapsed umbilical cord until delivery can take place.

fluid gush or long after the membranes rupture. Interruption in blood flow through the cord interferes with fetal oxygenation and is potentially fatal.

Etiology

Prolapse of the umbilical cord is more likely when the fit is poor between the fetal presenting part and the maternal pelvis. When the fit is good, the presenting part fills the pelvic opening, leaving little room for the cord to slip down. Although prolapse of the cord is possible during any labor, it is more likely if the following conditions are present:

- A fetus that remains at a high station
- A very small fetus
- Breech presentations (the footling breech is more likely to be complicated by a prolapsed cord because the feet and legs are small and do not fill the pelvis well)
- Transverse lie
- Hydramnios (often associated with abnormal presentations; also, the unusually large amount of fluid exerts more pressure to push the cord out)

Manifestations

Prolapse may be complete, with the cord visible at the vaginal opening. A prolapsed cord may not be visible but may be palpated on vaginal examination as it pulsates synchro-

nously with the fetal heart. An occult prolapse of the cord is one in which the cord slips alongside the fetal head or shoulders. The prolapse cannot be palpated or seen but is suspected because of changes in the FHR, such as bradycardia or variable decelerations. A prolapsed cord may occur with membrane rupture when a woman is not in the hospital, usually if her fetus is very small.

Therapeutic Management

Medical and nursing management often overlap, as they do in many emergency situations. The nurse, birth attendant, or a physician resident may be the first to discover cord prolapse. Birth is almost always cesarean unless vaginal delivery can be accomplished more quickly and less traumatically. Because many variations in the severity of cord prolapse exist, medical and nursing actions to promote fetal well-being may also vary.

The priority is to relieve pressure on the cord to restore blood flow after cord prolapse occurs. None of these interventions should delay the promptest possible delivery. Push the call light to summon help. Others should call the physician and prepare for birth. Notify neonatal nurses and the pediatrician or neonatologist to prepare for neonatal resuscitation.

Prompt actions are taken to relieve cord compression and increase fetal oxygenation:

Factors That Increase a Woman's Risk for a Prolapsed Umbilical Cord

Ruptured membranes *and*
- The fetal presenting part at a high station
- A fetus that poorly fits the pelvic inlet because of small size or abnormal presentation
- Excessive volume of amniotic fluid (hydramnios)

1. Position the woman's hips higher than her head to shift the fetal presenting part toward her diaphragm. Methods (Fig. 27-7) that may be used include:
   a. Knee-chest position
   b. Trendelenburg position
   c. Hips elevated with pillows, with side-lying position maintained
2. If elevation of the maternal hips does not result in an upward shift of the fetus to relieve cord compression, vaginal elevation of the presenting part using a sterile gloved hand may be required. Maintain this position until the physician orders it stopped, usually just before cesarean delivery, while minimizing added cord compression from the hand.
3. Avoid or minimize manual palpation or handling of the cord because possible cord vessel vasospasm or trauma may further reduce umbilical blood flow to and from the fetus.
4. Ultrasound examination may be used to confirm presence of fetal heart activity before cesarean delivery.

Give oxygen at 8 to 10 L/min by facemask to increase maternal blood oxygen saturation, making more oxygen available for the fetus.

Umbilical cord prolapse occurs with varying degrees of severity, and other options may be ordered by the physician. Prompt delivery of the viable fetus remains the priority, however. A tocolytic drug, such as terbutaline, may be ordered to inhibit contractions, increasing placental blood flow and reducing intermittent pressure of the fetus against the pelvis and cord. Warm saline–moistened towels retard cooling and drying of the cord that protrudes from the vagina if a delay in cesarean is required. Cooling causes vasospasm within the cord, further reducing blood flow to and from the placenta.

Prognosis for the woman is usually good because additional risks of umbilical cord prolapse are those associated with cesarean birth. Prognosis for the infant depends on how long and how severely blood flow through the cord has been impaired and on the gestational age. With prompt recognition and corrective actions, the infant usually does well.

Nursing Considerations

In addition to prompt corrective actions, the nurse must consider the woman's anxiety. The nurse must remain calm during this time and acknowledge the woman's anxiety. Explanations must be simple because anxiety interferes with the woman's ability to comprehend them. Her partner and family should be included as much as possible.

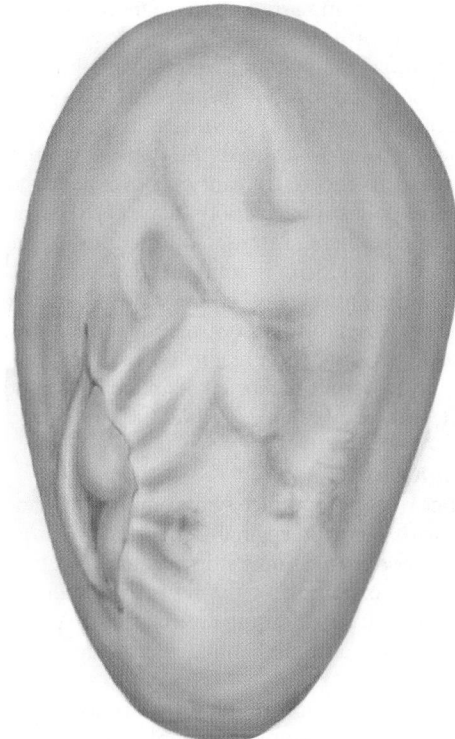

Figure 27-8 Uterine rupture in the lower uterine segment.

Uterine Rupture

Sometimes a tear in the wall of the uterus occurs because the uterus cannot withstand the pressure against it (Fig. 27-8). The three variations of uterine rupture are:

- *Complete rupture* is a direct communication between the uterine and peritoneal cavities.
- *Incomplete rupture* is rupture into the peritoneum covering the uterus or into the broad ligament but not into the peritoneal cavity.
- *Dehiscence* is a partial separation of an old uterine scar. There may be little or no bleeding. There may be no signs or symptoms, and the rupture ("window") may be found incidentally during a subsequent cesarean birth or other abdominal surgery.

Etiology

Although uterine rupture is rare, dehiscence is not unusual. Uterine rupture is associated with previous uterine surgery, such as cesarean birth or surgery to remove fibroids. The risk for rupture in a woman who has had a prior cesarean birth depends on the type of uterine incision. The risk for rupture is greater in women with a classic incision (vertical into the upper uterine segment) than in women with a low transverse incision. For this reason, vaginal birth after cesarean (VBAC) is not recommended for women who have had a previous birth through a classic cesarean incision (see Fig. 20-9 [types of uterine incisions]). The decision about choosing a VBAC is made by the woman and her physician because of the benefits as well as potential problems associated with vaginal birth that follows a previous cesarean.

Rupture of the unscarred uterus is more likely for women of high parity with a thin uterine wall, women sustaining blunt abdominal trauma, and women with intense contractions, especially if fetopelvic disproportion is present. Excessively strong (hypertonic) contractions may cause the intrauterine pressure to exceed the tensile strength of the uterine wall. If the fetus cannot be expelled downward through the pelvis, contractions may push it through the lower uterine segment. Intense contractions are more likely to occur when oxytocin is administered to stimulate labor, but uterine stimulation may be needed for a variety of reasons during labor. Misoprostol is not recommended for a woman with VBAC. A drug such as prostaglandin, often given to soften the firm cervix before labor induction, is not recommended (AAP & ACOG, 2002; ACOG, 1999).

Manifestations

Dehiscence does not produce symptoms initially and may not interfere with labor or vaginal delivery if the area is small. However, labor progress may stop because the open area prevents efficient expulsion of the fetus. Intrauterine pressures may have little change during contractions. A larger area of dehiscence may cause abdominal pain that persists despite analgesic.

Manifestations of uterine rupture vary with the degree of rupture and may mimic other complications. Possible signs and symptoms of uterine rupture include:

- Abdominal pain and tenderness. The pain may not be severe; it may occur suddenly at the peak of a contraction. The woman may describe a feeling that something "ripped" or "gave way."
- Chest pain, pain between the scapulae, or pain on inspiration. Pain occurs because of the irritation of blood below the woman's diaphragm.
- Hypovolemic shock caused by hemorrhage: falling blood pressure, tachycardia, tachypnea, pallor, cool and clammy skin, anxiety. Signs of hypovolemia may not occur until after birth, and the fall in blood pressure is often a late sign of the hemorrhage.
- Signs associated with impaired fetal oxygenation, such as late decelerations, reduced variability, tachycardia, and bradycardia.
- Absent fetal heart tones with a large disruption of the placenta.
- Cessation of uterine contractions.
- Palpation of the fetus outside the uterus (usually occurs only with a large, complete rupture). The fetus is often dead if the placenta is involved.

If the rupture is incomplete, blood loss is slower and signs of shock, chest pain, or shoulder pain may be delayed. Complete rupture results in massive blood loss. Signs of shock and pain develop quickly. External bleeding may not be impressive because most of the blood is lost into the peritoneal cavity.

Therapeutic Management

Initial management is to stabilize the woman and fetus and to perform cesarean delivery. If the rupture is small and the woman wants other children, the uterus may be repaired. A woman with a large uterine rupture requires hysterectomy. Blood is replaced if needed.

Nursing Considerations

The nurse must be aware if the woman is at increased risk for uterine rupture and must stay alert for the signs and symptoms. Administer oxytocin cautiously to reduce the likelihood of excessive contractions. Keep in mind that hypertonic contractions can occur in either a stimulated or an unstimulated labor, and monitor for their presence. Notify the birth attendant if hypertonic contractions occur.

Uterine rupture may not be detected before birth. If postpartum bleeding is excessive and the fundus is firm, injury to the birth canal, including uterine rupture, is possible. Bleeding may be concealed if the ruptured area bleeds into the broad ligament. In this case, signs of hypovolemic shock are likely to develop quickly.

Uterine Inversion

An inversion occurs when the uterus completely or partly turns inside out, usually during the third stage of labor. Such an event is uncommon but potentially fatal.

Etiology

Often no single cause is identified. Predisposing factors are:

- Pulling on the umbilical cord before the placenta detaches from the uterine wall
- Fundal pressure during birth
- Fundal pressure on an incompletely contracted uterus after birth
- Increased intraabdominal pressure
- An abnormally adherent placenta
- Weakness of the uterine wall
- Fundal placenta implantation

Manifestations

The birth attendant notes that the uterus is either absent from the abdomen or a depression in the fundal area is present. The interior of the uterus may be seen through the cervix or protruding into the vagina. Massive hemorrhage, shock, and pain quickly become evident. The woman has severe pelvic pain.

Therapeutic Management

Quick action by nursing and medical personnel is required to reduce maternal morbidity and mortality rates. The physician tries to replace the uterus through the vagina into a normal position. If that is not possible, laparotomy with replacement is done. Hysterectomy may be required, and several units of blood are usually ordered immediately.

Two intravenous lines are established to allow rapid fluid and blood replacement. General anesthesia or a tocolytic drug is often needed to relax the uterus enough to replace it. After the uterus is replaced, oxytocin is given to contract the uterus and control blood loss. *Oxytocin is not given until the uterus is repositioned to avoid trapping the inverted fundus in the cervix.*

Nursing Considerations

Nursing care during the emergency supplements that of other staff members. Postpartum nursing care is directed toward observing and maintaining maternal blood volume and correcting shock. The woman may be transferred to the intensive care unit.

Assess the uterine fundus for firmness, height, and deviation from the midline. Initially, frequent maternal vital signs checks are set on an electronic monitor that can maintain observation of hemodynamic factors. After postbirth outcomes stabilize, the assessment frequency of the woman's hemodynamic status is gradually reduced to a standard recovery room frequency while continuing observation for other complications that may be less obvious. Observe for tachycardia and a falling blood pressure, which are associated with hypovolemic shock. Cardiac dysrhythmias may occur because of severity of hypovolemia and also secondary effects from drugs to manage the complications.

An indwelling catheter is often inserted to observe fluid balance and to keep the bladder empty so that the uterus can contract well. Assess the catheter for patency, and record intake and output. Urine output should be at least 30 ml/hr. A fall in urine output may indicate hypovolemia or an obstructed catheter.

The woman is allowed nothing by mouth until her condition stabilizes. She can usually receive fluids and progress to solid foods quickly if uterine inversion does not recur. It may recur in a future pregnancy, however, if conditions favor its development.

Anaphylactoid Syndrome

Pregnancy-related anaphylactoid syndrome, often called *amniotic fluid embolism,* occurs when amniotic fluid is drawn into the maternal circulation and carried to the woman's lungs. Fetal particulate matter (skin cells, vernix, hair, meconium) in the fluid obstructs pulmonary vessels. Failure of the right ventricle occurs early and can lead to hypoxemia. Left ventricular failure follows. Abrupt respiratory distress, depressed cardiac function, and circulatory collapse may occur rapidly. Disseminated intravascular coagulation (see Chapter 26) is likely because thromboplastin-rich amniotic fluid interferes with normal blood clotting. This infrequent disorder is often fatal, possibly having 50% maternal death rate during the acute episode. Survivors may have neurologic deficits (Clark, 2004; Gonik & Foley, 2004).

Entry of amniotic fluid containing fetal cells and other matter, such as vernix, is more likely if labor is very strong. High intrauterine pressure forces amniotic fluid into open uterine or cervical veins. The meconium that often accompanies a stressed fetus in such a labor adds to the particulate matter forced into the woman's circulation.

Although this disorder has been called *amniotic fluid embolism,* the newer name of *anaphylactoid syndrome* is preferred because of findings related to other complications. Other maternal conditions that are not characterized by leaking of amniotic fluids into her circulation include septic shock, preeclampsia, and cardiac disease. Other complications may be associated with this disorder, but are not fully known (Gonik & Foley, 2004).

Therapeutic management of a pregnancy-related anaphylactoid syndrome is primarily medical and includes (Clark, 2003; Gonik & Foley, 2004):

- Cardiopulmonary resuscitation and support
- Oxygen with mechanical ventilation
- Correction of hypotension
- Blood component therapy (e.g., fibrinogen, packed red blood cells, platelets, fresh frozen plasma) to correct coagulation defects

Trauma

Most trauma during pregnancy occurs because of accidents, assault, or suicide. Battering is a significant cause of maternal-fetal trauma during pregnancy. (The social and emotional issues of battering are addressed in Chapter 25.) Trauma may be blunt, such as that sustained in an automobile accident, or penetrating, such as gunshot and knife wounds. Burns and electrical injuries also may occur.

Although injury may not be fatal, infant neurologic deficits may be found after birth. Direct fetal trauma, such as skull fracture or intracranial hemorrhage, may occur from pelvic fracture, penetrating wounds, or blunt trauma. Indirect causes of fetal injury or death include abruptio placentae and disruption of the placental blood flow secondary to maternal hypovolemia or uterine rupture. The most common cause of fetal death is death of the mother.

The anatomic and physiologic changes of pregnancy make trauma care unique. During early pregnancy, the uterus is surrounded by the pelvis and is well protected from direct damage. As the uterus grows, it protrudes and becomes a large target for trauma. At the same time, it acts as a shield for other maternal organs such as the kidneys, often protecting them from direct trauma.

Normal alterations of pregnancy can affect the maternal and fetal outcomes after traumatic injury and can affect the interpretation of diagnostic studies that may be done. Pregnant women have a greater blood volume than nonpregnant women, which gives them a cushion against blood loss. However, the fetus may suffer if the woman hemorrhages because maternal blood is diverted from the placenta to increase her blood volume. Fetal hypoxia, acidosis, and death may then occur.

Maternal fibrinogen levels are higher during pregnancy (300 to 600 mg/dl). A decrease to lower levels is associated with abruptio placentae and may indicate that disseminated intravascular coagulation is developing.

Therapeutic Management

Care of the pregnant trauma victim first focuses on injuries that threaten her life. Management of the fetus depends on whether the fetus is living and on the gestational age. The fetus may be delivered by cesarean birth if it is mature enough to survive and if the maternal or fetal condition is likely to be improved by prompt delivery. The fetus that is dead or too immature to survive is not usually delivered unless delivery will improve the mother's outcome.

Nursing Considerations

Nursing care of the pregnant trauma victim also focuses first on maternal and then on fetal stabilization. A wedge is placed under one side of the mother to tip her uterus away from her major blood vessels. "Tipping" her to displace the uterus may prevent supine hypotension and further hemodynamic instability, also improving placental blood flow. Vital signs are taken as needed, based on the woman's condition. Vital signs and urine output (at least 30 ml/hr) provide information about the adequacy of her blood volume. Bloody urine suggests bladder or renal damage. Other nursing care is directed toward specific injuries and implementation of medical care.

Signs suggesting abruptio placentae (vaginal bleeding with uterine pain and tenderness) should be reported because this complication may occur with abdominal trauma. The uterine height may also increase as the uterus fills with blood.

Once the woman's condition is stable, nursing care intensifies for the fetus. External monitoring is appropriate if the fetus has reached a viable gestational age. Preterm labor may occur but may not be recognized if the woman is unconscious or if pain from injuries overshadows discomfort from contrac-

tions. Recurrent restlessness or moaning may accompany contractions. *The nurse should palpate the woman's uterus for contractions periodically because they may not be evident on the fetal monitoring strip, especially if the fetus is small.*

Although the nurse is usually anxious in an emergency situation too, it is important to keep a calm attitude. The woman and her family quickly pick up on the staff's anxiety, and consequently theirs escalates. To reduce fears of abandonment, the nurse should remain with the woman and, if possible, hold her hand. The nurse should speak in a low, calm voice.

KEY CONCEPTS

- Dysfunctional labor may occur because of abnormalities in the powers, the passenger, the passage, or the psyche. Combinations of abnormalities are common.
- Nursing care in dysfunctional labor focuses on prevention or prompt identification and action to correct additional complications: fetal hypoxia, infection, injury to the mother or fetus, and postpartum hemorrhage.
- Premature rupture of the membranes is associated with infection as both a cause and an effect.
- The early indications of preterm labor are often vague. Prompt identification of preterm labor enables the most effective therapy to delay preterm birth.
- Nursing care for the woman at risk for a very early preterm birth focuses on helping her delay birth long enough to promote fetal lung maturation with corticosteroids, allow transfer

- to a facility with an appropriate level of neonatal intensive care, or reach a gestation at which the infant's problems with immaturity are minimal.
- The main risk in prolonged pregnancy is reduced placental function. This may compromise the fetus during labor and may result in meconium aspiration in the neonate. Dysfunctional labor may occur as a fetus continues growing during the prolonged pregnancy.
- The key intervention for umbilical cord prolapse is to relieve pressure on the cord without compressing its blood vessels and to expedite delivery.
- Be aware of women at risk for uterine rupture, and observe for signs and symptoms: signs of shock, abdominal pain, a sense of tearing, chest pain, pain in the shoulder area, abnormal FHR patterns, cessation of contractions, and palpation of the fetus outside the uterus.

- Uterine inversion is often accompanied by massive blood loss and shock. Recovery care promotes uterine contraction and maintenance of adequate circulating volume.
- Anaphylactoid syndrome is more likely to occur when labor contractions are intense, allowing particulate matter to be forced into the mother's circulation. Once thought to result only from amniotic fluid entering the maternal circulation, this critical complication has also been associated with other complications such as maternal sepsis, preeclampsia, and cardiac disease.
- Medical and nursing care of the pregnant trauma victim focuses on stabilization of the mother first. Management of the fetus depends on gestational age and whether the fetus is alive. Abruptio placentae and uterine rupture are obstetric complications that may occur with direct abdominal trauma.

ANSWERS to Critical Thinking Exercise 27-1

1. When the fetus is in an occiput posterior position, back pain is usually persistent because the fetal head presses on the mother's sacrum with each contraction, often called "back labor." In addition, the fetal head has to rotate internally through a wider arc to reach an occiput anterior position for birth; this process prolongs labor in most women.

2. The nurse should take actions to make the woman more comfortable and to promote rotation of the fetal head to an occiput anterior position. The nurse should encourage the woman to change positions regularly. Positions that cause her uterus to fall forward reduce pressure on her sacrum and straighten the pelvic curve somewhat to encourage fetal rotation. Examples of these are

leaning forward while sitting, kneeling, standing, and a hands-and-knees position. Lunging toward her right side provides slightly more room on that side of her pelvis. A left side-lying position favors fetal rotation from the right occiput posterior position toward an occiput anterior position. Consult with the nurse-midwife if the woman wants analgesia or anesthesia.

REFERENCES and READINGS

Abbott, J.T. (1999). Emergency management of the obstetric patient. In G.N. Burrow & T.P. Duffy (Eds.), *Medical complications during pregnancy* (5th ed., pp. 225-236). Philadelphia: Saunders.

Alexander, J.M., McIntire, D.D., & Leveno, K.J. (2000). Forty weeks and beyond: Pregnancy outcomes by week of gestation. *Obstetrics & Gynecology, 96*(2), 291-294.

American Academy of Pediatrics (AAP), & American College of Obstetricians and Gynecologists (ACOG). (2002). *Guidelines for perinatal care* (5th ed.). Elk Grove Village, IL, and Washington, DC: Author.

American College of Obstetricians and Gynecologists (ACOG). (2003). *Dystocia and the augmentation of labor* (ACOG Practice Bulletin No. 49). Washington, DC: Author.

American College of Obstetricians and Gynecologists. (1999). *Induction of labor* (ACOG Practice Bulletin No. 10). Washington, DC: Author.

American College of Obstetricians and Gynecologists. (2000a). *Fetal macrosomia* (ACOG Practice Bulletin No. 22). Washington, DC: Author.

American College of Obstetricians and Gynecologists. (2000b). *Intrauterine growth restriction* (ACOG Practice Bulletin No. 12). Washington, DC: Author.

American College of Obstetricians and Gynecologists. (2000c). *Operative vaginal delivery* (ACOG Practice Bulletin No. 17). Washington, DC: Author.

American College of Obstetricians and Gynecologists. (2001). *Assessment of risk factors for preterm birth* (ACOG Practice Bulletin No. 31). Washington, DC: Author.

Bakewell-Sachs, S., & Blackburn, S. (2003). State of the science: Achievements and challenges across the spectrum of care for preterm infants. *Journal of Obstetric, Gynecologic, & Neonatal Nursing, 32*(5), 683-695.

Blackburn, S.T. (2003). *Maternal, fetal, & neonatal physiology: A clinical perspective*. Philadelphia: Saunders.

Bowes, W.A., & Thorpe, J.M. (2004). Clinical aspects of normal and abnormal labor. In R.K. Creasy, R. Resnik, & J.D. Iams (Eds.), *Maternal-fetal medicine: Principles and practice* (5th ed., pp. 671-705). Philadelphia: Saunders.

Clark, S.L. (2003). Critical care obstetrics. In J.R. Scott, R.S. Gibbs, B.Y. Karlan, & A.F. Haney (Eds.), *Danforth's obstetrics & gynecology* (9th ed., pp. 461-475). Philadelphia: Lippincott Williams & Wilkins.

Clark, S.L. (2004). Placenta previa and abruptio placentae. In R.K. Creasy, R. Resnik, & J.D. Iams (Eds.), *Maternal-fetal medicine: Principles and practice* (5th ed., pp. 707-722). Philadelphia: Saunders.

Cunningham, E. (2001). Coping with bedrest. *AWHONN Lifelines, 5*(5), 50-55.

Cunningham, F.G., Gant, N.F., Leveno, K.J., Gilstrap, L.C., Hauth, J.C., & Wenstrom, K.D. (2001). *Williams obstetrics* (21st ed.). New York: McGraw-Hill.

Curran, C.A. (2003). Intrapartum emergencies. *Journal of Obstetric, Gynecologic, & Neonatal Nursing, 32*(6), 802-813.

Davis, D. (2003). Amniotic fluid embolism: Exploring this rare but typically fatal condition. *AWHONN Lifelines, 7*(2), 126-131.

Flynn, K. (1999). Preterm labor and premature rupture of membranes. *High-Risk & Critical Care Intrapartum Nursing* (2nd ed., 102-122). Philadelphia: Lippincott.

Garite, T.J. (2004). Premature rupture of the membranes. In R.K. Creasy, R. Resnik, & J.D. Iams (Eds.), *Maternal-fetal medicine: Principles and practice* (5th ed., pp. 723-739). Philadelphia: Saunders.

Gennaro, S., & Hennessy, M.D. (2003). Psychological and physiological stress: Impact on preterm birth. *Journal of Obstetric, Gynecologic, & Neonatal nursing, 32*(5), 668-675.

Gilbert, E.S., & Harmon, J.S. (2003). *Manual of high-risk pregnancy & delivery* (3rd ed.). St. Louis: Mosby.

Goldenberg, R.L. (2002). The management of preterm labor. *Obstetrics & Gynecology, 100* (5 Pt. 1), 1020-1037.

Gonik, B., & Foley, M.R. (2004). Intensive care monitoring of the critically ill pregnant patient. In R.K. Creasy, R. Resnik, & J.D. Iams (Eds.), *Maternal-fetal medicine: Principles and practice* (5th ed., pp. 975-1004). Philadelphia: Saunders.

Iams, J.D., & Creasy, R.K. (2004). Preterm labor and delivery. In R.K. Creasy & R. Resnik (Eds.), *Maternal-fetal medicine: Principles and practice* (5th ed., pp. 498-531). Philadelphia: Saunders.

Jeffcoat, M.K., Geurs, N.C., Reddy, M.D., Cliver, S.P., Goldenberg, R.L., & Hauth, J.C. (2001). Periodontal infection and preterm birth: Results of a prospective study. *Journal of the American Dental Association, 132*(7), 875-880.

Kendrick, J.M., & Simpson, K.R. (2001). Labor and birth. In K.R. Simpson & P.A. Creehan (Eds.), *AWHONN's perinatal nursing* (2nd ed., pp. 298-377). Philadelphia: Lippincott.

Malone, F.D., & D'Alton, M.E. (2004). Multiple gestation: Clinical characteristics and management. In R.K. Creasy, R. Resnik, & J.D. Iams (Eds.), *Maternal-fetal medicine: Principles and practice* (5th ed., pp. 513-536). Philadelphia: Saunders.

Maloni, J.A. (1998). *Antepartum bedrest: Case studies, research & nursing care*. Washington, DC: Association of Women's Health, Obstetric, & Neonatal Nurses.

Maloni, J.A. (2000). *The prevention of preterm birth: Research-based practice, nursing interventions, and practice scenarios*. Washington, DC: Association of Women's Health, Obstetric, and Neonatal Nurses.

Maloni, J.A. (2001). Antepartum bedrest: Effect upon the family. *Journal of Obstetrics, Gynecologic, & Neonatal Nursing, 30*(2), 165-173.

Maloni, J.A. (2002). Astronauts & pregnancy bedrest. *AWHONN Lifelines, 6*(4), 318-323.

Maloni, J.A., Albrecht, S.A., Thomas, K.K., Halleran, J., & Jones, R. (2003). Implementing evidence-based practice: Reducing risk for low birth weight through pregnancy smoking cessation. *Journal of Obstetrics, Gynecologic, & Neonatal Nursing, 32*(5), 676-682.

Martin, J.A., Hamilton, B.E., Sutton, P.D., Ventura, S.J., Menacker, F., & Munson, M.L. (2003). Births: Final data for 2002. *National Vital Statistics Reports, 52*(10). Hyattsville, MD: National Center for Health Statistics. Retrieved Jan. 28, 2004, from www.cdc.gov/nchs/data/nvsr/nvsr52/nvsr52_10.pdf.

Moore, M.L. (2003). Preterm labor and birth: What have we learned in the past two decades? *Journal of Obstetrics, Gynecologic, & Neonatal Nursing, 32*(5), 638-649.

National Institutes of Health. (2000). Antenatal corticosteroids revisited: Repeat statement. *NIH consensus statement, 17*(2), August 17-18, 2000. Retrieved Feb. 2, 2004, from http://consensus.nih.gov/cons/112/112_statement.pdf.

Neumann, M., & Graf, C. (2003). Pregnancy after age 35. *AWHONN Lifelines, 7*(5), 422-430.

Poole, J., Sosa, M.E.B., Freeda, M.C., Kendrick, J.M., Luppi, C.J., Krening, C.F., Dauphinee, J.D., & Sosa, M.E.B. (2001). Common perinatal complications. In K.R. Simpson & P.A. Creehan (Eds.), *AWHONN's perinatal nursing* (2nd ed., pp. 173-296). Philadelphia: Lippincott.

Rao, P., & Andersen, H.F. (2003). Outcome of preterm premature rupture of membranes: A contemporary perspective. *American Journal of Obstetrics & Gynecology, 189*(6), S171.

Resnik, J.L., & Resnik, R. (2004). Post-term pregnancy. In R.K. Creasy, R. Resnik, & J.D. Iams (Eds.), *Maternal-fetal medicine: Principles and practice* (5th ed., pp. 663-669). Philadelphia: Saunders.

Schmidt, J. (1999). Prolonged pregnancy. *High-Risk & Critical Care Intrapartum Nursing* (2nd ed., 123-128). Philadelphia: Lippincott.

Segal, S.Y., Miles, A.M., Clothier, B., Parry, S., & Macones, G.A. (2003). Duration of antibiotic therapy after preterm rupture of fetal membranes. *American Journal of Obstetrics & Gynecology, 189*(3), 799-802.

Simkin, P. (2003). Maternal positions and pelves revisited. *Birth, 30*(2), 130-132.

Simpson, K.R., & Knox, G.E. (2001). Fundal pressure during the second stage of labor. *MCN: The American Journal of Maternal/Child Nursing, 27*(4), 245-248.

Thornberg, P. (2002). "Waiting" as experienced by women hospitalized during the antepartum period. *MCN: The American Journal of Maternal/Child Nursing, 26*(2), 86-92.

Tiedje, L.B. (2003). Psychosocial pathways to prematurity: Changing our thinking toward a life-course and community approach. *Journal of Obstetrics, Gynecologic, & Neonatal Nursing, 32*(5), 650-658.

Weiss, M.E., Saks, N.P., & Harris, S. (2002). Resolving the uncertainty of preterm symptoms: Women's experiences with the onset of preterm labor. *Journal of Obstetrics, Gynecologic, & Neonatal Nursing, 31*(1), 66-76.

Weitz, B.W. (2001). Premature rupture of the fetal membranes: Update for the advanced practice nurses. *MCN: The American Journal of Maternal/Child Nursing, 26*(2), 86-92.

Whitty, J.E., & Dombrowski, M.P. (2004). Respiratory diseases in pregnancy. In R.K. Creasy, R. Resnik, & J.D. Iams (Eds.), *Maternal-fetal medicine: Principles and practice* (5th ed., pp. 953-974). Philadelphia: Saunders.

28

The Woman with a Postpartum Complication

After studying this chapter, you should be able to:

◎ Describe the predisposing factors, causes, manifestations, and therapeutic management of postpartum hemorrhage.

◎ Explain major causes, manifestations, and therapeutic management of subinvolution.

◎ Describe three major thromboembolic disorders (superficial venous thrombosis, deep vein thrombosis, pulmonary embolism), together with their predisposing factors, causes, manifestations, and therapeutic management.

◎ Discuss the location, predisposing factors, causes, manifestations, and therapeutic management of puerperal infection.

◎ Describe two major mood disorders (postpartum depression, psychosis).

◎ Describe the role of the nurse in the management of women with postpartum complications.

◆ DEFINITIONS

atony Absence or lack of usual muscle tone.

dilation and curettage (D&C) Stretching of the cervical os to permit suctioning or scraping of the walls of the uterus. The procedure is performed in abortion, to obtain samples of uterine lining tissue for laboratory examination, and during the postpartum period to remove retained fragments of placenta.

embolus A mass that may be composed of a thrombus (blood clot) or amniotic fluid brought by the blood from another vessel and forced into a smaller one, thus obstructing circulation.

hematoma Localized collection of blood in a space or tissue.

hydramnios Excess volume of amniotic fluid (more than 2000 ml at term). Also called *polyhydramnios*.

hypovolemia Abnormally decreased volume of circulating fluid in the body.

hypovolemic shock Acute peripheral circulatory failure caused by loss of circulating blood volume.

placenta accreta Placenta that is abnormally adherent to the uterine muscle. If the condition is more advanced, it is called *placenta increta* (the placenta extends into the uterine muscle) or *placenta percreta* (the placenta extends through the uterine muscle).

psychosis Mental state in which a person's ability to recognize reality, communicate, and relate to others is impaired.

thrombus Collection of blood factors, primarily platelets and fibrin, that form a clot and may cause vascular obstruction.

Pregnancy and childbirth are natural functions from which most women recover without complication. However, nurses must be aware of problems that may occur and their effect on the family. The most common physiologic complications are hemorrhage, thromboembolic disorders, and infection. Psychogenic complications include postpartum depression and postpartum psychosis.

POSTPARTUM HEMORRHAGE

Postpartum hemorrhage is generally defined as blood loss that exceeds 500 ml after vaginal childbirth or 1000 ml after cesarean birth. However, this amount of blood loss is not un-usual during birth. Estimating blood loss is difficult, especially when bleeding is brisk or hemorrhage is concealed. Furthermore, blood loss during childbirth is frequently underestimated and constitutes only approximately half the actual loss (Cunningham et al., 2001). A drop in hematocrit of 10% after delivery or a need for blood transfusion is another definition that may be useful.

Postpartum hemorrhage complicates approximately 5% of deliveries (Katz & Wolfe, 2002). It is one of the leading causes of maternal morbidity and mortality. When hemorrhage occurs in the first 24 hours after childbirth, it is termed *early postpartum hemorrhage*. When it occurs after 24 hours, it is called *late postpartum hemorrhage*.

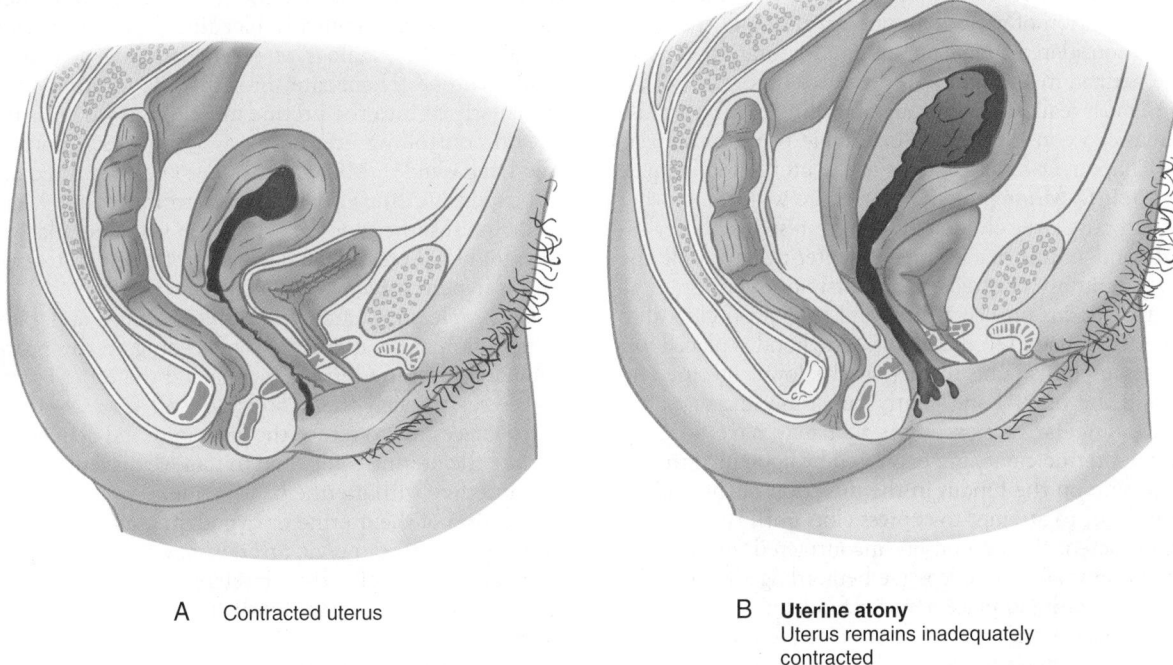

A   Contracted uterus

B   **Uterine atony**
Uterus remains inadequately
contracted

Figure 28-1 A, When the uterus remains contracted, the placental site is smaller, so bleeding is minimal. **B,** If uterine muscles fail to contract around the endometrial arteries at the placental site, hemorrhage occurs.

Early Postpartum Hemorrhage

The two major causes of early postpartum hemorrhage are uterine atony and trauma to the birth canal during labor and delivery. Abnormalities of the third stage of labor, such as placenta accreta (abnormal adherence of the placenta to the uterine wall) and inversion of the uterus, are described in Chapter 27.

Uterine Atony

Early hemorrhage is most often caused by uterine atony. *Atony* refers to lack of muscle tone that results in failure of the uterine muscle fibers to contract firmly around blood vessels when the placenta separates. The relaxed muscles allow rapid bleeding from the endometrial arteries at the placental site. Bleeding continues until the uterine muscle fibers contract to stop the flow of blood. Figure 28-1 illustrates the effect of uterine contraction on the size of the placental site and the amount of bleeding that occurs.

Predisposing Factors. Knowledge of factors that increase the risk for uterine atony can be used to anticipate and thus reduce excessive bleeding. Overdistention of the uterus from any cause (multiple gestation, a large infant, hydramnios) makes it difficult for the uterus to contract with enough firmness to prevent excessive bleeding. Multiparity results in muscle fibers that have been stretched repeatedly and these flaccid muscle fibers may not remain contracted after childbirth. Intrapartum factors include contractions that were barely effective, resulting in prolonged labor, or contractions that were excessively vigorous, resulting in precipitate labor. Labor that was induced or augmented with oxytocin is more likely to be followed by postdelivery uterine atony and hemorrhage. Retention of a large segment of the placenta does not allow the uterus to contract firmly and can result in uterine atony (Box 28-1).

> **BOX 28-1**
> *Common Predisposing Factors for Postpartum Hemorrhage*
>
> - Overdistention of the uterus (multiple gestation, large infant, hydramnios)
> - Multiparity (≥5)
> - Use of tocolytic drugs
> - Precipitate labor or delivery
> - Prolonged labor
> - Use of forceps or vacuum extractor
> - Cesarean birth or previous uterine surgery
> - Manual removal of the placenta
> - Previous postpartum hemorrhage
> - General anesthesia
> - Placenta previa, accreta, or low implantation
> - Drugs: oxytocin, prostaglandins, magnesium sulfate
> - Chorioamnionitis
> - Clotting disorders
> - Disseminated intravascular clotting

Manifestations. Major signs of uterine atony include:

- A uterine fundus that is difficult to locate
- A soft, or "boggy," feel when the fundus is located
- A uterus that becomes firm as it is massaged but loses its tone when massage is stopped
- A uterine fundus that is located above the expected level
- Excessive lochia

For the first 24 hours after childbirth, the uterus should feel like a firmly contracted ball roughly the size of a large grapefruit. It should be easily located at about the level of the umbilicus. Lochia should be dark red and moderate in amount. Saturation of more than one perineal pad (peripad) per hour is considered a large amount and saturation of more than one peripad in 15 minutes is excessive (Scoggin, 2000). The nurse must realize that although bleeding may be profuse and dramatic, a constant trickle or dribble is just as dangerous (see Chapter 21 for assessment of the uterus and lochia).

Therapeutic Management. Nurses are with the mother during the hours after childbirth and are responsible for assessments and initial management of uterine atony. If the uterus is not firmly contracted, the first intervention is to massage the fundus until it is firm and to express clots that may have accumulated in the uterus. One hand is placed just above the symphysis pubis to support the lower uterine segment while the other hand gently but firmly massages the fundus in a circular motion. Clots that may have accumulated in the uterine cavity are expressed by applying firm but gentle pressure on the fundus in the direction of the vagina. It is critical not to attempt to express clots until the uterus is firmly contracted. Pushing on an uncontracted uterus could invert the uterus and cause massive hemorrhage. Figure 28-2 illustrates correct hand placement for fundal massage.

If the uterus does not remain contracted after uterine massage or if the fundus is displaced, the problem may be a distended bladder. A full bladder lifts and displaces the uterus and prevents effective contraction of the uterine muscles. Nurses should assist the mother to urinate or should catheterize her, if necessary, to correct uterine atony caused by bladder distention.

Pharmacologic measures may also be necessary to maintain firm contraction of the uterus. A rapid intravenous (IV) infusion of dilute oxytocin (Pitocin) often increases uterine tone and controls bleeding. (See oxytocin drug guide, p. 447.) Analogs of prostaglandin $F_{2\alpha}$ (carboprost tromethamine [Hemabate, Prostin]) are often given intramuscularly or into the uterine muscle if oxytocin is ineffective in controlling uterine atony (Bowes & Thorp, 2004) (see Drug Guide). Misoprostol (Cytotec) given rectally is a less-expensive drug also used to control bleeding. Methylergonovine (Methergine) may be given intramuscularly, but it elevates blood pressure and should not be given to a woman who is hypertensive.

Other measures include uterine packing and bimanual compression of the uterus to stop bleeding. In this procedure, one hand is inserted in the vagina and the other compresses the uterus through the abdominal wall (Fig. 28-3). It may also be necessary to return the woman to the delivery area to explore the uterine cavity and to remove placental fragments that interfere with uterine contraction.

Ligation of the uterine or hypogastric artery or embolization (occlusion) of pelvic arteries may be necessary if other measures are not effective. Hysterectomy is a last resort to save the life of a woman with uncontrollable postpartum hemorrhage.

Hemorrhage requires prompt replacement of intravascular fluid volume. Lactated Ringer's solution and whole blood as well as other plasma extenders may be used. Enough fluid should be given to maintain urine flow of at least 30 ml/hr and preferably 60 ml/hr (Cunningham et al., 2001). The nurse is often responsible for obtaining properly typed and crossmatched blood and for inserting large-bore IV lines that are capable of carrying whole blood.

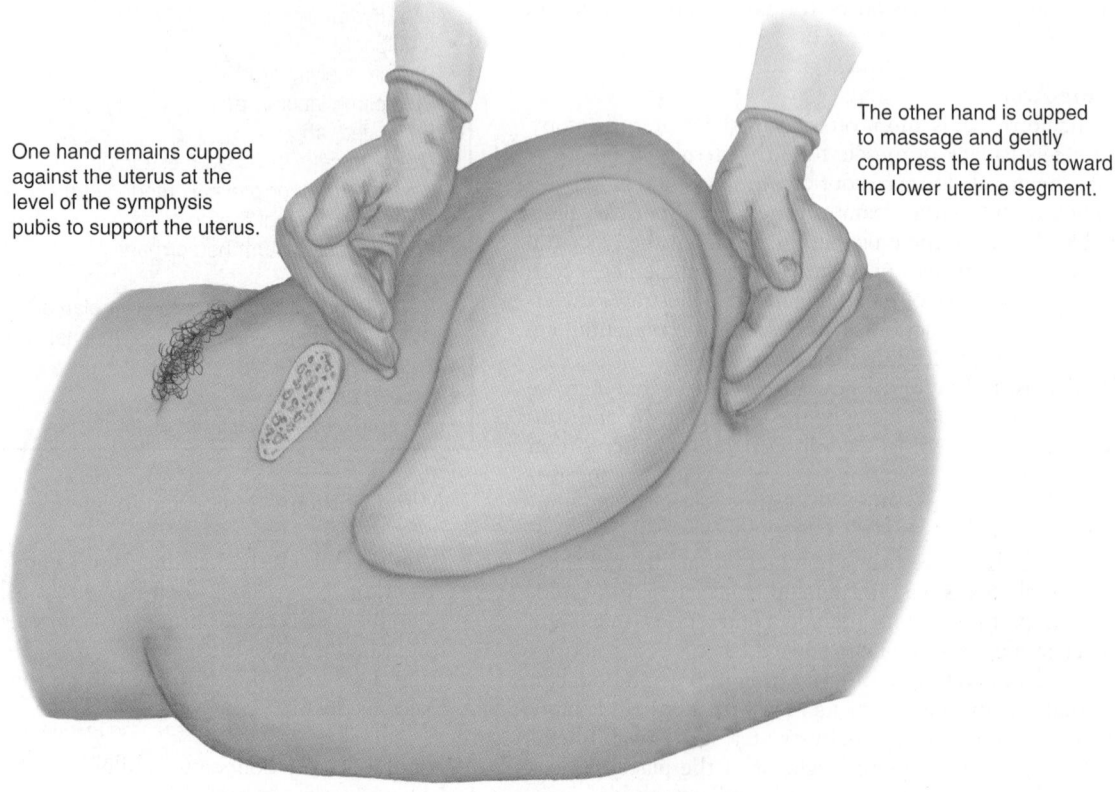

One hand remains cupped against the uterus at the level of the symphysis pubis to support the uterus.

The other hand is cupped to massage and gently compress the fundus toward the lower uterine segment.

Figure 28-2 Technique for fundal massage.

Trauma

Trauma to the birth canal is the second most common cause of early postpartum hemorrhage. Trauma can include vaginal, cervical, or perineal lacerations and hematomas.

Predisposing Factors. Many of the same factors that increase the risk for uterine atony also increase the risk for soft tissue trauma during childbirth. For example, trauma to the birth canal is more likely to occur if the infant is large or if labor and delivery occur rapidly. Induction and augmentation of labor and the use of assistive devices, such as a vacuum extractor or forceps, increase the risk for tissue trauma.

Lacerations. The perineum, vagina, cervix, and the area around the urethral meatus are the most common sites for lacerations. Cervical lacerations occur frequently when the cervix dilates rapidly during the first stage of labor. Lacerations of the vagina, perineum, and periurethral area usually occur during the second stage of labor, when the fetal head descends rapidly or when assistive devices are used to aid in delivery of the fetal head.

Lacerations of the birth canal should always be suspected if excessive uterine bleeding continues when the fundus is contracted firmly and is at the expected location. Bleeding from lacerations of the genital tract is often bright red, in contrast to the darker red color of lochia.

Hematomas. Hematomas occur when bleeding into loose connective tissue occurs while overlying tissue remains intact. Hematomas develop as a result of injury to soft tissue in spontaneous deliveries as well as in deliveries in which forceps or vacuum extractors are used. Hematomas may be found in vulvar, vaginal, or retroperitoneal areas.

Visible vulvar hematomas appear as discolored, bulging masses that are sensitive to touch. Hematomas in the upper vagina or retroperitoneal areas cannot be seen. Hematomas produce deep, severe, unrelieved pain and feelings of pressure. Formation of a hematoma should also be suspected if the mother demonstrates systemic signs of concealed blood loss, such as falling blood pressure or tachycardia, when the fundus is firm and lochia is within normal limits.

Therapeutic Management. When postpartum hemorrhage is caused by trauma to the birth canal, surgical repair is often necessary. The mother is returned to the delivery area, where surgical lights enhance visibility, and the laceration is repaired.

Small hematomas usually reabsorb naturally. Large hematomas, however, may require incision, evacuation of the clots, and location of the bleeding vessel so that it can be ligated.

Late Postpartum Hemorrhage

The most common causes of late postpartum hemorrhage are subinvolution (delayed return of the uterus to its nonpregnant size and consistency) and fragments of placenta that remain attached to the myometrium when the placenta is delivered. Clots form around the retained fragments, and excessive bleeding can occur when the clots slough away several days after delivery.

Late postpartum hemorrhage caused by retained placental fragments usually is preventable. The nurse-midwife or physician should carefully inspect the placenta at delivery to determine if it is intact. If a portion of the placenta is missing,

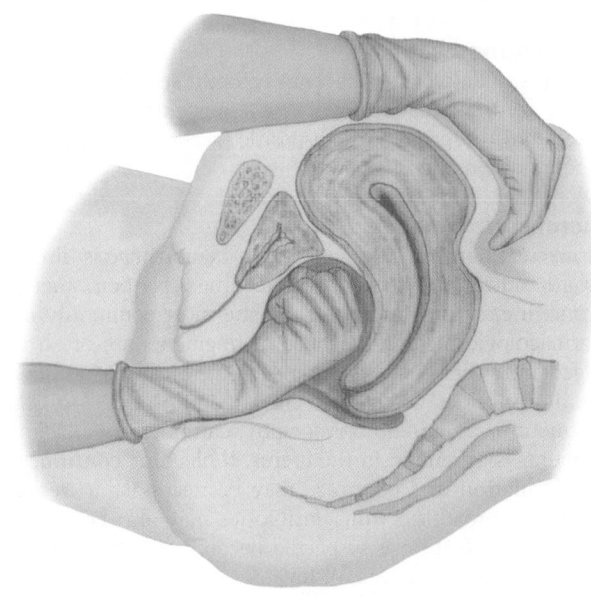

Figure 28-3 Bimanual compression. One hand is inserted in the vagina, and the other compresses the uterus through the abdominal wall.

Drug Guide

Carboprost Tromethamine (Hemabate, Prostin/15M)

Classification: Prostaglandin, oxytocic.

Action: Stimulates contraction of the uterus.

Indications: Used for the treatment of postpartum hemorrhage caused by uterine atony. Also used for abortion.

Dosage and Route: Postpartum hemorrhage: 150 mcg intramuscularly (IM). May repeat at 15- to 90-minute intervals.

Absorption: Metabolized by the liver and by enzymes in the lungs.

Excretion: Excreted primarily in urine.

Contraindications and Precautions: Contraindicated for women with hypersensitivity to carboprost or other prostaglandins; acute pelvic inflammatory disease; cardiac, pulmonary, renal, or hepatic disease. Use caution if woman has history of asthma, hypotension, hypertension, anemia, jaundice, diabetes, epilepsy.

Adverse Reactions/Side Effects: Excessive dose may cause tetanic contractions and laceration or uterine rupture. May cause uterine hypertonus if used with oxytocin. Nausea, vomiting, diarrhea, fever, chills, facial flushing, headache, hypertension, hypotension.

Nursing Considerations: Should be refrigerated. Give deep IM and aspirate carefully to avoid intravenous injection. Rotate sites if repeated. Monitor vital signs. Administer antiemetics and antidiarrheals as ordered.

Early Signs of Postpartum Hemorrhage

- An uncontracted uterus
- Large gush or slow, steady trickle of blood from the vagina
- Saturation of more than one peripad per hour
- Severe, unrelieved perineal or rectal pain
- Tachycardia

the health care provider can manually explore the uterus, locate the missing fragments, and remove them.

Late postpartum hemorrhage, which typically occurs without warning 7 to 14 days after delivery, can be dangerous for the unsuspecting mother. Families must be taught the proper way to assess the fundus and the normal duration of lochia. They must be instructed to notify their health care provider if bleeding persists or becomes unusually heavy.

Predisposing Factors

Attempts to deliver the placenta before it separates from the uterine wall, manual removal of the placenta, and placenta accreta are the primary predisposing factors for retention of placental fragments.

Therapeutic Management

Initial treatment for late postpartum hemorrhage is directed toward control of the excessive bleeding. Oxytocin, methylergonovine, or prostaglandins are the most commonly used pharmacologic measures. Placental fragments are often dislodged and swept out of the uterus by the bleeding, and if the bleeding subsides when oxytocin is administered, no other treatment is required. Sonography can identify placental fragments that remain in the uterus. If bleeding continues or recurs, dilation and curettage may be necessary to remove fragments. Broad-spectrum antibiotics may also be given if postpartum infection is suspected because of uterine tenderness, foul-smelling lochia, or fever.

▪ NURSING CARE

The Woman with Excessive Bleeding

Assessment

The initial postpartum assessment includes a chart review to determine whether factors such as prolonged labor, birth of a large infant, or assistive devices have increased the risk for the woman to bleed excessively.

Uterine Atony

Priority assessments for uterine atony include the fundus, bladder, lochia, vital signs, skin temperature, and color. Assess the consistency and the location of the uterine fundus. The fundus should be firmly contracted, at or near the level of the umbilicus and midline. If the fundus feels soft (boggy), the uterus is not firmly contracted and bleeding from the placental site is rapid and continuous. If the fundus is above the level of the umbilicus and displaced, a full bladder may be the cause of excessive bleeding. A full bladder lifts the uterus and impedes contraction, which allows excessive bleeding. The

accumulation of clots also expands the uterus, making contraction difficult and resulting in continued bleeding.

It is difficult to estimate the volume of lochia by visual examination of peripads. More accurate information is obtained by weighing peripads, linen savers, and if necessary, bed linens before and after use and subtracting the difference. One gram (weight) equals 1 ml (volume). When inspecting for blood loss, always ask the woman to turn on her side to be certain that large amounts of blood are not pooling undetected beneath her. Although bleeding may be profuse and dramatic, a continuous but small oozing of blood may lead to significant blood loss that becomes increasingly life-threatening.

Measure vital signs at least every 15 minutes to detect trends, such as tachycardia or a decrease in pulse pressure, that may reveal a deteriorating status in a woman with significant blood loss. Initially, the body compensates for excessive bleeding by constricting the peripheral blood vessels and shunting blood to vital organs. Therefore vital signs may remain normal although the woman is becoming hypovolemic.

The skin should be warm and dry; mucous membranes of the lips and mouth should be pink; and capillary return should occur within 3 seconds when the nails are blanched. These signs confirm adequate circulating volume to perfuse the peripheral tissue.

Trauma

If the fundus is firm but bleeding is excessive, the cause may be lacerations of the cervix or birth canal. Inspect the perineum to determine whether a laceration is visible in that area. Lacerations of the cervix or vagina are not visible, but bleeding in the presence of a contracted uterus suggests a laceration. This sign warrants examination of the vaginal walls and the cervix by the health care provider.

If the mother complains of deep, severe pelvic or rectal pain or if vital signs or skin changes suggest hemorrhage but excessive bleeding is not obvious, the cause may be concealed bleeding and the formation of a hematoma. Examine the vulva for bulging masses or discoloration of the skin. A hematoma may be developing in the vagina or in the retroperitoneal area, however, and will not be obvious when

---

CRITICAL THINKING EXERCISE 28-1

Dolores Navarra, a 26-year-old multipara, is admitted to the postpartum unit after rapid labor and the birth of her fourth infant 2 hours ago. The baby weighed 4000 g (8 lb, 13 oz). At the initial assessment, Dolores's fundus is firm, at the level of the umbilicus. Lochia is heavy, with occasional small clots expressed. Vital signs are unchanged from prenatal norms.

1. What are the "red flags" that suggest a potential problem or complication? What actions should the nurse take as a result?
2. The nurse observes that the fundus is soft and that lochia is excessive. What are the priority interventions? Why?
3. Within an hour, the fundus becomes boggy again and is located 3 cm above the umbilicus and displaced to the right. What is the priority nursing action? Why?
4. Dolores voids 500 ml. The fundus is difficult to locate, however, and lochia is excessive. What is the next nursing action? Why?

TABLE **28-1** Nursing Assessments for Postpartum Hemorrhage

Assessments	Abnormal Signs/Symptoms	Nursing Implications
Chart review	Presence of predisposing factors	Perform more frequent evaluations.
Fundus	Soft, boggy, displaced	Massage, express clots, assist to void or catheterize. Notify primary health care provider if measures are ineffective.
Lochia	Excessive bleeding (saturation of more than one pad in 15 minutes, steady trickle or profuse flow)	Assess for trauma, save and weigh pads, linen savers, and bed linens so estimation of blood loss will be more accurate. Notify physician or nurse-midwife.
Vital signs	Tachycardia, decreasing pulse pressure, falling blood pressure	Report signs of excessive blood loss.
Comfort level	Severe pelvic or rectal pain	Signs of hematoma, usually perineal or vaginal; examine vulva for masses or discoloration.
Skin	Cool, damp, pale	Signs of hypovolemia; vigilant assessment and management by entire health care team is necessary.

the vulva is examined. Table 28-1 summarizes assessments, abnormal signs and symptoms, and nursing implications.

Nursing Diagnosis and Planning

The collaborative problem postpartum hemorrhage is a potential complication that requires the efforts of the entire health care team to control the hemorrhage and prevent further complications, such as hypovolemic shock. Client-centered goals are inappropriate for this potential complication because the nurse cannot manage postpartum hemorrhage independently but must confer with the physicians or nurse-midwife for medical orders to treat the condition. Planning should reflect the nurse's responsibility to:

- Monitor for signs of postpartum hemorrhage.
- Perform actions that minimize postpartum hemorrhage and prevent hypovolemic shock.
- Consult with the health care provider if signs of postpartum hemorrhage are observed.

Interventions

Preventing Hemorrhage

Every nurse should be aware of factors that put the new mother at risk for postpartum hemorrhage. This knowledge alerts the nurse to be particularly vigilant in monitoring these women so that excessive bleeding can be anticipated and minimized.

When predisposing factors are present, assess frequently. Many hospitals and birth centers have a standard of care that calls for assessments every 15 minutes during the first hour after delivery, every 30 minutes for the next 2 hours, and hourly for the next 4 hours. This protocol, however, may not be adequate for the woman at known risk for postpartum hemorrhage, because bleeding occurs rapidly. A delay in assessment may result in a great deal of blood loss.

Collaborating With the Health Care Provider

Begin uterine massage to control bleeding. If bleeding is not promptly controlled, notify the physician or nurse-midwife. Weighing the blood-soaked pads and linen savers allow the nurse to report the amount of blood lost in a certain period.

In some hospitals or birth centers, protocols permit nurses to initiate specific laboratory studies, such as hemoglobin and hematocrit levels and typing and crossmatching of blood, so

that blood is available should transfusions be necessary. Many protocols also allow the nurse to start IV fluids while the health care provider is being informed of the mother's condition. These actions do not substitute for notifying the health care provider, but they do allow nurses to make initial interventions quickly.

Keep the woman on bed rest to increase venous return and maintain cardiac output. The Trendelenburg position may interfere with cardiac function and is not advised. Continue assessments, call for assistance, and save all pads, linen savers, and linen so that an accurate estimation of blood loss can be made. Assistance is necessary because one nurse must continue to massage the uncontracted uterus and perform and record assessments while the other notifies the health care provider of the mother's condition.

When notifying the health care provider, document the time and content of each communication. For example, "1300: Dr. X notified of difficulty maintaining uterine contraction and continued excessive bleeding. Requested Dr. X to see client. Orders received."

Administer medications and fluids ordered by the health care provider. Note the effects, and relay the information to the health care provider. If measures fail to control bleeding, notify the health care provider so that additional procedures can be initiated. These may include preparation for operative intervention (surgical preparation, consent signed for operative procedure, confirmation that blood replacement is available).

Providing Support for the Family

The unusual activity of the hospital staff may make the mother and her family anxious. Keeping family informed is one of the most effective ways of reducing anxiety.

Acknowledge the family's anxiety, and provide simple, appropriate explanations of the activity. "I know all this activity must be frightening. She is bleeding a little more than we would like, and we are doing several things at once."

Evaluation

- Does the fundus remain firm?
- Is lochia moderate?
- Do vital signs remain near predelivery levels?

HYPOVOLEMIC SHOCK

The pregnant woman can tolerate blood loss that approaches the volume of blood added during pregnancy, which is approximately 1 to 2 L (Cunningham et al., 2001). When more than this reserve is lost, hypovolemic shock can ensue. Hypovolemia endangers vital organs by depriving them of oxygen. The brain, heart, and kidneys are especially vulnerable to hypoxia and may sustain damage in a brief period.

Pathophysiology

During hypovolemic shock, the body compensates by constriction of peripheral blood vessels and release of catecholamines. This causes vasoconstriction, which increases the heart rate and blood pressure. As shock worsens, the compensatory mechanisms fail. Inadequate organ perfusion and decreased cellular oxygen for metabolism result in a buildup of lactic acid and the development of metabolic acidosis. Decreased serum pH (acidosis) results in vasodilation, which further increases bleeding. If circulating volume becomes insufficient to perfuse cardiac and brain tissue, the mother dies.

Manifestations

Tachycardia is one of the earliest signs of hypovolemic shock, and even gradual increases in the pulse rate should be noted. A decrease in blood pressure and narrowing of pulse pressure (difference between systolic and diastolic blood pressure) occur when the circulating volume of blood is sufficiently decreased. The respiratory rate increases as the woman becomes more anxious and attempts to take in more oxygen.

Skin changes also provide early cues. Vasoconstriction in the skin causes it to become pale and cool to the touch. As hemorrhage worsens, pallor increases and the skin becomes cold and clammy.

As shock progresses, changes also occur in the central nervous system. The mother becomes anxious, then confused, and finally lethargic when blood loss totals 30% to 40% of the total blood volume. Urine output also decreases from more than 30 ml/hr in early shock to less than 5 ml/hr when more than 40% of the blood is lost.

Therapeutic Management

The goals of therapy are to control bleeding and to prevent hypovolemic shock from becoming irreversible. A second IV line should be inserted with a large-bore (16-gauge) catheter capable of carrying whole blood. Sufficient fluid volume is infused to produce a urinary output of at least 30 ml/hr. The health care team makes every effort to locate the source of bleeding and to stop the loss of blood. Interventions may include uterine packing; ligation of the uterine, ovarian, or hypogastric artery; or hysterectomy.

Nursing Considerations

Immediate Care

One person should be assigned to evaluate and record vital signs, location and consistency of the fundus, amount of lochia, skin temperature and color, and capillary return every 3 to 5 minutes. Nurses often follow facility protocols that allow them to draw blood for hemoglobin, hematocrit, clotting studies, type, and crossmatch. In addition, a pulse oximeter should be applied to determine oxygen saturation of the blood. A urinary catheter is inserted so that hourly urinary output can be measured. The catheter is also necessary if a surgical procedure to control the hemorrhage is required. Oxygen may be administered to increase the saturation of fewer red blood cells.

Nurses are also responsible for administering fluids, whole blood, and medications as directed and for reporting on their effectiveness. In addition, nurses must make every effort to provide information and emotional support for the woman and her family.

Home Care

Nurses who work in home care or nurse-managed postpartum clinics must be aware that women who have had postpartum hemorrhage are subject to a variety of complications. In general, they are exhausted, and it may take weeks for them to feel well again. Anemia often results, and a course of iron therapy may be prescribed to restore hemoglobin level. Some women need extra assistance with housework and care of the new infant. Fatigue may interfere with bonding and attachment. Extensive blood loss increases the risk for postpartum infection, and the woman must be taught to observe for specific signs and symptoms.

SUBINVOLUTION OF THE UTERUS

Subinvolution refers to a slower-than-expected return of the uterus to its nonpregnant size after childbirth. Normally, the uterus descends at the rate of approximately 1 cm or one fingerbreadth per day. By 2 weeks, it is no longer palpable above the symphysis pubis. The endometrial lining has sloughed off as part of the lochia, and the site of placental attachment is well healed by 6 weeks after childbirth.

The most common causes of subinvolution are retained placental fragments and pelvic infection. Signs of subinvolution include prolonged discharge of lochia, irregular or excessive uterine bleeding, and sometimes profuse hemorrhage. Many women report pelvic pain or feelings of pelvic heaviness, backache, fatigue, and persistent malaise. On bimanual examination, the uterus feels larger and softer than normal for that point in time postpartum.

Therapeutic Management

Treatment is tailored to correct the cause of subinvolution. Oral methylergonovine maleate (Methergine) provides sustained contraction of the uterus. Infection responds to antimicrobial therapy.

Nursing Considerations

In most cases, subinvolution is not obvious until the mother has returned home after childbirth. For this reason, nurses must teach the mother and her family how to assess for the condition and how to recognize its occurrence.

The nurse should demonstrate how to palpate the fundus and how to estimate fundal height in relation to the umbilicus. The uterus should become smaller each day (by approximately one fingerbreadth). The nurse also explains the progressive changes from lochia rubra, to lochia serosa, and then to lochia alba (see Chapter 21).

The mother is instructed to report any deviation from the expected pattern or duration of lochia. A foul odor often indicates uterine infection. Additional signs include pelvic or fundal pain, backache, or feelings of pelvic pressure or fullness.

THROMBOEMBOLIC DISORDERS

The three most common thromboembolic disorders encountered during pregnancy and the postpartum period are superficial venous thrombosis, deep venous thrombosis, and pulmonary embolism. Superficial venous thrombosis usually involves the saphenous venous system and is confined to the lower leg. Deep venous thrombosis can involve veins from the foot to the iliofemoral region. It is a major concern because it predisposes to pulmonary embolism. Pulmonary embolism is a potentially fatal complication that occurs when the pulmonary artery is obstructed by a blood clot that was swept into circulation from a vein.

Incidence

The incidence of thromboembolic disease in pregnancy and the puerperium is approximately 1 per 1000 pregnancies and is divided equally between pregnancy and the puerperium (Cunningham et al., 2001). It remains a major cause of maternal death in the United States.

Etiology

A *thrombus* is a collection of blood factors, primarily platelets and fibrin, on a vessel wall. Once started, the thrombus can enlarge with successive layering of platelets, fibrin, and blood cells as the blood flows past the clot. Thrombus formation is often associated with an inflammatory process in the vessel wall, which is termed *thrombophlebitis*.

The three major causes of thrombosis are venous stasis, hypercoagulable blood, and injury to the intima (the innermost layer) of the blood vessel. Venous stasis and hypercoagulable blood are present in all pregnancies.

Venous Stasis
During pregnancy, compression of the large vessels of the pelvis and legs by the enlarging uterus causes venous stasis. Stasis is most pronounced when the pregnant woman stands for prolonged periods. It results in dilated vessels and the potential for continued pooling of blood postpartum. Prolonged time in stirrups during birth and repair of the episiotomy may also promote venous stasis and increase the risk for thrombus formation.

Hypercoagulation
Pregnancy also causes changes in the coagulation and fibrinolytic systems that persist in the postpartal period. During pregnancy, the levels of most coagulation factors are elevated. In addition, the fibrinolytic system (plasminogen activator and antithrombin III) is suppressed, which hinders clot disintegration (lysis). The net result is that factors that promote clot formation are increased to prevent maternal hem-

---

> **BOX 28-2**
> *Factors That Increase the Risk for Thrombosis*
>
> - Inactivity
> - Obesity
> - Cesarean birth
> - Smoking
> - History of previous thrombosis
> - Varicose veins
> - Diabetes mellitus
> - Prolonged time in stirrups in second stage of labor
> - Maternal age older than 35 years
> - Parity greater than 3

orrhage and factors that prevent clot formation are decreased, resulting in a higher risk for thrombus formation.

Blood Vessel Injury
Injury to the intima of the blood vessel occasionally occurs during cesarean births and could trigger a pelvic vein thrombosis. Thrombosis is nine times more likely to occur if the birth was cesarean (Laros, 2004).

Additional Predisposing Factors
Factors that create additional risk include varicose veins, obesity, a history of thrombophlebitis, using oral contraceptives before pregnancy, and smoking. Women older than 35 years or who are multiparas are also at increased risk (Box 28-2).

Superficial Venous Thrombosis
Manifestations
Superficial venous thrombosis is often seen in association with varicose veins and usually limited to the calf area. Signs and symptoms include swelling of the involved extremity as well as redness, tenderness, and warmth. It may be possible to palpate the enlarged, hardened vein. Women may experience pain when they walk, but some women have no signs at all.

Therapeutic Management
Treatment includes analgesics, rest, and elastic support. Elevation of the lower extremity improves venous return. Warm packs may be applied to promote healing. There is no need for anticoagulants unless the condition persists. After a period of bed rest, the woman may ambulate gradually if symptoms have disappeared. She should avoid standing for long periods and continue to wear support hose to help prevent venous stasis and a subsequent episode of superficial thrombosis. There is little chance of pulmonary embolism if the thrombosis remains in the superficial veins of the lower leg.

Deep Venous Thrombosis
Signs and symptoms of deep venous thrombosis are often absent or diffuse. If they are present, they are caused by an inflammatory process and obstruction of venous return. Leg swelling (more than 2 cm larger than the opposite calf), erythema, heat, tenderness, and edema are the most common signs.

It is a common belief that a positive Homans sign (presence of pain behind the knee when the foot is dorsiflexed) is an indicator of deep venous thrombosis in postpartum women, but Homans sign has proved to be of little value in the diagnosis because the sign may be absent in women who have a venous thrombosis. When present, the pain may be caused by a strained muscle or contusion.

Reflex arterial spasms may cause the leg to become pale and cool to the touch with decreased peripheral pulses. At one time, this condition was called *milk-leg*. Additional symptoms may include pain on ambulation, chills, general malaise, and stiffness of the affected leg.

Diagnostic Evaluation

Ultrasonography of the deep veins of the upper legs is most commonly used to detect alterations in blood flow diagnostic of deep venous thrombosis. Magnetic resonance imaging (MRI) may be used for pelvic veins. Impedance plethysmography, which measures changes in venous blood volume and flow, is less often used. Venography is an accurate method for diagnosing deep venous thrombosis but may cause pain, anaphylaxis, and radiation exposure (Clarke-Pearson, 2000).

Therapeutic Management

Preventing Thrombus Formation. Women who have had a previous deep vein thrombosis or pulmonary embolism are at risk to have another. During pregnancy, they may be placed on prophylactic heparin, which does not cross the placenta. Standard (unfractionated) heparin or a low molecular weight heparin such as enoxaparin (Lovenox) may be used. Heparin is discontinued during labor and birth and resumed 4 to 12 hours after childbirth (Bobrowski & Dzieczkowski, 2002).

During childbirth, stirrups should be padded to prevent prolonged pressure against the popliteal angle during the second stage of labor. It may also be possible to decrease the time in stirrups to no more than 1 hour.

To prevent thrombus formation after childbirth, the mother should ambulate frequently and as early as possible to prevent stasis of blood. If she is unable to ambulate, range-of-motion and gentle leg exercises, such as flexing and straightening the knee and raising one leg at a time, should begin within 8 hours after childbirth. In addition, the mother should avoid using pillows under her knees or the knee gatch on the bed because sharp flexion at the knees and pressure on the popliteal space cause pooling of blood in the lower extremities.

Antiembolism stockings or sequential compression devices are used for mothers with varicose veins, a history of thrombosis, or cesarean birth. The stockings should be applied before the mother gets out of bed, to prevent venous congestion when she stands. It is important that she understand the correct way to put on the antiembolism stockings because they can roll or bunch, slowing venous return from the legs if improperly applied.

Initial Treatment. The mother is placed on bed rest, with the affected leg elevated to decrease interstitial swelling and to promote venous return from that leg. She is allowed to ambulate gradually when all symptoms have disappeared and should wear elastic stockings. Anticoagulant therapy may be started with a continuous intravenous infusion or subcutaneous heparin injections to delay the clotting time of the blood and prevent extension of the thrombus. Activated partial thromboplastin time should be monitored, and the heparin dose should be adjusted to maintain a therapeutic level of 1.5 to 2.5 times the control (Laros, 2004). If enoxaparin is used, it is given subcutaneously and requires less frequent laboratory monitoring. The mother receives analgesics to control pain and antibiotic therapy, as necessary. Moist heat provides relief of pain and increases circulation.

Subsequent Treatment. The long-term management of deep venous thrombosis depends on whether the woman is pregnant or in the postpartum period. After several days of treatment with heparin, the postpartum woman is started on warfarin (Coumadin), which is often continued for 4 to 6 months or longer. Prothrombin time and the international normalized ratio (INR) are used to monitor coagulation time when warfarin is used. The INR corrects for variations in the potency of the thromboplastins used by different laboratories. An appropriate ratio for treatment of deep venous thrombosis is 2.0 to 3.0 (Bobrowski & Dzieczkowski, 2002).

Warfarin is contraindicated during pregnancy because of teratogenic effects and the risk for fetal hemorrhage. Therefore pregnant women are given heparin, which is administered by continuous infusion or subcutaneously. Heparin does not cross the placenta.

WOMEN
Want to Know

How Do I Prevent Thrombosis?

Methods to improve peripheral circulation help prevent the occurrence of thrombophlebitis. Especially important are these measures:

- Improve your circulation with a regular schedule of activity, preferably walking.
- Avoid prolonged standing or sitting in one position.
- When sitting, elevate your legs and avoid crossing them. This position increases the return of venous blood from the legs.
- Maintain a daily fluid intake of at least 2500 ml (approximately 2 1/2 quarts) to prevent dehydration and consequent sluggish circulation.
- Stop smoking.

▪NURSING CARE
The Mother with Deep Venous Thrombosis

Assessment

Assessment focuses on determining the status of the venous thrombosis. Palpate the pedal pulses to determine presence, equality, and strength. Inspect the leg for unusual warmth or redness, which indicates inflammation, and for unusual coolness or cyanosis, which indicates venous obstruction. Compare the affected and unaffected leg for size and color and measure the circumference to obtain an accurate estimation of the edema. Ask the woman about discomfort. Pain is caused by tissue hypoxia, and increasing pain indicates progressive obstruction.

Evaluate the laboratory reports of clotting studies. In addition to activated partial thromboplastin time, whole-blood partial thromboplastin time and platelets may be evaluated when heparin is used. Thrombocytopenia (low platelet count) is a concern when heparin is administered for a prolonged period. The INR is evaluated when the anticoagulant for the postpartum woman is changed to warfarin.

Nursing Diagnosis and Planning

The treatment of deep venous thrombosis includes the administration of anticoagulants for a prolonged period. As a result, the collaborative problem *hemorrhage secondary to anticoagulation therapy* is one of the most troubling potential complications. Planning should reflect the nurse's responsibility to:

- Monitor for signs of hemorrhage.
- Consult with the physician if signs of hemorrhage are observed.
- Perform actions that will minimize the risk for hemorrhage.

Interventions

Monitoring for Signs of Bleeding

At least twice a day, assess the mother for the appearance of bruising or petechiae. Instruct her to report the appearance of any bleeding: bloody nose, blood in urine, bleeding gums, or increased vaginal bleeding. The nurse must be alert to signs of hemorrhage, such as tachycardia, falling blood pressure, or other signs of shock that may indicate internal bleeding.

Unless frank hemorrhage is present, the usual treatment for excessive anticoagulation is to temporarily discontinue the anticoagulant. Protamine sulfate, the antidote for heparin, should, however, be available. The antidote for warfarin is vitamin K.

Explaining Continued Therapy

Carefully explain the treatment regimen, including the schedule of medication and possible side effects, such as unexplained fever, unusual fatigue, or sore throat (signs of agranulocytosis or diminished number of neutrophils). It is important to caution the mother not to "double up" if a dose is missed. The mother and another family member should learn how to inject heparin, if necessary.

Emphasize the importance of keeping the health care provider informed about any medications the mother takes, because oral anticoagulants are associated with many drug interactions. Common over-the-counter medications such as aspirin and nonsteroidal antiinflammatory drugs increase the risk for hemorrhage. The woman should understand that any unusual bleeding should be reported.

Suggest that the mother use a soft toothbrush and floss her teeth gently to prevent bleeding from the gums. She should postpone dental appointments until the therapy is completed. A depilatory to remove unwanted hair is safer than a razor during anticoagulant therapy. Remind the mother to avoid activities that may cause injury, and caution her about using alcohol, which inhibits the metabolism of oral anticoagulants.

Helping the Family Adapt to Home Care

Nurses often assist the family to adapt to home care. Assess the family structure and function to determine how prepared the family is to cope with the mother's illness. Determine the ages of the children and availability of family members or friends to help while the mother is confined to bed or on limited activity. Although the health of the mother is of primary importance, care must be taken that the attachment process between her and the infant progresses normally.

Evaluation

- Does the woman maintain therapeutic levels of her anticoagulant?
- Is she free from signs of unusual bleeding or other side effects of the medication?

PULMONARY EMBOLISM

Pathophysiology

Pulmonary embolism is a rare but dreaded complication of deep venous thrombosis. It occurs when fragments of a blood clot are carried to the lungs. The embolus occludes a vessel and obstructs the flow of blood into the lungs, either entirely or partially. If pulmonary circulation is severely compromised, death may occur within a few minutes. If the embolus is small, adequate pulmonary circulation may be maintained until treatment can be initiated.

Manifestations

Sudden, sharp chest pain, tachypnea, dyspnea, cough, pulmonary rales, and hemoptysis are the most common signs of pulmonary embolus. Arterial blood gas determinations show decreased partial pressure of oxygen, and chest radiography reveals areas of atelectasis and pleural effusion.

Therapeutic Management

Treatment of pulmonary embolism is aimed at dissolving the clot and maintaining pulmonary circulation. Heparin therapy is initiated and is continued throughout pregnancy if the embolism occurs at that time. During the postpartum, heparin can be switched to warfarin and continued for approximately 4 to 6 months (Laros, 2004). Oxygen is used to decrease hypoxia, and narcotic analgesics are used to reduce pain and apprehension. The woman is kept on bed rest, with the head of the bed slightly elevated to reduce dyspnea. Intensive care, support of ventilation, and other measures depend on her pulmonary status. Pulse oximetry should be initiated, and arterial blood gases should be evaluated.

Nursing Considerations

Monitoring for Signs

When caring for a woman with deep venous thrombosis, nurses look for early signs and symptoms of pulmonary embolism. Observation includes frequent assessment of respiratory rate and auscultation of breath sounds. Abnormalities, such as diminished or unequal breath sounds or coughing, should be reported immediately to the health care provider. Additional signs that require immediate attention include air hunger, dyspnea, tachycardia, pallor, and cyanosis.

Facilitating Oxygenation

Oxygen should be administered by tight facemask. The nurse should remain with the mother to allay fear and apprehension. The head of the bed should be raised to facilitate breathing. Narcotic analgesics, such as morphine, may be used to relieve pain.

Seeking Assistance

The woman's condition is precarious until the clot is lysed or until it adheres to the pulmonary artery wall and is reabsorbed. The primary nurse should call for assistance to initiate interventions. These include intravenous administration of heparin, continuous assessment of vital signs, and administration of any emergency drugs that may be needed. The woman who has pulmonary embolism requires critical care nursing skills and is usually transferred to an intensive care unit.

PUERPERAL INFECTION

Puerperal infection is a term used to describe bacterial infections after childbirth. Infection occurs in 3% of all women who have had vaginal births; it occurs in 15% to 20% of those who have had cesarean births with prophylactic antibiotics; and it occurs in 30% to 35% if cesarean birth is after prolonged labor and rupture of membranes without antibiotic prophylaxis (Duff, 2002; Gibbs, Sweet, & Duff, 2004). Until the advent of antibiotics, puerperal infection often resulted in death. Even today, it is one of the leading causes of maternal deaths.

The most common postpartum infections are metritis, wound infections, urinary tract infections, mastitis, and septic pelvic thrombophlebitis.

Definition

The definition of puerperal infection is a fever of 38° C (100.4° F) or higher occurring on at least 2 of the first 10 days after the first 24 hours following childbirth. Although a slight elevation of temperature may occur during the first 24 hours because of dehydration or the exertion of labor, any mother with fever should be assessed for other signs of infection.

Pathophysiology

Every part of the reproductive tract is connected to every other part, and organisms can move from the vagina, through the cervix, into the uterus, and out the fallopian tubes to infect the ovaries and the peritoneal cavity. The entire reproductive tract is particularly well supplied with blood vessels during pregnancy and after childbirth. Blood vessels or lymphatics can carry the infection to the rest of the body, which can result in life-threatening septicemia.

The normal physiologic changes of childbirth increase the risk for infection. During labor, the acidity of the vagina is reduced by the amniotic fluid, blood, and lochia, which are alkaline. An alkaline environment encourages growth of bacteria.

Necrosis of the endometrial lining and the presence of lochia provide a favorable environment for the growth of anaerobic bacteria. Many small lacerations, some microscopic in size, occur in the endometrium, cervix, and vagina during birth and allow bacteria to enter the tissue. Although the uterine interior is not sterile until 3 to 4 weeks after childbirth, infection does not develop in most women, partly because granulocytes in the lochia and endometrium prevent infection.

Etiology

Other factors may predispose a woman to infection (Table 28-2). Cesarean birth is a major predisposing factor. This is because of the trauma to the tissues, the incision that provides an entrance for bacteria, possible contamination during surgery, and foreign bodies such as sutures that can promote infection. In addition, women who must have a surgical delivery because of a problem that develops during labor may have other risk factors, such as prolonged labor, that raise the chances of infection. Colonization of the vagina with organisms also predisposes to the development of infection after childbirth.

Any trauma to maternal tissues increases the hazard of infection. Trauma may occur with rapid delivery, birth of a large infant, use of forceps or a vacuum extractor, or manual delivery of the placenta, as well as lacerations and episiotomies. Catheterization during labor increases the chance of introduction of organisms into the bladder and adds to the urinary tract trauma that occurs during normal childbirth.

With prolonged rupture of membranes during labor, organisms from the vagina are more likely to ascend into the uterine cavity, especially if more than 24 hours pass before delivery. A long labor or many vaginal examinations during labor increase the danger of infection. Each vaginal examination increases the possibility of contamination from gloves or from organisms in the vagina being pushed through the open cervix. Use of a fetal scalp electrode or intrauterine pressure catheter has the same effect. If part of the placenta remains inside the uterus after delivery, the tissue becomes necrotic and provides a good place for bacteria to grow.

Additional factors include postpartum hemorrhage, which causes loss of infection-fighting components of the blood such as leukocytes and leaves the mother in a weakened condition. Prenatal conditions such as poor nutrition or anemia interfere with the mother's ability to resist infection. Lack of knowledge of hygiene or lack of access to facilities that permit adequate hygiene increases the risk for postpartum infection.

Specific Infections

Metritis

Infections of the uterus have been called *endometritis*, *endomyometritis*, and *endoparametritis*. The preferred term is *metritis with pelvic cellulitis* because infection involves the decidua, myometrium, and parametrial tissues (Cunningham et al., 2001).

Etiology. Metritis is usually caused by organisms that are normal inhabitants of the vagina and cervix. Most infections are polymicrobial with both aerobic and anaerobic organisms involved. Organisms most often found include group B streptococci, enterococci, *Escherichia coli*, *Klebsiella pneumoniae*, *Proteus*, *Bacteroides*, and *Prevotella*. *Chlamydia trachomatis* is not a cause of early infection but is associated with late onset infections (Gibbs, Sweet, & Duff, 2004).

Manifestations. The major signs and symptoms of metritis are fever, chills, malaise, anorexia, abdominal pain and cramping, uterine tenderness, and purulent, foul-smelling lochia. Additional signs include tachycardia and subinvolution. In most cases, the signs and symptoms occur within the first 24 to 48 hours after delivery (Gibbs, Sweet, & Duff, 2004). When the causative organisms are group A beta-hemolytic streptococci, however, the lochia may be scant and odorless and the woman may exhibit no signs except fever.

TABLE **28-2** Risk Factors for Puerperal Infection

Risk Factor	Reason
History of previous infections (urinary tract infection, mastitis, thrombophlebitis)	May be more vulnerable to infectious process
Colonization of lower genital tract with pathogenic organisms	Infections usually caused by several microbes that have ascended to the uterus from the lower genital tract
Cesarean birth	Increased portals of infection
Trauma	Provides entrance for bacteria and makes tissues more susceptible
Prolonged rupture of membranes	Allows access for organisms to interior of uterus
Prolonged labor	Increases number of vaginal examinations and allows time for bacteria to multiply
Catheterization	Could introduce organisms into bladder
Excessive number of vaginal examinations	Increases chance that organisms from vagina or outside source are carried into the uterus
Retained placental fragments	Provide growth medium for bacteria and may interfere with flow of lochia
Hemorrhage	Loss of infection-fighting components of blood
Poor general health (excessive fatigue, anemia, frequent minor illnesses)	Increases vulnerability to infections and complications of labor
Poor nutrition (decreased protein, vitamin C)	Less able to repair tissue and defend against infection
Poor hygiene	Excessive exposure to pathogens
Medical conditions, such as diabetes mellitus	Decreases ability to defend against infections of any kind
Low socioeconomic status	More likely to have poor nutrition and inadequate prenatal care

Laboratory data may confirm the diagnosis. The results of a complete blood count may show an elevation of leukocytes, although leukocytes are normally elevated to as high as 30,000 during the early postpartum time (Cunningham et al., 2001). Continued elevations should lead to further evaluation. Specimens may be taken from the blood, endocervix, and uterine cavity for cultures. A catheterized urine specimen should also be obtained.

Therapeutic Management. Intravenous administration of antibiotics is the initial treatment for metritis. Broad-spectrum antibiotics, such as clindamycin plus gentamicin, are often used. Other drugs include ampicillin, cephalosporins, and metronidazole.

Improvement in clinical signs usually follows within 48 to 72 hours. Oral antibiotics are usually unnecessary after completion of intravenous treatment. Many physicians give a single dose of a prophylactic IV antibiotic to women having a cesarean birth or at particular risk for infection. The antibiotic is given during surgery just after the umbilical cord is clamped to avoid exposure of the infant to the drug. Other drugs include antipyretics for fever and oxytocics, such as methylergonovine, to increase drainage of lochia and promote involution.

Complications. If the infection spreads outside the uterine cavity, there may be infection of the fallopian tubes (*salpingitis*) or the ovaries (*oophoritis*), which could result in sterility. *Peritonitis* (inflammation of the membrane lining the walls of the abdominal and pelvic cavities) may occur and lead to formation of a pelvic abscess. In addition, the risk for pelvic thrombophlebitis is increased when pathogenic bacteria enter the bloodstream during episodes of metritis. Figure 28-4 illustrates complications of metritis.

Signs and symptoms that the infection is spreading may be similar to those of metritis, but more severe. Fever and abdominal pain will be particularly pronounced. Peritonitis may result in paralytic ileus and a distended, board-like abdomen with absent bowel sounds.

Nursing Considerations. The mother with metritis should be placed in a Fowler's position to promote drainage of lochia.

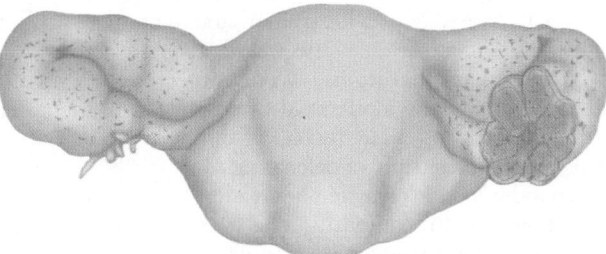

Salpingitis: Infection in fallopian tubes causes them to become enlarged, hyperemic, and tender.

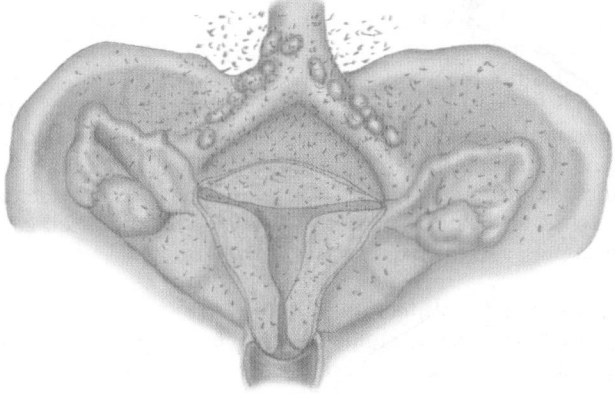

Peritonitis: Infection spreads through the lymphatics to the peritoneum; a pelvic abscess may form.

Figure 28-4 Areas of spread of uterine infection.

She may be medicated as needed for abdominal pain or cramping, which may be severe. The nurse should observe the mother for signs of improvement or new symptoms, such as nausea and vomiting, abdominal distention, absent bowel sounds, and severe abdominal pain. Comfort measures include warm blankets, cool compresses, cold or warm drinks, or a heating pad.

Teaching incorporates signs and symptoms of worsening condition, side effects of therapy, and the importance of adhering to the treatment plan and follow-up care. If the woman must be separated from her infant, a nursing diagnosis of Risk for Impaired Parenting related to separation from infant should be considered. If the mother is breastfeeding, she will need help to pump her breasts to establish and maintain lactation.

Wound Infection

Wound infections are common types of puerperal infection because any break in the skin or mucous membrane provides a portal for bacteria. The most common sites are cesarean surgical incisions; the perineum, where episiotomies and lacerations are common; and the vagina.

Manifestations. Signs of wound infection are edema, warmth, redness, tenderness, and pain. The edges of the wound may pull apart, and seropurulent drainage may be present. If the wound remains untreated, generalized signs of infection, such as fever and malaise, may develop as well. As with other puerperal infections, cultures may reveal mixed aerobic and anaerobic bacteria.

Therapeutic Management. An incision and drainage of the affected area may be necessary. Broad-spectrum antibiotics are ordered until a report of the organism is returned. Analgesics are often necessary, and warm compresses or sitz baths may be used to provide comfort and to promote healing by increasing circulation to the area.

Nursing Considerations. Wound infections are painful and annoying to the mother out of proportion to their size. Perineal infections cause discomfort during many activities, such as walking, sitting, or defecating.

Wound infections may require readmittance to the hospital or home health care visits. The woman requires reassurance and supportive care. If at home, she needs teaching about sitz baths, warm compresses, and frequent perineal care. She is taught to wipe from front to back and to change perineal pads frequently. Good handwashing techniques are emphasized. Adequate fluid intake and diet are important. Activity may be modified depending on the site, severity, and treatment of the wound infection.

The infant is not routinely isolated from the mother with a wound infection, but she must be advised to protect her infant from contact with contaminated articles, such as dressings. Anticipatory guidance should include teaching side effects of medication, signs of worsening condition, self-care measures, and the importance of handwashing.

Urinary Tract Infections

Etiology. During childbirth, the bladder and urethra are traumatized by pressure from the descending fetus. Insertion of a catheter, with its risk for infection, occurs at least once during many labors. After childbirth, the bladder and urethra are hypotonic, with urinary stasis and retention common problems. Residual urine and reflux of urine may occur during voiding. Women who had bacteria in the urine during pregnancy, often without symptoms, are at increased risk for postpartum urinary tract infections. Coliform bacteria such as *E. coli* are a common cause.

Manifestations. Symptoms typically begin on the 1st or 2nd postpartum day. They include dysuria (a burning pain on urination), urgency, and frequency of urination. A low-grade fever is sometimes the only sign. In some women, an upper urinary tract infection, such as pyelonephritis, may develop on the 3rd or 4th day, with chills, spiking fever, costovertebral angle tenderness, flank pain, and nausea and vomiting. If not promptly treated, this infection of the kidney pelvis may result in permanent damage to the kidney.

Therapeutic Management. Most urinary tract infections can be treated with antibiotics on an outpatient basis. Pyelonephritis during pregnancy may require IV hydration and IV administration of broad-spectrum antibiotics. If the postpartum woman is only moderately ill, she can be treated with oral antibiotics at home.

Nursing Considerations. The woman with a urinary tract infection must be instructed to take the medication for the entire time it is prescribed and not to stop when symptoms abate. In addition, she must drink at least 3000 ml of fluid each day to help dilute the bacterial burden and flush the infection from the bladder. Acidification of the urine inhibits multiplication of bacteria, and drinks that acidify urine, such as apricot, plum, prune, or cranberry juices, are frequently recommended. Carbonated drinks should be avoided because they increase urine alkalinity.

Teaching should also include measures to prevent urinary tract infections, such as proper perineal care, increasing fluid intake, and urinating frequently.

Mastitis

Mastitis, an infection of the lactating breast, occurs most often during the 2nd and 3rd weeks after childbirth, although it may develop at any time during breastfeeding. It usually affects only one breast.

Etiology. Mastitis is often caused by *Staphylococcus aureus*. The bacteria are most often carried on the hands of the mother or agency staff or in the mouth of the newborn. The organism may enter through an injured area of the nipple, such as a crack or blister, although there may be no obvious signs of injury. Soreness of a nipple may result in insufficient emptying of the breast because of pain during breastfeeding.

Engorgement and stasis of milk frequently precede mastitis, often when a feeding is skipped, when the infant begins to sleep through the night, or when breastfeeding is suddenly stopped. Constriction of the breasts from a bra that is too tight may interfere with emptying of all the ducts and may lead to infection. The mother who is fatigued or stressed or who has other health problems that might lower her immune system is also at increased risk for mastitis.

Manifestations. Initial symptoms may be flu-like with fatigue and aching muscles. Symptoms progress to include fever of 38.4° C (101.1° F) or higher, chills, malaise, and headache. Mastitis is characterized by a localized area of redness and inflammation (Figure 28-5).

Therapeutic Management. Antibiotic therapy and continued emptying of the breast by breastfeeding or breast pump constitute the first line of treatment. With early antibiotic treatment, mastitis usually resolves within 24 to 48 hours. Approximately 5% of women develop a breast abscess, which is treated with surgical drainage and antibiotics (Gibbs, Sweet, & Duff, 2004).

Supportive measures include application of heat or ice packs, breast support, and analgesics. The mother should continue to breastfeed from both breasts. If the affected breast is too sore, a breast pump can be used. Regular emptying of the breast is important in preventing abscess formation. If an abscess forms and ruptures into the breast ducts, breastfeeding on that side should be discontinued and a

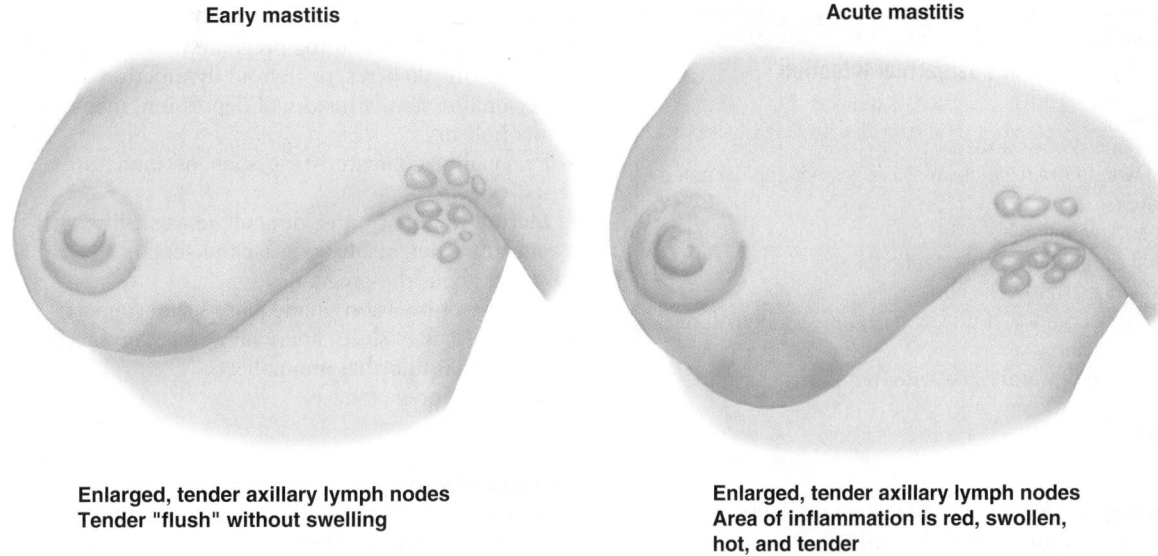

Early mastitis

Enlarged, tender axillary lymph nodes
Tender "flush" without swelling

Acute mastitis

Enlarged, tender axillary lymph nodes
Area of inflammation is red, swollen,
hot, and tender

Figure 28-5 Mastitis is an infection that usually occurs 2 to 3 weeks after childbirth in the breast of a woman who breastfeeds.

breast pump used to empty the breast temporarily. Milk obtained should be discarded (Lawrence & Lawrence, 1999).

Nursing Considerations. Because mastitis rarely occurs before discharge from the birth facility, the nurse must provide information for prevention. Measures to prevent mastitis include correct positioning of the infant and avoiding nipple trauma and milk stasis. The mother should breastfeed every 2 to 3 hours. She should avoid formula supplements and nipple shields, and she should change nursing pads when they are wet. She should also avoid continuous pressure on the breasts from tight bras or infant carriers.

Once mastitis occurs, nursing measures are aimed at increasing comfort and helping the mother maintain lactation. Moist heat promotes comfort and increases circulation. A shower or hot packs should be used before feeding or pumping the breasts. Cold packs can be used between feedings to reduce edema. The woman should complete the entire course of antibiotics to prevent recurrence or a breast abscess.

The breast should be completely emptied at each feeding to prevent stasis of milk, which can result in an abscess. If the mother is too sore to breastfeed on the affected side or if she is taking antibiotics that are contraindicated during lactation, she should be instructed to express the milk or use a pump to empty the breasts. Breastfeeding or pumping every 1 1/2 to 2 hours makes the mother more comfortable and prevents stasis. Starting the feeding on the unaffected side causes the milk-ejection reflex to occur in the painful breast and makes the process more efficient. Massage over the affected area before and during the feeding helps ensure complete emptying. The mother should stay in bed during the acute phase of her illness. Her fluid intake should be 3000 ml/day. Analgesics may be required to relieve discomfort.

The mother with mastitis is likely to be very discouraged and may need much encouragement. Some mothers decide to stop breastfeeding because of the discomfort involved. Weaning during an episode of mastitis may increase engorgement and stasis, leading to abscess formation or recurrent infection. Therefore the nurse should encourage the mother to continue breastfeeding.

Septic Pelvic Thrombophlebitis

Septic pelvic thrombophlebitis is the least common of the puerperal infections. It usually occurs 2 to 4 days after childbirth. It occurs when infection spreads along the venous system and thrombophlebitis develops. It is seen more often in women with wound infection and usually involves the ovarian, uterine, or hypogastric veins.

Manifestations. The primary symptom is pain in the groin, abdomen, or flank. Fever, tachycardia, gastrointestinal distress, and decreased bowel sounds may be present. Laboratory data may be used to exclude other diagnoses and usually include complete blood count with differential, blood chemistries, coagulation studies, and cultures. The only sign may be fever that does not respond to antibiotic therapy.

Therapeutic Management. Readmittance to the hospital is usually necessary. Treatment includes anticoagulation therapy with intravenous heparin and usually results in reduction of fever within 12 to 36 hours (Laros, 2004). Intravenous antibiotics are also given. Supportive care is similar to that for deep venous thrombosis and includes monitoring for safe levels of anticoagulation therapy and for signs and symptoms of pulmonary embolism.

▪ NURSING CARE
The Woman With an Infection

Assessment

Although all women are observed for indications of infection as part of routine nursing assessments, the nurse must practice increased vigilance for mothers who are at increased risk for infection.

Assessment focuses on signs that may be expected in infection, such as fever, tachycardia, pain, or unusual amount, color, or odor of lochia. Generalized symptoms of malaise and muscle aching may also be significant. Examine all wounds each shift for signs of localized infection, such as redness, edema, tenderness, discharge, or pulling apart of incisions or sutured lacerations. Ask the mother about difficulty emptying her bladder or discomfort related to urination.

Evaluate the mother's knowledge of hygiene practices that prevent infections, such as proper handwashing, perineal care, and handling of perineal pads. Also important are her knowledge of breastfeeding and the presence of problems that might result in breast engorgement and stasis of milk in the ducts. Examine the nipples for signs of injury that might provide a portal of entry for organisms.

Nursing Diagnosis and Planning

Because all women are at risk for infection after childbirth, most facilities have developed standards of practice that protect postpartum women from infection, and individual nursing care plans are usually not necessary. When predisposing factors increase the likelihood of infection, however, routine assessments and care may need to be modified and preventive measures intensified. In this case, the most relevant nursing diagnosis is

■ Risk for Infection related to the presence of significant risk factors.

The Nursing Care Plan: Postpartum Infection develops goals and interventions for this nursing diagnosis.

MOOD DISORDERS

Mood disorders are disturbances in function, affect, or thought processes that can affect the family after childbirth as severely as physiologic problems. They include postpartum blues, postpartum depression, and postpartum psychosis. Postpartum blues is a transient, self-limiting mood disorder, which is discussed in Chapter 21. Postpartum depression and postpartum psychosis are more serious disorders that disrupt the family and require intervention to resolve.

Postpartum Depression

Incidence
Postpartum depression (PPD) occurs in 15% to 20% of women (Hayashi & Zettelmaier, 2000). Many investigators believe that PPD is underdiagnosed and underreported. It usually develops within the first 3 months but may occur at any time during the first 12 months postpartum.

Etiology
The cause of PPD is unknown. Abrupt changes in hormone levels and the major life changes involved in childbirth may be involved. Factors believed to increase the risk for its occurrence include:

- Hormonal fluctuations that follow childbirth
- Medical problems during pregnancy, such as preeclampsia, preexisting diabetes, or thyroid dysfunction
- Personal or family history of depression, mental illness, or alcoholism
- Personality characteristics, such as immaturity and low self-esteem
- Marital dysfunction or difficult relationship with the significant other, resulting in lack of support
- Anger about the pregnancy
- Feelings of isolation, inadequate social support
- Fatigue, lack of sleep, financial worries, and birth of an infant who is ill or has anomalies
- Multifetal pregnancy
- Chronic stressors

Manifestations
The woman experiencing PPD shows less interest in her surroundings and a loss of her usual emotional response toward her family. Although she cares for the infant, she is unable to feel pleasure or love. She sees the infant as demanding and feels she is inept at mothering. The woman may have intense feelings of unworthiness, guilt, and shame. Generalized fatigue, complaints of ill health, and difficulty in concentrating or making decisions are also present. She often has little interest in food, may have weight changes, and experiences sleep disturbances. She may describe panic attacks, relentless obsessive thinking, and suicidal thoughts. Most of the symptoms are intensely and consistently present for at least a 2-week period.

Impact on the Family
Postpartum depression creates strain on the family's usual methods of coping and often causes difficulties in relationships. Stressors tend to be magnified, and as a result, family members may decrease their interactions with the depressed mother when she needs support the most. Communication is impaired because she gradually withdraws from contact with others. The decreased libido commonly associated with depression may also affect her relationship with her significant other.

Partners of depressed women report a sense of loss of the partner and the relationship they had known previously, feelings of loss of control, anger, and frustration. Fathers may take on household chores and child care that the depressed mother is unable to manage. They may also suffer from depression (Meighan, Davis, Thomas, & Droppleman, 1999).

Depressed mothers interact differently with their infants than do women who are not depressed. They appear tense, are more irritable, and feel less competent as mothers. They may not pick up on their infants' cues or smiles, thus failing to meet the infants' needs and to enjoy their positive feedback (Beck, 1995). Infants of depressed mothers tend to be fussier and more discontented, and they make fewer positive facial expressions.

Therapeutic Management
Early treatment of PPD is important because it shortens the length of depression. A combination of psychotherapy, social support, and medication may be used. The woman's partner and immediate family must be included in counseling sessions so they can develop an understanding of what the woman feels and needs.

Selective serotonin reuptake inhibitors are commonly prescribed medications. They have few side effects and have

Nursing Care Plan

Postpartum Infection

ASSESSMENT

Lisa Pyle, a thin, pale, 16-year-old primipara, is admitted to the postpartum unit after a cesarean birth. She was in labor for 16 hours before the birth, and her membranes were ruptured for 14 hours. She was catheterized twice during labor and now has an indwelling catheter. She plans to breastfeed her infant.

Nursing Diagnosis

Risk for Infection related to presence of favorable conditions for infections.

Goals/Expected Outcomes

Lisa will:
- Remain free of signs of infection during the postpartum period.
- Verbalize methods of prevention of infection and signs that infection may be present by discharge.

INTERVENTION	RATIONALE
1. Assess vital signs every 4 hours.	1. Temperature above 38° C (100.4° F) or tachycardia suggests an infectious process and should be reported.
2. Observe the surgical incision for redness, tenderness, or edema and note odor of lochia every 4 hours. Ask Lisa if she experiences frequency, urgency, or pain with urination when the catheter is removed.	2. Redness, pain, or swelling of the incision suggests wound infection. Foul odor of lochia suggests endometrial infection. Frequency, urgency, or painful urination may indicate urinary tract infection.
3. Instruct Lisa in hygienic practices to prevent infection: a. Careful handwashing before and after perineal care. b. Perineal cleansing after elimination. c. Changing peripads frequently. d. Wiping the perineum from front to back.	3. Handwashing is the most important defense against infection and its spread. Perineal cleansing helps prevent growth of bacteria. Frequent pad changes remove accumulated lochia, which provides an excellent culture for bacteria. Wiping from front to back prevents fecal contamination of the vagina.
4. Initiate measures to reduce the risk for urinary tract infection: a. Provide fluids of Lisa's choice when she is able to take them, and emphasize the importance of drinking 2500 to 3000 ml/day. b. Monitor bladder distention to prevent overfilling. Teach Lisa the importance of emptying her bladder every 2 to 3 hours during the first days after childbirth. c. Use methods to promote bladder emptying, such as running water in the shower or sink, running warm water over the perineum, and providing pain medication as needed.	4. Adequate hydration and frequent emptying of the bladder help prevent stasis of urine, which increases the risk for urinary tract infection. Relief of pain may allow the mother to relax enough to void. The sound of running water may stimulate the urge to void.
5. Assist Lisa in breastfeeding. Explain the reasons for proper positioning and frequent feedings.	5. Poor positioning and infrequent feedings may cause nipple trauma and engorgement and lead to mastitis.
6. Offer and encourage Lisa to eat well-balanced meals when she progresses to a regular diet. Emphasize the importance of a diet high in protein and vitamin C.	6. Adequate protein and vitamin C are necessary for healing damaged tissues.
7. Teach Lisa signs of infection that she should report to her health care provider. Include fever, chills, dysuria, increased incisional tenderness or drainage, and foul odor of the lochia.	7. Prompt recognition and reporting of signs of infection ensure early treatment and reduce further complications.

Evaluation

Lisa remains free of the signs and symptoms of infection throughout her hospital stay. She discusses measures that she will use to reduce the risk for infection when she is discharged from the hospital.

Additional Nursing Diagnoses to Consider

Activity Intolerance
Pain
Fatigue
Risk for Impaired Parenting

been used in breastfeeding mothers (Wisner, Parry, & Piontek, 2002). The breastfeeding infant should be monitored carefully by the pediatrician for signs of adverse reactions to medications (Burt et al., 2001). Other drugs include tricyclic antidepressants and hormones. Medication may be continued for 6 months or more. Electroconvulsive therapy may also be necessary.

■ NURSING CARE
The Woman With Postpartum Depression

Assessment

Assess all women for depression during pregnancy as well as after delivery. Assessment tools such as the Postpartum Depression Predictors Inventory may be helpful. This inventory identifies prenatal depression, life stress, social support, prenatal anxiety, satisfaction with marital relationship, history of depression, self-esteem, unwanted or unplanned pregnancy, marital status, socioeconomic status, child care stress, infant temperament, and maternity blues as factors that may predict the likelihood of a woman developing PPD (Beck, 2002a). In addition, screening for excessive fatigue in the first 2 weeks after childbirth may help identify women who will later develop postpartum depression and enable them to get early treatment (Bozoky & Corwin, 2002).

Observe for subjective symptoms, such as apathy, lack of interest or energy, anorexia, or sleeplessness. The mother's verbalizations of failure, sadness, loneliness, anxiety, or vague confusion are important cues. Assess for objective data, such as crying, sleeplessness, poor personal hygiene, or inability to follow directions. A tool such as the Postpartum Depression Screening Scale may be used to determine which mothers should be referred for further help (Beck & Gable, 2000, 2001).

Assess availability of family support. Single mothers or mothers with an absent or unavailable support system may feel increasingly isolated, leading to stress that they are unable to manage. Inappropriate expressions of blame or anger toward the partner and unmet expectations of the baby or the parenting role are sometimes present.

Nursing Diagnosis and Planning

A likely nursing diagnosis is

■ Risk for Ineffective Coping related to depression secondary to stressors associated with childbirth and parenting.
   Expected Outcomes: The new mother will verbalize feelings with the health care provider and the significant other throughout the postpartum period and will identify strengths and resources that are available during the postpartum period.

Interventions
Demonstrating Caring

Conveying a caring attitude is one nursing strategy to help mothers decrease their emotional distress and to guide them in regaining their well-being during the postpartum period. Acknowledge that the woman feels depressed, and reassure her that the condition is not her fault. It is an illness that can be treated and will end.

Providing Anticipatory Guidance

Provide all new mothers with anticipatory guidance about the early weeks at home. Emphasize the need for frequent contact with other adults so that the mother does not become isolated. Discuss the importance of maintaining continued communication with the partner or with a close friend who is available to provide support when loneliness or anxiety becomes a problem. Explain that adequate rest and nutrition can help the mother maintain energy and a feeling of health and well-being. Teach mothers the signs of postpartum depression and when they should seek help.

Helping the Mother Verbalize Feelings

Because women are expected to be happy after giving birth, many women do not discuss their negative feelings with others. When they do, friends or even health care workers may trivialize the problem by making comments such as "You'll get over it. After all, you have a beautiful baby."

Recommend that although some of her feelings may seem "unreasonable" (e.g., anger, guilt, shame), the woman should acknowledge the feelings to herself and insist that others recognize them as well. Discuss the realities of parenting and the fact that it is often exhausting. It may be helpful to rehearse some situations that may occur, such as a fussy baby or being home alone and feeling lonely, as a means to develop perspective and to find solutions before the situation occurs.

Enhancing Sensitivity to Infant Cues

Point out infant cues, and explain what they mean. Suggest measures that may enhance her sensitivity to infant cues. Kangaroo care (skin-to-skin) may help increase bonding and help the woman feel better about herself and her ability to care for the infant (Dombrowski, Anderson, Santori, & Burkhammer, 2001). Music, relaxation therapy, and massage techniques just before mother-infant interactions may be relaxing and increase her energy to care for the infant. St. John's wort is often used as an over-the-counter remedy to treat depression, but it has not been proven safe for use by lactating women.

Helping Family Members

Include the father in discussions about depression, and acknowledge his feelings. Offer practical suggestions of ways he can help manage the changes in their lives. Explain the impact of PPD on each family member.

Discussing Options and Resources

Ask the mother about stressors in her life that may be contributing to her depression. Help her plan ways to reduce common areas of stress. Assist her in identifying people who

---

CRITICAL THINKING EXERCISE 28-2

Aricella Nunez, a 23-year-old multipara, gave birth several days ago to her second baby. She is crying when the nurse makes a follow-up telephone call after discharge. Aricella says, "I don't know what's wrong with me. I can barely get out of bed in the morning, and I'm worn out just trying to take care of the kids." The nurse responds, "Oh, that's just the 'baby blues.' Just look at those beautiful babies, and you will feel better."
1. What assumption has the nurse made?
2. Is the nurse's response helpful for Aricella? Why or why not?
3. What would be a more therapeutic response?
4. What additional action should the nurse take?

are available to provide support. Suggest that she explain her anticipated needs to those people before the development of symptoms. In addition, give the mother telephone numbers for postpartum depression support groups in the area.

Evaluation

- Can the mother verbalize her feelings with others?
- Does she identify personal strengths and resources that will provide support during this time?

Postpartum Psychosis

Postpartum psychosis is a rare condition that causes psychiatric admission in 2 in 1000 postpartum women (Hayashi & Zettelmaier, 2000). It usually surfaces within 3 weeks of delivery. It may occur as bipolar disorder with manic and depressive episodes or as major depression consisting of depression without manic episodes. Women who have had one episode of postpartum psychosis are at risk for having another episode.

Women with bipolar disorder suffer from irritability, hyperactivity, euphoria, and grandiosity. They exhibit little need for sleep and are seldom aware they have a problem. The poor judgment and confusion they experience make self-care and infant care impossible and can be life-threatening for the mother and infant.

The depressions of the bipolar disorder and major depression are similar and are characterized by tearfulness, preoccupations of guilt, feelings of worthlessness, sleep and appetite disturbances, and an inordinate concern with the baby's health. Delusions about the infant being dead or defective are common. Hallucinations may also be present.

Assessment and management of postpartum psychosis are beyond the scope of maternity nurses, and mothers who experience these conditions must be referred to specialists for comprehensive therapy. Women with signs of postpartum psychosis need immediate medical attention, and hospitalization is usually necessary.

Women who have manic symptoms are usually treated with medications (lithium, carbamazepine, antidepressants, antipsychotics). Lithium is not recommended during pregnancy, but it may be resumed in the postpartum period if the mother is not breastfeeding. Women who have depressive symptoms must be assessed for suicidal potential and treated according to the severity of the threat. Antipsychotics and antidepressants are used for treatment, and careful monitoring is required because of the effect of hormonal imbalances on the mother's reaction to the prescribed medication.

KEY CONCEPTS

- Postpartum hemorrhage can sometimes be prevented by careful examination of factors that predispose to excessive bleeding.
- Overstretching of the muscle fibers during pregnancy or repeated stretching during past pregnancies predisposes to uterine atony and excessive uterine bleeding.
- Initial management of uterine atony focuses on measures to contract the uterus and provide fluid replacement.
- Soft tissue trauma (lacerations, hematomas) can cause rapid loss of blood even when the uterus is firmly contracted. Management involves repairing the trauma before excessive blood loss occurs.
- Compensatory mechanisms maintain the blood pressure so that vital organs receive adequate oxygen. When these mechanisms fail, hypovolemic shock follows.
- The process of uterine involution is delayed (causing subinvolution) when placental fragments are retained or when the inner lining of the uterus is infected (causing metritis).
- Subinvolution of the uterus develops after the mother goes home. The nurse teaches the

family the process of normal involution and the signs and symptoms that should be reported to the health care provider.

- Venous stasis that occurs during pregnancy, increased levels of coagulation factors, and decreased thrombolytic factors that persist into the postpartum period increase the risk for thrombus formation during the puerperium.
- Treatment for deep venous thrombosis includes anticoagulants, analgesics, and bed rest, with the affected leg elevated to decrease interstitial edema and improve venous return.
- Nurses who administer anticoagulant therapy assess the mother to determine whether her clotting time is within the recommended therapeutic range so that overmedication with anticoagulants does not result in bleeding.
- Pulmonary embolism is a complication of deep venous thrombosis that occurs when a clot is dislodged from the vein and carried by the blood to a pulmonary vessel, which may become completely or partially occluded.
- The risk for infection is increased with childbearing because there is open access to bac-

teria from the vagina through the fallopian tubes and into the peritoneal cavity. Increased blood supply to the pelvis and the alkalinization of the vagina by the amniotic fluid further increase the risk for metritis.

- Any break in the skin or mucous membranes during childbirth provides a portal of entry for pathogenic organisms and increases the risk for puerperal infection. Nurses must assess women for any signs of infections.
- Urinary stasis and urinary tract trauma increase the risk for urinary tract infection. Nurses must initiate measures to prevent urinary stasis.
- Nurses must provide information about the importance of completely emptying the breasts at each feeding and about measures to prevent nipple trauma to prevent mastitis.
- Postpartum depression is a disabling mood disorder that affects the entire family. Nurses help the woman acknowledge her feelings and assist her in identifying measures that will help her cope with the condition.

ANSWERS to Critical Thinking Exercise 28-1

1. Her history of multiparity, birth of a large infant, and rapid labor and delivery indicates that Dolores is at risk for postpartal hemorrhage. The nurse should assess the fundus, lochia, vital signs, and skin temperature and color more frequently.

2. Massage the fundus, and express clots that may have accumulated in the uterus. Mas-

sage stimulates uterine contractions that compress myometrial blood vessels and stop excessive bleeding. Continued assessment of the fundus and lochia is imperative.

3. Assist Dolores to void because a distended bladder lifts the uterus, making contraction more difficult and resulting in excessive bleeding.

4. Notify the physician or the nurse-midwife because excessive bleeding requires the combined efforts of primary health care providers and nurses to prevent postpartum hemorrhage.

ANSWERS to Critical Thinking Exercise 28-2

1. The nurse assumed that Aricella has the transient, self-limiting depression that occurs in most women who give birth. The nurse fails to obtain additional data that may indicate whether Aricella is experiencing postpartum depression and needs additional therapy.

2. The response is not helpful because it minimizes the feelings Aricella has expressed and it offers no measures for dealing with the feelings.

3. The nurse should acknowledge Aricella's feelings and ask questions that allow her to express those feelings fully.

4. The nurse must convey her genuine interest and caring. She can do this best by:
   a. Indicating that she is aware that something may be wrong.
   b. Sharing as much time as Aricella needs to express her feelings.
   c. Providing hope by reassuring Aricella that her feelings are not her fault and that the condition can be cured.
   d. Making appropriate referrals that try to provide as much continuity of care as possible.

REFERENCES and READINGS

American Academy of Pediatrics, & American College of Obstetricians and Gynecologists. (2002). *Guidelines for perinatal care* (5th ed.). Elk Grove Village, IL, and Washington, DC: Author.

Beck, C.T. (1995). The effects of postpartum depression on maternal-infant interaction: A meta-analysis. *Nursing Research, 44*(5), 298-304.

Beck, C.T. (2001). Predictors of postpartum depression. *Nursing Research, 50*(5), 275-285.

Beck, C.T., & Gable, R.K. (2000). Postpartum Depression Screening Scale: Development and psychometric testing. *Nursing Research, 49*(5), 272-282.

Beck, C.T., & Gable, R.K. (2001). Further validation of the Postpartum Depression Screening Scale. *Nursing Research, 50*(3), 155-164.

Beck, C.T. (2002a). Revision of the Postpartum Depression Predictors Inventory. *Journal of Obstetric, Gynecologic, and Neonatal Nursing, 31*(4), 394-402.

Beck, C.T. (2002b). Theoretical perspectives of postpartum depression and their treatment implications. *MCN: The American Journal of Maternal/Child Nursing, 27*(5), 282-287.

Benedetti, T.J. (2002). Obstetric hemorrhage. In S.G. Gabbe, J.R. Niebyl, & J.L. Simpson (Eds.), *Obstetrics: Normal and problem pregnancies* (4th ed., pp. 503-538). Philadelphia: Churchill Livingstone.

Biancuzzo, M. (2003). *Breastfeeding the newborn: Clinical strategies for nurses.* St Louis: Mosby.

Bobrowski, R.A., & Dzieczkowski, J.S. (2002). Anticoagulation. In S.B. Ransom, M.P. Dombrowski, M.I. Evans, & K.A. Ginsburg (Eds.), *Contemporary therapy obstetrics and gynecology* (pp. 142-146). Philadelphia: Saunders.

Bowes, W.A., & Thorp, J.M. (2004). Clinical aspects of normal and abnormal labor. In R.K. Creasy, R. Resnik, & J.D. Iams (Eds.), *Maternal-fetal medicine: Principles and practice* (5th ed., pp. 671-706). Philadelphia: Saunders.

Bozoky, I., & Corwin, E.J. (2002). Fatigue as a predictor of postpartum depression. *Journal of Obstetric, Gynecologic, and Neonatal Nursing, 31*(4), 436-443.

Burt, V.K., Suri, R., Altshuler, L., Stowe, Z., Hendrick, V.C., & Muntean, E. (2001). The use of psychotropic medications during breastfeeding. *American Journal of Psychiatry, 158*(7), 1001-1009.

Clarke-Pearson, D.L. (2000). Venous thromboembolic disease in pregnancy. In E.J. Quilligan & F.P. Zuspan (Eds.), *Current therapy in obstetrics and gynecology* (5th ed., pp. 368-371). Philadelphia: Saunders.

Cunningham, F.G., Gant, N.F., Leveno, K.J., Gilstrap, L.C., Hauth, J.C., & Wenstrom, K.D. (2001). *Williams obstetrics* (21st ed.). New York: McGraw-Hill.

Dietch, K.V., & Bunney, B. (2002). The "silent" disease: Diagnosing & treating depression in women. *AWHONN Lifelines, 6*(2), 140-145.

Dombrowski, M.A.S., Anderson, G.C., Santori, C., & Burkhammer, M. (2001). Kangaroo (skin-to-skin) care with a postpartum woman who felt depressed. *MCN: The American Journal of Maternal/Child Nursing, 26*(4), 214-216.

Duff, P. (2002). Maternal and perinatal infection. In S.G. Gabbe, J.R. Niebyl, & J.L. Simpson (Eds.), *Obstetrics: Normal and problem pregnancies* (4th ed., pp. 1293-1345). Philadelphia: Churchill Livingstone.

Gibbs, R.S., Sweet, R.L., & Duff, W.P. (2004). Maternal and fetal infectious disorders. In R.K. Creasy, R. Resnik, & J.D. Iams (Eds.), *Maternal-fetal medicine: Principles and practice* (5th ed., pp. 741-801). Philadelphia: Saunders.

Hauth, J.C. (2000). Postpartum hemorrhage. In E.J. Quilligan & F.P. Zuspan, *Current therapy in obstetrics and gynecology* (5th ed., pp. 317-320). Philadelphia: Saunders.

Hayashi, R.H., & Zettelmaier, M.A. (2000). Postpartum management. In S.B. Ransom, M.P. Dombrowski, S.G. McNeeley, K.S. Moghissi, & A.R. Munkarah (Eds.), *Practical strategies in obstetrics and gynecology* (pp. 321-325). Philadelphia: Saunders.

Higgins, P.G. (2000). Postpartum complications. In S. Mattson & J.E. Smith (Eds.), *Core curriculum for maternal-newborn nursing* (2nd ed., pp 637-655). Philadelphia: Saunders.

James, D.C. (2001). Postpartum care. In K.R. Simpson & P.A. Creehan, *AWHONN perinatal nursing* (2nd ed., pp. 446- 472). Philadelphia: Lippincott.

Katz, V.L., & Wolfe, H.M. (2002). Selective arterial embolization in the management of obstetric hemorrhage. In S.B. Ransom, M.P. Dombrowski, M.I. Evans, & K.A. Ginsburg (Eds.), *Contemporary therapy obstetrics and gynecology* (pp. 165-169). Philadelphia: Saunders.

Kennedy, H.P., Beck, C.T., & Driscoll, J.W. (2002). A light in the fog: Caring for women with postpartum depression. *Journal of Midwifery & Women's Health, 47*(5), 318-330.

Laros, R.K. (2004). Thromboembolic disease. In R.K. Creasy, R. Resnik, & J.D. Iams (Eds.), *Maternal-fetal medicine: Principles and practice* (5th ed., pp. 845-857). Philadelphia: Saunders.

Lawrence, R.A., & Lawrence, R.M. (1999). *Breastfeeding: A guide for the medical profession* (5th ed.). St. Louis: Mosby.

Maley, B. (2002). Out of the blue: Creating a postpartum depression support group. *AWHONN Lifelines, 6*(1), 62-65.

Matteson, P.S. (2001). *Women's health during the childbearing years: A community-based approach.* St. Louis: Mosby.

Meighan, M., Davis, M.W., Thomas, S.P., & Droppleman, P.G. (1999). Living with postpartum depression: The father's experience. *MCN: The American Journal of Maternal/Child Nursing, 24*(4), 202-208.

Normand, M.C., & Damato, E.G. (2001). Postcesarean infection. *Journal of Obstetric, Gynecologic, and Neonatal Nursing, 30*(6), 642-648.

Parry, B.L. (2004). Management of depression and psychoses during pregnancy and the puerperium. In R.K. Creasy, R. Resnik, & J.D. Iams (Eds.), *Maternal-fetal medicine* (5th ed., pp. 1193-1200). Philadelphia: Saunders.

Scoggin, J. (2000). Physical and psychological changes. In S. Mattson & J.E. Smith (Eds.), *Core curriculum for maternal-newborn nursing* (2nd ed., pp. 302-316). Philadelphia: Saunders.

Sorokin, Y. (2000). Obstetric hemorrhage. In S.B. Ransom, M.P. Dombrowski, S.G. McNeeley, K.S. Moghissi, & A.R. Munkarah, (Eds.), *Practical strategies in obstetrics and gynecology* (pp. 311-320). Philadelphia: Saunders.

Ugarriza, D.N. (2002). Postpartum depressed women's explanation of depression. *Journal of Nursing Scholarship, 34*(3), 227-334.

Vieira, T. (2003). When joy becomes grief: Screening tools for postpartum depression. *AWHONN Lifelines, 6*(6), 507-513.

Whitty, J.E., & Dombrowski, M.P. (2002). Respiratory diseases in pregnancy. In S.G. Gabbe, J.R. Niebyl, & J.L. Simpson (Eds.), *Obstetrics: Normal and problem pregnancies* (4th ed., pp. 1033-1064). Philadelphia: Churchill Livingstone.

Wisner, K.L., Parry, B.L., & Piontek, C.M. (2002). Postpartum depression. *New England Journal of Medicine, 347*, 194-199.

29

The High-Risk Newborn: Problems Related to Gestational Age and Development

After studying this chapter, you should be able to:

- Explain the special problems of the preterm infant.
- Identify common nursing diagnoses for preterm infants, and explain the nursing care for each.
- Describe the complications that may result from premature birth.

- Describe the characteristics and problems of the infant with postmaturity syndrome.
- Explain the effects of intrauterine growth restriction.
- Compare the problems of the large-for-gestational-age infant with those of the small-for-gestational-age infant.

apneic spells   Cessation of breathing for more than 20 seconds, or accompanied by cyanosis or bradycardia.

bronchopulmonary dysplasia   Chronic pulmonary condition in which damage to the infant's lungs requires prolonged dependence on supplemental oxygen.

compliance   Stretchability or elasticity of the lungs and thorax, which allows distention without resistance during respirations.

containment   A method of increasing comfort in infants by swaddling or other methods to keep the extremities in a flexed position near the body.

corrected gestational age   Gestational age that a preterm infant would be if still in utero. May also be called *developmental age*.

enteral feeding   Nutrients supplied to the gastrointestinal tract orally or by feeding tube.

intrauterine growth restriction   Failure of a fetus to grow as expected for gestational age.

large-for-gestational-age infant   An infant whose size is above the 90th percentile for gestational age.

low-birth-weight infant   Infant whose birth weight is less than 2500 g.

macrosomia   Infant birth weight more than 4000 g.

minimal enteral nutrition   Very small feedings designed to help the gastrointestinal tract mature. Also called *trophic feedings*.

necrotizing enterocolitis   Serious inflammatory condition of the intestines.

noncompliance   Resistance of the lungs and thorax to distention with air during respirations.

parenteral nutrition   Intravenous infusion of all nutrients known to be needed for metabolism and growth.

periventricular-intraventricular hemorrhage   Bleeding around and into the ventricles of the brain.

postmaturity syndrome   Condition in which a postterm infant shows characteristics indicative of poor placental functioning before birth.

postterm infant   An infant born after 42 weeks of gestation.

preterm infant   An infant born before the beginning of the 38th week of gestation. Also called *premature infant*.

pulse oximetry   Method of determining the level of blood oxygen saturation by sensors attached to the skin.

respiratory distress syndrome   Condition caused by insufficient production of surfactant in the lungs; results in atelectasis (collapse of the lung alveoli), hypoxemia (decreased O_2), and hypercapnia (increased CO_2).

retinopathy of prematurity   Condition in which damage to blood vessels often associated with oxygen use and proliferation of new vessels may cause decreased vision or blindness.

small-for-gestational-age infant   An infant whose size is below the 10th percentile for gestational age.

transcutaneous oxygen/carbon dioxide monitoring   Method of continuous noninvasive measurement of oxygen in the blood by transducers attached to the skin.

very-low-birth-weight infant   An infant weighing 1500 g or less at birth.

Maternity nurses identify and care for the immediate needs of neonates with gestational complications until they are transferred to the neonatal intensive care unit (NICU). Nurses also provide information and emotional care for parents. Neonatal intensive care is a nursing specialty requiring further study. Nurses who work in NICU nurseries have additional education and experience to prepare them for this role.

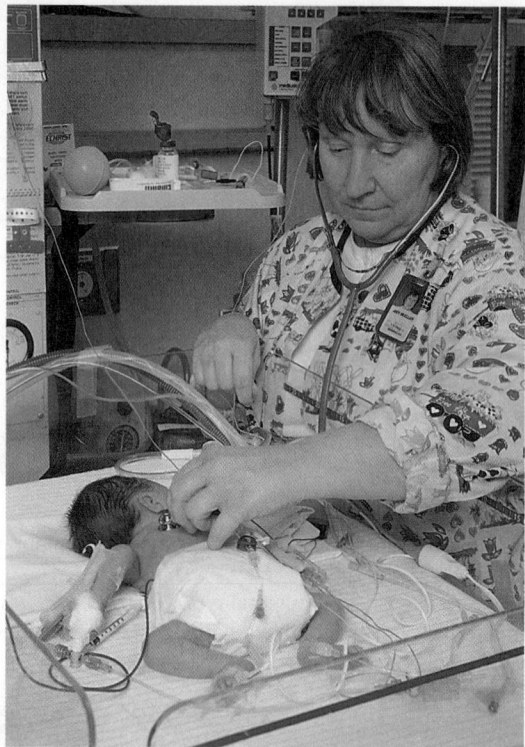

Figure 29-1 The infant in a neonatal intensive care unit (NICU) nursery is cared for by nurses with highly specialized skills.

CARE OF HIGH-RISK NEWBORNS

Approximately 9% of all newborns are sick enough at birth to require intensive care (Stoll & Kliegman, 2004b). Nurses care for minor illness in the normal newborn nursery, but more serious problems require care in specialized nurseries designed for that purpose (Fig. 29-1).

PRETERM INFANTS

Preterm infants (also called *premature infants*) are born before the beginning of the 38th week of gestation. The word *preterm* is sometimes confused with the term *low birth weight* (LBW), which refers to infants weighing 2500 g (5 lb, 8 oz) or less at birth. *Very-low-birth-weight* (VLBW) infants weigh 1500 g (3 lb, 5 oz) or less at birth. *Extremely-low-birth-weight* (ELBW) infants weigh 1000 g (2 lb, 3 oz) or less at birth. Although most of these infants are preterm, others are full-term and have failed to grow normally while in the uterus, a condition called *intrauterine growth restriction* (IUGR).

Incidence and Etiology

Scope of the Problem

Advances in technology have resulted in infant survival at much lower birth weights than ever before. The number of early births, however, is not decreasing. In 2002, 12% of births were preterm and 7.8% of newborns weighed less than 2500 g. Prematurity and low birth weight are the second leading causes of infant death (Arias, MacDorman, Strobino, & Guyer, 2003).

In terms of medical expense, lost potential, and suffering of infants and their parents, preterm birth is extremely costly.

Causes

The exact causes of preterm birth are not known, but all risk factors in pregnancy are potential causes of complications for the newborn as well (see Chapter 13).

Prevention

Prevention of preterm birth is best accomplished by provision of adequate prenatal care for every pregnant woman to identify and treat risk factors as early as possible. Teaching women signs of preterm labor will help them seek care when halting the labor is still a possibility (see Chapter 27).

Characteristics of Preterm Infants

Preterm infants vary by gestational age. For example, the appearance and problems of infants born at 34 weeks' gestation are different from those of infants born at 26 weeks' gestation. Some characteristics, however, are common to all preterm infants.

Appearance

Preterm infants appear frail and weak, and they have underdeveloped flexor muscles and muscle tone. Their extremities are limp, and they typically lie in an extended position (see Fig. 22-24).

Preterm infants lack subcutaneous fat, which makes their thin skin appear red and almost transparent, with blood vessels clearly visible. The nipples and areola may be barely perceptible, whereas vernix caseosa and lanugo may be abundant. Plantar creases are absent in infants of less than 32 weeks' gestation (see Fig. 22-31).

The pinna of the ear is soft and flat, lacking the rolled-over look of full-term ears (see Fig. 22-32). In the female infant, the clitoris and labia minora appear large and are not covered by the small, separated labia majora. The male infant may have undescended testes, with a small, smooth scrotal sac (see Figs. 22-33 and 22-34).

Behavior

Behavior varies according to gestational age. In general, preterm infants have little excess energy for maintaining muscle tone. They are easily exhausted from noise and routine activities. Their response is varied, including lowered oxygenation levels and behavior changes. The cry is feeble.

Assessment and Care of Common Problems

Preterm infants are prone to problems that affect all systems and body processes.

Problems With Respiration

Problems of the respiratory system are a major concern because preterm newborns have immature lungs. The presence of surfactant in adequate amounts is of primary importance. Surfactant reduces surface tension in the alveoli and prevents their collapse with expiration. Infants born before surfactant production is adequate develop respiratory distress syndrome (see p. 739). In addition, preterm infants have a poorly developed cough reflex and narrow respiratory passages, which increase the risk for respiratory problems.

Assessment. The infant's respiratory status must be observed constantly. The lungs are assessed for adventitious breath sounds or areas of absent breath sounds. The Silverman-Andersen index is a useful tool for evaluating the degree of respiratory distress (Fig. 29-2).

The nurse differentiates periodic breathing from apneic spells. Periodic breathing is the cessation of breathing for 5 to 10 seconds without other changes. The average respiratory rate is 30 to 40 breaths per minute (Hagedorn, Gardner, & Abman, 2002). Apneic spells last more than 20 seconds or are accompanied by cyanosis or bradycardia. They are common in preterm infants, increasing in incidence with lower gestational age. Apnea without an identified cause in a preterm infant is called *apnea of prematurity* and generally improves as the infant matures. The infant may require gentle stimulation or bag-and-mask ventilation.

The nurse observes the effort required for breathing and the location and severity of retractions. Retractions are particularly noticeable in the preterm infant, whose weak chest wall is drawn in with each inspiration. The excessive compliance (elasticity) of the chest cage during retractions may interfere with full expansion of the lungs.

Grunting may be an early sign of respiratory distress syndrome. It closes the glottis and increases the pressure within the alveoli. This process keeps the alveoli partially open between breaths and increases the amount of oxygen absorbed.

Nursing Interventions. Interventions focus on collaborating with other team members, such as the respiratory therapist, to manage technical equipment and facilitate removal of secretions.

Working With Respiratory Equipment. An oxygen hood is often used for infants who can breathe alone but who need extra oxygen. The hood is a plastic dome that fits over the infant's head or head and upper body. The infant breathes the higher levels of oxygen within the hood, and the device does not interfere with access to the rest of the infant's body for care (Fig. 29-3).

Oxygen may also be given by nasal cannula to the infant who breathes well alone. After discharge, many preterm infants continue to receive oxygen via nasal cannula at home. Oxygen must be humidified to prevent insensible water loss and drying of the delicate mucous membranes. It is warmed to maintain body temperature.

Continuous positive airway pressure may be necessary to keep the alveoli open and improve expansion of the lungs. It can be delivered with nasal prongs or an endotracheal tube. The infant may need conventional mechanical ventilation, or high-frequency ventilation may be used to provide very fast, frequent respirations with less pressure and volume. This helps prevent injury to the tissue from pressure (barotrauma) and volume (volutrauma). Inhaled nitric oxide, extracorporeal membrane oxygenation, and partial liquid ventilation are newer, very high technology methods used for infants with severe respiratory problems.

When oxygen is administered, the level of oxygen in the infant's blood must be monitored. Arterial blood may be drawn for testing arterial oxygen levels. Pulse oximetry or transcutaneous monitoring may also be used. They are less invasive and provide continuous information about oxygen partial pressure (PO_2) levels through sensors attached to the skin.

The nurse must observe the infant's increasing or decreasing dependence on breathing assistance and need for oxygen. The infant's response to activity that may increase oxygen need, such as handling, feeding, and linen changes, may require changes in settings on equipment to meet the infant's needs. Oxygen flow is increased when suctioning is necessary.

Positioning the Infant. The infant should be placed in a side-lying or prone position to facilitate drainage of respiratory secretions and regurgitated feedings. The prone position is not recommended for normal newborn infants because it is associated with an increased incidence of sudden infant death syndrome (SIDS). In the preterm infant, however, the prone position increases oxygenation and lung compliance and reduces energy expenditure (Lefrak & Lund, 2001). Supine positioning for sleep is begun when respiratory concerns are less and before the infant is discharged.

Frequent position changes help air passages drain and prevent stasis of secretions. Infants should be repositioned every 2 to 3 hours when other care is given to help dependent areas of the lungs drain into the main bronchi.

Suctioning Secretions. The nurse checks equipment at the beginning of each shift to ensure that it is available and functioning properly at all times. The infant is suctioned only as necessary when the need becomes apparent. Suction should always be gentle to avoid traumatizing the delicate mucous membranes. Trauma could cause edema, which could further decrease the size of the air passages and lead to more respiratory difficulty.

In addition, suctioning decreases oxygenation during the procedure and may cause changes in heart rate, blood pressure, and cerebral blood flow, and suction provides an entry for organisms. Increased oxygen should be provided before and after each suction attempt. The mouth is suctioned before the nose because stimulation of the nares causes reflex inspiration that could cause aspiration of fluids in the infant's mouth (Hagedorn et al., 2002).

Maintaining Hydration. Adequate hydration is essential to keep secretions thin so that they can be removed by drainage or suction. If infants become dehydrated, secretions will become thick and viscous and could obstruct tiny air passages. Fluid intake should be increased, within the limits of the overall treatment plan, if secretions seem to indicate even minimal dehydration. Small amounts of saline may be administered through endotracheal tubes just before suctioning to thin secretions.

Problems With Thermoregulation

Although heat loss can be a problem for full-term infants, it is even more significant for preterm infants. They have thin skin and little subcutaneous (white) fat for insulation. Less brown fat is present for nonshivering thermogenesis. Preterm infants' body surface area is proportionately larger than that of full-term infants, and their extended extremities increase exposure. The temperature control center of the brain of preterm infants is less mature and may be further impaired by asphyxia. These conditions all contribute to heat loss.

Complications of heat loss are more likely in the preterm infant than in the full-term infant. They include hypo-

| Grade | 0 | 1 | 2 |

CHEST/ABDOMINAL MOVEMENT

INTERCOSTAL SPACES

XIPHOID AREA

NARES

EXPIRATORY SOUND

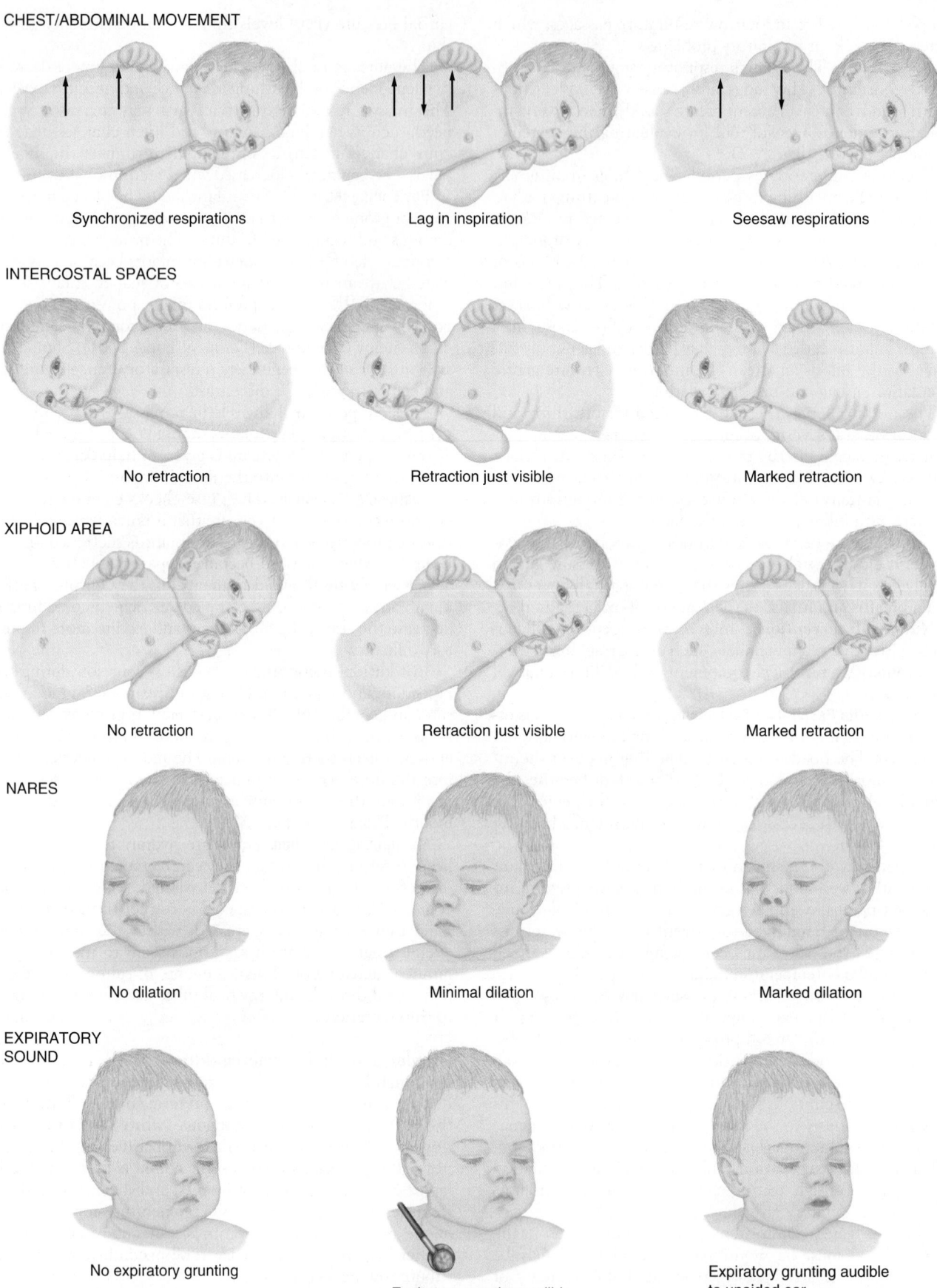

CHEST/ABDOMINAL MOVEMENT: Synchronized respirations / Lag in inspiration / Seesaw respirations

INTERCOSTAL SPACES: No retraction / Retraction just visible / Marked retraction

XIPHOID AREA: No retraction / Retraction just visible / Marked retraction

NARES: No dilation / Minimal dilation / Marked dilation

EXPIRATORY SOUND: No expiratory grunting / Expiratory grunting audible by stethoscope / Expiratory grunting audible to unaided ear

Figure 29-2 Assessment of respiratory distress. The Silverman-Andersen index is used to score the infant's degree of respiratory difficulty. The score for individual criteria matches the grade, with a total possible score of 10 indicating severe distress. (Modified with permission from Silverman, W., & Andersen, D. [1956]. A controlled clinical trial of effects of water mist on obstructive respiratory signs, death rate, and necropsy findings among premature infants. *Pediatrics, 17*[4], 1-9).

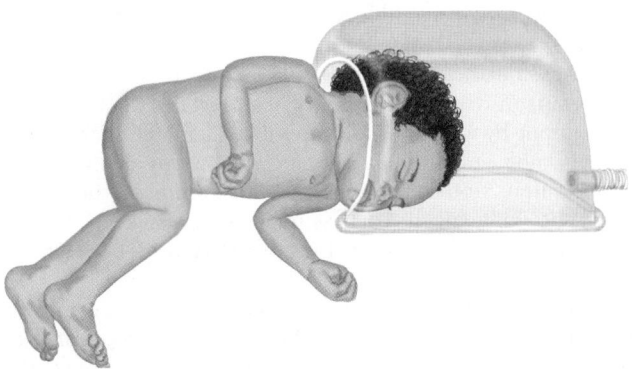

Figure 29-3 The oxygen hood is one way of delivering oxygen to an infant who can breathe unassisted.

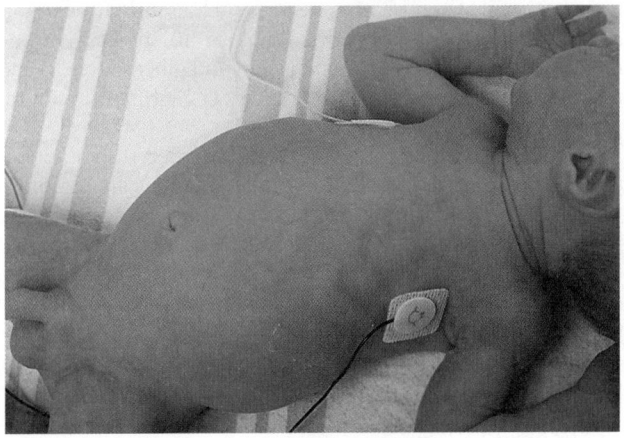

Figure 29-4 This preterm infant has mildly mottled skin and slight abdominal distention and retractions.

glycemia, metabolic acidosis, pulmonary vasoconstriction, and impaired surfactant production.

Assessment. The infant's temperature is monitored continuously by a skin probe, which is attached to the heat control mechanism of the radiant warmer or incubator. The abdominal skin temperature is usually maintained at 36° to 36.5° C (96.8° to 97.7° F). The infant's temperature as shown on the monitor should be recorded every 30 to 60 minutes initially and every 3 to 4 hours when the infant is stable. The nurse should assess the axillary temperature every 4 to 8 hours and compare it with the heat control reading to ensure that the machinery is functioning properly.

The axillary temperature for a preterm infant should remain between 36.3° and 36.9° C (97.3° and 98.4° F) (Blake & Murray, 2002.) If the infant has accumulated brown fat, a normal axillary temperature when the monitor shows a decreased skin temperature may indicate that brown fat in the axillary space is being used to maintain the infant's core temperature.

Indications of inadequate thermoregulation include poor feeding or intolerance to feedings in an infant who previously had little difficulty, lethargy, irritability, poor muscle tone, cool skin temperature, and mottled skin (Fig. 29-4). Hypoglycemia and respiratory distress may be the first signs that the infant's temperature is low. Because temperature instability may be an early sign of infection, the nurse should assess for other evidence that infection may be present.

! CRITICAL **TO REMEMBER**

Signs of Inadequate Thermoregulation

- Axillary temperature <36.3° C or >36.9° C (<97.3° or >98.4° F)
- Abdominal skin temperature <36° C or >36.5° C (<96.8° or >97.7° F)
- Change in feeding behavior
- Lethargy
- Irritability
- Decreased muscle tone
- Cool skin temperature
- Mottled skin
- Signs of hypoglycemia
- Signs of respiratory difficulty

Nursing Interventions. Maintenance of heat in preterm infants involves the same basic nursing care principles as for the full-term infant (see Chapter 23). These principles, however, must be adapted to meet the needs of the preterm infant.

Maintaining a Neutral Thermal Environment. A neutral thermal environment is especially important to prevent the need for increased oxygen to maintain body temperature. Radiant warmers or incubators are used until infants can maintain normal body temperature alone. Because they produce less heat and lose more heat than larger or older preterm infants, smaller, less mature infants need more warmth to maintain body heat.

Infants needing many procedures are usually placed under the open radiant warmer to make it easier to see them and work with equipment. Air currents around an unclothed infant can, however, cause heat loss by convection despite the heat generated by the warmer. Doors near the warmer should be closed and traffic kept to a minimum to decrease convective heat loss further. The infant should receive only warmed oxygen, because thermal receptors in the face are very sensitive to cold. Cold oxygen could quickly lead to cold stress.

Equipment or caregivers should not come between the infant and the heat source, preventing heat from reaching the infant. A transparent plastic blanket over the infant allows heat from the warmer to pass across to the infant and decreases exposure to drafts and insensible water loss while maintaining visibility of the infant's body parts.

Incubators are used for infants who do not need to be under radiant warmers. Warmed air is circulated to provide heat. Humidity may also be added if needed. When infants are in incubators, nurses should keep portholes and doors closed as much as possible. A significant amount of heat is lost every time the incubator is opened, and it takes time to build up again. On removal from the incubator for procedures or holding, the infant should be wrapped in heated blankets and head coverings should be used. To retain heat inside the incubator, the doors should be closed while the infant is out of it.

Although temperature loss is the most common concern, overheating is also a problem for preterm infants. Overheating may occur when heating devices such as radiant warmers are set too high. Overheating leads to an increase in the metabolic rate, with increased oxygen and glucose needs, and insensible water losses. Alarms to detect high and low temperatures should always be turned on.

Although temperature regulation in preterm infants is usually provided in incubators until infants can maintain their own temperature, warmth can also be provided by the parents holding them. Adequate temperature is maintained in stable infants during kangaroo care (see p. 737) or even when infants are swaddled and held close to the parent's body (Mellien, 2001).

Weaning to an Open Crib. Preparation of infants for moving to open cribs should begin early. When stable, an infant can be dressed in a shirt, diaper, and hat while in the incubator. Clothing conserves heat and helps infants adjust to a different temperature on the face than the rest of the body. Infants who weigh about 1500 g (3 lb, 7 oz.), who have a consistent weight gain for 5 days, who have no medical complications, and who are tolerating enteral feedings can begin gradual weaning from external heat (Blake & Murray, 2002).

Each NICU has its own protocol for the weaning process. The incubator temperature is usually decreased gradually. The heat is increased if the infant's temperature falls below the desired range. If the temperature remains stable, the process can continue the next day.

When the infant is ready for transfer to an open crib, double-wrapping with warm blankets at first will help insulate body heat. The temperature is assessed at gradually increasing intervals until the infant is on a routine schedule. A blanket is added for a low temperature, but if the temperature does not rise to normal, the infant is returned to the incubator.

Nurses should observe the infant carefully during the first few days after transfer to an open crib. Signs that may indicate inadequate thermoregulation include decreased weight gain, poor feeding, or increased requirement for oxygen.

Problems With Fluid and Electrolyte Balance

Preterm infants lose fluid very easily. The rapid respiratory rate and the use of oxygen can increase fluid loss from the lungs. Their thin skin is more permeable than the skin of term infants. The large surface area, in proportion to body weight, and lack of flexion further increase insensible water losses. Radiant warmers and the heat from phototherapy lights cause even more fluid loss through the skin. Radiant warmers heighten insensible water losses by 40% to 50%, compared with water loss in an incubator (Blake & Murray, 2002).

Development of the kidneys is not complete until approximately 35 weeks of gestation. The ability of the kidneys to concentrate or dilute urine is poor before that time, causing a fragile balance between dehydration and overhydration. With variation according to size and gestational age, the fluid needs of preterm infants range from 90 to 140 ml/kg per day on the 2nd and 3rd days of life with more needed by extremely-low-birth-weight infants. Normal urinary output is 2 to 5 ml/kg per hour (Berry, Adcock, & Starbuck, 2002).

The kidneys' regulation of electrolytes is also a problem. Preterm infants need higher intakes of sodium because the kidneys do not reabsorb it well. If they receive sodium, however, they may be unable to increase sodium excretion adequately and are susceptible to sodium and water overload as a result.

Assessment. Monitoring intake and output of fluids is important in determining fluid balance. The infant's intake and output by all routes are carefully calculated. Parenteral, feeding tube, and oral fluids are included when measuring intake. Output from regurgitation, stools, drainage tubes, and urine should be measured. The nurse must also keep track of the amount of blood taken for laboratory tests because the loss can be substantial.

Urinary Output. There are several methods of measuring urinary output. Plastic bags that adhere to the perineum are not suitable for the preterm infant because they may damage the fragile skin. Weighing diapers is less invasive to the infant. The weight of dry diapers is subtracted from the weight of wet diapers to determine the amount of urine excreted. One gram is equivalent to 1 ml of urine. Humidification, however, may add moisture to the diaper, and a radiant warmer may cause evaporation of urine on the diaper. When precise measurement is essential, diapers can be fastened instead of placing them open under the infant.

Specific gravity should be checked to determine if urine is more concentrated or dilute than expected. Urine is collected by placing cotton balls at the perineum. The specific gravity should range between 1.002 and 1.010 (Berry et al., 2002).

Weight. Changes in the infant's weight can give an indication of fluid gain or loss, especially if the changes are sudden and greater than would be expected. The undressed infant should be weighed daily at the same time with the same scale. Very small infants are often placed in a bed that has a scale on it so that they are not disturbed for daily weighing. They may be weighed twice a day to monitor their fluid status more closely.

Signs of Dehydration or Overhydration. The nurse should observe for signs that indicate that the infant has received too little or too much fluid. Early signs of dehydration include decreased urine output (<2 ml/kg/hr) and increased specific gravity. Weight losss may exceed that expected for the infant's age and general condition. Dry skin or mucous membranes, sunken anterior fontanel, and poor tissue turgor are late signs. Changes in the blood include increased sodium, protein, and hematocrit levels resulting from decreased plasma volume.

Signs of overhydration include increased output of urine (>5 ml/kg/hr) with a below-normal specific gravity. Edema and weight gain occur from retention of fluids. Bulging fontanels, moist breath sounds, and decreased blood sodium, protein, and hematocrit levels are also present. Complications of excess fluid may include patent ductus arteriosus and congestive heart failure.

Nursing Interventions. The nurse must carefully regulate intravenous (IV) fluids using infusion control devices that administer 1 ml/hr or less to help prevent fluid volume overload. Intravenous medications should be diluted in as little fluid as is consistent with safe administration of the drug and should be included when measuring intake. Starting IV lines on infants with poor veins is a lengthy, difficult procedure. Infants must be restrained as necessary to prevent infiltration. If they infiltrate, some fluids cause extensive damage as a result of tissue sloughing. The site should be assessed at least every hour for signs of infiltration. Many infants have central ve-

CRITICAL TO REMEMBER

Signs of Fluid Imbalance in the Newborn

DEHYDRATION
- Urine output <2 ml/kg/hr
- Urine specific gravity >1.010
- Weight loss greater than expected
- Dry skin and mucous membranes
- Sunken anterior fontanel
- Poor tissue turgor
- Blood: elevated sodium, protein, and hematocrit levels

OVERHYDRATION
- Urine output >5 ml/kg/hr
- Urine specific gravity <1.002
- Edema
- Weight gain greater than expected
- Bulging fontanels
- Blood: decreased sodium, protein, and hematocrit levels
- Moist breath sounds
- Difficulty breathing

nous catheters or umbilical lines that must be assessed for infection or position changes. Small blood transfusions may be necessary to replace blood drawn for frequent laboratory tests.

Problems With the Skin

Preterm infants have fragile, permeable, easily damaged skin. They often have endotracheal tubes, IV lines, electrodes, and other equipment that must be maintained in place, but adhesive tape can be very damaging to the skin, especially during removal. Preparations used to disinfect the skin before invasive procedures can be damaging to fragile skin and may be absorbed.

Assessment. The nurse should frequently assess the condition of the infant's skin and note any changes. The infant's response to products used for cleansing and disinfection should be noted.

Nursing Interventions. Tape should be used as little as possible. Tape that is specially prepared to be less traumatic on removal is available. Backing tape with cotton, waiting more than 24 hours to remove it, and using gauze wraps decrease skin damage. Semipermeable dressings and products that use pectin or hydrogel adhesive are less disruptive to the skin surface. They can be removed with water or mineral oil.

The nurse should avoid the use of chemicals that can injure the skin or may be absorbed through it. Povidone-iodine or chlorhexidine is often used. It should be removed with sterile water after the procedure. Alcohol should not be used (Association of Women's Health, Obstetric, and Neonatal Nurses [AWHONN], 2001).

Sterile water should be used for bathing infants less than 32 weeks' gestational age. Stable preterm infants may be immersed in water for bathing if there are no contraindications. Petrolatum-based emollients can help reduce fissures in dry skin and transepidermal water loss (AWHONN, 2001).

Infants and their equipment should be positioned to avoid undue pressure on the skin. Frequent position changes are important but should be based on the infant's ability to tolerate changes.

Problems With Infection

The incidence of infection in preterm infants is three to ten times greater than that in full-term newborns (Stoll, 2004). Many preterm infants have one or more episodes of sepsis during their hospital stays. Factors contributing to the high rate of infection include exposure to maternal infection, lack of transfer of immunoglobulin G from the mother during the third trimester, and immature immune response to infection.

Preterm infants are often exposed to situations that may cause infection. They are subject to many invasive procedures such as insertion of IVs and drawing of blood specimens. A prolonged stay in the hospital increases the likelihood of acquiring an infection from multiple exposures to organisms.

Assessment. The nurse should be alert for signs of infection at all times (see Chapter 30).

Nursing Interventions. Nursing care involves scrupulous cleanliness and maintaining the infant's skin integrity. Even the normal flora on the hands of caretakers may cause sepsis. Therefore parents and staff members should thoroughly wash their hands and arms before handling infants. Exposure to staff or family members who have contagious diseases should be prevented.

Early signs of infections should be identified (see Chapter 30, p. 755) and reported so that treatment may begin. The nurse carefully notes the infant's response to treatment because some organisms become resistant to antibiotics. Other nursing care is discussed in Chapter 30.

Problems With Pain

Infants in the NICU undergo many painful procedures each day. Caregivers once thought that newborns, particularly preterm infants, were neurologically too immature to feel pain. It is now recognized that pain stimuli cause physiologic and behavioral changes in infants.

Pain can have numerous untoward effects. For example, increases in intracranial pressure resulting from pain may elevate the risk for intraventricular hemorrhage (Blackburn, 2003b). In addition, infants repeatedly exposed to pain may respond to touch or other nonpainful stimuli as if they were in pain (Agarwal, Hagedorn, & Gardner, 2002). The long-term effects of pain in the neonate are not yet fully understood. The American Academy of Pediatrics and the Canadian Paediatric Society recommend that environmental, nonpharmacologic, and pharmacologic interventions be used to prevent, reduce, or eliminate pain in neonates (2000).

Assessment. The nurse must assess the infant's response to painful stimuli. Assessment tools are available to evaluate physiologic and behavioral responses to pain in term and preterm infants.

Physiologic responses include changes in heart rate and respirations, increased blood pressure, and decreased oxygen saturation. Hormonal and metabolic changes occur as well. However, physiologic changes may be unpredictable and cannot be used alone to assess pain.

Behavioral changes include high-pitched, intense, harsh crying. Infants who are intubated or too weak to cry have a

CRITICAL TO REMEMBER

Common Signs of Pain in Infants

- High-pitched, intense, harsh cry; whimpering
- "Cry face"
- Eyes squeezed shut
- Mouth open
- Grimacing, bulging or furrowing of the brow
- Tense, rigid muscles or flaccid muscle tone
- Rigidity or flailing of extremities
- Color changes: red, dusky, pale
- Increased or decreased heart rate
- Increased respirations or apnea
- Increased blood pressure
- Decreased oxygen saturation

"cry face," a facial expression of crying without the sound of a cry. Infants who have been exposed to prolonged or repeated pain may no longer be able to show behavioral changes but still may be experiencing pain.

Nursing Interventions. Nurses should prepare infants for potentially painful procedures by waking them slowly and gently and using containment. Containment simulates the enclosed space of the uterus and is comforting to infants. It involves keeping the extremities in a flexed position near the body by swaddling, nesting, or positioning devices or the nurse's hands. At least one of the infant's hands should be near the mouth for sucking.

Comfort measures help the infant cope with short-term, mild pain and reduce agitation. They include using a pacifier or the infant's hand for nonnutritive sucking. Sucrose placed on the pacifier or given by mouth may increase pain relief. Talking softly, restraining the extremities to prevent flailing, holding, and rocking are other measures. Measures should be adapted according to infants' responses.

The nurse should discuss the infant's pain with the primary care provider to ensure that medications are available for long-term and more severe pain. Opioids, such as fentanyl, can be tolerated by preterm infants. Non-narcotic analgesics such as acetaminophen or nonsteroidal antiinflammatory drugs may be used alone or to potentiate opioids. Sedatives are effective for agitation but do not treat pain. Regional or general anesthesia is used during surgery.

The nurse gives ordered medications before painful procedures and when the infant demonstrates signs of pain. To determine the need to increase or decrease the dosage, the nurse carefully notes the infant's response frequently. Analgesics may be given continuously or on an as-required (PRN) basis.

Clinical Pathways

Preterm infants may remain in the NICU for many days, at a cost of thousands of dollars each day. Clinical pathways are methods to ensure care that allows discharge as soon as possible. The pathways list the care infants will need along a time line and the expected outcomes of that care. Different pathways are created to meet the needs of different types of infants, such as infants with various complications of prematurity.

NURSING CARE

The Preterm Infant

Preterm infants commonly have difficulty with stress from the NICU environment and obtaining adequate nutrition. Their parents may have difficulty with bonding.

ENVIRONMENTALLY CAUSED STRESS

Preterm infants are often exposed to bright lights and a noisy environment. Although the recommended hourly maximum level of background and transient noise is 50 decibels with a transient maximum level of 70 decibels, higher levels of noise do occur in NICUs (Consensus Committee to Establish Recommended Standards for Newborn ICU Design, 2002). The sounds of alarms, ventilators, incubators, doors, and people create a noise level that may increase the risk of hearing loss and other complications. In addition, stimulation of any kind can cause increased energy expenditure by the preterm infant. Infants are subjected to numerous procedures and often disturbing handling many times each day. Noise and routine nursing interventions are often accompanied by changes in heart rate, oxygen saturation levels, and behavior states.

Although touch is generally thought to be comforting to infants, it is often associated with painful events for preterm infants. This can cause infants to develop touch aversion, a negative response to touch of any kind.

Preterm infants undergo multiple assessments, procedures, and treatments that often cause frequent interruptions of sleep and may interfere with the development of normal sleep-wake cycles. Energy used coping with an overstimulating and stressful environment may be unavailable for normal growth and development.

Assessment

Assess the amount of noise to which the infant is exposed. Determine how often interruptions occur and how the infant responds to different types of care. Assess the infant's ability to tolerate activity and noise. Overstimulation results in changes in oxygenation and behavior.

Nursing Diagnosis and Planning

A nursing diagnosis appropriate for preterm infants having difficulty enduring the multiple stimuli in their environment is

- Disorganized Infant Behavior related to stress from an overstimulating environment.

    Expected Outcomes: The infant will show decreasing signs of overstimulation during routine activity, as evidenced by fewer respiratory changes during handling and increased periods of relaxed behavior or sleep.

Interventions

Interventions are focused on providing developmentally supportive nursing care that meets the preterm infant's ability to tolerate stimulation. Developmental care keeps stressors in the environment to a minimum based on the infant's physiologic and behavioral responses.

Scheduling Care

Schedule periods of undisturbed rest to allow the infant to recover from treatments. Avoid waking an infant during the short quiet sleep phase. If the infant must be awakened, try to wait until the infant is in an active sleep phase and more

---

! CRITICAL TO REMEMBER

Signs of Overstimulation in Preterm Infants

OXYGENATION CHANGES
- Increase or decrease in pulse and respiratory rate
- Cyanosis, pallor, or mottling
- Flaring nares
- Decreased oxygen saturation levels

BEHAVIOR CHANGES
- Stiff, extended arms and legs
- Fisting of the hands or splaying of the fingers
- Alert, worried expression
- Turning away from eye contact
- Hiccupping
- Regurgitation
- Coughing
- Yawning
- Fatigue

---

easily aroused. Arrange routine care to correspond with the infant's awake periods and avoid disturbing rest. Decrease the frequency of taking vital signs and other routine care as soon as possible. Even the handling involved in routine sponge bathing may cause stress in small infants. Routine daily baths are unnecessary and should be avoided. One study showed baths can be postponed as long as 4 days without an increase in infection (Franck, Quinn, & Zahr, 2000).

Group care so that several tasks are performed at one time to provide a longer period of rest between care activities. Be alert, however, to the infant's signs of stress. Too many activities may be more than the infant can tolerate. If the infant shows signs of overstimulation, allow short rest periods within grouped activities or during long or painful procedures. Coordinate diagnostic tests and other care given by other health care workers to ensure the infant is not stressed.

Reducing Stimuli
Keep noise around the infant as low as possible. Place incubators away from traffic and congestion of people, and avoid talking near the incubator. Incubator covers help lower sound inside the incubator. Set alarm volumes on low, and respond quickly when they sound. Open and close incubators and cupboards gently. Do not place objects on top of the incubator or use it as a writing surface, because this increases the noise inside. Teach parents to avoid tapping on the incubator.

The lights that are on 24 hours a day in the nursery may interfere with the development of sleep cycles. Position the incubator so that the infant is not facing bright lights, and drape blankets or incubator covers over the back and ends to decrease light further. Use dimmer switches to vary the intensity of lights as needed. Place infants in a prone position to help them avoid looking at ceiling lights.

Promoting Rest
When possible, schedule "quiet periods" when lights and noise in the unit are kept to a minimum to promote rest. Rest periods should be at least an hour in length to allow preterm infants to complete a sleep cycle (Gardner & Goldson, 2002).

Scheduled naps when infants are disturbed as little as possible may help increase sleep, decrease waking, and lead to longer uninterrupted sleep. Naps may also help the infant begin to differentiate day and night sleeping patterns. Lights should be lowered at night to help develop circadian rhythms.

Contain the infant's arms and legs to promote flexion and reduce energy loss from flailing extremities. Provide a "nest" with blankets or positioning devices placed around the infant for boundaries. Use the prone position to increase quiet sleep periods. In the side or supine position, arrange the infant's arms and legs in a flexed position, with the hands near midline to allow hand-to-mouth activity and sucking.

Stroking and gentle massage may be calming for stable preterm infants. It may help increase weight gain and help involve parents in care of the infant (Beachy, 2003). However, it may be overstimulating to unstable infants and should not be used for them.

Promoting Motor Development
Preterm infants may have musculoskeletal and developmental problems from prolonged immobilization and the effects of gravity on their immature neuromuscular system. Because the extensor muscles mature before the flexor muscles, the infant tends to remain in an extended, "frog-leg" position. Shoulder retraction, abduction and external rotation of the lower extremities, and lateral flexion of the arms may result. When possible, position the infant in a side or prone position with the extremities flexed and the hands positioned near the mouth to allow the infant to suck the hands for comfort. Turn the infant every 2 hours, avoiding the supine position, and use blankets or positioning devices to maintain flexion.

Individualizing Care
The ability to tolerate stress varies with each infant. Adapt general care according to the infant's ability to tolerate it. When possible, the same nurse should care for the infant each day to provide consistency in care and handling techniques. Even positive stimuli, such as soft music or soft talking, can overstimulate the infant. Use these measures judiciously according to the infant's tolerance level.

Infants often require extra energy to adjust to changes in care. Observe how well an infant tolerates changes such as moving from assisted to more independent breathing or introduction of new feeding methods. Increase rest periods during these times.

Communicating Infants' Needs
Use the nursing care plan, Kardex, and shift reports to inform other caregivers of techniques that are especially effective for certain infants. Explain all techniques to parents.

Evaluation
- Does the infant display signs of overstimulation less often?

NUTRITION
Preterm infants are born before they are able to accumulate stores of nutrients. Full-term newborns have reservoirs of calcium, iron, and other nutrients, but these are lacking in preterm infants. Fat stores are minimal or absent, and glucose reserves are used up soon after birth. Low blood glucose levels develop very rapidly and must be prevented or treated quickly because the brain needs a steady supply of glucose.

Preterm infants need approximately 105 to 130 kcal/kg per day (Kleinman, 2004). This amount varies according to activity, illness, and other factors. These infants also need increased amounts of protein, iron, calcium, and phosphorus. The average healthy preterm infant should gain approximately 15 to 20 g/kg/day (Anderson, Johnson, Townsend, & Hay, 2002).

The gastrointestinal tract of preterm infants does not absorb nutrients as well as that of full-term infants. Although they digest protein fairly well, preterm infants have insufficient bile acids and pancreatic lipase to absorb fat adequately. They have some lactase deficiency but digest glucose and sucrose adequately. Although their smaller stomach capacity limits the volume that they can tolerate at each feeding, preterm infants require supplementation because they need more of many nutrients per kilogram than do full-term infants.

Assessment

Feeding Tolerance
Assess how well the infant tolerates feedings, whether by feeding tube or nipple. Aspirate the stomach contents to measure the residual amount in the stomach every 2 to 4 hours before feedings. This procedure helps determine whether the stomach is emptying and prevents overdistention. If the residual measures more than 2 to 4 ml/kg or is equal to the volume given over an hour for continuous feeding, the amount is excessive (Anderson et al., 2002). An excessive residual may indicate that the amount, the type, or the formula flow rate needs changing.

Practice varies on whether to replace gastric residuals (Wyckoff, McGrath, Griffin, Malan, & White-Traut, 2003). Unless they are bloody, have large amounts of mucus, or are otherwise abnormal, residuals are often replaced to prevent loss of electrolytes. The next feeding may be reduced by the amount of the residual. If residuals are not replaced, observe carefully for signs of electrolyte imbalance.

Vomiting or frequent regurgitation may indicate that the feedings are too large. Vomitus or residuals containing bile may be a sign of intestinal obstruction. Diarrhea may be caused by rapid advancement of the feeding or intolerance to the type of formula.

Observe for signs of intestinal complications. Obtain objective data about abdominal distention by using a tape to measure abdominal girth at the level of the umbilicus every 4 hours. Stools may be tested for reducing substances, which indicate malabsorption of carbohydrates. Also check for occult blood. Report signs of feeding intolerance to the physician or nurse practitioner because they may be early indications of complications, such as ileus, sepsis, obstruction of the gastrointestinal tract, or necrotizing enterocolitis.

Readiness for Nipple Feeding
During gavage feedings, watch for signs that nipple feeding may soon be possible. These include rooting, respiratory rate below 60, and an increasing ability to tolerate holding and handling. Although sucking on the gavage tube, a finger, or a pacifier may be a sign of readiness, it is not enough. Infants must also have an intact gag reflex or they are more likely to aspirate feedings. Note whether the infant gags on the tube or a gloved finger inserted into the mouth.

When the infant begins to feed by nipple, assess coordination of suck and swallow and observe for aspiration. Frequent choking, gagging, or cyanosis during feedings may indicate that the infant cannot coordinate sucking, swallowing, and breathing well enough for nipple feeding.

! CRITICAL TO REMEMBER

SIGNS OF READINESS FOR NIPPLE FEEDINGS

- Rooting
- Sucking on gavage tube, finger, or pacifier
- Able to tolerate holding
- Respiratory rate <60 breaths per minute
- Presence of gag reflex

SIGNS OF NONREADINESS FOR NIPPLE FEEDINGS

- Respiratory rate >60 breaths per minute
- No rooting or sucking
- Absence of gag reflex
- Excessive gastric residuals

ADVERSE SIGNS DURING NIPPLE FEEDINGS

- Tachycardia
- Bradycardia
- Increased respiratory rate
- Markedly decreased oxygen saturation level
- Apnea
- Cyanosis
- Coughing
- Choking
- Gagging
- Falling asleep early in feeding
- Feeding time more than 20 to 30 minutes

Some infants are so weak that the usual signs of aspiration are minimal or absent.

Assess the respiratory rate before and during feedings. When the respiratory rate is 60 breaths per minute or faster before feedings, gavage feed to prevent aspiration. Observe for signs that the effort of nipple feeding requires too much energy and oxygen for the infant.

Nursing Diagnosis and Planning

The nursing diagnosis that addresses the nutritional problems of the preterm infant is

- Risk for Imbalanced Nutrition: Less Than Body Requirements related to uncoordinated suck and swallow and fatigue during feedings.

   Expected Outcomes: The infant will take in adequate amounts of breast milk or formula to meet nutrient needs for age and weight and will gain 15 to 20 g/kg/day. The actual amount of feedings and weight gain vary according to the infant's gestational age and other conditions. What is appropriate for a particular infant can be discussed with the physician or nurse practitioner.

Interventions

Administering Parenteral Feedings
The nurse manages the administration of parenteral nutrition, which may be necessary for very immature infants because of respiratory problems, limited gastric capacity, and reduced peristalsis. Parenteral nutrition is the intravenous infusion of solutions containing the major nutrients known to be needed for metabolism and growth. It provides calories, amino acids, fatty acids, vitamins, and minerals in amounts adapted to the needs of infants. It is continued, in decreasing amounts, until the infant is able to tolerate full enteral feedings.

Administering Enteral Feedings

Enteral feedings (feeding into the gastrointestinal tract, orally or by feeding tube) are usually begun within the first few days with *minimal enteral nutrition* (also called *trophic feedings*) in which a few milliliters of feeding are given at a time. This helps prime the gastrointestinal tract and promotes maturation and gastric hormone and enzyme production and increases later feeding tolerance and weight gain (Anderson et al., 2002). Human milk is preferred if it is available. Feedings are gradually increased according to the infant's tolerance.

Preterm infants need special formulas or fortified breast milk. Special formulas are adapted to meet the need for easily digestible, concentrated nutrients in a smaller volume of fluid. Preterm infants may need 24 kcal/oz (instead of 20 kcal/oz used for the full-term infant) to meet their requirements. Preterm formulas contain added calcium, phosphorus, and vitamins. Medium-chain triglycerides form 40% to 50% of the fat. The addition of long-chain polyunsaturated fatty acids may be especially important for brain growth and the blood vessels (Brooks, Mitchell, & Steffenson, 2000). Additional components may be added to formulas to meet the needs of individual infants. Breast milk fortifiers add needed nutrients to breast milk.

Administering Gavage Feedings

Gavage feedings are usually started before oral feedings for preterm infants (see Procedures 37-9 and 37-10). A small, soft catheter is inserted through the mouth or nose at each feeding for intermittent (bolus) feedings every 2 to 3 hours. An indwelling catheter may also be used to provide for intermittent or continuous feedings.

Inserting the catheter at each feeding may be more traumatic than leaving it in place. Frequent oral placement may cause vomiting or increase infant aversion to oral stimuli, which may lead to difficulty with oral feedings later. Vagal stimulation during insertion may cause apnea and bradycardia. Nasal placement is often used but may interfere with air flow through the infant's small nasal passages.

Intermittent bolus feedings provide a more normal feeding pattern with periodic stimulation of gastric hormones and enzymes. Continuous feedings may be better for very small infants, those with severe respiratory problems, and infants who have large residuals with bolus feedings. However, continuous feedings have a higher risk of aspiration because the infant is not attended at all times during the feeding. In addition, bacteria counts in the milk or formula may become too high, and fats tend to adhere to the tubing during continuous feeding.

Pacifiers are often used during gavage feedings. Preterm infants have been exposed to aversive stimulation around the mouth, such as intubation and suctioning. As a result, they may react negatively to any additional oral stimulation, thus interfering with feedings. Allowing the infant to use a pacifier during gavage feedings provides positive oral stimulation and helps associate the comfortable feeling of fullness with sucking. Nonnutritive sucking also increases later success in oral feedings and decreases length of hospital stay.

Administering Oral Feedings

The ability to feed orally and gaining weight are important milestones because they are often among the criteria for discharge from the hospital. Oral feedings are often begun when the infant reaches what would be 32 to 34 weeks of gestation

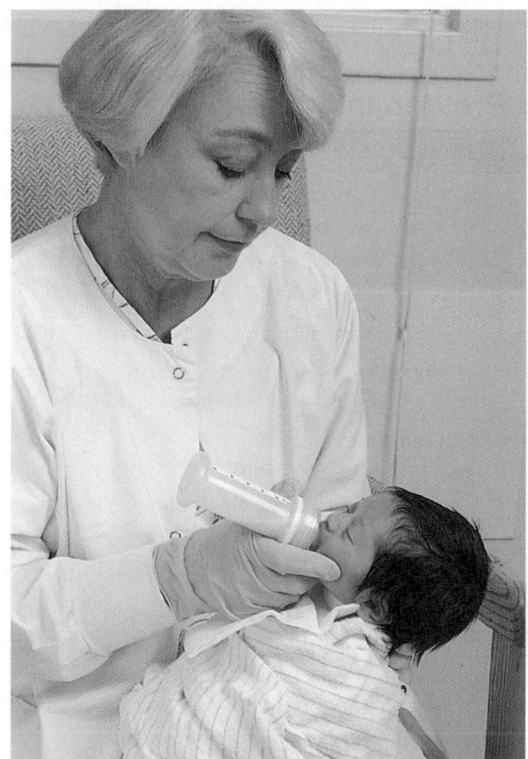

Figure 29-5 The nurse positions her hands to provide cheek and jaw support for feeding this preterm infant.

(Fig. 29-5). At this age many infants have the ability to coordinate sucking and swallowing with breathing (Kleinman, 2004). They also have a functional gag reflex. However, even if sucking, swallowing, and breathing are coordinated, oral feeding may cause the very weak infant to expend too much oxygen and glucose. When sucking is uncoordinated or takes too much energy, the infant must receive gavage feedings.

The first nipple feedings may be only a few milliliters once a day, completed by gavage. Placing the gavage tube before beginning oral feedings helps prevent regurgitation stimulated by passing the catheter. Gradually increase the amount and frequency of oral feedings until the infant feeds by breast or bottle once a shift, then every second or third feeding, and eventually every feeding.

Preparing for Feedings Provide for heat maintenance during feeding times. When infants have stable temperature maintenance, wrap them in warm blankets and hold for feedings.

Nipple feedings involve a greater expenditure of energy by the infant than gavage feedings. Allow a period of rest before and after feedings. Use of a pacifier before feedings to help bring the infant to an alert state will improve feeding success.

Infants may be fed on a schedule such as every 3 hours or when they begin to show hunger cues such as sucking on fingers or crying. Infants who receive cue-based feedings may sleep better and be able to attain full nipple feedings earlier than infants who receive scheduled feedings (McCain & Gartside, 2002).

Giving Bottle Feedings Nursing interventions for bottle feeding the preterm infant are presented in Nursing Care Plan: The Preterm Infant.

Nursing Care Plan

The Preterm Infant

ASSESSMENT

Giovanni was born at 33 weeks' gestation and now weighs 1800 g (4 lb). He breathes on his own with oxygen by hood. Giovanni needs many treatments throughout the day. He demonstrates pallor and increased respiratory rate when tired. Noises often cause a drop in oxygen saturation. When held or disturbed for care, Giovanni may stiffen and extend his arms with the fingers splayed. He sleeps most of the time when he is undisturbed.

Nursing Diagnosis

Activity Intolerance related to weakness, fatigue, and possible overstimulation.

Goals/Expected Outcomes

Giovanni will:
- Not show signs of overstimulation (increased respirations, pallor, decreased oxygen saturation level, stiffening of arms and legs, splaying of fingers) as a result of normal activity.
- Increase tolerance to activity gradually, as demonstrated by fewer signs of fatigue or stress.

INTERVENTION	RATIONALE
1. Whenever possible, arrange to provide routine care to correspond with Giovanni's natural awake periods.	1. Preterm infants need undisturbed sleep to promote growth.
2. Schedule periods of uninterrupted rest, especially before and after energy-draining activities.	2. Infants tolerate activities best when they begin in a rested state and are allowed to recover from them before other activities are necessary.
3. Experiment with grouping care to determine the number and combination of care activities that Giovanni tolerates best.	3. Grouping accomplishes more tasks at once so that longer rest periods are possible between tasks. Too many activities, however, may cause too much fatigue.
4. Assess the infant's stress signs before beginning care activities. Reassess frequently during each period of care and again after care to determine the infant's response.	4. Careful assessment helps the nurse individualize nursing care to the changing needs of the infant.
5. Observe carefully to determine which activities bring about signs of overstimulation and fatigue. Stop activities and allow short periods of rest, if possible.	5. Careful observation allows the nurse to be sensitive to the infant's ability to tolerate care.
6. Reduce the noise level around Giovanni. Avoid talking unnecessarily; open and close doors softly; keep alarm volumes low.	6. Noise may be overstimulating and result in increased oxygen need.
7. Place Giovanni prone and facing away from bright lights. Partially cover the incubator to keep out light but allow visibility of infant.	7. Continuous lighting interferes with the infant's sleep. Reducing light in the infant's face will increase rest.
8. Use blanket rolls and positioning devices to form "boundaries" around Giovanni and keep his extremities flexed.	8. Because it is similar to the small space of the uterus, enclosed space promotes rest and comfort.
9. Collaborate with other nurses to determine what works best to decrease Giovanni's fatigue. Tape signs on the bed to provide this information to parents and others.	9. All caregivers should have information available to help meet the infant's needs consistently.
10. Explain to the parents Giovanni's needs for rest and low stimulation. Suggest ways that they can interact appropriately to meet Giovanni's needs, and point out signs that he is receiving too much stimulation. Ask for their input.	10. Parents who are informed can care for the infant appropriately and feel that they are members of the team and are parenting their child by learning his needs.

Evaluation

Giovanni gradually shows increased ability to tolerate progressive activity with fewer episodes of overstimulation. His respirations and oxygen saturation levels remain stable, and he rarely stiffens his arms and legs during activity.

Nursing Care Plan

The Preterm Infant—cont'd

ASSESSMENT

Two or three times a day, Giovanni receives feedings by nipple supplemented by gavage when he becomes too tired. The feeding plan is for him to receive 120 kcal/kg/day to meet his needs. Giovanni has occasional episodes of increased respirations or short cyanotic spells when fed. He sometimes takes only half the feeding before falling asleep and must receive the rest by gavage. Giovanni's mother has decided to formula feed.

Nursing Diagnosis

Ineffective Infant Feeding Pattern related to muscle weakness and fatigue during feedings.

Goals/Expected Outcomes

Giovanni will:
- Take 216 kcal/day to meet his needs at a weight of 1800 g.
- Gain 27 to 36 g daily.
- Complete nipple feedings without signs of excessive fatigue (e.g., increased respiratory rate, falling asleep during feeding).

INTERVENTION

1. Schedule nursing care to provide a rest period before and after nipple feedings. Feed the infant before he begins to show signs of hunger such as trying to suck on his hands or rooting and before he begins to cry with hunger.

2. Use a feeding container (e.g., a Volutrol) on which each milliliter is marked. Place the container in warm water to heat milk to room temperature or slightly warmer. Do not use a microwave oven to warm.

3. Determine the type of nipple that works best for Giovanni. Choose between various sizes and consistencies.

4. Wrap Giovanni in warmed blankets, and place a hat on his head. Feed him in the incubator or under the warmer if needed.

5. Position Giovanni at a 45° to 60° angle (or more upright) facing the nurse. Position the head slightly forward and the chin slightly down. Place a finger on each cheek and one under the jaw at the base of the tongue midway between the chin and the throat. Provide gentle pressure.

6. Feed slowly, and allow the infant to rest when he stops sucking. Do not move the nipple around in his mouth in an attempt to force the preterm infant to resume feeding before he or she is ready. Burp frequently.

7. Observe for coughing, gagging, cyanosis, apnea, and changes in heart rate, respirations, or oxygen saturation. Stop feeding, and allow the infant to recover. Evaluate the infant's ability to continue. Provide or increase oxygen if needed.

8. Reduce external stimuli during feedings if the infant shows signs of overstimulation.

RATIONALE

1. Nippling consumes a great deal of energy. Rest helps prevent excessive fatigue that might prevent the infant from completing the feeding. Crying increases energy needed.

2. Exact measurement of the amount taken is important to ensure that Giovanni receives required nutrients. Some infants take slightly warmed milk better. Microwaving provides uneven heating of formula and may cause the infant to be burned.

3. A low-flow nipple may be best at first so the infant does not receive more milk than he can manage. This would cause choking and interfere with breathing between sucking bursts. Later, the infant may be able to manage a nipple that allows a faster milk flow. Infants with very small mouths require smaller nipples.

4. A hat and blankets help maintain the temperature. If infants have difficulty with temperature maintenance, an incubator or warmer provides warmth during feedings.

5. Positioning the infant to face the nurse allows the nurse to observe the infant's suck response to feeding, and any regurgitation. A more upright position decreases the flow of formula. The finger position helps support the tongue and increases sucking strength.

6. Slow feeding is necessary because of the infant's decreased energy. Preterm infants need rest periods during feedings because they have difficulty regulating their breathing while feeding. They may swallow more air than full-term infants do because sucking is less efficient.

7. These signs show difficulty coordinating sucking, swallowing, and breathing, and possible aspiration. Some infants have prolonged bursts of sucking without stopping to breathe and need to have the nipple removed so they will rest and resume breathing. Feeding requires more oxygen intake.

8. Too many stimuli may exhaust the infant and prevent optimal feeding behaviors.

Continued

Nursing Care Plan

The Preterm Infant—cont'd

INTERVENTION	RATIONALE
9. Assess for signs of overfatigue: falling asleep during feedings, feedings lasting more than 20 to 30 minutes, increased respirations.	9. Feedings may require more energy than the infant has available. Infants who are overfatigued are more likely to aspirate. Calories may be used for feeding instead of for growth.
10. Finish feeding by gavage if necessary.	10. Completing the feeding by gavage conserves energy, prevents aspiration, and ensures the infant receives the desired nutrient intake.
11. After feeding, position Giovanni on the right side or prone with his head elevated approximately 30°.	11. If regurgitation occurs, fluid will run out of the mouth easily so that the infant will not aspirate it. The right-side position and elevation of the head allow gravity to help empty the stomach.
12. Involve parents as soon as possible in giving feedings. Teach them to assess feeding cues and the infant's response to feedings. Help them learn the infant's usual pattern of sucking, swallowing, and breathing and to watch for changes such as milk dribbling out of the infant's mouth or breathing irregularities that indicate a need to stop the feeding temporarily.	12. Feeding allows parents to participate in the infant's care. Their comfort with feedings and learning about the infant's responses will help them prepare for discharge.

Evaluation

Giovanni consumes an average of 220 calories and gains an average of 31 g daily. He gradually takes more of his feeding by nipple and rarely needs gavage feeding to finish. His respiratory rate remains less than 60 breaths/minute, and he stays awake for the entire feeding.

Additional Nursing Diagnoses to Consider

Ineffective Thermoregulation
Ineffective Airway Clearance
Interrupted Family Processes
Risk for Caregiver Role Strain
Risk for Impaired Parenting
Risk for Infection
Pain

Facilitating Breastfeeding

Encourage mothers who would like to breastfeed. Contributing her milk helps the mother feel that she has something important to offer at a time when she may believe there is little she can do to help her baby. The immunologic benefits of breast milk are particularly important to the preterm infant who did not receive passive immunity during fetal life. Nutrients in breast milk are more easily digested and it provides antimicrobial components, enzymes, hormones, and growth factors important for the preterm infant. Although milk from mothers of preterm infants is higher in protein, fat, and electrolytes during the early weeks, it may be necessary to add fortifiers to meet total nutrient needs.

Breast milk may increase feeding tolerance, reduce infections and later allergies, enhance neurologic development, and help prevent necrotizing enterocolitis. In addition, breastfeeding may be less stressful than bottle feeding for preterm infants. Oxygenation levels are often higher during breast feeding because the infant can regulate breathing and suckling better than with bottle feeding.

Mothers who plan to breastfeed need help in maintaining lactation until the infant is mature enough to nurse. Help her begin to use a breast pump within the first 24 hours after birth, and give her sterile containers to store her milk. Tell her to place the milk in a refrigerator if the infant will receive it within 24 hours or in a freezer if it will be more than 24 hours before it is fed to the infant (Lemons, 2001). If fortifiers will be added to the milk, explain the higher needs of the preterm infant so the mother does not believe that something is wrong with her milk.

Ongoing support for the mother is important. Encourage the mother in her efforts in feeding, which may be difficult at first. Provide as much privacy as possible, using a separate room or screens. Help the mother feel comfortable holding the tiny infant and any attached equipment, such as monitor leads.

Adapt breastfeeding teaching to the needs of a very small infant. Show the mother how to use the cross-cradle hold (see Fig. 24-5), which allows the mother to see the infant well during latching-on and throughout the feeding. A supplemental nursing system, a device that holds expressed

CRITICAL THINKING EXERCISE 29-1

What are the major differences between feeding formula to a preterm infant and a full-term infant?

breast milk in a bag with a small tube attached to the mother's nipple, may be used to help infants receive more milk with less effort during early feedings.

Make the same observations of the infant during breast-feeding as during bottle feeding. Signs of fatigue, bradycardia, tachypnea, or apnea may show lack of readiness for breastfeed-ing. Be sure that the infant stays warm. The mother's body heat will help maintain the infant's temperature during feedings. Kangaroo care can often be combined with breastfeeding.

Making Ongoing Assessments

Continuously assess the infant's responses to all feeding meth-ods. Watch for signs of distress, especially when feedings are first initiated. Record the amount of breast milk or formula that the infant takes by gavage or bottle and compare it with the amount needed to meet nutrient needs for the infant's age and weight. Infants may be weighed on an electronic scale be-fore and after breastfeedings to determine intake. The weight allows supplementary gavage-feeding amounts to be calcu-lated based on the infant's oral intake of breast milk.

Weigh the infant daily at the same time with the same scale. Record the length and head circumference each week. Plot measurements on a growth chart for preterm infants to see if changes are within expected ranges. Weight increase not accompanied by increased length may be caused by edema and may be a sign of a complication such as conges-tive heart failure.

Observe changes in the infant's ability to take feedings. As the infant becomes more mature, less energy should be ex-pended during the feeding sessions. The infant will take the feedings more quickly and show fewer signs of fatigue, such as falling asleep during feedings.

Evaluation

- Does the infant consume adequate amounts of formula or breast milk to meet nutrient needs for age and weight?
- Is the pattern of weight gain approximately 15 to 20 g/kg/day?

PARENTING

The extended hospitalization of the preterm infant causes separation of the parents from their newborn, produces emotional trauma, and disrupts family life. It is stressful for parents to be unable to assume the parenting role they had expected, and they may state they do not feel like they are parents during this time. Although attachment begins dur-ing pregnancy, premature birth and prolonged hospitaliza-tion interfere with the process of continuing attachment after birth.

Preterm infants often look and behave very differently from those who are full term. When NICU care is required, parents may be unable to participate fully in infant care for sometimes prolonged periods. This interferes with parents' ability to learn their baby's unique characteristics such as the way the infant responds to stress and the methods of conso-

lation that work best. Separation and inability to assume the parenting role delay the development of the parent-infant re-lationship and may impair the parents' bonding. Nurses must evaluate the progress of bonding and assist parents to feel im-portant in caring for their infant.

Assessment

Assess for signs of parental attachment on the first and sub-sequent visits to the NICU nursery. Expect parents to be fear-ful at first but more able to focus on the infant as they get over the initial shock of preterm birth. Assess for common behaviors that show normal progression of attachment. These include talking about the infant in positive terms, making eye contact, pointing out physical characteristics, naming the infant, and calling the infant by name. When they can hold and participate in the care of the infant, ob-serve for gradual increase in comfort and skill. The parents should smile and talk to the infant and verbalize increasing confidence in their caretaking abilities.

Watch for signs that bonding is not occurring as expected. Determine if there are other stressors in the parents' lives that may interfere with their ability to visit and attach to the infant. The financial need to return to work, lack of trans-portation, or the need to care for other children may prevent parents from visiting as often as they would like.

After the critical period in the early days after birth, healthy preterm infants become more stable. They still re-quire specialized nursing care and hospitalization but gradu-ally need fewer technologic interventions. They are some-times called "growers" at this time. This is a time when parental participation in the infant's care should increase in preparation for discharge.

Nursing Diagnosis and Planning

For most parents of infants with problems at birth, the nurs-ing diagnosis is

- Risk for Impaired Parent/Infant Attachment related to sep-aration of parents from infant and lack of understanding about the preterm infant's condition and characteristics.
  Expected Outcomes: The parents will demonstrate bond-ing behaviors, including visiting frequently and interacting as appropriate for the infant's condition throughout the hospital stay. The parents will verbalize understanding of the preterm infant's condition and characteristics within 2 days and will express increasing comfort in participating in infant care within 1 week (as appropriate).

! CRITICAL TO REMEMBER

Signs That Bonding May Be Delayed

- Using negative terms to describe the infant
- Discussing the infant in impersonal or technical terms
- Failing to give the infant a name or to use the name
- Visiting or calling infrequently or not at all
- Decreasing the number and length of visits
- Showing interest in other infants equal to that in their own infant
- Refusing offers to hold and learn to care for the infant
- Showing a decrease in or lack of eye contact and in time spent talking to or smiling at the infant

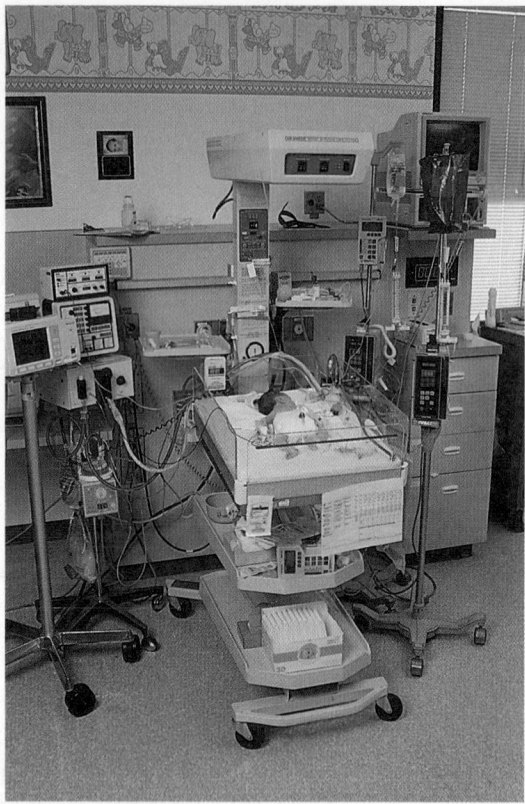

Figure 29-6 An infant in the neonatal intensive care unit (NICU) is surrounded by highly technologic equipment. This can be very frightening to parents at first. Preparation of parents before they visit is an important nursing responsibility.

Interventions

Making Advance Preparations

Preparing for threatening situations such as preterm birth helps parents cope with the actual event. Parents at higher risk for a preterm birth should visit the NICU nursery before delivery. If the mother is confined to bed, arrange for a nurse from the NICU to visit her. The father or another support person should tour the nursery so that he can discuss the nursery environment with the mother. Encourage the parents to ask questions they may have about how the infant will be cared for if it is born early.

Assisting Parents at Birth

After the birth, allow the parents to see and touch the newborn in the delivery room so that they have a realistic idea of the infant's appearance and condition and can begin bonding. If possible, allow the father to watch the initial care in the NICU. Explain what is happening and why. This attention allows him to see the intensive efforts made on behalf of his infant, increases his confidence in the staff, and enables him to give the mother a full description later. Support the father as well as the mother by using therapeutic communication during this difficult time.

If the infant must be transported to another facility, ask the transport team to visit the mother before leaving, if possible. The visit helps the parents feel connected to their infant and to the staff providing care. Leaving photographs with the mother is another way of helping her bond with the infant.

Supporting Parents During Early Visits

Take the mother to the NICU nursery as soon as she is able. If she is too sick to be with her infant, bring her photographs. Prepare parents before the first visit. Describe the equipment and its purposes, the various attachments to the infant, and the sounds of alarms (Fig. 29-6). Explain how the infant will look and behave. Table 29-1 provides specific steps that the nurse can follow to help parents become familiar with the NICU setting.

At first, stay with the parents during visits. When they are comfortable, allow them time alone with the infant so that they can interact in private. Answer questions and explain changes in the infant's condition and treatment. Parents may not know what questions to ask or may be too overwhelmed to ask questions. In this situation, the nurse can discuss questions that are common when parents first visit the NICU. Use therapeutic communication as the parents cope with their grief, guilt, and emotional turmoil.

Parents should touch the infant as soon as possible because touching helps promote attachment. They may be hesitant initially because of fear that they will interfere with equipment. Show them how to touch in ways appropriate for the infant, such as holding the infant's hand through the portholes of the incubator. Some parents may hesitate to touch because they are afraid of becoming attached to an infant whom they may lose. They need sensitive support from the nurse until they are ready to progress in their relationship with the infant.

Allow the parents to hold the baby as soon as possible. Holding the baby is particularly important to parents who may interpret it as a very positive sign of the infant's condition. Yet, it may be frightening too, especially if the infant is attached to various kinds of equipment. Help the parents find a comfortable position for themselves and the infant, and point out signs of a positive response from the infant.

Providing Information

An important role of the nurse is providing information to parents. In one study, 71% of parents felt nurses were the best source of information (Brazy, Anderson, Becker, & Becker, 2001). Encourage parents to ask questions about all aspects of their infant's condition and care. Although some mothers are not hesitant to ask questions, other mothers of NICU infants are fearful about asking for explanations because they are afraid that they might be seen as "difficult" parents and that this might jeopardize the infant's care (Hurst, 2001). Explain the equipment used to care for the infant. Interpret the information obtained from monitors and the meaning of alarms. Clarify all nursing care, its purpose, and the expected response. To help parents develop a realistic understanding of the infant's capabilities, point out how preterm infants are similar to and different from full-term infants.

Offer realistic reassurance about the infant's condition, emphasizing positive aspects while being truthful. If parents have misconceptions or did not understand a physician's explanations, clarify or ask the physician to go over specific information again. Translate medical terms into words the parents can understand. Use an interpreter if the parents do not understand English.

Repeat explanations, especially at first. Because of their emotional distress, parents are often unable to comprehend fully or remember what is said to them.

TABLE **29-1** Introducing Parents to the Neonatal Intensive Care Unit (NICU) Setting

Before Parents Visit the NICU	When Parents Visit the NICU
Describe the NICU environment. Include the noise of alarms, the busyness of the staff, the number of people and sick infants.	Help parents perform thorough handwashing while explaining the purpose.
Show parents photographs of the infant. These help prepare them but are not as overwhelming as seeing the infant in person.	Stay with the parents during their visit. Having a familiar person nearby will help them feel more comfortable while they adjust to this unfamiliar environment.
Describe the infant. Include the size, the lack of fat, the breathing, the weak cry. Explain that no sound of crying can be heard if the infant is intubated. Include some personal aspects: "He's a real fighter" or "She makes the funniest faces during her feedings."	Introduce them to the infant's nurse. Ask the nurse to explain some of the things being done for the infant.
	Provide parents with written information about the NICU so that they can take it home to read later.
Describe the equipment. Include ventilators, intravenous (IV) lines, and monitors. Explain how they look and how they are attached to the infant. Keep the explanations simple, without technical details.	Tell the parents that they will receive instruction on how to care for their infant in time. Encourage them to visit the infant as much as they can. Emphasize how important they are to their infant.
	Offer realistic encouragement based on the infant's condition.
	Provide an opportunity for the parents to express their concerns and feelings and to ask questions.

Offer written information in the parents' language about NICU policies and procedures. Explanations about visiting hours, who can visit, routines for handwashing, and the role of parents can be reinforced in writing and be available for later reading by parents who are overwhelmed.

Instituting Kangaroo Care

Begin kangaroo care (KC) as soon as possible. KC is a method of providing skin-to-skin contact between preterm infants and their parents. The infant, wearing only a diaper and hat, is placed under the mother's clothes between her breasts. A blanket is placed over the mother's clothes and the infant's back (Fig. 29-7). Mothers may breastfeed if they wish and the infant is able. Fathers may also participate in KC.

Explain the advantages of KC to parents, and elicit their participation. This method of care has been found safe for stable infants, even if intubated. It provides the developmental care so important for the preterm infant and is associated with improved infant growth and decreased length of hospital stay (Byers, 2003). The upright position of the infant against the parent's chest makes breathing easier. The containment of the extremities decreases purposeless movements that use oxygen and calories. Breastfeeding is facilitated, and the infant has more alert periods and increased deep sleep. The contact with the parent's skin maintains the infant's body temperature. In addition, KC provides an opportunity for parents to participate in the infant's care and helps increase parent-infant attachment and parents' feelings of confidence in caring for the infant (Gardner & Goldson, 2002).

Facilitating Interaction

Parents may feel rejected by the infant's lack of response or negative response during interactions. Explain to them that infants born at less than 34 weeks' gestation may not be able to cope with socialization. Interaction that is effective with full-term infants may be too stimulating for very young or sick preterm infants. Suggest forms of touch and interaction based on the individual infant's capacity. Quiet holding may be better until the infant can tolerate more stimulation.

Help parents understand the infant's behavior and cues. Teach parents signs of overstimulation, and explain that the

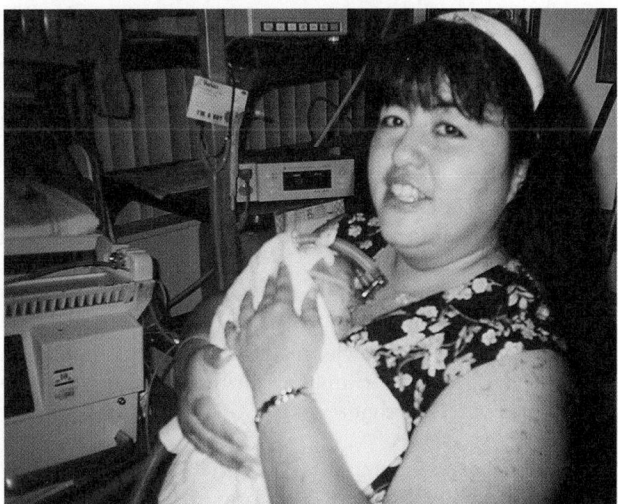

Figure 29-7 This mother holds her infant of 27 weeks' gestation under her clothes against her skin as she gives Kangaroo care.

infant needs a quiet rest period without stimulation when they occur. Discuss methods to avoid too much stimulation and ways to calm the infant. If several types of stimulation (e.g., rocking, eye contact, and talking) cause signs of distress, suggest they stop one or more activities until the infant has had a rest period. Show them how to position the infant with the hands near the mouth so the infant can suck on them as a self-comforting measure. When the infant is ready for more interaction, suggest appropriate types of stimulation.

Point out small signs of improvement and even minor strengths. Talk about normal preterm characteristics and emphasize individual characteristics that make this infant different from all others. The way the infant eats, reacts to sounds, or seems to get tangled in the monitor leads may help parents feel closer to their newborn.

Involve the parents in care of the infant as soon as possible to help them feel a sense of control (Fig. 29-8). At first, plan to change the linens in the incubator or radiant warmer when the parents are there so that they can hold their infant. As the

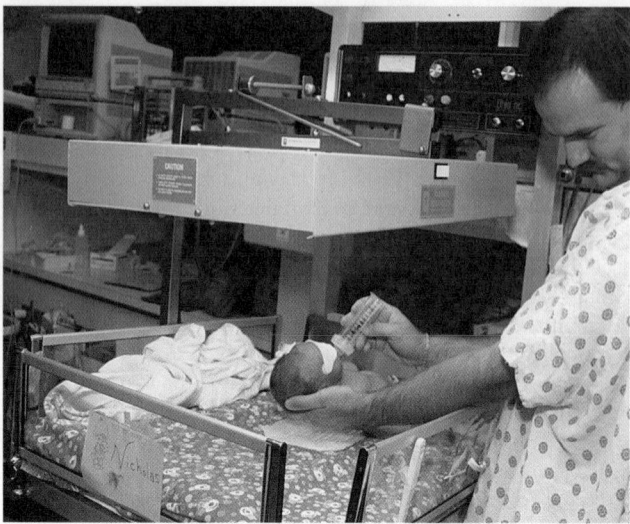

Figure 29-8 To promote family bonding with the infant, parents are involved as much as possible in the care of their infant. This father bottle feeds his infant in a radiant warmer.

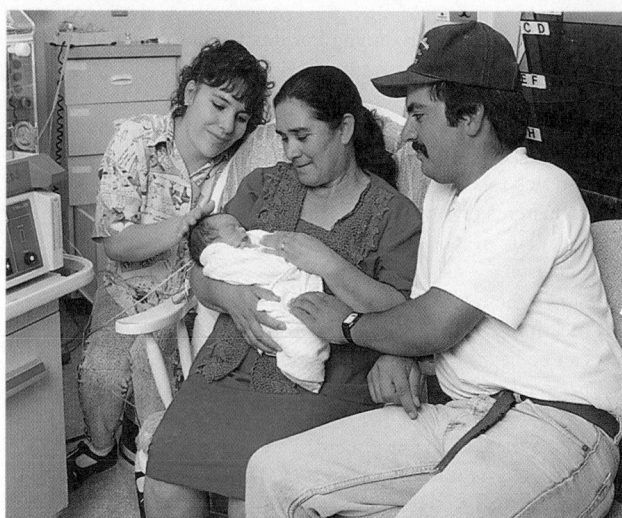

Figure 29-9 The parents look on while the grandmother holds the infant in the neonatal intensive care unit (NICU).

infant's condition improves, parents can develop skill in caring for the tiny infant by changing diapers, feeding, and bathing.

Increasing Parental Decision Making

Give parents the information they need to take an active part in decisions made about the infant's treatment plan. This knowledge will increase their feelings of control over a situation in which many parents feel they have little power. As parents become more knowledgeable and participate more in the caregiving, seek their input about how the infant is progressing and practices that seem to work best.

Alleviating Concerns

Invite parents to call the NICU at any time for information about their infant. Phone calls are especially beneficial for parents who cannot visit the infant because of distance or other reasons. Put them in touch with other parents who have had preterm infants, and refer them to parent groups. It is important to consider language and culture during this process. Talking with those who have faced the same problems can be very comforting. They can compare notes and get practical suggestions from an experienced parent's point of view.

Helping with Ongoing Problems

Parents may be unprepared for the inconsistent progress infants often make after surviving the risks of the early days. They expect steady progress once the infant can eat and breathe alone. Complications such as necrotizing enterocolitis or sepsis, however, can cause major setbacks at this time. To cope with a new crisis, parents need extensive support from the nurse. Use therapeutic communication techniques such as reflecting feelings to help them express and cope with their extreme disappointment. Give information about the infant's changing condition and what to expect in the days ahead.

Preparing for Discharge

Because infants go home very early, it is important that the parents understand the expected hospital course. If a clinical pathway is being used for the infant, give them a copy. They can chart the infant's achievement of major milestones in development and changes in care as the infant moves toward discharge. This information helps them prepare themselves and their home so they can provide the special care that their infant may need after discharge.

Begin early to teach parents and other caregivers any special procedures, treatments, and medications that the infant will need after discharge (Fig. 29-9). Observe the parents performing care until they are comfortable and can do it safely. Help them learn what is normal for their infant and how to recognize and respond to abnormal signs. Some hospitals have parents spend a night in a special "parent room," where they take over full 24-hour care of the infant yet still have help available if needed.

Help the parents determine what adaptations they will need to make at home for discharge. Utility companies should be notified if the infant is considered medically fragile. This notice ensures the family receives priority service in cases of power failure. Arrange home nursing services and delivery of special equipment before discharge.

Discuss what to expect in care of the infant after discharge. Many infants need feedings every 3 hours, day and night, to help them gain the 20 to 40 g a day expected after discharge (Sifuentes, 2000). Feedings may be time consuming, and parental fatigue resulting from sleep interruptions may be greater than they expected. Explore with parents what kind of help they might need in meeting the everyday requirements of the infant and the rest of the family. Help them identify where they might find assistance from family and friends.

Assist parents to form realistic expectations of the infant. For example, they should know that the infant will accomplish developmental tasks, such as crawling and walking, later than full-term infants. Parents should base expectations on the infant's developmental rather than chronologic age. Developmental age is the chronologic age minus the number of weeks the infant was born early.

Assist the parents to plan for integrating the new infant into the family. Meeting the needs of their other children in addition to the new responsibilities of caring for the preterm infant is a major source of worry. Encourage siblings who do not have infections to visit. Siblings should touch or hold the infant, if possible, to help them bond.

Before discharge, infants are often evaluated for apnea or bradycardia in the car seat the parents will use. Proper positioning with blanket rolls may be necessary because the infants may slump over, interfering with chest expansion. Some infants need car beds to allow them to ride in a recumbent position.

Evaluation

- Do the parents demonstrate common bonding behaviors?
- Do they verbalize understanding of the preterm infant's special needs and treatments?
- How active are the parents in caring for the infant?

ADDITIONAL COMPLICATIONS OF PRETERM INFANTS

Complications of prematurity increase as the infant's gestational age and birth weight decrease. Some complications, such as hyperbilirubinemia, are common to full-term and preterm infants and are discussed in Chapter 30. Complications most common in prematurity are discussed here.

Respiratory Distress Syndrome

Respiratory distress syndrome (RDS), also called *hyaline membrane disease*, is one of the most common problems of prematurity. It occurs most frequently in infants who are less than 30 weeks' gestation and weigh less than 1200 g (Hagedorn et al., 2002). It is also seen in birth asphyxia and infants of diabetic mothers because these conditions interfere with surfactant production. It occurs less frequently, however, when chronic fetal stress, such as in heroin addiction, preeclampsia, and prolonged rupture of membranes, causes the lungs to mature more quickly (Stoll & Kliegman, 2004a).

Pathophysiology

RDS is caused by insufficient production of surfactant, a phospholipid that lines the alveoli. Surfactant is first produced in the alveoli at 22 weeks' gestation. By 34 to 36 weeks' gestation, production of surfactant is usually great enough to enable the infant to breathe normally outside the uterus (Hagedorn et al., 2002).

Surfactant decreases surface tension to allow the alveoli to remain open when air is exhaled. It must be continuously produced as it is used. With too little surfactant, the alveoli collapse each time the infant exhales. The lungs become noncompliant or "stiff," and they resist expansion. Noncompliant lungs require a much higher negative pressure for the alveoli to open each time the infant inhales. This results in severe retractions with each breath because the chest wall is very compliant and the weak muscles of the chest wall are drawn inward. The resulting pressure on the lungs further interferes with expansion.

As fewer alveoli expand, atelectasis and hypoxia occur. This causes pulmonary vasoconstriction and decreased blood flow to the lungs because of the high resistance within the pulmonary blood vessels. Persistent pulmonary hypertension can result in a return to fetal circulation patterns, with opening of the ductus arteriosus. Acidosis and alveolar necrosis complicate the condition by interfering with surfactant synthesis. Hyaline membranes, consisting of a fibrous material with debris from necrotic cells, line the distal airways.

Lecithin, sphingomyelin, and phosphatidylglycerol are components of surfactant that can be detected by tests of amniotic fluid. These tests can predict whether the fetal lungs are mature enough for survival outside of the uterus (see Chapter 16). The incidence and severity of RDS may be reduced by giving the mother corticosteroids before birth (see Chapter 27).

Manifestations

Signs of RDS begin during the first hours after birth and include tachypnea, nasal flaring, retractions, and cyanosis. Grunting on expiration is characteristic and signifies physiologic efforts to maintain lung expansion. Breath sounds may be decreased, or rales may be present. Signs become worse and peak at 2 to 3 days and then begin to improve (Rodriguez, Martin, & Fanaroff, 2002). Blood gases show increased carbon dioxide levels and decreased oxygen. Acidosis develops as a result of hypoxemia. Chest radiographs show the "ground glass" appearance of the lungs that is characteristic of RDS.

Therapeutic Management

Surfactant replacement therapy is a common treatment to reduce the severity of RDS. Surfactant is instilled into the infant's trachea immediately after birth or as soon as signs of RDS become apparent. Improvement in breathing occurs in minutes. Infants treated with surfactant have higher survival rates, but it does not reduce other complications of prematurity such as bronchopulmonary dysplasia.

Other supportive treatment includes mechanical ventilation, correction of the acidosis, IV feedings, and care of other complications.

Nursing Considerations

The nurse observes for signs of developing RDS at birth and during the early hours of life. Changes in the infant's condition are constantly assessed. For example, diuresis may occur with improvement in the disease. Changes in ventilator settings may be necessary as the infant's ability to oxygenate increases. Observation for signs of common complications, such as patent ductus arteriosus and bronchopulmonary dysplasia, is important. The nurse must monitor the results of laboratory tests for abnormalities in blood gases and acid-base balance. Early signs of sepsis must be identified and reported. Other care is similar to general care for the preterm infant.

Bronchopulmonary Dysplasia (Chronic Lung Disease)

Bronchopulmonary dysplasia (BPD) or chronic lung disease (CLD) is a chronic condition that may occur when infants are treated with mechanical ventilation and oxygen. This treatment may cause damage to the lungs and result in prolonged dependence on supplementary oxygen. It is discussed in detail in Chapter 45.

Periventricular-Intraventricular Hemorrhage

Periventricular-intraventricular hemorrhage (PIVH) most often affects infants of less than 32 weeks' gestation or those who weigh less than 1500 g (Blackburn, 2003a). The first few days of life are the most common times for hemorrhage to occur.

Pathophysiology

PIVH results from rupture of the fragile blood vessels in the germinal matrix, located around the ventricles of the brain. It is most often associated with hypoxic injury to the vessels, increased or decreased blood pressure, and increased or fluctuating cerebral blood flow. Rapid blood volume expansion, hypercarbia, anemia, and hypoglycemia are other causes.

Hemorrhage is graded 1 through 4, according to the amount of bleeding. Grade 1 is a very small bleed at the germinal matrix, producing few if any clinical changes. Grade 2 hemorrhage extends into the lateral ventricles, and grade 3 causes distention of ventricles. Grade 4 hemorrhage causes ventricular dilation and extends into the surrounding brain tissue.

Grade 1 or 2 hemorrhage may result in little neurologic abnormality, but infants with grades 3 and 4 hemorrhages may have neurologic abnormalities and developmental delays. Those with grade 4 hemorrhage have a poor survival rate.

Manifestations

Signs of PIVH are determined by the severity of the hemorrhage. They may include lethargy, poor muscle tone, deterioration of respiratory status with cyanosis or apnea, drop in hematocrit level, decreased reflexes, full or bulging fontanel, and seizures. Subtle aberrations of eye position or movement may occur.

Therapeutic Management

Because some infants show no signs, early and repeated screening by ultrasonography is performed on preterm infants at risk for PIVH. Computed tomography (CT) may also be used to diagnose the condition. Serial ultrasonography may be used to determine progression of the problem.

Treatment is supportive and focuses on maintaining respiratory function and dealing with other complications. Hydrocephalus may develop from blockage of cerebrospinal fluid flow. Lumbar taps or a ventriculoperitoneal shunt (tube leading from the ventricles of the brain to the peritoneal cavity) may be necessary to drain the fluid.

Nursing Considerations

Many aspects of care may increase cerebral blood flow and blood pressure. These include mechanical ventilation, suctioning, and excessive handling. Even crying may produce changes in cerebral blood flow. Therefore the nurse must be alert for early signs of PIVH. Nursing care includes measurement of the head circumference daily and observation for changes in neurologic status, which may be subtle. Developmental care has been found helpful in preventing or minimizing the problem.

Parents need assistance to cope with the diagnosis and their concerns regarding long-term implications. They should learn how to assess for signs of increasing intracranial pressure from hydrocephalus and understand that follow-up care may include periodic ultrasound examinations.

Retinopathy of Prematurity

Retinopathy of prematurity (ROP), once called *retrolental fibroplasia*, may result in visual impairment or blindness in preterm infants. It occurs more often in infants weighing less than 1500 g.

Pathophysiology

ROP is caused by damage to immature blood vessels in the retina. The exact cause of the damage is unknown, but one cause may be high levels of oxygen.

However, ROP develops in some infants who never received supplementary oxygen. Prolonged ventilation, acidosis, sepsis, and shock have all been associated with ROP (American Academy of Pediatrics & American College of Obstetricians and Gynecologists [AAP & ACOG], 2002).

In ROP, immature blood vessels are damaged and new vessels proliferate to reestablish circulation. If the vessels extend into the vitreous humor, fluid leakage and hemorrhage occur. The result may be scarring, traction on the retina, and retinal detachment. However, the progress of pathology stops in more than 90% of infants and there is little visual loss (Olitsky & Nelson, 2004).

Therapeutic Management

Infants born at 28 weeks' gestation or less, those weighing 1500 g or less at birth, and those considered at risk should be screened 4 to 6 weeks after birth or at 31 to 33 weeks' corrected age to detect changes of the eye (AAP & ACOG, 2002). Cryotherapy and laser surgery have been used to destroy the proliferating blood vessels. Reattachment of the retina may also be necessary. Many infants have spontaneous regression with little or no impairment of vision.

Nursing Considerations

The nurse should check the pulse oximetry readings frequently for any infant receiving oxygen. Parents should be informed about ophthalmology tests and receive an explanation of the results. Eye examinations can be very stressful to the infant, and swaddling and rest periods should be provided as appropriate. Mydriatic eye drops given to dilate the eyes may cause apnea, bradycardia, and increased blood pressure. If surgery is performed, the eye is assessed for drainage. Ice packs may be used for edema, and pain medication should be given. Parental support is essential throughout the examinations and especially if damage to the eye is found.

Necrotizing Enterocolitis

Necrotizing enterocolitis (NEC) is a serious inflammatory condition of the intestinal tract that may lead to cellular death of areas of the mucosa of the intestines. It is discussed in Chapter 43.

POSTTERM INFANTS

Postterm infants are those who are born after the 42nd week of gestation. Their longer-than-normal gestation places them at risk for a number of complications.

Scope of the Problem

Approximately 12% of all pregnancies are considered postterm (Stoll & Kliegman, 2004b). In most cases, the fetus continues to be well supported by the placenta. Infants are usually of normal size or large for gestational age. Some may grow to more than 4000 g (8 lb, 13 oz), placing them at risk for birth injuries or cesarean birth.

In some cases, placental functioning decreases when pregnancy is prolonged. If placental insufficiency is present, decreased amniotic fluid volume (oligohydramnios) may occur. The fetus may not receive the appropriate amount of oxygen and nutrients and may be small for gestational age. This condition results in hypoxia and malnourishment in the fetus and is called *postmaturity syndrome*.

When labor begins, poor oxygen reserves may cause fetal compromise. The fetus may pass meconium as a result of hypoxia before or during labor, increasing the risk of meconium aspiration at delivery (see Chapter 30). Postterm infants have a higher perinatal mortality rate than infants born at term.

Assessment

Most infants will be normal at birth. If the infant is large, the nurse should assess for birth injuries and hypoglycemia.

The infant with postmaturity syndrome is unusually alert and wide-eyed and has a worried look. The infant may be thin and have loose skin with little subcutaneous fat. There is little or no lanugo and vernix caseosa, but the infant has abundant hair on the head and long nails. The skin is wrinkled, cracked, and peeling (Fig. 29-10). If meconium was present in the amniotic fluid, the cord, skin, and nails may be stained, indicating that meconium was present for some time.

Therapeutic Management

Therapeutic management focuses on prevention and symptomatic treatment. Labor is induced if signs of placental deterioration are present during fetal diagnostic testing. In cases of asphyxia or meconium aspiration, respiratory support is needed at birth (see Chapter 30).

Nursing Considerations

Signs of postmaturity syndrome in infants are noted during the initial assessment. Respiratory problems may necessitate continued assessment and care. Infants with any indications of postmaturity should be tested for hypoglycemia soon after birth and again an hour later. They need early and more frequent feedings to help compensate for the period of poor nutrition in utero.

Temperature regulation may be poor because fat stores were used for nourishment in utero. Extra blankets, frequent temperature assessment, and teaching parents about prevention of cold stress may be necessary throughout the hospital stay. Polycythemia increases the risk of hyperbilirubinemia.

SMALL-FOR-GESTATIONAL-AGE INFANTS

Small-for-gestational-age (SGA) infants are those who fall below the 10th percentile in size on growth charts. They have failed to grow in utero as expected, which is called *intrauterine growth restriction* (IUGR). The terms *SGA* and *IUGR* are often used interchangeably (as they are here) although not all infants who have had some growth restriction are SGA.

SGA infants may be preterm, full-term, or postterm. Infant mortality and morbidity increase steadily as growth restriction increases. Approximately one third of all LBW infants are full-term but SGA (Stoll & Kliegman, 2004b).

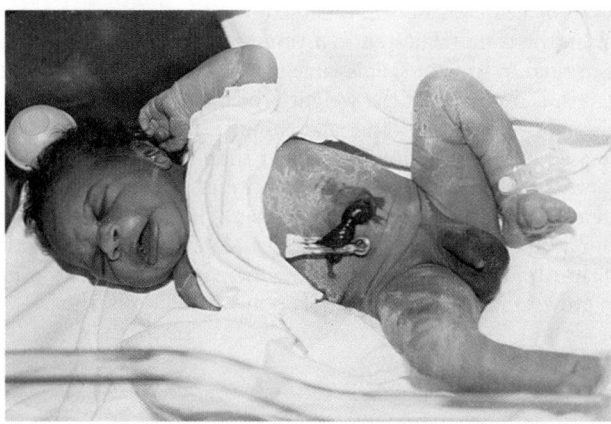

Figure 29-10 The postmature infant has no vernix and has dry, cracked, peeling skin.

Etiology

Many risk factors may cause an infant to be SGA. Congenital malformations, chromosomal anomalies, and fetal infections may cause IUGR. Poor placental function resulting from aging, small size, separation, or malformation may interfere with fetal growth. Illness in the expectant mother such as preeclampsia or severe diabetes restricts uteroplacental blood flow and decreases fetal growth. Smoking, drug or alcohol abuse, and severe maternal malnutrition also impair fetal growth.

Scope of the Problem

Infants affected with IUGR have higher perinatal morbidity and mortality rates than infants who are not growth restricted. Death may occur from asphyxia before or during labor because of poor placental functioning.

SGA infants are subject to many of the same complications as those who are preterm or postterm, depending on the cause and degree of growth restriction. Problems tend to be greatest in infants who are preterm in addition to being SGA.

Low Apgar scores, meconium aspiration, and polycythemia are increased in incidence in SGA infants. Hypoglycemia is common because of little storage of glycogen in the liver. Infants are prone to inadequate thermoregulation because subcutaneous and brown fat stores have been used to survive in utero.

Characteristics of Small-for-Gestational-Age Infants

The appearance of the SGA infant varies according to whether the cause of growth restriction began early or late in the pregnancy. Variation occurs because growth restriction affects the weight first. If it continues, the length and then the head size will eventually be affected.

Symmetric growth restriction may be caused by congenital anomalies or exposure to infections or drugs early in pregnancy. Although the infant's weight, length, and head circumference are all below the 10th percentile, the body is proportionate and appears normally developed for size. The total number of cells is decreased, and the infant may have long-term complications. These infants are often small throughout their lives.

Asymmetric restriction is caused by complications that begin in the third trimester. In asymmetric restriction, the head is normal in size but seems large for the rest of the body. The length is normal, but the weight is below the 10th percentile for gestational age. The abdominal circumference is decreased because the liver is smaller than normal. The infant appears long and thin. The loose skin has longitudinal thigh creases from loss of subcutaneous fat. The infant has sparse hair, a thin cord, dry skin, and the wide-eyed look associated with intrauterine hypoxia. These infants generally catch up in growth if they are adequately nourished after birth.

Therapeutic Management

Therapeutic management focuses on prevention with good prenatal care to identify and treat problems early. When growth restriction cannot be prevented, ultrasound examination may permit early discovery of the condition. Serial non-stress tests and biophysical profiles help determine if the infant should be delivered early, and preparation can be made for the expected complications at birth. Problems after birth are treated as they occur.

Nursing Considerations

Because the causes of growth restriction are so varied, care of the SGA infant must be adapted to meet the specific problems of the infant. When signs of growth restriction are present, the nurse must observe for the complications that commonly accompany it. The general appearance and measurements give an indication of the type of growth restriction that has occurred. Measurements of the head, chest, length, and weight are less than normal in the infant with symmetric growth restriction. If the restriction is asymmetric, the head circumference and length are normal and the abdominal circumference and weight are low.

The nurse should assess for hypoglycemia, especially in asymmetric growth-restricted infants. The brain of the infant is normal and needs large amounts of glucose, but the liver is small and has inadequate stores of glycogen. Caloric needs are greater than for a normal infant, making early and more frequent feedings important. Temperature regulation and respiratory support are added nursing concerns. Observation for jaundice is important in infants with polycythemia because a large amount of bilirubin may be released when the red blood cells break down.

LARGE-FOR-GESTATIONAL-AGE INFANTS

Large-for-gestational-age (LGA) infants are those who are above the 90th percentile on intrauterine growth charts. They may weigh more than 4000 g (8 lb, 13 oz) and are usually born at term, although they may be preterm or postterm. The preterm LGA infant may be mistaken for full-term but may have the same problems as other preterm infants.

Etiology

LGA infants may be born to multiparas, large parents, and members of certain ethnic groups known to have large infants. Diabetes in the mother may also cause increased size, as may erythroblastosis fetalis (see Chapter 30).

Scope of the Problem

The LGA infant is more likely to go through a longer labor, have injury during birth, or need a cesarean birth. Shoulder dystocia may occur because the shoulders are too large to fit through the pelvis. Fractures of the clavicle, damage to the brachial plexus or facial nerve, cephalhematoma, and bruising occur more often in these infants than in those of normal size. Congenital heart defects are more common, and the mortality rate is greater (Stoll & Kliegman, 2004b).

Therapeutic Management

Therapeutic management is based on identification of macrosomia (large size) during pregnancy by measurements of fundal height and ultrasound examination. Delivery problems may lead to the use of vacuum extraction, forceps, or cesarean birth. Specific treatment involves identification and treatment of birth injuries and complications as they arise.

Nursing Considerations

The nurse assists in a difficult delivery or cesarean birth resulting from dystocias when the infant is LGA. After birth, the infant is carefully assessed for injuries or other complications such as hypoglycemia (see p. 529) or polycythemia (see p. 761). Nursing care is geared to problems presented.

KEY CONCEPTS

- Preterm infants differ in appearance from full-term infants. Some differences include small size, limp posture, red skin, abundant vernix and lanugo, and immature ears and genitals.
- The lungs of preterm infants may lack adequate surfactant, which may cause the lungs to be noncompliant, increasing the amount of energy necessary for breathing and leading to atelectasis.
- Other factors that may increase respiratory problems are poor cough reflex, narrow respiratory passages, and weak muscles.

- Preterm infants should be positioned on the side or prone to increase drainage of respiratory secretions. Prone position decreases breathing effort and increases oxygenation.
- Preterm infants are subject to cold stress because they have thin skin with blood vessels near the surface, little subcutaneous (white) or brown fat, a large surface area, a limp position, and an immature temperature control center.
- It is important to maintain a neutral thermal environment at all times for infants. The nurse should prevent drafts, use warmed oxy-

gen, and keep incubator doors and portholes closed. When taken out of heating devices, the infant should be wrapped in warmed blankets and wear a hat.

- Preterm infants are subject to increased insensible water losses and have difficulty maintaining fluid balance. Their kidneys do not concentrate or dilute urine as well as those of full-term infants. Intake and output must be carefully measured.
- The fragile skin of a preterm infant is easily damaged. Adhesives or chemicals that could injure the skin should be avoided. Special

- products designed to prevent injury to the skin should be used.
- Preterm infants are subject to infections because they lack passive antibodies from the mother, have an immature immune system, have fragile skin, and are subjected to many invasive procedures.
- The nurse must watch carefully for signs of pain and use comfort measures, such as containment and pacifiers, and medications to alleviate it.
- Infants demonstrate that they are receiving too much stimulation by changes in oxygenation and behavior. The nurse should schedule care to allow rest periods, keep noise to a minimum, and teach parents to interact with the infant appropriately.
- Preterm infants lack nutrient stores and need more nutrients but do not absorb them well. They lack coordination in sucking and swallowing and fatigue easily.
- Signs indicating that an infant may be ready for nipple feeding include rooting, sucking on

a gavage tube or pacifier, presence of gag reflex, and respiratory rate less than 60 breaths per minute.
- The nurse can help the mother who wishes to breastfeed her preterm infant by teaching her how to use a breast pump and store her milk until the infant is ready to breastfeed. The nurse can provide privacy, give support, explain the infant's behavior, and answer questions about breastfeeding.
- Nurses can increase parents' comfort with their preterm infant by providing information about the infant's condition and characteristics, the NICU, equipment, and care. Spending time with parents during visits, offering therapeutic communication and realistic encouragement, and involving parents in care of the infant will also help with bonding.
- Preparation for discharge should be started early in the infant's hospital stay. Preparation allows parents to learn gradually and take on increasing responsibility in the care of the infant until they are comfortable with complete care.

- Common complications of preterm birth are RDS, BPD, PIVH, ROP, and NEC.
- Infants with postmaturity syndrome may appear thin, with loose skin folds; cracked, peeling skin; and meconium staining. They appear hyperalert and worried. They may have respiratory difficulties at birth and suffer from hypoglycemia and inadequate temperature regulation.
- Infants with IUGR may be SGA at birth. In symmetric growth restriction, the infant is proportionately small; in asymmetric growth restriction, the head and length are normal and the body is thin.
- LGA infants may have birth injuries such as fractures, nerve damage, or bruising as a result of their size. They may have hypoglycemia or polycythemia.

ANSWER to Critical Thinking Exercise 29-1

The preterm infant may need more frequent feedings with a special formula and smaller amounts. The preterm infant will take longer to feed, might need gavage feedings before introduction of a bottle or the breast, and is more prone to complications in feeding. See Nursing Care Plan: The Preterm Infant for interventions appropriate for bottle feeding the preterm infant.

REFERENCES and READINGS

Agarwal, R., Hagedorn, M.I.E., & Gardner, S.L. (2002). Pain and pain relief. In G.B. Merenstein & S.L. Gardner (Eds.), *Handbook of neonatal intensive care* (5th ed., pp. 191-218). St. Louis: Mosby.

Altimier, L.B. (2003). Management of the NICU environment. In C. Kenner & J.W. Lott (Eds.), *Comprehensive neonatal nursing: A physiologic perspective* (3rd ed., pp. 229-235). Philadelphia: Saunders.

American Academy of Pediatrics, & American College of Obstetricians and Gynecologists. (2002). *Guidelines for perinatal care* (5th ed.). Elk Grove Village, IL, and Washington, DC: Author.

American Academy of Pediatrics, & American Pain Society. (2001). The assessment and management of acute pain in infants, children, and adolescents. *Pediatrics, 108*(3), 793-797.

American Academy of Pediatrics, & Canadian Paediatric Society. (2000). Prevention and management of pain and stress in the neonate. *Pediatrics, 105*(2), 454-461.

Anderson, D.M. (2002). Feeding the ill or preterm infant. *Neonatal Network, 21*(7), 7-14.

Anderson, G.C., Chiu, S., Dombrowski, M.A., Swinth, J.Y., Albert, J.M., & Wada, N. (2003). Mother-newborn contact in a randomized trial of kangaroo (skin-to-skin) care. *Journal of Obstetric, Gynecologic, and Neonatal Nursing, 32*(5), 604-611.

Anderson, M.S., Johnson, C.B., Townsend, S.F., & Hay, W.W. (2002). Enteral nutrition. In G.B. Merenstein & S.L. Gardner (Eds.), *Handbook of neonatal intensive care* (5th ed., pp. 314-340). St. Louis: Mosby.

Arias, E., MacDorman, M.F., Strobino, D.M., & Guyer, B. (2003). Annual summary of vital statistics—2002. *Pediatrics, 112*(6 Pt. 2), 1215-1230.

Association of Women's Health, Obstetric, and Neonatal Nurses (AWHONN). (2001). *Evidence-based clinical practice guideline: Neonatal skin care*. Washington, DC: Author.

Beachy, J.M. (2003). Premature infant massage in the NICU. *Neonatal Network, 22*(3), 39-45.

Berry, D.D., Adcock, E.W., & Starbuck, A. (2002). Fluid and electrolyte management. In G.B. Merenstein & S.L. Gardner (Eds.), *Handbook of neonatal intensive care* (5th ed., pp. 283-297). St. Louis: Mosby.

Biancuzzo, M. (2003). *Breastfeeding the newborn: Clinical strategies for nurses* (2nd ed.). St. Louis: Mosby.

Blackburn, S.T. (2003a). Assessment and management of the neurologic system. In C. Kenner & J.W. Lott (Eds.), *Comprehensive neonatal nursing: A physiologic perspective* (3rd ed., pp. 624-660). Philadelphia: Saunders.

Blackburn, S.T. (2003b). *Maternal, fetal, and neonatal physiology* (2nd ed.). Philadelphia: Saunders.

Blake, W.W., & Murray, J.A. (2002). Heat balance. In G.B. Merenstein & S.L. Gardner (Eds.), *Handbook of neonatal intensive care* (5th ed., pp. 102-116). St. Louis: Mosby.

Bracht, M., Kandankery, A., Nodwell, S., & Stade, B. (2002). Cultural differences and parental responses to the preterm infant at risk: Strategies for supporting families. *Neonatal Network, 21*(6), 31-38.

Brazy, J.E., Anderson, B.M.H., Becker, P., & Becker, M. (2001). How parents of premature

infants gather information and obtain support. *Neonatal Network, 20*(2), 41-48.

Bremmer, P., Byers, J.F., & Kiehl, E. (2003). Noise and the premature infant: Physiological effects and practice implications. *Journal of Obstetric, Gynecologic, and Neonatal Nursing, 32*(4), 447-454.

Brooks, S.L., Mitchell, A., & Steffenson, N. (2000). Mothers, infants, & DHA: Implications for nursing practice. *MCN: The American Journal of Maternal/Child Nursing, 25*(2), 71-75.

Bruns, D.A., & McCollum, J.A. (2002). Partnerships between mothers and professionals in the NICU: Caregiving, information exchange, and relationships. *Neonatal Network, 21*(7), 15-23.

Byers, J.F. (2003). Components of developmental care and the evidence for their use in the NICU. *MCN: The American Journal of Maternal/Child Nursing, 28*(1), 174-181.

Cifuentes, J., Segars, A.H., & Carlo, W.A. (2003). Respiratory system management. In C. Kenner & J.W. Lott (Eds.), *Comprehensive neonatal nursing: A physiologic perspective* (3rd ed., pp. 348-362). Philadelphia: Saunders.

Colon, E.J. (2001). Culturally congruent care in the NICU. *AWHONN Lifelines, 5*(5), 60-64.

Consensus Committee to Establish Recommended Standards for Newborn ICU Design. (2002). *Recommended standards for newborn ICU design.* Retrieved Jan. 13, 2004, from www.nd.edu/~kkolberg/DesignStandards.htm.

Engler, A.J., Ludington-Hoe, S.M., Cusson, R.M., Adams, R., Bahnsen, M., Brumbaugh, E., Coates, P., Grieb, J., McHargue, L., Ryan, D., Settle, M., & Williams, D. (2002). Kangaroo care: National survey of practice, knowledge, barriers, and per-

REFERENCES and READINGS

ceptions. *MCN: The American Journal of Maternal/Child Nursing, 27*(3), 146-153.

Evans. R.A., & Thureen, P.J. (2001). Early feeding strategies in preterm and critically ill neonates. *Neonatal Network, 20*(7), 7-18.

Fanaroff, A.A., Martin, R.J., & Rodriguez, R.J. (2004). Identification and management of the high-risk neonate. In R.K. Creasy, R. Resnik, & J. Iams (Eds.), *Maternal-fetal medicine: Principles and practice* (5th ed., pp.1263-1301). Philadelphia: Saunders.

Franck, L.S., Bernal, H., & Gale, G. (2002). Infant holding policies and practices in neonatal units. *Neonatal Network, 21*(2), 13-20.

Franck, L.S., Quinn, D., & Zahr, L. (2000). Effect of less frequent bathing of preterm infants on skin flora and pathogen colonization. *Journal of Obstetric, Gynecologic, and Neonatal Nursing, 29*(6), 584-589.

Gardner, S.L., & Goldson, E. (2002). The neonate and the environment: Impact on development. In G.B. Merenstein & S.L. Gardner (Eds.), *Handbook of neonatal intensive care* (5th ed., pp. 219-282). St. Louis: Mosby.

Gardner, S.L., Snell, B.J., & Lawrence, R.A. (2002). Breastfeeding the infant with special needs. In G.B. Merenstein & S.L. Gardner (Eds.), *Handbook of neonatal intensive care* (5th ed., pp. 376-418). St. Louis: Mosby.

Hagedorn, M.I., Gardner, S.L., & Abman, S.H. (2002). Respiratory diseases. In G.B. Merenstein & S.L. Gardner (Eds.), *Handbook of neonatal intensive care* (5th ed., pp. 485-475). St. Louis: Mosby.

Hall, W.A., Shearer, K., Mogan, J., & Berkowitz, J. (2002). Weighing preterm infants before and after breastfeeding: Does it increase maternal confidence and competence? *MCN: The American Journal of Maternal/Child Nursing, 27*(6), 318-327.

Hill, A.S., Kurkowski, T.B., & Garcia, J. (2000). Oral support measures used in feeding the preterm infant. *Nursing Research, 49*(1), 2-10.

Holditch-Davis, D., Blackburn, S.T., & VandenBerg, K. (2003). Newborn and infant neurobehavioral development. In C. Kenner & J.W. Lott (Eds.), *Comprehensive neonatal nursing: A physiologic perspective* (3rd ed., pp. 236-284). Philadelphia: Saunders.

Hudson-Barr, D., Capper-Michel, B., Lambert, S., Palermo, T.M., Morbeto, K., & Lombardo, S. (2002). Validation of the Pain Assessment in Neonates (PAIN) scale with the Neonatal Infant Pain Scale (NIPS). *Neonatal Network, 15*(6), 15-21.

Hurst, I. (2001). Mothers' strategies to meet their needs in the newborn intensive care nursery. *Journal of Perinatal & Neonatal Nursing, 15*(2), 65-82.

Klaus, M.H., & Kennell, J.H. (2002). Care of the mother, father, and infant. In A.A. Fanaroff & R.J. Martin (Eds.), *Neonatal-perinatal medicine: Diseases of the fetus and infant* (7th ed., pp. 563-577). St. Louis: Mosby.

Kleinman, R.E. (Ed.). (2004). *Pediatric nutrition handbook* (5th ed.). Elk Grove Village, IL: American Academy of Pediatrics.

LeBlanc, M.H. (2002). The physical environment. In A.A. Fanaroff & R.J. Martin (Eds.), *Neonatal-perinatal medicine: Diseases of the fetus and infant* (7th ed., pp. 512-529). St. Louis: Mosby.

Lefrak, L., & Lund, C.H. (2001). Nursing practice in the neonatal intensive care unit. In M.H.

Klaus & A.A. Fanaroff (Eds.), *Care of the high-risk neonate* (5th ed., pp. 223-242). Philadelphia: Saunders.

Lemons, P.K. (2001). Breast milk and the hospitalized infant: Guidelines for practice. *Neonatal Network, 20*(7), 47-52.

Levy, G.D., Woolston, D.J., & Browne, J.V. (2003). Mean noise amounts in level II vs. level III neonatal intensive care units. *Neonatal Network, 22*(2), 33-38.

Loo, K.K., Espinosa, M., Tyler, R., & Howard, J. (2003). Using knowledge to cope with stress in the NICU: How parents integrate learning to read the physiologic and behavioral cues of the infant. *Neonatal Network, 20*(1), 31-37.

Ludington-Hoe, S.M., Ferreira, C., Swinth, J., & Ceccardi, J.J. (2003). Safe criteria and procedure for kangaroo care with intubated preterm infants. *Journal of Obstetric, Gynecologic, and Neonatal Nursing, 32*(5), 579-588.

Ludington-Hoe, S.M., & Swinth, J.Y. (2001). Kangaroo mother care during phototherapy: Effect on bilirubin profile. *Neonatal Network, 20*(5), 41-48.

McCain, G.C. (2003). An evidence-based guideline for introducing oral feeding to healthy preterm infants. *Neonatal Network, 22*(5), 45-50.

McCain, G.C., & Gartside, P.S. (2002). Behavioral responses of preterm infants to a standard-care and semi-demand feeding protocol. *Newborn and Infant Nursing Reviews, 2*(3), 187-193.

McGrath, J.M. (2001). Building relationships with families in the NICU: Exploring the guarded alliance. *Journal of Perinatal & Neonatal Nursing, 15*(3), 74-83.

Mellien, A.C. (2001). Incubators versus mothers' arms: Body temperature conservation in very-low-birth-weight premature infants. *Journal of Obstetric, Gynecologic, and Neonatal Nursing, 30*(2), 157-164.

Melnyk, B.M., Feinstein, N.F, & Fairbanks, E. (2002). Effectiveness of informational/behavioral interventions with parents of low birth weight (LBW) premature infants: An evidence base to guide clinical practice. *Pediatric Nursing, 28*(5), 511-516.

Merchant, J.R., Worwa, C., Porter, S., Coleman, J.M., & deRegnier, R.O. (2001). Respiratory instability of term and near-term healthy newborn infants in car safety seats. *Pediatrics, 108*(3), 647-652.

National Association of Neonatal Nurses. (2001). *Infant and family-centered developmental care guideline for practice.* Glenview, IL: Author.

Noerr, B. (2001). Sucrose for neonatal procedural pain. *Neonatal Network, 20*(7), 63-67.

Nystrom, K., & Axelsson, K. (2002). Mothers' experience of being separated from their newborns. *Journal of Obstetric, Gynecologic, and Neonatal Nursing, 31*(3), 275-282.

Olitsky, S.E., & Nelson, L.B. (2004). Disorders of the eye. In R.E. Behrman, R.M. Kliegman, & H.B. Jenson (Eds.), *Nelson textbook of pediatrics* (17th ed., pp. 2083-2126). Philadelphia: Saunders.

Paige, P.L., & Carney, P.R. (2002). Neurologic disorders. In G.B. Merenstein & S.L. Gardner (Eds.), *Handbook of neonatal intensive care* (5th ed., pp. 644-678). St. Louis: Mosby.

Pearson, J., & Anderson, K. (2001). Breast milk and the hospitalized infant: Guidelines for practice. *Neonatal Network, 20*(4), 43-48.

Pinelli, J., Symington, A., & Ciliska, D. (2002). Nonnutritive sucking in high-risk infants: Benign intervention or legitimate therapy? *Journal of Obstetric, Gynecologic, and Neonatal Nursing, 31*(5), 582-591.

Resnik, R., & Creasy, R.K. (2004). Intrauterine growth restriction. In R.K. Creasy, R. Resnik, & J. Iams (Eds.). *Maternal-fetal medicine: Principles and practice* (5th ed., pp. 495-512). Philadelphia: Saunders.

Rodriguez, R.J., Martin, R.J., & Fanaroff, A.A. (2002). Respiratory distress syndrome and its management. In A.A. Fanaroff & R.J. Martin (Eds.), *Neonatal-perinatal medicine: Diseases of the fetus and infant* (7th ed., pp. 1001-1011). St. Louis: Mosby.

Siegel, R., Gardner, S.L., & Merenstein, G.B. (2002). Families in crisis: Theroretic and practical considerations. In G.B. Merenstein & S.L. Gardner (Eds.), *Handbook of neonatal intensive care* (5th ed., pp. 725-753). St. Louis: Mosby.

Sifuentes, M. (2000). Well child care for preterm infants. In C.D. Berkowitz (Ed.), *Pediatrics: A primary care approach* (2nd ed., pp. 84-88). Philadelphia: Saunders.

Spicer, K. (2001). What every nurse needs to know about breast pumping: Instructing and supporting mothers of premature infants in the NICU. *Neonatal Network, 20*(4), 35-41.

Sredl, D. (2003). Myths and facts about pain in neonates. *Neonatal Network, 22*(6), 69-71.

Stoll, B.J. (2004). Infections of the neonatal infant. In R.E. Behrman, R.M. Kliegman, & A.M. Arvin (Eds.), *Nelson textbook of pediatrics* (17th ed., pp. 623-640). Philadelphia: Saunders.

Stoll, B.J., & Kliegman, R.M. (2004a). Respiratory tract disorders. In R E. Behrman, R.M. Kliegman, & H.B. Jenson (Eds.), *Nelson textbook of pediatrics* (17th ed., pp. 573-588). Philadelphia: Saunders.

Stoll, B.J., & Kliegman, R.M. (2004b). The high-risk infant. In R.E. Behrman, R.M. Kliegman, & H.B. Jenson (Eds.), *Nelson textbook of pediatrics* (17th ed., pp. 547-559). Philadelphia: Saunders.

Symanski, M.E., Hayes, M.J., & Kumar, A. (2002). Patterns of premature newborns' sleep-wake states before and after nursing interventions on the night shift. *Journal of Obstetric, Gynecologic, and Neonatal Nursing, 31*(3), 305-313.

Thoyre, S.M. (2001). Challenges mothers identify in bottle feeding their preterm infants. *Neonatal Network, 20*(1), 41-50.

Vandenberg, K.A. (2000). Supporting parents in the NICU: Guidelines for promoting parent confidence and competence. *Neonatal Network, 19*(8), 63-64.

Walden, M. (2001). *Pain assessment and management guideline for practice.* Glenview, IL: National Association of Neonatal Nurses.

Walden, M., & Franck, L.S. (2003). Identification, management, and prevention of newborn/infant pain. In C. Kenner & J.W. Lott (Eds.), *Comprehensive neonatal nursing: A physiologic perspective* (3rd ed., pp. 844-856). Philadelphia: Saunders.

Wyckoff, M.M., McGrath, J.M., Griffin, T., Malan, J., & White-Traut, R. (2003). Nutrition: Physiologic basis of metabolism and management of enteral and parenteral nutrition. In C. Kenner & J.W. Lott (Eds.), *Comprehensive neonatal nursing: A physiologic perspective* (3rd ed., pp. 425-447). Philadelphia: Saunders.

30

The High-Risk Newborn: Acquired and Congenital Conditions

◆ LEARNING OBJECTIVES

After studying this chapter, you should be able to:

- Describe the steps involved in neonatal resuscitation.
- Explain the common respiratory problems in the newborn.
- Explain the causes and significance of pathologic jaundice.
- Describe the nursing care of the infant with pathologic jaundice.
- Describe causes of neonatal infections and nursing care for infants with infections.
- Explain the effect of maternal diabetes on the newborn.
- Describe the effect of maternal substance abuse on the newborn.

◆ DEFINITIONS

asphyxia Insufficient oxygen and excess carbon dioxide in the blood and tissues.

bilirubin encephalopathy Brain damage resulting from deposits of unconjugated bilirubin in the brain tissue.

erythroblastosis fetalis Agglutination and hemolysis of fetal erythrocytes caused by incompatibility between the maternal and fetal blood types. In most cases, the fetus is Rh positive and the mother is Rh negative.

hydrops fetalis Heart failure and generalized edema in the fetus secondary to severe anemia resulting from destruction of erythrocytes.

kernicterus Staining of brain tissue caused by accumulation of unconjugated bilirubin in the brain.

meconium aspiration syndrome Obstruction and air trapping caused by meconium in the infant's lungs, which may cause severe respiratory distress.

neonatal abstinence syndrome A cluster of physical signs exhibited by the newborn exposed in utero to maternal use of substances such as heroin.

persistent pulmonary hypertension Vasoconstriction of the infant's pulmonary vessels after birth; may result in right-to-left shunting of blood flow through the ductus arteriosus, the foramen ovale, or both.

transient tachypnea of the newborn Condition of rapid respirations caused by inadequate absorption of fetal lung fluid.

In addition to the high-risk conditions related to gestational age discussed in Chapter 29, the newborn at risk may have acquired or congenital complications. Acquired conditions may be associated with prenatal complications or may occur at birth or shortly thereafter.

RESPIRATORY COMPLICATIONS

Respiratory distress is one of the most common problems of the neonate. It may be caused by asphyxia before, during, or after birth, disease of the respiratory system, and other conditions that affect the infant's ability to breathe. The nurse is responsible for identification and evaluation of respiratory status at birth and throughout the hospital stay.

Asphyxia

Asphyxia is a lack of oxygen and increase of carbon dioxide in the blood. It may occur in utero, at birth, or later. When asphyxia occurs at birth, it may be a continuation of asphyxia that began in utero or the result of other factors, such as preterm lungs with insufficient surfactant to function adequately.

If asphyxia occurs after birth, rapid respirations are followed by cessation of respirations (primary apnea) and a rapid fall in heart rate. Stimulation alone or with oxygen may restart respirations. If asphyxia continues without intervention, gasping respirations may resume weakly until the infant enters a period of secondary apnea. In secondary apnea, the oxygen levels in the blood continue to decrease, the infant loses consciousness, and stimulation is ineffective. Resuscitative measures must be initiated immediately regardless of whether primary or secondary apnea is present to prevent permanent damage to the brain or death.

Lack of oxygen to the cells leads to anaerobic metabolism and the production of lactic acid. Metabolic acidosis develops when available bicarbonate is no longer able to buffer the accumulating acids. A high partial pressure of carbon dioxide occurs in arterial blood ($PaCO_2$) and the partial pressure of oxygen (PO_2), pH, and bicarbonate levels are low. Vasoconstriction caused by low oxygen decreases blood flow to all or-

Drug Guide

Naloxone Hydrochloride (Narcan)

Classification: Opioid antagonist.

Action: Reverses central nervous system and respiratory depression caused by narcotics (opiates). Competes with narcotics at receptor sites.

Indications: Severe respiratory depression in the infant when the mother has received narcotics during labor.

Dosage and Route: Available in 0.4 mg/ml and 1 mg/ml. Dosage is 0.1 mg/kg. Given intravenously (IV), intramuscularly (IM), subcutaneously, or into an endotracheal tube. IV and endotracheal routes are preferred during resuscitation.

Absorption: Well absorbed by all routes. Onset of action is 1 to 2 minutes if given IV.

Excretion: Metabolized by the liver and excreted by kidneys.

Contraindications and Precautions: Duration of effect is 45 minutes if given IV, 45 to 60 minutes if given IM or subcutaneously. The dose may need to be repeated because the opioid may have a longer half-life than naloxone. If given to an infant of a mother addicted to drugs, it will cause withdrawal and may cause seizures. Resuscitative measures should be used as necessary.

Nursing Considerations: Note the strength of the medication available when calculating the dose. Prepare the syringe before birth by drawing up more than is needed. After birth, the excess is removed from the syringe and the amount is given according to the estimate of the infant's weight. Inject rapidly. Monitor for response, and be prepared to give repeated doses if necessary.

---

gans except the brain, myocardium, and adrenal glands. The ductus arteriosus and foramen ovale may remain open because of the low oxygen in the blood, high resistance to blood flow through constricted pulmonary vessels, and elevated pressure on the right side of the heart. Thus even circulating blood remains low in oxygen. Progression toward brain damage and death is rapid unless intervention is prompt.

Infants at Risk

Complications during pregnancy, labor, or birth increase the infant's risk for asphyxia. In addition, if the expectant mother receives narcotics shortly before birth, the infant may be too depressed at birth to breathe spontaneously. Naloxone (Narcan) may be given to these infants.

Neonatal Resuscitation

Although 90% of newborns have no difficulty with breathing at birth, approximately 10% require some help to begin respirations and 1% require extensive resuscitative measures (Kattwinkel, 2000). Therefore all personnel involved in deliveries should know how to perform resuscitative measures (Procedure 30-1). Equipment should be readily available and functioning properly at all times so that there is no delay in starting resuscitation. Nurses begin resuscitation measures as necessary and assist the physician in intubation, insertion of umbilical vein catheters, and administration of medications. Some nurses are taught to intubate infants in emergency situations.

Once the infant is stabilized, the nurse continues to assess for changes. Infants with asphyxia often have other complications. Communication with the parents is a vital nursing function. They need explanations, realistic reassurance, and continued support after the crisis.

Transient Tachypnea of the Newborn (Retained Lung Fluid)

Infants with transient tachypnea of the newborn (TTN) develop rapid respirations soon after birth. The condition, which resolves within a few days, is also called *retained lung fluid* and *respiratory distress syndrome, type II*. Risk factors include cesarean birth without labor, asphyxia, precipitous delivery, maternal analgesia, bleeding, and diabetes. Mild immaturity of surfactant production may also be a factor. Infants may be term or preterm.

Etiology

Although the exact cause of TTN is unknown, it is thought to result from a delay in absorption of fetal lung fluid by the pulmonary capillaries and lymph vessels. This causes decreased lung compliance and air trapping and produces signs similar to respiratory distress syndrome.

Manifestations

In TTN, rapid respirations develop within hours of birth. Retractions, nasal flaring, grunting, and mild cyanosis are also present. Chest radiography shows hyperinflation, streaking radiating from the hilum of the lungs showing interstitial fluid along the bronchovascular spaces, and presence of fluid in the fissures between the lobes and in the pleural space.

Therapeutic Management

Treatment is supportive and may include oxygen and intravenous or gavage feeding while tachycardia is high to prevent aspiration and conserve energy. Because the signs are similar to those of respiratory distress syndrome and sepsis, the infant is observed for those complications. Antibiotics may be given until sepsis is ruled out.

Nursing Considerations

After identifying signs, the nurse notifies the appropriate caregiver and carries out treatment. General nursing care is similar to that of the respiratory care of the preterm infant (see Chapter 29).

Meconium Aspiration Syndrome

Meconium-stained amniotic fluid occurs in 10% to 15% of births, and 5% of those infants develop meconium aspiration syndrome (MAS) (Stoll & Kliegman, 2004b). The condition occurs most often in postterm infants who have decreased amniotic fluid and are prone to cord compression. It also occurs

Procedure 30-1

Performing Resuscitation in Newborns

PURPOSE: To ensure adequate oxygenation of the neonate with asphyxia.

NOTE: Although this procedure is listed by steps, several steps may be performed at the same time. Resuscitation is performed as an integrated process rather than individual steps. Because two or more people often are working together, more than one step can be performed at a time.

1. Place the infant under a preheated radiant warmer immediately to prevent cold stress, which would increase oxygen need.
2. Position the infant with the neck in a neutral position or slightly extended ("sniffing") position so that the airway is open. Place a small blanket under the shoulders to help maintain an open airway. Avoid hyperextension or flexion of the neck, which may obstruct the airway.

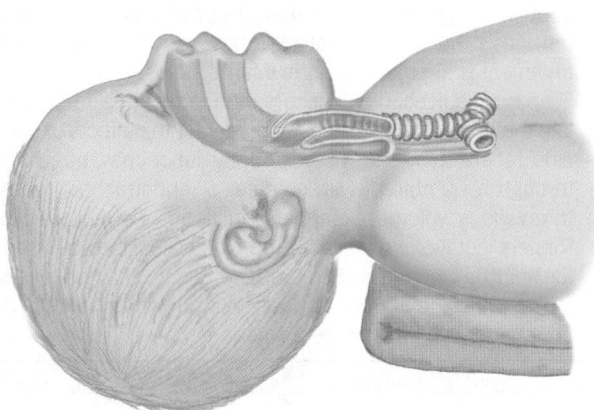

3. Suction the mouth and then the nose to remove mucus from the airways, if necessary. Infants often gasp when the nose is suctioned and may aspirate secretions from the mouth into the lungs. If meconium is present, an endotracheal tube may be used for suction. After suctioning, the endotracheal tube may be inserted at this time or later, if necessary, to provide an open airway.
4. Dry the infant to help prevent cold stress and increased oxygen need. (Drying is often performed simultaneously with the previous steps.) Stimulate the infant if necessary by gently rubbing the infant's back or body or flicking or slapping the soles of the feet. If two people are present, one can dry the infant while the other positions and suctions. The tactile stimulation of drying and suctioning the infant may cause spontaneous respirations. If the baby does not respond adequately, additional brief stimulation may be needed.
5. If no response occurs after stimulating once or twice, stop and initiate immediate resuscitation. Do not delay resuscitation to continue stimulating or until the Apgar scores are given. Resuscitation becomes more difficult the longer it is delayed.

6. Remove wet linens to decrease heat loss. Reposition the head if necessary because the infant has been moved. Give oxygen if necessary, and evaluate the respirations, heart rate, and color. If the heart rate is below 100 or respirations are absent or only gasping, resuscitation is necessary.
7. Give 100% oxygen if the infant is breathing but cyanotic to prevent damage to vital tissues. Holding the oxygen mask or tubing close to the infant's nose helps provide 100% oxygen rather than diluting it by combining with room air.
8. Evaluate the respirations, heart rate, and color to determine if further resuscitation is necessary to prevent hypoxic brain damage. Use a stethoscope or feel the pulsations at the base of the cord. Count the heart rate for 6 seconds and multiply by 10 to obtain the heart rate per minute. Positioning, clearing the airway, drying, stimulating, and providing oxygen should take no more than 30 seconds.
9. Begin positive-pressure ventilation with an appropriate-size bag and mask if the infant fails to breathe spontaneously with initial stimulation, has gasping respirations, or the heart rate is less than 100 beats per minute when respirations have begun. Positive-pressure ventilation ensures oxygen entry into the lungs.
10. Attach the bag to an oxygen source with 100% oxygen. Place the mask snugly over the infant's nose and mouth. Squeeze the bag gently to force air into the infant's lungs. Use a bag with a manometer to show the amount of pressure being used and a flow-control valve that can be adjusted to control the pressure delivered to the infant. Or use a bag with a pressure release valve that releases if the pressure is high enough to cause lung damage. The initial breaths require pressures of 30 to 40 cm H_2O to inflate the lungs. Less pressure is used for subsequent breaths but varies with the infant's condition. Great care must be taken to use a pressure that is high enough to inflate the lungs without causing damage from overinflation. More pressure is needed for the first breaths and diseased lungs.
11. Observe the rise and fall of the chest during ventilation. If the chest does not move, suction secretions and reposition the head and the mask. Ventilate the infant at a rate of 40 to 60 breaths per minute until the infant is breathing spontaneously and the heart rate is above 100 beats per minute. The airway must not be occluded by positioning or secretions.
12. If the heart rate is less than 60 beats per minute after 30 seconds of effective assisted ventilation, a second person should begin chest compressions while the first continues to ventilate the infant. Adequate ventilation causes improvement of bradycardia in most infants. Evaluation of the infant's status determines whether ventilation can be discontinued or chest compressions must be added for the infant to survive.
13. Compress the chest by placing the hands around the infant's chest with the fingers under the back to provide support and the thumbs over the lower third of the sternum (just above the xiphoid process). An alternate method is to use two fingers of one hand to compress the chest with the

Continued

Procedure 30-1

Performing Resuscitation in Newborns—cont'd

other hand under the back to provide support. Correct hand position compresses the heart but avoids or minimizes injury to the liver or spleen, fractures of the ribs, and pneumothorax. The alternative method may be necessary to allow access to umbilical vessels or for people with small hands.

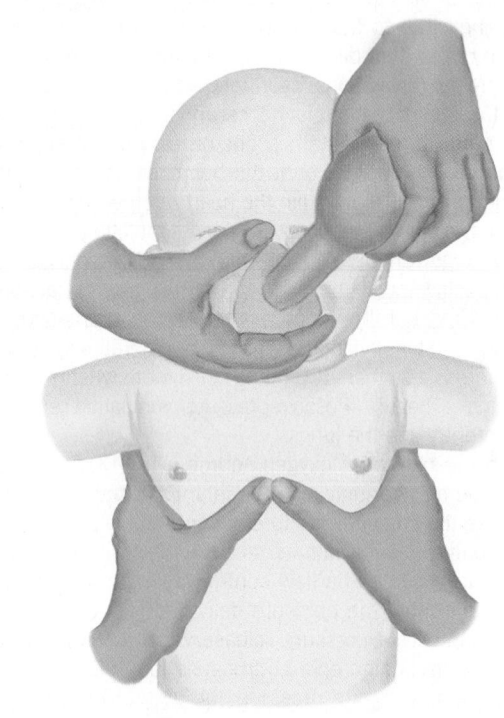

14. Compress the sternum to a depth of approximately one third of the anterior-posterior diameter of the chest and sufficient to cause a palpable pulse. The size of the infant determines the depth of compressions to avoid injury. The fingers should remain in contact with the chest between compressions so they do not have to be repositioned each time.

15. Use three compressions followed by one ventilation for a combined rate of compressions and ventilations of 120 each minute. This provides 90 compressions and 30 ventilations each minute. Pause for 1/2 second after every third compression for ventilation. Simultaneous compression and ventilation may interfere with adequate ventilation. The short pause allows air to enter the lungs.

16. Check the heart rate after approximately 30 seconds. If it is 60 beats per minute or more, discontinue compressions but continue ventilation until the heart rate is more than 100 beats per minute and spontaneous breathing begins. If the heart rate is less than 60 beats per minute, epinephrine will be necessary to stimulate the heart. If necessary, endotracheal intubation may be performed at this point if not performed previously. Periodic evaluation is necessary to ensure that treatment is appropriate to the infant's status.

17. Prepare medications, if necessary. Epinephrine to stimulate the heart and naloxone to counteract the effects of opioids received by the mother during labor may be given through an umbilical vein catheter or endotracheal tube. Intravenous volume expanders, including normal saline, Ringers lactate, or O-negative red blood cells, may be used for fluid or blood loss. Sodium bicarbonate may be given intravenously to correct acidosis, but only after prolonged arrest and with effective ventilation.

Data from Kattwinkel, J. (Ed.), American Academy of Pediatrics, & American Heart Association. (2000). *Textbook of neonatal resuscitation* (4th ed.). Elk Grove, IL: American Academy of Pediatrics and American Heart Association.

in term infants who have suffered intrauterine asphyxia. MAS causes obstruction of the airways, pneumonitis, and air trapping. It may lead to persistent pulmonary hypertension of the newborn.

Etiology

Although the normal fetus may pass meconium, MAS most often occurs when hypoxia causes increased peristalsis of the intestine and relaxation of the anal sphincter before or during labor. MAS develops when meconium in the amniotic fluid enters the lungs during fetal life or at birth. It may be drawn into the lungs if gasping movements occur in utero as a result of asphyxia and acidosis, or the meconium in the upper airways may be pulled deep into the respiratory passages when the infant takes the first breaths after birth.

Obstruction of the airways may be complete or partial. Atelectasis may result when small airways are completely obstructed. In partial obstruction, air can enter but not escape from the alveoli. During inhalation, the bronchioles expand slightly as air flows into them past the meconium. During exhalation, the passages constrict and meconium blocks movement of air out of the lungs.

This ball-valve mechanism results in air trapping. The overdistended alveoli may develop an air leak, with escape of air into the pleural cavity (pneumothorax) or mediastinum (pneumomediastinum). Surfactant production may be inhibited, increasing the respiratory distress. In addition, meconium is irritating to lung tissue and causes an inflammatory reaction and chemical pneumonitis. Persistent pulmonary hypertension may result.

Severe MAS develops in only a small number of newborns with meconium below the vocal cords. The addition of meconium to a lung damaged by asphyxia may increase the severity of the condition. Damage from asphyxia interferes with clearing of lung fluid and production of surfactant and causes pulmonary vasoconstriction that can result in a return to fetal circulation.

Manifestations

If meconium in the amniotic fluid is light, respiratory problems usually do not develop. Thick meconium, however, may cause serious respiratory pathology. Signs of mild to severe respiratory distress are present at birth, with tachypnea, cyanosis, retractions, nasal flaring, grunting, rales, rhonchi, and in severe cases a barrel-shaped chest from hyperinflation. Radiography shows atelectasis, consolidation, and hyperexpansion from air trapping.

Therapeutic Management

When thick meconium is noted in the amniotic fluid during labor, an amnioinfusion may be performed. This involves infusing normal saline into the uterus to decrease cord compression and to dilute thick meconium in the amniotic fluid.

At birth, the infant's mouth and pharynx are suctioned using wall suction as soon as the head is delivered and before delivery of the rest of the body. This helps prevent drawing the meconium from the upper air passages deep into the lungs during the infant's first breath. In depressed infants an endotracheal tube is inserted through a laryngoscope. The infant is suctioned with the endotracheal tube to remove thick meconium immediately after birth. If the infant is vigorous with a heart rate over 100, spontaneous respirations, and good muscle tone, intubation is not necessary (Miller, Fanaroff, & Martin, 2002).

Infants may need only warmed, humidified oxygen, or extensive respiratory support with a ventilator may be required. High-frequency ventilation may be used. Supportive care is given to meet the problems presented. Infants with severe MAS who do not respond to conventional treatment may benefit from extracorporeal membrane oxygenation (ECMO). ECMO, which is available in some hospitals, oxygenates the blood while bypassing the lungs to allow the infant's lungs to rest temporarily and recover.

Nursing Considerations

When meconium is noted in the amniotic fluid during labor, the nurse notifies the primary caregiver so that delivery care can be adapted as necessary. The nurse should ensure that equipment such as oxygen and suction is functioning properly and assists with care at delivery. After the infant's birth, nursing care is adapted as needed. Although meconium is sterile, lung damage promotes the growth of bacteria, and infants should be closely observed for infection.

Persistent Pulmonary Hypertension of the Newborn

Persistent pulmonary hypertension of the newborn (PPHN) is a condition in which the vascular resistance of the lungs does not decrease after birth and normal changes to neonatal circulation are impaired. For this reason, the condition is also called *persistent fetal circulation*.

Etiology

The cause of PPHN may be abnormal lung development or maternal use of nonsteroidal antiinflammatory agents or aspirin, or it may develop for unknown reasons. It is often associated with hypoxemia and acidosis from conditions such as asphyxia, meconium aspiration, sepsis, polycythemia, diaphragmatic hernia, and respiratory distress syndrome.

Inadequate oxygenation results in vasoconstriction, instead of the normal dilation, of the pulmonary artery and small pulmonary vessels, which causes increased resistance in the lungs. It also causes dilation instead of constriction of the ductus arteriosus. The elevated pulmonary vascular resistance causes a rise in pressure on the right side of the heart. This results in a right-to-left shunt of blood that flows through the foramen ovale and patent ductus arteriosus and bypasses the lungs, as occurs during fetal circulation. Metabolic acidosis causes more pulmonary vasoconstriction, making the condition even worse.

Manifestations

Infants with PPHN develop signs within the first 24 to 48 hours after birth. Tachypnea, respiratory distress, and progressive cyanosis often worsen with handling. Oxygen saturation and partial pressure of oxygen in arterial blood (PaO_2) are decreased, $PaCO_2$ is increased, and acidosis is present. Other signs may result from associated conditions.

Therapeutic Management

Management involves treating the underlying cause and relieving pulmonary vasoconstriction. Arterial pH may be increased with respiratory and drug therapy to cause pulmonary vasodilation. Sedation, high-frequency ventilation, surfactant therapy, and ECMO therapy may all be necessary. Inhalation of nitric oxide, which dilates pulmonary vessels, may be used to reduce the need for ECMO. Nursing care is similar to care of other infants with severe respiratory disease. Because infants become hypoxic with activity and other stimuli, handling and noise are kept to a minimum.

HYPERBILIRUBINEMIA (PATHOLOGIC JAUNDICE)

Jaundice is a common concern in caring for neonates. Conjugation of bilirubin and physiologic jaundice are discussed in Chapter 22. Pathologic jaundice is discussed here. When the bilirubin level reaches 5 mg/dl, jaundice is visible in the newborn's face. It moves down the body as bilirubin levels continue to rise (Stoll & Kliegman, 2004a). Jaundice is considered pathologic when it appears in the first 24 to 36 hours after birth; the direct bilirubin level is above 2 mg/dl; the total bilirubin concentration increases by more than 5 mg/dl per day or is higher than 12 mg/dl in a full-term infant or 10 to 14 mg/dl in a preterm infant; or persists after the second week of life (Stoll & Kliegman, 2004a).

Pathologic jaundice is a concern because it may lead to kernicterus. In kernicterus, bilirubin deposits cause yellowish staining of the brain, especially the basal ganglia, cerebellum, and hippocampus. It is more likely to occur in infants who have suffered sepsis, hypoxia, or respiratory acidosis, which impairs the blood-brain barrier and allows unconjugated bilirubin to enter the brain. Kernicterus causes bilirubin encephalopathy.

Although bilirubin encephalopathy is rare today because of improved treatment measures, the mortality rate of affected infants is high. Those who survive may have cerebral palsy, mental retardation, hearing loss, or more subtle long-term neurologic and developmental problems. The exact level at which bilirubin encephalopathy develops is unknown. It may occur when total bilirubin levels are more than 20 mg/dl in full-term infants and at lower levels in preterm infants or neonates with other complications.

Etiology

The most common cause of pathologic jaundice is hemolytic disease of the newborn from incompatibility between the blood of the mother and that of the fetus. The best known cause is Rh incompatibility, in which the Rh-negative mother forms antibodies when Rh-positive blood from the fetus enters her circulation (see Chapter 26). Antibodies may have developed during a previous pregnancy or after injury, abortion, amniocentesis, or a transfusion of Rh-positive blood. The antibodies cross the placenta and destroy fetal red blood cells. Excessive hemolysis causes erythroblastosis fetalis.

Infants with erythroblastosis fetalis are anemic from destruction of red blood cells. Severely affected infants may develop hydrops fetalis, a severe anemia that results in heart failure and generalized edema. Use of $Rh_O(D)$ immune globulin such as RhoGAM to prevent the mother from forming antibodies against Rh-positive blood has greatly decreased the incidence of erythroblastosis fetalis.

ABO incompatibility also causes pathologic jaundice. Mothers with type O blood have natural antibodies to types A and B blood. The antibodies cross the placenta and cause hemolysis of fetal red blood cells. The destruction, however, is much less severe than with Rh incompatibility and causes milder signs.

Other causes of pathologic jaundice include infection, hypothyroidism, glucuronyl transferase deficiency, polycythemia, glucose-6-phosphate dehydrogenase deficiency, and biliary atresia. Infants of diabetic mothers are more likely to develop pathologic jaundice, especially if they have macrosomia. Any condition that causes destruction of erythrocytes or impairment of the liver may result in pathologic bilirubin levels.

Therapeutic Management

The focus of therapeutic management is prevention of kernicterus. The cause is determined by history and diagnostic tests to identify infections or blood abnormalities. During pregnancy, an Rh-negative expectant mother will have an indirect Coombs test to identify the presence of antibodies against fetal blood. If the test is positive, amniocentesis may be performed to determine the fetal Rh factor and the degree of hyperbilirubinemia.

When infants are jaundiced, the cord blood is used for a Coombs test and to determine the infant's blood type. A positive Coombs test indicates that antibodies from the mother have attached to the infant's red blood cells. Serum bilirubin levels are followed closely for changes that indicate that treatment should be initiated or changed.

Because visual inspection for jaundice may be inaccurate, other noninvasive tests may be used. Reflectance photometers are hand-held devices that allow screening of transcutaneous bilirubin. End-tidal carbon monoxide (CO) is a test to measure the amount of carbon monoxide in the infant's breath. Carbon monoxide produced along with bilirubin when red blood cells break down is excreted by the lungs. Thus a high level of CO in expired air indicates increased production of bilirubin and helps predict infants who are at risk for excessively high bilirubin levels (Reiser, 2001; Stevenson, Vreman, Wong, & Contag, 2001).

Phototherapy

The most common treatment of jaundice is phototherapy, in which special lights are placed over the infant. During phototherapy, bilirubin in the skin absorbs the light and changes into water-soluble products, the most important of which is lumirubin. These do not require conjugation by the liver and can be excreted in the bile and urine.

Phototherapy can be delivered in several ways. The most common is a bank of fluorescent lamps or "bili lights" placed over the infant, who is usually in an incubator or under a radiant warmer. The infant wears only a diaper so that the skin is exposed to the lights. Patches are placed over the eyes to protect them from the lights. More than one bank of lights may be used if the bilirubin level is high. Blood is drawn frequently to monitor the serum bilirubin levels to determine the effectiveness of treatment and when it can be discontinued.

Other options for phototherapy include halogen lamps and fiberoptic phototherapy blankets. The infant can be swaddled with the blanket and does not require patches over the eyes. The blanket may be used alone or combined with phototherapy lights.

Side effects of phototherapy include frequent, loose green stools, resulting from increased bile flow and peristalsis. The stools may damage the skin and cause fluid loss. African-American infants may experience a tanning effect from the light. Bronze baby syndrome, a grayish brown discoloration of the skin and urine, occurs in infants with cholestatic jaundice in whom liver function and production or flow of bile are impaired. A macular skin rash may also occur. The color changes and rash disappear when phototherapy is completed. Some infants experience temporary lactose intolerance during therapy and need formula without lactose.

Home phototherapy allows the infant to go home yet continue treatment. Parents need extensive teaching on how to care for the infant receiving home phototherapy. Home visits by nurses are important to help ensure that the infant is making adequate progress and the parents understand how to provide care.

Exchange Transfusions

Exchange transfusions are seldom necessary but are performed when phototherapy does not reduce dangerously high bilirubin levels quickly enough. This treatment removes sensitized red blood cells, antibodies, and unconjugated bilirubin and corrects severe anemia.

Procedure. During the exchange transfusion, blood is removed and replaced with an equal amount of O-negative donor blood. Because the donor blood mixes with the infant's blood, approximately twice the infant's blood volume is administered. At the end of the transfusion, approximately 85% of the infant's red blood cells have been replaced.

When the level in the blood decreases, bilirubin from the tissues moves into the plasma. This rebound elevation of bilirubin may necessitate repeat transfusions, but phototherapy is generally adequate to resolve it.

Complications. Complications of exchange transfusions include electrolyte imbalance, infection, hypoglycemia, hypervolemia or hypovolemia, cardiac dysrhythmias, bleeding, and embolism. Samples of the blood are analyzed for complete blood count, bilirubin and calcium levels, and other tests as needed.

Role of the Nurse. The nurse's role during exchange transfusion is to prepare equipment, assess the infant during and after the procedure, and keep accurate records. A cardiac monitor is attached to the infant, and a radiant heater provides warmth. The nurse must clarify any misunderstandings that the parents may have about the treatment and help allay their anxiety.

PARENTS
Want to Know

Home Care for the Infant Receiving Phototherapy

- Dress the baby in only a diaper to expose as much skin as possible to the lights. Change your baby's position about every 2 hours so that the light reaches all areas of the body.
- Position the phototherapy or "bili" light at the proper distance from your baby according to the manufacturer's directions. Placing it too close to the infant could result in fever or burns. Placing it too far away will make the treatment ineffective.
- Close the baby's eyes and place patches over the eyes before positioning the infant under the lights. Check at least every hour to see that the patches remain in place. They must cover the eyes but not press on the nose because they can interfere with breathing. The patches should not press against the eyes.
- The infant may be removed from the lights for feedings, diaper changes, and other general care but should receive phototherapy for 18 hours every day (or the number of hours ordered by the physician). Hold and cuddle your infant during the time that the baby is out of the lights. When the infant is under the lights, you can talk to your baby. The sound of your voice will be comforting.
- If you are using a fiberoptic blanket, keep it next to the baby's skin at all times. Be sure the baby does not roll off the blanket. You may wrap the baby with a receiving blanket over the "bili" blanket and hold the baby for feedings and other care. It is not necessary to cover the infant's eyes if the blanket alone is used.

- Check your baby's temperature under the arm before every feeding. The temperature should remain between 97.7° and 99.5° F. If it is abnormal, see if the heat in the room is too low or high and if the "bili" light is out of position. Use warm blankets when you remove the baby from the warmth of the light. Call your physician if the baby has a temperature less than 97.7° or more than 100° F.
- Feed your baby every 2 to 3 hours because the phototherapy causes the baby to lose fluid from the skin and have loose stools. This could cause dehydration. The infant needs the protein in milk because it helps eliminate the bilirubin that causes the jaundice.
- Count your baby's wet diapers and stools. Increase the feedings if the baby has less than six wet diapers a day or if the urine appears dark.
- Keep a journal of the baby's temperature, feedings (time and amount), wet and dirty diapers, types of stools, and amount of time spent out of phototherapy.
- Keep all appointments for examinations or blood tests so that the baby's progress can be evaluated by your health care provider.
- Call the physician or home care nurse if you have questions about care, if the baby has a fever or appears sick to you, if the mouth seems dry, or if the urine is dark or less than normal.

■ NURSING CARE

The Infant With Hyperbilirubinemia

Although collaborative care of the infant with jaundice is an important part of the nurse's role, several nursing diagnoses are appropriate. Risk for Injury is one common finding. Infants are also at risk for increased fluid loss during phototherapy. The nursing diagnosis Risk for Deficient Fluid Volume is discussed in Nursing Care Plan: The Infant With Jaundice.

Assessment

Assess the level of jaundice every 8 hours by pressing the skin over a bony prominence and noting the color in the area before the blood returns. In infants with dark skin, assess the color of the conjunctiva of the eyes, palate, and mucous membranes of the mouth. Determine the areas of the body affected by the jaundice, and document carefully for comparison during future assessment. Jaundice begins at the head and moves down the body as the bilirubin levels rise. Monitor laboratory bilirubin levels for change.

Assess for risk factors that might further increase bilirubin levels. Note temperature fluctuations, hypoglycemia, and infection. Determine the infant's oral intake and number of stools.

Diagnosis and Planning

Nurses can do many things to prevent situations that might cause further rises in bilirubin. They must also protect the infant from injury from the light during phototherapy. The nursing diagnosis is

■ Risk for Injury related to preventable causes of further elevation of bilirubin or damage to the eyes secondary to phototherapy.

Expected Outcomes: The infant will avoid injury resulting from increased bilirubin or exposure of the skin or eyes to phototherapy lights.

Interventions

Maintaining a Neutral Thermal Environment

Prevent situations, such as cold stress or hypoglycemia, that could result in increased fatty acids in the blood caused by acidosis, thereby decreasing the availability of albumin-binding sites for unconjugated bilirubin. Prevent cold stress at birth and during all care by maintaining the infant in a neutral thermal environment. Check the infant's axillary temperature every 2 to 4 hours to identify an early decrease before it becomes a problem. Dress the infant in warmed clothes and blankets on removal from phototherapy lights.

Prevent elevation of the infant's temperature from exposure to the heat of the "bili" lights. Position the lights properly to prevent overheating the infant. Assess incubator or radiant warmer settings to be sure they are correct for the infant's needs.

Providing Optimal Nutrition

Ensure that the infant receives feedings every 2 to 3 hours, whether by breast or bottle. Frequent feedings prevent hypoglycemia, provide protein to maintain the albumin level in the blood, and promote gastrointestinal motility and prompt emptying of bilirubin from the bowel. Avoid offering water,

Nursing Care Plan

The Infant With Jaundice

ASSESSMENT

Holly, a 3-day-old, full-term infant born by cesarean, is jaundiced secondary to ABO incompatibility and is receiving phototherapy. She weighs 3.2 kg (7 lb, 1 oz), and her mucous membranes appear slightly dry. Skin turgor is good with quick recoil, and the anterior fontanel is flat. Urine appears slightly dark. Holly had three loose green stools with no water ring on this shift. She is a sleepy infant who takes formula poorly. Holly's mother, Valerie, appears tired and frustrated with Holly's slow eating behavior.

Nursing Diagnosis

Risk for Deficient Fluid Volume related to inadequate oral intake to meet needs of increased insensible water loss and frequent loose stools.

Goals/Expected Outcomes

Holly will:
- Take at least 320 to 480 ml of fluid per day (100 to 150 ml/kg/day) to meet normal needs.
- Show adequate hydration (moist mucous membranes, elastic skin turgor, flat fontanels, pale yellow urine, and at least 6 wet diapers/daily).

INTERVENTION	RATIONALE
1. Instruct Valerie to feed Holly every 2 to 3 hours. Feed Holly in the nursery at night or when Valerie needs rest, if she prefers.	1. Adequate intake of formula is necessary to meet the infant's nutrient and fluid needs and ensure excretion of bilirubin in the stools. The mother's needs for rest must be met without interfering with the infant's needs.
2. Explain to Valerie that Holly needs frequent feedings to help her pass stools that contain bilirubin that causes her jaundice.	2. The mother's understanding of the need and the reasons will increase her willingness to work with the infant.
3. Observe Valerie feeding Holly, and offer suggestions as needed. Show her how to waken the infant by unwrapping and gentle stimulation. Try warming the formula slightly. Use a pacifier or insert a gloved finger into Holly's mouth to elicit the suck reflex before feedings.	3. Observation of feedings may identify problems and interventions that work for this situation. A wide-awake infant is more likely to feed well. Some infants prefer warm milk. Nonnutritive sucking may help the infant suck effectively during feedings.
4. Tell the parents about the need for frequent feeding to provide added fluid, protein, and other nutrients.	4. Infants receiving phototherapy have a greater-than-normal insensible water loss. Albumin (protein) is necessary to carry bilirubin to the liver for conjugation. Heightened intestinal motility decreases absorption of nutrients.
5. Avoid offering water or dextrose water. Use formula instead.	5. Water supplements may decrease intake of formula. Formula increases excretion of bilirubin in stools, but water does not have the same effect.
6. If water loss appears excessive, weigh the diapers and check the specific gravity of the urine. Urine output should be 1 to 3 ml/kg/hr, which is a total of 76.8 to 230.4 ml/day. Specific gravity should be 1.001 to 1.020 for full-term infants.	6. Weighing the diapers and checking specific gravity will identify inadequate output and dehydration early. The wet diaper weight in grams minus the weight of a dry diaper equals the milliliters of urine.
7. Use therapeutic communication techniques to help Valerie vent her frustrations. Offer praise for her attempts to feed Holly.	7. Helping the mother deal with her feelings helps her meet the infant's needs. Praise increases her concept of herself as a "good mother."

Evaluation

Holly drinks a total of 450 ml (15 oz) of formula during 24 hours. Valerie is able to wake Holly, who begins to suck more vigorously. Holly's mucous membranes are moist, and there are 10 diapers with pale yellow urine during the 24 hours.

Additional Nursing Diagnoses to Consider

Impaired Skin Integrity
Anxiety
Impaired Parenting
Ineffective Thermoregulation

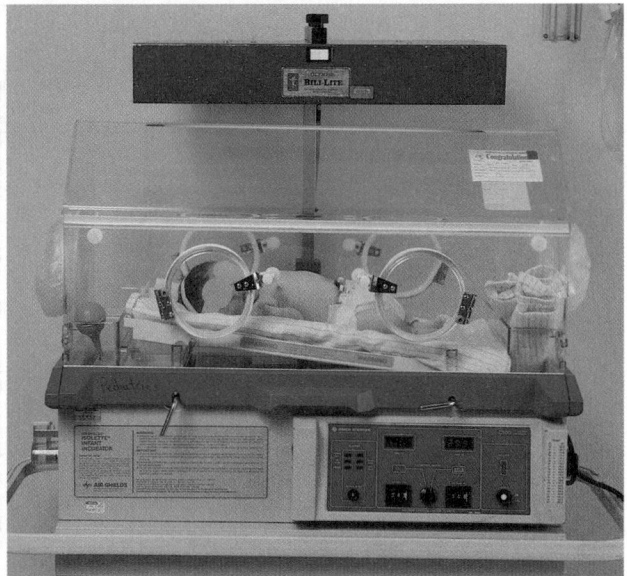

Figure 30-1 The infant receiving phototherapy is wearing eye patches to protect the eyes and is wearing a diaper to protect the gonads.

because the infant may decrease intake of milk, which is more effective in removing bilirubin from the intestines. If breastfeeding must be supplemented, use formula instead of water.

Protecting the Eyes

Provide patches to protect the eyes from retinal damage from the phototherapy lights (Fig. 30-1). To avoid abrasions to the cornea, close the infant's eyes before placing the patches. Check the position of the patches at least every hour. Infants can dislodge the patches so that they do not cover the eyes, press too hard on the eyes, or compress the nose and interfere with breathing. Observe for skin irritation around or under the patches at least every 4 hours.

Enhancing Response to Therapy

Expose as much skin as possible to the light. Remove all clothing except a diaper. Turn the infant frequently to expose all areas evenly and prevent skin irritation. If a fiberoptic blanket is used, check the position frequently. Infants sometimes need to be repositioned so that the blanket remains in contact with the skin.

Use a light meter to check the level of irradiance (energy output) to be sure the apparatus is functioning appropriately and to determine if the bulbs need to be replaced. Check laboratory reports of serum bilirubin levels to determine the effectiveness of treatment and when it can be discontinued.

Position the lights the proper distance away from the infant. Lights that are too close risk burning the skin. Lights too far away from the infant will not be effective in reducing jaundice. Halogen lights must be placed farther away from the infant than fluorescent lights to prevent burning. Follow the manufacturer's instructions about light placement. Although phototherapy increases insensible water loss from the skin, avoid the use of creams or lotions on the infant's skin because they might cause burning.

Explain care to parents, who may be frightened to see their infant in an incubator with the eyes covered. Explain-

CRITICAL THINKING EXERCISE 30-1

Why is it important to remove the patches from the eyes each time the infant is taken from the phototherapy lights for feeding or when parents visit?

ing the causes of jaundice and the purpose of phototherapy will decrease their worry. In addition, they will be more willing to hold their baby for only short times during feeding so that the therapy is not unduly interrupted.

Observe for other complications. Although bilirubin encephalopathy is rare today, monitor for signs that indicate its presence. These include lethargy, poor muscle tone, decreased or absent Moro reflex, high-pitched cry, opisthotonos, and seizures. Note the presence of rashes or changes in the color of the skin, and inform parents that they are not harmful and will disappear when phototherapy is discontinued.

Evaluation

- Is the infant free of signs of injury?
- Are the eyes protected from injury from the phototherapy lights?

INFECTION

Nurses must be constantly alert for signs of infection in neonates. Bacterial infection of the newborn affects 1 to 4 in every 1000 live births (Stoll, 2004). Infections can also be caused by viruses such as herpes, respiratory syncytial virus, or rotavirus, and by fungi such as *Candida albicans*.

Transmission of Infection

Newborns may acquire infection before, during, or after birth. Organisms such as rubella, cytomegalovirus, syphilis, and toxoplasmosis may pass across the placenta and cause infection during pregnancy. During labor and birth, organisms in the vagina such as group B streptococci and hepatitis B virus may enter the uterus after rupture of membranes or infect the infant during passage through the birth canal. Infection after birth occurs from contact with hospital staff members, contaminated equipment, or family members. An example is staphylococcal infections.

Some of the most common infections and their effects on the neonate are listed in Table 30-1. Other infections are discussed in Chapter 26.

Sepsis Neonatorum

Infection that occurs during or after birth may result in sepsis neonatorum, a systemic infection from bacteria in the bloodstream. Newborns are particularly susceptible to sepsis because their immune systems are immature and they react more slowly to invasion by organisms. Newborns and especially preterm infants have fewer antibodies and are unable to localize infection as well as older children. This inability allows the infection to spread easily from one organ to another. In addition, the blood-brain barrier is less effective in keeping out organisms, and central nervous system infection may result.

TABLE 30-1 Common Infections in the Newborn

Transmission	Effect on Newborn	Nursing Considerations
VIRAL INFECTIONS		
Cytomegalovirus Transplacental.	Most infants asymptomatic at birth. LBW, IUGR, enlarged liver and spleen, jaundice, mental retardation, hearing loss, blindness, epilepsy. May have no signs for months or years.	Major cause of mental retardation. Diagnosed by urine culture. May shed virus in saliva and urine for months. Antiviral drug therapy.
Hepatitis B Usually during birth through contact with maternal blood. Also transplacental, breast milk.	Asymptomatic at birth. LBW, prematurity. Most of those infected become chronic carriers. Risk of later liver cancer.	Wash well to remove all blood before skin is punctured for any reason. After cleaning, administer hepatitis B immune globulin and hepatitis B vaccine to prevent infection.
Herpes Usually during birth through infected vagina or ascending infection after rupture of membranes. Transplacental rarely. Transmission highest with primary infection.	Clusters of vesicles, temperature instability, lethargy, poor suck, seizures, encephalitis, jaundice, purpura. Death or severe neurologic impairment is likely with disseminated infection.	Contact precautions. Obtain lesion specimens for culture. High mortality and morbidity rate. Antiviral drugs improve outcome.
Human Immunodeficiency Virus/Acquired Immunodeficiency Syndrome Transplacental, during birth from infected blood and secretions, from breast milk. Transmission rate much lower if mother takes antiretroviral drugs during pregnancy and birth is by cesarean.	Asymptomatic at birth, signs usually apparent at 4 to 12 months. Enlarged liver and spleen, lymphadenopathy, failure to thrive, pneumonia, persistent candidal and bacterial infections.	Diagnosis may be delayed because of maternal antibodies. Some early tests available. Wash early and before skin is punctured to remove blood. Treat with antiretroviral drugs and prophylaxis against other infections.
Rubella Transplacental.	Asymptomatic or IUGR, cataracts, cardiac defects, deafness, mental retardation. Damage greatest in first trimester.	Contact precautions. Infant may shed virus for months after birth. Diagnosed by presence of antibody. No treatment.
Varicella Zoster Virus (Chickenpox) Transplacental.	Skin scarring, limb hypoplasia, eye and brain damage, IUGR, death. Damage greatest before the 20th week of gestation.	Immune globulin for infants of mothers infected just before or after delivery. Airborne isolation of infants with lesions.
OTHER INFECTIONS		
Group B Streptococcal Infection During birth or ascending after rupture of membranes.	Sudden onset of respiratory distress in infant usually well at birth, pneumonia, shock, meningitis. May have early or late onset.	Early identification essential to prevent death. Treatment of infected mothers during labor has decreased neonatal infection. IV antibiotics given to infected infants.
Gonorrhea Usually during birth.	Conjunctivitis (ophthalmia neonatorum), with red, edematous lids and purulent eye drainage. May result in blindness if untreated.	All infants receive prophylactic treatment. Erythromycin eye ointment most common. Infected infants are treated with antibiotics.
Chlamydial Infection During birth.	Conjunctivitis, pneumonia, otitis media.	Erythromycin or tetracycline eye ointment for prevention of conjunctivitis. Infection treated with erythromycin.
Candidiasis During birth.	White patches in mouth (thrush) that bleed if removed. Rash on perineum. May be systemic in preterm.	Administer nystatin drops or cream, and teach parents how to administer them. Assess mother for vaginal or breast infection. IV antibiotics for systemic infection.

TABLE **30-1** Common Infections in the Newborn—cont'd

Transmission	Effect on Newborn	Nursing Considerations
OTHER INFECTIONS—cont'd		
Toxoplasmosis Transplacental.	Asymptomatic or LBW, thrombocytopenia, enlarged liver and spleen, jaundice, anemia, seizures, microcephaly, hydrocephalus, chorioretinitis. Signs may not develop for years.	Consider in infants with IUGR. Confirmed by serum tests. Treatment: pyrimethamine, sulfadiazine, and folic acid.
Syphilis Transplacental.	Asymptomatic or enlarged liver and spleen, jaundice, lymphadenopathy, anemia, rhinitis, pink or copper-colored peeling rash, pneumonitis, osteochondritis, CNS involvement.	Diagnosed by blood and cerebrospinal fluid testing. Administer penicillin as ordered.

NOTE: Standard Precautions for infection control apply to all clients and are not listed above.
LBW, Low birth weight; *IUGR,* intrauterine growth restriction; *IV,* intravenous; *CNS,* central nervous system.

! CRITICAL TO REMEMBER

Signs of Sepsis in the Newborn

GENERAL SIGNS
Temperature instability (usually low)
Nurse's feeling that infant is not doing well
Rash

RESPIRATORY SIGNS
Tachypnea
Apnea
Respiratory distress—nasal flaring, retractions, grunting

CARDIOVASCULAR SIGNS
Color changes—cyanosis, pallor, mottling
Tachycardia
Hypotension
Decreased peripheral perfusion

GASTROINTESTINAL SIGNS
Decreased oral intake
Vomiting
Gastric residuals measuring more than half of previous feeding
Diarrhea
Abdominal distention
Hypoglycemia or hyperglycemia

CENTRAL NERVOUS SYSTEM SIGNS
Decreased muscle tone
Lethargy
Irritability
Bulging fontanel

SIGNS THAT MAY INDICATE ADVANCED INFECTION
Jaundice
Evidence of hemorrhage—petechiae, purpura, pulmonary bleeding
Anemia
Enlarged liver and spleen
Respiratory failure
Shock
Seizures

Etiology

Common causative agents of neonatal sepsis include coagulase negative staphylococci (e.g., *Staphylococcus epidermidis*), *Staphylococcus aureus*, enterococci, *Escherichia coli*, group B streptococci, *Haemophilus influenzae*, and *Listeria monocytogenes*. Sepsis may be divided into *early onset* and *late onset* according to when signs of disease begin.

Early-onset sepsis is acquired before or during birth, often from complications of labor such as prolonged rupture of membranes, prolonged labor, or chorioamnionitis. It usually begins in the first 24 hours but may begin up to 7 days after birth and has a more rapid progression than late-onset sepsis. The mortality rate is 5% to 20%. Multisystem involvement occurs, and pneumonia is a major cause of death (Edwards, 2002).

Late-onset sepsis generally develops after the first week of life. It is acquired during or after birth, before or after hospital discharge. It usually is a more localized infection, such as meningitis, and serious long-term effects can be common. The mortality rate is 5% (Edwards, 2002).

Therapeutic Management

Diagnostic Testing. Neonatal sepsis may be confused with other illnesses. For example, group B streptococcal pneumonia has the same initial symptoms as respiratory distress syndrome. Diagnostic testing helps identify sepsis and the organism responsible. A complete blood count with differential may show decreased total neutrophils, increased bands (immature neutrophils), an increased ratio of immature neutrophils to total neutrophils, and decreased platelets. Presence of elevated immunoglobulin M levels in cord blood or shortly after birth indicates that infection was acquired in utero, because this immunoglobulin does not cross the placenta. It often indicates transplacental infection.

The C-reactive protein may be elevated, a sign of an inflammatory process. Cultures of the blood, urine, cerebrospinal fluid, or any skin lesions may be obtained. Cultures of the nasopharynx, the cord, and gastric aspirate usually show colonization with organisms rather than infection. Chest radiography helps differentiate between respiratory distress syndrome and sepsis. Blood glucose levels should be checked because they may be unstable (high or low) in sepsis.

Treatment. Broad-spectrum antibiotics are given intravenously until culture and sensitivity results are available. Continued antibiotic therapy is based on culture results. Commonly used antibiotics for early-onset infection include ampicillin and an aminoglycoside such as gentamicin. If the organism is staphylococcus, a cephalosporin (such as cefotaxime) in combination with methicillin, nafcillin, or vancomycin is often used (Edwards, 2002). Intravenous immunoglobulins may also be used for some preterm infants.

Other care is supportive to meet the infant's specific needs. Infants may require oxygen and mechanical ventilation. The infant may need treatment for shock, hypoglycemia or hyperglycemia, electrolyte imbalances, and problems in temperature regulation.

Nursing Considerations

Assessment

Risk Factors. The nurse should identify infants at risk for infection. Mothers who have rupture of membranes longer than 18 hours have an increased risk of infection (Stoll, 2004). Other risk factors for sepsis include prolonged or precipitous labor, signs of infection before or during labor, and foul-smelling or meconium-stained amniotic fluid. The nurse needs to identify women known to have group B streptococcus and those who show signs of infection so they can be treated with antibiotics during labor to reduce risk to the infant.

Any infant in the neonatal intensive care unit (NICU) is at risk for nosocomial (hospital-acquired) infections, which occur more often in infants who require the specialized care of the NICU. These infants often have complications or conditions such as prematurity that make them more susceptible to infection. The risk of infection increases as gestational age and birth weight decrease. Preterm infants have not received maternal antibodies to help protect them from infection. In addition, they sometimes spend prolonged periods in the NICU, where they are exposed to many invasive procedures such as use of intravenous catheters and endotracheal tubes that increase their risk of infection. NICU infants may develop abnormal flora that may be carried by personnel from one infant to another and may be resistant to usual drug therapy (Saiman, 2002).

Signs of Infection. In the newborn, early signs of infection are often subtle and could indicate other conditions. There may be temperature instability (with a low temperature most common), respiratory problems, and changes in feeding habits or behavior. Other than the parents, the nurse is the only person who spends significant time with an infant and is therefore able to identify subtle changes in behavior. Experienced nurses may have a feeling that the infant is not doing well even before specific signs of infection are present. When this occurs, the nurse expands the assessment and watches carefully for the development of other signs. Early identification and treatment are important because infants can develop septic shock with little warning.

Nursing Interventions

Preventing Infection. Although it is not always possible to prevent infection, every effort should be made. The nurse should practice and teach parents to use careful handwashing or alcohol-based hand disinfectants before and after touching any infant. Equipment must be disinfected according to protocols. Meticulous sterile technique must be used during invasive procedures.

Transmission of infection to other infants in the nursery is prevented by handwashing, separation of infants' supplies, and Standard Precautions for infection control. Placing the infant in an incubator provides a physical separation between infected and well infants, similar to placing adults in isolation in private rooms.

Providing Antibiotics. The nurse must be knowledgeable about the specific antibiotics used and possible side effects. The nurse starts the intravenous fluids and ensures that medications are administered on time. If more than one antibiotic is ordered, the timing of administration must be coordinated to increase effectiveness. Laboratory analysis of peak and trough levels may be ordered to measure blood levels of the medications at times when they are expected to be at the highest and lowest points. Changes in dosage are based on the results of the laboratory tests. Antibiotics are usually continued for 10 to 14 days for sepsis and 21 days for meningitis.

Providing Other Supportive Care. Infants may be critically ill and need intensive nursing care. Nursing care involves use of oxygen or other respiratory support. Fluid balance maintenance, monitoring of the blood pressure, and hourly urine output measurements are important. Intravenous or gavage feeding may be necessary if the infant cannot take oral feedings. The nurse must be constantly alert for signs of other complications such as disseminated intravascular coagulopathy.

Supporting Parents. The infant with sepsis often appears healthy at birth but suddenly becomes critically ill. Parents experience shock, fear, and disappointment when their apparently healthy newborn is suddenly moved to the intensive care nursery. Or the preterm infant they thought was making good progress may suddenly develop a life-threatening illness. Parents benefit from a chance to talk about their feelings. Keeping the parents informed about the infant's treatments and changes in condition and involving them in care are essential.

INFANT OF A DIABETIC MOTHER

Scope of the Problem

The infant of a diabetic mother (IDM) faces many risks. Congenital anomalies are three times more likely in these infants (Stoll & Kliegman, 2004c). Anomalies occur in infants of mothers with pregestational diabetes when hyperglycemia is present during the early weeks of pregnancy when fetal organs are formed. Anomalies of the neural tube, heart, and kidney and caudal regression syndrome are most common. Cardiomegaly is common and may lead to heart failure. The incidence of anomalies is less if blood glucose levels remain within normal limits, especially before conception and in the early weeks of gestation.

Infants of mothers with long-term diabetes and vascular changes may be small for gestational age because decreased placental blood flow causes intrauterine growth restriction. Hypertension occurs more often in diabetic women and further compromises uteroplacental blood flow.

Macrosomia (birthweight >4000 g) (Figure 30-2) occurs in approximately one third of IDMs, even with good control of maternal glucose (Fanaroff, Martin, & Rodriguez, 2004). When the mother is hyperglycemic, large amounts of amino acids, free fatty acids, and glucose are transferred to the fetus. Insulin does not cross the placenta because the molecules are too large. The excessive glucose received by the fetus causes the fetal pancreas to secrete large amounts of insulin and leads to hypertrophy of the islet cells. Hypoglycemia may occur after birth, when the maternal supply of glucose is no longer available but the infant's high level of insulin production continues.

Insulin also acts as a growth hormone. The accelerated protein synthesis and the deposit of fat and glycogen in fetal tissues result in macrosomia. Macrosomic infants are at risk for trauma during birth, including fractures, cephalhematoma, and brachial plexus injury.

The IDM has a higher risk for asphyxia and respiratory distress syndrome (RDS). RDS occurs because high levels of insulin interfere with the production of surfactant. Hypocalcemia may result from decreased parathyroid hormone production. Magnesium levels may also be low. Polycythemia, a response to chronic hypoxia in utero, may result in hyperbilirubinemia as the large number of red blood cells break down after birth.

Characteristics of Infants of Diabetic Mothers

The macrosomic IDM has hypertrophy of the liver, adrenals, and heart. All organs except the brain are larger than normal. The length and head size are generally within the normal range for gestational age. Infants of diabetic mothers have a characteristic appearance. The face is round, the body is obese, and the skin is red (plethoric). The infant has poor muscle tone at rest but becomes irritable and may have tremors when disturbed. The small-for-gestational-age IDM is similar to infants who are SGA from other causes but is more likely to have congenital anomalies.

Therapeutic Management

Therapeutic management includes controlling the mother's diabetes to decrease complications in the fetus and newborn (see Chapter 26). If the infant is large, there may be shoulder dystocia or cephalopelvic disproportion and a cesarean birth may be required. Immediate care of respiratory problems and continued observation for complications determine treatment.

Nursing Considerations

Assessment

The IDM is assessed for signs of complications, trauma, and congenital anomalies at delivery and during the early hours after birth. Respiratory problems may be apparent at birth or de-

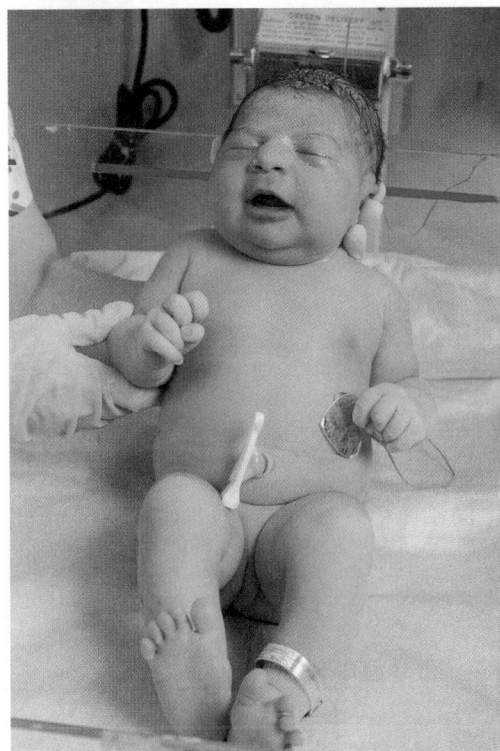

Figure 30-2 Macrosomia is common in infants of diabetic mothers.

velop later. The initial assessment may reveal injuries. For example, an infant who cries when an arm is moved or fails to move an arm may have a fractured clavicle or nerve damage.

Hypoglycemia occurs in 25% to 50% of infants of mothers with pregestational diabetes and 15% to 25% of those with gestational diabetes (Stoll & Kliegman, 2004c). The blood glucose level is screened according to hospital protocol. An example is screening every hour for 4 hours after birth and then every 4 hours twice or until the results are normal.

The most common sign of low glucose is jitteriness or tremors. Diaphoresis is uncommon in newborns but may occur with hypoglycemia. Rapid respirations, low temperature, and poor muscle tone are also common (see Chapter 22, p. 529). However, hypoglycemia may be present without observable signs.

Nursing Interventions

Infants should be fed early to prevent hypoglycemia and immediately if low blood glucose occurs. In some agencies, the infant is given a small amount of 10% dextrose (2 ml/kg), which is followed with 5 ml/kg of breast milk or formula. Giving larger amounts of dextrose is likely to stimulate increased insulin production and cause a rebound hypoglycemia. Gavage feeding may be used if the infant does not suck well or if the respirations are rapid. Infants whose glucose levels are not maintained with feedings or whose condition does not allow enteral feedings need intravenous dextrose to maintain balance and prevent damage to the brain.

The nurse must be alert for signs of other complications. Signs of respiratory distress syndrome or other respiratory complications may occur. Cold stress increases the need for oxygen and glucose, increasing hypoglycemia. Infants with polycythemia need adequate hydration to prevent sluggish

CRITICAL THINKING EXERCISE 30-2

The infant of a diabetic mother is jittery 1 hour after birth, and his glucose level is low. The infant weighs 4320 g (9.5 lb). The nurse, following nursery policy, prepares a feeding of 9 ml of 10% dextrose in water and 21 ml of formula. Why does the infant receive both the dextrose solution and formula instead of either of them alone?

blood flow and ischemia to vital organs. Hypocalcemia may be suspected if tremors continue.

Providing support to parents is important. They may not understand why their infant, who appears fat and healthy to them, needs close observation and frequent blood tests. The mother may have had a difficult pregnancy and may feel guilty, even if she followed a program of good diabetic control. Ample opportunity for discussion of feelings as well as information about the care of the infant is important.

PRENATAL DRUG EXPOSURE

Substance abuse affects the fetus at any time during pregnancy. Most drugs readily cross the placenta and cause a variety of problems. The effects of substance abuse on pregnancy, the fetus, and the neonate are discussed in Chapter 25. Neonatal abstinence syndrome (NAS), a disorder in which neonates demonstrate signs of drug withdrawal, is discussed here.

Identification of Drug-Exposed Infants

Maternal substance abuse may be identified before an infant is born, or it may be unknown to health professionals. A history of no prenatal care or the mother's behavior during labor may cause nurses to suspect substance abuse. When this occurs, the infant is observed closely for signs of prenatal drug exposure.

Neonatal abstinence syndrome occurs in infants who have suffered prenatal opiate exposure sufficient to cause withdrawal signs after birth. The syndrome is also seen in some infants exposed to other drugs such as codeine, tranquilizers, and sedatives. Infants with prenatal cocaine exposure may have signs similar to NAS such as irritability and poor sucking patterns, but these are thought to be caused by toxicity of the drug. These effects are not severe enough to require medication (Weiner & Finnegan, 2002).

Signs of drug exposure usually begin during the first 48 to 72 hours after birth for opiates, 2 to 3 days for cocaine, and within 3 to 12 hours for alcohol, depending on the time of the mother's last use. Polydrug use is common, and signs vary according to the drug or combination of drugs used but often include neurologic and gastrointestinal abnormalities. Some infants with prenatal drug exposure show no abnormal signs at all or do not show signs until after the first week.

Infants with NAS may be irritable and have hyperactive muscle tone and a high-pitched cry. Tremors may be present, but the blood glucose level is normal. Infants appear hungry and suck vigorously on their fists but have poor coordination of suck and swallow. Frequent regurgitation, vomiting, and

---

! CRITICAL TO REMEMBER

Signs of Intrauterine Drug Exposure

BEHAVIORAL SIGNS
Irritability
Jitteriness, tremors
Muscular rigidity, increased muscle tone
Restless, excessive activity
Exaggerated Moro reflex
Prolonged high-pitched cry
Difficult to console

SIGNS RELATING TO FEEDING
Uncoordinated sucking and swallowing
Frequent regurgitation or vomiting
Diarrhea

OTHER SIGNS
Poor sleeping patterns
Yawning
Nasal stuffiness, sneezing
Fever
Tachypnea
Apnea
Seizures
Diaphoresis
Excoriation

NOTE: Some infants with prenatal drug exposure have no abnormal signs at all, or signs may be delayed.

---

diarrhea are common. The infant's excessive activity, coupled with poor feeding ability, results in failure to gain weight. Various scoring systems are available to determine the number, frequency, and severity of behaviors associated with NAS. The score is helpful in determining the necessity of drug therapy to relieve effects of withdrawal. Infant behaviors are generally scored every 2 to 4 hours until low scores are obtained.

Congenital anomalies and other effects of prenatal drug exposure may be apparent at birth. Intrauterine growth restriction and prematurity are common. Infants are more likely to have respiratory distress at birth, jaundice, or sudden infant death syndrome. Infants with fetal alcohol syndrome have a characteristic appearance (see Fig. 25-3).

When drug exposure is suspected, a urine specimen is collected from the infant for analysis (see Procedure 37-3). Drugs are present in the newborn's urine for various lengths of time after the mother has used them. Some drugs last several days because of the infant's difficulty in excreting them, whereas others disappear very soon. Therefore it is important to obtain the first urine output from the infant, if possible. Meconium may also be tested for drugs because the drug is present for a longer period.

Therapeutic Management

Therapeutic management includes dealing with the complications common to drug-exposed infants during and after birth. Drug therapy may be necessary for approximately 50%

to 60% of these infants, who may have vomiting, diarrhea, marked irritability, and high scores on abstinence scales (Weiner & Finnegan, 2002). Medications commonly used include tincture of opium, phenobarbital, oral morphine, and diazepam (Valium). Paregoric is less often used because it has other ingredients that can be toxic. Medication dosage is gradually tapered until the infant no longer needs them. Although these drugs help relieve the signs of withdrawal, all have side effects that may be undesirable.

Gavage or intravenous feeding may be required because the infant's suck and swallow are uncoordinated. Some infants may need more than the normal caloric requirements because of their excessive activity. Involvement by social services is important to deal with the long-term effects of the drugs, placement of the infant after hospitalization, and follow-up with the mother or other caretaker to help provide for the infant's needs.

Nursing Considerations

The infant who has been exposed to drugs prenatally needs special care to cope with drug withdrawal. Care is focused on feeding, rest, and, if possible, enhancing parental attachment (Nursing Care Plan: The Drug-Exposed Infant).

Feeding

Feeding can be difficult and time consuming. The poor suck and swallow coordination of drug-exposed infants interferes with caloric intake, yet their increased activity increases caloric needs.

Assessment. The nurse should assess the infant's ability to coordinate sucking and swallowing with respirations. Changes in the frequency and amount of regurgitation or vomiting or the length of time it takes infants to finish feedings should be noted.

Nursing Interventions. Gavage feedings may be necessary to conserve the infant's energy and prevent aspiration if the infant is excessively agitated, cannot suck and swallow adequately, or has rapid respirations. When oral feedings are begun, infants may need jaw support similar to that used for preterm infants to help them suck more efficiently. Formula with 24 calories per ounce increases calorie intake. Infants should be swaddled during feedings to prevent excessive movement. Other types of stimulation such as rocking or talking should be minimized during feedings.

Rest

The excessive activity and poor sleep patterns of drug-exposed neonates interfere with their ability to rest.

Assessment. The infant's muscle tone, tremors, and tendency for excessive activity with and without being disturbed should be assessed. The degree of tremors and stimuli that increase or decrease irritability are important. The nurse also keeps track of the number of hours the infant sleeps after each feeding.

Nursing Interventions. Stimulation of the drug-exposed infant should be kept to a minimum by reducing noise and bright lights as much as possible. The nurse should organize nursing care to reduce handling and disturbances. A calm approach and slow, smooth movements during care help avoid startling the infant. If signs of overstimulation occur, the infants should be allowed to rest, if possible.

Swaddling the infant in a flexed position helps prevent startling and agitation. Nonnutritive sucking also helps quiet the infant. Skin excoriations from excessive activity or diarrhea may increase discomfort and agitation. They should be prevented if possible and treated promptly if they occur. Placing the infant in a prone position promotes better sleep.

Bonding

Infants who test positive for drugs may not be released to the mother until her ability to care for her infant safely has been assessed by social services or a court. She may be required to enter a drug rehabilitation program before she can obtain custody of the infant. After hospital discharge, the infant may receive care by family members approved by the court, in a foster home, or in an institution. The mother, however, will most likely gain custody of the infant eventually if she wishes, and attachment to the infant should be encouraged.

Assessment. The frequency of the mother's visits and her response to the infant may give an indication of her apparent interest in the infant. Bonding behaviors such as calling the infant by name and smiling at the infant should be noted.

Nursing Interventions. Because the mother may become the infant's primary caretaker, it is vital that nurses do whatever they can to enhance mother-infant bonding. Helping the mother feel welcome when she visits the infant provides a challenge. A friendly approach, however, will make the mother more likely to visit the infant and to accept teaching from the nurse.

The nurse can promote bonding by encouraging mothers to participate actively in infant care during visits. If the mother feels that the nurses trust her to care for the infant, her confidence may increase. Increased confidence may help increase the mother's effort to go through recovery to regain custody of her newborn.

The mother's participation also provides a chance for the nurse to assess the mother's infant care skills and areas in which further discussion of the newborn's needs will be helpful. In addition, it gives the nurse an opportunity to demonstrate parenting skills. Many mothers who use drugs have not had good parenting role models and do not know what to do. Frequent positive feedback about the mother's participation is also important.

The mother needs the same teaching given to all new parents, plus special techniques necessary to meet the needs of drug-exposed infants. The nurse should teach her about the newborn's special characteristics and help her take on more of the infant's care as she demonstrates readiness.

The mother needs to learn that infants are easily overstimulated and how to comfort them. Signs of overstimulation in drug-exposed infants have some similarities with those for the preterm infant. In addition, these infants cannot tolerate more than brief periods of interaction. They may not make eye contact, or they may avert their eyes after 30 to 60 seconds of social interaction. The nurse should teach the mother that the infant responds poorly to everyone so that she does not think that only she is being rejected.

The nurse can provide information and referral to any special programs available to help parents learn stimulation techniques appropriate for drug-exposed infants. Some withdrawal signs may continue for 2 to 6 months, and the mother needs to know how to deal with them (Weiner & Finnegan, 2002). If the mother cannot care for the newborn, the same

Nursing Care Plan

The Drug-Exposed Infant

Tracy was born at 38 weeks' gestation to Gloria, who was on a methadone maintenance program. During labor, Gloria admitted to using heroin several times during the last weeks of pregnancy.

ASSESSMENT

Tracy sleeps less than 1 hour after feedings. When she awakens, her high-pitched cry and agitation begin immediately. She wiggles out of her blankets, and her activity elicits the Moro reflex, which leads to more agitation. She is irritable and does not respond to caretaking activities as quickly as other infants.

Nursing Diagnosis

Disturbed Sleep Pattern related to agitation from own activity and irritability.

Goals/Expected Outcomes

Tracy will:

- Sleep for periods of 2 hours or more after feedings.
- Decrease crying by at least 1 hour a day within the first week.

INTERVENTION	RATIONALE
1. Place Tracy's crib in the quietest corner of the nursery. Place a sign nearby to remind others of the need for quiet in that area.	1. Drug-exposed infants are easily overstimulated by noise and activity.
2. Keep lights turned down as much as possible. Partially cover the crib with a blanket to decrease light.	2. Lowered lighting provides a more restful environment.
3. Keep Tracy tightly swaddled in a flexed position during sleep and feedings.	3. The drug-exposed infant's own movements can cause startling, awakening, and agitation.
4. Use a pacifier, and position her hands near her mouth.	4. Nonnutritive sucking may have a calming effect on the infant. Positioning the hands near the mouth allows the infant to self-comfort by sucking.
5. Organize nursing care so that Tracy is not disturbed unnecessarily, especially when sleeping.	5. Drug-exposed infants may have difficulty going back to sleep, if awakened.

Evaluation

Tracy gradually lengthens her sleep periods to 2 hours and decreases crying episodes within the first week.

ASSESSMENT

Gloria visits Tracy sporadically. She seems hesitant when she comes into the nursery and afraid to touch or care for Tracy. She asks, "Why does she cry so much?" When the nurse helps her hold Tracy, Gloria states, "I don't think she likes me."

Nursing Diagnosis

Impaired Parenting related to lack of understanding of the infant's characteristics and how to relate to an irritable infant.

Goals/Expected Outcomes

Gloria will:

- Visit at least every other day.
- Participate in Tracy's care by holding and feeding her.
- Make positive statements about her daughter.

INTERVENTION	RATIONALE
1. Show acceptance of Gloria when she comes to visit Tracy. Greet her, and provide her with an update on Tracy's progress.	1. A mother is more likely to visit her infant if she feels accepted by staff. The more she visits, the more she is likely to learn about parenting her infant.
2. Assist Gloria to hold and feed Tracy. Explain nursing actions such as placing the crib in a secluded area.	2. Participating in care of the infant helps the mother get to know her infant and gain comfort in providing infant care.

Nursing Care Plan

The Drug-Exposed Infant—cont'd

INTERVENTION	RATIONALE
3. Demonstrate comfort measures such as swaddling and rocking. Show her how to place a rolled blanket or positioning device around the infant to provide a feeling of security.	3. When the mother learns ways to comfort her infant, the positive response from the infant may increase bonding.
4. Explain common behavior in drug-exposed infants and that Tracy's stiff body posture and excessive activity are normal for her at this time. Point out signs such as gaze aversion that show Tracy is overstimulated.	4. Understanding that the infant's behavior is part of the infant's problem and is not caused by the mother's handling of her is reassuring to the mother.
5. Model ways of interacting with Tracy and calming her. Point out signs that Tracy is ready to interact. Suggest only one stimulus at a time, such as talking softly without rocking.	5. The mother learns appropriate interaction when she sees it performed by the nurse. Infants may need short time-outs before they are ready for more stimulation.
6. Point out positive points about Tracy, such as her long eyelashes or delicate fingers. Point out signs that show that Tracy is making progress.	6. The mother needs help to focus on positive aspects of the infant as well as the problems.
7. Explain the routine care of a newborn. Spread teaching out over Gloria's visits.	7. Mothers often need to learn the usual care of any newborn as well as the infant's special needs.
8. Give praise and encouragement frequently as Gloria works with Tracy.	8. The mother needs positive reinforcement and help to feel that she is capable of mothering her infant.
9. Use therapeutic communication techniques to help Gloria discuss her feelings as she cares for Tracy.	9. Mothers often find it frustrating to care for the drug-exposed infant. Helping them vent their feelings may increase their ability to cope with the infant's needs.
10. Discuss sources of support from family members or friends. Refer her to support groups in the community.	10. Ongoing support is necessary for the woman with addiction problems. Support for the mother will help her care more effectively for her infant.
11. If Gloria will have custody of Tracy, help her make plans for discharge. Discuss ongoing problems and concerns such as sudden infant death syndrome (SIDS).	11. Infants will have ongoing problems that will continue in the home setting. Infants exposed to heroin have an increased incidence of SIDS.

Evaluation

Gloria begins to visit more often, coming three or four times a week. She participates in care, begins to talk about her "pretty little girl," and discusses her plans for taking Tracy home with her.

Additional Nursing Diagnoses to Consider

Imbalanced Nutrition: Less Than Body Requirements
Interrupted Family Processes
Ineffective Coping
Impaired Skin Integrity
Disorganized Infant Behavior

interventions can be used to help the person who will take over care of the infant on hospital discharge.

Cocaine, amphetamines, and other drugs pass into breast milk. Trying to breastfeed an infant with poorly developed feeding skills may be too much stress for the mother who is trying to recover from addiction. Therefore mothers likely to continue drug use after delivery should be discouraged from breastfeeding. In some situations, however, breastfeeding may be acceptable. Women taking methadone may be allowed to breastfeed if they are not taking other drugs that are contraindicated as well (American Academy of Pediatrics, Committee on Drugs, 2001). If

the woman has a strong desire to breastfeed, the nurse should consult the health care provider.

POLYCYTHEMIA

Polycythemia is defined as a hematocrit above 65%. The increased viscosity of the blood causes an elevated resistance in the vessels and decreases blood flow. Organ damage from ischemia and microthrombi, congestive heart failure, renal vein thrombosis, PPHN, and necrotizing enterocolitis may result. Hyperbilirubinemia may occur from the excessive red blood cell breakdown after birth.

Causes

Polycythemia may occur when poor intrauterine oxygenation that occurs in intrauterine growth restriction, postmaturity, or maternal hypertension or diabetes causes the fetus to produce more erythrocytes than normal to compensate. Delayed clamping of the cord or a transfusion from one twin to another also may cause the condition.

Therapeutic Management

Treatment is primarily supportive but may include partial exchange transfusion. Blood is replaced with albumin or normal saline to decrease the total number of red blood cells.

Nursing Considerations

Infants may be plethoric (ruddy or dark red) but have no other signs, or they may have lethargy, jitteriness, cyanosis, respiratory problems, feeding disturbances, and hypoglycemia. Bilirubin levels should be monitored to determine if treatment for jaundice will be necessary. Infants must be hydrated adequately to prevent dehydration that would slow already-sluggish blood flow and increase ischemia to vital organs. If an exchange transfusion is performed, the nurse assists and watches for complications of the procedure.

HYPOCALCEMIA

Hypocalcemia is a total serum calcium concentration of less than 7.0 mg/dl. It is divided into *early onset* (less than 48 hours of age) and *late onset* (at about 1 week of age).

Etiology

Early-onset hypocalcemia occurs most often in IDMs and in infants with asphyxia, prematurity, and low birth weight. Late hypocalcemia is caused by maternal hyperparathyroidism or vitamin D deficiency, high-phosphate formula, low magnesium levels, and congenital hypoparathyroidism. Other causes of hypocalcemia include alkalosis, administration of bicarbonate or citrate-preserved blood, furosemide therapy, and renal disease.

Therapeutic Management

Laboratory testing of the serum calcium level determines the presence of the problem. Oral or intravenous calcium gluconate is given if feeding alone does not raise the calcium level. A cardiac monitor is necessary when intravenous calcium is given, because bradycardia can occur.

Nursing Considerations

The nurse must be alert for signs of hypocalcemia. These include irritability, tremors, poor feeding, high-pitched cry, tachycardia, apnea, muscle twitching, seizures, and electrocardiographic changes. The condition is often asymptomatic. Oral calcium should be given with feedings because it may cause gastric irritation. Intravenous calcium should be administered slowly and stopped immediately if bradycardia or dysrhythmia develops. The IV site should be assessed frequently because infiltration can cause necrosis and ulceration.

PHENYLKETONURIA

Phenylketonuria (PKU) is a genetic disorder that causes central nervous system damage from toxic levels of the amino acid *phenylalanine* in the blood. Mental retardation occurs in untreated infants and children.

Etiology

PKU is caused by a deficiency of the enzyme *phenylalanine hydroxylase*, which is necessary to convert phenylalanine to tyrosine for use. It is an autosomal recessive disorder (see Chapter 9).

Therapeutic Management

In the United States, all newborns are screened for this condition before or shortly after discharge from the birth facility. Positive screening tests are followed by other testing. Treatment is a low-phenylalanine diet. Small amounts of phenylalanine are allowed because it is a necessary amino acid. Early and continued treatment is necessary to prevent mental retardation.

Nursing Considerations

The nurse should see that the infant is screened for PKU at the appropriate time in the hospital. Screening performed before 24 hours of age should be repeated because the infant must have taken in enough protein for the test to be accurate.

Signs of untreated disease may begin with digestive problems and vomiting and later progress to seizures, musty odor of the urine, and mental retardation. Older children have eczema, hypertonia, hyperactive behavior, and hypopigmentation of the hair, skin, and irises.

The nurse assists parents in regulating the diet to meet the infant's changing phenylalanine needs. Parents can be reassured that good control helps promote normal infant growth and development (see Chapter 51).

KEY CONCEPTS

- Asphyxia before or during birth causes apnea, acidosis, pulmonary hypertension, and possible death. Neonatal resuscitation must be initiated immediately.
- Nurses must identify conditions that increase the risk of asphyxia, begin resuscitation promptly, and assist other members of the team during treatment. Continued follow-up of the infant and parental support are important.
- In transient tachypnea of the newborn, respiratory difficulty in full-term or preterm infants is caused by failure of fetal lung fluid to be absorbed completely. It usually resolves spontaneously with supportive care.
- In meconium aspiration syndrome, meconium enters the lungs before birth or during the first breaths after birth. It causes inflammation and blocks air flow.
- Pathologic jaundice appears in the first 24 hours of life and rises faster and to higher levels than physiologic jaundice. If untreated, it may

KEY CONCEPTS

result in damage to the brain from kernicterus.

- The nurse's role in phototherapy includes decreasing situations such as cold stress or hypoglycemia that might further elevate bilirubin levels, protecting the eyes, seeing that lights are used properly, observing for excessive fluid loss or skin impairment, ensuring adequate oral intake, and teaching parents.

- Infection can be transmitted to the neonate from the mother during pregnancy or birth or from the mother, family members, or agency staff after birth. Infections may have serious consequences.

- The IDM may have congenital anomalies, may be large or small for gestational age, and may have respiratory distress syndrome, hypoglycemia, hypocalcemia, and polycythemia.

- Nursing responsibilities in caring for IDMs include early identification and follow-up of complications, monitoring blood glucose levels, ensuring early and adequate feedings, and supporting parents.

- Infants with prenatal exposure to drugs may have congenital defects and behavioral and feeding abnormalities. They may have difficulty relating to others and fail to gain weight.

- Nursing care for infants with neonatal abstinence syndrome includes decreasing stimuli from lights, noise, or handling; increasing feeding abilities; and fostering the mother's attachment to and ability to care for her infant.

ANSWER to Critical Thinking Exercise 30-1

Patches hide the eye area, and irritation or infection might not be noticed immediately. The warm, dark, moist area under the patches provides a good breeding ground for organisms to grow. Removal of the patches at feedings allows inspection for signs of infection such as redness, edema, and drainage. Removal also allows a time of visual stimulation for the infant. Parental visits should be coordinated with feedings if possible so parents can see the infant's whole face while they visit. This will help the infant appear more normal to them and enhances attachment.

ANSWER to Critical Thinking Exercise 30-2

Giving infants fluids with high levels of sugar will provide glucose to begin to raise the blood glucose level, but if too much is given, there will be a rebound effect as a surge of insulin will cause more hypoglycemia. Giving formula alone would lengthen the time before glucose is available in the body. But giving formula along with a small amount of dextrose provides a source of glucose that will be metabolized more slowly without overstimulating insulin production.

REFERENCES and READINGS

American Academy of Pediatrics, Committee on Drugs. (2001). Transfer of drugs and other chemicals into human milk. *Pediatrics, 108*(3), 776-789.

American Academy of Pediatrics, & American College of Obstetricians and Gynecologists. (2002). *Guidelines for perinatal care* (5th ed.). Elk Grove Village, IL, and Washington, DC: Author.

Armentrout, D.C., & Huseby, V. (2003). Polycythemia in the newborn. *MCN: The American Journal of Maternal/Child Nursing, 28*(4), 235-241.

Association of Women's Health, Obstetric and Neonatal Nurses. (2003). *Standards for professional nursing practice in the care of women and newborns* (6th ed.). Washington, DC: Author.

Berkowitz, C.D. (2000). Infants of substance abusing mothers. In C.D. Berkowitz, *Pediatrics: A primary care approach* (2nd ed., pp. 486-495). Philadelphia: Saunders.

Blackwell, J.T. (2003). Management of hyperbilirubinemia in the healthy term newborn. *Journal of the American Academy of Nurse Practitioners, 15*(5), 194-198.

Cifuentes, J., Segars, A.H., & Carlo, W.A. (2003). Respiratory system management. In C. Kenner & J.W. Lott (Eds.), *Comprehensive neonatal nursing: A physiologic perspective* (3rd ed., pp. 348-362). Philadelphia: Saunders.

Cunningham, F.G., Gant, N.F., Leveno, K.J., Gilstrap, L.C., Hauth, J.C., & Wenstrom, K.D. (2001). *Williams obstetrics* (21st ed.). New York: McGraw-Hill.

Edwards, M.S. (2002). Postnatal bacterial infections. In A.A. Fanaroff & R.J. Martin (Eds.), *Neonatal-perinatal medicine: Diseases of the fetus and infant* (7th ed., pp. 706-745). St. Louis: Mosby.

Fanaroff, A.A., Martin, R.J., & Rodriguez, R.J. (2004). Identification and management of problems in the high-risk neonate. In R.K. Creasy & R. Resnik, *Maternal-fetal medicine* (5th ed., pp. 1263-1301). Philadelphia: Saunders.

Fike, D.L. (2003). Assessment and management of the substance-exposed newborn and infant. In C. Kenner & J.W. Lott (Eds.), *Comprehensive neonatal nursing: A physiologic perspective* (3rd ed., pp. 773-802). Philadelphia: Saunders.

Frank, C.G., Cooper, S.C., & Merenstein, G.B. (2002). Jaundice. In G.B. Merenstein & S.L. Gardner (Eds.), *Handbook of neonatal intensive care* (5th ed., pp. 443-461). St. Louis: Mosby.

Gagnon, A.J., Wagnorn, K., Jones, M.A., & Yang, H. (2001). Indicators nurses employ in deciding to test for hyperbilirubinemia. *Journal of Obstetric, Gynecologic, and Neonatal Nursing, 30*(6), 626-633.

Greene, C.M., & Goodman, M.H. (2003). Neonatal abstinence syndrome: Strategies for care of the drug-exposed infant. *Neonatal Network, 22*(4), 15-25.

Hagedorn, M.I., Gardner, S.L., & Abman, S.H. (2002). Respiratory diseases. In G.B. Merenstein & S.L. Gardner (Eds.), *Handbook of neonatal intensive care* (5th ed., pp. 485-475). St. Louis: Mosby.

Halamek, L.P., & Stevenson, D.K. (2002). Neonatal jaundice and liver disease. In A.A. Fanaroff & R.J. Martin (Eds.), *Neonatal-perinatal medicine: Diseases of the fetus and infant* (7th ed., pp. 1309-1350). St. Louis: Mosby.

Jones, C.W. (2001). Gestational diabetes and its impact on the neonate. *Neonatal Network, 20*(6), 17-23.

Kattwinkel, J., American Academy of Pediatrics, & American Heart Association. (2000). *Textbook of neonatal resuscitation* (4th ed.) Elk Grove, IL: American Academy of Pediatrics and American Heart Association.

Kenner, C. (2003). Resuscitation and stabilization of the newborn. In C. Kenner & J.W. Lott (Eds.), *Comprehensive neonatal nursing: A physiologic perspective* (3rd ed., pp. 210-227). Philadelphia: Saunders.

Lott, J.W., & Kenner, C. (2002). Assessment and management of immunologic dysfunction. In C. Kenner & J.W. Lott (Eds.), *Comprehensive neonatal nursing: A physiologic perspective* (3rd ed., pp. 550-579). Philadelphia: Saunders.

REFERENCES and READINGS

Maisels, M.J. (2001). Neonatal hyperbilirubinemia. In M.H. Klaus & A.A. Fanaroff (Eds.). *Care of the high-risk neonate* (5th ed., pp. 324-362). Philadelphia: Saunders.

Marcellus, L. (2002). Care of substance-exposed infants: The current state of practice in Canadian Hospitals. *Journal of Perinatal and Neonatal Nursing, 16*(3), 51-68.

Martin, R.J., Sosenko, I., & Bancalari, E. (2001). Respiratory problems. In M.H. Klaus & A.A. Fanaroff (Eds.), *Care of the high-risk neonate* (5th ed., pp. 243-276).Philadelphia: Saunders.

Merenstein, G.B., Adams, K., & Weisman, L.E. (2002). Infection in the neonate. In G.B. Merenstein & S.L. Gardner (Eds.), *Handbook of neonatal intensive care* (5th ed., pp. 462-484). St. Louis: Mosby.

Miller, M.J., Fanaroff, A.A., & Martin, R.J. (2002). Respiratory disorders in preterm and term infants. In A.A. Fanaroff & R.J. Martin (Eds.), *Neonatal-perinatal medicine: Diseases of the fetus and infant* (7th ed., pp. 1025-1049). St. Louis: Mosby.

Nash, P. (2001). Common neonatal complications. In K.R. Simpson & P.A. Creehan (Eds.), *AWHONN's perinatal nursing* (2nd ed., pp. 575-598). Philadelphia: Lippincott-Raven.

Reiser, D.J. (2001). *Hyperbilirubinemia: Identification and management in healthy term and near term newborns.* White Plains, NY: March of Dimes.

Rodriguez, R.J., Martin, R.J., & Fanaroff, A.A. (2002). Respiratory distress syndrome and its management. In A.A. Fanaroff & R.J. Martin (Eds.), *Neonatal-perinatal medicine: Diseases of the fetus and infant* (7th ed., pp. 1001-1011). St. Louis: Mosby.

Rubarth, L.B. (2003). The lived experience of nurses caring for newborns with sepsis. *Journal of Obstetric, Gynecologic, and Neonatal Nursing, 32*(3), 348-356.

Saiman, L. (2002). Risk factors for hospital-acquired infections in the neonatal intensive care unit. *Seminars in Perinatology, 26*(5), 315-321.

Shaw, N.M. (2003). Assessment and management of the hematological system. In C. Kenner & J.W. Lott (Eds.), *Comprehensive neonatal nursing: A physiologic perspective* (3rd ed., pp. 580-623). Philadelphia: Saunders.

Stevenson, D.K., Vreman, H.J., Wong, R.J., & Contag, C.H. (2001). Carbon monoxide and bilirubin production in neonates. *Seminars in Perinatology, 25*(2), 85-93.

Stoll, B.J. (2004). Infections of the neonatal infant. In R.E. Behrman, R.M. Kliegman, & H.B. Jenson (Eds.). *Nelson textbook of pediatrics* (17th ed., pp. 623-640). Philadelphia: Saunders.

Stoll, B.J., & Kliegman, R.M. (2004a). Digestive system disorders. In R.E. Behrman, R.M. Kliegman, & H.B. Jenson (Eds.). *Nelson textbook of pediatrics* (17th ed., pp. 588-599). Philadelphia: Saunders.

Stoll, B.J. & Kliegman, R.M. (2004b). Respiratory tract disorders. In R.E. Behrman, R.M. Kliegman, & H.B. Jenson (Eds.). *Nelson textbook of pediatrics* (17th ed., pp. 573-588). Philadelphia: Saunders.

Stoll, B.J., & Kliegman, R.M. (2004c). The endocrine system. In R.E. Behrman, R.M. Kliegman, & H.B. Jenson (Eds.). *Nelson textbook of pediatrics* (17th ed., pp. 613-616). Philadelphia: Saunders.

Weiner, S.M., & Finnegan, L.P. (2002). Drug withdrawal in the neonate. In G.B. Merenstein & S.L. Gardner (Eds.), *Handbook of neonatal intensive care* (5th ed., pp. 163-178). St. Louis: Mosby.

Wilbourne, P., Wallerstedt, C., Dorato, V., & Curet, L.B. (2000). Clinical management of methadone dependence during pregnancy. *Journal of Perinatal and Neonatal Nursing, 14*(4), 26-45.

31

Women's Health Care

◆ LEARNING OBJECTIVES

After studying this chapter, you should be able to:

◎ Explain examinations and various screening procedures that are recommended to maintain the health of women.
◎ Explain benign disorders of the breast, relate them to usual age of onset, and describe the diagnostic procedures used to rule out cancer of the breast.
◎ Describe the incidence, risks, pathophysiology, management, and nursing considerations of malignant breast tumors.
◎ Discuss the four most common menstrual cycle disorders.
◎ Explain management options for premenstrual syndrome (PMS) and premenstrual dysphoric disorder (PMDD), and nursing considerations.
◎ Discuss procedures, possible complications, and follow-up care related to induced abortion.

◎ Describe physical and psychological changes associated with menopause and options to alleviate uncomfortable changes.
◎ Discuss osteoporosis and measures to reduce severity.
◎ Discuss the major disorders associated with pelvic relaxation in terms of causes, treatments, and nursing considerations.
◎ Discuss the signs and symptoms, management, and nursing considerations for the most common benign and malignant disorders of the reproductive tract.
◎ Describe care of the woman with an infectious disorder of the reproductive tract, including sexually transmitted diseases, pelvic inflammatory disease, and toxic shock syndrome.

◆ DEFINITIONS

adjuvant therapy Additional treatment that increases or enhances the action of the primary treatment.

adnexa Accessory organs of the uterus, such as the fallopian tubes and ovaries.

amenorrhea Absence of menstruation. Primary amenorrhea is a delay of the first menstruation. Secondary amenorrhea is cessation of menstruation after its initiation.

atrophic vaginitis Inflammation that occurs when the vagina becomes dry and fragile, usually as a result of estrogen deficit after menopause.

autogenous graft Tissue moved from one part of the body to another part of the same person's body.

axillary tail Wedge of tissue extending from the breast into the axilla (also called the *tail of Spence*).

carcinoma in situ Malignant neoplasm in surface tissue that has not extended into deeper tissue.

climacteric Endocrine, body, and psychic changes occurring at the end of a woman's reproductive cycle. Also informally called *menopause*.

colposcopy Examination of the vaginal and cervical tissue with a colposcope for magnification of cells.

condyloma A wartlike growth of the skin seen on the external genitalia, in the vagina, on the cervix, or near the anus. Condyloma may be caused by human papillomavirus (condyloma acuminatum) or by syphilis (condyloma latum).

cryotherapy Destruction of abnormal tissue using extreme cold.

cystocele Prolapse of the urinary bladder through the anterior vaginal wall.

dysmenorrhea Painful menstruation.

dyspareunia Difficult or painful coitus in women.

dysplasia Abnormal development of tissue.

dysuria Painful urination, often associated with urinary tract infection.

endometrial hyperplasia Excessive proliferation of normal cells of the uterine lining; may be caused by administration of estrogen during the postmenopausal period.

endometriosis Presence of tissue resembling the endometrium outside the uterine cavity.

laparoscopy Insertion of an illuminated tube into the abdominal cavity to see contents, locate bleeding, and perform surgical procedures.

laparotomy Incision through the abdominal wall to examine the abdominal or pelvic organs.

mammogram Study of breast tissue using very-low-dose radiography; primary tool in the diagnosis of breast tumors.

menarche Onset of menstruation; usually occurs between 9 and 15 years of age (average age 12.4 yr).

menometrorrhagia Uterine bleeding that is irregular in frequency and excessive in amount.

menopause Permanent cessation of menstruation during the climacteric.

menorrhagia Excessive bleeding at the time of menstruation in duration, amount of blood lost, or both.

metrorrhagia Bleeding from the uterus at any time other than during the menstrual period.
osteoporosis Increased spaces (porosity) in bone; process greatly accelerates following menopause.
peau d'orange Dimpled skin condition that resembles an orange; associated with lymphatic edema and often seen over the area of breast cancer.

rectocele Herniation (protrusion) of the rectum through the posterior vaginal wall.
toxic shock syndrome Rare, potentially fatal disorder caused by toxin produced by *Staphylococcus aureus*; has been associated with improper use of tampons.

Nurses have an important role in primary and preventive care of women as it relates to routine assessments, screening procedures, and management of specific health concerns. The nurse acts as educator and advocate for women. Nurses explain screening and diagnostic procedures, clarify options so that women can make informed decisions about care, and provide support to women when they experience disruptions in their health.

HEALTH MAINTENANCE

Health maintenance refers to measures that can be taken to prevent or to detect specific diseases. Unfortunately, many women do not take advantage of recommended health maintenance procedures. Some seek care only when they have a problem. For others, the only health care they receive comes from a gynecologist or nurse practitioner. Therefore it is important that those who provide health care for women are familiar with principles of screening and counseling in areas that are not traditionally associated with gynecology, such as assessing risk factors for colon cancer and heart disease.

WOMEN'S HEALTH INITIATIVE

The Women's Health Initiative (WHI), started in 1991 by the National Heart, Lung, and Blood Institute of the National Institutes of Health, is a long-term national study focusing on prevention of four diseases that have a major impact on postmenopausal women of all races and socioeconomic backgrounds. Studies of these classes of disease include clinical trials, observational study, and community prevention measures. Internet information may be found at www.nhlbi.nih.gov/index.htm. The following diseases are the focus of the WHI studies:

- Cardiovascular disease
- Breast cancer
- Colorectal cancer
- Osteoporosis

Breast cancer and osteoporosis are covered in this chapter. For additional nursing information about these two diseases and about cardiovascular disease and colorectal cancer, see a medical-surgical nursing text.

Health History

The health history is most important in the determination of risk factors for a variety of conditions. The focus of a health history depends on the woman's age, but some topics need to be discussed with all women. Box 31-1 provides a summary of information that should be obtained.

Family history is essential to assess risk profiles. History of hyperlipidemia, heart disease, osteoporosis, and thyroid disease suggests screening tests, and examinations are needed. A list of family members who have had cancer and their ages when it was discovered provides important information about the risk of cancer, particularly breast and colon cancer.

Physical Assessment

A thorough physical examination is necessary to detect general health problems. Vital signs and weight are measured at each visit. Height is taken at the initial examination and yearly after that. Loss of height and abnormal curvature of the vertebral column (dorsal kyphosis or scoliosis) are important observations in evaluating osteoporosis.

The heart is auscultated at the initial visit to determine whether the rate and rhythm are normal and to detect heart murmurs. The extremities are observed for varicosities or edema, and pedal pulses are palpated. Palpation of the abdomen for tenderness, masses, or distention is an important part of the physical examination.

Additional assessments are necessary if the woman is at higher risk for disease. For instance, if she has a family history of diabetes mellitus, an oral glucose tolerance test may be indicated. If she has a history of multiple sexual partners or a sexual partner with multiple contacts, she may require testing for sexually transmitted diseases.

Preventive Counseling

Physical examination provides an excellent opportunity to counsel women about preventive care. Major preventable problems are obesity, inactivity, and smoking. Approximately 97 million adults in the United States weigh more than their most desirable weight. About 62% of women are overweight, having a body mass index (BMI) of 25 to 29.9, whereas 34% of women are obese, having a BMI of 30.0 or higher (Fried, Prager, MacKay, & Xia, 2003; National Institutes of Health: National Heart, Lung, & Blood Institute, 2004). Obesity is associated with diabetes, hypertension, and other chronic diseases, including some breast and reproductive cancers. Inactivity, often associated with being overweight, is associated with additional problems, such as osteoporosis, elevated levels of cholesterol, and coronary artery disease. Cigarette smoking is on the rise in young women, and smoking increases the risk for a wide variety of diseases, including cardiovascular problems and cancer. Counseling regarding diet should be offered, and positive behaviors, such as exercise and appropriate calorie intake, should be reinforced.

Infections, often sexually transmitted diseases, are a source of many health problems that should be reinforced in the nursing care of women. Use of latex condoms provides some

BOX 31-1
Health History

PERSONAL HISTORY

Demographic data (name, age, marital status or whether living with a partner of either sex)

Reason for seeking medical care (chief complaint)

Current and past state of health, previous surgeries

Height, weight, vital signs

Allergies (drugs, food, environmental allergens)

Medications, usual and reason for taking (over-the-counter; prescribed; illicit)

Use of complementary or alternative therapies, such as herbal or botanical preparations, acupressure

Habits (smoking, use of alcohol, drugs)

Appetite, usual dietary intake

Exercise pattern (type, frequency, duration)

Patterns of elimination (current or chronic problems)

Sleep and rest patterns

Degree of stress and stress management techniques

MENSTRUAL HISTORY

Age of menarche

Regularity, duration of menstrual cycle

Menstrual discomfort (time during cycles, intensity, relief measures)

Age at menopause, if applicable

OBSTETRIC HISTORY

Gravida, para, length of gestation, weight of infant at birth

Labor experience, medical interventions, and method of delivery

SEXUAL HISTORY

Sexual activity (one partner, multiple partners, age when first sexually active)

Method of contraception (satisfaction with method, adverse reactions, accuracy of use)

Previous sexually transmitted disease

Knowledge/practice of measures to protect self from sexually transmitted diseases

FAMILY HISTORY

Cardiovascular problems (anemia, hypertension, clotting disorders, stroke, heart attacks)

Cancer (breast, uterine, ovarian, bowel, lung)

Osteoporosis

PSYCHOSOCIAL HISTORY

Primary language, additional languages spoken or understood, ability to read

Marital status, employment, occupation, education (relevant to determine financial, social, and emotional support)

---

protection against transmission of viruses, such as human immunodeficiency virus (HIV) and human papillomavirus (HPV), which is strongly implicated as a risk factor for cervical cancer.

The history or physical examination may indicate other areas for which counseling is beneficial. These include the dangers of malignant melanoma with repeated exposure to ultraviolet rays of the sun. In addition, the health risks associated with alcohol and other substance abuse may be particularly important for some women. Domestic violence may be discovered, requiring counseling for the woman to deal with this complex social problem.

Screening Procedures

Screening procedures are important because early diagnosis allows early therapy while the pathologic process is still treatable. A variety of screening procedures are recommended for all women, including three screening procedures for early detection of breast cancer as well as vulvar self-examination and screening for cervical cancer. Other procedures are done based on the woman's age and risk status. Table 31-1 summarizes purposes for common screening procedures for women.

Breast Self-Examination

Most breast cancers are discovered by the woman herself. Yet only about half of all women examine their breasts each month. Breast self-examination (BSE, Box 31-2) should be performed monthly by all women older than 20 years.

Women should perform BSE approximately 1 week after the onset of menses, when hormonal influences on the breasts are at a low level. If the woman no longer menstruates, she may choose a day that is easy to remember and perform the test on that day every month. An example is the first day of the month.

Clinical Breast Examination

Clinical breast examination (CBE) performed by a health care professional may detect questionable areas that the woman misses during BSE. It should be routinely performed every 3 years for women ages 20 to 39 years and yearly for those 40 years or older. Some conditions need more frequent examinations because they are associated with a higher risk for breast cancer than the general population. The examination includes inspection and palpation.

Inspection. Follow these steps for breast inspection:

1. While the woman is in an upright position, the examiner inspects the breasts for size, symmetry, color, and skin changes. The nipples and areola are inspected for differences in size and color, unilateral retraction of a nipple, and asymmetric nipple direction, which may indicate an underlying tumor.
2. The woman raises her hands above her head, and the examiner inspects the sides and underneath portions of the breast for asymmetry and differences in color.
3. The woman places her hands on her hips and presses down to reveal skin dimpling or masses.

TABLE 31-1 Screening Procedures

Procedure	Purpose
Breast self-examination (BSE)	To assess monthly for breast changes or masses that might indicate breast tumors
Clinical breast examination (CBE)	To detect masses that women might miss
Mammography with additional imaging, such as ultrasonography, as needed 40 years or older (routine screening mammography)*	To detect breast lumps before they become palpable, promoting long-term survival. Diagnostic mammograms and other imaging may be started at a younger age for women having a higher risk for breast cancer or previous breast cancer or other disorders.
Cholesterol test	To detect blood levels that raise risk for heart disease; often combined with additional tests for high-quality screening, such as triglyceride level, high-density (HDL), and low-density (LDL) lipoprotein
Vulvar self-examination	To detect signs of precancerous conditions or infection
Pelvic examination	To confirm that no disease exists, or for early detection if disease does exist
Pap test	To detect abnormal cervical cytology as early as possible
Rectal examination	To check for hemorrhoids and lesions and to evaluate sphincter control
Fecal occult blood test	To detect blood in stool, an early sign of colon cancer
Urinalysis	To screen for diabetes and urinary infections

ADDITIONAL PROCEDURES MAY BE BASED ON RISK FACTORS

Procedure	Risk Factors
Sexually transmitted disease (STD) testing	Multiple sexual partners of the woman or her partner, history of STDs
Human immunodeficiency virus (HIV) testing	Seeking treatment for STDs, injection drug use, sexual partner who is HIV positive or bisexual or injects drugs, recurrent or persistent episodes of STDs such as candidiasis and herpes
Lipid profile	Diabetes, smoking, no estrogen use after menopause, family history of high cholesterol or coronary artery disease
Fasting glucose test	Overweight, history of gestational diabetes, family history of diabetes
Rubella antibodies	To assess immunity to rubella
Thyroid-stimulating hormone	Signs or strong family history of thyroid disease
Blood tests to evaluate genetic risk for reproductive cancers, such as BRCA1 and BRCA2, CA-125, or other indicated gene evaluation	To determine the degree of higher risk influenced by genetic alterations, improving options for therapy
Transvaginal ultrasound examination	Family history of ovarian cancer
Sigmoidoscopy or colonoscopy	Family history of bowel cancer or age >50 yr
Tuberculosis testing	To determine infection in a person at higher risk for tuberculosis

*American Cancer Society. (2003b). *Detailed guide: Breast Cancer: What are the risk factors for breast cancer?* Retrieved Feb. 17, 2004, from www.cancer.org/docroot/home/index.asp.

Palpation. Follow these steps for breast palpation:

1. With the woman in an upright position and while the arm is at the side and relaxed, each axilla is carefully palpated for enlarged or tender lymph nodes.
2. The woman lies in a supine position for palpation of the breasts. A small pillow or folded towel is placed under the shoulder, and the arm is placed at a 90-degree angle to stretch the tissue and thus flatten the breast. The examiner uses the flat part of the first three fingers to palpate the breast, rotating the fingers against the chest wall. Tissue that extends into the axilla, the tail of Spence, should also be palpated. The procedure is repeated on the opposite side. Normal breast tissue is described as firm, lumpy, nodular, tender, and thickened. Abnormal breast tissue is often likened to a raisin, watermelon seed, or grape. If a suspicious area is found, follow-up by mammography, often with related ultrasonography, is recommended.
3. The nipples are compressed to detect the presence of discharge. A sample of any discharge should be collected for culture and examination of cells.

Mammography

Mammography may be used either to screen for cancer or to assist in the diagnosis of a palpable mass in the breast. Mammography is the primary screening tool that can detect breast lumps long before they are large enough to be palpated. This procedure, often accompanied by ultrasound studies, allows early diagnosis and treatment and thus increases the chance of long-term survival.

The American Cancer Society (2003b) recommends yearly mammography to screen for breast cancer in women starting at age 40 years. Women at higher risk for breast cancer or with a suspicious growth in the breast may need mammography and other diagnostic studies at a younger age. Despite the value of screening mammography, many women have never had a mammogram. Reasons for this include expense, fear that x-ray exposure will cause cancer, fear of pain, and reluctance to hear "bad news."

Nurses provide information and reassurance to help the woman overcome her objections to the use of this valuable screening tool. Although mammography is relatively expensive, the cost is often covered by health insurance, and

WOMEN
Want to Know

How to Perform Breast Self-Examination

- Lie down. Flatten your right breast by placing a pillow under your right shoulder. If your breasts are large, use your right hand to hold your right breast while you do the examination with your left hand.

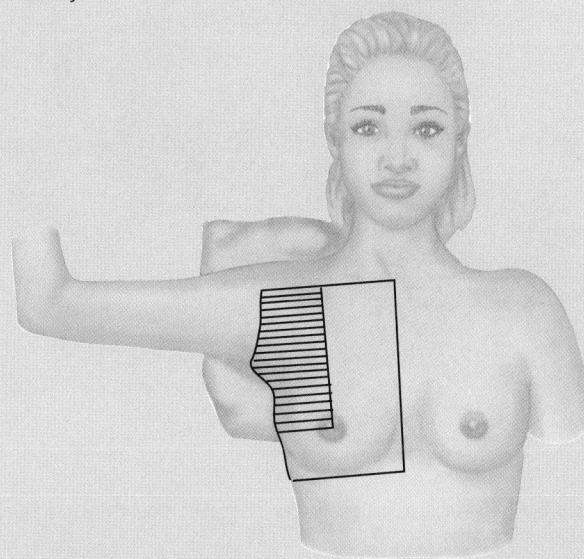

- Use the sensitive pads of the middle three fingers on your left hand and a massaging motion to feel for lumps or changes in the breast tissue.
- Press firmly enough to distinguish different breast textures: light pressure to feel tissues near the skin, medium pressure to feel slightly deeper, and firm pressure to feel tissues near the chest and ribs.
- Completely palpate or feel all parts of the breast and chest area. Be sure to examine the breast tissue that extends toward the shoulder. The amount of time required to completely palpate all the breast tissue depends on the size of the breast. Women with small breasts need at least 2 minutes to examine each breast. Larger breasts take longer.

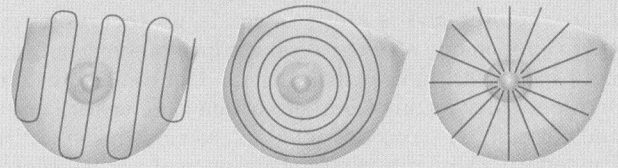

- Use the same routine or pattern to feel every part of the breast tissue. Any of three patterns can help you make sure you have covered your entire breast: the vertical strip, the circular pattern, and the wedge. Choose the method you find easiest. Evidence suggests the up-and-down pattern is the most effective to avoid missing breast tissue.
- When you have completely examined your right breast, examine the left breast with your right hand using the same method. Compare what you feel in one breast with the other.

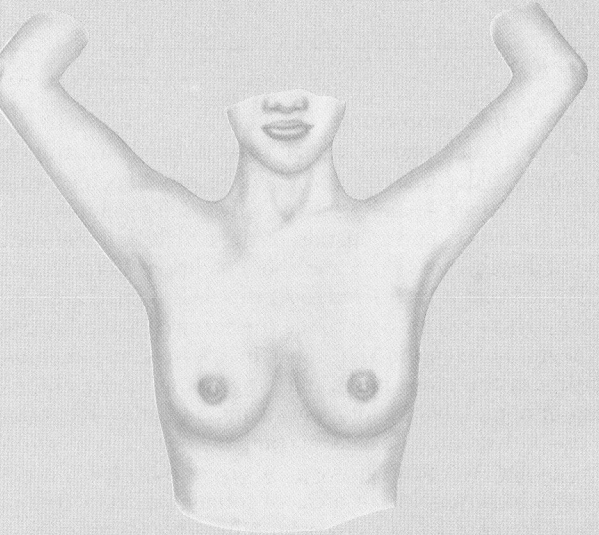

- You may also want to examine your breasts while bathing, when the skin is wet and lumps may be easily palpated.
- You can check your breasts in a mirror by raising your arms and looking for an unusual shape, dimpling of the skin, and any changes in the nipple.
- Examine each underarm, either when sitting or standing, by raising your arm slightly to better feel the area. Raising your arm high will tighten tissues in the area, reducing what you can feel.

Modified from the American Cancer Society (ACS) (2003). *How to perform a breast self-exam.* Available at the ACS website: http://www.cancer.org.

screening mammograms are frequently offered by the community at low cost. It is important to acknowledge that some discomfort occurs when the breast is compressed between two plates while the radiograph is taken. One measure that reduces discomfort is scheduling the mammography after a menstrual period, when the breasts are less tender. Knowledge that the risk of mammography is minimal to nonexistent because of the very-low-dose x-rays used may help women overcome some of their fear. Ultrasonography images may also be used if needed.

No screening test is 100% accurate. Therefore nurses must emphasize that the mammogram should be performed *in conjunction with* monthly BSE and recommended frequency of clinical breast examinations.

Vulvar Self-Examination

Vulvar self-examination should be performed monthly by all women older than 18 years and by those younger than 18 years who are sexually active. Vulvar self-examination is visual inspection and palpation of the female external genitalia to detect signs of precancerous conditions or infections.

The woman is instructed to sit in a well-lighted area and to use a hand-held mirror to see the external genitalia. She is taught to examine the vulva in a systematic manner, starting at the mons pubis and progressing to the clitoris, labia minora, labia majora, perineum, and anus. Palpation of the vulvar area should accompany visual inspection. New moles, warts or growths of any kind, ulcers, sores, changes in skin color, or areas of inflammation or itching should be reported to the woman's health care provider as soon as possible.

Pelvic Examination

The gynecologic assessment includes a pelvic examination. The woman is advised to schedule the examination about 2 weeks after her menstrual period and not to douche or have sexual intercourse for at least 48 hours before the examination. She is advised to avoid vaginal medications, douches, sprays, or deodorants that may interfere with a Papanicolaou (Pap) smear or other specimens obtained during the examination.

Before the examination, the procedure is carefully explained and the woman empties her bladder. She is placed in a lithotomy position, with a pillow under her head. If she wishes, she may assume a semi-sitting position and use a hand mirror so that she can observe the external genitalia and the examination. She is draped so that only the parts being examined are exposed.

Equipment needed for the pelvic examination includes gloves, a speculum of appropriate size, plus equipment to obtain test specimens needed, including a Pap test, also called a Pap smear. Additional equipment for collecting tissue specimens for Pap smear includes slides, cotton swabs, a fixative agent, and a cytobrush and spatula. Newer equipment for the Pap test transfers cervical cells to a liquid preservative. A stool specimen may be obtained by the examiner during the rectal examination, and a slide for this specimen should also

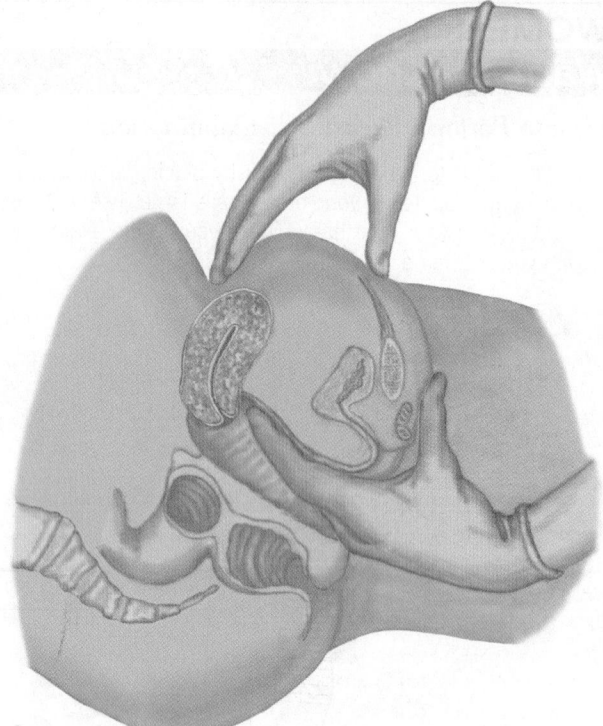

Figure 31-1 Bimanual palpation provides information about the uterus, fallopian tubes, and ovaries.

be available. Equipment to obtain specimens for suspected infection should also be available.

External Organs. The pelvic examination is conducted systematically and gently. The external organs are scrutinized for the degree of development or atrophy of the labia, the distribution of hair, and the character of the hymen. Any cysts, tumors, or inflammation of Bartholin's glands are noted. The urinary meatus and Skene's glands are inspected for purulent discharge. Perineal scarring caused by childbirth is noted.

Speculum Examination. A bivalve speculum of the appropriate size is used to inspect the vagina and cervix. The speculum is warmed with tap water or an electric warmer to reduce chilling and is gently inserted into the vagina. To avoid interference with test accuracy, lubrication is not used until specimens, such as those for the Pap test or a culture and sensitivity for infection, are obtained. The size, shape, and color of the cervix are noted. A sample is taken for the Pap test. In addition, a sample of any unusual discharge is obtained for microscopic examination or culture.

Bimanual Examination. The bimanual examination provides information about the uterus, fallopian tubes, and ovaries. The labia are separated, and the gloved, lubricated index finger and middle finger of the examiner's nondominant hand are inserted into the vaginal introitus.

The cervix is palpated for consistency, size, and tenderness to motion. The uterus is evaluated by placing the dominant hand on the abdomen with the fingers pressing gently just above the symphysis pubis so that the uterus can be felt between the examining fingers of both hands. The size, configuration, consistency, and motility of the uterus are evaluated (Fig. 31-1).

The ovaries are palpated between the fingers of both hands. Because ovaries atrophy after menopause, it is often impossible to palpate the ovaries of a postmenopausal woman.

The Pap Test

Purpose. Changes occur in cells of the cervix before cervical cancer develops. Cervical cytology, or the Pap test, is the most useful procedure for detecting precancerous and cancerous cells that may be shed by the cervix. Because infection with human papilloma virus (HPV) has been shown to be a contributor to cervical neoplasms, testing for this virus is often done during the pelvic examination process.

Procedure. A speculum is inserted into the vagina, and excess cervical mucus is wiped away. Samples of the superficial layers of the cervix and endocervix are obtained with a cytobrush and spatula or a broom-type sampling device.

Most lesions develop at the squamocolumnar junction (the border where developing squamous tissue meets the immature columnar epithelium). In postmenopausal women, the squamocolumnar junction recedes into the endocervix, making cervical specimens obtained by the cytobrush or broom-type device important. Cervical tissue is placed on slides that are then sprayed with or immersed in a fixative solution before being sent to the laboratory for analysis if the older Pap test technique is used. Specimens obtained with the broom-type device, such as those in the newer liquid-based Thin-Prep test for cervical cancer, are rotated in the liquid preservative to allow cells to disconnect from the collection device, thus flowing into the liquid.

Classification of Cervical Cytology. A meeting of professionals and patient advocates that was sponsored by the United States' National Cancer Institute created the Bethesda System 2001 to offer standard terminology for results of both the conventional Pap test and the liquid preparation (2004a). The Bethesda system consists of three elements: (1) a statement of specimen adequacy, (2) a general category for analysis (normal or abnormal), and (3) a descriptive diagnosis for abnormal cytology, whether results suggest malignancy or another disorder.

Categories for epithelial cell abnormalities include:

- Squamous cells:
  1. Atypical squamous cells of undetermined significance (ASCUS).
  2. Squamous intraepithelial lesion (SIL), which is subdivided into (a) low-grade, or LSIL (including cellular changes of HPV); and (b) high-grade, or HSIL (previously categorized as carcinoma in situ). The high-grade SIL is more likely to become cancerous without definitive treatment.
  3. Squamous cell cancer.
- Glandular cells:
  1. Atypical glandular cells of uncertain significance (AGCUS).
  2. Adenocarcinoma.

The woman's follow-up depends on the nature of the abnormality and whether it is persistent. Pap tests that have persistent ASCUS findings after a 3- to 6-month interval also usually are evaluated by a colposcopy. Suspicious lesions are examined with both colposcopy and biopsy.

Rectal Examination

The anus is inspected for hemorrhoids, inflammation, and lesions. The lubricated index finger is gently inserted, and sphincter tone is noted. A slide may be prepared to test for the presence of occult blood in stool.

Fecal occult blood testing (FOBT) is a useful screening measure for colorectal cancer. Special instructions are necessary to prevent false test results when materials for FOBT are sent home with the woman. She should be instructed to:

- Avoid aspirin and nonsteroidal antiinflammatory drugs (NSAIDs) such as ibuprofen or naproxen for at least 7 days before collecting the specimen.
- Avoid red meat, raw fruits and vegetables, horseradish, and vitamin C for 72 hours before testing.
- Collect a specimen from three consecutive stools.
- Return slides as directed within 4 to 6 days after the specimens are collected.

BREAST DISORDERS

Benign Disorders of the Breast

There are four relatively common benign disorders of the breast. The risk for each disorder is related to a specific age.

Fibroadenoma

Fibroadenomas are the most common benign tumors of the breast and are most common during the teenage years and the 20s. Fibroadenomas are composed of both fibrous and glandular tissue. They are felt as firm, rubbery, freely mobile nodules that may or may not be tender when palpated. Fibroadenomas do not change during the menstrual cycle. They are usually located in the upper, outer quadrant of the breast, and more than one may be present.

Treatment may involve careful observation for a few months. Persistence may require fine needle aspiration of the fibroadenoma to obtain cells for analysis. The aspiration may also collapse a cystic mass. If a specimen cannot be obtained, an excisional biopsy occasionally is required to determine if breast cancer, rare in adolescents, is present.

Fibrocystic Breast Changes

Fibrocystic breast changes are common breast changes during the reproductive years. Fibrosis, or thickening of the normal breast tissue, occurs in the early stages. Cysts form in the latter stages and are felt as multiple, smooth, well-delineated nodules that have a tender, moveable character. The lumpy, rubbery, or rope-like nodules often vary in size, from less than 1 cm to several cm. Fibrocystic changes are not cancerous, although atypical hyperplasia of the terminal breast ducts or lobules is associated with a greater risk for breast cancer. For women at higher risk for breast cancer, tissue specimens obtained by needle biopsy or an open surgical biopsy may be obtained to identify malignant changes (Gemignani, 2003; Hindle, 2000; Vail & Peterson, 2000).

Pain and tenderness (mastalgia) as the breasts respond to hormonal variations during the menstrual cycle are common symptoms. The pain is often bilateral and most apparent during the premenstrual phase of the normal cycle. Women with large pendulous breasts may have pain associated with stretching of breast ligaments (Gemignani, 2003).

Treatment for fibrocystic breast changes is based on the woman's symptoms. Nonsteroidal antiinflammatory drugs may provide adequate pain relief. Relaxation breathing and herbal therapy such as angelica or lady's mantle are thought to reduce estrogen levels. Evening primrose oil, 250 to 500 mg/day, is a botanical preparation that has been beneficial in reducing cyclic breast pain. Reducing intake of fat and caffeinated products may help some women relieve pain associated with their menstrual cycle (Fontaine, 2000; Huebscher, 2003; Vail & Peterson, 2000).

Ductal Ectasia

Ductal ectasia usually occurs as the woman approaches menopause. It is characterized by dilation of the collecting ducts, which become distended and filled with cellular debris. This initiates an inflammatory process resulting in:

- A mass that feels firm and irregular
- Enlarged axillary node
- Nipple retraction, pain, and discharge

These signs and symptoms are similar to those of breast cancer, and accurate diagnosis through biopsy is vital. Although ductal ectasia is benign, the ducts may be excised to prevent further discharge or to remove an abscess that results from infection.

Intraductal Papilloma

Intraductal papilloma develops most often just before or during menopause. It occurs when papillomas (small elevations or protuberances) develop in the epithelium of the ducts of the breasts, often under the areola. As the papilloma grows, it causes trauma and erosion within the ducts that result in serous or serosanguineous discharge from the nipple. Treatment consists of excision of the mass and ductal area, plus analysis of nipple discharge to rule out a malignant tumor. Regular follow-up after the excision is essential to identify any subsequent malignancy early.

Diagnostic Evaluation

When a lesion or lump is discovered in the breast, the physician must determine if it is benign or malignant. *Mammography* is used to locate and visualize suspicious areas of the breasts. However, mammography is not as effective a screening technique if breasts are dense such as in a younger woman or breasts that are dense because of changes associated with any disorder that is present. *Ultrasound* imaging differentiates fluid-filled cysts from solid tissue that is more likely to be malignant. For this reason, mammography and ultrasound examinations are often done together for improved diagnostic imaging. Variations of these visualization techniques are used to guide biopsy and excision of some small masses.

Options for biopsy vary with the type of lesion. *Fine needle aspiration biopsy* can be performed to remove fluid or small tissue fragments for analysis of the cells. *Core needle biopsy* uses a larger needle to obtain a cylinder of tissue from an area of abnormal breast tissue. *Open*, or *surgical*, *biopsy* is performed to obtain tissue for analysis and also to remove all or part of the lump of breast tissue. Other types of biopsy may be needed to obtain the most accurate tissue sample with

minimal trauma. Examples of conditions that may require a biopsy include:

- Suspicious mass that persists through a menstrual cycle
- Bloody fluid aspirated from a cyst
- Failure of the mass to disappear completely after fluid aspiration
- Recurrence of the cyst after one or two aspirations
- Solid dominant mass not diagnosed as fibroadenoma
- Serous or serosanguineous nipple discharge
- Nipple ulceration or persistent crusting
- Skin edema and erythema suspicious for inflammatory breast carcinoma
- Suspicious findings on mammography or ultrasonography
- Known or possible genetic abnormality that increases a woman's risk for breast cancer

Nursing Considerations

The nurse must acknowledge the anxiety that all women feel when a breast disorder is discovered. Furthermore, the apprehension continues for most women while they await a final diagnosis after biopsy. Some women may find it helpful to learn that most breast disorders are benign. However, as discussed, some benign disorders do increase the risk for later occurrence of cancer. For others, the most helpful intervention is to encourage them to express their concerns such as a genetic risk factor that increases their likelihood of developing cancer.

The nurse should reinforce medical explanations of procedures that are planned to diagnose the woman's breast disorder, such as ultrasound examination, mammography, needle biopsy, or surgical biopsy. Explanations should include what the procedures entail and how long the woman will have to wait for results to be known.

Malignant Tumors of the Breast

Incidence

The lifetime risk for a woman to develop breast cancer in the United States is one in eight. Although men develop breast cancer, the risk for women is 100 times greater than for men (American Cancer Society, 2003b). During 2001 the risk for development of invasive breast cancer was estimated to be over 190,000 among women in the United States (American Cancer Society, 2001). Breast cancer is the leading cancer among women of all races. However, in the United States, white women have a breast cancer rate that is 1.2 times higher than the rate for black women and 1.7 times higher than that for Asian/Pacific Islander women. However, African-American women have a higher risk of dying from breast cancer because they are more likely to be diagnosed at a later and more advanced stage. Asian, Hispanic, and Native American women have a lower risk for developing cancer. (American Cancer Society, 2003b; U.S. Cancer Statistics Working Group, 2003).

Predisposing Factors

Although the actual cause of breast cancer remains unknown, several factors are known to increase the risk for the development of breast and ovarian cancer or other diseases (see p. 770 [Box 31-2] and p. 787 [Box 31-4]). Mutations in two genes (*BRCA1* and *BRCA2*) thought to be responsible for most cases of familial breast cancer have been identified. Mutation of the *CHEK-2* gene has shown higher risk for development of breast cancer in both women and men. Study of genetic links to many types of cancers is ongoing. Because research has linked these and other genes to an increased risk for breast or other cancers, testing is offered to the woman having a higher risk or who has developed cancer at a younger age than expected.

Knowing risk factors is important to guide breast cancer screening and treatment processes so that a cancer is diagnosed at the earliest stage possible. It is also important for the nurse to convey to women that many breast cancers develop in women with no known risk factors, whereas other women with one or more risk factors do not develop breast cancer.

Pathophysiology

About 65% to 80% of the cases of breast cancer are infiltrating (invasive) ductal carcinoma, which originates in the epithelial lining of the mammary ducts. A cancer tumor becomes invasive when it is no longer confined to the duct and spreads to surrounding breast tissue. Another 10% to 14% of breast cancer cases are infiltrating lobular cancer, originating in the milk-secreting pockets of breast tissue. Growth of the tumor for common types of breast cancer occurs in irregular patterns and invades the lymphatic channels, eventually causing lymphatic edema and the dimpling of the skin that resembles an orange peel (peau d'orange) (Gemignani, 2003).

Cancer cells are carried by the lymph channels to the lymph nodes, and 40% to 50% of clients have involvement of axillary lymph nodes at the time of diagnosis. By the time a client consults a physician, breast cancer may be a systemic disease rather than being confined to the local tissue. Metastasis occurs when the malignant cells are spread by both blood and lymph systems to distant organs. The most common sites of metastasis are the lungs, liver, and bones.

Manifestations

When breast cancer becomes palpable, the woman or care-giver feels a breast lump, thickening, or distortion. Dimpling, nipple retraction, or changes in the skin or shape of the breast may occur. Most breast pain is benign. Changes on the mammogram or ultrasound images may occur before the cancer is palpable.

Staging

Although confirmation of malignancy is the first step in evaluating the woman with cancer, staging is necessary to understand the severity of the cancer. Staging is generally based on the tumor, node, and metastasis (TNM) system used to describe the cancer's anatomic extent. Stages of breast cancer progress from stage 1, indicating a small tumor without lymphatic involvement or metastases, to stage 4, which indicates spread to lymph nodes and metastases to other organs. The stages are often used to determine treatment, and they are useful guides to prognosis. The type of cancer cell, the presence of hormone receptors, and the proliferative rate of the breast cancer cells are also important factors in the rate of recurrence.

Therapeutic Management

The woman with breast cancer must choose from a variety of treatments offered. A combination of surgical excision and adjuvant therapy is often recommended. Radiation therapy of the breast is often done to minimize chances of recurrence or spread of the cancer.

Surgical Treatment. The surgical procedure depends on the type, stage, and location of the disease. The most common surgeries are (Gemignani, 2003; Kiebeck & Beller, 2000; Resnick & Belcher, 2002):

- *Breast conservation surgery* involves wide local excision (lumpectomy) of the malignant tissue to reach microscopically clear margins of healthy tissue surrounding the tumor. The excision can be performed without major cosmetic deformity. Varying numbers of axillary lymph nodes are usually removed to identify the stage of the woman's breast cancer.
- *Quadrantectomy* is a more extensive surgery for a breast tumor, removing a quadrant of tissue. Removal of the tumor involves resection of the skin and other tissue in the area to reach a microscopically clear margin of healthy tissue. Analysis of lymph nodes removed during the quadrantectomy allows staging of the cancer.
- *Simple mastectomy* is removal of the entire breast but not all axillary lymph nodes. Some lymph nodes may be removed for cancer staging, however. Simple mastectomy may be recommended for some women in whom prophylactic removal of the opposite breast is considered. It is also performed for elderly women who are poor operative risks and in whom no axillary involvement or distant disease is present.
- *Modified radical mastectomy* involves removal of breast tissue, axillary nodes, and some chest muscles. The pectoralis major and minor muscles, however, are preserved. This surgical procedure is recommended when a large primary lesion is found in a relatively small breast, radiation therapy is contraindicated, or a higher genetic risk for breast cancer exists. Breast reconstruction, ultimately the woman's choice, may be offered at the time of mastectomy. Timing of reconstruction is individualized by anticipated postoperative therapy and by the woman's choice.

Sentinel lymph node biopsy is a technique to remove a small number of key lymph nodes to evaluate cancer spread rather than removing most of the nodes in the area (axillary dissection). A radioactive suspension or a dye and often both materials are injected near the tumor site. The dye flows by the lymphatics toward the axillary nodes and is trapped by the first one or two lymph nodes, or the "sentinel" nodes, which are then removed for examination. Sentinel node biopsy may reduce the number of lymph nodes removed, reducing problems caused by lymphedema (see p. 775). A standard removal of nodes from the axilla, resulting in an average of 20 nodes, may be used if nodes are suspicious with palpation, if the tumor is large, or if a prior procedure has possibly disrupted the normal circulation of the lymphatic chain (Gemignani, 2003).

Adjuvant Therapy. Adjuvant therapy is supportive or additional therapy that may be recommended after the surgical procedure. Radiation therapy, chemotherapy, hormonal therapy, and immunotherapy are often recommended. The decision about whether to use adjuvant therapy is based on the woman's age, the stage of the disease, the woman's preference, and the hormone receptor status of the lesion. Radiation and chemotherapy are known to improve the chance of long-term survival after surgery for many cancers. Research is ongoing within many centers to determine the best uses for these adjuvant therapies when treating breast cancer.

Radiation Therapy. This therapy uses high-energy rays to destroy cancer cells remaining in the breast, chest wall, or underarm area. Radiation therapy follows many variations of surgical techniques to reduce the risk of cancer recurrence in the area. Radiation also is used to reduce problems from metastatic cancer, such as bone or brain lesions.

Chemotherapy. This therapy uses a combination of drugs best suited to kill proliferating cancer cells. Normal body cells, especially rapidly dividing cells such as those in the mouth, are also killed with chemotherapy but expected to regenerate. Supplemental drugs limit side or adverse effects, such as allergic reactions to the medication, nausea and vomiting, or diminished blood cells of specific types.

Hormonal Therapy. This therapy is used to block or alter estrogen or progesterone levels for women having tumors that are estrogen receptor (ER)– or progesterone receptor (PR)–positive. Tamoxifen (Nolvadex) is a common therapy that blocks estrogen by binding to estrogen receptors, including those on cancer cells. The drug is usually taken for 5 years. Hot flashes, vaginal dryness or an increased vaginal discharge, nausea, or anorexia may occur with tamoxifen therapy. Laboratory values for cholesterol and triglycerides may be elevated. Anastrozole (Arimidex) is a newer drug showing further improvement in survival over tamoxifen. Side effects for drugs are similar.

Raloxifene (Evista) is a drug for osteoporosis that also blocks the estrogen effects for the breast as well. Because of its estrogen-blocking effects, raloxifene is being studied in the Study of Tamoxifen and Raloxifene (STAR) research funded by the National Cancer Institute. For updated information see the Institute's website: http://cis.nci.nih.gov.

Immunotherapy. This is a biologically-based therapy that targets specific cell pathways that promote cancer growth. Approximately 25% of women with breast cancer have tumors that overexpress the HER2/neu, a protein that promotes growth of breast cancer cells. Trastuzumab (Herceptin) is a monoclonal antibody given to reduce overexpression by this protein.

Breast Reconstruction

Timing. Breast reconstruction to normalize the body's appearance is often an option for breast cancer treatment. Reconstruction options are discussed with the woman as other treatment plans are made. Immediate reconstruction appeals to many women because it quickly restores their breast contour and often makes them feel normal again. However, expected therapy for breast cancer may involve aspects for which later breast reconstruction is best. Some women prefer later reconstruction, even if not required, because it allows more time to learn options about reconstruction surgeries and about other ways she may enhance her appearance. The woman is able to physically heal from the mastectomy and to consider her personal values and desires about the added surgery.

Methods. Several methods of breast reconstruction are available. The *tissue expansion method* uses an empty silicone prosthesis fitted with a valve that can be accessed by percutaneous needle puncture. The bag is filled with saline in small increments to slowly expand the tissue. When the desired volume is attained, the incision is reopened, the device is removed, and the expander is exchanged for the appropriate implant. In some models, only the valve must be removed and the expander serves as the permanent implant (American Cancer Society, 2003a; Resnick & Belcher, 2002).

Tissue flap procedures move autogenous tissue from the back, abdomen, or buttocks to create a breast mound. Although these procedures do not always involve implants of a foreign substance as the tissue expansion method does, they involve at least two incisions: one at the breast and one at the site of the donor tissue. All women are not suitable for muscle flap grafts, particularly those with diabetes, connective tissue disorders, or smokers, because these procedures involve altering the blood supply to the transplanted tissue with the possibility of poor wound healing for these women. Thin women may not have sufficient tissue for transplant to the breast (American Cancer Society, 2003a; Gemignani, 2003; Resnick & Belcher, 2002).

Types of tissue flap procedures include:

- Transverse rectus abdominis muscle (TRAM) flap, which uses extra abdominal tissue in two common ways, as follows. A *pedicle flap* allows the tissue to remain attached to its original blood supply while it is tunneled under the skin to its site for breast reconstruction. The *free flap* involves removal of the tissue from its original site for attachment to the breast site. Because blood vessels are disconnected in free flap removal, microsurgery is required to reconnect the vessels and promote tissue preserving blood flow in the graft.
- Deep inferior epigastric artery perforator (DIEP) flap is a newer procedure that detaches skin and fat tissue from the lower abdominal area but does not use muscle in creating the new breast. Microsurgery is also required to connect blood vessels.
- Latissimus dorsi flap moves muscle and skin tissue from the upper back under the skin to the site of breast reconstruction. Weakness of the back, shoulder, or arm may persist after the surgery.
- Gluteal free flap uses surgical transfer of skin, fat, muscle, and blood vessels to recreate the breast.

Nipple/areola reconstruction improves the natural appearance in the reconstructed breast through a small skin graft. Tissue may be taken from the opposite nipple, from skin that covers the prosthesis mound, or from other body tissue. After the nipple has been reconstructed, tattooing promotes natural coloring to the nipple and areola (American Cancer Society, 2003a; Resnick & Belcher, 2002).

Psychosocial Consequences of Breast Cancer

The time from discovery to treatment of breast cancer is the most stressful time for many women. Factors that contribute to presurgery distress include a sense of uncertainty, inadequate information, the need to make difficult treatment decisions, and scheduling problems. Treatment usually involves consultations with one or more specialists, including a surgeon, a radiotherapist, a plastic surgeon, and a medical oncologist. When there are scheduling difficulties or conflicting opinions expressed by the health care team, the woman feels frustrated and confused.

Concerns frequently expressed during treatment for breast cancer include fear of recurrence and death, uncertainty about the quality of life, changes in body image, the effect on sexuality, and side effects of recommended therapy. For many women, the knowledge that they will lose their hair as a result of chemotherapy creates one of the most difficult situations in therapy.

Breast cancer can have psychological consequences not only for women but also for their significant others. Difficulties reported include sleep disturbances, eating disorders, and problems with work responsibilities. The marital relationship may be strained, primarily in the areas of sexual relations and communication about matters related to the illness. Women and their partners sometimes differ in regard to how much they want to discuss the illness. Some women have a great need to discuss their diagnosis, treatment, and fears of recurrence. Other women and many men view discussion of such fears as negative thinking that delays adjustment.

Nursing Considerations

The woman who is diagnosed with breast cancer depends on nurses for emotional support and accurate information. They must allow time for the woman to express her feelings and must convey a sense of empathic understanding by quiet presence, touch, and close attention to the woman's concerns. Many women feel that they have lost control and that their lives have been taken over by cancer and the recommended treatment. They may have concerns about family relationships and how their sexual partner will respond. Each woman should be allowed to express her fears and worries. Nurses must provide time and demonstrate genuine interest in the woman's concerns.

The anxiety that most women experience is reduced when procedures and care are clearly understood. Preoperative teaching should include significant others, to increase their ability to support the woman. Teaching should include the length of the hospital stay and what will happen during that time. The nurse should describe the dressings, drainage tubes, and appearance of the incision. Lymphedema of the arm on the same side as the mastectomy is possible because of blocked lymphatic vessels. Specific exercises such as arm lifts and pulley exercises may be necessary.

Discharge teaching focuses on the need for follow-up care and treatment. Some areas of concern are how to minimize the risk of wound infection, side effects of adjuvant therapy, and signs and symptoms that should be reported to the physician. Most women also benefit from information about such groups as Reach to Recovery and Encore, which provide support, information, and guidance after mastectomy.

Using nursing diagnoses to plan and implement care could ensure that care is complete. Relevant diagnoses might include:

- Fear related to uncertain outcome
- Disturbed Body Image related to loss of breast and temporary loss of hair during chemotherapy
- Interrupted Family Processes related to the woman's illness, changes in work and home activity, or inadequate information about the course of the disease
- Ineffective Sexuality Patterns related to concern about altered body structure

MENSTRUAL CYCLE DISORDERS

Although most menstrual cycle disorders are benign, all require comprehensive gynecologic assessment. Nurses must be knowledgeable about underlying processes, diagnostic procedures, and expected treatment so they can provide client advocacy, education, and supportive counseling.

Amenorrhea

Amenorrhea is normal before menarche, during pregnancy, during the puerperium and lactation, and after menopause. Amenorrhea at other times is abnormal, and it is called either *primary* or *secondary amenorrhea*, depending on when it occurs.

Primary Amenorrhea

Primary amenorrhea occurs if the girl passes the age by which menstruation has normally started, from 10 to 16 years. Ninety percent of girls have started menstruating if they have completed the sexual maturity rating 4 (SMR 4) (see Chapter 8). Primary amenorrhea is considered if onset of menstrual periods has not occurred, particularly if associated sexual changes have not taken place. Primary amenorrhea may be suspected if the girl is more than 1 year older than the ages at which her mother and sisters had menarche (Jenkins, 2004).

Etiology. The most common cause for primary amenorrhea associated with absence of breast or pubic hair development is Turner's syndrome. This syndrome occurs when girls have only one normal X chromosome. When the secondary sex characteristics are present, the cause may be incomplete development of the uterus, ovaries, and fallopian tubes. Intrauterine exposure to diethylstilbestrol is associated with abnormal development of the uterus. Other causes may include hormonal imbalances, systemic disease, and hypothalamic-pituitary abnormalities that result in inadequate secretion of gonadotropins. It may also be the result of excessive exercise, malnutrition, or eating disorders such as anorexia nervosa and bulimia, which cause a decrease in ovarian hormones.

Therapeutic Management. The success of medical management depends on the cause. Counseling for eating disorders and reducing excessive exercise may prove helpful. Hormone therapy may establish normal menses if the cause is hormone imbalance. Some conditions cannot be successfully treated. For example, if the cause is reproductive tract or congenital anomalies, normal menses and fertility may not be possible and psychological support becomes the most important therapy.

Secondary Amenorrhea

Secondary amenorrhea is the cessation of menstruation for 6 months or more in a woman who has established a pattern of menstruation, or absence for the duration of three normal cycles (Johnson, 2000). There may be a variety of causes, including systemic diseases such as diabetes mellitus, tuberculosis, hypothyroidism, or central nervous system lesions. Hormonal imbalances, strenuous aerobic exercise, poor nutrition, use of oral contraceptives, and ovarian tumors may also be causes.

Assessment includes a thorough medical and obstetric history and laboratory testing of hormone levels, as well as questions about eating habits, history of dieting, and current exercise pattern. Women are also questioned about their use of drugs, such as hormonal contraceptives, phenothiazines, and antihypertensives, which can cause secondary amenorrhea.

Medical treatment aims at identifying and correcting the underlying cause and will vary. Pregnancy testing is done for a sexually active woman, and medications that are potentially teratogenic must be withheld until pregnancy is ruled out. Other treatment may include testing levels of hormones related to the menstrual cycle, therapy to improve timing of the cycle, treatment of anovulation, and identification of other abnormalities that may be related to the disorder. Excess androgen levels may cause polycystic ovary syndrome (PCOS), characterized by acne, excess weight and body hair, as well as the anovulation that results in amenorrhea.

Nursing Considerations

Amenorrhea causes a great deal of concern for the young woman and her family, who may worry that it indicates a serious disease. Moreover, menstruation is a unique function of women, and absence of menstruation may provoke concerns about femininity and the ability to have children.

Teaching includes the importance of adequate nutrition and discouragement of rigorous dieting. The nurse should explain that, although exercise is beneficial, strenuous workouts or aerobic training can cause amenorrhea. Effective weight control may reduce factors related to polycystic ovary syndrome. The nurse also provides emotional support and explanation of proposed treatment.

Abnormal Uterine Bleeding

Abnormal uterine bleeding is bleeding that occurs with abnormal frequency, lasts an abnormal length of time, occurs irregularly, or is excessive in amount. Most abnormal bleeding occurs in cycles without ovulation, often near puberty and perimenopause. Complications of an unrecognized pregnancy, such as spontaneous abortion, must be considered when making the diagnosis (London, 2003; McGovern & Little, 2000).

Etiology

Common causes of abnormal bleeding fall into five basic categories:

1. Pregnancy complications, such as spontaneous abortion
2. Anatomic lesions, either benign or malignant, of the vagina, cervix, or uterus
3. Drug-induced bleeding, such as "breakthrough" bleeding that may occur in women who are on some oral contraceptives
4. Systemic disorders, such as diabetes mellitus, uterine myomas (fibroids), and hypothyroidism
5. Failure to ovulate (dysfunctional uterine bleeding)

Management

Evaluation of abnormal uterine bleeding may include a sensitive pregnancy test, coagulation studies, and tests to determine whether ovulation is occurring. Hormone and liver function tests plus tests to determine if the woman is anemic will often be done. Ultrasonography or hysteroscopy may be used to look for polyps and check the condition of the uterine lining.

A common hormone treatment is progestin-estrogen combination oral contraceptives that suppress ovulation and al-

low a more stable endometrial lining to form. Surgical therapy may include laparoscopy and possibly dilation and curettage (D&C) to remove polyps or to diagnose endometrial hyperplasia. Hysterectomy may be performed if the uterus is enlarged as a result of fibroids or adenomyosis (benign invasive growth of the endometrium into the muscular layer of the uterus) and if the woman does not want more children. Laser ablation may be used to permanently remove the endometrial lining without hysterectomy. Excessive uterine bleeding from any cause may warrant treatment for iron-deficiency anemia.

Nursing Considerations

Nurses are often responsible for encouraging women to seek medical attention promptly when irregular or prolonged bleeding occurs. Nurses also help the woman keep a record of the bleeding episodes and the amount of blood lost. This involves keeping a calendar and noting any vaginal bleeding (spotting, menses) that occurs in addition to the number of pads and tampons saturated each day.

The nurse teaches the importance of adequate nutrition and discourages rigorous dieting. For women who are concerned about amenorrhea, the nurse should explain that, although exercise is beneficial, excess workouts or aerobic training can cause amenorrhea. In addition, the nurse teaches methods to reduce stress and promote relaxation. Finally, nurses must provide support for women who fear that irregular bleeding indicates a serious disease, such as cancer. Offering false reassurance is unwise, but information about diagnostic procedures, such as pelvic examinations, Pap test, and other tests is helpful.

Pain Associated With the Menstrual Cycle

Cyclic pelvic pain must be distinguished from acute pelvic pain. Acute pelvic pain is sudden in onset, and it is not experienced with each menstrual cycle. It may indicate a serious disorder, such as ectopic pregnancy or appendicitis. On the other hand, cyclic pelvic pain occurs repetitively and predictably in a specific phase of the menstrual cycle. The most common causes of cyclic pelvic pain are mittelschmerz, primary dysmenorrhea, and endometriosis.

Mittelschmerz

Mittelschmerz ("middle pain") refers to unilateral pelvic pain that occurs midway between menstrual periods, or at the time of ovulation. The pain is caused by growth of the dominant follicle in the ovary or rupture of the follicle and subsequent spillage of follicular fluid and blood into the peritoneal space. The pain is fairly sharp and usually lasts from a few hours to 2 days, and slight vaginal bleeding may accompany the discomfort. Usually, explanation of the discomfort or mild analgesics are sufficient treatment.

Primary Dysmenorrhea

Primary dysmenorrhea refers to menstrual pain without an identified pathologic process. Commonly called *cramps*, primary dysmenorrhea affects at least half of all women and causes 10% to miss work or school (Dawood, 2000).

Manifestations. The pain of dysmenorrhea begins within hours of the onset of menses and is spasmodic or colicky in nature. It is felt in the lower abdomen but often radiates to

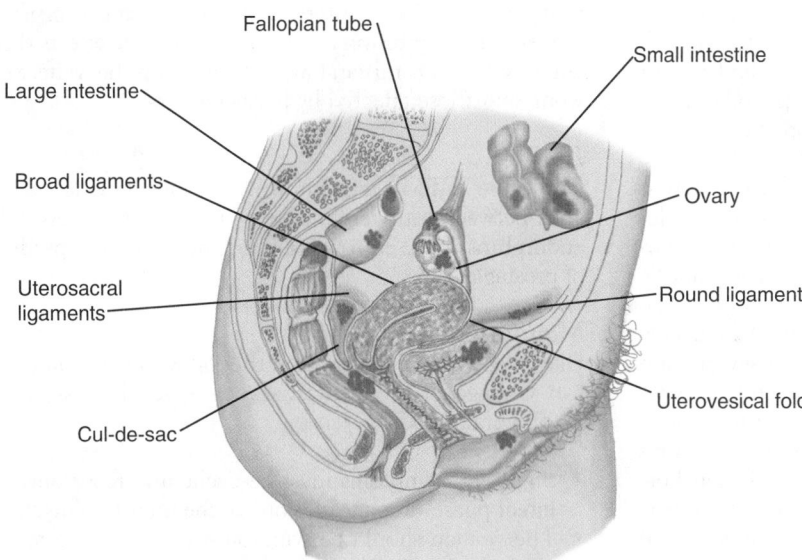

Figure 31-2 Common sites of endometriosis.

the lower back or down the legs. Primary dysmenorrhea occurs in ovulatory cycles, and it is most common in young, nulliparous women. Pelvic examination is usually normal.

Etiology. One of the most confusing aspects of primary dysmenorrhea has been why it is experienced by some but not all women. Some women produce excessive endometrial prostaglandins during the late luteal phase of the menstrual cycle. The prostaglandins (particularly E_2) diffuse into endometrial tissue and cause abnormal uterine muscle contractions, uterine ischemia, and hypoxia. This process accounts for the cramping uterine pain as well as symptoms that often accompany it, such as diarrhea, nausea, and vomiting.

Therapeutic Management. Oral contraceptives and NSAIDs, such as ibuprofen (Advil, Motrin) and naproxen (Naprosyn, Anaprox), provide effective dysmenorrhea relief by reducing secretion of prostaglandin in endometrial tissue. For best pain management using NSAIDs, the drug should be taken around the clock for 48 to 72 hours, starting at the onset of menstrual flow.

Endometriosis

Endometriosis occurs when endometrial tissue is present outside the uterus. It is estimated that as many as 15% of women, often in their 20s and 30s, are affected (Schenken, 2003; Surrey, 2000).

Etiology. The cause of endometriosis remains unknown. One theory is that retrograde menstruation (reflux of menstrual flow through the fallopian tubes) causes endometrial cells to attach to nearby structures and proliferate, creating spots of endometrial tissue. Endometriosis may also represent an autoimmune process. Delayed childbearing, also associated with endometriosis, often occurs among women of upper economic status because they more often delay pregnancy (Scheneken, 2003; Surrey, 2000).

Pathophysiology. Endometrial tissue outside the uterus responds to stimulation from estrogen and progesterone in the same manner that tissue inside the uterus responds. That is, it grows and proliferates during the follicular and luteal phases of the cycle and then sloughs during menstruation.

The menstruation from endometriosis lesions, however, occurs in a closed cavity, which causes pressure and pain on adjacent tissue. In addition, prostaglandins secreted by the endometriosis lesions irritate nerve endings and stimulate uterine contractions that further increase pain. Moreover, cyclic bleeding into the pelvic cavity initiates chronic inflammation that may cause scarring and adhesions and make conception and implantation difficult. The most common sites of endometriosis lesions are illustrated in Figure 31-2.

Manifestations. The two major symptoms of endometriosis are cyclic pain and infertility. The pain of endometriosis differs from that of primary dysmenorrhea. Endometriosis pain is deep, unilateral or bilateral, and either sharp or dull. It is constant, as opposed to the spasmodic or colicky pain of primary dysmenorrhea. Dyspareunia (painful intercourse) is typical, particularly with deep penetration. Rectal pain is common, especially during defecation. Diarrhea, constipation, and sensations of rectal pressure or urgency are other common symptoms of endometriosis. Although the cause of infertility is not completely understood, pelvic adhesions and tubal disease caused by chronic inflammatory changes are certainly contributing factors.

Therapeutic Management. Treatment may be either medical or surgical, and the therapy chosen must weigh the need for pain relief and the desire to maintain fertility against the side effects that accompany many treatment regimens. Growth of endometriosis tissue depends on adequate production of ovarian hormones during the menstrual cycle.

Continuous oral contraceptives suppress endometrial tissue proliferation, particularly in a woman who desires pregnancy after endometriosis treatment is complete. Progestins such as medroxyprogesterone acetate (Depo-Provera) or norethindrone (Micronor) directly inhibit growth of the excessive endometrial tissue.

Both the testosterone derivative danazol (Danocrine) and GnRH agonists such as leuprolide acetate (Lupron) and nafarelin (Synarel) interfere with hormones needed for ovulation and the menstrual cycle, creating a "pseudomenopause" while taken. The woman may have hot flashes, vaginal dryness, insomnia, decreased libido, and reduced bone density. In addition, danazol may produce masculinizing effects, such as deepening of the voice, facial and body hair, and weight gain. The woman takes the drug for a varying period of time, often between 3 and 6 months, depending on the drug and the degree of her endometriosis.

Surgical treatment of endometriosis may have different options because of the varied size, number, and location of lesions, the age of the affected woman, and whether endometriosis contributes to her infertility. Laparoscopy may be performed for lysis of adhesions and laser vaporization of the lesions of endometriosis. This procedure is used especially when infertility is a problem. For women with severe pain who no longer wish to have children, a hysterectomy, sometimes including bilateral salpingo-oophorectomy to remove both fallopian tubes and ovaries, and excision of all lesions offer relief. Removal of both ovaries causes loss of their hormone production, resulting in an early menopause. Postoperative hormone replacement therapy may be recommended if endometriosis lesions are removed.

Nursing Considerations

Dysmenorrhea varies from mild "menstrual awareness" to incapacitating pain that affects the quality of life for many days of each month. Too often the pain is belittled ("It's just cramps"). One of the most important nursing actions is to acknowledge the pain in a supportive manner.

The nurse should suggest non-pharmacologic pain-relief measures, such as frequent rest periods, application of heat to the lower abdomen, moderate exercise, and a well-balanced diet. The woman should avoid scheduling stress-provoking situations during the menstrual period. The nurse should counsel the woman about expected effects of over-the-counter (OTC) or prescribed medications. The woman should also be instructed about side or adverse effects specific to the medications recommended that should be reported.

The nurse should allow time for the woman to express her concerns about the therapy. The woman should be taught expected effects for drugs given for endometriosis and about the drug's precautions and any side or adverse effects that may occur. Some women benefit from information about measures that promote sleep and relaxation, and, most important, from the knowledge that someone is available to provide support and guidance when needed. A woman may demonstrate emotional distress if she has not had all the children she desires but must decide whether to have a hysterectomy to reduce physical pain that simpler measures have not relieved.

Premenstrual Syndrome

Premenstrual syndrome (PMS) is a group of symptoms that occur during the second half of the menstrual cycle and cause varied types and severity of problems in a woman's work and relationships with others (Box 31-3). As many as 85% of women are affected with PMS. Of these women, about 5% to 10% have more severe symptoms that interfere with their work or social life, many of which are psychiatric in nature, known as *premenstrual dysphoric disorder* (PMDD) (Pritham, 2002; Reid, 2003). Once thought to be trivial problems, PMS and PMDD can significantly impair a woman's work produc-

tivity and her social interactions. Severe anger, aggression, anxiety, and depression are serious psychiatric effects that occur with PMDD and can have an impact on the welfare of the woman or those affected by her behaviors.

Etiology

The cause of PMS is unknown. Theories include an imbalance between estrogen and progesterone, low levels of beta-endorphins, low serotonin levels, and abnormal production of prostaglandins.

Manifestations

Diagnosis of PMS depends on the following criteria (American College of Obstetricians and Gynecologists [ACOG], 2000; Baram, 2000):

- Signs and symptoms must be cyclic and recur during the luteal phase (after ovulation) of the menstrual cycle.
- The woman should be symptom-free during the follicular phase (before ovulation) of the menstrual cycle, and the cycle must include 7 symptom-free days.
- Symptoms must be severe enough to impact the woman's work, lifestyle, and personal relationships.
- Diagnosis should be based on *prospective* symptom recording by the woman, meaning that symptoms are recorded as they occur rather than recalling symptoms that occurred in the past.

Figure 31-3 illustrates one type of calendar or diary the woman can use to record her PMS/PMDD symptoms and their severity. Other records may include additional factors such as appetite and food cravings, life events, how the symptoms affect her lifestyle, and her psychosocial reactions.

Premenstrual syndrome puts a consistent strain on family relationships because major symptoms recur monthly. Clinical descriptions of severe family disruptions include increased family conflict, disrupted communication, and decreased family cohesion. Of particular concern is the group of women who report symptoms of loss of control, child battering, self-injury, and increased accidents.

Therapeutic Management

Treatment of PMS is based on the symptom profile of each woman after ruling out other problems, especially psychiatric diagnoses such as depression. Varied dietary measures may provide relief. Vitamin B$_6$ (pyridoxine), which is an important cofactor in the synthesis of neurotransmitters that influence mood, may be prescribed but has not proved effective. Low doses of 100 mg/day are considered safe, but the woman should be cautioned that excessive doses of vitamin B$_6$ may cause peripheral neuropathy. Other trials have shown that supplements of calcium (1200 mg/day) have some effectiveness and magnesium (200-400 mg/day) is minimally effective. Carbohydrate-rich food and beverages may improve the mood and reduce food cravings in some women. Reducing caffeine and taking vitamin E (400 international units [IU]/day) during the luteal phase of the cycle may reduce breast pain (mastalgia) in some women (ACOG, 2000; Baram, 2000; Reid, 2003).

Women with physical, emotional, and cognitive symptoms may be prescribed antidepressant medications, oral con-

Calendar for PMS Symptoms

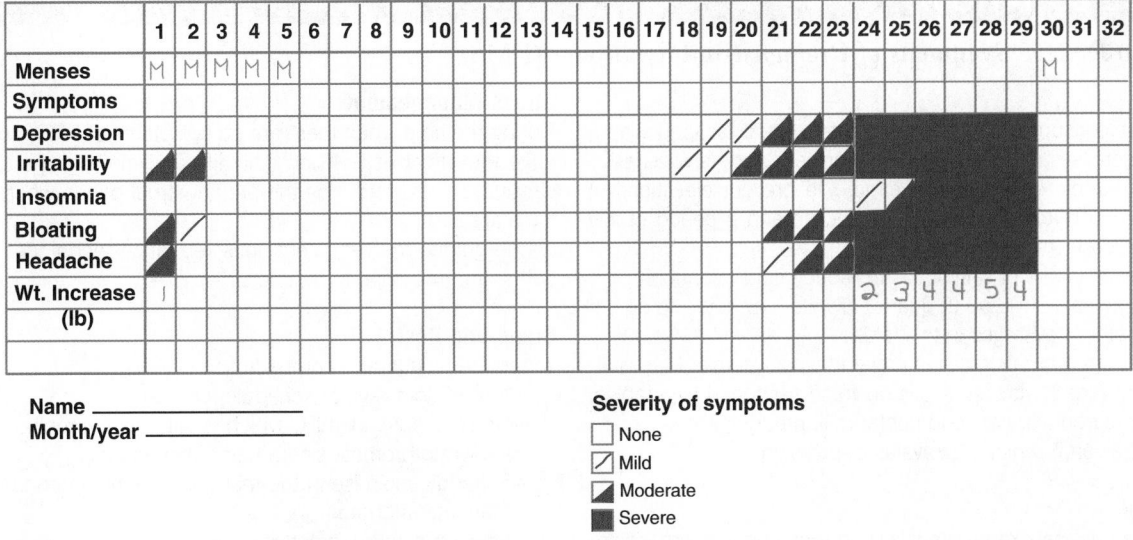

	1	2	3	4	5	6	7	8	9	10	11	12	13	14	15	16	17	18	19	20	21	22	23	24	25	26	27	28	29	30	31	32
Menses	M	M	M	M	M																									M		
Symptoms																																
Depression																																
Irritability																																
Insomnia																																
Bloating																																
Headache																																
Wt. Increase (lb)	1																							2	3	4	4	5	4			

Name _____
Month/year _____

Severity of symptoms
☐ None
◩ Mild
◪ Moderate
■ Severe

Figure 31-3 The woman uses a diary to record occurrence and severity of premenstrual symptoms.

traceptives to suppress ovulation, or both. Danazol taken in low doses relieves mastalgia, but higher doses may be required for the drug to relieve other PMS symptoms. Preferred antidepressants are selective serotonin reuptake inhibitors (SSRIs) such as fluoxetine (Prozac), sertraline (Zoloft), or paroxetine (Paxil), although tricyclic antidepressants may also be useful. Short-acting drugs to reduce anxiety, such as alprazolam (Xanax) or buspirone (BuSpar), have also shown benefit (ACOG, 2000; Baram, 2000; Reid, 2003).

Nursing Considerations

Many women experience some of the symptoms and diagnose themselves as having PMS. Nurses must discourage this practice because serious systemic disease can be missed if the criteria for diagnosis are ignored. Nurses should recommend that the woman consult with her health care provider so that a complete history and physical examination can be performed to rule out other causes.

Once the diagnosis of PMS is confirmed, nurses can educate the family about lifestyle changes that may help. Nurses should acknowledge that dietary changes are particularly difficult because many women crave salty or sweet foods, which should be restricted. Women also benefit from education about expected cyclic changes. As they learn to predict the pattern of symptoms and gain a sense of control over them, the symptoms often diminish.

Education and support must be expanded to include the family. When the woman exhibits symptoms of PMS, family members often respond by withdrawing or confronting the woman. Family members should also be encouraged to express their feelings so that anger and resentment within the family can be diminished.

Nurses must help the woman make concrete arrangements to obtain relief when she feels she is losing control or when she fears that she may harm herself or a child. A neighbor, friend, or family member should be identified to provide immediate relief, without questions or explanations, when the woman feels she is losing control.

BOX 31-3
Symptoms of Premenstrual Syndrome (PMS)

PHYSICAL SYMPTOMS
Headache, dizziness
Abdominal bloating or swelling; swelling of extremities
Weight gain
Breast tenderness
Hot flashes
Abdominal cramps
Generalized muscle and joint pain
Fatigue
Appetite changes: binge eating, food craving
Sleep changes: excessive or insomnia
Reduced sexual interest

BEHAVIORAL SYMPTOMS
Depression or sadness
Feelings of hopelessness
Marked anxiety
Confusion, forgetfulness, poor concentration
Accident prone
Irritability and anger
Emotional lability: tearfulness or crying easily, loneliness, mood instability
Reduced interest in normal daily activities
Social avoidance
Lethargic or energetic

WOMEN
Want to Know

How to Relieve Symptoms of Premenstrual Syndrome (PMS)

Diet

Decrease consumption of caffeine (coffee, tea, colas, chocolate), which increases irritability, insomnia, anxiety, and nervousness.

Avoid simple sugars (cake, candy) to prevent elevations of blood glucose followed by a rapid decline and a period of low blood glucose (hypoglycemia).

Decrease intake of salty foods to reduce fluid retention.

Drink at least 2000 ml (2 quarts) of water per day, and do not include other beverages in this total.

Eat six small meals a day to prevent hypoglycemia. Plan well-balanced meals with emphasis on fresh fruits and vegetables, complex carbohydrates, and nonfat milk products.

Avoid alcohol, which aggravates depression.

Exercise

Increase physical exercise to relieve tension and to decrease depression. Aerobic activity, such as jogging or walking, several times a week is recommended.

Stress Management

During the time when there are no symptoms of PMS, acknowledge the effect of PMS on daily life and make plans to avoid stressful situations during the premenstrual period when symptoms are acute.

Use guided imagery, conscious relaxation techniques, warm baths, and massage to reduce stress.

Sleep and Rest

To reduce fatigue and combat insomnia:
—Adhere to a regular schedule for sleep.
—Drink a glass of milk, which is high in tryptophan and is known to promote sleep, before bedtime.
—Schedule exercise in the morning or early afternoon rather than late afternoon.
—Engage in relaxing activities, such as reading, before bedtime, and avoid excitement at this time.

MEDICAL TERMINATION OF PREGNANCY

Induced abortion is a voluntary method of terminating a pregnancy. It may be performed to preserve the health of the mother, to prevent the birth of an infant with severe genetic defects, or to end a pregnancy caused by rape or incest. A woman may also choose to terminate a pregnancy for economic or social reasons. Abortions involve social and ethical implications (see Chapter 1).

Methods of Abortion

The technique used to terminate a pregnancy depends on the length of gestation. Abortion techniques based on medications may be options within 7 weeks of the woman's last menstrual period. Inducing uterine contractions with specific medications to end pregnancy early makes the process more private, eliminates risks such as uterine trauma or perforation, and does not require anesthesia. Medications used include:

• Mifepristone (Mifeprex, or RU486), an anti-progesterone drug, is followed by misoprostol (Cytotec), a prostaglandin drug commonly used to reduce gastric acid secretion. Oral or vaginal use of misoprostol in medical abortion is unlabeled by the manufacturer. The woman receives an initial dose of 600 mg mifepristone orally. Oral or vaginal misoprostol 400 mcg follows in 48 hours to promote expulsion if pregnancy has not ended. The woman usually expels the young pregnancy within 14 days of her first visit. Newer regimens may use a combination of mifepristone 200 mg followed by a client-administered dose of vaginal misoprostol 800 mcg and may be prescribed up to 9 weeks of gestation (Taylor & Hwang, 2003/2004; Trupin, 2003; U.S. Food and Drug Administration [FDA], 2000).
• Methotrexate (Folex, Mexate) is an antimetabolite also used to treat certain types of cancer. Although not FDA-

approved for medical abortion, individualized doses have been successfully used for medical pregnancy termination. Misoprostol may be prescribed to enhance expulsion of uterine contents (Taylor & Hwang, 2003/2004; Trupin, 2003).

Surgical abortion techniques are needed if the woman has been pregnant for over 7 weeks or if her medical abortion failed and she still desires pregnancy termination. Through 12 weeks' gestation, vacuum aspiration with curettage is the method of choice. The cervix is dilated after locally injecting anesthetic in the area, and a plastic cannula is inserted into the uterine cavity. The contents are aspirated with negative pressure, and the uterine cavity may be scraped with a curet to ensure that the uterus is empty. Cramping may last 20 to 30 minutes after the procedure is completed. Complications may include uterine perforation, hemorrhage, cervical lacerations, and adverse reactions to the anesthetic agent.

For second-trimester abortions, *dilation with removal of the fetus and placenta* is generally performed. The procedure is similar to vacuum curettage but requires greater cervical dilation and a larger aspirator because the products of conception have grown in size and must be removed gradually. Dilation begins with insertion of laminaria, rounded cone-shaped materials that absorb water, into the cervix 24 hours before the procedure. The laminaria draw fluid from the cervical canal and expand, causing the cervix to dilate slowly and with minimal trauma. If needed before aspiration and removal of the products of pregnancy, additional cervical dilation is done.

Medical methods exist for abortion in the second trimester, but these involve labor. Retention of the placenta often occurs, requiring a dilation and curettage to fully clean the uterus. Laminaria are inserted about 12 hours before the procedure to start cervical dilation. Prostaglandin E_2, which stimulates contractions, may be given via vaginal suppository or intraamniotic infusion. Oxytocin is not effective at starting labor because of the early gestation, but it may shorten labor after it has been established by other methods. Because of the emotional distress caused by the longer procedure and the increased risks involved, medical termination of pregnancy is not often chosen in the second trimester.

Nursing Considerations Related to Induced Abortion

The nurse's role in caring for women seeking induced abortion is to provide physical and emotional support and information. The nurse may take a history and collect specimens for laboratory testing. Counseling and emotional support are nursing responsibilities. The nurse should reinforce instructions about returning to the clinic and provide information for self-care. They should teach the woman signs of complications such as excessive bleeding or infection. Nurses may teach use of a recommended contraceptive method after the pregnancy has ended. Rh-negative women should receive $Rh_o(D)$ immune globulin (RhoGAM) if they do not have a preexisting sensitivity to Rh-positive blood.

MENOPAUSE

Menopause simply means "the end of menstruation." Many people, however, use the term to indicate all changes that occur at the end of the reproductive period. The entire process, frequently called the *change of life*, is correctly termed the *climacteric*. *Premenopause* refers to the early part of the climacteric, before menstruation ceases but after the woman experiences some of the climacteric symptoms, such as irregular menses. *Perimenopause* includes premenopause, menopause, and at least 1 year after menopause. *Postmenopause* refers to

the phase after menopause, when menstrual periods have ceased altogether.

Once a woman is postmenopausal, *unplanned bleeding should always be investigated as soon as possible* because it is highly suggestive of endometrial cancer. Women who take estrogen and progesterone sequentially have planned bleeding when they stop taking the drugs, usually once a month. This allows the uterine lining to be sloughed and prevents endometrial hyperplasia.

Age at Menopause

The woman's reproductive function falls during the climacteric, from about 45 to 50 years of age, as the ovarian hormones decline and then cease. Menopause occurs at the time of the woman's final period during the climacteric. If therapeutic, menopause can be created artificially at any age, through surgical removal of the ovaries or their destruction by radiation therapy, often related to treatment for cancer. Young women who experience artificial menopause often have more symptoms associated with menopause than do women who go through the natural process gradually.

Women can now expect to live another 30 years after menopause at the expected age. During this period, they must deal with physical, psychological, and social changes that often require a reevaluation of their primary roles and restructuring of personal goals.

Physiologic Changes

During the premenopausal period, the ovaries are less responsive to gonadotropins. Although increased amounts of follicle-stimulating hormone are secreted, ovulation is sporadic and menstrual periods are irregular. With progressive aging, the ovaries become unresponsive, even to high levels of gonadotropins, and ovulation, menstruation, and the secretion of ovarian hormones (estrogen and progesterone) cease. Menstrual periods become less frequent as menopause approaches.

When estrogen levels decline, the organs of reproduction undergo regression. The labia become thin and pale. The vaginal mucosa atrophies, and vaginal tissue loses its lubrication and is easily traumatized. Dyspareunia is not uncommon, and bacterial invasion of the epithelium may lead to frequent vaginal infections. This process is called *atrophic vaginitis*. Breasts become smaller, and atrophy of the uterus and ovaries occurs. A concurrent benefit is that uterine myomas (fibroids) and endometriosis lesions also atrophy. Estrogen deficit can also result in atrophic changes in the bladder and urethra that may give rise to loss of urethral tone and frequent atrophic cystitis.

In addition, absence of estrogen is associated with an adverse change in serum lipids. Low-density lipoproteins, which carry cholesterol to blood vessels, increase. High-density lipoproteins, which carry cholesterol to the liver and protect against the development of coronary artery disease, decrease.

Most menopausal women experience hot flashes or flushes, which are the result of vasomotor instability. The cause of vasomotor instability is unknown, but it is closely associated with increased secretion of gonadotropins. Hot flashes are characterized by a sudden feeling of heat or burning of the skin, followed by perspiration. They occur more frequently during the night, causing fatigue from interrupted sleep.

Psychological Responses

Psychological and social changes also accompany menopause, and individual responses vary widely. Many women are relieved that their childbearing and child-rearing tasks are coming to an end. Other women grieve that the possibility of childbearing is past, especially if they are childless.

Some symptoms do not have a physiologic explanation, but they are no less real to women who experience them. Depression, mood swings, irritability, and agitation are common climacteric complaints. Insomnia and fatigue are frequently mentioned as major problems.

One of the most puzzling aspects of menopause is the wide variation in both physical and psychological symptoms that women experience. For some women, the only changes are mild, infrequent hot flashes and amenorrhea. Other women experience severe, debilitating hot flashes, atrophic vaginitis, and multiple psychological symptoms, such as irritability and prolonged depression.

Therapy for Menopause

Although many women comfortably undergo the age-associated changes of menopause, others seek assistance for their individual discomforts such as hot flashes, interrupted sleep, or vaginal dryness. The psychological perception that increasing reproductive hormones would slow the aging process and promote a more youthful appearance strengthened replacement therapy during the climacteric. Additional beneficial effects were thought to be a reduction in cardiovascular disease, colorectal cancer, breast cancer, and osteoporosis as well as other medical-surgical conditions associated with aging.

As greater research results emerged, including that of the Women's Health Initiative (WHI), additional risk factors as well as benefits of hormone therapy emerged. Two groups of perimenopausal women were included in the hormone studies of the WHI research:

- Estrogen and progesterone have been given to women with a uterus. Combining progesterone with estrogen therapy prevents uterine hyperplasia, a precursor to uterine cancer, in this group.
- Estrogen therapy alone has been given to women who have had a hysterectomy, because uterine hyperplasia is not a risk.

The combination of estrogen and progesterone replacement is usually called *hormone replacement therapy*, or *HRT*, whereas the estrogen-only replacement therapy may be called *ERT*. It is common to see HRT used for either or both therapies, however.

Other hormone replacement research studies were being done as the WHI study continued, and increasing evidence emerged that estrogen plus progesterone therapy significantly increased risks of some disorders, primarily breast cancer and heart disease. Therefore the estrogen-progesterone arm of the study was stopped in 2002. The estrogen-only arm of the study continues because risk levels in this group have not shown the higher levels that the estrogen-progesterone group showed. The WHI hormone study, now having a single arm, continues until 2005 unless excessive risk factors also cause this half of the hormone-replacement study to be discontinued.

Although once routinely prescribed to reduce the annoying changes of menopause for many women, the decision about hormone therapy is more complex because both the benefits and risks associated with a prescribed hormonal drug must be considered. In addition, complementary therapy often has a greater usefulness for women having milder menopausal changes.

Some women do not qualify for hormone therapy. For example, women who have breast cancer or blood coagulation disorders do not qualify. Women who had breast cancer before the climacteric often should not take hormone therapy because their risk of cancer recurrence is higher than that of the general population. Smoking, hypertension, diabetes, cardiovascular disease, and renal or liver disease are often contraindications for hormone therapy, whether therapy includes both estrogen and progesterone or estrogen only.

Nursing Considerations Related to Menopause

Nursing care focuses on helping women understand the physical and psychological changes that may occur during the perimenopause. If the woman chooses hormone therapy, nurses must reinforce both the prescribed regimen as well as the risks and benefits of the therapy. For instance, women should be told that although hormone replacement therapy effectively treats atrophic vaginitis and reduces dyspareunia, it may not correct the loss of libido that some women experience.

If hormone replacement therapy is contraindicated or not chosen by the woman, nurses may often provide information about measures to reduce problems and promote comfort:

- Using water-soluble lubricants, such as K-Y Liquid, Lubrin, Replens, or K-Y Silk-e to relieve vaginal dryness and dyspareunia. Oil-based lubricants should not be used because they adhere to the mucous membrane for long periods and provide a medium for bacterial growth.
- Discussing alternatives to estrogen, such as botanical preparations, if the woman does not want estrogen replacement therapy. The woman should discuss these with her health care provider because some have side or adverse effects or interactions with other drugs.
- Doing Kegel exercises to increase muscle tone around the vagina and urinary meatus and counteract the effects of genital atrophy.
- Drinking at least eight glasses of water a day to decrease the concentration of urine, to flush urine from the bladder, and to reduce bacterial growth, thereby preventing atrophic cystitis.
- Wiping from front to back after urination and defecation to reduce the transfer of bacteria from the anus to the urinary meatus and to help prevent cystitis.

Osteoporosis

Osteoporosis is one of the greatest hazards of the postmenopausal years, yet bone loss begins well before menopause in most women. It is characterized by reduced bone density, leaving the bones porous, fragile, and susceptible to fractures. The vertebrae and hips are the most common sites of fractures, with wrists, forearms, feet, and toes also having fractures from osteoporosis. In the United States, 1.5 million osteoporosis-related fractures occur yearly, with women having the highest risk. More osteoporosis-related fractures are expected as the age of the U.S. population rises (Bennett, 2003; Schenken, 2003).

Predisposing Factors

The combination of peak bone density and the rate of bone loss influences the severity of osteoporosis. Small-boned, fair-skinned white women of northern European extraction and Asian women are at greatest risk for osteoporosis, but African-American and Hispanic women are also at risk. Other risk factors may include a family history of the disease, late menarche, early menopause, and a sedentary lifestyle. Women who smoke, drink alcohol, or consume excessive amounts of caffeine also have an increased risk for osteoporosis. Drug intake such as corticosteroids, some anticonvulsants, heparin, lithium, or aluminum antacids may also reduce bone density. Inadequate lifetime intake of calcium or vitamin D is a risk factor because reaching one's peak bone mass near age 30 does not occur Bennett, 2003; Cedars & Evans, 2003; Evans & Dumesic, 2000).

Manifestations

Osteoporosis has been called the "silent thief" because it takes place gradually throughout the course of many years without symptoms. The first noticeable signs are loss of height and back pain that occurs when the vertebrae collapse. Later signs include the "dowager's hump," which occurs when the vertebrae can no longer support the upper body in an upright position. Secondary to this, the waistline disappears and the abdomen protrudes because the rib cage moves closer to the pelvis. Depending on the number of fractures, several inches of height may be lost. Figure 31-4 illustrates progressive changes in posture associated with osteoporosis.

Diagnosis of osteoporosis depends on history and physical examination. Bone mineral analysis may be performed if results will influence the decision to use hormone replacement therapy. Conventional radiography is of little help because more than 30% of the bone mass must be lost before changes are apparent. Dual-energy x-ray absorptiometry (DEXA) is a highly accurate, fast method of diagnosis that involves low exposure to radiation.

Prevention and Therapeutic Management

The major goal of treatment is to prevent or slow osteoporosis and to stabilize remaining bone mass. Although research has upheld estrogen therapy to reduce osteoporosis by inhibition of bone resorption, fewer women are choosing the hormone because of its potential adverse effects.

Drug Therapy. Other drug categories to reduce osteoporosis include:

- Calcitonin (Calcimar, Miacalcin), a synthetic thyroid hormone usually prescribed as a daily nasal spray.
- Biophosphonates, which inhibit osteoclasts, reducing bone turnover. Alendronate (Fosamax) has been evaluated extensively, showing significant reduction of osteoporosis-related fractures. Risedronate (Actonel) is a newer drug with similar effects. Alendronate and risedronate may be prescribed in daily or weekly doses. Biophosphonates may be contraindicated for women with ulcers or an inflammatory gastrointestinal disease such as dysphagia or esophagitis.
- Raloxifene (Evista), a selective estrogen receptor modulator, or SERM, that binds to estrogen receptors to reduce bone loss. Because of the combined estrogen agonist and

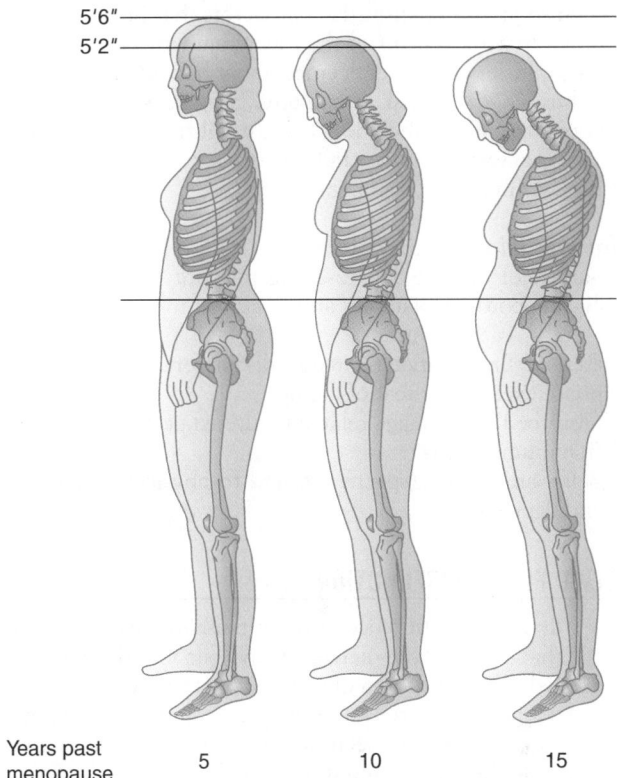

5'6"
5'2"

Years past menopause   5   10   15

Figure 31-4 With progression of osteoporosis, the vertebral column collapses, causing loss of height and back pain. *Dowager's hump* is the term used for this curvature of the upper back.

estrogen antagonist effects of SERMs, raloxifene is being studied to see if its effects also improve cardiac health without raising breast or uterine cancer risks.

Calcium and Vitamin D. Although calcium does not prevent bone loss, other therapies cannot be effective if calcium is deficient. A woman older than 50 years needs 1200 mg of calcium daily, and the woman 65 years or older needs 1500 mg/day. Daily calcium supplements are recommended because it is difficult to ingest these quantities through food intake only. Vitamin D is necessary for calcium to be absorbed from the intestine. Supplemental vitamin D, 400 to 800 units, is recommended for many women (Cedars & Evans, 2003; Curry & Hogstel, 2002).

Exercise. Weight-bearing and resistance exercises have been shown to increase bone density and build muscle mass in women. Walking, hiking, stair climbing, and dancing are examples of weight-bearing exercises. Use of free weights or weight machines build muscle mass and increase bone strength. High-impact exercises should be avoided if fragile vertebrae exist. At least 30 minutes of therapeutic exercise is needed. Other exercises, such as swimming or water-based exercises, often improve cardiovascular and respiratory fitness while managing weight, although their primary use is not to limit bone loss.

Nursing Considerations

Nurses often counsel women about lifestyle factors that contribute to bone loss, such as cigarette smoking, excessive alcohol or caffeine intake, and the importance of following the recommended medical regimen. Adolescents and young women should be counseled about factors that impair as well as promote achievement of their ideal amount of peak bone density. Nurses are also concerned about how to prevent falls and thus reduce the risk of fractures. Suggestions to increase safety in the home include adequate lighting and avoiding objects that might increase falls, such as loose electrical cords or rugs with nonskid backing.

Nursing Diagnoses

A variety of nursing diagnoses are relevant for the woman with osteoporosis. Examples are:

- Activity Intolerance related to discomfort, lack of appropriate exercise, or fear of falling
- Disturbed Body Image related to altered posture and functional limitations
- Self-Care Deficit (specify) related to physical limitations and depression

PELVIC FLOOR DYSFUNCTION

Pelvic floor dysfunction occurs when muscles, ligaments, and fascia that support the pelvic organs become damaged or weakened. This relaxation of pelvic support allows the pelvic organs to prolapse into, and sometimes out of, the vagina. Pelvic disorders usually occur in the perimenopausal period and may be the delayed result of traumatic childbirth.

Vaginal Wall Prolapse

The vagina may prolapse at either the anterior or posterior wall. Anterior wall prolapse involves the bladder and urethra and is called *cystocele*. Prolapse of the posterior wall produces *enterocele* or *rectocele*. A woman may have both anterior and posterior vaginal wall prolapse.

Cystocele

When the weakened upper anterior wall of the vagina is no longer able to support the weight of urine in the bladder, cystocele develops (Fig. 31-5, A). The bladder protrudes downward into the vagina, resulting in incomplete emptying of the bladder and consequent cystitis. Urethral displacement may occur when the urethra bulges into the lower anterior vaginal wall, producing stress incontinence. Stress incontinence is the loss of urine that occurs with a sudden increase in intraabdominal pressure from sneezing, coughing, lifting, or other sudden, jarring motions.

Enterocele

Enterocele refers to prolapse of the upper posterior vaginal wall between the vagina and rectum. This condition is almost always associated with herniation of the pouch of Douglas (a fold of peritoneum that dips down between the rectum and the uterus) and may contain loops of bowel (Fig. 31-5, B). Enterocele often accompanies uterine prolapse.

Rectocele

Rectocele occurs when the posterior wall of the vagina becomes weakened and thin. When the woman strains at defecation, feces are pushed against the thin wall, causing further stretching, until finally the rectum protrudes into the vagina (Fig. 31-5, C). Many rectoceles are small and produce few symptoms. If the rectocele is large, the woman may have difficulty emptying the rectum. Some women facilitate bowel elimination by applying digital pressure on the posterior vaginal wall to keep the rectocele from protruding during a bowel movement.

Uterine Prolapse

Uterine prolapse occurs when the cardinal ligaments, which support the uterus and vagina, are stretched during pregnancy and do not return to normal after childbirth. As the ligaments stretch, the uterus may sag backward and downward into the vagina. Figure 31-6 illustrates three levels of uterine prolapse, from first degree, in which the uterus remains in the vagina, to third degree, in which the cervix protrudes through from the vagina. Detailed staging, from stage 0 through stage IV, provides details about the amount and direction of vaginal wall shape alterations and the descent in specific areas of the vagina (DeLancey & Strohbehn, 2003).

Manifestations

Symptoms usually become obvious during the menopausal period, when decreased estrogen causes atrophic changes in the supporting structures. Symptoms include feelings of pelvic fullness, a dragging sensation, pelvic pressure, and fatigue. Low backache and a feeling that "everything is falling out" are sometimes described.

Symptoms relate to the affected area and the level at which support has decreased. For instance, urinary frequency, urgency, and incontinence often occur in women with cystocele because the support of their urethra and lower vaginal wall has decreased. Constipation, flatulence, and difficulty defecating are major symptoms of rectocele. Regardless of the structures involved, symptoms become worse after prolonged standing and are relieved by lying down. Symptoms of uterine prolapse are produced by the weight of the descending structures and may include pelvic pressure, backache, and fatigue. Cervical ulceration and bleeding occur if the cervix protrudes from the vaginal introitus. Some women fear their symptoms are caused by cancer in the affected structures.

Therapeutic Management

Treatment of disorders related to pelvic floor dysfunction depends on the woman's age, physical condition, sexual activity, and degree of prolapse. Surgical procedures provide the most satisfactory therapy for women who have significant discomfort. The most common procedures are the anterior and posterior colporrhaphy. The anterior colporrhaphy, performed for a cystocele, involves suturing the pubocervical fascia to support the bladder and urethra. For a rectocele, a posterior colporrhaphy (suturing the fascia and perineal muscles that support the perineum and rectum) is performed.

Surgical treatment for prolapse of the uterus is individualized to best correct both the degree and location of uterine prolapse. An anterior and posterior colporrhaphy may be effective for a first-degree prolapse. Treatment for more severe prolapse may include vaginal hysterectomy, in which the uterus is removed through the vaginal canal rather than through an abdominal incision. Vaginal hysterectomy may be combined with anterior and posterior colporrhaphy to improve vaginal support for the bladder or rectum.

Cystocele

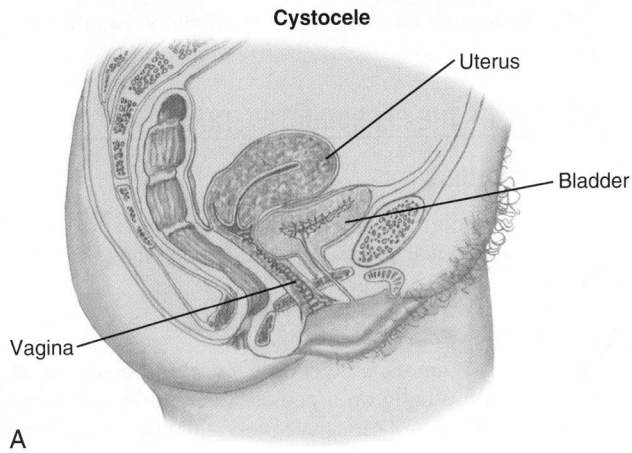

A

Enterocele

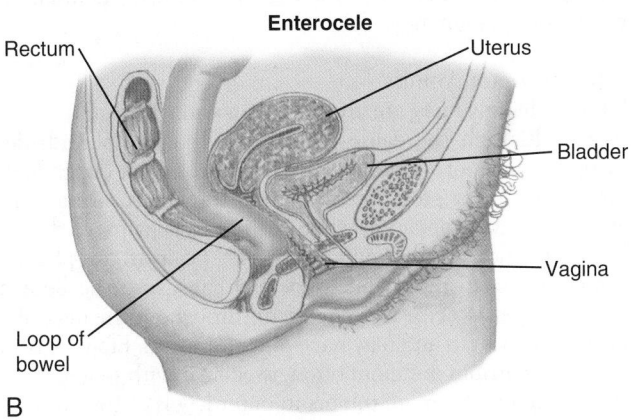

B

Rectocele

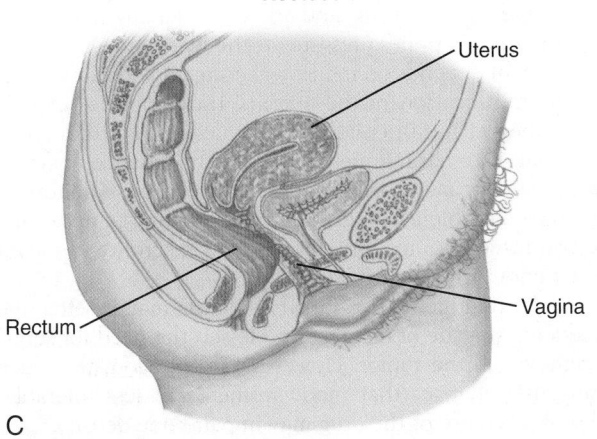

C

Figure 31-5 Three types of vaginal wall prolapse. **A,** Note bulging of bladder into the vagina. **B,** Note loop of bowel between rectum and uterus. **C,** Note bulging of rectum into vagina. More than one type of vaginal wall prolapse may exist in the same woman.

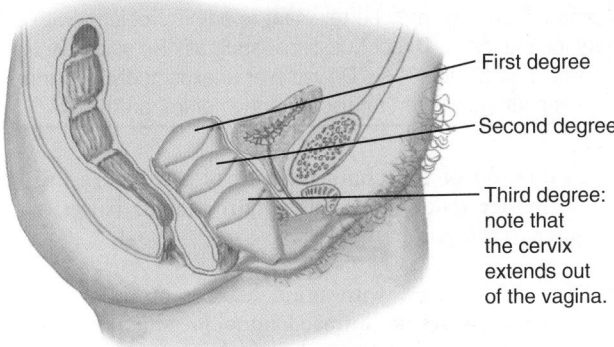

Figure 31-6 Three degrees of uterine prolapse.

or infection. Teaching the woman to insert the pessary and remove it nightly reduces discharge. Topical or systemic estrogen treatment may be indicated for the woman (DeLancey & Strohbehn, 2003).

Nursing Considerations
Pelvic Exercises. Kegel exercises strengthen the pubococcygeus muscle, which surrounds the urethra, vagina, and rectum and provides support for the pelvic floor. Before teaching Kegel exercises, the nurse should ask the woman to try to contract the pubococcygeus muscle while urinating. If she can stop the stream of urine, she is able to perform the exercise. After verifying that the woman can perform Kegel exercises, the nurse should teach her to perform them as recommended but not while urinating.

Kegel exercises involve conscious contracting and relaxing of the pelvic muscles. Only the pelvic muscles should be used; the abdomen, thighs, and buttocks should *not* tighten. Women should be taught to exhale and keep the mouth open to avoid bearing down when contracting the pelvic muscles for at least 3 seconds, building to a maximum hold of 10 seconds, and then gradually relaxing the muscle contraction. A minimum of 10 seconds of muscle relaxation should follow the pelvic muscle contractions. Variations exist about how frequently to repeat pelvic muscle contractions each day, but from 24 to 45 daily repetitions are beneficial. To maintain pelvic muscle tone, the woman should continue Kegel exercises for the rest of her life (Newman, 2003b; Sampselle, 2003).

Graduated weight cones may be used as an adjunct to pelvic muscle exercise. Incrementally weighted cones are inserted into the vagina, and the woman attempts to hold the weights in place. As the weight of the cones increases, the resistance against which the pelvic muscles contract increases, thereby strengthening the pelvic muscles (Wyman, 2003).

Measures that help reduce the symptoms of pelvic relaxation may also prove helpful. These include lying down with the legs elevated or assuming a knee-chest position for a short time several times a day. Additional teaching includes measures to prevent constipation.

Urinary Incontinence. Nurses must acknowledge the reluctance many women feel about discussing incontinence and help them overcome these feelings and seek medical intervention.

If surgery is contraindicated, a pessary (a device to support pelvic structures) may be inserted into the vagina. The pessary must be inspected and changed frequently by a physician or nurse practitioner to prevent vaginal discharge, ulceration,

Women of any age may be reluctant to admit problems with urinary incontinence. Direct questions, such as "Do you have trouble with your bladder?" or "Do you ever unexpectedly lose urine?" may encourage women to discuss urine control problems.

Evaluation of the characteristics of a woman's urinary incontinence guides treatment. Three major patterns are (Fenner, 2003; Sampselle, 2003):

- *Stress incontinence*, with urine leakage occurring as the woman increases her intraabdominal pressure. Examples of times when intraabdominal pressure may increase sufficiently include coughing, sneezing, laughing, or physical exertion such as picking up a full shopping bag or heavier load.
- *Urge incontinence*, characterized by urine leakage that accompanies a woman's strong need to void promptly.
- *Mixed incontinence*, in which a woman's urine leakage has associated factors from both the stress and urge incontinence patterns.

Overactive bladder (OAB) may occur with both urge and mixed incontinence. OAB is characterized by frequent sensations of urgency and nocturia and may accompany neurologic, anatomic, or structural disorders.

Several evaluation processes may be done to best evaluate the type of urinary incontinence and choose the best corrective actions. In addition to physical examination, the woman may be asked to keep a daily record of her urinary pattern and sensations. Additional tests may include those that identify leakage patterns and specialized testing of urinary tract functions.

Continence may be enhanced by teaching health promotion activities, such as Kegel exercises and bladder training. Kegel exercises are designed to improve the strength of the pelvic floor as described earlier and also to help the woman intentionally contract pelvic muscles to control urine leaking. Bladder training helps the woman decrease the frequency of urination during waking and sleeping hours (Sampselle, 2003). Women may benefit from biofeedback, electrical stimulation, or physical therapy. Surgery may be necessary to reposition or stabilize the bladder neck and proximal urethra.

Women often benefit from knowing about some of the commercial products that protect the skin and prevent odor. These products are made of material that traps urine and prevents constant contact with the skin.

Women often restrict fluids, believing that this will decrease urinary incontinence. Restricting fluids may actually make the condition worse because the bladder does not fill to its normal capacity. Furthermore, decreased fluid intake can lead to highly concentrated urine that can irritate bladder mucous membranes and increase the urge to void. Alcohol and caffeine can also irritate the bladder and worsen incontinence. Obesity is associated with urinary incontinence, increasing the benefits for a woman to achieve her ideal weight range.

Drug treatment may enhance bladder control. Drugs that may be prescribed include (Newman, 2003a):

- Vaginal estrogen using a cream, tablet, or vaginal ring to reduce atrophy of the urinary and vaginal areas
- Anticholinergic drugs, including their long-acting versions, such as oxybutynin or tolterodine.

Other drugs are being studied for possible use in improving bladder control.

DISORDERS OF THE REPRODUCTIVE TRACT

Benign Disorders

The most common benign conditions of the reproductive tract include cervical polyps, uterine leiomyomas (fibroids), and ovarian cysts.

Cervical Polyps

Polyps are small tumors, usually only a few millimeters in diameter, that are usually on a pedicle (a stemlike structure). They are caused by proliferation of cervical mucosa, and they often cause intermittent vaginal bleeding.

Cervical polyps are surgically removed in an outpatient setting, and the specimen is sent for pathologic examination to rule out malignancy.

Uterine Leiomyomas

Uterine leiomyomas are the most common gynecologic tumors. Although the cause is unknown, uterine fibroids develop from smooth muscle cells and are estrogen dependent. As a result, they grow rapidly during the childbearing years and may be very apparent when the uterus is palpated during late pregnancy. During menopause they begin to atrophy, although estrogen replacement therapy can cause the benign tumors to persist. Fibroids may occur throughout the muscular layer of the uterus and may have different forms. Fibroids near the endometrium are more often associated with heavy menstrual bleeding than are tumors in outer levels of the uterus.

Uterine fibroids usually produce no symptoms, but increased uterine size, pelvic pain, and excessive menstrual bleeding may occur. Excessive bleeding may result in anemia, weakness, and fatigue. Additional symptoms include feelings of pelvic pressure, bloating, and urinary frequency that occurs when the tumor applies pressure on the bladder.

Treatment depends on multiple factors, including the size, number, and location of the fibroids, the symptoms experienced, whether future childbearing is desired, and how near the woman is to natural menopause. In the absence of symptoms, treatment may consist of observation only. If abnormal bleeding is a problem, surgical intervention may be necessary. The two most common surgeries are myomectomy (removal of the tumor only) and hysterectomy.

Medical treatment with GnRH agonists may be effective in reducing the size of myomas and lessen the need for surgical removal of the tumor. However GnRH agonists induce menopausal changes that many women find less tolerable, and prolonged use of the drug may impair bone density.

Ovarian Cysts

An ovarian cyst may be either follicular or luteal. If the ovarian follicle fails to rupture during ovulation, a follicular cyst may develop. These cysts are usually asymptomatic, and they usually regress during the subsequent menstrual cycle. A lutein cyst may develop if the corpus luteum becomes cystic and fails to regress. A lutein cyst is more likely to cause pain and some delay in the next menstrual cycle. Occasionally, an ovarian cyst can rupture or twist on its pedicle and become infarcted, causing pelvic pain and tenderness.

! CRITICAL TO REMEMBER

Symptoms That Must Always Be Investigated

- Irregular vaginal bleeding
- Unexplained postmenopausal bleeding
- Unusual vaginal discharge
- Dyspareunia
- Persistent vulvar or vaginal itching
- Elevated or discolored lesions of the vulva
- Persistent abdominal bloating or constipation
- Persistent anorexia or vomiting
- Blood in stools

BOX 31-4
Risk Factors for Cancer of the Reproductive Organs

UTERUS
African-Americans: higher risk for leiomyosarcoma
Obesity
Nulliparity
Middle-aged and elderly
Late menopause (>52 yr)
Diabetes mellitus
Breast, colon, or ovarian cancer
Estrogen replacement therapy

CERVIX
Human papilloma virus (HPV) infection
Sexual risks: young age at start of intercourse (<20 yr), multiple sexual partners, uncircumcised male partners
Many pregnancies
Obesity
Diet low in fruits and vegetables
Smoking
Lower socioeconomic status (may be related to infrequent gynecologic examinations)
History of sexually transmitted diseases, such as chlamydia or human immunodeficiency virus (HIV) infection

OVARIES
Menses started at <12 yr
No child or first child after 30 yr
Late menopause (>55 yr)
Infertility; infertility drugs
Family history of ovarian, breast, or colorectal cancer
Personal history of breast cancer

Treatment depends on differentiating a cyst from a solid ovarian tumor that may indicate cancer. If the woman is in her childbearing years, when the risk of ovarian cancer is less, the physician may wait until after the next menstrual cycle and examine the woman again. Transvaginal ultrasound examination is useful to determine if it is a fluid-filled cyst or a solid tumor. Laparoscopy or laparotomy may be performed to remove the cyst from the ovary for examination by a pathologist.

Malignant Disorders

The primary sites for cancer in the female reproductive organs are the cervix, uterus, and ovaries. Although cancer can occur at any age, the incidence increases with age. Risk factors associated with cancer of the reproductive area are summarized in Box 31-4.

Manifestations
Cancer of the reproductive organs may not be diagnosed until it is advanced because few symptoms are experienced in the early stages. When symptoms occur, they are often nonspecific and could be caused by other conditions. Cancer of the ovaries is particularly difficult to diagnose because the condition may remain "silent" until far advanced, when the chance of long-term survival is greatly reduced.

Diagnostic Evaluation
A variety of screening and diagnostic procedures are useful in early detection that improve long-term survival among women with reproductive cancer. Screening tests include periodic pelvic examinations, Pap tests, and ultrasonography. Serum tests for tumor markers such as CA-125 identify if ovarian or other cancers may have spread beyond their primary site. Genes linked to other cancers, such as BRCA1 or BRCA2 (see p. 772), may lead to more diagnostic procedures than if the higher genetic risk is not apparent. Diagnostic procedures include endometrial sampling and colposcopy, which can identify patterns of abnormality near the cervical os, where most cancers of the cervix develop.

Therapeutic Management
Treatment of cervical, endometrial, or ovarian cancer is based on the location and extent of the disease in the organs and the woman's desire to bear more children. The extent of surgical treatment for these cancers varies with the tumor's size, degree of malignancy, and spread beyond the primary site of the tumor. Chemotherapy and radiation oncology therapy supplement treatment for many invasive cancers. Drugs such as anastrozole (Arimidex) and exemestane (Aromasin), aromatase inhibitors, may reduce estrogen secretion that increases cancer growth in most breast and reproductive organs.

Cervical Cancer. A lesion of early cervical cancer is usually squamous intraepithelial lesion (SIL). Early treatment of cervical cancer may consist of cryosurgery, destruction of abnormal tissue by laser, loop electrosurgical excision procedure, or surgical conization of the cervix. Regular surveillance following cervical cancer therapy is recommended to identify recurrence, particularly in the woman who had a high-grade SIL, whose risk for repeated cervical cancer is greater.

Treatment for advanced cervical cancer usually consists of a total abdominal hysterectomy and bilateral salpingo-oophorectomy. Treatment may include adjuvant therapy with radiation or chemotherapy. Survival results are similar, but the woman retains ovarian function with a hysterectomy alone (Kohler & DiSaia, 2000).

Endometrial Cancer. Treatment for endometrial cancer is often complicated by the fact that women with the disease are often elderly, obese, and diabetic (Berchuck & Cirisano, 2000). The highest cure rate is with surgery (hysterectomy and salpingo-oophorectomy), but poor surgical candidates may be treated only with chemotherapy and/or radiation therapy.

Ovarian Cancer. Surgery, possibly involving removal of the healthy ovary as well as the ovary affected with cancer, is an essential part of therapy and may be curative for women in the earliest stages of ovarian cancer. Surgery for more advanced ovarian cancer improves diagnostic information, allows more accurate staging, and permits surgical reduction of the cancer. Chemotherapy is required after surgery for all but the very early cancers, and newer drugs have improved the 5-year survival rate to about 50% (Cass & Karlan, 2003).

INFECTIOUS DISORDERS OF THE REPRODUCTIVE TRACT

Candidiasis

Candidiasis, also known as *moniliasis* and *yeast infection*, is the most common form of vaginitis. The cause is believed to be related to a change in vaginal pH that allows accelerated growth of *Candida albicans*, a yeast-like fungus commonly found in the digestive tract and on the skin. Some conditions, such as pregnancy, diabetes mellitus, oral contraceptive use, and systemic antibiotic therapy, result in changes in vaginal pH and flora that favor accelerated growth of *C. albicans*. Though not considered a sexually transmitted disease, recurrent candidiasis in sexually active women may occur. A small number of male partners may have erythema and itching of their glans penis (balanitis).

The main symptoms for candidiasis are vaginal and perineal itching. Vulvar and vaginal tissues are inflamed, causing burning on urination. Vaginal discharge is white with a typical "cottage cheese" appearance. Diagnosis is made by identifying the spores of *C. albicans*.

Treatment may consist of nonprescription or prescription medications. Medications available without prescription include butoconazole, miconazole, clotrimazole, nystatin, terconazole, or tioconazole by vaginal application. The duration for most of the nonprescription medications for candidiasis ranges from 3 to 7 days, depending on the specific medication. Women should be advised to seek medical attention with the first infection or if the infection persists or recurs frequently. Oral fluconazole is a prescription medication for candidiasis. Recurrent yeast infections that resist treatment are associated with diabetes mellitus or HIV infection.

Sexually Transmitted Diseases

Sexually transmitted diseases are transmitted through sexual activity. For some diseases, such as gonorrhea and chlamydial infection, sexual activity is almost the only method of transmission. For other diseases, such as bacterial vaginosis, sexual activity may or may not be the mode of transmission. A woman may have more than one sexually transmitted disease at a time.

Incidence

Sexually transmitted diseases are epidemic today, with the highest incidence among adolescents and young adults. Because the vagina and microscopic tears in mucosa from in-

tercourse provide favorable conditions for infection, women are twice as likely as men to be infected by a sexually transmitted disease (Centers for Disease Control and Prevention [CDC], 2002).

Methods of contraception have a significant impact on the risk for sexually transmitted diseases. The best protection is the use of condoms. Barrier methods, such as the diaphragm and cervical cap, are less effective than the condom in preventing sexually transmitted diseases, but they provide some protection for the upper genital tract. Other methods may prevent pregnancy but do not prevent exposure to sexually transmitted diseases.

Major concerns include:

- The vulnerability of women to sexually transmitted diseases
- The resistance of some organisms to antibiotics
- The relationship between HIV infection and other sexually transmitted diseases
- Failure of asymptomatic people to seek treatment when their sexual partner is infected

See Chapter 26 for the impact of sexually transmitted diseases on pregnancy and the fetus.

Types of Sexually Transmitted Diseases

Trichomoniasis

Trichomoniasis is caused by *Trichomonas vaginalis*, a protozoon that thrives in an alkaline environment. The presenting symptoms include a purulent vaginal discharge that is thin or frothy, malodorous, and yellow-green or brownish gray in color. The pH of the discharge is usually greater than 4.5. Vulvar itching, edema, and redness may also be present. The diagnosis is made by identifying the organism in a wet mount preparation.

The treatment of choice is metronidazole (Flagyl, Protostat), 2 g in a single oral dose. Alcohol ingestion when taking metronidazole may result in a disulfiram-like (Antabuse) reaction. Women should be advised to avoid using alcohol during treatment with metronidazole and for 24 hours after treatment is complete.

Sexual partners should refrain from intercourse until a cure is established. Reinfection may result when the woman's partner is not treated. In particular, emphasize that all sexual partners should be treated and that condoms should be used with a new partner.

Bacterial Vaginosis

This infection, previously referred to as *nonspecific vaginitis*, is associated with organisms that replace normal lactobacilli with *Gardnerella vaginalis* or *Mycoplasma hominis* or with anaerobic bacteria, such as *Prevotella* or *Mobiluncus*. Causes of the bacterial proliferation are not known, although tissue trauma and vaginal intercourse have been identified as contributing factors. Multiple partners, douching, and lack of vaginal lactobacilli are associated with bacterial vaginosis.

Chief signs and symptoms are a thin, grayish white vaginal discharge that typically exudes a fishy odor. The diagnosis is made by preparing a saline wet mount and identifying characteristic clue cells (epithelial cells with numerous bacilli clinging to their surface).

Treatment for bacterial vaginosis is directed toward reestablishing the balance of flora in the vagina. Metronidazole has been shown to relieve symptoms and to improve vaginal flora. Clindamycin is an alternative treatment. The woman should refrain from sexual intercourse until cured, or her partner should use a condom. Treatment of her male partner has not been shown to be beneficial (CDC, 2002).

Chlamydial Infection

The incidence of infection by the gram-negative bacterium *Chlamydia trachomatis* is particularly high in the sexually active teen and young adult populations. Chlamydial infection is often asymptomatic in men and women, which makes diagnosis and control of the disease difficult. The woman exhibits symptoms similar to those of gonorrhea, such as a yellowish vaginal discharge and painful urination. Gonorrhea and chlamydial infections often coexist.

Untreated, chlamydial infection ascends from the cervix to involve the fallopian tubes, and it is one of the chief causes of tubal scarring that results in pelvic inflammatory disease (PID), infertility, or ectopic pregnancy. Treatment is usually directed to eradicate both chlamydia and gonorrhea, since the two often coexist. Treatment options include azithromycin (Zithromax), doxycycline (Vibramycin), ofloxacin (Floxin), levofloxacin (Levaquin), and erythromycin. Treatment of all sexual partners is essential to prevent recurrence. Use of condoms until a cure is established is essential as well.

Gonorrhea

Gonorrhea is an infection of the genitourinary tract that is caused by the gonococcus *Neisseria gonorrhoeae*. Gonorrhea is often asymptomatic in women, but symptoms that do occur may include purulent discharge, dysuria, and painful intercourse. Diagnosis is based on a positive culture for the gonococcus. Gonorrhea, as is chlamydia, is associated with PID, which increases the risk of tubal scarring and can result in infertility or ectopic pregnancy.

Dual treatment of gonorrhea and chlamydia infections is often routine. Additional drugs to those previously discussed for chlamydia with gonorrhea infections include cefixime (Suprax), ceftriaxone (Rocephin), and ciprofloxacin (Cipro). All sexual partners should be treated simultaneously, and intercourse should be avoided or the man should use a condom until a cure is confirmed.

Syphilis

Syphilis is caused by the spirochete *Treponema pallidum*, and it is divided into primary, secondary, and tertiary stages. The first sign of primary syphilis is a painless chancre that develops on the genitalia, anus, or lips or in the oral cavity. At this time, diagnosis is made by identifying the spirochete on dark-field microscopy in material scraped from the base of the chancre. A serologic test is generally negative in the primary stage. If untreated, the chancre heals in about 6 weeks. The disease is highly infectious at the primary stage.

Although the chancre disappears, the spirochete lives and is carried by the blood to all parts of the body. About 2 months after the initial infection, infected people exhibit symptoms of secondary syphilis, including enlargement of the spleen and liver, headache, anorexia, and a generalized maculopapular skin rash. Skin eruptions, called *condylomata lata*, may develop on the vulva during this time. Condylomata lata resemble warts; they contain numerous spirochetes and are highly contagious. Serologic tests are generally positive at this time.

If untreated, the disease enters a latent phase that may last for several years. Tertiary syphilis, which follows the latent phase, may involve the heart, blood vessels, and central nervous system. General paralysis and psychosis may result.

In addition to identification of the spirochete in material scraped from a chancre, diagnosis is also made by serology. The usual screening test is the Venereal Disease Research Laboratory (VDRL) serum test, which is based on the presence of antibodies produced in response to the infection. The rapid plasma reagin (RPR) and fluorescent treponemal antibody absorption (FTA-ABS) tests are more specific and are commonly performed to confirm a positive VDRL.

The best treatment of all stages of syphilis is with penicillin. Ceftriaxone and doxycycline are second options for women who cannot take penicillin. Tetracycline may be given to some women if they are not pregnant. A woman who is allergic to penicillin can be admitted to the hospital for desensitization to penicillin and followed by administration of the drug.

Herpes Genitalis

Herpes genitalis is a sexually transmitted disease caused by the herpes simplex virus (HSV). Two types of HSV have been identified: type 1 and type 2. HSV 2 usually causes genital lesions and HSV 1 usually causes oral-pharyngeal infection. However, either organism may infect the less-frequent location. Transmission occurs through direct contact with an infected person and the partner often is not yet aware of having an HSV infection. Diagnostic tests to detect either HSV antigen are most accurate before HSV lesions begin healing. Some diagnostics distinguish between HSV 1 and HSV 2, whereas others are less specific.

Within 2 to 12 days after the primary infection, vesicles (blisters) appear in a characteristic cluster on the vulva, perineum, or perianal area. The lesions of the primary infection may cause severe vulvar pain and tenderness as well as dyspareunia. Lesions may also occur on the cervix or in the vagina. With primary infection, the woman may also experience flu-like symptoms, including fever, general malaise, and enlarged lymph nodes. The vesicles rupture within 1 to 7 days and form ulcers that take an average of 7 to 10 days to heal.

When symptoms abate, the virus remains dormant in the nerve ganglia and periodically reactivates, particularly in times of stress, fever, and menses. Recurrent episodes are seldom as extensive or painful as the initial episode but they are just as contagious. Diagnosis is often based on clinical signs and symptoms and confirmed by viral culture of fluid from the vesicle. No cure exists, but the antiviral drugs acyclovir, famciclovir, and valacyclovir help reduce or suppress symptoms, shedding, and recurrent episodes. Women should be advised to abstain from sexual contact while the lesions are present. If it is an initial infection, they should continue to abstain until they become culture-negative, because prolonged viral shedding may occur in such cases.

Condylomata Acuminata

Condylomata acuminata, also known as *venereal* or *genital warts*, are caused by human papilloma virus, or HPV. The dry, wartlike growths may be small, discrete, and asymptomatic, or they may cluster and resemble cauliflower. Common sites include the vagina, labia, cervix, and perineal area.

Condylomata acuminata are of particular concern because of the association of HPV with some degrees of cervical cancer. Colposcopy, examination by a magnifying instrument called the *colposcope*, is generally recommended to evaluate abnormal cervical tissue and to identify HPV. Women with HPV are advised to have Pap tests more frequently to detect cervical dysplasia.

The goal of treatment is to remove the warts, which easily transmit the virus back and forth between sexual partners. Treatment is determined by the site and extent of the warts and the woman's preference. Treatment options that involve application of medication directly to the warts include podophyllin solution or gel, imiquimod cream, trichloroacetic acid (TCA), and bichloroacetic acid (BCA). More extensive warts or those that do not respond to topical therapy may require removal by cryotherapy, electrodessication, electrocautery, or laser. Interferon, an antineoplastic drug, is sometimes used to treat condylomata acuminata in women older than 18 years who have not responded to conventional therapy.

The woman must understand that none of these treatments eradicate the virus and that she may have recurrences. Furthermore, all sexual partners must be treated. Sexual contact should be avoided until all lesions are healed, and the use of condoms is recommended to reduce transmission.

Acquired Immunodeficiency Syndrome

Acquired immunodeficiency syndrome (AIDS), caused by HIV, remains the most devastating sexually transmitted disease in the world today, although new treatments have improved the outlook considerably. Human immunodeficiency virus has been isolated from blood, semen, vaginal secretions, urine, saliva, tears, cerebrospinal fluid, amniotic fluid, and breast milk. The primary modes of transmission are intimate contact with infected bodily secretions, exposure to infected blood and blood products, and perinatal transmission from mother to infant.

HIV testing is offered to all pregnant women and to high-risk groups such as those who are poor or who use injectable drugs. However, a woman's risk for infection through a heterosexual relationship has surpassed the risk that her HIV infection stems from injectable drug use. Diagnosis of another sexually transmitted disease is an indication to offer HIV testing, as is the client who has infections such as herpesvirus or repeated candidiasis, which were previously discussed (CDC, 2002; Minkoff & Gibbs, 2003).

No medications have been shown to cure HIV and AIDS. Research continues about the benefits and safety of drug regimens that interrupt production of the virus. Zidovudine (a reverse transcriptase inhibitor) is a familiar drug having substantial safety for the fetus during pregnancy. However, combined drug therapy often benefits the HIV-infected woman and may have acceptable safety for her fetus. Protease inhibitors, such as indinavir or saquinavir, block the enzyme crucial to one step in the reproductive cycle of HIV. See Chapters 26 and 30 for a discussion of HIV and AIDS management in pregnant women and neonates. Updated guidelines for HIV and AIDS treatment in the pediatric, adult, and perinatal groups may be found at the AIDS Info website, a service of the National Institutes of Health: http://aidsinfo.nih.gov/guidelines.

Nursing Considerations

In their role as teachers and counselors, nurses can play a major part in preventing the spread of sexually transmitted diseases as well as in treating specific infections. For best client care, nurses must:

- Teach the signs and symptoms that require medical attention
- Explain diagnostic or screening tests
- Reinforce information for effective treatment and prevention measures

Pelvic Inflammatory Disease

Pelvic inflammatory disease (PID), infection of the upper genital tract that may cause chronic pelvic pain, is a serious health problem in the United States. It is estimated that PID develops in 1 million women each year, and a large proportion of those have complications such as infertility and ectopic pregnancy. More than 150 women die annually from PID or its complications (STD Prevention, 2003/2004).

Etiology and Pathophysiology

The primary sources of infection are *C. trachomatis* and *N. gonorrhoeae*. These sexually transmitted organisms invade the endocervical canal and cause cervicitis. Bacteria ascend and infect the endometrium, fallopian tubes, and pelvic cavity. The chronic inflammatory response is responsible for extensive tubal scarring and peritubal adhesions, which interfere with conception and with transport of the fertilized ovum through the obstructed fallopian tubes. Cytomegalovirus (CMV) and a number of common vaginal organisms, such as *G. vaginalis*, may also be found in women with PID. Because the fallopian tubes are often infected, a woman's risks for ectopic pregnancy or infertility are increased.

Manifestations

Some women with PID are asymptomatic or have subtle, mild symptoms. Others experience pelvic pain, fever, purulent vaginal discharge, nausea, anorexia, and irregular vaginal bleeding. Findings during physical examination may include abdominal or adnexal tenderness and pain of the uterus and cervix when they are moved during bimanual examination (cervical motion tenderness). Laboratory evaluation may reveal a marked leukocytosis and increased sedimentation rate. A urinalysis is needed to rule out urinary tract infection. Cultures for *N. gonorrhoeae*, *C. trachomatis*, or other suspected infectious organism help diagnose and best treat PID.

Therapeutic Management

Women with serious infection, as manifested by fever, abdominal pain, and leukocytosis, may be admitted to a hospital. They are treated initially with intravenous combinations of antibiotics such as cefoxitin or cefotetan plus doxycycline,

WOMEN
Want to Know

About Sexually Transmitted Diseases

What are the most common symptoms of sexually transmitted diseases (STDs)?
- Unexpected, nonbloody vaginal discharge (increased amount, unusual color, or odor) or vaginal bleeding.
- Vulvar itching or swelling.
- Pelvic pain, including painful intercourse, painful urination, and abdominal tenderness.
- Skin eruptions or changes (rashes, ulcers, warts, blisters).
- Flu-like symptoms (fever, swollen or painful lymph glands, loss of appetite, nausea or vomiting).
- Presence of symptoms in a sexual partner, even though symptoms are absent in the woman.

What are common methods of diagnosis?
- Culture (vaginal discharge, cervix, lesions) to identify organism; often combined with sensitivity to determine best medication therapy.
- Blood test (serology) to determine if antibodies for specific diseases are present.
- VDRL, RPR, or FTA-ABS test for syphilis, test for human immunodeficiency virus (HIV).
- Genetic tests from blood samples, such as visualization of chromosomes, analysis to identify abnormal sequences in genes or abnormal levels of genes associated with a specific disorder.

How can STDs be prevented?
- Limit number of sexual partners.
- Establish monogamous relationship with uninfected partner.
- Use mechanical and chemical barriers such as a latex condom with every act of intercourse
- Remember that one episode of an STD offers no protection from future infection.
- Make sure partner is simultaneously treated to prevent reinfection.

What are the most important things to know about the treatment?
- The entire course of medication must be completed even if symptoms subside.
- Comply with follow-up care as the health care provider recommends.
- Sexual intercourse should be avoided until free of active infection.
- Partner must be examined, treated, and a follow-up evaluation performed before sexual intercourse is resumed.
- Side effects of medications, such as skin rashes, difficulty breathing, or headaches, should be reported.
- Not all STDs can be cured (herpes, AIDS, venereal warts), and treatment is aimed at slowing the disease and preventing complications.

Are there measures that provide comfort and prevent secondary infections?
- Keep the vulva clean but avoid strong soaps, creams, and ointments unless prescribed by health care provider.
- Keep the vulva dry. A hair dryer turned on low may help.
- Wear absorbent cotton underwear and avoid pantyhose and tight pants as much as possible.
- Take analgesics (e.g., ibuprofen or acetaminophen) as directed by health care provider.
- Cool or tepid sitz baths may provide relief from itching.
- Wipe vulva from front to back after urination or defecation and then carefully wash hands.

VDRL, Venereal Disease Research Laboratory; *RPR,* rapid plasma reagin; *FTA-ABS,* fluorescent treponemal antibody absorption; *AIDS,* acquired immunodeficiency syndrome.

---

or clindamycin plus gentamicin. Intravenous antibiotic treatment can usually be changed to oral treatment after 48 hours, and the total duration of antibiotic therapy should be 14 days. Surgery may be needed for women who have a pelvic abscess or other persistent problems. Outpatient treatment is appropriate for many women who are able to comply with the recommended regimen (CDC, 2002).

Nursing Considerations

Nurses can play an important role in preventing PID by teaching women how to prevent sexually transmitted diseases. Primary prevention involves avoiding exposure to these diseases or preventing acquisition of infection during exposure. Measures include limiting the number of sexual partners and avoiding intercourse with those who have had multiple partners. Barrier methods (such as latex condoms) used consistently and correctly during all sexual activity reduce some sexually transmitted diseases.

Secondary prevention for PID involves preventing a lower genital tract infection from ascending to the upper genital tract. Nurses should advise women to seek medical attention promptly after having unprotected sex with someone suspected of having a sexually transmitted disease and when unusual vaginal discharge or genital lesions are apparent. Additional measures include taking medication as prescribed and returning for follow-up evaluation. Periodic medical evaluations may be recommended for a woman who is asymptomatic yet engages in sexual activity that increases risk.

Toxic Shock Syndrome

Although toxic shock syndrome is rare, it is a potentially fatal condition caused by toxin-producing strains of *Staphylococcus aureus.* The toxin produced alters capillary permeability, which allows intravascular fluid to leak from the blood vessels, leading to hypovolemia, hypotension, and shock. The toxin also causes direct tissue damage to organs and precipitates serious defects in coagulation.

If toxin-producing strains of *S. aureus* inhabit the vagina, certain factors increase the risk that the toxin will gain entry into the bloodstream. These include the use of high-absorbency tampons during menstruation and barrier methods of contraception (cervical cap or diaphragm), both of which may trap and hold bacteria if left in place for a prolonged time. Persons having had nasal surgery or previous *S. aureus* wound infections also have a greater risk.

Symptoms of toxic shock syndrome include a sudden spiking fever and flu-like symptoms (headache, sore throat, vomiting, diarrhea), hypotension, a generalized rash resembling sunburn, and skin peeling from the palms of the hands and the soles of the feet 1 to 2 weeks after the onset of the illness.

Treatment consists of fluid replacement, administration of vasopressor drugs, and antimicrobial therapy. Corticosteroids may be used to treat skin changes.

Nursing Considerations

Nurses are often responsible for providing information that may help prevent toxic shock syndrome and should instruct women to do the following:

- For tampon use:
  —Wash the hands thoroughly to remove bacteria before inserting tampons.
  —Change tampons at least every 4 hours to prevent excessive bacterial growth on the tampon.
  —Do not use super-absorbent tampons at any time because they may be left in the vagina for a prolonged period, allowing bacteria to proliferate.
  —Use pads rather than tampons during hours of sleep, which usually exceed the 4-hour segments of tampon use.
- For diaphragm use:
  —Wash the hands thoroughly before inserting the diaphragm.
  —Do not use a diaphragm during menstrual periods.
  —Remove the diaphragm within the time recommended by the health care provider.

KEY CONCEPTS

- *Health maintenance* refers to examinations and screening procedures that allow early detection of specific conditions, such as breast or cervical cancer, and allow for prompt treatment that increases the chance of long-term survival.
- A major role of nurses is to explain screening procedures and to encourage women to have them on a regular basis. The most common screening procedures include breast self-examination, clinical breast examination, mammography, and often ultrasound examinations for breast cancer; vulvar self-examination to detect precancerous conditions or infections; pelvic examination to detect abnormalities of the uterus or ovaries; Pap test for cervical cancer; and screening for fecal occult blood.
- Disorders of the breast may be benign, such as fibrocystic changes that occur in relation to the menstrual cycle, or malignant. The discovery of any breast disorder creates anxiety in women, and nurses must be prepared to explain diagnostic procedures.
- Breast cancer develops in one in eight women in the United States. Besides gender, the greatest risk factors are advancing age and prior history of breast cancer. Additional factors may include family history of breast cancer, specific genetic abnormalities, and previous uterine, ovarian, or colon cancer.
- Management of breast cancer includes surgical removal of the tumor plus varying amounts of surrounding tissue and lymph nodes. Adjuvant therapy includes radiation, chemotherapy, and drugs such as hormonal

therapy or immunotherapy that block factors that promote growth of cancer cells.
- Breast reconstruction is an integral part of the surgical options related to breast cancer. Types of reconstruction methods include tissue expansion procedures, in which fluid-filled prostheses are placed, and tissue flap procedures, in which a variety of the woman's own tissue may be used to create a graft for a new breast. Some women may receive a combination of tissue expansion and tissue flap procedures for best reconstruction.
- Nursing care for women with cancer of the breast focuses on providing emotional support and accurate information.
- Menstrual cycle disorders include amenorrhea, abnormal uterine bleeding, cyclic pelvic pain, and PMS. Some of the disorders, such as PMS, respond to lifestyle alterations such as changes in diet, exercise habits, and stress management.
- Induced abortion may be performed by medical or surgical methods, and each method is associated with social and ethical conflicts.
- The *climacteric,* a period of time that precedes the final menstrual period that denotes menopause, is a combination of endocrine, somatic, and psychic changes that occur at the end of the reproductive cycle. A state of estrogen deficit accelerates during the climacteric and can result in bone loss (osteoporosis).
- Hormone replacement therapy may be prescribed to manage the symptoms of estrogen deficit, such as hot flashes and atrophic vaginitis, and to decrease osteoporosis. How-

ever, adverse effects of estrogen-progesterone therapy have been found to include a greater risk for cardiovascular disease as well as for breast and uterine cancers. For women who decline or should not take hormone replacement, including estrogen-only medications, alternative measures are needed to control the symptoms of menopause.
- Relaxation of pelvic support structures, often occurring because of childbirth trauma, becomes troublesome as the woman ages and her falling estrogen levels cause genital atrophy.
- Benign disorders of the reproductive tract include cervical polyps, uterine leiomyomas (fibroids), and ovarian cysts. Malignant disorders include cancer of the cervix, uterus, and ovaries.
- Although some infections of the reproductive tract are related to a change in the pH or the flora of the vagina, such as candidiasis, many are transmitted by sexual contact.
- Pelvic inflammatory disease is often a complication of sexually transmitted diseases, particularly chlamydial infection or gonorrhea. PID can result in infertility or ectopic pregnancy because the fallopian tubes become scarred by inflammation during the infection.
- Toxic shock syndrome is a life-threatening condition resulting from infection with toxin-producing strains of *S. aureus*. The infection is believed to be related to use of high-absorbency tampons, cervical caps, and diaphragms that trap and hold bacteria in nutrient-rich menstrual blood for an extended time.

REFERENCES and READINGS

Adams, K. (2002). Confronting cervical cancer: Screening is the key to stopping this killer. *AWHONN Lifelines, 6*(3), 216-222.

American Cancer Society. (2001). *Breast cancer facts & figures 2001-2002.* Retrieved Feb. 17, 2004, from www.cancer.org/docroot/home/index.asp.

American Cancer Society. (2003a). *Breast reconstruction after mastectomy.* Retrieved Feb. 19, 2004, from www.cancer.org/docroot/home/index.asp.

American Cancer Society. (2003b). *Detailed guide: Breast Cancer: What are the risk factors for breast cancer?* Retrieved Feb. 17, 2004, from www.cancer.org/docroot/home/index.asp.

American Cancer Society. (2003c). *How to perform a breast self exam.* Atlanta: Author. Retrieved Feb. 15, 2004, from www.cancer.org/docroot/home/index.asp.

American Cancer Society. (2003d). *Ovarian cancer.* Retrieved Feb. 23, 2004, from www.cancer.org/docroot/home/index.asp.

American Cancer Society. (2003e). *Updated cancer screening guidelines released: More advice for older women and women at increased risk.* Atlanta: Author. Retrieved Feb. 15, 2004, from www.cancer.org.docroot/home/index.asp.

American Cancer Society. (2003f). *Uterine sarcoma.* Retrieved Feb. 23, 2004, from www.cancer.org/docroot/home/index.asp.

American Cancer Society. (2004a). *ACS cancer detection guidelines.* Atlanta: Author. Retrieved Feb. 16, 2004, from www.cancer.org/docroot/home/index.asp.

American Cancer Society. (2004b). *Cervical cancer.* Retrieved Feb. 23, 2004, from http://documents.cancer.org/115.00/115.00.pdf.

American College of Obstetricians and Gynecologists (ACOG). (2000). *Premenstrual syndrome* (ACOG Practice Bulletin No. 15). Washington, DC: Author.

Association of Women's Health, Obstetric, and Neonatal Nurses. (2003). *Standards for professional nursing practice in the care of women and newborns* (6th ed.). Washington, DC: Author.

Baram, D.A. (2000). Premenstrual syndrome. In E.J. Quilligan & F.P. Zuspan (Eds.), *Current therapy in obstetrics and gynecology* (5th ed., pp. 139-143). Philadelphia: Saunders.

Berchuck, A., & Cirisano, F.D. (2000). Endometrial carcinoma. In E.J. Quilligan & F.P. Zuspan (Eds.), *Current therapy in obstetrics and gynecology* (5th ed., pp. 207-210). Philadelphia: Saunders.

Bennett, B. (2003). The lowdown on osteoporosis: What we know and what we don't. *The NIH Word on Health.* Retrieved Feb. 21, 2004, from www.nih.gov/news/WordonHealth/dec2003/osteo.htm.

Boyer, L.E., Williams, M., Callister, L.C., & Marshall, E.S. (2001). Hispanic women's perceptions regarding cervical cancer screening. *Journal of Obstetrics, Gynecologic, & Neonatal Nursing, 30*(2), 240-245.

Brucker, M.C., & Youngkin, E.Q. (2002). What's a woman to do? Exploring HRT questions raised by the Women's Health Initiative. *AWHONN Lifelines, 6*(5), 408-417.

Burns, M. (2003). Physical assessment. In E.T. Breslin & V.A. Lucas (Eds.), *Women's health nursing: Toward evidence-based practice* (pp. 301-342). Philadelphia: Saunders.

Cass, I., & Karlan, B.Y. (2003). Neoplasms of the ovary and fallopian tube. In J.R. Scott, R.S. Gibbs, B.Y. Karlan, & A.F. Haney (Eds.), *Danforth's obstetrics and gynecology* (9th ed., pp. 971-1006). Philadelphia: Lippincott Williams & Wilkins.

Cedars, M.I., & Evans, M. (2003). Menopause. In J.R. Scott, R.S. Gibbs, B.Y. Karlan, & A.F. Haney (Eds.), *Danforth's obstetrics and gynecology* (9th ed., pp. 721-737). Philadelphia: Lippincott Williams & Wilkins.

Centers for Disease Control and Prevention (CDC). (2002). Sexually transmitted diseases treatment guidelines 2002. *Morbidity and Mortality Weekly Reports, 51*(RR-6), 1-84. Retrieved Feb. 23, 2004, from www.cdc.gov/std/treatment/3-2002TG.htm.

Centers for Disease Control and Prevention, Division of Bacterial and Mycotic Diseases. (2003). Toxic shock syndrome. Retrieved Mar. 1, 2004, from www.cdc.gov/ncidod/dbmd/diseaseinfo/toxicshock_t.htm.

Cervical cancer screening: Testing can start later, occur less often under new ACOG recommendations. (Dec. 2003/Jan. 2004). *AWHONN Lifelines, 7*(6), 512-514.

Coombes, R.C., Hall, E., Gibson, L.J., et al. (2004). A randomized trial of exemestane after two to three years of tamoxifen therapy in postmenopausal women with primary breast cancer. *New England Journal of Medicine, 350*(11), 1081-1092.

Culver, S.M., & Martens, M.G. (2000). Pelvic inflammatory disease. In E.J. Quilligan & F.P. Zuspan (Eds.), *Current therapy in obstetrics and gynecology* (5th ed., pp. 125-131). Philadelphia: Saunders.

Cummings, S. (2001). Weighing the risks: Genetic counseling for hereditary breast and ovarian cancer. *AWHONN Lifelines, 5*(3), 42-47.

Curry, L.C., & Hogstel, M.O. (2002). Osteoporosis: Education and awareness can make a difference. *American Journal of Nursing, 102*(1), 26-32.

Dawood, M.Y. (2000). Dysmenorrhea. In E.J. Quilligan & F.P. Zuspan (Eds.), *Current therapy in obstetrics and gynecology* (5th ed., pp. 31-36). Philadelphia: Saunders.

DeLancey, J.O.L., & Strohbehn, K. (2003). Pelvic organ prolapse. In J.R. Scott, R.S. Gibbs, B.Y. Karlan, & A.F. Haney (Eds.), *Danforth's obstetrics and gynecology* (9th ed., pp. 791-817). Philadelphia: Lippincott Williams & Wilkins.

Eisenbach, D.A. (2003). Pelvic infections and sexually transmitted diseases. In J.R. Scott, R.S. Gibbs, B.Y. Karlan, & A.F. Haney (Eds.), *Danforth's obstetrics and gynecology* (9th ed., pp. 581-603). Philadelphia: Lippincott Williams & Wilkins.

Evans, M., & Dumesic, D.A. (2000). Menopause. In E.J. Quilligan & F.P. Zuspan (Eds.), *Current therapy in obstetrics & gynecology* (5th ed., pp. 108-113). Philadelphia: Saunders.

Faro, S. (2000). Sexually transmitted diseases. In E.J. Quilligan & F.P. Zuspan (Eds.), *Current therapy in obstetrics & gynecology* (5th ed., pp. 161-169). Philadelphia: Saunders.

Fenner, D.E. (2003). Incontinence. In J.R. Scott, R.S. Gibbs, B.Y. Karlan, & A.F. Haney (Eds.), *Danforth's obstetrics and gynecology* (9th ed., pp. 845-867). Philadelphia: Lippincott Williams & Wilkins.

Fontaine, K.L. (2000). *Healing practices: Alternative therapies for nursing.* Upper Saddle River, NJ: Prentice Hall.

Freid, V.M., Prager, K., MacKay, A.P., & Xia, H. (2003). *Health, United States, 2003.* Hyattsville, MD: National Center for Health Statistics.

Fritz, M.A. (2003). Amenorrhea. In J.R. Scott, R.S. Gibbs, B.Y. Karlan, & A.F. Haney (Eds.), *Danforth's obstetrics and gynecology* (9th ed., pp. 625-641). Philadelphia: Lippincott Williams & Wilkins.

Furniss, K. (2000). Tomatoes, Pap smears, and tea? Adopting behaviors that may prevent reproductive cancers and improve health. *Journal of Obstetric, Gynecologic, and Neonatal Nursing, 29*(6), 641-652.

Gemignani, M.L. (2003). Disorders of the breast. In J.R. Scott, R.S. Gibbs, B.Y. Karlan, & A.F. Haney (Eds.), *Danforth's obstetrics and gynecology* (9th ed., pp. 889-910). Philadelphia: Lippincott Williams & Wilkins.

Halcón, L.L., Lifson, A.R., Shew, M., Joseph, M., Hannan, P.J., & Hayman, C.R. (2002). Pap test results among low income youth: Prevalence of dysplasia and practice implications. *Journal of Obstetric, Gynecologic, & Neonatal Nursing, 31*(3), 2002.

Hindle, W.H. (2000). Mastalgia and fibrocystic changes of the breast. In E.J. Quilligan & F.P. Zuspan (Eds.), *Current therapy in obstetrics & gynecology* (5th ed., pp. 494-495). Philadelphia: Saunders.

Huebscher, R. (2003). Natural, alternative, and complementary health care. In E.T. Breslin & V.A. Lucas (Eds.), *Women's health nursing: Toward evidence-based practice* (pp. 97-132). Philadelphia: Saunders.

Huff, B.C. (2000). Screening for cervical cancer: It's time to check your Pap technique. *AWHONN Lifelines, 4*(3), 53-55.

Hurt, W.G. (2000). Urinary incontinence. In E.J. Quilligan & F.P. Zuspan (Eds.), *Current therapy in obstetrics and gynecology* (5th ed., pp. 176-180). Philadelphia: Saunders.

Jenkins, R.R. (2004). Menstrual problems. In R.E. Behrman, R.M. Kliegman, & H.B. Jenson (Eds.), *Nelson textbook of pediatrics* (17th ed., pp. 663-667). Philadelphia: Saunders.

Johnson, C.A. (2000). Amenorrhea. In B.E. Johnson, C.A. Johnson, J.L. Murray, & B.S. Apgar (Eds.), *Women's health care handbook* (2nd ed., pp. 115-117). Philadelphia: Hanley & Belfus.

Kanusky, C. (2003). Health concerns of women in midlife. In E.T. Breslin & V.A. Lucas (Eds.), *Women's health nursing: Toward evidence-based practice* (pp. 628-683). Philadelphia: Saunders.

Kiebeck, D., & Beller, F.K. (2000). Breast cancer: Principles of therapy. In E.J. Quilligan & F.P. Zuspan (Eds), *Current therapy in obstetrics & gynecology* (5th ed., pp. 456-461). Philadelphia: Saunders.

Kohler, M.F., & DiSaia, P.J. (2000). Cervical carcinoma. In E.J. Quilligan & F.P. Zuspan (Eds.), *Current therapy in obstetrics and gynecology* (5th ed., pp. 204-207). Philadelphia: Saunders.

Lemaire, G.S. (2004). More than just menstrual cramps: Symptoms and uncertainty among women with endometriosis. *Journal of Obstetric, Gynecologic, and Neonatal Nursing, 33*(1), 71-79.

London, S.N. (2003). Abnormal uterine bleeding. In J.R. Scott, R.S. Gibbs, B.Y. Karlan, & A.F. Haney (Eds.), *Danforth's obstetrics and gynecology*

REFERENCES and READINGS

(9th ed., pp. 643-651). Philadelphia: Lippincott Williams & Wilkins.

McCrink, A. (Dec. 2003/Jan. 2004). Evaluating the female pelvic floor: Understanding and treating prolapse, incontinence in women. *AWHONN Lifelines, 7*(6), 516-522.

McEvoy, M., Chang, J., & Coupey, S.M. (2004). Common menstrual disorders in adolescents. *MCN: The American Journal of Maternal/Child Nursing, 29*(1), 41-49.

McGovern, P.G., & Little, A.B. (2000). Dysfunctional uterine bleeding. In E.J. Quilligan & F.P. Zuspan (Eds.), *Current therapy in obstetrics and gynecology* (5th ed., pp. 27-31). Philadelphia: Saunders.

McKeon, V.A. (2002). Exploring HRT: Gauging the benefits, risks, and unknowns of hormone replacement therapy. *AWHONN Lifelines, 6*(1), 24-31.

Minkoff, H.L., & Gibbs, R.S. (2003). Obstetric and perinatal infections. In J.R. Scott, R.S. Gibbs, B.Y. Karlan, & A.F. Haney (Eds.), *Danforth's obstetrics and gynecology* (9th ed., pp. 339-364). Philadelphia: Lippincott Williams & Wilkins.

National Cancer Institute. (2004a). *Breast cancer (PDQ®) Treatment.* Retrieved Feb. 18, 2004, from www.cancer.gov/cancerinfo/pdq/treatment/breast/healthprofessional/.

National Cancer Institute. (2004b). *Final: Bethesda system 2001.* Retrieved Feb. 16, 2004, from http://bethesda 2001.cancer.gov.terminology.htm.

National Institutes of Health: National Heart, Lung, & Blood Institute. *Clinical guidelines on the identification, evaluation, and treatment of overweight and obesity in adults: Executive summary.* Retrieved Feb. 13, 2004, from www.nhlbi.nih.gov/guidelines/obesity/ob_xsum.htm.

Newman, D.K. (2003a). Pharmaceutical review: Drugs used to treat incontinence. *American Journal of Nursing, March*(Suppl.), 48.

Newman, D.K. (2003b). Stress urinary incontinence in women. *American Journal of Nursing, 103*(8), 46-55.

Newman, D.K., & Giovannini, D. (2002). The overactive bladder: A nursing perspective. *American Journal of Nursing, 102*(6), 36-45.

Nichols, D.H. (2000). Disorders of pelvic support. In E.J. Quilligan & F.P. Zuspan (Eds.), *Current therapy in obstetrics and gynecology* (5th ed., pp. 22-27). Philadelphia: Saunders.

Pritham, U.A. (2002). Managing PMS & PMDD: Exploring new treatment options. *AWHONN Lifelines, 6*(5), 430-437.

Reid, J. (2001). Women's knowledge of Pap smears, risk factors for cervical cancer, and cervical cancer. *Journal of Obstetric, Gynecologic, & Neonatal Nursing, 30*(3), 299-305.

Reid, R.I. (2003). Premenstrual syndrome. In J.R. Scott, R.S. Gibbs, B.Y. Karlan, & A.F. Haney (Eds.), *Danforth's obstetrics and gynecology* (9th ed., pp. 653-662). Philadelphia: Lippincott Williams & Wilkins.

Resnick, B., & Belcher, A.E. (2002). Breast reconstruction: Options, answers, and support for patients making a difficult personal decision. *American Journal of Nursing, 102*(4), 26-33.

Sampselle, C.M. (2003). Behavioral interventions in young and middle-aged women. *American Journal of Nursing, March*(Suppl.), 9-19.

Sandau, K.E. (2002). Free TRAM flap breast reconstruction. *American Journal of Nursing, 102*(4), 35-43.

Schenken, R.S. (2003). Endometriosis. In J.R. Scott, R.S. Gibbs, B.Y. Karlan, & A.F. Haney (Eds.), *Danforth's obstetrics and gynecology* (9th ed., pp. 713-720). Philadelphia: Lippincott Williams & Wilkins.

Sellers, J.B. (2003). Health care for older women. In E.T. Breslin & V.A. Lucas (Eds.), *Women's health nursing: Toward evidence-based practice* (pp. 684-760). Philadelphia: Saunders.

Sharp, B.A.C., Taylor, D.L., Thomas, K.K., Killeen, M.B., & Dawood, M.Y. (2002). Cyclic perimenstrual pain and discomfort: The scientific basis for practice. *Journal of Obstetric, Gynecologic, and Neonatal Nursing, 31*(6), 637-649.

Skillman-Hull, L. (2003). Adolescent women's health. In E.T. Breslin & V.A. Lucas (Eds.), *Women's health nursing: Toward evidence-based practice* (pp. 432-552). Philadelphia: Saunders.

Spencer, J.W., & Jacobs, J.J. (2003). *Complementary and alternative medicine: An evidence-based approach.* St. Louis: Mosby.

STD prevention: Pelvic inflammatory disease (PID). (Dec. 2003/Jan. 2004). Retrieved Feb. 24, 2004, from www.cdc.gov/std/PID/STDFact-PID.htm.

Surrey, E.S. (2000). Endometriosis and adenomyosis. In E.J. Quilligan & F.P. Zuspan (Eds.), *Current therapy in obstetrics and gynecology* (5th ed., pp. 44-47). Philadelphia: Saunders.

Taylor, D., & Hwang, A.C. (Dec. 2003/Jan. 2004). Mifepristone for medical abortion: Exploring a new option for nurse practitioners. *AWHONN Lifelines, 7*(5), 524-529.

Taylor, R.R., & Birrer, M.J. (2000). Ovarian cancer. In E.J. Quilligan & F.P. Zuspan (Eds.), *Current therapy in obstetrics and gynecology* (5th ed., pp. 217-220). Philadelphia: Saunders.

Teschendorf, M. (2003). Women during the reproductive years. In E.T. Breslin & V.A. Lucas (Eds.), *Women's health nursing: Toward evidence-based practice* (pp. 553-627). Philadelphia: Saunders.

Trupin, S.R. (2003). Induced abortion. In J.R. Scott, R.S. Gibbs, B.Y. Karlan, & A.F. Haney (Eds.), *Danforth's obstetrics and gynecology* (9th ed., pp. 561-580). Philadelphia: Lippincott Williams & Wilkins.

U.S. Cancer Statistics Working Group. (2003). *United States cancer statistics: 2000 incidence.* Atlanta, GA: Department of Health & Human Services, Centers for Disease Control & Prevention, and National Cancer Institute. Retrieved Feb. 17, 2004, from www.cdc.gov/cancer/npcr/uscs/pdf/USCS_Report_2000.pdf.

U.S. Food and Drug Administration. (2000). *FDA approves mifepristone for termination of pregnancy.* Retrieved Feb. 20, 2004, from www.fda.gov/fdac/features/2000/600_ru486.html.

U.S. Preventive Services Task Force. (2003). Screening for osteoporosis in postmenopausal women: Recommendations and rationale. *American Journal of Nursing, 103*(1), 73-75, 79.

Vail, B.A., & Peterson, M. (2000). Breast lumps. In B.E. Johnson, C.A. Johnson, J.L. Murray, & B.S. Apgar (Eds.), *Women's health care handbook* (2nd ed., pp. 320-324). Philadelphia: Hanley & Belfus.

Wilkinson, E.J. (2003). Benign vulvovaginal disorders. In J.R. Scott, R.S. Gibbs, B.Y. Karlan, & A.F. Haney (Eds.), *Danforth's obstetrics and gynecology* (9th ed., pp. 605-623). Philadelphia: Lippincott Williams & Wilkins.

Wyman, J.F. (2003). Treatment of urinary incontinence in men & women. *American Journal of Nursing, March*(Suppl.), 26-31.

Zimmerman, V.L. (2002). BRCA gene mutations and cancer: Preventive strategies benefit patients at risk. *American Journal of Nursing, 102*(8), 28-36.

32

Communicating with Children and Families

◆ **LEARNING OBJECTIVES**

After studying this chapter, you should be able to:

◎ Describe six components of effective communication with children.
◎ Describe communication strategies that assist nurses in working effectively with children.
◎ Explain the importance of avoiding communication pitfalls in working with children.

◎ Describe effective family-centered communication strategies.
◎ Describe effective strategies for communicating with children with special needs.

◆ **DEFINITIONS**

active listening Listening empathically to gain a better understanding of both the actual and the implied message.

empathy Seeing from another's perspective while remaining objective.

empowerment Provision of appropriate tools (education, information, support) to individuals that enable them to participate fully in decision making.

preparation Provision of information before procedures, treatments, or events; facilitates coping.

professional boundaries Limits separating professional from personal relationships; observed in work settings.

self-esteem Personal value that individuals place on themselves.

sensory information Information gained from sight, taste, touch, smell, and hearing.

win-win solution Solution to a problem, such as the resolution of a conflict, that both parties can support as a common goal.

To effectively work with children and their families, nurses must develop keen communication skills. Parents and other family members play a crucial role in the lives of pediatric clients. To identify mutual goals and facilitate positive outcomes, nurses need to establish rapport with the family. An awareness of body language, eye contact, and tone of voice must accompany good verbal communication skills when listening to children and their families. The same awareness helps nurses assess their own communication styles.

COMPONENTS OF EFFECTIVE COMMUNICATION

Communication is much more than words going from one person's mouth to another person's ears. In addition to the words themselves, the tone and quality of voice, eye contact, physical proximity, visual cues, and overall body language convey messages. In choosing communication techniques to be used with children and families, the nurse considers cultural differences, particularly in regard to touch and personal space (see Chapter 3).

Touch

Touch can be a positive, supportive technique that is effective from birth through adulthood. Touch can convey warmth, comfort, reassurance, security, trust, caring, and support.

In infancy, messages of love, security, and comfort are conveyed through holding, cuddling, gentle stroking, and patting. Infants do not have cognitive understanding of words they hear, but they sense the emotional support and they can feel, interpret, and respond to gentle, loving, supportive hands caring for them. Toddlers and preschoolers find it soothing and comforting to be held and rocked, as well as stroked gently on the head, back, arms, and legs (Fig. 32-1).

School-age children and adolescents appreciate giving and receiving hugs as well as getting a reassuring pat on the back or a gentle hand on their hand. The nurse, however, needs to request permission for any contact beyond a casual touch.

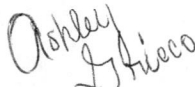

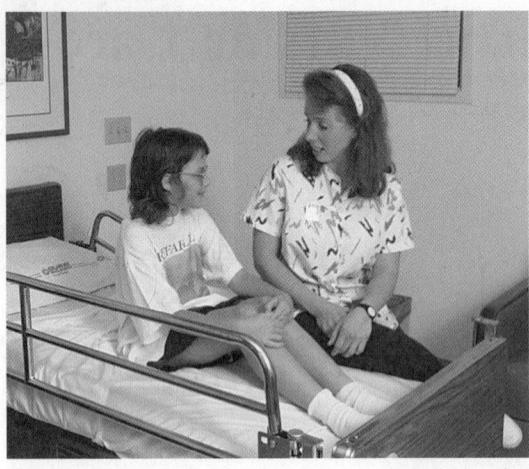

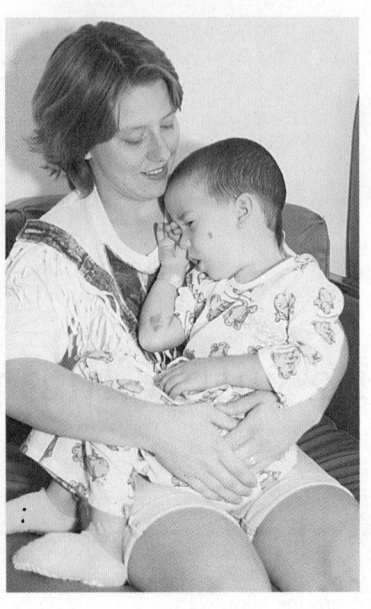

A child can communicate more easily with a nurse who is at eye level and at a comfortable conversational distance. The nurse may need to squat or even sit on the floor to talk with very young children.

Touch is a powerful means of communicating. Toddlers and preschoolers often find touch in the form of cuddling and stroking to be soothing. Even older children who prize their independence find that a parent's hug or pat on the back helps them feel more secure.

Figure 32-1 Communication with children is enhanced by direct eye contact and by body language that conveys attentiveness and openness.

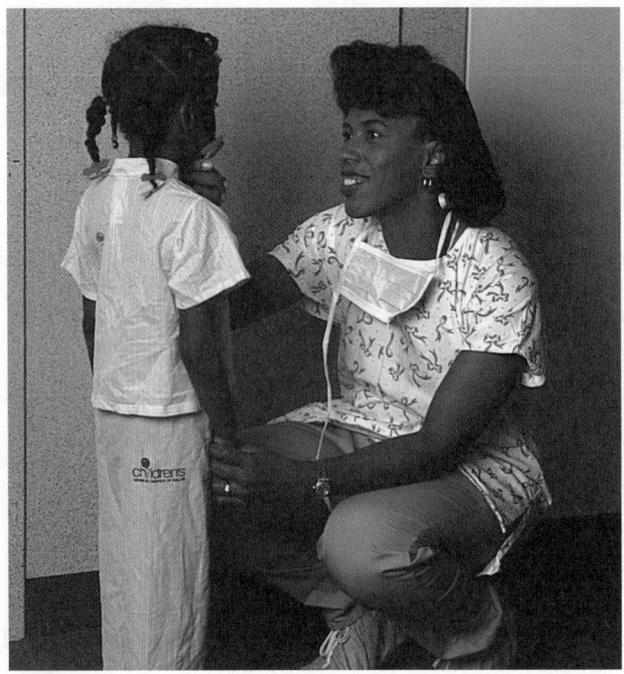

Figure 32-2 For effective communication, the nurse needs to be at the child's eye level.

Physical Proximity and Environment

Children's familiarity and comfort with their physical surroundings affect communication. Normally, children are most at ease in their home environments. Once they enter a clinic, emergency department, or patient care unit, they are in an unfamiliar environment and they experience heightened anxiety. Hospital and clinic staff members have a tremendous advantage in knowing their clinic or unit as a familiar workplace. Nurses can gain a better picture of what a child is experiencing by trying to place themselves in the child's position and imagining the child's first impression of the triage desk, the reception desk, the admitting office, the treatment room, and the hospital room. The child's perspective is probably very different from an adult's. Creating a supportive, inviting environment for children includes the use of child-size furniture, colorful banners and posters, developmentally appropriate toys, and art displayed at a child's eye level.

Individuals have different comfort zones for physical distance. The nurse should be aware of differences and move cautiously when meeting new children and families, respecting each individual's personal space. For example, standing over the child and family can be intimidating. Instead, the nurse should bring a chair and sit near the child and family. This action puts the nurse at eye level. If a chair is not accessible, the nurse may also stoop or squat. The important part is to be at eye level while remaining at a comfortable distance for the child and family (Fig. 32-2).

The nurse should not overlook privacy or underestimate its importance. A room should be available for conducting private conversations away from roommates or family members and visitors. Privacy is particularly critical when working with adolescents, who typically will not discuss sensitive topics with parents present. The nurse's skill and ease with parents of adolescents will increase the adolescents' trust in the nurse. Hallway conversations, particularly outside a child's room, should be avoided because children and parents may overhear only some words or phrases and misinterpret their meaning. Overhearing may lead to unnecessary stress and mistrust between the health care providers and the child or family.

Listening

Messages given must be received for communication to be complete. Therefore listening is an essential component of the communication process. By practicing active listening skills, nurses can be effective listeners. *Active listening* skills include the following.

• *Attentiveness*

The nurse should be intentional about giving the speaker undivided attention. Eliminating distractions is important, whenever possible. For example, the nurse should maintain eye contact, close the door, and eliminate potential distractions (e.g., TV, computer, video games).

• *Clarification Through Reflection*

Using similar words, the nurse should express back to the speaker what was heard and understood about the content of the message. For example, when the child or family member says, "I hate the food that comes on my tray," a reflective response would be, "You are unhappy with the food you've been given?"

• *Empathy*

The nurse should identify and acknowledge feelings expressed in the message. For example, if a child is crying after a procedure, the nurse might say, "I know it is uncomfortable to have this procedure. It is okay to cry. You did a great job holding still."

• *Impartiality*

To understand and avoid prejudicing what is heard with personal bias, the nurse should listen with an open mind. For example, if an adolescent expresses concern that she is having difficulty with relationships at school and that she feels disconnected socially because she is a lesbian, the nurse should remain a supportive listener. The nurse can then help her identify ways to connect with peers and interact with her as with all children, regardless of the nurse's personal values and beliefs.

Nurses must role model effective listening so children also learn listening skills. There are many ways in which thoughts and feelings are expressed by children to communicate their needs, opinions and wishes. The nature and form of these expressions will change significantly as children develop from infancy through childhood to adolescence (McPherson & Thorn, 2000). It is important to recognize individual growth and development attributes to enhance comprehension of your message.

To enhance the effectiveness of communication and maximize normal language patterns that contribute to language development, the nurse should focus on talking *with* children rather than *to* them and should develop conversations with children.

The nurse must be prepared to listen with the eyes as well as the ears. Information will not always be audible, so the

nurse must be alert to subtle cues in body language and physical closeness. Only then can one fully understand the messages of children. For example, when the nurse enters the room to complete an initial assessment of a 4-year-old child and observes the child turning away and beginning to suck her thumb, the child is communicating about her basic security and comfort level, even though she has not said a word.

Visual Communication

Eye contact is a communication connector. Making eye contact helps confirm attention and interest between the individuals communicating. Eye contact can be uncomfortable, however, for people in some cultures. For example, Asian-Americans believe that making eye contact is rude; some Latino cultures believe in the "evil eye" (Stein, 2000).

Clothing, physical appearance, and objects being held are visual communicators. Children may react to an individual's presence based on a white lab coat, a bushy beard, a syringe, or a video game in hand. The nurse needs to think ahead and anticipate visual stimuli a child may find startling as well as those that may be pleasing and make appropriate adjustments when possible. For example, it is a routine practice for nurses to bring a medication in a syringe for insertion into an intravenous (IV) line. Unless the purpose of the syringe is immediately explained, children might immediately assume they are about to receive an injection.

Some children, as well as some adults, are visual learners. They learn best when they can see or read instructions, demonstrations, diagrams, or information. Using various methods of presenting and sharing information will increase comprehension.

Concepts can be presented more vividly by using photographs, videotapes, dolls, computer programs, charts, or graphs than by using written or spoken words alone. The nurse needs to select teaching tools and materials that appropriately match the child's growth and developmental level.

Tone of Voice

The spoken word comes to mind most often when communication is the topic. Communication, however, consists of not only what is said but also the way it is said. The tone and quality of voice often communicate more than the words themselves.

Because infants' cognitive understanding of words is limited, their understanding is based on tone and quality of voice. A soft, smooth voice is more comforting and soothing to infants than a loud, startling, harsh voice. Infants can sense from the tone of voice whether their caregiver is angry or happy, frustrated or calm. The nurse can assess how aware of and sensitive to these messages infants are by observing their body language. Infants are relaxed when they hear a calm, happy caregiver and tense and rigid when they hear an angry, frustrated caregiver.

Children can detect anger, frustration, joy, and other feelings that voices convey, even when the accompanying words are incongruent. This incongruity can be very confusing for children. The nurse should strive to make words and their intended meanings match.

Verbal communication extends beyond actual words. All audible sounds convey meaning. An infant's primary mode of

---

> ### ! CRITICAL TO REMEMBER
>
> **Tips to Enhance Listening and Communication Skills**
>
> - Children understand better than they can talk.
> - To develop conversations with children, ask open-ended questions rather than questions requiring *yes* or *no* responses.
> - Comprehension is increased when the nurse uses different methods to present and share information.

TABLE 32-1 Open and Closed Body Postures	
Open	**Closed**
Leaning toward other person	Leaning away from other person
Arms loose at the sides	Arms folded across the chest
Frequent eye contact	No eye contact
Hands moving freely	Hands on hips
Soft stance, body swaying slightly	Rigid stance
Head up	Head bowed
Calm, slow movements	Constant motion, squirming
Smiling, friendly facial cues	Frowning, negative facial cues
Conversing at eye level	Conversing at diagonal eye level

⚠ CRITICAL TO REMEMBER

Communicating With Families

- Include all involved family members. One essential step toward achieving a family-centered care environment is to develop open lines of communication with the family.
- Encourage families to write down their questions.
- Remain nonjudgmental.
- Give families both verbal and nonverbal signals that send a message of availability and openness.
- Respect and encourage feedback from families.
- Families come in various shapes, sizes, colors, and generations.
- Avoid assumptions about core family beliefs and values.
- Respect family diversity.

audible communication is crying. Crying is a cue to check basic needs, including hunger, pain, discomfort (e.g., wet diaper), or temperature. Cooing and babbling, also heard during the first year of life, generally convey messages of comfort and contentment. As children develop and mature, they will have increasing vocabularies to verbally express their ideas, thoughts, and feelings.

The choice of words is critical in verbal communication. The nurse should avoid talking down to children but should not expect them to understand adult words and phrases. Technical health care terms should be used selectively, and jargon should be avoided (see Table 32-4).

Body Language

From the gentle caress of holding an infant to sitting and listening intently to an adolescent's story, body language is a factor in communication. An open body stance and positioning invite communication and interaction, whereas a closed body stance and positioning impede communication and interaction.

Using an open body posture improves the nurse's understanding of children and the children's understanding of the nurse. Nurses need to learn to read children's body language and should become more aware of their own body language. Table 32-1 compares open and closed body postures.

Timing

Recognizing the appropriate time to communicate information is a developed skill. A distraught child whose parents have just left for work is not ready for a diabetic teaching session. The session will be much more productive and the information better understood if the child has a chance to make the transition. The convenience of a schedule should be secondary to meeting a child's needs.

FAMILY-CENTERED COMMUNICATION

Any discussion about effective ways to communicate with children must also include a discussion of effective communication with families. *Family-centered care* emphasizes that the family is intricately involved in the care of the child. Family-centered care is achieved when health care professionals can create partnerships with families, recognizing that

the family is essential to the child and that the family has the right to participate fully in planning, implementing, and evaluating the child's plan of care.

Commitment to family-centered care means that the nurse respects the family's diversity. Children and parents live in a variety of family structures. An expanded definition of family is required in the twenty-first century, because *family* no longer refers to only the intact, nuclear family in which parents raise their biologic children. Family is more accurately described as individuals, related biologically or through sustaining social commitments and represented by similar or different generations and genders, who provide mutual socialization, nurturing, and emotional support (Lerner, Sparks, & McCubbin, 2000). Therefore adolescent parents, extended families with aunts or cousins parenting, intergenerational families with grandparents parenting, blended families with stepparents and stepsiblings, gay or lesbian parents, foster parents, group homes, and homeless children all qualify as contemporary family structures. The nurse should be prepared to identify the foundational strengths in all family structures (see Chapter 3). Family-centered care also means that the nurse truly believes that the child's care and recovery are greatly enhanced when the family fully participates in the child's care (Fig. 32-3).

Establishing Rapport

Critical to establishing rapport with families is the nurse's ability to convey genuine respect and concern during the first encounter. A nonjudgmental approach and willingness to assist family members in effectively caring for their child demonstrate the nurse's interest in their well-being.

Availability and Openness to Questions

A nurse who does not take time to see how a child and family are doing—such as a nurse who leaves a room immediately after a treatment or administration of a medication—will not encourage or invite families to ask questions. Families want and need unrushed and uninterrupted time with the nurse. Sometimes this time can be made available only by purposefully scheduling it into the day. Encouraging families to write down their questions will enable them to take full advantage of their time with the nurse.

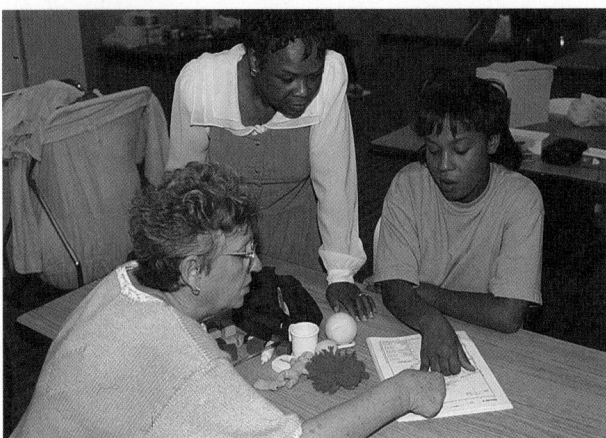

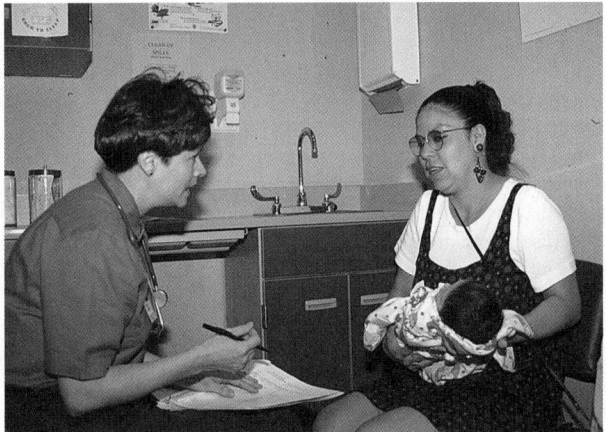

◄ The nurse explains a child's test results to his mother and grandmother. Including all important family members in the child's health care reflects a commitment to family-centered care. (Courtesy The University of Texas at Arlington School of Nursing.)

This nurse practitioner has learned Spanish to communicate better ▶ with her many Spanish-speaking clients. Speaking with family members in their own language encourages the family to remain in the health care system. The nurse is also using eye contact and has positioned herself at the mother's eye level. (Courtesy Parkland Health and Hospital System Community Oriented Primary Care Clinic, Dallas, TX.)

Figure 32-3   The child's ongoing helath care, both preventive and during illness, is enhanced by participation of the family.

The nurse might encourage use of time by saying, "I know you have a lot of questions and are very anxious to learn more about your son's condition. I have another patient who has an immediate need, but I will be available in 10 minutes to meet with you. In the meantime, here is a parent handbook that gives general information about seizures. Please feel free to review it and write down any questions that we can discuss when I return."

Family Education and Empowerment

Educating parents about their child's condition, ensuring their continued involvement in planning and evaluating the plan of care, and teaching them the skills to participate em-

power the family. Families need support as they gain confidence in their skills, and they need guidance to assist them as they navigate through the health care experience. Communication is enhanced when families feel competent and confident in their abilities.

Effective Management of Conflict

When conflict occurs, it should be addressed in an expedient manner to prevent further breakdown in communication. Box 32-1 provides strategies for managing conflict, and Table 32-2 discusses the importance of choosing words carefully to make families feel welcome and to further facilitate family-centered care.

BOX 32-1
Strategies for Managing Conflict

- *Understand the parents' perspective (walk in their shoes).* Imagine yourself as the parent of a child in a hospital where your values and beliefs are exposed and scrutinized. Try to understand their perspective better by encouraging them to share it.
- *Determine a common goal, and stay focused on it.* Determine the agreed-on result, and work toward it. By staying focused on a common goal, the parties involved are more likely to find workable strategies to achieve the identified goal.
- *Seek win-win solutions.* Conflict should not be about who is right and who is wrong. Effective conflict management focuses on finding a solution whereby both people "win." By establishing a common goal, both parties win when this goal is achieved.
- *Listen actively.* Critical to resolving situations of conflict is the ability to listen and understand what the other person is saying and feeling. In active listening, the receiver actively and empathically listens to gain a better understanding of the actual and the implied message.

- *Openly express your feelings.* Talking about feelings is much more constructive than acting them out.

The nurse might say, "I am very concerned about Jamie's safety when you leave his side rails down."

- *Avoid blaming.* Each party owns part of the problem. Pointing fingers and blaming others will not solve the problem. Instead, identify the part of the problem that each party owns and work together to resolve it. Seek win-win solutions.
- *Summarize the decision.* At the end of any discussion, summarize what has been decided and identify who is responsible for follow-up. This process ensures that everyone is clear about the decision and facilitates accountability for implementing solutions.

TABLE 32-2 Choosing Words Carefully

Poor Words	Rationale	Better Words	Rationale
Policies allowed or *not permitted*	Convey attitude that hospital personnel have authority over parents in matters concerning their children	*Guidelines, working together, welcome*	Convey openness and appreciation for position and importance of families
Noncompliant, uncooperative, difficult (when referring to parents and other family members)	Imply that health care providers make the decisions and give instructions that families must follow without input	*Partners, colleagues, joint decision makers, experts about their child*	Acknowledge that families bring important information and insight and that families and professionals form a team
Dysfunctional, in denial, overprotective, uninvolved, uncaring (labeling families)	Pronounce a judgment that may not incorporate a full understanding of a family's situation, reactions, or perspective	*Coping* (describing family's reactions with care and respect)	Leaves room to build a more complete and appreciative understanding of families over time

Feedback From Children and Families

The nurse must be alert for verbal as well as nonverbal cues. Routinely checking with family members about their experiences, satisfaction with communications, teaching sessions, and health care goals is an effective way to ensure that health care providers obtain appropriate feedback. To enhance the delivery of care, the nurse should explain how this feedback will be used. The nurse should listen and observe carefully to make sure that what family members are saying is truly what they are feeling.

For example, while one nurse was teaching the mother of a 2-year-old who was recently diagnosed with diabetes mellitus, the mother reported that although she was the primary caregiver of her child, the child's grandmother frequently cared for the child while the mother was at work. The nurse therefore notified the other team members and altered the teaching plan for diabetes care to include the child's grandmother.

Spirituality

Children have rich spiritual lives although they do not use the same vocabulary as adults to describe them.

Spiritual care is a vital support for many children. Children coping with acute illness or injury may be facing fear, anger, and guilt. These are powerful emotions that can lead to feeling isolated from one's Higher Power, family members, and friends. For children with chronic disease or disability, it is important to remember that sustained spiritual support is critical. Childhood chronic conditions often have lifetime implications (Grossoehme, 1999). Children can be assisted in maintaining their rituals, whether they are bedtime prayers, songs, or blessings at meals. A resource to pursue in most hospital or medical center settings is the pastoral care or chaplain's department.

Transcultural Communication: Bridging the Gap

Conflict can arise when the nurse comes from a cultural background different from that of the child and family. Such differences could influence the approach to care. As the demographics in the United States continue to change, health care professionals will be challenged to become more transcultural in their approach to clients if they want to continue to be effective in their relationships with children and families. Health care professionals need to be aware of their own values and beliefs and need to recognize how these influence their interactions with others. They also need to be aware of and respect the child's and family's values and beliefs. In working with children and families, the initial assessment should address values, beliefs, and traditions. The nurse can then consider ways in which culture might affect communication style, methods of decision making, and other behaviors related to health care practices.

During the initial interview, the nurse should ascertain the following information related to the child and family:

- *Decision-making practices:* Are decisions made by individuals or collectively as a group?
- *Child-rearing practices:* Who are the primary caregivers? What are their disciplinary practices?
- *Family support:* What is the family structure? To whom do the patient and family turn for support?
- *Communication practices:* How is the information communicated to the rest of the family?
- *Health and illness practices:* Do family members seek professional help or rely on other resources for treatment and advice?

Once this information is obtained, the nurse can use this knowledge to individualize the treatment plan and approach for the child's and family's needs. For example, if the parents of a child with an Orthodox Jewish religious background request a kosher diet, the nurse facilitates the routine delivery of kosher meals and communicates the family's wishes to the rest of the team members so that they can also respect the family's customs. If the family of a child who suffered a severe brain injury requests the services of a healer, the nurse enables the family to arrange the visit. Coordinating the child's daily schedule to provide an uninterrupted visit with the healer is one aspect of family-centered care. When the nurse communicates the family's cultural preferences to other members of the health care team, communication and holistic care are enhanced.

BOX 32-2
Warning Signs of Overinvolvement ✿

- Buying gifts for individual children or families
- Giving out a home phone number
- Competing with other staff for the child's or family's affection
- Inviting the child or family to social gatherings
- Accepting invitations to family gatherings (e.g., birthday parties, weddings)
- Visiting or spending time with the child or family during off-duty time
- Revealing personal information
- Lending or borrowing money
- Making decisions for the family about the child's care

THERAPEUTIC RELATIONSHIPS: DEVELOPING AND MAINTAINING TRUST

Trust is important in establishing and maintaining therapeutic relationships with families. Families and nurses communicate more easily and collaborate better within a climate of reciprocal trust (Lynn-McHale & Deatrick, 2000). Becoming overly involved with the child or family can inhibit a reciprocal relationship. Because nurses are caring, nurturing people and the profession demands that nurses sometimes become intimately involved in other people's lives, maintaining the balance between appropriate involvement and professional separation is at times very difficult. Overinvolvement can be a type of controlling behavior that interferes with a reciprocal, trusting relationship (Lynn-McHale & Deatrick, 2000). Box 32-2 delineates behaviors that indicate overinvolvement. The nurse who becomes too emotionally involved loses effectiveness as an objective professional resource.

Family members may display feelings of incompetence, fear, and loss of control by expressing anger, withdrawal, or dissatisfaction. Most important in working with these families is to promote the parents' feelings of competency through education and empowerment. The nurse should keep parents well informed of the child's care through frequent phone calls and involvement in decision making. The nurse should promote their confidence, enhance their self-esteem, and foster their independence by teaching them the skills necessary to care for their child.

Nurses must be able to recognize their own personal and professional needs. Awareness of the motives for one's own actions will greatly enhance the nurse's ability to understand the needs of children and families and to give families the tools to manage care effectively.

▪ NURSING CARE

Communicating With Children and Families

Assessment

A comprehensive needs assessment of the child and family elicits information about problem-solving skills, cultural needs, coping behaviors, and the child's routines. Any assessment requires the nurse to obtain information from the child as well as the family.

⚠ CRITICAL TO REMEMBER

Maintaining a Therapeutic Relationship

Maintaining professional boundaries requires that the nurse constantly be aware of the fine line between empathy and overinvolvement.

The nurse might say, "Mrs. Brown, I value your input as well as your child's. Hearing Michael explain his understanding of his diabetic dietary restrictions in his own words will help us gain better insight into how best to manage his care. Let's take a few minutes to hear from Michael, and then we can talk about your perspective."

Assessment enables the nurse to develop better insight by gathering information from multiple perspectives and facilitates the development of a more comprehensive plan of care. A thorough assessment of the child's communication skills presumes the nurse understands developmental milestones and can relate comprehension and communication skills to the child's cognitive and emotional development and language abilities. During the initial assessment of the child and family, the nurse should also describe routines and provide information about what the child and family can expect during their visit.

Nursing Diagnosis and Planning

The nursing assessment may suggest diagnoses that affect communication but that arise from the child's encounter with the health care system. Other diagnoses are related to the child's and family's communication abilities.

- Anxiety related to potential or actual separation from parents (e.g., a 4-year-old who becomes withdrawn and unable to cooperate with an office hearing test when separated from her mother).
  Expected Outcomes: The child verbalizes the cause of the anxiety and more readily communicates with the health professional. The child exhibits posture, facial expressions, and gestures that reflect decreased distress.

- Fear related to a perceived threat to the child's well-being and inadequate understanding of procedures or treatments (e.g., a 7-year-old scheduled for tonsillectomy who wonders where his throat will be cut to remove his tonsils).
  Expected Outcomes: The child talks about fears and accurately describes the procedure or treatment.

- Hopelessness related to a deteriorating health status (e.g., an 11-year-old in isolation with prolonged illness and uncertain prognosis).
  Expected Outcomes: The child verbalizes feelings and participates in care. The child makes positive statements, maintains eye contact during interactions, and has appetite and sleep patterns that are appropriate for age and physical health.

- Powerlessness related to limits to autonomy (e.g., a 3-year-old with a C6 spinal fracture as a result of a motor vehicle trauma).
  Expected Outcomes: The child expresses frustrations and anger and begins to make choices in areas that are controllable. The child asks appropriate questions about care and treatment.

TABLE 32-3 Developmental Milestones and Their Relationship to Communication Approaches

Development	Language Development	Emotional Development	Cognitive Development	Suggested Communication Approach
INFANTS (0-12 MO)				
Infants experience the world through the senses of hearing, seeing, smelling, tasting, and touching.	Crying, babbling, cooing. Single-word production. Able to name some simple objects.	Dependent on others; high need for cuddling and security. Responsive to environment (e.g., sounds, visual stimuli). Distinguish between happy and angry voices as well as between familiar and strange voices. Beginning to experience separation anxiety.	Interactions largely reflexive. Beginning to see repetition of activities and movements. Beginning to initiate interactions intentionally. Short attention span (1-2 min).	Use calm, soft, soothing voice. Be responsive to cries. Engage in turn-taking vocalizations (adult imitates baby sounds). Talk and read regularly to infants. Prepare infant as you are about to perform care; talk to infant about what you are about to do. Use a slow approach and allow child time to get to know you.
TODDLERS (1-2 YR)				
Toddlers experience the world through the senses of hearing, seeing, smelling, tasting, and touching.	Two-word combinations emerge. Participate in turn-taking in communication (speaker/listener). "No" becomes a favorite word. Able to use gestures and verbalize simple wants and needs.	Strong need for security objects. Separation/stranger anxiety heightened. Participate in parallel play. Thrive on routines. Beginning development of independence: "Want to do by self." Still very dependent on significant adults.	Experiment with objects. Participate in active exploration. Begin to experiment with variations on activities. Begin to identify cause-and-effect relationships. Short attention span (3-5 min).	Learn the toddler's words for common items, and use them in conversations. Describe activities and procedures as they are about to be done. Use picture books. Use play for demonstrations. Be responsive to child's receptivity toward you, and approach cautiously. Preparation should occur immediately before the event.
PRESCHOOL CHILDREN (3-5 YR)				
Preschool children use words they do not fully understand, nor do they accurately understand many words used by others.	Further development and expansion of word combination (able to speak in full sentences). Growth in correct grammatical usage. Use pronouns. Clearer articulation of sounds. Vocabulary rapidly expanding; may know words without understanding meaning.	Like to imitate activities and make choices. Strive for independence but need adult support and encouragement. Demonstrate purposeful attention-seeking behaviors. Learn cooperation and turn-taking in game playing. Need clearly set limits and boundaries.	Begin developing concepts of time, space, and quantity. Magical thinking prominent. World seen only from child's perspective. Short attention span (5-10 min).	Seek opportunities to offer choices. Use play to explain procedures and activities. Speak in simple sentences, and explore relative concepts. Use picture and story books, puppets. Describe activities and procedures as they are about to be done. Be concise; limit length of explanations (5 min). Engage in preparatory activities 1-3 hr before the event.

TABLE **32-3** Developmental Milestones and Their Relationship to Communication Approaches—cont'd

Development	Language Development	Emotional Development	Cognitive Development	Suggested Communication Approach
SCHOOL-AGE CHILDREN (6-11 YR)				
School-age children communicate thoughts and appreciate viewpoints of others. Words with multiple meanings and words describing things they have not experienced are not thoroughly understood.	Expanding vocabulary enables child to describe concepts, thoughts, and feelings. Development of conversational skills.	Interact well with others. Understand rules to games. Very interested in learning. Build close friendships. Beginning to accept responsibility for own actions. Competition emerges. Still dependent on adults to meet needs.	Able to grasp concepts of classification, conversation. Concrete thinking emerges. Become very oriented to "rules." Able to process information in serial format. Lengthened attention span (10-30 min).	Use photographs, books, diagrams, charts, videos to explain. Make explanations sequential. Engage in conversations that encourage critical thinking. Establish limits, and set consequences. Use medical play techniques. Introduce preparatory materials 1-5 days in advance of the event.
ADOLESCENTS (12 YR AND OLDER)				
Adolescents are able to create theories and generate many explanations for situations. They are beginning to communicate like adults.	Able to verbalize and comprehend most adult concepts.	Beginning to accept responsibility for own actions. Perception of "imaginary audiences." Need independence. Competitive drive. Strong need for group identification. Frequently have small group of very close friends. Question authority. Strong need for privacy.	Able to think logically and abstractly. Attention span up to 60 min.	Engage in conversations about adolescent's interests. Use photographs, books, diagrams, charts, and videos to explain. Use collaborative approach, and foster and support independence. Introduce preparatory materials up to 1 wk in advance of the event. Respect privacy needs.

The nurse caring for 8-year-old Jermaine observes him lying in his bed with his back facing the door. He is crying, although he quickly wipes his eyes when he sees the nurse at the door. Jermaine has been hospitalized because of leukemia. He lives in a small community 350 miles from the hospital. His parents visit on the weekends.
1. Identify two things that might be upsetting Jermaine.
2. What strategies could you use to encourage Jermaine to talk about his feelings related to the problems you have identified?

■ Impaired Verbal Communication related to physiologic barriers or cultural and language differences (e.g., a 17-year-old adolescent who has had her jaw wired subsequent to orthodontic surgery).
Expected Outcomes: The child with a physiologic barrier to communication effectively uses alternative communication methods. The child and family who speak and understand a different language appropriately communicate through an interpreter.

Interventions

Nurses working with children should determine the best communication approach for each child individually, based on the child's age and developmental abilities. Table 32-3 presents an overview of developmental milestones related to communication skills in children and some approaches to facilitate successful interactions.

Play

Play can greatly facilitate communicating with children. Approaching children at their developmental level with familiar forms of play increases their comfort and allows the nurse to be seen in a more positive, less threatening role.

Because play is an everyday part of children's lives and a method they use to communicate, they are less likely to be inhibited when participating in play interactions. Through play, children may express thoughts and feelings they may be

BOX 32-3
Storytelling Strategies

- Capture a story on paper or on videotape as told by a child or group of children.
- Tell a "yarn story" with two or more people. A long piece of yarn with knots tied at varied intervals is slid loosely through the hands of the teller until a knot is felt, at which time the yarn is passed to the next person, who continues the story.
- Initiate a game of sentence completion, either oral or written, with sentences beginning "If I were in charge of the hospital . . . ," "I wish . . . ," "When I get home I will . . . ," or "My family . . . ."
- Read stories with themes related to issues a child is facing. The children's section of the local public library is an excellent resource.

unable to verbalize (see Chapters 5 through 8 for normal play activities and Chapter 35 for therapeutic play).

Storytelling

Storytelling is an innovative and creative communication strategy. It is also a skill that can be acquired and refined through practice. Familiarity with stories and frequent practice in storytelling increase a nurse's confidence and competence as storyteller. Storytelling can be a routine part of a nurse's day. Its purposes range from establishing rapport to approaching uncomfortable topics, such as loss, death, fear, grief, and anger. In storytelling, there is a teller and a listener. In individual situations, the child may be the teller or the listener, although in a shared story, adult and child may each take a turn in both roles (Box 32-3).

Explaining Procedures and Treatments

Preparation before a procedure, which includes explaining the reasons for the procedure and the expected sequence of events and outcomes, can greatly reduce a child's fears and anxieties. Preparation enables the child to experience some mastery over events, gives the child time to develop effective coping behaviors, and fosters trust in those caring for the child. Adequate preparation is the key to helping a child have a successful, positive health care experience.

In general, the younger the child, the closer in time to the event should the child be prepared for it. For example, a 3-year-old will generally be very anxious and therefore should be prepared immediately before, whereas teenagers would benefit from a longer preparation time so that they can develop strategies for dealing with the situation. Table 32-3 gives age-related attention span guidelines.

Key elements for communicating complete and accurate information are as follows (Gaynard et al., 1998):

- *Learn the procedure*. To explain a procedure adequately, the nurse must understand what is involved. What pieces of equipment will be used? Where will the procedure take place? Essentially, the nurse needs to learn what the child can expect to happen during the procedure.
- *Determine what information to share with the child and family*. The preparation should include information only about

what the child will experience or perceive directly. Consultation with the family will allow the nurse to learn words and terminology used by the child. Table 32-4 offers other concrete suggestions of appropriate language for nurses to use in working with children.

- *Provide sensory information*. Allowing children to see, hear, feel, taste, smell, and experience similar sensations during their preparation will greatly enhance their preparedness and diminish their anxieties. For example, in preparing a child for an IV line insertion, the nurse can show the child the catheter or explain the purpose of the tourniquet and allow the child to put it on or to put it on the arm of a doll, if the child so desires. The nurse should let the child smell an alcohol swab and feel its coolness when applied to the skin. Showing the child the treatment room and allowing the child to sit on the treatment table where the procedure will be performed are effective ways to convey information.
- *Explain the sequence of events*. Preparation includes a description of the sequence in which events will occur. Recognizing the procedure as a series of sequential steps allows children to anticipate appropriately and gives them a sense of control as well as a better understanding of the number of steps to expect before the procedure is over.
- *Explain how long the procedure will last*. Whenever possible, the nurse should allow the child to have simulated play experiences. Inviting the child to perform the procedure on a doll or stuffed animal is often effective and gives the child a real sense of time as well as firsthand experience with the sequence of events. If a concrete demonstration is not possible, the nurse should explain the timing in terms that the child can understand; for example, the nurse might say, "The procedure will last as long as it takes to sing your favorite song."
- *Monitor accuracy of information (feedback)*. Feedback can be used to modify or reinforce future preparation sessions. Feedback also allows the nurse to correct any misunderstandings the child may have and provides an opportunity for the child to process verbally and express feelings about the experience.

Open, honest communication about treatments and procedures and attentiveness to the learning needs of the child will greatly facilitate achievement of the treatment goals.

Strategies for Enhancing Self-Esteem

Coopersmith (1967) defined self-esteem as a "personal judgment of worthiness that is expressed in the attitudes the individual holds toward himself or herself." Communication practices play an important role in the development of children's self-esteem. Nurses are in an excellent position to model communication practices that enhance self-esteem. Table 32-5 compares helpful and harmful communication practices.

The words adults choose, their tone of voice, and the place and timing of message delivery all influence the child's interpretation of the message. The interpretation may be positive, negative, or neutral. To enhance the child's self-esteem, adults should strive for positive language. Being attentive, engendering trust, demonstrating affection, and affirming goodness and talents are communication practices that contribute to building self-esteem (McClowry, 2003).

Stroke - in adult because they need to relearn things

TABLE 32-4 Considerations in Choosing Language

Potentially Ambiguous	Concrete Explanation
"The doctor will give you some dye." *To make me die?*	"The doctor will put some medicine in the tube that will help her see your _____ more clearly."
Dressing, dressing change. *Why are they going to undress me?* *Do I have to change my clothes?*	Bandages; clean, new bandages.
Stool collection. *Why do they want to collect little chairs?*	Use child's familiar term, such as "poop," "BM," or "doody."
Urine. *You're in?*	Use child's familiar term, such as "pee."
Shot. *When people get shot, they're really badly hurt.*	Describe giving medicine through a (small, tiny) needle.
CAT scan. *Will there be cats?*	Describe in simple terms, and explain what the letters of the common name stand for.
PICU. *Pick you?*	Explain as above.
ICU. *I see you?*	Explain as above.
IV. *Ivy?*	Explain as above.
Stretcher. *Stretch her? Stretch whom?*	Bed on wheels.
Special; funny (words that are usually positive descriptors). *It doesn't look/feel special to me.*	Odd, different, unusual, strange.
Gas, sleeping gas. *Is someone going to pour gasoline into the mask?*	"A medicine, called an anesthetic, is a kind of air you will breathe through a mask like this to help you sleep during your operation so you won't feel anything. It is a different kind of sleep." (Explain differences.)
"The doctor will put you to sleep." *Like my cat was put to sleep? It never came back.*	"The doctor will give you medicine that will help you go into a very deep sleep. You won't feel anything until the operation is over. Then the doctor will stop giving you the medicine, so you can wake up."
"Move you to the floor." *Why are they going to put me on the ground?*	Unit, ward. (Explain why the child is being transferred, and where.)
OR (or treatment room) table. *People aren't supposed to get up on tables.*	A narrow bed.
"Take a picture." (X-ray, CT, and MRI machines are far larger than a familiar camera, move differently, and don't yield a familiar end product.)	"A picture of your insides." (Describe appearance, sounds, and movement of the equipment.)
"Flush your IV." *Flush it down the toilet?*	Explain.

Words can be experienced as "hard" or "soft" according to how much they increase the perceived threat of a situation. For example, consider the following word choices:

Harder	Softer
"This part will hurt."	"It (you) may feel (or feel very) sore, achy, scratchy, tight, snug, full, or _____ (other manageable, descriptive term)." (Words such as scratch, poke, or sting might be familiar for some children and frightening to others.)
"The medicine will burn."	"Some children say they feel very warm."
"The room will be very cold."	"Some children say they feel very cold."
"The medicine will taste (or smell) bad."	"The medicine may taste (or smell) different from anything you have tasted before. After you take it, will you tell me how it was for you?"
"Cut," "open you up," "slice," "make a hole."	"The doctor will make an opening." (Use concrete comparisons, such as "your little finger" or "a paper clip" if the opening will indeed be small.)
"As big as _____" (e.g., size of an incision or of a catheter).	"Smaller than _____."

Continued

TABLE 32-4 Considerations in Choosing Language—cont'd

Harder	Softer
"As long as _____" (e.g., for duration of a procedure).	"For less time than it takes you to _____."
"As much as _____."	"Less than _____."
(These are open-ended and "extending" expressions.)	(These expressions help confine, familiarize, and imply the manageability of an event or of equipment.)

The unfamiliar usage or complexity of some common medical words or expressions can be confusing and frightening.

Potentially Ambiguous	Concrete Explanation
"Take your vitals" (or "your vital signs").	"Measure your temperature," "see how warm your body is," "see how fast and strongly your heart is working." (Nothing is "taken" from the child.)
Electrodes, leads.	"Sticky like a Band-Aid, with a small wet spot in the center, and small strings that attach to the snap (monitor electrodes); paste like wet sand, with strings with tiny metal cups that stick to the paste (EEG electrodes). The paste washes off easily afterward; the strings go into a box that will make a picture of how your heart (or brain) is working." (Show child electrodes and leads before using. Let child handle them and apply them to a doll or to self.)
"Hang your (IV) medication."	"We will bring in a new medicine in a bag and attach it to the little tube already in your arm. The needle goes into the tube, not into your arm, so you won't feel it."
NPO.	"Nothing to eat. Your stomach needs to be empty." (Explain why.) "You can eat and drink again as soon as _____." (Explain with concrete descriptions.)
Anesthesia.	"The doctor will give you medicine—you may hear it called 'anesthesia.' It will help you go into a very deep sleep. You will not feel anything at all. The doctor knows just the right amount of medicine to give you so you will stay asleep through your operation. When the operation is over, the doctor stops giving you that medicine and helps you wake up."

NOTE: Words or phrases that are helpful to one child may be threatening for another. Health care providers must listen carefully and be sensitive to the child's use of and response to language.
Modified with permission of the Child Life Council, Inc., 11820 Parklawn Drive, Rockville, MD 20852-2529, from Gaynard, L., Wolfer, J., Goldberger, J., Thompson, R., Redburn, L., & Laidley, L. (1998). *Psychosocial care of children in hospitals: A clinical practice manual from ACCH Child Life Research Project.* Rockville, MD: The Child Life Council, Inc.

Evaluation

Even though evaluation is traditionally thought of as a closure activity, evaluation should be a continuous activity throughout the nursing process. Keep expected outcomes visible, and assess if they are being realized. Are the outcomes attainable? Could the wrong nursing diagnosis have been made? Adjust the plan of care as needed.

COMMUNICATING WITH CHILDREN WITH SPECIAL NEEDS

The opportunity to interact with children who have special communication needs presents an exciting challenge for nurses. To identify successful alternative methods of commu-

> ! CRITICAL TO REMEMBER
>
> **Communicating With Children With Special Needs**
>
> In working with children with special needs, the nurse must carefully assess each child's physical, mental, and developmental abilities and determine the most effective methods of communication.

nication, the nurse needs to learn particular techniques for working with children and families. Alternative methods of communicating are critical. Children need to express their wants and needs accurately. Through adequate preparation and reassurance, the nurse can offer the child comfort and understanding. Successfully meeting this challenge is a rewarding experience for the nurse and a positive, supportive experience for the child and family.

The Child With a Visual Impairment

For the child with a visual impairment, the nurse can:

- Obtain a thorough assessment of the child's self-help skills and abilities (i.e., toileting, bathing, dressing, feeding, mobility).
- Orient the child to the surroundings. Walk the child around the room and unit several times, indicating landmarks (e.g., doors, closets, bedside tables, windows) while guiding the child by the hand or by the way the child prefers. Explain sounds that the child may frequently hear (e.g., monitors, alarms, nurse call bells).

TABLE **32-5** Self-Esteem in Children: Communication Practices

Techniques to Enhance Self-Esteem	Practices That Harm Self-Esteem
Praise efforts and accomplishments.	Criticize efforts and accomplishments.
Use active listening skills.	Be too busy to listen.
Encourage expression of feelings.	Tell children how they should feel.
Acknowledge feelings.	Give no support for dealing with feelings.
Use developmentally based discipline.	Use physical punishment.
Use "I" statements.	Use "you" statements.
Be nonjudgmental.	Judge the child.
Set clearly defined limits, and reinforce them.	Set no known limits or boundaries.
Share quality time together.	Give time grudgingly.
Be honest.	Be dishonest.
Describe behaviors observed when praising and disciplining.	Use coercion and power as discipline.
Compliment the child.	Belittle, blame, or shame the child.
Smile.	Use sarcastic, caustic, or cruel "humor."
Touch and hug the child.	Avoid coming near the child, even when the child is open to touching, holding, or hugging. Touch and hold only when performing a task.
Rock the child.	Avoid comforting through rocking.

- Encourage the parents to stay with the child. They can facilitate communication and greatly enhance the child's comfort in this unfamiliar environment.
- Keep furniture and other items in the same consistent place. Consistency aids in the child's orientation to the room, fosters independence, and promotes safety.
- Keep the nurse call bell in the same place and within the child's reach.
- Identify yourself when entering the room, and tell the child when you are departing.
- Carefully and fully explain all procedures.
- Allow the child to handle equipment as the procedure is explained.

- Do not shout or exaggerate speech. This behavior distorts the face and can be very confusing. Rather, speak in a normal tone and at a regular pace.
- Remember that nonverbal communication can speak as loud as, if not louder than, speech (e.g., a frown or worried face can say more than words).
- When performing a procedure that requires standing behind the child, such as when giving an enema or assisting with a spinal tap, have another person stand in front of the child and explain the procedure as it is being performed.
- Whenever possible, use play strategies to help communicate and demonstrate procedures (see Table 32-3).

The Child With a Hearing Impairment

For the child with a hearing impairment, the nurse can:

- Thoroughly assess the child's self-help skills and abilities.
- Identify the family's method of communication, and if possible, adopt it.
- Encourage a family member to stay with the child at all times to decrease the stress of hospitalization and facilitate communication.
- If sign language is used, learn the most frequently used signs and use them whenever able. Keep a chart of signs near the child's bed.
- Develop a communication board with pictures of most commonly used items or needs (e.g., television, cup, toothbrush, toilet, shower).
- Determine whether the child uses a hearing aid. If so, make sure the batteries are working and the hearing aid is clean and intact.
- When entering the room, do so cautiously and gently touch the child before speaking.
- Always face the child when speaking. If the child is a lip reader, face-to-face visibility will greatly enhance the child's ability to understand.

The Child Who Speaks Another Language

For the child who speaks another language, the nurse can:

- Thoroughly assess the child's abilities in speaking and understanding both languages.
- Ask family members if they would like an interpreter, and involve them in the selection.
- Identify an interpreter, perhaps another adult family member, friend of the family, or other individual with proficiency in both languages. Other children should not be used as interpreters.
- Use an interpreter whenever possible but especially when explaining procedures, determining understanding, teaching new skills, and assessing needs.
- Use a communication board with the names of items printed in both languages.
- Learn the words and names of commonly used items in the child's language, and use them whenever possible. Using the familiar language not only aids in communication but also demonstrates sincere interest in learning the language and respect for the culture.
- Learn as much about the child's culture as possible, and develop plans of care that demonstrate respect for the culture.

Sincere attempts to learn to communicate with the child and family demonstrate your concern for their well-being.

- Use play strategies whenever possible. Play seems to be a universal language.

The Child Who Is Aphonic

For the child who is aphonic, the nurse can:

- Thoroughly assess the child's self-help skills and abilities. Determine the child's and family's methods of communicating, and adopt these as much as possible.
- Encourage parents to stay with the child to decrease anxiety and foster communication.
- Determine whether the child uses sign language or augmented communication devices. Use a communication board if appropriate.
- Be attentive to and maximize the child's nonverbal communication. Facial grimaces, frowns, smiles, and nods are effective means of communicating responses and expressing likes and dislikes.
- If appropriate, encourage the child to use writing boards (dry erase, chalk, pads of paper) to write needs, wants, questions, and concerns.

The Child With a Profound Neurologic Impairment

Because hearing, vision, and language abilities are often hard to determine in the child who is profoundly neurologically impaired, assume the child can hear, see, and comprehend something in what is said. Use a friendly tone of voice that conveys warmth and respect. For the child with a profound neurologic impairment, the nurse can:

- Address the child when entering and exiting the room. Gently touch the child while saying the child's name.

- Speak softly, calmly, and slowly to allow the child time to process what you are saying.
- While in the room with the child, talk to the child. Do not talk as if the child were not there.

The nurse might say, "Jenny, I am going to wash your arm now," or "Jenny, now I am going to take your temperature by putting the thermometer under your arm." Identifying an assistant, the nurse might say, "Jenny, Kristi, another nurse, is here to help me lift you into your chair."

- Talk to the child about activities and objects in the room, things that the child might see, hear, smell, touch, taste, or sense.

For example, the nurse might say, "It is a sunny day today; can you feel the warm sun shining on you through the window?"

- When asking the child questions, allow the child adequate time to respond. Be careful to ask questions only of children who are capable of responding.
- Ascertain the child's ability to respond to simple questions. Some children can respond to *yes* or *no* questions by squeezing a hand or blinking their eyes (once for *yes* and twice for *no*).
- Be extremely attentive to any signs or gestures (e.g., facial grimaces, smiling, eye movements) that may convey responses to likes or dislikes. Signs or gestures may be the child's only means of communicating.

As with all children with special communication needs, thoroughly document and communicate to others who interact with the child any special techniques that work. Providing information will greatly enhance continuity and more fully facilitate the child's ability to communicate.

KEY CONCEPTS

- Components of effective communication with children involve verbal as well as nonverbal interactions. Essential components include touch, physical proximity, environment, listening, eye contact, visual cues, pace of speech and tone of voice, and overall body language.
- Nurses should determine the best communication approach for an individual child, based on the child's age, developmental abilities, and cultural preferences. Strategies include play and storytelling, explaining procedures

and treatments, and modeling communication practices that enhance self-esteem.
- Communication pitfalls, such as using jargon, talking down to children or beyond their developmental level, and avoiding or denying a problem, can lead to a breakdown in the relationship between the nurse and the child and family.
- Family-centered communication strategies include establishing rapport, identifying needs, establishing expectations, being available and open to questions, family education,

empowerment, obtaining feedback from children and families, promoting effective conflict management, learning techniques for transcultural communication, and maintaining professional boundaries.
- In working with children with special needs, the nurse should carefully assess each child's physical, mental, and developmental abilities and determine the most effective methods of communication.

1. Two areas that the nurse should explore are Jermaine's feelings about separation from his family and issues related to having leukemia, including the discomfort, treatment, and prognosis.

2. School-age children often do not readily discuss their feelings. The nurse needs to build trust with the child. Involving the child in a board game can be a useful strategy to help the child relax. As the game progresses, the nurse can begin to talk with the child, using a lead-in such as, "You seem very quiet today" or "You seemed upset when I came into your room." The child can choose to validate or deny the nurse's observation.

Another approach would be to say, "If you could have one wish today, what would it be?" Some children will use this as an op-portunity to describe what they would like to change. The nurse can cue into this disclosure. It is important to remember that all children are different and what works for one child may not work for another. Every nurse caring for children needs to understand growth and development and learn related communication techniques.

REFERENCES and READINGS

Ahman, E., & Lawrence, J. (1999). Exploring language about families. *Pediatric Nursing, 25*(2), 221-224.

Barnes, L.L., Plotnikoff, G.A., Fox, K., & Pendleton, S. (2000). Spirituality, religion, and pediatrics: Intersecting worlds of healing. *Pediatrics, 106*(Suppl. 4), 899-908.

Blackwell, P. (2000). The influence of touch on child development: Implications for intervention. *Infants and Young Children, 13*(1), 25-39.

Boggs, K. (1999). Communicating with children. In E. Arnold & K.U. Boggs (Eds.), *Interpersonal relationships: Professional communication skills for nurses* (3rd ed., pp. 405-429). Philadelphia: Saunders.

Cooper, C. (2001). *The art of nursing.* Philadelphia: Saunders.

Coopersmith, S. (1967). *The antecedents of self-esteem.* San Francisco: Freeman.

Darley, M. (Ed.). (2002). *Managing communication in health care.* London: Harcourt.

Deering, C.G., & Jennings, D. (2002). Communicating with children and adolescents. *American Journal of Nursing, 102*(3), 34-42.

Dernocoeur, K. (2000). Street smarts. Parents: The secondary patients. *Emergency Medical Services, 29*(6), 24-26.

Dokken, D.L., & Sydnor-Greenberg, N. (2000). Family focus. C.A.L.M.: A model for enhancing effective communication between parents and professionals. *Journal of Child and Family Nursing, 3*(5), 379-383.

Gaynard, L., Wolfer, J., Goldberger, J., Thompson, R., Redburn, L., & Laidley, L. (1998). *Psychosocial care of children in hospitals: A clinical practice manual from ACCH Child Life Research Project.* Rockville, MD: The Child Life Council.

Grossoehme, D.H. (1999). *The pastoral care of children.* New York: Haworth Pastoral Press.

Leavitt, L.A. (2002). When terrible things happen: A parent's guide to talking with their children. *Journal of Pediatric Health Care, 16*(5), 272-274.

Lerner, R., Sparks, E., & McCubbin, L. (2000). Family diversity and family policy. In D. Demo, K. Allen, & M. Fine (Eds.), *Handbook of family diversity* (pp. 380-401). New York: Oxford University Press.

Lynn-McHale, D., & Deatrick, J. (2000). Trust between family and healthcare provider. *Journal of Family Nursing, 6*(3), 210-230.

Macnab, A., Thiessen, P., McLeod, E., & Hinton, D. (2000). Parent assessment of family-centered care practices in a children's hospital. *Children's Health Care, 29*(2), 113-128.

Manworren, R.C., & Woodring, B. (1998). Evaluating children's literature as a source for patient education. *Pediatric Nursing, 24*(6), 548-553.

McClowry, S.G. (2003). *Your child's unique temperament: Insights and strategies for responsive parenting.* Champaign, IL: Research Press.

McPherson, G., & Thorne, S. (2000). Children's voices: Can we hear them? *Journal of Pediatric Nursing, 15*(1), 22-29.

McSherry, W. (2000). *Making sense of spirituality in nursing practice.* London: Harcourt.

Melnyk, B.M., Feinstein, N.F., Tuttle, J., Moldenhauer, Z., Herendeen, P., Veenema, T.G., Brown, H., Gullo, S., McMurtrie, M., & Small, L. (2002). Mental health worries, communication, and needs in the year of the U.S. terrorist attack: National KySS survey findings. *Journal of Pediatric Health Care, 16*(5), 222-234.

Newton, M. (2000). Family-centered care: Current realities in parent participation. *Pediatric Nursing, 26*(2), 164-168.

Osborne, H. (2001). In other words . . . start where they are: Communicating with children and their families about health and illness. *On Call, 4*(3), 46-47.

Reinbartsen, D.R. (2000). Preverbal communicative competence: An essential step in the lives of infants with severe physical impairment. *Infants and Young Children, 13*(1), 49-59.

Ryan-Wenger, N. (2001). Use of children's drawings for measurement of developmental level and emotional status. *Journal of Child and Family Nursing, 4*(2), 139-149.

Stein, M. (2000). The development-based office: Doing more with each visit. In S. Dixon & M. Stein, *Encounters with children* (3rd ed., pp. 47-64). St. Louis: Mosby.

Sydnor-Greenberg, N., & Dokken, D.L. (2001). Family focus. Communication in health care: Thoughts on the child's perspective. *Journal of Child and Family Nursing, 4*(3), 225-230.

Tates, K., Meeuwesen, L., Elbers, E., & Bensing, J. (2002). "I've come for his throat": Roles and identities in doctor-parent-child communication. *Child: Care, Health, & Development, 28*(1), 109-116.

Walker, C.L., Wells, L.M., Heiny, S.P., & Hymovich, D.P. (2002). Family-centered psychosocial care. In C.R. Baggott, K.P. Kelly, D. Fochtman, & G.V. Foley (Eds.), *Nursing care of children and adolescents with cancer.* Philadelphia: Saunders.

Wissow, L.S., & Kimel, M.B. (2002). Assessing provider-patient-parent communication in the pediatric emergency department. *Ambulatory Pediatrics, 2*(4), 323-329.

33

Physical Assessment of Children

◆ LEARNING OBJECTIVES

After studying this chapter, you should be able to:

- ◎ Apply principles of anatomy and physiology to the systematic physical assessment of the child.
- ◎ Describe the major components of a pediatric health history.
- ◎ Identify the principal techniques for doing a physical examination.
- ◎ Use a systematic and developmentally appropriate approach for examining a child.

- ◎ Describe the general sequence of the physical examination of the infant, the young child, the school-age child, and the adolescent.
- ◎ Describe normal physical examination findings.
- ◎ List common terms used to describe the findings on physical examination.
- ◎ Record physical examination findings in a systematic way.

◆ DEFINITIONS

auscultation Elicitation and evaluation of sounds produced by the body, frequently by using a stethoscope to magnify body sounds.

circumduction Circular movement of a limb or an eye.

crepitation A dry, crackling sound or sensation.

development Changes that occur over time in function and psychosocial and cognitive behavior.

fasciculation A small, local, involuntary muscular contraction visible under the skin.

fremitus A vibration perceptible on palpation or auscultation.

growth Measurable physical and physiologic changes that occur over time.

history The aggregate of subjective data that describe past and present health status.

inspection Careful observation to identify physical findings.

obtund To render dull or blunt.

palpation The use of touch to determine factors such as texture, temperature, moisture, and organ size and location.

percussion Tapping of the body to determine the density, location, and size of organs.

systematic assessment Organized method of collecting data.

Nurses perform physical assessments of infants and children in various settings—the clinic, the hospital, the school, and the home. The physical examination may be part of a well-child assessment, it may be the admission examination when a child enters the hospital, or it may be part of an initial assessment for home health care. The physical examination provides objective and subjective information about the child. It allows health care providers to determine the child's health status and make judgments about the need for nursing care.

GENERAL APPROACHES TO PHYSICAL ASSESSMENT

As when providing any nursing care for infants and children, the nurse applies knowledge of growth and development when preparing the child and performing the examination. Parents should be involved as much as possible, and the child should be encouraged to handle and play with instruments that are safe and clean, such as the stethoscope.

The physical examination is often the first direct contact between the nurse and the child. Establishing a trusting relationship between the child and the examiner is important. Throughout the examination the nurse should be sensitive to the cultural needs of and differences among children. Providing a quiet, private environment for the history and physical examination is important. The classic systematic approach to the physical examination is to begin at the head and proceed through the entire body to the toes. When examining a child, however, the examiner tailors the physical assessment to the child's age and developmental level.

! CRITICAL TO REMEMBER

Adapting the Physical Examination to the Child

The classic systematic approach to the physical examination is to begin at the head and proceed to the toes. For children, painful or frightening procedures should be left until last. Involving parents by asking them to hold or stand by the child can decrease children's anxiety and assist them in relaxing.

Infants 1 to 6 Months

Infants ages 1 to 6 months are responsive to human faces, are increasingly interested in their environment, and do not mind being undressed (see Chapter 5). Their examination should therefore be relatively easy. If the infant is nursing or asleep in the parent's arms, auscultate the heart, lungs, and abdomen without waking the baby. If the baby is awake, lay the baby on the examining table with the parent close by. As body parts are examined, incorporate evaluation of the primitive reflexes—palmar grasp, plantar grasp, placing, stepping, and tonic neck reflexes. Leave all uncomfortable procedures, such as abduction of the hips, speculum examination of the tympanic membranes, and eliciting the Moro reflex, until last. Before beginning the examination, undress the infant, leaving the diaper on a male child. Refocus an unhappy infant by calmly talking in a soft voice, distracting with a rattle, or offering a pacifier.

Infants 6 to 12 Months

For an older infant, follow the same procedures used for the infant from birth to 6 months but keep in mind that infants 6 months and older experience stranger anxiety and so are more difficult to examine. Distracting a child of this age with a toy or object may be useful. It is easier to do as much of the examination as possible with the child held on the parent's lap. Leave ear, oral, and other uncomfortable procedures until last.

Toddlers

Toddlers are the most challenging to examine because they are least likely to cooperate (see Chapter 6). To form a supportive relationship with the parent and toddler, the examiner begins by sitting or standing next to the parent. To facilitate relaxation, the examiner can provide a few toys and books and encourage the child to explore. Allowing the child to handle objects used during the examination can decrease fears. Communicating with the child, using age-appropriate words to describe what is about to be done, can also help decrease fear.

Portions of the examination can be done before the child is totally undressed. The order of the examination is flexible, and painful or frightening procedures should be left to last. Resistance and crying are common with toddlers. Assure the parent that the child's response to the examination is normal. The parent is the best assistant and can be asked, if willing, to hold the child's outstretched arms against the child's head or abdomen while the examiner's body immobilizes the lower half of the child's body.

Preschoolers

The preschool child is usually more cooperative, but these children still like to have their parents nearby (see Chapter 6). Preschool children are happy to show nurses that they can undress themselves. They can also be expected to cooperate. The nurse may proceed with the examination from the head to the toes but should still save the more invasive procedures, such as the speculum ear examination and the oral examination, until the end of the examination. The examiner can reinforce the child's interest by allowing the child to participate in the examination and by praising the child for cooperating.

School-Age Children

To establish trust with the school-age child, the examiner asks the child questions the child can answer. Children in elementary school will talk about school, favorite friends, and activities (see Chapter 7). Older school-age children may have to be encouraged to talk about their school performance and activities. The examiner encourages the parent to support and reinforce the child's participation in the examination.

The examination proceeds from head to toe. Children of this age prefer a simple drape over their underpants or a colorful examination gown, and the examiner should be sensitive to the child's modesty. The examination is a wonderful opportunity to teach the child about the body and personal care. The nurse answers questions openly and in simple terms.

Adolescents

Adolescents are most comfortable with a straightforward, uncondescending approach (see Chapter 8). Decisions about who should be present during the examination should be openly discussed with the adolescent. In most cases adolescents should be examined without the parent present. However, the parent should be given the opportunity to talk to the nurse about any concerns. The order of the examination is the same as for the school-age child.

It is best to incorporate the genital examination into the middle of the examination. If possible, proceed from the abdominal examination to the genital examination, to allow ample time for questions and discussions about this part of the examination. The physical examination is a wonderful opportunity to assure the pubertal child about normal developmental stages and to answer concerns children this age frequently have about what is happening to their bodies. The adolescent is expected to undress and wear a gown. The adolescent is draped appropriately during the examination.

TECHNIQUES FOR PHYSICAL EXAMINATION

When performing the physical assessment, the nurse uses the four basic techniques of inspection, palpation, percussion, and auscultation, in that order. During the abdominal examination, the sequence is altered: inspection is performed first, and then auscultation, percussion, and palpation. The sequence of the abdominal examination is changed so as not to alter bowel sounds before determining their presence and characteristics. Percussion is performed to determine the size of abdominal organs before palpation.

Health Screening for a 2-year-old

Community-based clinics promote optimal health in their clients. Children and their parents can develop an ongoing relationship with a provider, which encourages them to return for needed care in both health and illness. This 2-year-old girl is having a routine checkup at the clinic today.

Communication and enlisting the trust of the child are vital elements in a successful physical examination. The girl remains in the security of her mother's arms as the nurse assesses her head. The little girl's anterior fontanel is not quite fully closed. The nurse reassures her mother that, although the fontanel is usually closed by 18 months of age, her child's open fontanel likely represents a normal variation. Note that the nurse is at the mother's eye level and makes eye contact with her, promoting effective communication.

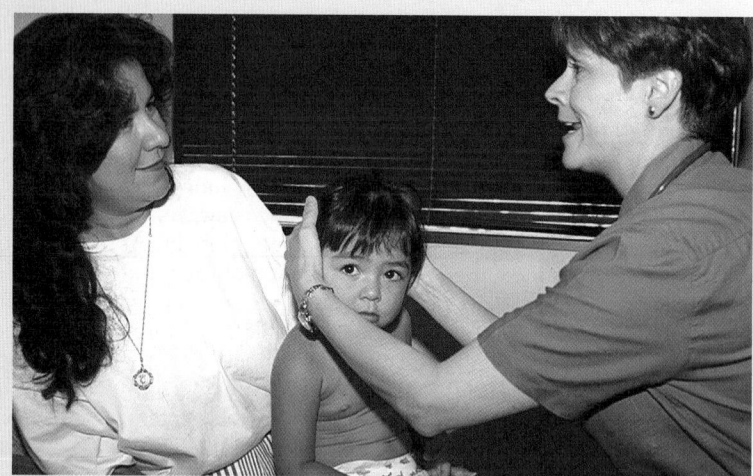

The nurse examines the child's feet for the presence of normal or abnormal reflexes and for straightness.

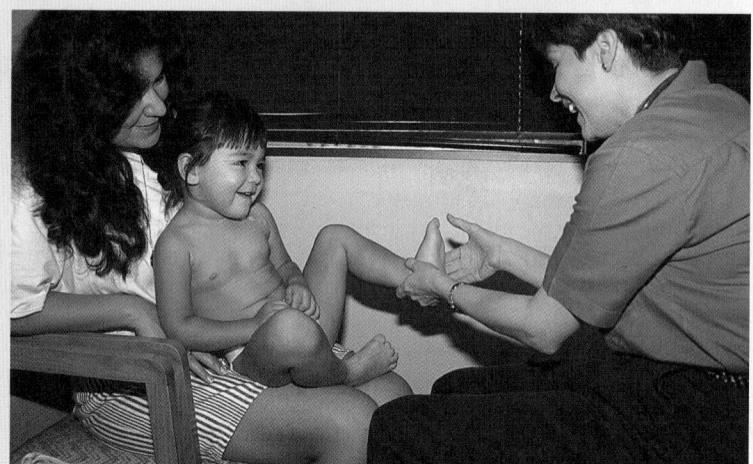

To limit the child's stress, the nurse creates an "examination table" by placing her knees next to the mother's knees. The child then lies across their laps as the nurse examines her thorax and abdomen.

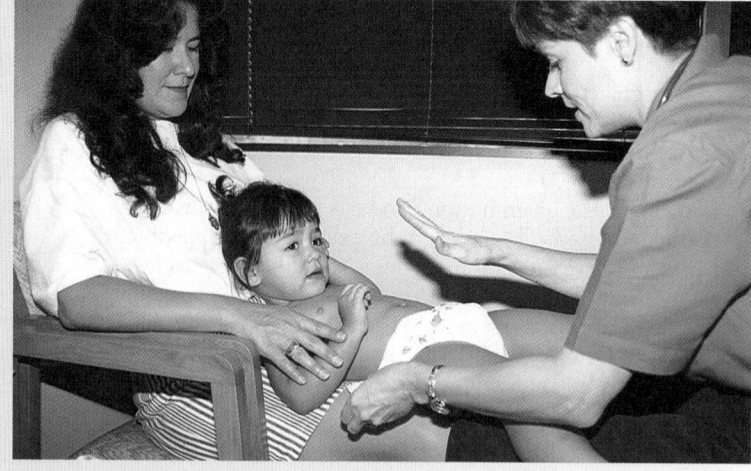

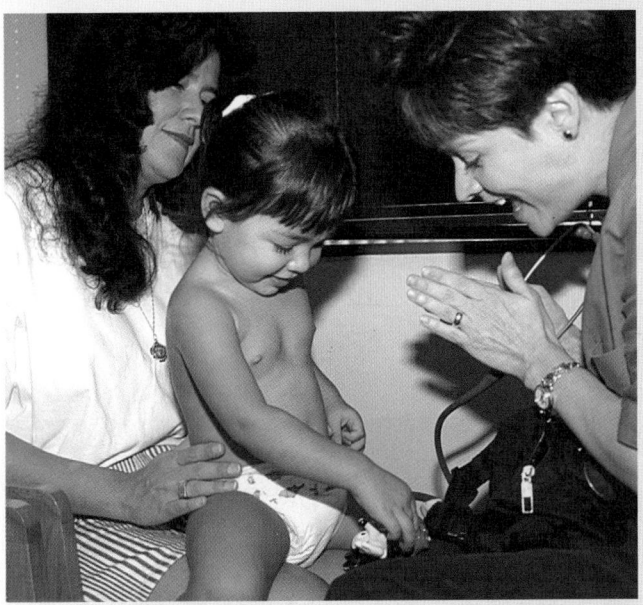 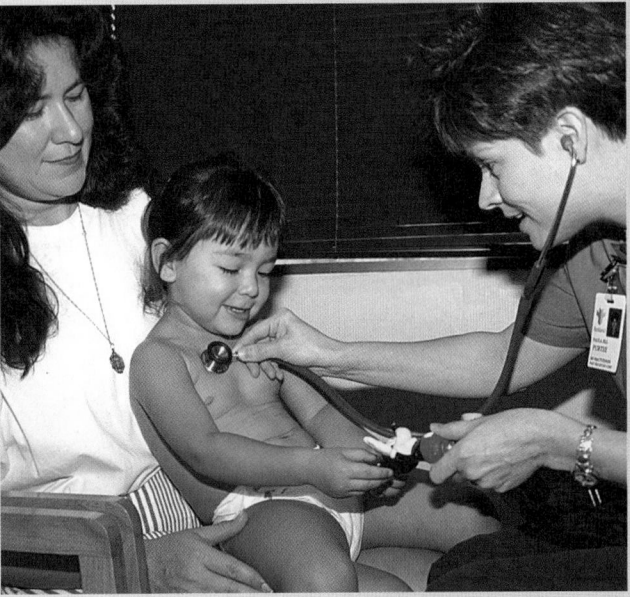

Allowing the child to check Mickey Mouse with a stethoscope before the nurse auscultates her chest enlists the child's cooperation and reduces her stress. This effort is especially important for assessments that are best done when the child is quiet. As the nurse auscultates her chest, the child is distracted by handling Mickey. Toddlers must be prepared for procedures immediately before they occur because a toddler's attention span is so short.

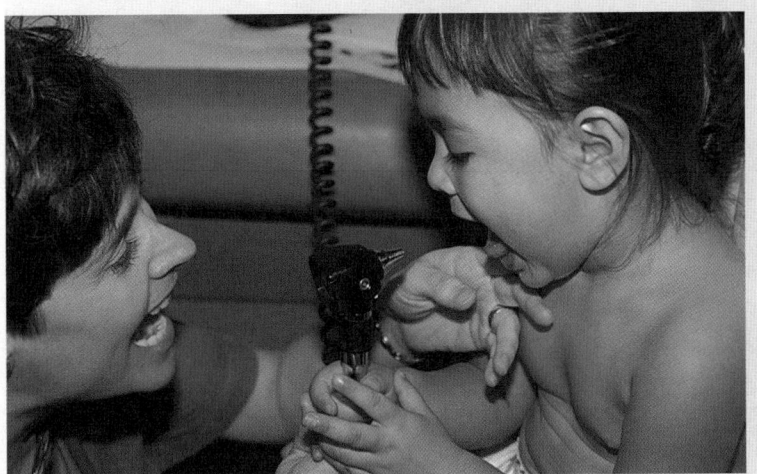

"Pant like a puppy!" the nurse tells the child as she examines her mouth and throat. Incorporating play and fun into examinations promotes the child's trust in the nurse as well as enlists her cooperation.

Continued

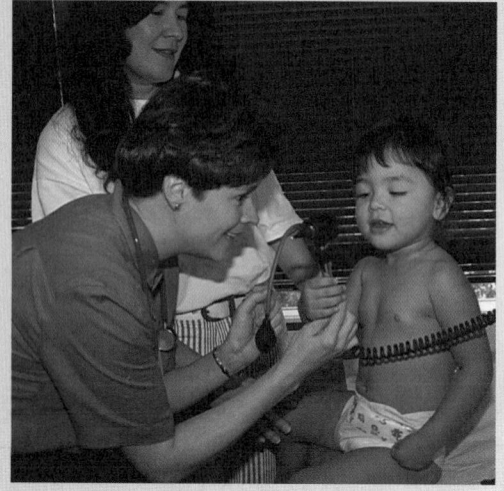

As in other examinations, the nurse helps the child examine the otoscope just before she uses it to examine her ears.

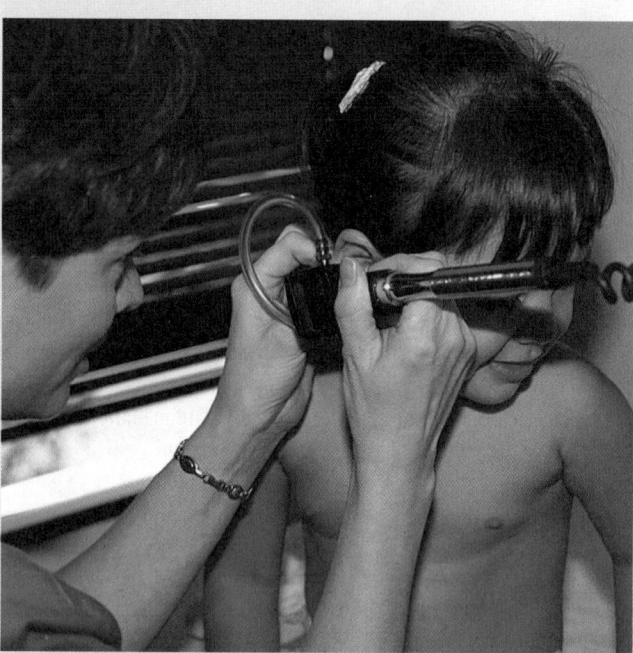

The nurse deftly examines the child's ears, pulling her pinna down and back. Ear examinations are especially important during the toddler years to identify fluid accumulation in the middle ear, which can interfere with hearing and speech development.

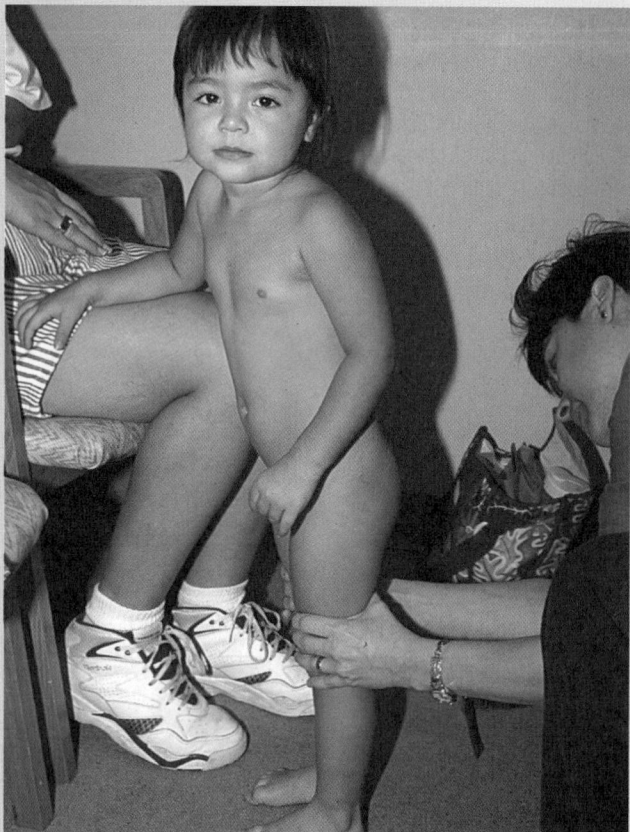

The nurse concludes the examination by checking the unclothed child for normal genital development, straightness of her spine and extremities, and evidence of previously undiagnosed hip dysplasia. To identify problems in motor development, the nurse observes the child's gait.

The nurse determines that this little girl's development is appropriate for her age. She is tall, like her mother, so the cherubic toddler appearance is less apparent than it might otherwise be. The nurse shares her findings as she does the examination and summarizes them for the mother at the end. Because the child is developing normally, she does not need to return to the clinic for a checkup until she is 3 years old.
(Photos courtesy Parkland Health and Hospital System Community Oriented Primary Care Clinic.)

Inspection

Most information is gathered during the physical examination by systematic and deliberate visual observations. The nurse first surveys an entire area of the body and then focuses on specifics, such as color, shape, size, or movement. Inspection can be both direct and indirect. Direct inspection relies on the examiner's senses of sight and hearing. Indirect inspection is accomplished with the use of special equipment, such as an otoscope, to examine a specific body area.

Palpation

During palpation, the nurse uses the sense of touch to make judgments about pulsations and vibrations and to locate structures and masses. Palpation allows the nurse to determine characteristics such as size, texture, warmth, mobility, and tenderness of various areas of the body.

Different parts of the hands are used to detect different characteristics. The fingertips are used to palpate the breast, lymph nodes, and pulses. The back of the hand is used to assess temperature. The palm of the hand is used to detect vibrations.

The type of palpation used is governed by the structure to be examined and the need to avoid any unnecessary discomfort to the child. Light palpation is accomplished by gently applying fingertip pressure to depress the skin surface approximately $1/2$ to $3/4$ inch and then moving the fingertips in a circular motion.

Deep palpation identifies abdominal structures such as the liver, spleen, and kidneys and detects abdominal masses. Deep palpation follows light palpation. The surface is depressed approximately $1^1/2$ to 2 inches to identify underlying masses and abdominal structures. Bimanual palpation is performed using both hands. The examiner superimposes one hand over the other to increase pressure or places one hand near the other to capture and trap a mass or structure between them, such as the kidneys or spleen.

Percussion

To percuss, the nurse uses quick, sharp tapping of the fingers or hands to produce sounds. Percussion is performed to locate the position, size, and density of underlying structures. The three basic methods are:

- *Mediate*, or *indirect*, *percussion*, in which the finger of one hand is placed against the body surface, and the finger of the other hand acts as the hammer
- *Immediate percussion*, performed by striking the finger of one hand directly against the body
- *Fist percussion*, in which the ulnar aspect of the fist is used to deliver a firm blow directly to the area

The method used depends on the area to be percussed. The nurse uses quick, light blows to create vibrations that

---

! CRITICAL TO REMEMBER

Using the Hands for Palpation

- Fingertips are used to palpate the breast, lymph nodes, and pulses.
- The back of the hand is used to assess temperature.
- The palm of the hand is used to identify vibrations.

BOX 33-1
Sounds Identified When Percussing

- *Flat:* high-pitched, soft-intensity sound elicited by percussing over solid masses, such as bone or muscle
- *Dull:* medium-pitched, medium-intensity sound elicited when percussing over high-density structures, such as the liver
- *Resonance:* low-pitched, loud-intensity sound elicited over a hollow organ, such as the lungs
- *Hyperresonance:* very low, very loud, with a booming quality heard over the lungs in young children
- *Tympany:* high-pitched, loud-intensity sound heard over air-filled body parts, such as the bowel or stomach

---

penetrate approximately 2 inches below the surface. Sounds identified by percussion are classified as *flat, dull, resonant, hyperresonant,* or *tympanic* (Box 33-1).

Auscultation

Auscultation entails eliciting and listening to body sounds created in the lungs, heart, blood vessels, and abdominal viscera. The most common way to auscultate is to use a stethoscope. Most auscultated sounds result from air or fluid movement within the body. The diaphragm of the stethoscope is most effective in assessing high-pitched sounds, such as heart and breath sounds. The bell of the stethoscope is most effective in hearing low-pitched sounds, such as blood pressure and vascular sounds. Auscultation requires a quiet environment. The nurse places the stethoscope on the skin in the appropriate area. Sounds heard are described according to pitch, intensity, duration, and quality.

Smell

While examining the child, the nurse uses the sense of smell to detect general body odors, common in children who are neglected or dirty. Odor may also indicate infection. Odors from the mouth, urine, or feces can be important. In particular, some diseases are characterized by odors coming from the mouth (Seidel, Ball, Dains, & Benedict, 2003).

SEQUENCE OF PHYSICAL EXAMINATION

General Appearance

During the first contact with the child and parent, the examiner forms an initial impression by making a general survey. The nurse determines the child's age, gender, and race and identifies clues concerning the child's behavior and health status. Because each child is a unique human, individual differences in behavior and health status related to growth and development will be evident. During the general survey, the examiner continually notes the parent-child interaction and the way the parent responds to the child's needs and behavior. Physical and emotional neglect as well as inadequate parental supervision for the child's age may be subtle or overt. These, together with other indicators of the child's health status, may provide clues to distress or abuse (Box 33-2).

History Taking

Taking an accurate history is the single most important component of the physical examination. Practitioners obtain three different types of health histories: the complete, or initial, history; the well, interim history; and the episodic, or problem-oriented, history.

In the *complete*, or *initial*, *history* (Box 33-3), data are gathered about the child from the time of conception to the child's current status. The *well, interim history* includes data gathered about the child from the last well visit to the current visit. When doing a well, interim history, the examiner assumes that a database is in place. In a *problem-oriented*, or *episodic*, *history* (Box 33-4), information is gathered about a

---

BOX 33-2
Potential Indicators of Child Abuse

- *Dress:* inappropriate for the weather; ragged or excessively dirty
- *Grooming and personal hygiene:* dirty teeth; broken and dirty fingernails; matted and dirty hair
- *Posture and movements:* crouching in a corner; slow, concentrated movements
- *Body image distortion:* being thin but describing self as fat
- *Speech and communication:* answering questions in words of one syllable; looking to others to respond first; seeking approval for answers
- *Facial characteristics and expressions:* fearful, anxious, tearful, sad, or angry expressions
- *Psychologic state:* labile, demanding, bizarre, overly dramatic, or condescending

---

CRITICAL THINKING EXERCISE 33-1

Ann Maloney, a 17-year-old single mother, brings her 6-month-old daughter, Kerrie, to the clinic. This is Kerrie's first visit. Ms. Maloney had made several earlier appointments for Kerrie but was always unable to keep them. She states, "I am very busy trying to work and care for Kerrie. I have had to miss work because Kerrie has had lots of colds. I hate to take time off when she is well. My supervisor at work said that it was important for her to have her immunizations and a physical examination. I guess I messed up."
1. What assumptions could the nurse make about Ms. Maloney?
2. How should the nurse respond to Ms. Maloney's comment?
3. How can the nurse best act as an advocate for both Kerrie and her mother?

BOX 33-3
The Complete History

The complete or initial history includes:
1. *Statistical information:* Name, age, address, telephone number, Social Security number, names of parents or guardians, and source of support.
2. *Client profile:* Times the child eats and sleeps, educational level, developmental level, race and nationality, religion, economic status, and health status perception. If an interpreter is used to gather the health history, the person's name is included in the record, usually in this section of the history. Also included is a statement about the reliability of an informant, such as an older sibling who answers questions concerning a younger sibling or an aunt or uncle who answers questions regarding a child visiting him or her.
3. *Health history:* Birth history, growth and development, common childhood illnesses, immunizations, previous hospitalizations, accidents or injuries, and allergies or allergic reactions and exact symptoms the allergy produced. The person taking the history should ask about medications taken daily or for an acute episode of an illness and should list all medications being taken, including dose and frequency. The parent should name both prescription and over-the-counter medications. The examiner also asks if the child has ever had a blood transfusion or has received any blood products. For any hospitalizations, serious illnesses, and injuries, the nurse should obtain the following information:
   a. Reason for admission
   b. Place of admission
   c. Length of stay
   d. Surgical procedures
   e. Outcomes
   f. Other

4. *Family history:* Information concerning the health status of the child's mother, father, siblings, and specific blood relatives such as aunts, uncles, and grandparents. If any are deceased, the history includes the age and cause of death. The purpose is to determine constitutional and hereditary factors that are likely to affect the child's health.
5. *Lifestyle and life patterns:* The child's interaction with the social, psychologic, physical, and cultural environment. Growth and development; use of street drugs, alcohol, and tobacco; roles and relationships; and family life information are all important.
6. *Review of systems:* A systematic review of the major anatomic and physiologic parts. A head-to-toe review focusing on the health function and maintenance of each body part should occur in this order:
   a. General appearance
   b. Head
   c. Hair
   d. Face
   e. Eyes
   f. Ears
   g. Nose and sinuses
   h. Mouth
   i. Throat
   j. Neck
   k. Lungs
   l. Heart
   m. Breasts
   n. Abdomen
   o. Kidneys and bladder
   p. Bowels, rectum, and anus
   q. Genitals
   r. Extremities

BOX 33-4
Problem-Oriented History

- *Chief complaint:* Use the child's own words.
- *Body location:* Place the problem somewhere on the body.
- *Quality:* Define what the problem is like for the child.
- *Quantity:* Describe the intensity of the problem for the child.
- *Chronology:* Determine when the problem began, the periodicity and frequency, and the course of symptoms.
- *Setting:* Identify where the problem occurs.
- *Aggravating and alleviating factors:* Find out what makes the problem better or worse.
- *Associated manifestations:* Document other related information.
- *Treatment:* Document what has been used to treat the problem. Be sure to ask about complementary therapies as well as traditional approaches.

current problem. Information about the specific problem is then added to the existing database.

Recording Data

The information gathered during the history is documented concisely to provide all necessary information from pregnancy to the child's current status. Milestones in growth and development, immunizations, and family status are always included in the child's history.

Vital Signs

Vital signs are taken on every child at every visit in ambulatory settings and are monitored throughout the day in a hospitalized child. Assessment of vital signs (temperature, pulse, respirations, blood pressure) is an important way to measure and monitor vital body functions. Measuring vital signs provides the basis for decisions concerning the child's overall health and illness. In children, changes in vital signs are important signs of changes in health status. Table 33-1 describes normal vital signs by age, and Chapter 37 details the procedure for taking vital signs in children.

Temperature

The method for measuring children's temperature may vary from one setting to another. Some parents are comfortable taking a rectal or axillary temperature. Health care providers may use a tympanic membrane sensor, an electronic, or a digital thermometer. Currently, parents are encouraged to take axillary rather than rectal temperatures. Reasons for the recommendation are the invasive nature of rectal temperature measurements, the risk of injury, and their questionable accuracy with febrile children, because feces retain body heat for hours after a fever has diminished. Axillary temperatures, when taken correctly, provide accurate information concerning changes in the child's health status.

Tympanic temperature measurements are frequently used in health care agencies because they can be performed quickly and involve less cross contamination; however, they may not be as accurate in detecting fever in infants and young children (Houlder, 2000). When recording a tympanic

TABLE **33-1** Normal Vital Signs by Age

Age	Temperature*		Pulse Rate (beats/min)	Respiratory Rate (breaths/min)	Blood Pressure Range (mm Hg)
	Degrees Fahrenheit	Degrees Celsius			
Newborn	96.8-99 (axillary)	36-37.2 (axillary)	120-160	30-60	Systolic: 60-99† Diastolic: 30-62†
4 yr	97.5-98.6 (axillary)	36.4-37 (axillary)	80-125	20-30	*Girls* Systolic: 101-111 Diastolic: 63-71 *Boys* Systolic: 102-115 Diastolic: 62-71
10 yr	97.5-98.6 (oral)	36.4-37 (oral)	70-110‡	16-22	*Girls* Systolic: 112-122 Diastolic: 73-80 *Boys* Systolic: 110-123 Diastolic: 73-82
16 yr	97.5-98.6 (oral)	36.4-37 (oral)	55-90	15-20	*Girls* Systolic: 120-130 Diastolic: 79-86 *Boys* Systolic: 125-130 Diastolic: 79-87

*The normal range of the child's temperature will depend on the method used. Temperatures exhibit circadian rhythms at all ages.
† Taken with Doppler.
‡After age 12 yr, a boy's pulse is 5 beats/min slower than a girl's.

temperature, the nurse notes the side on which the temperature was elicited. Variation can occur from one ear to the other on the same child.

An oral thermometer may be used with older children, usually at 5 or 6 years old. For oral temperature measurements, an electronic thermometer is unbreakable and registers quickly but it may not be available (see Chapter 37 for a discussion of various methods of assessing temperature).

Pulse

Apical pulse rates are taken in children younger than 2 years and in any child who has an irregular heart rate or known congenital heart disease. Radial pulse rates may be taken in children older than 2 years. To compensate for normal irregularities, the nurse counts the pulse for 1 full minute. Chapter 37 details the procedure for measuring pulse.

Arterial pulses are palpated to determine pulse rate and rhythm and to evaluate blood flow, arterial wall elasticity, and vessel patency. To determine the position of the heart in the anterior precordium, the nurse palpates the apical impulse in infants and children younger than 6 years. In the acute care setting, an apical impulse is always palpated on every child and the location of the apical impulse is noted. Simultaneously, the examiner palpates and compares femoral, radial, and carotid pulses on children of any age. The nurse may also compare a carotid pulse with a femoral or radial pulse for equality of pulses. In infants, the nurse notes the pulsating anterior fontanel. The pulse may be increased significantly above normal in infants and children with anxiety, fever, exercise, inflammatory illnesses, shock, or heart disease. The resting heart rate changes with increasing age.

The rhythm of the heartbeat is assessed for equal spacing between consecutive beats. Irregular cardiac rhythms are not uncommon in children and are often related to changes in rhythm that occur in response to respiratory inspiration and expiration.

Respirations

The nurse observes the rate, depth, and ease of respiration in the child. Respirations vary with age. The respiratory rate, like the heart rate, is significantly influenced by emotion and exercise. In infants, the rate may be determined by observing abdominal excursion. In toddlers and older children, the nurse observes thoracic excursion. Because the movements are irregular, the rate should be assessed for 1 minute in infants and young children. Respirations are best counted when the child is not paying attention to the examiner. Respirations should be counted while the examiner continues to keep fingers on a pulse or the stethoscope on the chest, as though checking the pulses. This effort will ensure that the child is unaware that the examiner is counting respirations.

The depth and rhythm of respirations are determined subjectively and compared with norms for a particular age-group. The ease or difficulty of respirations is a somewhat subjective observation. Respirations should be quiet and appear effortless. Stridor—a crowing noise heard on inspiration and heard louder over the neck—is worrisome in a child and may be a sign of croup or epiglottitis (see Chapter 45). Inspiratory stridor indicates a partial obstruction of the airway. Continuous inspiratory and expiratory stridor may be related to delayed development of the cartilage in the tracheal rings or to a relatively small larynx.

Blood Pressure

Blood pressure measurements are taken on all children at every ambulatory visit; in an acute care setting, blood pressure is measured at least daily, and often more frequently, depending on the child's condition. The appropriate-size cuff must be used to auscultate the blood pressure. Blood pressure measurements in healthy ambulatory children are compared with standard norms (see Table 33-1 for the effects of age on vital signs). In children, blood pressure is more closely correlated to height than it is to age. (See Appendix G for blood pressures values for boys and girls by percentiles of height) Three abnormal blood pressures readings obtained at different times should be obtained before determining that a child has hypertension. Blood pressure is monitored more closely on any child suspected of having a condition that affects blood pressure, such as hypertension, cardiovascular disease, kidney disease, or liver disease (Flynn, 2003).

The size of the cuff is important. Cuffs that are too small will cause falsely elevated values; those that are too large will cause inaccurate low values (see Chapter 37 for determining appropriate cuff size). Several determinations may be needed to obtain values unaffected by anxiety. Instructing the child that the "balloon" will gently squeeze the arm or give the arm a "hug" will usually decrease anxiety. To alleviate anxiety, the child can also assist with taking a blood pressure on a doll, a stuffed animal, or the parent.

Anthropometric Measurement

Anthropometrics entails measuring the human body and assessing nutritional status as well as growth and development. Weight, height, and head circumference are always measured in children and are compared with averages for age-group and gender. The amount of body fat should be measured based on the body mass index (BMI), which is calculated using a simple formula:

$$BMI = \frac{Weight\ (kg)}{Height\ (m)^2} \quad OR \quad BMI = \frac{Weight\ (lbs) \times 703}{Height\ (in)^2}$$

BMI tables can be accessed at *www.cdc.gov/nccdphp/dnpa/bmi/00binaries/bmi-tables.pdfhildren*. Midarm muscle circumference, skinfold thickness, and weight provide information about three body tissues (subcutaneous tissue, muscle, fat) altered by nutrition. Anthropometric measurements are most valuable when they are evaluated serially so that trends can be monitored.

Measuring height and weight are routine procedures that provide valuable information about the health of a child. Children grow and develop rapidly, and this growth and development must be constantly evaluated. Physical measurements of a child reflect the rate of growth; a failure in growth,

---

! CRITICAL TO REMEMBER

Importance of Anthropometric Measurements

Anthropometric measurements reflect any change in the growth pattern and may be the first clue to a serious problem. Measurements must be taken at every health care visit from birth to adulthood. A child's falling off his or her own growth curve is a significant indicator of changing health status.

an acceleration in growth, or any change in growth pattern may be the first clue to serious problems. A child's falling off the child's own growth curve is the most significant indicator of changing health status. Measurements must be correct and accurate and are taken at every visit from birth to adulthood.

Height

The methods of measurement of a child vary with age. Length of infants and toddlers is best measured with the child lying down on a flat measuring board. This method is used until the child is able to stand independently. The child's head is held securely to the headboard, and the movable foot-board is stretched to touch the child's heel. If a measuring board is not available for the infant and young child, it is possible to position the child's body on a flat surface, mark the point where the heel touches the surface, and then mark the point where the top of the head is lying on the surface, taking care to ensure that the child's legs and body are straight on the surface. The examiner then removes the child and measures the distance between the two points with a measuring tape. Measuring the length of the child in this manner is not as accurate as using a measuring board.

When a child is able to cooperate and stand without support, around age 2 years, the examiner stands the child in stocking feet next to a standard measuring tape that begins at the child's heel and is not displaced by room molding. A flat, hard surface is used to reach from the top of the child's head to the tape so that the examiner does not guess or add height because of the hair. If this is the first standing measurement, there may be a slight discrepancy from the lying measurement.

Once the measurement is taken, it must be plotted on a standardized growth chart appropriate for length or height measurement (see Appendix E). Height and weight are evaluated by determining whether the child is following a predictable percentile curve on a growth chart. Height and weight are related to hereditary factors and will vary from child to child.

Weight

The method and equipment for weighing vary with the child's age. All scales must be balanced first before weighing. Infants are placed in a lying position on a regular baby scale with all their clothing removed. Older children who are able to stand or walk without support may be weighed on the adult standing scale. On the older child, remove all clothing except underwear. Like height, weight is plotted on a standardized growth chart (see Appendix E).

Head Circumference

Head circumference is measured on all children from birth to age 36 months and plotted on a standard growth chart on all visits. Children older than 3 years with any questionable head size—megalocephaly or microcephaly—should have their head circumference measured at every visit. To measure the head circumference, a nonstretching measuring tape is wrapped above the supraorbital ridges and over the most prominent part of the occiput (Fig. 33-1).

The head circumference is plotted on a standardized growth chart. During the first year of life, the head circumference normally increases by 0.4 inch (1 cm) each month. Head circumference can reflect an abnormal rate of development, give some indication of nutritional status, and possibly indicate tumor growth.

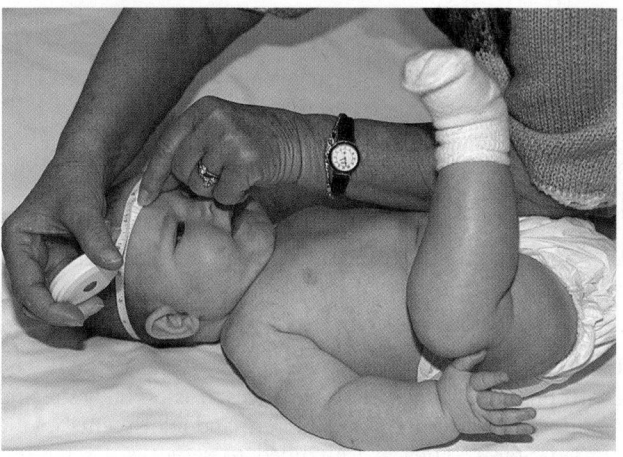

Figure 33-1 Measuring head circumference. The head circumference is measured from birth through age 36 months. The nurse uses a nonstretching tape and measures in a "hat band" position, just above the eyebrows and around the occipital prominence in the back. Chest circumference is also routinely measured in the newborn and is usually smaller than the newborn's head circumference. (Courtesy The University of Texas at Arlington School of Nursing.)

Chest Circumference

Chest circumference is routinely measured only in the newborn. The newborn's head circumference is larger than the chest circumference. Chest circumference is almost equal to head circumference after age 1 year. To measure chest circumference, the measuring tape is wrapped around the chest at the nipple line. The measurement is taken between inspiration and expiration.

Midarm Circumference

Midarm circumference reflects muscle mass and fat. To measure midarm circumference, the midpoint on the arm between the acromial process and the olecranon process is determined. Then, with the arm hanging loosely at the side, the child's arm is measured at the midpoint with a tape measure. The measurement is recorded in centimeters. With a decrease in fat or muscle atrophy, the midarm circumference decreases. It will increase with weight gain.

Triceps Skinfold

Triceps skinfold thickness indicates total body fat, because at least half of body fat is directly below the skin. Metal calipers are used to obtain this measurement. On the nondominant arm, the midpoint of the arm is determined using the same method as is used for measuring midarm circumference. With the arm hanging loosely at the side, a fold of skin at the midpoint on the posterior aspect of the arm is grasped. To avoid error, the child is asked to flex the arm muscle after the examiner grasps the skin. If contraction is felt, muscle as well as fat has been grasped. The examiner applies the caliper and takes a reading after waiting 3 seconds. Fat stores decrease with long-term undernutrition and malnutrition.

Use of Growth Charts

An accurate record of an infant's or child's overall pattern of growth is best determined by serial measurements over months or years. The National Center for Health Statistics

TABLE **33-2** Body Mass Index (BMI)

BMI	Description	Percent
<27.5	Normal	65.2
27.5-30.0	Mild obesity	9.0
>30.0-40.0	Moderate obesity	20.5
>40.0	Morbid obesity	5.2
Total		99.9

BOX 33-5
Skin Color Terminology

- *Vitiligo:* areas of depigmentation
- *Nevi:* areas of increased pigmentation
- *Jaundice:* a yellow discoloration of the skin, best seen in the sclera of the eyes
- *Cyanosis:* a blue discoloration of the skin, best seen in all races in the mucous membranes of the mouth, particularly under the tongue
- *Carotenemia:* an orange color of the skin, best seen on the soles of the feet and palms of the hands
- *Pallor:* loss of skin color
- *Erythema:* diffusely red
- *Mottling:* discolored areas of the skin

! CRITICAL TO REMEMBER

Skin Inspection in Dark-Skinned Children

- Erythema: dusky red or violet
- Cyanosis: black or dusky
- Jaundice: diffusely darker than the child's normal color

(NCHS) publishes growth charts (see Appendix E). The charts provide a single set of references to assess body size and monitor growth in infants, children, and adolescents in the United States. They are intended to serve as a reference rather than as growth standards or clinical ideals to be achieved.

National survey data for all racial and ethnic groups are combined to develop the growth charts. Racial and ethnic differences in growth appear to be attributable primarily to environmental influences. Special growth charts for premature infants, children with genetic alterations, such as Down syndrome, and cultural variations such as Asian children, are now available from the American Academy of Pediatrics.

The recently revised charts include these components:

- Infant charts for birth to age 3 years relate length, weight, and head circumference to age and relate weight to length.
- Charts for ages 2 through 19 years relate stature, weight, and BMI to age. BMI has been recommended for evaluating and tracking overweight children and adolescents. The 85th percentile line helps identify children at risk for overweight.

Separate charts exist for boys and girls.

To plot on a growth chart, the exact age of the child is determined on the chart's horizontal axis. The corresponding measurement is marked on the chart's vertical axis. The chart is marked where the two lines intersect. The percentile lines on these charts indicate the number of children expected to fall above and below the child's measurement.

Weight and height measurements above the 97th percentile or below the 3rd percentile on a standard growth chart may indicate a growth disturbance and need further investigation. BMIs at or above the 95th percentile in children older than 2 years indicate obesity (Story, Holt, & Sofka, 2002) (Table 33-2).

Generally, black children weigh less than white children during the first 2 years of life, but as they grow they tend to be taller and heavier than white children of the same age. Asian children are found to be shorter and lighter than white counterparts.

Skin, Hair, and Nails

Skin

Skin assessment includes inspection and palpation. The entire skin surface is examined for color, texture, turgor, and presence of lesions. This examination may be combined with assessment of other areas of the body.

Inspection. The nurse observes the color and pigmentation of the skin. Skin color reflects the amount of melanin and can range from pink to black (Box 33-5). In dark-skinned infants and children, erythema will appear dusky red or violet; cyanosis will appear black; and jaundice will appear diffusely darker. In dark-skinned infants and children, it is best to determine the normal skin color and then compare any color change with the normal color. Color changes to the skin may be related to sun exposure or tattooing.

Palpation. The examiner palpates the skin to assess moisture, temperature, texture, turgor, edema, and lesions.

Moisture is assessed by lightly stroking the skin surface and body creases. The external skin on exposed areas is normally dryer than unexposed areas of the skin.

Temperature is assessed by using the back of the hand, because it is more sensitive to skin changes. The two sides of the child's body are compared with each other.

Normal *texture* of the skin is described as being smooth and soft. Scars or excessive scar tissue should be noted.

Turgor is assessed by grasping the skin between the thumb and index finger and quickly releasing it (Fig. 33-2). The skin normally returns to place without excessive skin markings. Skin that "tents" when released indicates dehydration. The abdomen and upper arm are the best places to test for tissue turgor on a child.

Edema, the accumulation of excessive salt and water in the interstitial spaces, is identified by pressing the thumb into areas of the body that may appear puffy. The extremities and buttocks are classic areas to palpate for edema in the child. Periorbital edema is observed on the eyelids.

Lesions are identified, noting configuration, distribution, color, and size. Skin lesions are identified as primary lesions, arising from normal skin (e.g., freckle), or secondary lesions, resulting from an alteration of a primary lesion (e.g., scab). Configuration of a skin lesion refers to the arrangement or position of several lesions in relation to each other or to the arrangement of a single lesion. Distribution refers to the body location and the symmetry or asymmetry of lesions.

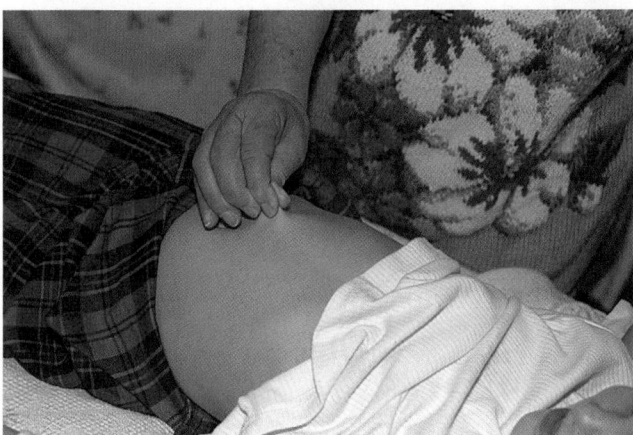

Figure 33-2 Skin turgor is best tested by grasping the abdominal skin between the thumb and forefinger and quickly releasing it. "Tenting" (persistent elevation of the skin when released) suggests dehydration. (Courtesy The University of Texas at Arlington School of Nursing.)

Hair

Hair normally covers the entire body except for the palms, soles, and parts of the genitalia. Hair is examined for texture, changes in color, unusual distribution, and cleanliness.

Scalp hair has a wide range of normal textures, including straight, curly, or kinky. The hair is usually shiny, silky, and strong. The examiner should keep in mind the age and development of the child. Fine, downy hair is normal for a newborn, whereas in an older child it would lead the examiner to consider nutrition and endocrine abnormalities. Brittle hair, identified when the hairs break off easily when bent between the fingers, also might indicate endocrine and nutrition abnormalities.

The color of the hair is genetically determined and may be anything from pale blond to black. Changes in color may be caused by depigmentation, hereditary factors, or chemicals applied to the hair. Hair texture varies widely with race.

The distribution of the hair over the head is identified. In most children, the hair begins in a whorl and then is distributed over the head. Some children may have more than one whorl. Scalp hair does not grow beyond the nape of the neck or down to the eyebrows. *Hirsutism* is defined as excessive hair growth; *alopecia* is unusual hair loss.

The hair is separated and examined for cleanliness, signs of trauma, lesions, or scaling. The scalp should be clean and free of any infestations. Most cases of head lice (*pediculosis capitis*) are first detected when one or more children are seen scratching their heads. Closer observation may reveal nits adhering to the hairs. Depending on their distance from the scalp, usually these are the whitish to sand-colored empty shells of eggs that have hatched (see Chapter 49 for further discussion of the integumentary system).

Nails

Nails are inspected and palpated for shape and contour. The nail surface is normally flat or slightly convex. The edges of the nails should be smooth, rounded, and clean. Clubbing of fingernails can be identified by looking at the index finger; the angle at the nail base and the finger should be less than 160 degrees. On palpation, the base of the fingernail should be firm. On touching the index fingernails back to back, a diamond of light below the knuckle and above where the fin-

gernails touch will be present. In early clubbing, the diamond shape is decreased or not apparent (see Chapter 46).

Pressing and releasing on the nail edge assesses capillary refill; the nail will blanch, and then color will return to the nail within 1 to 2 seconds. A capillary refill time of more than 2 seconds may be caused by anemia, peripheral edema, vasoconstriction, or decreased cardiac output as a result of hypovolemia, shock, or congestive heart failure (Jarvis, 2000).

Lymph Nodes

Lymph nodes are inspected and palpated. Lymph tissue is found all over the body and must be evaluated as the examiner assesses body systems. Always assess for enlarged lymph nodes in the head and neck, the supraclavicular area, the axillary region, the arms, and the inguinal region (Fig. 33-3). At the time these areas are examined, the lymph nodes are assessed as well. When an enlarged lymph node or a mass is found during examination, its characteristics should be described (Box 33-6).

To palpate for most lymph nodes, the examiner uses the distal portion of the fingers and gently but firmly moves the fingers in a circular motion to determine the node's characteristics and mobility.

Lymph nodes that are enlarged, warm, and firm and fluctuant are a sign of infection. Lymph nodes that are small, firm, and shotty (freely palpable and very small) are often palpable in healthy infants and children, up to the age of 12 years, in the cervical, axillary, inguinal, and occipital areas (Fox, 2002). An enlarged supraclavicular lymph node on the left in

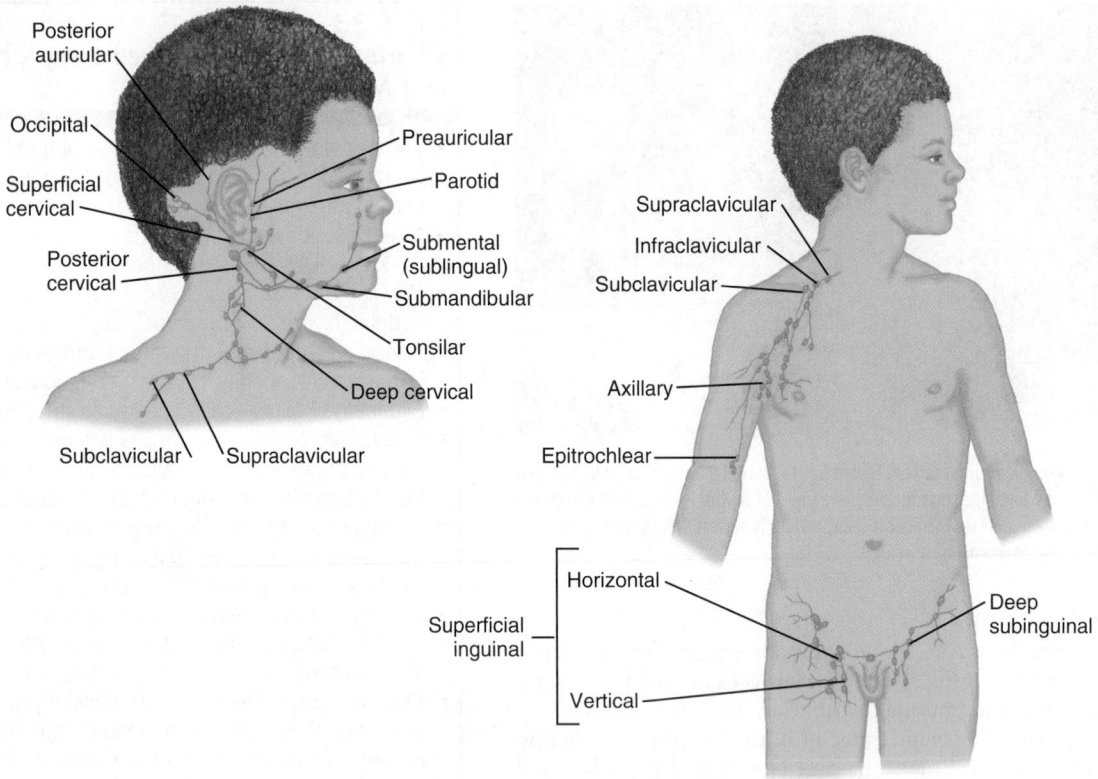

Figure 33-3 Location of superficial lymph nodes.

> **BOX 33-7**
> *Head Shape Terminology*
>
> - *Normocephalic:* normal-size head
> - *Microcephalic:* head small for body size and age
> - *Macrocephalic:* abnormally large head
> - *Bossing:* frontal enlargement

young children is called the *sentinel node* because it may suggest a Wilms tumor or other neoplastic disease.

Head, Neck, and Face

Head

The head is inspected and palpated. To examine the head, the examiner must see and feel. The head is evaluated from the front, the back, and the sides. The head is examined for symmetry, paralysis, weakness, and movement (Box 33-7).

Symmetry is assessed by looking at and feeling the entire head. If any lumps or bumps are seen or felt, the examiner notes their exact location and size and density. The suture lines in infants should be palpated. Sutures are felt as prominent ridges in the newborn but usually flatten by 6 months.

Paralysis and weakness of the head are directly related to the condition of the neck muscles. That is, paralysis and weakness of the head will occur with paralysis or weakness of the neck muscles.

Head movement is evaluated by observing the child move the head. Head control is observed with the child in a lying position and while the examiner grasps the child's hands and pulls the infant into a sitting position. An infant younger

than 4 months may show some head lag, but the infant in an upright position should be able to maintain the head upright for several seconds. Head lag after age 6 months may indicate poor muscle development. The head should be put through a full range of motion by asking the older child to look up, down, and sideways. After age 4 months, inability to move the head or to hold the head in an upright position may be related to paralysis or weakness of the neck muscles.

The fontanels are inspected and palpated for size, tenseness, and pulsation (Fig. 33-4). The posterior fontanel is closed by age 2 to 3 months. The anterior fontanel should be soft and flat when the child is sitting. Measure the width and length of an open anterior fontanel. The anterior fontanel should be less than 5 cm in length and width after age 12 months and should be completely closed by age 12 to 18 months. A sunken fontanel is associated with dehydration, and a bulging fontanel can be associated with increased intracranial pressure. A bulging fontanel is normally seen when an infant cries, coughs, or vomits.

Neck

In the child, the neck is inspected and palpated for symmetry, size, and shape, which is directly related to the use or disuse of the neck muscles. The infant's neck is relatively short and lengthens as the child grows. View the neck from the front, the back, and both sides. Webbing of the neck—the presence of an extra fold of skin posteriorly—is associated with some chromosomal abnormalities such as trisomy 21, or Down syndrome.

The neck is mobile and supple. While palpating the child's neck, the thyroid gland is palpated by identifying the isthmus of the thyroid across the trachea. To identify an enlarged thyroid in a child, the examiner gently displaces the thyroid gland laterally and palpates thyroid tissue with the

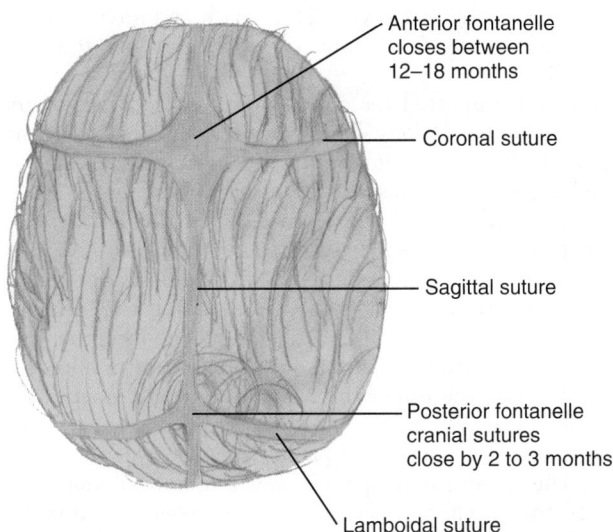

Figure 33-4 Fontanels are inspected and palpated for size, tenseness, and pulsation.

opposite thumb and fingers. The lobe may be more palpable when the child swallows.

Face

The child's face is inspected and palpated for dysmorphic features. Spacing and symmetry of facial features are noted. The face is observed for any changes in color or the presence of edema, such as cellulitis. The eyes are examined for size, position, and configuration. *Hypertelorism* is a condition in which the eyes are unusually widely spaced; in *hypotelorism*, the eyes are unusually close together. The child's nostrils should be oval in shape and equal in size, with no evidence of a hypoplastic philtrum (shallow crease or absence of a crease below the nose). The lips should be equal on either side of the midline. The child's ears are inspected for alignment. Low-set ears are identified when the auricle of the ear does not cross or touch the eye-occiput line. The position of the auricle should be almost vertical, with no more than a 10-degree lateral posterior angle (Fig. 33-5).

The functions of cranial nerve V (trigeminal nerve) and cranial nerve VII (facial nerve) are evaluated while assessing the face. Cranial nerve V is evaluated by observing chewing or sucking, which demonstrates the strength of the temporomandibular joint, and by touching the child's forehead and cheeks with a piece of cotton. The child should move the head or bat the object away. Cranial nerve VII is evaluated by having the child frown, smile, or make a face while the examiner observes for symmetry of movement. Having the child puff out the cheeks or whistle also allows the examiner to evaluate cranial nerve VII (Jarvis, 2000).

Nose, Mouth, and Throat

Nose

The examiner should wear gloves when doing the nasal examination. Note any drainage coming from the nose. Describe the amount, color, and consistency.

The external nose is inspected and palpated. Patency can be determined by occluding one nostril and having the child sniff. Repeat on the other side. The external nose is observed

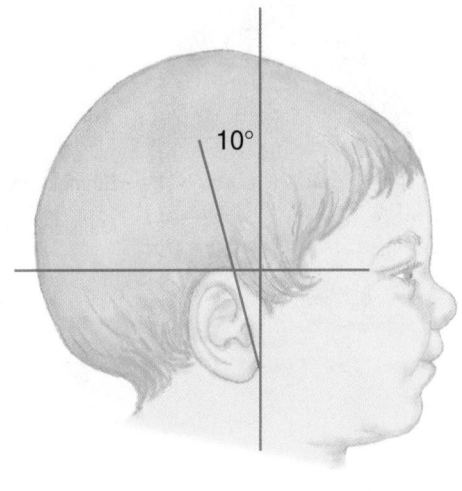

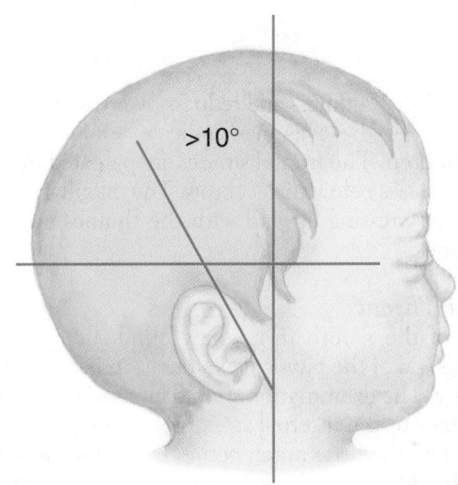

Figure 33-5 The child's ears are inspected for alignment. Low-set ears could indicate mental retardation or renal anomalies.

for symmetry, deformity, inflammation, or skin lesions. The "allergic salute," frequent wiping of the nose because of drainage, produces a transverse crease on the child's nose and indicates that the child has allergies. Palpate the entire external nose for septal deviation or other deformities. The sense of smell is mediated by cranial nerve I. This function can be evaluated by having the child close the eyes, occlude one nostril, and identify familiar odors, such as cinnamon, peppermint, orange, or cherry.

The nasal cavity can be examined by using a short, wide-tipped speculum on the otoscope and inserting it into the nasal vestibule, being careful not to put pressure on the nasal septum. The nasal mucosa is inspected for color and moisture. The nasal mucosa is normally smooth and moist, with a bright pink color. In children with allergies, the mucosa is pale and appears boggy. With infectious diseases, the mucosa is erythematous and swollen; the nasal drainage may be yellow or green. The nasal septum is examined for intactness and for any deviation.

The *frontal* and *maxillary sinuses* are inspected and palpated (Fig. 33-6). The areas over the sinuses are examined for

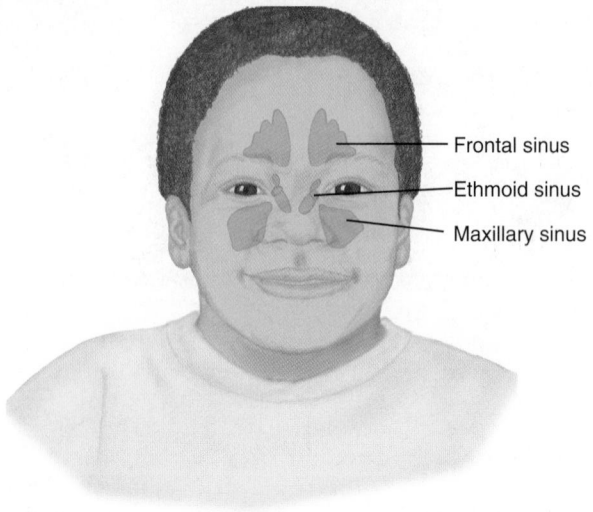

Figure 33-6 The frontal, ethmoid, and maxillary sinuses.

color and swelling. Puffiness and redness over the sinuses and dark circles under the eyes may indicate an inflammatory process in children. The frontal sinuses are palpated by pressing over the sinuses below the eyebrow. The maxillary sinuses are palpated by pressing upward with the thumbs under the maxillary bones.

Mouth and Throat

Assessment of the mouth in a young child should be performed at the end of the physical examination because it may create anxiety. The examination should proceed from the anterior structures to the internal structures of the mouth.

The *philtrum*, the little notch between the nose and upper lip, should be intact. In children with dysmorphic features, the philtrum is absent or shallow.

The examiner should wear gloves when doing the oral examination. A tongue blade and a good penlight assist with visualization of the oral cavity. The mouth and internal structures are examined using inspection, palpation, and the sense of smell.

Lips are inspected for color, moisture, cracking, or the presence of any lesions. The alveolar frenulum, which attaches the lips to the gums, should be intact. The lips are palpated to identify any masses.

The *buccal mucosa* is examined by holding the cheeks open with a tongue blade and examining for color, nodules, or lesions. Significant mouth odors should be noted. For many children, this part of the examination can be unpleasant. To facilitate the child's cooperation, the examiner may want to demonstrate on a doll or on the parent or allow the child to place the tongue blade in the parent's mouth. The buccal mucosa should be pink, smooth, and moist. Dark-skinned children may have patchy areas of hyperpigmentation. The opening of the *parotid gland* is found as a small dimple on the buccal mucosa opposite the upper second molar. The entire surface of the buccal mucosa is palpated for changes in consistency or masses.

Teeth are inspected for number, cavities, tooth formation, and occlusion. The number and characteristics of the teeth will change with growth and development (Fig. 33-7). The eruption of deciduous teeth begins around the 6th month of extrauterine life; all 20 deciduous teeth are present by age 30 months. Have the child bite down, and gently part the lips and note the position of the teeth. The upper teeth slightly override the lower teeth. The color and shape of each tooth should be noted. The crown is white, with some variation from person to person. Permanent teeth are larger and have a darker color than deciduous teeth. Brown or black discoloration of the teeth is usually caused by dental caries. Long-term use of certain medications (i.e., tetracycline, iron) may stain teeth. With excessive fluoride ingestion, the enamel of the permanent teeth may appear mottled. The shape of the tooth is determined by age, development, and the amount of wear.

The gums (*gingivae*) are inspected and palpated for color and swelling. The gum surface has a pink, stippled appearance and feels firm. Dark-skinned children may have a dark-pigmented line along the gingival margin.

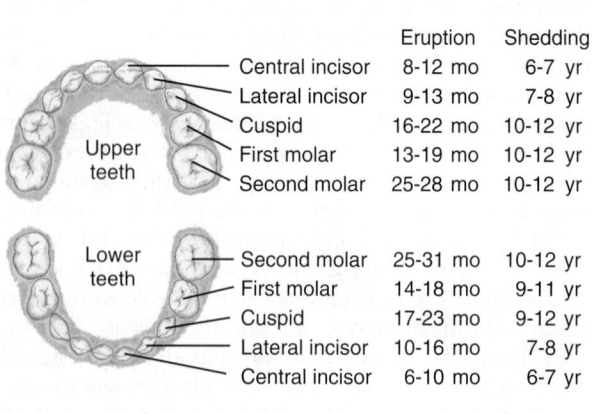

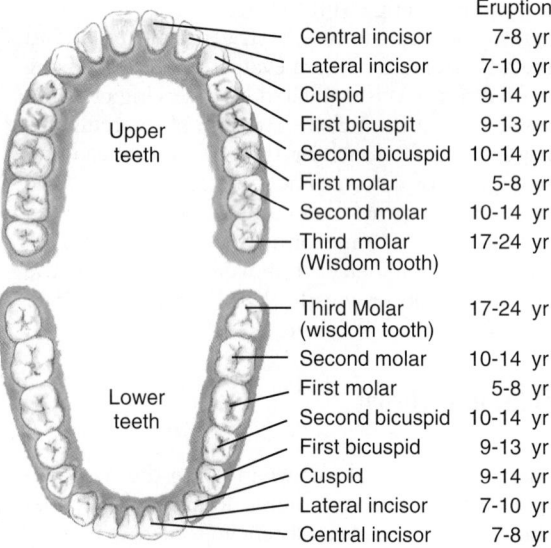

Figure 33-7 Sequence of eruption of primary and secondary teeth.

The floor of the mouth can be inspected by asking the child to lift the tongue to the roof of the mouth. Observe the frenulum, sublingual ridge, and Wharton's ducts, which lie on either side of the frenulum. The color of the floor of the mouth is pink.

The tongue is inspected and palpated. The dorsum of the tongue should appear dull red, moist, and glistening, with a white coat. The anterior portion of the tongue should have a slightly roughened appearance with papillae and small fissures. The tongue is palpated for indurations or ulcerations. While palpating the mouth of a young child, biting can be prevented by holding the child's cheeks.

Cranial nerve XII (*hypoglossal nerve*) is examined by asking the child to stick out the tongue as though licking a lollipop and observe for any deviation of the tongue to one side. The examiner can determine the strength of the tongue by placing a finger to the side of the child's cheek and asking the child to press the tongue against the examiner's finger. The tongue should feel equally strong on each side.

The hard palate, soft palate, and uvula are examined by asking the child to tilt the head back. The examiner inspects the hard palate for shape and color. The hard palate is whitish and convex, with transverse rugae. The examiner palpates the hard palate for the height of the arch and intactness. The examiner can allow the infant to suck on a gloved finger while palpating the hard palate to determine the strength of the sucking reflex. The soft palate is continuous with the hard palate and is concave and pinker in color. The uvula varies in length and thickness and is located in midline as a continuation of the soft palate. Cranial nerves IX (*glossopharyngeal nerve*) and X (*vagus nerve*) are evaluated at this time. The child is asked to say "ah"; normally, the soft palate and the uvula rise symmetrically and phonation of "ah" is understood.

A tongue blade is used to depress the tongue and observe the oropharynx. This action can be unpleasant for the child. To minimize discomfort, the examiner slides the tongue blade along the side of the tongue until reaching the soft palate and then compresses the tongue to elicit the gag reflex (cranial nerve X) and observes the back of the throat. The tonsillar pillars are inspected with particular notation of size and color of tonsils. The tonsils are pink in color.

The size of tonsils varies; large tonsils are common in young children. Tonsils may have crypts where food particles collect. With inflammatory processes, the crypts may contain exudate. A child whose parents comment on the child's snoring or waking up by snoring may have grossly enlarged tonsils. The posterior wall of the pharynx should be smooth and glistening pink; the wall may have small, irregular spots of lymphatic tissue and small blood vessels (Seidel, Ball, Dains, & Benedict, 2003).

Eyes

The eyes are inspected and palpated, as well as evaluated for visual acuity and extraocular muscle function.

Visual Acuity

Visual acuity can be difficult to evaluate in a young child. Acuity develops over time, and evaluation requires the child's cooperation. Items needed for evaluating visual acuity in a child are an eye cover and vision charts (Box 33-8). The chart cho-

sen will be determined by the child's age and development. The infant from birth to age 1 or 2 months gazes at black-and-white contrasting figures and faces. At age 4 weeks or older, an infant fixes on a brightly colored object and follows it.

Depending on verbal ability, children age 2 years may be able to use Allen cards to identify pictures from a distance of 15 feet. Each eye is tested separately. The child should be able to name three of seven cards in a maximum of five tries.

Preschool children can be tested using the HOTV chart at 10 feet. A card with *H, O, T,* and *V* is given to the child to hold. One eye is covered, and the child is instructed to match the letters on the held card with the chart at 10 feet with the uncovered eye. The child holds the letters, or they are placed on a table directly in front of the child.

Older children's visual acuity can be tested using the Snellen chart, placed on a wall 20 feet away from the child. The chart should have no glare and should be well illuminated. No other materials should be around or near the chart. Test both eyes together first, and then test each eye separately. If the child has corrective lenses, the procedure should be repeated with the corrective lenses on. Unless the child is known to have very poor vision, testing is begun at the line on the chart for 40 feet. To determine at what level the child cannot see, the examiner finds the distance at which the child misses half plus one of the symbols on a line of the chart. The visual acuity is then designated as the smallest line at which the child is able to identify more than half the symbols on the line. For corrective lenses, the examiner notes the last date the child was examined for a prescription. Findings are recorded by noting the distance of the line correctly read for both eyes (i.e., right eye 20/20, left eye 20/20). This annotation means that the child has correctly interpreted the letters on the chart for 20 feet at a distance of 20 feet, which matches what the average child can see at that distance. If the child correctly identifies the letters on the line labeled *40 feet,* that child can see at 20 feet what the average child can see at 40 feet. Visual acuity changes with age and varies according to the test used. Normal ranges are:

- *Birth:* fixates on objects (8 to 12 inches), 20/100 to 20/150
- *4 months:* 20/50 to 20/80
- *1 year:* 20/40 to 20/70
- *4 years:* 20/30 to 20/40
- *5 years:* 20/20 to 20/30

Color Vision

Color vision deficit, less correctly termed *color blindness,* is an inherited recessive X-linked trait that, in varying degrees, may affect the child's ability to discern traffic lights, brake lights, and color-coordinated clothing. Color discrimination occurs through integration of information from the cone pigments in the retinal layers of the eye. The genes for some colors are located on the X chromosome, and because boys have only one X chromosome, they are more likely to have color vision deficit. Color vision deficit may affect learning if the learning is color-related. The condition is very rare in females but affects 8% to 10% of males.

Color vision is evaluated using Ishihara charts—a series of polychromatic cards. These cards have a pattern of colored pictures embedded in the charts. Children between ages 4 and 8 years are tested once and are asked to touch or identify

BOX 33-8
Types of Eye Charts

- *Snellen chart:* A standardized chart with graduated letters for testing far vision of children at 20 feet. Used with children older than 6 years.
- *Tumbling E (Snellen E):* A standardized chart using the letter E in various directions that is used with preschoolers ages 3 to 6 years to test far vision at 20 feet. Also available for a distance of 10 feet.
- *Preliterate chart:* A standardized chart with pictures used with children ages 3 to 6 years to test far vision at a distance of 20 feet.
- *HOTV chart:* A standardized chart with letters H, O, T, and V in graduated sizes. Designed for use at 10 feet with children ages 3 to 6 years.

- *Allen cards:* Picture cards of familiar objects for testing children ages 2½ years and older. Vision is tested at a distance of 15 feet. If the child is cooperative, Allen cards may be used in children as young as 24 months.
- *Jaeger chart:* Standardized chart with graduated letters for testing near vision at 12 to 14 inches from the eyes. Used with children older than 6 years.
- *Ishihara chart:* A series of polychromatic cards with a pattern of dots printed against a background of many colored dots. Designed to test for color vision between ages 4 and 6 years.

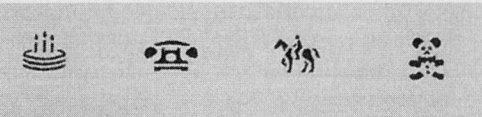

Allen cards for testing preliterate children. (From Cassin, B. [1995]. *Fundamentals for ophthalmic technical personnel* [p. 160]. Philadelphia: Saunders.)

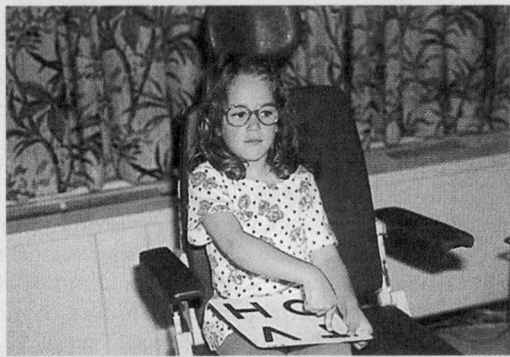

HOTV chart for children ages 3 to 6 years. The letters *H, O, T,* and *V* are presented at a distance, and the child points to the corresponding letter on the card resting on her lap. (From Goldbloom, R.B. [2003] *Pediatric clinical skills* [3rd ed., p. 138]. Philadelphia: Saunders.)

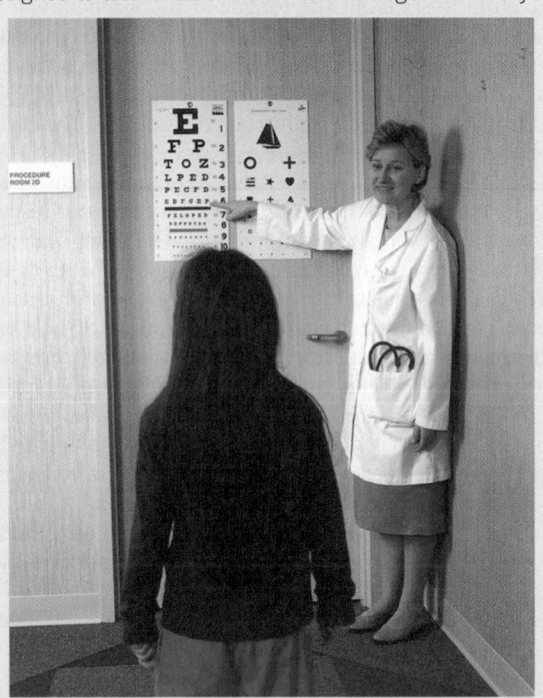

The standard Snellen E chart can be used for an older child who can read letters. The picture chart to the right of the Snellen chart can be used to assess vision in 3- to 6-year-olds. (From Jarvis, C. [2000]. *Physical examination and health assessment* [3rd ed., p. 307]. Philadelphia: Saunders.)

the embedded patterns. A child with this deficit cannot see the patterns against the field of color.

Peripheral Vision
Visual fields are evaluated in older children to identify peripheral vision. The examiner's face is positioned directly in front and on the level of the child, about 2 feet away. The visual fields should roughly mirror the examiner's. The examiner covers one eye and has the child mimic by covering the opposite eye. Slowly a puppet or some other test object is brought from the periphery into the child's field of vision. The object should come from a position slightly behind the child's head, and the child is asked to say "now" when the object is in view (Fig. 33-8). Testing for visual acuity and visual fields evaluates cranial nerve II, the optic nerve, which mediates vision.

Binocular Vision and Strabismus
Extraocular muscle function is evaluated to test binocular vision and the presence of strabismus. Strabismus, or "crossed eyes," is the abnormal or incomplete development of binocular visual alignment. Three tests are performed: the corneal light reflex (Hirschberg) test; field-of-vision test; and cover/uncover (alternate cover) test.

Corneal Light Reflex Test. The corneal light reflex is assessed by shining a light directly onto the irises from a distance of about 40.5 cm (16 in). The reflection of the light should appear in exactly the same spot on both eyes. If the light falls off center in one eye, the eyes are malaligned. Children with *epicanthal folds*—vertical folds that partially or completely cover the inner canthi (Fig. 33-9)—may give a false impression of malalignment (pseudostrabismus).

Field-of-Vision Test. The six cardinal fields of vision are tested by holding the child's chin so that the head does not move and asking the child to follow a puppet or a familiar object held approximately 12 inches away from the face as the object is moved to each of the six cardinal positions. As the object is moved to the margins of each cardinal position, the examiner holds it momentarily in that position before proceeding back to the center. The eyes will track in a parallel fashion to each position. As the eyes are

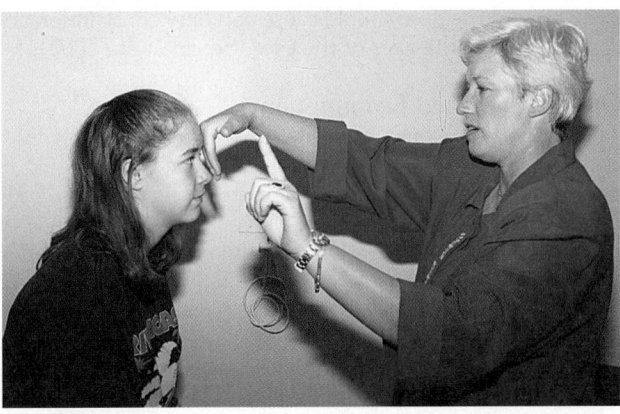

Figure 33-8 Visual fields (cranial nerve II) are tested in each eye separately. One eye is covered as the child stares straight ahead. An object is slowly moved from the side of the head into the field of vision. The child says "now" when first seeing the object.

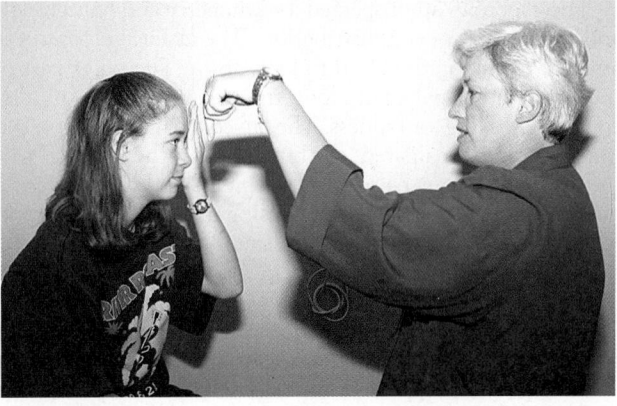

Figure 33-10 The cover/uncover test detects small degrees of deviated eye alignment. With one eye covered, the child gazes straight ahead with the uncovered eye. The cover is then removed, and the eye should continue to stare straight ahead. Movement in either eye suggests muscle weakness. Extraocular muscle function is controlled by cranial nerves III, IV, and VI.

in the margins of each position, the examiner can note *end-stage nystagmus*, a gentle oscillation of the eye, which is considered normal. Children younger than 2 to 3 years may not be able to cooperate with this test.

Cover/Uncover Test. The cover/uncover test is used to detect deficits in binocular vision by interrupting fusion of the eyes as they gaze at a fixed object. One eye is covered with an opaque card while the child stares straight ahead, at which time the examiner observes the uncovered eye. A steady, fixed gaze is maintained by the uncovered eye. Next the covered eye is uncovered and observed for any movement; it should continue to stare straight ahead (Fig. 33-10).

The procedure is repeated with the opposite eye. Any movement in either eye in the process of covering or uncovering may indicate muscle weakness.

Testing for extraocular muscle function in children younger than 5 years is critical to identifying any muscle imbalance,

so that it can be corrected at an early age to preserve vision. Extraocular muscle function evaluates three cranial nerves: cranial nerve VI, the *abducent* nerve, which innervates the lateral rectus muscle (responsible for abducting the eye); cranial nerve IV, the *trochlear* nerve, which innervates the superior oblique muscle (responsible for down and inward movement of the eye); and cranial nerve III, the *oculomotor* nerve, which innervates the superior, inferior, and medial rectus and the inferior oblique muscles (Seidel et al., 2003).

External Eye

The external eye is evaluated for position and placement (see Fig. 33-9). The examiner notes whether the eyes are set wide apart or close together. Epicanthal folds are seen in Asian children and in some non-Asian children as well. The slant of the eyes is determined by drawing an imaginary line across the inner canthi (see Fig. 33-9).

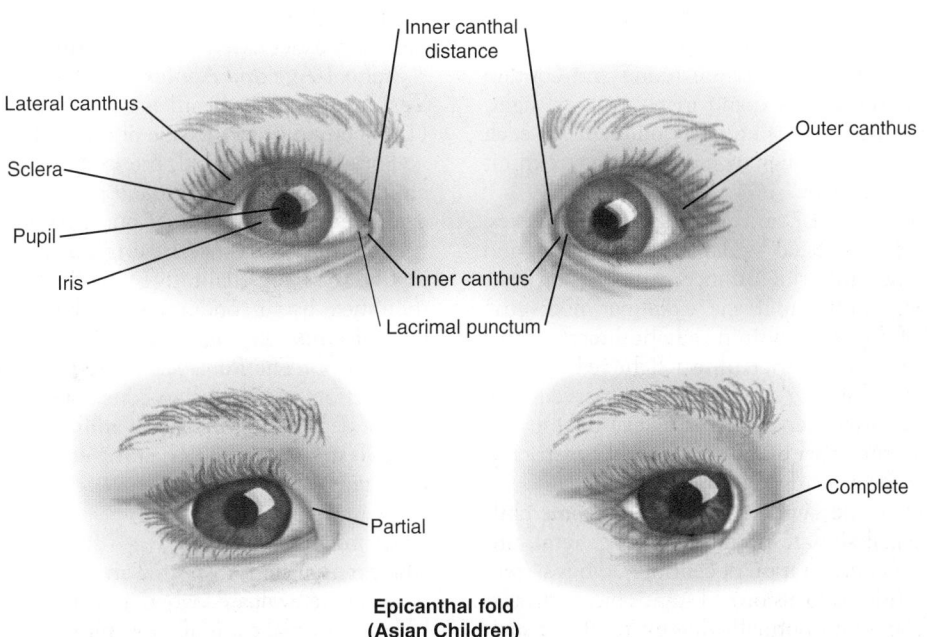

**Epicanthal fold
(Asian Children)**

Figure 33-9 External structures of the eye.

The eyebrows are inspected for symmetry and hair growth and eyelashes for even distribution. The *lacrimal apparatus* is assessed by asking the child to look down. The outer part of the upper lid is palpated along the bony orbit for any discomfort, swelling, or redness. The *punctum* (tear duct) on the inner canthus is palpated for obstruction in the infant.

The eye globe is palpated for firmness and can be gently pushed into the orbit without causing discomfort. Palpation of the eye may cause anxiety in small children and should not be done unless there is a serious concern about the size of the eye.

Eyelids are inspected for color, swelling, discharge, and lesions. Note the position of the eyelids on the globe. With the eyelids open, the upper lid normally falls below the superior limbus but does not cover any of the pupil. The lower lids normally fall just at the inferior limbus. The limbus is the point where the sclera of the eye meets the color portion of the iris. When closed, the eyelids approximate each other completely, without tremor, fasciculations, or tics.

The *conjunctiva* has two portions to evaluate. The palpebral portion of the conjunctiva lines the lids. The palpebral conjunctiva is examined by pulling down as the child looks up. It is normally clear, with a pink color, and may have several small blood vessels visible. The upper lid can be inspected by everting the upper eyelid over a cotton-tipped applicator. Eversion of the upper eyelid is not normally done because eye manipulation may cause apprehension in a child. The bulbar portion of the conjunctiva is transparent and lies over the sclera, allowing the white of the sclera to be clearly visible.

The following anterior structures of the eye are inspected: sclerae, cornea and lens, anterior chamber, and irises. The sclerae are white. The sclera of dark-skinned children may have gray-blue or "muddy" color variations. Dark-skinned children may have small brown macules around the limbus (where the iris meets the sclera). These variations are normal. The corneas are clear, transparent, and very sensitive. Shining a light obliquely across the cornea highlights any abnormal irregularities on the corneal surface. The examiner illuminates the anterior chamber by shining a light across the eye from the temporal side to illuminate the entire iris without producing a shadow. The irises are round and contain muscle fibers that contract or expand in response to light. The pigmentation of the irises is uniquely different for each individual. The irises are similar in color but may exhibit some variation between them.

Pupils appear round, regular, and of equal size in both eyes. The *pupillary light reflex* is tested by darkening the room and asking the child to gaze into the distance. A light is brought from the side (temporally), and the examiner notes the change in the size of the pupil. Shining a light directly into a pupil causes the pupil to constrict (direct light reflex). The procedure is repeated while the opposite eye is observed. The opposite eye constricts (consensual light reflex) in response to the light shone in the other eye. Pupils should constrict at equal speeds and to the same degree.

Pupil size should be the same in both eyes. In some children, pupils of unequal size are normal, but in general, unequal pupils call for a consideration of central nervous system injury. Asking the child to focus on a distant object can test accommodation. The pupils normally dilate. An object such as a puppet or a finger brought into the line of vision about 7 to 8 cm from the nose should cause pupillary constriction and convergence of the axes of the eyes (Seidel et al., 2003).

Ophthalmoscopic Examination

The ophthalmoscopic examination requires a cooperative child, practice, and patience. Lights in the room should be dim. Most children enjoy playing with the light of the "flashlight," and watching the light as you move it around the room facilitates cooperation. Minimally, all practitioners view the red reflex, but the procedure requires demonstration and practice. When the ophthalmoscope is placed in front of the pupil and the light hits the lens, a red color is reflected from the retina to the examiner. The retina, choroid, optic disc, macula, fovea centralis, and retinal vessels are also visible with the ophthalmoscope.

Ears

Assessment of the ears includes testing for hearing acuity, inspection and palpation of the external ear, and examination of the internal ear using the otoscope.

Hearing Acuity

Infant Assessment. Infants born in a hospital are tested for response of the acoustic nerve at the time of birth. In an infant, hearing is assessed by asking the parent to speak to the infant from behind and observing the infant's response to the parent's voice. The examiner can stand behind the infant and ring a bell or make a sound the infant is familiar with and observe the infant turning to locate the sound. A very young infant, younger than 4 months, may demonstrate a startle reflex to loud sounds.

Preschool and School-Age Assessment by Audiometry. In preschool and school-age children, the audiometer gives a precise (quantitative) assessment of the child's ability to hear. The child is placed in a soundproof room and is asked to identify tones played at a level the child can hear. With the audiometer, two tests are used to evaluate hearing: the sweep test and the pure tone hearing test. The *sweep test* is used to screen for hearing losses. The *pure tone test* is used to determine the exact extent of the hearing loss.

School-Age and Adolescent Assessment: The Whisper Test. A whisper is heard as the examiner stands about 0.3 m (1 ft) behind or to the side of the child.

For a preschool child, the examiner stands in front of the child approximately 0.6 to 0.9 m (2-3 ft) and gives the child a command such as "Please put the toy on the floor."

Conduction Tests (Tuning Fork Hearing Tests). Tuning fork tests are qualitative tests done to determine the ability to hear by air conduction and by bone conduction. In the normal child, air conduction of sound is greater than bone conduction. The *Rinne hearing test* is used to determine if air conduction is greater than bone conduction. The *Weber hearing test* determines the child's ability to hear by bone conduction. Testing the child's hearing evaluates cranial nerve VIII (*acoustic nerve*).

External Ear

The external ear is inspected and palpated. Ear placement and position are evaluated when assessing the face (see Fig. 33-5), but the external ear is also examined for any malformations or unusual markings (Fig. 33-11). Any discharge coming from the auditory meatus is noted, and its amount and characteristics are described. Soft, yellow-brown cerumen (ear wax) is normally seen in the external auditory meatus.

The bony prominence of the mastoid process behind the ear is palpated for tenderness. The auricles are gently pulled to determine if discomfort is created.

Otoscopic Examination

The *tympanic membrane* is examined, using the otoscope (Fig. 33-12). Many children may be apprehensive about this examination. If necessary, a small child is positioned on the parent's lap and the child's arms are secured. The examiner uses the largest speculum that will fit comfortably into the ear canal. In a child younger than 3 years, the ear canal is straightened by pulling the pinna of the ear down and back. If a child is 3 years old or older, the pinna is pulled up and back. As much of the canal as possible should be visible before inserting the speculum into the auditory meatus.

The canal is inspected for any lesions and for cerumen. The tympanic membrane is inspected for landmarks, color, and mobility. A puff of air is injected into the canal with an insufflation bulb, and the tympanic membrane is observed for movement. Normally, the tympanic membrane moves inward with a slight puff and outward with a slight release.

Thorax and Lungs

Assessment of the thorax and lungs consists of inspection, palpation, percussion, and auscultation, in that order. To assist with localizing findings on the thorax, anatomic landmarks such as the ribs and intercostal spaces are identified and imaginary lines are drawn on the surface (Fig. 33-13).

Location of lung tissue depends on the age and development of the child. In an infant, lung tissue on the anterior chest can be located from the apex, above the clavicle, to the level of the fifth rib in the midclavicular line. By age 6 years, lung tissue is assessed from the apex to the level of the sixth rib in the midclavicular line. Laterally, lung tissue is assessed from the axilla to the level of the eighth rib. Posteriorly, lungs are assessed from the level of the first thoracic vertebra to the tenth thoracic vertebra.

Inspection

Remove the child's shirt or clothing covering the chest. In adolescent females, the breasts should be kept covered and exposed only when necessary. Inspection of the chest includes observing the child for any cough, stridor, grunting, hoarseness, snoring, wheezing, and type and amount of any sputum, if present. Respiratory rate and pattern are observed. In young children and infants, breathing is more diaphragmatic or abdominal (see Table 33-1 for the effect of age on vital signs). The chest wall should expand symmetrically during respiration. Respirations should be easy, regular, and without apparent distress. Rapid respirations, retractions, nasal flaring, and head bobbing may indicate respiratory difficulty.

Thoracic configuration is evaluated by determining the shape and symmetry of the chest from the front, sides, and back (Fig. 33-14). Two common alterations in structure in the anterior chest are *pectus carinatum* (pigeon chest) and *pectus excavatum* (funnel chest). *Scoliosis*, a lateral S-shaped curvature of the thoracic and lumbar vertebrae, is a common

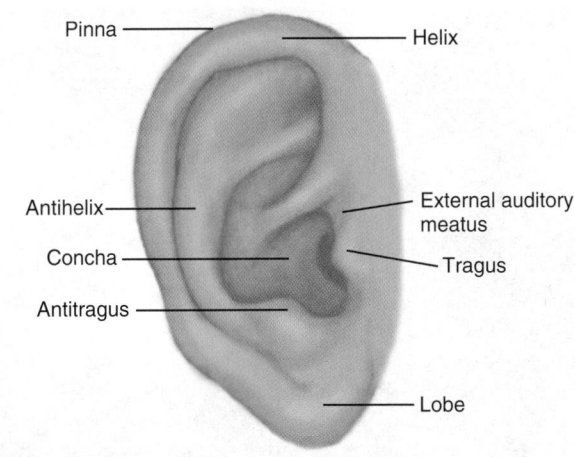

Figure 33-11 Landmarks of the external ear.

alteration of the posterior chest that may cause impaired pulmonary function.

Palpation

Palpation of the chest begins with the posterior chest. To alleviate fear in a young child, the examiner should stand in a position that allows the child visibility at all times. The posterior chest is palpated for areas of tenderness, tactile fremitus, and chest excursion.

To palpate for tenderness, the examiner touches the entire thorax with the palmar aspects of the fingers. This process elicits any points of discomfort or pain. The examiner notes any masses or edema (Fig. 33-15).

To evaluate for *tactile fremitus*, the examiner palpates the chest wall while the child says "ninety-nine." Vibrations felt on the chest wall are the result of vibrations produced in the vocal cords and transmitted to the chest wall through the respiratory tract.

Percussion of the chest is performed by advanced practitioners to determine changes in sound produced by the density of the underlying tissues.

Auscultation

Auscultating the chest with a stethoscope determines the characteristics of breath sounds. Breath sounds heard with the stethoscope are made by the flow of air through the respiratory tree and are characterized by intensity, pitch, quality, and duration.

It is best to listen to breath sounds with the child sitting upright if possible. Infants and toddlers can be held in the parent's lap; have the parent assist with removal of clothing and positioning of the child. The examiner's position is on the side of the child, allowing the child to observe the examiner's movements. Before touching the chest, the examiner allows the young child to hold or play with the stethoscope and warms the stethoscope before placing it on the child's chest.

An anxious or frightened child may cry during this part of the examination. Distracting the child or having the young child focus on another activity may facilitate listening. For the inconsolable child, the examiner listens to breath sounds between each cry. If the young child is sleeping or comfortable

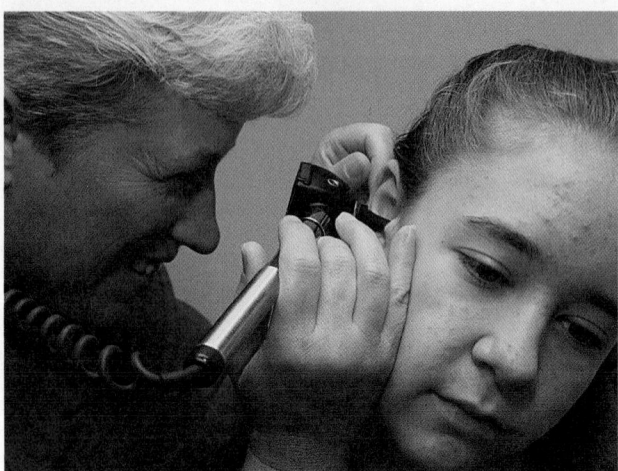

◀ To straighten the ear canal of a child older than 3 years, the nurse pulls the child's pinna up and back.

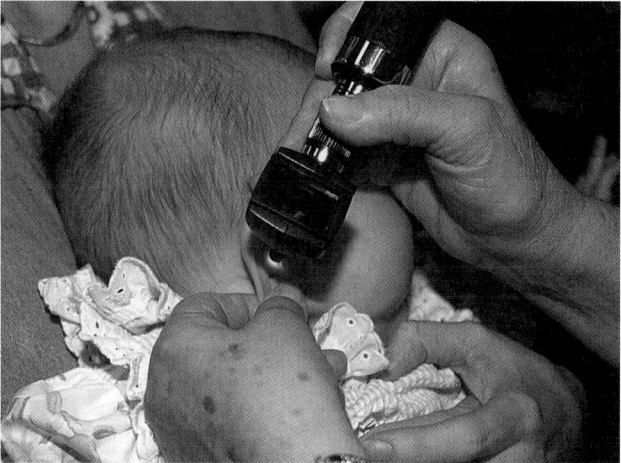

For children younger than 3 years, the pinna is pulled down and back. ▶

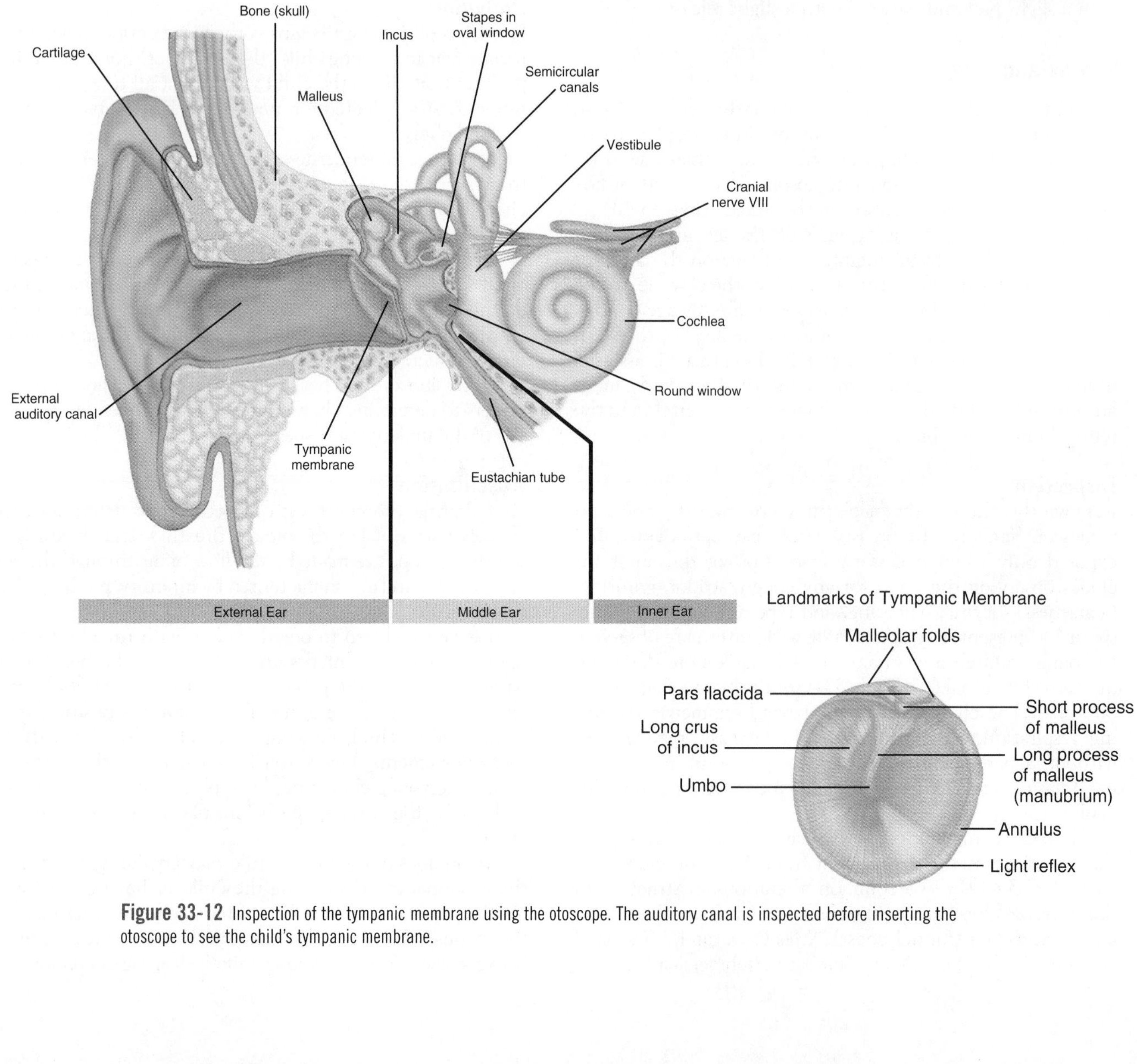

Bone (skull)

Stapes in oval window

Incus

Cartilage

Malleus

Semicircular canals

Vestibule

Cranial nerve VIII

Cochlea

External auditory canal

Round window

Tympanic membrane

Eustachian tube

External Ear	Middle Ear	Inner Ear

Landmarks of Tympanic Membrane

Malleolar folds

Pars flaccida

Short process of malleus

Long crus of incus

Long process of malleus (manubrium)

Umbo

Annulus

Light reflex

Figure 33-12 Inspection of the tympanic membrane using the otoscope. The auditory canal is inspected before inserting the otoscope to see the child's tympanic membrane.

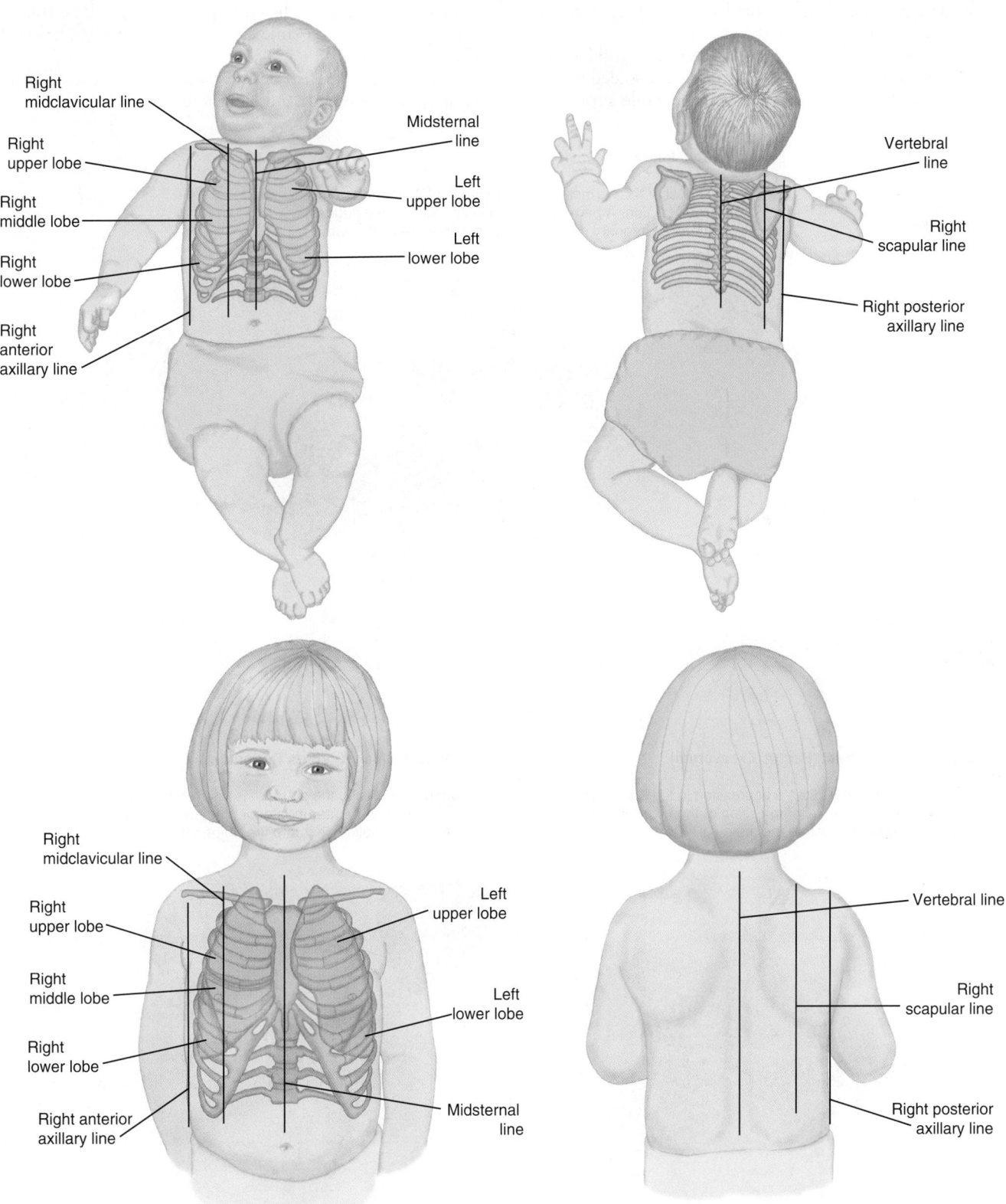

Figure 33-13 Anatomic landmarks of the thorax in infants and children.

in the parent's arms, the examiner listens to the chest first be-fore proceeding to the rest of the examination.

For listening to the posterior thorax, the child is posi-tioned with the head bent forward and hands folded in front. Having the child raise the arms overhead while sitting erect allows the examiner to listen laterally. To auscultate the an-terior chest, have the child sit erect with the shoulders back (Fig. 33-16).

The examiner begins on the posterior thorax and has the child open the mouth and breathe in and out while the ex-

Normal Infant

The chest of the normal infant is approximately round or barrel shaped in cross-section. A barrel chest in a child older than 6 suggests a chronic pulmonary disease such as asthma or cystic fibrosis.

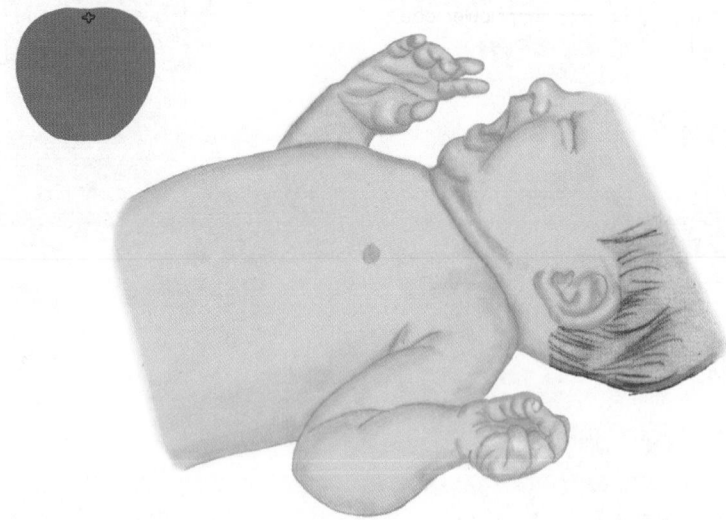

Funnel Chest (Pectus Excavatum)

A funnel chest has a depression in the lower portion of the sternum. Compression of the heart and great vessels may cause murmurs.

Pigeon Chest (Pectus Carinatum)

In pigeon chest, the sternum is displaced anteriorly, increasing the anteroposterior diameter. Grooves in the chest wall accentuate the deformity.

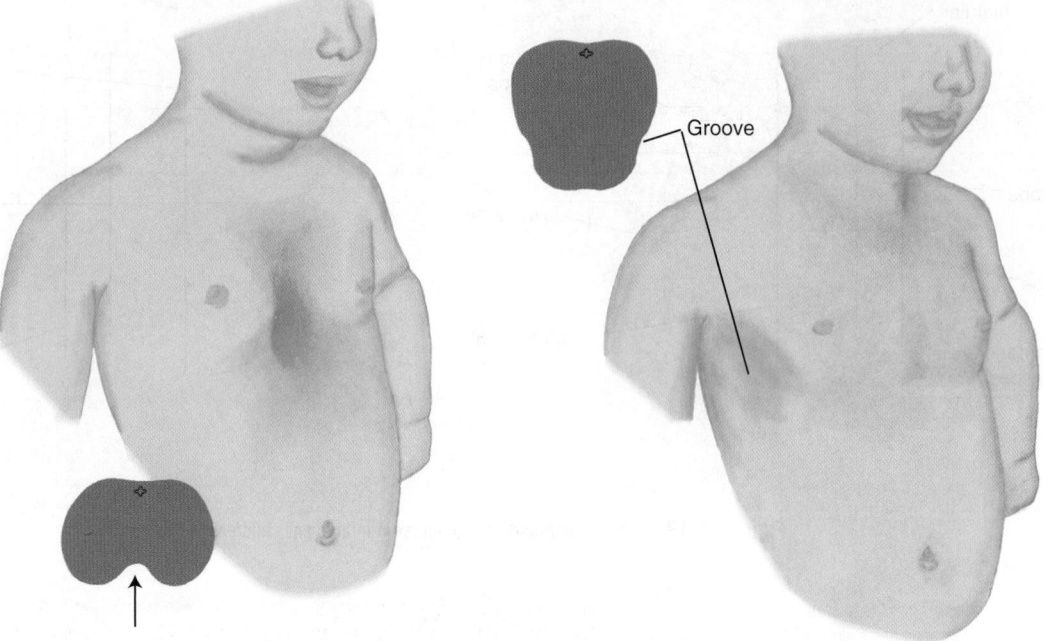

Figure 33-14 Common alterations in chest configuration.

aminer listens with the diaphragm of the stethoscope. Having the young child blow bubbles, pretend to blow out birthday candles, or blow a tissue increases breath sounds. Compressing the hand holding the stethoscope on the chest wall and placing the other hand on the opposite side of the chest accentuate expiration and make end-expiratory sounds (e.g., wheezes) easier to hear. The sequence for listening to breath sounds is posterior chest, right and left lateral chest, and anterior chest (Fig. 33-17).

Adventitious Breath Sounds

In addition to normal breath sounds, *adventitious sounds* may be audible with the stethoscope. Table 33-3 describes the origin and characteristics of adventitious sounds. Adventitious sounds are additional sounds heard in an abnormal clinical state. They are described by their quality. The examiner notes whether they are continuous or discontinuous and where they occur in the respiratory phase. The effects of coughing are also noted. When adventitious sounds are heard, they are described as to location, timing, and intensity.

Heart

The techniques for assessing the heart are inspection, palpation, and auscultation. The sequence of this examination depends on the age, growth, and development of the child being examined. For an infant or young child, the examiner may want to listen to the child's heart while the parent is holding the child, before doing other parts of the examination. Infants and children have varying degrees of dependence on parents and may be fearful of the examination. Per-

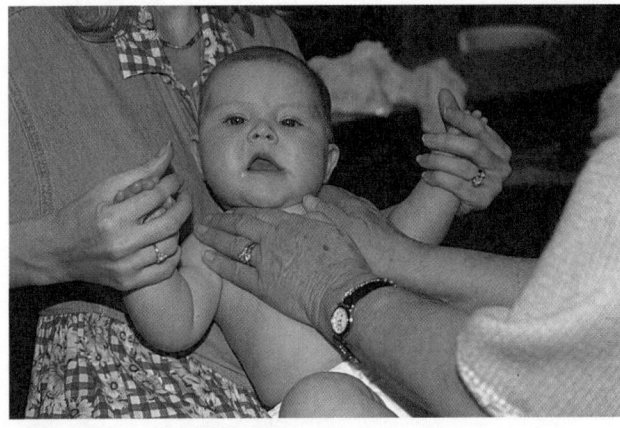

Figure 33-15 To identify areas of fremitus, tenderness, symmetry, and depth and equality of expansion, the nurse palpates the child's posterior and anterior chest. When palpating any area, warm hands increase the child's comfort. (Courtesy The University of Texas at Arlington School of Nursing.)

cussion of the heart indicates primarily the size and shape of the heart and is not routinely done. The heart is assessed with the child in a supine position, in a left lateral recumbent position, and in a sitting position while leaning forward slightly.

Inspection

The anterior chest is systematically inspected, with special attention paid to the following five areas: second right intercostal space (aortic area), second left intercostal space (pulmonic area), left sternal border (right ventricular area), fifth

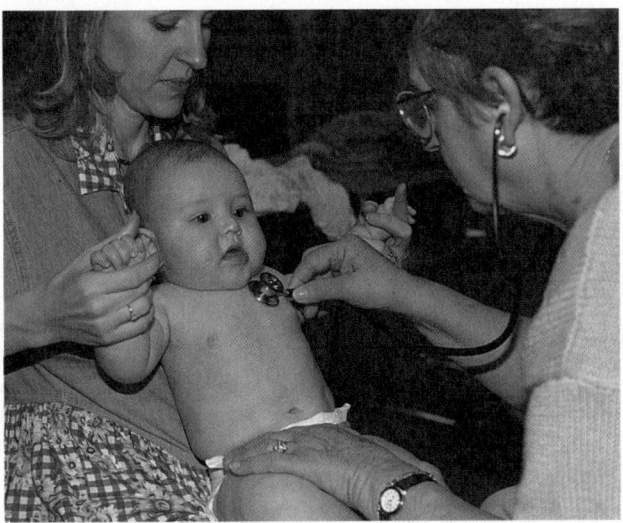

If the child is upset, the examiner may have to listen to breath sounds between cries. Keeping this child in the comfort of her mother's arms lessens her distress.

◀ Infants and toddlers can be held sitting upright in the parent's lap while the nurse listens to breath sounds.

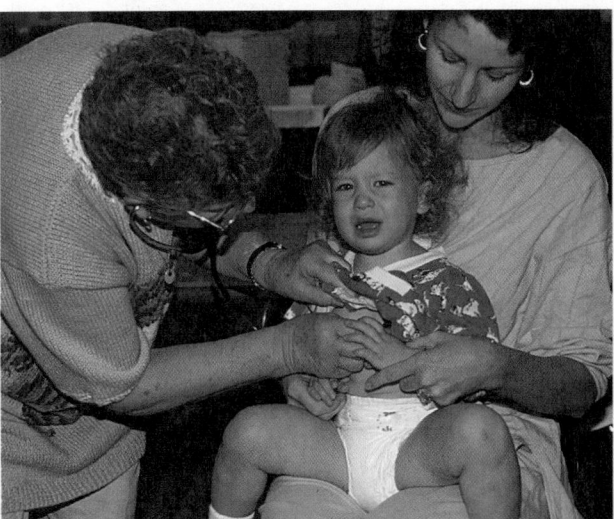

Figure 33-16 To hear heart and breath sounds, the nurse auscultates the child's chest with a stethoscope in an orderly way. Auscultation is most easily done when the child is quiet, so this part of the examination is best performed first if the child is quiet or asleep. To allay fears and make the examination more comfortable, the child can play with the stethoscope first and warm the instrument. The child also can be distracted with a toy while listening. (Courtesy The University of Texas at Arlington School of Nursing.)

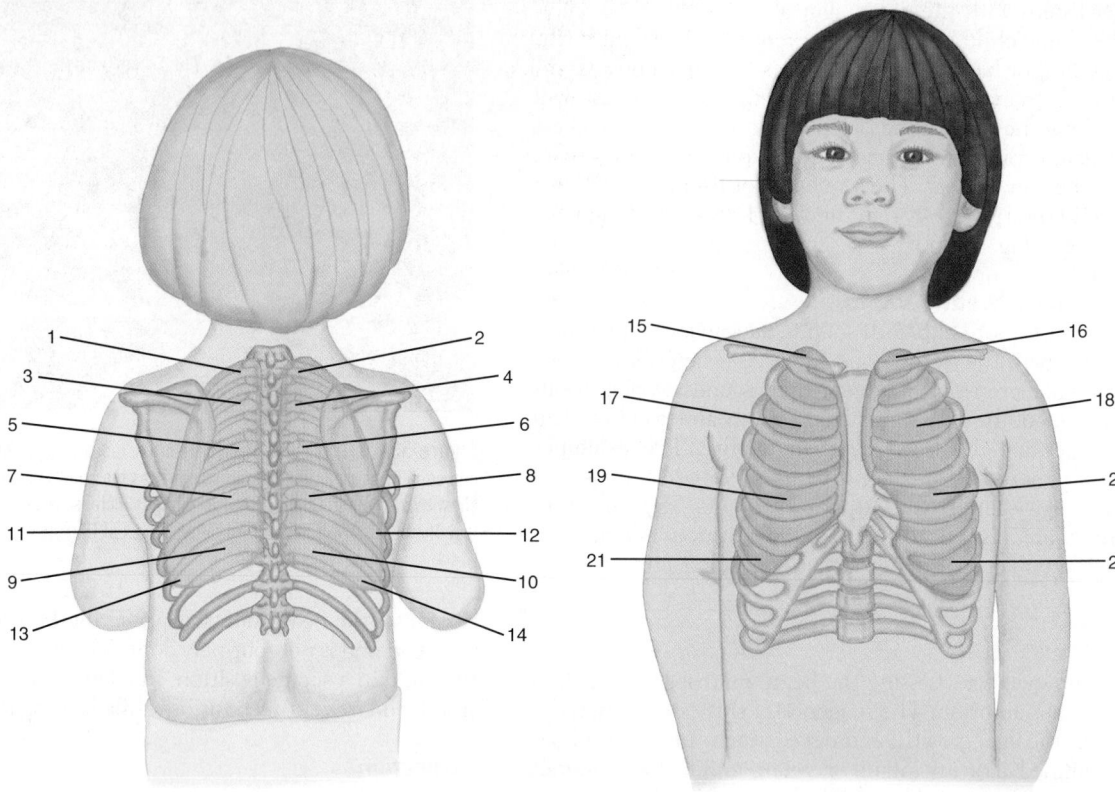

Figure 33-17 Sequence for listening to breath sounds.

left intercostal space in the midclavicular line (apex), and just below the xiphoid process (epigastric area). The areas will differ at different ages (Fig. 33-18). During infancy, the heart is more horizontal in the thorax, and the apex is one or two intercostal spaces above the fifth intercostal space and lateral to the midclavicular line. The second intercostal space is located by identifying the sternal angle. The second rib is attached to the sternum just below or at the sternal angle. The second intercostal space is below the second rib. Other ribs and intercostal spaces are identified by their relationship to the second rib.

The precordium (anterior chest overlying the heart and great vessels) is inspected for *bulges, lifts, heaves,* and *apical impulse.* The apical impulse is the light tapping of the anterior chest wall every time the heart beats. The location of the apical impulse will change gradually as the child matures and by age 7 years can be seen at the fifth intercostal space in the midclavicular line.

Palpation

The examiner palpates the precordium with the fingertips for the presence of any pulsations at each individual area (see Fig. 33-18). The examiner locates the apical pulse, sometimes identified as the *point of maximal impulse (PMI),* or the point where the light tapping of the heart is felt the best and varies with age. In a child younger than 7 years, the PMI is located in the fourth intercostal space, lateral to the midclavicular line. The PMI in a child older than 7 years is lo-

cated in the fifth intercostal space in the midclavicular line. Using the palmar aspect of the hand to feel for *thrills,* the examiner then palpates each individual area of the precordium. Thrills are palpable vibrations of the heart.

Auscultation

Auscultation of the heart is done by listening both with the bell and with the diaphragm of the stethoscope as the child is lying supine, in a left lateral recumbent position, and sitting up. To auscultate heart sounds, the examiner uses a systematic approach. Sounds heard with the stethoscope are predominantly produced with the closing of the heart valves. The four traditional areas for listening to heart sounds are the aortic valve area in the second right intercostal space, the pulmonic valve area in the second left intercostal space, the tricuspid valve area in the left lower sternal border, and the mitral valve area in the fifth intercostal space at the left midclavicular line (see Fig. 33-18). The position for listening to these areas depends on the age of the child. It is best to listen to heart sounds by inching the stethoscope across the precordium in a Z pattern, from the base of the heart across and down, or from the apex upward. All areas are auscultated with both the bell and the diaphragm of the stethoscope.

Sounds produced by the closing of the valves can be heard all over the precordium, so it will be necessary to concentrate on one heart sound at a time. The heart sounds are divided into two components—the first heart sound (S_1) and the second heart sound (S_2). S_1 is heard best

TABLE **33-3** Origin and Characteristics of Adventitious Breath Sounds

Sound	Description	Mechanism	Clinical Example
DISCONTINUOUS SOUNDS			
Crackles—fine (rales, crepitations); heard when fluid is in airways.	Discontinuous, high-pitched, short, crackling, popping sounds heard during inspiration and not cleared by coughing. You can simulate this sound by rolling a strand of hair between your fingers near your ear or by moistening your thumb and index finger and separating them near your ear. Described as discrete (short), discontinuous.	Inhaled air collides with previously deflated airways; airways suddenly pop open, creating crackling sound as gas pressures between the two compartments equalize.	*Late inspiratory* crackles occur with restrictive disease: pneumonia, congestive heart failure, and interstitial fibrosis. *Early inspiratory* crackles occur with obstructive disease: chronic bronchitis and asthma.
Pleural friction rub.	A very superficial sound that is coarse and low-pitched; it has a grating quality, as if two pieces of leather were being rubbed together. A pleural friction rub sounds just like crackles but close to the ear. It sounds louder if you push the stethoscope harder into the chest wall.	Caused when pleurae become inflamed and lose their normal lubricating fluid. Their opposing roughened pleural surfaces rub together during respiration. This sound is heard best in the anterolateral wall, where lung mobility is greatest.	Pleuritis, accompanied by pain with breathing. (Rub disappears after a few days if pleural fluid accumulates and separates pleurae.)
CONTINUOUS SOUNDS			
High-pitched wheeze heard with narrowing of the air passages from fluid, swelling, spasm, and tumors.	High-pitched, musical squeaking sounds that predominate in expiration but may occur in both expiration and inspiration. Coughing frequently will change the character of the sound.	Air squeezed or compressed through passageways narrowed almost to closure by collapsing, swelling, secretions, or tumors. The passageway walls oscillate in apposition between the closed and barely open positions. The resulting sound is similar to that produced by a vibrating reed.	Obstructive lung disease, such as asthma.
Low-pitched wheeze (sonorous rhonchi).	Low-pitched, musical snoring, moaning sounds. They are heard throughout the cycle, although they are more prominent on expiration and may clear somewhat by coughing.	Airflow obstruction as described by the vibrating reed mechanism. The pitch of the wheeze does not correlate with the size of the passageway that generates it.	Bronchitis.

NOTE: Although nothing in clinical practice seems to differ more than the nomenclature of adventitious sounds, most authorities concur on two categories: (1) discontinuous, discrete crackling sounds; and (2) continuous, coarse, or wheezing sounds.

at the apex of the heart, and S₂ is heard best at the base (see Fig. 33-18). S₁, phonetically described as *lub*, is produced by the closing of the mitral and tricuspid valves. S₂, phonetically described as *dub*, is produced by the closing of the aortic and pulmonic valves.

The physiologic splitting of S₂, an audible pause between the closing of the aortic and pulmonic valves, is frequently heard in children of all ages and is considered normal. Splitting of S₂ can be heard best at the pulmonic area because ejection times on the right side of the heart are slightly longer than on the left side. Splitting of S₂ is greatest at the peak of inspiration and decreases or goes away during expiration.

The routine for assessing heart sounds is the following sequence:

1. Identify the rate and rhythm.
2. Identify S₁ and S₂.
3. Assess S₁ and S₂ separately to determine where they are best heard.
4. Listen for extra heart sounds.
5. Identify murmurs.

Normal Rate and Rhythm. The normal rate of a child's heart is different at different ages (see Table 33-1). Children's

Cardiac Landmarks

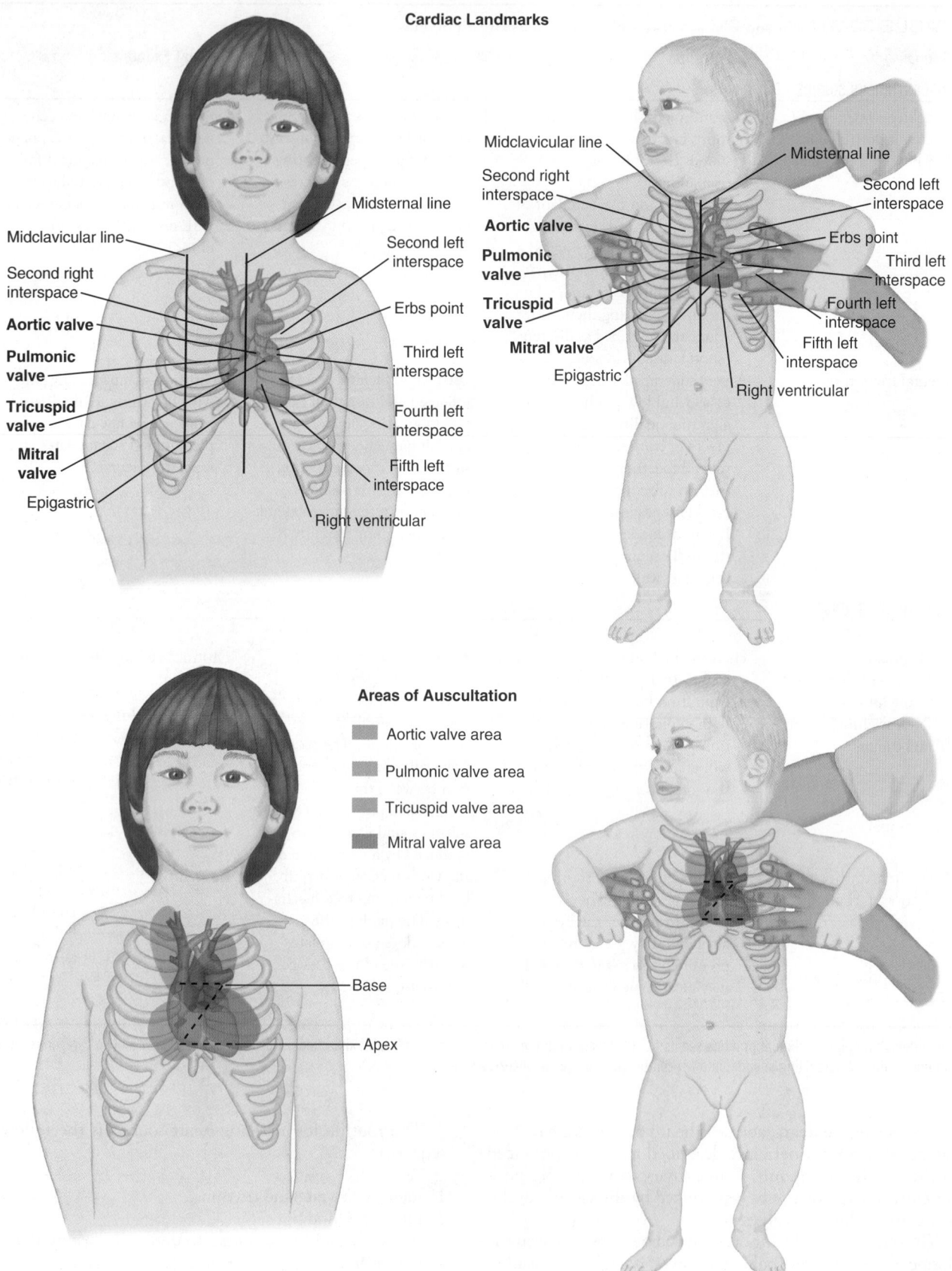

Midsternal line

Midclavicular line

Second right interspace

Aortic valve

Pulmonic valve

Tricuspid valve

Mitral valve

Epigastric

Second left interspace

Erbs point

Third left interspace

Fourth left interspace

Fifth left interspace

Right ventricular

Midclavicular line

Second right interspace

Aortic valve

Pulmonic valve

Tricuspid valve

Mitral valve

Epigastric

Midsternal line

Second left interspace

Erbs point

Third left interspace

Fourth left interspace

Fifth left interspace

Right ventricular

Areas of Auscultation

Aortic valve area

Pulmonic valve area

Tricuspid valve area

Mitral valve area

Base

Apex

Figure 33-18 Location of the heart within the thorax in the infant and the older child, showing landmarks and areas of auscultation.

heart rates often increase with inspiration and slow down during expiration. To decrease the irregular rhythm associated with respirations, the examiner has the child hold the breath as the examiner continues to listen.

Extra Heart Sounds, Including Murmurs. Extra sounds (sounds heard over and above the normal heart sounds) may be described as opening snaps, ejection clicks, mid-systolic to late systolic clicks, and murmurs. Snaps and clicks are short, high-pitched sounds heard with valve disorders and do not vary with respirations. *Murmurs* are blowing, swooshing sounds that occur because of some disruption in the blood flow into, through, or out of the heart. Innocent or functional heart murmurs are frequently heard in children. Innocent murmurs occur during systole, do not radiate, and change with position change. To describe and classify extra heart sounds, the nurse needs advanced training and practice.

Peripheral Vascular System

Arterial pulses are examined for decreased or absent pulses. Pulses are palpated, with the examiner noting the rate, rhythm, elasticity of the vessel wall, and equal force of bilateral pulses. The pulse force should be symmetric and should be the same for upper and lower extremities. Comparing opposite pulses is necessary in children. The examiner compares one femoral pulse with the opposite radial pulse for equality and compares one lower extremity pulse with an upper extremity pulse for equality. A diminished or absent femoral pulse, as compared with the radial pulse, may be the only finding in coarctation of the aorta in infants and children.

Breast

The examiner inspects and palpates breast tissue. Developmental differences occur in response to circulating hormones and affect the appearance of breast tissue. In infants of both genders, the breasts may appear engorged because of maternal estrogen crossing the placenta. *Thelarche,* or breast development, marks the beginning of puberty in preadolescent girls and can occur as early as age 8 years.

The examiner inspects the nipples for position and appearance. In infants, the nipple is flat and symmetric with darker areolar pigmentation. In preadolescent and adolescent girls, the Tanner sexual maturity rating is used to evaluate developmental levels (see Table 8-1). The nipples should be symmetric on the chest and should point in the same direction. Nipples may appear to be inverted or everted. An inverted nipple is significant if the inversion is of recent origin. The breast skin should be smooth and free of any dimpling. It is common to see some asymmetry during growth.

All adolescent girls should be taught how to do breast self-examination once they have reached menarche. Teaching self-examination to the adolescent and reinforcing its importance at every visit are important roles for the nurse. Many adolescents do not do breast self-examinations because of lack of knowledge or fear of finding something wrong. Once the adolescent is familiar with how her breasts look and feel, the natural and normal changes that occur in the breast as a result of hormonal fluctuations can be easily identified. Teach the adolescent girl to do breast self-examination 3 to 4 days after menses, because the breasts are least tender and sensitive at that time (Fox, 2002).

The examiner uses the same technique to palpate the breast tissue and the axilla of the adolescent boy. In the male, the examiner expects to feel a thin layer of fatty tissue overlying the muscle. During puberty, some boys experience *gynecomastia,* an enlargement of breast tissue, felt as a smooth, firm, movable disk. It frequently affects only one breast and can be temporary.

Abdomen

The child's comfort should be considered during the abdominal examination. An empty bladder, a warm room, and positioning the child supine on the examining table with a pillow under the head and the knees flexed enhance abdominal relaxation. For an infant or young child, most of the abdominal examination can be done while the child is lying in the parent's lap. For an older child, the genitalia and breasts are draped. The child or parent should be questioned about urinary and bowel patterns.

The abdomen is divided into four quadrants that correlate with underlying anatomic structures (Fig. 33-19). Because bowel sounds are disturbed by percussion and palpation, the sequence of techniques differs in abdominal assessment. The abdomen is first inspected, then auscultated, then percussed, and last palpated.

Inspection

Abdominal inspection assesses contour, symmetry, characteristics of the umbilicus and skin, pulsations or movement, and hair distribution. *Contour* is the profile of the abdomen from the rib margin to the pubic bone and is best determined by looking tangentially across the abdomen. The contour is described as flat, scaphoid, rounded, or protuberant (Fig. 33-20). The abdominal contour provides an overall indicator of nutritional state. The abdomen should be symmetric bilaterally. The examiner looks for distention, bulging, visible mass, or asymmetric shape.

The umbilicus is normally midline and inverted. There should be no signs of discoloration, inflammation, or hernia. Throughout the neonatal period, the umbilical cord is inspected for signs of infection or bleeding.

The skin of the abdomen is inspected for color and the presence of scars, lesions, and striae. A fine venous network may be seen in infants and small children.

Inspect the abdomen for pulsations and movement. In thin children, the examiner may see the pulsations from the aorta beneath the skin in the epigastric area. Most children have abdominal movement with respirations. Peristalsis of the abdomen should not be visible.

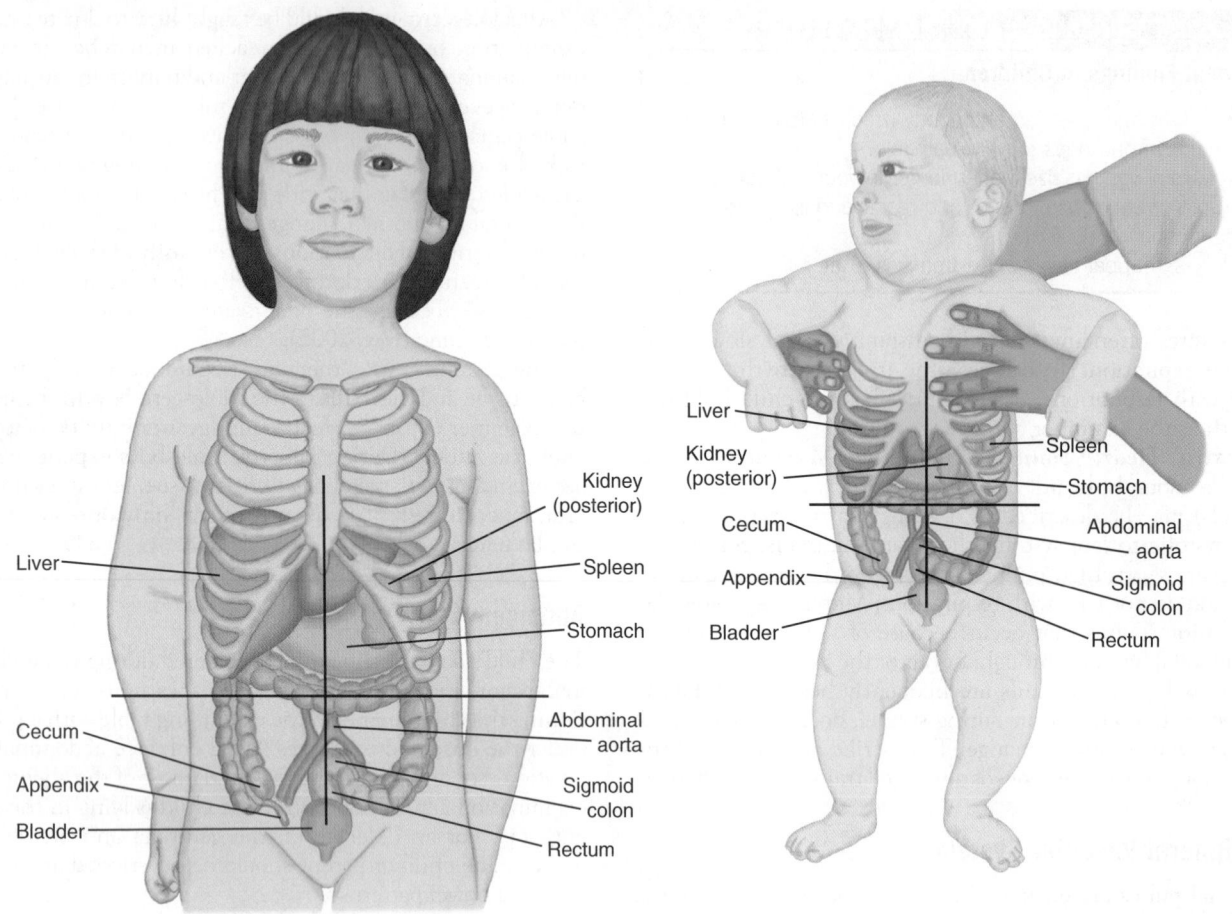

Figure 33-19 Abdominal quadrants and structures.

Auscultation

Auscultation of the abdomen follows inspection. The diaphragm of the stethoscope is held lightly against the skin to note the character and frequency of bowel sounds. Bowel sounds are high-pitched, gurgling sounds heard in all four quadrants. They are irregular and can occur from 5 to 34 times per minute. The examiner begins in the lower right quadrant and listens in all four quadrants. To determine that there are no bowel sounds, the examiner must listen for up to 5 minutes in an area where no bowel sounds are heard.

The bell of the stethoscope is used to listen for bruits over the aortic, renal, iliac, and femoral arteries. The examiner also listens in the epigastric region and around the umbilicus for a venous hum—a soft, low-pitched, continuous sound.

Percussion

Advanced practitioners perform abdominal percussion. The technique reveals tympany, liver span, and splenic dullness.

Palpation

Abdominal palpation can identify any mass or tenderness and determine the size, consistency, and location of certain organs. The examiner should have warm hands before palpating the abdomen. Palpation of the infant or young child can be done in the parent's lap by laying the child's head and thorax across the parent's legs and extending the child's ab-

domen and legs across the examiner's legs. Flex the child's knees to prepare the child for palpation of the abdomen.

Fear and anxiety may cause the child to resist when the examiner touches the abdomen. Distracting the young child with a toy or talking is helpful. Beginning with light palpation shows the child that palpation will not hurt.

Ask an older child who is anxious or ticklish to assist with this part of the examination. The child places a hand on the abdomen, and the examiner places a hand, with fingers touching the abdomen, on top of the child's hand and asks the child to push as the examiner pushes. This technique allows the child some control as the examination begins, and it reduces the sensation of tickling. To assist with relaxation of the abdominal muscles, the examiner can ask the child to take deep breaths.

The examiner begins with light palpation of all four quadrants using light, even pressure and pressing the palmar surface of the fingers no more than 1 cm into the abdomen. The hand is lifted while moving from area to area. Sudden jabs should be avoided. As the examiner circles around the abdomen, the abdomen should feel soft and smooth. Light palpation is useful in identifying areas of tenderness and muscular resistance. Guarding, resistance, or tenderness should alert the examiner to move cautiously with deeper palpation.

Tenseness can be either voluntary or involuntary. In a child, tenseness and rigidity may be caused by fear and anxi-

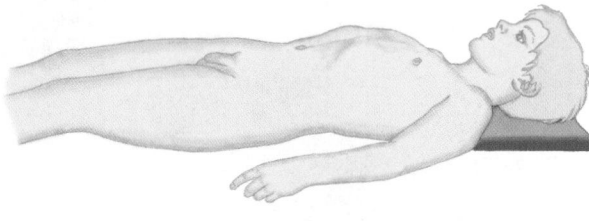

Flat: Thin child

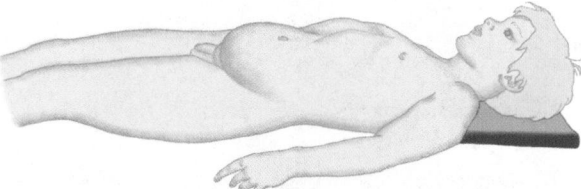

Rounded: Normal appearance of abdomen in a young child

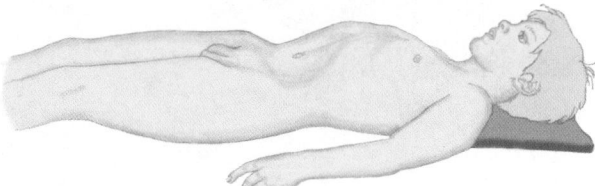

Scaphoid: Emaciated or malnourished child

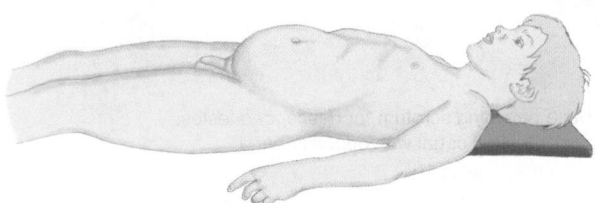

Protuberant: Recent distention with flatus; or extremely obese child. (If adolescent female, may indicate pregnancy.)

Figure 33-20 Abdominal contours. The contour of the abdomen provides an indication of the child's overall nutritional state.

ety. Distracting the child or waiting for the child to breathe will assist with determining whether the tenseness is voluntary or involuntary. The examiner gently indents the fingers into the abdominal wall during inspiration. With even pressure, the abdomen should feel soft. Rigidity, a constant, boardlike hardness, of the abdomen is usually associated with an acute inflammation of the peritoneum.

Using the same techniques, the examiner deeply palpates the abdomen. The examiner pushes down about 5 to 8 cm into the abdominal wall, beginning in the right lower quadrant. The entire abdomen is examined to identify palpable organs and masses.

To palpate the liver's edge, the examiner begins at the level of the umbilicus in the midclavicular line, using the side of the hand to indent the abdomen about 5 to 8 cm. With deep penetration of the abdominal wall, the hand is gently inverted toward the costal margin. Then the examiner progresses upward with the same maneuver until palpating the border of the liver. The edge of the liver is felt as soft and

smooth. The firm border moves downward when the child takes a deep breath. In infants and young children, the examiner can begin at the costal margin and, using the palmar aspects of the fingers, indent the abdominal wall about 5 to 8 cm. The examiner should move down from the costal margin until the hand falls off the edge of the liver border. In infants and toddlers, the liver edge may be palpated 1 to 3 cm below the costal margin.

While palpating the abdomen, the examiner checks skin turgor and palpates the femoral pulses and inguinal lymph nodes. Advanced practitioners palpate the spleen and kidneys to determine the presence and size of masses or enlargement.

When areas of tenderness are elicited during palpation, a special procedure for identifying rebound tenderness is used. A site away from the identified tenderness is chosen. The examiner places a hand perpendicular to the abdomen, pushes down slowly and deeply into the abdomen, and then lifts the hand quickly. With peritoneal inflammation, the sudden release of the pressure will cause severe pain and muscle rigidity.

The child is turned over, and the buttocks are inspected. The buttocks in children are full, with symmetric folds. No evidence of scars or ecchymosis should appear on the buttocks. The sacrococcygeal area is examined for any dimples or tufts of hair.

Male Genitalia

The approach to examining the male genitals will depend on the child's growth and development. In an infant, toddler, or young child, the nurse tells the child what will occur and then concurs with the parent or guardian that the nurse should proceed to examine the child's genitalia.

Adolescent boys are normally apprehensive about the genital examination. Concerns arise from modesty, fear of pain, negative judgment, or a previous uncomfortable experience. A matter-of-fact approach and direct communication will facilitate this part of the physical examination. The genital examination is performed during or immediately after the abdominal examination. In the adolescent, the physical examination should not conclude with the genital examination so as to allow further opportunity for communication. A good practice is to conclude the physical examination with the musculoskeletal and neurologic examination after the genital examination has been completed.

Gloves should be worn during every genital examination. The examiner begins by inspecting the penis. The size of the penis is directly related to age and to growth and development. In infants and young boys, the penis is approximately 2 to 3 cm. Genital hair distribution is noted. The adolescent shows a wide variation in normal development of the genitals. Tanner stages are used for determining the level of development in the adolescent (see Chapter 8).

The skin on the penis normally appears wrinkled, hairless, and without lesions. In the adolescent, a dorsal vein may be prominent. Any indurations on the penile shaft should be noted. In the circumcised male, the glans looks smooth and without lesions. In an uncircumcised infant, the glans may not be visible. By the time the male is age 5 to 6 years, the foreskin should be easily retractable behind the corona of the glans. The adolescent is asked to retract the foreskin himself.

The meatus is evaluated by compressing the glans between the thumb and forefinger anteroposteriorly. The adolescent

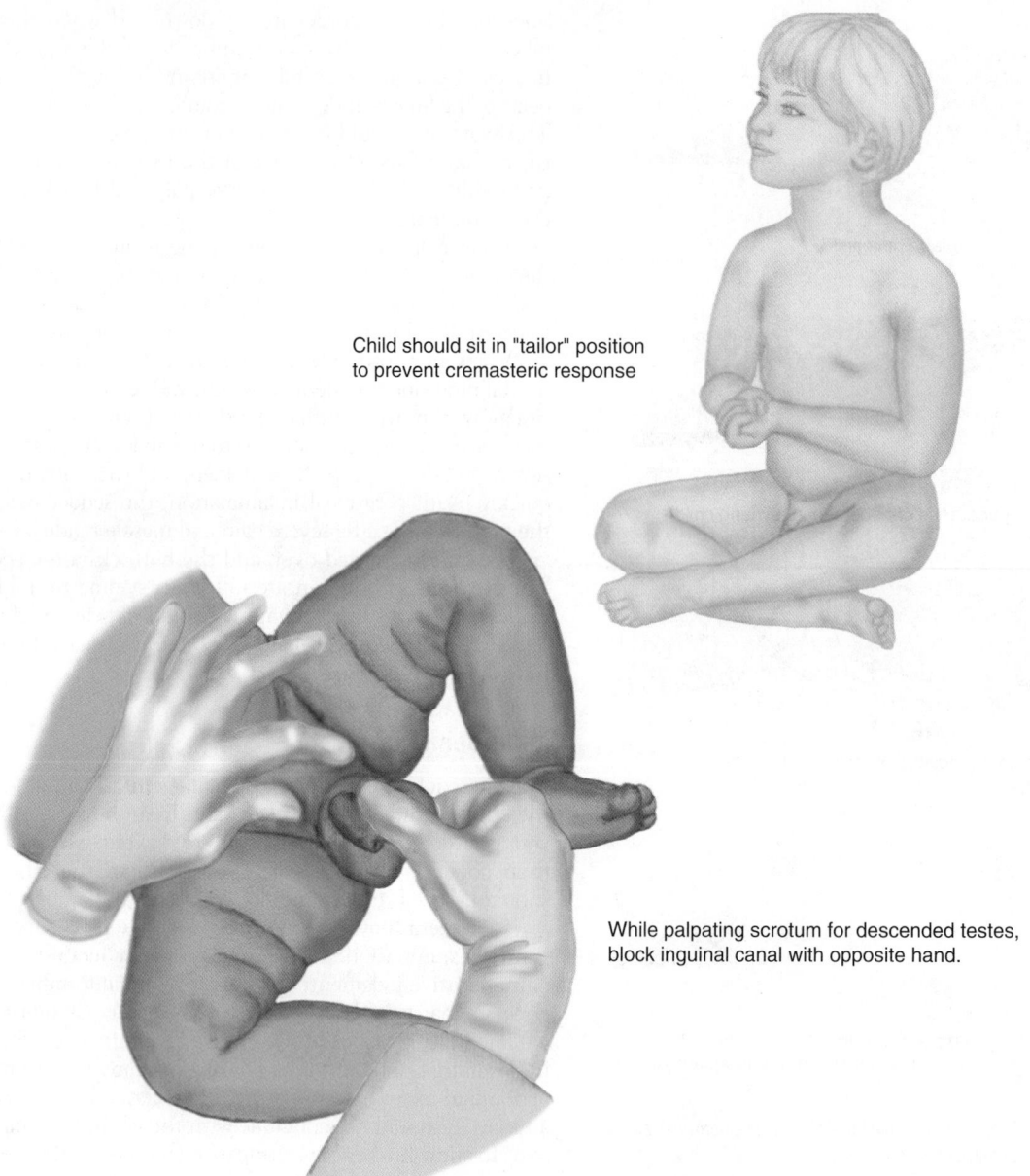

Child should sit in "tailor" position to prevent cremasteric response

While palpating scrotum for descended testes, block inguinal canal with opposite hand.

Figure 33-21 When a boy's scrotum is examined, the cremasteric reflex may cause the testes to withdraw into the inguinal canals. To prevent this reflex, the examiner can have the boy sit in a tailor position. The examiner uses one hand to block the inguinal canals and the other to palpate.

may be requested to compress the glans so that the examiner can see the meatus. The meatus in the male has a slitlike or tear-shaped configuration and is located on the ventral surface, just millimeters from the tip of the glans. The meatus opening is pink, smooth, and without discharge.

The scrotum is inspected for size and configuration, which changes with growth and development. In the infant or young boy, the proximal portion of the scrotum is wider and the distal portion narrower. In the adolescent boy, the proximal portion is narrower and the distal portion wider. Asymmetry of the scrotum is normal, with the left half slightly lower than the right. The scrotum is movable and,

to maintain optimal temperature of the testes, will move closer to or away from the body in response to environmental temperature.

The contents of the scrotum are palpated. The *cremasteric* reflex in young boys may cause the testes to withdraw into the inguinal canal, making palpation more difficult. If the boy is old enough, have him sit in a cross-legged, or "tailor," position, which will help prevent the cremasteric reflex by stretching the muscle, thereby preventing its contraction. In infants and young boys, before beginning the abdominal examination, the examiner warms the hands, blocks the inguinal canal with one hand, and palpates for the scrotal contents (Fig. 33-21). The examiner uses the thumb and first two fingers to palpate each testis and epididymis. The testes should be smooth, rubbery, and free of nodules. The size of the testes changes with growth and development. Tanner growth and development stages are used for appropriate interpretation. Because of the high incidence of testicular tumors in young men, adolescents should be taught to do testicular self-examination.

Female Genitalia

In general, the anogenital examination in prepubescent girls is limited to visual inspection and gentle palpation of the external area. Internal speculum examinations are not routine in prepubescent children. The appearance of the external genitalia in females varies from child to child and with growth and development. A relaxed, caring attitude will reassure both child and parent.

To safeguard privacy, reinforce modesty, and decrease anxiety, the child is draped appropriately. The examiner should communicate with the child what will be done and concur with the parent or guardian that it is appropriate to examine the genitalia. With the child in different positions, the genitals will differ in tone, relaxation, and appearance. Generally, the genitalia in young girls are examined with the child supine; the legs are gently drawn up onto the abdomen to expose the genitalia.

The examiner dons gloves and begins by inspecting the *mons pubis* and *labia majora*. The skin should be smooth and clean. The examiner notes the distribution of pubic hair. Tanner stages are used to determine appropriate growth and development (see Chapter 8).

In the newborn, the labia majora and minora may be edematous, with the *labia minora* often more prominent. In the infant, the *hymen* may protrude and may appear thick and vascular. The clitoris may appear relatively large. The hymen is centrally located and about 0.5 cm in diameter. The examiner determines whether the hymen has an opening.

In the young girl or adolescent, the labia majora may be gaping or closed, shriveled or full, and dry or moist, depending on the age and development of the child. The labia majora are usually symmetric (Fig. 33-22).

The examiner uses the fingers to gently spread the labia majora and then inspects and palpates the labia minora, the *clitoris*, the urethral orifice, and the *vaginal introitus*. The labia minora should appear symmetric, dark pink, and moist. On palpation, the tissue should be soft and homogeneous with no tenderness.

With the labia majora spread, the examiner can look superiorly and inspect the clitoris for size and length. The clitoris varies with growth and development. Progressing inferiorly, the examiner locates the urethral meatus, which may be close to or inside the vaginal introitus. The urethral meatus is usually in the midline and appears as a dimple posterior to the clitoris.

The vaginal introitus may be a thin, vertical slit or a large orifice with irregular edges, depending on the characteristics of the hymen. The hymen may or may not be stretched across the vaginal opening. By menarche, the opening should be at least 1 cm wide. The tissue is usually moist. The amount and characteristics of any vaginal discharge depend on the circu-

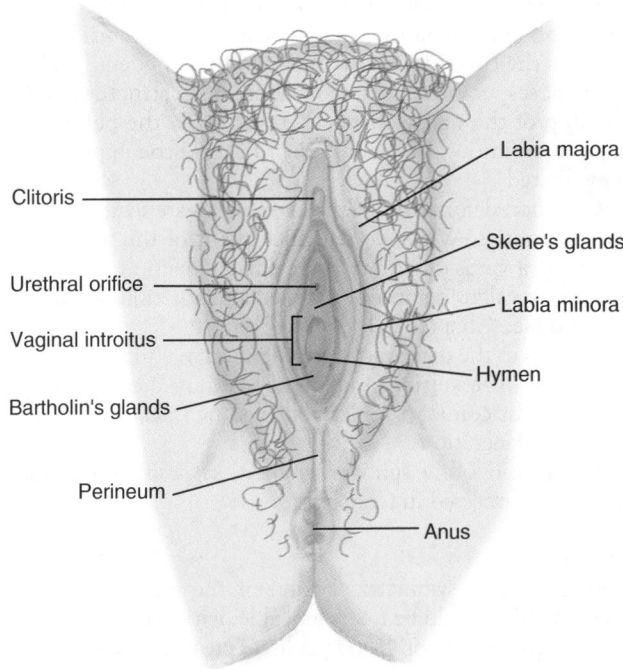

Figure 33-22 Postpubertal female genitalia.

lating hormones in the child. A normal vaginal discharge is odorless and may be cloudy or clear, thick or thin.

Normally, *Skene's glands*, located just inferior to the urethral meatus, are not seen or felt and have no discharge. Any discharge from Skene's glands indicates an infection. The examiner inspects and palpates *Bartholin's glands*, located in the posterolateral portion of the labia majora. Bartholin's glands should not be swollen or tender.

A speculum examination of the internal reproductive organs is not indicated for young girls. The adolescent girl has special needs during the genital examination, which is performed by advanced practitioners.

Musculoskeletal System

The musculoskeletal system is composed of the bones, joints, cartilage, ligaments, and muscles. Joint motions are defined as flexion, extension, abduction, adduction, internal rotation, external rotation, and circumduction. The musculoskeletal examination focuses principally on the upper and lower extremities and the spinal column. Musculoskeletal evaluation begins with observing the child during play or history taking. Observation of the child climbing, jumping, hopping, rising from a sitting position, and manipulating toys and other objects provides evidence of joint function, range of motion, bone stability, and muscle strength. Assessment of fine motor and gross motor ability is accomplished during the Denver II test for the child younger than 5 years (see Chapter 4 and Appendix F).

General inspection begins with visual scanning of the body using a *cephalocaudal* (head-to-toe) organization. The child can be examined in shorts or underwear. The examiner compares the two sides of the body for symmetry, contour, size, and involuntary movement. The examiner then inspects the two sides for areas of swelling or edema and for ecchymoses or other discolorations. The structural relationship of the feet to the legs, the hips to the pelvis, the upper extremities, the shoulder girdle, and the upper trunk is evaluated.

Common deformities of the extremities are *varus* and *valgus* deformities. With the reference point of the midline of the body, a varus deformity is a medial adduction or turning inward. A valgus deformity is a medial abduction or turning outward (see Chapter 50).

Injuries to the extremities are common in children and are caused by overexertion and strenuous movements. Sprains are the most common injury, followed by fractures, dislocations, and lacerations.

Deformities of the spine are *scoliosis*, *kyphosis*, and *lordosis*, which are discussed in Chapter 50.

Infants

During infancy, symmetric flexion of the arms and legs is noted. Limbs should be freely movable, with symmetry of the axillary, gluteal, femoral, and popliteal creases. The examiner inspects the hands, noting the shape, number, and position of the fingers and palmar creases. The clavicle should feel smooth, regular, and without crepitus. By age 2 months, the infant can lift the head while prone.

The examiner observes range of motion as the infant spontaneously moves the extremities. When the infant is lifted with the examiner's hands under the axillae, the infant with normal muscle strength wedges securely between the hands. The examiner checks the hips for congenital dislocation by comparing leg lengths. Place the baby's feet flat on the table, and flex the knees up. Look for the top of the knees to be the same height (Allis test). Posterior gluteal folds should be equal on both sides. The *Ortolani* and *Barlow maneuvers* are performed by a trained examiner on every visit until the infant is 1 year old (see Fig. 22-9).

Toddlers, Preschoolers, and School-Age Children

The examiner may want to start with the child's hands and arms by checking for range of motion and the presence of pain while the child is sitting. Children are willing to show their hands, so this is an excellent way to make contact with the child.

The child should stand so that the examiner can observe the posture from behind. The shoulders should be level and the scapulae symmetric. Lordosis is common in young children. Anteriorly, the examiner begins with the feet and observes for adduction and pronation of the foot. Pronation is common between ages 12 and 30 months because of the young child's broad-based stance. Adduction, or toeing in, is demonstrated when the child walks on the lateral side of the foot. Adduction tends to correct itself by age 3 years as long as the foot is flexible. *Genu varum* (bowleg) is present when a space of more than 2.5 cm is measured between the knees as the medial malleoli are held together. Genu varum is normal after the child has begun to walk and may persist until the child is 3 years old. *Genu valgum* means that more than 2.5 cm remains between the medial malleoli when the knees are held together. Genu valgum is present between ages 2 and 3½ years (see Chapter 50).

The child is instructed to stand on one leg and then the other while the examiner watches from behind. The iliac crest should stay level when the weight is shifted.

Adolescents

For adolescents, the examiner follows the sequence described for school-age children but with special attention to the spine. Adolescents frequently have kyphosis (see Fig. 50-9) caused by poor posture. Children ages 9 through 15 years should be screened for scoliosis (Box 33-9).

Range of Motion

The examiner notes the child's ability to perform active range-of-motion movements when the child is sitting, standing, and moving about the examination room. The equality of movement for each joint and for contralateral joints should be noted. There should be no pain, limitation of movement, spastic movement, joint instability, deformity, or crepitation during movement. Passive range-of-motion movements are performed on joints where limitations are noted. Passive range-of-motion movement is accomplished by the examiner anchoring the joint with one hand while the other hand slowly moves the joint to its limit. Active and passive ranges of motion should be the same.

Muscle Strength and Mass

The examiner assesses the strength of each muscle group. The child is asked to flex the muscle and then resist as opposing force is applied against flexion. Muscle tone should be firm on palpation. When appropriate, the evaluation of muscle strength is integrated with examination of the associated joint for range of motion. Evaluate the motor segment of cranial nerve V (*trigeminal nerve*) by applying opposing force to the temporalis muscle while the child clenches the teeth. Cranial nerve XI (*spinal accessory nerve*) is tested by assessing the strength of the sternocleidomastoid and trapezius muscles with rotation of the head from side to side and chin to shoulder.

When atrophy or hypertrophy is suspected, the examiner measures muscle mass. Muscles are best measured at their greatest circumference. With the joint used as a landmark, the distance from the joint to a point on the extremity is measured and compared with the opposite muscle. One measurement is not as significant as a series of measurements to determine changes in size of muscles.

Joints

The examiner palpates each joint for temperature, tenderness, swelling, crepitation, and masses. In children, fatigue, stiffness, or weakness, along with heat and redness, is frequently associated with disorders of the joints. Children will usually not move a joint if they are experiencing pain.

Gait

Assessment of gait and the ability to ambulate is an essential part of both the musculoskeletal and neurologic assessments. The developmental acquisition of the ability to walk follows a prescribed sequence in infants and toddlers (Table 33-4 and see Chapter 5).

Gait is assessed in two phases—stance and swing. The stance phase begins when the heel strikes the floor; then the

BOX 33-9
Screening Procedure for Scoliosis

To ensure early detection and treatment, children ages 9 through 15 years should be screened for scoliosis. At greatest risk are girls from 10 years old through adolescence.

The child should be unclothed or wearing only underpants so that the chest, back, and hips can be clearly seen. Have the child stand with her or his weight equally on both feet, legs straight, and arms hanging loosely at the sides. Observe for the following signs of scoliosis:

- Nonpainful lateral curvature of the spine
- A curve with one turn (C curve) or two compensating curves (S curve)
- Lateral deviation and rotation of each vertebra, observed better by looking at the ribs as well as the spinal column itself
- Unequal shoulder heights
- Congenital scoliosis visible in the infant lying prone; the condition is sometimes more prominent if the infant is suspended prone
- Unequal scapular prominences and heights. (Note that the muscle masses may be somewhat unequal, especially if the child uses one shoulder more than the other, as in carrying books. Look for bony, not muscular, prominence.)
- Unequal waist angles
- Unequal rib prominences and chest asymmetry
- Unequal rib heights when the child stands in Adam's position (see photograph)

The physical examination should also include:

- Observation for equal leg lengths
- Examination of the skin for hairy patches, nevi, café au lait spots, lipomas, dimples
- Neurologic examination
- Cardiac examination for Marfan syndrome

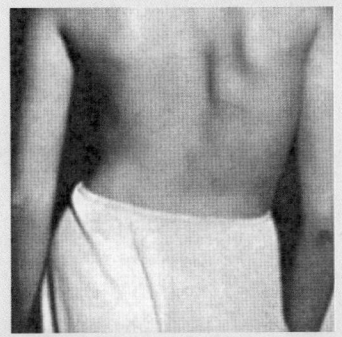

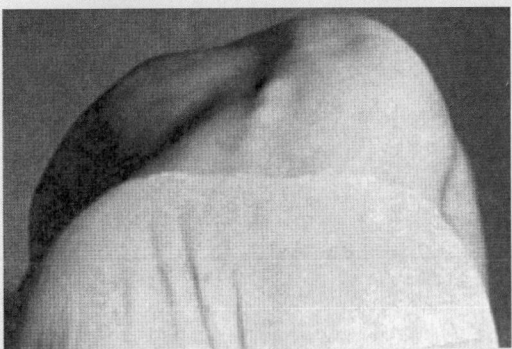

Adam's position with rib hump of structural scoliosis. Lateral curvature of thoracic and lumbar segments of the spine, usually with some rotation of involved vertebral bodies.

Functional scoliosis is flexible; it is apparent with standing and disappears with forward bending. It may be compensatory for other abnormalities such as leg-length discrepancy.

Structural scoliosis is fixed; the curvature is evident both when the individual stands and when the individual bends forward. Note the rib hump with forward flexion. When the child is standing, note unequal shoulder elevation, unequal scapulae, obvious curvature, unequal elbow level, and unequal hip level.

Data from Burns, C.E. (2000). Musculoskeletal disorders. In C.E. Burns, N. Barber, M.A. Brady, & A.M. Dunn (Eds.), *Pediatric primary care: A handbook for nurse practitioners* (p. 1147). Philadelphia: Saunders. Photographs from Delp, M.H., & Manning, R.T. (1981). *Major's physical diagnosis: An introduction to the clinical process* (9th ed., p. 450). Philadelphia: Saunders.

TABLE **33-4** Gross Motor Development in the Infant: Progression to Walking

Activity	Age
Raises head and holds position	2 wk to 2 mo
Moves all extremities, kicking arms and legs when prone	2 mo
Draws up knees and raises abdomen off table; rocks back and forth while up on hands and knees; rolls over	3-6 mo
Sits alone, using hands for support (tripod fashion)	By 7 mo
Lurches forward and pulls legs to chest in "inchworm" fashion, may move backward in same fashion; creeps and rolls	By 9 mo
Crawls in one-sided manner (moves arm and leg on same side of body, then other side)	6-9 mo
Crawls in regular fashion, alternating arm and opposite leg	6-9 mo
Begins to pull up	By 11 mo
Cruises: attempts to walk with support or holding on to something stable	By 12 mo
Momentarily lets go and maintains balance for a few seconds	Once comfortable standing and holding on
Takes first steps (a broad stance with arms flexed for balance)	Once standing balance accomplished
Sits from a standing posture	By 12 mo
Walks alone	By 15 mo

BOX 33-10
Specific Cerebral Function Tests

- *Sound recognition:* Can the child identify familiar sounds with the eyes closed?
- *Auditory and verbal comprehension:* Does the child answer questions and carry out instructions appropriate for age?
- *Recognition of body parts and sidedness:* Does the child recognize the parts of the body? Does the child know right from left?
- *Performance of skilled motor acts:* Can the child drink from a cup, button clothes, use a common tool?
- *Visual object recognition:* Can the child identify a familiar toy or object (e.g., wristwatch)?
- *Visual and verbal comprehension:* Can the child read appropriately and explain the meaning?
- *Motor speech:* Does the child imitate different sounds and phrases?
- *Automatic speech:* Can the child repeat series learned (e.g., nursery rhymes, days of the week)?
- *Volitional speech:* Does the child answer questions relevantly?
- *Writing:* Can the child write his or her name or the name of an object?

weight is transferred to the ball of the foot, and the toes push off the floor. The swing phase consists of acceleration, swing through, and deceleration.

Neurologic System

The purpose of the neurologic examination in the child and adolescent is to identify any nervous system malfunction and to ascertain the extent of nervous system development and functioning. In cases of neurologic deficit, the examiner needs to determine the degree, type, and location of nervous system lesions. In the child, the examiner determines the degree to which the nervous system is functioning so that the healthy portion of the nervous system can be used for habilitation or rehabilitation. For the child younger than 5 years, neurologic functioning is best evaluated by using the Denver II test (see Chapter 4 and Appendix F). For the child older than 5 years, adapt the sequence of the neurologic examination to the child's ability to understand and cooperate.

Testing cerebral function, cranial nerves, and cerebellar function gives a picture of nervous system functioning above the spinal cord. The child's age and development determine the sequence of the neurologic examination. The infant and younger child are not able to cooperate with neurologic testing. A review of developmental milestones attained helps establish the rate and consistency of development in the infant and younger child. The 3- or 4-year-old cooperates with testing when it is approached as a game.

Cerebral Function

The evaluation of cognitive function focuses on appearance, behavior, orientation, speech patterns, memory, logic, and affect. The examiner needs to obtain information from the primary caregiver about changes in the child's behavior, personality, appearance, and age-appropriate school performance. Evaluation of cognitive function in the older child and adolescent is based on observation of level of consciousness, awareness, thought processes, and communication.

The degree of response to sensory stimuli provides information about the older child's or adolescent's level of consciousness. The child is described as alert, lethargic, obtunded, stuporous, or comatose.

The older child and adolescent have the ability to understand, think, feel emotions, and appreciate sensory information about the self and surroundings. Awareness is evaluated by observing the older child's or adolescent's level of orientation in relation to person, place, and time. The normally functioning child is oriented to person, place, and time.

Thought processes include abstract thinking, problem solving (simple calculations and concentration), insight, memory (recent and remote), and judgment. The child's school performance may or may not be an accurate indicator of thought processes. Factors that may influence thought processes are attention span, communication, perceptual problems, and emotional withdrawal and depression.

Language ability is evaluated through speech patterns and comprehension. Question the child about reading and writing ability. Is the child's speech intelligible? Does the child answer questions appropriately for age and developmental level? The normally functioning child is able to speak fluently, name objects correctly, and write both name and address (Box 33-10).

Cranial Nerves

Assessment of the cranial nerves (Table 33-5) should be incorporated into the examination of the system each nerve affects. Games, such as making faces or performing tests on a parent or the examiner, will enhance cooperation.

Cerebellar Function

Proprioception, balance, and coordination are tested by having the child perform specific movements. The cerebellum controls balance and coordination. Proprioception evaluates laterality and orientation in space. The techniques used vary with the child's age and development. The child should attempt the technique and show continued improvement with maturation (Box 33-11).

Motor System

Muscle size, muscle tone, involuntary movements, and muscle strength are assessed during the musculoskeletal examination.

While the child is at rest, the muscles are inspected and palpated for size, consistency, and possible atrophy. The examiner notes symmetry of posture and of muscle contours and outlines.

Muscle tone is evaluated by palpating the muscles at rest and noting resistance to passive movement. The examiner inspects the muscles for involuntary movements. Muscle strength is tested first without resistance and then against resistance. Corresponding muscles are compared on each side. The examiner then tests the major joints for flexion, extension, and other movements.

TABLE **33-5** Assessing Cranial Nerves

CRANIAL NERVE	PROCEDURE
Cranial nerves are tested when the system in which they occur is assessed.	
I (olfactory nerve)	The child is asked to identify familiar odors with the eyes closed. Each side of the nose is tested separately.
II (optic nerve)	Visual acuity is tested using the Snellen chart, HOTV chart for young children, or the tumbling E chart for very young children. Each eye is tested separately and then both eyes together. If corrective lenses are worn, the eyes are tested both with and without correction.
III, IV, VI (oculomotor, trochlear, abducens nerves)	The child is asked to follow a toy or the examiner's finger as the object moves in all directions of gaze (six cardinal fields of gaze).
V (trigeminal nerve)	The child is asked to identify a wisp of cotton on the face. Corneal reflex is tested by observing for blinking when the examiner approaches the face closely. The masseter and temporal muscles' strength can be evaluated by having the child bite down on a tongue blade as the examiner tries to remove it.
VII (facial nerve)	The child is asked to imitate the examiner's frown, wrinkled forehead, smile, and raised eyebrow. The child tries to keep the eyes closed while the examiner attempts to open them, to test the strength of the eyelid muscles. The sensory portion of the facial nerve can be evaluated by having the child identify the taste of sugar and salt placed on the anterior part of the tongue on each side.
VIII (acoustic nerve)	Cochlear nerve tests are tests for hearing. Audiometric testing is a quantitative evaluation of hearing. The Weber (lateralization) and Rinne (air and bone conduction) tests are qualitative evaluations of hearing.
IX, X (glossopharyngeal nerve, vagus nerve)	The glossopharyngeal and vagus nerves are tested together. With a tongue depressor, the gag reflex is tested by touching the posterior pharyngeal wall. The palatal reflex is tested by stroking each side of the mucous membrane of the uvula. The side touched should rise. Normal function of the vagus nerve is revealed by the child's ability to swallow and to speak clearly.
XI (accessory nerve)	The examiner palpates and notes the strength of the trapezius and sternocleidomastoid muscles against resistance, or the child shrugs the shoulders against resistance.
XII (hypoglossal nerve)	The child is asked to stick out the tongue, and the examiner notes any lateral deviation when it is protruded. The strength of the tongue is assessed by having the child push against the examiner's finger pressed against the cheek with the child's tongue.

Sensory System

Sensory testing depends on the child's perception and interpretation of the stimuli and on the child's age and development. Sensory tests should first be done in an educational practice session before being done in a testing situation. Sensory testing compares both sides of the body, corresponding extremities, and the sensitivity of the distal and proximal parts of each extremity for each form of sensation. Sensory testing is performed to determine if sensory changes involve one entire side of the body, are *dermatomal* (along nerve pathways in the skin) in distribution, or are confined to the peripheral nerves (Box 33-12). In an older child, primary forms of sensation, such as superficial tactile, superficial pain, sensitivity to temperature, sensitivity to vibration, deep pressure pain, and motion and position, can be tested. Cortical and discriminatory forms of sensation require interpretation by the cerebral cortex. Cortical and discriminatory forms of sensation are evaluated by two-point discrimination, point localization, texture discrimination, *stereognostic* (touch recognition of objects) function, *graphesthesia* (identification of figures traced on the skin), and extinction phenomenon.

Reflex Status

Most brain growth occurs in the first year of life. Primitive reflexes in the newborn are inhibited when more advanced cortical functions and voluntary control take over as the child matures and grows. Commonly elicited reflexes are described and illustrated in Table 33-6.

Motor maturation proceeds in a cephalocaudal direction. The ability to elicit a reflex requires an intact afferent nerve fiber, functional synapses in the spinal cord, intact motor nerve fibers, functional neuromuscular junctions, and competent muscle fibers. The examiner compares the responses on the right and left sides, which should be equal. Diminished or hyperreflexic responses are reported for further evaluation.

Neurologic "Soft" Signs

Neurologic soft signs are findings that indicate the child's inability to perform certain activities related to the child's age. They may provide subtle clues to an underlying central nervous system deficit or neurologic maturation delay.

Although these findings may fall in a gray area, they should be recorded and reported when observed. Children

BOX 33-11
Cerebellar Function: Tests of Balance and Coordination

Balance and coordination are tested by having the child perform the following movements:

- *Finger-to-nose test.* Child performs first with one hand, then with the other; first with the eyes open, then with the eyes closed. Ask child first to touch her finger to her nose and then to your finger as you change the position of your finger. Repeat this action with increasing rapidity. The tests are performed with each hand.

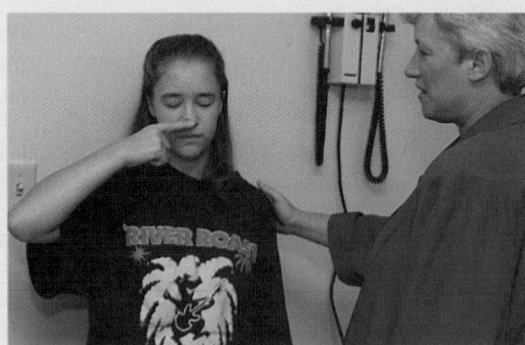

- *Rapid alternating movements.* Ask the child to rapidly pat his knee with the palms and backs of his hands by pronating and supinating the hands (*demonstrate first*). Ask the child to touch his thumb to each of his fingers in rapid succession (*demonstrate first*).

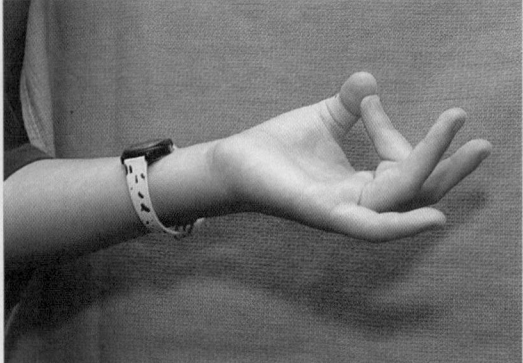

- Ask the child to stand erect, first with the eyes open and then with the eyes closed. Stand near the child to prevent injury if the child begins to fall.

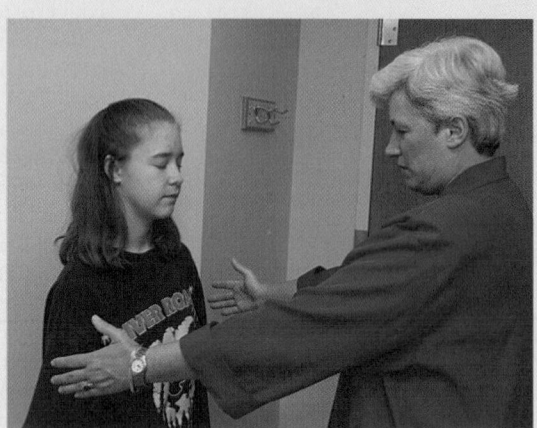

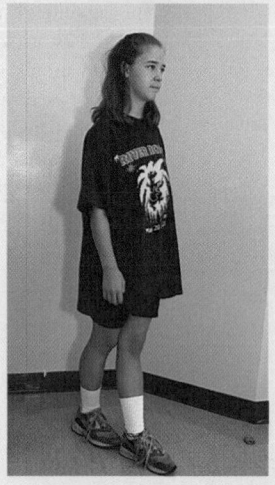

- Ask the child to walk in tandem fashion, placing her heel immediately in front of her opposite foot's toe and alternating while walking a straight line.

- Ask the sitting child to run each heel down the opposite shin. With the child lying down, ask the child to point to your hand with each big toe.

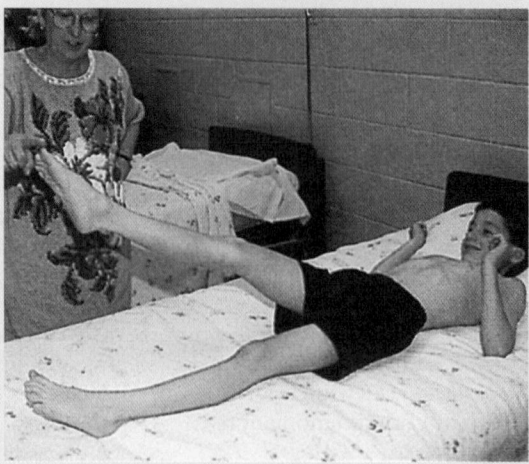

BOX 33-12
Tests for Evaluating Sensory Function

PRIMARY FORMS OF SENSATION

Check in sequence the hands, forearms, upper arms, trunk, thighs, lower legs, and feet for:

- *Superficial tactile sensation:* Touch the child with a wisp of cotton.
- *Superficial pain:* Touch the child with a pin or other sharp object. Be careful not to injure or frighten the child.
- *Sensitivity to temperature:* Touch the various parts of the child's body with test tubes containing warm and cold water. This test is infrequently done with children because of the difficulty of keeping water warm or cold enough for the child to distinguish the difference.
- *Sensitivity to vibration:* Hold a vibrating tuning fork to the bony prominences, noting the child's ability to perceive the vibration and tell you when the vibration stops.
- *Deep pressure pain:* Press the tip of your fingernail against the child's fingernail. The child will feel discomfort. You may also squeeze the Achilles tendon, calf, and forearm muscles, noting sensitivity.
- *Motion and position:* Hold the sides of the toes, thumbs, and fingers by grasping them between your index finger and thumb. Move the fingers and toes passively, and ask the child to tell you the final position of the digit.

CORTICAL AND DISCRIMINATORY FORMS OF SENSATION

These forms of sensation are complex somatic sensory impressions that require interpretation by the cerebral cortex. The following sensations can be evaluated, depending on the age and development of the child being tested:

- *Two-point discrimination:* Can the child differentiate between one and two points? With the child's eyes closed, various parts of the body are touched simultaneously with two sharp objects. Alternate touching the child with one point or two points. Different areas of the body differ in the distance by which the child can differentiate one from two points. This test is more appropriate for older children.
- *Point localization:* With the eyes closed, can the child locate the spot where the child was touched?
- *Texture discrimination:* Can the child recognize with the hands the difference in the feel of materials such as cotton, wool, and silk?
- *Stereognostic function:* Can the child identify familiar objects placed in each hand? Place several objects in a paper bag, and have the child identify them with each hand and show you the object.
- *Graphesthesia:* Can the child identify letters or numbers traced on the palm or back of the hand with a blunt point? Numbers are easier than letters for a young child to recognize.
- *Extinction phenomenon:* With the eyes closed, can the child identify touch on both sides? Touch opposite sides of the body in identical areas simultaneously. This test is used for older children only.

TABLE 33-6 Evaluating Common Reflexes

Reflex	Evaluation
Deep Tendon Reflexes	Evaluation elicited by tapping briskly on a tendon or a bony prominence, evoking a sudden stretching of certain muscles and their resulting contraction. For an adequate response, the limb should be relaxed and the muscle partially stretched. The reflex is stimulated by directing a sharp blow of the reflex hammer onto the muscle's insertion tendon.
Biceps Reflex	The child's arm should be flexed up to 45 degrees at the elbow. The biceps tendon in the antecubital fossa is palpated. The thumb is then placed on the biceps tendon, and a blow is struck on the thumb. The response is a visible or palpable flexion of the forearm.
Triceps Reflex	The arm is suspended by holding the upper arm and instructing the child to just let the arm "go limp." Alternatively, the forearm can be supported on the examiner's arm. The triceps tendon is struck directly just above the elbow. The response is extension of the forearm.

Continued

TABLE **33-6** Evaluating Common Reflexes—cont'd

Reflex	Evaluation
Brachioradialis Reflex	The child's arm is supported on the examiner's arm, and the elbow is flexed up to 45 degrees. The brachioradial tendon is struck with the reflex hammer 1-2 inches above the radial styloid process. The response is pronation and flexion of the elbow.

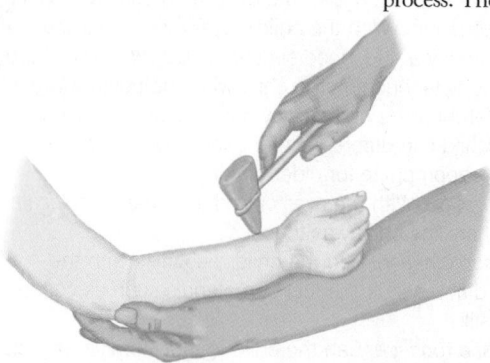

Patellar Reflex	The lower leg is allowed to dangle freely by flexing the child's knee up to 90 degrees. The examiner supports the upper leg with the hand and strikes the patellar tendon just below the patella. The response is extension of the lower leg.

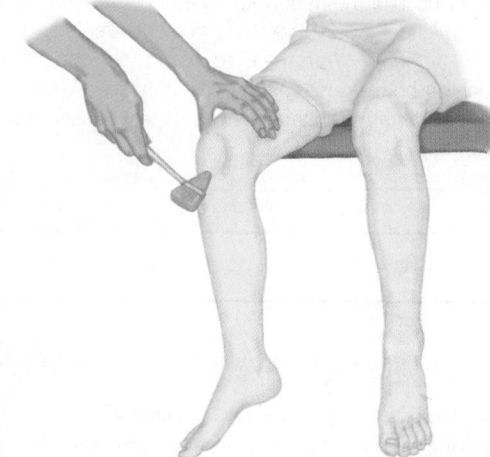

Achilles Reflex	The hip is externally rotated, and the foot is held in dorsiflexion. The Achilles tendon is struck directly. The response is plantar flexion of the foot. An alternative way to elicit this reflex is to have the child kneel on a chair with the toes pointing toward the floor; the examiner then strikes the Achilles tendon directly.

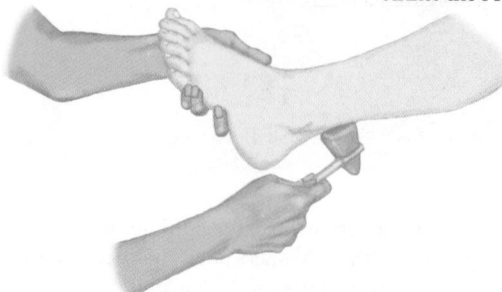

Clonus Reflex	Eliciting a *clonus*—a continued, rapid flexion and extension of the foot and hand—is attempted in children. Clonus is elicited by suddenly and briskly dorsiflexing the foot or hand and applying sustained and moderate pressure. No rhythmic oscillating movements should be palpated.
Superficial Reflexes	Tested by stroking the skin with an object that is moderately sharp but not sharp enough to break the skin. The receptors are in the skin rather than the muscles.

TABLE **33-6** Evaluating Common Reflexes—cont'd

Reflex	Evaluation
Upper and Lower Abdominal Reflexes and **Cremasteric Reflex** 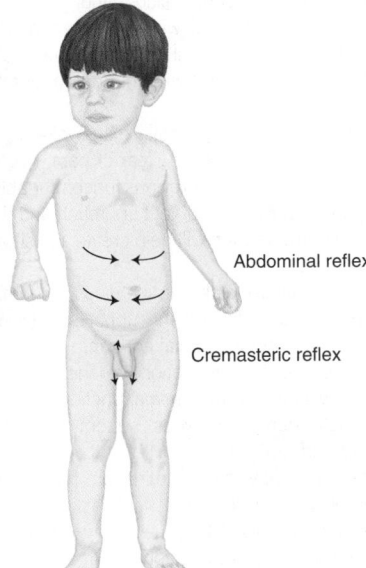 Abdominal reflex Cremasteric reflex	*Upper and lower abdominal reflexes:* While the child is in a supine position and with the abdomen exposed and knees slightly bent, the skin of the abdomen is stroked. Movement of stroking is from the side of the abdomen toward the midline at both the upper and lower abdominal levels. The response is ipsilateral contraction of the abdominal muscle with an observable movement of the umbilicus toward the side being stroked. *Cremasteric reflex:* In the male, light stroking of the inner aspect of the thigh causes the ipsilateral testicle to elevate. This reflex may cause withdrawal of the testicles into the inguinal canal when the abdomen is touched with very cold hands.
Plantar (Babinski) Reflex 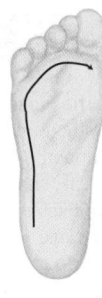	The lateral aspect of the sole of the foot, from the heel to the ball of the foot, is stroked in a movement curving medially across the ball. A fingernail or the wooden end of an applicator stick may be used. The response in an infant is dorsiflexion, fanning of the toes, and hyperextension of the great toe. Once a child is walking, the response is plantar flexion of the toes. Some children withdraw from this stimulus by flexing the hip and the knee.
Gluteal Reflex	When the buttocks are separated, the skin tenses at the gluteal area.

with multiple soft signs are often found to have learning problems (Seidel et al., 2003).

Children with soft neurologic signs need evaluation and monitoring because some children with other medical, mental, or emotional problems may also demonstrate neurologic soft signs (Box 33-13).

CONCLUSION AND DOCUMENTATION

When the physical examination has been completed, the examiner should ask the parents and child, if age-appropriate, whether they have any questions concerning the examination. Findings are documented in a complete and concise manner. Deviations from normal and risk factors should be identified and documented. Depending on the setting, referrals may be made.

BOX 33-13
Examples of Neurologic "Soft" Signs

- Short attention span
- Poor motor coordination
- Clumsiness
- Frequent falling
- Hyperkinesis, voluntary or involuntary
- Uneven perceptual development
- Incomplete laterality, with no side clearly dominant
- Language disturbances: articulation disorders, dyslexia
- Motor outflow (movements involving more muscles than intended)
- Mirroring movements of the extremities (e.g., both hands in motion when only one is performing a function)

KEY CONCEPTS

- A systematic approach to the physical examination is to begin at the head and proceed through the entire body to the toes. The physical examination is tailored to the child's age and developmental level.
- The order of the examination should be flexible, and intrusive and frightening procedures should be done at the end of the examination. The examiner should develop creative approaches to complete the physical examination for children of different ages.
- An accurate history is the single most important component of the physical examination. The history and physical examination provide both subjective and objective data for identifying health and illness.
- Vital signs should be assessed on every visit in ambulatory settings and monitored on a routine basis in the hospitalized child.
- Assessment of vital signs is an important way to measure and monitor vital body functions.
- Examination findings are recorded completely and concisely. Deviations from normal and risk factors should be identified, recorded, and, when appropriate, reported for further evaluation.
- Anthropometrics measure the human body and assess nutritional status as well as growth and development. These measures are of

- most value when they are taken serially so that trends can be evaluated.
- The skin is observed for color and palpated to determine moisture, temperature, turgor, edema, and lesions.
- The general appearance of the child is observed for signs of abuse, both physical and psychologic.
- Examination of the lymph nodes is incorporated into the examination when that part of the anatomy is being assessed.
- The head is inspected for symmetry, movement, control, and shape.
- The fontanels are inspected and palpated for size, tenseness, and pulsation.
- The eyelids, eyebrows, palpebral fissures, nasolabial folds, mouth, and nose are inspected for spacing and symmetry.
- The nasal mucosa is inspected for color and moisture.
- Assessment of the mouth in a young child should be performed at the end of the examination because it may cause anxiety.
- The chart chosen to evaluate visual acuity is determined according to the age and development of the child.
- Assessment of the thorax and lungs entails inspection, palpation, percussion, and auscultation.

- Auscultation of the heart is done by listening with both the bell and the diaphragm of the stethoscope with the child lying supine, in the left lateral recumbent position, and sitting up.
- An empty bladder, a warm room, and the child supine with a pillow under the head and the knees flexed will enhance abdominal relaxation.
- Examination of the genitalia may evoke concerns regarding modesty, fear of pain, negative judgment, or a previous uncomfortable experience. A matter-of-fact approach and direct communication will help create a positive experience.
- The musculoskeletal examination is predominantly directed toward the upper and lower extremities and the spinal column.
- The neurologic examination is done to identify any nervous system malfunction and to evaluate current nervous system development and functioning.
- When the physical examination has been completed, the examiner should ask the child and the parents if they have any questions concerning the examination.

ANSWERS to Critical Thinking Exercise 33-1

1. The nurse could assume that Ms. Maloney does not provide adequate care for her child. She might also assume that all teenage mothers lack the skills to be good parents. She might also assume that Kerrie has been neglected in other ways. In fact, however, Ms. Maloney may really be trying to meet all of Kerrie's needs but may not know what those needs are or how to meet them.

2. The nurse should display empathy and avoid displays of disapproval, perhaps by stating, "Children take a great deal of time and energy. You must be very busy trying to balance car-

ing for Kerrie and working. Let's take some time today to look at how we can help you."

3. The nurse can take a thorough history and determine Kerrie's health status from conception to the present. A head-to-toe assessment will provide baseline data. Assuming that no abnormalities are present, the nurse will want to focus on anticipatory guidance related to nutrition, immunizations, safety, and any age-related growth and development issues. While doing the assessment, the nurse role models activities that increase Kerrie's language, motor, sen-

sory, and psychologic skills. The nurse cannot provide care for Kerrie without meeting the needs of her mother. Support systems should be evaluated and, if weak, should be addressed. If Ms. Maloney understands she needs to bring Kerrie to the clinic for preventive care, she is more likely to give clinic visits a higher priority. Teaching is therefore critical. Because of the history of this case, the nurse should assist Ms. Maloney in making the next appointment while in the clinic and should follow up with a call before the visit.

REFERENCES and READINGS

Albert, D.M., & Jakobiec, F.A. (2000). *Principles and practice of ophthalmology* (2nd ed.). Philadelphia: Saunders.

Angel, T., Nigro, J., & Levy, M. (2000). Infestations in the pediatric patient. *Pediatric Clinics of North America, 47*(4), 921-935.

Barkauskas, V.H., Stoltenberg-Allen, K., Baumann, L.C., & Darling-Fisher, C. (2002). *Health and physical assessment* (3rd ed.). St. Louis: Mosby.

Bates, B. (1995). *A guide to physical examination* (6th ed.). Philadelphia: Lippincott.

Berkowitz, C. (2000). *Pediatrics: A primary care approach* (2nd ed.). Philadelphia: Saunders.

Boisvert, J.T., Reidy, S.J., & Lulu, J. (1995). Overview of pediatric arrhythmias. *Nursing Clinics of North America, 30*(2), 365-379.

Burg, F.D., Ingelfinger, J., Wald, E., & Polin, R. (1999). *Gellis & Kagan's current pediatric therapy*. Philadelphia: Saunders.

Burns, C., Barber, N., Brady, M., & Dunn, A. (2000). *Pediatric primary care: A handbook for nurse practitioner* (2nd ed.). Philadelphia: Saunders.

Chadwick, D.L., Berkowitz, D.D., Kerns, D., McCann, J., et al. (1989). *Color atlas of child sexual abuse*. Chicago: Year Book.

Coupey, S. (1997). Interviewing adolescents. *Pediatric Clinics of North America, 14*(6), 1349-1364.

Dinulos, J., & Graham, E.A. (1998). Influence of culture and pigment on skin conditions in children. *Pediatrics in Review, 19*(8), 268-275.

Erickson, B. (2003). *Heart sounds and murmurs across the lifespan* (3rd ed.). St. Louis: Mosby.

Estes, M.E.Z. (1998). *Health assessment and physical examination*. Albany, NY: Delmar Publishers.

Flynn, J. (2003). Recognizing and managing the hypertensive child. *Contemporary Pediatrics, 20*(8), 38-60.

Fox, J.A. (2002). *Primary health care of infants, children, & adolescents* (2nd ed.). St. Louis: Mosby.

Goldbloom, R. (2003). *Pediatric clinical skills* (3rd ed.). Philadelphia: Saunders.

Green, M. (1998). *Pediatric diagnosis*. Philadelphia: Saunders.

Greif, J., & Hewitt, W. (1998). The living canvas: Health issues in tattooing, body piercing, and branding. *Advances for Nurse Practitioners, 6*(6), 26-31, 82.

Heffernan, A.E., & O'Sullivan, A. (1998). Pediatric sun exposure. *Nurse Practitioner, 23*(7), 67-78.

Houlder, L. (2000). The accuracy and reliability of tympanic thermometry compared to rectal and axillary sites in children. *Pediatric Nursing, 26*(3), 311-314.

Jarvis, C. (2000). *Physical examination and health assessment* (3rd ed.). Philadelphia: Saunders.

Lyznicki, J.M., Young, D.C., Riggs, J.A., & Davis, R.M.; Council on Scientific Affairs, American Medical Association. (2001). Obesity: assessment and management in primary care. *American Family Physician, 63*(11), 2185-2196. (Review).

Martini, F.H. (1998). *Fundamentals of anatomy and physiology* (4th ed.). Englewood Cliffs, NJ: Prentice-Hall.

Mattoo, A. (1999). Measurement of blood pressure in children: Recommendations and perceptions on cuff selection. *Pediatrics, 104*(3), e30.

Moran, R. (2003). Breaking the cycle of childhood obesity. *The Clinical Adviso, Feb.*, 62-67.

Nagengast, S.L., Baun, M.M., Megel, M., & Leibowitz, J.M. (1997). The effects of the presence of a companion animal on the physiological arousal and behavioral distress in children during a physical examination. *Journal of Pediatric Nursing, 12*(6), 323-330.

National Center for Health Statistics. (2000). *Pediatric growth charts*. Available on-line: www.cdc.gov/growthcharts.

Nelson, L.B. (1998). *Harley's pediatric ophthalmology* (4th ed.). Philadelphia: Saunders.

Pelech, A. (1999). Evaluation of the pediatric patient with a cardiac murmur. *Pediatric Clinics of North America, 46*(2), 167-188.

Seidel, H.B., Ball, J., Dains, J., & Benedict, G.W. (2003). *Mosby's guide to physical examination* (5th ed.). St. Louis: Mosby.

Simon, C., & Janner, M. (1990). *Color atlas of pediatric diseases* (2nd ed.). Philadelphia: Decker.

Smith, K.M. (1997). The innocent heart murmur in children. *Journal of Pediatric Health Care, 11*(5), 207-214.

Snider, R.K. (Ed.). (1997). *Essentials of musculoskeletal care*. Rosemont, IL: American Academy of Orthopaedic Surgeons.

Story, M., Holt, K., & Sofka, D. (Eds.). (2002). *Bright futures in practice: Nutrition* (2nd ed.). Arlington, VA: National Center for Education in Maternal and Child Health.

Thibodeau, G., & Patton, K. (1999). *Anatomy and physiology* (4th ed.). St. Louis: Mosby.

Thomas, D. (1996). Assessing children: It's different. *RN, 59*(4), 38-45.

Weston, W.L., & Lane, A.T. (1991). *Color textbook of pediatric dermatology*. St. Louis: Mosby.

Wilson, C. (1999). Parental preparation of children for routine physical examinations. *Journal of Pediatric Nursing, 14*(5), 329-334.

Zitelli, B., & Davis, H. (2002). *Atlas of pediatric physical diagnosis* (4th ed.). St. Louis: Mosby.

34

Emergency Care of the Child

LEARNING OBJECTIVES

After studying this chapter, you should be able to:

◎ Describe general principles that encourage cooperation and help make examination and treatment of children in emergency settings more comfortable for the child and family.

◎ List the developmental issues that are significant when caring for infants, toddlers, preschool and school-age children, and adolescents.

◎ Compare the airway anatomy of a child with that of an adult, and explain the significance of the differences in managing the pediatric airway.

◎ Assess the early signs of shock in infants and children, recognizing that changes in heart rate and skin signs are more accurate signs of early shock than is decreased blood pressure.

◎ Define triage, and list the most important factors to assess when obtaining an overall ("across the room") impression of an infant's or child's condition.

◎ Describe the general guidelines for cardiopulmonary resuscitation in infants and children, and discuss what additional precautions and procedures are required for infants and children with traumatic injuries.

◎ List indications that suggest a child brought into the emergency care setting has been neglected or abused, and discuss the nurse's responsibility for reporting possible neglect or abuse.

◎ Identify several possible roles for nurses in preventing traumatic injuries, poison ingestions, and environmental injuries.

DEFINITIONS

ABCDEs Airway, Breathing, Circulation, Disability, and Exposure; critical components of the "primary assessment" that require assessment and interventions in the stabilization of a critically ill or injured child.

airway management Correct positioning of the airway, appropriate interventions used to ensure patency of the airway, and adequate oxygenation and ventilation.

cardiopulmonary resuscitation (CPR) Protocol performed when an individual's respiratory and cardiovascular systems require support to maintain vital functions; airway management, ventilation, and chest compressions are provided to improve tissue perfusion until definitive care is available.

dental emergency Injury or infection of a tooth or teeth occurring when the period of time to definitive care is critical for the survival of the tooth or to alleviate pain.

emergency Psychologic, medical, or traumatic condition that requires immediate care or care within 1 hour to prevent further deterioration.

envenomation Injection of venom by an animal (e.g., usually snakes, lizards, spiders, scorpions) into a human body.

environmental emergency Illness or injury occurring as a result of outside, or environmental, factors.

extracorporeal membrane oxygenation (ECMO) Temporary method of providing cardiovascular, pulmonary, and circulatory support for children for whom other methods of treatment are not effective.

hypothermia Cooling of body temperature to subnormal levels; temperature levels considered to be dangerous to infants and children are core body temperatures below 35.6° C (96° F).

ingestion Swallowing of a potentially toxic substance, such as inappropriate amounts or types of medication, petroleum products, insecticides, or toxic plants.

shock Inadequate tissue perfusion, usually caused by illness or injury, that results in respiratory or cardiovascular compromise.

submersion injury Injury resulting from a near-drowning incident; may be immediately apparent or may appear up to 48 hours after the submersion incident.

trauma Injury from an external cause, such as a motor vehicle collision, fall, gunshot wound, or stabbing; may be self-inflicted, may be deliberately inflicted or accidental, and may be physical or psychologic in nature.

trauma score Numeric score assessed by health care providers to determine the extent of trauma; usually results from adding, subtracting, dividing, or multiplying numbers representing physiologic parameters or specific types of injuries; used for field triage and assessed serially to determine whether a person's condition is improving or deteriorating; also correlated with survivability.

traumatic brain injury (TBI) One of the leading causes of death or permanent disability. Severity of injury may range from mild to severe. Any TBI can result in short-term and long-term disabilities.

triage Sorting process used to decide the urgency of an individual's illness or injury and allocate appropriate resources effectively; purpose is to ensure that the most seriously ill or injured people receive the appropriate level of care, before those with less urgent or emergent conditions.

GENERAL GUIDELINES FOR EMERGENCY NURSING CARE

Many factors affect the psychologic impact of an emergency on both the child and family. In addition to the expected fears children have at various developmental stages (e.g., separation, pain, altered body image), an overriding concern expressed by both children and parents in emergency settings is fear of the unknown. The suddenness with which the child and family come in contact with emergency personnel, the necessity for rapid assessment and intervention, and the relative seriousness of the child's condition can intensify a fearful response and overwhelm normal coping mechanisms. In addition, children and families are unfamiliar with the setting, the staff of the health care facility, the equipment, and the procedures. Emergency nurses can use some simple interventions to make examination and treatment of children in the emergency setting more comfortable for the child and for the family and to decrease the adverse psychologic effects of the experience.

Communicate an attitude of calm confidence. This attitude can be difficult to maintain when the situation is critical, but families in crisis look to nurses for reassurance and expect to see competent, professional behavior. Speak quietly and calmly to the child and parents, and remain firmly in charge. Remember to talk to the family often throughout the visit—silence is a form of communication that is easily misinterpreted. Keep the parents informed of any untoward delays. Acknowledge the child's and family's fears (Eckle & MacLean, 2001).

Establish a trusting relationship with the child and family. Make eye contact with the child and family when you speak to them. Call the child by name to personalize care. Treat the child and family kindly and gently. To establish a trusting relationship, check back with the family and provide periodic updates if the child and family are separated. When parents are confident that they are being kept informed, they are less likely to make demands for additional attention and information. When speaking to the child and family, use simple, nonmedical terms and remember that children (and sometimes adults) can have inaccurate ideas of how their bodies function and the location of body parts. Providing comfort measures to the family members also builds a trusting relationship. Protect their privacy, direct them to a public telephone or cafeteria, and provide space where they can talk quietly.

Encourage caregivers to stay with the child. Family-centered care recognizes the partnership between healthcare workers and family in ensuring the well-being of the child. Nursing care is driven by the needs of the family and client rather than controlled by healthcare providers. According to comfort levels and ability, include the parents as partners in their child's treatment. Unless the child does not want a parent in the room (e.g., some adolescents), a parent can help calm the child, and many examinations and procedures can be performed with the child on a parent's lap. Although having the family

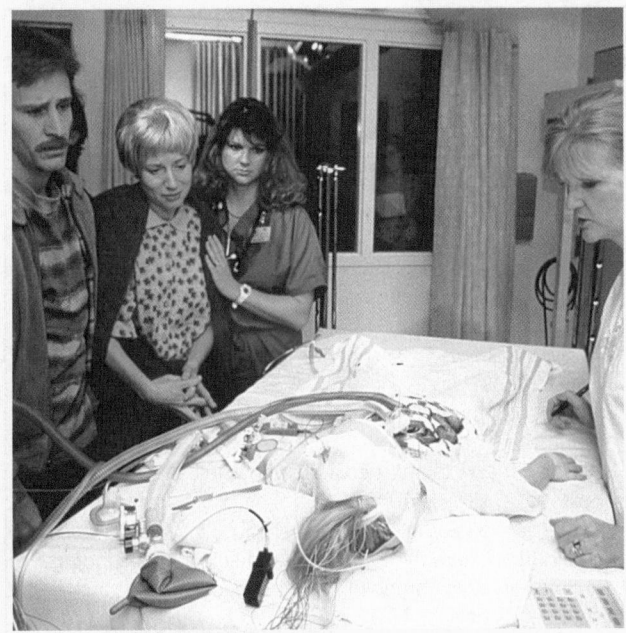

Encouraging parents to remain with their child in the emergency setting can bolster the family's coping. (Courtesy Cook Children's Medical Center, Fort Worth, TX.)

remain with the child can be calming and supportive, respect the family's right to leave if the child's condition or the painful nature of a procedure provokes more anxiety than the family member is able to handle.

For parents who do not know exactly how to be of assistance in these situations, it can help to explain how a parent might help, such as "I think he might stay calmer if you hold his hand and tell him a story while I clean this burn" or "Try counting to 10 with her while I start this intravenous line."

Whenever possible, designate one staff member as the child's caretaker and liaison to the parents. In the unfamiliar emergency setting, the child and family find that having one contact person is less confusing. Consistency is helpful in a crisis because the child and family may feel overwhelmed in the busy and sometimes confusing emergency department environment.

Tell the truth. To establish a trusting relationship, be as honest as possible. If a procedure will be painful, tell the child (usually briefly beforehand). Only then can the child believe health care providers when they say that a procedure will *not* be painful. When a painful procedure is completed, tell the child you are finished and there will be no more pain. Keeping a child informed of what will occur by describing sensations (e.g., "This will feel cold and wet as I clean your arm.") is more helpful than describing the actual procedure.

Provide incentives and rewards. Provide positive feedback when either the child or the parents are being help-

Pediatric Emergency Equipment

Airways:
   Oral: sizes 0-5
   Nasopharyngeal: sizes 12-30 French (Fr)
Endotracheal tubes:
   Cuffed: sizes 6.5-9
   Uncuffed: sizes 2.5-6
Tracheostomy tubes: sizes 00-6
Laryngoscope with blades:
   Straight: sizes 0-3
   Curved: sizes 2-3
Magill forceps
Oxygen equipment: infant, pediatric, and adult masks and cannulas
Bag-valve-mask: infant, pediatric, and adult sizes
Chest tubes: sizes 8-40 Fr
Flexible suction catheters: sizes 6-16 Fr
Pediatric peripheral IV equipment and solutions, including over-the-needle catheters: 14-24 gauge
Intraosseous device: 16-18 gauge
Nasogastric tubes: sizes 5-18 Fr
Urinary catheters: sizes 5-16
Length-based resuscitation tape
Defibrillator with adult and pediatric paddles
Monitors with pediatric-size electrodes and sensors
Blood pressure cuffs (neonatal, infant, child, and adult arm and thigh cuffs)
Heating source
Fluid warmer
Infrared lamp
Overhead warmer

Assess the child's unspoken thoughts and feelings. Try to determine what the child is thinking or feeling but not verbalizing. Encourage the child to express thoughts and feelings, because sometimes the child might be misinterpreting a situation or because the child might need to express emotions.

In some cases, however, the child's and family's coping mechanisms break down, causing inappropriate behavior. If violence or abusive behavior is an issue, you might need to obtain assistance from law enforcement or hospital security officers. For an emotional crisis that does not involve abusive or aggressive behavior, some simple rules apply:

- Encourage the person in crisis to move to a quiet place. Observers and stimuli from other sources tend to aggravate a crisis.
- Encourage the child or parent to talk about feelings as well as the "facts" of the situation. Use reflective statements.
- Avoid defensiveness, explanation, or justification of your own or others' behavior.
- Speak in simple sentences. Use sentences of no more than five words, with words no longer than five letters (e.g., "Let's sit down over here," "Let me help," "Please let go of that.").
- Set limits. Avoid "yes" or "no" responses. Rather than saying, "Will you take this medicine?" (the small child will probably say "NO!"), ask "Would you rather take the pink or the yellow medicine first?"

When interacting with families in distress, a good general rule is to try to listen rather than talk. Simply being present for children and families and empathizing with them are useful interventions. Help families identify specific problems and their effective coping mechanisms, and assist them to explore reasonable solutions.

When coping mechanisms break down entirely, however, some direction is necessary. Consulting social services, spiritual counselors (e.g., chaplain), or crisis intervention professionals can be helpful. Early intervention and support for appropriate coping mechanisms are far easier and less time-consuming than intervening after a child's or parent's emotional decompensation.

ful. Children from 3 to 12 years of age especially appreciate verbal praise and concrete rewards for good behavior, such as stickers, fancy bandages, or inexpensive toys (Emergency Nurses Association, 1998). Adults also appreciate being thanked for their patience and for their assistance in their child's care. All these techniques help create as positive an experience as possible.

Pediatric Emergency Medications

Medication	Use
Activated charcoal	Reduces drug absorption in toxic ingestions
Adenosine	Treats supraventricular tachycardia
Atropine sulfate	Treats symptomatic bradycardia
Bretylium tosylate	Treats ventricular tachycardia; ventricular fibrillation prophylaxis
Calcium chloride	Treats hypocalcemia, hypomagnesemia, hyperkalemia, and calcium channel blocker overdose
Dextrose (25%, 50%)	Treats hypoglycemia—a common complication of dehydration, sepsis, and resuscitation
Inotropic agents	Treat hypotension or hypoperfusion, severe congestive heart failure, or cardiovascular shock
Epinephrine (1:1000, 1:10,000)	Treats bradycardia or asystolic arrest
Lidocaine	Treats recurrent ventricular tachycardia, ventricular fibrillation, or ventricular ectopy
Naloxone hydrochloride	Reverses effects of some narcotics
Sodium bicarbonate (4.2%)	Treats severe acidosis associated with cardiac arrest, unstable hemodynamic status, hyperkalemia, or certain toxic ingestions

Very few experiences are as frightening to a family as a child's sudden illness or injury. Caring for children and families in the emergency setting therefore presents special challenges to the health care team. Nurses play an important role in emergency settings because they are most often responsible for the initial contact, triage, and continuing care throughout an emergency visit. The goals of emergency nursing care include not only addressing the child's physical problems but also supporting the child's and family's coping mechanisms and creating an atmosphere in which the family is valued and kept as intact as possible.

GROWTH AND DEVELOPMENT ISSUES IN EMERGENCY CARE

Emergency nursing care of children needs to address both the physiologic and psychologic differences in children in terms of age and development. Paying close attention to developmental issues assists in obtaining a more accurate assessment and can affect the course of care (see Chapters 5 through 8 for approaches to children of different ages). The nurse treats each child as an individual and avoids becoming judgmental when a child regresses to a "safer" developmental level. Although children of the same age-group are similar, past experiences, cultural differences, and maturity levels may result in a range of behaviors. One toddler might be much more mature than another, and one adolescent might lean more toward school-age behaviors than another (Box 34-1).

The Infant

An infant experiences the world through the senses; hunger, satiation, cold, warmth, quiet, and noise affect the infant's comfort or discomfort. An infant has not learned patience and has little tolerance for physical or emotional discomfort, including pain (see Chapter 39 for management of pain in infants and children).

Although infants are able to discriminate their parents from others, older infants (9 to 18 months of age) can exhibit signs of both separation and stranger anxiety. The nurse should allow the parent to hold the infant as much as possible for examination and treatment. This might not be possible in a critical situation, but nurses need to remember to reunite parent and child whenever feasible.

The Toddler

Toddlers are just beginning to explore the world and seem to have limitless energy and curiosity. They are also beginning to have a clearer image of themselves as autonomous and distinct humans. For this reason, they do not respond well to restrictions and tend to push any limits imposed. This tendency can be a problem in the emergency setting because some nursing care might involve securing and restraining the toddler, which makes the toddler feel vulnerable. The nurse should be sure to remove any restriction or restraint as soon as safety permits. Toddlers have little understanding of time, so procedures should be introduced just before they are initiated.

The Preschooler

The preschool child is talking and beginning to be more independent. This outward appearance of organization is somewhat misleading, however, because the preschool period is also the stage of fear and fantasy. Preschoolers are strong believers in cause-and-effect relationships and tend to blame themselves for illnesses and injuries.

The preschool child might be more willing than the toddler to be separated from parents, but the nurse should keep this separation as brief as possible. The nurse can include the parents in treatments and provide them with instruction on calming the child if they seem unsure. The nurse should not ask a parent to restrain the child, because this role may be confusing to the child and difficult for the parent.

The School-Age Child

School-age children are interested in learning and gradually acquire reasoning skills, including some abstract thinking. They are able to understand the cause of illness and injury and are much less likely to fantasize and exaggerate. School-age children have extensive vocabularies, and they can understand simple explanations of procedures. They are also able to make decisions about their own care. By this time, they have developed personal techniques to help them through painful times. The nurse helps them use coping techniques that work for them.

The Adolescent

Although adolescents are at varying stages of puberty, they begin to resemble adults in appearance. They are also beginning to explore the adult world and develop their own unique identities. The nurse needs to remember, however, that even though adolescents might appear physically mature, they might not be emotionally mature and they continue to require support. Coping with extraordinary changes in their physical appearance, they are often concerned with whether they are "normal" and whether others have similar thoughts and feelings.

Although this is an age of risk taking, which can make them prone to very serious injury, adolescents can be quite fearful of death. Although they are aware of the possibility of their own death, they avoid thinking about its reality. Adolescents consider themselves invincible, and many experience overwhelmingly emotions when a friend dies unexpectedly.

Adolescence is an age of extremes—teenagers might either exaggerate or underplay the seriousness of a condition. Sometimes it is difficult for the nurse to assess the full extent of an adolescent's illness or injury. Expert care of the adolescent requires sensitivity to both verbal and nonverbal cues. It is important to respect adolescents' privacy and approach them as one would an adult, giving them full attention and respect for their thoughts and feelings.

THE FAMILY OF A CHILD IN EMERGENCY CARE

Stress on the family results directly and indirectly from the child's illness or injury. The way a child perceives an illness or injury often is related to the parents' attitude, so caring for the child requires assessment of and intervention with the family.

BOX 34-1
Working With Children in Emergencies: Developmental Guidelines

INFANTS

Allow the use of a pacifier.

Use a quiet, soothing voice.

Touch, rock, or cuddle the infant. Holding the infant securely or swaddling a young infant can also be comforting.

Keep the infant warm; if the infant must be left undressed, use warming lights to ensure a comfortable temperature.

As much as possible, allay parents' fears so they will not be communicated to the infant.

Remember that infants experience pain (see Chapter 39 for pain interventions).

TODDLERS

Give treatments and perform procedures with the toddler sitting up on the stretcher or examining table or on the parent's lap.

Perform the most distressing or intrusive parts of the examination last.

Reassure family members as much as possible—the child will benefit from their confidence.

Allow the child to have familiar objects (transitional objects) such as a blanket, doll, or toy to help feel safe.

Keep frightening objects out of the child's line of vision. Also try to keep machines that make loud noises away.

Praise (e.g., "You are so brave.") and distraction (e.g., bubbles, puzzles) will decrease anxiety and increase cooperation.

PRESCHOOLERS

Explain a procedure or treatment a few seconds rather than minutes beforehand, because allowing the child time to think about it may result in frightening fantasies or exaggerations.

Talk to preschool children throughout procedures, describing the sensations they are feeling or will feel and telling them how they can help.

Distract the child with noises or bright objects. Counting with some preschool children might help calm them during procedures.

Avoid criticizing the preschool child for crying, struggling, or fighting during a procedure.

Reassuring a child that the child did try his or her best to cooperate will help to build a positive self-image.

Encourage the preschool child to talk about how the illness or injury occurred. If the child is inappropriately taking responsibility for the illness or injury, try to reassure that the child is not to blame for the situation.

Remember that preschool children can seem to understand more than they actually do. Health care providers often overestimate understanding in a child of this age, so be sure to explain things in words the child understands.

Use positive terms, such as "make better" and "help," and avoid more frightening terms, such as "shot" and "cut."

Use adhesive bandages over small wounds and injection sites. Preschool children might imagine their blood leaking out through puncture wounds.

SCHOOL-AGE CHILDREN

Offer simple choices whenever possible to help the child feel more in control. The school-age child is capable of deciding in which arm to have an injection or in which hand to hold a nebulizer. Talk directly to the child, explaining procedures in simple terms. When explaining treatments or care options to the parent, include the child.

Ask the child about the level of understanding, and allow time for questions.

Address the child's fears or concerns directly, rather than treating them as foolish or inconsequential.

Give rewards, such as a sticker or inexpensive toy, after a procedure, regardless of the child's behavior. Think of this gesture as a reward for undergoing the procedure, not as a judgment of "good" or "bad" behavior.

ADOLESCENTS

Preserve the adolescent's modesty; offer adolescents a choice as to whether they want their parents present when obtaining history and during the examination.

Consider the legal issues regarding the right to privacy for pregnant adolescents and adolescents with sexually transmissible diseases.

Provide an opportunity for questions.

Listen to the adolescent's concerns nonjudgmentally and without belittling the young person.

Developing a teasing relationship with an adolescent is often a temptation, but this has potential for harm—the adolescent is easily embarrassed.

Explain procedures or treatments carefully, and allow choices. Adolescents are capable of complex abstract thinking and can make intelligent and reasoned decisions about their own care.

The most common emotions experienced by parents of children cared for in emergencies are fear and anxiety. Past experiences may lessen or increase these emotions. Parents are afraid of the following possibilities:

- Their child might die. This fear is the greatest source of anxiety and can be present even when death is highly unlikely, such as in the case of minor illnesses or injuries.

This anxiety is often the underlying cause of parents' anger toward health care providers.

- Their child might experience pain. As a rule, parents try very hard to protect children from pain. Even when pain is necessary, it is difficult for parents to understand and accept.

- The child's body may be permanently altered. Parents often fear that their children will have permanent scars or body changes.

Parental guilt is another frequently seen emotion. Parents can feel guilty for the following reasons:

- They feel responsible for their child's illness or injury.
- They are submitting their child to a painful experience.
- They do not have enough knowledge to make educated decisions about their child's care.

In addition, parents might have had negative experiences with health care providers in the past or may have other concerns about siblings, financial arrangements, and work schedules.

The particular causes of stress for families in emergencies are unique to the circumstances and to the family involved. It is important for the nurse to ascertain who is the family (e.g., single parent, two parents, grandparent, other caregiver) and who are the decision makers (e.g., family members, religious leaders) and communicate accordingly. All the stressors combined could stretch parents' coping mechanisms to the limit and result in anger, withdrawal, or tearfulness. Stress also can manifest itself in hyperactivity—making numerous phone calls, repeating questions, and involving a large number of people.

Including family members in their child's care can reduce feelings of helplessness and promote positive coping mechanisms. It is of advantage to healthcare workers as well as family members if assessment and appropriate support are provided early, before problems occur.

EMERGENCY ASSESSMENT OF INFANTS AND CHILDREN

In the emergency setting, assessment of the ill or injured child must be rapid and accurate to identify abnormal findings quickly. In children, initial evidence of life-threatening conditions can be very subtle, with few signs of impending respiratory or cardiopulmonary arrest. It is particularly important to make as many initial observations as possible without touching the child, so that assessments can reflect the child's baseline, or resting condition. For an apparently stable infant or young child, most of the examination required for general triage can be performed with the child on the parent's lap. The nurse also observes the relationship between the parents and child during the examination process.

The triage nurse usually performs the initial observation in the emergency setting and decides the level of care needed for the child. Triaging is an important skill that improves with experience. The nurse bases much of the initial assessment on an overall sense of how the child looks (an "across the room" assessment)—sick or well. Because children do not try to cover up either how they feel or how they look, the nurse receives a fairly accurate impression of illness or wellness immediately.

Three essential factors combine to form a first impression: respiratory rate and effort, skin color, and response to the environment. Abnormalities are compared with the caregiver's perception ("Is this his normal color?"). If results of this assessment appear to be normal, the nurse completes a more thorough and in-depth evaluation. If the general impression is that the child is seriously ill, the nurse must intervene immediately and combine any additional evaluation with intervention.

> **! CRITICAL TO REMEMBER**
>
> **Initial Observations for Triage**
>
> - *Respiratory rate and effort: Is the child's breathing rapid or shallow, or is the child using accessory muscles? What is the child's position of comfort?* When children are having difficulty breathing, they use accessory muscles to help. Substernal, intercostal, or subclavicular retractions are all signs of serious breathing difficulties. Nasal flaring, head bobbing, grunting, stridor, upright position, and prolonged expirations signal increased work of breathing. A slow respiratory rate is of great concern; a child who seems to be breathing at a rate normal for an adult is almost certainly hypoventilating. This respiratory rate can signal imminent respiratory arrest. Observe for abnormal breath sounds, and assess oxygen saturation by pulse oximeter.
> - *Skin color: Is the child's skin pale, mottled, or cyanotic?* Abnormal skin color could result from the two greatest threats to a child's life: respiratory distress or failure and inadequate tissue perfusion (shock).
> - *Response to the environment: Is the child alert, interactive, crying, sleepy, or limp? Is the child smiling and able to play? Does the child make eye contact and interact appropriately?* Although response to the environment is more difficult to evaluate in the preverbal child, responsiveness is an important component of the assessment. A well child should look around, fixate on objects, and appear to recognize caretakers. An anxious-appearing child may be in respiratory distress; a flaccid, disinterested child may be in respiratory failure or frank shock.

Primary Assessment

Primary assessment, which is part of the initial triage assessment, consists of assessing the *ABCDEs*—*a*irway, *b*reathing, *c*irculation, level of consciousness (*d*isability), and *e*xposure. Because the two most common pathways to mortality in children are respiratory failure and shock, interventions include providing respiratory and circulatory support.

Airway Assessment

Although determining the etiology of respiratory distress or failure in an ill child ultimately will be important, more important is recognizing symptoms and signs of respiratory distress. In the emergency setting, initial treatment is the same regardless of the cause.

Because of some differences in airway anatomy and physiology, children are at greater risk of airway problems than are adults (Table 34-1). When assessing children's airways, the nurse pays particular attention to breath sounds (often audible to the naked ear) as well as snoring, stridor, wheezing, and grunting. Snoring is caused by obstruction in the upper airway (often the tongue relaxing against the posterior pharynx) and can be heard in a child with decreased mental status. Stridor is a high-pitched sound, heard on inspiration (laryngeal obstruction) or on both inspiration and expiration (midtracheal obstruction). Wheezing, a high-pitched, musical sound heard primarily on expiration, signals obstruction of the lower airway. Crackles or rales are fine, popping noises heard on inspira-

TABLE **34-1** Primary Assessment in Pediatric Emergencies

Assessment	Pediatric Differences	Nursing Implications
A—AIRWAY		
Patency, positioning for air entry, audible sounds, airway obstruction (blood, mucus, edema)	The child's airway is narrower than an adult's and more easily obstructed by foreign bodies, small amounts of mucus, or tissue edema. Infants are preferential nasal breathers for the first several months of life; therefore nasal secretions can cause respiratory compromise. Children are more susceptible to infectious respiratory diseases that contribute to risk of airway obstruction. Edema and mucus in a narrow airway cause incrementally more obstruction than in a wider one. The tongue is relatively large in relation to the oral cavity and can more easily fall into the airway in the unconscious child. Cartilage of the larynx is relatively soft, and the trachea is thinner and more flexible than an adult's. The larynx is higher and more anterior, increasing the risk of obstruction and aspiration. The submandibular area is softer and can be more easily compressed to occlude the airway. Deciduous teeth are poorly anchored and easily dislodged.	Allow the child to maintain a position of comfort, or manually position the airway (jaw thrust or head-tilt/chin-lift); encourage the child to avoid flexing or hyperextending the neck; use spinal immobilization and airway adjuncts as required.
B—BREATHING		
Increased or decreased work of breathing, nasal flaring, use of accessory muscles of respiration (retractions), rate, pattern, quality, oxygen saturation	The chest wall is thin, softer, and more compliant. Rib alignment is more horizontal. The younger child is more susceptible to respiratory distress and failure. Retractions commonly occur with respiratory distress and can compromise the ability to increase tidal volume. The diaphragm is the predominant muscle of respiration. Pressure above or below the diaphragm can impede respiratory effort. Infants and children have a higher metabolic rate and increased oxygen demand. Hypoxia occurs more rapidly.	Provide supplemental oxygen; initiate assisted ventilation with bag-valve-mask, and prepare for intubation as indicated; provide gastric decompression by use of orogastric or nasogastric tube; provide comfort measures.

Data from Bernardo, L. (1998). Multiple trauma. In M. Slota (Ed.), *Core curriculum for pediatric critical care nursing* (pp. 568-571). Philadelphia: Saunders; Emergency Nurses Association. (1998). *ENPC provider manual* (2nd ed., pp. 61-67). Park Ridge, IL: Author.

tion; they usually indicate that fluid is in the lungs, such as in pneumonia.

Breathing Assessment
The rate and depth of breathing, as well as breath sounds and the respiratory effort made by the child, indicate relative oxygenation. A rapid respiratory rate with shallow breathing indicates respiratory distress. Very slow breathing in an ill child is an ominous sign, indicating respiratory failure. A slowly breathing child might no longer have the energy for adequate ventilation. Increased work of breathing with quiet breath sounds may indicate an absence of air entry into lung fields. Abdominal breathing is normal in the infant or young child, so the nurse observes the rise and fall of the abdomen instead of the chest.

The use of accessory muscles for breathing invariably indicates respiratory distress. The chest wall of a child is rela-

tively weak and unstable, so retractions occur with increased work of breathing. Assessment of breathing includes observing the child for intercostal, substernal, suprasternal, supraclavicular, and infraclavicular retractions. As a child becomes exhausted, retractions might diminish, usually indicating respiratory failure. Nasal flaring with inspiration is another form of accessory muscle use. Grunting, a sound made by expiration against partially closed vocal cords, represents the body's effort to improve oxygenation by generating positive end-expiratory pressure and is a sign of hypoxemia.

The nurse observes the child's preferred body posture. A child in respiratory distress is upright with the jaw thrust forward, leaning forward on outstretched arms—the tripod position. This position helps to maximize airway opening and the use of accessory muscles of respiration.

Once the work of breathing has been carefully observed, listening to the chest provides some useful information. Chil-

TABLE **34-1** Primary Assessment in Pediatric Emergencies—cont'd

Assessment	Pediatric Differences	Nursing Implications
C—CIRCULATION		
Skin color, temperature, and capillary refill (<2 sec); rate and strength of peripheral and central pulses	The child's circulating blood volume per body weight is much larger than an adult's, even though actual blood volume is much smaller. Therefore small-volume losses have more severe circulatory consequences. A higher percentage of fluid is located in the extracellular compartment, causing more rapid fluid shifts. A higher metabolic rate and oxygen demand require an increased heart rate; tachycardia is the first compensatory mechanism for decreased oxygenation—*not* hypotension.	Control bleeding through application of direct pressure; obtain vascular access; initiate volume replacement; perform chest compressions; defibrillate or provide synchronized cardioversion; initiate drug therapy.
D—DISABILITY		
Level of consciousness or activity level; response to the environment (especially caregivers); pupillary response	A larger head/body ratio and weak neck muscles contribute to more serious head injury from shaking or impact. The anterior fontanel remains open until approximately age 18 mo. An open fontanel allows for expanded cranial volume, so signs of increased intracranial pressure, which indicate underlying brain injury, might be delayed. A thinner skull predisposes the child to more severe injury. Nerve myelinization is incomplete during infancy; unmyelinated tissue is more vulnerable to shearing injury.	Treat the underlying cause (e.g., signs of increased intracranial pressure; fluid or blood volume deficit; hypoxia); compare assessment with parent's perception (a deeply sleeping child may be difficult to arouse, which is "normal" to caregivers).
E—EXPOSURE		
To identify underlying injuries or additional signs of illness	Bulging fontanel, periorbital edema, unusual rashes, and edema or exudate in the pharynx can indicate a variety of severe childhood communicable diseases. Bruising, unusual burns, vaginal tearing, rectal bleeding, and discharge suggest child abuse.	Remove all clothing, including diapers; save any clothing needed for evidence; maintain an appropriately warm environment.

dren have small chests, and breath sounds can be transmitted throughout the chest. The nurse therefore auscultates a child's chest at both sides of the body at the midaxillary line and over the trachea to confirm equality of breath sounds and to distinguish upper from lower airway noises.

Normal respiratory rates for children vary by age and are faster than for adults (see Table 33-1). A respiratory rate over 60 breaths per minute, however, is abnormal for any age. Another important adjunct for respiratory assessment is the pulse oximetry reading (see Chapter 37).

Cardiovascular Assessment

Cardiovascular assessment includes observing the child's skin color and temperature, checking capillary refill, and assessing central and peripheral pulse rate and quality. A child can compensate more effectively for fluid loss, through increased heart rate and peripheral vasoconstriction, than an adult can. Tachy-

cardia and decreased peripheral perfusion are early signs of cardiovascular compromise in a child and require immediate intervention to prevent decompensation. Loss of circulating volume of 20% to 25% may initiate shock compensatory mechanisms without the child showing overt signs, such as altered mental status or hypotension (Caldwell & Ziglar, 2001). Hypotension is a late finding and suggests compensatory mechanisms are no longer adequate to maintain cardiac output.

Disability: Neurologic Assessment

The infant's or child's level of consciousness is an essential component of the primary assessment. Alteration in level of consciousness (irritability or agitation, lethargy, or inability to recognize caregivers) can be the first sign of respiratory compromise or worsening condition.

A rapid neurologic assessment consists of two components: (1) pupillary reactivity and size; and (2) a brief mental status

TABLE **34-2** Secondary Assessment in Pediatric Emergencies

Assessment	Nursing Implications
F—FULL SET OF VITAL SIGNS; FAMILY PRESENCE	
Evaluate the child's vital signs, including temperature, for abnormal findings; obtain weight in kilograms. Family presence: assess the needs of the family for support and inclusion in care.	Continuously monitor the child's vital signs, including temperature; weigh child, or obtain estimated weight if child's condition prohibits measured weight. Provide family support in a culturally appropriate way.
G—GIVE COMFORT MEASURES	
Discomfort is usually related to the underlying problem; use pain assessment scales for children.	Frequently monitor pain level and response to pain relief measures; include nonpharmacologic techniques for reducing pain.
H—HEAD-TO-TOE ASSESSMENT; OBTAIN HISTORY	
Perform a complete head-to-toe assessment, and obtain a history; during triage assessment, the head-to-toe (secondary) assessment may need to relate to the chief complaint.	Continuously monitor the child for changes in condition; assess for any unusual odors.
I—INSPECT THE BACK; ISOLATE	
Observe the back for obvious or hidden injuries; assess for communicable illness or susceptibility to illness (immunocompromised clients).	Reinspect the back as indicated; provide isolation as indicated.

Modified and reprinted with permission from Emergency Nurses Association. (1998). *ENPC provider manual* (2nd ed., pp. 68-75). Park Ridge, IL: Author.

assessment (*AVPU: a*lert; responds to *v*oice; responds to *p*ain; *u*nresponsive). More thorough and sophisticated means of assessment are used later if needed (see Chapter 52). Serial assessment is imperative. Progressive loss of consciousness may be a result of hypoxemia, hypoglycemia, increased intracranial pressure, or another life-threatening condition.

Exposure

Primary assessment ends with exposure, or removing the child's clothing to identify additional injuries or indicators of illness. The nurse needs to preserve the child's clothing appropriately if it will be needed for evidence in any potential civil or criminal proceeding. Infants and children have a larger body surface area/weight ratio, making them at risk for hypothermia. Maintaining body temperature by shivering increases metabolic needs, such as oxygen and glucose, and the child has limited reserves. Methods to assist the child maintain a normothermic state or to assist in warming include over-bed warmers and heat lamps, warmed intravenous (IV) fluids and humidified oxygen, removing wet clothes, and providing warmed blankets.

Secondary Assessment

After the primary assessment is complete and intervention (if necessary) has stabilized the child, the nurse begins the secondary assessment. Components of the secondary assessment include vital signs, assessing for pain, history and head-to-toe assessment, and inspection (Table 34-2).

Vital Signs

Vital signs are useful in the triage assessment of the child, but because age variations make their significance more difficult to interpret, they are not as reliable an indicator as in adult assessment. This variation is especially applicable to temperature. For example, an infant has an immature thermoregula-

tory system and might not have a fever or may even be hypothermic in the presence of infection, so the nurse needs to be alert for supporting signs. The nurse remembers that an alteration in one part of the vital signs may result in abnormal values in other parts. For example, an abnormally high heart rate and respiratory rate may be a result of hyperthermia, crying, pain, hypoxemia, or hypovolemia (see Chapter 37 for methods of obtaining a temperature).

When taking a child's vital signs, the nurse observes the respiratory rate first and then obtains the pulse; the nurse obtains the temperature and blood pressure last, because they can be the most upsetting for children. The nurse should be certain to use the correct-size blood pressure cuff and take both the respiratory and heart rates for 1 full minute, because subtle differences are important in the child. Normal respiratory and heart rates are faster than an adult's, whereas the blood pressure is lower on average (see Table 33-1 and Appendix H for normal vital signs by age). An accurate weight, as described subsequently, should be obtained at this time, and monitors such as cardiac or pulse oximeter should be applied as indicated.

History and Head-to-Toe Assessment

A brief history provides information about prior illness or injury that might affect the emergency care of the child. One format often used for pediatric clients is the mnemonic *AMPLE*:

A—allergies
M—medications taken and immunization history
P—prior illness or injury
L—last meal and eating habits
E—events leading up to this injury or illness (e.g., exposure to other children, mechanism of injury)

This mnemonic gives sufficient information to determine whether the child's medical history will play an important role in assessment and treatment of the current illness or injury. In emergency departments that care for children, a list of immunizations and the appropriate ages should be posted in a convenient location (see Appendix D).

After obtaining an appropriate history, the nurse begins to perform a head-to-toe assessment, documenting any findings that might affect the child's condition. Assessment findings are compared with the history to aid in diagnosis and to look for inconsistencies. The nurse inspects all body surfaces, looking for fractures, lacerations, contusions, and penetrating injuries. The nurse also observes the skin for petechiae or rashes. The presence and pattern of any pain are described. The nurse pays particular attention to signs of pneumothorax or hemothorax (e.g., decreased breath sounds on the affected side, signs of hypoxemia, signs of shock). The nurse then palpates the child's abdomen and auscultates for the presence of bowel sounds. Any sign of hematuria suggests genitourinary injury or infection. Blood found at the urinary meatus suggests disruptive injury of the lower urinary tract and that a urinary catheter should not be inserted.

Diagnostic Tests

Once the child has arrived in the emergency setting and has undergone initial assessment and interventions, many diagnostic tests assist in the evaluation process. Standard protocols for laboratory tests usually include a complete blood count (CBC) with differential count, serum electrolytes, bedside glucose, and urinalysis. Additional studies might be necessary for the child who has multiple trauma. These include coagulation profiles, blood urea nitrogen (BUN), creatinine, glucose, amylase, lipase, SGOT (serum glutamic-oxaloacetic transaminase, also known as *AST* [*aspartate aminotransferase*]), SGPT (serum glutamic-pyruvate transaminase, also known as *ALT* [*alanine aminotransferase*]), and blood type and crossmatch.

Radiologic films may be obtained, depending on the presenting problem and assessment data. Placement of a gastric tube, urinary catheter, or other device might be required.

Weight

Determining the weight of the child is essential in emergency care because all medication dosages and fluid amounts are calculated according to the child's weight in kilograms. The nurse weighs the child on an appropriate scale if possible. If not possible, the nurse obtains a weight history from the parent.

Another way to determine the child's weight and medication dosages is through the use of a length-based resuscitation tape, such as the Broselow tape. A length-based resuscitation tape is placed on a gurney or stretcher next to the child, and the child's length is measured. The length is keyed to emergency medication dosages, usually listed on the tape. The tape also indicates fluid bolus volumes, defibrillation energy levels, and sizes of the pediatric airway, bag-valve-mask, laryngoscope, endotracheal tube, gastric tube, urinary catheter, chest tube, and IV catheter.

When all else fails or in preparation for the arrival of a seriously ill or injured child, it is sometimes easiest to remember three estimated average weights for children younger than 10 years (Brownstein & Rivara, 2000) and estimate the child's weight from there:

1 year	10 kg
5 years	20 kg
10 years	30 kg

Parent-Child Relationship

Rapid triage assessment of the child also includes observation of the child in relation to the parents. If the relationship does not appear to be close, comfortable, and trusting, the nurse might want to explore further.

CARDIOPULMONARY RESUSCITATION OF THE CHILD

Airway and Breathing

Initial Assessment and Intervention

Whereas lethal dysrhythmias related to heart disease are the most common causes of cardiopulmonary arrest in adults, factors leading to shock and respiratory failure are the most common causes of cardiopulmonary arrest in children. Early recognition of and intervention for respiratory distress and compensated shock can be life-saving for the child. Assistance with ventilation and administration of fluids might prevent further deterioration in the child's condition. Once the child progresses to respiratory failure and shock, cardiopulmonary resuscitation (CPR) is necessary. Resuscitation of children requires attention to the differences between adults and children (see Table 34-1).

After appropriately opening and clearing the airway, the nurse looks for chest rise and listens and feels for exhaled breath against his or her cheek. When the child is not breathing or ventilation is not adequate after positioning the airway correctly, the nurse gives at least two slow breaths by means of a bag-valve-mask device, watching for the rise and fall of the chest. *The nurse should stop inflating the lungs when the chest just begins to rise and allow enough time for exhalation (longer than inhalation).* Endotracheal intubation by a provider skilled in the technique is necessary if the child cannot be ventilated adequately with these measures or if prolonged ventilation is anticipated. Ventilations should be given at a rate of 20/min, or approximately 1 breath every 3 seconds.

A pressure gauge attached to the bag-valve-mask device helps deliver breaths at the correct pressure, especially for infants and young children. Choosing the appropriate-size mask and the correct-volume bag is important. The mask should cover the child's mouth and nose but not place pressure on the eyes. A good fit ensures a seal around the face and under the chin. Gastric decompression by use of an orogastric or nasogastric tube is indicated during assisted ventilation.

Obstructed Airway Management

Inability to inflate the lungs suggests airway obstruction, a life-threatening emergency. When ventilation is not possible, the infant or child will die in a very short time.

Management of airway obstruction depends on the cause and on the child's age. Definitive treatment depends on diagnosis. Foreign body aspiration, for example, is a problem frequently seen in young children, with a large number of aspirations attributed to coins, small toy parts, and certain foods, particularly candy and gum (Centers for Disease Control and Prevention [CDC], 2002c). When a child is unable to ventilate adequately and aspiration of a foreign body is suspected as the cause, the nurse initiates maneuvers to remove the obstruction.

Although controversy remains about how to clear a foreign body from the airway, for children older than 1 year the American Heart Association recommends using the Heimlich maneuver for a conscious child and abdominal thrusts for the unconscious child. Lay rescuers are currently being taught to initiate CPR on the older child instead of abdominal thrusts.

! CRITICAL TO REMEMBER

Airway Obstruction in Children

When a child is in significant respiratory distress and the child is coughing or is able to breathe adequately despite partial obstruction, the child should be allowed to maintain *whatever position is comfortable* until specialized care is available. In the smaller child, this position may be in the parent's or caregiver's arms. The nurse remains with the child and encourages the child to remain calm by reassuring in a soothing manner.

The rescuer tries to visualize the foreign body for removal during the ventilation sequence (American Heart Association, 2000). Removal of a foreign body from an infant involves placing the infant in a downward-slant position and giving five back blows alternating with five chest thrusts. Blind finger sweeps to remove a foreign body are not recommended because of the risk of forcing the object farther down into the airway. A finger sweep can be used if the object is visible.

If obstruction continues after these maneuvers, subsequent actions might include direct laryngoscopy and use of a Magill forceps to remove the foreign body. Tracheostomy is used as a last resort. When the lower airway is obstructed because of a disease process, such as asthma, medication to open the airway might be necessary.

Circulation

The nurse feels for the pulse in the child older than 1 year by palpating the carotid artery. For an infant younger than 1 year, the nurse uses the brachial artery because the infant's relatively short, fat neck makes palpation of the carotid artery difficult. If no pulse is palpated or if the infant's heart rate is less than 60 beats per minute after 30 seconds of assisted ventilation, the nurse begins chest compressions at a rate of 100 compressions per minute (American Heart Association, 2000).

The nurse obtains venous access for fluid resuscitation and medication administration. If venous access through a peripheral vein cannot be obtained within 90 seconds, the next recommendation is an intraosseous line (placed in the anteromedial tibia or distal femur). Children should be given IV fluid (usually lactated Ringer's or normal saline solution), 20 ml/kg, as an initial bolus for symptoms of shock. The nurse administers additional boluses as needed after reassessing cardiovascular status and warms the solution before any rapid infusion.

Epinephrine is the drug of choice for management of cardiac arrest. It can be given through the endotracheal tube when necessary. Atropine diminishes vagally mediated bradycardia. Sodium bicarbonate is given on the basis of arterial blood gas results, and dextrose can be used on the basis of blood glucose results or for clients unresponsive to resuscitative efforts.

Although cardiac rhythm disturbances in children are rare, rapid heart rates can occur, including sinus tachycardia, supraventricular tachycardia, and ventricular tachycardia. Cardiac output is a function of stroke volume and heart rate. Because children are unable to increase stroke volume, they can increase cardiac output only by increasing their heart rate. As heart rates increase, cardiac filling time decreases and cardiac output falls.

Sinus tachycardia usually requires observation and determination of the cause (e.g., fever, shock, toxic ingestion). Vagal maneuvers (e.g., applying ice water to the face), cardioversion at 0.5 to 1.0 joules/kg, or adenosine might be necessary for symptomatic supraventricular tachycardia (heart rate >200 beats/min) (American Heart Association, 2000). Ventricular tachycardia in a child is usually the result of congenital abnormalities, toxic ingestion, or chronic cardiac disease and requires complex interventions.

Resuscitation of the child requires a team effort. Training and rehearsal, such as mock codes, are very helpful. Also helpful are national courses now available, such as the Pediatric Advanced Life Support (PALS) program provided by the American Heart Association and the Emergency Nursing Pediatric Course (ENPC) provided by the Emergency Nurses Association (Table 34-3).

Automatic external defibrillators (AEDs) are becoming increasingly more available in community settings. They are effective for correcting serious rhythm disturbances in adults, but have not been considered appropriate for use in the pediatric population because of the strength of the shock and their relative sensitivity for identifying shockable dysrhythmias in children. The Pediatric Advanced Life Support Task Force, International Liaison Committee on Resuscitation has updated recommendations for use of AEDs in the pediatric population (Samson, Berg, & Bingham, 2002). These recommendations state that AEDs can be used safely in children ages 1 to 8 years whose circulation is absent, especially if equipped with child-sized external pads and a pediatric shock dose level. Additionally, AEDs should be able to identify shockable rhythms with a high degree of accuracy (Samson, Berg, & Bingham, 2002). In the community setting, CPR should be performed for at least one minute before considering the use of an AED (Samson, Berg & Bingham, 2002).

THE CHILD IN SHOCK

Shock is an acute, complex, unstable physiologic state of inadequate oxygen delivery to tissues. Decreased tissue perfusion (circulation of blood through the vascular bed of tissue) leads to tissue hypoxia and ischemia, metabolic acidosis, and, if prolonged, irreversible tissue and organ damage (Caldwell & Ziglar, 2001). The etiology of shock can be classified into three major categories: hypovolemic, cardiogenic, and distributive (Tuite, 1997). Regardless of the etiology, the body will respond similarly to compensate for the alterations in perfusion and transport of oxygen and metabolic substrates that have occurred.

Etiology

Hypovolemic Shock

Hypovolemic shock is the most common cause of shock in children and is characterized by an overall decrease in circulating blood or fluid volumes. Hemorrhage, burns, and dehydration are the most common causes of hypovolemic shock. Blood loss can be caused by trauma or surgery; fluid and plasma losses can occur with vomiting and diarrhea, burns, and diabetic ketoacidosis.

Distributive Shock

Distributive shock is the result of an abnormality in the distribution of blood flow or inability of the body to maintain vascular tone through vasoconstriction.

TABLE **34-3** Basic Life Support Maneuvers in Infants and Children

Maneuver	Infant (<1 yr)	Child (1-8 yr)
Airway	Head-tilt/chin-lift (if trauma is present, use jaw thrust)	Head-tilt/chin-lift (if trauma is present, use jaw thrust)
Breathing:		
Initial	At least two breaths at 1-1$^1/_2$ sec/breath	Two breaths at 1-1$^1/_2$ sec/breath
Subsequent	20 breaths/min (approximate)	20 breaths/min (approximate)
Circulation: pulse check	Brachial, femoral	Carotid
Compression area	Lower half of sternum	Lower half of sternum
Compressed width	Two or three fingers; use (2) thumbs, encircling hands technique when there are two rescuers	Heel of one hand
Depth	Approximately one-third to one-half the depth of the chest	Approximately one-third to one-half the depth of the chest
Rate	At least 100/min	100/min
Compression/ventilation ratio	5:1 (pause for ventilation)	5:1 (pause for ventilation)
Foreign body airway obstruction	Back blows, chest thrusts	Heimlich maneuver

Modified from American Heart Association. (2000). *Basic life support for health care providers.* Dallas: Author. Copyright American Heart Association; updated from American Heart Association (2000). Guidelines for cardiopulmonary resuscitation and emergency cardiovascular care. *Currents in Emergency Cardiovascular Care, 11*(3), 1-30.

Septic shock is the most common form of distributive shock and occurs when microbial toxins (from bacteria, viruses, fungi, or rickettsiae) are present in the blood. These toxins cause a cascade of metabolic, hemodynamic, and clinical changes, resulting in impaired organ perfusion and hypotension. Despite major advances in vaccines in the past 2 decades, septic shock continues to be a frequent reason for admission to pediatric intensive care units. Organisms responsible for septic shock vary with age and immunocompetence, but include group B beta-hemolytic streptococci, Enterobacteriaceae, *Listeria monocytogenes*, *Staphylococcus aureus*, and *Neisseria meningitides* in neonates; *Haemophilus influenzae*, *Streptococcus pneumoniae*, *S. aureus*, and *N. meningitidis* in infants; and *S. pneumoniae*, *N. meningitidis*, *S. aureus*, and Enterobacteriaceae in children. Immunocompromised children are

Pathophysiology

of Shock

HYPOVOLEMIC SHOCK

Hypovolemic shock results from an abnormal decrease in circulating volume. Water constitutes a much greater portion of an infant's or child's body weight than it does an adult's, and because the bulk of fluid volume in young children is located primarily in the extracellular tissue spaces, infants and young children are more susceptible to hypovolemic shock. Infants, with their large body surface area and increased metabolic rate, also experience increased insensible fluid loss, thus compounding hypovolemia. Because of the small body size, even relatively small blood losses can result in hypovolemia.

When intravascular volume is reduced, the body initially compensates by increasing the peripheral vascular resistance, stroke volume, and heart rate and redistributing the blood flow to the vital organs (brain, heart). If a fluid resuscitation is not initiated within an appropriate time frame, altered sensorium and oliguria will be noted and hypovolemic shock will eventually result in irreversible tissue organ damage (Caldwell & Ziglar, 2001).

DISTRIBUTIVE SHOCK

Septic shock, the most common form of distributive shock, occurs when an invading organism infects a susceptible host, overwhelms the host's first and second lines of defense, and enters the bloodstream. The body's response to toxins or organisms in the blood, including endocrine, metabolic, and immunologic reactions, can result in inflammatory and coagulation abnormalities. Endotoxins, produced by lysis of bacteria, cause maldistributed blood flow, cardiac dysfunction, oxygen supply and demand imbalance, and metabolic alterations. The end result can be organ ischemia, multiple organ dysfunction syndrome, and death (Burns, 2003).

CARDIOGENIC SHOCK

Cardiogenic shock is characterized by low cardiac output and hypotension, which result in inadequate oxygen delivery to the tissues. Unlike hypovolemic shock, the compensatory mechanisms that occur in a child with cardiogenic shock can cause further myocardial dysfunction. These compensatory mechanisms redistribute blood away from the peripheral, splenic, and mesenteric circulation to help maintain the circulation to the vital organs: the heart and brain. Initially, compensatory mechanisms increase the heart rate, myocardial contractility, and vasoconstriction. Subsequent events result in sodium and fluid retention, producing a greater workload on the left ventricle (afterload). The increased workload causes increased oxygen demands on the myocardium in response to a depleted oxygen supply. This process leads to myocardial ischemia, which further depresses cardiac function, thereby establishing a vicious cycle.

An alteration in contractility, as seen in an injury to the myocardium and myocarditis, results in a decreased stroke volume and the ventricle is unable to eject blood.

BOX 34-2
Manifestations of Shock in Children

HYPOVOLEMIC SHOCK
Dry mucous membranes
Depressed fontanel
Cold, clammy skin
Oliguria
Poor skin turgor
Reduced capillary refill

DISTRIBUTIVE (SEPTIC) SHOCK: EARLY
Vasodilation
Extremities that are warm to the touch
Purpuric skin lesions
Tachypnea

SEPTIC SHOCK: LATE
Rapid, thready pulse
Cyanosis
Cold, clammy skin
Narrow pulse pressure
Oliguria or anuria

CARDIOGENIC SHOCK
Hepatomegaly
Cardiomegaly
Increased central venous pressure
Periorbital edema
Crackles
Diaphoresis
Oliguria
Reduced capillary refill
Reduced peripheral pulses

! CRITICAL TO REMEMBER
Hypotension in Children With Shock

Hypotension is a late sign of shock. The lower limits for systolic blood pressure in children are as follows:
- Infants younger than 1 month: 60 mm Hg
- Infants ages 1 to 12 months: 70 mm Hg
- Children older than 1 year: 70+ (2 times the child's age in years) mm Hg

more commonly affected by Enterobacteriaceae, *S. aureus*, Pseudomonadaceae, and *Candida albicans* (Butt, 2001). Infants and children with debilitating illnesses, clients in the intensive care unit for prolonged periods with many invasive lines, and those who are immunosuppressed are at greatest risk for development of septic shock.

Anaphylaxis, central nervous system or spinal injury, and drug intoxication are other forms of distributive shock, with profound inadequacies in tissue perfusion even in the presence of a normal or high cardiac output (Brownstein & Rivara, 2000).

Cardiogenic Shock
Cardiogenic shock occurs when myocardial function is impaired so that cardiac output is not sufficient to meet the body's metabolic demands. It is characterized by low cardiac output, decreased blood pressure, and poor tissue perfusion (Bengur & Meliones, 1998). The causes of cardiogenic shock include structural abnormalities related to congenital heart disease, infectious and noninfectious cardiomyopathies, trauma, ischemia, metabolic abnormalities, drug intoxication, and impaired cardiac function after intracardiac surgical repair.

Manifestations

Recognition of the clinical manifestations, with early intervention, is imperative for optimal treatment of shock (Box 34-2). In the early stages, the child is able to compensate with tachycardia, tachypnea, and vasoconstriction to maintain cardiac output. If the condition cannot be reversed, a decompensated state arises with altered perfusion (delayed capillary refill, weak pulses, cool extremities, hypotension) and profoundly altered mental status. Progression is cardiovascular collapse and death. Table 34-4 presents the general appearance of a child in shock.

Diagnostic Evaluation

The diagnosis of shock in infants and children is established chiefly on the basis of clinical manifestations and medical history. A chest radiograph may help differentiate cardiogenic shock from hypovolemic and distributive shock. In cardiogenic shock, the heart is usually enlarged and may show signs of pulmonary edema. In hypovolemic or distributive shock, the chest radiograph is usually normal or shows signs of infiltrates (indicative of pneumonia) and the heart is smaller than normal (indicative of a decrease in circulating volume). An echocardiogram can identify underlying structural cardiac disease.

Laboratory studies used in a differential diagnosis include blood cultures and cultures of other sites that may be the source of infection (e.g., spinal fluid, urine, sputum, wound drainage, indwelling lines), arterial blood gas values, glucose levels, electrolytes, BUN, creatinine levels, CBC, and coagulation studies.

Therapeutic Management

The therapeutic management of the child in shock includes basic life support (maintaining airway, breathing, and circulation) and treating signs and symptoms.

Monitoring with pulse oximetry and increasing ambient oxygen are indicated in most cases. If vascular access cannot be obtained, an intraosseous line can be used until the child is resuscitated, at which time the temporary intraosseous line can be replaced with an IV line.

Hypovolemic Shock
Once the airway, breathing, and circulation are established, the next priority is adequate vascular access. A crystalloid infusion of warm normal saline or lactated Ringer's solution should be initiated promptly. If hypovolemic shock is caused by hemorrhage and symptoms persist after 2 or 3 crystalloid

TABLE **34-4** Assessing a Child's General Appearance: "Looks Good" Versus "Looks Bad"

	"Looks Good"	"Looks Bad"
Color	Pink mucous membranes	Mottled color, "gray" or pale
	Consistent color over the trunk and extremities	
Skin perfusion	Warm	Cold (peripheral to proximal cooling)
	Brisk capillary refill (<2 sec)	Sluggish capillary refill (>2 sec)
Activity	Age-appropriate (may be frightened, unhappy, unwilling to be separated from parents)	Fretful, then lethargic
	Will engage in play	
Responsiveness	Age-appropriate	Irritable (early), then lethargic
		Decreased response to painful stimulus is worrisome
Infant feeding	Eats well	Weak suck
		Tires during feeding
		May have respiratory distress during feedings

Modified from Hazinski, M.F. (1990). Shock in the pediatric patient. *Critical Care Nursing Clinics of North America, 2*(2), 313.

boluses, consider infusion of 10 ml/kg of warmed, type-specific O-negative packed red blood cells (Caldwell & Ziglar, 2001).

Colloids (albumin) are protein-containing fluids that may be used in volume resuscitation after the initial treatment with crystalloids. Colloids are used primarily for dehydration or body fluid losses other than blood.

Distributive Shock

The therapeutic management of distributive shock involves restoring hemodynamic status with fluid resuscitation and promptly treating the underlying cause. Inotropic medications are used to manage the cardiovascular instability. Vasoconstrictors may be used to increase vascular tone and counteract the effects of toxins. Maintaining a secure, patent airway may be necessary if significant respiratory distress occurs. Surgery also might be indicated to eliminate the source of infection (e.g., an abscess) or to stabilize a central nervous system/spinal injury.

Cardiogenic Shock

The initial management of an infant or child with cardiogenic shock includes adequate oxygenation by maintaining both the airway and proper ventilation. Invasive monitoring of central venous pressure, arterial blood pressure, and pulmonary artery pressure helps to identify hemodynamic changes and subtle clinical signs and symptoms of decreased cardiac output (e.g., cyanosis, decreased skin temperature, delayed capillary refill).

With an excess of intravascular fluid volume, diuretics may be prescribed. Usually, furosemide (Lasix), 1 mg/kg, provides effective diuresis.

The heart rate must be in the normal range or higher than normal to improve the cardiac output. Children, especially infants younger than 6 months, have a decreased ability to increase stroke volume and thus depend much more on an increased heart rate to improve cardiac output. Pharmacologic therapy is the mainstay of medical treatment in children with cardiogenic shock. Frequently, a combination of pharmacologic agents is necessary to stabilize the child. Dobutamine, dopamine, and milrinone are the initial drugs of choice for treating cardiogenic shock.

Extracorporeal membrane oxygenation (ECMO) is a means of providing short-term circulatory and respiratory support for infants and children in whom other methods of treatment are not effective. Vital organ perfusion is maintained by ECMO to allow for recovery and/or stabilization required before definitive treatment, such as surgery, can be performed (Butt, 2001).

■NURSING CARE
The Child in Shock

Assessment

Nursing assessment of a child in shock should be thorough, with attention focused on the cardiopulmonary system and neurologic status. A changing level of consciousness is one of the first indicators of a worsening condition, and early identification and treatment of shock in infants and children are crucial to decreasing morbidity and mortality. Initial concerns are ensuring a patent airway and monitoring the child's respiratory effort to confirm adequate air exchange with good chest expansion. Central circulation is assessed by checking a brachial, carotid, or femoral pulse. Assessment of level of consciousness is performed serially to detect early changes.

Hypovolemic Shock

A child in hypovolemic shock may have a history of trauma, vomiting and diarrhea, or anorexia. The parent may report a decrease in wet diapers or explain that the child has not voided recently. With trauma, the child may demonstrate obvious signs of injury or bleeding or covert symptoms suggestive of blunt trauma.

The child in hypovolemic shock requires frequent assessment of vital signs, including blood pressure (every 15-60 min). Skin color, turgor, and temperature should be monitored very closely. The anterior fontanel (if present) should be assessed to determine whether it is depressed or full. A depressed fontanel may be a manifestation of dehydration, whereas a full or level fontanel usually suggests that fluid volume is adequate.

In addition, the nurse assesses and monitors the child's neurologic status closely. A depressed or deteriorating level of consciousness should be reported promptly. The nurse auscultates heart and lungs and palpates peripheral pulses. Capillary refill time, moistness of mucous membranes, and general muscle tone and strength should be assessed and urine output monitored closely. In very young children, weighing the diapers quantifies urine output. If the child has diarrhea, a urine bag or Foley catheter should be placed to monitor urinary output. The abdomen should be palpated and auscultated for the presence of bowel sounds. Abdominal injury must be ruled out, especially if the abdominal girth appears to be increasing, with evidence of abdominal distention. Any abnormal bruising or obvious trauma must be recognized quickly, because blunt abdominal trauma is the most common unrecognized cause of fatal injuries in children (Caldwell & Ziglar, 2001).

Distributive Shock

Early signs of distributive shock include hyperthermia or hypothermia. The temperature should be closely monitored. In early shock (the hyperdynamic phase), the skin is typically warm and flushed. In late shock (the hypodynamic phase), skin is ashen and cold. An exception is in the case of spinal injury, in which the body cannot maintain a normal temperature. Shock of any etiology may cause microcirculatory dysfunction leading to abnormal function of coagulation factors and platelets. Therefore the nurse observes the skin closely for signs of petechiae, oozing of blood from invasive lines, or purpuric lesions. The presence of petechiae that are spread diffusely over the body may indicate severe sepsis. In children, hypotension is a late sign of all types of shock.

Cardiogenic Shock

A child with cardiogenic shock requires close monitoring of the heart and lungs for adventitious sounds. The liver should be palpated and its size measured. The child's respiratory effort must also be assessed. Retractions, grunting, and nasal flaring may be apparent. Periorbital and peripheral edema or other signs of cardiac failure may be present. Close monitoring of the peripheral pulses and capillary refill is extremely important.

Nursing Diagnosis and Planning

The nursing diagnoses and expected outcomes that may be appropriate after assessment of the child with shock are
- Ineffective Tissue Perfusion (cardiopulmonary, cerebral, peripheral) related to decreased fluid volume (in hypovolemic shock); abnormal distribution of blood flow, metabolic acidosis, or both (in distributive shock); or decreased cardiac contractility (in cardiogenic shock).
  Expected Outcome: The child will maintain adequate tissue perfusion, as evidenced by strong peripheral pulses, appropriate skin turgor, normal capillary refill time, pink and warm mucous membranes and nail beds, vital signs within normal limits for age, and no evidence of dyspnea or altered mental status.
- Impaired Gas Exchange related to possible decreased pulmonary blood flow, increased interstitial fluid in alveoli, and inflammatory response of alveoli.
  Expected Outcome: The child will have adequate gas exchange, as evidenced by oxygen saturation level between 95% and 100% and normal arterial blood gas measurements.

- Risk for Infection related to invasive venous and arterial lines, indwelling catheters, presence of endotracheal tube, possible incisional wounds, and compromised state.
  Expected Outcome: The child will remain free from signs of infection, as evidenced by normal temperature, white blood cell count (WBC) within normal limits, no signs of redness or purulence from access sites, and negative blood cultures.
- Anxiety related to threat of a possible grave prognosis in a critically ill child.
  Expected Outcomes: The child and parent will verbalize symptoms of anxiety, seek information to ensure understanding of the condition, and demonstrate adequate coping skills.

Interventions

Interventions for the child experiencing shock are directed toward maintaining tissue perfusion by improving cardiac output, ensuring adequate oxygenation, preventing infection, and enhancing child and family coping.

Maintaining Tissue Perfusion

Careful and frequent observation of the child's cardiovascular status is essential. Take vital signs and assess circulation every 1 to 2 hours. After establishing an adequate IV access, administer appropriate fluid replacement. Carefully document intake and output, and report urine output that is abnormal for age (see Chapter 42) or any major discrepancy between intake and output. Weigh the child daily on the same scale. Report any rapid weight gain to the physician.

Because infants have high glucose requirements and low glycogen stores, alterations in glucose metabolism are frequently seen in response to stress. Monitor blood glucose levels every 2 to 4 hours.

Administer ordered medications by IV pump to ensure appropriate delivery of medication. Because vasoactive drugs can cause tissue necrosis if infiltration occurs in peripheral tissues, these agents are administered preferably through a central line.

Ensuring Oxygenation

Observe and record respiratory rate and effort, skin color, chest expansion, and aeration. Note signs of respiratory distress, and report them to the physician promptly. Administer oxygen as ordered, making sure the delivery mode is appropriate for the child's age. Monitor oxygen saturation, arterial blood gases, and hemoglobin levels. Maintain a patent airway, and have emergency endotracheal intubation and ventilation equipment available. Ensure normothermia and control pain and anxiety to decrease oxygen demands.

Preventing Infection

Because children in a compromised state are prone to infection, maintain strict aseptic technique when handling IV lines, invasive tubes, and incisional or puncture sites. Closely monitor the child's temperature, and report any rectal temperature greater than 38.1° C (100.5° F) or less than 36° C (96.8° F) (Jones, 1998). Observe secretions and body fluids, incisions, and puncture sites for erythema, edema, or purulence. Report positive culture results and elevated WBCs promptly. Administer ordered antipyretics, and ensure adequate caloric intake. If the child is unable to tolerate oral or nasogastric feedings, discuss alternative methods of feeding with the physician.

Enhancing Coping

Provide concise, accurate information to parents. Determine the child's developmental level and level of comprehension. Provide simple explanations of procedures before initiating them. Provide information in a calm, relaxed, and concerned manner. Answer all questions honestly. Be empathetic.

Allow the child and parents to express their feelings, concerns, and anxieties. Encourage the parents to participate in the child's care as appropriate (e.g., bathing, combing hair, feeding). This assistance provides them with some control. Be nonjudgmental in response to parents' actions. Use available resources (e.g., social worker, chaplain, other family members) to help calm parents who are exhibiting uncontrolled feelings.

Elicit the parents' perceptions of the event, and provide reassurance or clarify any misconceptions. Determine the availability of support systems, and encourage their use. Help the parents identify coping mechanisms that have been effective in the past, and encourage parents to determine whether these mechanisms may be effective during the current crisis.

Evaluation

- Does the child demonstrate pink mucous membranes, brisk capillary refill, alertness, responsiveness, and normal vital signs for age?
- Is the oxygen saturation at least 95% on room air, and are blood gas values within normal limits?
- Does the child demonstrate a normal breathing rate, pattern, and work of breathing?
- Is the child afebrile with negative culture results?
- Can the parents and child express their feelings to staff or significant others?
- Is the family demonstrating decreased anxiety by using available resources and effective coping mechanisms?

PEDIATRIC TRAUMA

Despite a 39% decline in unintentional injury deaths among children younger than 14 years from 1987 to 2000, injury is the leading cause of death for children (Wallis, Cody, & Mickalide, 2003). The Centers for Disease Control and Prevention (CDC) has consistently found that motor vehicle injuries are the leading cause of unintentional death in children younger than 18 years in the United States, followed by drowning and airway obstruction injury. Burns and poisoning are other major causes of unintentional death, whereas falls are the leading cause of nonfatal injuries requiring hospital emergency room treatment. The term *injury* is used in preference to accident when describing trauma because some trauma is not accidental and much of it is preventable.

Injury prevention and education have been credited with a decrease in unintentional deaths among children. Despite this, much more needs to be done. Successful prevention and education steps include motor vehicle safety restraints, firearm education, bicycle helmet programs, safety caps and locked medications, and eliminating potential hazards, such as old refrigerators and unfenced pools. Up-to-date educational resources can be obtained through organizations and

websites such as those offered by the National SAFE KIDS Campaign, the CDC, and the U.S. Consumer Product Safety Commission. When child victims of trauma are discharged from the emergency department, the nurse provides injury prevention information to the families. Injury prevention is also discussed at every well-child visit through adolescence (see Chapters 4 through 8).

Mechanism of Injury

Injuries can be categorized as *blunt, penetrating,* and *multiple trauma.* Knowing the mechanism of injury and recognizing anatomic and physiologic differences in the pediatric population help identify common injury patterns and predict the child's needs and outcomes.

Blunt Trauma

Blunt or penetrating force causes tissue trauma. Blunt trauma occurs more frequently than all other injuries combined. Injuries sustained from blunt trauma are often less apparent but can be more serious than those from penetrating trauma (Connors, 2001).

Motor Vehicle Trauma. A common cause of blunt trauma is acceleration-deceleration force, often from motor vehicle collisions or falls. Just before a motor vehicle collision, both the occupant and the vehicle are traveling at the same speed. When the vehicle meets an opposing force, the speed of both the occupant and the vehicle rapidly decelerate. When this change occurs, four collisions take place: (1) the moving vehicle collides with the opposing object; (2) the occupant's body collides with the interior portion of the vehicle; (3) the occupant's internal organs and tissues collide with rigid internal structures; and (4) loose objects in the vehicle become projectile forces (Emergency Nurses Association, 1998).

Unrestrained occupants in a motor vehicle collision have a higher incidence of injury than restrained occupants have because they are tossed around the interior of the vehicle or are ejected at the point of collision. This principle applies also to children riding unrestrained in the back of open pickup trucks; they become missiles ejected out of the vehicle into oncoming traffic or onto the road. Children who are held on an adult's lap during a motor vehicle collision can be instantly crushed between the rigid part of the automobile and the moving adult.

Child safety seats and safety belts, *when appropriately sized and correctly installed,* can prevent injury and save lives. Recently, childhood injuries and deaths have occurred as a result of airbag deployment. As of October 1, 2001, 137 children were killed by passenger airbags (National SAFE KIDS Campaign, 2003). Twenty-two of these deaths were among infants in rear-facing child safety seats in front of a passenger airbag. Approximately 88% of all children killed by passenger airbags were either unrestrained or improperly restrained at the time of death. The National Highway and Traffic Safety Administration (www.nhtsa.com) advises that all children younger than 12 years be placed in rear seats in all cars, especially those with passenger airbags, and that infants younger than 1 year and weighing less than 20 lb must ride in a rear-facing infant safety seat.

Pedestrian Injury. Pedestrian injuries in children are also a significant problem, with the largest number of incidences occurring in children 5 to 14 years of age (Wallis,

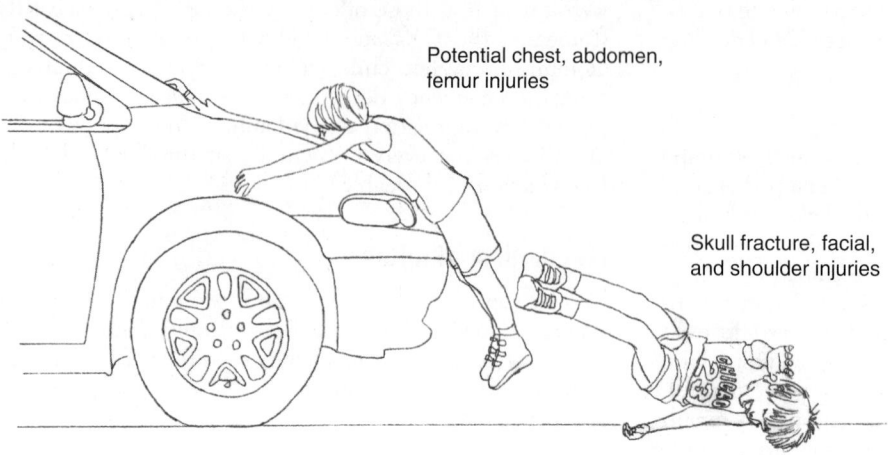

Potential chest, abdomen, femur injuries

Skull fracture, facial, and shoulder injuries

Figure 34-1 Waddell's triad of injuries.

Cody, & Mickalide, 2003). Most of these injuries occur during the daylight hours as the child darts out into the middle of the street between parked cars or stands unnoticed behind a vehicle backing out of a driveway.

When a child is hit by a motor vehicle, a triad of injuries, referred to as Waddell's triad, occurs (Fig. 34-1). This one traumatic event results in three different types of injuries:

1. After being struck by the bumper and hood of the car, the child sustains abdominal or thoracic injuries.
2. The child is then propelled into the air, lands on the ground, and sustains femur or other leg injury, as well as surface trauma.
3. As the child is propelled like a missile to the ground, the large size and weight of the child's head result in skull fracture or closed head injury to the contralateral side of the head.

Penetrating Trauma

Penetrating trauma includes stabbing, firearms, blasting, and impaling injuries. Damage to the body tissue can result from the penetrating object itself and secondarily from radiating energy forces along the pathway of the penetrating object. The severity of an injury depends on the location of impact and the type of object. For example, with gunshot wounds, what might seem like a fairly innocuous wound can actually be very severe, depending on factors such as projectile, fragmentation, type of tissue struck, and striking velocity. Injuries from a stab wound depend on length of the instrument, applied velocity, and angle of entry.

Multiple Trauma

A child with multiple trauma incurs injuries to more than one body system. A positive outcome for a child who has sustained multiple trauma depends on rapid assessment and intervention, which begin at the scene of the accident and continue through the trauma center emergency department, the critical care and acute care units, and the rehabilitation phase. Ideally, a critically injured child should be rapidly transported to a trauma facility with the personnel, equipment, and commitment to provide specialized care to children.

At the trauma center, and even in the emergency department of the community hospital, the presence of qualified trauma team members to assess and treat the trauma patient is crucial. A trauma team consists of skilled surgeons, other physicians, nurses, social workers, and other health professionals, each with a specific role and duties during trauma resuscitation. The team assembles after notification of pending arrival by emergency personnel and readies the trauma room with personnel and equipment.

All clients with multiple trauma require a rapid, complete, and thorough assessment to determine the extent of injuries. As with the ill child, assessment of a child with multiple trauma includes primary and secondary surveys, with concurrent appropriate interventions.

Primary Survey

The goal of the primary survey is to assess and manage life-threatening injuries. The primary assessment (see "Primary Assessment," p. 857) proceeds with the following additions.

Airway Assessment and Management. The priority is to open and maintain the airway, using the jaw-thrust maneuver to prevent movement of the cervical spine. The nurse inspects for loose teeth or other potential airway obstructions. Because the child's lower airway is narrow and easily obstructed by edema and mucus, oral suctioning might be required to keep the airway clear. A pediatric cervical collar and immobilization board secure a child when spinal cord injury is a concern (Fig. 34-2). To determine a correct fit, the cervical collar is measured for maximum stability: the chin must rest securely in the chin holder, with the collar below the ears and the lower end not extending below the upper part of the sternum. The cervical immobilization device and spinal immobilization device (long backboard) must remain in place until spinal injury has been ruled out.

In instances when an alert child is brought to the emergency setting in the carseat, the nurse places rolled towels on either side of the child's head and secures these with tape to maintain cervical immobilization without removing the child from the seat. The child can then remain in the carseat until radiographs have shown there is no injury to the cervical spine or unless a change in status is noted.

Breathing Assessment and Management. Pulse oximetry readings are an adjunct to evaluating ventilation and adequate oxygenation. Oxygen use in the child with multiple trauma is not contraindicated; therefore the nurse starts supplemental oxygen at a rate of 10 to 15 L/min by mask. If the

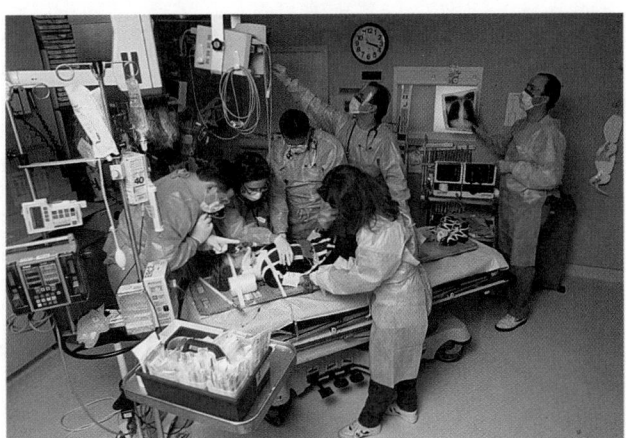

Figure 34-2 The child with multiple trauma injuries must remain on an immobilization board (long backboard) with a cervical immobilization device in place until being evaluated for spinal injuries. (Courtesy Children's Medical Center, Dallas, TX.)

child is alert and does not tolerate the mask, using blow-by oxygen with the tubing only or using a plastic cup attached to the end of the tubing might be less threatening to a child.

If ventilation is inadequate or absent, the nurse begins to ventilate the child (as described on p. 861), using a bag-valve-mask with a reservoir and high-flow oxygen. Using an oropharyngeal or nasopharyngeal airway maintains patency in a child with altered consciousness.

Endotracheal intubation might be needed for airway control and oxygenation in children with altered level of consciousness, lack of spontaneous respirations, or severe head injury. The nurse hyperventilates the child before this procedure and assists in evaluation of endotracheal tube placement after the procedure.

While observing the child for respiratory difficulty, the nurse checks the neck for jugular vein distention or tracheal deviation (the cervical collar can be opened for this assessment and then closed, keeping the neck in alignment). Because respiratory difficulty can be caused by chest injury, the nurse observes the chest for contusions, penetrations, abrasions, and paradoxical movement. A chest tube insertion or intervention for cardiac tamponade might be indicated for a penetrating chest injury, or an occlusive dressing may be taped on three sides for an open pneumothorax.

Severe facial trauma, although rare in children younger than 5 years, can be life-threatening, primarily because of the potential to obstruct ventilation—both fractures and soft tissue injury can cause narrowing of the airway. Facial trauma in children is treated as it is in adults. Nursing intervention includes ensuring an adequate airway and breathing, observing for possible progressive obstruction, and keeping the injured areas clean to prevent infection.

Circulation Assessment and Management. Cardiovascular assessment of the child focuses on early recognition and treatment of hypovolemia. Blood loss in children is usually caused by internal abdominal or chest injury, severe injuries to the extremities, or surface head trauma. As previously discussed, early indicators of shock in children are tachycardia, increased capillary refill time (>2 sec), mottled skin, agitation or apprehension, pallor, and cool extremities. Decreased level of consciousness, dusky skin color, clammy

extremities, bradycardia, and hypotension are late signs, indicating that cardiac arrest is imminent.

Cardiac monitoring and frequent cardiovascular assessments are necessary during the acute stage. During this stage, any external hemorrhage is noted and controlled and IV or other access to the circulatory system is obtained.

The nurse assesses extremities for fractures and decreased peripheral circulation and splints any suspected fracture, assessing peripheral circulation after applying any splint. Assessment includes motor (Can the child move the extremity? Is there pain?); circulatory (Is there good color, a strong pulse, and good capillary refill?); and neural function (Is sensation to the area intact? Is there any numbness or tingling in the extremity?). If neurovascular or circulatory compromise is present, immediate intervention is necessary.

Disability. During the primary survey phase, a brief neurologic examination is performed, establishing level of consciousness along with pupillary size and reactivity and muscle movement. AVPU can assess mental status. Sudden changes, such as agitation or somnolence, might indicate hypoxia or decreased cerebral perfusion.

Secondary Survey

After exposing the child by removing all the child's clothing and providing warming measures, the trauma staff assesses for pain, carefully inspects and documents all signs of injury by performing the head-to-toe assessment (including log rolling the child to inspect the back), and obtains a history of the injury.

Obtaining a History of the Injury. Determining the degree and severity of injuries is both an art and a science. Diagnosis depends on knowing the mechanism of injury as well as the presenting signs and symptoms. Nurses can obtain a comprehensive history by asking specific questions (Box 34-3). Thorough assessment depends on a systematic trauma evaluation, which takes place along with life-saving intervention.

Trauma Scoring. Various kinds of scoring, performed and documented by on-site emergency medical personnel and nursing staff, are used as an objective measure of the severity of the injury caused by a traumatic event and, sometimes, to decide the facility most appropriate for treating the child. Most scoring systems are for the assessment of injury to adults and do not take into account the anatomic differences of children (Box 34-4).

Assessing for Child Abuse. Child maltreatment can be a cause of injury (see Chapter 53 for an in-depth discussion

---

BOX 34-3
History of Injury Questions

FOR A VICTIM OF A MOTOR VEHICLE COLLISION
Was the child wearing a seatbelt or in a child's car seat?
What was the type of seatbelt (lap or lap and shoulder)?
What was the speed of the motor vehicle?
With what did the motor vehicle collide?
At what point on the motor vehicle was the location of impact?
Where was the victim seated in the motor vehicle?
How much damage was done to the motor vehicle?

FOR A VICTIM OF A FALL
How far did the child fall?
How did the child land (on what part of the body)?
On what type of surface did the child land?
Was the child's fall broken by any objects?

FOR A VICTIM OF A PENETRATING INJURY
How long and how wide was the blade of the knife?
How far away was the gun when it was fired?
What type of gun was used, and what was the caliber of the gun?

BOX 34-4
Trauma Scoring Systems

TRAUMA SCORE (TS)
Adult scoring tool sometimes used with children
Assesses respiratory rate and effort, blood pressure, and capillary refill
Includes the Glasgow Coma Scale (GCS)

REVISED TRAUMA SCORE (RTS)
Comprises the GCS, blood pressure, and respiratory rate

PEDIATRIC TRAUMA SCORE (PTS)
Adapted for the pediatric client
Assesses size, airway, central nervous system response, systolic blood pressure, open wounds, and skeletal fractures

---

of child abuse). Nurses working in emergency settings play an important role in both the assessment and reporting of child maltreatment. In acute care settings, there is rarely time to assess parent-child interactions or to observe at length the child's behavioral indicators, although these may provide important information. The following important indicators raise the suspicion of child maltreatment in the emergency setting:

- A history inconsistent with physical findings
- Activity reportedly leading to the trauma that seems inconsistent with the age and condition of the child
- Delay in seeking treatment for the trauma
- A history of other emergency visits.

Certain physical findings should also raise the level of suspicion:

- Bruises or fractures in various stages of healing noted on radiography
- Injuries rarely found in children (e.g., long bone or rib fractures) when the history is not appropriate for the injury
- Patterns of injury indicating that a specific object caused injury (e.g., belt marks, cigarette burns)

The nurse carefully assesses these indicators in the context of the injury and in relation to the affect of the child and family. The nurse also observes the family's reaction to the child and staff, keeping in mind that people behave very differently depending on culture, ethnicity, experience, and psychologic makeup. Above all, health care providers do not assume an investigative role—that is law enforcement's responsibility. Nurses are required to report suspicion of child maltreatment, however, and so must be careful to document any observations in detail. It might help to remember that more than 90% of parents who have abused their children feel ashamed of doing so but are unable to control the impulse. When child maltreatment is suspected, the intervention of child protective services is essential to ensure the safety of the child (and that of other children in the home) and to prevent additional injury.

Nursing Considerations

The Child and Family

The most critical aspect of nursing care of the child with traumatic injury is continuous assessment of respiratory, circulatory, and neurologic status. The nurse observes injured children for the early signs of shock and intervenes immediately to prevent rapid and irreversible deterioration. Preparing for the many procedures and examinations required and observing the equipment used for monitoring should not interfere with close and continuous observation of the child's signs and symptoms.

Nursing care of the child also requires care of the family. When the family arrives at the hospital, one staff member should become the contact person and should provide regular updates. Hospital staff supports family members when they visit their critically ill child. Information concerning their child's condition should be provided simply but completely, incorporating the family's educational and emotional status and readiness to learn. Family members are encouraged to touch and talk to their child if they so desire. Remember that informed consent must be obtained from the families of clients for all procedures, unless the intervention is required to save the child's life.

The Child During Recovery

Regardless of the cause of the injury, most children with traumatic injury do well unless the injuries are extremely severe. Their cardiovascular systems are strong and their bodies are growing, allowing them to compensate for even the most serious injuries. Even children with severe traumatic brain injuries (TBI) have far more favorable chances of recovery than do adults; however, any TBI can result in short-term and long-term disabilities (CDC, 2003b). Children and their families require nursing support to recover from both the physical and psychologic effects of trauma; the need for rehabilitation must be considered from the moment the child arrives in the emergency setting.

INGESTIONS AND POISONINGS

The term *poison exposure* is the ingestion of or contact with a substance that can produce toxic effects (CDC, 2003a). The combination of small weight and size, curiosity, lack of fear, and evolving mobility place all children at risk of injury or death from toxic exposure and ingestion. There are differences, however, in types of incident by age-group. Younger children (1 through 5 years of age) are indiscriminately curious and can innocently ingest a toxic substance in a matter of seconds. As children grow, they gradually learn from parents to avoid dangerous substances, but accidental ingestions and exposures still can occur. In adolescence, the risk is higher for deliberate ingestion.

Incidence

More than half of all poison exposures occurred among children younger than 6 years. The largest number of deaths from poisonings is in the adolescent age-group, with approximately half of the incidents deliberate (Litovitz, et al. 2001). More than 90% of all poison exposures occur in homes. Most poisonings occur as a result of oral ingestion. Ocular or dermal exposure, inhalation, parenteral exposure, and envenomation account for the remainder of poisoning incidents. Children are poisoned by plants; household and personal care products such as cosmetics, cleaning substances, and medicines; lead; and carbon monoxide. Adolescents have a much higher incidence of ingestion of psychopharmacologic drugs (tranquilizers, sedatives, anti-depressants, pain-relievers) and alcohol (Litovitz, et al. 2001).

Manifestations

Assessment and treatment of toxic exposure and ingestion go hand in hand. Although identification of the type and amount of the exposure is important, the child must initially be treated on the basis of physical signs and symptoms.

An accurate history of the ingestion is useful in planning care for the child. History given by the child, parent, friend, or caretaker might not always be accurate or complete—there are often areas of confusion, especially in cases of unwitnessed ingestions. The information obtained in the history of the ingestion is combined with the child's presenting physical assessment to provide a complete picture of the event and to plan treatment. Laboratory analysis in some cases may provide definitive diagnosis.

Most ingestions seen in emergency settings occur acutely, and the child is brought in immediately or when parents realize the event has occurred. An exception to this is lead poisoning. Although lead poisoning is relatively common, with an estimated 1 million children having elevated levels, it is rarely identified in the emergency setting. A child who has unusual neurologic signs or symptoms, neuropathy, or anemia that cannot be attributed to other causes might have lead poisoning. Elevated blood lead levels result primarily from exposure to lead-based paint or lead-contaminated dust and soil. Older miniblinds, improperly glazed pottery, folk remedies, and certain imported candies are also reported sources of lead poisoning (Childhood Lead Poisoning, 2002). A careful history can assist in the diagnosis of lead poisoning, but testing serum lead levels provides the only accurate diagnosis. The child with a markedly elevated lead level usually is admitted to the hospital. Chelation therapy, if needed, is administered on an inpatient basis to remove lead from the blood and tissue. When a child is found to have elevated lead levels, other children in the home should be tested as well because of the environmental nature of the ingestion.

Diagnostic Evaluation

In cases of known or suspected ingestion, laboratory tests can be performed to assess serum levels of the substance and the effect of the toxin on body systems. Regional poison control centers and clinical pharmacists should be included as members of the treatment team. Measurements of serum glucose level and toxicologic analysis of urine, serum, and stomach contents are the most common laboratory tests ordered for possible toxic exposure or ingestion. Blood gases and chest x-ray are required if the child is hypoventilating, has other respiratory difficulties, or has been exposed to hydrocarbon (e.g., gasoline) or bleach. Baseline liver enzymes and kidney function tests may be drawn if the suspected substance is known to be toxic to these organs.

Therapeutic Management

The first step in treatment of a toxic exposure or ingestion is to assess ABCs (airway, breathing, circulation) and to stabilize the child. Oxygen can be given and breathing supported with a bag-valve-mask device if necessary. If the child's level of consciousness is altered, endotracheal intubation may be necessary to protect the airway. When the child has ingested a sufficient amount of a substance to cause rapid deterioration in mental status, an intubation tray should be at the bedside even when the child is awake and alert. If the child is in shock or shows signs of compensated shock, IV fluid resuscitation is initiated. Cardiac rhythm disturbances can result from many ingested substances, so placement of a cardiac monitor and pulse oximeter is also indicated. Seizure precautions should be instituted in exposures to toxins with neurologic or metabolic side effects.

Care of the child who has been exposed to or ingested a toxic substance depends on the amount ingested and the toxicity of the ingested substance (Table 34-5). After initial

TABLE 34-5 Common Poisonous Substances

Substance	Pathophysiology	Clinical Manifestations	Treatment
ACETAMINOPHEN (TYLENOL, MANY OVER-THE-COUNTER PRODUCTS)			
Toxic dose: uncertain, do not exceed recommended levels. Seriousness of ingestion determined by amount ingested and length of time before intervention, and if it is an acute or accumulative toxicity. Other factors, such as decreased oral intake, have been linked with hepatotoxicity.	Metabolic by-products deplete liver glutathione and cause damage to hepatic cells. Children younger than 6 yr seem to be more resistant to development of hepatotoxicity than older children and adults.	*First stage* (first 24 hr): malaise, nausea, vomiting, sweating, pallor, weakness. *Second stage* (24-48 hr): latent period with a rise in liver enzymes (aspartate and alanine aminotransferase) and bilirubin; right upper quadrant pain; prolonged prothrombin time. *Third stage* (3-7 days): jaundice, liver necrosis, signs of hepatic failure. *Fourth stage* (5-7 days): recovery or progression to death.	Institute gastric lavage within 1 hr of ingestion, depending on amount ingested. Administer antidote: N-acetylcysteine (Mucomyst) as ordered. IV fluids. Sodium-restricted, high-calorie, high-protein diet.
SALICYLATES (ASPIRIN, MANY OVER-THE-COUNTER PRODUCTS, OIL OF WINTERGREEN)			
Toxic dose: single dose exceeding 200-280 mg/kg. Peak gastric absorption occurs within 2 hr of ingestion.	*First stage:* stimulation of respiratory center, leading to respiratory alkalosis. *Second stage:* loss of potassium; increase in metabolic rate; accumulation of ketones leading to metabolic acidosis, hypokalemia, and dehydration. Inhibition of prothrombin formation, decreased platelet levels and adhesiveness, capillary fragility (chronic poisoning).	GI effects: nausea, vomiting, thirst. CNS effects: hyperventilation, tinnitus, confusion, seizures, coma, respiratory failure, circulatory collapse. Renal effect: oliguria. Hematopoietic effects: bleeding tendencies. Metabolic effects: sweating, dehydration, fever, hyponatremia, hypokalemia, dehydration, hypoglycemia.	Perform gastric lavage; administer activated charcoal to decrease absorption. IV fluids, sodium bicarbonate (enhances excretion), potassium replacement; volume expanders as needed to support circulation. Vitamin K for bleeding tendencies (chronic poisoning). Glucose for hypoglycemia. Hemodialysis in severe cases if child unresponsive to therapy.
CORROSIVES (TOILET AND DRAIN CLEANERS, BLEACH, AMMONIA)			
Extent of damage depends on causticity of substance and amount ingested.	Severe chemical burns of mouth, throat, esophagus. "Splash" burns of eyes and skin. Alkali substances can continue to cause damage after initial contact. If damage is severe, long-term care is needed, including gastric button or tube, repeated esophageal dilations, and surgical repair of esophagus, sometimes with colon tissue transplant (done when child is older).	Whitish burns of mouth and pharynx, color darkens (red, swollen, oozing as ulcerations form and tissue erodes). Edema, difficulty swallowing, drooling. Respiratory distress, pain. Residual difficulty swallowing; subsequent healing of burns can produce esophageal strictures. Severe burns causing perforation can lead to vascular collapse and shock.	All medical personnel wear protective equipment; corrosives continue to burn. Do not induce vomiting: do not lavage. Activated charcoal may be given. Dilute with small amounts of water or milk (take care not to stimulate vomiting). Flood external areas with large amount of water. Endoscopy to diagnose esophageal burns. Possible gastrostomy, possible esophageal dilations to prevent strictures and to maintain patency of esophagus. IV fluids while NPO. Analgesics, steroids, antibiotics, nasogastric tube feedings.

IV, Intravenous; *GI*, gastrointestinal; *CNS*, central nervous system; *NPO*, nothing by mouth; *EDTA*, ethylenediaminetetraacetic acid.

TABLE **34-5** Common Poisonous Substances—cont'd

Substance	Pathophysiology	Clinical Manifestations	Treatment
HYDROCARBONS (GASOLINE, KEROSENE, PAINT THINNER, LIGHTER FLUID, TURPENTINE, FURNITURE POLISH)			
	Chemical pneumonitis from aspiration of hydrocarbon. Pneumonia and acute hemorrhagic necrotizing disease, usually in 24 hr.	Burning sensation in mouth and pharynx. Characteristic petroleum breath odor. Nausea, vomiting, anorexia, CNS depression, fever. Respiratory distress, wheezing.	Do not induce vomiting. Support ventilation; administer oxygen. IV fluids.
LEAD (PAINT CHIPS FROM OLDER HOMES, SOIL CONTAMINATED WITH LEAD, LEAD SOLDER USED IN PLUMBING, VINYL MINIBLINDS, IMPROPERLY GLAZED POTTERY)			
Diet high in fat and low in iron and calcium increases lead absorption. Serum lead level >10 mcg/dl: considered harmful; 10-15 mcg/dl: more frequent screening indicated; 15-20 mcg/dl: nutritional and educational interventions and environmental investigation; >20 mcg/dl: possible removal and treatment.	GI tract is major route of absorption. Lead is deposited in blood, bone, and soft tissue. Major toxic effects occur in bone marrow, nervous system, and kidney. Amount of lead ingested, size of the particle, and repeated ingestion over time contribute to severity of lead poisoning.	Symptoms may be vague with insidious onset. CNS effects: irritability, lethargy, hyperactivity, cognitive and perceptual-motor difficulties, clumsiness, seizures, coma, and death (associated with blood level of 100 mcg/dl). Hematopoietic effect: anemia. GI effects: anorexia, nausea, vomiting, constipation, lead line along gums. Skeletal effects: increased density of long bones, lead line in long bones. Renal effects: glycosuria, proteinuria, possible acute or chronic renal failure. Kidney damage is reversible early in the disease, but with continued lead exposure, permanent kidney damage may occur.	>25 mcg/dl: remove child from lead source, hospitalize if level is significantly higher. Administer chelating agents: succimer orally for lead level of 35-45 mcg/dl; EDTA for level >70 mcg/dl given IV over several hours for 5 days (causes lead to be deposited in bone and excreted by kidneys); bronchoalveolar lavage every 4 hr for six doses for level >70 mcg/dl. Monitor kidney function because EDTA is nephrotoxic; monitor calcium levels because EDTA enhances excretion of calcium. Provide adequate hydration. Calcium, phosphorus, and vitamins C and D. Anticonvulsants. Oral or intramuscular iron for anemia. Follow-up lead levels to monitor progress (lead is excreted more slowly than it accumulates in the body).
CARBON MONOXIDE			
Most often from improperly ventilated heaters; also from poorly ventilated vehicles. Cause of the exposure should be determined and eliminated.	An odorless, colorless gas that binds to receptors on hemoglobin more effectively than does oxygen, thereby causing hypoxia.	Headache, visual disturbances. Altered level of consciousness, cherry-red lips and cheeks, nausea, and vomiting.	100% oxygen by rebreathing mask. Serum carboxyhemoglobin levels, hyperbaric chamber treatment may be necessary for clients with high carboxyhemoglobin levels. Other interventions based on signs and symptoms.

stabilization, removing the poison, preventing its absorption, and limiting complications are primary goals. Several methods frequently used to treat toxic ingestions include removal of dermal and ocular toxins, dilution of the toxin, administration of activated charcoal, gastric lavage, and administration of an antidote.

Removal of Dermal and Ocular Toxins

Removing the child from a toxic environment, including removing contaminated clothes, brushing chemical powders from skin, and liberal washing, is mandatory with skin exposure (Hellman, 1998). Copious irrigation of the eyes with water or normal saline is imperative with an ocular exposure. In cases of exposure to an alkaline substance, irrigation proceeds until eyes return to a normal pH (see Chapter 55).

Diluting the Ingested Toxin

Administering water or milk can dilute the toxic effects of acid or alkali ingestion. These substances, when ingested, can cause burning of tissue along the gastrointestinal tract. Because these caustic substances continue to cause damage until neutralized, inducing emesis is contraindicated.

Administration of syrup of ipecac in the home setting is no longer recommended by the American Academy of Pediatrics (AAP, 2003). There are three rationales for the recommendation that ipecac not be kept in the home: 1. It doesn't completely remove the poison from the child's system, 2. Vomiting is uncomfortable for the child and can lead to intolerance of other approaches to treating the ingestion (e.g., administration of activated charcoal), and 3. Misuse of ipecac (e.g., by bulimic adolescents) (AAP, 2003). Parents are advised to call the poison control center immediately if they suspect their child has ingested a poisonous substance.

Gastric Lavage

Gastric lavage is used for gastric emptying in the first 1 to 2 hours after the ingestion. This method is selected when the toxic ingestion has potentially serious complications, such as seizures, decreased level of consciousness, respiratory or metabolic depression, and cardiac effects. Because of the danger of esophageal perforation, lavage should not be used after ingestion of corrosive substances. The nurse places the child on the left side, with the head lowered approximately 10 degrees in the Trendelenburg position. Depending on the size of the child, a 22 to 36 French orogastric tube is inserted. In comatose children, endotracheal intubation is recommended before beginning gastric lavage to protect the airway against aspiration of stomach contents. To prevent electrolyte disturbances, younger children are lavaged with normal saline or one-half normal saline. The nurse observes the returned fluid for any pill fragments or toxic substance and administers activated charcoal after completion of the lavage process if ordered. A specimen of lavage fluid may be sent to the laboratory for analysis in cases of an unknown substance.

Activated Charcoal

Activated charcoal is a charcoal substance with a porous surface that binds to the toxin and passes through the gastrointestinal system. Activated charcoal has become the recommended treatment for acute poisonings in the pediatric population, particularly for incidents in which identification of the poison is delayed. Activated charcoal can bind to the toxin at any point along the gastrointestinal tract. The longer the time between activated charcoal administration and the time the toxin was ingested, however, the less effective it will be. If the child has received ipecac, ongoing vomiting can delay administration and retention of activated charcoal.

Activated charcoal must have a stimulant, such as magnesium citrate, to counteract the side effect of constipation. Administering activated charcoal is a nursing challenge because the substance is unpalatable in both taste and appearance to young children. If gastric lavage has been performed, it is often easiest to administer the activated charcoal before removal of the gastric tube. In the toddler, having the child sit on a parent's lap and administering charcoal by oral syringe may be successful. Mixing the activated charcoal with chocolate milk or other flavoring sometimes makes it easier to drink. Placing the charcoal in a covered opaque or decorated container prevents the child from seeing the substance while drinking. Activated charcoal administration might be repeated to prevent reabsorption of the toxin from fluid secreted in the biliary tract. The dosage is usually 1 to 2 g/kg in children.

Antidotes

Specific antidotes can be used to inhibit the absorption of the toxin at the receptor site or reduce the concentration. Examples of commonly used antidotes are acetylcysteine (Mucomyst) for significant acetaminophen ingestion and naloxone (Narcan) for narcotics (see Table 34-5).

▪NURSING CARE
The Child Who Has Ingested a Toxic Substance

Assessment

Accurate and rapid assessment of the poisoned child can mean the difference between life and death. Assess ABCs. Take frequent vital signs. Initiate respiratory or circulatory support as needed. Because shock is a result of ingestion of many toxic substances, blood pressure, tissue perfusion, and urine output are carefully monitored. Observe and document the child's mental status frequently to determine any changes in level of consciousness. Assess changes in pupil size or reactivity as well as occurrence of seizures.

The nurse needs to take the responsibility for assessing the cause of poisoning. A poison exposure is extremely distressing to parents. Defer detailed questioning until the child's condition is stabilized. If the ingestion was purposeful, psychologic consultation and referral should be provided. In some cases, child abuse must be ruled out.

❗ CRITICAL TO REMEMBER
Assessment of Poison Ingestion

Obtain information about the following:
- Substance ingested if known
- Amount ingested (How many pills are missing?)
- Approximate time of ingestion
- Change in the child's condition
- Treatment administered at home

Nursing Diagnosis and Planning

The diagnoses that apply to the child and family are

■ Risk for Injury related to insufficient parental knowledge about first aid for toxic ingestion and accidental poisonings.
Expected Outcome: The parent will describe how to assess the child and access appropriate treatment if accidental poisoning occurs.

■ Ineffective Breathing Pattern related to effects of toxic substances.
Expected Outcome: The child will breathe in a way that maintains adequate oxygenation and ventilation, as evidenced by normal arterial blood gases and serum pH or pulse oximetry.

■ Risk for Deficient Fluid Volume related to effects of ingested substances, treatment modalities, or decreased fluid intake.
Expected Outcome: The child will maintain an hourly urine output appropriate for weight and age, with age-appropriate specific gravity.

■ Compromised Family Coping related to sudden hospitalization and emergency aspects of illness.
Expected Outcomes: The family will appropriately discuss the child's condition and treatment, verbalize feelings and concerns, and remain with the child as much as possible.

■ Risk for Poisoning related to insufficient parental knowledge about poisoning prevention.
Expected Outcome: The parent makes the necessary changes in the home environment to prevent future poisoning.

Interventions

Stabilizing the child is the nurse's priority in caring for the child who has ingested a poisonous substance. Nursing care also includes reducing the child's and the family's fear and anxiety, providing preventive teaching concerning the storage of poisons and supervision of children, and removal of the poison from the child's skin and mucous membranes to reduce further injury.

Parents usually are overwhelmed by feelings of guilt, fear, and anger when their child has ingested a poisonous substance. Providing an opportunity for them to express their feelings in a nonjudgmental atmosphere helps parents cope with this experience. Some aspects of treatment, such as placement of a gastric tube or support of ventilation, are disturbing and frightening to parents. Offer support by explaining treatment, including the parents in care (as appropriate), and informing them about the status of their child.

Ideally, nurses intervene with parents (and other caregivers such as grandparents, older siblings, and baby sitters) before a poison exposure occurs. Knowledge of safety and "safe proofing" the environment is important before the child becomes mobile. Discussion of safe storage of medications and other potentially toxic substances as well as age-appropriate supervision of children are essential aspects of poison prevention. Advise the parent to post the poison control phone number clearly and to call the poison center before treating the child. This and other injury prevention information should be readily available in daycare, primary care, and emergency care settings and should be given to families proactively. Education through community programs to prevent poisoning and reduce drug abuse should be directed to young children as well as to adolescents, parents, and caretakers. Simple ideas, such as not calling medication "candy," storing medication in the original containers, and labeling all cleaning products and containers should be encouraged.

Evaluation

• Do parents describe the appropriate actions to take in the event of a future poisoning?
• Are the child's oxygen saturation, blood gas measurements, and level of consciousness within normal limits?
• Is the child's hourly urine output appropriate for age and weight?
• Are family members remaining with the child and able to provide adequate support?
• Can parents and other caregivers describe poison prevention—common poisonous household hazards out of the child's reach, easily accessible poison control telephone number?

ENVIRONMENTAL EMERGENCIES

Active children are exposed to a variety of environmental hazards. Injuries from animal and snake bites, submersion injuries, and sun- and heat-related illnesses account for the majority of these hazards. This section focuses on animal, human, and snake bites; submersion injuries; and heat-related illnesses. Sunburn is discussed in Chapter 49.

Animal, Human, and Snake Bites

Etiology

Animal and Human Bites. Both animal and human bites involve soft tissue damage from crushing, lacerations, and puncture wounds. All animal bites have potential for infection. Although human bites are relatively rare, they carry the greatest risk of infection if they break the skin, particularly if they are on the scalp, face, hands, wrists, or feet. Serious injury can result from any type of bite, but most bites are not life-threatening.

Snake Bites. Envenomation of children on land is usually from snakes, scorpions, and spiders. Envenomation can also result from marine animals, such as jellyfish, sea urchins, and stingrays. Fatalities from envenomation are rare; most fatalities occur from snake bites.

Incidence

Animal bites in the pediatric age-group are most often from domestic animals and have the highest incidence in school-age boys. Most bites are from dogs, usually a dog familiar to the victim. Fatal dog attacks by pit-bulls, Akitas, chow-chows, rottweilers, German shepherds, huskies, and Alaskan malamutes are the most commonly reported (Calkins, 2001).

Cats are the most common family pets, and although a cat bite is less likely to cause serious injury initially, it is more likely to become infected than a dog bite. Bites from pet birds, rats, ferrets, pigs, hamsters, turtles, fish, alligators, snakes, horses, and many other animals have been seen in emergency settings, as have bites from a variety of wild animals, such as raccoons, skunks, and coyotes.

In the United States, the two groups of poisonous snakes are: pit vipers (Crotalidae) such as rattlesnakes, water moccasins, and copperheads; and coral snakes (Elapidae). Pit vipers are responsible for more than 95% of snake bites. Approximately 8000 venomous snake bites occur in the United States annually—about half of them in children (Bowman, 2003).

Manifestations

Animal and Human Bites. Because of the risk of infection, human bites are more serious and can be differentiated from dog bites by the distance between the canine teeth; in human bites the distance is generally greater than 3 cm. A human bite is horseshoe-shaped and rarely breaks the skin. Localized tissue damage and multibacterial infections are serious manifestations of animal and human bites. Dog bites run an additional risk because the massive force generated by their jaws can result in blunt force injury resulting in depressed skull fractures, chest wall destruction, and vascular injury (Calkins, 2001).

Snake Bites. To determine the cause of envenomation, medical staff in emergency settings should have some knowledge of the venomous snakes likely to be encountered in the surrounding geographic area.

Smaller children are usually bitten on the hand or foot, whereas older children are more commonly bitten on lower extremities, and more than half of snake bites occur when a person is purposely handling a known venomous snake (Bowman, 2003).

Regardless of whether the snake can be positively identified, treatment should be based on physical assessment and symptoms. These local signs and symptoms most commonly suggest envenomation:

- Bite marks that look like fang marks
- Burning at the site
- Ecchymosis and erythema
- Pain or numbness
- Progressing edema

The following systemic signs and symptoms suggest severe envenomation:

- Nausea, vomiting
- Sweating, chills
- Numbness, paresthesia of the tongue and perioral region
- Hypotension

Systemic signs and symptoms usually appear within 30 minutes or longer. When a substantial amount of venom has been injected and when treatment is delayed, envenomation can progress to coagulopathies, respiratory failure, renal failure, seizures, shock, and (rarely) death.

Therapeutic Management

Animal Bites. Emergency care for animal bites depends on the type of bite but usually includes thorough irrigation and débridement. Tetanus prophylaxis is given if the child's immunization is not up to date or if documentation is unavailable. Antibiotics are prescribed if there is a high probability of infection. Smaller bite wounds are often left open, rather than sutured, because puncture wounds and wounds closed with sutures have more potential for infection. Treatment of the child for rabies might be necessary, especially in cases of wild animal (e.g., raccoon, rat, skunk) bites.

Snake Bites. Three factors influence the severity of bite from a venomous snake:

- The child's age, size, and general health
- Size of the snake (larger snakes produce more venom)
- Location of the injury (peripheral injuries account for 90% of the bites and are less severe)

When assessing the child with a snake bite, identification of the type of snake is helpful, but this is not always possible. In most cases, an expert in the treatment of snake bites should be consulted. Traditional emergency treatments (e.g., use of a tourniquet, incision, and extraction of the venom; electric shock therapy; cryotherapy) are no longer recommended and can result in complications including increased tissue loss and infection (Bowman, 2003). First aid (after assessment and maintenance of the ABCs) now includes immobilization of the extremity in a position below the level of the heart; removal of clothes, rings, and other constricting items; and rapid transport to an emergency facility.

In the hospital setting, emergency management continues assessment and maintenance of the ABCs, insertion of an IV line if envenomation is suspected, laboratory studies including CBC, coagulation studies, electrolytes, creatinine phosphokinase, and urinalysis to assist in determination of need for antivenom therapy (Bowman, 2003). Children with no progression of symptoms after 6 hours may be discharged. Children with any progression of symptoms should be admitted to the hospital. In cases of moderate to severe envenomation, the negative side effects of antivenin must be weighed against the positive effects. Antivenin therapy is the mainstay of treatment for snakebites. Indications for administration include worsening injury, coagulation abnormalities, or systemic effects.

Nursing Considerations

With severe bites, significant envenomation, or anaphylaxis, nursing interventions for bites and envenomation begin with attention to the ABCs and support of vital functions. With envenomation, nursing care includes keeping the child as calm as possible to help prevent spread of the toxin or venom. Hospitals may not have sufficient antivenin for severe envenomation, so nurses should make sure that available protocols include the location of centers to contact for additional antivenin.

Carefully clean the injury site of all bites, and give tetanus prophylaxis if immunizations are not up to date. When the bite or envenomation is located on an extremity, immobilize the extremity. Measuring the circumference of the affected extremity every 20 to 30 minutes will track progression of the injury as well as results of treatment.

If antivenin is to be administered, obtain a careful history of allergies because the most common antivenins are made from horse serum. Antivenin is most effective if given within 4 to 6 hours after injury, but it may be repeated if coagulopathies or bleeding is present. Document the type and location of the injury, the length of time since the injury, and the signs and symptoms resulting from the injury. All children who require antivenin should be monitored in an intensive care setting. To assess hypersensitivity, a small test dose of antivenin is given intradermally before the full dose.

Education concerning avoiding snake habitats, wearing protective clothing, and avoiding provocative behavior around snakes should be emphasized.

In most states, notification of the local animal control agency is required for animal bites. Document rabies immunization status of the animal, if available, in nursing notes. Quarantine of the animal responsible for the attack might be necessary if the animal can be found.

Discharge instructions should include observation for signs and symptoms of infection and wound care. Provide injury prevention education to all families. Give parents information about how to teach their children to avoid animal bites, including avoiding strange animals and nonprovocative behavior in dealing with enraged animals.

Submersion Injuries (Near Drowning)

Known as the "silent event," submersion injury is the second leading cause of accidental death in children (CDC, 2003b). *Drowning* is submersion that results in asphyxia and death within 24 hours. If the child survives longer than 24 hours after submersion, the event is referred to as *near drowning*.

One of the most important nursing responsibilities related to drowning is prevention of injury, including water safety education and training, support of legislative efforts to pass drowning prevention measures, and teaching CPR. Nurses must emphasize the importance of adequate adult supervision when children are in or around water.

Etiology
Most drownings happen in residential swimming pools, although drownings can occur in any body of water, including hot tubs, spas, bathtubs, toilets, and even buckets. Open-water sites, such as lakes, rivers, and oceans, are more likely to be the site of accidents among teenagers. Alcohol is often a factor in teenage drownings because it alters judgment and increases risk-taking behaviors.

Incidence
Although death by drowning in the child younger than 14 years has decreased 37% from 1987 to 2000, 943 children in this age-group died in 2000 and an estimated 4700 children required emergency room treatment (Wallis, Cody, & Mickalide, 2003). The average age of more than half of drowning victims is younger than 4 years. Boys are two to four times more likely than girls to die from drowning. Drowning is more likely to occur in the summertime and on weekends. Southern and western states have higher drowning fatality rates.

Manifestations
The child's condition after near drowning varies with the extent of injury. Five factors contribute to the child's eventual prognosis: (1) age, (2) submersion time and water temperature, (3) elapsed time before resuscitation efforts are instituted, (4) neurologic status, and (5) arterial blood gas measurements (especially pH). The child with the poorest prognosis is younger than 3 years, has been submerged longer

---

Pathophysiology
of Submersion Injury

Hypoxia causes the injury to organ systems when drowning occurs. Drowning progresses in a predictable sequence of events. Drowning victims panic, struggle, and attempt to hold their breath. In doing so, they begin to swallow water, which is then vomited and aspirated. This process can cause laryngospasm, which leads to hypoxia, seizures, and death (called *dry drowning* because laryngospasm prevents large amounts of water from entering the respiratory system). If the child becomes unconscious before laryngospasm, hypoxia causes loss of airway reflexes and subsequent aspiration of large amounts of water (leading to *wet drowning*). As hypoxia and acidosis progress, cardiopulmonary arrest occurs. Swallowing large amounts of fresh water also causes electrolyte shifts into the intracellular spaces, resulting in hyponatremia and cerebral edema.

Submerged children lose body heat quickly in cold water because of their relatively large body surface area. Severe hypothermia offers some protection to the brain through the diving reflex, which is stimulated when the face is submerged in cold water. This neurologic reflex shunts blood away from the periphery, increasing blood flow to the brain and heart. The diving reflex is stronger in young children. Irreversible brain damage usually occurs after 4 to 6 minutes of submersion, but some children have had a complete recovery after lengthy submersion (10-40 min) in very cold water.

---

than 5 minutes, is comatose, has an arterial pH less than 7.10, and has not had resuscitative efforts within the first 10 minutes of the incident (Orlowski, 2001).

The child who is conscious with adequate respirations might have mild hypothermia, show slight pulmonary changes on radiography, and demonstrate minor blood gas alterations. Children who are unconscious (stuporous or comatose) demonstrate consequences related to whether respirations are present or absent. If respirations are adequate, the child might have mild to moderate hypothermia and mild to moderate respiratory distress with abnormal chest radiography and arterial blood gas results. The child who has required resuscitative efforts is in markedly poorer condition, with altered mental status, metabolic acidosis and other arterial blood gas abnormalities, electrolyte disturbances, possible seizures, or shock, and might develop disseminated intravascular coagulation. Death is the result of complete cardiopulmonary arrest or cerebral anoxic-ischemic injury. Most long-term sequelae of near-drowning are neurologic in origin (Orlowski, 2001).

Therapeutic Management
Prehospital Emergency Management. Treatment begins at the scene of the accident with rescue and removal from the water. The prehospital care the child receives can significantly affect the chances for a normal recovery. Prompt initiation of CPR and activation of the emergency medical system are imperative. The goal of prehospital care is to maintain adequate oxygenation and circulation, to minimize secondary organ damage, and to take proper precautions to stabilize possible cervical spine injuries.

Every child with submersion injury is considered hypoxic. When the brain is deprived of oxygen for even a short period, irreversible brain damage can occur. After the child's airway is opened, the nurse suctions the child's oropharynx to remove mucus and fluid and delivers 100% oxygen by mask or by bag-valve-mask in the child with inadequate respiratory rate or effort. It is important to avoid overinflation of the lungs to prevent a pneumothorax. Pulse oximetry may not be available in prehospital management or may be inaccurate in the child with hypothermia. Assessment of breath sounds, chest symmetry and rise and fall, and central color are more reliable indicators of adequate respirations.

Elevating the head of the bed to 30 degrees might help lower intracranial pressure but should be done only if no spinal injury or shock is present. Intubation should be considered for unconscious and nonbreathing children.

A cardiac monitor is used for ongoing assessment of heart rate and rhythm. Ventricular fibrillation or asystole that is unresponsive to resuscitative efforts can occur in the severely hypothermic (28° C) child. Resuscitative efforts continue while aggressive warming measures are instituted. Children have been successfully resuscitated up to 45 minutes after a cold-water immersion. Because the presence of a cardiac rhythm does not ensure perfusion of the tissues, the prehospital team assesses the child's cardiovascular status at regular intervals in addition to observing the rhythm on the cardiac monitor.

The wet clothes are removed, and the child is covered with warm blankets. Increasing the ambient temperature of the transport vehicle may be indicated. Rapid transport to the local emergency department or tertiary center is critical in the severely hypothermic child.

Two IV lines should be started immediately in critically ill children with submersion injuries. Because of the electrolyte and fluid shift into the intracellular space, children can become hypovolemic and fluid resuscitation is required. Adequate circulation is necessary to maintain organ perfusion. The rescuer may obtain blood for laboratory analysis while inserting the IV lines. Standard blood studies for the submerged child include CBC, serum electrolytes, BUN, creatinine level, and serum amylase. If the child is in shock or has experienced significant trauma, typing and crossmatching of 2 to 4 units of blood should be included.

Both air and water can be swallowed during a submersion incident. Air might also be forced into the stomach with resuscitative efforts. Because gastric distention resulting from air and water in the stomach can prevent full expansion of the lungs, a gastric tube should be inserted to decompress the stomach, ensure full respiratory excursion, and prevent aspiration of stomach contents from vomiting.

Hospital Management. Emergency care, on reaching the emergency department, continues the prehospital goals of maintaining adequate oxygenation and circulation, as well as initiation of other treatments based on laboratory and radiologic findings. Arterial blood gases may indicate the need to correct acidosis with sodium bicarbonate. Continued hypothermia is addressed by initiation of warmed IV fluids and oxygen, overhead lights, and warmed blankets. Fluid and electrolyte corrections can be instituted.

The child is admitted to the hospital for observation, even if in stable condition after initial rescue and emergency treatment.

▪NURSING CARE
The Child With a Submersion Injury

Nursing care of the child with a submersion injury requires obtaining an accurate history, ensuring adequate oxygenation and tissue perfusion, and maintaining body temperature.

Assessment

Assessment of the child with a submersion injury focuses on the respiratory system. Airway and breathing are the priorities. Observe the child for rate and depth of respiration, work of breathing, and any change in mental status. Cardiovascular assessment includes assessment of capillary refill and heart rate. Take the child's temperature as soon as possible to determine any hypothermia.

An accurate history of the injury is important although often difficult to obtain. Whether the submersion incident occurred in salt or fresh water is irrelevant for early treatment, but subsequent intensive care may vary somewhat depending on the immersion fluid.

Nursing Diagnosis and Planning

The diagnoses applicable to the child with a submersion injury are

- Impaired Gas Exchange (actual or potential) related to bronchospasm, aspiration of fluid, surfactant elimination, or pulmonary edema.
  Expected Outcome: The child will demonstrate normal oxygen saturation, blood gas measurements, and clear breath sounds.
- Risk for Imbalanced Fluid Volume related to electrolyte imbalances that cause volume shifts from interstitial to intravascular space.
  Expected Outcomes: The child will maintain hourly urine output appropriate for weight and age and vital signs within normal limits; electrolytes will return to normal.
- Hypothermia related to prolonged exposure to cold water.
  Expected Outcome: The child will maintain body temperature between 36.5° C and 37.4° C.
- Compromised Family Coping related to the child's critical status.
  Expected Outcomes: The family will verbalize feelings (including feelings of guilt and anger) and concerns appropriately, exhibit an attitude of confidence in care, and provide support to the child.

Interventions

After the initial assessment and emergency management have been completed, the nurse monitors for changes from the baseline, anticipates the development of complications, and implements therapeutic management.

Providing Respiratory Support

Because hypoxia is the primary problem, with potential for damage to all major organ systems, attention to the pulmonary system is a priority. Assess level of consciousness, and listen for adventitious breath sounds, which can signal the development of complications, such as pulmonary edema, atelectasis, or pneumonia. Persistent hypoxemia, dyspnea, tachycardia, and respiratory alkalosis can also signal these pulmonary complications. If the child is intubated, maintain the airway and observe for signs of tube displacement or pneumothorax.

Restoring Appropriate Circulatory Status

Cardiovascular monitoring includes measuring vital signs, pulses, level of consciousness, skin temperature, color, and urine output. The well-perfused child is alert with age-appropriate behavior and has a capillary refill time of less than 2 seconds and urine output of at least 1 ml/kg/hr. Maintain IV lines and administer fluid volume replacement as ordered.

Identifying and Preventing Neurologic Consequences

The neurologic system is monitored frequently. Common parameters include level of consciousness, pupillary response, movement of extremities, reflexes, and vital signs. Anticipate signs and symptoms of increased intracranial pressure up to 24 hours after the submersion event. Conventional measures to prevent increased intracranial pressure, such as positioning the head in the midline, elevating the head of the bed 20 to 30 degrees, preventing or managing elevated body temperature, and controlling pain and agitation, are instituted as ordered and as needed.

Restoring Fluid Balance

As a result of ingestion of large amounts of water during the near-drowning event, the child is at risk for development of alterations in fluid and electrolyte balance. Carefully monitor urine output, laboratory data, and physical signs and symptoms. Hyponatremia and water intoxication should be anticipated, particularly with a fresh-water submersion. Observe for changes in central nervous system functioning, especially seizures, as the serum sodium level drops.

Controlling Infection

The acutely ill child is at risk for local or systemic infection. Complications from organ damage, intubation and ventilation tubes, invasive monitoring lines, and urinary catheters are possible sources for infection. If infection is present, antibiotic therapy is started. Monitor the child's response to the therapy.

Maintaining Nutritional Status

In the gastrointestinal system, hypoxia leads to decreased blood supply to the bowel. Stress ulcers and gastrointestinal bleeding are not uncommon. Monitor gastrointestinal function in terms of what goes in (nothing by mouth [NPO], oral or enteral feedings), what goes on inside (bowel sounds, residual feedings), and what comes out (presence or absence of blood; amount, color, and consistency of stool).

The child's increased metabolic demands, along with disruption of gastrointestinal functioning, can result in a nutritional deficit. Implement nutritional therapy as ordered in the form of enteral feedings or total parenteral nutrition. If enteral feedings are ordered, monitor weight gain, residuals, amount and consistency of stools, and vomiting to ascertain tolerance of the feedings. If total parenteral nutrition is ordered, check the label with the order, administer

the fluid as ordered, monitor laboratory values, and assess for any side effects.

Providing Emotional Care for the Family

Because children brought to the emergency department with CPR in progress rarely have a positive outcome, an important element of nursing care is psychologic intervention and support for the child's family. The most important nursing interventions with the family of any critically ill or injured child initially include attention to the physical needs of the family and provision of information and hope.

Families should be encouraged to participate in the decision regarding their presence in the treatment area, especially if the child is likely to die and the family may not have an opportunity to see the child alive again. If the parents choose to be brought into the resuscitation room, one person should be their liaison, bringing them in, answering questions, and escorting them out at appropriate times.

Be honest with the family. If the child is in full arrest, a simple statement such as, "Your child (use the child's name if possible) is not breathing and has no heartbeat. We are supporting his breathing and helping his heart to beat right now." This statement is far better than "We're doing everything we can," which leaves much more room for doubt.

Parents react in many different ways, according to their cultures, religious beliefs, individual personalities, and past experiences. Remember that denial can be protective initially, and allow the family to accept information gradually. Ask family members if they want other family members or clergy contacted. Religious rites, including baptism, may be very important to families. A list of clergy from a variety of religions should be readily available for use by the nursing staff.

Providing hope for the family is always important. At times, the only hope may be that the child is not suffering, or did not suffer, and that the child is, or was, not alone. If the child survives the incident, the parents will have ample time to adjust to any adverse consequences, so it is not necessary to insist on their acceptance at this point. There have been many miraculous recoveries after lengthy submersions, although these are usually in very cold water. In the emergency setting, however, it is impossible to predict the ultimate outcome for a child. A realistically positive attitude, while acknowledging the strong possibility of long-term effects for the child, is the most reasonable approach.

! CRITICAL TO REMEMBER

Needs Expressed by Families of Critically Ill Children

The highest-ranked need identified for families in most research studies is the need for hope. Needs for privacy and comfort are also consistently identified as extremely important by the families of critically ill and injured children; these needs are usually ranked higher than the need for psychologic support from nursing staff. Another commonly cited need is to have a contact person to provide updates and answer questions.

TABLE **34-6** Heat-Related Illness

Type	Pathophysiology	Clinical Manifestations	Treatment
Overexertion	Body fluids are being lost through sweating; rapid breathing; increased metabolic demands	Dizziness; flushed skin; diffuse muscle cramps	Move to cool environment; offer oral fluids; loosen clothing
Heat exhaustion	Increased loss of body fluids; increased blood flow to the skin with resulting decreased blood flow to vital organs	Heavy sweating; nausea; vomiting; dizziness or fainting; exhaustion; headache; cramps; cool, moist, or flushed skin; core body temperature may be slightly elevated	Move to cool environment; apply cool, moist cloths to skin; remove clothing or change to dry clothing; offer oral fluids if no altered mental status or vomiting
Heat stroke	Thermoregulation is ineffective; sweating has stopped; vascular collapse and severe central nervous system abnormalities are noted because of hyperthermia and insufficient circulating volume	Hot, dry, red skin; change in level of consciousness or coma; rapid, weak pulse; rapid, shallow breathing; elevated core body temperatures: $\geq 105°$ F (40.6° C)	Emergency transport if not in an emergency setting; rapid cooling with moist, cool cloths and fans; administer oxygen by nonrebreather, or intubate for respiratory insufficiency; aggressive IV rehydration; intervene as needed to maintain vital functions

IV, Intravenous.

Evaluation

- Does the child demonstrate adequate oxygenation and independent breathing? Are lung sounds clear?
- Is the child's urine output appropriate for weight and age? Have electrolyte levels returned to normal?
- Is the child's body temperature between 36.5° C and 37.4° C?
- Do the parents verbalize their feelings and concerns appropriately, and do they provide appropriate support for the child?

Heat-Related Illnesses

Heat-related illnesses include sunburn, heat cramps, heat rash, heat exhaustion, and heat stroke. The most serious types are heat exhaustion and heat stroke, both of which can ultimately result in death.

Incidence

Children's anatomic and physiologic differences make them more susceptible to sun- and heat-related illnesses. About 80% of a person's sun and heat exposure occurs before 21 years of age. Few deaths from heat-related illnesses have been reported, but the majority of these involve very young or very old people. The majority of pediatric deaths are related to small children being left alone in closed vehicles. On the average, 25 children die each year as a result of being trapped in hot vehicles. Most of these children were age 3 years and younger (National SAFE KIDS, 2003). It is important to learn healthy habits such as use of sunscreen and adequate fluid intake early in life. This section focuses on heat-related illnesses; sunburn is discussed in Chapter 49.

Children involved in physical activity sweat less, create more heat in proportion to their body size, and adapt slower to warm environments than do adults (American Academy

of Pediatrics, 2000a). In addition, younger children have a greater body surface area/mass ratio, which causes their bodies to gain heat from the environment on a hot day. Obese children are vulnerable because of increased insulation. Active children may continue playing without feeling the need to drink adequate amounts of fluids even in extremely hot environments.

Manifestations and Therapeutic Management

Symptoms of heat-related illness are wide-ranging and, if left unrecognized or untreated, can quickly progress to heat exhaustion and the life-threatening state of heat stroke. Management of heat-related illness is dictated by the severity of symptoms. The first priority in all cases is to move the child to a cool place and start cooling measures such as loosening and removing wet clothes and applying cool clothes. Rehydration is instituted, either by oral fluids in cases of overexertion or by IV rehydration if the child is unable to tolerate the oral route. In cases of heat stroke, this is not sufficient. The child's temperature-controlling mechanisms are not working, the child is unable to sweat, and brain damage and death could result if the body is not cooled rapidly. Concurrent assessment and prompt stabilization of cardiopulmonary circulation are critical (Table 34-6).

Nursing Considerations

The nurse caring for a child with a heat-related emergency will assess and possibly intervene in stabilizing the ABCs, provide cooling measures aimed at progressively decreasing core temperature without causing shivering or increased metabolic demands, provide emotional support for the client and family, and provide education to promote healthy habits.

Depending on the severity of symptoms, the nurse will assess for respiratory compromise and intervene with the appropriate method of oxygen delivery. In the hospital setting, the child with heat exhaustion might benefit from cool oxygen blow-by or nasal cannula, whereas the child with heat stroke will require oxygen via nonrebreathing mask or even intubation in the case of an insufficient respiratory effort. The nurse performs serial assessments of circulation and disability to determine evaluation of IV fluid resuscitation.

As in other pediatric emergencies, the family should be involved early and to the extent they are comfortable. Family presence is encouraged, with the nurse or other member of the health care team available to provide clear explanations of procedures, answer questions, and provide support.

Involvement by the nurse in promoting healthy habits in the child and family is crucial. Young children should never be left alone in a vehicle, and they should be taught a car is not a toy. The danger of sun and heat exposure, along with adequate fluid intake, wearing light-colored, loose-fitting clothing, and adjustment of activity according to temperature and humidity levels are concepts the child, family, and community need to know and incorporate.

DENTAL EMERGENCIES

Incidence and Etiology

Injury to the teeth, particularly the anterior teeth, is common in children. Toddlers, because of their lack of coordination, receive dental injuries from falling from or onto furniture. School-age children are more likely to have their teeth injured on playgrounds and during sports activities. The first teeth begin to erupt at approximately 6 months of age. By approximately 2 years of age, a child has all 20 primary teeth. Permanent teeth come in at approximately 5 or 6 years of age. By adolescence, a child usually has the full complement of 32 permanent teeth, although the eruption of wisdom teeth might be somewhat delayed. Injury to primary and permanent teeth is considered equally serious.

Teeth are embedded in the bones of the maxilla and mandible. Injuries to teeth are usually divided into the following categories:

Concussion	The tooth is not displaced, but pressure may cause pain.
Subluxation	The tooth is moveable within the socket but is displaced less than 2 mm. There is no damage to the socket.
Intrusion	The tooth is pushed into its socket with injury to the underlying structures.
Extrusion	An upper tooth is dislodged downward from the socket, or a lower tooth is dislodged upward.
Luxation	The tooth is moved laterally with tearing of the periodontal ligament.
Avulsion	The tooth is no longer in the socket, and the socket itself might be damaged.

Therapeutic Management

Dental emergencies require specialized care, which is often difficult to obtain immediately. Survival of the tooth depends on the periodontal ligament attachment, so concussion, subluxation, lateral luxation, and extrusion, in which the periodontal ligament is still attached, have a better prognosis than complete avulsion of a tooth. Intrusion of a tooth might damage underlying structures to a greater extent and diminish chances for tooth survival.

Time is of the essence in caring for dental injuries. With injury to a child's mouth, the nurse observes for missing teeth. If a missing tooth cannot be found in the oral cavity, possible aspiration should be considered in the presence of dyspnea. To determine whether other teeth are loose or malpositioned, the nurse gently palpates (using Standard Precautions) the teeth for movement or encourages the child to check with the fingers or tongue. A tooth that is loose in the socket should not be removed. If the position is not correct, repositioning may be necessary when a specialist is available.

In general, primary teeth are not replanted because damage to the developing tooth bud can occur. Complete avulsion of a permanent tooth requires care of the socket and of the tooth itself. Survival of an avulsed tooth depends on prompt evaluation and replacement. Irreversible damage to the periodontal ligament because of dehydration of the open socket may occur after 60 minutes.

Emergency care by the dentist includes cleaning the tooth and socket, placing the tooth in the socket, and splinting the tooth. Tetanus immunization is given if needed, and an antibiotic may be prescribed.

Nursing Considerations

Parents should be instructed to keep the tooth moist. The tooth may be immersed in saline, water, milk, or a commercial tooth-preserving liquid. The tooth should not be cleaned or scrubbed. Although some recommend replacing the tooth in the socket immediately, a parent might replace the tooth

CRITICAL THINKING EXERCISE 34-3

Your friend's child is playing a soccer match at the local elementary school, and you have been invited to watch. During the match she trips and falls. Her mouth is bleeding profusely, and she appears to have been accidentally kicked in the mouth by another player.

1. What actions should you take if you are asked to help?
2. What actions will you take if you discover this child has lost one of her teeth?

backwards or the tooth or socket may not be clean or free of debris or clots and these problems would decrease the chances of tooth survival. The child should see a dentist, if possible, or should go to an emergency facility for care without delay.

Parents should be given careful discharge instructions and appropriate referrals for continuing care. When appropriate, reassure the family that first teeth are replaced by the second set of teeth and that there are many ways to ensure a good cosmetic outcome, even with loss of a permanent tooth, with good follow-up care.

KEY CONCEPTS

- Because of children's smaller sizes, the different equipment and dosages needed for their care, and age-related psychologic differences, nursing care of ill and injured children may seem more complicated than care of adults.
- Familiarity with the issues related to the child's growth and development, continuing education in pediatric emergency care, and careful organization of pediatric equipment, supplies, referrals, and reference lists can help to decrease anxiety in health care providers and improve the care of children in emergency settings.
- Airway management is the most critical element in pediatric emergency care. Emer-

gency assessment and triage should include airway assessment and intervention. Without adequate oxygenation and ventilation, clients have little hope of survival.

- Shock must be recognized early in the child and should always be considered a possibility when the heart rate increases, breathing increases, or changes occur in color, temperature, or moisture of the infant's or child's skin.
- Care of the family and the child's developmental stage should always be considered when providing nursing interventions in the emergency setting. The parents' reactions and the child's developmental factors affect compliance, cooperation, and anxiety levels.

- Trauma assessment of the child includes the standard primary and secondary survey and intervention but must also include assessment of skin signs, use of appropriate age-related tools for determining the level of consciousness, and prevention of or intervention for hypothermia.
- Injury prevention plays an important role in the nursing care of children. Motor vehicle injuries, ingestions, poisonings, and environmental injuries are largely preventable. Nurses can play an important role in offering anticipatory guidance and providing injury prevention materials and instruction to children and their families.

ANSWERS to Critical Thinking Exercise 34-1

Your primary assessment reveals: *Airway:* clear, with small amount of vomitus noted in corner of mouth; *Breathing:* rapid respirations, slightly shallow, no increased work of breathing; *Circulation:* pulses rapid, peripheral pulses slightly weak, skin pale, mottled, and cool, capillary refill 3 seconds, active bleeding and deformity noted in left lower extremity; *Disability:* eyes closed, responding to verbal stimuli.

The father states: "She was hit by a car going about 30 miles an hour. She flew up in the air about 20 feet. She was wearing her helmet. She cried immediately but is really sleepy now. This happened about 20 minutes ago. I just picked her up and ran. She had a snack about 2 hours ago. She has her shots, no allergies."

1. You would assess the ABCDs. *Airway:* Is the airway open? Any vomitus or other objects in the mouth? Is the child able to maintain her own airway? *Breathing:* Is she breathing? What is the rate and quality? Any increased work of breathing (e.g., retractions, grunting, head bobbing)? *Circulation:* What are the

central and peripheral pulses (rate, quality), skin color and temperature, and capillary refill? Any active bleeding? *Disability:* What is her level of consciousness?

2. History: What happened? When? Was there loss of consciousness? Was she wearing safety equipment? Does she have her immunizations? Allergies? When was the last time she ate or drank?

3. Hypovolemic shock from blunt trauma. Yes, this is an emergency because of her increased heart rate and respiratory rate and decreased level of consciousness. You do not know the extent of injuries at this time. The child is attempting to compensate to increase cardiac output. If not treated, uncompensated shock can ensue, which causes metabolic disturbances, organ damage, and other sequelae of decreased oxygenation, leading to coma and death.

4. You would do the following (in this order): stabilize the cervical spine while applying oxygen; apply heart monitor and pulse oximetry; obtain vascular access; apply pressure to bleeding site; assess and treat

pain; and provide support for the family. Next interventions include a fluid bolus of a crystalloid solution, 20 ml/kg; reassessment of effectiveness of interventions; assessment for extent of injuries; and stabilization of those injuries. You would expect laboratory studies (blood, urine); chest, cervical spine, and extremity x-rays; and cleaning and stabilizing of injuries. Intake and output (I&O) is accurately measured and recorded. Treatment is aimed at stabilization and maintenance of ABCDs, so oxygen, monitoring, rehydration, and determining extent of injuries are priorities of care. The father needs to be supported, with coping strategies and support systems assessed to decrease anxiety and provide comfort during the stressful time of having a seriously ill child.

5. You would expect color to improve with oxygenation and rehydration and heart rate and respiratory rate to slowly return to normal. Injuries would be stabilized and bleeding stopped. The father will express understanding of treatment and will actively help comfort and distract the child.

ANSWERS to Critical Thinking Exercise 34-2

1a. Heat exhaustion. The history of a hot, muggy day and outside activities. Physical symptoms: nausea, leg and arm cramps, dizziness, wet uniform, heavy sweating.

1b. Find shade or a car with air conditioning. Offer cool water or diluted sports drinks if not vomiting, have child change into dry clothes, caution child and family to avoid exertion, and check the other players for signs of overexertion.

1c. If unable to tolerate fluids, he needs to be taken to the hospital for intravenous (IV) hydration and observation.

2a. Possible heat stroke.

2b. Assess ABCDs. It would be expected that: the child's breathing is shallow; he is not sweating, and his skin is red, dry, and hot to touch; his pulse is weak, rapid, and thready; he is tachypneic; and he is lethargic or comatose.

2c. Recognize that this is an emergency and IMMEDIATELY CALL 911 or area emergency number. Move to cool room or air-conditioned car while awaiting ambulance. Remove wet clothes, apply cool wet cloths to body, and have fan blowing on child.

Monitor airway and breathing; assist if necessary. Maintain NPO status.

2d. Prehospital care will include high-flow oxygen, IV fluids, decreased ambient temperature in ambulance for continued cooling measures, ongoing assessment, and rapid transport to emergency department. The mother needs to decide if she wants to go in the ambulance or follow in a friend's car.

2e. Hospital care will continue prehospital care with advanced monitoring and testing. Hospital personnel will provide more information and allow the mother to be with the child if she is comfortable.

ANSWERS to Critical Thinking Exercise 34-3

1. First assess level of consciousness and ABCs. Initiate appropriate resuscitation if necessary. If the child is conscious and alert, observe her mouth carefully, being sure not to touch it without appropriate barrier protection.

2. If a tooth is missing, ask for help finding it. When it is found, your primary goal is to keep it moist to enhance eventual reimplantation. Milk, normal saline, or a commercially prepared tooth preservation solution is suggested. Do not try to replace the tooth in the socket. Alternatively, if a source of liquid

is not readily available, wrapping the tooth in a wet handkerchief is an acceptable way of transporting it. Advise that the child be seen by dental personnel within 2 hours.

REFERENCES and READINGS

Adams, J., Frumiento, C., Shatney-Leach, L., & Vane, D. W. (2001). Mandatory admission after isolated mild closed head injury in children: Is it necessary? *Journal of Pediatric Surgery, 36*(1), 119-121.

American Academy of Pediatrics. (2003). Poison treatment in the home [Electronic version]. *Pediatrics, 112*(5), 1182-1185.

American Academy of Pediatrics, Committee on pediatric Emergency Medicine and American College of Emergency Physicians, Pediatric Committee. (2001). Care of Children in the Emergency Department: Guidelines for Preparedness. *Pediatrics,* Vol. 107(4), 777-781.

American Academy of Pediatrics, Committee on Sports Medicine and Fitness. (2000a). Climatic heat stress and the exercising child and adolescent. *Pediatrics, 106*(1, Pt. 1), 158-159.

American Academy of Pediatrics, Committee on Sports Medicine and Fitness. (2000b). Intensive training and sports specialization in young athletes. *Pediatrics, 106*(1, Pt. 1), 154-157.

American Academy of Pediatrics: Committee on Drugs (2001). Acetaminophen Toxicity in Children. *Pediatrics, 108*(4), 1020-1024. Retrieved May 30, 2003, from American Academy of Pediatrics Web Site: http://www.aap.org/policy/0014.html

American College of Emergency Physicians, & American Academy of Pediatrics (2001). Care of children in the emergency department: Guidelines for preparedness. *Annals of Emergency Medicine, 37*(4), 423-427.

American Heart Association. (2000). Guidelines 2000 for cardiopulmonary resuscitation and emergency cardiovascular care. *Currents in Emergency Cardiovascular Care, 11*(3), 1-30.

Bengur, A., & Meliones, J. (1998). Cardiogenic shock. *New Horizons, 6*(2), 139-149.

Bernardo, L. (1998). Multiple trauma. In M. Slota (Ed.), *Core curriculum for pediatric critical care nursing* (pp. 551-594). Philadelphia: Saunders.

Boie, E., Moore, G., Brummett, C., & Nelson, D. (1999). Do parents want to be present during invasive procedures performed on their children in the emergency department? A survey of 400 parents. *Annals of Emergency Medicine, 34*(1), 70-74.

Bowman, M. J. (2003). From stingers to fangs: Evaluating and managing bites and envenomations. *TraumaReports, 4*(3), 1-9.

Brownstein, D., & Rivara, F. (2000). Emergency medical services for children. In R. Behrman, R. Kliegman, & H. Jenson (Eds.), *Nelson textbook of pediatrics* (16th ed., pp. 237-243). Philadelphia: Saunders.

Burns, J. P. (2003). Septic shock in the pediatric patient: Pathogenesis and novel treatments. *Pediatric Emergency Care, 19*(2), 112-115.

Butt, W. (2001). Septic shock. *Pediatric Clinics of North America, 48*(3), 601-625.

Caldwell, J., & Ziglar, M. (2001). Hemorrhagic Shock in Children. AJN. *EmergencyNursing Update 2001, Sept,* 25-30.

Calkins, C. M., Bensard, D. D., Partrick, D. A., & Karrer, F. M. (2001). Life-threatening dog attacks: A devastating combination of penetrating and blunt injuries. *Journal of Pediatric Surgery, 36*(8), 1115-1117.

Centers for Disease Control and Prevention (2002a). Heat-related deaths—four states, July-August 2001, and United States, 1979-1999. *MMWR Weekly, 51*(26), 567-570. Retrieved May 26, 2003, from CDC Web Site: http://www.cdc.gov/mmwr/preview/mmwrhtml/mm5126a2.htm

Center for Disease Control and Prevention (2002b). Injuries and deaths among children

left unattended in or around motor vehicles—United States, July 2000-July2001. *MMWR Weekly, 51*(26), 570-572. Retrieved May 26, 2003, from CDC Web Site: http://www.cdc.gov/mmwr/preview/mmwrhtml/mm5126a3.htm

Centers for Disease Control and Prevention (2002c). Nonfatal choking-related episodes among children—United States, 2001. *MMWR Weekly, 51*(42), 945-948. Retrieved May 26, 2003, from CDC Web Site: http://www.cdc.gov/mmwr/preview/mmwrhtml/mm5142a1.htm

Centers for Disease Control and Prevention (CDC) Web Site. (n.d.). *Poisonings.* Retrieved July 19, 2003, from CDC, National Center for Injury Prevention and Control Web Site: http://www.cdc.gov/ncipc/factsheets/poisoning.htm

Centers for Disease Control and Prevention. (2003b). *WISQARSTM (Web-based Injury Statistics Query and Reporting System).* Available online: http://webapp.cdc.gov/sasweb/ncipc/mortrate.html

Chameides, L., and Hazinski, M. (Eds.). (2000). *Textbook of pediatric advanced life support.* Dallas: American Heart Association.

Childhood Lead Poisoning Associated with Tamarind Candy and Folk Remedies—California, 1999-2000 (2002). *MMWR Weekly, 51*(31), 684-686. Retrieved May 26, 2003, from CDC Web Site: http://www.cdc.gov/mmwr/preview/mmwrhtml/mm5131a3.htm

Connors, J. M., Ruddy, R. M., McCall, J., & Garcia, V. F. (2001). Delayed diagnosis in pediatric blunt trauma. *Pediatric Emergency Care, 17*(1), 1-4.

Cosby, C. (1998). Pediatric emergencies. In L. Newberry (Ed.), *Sheehy's emergency nursing: Principles and practice* (4th ed.). St. Louis: Mosby.

Eckle, N., & MacLean, S. L. (2001). Assessment of family-centered care policies and practices for pediataric patients in nine US emergency

REFERENCES and READINGS

departments. *Journal of Emergency Nursing, 27*(3), 238-245, 313-318.

Eckle, N., Haley, K., & Baker, P. (Eds.). (1998). *Emergency nursing pediatric course provider manual.* Park Ridge, IL: Emergency Nurses Association.

Emergency Nurses Association. (1998). *ENPC provider manual* (2nd ed.). Park Ridge, IL: Author.

Hatton, S. (2000). Preventing heat related injuries. *On Trac (a Publication of the North Central Texas Trauma Regional Advisory Council), 4*(10), 1, 3-5. http://webapp.cdc.gov/cgi-bin/broker.exe

Hellman, M. (1998). Pediatric environmental emergencies. *Emergency Medical Services, 27*(7), 67-69, 83.

Huston, C. (1997). Dental luxation and avulsion. *American Journal of Nursing, 97*(9), 48.

Ilardi, D. (2003, May). After mild traumatic brain injury: helping school staff meet the needs of students and families. *School Nurse News*, 31-35.

Jacinto, S. J., Gieron-Korthals, M., & Ferreira, J. A. (2001). Predicting outcome in hypoxic-ischemic brain injury. *Pediatric Clinics of North America, 48*(3), 647-660.

Jewkes, F. (2001). Prehospital emergency care for children. *Archives of Disease in Childhood, 84*(2), 103-105.

Jones, G. (1998). Assessment criteria in identifying the sick sepsis patient. *Journal of Infection, 37*(Suppl. 1), 24-29.

Kane, B. E., Mickalide, A. D., Paul, H. A. (2001). *Trauma season: A national study of the seasonality of unintentional childhood injury.* Washington (DC): National SAFE KIDS Campaign.

Klinkhammer, B., & Andreoni, C. (1998). *Quick reference for emergency nursing.* Philadelphia: Saunders.

Kochanek, P. M., Clark, R. S., Ruppel, R. A., & Dixon, C. E. (2001). Cerebral resuscitation after traumatic brain injury and cardiopulmonary arrest in infants and children in the new millennium. *Pediatric Clinics of North America, 48*(3), 661-675.

Koschel, M. (2003). Is it child abuse? *American Journal of Nursing, 103*(4), 45-46.

Krug, S. (1998). The acutely ill or injured child. In R. Behrman & R. Kliegman (Eds.), *Nelson's essentials of pediatrics* (3rd ed., pp. 93-128). Philadelphia: Saunders.

Lipman, T. H. (2001). Toward evidence-based practice. Dog bites in children treated in a pediatric emergency department. *American Journal of Maternal Child Nursing, 26*(1), 55.

Litovitz, T. L., Klein-Schwartz, W., White, S., Cobaugh, D., Youniss, J., Omslaer, J., et al. (2001). 2000 Annual report of the American Association of Poison Control Centers Toxic Exposures Surveillance System. *American Journal of Emergency Medicine, 19*(5), 337-396.

Margolis, G. (1998). Immersion hypothermia. *Jems: Journal of Emergency Medical Services, 23*(9), 66-72, 74-80, 84-85.

National Center for Injury Prevention and Control. (n.d.). *Traumatic Brain Injury.* Retrieved May 26, 2003, from http://cdc.gov/ncipc/factsheets/tbi.htm

National SAFE KIDS Campaign and General Motors. (2003). *Keep your kids safe: Never leave your child alone* [Brochure]. Author.

National SAFE KIDS Campaign. (n.d.). *Sports/recreation: Why kids are at risk.* Retrieved May 26, 2003, from National SAFE KIDS Campaign Web Site: http://safekids.org

Newberry, L. (Ed.). (1998). *Sheehy's emergency nursing: Principles and practice* (4th ed.). St. Louis: Mosby.

Notredame, C., & Westcott, D. (2002). Pediatric poisoning. Retrieved November 25, 2002 from www.advancefornurses.com

Orlowski, J. P., & Szpilman, D. (2001). Drowning: Rescue, resuscitation, and reanimation. *Pediatric Clinics of North America, 48*(3), 627-646.

Samson, R., Berg, R., & Bingham, R. (2003). Use of automated external defibrillators for children: An advisory statement from the pediatric advanced life support task force, international liaison committee on resuscitation [Electronic version]. *Pediatrics, 112*(1), 163-169.

Sheer, B. (1999). Issues in summer safety: A call for sun protection. *Pediatric Nursing, 25*(3), 319-325.

Simon, B., Letourneau, P., Vitorino, E., & McCall, J. (2001). Pediatric minor head trauma: Indications for computed tomographic scanning revisited. *The Journal of Trauma: Injury, Infection and Critical Care, 51*(2), 231-238.

Soud, T. D., & Rogers, J. S. (1998). *Manual of pediatric emergency nursing.* St. Louis: Mosby.

Sztajnkrycer, M. J., & Bond, G. R. (2001). Chronic acetaminophen overdosing in children: Risk assessment and management. *Current Opinion in Pediatrics, 13*(2), 177-182.

Tuite, P. (1997). Recognition and management of shock in the pediatric patient. *Critical Care Nursing Quarterly, 20*(1), 52-61.

Wallis, A.L., Cody, B.E., Mickalide, A. D. (2003). *Report to the nation: Trends in unintentional childhood injury mortality, 1987-2000.* Washington (DC): National SAFE KIDS Campaign.

35

The Ill Child in the Hospital and Other Care Settings

After studying this chapter, you should be able to:
◎ Discuss the nurse's role in various settings where care is given to ill children.
◎ List common stressors affecting hospitalized children.
◎ Describe the child's response to illness.
◎ Discuss the stages of separation anxiety.
◎ Describe the factors that affect children's response to hospitalization and treatment.
◎ Discuss the psychologic responses of families to the illness of a child in the family.

◆ DEFINITIONS

denial   A defense mechanism in which unpleasant realities are kept out of conscious awareness.
egocentric   Preoccupied with one's own interests and needs.
regression   Defense mechanism in which conflict or frustration is resolved by returning to a behavior that was successful in an earlier stage of development.

separation anxiety   Distress and apprehension caused by being removed from parents, home, or familiar surroundings.
situational crisis   Unanticipated event that poses a threat to an individual's psychosocial or psychologic well-being.
therapeutic play   Guided play that promotes the child's psychophysiologic well-being.

Because of current trends in health care management, the care of ill children continues to move from the traditional acute hospital setting to community-based settings and the home. Hospitalized children are more acutely ill than in the past, and their stays are shorter. In addition, the hospitalized child is more likely to have a chronic or terminal disease or have special needs that require specialized care. These changes do not mean that the need for pediatric nurses has diminished; their role is ever-changing and expanding. Pediatric nurses will continue to care for children in hospitals, schools, clinics, and homes.

All children experience some form of illness. The ways in which stressors and developmental needs are addressed are important factors in resolving the immediate crisis and in dealing with future illnesses. The nurse is often the first person the child sees when the child enters the health care system, and the nurse spends more time with an ill child than does any other health care worker. The nurse therefore has a unique opportunity to influence that child's physical and emotional health.

SETTINGS OF CARE

The Hospital

Entering the hospital is somewhat like visiting a foreign country. The language, culture, activities, and expectations may be unfamiliar to the child and the family. The nurse acts as a "tour guide" and provides a safe environment, both physically and emotionally. Being the guide includes activities as diverse as explaining the jargon (e.g., NPO, IV, "vitals"), explaining procedures that are often painful, and facilitating the parents' access to hospital resources, such as social services, case managers, spiritual counselors, and ethics specialists. Above all, the nurse must educate the child and family about the disease process, its treatment, hospital procedures, and discharge issues.

Hospitalizations can be categorized according to length of stay, planned or unplanned admission, surgical or medical intervention, and outpatient (day) or inpatient status. Even though they overlap, these categories provide a framework for examining the child's experience.

Another variable is the type of facility. Children may be hospitalized in a pediatric hospital, on a pediatric unit within a general hospital, or in a general hospital that occasionally admits children. Pediatric units within a general hospital or hospitals that do not have a specific pediatric unit may not have as many child-oriented services as a pediatric hospital has. Special play areas and child-size equipment and fixtures often are not available in general hospitals. Staff members who routinely do not care for children may be less comfortable in that role.

The nurse in this situation is aware of these challenges and can provide support for the child and the family, for example, by taking extra time when the child is admitted to explain routines and procedures or by placing the child close to the nurses' station. This support might include moving a cot into the room for the parent and ordering special foods for the child. Sometimes it means removing part of the food from a tray that is about to be served so that the child is not overwhelmed by the large servings intended for an adult. Ultimately, it means being sensitive to the needs of the child and the family.

24-Hour Observation

Children become ill quickly and recover quickly. For this reason, they may need acute care for a short time, such as when they are dehydrated or are having an acute asthma episode. At the end of 24 hours, the child is evaluated to determine whether further hospitalization is needed or whether discharge with home care instructions is appropriate.

The nurse must prepare the child and family for discharge and assess the parents' ability to care for the child at home. Instructions should be written, and the parent should be encouraged to ask questions. The nurse informs the parent about when to notify the primary health care provider in the event the child's condition worsens. An awareness of cultural differences enhances the nurse's assessment ability. For example, is the parent smiling because of contentment, or is the parent embarrassed to ask a question? Are parents nodding because they understand or because they are too embarrassed to say they cannot read?

Emergency Hospitalization

Because of limited time for preparation, an emergency admission can be traumatic. The admission can be the result of trauma or acute sudden illness. The family may arrive at the hospital with little money, clothing, or other resources. Siblings may also be present, competing with the sick child for the parent's attention. In addition to caring for the sick child, the staff may be called on to help meet the family's basic needs for food, clothing, and a place to stay. A social service referral is appropriate in such situations.

Because of the intense level of activity in emergency departments, care of the family is often overlooked. The family may fear that the child will die or be permanently disabled. Although nurses may see many similar situations each day in which children do well, they must be sensitive to the family's fears, keep the family informed of the child's condition and care, and encourage a family member to stay with the child.

The time for preparing a child is usually limited in emergencies. Nurses must seize every opportunity to prepare children for the care they will receive. Holding and touching the child, talking softly, distracting the child, and involving the child in the procedure are methods of support used in emergencies. After the child is stable, the nurse returns and uses therapeutic communication to talk about the event. A child life specialist may also help the child express feelings. The use of dolls, puppets, and hospital equipment can aid children in communicating their feelings. (Chapter 34 provides more detailed information about caring for children and their families in an emergency setting.)

One 7-year-old boy was admitted to the medical-surgical unit after spending several hours in the emergency department because of acute asthma. Although his mother brought him to the hospital, she had his younger brother and sister with her and could not remain with him in the room. The boy remained quiet, but the nurse noticed that he watched every move she made. In such a case, the nurse might say, "Some kids say it's scary to come to the hospital and especially to be in the emergency room, with the bright lights and everyone rushing around. If you'd like, I can spend a little time with you and we can talk about being in the hospital."

Outpatient and Day Facilities

Outpatient facilities have evolved in an effort to keep children out of the hospital unless absolutely necessary. The outpatient facility may be part of a hospital, or it may be freestanding. The child arrives in the morning; undergoes a procedure, test, or surgery; and goes home by the evening. Common procedures performed during such admissions include tympanostomy tube placement, hernia repair, tonsillectomy, cystoscopy, and bronchoscopy.

This mode of care has three main advantages: (1) it minimizes separation of the child from the family; (2) it decreases the risk of infection; and (3) it decreases cost. A disadvantage is that outpatient facilities that are not connected to a hospital may not be equipped for overnight stays. If complications develop that require continued observation and treatment, the child may have to be transferred to a hospital. This situation can be upsetting to the child and the family.

Although the procedure may be short, teaching the child and the parent is as important as in the acute care setting. When possible, a tour of the facility before the procedure can decrease fear of the unknown. Parents have indicated that although they like the idea of outpatient care, taking a child home afterward can be frightening.

Assessing the parent can assist the nurse in deciding whether the parent is capable of handling the child's care at home or whether home health care is needed. Written instructions specific to the child and procedure are helpful and reassuring. At the very least, a follow-up phone call to the home should be required. Parents should also be encouraged to call the facility if they have any concerns, and they should be given other resources to contact after the facility closes. Families who live far from the health care facility may want to spend the night at a nearby hotel or consider an overnight admission.

Rehabilitative Care

After a serious illness or trauma, the child's ability to function may change. After the acute situation has resolved, the child may be admitted to a rehabilitation hospital. Staff members from nursing, medicine, physical therapy, occupational therapy, and other areas collaborate to develop a treatment plan in which the child, family, and health professionals work to help the child regain previous abilities. Children with neurologic injuries, such as head injuries, or children with serious burns may thrive in this environment, which usually resembles a home environment with facilities available for the child to relearn the activities of daily living.

Nurses in rehabilitative settings must balance nurturing and firm discipline as they help children reclaim independence. Parents often need encouragement and support because they are torn between doing for their child and watching the child struggle to function independently. Overprotection is a common reaction, and parents can be assisted in identifying the child's developmental need to master the environment. The focus should be on what the child can do rather than on the child's limitations.

The Medical-Surgical Unit

Children admitted to the hospital are usually acutely ill or have a chronic disease or disability that requires frequent, often long-term hospitalizations. (Care of the child with a chronic disease is discussed in Chapter 36.) The average length of hospital stay for the acutely ill child has shortened significantly, and the need for teaching has increased in proportion.

Preparation for a planned hospitalization is essential. Some hospitals provide an opportunity for the child to visit the hospital before admission, and many pediatric hospitals host preoperative parties or classes to introduce children to the strange sights and sounds during a surgical experience. Many children's books about the experience of illness and hospitalization are available in public libraries, but parents should check that these are up-to-date and present a realistic picture of the hospital experience (Manworren & Woodring, 1998). Some children's hospitals also have libraries. Parents should answer questions honestly and encourage the child to talk about the hospitalization. Videos may also be available for family members to view together and then discuss.

The Intensive Care Unit

When a child is admitted to the intensive care unit (ICU), both the child and the parents experience increased stress because of the seriousness of the admitting diagnosis and the high-technology, unfamiliar environment. In addition, the child often is experiencing pain, uncomfortable procedures, noise, and constant lighting. In many instances, the child cannot eat or talk. Meanwhile, the parents are experiencing a parent's worst fear—the possible loss of a child.

The child and family need intense emotional support. All the normal responses to hospitalization are magnified and need to be assessed. When possible, planned admissions to the ICU (e.g., for cardiac surgery) should be preceded by visits to the unit or special classes that provide information about special procedures and operations at a level the child can understand.

The parent should be encouraged to remain with the child and should be kept informed of the child's condition (Fig. 35-1). Procedures, equipment, and treatments should be explained, in appropriate language, to both the child and the parent. If the parent leaves and the child's condition changes or a new tube or piece of equipment has been added, the nurse should prepare the parent for the change before the parent sees the child. Nurses need to encourage parents to provide care and to touch their child as much as possible. The nurse's active listening is essential.

Siblings of the seriously ill, hospitalized child can easily be overlooked. Siblings may need to talk, be comforted, or have the hospital experience explained to them. Parents may feel pulled between the ill child and the rest of the family. Often family members want to help but do not know what to do. Suggesting that a grandparent or other relative relieve a parent so that the parent has time with the ill child's sibling can help both the parent and the child. Helping parents by discussing options can relieve stress and may lead to solutions. Inclusion of family members in the provision of care, such as

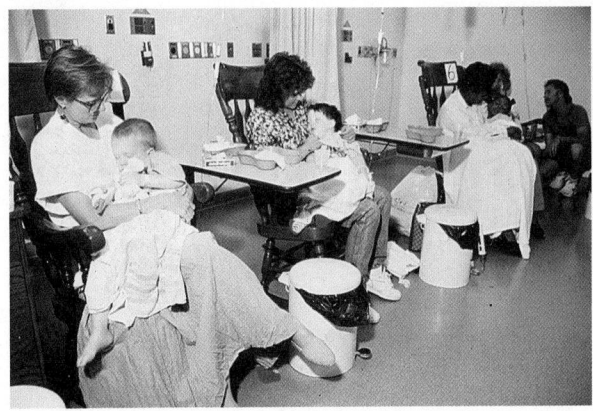

Figure 35-1 When nursing care centers on the family, hospital rules must be altered. These parents are holding their children and rocking them in a postanesthesia care unit, normally a place off-limits to those not on the staff. (Courtesy Cook Children's Medical Center, Fort Worth, TX.)

bathing and feeding, is important to both the family members and the child.

School-Based Clinics

The traditional areas of school health nursing that are still prevalent in many school systems include:

- *Health screening:* Vision, hearing, and growth checks can provide information about problems that may affect a child's ability to learn. When problems are identified, referral and follow-up services are provided.
- *Emergency care:* School nurses are the first to provide care for children involved in accidents, both on the playground and in the school building. Excellent assessment skills are necessary to determine the need for health care provider visits or emergency care.
- *Communicable disease management:* The nurse must assess children for illnesses that may be transmitted to other children, providing care and isolation until the parent can pick up the child from school and advice concerning the safe time for reentry into the school setting.
- *Health care advice:* The school nurse can be a source of referral for families in need of services.
- *Provision of specialized care for children with chronic health needs:* School attendance by children with many health care needs, including catheterization, gastric tube feedings, and suctioning, requires variation in the school nurse role to provide or supervise these specialized services.

School-based clinics have been part of health care for more than 25 years, but with the recent changes in health care delivery, this setting is now a site for expanding primary care. School-based clinics play an important role in providing care for children in remote rural communities and in underserved inner-city areas. School nurses, nurse practitioners, physicians, social workers, and other health care providers typically staff these clinics. This area of practice will continue to grow, and many believe that school-based clinics are the perfect setting for providing primary care for selected groups

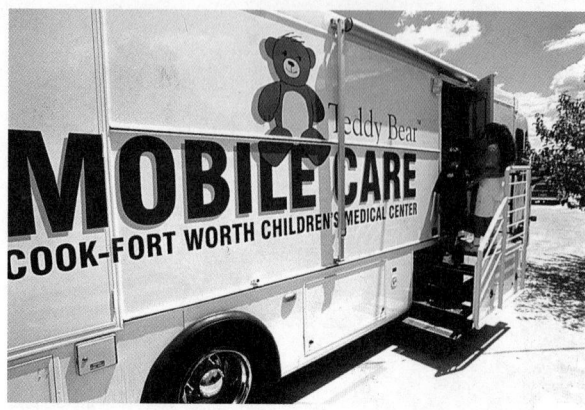

Figure 35-2 Nurses today help take health care on the road to provide services to those who otherwise might not obtain them. This mobile van is stationed at a public school, where it offers health screenings and prevention services to children. (Courtesy Cook Children's Medical Center, Fort Worth, TX.)

of children and adolescents because they are well situated to influence the health and well-being of underserved students (Kaplan et al., 1998).

Prevention remains the focus of school-based care as children learn health habits to prevent their developing acute problems. Nurses identify children who need immunizations and provide immunizations when necessary. Screening that once required referral can often be handled on site. Through school-based clinics, children can receive medical services in a timely manner and avoid expensive emergency visits. For example, a child who is experiencing an earache at school can be seen on site, treated, and sent home if warranted. The child's compliance with treatment can be monitored and a follow-up visit scheduled to determine whether treatment has been effective. Funding for school-based clinics is increasing, and they will continue to be a focus of health care delivery in the community.

Nurses in school-based clinics must be sensitive to parental concerns about certain topics in health care, especially areas related to sexuality (e.g., birth control, sexually transmissible diseases, abortion). Community involvement and support can dispel concerns and assist in setting guidelines for such clinics. School-based nurses must also be team members who act in collaboration with other health care workers and have a strong background in preventive health care as well as the ability to think critically.

The school-based clinic provides a setting for parental education in preventive health care, growth and development, anticipatory guidance, parenting skills, and care of acutely and chronically ill children. The nurse respects the rights and wishes of the parents, but respecting parents' wishes can be a challenge when the value systems of the health care provider and the parent differ. The pediatric nurse is a patient advocate but must exercise caution unless the child is being harmed. (Child abuse is discussed in Chapter 53.)

The nurse is an integral part of children's health education in the school system. The American Academy of Pediatrics recommends that health education is a priority and should be a required subject for all school children in kindergarten through grade 12. To be successful, health education programs should include active participation by the students in programs taught by qualified health educators and monitored by a school health committee. Activities should be fun, be integrated with appropriate school services, and include family and community involvement (Centers for Disease Control and Prevention [CDC], 1996).

Community Clinics

Community health clinics provide primary care for children and their families. In these settings, nurses, nurse practitioners, and physicians provide case management of illness and health promotion. Because most children enter this setting during illness, preventive health care is integrated into the child's acute care. Support services and groups (e.g., social services, a dental clinic, daycare) may be available in the same center, and referrals to medical specialists and other health care providers are also available.

Although many children seen at community health clinics are ill, nurses must use the opportunity to take a health history to assess immunization, nutrition, anticipatory guidance, and growth and development. If the child is ill at the time of the visit, the nurse can set an appointment for the child to return for immunizations or other care that cannot be given when the child is ill (see Appendixes C and D).

In some urban areas, nurses are involved in primary prevention and offer information and education about childhood immunization, the signs and symptoms of childhood illnesses, injury prevention, and parenting skills (Fig. 35-2).

Home Care

Pediatric home care is the provision of skilled care within the child's home. Nurses in this setting are part of a multidisciplinary team that usually includes physicians, physical therapists, speech therapists, occupational therapists, and social workers. Children cared for at home include those receiving respiratory therapy, having dressing changes, receiving total parenteral nutrition, or needing skilled care because of a chronic illness or an injury.

Nurses who work in home care should have previous hospital experience in their practice area. The nurse must be able to make independent decisions and think critically and should have good clinical, documentation, communication, and teaching skills. To meet the needs of each child and family, the nurse must understand various cultures and socioeconomic backgrounds.

Although the separation of child from family is not a problem in home health care, the child may experience many other effects of illness, such as fear of the unknown, loss of control, anger, guilt, and regression. In addition, care is taking place in the family's domain and the nurse is a guest in the home. Family members may have to adjust to unfamiliar noises and equipment, such as special beds, ventilators, or intravenous (IV) pumps, in their home. They may feel that they have lost their privacy and cannot "be themselves" because someone outside the family is frequently there. Awareness of siblings' needs is also a nursing goal in this setting.

<table>
<tr><td>

! CRITICAL **TO REMEMBER**

Children's Response to Illness

- Fear of the unknown
- Separation anxiety
- Fear of pain or mutilation
- Loss of control
- Anger
- Guilt
- Regression

</td><td>

BOX 35-1
Stages of Separation

- *Protest*: Child is agitated, resists caregivers, cries, and is inconsolable.
- *Despair*: Child experiences hopelessness and becomes quiet, withdrawn, and apathetic.
- *Detachment*: Child becomes interested in the environment, plays, and seems to form relationships with caregivers and other children. If parents reappear, the child may ignore them.

</td></tr>
</table>

The nurse's role as a teacher is especially important because many tasks that the nurse might perform in the hospital are delegated to the family, with the nurse monitoring the care. Here the nurse acts as a case manager and coordinator of care.

STRESSORS ASSOCIATED WITH ILLNESS AND HOSPITALIZATION

Age, cognitive development, preparation, coping skills, and culture influence a child's reaction to illness. Previous experience with the health care system and the parent's reaction to the illness also affect the child.

Each child is unique, so predicting reactions to an illness is often difficult. Much of the research on the effects of hospitalization on children has been based on adult assumptions of the child's experience and on children's self-reports. Several categories have been identified: separation, physical harm or body injury, fear of the unknown, uncertainty about limits and outcomes, and loss of control (Melnyk, 2000; Visintainer & Wolfer, 1975). Previous experience with hospitalization may or may not help a child cope with the current experience. Including the parent in the child's care enhances coping (Melnyk, 2000).

Although preschoolers and young school-age children experience separation anxiety, it is most significant in infants and toddlers, especially those ages 6 to 30 months. In times of stress, anxiety related to separation increases.

Each age-group has its own fears related to pain and injury. The past decade has seen an expansion of knowledge about pain and its treatment, negating many erroneous beliefs about children and pain. Children quickly learn to associate health care activities and professionals with pain and injury. The fear is usually focused on "shots." (Chapter 39 discusses issues related to pain.)

A child's feeling of having control over a situation has been shown to affect distress in reaction to medical events (LaMontagne, 1993). If children believe that they have personal control over a situation, they are more likely to feel confident and master a task, whether it is holding still while a needle is inserted or lying still while tomography is performed.

Although specific fears are related to the child's age, hospitalization puts all children at high risk for fears related to their unfamiliarity with the people, surroundings, and events. The child has not developed trust in the health care provider and therefore does not know what to expect. The child may have real or imagined fears: Will the nurse know when I am hungry or hurting? Will the nurse hurt me?

The Infant and Toddler

Separation Anxiety

Infants and toddlers, especially those between 6 and 30 months, experience separation anxiety. Separation is this age-group's major stressor, and it is traumatic to both the child and the parent. The child experiences several stages in reaction to the separation: *protest*, *despair*, and *detachment* (Box 35-1).

In the initial phase, known as *protest*, the child demonstrates distress by crying and rejecting anyone other than the parents (Fig. 35-3). The child appears angry and upset. During the *despair* phase, the child experiences hopelessness and becomes quiet and withdrawn. Crying decreases, and the child becomes apathetic. If separation from the parent continues, the child enters the *detachment* phase. During this phase, the child again becomes interested in the environment and begins to play. Nurses may misinterpret this phase as a positive sign that the child has adjusted to the hospitalization. In reality, the child has "given up." If the parents return during this stage, the child may ignore them and the parents may think that the child does not want to see them. The reaction, however, is a coping mechanism to protect the child from further emotional pain related to the separation.

Nurses in acute care settings see the first two stages of separation—protest and despair—much more frequently than the final stage, detachment, which is more common in long-term separations. Parents may misunderstand their child's behavior. They may even perceive the child's reaction as a behavior problem. Nurses need to reassure parents that this reaction is a normal response to separation and that most children will not suffer any permanent effects from the event. As understanding of separation anxiety has evolved, visiting times have changed from structured hours to more flexible rooming-in situations (see Fig. 35-3).

Most practitioners believe that if separation can be avoided, the child will be much more resilient during a hospitalization. Infants and toddlers go through the stages of separation. The older the children in this age-group, the more elaborate the protest. The child not only cries but also may cling to the parent, kick, and generally create a scene. Parents need to understand that this behavior is a sign of healthy parent-child attachment. The toddler may resist bedtime and eating and may have temper tantrums more frequently than normal for this age. Regression may occur in toileting and eating. Nurses need to explain to parents that regression is normal and encourage parents to

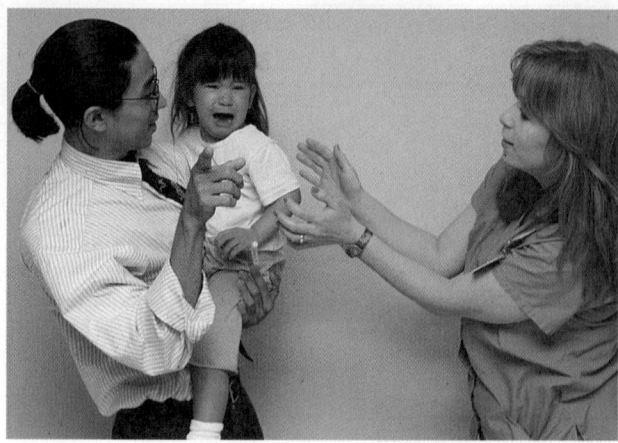

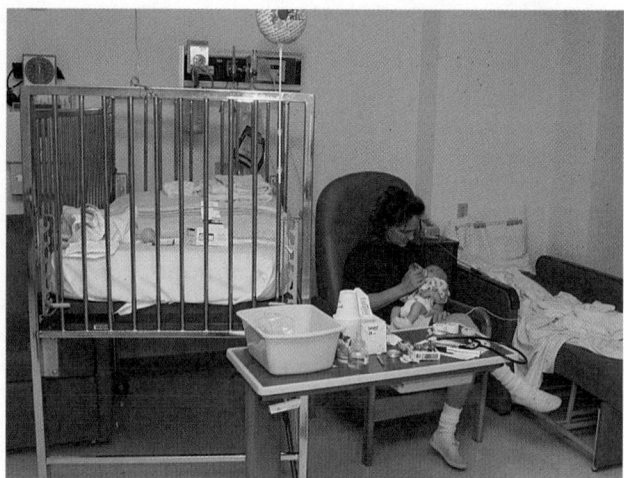

◀ Between the ages of 6 and 30 months, a child is expected to have separation anxiety. The child initially reacts with protest, as this girl is doing. If separation continues, the child becomes quiet and withdrawn (despair phase). In the final phase (detachment), the child may ignore the parents.

Hospitals try to reduce the stress of hospitalization for both parents and child ▶ by having rooming-in arrangements. Rooming-in promotes parental attachment and provides many opportunities to teach parents how to care for their child's needs.

Figure 35-3 Separation is one of the stressors of hospitalization that affects both child and parent. (Courtesy T.C. Thompson Children's Hospital, Chattanooga, TN.)

reinforce appropriate behavior while allowing the regressive behavior to occur.

A parent might ask whether someone needs to be with a hospitalized toddler all the time and may be especially concerned because the parents work and have other children. The nurse may respond, "We encourage parents to stay with their children when they are in the hospital. If you have to leave, however, we will spend time with your child and check on your child frequently. You may call us at any time, day or night. When you return, perhaps you could bring a favorite toy or stuffed animal and something that reminds the child of you. A picture or a piece of clothing (transition object) will make your child feel more secure because it is familiar."

Fear of Injury and Pain
Previous experiences, separation from parents, restraint, and preparation affect the reaction of infants and toddlers to pain and body injury. The young child views injury and pain concretely. Nurses who have worked with toddlers know that most toddlers react to any intrusive procedure, whether it is painful or not. (See Chapter 39 for a more extensive discussion of pain in infants and toddlers.)

Loss of Control
According to Erikson, the major task of the toddler period is developing autonomy. Control is a major issue with this age-group. The toddler experiences the environment through all the senses and loves to explore the environment. At the same time, toddlers need sameness (rituals, routines). Because of the changes in growth and development taking place in the toddler, familiar rituals and rou-

tines (e.g., those for eating, sleeping, playing) provide reassurance and stability.

Hospitalization, which has its own set of rituals and routines, can severely disrupt the toddler's life. The child may be confined to a crib, and the crib may have a cover over it. Because of safety issues, the child is not allowed to run in the halls. If the parents are unable to be with the child, the way the child is put to bed or bathed may be unfamiliar. Information obtained from parents about routines for feeding, going to bed, and playing can assist the nurse in maintaining usual and comforting routines. When children are unable to do things themselves, their sense of control and autonomy is weakened. They are frustrated and may have temper tantrums. Choices, even simple ones, can return some control to the child.

This lack of control is often exhibited in behaviors related to feeding, toileting, playing, and bedtime. The nurse should remember that each of these activities may have associated rituals and routines and that the child may also show some regression in these areas.

The Preschooler
Separation Anxiety
Separation anxiety occurs among preschoolers, but it is generally less obvious and less serious than in the toddler. Although the preschooler may already be spending some time away from parents at a daycare center or preschool, illness adds a stressor that makes separation more difficult.

The preschooler expresses the same protest as the toddler but tends to be less direct. The nurse may find a preschooler quietly crying because the parents have told the child to "act like a big boy (girl)." Children of this age may refuse to eat or take medications, and they may be generally uncooperative. They may repeatedly ask when their parents will be coming for a visit; with access to a phone, the child may constantly call the parents. All these behaviors are signs that the child is having difficulty coping with the situation.

Fear of Injury and Pain

The preschooler fears mutilation. The child who must have surgery affecting a limb or other body part experiences increased fear. The preschooler generally does not understand body integrity. Children of this age are also afraid of intrusive procedures, and because of their literal interpretation of words, they often imagine treatments to be much worse than they are. Finally, the child's active imagination can go wild during illness. The preschooler may believe that the illness occurred because of some personal deed or thought or perhaps just because the child touched something or someone. (The preschooler's specific reactions to pain are discussed further in Chapter 39.) *guilt + shame*

Loss of Control

The preschooler has attained a good deal of independence in self-care and has been given more independence at home, preschool, or daycare. Some children expect to maintain their independence in the hospital. For example, the preschooler may like to wander about the unit and may not be happy when restricted to the bed or room. Like the toddler, a preschooler likes familiar routines and rituals and may show some regression if not allowed to maintain some areas of control.

One 5-year-old boy refused to have his dressing changed by the nurse who cared for him during the previous day. She reported that he cried, pulled up the covers, and said that she was "mean." This behavior was unusual for him, and the nurse suspected that he had been told to do too many things and had not been given choices. In response, the nurse might say, "I know there have been many changes for you since you came to the hospital. Today, we are going to decide together what is going to happen. I see you have chosen a video to watch. Would you like me to change your dressing before you watch the video or after?" This approach gives the preschooler a choice and some control while maintaining boundaries.

Guilt and Shame

Because their thinking is egocentric and magical, preschoolers may believe that their illness is somehow related to a thought or deed. This belief can lead to feelings of guilt, shame, and increased stress at a time when the child has to cope with several other stressors. Because the child typically does not share these feelings with adults, parents and caregivers must be aware of the possibility of guilt and shame in this age-group.

The nurse's role is to assess the child for this type of thinking and, through therapeutic communication, assist the child in identifying unfounded fears and beliefs. The child may be able to relate perceptions of what is happening. The use of puppets, dolls, and drawings can help children deal with their feelings. A tremendous decrease in anxiety can result when the nurse helps the child identify a perceived punishment and then reassures the child that nothing the child did could cause the illness.

The School-Age Child

Separation

The school-age child is accustomed to periods of separation from parents, but just as in the preschooler, as stressors are added, the separation becomes more difficult. The younger school-age child may already have been experiencing separation anxiety related to starting school.

Older children may be more concerned with missing school and the fear that their friends will forget them. The need to adjust to an unfamiliar environment and the regression seen in ill children, however, increase the likelihood that some separation anxiety will take place.

Fear of Injury and Pain

The school-age child is concerned with body disability and death. The child is more relaxed about having a physical examination or having the eyes or an ear examined but is uncomfortable with any type of genital examination. These children want to know the reasons for procedures and tests, and they ask relevant questions about their illness. Because school-age children can understand cause and effect, they can relate actions to becoming ill. Their parents may tell them that if they do not get enough rest, wear warm clothes, or eat nutritious meals, they will get a cold. If they become ill, they associate their actions with the disease. (For further discussion of pain in the school-age child, see Chapter 39.)

Loss of Control

School-age children are "movers and shakers." They control their self-care and typically are highly social. They like being involved, and most fill their days with activities. Illness can change all these patterns. If children of this age have physical limitations, they can feel helpless and dependent (Fig. 35-4).

Friends are important to this age-group, and school-age children may think that their friends will forget them while they are ill. They are also accustomed to making choices about meals and activities. By capitalizing on the child's abilities and needs, the nurse can encourage children of this age to become involved in their own care. School-age children can select their own menus, assist with some treatments, keep their rooms neat, and visit with younger children when it is appropriate for both. With these opportunities for independence, children retain a sense of control, enhance their self-esteem, and continue to work toward achieving a sense of industry.

The Adolescent

Most complex

Separation

Adolescents often are unsure whether they want their parents with them when they are hospitalized. Some enjoy the freedom and the period of independence. Others, in response to the stress of illness, become more dependent and want their parents nearby. A third group cannot decide what they want, and this situation can be frustrating to parents. All these responses are consistent with the normal growth and development of adolescents.

Because of the importance of the peer group, separation from friends is a source of anxiety to the adolescent. Ideally, the peer group will support the ill friend. Some adolescents are reluctant to visit friends in the hospital, either because of their own health fears or because the reality of illness in

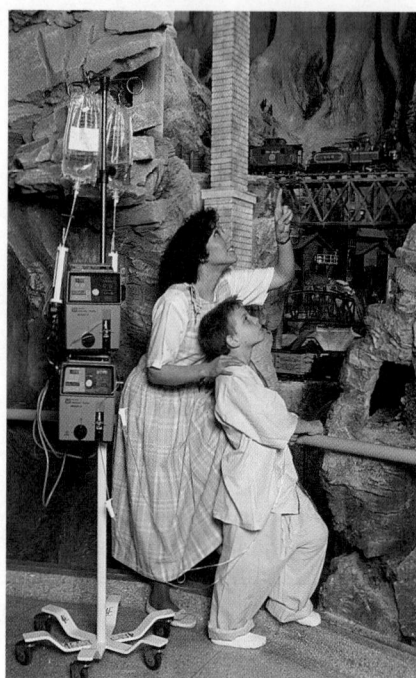

◀ This multilevel "trainscape" in a children's hospital provides children and adults alike with a welcome respite from real-life stresses. (Courtesy Children's Medical Center, Dallas, TX.)

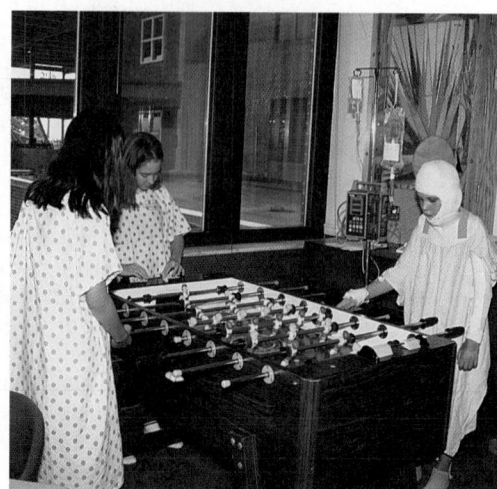

◀ Hospitalized teens need to interact with their peers, as they do when they are well. A lounge area that is separate from the playroom used by younger children fulfills this need.

Figure 35-4 Activities for the hospitalized child are important for growth and development, stress relief, socialization, and a sense of control.

someone their age is difficult for them to handle. Hospitalized adolescents may be upset if their friends simply go on with their lives, excluding them. Special activity areas and other opportunities for the adolescent to meet and interact with other hospitalized adolescents are important (see Fig. 35-4).

Fear of Injury and Pain

To the adolescent, appearance is crucial. Therefore illness or injury that changes adolescents' perceptions of themselves can have a major impact. Even children who have seemingly adjusted to a chronic disease in their earlier years may have difficulty during adolescence simply because they do not want to be different. The adolescent who has diabetes may not want to eat different foods or take time out from an activity for injections. Adolescents do not want attention drawn to them, so they may eat the wrong foods and skip their medication.

Adolescents may also give the impression that they are not afraid, even though they are terrified. Adolescents may think that being "cool" means being in control. They may question everything, or they may appear overly confident. Because of their concern with their bodies, they are guarded when any areas connected to sexual development are examined. Nurses need to be sensitive to adolescents' concerns and reassure them that they are normal, if in fact they are. Some adolescents also believe that they are invincible and that nothing can hurt them or cause death. This belief can cause them to take risks and to be non-adherent to treatment, because they may not see the consequences of their behavior. (Pain management is discussed in Chapter 39.)

Loss of Control

Control is important to the adolescent. Some challenges in caring for an ill adolescent stem from control issues, and understanding this issue is key when caring for adolescents. Giv-

ing the adolescent some control avoids endless power struggles. Behaviors exhibited in response to loss of control may include anger, withdrawal, and general uncooperativeness.

Control issues can cause a major conflict between adolescents and parents. Parents often feel like Ping-Pong balls as they are bounced back and forth by a child who wants help one minute and rejects it the next. Parents who do not understand growth and development can become frustrated and angry over such behavior. Educating the parents increases understanding and facilitates parent-child communication (Riesch et al., 2000).

Adolescents may also feel that they are losing control of their social lives as they sit on the sidelines of activities. Time to plan for the separation (e.g., scheduled surgery) allows a greater sense of control than an unplanned hospitalization (e.g., trauma).

Fear of the Unknown

The sights and sounds of the hospital can be frightening and confusing to the child. The child may have many questions: Why are the nurses wearing masks? Why does that alarm keep ringing? Am I dying? Why are they putting tubes in me?

The child's routines and rituals may have been disrupted, and the child may wonder what will happen next. Understanding these fears can assist the nurse in structuring care and teaching in a way that avoids unnecessary anxiety.

Regression

Children may regress in toileting or may cry for a bottle even though they have been weaned for several months. They may want more attention at bedtime or have temper tantrums. The

> **!** **CRITICAL** **TO REMEMBER**
>
> **Maintaining a Safe Place**
>
> A designated safe area can enhance the child's security. For example, intrusive procedures may cause discomfort or anxiety and might better be done in the treatment room rather than the child's room. The playroom should also be a place for playing, not treatments and administering medications. Nurses should consider the child's age, developmental level, coping skills, and parent/child preference when deciding where to perform procedures that may be painful or distressing.

Adapted from Fanurick, D., Schmitz, M., Martin, G., Koh, J., Wood, M., Sturgeon, L., & Long, N. (2000). Hospital room or treatment room: Where should inpatient pediatric procedures be performed? *Children's Health Care, 29*(2), 103-111.

older child may react to separation by clinging or crying or may have fears about shadows on the walls or noises in the halls.

Parents may be overly concerned about regression. They should be told that the child might continue the behavior at home. The child may need more emotional support while the parent slowly returns the child to normal routines. If the child has regressed in toileting, the parent should wait until the child has returned to a daily routine and then begin the toilet training again. Behavior that is appropriate for the child's age should be reinforced.

The nurse might explain, "I know that you are concerned because David has been soiling his pants since he has been in the hospital. This soiling is a normal reaction to the stress of being ill and in the hospital. When he returns home and things return to normal for him, he will resume his previous schedule."

FACTORS AFFECTING A CHILD'S RESPONSE TO ILLNESS AND HOSPITALIZATION

Each child responds to illness or hospitalization differently. The expression "perception is everything" certainly applies to the ill child. How children perceive the incident will affect their response before, during, and after the illness or hospitalization. How a child reacts is often related to the parents' response to the illness and the child's age, level of cognitive development, preparation, previous experiences, and coping skills.

If the child has had a previous illness or hospitalization, how that event unfolded and the child's response to it greatly affect the child's view of future occurrences. Children with chronic diseases who experience multiple hospitalizations have a different perception of illness from those who have an occasional cold (see Chapter 36). A visit to a pediatrician's office will show the wide range of responses children have. Some older children have more negative responses as they begin to associate certain people, colors, and surroundings with what was for them an unpleasant experience.

Age and Cognitive Development

Children's developmental level affects their reactions to illness. These differences should be considered when planning nursing care. Preparing a toddler for hospitalization or a procedure differs from preparing a school-age child. The content, the time frame, the setting, and the method of preparation are all based on the child's growth and development. Pediatric nurses must have a clear understanding of the cognitive abilities of each age-group (Box 35-2).

Parental Response to Illness or Hospitalization

Children have sharp observation skills and know when their parents are anxious and upset. This anxiety is transferred to the child, and the child's anxiety then increases. If the parents talk outside their child's room or within hearing range but in whispers, the child begins to imagine what the parents are saying. All children, but especially preschoolers, who have such active imaginations, can invent elaborate stories to explain what is happening.

The parent who does not answer the child's questions or who does not tell the truth for fear it will frighten the child only confuses the child and weakens the child's trust in the parent. The child wants to believe that someone is in control and that that person can be trusted. Some parents cannot be honest with their children because of their own fears and insecurities. The nurse needs to assess all these issues.

Preparing the Child and Family

Stress has been defined as a nonspecific response of the body to any demand made on it. Perceived stressors, the conditioning factors brought to the situation, and the coping mechanisms used to adapt, all affect each person's adaptation to a stress-producing situation (Selye, 1974). Preparing for an event (in this case, hospitalization) can decrease stress in several ways. During preparation, the child's and the parent's perceptions of the event can be explored. In addition, previous experiences that might affect the impending hospitalization and the use of previous coping strategies can be identified and discussed.

The depth and method of preparation vary among children and are based on an understanding of the child's individual needs. Variables that the nurse should consider include the child's age and developmental level, involvement of the family, timing, child's physiologic status and psychologic status, setting, sociocultural factors, and child's experiences with illness and hospitalization.

Preparation sessions should be planned. Teaching is more effective if the nurse and family develop trust. Honesty and language appropriate for the child's age are imperative. When possible, all the child's senses should be involved. The child should be allowed to see the intensive care area before being admitted, to take the blood pressure of a stuffed animal, or to handle the mask that will be used in surgery. The nurse should avoid using medical terms that children and their parents may not understand. Literal interpretation of some words may be confusing and scary to some children, especially preschoolers (see Chapter 6). Some children assume that certain procedures include pain. Explanation and the opportunity to handle equipment, when possible, can help children master the fear of hospitalization and treatment.

Coping Skills of the Child and Family

Coping is the process of contending with difficulties in an effort to overcome or work through them. How the child copes with illness or hospitalization is related to age, perception of the event, previous hospitalizations and encounters with the

BOX 35-2
Developmental Approaches to the Hospitalized Child

Neonate
- Anticipate needs, and fulfill them in a timely manner.
- Provide opportunities for nonnutritive (comfort) sucking and oral stimulation, using a pacifier.
- Provide swaddling, with the infant's hands drawn to the midline and close to the face. Use soft talking to soothe.
- If the infant is very ill, provide a quiet, soothing environment. Pay close attention to light and sound stimulation.
- When stimulation is appropriate, provide stimulation for each sense (e.g., mobiles, music, smell, soft stuffed animals). Use contrasting colors and textures.
- Watch for cues of overstimulation, such as eye avoidance, extension of arms, splaying of fingers, and "zoning-out" behavior.
- Before painful procedures, provide comforting touch and nonnutritive sucking. Follow painful procedures with tucking, holding, and cuddling.
- Model and share appropriate behaviors with family members regarding stimulation, touch, verbalization, and feeding.
- Provide consistent caregivers when parents are not available.
- Collaborate with parents on ways to provide them care.
- Involve the parents in the care of their infant as much as possible.
- Encourage parents to room-in if possible.

Infant
- For the younger infant, provide the same care given for neonate.
- The older infant will begin to anticipate painful procedures and fight. Use sheets and blankets to provide swaddling if necessary. Allow nonnutritive sucking for comfort.
- Expect regressive behavior, and inform parents to expect it and why.
- Limit the number of caregivers to whom the infant must adjust.
- Request that parents bring the infant's security object (e.g., blanket, stuffed animal).
- Encourage parents to be present during procedures.

Toddler
- Expect regression, and inform parents about behaviors.
- Follow home routines and rituals.
- Involve parents in the care of the toddler.
- Provide for rooming-in if possible.
- Allow opportunities for mobility when it can be done safely.
- Employ all possible methods of pain control when the child must have a painful procedure.
- Anticipate temper tantrums when the child's frustration level is high.
- Maintain a safe environment for the toddler's physical acting out and temper tantrums.
- Encourage the child to be independent (e.g., feed self, use potty chair, put on socks).
- Provide support when the toddler needs to be dependent (e.g., hold after a procedure, comfort if parents leave).
- Approach with a positive attitude ("I am going to give you your medicine.").

Preschooler
- Provide safe ways to act out aggression (e.g., with punching bags, painting, clay).
- Take time for communication. Answer questions with simple, concrete explanations. Explain all procedures honestly. Allow

for choices whenever possible.
- Expect egocentric behavior.
- Provide for a safe and secure environment (e.g., with a night light, view of others, objects from home).
- Be consistent.
- Ask the parents how the child usually copes in new situations.
- Tell the child that he or she did not cause the illness.
- Involve parents in care, and follow home routines.
- Place the child with other children of the same age if possible.
- Provide for play activities in the playroom and in the room.
- Accept regression if it occurs, and explain it to parents.
- Encourage the child to be independent (e.g., feeding, dressing, toileting).

School-Age Child
- Inform the child of limits, and enforce them (e.g., no water fights, wheelchair races, leaving the unit).
- Involve the child in planning and implementing care (e.g., allow child to choose from menu and assist with some procedures).
- Explain all procedures, and allow the child time for questions and answers. Use medical and scientific terminology and diagrams, body outlines, or anatomically correct dolls to explain the procedure.
- Accept regression, but encourage independence.
- Provide privacy.
- Encourage the child to assist in keeping the room and belongings in order.
- Assist the child in contacting friends. Encourage parents to contact the teacher and have school friends send cards and letters.
- If the child's condition supports visits and calls from friends, encourage this contact.
- Provide for the child's educational needs by encouraging parents to bring in work and by scheduling study times. If the child will have a prolonged period of hospital or home care, arrange for a teacher to work with the child. Some hospitals have a hospital-based teacher.

Adolescent
- Provide privacy for care and visiting.
- Encourage the adolescent to wear street clothes and perform normal grooming.
- Encourage questions about appearance and the effects of illness on the adolescent's future.
- Use scientific and medical terminology to prepare the adolescent for procedures.
- Use body outlines and diagrams, and give the rationale for the procedure.
- When possible, provide for a special activity area that is limited to adolescent use. Introduce the child to other adolescents on the unit.
- Encourage peers to call and visit if the adolescent's condition can tolerate this action.
- Assist parents in communicating, supporting, and guiding their adolescents by providing them with information about growth and development.
- Allow favorite foods to be brought in if the adolescent does not need a special diet.
- Approach the adolescent with caring, understanding, and acceptance.
- Provide for educational needs, as for a school-age child.

health care profession, support from significant others, and the child's and parent's coping skills.

Depending on age, children use words, behaviors, and physical actions to help them through stressful situations. The child may also cope by ignoring or negating the event. The younger child is more likely to use emotional expression, whereas the older child and adolescent are more likely to withdraw or practice more self-control behaviors. For example, whereas the younger child might scream and kick during a procedure, the older child might remain stoic and say that it did not hurt, even though it did. Some children try to appear brave and meet self-imposed or parental expectations.

Breathing (e.g., blowing bubbles, pinwheels, party blowers) or singing helps with relaxation and offers a focus for the child. Teaching coping mechanisms and practicing them before a procedure can help a child feel more in control as well as successful. Distraction (e.g., water wheels, games, books) and imagery (e.g., tapes, scenarios) for older children are effective tools for coping. Parents, nurses, and child life specialists may all serve as facilitators for these techniques.

Psychologic Benefits of Hospitalization

Some think that hospitalization causes only negative psychologic effects. The stress of illness and hospitalization can actually be growth-enhancing by promoting a child's coping skills and bolstering self-esteem. Children can increase their self-confidence as they overcome the anxiety related to hospitalization and perhaps master some self-care skills. They feel good about their recovery or increased ability to cope with any disability they have. In addition, hospitalization offers an opportunity for children to ask questions and obtain new information. Some even become interested in a career in health care while observing professionals caring for them. Hospitalization can also be an opportunity to teach parents about children's growth and development, improve parenting skills, and assess the child's immunization record.

PLAYROOMS IN HEALTH CARE SETTINGS

Hospitals and clinics often provide playrooms where children may go to play with toys, participate in age-appropriate arts and crafts, and socialize with other children. Children should always see this area as a safe place where procedures and treatments do not take place. Children, when their condition is stable, may be taken to the playroom in their beds and wheelchairs (Fig. 35-5). A separate activity area should be provided, when possible, for adolescents to listen to music, play video games, and visit with their peers.

Therapeutic Play

When a child is hospitalized, one component of the child's plan of care is the use of *therapeutic play*. Therapeutic play differs from normal play in its design and intent. Members of the health team guide it, and activities are planned to meet the physical and psychologic needs of the child. Therapeutic play can provide an emotional outlet, instruct, and improve physiologic abilities (American Academy of Pediatrics, 2000). Supervised play with medical equipment helps reduce fear and separate reality from fantasy.

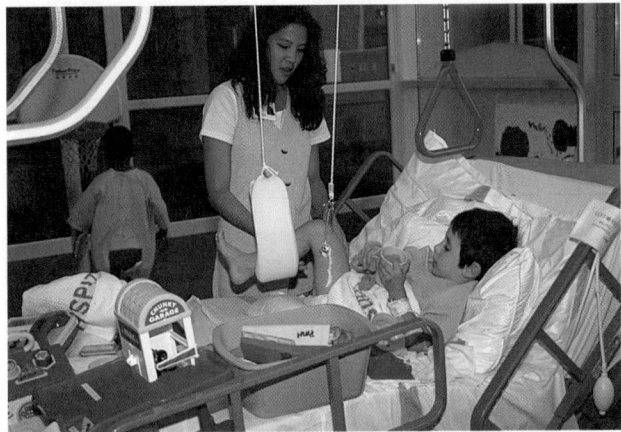

Figure 35-5 Being in traction is no reason not to enjoy the hospital's play facilities. To give him a change of surroundings and allow him to interact with her and with other children, the play therapist wheels this child in his bed to the playroom. Because his mobility will be limited for a significant period, providing diversion is especially important. (Courtesy Parkland Health and Hospital System, Dallas, TX.)

Child life specialists or play therapists are available in many hospitals and share their expertise in child growth and development and the use of play. Child life programs have as their goals maintaining normal living patterns, minimizing psychologic trauma, and promoting optimal development of the child and family. Nurses should also be involved in this type of activity, either in conjunction with the child life specialist or individually when a child life specialist is not available. Interpretations of the child's play behavior and some types of play therapy require guidance by a skilled health care worker.

Emotional Outlet Play

Emotional outlet play is often called *dramatic play*. During this type of play, the child acts out or dramatizes real-life stressors. These might include emotional stressors, such as abuse or neglect, or a painful physical stressor, such as a bone marrow aspiration. The hospitalized child who is separated from family and friends might use a wooden hammer and pegs to express anger over the separation. A child who has been sexually abused might not be able to communicate verbally the experience but may be able to use an anatomically correct doll to show what happened.

Many commercially crafted toys are available for dramatic play. Anatomically correct dolls and puppets are available. Some dolls have removable parts that enable the child to see the various organs of the body.

Children can express their inner beliefs and perceptions through drawing. A child may draw a very big bed with a tiny child on it surrounded by large, hovering adults or a huge syringe with a long needle. Children often express their thoughts and feelings through the use of paper and crayons or color markers (Fig. 35-6) (Ryan-Wenger, 2001).

Injection play is an appropriate intervention with the child who has to undergo frequent blood work, injections, IV therapy, or any other therapy involving syringes and needles. If a needle is used for this type of activity, safety is of the utmost

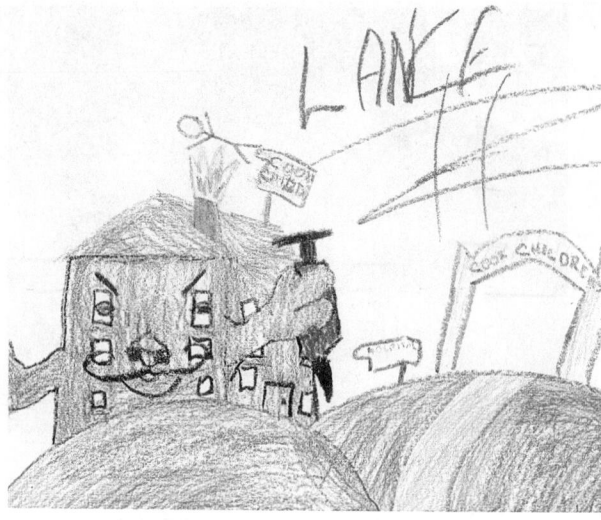

Art materials allow children to express their thoughts and feelings about ▶ health care problems.

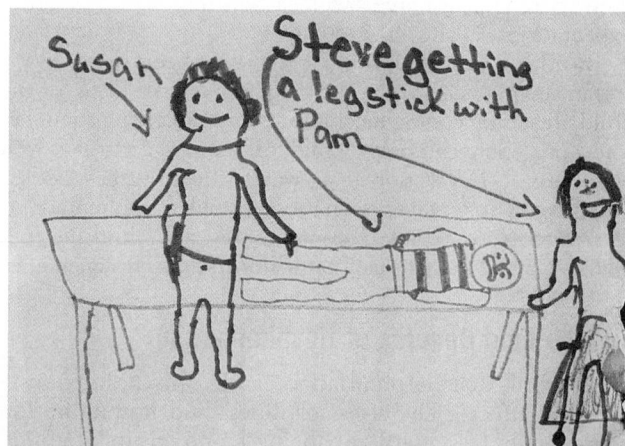

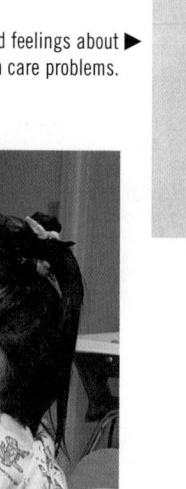

◀ Giving a doll an injection can help a child work through anxiety and anger about injections she may be receiving.

Figure 35-6 Therapeutic play can be used to teach children about medical procedures or help them work through their feelings about what has happened to them in the health care setting. Child life specialists or play therapists are often members of the team in children's hospitals to provide expert guidance for therapeutic play.

importance and the nurse should assess the child's growth and development level before using this type of directed play. An adult is always present if a needle is used. The child can give a doll an injection and can thereby work through anger and anxiety. Wooden hammers and pegboards, Nerf balls, and boxing gloves are all avenues for release of stress or anger.

Teaching Through Play

Play can also be used to teach. It can be used in preoperative teaching and teaching before a new, painful, or extensive procedure (see Fig. 35-6). The nurse assesses the child's cognitive level before this type of teaching, and the play should be appropriate to the child's level.

Hospital equipment is often used in this type of play. The nurse might demonstrate taking a blood pressure on the child's stuffed animal before putting the cuff on the child. A

breathing treatment might be "given" to the child's doll before the child is given the treatment. The nurse might use drawings and diagrams to explain procedures or surgery.

Some hospitals have preoperative visits during which children come to meet the people who will be taking care of them and see the physical surroundings. They may see the scrub gowns and masks worn by the surgical staff and visit a typical room. Children and parents can ask questions and meet other children and parents who are going through the same experience as they tour the area.

Enhancing Cooperation Through Play

Children with illnesses that require unpleasant or painful therapies often are uncooperative. Developing a plan that will stimulate and engage the child in the activity is a challenge. The nurse should include age-appropriate growth and development activities when planning care. The school-age child who loves competition and games is more likely to increase range of motion of an arm if points can be made each time the Nerf ball is thrown through the hoop.

Allowing the child to blow bubbles, a whistle, or a pinwheel or to simulate blowing out the nurse's penlight can enhance deep-breathing exercises. Range of motion can be accomplished by throwing Nerf balls, beanbags, and paper balls. The child who needs to increase intake can sometimes be motivated to drink more fluids if a graph shows the amount taken in and the child receives a reward when a selected goal is reached. Including the child in planning and identifying rewards and goals enhances motivation. Colorful stickers, baseball cards, small toys, and special pencils can be used as awards.

Unstructured Play

In addition to therapeutic play, the nurse encourages unstructured play in the hospital setting. Through unstructured play, children can control events, ideas, and relationships.

Hospitals without a special room set aside for play should be encouraged to provide developmentally appropriate toys, games, and books. These items can be kept in a special box accessible to the nursing staff.

Evaluation of Play

Therapeutic play should be reflected in the child's nursing care plan. During the evaluation step of the nursing process, the nurse looks at the outcome criteria to determine whether the goals have been met. The nurse is asking whether play enhanced the care of the child. Is the child coughing and deep breathing every 2 hours? Is the child relating feelings of fear over the separation from parents? Is the child eating or sleeping? If the client goals have been achieved, the interventions have been appropriate and effective.

ADMITTING THE CHILD TO A HOSPITAL SETTING

Taking the History

The admission procedure sets the tone for the hospitalization. It should not be a series of questions but rather a time of collaboration between the nurse and the family. The time the family has spent in the emergency department, the seriousness of the illness, and other family needs (e.g., other children with parents or left with neighbors) may affect the interview process.

The nurse can acknowledge the parent's concerns. For example, the nurse might say, "Mrs. Smith, I know you're concerned about your other children. Would you like to call your neighbor before I ask you some questions about Heidi and her illness?"

Most hospitals provide an admission interview form. Some of the information is essential for providing immediate care, and some can be collected later. By recognizing the family's needs, the nurse can structure each admission to fit that child and family. If the parent has entered the system through the emergency department, some of the questions may have previously been answered. By looking at the forms from other departments, repetition can be avoided, but data about aller-

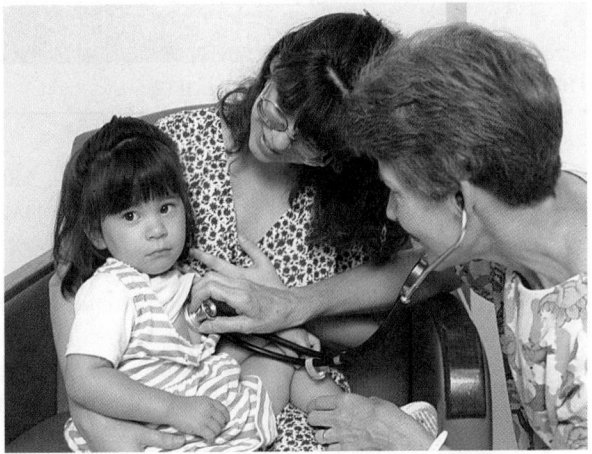

Figure 35-7 To reduce the stress of unfamiliar surroundings and people, the nurse assesses this child while the girl remains in the security of her mother's arms. (Courtesy T.C. Thompson Children's Hospital, Chattanooga, TN.)

gies, medications taken at home, the history of the illness, and other relevant details must be repeated.

Although hospitals have policies and procedures for admission, the routine may need to be altered because of the child's condition. For example, a severely dehydrated child should have an IV infusion started and a child in pain should be medicated before any other interventions are performed. On the other hand, the primary needs of the child and family may be emotional. A parent who has just been told that her child may have a terminal disease may have difficulty remembering the dates of the child's immunizations. In this situation, the nurse should provide the parent with support and assistance in mobilizing coping mechanisms and support systems rather than focusing on data gathering.

After the child and family are made comfortable (Fig. 35-7), the nurse obtains a thorough physical, health, and psychosocial history. This is followed by a detailed physical examination. For all types of admissions, the history is recorded on an admission data sheet. The format of the admission data sheet varies from hospital to hospital, but most admission forms ask for much of the same information: history; allergies; nutritional, sleep, elimination, and psychosocial information.

Physical Examination

Initial Inspection

The initial inspection determines the need for any immediate or emergency care that must be provided before other information can be obtained.

Baseline Data

The physical examination should be thorough, and special attention should be given to the body system involved in the child's admission. Many admission forms have an outline of the child's body on which the nurse should indicate any bruises, scratches, or other skin markings that provide specific objective data. (The process of interviewing, taking a history, and physical assessment is explained in Chapter 33.)

Data collected at admission are used to formulate nursing diagnoses and the child's plan of care and should be placed in the body of the child's chart—not at the back of the chart, where this information can be forgotten.

Nursing Care Plan

The Child in a Hospital Setting

FOCUSED ASSESSMENT

Assess the child for any problems related to the hospital admission by identifying pertinent historical data on the admission data sheet and analyzing the results of the physical examination. Important assessment areas that can cause problems for hospitalized children include:

- *Nutrition:* Assess the child's caloric intake, and compare it with the requirements for age and weight. Note any abnormalities after plotting and recording height and weight percentiles. Determine the child's favorite foods and customary rituals around mealtimes, in addition to cultural or religious dietary practices that may restrict a child's food choices.
- *Elimination:* Assess any regression the child may be experiencing in bowel or bladder control. Inquire about specific terms the child uses for elimination, and use these terms to provide comfort and assistance to the child. Although regression can be a normal response to the stress of hospitalization, it is distressing to the child and parent.
- *Sleep:* Understanding and communicating the child's usual sleep patterns and routines to others assist with planning care. Determine usual bedtime, hygiene practices used before sleep, and bedtime rituals (e.g., rocking, prayers, stories, snacks). Note any alterations in the number of hours the child is sleeping, and compare with the norm for the child's age.
- *Self-Care:* Assess and note the child's usual self-care activities (e.g., eating, bathing, dressing, brushing teeth). Alterations may indicate increasing anxiety or loss of control.
- *Emotional/Social Status:* Assess for signs of anxiety or fear related to the hospital setting (e.g., crying, temper tantrums, withdrawal, decreased communication). Assess the child's ability to keep in touch with peers. Note whether the child readily participates in unit activities.

Nursing Diagnosis

Imbalanced Nutrition: Less Than Body Requirements related to unfamiliar foods, separation from caregiver, strange environment, or disease process.

Expected Outcomes

The child will:
- Eat the appropriate number of calories and variety of nutrients according to age.
- Maintain prehospital weight.

INTERVENTION	RATIONALE
1. Identify the cause of the child's decreased intake.	1. Identifying the cause of any decreased appetite can assist in the elimination of the problem.
2. Encourage parents to bring foods from home and to be with the child during meals.	2. The parents' presence simulates the home environment and increases the likelihood that the child will eat.
3. Allow the child to select food from the menu. Communicate to other staff the types of foods the child particularly likes.	3. Allowing the child to select food gives the child control and provides an opportunity to select foods that the child likes and will eat.
4. Offer frequent, nutritious snacks, and encourage parents to do the same.	4. Children may eat junk food and then refuse nutritious foods offered at mealtimes.
5. Offer small portions. Use small dishes, cups, and glasses.	5. Children may be overwhelmed by large portions and refuse to eat any of the food. Child-size tableware, especially if appropriately decorated, is more appealing to children.
6. If parents cannot be available during meals, allow the child to eat with other children.	6. Older children may distract the child and decrease separation anxiety.
7. Request a dietary consultation.	7. Registered dietitians can assist in planning age-appropriate nutritious meals.

Evaluation

- Is the child's nutritional intake appropriate for age?
- Did the child maintain baseline body weight during hospitalization?

Nursing Care Plan

The Child in a Hospital Setting—cont'd

Nursing Diagnosis

Delayed Growth and Development, regression in toilet training or self-care skills, related to separation and hospitalization.

Expected Outcomes

The child will:
- Maintain usual self-care activities of feeding, toileting, dressing, and bathing. Any regression reverses quickly after discharge.

INTERVENTION	RATIONALE
1. Follow home routines of elimination.	1. Cooperation will increase and anxiety will decrease if the child's normal routine and rituals are maintained.
2. Do not scold the incontinent child.	2. If the incontinence is caused by anxiety, scolding will only increase the anxiety.
3. Explain to parents that some regression in all self-care activities is normal in hospitalized children and that most children resume their normal routines soon after discharge.	3. Parents may be concerned about the child's regression and may increase the child's anxiety by focusing on the child's incontinence.
4. Discourage parents from beginning toilet training during hospitalization.	4. Toilet training can be an additional stressor at a difficult time.
5. Encourage the child to participate in self-care according to developmental abilities.	5. Self-care increases the child's self-esteem and feeling of control.
6. Assist the child when the ability to perform self-care is limited because of fatigue, discomfort, or other factors related to the disease process.	6. The disease process may limit the child's ability, physically or mentally, to perform self-care.
7. Provide the necessary equipment for self-care, and place it within easy reach.	7. Accessible equipment decreases the complexity of providing self-care by making the environment easier to manipulate.
8. Offer choices and allow the child to make decisions when appropriate.	8. Choice increases the child's sense of control.

Evaluation
- Is the child able to feed, toilet, dress, and bathe at the same level as before the illness?
- Does the child readily participate in self-care activities?

Nursing Diagnosis

Disturbed Sleep Pattern related to unfamiliar environment, anxiety, or discomfort.

Expected Outcome

The child will:
- Sleep the appropriate number of hours for age.

INTERVENTION	RATIONALE
1. Plan care to allow time for periods of sleep. Care can be organized so that vital signs can be measured and other procedures performed when medication is given.	1. Planning allows for uninterrupted sleep. Children who are awakened a short time after they have fallen asleep often have difficulty going back to sleep.
2. Post a sign on the door when the child is asleep to prevent other staff and visitors from waking the child. Unplug the phone, turn off the television, close the door unless the child must be observed, and pull the blinds.	2. Environmental distractions can be major sleep interruptions.
3. If the parents are not with the child, explain that you will be nearby and will check during the night. Provide a night light.	3. Feelings of security are increased if the child understands that someone is watching.

Continued

Nursing Care Plan

The Child in a Hospital Setting—cont'd

Evaluation

■ Does the child take naps and sleep an appropriate amount of time based on age requirements?

Nursing Diagnosis

Anxiety related to fear of the unknown and separation from significant others and familiar surroundings.

Expected Outcomes

The child will:

■ Display decreased indicators of distress (e.g., crying, withdrawal, irritability).
■ Verbalize feelings of anxiety.
■ Play appropriately and maintain contact with peers.

INTERVENTION	RATIONALE
1. Orient the child and parent to the hospital and the routines of the unit.	1. Familiarity with the environment and its expectations will decrease anxiety related to fear of the unknown.
2. Prepare the child and parent for all procedures in an age-appropriate way.	2. Preparation for an event decreases anxiety and fear.
3. Encourage parents to stay with the child when possible and to be involved in the child's care.	3. The presence of parents supports the parental role and decreases the child's separation anxiety.
4. Hold, rock, and cuddle the infant or young child.	4. Holding and cuddling children increase feelings of security and trust.
5. If the parents cannot stay with the child, provide for a consistent caregiver.	5. Continuity of care provides the child with a consistent person with whom the child can develop a trusting relationship.
6. Follow home routines and rituals when possible.	6. Familiar routines help the child predict events and reduce anxiety caused by the unfamiliar setting.
7. Encourage the parents to be honest with the child when they leave and to inform the nurse where they can be reached and when they will return. Encourage the parents to call while they are away. Older children can talk on the phone with their parents.	7. Trust is increased when parents and caregivers are honest with the child. If parents just disappear, the child will feel anger, abandonment, and acute anxiety. By keeping open lines of communication, the parent's anxiety is decreased.

THE ILL CHILD'S FAMILY

Through family-centered care, the nurse considers and treats the child in the context of the family and recognizes the family as the primary and continuing provider of care for the child. Although the nurse sometimes must plan care without involving the family, it is difficult to do so.

Parents

A child's illness may cause a situational crisis for the family. If the illness leads to hospitalization, either planned or unplanned, the family's anxiety increases. Ill children become the parents' central focus. Four dimensions of support that nurses can provide for parents have been identified (Miles, Carlson, & Brunssen, 1999):

• Supportive communication and provision of information related to the child's illness, treatments, care, and related issues
• Parental support focused on respecting, enhancing, and supporting the parental role

• Emotional support to help the parents cope with their own emotional responses and needs related to the child's illness
• Caregiving support involving the quality of care provided to the child (Fig. 35-8)

Parents may wonder why their family is facing the crisis of a childhood illness or may believe that if they had sought treatment earlier, the child would not be so ill. A parent may have delayed taking a child with a low-grade fever and vague symptoms to a physician. If the symptoms were a sign of serious illness, the parent may feel guilty for not having sought care earlier.

Parents have varied responses to a child's illness. They may initially deny that their child is ill, especially if the illness is serious. The period of denial may be followed by anger. The anger may be directed at the nurse, at another family member, or sometimes at God. When the immediate crisis is over, a period of depression may occur. At this point, the parents are usually exhausted, both physically and psychologically. Often, they have been spending long hours at the hospital while working and trying to care for the other children in the family.

Nursing Care Plan

The Child in a Hospital Setting—cont'd

8. Encourage parents to bring transitional objects (e.g., blanket, teddy bear) and to provide reminders of themselves (e.g., pictures, scarf, handkerchief) if they cannot be with the child.
9. Take the child to the playroom and introduce to other children when appropriate, or plan play activities (reading, board games, drawing) for a child unable to leave the room.
10. For the older child, arrange for peer contact through visits, phone calls, and letters.

11. Offer choices and allow the child to make decisions when appropriate.
12. Encourage the older child to wear street clothes and to decorate the room.

13. Provide opportunities for the older child to express feelings about the illness and hospitalization; communicate with a child life specialist about the child's identified needs (e.g., anxiety, anger, boredom, lack of information).
14. Provide information to the parents about diagnosis, treatment, and prognosis. Attend to their needs for sleep and nutrition.

8. Transitional objects give the child a feeling of security. Both transitional objects and reminders of the parents comfort the child and help decrease the anxiety related to separation.
9. Other children provide a form of distraction and assist the child in adapting to the environment.

10. The older child may fear being forgotten by peers. By maintaining contact and sharing information with peers, the child maintains a sense of importance and security.
11. Choice increases the child's sense of control.

12. Normal attire gives the child an opportunity for self-expression and makes the child feel more comfortable in the environment.
13. Fear and anxiety may decrease if the child has an opportunity to communicate feelings, have them validated, and participate in problem-solving techniques.

14. The child is affected by parents' anxiety. Helping the parents cope will help decrease their anxiety, which will in turn decrease the child's anxiety.

Evaluation

- Is the child playing and communicating with other children and staff and showing decreased signs of distress?
- Is the child able to express feelings of anxiety either verbally or through play?

The nurse needs to be aware of parents' feelings and to listen closely to what is said. The nurse can then assist the parents in working through their feelings.

The parental role often changes when the child is admitted to the hospital. The parent who had been in control before the admission is now in an unfamiliar environment. Parents may be confused as to what they can and cannot do. Can they bathe their child? Can they even hold their child, or will they disturb the tubes? When the parent is not given permission to perform some of the care, both the child and the parent suffer.

The needs of fathers are sometimes forgotten. The father may come to the hospital only after he has spent a day at work and then, after a short visit, may need to go home to be with other children. He may not be there when the primary care physician makes rounds and therefore receives most of his medical information from someone else. The father may think that he needs to be the strong one in the family and not show his fear and anxiety. In some families, the mother works outside the home while the father stays with the child. In either case, an awareness of each parent's role will assist the nurse in identifying the individual needs of the parents.

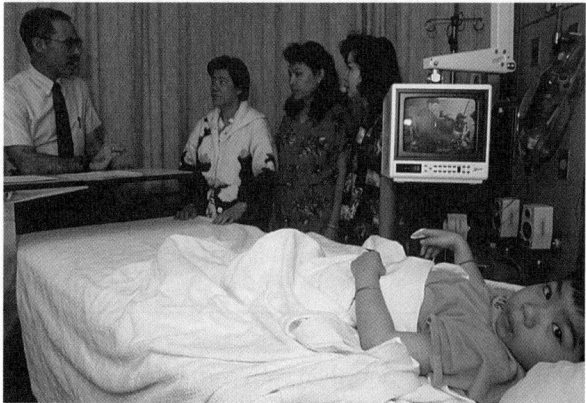

Figure 35-8 The family of a hospitalized child may not speak the prevailing language. Interpreters on call at many hospitals help such parents communicate with hospital personnel and provide a familiar link to the parents' and child's culture and language. (Courtesy Cook Children's Medical Center, Fort Worth, TX.)

Because of dual roles, long separations, increased stress, and numerous other factors, the parents' marriage may be strained. This situation is especially likely in marriages that

CRITICAL THINKING EXERCISE 35-1

Tommy, 4 years old, was admitted to the hospital with pneumonia. Tommy has cystic fibrosis. His family has recently moved to the area, and this is his first admission to your hospital. Tommy loves to play with his dinosaur collection and spends much of his day playing and watching his favorite videos. His mother visits for short periods during the lunch hour, and his father visits in the evening. Tommy cries when his parents leave. You mention to a colleague that you think Tommy's parents should spend more time with him. She responds, "We don't know what their other responsibilities are."
1. What other responsibilities might the family have?
2. What are some of the nursing interventions that would support a family with a child in the hospital?

PARENTS
Want to Know

Information for Discharge

After assessing the family's knowledge, provide the information families need to know to help the child's transition from hospital to home:

- Information about the illness or trauma and expected outcomes. Tell the parents when they should consult the primary care physician or nurse.
- Medications or treatments to be given at home and information about times, route, side effects, and any special care to be taken when giving the medication. Providing written information is valuable.
- Information about any special nutritional needs.
- Specific activities the child may, may not, and sometimes should participate in.
- The date when the child may return to school.
- The date to bring the child back to the hospital, clinic, or office for follow-up care.
- Information about any referral agency needed for the child or family.
- The unit phone number and primary nurse's name.

Explain, demonstrate, and request a return demonstration of any treatments or procedures that will be done at home. This teaching should be an ongoing process and not left until the time of discharge, because learning takes place at different rates.

BOX 35-3
Caring for the Siblings of an Ill or Hospitalized Child

Factors That Add to the Stress of Siblings
- Age younger than 10 years
- Emotional closeness to the hospitalized child
- Receiving only a limited explanation of the experience
- Fear of getting the illness themselves
- Being cared for outside their own home
- Perceiving that their parents are acting differently toward them
- Having a sibling who is progressively ill

Nursing Care Guidelines for Meeting the Needs of Siblings
- Encourage caregivers to have the ill child retell what happened. This experience may be uncomfortable for the adult, but it helps the sibling put the illness or accident in perspective.
- If the sibling has feelings of guilt, address the child's concerns directly. If the feelings of guilt continue, suggest a consultation with a counselor.
- Give parents educational materials, and show them how to use them with the sibling.
- Schedule a time for the sibling to visit. Prepare the sibling for the medical equipment and any changes in the ill child's appearance that may cause concern.
- If the sibling cannot visit, send photographs.
- Encourage the sibling to talk with the child on the telephone.

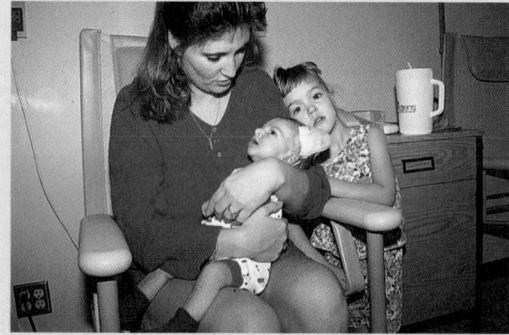

Her brother's repeated hospitalizations for problems associated with a diaphragmatic hernia have been difficult for this girl. Siblings of ill children may experience jealousy, insecurity, resentment, confusion, and anxiety. The nurse can help this child cope by paying attention to her when she is providing care to the infant. (Courtesy Children's Medical Center, Dallas, TX.)

Modified from Craft, M., Wyatt, N., & Sandell, B. (1985). Behavior and feeling changes in siblings of hospitalized children. *Clinical Pediatrics, 24*(7), 374-378.

are already at risk. Even when both partners are at the hospital, they may not have any time alone.

Many children have stepmothers and stepfathers. In such cases, both sets of parents need recognition, support, and education. How the family copes with the child's illness depends on its coping strategies. A family who is already in crisis or one without support systems (e.g., family, friends, church) will have more difficulty adjusting to the change than a family who is organized and adjusted. A family who deals successfully with the crisis is strengthened by the experience. (For further discussion of the effects of illness on the family, see Chapter 3. For a discussion of the family with a child with a chronic illness, see Chapter 36.)

Siblings

The illness or hospitalization of a brother or sister can be difficult for children. The ill child's siblings may experience jealousy, insecurity, resentment, confusion, and anxiety. Chil-

Nursing Care Plan

The Family With a Hospitalized Child

FOCUSED ASSESSMENT

Assess factors that affect a family's adjustment to illness and hospitalization; compare assessment with concerns expressed on the child's admission history. Was the admission an emergency? Were there previous admissions, and how did the parents perceive those hospitalizations? How serious is the illness or trauma? Are some factors unknown, such as the cause of the disease or the child's prognosis? Special attention should also be given to any information obtained in the admission interview.

Try to determine whether the parents and siblings are experiencing stress and how they are coping with hospitalization. Open-ended statements, such as "This must be difficult for you" may encourage communication in this crisis. Identify the parents' needs for sleep, nutrition, and information.

Nursing Diagnosis

Interrupted Family Processes related to the child's hospitalization and illness.

Expected Outcomes

The parents will:
- Participate in the child's care.
- Meet the needs of other family members.
- Use appropriate support systems.
- Identify ways to cope.
- Assist the child to move from a sick role to a well role.

INTERVENTION	RATIONALE
1. Orient the parents to the hospital, and provide information related to their physical needs (e.g., food, sleep, bathing).	1. The parents' physical needs must be met for them to meet the child's needs and their own emotional needs. Meeting their needs indicates support by the caregiver.
2. Encourage family members (parents, siblings) to express their feelings and to ask questions about the child's illness.	2. Expression decreases anxiety and clarifies misconceptions.
3. Provide the family with information about the child's condition, treatment, and support systems. Begin to prepare them for the child's discharge (see Parents Want to Know box).	3. Information gives parents a sense of control and decreases their anxiety.
4. Identify with the family the ways in which they are coping; support their parenting skills.	4. Individuals are not always aware of their coping mechanisms, and the nurse should help the family evaluate the effectiveness of theirs.
5. Refer the family to other professionals (e.g., social worker, clinical psychologist, clinical specialist, psychiatrist, clergy) when their problems are not within the scope of nursing.	5. Early identification of family problems can decrease the possibility of escalation of the problems. Collaboration with other health professionals can bring a holistic approach to the care of child and family.

Evaluation

- Are the parents able to participate in their child's care while meeting the needs of other family members?
- Do family members support each other and seek other resources when necessary?
- Are family members able to describe and use positive coping skills?
- Are the parents able to assist the child to move from a sick to a well role?

dren often have difficulty understanding why their ill sibling is getting all the attention and why their parents seem so preoccupied and have so little time for them. They may worry that if their sibling could get sick, so could they. Preschool children, who engage in magical thinking, may worry that they somehow caused the illness. All these thoughts and feelings are compounded by children's difficulty expressing their feelings (Box 35-3). Although some are at greater risk than others, many children hold everything inside. The amount of stress the sibling experiences varies according to the well child's age and developmental level, closeness of the sibling relationship, who is caring for the sibling while the ill child is hospitalized, how often the well sibling can visit, and the type of parental behavior changes perceived.

KEY CONCEPTS

- Pediatric nurses may care for children in the hospital, school, community, or home. Each setting requires special interventions.
- Common stressors affecting hospitalized children include fear of the unknown, separation anxiety, fear of pain or mutilation, and loss of control.
- Children may experience anger, guilt, and regression in response to illness.
- The stages of separation anxiety are protest, despair, and detachment.
- The more stressed children become, the more difficult it is for them to separate from their parents.

- A child's reaction to pain and fear of injury are related to the child's developmental stage, previous experiences, separation from parents, restraint, and amount of preparation.
- Children who feel that they have control over their illness and hospitalization are more likely to feel confident and be cooperative.
- Regression is a common response to illness and hospitalization. The child returns to an earlier form of behavior.
- How children react to illness and hospitalization is affected by their perception of the event, age, cognitive ability, preparation, previous experiences, coping skills, and parent's response.

- Nursing care of the ill child is directed toward meeting the child's needs related to self-care, separation anxiety, growth and development, diversion, family, control, and pain.
- Parents may experience guilt, denial, anger, and depression when their child is hospitalized.
- Therapeutic play can provide an emotional outlet, instruct, or improve physiologic abilities.
- Play can be incorporated into nursing care when the nurse is teaching or providing a therapeutic intervention that the child finds unpleasant or painful. Compliance increases when deep-breathing and range-of-motion exercises, for example, are made fun activities.

ANSWERS to Critical Thinking Exercise 35-1

1. Families' two most common responsibilities are care of other children and work. A family with a child with cystic fibrosis has the added responsibility of caring for a child with a chronic disease who may or may not have frequent hospitalizations. In addition, family members have the expenses associated with the treatment of the child and, in most cases, cannot afford to miss work. They also risk losing their jobs because of missing work when the child is ill. Families often must balance work, caring for other children, and providing for the needs of the ill child.

2. In most cases, families of ill children are doing the best they can and may not know of available resources that might support them both emotionally and financially. The nurse should review the history obtained on admission to seek additional information about this family. In addition, the nurse should talk with the parents when they visit to determine if they have a support system and if a social service consultation is appropriate. Because the family is new to the area, their needs will probably be greater than the needs of a family surrounded by extended family and friends. If other family members and friends, such as grandparents or church members, are available, the nurse can guide them in identifying ways in which they might assist the family. The staff's awareness that Tommy is often alone can mobilize staff to spend extra time with him. The child life department, if one is available, should also be consulted.

REFERENCES and READINGS

Agazio, J.G. (1997). Family transition through the termination of private duty home care nursing. *Journal of Pediatric Nursing, 12*(2), 74-84.

Als, H. (1996). *Newborn individualized developmental care & assessment program (NIDCAP) program guide.* Boston: National NIDCAP Center.

American Academy of Pediatrics Committee on Hospital Care. (2000). Child life services. *Pediatrics, 106*(5), 1156-1160.

Bossert, E. (1994). Factors influencing the coping of hospitalized school-age children. *Journal of Pediatric Nursing, 9*(5), 299-306.

Bradley, S., & Connell, J. (2000). Visiting children in hospital: A vision from the past. *Paediatric Nursing, 12*(3), 32-35.

Bricher, G. (1999). Paediatric nurses, children, and the development of trust. *Journal of Clinical Nursing, 8*(4), 451-458.

Carlson, K., Broome, M., & Vessey, J. (2000). Using distraction to reduce reported pain, fear, and behavioral distress in children and adolescents: A multisite study. *Journal of the Society of Pediatric Nursing, 5*(2), 75-85.

Carnevale, F.A. (1997). The experience of critically ill children: Narratives of unmaking. *Intensive and Critical Care Nursing, 13*(1), 49-52.

Centers for Disease Control and Prevention. (1996). Guidelines for school health programs to promote lifelong healthy eating. *MMWR: Morbidity and Mortality Weekly Report, 45* (RR-9), 1-33.

Clatworthy, S., Simon, K., & Tiedeman, M.E. (1999a). Child drawing: Hospital—An instrument designated to measure the emotional status of hospitalized school-aged children. *Journal of Pediatric Nursing, 14*(1), 2-9.

Clatworthy, S., Simon, K., & Tiedeman, M.E. (1999b). Child drawing: Hospital manual. *Journal of Pediatric Nursing, 14*(1), 10-18.

Craft, M., Wyatt, N., & Sandell, B. (1985). Behavior and feeling changes in siblings of hospitalized children. *Clinical Pediatrics, 24*(7), 374-378.

Dokken, D.L., & Sydnor-Greenberg, N. (1998). Family matters: Helping families mobilize their personal resources. *Pediatric Nursing, 24*(1), 66-69.

Dokken, D.L., & Sydnor-Greenberg, N. (2001). Communication in healthcare: The parents' perspective. *Journal of Child and Family Nursing, 4*(1), 71-75.

Dowling, J. (2002). Humor: A coping strategy for pediatric patients. *Pediatric Nursing, 28*(2), 123-131.

Dowling, J., & Fain, J. (1999). A multidimensional sense of humor scale for school-aged children: Issues of reliability and validity. *Journal of Pediatric Nursing, 14*(1), 38-42.

Elander, G., Hallstrom, I., & Runesson, I. (2002). Observed parental needs during their child's hospitalization. *Journal of Pediatric Nursing, 17*(2), 140-148.

English Long, E. (2003). Stress in families of children with sepsis. *Critical Care Nursing Clinics of North America, 15*, 47-53.

Fanurick, D., Schmitz, M., Martin, G., Koh, J., Wood, M., Sturgeon, L., & Long, N. (2000). Hospital room or treatment room: Where should inpatient pediatric procedures be performed? *Children's Health Care, 29*(2), 103-111.

Godshall, M. (2003). Caring for families of chronically ill kids. *RN, 66*(2), 30-35.

Griffin, T. (2003). Facing challenges to family-centered care. I: Conflicts over visitation. *Pediatric Nursing, 29*(2), 135-137.

Horn, J.D., Feldman, H.M., & Ploof, D.L. (1995). Parent and professional perceptions about stress and coping strategies during a child's lengthy hospitalization. *Social Work in Health Care, 21*(1), 107-127.

Instone, S. (2002). Developmental strategies for interviewing children. *Journal of Pediatric Health Care, 16*(6), 304-305.

Jacob, E., & Puntillo, K.A. (1999). Pain in hospitalized children: Pediatric nurses' beliefs and practices. *Journal of Pediatric Nursing, 14*(6), 379-391.

Kaplan, D.W., Brindis, C., Naylor, K.E., Phibbs, S.L., Ahlstrand, K.R., & Melinkovich, P. (1998). Elementary school based center use. *Pediatrics, 101*(6), e12-26.

Kristensson-Hallstrom, I., & Elander, G. (1997). Parents' experience of hospitalization: Different strategies for feeling secure. *Pediatric Nursing, 23*(4), 361-367.

LaMontagne, L. (1993). Bolstering personal control in child patients through coping interventions. *Pediatric Nursing, 19*(3), 235-237.

Lau, B. (2002). Stress in children: Can nurses help? *Pediatric Nursing, 28*(1), 13-18.

Lieber, M. (1997). Community-based pediatric experiences: Education for the future. *Journal of Pediatric Nursing, 12*(2), 85-88.

Lynn-McHale, D., & Deatrick, J. (2000). Trust between family and health care provider. *Journal of Family Nursing, 6*(3), 210-231.

Manworren, R.C., & Woodring, B. (1998). Evaluating children's literature as a source for patient education. *Pediatric Nursing, 24*(6), 548-553.

McClowry, S.G., Galehouse, P., Hartnagle, W., Kaufman, H., Just, B., Moed, R., & Patterson-Dehn, C. (1996). A comprehensive school-based clinic: University and community partnership. *Journal of the Society of Pediatric Nurses, 1*(1), 19-26.

McKlindon, D., & Barnsteiner, J.H. (1999). Therapeutic relationships: Evolution of the Children's Hospital of Philadelphia model. *MCN: The American Journal of Maternal/Child Nursing, 24*(5), 237-243.

Melnyk, B.N. (2000). Intervention studies involving parents of hospitalized young children: An analysis of the past and future recommendations. *Journal of Pediatric Nursing, 15*(1), 4-12.

Miles, M.S. (2003). Living with illness. Support for parents during a child's hospitalization. *American Journal of Nursing, 103*(2), 62-64.

Miles, M.S., Carlson, J., & Brunssen, S. (1999). The nurse parent support tool. *Journal of Pediatric Nursing, 14*(1), 44-50.

Mu, P., & Tomlinson, P. (1997). Parental experience and meaning construction during a pediatric health crisis. *Western Journal of Nursing Research, 19*(5), 608-636.

Nicastro, E.A., & Whetsell, M.V. (1999). Children's fears. *Journal of Pediatric Nursing, 14*(6), 392-402.

Riesch, S., Bush, L., Nelson, C., Ohm, B., Portz, P., Abell, B., Wightman, M., & Jenkins, P. (2000). Topics of conflict between parents and young adolescents. *Journal of Society of Pediatric Nurses, 5*(1), 27-38.

Ryan-Wenger, N.A. (2001). Use of children's drawings for measurement of developmental level and emotional status. *Journal of Child and Family Nursing, 4*(2), 139-149.

Selye, H. (1974). *Stress without distress*. New York: Lippincott.

Small, L. (2002). Early predictors of poor coping outcomes in children following intensive care hospitalization and stressful medical encounters. *Pediatric Nursing, 28*(4), 393-399.

Smit, E.M. (2000). Maternal stress during the hospitalization of the adopted child. *MCN: The American Journal of Maternal/Child Nursing, 25*(1), 37-42.

Visintainer, M., & Wolfer, J. (1975). Psychological preparation for surgical pediatric patient: The effect on children's and parents' stress response and adjustment. *Pediatrics, 56*(2), 187-202.

Webster, A. (2000). The facilitating role of the play specialist. *Paediatric Nursing, 12*(7), 24-27.

Yoos, H.L., & McMullen, A. (1996). Illness narratives of children with asthma. *Pediatric Nursing, 22*(4), 285-290.

36

The Child with a Chronic Condition or Terminal Illness

◆ LEARNING OBJECTIVES

After studying this chapter, you should be able to:

◎ Define chronic illness.
◎ Analyze the effects of a chronic illness on the child and family.
◎ Discuss the concerns and needs of the child and family dealing with a chronic illness.
◎ Compare the stages of death and dying.
◎ Apply the concepts of death and dying as they relate to the pediatric client.

◎ Explain the concerns and needs of the child and family facing an impending death.
◎ Analyze the nurse's response to death and dying in the pediatric population.
◎ Use the nursing process to describe nursing care of the chronically ill and dying child.

◆ DEFINITIONS

anticipatory grief   The processes of mourning, coping, interacting, planning, and psychosocial reorganizing that occur as part of the response to the impending death of a loved one.

chronic illness or condition   A condition or illness that is long-term and either is without cure or has a residual effect that limits activities of daily living.

chronic sorrow   Recurrent feelings of grief, loss, and fear related to the child's illness and the loss of the ideal, healthy child.

hospice care   A system of comprehensive care that provides support and assistance to clients and families affected by terminal illness; the purpose is to humanize the dying experi-

ence while providing the means for living as comfortably and as fully as possible; goals are accomplished by providing respectful, noninvasive care; pain and symptom control; and emotional, physical, psychologic, and spiritual support.

illness trajectory   The course of a chronic illness, including the work for and impact on the lives of all those involved.

normalization   Responses used to counteract an illness or abnormal behavior to maintain appropriate and valued social roles.

palliative care   Medical treatments or procedures that aim to promote comfort and quality of life rather than to cure the underlying disease.

Rapid advances in health care have changed the experience of chronic illness in childhood. Children with chronic illnesses are living longer, and an increasing number of children are living with illnesses previously considered to be fatal. Improvements in early diagnostic testing and treatment have enhanced quality of life as well as longevity.

CHRONIC ILLNESS DEFINED

A chronic illness or condition is one that is long-term. It does not resolve spontaneously, is usually without complete cure, and frequently has residual characteristics that limit activities of daily living (ADL) and require adaptation or special assistance. Box 36-1 lists some of the common chronic conditions of childhood. Severity varies among chronic conditions. Many, such as epilepsy, diabetes, or sickle cell disease, although not physically apparent, may

have a tremendous impact on the child and family. A chronic condition that is terminal but lasts only a short time may also have serious long-term effects on the surviving family. It is important to remember in the following discussions that although the first section will refer only to chronic conditions, this information applies to those conditions that are also terminal. The federal Maternal and Child Health Bureau's Division of Services for Children with Special Health Care Needs (Health Resources and Services Administration, 2003) developed the following definition regarding the special needs of chronically and terminally ill children for planning and advocacy purposes:

> Children with special health care needs are those who have or are at increased risk for a chronic physical, developmental, behavioral, or emotional condition and who also require health and related services of a type and amount beyond that required for children generally.

THE FAMILY OF THE CHILD WITH SPECIAL HEALTH CARE NEEDS

Impact on the Family

Improvements in technology, reimbursement provisions (insurance, state and federal funding), and allocation of health care resources have all affected the family's role in caring for the child with a chronic illness. Children with special needs can now be safely cared for in the home setting, with minimal periods of hospitalization. Such care, which includes psychosocial support, is the most desirable and cost-effective care for both child and family.

Although improved quality of life and longevity are positive developments, they do present certain difficulties. Despite health care advances, the child and family must live with a constant physical problem that requires consistent, ongoing attention and adaptation.

Chronic illness is stressful and can create situational crises for families. A situational crisis is an unexpected crisis for which the family's usual problem-solving abilities are not adequate. However, various studies show that some families reorganize and actually become stronger in response to a situational crisis. These families are considered resilient; that is, they are able to recover from adversities of a chronic illness. They do this through *normalization*, making necessary changes in their lives and adjusting to the presence of the chronic illness. They actively work on responses that will help counteract the illness and resulting abnormal behaviors to maintain social roles that are appropriate and valued.

Family resiliency implies present and future success at managing complex aspects of a crisis, such as having a child with a chronic condition (Patterson, 2002). Resilient families exhibit many important traits, but a predominant trait is family cohesiveness. This cohesion is achieved by active efforts to keep the family intact—by sharing not only the new responsibilities related to the chronic condition but also the routine, enjoyable activities of family life. Although family life may be altered by the crisis, resilient families successfully manage the family tasks of equitable economic support, socialization, and protection of the vulnerable family members (Patterson, 2002). Families accomplish this by developing protective factors to counteract the risk inherent with caring for a child with a chronic illness. Processes that enhance resilience include (Patterson, 2002):

- Reframing the situation to identify positive rather than negative aspects
- Successful coping that increases family self-efficacy, or the belief that the family can problem solve in new ways to meet the new challenges
- Maintaining high-quality communication patterns
- Being flexible
- Maintaining social integration
- Preserving family boundaries

Maintaining social integration involves balancing the needs of the family with the needs imposed by the child's condition, as well as reciprocal interactions with the community relative to the child's needs (Patterson, 2002). Resilient families are careful in allocating resources, including money, time, and energy, as they balance various needs. This

---

BOX 36-1
Common Chronic Conditions of Childhood

Asthma (reactive airway disease)
Bleeding disorders (e.g., hemophilia)
Bronchopulmonary dysplasia
Cancer
Cerebral palsy
Chronic renal failure
Congenital heart disease
Cystic fibrosis
Diabetes mellitus
Down syndrome
Epilepsy
Human immunodeficiency virus (HIV) infection and acquired immunodeficiency syndrome (AIDS)
Hydrocephalus
Juvenile rheumatoid arthritis
Lupus erythematosus
Muscular dystrophy
Neural tube defects
Phenylketonuria
Sickle cell disease

---

balance ensures that all children—ill and well—are not neglected or overindulged and that the condition-related needs of the ill child are balanced with normal growth and development needs and met without overprotection. In resilient families, the child's condition-related needs are incorporated into the family's daily life; they do not become the focus around which the activities of the entire family revolve. This integration helps achieve and maintain the family's new normality imposed by the illness. In such a family setting, baseball practices, school activities, ballet recitals, and other activities do not stop for either the ill child or the well sibling. Rather, care of the child, medical appointments, and treatments of the ill child are arranged around these activities, to the degree possible. When conflicts do arise, parents (or other family members or friends) alternate responsibility for maintaining the activities of both the ill child and well siblings.

Equitable allocation of care giving and encouraging parental involvement with each other and well siblings help maintain appropriate family boundaries. When either of the two parents becomes primarily involved in meeting the needs of the ill child, the parental relationship suffers. To keep these boundaries intact, resilient families pay specific attention to maintaining a positive parental relationship. They also work to avoid showing favoritism toward the ill child.

Single-parent families may encounter additional difficulties that heighten risk. Social support may not be inherent in the family structure, so these families are at increased risk for social isolation. Health care providers can refer single parents to support groups, put them in contact with other parents who have a child with a similar chronic condition, or organize group sharing experiences between parents experienced in the care of the child with a particular chronic condition and parents of newly diagnosed children. Organized programs can provide several services that help single parents, including providing information, enhancing confidence, and giving emotional support (Ireys, Chernoff, DeVet, & Kim, 2001).

Boundary problems of a different sort can arise when the need for outside care and assistance increases, such as the presence of home health or hospice personnel. Whether they are in the home around the clock or for various shifts throughout the week, external family boundaries can be negatively affected. However, difficulties can be minimized if family members adopt an assertive role in managing the child's care and, along with the health care personnel, work to maintain professional relationships and boundaries with caregivers.

Resilient families work consistently to ensure appropriate communication, which may be more difficult because of new, condition-related language (medical or otherwise), an increased need for problem solving–based communication, and most important, the need to express emotions. Accepting the validity of all emotions and learning suitable means of expressing them may be difficult. However, many families report that the experience of living with a chronic illness brings about positive life changes, such as increased empathy, increased family unity, and new meanings to life.

Even when positive meaning is attached to a child's chronic condition, much flexibility is required of family members with regard to family roles and expectations of family members. This flexibility is also required of the health care team, both for the benefit of the family and as a means of achieving a positive, collaborative relationship between the team and the family. The team becomes an integral part of family life. The quality of this relationship may affect how the entire family adapts to and copes with the child's condition.

For resilient families, coping is an active process that entails learning about their child's illness and available resources. These families do not sit idly by, letting others meet their child's needs. They are also the strongest advocates for their child. Subsequently, they have a tremendous need for any information concerning their child's condition. The nurse has an important role in helping families educate themselves and learn to meet their child's special health care needs.

At times of extreme stress, such as periods of unexpected physical setbacks, exacerbations, worsening, or relapse of the condition, as well as at the time of death, families may slip into less effective patterns of behavior and coping. Gentle reminders, support, and encouragement may be all the assistance that a resilient family needs to help members resume the behaviors that foster resiliency despite the many ongoing stressors and uncertainties of a chronic condition.

The Grieving Process

The most important aspect of a chronic illness is that it affects not only the ill child but also the entire family. This scope of concern necessitates consistent family-centered nursing care (see Chapter 3). All family members respond to a chronic condition. However, responses vary according to their age and developmental level, their relationship and involvement with the ill child, and any previous experiences with a health care problem.

Chronic and terminal conditions involve the loss of health and result in grief. Grief is a normal psychophysiologic process that occurs in response to a specific loss. A normal and frequent response to such conditions includes the five stages of dying noted by Elisabeth Kübler-Ross (1969). Her work identified the stages in relation to the anticipated death of an adult. However, they apply to children as well as adults and to the grief of not only a terminal illness but also a chronic condition. The ill child as well as family members may experience such stages.

The stages include denial, anger, bargaining, sadness or depression, and acceptance. During the first stage (*denial*), individuals react with disbelief and shock. Their feelings of "no, not me" and "no, not my loved one" occur whether they are explicitly told of the diagnosis or, in the case of the children, they figure it out on their own. *Anger* usually follows denial. This may include feelings of rage and resentment directed at themselves or at others. At this point, the questions of "why me?" and "why my loved one?" may also occur. Anger may recur at any time during the process of the illness. *Bargaining* then happens, whereby the individual attempts to postpone the inevitable. Although most bargaining is with a spiritual deity, bargaining with oneself or others may also take place.

Depression is the next stage. Such sadness may be either for past losses or those impending losses. Past losses may include physical losses, such as a change in appearance (e.g., hair loss), lifestyle changes, or changes in physical ability. Impending losses may include imminent loss of loved ones. It may also include preparing loved ones for the absence created by death.

The last stage is *acceptance*, whereby the individual is no longer depressed or angry. Although acceptance is not a happy stage, it is generally a time of comfort and peace.

Individuals need different periods of time to work through and resolve the feelings of one stage before proceeding to the next stage. The stages are not always experienced sequentially. Some fluctuation may recur across stages before acceptance and comfort are reached. Acceptance of a chronic illness can take place even in the presence of noticeable denial. Such denial might appear to be maintained throughout the course of the illness. Because children have less predictable and variable protective mechanisms, they may use denial frequently—more so than adults. An individual who has a positive, optimistic outlook and who focuses on concerns and tasks of the day rather than on fears about the condition may be using adaptive denial as a protective mechanism. This may assist in decision making, lowering distress and anxiety, and supporting daily functioning (Lugton & Kindlen, 1999).

The time frame for the presence of denial is important. Short-term, true denial, although often considered maladaptive, may truly be adaptive. It is generally experienced as a normal stage of grieving after the onset of a chronic or terminal illness. Persistence of such denial over the course of the illness, however, is maladaptive (Walker et al., 1993). It is important, though, to attempt to establish whether there is true, ongoing denial. Many times, what appears to be denial is just the individual's expression of the loss of their hopes for the ill child. This might be seen as a mother's talk of how beautiful her daughter will look as a bride. It might be a sibling's discussion as to how much fun he or she will have with the ill child next summer at camp. It is frequently very important for family to recognize and express the most difficult aspects of their impending loss, in order to grieve fully and appropriately. Another aspect of what appears to be denial is the expression of the faith that a miracle will occur and that the child will not die after all.

As adjustment to the condition progresses, many parents experience *chronic sorrow*, or the recurrent feelings of loss and fear related to the child's disorder and the loss of the ideal, healthy child (Edwards, Hertzberg, Hays, & Youngblood, 1999). Chronic sorrow is a normal process and may never resolve. However, there is adaptation to the presence of the illness. The family establishes a "new normal," and their life continues. It is important to note that chronic sorrow is not the same as chronic grief. Chronic grief refers to mourning after the death of an individual that is of excessive duration and interferes with the person's ability to return to normal living (Lugton & Kindlen, 1999).

The first step in supporting families and helping them deal with chronic sorrow is to listen and to recognize and acknowledge their emotions. The family can then be assisted to recognize the normality of such feelings and emotions themselves. Families should be gently encouraged to acknowledge and express feelings of chronic sorrow, to the degree at which they are comfortable. At the same time, however, they should be encouraged and assisted to verbalize and demonstrate realistic hopes and dreams.

Many organizations, both general and disease-specific, offer a wealth of information, support, and assistance to families of a child with a chronic or terminal illness. They offer much beyond the information related to the child's condition. The nurse should introduce the family to such services and, as necessary, assist them to use these services fully. Conversely, it is important to respect a family's decision not to use such support services if that is their decision.

Such supportive services may be particularly important when observation and assessment of family behaviors indicate problems that may necessitate referral to a mental health professional. In caring for children with a chronic or terminal illness and their families, one issue that is frequently overlooked is that death may occur unexpectedly and/or earlier than anticipated. This is an important but difficult issue to address with families. It should be done in the early stage of the condition to prepare them if the death does happen in an unexpected manner. It is important for the nurse to support children and their families through all stages of the grief process. Supporting the family requires understanding the family's current knowledge base, coping skills, and personal beliefs, as well as recognizing and attending to the grief-related problems that arise.

THE CHILD WITH SPECIAL HEALTH CARE NEEDS

Growth and Development Concerns

Children with chronic disorders have many different concerns and needs related to their conditions, not the least of which is successful navigation of the stages of growth and development. Children's responses to illness are influenced by their age at the onset of the disorder as well as growth and development considerations throughout the course of the illness. Nursing care is planned accordingly. (See Chapter 4 for a more complete discussion of the normal stages of growth and development.)

Often, chronic and terminal conditions span a number of years and developmental stages. Regardless of the stage, concerns related to self-esteem, self-reliance, and autonomy are prevalent among children with chronic conditions. Many will experience altered body awareness and body image as a result of physical changes related to the illness or treatment. These changes frequently have a negative impact on children's self-esteem. Control and autonomy may be decreased because of hospitalizations and treatment regimens that offer few decision-making opportunities for the child. Socialization activities and adjustment may be limited as a result of hospitalization and the side effects of the illness or treatment. Side effects, including altered appearance, decreased physical ability, or increased susceptibility to infection, may interfere with age-appropriate socialization. At times, it may not be a medical necessity (e.g., infection risk, bleeding risk) that keeps the child from participating but, rather, the child declines based on fears regarding his or her appearance or physical abilities.

Such factors may profoundly affect a child's acquisition of age-appropriate growth and developmental skills, especially throughout adolescence. An important goal is to minimize the effects of illness and hospitalization and to maximize the child's potential to the optimum degree possible. This is true regardless of the age or developmental stage, and it is important for the nurse to understand issues concerning self-esteem and autonomy in relation to each stage of growth and development (Box 36-2).

Despite the understanding and interventions of family and staff, a variety of consequences may occur frequently among children with a chronic condition or illness. Most are minimal, short-lived, and expected as a part of the "normal" course of a chronic condition. For example, among older infants and toddlers, stranger anxiety may be heightened or may reappear months after previous resolution.

Temporary regression may be seen with children of all ages, including adolescents. However, it is more prevalent among older infants through the young school-age years. Toddlers use regression frequently as they attempt to cope with the stress of a serious illness. Despite the normalcy of regression, it may be unsettling to child and family because it involves the loss of recently acquired skills or the reappearance of behaviors seen when the child was younger. Common regressive behaviors include reverting back to a bottle, pacifier or thumb sucking; a change in toileting skills; an increased incidence of bed-wetting; and an increased use of "baby talk" or communication techniques more appropriate for younger ages.

Another possible difficulty is a fluctuation in the child's age-appropriate communication patterns. Lack of communication or altered communication patterns with health care personnel may occur in the clinic or hospital setting, with regular patterns of communication resuming at home. Among older preschoolers, a lack of communication may be a form of withdrawal or an expression of stubbornness and a refusal to cooperate. This problem may also be seen in school-age children and adolescents and is usually related to issues involving independence and self-esteem. (Chapter 35 provides a more in-depth description of the impact of illness on the individual age-groups.)

Parental Responses to Developmental Issues

Regardless of the developmental stage or the number of years that a chronic illness has existed, the basic guidelines for child rearing still apply. As with the well child, discipline and

---

BOX 36-2
The Illness Experience: The Child and Adolescent

INFANT

Developmental task: Achievement of awareness of being separate from significant other.

Impact of illness: Potential distortion of differentiation of self from parents or significant others.

Cognitive age/stage: Sensorimotor (birth to 2 years).

Major fears: Separation, strangers.

Interventions: Provide consistent caretakers. Minimize separation from parents and significant others. Decrease parental anxiety, which is projected to infant. Maintain crib and nursery as "safe place" where no invasive procedures are performed.

TODDLER

Developmental task: Initiation of autonomy.

Impact of illness: Interference with or loss of developing sense of control, independence.

Cognitive age/stage: Preoperational (2 to 7 years): egocentric, magical, little concept of body integrity.

Major fears: Separation, loss of control.

Concept of illness: Phenomenism (2 to 7 years)—perceives external, unrelated, concrete phenomena as cause of illness (e.g., "being sick because you don't feel well"). Contagion—perceives cause of illness as proximity between two events that occurs by "magic" (e.g., "getting a cold because you are near someone who has a cold").

Interventions: Minimize separation from parents or significant others. Keep security objects at hand. Provide simple, brief explanations. Explain and maintain consistent limits. Encourage participation in daily care. Provide opportunities for play.

PRESCHOOLER

Developmental task: Creation of a sense of initiative.

Impact of illness: Interference with or loss of accomplishments, such as walking, talking, controlling basic body functions.

Cognitive age/stage: Preoperational thought—egocentric, magical, tendency to use and repeat words child does not understand, providing own explanations and definitions. Literal translation of words. Inability to abstract.

Major fears: Body injury and mutilation, loss of control, the unknown, the dark, being left alone.

Concept of illness: Phenomenism, contagion.

Interventions: Provide simple, concrete explanations. Advance preparation is important: days for major events, hours for minor events. Verbal explanations are usually insufficient, so use pictures, models, actual equipment, and medical play.

SCHOOL-AGE CHILD

Developmental task: Sense of industry.

Impact of illness: Potential feelings of inadequacy or inferiority if autonomy and independence are compromised.

Cognitive age/stage: Concrete operational thought (7 to 10 years).

Major fears: Loss of control, body injury and mutilation, failure to live up to expectations of important others, death.

Concept of illness: Contamination—perceives cause as a person, object, or action external to the child that is "bad" or "harmful" to the body (e.g., "getting a cold because you didn't wear a hat"). Internalization—perceives illness as having an external cause but being located inside the body (e.g., "getting a cold by breathing in air and bacteria").

Interventions: Provide choices whenever possible to increase the child's sense of control. Emphasize contact with peer group. Use diagrams, pictures, and models for explanations because thinking is concrete. Emphasize the "normal" things the child can do, because the child does not want to be seen as different. Reassure children that they have done nothing wrong; hospitalization, for example, is not punishment.

ADOLESCENT

Developmental task: Achieving a sense of identity.

Impact of illness: Potential alteration in or relinquishment of newly acquired roles and responsibilities.

Cognitive age/stage: Formal operational thought (11+ years): beginning of ability to think abstractly. Existence of some magical thinking (e.g., feeling guilty for illness) and egocentrism.

Major fears: Loss of control, altered body image, separation from peer group.

Concept of illness: Physiologic—perceives cause as malfunctioning or nonfunctioning organ or process; can explain illness in sequence of events. Psychophysiologic—realizes that psychologic actions and attitudes affect health and illness.

Interventions: Allow adolescent to be an integral part of decision making regarding care. Give information sensitively, because adolescents react both to the content of information and to the manner in which it is delivered. Allow as many choices and as much control as possible. Be honest about treatment and its consequences. Stress what the adolescent can personally do and the importance of cooperation and compliance. Assist in maintaining contact with peer group.

From Gibbons, M.B. (1993). Psychosocial aspects of serious illness in childhood and adolescence. In A. Armstrong-Dailey & S.Z. Goltzer (Eds.), *Hospice care for children* (Chapter 3). New York: Oxford University Press. Based on Bibace, R., & Walsh, M.E. (1980). Development of children's concepts of illness. *Pediatrics, 66,* 912-918.

---

consistency are very important. A very good example was the mother of a 3-year-old with cancer who would frequently remind both the ill child and her older sibling that cancer is no excuse for bad manners!

Experiencing a chronic illness is confusing, especially for children whose cognitive abilities are not sufficiently developed to allow understanding that could help them cope with the stress. When changes in a child's world begin to affect the only constant they know, their family, this is often reflected in the child's behavior. Negative behavior may result from the stress of the illness and/or from changes in the family and environment. Previously existing negative behaviors may worsen, making treatment and a positive relationship and cooperation with the health care team difficult. Future behav-

> ## ! CRITICAL TO REMEMBER
>
> **Goals for Chronic Care**
> ### GOALS FOR THE CHILD
> - To achieve and maintain normalization
> - To obtain the highest level of health and function possible—physically, emotionally, and psychosocially
>
> ### GOALS FOR THE FAMILY
> - To remain intact
> - To achieve and maintain normalization
> - To maximize function throughout the course of the illness

ior and long-term development may be affected as well. At the time their child is diagnosed, parents should be reminded about the importance of maintaining previous rules and expectations. The focus should continue to be on the accomplishment of developmental tasks rather than on the chronic condition (Clawson, 1996).

THE CHILD WITH A CHRONIC ILLNESS

The goal for any child with a chronic illness is to achieve and maintain the highest level of health and function possible—physically, emotionally, and psychosocially. The aim is similar for the family system, including parents or guardians, siblings, and extended family members. Goals for the entire family are to remain intact, achieve and maintain normalization, and maximize function throughout the illness. This necessitates a family-centered approach to nursing care.

The nursing process for the child with a chronic illness is ongoing for the duration of the illness. It may be more complex because of goals that are both physical and psychosocial. The psychosocial environment is significant in that it greatly influences the manner in which the child relates to others and copes with stress. In addition, the entire family is involved as well as the ill child. Care is provided over a span of years and must incorporate often-rapid changes in the child's growth and development. The nurse is prepared for a changing assessment, both physical and psychosocial, related to duration of care and fluctuations of the illness.

Planning and implementation of nursing care are based on several factors. The child's physical condition is the first consideration. It is not possible to generalize across broad categories of illnesses, such as cancer, respiratory conditions, or cardiac problems. Each illness will include specific implications, including subsequent disabilities. The child's growth and development across the span of the illness are also very important. In addition, the needs, coping mechanisms, and available resources of child and family are also influencing factors. Nursing care includes assisting the child and family to accept, understand, and incorporate the illness appropriately into each stage of growth and development, regardless of the child's age at diagnosis.

Ongoing Care

Evaluation as well as subsequent modification of planning and implementation of care will often take place on a daily basis because of the child's frequent physical changes. Unex-

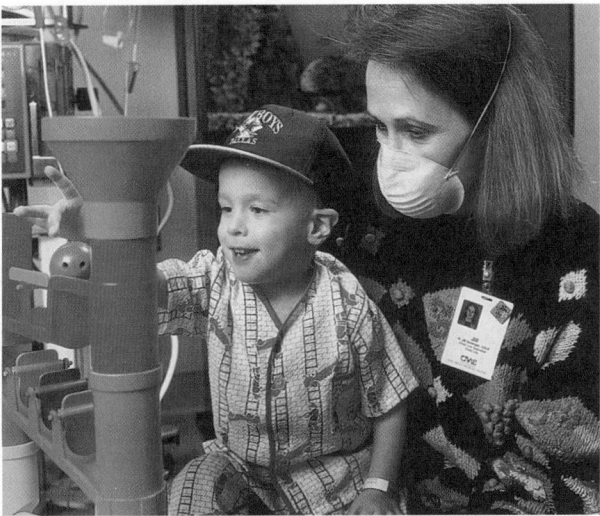

Figure 36-1 The nurse or a child life specialist can use therapeutic play, medical play, and therapeutic art to enhance self-expression, education, and growth and development. (Courtesy Norm Tindell for Cook Children's Medical Center, Fort Worth, TX.)

pected setbacks, such as an exacerbation, relapse, critical infection, an undesirable response to medication, lack of physical progress, or the need to undergo a medical or surgical procedure unexpectedly or sooner than anticipated, may be a standard part of the illness. Goals may have to be altered repeatedly. All of the changes may be stressful and difficult. This may be true even for the child and family who have been coping with an illness for a long period. Continuous support and reassurance are necessary throughout the illness.

Education

With an illness that continues for several years, numerous changes may occur because of the child's physical condition and/or the advancing age. Education involves child and family, addressing both physical and psychosocial issues. This ensures that the family has an accurate knowledge base to provide care at home. It also serves to assist in psychosocial needs of child and family.

One important consideration in relation to education and support for the ill child as well as siblings is use of a child life specialist (Fig. 36-1). The child life specialist uses methods that are educational, supportive, and therapeutic. These may include medical play, medical art, therapeutic play, and therapeutic art (see Chapter 35). All are similar in that they present the child with an opportunity for learning, increased expression of feelings, and coping methods for the difficult situations experienced as a result of their condition. The nurse may also use some of these techniques in daily care or when it is not possible for a child life specialist to be present. Child life services are used for siblings as well as for the ill child.

Communication

Communication with the ill child may be more difficult than physical care (see Chapter 32). Communication is the most important factor in establishing a good relationship with child and family. *Appropriate communication is based on the child's age and development and always involves honesty as well as compassion.* Following these principles can help decrease the child's fears and misunderstandings. This may also help increase the child's confidence in nurses and other members of the health care team. Increased cooperation with the therapeutic regimen is an additional benefit. If fears and misunderstandings are not alleviated at the beginning and caregivers do not gain the child's trust, establishing trust at a later date can be very difficult. This is particularly true when the nursing care involves unpleasant or painful medications and treatments.

To prevent misinterpretations and misunderstandings, the nurse can ask children to explain what they know and understand. The nurse should also strive to understand what the child is really asking. The classic example of miscommunication is the child who asks where she comes from and hears the entire story of reproduction, when all she really wanted to know was whether her family was from Texas or Oklahoma! Clarifying questions can help the nurse avoid providing more information than the child wants or can handle emotionally. Providing too much information may be overwhelming and frightening to the child. It may also inhibit future questions and interaction with the nurses.

Honesty and trust must be maintained at all times when caring for the child. These principles should be encouraged among the family and other members of the health care team. Complete honesty may cause problems for some individuals, family, or staff, especially when they face the difficult questions that often arise when caring for a chronically or terminally ill child. The most difficult and feared questions are usually centered on whether the child is going to die and why he or she became sick and is dying. These are followed closely by questions concerning the deaths of other children whom the child has known or with whom the child has developed a close relationship.

Children are often reluctant to question adults at all, much less to ask questions whose answers they fear. Many times the child already knows the answer, so the question is really a test concerning honesty and a point of reference in the child's relationship with the adult (parent or staff). As with adults, children need honesty to establish trust. They may not understand the use of dishonesty as a means of protecting them against emotional pain or unpleasantness. Once aware of dishonesty in an adult, children may feel that they cannot and will not trust the adults around them, whether parent or staff. Dishonesty may then have disastrous effects, particularly when one is trying to reassure the child and gain the child's cooperation. Often a chronic condition may progress to impending death, at which point the child's trust can be paramount to achieving comfort and peace.

For children with a chronic condition, honesty may increase their emotional pain to some degree. Conversely, it may help comfort them at the same time. Honest answers to a child's difficult questions are not always handled well by adults in the family. Realizing the importance of the child's trust, it is good practice for the nurse and family to understand and explore feelings about providing honest answers to the child's questions and establish and communicate guidelines up front. The family may give instructions about communication that bring about conflict for the nurse, both professionally and personally. The family may ask that the nurse answer deceitfully in regard to the serious nature of the illness or the fact that the child is expected to die. In many situations, a compromise is reached in that the nurse will not initiate conversations that may lead to the hard questions such

as whether the child is expected to die. However, if the child initiates the conversation and asks such questions directly, the nurse will reply honestly, in terms approved by the family. This may not work with some families. In such instances, it may be helpful to involve other members of the health care team to make communication decisions that best suit the needs of all involved. Such members might include physicians, child life specialist, the social worker, and those who provide pastoral care.

Care of the Parents

Parents of children with a chronic disease have some especially significant needs (Graves & Hayes, 1996):

- Obtaining information about the child's chronic condition and available services
- Receiving support through reading about how parents of a child with a similar condition manage day-to-day stress
- More time for themselves
- Opportunities to meet and talk with parents of children with similar conditions
- Assistance locating babysitters or respite care providers
- Assistance paying for food, housing, medical expenses, clothing, and other necessities
- Assistance with discussing problems and reaching solutions

Grief Education and Support

Nursing care should include education about the child's condition and treatment as well as education concerning the grief issues. The nurse assists all family members, including the child, to understand and express, in the manner most comfortable, their grief responses. Taking time to provide care and support in this area is as important as physical care. Many adults have not experienced illness or death before the child's diagnosis and are not accustomed to the idea of grief, much less grief as a normal, healthy process. Also, some family members may have had a previous experience with dying, death, and grief that they perceive to have been negative and very distressing. Both situations may increase support needs among the family.

The nurse educates the family about the importance of the grief process and provides opportunities for grieving. Such care may include conversations and time "being present" with family. Being present for all family members as the need arises entails the very important aspect of listening and/or sitting in silence. Many times family members do not need or want conversation; they just want to be with someone who knows their child and is familiar with what they might be experiencing. This may be true even for siblings. Children who just want to be with an adult may require only that the person sit with them while they play. The expression of emotions is recognized to be more beneficial for most individuals than holding the emotions inside. However, it is important to realize that for some, such expressions were not a normal or comfortable part of their life before their child's illness. It is unlikely that such patterns will be altered. The nurse accepts this choice while letting the family know that a caring individual is available at any time if the need for talking and sharing arises.

Cultural and Religious Beliefs

Culture and religion influence the meaning of illness and death as well as customs observed by the family. The family's explanation of the child's disease can be revealing and may lead to more culturally sensitive interventions (Sterling, Peterson, & Weekes, 1997). When faced with an unfamiliar culture or religion, the nurse becomes familiar with beliefs and practices used and honored by the family. The nurse and the entire health care team should communicate acceptance of such beliefs and standards. Team members cannot assume that an individual or family belongs to a particular religion or denomination solely on the basis of cultural background. In addition, they should not assume that the family adheres to all beliefs and practices of their chosen religion or denomination. If in doubt, the nurse should question the family, stressing that the questioning is an effort to provide the most comprehensive and appropriate care possible.

It is imperative that health care professionals deliver culturally sensitive care to families with chronically ill or disabled children. The meaning of chronic illness or disability to a family must be considered in light of that family's culture. Nurses need to avoid cultural stereotyping and appropriately communicate with families to determine personal meaning of the illness or disability (Banks, 2003). Many excellent resources can provide the nurse with appropriate information as to the impact of cultural and religious beliefs on illness and death, such as journals, research, textbooks, and the Internet. (See Chapter 3 for a more in-depth discussion about these issues.)

Referrals

To the degree possible, the nurse should endeavor to make sure that the physical, emotional, psychosocial, and intellectual needs of child and family are met. Also, nursing care includes assisting family members to provide for the child's physical and psychosocial needs themselves. Regardless of culture or religion, the nurse should not expect to be able to provide all the necessary support. This is related to a lack of both time and necessary expertise. At such times, the family should be referred to other personnel, such as members of the clergy, other spiritual counselors, and social workers. If these individuals cannot provide assistance, they are generally in a better position to refer the family to outside professionals or services. Members of the clergy generally have wider access to information on various religious beliefs as well as access to the necessary clergy from different religious sectors. The social work department will also be able to provide information concerning other helpful, necessary resources for the family. This information may include financial information, such as insurance and government assistance, housing and transportation assistance, and assistance with medical care and supplies.

Schooling

The face of public education and the child with special health care needs has changed dramatically. The Developmental Disabilities Act (PL 91-517) and subsequent amendments ensure a free public education for each child with a disability or other chronic condition. It also mandates that special education and support services be provided in the least restrictive environment for children 3 years and older. Consequently, children with a wide variety of physical needs are attending school with minimal difficulty or disruption. These needs range from the relatively simple needs (e.g., medication administration, respiratory treatments) to more extensive needs (e.g., gastrostomy tube feedings, tracheostomy tubes, ventilators). Facilitating the start of school or return to school for the child with special needs requires preparation and assistance

for the child, the family, and school personnel. In addition to child and family, those involved should include a nurse from the hospital or clinic, school nurse, teacher, and counselor and director of special education.

A specific, structured plan of care will be developed before the child's return to school. This will be accomplished by the school system through a legally mandated process referred to as an *individualized educational plan (IEP)* or *admission, review, and dismissal (ARD)*. This plan will be developed with input from the health care team, who are encouraged to attend the actual conference if possible. The plan includes cognitive and physical needs in regard to the child's school attendance. This plan includes those learning goals that might require alteration secondary to the special needs, as well as the specific task for achieving such goals. Both must be realistic in relation to the child's condition. The plan also addresses any special health care that is needed while the child is in school, such as medication, feedings, or other treatments. The planning conferences will be needed before the child is scheduled to start school for the first time after his or her condition is diagnosed. The IEP or ARD must take place at least once a year after that or when changes in the child's condition occur that will necessitate changes at school. Most schools now offer children the opportunity to attend school full-time as their condition allows and then change to homebound when necessary. Regardless of the type of school services the child is receiving, the hospital or clinic nurse may need to provide ongoing education and psychosocial support for the school nurse and other personnel, particularly if they are unfamiliar with the child's condition or the treatments it requires.

Special considerations are given in the school setting for a child who is experiencing immunosuppression, whether it is related to the disease itself or treatment. Preventing the infection that can occur with immunosuppression is a challenge in the school setting, regardless of the age of the child. Because of crowded conditions in school classrooms and the often poor infection control practices by children (e.g., good handwashing), preventing infection may be difficult. The school nurse should alert teachers to be particularly vigilant and notify the nurse if any infectious disease is present in the classroom. Families might also be reminded to notify the school if their child contracts certain serious illnesses such as chickenpox or strep throat. Such notification may or may not include information about the immunosuppressed child, as per the families' wishes. The school nurse can also use this as an opportunity to visit classrooms and present a health-teaching module on general infection prevention practices. It is important for the school nurse to obtain information about the specific signs of infection that accompany specific conditions or treatments, because these may differ from child to child. Information will also be required as to how to contact the child's health care team directly and quickly if problems are suspected.

Ongoing psychosocial support may also be necessary for the child and family in relation to school. Parents may experience mixed emotions regarding their child's return to school. They are likely to be pleased and excited that the child is well enough to attend school. At the same time, they may be concerned about the child's well-being during school hours, particularly about whether the special health care needs will be met appropriately. For those children with a terminal condition, parents may also experience a degree of sorrow in regard to being apart during what limited time they have with their child. The child's siblings may also experience similar feelings.

The nurse can best provide support, or refer to those who can, by maintaining ongoing communication with the family, recognizing that problems and concerns with school may vary over time. Referral to others such as a spiritual counselor, social worker, or mental health professional may also be helpful for the psychosocial support families are seeking.

Regardless of whether the child is transitioning into or reentering school, it is most important that all involved (child, family, health care and school personnel) understand how the condition or disability impacts the child's day. They must also recognize when the child's participation in an activity must be altered, as well as understand the need for adaptive tools or equipment (Edwards et al., 1999).

The Nurse as Liaison

The nurse is a liaison for the family in many different situations. The most important liaison work, however, is to link the family with other members of the health care team, particularly the physician. In this capacity, the nurse can help guarantee that family members receive accurate information and have an appropriate understanding of their child's condition as well as resulting psychosocial and physical needs. These efforts can facilitate the family's health care planning, help ensure a good relationship and appropriate communication with the health care team, and increase compliance with treatment.

Care of the Siblings

Sibling concerns and needs in relation to the chronic illness vary according to age and development in a similar way as the child experiencing the chronic illness. Fluctuations are common when the condition exists for several years. Siblings may experience many of the same anxieties and fears as their parents.

Regardless of whether they are past the age of magical thinking, siblings often have feelings of guilt as to their role in the ill child's condition. Many children with siblings have had thoughts of what life would be like without having to share material possessions and parental love with their sibling(s). When a sibling then becomes ill, the guilt and associated emotions may be overwhelming. The well sibling

should be reassured about the normalcy of such feelings and that the illness is not the result of anything that was said or done by them or anyone else.

Nursing care of the sibling involves education as to the ill child's condition, treatment, physical changes, disabilities, and expected disease progression. The sibling should always be kept up to date regarding changes in the ill child's condition. Ideally, from the standpoint of honesty, this means changes for good as well as bad. The same principles of honest communication apply to siblings as well as the child with the illness. However, what information is ultimately shared with siblings is at the parents' discretion. The hospital setting—rules, equipment, and personnel—must also be explained. As possible and suitable, according to the sibling's and parents' wishes as well as the sibling's growth and development, the sibling may also be allowed to participate in physically caring for the ill child.

As with the ill child, siblings may also regress in developmental stage and activities. Parents frequently do not expect such behavioral changes from a well sibling and may need to be reminded that in the presence of a stressful event, regression is a normal coping mechanism for all children, both ill and well.

The nurse can help the sibling understand that illness creates stress, which may result in difficult or painful emotions, such as anger and jealousy. Children need to know that these emotions are a normal part of life, although they are often perceived as negative and harmful. Children must be allowed to experience and, as they desire, express these feelings (Fig. 36-2). Whereas the physical and emotional needs of the ill child are generally well tended to, health care professionals and the family may too easily exclude siblings and neglect their psychosocial and emotional needs. Such oversight can lead to additional stress and problems that must be dealt with by the entire family. This in turn may negatively impact the ill child.

The nurse and family should include siblings as much as possible in the life and activities of the ill child, whether the child is hospitalized or receiving outpatient care. The family will require education and input from the health care team regarding the pros and cons of sibling involvement. Spiritual or cultural beliefs may affect this type of decision. Many families choose to minimize siblings' time and involvement in the medical setting as a means of keeping their lives as normal and uninterrupted as possible. Other families try to maintain the existing degree of closeness

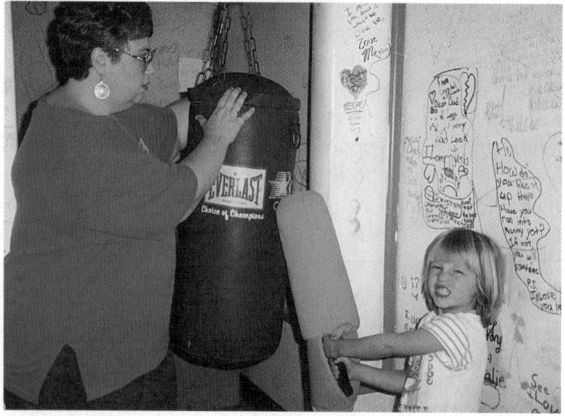

Figure 36-2 Chronic illness is stressful for the siblings of an ill child. Siblings' emotional needs may be overlooked. Siblings should be given the opportunity to express negative feelings, such as anger and jealousy, through therapeutic art and play as well as through physical outlets, such as striking a punching bag, as this little girl is doing.

! CRITICAL TO REMEMBER

Nursing Care for Children With Chronic Conditions and Their Families

- Caring for a child with a chronic condition means attending to the needs of the family system. Both parents and siblings may need additional support.
- The age and developmental level of the chronically ill child affect both the child's understanding and the family's needs. Goals may need to be revised frequently to meet the child's changing developmental needs.
- The nurse should listen carefully to the child's perception of the condition. A child's illness experience does not always match an adult's view of the physical limitations and emotional stress.

Nursing Care Plan

The Child with a Chronic Condition in the Community Setting

FOCUSED ASSESSMENT

Whether the child is at home, attending school, or in the hospital, assessment involves the entire family system and its existing coping and adaptive mechanisms. Note any inappropriate coping behaviors so suggestions and support for changing to healthy, beneficial mechanisms can be planned. As these areas are examined during the course of a chronic illness, the nurse needs to keep in mind the physiologic progression of the disease. As the condition progresses and the child's condition changes, so will the impact on the family and the work necessary to cope.

Explore the family's response to the child's illness and the family's recognition of the impact of illness on the entire family system. Discovering what each individual understands about the disease process and the treatment regimen can help determine whether misinformation or misinterpretation exists regarding information from the health care team. Explore and document the family's existing support system in the community. Such support not only helps with family coping but also may influence the family's beliefs, responses, and method of coping.

There must be a collaborative assessment of the child's development and abilities (physical, cognitive). This assessment involves the child, family, school personnel, and interdisciplinary health care team. This baseline assessment of skills and abilities may be done within the context of developing a school individual education plan or a plan for a hospital admission, and it helps to ensure consistency of expectations and gauge the level of assistance that will be needed. Psychosocial abilities to be assessed should include family patterns of communication and behavior, as well as emotional concerns.

The nurse should always assess *the child's perception* of physical changes and treatments, their effects, and their impact on the child's self-esteem, because issues of self-esteem, self-reliance, and autonomy are primary concerns for the child with a chronic illness. Even with apparently minor changes, altered body awareness and body image can lead to a negative impact on self-esteem. This assessment considers the special concerns of each developmental stage because these may change with the passing years. An 8-year-old child may be very comfortable with and well adjusted to a physical change or disability yet may experience difficulties with the same circumstances on becoming an adolescent. It is important for the school nurse to communicate assessment findings when the child moves to a new school level.

Nursing Diagnosis

Risk for Delayed Growth and Development related to the effects of chronic illness or disability.

Expected Outcomes

The child will:
- Experience minimal disturbance of normal growth and development (physical, cognitive, psychologic), as evidenced by minimal delays, documented by an age-appropriate developmental screening tool.
- Experience minimal disturbance of normal growth and development, as evidenced by ability to interact in an age-appropriate manner socially, physically, and cognitively to the degree allowed by the existing disability.
- Experience minimal disturbance of normal growth and development, as evidenced by ability to perform usual age-appropriate activities of daily living (ADL) as allowed by the existing disability.

INTERVENTION	RATIONALE
1. Educate the child and family about the physical conditions, expected physical changes or disabilities, and prescribed treatment. Education should be in a manner appropriate for the child's cognitive abilities rather than chronologic age.	1. Education encourages a sense of control and acceptance of the physical changes related to the condition, as well as increased cooperation with the prescribed treatment. Many children with a chronic condition are wise beyond their years, with a cognitive ability that does not necessarily correspond to their chronologic age. Among such children, even those as young as 6 years, may be able to knowledgeably discuss medical matters, such as laboratory values or the results of a diagnostic procedure.

Continued

Nursing Care Plan

The Child with a Chronic Condition in the Community Setting—cont'd

INTERVENTION	RATIONALE
2. Set reasonable goals for improving and maximizing abilities in relation to any existing disability. Goal setting should be a group effort involving the child, family, school, and interdisciplinary team.	2. Goal setting assists children and families to increase their abilities and self-esteem through successful accomplishment of tasks. Goal setting may also increase a sense of situational control.
3. Assist the child to develop a sense of pride in existing abilities and to gain incentive to expand the range of physical abilities.	3. Focusing on activities or skills once enjoyed can provide incentive for achieving them again. For example, the child with a prosthesis can strive toward once more becoming an accomplished skier, but on one leg! Alternatively, the child can establish a goal of learning to drive an automatic-shift instead of a standard-shift automobile, receiving a driver's license along with peers.
4. Encourage and provide opportunities for autonomy and situational control by offering as many choices as possible. Include the child in age-appropriate decisions regarding treatment. Work with the school-age child to modify a school routine to better fit the child's educational and social schedule.	4. Autonomy and situational control are often lost as a result of limitations imposed by the condition or treatment. The child often cannot have a say in accepting a treatment or determining the type of treatment received but can be made to feel a part of the decision-making process and planning. Situational control and autonomy are positively connected to self-esteem. Choices are not always possible, but when they are, no matter how small, they should be offered. Goal setting and the reasons for achieving the goal will be facilitated if the goal has meaning for the child—not just for the family or health care personnel.
5. Encourage and provide opportunities for the child to engage in normal, age-appropriate ADL and self-care. Provide assistive devices, and educate the child in their proper use. Have equipment that must be kept in a school health office available when the child needs it.	5. Self-care encourages independence and gives the child an opportunity to practice and improve abilities.
6. During hospital stays, provide regular street clothes (when possible) and items from home for grooming, eating, and recreation.	6. Personal items promote normalization despite an illness or disability and help minimize disturbances in the child's usual routines. Normalization also maintains and maximizes the child's sense of control.
7. Provide age-appropriate activities both in and out of the hospital, and encourage the child to continue regular peer interaction (e.g., sports, school clubs or activities, church, social groups) to the degree allowed by the child's physical condition or treatment. Advise the family to schedule clinic visits, treatments, and hospitalizations (if possible), so as not to interfere with social, school, or church events. During hospitalizations, support and encourage the completion of schoolwork, as well as peer visits and activities (Fig. 36-3). Include well peers in special events during hospitalizations.	7. Ongoing social connections encourage development and maintenance of age-appropriate activities and developmental skills. Social involvement also contributes positively to the child's self-esteem and autonomy. Peers' misunderstandings and fear regarding the child's condition or the medical setting can be counteracted by the school nurse's or child life specialist's visits to the classroom.
8. Encourage the child to participate in the general or disease-specific support groups found at most pediatric hospitals. Encourage participation in support groups, but accept the child's decision not to join if that is his or her choice. Disease-specific camps (e.g., for children with renal, endocrine, neurologic, pulmonary, hematologic, or oncologic conditions), where all campers share the same problem, are also available.	8. Tremendous and valuable support can be derived from peers who are experiencing a similar medical situation. Support groups can provide acceptance and understanding not frequently found among those who are well. It may be appropriate to offer the strongest encouragement to access a support group when the child is initially diagnosed (i.e., when fears and concerns are likely to be increased). Because comfort levels and the type of support needed vary, however, such support groups may not be the best or only answer for every child.

Nursing Care Plan

The Child with a Chronic Condition in the Community Setting—cont'd

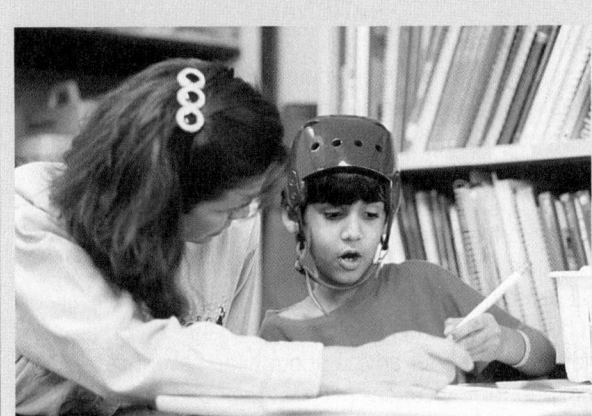

Figure 36-3 As more children with chronic conditions are living longer, more attend public school. Because these children are likely to be hospitalized frequently, however, hospitals often provide an area where teachers can help them keep up with their studies. (Courtesy Cook Children's Medical Center, Fort Worth, TX.)

Evaluation

- Does the child exhibit minimal developmental delays?
- Does the child exhibit age-appropriate social, physical, and cognitive interactions?
- Does the child perform age-appropriate ADL, as allowed by the existing disability?

Nursing Diagnosis

Disturbed Body Image related to actual or perceived physical differences or disabilities resulting from a chronic illness.

Expected Outcomes

The child will:

- Exhibit minimal disturbance of body image and will adapt to physical changes or disabilities caused by the illness, as evidenced by stating or demonstrating acceptance of change or loss and an ability to adjust to lifestyle changes.
- Experience grief resolution regarding the loss or change, as evidenced by returning to previous social involvement.

INTERVENTION	RATIONALE
1. Encourage and provide opportunities for the child to verbalize all feelings, positive and negative, regarding the illness, physical change, or disability. Emphasize the normality of negative emotions.	1. Negative emotions will occur. To assist the child progress to a positive, accepting attitude, these should be expressed and dealt with by the health care team and family in an accepting, nonjudgmental fashion.
2. Educate the child about physical changes or disability, expected limitations, or the progression of the disease, its duration, required assistive devices, and newly required self-care skills.	2. Misperceptions concerning physical changes or disability may hamper acquisition of a positive, accepting attitude; compliance with treatment; and the acquisition of new skills.
3. Encourage and assist the child to achieve as much independence as allowed by the physical change or disability. Provide specific suggestions to teachers and others in the community about how to facilitate the child's independence.	3. Independence in self-care promotes self-esteem and a sense of control. Communicating concrete suggestions for facilitating independence contributes to a more coordinated approach.
4. Provide constant reassurance about the child's self-worth and ability to be autonomous despite a physical change or disability. Teach the child and family the actual self-care skills necessitated by the physical change or disability.	4. An ongoing physical disability can cause poor self-esteem. It may also cause doubts regarding the child's ability to become and remain self-reliant and autonomous. These skills must be taught, encouraged, and supported.
5. Focus positively on the unchanged physical attributes of the child and the child's intact physical abilities. Teach and encourage the child, family, and others to do the same.	5. Achieving and maintaining a positive body image (with resulting increased self-esteem) is often difficult when physical changes have resulted from a condition, treatment, or use of an assistive device.

Continued

Nursing Care Plan

The Child with a Chronic Condition in the Community Setting—cont'd

INTERVENTION	RATIONALE
6. Assist the child to use aesthetic devices, such as wigs, special clothing, and makeup. Educate the child and family about more extensive measures, such as prosthetics and reconstructive surgery. Support any decision made about use of such measures.	6. Adults may consider physical changes, such as hair loss or scarring, to be minor when compared with limb loss or salvage, which results in disability. Children, however, often consider physical changes to be severe, resulting in negative emotions and poor self-esteem.
7. Teach and encourage positive, accepting attitudes about physical differences. Foster new ideas regarding what constitutes physical attractiveness. Advocate for legislation to assist children with chronic illness.	7. Minimizing or disguising physical changes is often necessary to foster a positive self-image. These adaptations may also be necessary to assist others to accept physical differences more easily. Many programs are available to help children adapt to physical changes. For instance, some offer advice about head coverings and makeup for the cancer patient (*Look Good, Feel Better,* a program of the American Cancer Society). Some provide fashion alternatives for those with braces or prosthetics. Disease-specific support groups provide information about available programs.
8. Refer the child or family to appropriate professionals to manage coping or adjustment difficulties requiring therapeutic intervention.	8. Some children experience serious problems, such as depression. Early intervention may lead to acceptance, adjustment, and resolution of such problems.

Evaluation

- Does the child openly verbalize feelings, both negative and positive, regarding the condition, physical changes, or disability?
- Does the child verbalize acceptance of the condition, physical changes, or disability?
- Does the child return to the previous social involvement?

Nursing Diagnosis

Interrupted Family Processes related to intermittent situational crisis of chronic illness.

Expected Outcomes

The child and family will:

- Experience normal family functioning, as evidenced by maintaining usual family routines, meeting developmental needs of all family members, and maintaining usual expectations for the ill child.
- Experience appropriate psychosocial adjustment, as evidenced by expressing feelings, identifying ways to cope effectively, and using appropriate support systems.

---

between sibling and ill child and may choose as complete involvement as possible. This may include the presence of siblings during the day and for overnight visits if allowed by the institution. Regardless of the type of involvement selected and the reasons behind it, the family's decision should be honored and supported.

When involvement that is more extensive is chosen, the nurse should ensure that the sibling has received appropriate education to decrease misunderstanding and fear. As with the ill child, medical play, therapeutic play, and therapeutic art are excellent means of educating, providing support, and alleviating fears and misunderstandings about the ill child's condition and medical treatment. This may also assist siblings to gain some understanding of their often intense and confusing emotional responses as well as how to express them in a healthy, appropriate manner.

Extensive sibling involvement may bring with it additional risks. The sibling may frequently be exposed to the ill child's intense physical and emotional experiences, which can certainly have emotional consequences for the sibling. Close attention from staff and family can help detect problems of this type if they occur. If problems become evident, appropriate team members, including nurses, physicians, child life specialists, clergy, and social workers, should provide support. As necessary, referrals can also be made to professional counseling services.

Nurses striving to teach, support, and include siblings in the hospital or clinic life of the ill child should collaborate with the child life specialist. This interaction can help the entire family discover, explore, and resolve feelings that might otherwise be problematic for both the ill child and the siblings.

Nursing Care Plan

The Child with a Chronic Condition in the Community Setting—cont'd

INTERVENTION	RATIONALE
1. Assist the family achieve a positive, realistic view of the child in relation to the condition by providing appropriate information. Describe ways the family can continue appropriate behavioral expectations for the ill child within the limits of the child's condition.	1. Education enables and encourages appropriate interaction with the health care team and compliance with treatment, in addition to decreasing fears and misconceptions.
2. Assist the family to identify fears and emotions pertaining to the child's illness. Emphasize that all feelings are normal and that appropriate verbalization is a positive and healthy part of coping.	2. Verbalization of feelings, with positive feedback, can help decrease stress and facilitate resolution of negative emotions.
3. Act as a role model for appropriate, accepting, positive attitudes and behaviors concerning the child.	3. Grief over the loss of a healthy child, discomfort with providing medical care, or a physical disability may hamper positive adjustment and acceptance. A positive role model may facilitate adjustment.
4. Refer the family or child to additional resources (e.g., social worker, clergy, professional counselor) when necessary (i.e., if problems are beyond the nurse's scope or if the family requests referral).	4. Situations requiring psychosocial assistance that is beyond the scope of nursing practice are not always indicators of family dysfunction requiring mental health intervention. When such intervention is indicated, however, early referral leads to a greater opportunity for positive outcomes.
5. Discuss with the family alternate approaches to maintaining usual routine.	5. By including some adaptations, families can maintain usual routines and meet the needs of all family members.

Evaluation

- Is the family able to maintain its usual routine and meet needs of all family members?
- Does the family treat the ill child as normally as possible to avoid overdependence?
- Do family members express their feelings? Has the family identified and utilized appropriate coping mechanisms, and are they using appropriate support systems?

The relationship between the ill child and sibling may be altered because of normal but unintentional feelings of resentment, jealousy, and competition as the ill child receives more attention. This change may be accentuated if the sibling spends extended time at the hospital, thus witnessing the extra attention given to the ill child. Siblings may experience guilt and shame about such feelings. The nursing staff, child life specialist, social worker, and chaplain can devote individual attention to the sibling separately from the ill child as a means of providing sibling support. The opportunity to verbalize emotions and interact with a caring, nonjudgmental individual may help siblings understand and accept the normality of their feelings. In addition, sibling support groups are a resource available at many hospitals.

The ill child often receives extra attention, including gifts, from family and friends during the course of the illness. Siblings may associate illness with such extra attention and gifts, subsequently experiencing real or imagined illnesses themselves as a bid for similar attention. An important aspect of sibling support is to encourage family and friends to also try to remember the sibling when they give gifts to the ill child. Remembering the siblings at special times, such as birthdays or special times of accomplishment, can also be helpful. Encouraging the parent to spend some time every day with each sibling is essential for maintaining emotionally positive relationships.

It is also important to maintain close contact with the sibling's school personnel and keep them up to date as to the current circumstances of the ill child. This can help personnel understand and support the sibling if behavioral issues are noted in school. It may also be helpful if increased absences are necessary because of problems with the ill child. Because the sibling's teacher and other personnel are generally not shared with the ill child, the sibling may turn more frequently to them for support than to members of the health care team. School personnel working with the sibling may need the same type of educational support as those working with the ill child. A school visit can be made and education provided to personnel as well as the sibling's peers and classmates. Family and members of the health care team determine the extent of information given to the children. As with school visits for the well child, education and support may best be provided by a nurse and child life specialist.

THE TERMINALLY ILL OR DYING CHILD

The Child's Concept of Death

An understanding of death and dying in relation to childhood is necessary when caring for the child approaching death. The established and accepted guidelines concerning children's concepts of death are based on the stages of growth and development. As Wass (1985) explains, these concepts correlate with age and cognition (Table 36-1). Intellectual, social, and psychologic life experiences will also affect a child's concept of death (Bowden, 1993).

Infants and Toddlers
Infants and toddlers view death in relation to the loss of a caretaker and the subsequent emptiness in their lives. They are also affected by the loss of comfort measures, as when they experience pain or cold. Consequently, time with primary caregivers is quite important. As they approach death, they often sense the severity of their condition through their parents' nonverbal communication. Children of this age may react to the dying process on the basis of the sadness, anger, and anxiety conveyed by their parents. Reactions will be expressed through crying, attachment to the primary caregiver, and separation anxiety.

Preschoolers
Preschoolers view death as a separation or departure and believe it to be only temporary. Death is also seen as reversible. Magical thinking and egocentricity at this age often lead to guilt and shame, because children may believe that their thoughts or actions caused the death. The child's first exposure to death frequently involves a dead animal, such as an insect, bird, or pet.

Preschoolers facing an impending death frequently view their condition as punishment for behaviors or thoughts. They respond with guilt, anger, sadness, and fear. Their self-imposed guilt may cause them to believe that others, including parents, see them as "bad" and are angry with them. Feelings are kept inside, and children this age may withdraw from everyone, including those whom they love and on whom they depend. Their anger at those they care about and the intensity of that anger frightens them. Great patience and understanding are required of their parents and nurses, particularly when emotions are labile and subject to frequent, acute changes. Indeed, all children feel greater security when adults maintain discipline and suitable, customary limits, especially when dying children are experiencing multiple changes and discrepancies in their daily life.

School-Age Children
By the school-age years, death begins to be understood as a sad and irreversible event, yet it still may be considered inevitable only for adults. By the age of 10 years or so, children begin to understand that they too can die. Some associated feelings of guilt often persist for school-age children. They may continue to believe that thoughts or actions can cause death or that death serves as a punishment for wrongdoing.

The school-age child has increased cognition and other resources necessary to cope with the dying process. However, these same abilities may lead to additional questions and fears. School-age children may wonder why they are ill and must die so young. Fear about the process of dying and what follows may also arise. Even in children who have a foundation of faith and spiritual beliefs, this fear may persist because they do not have a concrete knowledge of what it is like after a person dies. They may also fear being without the love and support of the parents they have always known. Moreover, school-age children may feel vulnerable and doubt their ability to cope with the knowledge of their impending death as well as the experience itself.

Adolescents
Most adolescents have a fully developed understanding of death as inevitable and irreversible. Because of an increasingly independent frame of reference, however, many adolescents view death as a distant event and may consider themselves invulnerable to death. Although adolescents may understand death and dying, they do not necessarily have an emotional acceptance. Adolescents who are attempting to separate from their parents often test and break rules as they strive for independence. This process may cause guilt for the dying child, especially when contemplating the spiritual aspects of life and death.

Adolescents may become isolated from their peers as a result of an illness. The terminal illness or disability of a peer

TABLE **36-1** The Child's Concept of Death		
Age	**Cognitive Stage**	**Concept**
Infancy and toddlerhood (0-2 yr)	Sensorimotor	Death as loss of the caretaker
Early childhood (2-7 yr)	Preoperational	Death as a reversible and temporary separation
Middle childhood (school-age; 7-12 yr)	Concrete operations	Death as sad and irreversible but not necessarily inevitable
Adolescence (12+ yr)	Formal operations	Death as inevitable and irreversible but often a distant event

forces adolescents to abruptly, unwillingly face and question their own mortality and wholeness. Discomfort with this possibility is often the cause of infrequent visits or a total lack of visits, even from close friends. Adolescents may also become isolated from caring adults, family, and staff because of feeling that adults do not understand them. Consequently, many feel lonesome and fear that they will die without the love and support that they need and desire. Realizing that they face death when their lives are just beginning, many adolescents respond with anger and sadness, particularly when they consider the adult experiences that will be denied them. This may contribute to the onset of depression.

Responses to Death and Dying

The process of dying, as well as the actual death of a child, is a unique and complex situation. The responses of all persons involved—child, family, staff—will be affected by various factors. These include personal and spiritual beliefs, previous experiences with illness and death, and experiences during the current illness and dying process. An individual's progression through the stages of grief and death is also important, as is the relationship with the dying child. At any given time, the child, parents, and siblings may all be experiencing a different stage of grief and expressing that grief in very different ways.

The Child's Response

A child who is dying wants to feel safe and does not want to be alone or in pain. These concerns are frequently more intense and problematic with school-age children and adolescents. The child's responses to death and dying will be multiple and varied, not always fully correlating with the child's chronologic growth, development, and cognition. The frequently traumatizing experiences of a chronic condition and its treatment tend to make children more mature and wise beyond their years. In addition, children with a terminal illness may reach a point where they consider their illness and treatment worse than death. Relief is frequently evident as the dying child works through the five stages of grief and dying. The responses and actions of the dying child may also be affected by the behaviors and feelings of those around them, particularly family and staff.

The child's response to dying and the resulting actions are often more precocious than would be expected, particularly among preschool children. Family or staff members often consider precocious actions and those of a spiritual nature to be inappropriate or unbelievable. They may possibly attribute these responses to physical alterations, such as a low hemoglobin level, altered neurologic status, or medications, such as analgesics or sedatives.

Spiritual beliefs may influence the child and be reflected in conversation and actions. Children may speak of seeing or even interacting with angels or the Higher Being recognized by their specific faith. They may also speak of going to heaven to be with the angels or other spiritual beings. In addition, children may speak of going to play or be with another child or relative who has already died. This type of conversation may take place anywhere from several weeks to days or hours before death, with children actually giving specifics as to when they will see or be with deceased individuals. Such behaviors are commonly referred to as *nearing death awareness*.

Dying children often experience a heightened sense of understanding and awareness, particularly as death nears. Many know specifically when they will die. As with adults, death often occurs after children have successfully achieved closure of some type. Closure may be a special event in their life or that of a loved one, such as a graduation, holiday, or birthday. Frequently, closure also involves resolution of unfinished business, such as interacting with a loved one who has been absent or apologizing for things they have said or done.

One concept of pediatric death that families may have difficulty understanding and accepting is "allowing" their child to die. As noted by Kübler-Ross (1983), children are afraid not of death but of abandonment. Children who are enveloped by hope, joy, and love may sustain their grasp on life. For most children, allowing them to die means giving the child permission to die. A predominant issue of childhood is that children should obey their parents. This assumption is based on the knowledge that parents know best and provide guidance for their child to do what is safe and correct. A child's death may not occur as smoothly until parents tell the child it is all right to die.

Accordingly, most children, particularly those who are younger, need verbal "permission" to die, as well as reassurance that it is safe to do so. Such reassurance should include a description of what and whom to expect as they die and in the time afterward. Children may also need reassurance that the family, friends, and loved ones who are left behind will grieve yet will be all right and that they will take care of each other. Equally important to children of all ages is the knowledge that loved ones will remember them always.

The Parents' Response

When a child is initially diagnosed with any condition that is life threatening, every parent faces and begins to cope with the *possibility* of the child's death. When they are informed that nothing more can be done medically, parents face the *reality* of their child's death. The stages of grief associated with the child's illness must now be experienced in relation to the child's death. Acceptance does not always occur. Some parents may find it difficult or unacceptable to discontinue treatment. They may choose to continue treatment of a curative rather than a palliative nature. Such a choice, however, does not always indicate denial. It may simply represent a belief system based on spiritual or personal convictions. Legally, emotionally, and psychosocially, the family's decision must be upheld and supported by members of the health care team.

Parents will exhibit the need to talk about their child and the experience of their child's illness and death. They talk to assimilate the experience, but more important, they talk to remember their child.

When a chronic condition has extended over time, the parents' initial reaction to their child's death is often relief that the child is no longer suffering and that the uncertainty of their situation has ended. Many times, this relief and feeling of peace may begin before death, when it is known to be inevitable and imminent. Such relief may evoke feelings of guilt. Support and explanations as to the normalcy of feeling relief may be necessary for parents. This might include a reminder that their feelings include

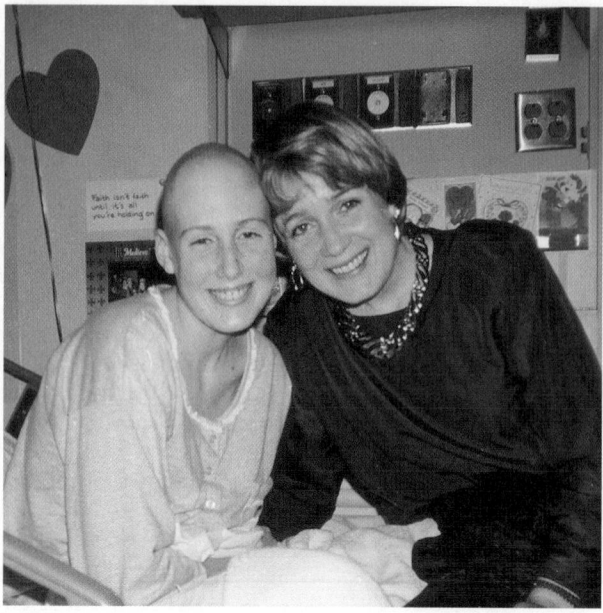

Figure 36-4 The family of the child with a terminal condition needs compassion and support from the nurse. Nursing care includes not only physical care but also support of the family's caregiving and assistance with the grieving process. (Courtesy Gwen Martin, Fort Worth, TX.)

relief that their child is no longer experiencing the illness along with the subsequent physical and emotional suffering. Relief at the death is followed by numbness, intense sadness, and a sense of profound loss and emptiness. The grief of a child's grandparent is similar to that of the parents yet, in a different manner, even greater. Grandparents must not only grieve for themselves at the loss of their grandchild. They also grieve for *their own child*, the parent who has experienced the death of a child.

The Siblings' Response

As with their responses to the illness itself, siblings' responses to death and dying, as well as their progression through the stages of grief, vary according to age and development. Although children usually experience all five stages of grief and dying, these may not necessarily occur in the given sequence. Frequently, children move between the stages in a seemingly random fashion, often experiencing a stage several times. This process is an appropriate coping mechanism for children's cognitive and developmental needs and abilities. Issues dealt with successfully earlier in the illness, such as concern over having caused the illness or death, may resurface. Without appropriate guidance and assistance, these issues may persist. Siblings may experience other emotions, many of which are the same as those experienced by their parents. In relation to their level of cognition and development, however, they may not be as well equipped to understand, to cope, and to work their way through the grieving process as smoothly and successfully.

Unresolved grief contributes to many problems in adult life. Because children work through the grieving process differently from adults, they often need assistance to complete the process. Such assistance does not necessarily mean professional counseling. Many grief support centers are now available that provide assistance for the child who has experienced the death of a loved one, including a sibling.

The most important aspect of providing support for the grieving child is to acknowledge that the loss of a sibling is just as *significant* as the parents' loss of their child. It is common practice for the health care team to send sympathy cards and other correspondence to parents after their child's death. This gesture can be taken an important step further by also addressing cards, phone calls, and other statements of sympathy to siblings individually. Such validation of their grief can be a first and important step in their successful navigation of the grieving process.

Caring for the Dying Child

Despite medical advances and current technology, many chronic disorders ultimately terminate in death. Providing nursing care to the child with a fatal illness who is nearing death as well as to family members requires a heightened level of understanding, compassion, and support. A family's coping abilities are often tested beyond measure. Nursing care includes assisting the family to withstand the tremendous pressures and to meet the emotional demands of the situation (Fig. 36-4).

Professional Boundaries

Caring for dying children involves certain potential stressors for all involved, including the nurses. An important aspect of self-care is for nurses to recognize and acknowledge such stressors for themselves. Caring for the child who is approaching death can be very rewarding, but it may also severely test the nurse's coping skills. Compassion is a must, but also essential are awareness and maintenance of professional boundaries. These boundaries are necessary for the nurse to provide clinically sound, compassionate care while maintaining emotional, physical, and spiritual health. To provide professional care and support, nurses must understand and accept their own feelings and beliefs about death. Unresolved difficulties may interfere with appropriate nursing care. Methods to provide good self-care and resolve emotional or spiritual difficulties might include meeting with the hospital pastoral care team or a personal spiritual counselor. Nursing support groups mediated by a member of the clergy, social worker, or counselor may also be helpful. Taking part in patient care conferences or ethics committee meetings may be useful to understand patient care decisions that the nurse does not understand or possibly does not support. This could serve to reassure the nurse that the family has had appropriate education and support in making difficult decisions. It also provides nurses with education and support as they care for the child in the midst of the decision-making process.

Communication

Staff and family must be aware of the dying child's communication needs and patterns. Such awareness requires openness and acceptance on the part of all involved. Nurses and parents should assure the child that they will not abandon or leave the child alone and that loved ones will always be present. Children should consistently be reassured that the illness and approaching death are not the result of anything they have said or done or something they did not say or do.

BOX 36-3
Resources on Death and Dying for Families and Health Professionals

INTERNET RESOURCES

Compassionate Friends (U.S.)—www.compassionatefriends.org—has brochures for parents and siblings in both English and Spanish. There are discussion support groups and chat rooms for siblings.

Baby Steps (Canada)—www.babysteps.com—has an extensive book list, sharing rooms, and grieving rooms.

BOOK SELECTIONS FOR CHILDREN

Alley, R.W. (1998). *Sad isn't bad.* St. Meinrad, IN: Abbey Press.

Buscaglia, L. (2002). *The fall of Freddie the leaf: 20th anniversary edition.* Thorofare, NJ: Slack Incorporated. (All ages)

Fitzgerald, H. (2000). *A guide for teenagers and their friends.* New York: Simon & Shuster. (Teens)

Simon, J. (2001). *This book is for all kids, but especially my sister Libby. Libby died.* Kansas City, MO: Andrews McMeel. (Preschool)

BOOK SELECTIONS FOR ADULTS

Coloroso, B. (2000). *Parenting through crisis: Helping kids in times of loss, grief, and change.* New York: Harper Collins.

Grollman, E.A. (1990). *Talking about death.* Boston: Beacon Press.

Ilse, S., & Leininger, L. (1985). *Grieving grandparents.* Maple Plain, MN: Wintergreen Press.

Rothman, J.C. (1997). *The bereaved parent's survival guide.* New York: Continuum Publishing.

BOOK SELECTIONS FOR NURSES

D'Avanzo, C., & Geissler, E. (2002). *Pocket guide to cultural assessment* (3rd ed.). St. Louis: Mosby.

Lipson, J., Dibble, S., & Miniarik, P. (1996). *Culture and nursing care: A pocket guide.* San Francisco, CA: University of California, San Francisco, School of Nursing.

Purnell, L., & Paulanka, B. (2003). *Transcultural health care: A culturally competent approach* (2nd ed.). Philadelphia: Davis.

Children must also be assured that none of their emotions and actions are wrong and that they are always loved and accepted. Children, parents, and siblings need assistance to understand their different, intense emotions, especially emotions such as anger and guilt, which are often perceived negatively. Parents, in particular, need opportunities away from the child to express their grief and anger. This opportunity helps minimize or prevent the child from feeling responsible for the parents' emotions. It also contributes to an environment that is as soothing, comfortable, and stress-free as possible, where parents can have uninterrupted time with their child and the opportunity to provide whatever level of physical care they wish to assume.

Regardless of age, most dying children will follow the rules and patterns of communication set by those closest to them. As death approaches, communication between child and family can decline in both extent and effectiveness. The nurse should take into account how communication was handled at previously stressful times, such as the time of diagnosis, relapse, or periods of disease exacerbation. Generally, what has been utilized in the past will continue to be effective during the dying process. The nurse should avoid blanket assumptions as to what will be the most appropriate or effective communication techniques for the family. Each circumstance should be carefully evaluated to assist the child and family experience the most effective, comfortable communication possible.

The most common issue that arises in relation to a child's impending death is whether to inform the child of the prognosis. The needs of the child, parents, and staff frequently conflict, but all must be considered, with the ill child's needs taking precedence. The suggested approach is to adopt a policy that allows the child to maintain open awareness and communication with those who choose to do so and are comfortable doing so. Such open acknowledgment makes it possible to meet children's need for someone to know and to acknowledge that they are dying. Simultaneously, it allows mutual pretense and decreased communication with those who prefer that approach. This flexible system has been found to be effective and is prevalent among many dying children and their caregivers.

Despite such flexibility, nurses may be caught between children who wish to talk about their death and parents who would forbid any such conversation. As the caregiver and primary advocate, the nurse should first meet the child's needs. Any skirting of the issues or dishonesty with the child may destroy the nurse-client relationship, possibly denying the child a much-needed source of comfort and support. The child is also likely to distrust the nurse as a result of such actions. This could be extremely detrimental in relation to the child's trust in the nurse's actions, especially giving medications for pain and symptom management. Nurses can inform the parents that they will not initiate any discussion with the child but that they need and intend to respond openly and honestly if and when the child initiates such a discussion. This policy allows nurses both to respect the wishes of the parents and to provide assistance or support when needed by the child.

Words are not always necessary to provide assistance and support. Presence—simply sitting with the child—or a light touch, such as holding a hand, may be all the child needs. The silence itself may be a therapeutic intervention, or it may help open the door for desired verbal communication.

The Family's Beliefs and Practices

To support parents appropriately during the difficult time surrounding the death of their child, nursing care must impart consistent respect and acceptance. This effort must occur regardless of any differences between the spiritual or cultural beliefs and practices of the family and those of the nurse (see Box 36-3 and Chapter 3).

The nurse will encounter different beliefs and practices surrounding death and the grieving process. These practices may include wearing prayer cloths; the laying on of hands; holy water or oil; viewing religious pictures, icons, or other objects; extemporaneous prayer gatherings; or the preparation and serving of certain foods. Some practices may be troublesome to deal with because of concern over whether they are in the best interest of the child or unsafe emotionally or physically. Each situation should be dealt with individually, carefully weighing the potential emotional or spiritual benefits against proven safety issues.

Many parents have difficulty moving from active treatment with a goal of cure to palliative care only. Palliative care promotes comfort and quality of life as opposed to cure. Parents' last-ditch attempts at cure may include the use of unproven medications or treatments, such as those used in other countries. Although difficult to justify in our world of U.S. Food and Drug Administration (FDA)–approved medical care, many of these attempts are not physically harmful to the child. Indeed, they may be emotionally beneficial to both parent and child, for such efforts affirm that everything possible was tried, a notion that may be very important to child and family. These efforts may also instill hope, which should not be taken from the child or parents under any circumstances. At times, however, such medication or treatment may be harmful to the child, as with painful intramuscular injections or treatments that may cause bleeding in a child with a low platelet count. In such instances, the staff may decide not to allow administration of the treatment. The decision and the rationale for it must be explained compassionately yet firmly, always noting that the decision was made in the best interest of the child.

Another area where the family's beliefs and practices as well as strong emotions come into play is deciding about a do-not-resuscitate (DNR) order. A DNR order means there is no initiation of cardiopulmonary resuscitation (CPR) or other interventions designed to initiate heartbeat and respiration after a cardiopulmonary arrest. Even in the face of acknowledging their child's impending death, many families experience a great deal of difficulty and uncertainty in relation to not having their child resuscitated. They may also change their mind several times regarding the DNR. Assisting families at this time includes educating them as to their choices, discussing their feelings about the matter, and exploring their wishes for their child. It may be helpful to remind parents that DNR does not mean withholding treatment *while the child is alive*. Rather, it involves not initiating treatment *after the child has died*. Parents are reminded that if a DNR order is chosen, they may change their mind and revoke the order at any time. Most important, they are continually reassured that the child's comfort remains the number-one priority, regardless of the DNR status.

Often, parents make treatment decisions that do not offer any hope of increased comfort and quality of life and are not based on cultural or spiritual beliefs. These decisions often do not seem to be in the best interest of the child. For instance, parents may refuse pain medication for their child because they feel the child will be more alert. They may request to continue treatments that are traumatic and offer no hope of long-term survival. The issue of pain medication may be more easily resolved than the question as to whether treatments should be continued or extraordinary means should be used to keep the child alive. These situations may cause emotional, spiritual, and professional distress for the nurse, particularly if the action conflicts with the nurse's beliefs and seems useless for the child. To provide the necessary appropriate care, the nurse must cope

with and resolve these situations. If unable to do so, the nurse should be given the option of not participating in the child's care. As mentioned, resolution of emotional, spiritual, or moral difficulties might include meeting with the hospital pastoral care team or a personal spiritual counselor. Nursing support groups mediated by a member of the clergy, social worker, or counselor may also be helpful. Taking part in patient care conferences or ethics committee meetings may be useful to understand patient care decisions that the nurse does not understand or possibly support. This could serve to reassure the nurse that the family has had appropriate education and support in making difficult decisions. It also provides the nurse with education and support when caring for the child in the midst of the decision-making process.

Pain Control

For all involved—child, family, staff—the most troubling and emotional issue relating to the dying child is usually pain control. The nurse educates the child and family regarding pain control and then provides constant, consistent reassurance that everything possible and appropriate will be done to guarantee the child's continued comfort. Families and older children may express concerns about addiction in the same breath as concerns that pain relief will not be adequate. Without belittling the feelings of those involved, the nurse should reassure the family that their concerns regarding addiction are unfounded in the current situation.

Child and family are reminded that when there is a physical reason and need for pain medication, such as with a terminal condition, addiction does not and will not occur. Questions regarding increasing doses of narcotics and addiction may arise just as frequently in the care of children as they do in the care of adults. The child and family should be informed that the pain associated with terminal conditions might escalate acutely and frequently, with a corresponding decrease in the child's response to narcotics. The nurse should also emphasize that any necessary increase in medication dosage or change in regimen will always occur in response to escalating pain. The child and family must always know and believe that pain will be handled in a manner that provides comfort as well as the optimal environment for meeting their psychosocial and spiritual needs. (For further information and discussion of pain control for children, see Chapter 39.) Education as to appropriate pain management, including myths and realities (see Chapter 39), should begin whenever pain medications are first used during the illness. Doing so can help ensure that education and information the family has already been given is simply being reinforced during the terminal phase of the illness.

Hospice Care

For many terminally ill children and their families, being outside the hospital environment, in either a home hospice program or at an inpatient hospice facility, may be the preferred choice for meeting their various needs during the dying process. *Hospice care* is a specialized, comprehensive system of care that provides support and assistance to the dying and their families in the last phase of a terminal illness. This phase is generally the last 6 months of a person's life.

The use of hospice care for children, either in a home setting or in an inpatient setting, is increasing. In part, this increase is the result of the wide range of support services offered by hospice programs. Although specialized nursing and physician support is the primary reason hospice care is feasible, it is only one component of the array of services available through a comprehensive hospice program. These include other team members: social workers, chaplains, home health aides, and volunteers. The physical support services include pharmacy prescriptions, supplies, and medical equipment that are delivered for use in the home. In general, death occurs peacefully for children, but home or an inpatient hospice facility may provide a more natural, comfortable, and relaxed backdrop than the traditional hospital setting. At home, children can have family, pets, friends, and the comfort of their own rooms and possessions close at hand. Inpatient hospice care may be provided in a freestanding setting or as a separate unit within an acute care setting. Families may choose an inpatient hospice for a variety of reasons:

- Physical care requirements and emotional burdens are too great for family caregivers to manage.
- The physical symptoms may require aggressive management, or the child may experience pain requiring intensive and complex medication control.
- The home may not be conducive to adaptations needed for the child's care (e.g., hospital bed, oxygen equipment, a private room).

Brief periods of inpatient hospice care may also be used to meet a family's respite care needs, providing an environment that is less threatening and more homelike than that available in a regular acute care setting.

Hospice care should always be offered to families, along with the information necessary for making an educated choice. Some families may choose home-based hospice care but later admit the child to a hospital during the final hours or days of life. This choice, which always remains available to families, may be based on fears about pain control, adequate physical care of the child, or handling the emotional aspect of a death at home. Parents may be particularly anxious as to how successfully they or siblings will cope with living in their home once a death has occurred there. This may lead to parents choosing hospitalization, even when their child prefers to die at home. It is beneficial for the health care team and family to discuss these fears early in the hospice experience. This will permit ample time to explore such fears and emotions, ideally leading to a choice that is acceptable and comfortable for child, siblings, and parents. In spite of such discussions, however, families may still elect hospitalization when death nears. The family's choices must be accepted and supported, regardless of the type or frequency of changes in decision making. Such changes may occur more frequently than anticipated, depending on the changing physical and emotional status of child and family.

The Dying Process and the Time of Death

The care needs of the dying child are much like those of the chronically or seriously ill child. Much of the care is directed by the physical, emotional, and spiritual needs of the child and family. The goal of nursing care is to provide comfortable, peaceful time for the child and family with minimal disruptions. Whether the death is occurring at home, in the hospital, or on an inpatient hospice unit, the child's room should be secluded, comfortable, and quiet. This type of sur-

roundings contributes significantly toward creating a meaningful time for the child and family.

Privacy for the Child and Family. Disruptions by staff and possibly even by friends or extended family should be discouraged and minimized to the extent desired by the child and family. Often, members of the immediate family will request private time with the dying child. Occasionally, this request may cause others, such as grandparents, to become distraught or to insist on spending time with the child. In a hospital or inpatient hospice setting, this response is less difficult to handle. In such an environment, the nurse can more easily treat the matter as a request that the nurse is appropriately responsible to enforce. The nurse then saves the family the responsibility of being the "bad guy." In the home environment, the nurse has no such authority yet still remains an advocate for child and family. Therefore the nurse attempts to communicate the family's wishes to others and should also work to educate others about the importance of meeting such wishes and needs for privacy.

Regardless of whether privacy is requested for emotional or spiritual needs, privacy is very important for physical reasons. The dying child's endurance will be greatly diminished, with increased needs for daytime napping and extended nighttime sleep. The child may also experience difficulties with sleep, such as sleep deprivation, frequent wakefulness, or nightmares. Privacy and careful control of the number and frequency of visitors will help ensure as much normalcy and quality in sleep as possible. The knowledge that loved ones are present or close by is also helpful. In the home or inpatient hospice setting, where privacy may not be as great a problem, open doors or an intercom system (e.g., a baby monitor) can help reassure the child that loved ones are always available.

Changes in Family Routines. The availability of loved ones becomes more important to the dying child, who will experience increasingly frequent and prolonged periods of sleep. Regardless of the duration—moments, minutes, or hours—intervals spent with the child can become treasured memories. The nurse should therefore facilitate family contact as much as possible. Special care must be taken to explain to siblings the reasons for rearranging life around the ill child's wakeful times. Siblings must also be allowed to have their time with the ill child. Most important, their feelings should be explored and emotional support provided.

Family Concerns About Oral Intake. The entire family often needs heightened emotional support with regard to nutrition and oral intake for the dying child. Disinterest in eating and drinking is a normal part of the dying process, yet diminishing nutritional needs can be one of the most difficult aspects of dying with which families must cope. Parents and siblings may worry that the child will starve to death and that hunger or thirst will add to other physical discomforts.

The nurse should remind the family that at a point before death—often days before or (rarely) weeks before—intake will cease as the child loses the ability to swallow. The family needs enhanced emotional support and reminders that lack of oral intake does not cause added discomfort for the dying child, even when it continues for an extended time. The family may also need to be educated that fluids may actually cause discomfort for the child, by increasing lung secretions. Such secretions can necessitate suctions, and the sounds of wet or rattling respirations can be emotionally distressing to the family. When kidney function is declining during the dying process, the child may also retain fluids. This can make the child uncomfortable and be visually distressing.

Fluids and Oral Care. Although the lack of oral intake is normal and contributes to the child's comfort, there are some important nursing implications in caring for the child. If the child has a dry mouth and thirst, small amounts of ice chips or fluids can be given when desired and requested by the child. It is important to note that thirst is usually experienced only minimally. It is almost unheard of to have children experiencing a degree of thirst that cannot be satisfied by the amount of fluid they are able to swallow.

In light of decreased swallowing function and the possibility of aspiration, water would appear to be the best choice. Given the terminal situation, however, physical and emotional comfort can be enhanced by meeting the child's requests. Many children continue to drink their favorite fluid, such as milk or root beer, until the time of death. A lack of strength or coordination may make drinking from a glass or straw difficult. In such cases, fluids can be introduced into the child's mouth easily and without spilling, using a medicine dropper or small syringe. A catheter-tip syringe may be an even better choice, because the child may find it easier to close the mouth around the syringe's wide opening and long tip, although care must be taken with such a wide opening not to deliver too much fluid and cause choking. Many older children also find it easy to drink from the "sippy cups" used to assist toddlers as they first learn to drink. These cups usually have easy-to-grip handles, a secure lid, and a small spout that requires little strength for drinking. Drinking from a cup may also give the child a small sense of independence and control, which are often lost in the process of dying.

If oral discomfort occurs because of lack of fluids, several interventions may prove useful and appropriate. Good oral care will help minimize any discomfort. Sponge swabs can be used to clean the lips and mouth, but lemon and glycerin swabs should be avoided because of the drying effect from the alcohol content. Dryness can be further minimized through the use of artificial saliva preparations, which can be swished if the child is able and then swallowed or spit out. These preparations may also be applied with the sponge swabs, along with agents to reduce inflammation or pain. Almost any type of lip balm or petroleum jelly products can be applied to dry, chapped lips. An important educational point will be to avoid lip products that have alcohol or fragrance, because these might be irritating if open areas are on the lips.

Good oral care will help minimize mouth odor and unsightliness, which may be distressing to the child and family. Providing oral care may also give the family a feeling of usefulness and an opportunity for much-needed physical contact with the child. Provision of physical care should therefore be encouraged in the amounts desired by family members and for as long as they wish, regardless of whether the child is alert enough to notice.

Responsiveness and Communication. A child's degree of awareness or wakefulness until the time of death is frequently an overwhelming concern for family members. This aspect of dying varies from person to person, in both children and adults. Many children will experience a "good" period of time (either a few hours or an entire day) immediately before they die. This time may involve more strength than seen recently, more wakefulness, or more interest in family life around them. Such periods may cause family members to experience inappropriate hope for recovery. It is important, therefore, to prepare and educate families about the possibility of this oc-

currence. The child may become unresponsive in the days or hours before death or may be intermittently responsive until the actual moment of death. The nurse should explain the possible variations to family members and remind them that hearing is the last sense to cease before death. For this reason, verbal communication and physical touch should be encouraged until death occurs, and even after as desired by the family.

Occasionally, personal fears or beliefs make such actions difficult. This may simply reflect a different comfort level in relation to the dying process, a different need for personal space, or different expression of emotions. The absence of either verbal communication or physical touch may not necessarily be emotionally harmful to either child or family. The nurse, however, should investigate the cause and offer assistance only when lack of interaction indicates a negative effect. No matter what the type or level of touch and communication, family members should be reassured that a heightened awareness of the presence of loved ones is common for a dying individual, regardless of age. This information may impart an added sense of comfort and security.

Indicators of Imminent Death. Security and comfort may also come from knowing that reliable physical indicators usually signal the time when death is imminent. This phase may last a few hours or a few days. The heart rate increases, with a concomitant decrease in the strength and quality of peripheral pulses. Blood pressure also decreases. Pulses and blood pressure may become difficult or impossible to palpate, a state that can last for hours. Cardiac changes generally occur before respiratory changes but not always. Even if mild respiratory changes occur without significant cardiac changes, the nurse should remember how quickly and acutely a cardiac transition could occur. In some cases, apparently innocuous respiratory variations, with normal heart rate and blood pressure, have been followed by death in less than 30 minutes.

Family members more readily notice respiratory changes, which usually follow a typical pattern that is both visible and audible. The force of the respiratory effort may decline, as evidenced by rapid, shallow respirations. An increased work of breathing, along with apnea, may also be evident. The respiratory picture may fluctuate between the two states. Respirations may cease after rapid, increasingly shallow breaths. Cessation may occur after a period of Cheyne-Stokes respirations. This is a cyclic period of slowing respirations with apnea, followed by a speeding up to peak, and then slowing and becoming apneic again. Such respirations are often referred to as *agonal*. This description may impart the belief that they are painful, and thus the term should be avoided around family members.

Respirations may become more audible and may be accompanied by an expiratory sigh, which often resembles moaning and may alarm family members because the sound seems to signal pain. If the child is otherwise without verbal or physical indications of pain, the family should be reassured that the child's pain level is well controlled. The nurse can reinforce this information by educating the family as to the cause of the sounds and noting their correlation with each breath. If a strong belief continues that the child is in pain, then pain medications should be given.

All these variations in respiratory patterns will result in either hypoxia or hypercapnia. If hypoxic agitation occurs, it is treated with oxygen, morphine, or both. The morphine may be given intravenously (IV) if there is such access, or a concentrated liquid form may be given sublingually. Both measures provide physical comfort for the child and emotional comfort for the family. If the nurse is uncertain whether the agitation results from hypoxia or pain, the child should be treated for pain as well. A rising carbon dioxide level may actually contribute to a peaceful and comfortable death through its sedative and analgesic qualities. Explaining this information may give the family an additional sense of comfort.

Continuing respiratory and cardiac changes may lead to cool extremities and cyanosis. These effects most often begin in the lower extremities and progress upward to the face. All these changes, although potentially distressing, are usually well handled by the family with adequate preparation and education.

Potentially most distressing is the noisy breathing caused by the rattling secretions in the upper airway. This rattling—often called the *death rattle*—occurs when the child has lost the strength and ability to clear airway secretions. Even with preparation, this sound can be extremely difficult for the family.

Pharyngeal suctioning can be helpful but may need to be done frequently and can be a source of discomfort for the child. Medications with a drying effect, such as diphenhydramine or scopolamine, are used to decrease the secretions. Until a prescribed medication takes effect, the child can be positioned on the side to facilitate drainage of the secretions. A cloth should be placed appropriately and the family prepared to expect secretions draining from the mouth. The child is very rarely aware of this respiratory occurrence, so the focus of care should be symptom management to ensure the emotional comfort of the family. When respirations have ceased, a short delay may occur before the heart stops beating. There may also be a final gasping noise after the respirations and heartbeat have stopped. Reassure the family that this sound is normal and not painful.

The Family After Death. After death has occurred, family members should have the opportunity to spend as much time with the child as they desire. They might want to spend time with their child before the body is cleaned. This should not be a problem, although it might be preferable to finish body preparation and cleaning first because of the drainage, bleeding, and spontaneous elimination of body wastes that often occur at the time of death. Before the body is bathed, families often appreciate the opportunity to make hand and foot prints or cut a lock of hair as a remembrance of the child. Family members should be invited to assist in the bathing if they so desire. This final act of physical care may be a special means of closure.

Frequently, siblings or other children are interested in this procedure. Adults may find such interest distressing, even if they themselves do not wish to participate. Encourage the family to allow the other children to participate, emphasizing that it may facilitate closure, as well as correct or prevent fears and misconceptions about death or the deceased child. The nurse should respect whatever decisions are made and offer an explanation as to what the care will involve, even if the family chooses not to participate. There may be certain times when the family's time with the child or ability to participate in after-death care may be limited, such as if an autopsy is to be performed. This does occur even in the case of a terminal condition, perhaps to learn from the child's condition, such as when the body has been donated for medical research. When this is the case, families should be given the exact information before death as to how much time they will have as well as how much involvement in after-death care will be possible.

The nurse should inform the family that the child can go to the funeral home either in a hospital gown or in personal clothes and should reassure the family that the clothes will be returned after the child is dressed for burial. If the family will not be participating in postmortem care, the period just after death is a good time to choose clothing and a personal item, such as a blanket or toy. These items will also be returned. Sibling participation in this process is another good closure activity. As family members prepare to hold the deceased child, the nurse reminds them that physical change after death may occur very quickly. Changes include cooling of the body, cyanosis or paleness, and stiffening. The nurse attempts to prevent further drainage of any body fluids, particularly if family members will be holding the child. The nurse prepares the family emotionally and provides towels if preventive measures are not possible or are ineffective.

The nurse should allow privacy for the family, promising to be close by and to return as needed or desired. The nurse always offers the support of clergy, even if there has been no such involvement previously. If personal clergy has not been identified or is not available, the nurse reminds the family of the availability of hospital or hospice personnel. If a funeral home has not been chosen, clergy and social services personnel are good sources for assistance.

The Nurse's Response to the Dying Child

Not all health care providers cope well with the reality of death. This limitation may hold serious implications for the nurse who chooses to work in an area where death is common. Caring for dying children and their families can be stressful and emotionally demanding. Even the nurse who works closely and frequently with dying children is not immune to the pressures and emotional responses experienced in such an environment. The demands of chronic or terminal illness may require increased emotional and psychosocial strength, as well as clinical expertise.

The nurse's response to the dying process and death of a child will correlate to a certain degree with the stages of grief and dying. The nurse who has become more accustomed to the reality and frequency of death may not experience each stage. Length of treatment and personal affinity often cause the nurse

---

! CRITICAL TO REMEMBER

Nursing Care for the Dying Child and the Child's Family

- The nurse should be available to assist both the dying child and the family but must not impose personal beliefs and expectations on either the child or the family members.
- The siblings of a dying child need time and attention. They too will experience grief and will need to resolve their feelings.
- Most family members need to talk about the experience of illness and death. Open communication helps support family resilience and helps family members remember the child after death.
- Caring for the dying child includes adequate pain control, oral care, ensuring privacy, and providing information on the signs of imminent death and what to expect in the immediate postmortem period.
- After death occurs, family members should have as much time as they desire with the child.

Nursing Care Plan

The Terminally Ill or Dying Child

FOCUSED ASSESSMENT

Nursing care of the dying child and the family is based on a complex set of issues. Circumstances affecting the child, parents, and siblings must be assessed and considered. Some of these circumstances include the family relationship to and involvement with the child; the child's cognition, developmental stage, and previous experiences with illness and death; and the family's and child's experiences during the current illness. The nurse also explores the individual's progression through the stages of grief and dying. Children and their families may have experienced these stages in relation to the grief caused by a chronic illness; now they must experience them in relation to the impending death.

Anxiety can negatively affect the child physically, exacerbating pain or bringing on other physical symptoms, such as dyspnea. Negative psychosocial effects may also exist for both the child and the family. Anxiety and concerns exhibited during the current illness should be assessed, particularly during times of increased stress, such as at diagnosis or during disease exacerbations or relapses. The nurse also assesses the coping and adaptive mechanisms of both child and family.

Nursing Diagnosis

Anticipatory Grieving related to the impending death of a child.

Expected Outcomes

The child and family will:

- Experience appropriate progression through the five stages of grief, as evidenced by verbalization of an understanding of the five stages of grief, expression of all emotions in an appropriate manner, and expression of feelings by each family member in a communication style most comfortable for the individual.
- Exhibit behaviors indicating acceptance of the child's impending death and will provide care and support—emotional, physical, and psychosocial—in the manner desired by the child.

INTERVENTION	RATIONALE
1. Explain the five stages of grief and their necessity for healthy grieving, including resolution to acceptance.	1. An understanding of the normal grieving process may be lacking. An explanation should facilitate grief progression and guide behaviors in each stage.
2. Identify the stage of grief being experienced, and provide each family member with the opportunity to verbalize feelings corresponding to that stage. Provide positive feedback for appropriate progression.	2. Verbalization of feelings and receiving positive feedback will guide behaviors and facilitate continuing progression.
3. Educate family about grief stage progression characteristic of children (the client and any siblings). Encourage patience with the extended time frame for a child's grief.	3. Understanding the ways in which children's coping mechanisms differ from those of adults will facilitate acceptance and understanding by parents.
4. Offer all family members the opportunity to verbalize and act out, as necessary, all emotions in an appropriate manner.	4. Venting of emotions helps decrease stress and helps facilitate resolution of anger.
5. Exhibit a nonjudgmental attitude toward and acceptance of verbalization and behaviors.	5. An attitude of acceptance will convey care and support. It will also encourage appropriate, needed expression of all emotions, both negative and positive.
6. Encourage open, honest communication with the child to the degree requested. Demonstrate appropriate communication techniques.	6. Appropriate communication with the child will provide comfort and support. It will also ease closure and resolution of problems for the client.
7. Offer family members the opportunity to participate in the child's physical care, as desired by both parties. Demonstrate care in a gentle, supportive fashion.	7. Many individuals fear the atmosphere of dying and the provision of physical care. Learning by example will lessen fears and enhance provision of care.

to become more involved with or closer to one child or another, a development that can lead to a more intense response or a delay in appropriate resolution of grief. In providing competent and caring nursing care, the nurse may have difficulty maintaining appropriate boundaries between personal involvement and professional care. A nurse who is compassionate yet can retain professionalism may be able to provide care more easily on a continuing basis in the area of terminal illness.

Regardless of the depth of involvement, level of professionalism, or the number of deaths encountered, however, every nurse who cares for dying children will experience loss and grief. Consequently, the nurse will need support through the

Nursing Care Plan

The Terminally Ill or Dying Child—cont'd

Evaluation

- Do the child (if cognitively able) and family verbalize an understanding of the five stages of grief and express all emotions in an appropriate manner and in a communication style most comfortable for each individual?
- Do the child and family exhibit behaviors that indicate acceptance of the impending death?
- Does the family provide physical, emotional, and psychosocial care and support in the manner and environment desired by the child?

Nursing Diagnosis

Anxiety related to the threat of impending death.

Expected Outcomes

The child and family will:

- Achieve anxiety control, as evidenced by open verbalization of all feelings and emotions and questions concerning the diagnosis and prognosis.
- Verbalize physical, emotional, and spiritual comfort.

INTERVENTION	RATIONALE
1. Educate the child and family about the terminal phase of illness, including what to expect physically, emotionally, and spiritually. Explain how needs will be met. Offer alternatives, such as hospice care.	1. Misconceptions may lead to increased fear and anxiety. Expression of feelings by family members may distress an otherwise comfortable child.
2. Assure the child and family that the child will be safe and comfortable and will not be alone. Provide frequent reassurance as needed.	2. Fears about the child's comfort and security are the most common. Frequent reassurances are often necessary as the disease or symptoms worsen.
3. Provide as much privacy as possible for the child dying in the hospital setting. Allow and encourage parents and siblings to stay with the child, as desired by the family. Regulate visitation by those outside the immediate family and friends as necessary.	3. Families may need extended time for closure. Although visitors may be well meaning, their increased visits as death nears may interfere with time needed by the family. Because of concerns over hurt feelings, the family may have difficulty regulating visitors. If so, the staff must help by regulating visitors as a means of ensuring the family's privacy.
4. Provide extensive opportunities for the family to care for the child. Teach family members the necessary physical skills. Allow the family to decline provision of care when it is physically distressing or painful.	4. Children are usually most comfortable when cared for by family members. In some instances, however, the child and family may be more comfortable and less anxious if the staff provides certain care.

Evaluation

- Do the child and family openly and appropriately verbalize all feelings, emotions, and questions concerning the diagnosis and prognosis?
- Do the child and family exhibit physical, emotional, and spiritual comfort?

difficult times. Both staff nurses and management must recognize this need. All must work together to provide mutual support through both active, organized support programs and simple acts of respect, concern, and care among colleagues. When a nurse begins working with dying children for the first time, having a more experienced nurse mentor may be very helpful.

This is true whether the nurse has many years experience or has experience working with dying adults. Parents caring for a dying child are frequently reminded that to provide such care they must care for themselves as well as they care for their child. This is equally true for the nurses who choose to care for children with chronic or terminal illnesses.

KEY CONCEPTS

- Children with chronic conditions are living longer, and more children are living with conditions that were once considered fatal. Despite improvements in quality of life and longevity, chronic illness is stressful and a situational crisis for families that requires ongoing attention and adaptation.

- The most important aspect of a chronic illness is that it affects the entire family, not just the child.

- Families dealing with chronic illness have many varied concerns and needs, including meeting the physical and emotional needs of the child, providing care for the rest of the family, and meeting financial burdens. The family must strive to meet the physical, emotional, psychosocial, and spiritual needs of each of its members.

- The stages of grief, as well as of death and dying, are applicable to pediatric clients but

with special considerations for both child and family. The child's concepts of death and dying are based on the child's stage of growth and development. These concepts are further affected by age, cognition, and experiences of life—intellectual, social, and psychologic. Both ill children and well siblings change in their understanding of death and dying.

- The dying child, like the dying adult, desires the comfort, safety, and presence of loved ones.

- Parents must move from *fearing* the child's death to *acknowledging* the child's impending death. For parents caring for a dying child, pain is the greatest concern.

- Although the grief of parents is often more intense, siblings' lesser cognitive abilities and changing developmental needs and capabilities can make the grief of siblings more difficult to address.

- Grief is similar for all families (adults and children); grief must be processed and the loss integrated. Loved ones must understand that the person who has died is gone, and they must experience the resulting emotions. Family members must reinvest in life and go forward with their lives.

- Nursing care of the terminally ill or dying child can be extremely stressful and demanding. It requires strict attention to one's own physical, emotional, and spiritual health. Care of the caregiver is imperative if the nurse is to provide physical and psychosocial care for families at such a difficult time.

ANSWER to Critical Thinking Exercise 36-1

The nurse can assist family members in problem solving and in using their coping skills. The family is educated as to the medical aspects of the disease and how to care for their child at home. Interpersonal communication

among family members and the development of social supports should be encouraged. Siblings should be included in the assessment of the family and incorporated into the plan of care for the family. Community

resources that support both child and family should be identified and the family assisted to access such support systems.

REFERENCES and READINGS

American Academy of Pediatrics Committee on Bioethics. (1994). Guidelines on forgoing life-sustaining medical treatment. *Pediatric Nursing, 20*(5), 517-521.

American Academy of Pediatrics Committee on Bioethics. (1996). Ethics and the care of critically ill infants and children. *Pediatrics, 98*(1), 149-152.

American Academy of Pediatrics Committee on Children With Disabilities. (1995). Guidelines for home care of infants, children, and adolescents with chronic disease. *Pediatrics, 96*(1), 161-164.

American Academy of Pediatrics Committee on Children With Disabilities. (1997). General principles in the care of children and adolescents with genetic disorders and other chronic health conditions. *Pediatrics, 99*(4), 643-644.

American Academy of Pediatrics Committee on Children With Disabilities. (2000). Policy statement: Provision of educationally related services for children and adolescents with chronic diseases and disabling conditions. *Pediatrics, 99*(2), 448-451.

Banks, M. (2003). Disability in the family: A life span perspective. *Cultural Diversity & Ethnic Minority Psychology, 9*(4), 367-384.

Bowden, V.R. (1993). Children's literature: The death experience. *Pediatric Nursing, 19*(1), 17-21.

Burke, S., Kauffman, E., Harrison, M., & Wiskin, N. (1999). Assessment of stressors in families with a child who has a chronic condition. *MCN: The American Journal of Maternal/Child Nursing, 24*(2), 98-106.

Carter, B.D., Kronenberger, W.G., Edwards, J.F., Marshall, G.S., Schikler, K.N., & Causey, D.L. (1999). *Psychological symptoms in chronic fatigue and juvenile rheumatoid arthritis. Pediatrics, 103*(5), 975-979.

Chernoff, R., Ireys, H., DeVet, K., & Young, K. (2002). A randomized controlled trial of a community-based support program for families of children with chronic illness: Pediatric outcomes. *Archives of Pediatrics & Adolescent Medicine, 56*(6), 533-540.

Clawson, J. (1996). A child with chronic illness and the process of family adaptation. *Journal of Pediatric Nursing, 11*(1), 52-61.

Cook, P. (1999). *Supporting sick children and their families*. St. Louis: Saunders.

Corbin, J.M., & Strauss, A. (1991). A nursing model for chronic illness management based upon the trajectory framework. *Scholarly Inquiry*

for Nursing Practice: An International Journal, 5(3) 155-172.

D'Avanzo, C., & Geissler, E.M. (2003). *Pocket guide to cultural health assessment* (3rd ed.). St. Louis: Mosby.

Edwards, P.A., Hertzberg, D.L., Hays, S.R., & Youngblood, N.M. (1999). *Pediatric rehabilitation nursing*. Philadelphia: Saunders.

Godshall, M. (2003). Caring for families of chronically ill kids. *RN, 66*(2), 30-35.

Graves, C., & Hayes, V. (1996). Do nurses and parents of children with chronic conditions agree on parental needs? *Journal of Pediatric Nursing, 11*(5), 288-299.

Hanson, W., Ridder, K., Liebergen, A., Olson, J., Barnard, M., & Tobin-Rommelhart, S. (1997). Outcomes of nursing interventions for siblings of chronically ill children: A pilot study. *Journal of Society of Pediatric Nurses, 2*, 127-137.

Health Resources and Services Administration, Maternal and Child Health Bureau. (2003). *Division of services for children with special health needs fact sheet*. Rockville, MD: U.S. Department of Health and Human Services.

Ireys, H., Chernoff, R., DeVet, K., & Kim, Y. (2001). Maternal outcomes of a randomized controlled trial of a community-based support program for families of children with chronic illness.

Archives of Pediatric and Adolescent Medicine, *155,* 771-777.

Kübler-Ross, E. (1969). *On death and dying.* New York: Macmillan.

Kübler-Ross, E. (1983). *On children and death.* New York: Macmillan.

Langton, H. (2000). *The child with cancer: Family centered care.* St. Louis: Saunders.

Lugton, J., & Kindlen, M. (Eds.). (1999). *Palliative care: The nursing role.* Philadelphia: Churchill Livingstone.

Olsen, S. (1999). Support, communication, and hardiness in families with children with disabilities. *Journal of Family Nursing, 5*(3), 275-292.

Patterson, J.M. (2002). Integrating family resilience and family stress theory. *Journal of Marriage and Family, 64,* 349-360.

Scott, L. (1998). Perceived needs of parents of critically ill children. *Journal of Society of Pediatric Nurses, 3*(1), 4-12.

Sterling, Y., Peterson, J., & Weekes, D. (1997). African-American families with chronically ill children: Oversights and insights. *Journal of Pediatric Nursing, 12*(5), 292-300.

Walker, C., Wells, L., Heiney, S. Hymovich, D., & Weeks, D. (1993). Nursing management of psychosocial care needs. In G. Foley, D. Fachman, & K. Mooney (Eds.). *Nursing care of the child with cancer.* Philadelphia: Saunders.

Wass, H. (1985). Concepts of death: A developmental perspective. *Issues in Comprehensive Pediatric Nursing, 8*(1-6), 3-25.

Williams, P., Williams, A., Graff, C., Hanson, S., Stanton, A., Hafeman, C., Liebergen, A., Leuenberg, K., Setter, R., Ridder, L., Curry, H., Barnard, M., & Sanders, S. (2003). A community-based intervention for siblings and parents of children with chronic illness or disability: The ISEE study. *The Journal of Pediatrics, 143*(3), 386-393.

Woodgate, R. (1998). Adolescents' perspectives of chronic illness: "It's hard." *Journal of Pediatric Nursing, 13*(4), 210-222.

37

Principles and Procedures for Nursing Care of Children

LEARNING OBJECTIVES

After studying this chapter, you should be able to:

◉ Describe how to prepare children and families for selected procedures frequently seen in an acute care setting and home care setting.

◉ Compare anatomic and physiologic differences in children and adults as they apply to selected procedures.

◉ Identify psychosocial considerations unique to children undergoing selected procedures.

◉ Describe techniques useful for eliciting cooperation from the child undergoing selected procedures.

◉ Describe step-by-step nursing actions and the reasons for performing selected procedures.

DEFINITIONS

antipyretic An agent that reduces or relieves fever.

apical pulse rate Heart rate determined by placing the stethoscope over the point of maximum intensity and counting for 1 minute.

auscultate To listen to body sounds (e.g., heart sounds, breath sounds).

enteral By way of the digestive system (e.g., enteral feeding).

epiglottitis Inflammation of the epiglottis (see Chapter 38).

informed consent A requirement, both legal and ethical, that the child and the parent or guardian completely understand

proposed procedures or treatments, including their benefits and risks.

lavage Wash.

pyrogens Substances that cause fever.

Standard Precautions Infection control guidelines developed by the National Center for Infectious Disease and the Hospital Control Practices Advisory Committee to prevent the spread of infectious organisms from blood, body fluids, secretions and excretions, mucous membranes, and nonintact skin.

Children need preparation before and accurate information about any procedure that is performed. This information is essential. It promotes a sense of security, decreases fear, elicits cooperation, and improves coping skills. Parents also need preparation, because their anxiety about a procedure may be transferred to the child.

Before preparing the child and family for any procedure, the nurse needs to plan how to carry out the procedure in the most effective manner. The nurse can implement strategies to help the child and parents through all phases of a procedure, including the anticipation and preparation for the pro-

cedure, the actual procedure, and the period after the procedure. Teaching before performing procedures also helps increase the child's and family's knowledge base.

PREPARING CHILDREN FOR PROCEDURES

Adequately preparing children and families for procedures, especially those that are painful, threatening, or invasive, necessitates a thorough, individualized assessment. This process should include an assessment of the child's age and developmental level, personality, existing level of knowledge, present level of understanding, past experience, coping skills, and family situation. The nurse can then match explanations and teaching to the specific needs of a child and family.

Explaining Procedures

Mentally reviewing the procedure before giving explanations is especially important if the procedure is seldom performed, new, or unfamiliar. Thinking about the procedure in advance

---

! CRITICAL TO REMEMBER

Standard Precautions

Always wash your hands and follow Standard Precautions before beginning any procedure. Wash your hands again when the procedure is finished.

BOX 37-1
Tips for Preparing and Supporting Children Undergoing Procedures

BEFORE THE PROCEDURE
- Offer the child ways to cope with pain or discomfort. For example, some children can use coping strategies, such as guided imagery. Others might listen to a radio, increasing the volume as the discomfort level increases. Give the child permission to cry or yell if necessary.
- Use developmentally appropriate words when discussing the procedure and expectations.
- Give the child as much choice as possible over what will happen. For example, when possible, the child might be allowed to choose an injection site or a site for intravenous (IV) catheter placement.
- Be sure the consent form has been signed, if applicable.
- Always wash your hands thoroughly before beginning any procedure, and follow Standard Precautions.

DURING THE PROCEDURE
- Talk to the child during the procedure if the child desires. If the child is using a coping strategy such as guided imagery, however, talking will be a distraction and will decrease the child's ability to cope with what is happening.

- Keep the child informed of the procedure's progress.
- Tell the child when the procedure is nearly completed and the "worst is over."

AFTER THE PROCEDURE
- *Praise* the child for *attempts* at cooperation even if the child did not do anything you asked. Trying counts! Specifically praise the child for accomplishing an expected task.
- Provide an opportunity for the child to vent feelings about the procedure. Remember that it is acceptable for feelings of anger to be expressed when appropriate. Tell the child that you understand if the child does not want to talk with you right now and that you will return later.
- If parents were not present during the procedure, reunite the child with the parents and allow them to provide comfort and support.
- Reward the child, using age-appropriate methods such as stickers.
- Record the preparation process and procedure performance, who performed the procedure, the child's tolerance of the procedure, and its outcomes.

---

provides an opportunity for the nurse to request sedation for the child, gather extra supplies, and obtain assistance as necessary. Gather all equipment to be used and check that it functions before beginning any procedure.

Explaining procedures includes demonstrating equipment and describing anything the child will feel, see, hear, and smell. Use words the child will understand, and use a developmentally appropriate approach. It helps to relate the experience to an object or situation familiar to the child or one in which the child is interested.

Appropriately timing the explanation is critical. Many children respond better to procedures if the explanation is given either just before the procedure or step by step as the procedure unfolds. Some older children and adolescents like to be prepared well in advance, in case they have questions that need answering. Advance preparation allows the child to express feelings about the procedure through role play. Often, parents can inform the nurse about the best timing for their child, so the nurse needs to question the parents about the best approach for their child. If possible, time should be allowed for questions and for the child to become familiar with the equipment (Box 37-1).

Also important for a child's successful coping with an invasive or painful procedure is the presence of someone the child trusts. Time spent establishing a trusting relationship with a child is time well spent. Trust in health care providers can enhance the child's unique coping strategies.

Before procedures, ensure the child's privacy by closing the door to the room and drawing a curtain around the bed or, optimally, by taking the child to a treatment room if it is appropriate and comfortable for the child and parent. The treatment room contains suitable equipment for invasive procedures and is a private area away from the "safe haven" of a child's room or the playroom (Fig. 37-1). Visitors should be asked to leave, and parents might also choose to leave at

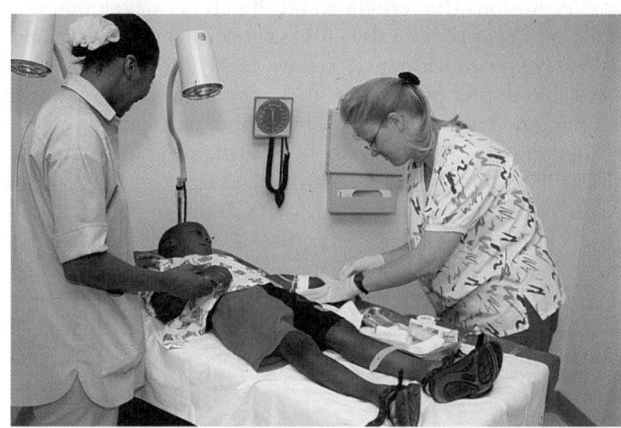

Figure 37-1 Because a child should feel that the hospital room is a safe place, a treatment room is used for invasive or painful procedures. The parent is present, not to restrain the child but to provide emotional support.

this point, although parental participation is supported and encouraged.

Telling children or parents what they can do to help gives them control and decreases potential feelings of powerlessness. For example, if the child must hold an extremity still for the placement of an intravenous (IV) catheter or for blood work, the child must know about this need *before* the procedure is begun.

You might say to the child, "We have talked about why you need to have an IV, but you need to know how important it is for you to hold your arm very still while we are putting the IV in. I will tell you everything that is going to happen so you can be prepared and know when to help. Do you think you can help us, or do we need to ask someone to help you remember?"

! CRITICAL TO REMEMBER

Preparation for Procedures

- A treatment room is the preferred location for performing painful procedures. It is a private area away from the "safe haven" of a child's hospital room, and it usually contains the necessary equipment for a variety of procedures (see Fig. 37-1).
- Ensure that a person the child trusts is there for support.
- Use terminology appropriate for the child's developmental level. Avoid using words or phrases that the child might misinterpret (e.g., dye, put to sleep, stick).
- Offer the child choices if appropriate.
- Tell the child and family how they can help with the procedure.
- Do not threaten punishment for lack of cooperation.
- Encourage parental participation in the procedure, but do not force an unwilling parent to stay.

Offer children choices when feasible. For example, let a child choose the type of colorful bandage that will cover an injection site or whether to have a procedure done before or after the next television show. Do not threaten children with punishment for not cooperating. Nurses need to have realistic expectations that are based on the child's developmental level and knowledge of the child's capacity for cooperation.

Involve parents as much as they desire, according to what is possible during procedures. For example, a child might be much more cooperative in taking oral medications if the mother administers them. Often, by explaining what the parents will be seeing and what they can do, the nurse helps them feel comfortable staying with and supporting their child. The nurse should recognize, however, that parents might be very uncomfortable remaining with their child during a painful or invasive procedure. Give parents permission to leave if they desire, and assure them that they will be called if they are needed or as soon as the procedure is completed.

Consent for Procedures

All surgical or diagnostic invasive procedures, particularly those that involve risk to the child, require *informed consent*. Some examples are lumbar puncture, chest tube insertion, and bone marrow aspiration. There are both legal and ethical requirements to inform the child, if appropriate, and the child's parents of the benefits and risks of the proposed procedure or treatment. Informed consent must be obtained from the parent or legal guardian *before* the procedure is performed.

Other procedures, such as IV line insertions, specimen collection, and medication and oxygen administration, are covered under the general consent to treat that is provided in signed form on admission. It is now also customary to obtain *assent* from children 7 years old and older. Assent means that the child has been fully informed about the procedure and concurs with those giving the informed consent. Laws on informed consent vary from state to state, so nurses should become familiar with the laws and policies of their institution. (See Chapter 1 for specific information related to legal issues.)

The person performing the procedure should obtain the consent. Nurses need to check that the consent form is signed and witnessed, and they need to answer questions relating to the procedure. Occasionally, an emergency or life-threatening situation arises in which it is not possible to contact the parent or legal guardian for consent. In such cases, administrative consent may be obtained to allow physicians to perform the indicated procedures. (Refer to Chapter 1 for legal issues related to informed and emergency consent provisions.)

HOLDING AND TRANSPORTING INFANTS AND CHILDREN

Infants can be held in several positions (Fig. 37-2). Before the infant is discharged from the hospital, the nurse teaches new parents how to hold the infant, and nurses working on children's units should hold infants in similar ways. Hold the infant securely, anticipating sudden movement; because infants younger than 4 months do not have well-established head control, supporting the head is essential. Cradle infants up to 2 to 3 months of age by holding them in a horizontal position, supporting the back, and grasping the thigh (see Fig. 37-2, A). When using the football hold, tuck the infant between your body and elbow, with your arm carrying the infant's body and your hand supporting the head (see Fig. 37-2, B). When carrying the infant upright, hold the infant erect against your chest (see Fig. 37-2, C). Rest the infant's buttocks on your forearm, and support the infant's head and shoulders with your other arm. Even for infants with well-developed neck muscles and head control, this extra support prevents the infant from falling backward should the infant make a sudden move. Advise parents who use a backpack or front-facing baby carrier to transport the infant at home to be sure that the infant's head is supported in the carrier at all times.

Hospitalized infants and children sometimes must be transported to other areas within a hospital unit or even outside the unit. A change in location might be a response to changes in the child's condition or might be done to increase parental involvement in the child's care (e.g., rooming-in). Children may also be transported for specialized care (e.g., rehabilitation) or for diagnostic testing. In addition, children might be transported to different areas on the same unit (e.g., treatment room, playroom).

The method of transportation will depend on the child's age, developmental level, and physical condition; the destination; safety factors; and whether specialized equipment is needed to accompany the child. Any special accommodations should be arranged before the time of the planned transfer.

Infants and toddlers can also be transported in their bassinet or crib. The rails should always be up, and for older infants and toddlers the protective top should be in place. Strollers and wagons can be used to transfer older infants and toddlers to other areas on the unit (see Fig. 37-2). Use safety belts, and make sure the sides of the wagon are raised. Do not leave an infant or toddler unattended. In all methods of transfer, equipment (e.g., IV pump, enteral feeding pump, oxygen) can be pushed or pulled along with the transporting vehicle or, in some cases, stored on a lower shelf of the transport vehicle. Do not place equipment in the transporting unit with infants or young children.

Transport older children in the same manner as adults (e.g., in wheelchairs or on stretchers with the side rails raised).

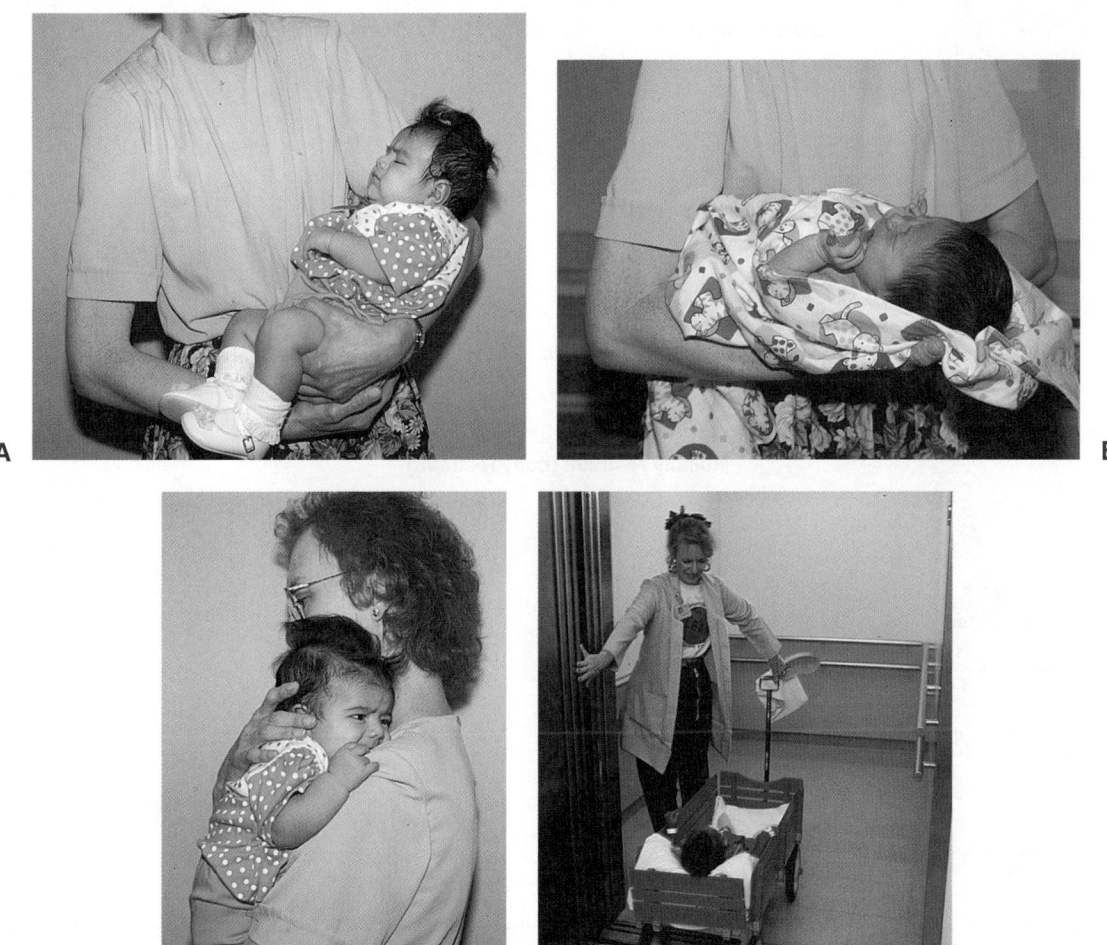

Figure 37-2 Methods of transporting infants and children. The nurse carries the infant securely, anticipating sudden movement. **A,** Cradle carry. **B,** Football hold. **C,** Over-the-shoulder carry, which can be used until the infant is 6 to 7 months. **D,** Transport can be fun for young children, especially when it is on wheels. (**A, B,** and **C** courtesy Parkland Health and Hospital System District Community Oriented Primary Care Clinic, Dallas, TX; **D** courtesy Cook Children's Medical Center, Fort Worth, TX.)

In some cases, such as for a child in traction, transporting the child in the bed is preferable. Alternatively, preschoolers may enjoy a ride in a wagon or other unconventional means of transport (see Fig. 37-2). As for younger children, remember to use safety belts, raised sides, and constant supervision.

USING RESTRAINTS

Safety is of paramount concern for all children, particularly infants and toddlers. Nurses and parents need to be especially vigilant about raising side (crib) rails and keeping small objects away from young children. *Always place your hand on an infant's or child's back or abdomen when the sides of the bed are down or when the child is in a high place; teach parents to do the same.* Keep small objects off bedside tables or any area within the child's reach.

Occasionally, to prevent trauma, temporarily restraining a child is necessary to suspend movement during certain procedures. In this instance, the restraint is removed as soon as the procedure is complete.

Some children are particularly active and prone to injury. Restraining the child might be the only option for maintaining the child's safety. All possible alternatives to restraint should be considered before applying the restraint. These alternatives might include using a sitter; behavior modification techniques, such as a time-out; or diversional activities, such as reading. If restraint is considered for unruly or dangerous behavior, the cause of the behavior should also be examined. Causes can include hypoxia (decreased oxygenation), sedation, adverse drug reactions, and mental illness.

The Omnibus Budget Reconciliation Act of 1987 states that restraints should be used only as a last resort for the protection of the client and others. The legislation further specifies that restraints should not be applied merely for the staff's convenience.

Physical restraints include items such as mitts, elbow restraints, and ankle and wrist restraints. Jacket restraints (safety vests), which might be used primarily to keep children in bed after surgery, are used with caution on a general children's unit because very active children can get twisted and

Elbow restraint

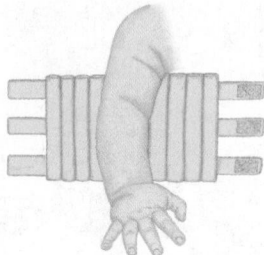

Prevents child from flexing and reaching face, head, IV and other tubes. Position so that it does not rub against the axilla.

Crib top bubble restraint

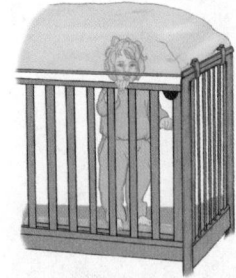

Prevents older infant and younger child from falling and climbing out of bed.

Mummy restraint (body restraint)

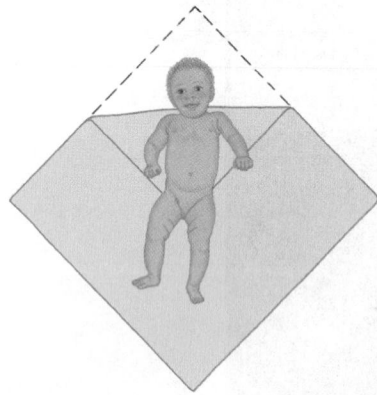

A restraint can be made from a sheet folded into a square of the appropriate size for the infant. Start by folding the top corner under the infant's shoulders and aligning the infant's head with the folded edge.

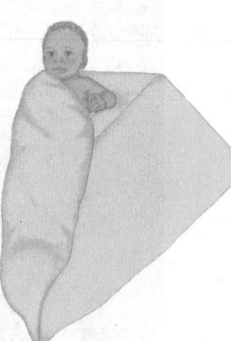

Fold one point of the sheet across the child and tuck it firmly behind the back.

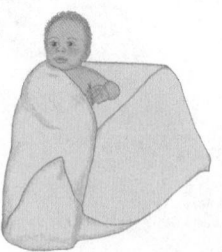

Fold the bottom corner of the sheet up to cover and restrain the infant's feet.

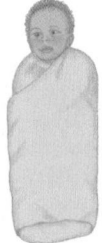

Fold the remaining corner over the child and tuck firmly behind the back.

Figure 37-3 Examples of pediatric restraints.

caught in the restraint. Most facilities require a physician's order stating why any restraint is needed and how long it will be in place. The restraint chosen should be the least restrictive device that will prevent injury. Less restrictive protective restraints include such mechanisms as a plastic bubble top placed over a crib. Examples of restraints used for children are illustrated in Figure 37-3.

Before placing the restraint, check the area to be restrained for any sign of compromised circulatory, integumen-

---

> **! CRITICAL TO REMEMBER**
>
> **Using Restraints**
>
> - Use the least restrictive restraint.
> - Choose the proper device for the child's condition.
> - Ensure proper fit of the device.
> - Tie knots that can be easily untied for quick access.
> - Secure ties to bed frames (not mattresses or side rails), to the frames of wheelchairs, or to another stable device.
> - Frequently check and record the child's neurovascular status, behavior, and general condition.

---

tary, and neurologic systems. Also note any orthopedic alterations. If these conditions exist, extra monitoring of the restrained extremity will be needed.

Preparing the Child and Family

When restraints are applied, the child and family should be told why the restraint will be used, where it will be applied, what movement it will prevent, and how long it will be in place. Tell the child and family how often a nurse will be coming in to check on the child. Have the call button readily available to older children so that they can call the nurse as needed. If possible, you need to consider and meet the child's developmental needs, such as thumb sucking. For example, an infant's or toddler's arm can be restrained so that the thumb can still be placed in the mouth.

Check the extremity distal to restraints for temperature, pulses, and capillary refill (CSM: Circulation, Sensation, Motion) every 15 minutes for 1 hour after initial placement. After that, check and record findings at least every hour and more often if the child is aggressive or extremely active. Remove restraints every 2 hours to allow for range-of-motion movement and repositioning and to offer the child food or the opportunity to use the bathroom.

Documentation

Record findings from hourly neurovascular checks and any other changes in the child's behavior or condition. Every 2 hours, record removal of restraints, range of motion, and position changes. Be particularly alert for skin irritation under the restraints.

INFECTION CONTROL

Standard Precautions, which are used in institutions and the workplace for infection prevention, apply to:

- Blood
- All body fluids, secretions, and excretions, except sweat, regardless of whether they contain visible blood
- Nonintact skin
- Mucous membranes

Two tiers of precautions are under this system. *Standard Precautions*, precautions in the first tier, apply in the care of all hospitalized clients without regard for diagnosis or presumed infectious state. Second-tier precautions apply in the care of specific clients and are referred to as *Transmission-Based Precautions*. They are for clients known or suspected to be infected by pathogens that are transmitted through air or droplet or through contact with dry skin or contaminated surfaces.

The complete guidelines for applying Standard Precautions, as well as those for applying Transmission-Based Precautions, are quite detailed and extensive. Each facility is responsible for making these guidelines available and implementing the precautions.

Implementing Precautions

It is important to remember that when Transmission-Based Precautions are in effect, the items with which the infected child comes in contact are also contaminated. These items include the bed, linens, IV pump, sink, and toys. Therefore the nurse who is going into the room to reset an IV pump, pick up soiled linens, and so forth must use whatever protective equipment is mandated by the type of precaution (gown, mask, gloves).

Children placed on Transmission-Based Precautions often need extra attention to avert boredom. They need more diversional activities, such as games or movies, and more psychosocial support. Young children, for example, may think that they are being punished. Visitors might hesitate to enter the child's room and may need additional support or reassurance from the nurse.

Family Teaching

Family education is crucial for effective infection control or prevention, and it is important to emphasize to parents, other visitors, and other health care providers that infection control precautions are important and must be followed closely. Parents often state that they are there to visit only their child

and do not understand the need to wear special clothing or equipment. The nurse needs to emphasize that some diseases, such as respiratory syncytial virus, can live on inanimate objects, such as clothing, for up to 48 hours and can spread throughout the hospital or to the home if infection control or prevention measures are not followed. Encourage family members to visit the child frequently because visits will decrease the child's sense of isolation. Advise the family that meticulous handwashing, both in the hospital setting and at home, is the best infection prevention intervention.

BATHING INFANTS AND CHILDREN

The nurse can use bath time as a time to help parents interact with their infants. When teaching a new parent how to bathe a baby, the nurse can model approaches that alert the parent to the baby's unique characteristics (Karl, 1999). Pointing out how the infant is reacting during various stages of the bath and demonstrating ways to calm or use consoling interventions not only provide the parent an opportunity to interact with the baby but also give the parent tools to use at home to help the infant self-console (Karl, 1999).

Strictly observing safety principles when bathing an infant or child can prevent falls, burns, or aspiration of water. When bathing an infant or a child in the hospital setting, be sure to take the opportunity to note any problems, such as altered skin integrity, surgical incisions, loss of sensation, abnormal skin color, bruising, paralysis, or any other condition that might warrant special consideration. Newborn infants can be immersed in water after the umbilical stump and circumcision sites (if applicable) have healed (see Chapter 23). The temperature of the bath water should not exceed 37.7° C (100° F)—that is, warm but not hot to the touch. If a bath thermometer is available, it should be used to check the temperature of the water. Otherwise, a temperature that is comfortable when tested on the inside of your wrist or elbow is appropriate.

Before bathing any child, assess the family's preferences and home practices. Factors to consider include the time of day usually set aside for the bath, bathing rituals, special equipment, any product allergies, and the type of bath preferred. You can also use this time to determine the amount of assistance needed and to address any learning needs related to hygiene. Because bathing is one of the few areas over which parents might be allowed to retain control when a child is hospitalized, it is important to allow them to make as many decisions as possible. Decision making also allows parents to maintain a part of the home routine with their child.

An infant who cannot sit unaided can be given either a sponge bath or a tub bath. Support the infant's body and head at all times during the bath (Fig. 37-4). Older infants and toddlers can be bathed in either a bedside tub or a regular bathtub. *Never leave an infant or small child unattended in the bath.* Older children can take showers if facilities are available. The nurse should use judgment in deciding how much supervision an older child needs while bathing. It is most important to provide privacy for the school-age child or adolescent.

Special Considerations

Bed baths are frequently used for hospitalized infants and children. When bathing a newborn or young infant, soap is not necessary. In fact, soap can be very drying to the skin if

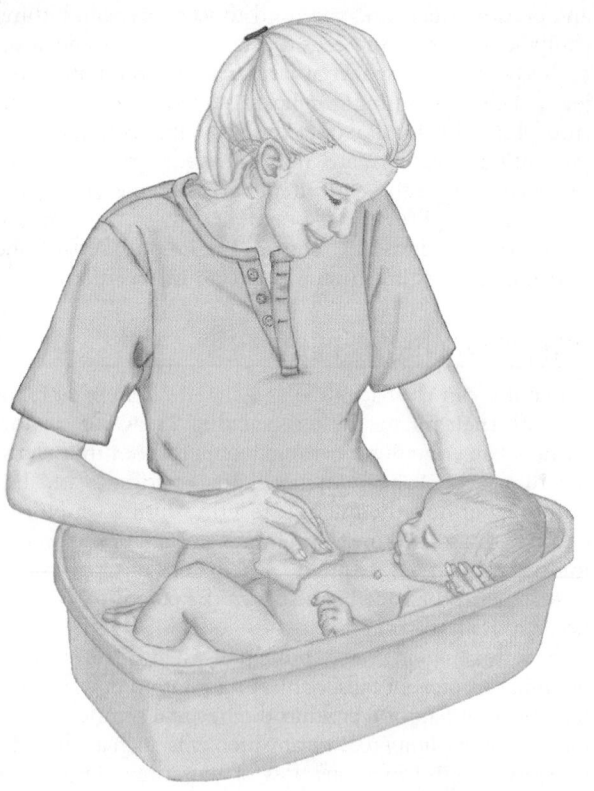

Using the hand to support infant's neck and head.

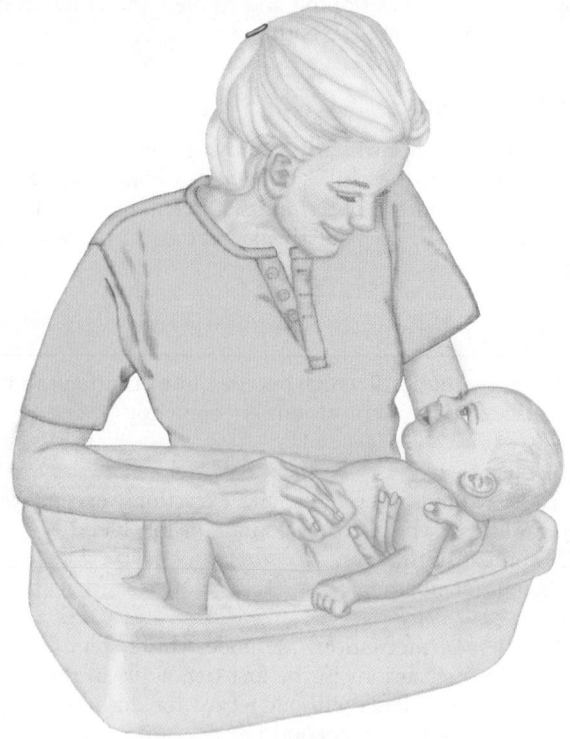

Using the arm to support infant's neck and head.

Figure 37-4 When giving an infant a tub bath, the nurse supports the infant's body at all times.

used too frequently. If soap is necessary or desired by the parent, use a gentle, nonalkaline soap.

To prevent chilling when giving a sponge bath, be sure to keep the infant covered with a cotton blanket. Cover the entire body except for the body part being washed or rinsed. Begin the bath with the face, and clean the diaper area last. Clean any eye discharge using a wet cotton ball, and clean from the inner canthus outward. Use a clean cotton ball for each eye. Outer ears can be cleaned with a wet face cloth.

If bathing an infant in a bathtub, line a plastic infant tub with a towel to provide comfort as well as traction to prevent slipping. To prevent accidental drowning should the infant slip out of your grasp, fill the tub with no more than 3 inches of water.

When finished with the infant bath, wrap the infant in a dry towel or cotton blanket. Using the football hold and holding the infant over the tub, shampoo the infant's head with baby shampoo. Be sure to shampoo over the fontanel. Avoid using talcum powder or cornstarch in the infant's diaper area. When these substances get moist, they provide a medium for organism growth. Talcum powder and cornstarch, if accidentally inhaled, also can cause severe respiratory consequences (Schmitt, 1999).

The technique for bathing a child differs little from that used for bathing an adult. The nurse performs the same assessment as with any client and provides assistance as necessary.

Adjust the room temperature to a comfortable setting, and draw the curtain around the bed. As with any bed bath, the nurse begins with the face and proceeds in a head-to-toe progression. Obtain fresh water when it is time to rinse the child.

As with the infant, drape the child adequately for privacy and warmth; and to prevent chilling, dry each body section as it is rinsed. The bath can be followed with application of lotion or deodorant if desired.

Some bathing restrictions might apply to children with surgical incisions, skin traction, IV catheters, casts, urinary catheters, artificial airways, and feeding tubes. Some children are also restricted in position and mobility. For example, children who have undergone orthopedic or neurosurgical procedures often must remain supine. Other children may be intolerant of position changes because of underlying physiologic conditions or injury. It is imperative to assess for these special needs before beginning the bath.

Documentation

Documentation includes the type of bath, child or family participation, procedure tolerance, and any abnormal findings noted, such as bruising, rashes, or excoriation. Any lotions or other skin preparations used also should be recorded.

Parent Teaching

General principles of hygiene and safety might need to be reinforced with some parents. (See Chapter 23 for instructions for care of the newborn infant.) Instruction in the use of special bathing equipment, such as infant bathtubs, safety bars, or tub grips, should be included as part of discharge teaching and preparation. After about 1 year of age, a child can be bathed safely in a regular tub. To prevent injury or accidental drowning, appropriate supervision should be maintained at all times. Advise parents never to leave an older infant or young child alone in the bath; the risk of drowning, even in small amounts of water, is high. Infant bath seats, which adhere to the floor of a regular bathtub by suction cups, can also be dangerous. The older infant can slip out of the sides of the seat, especially when the seat is wet, or the suction cups can accidentally release, tipping the seat over.

ORAL HYGIENE

To remove excess food and bacteria, wipe infants' gums gently with a wet cloth after each feeding. After teeth erupt, a soft, damp cloth, a piece of gauze, or a child's soft toothbrush can be used after each feeding and before bed. Until the parent is assured that the child can manage correctly and independently, young children will need supervision when performing oral care. Even then, reminders to brush might be necessary.

Children should brush their teeth at least twice daily with a child's soft toothbrush and a *small* (pea-sized) amount of toothpaste. Children may ingest excessive amounts of fluoride if they are allowed to use large amounts of toothpaste or if they eat the toothpaste. Using the recommended amount of toothpaste and encouraging the child not to swallow the toothpaste will prevent *fluorosis* (brown spots on the teeth caused by too much fluoride).

Flossing is useful for cleaning between teeth and maintaining healthy gums. The child should begin to floss when all the primary teeth are in or when the child's molars begin to touch.

Immunosuppressed children, in particular, need excellent oral hygiene. Soft toothbrushes, sponge-covered toothettes, or moistened gauze sponges can be used for dental care in the child who is at risk for gingival bleeding (see Chapter 48).

Discharge teaching in the area of oral hygiene is very important and often forgotten. Many parents do not realize that infants' gums and teeth can and should be cleaned. Children should have their first visit to a dentist by the time the first teeth erupt and no later than age 2½ years. Thereafter they should be seen on a regular basis (every 6 months) for checkups.

The risk of dental caries is increased if formula, milk, or other liquids remain in a child's mouth overnight. Allowing an infant to fall asleep drinking a bottle of one of these liquids can cause a condition known as *bottle mouth syndrome,* which results in severely decayed primary teeth. Discourage parents from putting a child to bed with a bottle of formula, juice, or sweetened liquid. If the child will not fall asleep without a bottle, advise the parent to use water only.

Good nutrition influences dental health and vice versa. Dental teaching often provides a means for educating the child and family about proper nutrition and health maintenance.

FEEDING

Mealtimes can be difficult for the hospitalized child. Changes in routine, diet, and surroundings, as well as dietary restrictions and illness, affect the child's ability and desire to eat. Refusing to eat might also be the only way the child can control the environment.

Assess the child's preferences and dislikes on admission and before ordering meals. Also note mealtime rituals and routines and cultural food variations. Serving favorite and preferred foods and offering nutritious snacks can ensure appropriate caloric intake.

The type and form of food chosen should be appropriate to the child's age and developmental status. (Refer to Chapters 5 through 8 for a discussion of food types appropriate for each age-group.) When planning meals, the nurse also considers whether the child has any special needs. For example, the child with an impaired gag reflex cannot tolerate the same foods as other children. Likewise, the child with nausea should not be offered favorite foods, because these foods may become associated with the nausea when the child is feeling better.

Feeding a hospitalized infant seldom differs from feeding an infant at home. Types of foods, feeding schedules, and routines should replicate home schedules and routines when possible. If the infant's bottle or nipple brand is not available in the hospital, ask the parents to bring what the infant uses at home. Encourage parents to feed their children or be present at mealtimes. Feeding reinforces the special bond that develops between child and parent.

Unless it is contraindicated by their medical condition, hold infants during feedings. Because of the risk of aspiration, *never prop a bottle (i.e., do not leave it on a pillow or rolled blanket next to the infant's mouth).* Frequent burping during and after feedings can reduce the incidence of regurgitation. Burp the infant by using the upright hold and gently patting or rubbing the infant's back. You can also seat the infant on your knees with your hand supporting the infant's chin. After feeding, position the infant on the right side to facilitate the flow of the feeding toward the lower end of the stomach and to allow any swallowed air to rise into the esophagus.

Toddlers and preschoolers often use food as a source of control. They might exhibit "food jags," during which they will eat only one or two items for a period of several days. They enjoy finger foods but are beginning to use spoons or forks fairly competently. Use colorful plates and cups to encourage a reluctant child to eat. Also, allow parents to bring the child's own cups or utensils from home to simulate the usual mealtime routines as closely as possible.

Cut foods into pieces appropriate in size and texture to decrease the risk of aspiration. Avoid foods such as hot dogs, popcorn, peanuts, and grapes, because if aspirated, these can occlude the airway. Do not allow young children to eat unsupervised. Secure them appropriately at a table, in a high chair, or in bed using an over-the-bed table during meals. "Roaming" while eating should be discouraged. Allow children to feed themselves if possible, and restrict the feeding time to 15 to 20 minutes. Discontinue the meal if the child begins to play with the food.

Older children and adolescents seldom have difficulty expressing their dietary preferences. Difficulty may arise, however, when children this age are placed on a restricted or special diet. For example, the diabetic child often has difficulty staying on a restricted diet in the face of peer pressure. Support and setting clear limits are often needed to ensure cooperation. Referral to a dietitian may be necessary to help the child make appropriate food choices.

Special Considerations

Keeping accurate intake and output (I&O) measurements might be necessary for some children. Measure and record all intake, both oral and parenteral. All output, including output from urine and stool; drainage from tubes, stomas, or fistulas; and emesis, is also measured and recorded. To measure urinary output in an untrained child, weigh each wet diaper and compare the weight with the weight of a dry diaper of similar size. One gram of weight equals approximately one milliliter of output.

Documentation

Recording the child's nutritional intake assists in determining the child's overall health. It is important to record not only food intake and preferences but also observations about the child's appetite and eating patterns. Particularly note abnormal eating habits in an older child or adolescent—the age at which eating disorders are prevalent.

Parent Teaching

Parental education is very important, particularly if the hospital admission is related to eating disorders or accidents, such as food aspiration. Carefully instruct parents about any food or fluid restrictions or special diets. For example, a child with *phenylketonuria (PKU)* or type 1 diabetes mellitus (see Chapter 51) is at high risk for injury if the diet is not followed closely.

VITAL SIGNS

The principles of measuring vital signs in children are similar to those for adults, with some modifications. Obtain vital signs when the infant or child is quiet. If this timing is not possible, record any activity that affects accurate measurement (e.g., crying, playing).

! CRITICAL TO REMEMBER

Measuring Vital Signs

- Temperatures should not be measured rectally in the immunosuppressed child or in any child who has had rectal surgery, diarrhea, or a bleeding disorder.
- Count respirations and measure the apical heart rate before taking other vital signs. Both of these signs are best measured on a sleeping child.
- Measure the apical heart rate for a full minute on any child younger than 2 years, on a child being assessed for the first time, on any child whose heartbeat is irregular, or on a child for whom treatment decisions are based on the heart rate.
- Observe the child's respiratory rate and effort for a full minute while the child is quiet. Abdominal movement is normally observed in infants and young children, whereas thoracic movement can be noted in older children and adolescents.
- Evaluate the quality of respirations, symmetry of chest movement with each breath, and any noisy respirations (e.g., crackles, wheezes, friction rubs). Observe the child for any signs of respiratory distress, such as nasal flaring, grunting, stridor, retractions, increased work of breathing, cyanosis, or apneic periods.
- Always use a manual cuff to verify electronically measured blood pressures that indicate hypertension or hypotension.

Measuring Temperature

Temperature is an objective and reliable indicator of illness, and measuring temperature is an integral part of assessing children. A child's temperature can be measured in a variety of ways. Oral, rectal, axillary, and tympanic temperatures can be measured using electronic, digital, or tympanic membrane thermometers. The American Academy of Pediatrics no longer recommends the use of thermometers containing mercury for children in hospital or home settings (Goldman, Shannon, & Committee on Environmental Health, 2001). Whatever temperature measurement method is chosen, the child's temperature should be measured at the same site and with the same temperature-measuring device to maintain consistency and allow for reliable comparison and tracking of temperatures over time. (See Table 33-1 for normal temperatures in children.)

Digital thermometers, which are electronic or run on a battery and measure the temperature quickly (usually in less than 30 sec), can be used to measure temperatures orally, rectally, or in the axillary area. To prevent cross contamination, use disposable covers for obtaining temperatures.

Tympanic temperature measurement is now frequently done in pediatric practice, on children's units in the hospital, and at home (Fig. 37-5). The advantage to tympanic temperature measurement is that the measurements are obtained quickly, usually within a few seconds. Recent research has suggested, however, that neither tympanic temperature nor axillary temperatures accurately measure fever in infants and young children (Craig, Lancaster, Taylor, Williamson, & Smyth, 2002; Houlder, 2000; Lanham, Walker, Klocke, & Jennings, 1999). For this reason it is recommended that mildly elevated tympanic or axillary temperatures be confirmed by rectal core temperature measurement (Houlder, 2000). For tympanic measurement to be accurate, the temperature probe must create a complete seal. Putting traction on the ear pinna (direction depending on the child's age) before probe insertion exposes the tympanic membrane and facilitates a seal.

Axillary temperatures should be measured in infants and children younger than 4 to 6 years and in any child who is uncooperative, immunosuppressed, neurologically impaired, or who has had oral surgery (see Fig. 37-5). Axillary temperatures are approximately 0.6° C (1° F) lower than the body's core temperature. To be accurate, a thermometer may need to remain in the child's axillary area for a longer time, so consider seating the child on your lap and reading a story or singing songs to help pass the time and help the child remain quiet.

Temperatures are measured orally in most children 6 years old or older, including adolescents. It is sometimes a challenge for the child to keep a thermometer in place. Encourage the child to keep the mouth closed around the thermometer (in a "kiss" position), and instruct the child not to

---

! CRITICAL TO REMEMBER

Measuring Temperature

- Follow an elevated tympanic or axillary temperature with a rectal core temperature measurement.
- Report any core temperature measurement of less than 36° C (96.8° F) or more than 38° C (100.4° F), especially in an infant under 2 months of age.

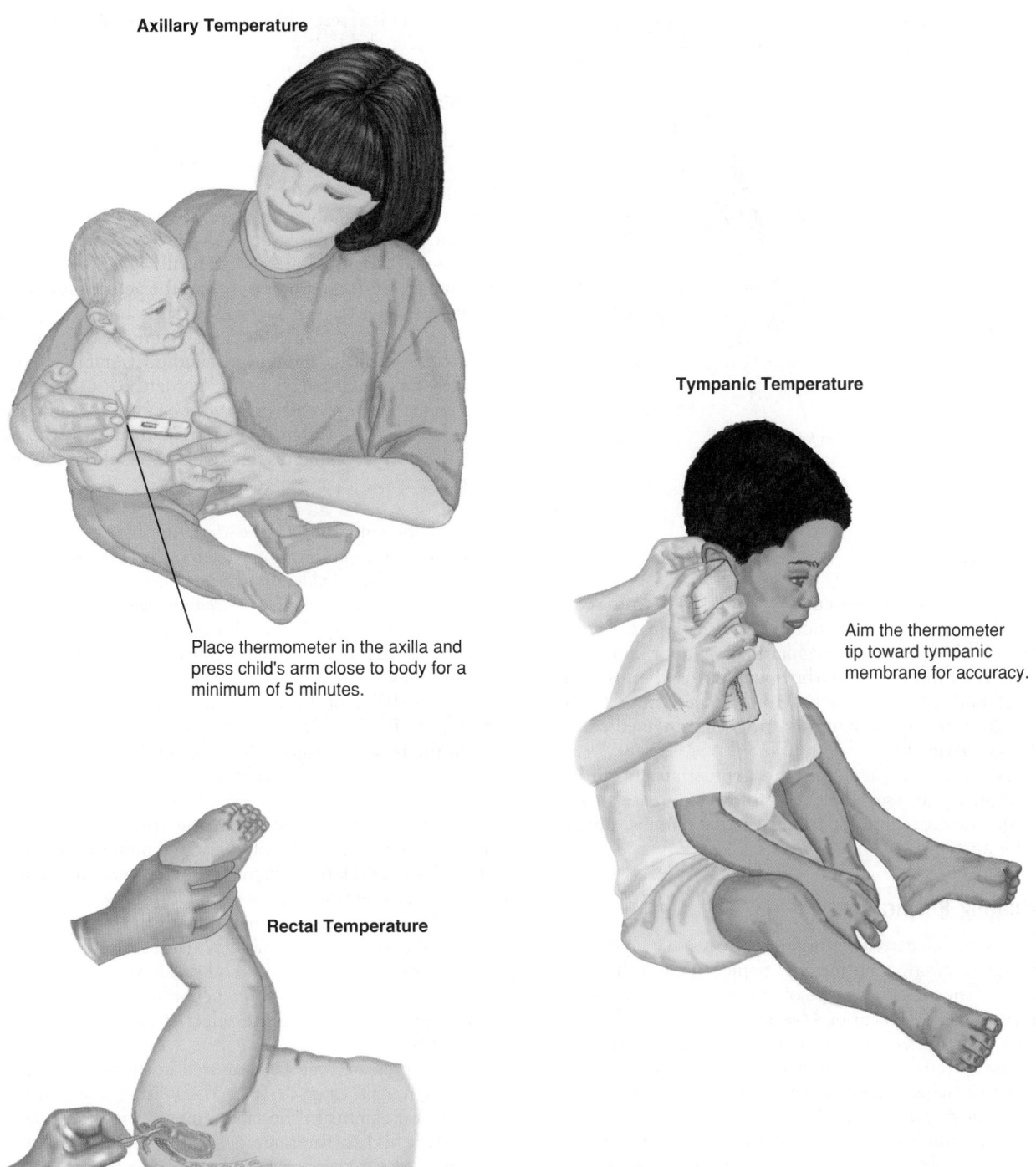

Axillary Temperature

Place thermometer in the axilla and press child's arm close to body for a minimum of 5 minutes.

Tympanic Temperature

Aim the thermometer tip toward tympanic membrane for accuracy.

Rectal Temperature

Insert lubricated thermometer no more than 1.25 cm in an infant, 2.5 cm in an older child.

Figure 37-5 Three methods of temperature measurement.

bite the thermometer. The child should avoid liquids for 30 minutes before the oral temperature measurement. Temperatures measured orally might be inaccurate because of oral intake, oxygen administration, nebulized treatments, or crying. Oral temperature measurement should not be used in any child who has had oral or tonsillar surgery or in whom epiglottitis is suspected.

Because of the risk of rectal perforation and the intrusive and upsetting nature of the procedure, temperatures are measured rectally only when no other route can be used or when it is necessary to obtain a core body temperature (see Fig. 37-5). Skin strips to measure temperature are not considered accurate but can be used in the home setting to estimate whether a child has a fever.

Apical pulse is lateral to the left midclavicular line (MCL) and fourth intercostal space (ICS) in children younger than 7 years and to the left MCL and fifth ICS in children older than 7 years.

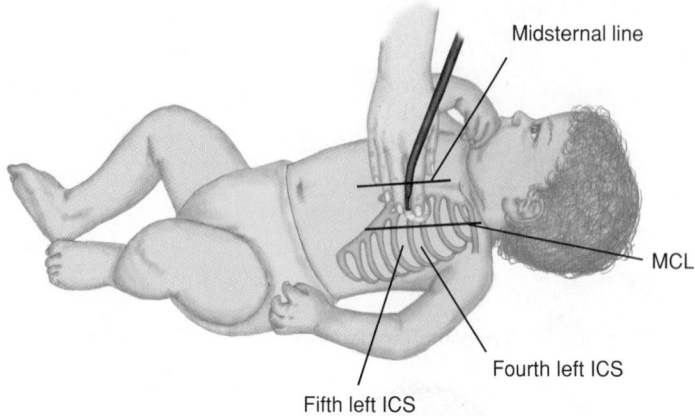

Figure 37-6 Locating the apical pulse.

Measuring Pulse

Apical pulse rate measurements (Fig. 37-6) are recommended for infants and children younger than 2 years and in any child who has an irregular heart rate or known congenital heart disease. Take the apical pulse when the child is quiet, and count for one full minute. Determine the apical heart rate before administering certain medications, such as digoxin.

Radial pulse measurements are appropriate for children older than 2 years (see Table 33-1 for normal pulse measurements). The procedure for taking a radial pulse is similar to that for an adult.

Evaluating Respirations

Infants often have irregular respiratory rates that change with stimulation, crying, and feeding. Some infants will initially exhibit a Cheyne-Stokes type of respiratory pattern, but this pattern should disappear by 4 weeks of age. Table 33-1 shows normal rates. When measuring respirations in an infant, observe the pattern of inspiration and expiration before auscultating; this helps determine any irregular rhythm. Measure the respiratory rate in an infant or young child by auscultating for one full minute. As with the apical pulse measurement, try to obtain the respiratory rate when an infant or young child is at rest. Either observe or auscultate respirations in the older child.

Measuring Blood Pressure

Blood pressure is assessed on hospital admission and may be assessed every shift, or more often if necessary. Unless a problem is suspected, however, blood pressure may not be assessed more than once per year during routine physical examinations.

Choosing the appropriate cuff size is extremely important, because an inappropriate cuff size will yield a blood pressure reading that is higher or lower than the actual pressure. Recommendations for the method of choosing an appropriate cuff size vary, and confusion exists among health professionals as to the most appropriate method (Arafat & Mattoo, 1999; Clark, Lieh-Lai, Sarnaik, & Mattoo, 2002). The *Update on the Task Force Report (1987) on High Blood Pressure in Children and Adolescents* (National Institutes of Health [NIH],1996) recommends that cuff size be selected in the following way:

- Find the midpoint of the right upper arm between the shoulder (acromion) and the elbow (olecranon).
- Holding the bladder of the cuff *lengthwise,* the bladder width should cover approximately 40% of the upper arm circumference (UAC) at this point.
- If measured this way, when you wrap the cuff around the arm to take the blood pressure, the bladder should encircle 80% to 100% of the arm without overlap.
- Palpate the brachial artery, and place the stethoscope bell on the brachial artery below the cuff.
- Measure the blood pressure with the arm at heart level.

If using a different site than the arm for blood pressure measurement, use 40% of the circumference of the site used. Commercially designated blood pressure cuffs are standardized widths. Choose the closest standard width to the 40% circumference measure, rather than the designated label on the cuff. Table 37-1 illustrates average bladder widths of commercial blood pressure cuffs. Blood pressure measurement will differ according to the measuring technique used and the site selected (see Appendix G for normal results).

Blood pressures can be measured in the upper arm, lower arm, thigh, calf, or ankle (Fig. 37-7). To ensure consistency, take measurements in the same limb, in the same place, and with the child in the same position. Remember that blood pressure measurements can differ depending on the site used.

TABLE **37-1** Standardized Blood Pressure Cuff Sizes				
Average Arm Circumference (cm)	Cuff Name	40% of Arm Circumference for Bladder Width (cm)	80% of Arm Circumference for Bladder Width (cm)	Average Standard Cuff Width (cm)
6	Newborn	3	5	*
10	Infant	4	8	6 (infant cuff)
17	Child	7	14	8 (infant or child cuff)
28	Small adult	11	22	11 (small adult cuff)
31	Adult	13	26	14 (adult cuff)

Modified from Arafat, M., & Mattoo, T. (1999). Measurement of blood pressure in children: Recommendations and perceptions on cuff selection, *Pediatrics, 104*(3), e30.
*Information not available.

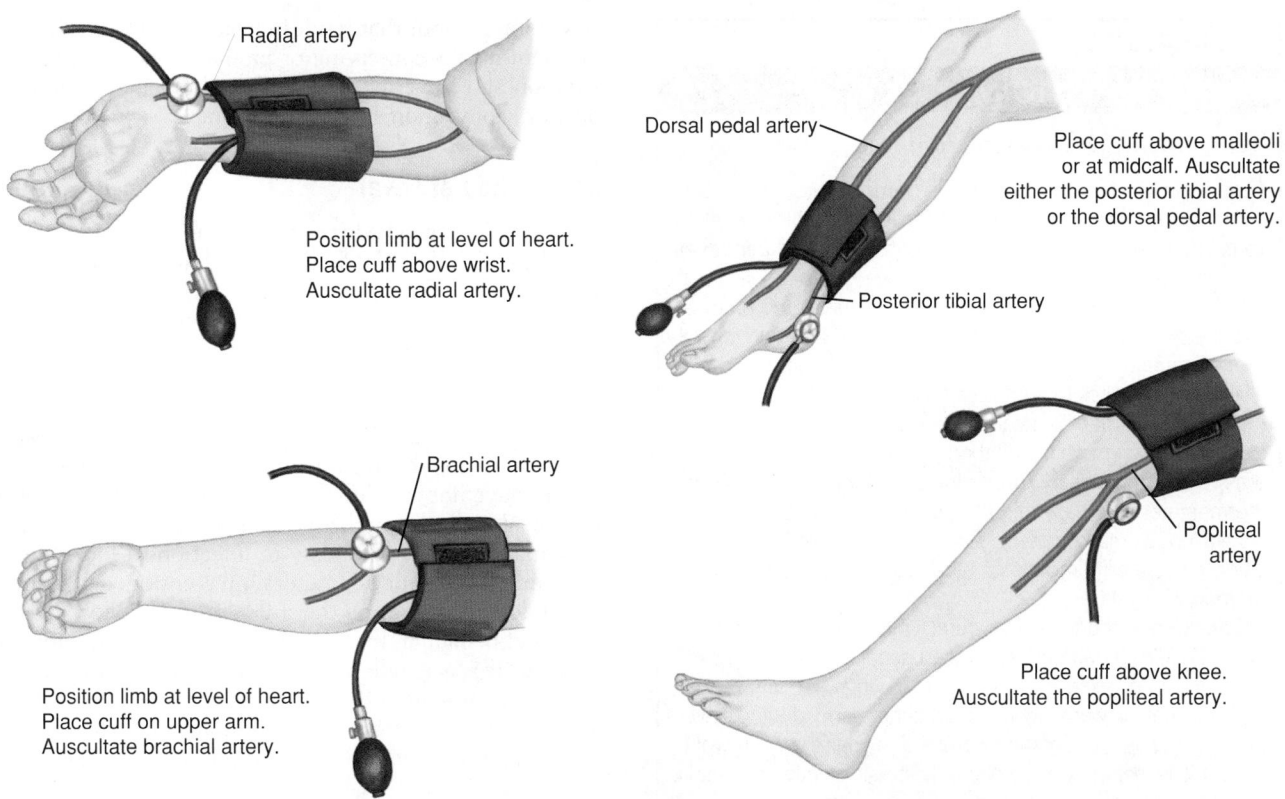

Figure 37-7 Blood pressures can be measured in the upper arm, lower arm, thigh, calf, or ankle. It is important that an appropriate-size cuff be used to obtain accurate results.

When using electronic devices to measure blood pressure, follow the manufacturer's guidelines closely to ensure accuracy. For most devices, the first reading is considered a "priming" reading and the second reading is considered the true blood pressure measurement.

The procedure for measuring blood pressure in children is similar to the procedure for adults. Recommendations state that the diastolic reading is the number at which sound is absent—not the number at which the sound quality changes (NIH, 1996). It might not be possible, however, to auscultate the diastolic pressure in young children. The systolic blood pressure sometimes can be heard down to a measurement of zero. In this case, record the blood pressure as the systolic number over pulse (e.g., 90/P).

When it is impossible to auscultate a blood pressure in infants and toddlers, you can palpate the pulse to obtain a systolic reading. Find the location of the pulse below the cuff with your index and middle fingers and inflate the cuff, as for an auscultated pressure. As the cuff deflates, note the point at which the pulse is first felt. Record this systolic measurement as if you had heard the systolic beat down to zero.

Documentation of Vital Sign Measurement

Record all vital signs in the child's medical record. Include the method used to measure the vital signs, the measurement obtained, and any action taken. Record and report core temperatures of less than 36° C (96.8° F) or more than 38° C (100.4° F). Record and report any other abnormal findings or findings that are significantly different for the individual child.

Preparing the Child and Family

Inform the child and family about the purpose of the procedure. Children who are fearful should be allowed to examine or handle the equipment while you explain how it is used.

You can tell young children that the blood pressure cuff feels like a "hug" or a "squeeze."

Many children have pretend medical equipment at home and might be familiar with the concept of taking vital signs.

Parent Teaching

Some parents may need to learn how to take the child's temperature at home. Demonstrate how to take the child's temperature, and then observe the parent perform the procedure. Make sure the parent is comfortable with the procedure and is able to read the thermometer accurately.

Some parents might need to be taught how to determine their child's heart rate accurately, as well as the acceptable range for their child. Special considerations relating to parents' notifying the physician may need to be made for children who are taking certain medications, such as digoxin.

If the child's condition requires home blood pressure monitoring, teach the procedure to the parent. You can provide helpful suggestions about the size of the cuff and methods to involve the child who might resist this procedure. For instance, parents might make a smaller cuff for the child's favorite doll or stuffed animal.

PARENTS
Want to Know

Temperature Measurement

Accurately measuring your child's temperature, along with other symptoms, helps your physician determine whether your child needs to be seen for assessment and treatment. Feeling your child's forehead can give you a clue as to whether the child's temperature should be measured but does not give accurate information about the child's body temperature. Temperature strips placed on the child's forehead also give only an approximate reading.

A variety of thermometer types are available at the drugstore. An inexpensive digital thermometer can be used to take oral, rectal, and axillary (under the arm) temperatures. Digital thermometers are easy to read because the numbers are displayed on a small screen. Pediatricians do not recommend using glass thermometers or other thermometers containing mercury for children.

The average body temperature, when measured orally, is 98.6° F (37° C). Mild increases can occur as a result of exercise, wearing excessive clothing, taking hot baths, hot weather, eating warm food, or drinking warm drinks. If you take your child's temperature and it is higher than you would expect it to be, encourage the child to sit quietly and retake the temperature in 30 minutes.

Your child has a fever if the temperature is greater than 100.4° F (38° C) when measured rectally, greater than 99.5° F (37.5° C) when taken orally, and greater than 99° F (37.2° C) when measured by the axillary method. If your infant is younger than 6 weeks, you should call your physician if the baby's rectal temperature is above 100° F (37.7° C).

In general, the height of the fever is not an indication of the seriousness of the illness. What is important is how your child is acting. If your child has a fever and is acting sick, notify your physician.

Special Considerations: Cardiorespiratory Monitors

Some children need cardiorespiratory monitoring so that heart rate, respiratory rate, blood pressure, and temperature can be measured continuously. Children who are acutely ill or who are undergoing procedures might be placed on a monitor to help health care providers detect subtle changes in the child's condition.

The procedure and indications for attaching a child to a cardiorespiratory monitor are no different from those for an adult. Monitors will sound an alarm to warn of changes in the child's cardiorespiratory status. Remember that false alarms can occur. *Always look at the child and perform an assessment before intervening.* A flat line on the electrocardiogram (ECG) does not always signal a cardiac arrest. It may be nothing but a loose monitor lead. Check the manufacturer's recommendations for attaching leads and monitoring selected vital signs.

FEVER-REDUCING MEASURES

The body's internal thermostat, the hypothalamus, attempts to keep the body's temperature between 36° and 38° C (96.8° and 100.4° F). This regulation is done through a complex se-

ries of interactions that result in heat gain or loss. The body's mechanisms for conserving or producing heat are vasoconstriction and shivering. Heat is lost through radiation, conduction, convection, and evaporation.

Description of Fever

Fever is defined as a body temperature above 38° C (100.4° F) rectally or 37.5° C (99.5° F) orally that results from an insult or disease during which the body's set-point temperature rises to a higher-than-normal level. After the cause of the fever is removed, the body resets its set point at the normal level.

The body's attempt to defend itself against illness is manifested by fever, which is triggered by endogenous *pyrogens* produced during the inflammatory response. Because research studies have not conclusively demonstrated whether fever is beneficial or detrimental, practitioners vary in their approach to managing fevers secondary to infections. Mild degrees of fever might or might not require intervention, depending on the underlying cause and the child's response. Most fevers are brief and benign and resolve when the underlying infection resolves. It is generally accepted that children with chronic cardiac or respiratory disease, those with neurologic disease, and those prone to febrile seizures should be treated for fever. Children with fevers of 40° C (104° F) or higher also should be treated.

Fever is uncomfortable, and children might become irritable. For every 1° C of temperature elevation, the body's metabolic rate increases 10% to 12%, resulting in increased insensible fluid loss, increased oxygen consumption, and increased stress on the cardiovascular system (Lorin, 2004). Regardless of the fever's cause, the child's comfort is the primary reason for treating a fever in a normally healthy child.

Medications and Environmental Management

Treatment can consist of environmental measures, antipyretics, or a combination of interventions. External cooling is one of the oldest and most common forms of fever management, particularly when the elevated temperature is caused by hyperthermia. Removing blankets and clothing and reducing the environmental temperature can reduce fever. Tepid sponge baths and the use of mechanical cooling blankets can reduce a moderate to high fever fairly quickly (Procedures 37-1 and 37-2). The challenge is to reduce the fever without causing shivering, which produces heat.

In febrile illnesses, the body attempts to resist external cooling, resulting in the need for antipyretics in addition to external cooling interventions. Fevers in children are treated with antipyretics, such as acetaminophen and ibuprofen (Drug Guide: Acetaminophen). Aspirin is avoided because of its association with Reye syndrome in children with viral illnesses such as influenza and varicella.

Children with elevated temperatures often experience loss of appetite. Dehydration can occur from decreased oral intake and increased insensible water loss through the lungs and the skin. Meet the need for adequate hydration by offering the child additional oral fluids. For those who refuse oral hydration or who are unable to take in adequate volume, consider the need for intravenous fluids.

Procedure 37-1

Giving a Cooling Bath

PURPOSE: To reduce fever.

1. Explain the purpose and the reason for selecting the intervention, using developmentally appropriate language. If possible, provide toys or some other distraction for the child. The parent can be present to help comfort or play with the child.
2. Gather the following equipment: tepid water (water temperature between 29° and 32° C [approximately 85° and 90° F]), cotton blankets, washcloths, and toys. The use of rubbing alcohol is contraindicated because of skin irritation, the risk of neurologic depression from the fumes or absorption through the skin, and too-rapid cooling, which can result in shivering.
3. Assist the infant or child to sit or lie in a position of comfort in the bed. Place the infant or child on a cotton bath blanket.

When Bathing the Child Outside a Tub

4. Using tepid water, wet the washcloths or towels and place them on the child, exposing one area at a time. Tepid water— not ice water—is used because it allows the body temperature to drop gradually, thus avoiding heat-producing responses, such as shivering, which are caused by too-rapid cooling. *If shivering occurs, the procedure should be terminated immediately.*

When the Child Is Placed in a Tub

5. Alternatively, the child can be placed in a tub of warm water, with cool water added until the desired temperature is reached. Gently pour or spray water over the child's back and chest. Continue this for 20 to 30 minutes. Use water toys to provide distraction during this nursing intervention. *Remember: An infant or young child should never be left unattended in the tub*

6. After the bath, dry the child. Dress the child in lightweight clothing or pajamas, and place in a dry bed.
7. Recheck the child's temperature approximately 30 minutes later to evaluate the effectiveness of the intervention.
8. Document in the nurses' notes the child's baseline vital signs, hydration status, general appearance, interventions used for fever reduction, the indications for the interventions, the duration, the child's response, and any problems identified. Also document any family teaching, as well as the degree of understanding the information given.
9. Take the opportunity to teach the parent how to care for a child with an elevated temperature. Provide information about how to take a temperature, how to read a thermometer, normal temperature range, administration of antipyretics, the use of tepid baths, and when to seek professional help. It is important to emphasize in your teaching that ice water and isopropyl alcohol should never be used for sponging or bathing the child with a fever.
10. Additional points to cover with parents include the importance of accuracy in dosing, the timing of doses, methods of administration, and appropriate medication choices when giving antipyretics. Parents need reassurance that fever is a common sign of illness and rarely poses a threat to the child's well-being.

Home Adaptations

To manage a fever at home, advise the parent to dress the child in lightweight clothing. Consult with the child's pediatrician before initiating tepid baths. If advised to use tepid baths, an infant tub or regular bathtub can be used. Advise the parent to keep the room at a comfortable temperature and discontinue the tepid bath if the child begins to shiver.

Procedure 37-2

Using a Cooling Blanket

PURPOSE: To reduce hyperthermia.

1. Using developmentally appropriate language, explain the purpose and the reason for using a cooling blanket. Encourage the parent to be present to help comfort or distract the child.
2. You will need the following equipment: a commercial cooling blanket, sheets or small blankets as needed, and a temperature probe.
3. Place the cooling blanket on the bed, and cover it with a sheet or thin blanket.
4. Connect the blanket to the cooling unit, and set the control mode (manual or automatic) and the desired blanket or body temperature. Temperature parameters should be set according to the manufacturer's recommendations and physician's orders.
5. Check the child's skin condition before, during, and after use of the blanket, and record the findings.

6. Cover the child lightly to maintain privacy and reduce shivering.
7. To prevent too-rapid cooling or overcooling, monitor the child's vital signs frequently. A temperature probe can be used to monitor the child's temperature continually during this cooling method.
8. To reduce shivering, wrap the child's extremities with towels or baby blankets.
9. Keep the child completely dry to reduce the risk of frostbite from dampness.
10. Reposition the child who is on a cooling unit frequently and gently to reduce the risk of skin breakdown.
11. Record the type of unit used, the control mode and temperature settings selected, and the condition of the child's skin before, during, and after use.

Drug Guide

Acetaminophen (Tylenol, Tempra, Panadol)

Classification: Non-narcotic analgesic and antipyretic.

Action: Unknown; may act on hypothalamic heat-regulating center.

Indications: Mild fever and pain relief.

Dosage and Route: Dosage is age- and/or weight-related; administered 4 or 5 times daily. Oral, rectal. Comes in a variety of oral preparations: infant drops (80 mg/0.8 ml), liquid or suspension (160 mg/5 ml), chewable tablets (80 mg/tab), caplets and chewables for older children (160 mg/tab), adult strength (325 mg/tab). Rectal suppositories in 80, 120, 125, 300, 325, and 650 mg.

Absorption: From the gastrointestinal tract; peak action in 1 to 3 hours.

Excretion: Duration approximately 4 to 5 hours.

Contraindications: Any previous sensitivity to the medication.

Precautions: Long-term use can cause liver damage. Other over-the-counter cold preparations can contain acetaminophen; if given concurrently they can increase the amount of acetaminophen above safe levels.

Adverse Reactions: Blood dyscrasias, hypoglycemia, rashes or urticaria, liver damage with prolonged use.

Nursing Considerations: Advise parents to be extremely careful not to confuse the liquid preparations; check the label very carefully before giving the medication. Never refer to this or any other medication as "candy." Acetaminophen overdose must be treated immediately to prevent hepatic toxicity. In clients performing home glucose monitoring, acetaminophen can affect glucose readings. Parents should not continue to give their children this medication for fever that lasts longer than 2 days without checking with the health care provider.

It is important to remember that infants who are being cared for in servocontrolled heating environments must be carefully monitored because of the potential for accidental dislodgment of the skin temperature probe. This problem can cause an increase in the heat production of the unit and a resulting increase in the infant's temperature. In addition, the insensible water loss in infants in these controlled units is greatly increased. These additional fluid losses must be considered when calculating fluid replacement.

Commercial Cooling Blankets

Commercial cooling blankets also can be used to control hyperthermia. These units, which can be controlled manually or automatically, lower the body temperature through cold transfer between the blanket and the child. Cooling unit operation varies among manufacturers. Therefore it is important to read the operating manual before using this equipment. Some cooling blankets may be reusable, but blankets designed for single client use are preferred. Shivering, frostbite, and skin breakdown are concerns when using a cooling blanket.

SPECIMEN COLLECTION

Specimens are collected from children for the same reasons they are collected from adults, but children often need more of an explanation of the reasons and procedure for specimen collection. All explanations should be given in age-appropriate language, and children should be prepared for any sensations that they might experience.

Regardless of the type of specimen to be obtained, use Standard Precautions. The use of gloves, gowns, masks, eye protection, and handwashing provides protection for individuals coming in contact with potentially infectious materials. The use of equipment for Standard Precautions will vary according to the degree of "potential splash." *Any time there is a chance for contamination, use Standard Precautions.* Follow procedures for handling biologic hazards as directed by individual facilities, on the basis of Standard Precautions.

Urine Specimens

Voided Specimens

Older children and adolescents often cooperate in the collection of urine specimens. Most can use a bedpan, urinal, or specimen cup with little difficulty. Younger children and preschoolers often have difficulty voiding on request. The nurse should take care to use familiar terms, such as "pee pee," "tinkle," or "potty," when telling the child what is needed. For younger children, it is helpful to have available a potty chair or collection "hat" that fits in the toilet. Parents can be very helpful in obtaining a specimen from children this age. Parents might also be successful obtaining specimens from older toddlers who are being toilet trained. Infants and young toddlers, however, are unable to void on request. Because they are not toilet trained, specimen collection devices are needed (Procedure 37-3).

If the specimen must be collected under special conditions (e.g., a midstream urine sample), the nurse carefully explains to the child what preparation is needed and verifies that the child understands all directions. An adult might need to accompany the child during the collection. A young child might be able to sit on the toilet but be unable to manipulate a specimen cup. The parent or nurse can hold the cup while the child voids. For a boy who wishes to stand while voiding, the cup can be held in the stream as he voids. If the specimen is to be carried to another room or down a hallway, provide a plastic bag or other container for transport.

If a midstream urine sample is needed and the child is at home, the nurse can describe the procedure to the parent over the telephone. The parent will need to boil a clean glass container and cover for 20 minutes in a covered pan. After letting the water cool, empty the water from the pan and carefully remove the container and the cover, being sure not to touch the inside of either. The urine is collected after the

Procedure 37-3

Urine Specimen Collection From the Incontinent Child

PURPOSE: To monitor urine output accurately or obtain a specimen for testing.

1. Before beginning the procedure, provide adequate privacy. The child may be more relaxed if a parent is present. If both blood and urine specimens need to be obtained from the incontinent child, position the collection bag *before* drawing the blood. Infants and toddlers often void during a painful procedure.

2. Obtain the following equipment: non-sterile gloves; urine collection bag; sterile specimen cup; mild soap, warm water, and a washcloth; diaper and towel; and label and requisition form.

3. Put on gloves, and clean the perineal area. Cleaning the perineum will remove any lotions or ointments and help the bag adhere:
   a. *For girls:* Clean from front to back and from the urinary meatus to the labia majora (in to out).
   b. *For boys:* Clean from the tip of the penis in a circular motion. *Do not* retract an infant's or young child's foreskin.

4. After the perineum has been cleansed, dry it thoroughly. The skin must be completely dry for the bag to adhere properly.

5. Remove the backing from the adhesive surface of the bottom half of the collection device.

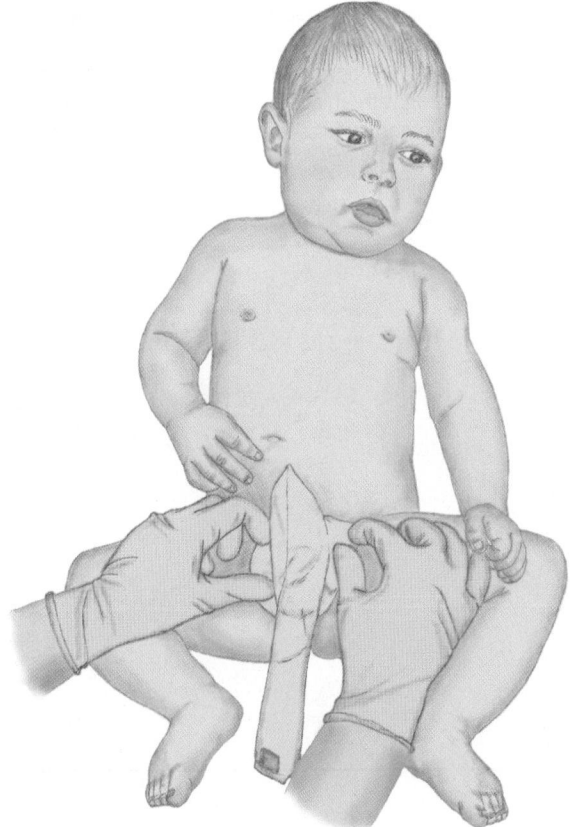

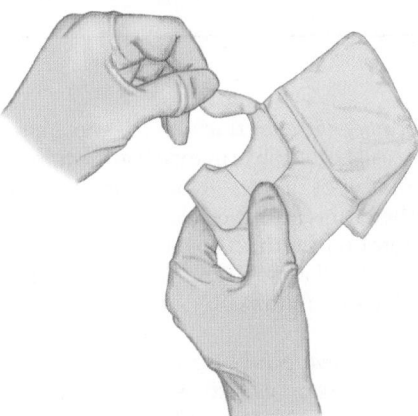

6. Place the child in a frog-leg position to eliminate skinfolds that may interfere with bag adherence. Apply the bag:
   a. *For girls:* Hold the perineum taut, and apply the adhesive portion of the bag, working outward. To keep the feces from contaminating the specimen, the narrow "bridge" on the adhesive patch must be placed on the tiny area of skin between the anus and the genitalia.

b. *For boys:* Place the penis and scrotum (if small enough) inside the bag.

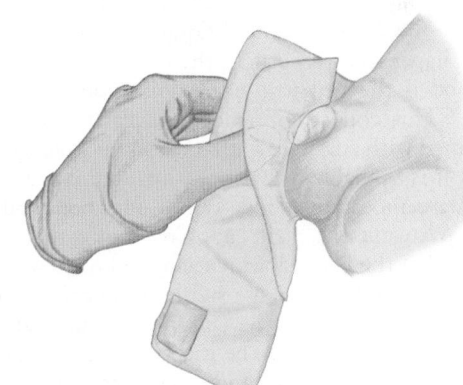

7. After the bag is attached, a diaper can be reapplied. Before replacing the diaper, cut a slit in the diaper and pull the end of the empty bag through the slit so that the bag protrudes from the diaper. This step reduces the chance of leaking and allows for observation of urine.

8. Check the bag every 30 minutes. Applying slight pressure over the suprapubic area or stroking along the older infant's spine will often induce voiding. As soon as urine is noticed in the bag, gently remove the bag from the perineum.

Continued

Procedure 37-3

Urine Specimen Collection From the Incontinent Child—cont'd

9. Transfer the urine into a sterile specimen cup. Most bags have a small tab that can be removed to allow the urine to be poured. If the bag does not have a tab, clean the outside of the bag with an alcohol pad and withdraw the urine with a needle and syringe for placement in the appropriate container.

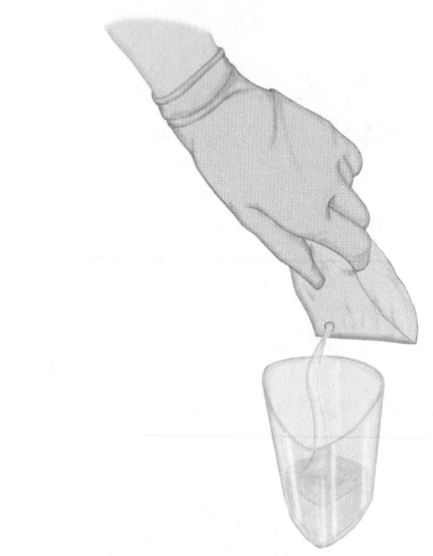

10. Label the urine specimen with the child's name and date and time of collection, and deliver it promptly, together with a requisition form, to the laboratory. Urine for culture that cannot be tested within 30 minutes should be refrigerated or placed in a sterile container with a preservative.
11. Record the collection of the specimen in the child's chart. Include the date and time of collection and the amount, color, and appearance of the urine.

Home Adaptations

If a urine specimen is to be obtained at home, give instructions to the parent and provide the appropriate equipment. Parents can keep the urine collected at home in the refrigerator until they are asked to bring it to the laboratory. The specimen should be kept chilled during transport (i.e., placed in a cooler or plastic bag packed with ice).

---

perineal area is cleaned (see Procedure 37-3). Advise the parent to place the specimen jar in a plastic bag and keep refrigerated until brought to the laboratory for testing.

Although many methods have been used to collect nonsterile urine from incontinent children (e.g., placing plastic wrap in a diaper to catch urine), the most reliable noninvasive method is the pediatric urine collection bag or urine "wee bag." This collection device is a plastic bag with an opening lined with adhesive so that it can be attached to the perineum. It is available in two sizes, infant and pediatric, to accommodate almost any child. Twenty-four-hour collection bags are also available. These bags have a tube that extends from the end of the bag, allowing each void to be removed.

Although some facilities use sterile urine collection bags to obtain a specimen for urine culture, this method of collecting urine is considered to be inappropriate to rule out a urinary tract infection. Bags can become contaminated with organisms usually present in the perineal area. Most physicians choose to use straight catheterization or suprapubic aspiration (inserting a needle through the skin and directly into the bladder) to obtain urine for culture from an incontinent child.

Urinary Catheterization

Catheterizing a child is different from catheterizing an adult because of the child's unique psychologic and developmental needs (Procedure 37-4). Pediatric catheterization kits often contain a completely closed collection system (with the catheter end already enclosed in the collection tube).

Choose a urinary catheter that is small enough so that it can be inserted easily into the urinary meatus but large enough to prevent leakage of urine. Avoid using feeding tubes as straight catheters because these could become coiled or knotted after insertion (Smith, 2003). Urinary catheters are available in sizes as small as no. 5 French (Fr) and can be matched to the child's age as follows:

- *Infants up to 1 year old:* No. 5 to 8 Fr
- *Children 1 to 5 years old:* No. 8 Fr
- *School-age children:* No. 8 to 12 Fr
- *Adolescents:* No. 10 to 14 Fr

Some facilities recommend pre-catheterization topical application and instillation of an anesthetic lubricant, such as 2% lidocaine hydrochloride, to diminish discomfort associated with catheterization (Gerard, et al, 2003). Some children, particularly those who undergo multiple urinary tract catheterizations (e.g., children with spina bifida), are at high risk for developing latex sensitivity. These children and other children with known or suspected latex allergy should be identified as early as possible, and latex-free catheters should be used.

Stool Specimens

Stool specimens are obtained to test for the presence of fat, blood, bacteria, parasites, or reducing substances in the stool. If a stool specimen from an incontinent child is needed, it of-

Procedure 37-4

Urinary Catheterization

PURPOSE: To obtain a sterile urine sample.

1. Prepare the child for the procedure by using age-appropriate methods. Explain what the child will feel and what the child can do to "help." It may be helpful to demonstrate the procedure on a teaching doll. Teach the child to take slow, deep breaths during the procedure, and have the child practice breathing before the procedure. Encouraging the child to sing also helps relax the appropriate muscles. The child might feel a need to urinate during the catheter insertion. Reassure the child that the feeling is normal. The assistance of another adult is often necessary with younger children.

2. Make sure the area is well lighted, and gather all necessary equipment. If equipment is not contained in the catheterization kit, bring the appropriate-size catheter, sterile gloves (extra pairs in case of contamination), specimen cup, sterile topical anesthetic lubricant, label, and requisition form. If the child is to have an indwelling catheter, bring a closed drainage bag.

3. The procedure is the same as for an adult, with the following additions:
   a. Take extra care to be gentle when cleansing the meatus or glans penis.
   b. Choose the appropriate-size catheter (see p. 948). Apply the lubricant according to manufacturer's directions.
   c. In girls, direct the catheter slightly upward and insert it gently through the meatus 1 to 2 inches (2.5 to 5 cm) or until urine appears. In boys, hold the penis at a 90-degree angle from the boy and gently insert the catheter 2 to 4 inches (5 to 10 cm) (longer in older boys) or until urine appears. Never force the catheter. The older child can assist in relaxing the external sphincter by bearing down.

4. When using an indwelling catheter, measure the distance from the catheter tip to the end of the balloon. Once urine is observed, insert the catheter an additional amount at least equal to this distance before inflating the balloon, or follow institution policy regarding insertion length. Research-based recommendations on insertion suggest inserting an indwelling catheter until urine is visualized and then inserting it an additional amount prior to inflating the balloon: 2 inches (5 cm) for girls, 3 to 4 inches (7.5 to 10 cm) for boys newborn to preschool, and 5 inches (12.5 cm) for older boys.* These distances reduce the risk of the balloon inflating in the urethra. Before inserting a Foley catheter, inflate and deflate the balloon to check for function and leaks.

5. Record the date and time the procedure was done, as well as the size of catheter used and the amount, color, and appearance of the urine. Note how the infant or child tolerated the procedure. Deliver the labeled specimen promptly, together with the requisition form, to the laboratory.

Home Adaptations

Catheterizing at home is usually a clean rather than sterile procedure and a procedure used for children who have spina bifida, neurogenic bladder, or incomplete bladder emptying. Some families choose to use a new, packaged catheter each time; however, this can be extremely expensive when a child has to be catheterized several times per day. The alternative is to thoroughly rinse, clean, and dry the catheters and keep them in a clean, covered container, or a plastic bag if the child is carrying the catheter in a pocket or pack. The parent needs to follow physician protocol for cleaning the perineum; this may include just mild soap and water or the use of povidone-iodine. The infant or young child can be catheterized on a changing table, allowing the urine to empty into a diaper or small container; the older child can be catheterized on the toilet. When teaching a girl how to self-catheterize, use a mirror to help her identify landmarks.

*Smith, A., & Adams, L. (1998). Insertion of indwelling urethral catheters in infants and children: A survey of current nursing practice. *Pediatric Nursing, 24*(3), 229-234.

---

ten can be scraped from a diaper and placed in an appropriate container. If the stool is watery, a specimen may be collected by placing a piece of gauze in the diaper to absorb some of the stool or by applying a "wee bag" over the anus.

A bedpan or a specimen collector that is designed to be placed in the toilet can be used to obtain a specimen from an older child. Because older children may be embarrassed about providing a stool sample, the nurse should use a calm, matter-of-fact manner when explaining why the specimen is needed and the procedure for handling the specimen.

Blood Specimens

Nurses use a variety of techniques to collect blood samples from children. Because blood collection is an invasive procedure, it should be performed in a treatment room if one is available.

Regardless of the sampling procedure used, most children find blood collection distressing. Some are concerned about the pain involved, and others fear the perceived loss of body fluid. The use of a eutectic mixture of local anesthetics (EMLA), a topical anesthetic cream, can reduce the child's discomfort. To be effective, EMLA must remain on the site for at least 45 minutes before the needle is inserted. (See Chapter 38 for a discussion of EMLA.)

In children who need long-term venous access for nutrition or medications and who have a central venous catheter or port in place, the nurse can obtain blood for laboratory studies from the central venous catheter or port. This procedure, however, may be performed *only* by specially trained, licensed personnel.

Venipuncture in children is often performed using a butterfly catheter (Procedure 37-5). The most commonly used sites are the veins of the hand and the antecubital area. Always follow Standard Precautions when collecting blood specimens or when assisting other personnel in collecting blood.

Procedure 37-5

Venipuncture

PURPOSE: To obtain a blood sample for laboratory testing with minimal trauma to the child.

1. As with any procedure, prepare the child using age-appropriate language. Be sure to include what the child will see and feel. Ask the parents whether it is better to prepare their young child in advance or to describe what you are doing as you are performing the procedure. It is often necessary to obtain help to restrain the child during the procedure. Parents might not wish to remain in the room.

2. Take the child to the treatment room. Have the following equipment available: 23- or 25-gauge butterfly catheter, gloves, alcohol or povidone-iodine (Betadine) swabs or pads, syringe or syringes, labels, appropriate collection containers, requisition form, and tourniquet. (NOTE: Most tourniquets are composed of rubber tubing that is 1/2 to 1 inch wide. Although rubber bands have been used as tourniquets in infants, these are not preferred because they may abrade the skin.)

3. Restrain the child by having one nurse place one gloved hand under the child's arm (usually at the shoulder) and the other gloved hand on the child's hand. The sampling nurse is then able to draw the blood with less likelihood of missing the vein. The vein of the antecubital area is commonly used for venipuncture in children.

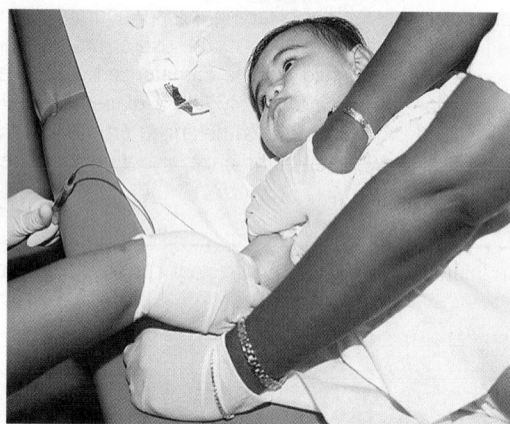

(Courtesy Parkland Health and Hospital System Community Oriented Primary Care Clinic, Dallas, TX.)

4. Put on gloves, and then apply a tourniquet tight enough to restrict blood flow toward the heart but not so tight as to cause pain or restrict arterial blood flow. Tourniquets are used to slow venous blood return to the heart and cause distention of the veins, thus making them more visible. To facilitate easy removal, the tourniquet should be looped when applied. To prevent hemoconcentration, a tourniquet should be left in place no longer than 2 minutes.

5. Lightly pat or rub the sample site to help the veins become more visible.

6. Using a circular motion, clean the site with alcohol and allow to dry. If the child is immunocompromised, use povidone-iodine (Betadine) to cleanse the skin instead of alcohol. Do not use both together, because they can damage the skin.

7. Insert the needle of the butterfly catheter into the vein, bevel side up.

8. When blood begins to flow into the catheter, avoid the temptation to place the syringe on the end of the catheter and attempt to speed up the blood flow by pulling back the plunger. Instead, to avoid venospasm wait until the blood reaches the end of the catheter, attach the syringe, and slowly draw the appropriate amount of blood into the syringe. The tourniquet can be released when blood begins to flow into the syringe.

9. After obtaining the required amount of blood, withdraw the needle and apply pressure to the puncture site until the bleeding has stopped. Fill the appropriate specimen tubes or containers. Be sure to dispose of needles and contaminated gauze properly.

10. Comfort the child, and offer praise for cooperation. Encourage the parent to provide comfort. Adhesive bandages are important because they help prevent bleeding from the puncture site. Specially colored or cartoon character bandages are available commercially and are appropriate for children's "boo-boos." The nurse can also give the child a reward, such as a sticker.

11. Label the specimen with the child's name; and record the date and time of collection, the amount of blood collected, the site used for puncture, and the reason blood was drawn (e.g., diagnostic test). Note the child's reaction to the procedure and the number of attempts made before a specimen was obtained.

Jugular and Femoral Venipuncture

Jugular venipuncture and femoral venipuncture are performed by a physician, with the nurse assisting and monitoring the child. If obtaining blood from one of the large superficial external jugular veins, place the child in a mummy restraint (see Fig. 37-3), allowing enough area at the top edge of the restraint to permit access to the jugular vein. If a restraint is not used, the arms and legs can be held by a second nurse. The child's head is hyperextended to the side opposite the site, over the edge of a table or a small pillow (Fig. 37-8). After the venipuncture, apply pressure to the site for 3 to 5 minutes or until bleeding stops. Care should be taken not to overextend the head to the point of causing airway problems.

If performing a femoral venipuncture, place the child supine in the frog-leg position to expose the groin area (see Fig. 37-8). One nurse stands above the child's head, holding the child's arms with the elbows and the legs with the hands. Place a cloth diaper over the infant's perineal area, tucked under the buttocks with the site exposed. The diaper protects the area in case the child urinates. Apply pressure to the site with a dry, sterile gauze square after the specimen is obtained.

Infant positioned for jugular venipuncture

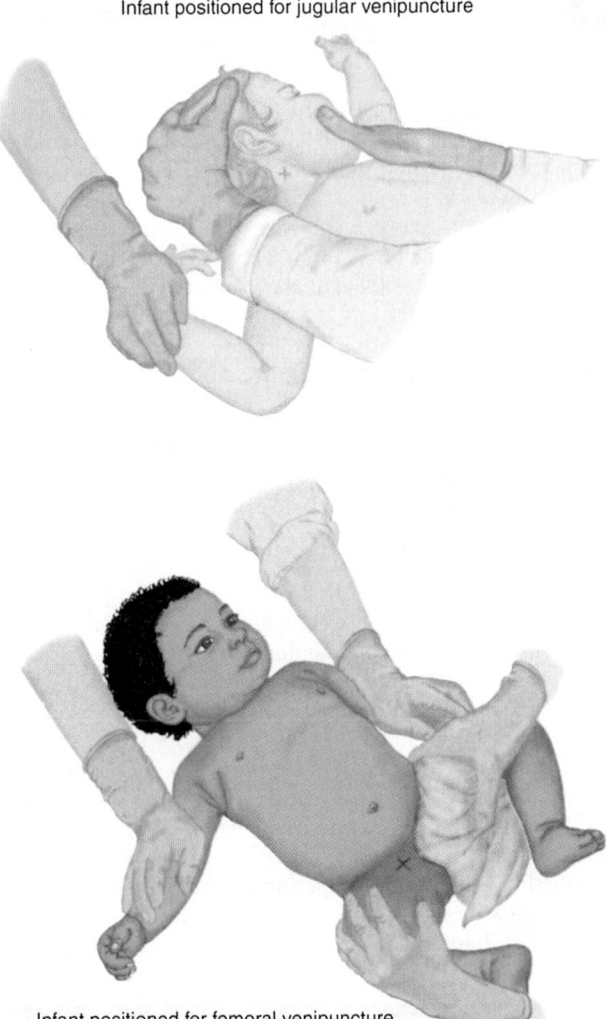

Infant positioned for femoral venipuncture

Figure 37-8 Two additional sites for obtaining blood specimens from infants and young children are the large superficial external jugular veins and the femoral veins.

Capillary Blood Sampling

When a small blood sample is needed, a disposable pediatric lancet (inserted 2.4 mm deep) can be used for a finger or heel puncture (Procedure 37-6). For finger punctures, the third (ring) finger of the nondominant hand should be used. Make the puncture just to the side of the finger pad rather than at the tip. There are fewer nerve endings, and the areas are highly vascular. The heel is used in infants; it is warmed first to increase blood flow. The heel is not used once the infant is walking because calluses make it more difficult to puncture.

Sputum Specimens

Sputum specimens are most frequently obtained to identify or rule out a respiratory infection. When obtaining any specimen, follow Standard Precautions. If splashing is anticipated, wear masks and goggles or protective eye wear in addition to gloves.

It is relatively easy to obtain sputum in the older child because most older children and adolescents can cough deeply and produce a sputum sample, which can then be placed in the

---

Procedure 37-6

Capillary Blood Sampling

PURPOSE: To obtain a small sample of capillary blood.

1. Prepare the child appropriately for the procedure using developmentally appropriate explanations (finger poke, "owie"). You can warm the site before proceeding or have the older child wash the hands in warm water.
2. Bring the child to the treatment room, where the following equipment should be available: disposable lancets or microlancets, alcohol or povidone-iodine (Betadine) swabs, sterile gauze pads, gloves, warm washcloth, specimen containers, and labels and requisition forms.
3. After putting on gloves and appropriately cleaning the site, make a puncture with the lancet across the fingerprint halfway between the center of the ball of the finger and its side. Use the third, or ring, finger of the nondominant hand. Do not use a bruised, edematous, or abraded finger, and avoid old puncture sites.

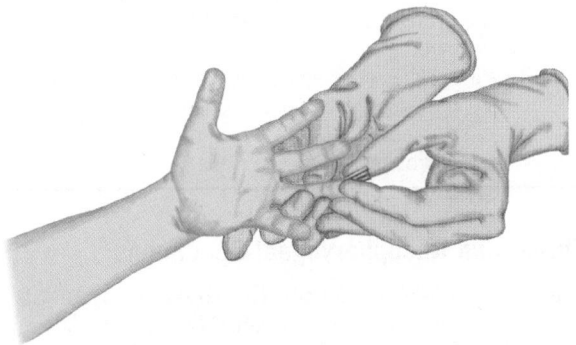

4. Wipe off the first drop of blood with a sterile gauze pad. To ensure adequate blood flow, you may gently massage the finger from its base to the tip.
5. Collect the blood in the appropriate container or containers. Apply pressure with sterile gauze until the bleeding stops. Apply a decorative Band-Aid if the child desires. Do not apply a Band-Aid on an infant.
6. Label the specimen with the child's name; and record the date, time, amount of blood collected, site used for the puncture, and reason the blood was drawn. Note the child's reaction to the procedure and whether more than one puncture was necessary. (For capillary sampling by heal stick, see Procedure 22-1.)

---

appropriate container. Specimens are easily obtained from children with artificial airways by attaching a mucus or suction trap to a suction catheter and suctioning the airway to obtain the specimen. A cough can be elicited by placing a suction catheter into the back of the throat in an infant or young child.

Because younger children and infants can seldom produce a deep cough on demand and often swallow those secretions, obtaining sputum samples in infants and young children often requires a nasal washing, or *lavage* (Procedure 37-7). Nasal washing is used particularly to obtain a sample for identifying respiratory syncytial virus (RSV) and pertussis.

Procedure 37-7

Nasal Washing

PURPOSE: To obtain a nasopharyngeal secretion sample from an infant or young child.

1. Prepare the child for the procedure by using developmentally appropriate language and describing any expected sensations (the procedure will make the child sneeze).
2. Gather the following equipment: butterfly catheter, syringe, sterile saline, gloves, goggles, sterile specimen container or pertussis kit, and labels and requisition form.
3. Ask for assistance restraining the child, or mummy-wrap an infant to restrain the arms and legs.
4. Cut the "butterfly" (needle and wings) off the butterfly catheter, and discard.
5. Attach a syringe (without needle) containing 1 to 3 ml of sterile saline to the catheter, and fill the catheter.
6. Put on gloves and goggles, and place the child in a supine position; gently place the catheter into one nostril.
7. Instill the saline into the nostril and immediately withdraw into the syringe, or aspirate secretions with a small sterile bulb syringe.
8. Place the saline or secretions into a sterile, labeled container.
9. Record the amount of saline instilled and the method of collection used. Note the date, time, amount, color, and consistency of secretions.

Throat and Nasopharyngeal Specimens

Throat cultures can identify the causative agent of "sore throats" or tonsillitis in children. Nasopharyngeal cultures are used mainly to identify pertussis (Procedure 37-8).

! CRITICAL TO REMEMBER

Throat Cultures

- Never attempt to obtain a throat specimen for culture in a child for whom a diagnosis of *epiglottitis* is suspected, because the procedure could precipitate sudden airway obstruction.
- Before obtaining a specimen for throat culture, assess for the presence of high fever of sudden onset, drooling, muffled voice, and erythema or exudate (signs of epiglottitis).

Cerebrospinal Fluid Specimens

Physicians perform lumbar punctures to examine the cerebrospinal fluid (CSF) for bacteria or abnormal cells, to measure pressure within the cerebrospinal cavities, or to inject certain medications (i.e., for pain control, to prevent or eradicate specific diseases, or as contrast agents for scans). A hollow spinal needle, inserted into the subarachnoid space between the third and fourth lumbar vertebrae, provides for fluid exit and collection. An attached stopcock and manometer are used to measure spinal fluid pressure.

Because a lumbar puncture is frequently performed when a child is acutely ill—with meningitis or leukemia, for example—this stressful procedure becomes even more stressful for the child and family. The nurse must provide a great deal of support and education for the child and family. The physician will explain what is planned and will obtain an informed consent from the parents or guardians. Only a physician or qualified nurse practitioner performs a lumbar puncture. The nurse assists by positioning, restraining, and monitoring the child (see Chapter 52).

Procedure 37-8

Throat or Nasopharyngeal Culture

PURPOSE: To obtain a specimen for culture.

1. Explain the procedure to the child in appropriate language. For a throat culture, explain that the child will need to look up toward the ceiling, open the mouth very wide, and might feel like coughing or gagging. Emphasize that the procedure does not hurt. For a nasopharyngeal swab, tell the child to look up and explain that you will be inserting the swab into the nose. The child will feel like sneezing. Do not do these procedures immediately after the child has taken medication, eaten, or had something to drink. Assistance may be needed to restrain a younger child.
2. Gather the following equipment: tongue depressor, throat or nasopharyngeal swab (cotton-tipped swab with a flexible wire extension), collection containers and labels (if not included with the swab), gloves, goggles, and sterile saline.
3. An older child can sit in a chair or sit upright in bed for the culture. A younger child should be placed supine on a bed or examining table.

Throat Culture

4. Put on gloves and goggles, and have the child open the mouth and say "Ahhh." Eliciting a cry from an infant will give optimal access to the pharyngeal area. Insert a tongue de-

pressor into the mouth with the nondominant hand so that it covers the anterior half of the tongue, and depress the tongue to allow observation of the pharyngeal area. Swab the area quickly, avoiding the tongue, buccal mucosa, and palate. If the child opens the mouth wide enough for adequate visibility, a tongue depressor might not be needed. Only one swab should be used for each culture.

Nasopharyngeal Culture

5. Ask the child to look up. Bend the wire so that, when the swab is inserted, the tip will go beyond the back of the nares and into the pharyngeal area. Dip the swab tip into saline, and gently insert it into one naris, down to the posterior nasopharynx. Leave it in place for several seconds, and then remove.
6. After the specimen is obtained, place the swabs in the appropriate culture media, and transport them to the laboratory.
7. If possible, offer the child cool fluids to drink after the procedure. Assist the parent to support and comfort the child during and after the procedure.
8. Record the date and time, the appearance of the specimen, and the child's response to the procedure.

Bone Marrow Aspirates

Bone marrow aspiration is performed to obtain specimens of marrow for diagnostic testing, for evaluation of response to treatment, or for transplantation (see Chapter 48). The most common site of bone marrow aspiration in the child is the posterior iliac crest. Other sites include the anterior iliac crest and the tibia.

Because the reasons for a bone marrow aspiration include ruling out serious disease, such as leukemia, or assessing the progress of cancer treatment, the child and family need a tremendous amount of support and preparation before the procedure.

GAVAGE AND GASTROSTOMY

Because some infants and children are unable to tolerate adequate oral nutrition, the physician might select an alternative method of feeding. *Enteral feedings* are an option for infants and children who are premature, ill, or injured or who have congenital anomalies, respiratory distress, swallowing disorders, or neurologic impairment or have previously undergone surgery. Feedings are given through an orogastric, nasogastric, or transpyloric tube or through a gastrostomy tube or button.

Tube Route and Placement

Placement of a gastrostomy tube or gastrostomy button is a surgical procedure performed by the surgeon. The nurse usually places an orogastric (OG), nasogastric (NG), or nasointestinal tube (Procedures 37-9 and 37-10). Nasogastric tubes are used most frequently because the tube is easier to stabilize with nasal placement than with oral placement and has decreased risk of inappropriate insertion into the respiratory tract. Because of increased mucus production caused by irritation from the tube, nasal placement can potentially interfere with respiratory function. Children with head or nasal anomalies or injuries and infants who are still preferential nose breathers (usually those 4 months old or younger) will need orogastric tube placement. A nasointestinal tube is more difficult to insert than an orogastric or nasogastric tube because it must exit the pyloric sphincter into the small intestine.

There is controversy regarding measurement of the length of the tube to be inserted. The two most common methods of measurement are (1) from the nose to the ear and to the end of the xiphoid process and (2) from the nose to the ear and to a point midway between the xiphoid process and umbilicus. Studies have examined the role that height and, in low-birth-weight infants, weight play in gastric insertion distance. Additional research is needed in this area.

Tube Selection

Many types and sizes of tubes are commercially available. Factors influencing the selection of feeding tubes include the child's age and size, the viscosity of the formula, the reason for the enteral feeding, and whether an infusion device will be used. A feeding tube of size 5 to 10 Fr is used in infants, and the size increases proportionately for older children. Selecting the smallest-bore tube for the infusion and a tube of soft material will decrease the child's discomfort.

Safety Issues Related to Tube Placement

Tube placement must be verified at the time the tube is inserted, any time feeding is interrupted, before each bolus feeding or medication administration, and every 4 to 8 hours during continuous feeding. Although auscultation is the most frequently used method for checking tube placement at the bedside, examination of aspirate and pH measurement of the aspirate are considered to be more reliable (Metheny & Titler, 2001). Insufflation of air (1 to 5 ml in infants and small children; 5 to 20 ml in adolescents) through the tube while auscultating over the epigastrium, stomach, or left upper quadrant for a distinctive "whooshing" or "gurgling" sound might indicate whether the tube is in the stomach. This sound is heard most readily in the left upper quadrant for nasogastric (NG) tubes and in the lower quadrant for nasointestinal tubes (Ellett & Beckstrand, 1999). Auscultation as a piece of confirmatory data relies on the nurse's experience, because a similar sound can be heard if the tube is placed in the respiratory tract.

Aspiration of enteral fluid can indicate the probability of the tube being in the stomach (pH of 5 or lower), particularly when accompanied by grassy green, brown, or mucoid-flecked, clear aspirate. Indications the tube is probably in the intestine would be an aspirate pH of 6 and yellow or brownish green aspirate (Metheny & Titler, 2001). A pH above 6, along with straw-colored fluid or mucus secretion (especially in a child with decreased level of consciousness; uncooperative or restless behavior; recent intubation or extubation; or decreased swallowing, cough, or gag reflexes), suggests respiratory tube placement (Metheny & Titler, 2001). Most research done on tube placement in adults and children emphasizes that *radiographic confirmation of tube placement is the only definitive method of correct positioning* (Ellett & Beckstrand, 1999; Metheny & Titler, 2001; Metheny, Wehrle, Wiersema, & Clark, 1998).

Do not assume that a feeding tube has remained in proper position just because the external position has not changed. Tubes can become dislodged with suctioning, retching, or vomiting.

Contraindications to Tube Placement

Determine any preexisting contraindications to the procedure, such as prior surgeries or trauma or congenital anomalies (e.g., choanal atresia, tracheoesophageal fistula, esophageal strictures) that could interfere with passage of the tube. If any of these findings are present, the physician might use fluoroscopy to guide the insertion. *Do not reinsert a dislodged tube that was placed during or through a surgical repair. Notify the surgeon if the tube becomes dislodged.*

Gastrostomy Feedings

The procedure for gastrostomy feedings is much the same as for orogastric, nasogastric, or nasointestinal feedings. As with any tube feeding, hold the infant or young child, when possible, to associate the feeding with pleasant sensations and socialization and to promote normal development and bonding.

Special considerations for children with gastrostomy tubes or buttons include skin and stoma care. Assess the site for abnormal findings, such as leakage, redness around the site,

Procedure 37-9

Feeding Tube Insertions

PURPOSE: To provide enteral nutrition.

1. Using developmentally appropriate language, explain the procedure to the child and family and assess their needs and concerns (e.g., previous experience with tube insertion, ability to assist with the procedure, need for restraint). Therapeutic play can be used to allay the child's and parents' fears related to the procedure.

2. Gather the following equipment before starting the procedure: feeding tube of appropriate size and type, ¼- or ½-inch hypoallergenic tape, 20-ml syringe, sterile water for oral use, stethoscope, water-soluble lubricating jelly (for nasal insertion only), pH reagent strips, gloves, feeding pump and setup (enteral feeding bag or burette), and the enteral fluid to be administered.

3. Position the child on the back or right side with the head of the bed elevated. To facilitate cooperation and decrease fear, a small child can be held in a parent's arms, with the child's head on the parent's shoulder. An older child may sit up in the bed. Restrain if necessary.

4. Wash your hands, and don gloves.

5. Measure the length of the catheter to be inserted, and mark with a waterproof marker or with tape:

    a. To place a nasogastric tube in a child, measure the distance from the tip of the nose to the earlobe and then down to the xiphoid process. Mark the total measurement on the tube.

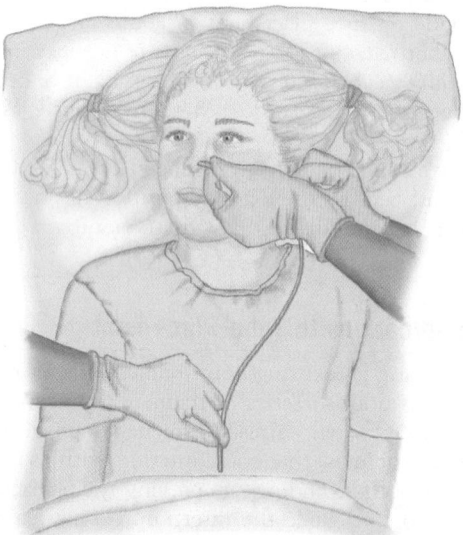

    b. To place an orogastric tube in an infant, measure the tube from the tip of the nose to the earlobe and to the midpoint between the end of the xiphoid process and the umbilicus. The total measurement, NEX (nose-ear-xiphoid), should be marked on the tube with tape or indelible marker.

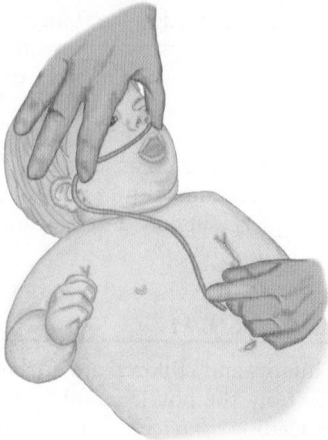

6. To facilitate passage through the nasopharynx, lubricate the tube with water or water-soluble lubricant. In neonates and for orogastric placement, use water only.

7. Insert the tube gently but firmly through the mouth or nose and down the throat. If you encounter obstruction or if the tube curls in the mouth, remove the tube and repeat this step. If the child gasps, coughs, gags, or turns cyanotic, withdraw the tube and wait for the response to subside before proceeding.

8. Continue to advance the tube gently to the predetermined mark. While advancing the tube, ask the cooperative child to swallow repeatedly when the tube reaches the pharynx, or give small sips of water through a straw if not contraindicated. Swallowing will ease insertion into the esophagus. Advance the tube 5 to 10 cm with each swallow. Giving an infant a pacifier will encourage swallowing. Direct the tube toward the back of the throat.

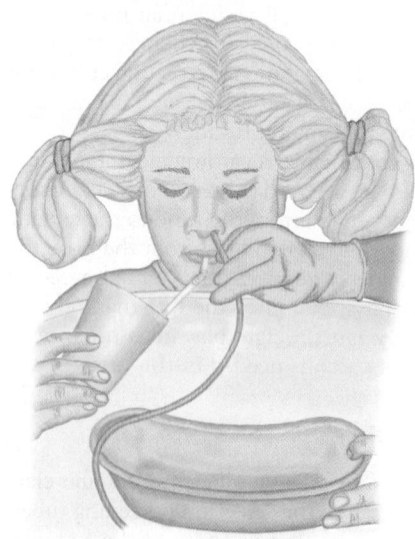

Procedure 37-9

Feeding Tube Insertions—cont'd

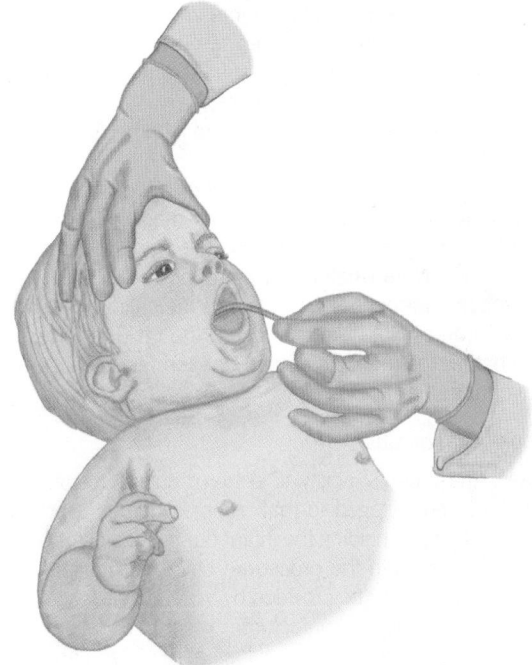

9. Temporarily secure the tube with tape to stabilize it while you check the tube position.
10. Attach the syringe to the end of the tube, and insufflate 1 to 5 ml (more for an older child or adolescent) of air while auscultating over the stomach area. Then, after withdrawing the air, attempt to aspirate the gastric contents for pH testing. Choking or soundless coughing may indicate placement in the trachea. Accidental placement of a small-diameter tube into the lungs may not be as apparent as with larger tubes, particularly if the child's cough or gag reflex is absent or suppressed, and radiographic confirmation of small-bore tube placement usually is necessary.*
11. Check the pH of the aspirate to confirm gastric or intestinal placement. (NOTE: Administration of antacid and gastric acid inhibitors will alter the pH of the aspirate, thus affecting the reliability of the pH test.*)
12. If a nasointestinal tube with a guide wire has been used, remove the guide wire by holding the tube at the child's nostril or the corner of the mouth and slowly removing it. To allow gravity to assist in the advancement of the tube into the duodenum, keep the child on the right side. A plain abdominal film will be ordered by the physician to confirm tube placement in the duodenum.
13. Once tube placement is confirmed, tape the tube securely in place and label the tube with the date and time of insertion. Refer to your facility's policy and procedure manual for recommended frequency of tube change. With indelible marker, mark the tube just below the insertion site. This will assist with future assessments of tube placement.
14. Record in the nurses' notes the size and type of tube used, route, placement, pH testing results, results of auscultation, date and time of insertion, child and family teaching, procedure tolerance, and any problems encountered.

Home Adaptations

If the child is to receive enteral nutrition at home, teach the parent how to insert and check placement of the tube. Describe comfort measures that may be helpful. Be sure to have the parent give a return demonstration before taking the child home. Make sure the parent has and knows how to read pH strips. Provide the parent with directions for reaching the health care provider if there is a question about tube placement.

* Metheny, N., & Titler, M. (2001). Assessing placement of feeding tubes. *American Journal of Nursing, 101*(5), 36-45.

Procedure 37-10

Administering Enteral Feedings (via the Orogastric, Nasogastric, or Nasointestinal Route)

PURPOSE: To provide adequate nutrition in a child who cannot tolerate oral feedings.

1. Using developmentally appropriate language, explain the procedure to the child and family. Assess their needs and concerns related to the procedure, such as previous experience with enteral feedings, ability to assist with the procedure, and need for restraint. Use therapeutic play to allay the child's and parent's fears related to the procedure.
2. The following equipment is needed: stethoscope, irrigation syringe, room-temperature formula and water, pacifier for neonates and infants, electronic feeding pump (for continuous tube feedings), and gloves.

Intermittent Feedings (Bolus)

3. Technique:
   a. Position the child, and remove the syringe or cap from the tube. Put on gloves.
   b. Check for proper tube placement (be sure the mark indicating insertion length is in its original place relative to the exit site), instill several milliliters of air, and aspirate for residual volume from the previous feed. Follow the facility's policy and procedure manual or physician's orders for disposition of residual volume.
   c. Remove the plunger from the syringe, and attach the syringe to the tube.

Continued

Procedure 37-10

Administering Enteral Feedings (via the Orogastric, Nasogastric, or Nasointestinal Route)—cont'd

d. Pour room-temperature formula into the syringe, and allow the feeding to flow slowly into the tube (usually over a period of 15 to 30 minutes). Raising or lowering the level of the syringe increases or decreases the flow of formula. Discontinue the feeding if signs of respiratory distress, cyanosis, abdominal distention, or vomiting occur. Notify the physician.

e. After the prescribed volume has been infused, rinse the tube with sterile water and clear the tube by injecting 1 to 5 ml of air.

f. Discard the used syringe, and close or clamp the tube unless otherwise indicated.

g. Leave the child lying on the right side with the head of the bed elevated for 30 to 60 minutes after the feeding.

Continuous Feedings

4. Technique:
   a. Position the child, and check tube placement. The aspirate will probably have the appearance of curdled milk if the tube is in the stomach or look bile-stained if in the intestine. Because feeding can alter aspirate pH, the pH is a less reliable indicator of placement when a child is on continuous feeds.*

b. Fill the feeding bag, volume-control set, or syringe and tubing with the prescribed formula.

c. Attach infusion tubing to the feeding tube, and begin the infusion at the prescribed rate.

d. Check tube placement and residual volumes every 4 to 8 hours.

e. To reduce the incidence of reflux and aspiration, keep the child positioned on the abdomen or right side.

5. If aspirate was present, record the amount, color, and consistency. Note whether it was re-fed or discarded. Note the type and amount of formula and the child's tolerance of the procedure. Note the position of the child after feeding and whether the tube is clamped or open (an open clamp allows venting of air).

Home Adaptations

Assess the parents' ability to perform enteral feedings. Parents should be encouraged to make this as normal a procedure as possible (e.g., by holding the infant during feedings). Ask the parent to demonstrate the procedure before discharge. Assistance with home care can be provided by a home health agency. Advise the parent to follow manufacturer's recommendations about discarding opened unused formula left at room temperature.

* Metheny, N., & Titler, M. (2001). Assessing placement of feeding tubes. *American Journal of Nursing, 101*(5), 36-45.

---

drainage, bleeding, and skin breakdown. Clean the skin around the tube insertion site with soap and water once or twice daily, depending on the condition, and with each spillage. To facilitate complete cleansing, rotate gastrostomy buttons in a full circle during cleaning.

Capped gastrostomy tubes extend several inches from the insertion site. Check to be sure that no tension is on the external tube. If necessary, coil the tube and tape near the exit site. Gastrostomy buttons are placed close to the skin surface. They have a one-way valve that eliminates the need for clamping and offers the added advantage of allowing children to participate in regular childhood activities. When feeding a child with a gastrostomy button, you might need to place extension tubing between the button and the feeding pump.

Watch for signs that the tube or button might need to be replaced. These signs include leaking, tube occlusion, malfunction of the antireflux valve, or abnormal tube position. Report these findings to the physician.

Many children are discharged home with gastrostomy tubes in place. Parents must be able to provide all required care. Parent teaching is a major part of the nursing care of a child with a feeding tube. Parents must know how to check tube position,

---

CRITICAL THINKING EXERCISE 37-1

Assessing feeding tube placement has historically been a nursing responsibility, even though the only totally accurate assessment measure is radiographic confirmation. Malpractice litigation has resulted from improperly placed tubes confirmed by unscientific methods.* A research study about tube placement in children† suggests that between 22% and 30% of feeding tubes were incorrectly placed (either too high in the esophagus or too low into the intestine).

1. What is the nurse's legal and ethical responsibility regarding feeding tube placement confirmation?
2. How does the nurse make the "best judgment" about what action to take if placement is questionable?

*Metheny, N., & Titler, M. (2001). Assessing placement of feeding tubes. *American Journal of Nursing, 101*(5), 36-45; †Ellett, M., & Beckstrand, J. (1999). Examination of gavage tube placement in children. *Journal of Society of Pediatric Nurses, 4*(2), 51-60.

! CRITICAL TO REMEMBER

Enteral Feedings

- Begin the feeding *only* after tube placement in the stomach has been properly verified.
- Discontinue feedings and notify the physician if signs of respiratory distress, cyanosis, abdominal distention, or vomiting occur.
- Provide a pacifier to infants so that they can associate sucking with feeding. Encourage older children to sit at a table during meals to promote the normal socialization associated with eating.
- To avoid accidental overfeeding should the infusion pump malfunction, use only an amount of formula appropriate for a 4-hour feeding. Discard any formula that has been opened for more than 4 hours.
- Follow the facility's policy or procedure manual or physician's orders regarding disposing of residual volumes and the prescribed frequency for changing feeding equipment.

how to administer feedings, how to care for the tube, what symptoms should be reported, and what to do if the tube becomes dislodged. Booklets are available to assist the family in the care of the child with a gastrostomy tube or button.

ENEMAS

Enemas are given when stool needs to be removed from the bowel because of severe constipation or in preparation for a diagnostic procedure or surgery. Giving an enema to an infant or child differs very little from the procedure for an adult. The differences are the type and amount of fluid administered and the distance that the enema tip is inserted into the rectum.

Enema Administration

Rectal damage and perforation can occur with improper insertion of the enema tip. Insert a lubricated tip gently 2.5 cm to 7.5 cm, depending on the age and size of the child. Commercially prepared single-use enemas come with a prelubricated tip of appropriate length.

Solutions and Volumes

The amount of the enema solution will vary with the age and size of the child. Unless the physician's orders specify a different amount, the values listed in Table 37-2 for volume of solution and depth of enema tip insertion into the rectum are recommended. Only isotonic solutions should be used with children. Plain tap water should never be used because it is hypotonic and can cause a rapid fluid shift and fluid overload.

After completing an enema administration, diaper the infant. Toddlers can use the bedpan or "potty" if possible. Older children and adolescents can use the bedpan or bedside commode or be assisted to the bathroom. Record in the nurses' notes or I&O sheet the date and time the enema was given, the type and amount of solution, the amount and characteristics of stool, any unusual findings (e.g., blood, mucus, foreign bodies, worms), and the child's tolerance of the procedure.

OSTOMIES

Urinary and fecal diversion may be needed when normal methods of elimination are temporarily or permanently halted. Some conditions requiring the creation of a fecal stoma include imperforate anus, Hirschsprung disease, necrotizing enterocolitis, some cases of intestinal atresia, intussusception, Crohn disease, and ulcerative colitis (see Chapter 43). The anatomic location of the stoma will dictate the consistency of the stool. The higher the stoma, the more liquid is the stool.

Urinary diversion is usually the result of obstructive uropathy, congenital anomalies, or occasionally neurogenic bladder (see Chapter 52). The ureters can be brought out

through the abdominal wall (ureterostomy) or connected to a segment of small bowel (ileal conduit).

Nursing care of the child with an ostomy focuses on minimizing the obstacles the child and family face in learning to care for the ostomy, maximizing skin integrity, encouraging the child and family to be actively involved in the treatment regimen, providing support and guidance, and making appropriate referrals to an enterostomal therapist or other support system. The actual management and care of pediatric ostomies differ little from that in adults with ostomies. The major difference is the need to use developmentally appropriate terminology to explain the procedure and care of the ostomy to the child and family. A teaching model, such as a doll with a stoma, can facilitate child and family education.

OXYGEN THERAPY

Hypoxemia, resulting from apnea or inadequate ventilation, occurs more rapidly in children than in adults because of children's higher metabolic rate and increased oxygen consumption. Because cardiopulmonary arrest in children can follow progressive respiratory distress, early recognition of subtle signs and symptoms of respiratory distress is a necessary skill for every nurse.

Oxygen is an essential body requirement for any energy-consuming activity or function. For infants and children who are unable to maintain a normal arterial oxygen pressure (PaO_2), supplemental oxygen might be needed. Because oxygen is a drug, a physician's order is needed for administration, except in an emergency situation. Follow your facility's policy for oxygen administration in emergencies.

Oxygen Delivery

Oxygen may be administered to children by nasal cannula, facemask (simple, nonrebreather, partial rebreather, Venturi, or aerosol), an oxygen hood, or an oxygen tent (Fig. 37-9). The method of delivery depends on the concentration needed and the child's ability to cooperate with the chosen method. In most facilities, a respiratory therapist is responsible for the setup, maintenance, and management of oxygen equipment. However, the nurse needs to have a working knowledge of the oxygen delivery system used.

The primary differences in oxygen delivery between children and adults are the size of the equipment and the teaching and emotional support needed for children receiving oxygen and their families. Usually, an oxygen hood is used to provide maximum oxygenation for neonates and infants. Older infants and young toddlers might better tolerate a nasal cannula, blow-by oxygen, or facemask. Oxygen delivery by nasal cannula, the blow-by method, or a facemask works well for toddlers and preschoolers. School-age children and adolescents prefer nonrebreather masks to achieve maximum oxygenation.

Children experiencing difficulty breathing might be less than cooperative when an attempt is made to place a mask or cannula on the face. Explain to the child and family in developmentally appropriate language what will happen, why the mask is needed, and how it will feel. Provide assistance, if needed, to keep the oxygen delivery system in place. Check the physician's orders for the percentage of oxygen to be delivered and the method of delivery.

A nasal cannula is a low-flow delivery system that is indicated for infants and children who need modest amounts of

TABLE **37-2** Recommended Volume and Depth for Enema Tip Insertion, by Age		
	Volume (ml)	**Depth of Insertion**
Infants	120-240	1 inch (2.5 cm)
2-4 yr	240-360	2 inches (5 cm)
4-10 yr	360-480	3 inches (7.5 cm)
11 yr and older	480-720	4 inches (10 cm)

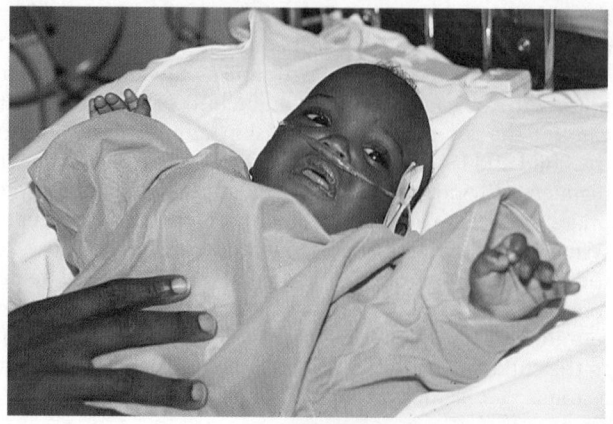
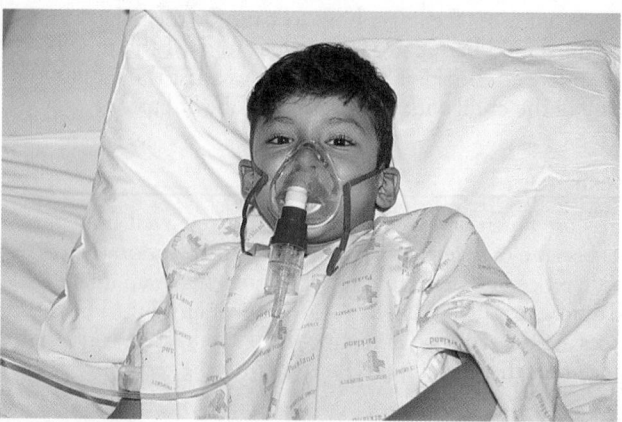
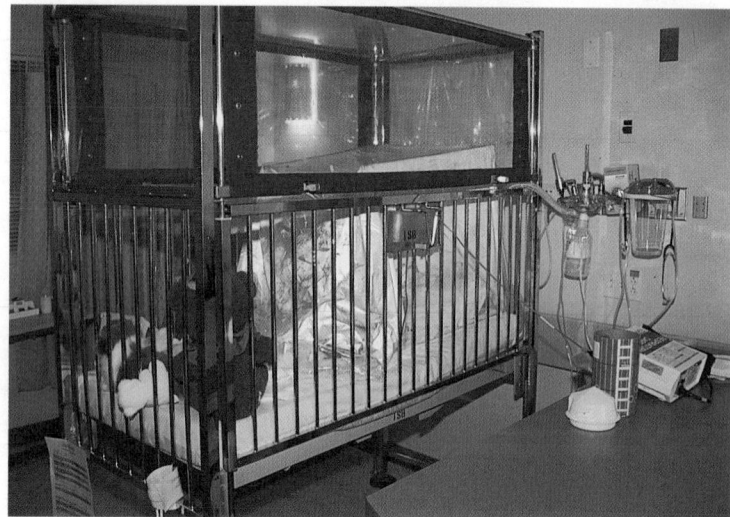

Figure 37-9 Administering oxygen to children differs from the procedure in adults in the choice and size of equipment and in the greater need to educate and support the child and family. **A,** Nasal cannula. **B,** Simple facemask. **C,** Oxygen mist tent. The bubble top prevents an older child from climbing over the crib rail. (Courtesy Parkland Health and Hospital System, Dallas, TX.)

supplemental oxygen (up to 40%). Flow rates should not exceed 6 L/min. The loop of the cannula can be enlarged to slip easily over the child's ears. Place the prongs in the nares, and tighten the loop. If the child is active, you can tape the cannula to the sides of the child's face to maintain proper position. Be aware, however, that a flow rate exceeding 6 L/min can irritate the nasopharynx and cause gastric distention and regurgitation without appreciably improving the child's oxygenation.

The simple facemask and the Venturi mask are indicated for infants and children who need modest amounts of supplemental oxygen (35% to 60%, or a flow rate of 6 to 10 L/min). The Venturi mask can be adjusted to deliver specific concentrations of oxygen (i.e., 24%, 28%, 35%, 40%, or 50%). You must maintain a minimum flow rate of 6 L/min to prevent rebreathing of exhaled carbon dioxide.

Partial and full nonrebreathing masks are simple facemasks with an attached reservoir that allows a portion of exhaled gas to remain in the bag and mix with oxygen. These masks supply oxygen concentrations of 50% to 60% at a rate of 10 to 12 L/min. A nonrebreather system can deliver almost 100% oxygen at a flow rate of 10 to 15 L/min.

Proper fit of an oxygen mask will ensure adequate oxygen delivery. When delivering oxygen by mask, it is important to select the correct-size mask to ensure a tight fit. Masks are available in preemie, newborn, infant, child, small adult, and adult

sizes. To determine proper size, check to see that the mask extends from the bridge of the child's nose to the cleft of the chin. Attach the mask to the humidified oxygen source, and adjust the flow rate to the prescribed level. Then place the mask over the child's face, and adjust the nose clip and head strap.

When humidified oxygen is required, such as to assist the child in mobilizing secretions, an oxygen hood or mist tent may be indicated. These devices are particularly useful in the treatment of croup, epiglottitis, pneumonia, and bronchiolitis (see Chapter 45). The mist moistens the airways, minimizes fluid loss from the lungs, and provides a cool environment, which aids in temperature reduction. Monitor the child's temperature frequently to prevent hypothermia, and be sure to keep the child in dry clothing and bedding.

When a hood or tent is used, it is difficult to deliver oxygen concentrations of more than 40%, because oxygen is heavier than air and will escape readily. Be certain to check that the sides and the end of the tent are securely tucked to prevent oxygen leakage. Also, remember that room air will be drawn into the tent any time the tent is entered, reducing the child's inspired oxygen concentration. Because of this, using a tent limits access to the child.

In addition, if humidified oxygen is used, the resulting mist limits both visual observation of the child and the child's ability to see out. The child might consequently feel

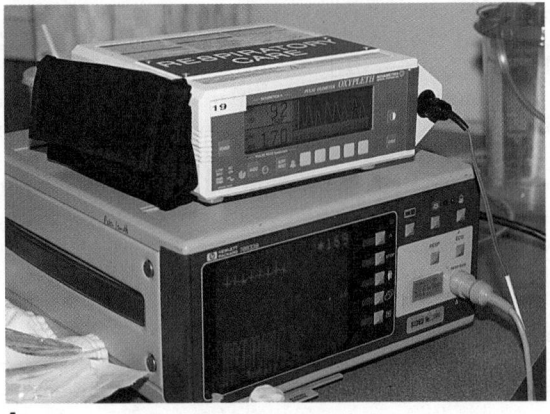 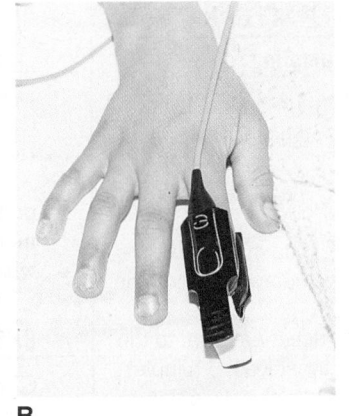 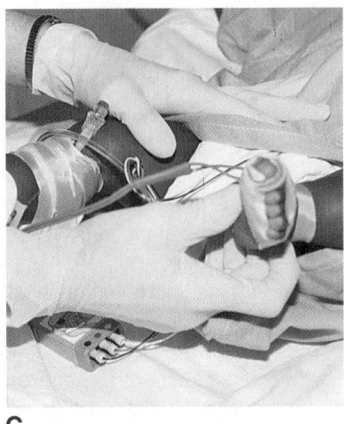

A   B   C

Figure 37-10 A, The pulse oximeter is a reliable, noninvasive way to measure blood oxygen saturation, allowing rapid adjustments in oxygen delivery to meet the child's needs. The sensor is applied to a child's finger (**B**) or an infant's toe (**C**) to permit information to be sent to the pulse oximeter. (**A** courtesy Parkland Health and Hospital System, Dallas, TX.)

isolated, and nursing creativity and ingenuity are needed to encourage the child to remain in the tent. If a concentration of inspired oxygen greater than 30% is required, another method of oxygen delivery will be more effective.

With the use of any oxygen administration system, safety is of great concern. Post "oxygen in use/no smoking" signs outside the child's door and over the bed. Although most health care facilities are nonsmoking facilities, remind parents and visitors that smoking is not allowed in the room. Toys that have the potential for producing a spark, including those that are battery-powered, should not be permitted near the oxygen.

Documentation

Record in the nurse's notes the date and time; the type of oxygen administration system used; the percentage of oxygen delivered and the flow rate; the child's vital signs, skin color, respiratory effort, and lung sounds; the child's response to the procedure; and any teaching done with the child or family.

Parent Teaching

Infants and children often receive home oxygen therapy. Educate parents or caregivers about the operation of equipment to be used at home, equipment cleaning, safety factors, cardiopulmonary resuscitation, and available support services.

ASSESSING OXYGENATION

Pulse oximetry is a sensitive, reliable, noninvasive means of measuring oxygen saturation (SaO_2) in the blood. Pulse oximetry measures the absorption of light waves as they pass through highly perfused areas of the body, providing the nurse with valuable information and acting as an early warning of hypoxemia. Pulse oximetry is a valuable method of assessing oxygenation status in acutely ill infants and children. It accurately identifies children whose oxygenation status is marginal (Fig. 37-10; Procedure 37-11).

Pulse oximetry has several advantages. It is noninvasive, requires no special site preparation, and in most cases yields

---

Procedure 37-11

Pulse Oximetry

PURPOSE: To assess the child's oxygen saturation.
1. Explain to the child and family the indication for the procedure, and describe the appearance of the sensor (e.g., "E.T., the extraterrestrial") to enhance cooperation.
2. Bring the oximeter and sensor (finger probe, adhesive probe, or ear clip) to the child's room. The sensor will differ, depending on whether the oximetry is intermittent or continuous.
3. Set the parameters for the alarm on continuous measuring oximeters.
4. Place the probe on the finger, toe, or foot. Avoid placing the probe on an extremity with an arterial line, blood pressure cuff, or intravenous (IV) line in place. Fingernail polish or artificial nails will need to be removed before placing the sensor. Do not wrap the sensor so tightly as to prevent venous flow and cause inaccurate readings.
5. Observe and record the pulse rate and oxygen saturation. The pulse rate on the oximeter should coincide with an api-

cal pulse or pulse rate on a cardiac monitor. If no pulse is detected, reposition the sensor.
6. To check the skin condition, remove the sensor from the site at least every 2 hours. If using a portable oximeter, be sure to clean the sensor with alcohol or the manufacturer's recommended cleaning solution.
7. Record the child's response to the procedure and the pulse oximetry reading obtained, the percentage of oxygen (if in use), and the activity level of the child. Report any abnormal findings to the physician (<95%, except in children with chronic cardiac or respiratory disease who might have a lower "normal" pulse oximetry value).
8. Inform parents that an alarm will sound if the child's oxygen saturation falls below the set parameters. The alarm might also sound if the child is particularly active or the sensor becomes dislodged.

! CRITICAL TO REMEMBER

Assisting With Arterial Blood Gas Sampling

- Position the child's wrist with the palm up but not hyperextended. Stabilize the extremity, allowing neither twisting of the wrist nor jerking of the shoulder.
- Do not hold the child's arm too tightly, because a tight grip occludes arterial blood flow.
- The skin is punctured at an angle of 15 to 45 degrees. When the needle is withdrawn, it is withdrawn slowly to decrease the incidence of arterial spasm.
- After the needle is withdrawn, apply direct pressure to the site using a sterile 2 × 2 gauze pad for at least 5 minutes.
- If the analysis is not to be done immediately, place the sample on ice.
- Record the puncture site and the child's activity level at the time of the sampling.

an accurate measurement of oxygenation status in the neonate, infant, child, or adult. Also, values are available immediately. Despite some limitations, pulse oximetry has significant benefit in the assessment and care of the ill child. The immediate feedback it provides can alert the nurse to changes in oxygenation that require immediate intervention.

Pulse oximeter measurements reflect the child's oxygen saturation and the perfusion status. Potential sources of error in measurements include an abnormal hemoglobin value (e.g., in hyperbilirubinemia or carbon monoxide poisoning), peripheral perfusion (e.g., in hypotension or hypothermia), ambient light interference, motion artifact, and skin breakdown from the adhesive used to secure the sensor. To eliminate the effects of ambient light, an opaque shield can be placed over the sensor site. Skin breakdown can be avoided by using a reusable sensor.

Under certain circumstances, capillary or arterial blood gases might need to be measured to establish correlation of oxygenation with pulse oximetry readings. Both capillary and arterial blood gas measurements are invasive. They measure the blood's oxygen content and the body's acid-base balance. Sampling can be done from indwelling arterial catheters or by arterial puncture.

The procedure for arterial blood sampling differs between the adult and pediatric populations. The differences include the sites used, the size of the equipment, the angle of entry, and the psychosocial interactions with the child and family. The preferred site in children is the radial artery, although alternatives (e.g., brachial artery) can be used. A capillary blood gas measurement provides similar information but is a less painful and less invasive procedure.

Because a respiratory therapist or trained nurse or other personnel must draw arterial blood for blood gas measurements, the novice nurse is responsible primarily for assisting with the procedure and restraining or comforting the child.

CHEST PHYSIOTHERAPY

Chest physiotherapy (CPT) includes postural drainage, chest percussion and vibration, and coughing and deep-breathing exercises. These techniques can mobilize and eliminate secretions, reexpand the lungs, and promote efficient use of the respiratory muscles, particularly in children with cystic fibrosis. CPT also may be used prophylactically in postoperative clients. Contraindications to this therapy include head injury, acute asthma, chest trauma with an unstable chest wall, osteogenesis imperfecta, and lung tumor.

In most health care facilities, CPT is the responsibility of the respiratory or physical therapist, but if respiratory therapy coverage is not available, the nurse performs this procedure (Procedure 37-12). Many children with chronic pulmonary disease receive this treatment at home, so the family must be educated in performing this aspect of the child's care. The goal of CPT is to prevent atelectasis and pneumonia.

Initiation of CPT requires a physician's order. The order should include the number of treatments per day, and it might specify the areas of the lungs to be treated. *Percussion* is rhythmic clapping with a cupped hand over the affected portion of the lung or the simulation of this movement using a percussion cup or mechanical percussor or vibrator. *Postural drainage* entails positioning the child to promote gravity-assisted drainage of the lungs. These two treatments are usually used in conjunction with each other and are carried out three or four times per day or more often if indicated. To decrease the risk of aspiration, treatments are performed before meals or $1\frac{1}{2}$ hours after meals. Children receiving continuous feedings should have their feeding interrupted 1 hour before the treatment. The "lost volume" can then be replaced in the interval before the next treatment.

Procedure 37-12

Chest Physiotherapy

PURPOSE: To mobilize secretions and facilitate effective airway clearance.

1. If the child and family are not familiar with chest physiotherapy (CPT), explain the procedure to them using developmentally appropriate language. Show them the equipment, and allow time for questions.
2. The following equipment is needed: a mechanical percussor, vibrator, or rubber cups (if being used instead of hands); stethoscope; towel or baby blanket; gloves; goggles; and tissues or collection container for sputum.
3. To provide a basis for determining response to the treatment, assess the child's baseline respiratory status before

beginning the procedure. Before the treatment, ask the child to cough or suction the trachea to remove secretions that might have accumulated in the trachea. Wear gloves and goggles for suctioning or the collection of sputum.

4. Place the child in a postural drainage position.
5. Gently but firmly clap the chest wall with cupped hands. The sound should be hollow. Percussion cups and mechanical vibrators may be used instead of the hand. If the child is young, has sensitive skin, or is otherwise more comfortable, percussion can be done with a very light blanket or gown covering the chest.

Procedure 37-12

Chest Physiotherapy—cont'd

Correct hand position for percussion

Cup the hand to trap a pocket of air that will transmit vibrations through the chest wall to the secretions that need to be dislodged.

Clap the cupped hand in rapid sequence over a lung segment. Elbow should be flexed and the wrist relaxed, while creating a rapid, popping action.

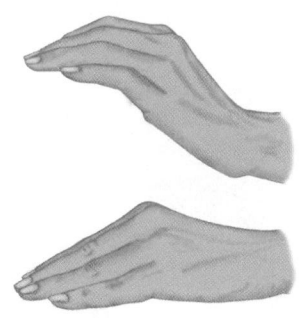

6. Reposition the child as needed to complete the procedure, maintaining each position for approximately 5 to 10 minutes. Ask the child to cough between positions.
7. Encourage the child to take deep breaths during the treatment. Expiration after these deep breaths will often stimulate coughing. Use toys, such as pinwheel toys and balloons (with close supervision), or engage the child in blowing soap bubbles to optimize deep breathing and stimulate coughing. Assist with removal of secretions if needed.
8. Assess the child's vital signs and breath sounds after therapy is completed. Record the following in the nurses' notes: the date and time of CPT; positions used for drainage and length of time each is maintained; chest segments percussed or vibrated; color, amount, and tenacity of any secretions produced; any complications and nursing actions taken; the child's response to and tolerance of the procedure; and any teaching done with the child and family and their degree of understanding of the teaching.

Home Adaptations

Determine the parent's ability to perform CPT at home. It can be done with the child on a regular bed, a couch, or the floor. A variety of devices (tilt tables, slant boards) are available to achieve the proper angle for the procedure. A piece of firm mattress foam purchased at an upholstery store, cut at an angle, and covered is an inexpensive alternative. Young children can achieve the appropriate positioning by lying over a large (3-foot size) ball or over a bean bag chair. Playing during the procedure makes the experience more pleasant for the child. Older children can perform some CPT techniques on themselves, particularly postural drainage and percussion of areas within reach. Observe the parents and child as they demonstrate the procedure. Provide written instructions for parents regarding the child's CPT needs. Teaching materials are available for families of children needing CPT performed at home. Assist the family in obtaining this literature, and refer them to appropriate financial resources if needed.

Chest physiotherapy for older children

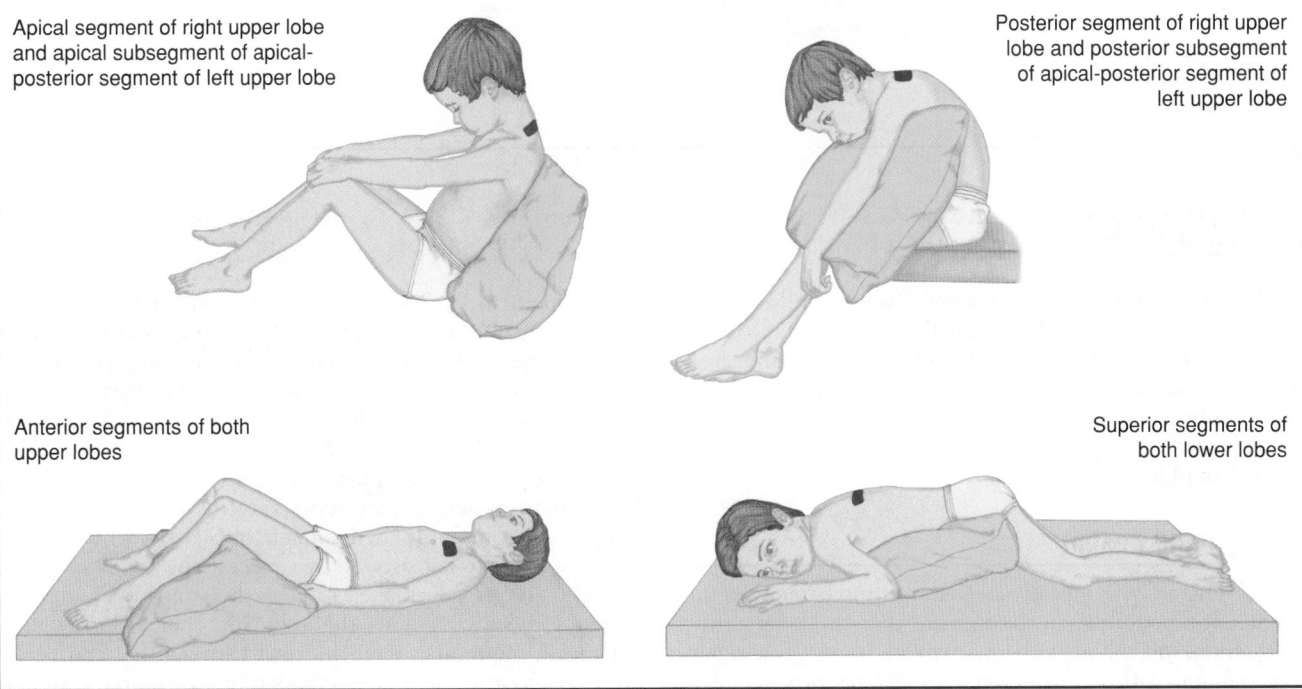

Apical segment of right upper lobe and apical subsegment of apical-posterior segment of left upper lobe

Posterior segment of right upper lobe and posterior subsegment of apical-posterior segment of left upper lobe

Anterior segments of both upper lobes

Superior segments of both lower lobes

Continued

Procedure 37-12

Chest Physiotherapy—cont'd

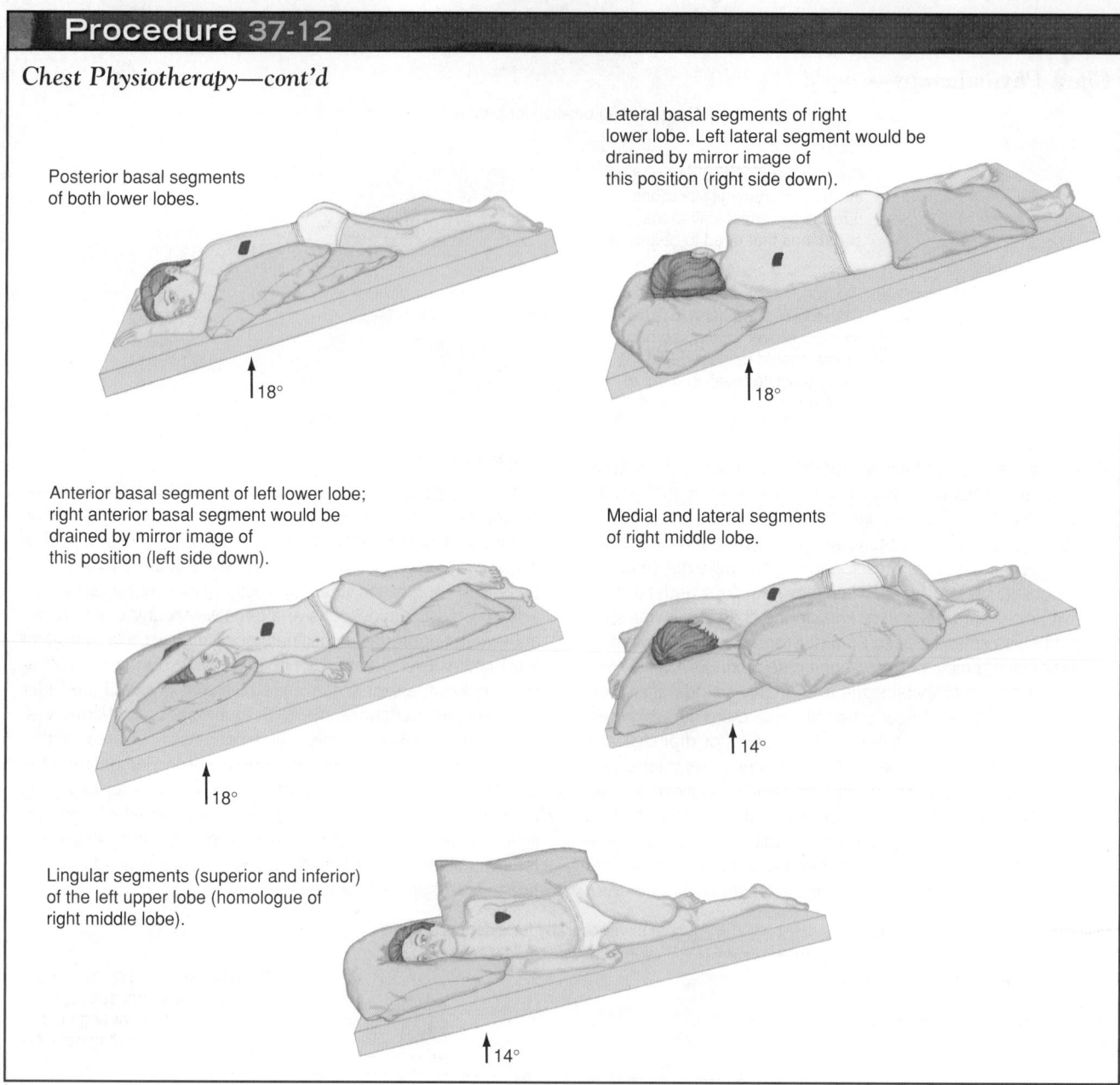

Posterior basal segments of both lower lobes.

18°

Lateral basal segments of right lower lobe. Left lateral segment would be drained by mirror image of this position (right side down).

18°

Anterior basal segment of left lower lobe; right anterior basal segment would be drained by mirror image of this position (left side down).

18°

Medial and lateral segments of right middle lobe.

14°

Lingular segments (superior and inferior) of the left upper lobe (homologue of right middle lobe).

14°

The length of the treatment depends on the child's ability to tolerate the procedure but is usually 20 to 30 minutes. Although there are several positions for postural drainage, it may not be necessary to use all of them at each session. Infants can be positioned on the lap using a pillow for the entire procedure. The pattern of postural drainage is similar to that for an older child.

TRACHEOSTOMY CARE

A *tracheostomy* is a surgically created opening (stoma) in the trachea. It is performed in children to bypass an upper airway obstruction, to facilitate pulmonary toilet, or to optimize mechanical ventilation. Tracheostomies can be either tempo-

rary or permanent. The use of tracheostomies for acute airway management has decreased because of the increased use of endotracheal intubation; tracheostomies continue to be used for long-term management of problem airways, particularly in children with bronchopulmonary dysplasia (see Chapter 45) (Carron, Derkay, Strope, Nosonchuk, & Darrow, 2000; Wetmore, Thompson, Marsh, & Tom, 1999).

Pediatric tracheostomy tubes vary in size and type. The tube most commonly used is made of Silastic, which is soft and flexible. It consists of two pieces: the outer cannula, which stays in the trachea to keep the stoma open; and an obturator, which guides the tube into place during tube changes. Some tubes have an inner cannula that can be removed for cleaning. Tracheostomy tubes with inner cannulas

Procedure 37-13

Suctioning a Tracheostomy Tube

PURPOSE: To maintain patency of the tracheostomy tube.

1. After using developmentally appropriate language to explain the procedure, its purpose, and other pertinent information to the child and parent, gather the following equipment: a sterile suction catheter of appropriate size, sterile gloves and goggles, normal saline solution, 3-ml syringe without needle for the required amount of normal saline, sterile container for normal saline, and equipment for ventilation.

2. Adjust the suction vacuum pressure to the prescribed level, and then put on the goggles. Pour normal saline into the sterile container, and open the syringe package. Put on sterile gloves.

3. Using sterile technique, instill normal saline (if being used) 0.5 to 2 ml, into the trachea to loosen secretions.

4. Insert the catheter the length of the tracheostomy tube (measure another tracheostomy tube the same size) *with suction off.*

5. Apply intermittent suction according to agency policy (policies differ as to whether to suction while entering the tracheostomy tube*). Withdraw the catheter using a twisting or twirling motion. Limit insertion and suctioning time to less than 5 seconds to prevent hypoxia. Holding your own breath during suctioning is a good reminder. If you need a breath, then the child probably does too.

6. Reoxygenate between suction catheter passes, and allow a sufficient recovery time after each pass. This time can include allowing the child to rest and take a few breaths, or it may involve "bagging" (giving oxygen by bag and mask). "Bagging" of children on ventilatory support is imperative.

7. Assess the child to determine whether secretions are still present. Auscultate to listen for air exchange. Repeat the procedure until the airway sounds clear, rinsing the suction catheter with normal saline between each insertion. Normal saline lavage may be used if thick secretions are encountered. Refer to your facility's procedure or policy manual regarding this controversial issue.

8. Assess the child's breath sounds and respiratory rate after suctioning to evaluate the effectiveness of suctioning.

9. Discard the suction tube and gloves in an appropriate container. Record in the nurses' notes the date and time the procedure was performed, the amount and characteristics of the secretions obtained, the character of the breath sounds before and after suctioning, the child's response to the procedure, and any teaching done with the child and family, as well as their level of understanding and their response to the teaching.

Home Adaptations

Tracheostomy suctioning at home is a clean rather than sterile procedure. The family will need a powered suction apparatus, catheters of appropriate size, normal saline and needleless syringe (if instillation is ordered), non-sterile gloves, boiled water, and the ordered catheter cleaning solution. The procedure for suctioning is as previously discussed, including presuctioning and postsuctioning assessments. Teach the parent to flush the catheter with boiled water, suction with air, and wipe the outer surface with alcohol or hydrogen peroxide.† Store the cleaned catheter in a clean, covered container.

The family will need much support and encouragement to feel comfortable with suctioning and tracheostomy care. The child can take baths, but care should be taken to prevent water from entering the trachea. Showers are not recommended. To avoid tracheal spasm, the tracheostomy can be covered loosely during cold or windy days.

---

*American Thoracic Society. (2000). Care of the child with a chronic tracheostomy. *American Journal of Respiratory and Critical Care Medicine, 161,*297-308.
† Suctioning of the patient in the home. (1999). *Respiratory Care, 44*(1), 91-98.

---

are often used for older children and for those who have increased mucus production.

Shiley single-lumen tracheostomy tubes are available in a variety of sizes (up to a no. 8 for an adult-size client). Tracheostomy tubes with inner cannulas are available in size no. 4 and larger.

Suctioning

In children with tracheostomies, secretions are removed from the airway by means of a catheter inserted into the airway. Using appropriate techniques and equipment for suctioning can prevent problems sometimes encountered during suctioning, such as hypoxia, tissue damage, and infection. Suctioning infants and children requires the use of a smaller suction catheter and lower suction settings than for the adult. Catheter sizes range from no. 5 Fr to no. 14 Fr, with smaller sizes used for smaller tubes. To avoid total airway occlusion, catheter size should be approximately half the inner diameter of the tracheostomy tube. Suction settings for tracheostomy care vary by age, as follows:

- *Neonates:* 60 to 80 mm Hg
- *Infants:* 80 to 100 mm Hg
- *Larger children:* 100 to 120 mm Hg

Assess and record the child's breath sounds, respiratory rate, and character of respirations every 4 hours. Suction the tracheostomy every 2 to 4 hours or as needed. Always use Standard Precautions (Procedure 37-13). Providing a humidified environment keeps secretions more liquid and easier to suction.

Stoma Care

Routine tracheostomy care (Procedure 37-14) includes assessing the stoma area for signs of infection and skin breakdown, changing tracheostomy ties, cleaning the tracheostomy site

Procedure 37-14

Cleaning and Care of the Tracheostomy Site and Inner Cannula

PURPOSE: To maintain a patent airway and prevent infection.

1. Using developmentally appropriate language, explain the procedure, its purpose, and other pertinent information to the child and parent. Some hospital facilities use videotapes and stoma dolls to demonstrate the procedure.
2. If the facility does not have a preassembled tracheostomy care kit, assemble the following: a small tray to hold the cleaning solution, cotton-tipped applicators, pipe cleaners or a brush for cleaning the inner cannula, forceps, tracheostomy ties, sterile dressing (optional), gauze pad, gloves (sterile and non-sterile), towel or blanket roll, hydrogen peroxide, sterile normal saline, and goggles.
3. To hyperextend the head and neck to expose the site, position the child with a towel or blanket under the shoulders.
4. Wash your hands, and open the tray, creating a sterile field.
5. Pour equal parts of normal saline and hydrogen peroxide in one small tray and normal saline in the other small tray. Use the large tray for holding cotton-tipped applicators, clean tracheostomy ties, and gauze pad.
6. Don non-sterile gloves and goggles, and remove the dressing around the tracheostomy if present. Discard the dressing and gloves according to agency policy. A dressing placed between the skin and the tube can increase the risk for skin breakdown because it will absorb any secretions. For this reason, it may not be used in some facilities. Assess the stoma for redness, drainage or discharge, and skin breakdown.
7. Don sterile gloves, and using cotton-tipped applicators moistened in half-strength hydrogen peroxide solution, clean the child's neck under the tracheostomy tube flanges and tracheostomy tape and allow to dry. If the child has a tracheostomy without an inner cannula, skip to step 11.
8. Unlock the inner cannula (if using a three-piece tracheostomy system) by rotating it counterclockwise. Remove the inner cannula and using pipe cleaners or a brush, quickly clean it in half-strength hydrogen peroxide solution. (Alternatively, it may be replaced with a new or extra inner cannula if available.) Rinse the cannula thoroughly in normal saline, and inspect it for cleanliness. Repeat the cleaning procedure if necessary.
9. To remove excess moisture, tap the cleaned inner cannula on the edge of the sterile container. Do not dry the outside of the inner cannula because moisture will act as a lubricant during reinsertion.
10. Reinsert the inner cannula into the tracheostomy tube, and lock it in place by rotating it clockwise.

NOTE: Some facilities require two people to change ties, in which case the following procedure is used. While the assistant (wearing sterile gloves and goggles) gently holds the tube in place, remove the existing tape from the flanges. Clean the skin under the ties, and inspect the skin for pressure sores from the ties.

11. Loop the new tracheostomy ties through the flange on one side of the tracheostomy (see p. 965). Bring the ties around the back of the child's neck, and tie them securely to the opposite flange. Ties are tight enough if only one finger can be inserted between the ties and neck. Tie the ties on the side, not the back, of the neck to prevent confusing the tracheostomy ties with bib ties and to avoid putting pressure on the back of the neck. Use triple knots to prevent accidental untying and dislodging of the tracheostomy. Clean and assess the skin under the ties.
12. Carefully cut and remove the soiled tracheostomy ties and any excess clean tracheostomy tape. Make sure the tracheostomy tube is secure before leaving the bedside.
13. Discard used supplies in appropriate receptacles. Record in the nurses' notes the date, time and type of procedure, the condition of the stoma and skin, any abnormal findings or complications and the nursing action taken, the child's tolerance of the procedure, and any child and family teaching done, as well as their understanding of and involvement in the care.

Home Adaptations

Assess the family's ability to perform the procedure. It might be necessary to engage the assistance of a home health agency if the family needs temporary assistance and support. Begin to teach tracheostomy care early in the child's hospitalization, and teach more than one family member how to do the care. All those caring for the child must also know cardiopulmonary resuscitation (CPR). Write clear instructions, and observe all caregivers perform the procedures. Return demonstrations of the technique are imperative. Advise the caregiver that $1/2$-inch width cotton seam binding, which can be found in fabric stores, makes acceptable tracheostomy ties.

and inner cannula, changing the tracheostomy tube, and suctioning. Clean the area around the tube at the time the tracheostomy ties are changed or more frequently if needed to keep the site clean and dry. Tracheostomy care can be given at various intervals but should be done at least every 8 hours. The tracheostomy tube is usually changed weekly. The tracheostomy tube is held in place with ties made of a durable, nonfraying material. These are changed daily or more frequently if they become soiled. *To prevent the tube from being accidentally dislodged while the ties are being changed,* *it is recommended that an assistant be present to hold the tube in place.*

Keep an extra tracheostomy tube of appropriate size at the bedside (or taped to the head of the bed) for easy access in an emergency. Because of the risk of aspiration and possible occlusion of the trachea, avoid giving the child small toys, toys with small parts, plastic bibs, and plastic bedding. In addition, do not use talcum powders and aerosol products near children with tracheostomies because of the risk of inhalation injury secondary to breathing the particles.

Caring for an Infant with a Tracheostomy

Caring for the child with a tracheostomy can involve several steps, including respiratory therapy treatments, suctioning, and changing the ties that secure the tube. Because many children are discharged from the hospital with a tracheostomy, their parents and other home caregivers must be taught these procedures.

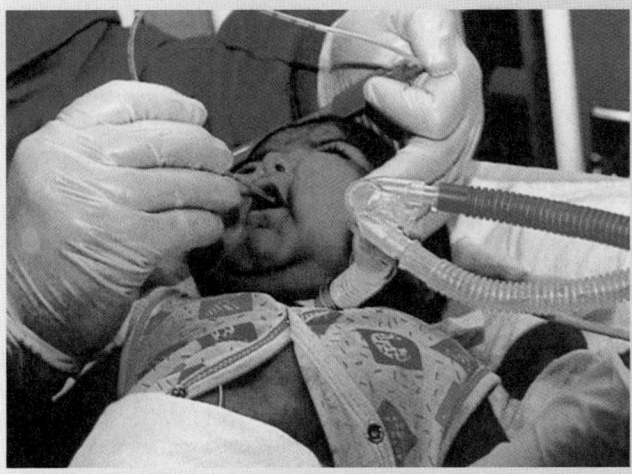

Often the oral cavity requires suctioning as well. The technique is similar to that for suctioning the tracheostomy: the catheter is inserted, and then suction is applied while the catheter is withdrawn.

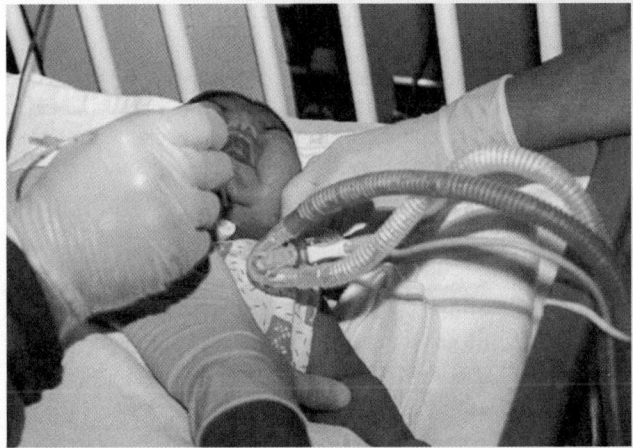

Secretions are removed from this infant's airway with a suction catheter. Appropriate techniques minimize problems with suctioning, such as hypoxia, tissue damage, or infection. The suction catheter is inserted into the tube with the suction turned off. After the appropriate length of tubing is inserted, suction is applied and the catheter is withdrawn using a twisting motion. Do not suction longer than 5 seconds at a time.

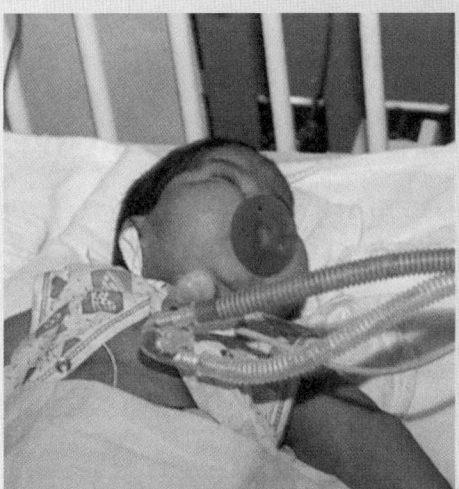

The infant who has a device such as a tracheostomy tube or a gastrostomy feeding tube still needs to suck. A pacifier fulfills this need. Because tracheostomy care is often tiring, the child should be allowed to rest afterward.

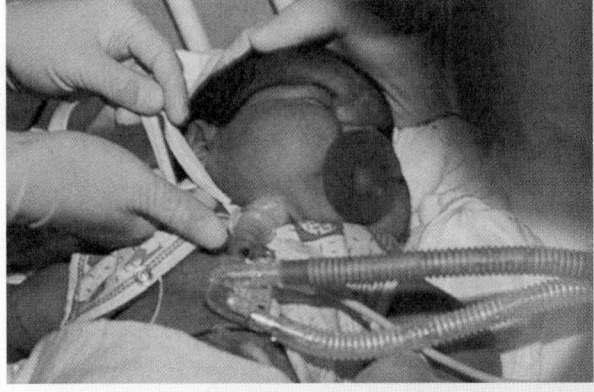

When changing the infant's tracheostomy ties, the nurse has an assistant hold the tube in place to reduce the chance that it will be displaced. The nurse makes sure the ties are snug but not too tight. When the new ties are in place, the nurse checks their snugness by inserting a finger beneath them.

Photos courtesy Parkland Health and Hospital System, Dallas, TX.

SURGICAL PROCEDURES

The child undergoing surgery has increased physical and psychologic needs. Although each surgical procedure is unique, a general body of knowledge relates to all children experiencing surgery. Surgery can be a very traumatic event for a child.

With the rising cost of health care, managed-care contracts, and the need for cost containment in health care, many surgeries are now done on an outpatient basis. Ambulatory, or same-day, surgery uses the same standards of care that apply to all routine hospital admissions but with the added benefit of lower cost.

Preparation for Surgery

A multidisciplinary approach should be used when preparing a child for surgery. Include the following: parents, nursing staff, child life specialist, physician, and any other specialists involved in the individual child's care. Preparation for outpatient procedures depends on the type of procedure to be done and the child's age and developmental level. Psychologic preparation for an outpatient experience is just as important as for an inpatient hospital experience. Indeed, much of the preparation is the same, regardless of whether the surgery will be done on an outpatient or an inpatient basis, and a multidisciplinary approach to teaching is appropriate for both settings.

Assess the child's and family's physical and psychosocial needs. Both the child and the family will be anxious, so the nurse needs to be a calming influence. Being aware of the stressors of surgery will guide the nurse in providing family-centered care. These stressors include:

- Separation from significant others, unfamiliar surroundings, and care by strangers
- Preoperative testing
- Pain
- Fear of mutilation or disfigurement
- Disruption in routine
- Anesthesia
- Lack of privacy
- Disability

Fear of the unknown is another common fear of children. By assessing the presence of these and other stressors, the nurse can develop a plan of care.

Preparing the child and family for surgery establishes a foundation of trust between the nurse and the family. Sched-

---

> ### BOX 37-2
> *Guidelines for Preoperative Fasting*
>
> 1. Fast from solid food and full liquids from the night before as directed. Some physicians allow a light breakfast early in the morning if surgery will be late in the afternoon (at least 6 hours after ingestion).
> 2. Stop breastfeeding at least 3 hours before the hospital arrival time. Unless otherwise instructed, stop formula feeding from the night before surgery.
> 3. Clear liquids, such as water, broth, ice pops, Jell-O, and clear juices can be taken up to 2 hours before time of arrival to the hospital.

---

ule formal sessions no more than 1 week before admission; younger children may need preparation closer to the operative day. Waiting too long to initiate preparation for surgery can give rise to fantasies and increase the child's fear. A preparation that is too close to surgery might not provide enough time to answer questions posed by the child or family so that they feel adequately prepared for the surgery.

Although preparation may vary from setting to setting, all teaching should be planned, should use a developmental approach, and should provide information that is simple and truthful. Many hospitals include a tour of the perioperative area. Conduct a review of the teaching on the day of the surgery. If a child life specialist participates in the preparation, that person should be present on the day of surgery.

The use of therapeutic play is an essential tool, both in preparation and perioperatively. (Therapeutic play is discussed in Chapter 35.) Keeping children busy is especially important if they have a waiting period before their scheduled surgery time. Provide age-appropriate toys in holding areas or in the child's room if that is the area where the child is waiting.

More and more often, parents are the primary educators for their child's surgical experience because of the increase in day surgery. Parents need to explain to the child as clearly as possible why the child is going to the hospital or surgery center and what will happen during the stay. Nurses can assist the parents in preparing their child. Books on hospitalization or surgery that are geared toward children help prepare them for the experience. Videotapes are also available.

Regardless of the procedure planned, some preoperative activities are routine. These include:

- No food or drink after a specified time
- A consent form for the procedure signed by the parent or guardian

In some instances, preoperative medication will be ordered. Reassure children that they will not be left alone and that they will not feel the procedure as it is done.

Because children are at greater risk for dehydration than adults, the period during which they can have nothing by mouth might be shorter. This period varies according to the protocol of the facility and the anesthesiologist (Box 37-2).

Some procedures require preoperative laboratory tests, such as a complete blood cell count, urinalysis, and chest x-ray. Most hospitals and surgical centers have preoperative checklists (similar to those used in adult care) that assist the nurse in documenting the child's preparation for the procedure. These lists usually include checking the child's identification, obtaining a signed consent form, laboratory results, administering preanesthetic medication, and other documentation. After the preanesthetic medication has been administered, the parent may hold the child or place the child on a stretcher with the side rails raised.

Preoperative Medication

Preoperative medication is used primarily to decrease anxiety in the child. In some settings, premedication is not used if the parents are present. It is becoming increasingly common for parents to be present during the induction of anesthesia. Many safe and painless premedication methods are now available (Box 37-3). After parents are asked to leave the child for surgery, the nurse keeps them informed of the anticipated length of the surgery and their child's status throughout the surgery.

Postanesthesia Care

After surgery, the child is taken to the post anesthesia care unit (PACU), or recovery room. There the nurse performs frequent assessments of the child's cardiorespiratory and circulatory systems until the child is fully awake. When the child awakens from surgery, it is important for the parent or parents to be present to comfort and calm the child. The child might also want a favorite toy or object. Providing warm blankets and a rocking chair as comfort measures can assist both the child and the parent. Pain medication should be provided as needed (see Chapter 39). Depending on the procedure performed, the child might be discharged from the hospital or admitted to an inpatient unit for the remainder of the hospital stay.

Postoperative Care

Most facilities have a specific protocol that is followed for postoperative care. After a surgical procedure, the child's vital signs are monitored frequently until they are stable. The surgical site is checked for drainage, and the child is assessed for pain. The use of patient-controlled analgesia (PCA) and the routine administration of analgesic afford effective pain control. Refer to Chapter 39 for a more detailed discussion of pain management in children.

Atelectasis, a common complication of surgery, can result from the effects of anesthesia combined with other factors, such as inadequate respiratory inflation from pain or decreased respirations associated with pain medications. Auscultate the lungs to determine any abnormal breath sounds or areas of diminished or absent sounds. In addition, encourage early ambulation, deep breathing, and coughing. Using incentive spirometers can increase respiratory movement. Games such as blowing cotton, a windmill, or bubbles can also facilitate air exchange for children unable or unwilling to use a spirometer.

Children generally recuperate more quickly in a familiar environment; as a result, they are discharged as soon as safely possible after surgery. Because of decreased lengths of stay, discharge planning begins at the time of admission. Using an organized plan of care, the discharge planner works closely with the child and family to identify needs and resources and then develops an efficient, cost-effective plan for meeting those needs.

Some children will need specialized care in the home after discharge from the hospital. The family's ability to provide some or all of the care will determine the extent of education provided before discharge and the need for involvement of a home health agency after discharge. The family and the nurse must identify the level of knowledge needed and any specific equipment or home modifications required to care for the child adequately at home. It is usually the responsibility of the home health agency to make the necessary arrangements for durable or disposable equipment. It is helpful, when possible, for equipment and supplies to be provided by the same agency that provides assistance with home nursing care. Some agencies also will provide education for the family before the child's discharge. To ensure the child and family the smoothest transition possible from hospital to home, these issues and del-

egation of responsibilities need to be addressed as soon as they are identified.

Nursing diagnoses frequently associated with the child undergoing surgery include:

- Anxiety and Fear related to separation from significant others, surgery, unfamiliar environment, and personnel
- Acute Pain related to the surgical incision
- Deficient Knowledge related to unfamiliarity with the procedure and expected outcomes
- Interrupted Family Processes related to the surgical procedure
- Risk for Deficient Fluid Volume related to NPO status before and after surgery, as well as to nausea and vomiting

ADDITIONAL INFORMATION

See Chapter 32 for assistance with communication challenges. Chapter 35 provides information on care related to hospitalization and separation, Chapter 39 discusses pain-related issues, and Chapter 42 presents nursing care as it relates to fluid balance. To deliver quality care, the nurse must identify the child's growth and developmental needs, along with the care needs associated with the disorder for which the surgery is being performed.

BOX 37-3
Pediatric Anesthesia Induction Techniques

PREMEDICATIONS—SEDATIVES
- Rectal midazolam
- Oral benzodiazepine or barbiturate or narcotic
- Intranasal benzodiazepine or ketamine
- Transmucosal (lollipop) fentanyl

INDUCTION AGENTS—SLEEP-INDUCING
- Barbiturates: rectal or intravenous (IV)
- Ketamine: intramuscular (IM) or IV
- Etomidate: IV
- Propofol: IV
- Potent inhalational agents

MODIFICATIONS OF MASK INDUCTION
- Give the child the option of sitting up, either in a chair or on a lap.
- Let the child hold the mask.
- Provide a choice of flavored gases.
- Conceal the breathing circuit—"Trojan horse."
  "Halothane Phone"—concealed in play phone.
  "Pungent Pacifier"—concealed behind a pacifier.
  "Sleepy Bear"—concealed with a stuffed animal.

MODIFICATIONS OF INTRAVENOUS INDUCTION
- Use a eutectic mixture of local anesthetics (EMLA) cream to place an IV cannula.
- Use a 25- or 27-gauge "butterfly" needle.
- Allow the child to push a syringe containing the appropriate dose of drug through a preexisting IV access line.
- Create diversions (e.g., have the child count backward from 100 or tell jokes or stories).

From Zuckerberg, A.L. (1994). Perioperative approach to children. *Pediatric Clinics of North America, 41*(1), 25.

KEY CONCEPTS

- Whenever possible, perform procedures in the treatment room, away from the child's room.
- Some procedures require informed consent. Children 7 years old and older must give assent to some procedures. Because laws on informed consent vary from state to state, nurses must be familiar with the laws and policies of their institution.
- Use developmentally appropriate and descriptive words when preparing children for procedures.

- Praise children for attempts at cooperation during a procedure even if they did not follow instructions. Praise them for accomplishing an expected task.
- Documentation of a procedure includes recording the preparation, who performed the procedure, the child's tolerance, the actual procedure, and outcomes.
- Follow Standard Precautions when collecting all specimens. Standard Precautions are used with all hospitalized clients and are not based on diagnosis or presumed infectious

state. Transmission-Based Precautions are used with clients known or suspected to be infected by pathogens that are conveyed by airborne or droplet transmission or by contact with dry skin or contaminated surfaces.
- Use restraints only as a last resort to protect the child and others.
- Because of children's developmental level and activity, be particularly conscious of safety measures when caring for children in a hospital setting.

ANSWERS to Critical Thinking Exercise 37-1

1. As a nurse, you are responsible to practice safely. This means checking the hospital policy and procedure manual before beginning any procedure and keeping current with evidence-based research. Because even experienced nurses disagree on the best approach to confirm feeding tube placement in children, using a combination of methods described in the literature increases the likelihood of an accurate assessment. Remember that the only truly accurate determination of placement is by radiography. In most institutions, nurses write procedures by committee. One way of ensuring that your institution's policy reflects evidence-based practice is to serve on the committee that periodically updates procedures.

2. If there is a question about tube placement (marginal pH measurements, questionable aspirate appearance), do not give an enteral feeding through the tube. Inform the physician about your findings. You can request that the physician order a radiographic confirmation. The tube may have to be removed and replaced.

REFERENCES and READINGS

Alsop-Shields, L. (2000). Perioperative care of children in a transcultural context. *AORN Journal, 71*(5), 1004-1020.

American Thoracic Society. (2000). Care of the child with a chronic tracheostomy. *American Journal of Respiratory and Critical Care Medicine, 161,* 297-308.

Arafat, M., & Mattoo, T. (1999). Measurement of blood pressure in children: Recommendations and perceptions on cuff selection. *Pediatrics, 104*(3), e30.

Attin, M., Cardin, S., Dee, V., Doering, L., Dunn, D., Ellstrom, K., Erickson, V., Etchepare, M., Gawlinski, A., Haley, T., Henneman, E., Keckeisen, M., Malmet, M., & Olson, L. (2002). An educational project to improve knowledge related to pulse oximetry. *American Journal of Critical Care, 11*(6), 529-534.

Bar-Mor, G. (1997). Preparation of children for surgery and invasive procedures: Milestones on the way to success. *Journal of Pediatric Nursing, 12*(4), 252-255.

Blazys, D. (1999). Gaining the trust of children. *Journal of Emergency Nursing, 25*(5), 387.

Bowen, W.H. (2002). Fluorosis: Is it really a problem? *Journal of the American Dental Association, 133*(10), 1405-1407.

Bowers, S. (2000). All about tubes. *Nursing 2000, 30*(12), 41-47.

Brenner, Z. (1999). Preventing postoperative complications. *Nursing 1999, 29*(10), 34-38.

Bryant, K., Davis, C., & Lagrone, C. (1997). Streamlining discharge planning for the child

with a new tracheotomy. *Journal of Pediatric Nursing, 12*(3), 191-192.

Carlson, D., & Mowery, D. (1997). Standards to prevent complications of urinary catheterization in children: Should and should-knots. *Journal of the Society of Pediatric Nurses: JSPN, 2*(1), 37-41.

Carpenter, K.H. (1998). Developing a pediatric patient/parent hospital preparation program. *AORN Journal, 67*(5), 1042-1046.

Carron, J.D., Derkay, C.S., Strope, G.L., Nosonchuk, J.E., & Darrow, D.H. (2000). Pediatric tracheotomies: Changing indications and outcomes. *Laryngoscope, 110,* 1099-1104.

Centers for Disease Control and Prevention. (2001). Recommendations for using fluoride to prevent and control dental caries in the United States. *Morbidity and Mortality Weekly Reports, 50*(RR14), 1-42.

Clark, J., Lieh-Lai, M., Sarnaik, A., & Mattoo, T. (2002). Discrepancies between direct and indirect blood pressure measurements using various recommendations for arm cuff selection. *Pediatrics, 110*(5), 920-923.

Craig, J., Lancaster, G., Taylor, S., Williamson, P., & Smyth, R. (2002). Infrared ear thermometry compared with rectal thermometry in children: A systematic review. *The Lancet, 360,* 603-609.

Ellett, M., & Beckstrand, J. (1999). Examination of gavage tube placement in children. *Journal of Society of Pediatric Nurses, 4*(2), 51-60.

Erwin-Toth, P. (2001). Caring for a stoma is more than skin deep. *Nursing 2001, 31*(5), 36-41.

Feldman, D., Reich, N., & Foster, J. (1998). Pediatric anesthesia and postoperative analgesia. *Pediatric Clinics of North America, 45*(6), 1525-1537.

Finkelstein, J., Christiansen, C., & Platt, R. (2000). Fever in pediatric primary care: Occurrence, management, and outcomes. *Pediatrics, 105*(1), 260-265.

Gelmetti, C. (2002). Skin cleansing in children. *Journal of the European Academy of Dermatology and Venereology, 15*(Suppl. 1), 12-15.

Gerard, L., Cooper, C., Duethman, K., Gordley, B., & Kleiber, C. (2003). Effectiveness of lidocaine lubricant for discomfort during pediatric urethral catheterization. *The Journal of Urology, 170*(2), 564-567.

Goldman, L., Shannon, M., & Committee on Environmental Health. (2001). Technical report: Mercury in the environment: Implications for pediatricians (RE 109907). *Pediatrics, 108*(1), 197-205.

Hanchett, M. (2002). Techniques for stabilizing urinary catheters. *American Journal of Nursing, 102*(3), 44-48.

Houlder, L. (2000). The accuracy and reliability of tympanic thermometry compared to rectal and axillary sites in young children. *Pediatric Nursing, 26*(3), 311-314.

Jeffery, K. (2002). Therapeutic restraint of children: It must always be justified. *Paediatric Nursing, 14*(9), 20-22.

Joyce, S. (1998). Tracheostomy care and tracheal suctioning. In J. Roberts & J. Hedges (Eds.),

Clinical procedures in emergency medicine (3rd ed., Ch. 5). Philadelphia: Saunders.

Karl, D. (1999). The interactive newborn bath. *MCN: The American Journal of Maternal/Child Nursing, 24*(6), 280-286.

Kohn-Keeth, C. (2000). How to keep feeding tubes flowing freely. *Nursing 2000, 30*(3), 58-59.

Krantz, C. (2001). Childhood fevers: Developing an evidence-based anticipatory guidance tool for parents. *Pediatric Nursing, 27*(6), 567-571.

Krause, M., & Hoehn, T. (2000). Chest physiotherapy in mechanically ventilated children: A review. *Critical Care Medicine, 28*(5), 1648-1651.

Lanham, D., Walker, B., Klocke, E., & Jennings, M. (1999). Accuracy of tympanic temperature readings in children under 6 years of age. *Pediatric Nursing, 25*(1), 39-42.

Liao, J., & Churchill, B. (2001). Pediatric urine testing. *Pediatric Clinics of North America, 48*(6), 1425-1440.

Lorin, M. (2004). Fever: Pathogenesis and treatment. In R. Feigin, J. Cherry, G. Demmier, & S. Kaplan (Eds.), *Textbook of pediatric infectious diseases* (5th ed., pp. 100-106). Philadelphia: Saunders.

McClosky, D. (2002). Catheter-related thrombosis in pediatrics. *Pediatric Nursing, 28*(2), 97-105.

McConnell, E. (2002). Clinical do's and don'ts providing tracheostomy care. *Nursing 2002, 32*(1), 17.

Metheny, N., & Titler, M. (2001). Assessing placement of feeding tubes. *American Journal of Nursing, 101*(5), 36-45.

Metheny, N., Wehrle, A., Wiersema, L., & Clark, J. (1998). Testing feeding tube placement: Auscultation vs. pH method. *American Journal of Nursing, 98*(5), 37-42.

Mowery, B., & Suddaby, B. (2002). Tracheostomy troubles. *Pediatric Nursing, 28*(2), 162.

National Institutes of Health. (1996). *Update on the task force report (1987) on high blood pressure in children and adolescents: A working group report from the national high blood pressure education program* (NIH Publication No. 96-3790). Bethesda, MD: Author.

O'Connor-Von, S. (2000). Preparing children for surgery: An integrative research review. *AORN Journal, 71*(2), 334-343.

Pagana KD, & Pagana, T. (2002). *Mosby's manual of diagnostic and laboratory tests* (2nd ed.). St. Louis: Mosby.

Schmitt, B. (1999). *Instructions for pediatric patients* (2nd ed.). Philadelphia: Saunders.

Siberry, G., Diener-West, M., Schappell, E., & Karron, R. (2002). Comparison of temple temperatures with rectal temperatures in children under two years of age. *Clinical Pediatrics, 41,* 405-414.

Smith, A., & Adams, L. (1998). Insertion of indwelling urethral catheters in infants and children: A survey of current nursing practice. *Pediatric Nursing, 24*(3), 229-234.

Smith, L. (2003). Which catheter? Criteria for selection of urinary catheters for children. *Paediatric Nursing, 15*(3), 14-18.

Splinter, W., & Schreiner, M. (1999). Preoperative fasting in children. *Anesthesia and Analgesia, 89*(1), 80-89.

Suctioning of the patient in the home. (1999). *Respiratory Care, 44*(1), 91-98.

Wetmore, R., Thompson, M., Marsh, R., & Tom, L. (1999). Pediatric tracheostomy: A changing procedure? *Annals of Otology, Rhinology and Laryngology, 108,* 695-699.

Worral, P., & Luke, S. (1998). Tympanic thermometry. *SPN News, 7*(2), 1.

38

Medicating Infants and Children

◆ DEFINITIONS

blood-brain barrier Selective anatomic or physiologic capillary obstruction that prevents potentially harmful substances, such as certain medications, radioactive ions, and viruses, from entering the parenchyma of the brain.

central venous access device Venous access device in which the catheter is placed centrally rather than peripherally, usually in the superior vena cava or jugular vein; used for long-term intravenous (IV) therapy.

eutectic mixture of local anesthetics (EMLA) Cream used to numb the skin at a depth of 0.5 mm; used before needle punctures.

implanted venous access device (IVAD, Infusaport) Surgically implanted port or reservoir in which the catheter tip is placed in the superior vena cava; used for long-term IV therapy.

intermittent infusion port IV catheter used to administer intermittent IV medications or fluids; remains clamped when not in use.

metered-dose inhaler Hand-held device that delivers "puffs" of medication for inhalation.

peripherally inserted central catheter (PICC) Central line that is inserted peripherally (usually through an antecubital vein) into the superior vena cava.

pharmacodynamics Behavior of medications at the cellular level.

pharmacokinetics The time and movement relationships of medications.

sustained-release medication Medication taken in a single dose but designed to dissolve slowly, releasing medication into the bloodstream over a specified period of time (usually 12 to 24 hours).

tunneled central line A surgically placed central line that is held in place by a Dacron cuff located in a subcutaneous tunnel; most commonly placed in the external jugular vein.

Medicating infants and children is one of the nurse's most important responsibilities. The nurse plays a key role in administering medications, supporting the child and family during the experience, and teaching the child and parents about pharmacologic aspects of the child's care. Although physicians or nurse practitioners prescribe medications, the nurse or caregiver is responsible for their administration. The nurse has a legal responsibility to administer medications safely and accurately. Safe administration of medications to children requires an understanding of the dosages of the medications used for children as well as the expected actions, possible side effects, and signs of adverse reactions or toxicity. Nurses should use reliable sources of information (e.g., pharmacists, drug handbooks, hospital formularies) when administering drugs that are unfamiliar or used infrequently and should question orders they do not understand before administering the medication.

Giving medications to children requires special skill. To gain the child's cooperation and to administer the medication in the least traumatic manner, the nurse needs to understand the physical characteristics and psychologic needs of children at each developmental level. The nurse should use developmentally appropriate strategies to handle children's fears, prevent injury, and enhance coping.

It is vitally important to provide parents with information about medications used in their child's treatment and to encourage parents to support their child during potentially uncomfortable experiences. Involving parents in the task of eliciting their child's cooperation not only makes the job easier but also gives the family a sense of self-management and control. If the parents will be asked to administer medications to their child at home, the nurse ensures that the parents are properly instructed before the child is discharged.

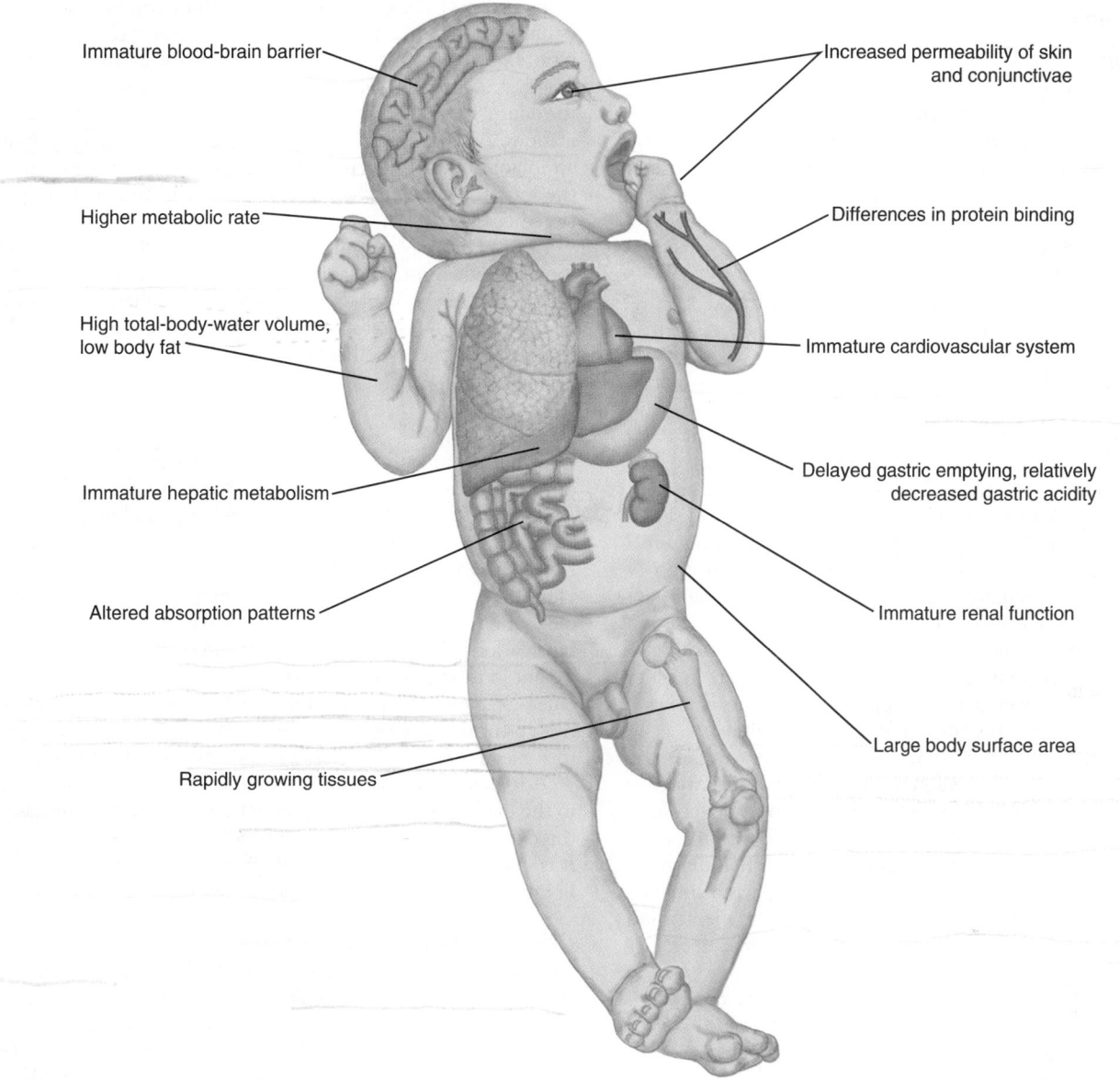

Immature blood-brain barrier

Increased permeability of skin and conjunctivae

Higher metabolic rate

Differences in protein binding

High total-body-water volume, low body fat

Immature cardiovascular system

Immature hepatic metabolism

Delayed gastric emptying, relatively decreased gastric acidity

Altered absorption patterns

Immature renal function

Large body surface area

Rapidly growing tissues

Figure 38-1 Physiologic differences between children and adults affect drug absorption, metabolism, distribution, and excretion. These differences are most extreme in the neonate.

Adherence to properly taking the full course of a medication continues to be a problem for children and adolescents (Blanchard, Primovic, & Leff, 1999; Staples & Bravender, 2002). Research has suggested that, after leaving the health care setting, parents remember only about half of the instructions they were given by health care personnel (Matsui, 1997). Medication administration times that fit into the family routine, medications that are palatable to the child, and clear, written instructions improve adherence (Matsui, 1997). Taking the time to explain to the child why the medication is needed may also improve cooperation (Blanchard, Primovic, & Leff, 1999). Any medication regimen should consider the developmental needs of the child or adolescent and should be presented to the child and family using a variety of educational and behavioral strategies. For example, strategies such as simple dosing schedules, personal interest expressed by the provider, and a variety of cues to help an older child remember to take the medication can be successful with increasing adherence (Staples & Bravender, 2002).

PHARMACOKINETICS IN CHILDREN

An understanding of pharmacokinetics and pharmacodynamics guides appropriate interventions in children. *Pharmacokinetics* refers to the actions of a drug (e.g., movement, biotransformation) within the human body over time, and *pharmacodynamics* is the behavior of a drug as it interacts with the biochemical and physiologic milieu of the body. The pharmacokinetic actions of absorption, distribution, metabolism, and excretion are influenced by the physiologic environment in which the drug moves, and this environment differs between adults and children (Fig. 38-1). The physiologic differences in body systems are most striking in the neonate.

Absorption

Oral Route

When a medication is given orally, several factors influence its absorption along the gastrointestinal (GI) tract. Because most medication absorption occurs in the small intestine, the drug must reach that location in a form suitable for maximum absorption. Four factors influence this process:

- Gastric acidity
- Gastric emptying time
- GI motility, or transit time through the GI tract
- Function of the pancreatic enzymes

Gastric Acidity. Infants' gastric secretions are less acidic than older children's or adults'. Secretions slowly increase in acidity during the first 2 years of life. Children, particularly infants, eat more frequently than adults and are more likely to have food and digestive enzymes present in their stomachs. Formula or milk can increase the alkalinity of gastric secretions, decreasing the absorption of medications that require a more acidic environment and enhancing the absorption of medications that require a more alkaline milieu. These factors can greatly affect serum drug levels.

Gastric Emptying. Gastric emptying is intermittent and unpredictable in infants but usually is slower than in older children. This slower pace can prolong the time it takes a medication to reach the intestinal absorption site.

Gastrointestinal Motility. Depending on whether the infant or young child has eaten recently, peristaltic activity in the intestine can be faster or slower than in the older child or adult. Infants up to 8 months of age tend to have prolonged motility. Certain adverse health conditions, such as diarrhea, can alter intestinal motility by increasing peristalsis. The longer the transit time in the intestine, the more medication is absorbed. Conversely, a shortened transit time decreases absorption.

Enzyme Activity. Pancreatic enzyme activity also is variable in infants for the first 3 months of life as the GI system matures. Medications that require specific enzymes for dissolution and absorption might not be digested to a form suitable for intestinal action.

Other Routes

Adequate absorption of medication administered intravenously (IV) depends on adequate peripheral perfusion. Medications given IV are immediately available for absorption into the child's bloodstream. The child's peripheral circulation is less reliable and more responsive to environmental changes than the adult's. As a result, vasoconstriction or vasodilation can occur and alter the absorption of a parenteral medication. Also, the cardiovascular system is less able to accommodate large or rapid changes in volume, and the child can develop fluid overload if volumes of IV infusions are not carefully monitored.

A child's muscle mass is less than an adult's. The infant's body weight is about 25% muscle, whereas the adult's is about 40%. Because of the smaller muscle mass in infants, fewer sites are available for intramuscular (IM) injections. Increased blood flow to muscle tissue is essential for adequate absorption. Blood flow to muscles in the young child is erratic and can affect the absorption of injected medications.

Infants and young children have a thinner outer skin layer (stratum corneum) and a larger body surface area (BSA)/weight ratio. Because the ratio of BSA to weight varies inversely with length, the infant has more surface area relative to weight than the adult. This difference affects the absorption of topical medications. Absorption of a similar dose of a topical medication in an infant and an adult is approximately three times greater in the infant because of the greater BSA and thinner skin layer (Reed & Gal, 2004).

Skin pH varies with age and can affect the absorption of topical medications. A child's skin is also more prone to irritation, making contact dermatitis and other allergic reactions more common. Irritated or open skin can enhance the absorption of topical medications.

Distribution

Distribution refers to the general and specific concentration of the medication in body fluids and tissues. The medication is distributed to body tissues through blood and body fluids.

Differences in Body Fluids

Fluid differences between children younger than 2 years and older children must be considered when determining dosages of medication. The body fluid content ranges from 75% of body weight in infants to 60% of body weight in children 2 years and older. Because of their greater fluid volume per weight, children need a higher dose per kilogram of a water-soluble medication to achieve the desired distribution effects (see Chapter 42).

A higher percentage of the young child's body fluid is located in the extracellular fluid compartment. During certain illnesses, this extracellular fluid can be lost rapidly, causing fluid depletion. It is important to adjust medication dosages accordingly in the ill infant or young child, to avoid overdosing or underdosing.

Differences in Fat Percentages

Percentages of fat also change as the child grows. Fat makes up about 16% of an infant's weight, although total body fat varies from child to child. This percentage increases in a 1-year-old but decreases during the preschool years. The percentage of body fat affects the distribution of fat-soluble medications in children. Because the body fat must be saturated with a fat-soluble medication before the drug becomes detectable in the blood, dosages often must be varied to achieve the desired effects.

Differences in Proteins

Medications bind to plasma proteins, mainly albumin, for distribution. Only free, unbound medication can be absorbed by the body. Because infants have lower levels of plasma proteins than do older children, more unbound drug circulates and is available for absorption. This increased concentration of unbound drug alters the amount of medication needed to maintain a therapeutic drug level.

Blood-Brain Barrier

The blood-brain barrier does not fully mature until the child is about 2 years old. This immaturity causes the barrier to be less selective and allows for distribution of medication into the central nervous system. As a result, encephalopathy can occur with some medications.

The relative immaturity of the neurologic system also can lead to paradoxic effects from certain medications. For example, medications that normally cause sedation in adults may have the opposite effect in many children and cause hyperactivity.

Metabolism

Most medications are metabolized in the liver. Because the metabolic enzyme systems are less mature in newborn and premature infants, they might not be able to properly metabolize all the medication in a prescribed dosage. Toddlers and preschoolers can have a much greater metabolizing capacity than adults do for certain drugs. For this reason, larger dosages or more frequent administration of certain drugs (e.g., pain medications) might be needed for young children, to achieve therapeutic results.

Excretion

Most medications are excreted through the renal system. The renal system also is immature at birth. The newborn's glomerular filtration rate is about 30% to 50% that of an adult's, and the renal tubules also function less efficiently. Adult rates are reached after approximately 1 year. Infants and young children cannot concentrate urine as well as older children or adults.

Because of renal immaturity, medications might not be filtered out of the circulating blood volume and excreted in the urine (the primary method of medication excretion). As a result, medications can circulate longer and reach toxic blood levels. Likewise, loss of fluid may decrease the child's ability to excrete medications. Therefore dehydration has a serious effect on drug serum levels.

Concentration

To administer appropriately therapeutic medication doses to children, nurses need to be aware of the importance of knowing the concentration of certain medications in serum. Maintaining serum levels within a safe therapeutic range maximizes the effect of a medication while reducing the risk of toxicity. When certain medications are used, the physician will order peak and trough serum levels to be measured to monitor medication concentration. The peak concentration is not necessarily the highest concentration but is the concentration of the medication after it has been distributed. The time at which a medication reaches peak concentration differs according to the specific medication but usually occurs a specified time after the medication has been administered.

The medication trough is the level at which the serum concentration is lowest. Trough levels usually are obtained just before the next medication dose. Knowing the usual therapeutic peak-and-trough range for a specific medication will assist the nurse in an accurate assessment of the child's response and the potential for toxic medication effects.

PSYCHOLOGIC AND DEVELOPMENTAL FACTORS

Growth and developmental principles and differences among age-groups must always be considered when medicating a child. Eliciting support from the parent usually eases any concern the child may have.

PARENTS
Want to Know

Medication Administration

Parents want to know how they can help their children when a procedure for administering medication is expected to be uncomfortable. They also become concerned if the child refuses to take a medication that is intended to help the child recover from an illness. Nurses should do the following to empower parents:

- Obtain the following information before administering the medication:
  —Medication allergies or sensitivities
  —The child's ability to take medications (e.g., can the child swallow pills?)
  —What method the parent usually uses to administer the medication (e.g., mixing it with certain foods)
- Give the parent a thorough explanation about the medication before administration. Include information about why the child needs the medication, any possible side effects, and how and where you expect to administer the medication.
- Allow the parent to administer certain medications if the child is more comfortable (e.g., oral, otic, ophthalmic). Check the medication "rights" before you allow a parent to administer a medication. Show the parent the most acceptable position for administering the particular medication.
- Encourage the parent who is concerned that a medication might not be effective or might be making the child ill to express these concerns. Parents know their children and often are aware of subtle changes long before hospital personnel notice them.
- Help the parent determine the best way to administer the child's medication at home. Recommend the use of positive reinforcements such as rewards or stickers to increase cooperation. Encourage the parent to explain to the child why the medication is needed and to be firm that the child takes the medication.

Always approach children at their developmental level and provide developmentally appropriate explanations about a medication procedure. To decrease feelings of powerlessness, give the child as many choices as possible.

Honesty, reward, and praise are important for gaining trust and cooperation. Give honest explanations, and tell the child when a procedure will be painful or uncomfortable. Also tell the child approximately how long the pain will last and what the child can do to help during that time. Use terms familiar to the child, such as "pinching" or "stinging."

Praising the child after the procedure for attempts at cooperation is important and helps gain trust and cooperation for future procedures. Do not scold a child for failure to cooperate.

Restraints are seldom necessary for administration of medications. It is appropriate to ask a parent or other staff member to assist with holding a child during an injection if the child's movements appear to jeopardize safe administration of the medication. Approaches include taking the child to a procedure room where another staff member assists in helping the child remember to hold still. Physical restraint devices, such as arm boards and mummy restraints, are occasionally necessary. It is important to explain that the staff person is helping the child remember to hold still. Do not threaten a child with restraint.

Rewards for good behavior often help the child feel better about the procedure. Rewards should always be safe and appropriate for the child's age. Stickers are a good choice for younger children. Older children might want a sticker or might choose a small toy or a privilege, such as watching a favorite video.

Infants

Infants are easier to medicate than toddlers but more difficult than children who can follow directions (see Chapter 5). Parents always need to know why the infant is receiving the medication. Because keeping a squirming infant still may be difficult, the nurse should get help in administering the medication if necessary. Maintaining a routine and cuddling and comforting the infant before and after the procedure are important interventions.

Toddlers and Preschoolers

Older toddlers (2 to 3 years) are prone to magical thinking and might view the administration of medication (especially if painful or intrusive) as punishment for "bad" thoughts (see Chapter 6). Give toddlers age-appropriate explanations, using play if possible. Allowing older toddlers to examine the equipment before the procedure might enhance cooperation. Because the toddler might react negatively to restraint, use as little restraint as possible and allow the toddler to sit on the parent's lap if the parent is willing. Praise and cuddling after

the procedure are important. Rewards, such as stickers, are useful for this age-group.

Preschoolers (3 to 5 years) continue to use magical thinking. They fear the unknown and painful procedures (see Chapter 6). This age-group benefits greatly from therapeutic play and participation. Allow as much control over the procedure, and offer as much choice as possible (e.g., "Do you want your medication with juice or milk?"). Ask preschoolers if they can hold still for a painful procedure; if they cannot, they usually will say so. Adhesive bandages are important to children in this age-group after an invasive procedure, such as an injection. Preschoolers believe that these bandages "make it better"—an example of magical thinking.

School-Age Children

School-age children (6 to 12 years) fear loss of control, pain, and injury. At this age, a child can understand more complex explanations (see Chapter 7). Provide as much choice as possible. School-age children often cooperate fully, even with painful procedures, but might need a source of distraction (e.g., a radio to turn up as pain increases, counting out loud for the length of pain time) and support (see Chapter 39). School-age children still need praise, and rewards (e.g., stickers) are appreciated.

Adolescents

Adolescents (11 to 21 years) fear separation from peers and loss of control (see Chapter 8). Persons in this age-group understand adult explanations and can assist in making decisions about their care. Often, however, adolescents exhibit a hyperresponse to procedures that can seem inconsistent with their age. It is important to praise their cooperation and find outlets for their frustration (e.g., drawing, writing).

CALCULATING DOSAGES

Medications for children usually do not have standard dosages. Instead, dosages are calculated based on the child's weight (milligrams per kilogram [mg/kg]). This practice usually is the most reliable method for precisely determining doses. For example, for a child weighing 10 kg, the daily dose of amoxicillin is 20 to 40 mg/kg, or 200 to 400 mg/day.

Dosages can also be calculated based on BSA (body surface area, milligrams per square meter [mg/m^2]) or according to other standardized methods (Fig. 38-2). To calculate medications on the basis of surface area, the following formula is used:

Approximate dose = BSA of child (m^2)/1.7 × adult dose

Administration Procedures

Because the margin of safety is minimal in pediatric patients, accuracy is a prime consideration when administering medications. Inaccurate dosage calculations can result in a tenfold or more dosage error if the decimal point is in the wrong place. Always check medication doses for accuracy in the following areas: (1) recommended dosage in mg/kg/day, (2) number of divided doses recommended (e.g., every 4 hours, three times a day [t.i.d.], every 12 hours), and (3) recommended route of administration. To further avoid errors, follow these procedures:

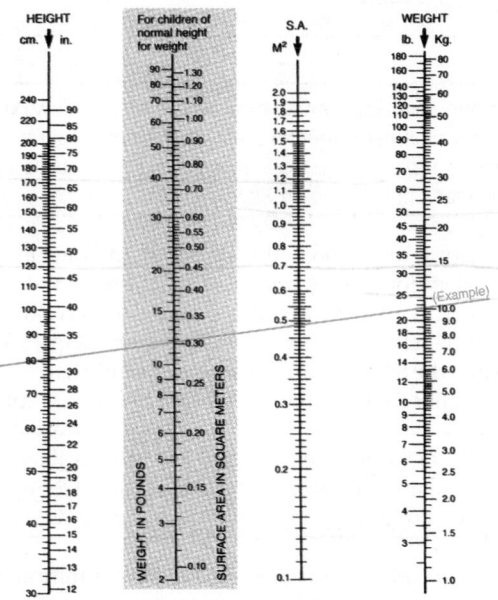

Figure 38-2 Nomogram for calculating body surface area, used for determining medication dosages for infants and children. *S.A.,* Surface area. (From Behrman, R.E., Kliegman, R.M., & Jenson, H. [2000]. *Nelson textbook of pediatrics* [16th ed., p. 2182]. Philadelphia: Saunders.)

- Adhere to the "six rights" of medication administration: right child, right drug, right dose, right time, right route, and right documentation.
- Check the orders to be sure that all information is correctly transcribed. Note any allergies.
- Always double-check medication calculations before administration. Be sure the child's weight is accurately recorded.
- Double-check calculations of medications provided by the pharmacy in a unit dose form. Consult with the physician or pharmacist if there is any question about a dose.
- Ask another nurse to double-check the following medications:
  - Insulin
  - Narcotics
  - Chemotherapy
  - Digoxin or other inotropic drugs
  - Anticoagulants
  - K+ and Ca++ salts

Many institutions also require two nurses to check any medication given by continuous infusion or by medication syringe pump.

Administering Oral Medications

The oral route is the most widely used and economic method of administering medications. It is also one of the least reliable methods of administration because absorption is affected greatly by the presence or absence of food in the stomach, gastric emptying time, GI motility, and stomach acidity. The oral route can be less predictable also because of medication loss to spillage, leaking, or spitting out.

Oral medications are available in liquid (elixir or suspension), tablet or capsule, chewable tablet, or sprinkle (powder) forms. If the child cannot swallow tablets or capsules, the nurse determines whether the medication is available in a liquid form and, if it is not, determines whether it can be crushed.

Before administering oral medications, the nurse assesses the child's gag reflex and ability to swallow. The oral form used should be tailored to the child's developmental level and ability to successfully take the form prescribed. An assessment of the way the child takes medications at home also helps determine the proper form. Some older infants and toddlers can successfully take crushed tablets but refuse liquid forms.

Medication Preparation

When preparing to administer an elixir or suspension, the nurse first ensures that the correct dose is drawn for administration. Physicians' orders often specify the dosage in milligrams, *not* milliliters, for liquid medications. It is important

to calculate the milliliter dose properly, based on the number of milligrams per milliliter in the liquid medication on hand.

Because tableware spoons vary in volume, use a calibrated spoon or dropper designed for medication administration. Calibrated syringes (preferably oral administration syringes) should be used for doses less than 5 ml or doses that are not in 5-ml increments. Pour larger volumes into calibrated plastic medicine cups. Avoid using paper measuring cups because their volumes tend to vary.

If a tablet is to be crushed and mixed with food or is available as a sprinkle or powder, mix it with a nonessential food, such as applesauce or pudding, not orange juice or formula. Giving medication with a favorite food can alter the flavor of the food. Avoid using syrup or other high-sugar substances. Never give infants medication or foods mixed with honey, because honey has been known to cause infantile botulism. Determine a medication's compatibility with food before giving it to the child. Mix any medication with a small amount (5 to 10 ml) of food or liquid, and give it to the child before a feeding, if not contraindicated.

Sustained-release tablets or capsules should never be crushed because their function is to release the medication slowly over a long period. Enteric-coated tablets (tablets covered with a substance that prevents the drug from dissolving until it reaches the intestine) can have an unpleasant taste or odor if crushed. Crushing also interferes with the function of the enteric coating.

Medication Administration

The method of administering oral medications differs according to the child's age and developmental level. Infants usually receive elixir or suspension forms of oral medications. Administer these with an empty nipple or oral syringe. First place the infant in an upright or semi-upright position. The position used for feeding the infant can be used for administering medications. Open the infant's mouth by applying gentle pressure to the chin or both cheeks. If using a nipple, place the nipple in the infant's mouth and add the medication to the empty nipple when the baby begins to suck. Unpleasant-tasting medications should not be given through a nipple because the taste can cause a future aversion reaction to the nipple, thus interfering with feeding.

If using an oral syringe or medicine dropper to administer the medication, place the syringe or dropper gently in the infant's mouth along the side of the cheek and squirt the medication in slowly as the infant sucks (Fig. 38-3). Aiming the medication toward the back of the throat is dangerous because it can cause choking and aspiration.

Toddlers and preschoolers can easily take liquid medications from an oral syringe or medicine cup. If the liquid medication has an unpleasant taste, offer to let the child take it through a straw. If a straw is used, cut the straw in half to avoid a loss of medication. Allowing children to take their own med-

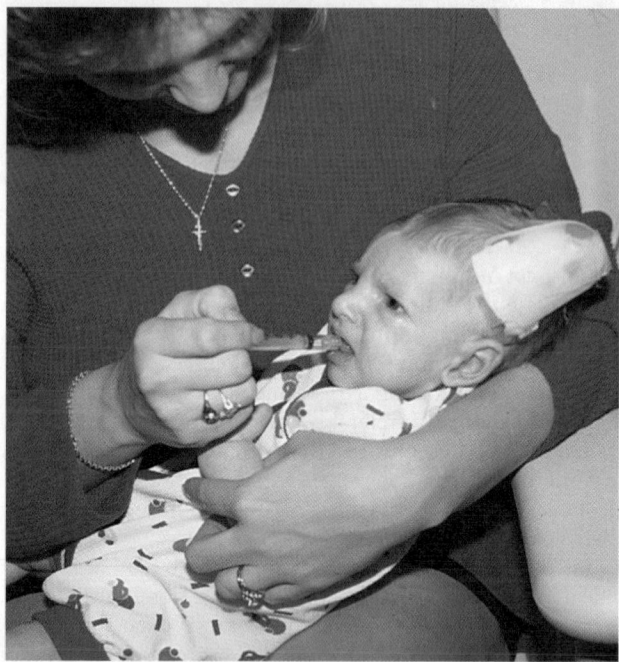

Figure 38-3 Administering an oral medication with an oral syringe to an infant. (Courtesy Parkland Health and Hospital System, Dallas, TX.)

ication, giving rewards as incentives, and providing choices that fit into the medication regimen enhance autonomy.

Preschoolers can usually manage chewable tablets without difficulty. Most older children can swallow tablets or capsules. The nurse, however, should determine whether the child can swallow pills. If not, the nurse should determine whether the medication can be crushed and mixed with food or a small amount of liquid. If the child cannot swallow tablets or capsules and the tablets or capsules cannot be crushed, the nurse needs to contact the pharmacy to identify another form for administration (elixir or suspension). If the child can swallow tablets and capsules, ask what the child prefers for the "chaser" (usually water or juice).

Administer oral medications with the child in an upright or slightly recumbent position. The nurse should always use the least amount of force or restraint possible to administer the medication safely and avoid choking and aspiration. The child who is reluctant to take a necessary medication can be positioned in the nurse's lap, as follows:

- Seat the child sideways on your lap, facing your dominant hand.
- Hug the child by bringing the arm closest to your body under your arm and around your waist or back.
- Bring your nondominant arm around behind the child's neck, and hold the child's free arm or hand with yours. This position cradles the child's head between your arm and body (see Fig. 38-3).
- If the child is very resistant, secure the child's legs between yours as well.

If the child vomits or spits up after the administration of medication, notify the physician. Another dose may need to be reordered depending on how long it has been since administration, the type of medication, and the amount vomited.

Alternative Oral Routes

Oral medications can be administered directly into the GI tract through a feeding tube. If the medication is to be administered through a feeding tube, verify tube placement before administration (see Chapter 37) and, depending on the type of tube (e.g., transpyloric), determine whether the tube is the proper route for the medication. After the medication is administered, flush the tube with water to ensure the medication has reached the GI tract and to prevent blockage in the tube.

Administering Injections

Injected medications are rapidly absorbed by diffusing into either plasma or the lymphatic system. Although injection results in faster and more reliable absorption than the oral route, injections are stressful and threatening to children and are not preferred. Injections are used most often for one-time doses of antibiotics (e.g., ceftriaxone for the initial treatment of severe infection), immunizations, iron administration, purified protein derivative (PPD) and allergy skin testing. Injections are potentially more dangerous in infants than in older children because of the infant's decreased muscle mass and variable blood flow to muscles.

Appropriately preparing the child for injections can reduce emotional and anticipatory concerns. Depending on the child's developmental level, explain the reason for the injection, any sensations the child might experience, and the length of time they are anticipated to last. Tell the child that the injection is not a punishment but is needed to make the child better or keep the child healthy. Practice counting, singing, deep breathing, or other distraction techniques with the child in advance.

Offer parents the option to leave if they feel unable to cope with the procedure; inform them when the procedure is completed. Most parents prefer to remain. Some are willing to help reassure the child or hold the child during the procedure.

To reduce the risk of injury, it is sometimes necessary to restrain the child before administering an injected medication. Restraint can be accomplished by swaddling the child or obtaining the assistance of another health care professional. Toddlers and older children often respond better to injections if parents can hold and comfort them during the procedure (Fig. 38-4). The parent, however, must feel confident in the ability to keep the child still enough to prevent injury.

Children perceive injections to be very painful. Even with the best preparation, it is hard for a child to understand that the pain of an injection lasts only seconds. Ice applied to the anticipated injection site for several minutes before the injection can numb the pain sensation, but it can also reduce blood flow to the area, interfering with absorption. Topical anesthetic agents, such as eutectic mixture of local anesthetics (EMLA) cream, also have been shown to be effective in reducing injection pain (see Chapter 39, p. 1003).

Children can be taught to deal with the pain of an injection using guided imagery, distraction, or other methods, such as taking a deep breath and blowing out the pain or turning the "pain switch" off (Kachoyeanos & Friedhoff, 1993).

Careful documentation of the injection is also important. Documentation includes recording the amount of medication injected and the site used. If the child will receive several injections, it is important to rotate sites to prevent tissue irritation and possible muscle atrophy and wasting. Federal vaccine regulations now require nurses to record the vaccine manu-

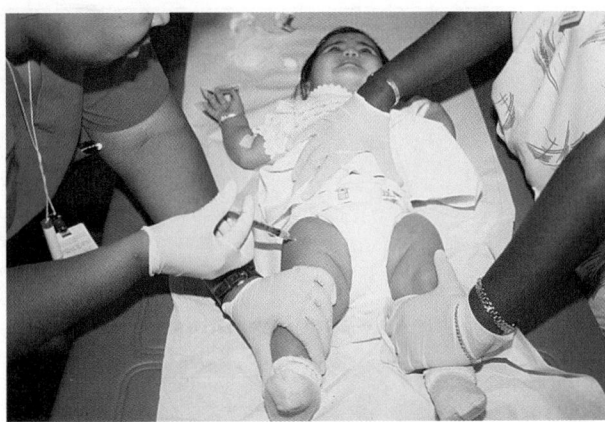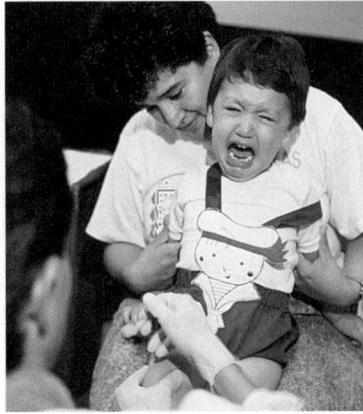

Figure 38-4 Two methods of restraint for intramuscular (IM) injection at the vastus lateralis site. (*Left,* Courtesy Parkland Health and Hospital System Community Oriented Primary Care Clinic, Dallas, TX. *Right,* Courtesy Cook Children's Medical Center, Fort Worth, TX.)

facturer and lot number for each immunization given, as well as any prior vaccine reaction the child might have incurred.

Preparing and Administering Intramuscular Injections

When filling a syringe for an injection, it is important to remember that most syringes and needle hubs contain approximately 0.2 ml of dead space. Therefore, to keep the dose accurate, do not flush the needle and hub after injection. On the rare occasion that a Z-track method is used (a method in which a small air bubble locks in the medication), the dead space in the hub of the needle must be taken into account so as not to overdose.

Select the site before the child is given an injection; the site should be soft, well vascularized, and healthy. It is important to avoid puncturing blood vessels, nerves, or bones and also to avoid injecting medications intended for IM administration into subcutaneous tissue. Inadvertent injection into any of these areas can result in accidental IV injection, pain, tissue sloughing, or nerve damage. The preferred IM injection sites in children are shown in Table 38-1.

TABLE **38-1** Preferred Intramuscular Injection Sites in Children

Site	Key Points	Site	Key Points
Vastus lateralis	Located on the anterior lateral thigh. Well developed at birth. Good choice for all age-groups but usually used in children younger than 3 yr. Able to tolerate larger volumes and not located near vital structures, such as nerves and blood vessels. To locate the appropriate site, divide the leg into thirds; give the injection into the middle outer third.	Dorsogluteal	Located by drawing a diagonal line between the posterior superior iliac spine and the greater trochanter of the femur. The dorsogluteal muscle is found above and lateral to this line. It develops with walking, so it should not be used until the child has been walking for at least 1 year. The child should be asked to "toe in" to avoid tensing the muscle. Can hold 1 to 2.5 ml but has the slowest and poorest absorption of all sites.
	Vastus lateralis		Dorsogluteal

Continued

TABLE 38-1 Preferred Intramuscular Injection Sites in Children—cont'd

Site	Key Points	Site	Key Points
Ventrogluteal	Located by placing the heel of the hand on the greater trochanter with fingers pointed toward the child's head. Place the index finger over the anterior superior iliac spine and the middle finger along the iliac crest posteriorly as far as possible to form a V. The injection is given in the center of the V. Site is safe for intramuscular (IM) injection in children older than 18 mo because it is free of major blood vessels and nerves. Can generally hold larger volumes (up to 2.5 ml in adolescents). Care should be taken to avoid bone and joint.	Deltoid	Use the part of the muscle located about two fingerwidths below the acromion process. This site is not used for injection in young children because the small muscle mass cannot hold large volumes of medication or medications that must be injected deep into muscle mass. This is the least painful site for injecting smaller volumes.

Ventrogluteal

Deltoid

Select an appropriate needle size (21 to 25 gauge) and length (¹/₂ to 1¹/₂ inches) for the injection. Use the smallest size and length that will *safely and comfortably* administer the medication. For example, a viscous medication is less painful when injected through a larger-gauge needle. Also, consider the amount of body fat, the distance to the muscle, the size of the muscle, the volume of medication, and the properties of the medication.

Safe volumes for IM injection range from 0.5 ml to 2.5 ml, depending on the age and size of the child. Wipe the injection site with a skin cleanser, and allow to dry. Insert the needle at a 90-degree angle with a quick darting motion. Pull back gently on the plunger to aspirate for blood. If blood is noted, withdraw the needle to avoid giving the medication IV. Change the needle and the site. If no blood is noted, give the injection slowly. Unless contraindicated, massage the injection site afterward.

Administering Subcutaneous Injections

A subcutaneous injection is given into the tissue that lies just below the skin. This type of administration is used for medications that provide a sustained effect (e.g., heparin, insulin). A subcutaneous injection should be given only into healthy tissue. If circulation is impaired (e.g., because of

---

! CRITICAL TO REMEMBER

Guidelines for Maximum Safe Volumes for Intramuscular Injections

Age	Deltoid	Ventrogluteal	Dorsogluteal	Vastus lateralis
Premature	—	—	—	0.5 ml
Neonate	—	—	—	0.5 ml
Infant	—	—	—	1 ml
Young child (3-6 yr)	—	1.5 ml	1 ml	1.5 ml
Older child (6-14 yr)	0.5 ml	1.5-2 ml	1.5-2 ml	1.5 ml
Adolescent (15 yr to adult)	1 ml	2-2.5 ml	2-2.5 ml	1.5-2 ml

CRITICAL THINKING EXERCISE 38-3

You need to immunize an infant with hepatitis vaccine. The infant's dose is 2.5 mcg. The type of vaccine you have on hand delivers 5 mcg/ml. How many milliliters will you give the infant?

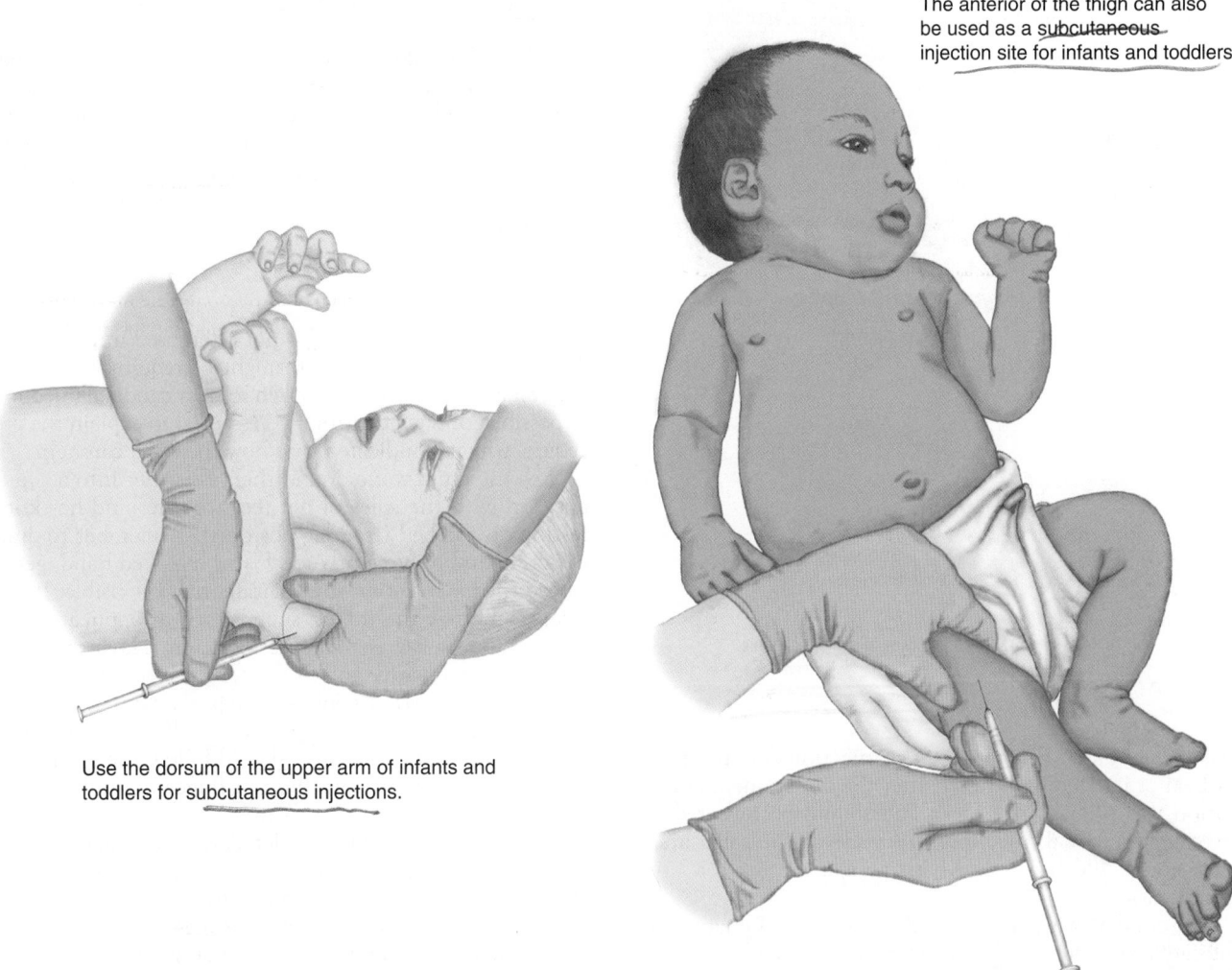

The anterior of the thigh can also be used as a subcutaneous injection site for infants and toddlers.

Use the dorsum of the upper arm of infants and toddlers for subcutaneous injections.

Figure 38-5 Two of the preferred subcutaneous injection sites in children. The fat pads above the iliac crests and hips may also be used.

edema, decreased temperature, shock), a subcutaneous injection should not be used because absorption will be altered.

Preferred subcutaneous injection sites are the fat pads located above the iliac crests, hips, lateral upper arms, and anterior thighs (Fig. 38-5). Children requiring frequent subcutaneous injections (e.g., children with type I diabetes mellitus) also use the abdomen, avoiding the 2-inch radius around the navel (Caffrey, 2003). Rotate sites to avoid the development of abscesses and to facilitate drug absorption. Record the site of the subcutaneous injection to avoid using the same site and causing tissue irritation.

Subcutaneous injections are usually given with a small (25- to 27-gauge), short (no more than 1/2- to 5/8-inch) needle to ensure that the medication is not inadvertently given IM. Insulin syringes come with even shorter, thinner needles (28 to 30 gauge; 5/16 inch). Volumes for subcutaneous injections are small, usually averaging 0.5 ml. Because the needle is so small and narrow, changing to a new needle after withdrawing medication through the stopper of a vial makes the injection more comfortable for the child.

Clean the site with alcohol, and allow it to dry. Pinch the tissue to raise the fatty tissue from the muscle. The angle of needle insertion is usually 45 degrees, although some practitioners insert the 1/2-inch or 5/16-inch needle at a 90-degree angle. Unless the child has little subcutaneous tissue, the short needle does not reach the muscle, even if it is inserted at a straight angle. Massage the insertion site after administration unless massage is contraindicated for the injected medication, such as heparin.

If subcutaneous injections are to be ongoing (e.g., insulin administration), pay special attention to client education. Older children and adolescents can usually learn to perform this procedure without difficulty.

Intradermal Injections

Intradermal injections enter just below the outer layer of skin, the epidermis, and usually on the inner aspect of the forearm or on the upper back. They are most often used for testing (e.g., allergy, PPD). The needle is small (25 to 27 gauge) and short (1/2 to 5/8 inch). The volume is also small (usually 0.1 ml). After cleaning the site with alcohol and allowing it to dry, turn the bevel of the needle up and insert gently at a 15-degree angle. The needle will barely penetrate the skin. Inject the medication to form a wheal (similar in appearance

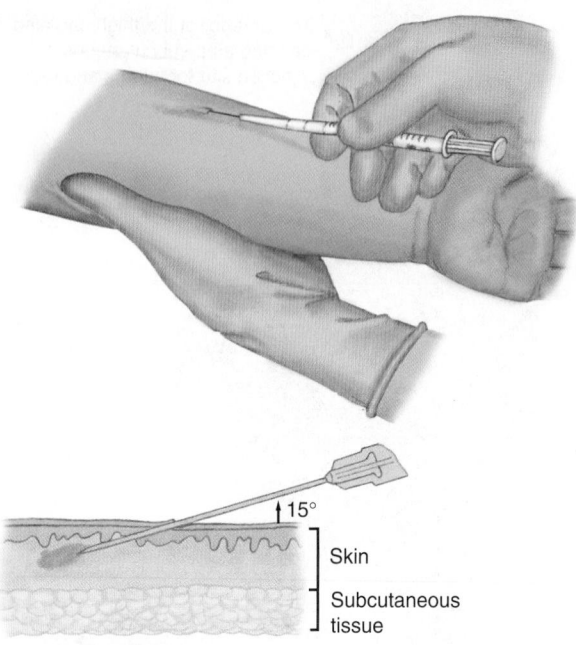

Figure 38-6 Intradermal injection site and technique.

to an insect bite) (Fig. 38-6). If the injection does not form a wheal or if bleeding is noted after the injection, administration was probably too deep and should be repeated. If several intradermal injections are made in the same area, each site should be marked with permanent ink for later identification.

The child who is to receive multiple injections might benefit significantly from carefully supervised needle play. In needle play, the child uses a syringe and needle to give shots to a doll. The nurse uses this play to prepare the child for injections and to help the child gain a sense of mastery over the experience of receiving an injection. The nurse offers a brief explanation of what will occur and why the child must receive an injection. Through therapeutic play, the child's anxiety is decreased.

Rectal Administration

The rectal route of administration is unreliable and is not used as often as other routes. It is most often reserved for times when a child cannot tolerate the oral route (e.g., because of nausea and vomiting). It has many possible complications, including the Valsalva response, rectal perforation, and other damage to the rectum or anus.

This route should not be used if the rectum is full of stool. Rectal administration is stressful for children because they fear intrusive procedures. Carefully prepare the child, and give an explanation about the procedure. Tell the child the reason the medication is being given in this form and what the child can do to help. The child is also told whether the suppository must be retained or expelled.

Position the child on the left side with the right leg flexed, and expose the rectal area sufficiently for visibility. Adequate draping is essential for preschool and older children. Often the child needs help to relax. Distraction and deep-breathing exercises can help the child relax the external sphincter. Lu-

bricate the suppository well with a water-soluble lubricant before inserting.

Advise the child to take a deep breath or bear down if possible to relax the sphincter further. Then gently insert past the internal sphincter. The child's rectal vault is not as long as an adult's, and the distance required to place medication is approximately 1 to 2 cm ($^1/_2$ to 1 inch). After insertion, hold the child's buttocks together until the urge to expel the suppository has passed.

Vaginal Administration

Although the vaginal route is not often used in infant, toddler, or preschool-age girls, it might be required for school-age or adolescent girls, most often to treat candidal infections or possibly for birth control. It is essential to explain the procedure, why it is indicated, and how the child can help.

Ask the child to void, and then assist her into a supine position with the soles of her feet together and her knees resting on the bed (frog-leg position). Remember to drape the child and provide privacy. Using a gloved hand, gently spread the labia so that the vaginal orifice is visible. If necessary, lubricate the tablet, suppository, or applicator with warm water or a water-soluble lubricant. Have the client take a deep breath, and then gently insert the vaginal tablet, suppository, or applicator approximately 9 to 10 cm ($3^1/_2$ to 4 inches) along the posterior wall of the vagina. To reduce discomfort, the nurse should follow the natural angle of the vagina by pointing the finger or applicator toward the sacrum.

After the procedure is completed, the child might need to remain in a supine position for a time. Older school-age children and adolescents can be taught to instill their own vaginal medications. It is important that these girls receive good education and give a return demonstration of the procedure, especially if the instillations are contraceptives.

Ophthalmic Administration

Instillation of ophthalmic preparations is a clean rather than sterile procedure (Procedure 38-1). Most pediatric ophthalmic solutions are available as either drops or ophthalmic ointment. If these preparations are refrigerated, allow them to warm to room temperature before instillation.

Before administering, note the expiration date and inspect the drops for color changes or cloudiness. Shake all suspensions well before instillation. Gently remove any exudate by wiping the child's eye with a sterile gauze pad from the inner to outer canthus. If exudates are dry or crusted, wipe with a warm, wet compress. Use a different pad for each eye.

Otic Administration

Otic procedures are clean rather than sterile procedures except in the case of a ruptured tympanic membrane (Procedure 38-2). Because cold ear drops can cause pain when they come in contact with the tympanic membrane, otic solutions should be allowed to warm to room temperature before administration.

Before administering ear drops, gently clean any exudate from the outer ear with sterile gauze. Because the risk of rupturing the tympanic membrane is high, never attempt to place anything inside the ear to clean the canal.

Procedure 38-1

Administering Ophthalmic Preparations

PURPOSE: To treat an eye infection, dilate pupils for diagnostic testing, or keep eyes moist.

1. Explain the purpose for the medication or lubricating drops. Tell the child how to help with the procedure. Explain that the child might experience blurred vision for a short time afterward.
2. Gather needed equipment: eye drops or ointment, gauze pads, and tissues. Wash your hands before proceeding. Wear gloves if contact with exudates is expected.
3. Assist the child into a supine position with the neck slightly hyperextended (e.g., by placing a rolled towel or small blanket under the shoulder blades).
4. If the drops are to be instilled into an infant's eyes, obtain assistance in restraining the child's arms and head or use a mummy wrap as necessary.
5. Instruct an older child to look upward, and gently pull the lower lid down and away from the eye.
6. Place the drops or a ribbon of ointment into the space between the eye and lower lid, taking care not to contaminate the end of the dropper or tube.
7. If both drops and ointment are ordered, the drops should be administered first. If they are placed after the ointment, they will not be absorbed.
8. Have the child look down as the lower lid is released. Encourage the child to close both eyes and keep them closed

for several seconds. Hand the child a tissue to gently blot any excess medication.

9. As with any procedure, praise the child for cooperation and assistance. Document the medication in the appropriate location.

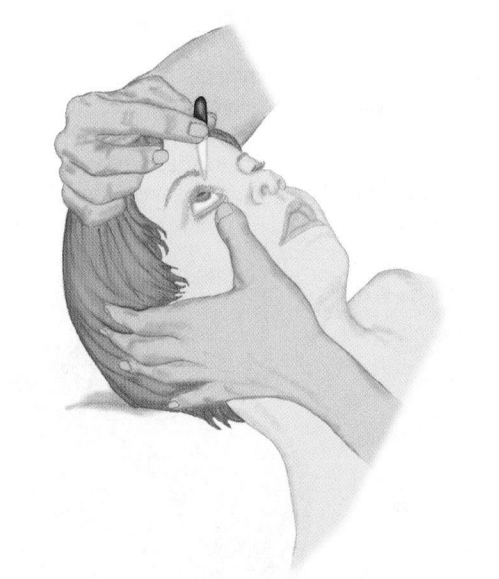

Nasal Administration

Although the mucous membrane route is generally used only for localized treatment, it has fairly rapid systemic absorption and may be used for the administration of certain systemic medications (e.g., antidiuretic hormone).

When administering nose drops to an infant, the nurse or parent removes any excess mucus by gently suctioning with a bulb syringe before administration. To make eating more comfortable, saline nose drops followed by gentle suction should be given 20 to 30 minutes before feedings.

Receiving nose drops is stressful for young children, who might feel that they are drowning during the instillation. A thorough explanation of what the child will feel, why the medication has been ordered ("to help unstop your nose"), and what the child needs to do to help is necessary. Assistance with restraint may be necessary with the young child, or mummy restraint or swaddling may be used.

Assist the child into a supine position, and hyperextend the neck slightly by placing a rolled towel or small blanket under the shoulder blades. Keeping the head in a midline position, instill the number of drops ordered into each naris. The head is kept in the same position to allow the drops to reach the ethmoid and sphenoid sinuses. Then briefly have the child turn the head slightly in each direction and back to midline to disburse the medication to the maxillary and frontal sinuses.

After the drops have been instilled, the child remains in a supine position for several minutes to allow the medication to be distributed to the sinuses. Instruct the child not to blow the medication out of the nose. Praise all efforts at cooperation.

Topical Administration

Because skin is relatively impermeable when intact and has a large surface area, topical administration of drugs is generally limited to localized treatment. If the medication is applied to abraded skin, over a large area, or over a long period, however, systemic effects can result. Solvents added to the medication to break down skin oils and occlusive dressings also increase absorption. Monitor the child carefully for systemic absorption effects.

As with all other procedures, explain what will be done, why it will be done, and what sensations the child will experience. Clean the skin gently to remove any exudate, scales, or other residue, and allow it to dry. To avoid contaminating the container, place the estimated amount of medication on a sterile pad. Wear gloves, and apply the ointment or cream as ordered or as recommended by the manufacturer. Cover the site afterward with a sterile pad if ordered. Encourage the child to avoid touching or scratching the area, and praise the child for cooperation.

Inhalation Therapy

Respiratory medications, used frequently in children, are delivered either by nebulizer or a metered-dose inhaler—a handheld device that delivers "puffs" of medication for inhalation. Although many inhaled medications have an unpleasant taste or smell, this route is a relatively nonthreatening form of medication delivery. Monitoring for desired therapeutic effects and systemic effects is essential because most medications used for inhalation have systemic side effects.

Procedure 38-2

Administering Otic Drops

PURPOSE: To treat inflammation or infection of the ear canal, relieve pain, or prevent otitis externa.

1. Explain any expected sensations to the child in developmentally appropriate terms (e.g., "It may sound like there is a butterfly flying inside your ear."), and describe how the child can help. Assistance in restraining a young child might be necessary.
2. Gather the following equipment: otic drops and cotton pieces. Wash your hands before the procedure.
3. Position the child lying down with the affected ear up or sitting with the head turned so the affected ear is up.
4. Brace the administering hand against the child's head above the ear.

5. If the child is 3 years or younger, pull the pinna of the ear back and down, holding near the lobe. If the child is older than 3 years, pull the pinna back and up.
6. Insert the required number of drops. Then gently massage the tragus (anterior portion) to ensure that the drops reach the tympanic membrane.
7. Pack cotton loosely into the canal, if ordered. Instruct the child not to remove the cotton or place anything inside the ear.
8. Keep the child on the unaffected side for several minutes after the administration. If medication is to be administered in both ears, the procedure should be repeated in the other ear after a wait of at least 1 minute.
9. Document the medication in the appropriate place.

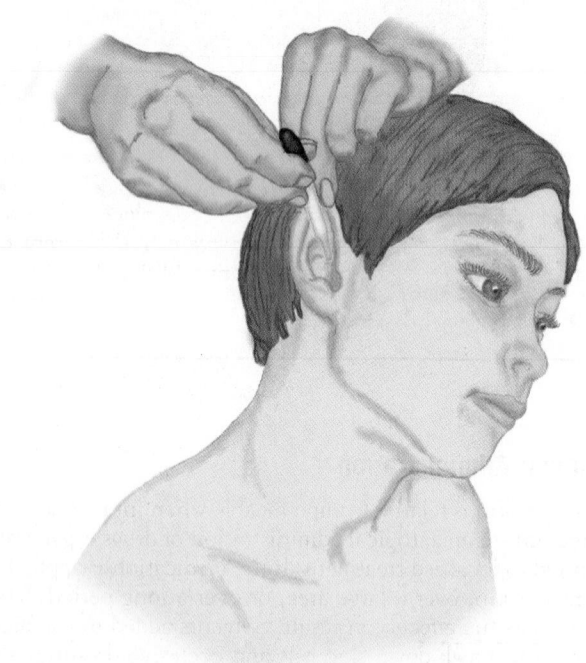

For a child older than 3 years, pull pinna up and back.

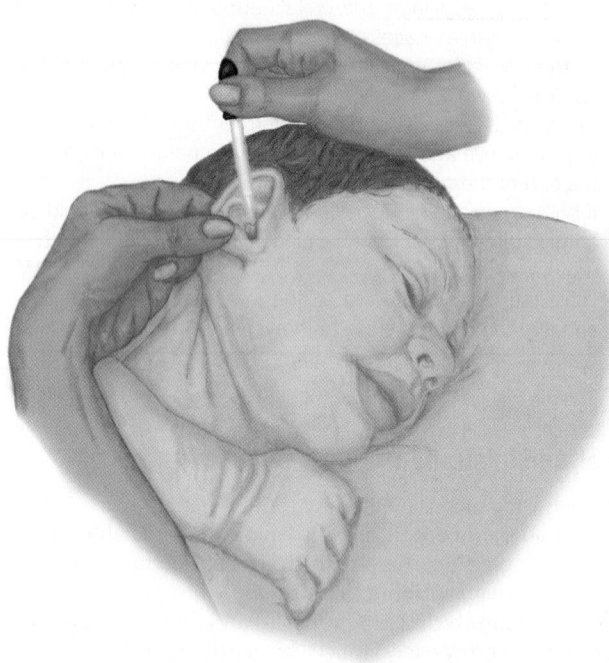

For an infant or a child younger than 3 years, grasp the pinna at the lobe and pull down and back.

Nebulized medications are diluted in normal saline and administered with a hand-held small-volume nebulizer (SVN or HHN). The SVN device aerosolizes the medication for the child to inhale. Medication can be delivered through a mask or through a plastic mouthpiece held between the lips or close to the face (Fig. 38-7). A mask is preferred for young children because they are seldom able to successfully hold a mouthpiece in place for the required length of time. Encourage the child to breathe deeply and slowly during the treatment.

Metered-dose inhalers offer an inexpensive, portable means of delivering inhaled medications. Many people, particularly children, have difficulty using a metered-dose inhaler correctly. The effectiveness of these medications is increased with the use of an inhalation aid, such as a spacer device. A spacer is a cylindric piece of hard or expandable plastic that attaches to the mouthpiece of the inhaler and is attached to a mouthpiece or mask. The child depresses the inhaler, and the medication enters the spacer, allowing the child time to deeply inhale the

medication. For people who cannot afford a commercial spacer, a small plastic commercial water bottle can be used; an opening large enough for the inhaler mouthpiece can be cut into the large end, and the bottle opening at the other end is small enough to fit into the child's mouth. (See Procedure 38-3 for directions to use a metered-dose inhaler.)

Although both forms of delivering inhaled medications are effective, the nebulized medication offers the advantage of delivery with supplemental oxygen to children in an acute episode of respiratory distress. Nebulized medications can also be delivered to an unconscious or intubated child by inserting the aerosol administration device in-line between the child and a bag-valve-mask.

Educating the parent and child is important to ensure the effectiveness of this form of medication delivery. The technique must be demonstrated and a return demonstration given. Use of the metered-dose inhaler should be reviewed at each return visit.

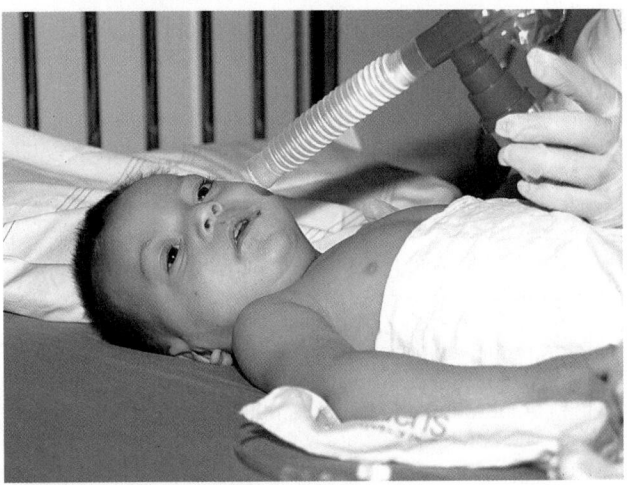

Figure 38-7 Administration of nebulized medication to an infant. (Courtesy Children's Medical Center, Dallas, TX.)

INTRAVENOUS THERAPY

IV therapy is widely used for children. Fluids and electrolytes, nutrition, blood products, and medications can be delivered by the IV route. When used to administer medications, IV therapy produces a steadier and more therapeutic blood level and is the only acceptable route of administration for some medications that might be irritating. The risks of IV therapy include possible fluid overload and possible complications with administration errors.

Intravenous Catheter Insertion

Typically, children's IV lines are infused through an over-the-needle catheter or a butterfly catheter. The type of catheter chosen often depends on hospital policy. Over-the-needle catheters are generally preferred because they are more flexible and stable, thus decreasing the risk of infiltration. Over-the-needle catheters come in even sizes (e.g., 22 and 24 gauge), and butterfly catheters are available in odd sizes (e.g., 23 and 25 gauge).

Venous access sites in children are shown in Figure 38-8. The rate and type of fluid to be infused, the projected length of time the IV line will be needed, and the availability of veins often determine site selection in children. The nurse also considers the child's developmental level. For example, placement of an IV line into a toddler's foot is often a poor choice because it inhibits walking, a newly learned skill. Avoid inserting an IV line into a dominant hand, if possible, because the site will interfere with activities of daily living. The hand, wrist, and antecubital sites are most frequently used in infants and children. Scalp veins are sometimes used in infants. Scalp veins have no valves and can be infused in either direction. IV catheters placed in this area can be adequately secured to allow the infant to move without dislodging the IV line.

Vein size and the kind of fluid to be infused also guide the choice of catheter. Generally, the smallest catheter through which fluids and medications can be safely infused should be used (often a 22- or 24-gauge catheter). For most children, a 20- to 24-gauge catheter provides adequate access.

Before an IV needle is inserted, explain the procedure to the child and parent. Include information about what will happen (what the child will see and feel) during each step of the procedure, why the catheter will be placed, where it will be placed (if possible), how long it will be in place (if known), and what function it will perform. Explain to the parent the purpose of both the IV therapy and any additional equipment (e.g., an infusion pump). Reassure the parent that once the IV catheter is in and stabilized, the child can be held as usual. Bring the child to the treatment room for the procedure.

Assess the child's ability to hold the affected extremity still during the procedure. Give children suggestions for coping with the discomfort and have them practice coping techniques in advance if possible. Nonpharmacologic interventions include guided imagery (e.g., putting on an imaginary magic glove that keeps the hand from hurting) and distraction (e.g., music, novelty toys, seek-and-find books). Pharmacologic interventions include ice and topical numbing gels or pastes, such as EMLA cream or ELA-Max. Buffered lidocaine injections, although used in some instances, can be threatening to children because they re-

---

Procedure 38-3

Using a Metered-Dose Inhaler

PURPOSE: To deliver medication directly to the respiratory system.

1. Verify the physician's order for medication or medications to be administered and number of puffs.
2. If one of the medications is an inhaled steroid, administer it last.
3. Explain the procedure to the child and parent or caregiver. It is often helpful to demonstrate the use of the inhaler and to explain specifically what the child is expected to do.
4. Place the inhaler in the spacer. Tell the child not to inhale too quickly or the spacer will whistle.
5. Tell the child to exhale ("big breath out") and place the spacer mouthpiece in the mouth or the spacer mask over the face. The child might be more comfortable holding the spacer and helping you.
6. Tell the child that you will squeeze the inhaler and release the medication into the spacer. Then direct the child to inhale ("big breath in") slowly. You may need to talk the child through this process.
7. Encourage the child to hold the breath for about 10 seconds or until you count slowly to 5.
8. Ask the child to exhale and then take another breath from the spacer and hold it for 10 seconds.
9. Repeat with another puff, if ordered. Praise the child for cooperation.
10. Rinse the inhaler adapter and spacer with cool water. Return the equipment to the medication room or designated area. Document.

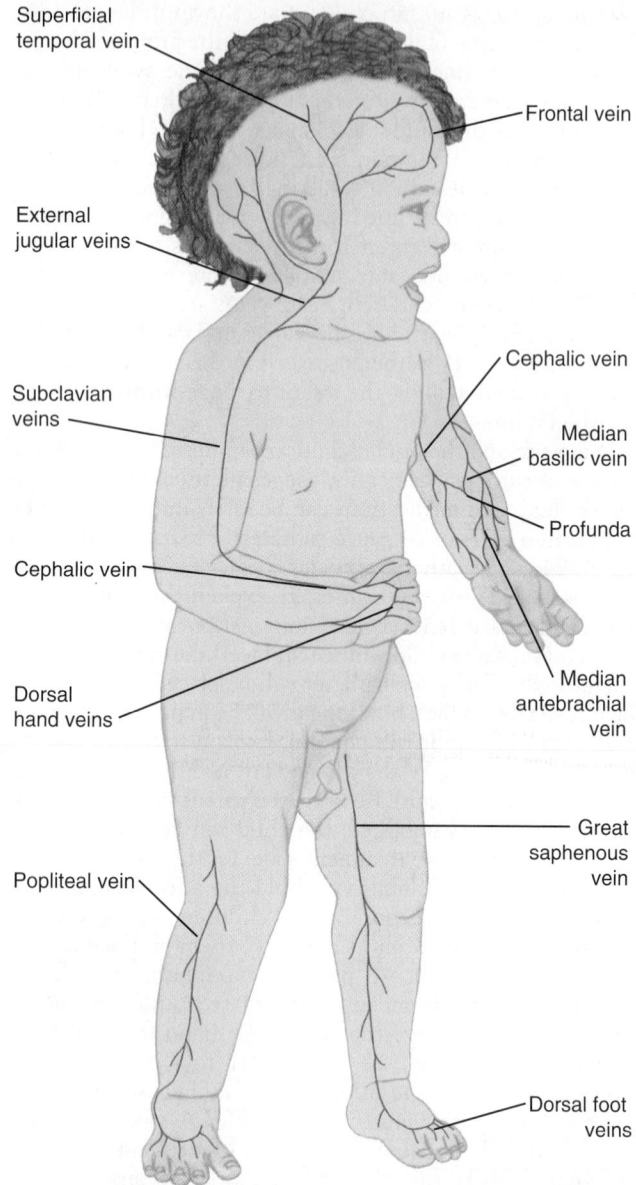

Figure 38-8 Venous access sites in children.

Labels on figure:
- Superficial temporal vein
- Frontal vein
- External jugular veins
- Subclavian veins
- Cephalic vein
- Median basilic vein
- Profunda
- Cephalic vein
- Median antebrachial vein
- Dorsal hand veins
- Great saphenous vein
- Popliteal vein
- Dorsal foot veins

the child during the procedure. Explain the procedure at each step. The nurse usually selects the IV site, beginning with the veins of the nondominant hand or forearm and moving proximally. As the catheter is inserted and the child experiences a "big sting" or "pinch," it might be helpful to advise the child to take a deep breath and blow out the pain.

Catheter placement is confirmed by a blood return, but a normal saline flush is needed to verify that there is no infiltration. After the catheter is placed, secure it in place with tape and a sterile, clear, occlusive dressing or tape and a small sterile dressing. The clear dressing allows for adequate visibility of the insertion site. In addition, secure the catheter extension tubing to the extremity with tape. Be sure to leave the plastic clamp accessible.

After fully stabilizing the IV catheter and tubing, you might need to prevent injury by securing the extremity to a well-padded arm board. This is particularly important for active children. Secure the extremity in an anatomic position to prevent nerve damage. You can further protect the catheter by using a plastic shield. This can be a medicine cup that is cut in half and taped on the edges or a commercially available device (Fig. 38-9). Document in the child's record the location of the IV line, the location and condition of the site, the type of access device used (length and gauge of catheter or butterfly), and the date and time inserted.

Intravenous Monitoring and Maintenance

To prevent fluid overload in children receiving IV therapy, IV fluids or medications are administered through an infusion pump that delivers a preset volume at an hourly rate (Fig. 38-10). Most infusion pumps are easily programmable with dose limits to prevent accidental fluid overload. If available, a pump with a tamper-proof design should be used.

quire a needle puncture of the skin. If the child is not able to hold still, obtain assistance before attempting to start the IV line. (See Chapter 39 for further discussion of pain management techniques.)

Have all the needed equipment ready in advance. Equipment includes an IV catheter of appropriate size, ordered IV solution, primed infusion set (most facilities now use needleless sets), extension tubing with a T-connector, tape, transparent occlusive dressing or other sterile dressing, a padded arm board, a tourniquet, alcohol pads, gloves, and blood-sampling tubes (if required). Povidone-iodine preparations might be necessary for immunosuppressed children. Bacteriostatic normal saline, 3 ml, is used to flush the catheter after any required blood samples have been obtained.

Encourage parents to remain with the child if they desire. Parents should not, however, be expected to restrain

This boy's IV line is secured well enough so he can pretend that ▶
he is a famous basketball star as he shoots baskets in the
playroom.

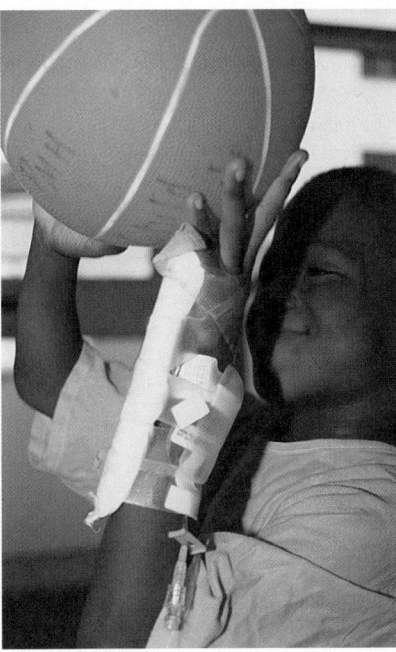

The foot is a useful site for the infant who is not walking or crawling.

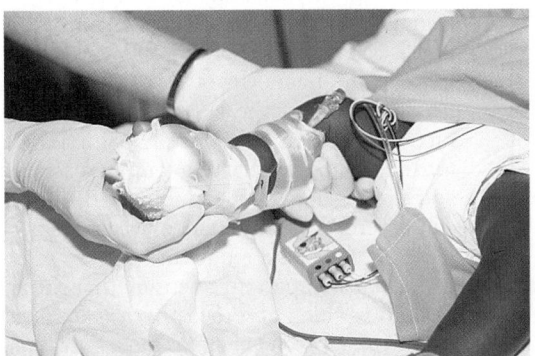

Figure 38-9 Because children's veins are fragile and intravenous (IV) lines can be difficult to place, the site must be well protected to prevent the child from removing the catheter and to tolerate the child's activity. Hand veins may be good for preschoolers and older children because IV lines placed here do not limit walking. A padded arm board gently limits movement of the foot or hand, reducing the risk of infiltration of the IV fluid. A plastic shield allows visibility of the site while protecting it. (Courtesy Parkland Health and Hospital System, Dallas, TX.)

In-line volume-control set. ▶

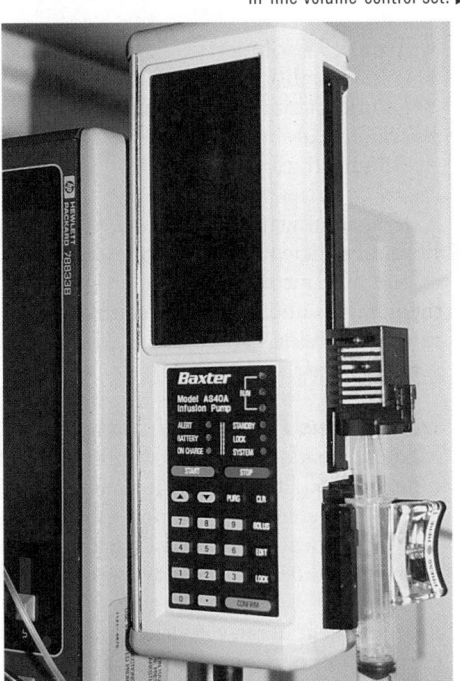

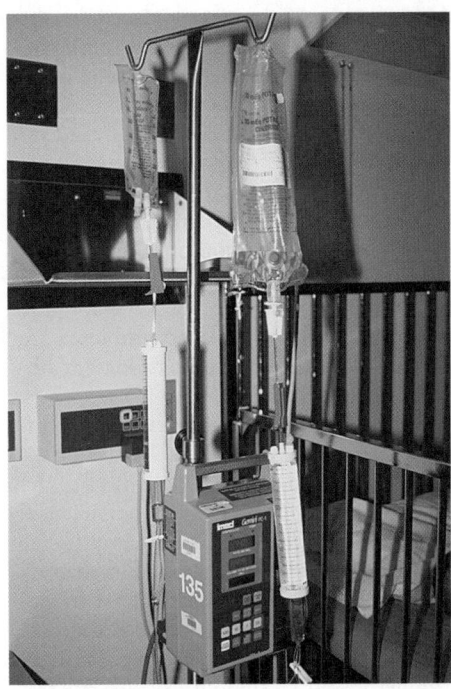

◀ Volumetric infusion pump.

Figure 38-10 Two types of infusion pumps. (Courtesy Parkland Health and Hospital System, Dallas, TX.)

BOX 38-1
Calculating Daily Maintenance Fluid Rates

[handwritten: If no loss of fluid going on such as trauma, etc. burn]

≤10 kg	100 ml/kg
10-20 kg	1000 ml + 50 ml/kg for each additional kg between 10 and 20 kg
20 kg	1500 ml + 20 ml/kg for each additional kg over 20 kg

The preceding formulas give the daily fluid requirements. To determine an hourly rate, take the total milliliters per day and divide by 24. For example:
1. A child weighing 15 kg should receive 1000 ml (1000 for the first 10 kg) + (50 × 5) (50 ml/kg for each 1 kg between 10 and 20) = 1250 ml/day.
2. The result is 1250 ml/24 hr = 52 ml/hr.

An additional safety feature, used in many institutions, is the in-line volume-control set and tubing (burette: Buretrol, Soluset, Metriset), which is used in place of regular IV tubing. A volume-control set usually has a 100- to 150-ml capacity (a 1- to 2-hour supply of fluid). The nurse programs the infusion pump to deliver only the amount in the volume-control set; the clamp between the burette and the IV container remains closed to prevent fluid from inadvertently dropping into the volume-control chamber. Medications can be mixed with an appropriate amount of fluid in the volume-control set by injecting the medication through the available port. The infusion pump is then set at a rate to infuse the amount in the burette over the correct time period.

To precisely administer very low volumes of fluid or medications, a volumetric infusion pump is used (Baxter, Bard). A syringe with the appropriate fluid volume or medication is attached to primed, low-volume tubing and placed in the pump. After connecting the tubing to the child, the nurse programs the pump to deliver the volume of fluid or medication in the syringe over a specified time period (see Fig. 38-10). Volumetric infusion pumps are used for both continuous and intermittent therapy and to deliver IV medications.

The nurse assesses and documents an IV site at least every hour (or according to institutional policy, if different) for signs and symptoms of infiltration or phlebitis. Using a transparent dressing over the IV site facilitates assessment. Feel the temperature of the site, observe for any redness or swelling, and assess for pain. If no problems are observed, chart that "no IV-related complications are observed" (Satarawala, 2000).

One way to assess for infiltration is by observing for symmetry in the size and shape of limbs or scalp. Gently touch the site to determine whether it is soft or taut or whether the scalp site is boggy. If signs of complications (e.g., edema, erythema, pain, blanching, coolness, streaking of the skin above the vein) are noted, discontinue the infusion immediately and notify the physician. Elevating the extremity can decrease edema. Dry heat can be applied if the infused solution or medication is neither a vesicant nor a sclerosing agent.

Unlike the situation with adults, children's IV sites are not changed every 72 hours because of the fragility of children's veins and the difficulty of finding a new site. Change IV fluid containers every 24 hours and tubing according to hospital policy. Many facilities require tubing to be changed every 48 to 72 hours. Many institutions, however, change total par-

enteral nutrition tubing every 24 hours in an attempt to decrease infection rates.

Infusion Rates and Methods

In most instances the physician orders an hourly IV fluid infusion rate. The nurse verifies the rate with the physician's order and documents on the child's flow sheet the type of solution, the location of the site, and the ordered rate. The rate is based on normal fluid maintenance requirements and additional fluids to replace deficits as needed. At some facilities, nurses can adjust the child's IV rate to infuse fluids in the required time frame. In other facilities, a physician's order is needed to adjust the IV infusion rate. Before adjusting the rate, the nurse must know the maintenance rates appropriate for the child's weight, to avoid increasing the rate too much and causing fluid overload. Box 38-1 illustrates how the nurse can determine maintenance fluid rates according to the formula for daily fluid requirements.

It is most important to ensure that the appropriate amount of fluid is being absorbed. *Even if the child is receiving fluids through an infusion pump, the nurse checks the fluid absorption at least hourly.* Pumps can malfunction, risking fluid overload if not meticulously checked.

Administering Intravenous Medications

IV medications can be administered as a continuous infusion (e.g., potassium chloride) or intermittently (e.g., antibiotics). Methods of administering IV medications include piggyback, push, and retrograde methods. It is imperative that the appropriate method is chosen to meet the needs of the child and fit any restrictions posed by the medication and fluid volume.

When administering IV solutions and medications to children, the nurse must consider the following:

- Type of IV solution
- Compatibility of the medication and IV solution
- Dilution volume of the medication
- Amount of flush needed
- Administration rate

The administration method, type of IV tubing used, and hospital policies and procedures determine some factors, such as the amount of flush needed. Information about specific medications and their reconstitution, compatible fluids, and rates of infusion can be obtained from pharmacists, drug inserts, or texts.

Intravenous Push Administration

Medications delivered by IV push are reconstituted, but not diluted in additional solution, and are pushed directly into the IV catheter using the port closest to the child. The volume of medication infused is small (usually <5 ml), and the effects (both desired and adverse) are immediate.

This method is used to give pain medications in the immediate postoperative period, administer sedatives, induce paralytic effects in ventilated patients, and administer other medications. To administer a medication by IV push, the nurse must first ensure that the medication can be administered safely in this way. Verify compatibility with the infusing solution (if there is a running IV line), and determine the administration rate (usually given in milligrams per minute). If hospital policy requires, check the medication with another nurse or physician before administering it. In explaining the procedure, reassure the child that the procedure is painless.

Before administering the medication, check the IV site for complications and the running IV line for patency. Clamp the IV tubing above the injection port closest to the child, and clean the port with alcohol. Use povidone-iodine (Betadine) if the line is a central access catheter or the child is immunosuppressed. If the medication is not compatible with the infusing IV fluid or if the medication is going into an intermittent infusion port, flush the tubing with approximately 2 to 3 ml of normal saline before and after administering the medication. Attach the medication syringe to the port, and administer the medication at the prescribed rate. Medications given by IV push are usually administered slowly and should not be administered faster than the rate the manufacturer or the formulary suggests. Remove the medication syringe, wipe the port with alcohol, and cover the port if the IV administration system requires a port cover.

Monitor the child carefully for the effects of the medication, including undesired side effects. Evaluate by monitoring the child's vital signs (including blood pressure) and reassessing frequently.

Intravenous Piggyback Administration

Medications given by piggybacking an IV line frequently are diluted in at least 20 ml of IV solution and administered over at least 15 minutes. These medications might be diluted by the pharmacy and sent to the nursing unit in a separate IV bag, or they can be prepared on the unit with a needleless mixing system, which allows the powdered medication to enter the diluent bag. The nurse can dilute reconstituted medications by injecting them directly into a volume-control set containing a predetermined amount of IV solution. Medications given by IV piggyback to children should be administered through an infusion pump to avoid infusing the medication either too rapidly or too slowly. If the medications are to be diluted in the volume-control set, the nurse notes the total amount of fluid (volume of medication plus volume in the burette) when setting the pump for the correct infusion rate.

When infusing medications by piggyback, the nurse must also flush the IV tubing with fluid to complete the delivery of the medication out of the IV tubing and into the child. The volume needed for the flush varies and must be added when accounting for the total volume infused. Generally, 16 to 20 ml is required to flush the IV tubing adequately, unless low volume tubing is used.

The total volume to be infused should be within safe limits for the child. For example:

- Vancomycin, 150 mg, is ordered for a 15-kg child. The child's maintenance hourly rate is 52 ml.
- The recommended concentration for administering vancomycin is 5 mg/ml. To achieve that concentration, 30 ml of fluid would be needed (150 divided by 5).
- Add a 20-ml flush, for a total volume of 50 ml to be administered over the course of 30 to 60 minutes.
- This amount is within the 52-ml hourly volume the child should be receiving.

Determine that the IV line is functioning and that the site is free of complications. Clean the injection port on the volume-

control set with alcohol, and add the medication to the required amount of diluent. Agitate the volume-control set gently to mix the medication and diluent. Set the pump to infuse the medication; the rate should be based on the volume actually in the volume-control set. It is important to set the pump to alarm when the volume is infused so that the nurse can return and add the volume needed to complete the flush. Label the volume-control set with the name of the medication added. Document what has infused. All flush and medication volumes must be added to recorded intake and calculated into the total volume limits to avoid fluid overload.

If the child does not have a running IV line but is receiving medication intermittently by piggyback, be sure to flush the IV catheter with saline before attaching the piggyback set. This procedure ensures patency of the line. In some instances, depending on hospital equipment, the medication and the regular IV infusion can be run concurrently, so long as the medication is compatible with the running IV fluid.

Intravenous Retrograde Administration

The IV retrograde method uses smaller volumes of both medication and flush and generally has a slightly shorter administration time than the piggyback method. The nurse clamps the IV tubing below the injection port nearest the child. After wiping the port with an appropriate cleansing solution, the nurse injects the medication into the port in a direction away from the child (retrograde), causing it to flow into the tubing above the injection port. The IV pump is then set to deliver the medication volume plus the amount of fluid needed to flush the IV tubing from the injection port to the child.

Some infusion pumps do not allow the pressure created by retrograde infusion. It is important for the nurse to be familiar with the type of infusion pump used and the facility's policy and procedure for retrograde administration.

Venous Access Devices

Intermittent Infusion Ports

Intermittent infusion ports (saline or heparin locks) allow drugs to be administered IV without the need for a running IV line. The intermittent infusion port is an IV catheter that is placed, flushed with normal saline or heparin to maintain patency, and then locked with a male adapter. The port is accessed when needed for fluid or medication infusion. Site observation and site care are the same as for any IV catheter.

The frequency of flushing is controversial and determined by hospital policy. Routine flushing with normal saline to maintain patency is performed every 6 to 12 hours. The device is flushed with saline before and after medication

---

CRITICAL THINKING EXERCISE 38-4

The doctor has ordered 1.4 g of intravenous (IV) ampicillin every 4 hours for your patient. You need to mix the ampicillin.
1. If you add 5 ml of normal saline to a 2-g vial of ampicillin, how many milliliters will you need to remove from the vial for the child?
2. You add the mixed ampicillin to 50 ml of the IV fluid to run in over the course of $\frac{1}{2}$ hour. How fast will you need to run the IV line to deliver the medication in the appropriate amount of time?

administration and with heparinized saline solution, if ordered, after blood is drawn or infused.

Central Venous Access Devices *Central venous access devices* are venous access devices in which the catheter is centrally placed directly into a major blood vessel. These devices are most often used to administer medications, blood products, IV fluids, and parenteral nutrition over the long term to chronically ill children. These devices can be tunneled or nontunneled central catheters and implanted infusion ports. *Percutaneously implanted central catheters (PICCs)* are also used for children who need IV access for a period longer than peripheral IV catheters can be adequately maintained. All central venous access devices need routine care (dressing changes, flushing) according to facility protocol. Because these devices enter the central venous system, all procedures are done using aseptic technique.

Tunneled central lines are surgically placed lines that are held in place by a Dacron cuff located in a subcutaneous tunnel. They are most commonly placed in an external jugular vein but may also be placed in the cephalic, axillary subclavian, femoral, saphenous, or internal jugular veins. The tip of the tunneled catheter is threaded until it rests at the junction of the superior vena cava and right atrium. Tunneled central lines are usually flushed with heparin at least every 24 hours and after blood is infused or drawn.

Short-term or nontunneled central catheters are most frequently placed in the subclavian or femoral veins. These lines involve the placement of a large-gauge catheter that is then sutured in place.

An *implanted venous access device* (IVAD, Infusaport) consists of a catheter that is connected to a port or reservoir. Like the tunneled catheter, the catheter tip rests at the junction of the superior vena cava and right atrium. The port is under the skin and is accessed with a noncoring needle placed through the skin into the port. The needle is then covered with a biooc-clusive dressing, and an extension set is attached to the end. When the port is no longer needed for infusions or obtaining blood specimens, it is flushed with heparin and the needle withdrawn. The child with an implanted port can participate in all typical childhood activities except those with a potential for high-impact contact with the chest (e.g., competitive football).

PICC lines are long catheters made of polyurethane or silicone and threaded through an introducer placed in the antecubital vein. They are usually placed by specially trained nurses and are frequently used for home antibiotic therapy. After the catheter is threaded so that the tip is located in the superior vena cava, the introducer is removed. The catheter is then covered with a biooclusive dressing, and placement is verified by x-ray. These catheters are usually left in place for several weeks to months. The major complications of this type of line are phlebitis, infection, and thrombosis (Klein, 2001).

ADMINISTRATION OF BLOOD OR BLOOD PRODUCTS

Education of the child and parent is essential whenever a transfusion is administered. Children and parents must receive all necessary information honestly, consistently, and at a developmentally appropriate level. Information includes why the transfusion is necessary, how long it will take, what the child will feel and hear, and the types of blood products to be used. Ask the parent or caregiver about the child's transfusion history and whether the child has ever experi-

enced a transfusion reaction. The nurse discusses the risks of receiving versus not receiving the blood product and explains each step as it is to be performed. It is important to use clear, concise, age-appropriate terminology.

Information about the types of blood products, the indications and procedures for their administration, and the identification and treatment of transfusion reactions is found in standard medical-surgical nursing texts. The key features of administration of blood products to children are:

- To prevent circulatory hypervolemia, packed red blood cells are usually administered to infants and children.
- Identify the child and verify blood (type, Rh factor, donor number, expiration date) with another nurse or physician.
- Take vital signs, including blood pressure, before administering blood. Then take vital signs every 15 minutes for the first 2 hours and every 30 minutes thereafter until the infusion is complete.
- Administer blood with normal saline (dextrose solutions cause hemolysis) on a piggyback setup, through an appropriate filter. If a central line is in place, other solutions can be administered concurrently through a different lumen (Fitzpatrick & Fitzpatrick, 1997).
- Use blood within 30 minutes of its arrival from the blood bank. Do not store blood in regular unit refrigeration. Return unused blood to the blood bank. Order only as much blood as can be used in 4 hours.
- The rate of infusion of packed red blood cells is approximately 2-3 ml/kg/hr over no more than 4 hours (Gunn & Nechyba, 2002). Run the infusion slowly for the first 15 minutes because many transfusion reactions are seen during this brief period. If the child has not displayed any signs of a reaction during this time, increase the rate to the ordered rate for the remainder of the dose.
- Cytomegalovirus-negative blood (blood that has tested negative for cytomegalovirus) is used for cytomegalovirus-negative, immunocompromised children; low-birth-weight neonates; bone marrow transplant recipients; and children younger than 2 years who are receiving chemotherapy.
- Blood that has been irradiated to prevent lymphocyte replication helps prevent graft-versus-host disease in immunocompromised children, such as bone marrow transplant recipients; it also is used in neonates.
- Although type and crossmatch should be less than 48 hours old, infants younger than 4 months rarely form red cell antibodies and therefore usually undergo a type and crossmatch only once. These results can be used until the infant reaches 4 months of age or is discharged from the hospital (Kevy & Gorlin, 1998).
- During the administration of blood or blood products, the child and parents should notify the nurse immediately if the child feels "bad" or has fever or chills, headache, nausea, pain at the needle site, or difficulty breathing. Children and parents often do not know how they are supposed to feel and will not notify the nurse of the signs and symptoms of a transfusion reaction. The child should not be left alone while receiving blood products.
- In neonates and small infants, auscultate the lungs before and frequently during a transfusion to detect signs of respiratory distress from fluid overload.
- If a reaction is suspected, stop the transfusion immediately and infuse normal saline through new tubing. Notify the physician. Continue to monitor vital signs. Monitor urine

output hourly, and send samples of the child's blood and urine to the laboratory.

- If the child's maintenance IV rate was decreased to avoid fluid overload, the blood sugar level must be monitored with reagent strips (Dextrostix) or another form of measurement because reducing the maintenance IV rate decreases the amount of IV glucose received by the child and may lead to hypoglycemia.
- After the transfusion, praise the child and family for their cooperation and help during the procedure.

CHILD AND FAMILY EDUCATION

Teaching children and their caregivers about medications is an essential part of therapy. Statistics about adherence suggest that approximately 50% of children taking medications for an acute condition complete their prescribed regimen. Adherence is higher in children taking medication for a chronic health problem (Matsui, 1997). In addition to factors such as forgetting to give a medication, refusal to take the medication because of unpleasant taste, and discontinuing a medication because symptoms have improved, lack of understanding about a medication and its effects is a major reason cited for nonadherence (Bartlett, Lukk, Butz, Lampros-Klein, & Rand, 2002; Blanchard et al., 1999; Staples & Bravender, 2002).

Teaching the family about medications begins with a thorough assessment that includes a list of all medications the child is currently taking, including over-the-counter medications. Any history of allergies to medications should be noted to prevent potential drug interactions.

Note as well any developmental needs or special learning needs, such as a hearing or speech disability, language barrier, or illiteracy. The nurse must make provisions to accommodate the child's special needs. For example, information should be presented in a variety of ways (e.g., spoken, written, illustrated). Written instructions should accompany any oral instruction.

Problem solve with the family before discharge from the hospital, clinic, or physician's office. This process includes devising acceptable schedules for medication administration, suggesting alternative methods of administering oral medications (e.g., crushing and mixing with food), and identifying foods that might be mixed with the medications.

Emphasize taking the medication as ordered. Particularly highlight finishing the full course of a prescribed antibiotic,

> ### PARENTS
> ## Want to Know
>
> ### Medication Administration at Home
>
> Address special medication problems before the child leaves the hospital or ambulatory care setting. Attention to this issue can help prevent medication errors or the child's and family's failure to follow the physician's order for home treatment. The parent and child (if old enough) will want to know:
> - Name of the medication (trade, generic)
> - Why it was prescribed
> - What it is supposed to do
> - How to take the medication (how much, how often, how long to take it, techniques for administering the medication)
> - Acceptable measuring device for home administration of medications (oral syringe, small medicine spoon, small medicine cup)
> - How to use calibrated droppers or syringes to measure and give the right amount of medication
> - Expected or potential side effects and what to do if they occur
> - When the nurse or physician should be notified of side effects
> - Any dietary restrictions
>
> If the child will need to take the medication during the school day, the health provider must give the parent a written order with the description of the medication, effects, side effects, and time of day the medication should be administered. This must be delivered to the school nurse, along with written permission from the parent for the medication to be administered and the medication in an original pharmacy container.

not changing dosages without consulting the physician, and returning for follow-up appointments.

Reinforce general safety information, such as keeping medications out of the reach of children and keeping all medications in their original containers. Evaluate your interventions by asking questions (scenarios work well), providing a demonstration, and asking for a return demonstration. Document all teaching and validation of understanding.

KEY CONCEPTS

- Standardized dosage ranges for many medications have not been established for children.
- Children's body proportions and composition differ from those of adults, and children's responses to medications differ accordingly.
- The nurse must incorporate principles of growth and development into medication administration.
- The margin of safety for medication administration is narrow for children.
- Oral medications should be administered using developmentally appropriate equipment.
- Injections are stressful to children and are not usually the first choice of administration route.

Take care to choose the appropriate site for the child's size and age, and use the shortest and smallest-gauge needle possible to ensure safe administration of the medication.
- The rate and type of fluid to be infused and the availability and accessibility of veins often determine the site selected for venipuncture.
- Children receiving IV infusions should receive their fluids through a pump that can be set to deliver a predetermined amount of fluid safely. A volume-control set can be used as well to decrease the chance of fluid overload.
- A baseline assessment must be performed before a blood product is administered to a

child. This assessment includes auscultating an infant's lungs so that signs of fluid overload during the transfusion are immediately recognized.
- As with any client, the infant or child receiving a transfusion needs to be carefully monitored throughout the procedure to assess effects and adverse reactions.
- Education of the child and parent is important to ensure that medications are administered to achieve therapeutic effects and avoid dangerous side effects.

ANSWERS to Critical Thinking Exercise 38-1

1. The nurse needs to emphasize the following to the father:
   a. Even though symptoms have disappeared, it is important for the child to take the entire amount of medication.
   b. The medication prescribed is the one best able to treat the child.
   c. Some children do react adversely to certain tastes, but there are methods of disguising the taste.
   d. Children of this age will react positively to expectations for compliance.

2. If, after a firm statement of expectation by the father for the child to take the medication, the child still refuses, suggest to the father that he try mixing the medication in a small (2-teaspoon) amount of a liquid (juice, soda) to disguise the taste. The nurse can also describe how to hold the child properly for administering an oral medication with control. If these methods do not work, the father should call back.

ANSWERS to Critical Thinking Exercise 38-2

1. 100 mg/5 ml = 150 mg/X ml;
   100 X = 750;
   X = 7.5 ml

2. 5 ml/1 tsp = 7.5 ml/X tsp;
   5 X = 7.5;
   X = 1½ tsp

ANSWER to Critical Thinking Exercise 38-3

5 μg/1 ml = 2.5 μg/X ml;
   5 X = 2.5;
   X = 0.5 ml

ANSWERS to Critical Thinking Exercise 38-4

1. 2 g/5 ml = 1.4 g/X ml;
   2 X = 7;
   X = 3.5 ml

2. 50 ml + 3.5 ml = 53.5 ml total fluid. Because you want to set the pump to deliver an hourly rate, you should do the following:

53.5 ml/30 min = X ml/60 min;
   30 X = 3210;
   X = 107 ml/hr

or

53.5 ml/.5 hr = X ml/1 hr;
   0.5 X = 53.5;
   X = 107 ml/hr

REFERENCES and READINGS

Bartlett, S., Lukk, P., Butz, A., Lampros-Klein, F., & Rand, C. (2002). Enhancing medication adherence among inner-city children with asthma: Results from pilot studies. *Journal of Asthma, 39*(1), 47-54.

Bell, E. (1999). Tastes of liquid medications: Pediatric implications. *Journal of Pediatric Pharmacy Practice, 4*(1), 43-50.

Blanchard, N., Primovic, J., & Leff, R. (1999). Compliance with pediatric medications. *Journal of Pediatric Pharmacy Practice, 4*(4), 181-185.

Britt, M., & Newman, M. (1999). Pediatric registered nurse usage and perception of EMLA. *Journal of the Society of Pediatric Nurses, 4*(3), 105-112.

Caffrey, R. (2003). Diabetes under control. Are all syringes created equal? *American Journal of Nursing, 103*(6), 46-49.

Camara, D. (2001). Minimizing risks associated with peripherally inserted central catheters in the NICU. *MCN: The American Journal of Maternal/Child Nursing, 26*(1), 17-22.

Ellenberger, A. (1999). Starting an I.V. line. *Nursing 1999, 29*(2), 56-59.

Fitzpatrick, L., & Fitzpatrick, T. (1997). Blood transfusion. *Nursing 1997, 27*(4), 34-42.

Fortescue, E.B., Kaushal, R., Landrigan, C.P., McKenna, K.J., Clapp, M.D., Federico, F., Goldmann, D.A., & Bates, D.W. (2003). Prioritizing strategies for preventing medication errors and adverse drug events in pediatric inpatients. *Pediatrics, 111*(4), 722-730.

Gunn, V., & Nechyba, C. (2002). *The Johns Hopkins Hospital Harriet Lane handbook*. St. Louis: Mosby.

Gura, K. (1999). Intravenous drug administration guidelines for pediatric patients. *Journal of Pediatric Pharmacy Practice, 4*(2), 80-100.

Heilskov, M.A., Johnson, K., & Miller, J. (1998). A randomized trial of heparin and saline for maintaining intravenous locks in neonates. *Journal of Society of Pediatric Nurses, 3*(3), 111-115.

Hodgson, B., & Kizior, R. (2004). *Saunders nursing drug handbook 2004*. Philadelphia: Saunders.

Kachoyeanos, M., & Friedhoff, M. (1993). Cognitive and behavioral strategies to reduce children's pain. *MCN: The American Journal of Maternal/Child Nursing, 18*(1), 14-19.

Kevy, S., & Gorlin, J. (1998). Red cell transfusion. In D.G. Nathan & S.H. Orkin (Eds.), *Hematology of infancy and childhood* (5th ed., pp. 1784-1801). Philadelphia: Saunders.

Klein, T. (2001). PICCs and midlines: Fine-tuning your care. *RN, 64*(8), 26-29.

Levine, S., Cohen, M., Blanchard, N., Frederico, F., Magelli, M., Lomax, C., et al. (2001). Guidelines for preventing medication errors in pediatrics. *Journal of Pediatric Pharmacology and Therapeutics, 6*, 426-442.

Matsui, D. (1997). Drug compliance in pediatrics. *Pediatric Clinics of North America, 44*(1), 1-14.

McCloskey, D. (2002). Catheter-related thrombosis in pediatrics. *Pediatric Nursing, 28*(2), 97-106.

Medical Economics Data Production Co. (1999). *Physicians' desk reference* (53rd ed.). Montvale, NJ: Author.

Millam, D., & Hadaway, L. (2000). On the road to successful I.V. starts. *Nursing 2000, 30*(4), 34-50.

Montgomery, L.A., Hanrahan, K., Kottman, K., Otto, A., Barrett, T., & Hermiston, B. (1999). Guideline for IV infiltrations in pediatric patients. *Pediatric Nursing, 25*(2), 167-179.

Mudge, B., Forcier, D., & Slattery, M.J. (1998). Patency of 24-gauge peripheral intermittent infusion devices: A comparison of heparin and saline flush solutions. *Pediatric Nursing, 24*(2), 142-145.

Mysak, T., & Carleton, B. (2000). Clinically significant pharmacokinetic differences between adult and pediatric patients: Review and case examples. *Journal of Pediatric Pharmacy Practice, 5*(6), 274-282.

Oakes, L., & Rosenthal-Dichter, C. (1998). Hematology and immunology. In M. Slota (Ed.), *Core curriculum for pediatric critical care nursing* (pp. 461-550). Philadelphia: Saunders.

Pena, B., & Krauss, B. (2000). Pediatric sedation: Seeing patients safely through. *Contemporary Pediatrics, 17*(8), 42-52.

Reed, M., & Gal, P. (2004). Principles of drug therapy. In R. Behrman, R. Kliegman, & H. Jenson. (Eds.), *Nelson textbook of pediatrics* (17th ed., pp. 2427-2432). Philadelphia: Saunders.

Satarawala, R. (2000). Confronting the legal perils of I.V. therapy. *Nursing 2000, 30*(8), 44-48.

Staples, B., & Bravender, T. (2002). Drug compliance in adolescents: Assessing and managing modifiable risk factors. *Pediatric Drugs, 4*(8), 503-513.

Vallino, L. (1998). I.V. HOUSE: Pediatric nurses contribute to refinement of IV protector. *Journal of Pediatric Nursing, 13*(3), 196-198.

Wong, D. (2003). Pain control. Topical local anesthetics. *American Journal of Nursing, 103*(6), 42-45.

39

Pain Management for Children

After studying this chapter, you should be able to:
◎ Define pain.
◎ Discuss the gate-control theory of pain.
◎ Discuss the myths and realities of pain.
◎ Discriminate between acute and chronic pain.
◎ Explain pain assessment in children according to developmental stages.

◎ Describe common pain assessment tools.
◎ Discuss non-pharmacologic and pharmacologic interventions that may be used for pain relief with children.
◎ Use the nursing process to describe nursing care of the child in pain.

◆ **DEFINITIONS**

AHRQ Agency for Healthcare Research and Quality, previously the *Agency for Health Care Policy and Research.* A federal agency established in 1989.

conscious sedation Medically controlled state of depressed consciousness that allows protective reflexes to be maintained, retains the child's ability to continuously maintain a patent airway independently, and permits appropriate response to physical stimulation or verbal command.

epidural Situated within the spinal canal, on or outside the dura mater; synonyms are *extradural* and *peridural.*

nociceptive Impulse giving rise to the sensation of pain.

pain An unpleasant sensory and emotional experience associated with actual or potential tissue damage or described in

terms of such damage (International Association for the Study of Pain, 1979).

pain threshold Level of intensity at which pain becomes appreciable or perceptible.

PCA Patient-controlled analgesia. Self-administration of an analgesic by a client instructed in how to do so; usually refers to self-dosing with an intravenous opioid.

TENS Transcutaneous electrical nerve stimulation. A method of producing electroanalgesia through electrodes applied to the skin.

Defining, identifying, and treating pain in children can be difficult. Infants and children are often unable or unwilling to communicate the presence, location, type, or intensity of pain. Parents may also be reluctant to acknowledge or help validate their child's pain, or they may be hesitant to allow suitable pain management secondary to fears related to the use of opioid and addiction. In addition, some physicians and nurses have inappropriate and outdated beliefs regarding pain and pain control in infants and children. Even with the comprehensive research and anecdotal experience over the past 10 to 15 years, the assessment and treatment of pain in children frequently remain inadequate (American Academy of Pediatrics [AAP], 2001).

Because of increased research on pain in children, the assessment of pediatric pain and the prescription and administration of analgesics have become more precise. The most

current resources and strategies for pain management, however, are not always implemented, emphasizing the continuing need for educating all health providers. Nurses, having frequent interaction with physicians and other health care workers, can make a significant difference in the pain management offered to infants and children. They can also play a vital role in providing education to other health care personnel as well as parents and children in regard to appropriate pain management.

Individual nurses vary in their ability to assess pain. Some of these differences have been linked to lack of education regarding pain, personal experiences with pain, personal assessment style, and practice setting (Franck, Greenberg, & Stevens, 2000). In addition, the behaviors of many health care professionals, including nurses, do not always correspond with the beliefs they report concerning pain assessment and management (Jacob & Puntillo, 1999).

DEFINITIONS AND THEORIES OF PAIN

There are many definitions of pain. In a commonly accepted definition, pain is whatever the experiencing person says it is, existing whenever the person says it does (McCaffery & Pasero, 1999). The International Association for the Study of Pain (1979, p. 249) defines pain as "an unpleasant sensory and emotional experience associated with actual or potential tissue damage, or described in terms of such damage." Both definitions underscore the fact that pain is subjective and personal.

Gate-Control Theory

Pain impulses travel between the initial site of injury and the brain, and certain mechanisms affect pain intensity. According to the gate-control theory, proposed by Melzack and Wall in 1965, a gating mechanism at the level of the dorsal horn in the spinal cord can facilitate or dampen the transmission of pain signals. Stimulation of the larger afferent nerves, which carry benign sensations, can blunt the transmission of pain signals. The gating mechanisms are influenced by the relative activity in the sensory fibers. Input from the large fibers closes the gate, whereas input from the small fibers opens it. For example, rubbing an injured part activates large-fiber activity, which decreases the ability of small-fiber activity to open the gate, thus decreasing the pain. The theory further postulates that cognitive processes, such as attention, emotion, and memory, influence the gating mechanism and have an impact on the transmission of pain. The gate-control theory lends support for the use of both physiologic and psychologic interventions in pain management.

Acute and Chronic Pain

Children may experience acute as well as chronic pain. The signs and symptoms seen with nursing assessment as well as prescribed treatment will differ based on whether the pain is acute or chronic. Acute pain usually has a sudden onset and continues for a limited time. Frequently, the acute pain experienced by children in the inpatient setting is procedural pain. Acute pain is experienced during and after procedures as well as after surgery, with fractures, and with other insults or injuries to the body. Chronic pain continues for an unpredictable period, is unlikely to resolve quickly, and usually affects the child's ability to live a normal life. Children with conditions such as juvenile arthritis, sickle cell disease, and cancer experience chronic pain. Improvements in pain management mean that children who experience pain related to a chronic condition are more comfortable and are able to spend less time in the acute care setting. They are also able to live their lives more normally in relation to school, play, and other activities of childhood (see Chapter 36). Nurses who work in the school, home health care, and hospice settings have more resources (e.g., knowledge, medication, equipment) to enable such pain-free, normal lives for these children.

RESEARCH ON PAIN IN CHILDREN

The past 2 decades have seen a tremendous increase in pediatric pain-related research, with information on acute and chronic pain being widely accessible in chapters of major texts as well as in entire texts devoted to pain. Articles appear frequently in various health care journals. There are also journals that focus exclusively on pain and pediatric pain. However, research on pain in neonates and infants is still limited.

In 1989 the Agency for Health Care Policy and Research (AHCPR), now renamed the Agency for Healthcare Research and Quality (AHRQ), was created to focus on the development of scientifically based practice guidelines for selected problems. Pain was a targeted area. The development of guidelines for the care of children experiencing pain was based on retrieval and review of articles related to postoperative, procedural, and trauma pain. The research studies tested pain assessment tools and pharmacologic and non-pharmacologic pain relief. Other studies included the description of pain in children, the development of pain assessment tools, and other issues related to pain in children. This work produced a document titled *Acute Pain Management Guidelines in Infants, Children, and Adolescents: Operative and Medical Procedures* (Agency for Health Care Policy and Research [AHCPR], 1992a). This guide remains the starting reference point for pediatric pain management, both for dosing as well as choice of medications.

Other bodies of research and development have yielded additional standards of care for both acute and chronic pain. These include numerous publications from the World Health Organization (WHO), the American Pain Society (APS) (see Appendix I on Evolve website), the American Academy of Pediatrics (AAP), and the International Association for the Study of Pain (IASP). The WHO three-step analgesic ladder was developed in the early 1980s to better treat cancer pain. These guidelines are a basis of care for children and adults, particularly for the use of multi-drug therapy. The APS developed guidelines for acute pain, cancer pain, juvenile arthritis (JA), as well as the acute and chronic pain associated with sickle-cell disease in 1999. In cooperation with the AAP, the APS issued recommendations for the assessment and management of acute pain in infants, children, and adolescents (AAP & American Pain Society [APS], 2001). In addition, the Joint Commission on Accreditation of Healthcare Organizations (JCAHO) added new standards that integrate pain assessment and management into their accreditation standards. The 2001 standards guarantee all hospitalized patients the right to developmentally appropriate, comprehensive assessment and management of pain from admission until discharge (Joint Commission on Accreditation of Healthcare Organizations [JCAHO], 2001). Pain management education is included in the standards as well (JCAHO, 2001).

Academic literature, research, and standards of care regarding pain management have increased significantly. Despite these advances in research, knowledge, and clinical expertise, vital improvements in pediatric pain management are still necessary. Needs include continued education of health care providers about appropriate, effective pain management, increased information about pain management in neonates and infants, and nurse-physician collaboration when managing pain in children. As new analgesics are introduced, their safety and efficacy for children should be tested, rather than depending on anecdotal use to guide use in the pediatric population.

MYTHS ABOUT PAIN AND PAIN MANAGEMENT IN CHILDREN

The two beliefs that are most likely to interfere with the provision of adequate pain relief in infants and children are fear of addiction and fear of respiratory depression. Table 39-1

TABLE **39-1** Pain and Pain Management in Children: Myths and Realities

Myth	
Neonates do not experience pain because of incomplete myelinization in the peripheral nerves and central nervous system (CNS).	Myelinization is not necessary for pain perception. Central and peripheral structures required for nociception are present and functional early in gestation. Therefore infants have the neurologic capacity for pain perception at the time of birth, even premature birth.[1]
Children have no memory of pain.	Feeding and sleeping differences have been reported in studies of infants who experienced pain, which suggests that the procedure had consequences extending beyond the event.[2]
There is a correct or given amount of pain for a specific injury or procedure-induced pain.	The amount of pain a child experiences varies and cannot be predicted because of cognitive, developmental, and emotional factors affecting the child.[3]
Children can easily become addicted to narcotic analgesics.	There is no identified characteristic of childhood physiology or development that indicates any increased risk of physiologic or psychologic dependence. The actual risk of addiction is very low.[4,5]
Narcotic administration can easily cause respiratory depression.	No data support the belief that children are at higher risk for respiratory depression than adults.[6] Respiratory depression is rare.[7]

[1]Franck, L.S., Greenberg, C.S., & Stevens, B. (2000). Pain assessment in infants and children. *Pediatric Clinics of North America, 47*(3), 487-512.
[2]Schechter, N.L. (1988). An approach to the child with pain. *Patient Care, 3,* 116-131.
[3]Chen, E., Joseph, M.H., & Zeltzer, L.K. (2000). Behavioral and cognitive interventions in the treatment of pain in children. *Pediatric Clinics of North America, 47*(3), 513-525.
[4]Agency for Health Care Policy and Research, Acute Pain Management Guideline Panel. (1992b). *Acute pain management: Operative or medical procedures and trauma. Clinical practice guideline* (AHCPR Publication No. 92-0032). Rockville, MD: Public Health Service, U.S. Department of Health and Human Services.
[5]Zeltzer, L., Bush, J., Chen, E. & Riveral, A. (1997). A psychobiologic approach to pediatric pain. Part II. Prevention and treatment. *Current Problems in Pediatrics, 27,* 264-284.
[6]Eland, J. (1990). Pain in children. *Nursing Clinics of North America, 25*(4), 871-884.
[7]Golianu, B., Krane, E.J., Galloway, K.S., & Yaster, M. (2000). Pediatric acute pain management. *Pediatric Clinics of North America, 47*(3), 559-587.

lists and refutes other prevalent myths about pain and pain management in children.

ASSESSMENT OF PAIN IN CHILDREN

Pain in children is multifactorial and subjective (AAP, 2001; Bishop-Kurylo, 2002) and is affected by gender, genetic variations, emotional status, temperament, developmental level, culture and ethnicity, previous pain experiences, type and duration of pain, and parental response to the child's pain. When assessing pain in a child or infant, the nurse considers all these factors. Assessing pain in infants and children is more difficult than in adults. Infants and young children do not have the language or cognitive abilities to communicate their pain. Their crying occurs for many reasons including hunger, sleepiness, and stranger anxiety. Accordingly, the nurse must use a combination of behavioral and physiologic signs to assess pain in this age-group (Bishop-Kurylo, 2002) (Box 39-1).

Although older children may be able to verbalize their discomfort, they are often afraid of the cure (injections) or they may have been told to "be brave." Increasingly, it is also seen that even children as young as 5 or 6 years may be fearful of taking pain medication because of the emphasis on "saying no" to drugs. Such an emphasis is meant to focus on illegal substances or inappropriate use of prescription medications. Despite this fact, some children translate this to mean they must shy away from using even appropriate and necessary pain medications. The nurse can depend on the current bank of literature, research, and standards of care in providing the education necessary to overcome such barriers to appropriate pain assessment and management.

Assessment According to Developmental Level

Neonates and Infants

Because neonates and young infants have immature central nervous systems, without myelinization of pain fibers, clinicians have long believed these children to be incapable of perceiving pain. Increasingly, however, research has challenged this assumption and demonstrated that neonates and infants do indeed experience pain (Bishop-Kurylo, 2002; McCaffery & Pasero, 1999; Stevens, Gibbins, & Franck, 2000). In addition, Franck, Greenberg, and Stevens (2000) note that research supports that the nociceptive processes between infants and adults differ in that in infants the primary transmission of pain impulses is along nonmyelinated C fibers, there is less precise pain signal transmission in the spinal cord, and there is a lack of descending inhibitory transmitters. For this reason, infants may actually perceive pain more intensely than adults or older children, secondary to immature descending control mechanisms, which would thus limit their ability to modulate the pain experience.

Given that infants are preverbal, the nurse's pain assessment should be based on behavioral, physiologic, and biochemical responses. Although biochemical measures indicate

BOX 39-1
Assessment According to Developmental Levels

NEONATE AND INFANT
- Changes in facial expression, including frowns, grimaces, wrinkled brow, expression of surprise, and facial flinching
- Increases in blood pressure and heart rate and decrease in arterial saturation
- High-pitched, tense, harsh crying
- Generalized or total-body response in neonate and young infant that becomes more purposeful as the infant matures
- May thrash extremities; may exhibit tremors
- Older infants: rub painful area, pull away, or guard the involved part

TODDLER
- Loud crying
- Verbalizes words that indicate discomfort ("ouch," "hurt," "boo-boo")
- Attempts to delay procedures perceived as painful
- Generalized restlessness
- Guards the site
- Touches painful areas
- May run from the nurse

PRESCHOOLER
- May think the pain is punishment for some deed or thought
- Crying, kicking
- Describes the location and intensity of pain (e.g., "ear hurts bad")
- Regression to earlier behaviors (loss of bladder and bowel control)
- Withdrawal
- Denies pain to avoid a possible injection
- May have been told to "be brave" and deny pain even though it is present

SCHOOL-AGE CHILD
- Able to describe pain and quantify pain intensity
- Fears body harm
- Has an awareness of death
- Stiff body posture
- Withdrawal
- Procrastinates or bargains to delay procedure

ADOLESCENT
- Perceives pain at a physical, emotional, and mental level
- Understands cause and effect
- Describes pain and quantifies pain intensity
- Increased muscle tension
- Withdrawal and decreased motor activity
- Uses words such as "sore," "ache," or "pounding" to describe pain

---

hormonal and metabolic changes in infants experiencing pain, such measures are difficult to obtain in the acute care setting. Behavioral indicators of infant pain are more easily assessed. These are detailed by multiple resources (Anand & Hickey, 1987; Craig, 1998; Franck, Greenberg, & Stevens, 2000; Grunau, Johnston, & Craig, 1990; McCaffery & Pasero, 1999) who note that such indicators include rapid changes of behavioral state, changes in sleep patterns, crying, fist clenching, grimacing, wrinkling of forehead, fussiness, and restlessness. Facial expression is considered the most reliable indicator of pain throughout populations of infants as well as children. Facial expression, in combination with short latency to onset of cry and a long duration of the first cry cycle, typifies infants' reactions to acute invasive procedures. Cries associated with pain may sound different from those associated with hunger, discomfort, and stress; these cries are higher-pitched, tense, and harsh. Parents and nurses may therefore be able to differentiate between the usual cries of infants and the cries of pain.

Motor movements associated with pain in the neonate and infant progress from a generalized body response to more purposeful movements. For example, infants ages 9 to 12 months can use their hands to push the nurse away if they perceive a painful action about to begin (Mills, 1989). The responses of neonates to painful stimuli are sometimes described as total-body responses (Fig. 39-1). The infant's extremities may thrash about, and some infants exhibit tremors. Older infants may rub the painful area, pull away, or guard the involved body part.

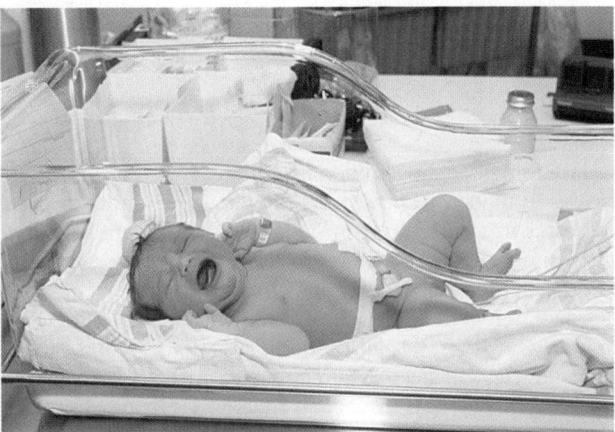

Figure 39-1 Neonates and infants have a total-body response to pain. Parents can usually distinguish the infant's cry of pain from other cries because it is tense, high-pitched, and harsh-sounding.

Franck, Greenberg, and Stevens (2000) note that an infant's behavioral state immediately before painful stimulation, such as sleep state, affects the vigorousness of the response. In addition, the responses of preterm infants are less vigorous than those of full-term infants. The nurse must be cognizant of this information to make an appropriate assessment of pain through observation of an infant's facial expressions, motor response, and cry.

CRITICAL THINKING EXERCISE 39-1

You are about to care for a 3500-g full-term neonate who is status 24 hours postoperative fundoplication and gastrostomy device placement. The nurse who has been caring for Tanika reports that Tanika has slept for short periods throughout the shift, sucks vigorously on her pacifier, and occasionally cries. The nurse notes that she has not medicated Tanika for pain because she does have periods when she sleeps for 15 to 30 minutes. Her blood pressure is 98/74, pulse 170, and respirations 50/min.

1. What would be your first nursing action?
2. What principles related to pediatric pain control would apply to this infant?

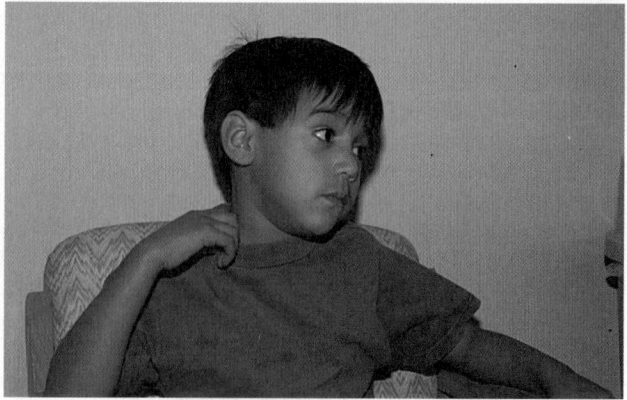

Figure 39-3 School-age children may withdraw and become very quiet when they are ill or in pain. Note how dull this boy appears. Although he has asthma, his mother knew something else was wrong because he was unusually quiet and withdrawn. (Courtesy Parkland Health and Hospital System Community Oriented Primary Care Clinic, Dallas, TX.)

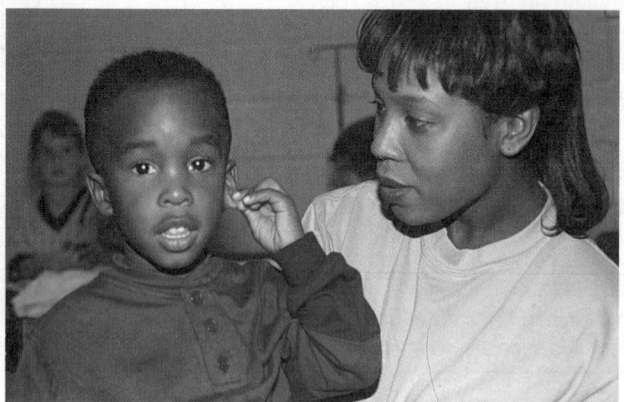

Figure 39-2 Toddlers and preschoolers may express pain by guarding or touching the painful area. Pulling on the ear is a characteristic expression of ear pain that accompanies otitis media. (Courtesy The University of Texas at Arlington School of Nursing.)

Physiologic changes are also more easily assessed. Increases in blood pressure, heart rate, and respiratory rate and decreases in arterial oxygen saturation have been associated with pain in neonates, although these changes can be linked to other alterations in the infant's body as well, such as agitation. Crying may also affect the infant's physiologic response. Rawlings, Miller, and Engel (1980) reported that oxygenation will decrease in response to pain but may increase after vigorous crying, so that data can be confusing. Distinguishing between pain and agitation is sometimes difficult. If an infant is simply agitated, yet is treated for pain, the cause of the agitation will be unchecked, the intervention is inappropriate, and the agitation will likely increase. The nurse should realize that physiologic changes are just one part of the assessment of pain in the neonate and infant and should suspect that an infant is in pain before physiologic changes occur.

Toddlers

The toddler experiencing pain tends to cry longer than the infant. As verbal abilities become more advanced, the toddler can verbally express displeasure when a painful experience occurs. The toddler asks for parents, verbalizes words

that indicate discomfort ("ouch," "hurt"), and may attempt to delay the nurse's attempts to do a procedure judged as painful. The older toddler can often localize the pain and point to the body part that hurts.

Generalized restlessness, guarding the site, and touching the painful area are signs of pain in the toddler (Fig. 39-2). The toddler may associate discomfort with a particular procedure, such as a dressing change, and may run from the nurse when approached. The toddler's face may show anger and fear. The child may avoid eye contact or look sad. In response to discomfort and pain, the toddler may also demonstrate regression to earlier, more comfortable behaviors.

Preschoolers

Preschoolers are egocentric. Relating only to the present, they cannot associate discomfort with any positive outcome. For example, the preschooler will not understand how débriding a painful burn will ultimately have a positive effect. The child who is unable to understand why an uncomfortable procedure might be positive may find pain disorienting and be affected more profoundly than an older child (Schechter, 1988).

Preschoolers tend to think pain will magically go away and that they are being punished for some previous thought or deed. They also fear body mutilation; males in this age-group fear castration. Preschoolers may deny pain to avoid an injection. The preschooler may cry and kick to avoid a procedure perceived as painful. Preschoolers may also regress to earlier, more comfortable behaviors as a response to pain or may withdraw and not participate in activities on the unit. These children can, however, describe the location and intensity of pain.

School-Age Children

School-age children can describe pain and relate it to a body part as well as quantify the pain intensity. They are beginning to understand the need for painful procedures. They fear body harm and have an awareness of death. Therefore they may appear to overreact to illness or injury. As in all age-

Assessing Pain in Children

- The use of a pain assessment tool is imperative in the assessment of pain in children and the evaluation of pain management interventions. The tool is part of the child's chart.
- If the child is unable to express or quantify pain, use parents as one of the first resources to assess the child's pain and response to interventions.
- Behavioral changes, such as guarding, body position, crying, altered facial expression, and changes in activity level may or may not be present.*
- Physiologic changes are only one source of information when assessing pain in the neonate or infant and should not be relied on before intervening. Other states, such as fear and anxiety, may also cause physiologic changes. Because physiologic changes tend to occur during the acute period and then return to normal, they may not be valid indicators of chronic pain.

*Children's Hospital, Boston. (2002). *Reference tool: Pain assessment tools.* Boston, MA: Author.

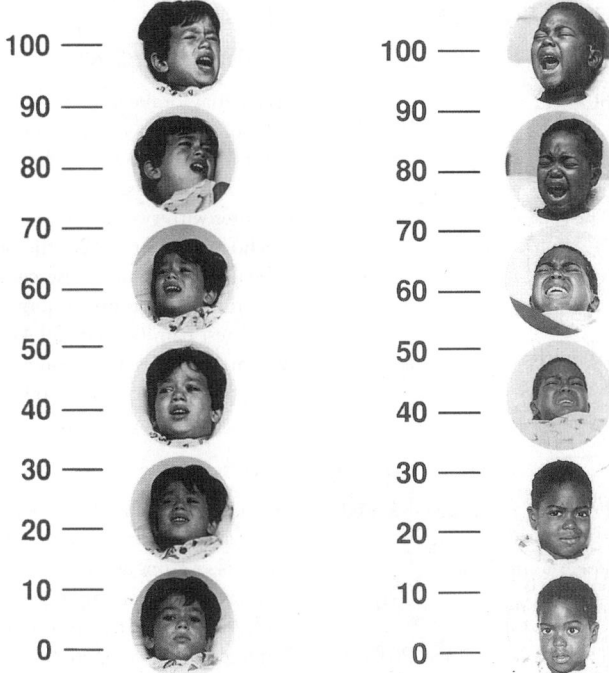

Figure 39-4 A, The Hispanic (Latino) version of the Oucher pain scale. **B,** The African-American version. (**A,** Developed and copyrighted by Antonia M. Villarruel, R.N., Ph.D., & Mary J. Denyes, R.N., Ph.D., 1991. **B,** Developed and copyrighted by Mary J. Denyes, Ph.D., R.N., FAAN [Wayne State University], & Antonia Villarruel, Ph.D., R.N., FAAN [University of Pennsylvania] at the Children's Hospital of Michigan in 1990. Cornelia P. Porter, Ph.D., R.N., & Charlotta Marshall, M.S.N., R.N., contributed to the development of this scale.)

groups, the school-age child remembers previous pain experiences, which will affect the child's response. The child's culture, gender, and cognitive abilities will also affect the pain experience.

Nonverbal cues are very important in school-age children. The child may exhibit a stiff body posture, may withdraw, or may be found quietly sobbing (Fig. 39-3). If the school-age child resists a treatment, cries loudly, or otherwise acts in an aggressive manner, the child may later deny the behavior. School-age children may also attempt to procrastinate or bargain to delay a painful procedure. As with younger children, the school-age child may demonstrate regressive behaviors when experiencing pain.

Adolescents

Adolescents can think abstractly and understand cause and effect. They can describe and quantify pain intensity as well as their feelings about pain. They can also discuss the strategies that help manage their pain. They are able to perceive and understand pain at a physical, emotional, and mental level. Having these abilities does not mean the adolescent will exercise them. Adolescents are often confused by control issues and are uncertain of their role as they move from childhood to adulthood. Regression may also occur at this age in relation to pain.

Because adolescents are egocentric, they tend to think that others also focus on their behavior and so may suppress manifestations of pain. In addition, they may not report pain because they believe that the nurse is aware of when they hurt and so they expect they will receive the medication as they need it. Adolescents tend to exhibit fewer outward signs of pain than young children. Signs observed in the adolescent include increased muscle tension, withdrawal, and decreased motor activity. Hospitalized adolescents use words such as "sore," "like an ache," "pounding," and "miserable" to de-

scribe pain. They complete the statement, "When I have pain, I most often feel . . ." with "sick to my stomach," "scared," "angry," "like crying, but I don't," "like hitting someone," and "like screaming" (Savedra, Tesler, & Wegner, 1988).

Assessment Tools

A number of valid and reliable pain assessment tools enable the nurse to make a more accurate pain assessment. Both self-report and behavioral instruments are available. Children benefit when a pain assessment tool is used because they are given a simple and effective way to communicate the pain they are experiencing. Assessment tools provide more objective data, decreasing the chance that more discreet signs of pain will be overlooked. Unfortunately, they are not always used consistently and appropriately in the clinical setting.

An assessment tool should be selected according to the child's age and developmental abilities. The crucial factors in regard to a pain assessment tool are that it is appropriate for the child's age and that an effective plan can be made utilizing the information gathered from the assessment. A variety of tools are available for infants and the preverbal or nonverbal child, such as those who are neurologically unresponsive, developmentally delayed, or unable to speak because of medical treatment such as intubation. Tools for

TABLE **39-2** Pain Assessment Tools

Tool	Description	Age
FLACC[1]	Five behavioral categories—Face, Legs, Activity, Cry, Consolability—each scored from 0 to 2, resulting in a total score of 0 to 10. A higher score indicates higher pain or distress.	Infants and preverbal or nonverbal children.
The Oucher[2-5]	A poster with two scales: one is numeric, for use by children who can count to 100; the other is a photographic scale to be used by children who cannot count to 100. The bottom picture (or 0) is no pain; the top picture (or 100) is the greatest pain (see Fig. 39-4).	3-12 yr.
FACES Pain Rating Scale[6]	Six cartoon faces with a number under each, ranging from a happy face (0 or No Hurt) to a crying face (5 or Hurts Worst) (see Fig. 39-5).	3 yr and older. It may be more helpful if the child is able to understand number order or "greater than." This is usually seen in children of kindergarten or school age.
FACES Pain Scale—Revised[7]	Six faces with neutral to gradually increasing painful expressions, corresponding to an analog scale of 0 to 10.	4 yr and older.
Poker Chip Tool[8]	Four poker chips are used; each chip represents a piece of hurt. One poker chip represents a little hurt, and four chips represent the most hurt the child could have.	4-12 yr.
The Adolescent and Pediatric Pain Tool: APPT[9,10]	Three-part tool composed of a body outline, an intensity scale, and a pain descriptor word list (see Fig. 39-6).	8-17 yr.
Visual Analog Scale (VAS)	Usually a 10-cm line with one end representing "no pain" and the opposite end "the worst pain."	Older school-age children and adolescents. May be used by younger school-age children, but less abstract tools are more appropriate.
Numeric Rating Scale (NRS)	Uses numbers (e.g., 0 to 10 or 0 to 100) to indicate increasing pain.	Child must know numbers.

[1]Merkel, S., Voepel-Lewis, T., & Malviya, S. (2002). Pain assessment in infants and young children: The FLACC scale: A behavioral tool to measure pain in young children. *American Journal of Nursing, 102*(10), 55-58.

[2]Beyer, J. (1984). *The Oucher: A user's manual and technical report.* Evanston, IL: Judson Press.

[3]Beyer, J., & Aradine, C. (1986). Content validity of an instrument to measure young children's perceptions of the intensity of their pain. *Journal of Pediatric Nursing, 1*(6), 386-395.

[4]Beyer, J., Denyes, M., & Villarruel, A. (1992). The creation, validation, and continuing development of the Oucher: A measure of pain intensity in children. *Journal of Pediatric Nursing, 7*(5), 335-346.

[5]Beyer, J.E., & Knott, C.B. (1998). Construct validity estimation for the African-American and Hispanic versions of the Oucher Scale. *Journal of Pediatric Nursing, 13*(1), 20-31.

[6]Wong, D.L., Hockenberry-Eaton, M., Wilson, D., Winkelstein, M.L., & Schwartz, P. (2001). *Essentials of pediatric nursing* (6th ed.). St. Louis: Mosby.

[7]Spagrud, L., Piira, T., & Von Baeyer, C. (2003). Children's self-report of pain intensity. *American Journal of Nursing, 103*(12), 62-64.

[8]Hester, N.O. (1979). The preoperational child's reaction to immunization. *Nursing Research, 4*(28), 250-254.

[9]Savedra, M.C., Tesler, M.D., Holzemer, W.L., Wilkie, D.J., & Ward, J. (1989). Pain location: Validity and reliability of body outline markings by hospitalized children and adolescents. *Research in Nursing and Health, 12,* 307-314.

[10]Savedra, M.C., Tesler, M.D., Holzemer, W.L., & Ward, J. (1992). *Adolescent and pediatric pain tool: User's manual.* San Francisco: University of California, San Francisco, School of Nursing.

infants and preverbal children usually are based on behavioral cues (e.g., facial expression, motor responses, intensity of cry). Children verbalize words for pain by approximately 18 months of age, and cognitive development is sufficient for reporting the extent of pain by 3 to 4 years of age. Self-report tools are effective in children older than 3 years. The Oucher, the Poker Chip Tool, and the FACES Scale are examples of tools for preschoolers and school-age children (Table 39-2). For some children, the African-American or Latino versions of the Oucher pain scale provide more culturally sensitive assessment (Fig. 39-4). Matching the tool to the child's race and ethnicity can provide better information about pain experienced by children

from nonwhite populations and so promote better pain control for these children (Beyer & Knott, 1998).

School-age children can understand concepts of order and number and can use numeric rating scales, horizontal word-graphic rating scales, and visual analog scales. Table 39-2 describes pain assessment tools and lists the appropriate age or developmental level for each tool (Figs. 39-5 and 39-6). To avoid confusing the child and to obtain appropriate, consistent data, the same scale should be used each time the child is assessed. Ideally, the child should be taught how to use the tool before pain is experienced (e.g., preoperatively). Obviously, in emergencies, such preparation will not be possible. Appropriate use of any tool is essential. Using a tool in a way

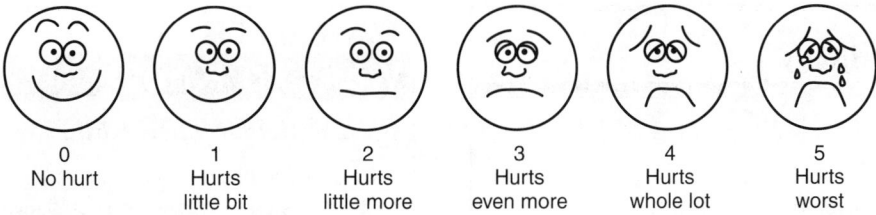

0
No hurt

1
Hurts
little bit

2
Hurts
little more

3
Hurts
even more

4
Hurts
whole lot

5
Hurts
worst

Figure 39-5 FACES Pain Rating Scale. *Instructions:* Explain to the child that each face is for a person who feels happy because he has no pain (hurt) or sad because he has some or a lot of pain. *Face 0* is very happy because he doesn't hurt at all. *Face 1* hurts just a little bit. *Face 2* hurts a little more. *Face 3* hurts even more. *Face 4* hurts a whole lot. *Face 5* hurts as much as you can imagine, although you don't have to be crying to feel this bad. Ask the child to choose the face that best describes how he is feeling. Recommended for persons age 3 years and older. (From Wong, D.L., Hockenberry-Eaton, M., Wilson, D., Winkelstein, M.L., & Schwartz, P. (2001). *Essentials of pediatric nursing* (6th ed.). St. Louis: Mosby.)

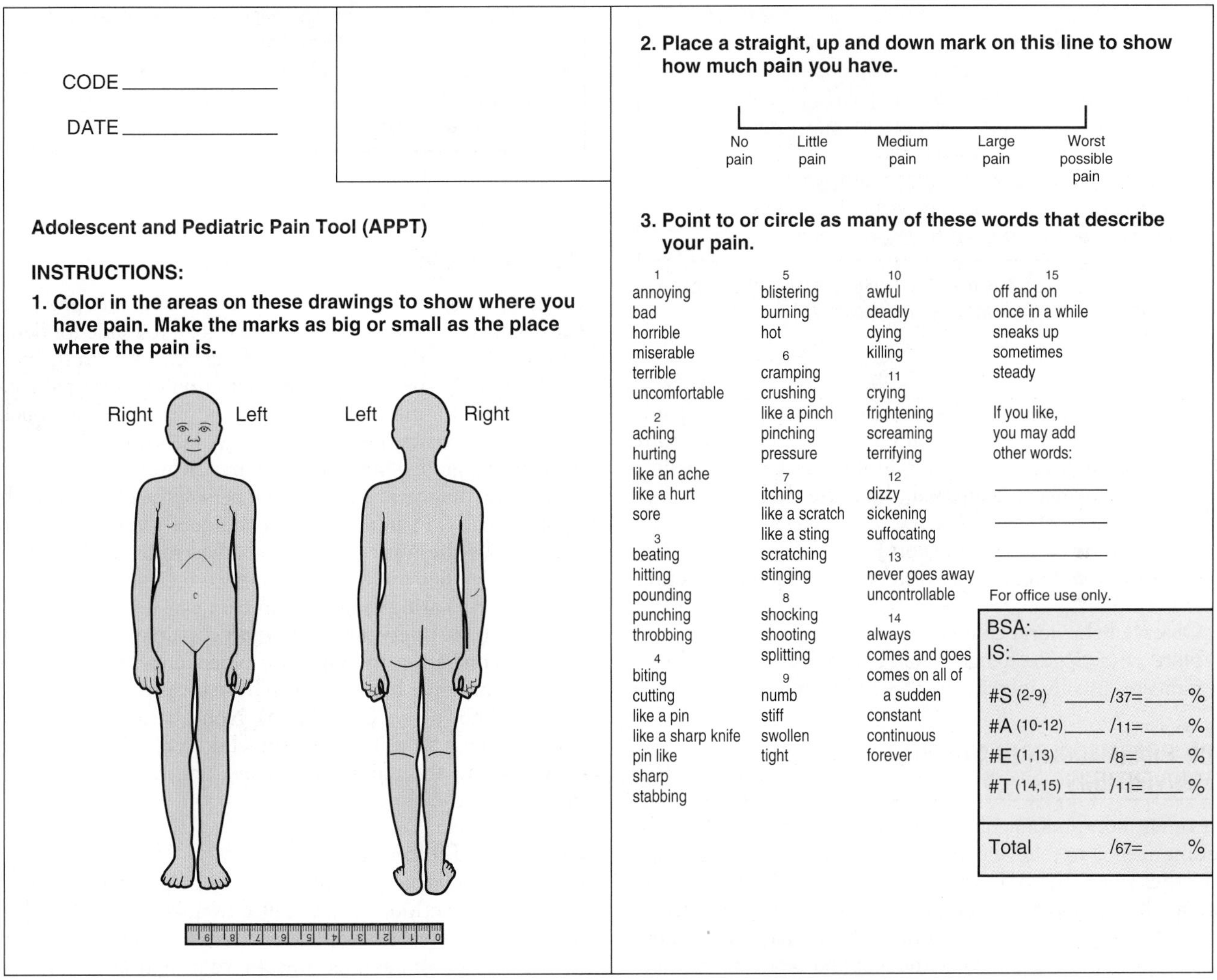

CODE _____

DATE _____

Adolescent and Pediatric Pain Tool (APPT)

INSTRUCTIONS:

1. **Color in the areas on these drawings to show where you have pain. Make the marks as big or small as the place where the pain is.**

Right   Left   Left   Right

2. Place a straight, up and down mark on this line to show how much pain you have.

| No pain | Little pain | Medium pain | Large pain | Worst possible pain |

3. Point to or circle as many of these words that describe your pain.

1	5	10	15
annoying	blistering	awful	off and on
bad	burning	deadly	once in a while
horrible	hot	dying	sneaks up
miserable	6	killing	sometimes
terrible	cramping	11	steady
uncomfortable	crushing	crying	
2	like a pinch	frightening	If you like,
aching	pinching	screaming	you may add
hurting	pressure	terrifying	other words:
like an ache	7	12	
like a hurt	itching	dizzy	_____
sore	like a scratch	sickening	
3	like a sting	suffocating	_____
beating	scratching	13	
hitting	stinging	never goes away	_____
pounding	8	uncontrollable	
punching	shocking	14	
throbbing	shooting	always	
4	splitting	comes and goes	
biting	9	comes on all of	
cutting	numb	a sudden	
like a pin	stiff	constant	
like a sharp knife	swollen	continuous	
pin like	tight	forever	
sharp			
stabbing			

For office use only.

BSA: _____		
IS: _____		
#S (2-9) _____ /37= _____ %		
#A (10-12) _____ /11= _____ %		
#E (1,13) _____ /8= _____ %		
#T (14,15) _____ /11= _____ %		
Total _____ /67= _____ %		

Figure 39-6 Adolescent and Pediatric Pain Tool, appropriate for use with 8- to 17-year-olds. (From Savedra, M.C., Tesler, M.D., Holzemer, W.L., & Ward, J.A. [1992]. *Adolescent and Pediatric Pain Tool: User's manual.* San Francisco: University of California, San Francisco, School of Nursing. Copyright © 1989, 1992. For original tools, write or call 415-476-4040.)

other than the developer intended may invalidate the pain assessment.

In assessing pain and obtaining the pain history, the nurse should first question children to determine which word or words they use for pain. Such words must be used consistently in any future discussions with a child regarding pain. This chapter will refer to either pain or hurt, with the understanding that the child's word of choice (e.g., "owie," "ouchie") is always used by the nurse. In questioning the parents, one of the first issues the nurse should address is the presence of fam-

BOX 39-2
Pain Experience History

CHILD FORM
Tell me what pain is.
Tell me about the hurt you've had before.
Do you tell others when you hurt? If yes, who?
What do you do for yourself when you are hurting?
What do you want others to do for you when you hurt?
What don't you want others to do for you when you hurt?
What helps the most to take your hurt away?
Is there anything special that you want me to know about you
   when you hurt? (If yes, have child describe.)

PARENT FORM
What word or words does your child use in regard to pain?
Describe the pain experiences your child has had before.
Does your child tell you or others when hurting?
How do you know when your child is in pain?
How does your child usually react to pain?
What do you do when your child is hurting?
What does your child do when hurting?
What works best to decrease or take away your child's pain?
Is there anything special that you would like me to know
   about your child and pain? (If yes, describe.)

Modified from Hester, N.O., & Barcus, C.S. (1986). Assessment and management of pain in children. *Pediatrics: Nursing Update, 1,* 2-8.

ily, cultural, or spiritual beliefs and practices regarding pain. Box 39-2 describes how to obtain a pain history from both child and parent. After pain terminology and special beliefs or practices have been addressed, the nurse should:

- Question the child (pain history).
- Question the parent (pain history, other factors affecting the child).
- Observe behavioral changes.
- Note physiologic changes (pulse, blood pressure, and respirations usually increase and then return to normal).

NON-PHARMACOLOGIC AND PHARMACOLOGIC PAIN INTERVENTIONS

At times, non-pharmacologic interventions may be the only action needed to relieve certain types and intensities of pain. At other times, the only way to break the cycle of pain is to use a pharmacologic agent. The nurse's assessment determines the appropriate intervention. If pharmacologic interventions are determined to be the first and best option, non-pharmacologic interventions may always be offered along with the chosen analgesic. Doing so may offer the child a sense of accomplishment and control that can replace the sense of helplessness that often accompanies the presence of pain. In addition, Rusy and Weisman (2000) note that children are highly responsive to pain management strategies that involve use of their imagination as well as their sense of play and that use of non-pharmacologic or complementary therapies may reduce the amount of medication required to treat pain.

PARENTS Want to Know

Pain Relief for Their Child

- Parents are given a pain assessment tool together with instructions on its use. They should give a return demonstration.
- The dose, route, and schedule of any pain medication to be given are explained to the parents verbally and in writing.
- Non-pharmacologic interventions that are appropriate and comforting for the child's particular pain (e.g., massage, warm or cold compresses, repositioning) are explained and demonstrated.
- Parents are instructed to notify the primary health care provider if pain-relief interventions are ineffective or if the child shows behavior or physiologic changes not consistent with the expected outcomes for the child.
- Parents are given a phone number where they can contact a nurse if they have any questions about their child's condition once the child is back in the home setting.

Non-pharmacologic Interventions

Parents play a very important role in assessing and providing pain management for children. They are a resource for determining what methods of pain relief were effective in the past. They can help the nurse assess their child's current pain status and need for intervention. Repositioning, holding, touching, massage, warm or cold compresses, breathing techniques, distraction, guided imagery, and muscle relaxation are all techniques that can be used by the person the child trusts the most—usually a parent. Many techniques require initial instruction by the nurse or other qualified individual but then are easily learned and put into practice by a parent.

The nurse caring for a child in pain can also provide non-pharmacologic interventions as a part of pain management. In addition, preparing the child for procedures and treatments can help minimize or relieve pain by reducing anxiety and fear of the unknown (see Chapter 35). Non-pharmacologic interventions must be suitable for the child, considering stage of development, the child's personality, and the circumstances surrounding the child.

Breathing Techniques
Regulated breathing techniques can help provide a focal point for distraction, produce relaxation, be a simple mode of biofeedback, or be a component of imagery. The child is instructed about and assisted to achieve a rhythmic pattern of breathing. This pattern must also be easily sustainable. Parents can demonstrate and participate in the breathing technique themselves.

Distraction
Distraction can be one of the more effective adjuvants for pain management (Fig. 39-7). It is also one of the most simple to accomplish. Distraction works by refocusing the child from the pain to something else. It does not imply total pain relief, and children experiencing severe pain may not be able

to be distracted. The child's ability to use distraction does not mean that the child is not experiencing pain. Children may distract themselves to "forget" their pain, but the child's watching television, playing, or reading does not mean the child is pain-free. The form of distraction should be appropriate for the child's developmental level.

Distraction may be accomplished with blowing bubbles, looking through a kaleidoscope, music, stories, number games, video games, board games, watching a video, or even doing multiplication tables or spelling words. If a child has a favorite doll or stuffed animal, it may be used to create a story or a game. Children love to talk about their pets, and the nurse can ask the child to tell a favorite story about the pet. Another distraction technique is to allow the child to help by handing, opening, or holding objects. This technique should be used only when it is safe and there is no danger of contamination of materials or of a site.

For example, a child brought to the emergency department after an accident is invariably frightened. Even if the injury is minor by emergency department standards, the fear and pain are real to the child. Using distraction, the nurse can decrease both anxiety and pain. Although each child is different, cues or verbal instruction from the child and the parent can indicate whether the nurse should hold the child's hand, touch the child's head, or provide some other interventions that are appropriate and comforting for the child.

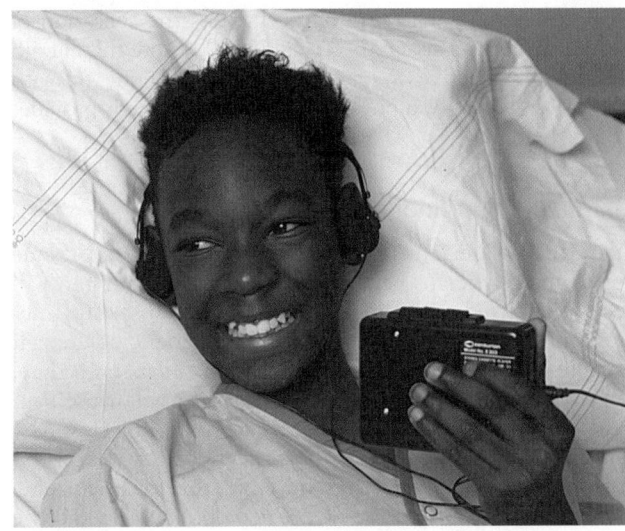

Figure 39-7 Distraction effectively reduces pain by helping the child refocus attention. This boy listens to the radio through earphones, allowing him to be distracted without annoying others. (Courtesy Children's Medical Center, Dallas, TX.)

Once both the child and nurse can communicate personally, the nurse might say, "I see you have a baseball shirt on. Do you play baseball?" If the child expresses an interest in the game, the nurse can continue, "Which team is your favorite? What was the most exciting play you saw this year? Have you been to a game?" The nurse should be comfortable with the topic because the child will sense a lack of genuine interest. If it is appropriate based on the child's developmental level and degree of egocentricity, the nurse might interject a personal note: "I love baseball also. When I was a child, it was my biggest treat to go with my father to see the St. Louis Cardinals play." This conversation could go on for 10 to 15 minutes, certainly long enough for sutures to be put in or other minor procedures completed. The child will not be focusing as much on the procedure as on baseball. The topic should be of interest to the child, because the important idea is to focus the child on something other than the injury and procedure.

Guided Imagery
Guided imagery is a process involving relaxation and focused concentration on mental images. The child can be encouraged to think of a favorite place and imagine the sounds, sights, and smells of that place. The nurse, in a quiet, soothing voice, can guide the child on a "make-believe" trip. Breathing techniques can also relax the child. The child is instructed to take several slow, deep breaths while thinking pleasant thoughts. Children often need guidance, and the nurse may suggest remembering a birthday or a special time with family, friends, or a pet.

Biofeedback
Biofeedback provides visual or auditory evidence that physiologic changes are taking place. Special instruments detect and magnify body states that a person cannot usually notice.

It also helps the person bring them under control. Visual feedback involving changes in colors or numbers or involvement in computer games is an effective way to use this technique. Biofeedback gives the child a response that can be seen instantly and can keep the child interested. Biofeedback does require specialized equipment and trained instructors and is more often useful for chronic pain as opposed to acute pain (Rusy & Weisman, 2000).

Progressive Muscle Relaxation
Children can achieve relaxation, decrease anxiety, and decrease pain by identifying and decreasing body tension that can accompany pain. They are taught a progressive, systematic, purposeful relaxation of their body, part by part. This involves tensing and relaxing specific muscles, usually beginning with the arms and moving down the body. Learning this method can require a degree of skill and ability to practice frequently that may be seen only with older children.

Hypnosis
Hypnosis is a form of focused and narrowed attention, an altered state of consciousness, or a trance, often accompanied by relaxation. Hypnosis is effective in relieving pain and symptoms in children undergoing painful procedures associated with cancer, burns, and sickle-cell disease (Cravero, Manzi, & Rice, 1998). Hypnosis has also been shown to have positive effects on children undergoing surgery (Jones, 1997; Lambert, 1996). Typically, a licensed psychologist or health care personnel who have undergone special training perform hypnosis. Children can be taught self-hypnosis. Hypnosis and self-hypnosis are being used with increasing frequency and positive results among children.

Transcutaneous Electrical Nerve Stimulation
In transcutaneous electrical nerve stimulation (TENS), a unit with electrodes delivers small amounts of electrical energy to the skin. The stimulation interferes with the trans-

mission of pain signals and helps suppress the sensation of pain in that area. Rusy and Weisman (2000) note that TENS has proven effective in pain management, alone or with analgesics. Typically, a physical therapy department provides TENS therapy.

Pharmacologic Interventions

Many nurses are reluctant to administer analgesics. Some nurses and physicians believe, incorrectly, that children will become addicted to the analgesic. Others fear respiratory depression or do not believe the child is experiencing enough pain to justify analgesic administration. If a procedure, surgery, or trauma causes pain in an adult, it will cause pain in a child and analgesic medications are necessary. However, it is important to ensure that the correct dose of analgesic is ordered and administered. In some cases, the analgesic being administered is not ordered at the appropriate dose and the child still experiences untreated, unwarranted pain. Not one analgesic or combinations of analgesics will be ideal for all circumstances of pain management. Analgesic therapy must have a predictable, prompt onset of action, a brief duration of action, negligible side effects, and an appropriate reversal agent.

Administration of Analgesics

Analgesics can be administered by various routes—oral, rectal, intranasal, topical, transdermal, intravenous (IV), intramuscular (IM), subcutaneous, and epidural. (See Chapter 38 for a discussion of the common routes.)

  Patient-Controlled Analgesia. One of the most effective ways of administering analgesic is using a patient-controlled analgesia (PCA) pump. The pump administers an IV bolus of pain medication either with or without a continuing infusion of the same medication. PCA can be used in a child as young as 5 years who is developmentally normal (McCaffery & Pasero, 1999). In some institutions, children younger than 5 years use PCA with parents or nurses activating the pump for them. Further research and anecdotal experience are needed on the use of PCA in children younger than 5 years.

  When the child needs pain medication, a small dose of the medication is received after a button connected to the pump is pushed (Fig. 39-8). After each dose, there is "lock-out" time during which the pump will not release the medication even if the button is pushed. The pump also has a maximum amount of medication that can be given over a designated

period—usually 1 hour. If the maximum amount of medication for the time has been reached, the pump will not release medication even if the button is pushed.

  After checking to ensure that all doses are within appropriate range, two registered nurses (RNs) must check the bag or syringe of opioid before hanging it. After a PCA pump is programmed, it must then be double-checked by a second RN. Box 39-3 gives an example of orders for a PCA infusion. The opioid bag or syringe is locked into the PCA pump, and the pump itself is locked to the IV pole. Typically, the PCA tubing is special tubing that does not have IV port access.

  The child is monitored frequently to ensure that pain control is effective and that the equipment is functioning correctly. The nurse should also carefully monitor the child for signs of overmedication (especially depressed respiratory rate or inability to rouse) and the side effects that may accompany opioid administration. Vital signs should be assessed every 15 to 30 minutes when PCA therapy is first initiated and then every 2 to 4 hours thereafter. Some institutions require hourly documentation of respiratory rate.

  In addition, many institutions' policies require that children receiving PCA therapy be placed on continuous pulse oximetry, cardiac and respiratory monitoring, or both. Oxygen, a bag and mask, and naloxone (Narcan) should be readily available. Naloxone will reverse the opioid-related analgesia as well as the respiratory depression. For this reason, it is administered slowly until respiratory depression is first noted to be reversed. It has a short half-life and so may need to be repeated every 30 to 60 minutes. Many institutions will mandate that naloxone must be given in the presence of a physician because too-rapid infusion can result in cardiac arrest.

  Frequent pain assessment is also necessary. This is usually every 4 hours as well as with any bolus dose and subsequent reassessment as to the bolus's effectiveness. Charting will include hourly documentation as to the number of boluses received

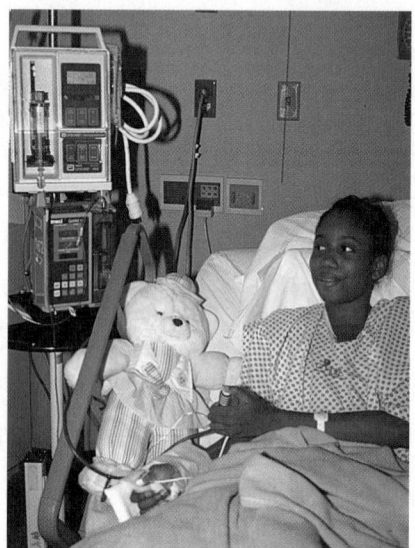

Figure 39-8 Patient-controlled analgesia (PCA) gives the older child greater control over pain management. The child presses the button when pain medication is needed, and the machine delivers a preprogrammed bolus through the intravenous (IV) line. The child cannot overdose because the controller has a lockout feature to prevent excess analgesic administration. (Courtesy Children's Medical Center, Dallas, TX.)

! CRITICAL TO REMEMBER

Disadvantages of Intramuscular Analgesics

- Altered tissue absorption leads to peaks and troughs in analgesia.
- Children quickly run out of suitable sites for injection.
- Intramuscular analgesics have a shorter duration of action than orally administered analgesics.
- Intramuscular analgesics are contraindicated in children with low platelet counts.
- Children hate intramuscular injections.
- Nurses dislike administering intramuscular injections.

Modified from Eland, J. (1990). Pain in children. *Nursing Clinics of North America, 25*(4), 871-884.

and possibly the number of bolus attempts made by the child. Total milligram dosages of the medication received will be noted anywhere from every hour to every 4 hours. This will be documented on the medication administration record.

Topical Anesthetic Cream. A topical anesthetic cream, lidocaine-prilocaine 5% cream (eutectic mixture of local anesthetics [EMLA]), can be used to reduce the pain associated with selected procedures, such as scheduled injections and immunizations, venipuncture, lumbar puncture, and bone marrow aspiration. Research related to the use of EMLA in the treatment of acute pain in neonates is ongoing. The main side effect is skin blanching or redness, which usually lasts a few hours. EMLA cream is applied to intact skin under an occlusive dressing at least 60 minutes before anesthesia is needed. The cream is applied in a mound, not rubbed in. The duration of anesthesia is at least 2 hours and not more than 4 hours. An EMLA disk is also available.

Parents may apply the cream at home before scheduled injections or drawing of blood to help decrease or eliminate pain. EMLA comes with directions in Spanish and English for use by parents. Care should be taken with small children to avoid their removing the dressing and rubbing the cream

in their eyes or eating the cream, which to some children may look like cake frosting. Even with the decreased or absent pain, children may still fear needles; therefore distraction or another non-pharmacologic method may remain necessary to help them through the painful procedure.

Nonsteroidal Antiinflammatory Drugs

Nonsteroidal antiinflammatory drugs (NSAIDs) are ibuprofen or aspirin-like drugs that reduce pain and inflammation. Ibuprofen, naproxen/naproxen sodium (Naprosyn, Anaprox) (see Chapter 50), ketorolac (Toradol), and choline magnesium trisalicylate (Trilisate) are some of the most commonly used drugs in this category. Because aspirin has been associated with Reye's syndrome, it is not recommended for children.

It is questionable whether acetaminophen can be classified as an NSAID at all, because it has a minimal antiinflammatory effect and does not inhibit prostaglandin. However, it is frequently listed with NSAIDs. The short-term use of acetaminophen is safe, even in neonates. It does not have the gastric side effects of aspirin, and although it can cause hepatic damage, this effect is usually related to overdosage. It is the drug of choice for treating fever in children in the United States and is the most commonly used analgesic for mild to moderate pain. However, ibuprofen may be the drug of choice for conditions where there is bone pain, such as may be seen with bone injuries, arthritis-like conditions, or certain types of cancer.

Opioids

Opioids are the cornerstone drugs in the management of most forms of moderate to severe acute and chronic pain, including postoperative pain, posttraumatic pain, the pain of sickle-cell vaso-occlusive crisis, and cancer pain. Some of the more commonly used opioids are codeine, fentanyl, hydrocodone, hydromorphone, meperidine, methadone, morphine, and oxycodone.

Opioids can be administered via most routes. However, the oral route should be used when it is appropriate and the child is able to take and tolerate oral opioids. Sustained-release forms of morphine and oxycodone are available that last for 12 hours. These are supplemented with a short-acting liquid for "break-through" pain. The use of these two forms of morphine and oxycodone can help ensure longer pain-free periods

---

BOX 39-3
Aspects of Patient-Controlled Analgesia (PCA) Orders

Medication/concentration:
_____

Mode: PCA only _____ PCA and basal infusion _____
Continuous infusion only _____
Doses:
- Bolus _____ mg by RN q _____ minutes or × _____ (recommended dose is 0.05 mg/kg/dose)
- PCA bolus _____ mg (recommended starting dose is 0.02 mg/kg/dose for morphine)
- Basal rate or continuous infusion _____ (recommended starting dose is 0.02 mg/kg/hr)

Lockout: _____ minutes (usual is 6-10 min PRN)
One-hour limit: _____ mg PCA and basal rate combined (usual is 0.075 mg/kg)

Drug Guide

Ibuprofen

Classification: Nonsteroidal antiinflammatory (NSAID), analgesic.

Action: Blocks prostaglandin synthesis.

Indications: Chronic, symptomatic rheumatoid arthritis and osteoarthritis; relief of mild to moderate pain.

Dosages and Route: By mouth (PO): 5-10 mg/kg/dose q6-8h. Do not exceed 40 mg/kg/24 hr. For juvenile arthritis: 30-50 mg/kg/24 hr. Medication comes in liquid form for young children.

Absorption: 80% absorbed from gastrointestinal (GI) tract; peak action in 1-2 hr.

Excretion: Excreted primarily in urine; some biliary excretion.

Contraindications: Contraindicated in children in whom urticaria, severe rhinitis, bronchospasm, angioedema, nasal polyps are precipitated by other NSAIDs; active peptic ulcer; bleeding abnormalities.

Precautions: Hypertension, history of GI ulceration, impaired hepatic or renal function, chronic renal failure.

Adverse Reactions: Heartburn, nausea, vomiting, epigastric or abdominal discomfort or pain, GI ulceration.

Nursing Considerations: Give on an empty stomach 1 hr before or 2 hr after meals. If GI intolerance, may be taken with meals or milk. If the child is unable to swallow a tablet, administer the medication in liquid form. Non-enteric-coated ibuprofen can be crushed and mixed with a very small amount (one tablespoon) of food or liquid before swallowing.

Drug Guide

Ketorolac

Classification: Nonsteroidal antiinflammatory (NSAID), analgesic.

Action: Blocks prostaglandin synthesis.

Indications: Short-term management of moderate pain.

Dosages and Route: Children older than 2 years intravenous (IV): 0.4-1 mg/kg one time, followed by 0.2-0.5 mg/kg/dose q6h, up to a maximum of 120 mg/24 hr.

Absorption: Absorbed fairly rapidly; peak action in 1 to 2 hr.

Excretion: Excreted in the urine; effects last 4-6 hr.

Contraindications: Contraindicated in patient in whom urticaria, severe rhinitis, bronchospasm, angioedema, nasal polyps are precipitated by other NSAIDs.

Precautions: Cautious use with history of ulcers, impaired hepatic or renal function.

Adverse Reactions: Drowsiness, dizziness, nausea, GI pain, hemorrhage.

Nursing Considerations: Do not administer longer than 5 days; monitor liver function studies, signs and symptoms of GI upset or bleeding.

Drug Guide

Acetaminophen

Classification: Analgesic, antipyretic.

Action: Unknown; thought to produce analgesia by blocking generation of pain impulses.

Indications: Mild pain or fever.

Dosages and Routes: By mouth (PO) or rectal suppository (PR): 10-15 mg/kg/dose q4-6h up to a maximum of 5 doses/24 hr.

Absorption: Rapid and almost complete absorption from gastrointestinal (GI) tract; less complete absorption from rectal suppository; peak effects in 1-1½ hr.

Excretion: 90%-100% of drug excreted as metabolites in urine; excreted in breast milk; effects last 4-6 hr.

Contraindications: Hypersensitivity to acetaminophen or phenacetin; administration to patients with anemia or hepatic disease; cautious use in arthritic or rheumatoid conditions affecting children younger than 12 yr; thrombocytopenia.

Adverse Reaction: Negligible with recommended dosage; rash.

Nursing Considerations: May be crushed. Chewable tablets need to be thoroughly chewed and wetted before swallowing. With high doses or long-term therapy, periodic tests of hepatic, renal, and hematopoietic function are advised. Caution the parent about giving other medications containing acetaminophen without medical advice. No more than 5 doses in 24 hr should be given to children unless prescribed by physician. Available in infant strength (drops). Be sure to advise parents to check the strength before administering liquid acetaminophen (Tylenol) to avoid overdosing.

for children, such as those experiencing cancer pain. The short-acting liquids may also be used for children who cannot effectively swallow tablets. When the oral route is contraindicated, an IV route, a subcutaneous route, or both can be used. IV and subcutaneous opioids may be given by bolus or continuous infusion, either separately or in combination with another analgesic or sedative agent. Morphine, fentanyl, hydromorphone, methadone, and meperidine can be given IV or subcutaneously.

The nurse should remember that opioids can produce sedation and respiratory depression in addition to analgesia. Other side effects can include constipation, pruritus, nausea, vomiting, cough suppression, urinary retention, and vasodilation. Although these side effects must be closely monitored, most children can tolerate these drugs if their dosages are adjusted. It has been noted that side effects such as pruritus, nausea, and sedation are inclined to be time-limited and will resolve spontaneously within 3 to 4 days. Until that time, antiemetics and antipruritics can be used to control such side effects.

Morphine is the preferred opioid for children. It reaches its peak effect 10 to 20 minutes after IV administration and 1 hour after oral administration. It can produce sedation along with the analgesia. If it occurs, maximum respiratory depression will happen 7 minutes after IV administration. Naloxone (Narcan) should be available to reverse the sedation or respiratory depression if necessary.

Fentanyl and its analogs (sufentanil, alfentanil) have a shorter duration of action than morphine and are 50 to 100 times more potent. Because much less histamine is released, these agents may cause less vasodilation and pruritus. The short duration of effect makes IV use of these drugs appropriate when a brief, painful procedure is to be performed (e.g., bone marrow aspirate, inserting a chest tube, changing a burn dressing) and when children are critically ill. Fentanyl should be administered in a closely monitored setting. Experience with the use of the fentanyl patch (Duragesic) is limited in children. Most often, it is used in adolescents whose weight is closer to that of an adult. The fentanyl patch is indicated for chronic pain. Transdermal fentanyl, 25 mcg/hr, is approximately equal to parenteral morphine at 15 mg/24 hr or oral morphine at 90 mg/24 hr.

Hydromorphone (Dilaudid) is very similar to morphine. It is approximately six times more potent than morphine. It may be used to control pain in cancer patients. Methadone is metabolized very slowly and therefore has a prolonged duration of action. It is absorbed well after both oral and IV administration. Because of its long duration, it must be carefully titrated according to pain level (moderate, minimal alert, minimal somnolent). It is equal in potency to morphine.

Meperidine (Demerol) should be used only for short-term pain control in children who have shown an allergy or intolerance to other opioids. It has no advantages to morphine. The duration of analgesia is shorter than with morphine.

Drug Guide

Morphine

Classification: Opioid analgesic.

Action: Binds with central nervous system (CNS) opiate receptors; alters physical and emotional response to pain.

Indications: Acute and chronic pain.

Dosages and Routes: Intermittent dose. By mouth (PO) or rectal: 0.2-0.5 mg/kg/dose q4-6h. Intramuscular (IM), intravenous (IV), subcutaneous (SC): 0.1-0.2 mg/kg/dose q2-4h, up to a maximum of 15 mg/dose. Continuous IV infusion: 0.01-.04 mg/kg/hr (average 0.06 mg/kg/hr). Begin with the lowest dose; increase up to 2 mg/kg/hr as required. Patient controlled: maintenance:

0.02 mg/kg/hr; increase if child requires more than 2 bolus doses per hour. Bolus at 0.02 mg/kg/dose at intervals of at least 10 min as needed (PRN).

Absorption: Variable absorption from the gastrointestinal (GI) tract; peak action 60 min PO, 20 min IV.

Excretion: Excreted primarily in the urine; 7%-10% excreted in bile. Effects last up to 7 hr.

Contraindications: Hypersensitivity to opioids, increased intracranial pressure, seizure disorders, chronic pulmonary disease, respiratory depression.

Precautions: Cautious use with cardiac dysrhythmias, reduced blood volume.

Adverse Reactions: Sedation, dizziness, euphoria, paradoxic CNS excitation, respiratory depression, hypotension, bradycardia, nausea, vomiting, constipation, urinary retention.

Nursing Considerations: Carefully and frequently assess respiratory status. Assess cough reflex; monitor intake and output (I&O) carefully for urinary retention and constipation.

Drug Guide

Fentanyl

Classification: Opioid analgesic.

Action: Narcotic agonist with actions similar to morphine and meperidine, but action is faster and less prolonged.

Indications: Moderate to severe pain, particularly for brief procedures or when children are critically ill or high risk. Transdermal fentanyl is for severe chronic pain only; experience with children is very limited.

Dosages and Routes: Intramuscular (IM) and intravenous (IV) intermittent doses: 1-2 mcg/kg/dose q30-60 min. IV patient-

controlled: maintenance 1 mcg/kg/hr continuous infusion, increased if the patient requires more than 2 bolus doses per hour. Bolus: 0.1-0.4 mcg/kg/dose at intervals of at least 5 min. Transdermal patch used only in children older than 12 years.

Absorption: Absorbed rapidly after IV administration, 6-8 hr transdermally.

Excretion: Excreted in the urine. Lasts 30-60 min IV; 72 hr transdermally.

Contraindication: Patients who have received monoamine oxidase (MAO) inhibitors within 14 days.

Precautions: Use cautiously in children with head injuries, increased intracranial pressure, respiratory problems, liver and kidney dysfunction.

Adverse Reactions: Sedation, dizziness, euphoria, seizures with high doses. Hypotension, bradycardia, circulatory depression, respiratory depression, bronchoconstriction.

Nursing Considerations: Watch carefully for signs and symptoms of respiratory distress, depression; have O_2, resuscitative equipment, and naloxone available.

Normeperidine, a metabolite of meperidine, has been associated with convulsions and dysphoria after as few as two doses. In addition, it has been shown to cause hallucinations and agitation. Meperidine is used minimally; it is most often used postoperatively and in combination with other medications for procedural pain.

The use of meperidine (Demerol), promethazine (Phenergan), and chlorpromazine (Thorazine), known as *DPT* (or "pediatric cocktail"), is discouraged. This combination is thought to be outdated and can cause significant adverse effects, including respiratory arrest, prolonged sedation, and decreased oxygen saturation (AAP, 1995). A combination of opioids and benzodiazepines is much safer.

Codeine is the most commonly given oral opioid for moderate pain. It is usually given in combination with acetaminophen or aspirin. It can cause constipation, nausea, vomiting, and pruritus. Oxycodone and hydrocodone have side effects similar to those with codeine and are given in combination with acetaminophen. However, oxycodone also comes as a sustained-release tablet and immediate-release solution.

Conscious Sedation   MRI, piccline, central line, radiology

Conscious sedation is a medically controlled state of depressed consciousness that allows protective reflexes to be maintained, retains the child's ability to continuously maintain a patent airway independently, and permits appropriate response to physical stimulation or verbal command (AAP, 2002). It generally is achieved using an amnesic, sedative, or both administered IV. With conscious sedation, children usually have little or no recollection of the procedure they have undergone.

Midazolam (Versed) is a short-acting drug that can be given by multiple routes—IV, intranasal, rectal, IM, oral, or sublingual. It can be used for conscious sedation as well as preoperative sedation and as an induction agent for general anesthesia. Advantages to using midazolam include minimal side effects, short duration of sedation, and ability to administer without an IV access. It may be used alone or in combination with other medications used for conscious sedation, including ketamine, fentanyl, and propofol. During and after conscious sedation, the child's vital signs, oxygen saturation, and level of consciousness should be closely monitored.

Drug Guide

Meperidine Hydrochloride

Classification: Opioid analgesic.

Action: Synthetic morphine-like compound.

Indications: Moderate to severe pain.

Dosage and Routes: By mouth (PO), intramuscular (IM), subcutaneous (SC) or intravenous (IV): 1-1.5 mg/kg/dose q3-4h; maximum dose 100 mg.

Absorption: 50%-60% from gastrointestinal (GI) tract, peak action in 1 hr, 30-50 min IM, 5-7 min IV.

Excretion: Excreted in the urine; effects last 2-4 hr.

Contraindications: Seizure disorders, acute abdominal conditions before diagnosis, MAO inhibitors.

Precautions: Cautious use in head injuries, increased intracranial pressure, asthma and other respiratory conditions. Impaired renal or hepatic function.

Adverse Reactions: Pruritus, dizziness, sedation, euphoria, respiratory depression, seizures, hypotension, bradycardia.

Nursing Considerations: Assess respiratory status carefully; abrupt discontinuation may result in morphine-like withdrawal symptoms.

Drug Guide

Codeine

Classification: Opioid analgesic.

Action: Binds with opiate receptors in the central nervous system (CNS); alters both perception of and emotional response to pain.

Indications: Mild to moderate pain.

Dosage and Routes: By mouth (PO), intramuscular (IM), subcutaneous (SC): 0.5-1 mg/kg/dose q4-6h; maximum dose 60 mg/dose.

Absorption: Readily absorbed from gastrointestinal (GI) tract, with peak action in 1-1½ hr.

Distribution: Crosses placenta; distributed into breast milk.

Excretion: Effects last approximately 4-6 hr; excreted in urine.

Contraindications: Hypersensitivity to codeine or other morphine derivatives; hepatic or renal dysfunction.

Precaution: Use cautiously in very young children.

Adverse Reactions: Primarily with CNS symptoms: dizziness, lightheadedness, drowsiness, sedation, lethargy, euphoria, agitation, restlessness, respiratory depression; GI: nausea, vomiting, constipation; genitourinary (GU): urinary retention.

Nursing Considerations: To reduce possibility of GI upset, administer PO codeine with milk or other food. Because dizziness and lightheadedness may occur, supervision of ambulation and other safety precautions may be necessary. Nausea is a common side effect; report if this is accompanied by vomiting. Change to another analgesic may be necessary.

Epidural Analgesia

Pain medication (usually an opioid, a local anesthetic, or both) can be administered through an epidural catheter inserted into the epidural space and secured to the child's back with an occlusive dressing. This form of administration is most useful for children undergoing abdominal, thoracic, and major orthopedic surgeries. Because the medication is administered directly to the nerves that transmit pain, smaller doses are required for pain control, with fewer side effects than usually associated with opioid administration.

Nursing care of the child with an epidural catheter is similar to that for a child receiving PCA therapy. The nurse monitors the child for adequate pain relief and the presence of undesired side effects (particularly decreased respirations), as well as for the complications that might accompany the catheter. The nurse avoids any action that would pull or place tension on the catheter. The nurse also monitors the catheter site frequently for slippage, bleeding, loss of cerebrospinal fluid, or a hematoma at the insertion site—a rare but serious complication that needs to be reported immediately. Other side effects include constipation, nausea, vomiting, urinary retention, motor block, and sensory block.

! CRITICAL TO REMEMBER

Administering Analgesics to Children

- The preferred route of administering analgesics to children is oral or intravenous (IV).
- Infants and children receiving IV and epidural opioids should be monitored by pulse oximetry.
- If respiratory depression occurs with opioid use, naloxone hydrochloride should be used for reversal if oxygen and stimulation of the child are ineffective.

Nursing Care Plan

The Child in Pain

FOCUSED ASSESSMENT

Regardless of setting (inpatient, clinic, home), the nursing assessment for the child in pain begins in the same way if the child is verbal. The child is questioned to determine what word or words are used for pain. Then the parents are questioned as to cultural or spiritual beliefs or practices that might have an impact on pain issues. The nurse should remember that parents are to be used as the first resource to help assess the child and the child's response to intervention. Then a pain history is taken from child and parent, including physical, emotional, and psychosocial factors that might affect the child in regard to pain.

The current pain is assessed as to onset, duration, location, intensity, and quality. An age-appropriate pain tool is used to assess the intensity of pain. The same tool is used consistently, and it becomes a part of the child's chart as a future reference. Behavioral and physiologic changes are noted also. If the child is preverbal or nonverbal, a behavioral assessment is completed along with use of an assessment tool designed for nonverbal children. Response to the interventions, pharmacologic and non-pharmacologic, is assessed again using pain tools, parents' input, and observation of behavioral and physiologic data.

Nursing Diagnosis

Acute Pain related to physical or biologic factors: edema, disease process, infection, invasive procedure, surgery, trauma.

Expected Outcomes

The child will:
- Experience a decrease in pain to an acceptable level, as evidenced by reduced pain level on an assessment tool, as well as a relaxed body posture and decreased crying, fussiness, restlessness, and facial grimacing.
- Return to the activity level experienced before the onset of pain.

INTERVENTION	RATIONALE
1. Observe and document behavioral and physiologic signs of pain in the child. Note both verbal and nonverbal responses. Assess vital signs.	1. Assessment of pain in children is based on behavioral and physiologic changes. Children may have difficulty verbalizing pain. The nurse will have to depend on behavioral changes alone to assess infants and other children who are nonverbal or unable to communicate clearly. Physiologic changes vary in response to pain and should be evaluated together with a behavioral assessment.
2. Assess for other factors that might be affecting the child: separation, fear, anxiety, loss of control, as well as spiritual or cultural beliefs regarding pain.	2. The child's perception of pain and ultimate reaction to pain may be influenced by other factors.
3. Monitor pain based on the child's developmental stage.	3. Infants and children at each developmental level have their own unique way of reacting to and coping with pain.
4. Use a developmentally appropriate pain assessment tool. The tool should be a part of the child's chart for easy reference.	4. Infants and children may have difficulty communicating about their pain. Assessment tools provide more consistent, objective, and quantitative information.
5. Question the child if possible to assess the onset, duration, location, and type of pain and what type of pain-relief measures works best.	5. Such factors will influence the choice of analgesic.
6. Note if the child's pain level is different when at rest, ambulating, playing, or during procedures.	6. Pain-relief measures can be improved by a thorough understanding of cause and effect.

Continued

Nursing Care Plan

The Child in Pain—cont'd

INTERVENTION	RATIONALE
7. Implement non-pharmacologic pain reduction strategies:	7. Non-pharmacologic pain management strategies can enhance pharmacologic measures and should be implemented before administering analgesics:
a. Distraction	a. Distraction interrupts the transmission of pain.
b. Relaxation techniques	b. Relaxation is also thought to interrupt pain.
c. Cutaneous stimulation, such as massage or warm or cold compresses	c. Cutaneous stimulation blocks pain transmission.
d. Quiet, calm environment	d. A quiet, calm environment is more conducive to rest and sleep, which enhance the effects of analgesia.
e. Repositioning	e. A change in position may relieve pressure or provide for a more relaxed, comfortable body.
f. Decreased environmental noise and light	f. A quiet, comfortable environment can have a soothing, relaxing effect on the child and parent.
g. Comfort measures (touch, holding, rocking)	g. Comfort measures can be provided by parents and decrease anxiety and the skeletal muscle tension that often accompanies pain.
8. Administer the appropriate analgesic. Give by oral or intravenous (IV) route. Avoid injections.	8. Non-narcotic analgesics are appropriate for mild to moderate pain. Narcotic analgesics should be given for moderate to severe pain. Children fear injections and may deny pain to avoid an injection.
9. Involve parents in care.	9. The presence of parents may reduce fear and anxiety and thus reduce the amount of pain experienced. Parents also know their child best and can assist in the assessment of pain and its management.
10. Record the response to both pharmacologic and non-pharmacologic pain reduction measures.	10. Documentation aids in determining the effectiveness of pain-relief measures as well as continuity in the management of pain.
11. Observe for side effects of medication.	11. Respiratory depression is the most serious side effect of opioids but is rare. Other side effects include sedation, nausea and vomiting, and constipation.

Evaluation

■ Does the child demonstrate decreased pain?
■ Has the child been able to return to the level of activity seen before the onset of pain?

KEY CONCEPTS

■ Pain is "an unpleasant sensory and emotional experience associated with actual or potential tissue damage or described in terms of such damage" (International Association for the Study of Pain, 1979).

■ The gate-control theory of pain postulates that gating mechanisms at the level of the dorsal horn can facilitate or inhibit pain transmission. The theory further states that stimulation of the larger afferent nerves, which carry benign sensations, can dull pain.

■ Two of the myths that interfere the most with the provision of adequate pain-relief medica-tion to infants and children are the fear of addiction and the fear of respiratory depression. Neither belief is supported by research.

■ Pain assessment in infants and children takes a multidimensional approach. The child and parent should be questioned, and behavioral and physiologic changes should be noted.

■ Both pharmacologic and non-pharmacologic measures should be used in the treatment of pain in children. Acetaminophen is used for mild to moderate pain and morphine is the opioid of choice for severe pain. Non-pharmacologic interventions include biofeedback, breathing techniques, distraction, guided imagery, hypnosis, progressive muscle relaxation, and TENS.

■ A pain assessment tool should be used for each child to effectively assess, implement, and document pain management. The tool should be developmentally correct for the child and must be used according to instructions for the results to be valid.

ANSWERS to Critical Thinking Exercise 39-1

1. An assessment to determine objective and subjective data should be performed. You will be looking for both behavioral (crying, facial expression, motor responses) and physiologic cues. When Tanika cries, describe the crying and duration. Note whether holding and cuddling can quiet her. If not, her behavior could be an indication of discomfort. Obtain current vital signs, and compare them with earlier signs. One clue from the nurse giving the report was that Tanika is not having periods of *uninterrupted* sleep. This information, together with the vital signs, type of surgery, and postoperative day, strongly indicates that Tanika should be medicated for pain. After completing the assessment, a review of the chart will determine patterns and a nursing judgment can be made. It should also be confirmed through documentation that pain medication was not given during the previous shift.

2. Research has shown that neonates do experience pain. Because they are preverbal, pain assessment is based on physiologic and behavioral responses. Physiologic and behavioral changes, plus an understanding of the type of surgery and postoperative day, are all valid indicators of pain in infants of this age.

REFERENCES and READINGS

Agency for Health Care Policy and Research, Acute Pain Management Guideline Panel. (1992a). *Acute pain management in infants, children, and adolescents: Operative and medical procedures. Quick reference guide for clinicians* (AHCPR Publication No. 92-0020). Rockville, MD: Public Health Service, U.S. Department of Health and Human Services.

Agency for Health Care Policy and Research, Acute Pain Management Guideline Panel. (1992b). *Acute pain management: Operative or medical procedures and trauma. Clinical practice guideline* (AHCPR Publication No. 92-0032). Rockville, MD: Public Health Service, U.S. Department of Health and Human Services.

American Academy of Pediatrics, Committee on Drugs. (1995). Reappraisal of lytic cocktail/Demerol, Phenergan and Thorazine (DPT) for the sedation of children. *Pediatrics, 95*(4), 598-602.

American Academy of Pediatrics, Committee on Drugs. (2002). Guidelines for monitoring and management of pediatric patients during and after sedation for diagnostic therapeutic procedures. *Pediatrics, 110*(4), 836-838.

American Academy of Pediatrics, Committee on Psychosocial Aspects of Child and Family Health, & American Pain Society. (2001). The assessment and management of acute pain in infants, children and adolescents. *Pediatrics 108*(3), 793-797.

American Pain Society. (1999a). *Guidelines for the management of acute and chronic pain in sickle cell disease.* Glenview, IL: American Pain Society.

American Pain Society. (1999b). *Principles of analgesic use in the treatment of acute pain and cancer pain* (4th ed.). Glenview, IL: American Pain Society.

Anand, K., & Hickey, P. (1987). Pain and its effects in the human neonate and fetus. *New England Journal of Medicine, 317*(21), 1321-1347.

Annequin, D., Tourniaire, B., & Massiou, H. (2000). Migraine and headache in childhood and adolescence. *Pediatric Clinics of North America, 47*(3), 617-632.

Beyer, J. (1984). *The Oucher: A user's manual and technical report.* Evanston, IL: Judson Press.

Beyer, J. (1989). *The Oucher: A user's manual and technical report.* Denver: University of Colorado Health Sciences Center.

Beyer, J., & Aradine, C. (1986). Content validity of an instrument to measure young children's perceptions of the intensity of their pain. *Journal of Pediatric Nursing, 1*(6), 386-395.

Beyer, J., Denyes, M., & Villarruel, A. (1992). The creation, validation, and continuing development of the Oucher: A measure of pain intensity in children. *Journal of Pediatric Nursing, 7*(5), 335-346.

Beyer, J.E., & Knott, C.B. (1998). Construct validity estimation for the African-American and Hispanic versions of the Oucher Scale. *Journal of Pediatric Nursing, 13*(1), 20-31.

Bishop-Kurylo, D. (2002). Pediatric pain management in the emergency department. *Topics in Emergency Medicine, 24*(1), 19-30.

Carlson, K.L., Broome, M., & Vessey, J.A. (2000). Using distraction to reduce reported pain, fear, and behavioral distress in children and adolescents: A multisite study. *Journal of the Society of Pediatric Nurses: JSPN, 5*(2), 75-85.

Chen, E., Joseph, M.H., & Zeltzer, L.K. (2000). Behavioral and cognitive interventions in the treatment of pain in children. *Pediatric Clinics of North America, 47*(3), 513-525.

Children's Hospital, Boston. (2002). *Reference tool: Pain assessment tools.* Boston, MA: Author.

Clark, L.M., & Manworren, R.C.B. (2001). Product alert. Immunizations: Could they hurt less? *Journal of Pediatric Health Care, 15*(6), 322-323.

Collins, J.J., Dunkel, I.J., Gupta, S.K., Inturrisi, C.E., Lapin, J., Palmer, L.N., Weinstein, S.M., & Portenoy, R.K. (1999). Transdermal fentanyl in children with cancer pain: Feasibility, tolerability and pharmacokinetic correlates. *Journal of Pediatrics, 134,* 319-323.

Craig, K.D. (1998). The facial display of pain in infants and children. *Pain Research and Management, 10,* 103-121.

Cravero, J.P., Manzi, D.J., & Rice, L.J. (1998). The management of procedure-related pain in the child. In M.A. Ashburn & L.J. Rice (Eds.), *The management of pain* (pp. 667-681). Philadelphia: Saunders.

Ely, B. (2001). Pediatric nurses' pain management practices: Barriers to change. *Pediatric Nursing (27)*5, 473-480.

Franck, L.S., Greenberg, C.S., & Stevens, B. (2000). Pain assessment in infants and children. *Pediatric Clinics of North America, 47*(3), 487-512.

Golianu, B., Krane, E.J., Galloway, K.S., & Yaster, M. (2000). Pediatric acute pain management. *Pediatric Clinics of North America, 47*(3), 559-587.

Grunau, R., Johnston, C., & Craig, K. (1990). Neonatal facial and cry responses to invasive and non-invasive procedures. *Pain, 42,* 295-305.

Gun, V., & Nechyba, C. (Eds.). (2002). *The Harriet Lane handbook* (16th ed.). St. Louis: Mosby.

Hamrin, V. (2002). Psychiatric assessment and treatment of pediatric pain. *Journal of Child and Adolescent Psychiatric Nursing, 15*(3), 106-114.

Henderson, C.W. (February 10, 2001). Techniques to help minimize children's suffering. *Pain and Central Nervous System Week,* 16-23.

Henry, D.B., & Foster, R. (2000). Burn pain management in children. *Pediatric Clinics of North America, 47*(3), 681-698.

Hester, N.O. (1979). The preoperational child's reaction to immunization. *Nursing Research, 4*(28), 250-254.

Hester, N.O., & Barcus, C.S. (1986). Assessment and management of pain in children. *Pediatrics: Nursing Update, 1,* 2-8.

Hodgson, B., & Kizior, R. (2004). *Saunders nursing drug handbook 2004.* Philadelphia: Saunders.

Hooke C., Hellsten, M.B., Stutzer, C., and Forte, K. (2002). Pain management for the child with cancer in end-of-life care: APON position paper. *Journal of Pediatric Oncology Nursing, 19*(2), 43-47.

International Association for the Study of Pain. (1979). Pain terms: A list with definitions and notes on usage. *Pain, 6,* 249.

Jacob, E., & Puntillo, K.A. (1999). A survey of nursing practice in the assessment and management of pain in children. *Pediatric Nursing, 25*(3), 278-286.

Joint Commission on Accreditation of Healthcare Organizations. *Pain standards for 2001.* Retrieved Dec. 19, 2003, from www.jcaho.gov.

Jones, C. (1997). Hypnosis and spinal fusion by Harrington rod instrumentation. *American Journal of Clinical Hypnosis, 19,* 155-157.

Joyce, B.A., Keck, J.F., & Gerkensmeyer, J. (2001). Evaluation of pain management interventions for neonatal circumcision pain. *Journal of Pediatric Health Care, 15*(3), 105-114.

Lambert, S.A. (1996). The effects of hypnosis/guided imagery on the post-operative course of children. *Developmental and Behavioral Pediatrics, 17,* 307-310.

Lewin, D.S., & Dahl, R.E. (1999). Importance of sleep in the management of pediatric pain. *Journal of Developmental and Behavioral Pediatrics, 20*(4), 244-252.

REFERENCES and READINGS

Liossi, C. (1999). Management of pediatric procedure-related cancer pain. *Pain Reviews, 6*(4), 279-302.

Liossi, C., & Hatira, P. (1999). Clinical hypnosis versus cognitive behavioral training for pain management in pediatric cancer patients undergoing bone marrow aspirations. *International Journal of Clinical and Experimental Hypnosis, 47*(2), 104-116.

Manworren, R.C.B. (2001). Pediatric nurses' knowledge and attitudes survey regarding pain. *Pediatric Nursing, 26*(6), 610-614.

McCaffery, M., & Pasero, C. (1999). *Pain clinical manual* (2nd ed.). St. Louis: Mosby.

Merkel, S., Voepel-Lewis, T., & Malviya, S. (2002). Pain assessment in infants and young children: The FLACC scale: A behavioral tool to measure pain in young children. *American Journal of Nursing, 102*(10), 55-58.

Mills, N. (1989). Pain behaviors in infants and toddlers. *Journal of Pain and Symptom Management, 4*, 184-190.

Ornstein, P.A., Manning, E.L., & Pelphrey, K.A. (1999). Children's memory for pain. *Journal of Developmental and Behavioral Pediatrics, 20*(4), 262-277.

Pietila, A., & Polkki, T. (2003). Hospitalized children's descriptions of their experiences with post-surgical pain relieving methods. *International Journal of Nursing Studies, 40*(1), 33-44.

Polkki, T. (2002). Nurses' perceptions of parental guidance in pediatric surgical pain relief. *International Journal of Nursing Studies, 39*(3), 319-327.

Rawlings, D., Miller, P., & Engel, R. (1980). The effect of circumcision on transcutaneous PO_2 in term infants. *American Journal of Diseases of Children, 134*, 676-678.

Rusy, L.M., & Weisman, S.J. (2000). Complementary therapies for acute pediatric pain management. *Pediatric Clinics of North America, 47*(3), 589-599.

Brent, A.S. (2000). The management of pain in the emergency department. *Pediatric Clinics of North America, 47*(3), 651-680.

Savedra, M.C., Holzemer, W.L., Tesler, M.D., & Wilkie, D.J. (1993). Assessment of postoperative pain in children and adolescents using the Adolescent Pediatric Pain Tool. *Nursing Research, 42*(1), 5-9.

Savedra, M.C., Tesler, M.D., Holzemer, W.L., & Ward, J. (1992). *Adolescent and pediatric pain tool: User's manual.* San Francisco: University of California, San Francisco, School of Nursing.

Savedra, M.C., Tesler, M.D., Holzemer, W.L., Wilkie, D.J., & Ward, J. (1989). Pain location: Validity and reliability of body outline markings by hospitalized children and adolescents. *Research in Nursing and Health, 12*, 307-314.

Savedra, M.C., Tesler, M.D., & Wegner, C. (1988). How adolescents describe pain. *Journal of Adolescent Health Care, 9*(4), 315-320.

Schechter, N.L. (1988). An approach to the child with pain. *Patient Care, 3*, 116-131.

Schechter, N.L. (1997). The status of pediatric pain control. *Child & Adolescent Psychiatric Clinics of North America, 6*(4), 687-702.

Spagrud, L., Piira, T., & Von Baeyer, C. (2003). Children's self-report of pain intensity. *American Journal of Nursing, 103*(12), 62-64.

Stevens, B., Gibbins, S., & Franck, L.S. (2000). Treatment of pain in the neonatal intensive care unit. *Pediatric Clinics of North America, 47*(3), 633-650.

White, K., Coyne, P., & Patel, U. (2001). Are nurses adequately prepared for end-of-life care? *Journal of Nursing Scholarship, 33*(2), 147-151.

Wilder, R.T. (2000). Local anesthetics for the pediatric patient. *Pediatric Clinics of North America, 47*(3), 545-558.

Willis, M., Merkel, S., Voepel-Lewis, T., & Malviya, S. (2003). FLACC behavioral assessment scale: A comparison with the child's self-report. *Pediatric Nursing, 29*(3), 195-199.

Wong, D.L., Hockenberry-Eaton, M., Wilson, D., Ahmann, E., & DiVito-Thomas, P.A. (1999). *Whaley & Wong's nursing care of infants and children.* St. Louis: Mosby.

Wong, D.L., Hockenberry-Eaton, M., Wilson, D., Winkelstein, M.L., & Schwartz, P. (2001). *Essentials of pediatric nursing* (6th ed.). St. Louis: Mosby.

World Health Organization (WHO) Expert Committee. (1998). *Cancer pain relief and palliative care in children.* Geneva, Switzerland: World Health Organization.

Yaster, M., Kost-Byerly, S., & Maxwell, L.G. (2000). The management of sickle cell disease. *Pediatric Clinics of North America, 47*(3), 711-746.

40

The Child with an Infectious Disease

1011

REVIEW OF DISEASE TRANSMISSION

Microorganisms exist throughout the environment. Most are harmless residents—a normal part of human flora. An organism that invades body tissue, causing tissue damage and disease, however, is a pathogen. For pathogens to invade a host, they must breach the normal host defenses, either by attaching to or penetrating the host. The power of these pathogens, known as their *virulence*, depends on their ability to overcome the host defense mechanisms. Thus a highly virulent organism can cause disease with relative ease.

Microorganisms can have one of several relationships with the host: *commensalism, mutualism,* or *parasitism.* Those that cause infectious disease are classified into five types: bacteria, viruses and rickettsiae, fungi, protozoa, and helminths.

Exogenous pathogens are transmitted from outside the body to the host by various mechanisms. Exogenous organisms exist in contaminated air, food, water, and body fluids and on objects contaminated by these substances. *Endogenous pathogens* are found within the human body. Microorganisms (normal flora) exist on the skin and in the nose, mouth, gastrointestinal tract, and urogenital tract. For example, *Staphylococcus epidermidis* inhabits the skin, and *Escherichia coli* is found in the intestines. These microorganisms are beneficial and play an important role in the body's defenses. They help prevent virulent pathogens from colonizing by maintaining an acidic pH environment to discourage pathogen attachment, by taking up epithelial space to prevent growth of pathogens, and by stimulating the immune system. However, situations may arise where these normally benign organisms become virulent and harmful to the host.

Chain of Infection

For a pathogen to maintain its infectious state, it must be transmitted to another host. Certain factors and conditions must be present for a disease (infection) to begin. These components and their relationships are often referred to as a *chain of infection.* The major variables in the chain of infection include the agent (organism), reservoir (environment in which the agent exists and multiplies), portal of exit (route by which the agent leaves the host), transmission mode, portal of entry (route by which the agent enters the new host), and host susceptibility (internal and external environmental factors that increase or decrease the likelihood the host will develop disease). Changes in any one variable result in a change in the presence, intensity, and frequency of the entire infectious disease process.

Microorganisms and Host Relationships

Commensalism: Host provides shelter and food for the organism; organism retains the ability to exist independently (e.g., nonpathogenic bacteria living in human intestines).
Mutualism: Host provides shelter and food for the organism; both benefit.
Parasitism: Host provides shelter and food; the parasite benefits, but the host may be harmed (e.g., a tapeworm living at the expense of its human host).

Transmission of Pathogens

Infection transmission occurs through several modes, or routes. For example, pathogens from the respiratory tract are shed through sneezing, coughing, and talking. If the pathogens survive in the air, they can infect others who inhale them *(airborne route).* Because this mode of transmission is relatively uncontrollable, infections can easily be spread in crowded conditions.

Pathogens may also be shed through fecal matter. When personal hygiene is poor and handwashing is not routinely practiced, pathogens have ample opportunities to enter through the mouth *(fecal-oral transmission).* Unclean hands can also contaminate food, which is then ingested.

In the urogenital tract, pathogenic transmission does not generally occur through infected urine. Rather, sexual activity involving direct mucosal contact is the most common means of transmission of sexually transmissible diseases (STDs) *(direct contact transmission).* If the mother's birth canal is infected, newborn infants can be infected by direct contact during birth. Saliva is another avenue of transmission, as is direct contact with infected skin. Pathogens can also be present in breast milk and can infect a nursing infant.

A tick, mosquito, mite, or animal can inject pathogens into the skin and blood of the host. Organisms carried in this way are considered to be *vector-borne.* For example, a certain species of mosquito carries the malaria parasite; likewise, certain bats carry the rabies microorganism.

Contamination by blood of an infected host can occur through transfusions, blood products, and the use of contaminated needles *(direct inoculation).* A pregnant woman can transmit such pathogens through the placenta. There can be other modes of transmission, such as through spores found in soil (tetanus).

Epidemiologic Investigations

Epidemiology is the study of the distribution of health and illness within a population and the factors that determine the population's health status. Recently, epidemiologic efforts have focused on identifying health-promoting factors, not just disease prevention (Clark & Spector, 2000). Nurses may not realize they are contributing to this process when they gather patient history information as part of the nursing assessment process. The data nurses collect help the entire health care team not only to identify, treat, and prevent disease processes but also to promote health. Moreover, the specific steps of the epidemiologic process mirror the steps in the nursing process and include defining the condition; determining the condition's natural history; identifying critical control points; and designing, implementing, and evaluating control strategies.

INFECTION AND HOST DEFENSES

The first stage of *infection* begins with *colonization* of the host by the pathogen. Microorganisms invade either by adhering to tissues or by invading cells. Initially, replication of the pathogen does not cause tissue damage and colonization can occur without development of a clinical infection. As the host "recognizes" the invasion, the defense system—the immune response—is activated. The two components of the immune response are the innate, nonspecific immune re-

TRANSMISSION OF PATHOGENS

Direct   **Indirect**

Droplets

Saliva

Blood

Urogenital   Fecal   Objects

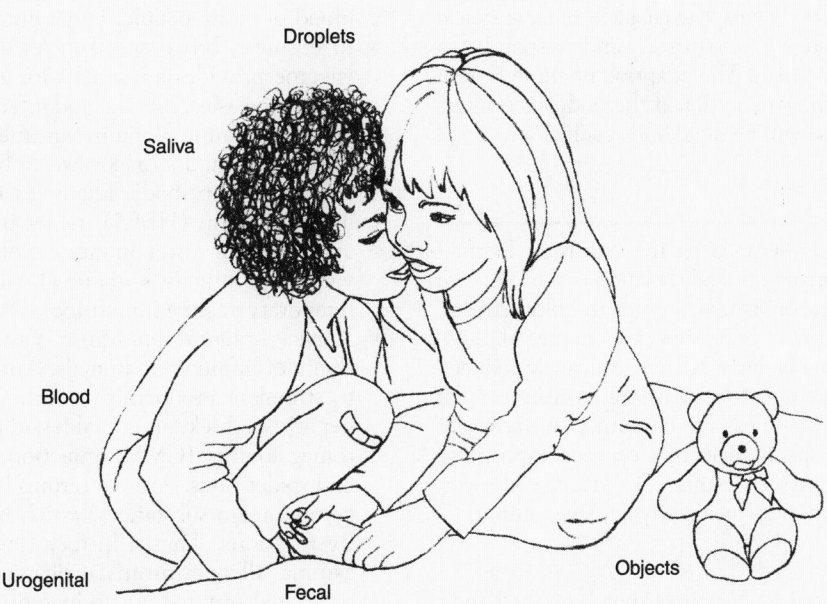

Animal/Insect

Animals with pathogens

Bites   Scratches

Feces

sponse and the adaptive, specific immune response: cell mediated and humoral (see Chapter 41).

The first lines of defense in the innate immune system are the skin and intact mucous membranes. The skin serves as a barrier, preventing colonization of most pathogens. The acid secreted in sweat and by sebaceous glands inhibits pathogenic invasion. Smooth muscle contraction and ciliary actions, such as those seen in bladder and bowel emptying and coughing and sneezing, provide for mechanical removal of pathogens. Physical and chemical barriers are provided by mucus production by goblet cells in mucous membranes. Nevertheless, the innate system may be unable to prevent the invasion. *Phagocytosis*, the process by which phagocytic cells digest and thereby destroy foreign microorganisms, can be overwhelmed. Large numbers of pathogens or their *toxins* can inhibit phagocytosis. When this process occurs, the *adaptive immune system* is activated. This system "recognizes" and responds to pathogens by destroying them. The adaptive immune system "imprints" on these pathogens so that if the body encounters them again, the response will be rapid and specific.

IMMUNITY

Immunity is the body's resistance to the effects of harmful agents. It occurs as an antigen-antibody reaction that takes place whenever a foreign agent or its toxins enter the bloodstream. Immunity can be either active or passive (see Chapter 41).

Some childhood diseases have been significantly reduced and some nearly eliminated through the administration of vaccines producing active or passive immunity. A variety of preparations of disease-specific vaccines can accomplish active or passive immunity (see Chapter 4). Vaccines also can produce artificially active or artificially passive immunity. These include:

- *Live or attenuated vaccines:* Vaccines that have had their virulence (potency) diminished so as not to produce a full-blown clinical illness. In response to vaccination, the body produces antibodies and causes immunity to be established. An example is the measles vaccine.
- *Killed or inactivated vaccines:* Vaccines that contain pathogens made inactive by either chemicals or heat. These vaccines, which are noninfectious, cause the body to produce antibodies. Their disadvantage is that they elicit a limited immune response from the body; therefore several doses are required. Examples include the Salk polio, rabies, and pertussis vaccines.
- *Toxoids:* Bacterial toxins that have been made inactive by either chemicals or heat. The toxins cause the body to produce antibodies. Examples include the diphtheria and tetanus vaccines.
- *Human immune globulin:* A vaccine made from the pooled blood of many people. Large numbers of donors are used to ensure a broad spectrum of antibodies. This type of vaccine provides antibodies for a variety of diseases, including measles, rubella, and infectious hepatitis. Disease-specific immune globulin vaccines are also available and obtained from donors known to have high blood titers of the desired antibody. Examples include hepatitis B immune globulin (HBIG), rabies immune globulin (RIG), and varicella-zoster immune globulin (VZIG). A disadvantage of human immune globulin is that it offers only temporary passive immunity.
- *Animal serums (antitoxins):* Vaccines derived from the serum of immunized animals. Antitoxin vaccines are used to stimulate production of antibodies. Examples include hepatitis, chickenpox, rabies, diphtheria, smallpox, cytomegalovirus (CMV) infection, botulism, snake bites, and spider bites. Animal serums have the disadvantage of being foreign substances, which may cause hypersensitivity reactions. Thus a history (including questions about asthma, allergic rhinitis, urticaria, and previous injections of animal serums) and skin sensitivity testing should always precede vaccine administration.

Infectious diseases are a major reason health care is sought for infants and children. Although most infections are not life-threatening, fatal complications can develop. The infant or child with an immature or compromised immune system is at increased risk for developing life-threatening complications. Moreover, a child's illness directly affects the family and caregivers. Absence from work for the parent of a sick child can threaten job security, and the accompanying missed income can be devastating for both single- and two-income families.

Nurses play a major role in preventing pediatric infectious diseases and decreasing the incidence of disability and death in both community and hospital settings. Regardless of their clinical setting, nurses must be able to confidently recognize the sometimes subtle signs and symptoms of infectious diseases in children and initiate appropriate treatment and nursing care. Nurses must also provide education about accessing appropriate community resources and limiting exposure of other children and community members. For example, in the community-based setting, the consequences of an unrecognized case of meningococcemia can be devastating and deadly. In the hospital setting, relatively mild diseases, such as chickenpox, may pose potentially fatal problems for the immunosuppressed child.

In addition, because of the growing number of uninsured and underserved children in the United States, nurses may well be the first and sometimes the only health care professionals to evaluate and treat children in community-based settings. School nurses are frequently required to notify parents and caregivers when their children have been exposed to infectious diseases. Figure 40-1 illustrates an example of a notification letter from a school nurse written to inform parents and caregivers about an exposure to fifth disease. Regardless of the particular type of infection, underlying principles of nursing care are similar.

VIRAL INFECTIONS

Viruses are small parasitic organisms with unique characteristics that cause them to be very different from other organisms. They contain only one type of nucleic acid—either deoxyribonucleic acid (DNA) or ribonucleic acid (RNA)—that prevents them from reproducing on their own. Instead, a host cell is needed to allow the virus to replicate.

The replication process begins with the virus first attaching itself to a host cell. After the initial attachment, a virus must invade the interior of the cell. Replication of the virus's nucleic material begins after the envelope and capsule (capsid) are shed and the nucleic material of the virus is released into the cell; the host cell then assists in the formation of the necessary nucleic material. New capsules are then formed and released into the host's cells. The infected host cell can respond to the viral invasion by cell death (lysis) and destruction, or the infected cells can remain alive and continue to function while new viral particles are slowly released. This slow release occurs in an asymptomatic person who is a carrier of the virus. Some viruses are selective about the cells to which they attach. For example, the human immunodeficiency virus (HIV) prefers to attach to the T cell.

A virus can also invade a host and remain dormant until a trigger stimulates the virus to begin replicating. Many triggering factors are not fully understood. However, some triggers have been identified. An example of this triggering effect is the effect of stress in herpes simplex (a viral disease) resulting in the formation of cold sores.

Nursing Considerations for the Child With a Viral Exanthem Infection

An *exanthem* is an eruption or rash on the skin. Several childhood infectious diseases are characterized by rashes with distinctive characteristics. Nurses need to be aware that rashes have more than one characteristic and obtain a detailed history of the characteristics of the rash, including its onset, initial location, and progression as well as any associated physical signs or symptoms. Specific characteristics of the rash should be documented, including color, elevation, pattern or shape, size (in centimeters), location and distribution on the body, and any drainage. Vital signs, including temperature, should be taken and recorded. Also record the child's general state of health, any recent exposures to illnesses, and any prescribed or over-the-counter medications and treatments taken and their results. The child's eyes, ears, nose, and throat should be examined for signs of inflammation, swelling, and secretions. Auscultate the lungs for any abnormal sounds, and palpate the child's spleen, liver, and lymph nodes, documenting any enlargement or tenderness.

Children with typical uncomplicated viral exanthems are usually cared for at home. Hospitalization is indicated when there are complications. High-risk (immunosuppressed) children and children with an infectious disease should not be cared for by the same nurse, to prevent any possible cross transmission by the nurse.

Whether the child is cared for in the hospital or at home, any specific isolation measures will be determined by the child's specific infectious disease process.

Rubeola (Measles)

Causative agent:	RNA virus
Incubation period:	8 to 12 days from exposure to onset of symptoms
Infectious period:	Ranges from 3 to 5 days before the appearance of the rash to 4 days after appearance of the rash
Transmission:	Transmitted between individuals by direct contact with infectious droplets or less frequently by airborne spread
Immunity:	Natural disease or live attenuated vaccine
Season:	Late winter and spring

Manifestations

The measles virus enters the body and slowly spreads. Respiratory symptoms appear after an average of 10 days. Typically, children have a prodrome period with fever and "the three Cs" (coryza [profuse runny nose], cough, conjunctivitis) that lasts between 1 and 4 days. Children are usually very ill during this time. *Koplik spots* appear approximately 2 days before the appearance of the rash (Fig. 40-2). Koplik

Text continued on p. 1020

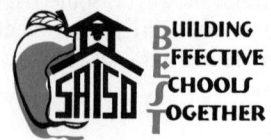

San Angelo Independent School District
HEALTH SERVICES
Ph: (915) 657-4049   Fax: (915) 657-4087

Susan Schultz, RN, BSN
Coordinator of Health Services

Dear Parent/Guardian:

Several students in our school district have been diagnosed as having Fifth Disease (Erythema Infectiosum). This is caused by a virus and can cause outbreaks, particularly among children, because the individual is infectious before symptoms appear. Symptoms are mild and it is usually recognized by a rash appearing on the cheeks resembling a "slapped cheek." There may also be a lacy rash on the trunk, arms and legs. Sometimes these characteristics are preceded by a low-grade fever, which lasts 5-7 days. No treatment is necessary. Children are no longer contagious and do not need to be excluded from school once the rash occurs.

Fifth Disease is generally a very mild disease. Please contact your primary care provider immediately if:

1. The rash becomes itchy

2. Your child develops a fever over 101°

3. You feel your child is getting worse

4. You have other concerns or questions

If you, a family member or a friend are pregnant and are exposed to a child with Fifth Disease, contact your obstetrician.

Please contact the nurse at your school if you have further questions or concerns.

Sincerely,

Susan Schultz, RN

Susan Schultz, RN, BSN
Coordinator, Health Services

Dr. Joe E. Gonzales, Superintendent • 1621 University • San Angelo, TX 76904

Figure 40-1 Sample notification letter from school nurse informing parents and caregivers about an exposure to an infectious disease. (Courtesy Susan Schultz, RN, BSN, Coordinator, Health Services, San Angelo Independent School District, San Angelo, TX.)

Nursing Care Plan

The Child with an Infection in the Community Setting

FOCUSED ASSESSMENT

Most infectious diseases in children and adolescents are self-limiting and rarely produce devastating illness. Thorough assessment is always indicated. Many infectious diseases present with subtle and common symptoms that may be difficult to identify. Because rashes and fever can suggest many diseases, the nurse needs to begin assessment by obtaining a complete history, including:

- Child's usual state of health
- Any signs or symptoms of developing disease (prodrome)
- Vital signs, especially body temperature
- Description of any skin lesions or rashes, including color, pattern, or shape; size, location, and distribution on the body; presence of any drainage or erythema; and any changes since initial eruption
- Any other family members, classmates, or playmates (friends) showing signs or symptoms
- Any other associated signs or symptoms (arthralgia, malaise, pain, vomiting, headaches)
- Medications or treatments tried and their effects

Nursing Diagnosis

Risk for Infection (cross contamination of self or others) related to insufficient knowledge of how to avoid the spread of infectious disease.

Expected Outcomes

Child's contacts will:
- Remain free from symptoms of infection.

Child will:
- Demonstrate absence of infection, as evidenced by vital signs within normal parameters, resolving lesions with no evidence of complications, and age-appropriate behavior.

Family and child (if age-appropriate) will:
- State symptoms of infectious disease and symptoms of secondary bacterial infections and appropriate disease-containment procedures.
- Verbalize understanding of written health promotion information, including contact information for local community agencies and resources.

INTERVENTION	RATIONALE
1. Teach the family and child (if old enough) the symptoms of secondary bacterial infections and complications of infectious diseases that should be promptly reported to their primary medical caregiver (e.g., redness, warmth, swelling, tenderness or pain, new onset of drainage or change in drainage from wound, increase in body temperature, malaise, abdominal pain, vomiting or diarrhea, enlarged glands, changes in skin lesions including sores or wounds that do not heal). Provide the phone number or numbers to call if complications occur.	1. Promptly recognizing and reporting signs and symptoms of secondary bacterial infections can decrease complications.
2. Teach the family and/or child about the underlying concepts of infection transmission, including how and to whom the infection should be reported (e.g., airborne, fecal-oral, direct contact).	2. Understanding promotes cooperation with infectious disease containment issues, policies, and procedures (e.g., child with chickenpox may not return to daycare or school until the 6th day after onset of rash or sooner if all lesions have dried and crusted).
3. Emphasize importance of and encourage the child and family to complete the full course of any prescribed medication, unless experiencing adverse side effects.	3. Providing information and encouragement promotes understanding and compliance.

Continued

Nursing Care Plan

The Child with an Infection in the Community Setting—cont'd

INTERVENTION	RATIONALE
4. Role model and teach the child and family preventive behaviors, such as frequent and meticulous handwashing, disposal of used dressings to prevent spread of infectious disease to others, proper disposal of tissues, and covering the mouth when coughing or sneezing. (Follow Standard Precautions guidelines during any contact with blood, mucous membrane, nonintact skin, or any body substance except sweat; use goggles, gloves, and gowns when appropriate; help the family access these if needed.)	4. Demonstration and active participation are more effective teaching strategies (parents will retain better if they "use" the instruction) than verbal instruction alone. Nurses must assume all people are carrying bloodborne pathogens such as human immunodeficiency virus (HIV) or hepatitis B or C (HBV, HCV). Standard Precautions apply to everyone.
5. Review the infectious disease and plan of care for the child, including provision of rest, proper nutrition, fever control, and when the child can resume normal activities. Provide written information about the child's plan of care, including any instructions for treatment, medication administration, and any scheduled follow-up visits with the child's primary health care provider.	5. Providing information and encouragement promotes understanding and adherence to treatment plan.
6. Provide health promotion information and education (e.g., routine immunization schedule) for the family and child. Refer the family and child to local community agencies (health departments, clinics) as appropriate.	6. Maintenance of an ongoing relationship with a primary care provider provides continuity of care and methods for access to care for the well and sick child as needed.

Evaluation

- Have any of the child's contacts contracted the disease?
- Is the child free from infection, afebrile, and exhibiting age-appropriate behavior?
- Have the parents and/or child verbalized an understanding of the infectious process and disease-containment procedures?
- Is the family and/or child cooperative with written contact information and accessing follow-up and preventive health care and appropriate community resources?

Nursing Diagnosis

Ineffective Health Maintenance related to insufficient knowledge about how to obtain needed information about infectious disease and its management.

Expected Outcomes

The child and family will:
- Follow an agreed-on infection control plan.
- Meet goals for health maintenance.

INTERVENTION	RATIONALE
1. Teach the family or child skin and wound assessment and ways to monitor for signs and symptoms of infection, complications, and healing.	1. Early assessment and intervention help prevent serious problems from developing (e.g., sexually transmissible diseases [STDs] in the adolescent female can result in sterility). Providing information and encouragement promotes understanding and compliance with treatment plan, thus preventing secondary infection or adverse consequences from infection.
2. Provide written instructions for comfort and prevention of secondary infections according to the child's specific condition.	2. Providing information and encouragement promotes understanding and cooperation with treatment plan.
3. Teach adolescents health-promoting and health-seeking behaviors to reduce the risk of contracting an STD; this includes a description of the direct contact transmission mode and recognition of complications.	3. Providing information and establishing a nonjudgmental environment encourage future health-seeking behaviors. Long-term complications (e.g., sterility, chronic abdominal pain from untreated STDs) can be avoided with early detection, treatment, and appropriate follow-up care.

Nursing Care Plan

The Child with an Infection in the Community Setting—cont'd

INTERVENTION	RATIONALE
4. Screen for STDs as appropriate (e.g., a prepubescent female with signs and symptoms of an STD). For prevention, teach children that it is not all right for someone to look at or touch their private parts.	4. Signs and symptoms of problems with the genital area (itching, rash, vaginal discharge) should always be explored by the nurse with a complete history of symptoms to rule out sexual abuse, especially in a prepubescent female. Sexual abuse of a child is a reportable offense and must be ruled out.
5. Provide health promotion information and education (e.g., Papanicolaou [Pap] smears for sexually active adolescents). Refer the family or child to local community agencies (health departments, clinics) as appropriate.	5. Maintenance of an ongoing relationship with a primary care provider provides continuity of care and methods for access to care for health promotion and disease prevention.

Evaluation

- Do the child and family follow the agreed-on infection control plan?
- Are they able to meet goals for health maintenance?

Nursing Diagnosis

Risk for Ineffective Thermoregulation related to infection.

Expected Outcome

The child will:
- Be afebrile and exhibit age-appropriate behavior.

INTERVENTION	RATIONALE
1. Teach the family and/or child normal temperature parameters (e.g., What is a fever?) and temperature-monitoring techniques (see age-appropriate guidelines in Chapter 37).	1. Consistently monitoring and promptly recognizing and reporting signs and symptoms of hyperthermia complications promote prevention and early intervention and can decrease the potential for disability or death.
2. Teach the family the signs and symptoms of hyperthermia and the complications that should be promptly reported to their primary medical caregiver (e.g., visual disturbances, headache, nausea, vomiting, muscle flaccidity, absence of sweating, delirium, coma). Provide the phone number(s) to call if complications occur.	2. Understanding promotes cooperation and compliance with the child's treatment and care plan.
3. Teach the family about specific comfort measures (cool environment, light clothing, tepid baths) and medication administration (antipyretics) for hyperthermia. Teach parents the appropriate use of antipyretics (see Chapter 37). Use acetaminophen and/or ibuprofen as directed for fever control. Avoid aspirin products because of possibility of developing Reye's syndrome (see Chapter 52). Check all over-the-counter medicines to be sure they do not contain aspirin or salicylate. Provide written information that explains the various preparations available (drops, suspension, chewable tablets, suppositories) and the appropriate dose and administration intervals for their child. For example: The dosage of acetaminophen for a 25-lb child is 160 mg. Any one of the following can be given every 4-6 hours as needed for fever or discomfort: • Concentrated drops (80 mg in 0.8 ml) = 0.8 ml + 0.8 ml = 1.6 ml • Suspension liquid (80 mg in ½ tsp) = 1 tsp • Children's chewable (80 mg each) = 2 tablets • Suppository (80 mg each) = 2 suppositories	3. Appropriate teaching not only promotes cooperation and adherence to the child's treatment and care plan but also can prevent innocent administration of readily available, potentially lethal over-the-counter medication to a child with a viral illness. Providing information and creating awareness of self-care steps the family or adolescent can take to maintain or regain health promotes positive health-seeking behaviors. Because of the many different formulations of both of these over-the-counter medications, parents are frequently confused and inadvertently give the wrong dose, sometimes resulting in overdosing or underdosing and inadequate fever control.

Continued

Nursing Care Plan

The Child with an Infection in the Community Setting—cont'd

INTERVENTION	RATIONALE
4. Teach the importance and specific techniques for maintaining adequate hydration (monitoring the child's intake and output, frequently offering cool liquids, Popsicles).	4. Maintaining adequate hydration will help maintain a normal body temperature. An elevated temperature is associated with increased metabolism and fluid use.
5. Provide written health promotion information and education about fever control and when to access the health care system.	5. Maintenance of ongoing relationship with primary care provider provides continuity of care and methods for access to care for well and sick child care as needed.

Evaluation

- Has the child maintained a body temperature within normal parameters?
- Is the child's behavior within normal parameters for age?

Nursing Diagnosis

Fatigue related to discomfort associated with the infectious disease.

Expected Outcome

The child will experience:

- An increase in comfort level and energy, as evidenced by verbalization of decreased discomfort, a relaxed body posture, ability to rest appropriately, decreased crying and irritability, and an interest in age-appropriate activities.

INTERVENTION	RATIONALE
1. Teach and provide written information for comfort measures (cool environment; Aveeno baths; lightweight, cool clothing); treatments (monitoring the child's temperature); or medication administration (antipruritics, antipyretics).	1. Appropriate teaching promotes cooperation and compliance with the child's treatment and care plan. Maintaining adequate hydration will help maintain a normal body temperature. An elevated temperature is associated with increased metabolism and fluid use.
2. Encourage bed rest and energy conservation during healing process of an infectious disease. Provide age- and energy-appropriate activities, depending on the child's level of wellness.	2. Bed rest and energy conservation promote the healing process and provide comfort to children with discomfort, pain, or fever. Non-pharmacologic techniques, such as distraction, provide diversion.
3. Teach the child's family personal hygiene principles to promote the healing process and maintain health after the infectious disease process. Keep the child's skin clean, and change linens and clothing frequently. Wash clothes and linen in mild detergent, and double rinse.	3. Clean clothing helps prevent the spread of secondary infections. Double rinsing reduces the potential irritants in the clothing, thereby minimizing irritation.

spots are small, blue-white spots with a red base that cluster near the molars on the buccal mucosa. These spots last approximately 3 days, after which they slough off. As prodromal symptoms reach a peak, the exanthem appears and is characterized by a deep-red, macular rash that usually begins on the face and neck and spreads down the trunk and extremities to the feet. The rash blanches easily with pressure and will gradually turn a brownish color. The duration of the rash is about 6 to 7 days.

A partially immune child, such as an infant younger than 9 months who has passively acquired maternal antibodies or a child given immune gamma globulin, may contract modified measles. The prodromal period is shorter, and the symptoms are minimal, with few to no Koplik spots. The rash progression follows the pattern of regular measles.

Complications

Because of respiratory involvement, secondary bacterial infections, such as otitis media, bronchopneumonia, and laryngotracheobronchitis (croup), can occur, especially in infants and younger children. Central nervous system (CNS) complications including acute encephalitis are rare but can occur.

Therapeutic Management

The treatment of measles is symptomatic, whether the child is hospitalized or remains at home. If hospitalized, the child will require airborne isolation precautions. During the febrile period, the child should be restricted to quiet activities and bed rest.

The World Health Organization and the United Nations International Children's Emergency Fund recommend admin-

Nursing Care Plan

The Child with an Infection in the Community Setting—cont'd

Evaluation

- Has the child experienced relief from discomfort by demonstrating a relaxed body posture, an interest in age-appropriate play, and verbalization of an increased comfort level?

Nursing Diagnosis

Social Isolation related to the confinement for the duration of the communicable disease.

Expected Outcomes

The child and family will:
- Describe the reasons for isolation and will incorporate the resulting restrictions into their home management.

The child will:
- Participate in age-appropriate activities within the restrictions imposed.

The family will:
- Contact community agencies for assistance if appropriate.

INTERVENTION	RATIONALE
1. Encourage the family and child to maintain contact with friends and family by telephone, mail, or e-mail while the child is isolated.	1. Maintaining contact with family and friends helps the family adjust to activity limitations, reduces boredom, and provides emotional support.
2. Provide written information to family about age- and energy-appropriate activities.	2. Providing age-appropriate activities prevents boredom and promotes normal growth and development.
3. Provide information about community resources for respite and/or sick child care.	3. Providing resources for family not only provides for caregiver relief but also could result in the family's primary wage earner (especially in single-parent families) returning to work with less loss of income and decrease in the financial burden on the family.

Evaluation

- Can the child and family describe the reasons for the isolation, and have they incorporated the appropriate restrictions?
- Is the child engaging in age-appropriate activities?
- Is the family able to maintain contact with family and friends?
- Have support systems been mobilized, both within the family and in the community?

---

istration of vitamin A to all children diagnosed with measles in communities where vitamin A deficiency is a recognized problem or where the measles case fatality rate is 1% or greater. In the United States, low blood levels of vitamin A have been found in children with more severe cases of measles. Although vitamin A deficiency is not recognized as a major problem in the United States, the American Academy of Pediatrics (AAP, 2003d) has recommended that vitamin A supplementation should be considered in the following circumstances:

- Children ages 6 months to 2 years who are hospitalized with complications (pneumonia, croup, diarrhea)
- Children older than 6 months with measles who are not already receiving vitamin A supplementation and who have the following risks: immunodeficiency, evidence of

vitamin A deficiency, impaired intestinal absorption, moderate to severe malnutrition, or recent immigration from an area with high mortality from measles

Parenteral and oral formulations of vitamin A are available in the United States. The recommended dosage is:

- Children 6 months to 1 year of age should receive a single dose of 100,000 international units orally.
- Children 1 year and older should receive a single dose of 200,000 international units orally.
- Additional doses are recommended at 24 hours and again 4 weeks later for children with ophthalmologic evidence of vitamin A deficiency. Vitamin A toxicity is rare and usually associated only with extremely large doses (>1 million international units) (AAP, 2003d).

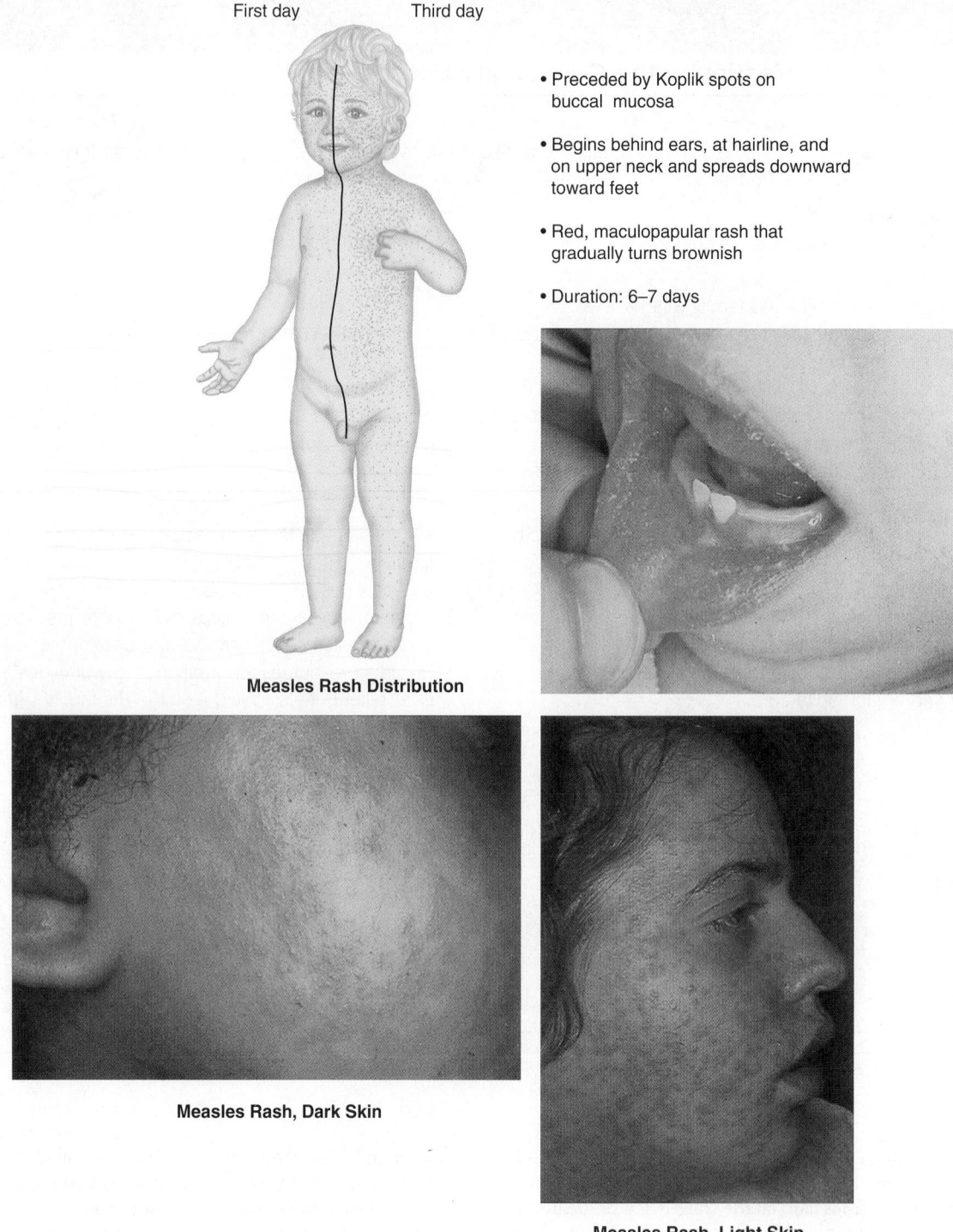

First day   Third day

- Preceded by Koplik spots on buccal mucosa

- Begins behind ears, at hairline, and on upper neck and spreads downward toward feet

- Red, maculopapular rash that gradually turns brownish

- Duration: 6–7 days

Measles Rash Distribution

Measles Rash, Dark Skin

Measles Rash, Light Skin

Figure 40-2 Rubeola (measles) lesions and rash distribution. (Photos from Feigin, R.D., & Cherry, J.D. [Eds.]. [1998]. *Textbook of pediatric infectious diseases* [4th ed.]. Philadelphia: Saunders; Hurwitz, S. [1993]. *Clinical pediatric dermatology: A textbook of skin disorders of childhood and adolescence* [2nd ed.]. Philadelphia: Saunders.)

Children can be protected against measles and other vaccine-preventable diseases by receiving *all* their routine immunizations during their routine well-child checkups. Two doses of measles, mumps, and rubella vaccine (MMR) are required to be fully protected. The first MMR is recommended routinely at 1 year of age. The second dose of MMR is rec-ommended at 4 to 6 years but may be administered during any visit if at least 4 weeks has elapsed since the first dose and both doses are administered beginning at or after 12 months of age. Children who have not previously received their second MMR dose should complete the schedule no later than their 11- to 12-year health maintenance visit.

First day   Third day

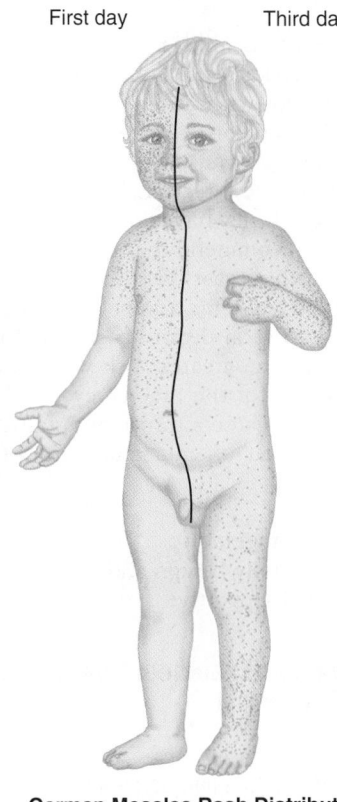

• Begins on face, neck, and scalp and spreads downward to entire body. Fades on face as it spreads to trunk.

• Pinkish, maculopapular

• Reddish, pinpoint petechiae may occur on soft palate (Forscheimer's sign).

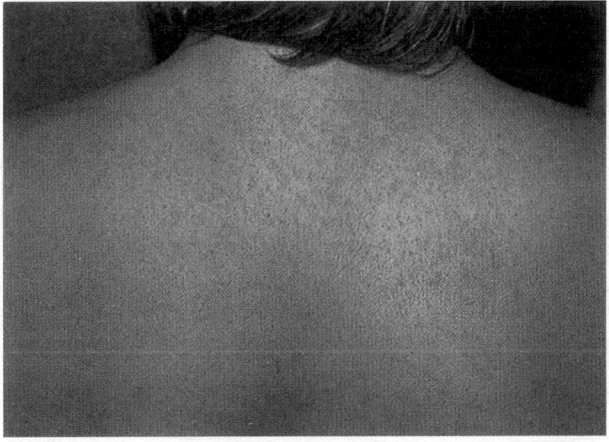

German Measles Rash Distribution

Figure 40-3 Rubella (German measles) lesions and rash distribution. (Photo from Hurwitz, S. [1993]. *Clinical pediatric dermatology: A textbook of skin disorders of childhood and adolescence* [2nd ed.]. Philadelphia: Saunders.)

Rubella (3-Day Measles, German Measles)

Causative agent:	RNA virus
Incubation period:	14 to 21 days
Infectious period:	Ranges from 7 days before onset of symptoms to 14 days after appearance of the rash
Transmission:	Airborne particles or direct contact with infectious droplets, transplacental transmission; small number of infants with congenital rubella continue to shed the virus for months after birth
Immunity:	Natural disease or live attenuated vaccine
Season:	Late winter and early spring

Manifestations

Rubella is usually a mild disease for children and adults. The virus enters the host, producing a rash after about 14 to 16 days. Young children are often asymptomatic until the appearance of the rash. Older children may complain of profuse nasal drainage, diarrhea, malaise, sore throat, headache, low-grade fever, polyarthritis, eye pain, aches, chills, anorexia, and nausea. Children of all ages usually have impressive posterior cervical, posterior auricular, and occipital lymphadenopathy.

The rash presents as a pinkish rose maculopapular exanthem that begins on the face, scalp, and neck (Fig. 40-3). It spreads downward to include the entire body within 1 to 3 days. As the rash spreads to the trunk, the rash on the face begins fading. Petechiae (spots), which are reddish and pinpoint, may occur on the soft palate. Their appearance is sometimes referred to as *Forschheimer's sign.*

Complications

Rubella has relatively few complications. The most common are arthritis and arthralgia, which occur more often in adult women than in children or adolescents. Mild thrombocytopenia may also occur but is usually self-limiting and of short duration. A rare complication is encephalitis, which is usually less severe than measles-related encephalitis.

The importance of recognizing and respecting this viral illness is not the morbidity of the disease itself but rather the consequences that can occur to a fetus during maternal infection. The most devastating form of rubella is congenital rubella that occurs after maternal infection. The risk for damage to the developing fetus is greatest in the early weeks of the pregnancy. Kenner and Lott (2003) report when infants born to mothers who were infected during the first 8 weeks of gestation were followed for 4 years, 85% were affected. When infection occurred in the 9th through 12th week of gestation, the risk of infant anomalies dropped to 52% and the risk of defects virtually disappeared after the 20th week of gestation.

! CRITICAL TO REMEMBER

Congenital Rubella

The rubella virus can cross the placenta and infect the fetus, causing fetal death or abnormalities.

Congenital rubella can result in growth retardation, cataracts, retinopathy, and cardiac anomalies. The most common complication is sensorineural deafness. Some manifestations may not be present at birth but may develop at a later time, including mental retardation, diabetes mellitus, thyroid disorders, and encephalopathy.

Therapeutic Management

Treatment is generally supportive and symptomatic, with the disease being self-limiting. Children with postnatal rubella should be excluded from school or child care for 7 days after the onset of the rash. Infants with congenital rubella should be considered contagious until they are at least 1 year old, unless nasopharyngeal and urine cultures are repeatedly negative for the rubella virus. Parents should be made aware of the potential risks their infants pose for pregnant women with whom they come into contact (AAP, 2003h). Primary prevention of rubella can be accomplished through administration of the rubella vaccine in combination with measles and mumps vaccine (MMR) as previously discussed.

Erythema Infectiosum (Parvovirus B19, Fifth Disease)

Causative agent:	Parvovirus B19
Incubation period:	4 to 14 days but can be up to 21 days
Infectious period:	Unknown but thought to extend from the prodromal period until the rash appears
Transmission:	Airborne particles, respiratory droplets, blood, blood products, transplacental transmission
Immunity:	Natural disease is thought to provide antibodies for immunity
Season:	Winter and spring

This disease is most common in children ages 5 to 14 years but may also occur in adults.

Manifestations

Fifth disease is a relatively mild systemic disease. Typically, the child may appear well but presents with an intense, fiery red, edematous rash on the cheeks, which gives a "slapped cheek" appearance (Fig. 40-4), or the history of a rash that "comes and goes." Before the appearance of the rash, many children are asymptomatic or have nonspecific symptoms, such as headache, runny nose, malaise, and mild fever. Approximately 1 to 4 days after the facial rash appears, an erythematous, maculopapular, lacy rash appears on the trunk and extremities. The rash fades with a central clearing area, resulting in a lacy appearance. The rash may last 2 to 39 days and reappear when aggravated by environmental factors, such as heat, exercise, warm baths, rubbing of the skin, and stress.

Complications

Because the disease is mild, there are usually no reported complications, especially in children. A careful history should be obtained, with an emphasis on identifying any pregnant family members, teachers, or friends, to prevent intrauterine infection and mortality. Pregnant women are at risk for intrauterine infection. Many school districts notify pregnant staff if they have been exposed to a child with fifth disease and recommend that they contact their health care provider. Fifth disease has resulted in fetal death, but parvovirus-associated fetal anomaly has not been established. The risk of fetal death is estimated to be between 2% and 6%, with the greatest risk when infection occurs during the first half of the pregnancy (AAP, 2003c). Parvovirus 19 also can cause a transient aplastic crisis in children with sickle cell anemia and some other hemoglobinopathies.

Therapeutic Management

The disease is generally benign and self-limiting. Treatment is symptomatic and supportive.

Roseola Infantum (Exanthem Subitum, Sixth Disease, 3-Day Fever)

Causative agent:	Human herpesvirus 6 (HHV-6)
Incubation period:	Unknown but estimated to be 9 to 10 days
Infectious period:	Unknown but thought to extend from the febrile stage to the time the rash first appears
Transmission:	Most likely by contact with secretions (saliva, cerebrospinal fluid [CSF]) of asymptomatic close contacts
Season:	Throughout the year without a distinctive seasonal pattern

Manifestations

Roseola was the sixth childhood exanthem identified. Although HHV-6 appears to be the major causative agent, other viruses have been linked to the disease. Most clinical cases of roseola occur in children 6 to 18 months old. The child has a sudden high fever (39.4° to 41.1° C [103° to 106° F]), malaise, and irritability but may remain active and alert. An intermittent or constant fever may persist for 3 to 5 days. The child may also have a mild cough, runny nose, abdominal pain, headache, vomiting, and diarrhea. After 3 to 5 days the fever subsides, and within several hours to 2 days a rash appears. The rash consists of rose-pink maculopapules or macules that blanch with pressure (Fig. 40-5). The rash occurs predominantly on the neck and trunk and may be surrounded by a whitish ring. Normally, it persists for 24 to 48 hours before fading.

Complications

Complications associated with roseola are uncommon. Seizures related to the high fever may occur. Rare cases of encephalitis, hemiplegia, paresis, and mental retardation have been reported.

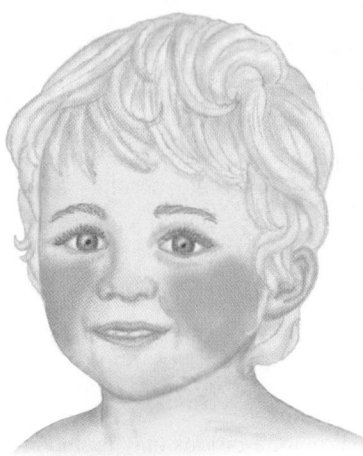

- Presents with fiery red edematous rash on cheeks—"slapped cheek" appearance

- Followed in 1–4 days by erythematous maculopapular lacy rash on trunk and extremities

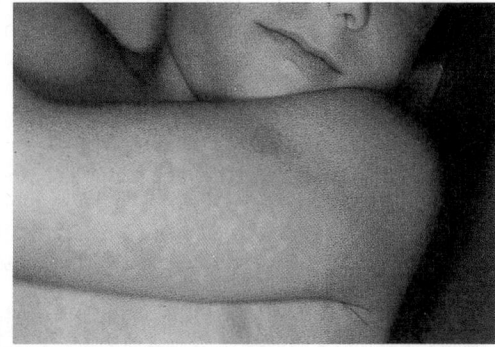

Erythema Infectiosum: "Slapped Cheek" Appearance

Rash

Figure 40-4 Erythema infectiosum lesions and rash distribution. (Photo from Hurwitz, S. [1993]. *Clinical pediatric dermatology: A textbook of skin disorders of childhood and adolescence* [2nd ed.]. Philadelphia: Saunders.)

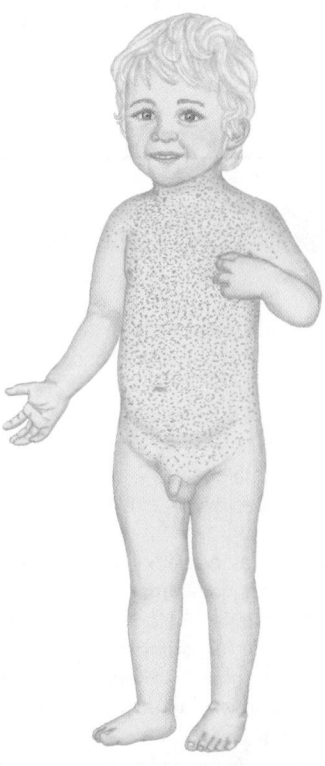

- Rash appears several hours to 2 days after fever subsides.

- Erythematous maculopapular or macular, may be surrounded by whitish ring

- Blanches with pressure

- Predominantly on neck and trunk

- Usually persists for 24–48 hours

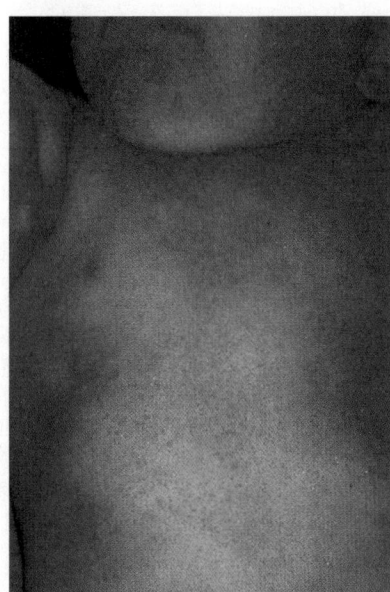

Roseola Infantum Rash Distribution

Figure 40-5 Roseola infantum lesions and rash distribution. (Photo from Hurwitz, S. [1993]. *Clinical pediatric dermatology: A textbook of skin disorders of childhood and adolescence* [2nd ed.]. Philadelphia: Saunders.)

Therapeutic Management

Treatment is symptomatic. Family members should be taught about fever control management.

Generally, fever can be controlled with antipyretic medications, tepid sponge baths, decreased clothing, environmental temperatures, and increased fluid intake. Temperature monitoring, medication administration (prescription and over-the-counter), and other comfort measures should be discussed. The nurse should make sure the child's family has access to a thermometer and knows how to use it. In addition, parents should be given information regarding the absolute avoidance of any form of aspirin (including over-the-counter medications containing salicylates) because of the potential risk of developing Reye's syndrome (see Chapter 52). Anticipatory guidance should include alerting the parent to the possibility of febrile seizures (caused by the sudden high fevers) and teaching about seizure precautions (especially if the child has a history of previous febrile seizures) (Parents Want to Know box).

Parents' understanding of the care necessary for their child is important. Parents need to be educated about immunizations and measures to prevent the spread of infectious diseases. They should also be taught to recognize the signs and symptoms of complications so that they can seek medical treatment when warranted. Providing parents with written instructions that they can refer to at home may prove helpful.

Mumps

Causative agent:	Paramyxovirus
Incubation period:	Usually 16 to 18 days but may extend to 25 days
Infectious period:	From 7 days before swelling to 9 days after onset
Transmission:	Airborne droplets, salivary secretions, possibly urine
Immunity:	Natural disease or live attenuated vaccine
Season:	Late winter and spring

Manifestations

Prodromal manifestations may include fever, muscular pain, headache, and malaise. The classic clinical sign of parotid glandular swelling (parotitis) often follows these, although a substantial number of individuals experience no such swelling. When parotid swelling does occurs, it may be accompanied by fever.

Complications

Mumps generally affects the salivary glands but can involve multiple organs. The most common complication is aseptic meningitis, with the virus identified in the CSF. Signs of CNS involvement include nuchal rigidity, lethargy, and

---

PARENTS
Want to Know

How to Care for Their Child With a Viral Exanthem

- For elevated temperature, the child's activity should be restricted to age-appropriate, quiet activities and bed rest. As the fever decreases, the activity level can be gradually increased to a normal level.
- Generally, fever can be controlled with acetaminophen or ibuprofen or both (no aspirin products because of the possible risk of developing Reye's syndrome), sponge baths, decreased clothing, decreased environmental temperature, and increased fluid intake. Bed linens may need to be changed frequently during periods of high fevers. Over-the-counter antipyretic acetaminophen comes in several different formulations. It is important to read the label carefully and ask your primary care provider if you have any questions regarding medication administration. Seizure precautions should be taken if your child has had a seizure previously.
- The amount of skin irritation and discomfort will vary. Lukewarm baths using colloid preparations (Aveeno) or baking soda (1/2 cup in tub of water) may help relieve itching. Soothing lotions (Lubriderm, Curel, Moisturel) may also provide comfort. Avoid the use of topical corticosteroids unless ordered by your primary care provider. Use superfatted soaps for sensitive skin (Dove, Basis, Neutrogena, Aveeno). Fingernails should be short. If the child continues to scratch, cotton mittens or socks can be applied to the child's hands. It is es-

sential to maintain the integrity of the skin and prevent any secondary infections. If secondary infections occur, antibiotic therapy might be necessary.
- Administer antihistamines or antipruritics as prescribed.
- Dress your child in lightweight clothing that is not irritating. Avoid wool and scratchy materials.
- Coughing can be managed with cool humidification of the room and antitussives.
- For arthralgia, antiinflammatory medications may be used. Involvement of weight-bearing joints may warrant bed rest.
- Some viral exanthems cause photophobia. In such cases, keeping the room dimly lit or providing sunglasses for the child may be helpful. If the child has conjunctivitis, secretions or crust should be removed with tepid water and a clean cloth to prevent contamination.
- Fluid intake is important for successfully managing febrile stages of the disease. Encourage your child to drink cool liquids frequently. If the child's mucous membranes are involved, soft, bland foods may be beneficial.
- As your child progresses through the stages of illness, it will be necessary to provide diversional activities during the period of isolation. Choose activities that your child likes and can participate in without becoming unduly tired.

vomiting. Individuals with these manifestations usually recover completely. A less common CNS complication is meningoencephalomyelitis manifested by fever, headache, nausea, vomiting, nuchal rigidity, and changes in sensorium. These complications are treated symptomatically and generally have an uneventful recovery period.

The potential complication of most concern to parents is orchitis (inflammation of a testis). Orchitis is a common complication in adolescents, with sterility occurring rarely. Although deafness does not occur frequently, mumps can cause hearing impairment. Other rare complications include pancreatitis, nephritis, thyroiditis, myocarditis, arthritis, and mastitis.

Therapeutic Management

Uncomplicated mumps may require only symptomatic care. Droplet Precautions are indicated until 9 days after the onset of the parotid swelling. Parents should be given educational information regarding the absolute avoidance of any form of aspirin (including over-the-counter medications containing salicylates) because of the potential risk of developing Reye's syndrome.

Orchitis requires bed rest, intermittent application of ice packs, emotional support, and diversional activities. CNS complications require neurologic evaluations and vital sign measurement as indicated by the child's condition when the complications require hospitalization.

Nursing Considerations

The nurse needs to obtain a history of the onset of symptoms, examine the child's ears and throat, and perform a neurologic assessment. The child's vital signs (including temperature), usual state of health, and characteristics of the lymph nodes in the neck should be documented. In boys, an examination of the testes should be included in the initial assessment.

Typically, children with mumps are not hospitalized unless they have complications. Therefore good handwashing technique should be taught to the child, the family, and close contacts to prevent transmission. Hospitalized children will be placed in isolation according to the facility's policies.

Primary prevention of mumps can be accomplished through administration of the mumps vaccine in combination with measles and rubella vaccine (MMR) as previously discussed.

Varicella-Zoster Infections (Chickenpox, Shingles)

Causative agent:	Varicella-zoster virus
Incubation period:	10 to 21 days
Infectious period:	1 to 2 days before the onset of rash until all lesions are dried (crusted over), usually 5 to 7 days
Transmission:	Direct contact, droplet, airborne particles
Immunity:	Natural disease of varicella; same virus causes zoster, and child may contract zoster at a later time; varicella vaccine
Season:	Late winter through early spring

Primary infection with the varicella-zoster virus causes chickenpox. Before a vaccine was available, this was one of the most common childhood diseases in children 5 to 9 years old. Zoster (shingles), which is the reactivation of the latent varicella-zoster virus, occurs most frequently in the elderly population but can occur also in children, especially adolescents and young adults. Generally, varicella and zoster in children are not life-threatening. However, varicella is a major risk factor for severe invasive group A streptococcal disease (AAP, 2003k). Secondary bacterial infections, frequently group A streptococcal disease, can occur and are considered life-threatening complications. Severe, sometimes fatal cases of varicella have been reported in otherwise healthy children who have received short courses of steroids (for asthma and other chronic illnesses) before becoming infected with the disease. Children who are immunosuppressed and contract varicella are at risk for developing serious, potentially fatal complications.

Manifestations

Varicella. During the 24 to 48 hours before the appearance of lesions, symptoms may include a slightly elevated body temperature, malaise, and anorexia. The macular rash generally first appears on the trunk and scalp (Fig. 40-6). The lesions may be in various stages of development, beginning as macular and developing into a red papular rash. The lesions soon become teardrop vesicles with an erythematous base. The vesicles then become pustular, after which they begin to dry and develop a crust. The lesions appear in crops, beginning on the trunk and scalp and moving (sparsely) to the extremities. These crops of lesions generally appear in three successive eruptions over a period of 3 to 4 days. The number of lesions will vary from child to child, but children in the household with secondary cases generally have more extensive rashes than does the child with the primary case. The lesions may appear on the mucous membranes in the mouth, genital area, and rectum. Second attacks are rare and are more common in immunocompromised children.

Zoster (Shingles). During the primary infection with varicella, the varicella-zoster virus enters the sensory nerve ending and the dorsal root ganglion and establishes a latent infection. Activation of the infection causes zoster (shingles). Zoster manifests with pain and tenderness along the involved nerve and surrounding skin for approximately 2 weeks before the appearance of the rash. The intensity of the pain can range from an unpleasant, abnormal sensitivity to touch to burning, tingling, itching, sharp knifelike prickling, or even deep pain. Unilateral crops of lesions appear along the nerve. These macules and papules progress through the same stages as varicella. There may be enlargement and tenderness of the lymph nodes in the same region.

Zoster is generally thought to be a disease of elderly people, but it can occur also in children, especially those who are immunocompromised, have HIV infection, were exposed in utero, or were infected before their second birthday (AAP, 2003k).

Complications

The most common complication of varicella-zoster virus infection is secondary bacterial infection of the skin lesions. Staphylococci and group A beta-hemolytic streptococci are

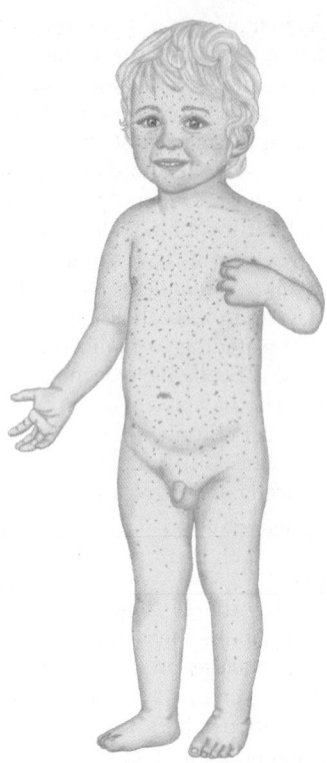

- Macular rash 24–48 hours following slight fever, malaise, anorexia

- Lesions appear in "crops," first on trunk and scalp, then moving sparsely to extremities. May appear in mucous membranes (mouth, genital area, rectum).

- Generally 3 successive eruptions over 3–4 days

- Lesions begin as a macular rash, develop into a red papular rash, then move quickly into teardrop vesicles with erythematous base. Vesicle becomes pustular and begins drying, and a crust develops.

- Rash varies from child to child

Chickenpox Rash Distribution

Chickenpox

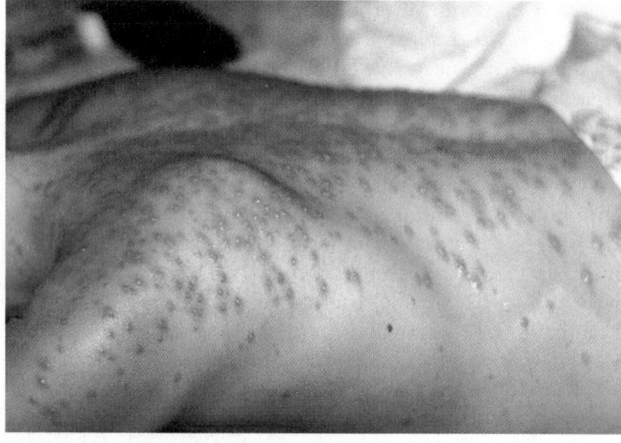

Shingles

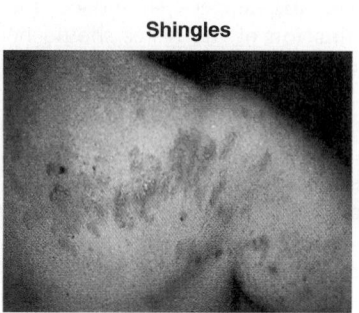

Figure 40-6 Chickenpox and shingles lesions and rash distribution. (Shingles photo from Moschella, S.L., & Hurley, H.J. [1992]. *Dermatology* [3rd ed.]. Philadelphia: Saunders.)

the usual causative agents. CNS complications have been associated with mild to severe varicella infections. Encephalitis with ataxia, tremor, and nystagmus may occur in the first week. The prognosis is generally good unless CNS involvement is severe, usually manifested by convulsions and coma. Children with these complications may have future CNS difficulties, including seizures, mental retardation, or behavior disorders.

Varicella pneumonia, a common complication in adults, rarely occurs in children. Reye's syndrome has been known to occur after varicella infection (see Chapter 52). Corneal involvement may occur if lesions involve the eye.

Complications of zoster are rare but may involve the same difficulties with secondary infections that occur with varicella.

Parents should be given educational information regarding the absolute avoidance of any form of aspirin (including over-the-counter medications containing salicylates) because of the potential risk for developing Reye's syndrome.

Therapeutic Management
Treatment is symptomatic and supportive for the healthy child. Oral acyclovir is not recommended for routine use in otherwise healthy children with varicella. However, varicella and zoster can be treated with intravenous (IV) or oral an-

tiviral drugs (acyclovir being the most common). The decision to use these medications, along with the duration and route, is determined individually by the primary health care provider. Antiviral drugs have a limited "window of opportunity" to affect the infection's outcome and, if administered, should be started as soon as symptoms are present. Oral acyclovir should be considered for those at high risk for moderate to severe varicella (>12 years of age, persons with chronic illnesses, persons receiving long-term aspirin therapy or short courses of steroids) (AAP, 2003k).

In the hospital setting, children with varicella or zoster infections should be placed in strict isolation. The nurse assigned should not simultaneously care for immunocompromised clients, to decrease the risk of varicella transmission. Early initiation of IV acyclovir therapy (within 24 hours of onset of rash) is recommended for immunocompromised clients.

For children at high risk for developing severe varicella or zoster, varicella-zoster immune globulin (VZIG) should be given within 96 hours for maximum effectiveness. Immunocompromised children, newborns of mothers having active varicella infections at the time of birth or with siblings at home with active varicella infection, and HIV-positive children are considered to be at increased risk.

Primary prevention of varicella includes screening and administering the vaccine at routine well-child visits. Varicella vaccine (one dose) is recommended at any visit on or after the first birthday for all susceptible children without a reliable history of actual disease or immunization. Susceptible children 13 years or older should receive two doses of vaccine, given at least 4 weeks apart.

Nursing Considerations

The nurse needs to obtain a detailed history of the onset of symptoms and examine the skin lesions. The appearance, distribution, and stages of the lesions should be documented. The child's vital signs (including temperature) and a general physical assessment should also be noted.

Community-based care of children with varicella can be challenging. Parents and caregivers should be given educational information regarding disease transmission, supportive care, school or daycare attendance policies, and any available community resources (sick child care). Missing work can be especially difficult for single, working parents and can affect their job security.

Hospitalized children with varicella infections are placed in strict isolation, which requires that the nurse wear a mask, gown, and gloves for all contacts with the child. All contaminated materials must be bagged and labeled before reprocessing. Hands should be washed after contact with the child and before contact with another client. Hospitalized children

who have been exposed to varicella should be kept in strict isolation for 8 to 21 days after the onset of rash in the infected individual. At birth, neonates with mothers who have active varicella infections should be placed in strict isolation. In addition, Airborne Precautions and Contact Precautions should be in effect for children with zoster infections.

The nurse needs to educate parents of children with varicella about skin care to prevent secondary bacterial infections and emphasize the importance of absolute avoidance of any form of aspirin (including over-the-counter medications containing aspirin). Resource identification to provide a plan for access to acute or follow-up well-child visits should be discussed, along with any community child-care alternatives.

Smallpox (Variola)

Worldwide eradication of smallpox (variola) was declared in 1980. The last naturally occurring smallpox case was in Somalia in 1977, followed by two cases attributable to laboratory exposure in 1978. The United States discontinued routine childhood immunization against smallpox in 1971 and routine immunization of health care workers in 1976. The U.S. military continued to immunize military personnel until 1990. Since 1980, the vaccine has been recommended only for people working with non-variola orthopoxviruses (AAP, 2003j). There is increasing concern that the virus and the expertise to use it could be used as a bioterrorism weapon. This concern is the reason that smallpox is included in this discussion of infectious diseases.

Causative agent:	Smallpox (variola virus)
Incubation period:	Averages 12 days, with a range of 7 to 17 days
Infectious period:	As the rash in the mouth breaks down, a skin rash becomes visible and the client is the most contagious during this time and remains contagious until all of the lesions have scabbed over and the scabs have dried and fallen off.
Transmission:	Transmitted through direct and prolonged face-to-face contact with an infected person; less commonly, smallpox can also be transmitted through contact with contaminated objects
Immunity:	Live vaccinia virus
Season:	Not confined to a particular season

Manifestations

Smallpox is an acute, contagious disease that can sometimes be fatal. The prodrome of the illness begins abruptly with fever, malaise, headache, muscle pain, prostration, and often nausea, vomiting, and backache. Fever is usually at least 101° F but can be higher. The client usually appears quite ill. About day 4 of the illness, the first signs of rash appear as red spots in the mouth and on the tongue, which develop into sores and break open. As the rash in the mouth breaks down, a skin rash becomes visible. The client is most contagious during this time. The skin rash typically appears first as a few macules, known as "herald spots," on the face, par-

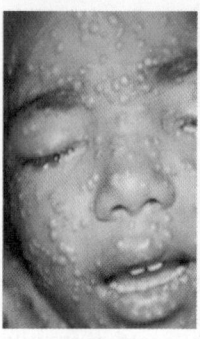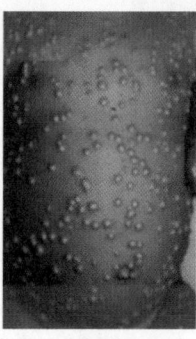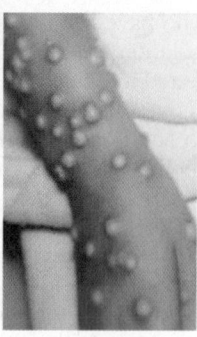

Figure 40-7 Lesions of variola are at the same stage of development on all body parts. (Photos from Centers for Disease Control and Prevention. [2002]. *Evaluating patients for smallpox*. Atlanta, GA: Author.)

ticularly on the forehead. Within a few days of rash onset, clients with smallpox develop a distinctive generalized vesicular rash (Fig. 40-7). By the 3rd or 4th day of illness, the temperature usually falls and the client feels somewhat better. The rash progresses into pustules, which then form scabs. By the end of the 2nd week, the pustules have all scabbed over. The person continues to be contagious until all the scabs have dried and fallen off.

Therapeutic Management

Variola virus can be detected in vesicular or pustular fluid by culture or polymerase chain reaction assay. Variola diagnostic testing is conducted only at the Centers for Disease Control and Prevention (CDC) but may be expanded in the future. If a client is suspected of having smallpox, Standard Precautions, Contact Precautions, and Airborne Precautions should be implemented immediately and the state and/or local health departments should be alerted at once. Postexposure immunization (within 3-4 days of exposure) provides some protection against disease and significant protection against a fatal outcome. A smallpox immunization plan has been implemented in the United States (www.bt.cdc.gov). The plan does not include immunizing children. However, children may be at risk of complications related to coming in contact with vaccinated individuals (Onieal, 2003). Additional information can be found at CDC website: www.cdc.gov/smallpox. Further discussion about the smallpox vaccine can be found in Chapter 4.

Cytomegalovirus

Causative agent:	Human cytomegalovirus (CMV)
Incubation period:	Unknown, except for 3 to 12 weeks after blood transfusions and 4 weeks to 4 months after organ (tissue) transplantation
Transmission:	Saliva, urine, blood, semen, cervical secretions, breast milk, organ transplants
Immunity:	None, although CMV immune globulin, used only in seronegative transplant clients, has had moderate effectiveness
Season:	Can occur during any season

CMV infection is a common cause of congenital infection in infants. A child may become infected with the virus during the prenatal, perinatal, or postnatal period. Congenital infection has a wide variety of manifestations but those who are affected are usually asymptomatic. Some congenitally infected infants who are asymptomatic at birth are later found to have hearing loss or a learning disability. Approximately 10% of infants with congenital CMV infection have profound involvement, evident at birth (AAP, 2003a).

Signs and symptoms in the infant can include jaundice, lethargy, seizures, enlarged spleen and liver, petechial rash, respiratory distress, microcephaly, and intracerebral calcifications. Complications include mental retardation, hearing loss, blindness, and learning disabilities. Some of these conditions may not be apparent until the child is older. The child can continue to shed the virus for up to 5 years.

During the postnatal period, the infant may acquire CMV from a maternal or nonmaternal source. The virus can be transmitted through the breast milk of an infected mother. Blood transfusions, which can be numerous in the premature infant, can also be a source of CMV infection. Children who are not infected congenitally or perinatally often acquire the virus during their toddler or preschool years. Because of sexual activity, the teen years may be another period of acquisition. Affected adolescents are generally asymptomatic but can present with a mononucleosis-like syndrome with fever, hepatosplenomegaly, mild hepatitis, and absence of heterophil antibody.

Therapeutic Management

Specific therapy for CMV is still in the experimental stage but includes immunoglobulin therapy, vaccines, and chemotherapy. Intravenous immunoglobulin therapy provides passive immunity to at-risk infants but not to those already infected. Limited research has been performed on two live attenuated vaccines that could, theoretically, prevent vertical transmission of CMV. Chemotherapy offers the most promise for treatment of neonatal CMV infection, but it has so far not been shown to be clinically effective or improve outcomes (Kenner & Lott, 2003). An antiviral drug (ganciclovir) has been beneficial in treating acquired or recurrent retinitis in the immunocompromised client. Experience with this drug in the pediatric population has been limited, and more research is needed (Kenner & Lott, 2003). Toxicity and associated immunosuppression are major concerns with use in the neonatal population (Stagno, 2001).

Nursing Considerations

The nurse needs to obtain a history of the child's symptoms and possible exposures. Children with congenitally acquired CMV may develop a wide range of manifestations, so nursing care will vary according to the child's specific needs. When developmental delays, mental retardation, neurologic deficits, or hearing losses occur, the nurse can help coordinate the health care team's efforts to meet the child's needs. Parents will need support and education in caring for a child with developmental deficits. The nurse will play a key role in identifying the need for referral and any resources available in the community, including parental support groups.

Epstein-Barr Virus (Infectious Mononucleosis)

Causative agent:	Epstein-Barr virus (EBV, a herpes-like virus)
Incubation period:	4 to 7 weeks
Infectious period:	Unknown; commonly, the virus is shed before clinical onset of disease until 6 months or longer after recovery; asymptomatic carriers are common
Transmission:	Saliva, intimate contact, blood
Immunity:	Natural disease
Season:	Can occur during any season

The primary sites of infection in mononucleosis are the epithelial cells and the B lymphocytes. EBV has been well recognized as the causative agent in infectious mononucleosis. It has also been associated with other diseases, especially outside North America. It has been identified as a co-factor in Burkitt's lymphoma, often seen in Africa, and in cases of nasopharyngeal carcinoma seen in China and Southeast Asia. EBV alone cannot cause the lymphomas or the carcinoma, but it acts in association with other factors.

Manifestations

Infectious mononucleosis typically occurs in otherwise healthy individuals, most commonly in older children and young adults. Clinical signs include fever, exudative pharyngitis, lymphadenopathy, and hepatosplenomegaly. The severity of the clinical signs can range from asymptomatic and mild to severe and fatal. Some children develop a maculopapular rash. Children may complain of malaise, headache, fatigue, nausea, and abdominal pain. The acute illness usually lasts 2 to 4 weeks and is followed by a gradual recovery. The prognosis is generally excellent if there are no complications.

Complications

The risk of splenic rupture associated with EBV infection occurs most frequently during the 2nd week of the illness. Swelling of the pharynx and tonsils can be severe enough to compromise respiration. The outcome of these complications depends on the severity of the infection and the course of the complications.

Therapeutic Management

The illness is generally self-limiting; therefore treatment is supportive. Complications are addressed with appropriate medical treatment. Steroids may be indicated for tonsillar swelling associated with complications. Strenuous physical activity and contact sports should be avoided during the acute illness and as long as the spleen is enlarged, to minimize the risk of splenic rupture.

Nursing Considerations

The history should include presenting signs and symptoms. Physical examination of the pharynx should be performed, with documentation of any redness or swelling. Note any rashes, including a description of their distribution and appearance. The spleen and liver should be evaluated for enlargement. The child's body temperature should be recorded and nutrition and hydration status evaluated.

PARENTS Want to Know

How to Care for Their Child With Infectious Mononucleosis

- Bed rest is indicated during the acute stage of the illness.
- Acetaminophen may be useful in controlling discomfort secondary to fever and enlarged tonsils.
- Activity restrictions include no contact sports of any type, including no roughhousing at home with siblings or friends, to protect the child's enlarged spleen from rupture. With improvement in clinical signs, the child should be allowed to resume normal activities as tolerated.
- The parents and child need to be prepared for a slow and gradual recovery. Fatigue may continue, necessitating a gradual return to school activities.
- Hydration should be monitored and encouraged.
- In children with a sore throat, soothing liquids, bland foods, and milk shakes may be better tolerated than a regular diet.
- Anxiety related to missed schoolwork should be anticipated. Home-bound school programs should be arranged if the child will be absent from school for a prolonged period.
- The parents should have an understanding of the disease and the usual course of recovery. They may need support in exploring options for caring for their child during a lengthy recovery period, including referrals for alternative child-care arrangements, to decrease lost income and maintain job security.

Because EBV infection is self-limiting, nursing care is mainly supportive. Most children are cared for at home. Hospitalization for hydration therapy may be necessary if the child is unable to swallow. Care in both settings involves bed rest, hydration, and relief of discomfort.

Education and reinforcement regarding the importance of avoiding contact sports, including roughhousing at home with family and friends, should be given to older children or adolescents to help them understand the risks involved (Parents Want to Know box).

Poliomyelitis

Causative agent:	Poliovirus (an enterovirus)
Incubation period:	3 to 6 days for abortive poliomyelitis; 7 to 21 days for paralytic poliomyelitis
Infectious period:	Shortly before and after the onset of clinical illness when the virus is in the throat and in high concentration in feces; the virus is shed in the pharynx for 1 week after onset and in the feces for several weeks to months
Transmission:	Fecal-oral, oral-oral (respiratory)
Immunity:	Inactivated poliovirus (IPV) and oral poliovirus (OPV) vaccines
Season:	Summer and fall

The three forms of poliovirus are Brunhilde, Lansing, and Leon. The virus, which enters the body through either ingestion or inhalation, has a preference for the CNS, affecting only certain cells, such as the anterior horn cells of the spinal cord.

Manifestations

The initial signs and symptoms of poliomyelitis are fever, malaise, anorexia, nausea, headache, sore throat, and generalized abdominal pain. This stage, referred to as *abortive poliomyelitis*, is generally so mild and brief that it may go unrecognized. The second stage is *nonparalytic poliomyelitis*. The signs and symptoms are the same as in the abortive stage but are more intense, with soreness and stiffness of the trunk, neck, and limbs. Without further progression to paralysis, the temperature will fall and the meningeal symptoms will decrease. Recovery may begin within 3 to 10 days. In the third (*paralytic*) stage, flaccid paralysis is the most obvious sign. With paralysis, muscles deteriorate and atrophy. Distribution of signs and symptoms may be asymmetric. Generally, the lower extremities and the large muscle groups are affected. There may also be cervical involvement, which is called *bulbar polio*. This is the most life-threatening form of polio because it affects the respiratory and vasomotor centers. Damage to the respiratory center can result in inability to breathe.

Therapeutic Management

Poliomyelitis has no specific treatment. Rather, treatment is specific for each child's needs. For paralytic polio, hospitalization may be necessary. In children with respiratory paralysis, mechanical ventilation is necessary. Physical therapy helps maintain muscle integrity and prevent contractures.

The prognosis for polio depends on the severity of nerve damage. It may be months before the full extent of damage and the probable degree of recovery can be determined.

Primary prevention of polio includes administering the vaccine at routine well-child visits. The two types of poliovirus vaccines are inactivated vaccines (IPV) given parenterally (subcutaneously [SC] or intramuscularly [IM]) and live-virus vaccine (OPV) given orally. Inactivated poliovirus vaccine is now the only poliovirus vaccine available in the United States. OPV can cause vaccine-associated paralytic poliomyelitis (VAPP). Before the expanded use of IPV vaccine in the United States, the overall risk of VAPP was approximately 1 case in 2.4 million doses of OPV vaccine distributed. The American Academy of Pediatrics (AAP, 2003e) recommends a four-dose, all-IPV vaccine schedule for routine immunization of all infants and children in the United States (see Chapter 4 and Appendix D).

Nursing Considerations

The nurse should obtain a history of symptoms along with an immunization history. It is important to also obtain a family immunization history to identify any unvaccinated adult family members.

In immunocompromised children, it is also important to obtain a history of contact with anyone who recently received the active polio vaccine. The child should be observed for neurologic symptoms and respiratory distress, and the body temperature should be recorded.

The primary focus of nursing should be preventive, because the development and use of the polio vaccine have drastically reduced the incidence of polio. In addition, the

American Academy of Pediatrics (AAP, 2003e) recommends the use of inactivated poliomyelitis vaccine for the prevention of vaccine-acquired poliomyelitis cases.

For the child with paralytic polio, hospitalization may be necessary and nursing care should focus on preventing muscle and skeletal deformities. Active and passive range-of-motion exercises are indicated. Constipation is common, and fluid intake and nutrition should be monitored. If mechanical ventilation is indicated, the nursing care is the same as for any child on ventilatory support.

Nursing care of children with abortive polio focuses on reducing the parents' and child's fear and on minimizing muscular deformities. The child can be treated at home with analgesics, sedatives, and bed rest until the fever subsides. Nonparalytic polio can also be treated at home.

Rabies

Causative agent:	Rhabdovirus
Incubation period:	5 days to more than 1 year; incubation can extend to 6 years, but the average is 2 months
Infectious period:	10 days (if the animal is still healthy, rabies is unlikely); however, bats may harbor the virus for a longer period
Transmission:	Bites with contaminated saliva, scratches from claws of infected animals, airborne transmission in laboratory settings and in bat-infested caves, transplantation of corneas from undiagnosed donors
Immunity:	Human diploid cell vaccine (HDCV)
Season:	Can occur during any season

Rabies is caused by a virus that can infect any warm-blooded animal. In the United States, the reservoir consists of skunks, bats, raccoons, foxes, squirrels, and woodchucks. Dogs and cats may also be reservoirs, but the use of animal vaccines makes them a less common source of infection.

Manifestations

The rhabdovirus results in a slowly developing infection. The virus travels up the axons of the motor or sensory neurons to the brain. For this reason, bites that occur on the feet or lower extremities are associated with longer incubation periods than bites on the face. Incubation periods are shortened in children.

When left untreated, the virus will cause vague signs and symptoms. The child may complain of not feeling well. The child may have a sore throat, headache, fever, discomfort at the site of the bite, hyperactivity, anxiety, muscle spasms, or convulsions. The decreased ability to swallow results in drooling or aspiration, which explains the use of the term *hydrophobia* in connection with rabies. Once the disease has established itself, it is fatal. Once symptoms appear, the disease generally lasts 5 to 6 days before progressing to death.

Therapeutic Management

The focus of rabies management is preventive and includes educating adults and children to avoid touching and petting strange animals, especially those in unusual settings exhibiting strange behaviors. When an animal bites a child, a determination must be made as to whether to treat that child. Factors to be considered include the geographic area, type of animal, circumstances of the bite, and animal's vaccination record. If the animal is available, it can be observed for 10 days or killed for microscopic examination of the brain.

The bite wound should be cleaned with copious amounts of soap and water. Human rabies immune globulin (HRIG) is given. One half of the dose is infiltrated locally around the wound, and the other half is administered intramuscularly. The vaccine (HDCV) should be administered as early as possible after exposure, preferably within 48 hours. The injection is given into the deltoid muscle on days 3, 7, 14, and 28. Rabies vaccine is the only vaccine that can be given after exposure and result in successful vaccination.

Nursing Considerations

A complete history of the event should be obtained, including the type of animal involved, identification of the animal as wild or domestic, immunization record of the animal, and the present location of the animal (if known). This information will determine the course of action. The wound should be examined and a description noted in the child's record.

For the child who will undergo a complete series of vaccinations, the nurse may use a variety of distraction techniques (e.g., counting, singing). Allowing the child to administer injections to a doll may help relieve some anxiety associated with multiple injections. For the older child, an explanation of the injection process and reasons for treatment may be adequate.

Primary prevention of rabies includes anticipatory guidance focusing on teaching children to avoid petting or touching unknown animals.

For the child who develops rabies, nursing actions are supportive, including support of the child and family through the dying process (see Chapter 36). The child will be in strict isolation, and Standard Precautions will be instituted. The family will need support in preparing for the child's inevitable death and in coping with feelings of guilt.

BACTERIAL INFECTIONS

Bacteria are abundant in the environment, yet relatively few cause diseases that have an impact on humans. Bacteria are organisms that contain both DNA and RNA. They lack a nuclear membrane but have a complex cell wall. The properties of the cell wall determine the bacterium's classification as either gram-positive or gram-negative. Gram-positive bacteria have a thicker wall that helps resist bile activity, drying, and other environmental factors. Gram-positive bacteria can cause chronic inflammation of dermal tissue, fever, and shock. Gram-negative bacteria have a thinner cell wall.

Outside the cell wall, many bacteria have flagella, which help propel the bacteria through their environment. They may also have pili—rigid projections that assist in attachment to the host cell or other bacteria. The capsules help hide the bacteria's presence from the host and make phagocytosis by the host cell more difficult.

Bacteria excrete toxins. Exotoxins are highly poisonous substances that cause cell damage by cell lysis, inhibition of protein synthesis, or interference with passage of nerve impulses. Endotoxins, which are a portion of the gram-negative cell, cause fever, shock, and disseminated intravascular coagulation (DIC) (see Chapter 26).

! CRITICAL TO REMEMBER

Classification of Bacteria

Bacteria are classified by three characteristics:
- Shape (rods or cocci)
- Reaction on Gram stain (positive or negative)
- Ability to grow in the presence of oxygen (aerobic or anaerobic)

Diphtheria

Causative agent:	*Corynebacterium diphtheriae* (a gram-positive, nonmotile bacillus)
Incubation period:	2 to 7 days
Infectious period:	Ranges from 2 weeks or less up to several months in an untreated individual
Transmission:	Contact with carrier or disease, droplets
Immunity:	Vaccine with boosters, passive immunity from maternal antibodies, natural disease
Season:	Fall and winter

Manifestations

Nasal manifestations of diphtheria include discharge of foul-smelling mucopurulent material. Low-grade fever is common. Thin, gray membranes appear on tonsils and pharynx, causing "bull neck," or neck edema.

Therapeutic Management

Treatment includes the administration of diphtheria antitoxin intravenously and antibiotics.

Primary prevention of diphtheria can be accomplished through administration of the diphtheria vaccine in combination with tetanus and acellular pertussis (DTaP). Immunization of children ages 2 months to 7 years should consist of five doses of the DTaP vaccine (see Chapter 4 and Appendix D). For children older than 7 years, Td vaccine should be administered. After the initial childhood immunization series is completed, a booster dose of diphtheria and tetanus toxoids (given as Td) is recommended at 11 to 12 years of age and should be given no later than age 16 years (AAP, 2003b).

Nursing Considerations

The nurse should obtain a history of symptoms, along with an immunization history. The nurse should teach parents and give them information about monitoring for any increased respiratory efforts, mode of transmission, and prevention of spread of the disease to family and close contacts. Nursing care of the hospitalized child with diphtheria involves Droplet Precautions, bed rest, and monitoring the child's respiratory status (patency of the airway).

The primary focus of nursing should be preventive, because the development and use of the diphtheria vaccine have drastically reduced the incidence of diphtheria in the United States. In addition, the American Academy of Pediatrics (AAP, 2003b) recommends the use of DTaP (diphtheria vaccine with tetanus and acellular pertussis vaccines) for the prevention of any adverse reactions to the whole-cell pertussis vaccine available as DTP.

CATARRHAL
Duration: 1-2 weeks
Symptoms: Symptoms of upper respiratory tract infection (rhinorrhea, lacrimation, mild cough, low-grade fever).

PAROXYSMAL
Duration: 2-4 weeks or longer
Symptoms: Increased severity of cough. Repetitive series of coughs during a single expiration, followed by massive inspiration with a whoop. Cyanosis, protrusion of tongue, salivation, distention of neck veins. Coughing spells may be triggered by yawning, sneezing, eating, or drinking. Coughing may induce vomiting.

CONVALESCENT
Duration: 1-2 weeks
Symptoms: Episodes of coughing, whooping, and vomiting that decrease in frequency and severity. Cough may persist for several months.

Pertussis (Whooping Cough)

Causative agent:	*Bordetella pertussis* (a gram-negative bacillus)
Incubation period:	6 to 20 days
Infectious period:	Catarrhal stage (1 to 2 weeks) until the 4th week
Transmission:	Direct contact or respiratory droplets from coughing
Immunity:	Bacteria or vaccine, both of which provide varying degrees and duration of immunity against pertussis
Season:	Can occur during any season

Manifestations

The three stages of pertussis are catarrhal, paroxysmal, and convalescent (Box 40-1).

Complications

The most common complication of pertussis is pneumonia. There may be varying degrees of other respiratory complications, ranging from atelectasis to interstitial or subcutaneous emphysema to pneumothorax. Approximately 90%

! **CRITICAL TO REMEMBER**

Immunity to Pertussis

Because infants do not receive maternal immunity to pertussis, they are very susceptible to pertussis. Pertussis is a highly contagious illness that is associated with a high infant mortality rate.

---

of the deaths attributable to pertussis are related to respiratory complications. Anoxia can lead to CNS involvement. Malnutrition and dehydration may result from extensive vomiting and can be very dangerous, especially for infants. Other complications include otitis media, ulcers of the frenulum of the tongue, epistaxis, hernia, and rectal prolapse.

Therapeutic Management

Primary prevention of pertussis can be accomplished through administration of the pertussis vaccine in combination with tetanus and diphtheria vaccines (DTaP) as previously described.

Erythromycin, if given early in the course of the disease, will eliminate the organism from the nasopharynx within a few days, thereby reducing communicability. Erythromycin is also given to all nonimmune close contacts, which include most children older than 13 years, because the immunity conferred by the childhood immunization declines by that age. Corticosteroids and albuterol have been used to reduce paroxysmal coughing.

Hospitalization and supportive care for the infant may be necessary to monitor airway patency, whereas older children can usually be cared for at home. Respiratory status is monitored with a cardiopulmonary monitor and pulse oximeter. Droplet Precautions are observed.

Nursing Considerations

The nurse should obtain a complete immunization history and any recent known exposures to illnesses. Documentation should also include the parent's description of any respiratory events before admission and indicators such as coughing, secretions, cyanotic episodes, and the child's activity level. Assessment of the child's respiratory, fluid, nutrition, output, and neurologic status should be done.

The child's respiratory status needs monitoring with a cardiopulmonary monitor and pulse oximeter. If the child is hospitalized, the limits of the monitor should be checked frequently. Explain any monitoring devices to the child (if age-appropriate) and parents to help alleviate anxiety. Suction and oxygen equipment should be readily available. Supplemental oxygen therapy could be ordered if the child's oxygen saturation falls below an acceptable range (especially during any coughing episodes). If the child needs oxygen therapy, parents should receive instructions about any oxygen equipment and the timing and possible length of treatment. Some children will need additional oxygen only during the paroxysmal spells.

Because the child's coughing paroxysms may be triggered by noises or frightening experiences, a quiet environment and a calm, reassuring approach should be used when caring for the child and supporting the parents. Paroxysmal episodes should be monitored for any drop in oxygen saturation levels. Parents and children will need additional support and reassurance that assistance is near and ready if needed during the child's coughing spells, because these episodes can be extremely frightening.

The infant's nutritional status should be closely monitored. Small, frequent feedings may benefit infants if the feeding process becomes exhausting. Should the child's intake be insufficient, nutritional support (gavage or parenteral nutrition) may be needed to prevent dehydration or weight loss. If the child has vomiting episodes when coughing, frequent oral care will be necessary.

Nursing care activities should be clustered, if possible, to allow the child and parent or parents to rest. Diversional activities should be age-appropriate. Parents may need emotional support to deal with feelings of guilt, especially if they chose not to immunize their child.

Scarlet Fever (Scarlatina)

Causative agent:	Group A beta-hemolytic streptococci
Incubation period:	1 to 7 days (average 3 days)
Infectious period:	Acute stage until 24 hours after antimicrobial therapy has begun
Transmission:	Airborne (inhalation or ingestion), direct contact
Immunity:	None
Season:	Late fall, winter, and spring

Manifestations

Abrupt fever, vomiting, headache, abdominal pain, pharyngitis, and chills may characterize the onset of scarlet fever. The fever reaches a peak by the 2nd day and returns to normal within 5 to 6 days. Within 24 hours a red, fine, papular rash appears in the axillae, groin, and neck. The rash then spreads peripherally to cover the entire body (Fig. 40-8). The rash will blanch on pressure except in areas of deep creases (Pastia's sign). Desquamation begins on the face at the end of the 1st week, and flaking proceeds down the trunk. This process may continue for up to 6 weeks. The tongue is initially coated with a white, furry covering with red projecting papillae (so-called *white strawberry tongue*). By the 4th day the white strawberry tongue sloughs off, leaving a red, swollen tongue (so-called *strawberry tongue*). The tonsils are edematous and may be covered with a gray-white exudate, which may spread to the pharynx. Petechial hemorrhages cover the soft palate.

Complications

Complications generally result from extension of the streptococcal infection. They may include sinusitis, otitis media, mastoiditis, peritonsillar abscess, bronchopneumonia, meningitis, osteomyelitis, rheumatic fever, and glomerulonephritis.

Therapeutic Management

The preferred treatment for any streptococcal infection is penicillin. Children allergic to penicillin can be given erythromycin. Supportive care for symptoms is indicated. Laboratory confirmation (generally by a throat culture) is recommended for children with sore throats because of the similarity of symptoms between viral and group A strep throats. Children with streptococcal infections (throat, skin) may return to school or daycare 24 hours after beginning antibiotics when they are no longer considered contagious. Droplet Precautions should be observed also until the child has been on antibiotics for 24 hours.

Nursing Considerations

The nurse should obtain and document a complete history of symptoms. The nurse should also assess the child's throat, tongue, rash, nutritional and fluid intake, vital signs, and

> ## PARENTS
> ## Want to Know
>
> ### How to Care for Their Child With Scarlet Fever
>
> - It is necessary to give the entire course (usually 10 to 14 days) of the antibiotic to destroy all the bacteria and decrease the risk of complications. If a partial course of antibiotics is given (antibiotic stopped by parent when child is feeling better), the bacteria can become resistant and fail to be eradicated with subsequent attempts.
> - Cool drinks and liquid refreshments (Popsicles, milk shakes) may be soothing and will help to maintain hydration.
> - Acetaminophen, ibuprofen, throat lozenges, antiseptic throat spray (e.g., Chloraseptic), and cool mist may be used to relieve discomfort.
> - Encouraging quiet activities will help prevent fatigue.
> - In providing oral care, acidic preparations should be avoided. Saline rinses may provide comfort and promote hygiene.
> - A soft, bland diet should be offered.
> - Call your primary health provider if your child develops drooling or great difficulty swallowing or acts very sick. After 48 hours of antibiotic therapy, your child should not have a fever.
> - Your child is no longer contagious after 24 hours of antibiotic therapy. The rash is not contagious.

level of general wellness. Any history of sensitivity to penicillin should be thoroughly explored and prominently noted on the child's records.

Generally, children with scarlet fever are cared for at home. Comfort measures include encouraging fluids (especially cool, nonacidic liquids) and administering antipyretics for fever control.

Analgesics may be given for discomfort, and antipruritic comfort measures may be necessary. Parents should understand the typical course of disease and any treatment measures, including the importance of completing the full course of any antibiotics prescribed (to prevent growth of resistant bacteria). Bed rest and quiet activities may be beneficial during the acute stage (Parents Want to Know box).

Children with severe symptoms and complications may, however, need hospitalization and supportive care. In such cases, vital signs, especially body temperature, should be monitored.

RICKETTSIAL INFECTIONS

Rickettsiae are small, parasitic bacteria that are transmitted to humans by blood-sucking arthropods. A vertebrate is not necessary for the survival of the bacteria, and the host arthropod appears not to be affected adversely by the rickettsiae. Replication of the rickettsiae in the new host cell causes cell death, which may be accompanied by vasculitis with thrombosis, increased permeability, tissue edema, hemorrhage, circulatory failure, and meningoencephalitis. Rickettsial diseases cannot be transmitted from person to person.

First day   Third day

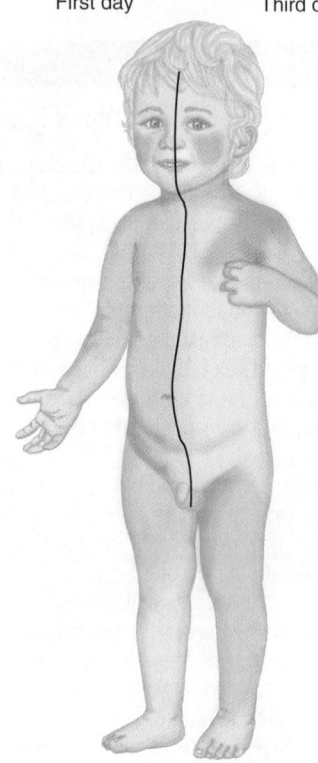

**Scarlet Fever Rash
Distribution**

- Red, fine, papular rash
  appears within 24 hours of
  fever and other symptoms.
  In dark skin, the rash is often
  seen as punctate papular elevations.

- Begins in axillas, groin, and
  neck and spreads to cover
  entire body

- Desquamation begins on face
  at end of first week, and flaking
  proceeds down trunk. May
  continue up to 6 weeks.

- Tongue: Initially presents with
  white, furry coat with red
  projecting papillae (white strawberry
  tongue). By the 4th day, the white
  sloughs off, leaving a red swollen
  tongue (strawberry tongue).

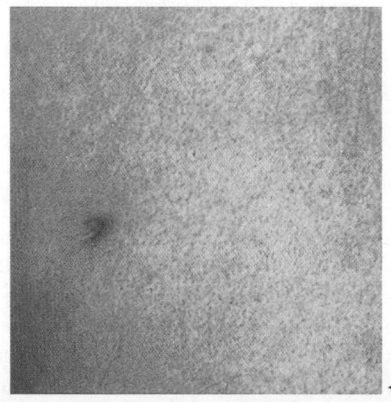

◄ **Rash, Light Skin**

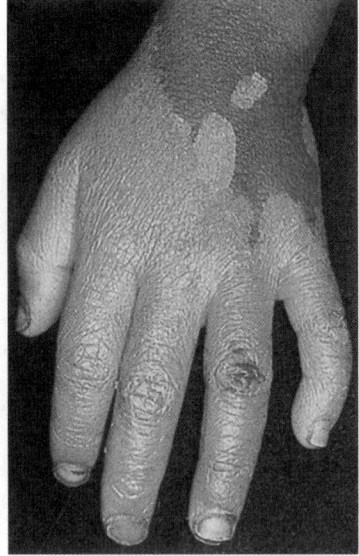

Desquamation, Dark Skin

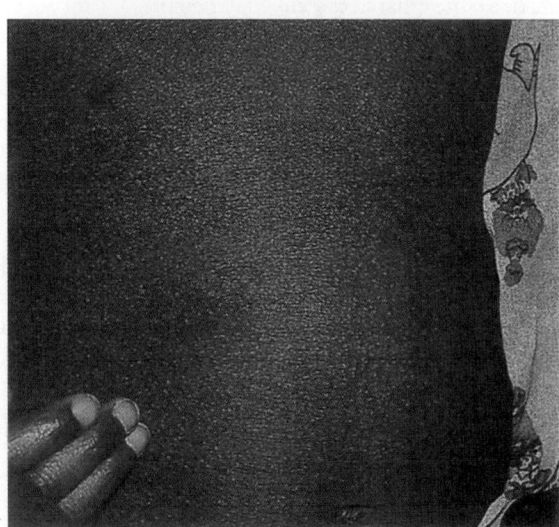

Rash, Dark Skin ►

Figure 40-8 Scarlet fever rash distribution and appearance. Note the characteristic skin peeling. (Photos from Hurwitz, S. [1993]. *Clinical pediatric dermatology: A textbook of skin disorders of childhood and adolescence* [2nd ed.]. Philadelphia: Saunders.)

Rocky Mountain Spotted Fever

Causative agent:	*Rickettsia rickettsii*
Reservoir:	Wild rodents, dogs
Vector:	Tick (wood, dog, Lone Star)
Incubation period:	2 to 14 days (average 7 days)
Transmission:	Bite of infected tick
Season:	April through October

Manifestations

The onset of Rocky Mountain spotted fever is marked by nonspecific signs and symptoms, such as headache, fever, anorexia, and restlessness. Generally, on the 3rd day a characteristic maculopapular or petechial rash appears. This rash begins on the extremities (usually the wrists/palms and ankles/soles) and spreads to the rest of the body. As the rash progresses, hemorrhagic and necrotic lesions can appear. Gangrene of the distal parts of the body can result from thrombosis. Edema develops, beginning in the periorbital area and progressing to a generalized edema of the body and extremities. Delayed treatment can lead to a mortality rate of 25%.

Therapeutic Management

With early detection in children (within 5 days of the beginning of the illness), the likelihood of positive resolution increases. Doxycycline is the drug of choice; chloramphenicol is an alternative. Chloramphenicol and tetracycline are both used less frequently because of the side effects (including staining of teeth) in children younger than 8 years. If vascular damage has already occurred, however, the drugs may not alter the course of the disease. Treatment before day 5 of illness in children with clinical signs and symptoms is more likely to achieve a good outcome. There is no licensed vaccine in the United States or role for antibiotics in the prevention of Rocky Mountain spotted fever.

Nursing Considerations

The assessment of children presenting with symptoms indicating Rocky Mountain spotted fever should include obtaining a complete history of skin eruptions, medications taken, exposure to infectious diseases, and recent hiking or other activities in wooded areas. Any rashes or skin lesions should then be examined, with documentation of distribution and morphology. The child's vital signs, especially body temperature, should also be assessed and noted.

Hospitalized children will require supportive care for their presenting symptoms. Straws should be used, and the mouth should be flushed if tetracycline is administered because it can stain the teeth. Parents should be cautioned to give the full course of any antibiotic to decrease the risk of complications and ensure that the disease is eradicated.

Education in the control measures for prevention of tick-borne infections is vital (Box 40-2).

BORRELIA INFECTIONS

Borrelia is a genus of spiral bacteria that are transmitted to humans by arthropods. The diseases caused by *Borrelia* are relapsing fever and Lyme disease.

> **BOX 40-2**
> *Preventive Measures to Avoid Insect and Tick Bites*
>
> - Children should wear tightly woven clothing consisting of long pants, long-sleeved shirts, long socks, and a hat when in woods and grassy areas. Pants should be tucked into socks. Clothing should also be light-colored so ticks are easily visible.
> - Paths should be followed and dense areas avoided if possible. Avoid known tick-infested areas.
> - Insect repellents that contain diethyltoluamide (DEET) and permethrins should be used; apply before any possible exposure and every 1 to 2 hours sparingly according to manufacturer's directions. Care should be taken to avoid contact of repellent with the child's eyes or mouth. The repellent should not be applied to the hands to avoid contact with the eyes and mouth. Wash hands and skin after the child goes indoors.
> - Repellents should be used with caution in infants because of the risk of encephalopathy.
> - Insect repellent should not be applied to wounds or irritated skin.
> - The body (especially exposed hairy regions) should be inspected periodically for ticks, which may resemble small moles or blood blisters. Early removal can prevent transmission of disease from an infected tick.
> - Ticks should be removed with tweezers. The tick should be removed as close to the skin as possible.
> - Care should be taken to avoid handling the tick with bare hands or crushing the tick's body.
> - Ticks may be preserved in alcohol for later identification.
> - Pets should be kept free of ticks by dipping and spraying during tick season. Yards should be kept free of brush and undergrowth.

Relapsing Fever

Relapsing fever is spread from person to person by lice or ticks. The bacteria are introduced into a bite wound when the bite is rubbed. This infection is spread when people fail to wash thoroughly and do not change clothes.

Tick-borne relapsing fever (*Borrelia hermsii*, *Borrelia turicatae*) results from tick exposures in rodent-infested cabins in western mountainous areas of the United States, including state and national parks. *Borrelia turicatae* infections occur less frequently, with the majority in Texas.

Manifestations

The sudden onset of high fever, shaking chills, sweats, headache, muscle and joint pains, and progressive weakness characterizes relapsing fever. A macular rash on the trunk and petechiae of the skin and mucous membranes may occur.

Therapeutic Management

Several antibiotics provide effective treatment. These include penicillin, tetracycline, erythromycin, and chloramphenicol in children older than 8 years. For children younger than 8 years and for pregnant women, penicillin or erythromycin is the preferred drug.

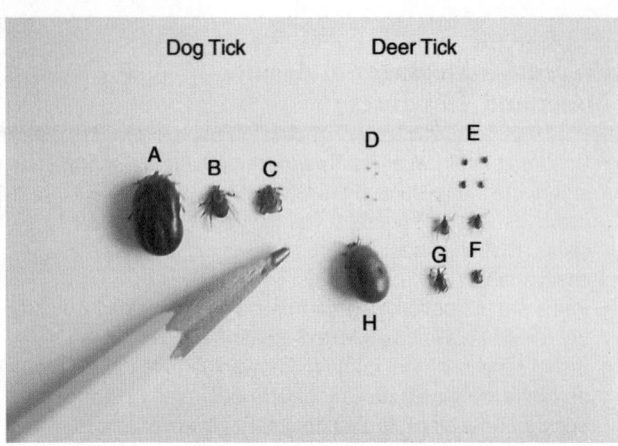

Figure 40-9 Dog (wood) ticks and deer (black-legged) ticks compared with a pencil. Dog ticks: *A*, Engorged female; *B*, female; *C*, male. Deer ticks: *D*, Larvae; *E*, nymphs; *F*, males; *G*, females; *H*, engorged female. (Courtesy Lyme Disease Foundation, www.lyme.org.)

Nursing Considerations

Assessment should include a complete history of rash onset and characteristics, medications taken, and living environment, including available bathing and washing facilities. Fever, headache, and arthralgias should be treated with antipyretics and analgesics. Antibiotics should be given as ordered. Education includes personal hygiene, the use of pediculicides, and eradication methods.

Lyme Disease

Lyme disease is spread by tick bites and is the most frequently reported vector-borne disease in the United States (AAP, 2000). Lyme disease is a multisystem illness that affects the skin and the musculoskeletal, cardiovascular, and nervous systems.

Causative agent:	*Borrelia burgdorferi* (spirochete)
Vector:	Tick (Fig. 40-9)
Incubation period:	3 to 32 days
Transmission:	Bite of infected tick (person-to-person transmission not possible)
Season:	April to October

Manifestations

The manifestations of Lyme disease can be divided into three stages (early localized, early disseminated, late disseminated). In the first stage (early localized), the skin lesions are most prominent; in the second stage (early disseminated), cardiac and neurologic findings are prominent; and in the third stage (late disseminated), arthritis is the main manifestation (Wade, 2000).

In the early localized stage of Lyme disease, local reactions to an infected tick bite occur, along with vague, flu-like symptoms (headache, chills, fatigue, vague muscle aches and pains). An erythematous macula or papule forms at the site of the tick bite within 3 to 30 days (Fig. 40-10). This rash can enlarge to 16 to 68 cm in diameter, with a clearing in the center (erythema migrans, bull's eye rash). It may itch, prickle, or burn. The rash generally lasts for 3 weeks, during which time it gradually fades.

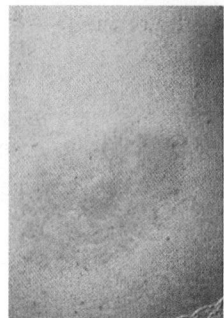

Figure 40-10 Characteristic lesion of Lyme disease. (From Larson, W.G., Adams, R.M., & Maibach, H.I. [1991]. *Color text of contact dermatitis*. Philadelphia: Saunders.)

In the early disseminated stage (generally 1 to 4 months after the bite), neurologic symptoms may be the first to occur. CNS symptoms may include severe headaches with myelitis, nausea, vomiting, facial nerve paralysis (Bell's palsy), forgetfulness or decreased concentration, and cerebral ataxia. General lymphadenopathy and joint and muscle pain may also be present. Lyme arthritis generally affects the large joints, with the knee being the most often involved. Cardiac disease is usually brief and uncommon in children. The signs and symptoms generally resolve over a few days, but many individuals have recurrences. Skin lesions may recur but are smaller and more diffuse than the initial ones.

Symptoms of late disseminated Lyme disease (occurring months to years after the initial infected tick bite) occur intermittently and include chronic arthritis, profound fatigue, and chronic neurologic manifestations. The debilitating effects frequently affect a child's ability to participate in normal activities (e.g., sports) because of extreme fatigue or cardiac complications.

Therapeutic Management

Primary prevention of Lyme disease includes anticipatory guidance and information about routine preventive measures to avoid insect bites. A vaccine that had been approved for use in the United States in those between the ages of 15 and 70 years has been withdrawn from the market by the manufacturer. Currently, no other vaccine for Lyme disease is available (Shapiro, 2003).

Early detection and antibiotic treatment in any of the disease's stages are highly effective and are usually highly successful in positively affecting the course of the disease (Shapiro, 2003). In addition, disease identified in early stages and treated with antibiotics does not progress to the more debilitating stages. The characteristic rash of Lyme disease linked to other symptoms leads to a diagnosis except in cases where the child has atypical manifestations of the disease (e.g., one septic joint, usually the knee).

Presently, treatment for early-localized disease involves the use of doxycycline for children older than 9 years and amoxicillin for children younger than 9 years and pregnant or lactating women, with the course of treatment lasting 14 to 21 days. For those allergic to penicillin, cefuroxime axetil and erythromycin are alternate drugs. For early disseminated and late Lyme disease with additional systemic complications (persistent or recurrent arthritis, carditis, meningitis, encephalitis), IV or IM ceftriaxone or penicillin is indicated.

TABLE **40-1** Common Helminths

Class and Typical Agent	Transmission	Manifestations	Diagnosis	Treatment
Roundworm (*Ascaris lumbricoides*)	Ingestion of eggs from contaminated soil or food, transfer to mouth from fingers, toys, or other vectors	Abdominal pain or distention, abdominal obstruction, vomiting with bile staining, pneumonitis	Fecal smear	Mebendazole Pyrantel pamoate
Pinworm (*Enterobius vermicularis*)	Ingestion or inhalation of eggs, transfer from hands to mouth	Nocturnal anal itching, sleeplessness	Scotch tape test and microscopic examination	Pyrantel pamoate Mebendazole
Tapeworm (*Taenia saginata*)	Ingestion from handling or eating infected beef or pork	Asymptomatic, segments of worms seen in stool, abdominal pain, nausea, anorexia, weight loss, insomnia	Fecal smear or microscopic examination	Praziquantel (safety under age 4 yr not established, and use is investigational)
Hookworm (*Necator americanus*)	Skin penetration from direct contact with contaminated soil	Dermatitis, anemia, pneumonitis, blood loss, malnutrition	Fecal smear or microscopic examination	Pyrantel pamoate

Nursing Considerations

Assessment should include a complete history of rash onset and characteristics; medications taken; recent exposures to infectious diseases; and recent hiking, working (forestry, farming, outdoor construction or maintenance), or vacationing (camping [e.g., Boy or Girl Scouts], hunting) in a known endemic area or heavily wooded area. Rashes should be examined for characteristics and distribution and documented (Wade, 2000).

Fever, headache, and arthralgia should be treated with antipyretics and analgesics. Parents should have a complete understanding of the course of treatment including the importance of administering medication, including antibiotics, as prescribed. The importance of completing the entire course of antibiotic treatment should be stressed. Generally, affected children will be treated at home. Parental and caregiver education is important to prevent further exposures and to facilitate early recognition of disease symptoms.

HELMINTHS

Helminths are worms that live as parasites. The three groups with the greatest impact on humans are tapeworms, flukes, and roundworms (Table 40-1). Children are more commonly infected than adults, primarily as a result of frequent hand-to-mouth activity and the likelihood of fecal contamination. Transmission may occur by oral-fecal ingestion, ingestion of contaminated tissue from another host, skin penetration, or the bite of a blood-sucking insect.

Therapeutic Management

Treatment consists of the administration of oral medications effective against a specific helminth. Treatment is provided to the entire family. Anticipatory guidance to prevent reinfestation and education about the prevention of the spread of disease (basic enteric isolation procedures) for the family and primary caregivers, along with personal hygiene and sanitary practices, are also necessary (Parents Want to Know box).

PARENTS
Want to Know

How to Prevent Parasitic Infections

- Handwashing (including under the fingernails) with soap and water should be done before eating or handling of food, as well as after using the toilet.
- Placing hands in the mouth and nail biting should be discouraged.
- Toilets or other appropriate bathroom facilities should be used for elimination.
- Toilets or bathroom facilities should be cleaned with agents containing bleach.
- Scratching the anal area with bare hands should be discouraged.
- Dogs and cats should be kept at a distance from play areas and sandboxes, and the latter need to be covered when not in use.
- Shoes should be worn when outside.
- All fruits and vegetables should be washed before being eaten.
- Diapers should be changed frequently and disposed of properly (out of children's reach).
- Swimming facilities that allow diapered children should be avoided.
- Only bottled water should be used during camping outings.

Nursing Considerations

A thorough history, including the child's general wellness, personal hygiene practices, availability of running water and bathing and laundry facilities, along with nutritional intake, should be obtained.

Most parasites are identified in fecal smears obtained from stool specimens. If the family or caregiver is to bring a stool specimen in for laboratory testing, the nurse needs to provide specific, clear instructions and provide a container if needed. Sample size and number, as well as proper storage, should be clearly explained. Stool specimens that have not been contaminated with urine are ideal. Obtaining urine-free specimens may be difficult, especially in infants or very young children. Plastic wrap can be placed over the toilet bowl or a potty chair, or specimens can be collected from a diaper using a clean tongue blade and placing in a container. The container should be marked with the child's name and the date and time of collection. It should then be refrigerated until it is delivered to the laboratory.

Education for the parents and primary caregivers should focus on medication administration, primary prevention of future reinfestations, and resource identification with referral to available community and social services for any basic living needs (running water, bathing facilities). The rationale for evaluating and treating the entire family for infection and the usual mode of transmission must be discussed to prevent future reinfestation or cross contamination of family members. Anticipatory guidance regarding primary prevention and teaching about prevention (personal hygiene and health habits) should be covered with the child's family. The nurse should help the family identify any resources (access to care, social services) necessary and initiate referral if appropriate.

FUNGAL INFECTIONS

Fungi are free-living organisms that can be found throughout the environment. Some species of fungi are part of the normal human flora, especially those in the mouth, intestine, vagina, and skin. A fungus is transmitted through inhalation or penetration of tissue as a result of trauma. Fungi grow very slowly, so clinical symptoms may appear only after a prolonged period. They are aerobic, can grow in a wide range of temperatures, and are resistant to most antibiotics. They exist in two forms: *molds* and *yeasts*.

Infections caused by fungi are classified into four groups:

- Opportunistic—secondary to a defect in host immunity
- Systemic—involving deep tissues and organs
- Subcutaneous—limited to deep subcutaneous tissue
- Superficial—limited to skin, hair, and nails

Common fungal infections include tinea capitis, tinea pedis, and candidal infections (see Chapter 49).

SEXUALLY TRANSMISSIBLE DISEASES

The rates of infection of many sexually transmissible diseases (STDs), or diseases transmitted through sexual activity, are highest among adolescents. Those adolescents at highest risk are male homosexuals, sexually active heterosexuals, younger sexually active adolescents, and IV-drug users. Adolescents are at greater risk because they have frequent unprotected intercourse, are biologically more susceptible to infection, and face multiple obstacles to access to health care (Eissa & Cromwell, 2003). Often, adolescents lack knowledge of methods for preventing STDs. Moreover, the use of drugs and alcohol makes unsafe, unprotected sex more likely to occur. In addition, adolescents' inherent developmental stage and

---

TEENAGERS Want to Know

About Sexually Transmissible Diseases

- Sexually transmissible diseases (STDs) are diseases that can be transmitted through body fluids (semen, vaginal fluids, blood).
- Not all STDs have symptoms. Many people with chlamydia (an STD infection) do not have *any* symptoms. It is possible to transmit an STD that you do not know you have to someone else.
- STDs can be painful, ugly, and dangerous to those who have them. Some can even cause sterility, neurologic (brain) damage, cancer, or death.
- STDs can infect anyone, regardless of race, religion, sexual preference, social status, or gender.
- Because many STDs can be transmitted not only through sexual intercourse but also through skin-to-skin contact, even the most careful individuals can be susceptible to infections.
- Some STDs, such as gonorrhea, chlamydia, and syphilis, can be cured fairly easily by completing a course of medication. Others, such as herpes, genital warts, and human immunodeficiency virus (HIV), cannot be cured, although some treatments are available to reduce their symptoms.
- Abstinence is the *only* 100% effective way to prevent both pregnancy and STD transmission.
- Abstinence means never engaging in any form of sexual contact with a partner.
- Deciding if and when to have sex is an important issue to think about.
- No one should ever be pressured to have sex.
- If you choose to have sex, using a male or female condom can reduce *(not eliminate)* your chances of acquiring or passing on an STD.
- Some symptoms that might mean you have an STD are unusual discharge, swelling, pain, sores, or a rash in your genitals; unusual nonmenstrual bleeding; pain when you urinate or have a bowel movement; or a sore throat for several weeks.
- If you are sexually active and note any of these symptoms, see your primary health care provider as soon as possible. Detecting and treating an STD early will decrease the chances of permanent damage.

---

sense of invulnerability lead to risky behavior and risk taking (Teenagers Want to Know box).

Neonates are at risk for transplacental transmission of STDs from an infected mother or from direct contamination during the birthing process. Children who acquire STDs after the neonatal period should be highly suspect of being sexually abused. These children may present without the typical genital symptoms but with a variety of physical or behavioral complaints. Related changes in behavior may include insomnia, eating disorders, bed wetting, or emotional withdrawal. A careful, complete history and physical examination are required. The examination should include inspection of oral, anal, and genital mucosa for any signs of trauma or infection. Because obtaining a complete history may be difficult, children should undergo a complete laboratory evaluation and all potentially infected areas should be cultured if sexual abuse is suspected.

Gonorrhea

Causative agent:	*Neisseria gonorrhoeae* (gram-negative diplococcus)
Incubation period:	2 to 7 days
Transmission:	Intimate contact (perinatally, through sexual abuse, by sexual intercourse)

Gonorrhea may be transmitted three different ways:

- *Perinatally:* Transmission can occur during birth of a neonate whose mother is infected or with premature rupture of the membranes. The neonate can acquire the disease through aspiration of vaginal secretions, which leads to sepsis; through direct contact through the conjunctiva; or through direct contact through attachment of a fetal scalp electrode.
- *Sexual abuse:* Any child with a positive culture and without a prior history of voluntary sexual behavior should be considered a potential sexual abuse victim until proven otherwise. Transmission through sexual play with children has been documented but is rare. Almost all children diagnosed with gonorrhea at the age of 1 year or older have experienced sexual abuse.
- *Voluntary sexual activity:* This route of transmission remains the primary route of infection among adolescents. Sexual abuse should not, however, be excluded as a possibility.

Manifestations

Ophthalmia neonatorum is the most common type of gonorrheal infection in the infant, presenting 1 to 4 days after birth. A thick, purulent discharge from the eyes may be present and, if not treated promptly, will progress to corneal ulceration, rupture, and blindness. Ophthalmia neonatorum has been controlled through prophylactic treatment with an ophthalmic antibiotic given immediately after birth. In older children, ophthalmic infection can be the result of self-inoculation from the genital site.

Girls with gonorrheal infection may present with a purulent vulvovaginitis, whereas boys often have urethritis. A history of purulent discharge with burning during urination is often elicited. Adolescent girls may present with cervicitis, urethritis, perihepatitis, and salpingitis. Gonorrhea in adolescent and younger females may progress to pelvic inflammatory disease (PID). PID is the most common cause of infertility in young women (Eissa & Cromwell, 2003).

Therapeutic Management

Because syphilis and chlamydial infection are also often present in individuals with gonorrhea, testing should take place for those diseases. Penicillin-resistant *N. gonorrhoeae* strains have influenced the choice of therapy. Currently, the drug of choice for gonorrhea is a third-generation cephalosporin, such as ceftriaxone. Ceftriaxone is effective in treating syphilis but not chlamydial infections. It is recommended therefore that a course of tetracycline or doxy-

cycline be administered in conjunction with ceftriaxone for those with chlamydial infection. Sexual partners should be treated.

Syphilis

Causative agent:	*Treponema pallidum*
Incubation period:	Acquired primary infection—10 to 90 days (average 21 days)
Transmission:	Intimate contact, transplacentally, or sexually

Congenital syphilis may be transmitted transplacentally by an infected mother at any time during pregnancy or birth. Acquired syphilis is contracted through sexual contact. In children, syphilis diagnosed after the neonatal period can almost always be linked to sexual abuse.

Manifestations

Infants with congenital syphilis may be asymptomatic or may exhibit signs and symptoms within the first 3 months of life. The classic signs are rhinitis, a maculopapular rash, and hepatosplenomegaly. Diagnostic radiographs may show osteochondritis, periosteitis, or metaphyseal changes, especially in the long bones of the femur and humerus. Late manifestations are a result of the scarring from the systemic disease process. The bones, teeth, eyes, and eighth cranial nerve are involved. The teeth are notched (Hutchinson's teeth), and hearing loss can occur suddenly around the age of 8 to 10 years. Acquired syphilis has the same clinical course in children as in adults (see Chapter 31).

Therapeutic Management

Syphilis responds well to a single dose of benzathine penicillin G intramuscularly (the preferred treatment for children and adults). Aqueous crystalline penicillin G or procaine penicillin is effective with congenital syphilis. Acquired syphilis can be treated with benzathine penicillin G. Tetracycline and doxycycline are options for the client older than 8 years but should not be used in younger children because of the greater risks of permanent tooth staining. In addition, the effectiveness of drugs other than penicillin and tetracycline remains unproven. When follow-up cannot be guaranteed, especially for children younger than 8 years, consideration should be given to hospitalizing the child and consulting a specialist (for potential desensitization followed by penicillin G administration) (AAP, 2003i).

Education regarding potential long-term effects of partially or untreated syphilis must be discussed. Resources should be available and care should be accessible to ensure completion of treatment and eradication of disease.

Chlamydial Infection

Causative agent:	*Chlamydia trachomatis, Chlamydia psittaci, Chlamydia pneumoniae*
Incubation period:	7 to 21 days
Transmission:	During birth if mother is infected, through sexual activity

Chlamydial infection has become one of the most prevalent STDs. Infants are infected during the birthing process. Chlamydial infection can cause morbidity in the infant and is responsible for neonatal eye infections and interstitial pneumonia.

Manifestations

Many people with a chlamydial infection have few or no symptoms. As a result, the disease may go undiagnosed until complications develop.

Neonatal conjunctivitis manifests with a watery discharge that becomes purulent. Eyelids are edematous, and the conjunctiva may become inflamed. Mucoid rhinorrhea may be associated with the infection. Many infants with conjunctivitis will develop infection of the nasopharynx, which can progress to pneumonia. These infants may have a history of a cough and congestion. Long-term abnormalities of pulmonary function may result in chronic respiratory problems.

Urethritis with dysuria, urinary frequency, or mucopurulent discharge may indicate chlamydial infection. Any identification of this organism in presexual children indicates possible child abuse.

Therapeutic Management

In infants with conjunctivitis or pneumonia, a 14-day course of oral erythromycin is recommended. For uncomplicated genital tract infection, azithromycin is effective for children younger than 8 years and doxycycline may also be used for older children and teenagers.

Trichomoniasis

Causative agent:	*Trichomonas vaginalis* (flagellated protozoan)
Incubation period:	4 to 28 days (average 1 week)
Transmission:	Perinatal contact during delivery, sexual activity

Manifestations

Infections with *Trichomonas* are frequently asymptomatic. Only 25% to 50% of female clients with trichomoniasis will exhibit symptoms. Most male clients are asymptomatic. When symptoms occur, they may include dysuria, vaginal itching and burning (in females), and a frothy, yellowish green, foul-smelling discharge. Infected mothers can infect their newborn infants during birth. Children with a positive culture for *Trichomonas* should be investigated for possible sexual abuse.

Therapeutic Management

A single dose of metronidazole (Flagyl, Protostat) is the treatment of choice for adolescents and adults; it has an approximate cure rate of 95%. For prepubertal girls, the drug is given in two or three divided doses. Sexual partners should also be treated. Metronidazole should not be used during the first trimester of pregnancy.

Education regarding the potential presence of other STDs should be thoroughly discussed, especially with the adolescent client, in a respectful and confidential manner.

Human Papillomavirus

Causative agent:	Human papillomavirus (HPV)
Incubation period:	4 weeks to many months
Transmission:	Direct sexual contact, perinatal contact during delivery

Human papillomavirus is responsible for the common wart and for venereal warts (condylomata acuminata). These anogenital warts may be contracted through direct sexual contact or perinatally during the delivery process. Children with anogenital warts should be investigated for sexual abuse. A person can get warts through autoinoculation from other body sites. A break in skin integrity is necessary for infection to occur.

Manifestations

Anogenital warts begin as small papules that grow into soft, clustered lesions. They are found in moist areas, such as the labia minora, vagina, cervix, anus, rectum, and glans penis. Most warts in children resolve within several years.

Therapeutic Management

Treatment can include surgery, cryotherapy, electrocautery, and laser therapy or chemical ablation. For sexually active individuals, transmission can be decreased by the use of condoms.

Herpes Simplex Virus

Causative agent:	Herpes simplex virus, type 2 (see Chapter 49 for a discussion of HSV 1)
Incubation period:	2 to 20 days
Transmission:	Direct sexual contact with an infected person

Herpes simplex virus, type 2, is the cause of genital herpes. Genital herpes is one of the most frequently seen STDs in the United States. It is especially problematic because an infected mother can transmit it to her newborn during vaginal delivery, causing multisystem disease. Women with active

---

CRITICAL THINKING EXERCISE 40-1

Adolescents with a sexually transmissible disease (STD) may seek out school or community-based health care. Their complaints may be vague, with generalized feelings of malaise or fever; or specific, with complaints of painful urination or vaginal or penile discharge. Often they hope that the nurse will ask about sexual activity because they feel they cannot trust other adults. What challenges does the nurse face when caring for these adolescents?

HSV infection as labor and delivery approach may be advised to have a cesarean delivery.

Manifestations

At the initial infection, lesions occur in the genital area, usually on the vulva, perineum, or perianal area. However, lesions may also occur in the vagina and on the cervix, areas where they cannot be seen. Pain and tenderness in the affected area may coincide with lesion eruption. Vesicles erupt, rupture, and then ulcerate over the course of 1 to 7 days. The virus is shed for 2 to 3 weeks. Occasionally, flu-like symptoms (fever, malaise, enlarged lymph nodes) can accompany vesicular eruption. After the acute phase has passed, the virus can remain dormant in the nerve ganglia, where it can reappear later in response to stressful triggers.

Therapeutic Management

Viral culture from vesicular fluid can confirm the diagnosis. There is no cure for HSV 2, but administration of acyclovir (Zovirax) can diminish symptoms and reduce shedding time. Infected neonates are treated with parenteral acyclovir; those with ocular involvement receive a topical ophthalmic drug as well. Infected individuals should refrain from all sexual contact until the lesions have healed completely. Because shedding time in an initial infection is prolonged, abstinence is recommended for several weeks.

Nursing Considerations

Prevention, early identification, and treatment are the goals of nursing care associated with any STD. The nurse plays a key role in educating young people about STDs. Often, the school nurse is the health care professional whom adolescents feel they can trust, so school nurses may be the care providers in the best position to educate this population. Establishing rapport with the teenager with a nonjudgmental approach and reassurance of confidentiality is key. The nurse must be aware of symptoms and assist in identifying those adolescents who are at risk for STDs. Encouraging abstinence in those who are not sexually active and condom use in sexually active adolescents is a way to prevent STDs. The nurse may be the one to assume responsibility for helping the adolescent obtain proper medical treatment and gain an understanding of the importance of completing the entire course of medication as well as treatment of partners.

KEY CONCEPTS

- Microorganisms that cause infectious disease are classified as bacteria, viruses, fungi, protozoa, and helminths.
- The skin is the first line of defense in the innate immune system.
- Infectious diseases can be transmitted by direct contact with another infected person, by contact with animal or insect carriers, by ingestion of contaminated food or water containing the pathogens, and by contact with a contaminated object.
- Exogenous pathogens are transmitted by direct contact, by animal or insect contact, through contaminated water or food, or by contact with a contaminated object.
- Vaccines can be live or attenuated, killed or inactivated toxoids, human immune globulin, or animal serums or antitoxins.

- Assessment of the child with an infectious disease includes a thorough history (recent exposure, other family members or friends exhibiting signs or symptoms) and documentation of the type, configuration, and distribution of lesions; the child's temperature; and any associated signs and symptoms.
- Children with infectious diseases usually can and should be cared for at home.
- Neonates with sepsis frequently display subtle signs and symptoms. Recognition and sensitivity on the part of the nurse can lead to early and life-saving interventions.
- Children who acquire an STD after the neonatal period should always be evaluated for possible sexual abuse.
- Gonorrhea can be transmitted during delivery of a neonate or with premature rupture of the membranes, through sexual abuse, and through voluntary sexual activity.

- Abstinence is the only 100% effective way to prevent both pregnancy and STD transmission. Sexually active individuals need to use barrier protection to prevent STDs.
- Not all STDs have symptoms. Many people with chlamydia (an STD infection) do not have any symptoms. It is possible to transmit an asymptomatic STD.

ANSWERS to Critical Thinking Exercise 40-1

Frequently, the community-based or school nurse is the only health care provider to have an ongoing relationship with an adolescent. The school nurse's vital role in risk assessment for STDs is challenging. Two major challenges are involved:

- Establishing rapport and providing educational information in an easily understood, nonjudgmental manner. This includes maintaining confidentiality and providing guidance and referral to community resources. All 50 states in the United States allow minors to give their own consent for confidential STD diagnosis and treatment (AAP, 2003i).
- Striking a balance between school district policies and guidelines for distributing sex education materials to students in the school setting and the nurse's personal philosophy about what teens should know. Some school districts, under pressure from parents, do not allow school nurses to give any information to students about STD and pregnancy prevention. In this instance, the school nurse may need to advocate for adolescents' rights to have appropriate information.

REFERENCES and READINGS

Ackley, B.J., & Ladwig, G.B. (Eds.). (2002). *Nursing diagnosis handbook: A guide to planning care* (5th ed.). St. Louis: Mosby.

American Academy of Pediatrics. (2003a). CMV. In L.K. Pickering (Ed.), *Red Book: 2003 Report of the Committee on Infectious Diseases* (26th ed., pp. 259-262). Elk Grove Village, IL: American Academy of Pediatrics.

American Academy of Pediatrics. (2003b). Diphtheria. In L.K. Pickering (Ed.), *Red Book: 2003 Report of the Committee on Infectious Diseases* (26th ed., pp. 263-266). Elk Grove Village, IL: American Academy of Pediatrics.

American Academy of Pediatrics. (2003c). Fifth Disease—Human parvo 19. In L.K. Pickering (Ed.), *Red Book: 2003 Report of the Committee on Infectious Diseases* (26th ed., pp. 459-461). Elk Grove Village, IL: American Academy of Pediatrics.

American Academy of Pediatrics. (2003d). Measles. In L.K. Pickering (Ed.), *Red Book: 2003 Report of the Committee on Infectious Diseases* (26th ed., pp. 419-429). Elk Grove Village, IL: American Academy of Pediatrics.

American Academy of Pediatrics. (2003e). Poliomyelitis. In L.K. Pickering (Ed.), *Red Book: 2003 Report of the Committee on Infectious Diseases* (26th ed., pp. 505-509). Elk Grove Village, IL: American Academy of Pediatrics.

American Academy of Pediatrics. (2003f). Preventing tickborne infection. In L.K. Pickering (Ed.), *Red Book: 2003 Report of the Committee on Infectious Diseases* (26th ed., pp. 186-187). Elk Grove Village, IL: American Academy of Pediatrics.

American Academy of Pediatrics. (2003g). Rabies. In L.K. Pickering (Ed.), *Red Book: 2003 Report of the Committee on Infectious Diseases* (26th ed., pp. 514-521). Elk Grove Village, IL: American Academy of Pediatrics.

American Academy of Pediatrics. (2003h). Rubella. In L.K. Pickering (Ed.), *Red Book: 2003 Report of the Committee on Infectious Diseases* (26th ed., pp. 536-541). Elk Grove Village, IL: American Academy of Pediatrics.

American Academy of Pediatrics. (2003i). Sexually transmitted diseases in adolescents and children. In L.K. Pickering (Ed.), *Red Book: 2003 Report of the Committee on Infectious Diseases* (26th ed., pp. 157-167). Elk Grove Village, IL: American Academy of Pediatrics.

American Academy of Pediatrics. (2003j). Smallpox. In L.K. Pickering (Ed.), *Red Book: 2003 Report of the Committee on Infectious Diseases* (26th ed., pp. 554-558). Elk Grove Village, IL: American Academy of Pediatrics.

American Academy of Pediatrics. (2003k). Varicella. In L.K. Pickering (Ed.), *Red Book: 2003 Report of the Committee on Infectious Diseases* (26th ed., pp. 672-686). Elk Grove Village, IL: American Academy of Pediatrics.

American Academy of Pediatrics, Committee on Infectious Diseases. (2000). Prevention of Lyme disease. *Pediatrics, 105,* 142-147.

American Academy of Pediatrics, Committee on Psychosocial Aspects of Child and Family Health. (2002). *Guidelines for health supervision.*

Elk Grove Village, IL: American Academy of Pediatrics; 1997 (updated 2002).

Behrman, R.E. (Ed.). (2001). *Nelson textbook of pediatrics—pocket companion* (16th ed.). Philadelphia: Saunders.

Berkowitz, C.D. (2000). *Pediatrics: A primary care approach.* Philadelphia: Saunders.

Burg, F., Ingelfinger, J., Polin, R., & Gerson, A. (Eds.). (2002). *Gellis & Kagan's current pediatric therapy* (17th ed.). Philadelphia: Saunders.

Butt, W. (2001). Septic shock. *Pediatric Clinics of North America, 48*(3), 601-624.

Centers for Disease Control and Prevention. (2000). Gonorrhea incidence in the United States with associated risk factors and potential implications. *MMWR: Morbidity and Mortality Weekly Report, 49*(RR-1), 538-543.

Centers for Disease Control and Prevention. (2002). Sexually transmitted diseases treatment guidelines—2002. *MMWR: Morbidity and Mortality Weekly Recommendations and Reports 2002, 51*(RR-6), 1-80.

Chamberlain, L.J. (2003a). Bacterial meningitis is less prevalent but still dangerous. *Infectious Diseases in Children, 16*(5), 55.

Chamberlain, L.J. (2003b). Varicella epidemiology may be changing. *Infectious Diseases in Children, 16*(5), 15-19.

Choma, K. (2003). ASC—US HPV testing. *American Journal of Nursing, 103*(2), 42-50.

Clark, M.J., & Spector, R. (2000). *Nursing in the community: Dimensions of community health nursing* (3rd ed.). Upper Saddle River, NJ: Prentice Hall Health.

Colyar, M. (2003). Testing for sexually transmitted diseases. *Advance for Nurse Practitioner, 11*(5), 28-31.

Eftychiou, V. (2003). Sexually transmitted disease treatment update: A closer look at the CDC guidelines. *Advance for Nurse Practitioners, 11*(1), 43-45.

Eissa, M., & Cromwell, P. (2003). Diagnosis and management of pelvic inflammatory disease in adolescents. *Journal of Pediatric Health Care, 17*(3), 145-147.

Jarvis, C. (2003). *Physical examination and health assessment* (4th ed.). Philadelphia: Saunders.

Johnson, M., Maas, M., & Moorhead, S. (2000). *Nursing outcomes classification (NOC)* (2nd ed.). St. Louis: Mosby.

Kenner, C., & Lott, J.W. (2003). *Comprehensive neonatal nursing: A physiologic perspective* (3rd ed.). Philadelphia: Saunders.

Mack, T. (2003). A different view of smallpox and vaccination. *New England Journal of Medicine, 348*(5), 460-463.

Mauldon, M. (2000). Amenorrhea in adolescents: Sorting out the clinical picture. *Advances for Nurse Practitioners, 8*(7), 44-51.

McCloskey, J.C., & Bulechek, G.M. (Eds.). (2000). *Nursing interventions classification (NIC)* (3rd ed.). St. Louis: Mosby.

Merenstein, G.B., & Gardner, S.L. (2002). *Handbook of neonatal intensive care* (5th ed.). St. Louis: Mosby.

Onieal, M.E. (2003). Smallpox update: Educate yourself. *Advance for Nurse Practitioners, 11*(2), 70.

Parks, D.K., Yetman, R.J., Moyer, V., & Kennedy, K. (2000). Early-onset neonatal group B streptococcal infection: Implications for practice. *Journal of Pediatric Health Care, 14*(6), 264-269.

Pearson, L. (2000). *Healthy People 2010* and protecting children. *Nurse Practitioner, 25*(7), 12-17.

Pender, N.J., Murdaugh, C., & Parsons, M. (2001). *Health promotion in nursing practice* (4th ed.). Stamford, CT: Appleton & Lange.

Reddy, D.M., Fleming, R., & Swaiin, C. (2002). Effect of mandatory parental notification on adolescent girls' use of sexual health care services. *Journal of American Medical Association, 288*(6), 710-714.

Revell, M.G., & Gerna, G. (2002). Diagnosis and management of human cytomegalovirus infection in the mother, fetus, and newborn infant. *Clinical Microbiology Review, 15*(4), 680-715.

Shapiro, E. (2003). Lyme disease: The great intimidator. *Infectious Diseases in Children, 16*(6), 44-48.

Smallpox fact sheet. (2002). Available online at www.bt.cdc.gov/agent/smallpox/overview/diseasefacts.asp.

Smallpox vaccine fact sheet. (2002). Available online at www.bt.cdc.gov/agent/smallpox/vaccination/facts.asp.

Sparbel, K.J.H., & Anderson, M.A. (2000). *Journal of Nursing Scholarship, 32*(2), 131-136.

Stagno, S. (2001). Cytomegalovirus. In J.S. Remington & J.O. Klein (Eds.), *Infectious diseases of the fetus and newborn infant* (5th ed.). Philadelphia: Saunders.

Trossman, S. (2003). The return of the smallpox vaccination: Nurses report on plans, concerns. *The American Nurse, 35*(2), 1-3.

U.S. Department of Health and Human Services. (2000). *Healthy People 2001.* Washington, DC: Author. Full text available at http://books.nap.edu/html/healthy3.

Wade, C.F. (2000). Keeping Lyme disease at bay: An integrated approach to prevention. *American Journal of Nursing, 100*(7), 31.

Weis, B. (2001). HIV in adolescents: Prevention and identification are pivotal. *Advance for Nurse Practitioners, 9*(3), 44-50.

Weigand, J. (2003). Pushing the edge of viability: Treatment dilemmas in neonatology. *Advance for Nurse Practitioners, 11*(5), 59-62.

Wexler, D.L. (2003). *Needle Tips and the Hepatitis B Coalition News, 13*(1). Also available at www.immunize.org.

Wong, D.L., Hockenberry-Eaton, M., Wilson, D., Winkelstein, M.L., & Schwartz, P. (2001). *Wong's essentials of pediatric nursing* (6th ed.). St. Louis: Mosby.

The Child with an Immunologic Alteration

After studying this chapter, you should be able to:

◉ Describe how the immune system attempts to maintain homeostasis of the internal and external environment and what happens when it over-functions or under-functions.

◉ Explain how neonates acquire active and passive immunity.

◉ Delineate how to prevent the spread of organisms in children with an immunodeficiency.

◉ Describe how to care for and support children with human immunodeficiency virus (HIV) and their families throughout the entire spectrum of illness.

◉ Outline critical information needed by families with children receiving long-term corticosteroid therapy.

◉ Describe nursing interventions to help prevent the sudden death of a child having an anaphylactic reaction.

◆ DEFINITIONS

active immunity Protection that forms in response to exposure to natural antigens or vaccines; protection can last months, years, or a lifetime.

allergy A hypersensitivity reaction in various body systems resulting from the immune system's response to exposure to an irritant (allergen).

antibody A protein that the immune system produces to bind to specific antigens and eliminate them from the body.

antigen A substance that possesses unique configurations enabling the immune system to recognize it as foreign.

autoimmune disease Disease that occurs when the immune system produces antibodies—called *autoantibodies*—against cells of the body.

complement An accessory system to a humoral response that is composed of serum proteins that facilitate enzyme action and antigen death.

immune (lymphoreticular) system The body's internal defense against foreign substances, such as bacteria, viruses, parasites, and fungi.

immunodeficiency A defect in the immune system leading to increased susceptibility to multiple and repeated infections.

leukocytes White blood cells, whose chief function is to protect the body against foreign substances; includes five types: lymphocytes, monocytes, neutrophils, eosinophils, and basophils.

lymphocytes The primary white blood cells of the immune system (e.g., B lymphocytes or B cells; and T lymphocytes or T cells).

nonspecific immune functions Protective barriers, such as chemicals, interferon, inflammation, and phagocytosis, that are activated in the presence of an antigen but are not specific to that antigen.

passive immunity Protection that occurs when serum containing an antibody is given or transmitted to a person who does not have that antibody.

specific immune functions Humoral (B cell and antibody production) and cell-mediated (T cell) responses that are activated in a highly discriminatory way to antigens that survive in the body.

REVIEW OF THE IMMUNE SYSTEM

The body's network of first-line, or external, defenses—intact skin and mucous membranes and processes such as sneezing, coughing, and tearing—helps keep it free of disease. When a foreign substance penetrates first-line defenses, the immune or internal defense system provides secondary and tertiary protection through nonspecific and specific responses. The immune system is able to distinguish the body's own cells, or self, from foreign substances, or nonself; activate a response to detect and destroy foreign substances; suppress a response against the self; and memorize and store information.

Foreign substances, or antigens, possess unique configurations that mark them as foreign. The immune system first re-

sponds to the invader through nonspecific immune functions. If the antigen survives the action of the nonspecific response, the immune system initiates specific immune functions. It begins producing proteins called *antibodies* or *immunoglobulins*. Each antibody is specific for a particular antigen, contains sites that are complementary, and can combine with the antigen. This combination of antigen and antibody is called the *antigen-antibody complex* or *immune complex*. The immune complex acts to destroy the antigen.

The major organs and tissues of the immune system include the bone marrow, thymus, spleen, lymph nodes, and lymphoid tissue. Both the circulatory system and the lymphatic system connect these organs and tissues to one another. Specific types of cells are also important to the immune system.

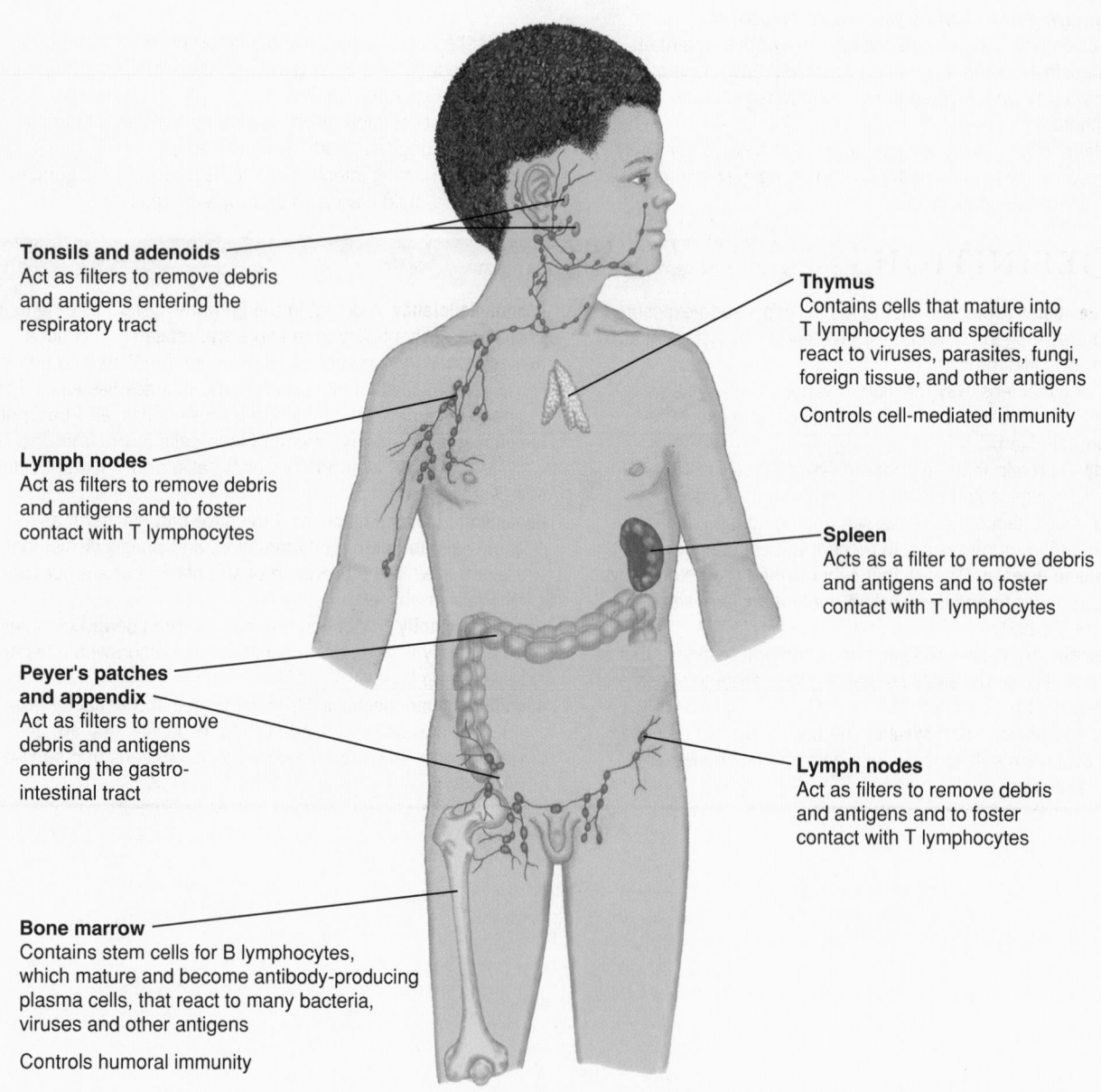

Tonsils and adenoids
Act as filters to remove debris and antigens entering the respiratory tract

Lymph nodes
Act as filters to remove debris and antigens and to foster contact with T lymphocytes

Peyer's patches and appendix
Act as filters to remove debris and antigens entering the gastrointestinal tract

Bone marrow
Contains stem cells for B lymphocytes, which mature and become antibody-producing plasma cells, that react to many bacteria, viruses and other antigens

Controls humoral immunity

Thymus
Contains cells that mature into T lymphocytes and specifically react to viruses, parasites, fungi, foreign tissue, and other antigens

Controls cell-mediated immunity

Spleen
Acts as a filter to remove debris and antigens and to foster contact with T lymphocytes

Lymph nodes
Act as filters to remove debris and antigens and to foster contact with T lymphocytes

Major Organs and Tissues of the Immune System

Cells Involved in the Immune Response

Cell Type	Nonspecific Immune Response
GRANULOCYTES	
Neutrophils	First leukocytes to respond to tissue damage. Ingest and destroy antigens, especially bacteria, by phagocytosis. Increase in number during acute inflammation, bacterial infection, and necrosis. Immature neutrophils are called *bands*. Increased bands (shift to the left) indicate infection.
Eosinophils	Neutralize histamine. Increase in number during allergic reactions and infestation with parasitic worms.
Basophils	Secrete histamine, heparin, and serotonin in inflammation and immediate hypersensitivity reactions. Basophils located in tissue rather than in blood are called *mast cells*.
AGRANULOCYTES	
Monocytes/Macrophages	Monocytes are large phagocytic agranulocytes. In tissue, they are called *macrophages*. Monocytes ingest and introduce antigens into the circulation. Macrophages engulf bacteria and cellular debris to finish the cleanup process started by the neutrophils.

Cell Type	Specific Immune Response
B LYMPHOCYTES	
	Noncirculating, short-lived cells responsible for humoral immunity. As plasma cells, produce antibodies to bacteria. First responder to viral infection. Some become memory cells for recognition of specific antigens.
T LYMPHOCYTES	
	Responsible for cellular immunity. Interact with specific antigens on cell surfaces and directly attack invading microorganisms. Respond to viruses, fungi, parasites, and foreign tissue. T cell regulatory functions mobilize or deactivate the other cells in the immune system.
Helper (CD4+) T cells	Recognize antigens that have been processed and presented to them by B cells or macrophages. CD4+ cells secrete lymphokines that stimulate B cells to manufacture antibodies.
Suppressor T cells	Inhibit the actions of helper T cells and B cells. Help keep the immune system cells in check.
Cytotoxic T cells	Phagocytize target cells; make cells more vulnerable to chemical attack via production of lymphokines.

Data from Applegate, E.J. (1995). *The anatomy and physiology learning system: Textbook* (p. 300). Philadelphia: Saunders; Copstead, L.E. (1995). *Perspectives on pathophysiology* (p. 191). Philadelphia: Saunders; Hansen, M. (1998). *Pathophysiology: Foundations of disease and clinical intervention.* Philadelphia: Saunders.

Nonspecific Immune Functions

The body's innate immune system consists of nonspecific immune functions, which are protective barriers activated in the presence of an antigen but not specific to that antigen. Among these nonspecific immune functions are chemical barriers, such as bactericides and fungicides and enzymes in body secretions; interferon, a protein produced in response to viruses; and inflammation, increased capillary permeability, vasodilation, phagocytosis (cell eating), and elimination of cell products.

Phagocytosis can occur alone or as part of the inflammatory response. Phagocytes ingest the antigen and either survive or die. In dying, the phagocytes release additional chemicals that draw more phagocytes to the area.

Increased capillary permeability and vasodilation result in redness and edema. The products of phagocyte-antigen death include toxins that give rise to fever, pain, and purulence. As the antigens are destroyed, the toxins are cleared from the lymph nodes, which often become enlarged. If the immune response is effective, the inflammation subsides; if it is ineffective, fever follows.

Specific Immune Functions

If the antigen survives within the phagocyte, two types of specific immune functions can recognize and destroy it: humoral and cell-mediated. Both responses are closely related.

Lymphocytes (white blood cells) function in both types of immune response. Lymphocytes circulate in the blood and the lymphatic system. They make up 53% to 57% of white blood cells during the first year of life, when specific immunity develops rapidly, but they make up only 25% to 30% after 12 months of age. Two classes of lymphocytes are involved in the immune response: B lymphocytes (B cells); and T lymphocytes (T cells).

B cells, which promote the humoral response, originate in the bone marrow or liver but mature in the lymphoid tissue, becoming plasma cells. When exposed to antigens, some of the plasma cells produce antibodies, whereas others become memory cells. Antibodies are classified as immunoglobulins G, M, A, D, and E, often abbreviated IgG, IgM, IgA, IgD, and IgE. Immunoglobulins bind to antigens and facilitate their destruction.

T cells, which are responsible for the cell-mediated response, originate in the bone marrow and mature in the thymus, where they react specifically to viruses, fungi, parasites, foreign tissue, and other antigens. The three types of T cells are: suppressor T cells, cytotoxic cells, and helper T cells or CD4+ cells.

Natural killer cells, or large granular lymphocytes, can directly destroy tumor cells and other antigens. They are not antigen-specific (Rote, 2002).

The Humoral Response

The humoral response involves chiefly B cells, although the cooperation of helper T cells is almost always necessary. Macrophages ingest antigens and introduce them into the

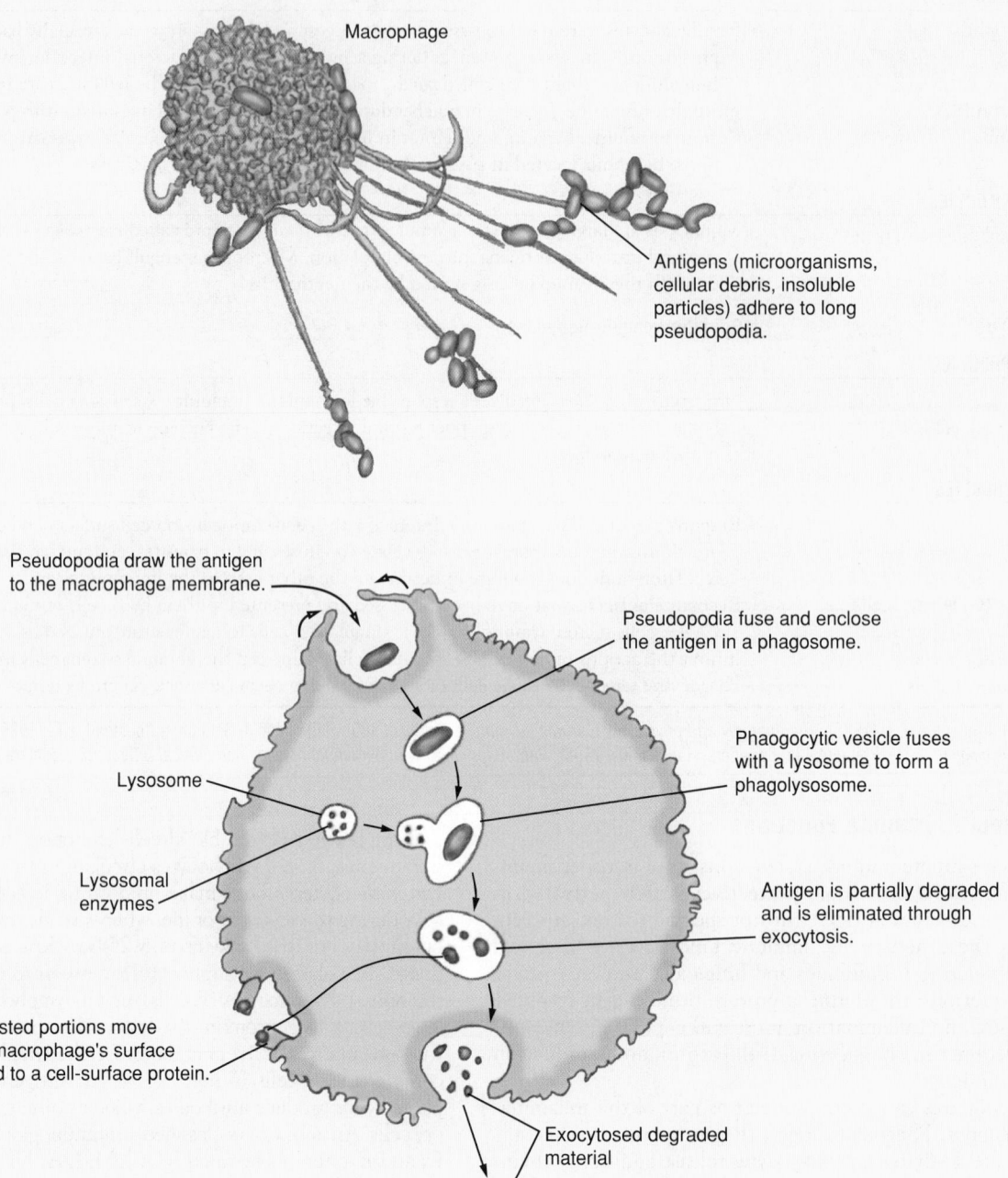

Macrophage

Antigens (microorganisms, cellular debris, insoluble particles) adhere to long pseudopodia.

Pseudopodia draw the antigen to the macrophage membrane.

Pseudopodia fuse and enclose the antigen in a phagosome.

Phaogocytic vesicle fuses with a lysosome to form a phagolysosome.

Lysosome

Lysosomal enzymes

Antigen is partially degraded and is eliminated through exocytosis.

Undigested portions move to the macrophage's surface coupled to a cell-surface protein.

Exocytosed degraded material

circulation. In response, the B cells and helper T cells interact. The helper T cells secrete substances that cause B cells to multiply and differentiate into plasma cells, which produce vast quantities of antibodies specific to the antigen. These antibodies combine with the antigens to form immune complexes. The antibodies either destroy the antigens or activate an accessory system called *complement*, a series of serum proteins involved in enzyme action and antigen death. Suppressor T cells reduce the production of antibodies after the antigens are eliminated from the body (Rote, 2002).

Pediatric Differences in the Immune System

The organs of the immune system mature during infancy and childhood:

- Lymphoid tissue increases in mass during infancy and early childhood. It reaches adult size by 6 weeks of age, grows larger during the prepubertal years, and involutes at puberty.
- The thymus reaches its peak mass before puberty and then involutes.
- The spleen reaches its full size during adulthood.
- The number of Peyer's patches increases until the adult mean is exceeded during adolescence.

Immaturity of the immunologic system places the infant and young child at greater risk for infection:

- The infant has a limited capacity to mount an antibody response. The ability to respond to infections develops gradually as the infant acquires immunity actively and passively.
- Because of the immaturity of the inflammatory response in neonates, the more common signs and symptoms of infection (e.g., fever) are less pronounced, making diagnosis more difficult.
- Neonates' diminished nonspecific immune response allows a more rapid spread of infection, leading potentially to sepsis.
- The term newborn receives an adult level of IgG as a result of transplacental transfer from the mother. This level begins to disappear during the first 6 to 8 months, causing a physiologic drop in IgG.

- Premature infants are more susceptible to neonatal infections because of lower levels of transplacental transfer of IgG from the mother and a more severe physiologic drop in IgG.
- IgM, IgE, and IgD are normally in low concentration at birth. IgM, IgE, IgA, and IgD do not cross the placenta. The immunoglobulins reach adult levels at different ages*:
  —IgM: 1 year
  —IgA: 6 to 7 years
  —IgG: 7 to 8 years
  —IgE: 6 to 7 years
- Absolute lymphocyte counts reach a peak during the first year. Helper T cells reach adult levels by 6 years of age.
- Passive placental transfer of IgG may affect infants' response to active immunization (i.e., pertussis and/or diphtheria).
- Immature or inexperienced immune cells affect the reliability of delayed hypersensitivity skin reactions. For this reason, allergy skin tests are not routinely used with infants.

Disorders of the immune system present differently in children than in adults:

- Primary immunodeficiencies typically present in the first 6 months of life.
- HIV infection, the major secondary immunodeficiency in children, typically (1) infects an infant through the mother, not sexually; (2) is diagnosed by measuring an aspect of the virus, not antibodies as in adults; and (3) has a shorter latency period in infants, with several different AIDS-defining illnesses.

*Buckley, R. (2000). T-, B-, and NK-cell systems. In R. Behrman, R. Kliegman, & H. Jenson (Eds.), *Nelson textbook of pediatrics* (16th ed., pp. 590-595). Philadelphia: Saunders.
Ig, Immunoglobulin; *AIDS,* acquired immunodeficiency syndrome.

The Cell-Mediated Response

A cell-mediated response is also initiated by macrophages presenting antigens. Once activated, helper T cells secrete substances that spur additional T cells to grow. One set of T cells, called *cytotoxic T cells,* tracks down and kills viruses, tumor cells, and other pathogens. Suppressor T cells draw the immune response to a close (Rote, 2002).

Development of Immunity

The normal fetus can produce IgM by 20 to 24 weeks of gestation. The neonate's immune protection comes from prenatal transfer of maternal antibodies (IgG) and breast milk transfer of IgA. Gradually, the normal newborn's own humoral and cell-mediated responses to infections begin; immunity is acquired both actively and passively.

Active Immunity

When the body reacts to an antigen through either a humoral or a cell-mediated response, it is developing active immunity. Active immunity is long-lived and measured in months, years, or even a lifetime; it follows exposure to environmental antigens or vaccines. Immediately after exposure, there is a latency period when antibody levels are low. When

the body recognizes the antigen as foreign, it makes antibodies. The first antibodies produced are predominantly IgM and subsequently IgG. After a second exposure to the antigen, antibodies appear at a faster rate and the latency period is shortened or nonexistent. The antibody levels remain high and persist for much longer periods. The predominant antibody in a secondary response is IgG.

Infants receive specific live or attenuated vaccines on a recommended schedule to induce immunity against the antigens in the vaccine (see Appendix D).

Passive Immunity

Passive immunity results from antibody transfer from one person to another. Transfer of antibodies from a woman to her fetus is an example of passive immunity. The fetus receives maternal IgG antibodies across the placenta and becomes protected against many infections. Most maternal antibodies dissipate in the infant by 6 to 9 months of age, but some persist for up to 18 months. The duration depends on the level of a particular antibody in the maternal plasma. Protection against measles, for example, may last through the 2nd year of life, whereas protection against certain bacterial infections may last only 1 to 2 months. The reason neonates are so susceptible to infections by bacteria such as *Escherichia coli* is that the respective antibodies do not cross the placenta.

COMMON LABORATORY AND DIAGNOSTIC TESTS OF IMMUNE FUNCTION

Immunodeficiencies

A variety of laboratory tests evaluate immune system function. Laboratory evaluation determines intactness of its major functions: B cell immunity, T cell immunity, and phago-

cytosis. Many values vary significantly with age, especially during infancy. Among these are the differential in the complete blood cell count, the amount of various immunoglobulins, the lymphocyte surface antigen count (e.g., CD4+ count), and the total lymphocyte count.

Allergy

Measurement of eosinophilia and IgE levels, along with a radioallergosorbent test and skin testing, is helpful in diagnosing allergic reactions.

Immunoglobulin Function and Pediatric Implications

Immunoglobulin (Ig) Type	Percent (%) of Total Ig*	Function and Pediatric Significance	Location
IgG	70-80	Contains most antibodies against bacteria, viruses, and fungi in blood and body spaces. Crosses the placenta; provides maternal antibody protection to infants. Responsible for Rh reactions. IgG response is longer and stronger than that of the other immunoglobulins.	Appears in all internal body fluids; present in majority of B cells.
IgM	5-10	Produced 48-72 hr after an antigen enters the body and remains in the blood. First immunoglobulin produced in response to bacterial and viral infections. Responsible for transfusion reactions in the ABO blood typing system. Does not cross placenta, so values are low in newborns. However, IgM is produced early in life, and level increases after 9 mo of age. Presence in cord or infant blood may mean infection in utero or newborn period.	Appears mostly in intravascular serum. Attached to B cells; released into plasma during immune response.
IgA	10-15	Prevents infection across mucous membranes (local immunity). Especially important in antiviral protection. Passes to newborn in breast milk. Those having congenital IgA deficiency are prone to autoimmune disease.	Appears in body fluids (nasal and respiratory secretions, saliva, tears, breast milk).
IgE	0.004	Leads to release of histamines producing an allergic response. Elevation may indicate allergy in children. Plays a role in defense against parasites.	Appears in serum. Found on the surface membranes of basophils and mast cells. Produced by plasma cells in mucous membranes and tonsils.
IgD	0.2	Poorly understood. Thought to influence B cell differentiation.	Appears in small amounts in serum. Attached to B cells.

Data from Applegate, E.J. (1995). *The anatomy and physiology learning system: Textbook* (p. 300). Philadelphia: Saunders; Copstead, L.E. (1995). *Perspectives on pathophysiology* (p. 191). Philadelphia: Saunders; Sandberg, E., & Shearer, W. (1996). Normal immune responses. In C.W. Bierman, D. Pearlman, G. Shapiro, & W. Busse (Eds.), *Allergy, asthma, and immunology from infancy to adulthood*. Philadelphia: Saunders.
*Normal immunoglobulin values differ for age.

Laboratory and Clinical Screening Tests for Allergy

Test	Findings Suggestive of Allergy
CBC, differential	Excess eosinophils (>5% of WBCs)
Total eosinophil count	>750 eosinophils
Nasal smear	Excess eosinophils
Serum IgE	Elevated for age
RAST, antigen-specific IgE	Increase in antigen-specific IgE in the serum
Skin testing	Urticarial wheal appears on skin within $1/2$ hr after administration of selected potential allergens; reaction can be immediate or delayed and can even include anaphylaxis

Modified from Centers for Disease Control and Prevention. (1994, Sept. 30). *MMWR: Morbidity and Mortality Weekly Report, 43*(RR-12), 1-10.
CBC, Complete blood cell count; *IgE,* immunoglobulin E; *RAST,* radioallergosorbent test.

Common Laboratory and Diagnostic Tests of Immune Function

Test	Function	Nursing Considerations
Serum immunoglobulins (IgG, IgM, IgA, IgE)	Tests humoral immunity. Measures levels of immunoglobulins by separating them through immunoelectrophoresis.	Immunization and toxoids received in the last 6 mo as well as blood transfusions, tetanus antitoxin, and gamma globulin received in the last 6 wk can affect results and should be noted on the laboratory requisition. Total immunoglobulins tend to be elevated in early months and then decrease over the first year of life. These also may be unusually high early in human immunodeficiency virus (HIV) infection and then decrease.
Lymphocyte surface antigen	Determines the types and subtypes of lymphocytes present in blood. Names of lymphocyte surface antigens are based on "clusters of differentiation" (CDs). CD antigens on a leukocyte allow its identification. The two most commonly used surface antigens and the cell types they identify: CD4: helper T cells CD8: suppressor T cells	To determine the number of a particular type of cell, a complete blood cell count (CBC) must also be done.
Serum antibody titer to antigens in vaccines received (e.g., D, T)	Tests humoral immunity.	Tests antibody level to specific antigens.
Skin tests to mumps, tuberculin, tetanus, *Candida*	Tests cell-mediated immunity.	Measures the immune system's ability to develop antibody to foreign substances.
Differential white blood cell count (WBC)	Part of the CBC, composed of five types of WBCs (leukocytes): neutrophils, eosinophils, basophils, monocytes, and lymphocytes. The differential WBC count is expressed in number per cubic millimeter (mm^3) and as a percent of the total number of WBCs.	These tests measure whether immune cells can ingest and destroy foreign substances.
Allergy skin tests	On administration of antigen into the skin to test either immediate or delayed-type hypersensitivity.	Because anaphylactic reactions can occur even in the presence of minimal allergen exposures, emergency equipment and medications should be immediately available.
Radioallergosorbent test (RAST)	Measures the quantity and increase of antigen-specific IgE present in the serum. Exact quantities of antibodies to pollens, foods, etc., can be tested.	More expensive than traditional allergy skin testing but provides precise information without risk for hypersensitivity reaction.

Data from Corbett, J.V. (1992). *Laboratory tests and diagnostic procedures with nursing diagnoses.* East Norwalk, CT: Appleton & Lange; Kee, J.L. (1991). *Laboratory and diagnostic tests with nursing implications.* East Norwalk, CT: Appleton & Lange; Taeusch, H.W., Christiansen, R.O., & Buescher, E.S. (1996). *Pediatric and neonatal tests and procedures.* Philadelphia: Saunders.
Refer to Appendix H for normal values.

Immunologic alterations typically are chronic, lasting from months to years and interfering with a child's life. Physical signs range from simple, such as impaired skin integrity, to complex, such as overwhelming infection. Intervals of wellness, relapses, and sometimes a decline in health should be expected. Repeated office visits and hospitalizations, disruptions in family routines, altered social interactions, and emotional and financial strain often are coupled with anxiety about the future.

Initially, the nurse helps the family adjust to a new, often devastating diagnosis. Care during the acute phase of the illness may be critical in nature, as underlying organisms are diagnosed and treated and fevers and pain are controlled. Once the acute crisis has resolved, the nurse prepares the family for discharge by teaching home management and identifying community resources and referrals for ongoing support. The nurse also teaches the family how to prevent the spread of microorganisms through infection control practices at home and describes parameters for when to call the physician. The nurse discusses ways to maintain the child's skin integrity—the body's first line of protection against microorganisms—and recommends a diet that supports immune cell growth. The nurse must keep abreast of current information because the field of immunology continues to evolve. Nurses also play a vital role in advocating for children with conditions such as human immunodeficiency virus (HIV) infection.

Despite all efforts, rehospitalization is often inevitable. The family is an integral part of the multidisciplinary team, keeping the physicians, nurses, and social workers informed of changes in the child's condition, administering medications, providing respiratory care, and often making difficult decisions about continued treatment and comfort.

THE CHILD WITH AN IMMUNODEFICIENCY

A deficiency in one or more components of the immune system results in an immunodeficiency disorder. Immunodeficiency disorders can be inherited, acquired through infection or other illness, or produced as a side effect of certain medications.

Some children are born with defects in their immune system. Children born with defects in the humoral system are unable, or only partially able, to produce antibodies, thus making them susceptible to bacterial infections. Other children are born with an abnormal thymus, which affects T cell production. These children are more susceptible to viral and fungal infections as well as to certain cancers. In rare cases, children demonstrate deficiency in both B cells and T cells, a condition termed *severe combined immunodeficiency disease (SCID)* (Box 41-1). The most devastating acquired immunodeficiency is HIV infection, which destroys helper T, or CD4+, cells.

Medication can also cause certain acquired immunodeficiencies. For example, antibiotics can disrupt normal flora, making the body more susceptible to other microorganisms. Immunosuppressive agents and corticosteroids suppress components of the immune system, resulting in a decrease in the inflammatory response and an increased risk for bacterial invasion.

HUMAN IMMUNODEFICIENCY VIRUS INFECTION

HIV infection is an acquired cell-mediated immunodeficiency disorder that causes a wide spectrum of illness in children, ranging from no signs or symptoms to mild and moderate to severe

---

> ### BOX 41-1
> ### Clinical Findings Associated With Immunodeficiency
>
> **Frequently Present, Highly Indicative Signs**
> - Repeated or persistent respiratory tract infection
> - Repeated or persistent otitis media or sinusitis
> - Severe bacterial infections
> - Opportunistic infections, such as *Pneumocystis carinii* pneumonia or cryptosporidiosis
> - Poor response to appropriate therapy
>
> **Frequently Present, Somewhat Suggestive Signs**
> - Skin lesions
> - Failure to thrive or grow
> - Chronic diarrhea
> - Thrush
> - Hepatosplenomegaly
> - Anemia, thrombocytopenia, neutropenia
> - Small or absent lymph nodes, tonsils, and adenoids

signs and symptoms. Acquired immunodeficiency syndrome (AIDS) is the most advanced manifestation of this illness.

Etiology

HIV, present in an infected individual's blood or body fluids can enter an uninfected adult's or adolescent's body in several ways, including sharing of needles and/or syringes, engaging in unprotected sexual activity with an infected person where body fluids are shared, or receiving an infected blood product. Infected women can transmit the virus to a fetus across the placenta during pregnancy, to the infant at delivery, and to the young child through breastfeeding. The potential for such transmission was about 25% before 1994, when the Centers for Disease Control and Prevention (CDC) recommended identifying and treating HIV-positive pregnant women (Mofenson & Read, 1999). The transmission rate has dropped to as low as 8% in infants whose infected mothers received zidovudine (ZDV) during pregnancy and delivery and who themselves received zidovudine for 6 weeks after birth (Mofenson & Read, 1999). The Centers for Disease Control and Prevention (2002) states that in a longitudinal epidemiologic study conducted in the United States since 1990, transmission was observed in 20% of women with HIV-1 infection who received no antiretroviral treatment (ART) during pregnancy, 10.4% who received ZDV alone, 3.8% who received combination therapy without protease inhibitors, and 1.2% who received combination therapy with protease inhibitors (Table 41-3). The risk for transmission from mother to child remains multifactorial and includes, but is not limited to, factors such as high maternal viral load, prolonged rupture of membranes, prematurity, and low birth weight (Chen, Pau, & Piscitelli, 2000). The risk for children acquiring HIV infection through sexual abuse exists.

Historically, children, especially those with hemophilia, acquired HIV/AIDS through infected blood products. Most of those children have died, having been infected before widespread and accurate screening of donor blood. A small percentage of HIV-positive young adolescents are long-term

TABLE **41-1** Revised Human Immunodeficiency Virus Pediatric Classification System: Immune Categories Based on Age-Specific CD4+ T Cell Count and Percentage*

Immune category	<12 Mos		1-5 Yrs		6-12 Yrs	
	No./mm³	(%)	No./mm³	(%)	No./mm³	(%)
Category 1: No suppression	≥1500	(≥25%)	≥1000	(≥25%)	≥500	(≥25%)
Category 2: Moderate suppression	750-1499	(15%-24%)	500-999	(15%-24%)	200-499	(15%-24%)
Category 3: Severe suppression	<750	(<15%)	<500	(<15%)	<200	(<15%)

From, Working Group on Antiretroviral Therapy and Medical Management of HIV-Infected Children. (2004). *Guidelines for the use of antiretroviral agents in pediatric HIV infection.* Table 1. Retrieved April 21, 2004 from www.aidsinfo.nih.gov.

survivors of perinatally acquired infection. Currently, the median age of perinatally infected children enrolled in the Pediatric Spectrum of HIV Disease study from four U.S. sites is 14.8 years (Frederick et al., 2000).

Incidence

In the United States through 2001, approximately 9100 children younger than 13 years have been diagnosed with AIDS. Perinatal transmission accounts for 91% of the pediatric cases; 7% are attributed to contaminated blood transfusions. Between 1988 and 1993, there were 6000 to 7000 infants born to HIV-infected women; more than 1500 of these infants became infected. Subsequent to 1994 the perinatal infection transmission has decreased by two-thirds. The highest incidence of HIV infection is in African-American and Latino children (CDC, 2002). Half of all new HIV infections in the United States occur in young people between the ages of 13 and 24 years. Insofar as the known median HIV incubation period in adults is 10 years, young adults (ages 20-29 yr) who are infected with HIV probably became infected in their teens (Futterman, Chabon, & Hoffman, 2000). HIV infection is the tenth leading cause of death in 15- to 24-year-olds and is no longer in the top 10 leading causes of death in young children (CDC, 2000).

Manifestations

HIV infection in children and adults differs in several ways (Yogev & Chadwick, 2004):

- The progression of HIV infection to AIDS is faster in infants and young children; most untreated infants develop symptoms associated with HIV infection by 1 year of age and many young children with AIDS die before age 2 years. One factor contributing to the rapid progression in children is a higher viral load.
- Signs in children may include physical and developmental failure to thrive.
- Children experience early opportunistic infections (e.g., chronic oral candidiasis), a greater number of bacterial infections from childhood illnesses, and lymphoid interstitial pneumonitis (LIP), a condition in which the child may be asymptomatic or may experience parotid gland enlargement, hypoxia, and digital clubbing.
- *Pneumocystis carinii* pneumonia (PCP) in children with perinatally acquired HIV infection can occur early in infancy, with the average age at onset being between 3 and 6 months.

The CDC classifies the clinical manifestations of HIV infection as mild, moderate, or severe in children younger than 13 years (CDC, 2003) (see Table 41-1). Mild signs of the illness may be nonspecific and include lymphadenopathy; hepatomegaly; splenomegaly; dermatitis; parotitis; and recurrent or persistent upper respiratory infection, sinusitis, or otitis media. In moderate disease, some signs are considered to be important if they persist or recur, particularly anemia, neutropenia, or thrombocytopenia; diarrhea; fever for longer than 1 month; herpes simplex; and oral candidiasis in children older than 6 months. Other signs of moderate infection include bacterial meningitis, pneumonia, or sepsis (one episode); cardiomyopathy; complicated chickenpox; herpes zoster; hepatitis; nephropathy; LIP; and toxoplasmosis onset before age 1 month. In addition to LIP, the most common indicators of AIDS in children younger than 13 years are serious bacterial infections (multiple or recurrent), PCP, cytomegalovirus (CMV), encephalopathy, and wasting syndrome (seen most commonly in African children) (Yogev & Chadwick, 2004).

Diagnostic Evaluation

Because most HIV infections in infants and children occur as a result of perinatal transmission, HIV-positive pregnant women must be identified, educated, and treated. Early identification and treatment of women reduce the HIV transmission rate and enable early diagnosis for infected infants.

Traditional HIV antibody measurement by enzyme-linked immunosorbent assay (ELISA) or Western blot assay is not accurate in infants younger than 18 months because of the persistence of maternal antibodies.

Viral diagnostic tests (culture, DNA polymerase chain reaction [PCR], RNA assay) can definitively diagnose most HIV-infected infants as early as 1 month of age and nearly all infected infants by 6 months of age. Initial diagnostic testing of HIV-exposed infants is done before the infant is 48 hours old. A positive result is confirmed as soon as possible by viral assay on a second specimen. HIV-exposed infants are re-tested at 1 to 2 months and again at 3 to 6 months (Table 41-2). Testing at age 14 days also may be advantageous for early detection of infection. HIV-exposed infants should be evaluated by, or in consultation with, a specialist in HIV infection (Working Group on Antiretroviral Therapy and Medical Management of HIV-Infected Children, 2004).

Pathophysiology

of HIV Infection

HIV is a retrovirus composed of RNA and an enzyme, reverse transcriptase, which plays a key role in viral replication. HIV gains entry into a CD4+ cell by direct fusion of the viral envelope to CD4+ receptors on the cell surface. Within the CD4+ cell, reverse transcriptase causes the synthesis of HIV DNA. This integrates with the CD4+ cell's DNA. The HIV virus then uses the CD4+ cell to make more of itself. The new viruses assemble at the host cell's surface. As they bud through the cell membrane, the viruses mature, are released, and can infect other CD4+ cells. The most critical result of HIV entry into the CD4+ cell is cell incapacitation and death.* Because CD4+ cells primarily enhance cell-mediated immunity, severely infected infants and children will exhibit symptoms of viral or fungal infection. In addition, CD4+ helper cells interact with the humoral immune response. Immunoglobulins become nonfunctional, making the child extremely vulnerable to bacterial infections.

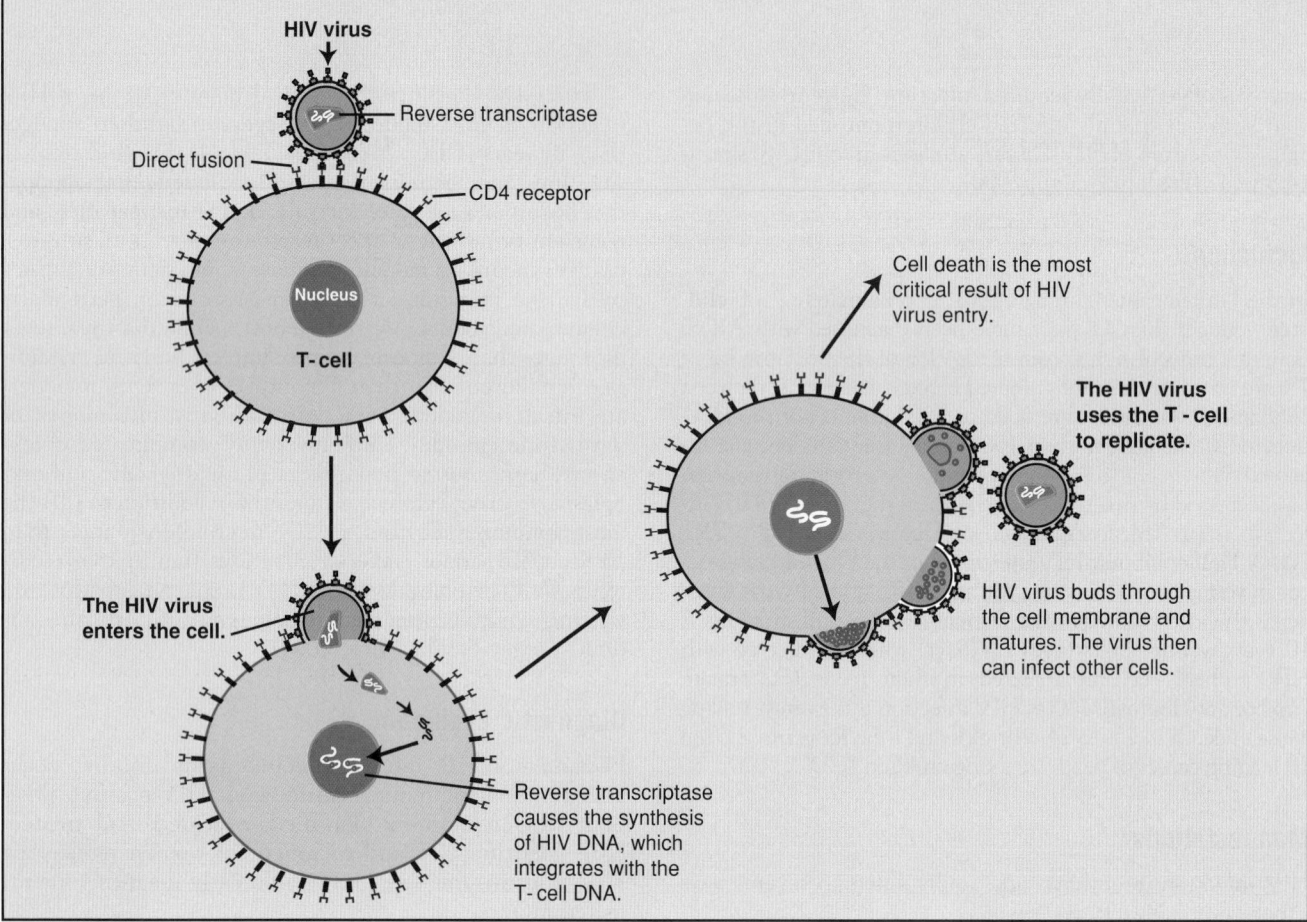

*Rote, N. (2002). Immunity. In K. McCance & S. Huether (Eds.). *Pathophysiology: The biologic basis for disease in adults and children* (4th ed., pp. 168-196). St. Louis: Mosby.
HIV, Human immunodeficiency virus; *RNA,* ribonucleic acid; *DNA,* deoxyribonucleic acid.

CD4+ counts and HIV ribonucleic acid (RNA) assays are useful tools to assess an infected young child's immune status, response to therapy, risk for disease progression, and need for PCP prophylaxis after 1 year of age. CD4+ counts are measured every 3 months. It is important to note that pediatric CD4+ lymphocyte counts vary by age and that determination of the level of immune function or suppression of children infected with HIV is based on the child's age (Working Group on Antiretroviral Therapy and Medical Management of HIV-Infected Children, 2004).

Therapeutic Management

HIV-Exposed Infants

In addition to intravenous (IV) ZDV in the mother during labor, infants of known HIV-positive mothers should receive oral ZDV therapy within 6 to 12 hours after birth. This continues for 6 weeks. Some women may not be identified as being HIV infected until delivery. There are still prophylactic options for the newborn. The Perinatal HIV Guidelines Working Group (2003) describes clinical situations and

TABLE 41-2 Testing for the Presence of HIV

Infants With Negative Viral Diagnostic Tests by 48 Hours of Age	Infants With Positive Viral Diagnostic Tests by 48 Hours of Age
Retest at 1-2 mo	Repeat the test as soon as possible after initial testing.
	CD4+ lymphocyte count and HIV viral load as soon as possible after the first positive test.
Retest at 3-6 mo	Determine sequential CD4+ lymphocyte counts every 2-3 mo.
HIV infection can be reasonably excluded in children with (1) two or more negative virologic tests at or after age 1 mo., with one of those tests performed at or after 4 mo., or (2) two or more negative HIV IgG antibody tests performed at age >6 mo with an interval of at least 1 mo between the tests also can be used to reasonably exclude HIV infection among children with no clinical evidence of HIV infection. HIV can be definitively excluded if HIV IgG antibody is negative in the absence of hypogammaglobulinemia at age 18 mo and if the child has both no clinical symptoms of HIV infection and negative HIV virologic assays.	HIV infection is diagnosed from two positive virologic tests performed on separate blood samples. HIV DNA PCR is the preferred virologic method for diagnosing HIV infection during infancy.

Data from Working Group on Antiretroviral Therapy and Medical Management of HIV-Infected Children. (2004). *Guidelines for the use of antiretroviral agents in pediatric HIV infection.* Retrieved April 21, 2004 from www.aidsinfo.nih.gov.
HIV, Human immunodeficiency virus; *IgG,* immunoglobulin G; *DNA,* deoxyribonucleic acid; *PCR,* polymerase chain reaction.

TABLE 41-3 Pediatric AIDS Clinical Trials Group (PACTG) 076 Zidovudine (ZDV) Regimen

Time of ZDV Administration	Regimen
Antepartum	Oral administration of 100 mg ZDV five times daily,* initiated at 14-34 weeks' gestation and continued throughout the pregnancy.
Intrapartum	During labor, intravenous administration of ZDV in a 1-hour initial dose of 2 mg/kg body weight, followed by a continuous infusion of 1 mg/kg body weight/hour until delivery.
Postpartum	Oral administration of ZDV to the newborn (ZDV syrup at 2 mg/kg body weight/dose every 6 hours) for the first 6 weeks of life, beginning at 8-12 hours after birth.†

Data from Perinatal HIV Guidelines Working Group. (2003). *U.S. Public Health Service Task Force recommendations for use of antiretroviral drugs in pregnant HIV-1-infected women for maternal health and interventions to reduce perinatal HIV-1 transmission in the United States.* Table 1. Retrieved April 21, 2004 from www.aidsinfo.nih.gov
*Oral ZDV administered as 200 mg three times daily or 300 mg twice daily is currently used in general clinical practice and is an acceptable alternative regimen to 100 mg orally five times daily.
†Intravenous dosage for full-term infants who cannot tolerate oral intake is 1.5 mg/kg weight intravenously every 6 hours. ZDV dosing for infants <35 weeks' gestation at birth is 1.5 mg/kg/dose intravenously, or 2.0 mg/kg/dose orally, every 12 hours, advancing to every 8 hours at 2 weeks of age if >30 weeks' gestation at birth or at 4 weeks of age if <30 weeks' gestation at birth.
AIDS, Acquired immunodeficiency syndrome.

therapeutic recommendations for women in the following categories:

- HIV-1–infected pregnant women who have not received prior antiretroviral therapy
- HIV-1–infected women receiving antiretroviral therapy during the current pregnancy
- HIV-1–infected women in labor who have had no prior therapy
- Infants born to mothers who have received no antiretroviral therapy during pregnancy or intrapartum (Table 41-3).

Discussion about treatment options and recommendations should not be threatening. The mother makes the final decision about the use of antiretroviral medications. Women who

CRITICAL THINKING EXERCISE 41-1

Some states in the United States have begun considering mandatory human immunodeficiency virus (HIV) antibody testing of newborns. This test is done at the same time as the other mandatory newborn screenings (e.g., phenylketonuria, sickle cell disease). Because recent HIV medication protocols have produced a marked decrease in the perinatal infection transmission rate and because very early treatment of HIV-infected infants has been shown to prolong intact immune status, universal HIV testing appears warranted.

What are the major issues, positive and negative, that legislators should consider before approving legislation for mandatory universal HIV testing for infants?

decide not to accept treatment with ZDV or other drugs should not face punitive action or denial of care (Perinatal HIV Guidelines Working Group, 2003).

Because PCP can affect an infant as young as 2 months, PCP prophylaxis is initiated when an exposed infant is 4 to 6 weeks old, regardless of HIV status. Treatment with trimethoprim-sulfamethoxazole usually continues until the infant is 1 year old or is determined to be HIV-negative, usually by 6 months of age (U.S. Department of Health and Human Services, Panel on Clinical Practices for the Treatment of HIV Infection, 2000).

HIV-Infected Infants and Children

The Working Group on Antiretroviral Therapy and Medical Management of HIV-Infected Children updates treatment recommendations regularly. Guidelines for antiretroviral treatment of infants and children infected with HIV are based on the following concepts (2004):

- To prevent perinatal transmission of HIV, prenatal HIV identification, counseling, and testing with consent should be the standard of care for all pregnant women in the United States.
- Participation in clinical trials offers the best means of determining safe and effective therapies for HIV-infected pregnant women, exposed and infected infants, and infected children and adolescents.
- Collaboration between pharmaceutical companies and the federal government should ensure that medications suitable for administration to infants and children are available at the time that new agents are being evaluated in adults.
- While clinical trials of antiretroviral drugs are needed to determine the impact drugs have on manifestations of HIV specific to children, including growth, development, and neurologic disease, the absence of such clinical trials does not preclude the use of any approved antiretroviral drug in children.
- Because management of HIV infection in the child and adolescent population is rapidly changing and increasingly complex, a specialist in the treatment of pediatric and adolescent HIV infection should manage care or be consulted regularly.
- Effective management of the complex and diverse needs of HIV-infected infants, children, adolescents, and their families requires a comprehensive and multidisciplinary team approach.
- Assays to measure HIV RNA and CD4+ cell levels should be made available to monitor and modify antiretroviral treatment in infected individuals of all ages.
- Adherence to therapy is affected by the following:
  —Availability and palatability of pediatric formulations
  —Impact of the medication schedule on quality of life, including number of medications, frequency of administration, ability to co-administer with other prescribed medications, and need to take with or without food
  —Ability of the child's caregiver or the adolescent to administer complex drug regimens and availability or resources that might be effective in facilitating adherence
  —Potential for drug interactions
- The choice of antiretroviral regimens should include consideration of factors associated with possible limitation of future treatment options, including the presence of or potential for the development of antiretroviral resistance.

HIV resistance assays have proven useful in guiding initial therapy and in changing failing regimens, but expert clinical interpretation is required.

- Because growth failure and neurodevelopmental deterioration may be specific manifestations of HIV infection in children, growth and developmental monitoring is essential in the care of HIV-infected infants and children. Nutritional-support therapy is an intervention that affects immune function, quality of life, and bioactivity of antiretroviral drugs.

The goal of antiretroviral therapy is to maximally suppress viral replication reflected by an undetectable (<400) viral load. This is an attempt to preserve immune function and to delay disease progression. Therefore, an aggressive approach is to offer individuals a combination of drugs, referred to as *highly active antiretroviral therapy (HAART)*. Currently, 16 antiretroviral agents representing three different classes of compounds are available to treat HIV infection. The Food and Drug Administration has approved 11 of these for pediatric use. Nucleoside analog reverse transcriptase inhibitors (NRTIs) and non-nucleoside reverse transcriptase inhibitors (NNRTIs) target the HIV reverse transcriptase enzyme, and protease inhibitors (PIs) block the function of viral protease, a critical enzyme for the completion of the viral replicating cycle (Khoury & Kovacs, 2001). An individual's antiretroviral drug regimen may be changed in response to worsening immune function, medication intolerance or toxicity, or the development of a newer and better regimen.

When to initiate antiretroviral therapy is a major area of concern. The Working Group on Antiretroviral Therapy and Medical Management of HIV-Infected Children (2004) recommends that combination therapy should be offered to all HIV-infected infants and children who exhibit clinical signs of infection or whose immune status is suppressed. Experts disagree about whether to treat asymptomatic infants with normal immune status who are younger than 1 year of age. Many suggest that all HIV-infected infants be treated, and others recommend that treatment decisions for infected infants older than 6 months be made in light of clinical and immune status and adherence risks (Working Group on Antiretroviral Therapy and Medical Management of HIV-Infected Children, 2004).

Children older than 1 year of age who have AIDS or severe immune suppression should be treated, and treatment is considered also for those with less severe symptoms or immune suppression. Treatment of asymptomatic children older than 1 year can be deferred if immune status is normal, the child has a low viral load, and there are medication adherence risks (Working Group on Antiretroviral Therapy and Medical Management of HIV-Infected Children, 2004). If the latter option is chosen, the child should have frequent monitoring of virologic, immunologic, and clinical status to ensure that these parameters remain stable in the absence of antiretroviral therapy.

Special Considerations for Adolescents

Long-term survivors of perinatally acquired HIV infection are now becoming teenagers. Whereas some of these teens continue to enjoy relatively good health, others may have advanced HIV disease, which may interfere with their normal daily activities, such as going to school or participating in sports. These limitations may have an impact on their quality of life and should be assessed at each visit. Another unique consideration is that many of these adolescents have one or more family members who also are infected or may now be deceased (Steele, 2000). Newly diagnosed behaviorally infected adolescents contrast greatly with the long-term survivors of perinatal infection. These adolescents are typically healthy with normal immune systems and may not be aware that they are infected. Most enter the health care system because of other sexually transmitted diseases (STDs) or pregnancy.

It is critical that the adolescent be involved in decision making. This includes an in-depth discussion about antiretroviral therapy options. According to Steele (2000), the goal for any treatment regimen should include maximizing adherence; this goal is related to the number of pills and capsules in the regimen and the side effects of the drugs. Combination antiretroviral therapy for infected adolescents is similar to therapy for infected children, but dosages are based on Tanner stage of puberty, not age. Dosages for adolescents in Tanner stage 1 or 2 are based on pediatric dosages, whereas those for adolescents in Tanner stage 5 are based on the adult dosage. Adolescents at other Tanner stages need to have dosages monitored and adjusted for effectiveness (Working Group on Antiretroviral Therapy and Medical Management of HIV-Infected Children, 2004).

In addition to antiretroviral therapy, aggressive treatment of infections is essential. Ensuring appropriate immunizations (Table 41-4), monitoring growth and development, providing nutritional support, and referring for multidisciplinary care are additional therapeutic interventions. It is important to counsel sexually active teenagers about preventing pregnancy and the transmission of HIV.

Additional Issues Related to HIV

Medication Adherence. Most important for successful treatment of HIV-infected children and adolescents is meticulous adherence to the medication regimen. Failure to follow the regimen can result in the development of drug resistance and subsequent treatment failure. It is critical to educate and reinforce medication adherence at every visit. Palatability of the medication, ability to meld the medication schedule with existing routines, denial, guilt, and embarrassment about the diagnosis are all barriers to appropriate cooperation with the regimen. Education at an early age about pill taking can be a great help in eliminating the hard-to-take liquid formulations of medication.

Multigenerational Problems. Pediatric HIV infection requires specific and ongoing management in both primary and specialty care practices. Because children may experience a wide spectrum of manifestations of HIV-associated problems, the nurse, as a collaborator on the therapeutic management team, must be able to identify areas of concern and develop strategies that allow for individual approaches to health care. These should incorporate the family's belief systems; cultural influences; and knowledge of the disease process, its symptoms, and treatment options. Many families affected by the disease have limited financial resources or emotional support systems. As a result, the nurse may consult with a social worker to ensure that basic needs, such as food, housing, and transportation, are met (Boland, 2000).

One of the unique aspects of perinatal HIV infection is the multigenerational nature of the disease, in which both

the mother and child may be infected. An important but difficult area to be addressed is future planning. This can include exploring the efficacy of standby guardianship, kinship care, or foster and adoptive placement. In addition, for children with advanced HIV disease, families have to make difficult decisions about an infected child's ongoing care. Should aggressive treatment continue, or should the goal of treatment be to make the child comfortable? These decisions are best made in consultation with a multidisciplinary team.

Issues such as disclosure and do-not-resuscitate (DNR) orders will need to be explored when the time is right for each individual family. For example, when trust is established, families may talk about their feelings about disclosure. Some choose to share the diagnosis with a trusted friend. For many, however, keeping the secret is a way of life. The nurse can be a resource for facilitating a child learning about personal HIV infection status. The nurse can listen as the family discuss when and how to tell the child. (See Appendix I on Evolve website for a list of support organizations for families affected by HIV infection.)

Text continued on p. 1066

TABLE 41-4 Recommendations for Routine Immunization of HIV-Infected Children in the United States

Vaccines	Known Asymptomatic HIV Infection	Symptomatic HIV Infection
Hepatitis B	Yes	Yes
DTaP	Yes	Yes
IPV[1]*	Yes	Yes
MMR	Yes	Yes[2]
Hib	Yes	Yes
Pneumococcal[3]	Yes	Yes
Influenza[4]*	Yes	Yes
Varicella[5]	Consider	Consider
BCG	No	No
Hepatitis A[6]	See text	See text

Data from American Academy of Pediatrics. (2003). *Red Book 2003: Report of the Committee on Infectious Diseases* (25th ed.). Elk Grove Village, IL: Author.
NOTE: Always check the most current immunization schedule. Administer immune globulin after measles exposure and varicella-zoster immune globulin after chickenpox exposure, unless administered during the previous 2 wk. Administer tetanus immune globulin in the management of tetanus-prone wounds.
*Including siblings and other family members.
HIV, Human immunodeficiency virus: *DTaP*, diphtheria and tetanus toxoids and acellular pertussis; *IPV*, inactivated poliovirus; *MMR*, live-virus measles-mumps-rubella; *Hib*, Haemophilus influenzae type b conjugate; *BCG*, bacille Calmette-Guérin.
[1]Only IPV vaccine should be used for HIV-infected children, HIV-exposed infants whose status is indeterminate, and household contacts of HIV-infected people.
[2]Severely immunocompromised HIV-infected children should not receive MMR vaccine.
[3]Pneumococcal vaccine should be administered to all age-appropriate HIV-infected children. Children who are older than 2 months of age should receive pneumococcal vaccine at the time of diagnosis. Reimmunization after 3 to 5 years is recommended in either circumstance.
[4]Influenza vaccines should be provided each autumn for HIV-exposed infants 6 months of age and older, HIV-infected children and adolescents, and household contacts of HIV-infected people.
[5]Consider for HIV-infected children in Centers for Disease Control and Prevention class N1 and A1
[6]Two doses 6-12 months apart after 2 years of age.

PARENTS AND CAREGIVERS
Want to Know

How to Care for the Child With an HIV Infection

Review the following information and health practices at the time of initial testing and subsequent visits.

Transmission

HIV can be spread by:
- Unprotected sexual activity
- Sharing of needles
- An infected mother to her baby
- Breastfeeding
- Open wounds (if there is blood-to-blood contact)

HIV cannot be spread by:
- Sharing knives, forks, spoons, or cups
- Using the same toilet seats, bathtubs, or showers
- Coughing or sneezing
- Hugging, holding, or touching people

Prevention

The best way to prevent the spread of HIV is to:
- Abstain from sex and from sharing needles, or
- Use latex condoms with nonoxynol 9, and
- Wash needles in a 1:10 bleach solution

The best way to prevent pregnancies is to:
- Abstain from sex, or
- Use a latex condom
- Use birth control pills
- Undergo tubal ligation

If infected with HIV, follow these precautions:
- Do not breastfeed
- Do not donate blood, sperm, or organs

Testing

- The most common HIV tests used for older children and adults are the ELISA and the Western blot assay, which measure levels of antibodies to the virus.
- The most common HIV tests used for infants and children younger than 18 months are the HIV DNA polymerase chain reaction and HIV RNA assays, which detect the presence of the virus itself.
- CD4+ counts indicate how well the immune system is working.

Illness (AIDS)

Children with HIV infection might initially be asymptomatic. Mild and moderate symptoms include:
- Persistent upper respiratory and ear infections
- Thrush
- Skin conditions
- Vomiting and diarrhea
- Enlarged liver, spleen, lymph nodes, and parotid gland
- Growth and development problems
- LIP—a rare lung disease

Some severe symptoms of the illness include:
- Opportunistic infections, such as PCP and CMV
- Recurrent bacterial infections, such as sepsis and meningitis
- Severe developmental delay
- Wasting syndrome

Medications

- Adherence to schedule
- Proper administration
- Safe and proper storage
- Side effects

Home Care

Offer a high-calorie, high-protein diet:
- Mix formula as directed.
- Do not add extra water or cereal to formula.
- Give supplemental vitamins and minerals as ordered.

Practice basic infection control measures and follow Standard Precautions, including the following practices:
- Avoid touching blood.
- Do not share toothbrushes, pierced earrings, razors, or nail clippers.
- Use a barrier when caring for a cut or bloody nose.
- Cover open sores.
- Leave scabs alone.
- Wipe up blood spills with a paper towel, wash the area with soap and water, rinse with bleach and water, and air-dry.
- Wrap disposable materials soiled with blood in newspaper, tie off in a plastic bag, and throw away in a plastic-lined trash can.
- Wash hands with soap and water if you touch blood.
- Rinse blood-soiled clothing with hydrogen peroxide or cold water, and then wash as usual.
- Allow blood to air-dry on dry-clean-only clothing.

Keep your child's immunizations up to date. Your child should also receive:
- Pneumococcal vaccine at 2 years of age, if not given during infancy
- Flu shot each fall
- Immune globulin after measles exposure
- Varicella-zoster immune globulin after chickenpox exposure
- Tetanus immune globulin for tetanus-prone wounds

Call the physician if any of the following symptoms occur:
- Fever higher than 101° F
- Vomiting and diarrhea
- Decreased appetite, difficulty swallowing, drooling
- Rashes, bumps, lumps, or sores on the skin
- Coughing or chest congestion
- Ear pain, pulling on the ears, or drainage from the ears
- Wounds that will not heal
- Exposure to measles or chickenpox

Give prophylaxis against PCP and antiretroviral drugs as ordered.

HIV, Human immunodeficiency virus; *ELISA,* enzyme-linked immunosorbent assay; *DNA,* deoxyribonucleic acid; *RNA,* ribonucleic acid; *AIDS,* acquired immunodeficiency syndrome; *LIP,* lymphoid interstitial pneumonitis; *PCP, Pneumocystis carinii* pneumonia; *CMV,* cytomegalovirus.

Nursing Care Plan

The Child With HIV Infection

FOCUSED ASSESSMENT

Nurses play a critical role in the care of the child and family with human immunodeficiency virus (HIV) infection in a variety of settings, including hospital, home, school, and daycare. In each of these settings, the nurse has an opportunity to listen, educate, and support the child and family through the maze of HIV care. Many children with HIV infection experience normal health. When the immune system becomes more compromised and symptoms develop, hospitalization may become necessary. Therapeutic management focuses on the prevention of potential serious infections (primary prophylaxis), the treatment of serious bacterial and opportunistic infections that might affect multiple organs and systems when they occur, and the prevention of recurrence of serious infections (secondary prophylaxis). The nurse should engage the family in a helping relationship and put aside biases regarding mode of transmission so that they do not interfere with listening, supporting, and providing care. The nurse should use an interpreter, if needed, to provide culturally sensitive care.

When an HIV diagnosis has been made, assess what the family understands about the HIV-related spectrum of illness, including immunologic status and special immunization considerations. Under certain circumstances, the use of monthly intravenous immune globulin (IVIG) may be recommended. Specific circumstances in which IVIG should be considered include children with hypogammaglobulinemia, recurrent serious bacterial infections, treatment of parvovirus B19 infections and treatment of thrombocytopenia; and single-dose administration of IVIG for measles exposure.* Assess the child's growth and development according to age-appropriate parameters, and ask the caregivers about any fever, nausea, vomiting, diarrhea, ear pulling, or changes in appetite, sleep pattern, or behavior that might suggest secondary infections. Other nursing assessment factors include determination of co-infection with other viruses/organisms, such as cytomegalovirus (CMV), *Cryptococcus,* and *Toxoplasma,* which could cause significant problems for children with advanced HIV disease.

Focus the physical examination on indicators of an infection:

- *Hydration status:* Assess the skin for turgor and the mucous membranes for moistness, drying, or cracking; confirm the absence or presence of tears; in infants, determine whether the anterior fontanel is palpable and soft; measure intake, urine output, and specific gravity.
- *Respiratory status:* Listen and observe for nasal flaring, retractions, cough, difficulty breathing, tachypnea, grunting, wheezing, rhonchi, and decreased breath sounds.
- *Mouth lesions:* Observe for white patches on the tongue or inside the cheeks or blisters on the lips.
- *Skin lesions (especially in the diaper area):* Observe for blotchy, red, flat areas, blistering, or dryness.

Assess pain by obtaining a self-report from the child, using faces, numbers, or color scales when appropriate; by observing the child's speech, facial expressions, body movements, and responses; and by talking with the family.

Nursing Diagnosis

Deficient Knowledge about the natural history of pediatric HIV disease, potential complications associated with HIV infection, and current treatment modalities related to emotional reaction to the diagnosis.

Expected Outcome

The family will:

- Demonstrate knowledge acquisition, as evidenced by explaining what has been taught about HIV infection and playing an active role in determining the plan of care for the child.

INTERVENTION	RATIONALE
1. Determine the family's knowledge about HIV infection and treatment modalities.	1. Teaching needs to begin at the family's level of understanding. It is important to note that because 90% of HIV-infected children are perinatally infected, the nurse may also be educating parents about their own disease process.
2. Teach the family about HIV infection, its signs and symptoms, progression, and treatment.	2. Knowledge and understanding of HIV may increase cooperation and adherence to the often-complicated treatment regimens that are necessary to achieve viral suppression and will also serve to reduce anxiety.

*American Academy of Pediatrics. (2003). *2003 Red Book: Report of the Committee on Infectious Diseases* (26th ed.). Elk Grove Village, IL: Author.

Continued

Nursing Care Plan

The Child With HIV Infection—cont'd

INTERVENTION	RATIONALE
3. Identify the family's area of concern (e.g., a new diagnosis, fear of transmission by casual contact within the family).	3. Addressing family concerns decreases misinterpretation. First educate about the lack of transmission by household contact and correct any myths or misperceptions that may exist.
4. Use teaching strategies that will maximize potential for success (e.g., medication sheet that details medication name, dosage, how often to give, why the child is on the medication, and hints for administering bad-tasting medication).	4. Written information may assist the family to ensure that the correct medication regimen is being followed.
5. Educate the family about what signs or problems necessitate calling the health care provider for management advice.	5. Early identification of potential problems may prevent serious complications from developing.

Evaluation

- Can the family describe the natural history of HIV, systems affected by HIV, and current treatment modalities?
- Can the family administer the correct dosages of medications at the appropriate times?
- Does the family readily participate in developing and carrying out a plan of care for the child?
- Does the family contact health care providers when the child is ill and in need of services?

Nursing Diagnosis

Risk for Infection related to cell-mediated immunodeficiency.

Expected Outcomes

The child will:
- Be free of secondary and opportunistic infections.
- Have up-to-date immunization status.

INTERVENTION	RATIONALE
1. Follow basic infection control and Standard Precautions.	1. Children with HIV are susceptible to infections. Standard Precautions protect caregivers from infection.
2. Administer antimicrobial therapy as ordered; monitor the child for side effects and signs and symptoms of infection.	2. Children with HIV mount a poor antibody response. Common pathogens include *Salmonella, Shigella, Campylobacter, Yersinia, Giardia lamblia, Isospora belli,* and *Cryptosporidium.*
3. Administer antipyretics for fever as ordered. Monitor for effects, and notify the physician if fever does not resolve. Offer fluids. Organize care to allow for rest periods.	3. Children with HIV may have fevers that can be exacerbated by fluid loss from increased respiratory effort that accompanies increased activity.
4. Administer IVIG as ordered. Monitor the child for side effects. Notify the physician, and adjust the rate as ordered.	4. IVIG may prevent serious bacterial infections and hospitalizations; however, it does not affect the child's overall survival rate.
5. Reinforce principles of infection control (see Parents and Caregivers Want to Know box, p. 1068), appropriate immunization schedules, and indications for calling a physician (see Parents and Caregivers Want to Know box, p. 1058). Teach families how to administer medications and how to take the child's temperature, as well as when to administer antipyretics at home.	5. The best way to prevent the spread of organisms at home is through good handwashing. All household members receive influenza vaccine. If the child with HIV is exposed to measles or chickenpox, the family must notify the physician immediately.

Evaluation

- Is the child free of secondary and opportunistic infections?
- Is the child afebrile?
- Are the child's and family's immunizations up to date?
- Can the family describe signs and symptoms of infection and when to call the physician?

Nursing Care Plan

The Child With HIV Infection—cont'd

Nursing Diagnosis

Imbalanced Nutrition: Less Than Body Requirements related to inadequate caloric intake and altered gastrointestinal function.

Expected Outcomes

The child will:
- Eat foods from the recommended food groups, consuming enough calories to meet metabolic and growth needs.
- Be free of painful oral lesions that interfere with eating.
- Maintain growth parameters for age.

INTERVENTION	RATIONALE
1. Offer foods high in protein and calories; give vitamin and mineral supplements; consult with a dietitian if there are any problems with food choices.	1. Children with HIV are often small in stature and size. Malabsorption and diarrhea can exacerbate problems with slow weight gain.
2. Inspect the mouth for the presence of oral lesions or thrush. Administer antifungal medications as ordered, and notify the physician of any changes.	2. Mouth sores can interfere with eating. Early diagnosis and treatment of *Candida,* herpes simplex virus (HSV), and other infections may reduce pain and allow for increased food intake.
3. Offer licks of a Popsicle or ice before meals.	3. Cold may numb the mouth when sores are present.
4. Allow older children to use a straw.	4. A straw keeps liquids from touching sore spots.
5. Offer soft, bland, lightly seasoned foods that are room temperature, nutritious, and easy to eat.	5. Spicy or salty foods and hot or cold temperatures can aggravate mouth sores. Favorite foods can be mashed, ground, or pureed to facilitate consumption.
6. Offer six small meals per day. Increase calories by adding milk, butter, or cheese to potatoes, eggs, casseroles, vegetables, soups, and gravies; by using sauces on rice, noodles, and potatoes; and by offering shakes.	6. There may be times children just do not have an appetite. Allow them to eat the food they want, but attempt to increase calories.
7. Offer bland, low-fiber, nonirritating foods, as ordered, along with Pedialyte, Gatorade, or cranberry juice.	7. Children with HIV often have abdominal cramps and diarrhea because of secondary infections.
8. Encourage the family to visit at mealtimes, or assign a consistent person to feed the child at a set time.	8. Children tend to eat better in the presence of family or a familiar trusted person.
9. Weigh the child every morning, and review caloric intake every 24 hours. Measure specific gravity at every void; compare consistency of stools; obtain specimens as ordered.	9. It is important that the child follow his or her individual growth curve, even if small for age.
10. Begin tube or parenteral feedings as ordered.	10. Alternative feeding techniques are necessary when the child is not gaining weight or is deviating from the established growth curve because of mouth or esophageal lesions, malabsorption, or neurologic findings.
11. Review with the family how to reconstitute formula at home, give vitamins, increase protein and calories, and adjust intake based on oral lesions and evidence of malabsorption. Teach families how to give alternative foods as ordered. Refer to visiting nurse if needed.	11. Proteins and calories are important to immune cell function. Because some families may add water to formula to make it last longer and other families may add cereal to increase calories, it is important to reinforce formula preparations.

Evaluation
- Is the child eating from all recommended food groups?
- Is the child growing according to normal and individual parameters?
- Is the child free from oral lesions?

Nursing Diagnoses

Impaired Gas Exchange related to secondary or opportunistic infections; Ineffective Airway Clearance related to ineffective cough or fatigue.

Continued

Nursing Care Plan

The Child With HIV Infection—cont'd

Expected Outcomes

The child will:
- Demonstrate clear breath sounds.
- Have normal pulse and respiratory rates for age.
- Breathe comfortably with minimal exertion.
- Have an oxygen saturation measurement within normal limits.

INTERVENTION	RATIONALE
1. Maintain oxygen therapy as ordered, and monitor pulse oximetry values.	1. Changes in the child's pulse oximetry values or clinical condition may indicate a need for a change in oxygen therapy.
2. Administer *Pneumocystis carinii* pneumonia (PCP) prophylaxis or treatment as ordered, with a large glass of water or juice; monitor the child for side effects.	2. Specific sulfonamides, such as trimethoprim-sulfamethoxazole, can help prevent or treat PCP. PCP causes dyspnea, tachypnea, cyanosis, and a nonproductive cough.
3. Administer corticosteroids, as ordered, with food or milk (see p. 1069). Monitor the child for side effects.	3. Corticosteroids are used to treat lymphocytic interstitial pneumonia (LIP).
4. Perform chest physiotherapy as ordered. Turn and position the child every 2 to 3 hours; elevate the head of the bed. Encourage the child who is able to get out of bed to do so frequently. Have the child practice coughing and deep breathing using an incentive spirometer. Obtain a sputum sample for culture as ordered.	4. Changing position and getting out of bed, even if the child is simply held upright in someone's arms, allow for lung expansion and help prevent atelectasis of dependent lung segments.
5. Instruct the parents how to administer trimethoprim-sulfamethoxazole (and steroids as ordered) at home; teach the family chest physiotherapy and coughing and deep-breathing exercises for the child, as well as how to administer aerosol treatments at home. Arrange for oxygen tanks and nebulizers as ordered. Nebulizer pieces are cleaned with warm water after each treatment and left to air-dry. They are soaked in white vinegar and water for 30 minutes at the end of the day.	5. PCP prophylaxis is usually taken twice daily for 3 days per week. Nebulizer treatments help to open the airway before chest physiotherapy.

Evaluation

- Have the child's breath sounds improved on auscultation?
- Does the child have normal pulse and respiration for age?
- Does the child breathe effortlessly when at rest?
- Can the child expectorate upper airway secretions?
- Is the child's pulse oximetry value more than 95%?

Nursing Diagnosis

Risk for Impaired Skin Integrity related to cellular immunodeficiency.

Expected Outcomes

The child's:
- Skin will be clean, dry, and intact.
- Throat and mouth will be free of sores or inflammation.

INTERVENTION	RATIONALE
1. Use mild soap. Offer liquids throughout the day. Apply moisturizers like Eucerin or Cetaphil to the skin. Avoid tight braids or ponytails. Use salve to keep lips moist.	1. Children with HIV may have very dry skin, scalp, and lips. Lubricants reduce dryness. Tight hairstyles stress the skin.
2. Clean open sores with warm water; pat dry or air-dry. Apply antibacterial or antiviral agents as ordered; cover with a nonadherent pad. Monitor the effectiveness of treatment.	2. Children with HIV may develop herpes lesions on the skin or in the mouth. Acyclovir is often ordered.

Nursing Care Plan

The Child With HIV Infection—cont'd

INTERVENTION	RATIONALE
3. Clean the child's teeth two or three times each day with a soft brush. For infants, clean the mouth with a cotton swab and plain water.	3. The skin inside the mouth must be kept clean to prevent infections and dental caries. A soft brush decreases injury to gums.
4. Using a cotton swab, clean the mouth and apply an oral antifungal agent. Do not offer food or drink for 30 minutes after application. Monitor the effects of treatment.	4. Children with HIV often develop a fungal infection from *Candida albicans,* which causes pain with swallowing and can spread down the esophagus. Nystatin is used initially, followed by ketoconazole.
5. Use extra care to keep the diaper area smooth and soft. Change diapers as soon as they are wet. Clean the area with warm water, and then pat dry or air-dry. Do not use wipes if the child is sensitive to them.	5. Some brands of disposable diapers and wipes may be irritating to the skin; moistness contributes to skin breakdown.
6. Leave the diaper area open to the air. Avoid wiping (squeeze a wet cloth over the bottom to wash away stool). Pat dry or air-dry (do not rub). Apply a thin layer of antifungal agent as ordered, and monitor its effectiveness. Handle the child gently. Loperamide (Maalox), applied topically, and colloidal oatmeal baths are effective if skin breakdown is severe.	6. Children with HIV often develop fungal infections in the diaper area. Nystatin powder is used if the rash is wet and weepy. Nystatin cream allows the skin to breathe.
7. Reinforce techniques to be used at home for meticulous mouth and skin care. Mouth care includes inspecting for white patches, blisters, and sores that recur and persist despite meticulous treatment and care. Skin care of the diaper area is especially important. Teach the family how to apply topical antifungal agents.	7. The skin and mucous membranes are the body's first line of defense against infecting microorganisms that challenge the immune system.

Evaluation

- Is the child free of further skin breakdown?
- Are the child's skin lesions and open sores healing?

Nursing Diagnosis

Delayed Growth and Development related to the effects of the virus on the neurologic system, chronicity of the illness, separation from family, and hospitalization.

Expected Outcome

The child's motor, cognitive, and psychosocial development will:
- Reach maximum potential, as measured by appropriate tools and scales.

INTERVENTION	RATIONALE
1. Encourage the family to visit the child as often and as long as possible. Supplement family visits with visits from volunteers.	1. Personal interaction is essential to prevent withdrawal and promote language and motor skills.
2. Administer antiretroviral drugs as ordered. Monitor the child for side effects.	2. HIV can infect brain cells. Opportunistic organisms, such as CMV and *Toxoplasma,* can cause brain infections. Thrombocytopenia can cause internal bleeding. As a result, some children with progressive disease exhibit developmental delay. Many children taking antiretroviral drugs, however, have achieved developmental milestones after a previous delay and have gained weight.
3. Interact with the child according to the child's developmental level. Provide safe, age-appropriate toys; integrate physical, occupational, and speech therapy techniques into the child's activities of daily living and play. Use a child life specialist to decrease the child's anxiety about medical procedures. Assess the child each week for changes in any aspect of development.	3. Developmental delay is a manifestation in HIV-infected children; motor impairment may become more profound as the disease progresses.

Continued

Nursing Care Plan

The Child With HIV Infection—cont'd

INTERVENTION	RATIONALE
4. Reinforce physical and occupational therapy techniques, but not to the point of pain. Encourage the family to follow speech therapy instructions, especially those that enhance receptive language skills.	4. As a child begins to lose motor function, the family continues to feel hopeful when general comprehension persists.

Evaluation

- Are all aspects of the child's development within normal limits?
- Is the child's communication appropriate for age?

Nursing Diagnoses

Acute Pain and Chronic Pain related to the treatments, procedures, and effects of the disease process.

Expected Outcomes

The child will:

- Be able to communicate where any pain is located.
- Participate in activities to the maximum extent.
- Be comfortable, as evidenced by ability to participate in activities and obtain appropriate rest.

INTERVENTION	RATIONALE
1. Continuously anticipate, assess, recognize, and treat pain appropriately. Use developmentally appropriate pain assessment scales, and document pain rating every 2 to 4 hours.	1. Pain management requires a multidisciplinary input: the caregiver reports pain to the physician, who may order analgesics. Refractory pain may require referral to pain service.
2. Offer acetaminophen and nonsteroidal antiinflammatory drugs (NSAIDs) for mild pain; add codeine for moderate pain and morphine or methadone for severe pain.	2. A "ladder" approach to analgesia has proved effective in managing pain.†
3. Plan care so that rest periods are possible and everything that requires touching is done at once. Line the bed with soft blankets or cushions or a partially inflated mattress. Alternate the child's positions, using the palms of your hands for lifting. Keep the environment clean, speak in gentle tones, play quiet music, dim the lights. Apply mild heat, and offer a warm bath.	3. Organizing care, environmental control, and distraction are important non-pharmacologic interventions for managing pain.
4. Teach deep-breathing exercises and use distraction techniques (e.g., imaging, singing, watching television, reading a story) to manage pain.	4. Giving children power to help control pain can help lessen it.
5. Teach the family how to administer analgesics and use non-pharmacologic interventions for managing pain at home. Remind the family to call the physician if the pain cannot be controlled.	5. Children should not have to be in pain. There is always something that can be done. Families know their children best and are positioned to assess and manage pain at home with much support.

Evaluation

- Has the child's pain improved, as evidenced by improved relaxation and ability to sleep and absence of crying and expressed discomfort?
- Is the child able to participate in age-appropriate activities?

Nursing Diagnosis

Anxiety (primary caregiver) related to fear of disclosure.

---

†Oleske, J. (1995, June). *Pain in pediatric HIV disease: Meeting the challenge.* Plenary session at a workshop c-sponsored by the National Pediatric and Family HIV Resource Center, Greenbelt, MD.

Nursing Care Plan

The Child With HIV Infection—cont'd

Expected Outcomes

The family will:
- Share the diagnosis with health care professionals who need to know.
- Move through the stages of disclosure and will feel comfortable sharing their feelings about the diagnosis with one significant person.
- Answer the child's questions honestly and share the diagnosis when the time is right.

INTERVENTION	RATIONALE
1. Listen quietly when the family talks about the diagnosis of HIV. Note their stage of disclosure (secrecy, exploratory, readiness, or full disclosure).	1. Sharing the diagnosis occurs on a continuum, with secrecy at one end and full disclosure at the other. Families initially may want to keep their feelings about the diagnosis private. However, a time may come when they wish to talk; the nurse should develop rapport and gain trust.
2. Encourage the family to share the diagnosis with health care professionals.	2. Health care professionals who plan and coordinate care need to know the diagnosis.
3. Help family members decide who else needs to know the child's diagnosis; ask them to name one person with whom they wish to share the diagnosis. Encourage peer support groups when the family is ready.	3. Although many people would like to know the diagnosis, only a handful need to know. Ask families to consider the following when choosing whom to tell: the child's age, clinical condition, and health care requirements; the likelihood that bloody injuries will occur; the use of Standard Precautions.
4. Encourage the family to be honest with the child and to explain the reason for physicians' visits and procedures.	4. When to tell the child the diagnosis is a personal choice, but families need to understand that children will worry more if no one talks with them or if they sense dishonesty.
5. Encourage the family to listen to the questions the child is asking and to answer the questions briefly, using words the child can understand. Look for readiness cues that indicate the child wants to know more.	5. It is important for families to understand what their children are asking and to answer their questions, keeping responses short and simple.
6. Encourage the family to speak with a health care professional when the child asks questions that are difficult to answer. Suggest that the parent seek counseling to help find the appropriate language for answering the child.	6. Role playing is a useful technique that allows families to practice potential responses to difficult questions. The nurse can offer to accompany them if they decide to share the diagnosis.
7. Promote normal routines at home.	7. Children with HIV infection can go to school, church, and parties; play sports and games; and develop or maintain friendships.

Evaluation

- Is the family able to share the diagnosis with all appropriate health care professionals and at least one significant person?
- Does the family appear to be moving through the stages of disclosure and seeking out support from peers?
- Is the family able to seek social and health services for which they qualify based on their HIV/acquired immunodeficiency syndrome (AIDS) status?
- Can family members answer the child's questions in a developmentally appropriate way?

Nursing Diagnosis

Ineffective Therapeutic Regimen Management: Noncompliance related to lack of support systems or denial of the illness.

Continued

Nursing Care Plan

The Child With HIV Infection—cont'd

Expected Outcomes

The mother will:
- Keep her health care appointments.

The family will:
- Work toward accepting the diagnosis.
- View themselves as valued members of the health care team.

The child will:
- Adhere to the medication regimen.

INTERVENTION	RATIONALE
1. Use language that shows respect. Offer information in a language that can be understood by the child and family. Use a translator as needed.	1. Families affected by HIV do not want their children called *innocent victims* or *AIDS babies,* nor do they want to be judged as promiscuous or substance abusers. Labels can create barriers, which can result in noncompliance with health care recommendations.
2. Encourage the mother to keep her own health care appointments.	2. HIV-infected women often neglect their own health care needs as they attend to those of their children.
3. Accept the parents' use of denial during periods of emotional respite. Refer for counseling to assist with the grieving process.	3. The diagnosis of HIV brings a series of losses, including the loss of the future and all that the future holds for a child. Denial is a coping mechanism.
4. Maintain realistic hope when possible.	4. With new prophylaxis for HIV-positive pregnant women and their infants, fewer than 5% of all seropositive babies actually develop HIV infection, and antiretroviral treatments have been successful in preserving immune function.
5. Refer the family to social services for assistance with finances, transportation, food, housing, clothing, medical care, and respite care as needed.	5. Although some women with HIV infection are judged to be uncaring because of missed appointments or because their child fails to gain weight, many simply lack the basic resources for compliance.
6. Teach the family how to give antiretroviral agents at home, keep a log, and adjust the schedule to accommodate school schedules. Monitor medication adherence every visit. Suggest ways to make medications more palatable to children (e.g., by using liquid forms or mixing with foods).	6. The antiretroviral regimen may include a combination of three drugs in addition to the other medications a child is taking. A daily log helps families keep track.

Evaluation

- Is the mother able to take care of herself?
- Has the patient or caregivers been able to move from denial to anger to acceptance of the diagnosis?
- Are the primary caregivers active, participatory, and valued members of the health care team?
- Does the child adhere to the medication regimen?

CORTICOSTEROID THERAPY

Corticosteroids, given as part of a treatment regimen, act as natural products of the adrenal glands, reducing local and systemic inflammatory symptoms.

Incidence

Topical steroids are applied to the skin or mucous membranes to reduce edema and redness and to counteract itching. They may be used to treat ophthalmic reactions and skin conditions such as eczema. Hydrocortisone cream is one example of a topical steroid. *Systemic steroids* reduce the inflammatory symptoms of generalized allergic reactions (e.g., asthma, hives, severe contact dermatitis). Systemic steroids are also given increasingly to treat malignant or autoimmune disorders. An example of a systemic steroid is prednisolone (Drug Guide, p. 1068).

Inhaled corticosteroids (ICS) produce a very strong local action and can control symptoms in children with asthma and allergic rhinitis. An example of an aerosol steroid is beclomethasone (see Chapters 45 and 49). Studies have varied as to

Nursing Care Plan

The Adolescent With HIV Infection

FOCUSED ASSESSMENT

Irrespective of the mode of acquisition, adolescent patients with human immunodeficiency virus (HIV) infection pose unique and important challenges for nurses. In addition to providing education and support surrounding normal adolescent growth and development, special attention must be directed to ensuring that the adolescent possesses an understanding of the disease process, risk-taking behaviors that could potentially transmit the virus to others, and how to prevent such occurrences. The adolescent's understanding of the importance of regular medical follow-up must also be assessed. It is critical that the adolescent be involved in all aspects of decision making.

Nursing Diagnosis

Deficient Knowledge about the effect of HIV on adolescents, current treatment options available, and prevention of transmission of virus to others.

Expected Outcome

The adolescent and family will:
- Explain in their own words what has been taught about HIV infection, including potential treatment regimens, goals of preserving or restoring immune function, and issues related to adolescent risk taking and adolescent sexuality.

INTERVENTION	RATIONALE
1. Determine the adolescent's and family's knowledge related to HIV infection.	1. Teaching needs to be geared toward the adolescent's cognitive and emotional readiness to learn about HIV, its treatment, and prevention of complications.
2. Identify specific concerns of the adolescent, and address them first.	2. Acknowledging the adolescent's concerns may help allay fears and anxiety and help begin to develop a trusting relationship.
3. Educate the adolescent about potential symptoms and problems to report to the health care provider.	3. Early identification of problems may prevent development of serious complications.
4. Establish readiness to adhere to medication regimen.	4. Adherence to medication regimens is critical to prevent development of viral resistance.
5. Discuss high-risk behaviors that could result in transmission of HIV to others and methods of prevention of transmission (e.g., sexual activity, IV drug use).	5. Frank discussions may empower the adolescent to assume responsibility for reducing the risk for transmission to others by encouraging safer behaviors in sexual practices and drug use.
6. Offer participation in peer support groups.	6. The adolescent may benefit from sharing thoughts and feelings about living with HIV, difficulties in taking medications, and so on with others.

Evaluation

- Can the adolescent and family explain what HIV is and its treatment goals?
- Can the adolescent describe appropriate measures to reduce disease transmission to others?

---

whether long-term use of ICS results in growth delay, with the general consensus being that there may be an initial period of growth delay but little effect on eventual height (Randell, Donaghue, Ambler, Cowell, Fitzgerald, & VanAsperen, 2003; Salvatoni, Piantanida, Nosetti, & Nespoli, 2000).

Pathophysiology

Corticosteroids have many different effects but are usually prescribed for their antiinflammatory or immunosuppressive properties. As antiinflammatories, they inhibit chemical me-

diators and the occurrence of edema, capillary dilation, phagocytic activity, and the migration of leukocytes associated with the inflammatory response. As immunosuppressives, they decrease monocyte and macrophage differentiation and block lymphokine production, leading to T cell inhibition.

The side effects of steroids vary widely with the child and the medication. Generally, the higher the dose and the longer the medication is taken, the more serious are the side effects. More knowledge about reactions and a broader selection of steroids and alternatives have significantly reduced untoward reactions in recent years.

PARENTS AND CAREGIVERS
Want to Know

About Basic Infection Control for the Child With Immunodeficiency

Review the following basic infection control practices for the child with immunodeficiency.

To prevent contact with germs:
- Keep immunizations up to date.
- Keep child home when sick.
- Turn away when someone coughs or sneezes.
- Do not share cups, bottles, plates, utensils, drinks, or pacifiers.
- Do not kiss babies on the mouth.
- Do not use fingers as a pacifier.
- Discard unused refrigerated formula after 24 hours.
- Change diapers—away from food areas—every 2 to 3 hours or sooner if the baby has a stool.
- Dispose of trash daily.

To create a barrier to germs if contact is unavoidable:
- Cover your mouth when coughing or sneezing.
- Use a tissue to wipe nose.
- Cover unused food and formula, and refrigerate.
- Keep a bowl close by if feeling nauseated.

- Fold soiled disposable diapers inward and tab.
- Discard dirty diapers and used tissues in a tightly covered, plastic-lined container.
- Cover sandboxes when not in use.

To kill germs if contact is made:
- Wash hands (using friction) with soap and warm water for 15 seconds before eating and after using the bathroom, wiping noses, changing diapers, cleaning up vomit, or catching a sneeze.
- Provide meticulous skin and mouth care.
- Carefully wash all fruits and vegetables that are to be eaten raw.
- Cook food well, especially meat, fowl, and eggs.
- Wash eating utensils, baby bottles, nipples, and pacifiers with soap and hot water or in the dishwasher.
- Rub the inside of the nipple with salt and rinse well if slimy.
- Clean kitchen and bathroom surfaces, shelves, pails, trash cans, and mops routinely.
- Clean litter boxes, bird cages, and turtle homes frequently and carefully.

Modified from Ward-Wimmer, D., & Riley, M.W. (1991). *Caring at home: A guide for families.* Washington, DC: The Child Welfare League of America.

Drug Guide

Prednisolone (Pediapred, Prelone)

Classification: Corticosteroid.

Action: Decreases inflammation; suppresses the immune response; affects bone marrow and the metabolism of proteins, carbohydrates, and fats.

Indications: Given for severe allergic and inflammatory conditions (e.g., asthma, eczema, juvenile arthritis), immunosuppression, and some autoimmune disorders.

Dosage and Route: Pediatric, oral (PO): 0.5-2 mg/kg daily in divided doses; comes in syrup (15 mg/5 ml) or tablets (1 mg, 5 mg, 25 mg).

Absorption: Rapid absorption from the gastrointestinal tract.

Excretion: Half eliminated in 2-4 hr; metabolized in the liver and excreted in the urine.

Contraindications: Do not give if the child has a systemic fungal infection or is sensitive to any of the ingredients.

Precautions: Children taking prednisolone are more prone to infection. Avoid exposure to measles or chickenpox while on prednisolone; immunize the child with live virus vaccines (measles, mumps, rubella [MMR]; varicella) before beginning corticosteroid treatment. Avoid giving with nonsteroidal antiinflammatory drugs (NSAIDs) or aspirin because it may increase the risk for gastrointestinal bleeding.

Adverse Reactions: Gastrointestinal distress, cushingoid state (moon face, buffalo hump), delayed wound healing, skin eruptions, carbohydrate intolerance, fluid retention, growth delay in children. *Acute adrenal insufficiency can occur when the child is under stress or if the medication is withdrawn abruptly. Do not discontinue this medication without tapering the dose.*

Nursing Considerations: Teach the parent to have the child take the medication with food or milk. Store the medication in a cool, dry location. Teach the parent to notify the doctor if the child exhibits any of the following: fever, other signs of infection, fatigue, muscle weakness, sudden weight gain, severe gastric irritation, slow wound healing, or growth delay, or if the child is experiencing increased stress.

Manifestations

Clinical manifestations of excess topically administered steroids include skin atrophy, delayed wound healing, telangiectasis or dilation of the cheek blood vessels, striae, and excess absorption leading to any of the clinical manifestations of systemic use.

Some clinical manifestations of excess steroid administered systemically include:

- Edema, particularly in the face
- Gastrointestinal irritation, even bleeding
- Bruising and delayed wound healing
- Susceptibility to infections

- Growth limitations
- Hypertension
- Loss of muscle mass
- Increased appetite and weight gain
- Amenorrhea
- Pancreatitis
- Joint pain and osteoporosis (may lead to bone fractures)
- Cataracts

Diagnostic Evaluation

The diagnosis of corticosteroid excess is suspected when clinical manifestations appear and is confirmed by administering a bolus of adrenocorticotropic hormone (ACTH) to the child. ACTH challenges the adrenal gland to respond to pituitary stimulation. If serum cortisol levels do not rise after administration of ACTH, adrenal suppression (cortisone excess) is present.

Therapeutic Management

Every effort is made to prevent corticosteroid excess by observing the following:

- Short-term, high-dose therapy (for 1 week or less) is preferred over long-term therapy if there is a strong indication for the use of steroids.
- If long-term use is necessary, alternate-day administration may be prescribed.
- At the time of an acute infection or surgery, supplementary steroids are indicated for children who have received them over a long period.

Because of immunosuppression, killed-virus vaccines are substituted for live-virus vaccines for children receiving high-dose or long-term steroids.

▪ NURSING CARE
The Child Receiving Corticosteroids

Assessment

Assessment of a child receiving long-term steroid therapy includes measuring height, weight, and blood pressure at each visit. In addition, the nurse observes the child for facial puffiness, abdominal pain, increased appetite, blurred vision, and increased thirst or urination. Families may report recent illnesses, bruising, or delayed wound healing.

Nursing Diagnosis and Planning

The nursing diagnoses and expected outcomes that may be appropriate following assessment of a child receiving corticosteroid therapy are

- ▪ Ineffective Therapeutic Regimen Management: Noncompliance related to associated complications.
  Expected Outcome: The child will take all medications as directed.
- ▪ Disturbed Body Image related to changes caused by treatment.
  Expected Outcome: The child will share feelings about any changes in appearance.
- ▪ Risk for Infection related to immunosuppression.

Expected Outcome: The child will be afebrile and free of signs of secondary infections.
- ▪ Risk for Injury (adrenal insufficiency, delayed wound healing) related to insufficient knowledge.
  Expected Outcomes: The child will not experience injury as a result of too rapid withdrawal of medication or delayed wound healing. The parent can explain the reason for not withdrawing the medication abruptly.
- ▪ Risk for Delayed Growth and Development related to growth suppression and muscle wasting.
  Expected Outcome: The child will continue to grow according to his or her own height and weight curve.

Interventions

The nurse should provide the family with written instructions that specifically state what to do if a dose is missed and when to decrease dosages. In general, if a dose is missed, the child should take it as soon as it is remembered; if it is almost time for the next dose, skip the dose altogether. The nurse should emphasize not to discontinue corticosteroid therapy abruptly.

The child needs to take the medication with foods or milk to minimize the risk for gastrointestinal bleeding. Because the child's appetite may be increased, encouraging low-calorie snacks throughout the day is appropriate. (The nurse should remind the family that salt may increase fluid retention.) Liquid forms of systemic corticosteroids can seem unpalatable to children. In this instance, the child may prefer a crushed tablet that has been put in a very small amount of a sweet food, or the liquid can be mixed with a sweet drink. Be sure to tell parents to mix the medication in 1 teaspoon or less of food or only a small amount of liquid to ensure the child receives all the medication.

Changes in appearance are temporary and reversible. The nurse can compare changes in appearance and weight gain at each visit and encourage expression of the child's feelings. Weight and height monitoring of the child receiving long-term corticosteroid therapy is important; fluid retention can mask muscle wasting and growth suppression.

Corticosteroids can also mask infections. The family should be instructed to call the physician in the event of temperature elevation, cough, runny nose, ear tenderness, decreased appetite, nausea, vomiting, diarrhea, or behavioral change, or even if the child just "does not seem right." The child's skin should be checked routinely for bruising and signs of wound infection, and lesions that do not resolve as expected should be reported. The family should not treat the child with over-the-counter products without consulting the physician. The child receiving long-term therapy should avoid others who are sick; parents should promptly report any exposure to a communicable disease, such as measles or chickenpox, to the health care provider.

Potential environmental hazards and accident prevention strategies based on the child's developmental age should be emphasized. If the child gets a cut, the parent may hold gentle pressure to the site for 3 to 5 minutes to stop the bleeding and prevent hematoma formation. The child should wear a Medic-Alert bracelet stating the key clinical manifestations of corticosteroid excess or adrenal insufficiency.

Evaluation

- Is the child taking corticosteroids as directed?
- Is the child able to express feelings about any changes in appearance?

! CRITICAL TO REMEMBER

The Child Taking Oral Corticosteroids

Long-term corticosteroid therapy causes adrenal insufficiency because exogenous (outside the body) use reduces the need for endogenous (within the body) production. Abrupt cessation of corticosteroid use without allowing for a gradual increase in adrenal production can cause insufficiency.
- Gradually taper the dose to allow for a gradual return of adrenal function.
- Carefully monitor the child during the taper for the following: fatigue, muscle weakness, joint pain, dizziness, anorexia, nausea.
- Supplemental glucocorticoids might be necessary during times of increased stress to prevent adrenal insufficiency.

- Does the child remain afebrile and free of any signs of secondary infection?
- Are any wounds healing at a normal rate?
- Is the child experiencing any signs of adrenal insufficiency, and can the parent explain why the medication should not be withdrawn abruptly?
- Is the child growing at a rate appropriate for age as measured on a standard growth chart?

IMMUNE COMPLEX AND AUTOIMMUNE DISORDERS

Immune Complex Disorders

Immune complexes are clusters of interlocking antigens and antibodies. Under normal conditions, immune complexes are removed from the blood. In some circumstances, however, immune complexes continue to circulate. Eventually they become trapped in the tissues of the kidneys, lungs, skin, joints, or blood vessels. There they set off reactions that lead to tissue inflammation and damage.

Deposition of immune complexes is considered to be a precipitator for several different conditions in childhood. Both Kawasaki disease (see Chapter 46) and acute poststreptococcal glomerulonephritis (see Chapter 44) are thought to be caused by immune complex deposition in tissue.

Autoimmune Disorders

Sometimes the immune system's ability to differentiate self from nonself breaks down and the body begins to make antibodies against its own cells, tissues (particularly connective tissue), and organs. Such antibodies are known as *autoantibodies*. Autoantibodies are common in conditions such as rheumatic fever (see Chapter 46), juvenile arthritis (see Chapter 50), and systemic lupus erythematosus.

It is still unclear what initiates an autoimmune response. Several theories have been proposed:

- Activation of immature B cells that do not develop antigen-specific receptors
- Alteration of normal tissue cells by infection or another process, which causes them to become antigenic
- Similarity between the structures of some infectious organisms and self-antigens, causing a cross-reaction
- Genetic predisposition of defective immune regulation

The response is exacerbated by a malfunction of helper T and suppressor T cells, when there are too many helper cells and not enough suppressor cells to turn off the immune response. Some autoimmune disorders also manifest with increased tissue deposits of immune complexes.

SYSTEMIC LUPUS ERYTHEMATOSUS

Systemic lupus erythematosus (SLE) is a chronic, multisystem, autoimmune disease characterized by inflammation of the connective tissue. SLE varies in severity and is marked by remissions and exacerbations.

Etiology

Although the etiology of SLE is not known, genetic, environmental, hormonal, and immune response factors are likely to be responsible. Environmental factors can include exposure to the sun, ultraviolet light, stress, fatigue, viruses, bacteria, certain medications, and some food additives. Exacerbations can occur with the use of birth control pills, menses, pregnancy, and the postpartum period (O'Neil, 1998).

Incidence

The overall incidence of SLE in the United States is up to 250 cases per 100,000 population (Klein-Gitelman & Miller, 2004). The condition is relatively rare in young children. In young children, the female to male ratio is 4:1; after puberty, this ratio increases to 8:1 (Klein-Gitelman & Miller, 2004). Onset in girls is most common between the ages of 9 and 15 years. More African-American, Hispanic, and Asian children are affected than white children.

Manifestations

Malaise, arthralgia, and recurrent fever of unknown etiology frequently are among the early manifestations of SLE. The symptoms, however, depend on what organs the immune complexes affect and can include (Klein-Gitelman & Miller, 2004; Rote, 2002):

- Malar butterfly rash—a fixed, red, flat or raised rash over the cheeks and bridge of nose (Fig. 41-1)
- Discoid rash—red, round, raised patches that spread
- Photosensitivity—skin rash from sun exposure
- Oral and nasal ulcers—usually painless lesions
- Arthritis—painful, swollen joints with edema
- Pleuritis, pericarditis, or peritonitis
- Renal disorder—protein, casts, or red cells in urine
- Neurologic disorders—headaches, personality changes, seizures, or psychosis
- Hematologic disorders—anemia, leukopenia, lymphoma, or thrombocytopenia
- Immunologic disorders
- Positive antinuclear antibody (ANA) assay

A child with SLE also might experience weight loss, growth impairment, headache, and memory problems. Occasionally, children will have Raynaud's phenomenon, in which the digits of the hands and feet suddenly change color (mottled to white to blue) in response to cold. The most se-

Pathophysiology

Systemic Lupus Erythematosus

Many abnormalities in the immune system are associated with systemic lupus erythematosus (SLE). Autoantibodies, referred to as *antinuclear antibodies (ANA),* act against DNA and other cell nucleus components. Abnormal immune complex formation and nonspecific activation of B lymphocytes cause an increase in immune globulins, a process that triggers autoantibodies. This response is exacerbated by a reduction in the number of suppressor T cells. These autoantibodies produce inflammation and damage tissues and organs, including the skin, joints, heart, lungs, kidneys, brain, and circulatory vessels.

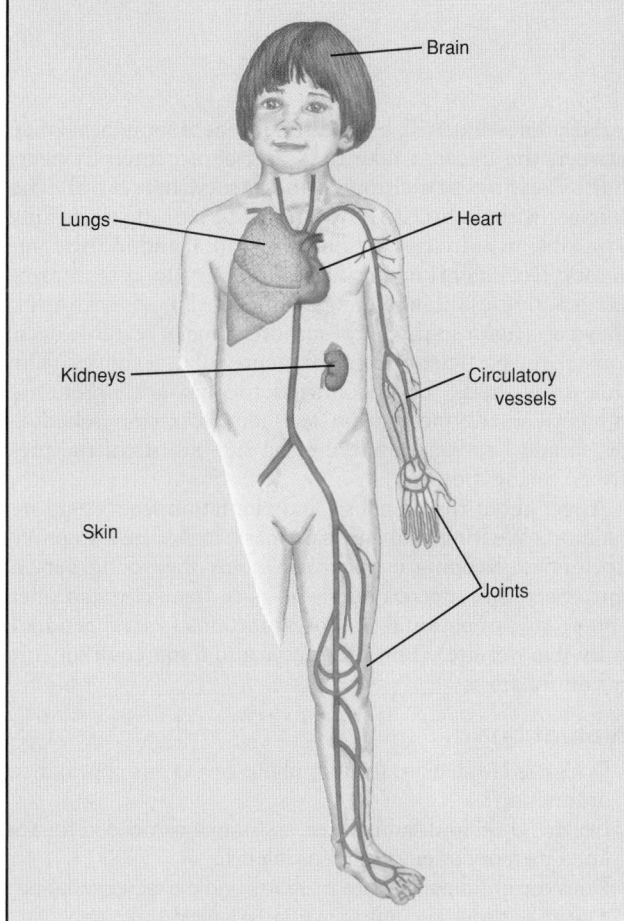

Brain

Lungs

Heart

Kidneys

Circulatory vessels

Skin

Joints

DNA, Deoxyribonucleic acid.

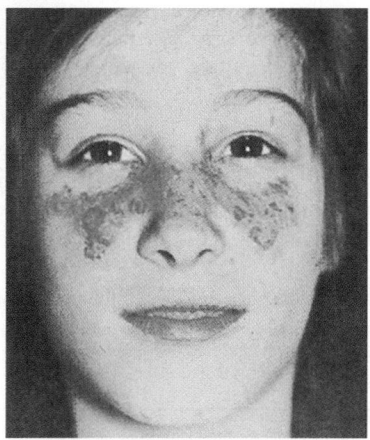

Figure 41-1 The butterfly rash of systemic lupus erythematosus. (From Behrman, R.E., Kliegman, R.M., & Arvin, A.M. [1996]. *Nelson textbook of pediatrics* [15th ed.]. Philadelphia: Saunders. Color Plate Fig. 150-1.)

levels, gamma-globulin levels, and the erythrocyte sedimentation rate might be elevated. Complement levels (C3 and C4) can be decreased. Pathologic changes compatible with SLE may be confirmed by electrocardiography, computed tomography, and magnetic resonance imaging and by skin and renal tissue biopsies demonstrating immune complexes.

Therapeutic Management

The treatment of SLE is tailored to the organ system or systems affected and is aimed at preventing exacerbations and complications. The goal of treatment is to use the least amount of pharmacologic intervention needed. Helping the child and family develop long-term coping strategies is important.

Systemic corticosteroids are most often given to control the inflammatory response. When steroid treatment is not effective or renal progression is rapid, cyclophosphamide (Cytoxan) might be considered. NSAIDs, excluding ibuprofen, are sometimes used to treat arthritis, serositis, and febrile attacks. Because they can cause liver damage, they are used with caution and careful monitoring. Children with renal and neurologic disorders generally receive anticonvulsant and antihypertensive therapy, whereas those with skin lesions and joint problems take antimalarial drugs, such as hydroxychloroquine (Plaquenil). Killed-virus vaccines rather than live-virus vaccines are used in affected children. A low-salt diet may reduce fluid retention and prevent elevated BUN levels; a low-protein diet helps preserve renal function.

The long-term prognosis for children with SLE is positive; the 10-year survival rate is 95% (Szer & Athreya, 2002). Close monitoring is essential for positive outcomes.

■ NURSING CARE

The Child With Systemic Lupus Erythematosus

Assessment

During a period of disease exacerbation, a child can become acutely ill. The nurse should monitor the child's vital signs, mobility, activity level, and pain and should complete a neurologic examination that assesses for decreased sensation,

rious complications of SLE include renal disease and neurologic problems.

Diagnostic Evaluation

The presence of four or more of the clinical manifestations just listed, whether or not they occur simultaneously, is suggestive of SLE. In addition, a number of tests can be used to diagnose and monitor the progress of SLE. A positive ANA test and the presence of anti–deoxyribonucleic acid (DNA) antibody are highly suggestive of SLE but can occur also in other autoimmune disorders. Blood urea nitrogen (BUN)

TABLE 41-5 Classification of Allergic Reactions

Type	Pathophysiology	Examples
I Immediate (anaphylactic) hypersensitivity	IgE attaches to mast cells and basophils, causing rupture and release of all contents (i.e., histamines).	Allergic rhinitis, acute anaphylaxis, hives, eczema, asthma
II Cytotoxic hypersensitivity	An allergen (e.g., red blood cell) stimulates IgE or IgM to react and mobilize complement to destroy the allergen.	Transfusion reaction after receiving incompatible blood
III Arthus hypersensitivity (immune complex)	Immune complex is formed and can destroy tissues.	Serum sickness, glomerulonephritis
IV Delayed cell-mediated hypersensitivity	An allergen reacts with T lymphocytes, and these lead other cells to produce damage.	Contact dermatitis (e.g., poison ivy)

IgE, Immunoglobulin E; *IgM*, immunoglobulin M.

weakness in the extremities, and changes in behavior. Of equal importance is evaluation of the effect of living with a chronic illness on a young child's self-image and interaction with peers.

Nursing Diagnosis and Planning

The nursing diagnoses that apply to the child with SLE are
- Disturbed Body Image related to changes secondary to the disease process and treatments.
  Expected Outcome: The child will share feelings about altered appearance or function.
- Powerlessness related to memory and emotional alterations.
  Expected Outcome: The child and family will seek assistance in managing memory or emotional problems.
- Activity Intolerance related to the effects of the disease process.
  Expected Outcome: The child will participate in activities to the extent possible.
- Chronic Pain related to arthritis and numbness of the hands and feet.
  Expected Outcome: The child will be free of pain, demonstrating an acceptable level on an age-appropriate pain assessment tool and the ability to gain appropriate rest and participate in age-appropriate activities.
- Ineffective Therapeutic Regimen Management: Nonadherence related to associated complications and developmental level.
  Expected Outcome: The child will take all medications as directed and describe the medication plan and any medication side effects.

Interventions

The nurse needs to help the child and family understand the importance of drug therapy and activity restriction during acute exacerbations. Avoiding triggers that cause exacerbations is essential (e.g., avoiding exposure to sun or avoidable sources of infection). Wearing an appropriate sunscreen is a necessity (sun protection factor [SPF] above 15, waterproof, para-aminobenzoic acid [PABA]–free, ultraviolet A [UVA]– and ultraviolet B [UVB]–protective). Raynaud's phenomenon can be prevented by dressing warmly in cold weather, paying particular attention to hat, gloves, and warm socks.

An adolescent will have difficulty achieving a balance between the need to take risks and be accepted by peers and the realities of a chronic illness (see Chapter 36). The teenager with a chronic illness needs to participate as fully as possible in activities at home, at school, and in the community. Documenting episodes of fatigue along with associated activities allows young people to gain some control. They can then use this information to make sensible decisions about participation in extracurricular activities. The adolescent should be encouraged to plan an appropriate and convenient medication self-administration schedule and should be able to describe the side effects of the prescribed medications.

Anger about the diagnosis and alienation from peers are common. Wearing makeup can mask rashes and improve appearance. Keeping a diary also helps the young person vent anger. An affected peer who is in remission can offer support, as can national SLE organizations (see Appendix I on Evolve website). The Internet is also a source of support and information.

Evaluation

- Does the child share feelings about her or his appearance or function?
- Do the child and family seek assistance as needed for related memory or emotional problems?
- Does the child participate in sports and extracurricular activities without becoming overly fatigued?
- Is the child free of pain as documented on an age-appropriate pain assessment tool?
- Is the child taking all medications as directed, and can the child describe the medication plan as well as side effects from the medications?

ALLERGIC REACTIONS

Allergy is the immune response to an antigen called an *allergen* that causes a hypersensitive reaction in various body systems. This hypersensitive reaction occurs with a second exposure to an antigen and can be immediate or delayed. The classification of allergic reactions often reflects the pathophysiology of each type (Table 41-5). In most children with allergies, there is a genetic link. Common allergic conditions

TABLE **41-6** Common Allergic Conditions in Children

Allergens	Manifestations	Diagnosis
INHALANTS		
Pollen, dust, mold, dander	Sneezing; red, itchy nose, eyes, pharynx, and palate; edematous nasal passages; tongue clicking; runny or congested nose; mouth breathing; chronic cough; dark circles under eyes; nose wrinkling; pale, boggy nasal mucous membranes	Allergic rhinitis
APPLICANTS		
Heat, cold, wool, cosmetics, solutions for hair permanents, sunscreens, plants, grasses	Well-defined red, raised skin or mucosal lesions	Hives Contact dermatitis
FOODS		
Milk, wheat, eggs, strawberries, tomatoes, oranges, chocolate, nuts, shellfish	Intestinal cramping, nausea, vomiting, diarrhea Bronchospasm Red patches on cheeks, face, wrists, neck, hands, extremities; swelling; itching; weeping; scales and crust Well-defined red, raised skin or mucosal lesions Vascular headaches	Colic Asthma Eczema Hives Migraines
MEDICINES		
Penicillin, cephalexin, immunizations, allergy immunotherapy, chemotherapy	Redness, swelling, pain Weakness, restlessness, edema, laryngospasm, cardiovascular collapse	Local inflammation Anaphylaxis
INSECTS		
Stings of bees, wasps, hornets	Redness, swelling, pain Weakness, restlessness, edema, laryngospasm, cardiovascular collapse	Local inflammation Anaphylaxis

include allergic rhinitis, hives, eczema, asthma, colic, and migraines (Table 41-6).

Allergic rhinitis is an immediate hypersensitivity reaction to allergens trapped by the hairs and mucus that line the inside of the nose (see Chapter 45). Anaphylaxis is a life-threatening allergic response. Allergic reactions are related to the antibody IgE.

ANAPHYLAXIS

Anaphylaxis, a severe, immediate hypersensitivity reaction to an excessive release of chemical mediators, affects the entire body.

Etiology

Food allergy has become the primary cause of anaphylaxis in children (Sampson & Leung, 2004). Other causes include penicillin or other antibiotics, insect stings, immunizations, allergy immunotherapy (desensitization), chemotherapeutic agents, blood products, and diagnostic contrast media. Peanuts (including peanut butter) and tree nuts (e.g., cashew, almond, walnuts, pecans, pistachios) are particularly potent substances, causing anaphylaxis in increasing numbers. Other frequently seen food allergies include milk, eggs, wheat, shellfish, and other fish. Anaphylactic reactions to products containing latex have increased in incidence, especially among children with spina bifida (see Chapter 52) and children with abnormalities of the urinary tract.

Incidence

Approximately 6% to 8% of children younger than 3 years in the United States experience severe allergic reactions to foods (Sampson & Leung, 2004). In many cases, previous exposure to the allergen is undocumented, so the child experiences anaphylaxis presumably on first documented exposure. For example, studies suggest that exposure to peanut allergens can occur in a breastfeeding child whose mother has a high intake of nuts (Jackson, 2002), but the child only experiences anaphylaxis when peanut butter is introduced into the diet at about age 2 years. In the child who is allergic to peanuts or other nuts, anaphylactic reaction can occur with exposure to nut oils, surfaces contaminated with nuts, shell fragments, or cooking and serving utensils used previously for nut products.

The incidence of anaphylaxis in the United States from all causes is considered to be 30/100,000 (Sampson & Leung, 2004).

Manifestations

The onset of anaphylaxis is sudden, usually occurring within seconds to minutes after exposure to an allergen. Initial symptoms of impending anaphylaxis include:

- Sneezing
- Tightness or tingling of the mouth or face, with subsequent swelling of the lips and tongue

Pathophysiology

Anaphylaxis

Anaphylaxis occurs when an allergen binds with immunoglobulin E (IgE) on mast cells and basophils, causing degranulation and release of histamines and other chemical mediators. Histamine action precipitates respiratory signs of bronchoconstriction with bronchospasm and edema (especially laryngeal edema) from increased vascular permeability. Other systems most affected during an anaphylactic response include gastrointestinal (itchiness and tingling along the gastrointestinal tract, vomiting, diarrhea, pain) and integumentary (urticaria). Anaphylaxis can lead to circulatory collapse and death if not promptly managed. An allergen that has previously provoked a response, or one that has not, can cause anaphylaxis.

- Severe flushing, urticaria, and itching of the skin, especially on the head and upper trunk
- Rapid development of erythema
- A sense of impending doom

These symptoms might be followed by gastrointestinal and respiratory symptoms, which include nausea, vomiting, diarrhea, and cramping, as well as rhinorrhea, stridor, wheezing, and hoarseness.

The most serious features of anaphylaxis are laryngospasm, edema, cyanosis, hypotensive shock, vascular collapse, and cardiac arrest. Several hours after the initial phase of anaphylaxis resolves, a second, or biphasic, reaction can occur. This second reaction can be as severe as the initial reaction, affects similar body systems, and can occur up to several days after the initial episode. The average time of onset of a biphasic reaction is 1.3 to 28.4 hours (Lee & Greenes, 2000).

Diagnostic Evaluation

Anaphylaxis occurs suddenly, allowing no time for diagnosis. The etiology is determined later by obtaining a history of the exposure. Serum studies may reveal an elevated IgE for the agent of exposure. In some cases the allergen can be confirmed by skin tests or radioallergosorbent test (RAST).

Therapeutic Management

Treatment of anaphylaxis must begin immediately, because it may be only a matter of minutes before the child experiences shock. In the community setting, immediately activate the emergency response system. Injectable epinephrine is the first drug of choice in the acute treatment of anaphylaxis; the earlier the epinephrine is administered, the lower the likelihood of a biphasic reaction (Lee & Greenes, 2000). In addition to epinephrine, oral diphenhydramine and a histamine inhibitor (e.g., cimetidine) may be indicated.

Epinephrine (0.01 mg/kg/dose of 1:1000 concentration) is administered to children with suspected anaphylaxis. Chil-

dren with known severe allergic reactions need to have an EpiPen or other preloaded, automatic delivery system available at all times. The EpiPen (0.3 mg) is appropriate for children who weigh more than 66 lb., whereas the EpiPen Jr. (0.15 mg) can be administered to children who weigh at least 22 lb. (Sampson, 2003).

In a hospital or emergency setting, managing anaphylactic shock includes the following:

- Ensure an adequate airway, possibly by endotracheal intubation (see Chapter 34).
- Administer epinephrine. If reaction is caused by an insect sting, place a tourniquet proximal to the site of the sting and administer epinephrine in the uninvolved extremity and in the area of reaction, with repeat dosing within 5 to 10 minutes.
- Administer oxygen if available.
- Administer corticosteroids and antihistamines as ordered.
- Keep the child warm and lying flat or with feet slightly elevated.
- Start an intravenous (IV) line.

Children who have experienced life-threatening insect sting anaphylaxis and demonstrate venom-specific IgE antibodies on skin studies or RAST are candidates for venom immunotherapy. All children experiencing episodes of anaphylaxis in the community should be transported by ambulance to an emergency facility (see Chapter 34) and kept for observation at least 4 hours after the episode is resolved.

◾ NURSING CARE
The Child With Anaphylaxis

Assessment

The child should be monitored closely for airway obstruction and vascular collapse during the acute phase of anaphylaxis. Assessment includes noting airway patency, respiratory rate and effort, heart rate, peripheral pulses, capillary refill time, oxygen saturation, urine output, and level of consciousness. After emergency efforts, the nurse can try to determine the cause of the attack by correlating when the symptoms first occurred with foods ingested, medications administered, and the possibility of an insect sting.

Nursing Diagnosis and Planning

The nursing diagnoses that apply to the child with anaphylaxis and to the family are

- Ineffective Breathing Pattern and Decreased Cardiac Output related to an excessive hypersensitive reaction to an allergen.
  Expected Outcome: The child will maintain a patent airway and adequate cardiac output (short term).
- Deficient Knowledge about allergens and prevention through risk reduction related to inexperience.
  Expected Outcome: The child and family will describe the child's allergic reaction and initiate a management plan for avoiding allergens and treating reactions (long term).

Interventions

Initially, the nurse maintains an adequate airway by administering oxygen and assisting with aerosol treatments and intubation as necessary. A laryngoscope, intubation tray, and tracheostomy kit should be available, and the code cart should be nearby. In the case of an insect sting or injected medication, a tourniquet applied to the affected extremity just proximal to the site might help confine the allergen. It is important to have IV access, with a large-bore needle, in at least one site, preferably two, for medication administration. The nurse administers IV fluids, epinephrine, corticosteroids, and antihistamines as ordered and informs the physician of the child's improvement or deterioration. Extra fluids (crystalloids or colloids) and plasma expanders should be administered if the child shows signs of vascular collapse (see Chapter 34).

Because epinephrine causes vasoconstriction and an increase in cardiac output, a child receiving the drug might experience heart palpitations and tachycardia. This is frightening and aggravated by the emergency nature of the situation. The nurse should offer gentle reassurance to the child and provide the family with frequent reports about the child's condition.

After an initial anaphylactic episode, the nurse should assure the child and family that they were not at fault for the anaphylactic reaction and discuss how to prevent recurrences. Any child who has experienced anaphylaxis should have and learn to use an injectable epinephrine. The Epi-Pen Jr. for children delivers 0.15 mg of epinephrine through a spring-loaded injector, and the Epi-Pen provides 0.3 mg of epinephrine. The dose chosen by the provider is based on the child's weight. Teach the parent or child to hold the injector against the skin of the upper outer region of the child's thigh for 10 seconds after administering the injection to deliver the medication completely. The Epi Pen can be injected through clothing. A Medic-Alert bracelet alerts others to the child's allergy.

Caring for the child at school presents an additional challenge. The school nurse must be aware of and communicate to appropriate others information about any child who has experienced anaphylaxis. Policies about storage of and access to the Epi-Pen in the school setting differ in each school district. Some school districts train non-medical personnel to administer the epinephrine if the child goes on a field trip; other school districts require a parent of a child who cannot self-administer epinephrine to accompany the child on a field trip. It is necessary for the school nurse to notify teachers and school nutrition personnel if a child or children in the school have allergies to peanuts or other foods. In some instances, the child may be so highly allergic that lunch needs to be eaten in the school health office, away from even the odor of peanut butter. Most commercial fast-food establishments post signs if pastries or other foods contain peanuts or other allergenic substances.

Evaluation

- Is the child awake and alert with adequate oxygenation and a patent airway?
- Are the child's vital signs within normal limits for age?
- Is the family taking appropriate steps to reduce the risks of another anaphylactic reaction?
- Do the child, family, and other appropriate adults demonstrate the proper use of the insect sting kit?

CHILDREN
Want to Know

How to Prevent Insect Stings

- Select clothes with white or khaki colors, not dark or brightly decorative ones.
- Wear fitted clothes with long sleeves, pants, and shoes.
- Use unscented soaps, lotions, and deodorants.
- Apply insect skin protection.
- Avoid orchards, flowers, blooming trees, and shrubs.
- Stay away from picnic areas.
- Keep out of the garden.
- Keep car windows closed while driving.
- Place screens on all windows.
- Cover all garbage cans.
- Move away slowly from approaching insects.

PARENTS
Want to Know

About Communicating With the School About Peanut Allergies

- If your child has had a severe reaction to peanuts or other nuts, it is important for you to talk to your health care provider about whether the child should have medication available at home and school.
- Epinephrine, the medication that relieves a severe allergic reaction, is available in an easy-to-use automatic injector, which older children can self-administer and teachers or other school personnel can be taught to administer.
- Important things to remember when using automatically injected epinephrine are:
  1. If using an Epi-Pen, the injection can be given through the child's clothing.
  2. After starting the injection, you must continue to hold the Epi-Pen against the child for at least 10 seconds for all the medication to be delivered.
- Your child should have an allergy action plan readily available at school. You can obtain a sample action plan from www.foodallergy.org.
- Talk to the school nurse about the severity of your child's reaction, and work with the nurse to create a way your child can avoid contact with peanuts while not singling the child out for special attention.

Many school districts have policies that prohibit sharing of food or eating food on school buses. Other practices available at certain schools include peanut-free classrooms and a peanut-free area in the school cafeteria. Your school nurse can help you decide what modifications are appropriate for your child.

KEY CONCEPTS

- The immune system maintains homeostasis of the internal and external environment through nonspecific functions (inflammation, phagocytosis) and specific functions (humoral and cell-mediated immunity). Any derangement results in an immunologic imbalance whereby the immune system either under-functions or over-functions.

- When the immune system under-functions, susceptibility to infections is increased (immunodeficiency). When the immune system over-functions, it produces antibodies against cells of the body in autoimmune disease or against external sensitizing agents, forming the basis for allergies.

- The immune response is produced either actively or passively. Active immunity means the body has reacted to antigens in nature or vaccines. The effect of active immunity lasts months to a lifetime. Passive immunity results from antibody transfer from a person with active immunity to a person who does not have that antibody. The effect of passive immunity is transitory.

- Children with acquired or congenital immunodeficiency are vulnerable to bacterial and viral infections. The best way to prevent the spread of organisms is to wash hands routinely and to follow basic infection control practices, based on three principles: (1) prevent contact with organisms; (2) create barriers if contact is unavoidable; and (3) kill organisms if contact is made.

- HIV infection is the best-known acquired immunodeficiency disease. It causes a wide spectrum of illness in children, ranging from no symptoms to mild and moderate symptoms to severe symptoms.

- Standard treatments for HIV infection include a modified immunization program, antiretroviral therapy, PCP prophylaxis, and the aggressive use of antibiotics.

- For children with HIV, nurses have the challenging tasks of promoting normal growth and development, preventing infections, providing comfort, and respiratory management. In addition, nurses must support families in dealing with a stigmatizing illness that is ultimately terminal.

- Adolescents who acquired HIV when they were born are now reaching teen years. Nurses must discuss issues of infection transmission and medication compliance with these teens.

- Corticosteroids have immunosuppressive and antiinflammatory properties. Tapering the dose during both long-term and short-term therapy regimens allows for the gradual return of adrenal function.

- Emergency treatment takes priority in an anaphylactic reaction, because it is only a matter of minutes before the child will go into shock. In a community setting, epinephrine is administered to children with a known prior anaphylactic episode and the emergency service system is activated. Initially, the goal is to maintain an adequate airway, sometimes necessitating endotracheal intubation. This is followed by the administration of epinephrine.

ANSWERS to Critical Thinking Exercise 41-1

Negative Considerations

Human immunodeficiency virus (HIV) antibody testing in infants younger than 18 months is unreliable because antibodies (indicating infection) are passed from the mother to the child. HIV antibody testing in infants only indicates the HIV infection status of the mother. Several problems are associated with this:

- The mother might not know or suspect she is HIV-positive.
- Her denial on learning of her diagnosis might delay her and the baby's treatment.

- Early discharge of mother and infant from the hospital complicates follow-up.
- Some infants are not brought for well-child care, and the mother does not receive the information.
- HIV testing without consent might violate the mother's rights.

Positive Considerations

HIV testing allows for early identification and treatment of potentially infected infants and their mothers. This is especially important for *Pneumocystis carinii* pneumonia (PCP) prophylaxis initiation and treatment with combination antiretroviral agents. The Centers for Disease Control and Prevention (CDC) has recommended education about voluntary HIV testing for pregnant women. If the nurse's first contact with an infant, particularly the infant of a high-risk mother, is after delivery and HIV testing was not done during pregnancy, HIV testing should be offered for both the mother and the newborn.

REFERENCES and READINGS

American Academy of Pediatrics. (2003). *2003 Red Book: Report of the Committee on Infectious Diseases* (26th ed.). Elk Grove Village, IL: Author.

Behrman, R., Kliegman, R., & Jenson, H. (Eds.). (2004). *Nelson textbook of pediatrics* (17th ed.). Philadelphia: Saunders.

Boland, M. (2000). Caring for the child and family with HIV disease. *Pediatric Clinics of North America, 47*(1), 189-202.

Buckley, R. (2000). T-, B-, and NK-cell systems. In R. Behrman, R. Kliegman, & H. Jenson (Eds.), *Nelson textbook of pediatrics* (16th ed., pp. 590-595). Philadelphia: Saunders.

Butz, A., Joyner, M., Friedman, D., & Hutton, N. (1998). Primary care for children with human immunodeficiency virus infection. *Journal of Pediatric Health Care, 12*(1), 10-19.

Centers for Disease Control and Prevention (CDC). (1994). Recommendations for the use of zidovudine to reduce perinatal transmission of HIV. *MMWR: Morbidity and Mortality Weekly Report, 43*(11), 285-287.

Centers for Disease Control and Prevention. (1995). 1995 revised guidelines for prophylaxis against PCP for children infected with or perinatally exposed to HIV. *MMWR: Morbidity and Mortality Weekly Report, 44*(RR-4), 1-11.

Centers for Disease Control and Prevention. (1998). Guidelines for the use of antiretroviral agents in pediatric HIV infection. *MMWR: Morbidity and Mortality Weekly Report, 47*(RR-4), 1-31.

Centers for Disease Control and Prevention. (1999). *HIV and its transmission.* Retrieved July 13, 2003, from Centers for Disease Control and Prevention: www.cdc.gov/hiv/pubs/facts/transmission.htm.

Centers for Disease Control and Prevention. (2000). *Leading causes of death report.* National Center for Health Statistics (NCHS) Vital Statistics System. Office of Statistics and Programming, National Center for Injury Prevention and Control.

Centers for Disease Control and Prevention. (2002). *Divisions of HIV/AIDS prevention.* Retrieved July 13, 2003, from Centers for Disease Control and Prevention: www.cdc.gov/hiv/stats/hasr1302/table5.htm.

Centers for Disease Control and Prevention. (2003). Guidelines for the use of antiretroviral agents in pediatric HIV infection. *MMWR: Morbidity and Mortality Weekly Report, 47*(RR-4), 1-31.

Chen, F., Pau, A.K., & Piscitelli, S.C. (2000). Update on preventing vertical transmission of HIV type 1. *American Journal of Health Systems and Pharmacies, 57*(17), 1616-1623.

Deatrick, J.A., Lipman, T.H., Thurber, F., Ash, L., Carlino, H., McKnight, H., & Rutstein, R.M. (1998). Nutritional assessment for children who are HIV-infected. *Pediatric Nursing, 24*(2), 137.

Elder, M. (2000). T-cell immunodeficiencies. *Pediatric Clinics of North America, 47*(6), 1253-1275.

Fahrner, R., & Manio, E. (2000). HIV infection and AIDS. In P. Jackson & J. Vessey (Eds.), *Primary Care of the Child With a Chronic Condition* (3rd ed., pp. 538-558). St. Louis: Mosby.

Fleisher, T., & Ballow, J. (2000). Immune function. *Pediatric Clinics of North America, 47*(6), 1197-1210.

Frank, S., Esch, J., & Margeson, N. (1998). Mandatory HIV testing of newborns: The impact on women. *American Journal of Nursing, 98*(10), 49-51.

Frederick, T., Thomas, P., Mascola, L., Hsu, H.W., Rakusan, T., Mapson, C., Weedon, J., & Bertolli, J. (2000). Human immunodeficiency virus–infected adolescents: A descriptive study of older children in New York City, Los Angeles County, Massachusetts, and Washington, DC. *The Pediatric Infectious Disease Journal, 19,* 551-555.

Futterman, D., Chabon, B., & Hoffman, N. (2000). HIV and AIDS in adolescents. *Pediatric Clinics of North America, 47*(1), 171-188.

Jackson, P. (2002). Peanut allergy: An increasing health risk for children. *Pediatric Nursing, 28*(5), 496-500.

Khoury, M., & Kovacs, A. (2001). Pediatric HIV infection. *Clinical Obstetrics and Gynecology, 44,* 243-275.

Klein-Gitelman, M., & Miller, M. (2004). Systemic lupus erythematosus. In R. Behrman, R. Kliegman, & H. Jenson (Eds.). *Nelson textbook of pediatrics* (17th ed., pp. 809-813). Philadelphia: Saunders.

Klunklin, P. & Harrigan, R. (2002). Child-rearing practices of primary caregivers of HIV-infected children: An integrated review of the literature. *Journal of Pediatric Nursing, 17*(4), 289-296.

Lee, J., & Greenes, D. (2000). Biphasic anaphylactic reactions in pediatrics. *Pediatrics, 106*(4), 762-767.

Lindegren, M., Steinberg, S., & Byers, R. (2000). Epidemiology of HIV/AIDS in children. *Pediatric Clinics of North America, 47*(1), 1-20.

Michaels, M., & Green, M. (1999). General principles of immunosuppression in transplantation. In F. Burg, E. Wald, J. Ingelfinger, & R. Polin (Eds.), *Gellis & Kagan's current pediatric therapy* (16th ed.). Philadelphia: Saunders.

Mofenson, L., & Read, J. (1999). Human immunodeficiency virus infection. In F. Burg, E. Wald, J. Ingelfinger, & R. Polin (Eds.), *Gellis & Kagan's current pediatric therapy* (16th ed.). Philadelphia: Saunders.

Moye, J. (1995, June). *Update: Prophylaxis of opportunistic infections in pediatric HIV disease.* Paper presented at a workshop co-sponsored by the National Pediatric and Family HIV Resource Center, Greenbelt, MD.

Munoz-Furlong, A. (2003). Daily coping strategies for patients and their families. *Pediatrics, 111*(6), 1654-1662.

Newshan, G., & Hoyt, M. (1998). Use of combination antiretroviral therapy in pregnant women with HIV disease. *MCN: The American Journal of Maternal/Child Nursing, 23*(6), 307-312.

Oleske, J. (1995, June). *Pain in pediatric HIV disease: Meeting the challenge.* Plenary session at a workshop c-sponsored by the National Pediatric and Family HIV Resource Center, Greenbelt, MD.

O'Neil, K. (1998). Systemic lupus erythematosus. In L. Finberg (Ed.), *Saunders manual of pediatric practice.* Philadelphia: Saunders.

Pagana, K.D., & Pagana, T. (2002). *Mosby's manual of diagnostic and laboratory tests.* St. Louis: Mosby.

Perinatal HIV Guidelines Working Group. (2003). *U.S. Public Health Service Task Force recommendations for use of antiretroviral drugs in pregnant HIV-1-infected women for maternal health and interventions to reduce perinatal HIV-1 transmission in the United States.* Retrieved April 21, 2004 from www.aidsinfo.nih.gov

Randell, T., Donaghue, K., Ambler, G., Cowell, C., Fitzgerald, D., & VanAsperen, P. (2003). Safety of the newer inhaled corticosteroids in childhood asthma. *Pediatric Drugs, 5*(7), 481-504.

Rote, N. (2002). Immunity. In K. McCance & S. Huether (Eds.). *Pathophysiology: The biologic basis for disease in adults and children* (4th ed., pp. 168-196). St. Louis: Mosby.

Salvatoni, A., Piantanida, E., Nosetti, L., & Nespoli, L. (2000). Inhaled corticosteroids in childhood asthma. *Pediatric Drug, 5*(6), 351-361.

Sampson, H. (2002). Peanut allergy. *New England Journal of Medicine, 346*(17), 1294-1299.

Sampson, H. (2003). Anaphylaxis and emergency treatment. *Pediatrics, 111*(6), 1601-1609.

Sampson, H. & Leung, D. (2004). Adverse reactions to foods. In R. Behrman, R. Kliegman, & H. Jenson (Eds.). *Nelson textbook of pediatrics* (17th ed., pp. 789-792). Philadelphia: Saunders.

School guidelines for managing students with food allergies. (2003). Retrieved Sept. 21, 2003, from www.foodallergy.org/school/guidelines.html.

Schwartz, S. (2000). Intravenous immunoglobulin treatment of immunodeficiency disorders. *Pediatric Clinics of North America, 47*(6), 1355-1370.

Shea, K. (2002). Human immunodeficiency virus and acquired immune deficiency syndrome. In J. Fox (Ed.), *Primary health care of infants, children, and adolescents* (2nd ed., pp 796-815). St. Louis: Mosby.

Sicherer, S., Munoz-Furlong, A., & Sampson, H. (2003). Prevalence of peanut and tree nut allergy in the United States determined by means of a random digit dial telephone survey: A 5-year follow-up study. *The Journal of Allergy and Clinical Immunology, 112*(6), 1203-1207.

Sicherer, S., Noone, S., & Forman, J. (2000). Use assessment of self-administered epinephrine among food-allergic children and pediatricians. *Pediatrics, 105*(2), 359-363.

Simons, F., Gu, X., Johnston, L., & Simons, K. (2001). Can epinephrine inhalations be substituted for epinephrine injection in children at risk for systemic anaphylaxis? *Pediatrics, 106,* 1040-1044.

Sofat, N., & Higgens, C. (2001). Diagnostic issues in systemic lupus erythematosus. *Postgraduate Medicine, 77*(906), 266.

Steele, R. (2000, Oct.). *What are the special needs of adolescent patients with HIV/AIDS?* Paper presented on Day 1 at the annual meeting of the American Academy of Pediatrics.

Students with chronic illness: Guidance for families, schools, and students. (2003). *Journal of School Health, 73*(4), 131-132.

Szer, I.S., & Athreya, B. (2002). Systemic lupus erythematosus in children. In F. Burg, J. Ingelfinger, R. Polin, & A. Gershon (Eds.). *Gellis & Kagan's current pediatric therapy* (17th ed., pp. 754-757). Philadelphia: Saunders.

U.S. Department of Health and Human Services, Panel on Clinical Practices for the Treatment of HIV Infection (2000, Jan. 7). *Guidelines for the use of antiretroviral agents in pediatric HIV infection.* Available on-line: www.hivatis.org.

U.S. Department of Health and Human Services, Panel on Clinical Practices for the Treatment of HIV Infection (2001, April 23). *Guidelines for the use of antiretroviral agents in HIV-infected adults and adolescents.* Available on-line: www.hivatis.org.

Waugh, S. (2003). Parental views on disclosure of diagnosis to their HIV positive children. *AIDS Care, 15*(2), 169-176.

Working Group on Antiretroviral Therapy and Medical Management of HIV-Infected Children. (2004). *Guidelines for the use of antiretroviral agents in pediatric HIV infection.* Retrieved April 21, 2004 from www.aidsinfo.nih.gov.

Yogev, R., & Chadwick, E. (2004). Acquired immunodeficiency syndrome (human immunodeficiency virus). In R. Behrman, R. Kliegman, & H. Jenson (Eds.). *Nelson textbook of pediatrics* (17th ed, pp. 1111-1121). Philadelphia: Saunders.

42

The Child with a Fluid and Electrolyte Alteration

◆ LEARNING OBJECTIVES

After studying this chapter, you should be able to:

- ◉ Identify the regulatory mechanisms that maintain fluid and electrolyte balance in the body.
- ◉ Compare those differences in body fluid and electrolyte composition and regulation between infants/children and adults that make infants and children more vulnerable to imbalances.
- ◉ Describe dehydration and acid-base imbalance.

- ◉ Differentiate among the various types of acid-base disturbances.
- ◉ Describe the processes of diarrhea and vomiting.
- ◉ Integrate assessment findings with nursing implementation to determine the success of therapy.
- ◉ Describe nursing interventions to prevent fluid and electrolyte imbalances.

◆ DEFINITIONS

acidosis Abnormal accumulation of acid in or loss of base from the body, with pH less than 7.35.

alkalosis Abnormal accumulation of base in or loss of acid from the body, with pH more than 7.45.

anuria Absence of urine formation; usually indicative of kidney failure but may be secondary to severe dehydration.

extracellular fluid (ECF) Fluid found outside the cell, composing approximately one third of the body's fluid in older children and about one half of the body's fluid in infants.

hypernatremic (hypertonic) dehydration State in which the sodium concentration is above that of normal body fluids (i.e., >150 mEq/L).

hyponatremic (hypotonic) dehydration State in which the sodium concentration is below that of normal body fluids (i.e., <130 mEq/L).

interstitial fluid Extracellular fluid surrounding the cell, including lymph fluid.

intracellular fluid (ICF) Fluid found within the cells, composing approximately two thirds of the body's fluid in older children and about one half of the body's fluid in infants.

intravascular fluid Extracellular fluid contained within a blood vessel (e.g., plasma).

isonatremic (isotonic) dehydration State in which the sodium concentration is practically identical to that of body fluids (i.e., between 135 and 145 mEq/L).

oliguria Diminished urine output.

REVIEW OF FLUID AND ELECTROLYTE IMBALANCES IN CHILDREN

Characteristics unique to children affect fluid and electrolyte balance. Infants and young children are more vulnerable than adults to changes in fluid and electrolyte balance. Under normal conditions, the amount of fluid ingested during a day should equal the amount of fluid lost through sensible water loss (e.g., urine output) and insensible water loss (via the respiratory tract and skin). Insensible water loss per unit of body weight is significantly higher in infants and children. The faster respiratory rates of infants and young children also result in higher evaporative water losses. Any condition that prevents normal oral fluid intake (e.g., vomiting) or results in fluid losses (e.g., diarrhea, hyperventilation, burns, hemorrhage) is especially significant because it depletes the body's store of water and electrolytes much more rapidly in infants and young children than in adults.

Body water is located in two major compartments: within the cell, in the intracellular compartment; and outside the cell, in the extracellular compartment. These two compartments are separated by the cell membrane, across which body fluid is continually exchanged. Extracellular fluid (ECF) is located in several places: in interstitial spaces (surrounding the cells, e.g., lymph fluid); intravascularly (within the blood vessels or plasma); and transcellularly (e.g., cerebrospinal fluid, pericardial fluid, pleural fluid, synovial fluid, sweat, digestive secretions). A child is more likely to lose ECF than intracellular fluid (ICF). ECF is lost first when fluid loss occurs (e.g., through illness, trauma, fever). The intracellular compartment is more difficult to dehydrate.

In the neonate, approximately 40% of body water is located in the extracellular compartment, compared with 20% in the adolescent and adult. In the infant, one half of the ECF may be exchanged, compared with an adult exchange of one sixth of the ECF in a similar time. Because approximately 50% of this ECF is exchanged daily in an infant, dehydration can occur very suddenly and rapidly if fluid intake is inadequate or fluid losses are excessive. Because of the infant's higher metabolic rate, the rate of water turnover is rapid. Depletion of ECF, often caused by gastroenteritis, is one of the most common problems among infants and young children. In adults and older children, because a greater proportion of fluid is located in the intracellular compartment, severe fluid depletion does not occur as rapidly. Maturity in body space distribution is usually reached around age 3 years.

Body fluids are basically composed of two elements, water and solutes. *Water* is the primary constituent, with the infant's weight being approximately 75% water to the adult's 55% to 60%. In general, the volume of total body water to total body weight decreases with increasing age. An inverse relationship exists between total body water and total body fat. Compared with adults, neonates, particularly premature infants, have a lower proportion of fat.

Solutes are composed of both electrolytes and nonelectrolytes. Most of the body's solutes are electrolytes, primarily sodium (Na^+), potassium (K^+), chloride (Cl^-), calcium (Ca^{++}), and magnesium (Mg^{++}). The primary electrolyte of the ECF is sodium; potassium and magnesium are the primary electrolytes in the ICF. The extracellular compartment contains more sodium and chloride during infancy, which increases the vulnerability of infants to electrolyte imbalances. Changes in the concentration of these electrolytes may result in cellular dysfunction and illness. Problems of fluid and electrolyte balance involve both water and electrolytes; thus treatment includes replacement of both, calculated according to serum electrolyte laboratory values.

Pediatric Differences Related to Fluid and Electrolyte Balance

Infants
- Because of the higher percentage of water in the extracellular fluid (ECF), infants can lose fluids equal to their ECF within 2 to 3 days.
- Infants are less able to concentrate urine because of immature renal function.
- Infants have a higher rate of peristalsis than do older children.
- Infants have an immature lower esophageal sphincter, which makes them more prone to gastroesophageal reflux, which can lead to dehydration and electrolyte disturbances.
- Infants have a harder time compensating for acidosis because of their decreased ability to acidify urine.

Infants and Young Children
- Infants and young children have a higher metabolic turnover of water relative to adults because of a higher metabolic rate. (If losses are not replaced rapidly, imbalance occurs.)
- Infants and young children are unable to verbalize or communicate thirst.

Infants and Children
- In comparison with adults, infants and children have a proportionately greater body surface area in relation to body mass, resulting in a greater potential for fluid loss via the skin and gastrointestinal tract.
- Infants and children have a higher proportionate water content (premature infants have 90%; full-term infants 75% to 80%; preschool children 60% to 65%; and adolescents and adults approximately 55% to 60%), with a larger proportion of fluid in the extracellular space.
- The immune system of infants and children is not as robust as an adult's immune system, rendering young children more susceptible to infectious diseases, fever, gastroenteritis, and respiratory infections, all of which can result in fluid and electrolyte disturbances and fluid-volume deficit.
- Infants and children are at higher risk because of increased exposure to infections in a daycare or nursery setting.

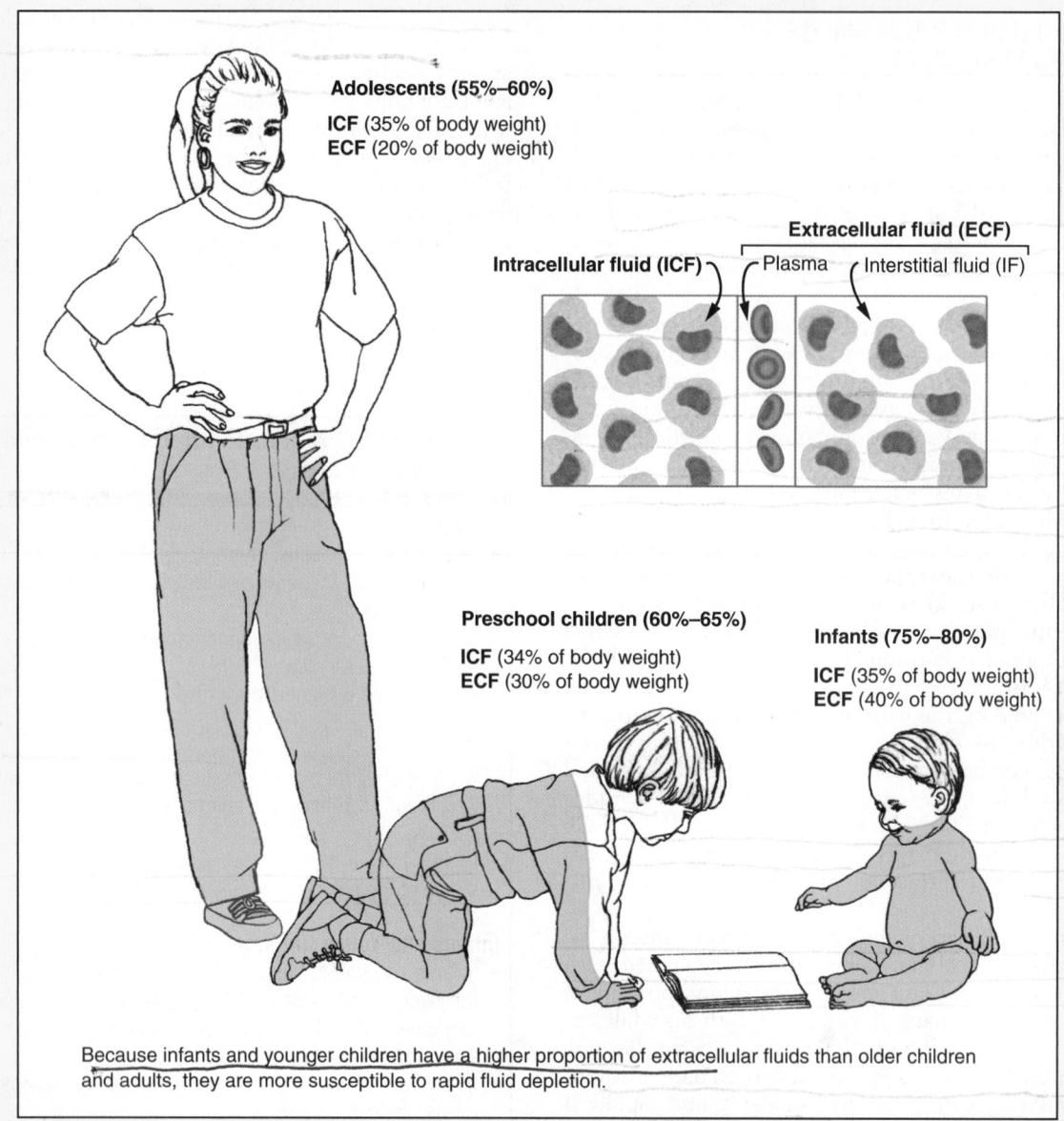

Adolescents (55%–60%)
ICF (35% of body weight)
ECF (20% of body weight)

Extracellular fluid (ECF)
Intracellular fluid (ICF)   Plasma   Interstitial fluid (IF)

Preschool children (60%–65%)
ICF (34% of body weight)
ECF (30% of body weight)

Infants (75%–80%)
ICF (35% of body weight)
ECF (40% of body weight)

Because infants and younger children have a higher proportion of extracellular fluids than older children and adults, they are more susceptible to rapid fluid depletion.

ALTERATIONS IN ACID-BASE BALANCE IN CHILDREN

Alterations in acid-base balance can affect cellular metabolism as well as enzymatic processes. The body's ability to regulate this status is crucial. Children can experience acid-base imbalance as a result of many pathologic conditions. The pH, or measure of acidity or alkalinity of body fluids, is regulated within a narrow range (normal blood pH is 7.35 to 7.45). Maintenance of serum pH within normal limits is crucial to maintaining cellular function, enzyme activity, and neuromuscular membrane potentials. Chemical buffers, the respiratory system, and the kidneys work together to keep the blood pH within normal range. Acid is constantly produced as a by-product of metabolism. The body attempts to maintain blood pH within normal limits by reducing the buildup of acid. Chemical and cellular buffer systems minimize the effect of alterations in blood pH by neutralizing excess acids and bases that accumulate in body fluids. Two of the most significant buffers are bicarbonate and proteins. Bicarbonate, the most important buffer for plasma and interstitial fluids, is

responsible for most ECF buffering and can exert its effects relatively quickly (within minutes).

When alterations in pH become too much for the buffer systems to handle, compensatory mechanisms in the respiratory and renal systems are activated. The lungs remove carbon dioxide from the blood, reducing the amount of carbonic acid and raising the blood pH. The respiratory system works rapidly to compensate for acid-base disturbances. If the blood pH drops below normal (causing *acidosis*), the respiratory rate and depth will increase, removing carbon dioxide and raising

> ### ! CRITICAL TO REMEMBER
> **Treatment Goals in Acid-Base Imbalance**
>
> The treatment of metabolic acid-base disturbance is oriented toward correcting the underlying problem. The treatment of respiratory imbalance is directed toward reestablishing alveolar ventilation.

Overview of Fluid and Electrolyte Disorders

Disorder	Precipitating Events	Clinical Manifestations
Hyponatremia (sodium <130 mEq/L)	Fever Increased water intake without electrolytes Decreased sodium intake Diabetic ketoacidosis Burns and wounds SIADH Malnutrition Cystic fibrosis Renal disease Vomiting, diarrhea, nasogastric suction	Neurologic: • Usually do not show signs until sodium reaches 125 mEq/L • Behavioral changes: irritability, lethargy, headache, dizziness, apprehension Cardiovascular: • Increased heart rate • Decreased blood pressure • Cold, clammy skin Muscle cramps (especially abdominal) Nausea
Hypernatremia (sodium >150 mEq/L)	Water loss or deprivation High sodium intake Diabetes insipidus Diarrhea Fever Hyperglycemia Renal disease	Intense thirst Oliguria Agitation, restlessness Flushed skin Peripheral and pulmonary edema Dry, sticky mucous membranes Nausea and vomiting Serum sodium 150 mEq/L: disorientation, seizures, hyperirritability when at rest
Hypokalemia (potassium <3.5 mEq/L)	Stress Starvation Malabsorption Excessive loss of GI fluids through vomiting, diarrhea, sweat, nasogastric tube Administration of diuretics (especially furosemide, ethacrynic acid, thiazide diuretics) IV fluids without added potassium Administration of corticosteroids Diabetic ketoacidosis	Muscle weakness, paralysis Leg cramps Decreased bowel sounds Weak and irregular pulse, tachycardia or bradycardia, cardiac dysrhythmias Hypotension Ileus Irritability, fatigue
Hyperkalemia (potassium >5 mEq/L)	Increased intake of potassium (e.g., salt substitutes) Decreased urine excretion Kidney failure Metabolic acidosis Hyperglycemia Potassium-sparing diuretics Dehydration (severe) Too rapid IV administration of potassium Burns	Irritability, anxiety Twitching, hyperreflexia Weakness, flaccid paralysis Nausea, diarrhea Bradycardia Cardiac arrest (concern if potassium >8.5 mEq/L) Apnea, respiratory arrest
Hypocalcemia (calcium <8.5 mg/dl, ionized calcium <4.5 mg/dl)	Inadequate intake of calcium Vitamin D deficiency Renal insufficiency Calcium losses (e.g., infection, burns) Alkalosis Administration of diuretics Hypoparathyroidism	Numbness and tingling of fingers, toes, nose, ears, circumoral area Hyperactive reflexes, seizures Muscle cramps, tetany Laryngospasm Lethargy and poor feeding in the newborn Positive Trousseau's and Chvostek's signs Hypotension Cardiac arrest
Hypercalcemia (calcium >11.0 mg/dl, ionized calcium >5.5 mg/dl)	Milk-alkali syndrome (chronic ingestion of calcium carbonate antacids or milk) Excessive IV or oral calcium administration Acidosis Prolonged immobilization Hypoproteinemia Renal disease Hyperparathyroidism Hyperthyroidism	Lethargy, weakness, anorexia Thirst Itching Behavioral changes: confusion, personality change, stupor Nausea, vomiting, constipation Bradycardia, cardiac arrest

SIADH, Syndrome of inappropriate secretion of antidiuretic hormone; *GI,* gastrointestinal; *IV,* intravenous.

CLINICAL REFERENCE

Assessment of Fluid and Electrolyte Disturbances

Parameter Evaluated	Clinical Manifestations	Possible Fluid or Electrolyte Disturbance
Heart rate	Rapid, weak, thready	Fluid volume deficit
	Rapid, bounding	Fluid volume excess
	Weak, irregular, slowing	Severe hyperkalemia
	Weak, irregular, rapid	Severe hypokalemia
Respirations	Rapid, deep	Metabolic acidosis
	Slow, shallow	Metabolic alkalosis
Blood pressure	Increased	Fluid volume excess
	Decreased	Late stages of shock, fluid volume deficit, hypokalemia or hyperkalemia, hyponatremia
Skin	Poor elasticity	Fluid volume deficit
	Pallor	Fluid volume deficit
	Cool to touch	Fluid volume deficit, increased or decreased sodium
	Poor capillary refill	Fluid volume deficit
	Edema	Fluid volume excess (usually)
Mucous membranes	Dry	Fluid volume deficit
Salivation and/or tearing	Decreased	Fluid volume deficit
Behavioral changes	Lethargy	Fluid volume deficit
	Irritability	Fluid volume deficit
	Increased restlessness	Hyperkalemia
	Coma	Markedly increased acidosis or alkalosis
Sensorium changes	Thirst	Fluid volume deficit, increased sodium and/or calcium
	Tingling in extremities	Hypocalcemia, alkalosis
	Abdominal cramps	Hyponatremia, hyperkalemia
	Muscular cramps	Hypocalcemia, hypokalemia
	Lightheadedness or dizziness	Respiratory alkalosis
	Nausea	Hypercalcemia, hypokalemia, or hyperkalemia
Neurologic changes	Hypotonia	Hypokalemia, hypercalcemia
	Weakness	Metabolic acidosis
	Hypertonia:	
	• Positive Chvostek's sign	Hypocalcemia
	• Tremors, cramps, tetany	Hypocalcemia, alkalosis

Data from Kee, J.L., & Paulanka, B.J. (2000). *Fluid and electrolytes: Clinical applications* (Chapters 2, 3, 6-8, 13, 14). Albany, NY: Delmar; Behrman, R., Kliegman, R., & Jenson, H.B. (2000). *Nelson textbook of pediatrics* (Chapters 45-49). Philadelphia: Saunders.

Common Laboratory and Diagnostic Tests for Fluid and Electrolyte Imbalance

Test	Description	Indications	Normal Findings	Nursing Considerations
Urine osmolality	24-hour urine collection or random test	Altered fluid status	300-900 mOsm/kg	No preparation Done by nurse
Urine sodium	24-hour urine collection or random urine specimen	Altered fluid status, hyponatremia	50-130 mEq/L	No preparation Done by nurse
Urine specific gravity	Random urine specimen	Altered fluid status	1.002-1.030	No preparation Done by nurse
Urea nitrogen	Random blood specimen	Altered fluid status Renal function	5-18 mg/dl	No preparation Draw blood needed for sample
Serum osmolality	Random blood specimen	Altered fluid status Measures solute concentration of blood	275-295 mOsm/kg	No preparation Draw blood needed for sample

Acid-Base Disturbances: Principal Causes, Clinical Manifestations, and Treatment

Condition	Principal Causes	Clinical Manifestations	Principal Treatment Methods
Metabolic acidosis	Ketoacidosis (DKA, alcohol-induced ketoacidosis) Increasing metabolic rates from fever, RDS, seizures Interference with normal metabolism: ketosis, tissue hypoxia Loss of bicarbonate from diarrhea, ileostomy, or fistula drainage Acute and chronic renal failure ECF expansion and decreasing HCO_3^- concentration	Increasing heart rate, dysrhythmias (fibrillation) Hyperventilation Kussmaul respirations Cold, clammy skin (mild to moderate acidosis) Warm, dry skin (severe acidosis) Level of consciousness changes from fatigue and confusion to stupor and coma	Identify and treat the underlying disorder Provide $NaHCO_3$, K^+ replacement, and mechanical ventilation as indicated
Metabolic alkalosis	Volume depletion related to various conditions, such as vomiting, pyloric stenosis, gastric drainage, and diuretics Increased alkali intake Medical conditions, such as cystic fibrosis	Dysrhythmias (atrioventricular with prolonged QT interval) Increasing heart rate Decreased respiratory rate and depth Change in level of consciousness from apathy and confusion to stupor Muscular weakness	Treatment depends on underlying cause; mild to moderate alkalosis usually does not require treatment Use of fluids with NaCl and KCl, along with isotonic saline, an H_2-receptor antagonist (e.g., cimetidine) to decrease gastric hydrochloric acid, acidifying agents, and potassium-sparing diuretics (e.g., spironolactone [Aldactone], mannitol)
Respiratory acidosis	Pulmonary disease (BPD, RDS, asthma, cystic fibrosis, croup) Airway obstruction Chest conditions, such as flail chest, pneumothorax Acute and chronic respiratory failure Neuromuscular abnormalities such as Guillain-Barré syndrome, toxins, drugs, paralysis CNS depression from sedative overdose, trauma, anesthesia	Increasing heart rate Dysrhythmias with hypotension Increasing rate and depth of respirations, forceful use of accessory muscles with retraction and cyanosis Increasing intracranial pressure	Correction of ventilation problem: use of oxygen, intubation, mechanical ventilation, $NaHCO_3$
Respiratory alkalosis	Hyperventilation from CNS stimulation, such as emotions, fear, hysteria, pain, salicylate poisoning Decreased lung compliance and hypoxemia from conditions such as pulmonary edema, CHF, pneumonia, asthma, pulmonary emboli Pregnancy Compensation from metabolic acidosis Sepsis	Dizziness, paresthesias, lightheadedness, diaphoresis Dysrhythmias (changes in ST-T wave)	Mild to moderate respiratory alkalosis usually does not require specific treatment For hyperventilation-induced conditions, provide oxygen, rebreathing oxygen masks, breathing into a paper bag, psychological reassurance Institute mechanical ventilation if condition is severe Give sedatives or tranquilizers for anxiety-induced condition, acetazolamide to prevent motion sickness

DKA, Diabetic ketoacidosis; *RDS,* respiratory distress syndrome; *ECF,* extracellular fluid; *HCO_3^-,* bicarbonate; *$NaHCO_3^-$,* sodium bicarbonate; *K^+,* potassium; *NaCl,* sodium chloride; *KCl,* potassium chloride; *BPD,* bronchopulmonary dysplasia; *CNS,* central nervous system; *CHF,* congestive heart failure.

Mechanisms of Acid-Base Disturbances*

Principal	Primary Disturbance	Principal Compensatory Response
Metabolic acidosis	Decreasing HCO_3^-	Hyperventilation causes decreased $PaCO_2$
Metabolic alkalosis	Increasing HCO_3^-	Hypoventilation causes increased $PaCO_2$
Respiratory acidosis	Increasing $PaCO_2$	Release of HCO_3^- and increased renal reabsorption of HCO_3^-
Respiratory alkalosis	Decreasing $PaCO_2$	Decreased renal reabsorption of HCO_3^-

*Important items to remember when acid-base compensation occurs:
- Normal values from which to interpret blood gases: $PaCO_2$ = 35-45 mm Hg; pH = 7.35-7.45; Bicarbonate = 22-26 mEq/L.
- When metabolic compensation occurs, assume origin in respiratory alteration.
- When respiratory compensation and release of tissue buffers occur, assume metabolic origin.

Modified from Kee, J.L., & Paulanka, B.J. (2000). *Fluid and electrolytes: Clinical applications* (Chapters 2, 3, 6-8, 13, & 14). Albany, NY: Delmar.
HCO_3^-, Bicarbonate; $Paco_2$, partial pressure of carbon dioxide in arterial blood.

Selected Laboratory Values for Acid-Base Disturbances

Test	Metabolic Acidosis	Metabolic Alkalosis	Respiratory Acidosis	Respiratory Alkalosis
ABG: pH	<7.35	>7.45	<7.35	>7.45
$PaCO_2$ (mm Hg)	<40	>45	>45	<35
PaO_2 (mm Hg)	WNL or slightly decreased	Decreased	Decreased	Decreased
HCO_3^-, (mEq/L)	<22	>26	WNL or slightly increased	Decreased
K^+(mEq/L)	>4.0	Decreased	WNL	Slightly decreased
Na^+(mEq/L)	Varies according to condition	Decreased	WNL	Slightly decreased
Cl^- (mEq/L)	Usually increased	Decreased	WNL	Slightly decreased

ABG, Arterial blood gas; *WNL*, within normal limits; *Paco₂*, partial pressure of carbon dioxide in arterial blood; *Pao₂*, partial pressure of oxygen in arterial blood; HCO_3^-, bicarbonate; *K⁺*, potassium; *Na⁺*, sodium; *Cl⁻*, chloride.

blood pH. Conversely, in the presence of alkalosis, the respiratory rate and depth decrease, thus lowering blood pH.

Kidneys regulate bicarbonate and remove hydrogen ions from the blood. If the blood is too alkaline, the kidneys conserve hydrogen ions, thus lowering blood pH. In the presence of acidosis, the kidneys excrete hydrogen ions and conserve bicarbonate, raising blood pH. Renal compensatory processes work more slowly than respiratory mechanisms—usually within 1 to 2 days. If compensatory mechanisms are ineffective, acid-base imbalances occur. When a dysfunction results in decreased hydrogen ion concentration in the blood, the arterial pH increases (causing *alkalosis*). When a dysfunction results in an increase in hydrogen ions, the arterial pH decreases (causing *acidosis*).

DEHYDRATION

Dehydration, or fluid loss in excess of fluid intake, is common in infants and children. Decreased fluid intake or increased fluid loss may cause it. Dehydration produces both fluid and electrolyte deficiencies. Dehydration is classified as isonatremic, hyponatremic, or hypernatremic (Table 42-1), according to the status of the serum sodium concentration. In *isonatremic dehydration*, the most common type of dehydration in children, water and electrolytes are lost in approximately the same proportion as they exist in the body, and serum sodium levels remain within the normal range of 135 to 145 mEq/L. In *hyponatremic dehydration*, the electrolyte loss is greater than the water loss, resulting in a serum sodium concentration of less than 130 mEq/L. In *hypernatremic dehydration*, the water loss is greater than the electrolyte loss and the serum sodium concentration is above 150 mEq/L.

[handwritten annotations: nephritis, adrenal insufficiency, diuretics, suctioning (gastric), burns]

TABLE **42-1** Types of Dehydration: Etiology, Clinical Manifestations, and Laboratory Values *[handwritten: burns]*

Isonatremic Dehydration	Hyponatremic Dehydration	Hypernatremic Dehydration
ETIOLOGY *[handwritten: best of the bad]*	*[handwritten: should recover from]*	*[handwritten: crabby]*
Vomiting, diarrhea	**Renal Losses**	**Renal Losses**
Insensible fluid loss via respiratory and integumentary systems	Diuretics, hyperglycemia, nephritis, adrenal insufficiency	Diuretics, diabetes insipidus, adrenal insufficiency
Decreased oral intake with increased activity	**Extrarenal Losses**	**Extrarenal Losses**
	Vomiting, diarrhea, third spacing, burns, tube drainage	Vomiting, diarrhea
	Other	**Other**
	CHF, SIADH, nephrosis; administration of large amounts of electrolyte-free solutions (plain water) during illness or postoperatively	Fever, increased sodium in formula, diet, or tube feeding; administration of hypertonic sodium IV fluids
CLINICAL MANIFESTATIONS		
Mild thirst	Increased thirst	Thirst very increased
Skin turgor poor	Skin turgor very poor	Skin turgor fair
Dry skin	Skin usually clammy	Skin texture thickened or "doughy"
Decreased urine output	Decreased urine output	Decreased urine output
Dry mucous membranes	Mucous membranes dry to slightly moist	Mucous membranes parched
Skin temperature cold	Skin temperature cold	Skin temperature cold ↔ hot
Body temperature afebrile ↔ febrile	Body temperature afebrile ↔ febrile	Body temperature afebrile ↔ febrile
Lethargy	Very lethargic, possible seizures	Lethargic, hyperirritable with stimulation
LABORATORY VALUES		
Serum sodium: 130-150 mEq/L	**Renal Losses**	**Renal Losses**
	Serum sodium <130 mEq/L	Serum sodium >150 mEq/L
Urine		
Sodium usually within normal limits	Urine sodium increased	Urine sodium increased
Specific gravity slightly elevated	Urine specific gravity decreased	Urine specific gravity decreased
Osmolality usually within normal limits	Urine osmolality decreased	Urine osmolality decreased
Volume usually within normal limits or slightly decreased	Urine volume increased	Urine volume increased
	Extrarenal Losses	**Extrarenal Losses**
	Serum sodium <130 mEq/L	Serum sodium >150 mEq/L
	Urine sodium decreased	Urine sodium decreased
	Urine specific gravity increased	Urine specific gravity increased
	Urine osmolality increased	Urine osmolality increased
	Urine volume decreased	Urine volume decreased
	Other	**Other**
	Serum sodium <130 mEq/L	Serum sodium >150 mEq/L
	Urine sodium decreased	Urine sodium decreased
	Urine specific gravity increased	Urine specific gravity increased
	Urine osmolality increased	Urine osmolality increased
	Urine volume decreased	Urine volume decreased

Data from Behrman, R.E., Kliegman, R.M., & Jenson, H.B. (Eds.). (2000). *Nelson textbook of pediatrics* (16th ed.). Philadelphia: Saunders.
CHF, Congestive heart failure; *SIADH,* syndrome of inappropriate secretion of antidiuretic hormone; *IV,* intravenous.

[handwritten: can seize]

Pathophysiology

Of Dehydration

In the early phases of dehydration, fluids, with some electrolytes, are lost from the extracellular fluid (ECF). If the fluid loss continues, loss of intracellular fluid (ICF) can occur. Dehydration can lead to shock (see Chapter 34).

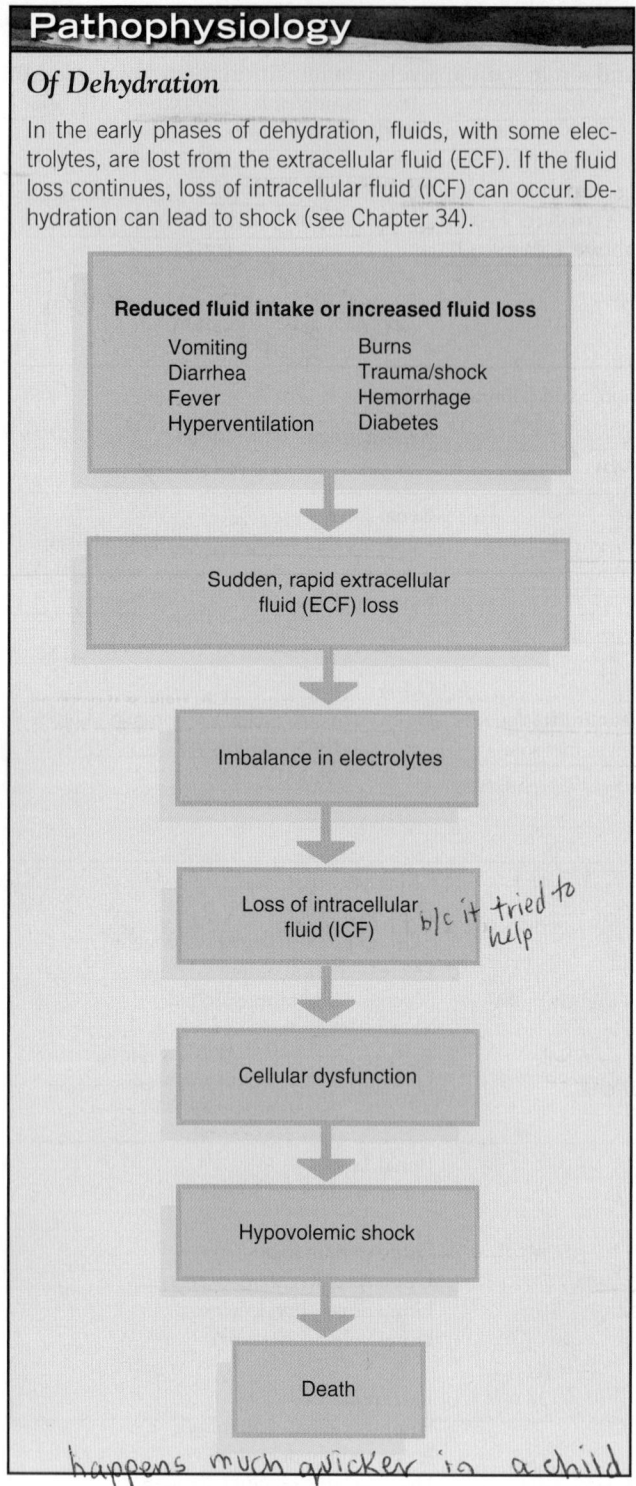

Reduced fluid intake or increased fluid loss

Vomiting	Burns
Diarrhea	Trauma/shock
Fever	Hemorrhage
Hyperventilation	Diabetes

Sudden, rapid extracellular fluid (ECF) loss

Imbalance in electrolytes

Loss of intracellular fluid (ICF) *b/c it tried to help*

Cellular dysfunction

Hypovolemic shock

Death

happens much quicker in a child

Etiology and Incidence

Dehydration has many varied causes. Common alterations that may lead to dehydration reflect disturbances in the following systems:

- Gastrointestinal tract: vomiting, diarrhea, pyloric stenosis, malabsorption
- Endocrine system: fever, diabetes mellitus, cystic fibrosis
- Skin: burns

! CRITICAL TO REMEMBER

Signs of Impending Shock in the Dehydrated Child

Because of the child's ability to compensate and maintain an adequate cardiac output, changes in heart rate, sensorium, and skin color are earlier indicators of impending shock than is blood pressure.

- Lungs: tachypnea
- Kidneys: renal failure
- Heart: congestive heart failure

Any age-group can be affected, but neonates and infants, as discussed previously, are especially vulnerable to the effects of dehydration.

Manifestations

For infants and young children with isonatremic dehydration, the fluid deficit is described as mild, moderate, or severe dehydration, depending on the percentage of body weight lost:

- *Mild dehydration:* 4% to 5% loss of body weight; fluid volume loss of less than 50 ml/kg
- *Moderate dehydration:* 6% to 10% loss of body weight; fluid volume loss of 50 to 100 ml/kg
- *Severe dehydration:* 10% or more loss of body weight; fluid volume loss of 100 ml/kg or more

One milliliter of body fluid is approximately equal to 1 g of body weight, so a weight loss or gain of 1 kg (2.2 lb) in 24 hours represents a 1-liter fluid loss or gain.

Older children have a lower total body water content and extracellular fluid volume than do infants and younger children. Therefore an equivalent percentage of body weight lost from dehydration represents a more severe fluid depletion in the older child. Isonatremic dehydration in the older child is classified as *mild* if 3% of body weight is lost, *moderate* if 6% of body weight is lost, and *severe* if 9% of body weight is lost.

The signs and symptoms associated with degree of isonatremic dehydration are listed in Table 42-2. As with impending shock, the most essential manifestations are changes in heart rate, behavior or sensorium, urine output, skin qualities, and, in infants, fontanels.

Diagnostic Evaluation

Key factors to consider in determining the type and severity of dehydration include:

- A history of acute or chronic fluid loss
- Clinical manifestations
- Weight of the child
- Serum electrolyte values

Therapeutic Management

Management is directed toward correcting the fluid and electrolyte imbalance and then treating the causative factors. Oral rehydration therapy (ORT) is the preferred treatment of fluid

TABLE **42-2** Assessment of the Severity of Dehydration

Clinical Signs	Mild	Moderate	Severe
Weight loss	4%-5%	6%-10%	>10%
Vital Signs:			
Pulse	Normal	Increased	Increased and weak
Blood pressure	Normal	Normal to low	Very low, orthostatic, shock
Respiratory rate	Normal	Normal to deep	Rapid and deep
General Appearance:			
Infants	Fussy, thirsty, alert	Fussy, restless, thirsty, lethargic but arousable	Drowsy to comatose, not arousable, gray color, limp, cold, and sweaty
Older children	Thirsty, restless, alert	Thirsty, restless, postural hypotension	Apprehensive, comatose, cold, mottled skin, cyanotic
Mucous membranes	Normal to slightly dry	Dry	Parched
Anterior fontanel	Normal	Sunken	Markedly depressed
Eyes	Normal	Sunken	Markedly sunken
Capillary refill	<3 sec	3-5 sec	>5 sec
Skin turgor (see Fig. 42-1)	Normal	Decreased (may have a doughy feel in hypernatremic dehydration)	Tenting (may have a doughy feel in hypernatremic dehydration)
Urine output	Mildly decreased, diaper may be dry	Decreased, diaper is dry, concentrated urine with specific gravity of 1.020-1.030	Decreased, diaper is dry, decrease in the number of diapers changed during the day, concentrated urine with specific gravity >1.030

Modified from Dabbagh, S., Atiyeh, B., Fleischmann, L.E., & Gruskin, A.B. (1999). Fluid and electrolyte therapy. In F.D. Burg, J.R. Ingelfinger, E.R. Wald, & R.A. Polin (Eds.), *Gellis & Kagan's current pediatric therapy* (16th ed.). Philadelphia: Saunders.

and electrolyte imbalances in children with mild to moderate dehydration if the child is awake, alert, and able to take fluids by mouth. Examples of oral rehydration formulas are the World Health Organization's (WHO's) solution (Rehydralyte), Pedialyte, and Infalyte. Rehydralyte, or the WHO's solution, is the best source of oral rehydration, but Pedialyte and Infalyte are also excellent choices (Straughn & English, 1996). Electrolyte or sports drinks (e.g., Gatorade) have long been accepted oral rehydration formulations for older children. Recent studies suggest that sports drinks are not the best solutions for rehydration and may in fact worsen diarrhea because of their high percentage of sugar and carbohydrates. These supplements greatly increase the osmotic load in the intestines and further aggravate diarrhea (Santosham, 2002). Suggested rehydration for children with mild to moderate dehydration is 50 to 100 ml/kg of ORT over 4 hours and the hydration status should be reevaluated frequently (Berman, 2003). Most regimens encourage maintenance for 4 to 6 hours.

If the child is severely dehydrated or unable to take fluids by mouth and ongoing fluid replacement is needed, parenteral fluid and electrolyte therapy is initiated. Initial therapy is aimed at treating or preventing shock. Lactated Ringer's solution or 0.9% sodium chloride solution is the fluid of choice for rehydration and restoration of circulation. Sodium chloride (0.9%) solution may be ordered initially in boluses, depending on the calculated fluid losses. The remainder of the fluid losses is provided by 5% dextrose in 0.45 normal saline and maintenance therapy is provided by 5% dextrose in 0.2 normal saline at 1.5 times the hourly maintenance rate (Roberts, 2001). If necessary, potassium is added to the IV solution once urine output is adequate. See Box 42-1 for daily fluid requirements by body weight and age-appropriate urine output.

BOX 42-1
Maintenance Fluid Requirements and Minimum Urine Output

Daily Fluid Requirements by Body Weight

≤10 kg:	100 ml/kg
10-20 kg:	1000 ml + 50 ml/kg for each additional kilogram between 10 and 20 kg
>20 kg:	1500 ml + 20 ml/kg for each additional kilogram over 20 kg

Minimum Urine Output by Age-Group

Infants and toddlers:	>2-3 ml/kg/hr
Preschoolers and young school-age children:	>1-2 ml/kg/hr
School-age children and adolescents:	0.5-1 ml/kg/hr

The type of dehydration determines the rate of administration of replacement fluids. For the child with isonatremic or hyponatremic dehydration, lost fluids are replaced over 24 hours (in addition to the child's maintenance fluid requirements). Half the amount of estimated fluid loss is replaced over the first 8 hours and the remaining half over the next 16 hours (Roberts, 2001). With hypernatremic dehydration, lost fluids are replaced more slowly, over 48 hours, to prevent a sudden decrease in serum sodium level. Potassium losses must also be replaced; this process should proceed slowly to avoid hyperkalemia. Potassium replacement should begin only after urine

! CRITICAL TO REMEMBER

Guidelines When Administering Potassium

- Do not administer potassium chloride if urine output is not age-appropriate. See Box 42-1 for adequate urine output.
- *Never* give potassium by intravenous (IV) push.
- Give no more than 40 mEq/L, at a rate no faster than 1 mEq/kg/hr.
- Always check the dose and dosage calculations of potassium chloride. (Incorrect placement of a decimal point can result in a dose lethal to a child.)
- To avoid the risk of inadequate mixing, add potassium chloride to IV fluids with the plastic IV bag in the upright (non-infusion) position rather than in the down (infusion) position. (Inadequate mixing could result in the child's receiving an excessive amount of potassium chloride in the first few minutes.)
- Because of irritation of the vessel walls and potential phlebitis, IV solutions containing more than 30 mEq/L of potassium chloride should not be given via a peripheral IV line.

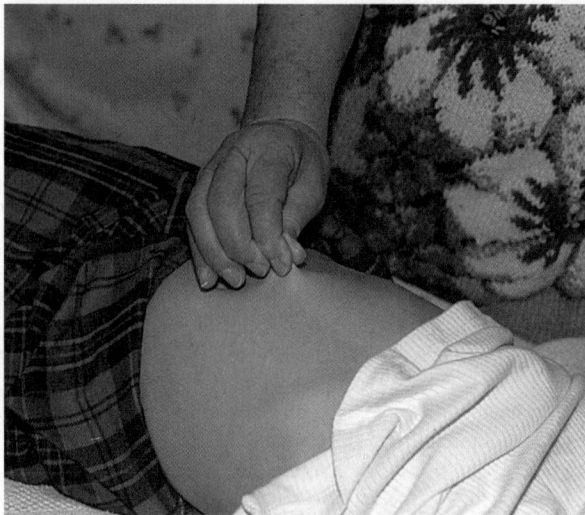

Figure 42-1 Testing skin turgor. Turgor refers to the elasticity of the skin, which is affected by the extent of hydration. The nurse tests turgor by gently grasping the skin. When the skin is released, it should instantly spring back into place; if it does not, tissue turgor is considered poor. (Courtesy The University of Texas at Arlington School of Nursing.)

output is adequate (see Box 42-1) and should be administered with extreme caution. If the child is anuric, potassium is retained, causing elevated potassium levels.

■ NURSING CARE

The Child Experiencing Dehydration

Assessment

Because dehydration can develop very quickly in infants and young children, the nurse must be alert for early signs of dehydration in children with conditions in which fluid losses are likely to occur, such as diarrhea, vomiting, burns, diabetes, trauma, and fever. The condition of infants and young children can change rapidly when fluid and electrolyte imbalances occur.

The general appearance of the child should be assessed, as well as specific parameters:

- *Intake and output:* Measure all fluid intake and losses accurately (including vomitus, urine, stools, nasogastric drainage, wound drainage). The practitioner must also consider insensible water loss.
- *Urine output and specific gravity:* Output of less than 2 to 3 ml/kg/hr in infants and toddlers, 1 to 2 ml/kg/hr in preschoolers and young school-age children, and 0.5 to 1 ml/kg/hr in school-age children or adolescents, or a specific gravity above 1.020 may indicate dehydration. Glucose, large amounts of protein, and radiographic dyes, however, elevate the specific gravity and may interfere with its accuracy.
- *Weight:* Weight is a crucial indicator of fluid status. Accurate measurements of the weight of the unclothed child, using the same scale at the same time of day, are essential. Changes in weight related to changes in intravenous (IV) lines or dressings should be identified by recording "with IV." Weight gain during illness may indicate fluid reten-

tion or pulmonary or generalized edema. The weight should be rechecked, and the child should be assessed for pulmonary crackles and periorbital edema.

- *Stools, vomitus:* Frequency, type, amounts, and consistency should be assessed and recorded.
- *Sweating:* Estimate from dampness of clothing and linen.
- *Serum electrolytes:* See p. 1081.
- *Skin:* Assess color, temperature, turgor (Fig. 42-1), moisture, and capillary refill.
- *Mucous membranes and presence of tears:* Dry or sticky mucous membranes and the absence of tears indicate dehydration. Absence of tears is not significant in an infant younger than 2 to 4 months because infants of this age often do not manufacture tears.
- *Anterior fontanel:* A sunken or depressed fontanel in infants indicates dehydration. Cranial suture lines may also become prominent with dehydration.
- *Vital signs:* Fever increases the metabolic rate and fluid requirements. With dehydration, the pulse is rapid, weak, and thready. An increase in the respiratory rate compensates for metabolic acidosis, which often accompanies dehydration. Blood pressure may be decreased in moderate and severe dehydration, but it is a late sign of hypovolemia.
- *Behavior:* Irritability, lethargy, confusion, or seizures may be present. The child's cry may be high-pitched and weak.

Nursing Diagnosis and Planning

- Deficient Fluid Volume related to gastric or intestinal infection or inflammation, hemorrhage, burns, or failure of fluid regulatory mechanisms.

  Expected Outcome: The infant or child will display adequate fluid volume, as evidenced by age-appropriate urine output, age-appropriate urine specific gravity, elastic skin turgor and moist mucous membranes, serum pH and electrolyte levels within normal limits, and weight gain.

fontanels
absence of tears

PARENTS
Want to Know

About Dehydration

Signs and Symptoms of Dehydration

Parents should be taught to watch for the following signs and symptoms of dehydration:

- Fewer wet diapers (especially no wet diaper for more than 6 to 8 hours)
- No tears when crying if older than 2 to 4 months
- Inside of mouth dry or sticky
- Irritability; high-pitched cry
- Difficulty in awakening
- Increased respiratory rate or difficulty breathing
- Sunken fontanel, sunken eyes with dark circles
- Abnormal skin color, temperature, or dryness

  Because a young child's condition may worsen faster than an older child's, parents of infants younger than 6 months should seek professional assistance early.

Oral Rehydration Therapy

Parents must understand that giving plain water alone or in large amounts can be extremely dangerous because it does not contain needed electrolytes. Instead, commercially available oral rehydration solutions, such as Rehydralyte, Infalyte, or Pedialyte, should be given.

Pathophysiology

Of Diarrhea

Increased motility and rapid emptying of the intestines result in impaired absorption of nutrients and water, as well as electrolyte imbalance. Water, sodium, potassium, and bicarbonate are drawn from the extracellular space into the stool, resulting in dehydration, electrolyte depletion, and metabolic acidosis.

  Diarrhea occurs when there is excess fluid in the small intestine. This condition can result from a number of processes:

- Bacterial toxins stimulating active transport of electrolytes into the small intestine: cells in the mucosal lining of the intestines are irritated and secrete increased amounts of water and electrolytes.
- Organisms invading and destroying intestinal mucosal cells, decreasing intestinal surface area, and impairing the intestine's capacity to absorb fluids and electrolytes.
- Inflammation, which decreases the intestine's ability to absorb fluid, electrolytes, and nutrients. This condition occurs in malabsorption syndromes.
- Increased intestinal motility, resulting in impaired intestinal absorption.

Interventions

Teach parents how to prevent dehydration. Parents should be taught to give infants and young children extra fluids during hot weather, to avoid overdressing, and to encourage frequent rest periods during high-energy playtimes. During minor illness, providing additional fluids to a child with fever may prevent the development of more serious problems. Teach parents how to identify the early signs and symptoms of dehydration, and instruct them to seek professional help if these signs and symptoms should occur.

  Also, teach parents how to replace fluids when the child is mildly dehydrated. Oral rehydration formulations, such as Rehydralyte, Infalyte, or Pedialyte, contain the appropriate concentration of electrolytes and should be used when fluid is the child's only intake for a prolonged period or in times of decreased intake. Parents need to understand that giving plain water alone or in large amounts can be extremely dangerous, and why.

  When caring for the hospitalized child with fluid and electrolyte imbalance, the nurse assumes the responsibility of continuously monitoring the child's condition and administering oral and IV fluids safely (see Chapter 38 for a discussion of IV therapy). When caring for children with conditions such as fever, burns, diarrhea, vomiting, or trauma, the nurse must continuously assess for signs of dehydration.

Evaluation

- Is the child alert?
- Is urine output appropriate for age with a specific gravity of 1.002 to 1.030?
- Is the skin elastic and soft?

- Are the mucous membranes moist?
- Are serum pH and electrolyte levels within normal limits?

DIARRHEA

Diarrhea, one of the most common disorders in childhood, is defined as an increase in the frequency, fluidity, and volume of stools. In the United States, children younger than 5 years experience 2.2 to 3.3 episodes of diarrhea per year, with 49.4 hospitalizations for every 10,000 children annually (Berman, 2003). Diarrhea accompanies many childhood disorders. Diarrhea in children may be acute or chronic, inflammatory or noninflammatory. Diarrhea caused by infection is usually called *gastroenteritis*. Viral gastroenteritis is the cause of approximately 80% of all cases, making it the most common cause of diarrhea in children older than 1 year.

  If not treated, acute diarrhea can lead to dehydration, electrolyte imbalance, and hypovolemic shock. Acute diarrhea can be life-threatening in infants and small children if gastrointestinal fluid losses are not adequately replaced.

Etiology and Incidence

There are many causes of both acute and chronic diarrhea (Table 42-3). Diarrhea with ensuing dehydration is the leading killer of children worldwide and is a major cause of morbidity, as well as a primary sign of many other conditions. In the United States, diarrhea accounts for approximately 3.7 million acute-care visits by children younger than 5 years, with 220,000 hospitalized annually (Atherly-John, Cunningham, & Crain, 2002). It can be either a short-term or a long-term condition. In infants and young children, diarrhea can be life-threatening if the losses are not replaced.

TABLE **42-3** Causes and Manifestations of Diarrhea in Infants and Children

Causes of Diarrhea	Manifestations
Intestinal infection: Bacterial (*Campylobacter jejuni*,* *Salmonella*,* *Shigella*,* *Escherichia coli*) Viral (rotavirus;* cause of more than 50% of cases of acute diarrhea in children; enteric adenovirus) Parasitic (*Giardia lamblia*,* *Cryptosporidium**—high incidence of both in daycare centers) Fungal overgrowth	Watery stools containing mucus and possibly blood Pain, cramps, nausea, vomiting, fever (over 101.6° F [38.7° C] with bacterial infection); risk of dehydration, electrolyte imbalance, and shock
Food intolerance (lactose intolerance, overfeeding, introduction of new foods)	Diarrhea, increased mucus in stools, flatus, pain after ingestion of lactose or offending food
Malabsorption (cystic fibrosis, disaccharide deficiencies, celiac disease)	Diarrhea, cramps, distention, steatorrhea occurring after meals May experience anorexia, weight loss, fatigue
Medications (antibiotics, chemotherapy)	Diarrhea after administration of medications, which usually stops when medications are discontinued
Colon disease (ulcerative colitis, Crohn's disease, enterocolitis)	Inflammation and ulceration of intestinal walls, increased motility May have 10-20 stools per day Abdominal pain, fever, chills, anorexia, weight loss
Irritable bowel syndrome	Diarrhea alternating with constipation or normal bowel function Pain, distention, nausea may be present
Intestinal obstruction (including intussusception)	Partial obstruction may result in diarrhea caused by increased intestinal motility Pain, nausea, and sometimes bloody stool; may note mucus in stools
Emotional stress (anxiety, fatigue)	Increased motility
Infectious disease (otitis media, upper respiratory infection, urinary tract infection)	Diarrhea frequently accompanies other infections

*Most common causative organisms.

Manifestations

Diarrhea may manifest either quickly or insidiously. Its manifestations include:

- *Integumentary:* dry, hot skin; changes in skin texture and turgor; dry mucous membranes
- *Small intestine:* cramps, nausea, vomiting; large-volume stools, light in color, loose to watery in texture; stools that tend to be soupy, greasy, or foul-smelling
- *Large intestine:* the urge to defecate with insignificant stool present; mushy, jellylike, or even bloody fecal matter; stool that is usually dark in color; stool that is rarely foul-smelling
- *Other:* increased heart and respiratory rates, decreased tearing, fever

Diagnostic Evaluation

Most infectious causes of diarrhea are self-limiting, making comprehensive testing of minor cases of diarrhea impractical. Because of the different possible causes, the diagnostic workup is frequently geared toward ruling out infectious agents as well as anatomic and physiologic reasons, such as allergies, food intolerance, and bowel problems. Tests to be performed after an initial history has assessed for food intolerance, stress, or school- or work-related problems include:

- *Stool:* cultures (for bacteria, ova, parasites, rotavirus), pH, red blood cells, leukocytes, glucose (Clinitest), blood (guaiac test or Hemoccult)

- *Blood tests:* especially blood cell counts, electrolytes, blood urea nitrogen, glucose, and blood cultures (if an infectious agent is suspected)
- *X-rays:* check for possible bowel abnormalities

Therapeutic Management

The treatment of diarrhea is aimed at restoring fluid and electrolyte balance and returning the bowel to normal function. Preventing the spread of infection to others is an important component of care, with meticulous handwashing being critical. Parents must be informed of specific fluid intake requirements and signs of dehydration, which would signal a worsening of the child's condition. Treatment of diarrhea and prevention of dehydration include replacing fluids, providing early feedings, and close monitoring and observation. Infants should continue to be given breast milk or regular-strength formula. Infants with more severe diarrhea may require a lactose-free formula until they recover (Berman, 2003). The continued feeding of a normal diet can prevent dehydration, reduce stool frequency and volume, and hasten recovery. It does not prolong diarrhea, and there is evidence that it may reduce the duration of diarrhea. Normal diets replace much-needed nutrients lost during diarrheal events; not continuing a normal diet could lead to altered growth or malnutrition, particularly in children from some underdeveloped countries (Santosham, 2002).

ORT is the preferred treatment of fluid and electrolyte losses caused by diarrhea in children with mild to moderate dehydration. Oral rehydration solutions, such as Rehydralyte, Infalyte, or Pedialyte, may be given. Rice-based oral rehydra-

TABLE **42-4** Oral Replacement Therapy in Children With Vomiting or Diarrhea

	Not Dehydrated	Mild Dehydration	Moderate Dehydration	Severe Dehydration
Oral replacement therapy (ORT)	Not necessary unless not taking other fluids well	50 ml/kg of ORT plus replace ongoing losses over a 4-hr period	100 ml/kg of ORT plus replace ongoing losses over a 4-hr period	Intravenous (IV) therapy: bolus of 20 ml/kg of normal saline or lactated Ringer's
Ongoing losses	10 ml/kg of ORT for each stool or emesis Volume is estimated and replaced	10 ml/kg of ORT for each stool or emesis Volume is estimated and replaced	10 ml/kg of ORT for each stool or emesis Volume is estimated and replaced	
Feeding	Continue age-appropriate diet	Resume age-appropriate diet as soon as dehydration is corrected	Resume age-appropriate diet as soon as dehydration is corrected	Begin ORT when child is stable and alert; keep IV line in place until child is drinking well; resume age-appropriate diet as soon as dehydration is corrected
Reevaluate hydration, and estimate ongoing fluid losses	As necessary	Every 2 hours	Every hour	Continuous evaluation; must evaluate after each bolus of IV solution

Modified from American Academy of Pediatrics, Provisional Committee on Quality Improvement, Subcommittee on Acute Gastroenteritis. (1996). The management of acute gastroenteritis in young children. *Pediatrics, 97*(3), 424-435; Burkhart, D.M. (1999). Management of acute gastroenteritis in children. *American Family Physician, 60*(9), 2555-2563.

tion solutions increase the absorption of salt, water, and glucose from the intestine and may be more beneficial than glucose-based oral rehydration solutions (Misra & Ament, 1998). These solutions are not the same as rice water or commercial products that derive their carbohydrates from glucose polymers purified from rice.

The oral rehydration solutions have changed from the days of homemade recipes (mixtures of water, salt, sugar, and cereals) to today's commercially available, lower-osmolality fluids. Because of their osmotic effect, the high carbohydrate content in fluids such as apple juice, sports drinks, or colas may further aggravate diarrhea and cause additional fluid loss. In addition, Gatorade and other sports drinks do not provide the electrolytes needed to replace the losses in stool during severe diarrhea.

Children and infants who have diarrhea and are not dehydrated should continue to be fed age-appropriate diets. Those needing rehydration should be fed age-appropriate diets as soon as they have been rehydrated (American Academy of Pediatrics Provisional Committee on Quality Improvement, 1996). If adding milk to the diet increases diarrhea, transient lactose intolerance may be considered, although it is not as common as was once thought. If lactose intolerance is present, it may be necessary to give the infant a soy formula until the deficiency resolves, usually within several weeks (Berman, 2003). Common foods that are especially well tolerated during diarrhea are bland but nutritional foods, including complex carbohydrates (e.g., rice, wheat, potatoes, cereals), yogurt, cooked vegetables, and lean meats. Fatty foods and foods high in simple sugars (e.g., tea, juices, soft drinks) should be avoided. This recommendation is a change from the formerly recommended BRAT diet, which consisted of bananas, rice, applesauce, and toast. The BRAT diet can be tolerated but is low in energy, density, fat, and protein.

For infants with mild to moderate diarrhea who have not become dehydrated, ORT is started at home (Table 42-4). Breastfeeding should be continued. If an infant or child has become mildly to moderately dehydrated and requires a visit to a clinic or emergency department, oral rehydration solution is recommended. Children with mild dehydration should be given ORT, 50 ml/kg, plus replacement of continuing losses during a 4-hour period. Replacement of continuing losses is accomplished by giving 10 ml/kg for each stool. Hydration and replacement losses should be reevaluated at least every 2 hours. Children with moderate dehydration should be given ORT, 100 ml/kg, plus replacement of continuing losses during a 4-hour period. At the end of each hour of rehydration, hydration and replacement losses should be assessed.

Feeding of solids or formula is started as soon as the child is rehydrated. Children should be encouraged to eat frequently—every 3 to 4 hours. Parents should be instructed that although stool output may increase, feeding will not prolong diarrhea and the child will be absorbing necessary nutrients and calories. For a child with severe dehydration and ongoing losses, ORT is not recommended. Such children are usually admitted to a hospital for observation and IV therapy. See Box 42-1 for IV fluid requirements.

If bacteria, parasites, or fungi cause the diarrhea, other types of medication along with antibiotics may be ordered. The use of antidiarrheal medication is not recommended in children because of the binding nature of these products and the potential for toxicity. Antidiarrheal medications have not been found to shorten the course of the diarrhea, and in

CRITICAL THINKING EXERCISE 42-1

Mrs. Peters calls the clinic about 8-month-old David. She states that David has had diarrhea for 2 days and that she does not know what to do. She also states that her neighbor said she should stop breastfeeding and give David clear liquids. Mrs. Peters tells you that she is afraid she may have done something to cause David to get sick.

1. What questions should you ask Mrs. Peters about her infant?
2. What teaching can you do to help Mrs. Peters?

cases where the diarrhea is caused by pathogens, they may increase fluid and electrolyte loss by interfering with the body's attempt to rid itself of the organism and allowing the pathogen to remain in the body longer.

Prognosis

Most children experiencing diarrhea and subsequent dehydration usually have a relatively quick recovery, provided that the cause of the diarrhea is determined and therapy is started as soon as possible.

PARENTS
Want to Know

About Caring for a Child With Diarrhea

Diet
Diet depends on the age of the child and the severity of the diarrhea.

Mild Diarrhea (Mushy Stools) in Children of any Age
Continue with an age-appropriate diet. Continue breastfeeding, formula, or milk. Encourage increased intake of fluids and extra water. Avoid fruit juices, because they may worsen diarrhea. Provide bland but nutritious foods. Avoid raw fruits and vegetables and fatty or spicy foods.

Moderate Diarrhea (Watery or Frequent Stools) in Children Younger than 1 Year
Provide oral rehydration solutions for 6 to 24 hours. Infalyte, Pedialyte, Rehydralyte, or other similar commercially prepared oral rehydration solutions should be given. Juices should be avoided, because they may increase diarrhea.

After the infant has been receiving oral rehydration solutions for 6 to 24 hours, regular formula can be resumed. If the diarrhea was severe or if the diarrhea does not improve after 3 days on regular formula, the infant should be given soy formula (Isomil, ProSobee) instead of cow's milk formula. Soy formula should be continued until the diarrhea is gone for 3 days.

Solids may be given after liquids are fully tolerated. Foods include the ABCs (applesauce, bananas, strained carrots), mashed potatoes, rice cereal, yogurt, and other bland foods.

Breastfeeding should not be discontinued because of diarrhea. Offer more frequent feedings, and if urine decreases, offer oral rehydration solutions in addition to breastfeeding.

Moderate Diarrhea (Watery or Frequent Stools) in Children Older than 1 Year
- Give oral rehydration solutions for 6 to 24 hours.
- After oral rehydration solutions, provide foods that are appropriate for your child's age and that are nutritional, bland, and high in starch. Suggested foods include breads, crackers, rice, mashed potatoes, noodles, yogurt, cooked vegetables, and lean meats.
- Avoid raw fruits and vegetables, beans, spices, and fatty foods.
- Avoid sports drinks, colas, and apple juice.

Preventing the Spread of Infection
Infectious diarrhea is very contagious. Some of the infectious agents can live on toys, water fountains, and other inanimate objects for several days. Thorough handwashing after diaper changing or using the toilet is crucial to prevent others in the household from getting diarrhea. All family members should be taught the importance of thorough and frequent handwashing. Diapers should be changed on a surface designated for that purpose and *not* on the kitchen counter where food is prepared. Changing areas should be cleaned with disinfectant after each diaper change.

Skin Care
To prevent breakdown of the sensitive skin in the diaper area, diarrhea stools should be completely washed off with mild soap and water after each bowel movement. (Washing the child under running water in the bathtub makes the job easier. The tub should be cleaned with disinfectant before anyone else uses it.) The skin should be patted dry and a layer of A & D ointment or other protective or "barrier" ointment applied.

Changing diapers immediately after bowel movements is important to prevent skin breakdown. The use of commercial baby wipes should be avoided, because they may further irritate and cause additional breakdown of the skin. To prevent overflow of diarrhea from the diaper, diapers should be applied snugly.

When to Call the Physician
Call the physician immediately if any of the following occurs:
- The child does not urinate for longer than 6 hours.
- Crying produces no tears, or the mouth becomes dry.
- The infant's fontanel appears sunken.
- Blood appears in the diarrhea, or the diarrhea becomes severe (e.g., a bowel movement every hour for more than 8 hours, or more than 10 watery bowel movements in 1 day).
- Severe abdominal cramps occur.
- The child becomes dizzy when standing.
- The child starts acting very sick.
- Fever over 100° F (37.8° C) has been present for more than 72 hours.
- Mild diarrhea lasts more than 1 week.

Modified from American Academy of Pediatrics, Provisional Committee on Quality Improvement, Subcommittee on Acute Gastroenteritis. (1996). The management of acute gastroenteritis in young children. *Pediatrics, 97*(3), 424-435; Schmitt, B.D. (1999). *Instructions for pediatric patients* (pp. 72-73). Philadelphia: Saunders.

Nursing Care Plan

The Child With Diarrhea

FOCUSED ASSESSMENT

The child's condition and hydration status should be the first area of assessment. The concern about dehydration is the potential for shock. The child and family should be questioned about possible food allergies, intolerance of foods, food eaten over the past 24 hours, and outbreaks of diarrhea in the nuclear or extended family or daycare setting. If diarrhea is present, stools should be assessed for amount, color, consistency, and time—abbreviated as ACCT—and odor. When assessing and monitoring for ACCT, note the quantity and quality of the stool, its color (e.g., green, brown, black, clear, blood-tinged), consistency (watery, loose), the presence of mucus, and the length of time since the stool's consistency has changed.

Other ongoing assessments include monitoring intake and output; assessing the current weight and comparing it with the last known weight; assessing for thirst, along with skin turgor and texture and mucous membranes; and monitoring the child's level of activity. If diarrhea is severe, it may be necessary to apply a urine bag to measure urine output and to obtain urine to measure specific gravity. Skin integrity must be monitored if a urine bag is to be used. Observe the skin in the perineal and perianal area for color, texture, lesions, and/or drainage with each diaper change. Assess family members' knowledge of the transmission of infection by questions or testing. Observe family members using Contact Precautions. Ask family if any members have developed cramping or diarrhea.

NUTRITIONAL ASSESSMENT

- Assess the child's weight on admission and daily, using the same scale, at the same time of day, and after removing the child's clothes. Older children may wear underwear.
- Monitor the child's intake and output at least every 8 hours. Urine output should be at least 2 ml/kg/hr for infants and toddlers and 1 ml/kg/hr for school-age children. Older children have lower minimum requirements.
- Assess serum electrolytes, calcium, vitamins B_{12}, and K, folic acid, and zinc levels if ordered.
- Assess and record bowel sounds and any abdominal distention. Peristalsis (as evidenced by bowel sounds) is necessary for the child to tolerate oral feedings. Hyperactive bowel sounds may indicate excessive peristalsis. Measuring abdominal circumference assesses abdominal distention.

Nursing Diagnosis

Deficient Fluid Volume related to increased stool output.

Expected Outcome

The child will:
- Maintain fluid balance within normal limits, as evidenced by age-appropriate urine output, capillary refill time less than 2 seconds, elastic skin turgor, moist mucous membranes, and weight gain.

INTERVENTION	RATIONALE
1. Weigh the unclothed child carefully on admission and daily on the same scale and at the same time each day.	1. Weight is a useful indicator of fluid status. Weighing in the same clothing, on the same scale, and at the same time of day prevents misinterpretation of weight fluctuation.
2. Monitor and document intake and output hourly. Monitor urine color every 4 hours and specific gravity when appropriate. Weigh diapers after each voiding and liquid stool. (Each gram of diaper weight is equivalent to 1 ml of urine.) Assess and record the amount, frequency, color, and consistency of stools. Notify physician with signs of dehydration.	2. Urine output should be at least 2 ml/kg/hr for infants and toddlers and 1 ml/kg/hr for school-age children. Older children have lower minimum milliliter per kilogram requirements.
3. Monitor vital signs at least every 4 hours or more frequently as indicated. Temperature should not be taken rectally. Report abnormalities to physician.	3. Dehydration can quickly lead to shock in infants and small children. Using a rectal thermometer can stimulate peristalsis and cause more diarrhea. Fever can be both a cause and a sign of dehydration.
4. Assess for signs of dehydration (dry mucous membranes, decreased tearing, sunken fontanel) frequently.	4. Such signs are often the first signs of dehydration.
5. Administer oral and intravenous (IV) fluids as ordered. Check the IV line for patency and infiltration every hour.	5. Excessive output without replacement leads to fluid deficit and electrolyte imbalances.

Continued

Nursing Care Plan

The Child With Diarrhea—cont'd

INTERVENTION	RATIONALE
6. Administer medications as ordered.	6. Medications may be administered to treat the cause of the diarrhea as well as assist in minimizing possible sequelae.
7. Send stools to laboratory for culture and other ordered tests. Perform tests for guaiac, pH, and reducing substance. Monitor laboratory reports (electrolytes, pH, hematocrit, serum albumin, urine specific gravity). Notify physician of abnormal laboratory values.	7. Laboratory reports are monitored to evaluate response to therapy.
8. Implement measures to reduce fever (give antipyretics as ordered).	8. See Chapter 37 for a discussion of care of the child with fever.
9. Parent teaching: Because diarrhea is often treated at home, parents need clear, specific instructions in caring for their sick child (See Parents Want to Know box, p. 1092).	9. Limiting fluids can be dangerous, especially in infants and small children. Severe dehydration can develop quickly in a fluid-restricted infant with diarrhea. The main goal is to prevent dehydration by giving enough oral fluids to stay abreast of fluid loss through diarrhea. A common myth is that the bowel should be "put to rest" by restricting food and fluids.

Evaluation

- Are weight, urine output, and specific gravity within normal limits for age?
- Is capillary refill less than 2 seconds?
- Is skin turgor elastic, and are mucous membranes moist?

Nursing Diagnosis

Impaired Skin Integrity related to exposure to stool.

Expected Outcome

The child will:

- Have no sign of skin breakdown, as evidenced by intact perineal and perianal skin, or will exhibit signs of healing on affected or excoriated areas.

INTERVENTION	RATIONALE
1. Attempt to reduce peristalsis, and avoid solutions or foods irritating to mucosal lining.	1. External stimuli aggravate the condition.
2. Gently wash diaper area with warm water and mild soap after each stool, and pat dry thoroughly. Care must be taken not to cause further damage to the skin. Apply medicated ointment or cream as ordered. Do not use plastic pants if hydrocortisone cream is used.	2. Thorough and consistent skin care decreases the risk of skin breakdown. Commercial cleaning wipes often contain alcohol or perfume and may cause irritation and pain. Plastic can increase absorption of medication.
3. Before applying ointments, expose affected area to air as much as possible (but not with explosive diarrhea). Keep clothing and linen clean and dry.	3. Exposure of skin to air decreases irritation and promotes healing.
4. Use protective moisture barriers, such as creams or ointments.	4. Barrier creams are useful for protection from diarrhea stools.
5. Measure axillary or tympanic temperatures only. Do *not* take rectal temperatures.	5. Inserting a thermometer in the rectum stimulates peristalsis and may further damage excoriated tissue.
6. Turn the child every 2 hours, and protect reddened bony prominences. Use prophylactic pressure-relieving devices in bed and chairs.	6. Decreasing pressure on irritated skin promotes healing.
7. Teach parents skin care routines.	7. Parent involvement is necessary to provide ongoing care of the child.

Nursing Care Plan

The Child With Diarrhea—cont'd

Evaluation

- Have signs of excoriation, redness, blisters, pruritus, and infection been reduced or eliminated?

Nursing Diagnosis

Risk for Infection (in others) related to lack of knowledge about transmission prevention.

Expected Outcome

Family members will:
- Show no signs of infection.
- Demonstrate correct precaution technique (Contact Precautions).

INTERVENTION	RATIONALE
1. Practice careful handwashing. Wear gloves when caring for the child. Isolate the child according to institution policy.	1. Good handwashing and adherence to isolation guidelines help prevent nosocomial infection.
2. Instruct family and visitors in proper handwashing, and observe a return demonstration. Determine parents' understanding of the need for precautions. Discuss the importance of maintaining precautions, and explain precaution technique. Teach parents how to contain organisms, and demonstrate techniques to prevent spread. Offer explanations using simple, accurate terminology appropriate to the parents' level of understanding. (See Chapter 37 for a further discussion of precautions.)	2. If precaution measures are not maintained, infection may spread to the family and others.
3. Dispose of linen and other soiled items correctly.	3. Proper disposal of contaminated articles decreases the risk of spread of infection.
4. Clean toys, desk, trays, and other equipment at least daily and after contact with stools.	4. Proper cleaning of contaminated articles decreases the risk of spread of infection.

Evaluation

- Are family members free of infection?
- Do family members demonstrate an understanding of isolation technique on a consistent basis?

Nursing Diagnosis

Imbalanced Nutrition: Less Than Body Requirements related to decreased intake and inability of body to absorb fluid.

Expected Outcome

The child will:
- Tolerate the diet, as evidenced by weight gain and no recurrence of diarrhea.

INTERVENTION	RATIONALE
1. When ordered, begin oral rehydration solutions (Rehydralyte, Pedialyte, Infalyte). Discourage the use of Popsicles and other sugary drinks.	1. Fluids high in sugar have high osmotic activity and may increase diarrhea. Frozen electrolyte pops can be used for the child who refuses liquid solutions.
2. Offer oral rehydration solution in small, frequent feedings (beginning with 5 to 15 ml every 10 min). If tolerated, the volume can be gradually increased.	2. Fluids should be offered in small amounts at first to prevent gastric distention and vomiting.
3. Give liquids at room temperature.	3. Cold liquids stimulate peristalsis.
4. Apple juice, sports beverages, and colas should be avoided during oral rehydration therapy.	4. These beverages have low electrolyte concentrations for oral rehydration therapy and high carbohydrate content.
5. After rehydration, introduce age-appropriate foods that are bland but nutritional and include complex carbohydrates.	5. Once rehydration has been achieved, an age-appropriate diet provides necessary nutrients.
6. Keep room as odor-free as possible. Provide oral hygiene.	6. Minimizing unpleasant stimuli increases intake and feelings of well-being.

Evaluation

- Can the child retain food and fluids?
- Are normal bowel elimination patterns present?
- Has the child maintained or shown an increase in weight?

VOMITING *prevent aspiration*

Vomiting is the forcible ejection of stomach contents through the mouth. It involves a complex reflex associated with sweating, salivation, and often tachycardia (all symptoms of autonomic nervous stimulation). Other terms that may be used to differentiate vomiting episodes include *spitting up* (or *chalasia*, which is a normal process during infancy), *regurgitation* (associated with gastroesophageal reflux or overfeeding), and, if severe, *projectile vomiting* (usually indicative of obstruction, tumor, pyloric stenosis, or increasing intracranial pressure). Isolated incidents of vomiting are usually of little concern. The consequences of persistent or prolonged vomiting, however, can be serious.

Etiology

Vomiting, which occurs frequently in children, is usually a sign of some other underlying problem or disease. Vomiting has many possible causes. Some of them are infections, obstructions, motion sickness, metabolic alterations, and psychologic alterations. If vomiting occurs in association with diarrhea, it may be related to gastroenteritis. Vomiting can also result from allergic reactions, as a side effect of medications (e.g., chemotherapy), as a toxic effect of medications or ingested substances, and from certain eating disorders.

Pathophysiology

Of Vomiting

Vomiting is under the control of the emetic center, located in the reticular core of the medulla (in the brainstem). The emetic center receives stimuli from one of three sources:

- From the vagal and sympathetic afferent nerves, such as the stimulation of irritation, distention, obstruction, or inflammation
- Chemically, from drugs (e.g., ipecac, other opioids), cerebral hypoxia, inner ear disturbances, or increased intracranial pressure
- From the higher cortical centers, with stimuli such as sights, odors, and fright or fear

The mechanism of vomiting occurs in the presence of several complex reflexes:
- Autonomic nervous system discharge, which causes salivation, sweating, pallor, and an increased heart rate
- Contraction of the stomach antrum and duodenum
- Relaxation of the remainder of the stomach, esophagus, and sphincters
- Closure of the glottis and soft palate
- Contraction of the diaphragm and abdominal muscles, which increases intraabdominal pressure and compresses abdominal contents, thus propelling them into the esophagus and out the mouth

Manifestations

Sour milk curds without green or brown color and undigested food from the stomach are manifestations of vomiting. Green emesis usually indicates the presence of bile and possible intestinal obstruction below the ampulla of Vater. A fecal odor indicates lower intestinal obstruction or peritonitis. Emesis may be blood-tinged, or the color may be bright red or look like coffee grounds. Bright red blood indicates that the blood has not been in contact with gastric juices.

The force of vomiting varies. Regurgitation, a backward flow of undigested food, could be caused by overfeeding. Forceful vomiting could indicate some obstruction. Projectile vomiting may indicate obstruction, tumor, or increased intracranial pressure.

Diagnostic Evaluation

Vomiting in children is usually of brief duration and not severe. If vomiting continues and the child starts to look deficient in fluid or electrolytes, however, the following tests may be indicated:

- Complete blood cell counts and electrolyte studies, blood urea nitrogen, glucose levels, and urine tests
- Radiographic studies (if an obstructive or neurologic process is suspected)
- Blood cultures (if an infectious disease is suspected)
- Arterial blood gas determinations

Therapeutic Management

The primary focus of managing vomiting is detecting and treating the cause, with the secondary intent of preventing complications. ORT, as indicated for the treatment of diarrhea (see Table 42-4), is also appropriate for the vomiting child and may be given in small, frequent amounts. The time intervals and volume depend on the child's weight and age. Even with continued vomiting, most children can maintain hydration with small frequent feedings of an oral rehydration formulation. Maintenance ORT and replacement of continuing losses from emesis are necessary. The practitioner and parents must estimate the volume of emesis and replace. Reevaluation and continuing loss replacement should be done every 1 to 2 hours for a mild to moderately dehydrated child. As the vomiting decreases in frequency, the amount

---

! CRITICAL TO REMEMBER

Caring for the Child Who Is Vomiting

Nursing care of the child who is vomiting is directed toward:
- Observing and reporting vomiting
- Assessing for associated problems, such as dehydration
- Implementing measures to reduce the vomiting
- Recording accurate intake and output
- Evaluating the effectiveness of therapy
- Preventing aspiration

and interval between feedings can increase. If the vomiting is severe or prolonged in neonates and young infants, however, IV therapy is initiated. Most children will respond well, but some will need antiemetics.

Once the vomiting has ceased, liquids or foods should be reintroduced gradually, as tolerated. The mouth should be rinsed and the teeth brushed after vomiting, to rid the mouth of the hydrochloric acid as well as to freshen the mouth.

▪NURSING CARE
The Vomiting Child

Assessment

Major concerns with vomiting are dehydration and fluid and electrolyte imbalance; therefore it is essential that hydration status be carefully assessed, including accurate monitoring of intake and output, weight, fontanels in infants, skin turgor, eyes, skin, and heart and respiratory rates.

Determine and describe the type and force of vomiting (i.e., "spitting up" as opposed to regurgitation, forceful vomiting, or projectile vomiting), as well as the character (using the acronym ACCT: amount, color, consistency, time) of the vomitus. Because vomiting is often associated with gastric distention, the relationship, if any, with infant feeding should be assessed (e.g., poor feeding techniques, failure to bubble or burp, regurgitation with burp or "wet burp," improper positioning).

Nursing Diagnosis and Planning

The following nursing diagnoses and expected outcomes may be appropriate in the treatment of the vomiting child:

■ Deficient Fluid Volume related to increased loss of gastrointestinal contents.
   Expected Outcomes: The child will maintain fluid balance within normal limits, as evidenced by age-appropriate fluid intake, and will have age-appropriate urine output, a capillary refill time of less than 2 seconds, elastic skin turgor, and moist mucous membranes.
■ Imbalanced Nutrition: Less Than Body Requirements related to vomiting.
   Expected Outcomes: The child will maintain electrolyte balance within normal limits, as evidenced by adequate amount of calories absorbed, steady weight gain or lack of weight loss, and lack of vomiting.

Interventions

The vomiting child should be placed in an upright or side-lying position to prevent aspiration. Nursing interventions are frequently determined by the cause of the vomiting and therefore may be very specific. For example, if the vomiting is found to be caused by incorrect feeding techniques or solutions, the nurse's role is to educate the family regarding appropriate feeding techniques (e.g., adequate bubbling and burping as well as positioning after the feeding) and preparation of formulas.

Once the cause of vomiting has been determined, nursing interventions are directed toward ensuring a continued reduction in the vomiting. In reintroducing oral fluids and feedings for the child who is vomiting, start with an appropriate electrolyte-containing solution. Offer an oral rehydration solution in small, frequent feedings to avoid gastric distention. If the child has repeated vomiting or vomits large volumes, the physician should be notified so that IV therapy can be considered. If fluids are tolerated, the volume can be gradually increased. If oral fluids are well tolerated, solid foods may be added.

Another important consideration is education for the child and family about avoiding certain foods (e.g., fatty, acidified, or seasoned foods), as well as minimizing stimuli such as stress, anxiety, or unfavorable-smelling foods, which might lead to nausea and subsequent vomiting. Antiemetic medications, decreased stimuli, and avoidance of food or activities that might tend to upset the stomach, either directly or by association, may be helpful in decreasing nausea and vomiting.

Evaluation

• Is the child taking age-appropriate amounts of fluid without vomiting?
• Is the child's urine output age-appropriate?
• Is the child's skin turgor elastic, with a capillary refill time of 2 seconds or less?
• Does the child have moist mucous membranes?
• Are the child's serum sodium and potassium levels within normal limits?
• Is the child tolerating an age-appropriate diet?

KEY CONCEPTS

■ Infants and children are at a much greater risk than adults for fluid and electrolyte disturbances.
■ The three mechanisms by which acid-base balance is maintained are chemical buffering, respiratory control of carbon dioxide, and renal regulation of bicarbonate and secretion of hydrogen ions.
■ The two major forms of acid-base disturbance are acidosis and alkalosis, either of which may be respiratory or metabolic.

■ The treatment of metabolic disturbances is directed toward correcting the underlying problem. Interventions for respiratory alterations are implemented toward reestablishing alveolar ventilation.
■ Dehydration may be classified as isonatremic (the most common form), hyponatremic, or hypernatremic.
■ Monitoring of intake and output, vital signs, and level of activity (or sensorium) is crucial

in appropriately assessing the child with a fluid or electrolyte disturbance.
■ Diarrhea can lead to loss of bicarbonate (and subsequently to acidosis).
■ Oral rehydration therapy is indicated for the child with diarrhea, dehydration of any degree, and vomiting.

ANSWERS to Critical Thinking Exercise 42-1

1. When taking a history related to diarrhea, it is very important that you have accurate information. One person's definition of diarrhea may be very different from the next. David may indeed have severe diarrhea, or he may have just an increase in stools. Ask Mrs. Peters the following questions:

   - How long has David had diarrhea?
   - How many stools has he had? What is the color, amount, and consistency of the stools?
   - How many wet diapers has David had in the last 24 hours?
   - Is David playing and acting normally?
   - What is David's temperature?
   - When David cries, does he have tears?
   - Has David been in a daycare setting or church nursery?
   - Does anyone else in the family have diarrhea?
   - What solids does David eat?

2. On the basis of Mrs. Peters' response, you can develop a teaching plan. Three areas need to be addressed: diet, infection control, and emotional support. Although you may think diet and infection control are pri-

orities, until Mrs. Peters is less anxious she will not be able to give full attention to the information you are about to give her. For that reason, you should provide emotional support and assurance.

Emotional Support

Mrs. Peters seems to be blaming herself for David's illness. Provide an environment that encourages her to talk about her feelings. The use of therapeutic communication will build trust and allow her to share her concerns. You can commend her for breastfeeding and point out that breastfeeding provides extra help in fighting infections. Because David is now 8 months old the antibodies that Mrs. Peters passed to him during her pregnancy are gone, and he is more susceptible to infections. As you talk with Mrs. Peters, you are constantly assessing her emotional needs and responding to her questions.

Diet

Mrs. Peters should continue breastfeeding David. If he shows no signs of dehydration, an age-appropriate diet of solids should be continued. Fruit juices and raw fruits and vegetables

should be discontinued because they may increase the diarrhea. If David is mildly dehydrated, Mrs. Peters should be encouraged to breastfeed at more frequent intervals. If urine output is decreased, she can also add an oral rehydration solution for 6 to 24 hours. David can be given a regular diet that is age-appropriate as soon as he is rehydrated. Foods given should be nutritional and include complex carbohydrates. Suggested foods include cereal, mashed potatoes, strained bananas, strained carrots, and applesauce. Mrs. Peters should be given instructions regarding signs of dehydration, as well as when she should notify David's primary health provider if his condition worsens.

Infection Control

Instructions should also cover handwashing and infection control. Instruct Mrs. Peters in the disposal of contaminated linens and other soiled items. Instruct her in the cleaning of areas where diapers are changed and where children play with toys. Instruct her to clean the bathtub after use. Reinforce the importance of not sharing toys among children who have diarrhea.

REFERENCES and READINGS

American Academy of Pediatrics, Provisional Committee on Quality Improvement, Subcommittee on Acute Gastroenteritis. (1996). The management of acute gastroenteritis in young children. *Pediatrics, 97*(3), 424-435.

Atherly-John, Y.C., Cunningham, S.J., & Crain, E.F. (2002). A randomized trial of oral vs. intravenous rehydration in a pediatric emergency room. *Archives of Pediatric Adolescent Medicine, 156*, 1240-1243.

Behrman, R., Kliegman, R., & Jenson, H.B. (2000). *Nelson textbook of pediatrics* (16th ed.). Philadelphia: Saunders.

Berman, J. (2003). Heading off the dangers of acute gastroenteritis. *Contemporary Pediatrics, 20*(7), 57-68.

Bohn, D. (2000). Problems associated with intravenous fluid administration in children: Do we have the right solutions? *Current Opinion in Pediatrics, 12*, 217-221.

Burkhart, D.M. (1999). Management of acute gastroenteritis in children. *American Family Physician, 60*(9), 2555-2563.

Dabbagh, S., Atiyeh, B., Fleischmann, L.E., & Gruskin, A.B. (1999). Fluid and electrolyte therapy. In F.D. Burg, J.R. Ingelfinger, E.R. Wald, & R.A. Polin (Eds.), *Gellis & Kagan's current pediatric therapy* (16th ed.). Philadelphia: Saunders.

Eliason, B.C. & Lewan, R.B. (1998). Gastroenteritis in children: Principles of diagnosis and treatment. *American Family Physician, 58*(8), 1769-1776.

Endsley, S., & Galbraith, A. (1998). Are you overlooking oral rehydration therapy in childhood diarrhea: It's not just for use in developing countries. *Postgraduate Medicine, 104*(4), 159-171.

Fann, B.D. (1998). Fluid and electrolyte balance in the pediatric patient. *Journal of Intravenous Nursing, 21*(3), 153-159.

Farthing, M.J.G. (2002). Oral rehydration: An evolving solution. *Journal of Pediatric Gastroenterology and Nutrition, 34*, 564-567.

Fuchs, G.J. (2001). A better oral rehydration solution? *BMJ, 323*, 59-60.

Fuchs, G. J. (2002). Reduced osmolarity oral rehydration solutions: New and improved ORS? *Journal of Pediatric Gastroenterology and Nutrition, 34*(3), 252-253.

Hugger, J., Harkless, G., & Rentschler, D. (1998). Oral rehydration therapy for children with acute diarrhea. *Nurse Practitioner, 23*(12), 52-64.

Kee, J.L., & Paulanka, B.J. (2000). *Fluid and electrolytes*. Albany, NY: Delmar.

Lam, W.H. (1998). Fluids in paediatric patients. *Care of the Critically Ill, 14*(3), 93-96.

Liacouras, C.A., & Baldassano, R.N. (1998). Is it toddler's diarrhea? *Contemporary Pediatrics, 15*(9), 131-144.

McVerry, M., & Collin, J. (1998). Managing the child with gastroenteritis. *Paediatric Nursing, 10*(8), 29-35.

Misra, S., & Ament, M.E. (1998). Gastrointestinal tract infections. In R.D. Feigin & J.D. Cherry

(Eds.), *Textbook of pediatric infectious diseases* (4th ed.). Philadelphia: Saunders.

Nager, A.L., & Wang, V.J. (2002). Comparison of nasogastric and intravenous methods of rehydration in pediatric patients with acute dehydration. *Pediatrics, 109*(4), 566-572.

Ozuah, P.O., Avner, J.R., & Stein, R.K. (2002). Oral rehydration, emergency physicians, and practice parameters: A national survey. *Pediatrics, 109*(2), 259-261.

Roberts, K.B. (2001). Fluid and electrolytes: Parenteral fluid therapy. *Pediatrics in Review, 22*(11), 380-387.

Santosham, M. (2002). Oral rehydration therapy. *Archives of Pediatric Adolescent Medicine, 156*, 1177-1179.

Schmitt, B.D. (1999). *Instructions for pediatric patients*. Philadelphia: Saunders.

Siberry, G.K., & Iannone, R. (2000). *The Harriet Lane handbook*. St. Louis: Mosby.

Straughn, A. & English, B. (1996). Oral rehydration therapy: a neglected treatment for pediatric diarrhea. *MCN: The American Journal of Maternal/Child Nursing, 21*, 144-146.

Wetzel, G.V. (1999). Red flags in common pediatric symptoms. *MCN: The American Journal of Maternal/Child Nursing, 24*(1), 37-45.

Willock, J., & Jewkes, F. (2000). Making sense of fluid balance in children. *Paediatric Nursing, 12*(7), 37-42.

43

The Child with a Gastrointestinal Alteration

◆ LEARNING OBJECTIVES

After studying this chapter, you should be able to:

- Describe the development of the gastrointestinal (GI) system and its relationship to selected congenital defects.
- Describe the anatomy and physiology of the GI system in the infant and child.
- Describe the common diagnostic and screening tests used to detect alterations in GI function.
- Discuss and display an understanding of the pathophysiology, etiology, clinical manifestations, diagnostic evaluation, and therapeutic management of cleft lip and palate, esophageal atresia, tracheoesophageal fistula, diaphragmatic and hiatal hernias, gastroesophageal reflux, pyloric stenosis, and ulcers.
- Discuss and display an understanding of the pathophysiology, etiology, clinical manifestations, diagnostic evaluation, and therapeutic management of the following disorders: lactose intolerance, celiac disease, Hirschsprung's disease,

abdominal wall defects, constipation, irritable bowel syndrome, necrotizing enterocolitis, imperforate anus, intussusception, Crohn's disease, ulcerative colitis, appendicitis, infectious gastroenteritis, biliary atresia, hepatitis, and cirrhosis.
- State expected nursing diagnoses for GI alterations.
- Use the nursing process to develop nursing care plans and teaching guidelines for the child with GI alterations.
- Develop guidelines for home care for the child with GI alterations.
- Implement child and family teaching.
- Develop nursing implications for common medications used with the child with GI alterations.
- Demonstrate critical thinking skills to manage a given patient care situation.

◆ DEFINITIONS

achalasia Failure of smooth muscle fibers of the GI tract to relax, resulting in a functional obstruction and difficulty in passage of food and chyme along the GI tract.

atresia Absence or abnormal closure of a normal body orifice or passage.

azotemia The presence of urea and other nitrogenous bodies in the blood; an elevated blood urea nitrogen (BUN) or creatinine level.

dysphagia Inability to swallow or difficulty in swallowing.

encopresis Incontinence of feces.

fistula Abnormal passage or communication between two organs or tissues.

fundoplication A 270- to 360-degree wrap of the stomach fundus around the distal esophagus to tighten the lower esophageal sphincter and prevent gastric reflux.

hematemesis Vomiting of bright red blood or of denatured blood that looks like coffee grounds; usually represents a bleeding source proximal to the jejunum.

melena Rectal passage of black, tarry stools, indicating denatured blood from the upper GI tract.

occult bleeding Bleeding in such minute quantity that it can be recognized only by microscopic or chemical means.

peristalsis Progressive, wavelike movements caused by contraction and relaxation of the longitudinal and circular muscles of the GI tract; propels a bolus of food or fluid forward.

projectile vomiting Vomiting that is projected with force, perhaps 2 to 4 feet away from the mouth; may be preceded by deep gastric left-to-right peristaltic waves, characteristic of pyloric stenosis.

pylorus The distal opening of the stomach where the stomach contents pass into the duodenum; the pylorus is surrounded by muscle bands.

tenesmus Ineffective, painful, or continuous urge to defecate.

REVIEW OF THE GASTROINTESTINAL SYSTEM

Upper Gastrointestinal System

The upper gastrointestinal (GI) system includes the mouth, esophagus, and stomach. Its primary functions are to take in food and fluids, begin the digestive process, and propel food into the intestines, where nutrients are absorbed. The *mouth*, or buccal cavity, is the entrance to the GI tract. Here food is broken up and mixed with saliva. This process starts the digestion of carbohydrates. The submandibular, parotid, and sublingual glands secrete saliva in response to the smell, taste, or thought of food. The tongue contains taste buds that distinguish salt, sweet, sour, and bitter sensations. The tongue is essential for swallowing.

At birth, the *esophagus* measures approximately 10 cm in length; it lengthens to 18 to 25 cm by adulthood. The upper third of the esophagus consists of striated voluntary muscle; the lower two thirds consists of smooth muscle. The upper esophageal sphincter (UES) prevents the reflux of esophageal contents into the pharynx and lungs and prevents esophageal distention during respiration; the lower esophageal sphincter (LES, cardiac sphincter) prevents the reflux of gastric contents into the lower esophagus.

Swallowing is under both voluntary and involuntary control. As food is chewed, it forms a small bolus, or mass; the tongue propels the bolus toward the oropharynx. The presence of this mass in the oropharynx stimulates the medulla, causing the soft palate to rise. The nasal passages close, the pharyngeal muscles contract, the larynx closes, and respiration is inhibited. As a result of these processes, food is propelled to the esophagus. Through peristalsis, the bolus moves on to the LES, the muscle relaxes, and the bolus enters the stomach.

The *stomach* lies in the epigastric, umbilical, and left hypochondrial regions of the abdomen. It is a muscular pouch, shaped somewhat like a gourd, where the bolus is re-

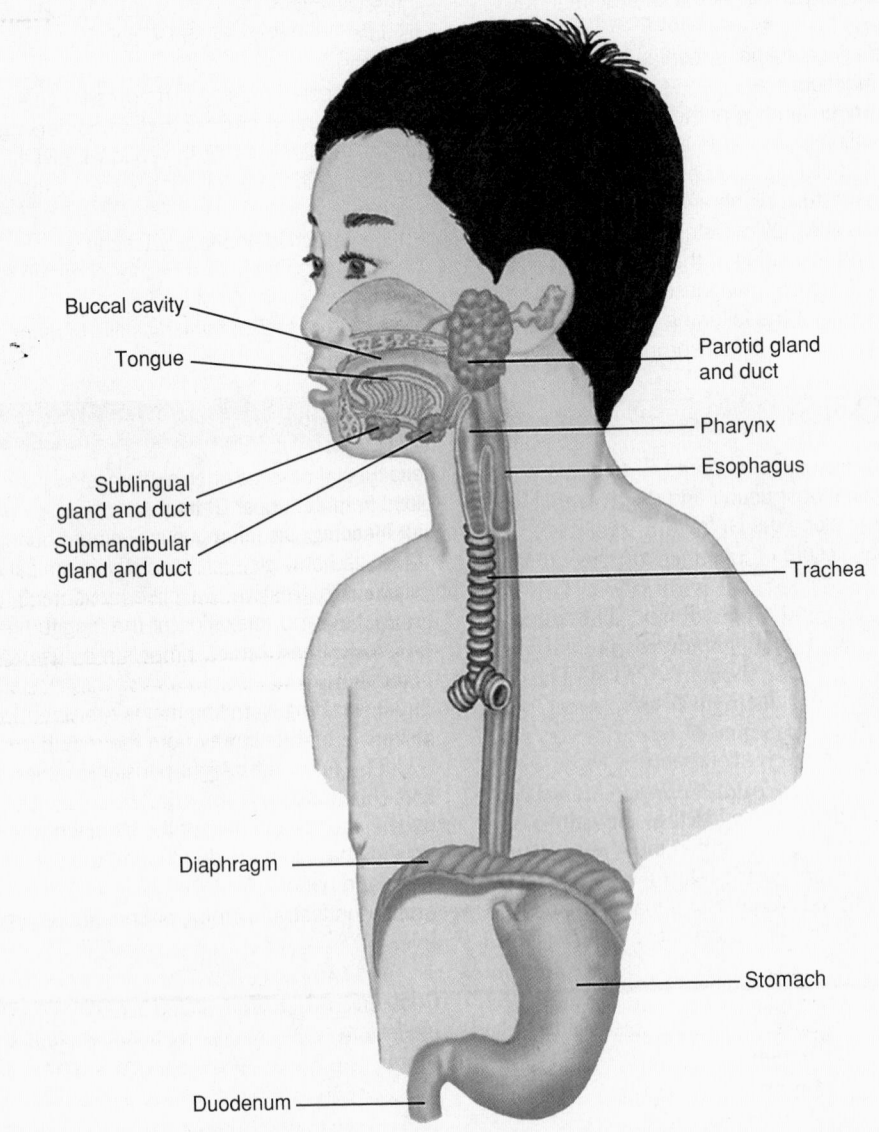

Buccal cavity

Tongue

Sublingual gland and duct

Submandibular gland and duct

Parotid gland and duct

Pharynx

Esophagus

Trachea

Diaphragm

Stomach

Duodenum

Anatomy of the Upper Gastrointestinal Tract

ceived. As the LES and the pylorus contract, the stomach muscles churn the contents. The contents mix with the digestive juices to form chyme. The chyme moves on to the pylorus and into the duodenum.

A mucus-bicarbonate barrier in the stomach provides a thick layer of mucus and a buffer zone to neutralize acid. Stomach acids diffuse slowly through this layer toward the gastric wall. They are neutralized by bicarbonate ions from the surface epithelial cells. Thus a neutral pH is maintained at the gastric epithelial surface.

Lower Gastrointestinal System

The lower GI system includes the duodenum, liver, gallbladder, pancreas, jejunum, ileum, cecum, appendix, ascending colon, transverse colon, descending colon, sigmoid colon, rectum, and anus. The primary functions of the lower GI tract are to digest and absorb nutrients, to detoxify and excrete unwanted waste, and to aid in fluid and electrolyte balance.

The *duodenum,* the first part of the small intestine, extends from the pylorus to the jejunum. Partially digested chyme from the stomach enters the duodenum, where pancreatic enzymes and bile are excreted to further break down fats, carbohydrates, and proteins. The *pancreas* is an oblong gland lying behind the stomach that secretes enzymes to digest food and secretes glucagon and insulin to control motility and absorption.

The *liver,* the largest organ in the body, is located under the right diaphragm. The liver lies predominantly in the right upper quadrant, with the left lobe extending into the left upper quadrant. It is divided into two lobes separated by the falciform ligament. Within each lobe are numerous lobules, which form the functional units of the liver.

The liver is unique in that it is supplied with blood from two sources: (1) the hepatic artery, which supplies oxygenated blood; and (2) the hepatic portal vein, which supplies deoxygenated blood with absorbed nutrients from the GI tract. The liver has numerous functions, including phagocytosis, bile production, detoxification, glycogen storage and breakdown, and vitamin storage. The production of bile is essential for the absorption of fat and the excretion of the end products of blood cell breakdown. The primary function of the *gallbladder,* a saclike structure attached to the underside of the right lobe of the liver, is to store bile for secretion into the duodenum when stimulated by the presence of fat in its lumen.

The *jejunum* and *ileum* form the remainder of the small intestine. Absorption of all nutrients and vitamins occurs here through the villi and microvilli by the processes of diffusion and active transport. Absorption of vitamin B_{12} occurs only in the terminal ileum.

The large intestine starts with the *cecum.* This blind pouch, 2 to 3 inches long, begins at the ileocecal valve, which prevents reverse peristalsis into the small intestine. Attached to it is the *appendix,* a wormlike tube about 3 inches long. The open end of the cecum attaches to the remainder of the colon, which is divided into four sections: the *ascending, transverse, descending,* and *sigmoid colon.* One major function of the large intestine is water reabsorption, which occurs mostly in the cecum and as-

---

Pediatric Differences in the Gastrointestinal System

- Infants have minimal saliva.
- Swallowing is not under voluntary control until 6 weeks.
- Infants and children have less stomach capacity:

Age	Stomach Capacity (ml)
Newborn	10-20
1 wk	30-90
2-3 wk	75-100
1 mo	90-150
3 mo	150-200
1 yr	210-360
2 yr	500
10 yr	750-900
16 yr	1500
Adult	2000-3000

reduce reflux

- The stomach lies transversely and is horizontal in infants' abdomens; the abdomen is round in infants and toddlers.
- Peristaltic waves may reverse in infancy, causing regurgitation and vomiting. Peristalsis is faster; food remains in the stomach for a shorter period.
- Hydrochloric acid concentration is low until school age.
- Fever increases the rate of propulsion.
- The immature neonatal liver is not yet efficient in its detoxifying ability, which results in less vitamin and mineral breakdown than in older children.
- The large intestine is relatively short, with less epithelial lining to absorb water from a fecal mass. As a result, stools have a soft consistency and peristalsis is more rapid.

Major Digestive Enzymes ✳		
Location	**Enzyme**	**Function**
Mouth	Amylase	Converts complex carbohydrate to simple carbohydrate
Stomach	Pepsin	Converts proteins to proteases
Small intestine	Enterokinase	Activates trypsin
	Peptidases	Convert peptides to amino acids
	Sucrase, maltase, lactase	Convert disaccharides to monosaccharides
Pancreas	Trypsin	Converts peptides to amino acids
	Lipase	Converts fat to fatty acids and glycerol
	Amylase	Converts carbohydrates to disaccharides
Liver, gallbladder	Bile	Emulsifies fat, allowing the lipase to function
		Increases fat and fat-soluble vitamin absorption

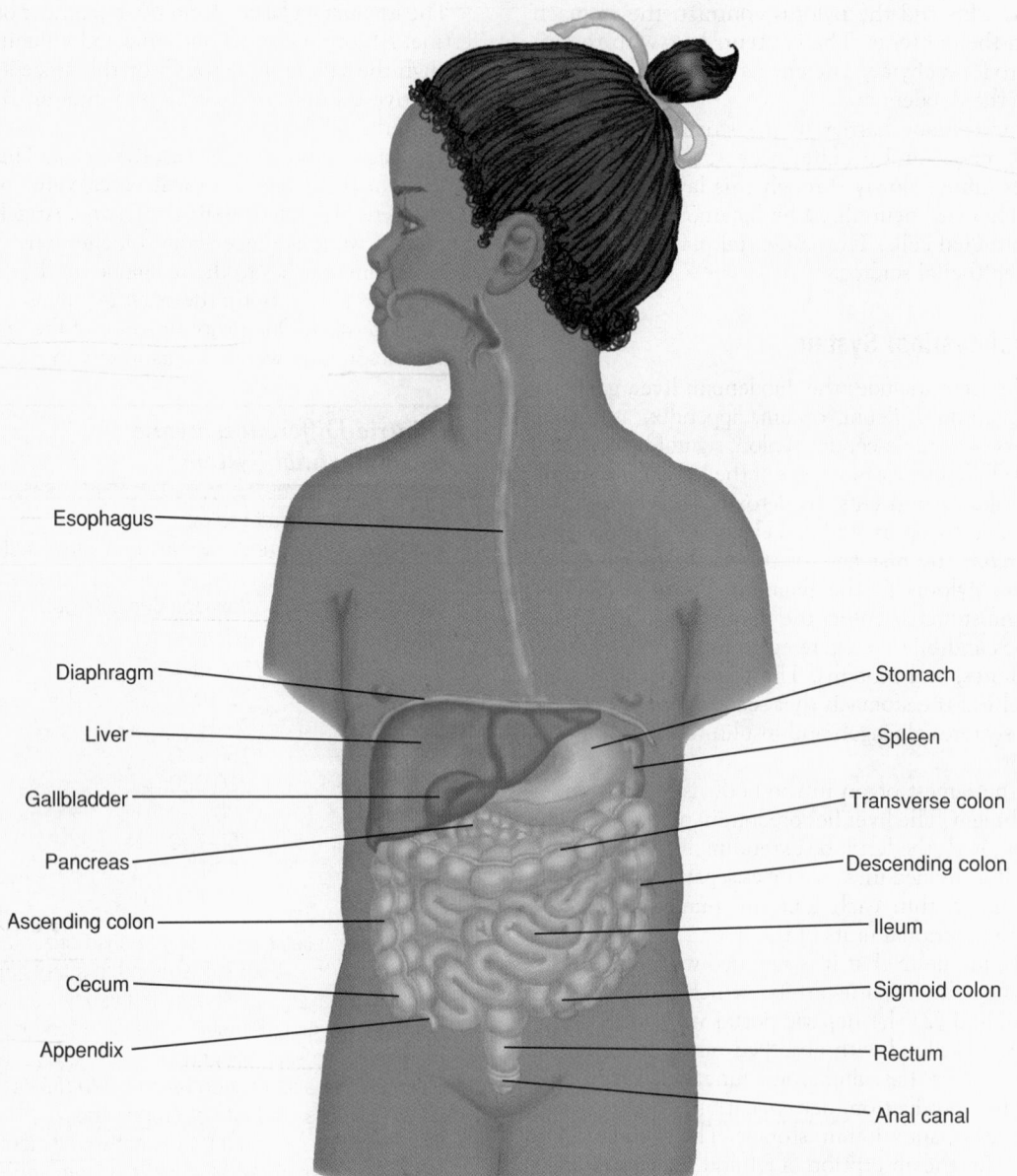

Esophagus

Diaphragm

Liver

Gallbladder

Pancreas

Ascending colon

Cecum

Appendix

Stomach

Spleen

Transverse colon

Descending colon

Ileum

Sigmoid colon

Rectum

Anal canal

Anatomy of the Lower Gastrointestinal Tract

cending colon. Intestinal bacteria ferment the remaining carbohydrates and aid in the synthesis of vitamins B and K. Final breakdown of bile occurs here. Mucus secretion and peristalsis of wastes are also important functions.

The *rectum* is the last 7 to 8 inches of the intestine, and the *anal canal* refers to the last 1 to 2 inches. Stool is stored in the rectum until distention of the rectal walls initiates the defecation reflex—the final stage of the GI processes.

Prenatal Development

The primitive gut is formed from the endoderm in the first 4 weeks of embryonic development. The primitive gut then gives rise to three sections of the GI tract, each having an individual blood supply and rate of development:

- *Foregut*—from pharynx to duodenum, including the liver, pancreas, and biliary tract
- *Midgut*—from duodenum to transverse colon
- *Hindgut*—descending colon, rectum, and anal canal

Problems in the development of each of these three sections give rise to specific malformations and disease states. Anatomically, development is complete at birth, but physiologically, the neonate's GI tract is immature.

Fetal swallowing, intestinal motility, and defecation are detectable in the second trimester of gestation, but the most rapid and extensive development of the GI system occurs in the third trimester. The newborn must be able to adapt from total parenteral nutrition to total enteral nutrition because the placenta no longer performs nutrient exchange and waste removal.

Common Laboratory and Diagnostic Tests for GI Disorders

Test	Description	Normal Findings	Indications	Preparation and Nursing Considerations
STOOL				
Culture and sensitivity	Organisms from a small sample of stool are grown in culture media.	Normal GI flora	To identify infectious organisms and determine their antibiotic sensitivity.	No patient preparation is necessary. The sample is delivered to the laboratory immediately; it must be kept free from contamination.
Reducing substances (Clinitest)	Stool is diluted with water and then tested for undigested carbohydrates using Clinitest tablets.	Negative	Used to diagnose malabsorption syndromes.	No preparation is necessary. The test is done by the nurse, who checks for a color change in the solution.
Occult blood (guaiac, Hematest)	Stool is smeared on filter paper and prepared with solution.	Negative	Used in inflammatory conditions, bowel necrosis.	No preparation is necessary. The test is done by the nurse; a blue color is positive.
Ova and parasites (O&P)	Stool is examined microscopically for presence of parasites or their eggs.	Negative	To identify enteric parasites in child with diarrhea or abdominal pain.	No patient preparation is necessary. Sample must be free from water or urine contamination. The sample is delivered to the laboratory either fresh or in preservatives. Barium, antacids, mineral oil, and antibiotics may interfere with results. 1-3 samples collected.
URINE				
Urobilinogen	Dipstick or laboratory analysis is performed to determine bile by-products in urine.	Negative	Levels determined in hepatic dysfunction and obstruction.	No preparation is necessary. The test is done by the nurse.
BLOOD				
Liver function tests	Serum levels are measured to give an indication of liver function.	AST: <9 yr, 15-55 U/L; >9 yr, 5-45 U/L ALT: 5-45 U/L Total bilirubin: 0.2-1.0 mg/dl Ammonia: 29-70 mcg/dl children; 90-150 mcg/dl newborns	Studies are performed when liver problems are suspected.	No preparation is necessary. Venipuncture is performed.
ENDOSCOPY				
Fiberoptic upper GI endoscopy	Study allows direct viewing of the lining of the esophagus, stomach, and proximal duodenum. It also provides a means to obtain material for biopsies and cultures.	Normal mucosa	Used to rule out various upper GI tract disorders.	Preparation includes teaching, keeping the child on NPO status for at least 6 hr before the examination, providing conscious sedation, and monitoring the child's respiratory function during sedation.

GI, Gastrointestinal; *AST,* aspartate aminotransferase; *ALT,* alanine aminotransferase; *NPO,* nothing by mouth.

Continued

CLINICAL REFERENCE ■

Common Laboratory and Diagnostic Tests for GI Disorders—cont'd

Test	Description	Normal Findings	Indications	Preparation and Nursing Considerations
ENDOSCOPY—cont'd				
Colonoscopy	The colon is viewed directly using a fiberoptic scope and camera inserted rectally.	Normal mucosa, patent bowel	Performed to detect mucosal changes and abnormalities in the lumen of the colon.	Preparation includes teaching, keeping the child on NPO status, bowel cleansing, and providing conscious sedation.
Biopsy (gastric, jejunal, rectal, liver)	A small piece of tissue is removed for analysis.	No abnormal tissue	Study determines the amount of mucosal inflammation and the absence of ganglion cells.	Preparation includes teaching, bowel cleansing, and providing sedation or anesthesia if the procedure is done percutaneously (liver).
RADIOLOGIC EXAMINATIONS				
Abdominal flat plate	Anterior and posterior radiographs are obtained.		Radiographs demonstrate stool and gas patterns, inflammation, and patency of the GI tract. It is commonly performed in cases of abdominal pain, imperforate anus, intussusception, and appendicitis.	Usually no preparation is necessary other than teaching.
Barium swallow examination	Radiopaque contrast medium or air (or both) is swallowed.	Normal swallowing, no anatomic defects	Study identifies esophageal abnormalities, swallowing difficulties, and sphincter function.	Preparation includes teaching and keeping the child on NPO status for 2-4 hr before the examination. Adequate fluids are essential after the examination to prevent barium impaction.
Upper GI examination	Radiopaque contrast material is swallowed or inserted by NG tube.	Normal gastric emptying, no abnormalities	Study outlines the stomach and pyloric canal and can be used to determine gastric emptying time.	Preparation includes teaching and keeping the child on NPO status for 4 hr before the examination. Adequate fluids are essential after the examination to prevent barium impaction.

Common Laboratory and Diagnostic Tests for GI Disorders—cont'd

Test	Description	Normal Findings	Indications	Preparation and Nursing Considerations
RADIOLOGIC EXAMINATIONS—cont'd				
Barium enema, air-contrast barium enema examination	Radiopaque contrast material or air (or both) is placed in the large intestine via the rectum.		Study used to identify abnormalities on the surface of the bowel lumen and to determine bowel patency. It also provides hydrostatic reduction of intussusception.	Preparation includes teaching, keeping the child on NPO status, and bowel cleansing. Adequate fluids are essential after the examination to prevent barium impaction.
CT scan	Oral radiopaque contrast material often used. May also use IV or rectal contrast.	Normal anatomy without evidence of inflammation	Used to identify inflammatory conditions, appendicitis.	No patient preparation other than teaching. Sedation may be used if child unable to remain still. Can be completed in less than 15 min.
OTHER				
Ultrasound	Study uses sound waves noninvasively to image anatomy and inflammation.		Performed to identify anatomic abnormalities and inflammatory conditions.	Preparation includes teaching. For pelvic ultrasound, a full bladder is needed to improve imaging of pelvic organs.
Breath hydrogen test	Carbohydrate solution is given PO and exhaled. Breath samples are collected over 3 hr.	Less than 20 ppm above baseline	Used to diagnose maldigestion or malabsorption syndromes. Inadequately digested carbohydrate produces hydrogen when acted on by GI flora.	Nursing preparation entails teaching about the procedure. The child prepares by fasting for 4$\frac{1}{2}$ hr. The study is noninvasive. A facemask may be worn to collect expired air.

CT, computed tomography; *IV,* intravenous; *ppm,* parts per million.

hildren with GI alterations and their families have many special needs. Some GI problems begin at birth, with life-threatening consequences. Some require the parents to accept their child's altered appearance. Other problems develop after birth and provide long-term challenges in management and treatment. Sudden, unexpected surgery may be necessary. GI alterations cause anxiety and affect nutrition, elimination, respiratory status, skin integrity, body image, family processes, growth and development, and educational needs.

Upper and lower GI conditions can be categorized as follows:

- Developmental problems, such as cleft lip and palate, hernias, esophageal atresia, tracheoesophageal fistula, imperforate anus, and abdominal wall defects
- Problems affecting motility, such as gastroesophageal reflux, constipation, encopresis, and irritable bowel syndrome
- Inflammatory or infectious conditions, including ulcers, gastroenteritis, appendicitis, inflammatory bowel disease, and necrotizing enterocolitis
- Obstructive disorders, such as pyloric stenosis, intussusception, and Hirschsprung's disease
- Malabsorptive conditions, such as lactose intolerance and celiac disease
- Hepatic disorders, such as hepatitis, biliary atresia, and cirrhosis

Disorders that involve the liver and biliary tract may be the result of congenital malformations or acquired infection. Because the liver is important to metabolism, alterations in its function can affect many body systems, including the cardiovascular, integumentary, renal, neurologic, hematologic, and immunologic systems. These disorders can also have significant effects on growth and development. Nursing care may involve nutritional support, infection control, developmental stimulation, family support, and intensive physiologic care during a period of crisis or transplantation.

DISORDERS OF PRENATAL DEVELOPMENT

Cleft Lip and Palate

Cleft lip, cleft palate, and cleft lip and palate are separate anomalies that are closely related in etiology, pathophysiology, and nursing care. These distinct problems are all abnormal openings in the lip or palate. The defects may occur unilaterally (on either side) or bilaterally and are the most common congenital craniofacial deformity.

Incidence

The incidence ranges from 1 in 750 births for cleft lip and palate to 1 in 2500 births for cleft palate. Cleft lip is seen predominantly in males and cleft palate in females. The incidence of cleft is higher in Asians and lowest in African Americans (Behrman, Kleigman, & Jenson, 2004). Cleft lip and palate accounts for 35% to 40% of these facial malformations. Approximately 15% of affected infants have other associated defects.

Manifestations and Diagnostic Evaluation

Cleft lip has the following manifestations: a notched vermilion border, variably sized clefts that involve the alveolar ridge, and dental anomalies (usually deformed, super-

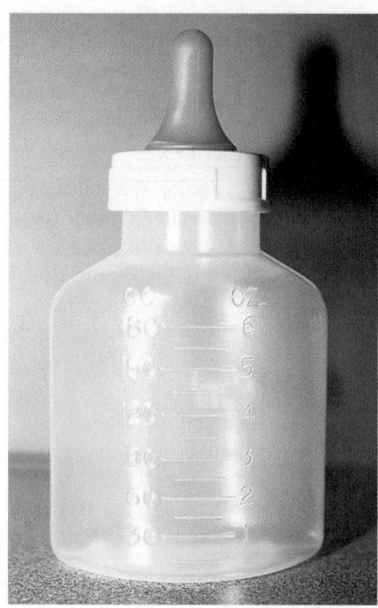

Figure 43-1 Before and after repair of a cleft lip or palate, special feeding techniques are essential for adequate nutrition. A feeder with compressible plastic sides allows the person feeding the baby to gently squeeze the sides of the bottle to help eject the breast milk or formula. A slightly longer nipple allows the milk to be swallowed with less chance of entering the nasopharynx and yet is not so long that it stimulates the gag reflex.

numerary, or absent teeth). Cleft palate includes nasal distortion, midline or bilateral cleft with variable extension from the uvula and soft and hard palates, and exposed nasal cavities.

The diagnosis of cleft lip and cleft palate is based on observation at birth and complete examination in the neonatal period. Diagnosis may also be made in utero with ultrasound. Cleft lip is readily diagnosed through inspection of the lip. The first sign of cleft palate may be formula coming from the nose. A gloved finger placed in the mouth to feel the defect or visual examination with a flashlight will confirm the diagnosis.

Therapeutic Management

Management is based on the severity of the defect. A number of professionals are involved in this process, including surgeons; nurses; geneticists; psychologists or psychiatrists; ear, nose, and throat specialists; audiologists; and occupational and speech therapists. Orthodontists and plastic surgeons become involved in the lengthy management. Pediatricians provide ongoing child health care.

The first intervention involves modifying feeding techniques as needed to allow adequate growth. Use of special feeding techniques, obturators, and unique nipples and feeders can usually accomplish this goal and provide for early discharge with parents (Fig. 43-1).

Cleft lip repair is usually performed by age 3 to 6 months. Early repair may improve bonding and makes feeding much easier. The surgical technique involves the use of a staggered suture line to minimize scarring. Some cosmetic modifications may be needed again at age 4 to 5 years.

Cleft palate repair is individualized and based on the degree of deformity and size of the child. Closure is completed

Text continued on p. 1112

Pathophysiology

of Cleft Lip and Palate

Cleft lip and cleft palate occur from embryonic developmental failures related to multiple genetic and environmental factors. These developmental failures result in an abnormal opening in the lip, palate, and, sometimes, nasal cavity. Cleft lip results when the medial nasal and maxillary processes fail to join at 6 to 8 weeks of gestation. Cleft palate results from failure of the pri-

mary palatal shelves, or processes, to fuse at 7 to 12 weeks of gestation.

Each of these abnormalities appears as a distinct malformation, but they may also appear together. Achieving suction during feedings may be impossible, and fluids may enter the nose, putting the child at risk for aspiration, feeding difficulties, and respiratory distress.

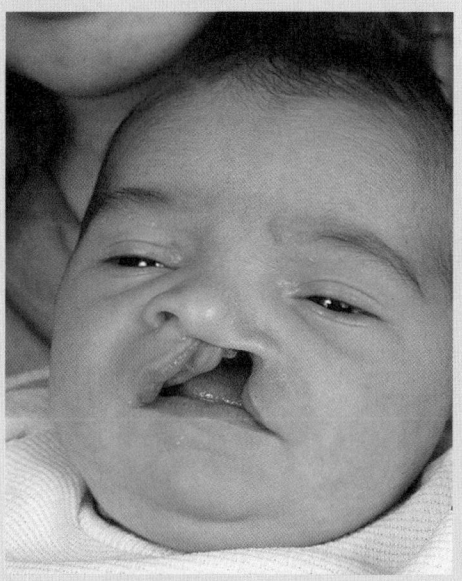
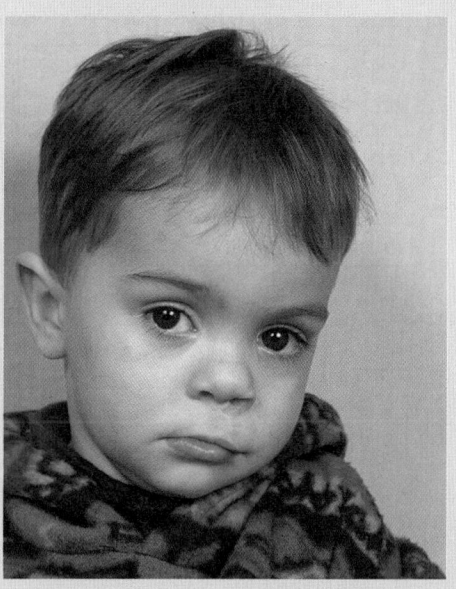

A   **B**

Child born with a cleft lip and palate, before (**A**) and after (**B**) repair. Repair of facial clefts usually requires multiple surgeries at different stages in the child's growth. Early repair of a cleft lip facilitates parent-infant bonding and improves feeding. Results are generally quite good with today's surgical, orthodontic, and speech therapy techniques. (Courtesy Children's Medical Center, Dallas, TX.)

PARENTS
Want to Know

About Home Care of the Child With Cleft Lip or Palate

Your infant may require a special feeding method to maximize growth while waiting for surgery, and you may need to practice the feeding method to be used after surgery until the incision heals. The feeding method you use will be based on what works for your child and what your physician recommends. In general:

- Breastfeeding may be possible if your child has a small cleft lip or palate.
- A compressible bottle will prevent your child from having to suck because the breast milk or formula can be squeezed into the mouth.
- A longer nipple may allow the milk to be swallowed without entering the nose. It must not be so long that it causes gagging. Making a larger hole or "cross-cutting" a nipple may also be effective.
- A syringe with a rubber tip may also be used, especially after surgery.
- Try to keep your child in an upright position during feedings to allow gravity to assist in the feeding and decrease the chance that your child might choke.
- Burp frequently because excess air is often swallowed.

After surgery, elbow restraints (no-no's) may be used so that your baby cannot touch the stitches. Follow these recommendations:

- Do not apply the restraints too tightly. They should be loose but still prevent elbow bending.
- Remove no-no's every 2 hours for 10 to 15 minutes, and play games with your child that encourage movement of the elbows. Look for any skin irritation every time you remove the no-no's.
- Remove only one no-no at a time.

Position your child for sleep using blankets to prevent rolling onto the abdomen so the child cannot rub the stitches on the linens. An infant seat may be used.

Do not brush your child's teeth for 1 to 2 weeks after surgery. Feeding a small amount of water after meals will help keep the teeth clean. Clean your child's lip as recommended by your physician. Use a cotton swab, and use a gentle rolling motion down the suture line. Apply antiinfective ointment using the same technique.

Make use of the many support professionals in following your child for speech, hearing, dental, or orthodontic problems.

Contact the American Cleft Palate-Craniofacial Association and the Cleft Palate Foundation at (919) 933-9604 or www.cleft.com for further information.

Nursing Care Plan

The Child With a Cleft Lip or Palate

FOCUSED ASSESSMENT

Cleft lip and cleft palate are readily apparent at birth, and the degree of involvement should be documented during the newborn examination (see Chapter 22). After identifying this condition, assess the infant's ability to suck, swallow, and breathe without distress and handle normal secretions. Because the occurrence of cleft lip and palate is usually unexpected and its appearance can be frightening to parents and families, assess and record parents' reactions as well as their interactions with the neonate.

Parents of an infant with a cleft lip or palate may need help to resolve feelings about their infant's appearance. The parents might need to deal with many questions from family members, stares from strangers, and expressions of pity from other new parents. Providing information about the etiology of the defect and showing them pictures of other children before and after surgical repair can give them some relief from these fears and concerns. In addition, modeling and encouraging bonding through touching, holding, and examining their newborn can be very reassuring. Pointing out the newborn's positive attributes can help decrease the focus on the defect. For example, emphasize how alert the baby is or the infant's responsiveness or beautiful eyes.

Nursing Diagnoses

Imbalanced Nutrition: Less Than Body Requirements related to inability to suck and to the surgical repair.
Deficient Knowledge about feeding techniques and surgery related to unfamiliarity with the information.

Expected Outcomes

The child will:
- Drink the desired amount of fluid within 30 minutes.
- Be content during and after feeding.
- Gain weight and height according to the normal growth curve.

The parents will:
- Express satisfaction with progress of feedings.
- Understand expected preoperative and postoperative feeding techniques.

INTERVENTION	RATIONALE
1. Describe the degree of cleft and impairment of sucking.	1. Infants with cleft lip alone or simple cleft dental arch may be successful with breastfeeding or bottle-feeding without modifications.
2. Keep care and teaching simple and as closely related to normal infant feeding as possible.	2. Nutrition, parent-infant relationship, and compliance may be improved if normal techniques can be used.
3. Provide alternative assistive feeding devices as needed and ordered. Some infants may be able to breastfeed successfully.	3. Techniques and equipment vary among institutions. Use what is available and effective for each child. Encourage breastfeeding first.
4. Burp frequently, and hold the infant in a more upright position.	4. Burping minimizes air swallowing and gastrointestinal (GI) flatus and minimizes risk of aspiration.
5. Document the feeding program in written form for parents to use at home, and provide the plan to other health professionals.	5. Documentation provides consistency at home and at other times, when the family is in contact with numerous medical professionals treating the child.
6. Provide emotional support and positive reinforcement to parents as they learn to feed their child.	6. Self-care and bonding are improved when parents can assume total care.
7. Keep an accurate record of the child's growth by using a growth chart.	7. A chart identifies growth changes early, when intervention can be most effective.
8. Explain preoperative and postoperative procedures: oral feedings withheld for 6 hours, placement of intravenous (IV) lines, use of arm restraints, appearance of repair in the immediate postoperative period (see Parents Want to Know box, p. 1107).	8. Explanation decreases parental anxiety and encourages involvement.

Nursing Care Plan

The Child With a Cleft Lip or Palate—cont'd

9. Postoperatively:
   a. Keep straws, pacifiers, spoons, or fingers away from the child's mouth for 7 to 10 days. Do not take temperatures orally.
   b. Advance the child's diet as ordered and tolerated from clear liquids to a normal *soft* diet within 48 hours.
   c. After repair of a cleft lip, resume preoperative feeding techniques.
   d. After repair of a cleft palate, provide short nipples that do not rest on palatal sutures; give baby food or baby food mixed with water.

9. For postoperative care:
   a. Avoiding contact with the incision site reduces stress on surgical repair and prevents accidental tearing of very fine sutures.
   b. A normal diet minimizes nutritional deficits and stress on the child. No foods that can tear surfaces are offered.
   c. Little evidence shows that sucking causes excess suture stress.
   d. Prevents direct contact with surgical site.

Evaluation

- Is the infant following the appropriate growth curve?
- Is the infant happy and content during and after feedings?
- Do the parents express satisfaction with the feeding technique used and the time required to complete a feeding?
- Can the parents explain and demonstrate expected preoperative and postoperative care?

Nursing Diagnosis

Interrupted Family Processes related to the emotional reaction to an infant with a visible defect.

Expected Outcomes

The parents will:
- Demonstrate positive behaviors toward the infant.
- Access appropriate support.

INTERVENTION	RATIONALE
1. Encourage parents to discuss their fears, concerns, and negative emotions.	1. Grief, anxiety, confusion, guilt, denial, and anger are not uncommon and should be expressed.
2. Encourage touching and holding.	2. Contact encourages bonding and prevents a delayed attachment.
3. Make appropriate referral to a cleft lip and palate team of nurses, physicians, and other specialists as soon as possible.	3. A health care team can provide accurate information and begin to outline a plan of action.
4. Express acceptance of the baby by modeling feeding and close physical contact.	4. These interventions assist parents with the adaptation process.
5. Refer parents to community resources and parent groups (see Appendix I on Evolve website).	5. Sharing with others in similar situations facilitates acceptance and adaptation.
6. Encourage parents to share concerns about long-term care and emotional and financial stress.	6. Long-term concerns require extensive follow-up and can strain many families' resources. Identifying concerns early can increase problem-solving options.

Evaluation

- Can the parents identify their infant's positive characteristics?
- Do the parents hold, cuddle, and make eye contact with the infant?
- Have the parents sought personal, community, or national support?

Nursing Diagnoses

Impaired Skin Integrity related to the surgical repair.
Risk for Infection related to the surgical repair and aspiration.

Continued

Nursing Care Plan

The Child With a Cleft Lip or Palate—cont'd

Expected Outcomes

The repair site will:
- Heal without complications.

The infant will:
- Show no signs of infection as evidenced by a clean and intact suture line, absence of fever, and clear breath sounds.

INTERVENTION	RATIONALE
1. Clean the lip repair site according to physician protocol. Many physicians recommend cleaning with sterile water using a cotton swab or saline after feeding and as ordered. Use a rolling motion vertically down the suture line. Have parents demonstrate this cleaning technique.	1. The procedure decreases the medium for bacterial growth, decreases crusting, and minimizes scarring.
2. Apply antiinfective ointment as ordered.	2. Antiinfective ointment prevents infection, crusting, and scarring.
3. Use elbow restraints (no-no's) to keep the child from touching the repair site. Continue for 6 to 8 days. Remove every 2 hours for 10 to 15 minutes. Remove restraint from only one elbow at a time, with a parent or nurse in constant attendance.	3. Elbow restraints prevent accidental rupture or tear of sutures. Periodically removing restraints promotes contact with the child, decreases anxiety, and allows the nurse to assess skin integrity and circulation.
4. Do not brush the child's teeth for 1 to 2 weeks.	4. Avoiding brushing prevents accidental tear of palatal sutures.
5. Keep the child in a supine position, on the side opposite to the repair, or in an infant seat.	5. Careful positioning prevents contact of suture lines with bed linens.
6. Observe for redness, swelling, excessive bleeding, drainage, respiratory distress, or fever.	6. Signs of infection must be identified early because additional inflammation can increase scarring.
7. To clean the palate repair site, rinse the child's mouth with water after feedings.	7. Rinsing after feeding removes food and residual sugars from suture lines, reducing the risk of infection.
8. Encourage the parents to hold and cuddle the child as the child desires.	8. Crying puts additional stress on the suture line.
9. Maintain lip protective devices if ordered.	9. Protective devices prevent separation of lip suture lines.

Evaluation

- Is the suture site clean, dry, and without redness, heat, or drainage?
- Is the suture site intact and healing without crusting or excessive scarring?
- Is the infant afebrile and demonstrating clear breath sounds?

Nursing Diagnosis

Acute Pain related to the surgical incision and elbow restraints.

Expected Outcome

The child will:
- Be free from pain.

INTERVENTION	RATIONALE
1. Describe and document pain using appropriate tools (see Chapter 39).	1. Infants and young children do not react to pain in typical adult ways, and alternative observations are needed to validate assessment findings. Parents are the best resource to validate the nurse's assessment of their infant.
2. Provide comfort measures, especially holding, rocking, and parental voices.	2. Comforting increases parental involvement, relieves discomfort, and reduces stress on sutures caused by crying.
3. Provide analgesics and sedatives on a regular basis as ordered. Pain should decrease significantly after 24 to 48 hours.	3. Medication can prevent peaks of pain that cannot be managed appropriately.
4. Report pain not managed by usual means.	4. Pain may indicate hematoma formation or other complications of the repair.

Nursing Care Plan

The Child With a Cleft Lip or Palate—cont'd

Evaluation

- Does the child participate in age-appropriate activities?
- Is the child responding well to pain medication?
- Does the child appear relaxed and content at rest?
- Does the parent describe a child who is not in pain?

Nursing Diagnosis

Ineffective Health Maintenance related to the need for long-term care.

Expected Outcomes

The parents will:
- Seek continued follow-up care to evaluate and manage long-term complications.

The child will:
- Demonstrate normal speech and hearing.

INTERVENTION	RATIONALE
1. Make appropriate and early referrals for any problems with speech impairment or language-based learning disabilities.	1. Speech and language-learning impairments are common complications of cleft lip and palate. Early intervention minimizes harm.
2. Monitor for recurrent or chronic otitis media. Schedule frequent hearing tests.	2. Because of craniofacial deformities, otitis media can occur frequently and must be treated to prevent language and learning problems.
3. Encourage early speech attempts. Arrange speech therapy as needed.	3. Cleft palate can make speech difficult to understand, and the child may feel self-conscious about speech errors. Practice improves development.
4. Encourage good dental care.	4. With abnormalities of teeth and the alveolar ridge, malocclusion and dental caries are a major concern.

Evaluation

- Do the parents continue to seek follow-up care (ear, nose, and throat [ENT]; speech therapy; dental)?
- Does the child demonstrate age-appropriate speech?
- Does the child have normal hearing?
- Does the child have normal dentition?

Nursing Diagnosis

Anxiety (parental) related to special care needs and surgery.

Expected Outcomes

The parents will:
- Express concerns and fears.
- Express control over special care needs.

INTERVENTION	RATIONALE
1. Use a calm, reassuring, accepting approach with the infant and family.	1. Being calm and accepting encourages communication and reinforces to parents that their child is worthwhile.
2. Explain all procedures and their rationale including sensations likely experienced by their child.	2. Uncertainty and loss of control contribute to increased levels of anxiety.
3. Listen actively to parents and their concerns. Encourage verbalization of feelings, perceptions, and fears.	3. Talking and sharing may decrease anxiety.
4. Encourage parents to stay with their child in the immediate preoperative and postoperative periods.	4. Staying with the child encourages parent participation and control over as much as possible.

Evaluation

- Do the parents express concerns and fears?
- Do the parents seek information to decrease anxiety?
- Do the parents demonstrate ability to care for their child?
- Do the parents express confidence in their ability to deal with the situation?

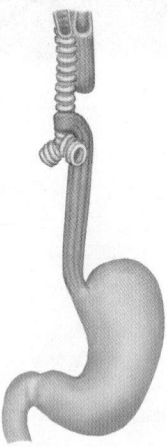

Esophageal Atresia With Distal TEF

Incidence: 85%–88%
Clinical Manifestations: Feeding causes regurgitation and coughing. Constant flow of saliva. Gastric distention.
Diagnostic Findings: Contrast reveals blind pouch. Air on abdominal x–ray.
Surgical Treatment: One-stage surgical repair to ligate fistula and anastomose esophagus

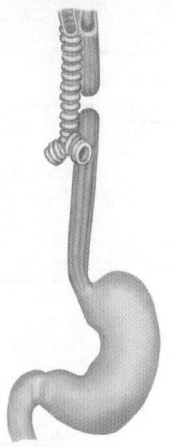

Esophageal Atresia Without Fistula

Incidence: 6%–8%
Clinical Manifestations: Excess oral secretions. Regurgitation of feedings.
Diagnostic Findings: Blind pouch. No air in abdomen.
Surgical Treatment: Two-stage repair: (1) Gastrostomy and cervical esophagostomy; (2) colon interposition to create patent esophagus

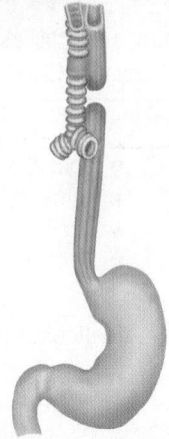

Proximal Esophageal Fistula With Trachea; Distal Segment Has No Communication

Incidence: 1%
Clinical Manifestations: Excessive oral secretions. Immediate respiratory distress with oral intake.
Diagnostic Findings: PO contrast outlines tracheal tree. No air in abdomen.
Surgical Treatment: One- or two-stage repair depending on length of separation

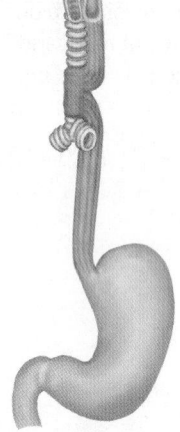

Proximal and Distal Esophageal Fistulas With Trachea

Incidence: 1%
Clinical Manifestations: Excessive secretions. Respiratory distress with feedings.
Diagnostic Findings: PO contrast outlines tracheal tree. Air in abdomen.
Surgical Treatment: Ligation of fistulas and anastomosis of esophagus

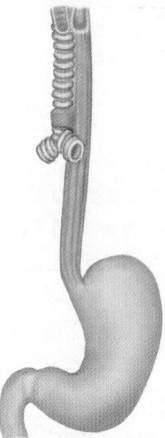

TEF Without Atresia (Also Called "H Type")

Incidence: 4%
Clinical Manifestations: Minimal symptoms unless regurgitation occurs. Choking, coughing. Abdominal distention.
Diagnostic Findings: Bronchoscopy demonstrates fistula.
Surgical Treatment: Ligation of fistula

Figure 43-2 Types of esophageal atresia and tracheoesophageal fistulas (TEFs).

between ages 6 and 24 months. Most teams recommend repair by 1 year. Earlier closure facilitates speech development.

Concurrent treatment of altered dentition, recurring otitis media, speech dysfunction, emotional issues, and cosmetic concerns completes the ongoing therapy. Children with cleft palate are at high risk for developing chronic otitis media. Parents should be aware of this risk so that otitis media can be diagnosed early to decrease the chance of long-term scarring and hearing loss (Resnick & Zarem, 1999).

Esophageal Atresia With Tracheoesophageal Fistula

Esophageal atresia and tracheoesophageal fistula (TEF) are congenital malformations in which the esophagus terminates before it reaches the stomach and/or a fistula is present that forms an unnatural connection with the trachea. Figure 43-2 reviews types of TEF.

Etiology and Incidence

The cause of TEF and esophageal atresia is unknown. Esophageal atresia with or without TEF occurs in 1 in 2000 to 4500 births with no difference in the genders. From 30% to 50% have other associated anomalies of the cardiac, GI, and central nervous systems. Prematurity and low birth weight are frequent concomitant problems that have a significant impact on long-term prognosis.

Manifestations

- Failure to pass suction catheter, nasogastric (NG) tube at birth
- Excessive oral secretions
- Vomiting
- Abdominal distention
- Airless, scaphoid abdomen (atresia without fistula)

Diagnostic Evaluation

A history of maternal polyhydramnios is a significant prenatal clue. If TEF is suspected prenatally, diagnosis can be made at the ideal time—in the delivery room. Atresia should be suspected if an NG tube cannot be passed 10 to 11 cm beyond the gum line. This suspicion is confirmed with an abdominal x-ray film that will identify a proximal esophagus dilated with air (atresia) or abdominal distention (fistula). The radiologist can identify the specific type of defect after instilling less than 1 ml of a water-soluble contrast medium into the NG tube and documenting its movement into the tracheal tree and the proximal pouch. This is then withdrawn from the pouch to minimize the risk of aspiration. Bronchoscopy and endoscopy are also used to identify and assess fistulas.

Therapeutic Management

Keeping the infant supine with the head of the bed elevated decreases the chance of gastric secretions entering the lungs. An NG tube must be in place and aspirated every 5 to 10 minutes to keep the proximal pouch clear of secretions. Intravenous (IV) fluids are essential. Normal newborn care is appropriate, with special attention to keeping the infant warm and oxygenated.

Surgical repair is the mainstay of treatment. Initial repair includes the ligation of the fistula and end-to-side anastomosis of the atresia to decrease the severity of stricture formation. If the gap between the two parts of the esophagus is too large, a staged repair is necessary and a gastrostomy tube (G-tube) and cervical esophagostomy are placed. Later anastomosis, colon interposition, and dilation can be expected. Evaluation and treatment of esophageal motility dysfunction, gastroesophageal reflux, strictures, bronchitis, and pneumonia may occur as the child grows.

Pathophysiology

of Esophageal Atresia and Tracheoesophageal Fistula

Tracheosophageal fistula (TEF) is the result of an embryonal failure to differentiate the foregut into the trachea and esophagus and the incomplete fusion of them into distinct organs. The failure occurs between the 4th and 5th week of pregnancy and is manifested in several ways (see Fig. 43-2).

The presence of a fistula between the esophagus and trachea causes oral intake to enter the lungs or large amounts of air to enter the stomach. Coughing, choking, and severe abdominal distention can occur. Eventually, aspiration pneumonia and severe respiratory distress will develop in the untreated child, and death may occur without surgical intervention. Esophageal atresia occurring by itself causes respiratory distress secondary to aspiration of saliva and any oral fluids that may be given before diagnosis.

NURSING CARE

The Infant With TEF

Assessment

The infant with TEF is at constant risk for aspiration. Assessment for respiratory distress in the immediate period after birth is essential. The nurse must examine the infant for excessive oral secretions, choking, and cyanosis. Difficulty swallowing, regurgitation, vomiting, and unexplained cyanosis after an initial feeding in the infant who is not diagnosed at birth are important assessment findings that must be reported to the physician immediately. Abdominal distention should be measured and the infant continually assessed for distress (vital signs, respiratory effort, nasal flaring, retractions, cyanosis). A newborn assessment should be completed with special attention to identifying any concomitant congenital defects.

Family assessment of anxiety levels, fears, concerns, and knowledge level will provide important information for planning nursing care and teaching.

Nursing Diagnosis and Planning

The nursing diagnoses and expected outcomes that are appropriate after assessment of the infant with TEF are

- Risk for Aspiration related to TEF.
  Expected Outcome: The infant will not aspirate, as evidenced by control of oral secretions without coughing, cyanosis, or adventitious breath sounds.
- Imbalanced Nutrition: Less Than Body Requirements related to possible feeding difficulties.
  Expected Outcome: The infant will gain weight and follow growth chart at appropriate level.
- Risk for Impaired Skin Integrity related to G-tube and esophagostomy.
  Expected Outcome: The infant will maintain skin integrity, as evidenced by intact skin around the G-tube and esophagostomy.

- Risk for Infection related to surgical repair.
  Expected Outcome: The infant will have surgical site, G-tube site, and esophagostomy free from infection, as evidenced by clean, intact skin without drainage, exudate, or redness.
- Acute Pain related to surgical repair.
  Expected Outcome: The infant will be free from pain, as evidenced by resumption of normal activities, ease of comforting, and relaxed facial features.
- Anxiety (parental) related to neonatal surgical emergency.
  Expected Outcome: The parents will express feelings and concerns.
- Deficient Knowledge related to home care needs and follow-up care.
  Expected Outcome: The parents will demonstrate safe G-tube feedings and esophagostomy care.

Interventions

Nursing interventions are different in the preoperative and postoperative periods. In the immediate period after birth, placing the newborn in a radiant warmer and administering humidified oxygen are essential to relieve respiratory distress. The child is prepared for surgery, remains on nothing-by-mouth (NPO) status, and is hydrated with IV fluids. Maintaining thermoregulation and fluid balance is essential, so monitoring temperature and other vital signs, using radiant warmers, and keeping accurate intake and output records are important.

It is essential to minimize the risk of aspiration. Using a chalasia board that helps keep the child at a 30-degree angle while supine can be useful to decrease reflux. Placing a suction catheter in the proximal pouch and mouth will keep secretions to a minimum. Maintaining constant assessment of respiratory status is essential. Even after surgical repair, these children are prone to gastroesophageal reflux.

In the immediate postoperative period, monitoring respiratory status, supporting fluid balance and nutrition, maintaining thermoregulation, providing pain relief, monitoring for infection, and promoting bonding with parents take priority. The child will likely have a chest tube in place. Patency must be maintained, suction monitored, and output documented. Respiratory rate, effort, and the presence of abnormal breath sounds should be documented. Thermoregulation can significantly affect respiratory status in the newborn, so monitoring and maintaining temperature with a radiant warmer may be needed.

IV fluid, antibiotics, and parenteral nutrition may be ordered. The nurse must maintain patency of the IV line;

monitor intake and output; and assess for signs of fluid and electrolyte alterations including sunken fontanel and increased urine specific gravity measurements. Daily weights and measurement of head circumference can aid in assessing growth. Pain medications must be administered as needed based on objective assessment measures used in each institution.

If a cervical esophagostomy has been performed as the first stage of a surgical repair, keep it covered with gauze to absorb saliva and provide skin care. Frequent cleaning with half-strength hydrogen peroxide and assessing for redness, breakdown, or exudate are essential because this wet area easily can become macerated and infected. Referral to an enterostomal therapist can be helpful in teaching parents esophagostomy care.

In the immediate postoperative period, the gastrostomy tube is elevated to allow gastric contents to pass to the small intestine and air to escape; this promotes comfort and decreases risk of leakage at the anastomosis. A pacifier satisfies sucking needs, provides early training in swallowing, makes later feeding easier, and provides comfort through distraction. Pacifiers should not be offered until the child can tolerate oral secretions.

Numerous types of G-tubes are available for placement, either percutaneously or during surgery. Among these are traditional gastrostomy tubes and Foley catheters, which are anchored in place by means of an air- or saline-inflated balloon, as well as more innovative tubes that use a variety of means for anchoring, depending on manufacturer (Fig. 43-3). Tube selection is usually made by the physician, but long-term successful care and use of the tube are nursing and parental responsibilities.

Parents should be taught the techniques of G-tube feeding and care. Skin care at the site may include cleaning with half-strength hydrogen peroxide, rotating the tube, and using a skin barrier product, as well as other ostomy skin care products. Redness, exudate, pus, heat, or leakage of formula should be reported.

Parent education and support are critical components. These should include discussing feelings and anxieties, providing information about home care, practicing with special techniques, providing stimulation, and using appropriate resources, such as enterostomal therapists and dietitians.

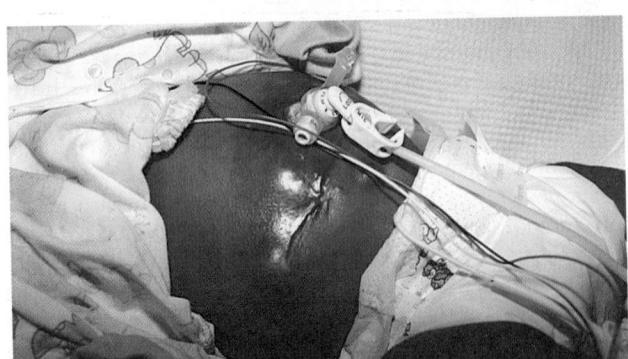

Figure 43-3 The skin level gastrostomy button is good for children who require long-term gastrostomy feeding. It is relatively flat, reduces skin breakdown, increases comfort, and is fully immersible in water. (Courtesy Parkland Health and Hospital System, Dallas, TX.)

! CRITICAL TO REMEMBER

Assessing and Managing the Child With Esophageal Atresia and Tracheoesophageal Fistula

Any child who exhibits the "3 Cs" of Coughing, Choking with feedings, and Cyanosis should be suspected of tracheoesophageal fistula (TEF). Esophageal atresia and TEF represent a critical neonatal surgical emergency. While the baby is awaiting transfer to a neonatal unit and surgery, management centers on prevention of aspiration.

Evaluation

- Can the child coordinate sucking and swallowing?
- Is the child tolerating oral feedings without choking, coughing, or cyanosis?
- Is the child growing according to growth chart?
- Is the surgical site clean, dry, intact, and free of redness, drainage, or exudate?
- Is the skin intact without breakdown around the gastrostomy tube and esophagostomy?
- Is the child resting contentedly without pain medication?
- Can the parents explain the need for the surgical procedure?
- Do parents demonstrate appropriate care of the gastrostomy tube or esophagostomy?
- Have parents assumed all care responsibilities?

Upper Gastrointestinal Hernias

A hernia is an abnormal protrusion of part of an organ or tissue through the structures that normally contain it. Hernias can be either congenital or acquired. Some hernias can be reduced, whereas others become incarcerated and cannot be returned by manipulation. A medical emergency occurs when a hernia becomes strangulated and blood supply is cut off. This condition can occur suddenly and requires immediate treatment. The most common hernias of the upper GI tract are discussed in Table 43-1.

Other Developmental Disorders

Table 43-2 discusses other developmental disorders of the upper and lower GI tracts.

Text continued on p. 1119

TABLE 43-1 Upper Gastrointestinal Hernias

Description	Clinical Manifestations	Therapeutic Management	Nursing Management
HIATAL HERNIA			
Protrusion of a portion of the stomach through the esophageal hiatus of the diaphragm	Vomiting Coughing, wheezing, short periods of apnea Failure to thrive	Medical management similar to that for the child with reflux Surgical repair of defect	Monitor intake and output, document vomiting, observe for respiratory distress, provide routine postoperative care for GI surgery. Teach parents about surgery and medical treatment of reflux.
CONGENITAL DIAPHRAGMATIC HERNIA (CDH)			
Opening in the diaphragm through which abdominal contents herniate into the thoracic cavity during prenatal development *and* some degree of pulmonary hypoplasia, determined by the timing and size of the herniation Mortality: 50%-80%; 40% if ECMO used Degree of pulmonary hypoplasia determines outcome Incidence: 1 in 2200-5000 live births	Clinical findings depend on severity of defect and may include: • Abdominal organs in chest (by fetal ultrasonography) • Diminished or absent breath sounds on affected side • Bowel sounds that may be heard over the chest • Cardiac sounds that may be heard on the right side of the chest • Respiratory distress developing soon after birth: dyspnea, cyanosis, nasal flaring, tachypnea, retractions • Scaphoid abdomen	If diagnosed prenatally, mother moved to tertiary care center before delivery In utero surgery may be performed *Neonatal emergency* NG intubation with suction Ventilate with high-frequency ventilation; manage acidosis with bicarbonate and ventilation ECMO Inhaled nitric oxide Liquid ventilation Manage pulmonary hypertension, inhaled nitric oxide may be used Surgical reduction of hernia after physiologically stable May wait 6-18 hr after birth Respiratory support, ECMO until lungs functioning after surgery	Identify clinical findings, and report immediately. Place child in semi-Fowler position on affected side with head of bed elevated. Maintain patency of NG tube. Monitor IV fluids. Maintain mechanical ventilation, ECMO, chest tubes, assess oxygenation. Do not use facemask/bag for ventilatory support because air can enter stomach and further impair respiratory function. Provide minimal stimulation. Provide routine postoperative care. Monitor for signs of infection, respiratory distress, and feeding difficulties; report to physician. Support family mourning loss of perfect child. Provide clear, truthful information. Encourage the parent to see and touch the infant. Provide referral to support groups. Provide discharge teaching. Use prescribed feeding techniques.

GI, Gastrointestinal; *ECMO,* extracorporeal membrane oxygenation; *NG,* nasogastric; *IV,* intravenous.

PARENTS
Want to Know

About Home Care of the Child With Esophagostomy or Gastrostomy Tube

Your child's esophagostomy will require special but simple care:
- Cover the stoma with gauze.
- Change gauze frequently to prevent constant wetness.
- Clean with half-strength peroxide daily.
- Use skin barriers, such as Skin-Prep protective dressing, to prevent breakdown.
- Look at the stoma daily, and observe for redness, drainage, swelling, and pain. Call your physician if these develop.
- Call your enterostomal therapist for support or help.

Remember to use a pacifier or small amounts of fluid in a bottle to allow your baby to practice swallowing. This should be done every day.

Your child's gastrostomy tube will also require special care depending on the type of tube that is used. Your nurse and physician will help you learn these skills:
- For a new gastrostomy, clean the site daily with half-strength peroxide, rinse with water, and apply antimicrobial ointment. Rotate the tube every day.

- After 1 to 2 weeks, soap and water and tub baths may be used to clean the site. Stomahesive powder may be used to decrease moisture.
- Keep the tube open in the postoperative period.
- While the site is healing, make sure it is stabilized by using a Hollister tube drainage attachment, nipple with gauze at the base, or silicone retention disks as determined by the tube used.
- When the tube is well healed, it can be secured with tape or OpSite.
- Use skin barriers around the stoma to prevent breakdown.
- Report any drainage, leakage of formula, redness, or pain to your physician.
- Ask your enterostomal therapist for help in making the best choices for your child.

TABLE 43-2 Developmental Gastrointestinal Defects

Imperforate Anus	Gastroschisis	Omphalocele	Umbilical Hernia
PATHOPHYSIOLOGY, ETIOLOGY, AND CLINICAL MANIFESTATIONS			
Incomplete development or absence of the anus in its normal position in the perineum. Defect can be high (above the levator ani muscle) or low (below the levator ani muscle). Symptoms include failure to pass meconium stool, absence of anorectal canal, presence of an anal membrane, external fistula to the perineum. Condition is diagnosed during the newborn examination with radiography, ultrasound, or CT used to determine the level of the lesion and associated anomalies.	Embryonal weakness in abdominal wall causes herniation of gut on one side of umbilical cord during early development, most commonly on right side. Viscera are outside the abdominal cavity and are not covered with the sac.	Large herniation of gut into umbilical cord. Viscera are outside the abdominal cavity but inside translucent sac, covered with peritoneum and amniotic membrane.	Imperfect closure of umbilical ring allows gut to push outward at umbilicus during straining and crying. Viscera are inside the abdominal cavity and under the skin. The hernia is usually 1-3 cm and easily reduced.
INCIDENCE			
1 in 4000-5000 live births. More common in males.	1 in 4000 live births.	1 in 5000 to 10,000 live births.	Most common in low-birth-weight and African-American infants.

CT, Computed tomography.

TABLE **43-2** Developmental Gastrointestinal Defects—cont'd

Imperforate Anus	Gastroschisis	Omphalocele	Umbilical Hernia
ASSOCIATED ANOMALIES			
Genitourinary, sacral, or additional GI anomalies.	Prematurity. Malrotation of intestines. Decreased abdominal capacity. Atresia, stenosis rare. Higher incidence of Meckel's diverticulum. Other anomalies rare.	Malrotation of intestines. Decreased abdominal capacity. Atresia, stenosis common. Higher incidence of Meckel's diverticulum. Cardiac, genitourinary, or chromosomal anomalies in one third to one half of cases. Associated with Beckwith's syndrome (hypoglycemia, macrosomia, macroglossia).	Commonly occurs in children with Down syndrome, hypothyroidism, Hurler's syndrome.
MORBIDITY AND MORTALITY			
Prognosis depends on the level of the lesion. Complete continence may be impossible.	Mortality 10%-15%.	Mortality 20%-30%. Common complications include sepsis and intestinal obstruction.	Minimal.
THERAPEUTIC MANAGEMENT			
Anal stenosis is treated with repeated dilation. All other defects require surgical intervention. High defects may require a colostomy and bowel pull-through procedure.	IV and NG tubes are placed immediately. Total parenteral nutrition is provided. Synthetic material (Silastic) is used to cover the gut in a sac (if the sac has ruptured or the omphalocele is large). If defect is large, the sac is suspended over the child's abdomen and gravity is used to return the gut slowly to the abdominal cavity over 28 days or longer. The defect is closed surgically after all contents have been returned to the abdominal cavity. Even if the defect is small, immediate surgical repair may be done in several stages. If the condition is diagnosed prenatally, surgical delivery is recommended. Necrotic bowel may need to be removed surgically.	Same as for gastroschisis.	Most umbilical hernias disappear spontaneously by 1 yr. No surgical repair is necessary unless the hernia causes symptoms, persists past age 5 yr, becomes strangulated, or continues to grow.

GI, gastrointestinal; *NG,* nasogastric; *IV,* intravenous.

Continued

Sterile latix
free glove kid

TABLE 43-2 Developmental Gastrointestinal Defects—cont'd

Imperforate Anus	Gastroschisis	Omphalocele	Umbilical Hernia
NURSING CARE			
Report any skin dimples or the presence of stool in the urine or vagina.	Thermoregulation is critical because significant heat loss can occur through the exposed intestines. Use warmers, and monitor the child's temperature.	Same as for gastroschisis.	Binding is not effective in reducing or minimizing the bulge.
Determine anal patency if meconium is not passed in the first 24 hr after birth.	Use sterile technique in dealing with the defect. Immediately cover with warm, moist, sterile gauze; and wrap with plastic to keep moist.		Monitor for changes in size of hernia.
Assess for other GI or GU anomalies.	Minimize movement of the infant and handling of the intestines.		Assess for changing bowel sounds and an irreducible mass, which may indicate strangulation.
Facilitate bonding.	Assess for circulatory compromise, obstruction, sepsis: monitor temperature, pulses, capillary refill time, skin color, changes in respiratory patterns, heart rate.		
Provide appropriate postoperative care, including care of the colostomy.	Observe for respiratory distress secondary to high intraabdominal pressure as the gut returns to the peritoneal cavity.		
	Fluid-volume management is a crucial nursing responsibility: monitor intake and output and daily weights, assess fontanels, monitor electrolytes, maintain IV line.		
	Postoperatively, monitor and manage ileus, which commonly lasts for 2-4 wk: maintain NG tube for decompression, monitor bowel sounds and stools, measure abdominal girth.		
	Maintain parenteral nutrition to sustain growth.		
	Offer pacifier to meet sucking needs.		
	Provide emotional support for parents as they deal with the loss of the "perfect child."		
	Encourage parents to provide care as they are able, to talk to and touch infant, and to hold the infant, when appropriate.		

GU, genitourinary.

TABLE **43-2** Developmental Gastrointestinal Defects—cont'd

Imperforate Anus	Gastroschisis	Omphalocele	Umbilical Hernia
TEACHING AND HOME CARE			
Teach parents colostomy care. Demonstrate anal dilation (use only prescribed dilator, insert no more than 1-2 cm, and use a water-soluble lubricant). Refer parents for counseling and support: March of Dimes Birth Defects Foundation, (914) 428-7100, www.modimes.org. Provide guidance for toilet training.	Encourage parents to hold, cuddle, and bond with infants as soon as possible. Provide developmental stimulation for long-term hospitalization. Assist parents in dealing with feelings of guilt and disappointment. Use pictures to help parents understand the defect. Contact national support groups and community resources (March of Dimes). Teach parents signs of bowel obstruction: vomiting, pain, irritability, anorexia, firm abdomen. Provide follow-up from nutritional support personnel as needed.	Same as for gastroschisis.	Teach parents signs of strangulation: vomiting, pain, irreducible mass at umbilicus. Contact physician immediately if strangulation is suspected.

MOTILITY DISORDERS

Gastroesophageal Reflux

Gastroesophageal reflux (GER) is regurgitation of gastric contents back into the esophagus. GER is a normal physiologic phenomenon; all adults and infants experience reflux periodically, especially after meals. Reflux can be divided into three types: physiologic, functional, and pathologic (Box 43-1).

Etiology

Many factors contribute to the development of GER. Neurologic impairment, such as cerebral palsy, Down syndrome, and head injury, may affect the transmission of neural signals to the lower esophageal sphincter. Delayed gastric emptying of a liquid meal because of distention may also contribute. Partial or incomplete swallowing dysfunctions or drugs such as theophylline or caffeine can also trigger LES relaxations. Increased intraabdominal pressure incurred while straining, crying, coughing, or slumping tends to promote increased episodes of GER. These postural effects are most likely primary contributing factors in infants. Obesity and hiatal hernias also promote GER. Finally, during the first 6 months of life, the LES pressure undergoes maturational development. Because infants have a short abdominal LES, they experience GER more often. As the infant grows, the LES matures and the reflux improves. The prognosis is likely related to the severity of symptoms. Reflux from maturational causes will likely resolve by 1 to 2 years of age.

Incidence

Pathologic GER occurs in about 3% of all newborns. Boys are affected three times more than girls, and premature infants are affected more than full-term infants. Almost all

---

BOX 43-1
Types of Gastroesophageal Reflux

Physiologic
Infrequent emesis
Parents may not be concerned or may think it is normal
Rarely occurs during sleep

Functional
Painless, frequent emesis after meals
No failure to thrive
40% asymptomatic by 3 months
70% asymptomatic by 18 months
Medical management very effective

Pathologic
Failure to thrive
Aspiration pneumonia
Apnea, coughing, and choking
Frequent emesis, amount varies
Often requires surgery

Data from Mason, D. (2000). Gastroesophageal reflux in children: A guide for the advanced practice nurse. *Nursing Clinics of North America, 35*(1), 15-35.

---

infants with GER will have symptoms by age 6 weeks. In the absence of therapy, 2% to 5% will die of respiratory complications and 3% to 5% will develop significant esophageal scarring that will require medical and surgical management.

Pathophysiology

of Gastroesophageal Reflux

The lower esophageal sphincter (LES), a zone of tonically contracted smooth muscle surrounding the distal esophagus, is innervated by vagal nerves and receives signals from multiple organs. A defect in this neural control may result in a dysfunctional LES with periods of transitory spontaneous relaxation. These periods of relaxation allow gastric contents to reflux back into the esophagus.

In addition, the esophagus traverses both the abdominal and thoracic cavities, with the LES positioned strategically between the two. Most of the LES is abdominal. The greater the length of intraabdominal esophagus, the more competent this valve becomes. Any condition that shortens the abdominal segment of the LES will increase the likelihood of reflux.

Manifestations and Diagnostic Evaluation

Vomiting or spitting up after a meal, hiccupping, and recurrent otitis media related to pooled secretions in the nasopharynx during sleep are the hallmarks of all types of GER. In addition, the infant with pathologic GER can experience weight loss, failure to thrive, irritability, discomfort, and abdominal pain. Severe GER can result in hematemesis or melena and anemia. Frequently, respiratory illness is associated with GER, and the child may experience coughing, choking, wheezing, pneumonia, apnea, or bradycardia.

A variety of chronic and acute illnesses have been associated with GER. It is necessary to confirm the presence of GER only after other major conditions have been ruled out. Diagnostic tests include barium swallow examination, upper GI study, fiberoptic endoscopy, esophageal manometry, ambulatory pH studies, and gastroesophageal scintigraphy (radionuclide scan), ultrasound, and chest computed tomography (CT).

Therapeutic Management

Therapy for GER is based on the severity of symptoms and includes dietary alterations, positional changes, medications, and surgery. Many infants suspected of functional GER are treated conservatively, without time-consuming and costly diagnostic testing.

Diet. Small, frequent feedings of predigested formulas, such as Nutramigen or Pregestimil, will reduce the amount of formula in the stomach, decrease distention, and minimize reflux. These smaller, more frequent feedings with frequent burping are often tried as the first line of treatment. Feedings thickened with rice cereal may reduce episodes of emesis but do not affect reflux time. In fact, thickened feedings actually may increase the risk of GER by delaying gastric emptying time. However, thickened feedings do tend to decrease crying and the number of episodes of vomiting (Mason, 2000). Concentrated formulas and NG tube feedings provide nutritional supplementation for the child with failure to thrive. Caffeine and fatty foods lower LES pressure and should be eliminated.

Positioning. Much attention has been given to the best positioning for GER. Although prone positioning more effectively reduces reflux, current recommendations from the American Academy of Pediatrics and the North American Society for Pediatric Gastroenterology and Nutrition (Rudolph et al., 2001) are that infants younger than 12 months should be placed supine to sleep to reduce the risk of sudden infant death syndrome (SIDS), even if an infant is diagnosed with GER. The only exception to this recommendation would be if the risk of death from aspiration or other complications of GER greatly outweighed the increased risk from the prone positioning (Rudolph et al., 2001).

Medications. Although the Food and Drug Administration (FDA) has not approved most medications used in the treatment of GER for children, their use in children is quite common. Medications are not usually added to the treatment protocol until pathologic reflux has been determined (Mason, 2000). Antacids for symptom relief, H_2-receptor antagonists (e.g., cimetidine, ranitidine) to decrease acid secretion, mucosal protectants (e.g., sucralfate) for barrier protection, proton pump inhibitors (e.g., omeprazole) to suppress gastric acid secretion, and prokinetic agents (e.g., metoclopramide) to accelerate gastric emptying may be used.

Treatment of Acute Bleeding. Bleeding is a complication of long-standing GER and esophagitis. Stomach lavage (washing) via an NG tube is commonly performed to evacuate blood and blood clots during an episode of upper GI bleeding. The use of iced saline lavage to stop bleeding is no longer advocated. Radiologic procedures or surgery to coagulate bleeding vessels may be needed.

Surgery. Up to 15% of infants with GER will require fundoplication. A 270-degree to 360-degree wrap to the stomach fundus is made around the distal esophagus. This procedure tightens the LES and prevents gastric reflux. Gas bloat syndrome may develop because of the child's inability to burp, and a gastrostomy tube may be temporarily needed for gastric decompression.

Constipation and Encopresis

Constipation is the infrequent and difficult passage of dry, hard stools. A major concern with constipation is the development of encopresis, or fecal incontinence. Encopresis is repeated and involuntary defecation in a child older than 4 years who has normal colon and rectal anatomy. With encopresis, children often complain that soiling occurs without warning. Parents find the situation frustrating, and soiling often becomes a major issue between parent and child. Often encopresis causes children to feel ashamed or embarrassed, and they may avoid situations in which embarrassment might be heightened, such as spending the night with a friend or even going to school. If the condition persists over a long period, it usually affects the child's self-esteem and may impair social relations. Often, the parents experience guilt and shame or revulsion, disgust, or anger, and they may project these feelings onto the child.

Etiology and Incidence

Constipation can have many causes, such as changes in diet, dehydration, lack of exercise, emotional stress, certain drugs, pain from anal fissure, or excessive milk intake. If the child has no neurologic or anatomic disorders, encopresis is usually the result of recurrent fecal impaction and an enlarged rectum caused by chronic constipation. Factors predisposing to

Nursing Care Plan

The Infant With Gastroesophageal Reflux in the Community Setting

FOCUSED ASSESSMENT

Nursing assessment begins with a thorough history, including the amount and frequency of feedings, changes in formula, and position during feedings. The frequency and pattern of emesis should be recorded, including documentation of whether it is projectile, is painful, or contains blood. A medical history of frequent respiratory problems or pneumonia, apnea, choking, or cyanosis should be gathered. Observing the child during a feeding can provide critical information about choking, gagging, coughing, color change, and comfort during feeding.

Plot the child's length, weight, and head circumference on a growth chart. Assess the infant for *Sandifer's movements,* unusual postural habits that may be observed in infants with severe reflux-induced esophagitis. These typically irritable infants may demonstrate head cocking, arching, and arm thrashing. Drawing the head to one side may relieve pain by keeping gastric secretions from entering the esophagus or mouth. If a history of respiratory symptoms is present, assess the infant for abnormal breath sounds or retractions.

Assessment of the family should not be overlooked. Assessment should include observations of parent-child interactions and feeding styles and a discussion of feelings and concerns about the child who vomits frequently, is difficult to feed, and may have failure to thrive.

Nursing Diagnoses

Risk for Aspiration related to GER.
Impaired Swallowing related to esophagitis.
Acute Pain related to esophagitis.

Expected Outcomes

The infant will:
- Maintain a patent airway, without signs of aspiration or respiratory distress.
- Swallow effectively without choking, coughing, or cyanosis.
- Remain free from the discomfort of esophageal irritation, as evidenced by calm appearance, ability to sleep well, and participation in usual play activities.

The parents will:
- Demonstrate cardiopulmonary resuscitation (CPR).

INTERVENTION	RATIONALE
1. Provide continuous cardiac and/or apnea monitoring.	1. Monitoring reduces risk of silent apnea or respiratory distress.
2. Provide repeated instructions, written materials, home health visits, and emotional support in managing monitoring.	2. Parents of infants with gastroesophageal reflux (GER) may feel overwhelmed by doubt and anxiety over their ability to care for their child. This support can significantly increase their competency.
3. Train all caretakers in infant CPR.	3. Apnea is a serious complication of GER, and all caretakers must be able to provide support as needed.
4. Have parents keep a log of episodes of apnea, bradycardia, or color change.	4. Because this is a home care issue, accurate parental reporting is essential.
5. Position infant on right side after feeding, and minimize handling of infant after feedings. Position supine for sleeping.	5. Proper positioning reduces the risk of aspiration.
6. Encourage parents to offer pacifiers so that infant can "practice" swallowing.	6. Pacifier use decreases crying and reflux episodes and may increase clearance of refluxed stomach contents.

Evaluation

- Is the child's airway patent, without choking, coughing, cyanosis, or retractions?
- Have the parents and all caregivers demonstrated infant CPR?
- Can the child swallow without incurring respiratory distress?
- Is the child content and comfortable during feedings, able to sleep appropriately, and able to participate in usual play activities?

Continued

Nursing Care Plan

The Infant With Gastroesophageal Reflux in the Community Setting—cont'd

Nursing Diagnoses

Deficient Fluid Volume related to reflux of stomach contents.
Imbalanced Nutrition: Less Than Body Requirements related to anorexia, reflux, and dysphagia.

Expected Outcomes

The infant will:
- Retain feedings with regurgitation of less than 10 ml.
- Maintain and gain weight according to growth charts.

INTERVENTION	RATIONALE
1. Explain to parents that several different formula and feeding routines may need to be tried before success is found.	1. Frustration will be avoided if parents know that this may be a trial-and-error process with their infant.
2. Feed infant small, frequent feedings with predigested formulas or breast milk.	2. This reduces amount of formula or breast milk in stomach, decreases distention, and minimizes reflux.
3. Try thickened formula or breast milk by adding 1 to 3 teaspoons of rice cereal per ounce.	3. Thickened formula is more difficult to reflux high into the esophagus.
4. Show parents how to cross-cut nipples to improve feeding of thickened formulas. Several tries may be necessary to determine what works best for their infant.	4. Nipple holes must be enlarged, or baby will not be able to exert enough force to receive formula. Too large a hole can increase risk of aspiration.
5. Use thickened feedings only with infants who are not on solid foods. Give toddlers solids first, followed by liquids.	5. This decreases the chance of reflux or aspiration.
6. Eliminate chocolate and caffeine from the diets of older children. Offer alternative treats.	6. Caffeine relaxes the lower esophageal sphincter.
7. Help parents position infants properly after feedings. Side-lying is preferred. Older children should remain in an upright position, standing or sitting, while awake.	7. Proper positioning assists in preventing reflux.
8. Have parents keep a log of feeding successes and any reflux.	8. Success of interventions relies on accurate information from parents. A log eliminates the need to remember details.
9. Teach parents signs of dehydration: sunken fontanels, decreased number of wet diapers, no tears when crying. Have them call immediately if child becomes dehydrated.	9. Early detection is essential.

Evaluation

- Can the child retain feedings with regurgitations of less than 10 ml?
- Is the child growing according to growth charts?
- Is the child well-hydrated as evidenced by flat fontanels, good skin turgor, moist mucous membranes, and adequate urine output for age?

---

encopresis include inadequate or inconsistent toilet training or some type of psychologic stress, such as starting school or the birth of a sibling.

Constipation can affect any child at any time. Encopresis generally affects 3- to 7-year-olds with three to six times more boys than girls affected. The incidence of encopresis is higher in lower socioeconomic classes and among children with learning disabilities.

Manifestations

Constipation. The principal symptoms of constipation are absence of stool, abdominal pain and cramping without distention, and palpable, movable fecal masses with large amounts of stool in an enlarged rectum. The child may also experience diarrheal overflow; normal or decreased bowel sounds; malaise, anorexia, and headache; nausea and vomiting; or anal fissure.

Encopresis. Children with encopresis have evidence of soiled clothing and fecal odor without apparent awareness. Anal irritation leads to scratching or rubbing of the anal area. Social withdrawal and avoidance of extended contact with others (e.g., overnight stays, camp) are common. Children with constipation or encopresis often have a higher incidence of urinary tract infections and urinary incontinence than those without encopresis (Loening-Baucke, 1997).

Nursing Care Plan

The Infant With Gastroesophageal Reflux in the Community Setting—cont'd

Nursing Diagnoses

Deficient Knowledge related to unfamiliarity with the disease process, home care, and medications.

Anxiety (parental) related to special needs of infant and possible need for surgery.

Impaired Home Maintenance management related to complex, long-term care.

Expected Outcomes

The parents will:

- Explain GER and the reasons for diagnostic tests, medications, dietary changes, and surgery.
- Demonstrate effective coping mechanisms for dealing with the long-term consequences of GER.
- Express confidence in their ability to deal with their infant's special needs.

INTERVENTION	RATIONALE
1. Teach parents about each medication their child is taking, including mechanism of action, dosage, times, relationship to feedings, side effects.	1. Parent education is essential for appropriate home care.
2. Help parents rearrange mealtimes so that medications can be given correctly.	2. Some medications must be given in relation to meals to have maximum effect.
3. Encourage parents to continue medications for the full period and not to discontinue them if their child improves.	3. This is a long-term problem that may require several months to resolve. Esophagitis may be present after reflux has resolved.
4. Help parents modify positioning at home, using supplies that are readily available.	4. What works in the hospital may be difficult to achieve at home without special equipment. Parents will need support and suggestions to make these modifications work in their own homes.
5. Encourage parents to practice medication administration, positioning, feeding techniques, and assessment with supervision until they are confident in their abilities to provide total care for the infant.	5. Return demonstration and positive reinforcement can significantly increase compliance at home and decrease parental anxiety.
6. Allow and encourage parents to share their concerns and worries.	6. This decreases anxiety.
7. Provide community referral as needed.	7. Support and continued communication with other parents and children experiencing the same stresses can increase coping.

Evaluation

- Is the child receiving medications as prescribed at the correct times and in the correct dosage?
- Can the parents explain GER and the reasons for positioning and dietary modifications?
- Have the parents assumed all care responsibilities?
- Do the parents demonstrate correct feeding techniques?
- Have the parents expressed their concerns and feelings related to caring for their child?
- Are the parents demonstrating confidence in their abilities to care for the many needs of their child?

Diagnostic Evaluation

Abdominal radiographs may demonstrate an enlarged rectum with large amounts of stool and gas. The definitive diagnostic procedure is a rectal examination. This is rarely performed because of its emotional impact on the child and the possibility of pain from anal fissure. A thorough history is usually sufficient for the diagnosis.

Therapeutic Management

The best form of treatment is preventing development of the chronic problem through appropriate diet, exercise, and regular toileting habits. Education about "normal" bowel function can prevent a psychogenic component from compounding the problem. The focus of management is to remove the impaction, retrain the rectum to be aware of when it is full, and help the child overcome the pain-retention cycle.

Treatment usually involves three phases:

1. Disimpaction:
   a. Enemas until impaction is cleared; use Fleet, 1 oz/5 kg; if the child is over 20 kg, use an adult size
   b. Stool softener or laxative
2. Maintenance:
   a. Mineral oil, 2 ml/kg b.i.d., up to 180 to 240 ml/day for children older than 1 year; the dosage is adjusted de-

Pathophysiology
of Constipation and Encopresis

When stool passes into the rectum, distention of the walls stimulates mass peristaltic movements in the bowel. This process is called the *defecation reflex*. If defecation is not desired, the external sphincter contracts and voluntary retention of stool occurs. As the stool remains in the rectum, the rectum relaxes and the defecation reflex wanes. Water reabsorption from the colon continues, resulting in hard, dry stool that is difficult to pass. The eventual passage of that stool may result in pain or anal fissures. If retention of stool continues, more fissures may develop or become worse, so that eventually even soft stool may produce pain. A cycle of pain develops whereby the stool is retained to avoid pain but the retention leads to even more difficult defecation. Over time, the rectum becomes enlarged. An enlarged rectum can result in failure to control the external sphincter, which in turn results in encopresis.

pending on results achieved. Mineral oil may be contraindicated in children who resist taking it or who vomit frequently after it is taken; aspiration of mineral oil can lead to aspiration pneumonia in these children (Coughlin, 2003).

  b. Lactulose (10 g/15 ml), 1 or 2 ml/kg b.i.d or milk of magnesia (according to physician direction) for children older than 6 months and younger than 1 year.

  c. Dietary changes, including limiting milk intake, increasing water intake, and increasing residue

3. Changing the retention habit:

  a. Sitting on the commode for 5 to 10 minutes approximately 20 to 30 minutes after meals

  b. Keeping a behavioral chart with positive rewards (daily stars may be helpful)

  c. Avoiding negative reinforcement

  d. Biofeedback may be a useful tool to reteach the feeling of rectal fullness

The goal is for the child to pass two or three soft stools per day without pain within the first month. Medications are withdrawn slowly over 3 to 6 months after the fear of pain has been lost.

For infant constipation, rectal stimulation is discouraged. For example, rectal thermometers and glycerin suppositories should not be used. Barley cereal can be substituted for rice cereal. Fructose, such as prune juice, or lactulose can help. High-fiber fruits and vegetables will also decrease constipation.

■ NURSING CARE
The Child With Constipation or Encopresis

Assessment

Obtain a thorough history of the soiling events, including frequency, intensity, and duration. Because parent-child relationships are often strained, it is often helpful to interview the parents and child separately to reduce the child's embarrassment. The nurse can explain to parents that a medical history and examination will be performed to rule out organic causes of the chronic constipation, such as Hirschsprung's disease.

Nursing Diagnosis and Planning

The nursing diagnoses and expected outcomes that may be appropriate after assessing for constipation or encopresis in the child are

- Constipation or Bowel Incontinence related to inconsistent patterns of elimination, anxiety, or pain during elimination.
  Expected Outcome: The child will have normal bowel function, as evidenced by the passage of soft stools without pain or incontinence, maintenance of a well-balanced diet high in fiber and sufficient fluid intake, and decreased reliance on laxatives.
- Compromised or Disabled Family Coping related to persistent stress, guilt, and embarrassment about the child's elimination difficulty.
  Expected Outcomes: The family will function effectively as a unit, openly discuss problems, and develop a plan to achieve control over incontinence.
- Social Isolation related to embarrassment, peer teasing, and odor from bowel incontinence.
  Expected Outcomes: The child will verbalize positive, realistic feelings about self and verbalize appropriate ways to achieve control over bowel incontinence.
- Impaired Skin Integrity related to poor hygiene in anal area, bowel incontinence, and lack of knowledge.
  Expected Outcome: The child will maintain skin integrity, as evidenced by clean, intact skin.

Interventions

Because constipation and encopresis represent a continuum of the same problem, a variety of approaches can be tried as needed to deal with the problem. Simple constipation may resolve with only dietary changes or changing a habit of retention. Severe encopresis may require that all interventions be continued for 3 to 6 months.

Overcoming Withholding

Before bowel retraining can begin, the child's bowel must be evacuated of all hard stool and impactions. This goal is best accomplished with the use of appropriate-size Fleet or isotonic enemas every 12 hours until the impaction is cleared, usually within 48 hours. Teach parents to administer enemas at home. During this time, the child should be monitored for hypernatremia or hyperphosphatemia, which could result from repeated use of Fleet enemas (see Chapter 37 for a discussion of enema administration).

After bowel cleansing has been achieved, the child older than 1 year may be started on mineral oil (Abel, 2001). Lactulose or milk of magnesia may be used in infants at least 6 months old but younger than 12 months. Mineral oil is best tolerated when it is given chilled or mixed with cold drinks. Mixing the oil with ice cream or chocolate milk, blending it with ice cubes and fruit juice, or chilling it helps to disguise the taste. It is not unusual for the child to leak oil when dosages are high, and parents and children need to be aware that leakage does not constitute encopresis. At the end of this intervention, the child should be passing soft stool without pain or incontinence.

Dietary Changes

Dietary modifications are used as a part of the treatment. Increasing water and fiber intake by offering granola bars, dried fruits, whole-grain cereals, and fresh vegetables with low-fat dip can increase the bulk in stool and make it easier to pass. Decreasing sugar and milk intake will also help keep stools soft. Advise supplementing with fat-soluble vitamins when mineral oil is being used because the oil can theoretically interfere with vitamin absorption in the small intestine.

Changing the Retention Habit

To help reestablish a normal bowel habit, the child should sit on the toilet for 5 to 10 minutes after breakfast and dinner. This routine will allow the normal gastrocolic reflex to assist with defecation and will eliminate the need to be involved with retraining during school hours. Star charts and small prizes may be helpful in rewarding success. These interventions are continued for at least 3 to 6 months, during which the rectum will resume its normal size and the child will relearn to attend to the defecation reflex. If fecal impaction occurs at any time, enemas are again administered and the dosage of mineral oil is adjusted.

Emotional Support

Allow the child and parents to express their feelings of success and failure with the ongoing program. To minimize the damage to the child's self-esteem, encourage self-care as much as possible. To decrease embarrassment, it is helpful for school-age children to have a complete change of pants and underwear at school, should leakage or an accident occur. Age-appropriate support groups may be available in a center with a large population or encopresis clinic.

Teaching is a major intervention. Encouraging the child and parents to share feelings of embarrassment is equally important. Allow the child to verbalize any concerns, and provide developmentally appropriate anatomic information to assist with understanding the etiology of the problem. Using drawings and books may be an effective way to begin this sharing of feelings and information. Relieving the child of shame and embarrassment may improve cooperation with the plan of care.

Home Care

Because this condition is managed at home, teaching parents is a critical intervention. The parents need to understand the correct way to administer enemas (see Chapter 37). They also need support in implementing and documenting the child's successes and setbacks. The child and parents need encouragement to continue, even when the successes seem few. This problem develops over time and takes time, patience, and perseverance to resolve.

Evaluation

- Is the child passing soft stools without pain?
- Does the food diary indicate a well-balanced, high-fiber diet?
- Is the child experiencing any incontinence?
- Are enemas, laxatives, or mineral oil still needed?

- Is the child experiencing success with bowel control as a result of implementation of a family-designed plan?
- Does the child more readily participate in age-appropriate activities and express increasing control over bowel incontinence?
- Is the skin in the anal area clean and intact?

Irritable Bowel Syndrome

Irritable bowel syndrome (IBS) is the result of increased intestinal motility, which can lead to spasm and pain.

Etiology and Incidence

Stress and emotional factors are thought to be the most common causes of this disorder. Theoretically, an abnormality in the autonomic nervous system accounts for the changes in motility and secretion, but this hypothesis has not been adequately proven (Carlson, 1998). In infants, it may be related to a lactase deficiency. It is not associated with any psychopathology.

Irritable bowel syndrome occurs after infancy and is most common in toddlers (in whom it is sometimes called *chronic nonspecific diarrhea of childhood*) and adolescents. The condition tends to occur in families with a history of other bowel disturbances or infantile colic. The condition tends to resolve by late adolescence but is sometimes present in adults.

Manifestations and Diagnostic Evaluation

Manifestations of irritable bowel syndrome include diffuse abdominal pain unrelated to meals or activity; alternating constipation and diarrhea, with undigested food and mucus present in the stool; and normal growth.

The diagnosis is based on the elimination of major GI pathologic conditions, including Crohn's disease, giardiasis, lactose intolerance, and genitourinary abnormalities. Abdominal ultrasound, stool for ova and parasites (O&P) and cultures, abdominal radiography, and a complete gynecologic assessment are often ordered.

Therapeutic Management and Nursing Considerations

There is no definitive treatment for this poorly understood functional bowel problem. Management is aimed at decreasing symptoms. The primary nursing intervention should be reassurance that it is a self-limiting, intermittent problem.

Unless lactose intolerance is suspected, no dietary modifications are required other than the maintenance of a healthy,

---

Pathophysiology

of Irritable Bowel Syndrome

The precipitating factors in irritable bowel syndrome are unknown but result in two distinct problems. The first is *disorganized contractility*, which causes spasmodic peristaltic rushes and lulls. This disorganization causes alternating diarrhea and constipation with intermittent abdominal pain. The second component is *excess mucus production in the lumen of the bowel*. This produces maldigestion and the passage of incompletely digested food and nutrients.

well-balanced, moderate-fiber diet. Encourage the child to eat slowly and not to drink carbonated beverages. Because carbohydrate malabsorption from fruit juice may also trigger symptoms in some children, eliminating juice or changing from apple to white grape can help eliminate symptoms (Moukarzel, Lezicka, & Ament, 2002).

Medications are not usually used in the treatment but pH dependent, enteric-coated peppermint oil capsules have been used successfully in initial trials to reduce IBS pain (Kline, Kline, DiPalma, & Barbero, 2001).

Family and psychosocial assessment may reveal a family that is worried about a serious life-threatening disease and is very focused on the bowel habits of the child. The family may not be reassured by the normal findings on a physical and developmental examination.

The primary nursing interventions are teaching and reassurance. Health promotion activities, such as exercise, balanced nutrition, and school activities, have the best influence on the disease. Because of the associated psychosocial component, referral to mental health and family counseling services can be effective in cases that are unresponsive to other measures. The child and family will express feelings and concerns that will assist in evaluating the interventions.

INFLAMMATORY AND INFECTIOUS DISORDERS

Ulcers

A peptic ulcer is an area of sharply circumscribed loss of the mucosa, submucosa, or muscular tissue occurring in areas of the digestive tract exposed to acid and pepsin. Peptic ulcers can be primary or secondary, gastric or duodenal. Primary, or idiopathic, ulcers occur in the absence of underlying systemic disease. Secondary, or stress, ulcers are acute and are found in conjunction with other illnesses, such as shock, respiratory failure, sepsis, hypoglycemia, severe burns, or intracranial lesions.

Gastric ulcers occur in the stomach, particularly the gastric antrum, and are uncommon in childhood. Duodenal ulcers occur in the pylorus or duodenum, are often chronic, frequently lead to complications, and are the most commonly encountered ulcers in children.

Etiology

Known factors that can alter the mucus-bicarbonate barrier in children include:

- *Excessive acid secretion:* Zollinger-Ellison syndrome or gastrinoma may cause excess acid secretion and multiple ulcers. Hyperparathyroidism may also contribute to increased acid secretion.
- *Bile salts:* Bile breaks down the adherent mucous structure of the gastric-duodenal lining and exposes the mucosa to acid.
- *Lack of prostaglandins:* Prostaglandins augment both the mucous gel lining and bicarbonate secretion. Deficiencies in mucosal prostaglandins may cause impairment of the mucus-bicarbonate barrier.
- *Genetic factors:* Duodenal ulcers show a familial tendency. This, together with environmental factors, may predispose children to ulcer formation. An association between ulcer activity and type O blood has also been noted.

- *Bacteria: Helicobacter pylori* is a gram-negative spiral bacterium that has been identified in the gastric antrum of children with duodenal ulcer. It infects most adults with ulcer disease and acts by weakening the gastric mucosal barrier and allowing acid and peptic digestion of the susceptible mucosa.
- *Psychological factors:* The importance of psychological factors is questionable. They likely influence exacerbations or complications but not initial ulcer activity.
- *Stress:* Stress accounts for at least 80% of secondary ulcers encountered during infancy and early childhood. They tend to be acute and occur in seriously ill children.
- *Diet:* Diet does not seem to influence the development of ulcer disease in children. Although certain foods may cause indigestion, no convincing data show that dietary factors cause, perpetuate, or reactivate ulcers, especially duodenal. Colas, teas, and chocolate do, however, increase acid secretions and may be contributing factors.
- *Medications:* Many medications, such as aspirin, nonsteroidal antiinflammatory agents, and indomethacin, as well as tobacco and alcohol, are known to adversely affect the gastroduodenal mucosa in adults but appear to have little importance in pediatric ulcer disease.

Incidence

The true incidence of peptic ulcer disease in children is unknown because ulcers often spontaneously heal before a diagnosis is made. The average age for ulcer activity is 11 to 12 years, with boys affected two to three times more than are girls. Duodenal ulcers occur more frequently in children older than 6 years. *H. pylori* gastritis has been found in 90% to 100% of children with duodenal ulcers (Wyllie, 2004). Stress ulcers account for 80% of ulcers occurring during infancy and early childhood, affect both genders, and are equally distributed between the stomach and duodenum.

Manifestations and Diagnostic Evaluation

Manifestations of ulcer disease in children are burning, cramping pain when the stomach is empty; awakening during the night or early morning complaining of abdominal discomfort; and vomiting in children younger than 6 years. Hematemesis and melena are common in infants and young children.

Fiberoptic upper endoscopy is the diagnostic tool of choice for all children, including neonates. Endoscopy not only provides direct visual observation of the lining of the esophagus, stomach, and proximal duodenum but also is a

Pathophysiology

of Ulcers

A thick mucus-bicarbonate barrier, a layer of mucus that provides a buffer zone for acid neutralization, lines the stomach and duodenum. Stomach acids diffuse slowly through this layer toward the gastric wall but are encountered and neutralized by slowly diffusing bicarbonate ions liberated from surface epithelial cells. The establishment of a neutral pH at the gastric epithelial surface provides protection from the combined effects of acid and pepsin. Ulcers result when any imbalance in the process occurs and erosions develop on the surface of the gastric or duodenal mucosa.

PARENTS
Want to Know

About Care of the Child With an Ulcer

Parents need to understand the pathophysiology, causes, diagnosis, and therapeutic management of ulcers. When explaining these to the parent and older child, follow these guidelines:

- Emphasize the relationship of the ulcer to acute illness.
- Help the older child identify sources of excess stress that can be modified.
- Teach stress reduction activities, such as relaxation and exercise, and refer parents to support groups.

Directions for administering medications include:

- Do not administer antacids within 1 hour of other anti-ulcer medications.
- Do not stop medications when symptoms improve; continue for the full prescribed course.
- Do not use aspirin or other nonsteroidal antiinflammatory drugs, because they may cause bleeding.
- Do not use over-the-counter medications without your physician's knowledge.

- Do not add other drugs, because your child's metabolism and absorption may be altered by ulcer medications.

Help parents make changes in diet as prescribed by teaching the following:

- If your child has a poor appetite, provide a well-balanced diet with many choices.
- Seek assistance from dietary services as needed.
- Provide meals and snacks every 2 to 3 hours.
- Make sure your child avoids coffee, chocolate, and caffeine and any other foods that might cause discomfort.

Instruct parents to call their physician if their child experiences any of the following problems:

- "Coffee grounds" vomitus
- Weight loss
- Tarry stools
- Increased pain
- Diarrhea
- Vomiting

---

means for obtaining biopsy or culture material. Ultrasound may be performed to rule out gallstones, tumors, or mechanical obstruction. The fecal occult blood test may be done to check for GI bleeding.

Therapeutic Management

Medical management is the most common treatment for ulcer disease in children. Factors considered in ulcer treatment include drug safety, symptom relief, patient and parent compliance, and the prevention of complications or ulcer recurrence. A bland diet with milk and small, frequent feedings was long thought to be the mainstay of ulcer therapy. It has been shown, however, that the protein and calcium in milk actually stimulate more acid secretions than they buffer. A regular diet low in caffeine is now generally prescribed because caffeine is a potent stimulant of acid secretion and exacerbates GER. A diet high in fiber and polyunsaturated oils may also play a role in ulcer prevention.

Medications are now considered the first line of treatment. They include antibiotics, antacids, H_2-receptor antagonists, and mucosa-protective agents. Vaccines to prevent *H. pylori* infections are currently under development.

Surgery is indicated for the management of ulcer complications, such as hemorrhage, perforation, or obstruction. Vagotomy, pyloroplasty, ligation of a bleeding vessel, or closure of a perforation may be performed.

If the child is actively bleeding, an NG tube is inserted to remove blood, decompress the stomach, and estimate blood loss. IV fluids, oxygen, blood replacement, and vasoactive drugs, such as vasopressin (Pitressin), may be given. Balloon tamponade with a Sengstaken-Blakemore tube may be indicated. Blood or clots are removed with room-temperature gastric lavage. The use of iced saline lavage to stop GI bleeding is no longer advocated because it increases bleeding and clotting times and prolongs the prothrombin time. It also imposes a risk of hypothermia on an already compromised child.

The long-term prognosis for children diagnosed with peptic ulcer disease remains controversial. Marked improvement in symptoms, however, is noted with the use of H_2-receptor blockers and other medications. Without adequate treatment, peptic ulcer disease frequently persists into adult life.

Nursing Considerations

Nursing assessment of the child with peptic ulcer disease begins with a thorough history, including a family history of ulcer disease, past episodes of abdominal pain, or recent stressful events in the home, school, or community. A complete assessment of pain includes a description of the nature of the pain and its location; its relationship to meals, defecation, or voiding; episodes of nocturnal pain; and medications used to effectively relieve the pain. The child is examined for the presence of epigastric tenderness, nausea, vomiting, abdominal distention, hematemesis, melena, or recent changes in appetite or eating habits.

All stools and emesis fluid should be checked for the presence of blood. Bowel sounds are auscultated for 5 minutes. If vomiting is present, the child is assessed for signs of dehydration. If bleeding is observed, the child is monitored for changes in vital signs and the physician is notified immediately. Finally, the nurse assesses family members for their understanding of the disease, the presence of a viable support system, and their ability to participate in their child's care.

Providing Information. The major focus of nursing interventions is teaching. The nurse reviews pathophysiology, medication administration, and diet and assesses for complications.

Preparing the child for diagnostic tests also is an important nursing intervention. Because fiberoptic endoscopy is often performed, the child must be prepared for conscious sedation. Keeping the child on NPO status for at least 6 hours, maintaining an IV line, and monitoring vital signs and respiratory function during the procedure are nursing responsibilities. Upper GI examinations and ultrasonography may also be performed.

Home Care. Ulcers are managed almost exclusively in the home environment, so teaching, follow-up, and home health referral are essential. The correct use of medications and dietary modifications are parental responsibilities that may require educational materials, emotional support, help with time organization, and encouragement to continue even when symptoms are relieved.

Infectious Gastroenteritis

Infectious gastroenteritis is caused by a group of viruses, bacteria, and parasites capable of causing serious communicable diarrhea, massive fluid and electrolyte loss, sepsis, and death (for further discussion of fluid and electrolyte alterations, see Chapter 42).

Etiology

Ingestion of contaminated food or water and person-to-person contamination are the most frequent causes of infectious gastroenteritis in the United States. High-risk groups include children in daycare centers, preschools, and long-term care facilities and those infected with the human immunodeficiency virus (HIV). *Giardia* is the most common pathogen seen in children in daycare settings, and rotavirus is the most common GI pathogen seen in infants and young children (Cohen & Laney, 1999; Wald, 1999). In most cases the pathogen is not identified (Table 43-3).

Incidence

Gastroenteritis is one of the most common outpatient infectious diseases in children. In children younger than 5 years in the United States, more than 20 million cases of diarrhea occur each year. Infections peak in the summer and have an equal gender distribution. Despite the usually self-limiting nature of the condition, each year approximately 300 to 400 children in the United States and more than 4 million worldwide die from GI illness (Cohen & Laney, 1999).

Pathophysiology

of Infectious Gastroenteritis

As the pathogen adheres to the mucosa of the intestine, it is no longer affected by peristaltic waves and is not removed from the site. Epithelial invasion occurs, causing an inflammatory response and epithelial cell death. This leads to ulcerations, pseudomembranes, bleeding, and possibly sepsis. As the pathogens multiply, they may produce toxins. Enterotoxins (e.g., cholera, *Shigella*) cause fluid and electrolyte shifts that result in increased secretion into the intestine and simultaneous decrease in absorption secondary to edema. The absorptive capacity of the colon is exceeded, and massive diarrhea and dehydration result. Cytotoxins (e.g., *Salmonella*) produce local edema, malabsorption, and dehydration. Some pathogens are also capable of producing neurotoxins (e.g., *Shigella*) that act outside the gastrointestinal (GI) tract.

Manifestations

Gastroenteritis will likely manifest with diarrhea of varying amount and consistency, vomiting, and abdominal pain. In addition, the child might experience tenesmus and fever. Dehydration is a severe consequence of gastroenteritis and occurs mainly in children younger than 2 years. A history of travel to other regions of the world can provide clues to the causative organism.

Diagnostic Evaluation

A definitive diagnosis can be made when a rectal or stool culture yields a pathogen, but these cultures are expensive and result in many false-negative findings. Ova and parasites are more reliably found. Usually only children who appear to be in a toxic condition or have bloody stools, abdominal pain, or tenesmus undergo a diagnostic work-up. The presence of white blood cells (WBCs) and blood in the stool can support the presumptive diagnosis based on clinical findings. Blood cultures may also be needed in the acutely ill infant and young child. An unprepared sigmoidoscopy can be useful in determining the amount of mucosal involvement, in obtaining more reliable samples for culture, and in the diagnosis of the disease.

Therapeutic Management

The priority therapy is to replace water and correct acid-base or fluid and electrolyte disturbances with IV fluids or oral (PO) electrolyte replacement liquids. The rate of replacement may be as high as 50 to 100 ml/kg over 4 to 6 hours (1 to 2½ times maintenance requirements). Because diarrheal fluid is high in sodium, potassium, and bicarbonate, oral rehydration solutions should be used to match losses (see Chapter 42). Hospitalization for treatment is not uncommon, especially for the infant or small child, to allow for continued assessment and management of symptoms or sepsis. Antimicrobial therapy is useful in cases of infection with *Shigella* and *Giardia*, and in some cases of infection with *Salmonella, Clostridium difficile,* and *Escherichia coli* but not for rotavirus infection. Rotavirus immunization is still undergoing study because of complications associated with the vaccine.

▪NURSING CARE
The Child With Infectious Gastroenteritis

Assessment

Obtain an adequate history of the event, including the length of symptoms, the frequency and consistency of stools, and the presence of blood or mucus in stools. Noting the amount, color, consistency, and time (ACCT) of each stool or episode of vomiting is a consistent way to document findings. The concurrent appearance of symptoms in other members of the family can be helpful in the diagnosis. Any travel to other countries or wilderness areas should be recorded. Evaluating formula and food preparation at home and in daycare facilities as well as examining sanitation and hygiene in these places can provide valuable information.

The child may appear moderately to severely dehydrated with hyperactive bowel sounds and severe diarrhea, which is

TABLE 43-3 Characteristics of Infectious Gastroenteritis

Infectious Agent	Characteristics	Clinical Manifestations	Diagnostic Findings	Treatment
Shigella (enteroinvasive with cytotoxin)	Incubation period 1-7 days Most common in summer Fecal-oral spread Remains communicable for 1-3 wk	Symptoms last 5-10 days Diarrhea begins as watery, progresses to small, bloody, with mucus Severe abdominal pain High fever Neurologic symptoms (headache, nuchal rigidity, convulsions) Risk for sepsis, hemolytic uremic syndrome, rectal prolapse, DIC	Blood, mucus, WBCs in stool Positive culture in some cases	Bactrim, 8-10 mg/kg/day × 5 days, OR Ampicillin, 50-100 mg/kg/day × 5 days Contact Precautions Identify source if possible
Salmonella (enteroinvasive)	Incubation 6 hr to 3 days Most common in summer, fall Usually food-borne Infectious for duration of illness and variable period afterward	Symptoms last 2-5 days Rapid onset Secretory diarrhea Abdominal pain, nausea, vomiting common	Blood and PMNs in stool	For infants younger than 12 wk, same as for *Shigella* Contact Precautions Identify source if possible
Escherichia coli (enteroinvasive with enterotoxin)	Variable incubation Most common in summer Food-borne most common	Green, watery, secretory diarrhea May cause hemorrhagic colitis Fever	Blood and PMNs in stool	Same as for *Shigella* Contact Precautions
Campylobacter	Incubation 1-8 days Most common in infants and adolescents	History of consumption of contaminated shellfish Severe abdominal pain Foul-smelling, watery diarrhea	Blood and PMNs in stool	Possibly treated with erythromycin for 7 days Contact Precautions
Giardia lamblia	Most common cause of parasitic diarrhea Spread in water	Afebrile Abdominal distention, flatulence Variable diarrhea	Ova and parasites found in stool but no blood or PMNs Parasites found on duodenal biopsy	Metronidazole (Flagyl) for 7 days Contact Precautions Treat all unknown water sources with chlorine/iodine before drinking
Rotavirus	Incubation 1-3 days Common in winter months Accounts for 50% of cases of acute diarrhea in children	Symptoms usually last 2-6 days History of preceding or concurrent respiratory illness	Virus in stool detected by enzyme immunoassay	No pharmacologic treatment Contact Precautions
Clostridium difficile	Antibiotic-associated Most common nosocomial diarrhea	Fever for 24-48 hr Diarrhea develops after antibiotic treatment	Blood and PMNs in stool	Cholestyramine used to enhance mucosal recovery and decrease length of diarrhea Possibly treated with vancomycin or metronidazole (Flagyl) for 10 days

WBCs, White blood cells, *DIC,* disseminated intravascular coagulation; *PMNs,* polymorphonuclear leukocytes.

often bloody. Blood in the stool usually appears after the maximum fluid loss has occurred and can be useful in determining the stage of illness. The presence of abdominal pain, vomiting, tenesmus, and fever should be assessed. Headache, nuchal rigidity, irritability, and seizures are important symptoms of the neurotoxic effects of *Shigella*.

Assessment of hydration status is critical. Poor urine output, high urine specific gravity, poor skin turgor, dry mucous membranes, crying without producing tears, a sunken or depressed fontanel in infants, and skin tenting can occur quickly with the large amount of fluid lost through diarrhea. Loss of bicarbonate from severe diarrhea and dehydration makes metabolic acidosis a major concern. The compensatory mechanisms of increased respiratory rate and effort are important to document.

Nursing Diagnosis and Planning

The nursing diagnoses and expected outcomes that may be appropriate for the infant or child with gastroenteritis are

- Deficient Fluid Volume related to severe diarrhea.
  Expected Outcomes: The child will be adequately hydrated without electrolyte disturbance, as evidenced by moist mucous membranes; good skin turgor; urine output appropriate for age; return to normal weight; and normal serum sodium, potassium, and bicarbonate levels; and the child will have soft, formed stools without diarrhea, blood, or mucus.
- Risk for Infection related to exposure of family members and others to infectious agents.
  Expected Outcome: The child will not transmit pathogens to others.
- Acute Pain related to hyperactive motility.
  Expected Outcome: The child will be free from abdominal pain, as evidenced by a return to normal activity and no complaints of pain.
- Deficient Knowledge related to inadequate information about the disease and its control.
  Expected Outcomes: The parents will describe how to prevent transmitting the condition to others and will use Standard and Contact Precautions when handling the child's excretions.
- Imbalanced Nutrition: Less Than Body Requirements related to malabsorption.
  Expected Outcomes: The child will resume a normal diet and will regain weight lost during the acute phase within 1 week after symptoms abate.
- Risk for Impaired Skin Integrity related to skin contact with feces and the necessity for frequent cleansing.
  Expected Outcome: The child will maintain skin integrity, as evidenced by clean, dry, intact skin without redness, drainage, or breakdown.

Interventions

Maintaining Fluid Balance

Critical nursing interventions are related to the fluid volume deficit. Oral or parenteral rehydration with correction of acid-base imbalances is essential to establish homeostasis. Accurate intake and output and weight measurements are important. Monitoring skin turgor, urine output, and serum electrolyte levels will provide evaluation criteria in this area (see Chapter 42 for a further discussion of fluid and electrolyte alterations).

Decreasing Risk

Providing safety, assessing neurologic symptoms, and monitoring for seizures are also priorities for the child with *Shigella* infection. Preventing the spread of infection remains a critical nursing intervention. Thorough handwashing is a must. Contact Precautions must be strictly enforced for all staff and family members to minimize the risk of infection. These precautions must be maintained at home for up to 2 weeks or for less time if antibiotics are given. Pain and fever may be treated with acetaminophen, but symptomatic treatment with antidiarrheals is not recommended because it tends to increase the length of symptoms. Symptomatic care of the febrile child includes tepid sponging and light dressing.

Parents and children will need to be taught these interventions and given information about the disease process during this period. Depending on the organism causing the gastroenteritis, follow-up by the public health department may be necessary. Organisms such as *Salmonella* and *E. coli* can be found in food and present a significant public health concern. A dietary recall for possibly contaminated foods can be important in establishing the cause and minimizing the risk of spread to the public.

Home Care

The most important intervention that can be implemented at home is proper rehydration to prevent the need for hospitalization and IV therapy (see Chapter 42 for a discussion of oral rehydration fluids and care for the child with diarrhea). After rehydration has been successful and symptoms have subsided, feeding should resume.

Dietary changes for vomiting and diarrhea may not be necessary if the child does not demonstrate dehydration. Breast milk may be offered as needed, and formula should be given full strength. Oral rehydration therapy (ORT) may also be used. Rehydration with ORT solution should begin with 100 ml/kg over 4 hours and 10 ml/kg given to replace each stool (Larson, 2000). These are not well tolerated by small children, but adding sugar should not be encouraged. Vomiting does not prevent oral rehydration because the child can be successfully rehydrated with 5 to 10 ml of rehydrating solution every 2 minutes. When diet is continued, fats and high sugar concentrations should be avoided. Complex carbohydrates, starches, lean meats, and vegetables should be encouraged.

Children who demonstrate mild or moderate dehydration may require ORT at a rate of 50 to 100 ml/kg over 4 to 6 hours in addition to replacement of 10 ml/kg per stool. Regular diet may be resumed as just described once the fluid deficit has been corrected. Severe dehydration may require parenteral therapy and hospitalization.

Preventing the spread of infection is also essential for home care. Good handwashing; the disinfection of contaminated linens, clothes, and diapers; and the use of surface disinfectant sprays are important preventive measures.

Evaluation

- Has the child returned to pre-infection weight within 1 week after symptoms subside?
- Does the child have good skin turgor, moist mucous membranes, and a urine specific gravity of less than 1.030?
- Does the child have a serum sodium level of 138 to 145 mmol/L and a serum potassium level of 3.5 to 5 mmol/L?

PARENTS
Want to Know

About Care of the Child With Infectious Gastroenteritis

If your child has infectious gastroenteritis, you must:

- Wash your hands frequently and thoroughly, and insist that your child do so as well. Always wash your hands after changing diapers.
- Allow your child to use a separate bathroom if available.
- Continue to follow these measures for several weeks because bacterial diarrhea may be communicable for several weeks after symptoms disappear.
- Administer oral fluids using appropriate rehydration solutions (e.g., Rehydralyte) in small, frequent amounts (every 30 min). If your child is vomiting, administer 1 teaspoon of fluid every 5 to 10 minutes. Give ½ cup for each watery stool.
- Do not give your child fruit juices, cola, sports drinks, tea, or Kool-Aid.
- Continue to feed your child but avoid high-fat or high-sugar foods. Breast milk and formula may be continued.
- Do not give over-the-counter medications without notifying your physician.

Call your physician if:

- Your child is younger than 6 months.
- Your child has a fever.
- Diarrhea worsens.
- Diarrhea has blood in it.
- Vomiting increases, or your child cannot keep down any fluid.
- Your child complains of severe abdominal pain.
- Your child shows signs of dehydration, such as no tears, sunken eyes, or decreased urination.

Pathophysiology

of Appendicitis

Obstruction of the appendix allows normal mucus secretions to accumulate in the appendix, producing distention. Distention eventually causes occlusion of the capillaries and engorgement of the walls of the appendix. Microabscesses form and can progress to abscesses and fistulas. Perforation occurs as a result of tissue breakdown and swelling. Bowel contents then contaminate the mesenteric bed and peritoneum, leading to peritonitis and sepsis.

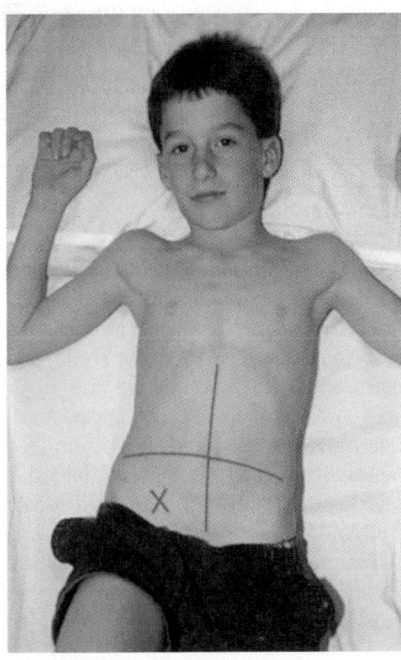

Figure 43-4 McBurney's point is midway between the right anterior superior iliac crest and the umbilicus. It is usually the location of greatest pain in the child with appendicitis. (Courtesy The University of Texas at Arlington School of Nursing.)

- Is the child passing soft, formed stools without diarrhea, blood, or mucus?
- Are other family members free from infectious diarrhea, and is the family following the appropriate precautions to prevent transmission?
- Is the child complaining of abdominal pain?
- Does the child guard the abdomen during palpation?
- Are parents and staff at the daycare facility practicing infection control procedures, if appropriate?
- Can the child tolerate an age-appropriate regular diet?
- Is the child's skin intact and free from irritated areas?

Appendicitis

Appendicitis is the inflammation and infection of the vermiform appendix, a small lymphoid, tubular, blind sac at the end of the cecum. It is the most common cause of emergency surgery in children and adolescents.

Etiology and Incidence

Common causes of obstruction and subsequent appendicitis include lymphoid swelling related to viral infection, impacted fecal material, foreign bodies, and parasites. In most cases no definitive cause can be identified at the time of surgery.

Appendicitis occurs with equal frequency in both genders, with most cases occurring during adolescence and early adulthood. Annually, approximately 80,000 children in the United States undergo surgery to remove the appendix (Mattei, Stevenson, & Ziegler, 1999). Appendicitis is uncommon in children younger than 4 years, but in young children it is associated with a very high frequency of perforation, most likely related to the difficulty in establishing the diagnosis. In more than 70% of children younger than 2 years, the appendix will have perforated by the time of the initial visit (Pena, Taylor, & Lund, 2000).

Manifestations and Diagnostic Evaluation

The cardinal symptom of appendicitis is pain, progressing in intensity and localizing to the right lower quadrant at McBurney's point (Fig. 43-4). Associated signs and symptoms include nausea and vomiting, anorexia, diarrhea or constipation, and fever and chills. If the appendix perforates, the child will initially experience relief of pain. Other signs and symptoms will worsen, so that the child will appear acutely ill with high fever and signs of dehydration.

The diagnosis is usually based on the classic abdominal findings of pain localizing at McBurney's point, guarding, rebound tenderness, nausea, vomiting, and fever. A WBC count of 15,000 to 20,000/mm^3 can support the clinical findings. A quick, safe, and accurate diagnosis can usually be made with ultrasound, which shows an enlarged, incompressible appendix that may be fluid-filled and locally inflamed. CT of the abdomen is considered the most accurate radiologic study when used with contrast in the rectum. However, it is usually reserved for those cases that are more difficult to diagnose (Pena, Taylor, & Lund, 2000).

Therapeutic Management

The definitive treatment for appendicitis and suspected appendicitis is appendectomy. Preoperatively the child is managed with fluid therapy, immobilization to control pain, NPO status, and antibiotics. The procedure may be done laparoscopically or through an open abdominal approach if perforation is suspected.

■ NURSING CARE

The Child With Appendicitis

Assessment

The nursing assessment will reveal a history of pain, fever, vomiting, and diarrhea or constipation. The physical examination discloses abdominal tenderness and guarding. The child may assume a supine position with the right leg flexed to decrease tension on the abdominal wall. The nurse must be keenly aware of the symptoms of perforation, including a sudden relief from pain followed by an increase in pain, rigid abdomen, and early shock symptoms. Behavioral changes and refusal to eat are important indicators in infants.

Assess anxiety in the child and family members, who are most likely facing unexpected surgery. Because of the pain, the child may be uncooperative with abdominal assessment.

The parents may have financial concerns related to the unplanned surgery.

Nursing Diagnosis and Planning

The nursing diagnoses and expected outcomes that may be appropriate after assessing the child with appendicitis are

- Acute Pain related to abdominal inflammation and surgical incision.
  Expected Outcome: The child will be free from pain, as evidenced by resumption of normal activity and movement with no complaints of pain.
- Risk for Infection related to rupture and surgery.
  Expected Outcomes: The child will have a clean, dry surgical incision that is free from redness, heat, or exudate, and the child will be afebrile with a WBC count of 5,000 to 15,000/mm^3.
- Deficient Fluid Volume related to vomiting or diarrhea.
  Expected Outcome: The child will be well hydrated, as evidenced by moist mucous membranes, good skin turgor, and hourly urine output appropriate for age (see Chapter 42).
- Anxiety related to unplanned surgery.
  Expected Outcomes: The parent or child will express feelings about surgery and will verbalize the need for emergency hospitalization.

Interventions

Uncomplicated Appendicitis

On admission, vital signs should be taken to monitor for sepsis or shock. Institute comfort measures, including topical cold application, pain medications, and encouraging positions of comfort. Enemas or laxatives should not be administered. No heat should be applied to the abdomen because it may increase the chance of perforation secondary to vasodilation. IV fluid therapy is started to prepare the child for surgery and correct any existing acid-base disturbance related to vomiting and diarrhea.

If the procedure is performed by laparoscopy, the nurse can expect the child to be discharged within 24 hours. Open surgery may be followed by several days of recovery in the hospital. After either operation, the child will be on NPO status until bowel function has returned.

Ruptured Appendix

The child with a ruptured appendix needs special care (Fig. 43-5). If perforation is suspected, prepare the child for NG tube insertion. The NG tube provides decompression before surgery and allows gastric content drainage postoperatively. The child will need IV antibiotics, which may be started preoperatively. For the child with a perforation, IV antibiotics are continued and hospitalization may last 5 to 14 days. During this time and after the NG tube is removed, the diet should be advanced gradually as tolerated so that the child can tolerate a normal diet without vomiting or diarrhea.

Depending on the extent of the peritonitis, the child is likely to have postoperative incisional drains. These drains may be attached to suction, and aseptic technique and maintenance of patency are essential. Carefully document the drainage amount each shift. The wound is often left open and treated with sterile wet-to-dry (saline-soaked gauze) dressings and wound irrigation with antibacterial solutions.

APPENDECTOMY-PERFORATED
(Uncomplicated-without multi-system problems)
ICD-9 Codes 540.0 and 540.1

Expected LOS-5 Days
D#.#=Key interventions for this study.

Examples of appropriate Co-morbidities
Otitis Media
Acute Sinusitis
Pharyngitis
chronic illness not in active stage

Examples of Co-morbidities that are not appropriate:
HIV
Pneumonia
Sickle Cell
Hemophilia
Immuno-compromised patients
cardiac patients
reflux
oncology diagnoses

Refer to Variance Sheet for Recording

Aspect of Care	Admission Day	Day 2	Day 3	Day 4	Day 5
	Date__ Unit __ ED/OR ____	Date__Unit __	Date__Unit __	Date__Unit __	Date__Unit __
DAILY OUTCOME			Ambulating	NG tube out	Afebrile Discharge *(D 7.1 If not d/c by Day 7. record on tracking sheet)*
TESTS	CBC BUN, Cr Sonogram (if ind)	BUN,Cr		CBC (+/-)	CBC (+/-)
CONSULTS	Surgeon		Consider Home Health		
FLUID/ELECTROLYTE MANAGEMENT	Strict I&O	Strict I&O	Routine I&O	Routine I&O	Routine I&O
TREATMENTS/ PROCEDURES	Appendectomy NG Irrigation Wound Care	NG Irrigation Wound Care	NG Irrigation Wound Care	Wound Care	Wound Care
MEDICATIONS	IV (pump, site check) *D1.1 Gentamicin w/ Clindamycin q 8 hrs. +/-Ampicillin q 6 hrs +/- Mefoxin q 6 hrs.* Methadone or morphine for pain.	IV (pump, site check) *D2.1 Gentamicin w/ Clindamycin q 8 hrs. +/-Ampicillin q 6 hrs +/- Mefoxin q 6 hrs.* Methadone or morphine for pain.	IV (pump, site check) *D3.1 Gentamicin w/ Clindamycin q 8 hrs. +/-Ampicillin q 6 hrs +/- Mefoxin q 6 hrs.* Methadone or morphine for pain.	IV (pump, site check) *D4.1 Gentamicin w/ Clindamycin q 8 hrs. +/-Ampicillin q 6 hrs +/- Mefoxin q 6 hrs.* Methadone or morphine for pain.	Hep lock *D5.1 Gentamicin w/ Clindamycin q 8 hrs. +/-Ampicillin q 6 hrs +/- Mefoxin q 6 hrs.* Methadone or morphine for pain Analgesics p.o. if tol.
CLINICAL SUPPORT	NPO Parent Support Bed/Chair Extra Patient Checks Routine Safety	NPO Parent Support Chair Routine Safety	NPO Parent Support Ambulate Routine Safety	NPO/Cl liq (+/-) Parent Support Ambulate Routine Safety	Full liq/Regular Parent Support Ambulate Routine Safety Pain Control Wound Care Activity Follow-up Visit

Original 7/22/1994   Revised 11/2/1995 5/1/97

Disclaimer: This clinical pathway is provided as a general guideline for use by physicians and staff in planning the care and treatment of patients and their families. **It is not intended to be and does not establish a standard of care.** Each patient's care is individualized according to specific needs.

Cook Children's Medical Center
M:\WPFILES\PATHWAYS\APPYPERF.WPD

This pathway is not a permanent part of the patient's medical record.

Figure 43-5 Clinical pathway for a child undergoing an appendectomy. (Courtesy Cook Children's Medical Center, Fort Worth, TX.)

Round-the-clock opioid analgesics provide relief from incisional pain and from pain caused by frequent dressing changes (see Chapters 38 and 39). Continued reassessment of abdominal pain is essential for evaluating the presence of abscess or fistula.

Monitor vital signs, including temperature, every 2 to 4 hours. NG suction will likely be continued postoperatively until normal bowel sounds return. Positioning the child to facilitate drainage and minimize the spread of infection into the upper abdomen should be done by elevating the head of the bed or having the child lie on the operative side.

Home Care

After surgery and discharge, parents must be prepared to assume responsibility for the child's care. The surgical incision and any drain sites must be assessed for redness, drainage, dehiscence, or suture infections. Report any problems to the physician. Parents should advance the child's diet slowly, beginning with liquids and soft foods and progressing to the child's normal diet if tolerated without nausea or vomiting. Teach parents to watch for vomiting, abdominal pain, or distention as possible signs of bowel obstruction or peritoneal infection.

Evaluation

- Does the child complain of pain?
- Does the child demonstrate guarding on abdominal palpation?
- Has the child returned to normal activity level?
- Is the surgical incision clean, dry, and free from redness, heat, purulent drainage, or dehiscence?
- Is the child afebrile, with a WBC count of 5,000 to 15,000/mm^3?
- Is the child tolerating an age-appropriate regular diet without vomiting, diarrhea, or increased abdominal pain?
- Are the child and parents able to express relief from anxiety?

Inflammatory Bowel Disease

Inflammatory bowel disease is a chronic inflammatory condition of the small or large intestine. It includes two distinct conditions: ulcerative colitis and Crohn's disease. Ulcerative colitis affects only the colon and involves both the mucosal and submucosal layers of the intestine. Crohn's disease can occur anywhere in the GI tract, from the mouth to the anus, and is transmural, involving all layers of the intestine.

Pathophysiology

of Inflammatory Bowel Disease

The triggering factor, whether viral, allergic, or immunologic, causes the bowel to "respond" as if to an injury and results in capillary vasoconstriction and histamine release within the bowel. The histamine has two effects on the bowel. The first is *vasodilation,* which results in swelling that can cause malabsorption by distorting the surface area of the villi. Swelling then produces cell death and ulceration, which can progress to the development of fissures, strictures, fistulas, adhesions, and bowel obstruction. The second effect of histamine release is *increased capillary permeability,* which results in increased fluid in the intestine and subsequent diarrhea. Crohn's disease affects all layers of the bowel; ulcerative colitis affects the mucosa and submucosa only.

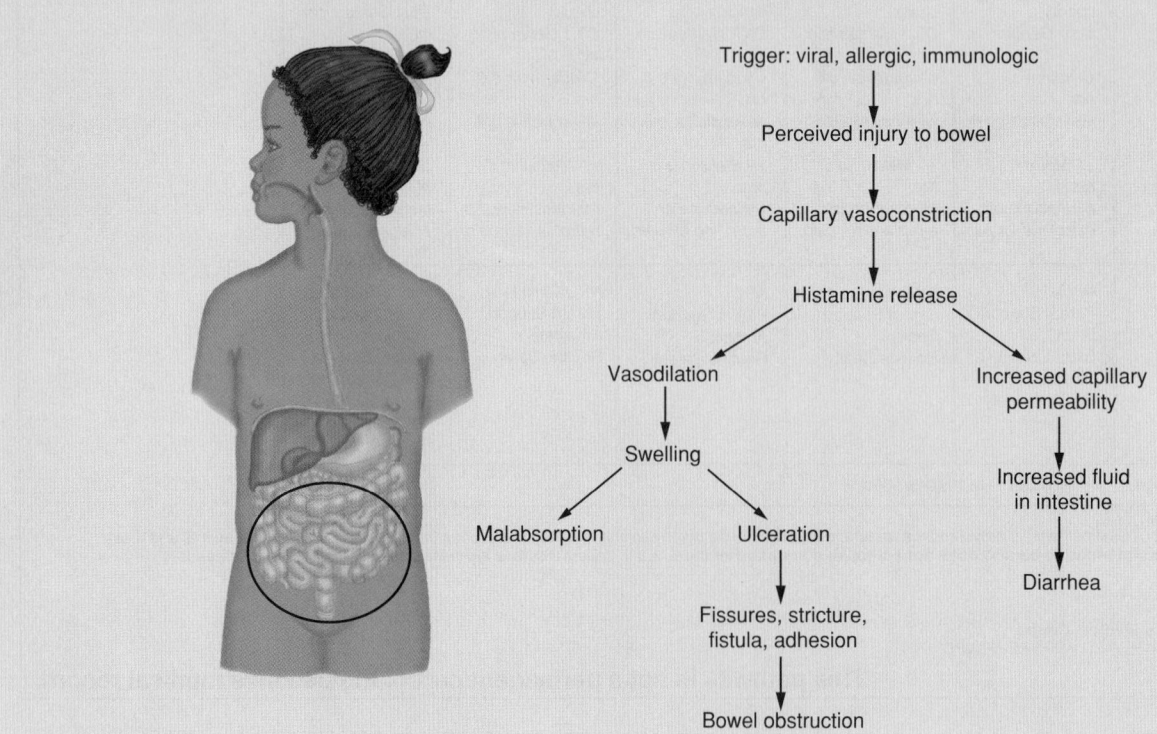

Etiology

The exact cause of inflammatory bowel disease is not known. Several triggers have been identified, including viral and other infectious agents, food allergies, vasculitis, increased intestinal permeability, immunologic dysfunction, and genetic factors. Increasing evidence demonstrates a connection between an individual with inflammatory bowel disease in a stressed state generating an immune response that affects the disease outcome (Anton, 1999).

Incidence, Manifestations, and Diagnostic Evaluation

The incidence, manifestations, and diagnostic evaluation for both ulcerative colitis and Crohn's disease are summarized in Table 43-4.

Therapeutic Management

Management for inflammatory bowel disease is multidimensional and includes medication, dietary and nutritional support, and symptomatic treatment. Pharmacologic treatment includes antiinflammatory, antibacterial, antibiotic, and immunosuppressive drugs. The principal medications used to treat inflammatory bowel disease include:

- 5-Aminosalicylic acid (5-ASA) medications, such as sulfasalazine
- Corticosteroids, such as prednisone
- Immune modulating agents, such as azathioprine, 6-mercaptopurine (6-MP), methotrexate, and cyclosporin A

- Monoclonal antibodies, such as infliximab
- Antibiotics, such as metronidazole (Flagyl) and ciprofloxacin

Monoclonal antibodies are a new approach in these diseases. Infliximab (Remicade) has been approved for treatment of Crohn's disease. It binds to tumor necrosis factor–alpha to decrease inflammation and increase intestinal healing.

5-ASA and 6-MP are first-line immunosuppressants that allow selected patients with Crohn's disease to avoid steroids and their side effects (Aranda & Horgan, 1998).

For ulcerative colitis, avoidance of milk products and ingestion of a hypoallergenic, low-fiber, low-fat, low-residue, high-protein, elemental diet can be useful. Elemental diets may be as useful as corticosteroids in inducing remission in children (Rayhorn & Rayhorn, 2002). These diets may include Tolerex, Vivonex, Peptamen, or Modulen. Nutritional therapy is a useful component with no side effects. Total parenteral nutrition (TPN) may be needed during acute flareups or surgery to maintain nutritional support. Total colectomy is the only true cure.

Crohn's disease is best managed before permanent structural changes have developed. Malnutrition is a common problem and can involve protein, fat, carbohydrate, and vitamin deficiencies. Nutritional support and teaching are essential. Surgery is not curative but may be necessary to treat abscesses, fistulas, or chronic recurrent obstruction. Bowel resection is the usual procedure.

TABLE 43-4 Crohn's Disease and Ulcerative Colitis

	Crohn's Disease	Ulcerative Colitis
Pathophysiology	Affects entire gastrointestinal (GI) tract, most common in the terminal ileum	Involves only colon, starting at the rectum and moving upward
	Transmural involvement	Mucosa and submucosa only
	Cobblestone appearance of mucosa	Mucosa lacking in most cases
	Fistulas common	Fistulas rare
	Remissions and exacerbations	Remissions uncommon
Diagnostic evaluation: colonoscopy, rectoscopy, barium enema, biopsy	"Skip" lesions with deep fissures and granulomas	Continuous spreading with superficial ulceration
	Normal	No normal mucous membrane
Incidence	5 per 100,000 and increasing	5 per 100,000
	Equal gender distribution	Equal gender distribution
	Not seen in infants; peaks in teens, early 20s	Peaks between ages 15 and 40 yr
	Clusters in families	Clusters in families
	Associated with higher standard of living	Affects whites more than others
Clinical manifestations	Abdominal pain	Abdominal pain unusual
	Diarrhea, nonbloody	Diarrhea, occasionally with hemorrhage and anemia
	Fever	No masses
	Palpable abdominal mass	Moderate weight loss
	Anorexia and severe weight loss	Mild growth impairment
	Significant growth impairment	Perianal and anal lesions rare
	Perianal and anal lesions	Fistulas and obstructions rare
	Fistulas and obstructions	Risk of toxic megacolon
	Extraintestinal symptoms (arthralgia, arthritis)	
Morbidity and mortality	Life expectancy not reduced	12%-15% mortality
	50%-70% will eventually require surgery for obstruction or fistula	10% chance of cancer after 10 yr
	Surgery does not cure disease	Removal of colon cures intestinal disease

■ NURSING CARE
The Child With Inflammatory Bowel Disease

Assessment

Recurrent or chronic diarrhea is the primary finding in the nursing history of a child with inflammatory bowel disease. The major assessment findings are related to this diarrhea and the associated malabsorption that occurs. Weight loss, dehydration, anorexia, growth failure, vitamin deficiencies, and anemia are common. The severity of the GI symptoms and the amount and length of steroid use will have a significant influence on a child's growth rate. Remissions and exacerbations of symptoms are common. Frank bleeding is possible in ulcerative colitis. Intermittent cramping discomfort exacerbated by eating is common in Crohn's disease. The child with Crohn's disease may complain of oral lesions and perianal skin breakdown.

Inflammatory changes also can occur outside the GI system. Arthralgia and arthritis, especially of the lower extremities, can cause discomfort and mobility problems.

Depression, anxiety, fears about social interactions, and low self-esteem occur and are most likely related to the need to have quick access to restrooms at all times and to be close to home should an accident occur. The chronic nature of this condition and its unknown prognosis can lead to family stress and tax the family's financial resources and support systems. Assessment should include questions about family and peer support, resources, and knowledge about the disease.

Nursing Diagnosis and Planning

The nursing diagnoses and expected outcomes that may be appropriate for the child with inflammatory bowel disease and for the child's family are

- Imbalanced Nutrition: Less Than Body Requirements related to chronic malabsorption.
  Expected Outcomes: The child will have acceptable bowel patterns, as evidenced by passing no more than four stools per day and being free from nocturnal diarrhea; and the child will receive adequate nutrition, as evidenced by normal hemoglobin values and normal growth that follows the growth curve.
- Acute Pain related to cramping.
  Expected Outcome: The child will be free from abdominal pain, as evidenced by resumption of normal activity and no complaints of pain.
- Chronic Low Self-Esteem related to chronic diarrhea and colostomy.
  Expected Outcome: The child will have a positive self-concept, as evidenced by leading an active lifestyle without depression.
- Delayed Growth and Development related to malnutrition, chronic illness, and steroid use.
  Expected Outcome: The child will meet normal developmental milestones, as evidenced by progress on standard developmental screenings.
- Disturbed Body Image related to weight loss, water retention from steroid therapy, and colostomy or ileostomy.
  Expected Outcome: The child will state reasons for changes in body appearance and will share concerns about changes with family and support personnel.

- Anxiety related to chronic diarrhea and risk for surgery.
  Expected Outcomes: The child will express concerns about the future and will contact support services as needed.
- Deficient Knowledge related to management of chronic disease.
  Expected Outcomes: The child will explain day-to-day management of disease and will demonstrate ability for self-care that is age-appropriate.

Interventions

Nursing interventions focus on maintaining pharmacologic interventions, developing long-term nutritional management, educating, and providing emotional support.

Medications

Teaching appropriate administration of medications is an important nursing role. Enemas are used before critical diagnostic tests and as a method of medication administration. Any child who will be taking steroids (see Chapter 41) needs to understand the importance of regular administration. Steroids should be given with food or antacids if GI distress becomes a problem. The steroids, although beneficial in suppressing symptoms, may actually exacerbate the growth delays associated with inflammatory bowel disease.

Nutritional Management

Nutritional support varies with the disease and the child's tolerance of changes. In general, maintaining a low-fiber, low-residue, low-fat, milk-free elemental diet provides some relief, although strict restrictions do not alleviate symptoms. A balanced, nutritious diet is recommended, as are vitamin, iron, and folate supplements.

During acute flare-ups or surgery, TPN and lipids may be needed to restore a seriously malnourished child. These interventions do not change the course of the inflammation in the bowel but will provide essential nutritional support. Elemental diets, which can be absorbed without significant digestion, may be used during acute episodes of Crohn's disease to allow the bowel to rest. NG or gastrostomy tube feedings during the night may be necessary during puberty to prevent further growth impairment (see Chapter 37).

Continued assessments of nutritional status, growth patterns, and development are important elements of nursing care for children with this chronic problem. Assessing the number of stools, nutritional status, weight, developmental milestones, and pain will help in evaluating the child's response to treatment.

Family Education and Support

Appropriate community resources can provide education and support. The Crohn's and Colitis Foundation of America will supply educational materials and give the child and family information on local resources and support groups (see Appendix I on Evolve website). Long-term nursing care can be improved by providing consistent caregivers and encouraging the child to form relationships. Self-care and management should be major goals in working with children with inflammatory bowel disease, as with other chronic diseases.

The parents and child will be assuming responsibility for home care. Because Crohn's disease is a long-term health problem with numerous medical, pharmacologic, and surgical interventions required, family support and financial resources can be strained to the limit. National and local support groups may be able to give essential support to the family in these areas. In addition, emotional support for caregivers becomes very important.

Another important resource for children with inflammatory bowel disease is Camp MAGIC, Inc. MAGIC stands for Many Adventures at GI Camp. They can be contacted at the following address: Camp MAGIC, Children's Medical Center of Dallas, 1935 Motor Street, Dallas, TX 75235.

Home Care

Home care is a mainstay of treatment. Teaching parents to administer steroids, including providing information on their inherent side effects and the importance of not discontinuing their use abruptly, should be a high priority. Also teach techniques of enema administration and skin care for perianal lesions. Keeping nutrition diaries can provide useful information. TPN may be administered at home, and parents need complete instructions.

In addition, helping children and parents know when to seek care is important. Sudden exacerbations of symptoms, weight loss, blood loss, and severe abdominal pain should be reported to health care professionals. Stress management, such as exercise, may increase the quality of life and may help modulate the disease (Anton, 1999).

Evaluation

- Is the child free from nocturnal diarrhea?
- Is the child passing fewer than four stools per day?
- Is the child gaining weight appropriately and following the growth chart?
- Is the child's hemoglobin value between 11 g/dl and 16 g/dl?
- Does the child complain of abdominal pain?
- Does the child participate in age-appropriate activities without evidence of depression?
- Is the child's development normal for age?
- Is the child able to share body image concerns with appropriate family members?
- Has the child or family sought external support through appropriate referral groups?
- Do the child and parent demonstrate appropriate skills for day-to-day management and make appropriate future plans for long-term management of disease?
- Do the child and family seek help when exacerbations occur?
- Does the child manage self-care as age-appropriate?

OBSTRUCTIVE DISORDERS

Hypertrophic Pyloric Stenosis

Pyloric stenosis results when the circular area of muscle surrounding the pylorus hypertrophies and obstructs gastric emptying. This condition is one of the most common surgical disorders of early infancy.

Etiology and Incidence

The exact cause of pyloric stenosis remains unknown, but muscular hypertrophy is not present at birth. Pyloric stenosis may be associated with other GI anomalies, such as malrota-

tion, short-gut syndrome, esophageal and duodenal atresia, anorectal anomalies, hiatal hernia, and GER. Heredity and family predisposition seem to increase the risk of pyloric stenosis.

The incidence of pyloric stenosis is 3 in 1000 births. First-born children and offspring of an affected parent are at highest risk. Males are affected five times more often than females, and full-term infants are affected more often than premature infants (Phillips, 1999). The incidence is also higher in white infants than in African-American or Asian infants.

Manifestations

Progressive projectile, non-bilious vomiting in a previously healthy infant is the major manifestation of pyloric stenosis. The vomitus may become blood-tinged if esophageal irritation occurs. A movable, palpable, firm, olive-shaped mass is felt in the right upper quadrant. This mass is most easily palpated when the stomach is empty and the infant is relaxed. Deep gastric peristaltic waves from left upper quadrant to right upper quadrant may be visible immediately before vomiting. The infant will be irritable and hungry a short time after being fed. If the condition progresses, the infant may become dehydrated and experience metabolic alkalosis.

Diagnostic Evaluation

The diagnosis is based on a history of vomiting, visible peristaltic waves, and a palpable pyloric mass. When the mass cannot be palpated, radiography and ultrasonography are helpful. A flat plate of the abdomen will show a narrow pylorus with a dilated stomach and the absence of gas distal to the pylorus. Ultrasonography can confirm the presence of a pyloric mass. A barium swallow examination will disclose the long, narrow pyloric canal and detect delayed gastric emptying. Laboratory findings may indicate metabolic alkalosis as a result of vomiting, including decreased serum potassium and sodium levels, increased pH and bicarbonate, and a decreased chloride level. Indirect bilirubin may be elevated.

Therapeutic Management

Because pyloric stenosis is usually diagnosed early, few infants are seen in advanced stages of dehydration, malnutrition, and alkalosis. If present, these conditions must be corrected before surgery. An infant who is slightly dehydrated with a total serum or plasma carbon dioxide (CO_2) of 25 mEq/L or less or an infant who is moderately dehydrated with a CO_2 of 26 to 35 mEq/L is managed with replacement parenteral fluids and electrolytes and an NG tube for stomach decompression. Once the stomach is empty, most infants will stop vomiting. Surgery is usually delayed 24 to 48 hours until fluid and electrolyte deficits and the acid-base balance are corrected. Severely dehydrated and malnourished infants with CO_2 levels above 35 mEq/L may need a 3- to 5-day course of IV fluids, electrolyte replacement, and infusions of plasma or packed red blood cells (RBCs) before surgical repair.

It is universally agreed that a *pyloromyotomy*, an incision of the pyloric muscle to release the obstruction, is the definitive treatment. Pyloromyotomy is not considered an emergency procedure but is usually performed without delay in well-hydrated infants.

Pathophysiology

of Hypertrophic Pyloric Stenosis

Pyloric spasms cause milk curds to be propelled against a narrowed pyloric channel and subsequently irritate its sensitive mucosal lining. Edema of the pyloric mucosa results. This edema further reduces the size of the pyloric canal and creates resistance to the flow of milk. To promote gastric emptying and compensate for this resistance, the pylorus contracts with more force and gradually enlarges. This enlarged pyloric muscle slowly begins to constrict the pyloric channel, and when the mucosal edema subsides, the resistance to flow still remains. A vicious cycle develops and progresses to a high-level obstruction of the pyloric canal.

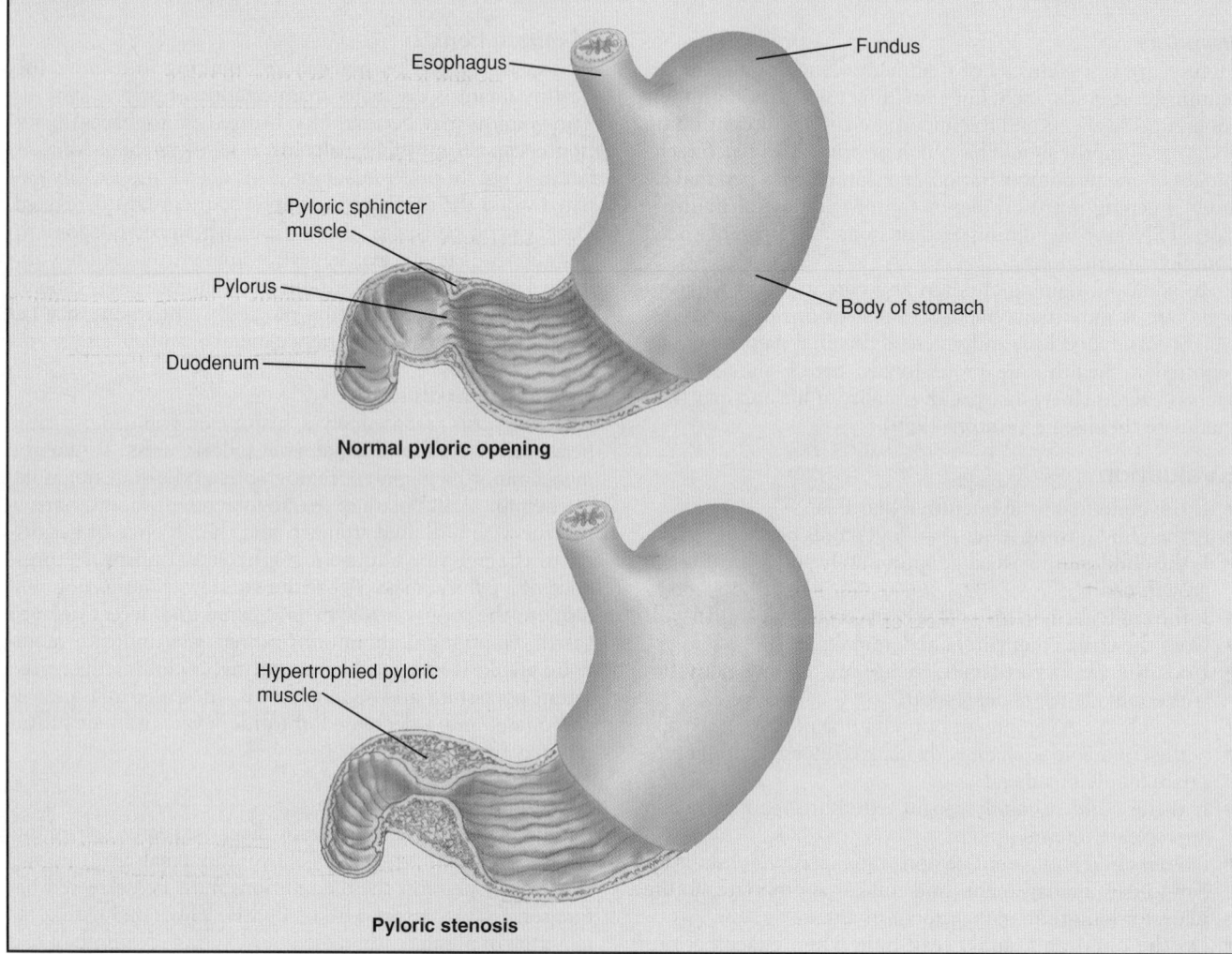

Normal pyloric opening

Pyloric stenosis

■ NURSING CARE

The Child With Hypertrophic Pyloric Stenosis

Assessment

Hypertrophic pyloric stenosis is suspected in infants who present with a history of projectile vomiting, especially after meals. A thorough nursing history includes the infant's feeding schedule with the type, amount, and frequency of fluid taken. Determine and document the relationship of feedings to vomiting. Vomiting is assessed for frequency, amount, color, and consistency, as well as projection.

Assess for signs of dehydration, such as the absence of tears, a weak cry, a depressed fontanel, poor skin turgor, and dry mucous membranes. Signs of potassium, sodium, and chloride depletion should be noted. The abdomen is checked for distention, tenderness, bowel sounds, the presence of a pyloric mass, or gastric peristaltic waves. Assess family members for their understanding of the disorder, a viable support system, and the ability to participate in their child's care.

Nursing Diagnosis and Planning

The nursing diagnoses and expected outcomes that are appropriate after assessment of the child with hypertrophic pyloric stenosis are

■ Deficient Fluid Volume related to vomiting.

　Expected Outcomes: The infant will have a balanced intake and output, be free of signs of dehydration, and have a urine output greater than 2 to 3 ml/kg/hr.

Gathering Information From a Parent About Infant Vomiting

Eliciting a description of the amount and characteristics of vomiting can be difficult because descriptive terms are non-specific and estimation of amounts is very inconsistent. Useful questions might include:
- Could you wipe the vomitus off the child with a diaper or cloth?
- Did it require a change of clothes for the infant or caregiver?
- If it was on a bed or sheet, how big a circle did it make?
- If it was on the floor, how big a circle did it make?
- Did it happen after every feeding?
- Did it look like what was just eaten, or was it curdled?
- What color was it?
- Did it appear to be under force and projected away from the child?

Encouraging the parents to keep a written record of answers to these questions can provide essential assessment information.

- Imbalanced Nutrition: Less Than Body Requirements related to persistent vomiting.
   Expected Outcomes: The infant will tolerate regular feedings and will continue to show growth according to a growth chart.
- Impaired Skin Integrity and Risk for Infection related to a surgical incision.
   Expected Outcome: The infant will have a clean, dry, intact incision without redness or exudate.
- Deficient Knowledge related to insufficient information about the need for surgery or about pyloric stenosis.
   Expected Outcomes: The parents will describe pyloric stenosis and the expected preoperative and postoperative care and will assume total care of the infant before discharge.
- Acute Pain related to surgery.
   Expected Outcomes: The child will not exhibit guarding to palpation and will be calm and content in parent's arms. The parent will be confident that the infant is pain-free.
- Anxiety (parental) related to need for hospitalization and surgery.
   Expected Outcomes: The parent will express feelings about the surgery and will list the reasons the infant needs to be hospitalized.

Interventions

Preoperative Care

Preoperatively, the infant is on NPO status and is stabilized with IV fluids and electrolytes. Measuring the vital signs, weighing the infant daily, and monitoring laboratory values and intake and output are essential nursing interventions. Intake and output should include all IV and PO fluids, blood products, emesis, urine output, stools, and NG drainage. Keep the dehydrated infant warm and quiet. The nurse should provide oral care because membranes are more susceptible to breakdown in their dehydrated state.

Elevate the head of the bed to reduce the risk of aspiration. Use blankets or towel rolls to maintain desired position.

The NG tube should be patent and properly positioned. Record the amount, color, and type of drainage. Assess for respiratory distress.

Explain procedures and plans to parents. Encourage their participation in holding and caring for their infant.

Postoperative Care

Postoperatively, the care varies with each surgeon. Most surgeons remove the NG tube immediately and order feedings within the first 4 to 6 hours after surgery if bowel sounds are normal. Because gastric peristalsis is normally depressed for 12 to 18 hours after the pyloromyotomy, others delay feedings for 24 hours and leave the NG tube in place.

Feeding is started with small amounts of an oral electrolyte solution, such as Pedialyte, and the amount is slowly increased. Formula is offered in half-strength concentrations and advanced to full strength within 48 hours after surgery. If the child is receiving breast milk, dilution is not necessary. Feedings are not advanced until the child can tolerate the previous amount without vomiting. IV fluids are continued until the infant is taking and retaining sufficient amounts of formula or breast milk. Many infants experience some vomiting during the early postoperative periods, but vomiting is usually temporary and without complications.

Ad lib feedings within 6 hours postoperatively are now being recommended to decrease time to full diet and discharge, but these protocols vary within institutions (Morash, 2002).

Postoperative nursing care follows the same guidelines as preoperative care, with accurate monitoring of all vital signs, laboratory values, respiratory problems, and hydration. In addition, the nurse assesses the small surgical incision for redness, swelling, or drainage. Encourage parents to participate as much as possible in their infant's care, but they may need emotional support in the unfamiliar environment of the hospital.

Home Care

Because symptoms normally abate in the immediate postoperative period, parents may find taking care of their infant much easier than it had been before repair. They need to be instructed, however, to report any excessive vomiting, abdominal tenderness, fever, incisional redness, or drainage. If the child is discharged before the diet has been advanced to full strength, written instructions for advancing the diet are essential.

Evaluation

- Does the child have a flat fontanel, good skin turgor, moist mucous membranes, a urine specific gravity of less than 1.030, and a sodium level within normal limits?
- Is the child tolerating oral feedings without vomiting?
- Has the child's weight returned to pre-illness level within 1 week?
- Is the surgical site clean, dry, intact, and without drainage or redness?
- Can the parents explain the need for surgery and routine preoperative and postoperative care?
- Is the child calm, content, and free from pain?
- Have the parents assumed all care responsibilities at home without assistance?

Andrew, age 5 weeks, is seen in the outpatient clinic of a large hospital. This is his first visit to the clinic since birth. Andrew's mother states that Andrew is her first child and that she has been concerned that Andrew "spits up" so much. She states she called the clinic about 2 weeks ago, but the nurse told her that all babies spit up and that she could talk with someone when she came in for Andrew's 1-month checkup. She missed the appointment because she could not get a ride to the clinic. She further states that the "spitting up" has increased, and for the past 2 days she has not been sure whether Andrew was keeping any of his feedings in his stomach; also, he has been very fussy. After several unsuccessful attempts to speak to someone at the clinic by phone, she decided to bring Andrew in to be seen.

1. What will be your priority nursing action?
2. Identify two issues that you should address with Andrew's mother related to seeking care when health care information is needed.

Intussusception

Intussusception is an invagination of a section of the intestine into the distal bowel that causes bowel obstruction. In children, this condition most often occurs as a section of terminal ileum telescopes into the ascending colon through the ileocecal valve. It is the most common cause of bowel ob-struction in children younger than 2 years (Wyllie, 2004). Although relatively rare, it does represent a pediatric emergency with classic assessment findings.

Etiology and Incidence

In young children, the cause of intussusception is unknown. Contributing factors include a preexisting upper respiratory tract infection or other viral infection. A pathologic condition within the colon, such as a mass or anatomic defect, is the most likely cause in children older than 6 years.

Intussusception generally affects infants and young children, with most cases occurring before age 2 years, but rarely before 3 months. This incidence is 1 to 4 per 1000 births, but the condition is more common in children with celiac disease and cystic fibrosis (Wyllie, 2004). The male-to-female ratio is 4:1. Recurrence is a risk.

Manifestations and Diagnostic Evaluation

Intussusception occurs in children who are well-nourished and without a history of GI problems. Paroxysms of pain occur, subside, and recur during the first several hours and then progress to a more constant severe pain. The child may vomit. The classic signs of intussusception are:

- Passage of bloody mucus ("currant jelly") stool and diarrhea, which may not occur until the postoperative period
- A sausage-shaped abdominal mass

Pathophysiology

of Intussusception

As the bowel telescopes inside itself, obstruction develops. In addition, the mesenteric vessels become trapped between the walls of the two layers, and ischemia occurs. This pressure on the bowel leads to bleeding and "currant jelly" stools. Mesen-teric ischemia also causes edema and possible strangulation or infarction of the bowel, which can progress to perforation, peritonitis, sepsis, shock, and death.

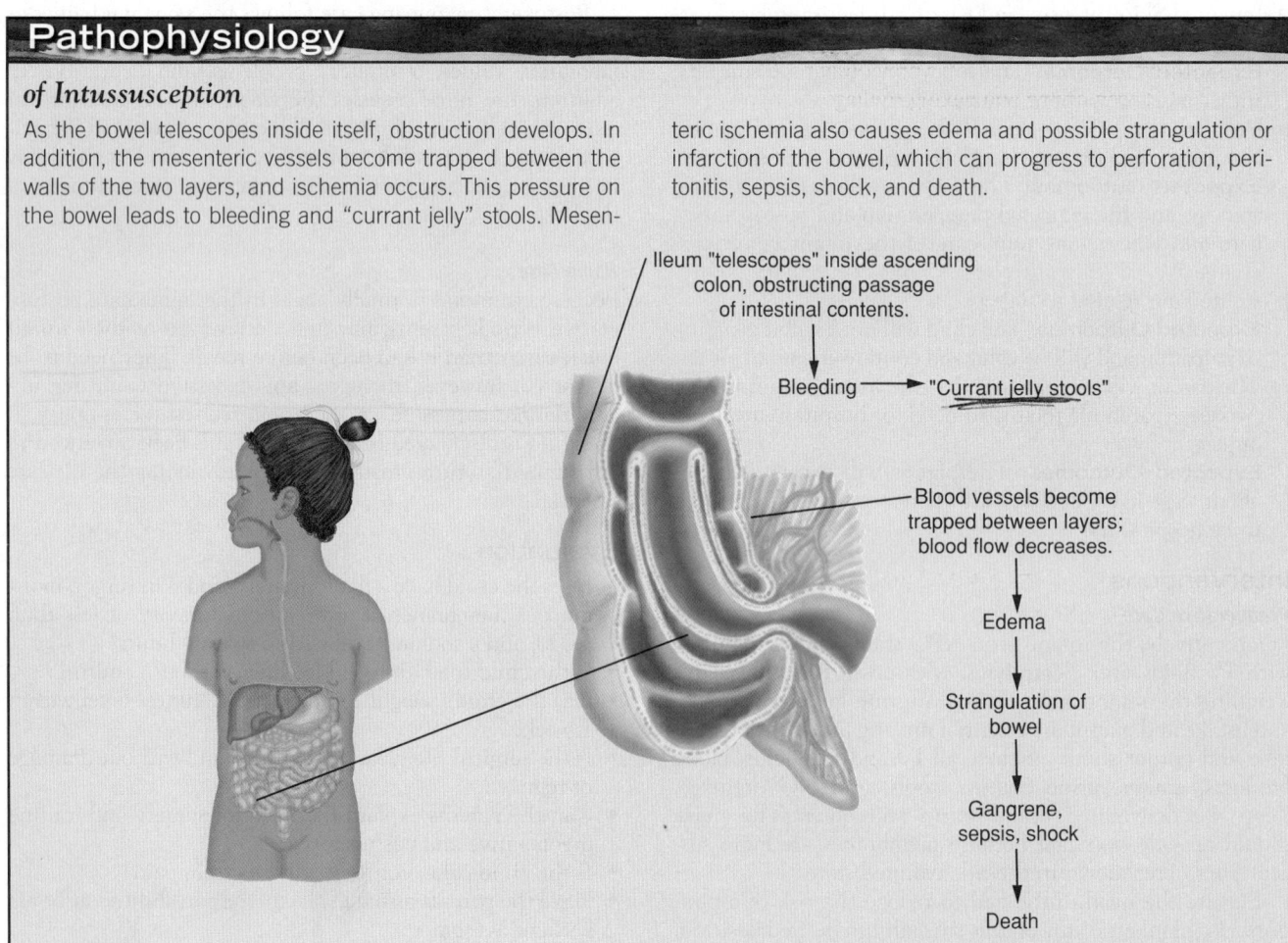

Ileum "telescopes" inside ascending colon, obstructing passage of intestinal contents.

Bleeding ⟶ "Currant jelly stools"

Blood vessels become trapped between layers; blood flow decreases.

↓

Edema

↓

Strangulation of bowel

↓

Gangrene, sepsis, shock

↓

Death

Symptoms of shock and sepsis are present if obstruction has been present for longer than 12 to 24 hours. The child may be listless. Older children may present with pain without other symptoms.

Abdominal radiographs may show abnormal gas patterns related to the bowel obstruction or a soft tissue mass. Ultrasonography is useful in identifying the location of the intussusception and the amount of edema in the area. A definitive diagnosis can be made and treatment provided simultaneously with a barium enema or air enema examination.

Therapeutic Management

The goal of treatment is to restore the bowel to its normal position and function as quickly as possible. In children who do not show symptoms of shock or sepsis, attempts at hydrostatic reduction are made with a barium or air enema until free flow of barium into the terminal ileum is evident. This procedure can be done in approximately 80% of cases. Ultrasound-guided isotonic saline enema may also be used (Wyllie, 2004). If reduction fails or findings indicate damage to the bowel, immediate surgery is performed. If the intussusception is detected and reduced within 24 hours, morbidity is minimal. Laparoscopy is now being used if enema fails to reduce the intussusception except where bowel necrosis is present.

▪ NURSING CARE
The Child With Intussusception

Assessment

The nursing history typically reveals a previously healthy infant who suddenly began crying and flexing the legs in severe pain. This problem may resolve, only to recur a short time later and become more constant. Assess any child with these signs for indicators of bowel obstruction: vomiting, nausea, distention, and hypoactive or hyperactive bowel sounds. A palpable abdominal mass and passage of "currant jelly" stools will help confirm the diagnosis. Assess the child's hydration status on admission. Fever, an increased heart rate, changes in level of consciousness or blood pressure, and respiratory distress should be reported immediately as possible indicators of sepsis or peritonitis.

Nursing Diagnosis and Planning

The nursing diagnoses and expected outcomes that may be appropriate for the child with intussusception and the family are

- Ineffective Tissue Perfusion (GI) related to bowel compression.
  Expected Outcome: The child will have a patent bowel, as evidenced by the passage of soft, formed, Hematest-negative stools.
- Acute Pain related to bowel obstruction and surgery.
  Expected Outcomes: The child will be free from abdominal pain, as evidenced by age-appropriate play and activity, and will not exhibit guarding during palpation.
- Deficient Fluid Volume related to vomiting and diarrhea.
  Expected Outcomes: The child will tolerate age-appropriate food and fluids without vomiting or recurrence of symptoms and will be free from fluid and electrolyte disturbances, as evidenced by return to normal weight, moist mucous membranes, good skin turgor, and normal serum sodium level and hematocrit.

- Deficient Knowledge related to possibility of surgery and the need for immediate intervention.
  Expected Outcomes: The parents will verbalize an understanding of the need for immediate intervention and will explain the mechanisms of intussusception and hydrostatic reduction.
- Anxiety (parental) related to the child's hospitalization or possible surgery.
  Expected Outcomes: The parents will express concerns and fears and will seek appropriate support as needed.
- Disturbed Sleep Pattern related to colicky abdominal pain.
  Expected Outcome: The child will return to normal sleep patterns.

Interventions

Once the diagnosis is made, immediate plans are made to admit the child to the hospital for hydrostatic reduction. Prompt assessment for dehydration, shock, or sepsis is essential, including documenting mental status, capillary perfusion, and urine output. The child is given IV fluids, and an NG tube is inserted if distention is present. During reduction, pain medications or sedation may be needed to decrease spasm. After reduction, clear liquids are started and the diet is advanced gradually as tolerated.

Observe for the passage of barium, and note the characteristics of stool. Also note the recurrence of previous symptoms of bowel obstruction; the risk of recurrence after nonsurgical reduction is about 10%. Resumption of a normal diet and normal activity and the passage of stool without blood will indicate a successful outcome. If hydrostatic reduction is unsuccessful, the child must be prepared for abdominal surgery or laparoscopy. If hydrostatic reduction is unsuccessful, continue to monitor for return of normal bowel function because spontaneous resolution could occur, eliminating the need for surgery.

Postoperatively, the child is kept on NPO status until bowel function returns. NG suction and IV therapy, pain medications, maintenance of respiratory function, frequent assessment, and meeting developmental needs remain nursing responsibilities.

During this difficult time for parents, relieving their anxiety by providing appropriate information is essential. This effort should include a description of the pathophysiology of intussusception, the usefulness of hydrostatic reduction, and the expected recovery care for their child, including the need for IV fluids, NG suction, and frequent vital sign checks and assessments. In addition, emotional support can be provided by encouraging them to participate in their child's care, listening to their concerns, and encouraging expression of their feelings during this stressful time.

To help parents understand intussusception, use a hospital glove. As you press one finger (representing the terminal ileum) into the inflated glove (the distal colon) and cause it to go inside itself, the parents can visualize the telescoping. The same mechanism can show how hydrostatic reduction works. As you press on the glove (the distal portion) with your hand, you can see and feel how the telescoped portion is pushed back to its normal position.

Evaluation

- In the preoperative period, does the child achieve moist mucous membranes, good skin turgor, and a urine specific gravity of less than 1.030?

Pathophysiology

of Hirschsprung's Disease

Ganglia provide parasympathetic innervation of the colon. In Hirschsprung's disease, ganglia are absent from a variable length of colon extending proximally from the anus. Adequate peristalsis cannot occur in the affected colon, leading to a tonic contraction of the lumen. This produces a functional bowel obstruction, chronic constipation, and the passage of ribbonlike stools. It can lead to a complete bowel obstruction. Because of the constriction of the lumen, huge amounts of feces and gas collect proximal to the aganglionic portion, resulting in a gross enlargement of this segment. The enlarged segment of colon is actually normal in its function.

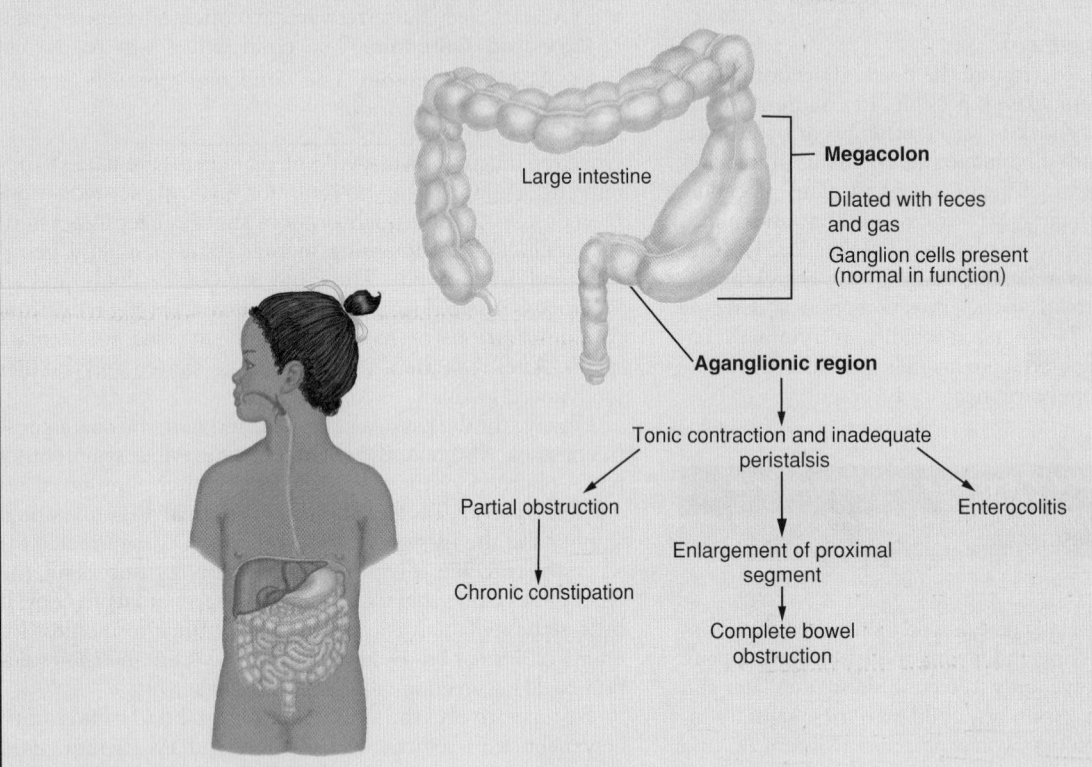

Large intestine

Megacolon

Dilated with feces and gas

Ganglion cells present (normal in function)

Aganglionic region

Tonic contraction and inadequate peristalsis

Partial obstruction

Chronic constipation

Enlargement of proximal segment

Complete bowel obstruction

Enterocolitis

- Is the child passing soft, formed, Hematest-negative stools?
- Does the infant guard the abdomen during palpation?
- Is the child demonstrating age-appropriate activity levels, sleep patterns, and play?
- Is the child tolerating age-appropriate food and fluids without vomiting or recurrence of symptoms?
- Can the parents explain the rationale for hydrostatic reduction?
- Are all the parents' questions answered to their satisfaction?
- Are the parents able to resume care of their infant without stressor anxiety?
- Has the child returned to normal sleep patterns?

Volvulus

Volvulus is a condition caused by a malrotation or twisting of the bowel that causes a bowel obstruction. It is the result of a defect in fetal development in which the midgut, which normally rotates 270 degrees around the superior mesenteric artery, fails to rotate and fixes itself to the abdominal wall.

Affected infants usually manifest pain, bilious vomiting, and other signs of bowel obstruction. Surgery is essential to prevent bowel ischemia. The nursing care is similar to that for the child with intussusception who has undergone surgery.

Hirschsprung's Disease

Also known as *congenital aganglionosis* or *megacolon*, Hirschsprung's disease is the result of an absence of ganglion cells in the rectum and, to varying degrees, upward in the colon. Eighty-five percent of cases affect the rectosigmoid region (Klein & Burd, 1999). Hirschsprung's disease accounts for 20% to 25% of all neonatal GI obstructions.

Etiology and Incidence

The disease is a result of embryonic failure of migration of the hindgut ganglion cells to the most caudal portion of the GI tract, the rectum. The initiating factor in this failure is unknown.

Hirschsprung's disease occurs in 1 in 5000 live births, with a 4:1 male-to-female ratio. It has a strong hereditary component and a higher incidence in children with Down syndrome.

Manifestations and Diagnostic Evaluation

Delayed passage or absence of meconium stool in the neonatal period is the cardinal sign of Hirschsprung's disease. Any child who fails to pass meconium within the first 24 hours and who is prone to constipation or stool infrequency in the first month after birth is suspected of having Hirschsprung's disease. The neonate, infant, or older child may exhibit signs of bowel obstruction, abdominal pain and distention, vomiting, and failure to thrive. Chronic constipation beginning in the first month of life results in pelletlike or ribbon stools that are foul-smelling.

A rectal examination will reveal a tight internal sphincter and the absence of stool, followed by an often explosive release of gas and feces related to the sudden but transient increase in rectal size. Barium enema examination will demonstrate an abrupt change in the size of the colon from a very distended ganglionic proximal portion to the contracted, saw-toothed appearance in the aganglionic distal portion, with a transitional zone of tapered bowel between them. Significantly, the child will fail to evacuate barium after the examination. The definitive diagnosis is made by rectal biopsy. During biopsy, a small core or punch sample that contains all layers of the bowel mucosa is removed. Absence of ganglionic cells in the sample confirms the diagnosis of Hirschsprung's disease.

Therapeutic Management

Treatment for mild to moderate Hirschsprung's disease is based on relieving the chronic constipation with stool softeners and rectal irrigations. Treatment for moderate to severe Hirschsprung's disease involves removing the aganglionic portion of the intestine in a two-step surgical intervention. In the neonatal period, performing a temporary colostomy with the most distal section of normal bowel relieves the obstruction. A complete surgical repair is delayed until the child weighs 8 to 10 kg (18 to 20 lb), at which time a pull-through procedure is performed to excise all aganglionic portions of the bowel and reanastomose the normal bowel to the anal canal. The colostomy is closed during this procedure, and normal bowel function returns shortly thereafter. If the child is older before diagnosis and surgery, the physician will most likely wait 3 or 4 months before the pull-through procedure.

If diagnosis is made early enough before the bowel becomes severely dilated, a one-stage pull-through procedure may be used that eliminates the necessity of a temporary colostomy. In addition, some medical centers are now performing this surgery using minimally invasive or laparoscopic techniques that have less morbidity and shorter recovery times.

■ NURSING CARE
The Child With Hirschsprung's Disease

Assessment

The child with Hirschsprung's disease will have constipation that has been present since the neonatal period and frequent passage of foul-smelling ribbonlike or pellet stools. Nutritional status should be assessed because malnutrition can develop secondary to extreme distention or enterocolitis. Thin extremities, abdominal distention, and a history of poor feeding should be noted.

If the child is acutely ill on presentation, enterocolitis must be suspected. *This is a life-threatening complication and, if it is suspected, must be reported immediately!* Document the assessment of bowel sounds and abdominal distention, the frequency of vomiting and diarrhea, and changes in abdominal circumference. Assess temperature using a route other than rectal.

Assess family members' concerns and their methods of dealing with the problem. This disease can drain family and financial resources during the diagnosis and surgical treatment. Mild disease may not be diagnosed until the child is older. Assessing the older child's feelings about chronic constipation and its treatment is important.

Nursing Diagnoses and Planning

The nursing diagnoses and expected outcomes that may be appropriate for the child with Hirschsprung's disease are

- Constipation related to aganglionic bowel and inadequate peristalsis.
  Expected Outcome: The child will pass soft, formed stools without retention.
- Risk for Deficient Fluid Volume or Excess Fluid Volume related to surgical preparation.
  Expected Outcome: The child will be free from fluid or electrolyte disturbances related to bowel cleansing.
- Impaired Skin Integrity related to colostomy and surgical repair.
  Expected Outcomes: The surgical and colostomy sites will be clean and free from exudate, redness, or drainage; the colostomy site will be intact without bleeding or skin irritation.
- Risk for Infection related to surgical repair.
  Expected Outcome: The child will be afebrile without signs of infection at the site.
- Imbalanced Nutrition: Less Than Body Requirements related to GI surgery.
  Expected Outcomes: The child will have normal bowel sounds, will pass stool, and will tolerate a regular diet.
- Acute Pain related to surgical incisions.
  Expected Outcomes: The child will be free from pain and will be able to participate in usual activities of daily living.
- Deficient Knowledge related to incomplete information about the need for surgery, irrigation, or care of the ostomy.
  Expected Outcomes: The parent will state the necessity of rectal irrigations or surgical intervention; the parent or child will assume responsibility for care of the ostomy.
- Disturbed Body Image related to colostomy and irrigations.
  Expected Outcome: The child and family will express feelings about irrigations, ostomy care, and the impact the condition has had on the child's body image.
- Anxiety (parental and child) related to the loss of the perfect child or need for surgery.
  Expected Outcomes: The parent will express fears and concerns and will seek support as needed.

Interventions

Preparing the Child for Surgery

The nurse closely monitors and records the child's bowel elimination pattern. Isotonic saline enemas are administered preoperatively until the return is clear (see Chapter 37). An alternative bowel-cleansing regimen is to administer a polyethylene glycol-electrolyte lavage solution (GoLYTELY) orally or through the NG tube. This regimen is used only in children older than 5 years and is given at a dosage of 25 to 40 ml/kg/hr. After bowel cleansing, keep the child on NPO status until surgery. Provide IV fluids as needed, and keep strict intake and output records.

Preventing Infection and Maintaining Skin Integrity

Neomycin 1.0% solution given by rectum or stoma is administered preoperatively to sterilize the bowel for surgery. Additional sterilization is provided by IV antibiotics, which also prevent infection at the surgical incision site. Monitor vital signs carefully, and measure the child's abdominal circumference with each vital sign measurement. Use tympanic or axillary methods for taking the temperature to avoid traumatizing the rectal mucosa. Monitor the surgical site for redness, swelling, and purulent drainage.

If the child has a colostomy, monitor the stoma site for bleeding and impaired skin integrity. After a pull-through procedure, which pulls the healthy bowel to the anal opening, monitor the anal site carefully for redness, discharge, and the presence of stool. To prevent skin breakdown, provide meticulous skin care of abdominal, perineal, and ostomy sites by changing dressings and appliances as needed. Use the appropriate-size hypoallergenic ostomy supplies. Encourage the parent and child to begin ostomy care as soon as possible.

Maintaining Nutritional and Hydration Status

Postoperatively, keep the child on NPO status until bowel sounds return or the child passes flatus; set the NG tube to intermittent suction until peristalsis returns. Monitor the child for signs of dehydration and acid-base disturbances. Begin advancing the diet from clear liquids to a regular diet as ordered. To prevent dehydration, keep the child on IV fluids until the child tolerates oral fluids well.

Relieving Pain

Provide pain medications on a regular basis as ordered. Most school-age children can use patient-controlled analgesia for effective pain control (see Chapter 39). The nurse should encourage the parents to institute non-pharmacologic pain control measures, such as repositioning, back rubs, music, holding, rocking, massage, and quiet talking. If pain is not controlled by usual means, the child may be experiencing a bowel obstruction or infection.

Providing Education and Relieving Anxiety

Before the time of scheduled surgery, the parents may need to manage rectal irrigations at home. It is necessary for the parent not only to learn the procedure but also to observe for distention and signs of obstruction. Encourage the parents to express any concerns they may have about the need for irrigations or their ability to perform them. Teach the parents and child about the surgery and recovery process. If the child is to have a colostomy, it is helpful for the child and parents to see and manipulate the equipment.

Postoperatively, encourage preschoolers and young school-age children to draw pictures, use dolls, and play to express concerns about body appearance, irrigations, and the colostomy. Teach colostomy care in the immediate postoperative period, and encourage the parents to participate in the child's care as quickly as possible in the supervised setting. Promote self-care as soon as possible for the older child. Referral to an enterostomal therapist can be helpful. The nurse also can refer the family to support groups for children with ostomies.

Provide parents time to share their fears, concerns, and questions. Active listening is a critical nursing intervention. Referral to community resources may be very useful (see Appendix I on Evolve website).

Evaluation

- Does the child pass soft, formed stools without retention after completion of the surgical correction?
- Has the child tolerated the bowel-cleansing regimen without signs of fluid and electrolyte imbalance, as evidenced by moist mucous membranes, good skin turgor, and an hourly urine output appropriate for age?
- Is the child afebrile, and are surgical sites free from redness, purulent drainage, excess heat, and dehiscence?
- Is the colostomy or anal pull-through area free from bleeding and skin breakdown?
- Are bowel sounds active and present in all four quadrants, and is the child tolerating a developmentally appropriate diet without vomiting or diarrhea?
- Does the child appear to be free of pain, as evidenced by the ability to sleep comfortably and participate in appropriate play activities when awake?
- Can the parents and child demonstrate all procedures needed for appropriate care?
- Is the child able to express feelings about body changes related to treatments or procedures?
- Are the parents calm and able to resume all care of their child without anxiety?

MALABSORPTION DISORDERS

Lactose Intolerance

An inability to tolerate lactose, the sugar found in dairy products, is the result of an absence or deficiency of lactase, an enzyme found in the secretions of the small intestine and needed for the digestion of lactose. The two types of lactose intolerance are congenital and developmental. Congenital lactose intolerance, which is very rare, appears at birth, with a complete absence of lactase. Developmental lactose intolerance, which is more common, is a deficiency of lactase that appears in early to late childhood.

Etiology and Incidence

Most cases of lactose intolerance are the result of inadequate levels of lactase. The exact reason for this deficiency is unknown. The condition is likely to be more severe during and after other illnesses affecting the GI mucosa, such as viral gastroenteritis or food poisoning.

The condition appears to have an ethnic association, with a 50% to 90% incidence in Asians, Arabs, Jews, African Americans, and southern Europeans.

Pathophysiology

of Lactose Intolerance

An absence or deficiency of lactase leads to inability to digest lactose and the subsequent accumulation of lactose in the lumen of the small intestine. As a result, water is drawn into the colon, resulting in watery osmotic diarrhea containing undigested lactose. In addition, GI bacteria break down lactose and release hydrogen, which causes excess gas production, bloating, and abdominal pain.

[handwritten: celiac disease-wheat barley oats can't have]

Manifestations and Diagnostic Evaluation

Manifestations of lactose intolerance include diarrhea that is frothy but not fatty, abdominal distention, cramping abdominal pain, and excessive flatus. The symptoms are not usually seen until lactase activity begins to decrease after age 3 years or during other GI insults. If the child has congenital lactose intolerance, symptoms will be immediate and may be severe.

A history of improvement after a lactose-free diet has been implemented provides a presumptive diagnosis. The finding of 1+ or greater sugar values on Clinitest examination of the stool can support the diagnosis. Breath hydrogen testing may indicate the amount of lactase available by indirectly measuring the amount of undigested carbohydrate.

Therapeutic Management

The treatment for lactose intolerance is removal of lactose from the diet. In most cases, total elimination is unnecessary. Removing milk as the beverage of choice can provide enough relief from symptoms. Additional dietary changes may be necessary to provide adequate sources of calcium and, in the infant, protein and calories. Formulas that do not contain lactose (Isomil, Nursoy, Nutramigen, ProSobee, and other soy-based formulas) may be given to the infant suspected of having lactose intolerance. Breastfeeding mothers are urged to eliminate lactose products from their diet.

These dietary changes can be supplemented with the use of commercial lactase preparations (Lactaid, Dairy Ease, Lac-Dose) that can be taken with lactose-containing food to provide adequate lactase levels and variable relief from symptoms.

[handwritten: Also can't have stuff w/ Calcium egg yolk,]

■ NURSING CARE

The Child With Lactose Intolerance

Assessment

Assessment will reveal a healthy-looking child with episodic abdominal pain and occasional diarrhea without any nutritional deficiencies or other health problems. If the problem is congenital and thus likely to be more severe, diarrhea may be a major concern. The neonate or infant may appear extremely dehydrated, with severe diarrhea and weight loss. The child and family may or may not be able to correlate symptoms with food intake.

Nursing Diagnosis and Planning

The nursing diagnoses and expected outcomes that may be appropriate for the infant or child with lactose intolerance are

■ Acute Pain related to bloating and flatus.
   Expected Outcomes: The child will be free from abdominal pain, as evidenced by developmentally appropriate play and activity; the child will have normal bowel sounds with a soft abdomen that is not painful during palpation.
■ Diarrhea related to maldigestion.
   Expected Outcome: The child will have soft, formed stools.
■ Deficient Knowledge related to incomplete understanding about needed dietary changes.
   Expected Outcome: The child will take in a minimum of 800 mg of calcium per day, as reported in the dietary history. The family will state foods to be avoided or pro-

PARENTS
Want to Know

About Care of the Child With Lactose Intolerance

- It is necessary for your child to avoid all high-lactose foods (e.g., milk, ice cream). If you are unsure about whether a food contains lactose, examine labels for milk or milk products.
- You can use soy-based, lactose-free formulas as needed for your infant (Isomil, Nursoy, Nutramigen, ProSobee). If you are breastfeeding, limit your own intake of dairy products.
- You or your older child can obtain calcium through other foods besides milk. They include egg yolk, green leafy vegetables, dried beans, cauliflower, and molasses. Calcium supplements are also available.
- Once your child's symptoms have disappeared, you can gradually add yogurt, hard cheeses, and small amounts of milk to assess tolerance.
- If you are having difficulty determining what foods are lactose-free or need help finding tasty recipes using lactose-free foods, ask for a dietary consultation.

vided in small amounts and will provide adequate calcium sources in diet and select appropriate lactase products.

Interventions

The principal nursing intervention is teaching. Symptoms are often relieved after a lactose-free diet is followed for a short period. Foods containing small amounts of lactose may be added gradually after this time to assess the child's reaction. If small amounts of milk are tolerated, it is useful to offer food or lactase preparations simultaneously with milk. These simple changes can offer instant relief.

After diagnosis and initial management, this condition is often perceived to be only a minor nuisance. Emotional support for the family, however, may be needed. Referring the family to self-help and information groups and encouraging family members to share successes and concerns are important nursing interventions.

Evaluation

- Is the child happy, content, and free of excess gas and bloating?
- Can the parent state what foods it is essential to avoid?
- Are the child's stools normal and formed?
- Does the food diary indicate an intake of at least 800 mg of calcium daily for a child age 1 to 10 years?
- Does the parent express satisfaction with control of the child's condition?

Celiac Disease

Celiac disease, also known as *gluten enteropathy* or *tropical sprue*, results from the inability to digest fully the gliadin or protein part of wheat, barley, rye, and oats. This is a lifelong deficiency requiring dietary modification to prevent chronic maldigestion and malabsorption.

Pathophysiology

of Celiac Disease

Gluten—the protein found in rye, oats, barley, and wheat—breaks down into gliadin and other by-products. Celiac disease results from an inability to digest gliadin. This results in the accumulation of glutamine in the intestine, which has a toxic effect on the mucosal cells. This leads to atrophy of the villi and a marked decrease in the absorptive surface. Malabsorption of fats, carbohydrates, and vitamins develops. *Celiac crisis* is a result of sudden accumulation of glutamine and the subsequent destruction of the mucosal cells, causing severe diarrhea and dehydration.

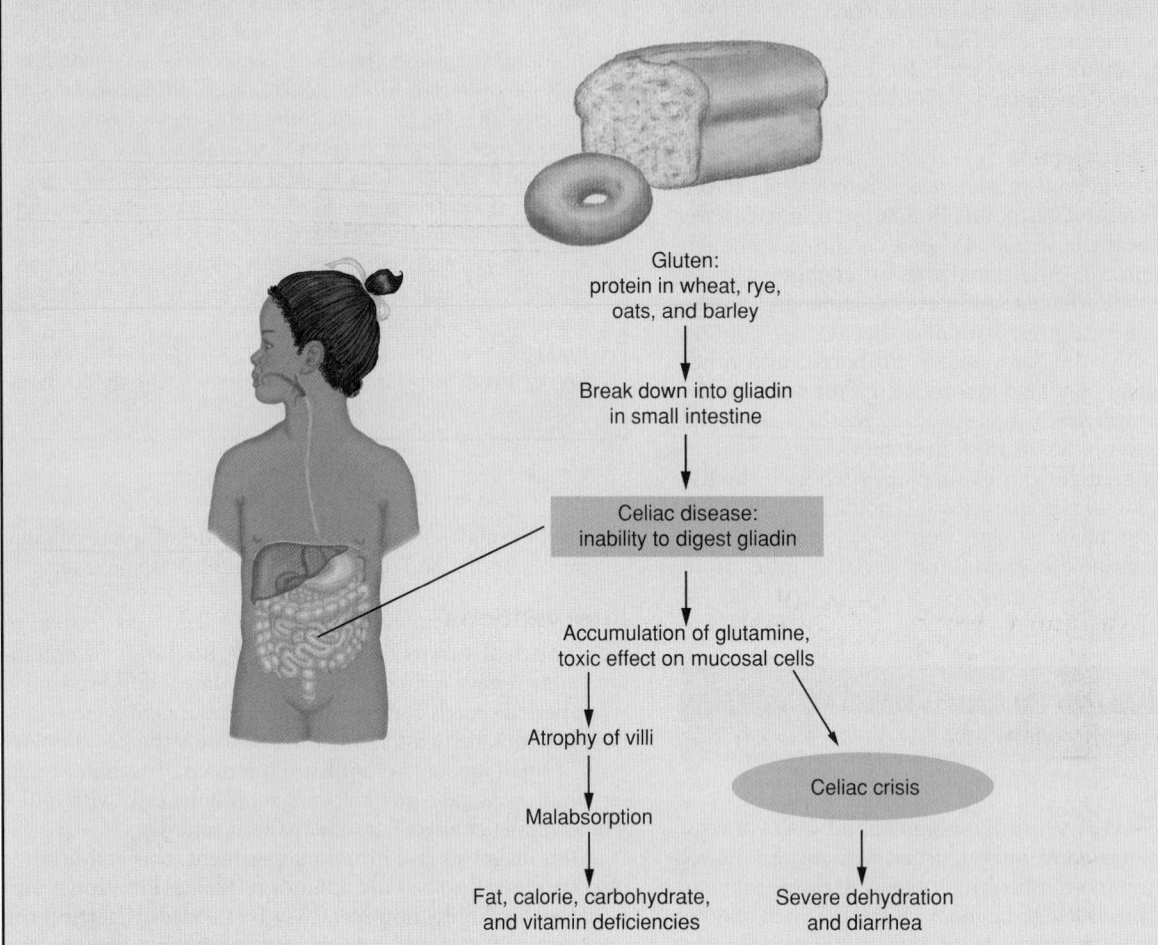

Gluten:
protein in wheat, rye,
oats, and barley

Break down into gliadin
in small intestine

Celiac disease:
inability to digest gliadin

Accumulation of glutamine,
toxic effect on mucosal cells

Atrophy of villi

Celiac crisis

Malabsorption

Fat, calorie, carbohydrate,
and vitamin deficiencies

Severe dehydration
and diarrhea

Etiology and Incidence

Celiac disease is considered genetic. From 80% to 90% of children with celiac disease have the genetic marker HLA-B8, a human leukocyte antigen complex located on chromosome 6. This chromosomal variation results in the inability to digest gliadin, causing severe GI mucosal changes that continue on exposure to gluten.

The incidence of celiac disease varies in different regions. In the United States the incidence is about 1 in 1000 live births. The incidence is much higher in Europe. Siblings and children of affected individuals are at highest risk for the disease (Garcia-Careaga & Kerner, 2004).

Manifestations

The major manifestations in the child with celiac disease include diarrhea and growth failure. The child's growth usually is below the 25th percentile on growth charts.

The child may also experience abdominal distention, vomiting, anemia, irritability, anorexia, muscle wasting, edema, anemia, and folate deficiency. Symptoms are not seen until 3 to 6 months after the introduction of grains to the diet, usually at age 9 to 12 months. The child in celiac crisis exhibits profuse, watery diarrhea and vomiting.

Diagnostic Evaluation

The serum antigliadin antibody (AGA) assay is a diagnostic test that allows continued assessment and evaluation of dietary changes. In the past, this test required specialized laboratory equipment. Now, the strip AGA test requires only a single drop of blood, and results can be determined quickly and inexpensively. Its ease of use makes the diagnosis of celiac disease simpler and more cost-effective. A newer, more accurate test measures tissue transglutaminase (tTG) through enzyme-linked immunosorbent assay (ELISA). The test is also effective in evaluating the adequacy of dietary changes. Jejunal biopsy will unequivocally identify ulcerations in the GI tract. Monitoring the reaction to a gluten-free diet supports the diagnosis. Symptoms are often relieved in 1 week by removal of gluten from the diet.

Further diagnostic testing may include the breath hydrogen excretion test to identify the amount of carbohydrate malabsorption occurring. This test is not specific for sprue. D-Xylose testing indicates the amount of mucosal damage; the remaining absorptive surface can be estimated.

Therapeutic Management

Dietary management is the mainstay of treatment. All wheat, rye, barley, and oats should be eliminated from the diet and replaced with corn and rice. To correct deficiencies, vitamin supplements, especially with fat-soluble vitamins and folate, may be needed in the early period of treatment.

Dietary restrictions are likely to be lifelong, although small amounts of grains may be tolerated after the ulcerations have healed. It is difficult for adolescents to maintain a gluten-free diet without having an unbalanced diet high in protein and fat. An adolescent on a strict gluten-free diet still has a risk for dietary imbalance, and supplements or support from dietary services is essential for maintenance.

Occasionally the nurse is the first to see a child in celiac crisis. Celiac crisis causes profuse, watery diarrhea and vomiting and can quickly lead to severe dehydration and metabolic acidosis. The cause of the crisis, usually an infection or a hidden source of gluten, must be identified. The child is given fluids IV to correct fluid and acid-base imbalance, albumin to treat shock, and corticosteroids to decrease severe mucosal inflammation.

■NURSING CARE
The Child With Celiac Disease

Assessment

Assessment of the infant with celiac disease usually reveals an irritable, malnourished infant who exhibits failure to thrive by 9 to 12 months. Any child with diarrhea, especially one with foul-smelling, fatty stools and significant growth delays, should be suspected of having this disorder. A noticeable decline in the child's rate of growth as charted on the growth curve, associated with the addition of grains to the diet, is essential supportive evidence.

Abdominal assessment will reveal distention and ascites with an increasing girth; observation will identify other signs of malnutrition, such as thin, edematous extremities; pallor; and muscle wasting. Anemia is a common finding.

The child who presents with severe diarrhea, foul-smelling stools, vomiting, poor perfusion, edema, or changes in vital signs (shock or metabolic acidosis) should be referred for emergency care of celiac crisis.

Nursing Diagnosis and Planning

The nursing diagnoses and expected outcomes that may be appropriate for the infant or child with celiac disease are
■ Imbalanced Nutrition: Less Than Body Requirements related to malabsorption.
    Expected Outcome: The infant or child will have soft, formed stools without diarrhea.

PARENTS
Want to Know

About Care of the Child With Celiac Disease

- You must eliminate all wheat, rye, barley, oats, and hydrolyzed vegetable protein from your child's diet. This includes most pasta, baked products, and many breakfast cereals.
- You may be able to find gluten-free substitutes at specialized stores.
- You can substitute corn, rice, or millet as grains. These can be obtained as flour for baking.
- Your child should take vitamin supplements, especially folate and fat-soluble vitamins, because these vitamins will be hard to provide in your child's diet.
- You will need to read all labels on foods and medications carefully to avoid any unknown additives.
- When your child is old enough to understand, you will need to help your child make appropriate food choices. This can be difficult for an older child or adolescent because popular foods often contain ingredients that will make your child's condition worse. Encourage your child to talk with a nutritionist to plan a diet that is appropriate and not too different from the diet of peers.

Support groups are available to provide information and resources (see Appendix I on Evolve website).

■ Acute Pain or Chronic pain related to abdominal distention.
    Expected Outcome: The infant or child will be free from abdominal pain, as evidenced by age-appropriate play and activity.
■ Delayed Growth and Development related to malnutrition.
    Expected Outcome: The infant or child will return to and follow a normal growth pattern according to a growth chart.
■ Deficient Knowledge related to dietary changes.
    Expected Outcomes: The family will offer appropriate foods to the infant or child, as evidenced by a food diary, will state the need for lifelong dietary changes, and will seek emotional and educational support as needed.
■ Deficient Fluid Volume related to celiac crisis.
    Expected Outcome: The infant or child will be adequately hydrated, as evidenced by moist mucous membranes and good skin turgor.

Interventions

The most important nursing intervention is teaching parents to modify their child's diet. Pain will likely be relieved quickly by eliminating gluten in the diet. Involvement of nutritionists in teaching and follow-up is helpful. Careful and consistent follow-up will be necessary to ensure the infant resumes a normal growth and development pattern as soon as possible. When the child has normal stools without diarrhea and resumes a normal growth pattern, teaching will have been effective.

Because celiac disease is a lifelong condition, support groups can be useful in managing the problem. The American Celiac Society is an excellent source of information and

TABLE **43-5** Differentiation of Viral Hepatitis

Type/Etiology	Transmission	Incubation	Clinical Manifestations	Recovery Prognosis
Hepatitis A virus (HAV), previously called *infectious hepatitis*	Fecal-oral Food or water contaminated with HAV	15-50 days (average 28 days) Most contagious 1-2 wk before symptoms Onset at 28-30 days	Mild, flu-like symptoms 70% of children asymptomatic No jaundice in children Adolescents: fever, malaise, anorexia, nausea, jaundice	Good prognosis Carriers do not occur Recovery provides life-long immunity
Hepatitis B virus (HBV), previously called *serum hepatitis*	Blood and blood products Secretions Prenatally, perinatally Sexual contact Breast milk	15-180 days (average 90 days)	Same as HAV Severity ranges from asymptomatic to fatal fulminant infection Anicteric or asymptomatic most common in children 90% of infected neonates will develop chronic carrier state	Generally a full recovery except in chronic carriers 40%-90% of infected children <10 yr old develop chronic carrier state and are predisposed to cirrhosis and hepatocellular cancer
Hepatitis C virus (HCV), non-A, non-B hepatitis	Blood and blood products Perinatally	14-115 days (average 45 days)	Same as HAV	85% progress to chronic hepatitis 5%-20% develop cirrhosis or cancer
Hepatitis delta virus (HDV), occurs only in patients with acute or chronic HBV infection	Blood and blood products More common in Mediterranean countries and among intravenous (IV) drug users and hemophiliacs	21-90 days	Occurs with HBV and causes it to be more severe	More likely to develop fulminating hepatitis than other strains
Hepatitis E virus (HEV), enterically transmitted non-A, non-B hepatitis	Fecal-oral More common in adults	15-60 days (average 40 days)	Epidemic with characteristics of HAV Uncommon in developed countries	High incidence of mortality in pregnant women Children usually asymptomatic

Data from Aach, R. (1998). Viral hepatitis due to hepatitis viruses A-E and GB virus. In R. Feigin & J. Cherry (Eds.), *Textbook of pediatric infectious diseases* (4th ed.). Philadelphia: Saunders; Selekman, J. (1999). Hepatitis update. *Pediatric Nursing, 25*(5), 542-546.

support (see Appendix I on Evolve website). Referral to this group and other family support organizations is essential. Encourage the parents to share their fears and concerns about the chronic nature of the disease and its impact on family life.

Evaluation

- Does the child have soft, formed stools without diarrhea or signs of dehydration?
- Is the child participating in age-appropriate activities?
- Has the child resumed a normal growth pattern according to a growth chart?
- Is the family able to verbalize an understanding of the child's dietary and emotional needs?
- Does a food diary indicate an intake of approximately 100 kcal/kg for the infant and for the child up to age 3 years?
- Do the parents use available support and education groups?
- Do the parents express satisfaction with the way they are coping with dietary changes?
- Does the child have good skin turgor, moist mucous membranes, and a urine output appropriate for age (see Chapter 42)?

HEPATIC DISORDERS

Viral Hepatitis

Hepatitis is an acute or chronic inflammation of the liver caused by several different viruses and some toxins or disease states. Although each type of hepatitis is unique, assessment findings and treatment have many similarities.

Etiology

The most common causes and modes of transmission of viral hepatitis are discussed in Table 43-5. Rubella, cytomegalovirus (CMV), herpes simplex virus, and Epstein-Barr virus may also occasionally produce hepatitis in children.

In children, hepatitis A virus (HAV) is highly contagious and spreads readily in households and daycare centers. Infection with hepatitis B virus (HBV) can be transmitted perinatally. The incidence of HBV infection transmitted by blood transfusions has decreased in recent years as a result of improved blood product screening procedures. Contaminated body fluids splashed into the mouth or eyes can cause HBV infection. HBV can survive in the dried state for 1 week or longer, and percutaneous contact with contaminated objects can transmit infection.

Incidence

More than 60,000 cases of hepatitis are reported each year. Because the virus may be excreted for 2 to 3 weeks before the appearance of clinical signs and for 2 to 3 weeks afterward, outbreaks are common wherever good handwashing is not practiced.

In the United States and other Western industrialized countries, HBV infection occurs most often in adolescents and adults. The incidence of hepatitis B infection in the United States has declined over the past 10 years to 2.8/100,000 in adults and 0.3/100,000 in children (Centers for Disease Control and Prevention [CDC], 2004). In developing countries where sanitation is poor, HBV occurs most often in infants and children younger than 5 years. In the United States, perinatal exposure to a hepatitis B positive mother is the major cause of infection in young children (Snyder & Pickering, 2004). The incidence of Hepatitis A is 4/100,000 (CDC, 2003).

Manifestations

In infants and preschool-age children, HAV infection usually causes no symptoms or causes mild, nonspecific symptoms, such as anorexia, malaise, and easy fatigability. In adults, the disease causes the more severe symptoms of nausea, jaundice, and malaise. Because most children with HAV infection are asymptomatic or have mild, nonspecific symptoms, the disease may not be diagnosed until an outbreak of hepatitis occurs. Thus spread of HAV infection in a daycare center often occurs before the initial case is identified.

HBV infection may cause a wide range of clinical manifestations, from asymptomatic infection to fatal acute fulminant hepatitis. Symptomatic acute hepatitis occurs in two stages: the anicteric (without jaundice) phase; and the icteric (jaundiced) phase.

During the anicteric phase, manifestations include anorexia, nausea and vomiting, right upper quadrant or epigastric pain, fever, malaise, fatigue, depression, and irritability. The anicteric phase lasts approximately 5 to 7 days. During the icteric phase, manifestations include jaundice, urticaria, dark urine, and light-colored stools. The child begins to feel better as jaundice becomes more apparent. Acute fulminating hepatitis is marked by bleeding problems, encephalopathy, ascites, and acute hepatic failure. Fulminant hepatitis is caused primarily by hepatitis B and hepatitis C.

The symptoms and clinical changes should return to normal within 3 months of onset. If not, a chronic state should be suspected. Infection with hepatitis B, hepatitis D, and hepatitis C viruses (HBV, HDV, and HCV) can result in chronic hepatitis and cirrhosis. Chronic HBV infection can also cause hepatic carcinoma.

Diagnostic Evaluation

A history of exposure to jaundiced individuals, confirmed outbreaks in daycare centers, or percutaneous exposure to blood or body fluids should raise the suspicion of hepatitis. Although no liver function test is specific for hepatitis, tests of liver function, especially aspartate transaminase (AST), alanine transaminase (ALT), and bilirubin levels and sedimentation rate, can indicate liver damage caused by hepati-

Pathophysiology

of Viral Hepatitis

Hepatitis viruses cause necrosis of the parenchymal cells of the liver. The inflammatory response causes swelling and blockage of the drainage system in the liver. Biliary stasis and further destruction of the hepatic cells occur. Because the liver cannot excrete bile into the intestine, bile appears in the blood (causing hyperbilirubinemia), urine (as urobilinogen), and skin (causing hepatocellular jaundice).

Hepatitis infection may result in asymptomatic or mild illness, in which complete regeneration of liver cells occurs within 2 to 3 months. More severe forms of hepatitis include (1) fulminant hepatitis, in which hepatic necrosis and death can occur within 1 to 2 weeks, and (2) subacute, or chronic, hepatitis, which can result in permanent scarring of the liver and impaired liver function. Chronically infected persons are carriers of the disease and are at increased risk for developing chronic liver disease (e.g., cirrhosis, chronic persistent hepatitis) or liver carcinoma later in life.

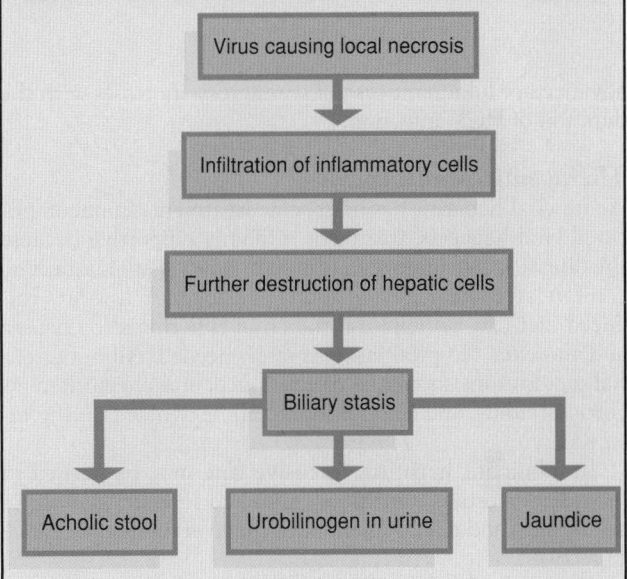

tis. Serum bilirubin levels peak 5 to 10 days after jaundice appears. A history and the course of the disease are essential in making the appropriate diagnosis.

Hepatitis is diagnosed by identification of the antigens (HBsAg, HBeAg) responsible for the disease or the antibodies (anti-HAV, anti-HBc, anti-HBe, anti-HBs, or anti-HCV) that develop as a result. Immunoglobulin M (IgM) anti-HAV antibodies are present at the onset of illness. They usually disappear within 6 months but may persist for 12 months. IgG anti-HAV antibodies develop shortly after IgM anti-HAV antibodies do. The presence of IgG without IgM anti-HAV antibodies indicates past infection (Aach, 1998). HCV serologic assays are used mainly to detect chronic hepatitis C because they remain negative for at least 1 to 3 months after onset of the illness (Aach, 1998).

Liver biopsy may be needed to evaluate the chronic active forms of the disease and to determine the extent of damage in

TABLE 43-6 Hepatitis Prophylaxis

Infective Agent	Prevention of Spread	Immunization	Postexposure Prophylaxis

Hepatitis A virus (HAV)	Handwashing
	Gloves
	Identifying infected food
	  handlers
		Vaccine 80%-98% effective
		Given as two injections at
		  age 2 yr and 6-18 mo later
		Recommended only for spe-
		  cific populations in high
		  risk areas
			Within 2 wk, give hepatitis A im-
			  mune globulin (HAIG), 0.02 ml/kg
			  intramuscular (IM)

Hepatitis B virus (HBV)	Sterilization of needles
	Blood Precautions
	Gloves
		Vaccine 80%-90% effective
		Three injections at 0, 1, and
		  6-18 mo
		Recommended for all infants,
		  children, and adolescents
			For neonates of infected mothers,
			  give hepatitis B immune globulin
			  (HBIG) within 12 hr of birth
			  followed by vaccines
			HBIG, 0.06 ml/kg, within 24 hr of
			  any percutaneous exposure

Hepatitis C virus (HCV)	Standard Precautions	None	None

Hepatitis delta virus (HDV)	Same as for HBV	Protecting from HBV will
		  protect because HDV
		  cannot exist alone
			None

Hepatitis E virus (HEV)	Standard Precautions	Vaccine under animal trials	None

advanced or fulminant cases. Liver fibrosis increases with the duration of HCV infection.

Therapeutic Management

Acute viral hepatitis has no specific treatment. In uncomplicated viral hepatitis, treatment is mainly supportive because the disease is self-limiting. Treatment is aimed at maintaining comfort and adequate nutritional balance. A low-fat, balanced diet can be helpful if the child is bothered by nausea and anorexia. Hospitalization is rarely needed. All nonessential medications should be discontinued, and chemotherapy, corticosteroids, and alcohol should all be avoided during infection.

In fulminant hepatitis, intensive care may be needed to provide hemostasis, nutritional and fluid support, neurologic assessment, and management until the liver has had a chance to recover.

Hepatitis A. Control of further spread is essential. Because HAV can survive on contaminated objects for weeks, good handwashing and thorough disinfection of diaper-changing surfaces are imperative. Children and adults who have had direct contact with a person infected with HAV should receive immune globulin (IG) as soon as possible after exposure. A vaccine has been developed to prevent HAV infection, and immunization is recommended for daycare workers, homosexually active males, military personnel, children with hemophilia or chronic liver disease, and travelers to areas of high endemicity. Cases of hepatitis should be promptly reported to local public health officials. Testing for IgM anti-HAV antibodies should be done in suspected cases of infected daycare center employees and household contacts of infected persons (American Academy of Pediatrics, Committee on Infectious Diseases, 2000).

Hepatitis B. Children with acute or chronic HBV infection should be cared for with scrupulous Standard Precautions. The most effective means of preventing HBV infection is immunization with hepatitis B vaccine. Hepatitis B vaccination is recommended beginning in infancy as part of the routine childhood immunization schedule and for all unimmunized children before they reach adolescence. Other persons who should receive hepatitis B immunization include IV drug users, health care and residential facility workers, household contacts and sexual partners of HBV carriers, inmates of correctional facilities, and international travelers. Hepatitis B immune globulin (HBIG) is effective in preventing HBV infection if given within 2 weeks after exposure. It is possible to prevent hepatitis D by preventing hepatitis B (Table 43-6).

▪NURSING CARE
The Child With Viral Hepatitis

Assessment

The nursing history may identify a source of infection. In children, flu-like symptoms of fever, malaise, anorexia, fatigue, and nausea may be the *only* symptoms of viral hepatitis. Abdominal assessment may disclose right upper quadrant tenderness and hepatomegaly. Stools will be pale and clay-colored, and urine may be dark and frothy. Jaundice, if present, is best assessed in sclera, nail beds, and mucous membranes and usually follows a cephalocaudal progression. In HBV infection, arthralgias may be the presenting complaint.

Fulminant hepatitis will likely manifest as acute hepatic failure with associated encephalopathy, bleeding, fluid retention, ascites, and an icteric appearance.

Nursing Diagnosis and Planning

The nursing diagnoses and expected outcomes that may be appropriate after assessing the child with viral hepatitis and the child's family are

■ Imbalanced Nutrition: Less Than Body Requirements related to anorexia.

   Expected Outcomes: The child will tolerate an age-appropriate diet without weight loss, vomiting, or abdominal pain and will return to a normal activity level.

- Risk for Infection related to exposure of family members to infectious agents.
  Expected Outcomes: The family will practice good handwashing and other necessary isolation procedures and will remain free from infection.
- Risk for Injury related to fulminant hepatitis.
  Expected Outcome: The child will return to pre-illness weight and activity level.
- Deficient Knowledge related to incomplete information about home care and long-term prognosis.
  Expected Outcome: The parents will verbalize a basic understanding of hepatitis and the importance of treatment and prevention.

Interventions

Unless fulminant hepatitis develops, children are usually treated at home, so parental education is crucial. Teaching parents the importance of a nutritious, low-fat diet as tolerated by the child, rest, and general supportive care is important. The child with hepatitis is often anorexic. Several small meals and snacks throughout the day are better tolerated than regular portions at mealtimes.

Fatigue and malaise can last for several weeks. Adequate rest and sleep are important for recovery. Because HAV is not infectious within 1 week after the onset of jaundice, the child may return to school at that time if well enough.

Child and Parent Teaching

Teach the parents the danger signals that could indicate a worsening of the child's condition—specifically, changes in neurologic status, bleeding, and fluid retention. Jaundice may worsen before it resolves, and parents should be prepared for this possibility. Also, teach parents not to give their child any over-the-counter medications, because impaired liver function may result in inadequate metabolism and excretion of the medication. Caution adolescents not to drink alcohol during the illness or recovery period.

Preventing the spread of infection is an essential intervention for HAV. Prevention should include the use of Contact Precautions for at least 1 week after the onset of jaundice and excellent handwashing. Handwashing is the most important preventive measure. Teach family members to institute appropriate precautions and to clean exposed household surfaces with bleach. Diapers should not be changed on or near surfaces used for preparing or serving food. Explain to family members the ways in which HAV (fecal-oral route) and HBV (parenteral route) are spread to others. Provide education about the recommendations concerning hepatitis A and hepatitis B vaccination (see Appendix G).

If the child has HBV infection, especially neonatal HBV, prepare the parents for the possibility of a chronic carrier state and the development of cirrhosis and hepatocellular cancer in later years. If a child or adolescent with HBV infection has a history of illicit IV drug use, the nurse has the responsibility of teaching the dangers of such behaviors, including the risk of transmission of hepatitis and other infections. The youth should be assisted to obtain counseling through a drug program.

Home Care

Children with hepatitis are almost always managed at home. Nursing interventions include teaching parents handwashing skills, the use of gloves, and disinfection of contaminated surfaces and articles. Parents should be taught to monitor for complications, provide a well-balanced, low-fat diet, and monitor other family members for infection. All children in the family should be immunized against hepatitis.

Evaluation

- Has the child maintained a weight within 5% of the pre-illness weight?
- Is the child free of vomiting?
- Is the child participating in age-appropriate activities and play?
- Do family members practice good handwashing and adhere to procedures?
- Has the spread of hepatitis to other family members been avoided?
- Have all family members been immunized as appropriate?
- Can the parents explain the symptoms to watch for in other family members?

Biliary Atresia

Biliary atresia refers to the obstruction or absence of the extrahepatic bile ducts. At birth, the liver structure itself is normal without inflammation, but the structural problem leads to significant cellular damage and eventual liver failure and death.

Etiology and Incidence

The cause of biliary atresia is unknown. Because the problem originates during the prenatal period, viruses, toxins, and chemicals cannot be ruled out. The condition is unlikely to recur within the same family.

Extrahepatic biliary atresia occurs in 1 in 10,000 to 15,000 births, with a slightly higher incidence in females than in males (A-Kader & Balistreri, 2004). It is the major indication for liver transplantation in children.

Manifestations

The child is apparently healthy at birth. Developing manifestations, however, include acholic stools (light in color because of the absence of bile pigment), bile-stained urine, and hepatomegaly.

Diagnostic Evaluation

Investigations of liver function (bilirubin, aminotransferases [ALT, AST]) and clotting studies (prothrombin time, partial thromboplastin time [PT, PTT]) are useful screening tools. Any newborn with conjugated hyperbilirubinemia should be evaluated completely. To rule out inborn errors of metabolism, such as galactosemia and alpha$_1$-antitrypsin deficiency, which can produce similar initial findings, metabolic screens are essential in these children. Hepatitis and other viral titers are also necessary so that neonatal hepatitis can be eliminated as the source of dysfunction. Urine and stool should be examined and urobilinogen levels determined as an indication of the degree of obstruction.

Percutaneous liver biopsy can provide a definitive diagnosis if bile plugs, edema, and fibrosis are found in the presence of normal hepatic lobular structure (A-Kader & Balistreri, 2004). Cholangiography may be used to determine the extent of atresia.

Pathophysiology

of Biliary Atresia

Obstruction of the extrahepatic bile ducts causes obstruction of the normal flow of bile out of the liver and into the gallbladder and small intestine. As a result, bile plugs form, causing bile to back up in the liver. This process causes inflammation, edema, and hepatic degeneration. Eventually the liver becomes fibrotic, and cirrhosis and portal hypertension develop, leading to liver failure. The gradual degeneration of the liver causes jaundice, icterus, and hepatomegaly. Because bile is not present in the intestine, fat and fat-soluble vitamins cannot be absorbed. This condition leads to malnutrition, deficiencies in fat-soluble vitamins, and growth failure.

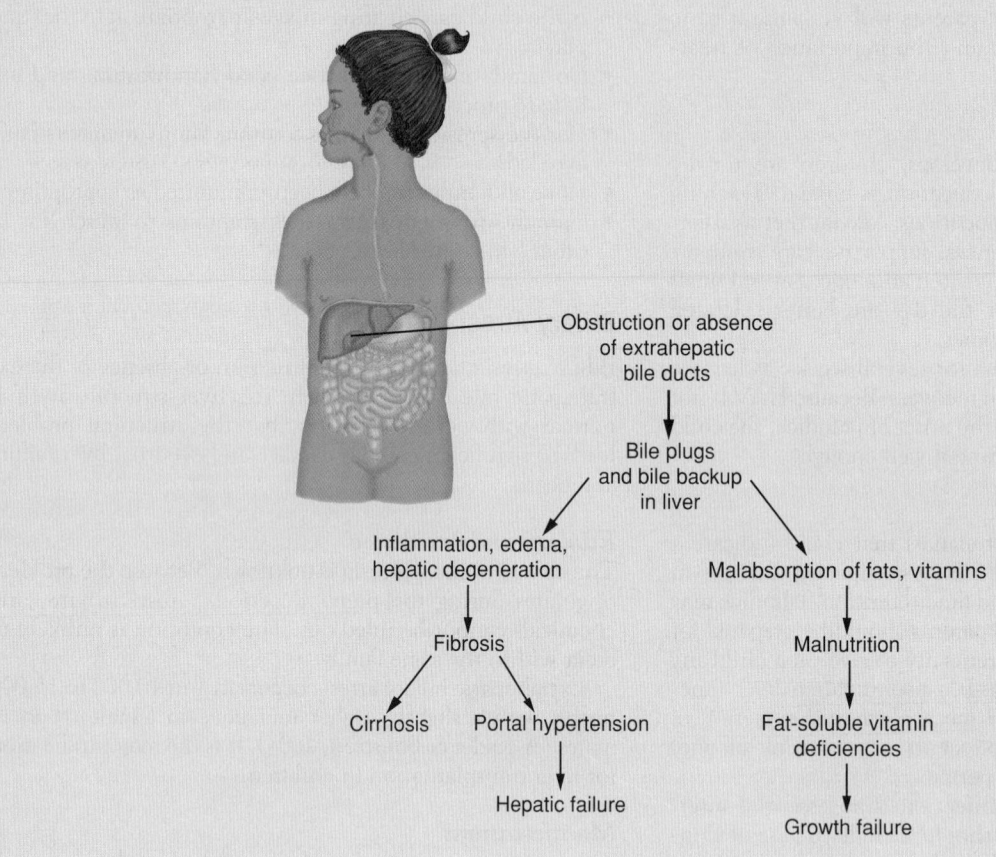

Obstruction or absence of extrahepatic bile ducts

→ Bile plugs and bile backup in liver

Inflammation, edema, hepatic degeneration → Fibrosis → Cirrhosis / Portal hypertension → Hepatic failure

Malabsorption of fats, vitamins → Malnutrition → Fat-soluble vitamin deficiencies → Growth failure

Therapeutic Management

During and after exploratory laparotomy, the size of the lesion can be identified and drainage can be attempted. If no correctable lesion is found, a hepatic portoenterostomy (Kasai procedure) will be performed to allow bile to drain from the liver. This procedure allows bile to flow directly into the intestine through an anastomosis of the jejunum to the porta hepatis, the point at which the hepatic ducts join to form the common bile duct. The Kasai procedure does provide some long-term benefits, but hepatic dysfunction will persist. The main goal of the procedure is to allow growth and development of the child until liver transplantation can be performed.

The medical management of the child involves managing the malnutrition and providing symptom relief. Medium-chain triglyceride (MCT) oil added to formula to increase calories or TPN provides essential nutrition. Vitamin malabsorption must be treated to prevent night blindness (vitamin A), neuromus-cular degeneration (vitamin E), rickets (vitamin D), and hypo-prothrombinemia (vitamin K). Assessment for and treatment of portal hypertension with its concomitant problems of ascites and variceal bleeding must be instituted. Controlling bleeding, restricting salt, and using diuretics are important in managing portal hypertension.

Nursing Considerations

During the early phase of disease, in the first months of life, the infant with biliary atresia will appear jaundiced, with mild hepatosplenomegaly and increased abdominal girth. As the disease progresses, the child may appear thin, with failure to thrive, marked jaundice, and evidence of rickets secondary to chronic vitamin D deficiency. Pruritus becomes a major problem; the child may develop skin infections or xanthomas (lipid deposits in the skin) secondary to retention of cholesterol in the skin.

After the Kasai procedure, the child needs to be assessed for evidence of portal hypertension, which may include the development of ascites and GI bleeding. Even after repair, it would not be unusual to find acholic stools and bile-stained urine.

Psychosocial and family assessment should have a high priority. Biliary atresia is a life-threatening, chronic problem that requires surgical intervention, contacts with numerous health care personnel, repeated hospitalizations, and eventually an extended wait for a transplant. The nurse gathers information about family and financial resources, emotional support available, and the feelings of the child and family about the progress and management of the disease.

Nursing interventions are directed toward six major areas: nutritional support, skin care, developmental stimulation, continued assessment, education, and emotional support.

Nutritional Support. Providing adequate calories, aiding in vitamin supply and absorption, and preventing hepatic encephalopathy are important goals. Calorie counts, daily weights, and abdominal girths are important assessments and will provide the data necessary to improve nutritional support. Concentrating calories with the use of Polycose and providing MCT supplements that do not require the presence of bile salts to digest will significantly change the nutritional status of the child. NG tube feeding or TPN may become necessary at times. Supplements of vitamins A, D, E, and K as well as calcium, phosphate, and zinc are essential for adequate nutrition. Protein may need to be limited to avoid the development of hepatic encephalopathy. Using growth charts and weighing on a monthly basis will provide evaluation criteria.

Skin Care. Bile acid binders, such as cholestyramine, aid in the excretion of bile salts and decrease pruritus and the development of xanthomas (A-Kader & Balistreri, 2004). Colloidal oatmeal baths (Aveeno) can relieve severe itching. Preventing skin breakdown from severe scratching is essential. Wearing gloves during sleep and applying soothing lotions and creams for dry skin may prevent infection.

Developmental Stimulation. Teaching parents activities to provide developmental stimulation and using resources available through physical and occupational therapy are essential nursing responsibilities. As the child awaits a transplant, efforts should be made to facilitate as much development as possible by providing stimulation for gross and fine motor skills and social and emotional growth. Routine screening tests can document developmental growth and help evaluate interventions.

Continued Assessment. Continued assessment for the development of portal hypertension is vital. The parents must be taught to watch for GI bleeding and the development of severe edema and ascites. Should any of these occur, sodium restriction, diuretics, IV albumin, and hospitalization may become necessary.

Family Education and Support. The family has many educational needs, and the nurse needs to help family members understand the disease process, deal with nutritional changes, manage skin care, assess for danger signs, and enhance the child's development. National resources are available to help these families. The Children's Liver Foundation can provide programs, educational materials, and referral to support groups as needed (see Appendix I on Evolve website).

The nurse plays a critical role by listening to parental concerns, providing resources and support, and encouraging participation and involvement. Provide information about daily care, and focus the parents' attention on the future liver transplant and its long-term care and treatment. Because transplantation usually occurs within the first 2 years of life, age-appropriate explanations for the toddler are also indicated.

The child and family should be prepared for the eventual need for a liver transplant and the possible death of the child. The life-threatening condition requires numerous hospitalizations, and the many diagnostic tests place immense stress on families. Arranging the educational and emotional support needed by family members so that they can manage their child until liver transplantation becomes possible is a critical nursing intervention.

Home Care. The parents must be able to assume all home care responsibilities. They need to be able to monitor growth and nutritional intake, mix special formulas, manage NG feedings, provide skin care, and give medications. Their ability to assess for GI bleeding, ascites, edema, and skin infections is critical so that treatment can begin as soon as possible.

Cirrhosis

Cirrhosis is a chronic, degenerative condition of the liver that results in the development of bands of fibrous tissue, firm nodules, and connections between the central and portal areas of the liver. This scarring causes irreversible damage to the liver.

Etiology

Cirrhosis in children usually results from chronic liver disease, such as hepatitis B infection or biliary atresia. Sickle cell disease, inborn errors in metabolism such as alpha$_1$-antitrypsin deficiency and disturbances in copper metabolism, cystic fibrosis, and Wilson's disease are also possible causes in children.

Incidence

Cirrhosis is uncommon in children, but as the life span of children with chronic disease continues to rise, it will become more common. Children with biliary atresia, chronic hepatitis, cystic fibrosis, or sickle cell disease are at risk.

Pathophysiology

of Cirrhosis

Stasis of bile causes inflammation and hepatomegaly. If this continues, destruction of the liver begins. As the liver attempts to heal itself, fibrotic regeneration and nodules develop and function is impaired. This scarring can cause altered hepatic blood flow and decreased liver cell function. Changes in hepatic blood flow can cause scarring and collapse of the hepatic vasculature, increased vascular resistance, and eventually portal hypertension. As the liver cells decrease in function, more die and the liver cannot produce necessary proteins or bile, causing malabsorption and malnutrition. As liver cells continue to die, the cycle is repeated.

Manifestations

The symptoms are often nonspecific, vague, and slow to develop. They result from either liver cell failure or portal hypertension. Liver cell failure results in jaundice, intense pruritus, steatorrhea, distention, edema, anemia, bleeding tendencies, anorexia, frequent infections, and poor growth. Portal hypertension may present as splenomegaly, varices, or GI bleeding. Both liver cell failure and portal hypertension contribute to the development of ascites.

Diagnostic Evaluation

Because the most likely cause of cirrhosis in children is chronic biliary obstruction, evaluation is based on the history of preexisting conditions, including biliary atresia and hepatitis. The presence of clinical manifestations of chronic liver disease and the history of one of these conditions are used for a presumptive diagnosis. Liver function tests, such as bilirubin, aminotransferases, ammonia, albumin, cholesterol, and prothrombin time, support the diagnosis. Definitive diagnosis is a liver biopsy, which will identify fibrous scarring and changes of hepatic vasculature.

Therapeutic Management

Because there is no effective treatment to halt the progression of cirrhosis, management is aimed at relieving the cause if possible. Any infectious agents should be treated and obstructive causes repaired. Supportive care, including rest, nutritional support, fluid management, and relief of symptoms, is included. Management of life-threatening complications, especially bleeding varices, ascites, and hepatic encephalopathy, takes priority in medical management. Monitoring liver function is important to evaluate the child for eventual liver transplantation. Definitive therapy is a liver transplant.

Nursing Considerations

History and general appraisal will likely reveal a child with a history of failure to thrive and of chronic biliary obstruction or hepatitis B infection. The child may present with varying degrees of distress and discomfort. Many children will present with vague complaints or be asymptomatic. The earliest findings are likely to be anorexia, nausea, indigestion, fatigue, and right upper quadrant (RUQ) pain or fullness. Monitoring height and weight using a growth chart, gathering information on a typical day's food intake, and assessing sleep habits and activity levels can help identify these more general problems and provide essential supportive evidence.

Abdominal palpation will likely reveal splenomegaly and RUQ tenderness or hepatomegaly. Distended superficial veins; tight, shiny skin; and edema may be present. Jaundice and pruritus may be detected, especially if the cirrhosis is the result of biliary obstruction. A complete skin assessment, including nail beds and sclera, will identify jaundice at its earliest stages. The skin should be examined for breakdown or infection caused by intense scratching. The amount and location of edema should also be noted. This skin assessment may also reveal bruises related to thrombocytopenia and pale color related to anemia. A stool specimen may be useful in identifying the degree of bile obstruction and malabsorption.

The most critical assessment needs to be centered on detecting signs of the three major complications of cirrhosis: ascites, varices, and encephalopathy. The child who presents with significantly increased abdominal girth, edema, bloody emesis, or changes in level of consciousness should be referred for emergency medical care of these life-threatening complications.

The goal of nursing care is to sustain the child in optimum condition until a liver transplant can be achieved. The care can be divided into four areas: nutritional support, skin care, prevention of complications, and developmental and parental support.

Nutritional Support. Providing optimum nutrition for the child to grow and develop is a major nursing intervention. The diet needs to be high-carbohydrate, high-calorie, normal-protein, and low-fat. Protein may need to be limited in case encephalopathy develops. Because anorexia can be a problem, creative food options, NG tube feedings, and TPN may be needed. These changes put minimal stress on the liver while meeting the growth requirements of the child. In addition, sodium restriction can help prevent edema. Multivitamins with vitamins A, D, E, and K supplements are essential. Vitamin K injections may be needed. Monitoring the child's weight on a daily and weekly basis and recording intake and output can provide critical information about edema and growth. Support from dietary personnel can be valuable when working with and teaching these families.

Skin Care. Pruritus can be intense in the child with cirrhosis. Continued assessment for open lesions, scratch marks, and bleeding is essential. Colloidal oatmeal baths and topical antipruritic lotions, such as calamine, may provide temporary relief. Drugs are not usually an option for itch relief because impaired liver function affects metabolism of drugs. Use of sedatives, opioids, acetaminophen (Tylenol), and alcohol is strictly avoided. Keeping the nails trimmed short or wearing cotton gloves during sleep can minimize damage to the skin from scratching. Ease of bruising should also be noted.

Prevention of Complications. The following are critical interventions:

- *Infection.* Prevent exposure to infection. Monitor for fever, and report immediately.
- *Ascites.* Monitor for edema, give diuretics as ordered, maintain low-sodium diet, and give albumin as ordered. The child will likely have to be hospitalized for treatment; monitoring intake and output and weight, maintaining fluid balance, and monitoring abdominal girth and distention are nursing concerns.
- *Bleeding.* Administer stool guaiac tests, avoid injections, give vitamin K as ordered, and protect from injury. Identify bleeding as soon as possible. While the child is hospitalized, nursing care involves transfusing blood or blood products safely, maintaining fluid balance, monitoring pulse and blood pressure, administering oxygen therapy, and assisting with endoscopic sclerotherapy or the placement of a Sengstaken-Blakemore tube for compression of bleeding esophageal varices.
- *Encephalopathy.* This results from a buildup of ammonia in the blood from the incomplete breakdown of protein. Limiting protein in the diet, giving lactulose as ordered to decrease the GI bacteria that produce ammonia, administering antibiotics as ordered, and monitoring changes in behavior and level of consciousness are nursing responsibilities.

Developmental and Parental Support. Children with cirrhosis are chronically ill and require much time and effort to maintain optimum health. Providing developmental stimulation on a daily basis is essential, and parents need education and support services to achieve this. In addition, parents need to be educated about the disease, its prognosis, the feasibility of a liver transplant, and the risk of complications. As the parents cope with the potential loss of their child, community resources and national support groups, such as the Children's Liver Foundation, are helpful.

Home Care. The focus of home care is teaching. Because the child will be cared for at home unless a serious complication arises or the child is hospitalized for a liver transplant, parents need much information. Helping the parents develop meals and snacks that meet special nutritional needs on a day-to-day basis can be difficult, and dietary personnel can provide invaluable information. Preventing infection is something parents can control somewhat by sheltering the children from infected individuals as much as possible. The most critical intervention is helping parents identify when they should seek help, specifically if the child develops GI bleeding, changes in level of consciousness, or severe edema. The healthier the child can remain, the better the child and family can focus on developmental skills and preparation for liver transplant.

KEY CONCEPTS

- The GI system is formed in the first 4 weeks of embryonic development. Congenital defects can be traced to this period.
- The GI system is anatomically fully developed at birth but physiologically immature, affecting enzymes, sphincter tone, permeability, secretion, and reabsorption.
- Assessment of GI distress is very difficult in small children and must include a thorough history, physical assessment, and general appraisal of the child's distress, as well as the parent's perception of the child's pain.
- Fluid balance is very quickly affected if the child is experiencing vomiting, diarrhea, or anorexia, so the nurse must assess changes quickly and completely.
- Gastroesophageal alterations often place the child at risk for respiratory distress secondary to aspiration and compression of the abdomen into the pulmonary spaces. Assessment of respiratory function and maintaining the airway are critical interventions.
- Medications play a crucial role managing some upper GI alterations, so the nurse must be aware of dosages, indications, side effects, and teaching needs.
- The emotional needs of the parents need to be addressed quickly if the child has a congenital condition.
- Surgery to repair congenital defects and obstructive conditions requires nursing care similar to that for an adult but with special emphasis on nutrition, fluid status, pain control, parental involvement, and the developmental level of the child.
- Parental anxiety must be addressed with every GI alteration because it can have a significant effect on the child.
- Using appropriate Standard Precautions is essential to prevent the spread of infection in children with GI disorders.
- Some malabsorptive GI disorders are managed by simple dietary changes.
- Home care and teaching have a high priority because parents must have the necessary information to care for their child during the management of GI alterations.
- Community and home health resources are a critical part of nursing care for the child with GI alterations.

ANSWERS to Critical Thinking Exercise 43-1

1. An accurate history is essential to identify the cause of Andrew's problem and any pathophysiologic process that is occurring. Guide Andrew's mother in carefully describing the frequency, amount, and character of the emesis. Ask about the relationship of feeding to vomiting, and determine whether the vomiting is projectile. A comparison of birth weight and current weight will determine whether Andrew is receiving normal nutrition to support weight gain and will assist in an assessment for dehydration. Assess the skin turgor, the fontanels, mucous membranes, and alertness appropriate for his age.

2. Parents, especially first-time parents, often are uncertain of when to seek health care advice. The nurse's responsibility is to set a tone that encourages questions and to give guidelines as to when to seek help. Andrew's mother had called the clinic, but either she did not give an accurate description of the problem or the nurse did not ask the questions that would have made that happen. Access to health care is often limited because clients do not have transportation and do not live near public transportation. Nurses can assist clients to identify resources that are more accessible or resources that assist them in other ways (e.g., financial aid, childcare). Stories of frustration told by parents seeking access to care should be a red flag for change within the system. Some clinics have hotlines that parents can use. Nurses can also manage caseloads of clients and track both preventive and acute care of those clients assigned to them. This process enables them to identify infants and children who are not receiving preventive care, monitor those receiving acute care, and respond to cues that additional intervention is needed.

REFERENCES and READINGS

Aach, R. (1998). Viral hepatitis due to hepatitis viruses A-E and GB virus. In R. Feigin & J. Cherry (Eds.), *Textbook of pediatric infectious diseases* (4th ed., pp. 612-640). Philadelphia: Saunders.

Abel, E. (2001). Managing constipation in a pediatric patient: It is more than a simple problem. *Clinical Excellence for Nurse Practitioners, 5*(4), 211-217.

Ackley, B., & Ludwig, G. (2002). *Nursing diagnosis handbook* (5th ed.). St. Louis: Mosby.

A-Kader, H., & Balistreri, W. (2004). Cholestasis. In R. Behrman, R.M. Kliegman, & H. Jenson (Eds.), *Nelson textbook of pediatrics* (17th ed., pp. 1314-1319). Philadelphia: Saunders.

American Academy of Pediatrics, Committee on Infectious Diseases. (2000). *Report of the Committee on Infectious Diseases: 2000 Red Book* (25th ed.). Elk Grove Village, IL: American Academy of Pediatrics.

American Academy of Pediatrics, Task Force on Infant Position and SIDS. (1992). Positioning and SIDS. *Pediatrics, 89,* 1120-1126.

Anton, P. (1999). Stress and mind-body impact on the course of inflammatory bowel disease. *Seminars in Gastrointestinal Disease: Problem-Solving Approach for Clinical Diagnosis and Management, 10*(1), 14-19.

Aranda, R., & Horgan, K. (1998). Immunosuppressive drugs in the treatment of inflammatory bowel disease. *Seminars in Gastrointestinal Disease: Problem-Solving Approach for Clinical Diagnosis and Management, 9*(1), 3-9.

Baron, M. (2002). Crohn disease in children. *American Journal of Nursing, 102*(10), 29-34.

Behrman, R., Kliegman, R., & Jenson, H. (Eds.). (2004). *Nelson textbook of pediatrics* (17th ed.). Philadelphia: Saunders.

Belkengren, R., & Sapala, S. (2001). Pediatric management problems: Gastroesophageal reflux disease. *Pediatric Nursing, 27*(5), 525.

Berkowitz, C. (2000). *Pediatrics: A primary care approach* (2nd ed.). Philadelphia: Saunders.

Boxel, A., & Puhl, P. (2001). Assessing gut pain. *RN, 64*(4), 39-42.

REFERENCES and READINGS

Braby, J. (2001). Current and emerging treatment for congenital diaphragmatic hernia. *Neonatal Network: Journal of Neonatal Nursing, 20*(2), 5-15, 32-35.

Burg, F., Ingelfinger, J., Polin, R., & Gershon, A. (2002). *Gellis and Kagan's current pediatric therapy* (17th ed.). Philadelphia: Saunders.

Carlson, E. (1998). Irritable bowel syndrome. *Nurse Practitioner, 23*(1), 82-89.

Castiglia, P. (2001). Growth and development: Constipation in children. *Journal of Pediatric Health Care, 15*(4), 200-202.

Centers for Disease Control and Prevention. (2004). Incidence of hepatitis B – United States 1990-2002. *Morbidity and Mortality Weekly Report, 52*(51), 1252-1254.

Centers for Disease Control and Prevention. (2003). Summary of notifiable diseases United States, 2001. *Morbidity and Mortality Weekly Report, 50*(53), 1-108.

Cohen, M., & Laney, D.W. (1999). Infectious diarrhea. In R. Wyllie & J. Hyams (Eds.), *Pediatric gastrointestinal disease* (2nd ed., pp. 348-370). Philadelphia: Saunders.

Coughlin, E. (2003). Assessment and management of pediatric constipation in primary care. *Pediatric Nursing, 29*(4), 296-302.

D'Agostino, J. (2002). Common abdominal emergencies in children. *Emergency Clinics of North America, 20*(1), 139-153.

DiPalma, J., & Gremse, D. (2001). Chronic constipation in children: Rational management. *Consultant, 41*(13), 1723-1732.

Duncan, S. (2000). Educating women about hepatitis. *MCN: The American Journal of Maternal/Child Nursing, 25*(2), 107.

Feldman, M., Friedman, L., Sleisenger, M., & Scharschmidt, B. (2002). *Sleisenger & Fordtran's gastrointestinal and liver disease: Pathophysiology, diagnosis and management.* Philadelphia: Saunders.

Gallarte, R. (2002). Rotavirus: Prevalent cause of viral gastroenteritis in young children. *Journal of Continuing Education Topics and Issues, 4*(1), 43-46.

Garcia-Careaga, M. & Kerner, J. (2004). Malabsorptive disorders. In R. Behrman, R.M. Kliegman, & H. Jenson (Eds.), *Nelson textbook of pediatrics* (17th ed., pp. 1257-1272). Philadelphia: Saunders.

Ghisham, F. (2004). Chronic diarrhea. In R. Behrman, R. Kliegman, & H. Jenson (Eds.), *Nelson textbook of pediatrics* (17th ed., pp. 1276-1281). Philadelphia: Saunders.

Gulanick, M., & Myers, J. (2002). *Nursing care plans: Nursing diagnosis and intervention* (5th ed.). St. Louis, Mosby.

Johnson, M., Maas, M., & Moorhead, S. (2000). *Nursing outcomes classification* (2nd ed.). St. Louis: Mosby.

Jones, M. (2002). Prenatal diagnosis of cleft lip and palate: Detection rates, accuracy of ultrasonography, associated anomalies, and strategies for counseling. *Cleft Palate-Craniofacial Journal, 39*(2), 169-173.

Jones, S. (2003). A clinical pathway for pediatric gastroenteritis. *Gastroenterology Nursing, 26*(1), 7-20.

Kinservik, M., & Friedhoff, M. (2000). Control issues in toilet training. *Pediatric Nursing, 26*(3), 267-274.

Klein, M., & Burd, R. (1999). Hirschsprung's disease. In R. Wyllie & J. Hyams (Eds.), *Pediatric gastrointestinal disease* (2nd ed., pp. 489-498). Philadelphia: Saunders.

Kline, R., Kline, J., DiPalma, J., & Barbero, G. (2001). Enteric-coated pH-dependent peppermint oil capsules for the treatment of irritable bowel syndrome in children. *Journal of Pediatrics, 138*(1), 125-128.

Larson, C. (2000). Evidence-based practice: Safety and efficacy of oral rehydration therapy for the treatment of diarrhea and gastroenteritis in pediatrics. *Pediatric Nursing, 26*(2), 177-179.

Loening-Baucke, V. (1997). Urinary incontinence and urinary tract infection and their resolution with treatment of chronic constipation and urinary symptoms. *Pediatrics, 100,* 288-232.

Martin, L. (2001). Pediatric update: Implementing a critical pathway for oral rehydration of mild to moderate dehydration of children. *Journal of Emergency Nursing, 27*(6), 597-601, 614-618.

Marx, G., Seidman, E., Martin, S., & Deslandres, C. (2002). Outcome of Crohn's disease diagnosed before two years of age. *Journal of Pediatrics, 140*(4), 470-473.

Mason, D. (2000). Gastroesophageal reflux in children: A guide for the advanced practice nurse. *Nursing Clinics of North America, 35*(1), 15-35.

Mattei, P., Stevenson, R., & Ziegler, M. (1999). Appendicitis. In R. Wyllie & J. Hyams (Eds.), *Pediatric gastrointestinal disease* (2nd ed., pp. 466-471). Philadelphia: Saunders.

McCloskey, J., & Bulechek, G. (2000). *Nursing interventions classification* (3rd ed.). St. Louis: Mosby.

McGinley, M. (2001). Management of encopresis and the parent's role. *Nursing Times, 97*(20), 55-58.

Mitchell, J., & Wood, R. (2000). Management of cleft lip and palate in primary care. *Journal of Pediatric Health Care, 14*(1), 14-19.

Morash, D. (2002). An interdisciplinary project that changed practice in feeding methods after pyloromyotomy. *Pediatric Nursing, 28*(2), 113-120.

Moukarzel, A., Lezicka, H., & Ament, M. (2002). Irritable bowel disease and nonspecific diarrhea in infancy and childhood: Relationship with juice carbohydrate malabsorption. *Clinical Pediatrics, 41*(3), 145-50.

Nager, A., & Wang, V. (2002). Comparison of nasogastric and intravenous methods of rehydration in pediatric patients with acute dehydration. *Pediatrics, 109*(4), 566-572.

Nechyba, C., & Gunn, V. (2002). *The Harriet Lane handbook: A manual for pediatric house officers* (16th ed.). St. Louis: Mosby.

Negai, B., & Feldstein, V. (2003). Ultrasound of the acute pediatric abdomen. *Applied Radiology, 32*(3), 13-19.

Nurko, S., Baker, S., Colletti, R., Croffie, J., DiLorenzo, C., Ector, W., & Liptak, G. (2001). Managing constipation: Evidence put to practice. *Contemporary Pediatrics, 18*(12), 56-69.

Nurko, S., Garcia-Aranda, J., Worona, L., & Zlochistry, O. (2000). Cisapride for the treatment of constipation in children: A double-blind study. *Journal of Pediatrics, 136*(1), 35-40.

Orenstein, S.R. (1999). Gastroesophageal reflux. In R. Wyllie & J. Hyams (Eds.), *Pediatric gastrointestinal disease* (2nd ed., pp. 164-188). Philadelphia: Saunders.

Paton, E. (2003). Pediatric update: A 3-month-old with blood in the stool—A case scenario. *Journal of Emergency Nursing, 29*(1), 68-71.

Pena, B., Taylor, G., & Lund, D. (2000). Appendicitis in children: New insights into an old problem. *Patient Care, 34*(5), 183-188.

Phillips, J.D. (1999). Abdominal surgical emergencies. In R. Wyllie & J. Hyams (Eds.), *Pediatric gastrointestinal disease* (2nd ed., pp. 138-146). Philadelphia: Saunders.

Rayhorn, N., & Rayhorn, D. (2002). Inflammatory bowel disease: Symptoms in the bowel and beyond. *Nurse Practitioner, 27*(11), 13-29.

Resnick, J., & Zarem, H. (1999). Diseases and injuries of the oral region. In F.D. Burg, J.R. Ingelfinger, W.R. Wald, & R.A. Polin, *Gillis and Kaman's current pediatric therapy* (16th ed., pp. 1029-1032). Philadelphia: Saunders.

Rudolph, C., Mozur, L., Liptak, G., Baker, R., Boyle, J., Colletti, R., Gerson, W., & Werlin, S. (2001). Guidelines for the evaluation and treatment of gastroesophageal reflux in infants and children. *Journal of Pediatric Gastroenterology and Nutrition, 32* (Supplement 2), S1-S31.

Ruemmele, F., Roy, C., Levy, E., & Seidman, E. (2000). Nutrition as primary therapy in pediatric Crohn's disease: Fact or fantasy? *Journal of Pediatrics, 136*(3), 285-291.

Sandberg, D., Magee, W., & Denk, M. (2002). Neonatal cleft lip and palate repair. *AORN Journal, 75*(3), 490-501.

Selekman, J. (1999). Hepatitis update. *Pediatric Nursing, 25*(5), 542-546.

Snyder, J. & Pickering, L. (2004). Viral hepatitis. In R. Behrman, R.M. Kliegman, & H. Jenson (Eds.), *Nelson textbook of pediatrics* (17th ed., pp. 1324-1332). Philadelphia: Saunders.

Troncone, R., & Auricchio, S. (1999). Celiac disease. In R. Wyllie & J. Hyams (Eds.), *Pediatric gastrointestinal disease* (2nd ed., pp. 306-314). Philadelphia: Saunders.

Vitito, L. (2000). Self-care interventions for the school-aged child with encopresis. *Gastroenterology Nursing, 23*(2), 73-77.

Wald, E., & Marcy, M. (2002). Infections in day care environments. In F. Burg, J. Ingelfinger, R. Polin, & A. Gershon (Eds.), *Gellis and Kagan's current pediatric therapy* (17th ed., pp. 216-223). Philadelphia: Saunders.

West, K., & Grosfeld, J. (1999). Intussusception in infants and children. In R. Wyllie & J. Hyams (Eds.), *Pediatric gastrointestinal disease* (2nd ed., pp. 472-478). Philadelphia: Saunders.

Wyllie, R. (2004). Ileus, adhesions, intussusception, and closed-loop obstructions. In R. Behrman, R.M. Kliegman, & H. Jenson (Eds.), *Nelson textbook of pediatrics* (17th ed., pp. 1241-1243). Philadelphia: Saunders.

44

The Child with a Genitourinary Alteration

◆ LEARNING OBJECTIVES

After studying this chapter, you should be able to:

◎ Describe the anatomy and physiology of the infant's and child's genitourinary system.

◎ Describe the most common diagnostic and screening tests used to assess alteration in genitourinary function.

◎ Discuss frequently seen alterations in the genitourinary system.

◎ Use the nursing process to assess, plan, and provide nursing care to children with common genitourinary alterations.

◎ Develop home care guidelines for the child experiencing a genitourinary alteration.

◆ DEFINITIONS

arteriovenous fistula A connection between an artery and vein, usually for the purpose of hemodialysis.

arteriovenous graft A U-shaped plastic tube inserted between an artery and vein, usually for the purpose of hemodialysis.

dysuria Pain on urination.

edema Presence of abnormally large amounts of fluid in the intercellular tissue spaces of the body.

frequency Urination at short time intervals.

hypercalciuria Excessive calcium in the urine.

hyperlipidemia High cholesterol and triglyceride levels in the blood.

hypoalbuminemia Low albumin levels in the blood.

proteinuria Protein in the urine.

urgency Sudden urge to urinate.

REVIEW OF THE GENITOURINARY SYSTEM

The urinary system consists of the kidneys and ureters, or the upper urinary tract; and the bladder and urethra, or the lower urinary tract. The child's genitourinary system differs in structure and function from an adult's in several ways.

Structure

The bean-shaped kidneys lie one on each side of the spinal column. In an adolescent or adult, the kidney is approximately the size of a fist; in an infant, the size of the kidney is small but proportionally larger. The upper portion of the left kidney lies near the twelfth rib, with the right kidney slightly lower. The *hilum*, the indentation in the kidney, is the area where the blood vessels, lymphatics, nerves, and *ureter* enter the kidney.

A thin, fibrous capsule encases the kidney. The outer region of the kidney is the cortex, and the inner region is the medulla; both can be observed with the kidney dissected longitudinally. The cortex contains the glomeruli and tubules, whereas the medulla contains the renal pyramids. The renal pelvis, located in the area of the hilum, is an extension of the upper end of the ureter.

The ureters extend downward from the kidney and enter the bladder wall. As the bladder fills with urine, it compresses the distal ureters, preventing urine reflux. The bladder is a muscular vessel with a rich blood supply. The infant and child's bladder capacity is approximately equal to 10 ml/kg of body weight (Chandra, 1999). The urethra leads from the bladder and contains an internal sphincter and an external sphincter, which control urination. Boys have a longer urethra than do girls.

The *nephron* is the kidney's functional unit. It consists of Bowman's capsule, glomerulus, proximal tubule, loop of Henle, distal tubule, and collecting duct. Each kidney contains approximately 1 million nephrons.

Blood enters the kidney through the renal arteries, which branch off the abdominal aorta. The renal artery divides and subdivides, eventually culminating in the afferent arterioles, which feed into the glomerular capillaries. The glomerular capillaries empty into the efferent arterioles.

Peritubular capillaries surround the proximal tubule, the loop of Henle, and the distal tubules. The capillaries drain into the venous system. Blood returns to the heart through the renal vein, which enters the inferior vena cava.

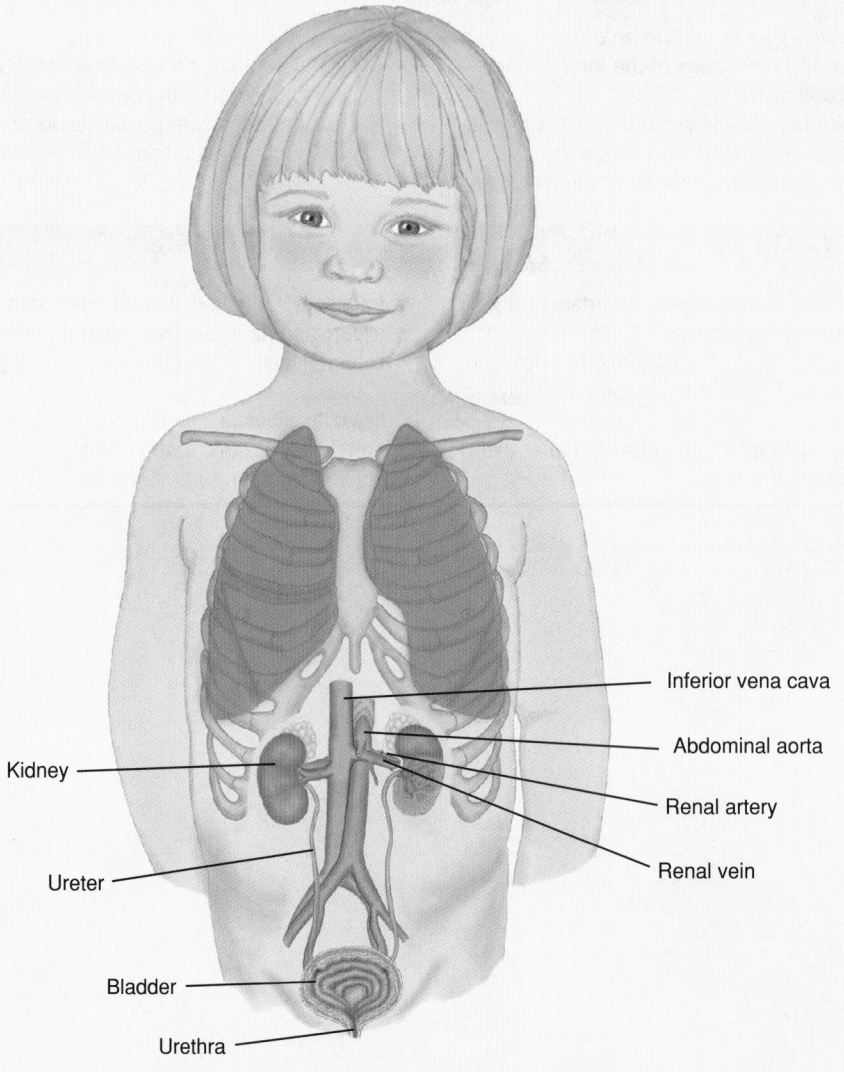

Anatomy of the Genitourinary System

Pediatric Differences in the Genitourinary System

- In a healthy infant, the kidneys operate at a functional level appropriate for body size; however, function is reduced when the infant is under stress.
- By 6 to 12 months of age, kidney function is nearly like that of the adult.
- In premature infants, the reabsorption of glucose, sodium, bicarbonate, and phosphate is reduced.
- The young infant's kidneys cannot concentrate urine as efficiently as those of older children and adults because only 20% of the nephrons have long enough loops of Henle to reach the inner medulla, where concentration and reabsorption occur.* After the first few weeks of life,

the kidneys' acidifying ability reaches the adult level. With acidosis, however, there is only a small increase in acid secretion and susceptibility to acidemia rises.
- The newborn's bladder, which is in the lower abdominal cavity, gradually sinks into the pelvic cavity during early childhood.
- Young children have shorter urethras, which can predispose them to urinary tract infection.
- Children usually achieve complete bladder control by approximately 4 to 5 years of age.†
- Unlike adults, most children with acute renal failure regain normal function.

*Hansen, M. (1998). *Pathophysiology: Foundations of disease and clinical intervention.* Philadelphia: Saunders.
†Tobias, N.E. (2000). Management of nocturnal enuresis. *Nursing Clinics of North America, 35*(1), 37-60.

Function

The kidneys maintain fluid and chemical balance through glomerular filtration, tubular reabsorption, and secretion. The kidney also has important hormonal functions:

- Production of *renin*, which helps with the regulation of blood pressure. Release of renin is stimulated primarily by decreased pressure in the afferent arterioles of the glomerulus.

- Production of *erythropoietin*, which stimulates red blood cell (RBC) production by the bone marrow.
- Metabolism of vitamin D to its active form, which is important in calcium metabolism.

Adequate renal function is important to the function of other body systems. When assessing a child for a possible genitourinary dysfunction, the nurse should consider such nonspecific assessment data as altered growth, skeletal anomalies, hypertension, skin lesions, and immune dysfunctions.

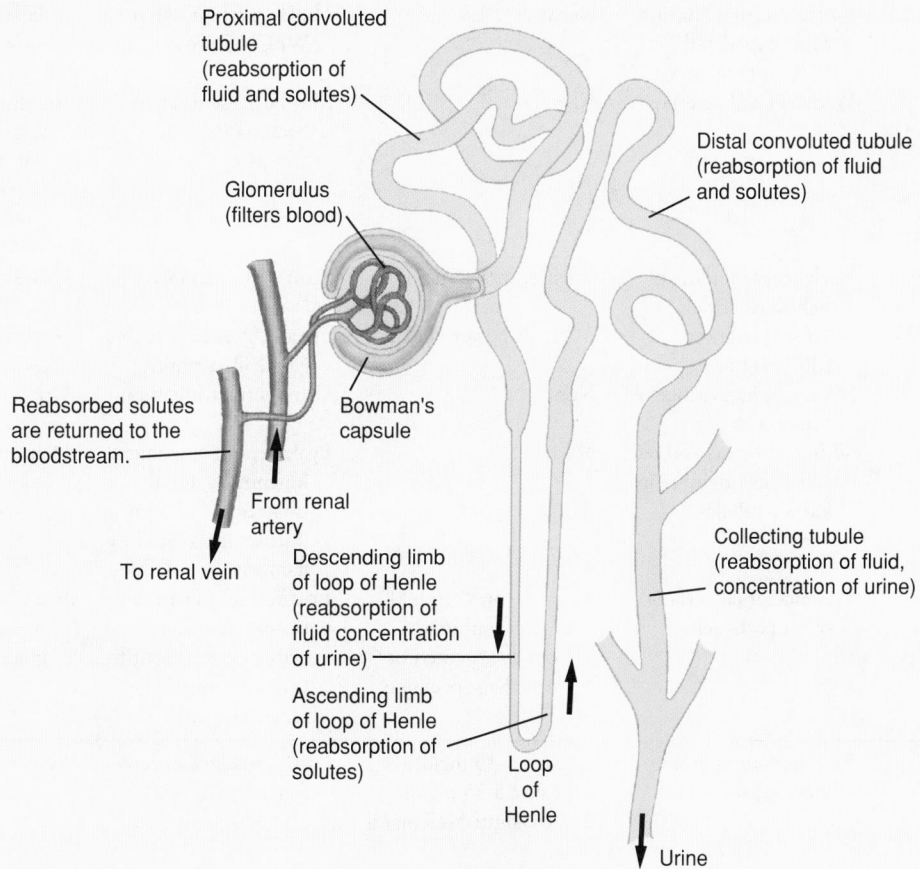

The Nephron

- Proximal convoluted tubule (reabsorption of fluid and solutes)
- Glomerulus (filters blood)
- Distal convoluted tubule (reabsorption of fluid and solutes)
- Reabsorbed solutes are returned to the bloodstream.
- Bowman's capsule
- From renal artery
- To renal vein
- Descending limb of loop of Henle (reabsorption of fluid concentration of urine)
- Ascending limb of loop of Henle (reabsorption of solutes)
- Collecting tubule (reabsorption of fluid, concentration of urine)
- Loop of Henle
- Urine

Common Laboratory and Diagnostic Tests for Genitourinary Disorders

Test	Description	Normal Findings	Indications	Nursing Considerations
URINALYSIS (UA)				
Specific gravity	Measurement of concentration of urine	1.002-1.030	Provides information regarding hydration and renal concentration ability	Specific gravity is higher if protein or glucose is present
pH	Determines acidity and alkalinity	4.6-8.0	Increases in urinary infections	Affected by diet
Protein	Detection of protein in urine	Negative	May be first indication of renal disease	Early-morning specimens preferable because they are more concentrated
Glucose	Detection of glucose in urine	Negative	Screens or confirms diabetes and monitors effectiveness of diabetes control; may be present in child with weight loss, dehydration, infection, renal disease	Nonspecific, needs further evaluation
Ketones	Formed in liver and completely metabolized; alteration in carbohydrate metabolism leads to excessive ketone production	Negative	Mainly associated with diabetes; may be present with fever, anorexia, diarrhea, fasting, starvation, prolonged vomiting	Children are more prone to development of ketonuria
Leukocyte esterase	Enzyme released during white blood cell (WBC) breakdown	Negative	May be present when WBCs in urine	Indicates possible urinary tract infection
Nitrites	Produced by bacteria	Negative	May be present when bacteria in urine	In infant and child, bacteria may not be present in bladder long enough to produce sufficient nitrites to yield positive results
White blood cells (WBCs)	Microscopic finding of WBCs in urine	0-2/high-power field	Seen with infection	Urine culture indicated
Red blood cells (RBCs)	Microscopic finding of RBCs in urine	0-2/high-power field	Trauma, stones, infection, glomerulonephritis	Normal in menstruating females
Bacteria	Microscopic presence of bacteria in urine	None	Urinary tract infection	Urine culture indicated
Casts	White cell casts and red cell casts originate in kidney tubules	None	Pyelonephritis, glomerulonephritis, renal infarction, collagen disease, interstitial inflammation of kidney	Helps in diagnosis
Urine culture and sensitivity	Presence of bacteria or other pathogens	Negative or < 100,000 colonies/ml urine from clean-catch or sterile bag specimen	Isolation and identification of pathogens in urinary tract; identification of antibiotic sensitivity	See Chapter 37 for specimen collection guidelines
SERUM STUDIES				
Blood urea nitrogen (BUN)	End product of protein metabolism	0-6 mo: 4-15 mg/dl 6-24 mo: 5-15 mg/dl 2 yr to adult: 5-25 mg/dl	Gross indicator of renal function	Increases in renal insufficiency

Common Laboratory and Diagnostic Tests for Genitourinary Disorders—cont'd

Test	Description	Normal Findings	Indications	Nursing Considerations
SERUM STUDIES—cont'd				
Serum creatinine (Cr)	By-product of muscle metabolism; production is constant as long as muscle mass remains constant	0-2 wk: 0.2-0.8 mg/dl 2 wk to 2 yr: 0.2-0.4 mg/dl 2-4 yr: 0.3-0.6 mg/dl 4-6 yr: 0.4-0.8 mg/dl 6-10 yr: 0.4-0.8 mg/dl 10-12 yr: 0.5-1.0 mg/dl *Female:* 12 yr to adult: 0.5-1.1 mg/dl *Male:* 12 yr to adult: 0.6-1.2 mg/dl	Increases in renal insufficiency	Should be assessed before giving nephrotoxic chemotherapeutic agents
Serum osmolality	Measurement of concentration of blood, determined by solute in blood	275-295 mOsm/kg	Indication of fluid and electrolyte balance	Helpful in evaluating hydration status, liver disease, antidiuretic hormone function
RADIOGRAPHY				
Kidney, ureter, bladder (KUB), flat plate scout film	Abdominal radiograph	Normal abdominal structures	Diagnoses renal stones; done before renal studies	No discomfort
Cystoscopy	Bladder and urethra examined with cystoscope—a tubular, lighted, telescopic lens	Normal appearance	Examination of bladder and lower tract; visualization of tumor and stones; removal of small stones; biopsy of bladder or tumors; fulguration of bladder tumors and posterior urethral valves	Usually performed with child under general anesthesia; little pain involved; encourage fluids; assess ability to void after procedure
IMAGING STUDIES				
Computed tomography (CT scan)	Computerized calculations revealing a pattern of shades	Normal appearance	Renal tumors	Sedation may be required; child lies on back and should be still; oral contrast material may be administered; child is usually on nothing-by-mouth (NPO) status because of sedation or oral contrast material
Voiding cystourethrogram (VCUG)	Contrast dye instilled in bladder; child or infant voids after bladder is full; serial films taken	Negative for reflux and dilation of posterior urethra, complete bladder emptying	Detects reflux of urine into ureters and its severity; detects bladder-emptying problems; detects urethral problems	Can be done in nuclear medicine department to decrease radiation exposure; procedure is invasive; provide support and diversionary activities for child
Dimercaptosuccinic acid (DMSA) renal scan	Injection of radioactive agent technetium-99m (^{99m}Tc)-DMSA to allow visualization of kidney structures and function; serial films taken	Prompt uptake and excretion of radioactive agent	Evaluates blood flow and renal function; assess renal scarring; identifies pyelonephritis	Minimal radiation exposure; child must remain still for procedure

Continued

Common Laboratory and Diagnostic Tests for Genitourinary Disorders—cont'd

Test	Description	Normal Findings	Indications	Nursing Considerations
IMAGING STUDIES—cont'd				
Renal ultrasound	Noninvasive; high-frequency sound waves directed at kidneys, ureters, and bladder	Normal size, shape, position, function of kidneys	Assesses position, size, and contour of kidneys, ureters, bladder; detects obstruction and stones; localizes for renal biopsy	Child lies on abdomen; if for transplantation, child lies on back
Intravenous pyelogram (IVP)	Intravenous injection of contrast material concentrates in urine and is seen in kidneys and urine; serial radiographic studies are done; a postvoid film is done after child has emptied the bladder	Normal appearance; activity in kidneys by 2-5 min; no residual urine on postvoid film	Determines bladder's ability to empty completely; provides information about kidneys, ureters, and bladder anatomy; identifies masses that compress urinary system	Child should be on NPO status for a period of time in preparation for receiving contrast material; assess child for hypersensitivity to contrast material; contraindications include decreased renal function
URODYNAMIC STUDIES				
	Invasive test involving urethral and rectal catheters and perineal surface electrodes; measures urine flow, bladder capacity, sensation, sphincter function, bladder pressures; measures voluntary and involuntary contractions	Normal bladder function	Voiding dysfunction, abnormal urinary tract	Inform child and family of procedure; provide support for child throughout procedure; provide diversionary activities

Genitourinary alterations in children encompass a wide range of conditions, from a single acute urinary tract infection (UTI) to end-stage renal disease (ESRD). The effects of illness on the child and family depend on the nature of the illness as well as its severity and prognosis. Nursing care also varies. A child in an acute phase of nephrotic syndrome is hospitalized. Less severe genitourinary disorders may be treated at home. There, the nurse can teach administration of an intravenous (IV) antibiotic or monitor adherence to a treatment plan.

ENURESIS

Children with difficulties in urinary control are defined as having enuresis. Nocturnal enuresis occurs at nighttime during sleep, whereas diurnal enuresis occurs during the day, or in waking hours. Primary enuresis is defined as never having experienced a period of dryness, whereas secondary enuresis occurs when a 6- to 12-month period of dryness has preceded the onset of wetting (Tobias, 2000).

Etiology

Although there is no single cause for enuresis, several risk factors have been implicated. Physical factors include decreased bladder capacity, underlying urinary tract abnormalities, neurologic alterations, obstructive sleep apnea, constipation, urinary tract infection, pinworm infestation, diabetes mellitus, and voiding dysfunction. Emotional factors related to increased stress can contribute to secondary enuresis. These factors include family disruption, inappropriate pressure during toilet training, inadequate attention to voiding cues, and decreased self-esteem. Sexual abuse must be considered in a child with secondary enuresis.

Incidence

Primary nocturnal enuresis is common, affecting approximately 3% to 7% of children at 5 years of age and decreasing to 2% to 3% of children older than 8 years (Boris & Dalton, 2004). It occurs more frequently in boys and in children with a family history of bed-wetting. Most children eventually outgrow bed-wetting without therapeutic intervention. Some children experience diurnal enuresis without nocturnal enuresis; this usually is related to waiting until the last minute to void and not being able to access a bathroom quickly (Boris & Dalton, 2004). Children with both nocturnal and diurnal enuresis are at increased risk for genitourinary abnormalities (Boris & Dalton, 2004). Primary enuresis often resolves spontaneously.

Manifestations

Nocturnal Enuresis   only at night

Children with an ongoing history of bed-wetting are not able to sense bladder fullness and do not awaken to void. Because physical maturation varies, nocturnal enuresis is not a matter for excessive concern until the child is older than 6 years or experiences markedly decreased self-esteem.

Pathophysiology

of Enuresis

Control of urination is related to the maturity of the central nervous system. By 5 years of age, most children are aware of bladder fullness and are able to voluntarily control voiding. Children usually achieve daytime urinary control first, with nighttime dryness occurring later. Girls seem to master this earlier than boys. Children who have primary nocturnal enuresis may have delayed maturation of this portion of the central nervous system.

A child with secondary nocturnal enuresis or with problems of daytime control and complaints of dysuria, urgency, or frequency should be evaluated for other conditions. Bladder infections can give rise to such symptoms. Excessive calcium loss in the urine can irritate the bladder and cause painful urination, urgency, frequency, or wetting. Secondary enuresis accompanied by excessive thirst and weight loss may indicate the onset of diabetes mellitus. Children whose bladders are very sensitive to urine volume may experience uninhibited bladder contractions. Moderate to large amounts of urine in the bladder give rise to strong contractions of the bladder muscle. Anatomic abnormality in these cases is rare.

Diurnal Enuresis

Children experiencing urgency, frequency, and inappropriate wetting during the day may be seen rushing to the bathroom or tightly crossing their legs. Often these children cannot sit still and exhibit a constant odor of urine.

Diagnostic Evaluation

The diagnosis of enuresis is based on the history and presenting clinical symptoms. Urinalysis and urine culture can rule out possible UTI. Urine specific gravity and glucose measurement test for underlying diabetes. In addition, the child's urine should be checked for excessive calcium and a pinworm preparation should be done to exclude infestation.

If the child is experiencing daytime enuresis, voiding dysfunction with urge incontinence is explored. Measures of urine flow and bladder capacity and bladder ultrasound may be indicated. Children with UTIs should have a work-up for underlying structural abnormalities.

Therapeutic Management

Treatment of primary nocturnal enuresis may begin with general interventions, such as explaining theories underlying the problem in terms the child can understand. The child is reassured that, with assistance, the problem can resolve. Commonsense approaches of limiting fluids after supper and voiding just before bedtime are encouraged. Also, the child can be trained to use imagery: thinking about what a full bladder feels like and picturing waking up and going to the bathroom. This imagery is done as the child lies in bed before drifting off to sleep. The child should keep a record of the number of dry and wet nights to measure progress (Jalkut, Lerman, & Churchill, 2001).

Reward systems assume bed-wetting is a voluntary behavior and have had varying results for the child with primary nocturnal enuresis. The child may be given a roll of favorite stickers to mark the dry nights on the calendar. The family decides on a special reward or outing when the child has achieved a certain number of consecutive dry nights.

Behavioral conditioning using alarms has been successful in the older child with nocturnal enuresis. A device worn on the child's pajamas contains a moisture-sensitive alarm. As the child starts to void, the alarm goes off, awakening the child. The alarm system must be used consistently over several months to evaluate its effectiveness.

Imipramine hydrochloride, a tricyclic antidepressant, has been used effectively to treat nocturnal enuresis, although the mechanism of action is not completely understood. Because of the overdose potential with this medication, parents should be cautioned about safe storage. Desmopressin acetate (1-deamino-8-D-arginine vasopressin [DDAVP]) has also been helpful because of its antidiuretic effect. DDAVP is a nasal spray and particularly useful for periodic management of enuresis, such as when the child attends a sleep-over at another child's house.

Voiding frequently to keep urine volume in the bladder low may benefit children who are affected by uninhibited bladder contractions during the day. The use of an anticholinergic, such as oxybutynin chloride, which relaxes the smooth muscle of the bladder, can be helpful for children with diurnal enuresis related to underlying bladder instability or small bladder capacity. Biofeedback may also help children with diurnal enuresis, particularly those with dysfunctional voiding.

■ NURSING CARE
The Child With Enuresis

Assessment

The nurse should obtain a full set of vital signs and assess the child and parent for their understanding of enuresis, including the interventions they have already tried. The nurse asks the child and parent to describe voiding and bowel elimination patterns, establishing whether the enuresis is primary or secondary. The nurse should also ask if the child participates in social activities with peers, such as sleep-overs, and if the child is concerned about the problem of wetting. Therapy is much more successful for the older child than for the younger child, who may not be bothered by bed-wetting. The nurse should assist the child in obtaining a urine specimen. The physical examination includes assessment for signs of sexual abuse or visible genital abnormalities. It also is important to observe the lower spine for the presence of a dimple or hair tuft that might suggest spina bifida occulta (see Chapter 52).

Nursing Diagnosis and Planning

The nursing diagnoses and expected outcomes that may be appropriate following assessment of the child with enuresis are

- Situational Low Self-Esteem related to bed-wetting or urinary incontinence.
  Expected Outcome: The child will demonstrate positive self-esteem, as evidenced by a realistic description of the problem and positive self-statements.

- Impaired Social Interaction related to bed-wetting or urinary incontinence.
  Expected Outcome: The child will participate in age-appropriate activities such as sleep-overs and overnight camp.
- Compromised Family Coping related to negative social stigma and increased laundry load.
  Expected Outcomes: The family will identify strengths and will describe positive problem-solving strategies.
- Risk for Impaired Skin Integrity related to prolonged contact with urine.
  Expected Outcome: The child will have no rashes or redness in the perineal area.

Interventions

Enuresis can be a frustrating problem for both the child and family. The nurse can help by providing them with correct information about causes and therapeutic approaches. It is important that the family choose the treatment that will best meet its needs. Follow-up to determine the effectiveness of treatment is essential, because becoming dry can be a long process and the nurse is instrumental in providing support to the child and family over the entire course of therapy.

Evaluation

- Is the child able to describe ways to manage the condition?
- Is the child verbalizing a decrease in stress related to the enuresis, and does the child make positive self-statements?
- Is the child showing an increased interest in peer activities?
- Is the family able to identify its strengths and demonstrate appropriate problem solving?
- Is the child experiencing increased dry nights, and does the child's skin remain intact?

URINARY TRACT INFECTIONS

UTIs, which are characterized by the presence of bacteria in the urine along with systemic signs of infection, are commonly seen in children. In fact, they result in significant morbidity in infants and children (Chon, Lai, & Shortliffe, 2001). These infections can have long-term complications that include renal scarring with decreased renal function, high blood pressure, and, rarely, ESRD.

Etiology

UTIs, except in newborn infants, are caused by bacteria ascending from outside the urethra into the bladder and from there into the upper urinary tract. Bacteria in the blood, which seed in the kidney, can cause UTIs in newborn infants.

Fecal bacteria cause most UTIs. *Escherichia coli* is implicated in approximately 80% of affected infants and children. Other bacteria known to cause UTIs are group B streptococci, *Klebsiella pneumoniae*, *Proteus* species, *Enterobacter* species, enterococci, and *Staphylococcus* species. Viruses and fungi, specifically *Candida* species, can rarely cause infections.

The following conditions predispose the infant or child to UTI:

- Urinary tract obstructions, which can be congenital or acquired. These include strictures, ureteropelvic narrowing, or other urinary tract anomalies. *Hydronephrosis* is dilation of the renal pelvis, usually caused by ureteropelvic junction obstruction. *Phimosis*, which is a narrowing of the prepuce opening, prevents the foreskin from being retracted.
- Voiding dysfunction resulting in urinary stasis. Conditions contributing to incomplete bladder emptying include neurogenic bladder and bladder instability. Constipation that causes pressure on the bladder can inhibit complete bladder emptying.
- Anatomic differences. Young girls have a short urethra, which expedites bacterial transit.
- Individual susceptibility to infection. Some infants and children experience UTIs without any structural abnormality and may be more prone to bacterial adherence to epithelial cells in the urinary tract (Bartkowski, 2001).
- Reflux. A primary contributing factor to upper UTI, or pyelonephritis, is vesicoureteral reflux (VUR).
- UTIs in toddler-age girls is more frequent during toilet training, most probably due to urinary retention or incomplete bladder emptying (Elder, 2004). It is generally accepted, however, that bacterial colonization of the prepuce of uncircumcised infants can increase the risk of UTI in infant boys younger than 1 year.
- Sexually active adolescent girls are at risk for UTIs.

Incidence

Infections during infancy are seen more frequently in boys, particularly before the age of 6 months in uncircumcised boys; after age 1 year, the incidence is substantially higher in girls. Current recommendations include obtaining a urinalysis on the child with fever of unknown origin and obtaining urine cultures on the infant or young child 2 to 24 months of age with unexplained fever (American Academy of Pediatrics, 1999).

The overall prevalence of UTIs in the United States is 3% to 5% in girls and 1% in boys (Elder, 2004). Shaw, Gorelick, McGowan, Yakscoe, & Schwartz (1998) concluded that the incidence of UTI is greater than previously estimated because children younger than 2 years who present with a febrile respiratory or gastrointestinal illness frequently have a coexisting undiagnosed UTI. Because scarring with reduced renal

---

Pathophysiology

of Urinary Tract Infections

Fecal bacteria colonize the perineal area or under the prepuce of uncircumcised infant boys. Bacteria adhere to epithelial cells in the urinary tract and then ascend through the urethra into the bladder, causing a bladder infection, or *cystitis*. In most circumstances, the bladder is emptied on a regular basis, which decreases the opportunity for bacterial growth. In children with incomplete bladder emptying, bacteria grow in the residual urine.

Bacteria ascending from the bladder into the ureters and up into the renal parenchyma cause pyelonephritis. Pyelonephritis is more frequently seen in children with vesicoureteral reflux (VUR) but can occur in its absence.

Scarring, as an inflammatory consequence of pyelonephritis, is more frequently seen in infants younger than 1 year and is a significant cause of hypertension during childhood. Scarring causes decreased arterial perfusion to the kidney, mimicking volume depletion. This triggers the renin-angiotensin mechanism to increase aldosterone release and cause sodium and fluid retention. The subsequent increase in circulating blood volume results in hypertension.

Pathophysiology

of Hydronephrosis

Obstruction at the ureteropelvic junction or other parts of the ureter causes dilation of the kidney. As the renal dilation increases, the risk of renal parenchymal damage and decreased renal function increases as well. In some instances, the obstruction is only partial, causing an initial dilation but no progressive renal function loss. Hydronephrosis can be associated with vesicoureteral reflux (VUR).

Ultrasonography has facilitated prenatal diagnosis of hydronephrosis. Many infants diagnosed prenatally have had spontaneous resolution of the condition.

---

function can result from missed UTIs, the study authors suggest considering UTI in any young child who presents with a febrile illness (Shaw et al., 1998). VUR is a frequently seen underlying anatomical abnormality in children with UTIs. Caucasian girls are affected much more frequently than African-American girls.

Manifestations

Clinical manifestations of UTI vary widely; factors include the child's age, gender, underlying anatomic or neurologic abnormalities, and frequency of recurrence. Signs in the young child and infant are more vague and nonspecific. *Fever* (38° C [100.4° F]) without a focus for infection in infants and young children 2 to 24 months of age suggests a UTI.

An abdominal mass can suggest hydronephrosis in an infant. Other signs and symptoms of hydronephrosis are similar to those for an infant with a UTI (Box 44-1).

Pathophysiology

of Vesicoureteral Reflux

A valvelike mechanism at the junction of the ureter and bladder prevents urine from refluxing into the ureters. As urine fills the bladder or as the bladder contracts during voiding, pressure in the bladder occludes the opening to the ureter. When a defect occurs at the vesicoureteral junction, vesicoureteral reflux (VUR) results. The defect at the vesicoureteral junction is considered a congenital abnormality, although transitory VUR associated with a lower urinary tract infection is also possible.

In VUR, two mechanisms contribute to urinary tract infection (UTI). Bacteria in the urine can be carried up to the kidney, causing pyelonephritis and renal damage with scarring. Also, urine that has refluxed into the lower ureter can return to the bladder, leaving a urine residual that becomes a medium for bacterial growth.

The severity of VUR determines the potential risk for pyelonephritis and kidney damage. The International Classification of Reflux grades reflux on a scale of I through V. Grade I describes reflux into the ureter only with no dilation. Grade V, the most severe, includes gross dilation and reflux involving the kidney.

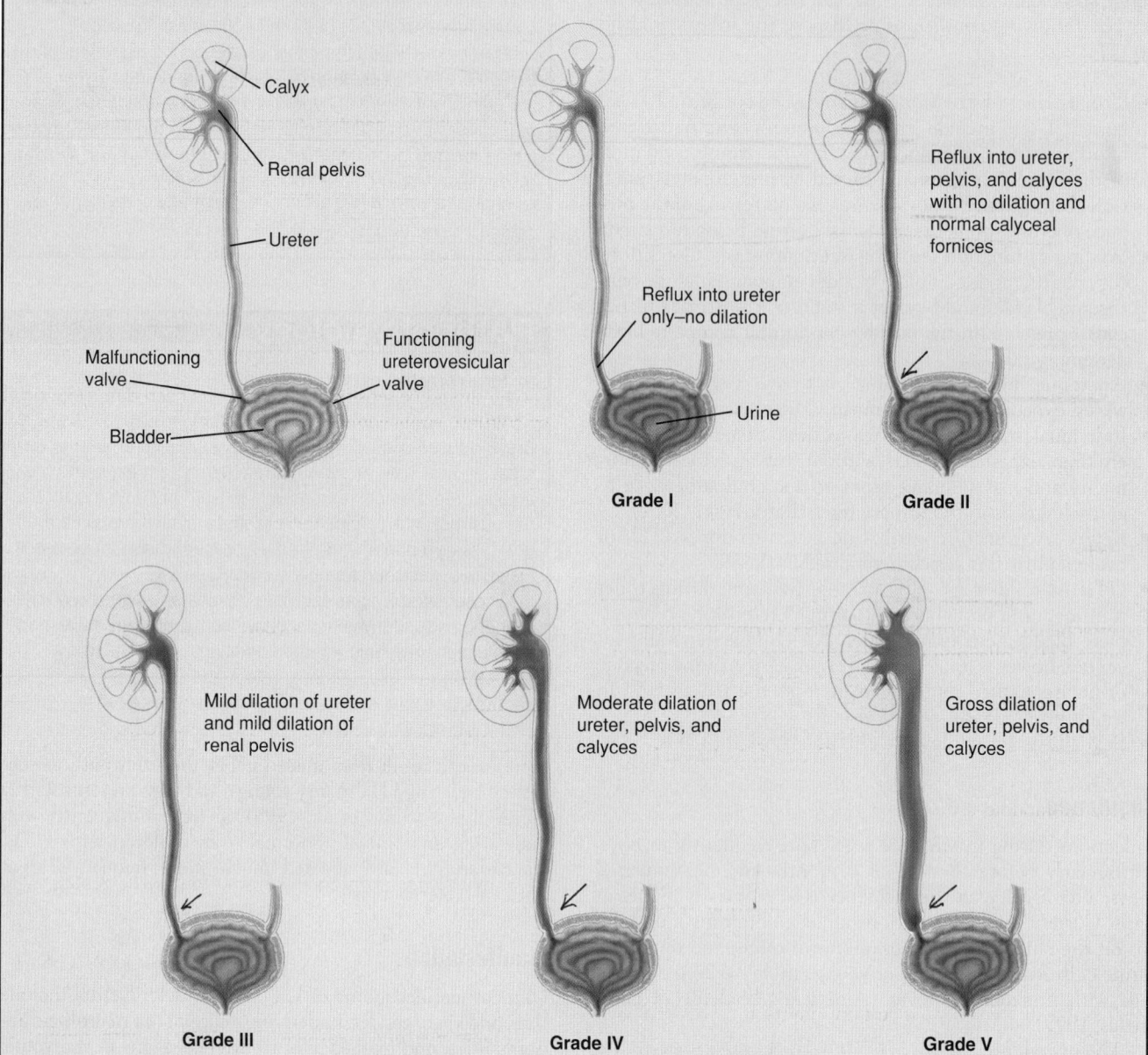

Calyx

Renal pelvis

Ureter

Malfunctioning valve

Functioning ureterovesicular valve

Bladder

Grade I

Reflux into ureter only—no dilation

Urine

Grade II

Reflux into ureter, pelvis, and calyces with no dilation and normal calyceal fornices

Grade III

Mild dilation of ureter and mild dilation of renal pelvis

Grade IV

Moderate dilation of ureter, pelvis, and calyces

Grade V

Gross dilation of ureter, pelvis, and calyces

where ureters enter the bladder (the opening size)

Diagnostic Evaluation

Bacteria in the urine establish a diagnosis of UTI. Symptoms of UTI in the absence of bacteriuria can be caused by perineal inflammation, vaginitis, pinworms, or chemical irritation from bubble baths.

Routine urinalysis that demonstrates hematuria, presence of white blood cells (WBCs), and positive nitrites can suggest a UTI. Urinalysis should be performed on a first morning urine specimen to be most accurate.

Urine culture is the single determining diagnostic study for a UTI. Any bacterial growth of a single-strain bacterium ex-

BOX 44-1 ●
Manifestations of Urinary Tract Infection in Infants and Children

Infants
Nonspecific
Fever or hypothermia in neonate
Irritability
Dysuria as evidenced by crying when voiding
Change in urine odor or color
Poor weight gain
Feeding difficulties

Children
Abdominal or suprapubic pain
Voiding frequency
Voiding urgency
Dysuria
New or increased incidence of enuresis (bed wetting)
Fever — does not happen right away

Children with Pyelonephritis
Same symptoms as for children with uncomplicated urinary
   tract infection plus
High fever, chills
Back pain
Costovertebral angle tenderness
Nausea and vomiting
Appears sick

! CRITICAL TO REMEMBER

Evaluation After a Documented Urinary Tract Infection

Radiologic studies are indicated for infants and children who are likely to experience renal damage associated with structural abnormalities. Studies can diagnose underlying abnormalities as well as monitor the extent of potential renal scarring. The following recommendations guide the necessity for follow-up:
- Radiographic imaging studies for at-risk infants and children (all boys with urinary tract infections [UTIs] and all girls younger than 5 years) after the first UTI. Evaluation of older girls with recurrent UTIs.
- Renal ultrasound before discharge in all infants and children hospitalized for treatment of a febrile UTI or suspected pyelonephritis.
- Voiding cystourethrogram (VCUG) or isotope cystogram for at-risk children when symptoms have disappeared and the urine culture is negative. Some practitioners prefer to wait 4 to 6 weeks after the resolution of the UTI to allow transitory vesicoureteral reflux (VUR) to resolve.
- Renal scan for children diagnosed with VUR and children with suspected pyelonephritis.
- Evaluation of children after the first UTI who have hypertension, have a family history of urinary tract abnormalities, or exhibit delayed growth.

---

ceeding 10^5 colony-forming units/ml of a clean-catch urine establishes a diagnosis of UTI. Obtaining a sterile urine sample is difficult in children, especially children who are not yet toilet-trained. A child who can void on demand can provide a midstream clean-catch urine specimen. In infants and children who are not toilet-trained, a sterile pediatric urine collection bag attached to the perineum can collect a urine specimen (see Chapter 37). Collecting urine by this method is less invasive but not as accurate as by other methods, and the urine specimen must be plated as quickly as possible. If the urine cannot be plated within 10 minutes of collection, it should be refrigerated.

When accurate determination of bacteria is the goal, more intrusive methods of bladder catheterization (see Chapter 37) or suprapubic aspiration are the collection methods of choice. If suprapubic aspiration is necessary, the area above the pubis is cleaned with an antiseptic solution, a needle attached to a syringe is inserted at a 90-degree angle into the bladder, and urine is aspirated. If catheterization or suprapubic aspiration is used to obtain a urine culture, the growth of any bacteria indicates infection.

More intensive evaluation for underlying structural abnormalities is necessary for certain infants and children with UTIs. Evaluative studies include ultrasonography to detect dilation secondary to obstruction and a voiding cystourethrography or radionuclide cystography to detect VUR.

Therapeutic Management

A 3- to 5-day course of oral antibiotics is the treatment of choice for an uncomplicated UTI without systemic symptoms (Chon, Lai, & Shortcliffe, 2001; Elder, 2004). The antibiotic chosen should be sensitive to the specific bacterium (identified by culture), easily administered, and have minimal adverse effects. Oral trimethoprim-sulfamethoxazole and cephalosporins are frequently used. A follow-up urine culture evaluates treatment success.

Children with pyelonephritis require initial treatment with parenteral antibiotics followed by oral antibiotic treatment. The older child who does not need hospitalization can receive daily intramuscular ceftriaxone for 1 to 2 days, followed by 10 to 14 days of oral antibiotics (Bartkowski, 2001). Infants and children admitted to the hospital for treatment usually receive an IV ampicillin or cephalosporin and an aminoglycoside (e.g., gentamicin). Oral antibiotics may follow this initial treatment.

When anatomic abnormalities are detected or UTIs recur, prophylactic antibiotic therapy might be initiated. Prophylactic antibiotics also are given to children after their initial course of treatment while they are waiting for imaging studies to confirm an underlying structural abnormality.

Because the majority of children with grades I through III VUR experience spontaneous resolution of the reflux, most physicians choose nonsurgical management of this condition (Elder, 2004). Children are given prophylactic antibiotics and screened for UTI every 2 to 4 months and when febrile. Cystography every 12 to 18 months monitors the progress of resolution.

A new first-line treatment for children with long-term vesicoureteral reflux is the endoscopic injection of bulking material into the submucosa of the affected ureter. The material, Deflux injectable gel, builds a protective wall inside the ureter to prevent the backflow of urine (Lackgren, Wahlin, Skoldenberg, & Stenberg, 2001). Children with grade III or greater after treatment receive up to two more implantations of Deflux, and those with persistent reflux are referred for open surgery.

Surgical intervention, or reimplantation of the ureters into the bladder, is indicated for persistent severe grades IV and V reflux. Other indications for surgical treatment include frequent UTIs, presence of renal scarring, or noncompliance with antibiotic therapy. Nonsurgical treatment of the child with hydronephrosis is similar to that for the child with VUR. Surgery is required for children with complete obstruction.

■NURSING CARE
The Child With a Urinary Tract Infection

Assessment

The nurse obtains a history of signs and symptoms of UTI from the child and family, which will vary according to age. Determining bowel elimination patterns is important as well, because constipation can increase the risk for UTI in certain children.

Physical assessment includes temperature, blood pressure, abdominal examination for masses, examination for costovertebral angle tenderness, and examination for genital abnormalities. It is important to obtain a urinalysis and urine culture before initiating antibiotics.

Nursing Diagnosis and Planning

The nursing diagnoses and expected outcomes that apply to the child with UTI and family are

■ Risk for Injury to the kidney related to complications from the infectious process.
  Expected Outcome: The child will be free of recurrent UTIs, as evidenced by the absence of voiding frequency and urgency, dysuria, and fever and the presence of a negative urine culture.
■ Deficient Fluid Volume related to decreased intake and increased fluid loss from fever.
  Expected Outcome: The child will maintain adequate intake of fluids and electrolytes for age, as evidenced by an output normal for age (see Chapter 42).
■ Deficient Knowledge related to incomplete understanding of the disease process, diagnostic tests, antibiotic administration, and preventive measures for UTI.
  Expected Outcomes: The parent or child will explain the disease process, diagnostic tests, and preventive measures for UTIs. The family will follow through with appropriate follow-up care, including antibiotic administration and imaging studies, if recommended.

Interventions

Infants admitted to the hospital with fever of unknown origin often are evaluated to rule out a focal infection or septicemia, even though UTI is one of the most frequent causes of fever in infants. The evaluation includes blood studies and cultures, lumbar puncture, and urinary catheterization or suprapubic aspiration for urine culture. The parent already is anxious about the infant, so it is imperative that the nurse inform the parent about why procedures are being done. An IV line is established at the time of the septic work-up because parenteral antibiotics are given while waiting for laboratory results and for several days thereafter if the child has a UTI.

Allow the parent to express concerns, and provide reassurance about the infant's condition. Try to incorporate the infant's routine in care: the mother can continue to breast-feed, ensuring that the IV site is protected as she holds the infant. If the breastfeeding mother is unable to remain with the infant, she will need to pump her breasts. Allowing parents to participate in the infant's care provides them a measure of control in an uncertain situation. The infant with a documented UTI will require a renal ultrasound at the earliest convenient time.

Nursing care of the child who is not hospitalized includes ensuring administration of antibiotics, promoting comfort, maintaining good hydration, preparing the child and parent for diagnostic procedures, and monitoring for response to treatment and complications.

Give the child and family information on the prevention of UTIs. Advise them to adhere to any treatment and recommended follow-up studies. Without causing anxiety, emphasize that repeated UTIs can contribute to renal damage, so prevention is especially important. For older children, once-daily antibiotics are best administered at bedtime because of urinary stasis during the night.

Good hydration is important, especially if the child has been febrile, nauseated, vomiting, or feeding poorly. Encourage oral fluids if possible. IV hydration may be required, especially for young infants. Observe the child for signs of dehydration: poor skin turgor, dry mucous membranes, a sunken fontanel, decreased output, and decreased peripheral perfusion. Daily weights, intake and output, and urine specific gravity are indicators of hydration. Acute renal infection with resulting renal impairment can alter the kidney's ability to concentrate urine, leading to falsely low specific gravity readings (AAP, 2000).

For children with VUR, explain the treatment plan, including medical or surgical management, to the parent and child in a simple, age-appropriate manner. If medical management is elected, both parent and child should understand treatment may last for years and adherence is important. Follow-up includes antibiotic therapy, urine cultures, renal function tests (blood urea nitrogen [BUN], serum creatinine), blood pressure monitoring, and imaging studies.

If surgical treatment is required, give the parent and child information regarding the procedure as well as preoperative and postoperative care. They need to understand that an inpatient hospitalization is required. Medications are given for pain and bladder spasms, which frequently occur after surgery. Follow-up care involves prophylactic antibiotics until a postsurgery cystogram indicates that the VUR has been corrected.

Evaluation

- Is the child free of frequency and dysuria?
- Is the urine culture negative?
- Is the child taking fluids based on expected amounts for age, and is the child's urine output adequate (see Chapter 42)?
- Has the child received follow-up diagnostic testing and antibiotic therapy?
- Can the parent or child describe symptoms of recurrence and measures to take if infection occurs?

CRYPTORCHIDISM

Cryptorchidism (undescended or hidden testes) occurs when one or both testes fail to descend through the inguinal canal into the scrotal sac.

CHILD AND FAMILY
Want to Know

How to Manage and Prevent Urinary Tract Infections

If your child has been diagnosed with a urinary tract infection, it is most important for you to:

- Give your child the prescribed medication for the full number of days your physician or nurse practitioner recommends. Some children need to continue on a lower dose of the antibiotic after the initial treatment is finished.
- Take a follow-up urine culture to the laboratory if your physician or nurse practitioner has requested one. Use a sterile container to collect the urine. If the laboratory has not given you a sterile plastic container, you can use a glass container with a cover that has been sterilized. Make sure the urine stays refrigerated or in a cooler while you take it to the laboratory.
- Keep the appointment if the physician or nurse practitioner has ordered some follow-up studies of your child's urinary system. These studies can help diagnose a structural problem with your child's urinary system or monitor the kidney for any problems.
- Call your physician or nurse practitioner if your child has a fever or symptoms that make you think the infection has returned.

Preventing a urinary tract infection from recurring is important because repeated infections can cause kidney damage. Some suggestions that can help prevent a urinary tract infection are to:

- Wipe babies and teach young girls to wipe from front to back after going to the bathroom. This takes any germs away from the opening that leads into the urinary system. Be sure to keep the foreskin on uncircumcised baby boys as clean as possible.
- Encourage your toilet-trained child to avoid "holding" urine and to urinate at least four times per day, emptying the bladder completely.
- Give your child lots of fluids throughout the day to help flush out the bladder.
- Avoid dressing your child in tight clothing or diapers. Use cotton underwear, rather than synthetic fabric.
- Avoid bubble baths, which can irritate your child's urinary system.
- Emphasize proper hygiene if your daughter is sexually active, and encourage her to urinate immediately after having sexual intercourse.

Incidence

Cryptorchidism is a common urologic problem. Because of the relatively late timing of this developmental process during intrauterine life, premature infants have a higher incidence of undescended testes. Approximately 4% of normal healthy boys have undescended testes at birth (Elder, 2004). Most infants have spontaneous descent of their testes during the first year of life. Children with undescended testes are at increased risk for testicular malignancy.

Manifestations

Testes that are not palpable or not easily guided into the scrotum as well as a previously descended testis that ascends into an extrascrotal position are manifestations of cryptorchidism.

Diagnostic Evaluation

One or both testes may be undescended. If the testis is not palpable, in some instances ultrasound, computed tomography (CT) scan, or magnetic resonance imaging (MRI) can determine its location. The missing testis may be found at any point along the process vaginalis, may be located in the abdomen, or may follow an aberrant course and come to lie in the inguinal area, base of the penis, or perineum (Docimo, Silver, & Cromie, 2000).

Location of an intraabdominal testis may require surgical exploration by laparoscopy. When neither testis can be palpated, the child is evaluated for their presence by hormonal stimulation and measurement of testosterone response. Elevated follicle-stimulating hormone and luteinizing hormone levels accompanied by absent testosterone indicate testicular absence. True absence of both testes is rare.

Pathophysiology
of Cryptorchidism

In normal fetal development, the testes begin their descent from the abdomen between 26 and 28 weeks' gestation. The exact reason for failure of the testes to descend is not known. It is generally agreed that endocrine, mechanical, and neural factors all play significant roles.* Sperm production is decreased in the undescended testis, and risk is increased for development of a malignancy when the child reaches adulthood. Inguinal hernias are commonly associated with cryptorchidism.

*Pillai, S., & Besner, G. (1998). Pediatric testicular problems. *Pediatric Clinics of North America, 45*(4), 813-830.

Therapeutic Management

Initially, the infant with cryptorchidism is managed by observation, because spontaneous descent of the testes during the first year of life is common. Medical or surgical treatment may be instituted after the child's first birthday. Human chorionic gonadotropin (hCG), the pituitary hormone that stimulates the production of testosterone, may be prescribed. It has shown limited success in stimulating the testis to descend.

The treatment of choice is surgical correction, or orchidopexy. The testis is brought down and sutured in place. The most common complications from this surgery are bleeding and infection. The purpose of therapy is to preserve testicular function, provide a normal-appearing scrotum, and enable the child to perform testicular self-examinations as he matures, to screen for malignancy. A testicular prosthesis can be considered for the child with an absent testis on one side.

physical assessment — warm room so they are relaxed

! CRITICAL TO REMEMBER

Assessing for Cryptorchidism

Testes can retract into the inguinal canal if the infant is upset or cold. The cremasteric reflex, or testicular retraction in response to tactile stimulation to the front inner thigh, can lead to a false diagnosis of cryptorchidism.
- Examine the infant in a warm environment. Be sure the infant is calm before the examination.
- Warm your hands before touching the infant.
- Milk the testis downward from the groin, and document its distal point.
- Examine the older child in both a sitting and a frog-leg position.
- Most testes descend by the time the infant is 1 year of age.

▪NURSING CARE

The Child With Cryptorchidism

Assessment

A physical examination should be performed, with careful attention given to the genitalia. Assess the parents' knowledge of undescended testes and the importance of treatment.

Nursing Diagnosis and Planning

The nursing diagnoses and expected outcomes that apply to the child with cryptorchidism and the family are

- Deficient Knowledge (parental) related to cause and management of cryptorchidism.
  Expected Outcome: The parents will be able to explain cryptorchidism, its management, and possible sequelae.
- Effective Therapeutic Regimen Management (individual) related to possible decreased fertility and increased risk of testicular malignancy.
  Expected Outcomes: The parents will help the child learn to perform regular testicular self-examination during adolescence and the individual will seek referral for fertility testing as warranted.

Interventions

Nursing care should be directed at educating parents and providing them with information and resources. If the child has bilateral undescended testes or absence of testes, referrals to a counselor, psychologist, or subspecialist may be appropriate. The nurse provides routine postoperative care after orchidopexy, paying particular attention to voiding patterns, pain and swelling, and signs of bleeding or infection.

Evaluation

- Are the parents able to explain cryptorchidism and its management?
- Do the parents state their responsibilities to guide their child when he is an adolescent to perform regular testicular self-examination and to seek fertility testing if appropriate?

HYPOSPADIAS AND EPISPADIAS

Hypospadias is a congenital anomaly in which the actual opening of the urethral meatus is below the normal placement on the glans of the penis (Fig. 44-1). The degree of misplacement of the urethral opening can vary. The urethra may

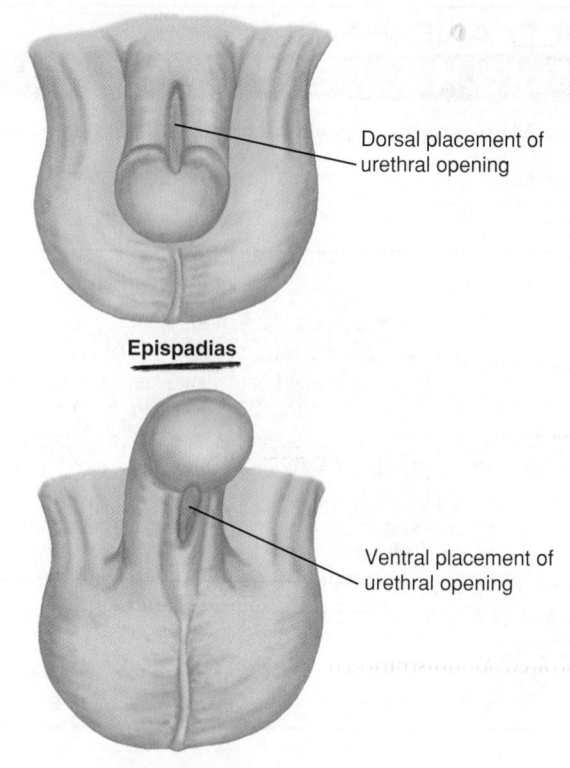

Epispadias

Dorsal placement of urethral opening

Ventral placement of urethral opening

Hypospadias

Figure 44-1 Epispadias and hypospadias are congenital anomalies in which the urethral opening is above or below its normal location on the glans of the penis. Stenosis of the opening could occur, leading to possible urinary tract infections or hydronephrosis. Hypospadias might interfere with fertility if left uncorrected.

open only slightly ventral to the glans or as far back as the penoscrotal junction. *Chordee,* or downward curvature of the penile shaft, can accompany hypospadias. Associated anomalies may include undescended testes and inguinal hernias. Dorsal placement of the urethral opening, or epispadias, also may occur but is less common.

Etiology and Incidence

Hypospadias, including minor degrees, occurs in 2 of every 500 male children (Dolk, 1998). Risk is increased if either the father or a sibling has the anomaly. Testes are undescended in 10% of affected children, and risk for inguinal hernias is increased. Epispadias is extremely rare and is often associated with bladder exstrophy.

Manifestations and Diagnostic Evaluation

Ventral or dorsal placement of the urethral opening, altered urinary stream, and chordee are physical manifestations of hypospadias. Diagnosis is based on physical examination.

Therapeutic Management

Correction of hypospadias is accomplished by surgical intervention, which is usually done in one stage and on an outpatient basis. The surgeon releases the chordee, lengthens the urethra, positions the meatus at the penile tip, and reconstructs the penis. The surgical procedure should be done before the age of toilet training because the location of the

Pathophysiology

of Hypospadias

Hypospadias occurs from incomplete development of the urethra in utero. The exact cause of the defect is not known but is thought to be related to genetic, environmental, and hormonal influences.*

The displacement of the urethral meatus does not usually interfere with urinary continence. Stenosis of the opening, however, would give rise to partial obstruction of out-flowing urine. Further, ventral placement of the urethral opening might interfere with fertility in the mature man if left uncorrected.

*Langer, J., & Coplen, D. (1998). Circumcision and pediatric disorders of the penis. *Pediatric Clinics of North America, 45*(4), 801-812.

meatus may make it difficult for the child to urinate standing up. Surgery is usually done when the child is between 6 and 12 months of age, and with newer microsurgery techniques, the surgery can be done earlier. Studies in infants have demonstrated administration of hCG for a 5-week period preoperatively significantly increases the penile length proximal to the meatus, thus advancing the meatus distally to decrease the severity of the defect (Koff & Jayanthi, 1999). Infants with hypospadias should not be circumcised because the foreskin may be used in the surgical reconstruction. After surgery, the child has some type of temporary urinary diversion to allow for healing of the meatus. Indwelling urinary catheters or urethral stents are commonly used. In addition, the child's activity must be restricted for several days. These treatments are tolerated better by the younger child. The goal of surgery is to make urinary and sexual function as normal as possible and to improve the cosmetic appearance of the penis.

Surgical correction of the child with epispadias can include bladder neck reconstruction and lengthening of the penis and urethra.

■NURSING CARE

The Child With Hypospadias

Hypospadias is usually discovered during the newborn examination. In the infant with hypospadias, palpate the abdomen for a distended bladder or enlarged kidneys. Assess urinary function by observing the urinary stream if possible. For the older infant with hypospadias, question the parents about UTIs, quality of urinary stream (whether it is steady or intermittent), dribbling, or family history of genitourinary problems. Assess the parents' understanding of hypospadias and the surgical procedure and follow-up care necessary for correction.

Nursing Diagnosis and Planning

The nursing diagnoses and expected outcomes that apply to the child with hypospadias and the family are
- Deficient Knowledge (parental) related to diagnosis of hypospadias, surgical procedure, and postoperative care.
  Expected Outcomes: The parents will describe hypospadias and the reason for surgical correction. The parents will actively participate in the postoperative care.

- Risk for Infection related to indwelling catheter.
  Expected Outcome: The child will remain free of UTI, as evidenced by normal urinalysis and culture and absence of fever.
- Acute Pain related to surgery.
  Expected Outcome: The child will exhibit infrequent episodes of crying and normal sleep patterns.
- Impaired Physical Mobility related to surgical procedure on the penis.
  Expected Outcome: The child will tolerate activity restriction, as evidenced by participating in developmentally appropriate bedside play.

Interventions

The nurse should provide parents with detailed preoperative teaching and encourage them to participate in the postoperative care of their child. The child has a pressure dressing to decrease edema, which is removed by the physician after approximately 4 days. Some infants have a stent that drains directly into the diaper, whereas others require a closed drainage bag system. The parents should be able to demonstrate proper care of the catheter or stent before discharge.

The nurse advises parents to encourage the child to drink frequently. High fluid intake is necessary to maintain hydration and free flow of urine. Teach the parent to monitor the child's temperature and observe urine for cloudiness or foul smell. Any signs of a UTI should be reported immediately. Postoperative prophylactic antibiotics are usually prescribed.

The parent should provide the child with a variety of quiet diversional activities, being careful not to traumatize the site. The child can receive medication as ordered for pain. The parent can provide environmental stimulation and a feeling of mobility by transporting the child in a carriage, wagon, or cart. Encourage parents to bring favorite toys or music to help the child feel less anxious.

Evaluation
- Can the parents explain the surgical procedure and postoperative care of their child?
- Are the parents participating in the care of their child?
- Is the child afebrile, and are the child's urinalysis and culture within normal limits?
- Is the child happy, comfortable, and able to sleep?
- Is the child participating in age-appropriate play within restrictions?

MISCELLANEOUS DISORDERS AND ANOMALIES OF THE GENITOURINARY TRACT

Other disorders and anomalies associated with the genitourinary tract are described in Table 44-1. Most of them require surgical correction as noted. For both psychological and mechanical reasons, these defects are usually corrected at a young age; some may require more than one surgery.

ACUTE POSTSTREPTOCOCCAL GLOMERULONEPHRITIS

The term *glomerulonephritis* refers to a group of kidney disorders characterized by inflammatory injury in the glomerulus. Infection or a systemic disease process, such as lupus erythematosus (see Chapter 41) or Schönlein-Henoch purpura (an autoimmune vasculitis), can cause glomerular inflammation. Acute glomerulonephritis refers to disorders that occur suddenly, are

TABLE 44-1　Miscellaneous Disorders and Anomalies of the Genitourinary Tract

Disorder or Anomaly	Therapeutic Management
Hydrocele: Painless swelling of the scrotum caused by a collection of fluid.	In the majority of infants, there is no indication for surgery within the first 12-24 months.[1] Some experts indicate repairing if, in the absence of a hernia, it is readily reducible by examination, progressively enlarging, or persisting as years pass.
Phimosis: Inability to retract the prepuce at an age when it should be retractable (usually 3 yrs).	Accumulation of sebaceous gland secretions and mild cases can be corrected through cleaning and gentle manual retraction. More severe cases require surgical enlargement of the phimotic ring or circumcision.
Testicular torsion: Rotation of the testicle that interrupts its blood supply, causing irreparable testicular damage if not corrected quickly. Manifests by sudden onset of severe, progressive scrotal pain, erythema, and edema. More common in adolescents and infants.	This is a surgical emergency. Surgery straightens and fixates the affected testicle and fixates the other testicle as well, to prevent torsion on the opposite side. If the affected testicle is necrotic, it is removed.
Bladder exstrophy: The extrusion of the urinary bladder to the outside of the body through a developmental defect in the lower abdominal wall. Associated with other genital anomalies, including a wide symphysis pubis.	Protect the exposed bladder tissue by covering it with nonadhering plastic wrap until surgical reconstruction. Surgical management is done in several stages, which include closing the abdominal defect and reconstructing the bladder and genitalia to allow the child to achieve urinary continence. It is important to address attachment issues with parents, who might be overwhelmed by their infant's appearance. Preventing urinary tract infection is essential.
Ambiguous genitalia: *Female pseudohermaphroditism:* Normal internal structures; is potentially fertile. Most common disorder of sexual differentiation, accounting for 60%-70% of all cases. May be associated with an inborn error in the biosynthesis pathway of cortisol.[2] *Male pseudohermaphroditism:* In some types of this disorder, fetal testes do not receive stimulation to produce testosterone. *True hermaphroditism:* Infant has both ovarian and testicular tissues, with abnormal internal and external genital structure. *Anatomic disruption of normal female or male structures:* The mechanism is neither hormonal nor chromosomal.	Cases require special attention, because life-threatening biochemical imbalances can be associated with this condition.[3] Traditionally, potential sexual function, fertility, and the cosmetic appearance of reconstructed genitalia have solely dictated gender assignment. However, new outcome data suggest gender identity is influenced by androgens and sexual dimorphism of the brain and the external virilization is related to the degree of masculinization of the brain.[4] An external and internal masculinization scoring system provides a standardized format to summarize clinical features in newborn infants.[5] It is strongly implied that the prediction of the degree of masculinization of the brain will predict the likelihood of a child accepting his or her gender assignment. Decisions must be made cautiously.[6-8] A genetic workup is indicated because many of these conditions are inherited or autosomal recessive or X-linked traits. Psychological support should also be provided regularly from birth onward.

[1]McCabe, A.J., Martin, D., & Glick, P.L. (2000). Insights. An "owl's eyes" view of hydroceles. *Journal of Pediatrics, 137*(2), 286.

[2]American Academy of Pediatrics, Committee on Genetics. (2000). Evaluation of the newborn with developmental anomalies of the external genitalia. *Pediatrics, 106*(1 Pt. 1), 138-142.

[3]McCormack, K. (1999). A very special baby: Managing a baby with congenital adrenal hyperplasia. *Journal of Neonatal Nursing, 5*(2), 19-25.

[4]Reiner, W.G. (1999). Assignment of sex in neonates with ambiguous genitalia. *Current Opinion in Pediatrics, 11*(4), 363-365.

[5]Ahmed, S.F., Khwaja, O., & Hughes, I.A. (2000). The role of a clinical score in the assignment of ambiguous genitalia. *BJU International, 85*(1), 120-124.

[6]Beh, HG., & Diamond, M. (2000). An emerging ethical and medical dilemma: Should physicians perform sex assignment surgery on infants with ambiguous genitalia? *Michigan Journal of Law, 7*(1), 1-63.

[7]Creighton, S.M., Minto, C.L. & Steele, S.J. (2001). Objective cosmetic and anatomical outcomes at adolescence of feminizing surgery for ambiguous genitalia done in childhood. *Lancet, 358*(9276), 124-125.

[8]Hermer, L. (2002). Paradigms revised: Intersex children, bioethics & the law. *Annals of Health Law, 11*, 195-236.

self-limiting, and resolve completely. Acute poststreptococcal glomerulonephritis is the most common type and is characterized by hematuria, proteinuria, edema, and renal insufficiency.

Etiology and Incidence

Acute poststreptococcal glomerulonephritis occurs as an immune reaction to a group A beta-hemolytic streptococcal infection of the throat or skin.

This disorder occurs most commonly in young school-age children, with a slightly higher incidence in boys. Incidence is higher in the winter and summer, when streptococcal infections are seen most frequently. Clinical symptoms of acute glomerulonephritis usually appear 8 to 21 days after a streptococcal infection (Lieberman, 2000).

Manifestations

Hematuria, which is a cardinal sign of poststreptococcal glomerulonephritis, ranges in severity from microscopic to gross, as evidenced by smoky or tea-colored urine. Edema, which is worse in the morning, affects primarily the eyelids and ankles. This can be accompanied by decreased urinary output. Hypertension can be severe. The child may be febrile.

Many children experience fatigue. Pulmonary edema can be a life-threatening complication.

Diagnostic Evaluation

what went on 3 wks. ago with child (at doctor)?

History, presenting symptoms, and laboratory results can establish the diagnosis of acute poststreptococcal glomerulonephritis. A urinalysis reveals macroscopic or microscopic hematuria with red cell casts, which indicate glomerular injury. Proteinuria is also present but not severe. Blood chemistry values are usually within the normal range. If renal insufficiency is severe, however, BUN and creatinine levels are elevated. Electrolyte disturbances, such as high serum potassium and low serum bicarbonate, can result from inadequate glomerular filtration.

The complete blood count usually demonstrates normal WBCs and mild anemia. The lower hemoglobin and hematocrit values reflect the dilutional effect of extra fluid in the blood as a result of decreased glomerular filtration.

Immunologic studies are important in diagnosing acute poststreptococcal glomerulonephritis. Serum complement (C3) may be low because of the fixation of complement in immune complexes. An antistreptolysin (ASO) titer, which indicates the presence of antibodies to streptococcal bacteria, or a streptozyme test can be elevated. The ASO titer might not be elevated in a streptococcal skin infection. Culture of the throat or skin lesion (if present) may be helpful for isolating the bacterium. Again, this is useful only if the infection is recent and the child has not received antibiotics. A renal biopsy may be indicated for two reasons: (1) for those children whose signs and symptoms are not characteristic of acute poststreptococcal glomerulonephritis; and (2) for those children whose symptoms do not improve as expected.

Therapeutic Management

There is no specific therapy for acute poststreptococcal glomerulonephritis. Supportive care and medical management are directed to the associated signs and symptoms and guided by the degree of renal dysfunction the child experiences. A 10-day course of antibiotic therapy may be required. Children with acute renal failure should be hospitalized to allow for fluid and electrolyte management until their renal function has stabilized.

Antihypertensive therapy may be necessary. This can be accomplished by limiting sodium and water intake or by administering diuretics or antihypertensive medication. The prognosis for children with acute poststreptococcal glomerulonephritis is excellent. The acute clinical episode is usually self-limiting, with diuresis signaling the beginning of resolution. Laboratory values usually return to baseline in 6 to 12 weeks. Most children experience a complete recovery.

■ NURSING CARE

The Child With Acute Poststreptococcal Glomerulonephritis

Assessment

Assess the child for presence of periorbital or lower extremity edema. Obtaining vital signs and monitoring daily weight are important for assessing the degree of fluid retention and hypertension. Be sure to use the appropriate-size blood pressure cuff for the most accurate blood pressure measurement (see Chapter 37). Monitor the child's level of fatigue and anxiety.

Pathophysiology

of Acute Poststreptococcal Glomerulonephritis

Acute glomerulonephritis after a streptococcal infection is thought to occur as a result of an immunologic response. The body responds to the *Streptococcus* bacteria by forming antibodies, which combine with the bacterial antigens to form immune complexes. As these antigen-antibody complexes travel through the circulation, they become trapped in the glomerulus and activate an inflammatory response in the glomerular basement membrane. Products of the inflammatory response damage the glomerular capillaries and reduce the size of the capillary lumen. This process causes a decrease in the glomerular filtration rate, leading to renal insufficiency. Sodium and fluid are retained, and the child exhibits edema and oliguria. In addition, injury to the capillary walls interferes with their permeability so that larger molecules and structures such as red blood cells (RBCs), casts, and proteins can pass through into the urine.

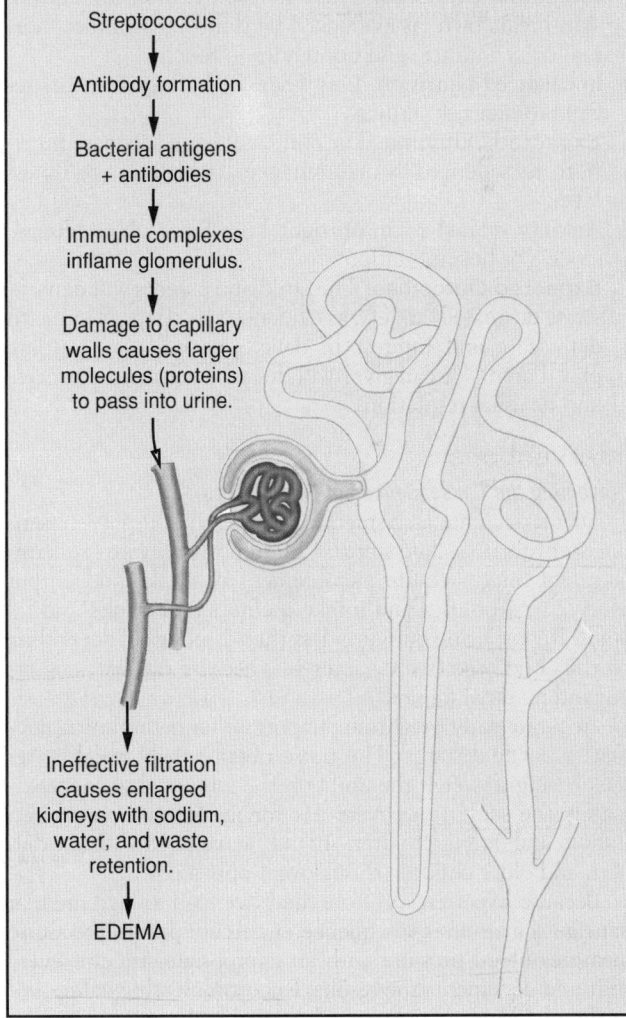

Streptococcus
↓
Antibody formation
↓
Bacterial antigens + antibodies
↓
Immune complexes inflame glomerulus.
↓
Damage to capillary walls causes larger molecules (proteins) to pass into urine.
↓
Ineffective filtration causes enlarged kidneys with sodium, water, and waste retention.
↓
EDEMA

Assess the respiratory system for presence of any respiratory difficulty, such as cough, increased respiratory rate, or increased work of breathing. Auscultate the breath sounds for crackles. Monitor laboratory values, especially urinalysis and serum electrolytes.

Determine what the child and family understand about the illness and reason for hospitalization. The parents may be anxious about permanent damage to the child's kidneys as a result of this condition.

Nursing Diagnosis and Planning

The nursing diagnoses and expected outcomes that apply to the child with acute poststreptococcal glomerulonephritis and the family are

- Risk for Imbalanced Fluid Volume related to retention of sodium and fluid and dietary fluid restriction.

  Expected Outcome: The child will maintain normal fluid status, as evidenced by urine output normal for age-group (see Chapter 42), moist mucous membranes, adequate skin turgor, normal blood pressure, no increase in weight, and no symptoms of respiratory distress.

- Risk for Activity Intolerance related to fatigue.

  Expected Outcome: The child will be rested, as evidenced by the ability to tolerate daily care and play activities.

- Risk for Impaired Skin Integrity related to edema and decreased activity.

  Expected Outcome: The child will exhibit no signs of skin breakdown, as evidenced by skin that is intact, normal color for race, and nontender to touch.

- Imbalanced Nutrition: Less Than Body Requirements related to diet restrictions.

  Expected Outcome: The child will have adequate nutrition, as evidenced by maintenance of weight at pre-illness level.

- Anxiety related to insufficient knowledge about disease process or hospitalization.

  Expected Outcomes: The child and parents will demonstrate decreased anxiety, as evidenced by cooperation with daily care and interest in developmentally appropriate play. Parents or caregiver will describe the disease process and its usual resolution.

Interventions

Preventing the Consequences of Fluid Excess

Frequent, accurate assessment of intake and output is essential for evaluating fluid status. Children with severe renal impairment might require measurement of intake and output every 2 to 4 hours. Fluid intake includes oral intake and IV fluids. Report urine output of less than 1 ml/kg/hr, depending on the child's age (see Chapter 42), because oliguria suggests impending renal failure.

Accurate daily weights are important for determining fluctuation in fluid status. The nurse obtains daily weights, remembering to weigh the child on the same scale at approximately the same time every day for maximum consistency. Infants and young children should be weighed without diapers, and older children should wear only a gown.

Because hypertension from fluid overload and glomerular damage is a severe consequence of this condition, the nurse measures blood pressure with an appropriate-size cuff every shift and documents the results. Report increasing values immediately. More frequent readings might be required if the child has significant hypertension or receives antihypertensive medication.

Auscultate breath sounds every shift, and document increased respiratory effort. Rapid respirations, retractions, nasal flaring, or crackles are signs of developing pulmonary edema, which can result from fluid overload.

Limit fluid intake if ordered. Limitation might be difficult if children are old enough to sneak drinks on their own or obtain them from people who are unaware of restrictions. The nurse should inform parents, visitors, and hospital staff of the need to limit fluids. Be sure to record the child's favorite fluids on the nursing care plan, so the child is able to enjoy the fluids given. Encourage the child to consume fluids gradually, rather than large amounts all at once. Provide the child with only the agreed-on amount for the period involved.

Excessive sodium can increase fluid retention. The nurse ensures that a low-sodium diet is followed if ordered. Inform parents and visitors of any dietary restrictions.

Providing Adequate Rest

If fatigue is a problem, it is important that the child has ample opportunity to rest. Children with glomerulonephritis may tire easily when first hospitalized, although most children participate in activities according to their level of fatigue. The nurse needs to arrange daily care so that the child has some uninterrupted time for sleep and naps. Encourage parents to bring a favorite sleep toy or blanket for the child, and allow for nap time and bedtime to coincide with the child's home schedule as much as possible. Try to follow home rituals. If the child is unable to limit activity, the nurse can limit play time to short periods and extend as the child's condition improves.

Maintaining Skin Integrity

Frequent position changes decrease pressure on bony prominences and help decrease edema in dependent areas. Encourage the child to change position at least every 2 hours during the day. If the child is experiencing edema of the lower extremities, elevate them with pillows when the child is sitting or lying in bed. Promote activity as the child improves because activity increases the circulation and promotes reabsorption of fluid from edematous areas.

To prevent skin breakdown, the nurse maintains good hygiene for the child by giving baths and cleaning the skin well after bowel movements and diaper changes. Using a small amount of lotion to massage the skin prevents dryness and promotes active circulation.

Maintaining Nutritional Status

Low-sodium foods taste different, and children may refuse to eat them. Offering low-sodium foods or treats different from those available in the hospital may encourage the child to eat. Consult with the dietary department about palatable low-sodium food and drinks. Allow parents to bring favorite foods from home if these foods comply with dietary restrictions.

A small fluctuation in weight can indicate fluid loss or gain or weight loss from decreased food intake. After obtaining the child's pre-illness weight, the nurse weighs the child daily to monitor for any fluid shifts or underlying weight loss. In addition, the nurse monitors the child for signs of dehydration (dry mucous membranes, listlessness, poor skin turgor, tachycardia) that would coincide with fluid restriction, diuresis, or diuretic administration.

Relieving Anxiety

Allowing parents and the child to voice their concerns provides support and a basis for evaluating their understanding of the disease process and prognosis. Reassure the family that most children recover from this condition with no residual effects. Encourage them to participate in the child's care, helping to make the child comfortable as well as providing suitable play activities and emotional support.

Information enables the child and parents to understand the course of the condition and anticipate procedures and events. Knowing what to expect helps decrease anxiety. It is especially important to provide information about the child's care at home because the child will be discharged quickly unless renal failure is a risk. If the child has been hypertensive or is to be discharged on antihypertensive medications, the nurse instructs parents on how to measure the child's blood pressure and emphasizes that blood pressure should be taken before medication administration. A blood pressure cuff of appropriate size and a stethoscope are ordered before discharge. The nurse explains the parameters for when to withhold medication or when to call the physician for high readings.

Evaluation

- Does the child demonstrate adequate urine output for weight and normal blood pressure for age?
- Are the child's mucous membranes moist, and does the child appear to be well-hydrated?
- Is the child's respiratory status stable?
- Has the child's weight changed from the pre-illness weight?
- Is the child able to tolerate usual activities for age?
- Is the child's skin intact, appropriate color for race, and nontender to touch?
- Is the child relaxed enough to cooperate with care activities and maintain interest in play?
- Do parents participate appropriately in the child's care, provide comfort to the child, and describe the disease process and care required?

NEPHROTIC SYNDROME

Nephrotic syndrome refers to a kidney disorder characterized by proteinuria, hypoalbuminemia, and edema. Nephrotic syndrome can be classified as primary or secondary. *Primary nephrotic syndrome*, or minimal change nephrotic syndrome (MCNS), results from a disorder within the glomerulus of the kidney and is the most common type seen in children. A child also can acquire nephrotic syndrome secondary to a systemic disease, such as hepatitis, systemic lupus erythematosus, heavy metal poisoning, or cancer.

occurs ages 2-6

Etiology

The cause of primary nephrotic syndrome is not fully understood, but it can arise from one of four types of renal lesions. Success in controlling the disease by the use of immunosuppressive drugs suggests the possibility of an immunologic component. In most children, minimal alterations of the glomerulus are seen on histologic examination. Accordingly, the most common disorder is termed *minimal change nephrotic syndrome* and accounts for almost 85% of childhood nephrotic syndrome (Vogt & Avner, 2004). Nephrosis develops in others as a result of focal segmental glomerulosclerosis or, more rarely, because of membranoproliferative glomerulonephritis or mesangial proliferation.

Incidence

Primary nephrotic syndrome occurs most frequently in children between ages 2 and 6 years. The incidence is slightly higher in boys. The prognosis for children with MCNS is very good. Manifestations of the disease usually decrease with age, so relapses are rare in adolescence. Focal segmental glomerulosclerosis carries a poorer prognosis; the disease is progressive and often results in ESRD.

! CRITICAL TO REMEMBER

Differences Between Children With Glomerulonephritis and Children With Nephrotic Syndrome

The signs and symptoms of glomerulonephritis and nephrotic syndrome in children can be confusing. It is important for nurses to be able to discriminate between the two. Remember the following:

The Child with Poststreptococcal Glomerulonephritis
Manifestations
- Hematuria—cola-colored urine
- Hypertensive
- Edema—abrupt onset, mild periorbital or lower extremity
- Usually young school-age child

Laboratory Findings
- Red blood cells, casts, small amount of protein in urine (0 to 2+)
- Normal serum albumin, cholesterol, triglycerides; decreased or normal hemoglobin and hematocrit
- Altered electrolytes, elevated blood urea nitrogen or creatinine
- Elevated antistreptolysin (ASO) titer or streptozyme, decreased complement

Management
- Supportive
- Administration of antihypertensives and diuretics; antibiotic treatment for active streptococcal infection
- Low-salt diet

The Child with Nephrotic Syndrome
Manifestations
- Proteinuria—frothy urine
- Edema—insidious onset, massive edema from shift of fluid into interstitial spaces, worsens during the day
- Hypovolemia
- Normotensive
- Pallor, fatigue
- Toddler or preschool-age child

Laboratory Findings
- Proteinuria (3+ to 4+), possible microscopic hematuria
- Hypoalbuminemia (<2.5 g/dl), elevated cholesterol and triglycerides, elevated hemoglobin, hematocrit, platelets
- Normal serum electrolytes, complement levels, ASO titer

Management *steroids*
- Prednisone to initiate remission—0 to trace protein in urine for 5 to 7 days
- Diuretics, possible albumin administration
- Antibiotics to prevent infection
- No-added-salt diet

Manifestations

Manifestations of primary nephrotic syndrome include edema, anorexia, fatigue, abdominal pain, respiratory infection, and increased weight. Unlike the child with glomerulonephritis, the child with nephrotic syndrome usually has normal blood pressure.

Edema is usually first noted in the periorbital spaces and dependent areas of the body; its onset is often insidious. Children often awaken with facial edema and, as the day progresses, become noticeably edematous in their abdomen, gen-

Pathophysiology

of Nephrotic Syndrome

Primary nephrotic syndrome occurs from an insult to the glomerular basement membrane. Damage to the membrane causes increased permeability and loss of substances that would normally prevent negatively charged proteins from crossing the membrane. Negatively charged proteins, particularly albumin, are cleared at an increased rate, resulting in loss of plasma proteins and proteinuria. Proteinuria is essential for the diagnosis of nephrotic syndrome.

Blood albumin values are low (hypoalbuminemia) because of the loss of albumin through the defective glomerulus and the liver's inability to synthesize proteins to balance the loss. Decreased levels of albumin reduce the plasma oncotic pressure so that the intravascular fluid moves into the interstitial spaces. This shifting of fluid reduces the intravascular volume, causing hypovolemia and subsequent decreased renal blood flow. In an effort to increase blood volume, the kidney stimulates renin production. Renin causes increased excretion of aldosterone, resulting in renal tubular reabsorption of sodium,

which in turn causes water retention. The net effect of this phenomenon is edema.

In addition, the serum values of cholesterol and triglycerides are elevated. This change is thought to result from increased stimulation of lipoprotein production because of the decrease in oncotic pressure. Loss of immunoglobulins into the urine is common in nephrotic syndrome. Most notably, levels of immunoglobulin G (IgG) are decreased, which makes these children more susceptible to infection. Before the use of antibiotics, infection was a frequent cause of death in these children.

Children with nephrotic syndrome are in a hypercoagulable state, predisposing them to venous thrombosis. This tendency occurs as a result of several factors, including decreased intravascular volume (hypovolemia), which causes increased concentration of red blood cells (RBCs) and platelets and slowing of circulation. Urinary loss of proteins that inhibit coagulation also contributes to the risk of thrombus formation.

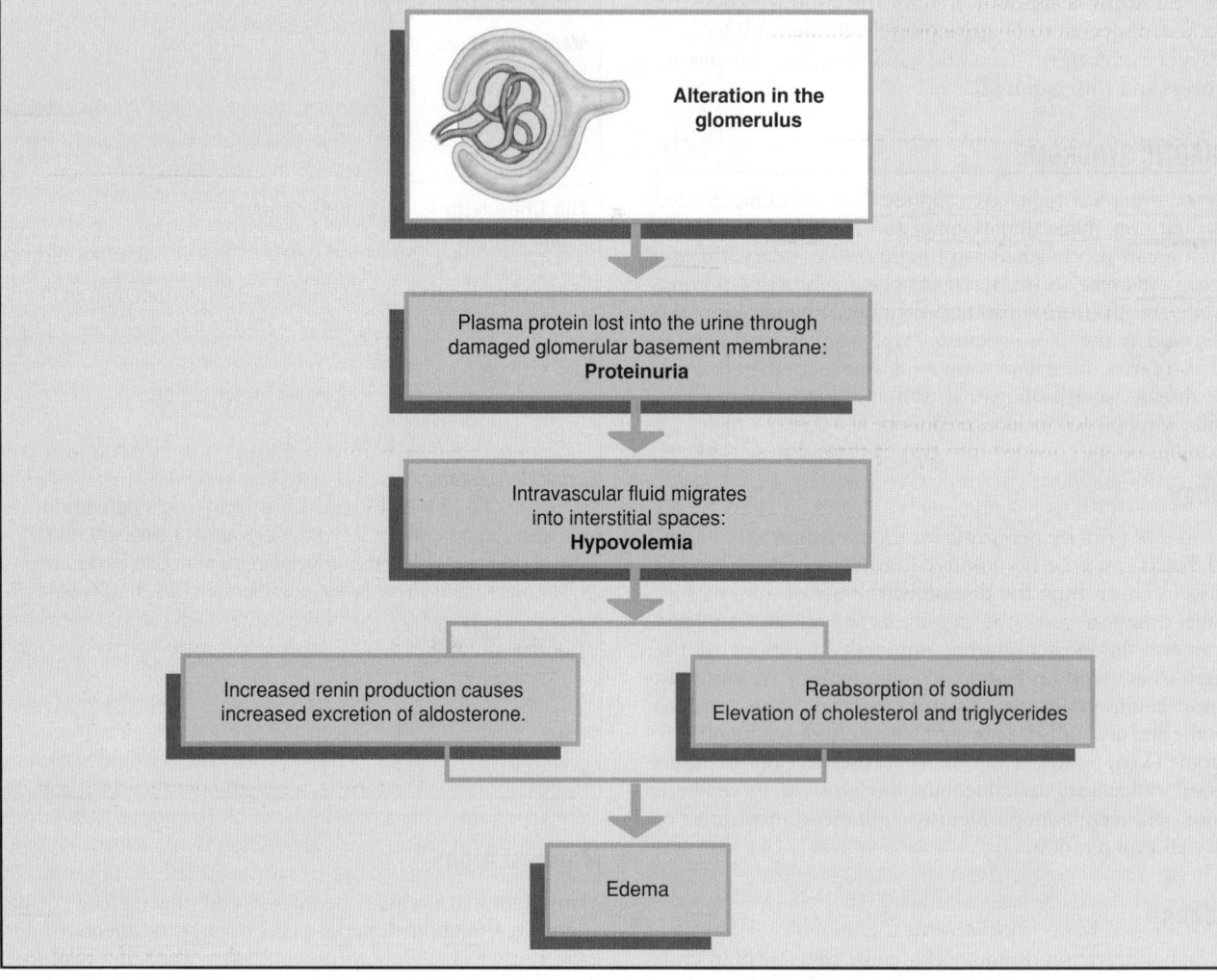

ital area, and lower extremities. The pitting edema is most noticeable over the bony prominences of the lower extremities. Abdominal pain can occur from the presence of extra fluid in the peritoneal area. Edema of the bowel may cause decreased absorption of nutrients and diarrhea. Many children are misdiagnosed with allergies because of periorbital edema and respiratory symptoms.

Diagnostic Evaluation

Nephrotic syndrome can be diagnosed based on the clinical presentation, age of the child, and laboratory results. Urinalysis demonstrates protein (3+ to 4+), and the urine appears dark and frothy. Microscopic hematuria may be present. Serum cholesterol, triglycerides, hematocrit, and hemoglobin are elevated. Serum albumin is markedly decreased (<2.5 g/dl). The child has normal electrolytes and a negative ASO titer or streptozyme test. Serologic tests for hepatitis, human immunodeficiency virus, and syphilis as well as antinuclear antibody titers are done to rule out underlying systemic disease.

Because of an atypical presentation (a child older than 10 years or having gross hematuria or hypertension), a kidney biopsy might be done if a lesion other than MCNS is suspected. A biopsy is also indicated for the child who does not respond as expected to pharmacologic treatment.

Therapeutic Management

It is not unusual for the child with primary nephrotic syndrome to be hospitalized briefly during the initial onset of the disease to provide palliative treatment for the edema, perform necessary diagnostic testing, and initiate therapy. Parents also may be educated about the disease process and necessary home care. Before treatment begins, the child is tested for exposure to tuberculosis and varicella because treatment suppresses the immune system.

Remission Induction

Therapy for remission includes prednisone at a dose of 2 mg/kg/day (maximum 60 mg) divided into two or three doses. This regimen is continued until the child is in remission (zero to trace urine protein for 5 to 7 consecutive days). Steroids usually are continued at the same daily dose for 4 to 6 weeks. After the initial treatment, the child's dose is decreased and changed to an alternate-day schedule and then slowly tapered.

In the event of a relapse, steroid therapy is less prolonged. Once remission is achieved, dosing decreases to alternate days and is tapered more quickly. This is done to minimize prednisone side effects (see Chapter 41).

Some children respond to steroids quickly and achieve remission in 5 to 7 days, whereas others may not respond for 4 weeks. If proteinuria continues beyond 8 weeks of daily steroid therapy, the child is said to be steroid-resistant and a kidney biopsy is done to determine the exact nature of the disease. Children who initially respond to steroid therapy but have relapses while on a tapering schedule or shortly after stopping steroids are said to be *steroid-dependent* (Fig. 44-2). These children may benefit from a course of an alkylating agent, such as cyclophosphamide or chlorambucil. The risks and benefits of this therapy must be carefully considered, and the parents should be informed of all possible side effects. A kidney biopsy is usually

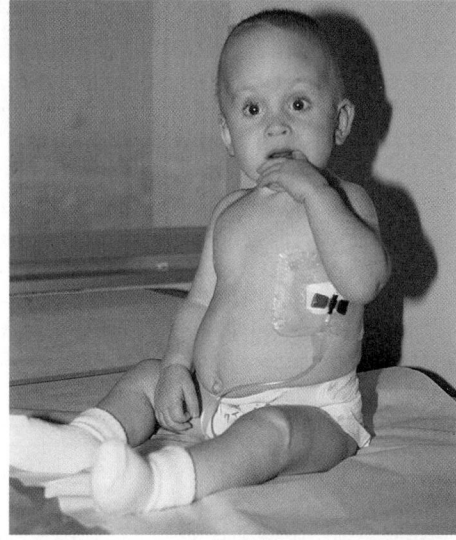

Figure 44-2 This child has nephrotic syndrome that is in remission. She previously received steroid therapy and is now receiving cyclosporine chemotherapy to control the process. During the acute phase of the nephrotic syndrome, the child may have massive edema because blood proteins are lost in the urine. Skin pallor is also common. (Courtesy Children's Medical Center, Dallas, TX.)

done before starting therapy. The use of cyclosporine in children who remain steroid-dependent despite a course of an alkylating agent has proven to be effective in maintaining remission.

Additional Therapy

A no-added-salt diet is indicated. The caregiver should not use salt when cooking; the child should not be permitted to use the salt shaker; and the caregiver should avoid serving high-sodium foods, such as pickles, salted chips, and cured meats. If edema is severe or if the child is hypertensive, sodium intake may be further restricted and the child may be placed on fluid restriction.

Diuretic therapy is initiated until urinary protein loss is controlled. If the edema is marked and causes the child to have decreased mobility, poor oral intake, or decreased urine output, salt-poor albumin may be given intravenously. Albumin helps restore normal plasma osmotic pressure and promotes the movement of interstitial fluid back into the intravascular compartments. Furosemide is given intravenously after the albumin infusion to enhance diuresis and decrease the chance of fluid overload.

Oral penicillin is frequently given to reduce the likelihood of developing an infection. Severe edema in the lower extremities can give rise to cellulitis because of fluid stasis and poor circulation. Peritonitis, a severe complication, can develop from stasis of ascitic fluid, which is an excellent culture medium for organisms such as *Streptococcus pneumoniae*. Live-virus vaccines are contraindicated in children receiving steroid therapy. In addition to routine killed-virus vaccines, the child should receive pneumococcal vaccine to prevent pneumococcal infection in the event of a relapse. It may also be beneficial for the child with nephrotic syndrome to receive an influenza vaccine each year because an exacerbation of the disease can occur after an infection.

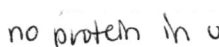

Nursing Care Plan

The Child With Nephrotic Syndrome

FOCUSED ASSESSMENT

The nurse should monitor the child's vital signs for early signs of infection or hypovolemia. Carefully document the child's fluid intake and urine output, and obtain accurate daily weights. Nursing care should include assessing the amount of edema present in the child each shift, specifically in the periorbital areas, abdomen, genitalia, and lower extremities.

Monitor laboratory results to check urine daily for protein. The nursing history should include the child's immunization status and known recent exposures to communicable diseases. Assessment of the family's understanding of the disease process and treatment is important so that the nurse can make appropriate referrals and provide the parents with information.

Nursing Diagnosis

Risk for Impaired Skin Integrity related to edema and decreased circulation.

Expected Outcome

The child will:
- Remain free from skin breakdown, as evidenced by the absence of redness, tenderness to touch, and ulceration.

INTERVENTION	RATIONALE
1. Ensure that the child changes position every 2 hours.	1. Frequent position change decreases pressure on body parts and helps relieve edema in dependent areas.
2. Maintain good hygiene by giving daily baths and changing linen daily. Use non-alcohol-based lotion for dry skin.	2. Body secretions and debris on linens can irritate the skin. Gentle massage when bathing and applying lotion helps increase circulation.
3. Support or elevate edematous body parts with pillows while the child is in bed or sitting in a chair.	3. Edema is gravity-dependent. Elevation helps move fluid away from dependent body parts.
4. Promote physical activity, as the child is able to tolerate, by providing developmentally appropriate play activities.	4. Increased activity helps promote circulation.

Evaluation

- Is the child's skin intact without redness or tenderness?

Nursing Diagnosis

Risk for Infection related to urinary loss of gamma globulins and immunosuppressive therapy.

Expected Outcome

The child will:
- Be free of signs of an infection, as evidenced by normal white blood cell (WBC) count, normal body temperature, and absence of abdominal pain and cough.

INTERVENTION	RATIONALE
1. Screen visitors for signs of infection, such as upper respiratory symptoms, sore throats, or exposure to communicable diseases.	1. Communicable diseases, especially varicella, pose a serious threat because the child receiving immunosuppressive therapy is not able to respond appropriately to infection.
2. Administer antibiotics as ordered.	2. Antibiotics are usually given for peritonitis prophylaxis during the edematous phase.
3. Use good handwashing techniques, and instruct family members to do the same.	3. Handwashing helps decrease transmission of germs.
4. Monitor child for fever, cough, sore throat, or complaints of abdominal pain each shift. Monitor laboratory values.	4. Frequent monitoring ensures early detection of infectious processes. Abdominal pain can be an indication of peritonitis.

Evaluation

- Does the child maintain normal body temperature and exhibit normal laboratory values?
- Is the child free from cough, pain, or other signs of infection?

Nursing Care Plan

The Child With Nephrotic Syndrome—cont'd

Nursing Diagnosis

Risk for Deficient Fluid Volume (intravascular) related to proteinuria, edema, and effects of diuretics.

Expected Outcome

The child will:
- Maintain adequate fluid volume, as evidenced by normal blood pressure measurement, urine output appropriate for age, and normal hematocrit and hemoglobin.

INTERVENTION	RATIONALE
1. Monitor vital signs, including blood pressure and pulse, every shift. Report variance from baseline.	1. Low blood pressure and increased heart rate are signs of hypovolemia. Blood pressure may be elevated because of renin release.
2. Monitor intake and output every shift. Report if child has output of less than 1 to 2 ml/kg/hr of urine (see Chapter 42).	2. Accurate intake and output measurement is essential for evaluating fluid status.
3. Monitor laboratory values, particularly hemoglobin and hematocrit.	3. Increasing values of hemoglobin, hematocrit, and platelets may indicate hemoconcentration or low intravascular volume.
4. Observe for signs of dehydration, such as appearance of mucous membranes, capillary refill, and level of activity. (Capillary refill may be altered because of edema; assess in non-edematous area.) Report positive findings.	4. The pathophysiology of nephrotic syndrome may predispose the child to decreased intravascular volume. This condition is compounded by the use of diuretics.

Evaluation

- Are the child's vital signs and hematocrit and hemoglobin within normal limits?
- Is the urine output normal for age-group (see Chapter 42)?
- Does the child have moist mucous membranes and good skin turgor?

Nursing Diagnosis

Excess Fluid Volume related to decreased excretion of sodium and fluid retention.

Expected Outcome

The child will:
- Not demonstrate fluid overload, as evidenced by stable daily weights and normal respiratory pattern.

INTERVENTION	RATIONALE
1. Monitor intake and output each shift.	1. Accurate intake and output are essential for evaluating fluid status.
2. Obtain accurate daily weights. Weigh child on same scales, at same time each day, in a gown only.	2. Daily weights are necessary to detect changes in fluid status. Clothing or presence of wet diaper can alter weight. Readings of weight can vary from scale to scale and time of day.
3. Adhere to no-added-salt diet, and fluid restriction if ordered.	3. Excessive sodium intake can increase amount of water retention. If the child is hyponatremic, fluid restriction may be indicated (Vogt & Avner, 2004)
4. Measure and record abdominal girth each day. Ensure accuracy by measuring in the same area each time.	4. Edema commonly occurs in the abdomen.
5. Monitor blood pressure at least once each shift.	5. Increased total-body fluid volume and concurrent steroid therapy can result in increased blood pressure.
6. Administer diuretics as ordered. Ensure adequate potassium intake.	6. Diuretics may aid in the elimination of excessive fluid. Diuretics can increase excretion of potassium.
7. Monitor pulmonary status by listening to breath sounds for crackles and observing for signs of increased work of breathing and presence of cough.	7. Fluid overload can result in pulmonary edema.

Continued

Nursing Care Plan

The Child With Nephrotic Syndrome—cont'd

Evaluation

- Does the child maintain a stable weight?
- Is the child free from respiratory distress?

Nursing Diagnoses

Anxiety (parental) related to hospitalization of child and caring for a child with a chronic disease. Deficient Knowledge about home management related to anxiety or incomplete understanding.

Expected Outcomes

The parents will:

- Demonstrate decreased anxiety, as evidenced by participating in the care of their child and explaining the normal course of the disease process.
- Be able to explain principles of home management.

INTERVENTION	RATIONALE
1. Allow parents to verbalize frustration and fears. Encourage them to ask questions, and provide them with information about nephrotic syndrome and its treatment.	1. Verbalization of fears is often therapeutic in itself. Information helps decrease anxiety because people often fear the unknown.
2. Incorporate the parents' help in the daily care of the child. Have them practice using Albustix, taking blood pressures, and assessing edema.	2. Nephrotic syndrome can be a chronic condition and is usually managed at home. It is important for the parents to feel comfortable with caring for their child.
3. Arrange for a dietary consultation.	3. Steroid therapy stimulates appetite. Children should be informed about low-calorie snacks and portion size. Encourage the parent to cook without salt and remove the salt shaker from the child's access.
4. Teach parents how to maintain a daily calendar of protein readings, how to do a daily weight, what medications are appropriate for the child, and how to prevent infection. Encourage parents to report any exposure to communicable disease.	4. Providing appropriate information allows the family to manage the child's care. The child's urine protein results are monitored for signs of relapse. It is important to check with the nephrologist before giving the child any over-the-counter medications because some medications can aggravate hypertension. Children receiving steroids are unable to respond appropriately to viral or bacterial infections and may require additional treatment.

Evaluation

- Can the parents describe their child's condition and required treatment?
- Do the parents actively participate in the child's care?
- Do the parents accurately demonstrate procedures necessary to do at home?

ACUTE RENAL FAILURE

Acute renal failure is defined as the sudden, severe loss of kidney function. In acute renal failure, the kidneys can no longer filter waste products, regulate fluid volume, or maintain chemical balance. Most children with acute renal failure regain renal function.

Etiology and Incidence

Possible causes of prerenal failure are dehydration, perinatal asphyxia, hypotension, septic shock, hemorrhagic shock, and renal artery obstruction. Nephrotoxins (e.g., aminoglycosides, contrast dye), ureterovesical obstruction, hemolytic uremic syndrome (HUS), glomerulonephritis, and pyelonephritis cause intrarenal acute renal failure. Postrenal acute renal failure is associated with structural abnormalities, such as ureteropelvic obstruction, ureterovesical obstruction, posterior ure-

thral valves, neurogenic bladder, and outlet obstruction by stones, tumor, or edema.

[handwritten annotation: hemolytic uremic syndrome]

HUS is the most frequent cause of acute renal failure in children. It is an acute disorder characterized by anemia, thrombocytopenia, and acute renal failure. Children with HUS become infected by *E. coli* in improperly cooked meat or contaminated dairy products. Acute renal failure in the child is uncommon.

Manifestations

Manifestations of acute renal failure include electrolyte imbalances, fluid imbalances, increased BUN and serum creatinine, acid-base imbalances, and nonspecific manifestations, such as poor feeding or decreased appetite, vomiting, lethargy, seizures, and pallor. In children with HUS, gastrointestinal illness characterized by abdominal pain, fever, vomiting, and bloody diarrhea may be present.

Pathophysiology

of Acute Renal Failure

Acute renal failure is categorized as prerenal, intrarenal, or postrenal. *Prerenal acute renal failure* is the result of decreased perfusion of the kidney. The kidney must have adequate blood flow for effective functioning. The decreased blood flow and subsequent ischemia cause cellular swelling and injury and possible cell death. *Intrarenal acute renal failure* is the result of actual ischemic damage to kidney tissue. *Postrenal acute renal failure* is the result of obstruction of urine outflow. The obstruction increases pressure within the kidney, which decreases renal function.

Impaired perfusion markedly decreases the glomerular filtration rate, triggering oliguria (markedly decreased urine output), azotemia (elevated blood levels of urea, creatinine, and uric acid), and associated electrolyte imbalances. Tissue injury further magnifies the damage and the decreased perfusion.

As the underlying problem is treated, recovery of the renal endothelial and tubular cells begins and renal function gradually returns. Because the glomerular filtration rate returns to normal faster than the tubular transport mechanisms, the child begins to diurese large amounts of dilute urine.

The danger for dehydration is high at this time.* Renal function gradually returns to normal.

*Hansen, M. (1998). *Pathophysiology: Foundations of disease and clinical intervention.* Philadelphia: Saunders.

gastro enteritis

Pathophysiology

of Hemolytic Uremic Syndrome

Most affected children have an associated prodrome of gastrointestinal symptoms, including bloody diarrhea, which suggests that an infectious agent may be the cause of HUS. Nearly all cases are the result of an antecedent infection by Shiga's toxin-producing strains of *Escherichia coli,* especially the O157:H7 serotype.* Two important characteristics of *E. coli* O157:H7 contribute to the development of HUS. First, because this bacterium attaches itself to the intestinal mucosa, its clearance through normal intestinal peristalsis is decreased, allowing the bacteria to grow and multiply. Second, the bacteria produce a toxin that damages the endothelial cells of capillary walls, and the subsequent inflammatory response results in occlusion of capillaries. This is especially significant in the renal glomeruli. The occlusion of glomerular vessels decreases filtration and results in acute renal failure. However, it is important to understand that the vascular process seen in HUS can affect any organ. Anemia results from fragmentation of red blood cells (RBCs), which are damaged as they try to pass through the occluded vessels and are removed from circulation by the spleen. Thrombocytopenia occurs because the platelets get trapped within the small vessels.

*Slutsker, L., Ries, A.A., Maloney, K., Wells, J.G., Greene, K.D., & Griffin, P.M. (1998). A nationwide case-control study of *Escherichia coli* O157:H7 infection in the United States. *Journal of Infectious Disease, 177,* 962-966.

Diagnostic Evaluation

Determining the underlying cause of acute renal failure is very important. If the underlying cause can be reversed, renal function usually returns to normal.

History

The history often gives an indication of the underlying cause of the acute renal failure. Vomiting, diarrhea, and fever may indicate dehydration and prerenal acute renal failure. It is necessary to ascertain any recent history of bloody diarrhea that might suggest HUS.

Fluid Status

Acute renal failure is usually associated with dehydration and oliguria (urine output <1 ml/kg/hr). Urine output might be normal or increased (see Chapter 42).

Laboratory Data

Serum creatinine and BUN levels are increased. BUN, an end product of protein catabolism, may reflect the nutritional status of the child. Metabolic acidosis can occur, as indicated by low serum bicarbonate. Serum potassium may be increased. Serum sodium may be increased or decreased, depending on fluid status. The child with HUS exhibits hemolytic anemia, thrombocytopenia, hematuria, urine casts, proteinuria, and *E. coli* by stool culture.

Physical Examination

The child may be hypertensive. Edema secondary to decreased urine output and fluid overload may be present. The child may be in respiratory distress secondary to fluid overload.

Imaging Studies

Renal ultrasound may help with diagnosis of obstruction and postrenal acute renal failure. Renal scan can be helpful in determining the cause of renal failure. It can assess blood flow, function, and obstruction.

Therapeutic Management

Many children in acute renal failure are managed without dialysis. Management includes the following principles.

Fluid Imbalances

Fluid balance is an important component of the management of a child with acute renal failure. If the child is dehydrated, careful fluid replacement is essential. Fluid restriction is necessary for a child who has decreased or absent urine output and is adequately hydrated or experiencing fluid overload. Fluid intake is carefully calculated to replace insensible fluid loss and urinary output. Maintaining fluid restriction can be difficult for some children. It is helpful to give small amounts more frequently, rather than a large amount occasionally. Older children can participate in decision making about the kind and frequency of fluids.

Electrolyte Imbalances

Potassium. Most children with acute renal failure have a high potassium level, requiring intervention when the serum potassium level reaches 6 mEq/L. Potassium is restricted from the diet and IV fluids. Interventions to remove potassium include instituting gastric suction; administration of an exchange resin, such as Kayexalate; or administration of sodium bicarbonate, glucose, and insulin.

> **! CRITICAL TO REMEMBER**
>
> **Indications for Dialysis in Acute Renal Failure**
>
> - Severe fluid overload
> - Pulmonary edema or congestive heart failure secondary to fluid overload
> - Severe hypertension
> - Metabolic acidosis not responsive to medications
> - Hyperkalemia not responsive to medications
> - Blood urea nitrogen greater than 120 mg/dl

Sodium. The sodium level may be elevated or decreased. It is more common for the level to be decreased, because of water overload. Fluid restriction helps improve the serum sodium level. Any replacement sodium is adjusted to maintain a normal sodium level.

Acid-Base Imbalances. Children with acute renal failure are unable to excrete hydrogen ions and ammonia through the kidney and develop metabolic acidosis (low serum bicarbonate). Additional sodium bicarbonate can be administered orally or intravenously.

Nutrition

Children with acute renal failure are at risk for malnutrition (Somers, 2002). The underlying principle of nutritional therapy for these children is to provide maximum calories and protein within the fluid restrictions. Foods should be low in sodium and potassium.

Dialysis

Dialysis is a process of removing waste products and excess body fluid and regulating electrolytes and minerals. Two types of dialysis are hemodialysis and peritoneal dialysis.

Nursing Considerations

Most children with acute renal failure are cared for in special care units. Principles of nursing care include (1) monitoring and maintaining fluid, electrolyte, and acid-base balance; (2) preventing infection; (3) providing adequate nutrition; (4) reducing parent and child anxiety; and (5) teaching about dialysis (Box 44-2).

CHRONIC RENAL FAILURE AND END-STAGE RENAL DISEASE

Chronic renal failure is an irreversible loss of kidney function that occurs over months to years. It can be managed conservatively with medications and diet restrictions. Chronic renal failure progresses to ESRD, which is the permanent, irreversible loss of kidney function that can no longer be managed conservatively to maintain life and health. Dialysis or transplantation is required to treat ESRD. Treatment usually occurs when only 5% to 10% of kidney function remains.

Etiology

The causes of chronic renal failure in children are different from those in adults. The most common causes, especially in younger children, are congenital anomalies, such as obstruction, VUR, and renal dysplasia. Chronic renal failure can de-velop in children from diseases such as glomerulonephritis, pyelonephritis, and HUS. In general, secondary causes of ESRD, such as diabetes and high blood pressure, are not seen in children.

Incidence

The incidence of chronic renal failure with ESRD among children younger than 19 years is approximately 18 in 1 million (Vogt & Avner, 2004). The incidence is higher in adolescents, in boys, and in Caucasians.

Pathophysiology

Regardless of the cause of kidney damage, chronic renal failure progresses to ESRD. The exact mechanisms are unclear. Negative contributing factors include ongoing immunologic injury, hyperfiltration (the overwork of the remaining nephrons), high dietary protein and phosphorus intake, persistent proteinuria, and hypertension.

Manifestations

Manifestations of chronic renal failure and ESRD include electrolyte imbalance, fluid imbalance (dehydration or fluid overload), acid-base imbalance, renal bone disease (osteodystrophy) and rickets, anemia, poor growth, hypertension, fatigue, decreased appetite or poor feeding, nausea and vomiting, and neurologic symptoms from accumulation of wastes.

Diagnostic Evaluation

Chronic renal failure may present nonspecifically. Physical examination may reveal short stature and failure to thrive. The child may be hypertensive. Blood work reveals electrolyte abnormalities (varying according to the underlying disease process), calcium and phosphorus abnormalities (decreased calcium and bone calcium resorption, elevated serum phosphorus), or anemia. Rising creatinine and BUN suggest ESRD. Creatinine clearance testing measures the ability of the renal system to excrete metabolic products. Bone radiographs diagnose renal osteodystrophy. The child may have normal fluid volume, be dehydrated, or have fluid overload.

The history may or may not include known renal disease. Diagnostic tests may be performed to determine etiology and prognosis. These may include a voiding cystourethrogram (VCUG), renal ultrasound, renal scan, and renal biopsy.

Therapeutic Management

Chronic Renal Failure

The diet of a child with chronic renal failure is modified secondary to the decreased ability of the kidney to regulate fluids, electrolytes, minerals, and waste products. This might include the following restrictions: salt and fluid to prevent fluid overload and hypertension, protein because of the kidneys' inability to remove waste products, phosphorus to help prevent bone disease, and potassium because of the kidneys' inability to remove it.

BOX 44-2
Dialysis

Dialysis is a process of removing waste products and excess body fluids and regulating electrolytes and minerals. It is sometimes necessary in acute renal failure. When chronic renal failure progresses to end-stage renal disease, dialysis or kidney transplantation is required. The two types of dialysis are hemodialysis and peritoneal dialysis.

∗ Know diffences

Hemodialysis

Hemodialysis cleanses the blood by circulating it through a special filter called an *artificial kidney.* Blood is pumped through the artificial kidney and returned to the body. Hemodialysis occurs through a vascular access, such as a double-lumen central line or an arteriovenous fistula or shunt. The access is surgically placed. Children who receive long-term dialysis usually receive treatments three times per week for 3 to 4 hours each time.

The major complications of hemodialysis include access infection and access obstruction. In addition, school, peer, and family life are disrupted because of the treatment schedule. However, children treated with hemodialysis in a specialized pediatric unit can thrive. In infants and small children, hemodialysis is technically more difficult and fluid and electrolyte shifts are more pronounced.

Hemodialysis is more efficient and requires less time than peritoneal dialysis. In addition, the family has less responsibility.

Peritoneal Dialysis

In peritoneal dialysis, fluid enters the peritoneal cavity through a catheter, which may be placed in the child at the bedside or in the operating room. The dialysis fluid remains in the cavity for a prescribed time, during which waste products, chemicals, and fluid pass through the peritoneal membrane into the fluid. The fluid is then drained, and the process is repeated.

In children receiving long-term dialysis, the exchanges can be performed overnight with an automated cycler or they can be done manually four or five times per day. The treatments usually are performed at home.

Peritoneal dialysis is technically easier than hemodialysis. Advantages over hemodialysis include more independence for the child and family and a more stable physiologic state because of frequent dialysis. The disadvantages include the risk of infections (peritonitis, catheter exit site) and family and child fatigue from treatment demands.

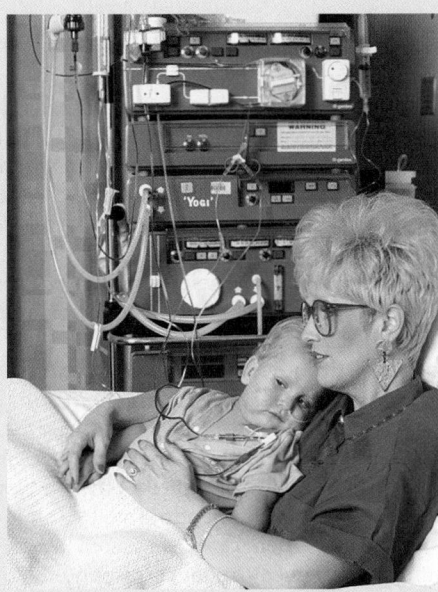

Child receiving hemodialysis. Family members should participate in the child's care as much as possible.

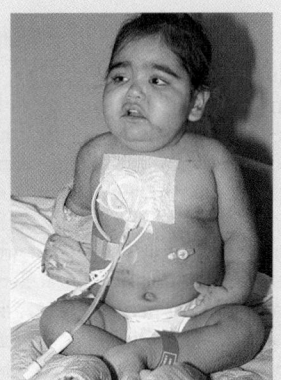

◀ Peritoneal dialysis. Implanted lines allow instillation of the dialyzing fluid into this child's peritoneal cavity. This child has rejected a transplanted kidney and receives peritoneal dialysis until another transplant will be attempted. She previously received steroids in an attempt to control rejection, which accounts for the characteristics typical of Cushing's syndrome.

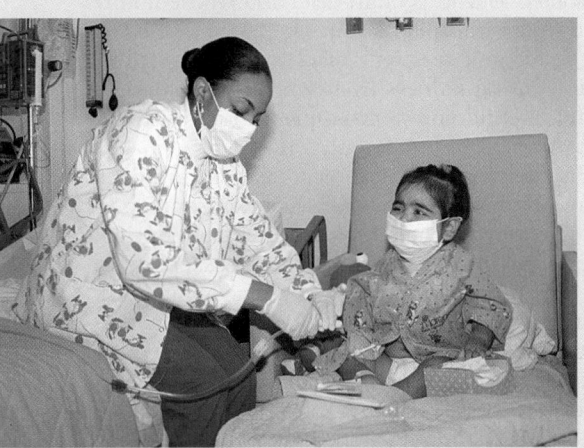

Infection of the peritoneal cavity is the chief hazard of peritoneal dialysis. When the lines are open to begin or end the dialyzing cycle, both adult and child wear masks.

Photos courtesy Children's Medical Center, Dallas, TX.

Diuretics also are indicated to control fluid balance, and antihypertensives are given for hypertension. Sodium bicarbonate may be necessary to maintain acid-base balance. Vitamin D and phosphorus-binding medications may be helpful in preventing bone disease.

Children with chronic renal failure should receive all childhood immunizations and yearly influenza vaccine, unless immunosuppressive treatment precludes live virus vaccines. Immunization with live virus vaccines as soon as possible within the normal childhood schedule is desired because after kidney transplantation, the child will be taking immunosuppressants (Vogt & Avner, 2004).

Advances in the treatment of infants and children with chronic renal failure, such as recombinant erythropoietin and recombinant growth hormone, have improved the quality of life of these children (Vogt & Avner, 2004). Recombinant erythropoietin is used to treat anemia, thus avoiding repeated blood transfusions and improving the energy level. The use of recombinant growth hormone has significantly improved the growth of children with chronic renal failure (Chan, Williams, & Roth, 2002).

End-Stage Renal Disease

Once a child reaches ESRD, dialysis or kidney transplantation is required for health and life. The diagnosis of ESRD is made by monitoring serum creatinine, glomerular filtration rate, and the quality of the child's life. ESRD usually is diagnosed when the glomerular filtration rate decreases to about 10%.

Kidney Transplantation

Transplantation is the goal for most children with ESRD and offers the best opportunity to have a normal lifestyle. Unfortunately, transplantation is not a cure. Children who have received transplants must continue to take immunosuppressive medication, have blood tests, and keep clinic appointments.

Kidneys come from two types of donors: living donors and cadaveric donors. A living donor is someone in the child's family, such as a parent or grandparent. A person who donates must be in good health and have healthy kidneys. A cadaveric donor kidney is a healthy kidney obtained from someone who is brain-dead and whose family has consented to the transplantation. The blood and tissue types of the donor and recipient need to be compatible. Transplantations using kidneys from a relative have been more successful in children than transplantations using cadaveric kidneys.

Rejection is the most common complication of kidney transplantation. Immunosuppressive medications, taken to help prevent rejection, include cyclosporine, azathioprine, and prednisone. Other examples of immunosuppressive drugs include tacrolimus (Prograf), mycophenolate mofetil, and a new form of cyclosporine (Neoral).

As with all medications, immunosuppressive medications have side effects. When the immune system is suppressed, risk of infection is increased, related to the body's decreased ability to fight infection. Children with renal transplants should be monitored for infection and may take antiinfective medications routinely.

High blood pressure is also a complication of transplantation. Underlying renal disease, the transplanted kidney, or immunosuppressive medication side effects can cause high blood pressure.

■NURSING CARE

The Child With Chronic Renal Failure and End-Stage Renal Disease

Assessment

The assessment of the child with chronic renal failure or ESRD is directed toward clinical manifestations of the renal failure and its possible complications. Blood work is monitored for abnormalities and response to interventions. Monitoring hemoglobin and hematocrit assesses for potential anemia and assesses response to therapy in the child receiving recombinant erythropoietin. Serum calcium and phosphorus, alkaline phosphatase, and parathyroid hormone levels as well as bone radiographs are obtained to monitor for renal osteodystrophy.

The nurse assesses fluid status for fluid overload and dehydration by obtaining weight, monitoring blood pressure and heart rate, and observing and recording edema, skin turgor, mucous membranes, and fontanel.

Obtain accurate weights and height measurements regularly to assess growth and development. Ask the parent about the child's dietary and caloric intake. Information regarding attainment of development tasks, school performance, and peer relationships is helpful.

Nursing Diagnosis and Planning

The nursing diagnoses and expected outcomes that apply to the child with chronic renal failure and the family are

- Imbalanced Nutrition: Less Than Body Requirements related to decreased appetite and dietary restrictions.
  Expected Outcome: The child will receive adequate nutrition for growth and health as measured by appropriate growth for age.
- Deficient Knowledge about disease process, treatment, or diet restrictions related to anxiety or incomplete understanding of principles.
  Expected Outcome: The child or parents will be able to explain the disease process, its treatment, and dietary restrictions.
- Risk for Imbalanced Fluid Volume related to fluid and electrolyte shifts secondary to renal dysfunction.
  Expected Outcome: The child will exhibit no signs of fluid overload or deficit, as measured by weight, blood pressure, and absence of edema or signs of dehydration.
- Delayed Growth and Development related to restricted diet, chronic illness, and anemia.
  Expected Outcome: The child will attain maximum development according to normal growth and development measuring instruments.
- Interrupted Family Processes related to having a child with a chronic and potentially life-threatening disease.
  Expected Outcome: The child and family will achieve successful coping strategies, as measured by their ability to care for the child, meet the needs of other family members, and access appropriate support.
- Risk for Impaired Skin Integrity related to edema and poor nutrition.

Expected Outcome: The child's skin will not show signs of a break in integrity (redness, irritation, breaks).

Interventions

The care of the child with chronic renal failure or ESRD is complex and requires a multidisciplinary team. Maintaining adequate nutritional intake within the dietary restriction parameters is a challenge. The nurse individualizes the diet of the child with chronic renal failure and includes foods the child likes. Small, frequent meals may be helpful. Diet supplements may be necessary to meet caloric needs. Recombinant growth hormone may allow the child to have adequate growth.

Children with chronic renal failure and their families have multifaceted information requirements. The parents need information regarding diet, medications, potential effects of the renal failure, and its treatment. They need to be informed regarding treatment options, such as hemodialysis, peritoneal dialysis, and transplantation.

Provide appropriate fluid intake and ongoing assessment of fluid status. Instruct the child and family about fluid restriction and hydration assessment, such as weight, blood pressure, and appearance of edema.

Encourage the child to participate in school and age-appropriate activities. Parents may find it difficult to allow the child autonomy and will need support to do so.

The child with chronic renal failure and the family need support. They need opportunities to ask questions, verbalize feelings, and express concerns. Involving children in their own care and decisions regarding treatment is beneficial. Determine the family's prior successful coping strategies, and encourage family members to use those. A social worker, psychologist, or psychiatrist may provide additional support.

Evaluation

- Does the child maintain the age-appropriate growth percentile on a growth chart despite dietary restrictions?
- Can the parents and the child discuss the disease course and management and how well the child is adapting to diet restrictions?
- Is the child free of edema?
- Does the child have moist mucous membranes and adequate urine output (see Chapter 42)?
- Does the child continue to achieve age-appropriate developmental milestones?
- Is the family involved in the care of the child?
- Has the family demonstrated appropriate problem-solving strategies to meet the needs of all family members, and do they access appropriate support?
- Has the integrity of the child's skin been maintained?

KEY CONCEPTS

- The kidney reaches near-adult function at 6 to 12 months of age.
- Infants cannot concentrate urine as efficiently as older children and adults.
- Most children eventually outgrow enuresis with therapeutic intervention.
- The clinical manifestations of UTIs vary according to the child's age, underlying anatomic or neurologic abnormalities, and frequency of recurrence.
- Urinary tract infection is the most common clinical manifestation of VUR. Medical management includes low-dose prophylactic antibiotic therapy to prevent renal scarring.
- Nursing care of the child with a UTI includes giving information to the parents and child about perineal hygiene, increased fluid intake, emptying the bladder, and wearing cotton underwear.

- Most infants with cryptorchidism have spontaneous descent of their testes during the first year of life.
- The goals of surgery to correct hypospadias are to make urinary and sexual function as normal as possible and to improve the cosmetic appearance of the penis.
- Children with glomerulonephritis should be assessed for hypertension and the presence of any respiratory difficulty, such as cough, increased respiratory rate, and difficulty breathing, which may indicate fluid overload.
- Children at risk for fluid volume excess because of decreased urine output should be weighed daily on the same scale, at the same time, wearing only a gown. Infants should have their diapers removed.
- Children with edema should have their position changed at least every 2 hours and their

lower extremities elevated when they are sitting or lying in bed.
- Edema related to nephrotic syndrome is first noted in the periorbital spaces and dependent areas of the body. The child may awaken with facial edema; as the day progresses, edema becomes more noticeable. Prednisone usually induces a remission in the child with nephrotic syndrome.
- Most children with acute renal failure regain renal function.
- Children with chronic renal failure and ESRD and their families require multidisciplinary care and extensive nursing support.

ANSWERS to Critical Thinking Exercise 44-1

1. The nurse should first determine whether Thomas has ever been able to be dry at night. This information helps discriminate between primary and secondary nocturnal enuresis. Other information the nurse will need includes whether Thomas has experienced any excessive thirst or weight loss (signs of diabetes mellitus); whether he complains about anal itching (rule out pinworms); and whether he has a fever or other signs of a urinary tract infection. It would also be helpful to know what approach the parents used during toilet training and whether either parent had enuresis as a child.

2. After underlying problems have been ruled out, the nurse can reassure Mr. Sampson that nighttime wetting is not unusual in children of this age and the initial approach should be one of benign neglect. Focusing too much on the problem can create anxiety in the child and decreased self-esteem if the problem persists later into childhood. The nurse can suggest that the parents encourage Thomas to wear a disposable diaper or waterproof pull-up at night. They can explain to Thomas that lots of children this age need to be in pull-ups for a while and that it does not mean that he is a baby. When he has stayed dry, he can decide to try going without the pull-up. Putting a plastic draw sheet covered by a regular draw sheet over the middle portion of the bed can reduce the amount of laundry required and preserve the mattress.

REFERENCES and READINGS

Ackley, B.J., & Ladwig, G.B. (1999). *Nursing diagnosis handbook: A guide to planning care* (4th ed.). St. Louis: Mosby.

Ahmed, S.F., Khwaja, O., & Hughes, I.A. (2000). The role of a clinical score in the assignment of ambiguous genitalia. *BJU International, 85*(1), 120-124.

American Academy of Pediatrics. (1999). Practice parameter: The diagnosis, treatment, and evaluation of the initial urinary tract infection in febrile infants and young children. *Pediatrics, 103*(4), 843-852.

American Academy of Pediatrics, Committee on Genetics. (2000). Evaluation of the newborn with developmental anomalies of the external genitalia. *Pediatrics, 106*(1 Pt. 1), 138-142.

Anand, S.K. (2000). Urinary tract infections. In C.D. Berkowitz (Ed.), *Pediatrics: A primary care approach* (pp. 326-330). Philadelphia: Saunders.

Bartkowski, D. (2001). Recognizing UTIs in infants and children. *Postgraduate Medicine, 109*(1), 171-180.

Beh, H.G., & Diamond, M. (2000). An emerging ethical and medical dilemma: Should physicians perform sex assignment surgery on infants with ambiguous genitalia? *Michigan Journal of Law, 7*(1), 1-63.

Boris, N., & Dalton, R. (2004). Enuresis (Bedwetting). In R. Behrman, R. Kliegman, & H. Jenson (Eds. *Nelson textbook of pediatrics* (17th ed., pp. 74-75). Philadelphia: Saunders.

Chan, J.C.M., Williams, D.M., & Roth, K.S. (2002). Kidney failure in infants and children. *Pediatrics in Review, 23*(2), 47-60.

Chandra, M. (1999). Common voiding disorders. In F. Burg, E. Wald, J. Ingelfinger, & R. Polin (Eds.), *Gellis and Kagan's current pediatric therapy* (16th ed., pp. 837-840). Philadelphia: Saunders.

Chon, C.H., Lai, F.C., & Shortliffe, L.M.D. (2001). Pediatric urinary tract infections. *Pediatric Clinics of North America, 48*(6), 1441-1459.

Creighton, S.M., Minto, C.L., & Steele, S.J. (2001). Objective cosmetic and anatomical outcomes at adolescence of feminizing surgery for ambiguous genitalia done in childhood. *Lancet, 358*(9276), 124-125.

Davis, I.D., Bunchman, T.E., Grimm, P.C., Benfield, M.R., Briscoe, D.M., Harmon, W.E., Alexander, S.R., & Avner, E.D. (1998). Pediatric renal transplantation: Indications and special considerations. A position paper from the pediatric committee of the American Society of Transplant Physicians. *Pediatric Transplantation, 2*(2), 117-129.

Docimo, S.G., Silver, R.I., & Cromie, W. (2000). The undescended testicle: Diagnosis and management. *American Family Physician, 62*(9), 2037-2044.

Dolk, H. (1998). Rise in prevalence of hypospadias. *Lancet, 351*(9105), 770.

Elder, J. (2004). Urologic disorders in infants and children. In R. Behrman, R. Kliegman, & H. Jenson (Eds.), *Nelson textbook of pediatrics* (17th ed., pp. 1783-1826). Philadelphia: Saunders.

Elenberg, E. (2002). Enuresis and voiding dysfunction. In F. Burg, J. Ingelfinger, R. Polin, & A. Gershon (Eds.). *Gellis & Kagan's current pediatric therapy* (17th ed.; pp. 768-772). Philadelphia: Saunders.

Elenberg, E., & Travis, B. (2002). Urinary tract infection and perinephric/intranephric abscess. In F. Burg, J. Ingelfinger, R. Polin, & A. Gershon (Eds.). *Gellis & Kagan's current pediatric therapy* (17th ed.; pp. 772-777). Philadelphia: Saunders.

Flynn, J.T. (1998). Causes, management approaches, and outcome of acute renal failure in children. *Current Opinion in Pediatrics, 10*(2), 184-189.

Gill, F.T. (1998). Umbilical hernia, inguinal hernias, and hydroceles in children: Diagnostic clues for optimal patient management. *Journal of Pediatric Health Care, 12*(5), 231-235.

Goldberg, E. (1997). Physical assessment of children ages 1 to 10 years with renal disease. *ANNA Journal/American Nephrology Nurses' Association, 24*(2), 222-228.

Grady, R.W., Carr, M.C., & Mitchell, M.E. (1999). Complete primary closure of bladder exstrophy: Epispadias and bladder exstrophy repair. *Urologic Clinics of North America, 26*(1), 95-109.

Hansen, M. (1998). *Pathophysiology: Foundations of disease and clinical intervention*. Philadelphia: Saunders.

Hermer, L. (2002). Paradigms revised: Intersex children, bioethics & the law. *Annals of Health Law, 11*, 195-236.

Hoberman, A. (1999). Infections of the urinary tract. In F. Burg, E. Wald, J. Ingelfinger, & R. Polin (Eds.), *Gellis and Kagan's current pediatric therapy* (16th ed.). Philadelphia: Saunders.

Ingelfinger, J. (2002). Disorders of the bladder and urethra, ureter, and collecting system. In F. Burg, J. Ingelfinger, R. Polin, & A. Gershon (Eds.). *Gellis & Kagan's current pediatric therapy* (17th ed.; pp. 762-767). Philadelphia: Saunders.

Jalkut, M., Lerman, S., & Churchill, B. (2001). Enuresis. *Pediatric Clinics of North America, 48*(6), 1461-1488.

Johnson, M., Mass, M., & Moorhead, S. (2000). *Nursing outcomes classification* (2nd ed.). St. Louis: Mosby.

Kamil, E.S. (2000). Nephrotic syndrome. In C.D. Berkowitz (Ed.), *Pediatrics: A primary care approach* (pp. 553-559). Philadelphia: Saunders.

Kass, E., & Lundak, B. (1997). The acute scrotum. *Pediatric Clinics of North America, 44*(5), 1251-1259.

Kelleher, R. (1997). Daytime and nighttime wetting in children: A review of management. *Journal of Society of Pediatric Nurses, 2*(2), 73-82.

Koff, S.A., & Jayanthi, V.R. (1999). Preoperative treatment with human chorionic gonadotropin in infancy decreases the severity of proximal hypospadias and chordee. *Journal of Urology, 162*(4), 1435-1439.

Lackgren, G., Wahlin, N., Skoldenberg, E., & Stenberg, A. (2001). Long-term followup of children treated with dextranomer/hyaluronic acid copolymer for vesicoureteral reflux. *Journal of Urology, 166*, 1887-1892.

Langer, J., & Coplen, D. (1998). Circumcision and pediatric disorders of the penis. *Pediatric Clinics of North America, 45*(4), 801-812.

Lieberman, K.V. (2000). A practical guide to acute glomerulonephritis. *Office and Emergency Pediatrics, 13*(4), 151-154.

Lindert, A.K., & Shortliffe, L.M.D. (1999). Evaluation and management of pediatric urinary tract infections. *Urologic Clinics of North America, 26*(4), 719-728.

McCabe, A.J., Martin, D., & Glick, P.L. (2000). Insights. An "owl's eyes" view of hydroceles. *Journal of Pediatrics, 137*(2), 286.

McCloskey, J.C., & Bulechek, G.M. (2000). *Nursing interventions classification* (3rd ed.). St. Louis: Mosby.

McCormack, K. (1999). A very special baby: Managing a baby with congenital adrenal hyperplasia. *Journal of Neonatal Nursing, 5*(2), 19-25.

Mollohan, J. (1999). Exstrophy of the bladder. *Neonatal Network, 18*(2), 17-26.

Reiner, W.G. (1999). Assignment of sex in neonates with ambiguous genitalia. *Current Opinion in Pediatrics, 11*(4), 363-365.

Schnaper, W., Daouk, G., & Ingelfinger, J. (2002). Nephrotic syndrome. In F. Burg, J. Ingelfinger, R. Polin & A. Gershon (Eds.), *Gellis & Kagan's current pediatric therapy* (17th ed., pp. 798-804). Philadelphia: Saunders.

Shaw, K.N., & Gorelick, M.H. (1999). Urinary tract infection in the pediatric patient. *Pediatric Clinics of North America, 46*(6), 1111-1124.

Shaw, K.N, Gorelick, M., McGowan, K.L., Yakscoe, N.M., & Schwartz, J.S. (1998). Prevalence of urinary tract infection in febrile young children in the emergency department. *Pediatrics, 102*(2), e16.

Simckes, A. (1998). Nephrotic syndrome. In L. Finberg (Ed.), *Saunders manual of pediatric practice* (pp. 691-693). Philadelphia: Saunders.

Slutsker, L., Ries, A.A., Maloney, K., Wells, J.G., Greene, K.D., & Griffin, P.M. (1998). A nationwide case-control study of *Escherichia coli* O157:H7 infection in the United States. *Journal of Infectious Disease, 177*, 962-966.

Somers, M. (2002). Acute renal failure. In F. Burg, J. Ingelfinger, R. Polin & A. Gershon (Eds.), *Gellis & Kagan's current pediatric therapy* (17th ed., pp. 809-814). Philadelphia: Saunders.

Tobias, N.E. (2000). Management of nocturnal enuresis. *Nursing Clinics of North America, 35*(1), 37-60.

Vogt, B., & Avner, E. (2004). Conditions particularly associated with proteinuria. In R. Behrman, R. Kliegman, & H. Jenson (Eds.). *Nelson textbook of pediatrics* (17th ed., pp.1751-1762). Philadelphia: Saunders.

Wallace, M. (2003). What is new with renal transplantation [Electronic version]? *AORN, 77*(5), 945-958, 960-970.

45

The Child with a Respiratory Alteration

◆ LEARNING OBJECTIVES

After studying this chapter, you should be able to:

◎ Describe the differences in the anatomy and physiology of the infant or child's respiratory system that increase the risk for respiratory disease.

◎ Outline nursing care for a child with allergies to inhalants.

◎ Discuss the pathophysiology, clinical manifestations, and therapeutic management of common acute and chronic respiratory alterations.

◎ Identify the nursing care needs of infants and children with acute and chronic respiratory alterations.

◎ Develop guidelines for the home care of a child with an acute respiratory alteration.

◎ Identify common triggers of asthma symptoms.

◎ Apply measures that can be taken to prevent and treat asthma episodes.

◎ Identify teaching needs for children with asthma and their families.

◎ Describe the nursing care of the child with cystic fibrosis.

◎ Discuss measures to maintain adequate oxygenation, and provide appropriate developmental stimulation for the child with bronchopulmonary dysplasia.

◎ Describe the correct method of administering and evaluating tuberculosis skin tests.

◎ Identify ways to prevent the transmission of tuberculosis, and explain the importance of administering antituberculotic medications as prescribed.

◆ DEFINITIONS

atelectasis A collapsed or airless state of the lung that may involve all or part of the lung.

crackles An abnormal, discontinuous, nonmusical sound heard on auscultation, primarily during inhalation; also called *rales.*

dysphagia Difficulty swallowing.

dyspnea Difficulty breathing.

grunting A sound similar to a grunting noise that can be heard with or without a stethoscope.

hypercapnia Increased levels of carbon dioxide in the blood, as indicated by an elevated $Paco_2$ as determined by blood gas analysis.

hypocapnia Decreased levels of carbon dioxide in the blood.

hypoxemia Decreased levels of oxygen in the blood.

hypoxia Decreased oxygenation of cells and tissues.

nasal flaring A serious sign of air hunger demonstrated by widening of the nares to enable an infant or young child to take in more oxygen.

nasal polyps Semitransparent herniations of respiratory epithelium.

orthopnea Difficulty breathing except in an upright position.

retractions An abnormal movement of the chest wall during inspiration that may occur intercostally and substernally.

rhonchi Adventitious breath sounds caused by the passage of air through an airway obstructed by thick secretions; sounds do not clear with coughing.

stridor A shrill, harsh sound that can be heard during inspiration, expiration, or both; produced by the flow of air through a narrowed segment of the respiratory tract.

tachypnea Increased respiratory rate.

wheezing High-pitched, musical whistles that can be heard with or without a stethoscope; may be inspiratory or expiratory; caused by bronchial constriction or obstruction of the airway and commonly occurs in asthma.

REVIEW OF THE RESPIRATORY SYSTEM

The respiratory system consists of the nose, pharynx, larynx, trachea, bronchi, and lungs. It is further divided into the *upper respiratory tract* (nose, pharynx, larynx) and the *lower respiratory tract* (trachea, bronchi, lungs).

The Upper Airway

Air enters the body through the *nares*, or nostrils, two nasal cavities lined with mucous membrane. In older infants and children, air can also enter through the mouth into the *pharynx*, or throat. The *nasopharynx* is located immediately behind the nasal cavity; the *oropharynx* is located behind the mouth. The *laryngeal pharynx* lies below the oropharynx and opens into the larynx toward the front and into the esophagus toward the back.

The *larynx* is located between the pharynx and the trachea. The vocal cords are at the upper end of the larynx. The proximity of the upper esophagus to the upper respiratory system can put an individual at risk for inhaling food or liquids, but the *epiglottis* covers the larynx during swallowing and helps keep food out of the lower respiratory tract.

Cilia are hairlike processes that move mucus and fluid. Damage to cilia interferes with the removal of mucus from the respiratory tract. Ciliated mucous membranes line the larynx and filter dust and other particles from the air. The particles are then carried to the pharynx to be removed by sneezing, blowing, or coughing. After being filtered, the air that enters the respiratory system is humidified and warmed before proceeding into the lungs. The three types of tonsils are: the oval *palatine tonsils*, located on either side of the pharynx; the *lingual tonsil*, located below the palatine tonsils at the base of the tongue; and the *pharyngeal tonsils*, or *adenoids*, located at the nasopharyngeal border. The tonsils are composed mainly of lymphoid tissue. They help filter the circulating lymph of bacteria and other foreign material that enter the body, especially through the mouth and nose.

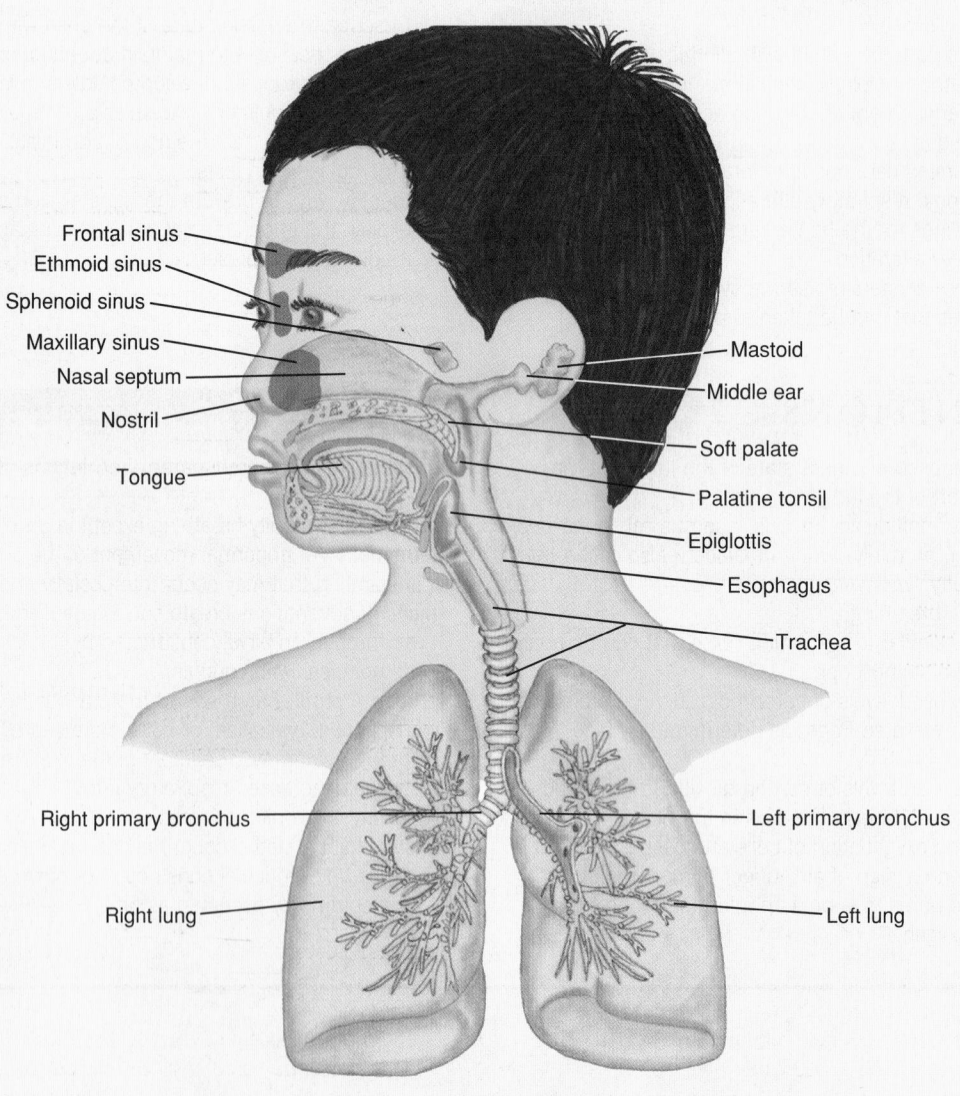

- Frontal sinus
- Ethmoid sinus
- Sphenoid sinus
- Maxillary sinus
- Nasal septum
- Nostril
- Tongue
- Mastoid
- Middle ear
- Soft palate
- Palatine tonsil
- Epiglottis
- Esophagus
- Trachea
- Right primary bronchus
- Left primary bronchus
- Right lung
- Left lung

Anatomy of the Respiratory System

The Lower Airway

The *trachea* conducts air between the larynx and the lungs. It divides into right and left main *bronchi* at its lower end, the *carina*. The right main bronchus is shorter and wider than the left. The main bronchi divide into *lobar bronchi*, *segmental bronchi*, and *bronchioles* and terminate in *alveoli*. Mucus-secreting goblet cells line the bronchi and protect the lungs from dust and bacteria.

The *lungs* are two conical structures within the thoracic cavity. The right lung has three *lobes* (upper, middle, lower); the left has two lobes (upper, lower). The *pleura* consists of two layers, the *parietal pleura* and the *visceral pleura*. The parietal pleura lines the entire thoracic cavity; the visceral pleura encases each lung. The pleura helps maintain lung stability. Negative pressure within the intrapleural space prevents the lungs from separating from the thorax. *Diffusion* of gases takes place in the lungs. Terminal bronchioles lack mucus-secreting goblet cells and cilia, and gas exchange does not take place here.

Distal to the terminal bronchioles are the alveoli, where most gas exchange occurs. Thinness of the alveolar walls aids in gas exchange. An almost solid sheet of capillaries is within the alveolar walls, so that the alveolar gases are proximate to the capillary blood.

Prenatal Respiratory Development

The respiratory system must mature before birth for the neonate to survive. The placenta performs oxygenation *in utero*, but to adapt to extrauterine life, the neonate must be able to inflate the lungs, establish continuous breathing, and transfer the gases needed to meet metabolic needs.

Postnatal Respiratory Changes

Postnatal changes in the respiratory system occur as follows:

1. Compression of the thorax during vaginal delivery forces out some fetal lung fluid.
2. Respirations are stimulated by hypoxemia; hypercarbia; cold, tactile stimulation; and a possible decrease in the concentration of prostaglandin E_2.
3. Inflation of the normal lung is complete within a few breaths, and most alveoli have expanded within the first hour of life.
4. Surfactant in the lung liquid lowers surface tension and facilitates lung expansion.
5. Pulmonary blood flow increases.
6. Closure of the foramen ovale and the ductus arteriosus (see Chapter 46) establishes the pulmonary and circulatory systems.

Gas Exchange and Transport

Two-way diffusion takes place between the walls of the alveoli. In *diffusion*, molecules move from an area of greater concentration to one of lesser concentration. Blood entering the lung capillaries is somewhat low in oxygen. Oxygen will diffuse from the alveoli, where its concentration is higher, into the blood. Similarly, carbon dioxide moves out of the blood and into the alveoli. Most oxygen that diffuses

Pediatric Differences in the Respiratory System

- Surfactant is lacking in premature infants. Infants born before 34 weeks' gestation have a higher risk for respiratory distress syndrome.
- Smaller lower airways and undeveloped supporting cartilage predispose the child to an increased risk for obstruction by mucus, edema, and foreign bodies. The neonate's airway is 50% smaller than that of adults. A premature infant has a more compliant chest wall and weaker respiratory muscles than those of a term infant.
- Lung size is proportional to body height. Therefore lung volumes and capacities do not vary from age to age.
- Infants are obligatory nose breathers; they have difficulty breathing through the mouth. If the infant has nasal congestion, breathing becomes more difficult.
- The diaphragm is the neonate's major respiratory muscle. Intercostal muscles are not well developed. Retractions are more common in the infant than in older children and adults.
- Brief periods of apnea (10-15 sec) are common in the neonate. The respiratory pattern may be irregular.
- Children's normal respiratory rate is higher than that of adults.
- An increased metabolic rate increases oxygen needs.
- Alveoli develop from approximately 20 million to 200 million by age 3 years. Alveolar development gradually decreases after age 3 years; few develop after age 8 years.
- The lung surface increases until 5 to 8 years. Actual lung growth continues into the adolescent years.
- Eustachian tubes are relatively horizontal, which increases the risk for bacteria entering the middle ear.
- Tracheal size approximately triples by adulthood.
- Tonsillar tissue is normally enlarged in early-school-age children.
- Infants and children use abdominal muscles to inhale until about age 5 to 6 years.
- The child's flexible larynx is more susceptible to spasm.

into the capillary blood in the lungs is bound to the hemoglobin of red blood cells. A small percentage is dissolved in plasma. For oxygen to enter the cells, it must separate from hemoglobin. Carbon dioxide diffuses into the blood from the tissues and is transported to the lungs by the blood. In this activity, hemoglobin is a buffer that enables blood to take up carbon dioxide without altering the blood pH significantly. The uptake and delivery of gases by the blood is a continuous process.

Ventilation occurs through *inspiration* and *expiration*. In inspiration, the diaphragm contracts and flattens, expanding the vertical dimension of the chest; the lung volume increases. In expiration the diaphragm and chest wall relax, decreasing thoracic volume. Intrathoracic pressure increases, and gas flows out of the lungs, taking with it the carbon dioxide that was delivered to the lungs by the blood. Ventilation of the lungs is intermittent. Inspired air is 21% oxygen; end-expired air is 16% oxygen and 35% carbon dioxide.

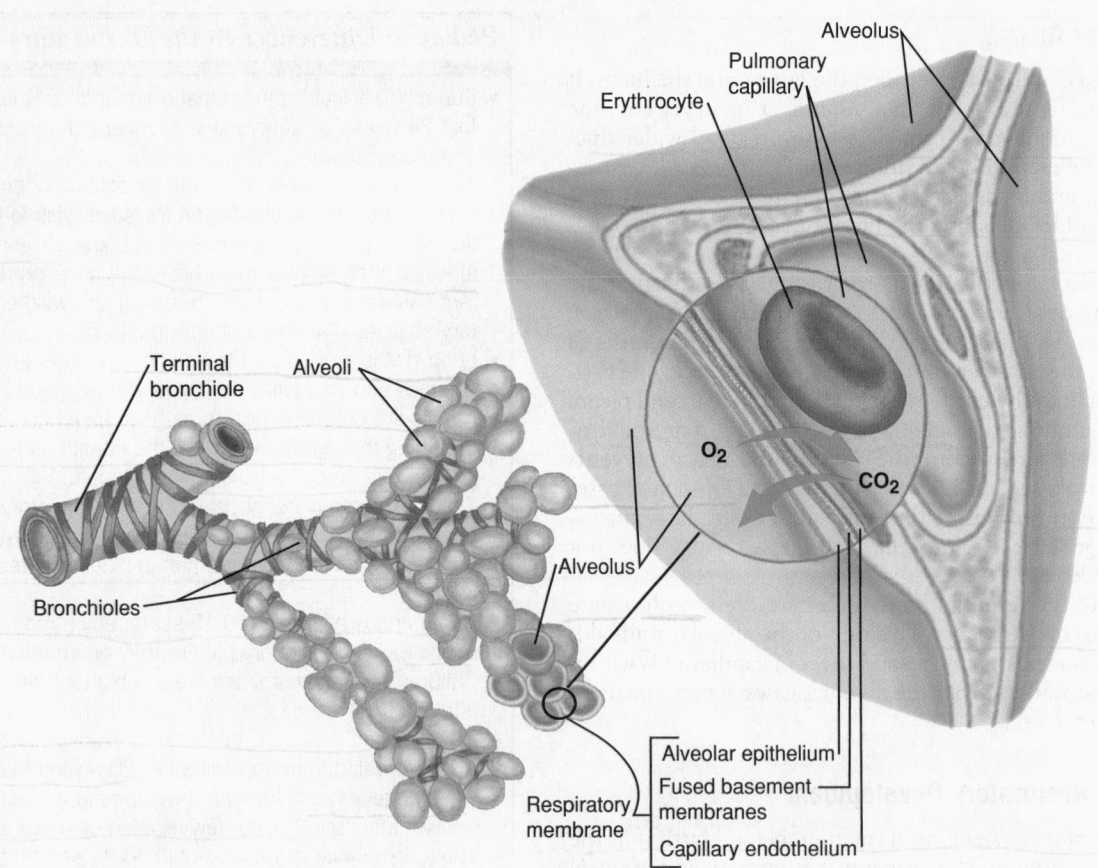

Labels on figure: Alveolus, Pulmonary capillary, Erythrocyte, Terminal bronchiole, Alveoli, Bronchioles, Alveolus, O_2, CO_2, Respiratory membrane, Alveolar epithelium, Fused basement membranes, Capillary endothelium

Mechanisms of Gas Exchange

DIAGNOSTIC TESTS

In most instances, respiratory tract disorders are diagnosed from the findings on physical examination and the clinical manifestations. Sometimes, however, specific diagnostic tests are needed.

Blood Gas Analysis

Arterial blood gas analysis plays an important role in the investigation of pulmonary function. Arterial blood gas values most frequently determined include PaO_2, $PaCO_2$, pH, and HCO_3^-. Arterial blood is more reliable than capillary or venous blood for these tests, especially in children with poor peripheral perfusion. Arterial blood gas values are used primarily to determine acid-base balance, not oxygen saturation (see Chapter 42).

Pulmonary Function Tests

Probably the most useful measures of ventilatory function are the *vital capacity* and the *expiratory flow rate*, both measured by spirometry. These tests can be performed in most children by age 6 years (Blonshire, 2000). Accurate measurements are difficult to obtain in younger children because they are unable to follow commands. Infant pulmonary function testing is now being performed at many institutions using conscious sedation (Godfrey, 2003). Pulmonary function tests assess the degree of pulmonary disease, the response to therapy, and the presence of restrictive or obstructive disease. They are also done to test the child's response to bronchodilators should pulmonary function be affected.

The child must be given instruction and practice in blowing, pushing, and holding respirations. The child should become familiar with the mouthpiece and the nose clip to feel comfortable with their use.

Pulse Oximetry

Pulse oximetry is a simple, noninvasive, intermittent or continuous method for measuring oxygen saturation for the purpose of determining the need for or response to oxygen therapy (see Chapter 37). The goal of treatment for most respiratory conditions is an oxygen saturation value greater than 95%. For children with chronic respiratory disease, however, a realistic goal may be slightly lower.

Transcutaneous Monitoring

Transcutaneous monitoring continuously checks oxygen and carbon dioxide concentrations in the body through an electrode placed on the child's skin. Electrode sites must be changed every 3 to 4 hours to prevent burning the skin, and the machine must be recalibrated each time electrodes are changed. The readings may not be accurate if tissue perfusion is poor.

Common Laboratory and Diagnostic Tests for Respiratory Disorders

Test	Description	Normal Findings	Indications	Nursing Considerations
Chest radiography, posteroanterior and lateral views	Shows airways, lungs, heart, great vessels.	Normal appearance of internal structures of the chest.	To detect respiratory disease of the lungs.	Assist in holding the child.
Computed tomography (CT)	Shows lesions in chest wall, pleural space, mediastinum, and lung parenchyma.	Normal cross section of lung tissue.	To image tumors or masses; to evaluate response to therapy aimed at defined lesions.	Assist with sedation and immobilization of the child. Withhold feedings 3-4 hr before the test because of frequent use of contrast medium.
Bronchoscopy	Provides viewing of tracheobronchial tree through a scope.	Normal appearance of tracheobronchial tree or successful removal of foreign body or mucous plugs.	To view a lesion and obtain biopsy material for culture; to remove a foreign body or mucous plugs.	Rigid bronchoscopy is usually performed with child under general anesthesia. Fiberoptic flexible bronchoscopy can be performed while the child is awake or sedated. Observe the child closely for signs of airway obstruction. Mist may be given to decrease swelling and edema.
Laryngoscopy	Provides direct viewing of larynx with a scope.	Normal appearance of larynx.	To identify cause of stridor and local abnormalities.	Mirror (indirect) laryngoscopy can be performed on children age 4 yr or older. In infants and younger children, direct laryngoscopy or transnasal laryngoscopy with flexible bronchoscope will give much better results. General anesthesia is usually required; topical anesthesia and mild sedation may be provided for a fiberoptic examination. Fluids and foods are withheld until the effects of local anesthetic have worn off and gag reflex has returned.
Cultures	Throat, blood, nasopharyngeal, sputum, induced sputum (hypertonic saline delivered via nebulizer).	No culture growth or normal flora only.	To isolate and identify pathogens.	See Chapter 37 for procedures.

Continued

Common Laboratory and Diagnostic Tests for Respiratory Disorders—cont'd

Test	Description	Normal Findings	Indications	Nursing Considerations
Radioallergosorbent test (RAST) for immunoglobulin E (IgE)	Measures quantity of IgE antibodies in serum after exposure to specific antigens.	If the child is not allergic to the antigen, IgE antibody is not detected. A test result is positive in relation to a specific antigen if the value is above 400% of control.	To identify specific allergens; systemic reactions to insect venom, drugs, and chemicals; to monitor response to desensitization procedures; also performed at the onset of asthma, hay fever, or dermatitis.	Prepare child for a peripheral blood sample to be drawn. Determine whether the child has undergone any radioisotope tests within the past week, because such tests may alter the results.
Pilocarpine iontophoresis (sweat test)	Measures sweat electrolyte concentration for diagnosis of cystic fibrosis (CF). Sweating is stimulated on the child's forearm with a small electrical current and pilocarpine; a sweat sample is then collected on preweighed, dry, sterile gauze or filter paper and the amounts of sweat sodium and chloride are measured.	*Normal chloride:* <40 mEq/L. *Suggestive of CF:* 40 mEq/L to 60mEq/L. *Positive for CF:* ≥ 60 mEq/L.	To diagnose cystic fibrosis.	No physical preparation is needed. Offer the parents and child support as they face the implications of a positive diagnosis. Inform the child and parents that the test is painless and that it is usually performed twice to ensure accurate results. Because an adequate amount of sweat is difficult to obtain from infants, the sweat test is usually unreliable in infants younger than 4 weeks.
Mantoux test	Skin test for tuberculosis (TB). Purified protein derivative (PPD), 5 TB units (0.1 ml), is injected intradermally into the volar surface of the forearm with a short, 26- to 27-gauge needle, beveled side up. A wheal 6-10 mm in diameter should appear during the injection. The site is checked in 48-72 hr by a health care professional. Results are recorded in millimeters (not simply as positive or negative). The reading is based on induration (hardness), not redness.	*Positive result:* in an area of induration ≥ 15 mm (in children 4 years of age and older); an area of induration ≥ 10 mm in children younger than 4 yr or at high risk for exposure; an area of induration ≥ 5 mm in the highest risk group. *Negative result:* Mantoux test cannot rule out the presence of TB, particularly in young infants.	To screen and test individuals suspected of having TB or of having been exposed to TB.	Test is fairly difficult to administer. After PPD is injected, withdrawal of the needle should be delayed 2-3 sec to minimize leakage of PPD at the puncture site. In most children, skin testing will elicit a positive reaction 3-6 wk after initial infection. Steroids and immunosuppressants given within 4-6 wk can cause false-negative skin test results. Positive tuberculin reactivity usually continues for the person's lifetime, even with treatment.

Respiratory alterations are the most common causes of illness in the infant and child. Upper respiratory disorders affect the ears, nose, pharynx, and larynx; lower respiratory disorders include those disorders that involve the trachea, bronchi, and lungs.

Infants and children younger than 3 years are at greater risk for developing respiratory infections than older children and adults because of their immature immune systems, smaller upper and lower airways, and underdeveloped supporting cartilage. Although most respiratory infections are self-limiting, infants and young children can quickly experience respiratory distress as mucus and edema obstruct their small airways.

Parents should be taught preventive measures, including adequate rest, good nutrition, and good hygiene, with an emphasis on handwashing. Even with the most careful hygiene and preventive practices, however, most children will experience some type of respiratory infection each year. School nurses often see children with respiratory problems in the school health office and may be the primary health caregivers for these children.

Most children can be cared for at home by their parents and do not need hospitalization. Those children who are hospitalized are being discharged from the hospital earlier in their recovery than in the past. The current health care environment underlies the need for nurses to teach parents good home care techniques, including careful observation and recognition of signs that indicate the need to contact health care providers. Parents, especially first-time parents, often are frightened by the sudden onset of respiratory symptoms, which may indicate a severe problem. Teaching them the signs and symptoms of serious illness will help them develop appropriate decision-making skills.

Children with chronic conditions have many special needs, and the child with a chronic respiratory disease is no different. Medications and treatments become a way of life for many of these children. Their activity level is often altered, and some may have a shortened life span.

The nurse plays an important role in the care of the child with a chronic respiratory disease. Beyond giving acute care to the hospitalized child, the nurse must coordinate and facilitate the child's long-term care. Because of advances being made in the treatment of chronic pediatric respiratory conditions, the treatment and care of children affected by these disorders are constantly changing and improving, requiring the nurse to stay current in these areas.

ALLERGIC RHINITIS

Allergic rhinitis is an inflammatory disorder of the nasal mucosa. It is usually seasonal, recurrent, and triggered by specific allergens (see Chapter 41). It is sometimes referred to as *seasonal allergic rhinitis, seasonal pollinosis,* or *hay fever.* Some children have symptoms year round (*perennial allergic rhinitis*).

Etiology and Incidence

Common causative agents of allergic rhinitis include dust mites, feathers, animal dander, mold spores, and pollens of trees, grasses, and weeds. There is usually a family history similar to that seen in individuals with atopic dermatitis and asthma. Unlike atopic dermatitis, however, allergic rhinitis does not predispose to the development of asthma.

Pathophysiology

of Allergic Rhinitis

Allergens (pollens, molds, spores, dust mites, animal dander) are deposited on the nasal mucosa, causing local inflammation and increased capillary permeability. Local immunoglobulin E (IgE) is produced, and sensitization of the respiratory tissues occurs. Mast cell mediators are released, producing vasodilation, mucosal edema, mucus secretions, stimulation of itch receptors, and a reduced threshold for sneezing.

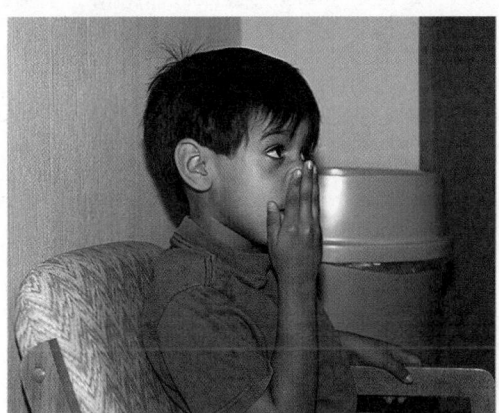

Figure 45-1 Children with allergic rhinitis often have dark circles under their eyes, called *allergic shiners,* and may be seen rubbing their noses upward with the palm—the "allergic salute." (Courtesy Parkland Health and Hospital System Community Oriented Primary Care Clinic, Dallas, TX.)

The onset of allergic rhinitis usually occurs during childhood but rarely before age 2 years. It is estimated that 20% to 40% of children have this type of allergic response (Milgrom & Leung, 2004).

Manifestations

The classic symptoms of allergic rhinitis are watery rhinorrhea, associated with itching of nose, eyes, ears, and palate; and paroxysmal sneezing. Additional signs and symptoms include the "allergic salute"—an upward rubbing of the nose with the palm of the hand, which can leave a crease below the bridge (Fig. 45-1); allergic shiners—dark circles under the eyes from congestion and edema; dry lips from mouth breathing; pale, boggy nasal mucous membranes; and nasal obstruction. Children with allergic rhinitis experience symptoms as long as they are exposed to the allergen.

It is important to distinguish allergic rhinitis from viral *nasopharyngitis* (the common cold), which is usually caused by a rhinovirus and is spread by droplet or by contact with contaminated items. Usually children with nasopharyngitis experience the associated symptoms of sore throat, fever, cough, and fatigue. The condition is self-limiting and usually resolves within 2 weeks. The quality of the nasal discharge in children with nasopharyngitis often changes from clear to cloudy or yellow. Management is supportive. Because young infants are obligatory nose breathers, the infant's blocked

PARENTS
Want to Know

How to Implement Environmental Modifications

To reduce your child's exposure to allergens, take the following measures:

Pollen and Dust
- Wash your child's sheets and blankets weekly in hot water.
- Avoid using wool and down blankets.
- Encase pillows and mattresses in dust-proof covers.
- Replace carpet with wood, tile, slate, or vinyl.
- Replace drapes and blinds with curtains and shades.
- Replace upholstered furniture with wood or plastic.
- Keep closet doors shut.
- Cover hot air vents with filters.
- Install air cleaners.
- Use multilayer vacuum bags.
- Clean with a towel treated to attract dust.
- Run an air conditioner.
- Keep household humidity at 40% to 50%.

Mold
- Clean with a mold inhibitor.
- Dry everyone's shoes thoroughly.

- Use a moisture remover in closets.
- Encourage your child to stay out of the basement.
- Replace foam rubber mattresses with inner spring mattresses.
- Run an air conditioner.
- Keep the humidity below 35%.
- Run a dehumidifier.
- Ventilate the house.
- Store firewood outside.
- Limit the number of indoor plants.

Dander
- Keep pets outside if possible.
- Ventilate the house.
- Install air cleaners.
- Encase mattresses and pillows in dust-proof covers.
  For further information, contact:
  Allergy & Asthma Network/Mothers of Asthmatics, Inc. Website: www.aanma.org. A patient site that provides information on asthma, products, kits, and books.

nasal passages can be relieved with instillation of normal saline drops followed by gentle bulb suction.

Diagnostic Evaluation

A thorough personal and family history usually elicit a description that suggests an allergic rather than infectious pattern. The nasal smear may demonstrate eosinophils. Allergy skin testing is done if signs and symptoms continue after treatment with medication. The radioallergosorbent test (RAST) is used only when skin testing is difficult because of generalized dermatitis, the child is very young, or the child is too ill for skin testing. A complete blood count might reveal elevated eosinophils, a finding associated with allergic manifestations.

Therapeutic Management

The treatment of choice is to eliminate the allergen from the child's environment (Berger, 2001). When this is impossible, as in the case of pollen in the air, medication can control symptoms. Finally, immunotherapy (allergy shots) may be considered for children whose condition is not responsive to either environmental modification or medication. Immunotherapy involves injecting the child with progressively larger doses of the allergen in an effort to reduce the magnitude of the body's allergic response. Injections are given once or twice a week until a maintenance dose is reached; monthly maintenance injections can continue for several years.

Antihistamines and/or intranasal corticosteroids are given to relieve symptoms. Antihistamines are most effective when given before or very early in an allergic episode. Because they can cause drowsiness, they should be given at night. Some of the newer antihistamines (e.g., loratadine, cetirizine, fexofenadine) are long-acting and require only one or two doses daily. A decongestant can be given in conjunction with an antihistamine if nasal congestion is a problem. Short-term topical intranasal corticosteroids (e.g., fluticasone, mometasone) are quite effective and seem to actually offer better relief than antihistamines and decongestants (Milgrom & Leung, 2004; Nielsen et al., 2001). It usually takes several days of treatment before the child feels the effects of topical corticosteroids. Children with severe symptoms that do not respond to treatment may be given systemic corticosteroids; relief is usually attained within 24 hours.

Nursing Considerations

Nursing care focuses on early identification of clinical signs and symptoms of allergic rhinitis and support of the therapeutic management of the condition. The nurse assesses and records the applicable history and helps the family identify allergens to which the child is sensitive. *environment*

Once the allergens are known, the nurse counsels parents regarding administration of medications, environmental control, and immunotherapy as appropriate. Drowsiness, the most common side effect of antihistamines, can usually be overcome if the child takes a combination antihistamine and decongestant or takes the medication at night. Some children experience dry mucous membranes or excitability. Warm water or saline irrigations of the nasal passages can be used to moisten mucous membranes, soften crusted secretions, and wash out irritants. Saline can be mixed by adding $1/4$ teaspoon of salt to a cup of warm water. Saline nose drops are also available without prescription.

When specific allergens have been identified, they should be eliminated or controlled. During the pollen season, the child should stay indoors as much as possible and the windows should be kept closed if the house is air-conditioned. After being outdoors, the child should shower and wash the hair to remove pollens from the body. Animals that have been outside may also be a source of contamination.

Receiving immunotherapy can be a traumatic experience for the child. It is often difficult for children to understand how an injection will help them. Allergy injections must be given in a physician's office because some children can experience an anaphylactic reaction to the allergy serum. Monitor the child closely (vital sign changes, difficulty breathing) for 20 to 30 minutes after the injection in case anaphylaxis develops. Keep emergency epinephrine ready.

SINUSITIS

Sinusitis, although not itself a serious disorder, can lead to life-threatening complications. Inflammation and infection of the sinuses can be acute or chronic.

Etiology and Incidence

Acute sinusitis often follows an upper respiratory tract viral infection. Children with chronic sinusitis often have allergic rhinitis or acute otitis media with effusion. Hypertrophied adenoids, immune deficiencies, and foreign body obstruction in the nose also predispose to sinusitis. Children with cystic fibrosis have a high incidence of sinusitis because of highly viscous mucous secretions and nasal polyps. The most common causative organisms are *Streptococcus pneumoniae*, *Haemophilus influenzae*, and *Moraxella catarrhalis*, and less frequently, group A *Streptococcus* species (Conrad & Jenson, 2002).

Sinus infections can occur in infancy as well as in childhood but are most common during the school-age years.

Manifestations

Sinusitis is characterized by signs and symptoms of a cold that do not improve after 14 days, low-grade fever, nasal congestion with purulent nasal discharge, halitosis, cough (which usually increases when the child is lying down), and headache, tenderness, and a feeling of fullness over the affected sinuses; young children may become irritable. Occasionally, children experience facial edema. Children with chronic sinusitis experience many of the same symptoms except that the cough is chronic and the headache is recurrent. The child's sense of taste or smell may be impaired, and the child may be fatigued.

Diagnostic Evaluation

Sinus radiographs show mucosal thickening, opacification, and air-fluid levels in children older than 1 year. Sinus radiographs are of no value in younger children because of their small sinuses. Computed tomography (CT) has become the gold standard for diagnosis of sinus disease because it provides detailed anatomic information. Because of the thick bone of the maxilla in the anterior part of the face and the small size of the sinus, transillumination of the sinuses is not useful.

Therapeutic Management

Antibiotics are the mainstay of treatment; amoxicillin or amoxicillin–potassium clavulanate (Augmentin) is used most frequently. In addition to antibiotics, treatment includes analgesics, hydration, the application of moist heat, and decongestants. The use of antihistamines in the treatment of sinusitis is controversial (Contopoulos-Ioannidis, Ioamidis, & Lau, 2003). Antihistamines may be used to treat allergy symptoms associated with chronic sinusitis, but they tend to impair sinus drainage by thickening secretions. Steroid nasal sprays may be used to reduce inflammation while avoiding the rebound effect of decongestant nose drops.

Obstructive deformities, such as enlarged adenoids or polyps, are surgically corrected. If orbital cellulitis develops, the child should be hospitalized immediately and parenteral antibiotic therapy begun.

Nursing Considerations

The nurse should assess the location of pain or fullness. Pain can occur in the forehead or over the cheek bones or upper teeth, or it may radiate to the top of the head. The nurse should inspect and palpate the face for edema, document any fever, and inspect the nose and throat for purulent discharge. The nasal mucous membranes are inspected for erythema and edema.

Nursing care focuses on teaching the parents antibiotic administration, comfort measures, how to monitor for response to treatment, and how to identify complications. Emphasize the importance of the child's taking the antibiotics as prescribed. Sinus drainage is facilitated by increasing the child's intake of clear fluids and by using a bedside humidifier.

Warm, moist compresses applied two or three times daily help decrease swelling and pain. Acetaminophen is given for fever and discomfort. Breathing warm mist in a hot shower or through hot, moist towels can help liquefy and mobilize nasal mucus, as can saline nose drops. The nurse teaches the parent to administer nose drops after the nasal passages have been gently cleaned. The amount, color, and consistency of nasal drainage should be noted and evaluated to determine whether the child is responding to treatment.

Carefully evaluate the child's response to treatment and the development of complications. Advise parents to contact the physician promptly if symptoms become worse, if the child experiences any periorbital redness or edema, or if the child does not seem to be feeling better after 3 to 4 days.

OTITIS MEDIA

Otitis media is one of the most common illnesses of infancy and childhood. The term *otitis media* refers to effusion and infection or blockage of the middle ear. *Acute otitis media* is effusion in the middle ear that occurs suddenly and is associated with other signs of illness. *Otitis media with effusion* refers to the presence of fluid behind the tympanic membrane without signs of infection. Otitis media with effusion often follows an episode of acute otitis media and usually resolves in 1 to 3 months.

Etiology

The bacterial pathogens that usually cause acute otitis media are *S. pneumoniae, H. influenzae,* and *M. catarrhalis.* Although viruses do not cause otitis media, they are thought to predispose the child to ear infection by altering host defenses and contributing to eustachian tube dysfunction. Allergies are also thought to precipitate otitis media.

Attendance at daycare centers predisposes children to otitis media. Infants younger than 1 year who attend daycare have a threefold risk for acquiring acute otitis media (Hoberman, Marchant, Kaplan, & Feldman, 2002). The risk for ear infections is up to three times higher in those who use a pacifier (Hanafin & Griffiths, 2002).

Bottle-feeding contributes to ear infection because of the position of the infant during feeding. Reflux of formula into the eustachian tube from the nasopharynx occurs when the infant swallows while supine. Breastfeeding offers some protection from ear infection by providing maternal antibodies and by decreasing the incidence of allergy; also, the more upright position of the infant while nursing is protective against ear infection.

Incidence

The incidence of otitis media peaks between ages 6 months and 6 years, with most episodes occurring in children younger than 3 years. Most initial episodes occur at about age 6 months, when maternal antibody levels decline. Early onset of acute otitis media (during infancy) increases the risk for recurrent episodes (Pelton, 2002).

By the end of the third year of life, 50% to 70% of all children have had at least one episode of acute otitis media. Most children younger than 5 years have two or three episodes of otitis media each year. Boys have a slightly higher incidence of otitis media than girls. Native-American and Eskimo children, especially infants, have higher otitis media–associated

outpatient and hospitalization rates than those for the general U.S. population of children (Curns et al., 2002). The incidence of otitis media is highest in winter and spring and lowest in the summer months.

Manifestations

Acute otitis media (AOM) is characterized by:

- Otalgia (earache); infants may pull their ears or roll their heads.
- A bulging, opaque tympanic membrane that usually looks red, with decreased mobility; diffuse light reflex; and obscured landmarks (Fig. 45-2).
- Drainage, usually yellowish green, purulent, and foul-smelling (indicates perforation of the tympanic membrane).

These signs and symptoms might also be accompanied by irritability, sleep disturbances, persistent crying in infants, fever, vomiting, anorexia, or diarrhea (especially in infants). Otitis media with effusion (OME) differs from acute otitis media in that there are no signs of acute infection. The tympanic membrane appears retracted and either dull gray or yellow, and an air-fluid level or air bubbles may be visible through the tympanic membrane. The mobility of the tympanic membrane is decreased, and landmarks are distorted. Associated signs and symptoms can be subtle and include:

- Tinnitus, popping sounds.
- Hearing loss (usually conductive) below 35 decibels, with delays in speech development possible from prolonged hearing loss; in the older child, hearing loss may manifest as behavior problems, poor school performance, disturbed sleep, irritability, and decreased responsiveness.
- Mild balance disturbances that may result in delays in motor skills.
- A flattened tracing and negative pressure on the tympanogram (a graphic representation of tympanic mobility and middle-ear pressure).

Diagnostic Evaluation

The diagnosis of otitis media is based on the history of signs and symptoms and pneumatic otoscopy. In pneumatic otoscopy, a small puff of air is blown into the ear canal through the otoscope; the examiner can discern the appearance and mobility of the tympanic membrane. In addition to pneumatic otoscopy, tympanometry can be used to confirm what was seen with the eye.

Therapeutic Management

The emergence of resistant organisms has created much discussion around the use of antibiotics to treat AOM because spontaneous resolution of the infection occurs in about 80% of children. In 2004, the American Academy of Pediatrics (AAP) issued two policy recommendations regarding identification and management of AOM and OME in healthy children ages 2 months to 12 years (AAP, 2004; American Academy of Family Physicians, American Academy of Otolaryngology-Head and Neck Surgery, American Academy of Pediatrics Subcom-

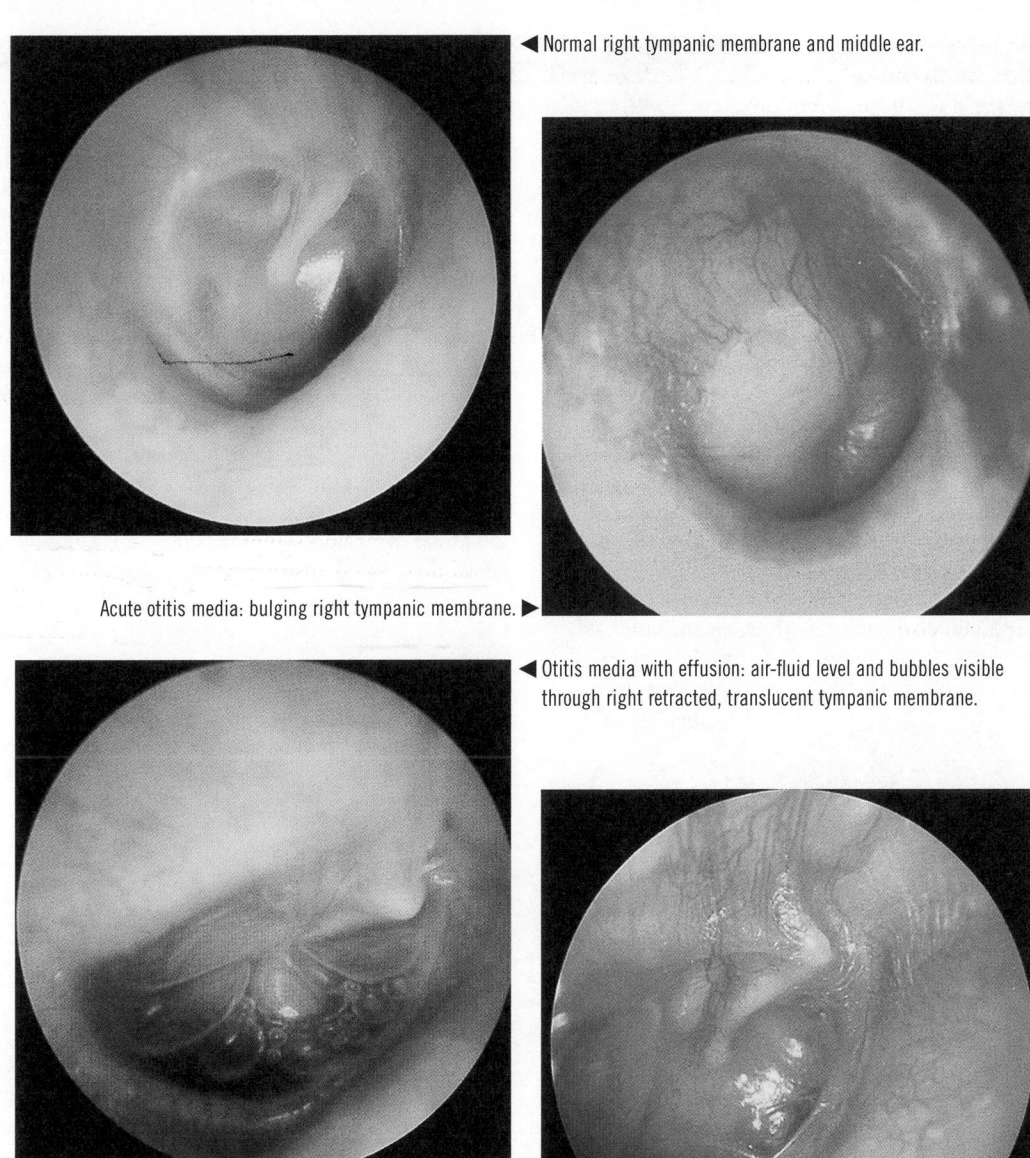

◀ Normal right tympanic membrane and middle ear.

Acute otitis media: bulging right tympanic membrane. ▶

◀ Otitis media with effusion: air-fluid level and bubbles visible through right retracted, translucent tympanic membrane.

Otitis media with effusion: severely retracted, opaque ▶ right tympanic membrane.

Figure 45-2 Appearance of tympanic membrane in otitis media as compared with normal tympanic membrane. (From Bluestone, C.D., & Klein, J.O. [1995]. *Otitis media in infants and children* [2nd ed.]. Philadelphia: Saunders.)

mittee on Otitis Media With Effusion, 2004). Recommendations include the following:

- Accurate discrimination between AOM and OME prior to treatment decisions
- Adequate pain relief for children with AOM
- Symptomatic treatment and observation for 48 to 72 hours after diagnosis as an alternative to initiating antibiotic therapy for selected children older than age 6 months with AOM
- Reassessment and treatment initiation for children with positive AOM after the 48 to 72 hour observation period
- Use of amoxicillin at a dose of 80 to 90 mg/kg/day for 5 to 10 days when treatment is indicated

- Encourage reduction of risk factors as a method for preventing AOM episodes
- Treat children with OME who are not at risk for hearing, language, or learning problems with 3 months of "watchful waiting"

Alternative antibiotics, such as erythromycin-sulfisoxazole (Pediazole), trimethoprim-sulfamethoxazole (e.g., Bactrim, Septra), cefaclor (Ceclor), cefixime (Suprax), or a macrolide (Zithromax), may be prescribed for penicillin-resistant organisms or in cases of penicillin allergy (Easton et al., 2003). The pneumococcal conjugate vaccine was recently approved for use in children and should be administered to all children

Pathophysiology
of Otitis Media

The immature anatomy of the child's middle ear and eustachian tube predisposes infants and toddlers to otitis media. When the eustachian tube is obstructed, as frequently occurs with enlarged adenoids or mucosal edema from an upper respiratory tract infection, effective drainage and ventilation of the middle ear cannot occur. Air that is normally present in the middle ear is absorbed by the blood, causing a vacuum or negative pressure in the middle ear. Fluid (effusion) accumulates within the middle-ear space, creating a medium for bacterial growth. After an upper respiratory tract infection, pathogens travel from the nasopharynx to the eustachian tube. In the presence of effusion, negative pressure in the middle ear draws mucus through the eustachian tube whenever the child cries, yawns, or sucks forcefully on a nipple. Purulent fluid accumulates in the middle-ear space, causing the pressure and pain of acute otitis media.

If the eustachian tube remains nonfunctional for a prolonged period, the fluid within the middle ear becomes thick and dark (glue ear). Mild temporary conductive hearing loss (see Chapter 55) often occurs in otitis media with effusion because of the decreased mobility of the ossicles and the tympanic membrane. Permanent conductive hearing loss can result from repeated episodes of otitis media and may interfere with the development of language and cognitive skills. Chronic otitis media with effusion is the most common cause of hearing loss in children.

Complications of otitis media include conductive hearing loss and sensorineural hearing loss. The infection of acute otitis media can spread to surrounding tissues, causing mastoiditis or intracranial complications such as meningitis or brain abscess. Inflammation and pressure from otitis media may result in *tympanosclerosis* (scarring of the tympanic membrane), perforation of the tympanic membrane, and *cholesteatoma* (pus and debris in the middle ear).

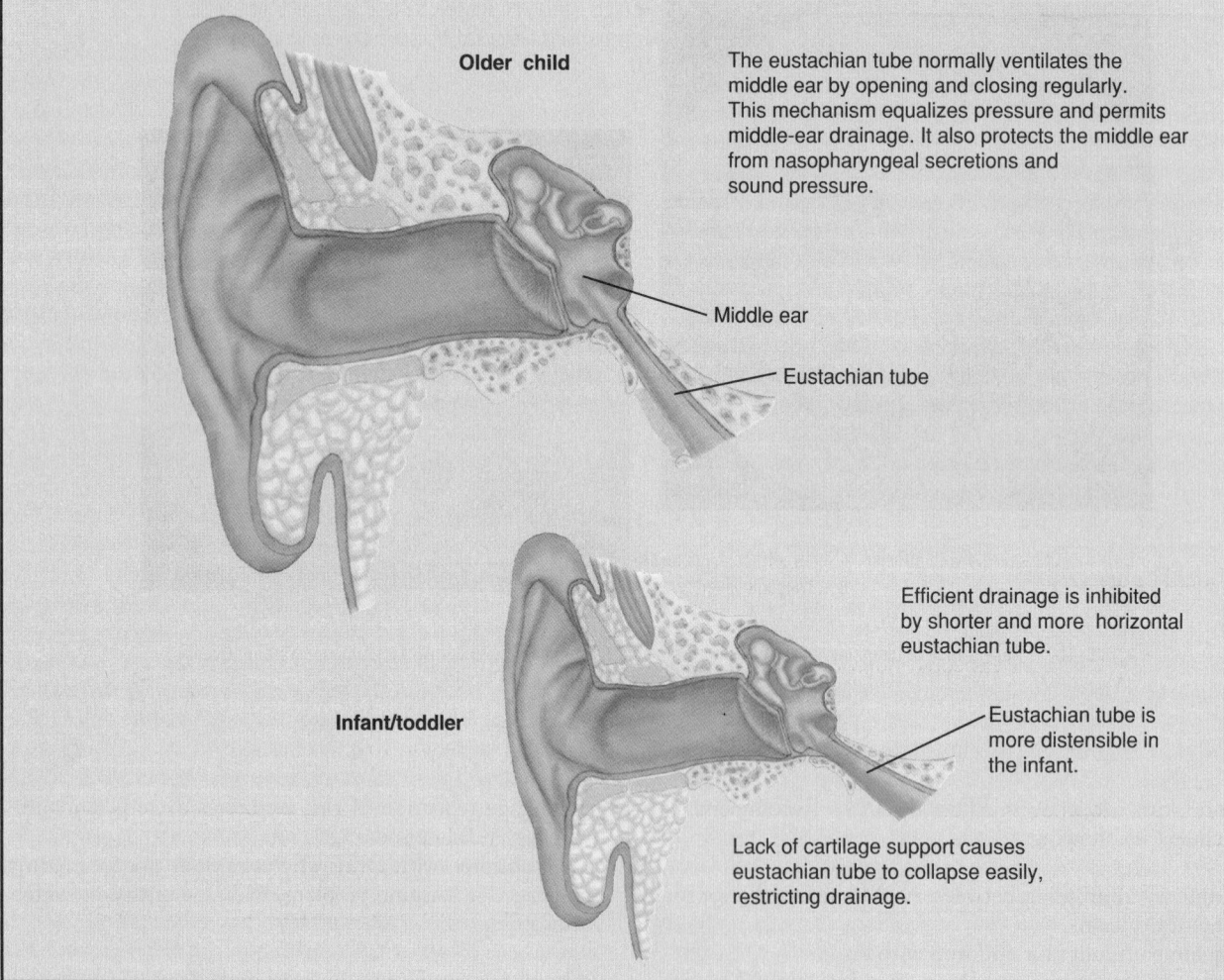

Older child

The eustachian tube normally ventilates the middle ear by opening and closing regularly. This mechanism equalizes pressure and permits middle-ear drainage. It also protects the middle ear from nasopharyngeal secretions and sound pressure.

Middle ear

Eustachian tube

Infant/toddler

Efficient drainage is inhibited by shorter and more horizontal eustachian tube.

Eustachian tube is more distensible in the infant.

Lack of cartilage support causes eustachian tube to collapse easily, restricting drainage.

younger than 2 years according to the recommended schedule (see Appendix D).

The usefulness of decongestants and antihistamines in the prevention and treatment of otitis media is controversial. Although these medications are widely prescribed, new policy recommendations do not support their use (American Academy of Family Physicians, American Academy of Otolaryngology-Head and Neck Surgery, American Academy of Pediatrics Subcommittee on Otitis Media With Effusion, 2004). Acetaminophen is given to help relieve pain and fever of acute otitis media.

In children with persistent ear infection despite antibiotic therapy or with otitis media with effusion that persists for more than 3 months and is associated with hearing loss, *myringotomy* with insertion of *tympanostomy tubes* (pressure-equalizing [PE] tubes) may be performed (Perkins, 2002). During this operation, mucoid material is removed from the middle ear and a tympanostomy tube is inserted through the tympanic membrane. A tympanostomy tube is a small polyethylene tube that is inserted into the middle ear to equalize the pressure on both sides of the tympanic membrane and to keep the ear aerated. Negative pressure in the middle ear is relieved, allowing the middle-ear mucosa to return to normal and growth of the eustachian tube to occur. The tube usually falls out spontaneously in 6 to 12 months. This period may provide enough time for the effusion process to resolve, but some children need repeated insertions of tympanostomy tubes because of persistent eustachian tube dysfunction. Tympanostomy tubes are inserted with the child under general anesthesia, usually in an outpatient surgery setting.

NURSING CARE
The Child With Otitis Media

Assessment

Ask the parent whether the child has had a recent upper respiratory tract infection or previous ear infections. Assess the child for fever and pain. Because signs of ear infection may be subtle in infants, the nurse should assess not only for obvious signs of ear pain, such as head rolling and pulling at the ear, but also for nonspecific findings, such as irritability, diarrhea, or decreased appetite. Older children may complain of pain or a feeling of fullness in the affected ear. The nurse examines the ear with a pneumatic otoscope, noting the color, mobility, and translucency of the tympanic membrane as well as the appearance of the external canal. The tympanic membrane should be inspected carefully for signs of perforation. The nurse obtains a culture of any drainage and notes the color, consistency, and odor. Hearing and language development should be assessed.

Nursing Diagnosis and Planning

The nursing diagnoses and expected outcomes that may be appropriate for the family and infant or child with otitis media are

- Acute Pain related to inflammation and pressure in the middle ear.
  Expected Outcomes: The child will be free of pain, as evidenced by sleeping through the night, not pulling at the ears, and crying less. The child's tympanic membranes will appear shiny and pearl-gray, with normal landmarks, a visible light reflex, and normal mobility on tympanography.
- Deficient Knowledge related to incomplete understanding of the disease process and treatment regimen.
  Expected Outcomes: The parents will demonstrate (1) methods of feeding the infant that decrease the risk for otitis media, (2) how to keep the child's ears dry if tympanostomy tubes are in place, and (3) ways to follow the treatment regimen, including administering the entire course of antibiotics.

- Risk for Imbalanced Body Temperature related to inflammation.
  Expected Outcome: The child will display a normal body temperature.
- Risk for Deficient Fluid Volume related to elevated temperature and decreased intake.
  Expected Outcomes: The child will have moist mucous membranes, good skin turgor, and appropriate intake and output for age.

Interventions

Teach the parents the importance of giving prescribed antibiotics on time and for the prescribed number of days. Because the child usually feels much better after a few days of medication, parents may believe that the antibiotics are no longer necessary and stop giving them. Increase adherence by giving written as well as oral instructions for administering medications. Providing a medication record form on which to record doses taken and a calibrated measuring device for liquid medications is also helpful.

The nurse also advises the parents to discard any unused antibiotic rather than save it and not to give the child an antibiotic without consulting the physician first.

Acetaminophen can be given to relieve discomfort. The child's fluid intake should be increased if fever is present. Advise the parents to notify the physician if the child's condition has not improved after 48 hours of observation without antibiotics, after 48 hours of antibiotic treatment without improvement in symptoms, or if there is drainage from the affected ear. If a follow-up visit is recommended, emphasize the importance of keeping the appointment.

The nurse can enhance medication adherence through specific teaching about administration of antibiotics. For example, the nurse might say, "After a few days, your child may seem to be well and show no signs of the ear infection. If you stop giving the antibiotic at that time, some of the germs that caused the otitis media might still be alive and your child can experience a relapse."

If the child is undergoing myringotomy with insertion of tympanostomy tubes, the nurse should prepare the child and parents as for any outpatient surgical procedure. Explain the procedure in clear terms, and answer questions simply and honestly.

Postoperatively, the child is monitored for ear drainage. A small amount of reddish drainage is normal for the first few days after surgery, but the parents should report any heavier bleeding or bleeding that occurs after 3 days. The parents should also be instructed to report any fever or increased pain. The child should avoid blowing the nose for 7 to 10 days.

Most physicians prefer that the child's ears be kept dry if tubes are in place, but some feel that a small amount of water in the ears is not harmful. Bath and lake water are potential sources of bacterial contamination, however, and chlorinated swimming pool water can be irritating to tympanic membranes with tubes. The usual recommendation is to place ear plugs or cotton balls covered with petroleum jelly in the ears during baths and shampoos. Swimming is allowed only with ear plugs and the physician's approval. Diving and swimming deep under water are prohibited. The size and appearance of the tympanostomy tubes should be described to the parents, and they should be reassured that if the tubes fall out it is not an emergency but that the physician should be notified.

Otitis media is usually a chronic problem, with frequent recurrences of infection and effusion. The nurse should teach the parents the early signs of ear infection and the importance of seeking care if these signs should occur. Because hearing impairment from middle-ear effusion can be very difficult for parents to detect, the child with chronic otitis media should undergo periodic hearing evaluations.

The nurse should teach parents methods to decrease the risk for recurrent otitis media, such as breastfeeding during infancy, discontinuing bottle-feeding as soon as possible, feeding the infant in an upright position, and refraining from giving a bottle to the infant in bed. Parents should be told not to smoke in the child's presence because passive smoking increases the incidence of otitis media.

Evaluation

- Is the child sleeping an appropriate amount of time for age with decreased episodes of crying or pulling at ears?
- Have otoscopic findings returned to normal?
- Did the parents complete the treatment regimen by giving the entire dose of the prescribed antibiotic, and are they able to demonstrate appropriate feeding methods?
- Were follow-up appointments kept to determine the resolution of the otitis media?
- Is the child afebrile?
- Does the child appear well-hydrated with moist mucous membranes and good skin turgor?

PHARYNGITIS AND TONSILLITIS

Pharyngitis, inflammation of the pharynx and surrounding lymphoid tissue, can be viral or bacterial in origin. Although pharyngitis is self-limiting and is a relatively minor disorder, streptococcal infections can have serious complications—among them, rheumatic fever and acute glomerular nephritis. *Tonsillitis* is the term commonly used to describe inflammation and infection of the two palatine tonsils. *Adenoiditis* refers to infection and inflammation of the pharyngeal tonsils, or adenoids, which are located above the palatine tonsils on the posterior wall of the nasopharynx. The purpose of these lymphoid tissues is to filter and protect the respiratory and digestive tracts from invasion by pathogens, but often the tonsils become a site for infection.

Etiology

Viral pharyngitis may be caused by adenoviruses, parainfluenza virus, influenza virus, coxsackieviruses, and respiratory syncytial virus. Group A beta-hemolytic *Streptococcus* accounts for approximately 5% to 10% of pharyngitis cases (Hayes & Williamson, 2001). Streptococcal pharyngitis is rare before age 3 years. Streptococcal infection is spread by close droplet transmission. Tonsillitis, like pharyngitis, may be bacterial or viral in origin. The most common bacterial agent is group A beta-hemolytic *Streptococcus*.

Incidence

The incidence of pharyngitis and tonsillitis peaks between ages 4 and 7 years, when most children begin preschool and elementary school and have increased exposure to microorganisms. Group A beta-hemolytic streptococcal infection oc-

Pathophysiology

of Pharyngitis

Pharyngitis often accompanies the common cold. Tonsillitis is usually present with pharyngitis. Infection and inflammation of the tonsils cause them to enlarge. The palatine tonsils may meet in the midline (i.e., kissing tonsils) and cause difficulty swallowing and breathing. If adenoids enlarge, they can obstruct the eustachian tubes, resulting in otitis media and hearing impairment. Hypertrophy of the adenoids can also block the passageway between the nose and the throat, causing mouth breathing or obstructive sleep apnea.

curs most frequently in the winter and is spread more readily in crowded living situations. The incidence of tonsillitis decreases during middle childhood as the lymphoid tissue undergoes normal shrinkage.

Manifestations

Signs and symptoms differ between viral and bacterial pharyngitis (Table 45-1). *The only reliable means of determining whether a case of pharyngitis is viral or bacterial in origin is with a throat culture.* Not all children with pharyngitis complain of a sore throat, particularly if they are of preschool age. Instead, the child may complain of a stomachache or simply refuse to eat. The child with tonsillitis demonstrates:

- Sore throat, which may be persistent or recurrent
- Tonsils enlarged and bright red; may be covered with white exudate or cryptic plugs — dents
- Difficulty swallowing
- Mouth breathing and an unpleasant mouth odor
- Enlarged adenoids, which may cause a nasal quality of speech, mouth breathing, hearing difficulty, otitis media, snoring, or obstructive sleep apnea

Older children and adolescents may experience a *peritonsillar abscess* associated with pharyngitis or tonsillitis. Peritonsillar abscess usually is unilateral, with the enlarged tonsil displacing the uvula to the opposite side. The child might refuse to talk or swallow because of severe pain that often radiates to the ear. There is a risk for airway obstruction and dehydration.

Diagnostic Evaluation

Rapid streptococcal antigen tests ("rapid strep test") can accurately screen for group A beta-hemolytic streptococcal infection, but if the child's symptoms suggest a streptococcal infection, culture of a throat specimen obtained by swab should be done simultaneously. Because rapid strep tests have an approximately 20% incidence of false-negative results, a throat culture should be done in symptomatic children with a negative rapid strep test. And because approximately 10% of children carry group A beta-hemolytic *Streptococci* in their throats, a positive throat culture is not proof of active infection.

TABLE 45-1 Comparison of Viral and Bacterial Pharyngitis	
Viral Pharyngitis	**Bacterial Pharyngitis**
Gradual onset	Abrupt onset (may be gradual in children <2 yr)
Sore throat (reaches a peak on the 2nd or 3rd day)	Sore throat (usually severe)
Erythema and inflammation of the pharynx and tonsils (may be slight), vesicles or ulcers on tonsils	Erythema and inflammation of the pharynx and tonsils
Fever (usually low grade but may be high)	Fever (usually high, 39.4° to 40° C [103° to 104° F], but may be moderate); begins early in illness and usually lasts 1-4 days
Hoarseness, cough, rhinitis, conjunctivitis, malaise, anorexia (early)	Abdominal pain, vomiting, headache
Cervical lymph nodes may be enlarged and tender	Cervical lymph nodes may be enlarged and tender
Usually lasts 3-4 days	Usually lasts 3-5 days

Therapeutic Management

During the acute phase of pharyngitis or tonsillitis, treatment is symptomatic, focusing on pain relief and rest. Acetaminophen or ibuprofen is used for pain; older children may find gargling with warm saline solution comforting. Cool, bland liquids are tolerated best because of the discomfort caused by swallowing solids or irritating liquids.

Antibiotics should be restricted to those children who test positive on antigen detection tests or cultures. Streptococcal pharyngitis is most commonly treated orally with penicillin given two or three times daily for 10 days. Recent studies have shown that shorter courses of antibiotics (amoxicillin, cephalosporins, azithromycin) were as effective or more effective than the traditional 10-day penicillin therapy because of superior compliance and adherence, lower incidence of side effects, improved patient/parent satisfaction, and lower drug costs (Brook, 2002). Erythromycin may be used in children who are allergic to penicillin. A single intramuscular dose of procaine penicillin and benzathine penicillin G might be considered in children for whom compliance is expected to be a problem. Children given penicillin therapy are noninfectious to others 24 hours after therapy is initiated.

Surgical removal of the tonsils, or tonsillectomy, is controversial. Although some physicians think that a tonsillectomy is warranted in cases of recurrent tonsillitis, the prevailing attitude is more conservative, and the procedure is generally reserved for cases of upper airway obstruction, peritonsillar abscess, obstructive sleep apnea, or other serious problems. Electrosurgical tonsillectomy is a newer technique using electromagnetic radiation to generate heat within tissue for cutting and coagulation. This technique may reduce the risk for bleeding and produce less patient discomfort than traditional surgical procedures (Maddern, 2002). Tonsillectomy is generally not performed in children younger than 3 years because of the tendency for remaining tonsillar tissues to hypertrophy. Contraindications to tonsillectomy include active infection and cleft palate (see Chapter 43). Surgical removal of the tonsils while they are infected can result in spread of the infecting organism and sepsis. In children with cleft palate, the tonsils help prevent air escape during speech. Adenoidectomy alone may be performed in cases of recurrent otitis media secondary to eustachian tube obstruction or for persistent nasal or airway obstruction.

Many parents believe that a tonsillectomy will solve their child's problems of frequent sore throats, mouth breathing, and poor weight gain. There is no evidence that a tonsillectomy reduces the incidence of recurrent pharyngitis. The nurse should be prepared to discuss the current treatment philosophy with parents and address their concerns. If tonsillectomy is chosen as the method of treatment, the procedure is often done in a day surgery setting.

Nursing Considerations

Assessment of the child with pharyngitis or tonsillitis includes inspecting the pharynx for erythema, exudate, or petechiae. The skin should be inspected for rash and color changes. Some children with streptococcal pharyngitis have a pink, sandpaper-like rash on the trunk (see Chapter 40). The child is questioned about the onset and location of throat, ear, or abdominal pain. The parent of a preverbal child may report that the child refuses to eat or begins to cry during feedings. The nurse also assesses the child's temperature and respiratory status and asks the older child or parent about the onset of symptoms and any known contact with streptococcal infection in the school or family. Also ask whether the child has been taking any antibiotics at home, because they will interfere with the results of the throat culture.

Measures to relieve throat discomfort include administering acetaminophen, warm salt water gargles (¼ teaspoon of salt per 8-ounce glass of water), and warm or cool compresses applied to the neck (Thomas et al., 2000). The child should not be forced to eat. Offer cool, bland liquids to prevent dehydration. Soft foods such as gelatin, soup, mashed potatoes, puddings, Cream of Wheat, and flavored ice pops appeal to children the best. Bed rest is advisable while the child has a fever. The nurse should advise the parent to call the health care provider if the child has difficulty breathing or increased difficulty swallowing or if the fever has lasted more than 3 days. If any family members develop a fever, sore throat, or headache, they should have a throat culture. Instruct the parents that leftover antibiotics from siblings or friends should never be used.

Moist mucous membranes and adequate urine output are signs of proper fluid balance. At the end of treatment, the child should be free of signs of infection and show no signs of complications of the disease.

NURSING CARE
The Child Undergoing a Tonsillectomy

Assessment: Preoperative Period

A complete history is taken, with special attention given to allergy symptoms, difficulty swallowing, or airway obstruction. The child is assessed for signs of active infection (fever, elevated white blood cell [WBC] count) and redness and exudate of the throat. The child should be questioned about the presence of pain in the throat or ears. Because the tonsillar area is so vascular, any bleeding history must be recorded and communicated to the primary physician.

Laboratory results (prothrombin time, partial thromboplastin time, platelet count, hemoglobin, hematocrit, urinalysis) are reviewed, and the child should be checked for loose teeth to decrease the risk for aspiration during surgery.

Nursing Diagnosis and Planning: Preoperative Period

The nursing diagnoses and expected outcomes that may be appropriate for the child undergoing a tonsillectomy and the child's family are

- Anxiety related to surgery.
  Expected Outcome: The child and parents will exhibit a decreased level of anxiety, as evidenced by relaxed body posture and involvement in play activities.
- Deficient Knowledge related to surgery and procedures.
  Expected Outcome: The child and parents will restate preoperative teaching.

Interventions: Preoperative Period

The nurse reassures the child that talking will not be a problem after surgery. Emphasize to the child that it is important to drink liquids after surgery, even though the child's throat will be sore (see also Chapter 42). Teach the child's family about postoperative pain assessment and appropriate analgesia administration, because many parents undermedicate their children. Undermedication can interfere with optimal postoperative recovery.

Evaluation: Preoperative Period

- Does the child demonstrate relaxed body posture and the ability to engage in play while waiting for surgery?
- Can the parents describe what to expect during the postoperative period?

Assessment: Postoperative Period

Immediately after surgery, the child should be assessed for bleeding and ability to swallow secretions. Postoperative hemorrhage is the most serious and life-threatening complication of tonsillectomy (Johnson, Elluru, & Myer, 2002). If bleeding occurs, the child is returned to surgery for recauterization. The rate and quality of respirations and breath sounds should be assessed. Vital signs, including blood pressure, should be monitored frequently (a common protocol is every 15 minutes for the first hour, hourly for 4 hours, and then every 2 to 4 hours for the next 24 hours). Suction equipment should be available, but do not suction unless there is airway obstruction. The child is assessed for bleeding (frequent swallowing; restlessness; a fast, thready pulse; or vomiting bright-red blood). When visually assessing the site for

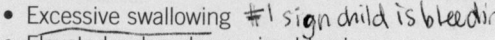

clots or bleeding, use a flashlight for illumination and avoid using a tongue depressor if at all possible. If a tongue depressor is necessary, use a sterile tongue depressor and keep it as forward in the mouth as possible.

Nursing Diagnosis and Planning: Postoperative Period

The nursing diagnoses and expected outcomes that may be appropriate for the child who has undergone a tonsillectomy and the child's family are

- Risk for Injury (hemorrhage) related to surgery.
  Expected Outcome: The child will experience minimal postoperative bleeding, as evidenced by vital signs within normal limits and absence of excessive swallowing, bright red vomitus, or restlessness.
- Ineffective Airway Clearance related to throat discomfort.
  Expected Outcome: The child will maintain a clear airway without jeopardizing the operative site.
- Acute Pain related to surgical removal of tonsils.
  Expected Outcomes: The child will describe relief from pain and will be able to rest.
- Risk for Deficient Fluid Volume related to difficulty swallowing and nothing-by-mouth (NPO) status before surgery.
  Expected Outcomes: The child will have adequate fluid intake for age and will experience minimal fluid loss.
- Deficient Knowledge related to home care.
  Expected Outcome: The parents will describe how to care for their child at home.

Interventions: Postoperative

The child should be placed in a prone or side-lying position to facilitate drainage. Although not all clinicians are in agreement, straws and forks may be withheld to prevent trauma to the surgical site. If bleeding occurs, the child is turned to the side and the physician notified.

Vomiting of old blood ("coffee grounds" emesis) is common. Antiemetics are given as ordered to decrease throat pain caused by retching. If vomiting occurs, keep the child on NPO status for 30 minutes and then resume clear liquids.

Non-aspirin analgesics (e.g., acetaminophen) are given as ordered. In some instances, the surgeon prescribes acetaminophen with codeine liquid to provide adequate analgesia. Adequate analgesia increases fluid intake. Some centers give the analgesic every 4 hours for the first 24 hours because throat discomfort is expected. An ice collar can be applied for comfort.

Provide clear, cool liquids when the child is fully awake. Avoid citrus drinks, carbonated drinks, and extremely hot or cold liquids because they may irritate the throat. Milk and milk

loose teeth? bad for anesthesia

PARENTS
Want to Know

About Caring for a Child After a Tonsillectomy

- Encourage your child to participate only in quiet activities for 1 week after surgery.
- Encourage abundant liquid intake. Avoid citrus juices, which irritate the throat, for 10 days.
- Avoid red liquids, which will give the appearance of blood if your child vomits.
- Add full liquids (cream soups, gelatin, puddings, other soups) on the second day and soft foods (mashed potatoes, soft cereals, eggs) as your child tolerates them. Avoid rough or scratchy foods (bacon, chips, popcorn), citrus foods, or spicy foods for 3 weeks.
- Encourage your child to chew and swallow, because this exercises pharyngeal muscles and promotes healing.
- Do not give your child any straws, forks, or sharp pointed toys that could be put in the mouth.
- Use acetaminophen for pain relief; your child may have a prescription for acetaminophen with codeine for sore throat. Do not use aspirin or any medicine containing aspirin because it might affect the clotting time of the blood.

- Pain should not persist past the first week. Notify your physician if pain persists.
- Discourage your child from coughing, clearing the throat, or gargling.
- Bad mouth odor is normal and may be relieved by drinking more liquids.
- Earache and slight fever are common.
- Call your physician for any bleeding, persistent earache, or fever over 101° F (38.3° C).
- Bleeding caused by tissue sloughing during the healing process can occur 7 to 10 days after surgery. Such bleeding requires immediate medical attention.
- To protect your child from catching a cold, keep the child away from crowds for 2 weeks.
- Your child may return to school when directed by the physician, usually in about 10 days.
- Bring your child for a follow-up appointment in 1 to 2 weeks.

CRITICAL THINKING EXERCISE 45-1

A recent study of postoperative pain management in children who had undergone a tonsillectomy revealed that most children in the study received inadequate pain relief at home.*
1. What factors may have contributed to this condition?
2. What effects might inadequate pain relief have on the child?

*Hamers, J.P., & Abu-Saad, H.H. (2002). Children's pain at home following (adeno) tonsillectomy. *European Journal of Pain, 6*(3), 213-219.

products (puddings, ice cream) can coat the throat, causing a need to clear the throat and thus increasing the risk for bleeding. Adequate fluid intake promotes healing and maintains hydration. The nurse teaches the parents the principles of home management and ensures that the child is retaining fluids before discharging the child from the surgical unit. Be sure to tell the parent to monitor the child for postoperative bleeding both within the first 24 hours and again 7 to 10 days after surgery.

Evaluation: Postoperative

- Does the child have minimal bleeding, nausea, and vomiting, and are vital signs within normal limits?
- Is the child taking clear liquids and avoiding liquids that irritate the throat?
- Are the child's complaints of pain and irritability minimal?
- Is the child's intake and urine output normal for age (see Chapter 42)?
- Can the parents describe home care measures?

LARYNGOMALACIA (CONGENITAL LARYNGEAL STRIDOR)

Flaccidity of the epiglottis and supraglottic aperture and weakness of the airway walls contribute to laryngomalacia,

the most common cause of inspiratory stridor in the neonatal period. Laryngomalacia may be caused by immature neuromuscular development in the airway.

Manifestations

Noisy, crowing inspiratory respiratory sounds (stridor) are present, with or without retractions. The infant usually does not become cyanotic despite the stridor. Stridor is usually present at birth but may begin as late as age 2 months. Symptoms increase when the infant is supine or when the infant is crying. The diagnosis is based on a thorough history and on findings on direct laryngoscopy.

Therapeutic Management

Symptoms usually resolve without treatment by age 18 to 24 months. In rare instances, endotracheal intubation or tracheostomy may be required.

Nursing Considerations

The nurse observes the neonate for stridor, retractions, and dyspnea, noting any signs of acute respiratory distress. Because some infants have feeding problems, the infant should be observed for feeding difficulties. The infant's respiratory status is assessed, and findings are recorded every 2 hours and as needed. Obstruction increases during crying when the child has a respiratory infection, and stridor increases when the child is supine with the neck flexed. Positioning with the neck hyperextended improves the child's breathing. A respiratory tract infection might place undue stress on the infant's system.

As part of discharge teaching, parents are taught the signs of respiratory distress so that they can monitor for changes that might indicate respiratory tract infection. If the bottle-fed infant has feeding difficulties, the parents can try using a smaller nipple. Smaller, more frequent feedings are sometimes better tolerated by infants with respiratory difficulties. Reassure the parents that the condition usually resolves by the time the child is 2 years old. The ability of parents to comfortably care for their child indicates the effectiveness of the discharge teaching.

CROUP

Croup refers to a group of conditions characterized by inspiratory stridor, a harsh (brassy or croupy) cough, hoarseness, and varying degrees of respiratory distress (Table 45-2). The major types of croup are acute spasmodic croup, laryngotracheobronchitis, bacterial tracheitis, and epiglottitis. Although epiglottitis is a type of croup, it is discussed separately because it is a bacterial infection with unique symptoms and treatment.

Etiology and Incidence

Parainfluenza viruses cause most cases of viral croup. The cause of acute spasmodic croup is unknown.

Laryngotracheobronchitis, the most common form of croup, usually affects infants and toddlers. Laryngotracheobronchitis is a common cause of airway obstruction in children ages 6 months to 6 years. The incidence of croup is higher in boys than in girls, and the disease occurs more often during the winter than in other seasons.

Acute spasmodic croup occurs most often in children ages 1 to 3 years. Spasmodic croup occurs more often in anxious and excitable children. There seems to be hereditary predisposition to spasmodic croup.

Bacterial tracheitis is less common than laryngotracheobronchitis and acute spasmodic croup. It progresses from an upper respiratory tract infection and may be confused with laryngotracheobronchitis because of similar manifestations. Treatment for laryngotracheobronchitis is not effective if the child has bacterial tracheitis.

The following discussion focuses on acute spasmodic croup and laryngotracheobronchitis, the most common types of croup leading to hospitalization.

Manifestations

Croup often begins at night and may be preceded by several days of symptoms of upper respiratory tract infection. The child with laryngotracheobronchitis may have a more gradual onset and a fever along with other signs and symptoms; occasionally the fever is as high as 40° C (104° F). Children with spasmodic croup do not have a fever. Other manifestations include:

- The sudden onset of a harsh, metallic barky cough; sore throat; inspiratory stridor; and hoarseness
- The use of accessory muscles (substernal, intercostal, suprasternal retractions) to breathe
- Frightened appearance
- Agitation
- Cyanosis

Symptoms are usually worse at night and better in the day; they may recur for several nights. Croup usually lasts 3 to 4 days.

TABLE 45-2 Comparison of Types of Croup				
	Acute Spasmodic Laryngitis (Spasmodic Croup)	**Acute Laryngotracheobronchitis (LTB)**	**Acute Epiglottitis**	**Acute Tracheitis**
Age usually affected	1-3 yr	3 mo to 3 yr	3-7 yr	1 mo to 6 yr
Location of swelling and inflammation	Subglottic (below the vocal cords)	Vocal cords, subglottic, and tissue below vocal cords, including bronchi	Supraglottic (above the vocal cords)	Mucosa of the upper trachea
Cause	Viral, emotional or genetic predisposition	Usually viral but may be bacterial	Bacterial (usually *Haemophilus influenzae,* type b)	*Staphylococcus* (most common)
Assessment	Sudden onset, usually at night	Gradual onset, usually at night	Sudden onset, which may rapidly progress to complete airway obstruction and death	Progresses from upper respiratory infection (1-2 days)
	Child awakens with harsh cough, inspiratory stridor, dyspnea, and hoarseness	Child awakens with harsh cough and inspiratory stridor	Sore throat, dyspnea, high fever	High fever
				Stridor
				Croupy cough
				Purulent secretions
Treatment	Humidity	Humidity	IV antibiotics	Humidified oxygen
	Increased fluids	Racemic epinephrine	Artificial airway	Antipyretics
	May treat at home	Intravenous (IV) fluids during respiratory distress	IV fluids	IV antibiotics
		Hospitalization may be necessary	Emergency hospitalization	May require intubation

Pathophysiology

of Croup

Croup is a viral infection of the upper airway. Although the entire upper, or nonreactive, airway is involved to some extent in all forms of croup, each type is named according to the anatomic area most severely involved. For example, laryngotracheobronchitis affects the larynx, trachea, and bronchi. In acute spasmodic croup, the larynx is the area of most severe inflammation.

In all forms of croup, mucosal inflammation and edema cause narrowing of the airway. This narrowing is more dangerous in infants and young children than in adults because of their small airway diameter and flexible larynx, which is more susceptible to spasm.

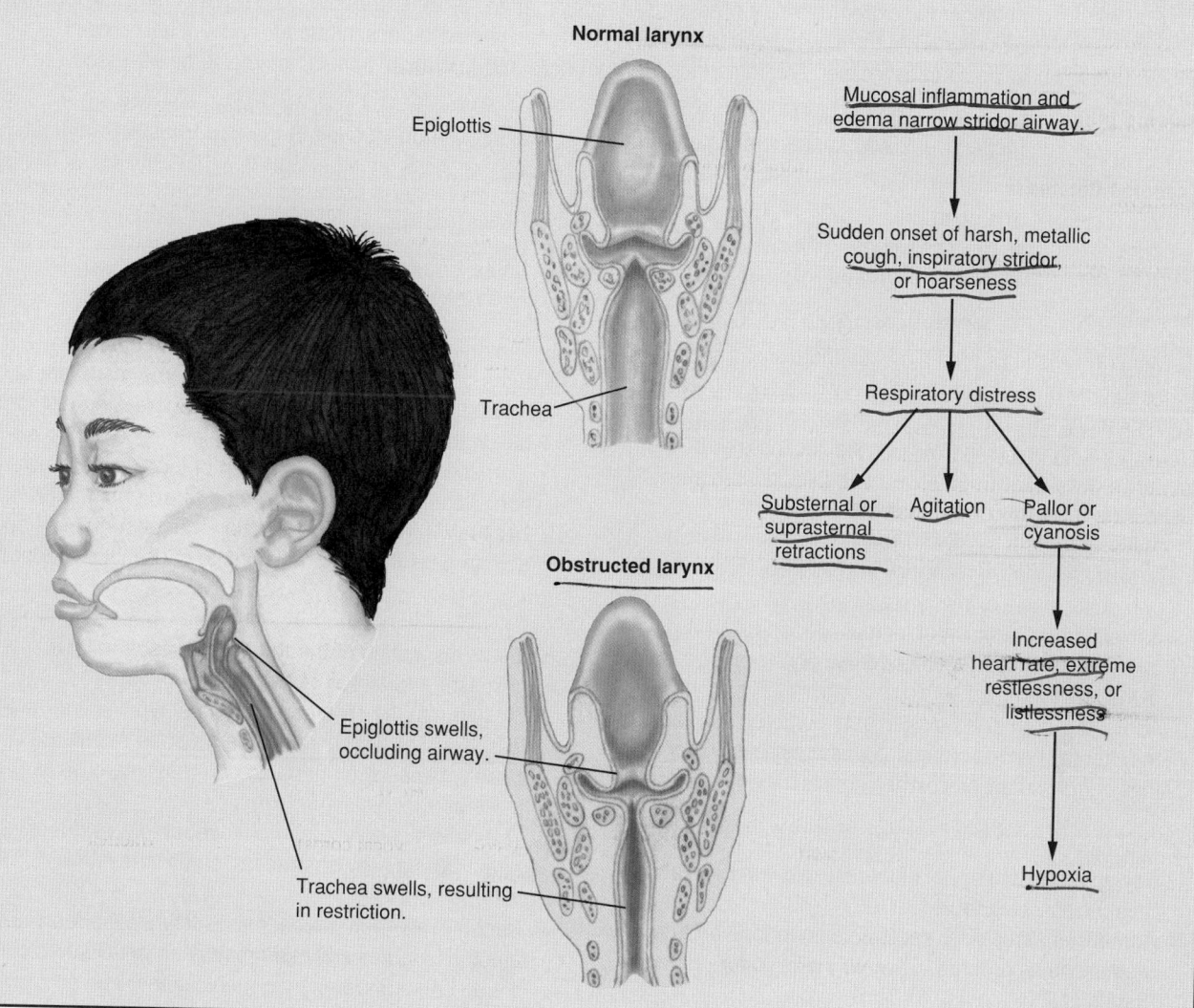

Normal larynx

Epiglottis

Trachea

Obstructed larynx

Epiglottis swells, occluding airway.

Trachea swells, resulting in restriction.

Mucosal inflammation and edema narrow stridor airway.

↓

Sudden onset of harsh, metallic cough, inspiratory stridor, or hoarseness

↓

Respiratory distress

Substernal or suprasternal retractions   Agitation   Pallor or cyanosis

↓

Increased heart rate, extreme restlessness, or listlessness

↓

Hypoxia

Diagnostic Evaluation

The diagnosis is made mainly from observation of clinical symptoms. Differentiation between viral croup and bacterial epiglottitis is very important, because treatment differs (Stroud & Friedman, 2001). However, the use of the *H. influenzae* type b (Hib) vaccine has reduced the incidence of epiglottitis. A croup score is often used to describe the severity of respiratory distress. Arterial blood gas values or pulse oximetry readings may be monitored to detect decreased PaO_2 levels.

Therapeutic Management

The goal of treatment is to maintain a patent airway. Children with acute spasmodic croup can usually be cared for at home. Treatment for acute spasmodic croup includes a calm approach and increased oral fluid intake if the child is not in respiratory distress. The benefits of providing mist, either from steam produced by hot running water in a closed bathroom or cool mist from a bedside humidifier, appear to provide more of a psychological effect than a physiologic one (Wright, Pomerantz, & Luria, 2002). If

bronchodilator — causes jitteryness can't sleep at night maybe

Nursing Care Plan

The Child With Croup

FOCUSED ASSESSMENT

A nursing history typically reveals a recent upper respiratory tract infection. Assess the child for inspiratory stridor, barking cough, hoarseness, and increased heart rate and respiratory rate. Record any signs of respiratory distress, such as the use of accessory muscles; substernal, intercostal, and suprasternal retractions; nasal flaring; restlessness and irritability; and pallor or cyanosis. Cyanosis, an increased heart rate and respiratory rate, extreme restlessness, or evidence of fatigue or listlessness may be signs of hypoxia and should be reported to the physician immediately. The lungs should be auscultated for adventitious breath sounds or areas of decreased breath sounds. Temperature and hydration status should also be assessed.

Nursing Diagnosis

Ineffective Airway Clearance related to mucosal swelling and obstruction of the upper respiratory tract.

Expected Outcomes

The child will:
- Breathe without difficulty.
- Have a heart and respiratory rate within normal limits for age.

INTERVENTION	RATIONALE
1. Monitor the child's breathing continuously for signs and symptoms of increased respiratory distress (increased respiratory rate, stridor at rest, nasal flaring, retractions, cyanosis, changes in level of consciousness or increased irritability, decreased or adventitious breath sounds, tachypnea). In addition: a. *Never* leave a child with respiratory distress alone. b. Measure vital signs hourly and as necessary. c. Monitor pulse oximetry readings. d. Notify the physician of increased respiratory distress. e. If epiglottitis is suspected, call a physician and do not inspect the throat.	1. The child must be monitored closely to detect early signs of worsening obstruction. Extreme restlessness, listlessness, cyanosis, and a rapid, increasing respiratory rate with an increased heart rate are signs of hypoxia. Increased stridor may be a sign of increasing inflammation. Decreased stridor may also be an ominous sign, because with severe obstruction, not enough air may be able to pass through the larynx to cause loud stridor. Visual inspection of the throat may result in laryngospasm and airway obstruction.
2. Administer humidified oxygen at the ordered flow rate; administer mist only if ordered. Monitor pulse oximetry readings or transcutaneous oxygen concentration frequently.	2. Oxygen may be ordered to alleviate hypoxia and restlessness. The child's condition must be monitored closely, because oxygen use can mask early signs of hypoxia and increasing obstruction.
3. Have emergency intubation equipment (e.g., intubation tray, oxygen, suction, manual-resuscitation bag-valve-mask) closely available.	3. The child's condition can change rapidly, and respiratory arrest from airway obstruction can occur.
4. Administer aerosolized racemic epinephrine and dexamethasone as ordered. Observe the child for response to medication. Monitor for tachycardia.	4. Racemic epinephrine decreases laryngeal edema. Dexamethasone has antiinflammatory action. Tachycardia is a side effect of adrenergic medications. The effect of racemic epinephrine lasts less than 2 hours. Children should be observed for recurrence of obstruction, which may occur within a few hours after administration of racemic epinephrine.
5. Keep the child as quiet as possible. Encourage parents to stay nearby or even to climb inside the mist tent (if used) with the child if the child is frightened and refuses to stay inside the tent. If the use of a tent or hood is causing distress, treatment may be more effective if the child is held by a parent and cool mist is directed toward the child's face. Maintain a calm, quiet environment. Provide a security object for the child. Observe the child closely, but disturb as little as possible.	5. Crying aggravates laryngospasm and increases hypoxia. A parent's presence is an effective supportive measure for frightened, agitated infants and children. Anxiety and crying increase the airway obstruction of croup.
6. Support the child in an upright position with the head of the bed elevated or with the child held by the parent.	6. An upright position facilitates respiration by decreasing pressure from abdominal contents on the diaphragm.

Nursing Care Plan

The Child With Croup—cont'd

Evaluation

- Are the child's respiratory rate and heart rate within normal limits for age, and is the oxygen saturation greater than 95%?
- Does the child have pink mucous membranes and nail beds and clear breath sounds with effective air movement?

Nursing Diagnosis

Risk for Deficient Fluid Volume related to inadequate oral intake and tachypnea.

Expected Outcome

The child will:
- Have adequate fluid intake for age and weight.

INTERVENTION	RATIONALE
1. Monitor the child's hydration status with intake and output measurements and urine specific gravity. Check mucous membranes, skin turgor, and presence of tears. Weigh the child daily on the same scale and at same time of day.	1. An increased respiratory rate causes insensible water loss. Difficulty swallowing leads to decreased intake.
2. Offer clear liquids as tolerated when the child no longer exhibits signs of respiratory distress.	2. Fluids are encouraged to decrease edema and the viscosity of secretions. Fluids may be given orally if stridor is mild and the child is not tachypneic. Increased oral fluids and a regular diet are offered as soon as the child's condition improves.
3. Give liquids at room temperature.	3. Cold liquids may increase respiratory distress.
4. Observe the child's ability to swallow, noting any respiratory distress.	4. Tachypnea and laryngospasm often cause dysphagia.
5. Administer intravenous (IV) fluids at ordered rate.	5. IV fluids may be ordered during the acute phase of croup to prevent dehydration. Oral fluids are contraindicated in the setting of severe respiratory distress because of the risk for aspiration and the increased stress put on the systems of the body.
6. Administer acetaminophen for fever as ordered. Monitor temperature every 4 hours.	6. Fever increases insensible water loss by increasing metabolic rate.

Evaluation

- Is the child taking adequate amounts of fluid?
- Does the child have urine output appropriate for age (see Chapter 42)?
- Does the child have urine specific gravity of 1.002 to 1.030?
- Does the child exhibit moist mucous membranes and good skin turgor?

Nursing Diagnosis

Fear related to dyspnea and hospitalization.

Expected Outcomes

The child will:
- Appear less fearful, as evidenced by resting quietly, crying less, and cooperating with nursing care as appropriate for age.

The parents will:
- Demonstrate decreased fear, as evidenced by their ability to assist the child to deal with stressors of hospitalization and illness.

Continued

Nursing Care Plan

The Child With Croup—cont'd

INTERVENTION	RATIONALE
1. Maintain a calm, restful environment. Organize nursing care so as to disturb the child as little as possible. Postpone unnecessary procedures until the child is in less distress. Allow periods of uninterrupted rest.	1. Fear and crying increase oxygen consumption and respiratory distress.
2. Encourage parents to touch and cuddle the child. Toddlers and infants like to be held when they are ill. If the child has a mist tent, parents should be told it is acceptable to sit inside the mist tent with their child. Children who are not in tents can be held in their parents' arms while mist is directed toward their faces.	2. A parent's presence is important in reducing fear in infants and young children.
3. Encourage parents' participation in care. Explain ways that they can make their child more comfortable, and tell them that their presence is important.	3. Parents' feelings of helplessness and anxiety are decreased when they are allowed to comfort and care for their child. Participation in the child's care also helps prepare the parents for discharge and home care.
4. Provide parents with breaks as needed, and assure them that their child will be cared for in their absence.	4. Caring for a child in the hospital is exhausting to parents. Fatigue magnifies feelings of anxiety and helplessness.
5. Allow the child to keep a favorite toy or blanket.	5. Familiar objects provide a sense of security for small children in the strange hospital environment.
6. Explain all treatments, equipment, and procedures to the child and parents.	6. Anxiety and fear related to lack of knowledge can be minimized by providing clear and timely explanations.
7. Allow the child and parents to ask questions and to discuss fears and concerns.	7. Cooperation is increased with understanding of the purpose of treatments. Parents are often very fearful because of the sudden onset and frightening nature of croup symptoms. Parents sometimes feel guilty for not having brought the child in for treatment sooner.
8. Use developmentally appropriate communication techniques (e.g., play, puppets).	8. A calm, empathic, caring approach is helpful in providing emotional support to the child and parents.

Evaluation

- Does the child exhibit decreased signs of agitation or being upset (less crying)?
- Does the child allow the nursing staff to provide comfort and support?
- Does the child demonstrate adequate rest and sleep patterns by not waking up during the night and showing no signs of fatigue or irritability?
- Can the child engage in age-appropriate play?
- Is the parent able to comfort the child?

Nursing Diagnosis

Deficient Knowledge related to the course of croup and home care.

Expected Outcomes

The parents will:
- Have accurate knowledge of croup symptoms.
- State they are comfortable in home management of croup.
- Seek assistance appropriately if symptoms become severe.

Nursing Care Plan

The Child With Croup—cont'd

INTERVENTION	RATIONALE
1. Determine the parents' level of understanding of croup and previous experiences in coping with the illness. Teach parents that once a child has had an attack, croup tends to recur. Teach parents that maintaining a stable environmental temperature and humidity and keeping the child well hydrated may help decrease the severity of attacks. Teach that croup is a viral infection, and avoiding large groups of people and practicing good health habits to prevent infection may decrease the risk for recurrence of croup.	1. Teaching about how to recognize and manage the condition increases parental control.
2. Teach parents the signs and symptoms of respiratory distress. Parents should be taught how to count respirations and how to assess for retractions and cyanosis: a. The child should be closely observed at all times for a worsening condition, which can occur rapidly. b. Parents should call the physician if any of the following occurs in the child: • Increased difficulty breathing or seems to be getting worse • Retractions (tugging in of the skin between, above, or below the ribs with inspiration) • Lips turn bluish or dusky • Breathing cool or warm mist does not improve symptoms in 20 minutes • Inability to drink much over the past 24 hours • Drooling or difficulty swallowing • Fever (over 39.4° C [103° F]) • Seems exhausted, listless, or very agitated	2. Knowing when to seek attention prevents more serious consequences of airway obstruction.
3. Explain the possible advantage of a humidified environment in treating croup symptoms. Ways to provide humidity include: a. Hold and cuddle the child in a steamy bathroom for at least 10 minutes or until symptoms are relieved; run all the hot water faucets full force with the door closed. b. Place a cool mist humidifier beside the child's bed. c. Take the child outside into the cool, moist night air; opening the freezer door can also be effective.	3. High humidity might help thin secretions and decrease swelling.
4. Explain the importance of adequate hydration and nutrition. If able, the child needs to drink two to four glasses (500 to 1000 ml) of fluids daily. Sips of warm fluids during a croup attack help relax the vocal cords and thin mucus.	4. Adequate hydration is important for thinning secretions. Adequate caloric intake helps replace calories expended fighting the infection.
5. Give acetaminophen for fever. Do *not* give cough syrup or cold medicines.	5. Acetaminophen is effective in reducing fever and will help the child feel more comfortable. Cough syrups and cold medicines can dry and thicken secretions.
6. If the episode resolves, the parents should put the child back to bed and check on the child periodically throughout the night. Instruct the parents to call the physician immediately if the child seems worse or does not improve in 48 hours.	6. Close observation is essential to detect worsening of croup symptoms. Worsening of symptoms will not necessarily awaken the child.

Evaluation

■ Can the parents explain the appropriate treatment of croup and when medical help is needed?

mist is used, cool mist humidifiers are recommended rather than steam vaporizers, which pose a danger of scald burns. Taking the child out into the cool, humid night air may relieve mucosal swelling.

Crying aggravates the airway obstruction. Children who develop stridor at rest, cyanosis, severe agitation or fatigue, or moderate to severe retractions or who are unable to take oral fluids should be seen in the emergency department.

Children with laryngotracheobronchitis, usually a more severe type of croup, are more often hospitalized than are those with acute spasmodic croup. Racemic epinephrine nebulized with oxygen may be given to decrease the laryngeal edema and bronchospasm. The child must be observed closely for changes in respiratory status and should not be treated with epinephrine on an outpatient basis because the effects of epinephrine are temporary. Children who receive epinephrine should be observed in the emergency department for at least 3 hours after treatment and should not be discharged if stridor or retractions are present.

Oral or parenteral corticosteroid therapy may be used in children with croup to reduce inflammatory edema and prevent destruction of ciliated epithelium. Nebulized budesonide may also be used. Antibiotics are not indicated unless a bacterial infection is present. Acetaminophen is given to reduce fever.

The benefits of mist tent or hood therapy remain controversial, particularly if placing the child in a tent increases agitation. Cool mist in the room may be more effective. Intravenous (IV) fluids are given until respiratory distress subsides and the child can take adequate fluids by mouth. Sedatives are contraindicated because they depress respirations and could mask restlessness, an early sign of hypoxia.

If signs of moderate or severe hypoxia develop, the child is intubated immediately and is transferred to an intensive care unit. Usually the tube remains in place from 3 to 5 days and is removed when the child can breathe around the tube.

EPIGLOTTITIS (SUPRAGLOTTITIS)

Epiglottitis, the acute inflammation and swelling of the epiglottis and surrounding tissue, is a life-threatening, rapidly progressive condition that may cause complete airway obstruction within a few hours of onset.

Etiology and Incidence

Epiglottitis is almost always caused by *H. influenzae*. Other organisms, such as *Staphylococcus aureus*, *Haemophilus parainfluenzae*, *S. pneumoniae*, and group A beta-hemolytic *Streptococci*, cause the infection less frequently. Viral epiglottitis is rare.

Epiglottitis occurs most often in children ages 3 to 7 years. The incidence is about equal in boys and girls. The incidence has decreased markedly with use of the Hib vaccine.

Manifestations

Unlike croup, epiglottitis has an abrupt onset with rapid progression of symptoms. Often parents report that the child was put to bed well and awakened with a severe sore throat and difficulty swallowing. The child demonstrates a high fever (39° to 40° C [102.2° to 104° F]) and appears to be in a toxic condition and very ill. The accompanying sore throat can progress to acute respiratory distress in a few hours. The child appears anx-

> **! CRITICAL TO REMEMBER**
>
> **Cardinal Signs and Symptoms of Epiglottitis**
> - **D**rooling
> - **D**ysphagia (difficulty swallowing)
> - **D**ysphonia (difficulty talking)
> - **D**istressed inspiratory efforts
>
> Do not examine or obtain material for culture from a child's throat if epiglottitis is suspected, because any stimulation with a tongue depressor or culture swab could trigger complete airway obstruction.
> Do not leave a child with epiglottitis unattended.

ious and frightened and may be irritable or lethargic. One of the classic signs of epiglottitis is that the child insists on sitting upright, often in a tripod position (leaning forward supported on the arms), with the chin thrust out and the mouth open. Respiratory symptoms include nasal flaring; suprasternal, substernal, and intercostal retractions; pale skin color to cyanosis (depending on the degree of airway obstruction); and tachycardia. The epiglottis appears edematous and cherry-red.

Diagnostic Evaluation

The most reliable diagnostic sign of epiglottitis is an edematous, cherry-red epiglottis. However, examination and visual observation of the epiglottis *are contraindicated* until emergency intubation equipment and qualified personnel are available to support the child in case of sudden airway obstruction. The child's WBC count is usually elevated (20,000 to 30,000/mm³).

Therapeutic Management

Treatment for epiglottitis should achieve a patent airway as quickly as possible. The child with epiglottitis has an edematous epiglottis, which can completely obstruct the airway at any time. Radiographs are best obtained at the bedside, where the child can be constantly monitored and emergency equipment is readily available. The danger of airway obstruction is so great that usually all invasive procedures, such as venipuncture, are postponed until the child is intubated. Once the airway is secured, the child is transferred to the intensive care unit. Oxygenation status is closely monitored with arterial blood gas values or pulse oximetry, and humidified oxygen is administered. Mechanical ventilation is sometimes instituted.

Throat and blood specimens are obtained for culture after the child is intubated. Antipyretics are given for fever. Antibiotics are administered IV until the child is extubated. Usually the child improves dramatically after 48 hours of antibiotic therapy and can be extubated at this time. The usual course of treatment is 7 to 10 days. Discharge occurs in about 3 to 7 days, and the child is sent home on a regimen of oral antibiotics.

Nursing Considerations

The nurse should continuously assess for signs of respiratory distress (stridor, nasal flaring, tachypnea, tachycardia, retractions, drooling, changes in level of consciousness, cyanosis).

Pathophysiology

of Epiglottitis

Epiglottitis is a bacterial form of croup. The epiglottis and surrounding structures become inflamed as bacterial infection invades the soft tissue. The epiglottis becomes edematous and cherry-red and may become so swollen that it completely covers the glottis and obstructs the airway. Secretions pool in the hypopharynx and larynx. As the disease rapidly progresses, swelling becomes so severe that the child is unable to swallow and begins to drool. The child's voice is muffled, and the throat is very sore. Inspiratory stridor, cough, and irritability are present. Complete airway obstruction can occur rapidly, resulting in hypoxia, acidosis, and death.

The onset of epiglottitis is usually sudden. The child may have had symptoms of a mild upper respiratory tract infection for a few days before symptoms began. Children with epiglottitis can progress from wellness to complete airway obstruction within 2 to 6 hours.

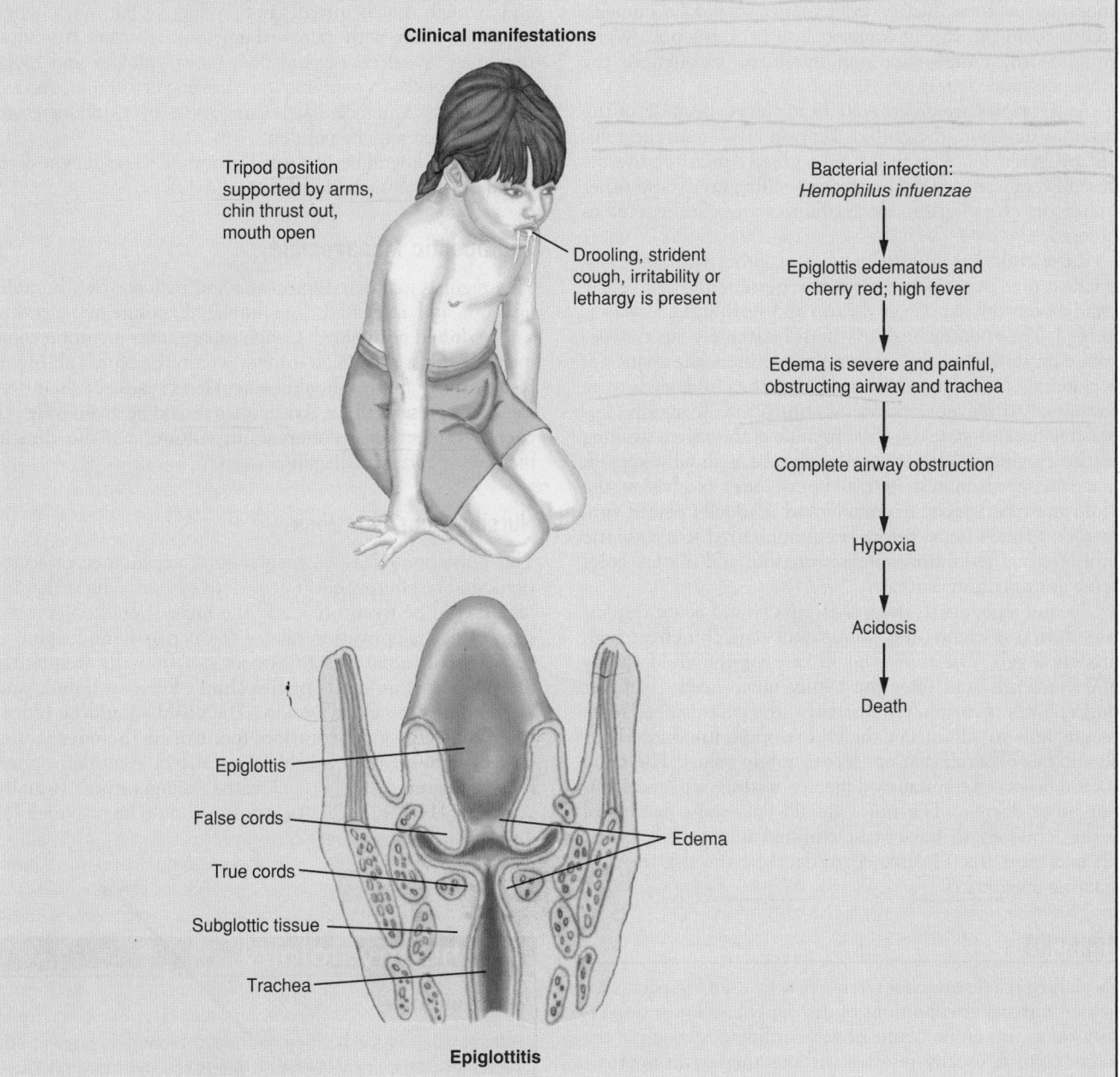

Clinical manifestations

Tripod position supported by arms, chin thrust out, mouth open

Drooling, strident cough, irritability or lethargy is present

Bacterial infection: *Hemophilus infuenzae*

↓

Epiglottis edematous and cherry red; high fever

↓

Edema is severe and painful, obstructing airway and trachea

↓

Complete airway obstruction

↓

Hypoxia

↓

Acidosis

↓

Death

Epiglottis

False cords

True cords

Subglottic tissue

Trachea

Edema

Epiglottitis

A sudden decrease in respiratory effort may be a sign of exhaustion and impending respiratory arrest. Arterial blood gas values and pulse oximetry findings are monitored. On pulse oximetry, the oxygen saturation should remain above 95%, with the PaO_2 between 80 and 100 mm Hg.

Maintenance of a patent airway is essential. The nurse should also keep the child as calm and quiet as possible. If temperature is taken, it should be by the axillary or tympanic route rather than the oral route. The child should be supported in a position of comfort, usually sitting straight up (orthopneic); never force the child to lie down. Children who are anxious and in respiratory distress are often less fearful on their parents' laps. Parents should be encouraged to hug and comfort their child. The parents' anxiety level must be assessed and controlled because their anxiety is easily transferred to the child.

Humidified oxygen is delivered in high concentrations. Oxygen therapy is usually less upsetting if the parent holds the oxygen tubing in front of the child's face. All procedures should be explained to the parent and child clearly, calmly, and according to the child's level of understanding.

Emergency intubation equipment (oxygen, laryngoscope, endotracheal tube, suction equipment) should be immediately available in case of complete airway obstruction. Worsening of the child's condition should be reported to the physician immediately.

Antipyretics are given rectally for fever. Because of the risk for aspiration, the child is kept on NPO status and fluids are given IV. The nurse must closely monitor the ordered IV rate as well as the urine specific gravity and other indicators of hydration. IV antibiotics are administered as ordered.

If the child has an artificial airway, either with an endotracheal tube or a tracheostomy, the nurse must observe the child closely for respiratory distress and suction the airway as needed. The endotracheal tube must be securely taped to decrease movement of the tube and to minimize the chance of accidental extubation. Once intubated, the child needs to be restrained to prevent accidental extubation. It may be impossible to reintubate the child because of the severe swelling of the epiglottis. The endotracheal tube is usually kept in place for approximately 24 to 40 hours. After extubation, the child must be watched carefully and is usually placed in a mist tent for 24 hours before being transferred to a pediatric unit. Normal respiratory rate and rhythm and normal color serve as evaluation criteria.

Because epiglottitis progresses rapidly and acute respiratory distress is frightening, both parents and child have high anxiety levels. The nurse should care for the child calmly and efficiently and offer the family much-needed support during hospitalization. On discharge, the parents need to be taught how to administer the child's oral antibiotics. They should be reassured that epiglottitis rarely recurs. The child should be free of respiratory difficulty, resting well, and without other distress. The nurse should encourage parents of young children to have their children immunized against *H. influenzae* (see Chapter 4) to decrease the risk for contracting epiglottitis.

BRONCHITIS

Bronchitis is a disease that rarely exists by itself but occurs together with other conditions of the upper and lower respiratory tracts. It can be confused with asthma. A cough is the major sign; it usually resolves without therapy in approximately 2 weeks.

Etiology and Incidence

Acute bronchitis is usually viral in origin. Rhinoviruses are the most common causative organisms. Other viruses thought to cause bronchitis include respiratory syncytial virus, influenza virus, parainfluenza virus, and adenovirus. Most bacterial infections occur secondary to a primary viral infection or some other airway problem. They may also occur secondary to foreign body aspiration. Air pollution has also been implicated in the disease.

The disorder is more common in young children and boys. It can occur anytime but is more common during the winter months than in other seasons.

Manifestations and Diagnostic Evaluation

Bronchitis is characterized by the gradual onset of rhinitis and a cough that is initially nonproductive but may change to a loose cough with increased mucus production. Auscultation may reveal coarse and fine, moist crackles and high-pitched rhonchi (resembling the wheezing of asthma). Associated symptoms include malaise, low-grade fever, and increased mucus, which may be purulent.

Chest radiographs are usually normal. The diagnosis is based on the clinical picture.

Therapeutic Management

Treatment is mainly symptomatic and includes rest, humidification, and increased fluid intake. Exposure to cigarette smoke should be avoided. Cough suppressants are not recommended unless the cough interferes with the child's ability to rest. Antihistamines should be avoided because of their drying effect on secretions. Antibiotics should be given only if a bacterial infection is confirmed by culture or if the clinical picture supports the diagnosis.

Nursing Considerations

The nurse should assess temperature, appearance of secretions, and respiratory effort every 2 to 4 hours. The child's intake should be monitored, and the nurse should observe for signs of sleep deprivation related to the persistent cough.

Advise the parents to encourage fluids by frequently offering small amounts of the child's favorite liquids and to humidify the child's room. The child should be monitored for signs of dehydration; monitoring includes taking daily weights if the child is hospitalized. Acetaminophen is administered for an elevated temperature (usually >38.3° C [101° F]). Quiet activities should be provided for diversion.

Pathophysiology

of Bronchitis

Inflammation of the trachea and major bronchi is present in bronchitis. Mucus production is increased, and the mucosa is congested. Because of nonspecific leukocytic migration, purulent secretions can occur even in the absence of a bacterial infection.

Acute bronchitis is a self-limiting disease. Chronic bronchitis in children may indicate an underlying chronic respiratory dysfunction.

BRONCHIOLITIS

Bronchiolitis, or inflammation of the bronchioles, is a significant cause of hospitalization in infants younger than 1 year (Barry, 2002). Respiratory syncytial virus (RSV) is the causative agent in more than 50% of cases.

Etiology and Incidence

Infants usually acquire the disease from an older child or adult, particularly a family member or daycare contact, who has a minor respiratory illness. RSV infection is easily communicable and is acquired mainly through contact with contaminated surfaces. Nosocomial outbreaks in pediatric hospitals are common. RSV can live on skin or paper for up to 1 hour and on cribs and other nonporous surfaces for up to 6 hours. Although it is not airborne, it is highly communicable. It is usually transferred by inadequately washed hands. Meticulous handwashing decreases the spread of organisms.

In addition to RSV, other causative organisms include *Mycoplasma*, parainfluenza virus, and some adenoviruses. RSV infection occurs in annual epidemics during the winter and early spring. The incidence peaks at age 6 months.

Pathophysiology

of Bronchiolitis

In bronchiolitis, edema and the accumulation of mucus and cellular debris cause obstruction of the bronchioles. Infants' bronchioles are very small and can become obstructed quickly. Airway resistance is increased during the inspiratory and expiratory phases of respiration because of the small air passages. Hyperinflation of the lungs results from air trapping because the bronchioles constrict during expiration. Atelectasis can occur if obstruction becomes complete and trapped air is absorbed.

Normal gas exchange is impaired, and the infant becomes hypoxic. Some infants develop mild respiratory alkalosis; more frequently, metabolic acidosis is observed.

The child with bronchiolitis is most acutely ill during the first 48 to 72 hours after the onset of the disease. Improvement usually occurs in a few days. Mortality is less than 1%, and hospitalization is rare.* Some infants' lung function studies remain abnormal for months.

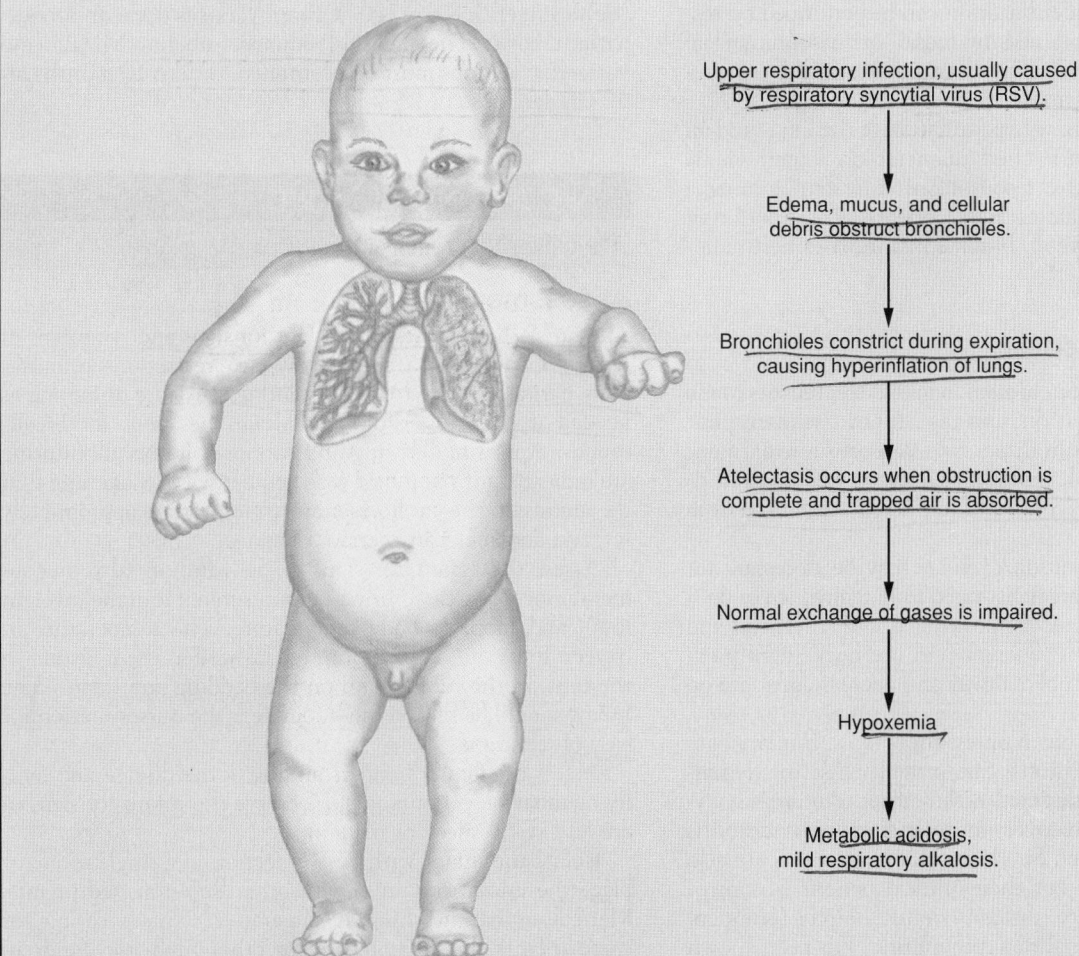

Upper respiratory infection, usually caused by respiratory syncytial virus (RSV).

↓

Edema, mucus, and cellular debris obstruct bronchioles.

↓

Bronchioles constrict during expiration, causing hyperinflation of lungs.

↓

Atelectasis occurs when obstruction is complete and trapped air is absorbed.

↓

Normal exchange of gases is impaired.

↓

Hypoxemia

↓

Metabolic acidosis, mild respiratory alkalosis.

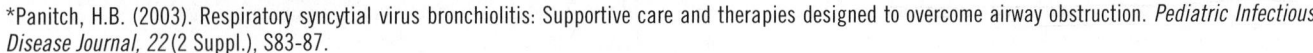

*Panitch, H.B. (2003). Respiratory syncytial virus bronchiolitis: Supportive care and therapies designed to overcome airway obstruction. *Pediatric Infectious Disease Journal, 22*(2 Suppl.), S83-87.

By age 2 years, nearly 100% of children will have had RSV (Panitch, 2001). Immunity does not occur, but the incidence and severity decrease with age.

Manifestations

A mild upper respiratory tract infection usually precedes the development of bronchiolitis. Serous nasal drainage, sneezing, low-grade fever, and anorexia are present for several days, followed by the onset of acute respiratory distress, manifested by the following signs and symptoms:

- Tachypnea—respiratory rates of 60 to 80 breaths/min
- Wheezing, crackles, or rhonchi
- Intercostal and subcostal retractions with or without nasal flaring
- Cyanosis

Feeding may be difficult because of increased respirations, which interfere with sucking and swallowing. The body temperature varies from hypothermic to as high as 41° C (105.8° F).

Diagnostic Evaluation

The clinical presentation and the age of the child suggest the diagnosis. Rapid virus identification can be performed on respiratory secretions obtained by nasal or nasopharyngeal washing (see Chapter 37). The diagnostic test is the enzyme-linked immunosorbent assay (ELISA).

Chest radiographs show hyperinflation of the lungs and an increased anteroposterior chest diameter on lateral views. There are scattered areas of consolidation in some infants, a finding attributable to atelectasis secondary to obstruction or inflammation of the alveoli. In some infants, the chest radiographs appear normal.

Therapeutic Management

Infants with mild bronchiolitis can be treated at home with fluids, humidification, and rest. Infants with respiratory distress are hospitalized for supportive treatment (Panitch, 2003). Cool, humidified oxygen is delivered to relieve dyspnea, hypoxemia, and insensible water loss from tachypnea.

Parenteral administration of fluids may be necessary for acutely ill infants who are dehydrated from tachypnea or poor intake. The infant should be positioned with the head and chest at a 30- to 40-degree angle and the neck slightly extended to maintain an open airway and decrease pressure on the diaphragm.

Antibiotics are not given unless there is a secondary bacterial infection. Some health care providers use inhaled albuterol, but this has not been shown either to increase oxygenation or to hasten recovery for infants with bronchiolitis (Smucny, Flynn, Becker, & Glazier, 2001). Steroids are also sometimes prescribed, but their clinical benefit is controversial because they are not consistently helpful (Kimpen, 2001). Nebulized adrenaline (epinephrine) has been shown to have significant effect with reduction in oxygen requirement, respiratory rate, and wheezing (Schindler, 2002).

Ribavirin (Virazole) is an antiviral respiratory drug that appears to interfere with ribonucleic acid (RNA) and deoxyribonucleic acid (DNA) synthesis, inhibiting viral replication. It is used primarily in hospitalized children with severe RSV and in high-risk children (those with congenital heart disease, chronic respiratory disease, prematurity, or immunodeficiency). Administration is via hood, facemask, or oxygen tent over 18 to 20 hours per day for a minimum of 3 days and a maximum of 7 days. The drug is most effective if administered within the first 3 days of the beginning of the disease. It is very expensive and has proved to be teratogenic in some animal studies, so pregnant health care workers or visitors should not be in the room where ribavirin is being delivered. Some caregivers experience headaches, burning nasal passages and eyes, and crystallized soft contact lenses. The use of ribavirin is controversial because a majority of studies have demonstrated neither dramatic nor cost-effective results (Kimpen, 2001).

RSV prevention is of the utmost importance to reduce hospitalizations for young, at-risk infants and children. Intravenous RSV immune globulin (RSV-IG, RespiGam) or intramuscular RSV monoclonal antibody (Synagis) administered monthly throughout the RSV season has significantly reduced the hospitalization risk for premature infants (<35 weeks' gestation) younger than 6 months and children younger than 24 months with chronic lung disease (Schlesinger & Koss, 2002). Prophylaxis is done on an outpatient basis. The measles, mumps, rubella (MMR) and varicella vaccines must be postponed for 9 to 10 months after the last dose of RSV-IG.

■NURSING CARE
The Child With Bronchiolitis

Assessment

The nurse should assess the infant for signs and symptoms of respiratory distress (tachypnea, dyspnea, retractions, cyanosis, nasal flaring) every 1 to 2 hours during the acute phase and as needed if changes occur. Auscultate the lungs for breath sounds. Apnea monitoring and cardiorespiratory monitoring are indicated for the infant with acute disease. Make sure that the alarms on the cardiorespiratory monitor are appropriately set, and document any periods of apnea.

Assess the infant for signs of dehydration (dry mucous membranes, decreased urine output, sunken fontanel, weight loss), and monitor body temperature. The temperature in oxygen tents should be monitored, as well as the moisture in the tent, in the tubing, and on the bedding and infant. The infant should be placed in a room near the nurses' station for easy observation.

Assess the family's understanding of the disease and family members' level of anxiety. Observe the infant for signs of anxiety, restlessness, or irritability.

Isolate the infant with RSV infection in a single room, or place the infant in a room with other RSV-infected infants. Meticulous handwashing is imperative. Nurses caring for these infants should not care for other high-risk children. Maintaining Contact Precautions (i.e., wearing a gown and gloves) reduces nosocomial transmission of RSV.

Nursing Diagnosis and Planning

The diagnoses and expected outcomes that may be appropriate for the infant with bronchiolitis and the infant's family are

■ Impaired Gas Exchange related to airway edema and increased mucus.
  Expected Outcome: The infant will have increased gas exchange, as evidenced by oxygen saturation above 95% on room air.
■ Ineffective Airway Clearance related to increased secretions.
  Expected Outcome: The infant will exhibit clear breath sounds and normal respiratory rate, depth, and rhythm.
■ Deficient Fluid Volume related to decreased intake and insensible loss.
  Expected Outcome: The infant will maintain adequate hydration, as evidenced by moist mucous membranes, a flat fontanel, urine output normal for age, and stable weight.
■ Ineffective Thermoregulation related to illness.
  Expected Outcome: The infant will demonstrate a body temperature within normal limits.
■ Anxiety related to hospitalization and the child's dyspnea.
  Expected Outcomes: The infant will demonstrate decreased anxiety, as evidenced by adequate sleep and stable vital signs. The parents will verbalize understanding of the infant's condition and be able to participate appropriately in the infant's care.

Interventions

Many hospitals are now using clinical pathways for children with respiratory disease. Figure 45-3 shows a clinical pathway for an infant with bronchiolitis. Even when using a clinical pathway, the nurse needs to focus on appropriate nursing interventions.

Facilitating Gas Exchange

The nurse monitors and documents the infant's vital signs and respiratory status every 1 to 2 hours or more often as needed. Particularly note the rate, quality, and depth of respirations along with any adventitious breath sounds and the presence of retractions. Close monitoring with a cardiorespiratory monitor or continuous pulse oximeter will ensure early identification of impending respiratory distress.

Monitor oxygen saturation, and administer humidified oxygen (at 35%-40% concentration) in the manner most comfortable for the infant (by tent, hood, mask, or nasal prongs) to decrease hypoxia and bronchial edema. Positioning the infant's head at a 30- to 40-degree upright angle with the neck slightly extended will maintain an open airway and ease respirations by decreasing pressure on the diaphragm. If the infant is in an oxygen tent, change the bedding and infant's clothes regularly to keep the infant dry. Toys that might cause static electricity are kept outside the tent; provide the infant with appropriate safe toys.

Scheduling periods of uninterrupted rest between care episodes decreases oxygen demand. Chest physiotherapy should be performed (it may require coordination with the respiratory therapy department) before or at least 1 hour after meals. The use of chest physiotherapy in infants is controversial because it might increase their stress and oxygen demand. Administer ribavirin if ordered.

Maintaining Fluid Balance

Most infants with bronchiolitis can take fluids orally; IV fluids are administered if respiratory distress is severe enough to risk aspiration. If the infant's nasal passages are blocked with mucus, instill saline nose drops (1 or 2 drops in each nostril, followed by gentle suctioning with a bulb syringe) before feeding. Offer the infant frequent, varied clear liquids (juices, Pedialyte, Ricelyte). Older infants may enjoy frozen electrolyte pops. The infant's hydration status (skin turgor, fontanel, mucous membranes) and electrolyte values are monitored, and daily weights and intake and output are documented.

Reducing Fever

The nurse monitors the infant's temperature every 2 to 4 hours and as needed. Control environmental temperature by maintaining the room temperature between 72° and 75° F, and dress the infant in light clothing. Fluid intake is encouraged, and liquid acetaminophen or ibuprofen is administered as ordered to reduce fever.

Decreasing Anxiety

Encourage the parent to stay with the infant when possible and to participate as much as possible in the infant's care. Hospital routines and all procedures and treatments should be explained to reduce fear of the unknown. Because adult anxiety can be transferred to the infant, maintain a calm environment and encourage parents to do the same. If the infant becomes anxious about being in an oxygen tent, the parent can hold the infant and direct the humidified oxygen toward the infant's face. If the infant remains in a tent, encourage the parent to play with the infant; the parent can get in the tent to maintain tactile contact with the infant. Parents need to be allowed to express concerns.

Evaluation

• Does the infant demonstrate adequate oxygenation (oxygen saturation >95%), clear breath sounds, and stable respiratory status?
• Does the infant have moist mucous membranes, good skin turgor, stable weight, a flat fontanel, and urine output of at least 1 to 2 ml/kg/hr? (For appropriate urine output in older children, see Chapter 42.)
• Is the infant's body temperature within normal limits?
• Does the infant demonstrate less crying or irritability and increased rest?
• Do the parents verbalize understanding of the disease, have a relaxed appearance, and demonstrate comforting behaviors toward the infant?

PNEUMONIA

Pneumonia is an inflammation of the lung parenchyma. It can occur as a primary or a secondary disease. Pneumonias can be classified by anatomic distribution or by the agents that cause them. Environment, immune system status, and the child's age are factors in the pathogenesis of the disease.

The two most common types of infectious pneumonia are *viral* and *bacterial* (Table 45-3). It is very difficult to differentiate clinically between viral and bacterial pneumonia. Viruses are the most common causative agents, but children with bacterial pneumonia tend to be more ill than are those

BRONCHIOLITIS & BRONCHIOLITIS (+) RSV
(Uncomplicated-without multi-system problems)
ICD-9 Codes 466.11 and 466.19

Expected LOS-3 Days
D#.#=Key interventions for this study.

Examples of appropriate Co-morbidities
Acute Pharyngitis
Acute Sinusitis NOS
Cellulitis
Other Specific Viral Infections
Otitis Media NOS

Examples of Co-morbidities that are not appropriate:
Asthma
Bronchopulmonary Dysplasia
Cardiac Conditions that extend the LOS
Cerebral Palsy
Cystic Fibrosis
Esophageal Reflux
HIV
Pneumonia
Respiratory Failure
Sickle Cell Anemia

Refer to Tracking Sheet for Recording

Clinical Pathway	Admission Day	Day 2	Day 3
Aspect of Care	Date__ Unit__ ED	Date__ Unit__	Date__ Unit__
DAILY OUTCOME		↓ nebs if tolerated ↓ O2 if tolerated	*Discharge*
TESTS	CBC <2 mo. CXR CBG if resp distress or ↑O2 requirements Possible: Pertussis preps Chlamydia preps Viral culture Blood Culture if fever (<2 mos)	CBG if distress (↓oxygenation) Serum electrolytes if indicated	
CONSULTS	Case Manager: Discharge needs and possible home nebulizer Specialist: Pulmonary or Infectious Disease consult if hi-risk*		Specialist if not improved
FLUID/LYTES MANAGEMENT	Possible IV fluids I/O	Hep lock if tolerating p.o.	
TREATMENTS/ PROCEDURES	*D1.0 Albuterol Nebs* Spot checks or Continuous oximeter if requiring 02 02 to keep Sat >92% Possible epi nebs CA monitor<2 mos or premature or severe respiratory distress Possible CPT	*D2.0 Albuterol or Epi Nebs* Wean 02 if tolerated Spot Check Oximetry w/vs	Albuterol or epi nebs *D3.0 Wean 02*
MEDICATIONS	*D1.2 Possible steroids (if hx recurrent wheezing)*	Review all IV meds and antibiotics	
CLINICAL SUPPORT	Diet p.o. if RR<60 Contact Isolation during season, even if viral studies are (-) or not ordered, gown and gloves when touching patient. R.T. to wear mask Education: Exposure (smoke) Follow-up Neb treatments	*D2.1 Diet p.o. if RR <60*	
Original 10/10/95	Rev. Date 11/9/95 5/1/97 8/18/97		

*AAP guideline-CHD, parenchymal lung disease, infants less than 6 weeks old, prematurity, immunodeficiency, severely ill (impaired gas exchange)

Disclaimer: This clinical pathway document is provided as a general guideline for use by physicians and staff in planning the care and treatment of patients and their families. It is not intended to be and does not establish a standard of care. Each patient's care is individualized according to their specific needs.

Cook Children's Medical Center
M:\WPFILES\PATHWAYS\AUGBRONC.WPD

Privileged and Confidential Committee Document
TEX.REV.CIV.STAT.ANN. art. 4995b x 5.0

This pathway is not a permanent part of the patient's medical record.

Figure 45-3 Clinical pathway for an infant with bronchiolitis. (Courtesy Cook Children's Medical Center, Fort Worth, TX.)

TABLE **45-3** Comparison of Types of Pneumonia

Type	Etiology and Incidence	Pathophysiology	Manifestations	Therapeutic Management
Viral	Most often caused by adenoviruses, influenza viruses, cytomegalovirus (mainly in neonates), and respiratory syncytial virus (RSV). Viruses cause 80% to 85% of all pneumonias. Most common in children younger than 3 yr.	Cell destruction with sloughing of cellular debris into lumen of terminal airways and alveoli causes patchy infiltrate that affects multiple lobes.	Low to high fever, cough, crackles, wheezing (more common with RSV), headache, malaise, myalgia, abdominal pain. Infiltrates seen on chest radiography. White blood cell (WBC) count < 20,000/mm³. Usually lasts 5-7 days.	Supportive. No antibiotics are prescribed. Severely ill infants and children may be hospitalized for oxygen and fluid therapy.
Bacterial and bacterial-like	Caused primarily by *Streptococcus pneumoniae* and *Staphylococcus aureus* in infants and children younger than 5 yr. Pneumococcal infection is major type in children older than 5 yr. Also may be caused by *Haemophilus influenzae* and group A streptococci. Other bacteria-like organisms include *Mycoplasma pneumoniae*, *Chlamydia pneumoniae*, and *Chlamydia trachomatis* (seen mainly in infants).	Alveoli fill with fluid and cells in a small segment or the entire lung. Bacteria enter the bloodstream via the pulmonary lymphatics. Vital capacity and lung compliance decrease as consolidation increases.	Preceded by upper respiratory infection. Abrupt onset of fever, chills, cough, decreased breath sounds, signs of respiratory distress (retractions, nasal flaring, tachypnea), restlessness, and apprehension. Symptoms may be vague in infants; older children can experience gastrointestinal symptoms, chest pain, and abnormal breath sounds. Onset of the bacterial-like pneumonias may be more insidious. Radiography reveals consolidation; WBC count is elevated.	Intravenous (IV) or oral antibiotic therapy, usually with penicillins, erythromycin (for penicillin-allergic children), or cephalosporins. Hospitalization for severely ill infants and children with oxygen and fluid therapy. Chest tube drainage of fluid or purulence from the pleural cavity may be necessary (particularly for children with staphylococcal pneumonia).

with viral disease (Bradley, 2002). Community-acquired pneumonia is a significant problem worldwide. Difficulties related to treatment in children have increased greatly because of the emergence of resistant bacteria (Esposito & Principi, 2002). Children with chronic and acute conditions, such as acquired immunodeficiency syndrome (AIDS), cystic fibrosis, congenital defects, and foreign body aspiration, are at increased risk for developing pneumonia. Opportunistic infections (*Pneumocystis carinii* pneumonia) may be associated with AIDS (see Chapter 41). Secondary pneumonia can result from aspiration of hydrocarbons contained in household products or lipids (e.g., mineral oil given to treat severe constipation).

■ NURSING CARE

The Child With Pneumonia

Assessment

Every 2 hours, assess the child's breath sounds, respiratory rate and rhythm, color, vital signs, and degree of restlessness. Immediately report any signs of respiratory distress, including dyspnea, tachypnea, cyanosis, use of accessory muscles of breathing, diminished breath sounds, and crackles. Also note any fever, tachycardia, malaise, anorexia, discomfort, and changes in condition.

Nursing Diagnosis and Planning

The nursing diagnoses and expected outcomes that may be appropriate for the child with pneumonia and the child's family are

■ Ineffective Airway Clearance related to bronchial obstruction.

  Expected Outcome: The child will have clear airways, as evidenced by the absence of abnormal breath sounds and dyspnea.

■ Ineffective Breathing Pattern related to increased mucus production.

  Expected Outcome: The child will demonstrate effective breathing, as evidenced by respiratory rate and rhythm within normal limits for age and absence of retractions.

■ Impaired Gas Exchange related to increased mucus and accumulation of exudate.

  Expected Outcome: The child will maintain adequate gas exchange, as evidenced by decreased restlessness,

About Home Management of the Child With Pneumonia

- Provide rest.
- Increase your child's fluid intake. Offer favorite fluids more frequently than usual, and be sure your child is urinating appropriate amounts. Warm liquids (lemonade, apple juice, Pedialyte, Ricelyte) help loosen secretions. Call your health care provider if the child's mucous membranes appear dry or if urination decreases.
- Administer acetaminophen for fever and discomfort.
- Use a cool mist humidifier, and follow the manufacturer's instructions for cleaning.
- Administer antibiotics as ordered, and give the correct dose and the entire prescribed amount.
- Avoid exposing your child to cigarette smoke.

appropriate oxygen saturation, and improved mucous membrane and nail bed color.

- Deficient Fluid Volume related to fever, decreased intake, and tachypnea.
  Expected Outcomes: The child will maintain fluid balance, as evidenced by moist mucous membranes, good skin turgor, urine output appropriate for age, and maintenance of age-appropriate weight.
- Deficient Knowledge related to the disease process and home care.
  Expected Outcome: The parents will explain the disease process and describe the child's care.
- Anxiety (parental) related to infant's dyspnea and hospitalization.
  Expected Outcomes: The parents will show a decrease in anxiety, as evidenced by decreased irritability and increased periods of rest. The parents will verbalize and demonstrate comfort and ease when caring for the child.
- Acute Pain related to coughing and difficulty breathing secondary to disease process.
  Expected Outcome: The child will have decreased pain, as evidenced by less irritability, verbalization of increased comfort (if age-appropriate), and a relaxed body posture.

Interventions

The severity of the illness and the cause of the disease direct the nursing care of the child with pneumonia. Some children will be cared for at home, whereas others will be hospitalized on a general pediatric unit or special care area.

For the hospitalized child, chest physiotherapy should be scheduled before meals and bedtime. Elevating the head of the bed and changing the child's position every 2 hours assist respiratory effort and promote pulmonary drainage. Older children may assume a position of comfort but still must change their position every 2 hours. The use of infant seats should be avoided because pressure may be placed on the diaphragm, thus actually decreasing lung expansion.

The older child should be assisted with coughing and deep breathing and splinting as necessary to ease discomfort. Oxygen should be humidified and monitored. Pulse oximetry aids in monitoring oxygen saturation and the ad-

equacy of air exchange. A cardiorespiratory monitor is used when available.

Oral or IV fluids are given as ordered. IV fluids may be indicated when oral intake increases the stress put on an already compromised body. The nurse monitors intake and output and observes for signs of dehydration (oliguria, poor skin turgor, dry mucous membranes, sunken fontanels, weight loss). Weight should be measured daily. The specific gravity of urine also is checked to monitor hydration status.

Because conserving energy aids oxygenation, nursing care is planned to provide for periods of rest. Quiet diversional activities, such as reading, puzzles, videos, and board games, are suggested. The nurse maintains a quiet and cool environment and limits visitors to allow the child maximum rest. Visits by anyone with an infection should be restricted.

Administer antipyretics (acetaminophen), antibiotics, and analgesics as ordered. Normal breathing may cause discomfort. If an analgesic is not ordered, the physician should be notified of any discomfort the child experiences. Splinting of the affected side by lying on that side may decrease discomfort. Diversional activities and manipulation of the environment are often effective for pain relief.

The family and child (if of appropriate age) need to receive information about the disease and its treatment. The nurse explains all procedures and treatments and encourages the parents to stay with their child and participate in the child's care. The nurse conveys empathy for the family's feelings and concerns. The nurse also teaches the family about home management of the infant or child.

Evaluation

- Are the child's vital signs and respiratory status within normal limits?
- Is the child's oxygen saturation greater than 95%?
- Does the child appear hydrated, with moist mucous membranes, good skin turgor, and adequate urinary output for age?
- Can the parents describe home care techniques?
- Do the parents appear relaxed, and are they able to fully participate in the child's care?
- Can the child comfortably participate in quiet activities and rest quietly when appropriate?

FOREIGN BODY ASPIRATION

Foreign body aspiration is seen most frequently in children ages 6 months to 5 years. Children who have objects in their mouths while they are playing, running, or laughing are at risk. Certain items have an increased incidence of aspiration by infants and children (Box 45-1).

BOX 45-1
Common Items of Aspiration

• Nuts	• Small toys
• Pins	• Chunks of food
• Screws	• Parts of toys
• Coins	• Hard candy
• Seeds	• Latex balloons
• Grapes	• Popcorn
• Bones	• Hot dogs
• Earrings	• Carrots

Etiology and Incidence

Children's curiosity, oral needs, and occasionally lack of supervision contribute to the occurrence of foreign body aspiration. Infants and children love to explore and investigate objects. Exploration often includes putting objects into their mouths. Children also have the uncanny ability to remove small parts from toys and to find other objects that parents thought were out of their reach (e.g., pins, screws, nuts, coins, earrings). Adults may give infants and small children foods they are not developmentally prepared to ingest (hard candy, popcorn, uncooked carrots, hot dogs, peanuts). Latex balloons account for a significant number of deaths from aspiration per year (Abdel-Rahman, 2000). One hospital review of 1160 children referred for foreign body aspiration found watermelon seeds to be the most common object at 39% (Eren, Balci, Dikici, Doblan, & Eren, 2003). Childhood aspiration can occur at any age, but most incidents occur in boys younger than 5 years, with a peak incidence at ages 1 to 3 years (Lima & Fischer, 2002). Forty percent of accidental deaths in the home are caused by foreign body aspiration.

Manifestations

Immediate signs and symptoms include sudden, violent coughing; gagging; wheezing; vomiting; brief episode of apnea; and possibly cyanosis.

After aspirating a foreign object, the child may remain asymptomatic for hours or weeks. If the object is not found and removed, signs and symptoms related to edema and increased irritation and obstruction may develop. Signs and symptoms of laryngeal and tracheal obstruction include choking, dysphagia, hoarseness, croupy cough, stridor, and possibly dyspnea with cyanosis. Coughing, wheezing, unilaterally decreased breath sounds, pneumonitis, and possibly respiratory arrest can indicate bronchial inflammation and obstruction.

Diagnostic Evaluation

The diagnosis is based on an accurate history and the clinical manifestations. Fluoroscopy and chest radiography are used to reveal the presence of a foreign object in the respiratory tract. Radiographs will reveal an opaque foreign body, and laryngoscopy or rigid bronchoscopy confirms the diagnosis and provides an avenue for removing the object.

Therapeutic Management

Foreign bodies are removed from the respiratory tract by direct laryngoscopy or bronchoscopy. After the procedure, the child should remain hospitalized for observation for laryngeal edema and respiratory distress. Antibiotics are unnecessary unless respiratory signs and symptoms suggest an infection. Cool mist and administration of bronchodilators and/or corticosteroids 24 to 48 hours after the removal of the foreign body may be indicated.

Nursing Considerations

The degree of obstruction should be assessed to determine the appropriate action to take. If the child is aphonic (not speaking) and not breathing, the nurse should follow the guidelines for managing an obstructed airway (see Chapter 34). Children

Pathophysiology

of Foreign Body Aspiration

Most foreign bodies become lodged in the bronchi. The right main bronchus is a more common site than the left main bronchus because of its anatomic development. Objects lodged in the larynx cause edema and inflammation. Bronchial obstruction manifests as obstructive emphysema, pneumonia, or atelectasis. Failure to remove obstructing foreign objects is almost always fatal. Most can be removed mechanically without complications; a delay in treatment can lead to aspiration pneumonia and airway trauma.

with a partially obstructed airway are observed for signs of increasing obstruction.

After the object has been removed, the child is observed for signs of obstruction caused by laryngeal edema and soft tissue swelling (restlessness, dyspnea). The child should be placed on a cardiorespiratory monitor.

Liquids are withheld until the child's gag reflex returns after anesthesia. Oral fluids should be started slowly and increased as the child tolerates the intake. Intake and output should be recorded. If the child refuses to drink because of a sore throat or is unable to take fluids orally, the physician should be notified so that IV fluids may be started. The parents' knowledge of respiratory distress is also evaluated before discharge.

Parental anxiety and guilt are common after an episode of aspiration. In addition to supporting the parents, the nurse assesses their knowledge of safety. Prevention is the key to reducing the incidence of aspiration. Safety is discussed at every well-child visit (see Chapters 5 through 8).

PULMONARY NONINFECTIOUS IRRITATION

Although we think of foreign body aspiration as the most common type of pulmonary noninfectious irritation in children, other forms of irritation may cause respiratory difficulties. These include acute (adult) respiratory distress syndrome (ARDS), passive smoking, and smoke inhalation. Respiratory distress syndrome in infants is discussed in Chapter 29.

Acute (Adult) Respiratory Distress Syndrome

Although there is not uniform agreement as to what constitutes ARDS, it is generally agreed that ARDS represents severe diffuse lung injury precipitated by a variety of illnesses. The mechanism of lung injury in children is similar to that of adults and usually occurs from 8 to 48 hours after the initial illness, which may be but is not limited to aspiration, trauma, drug ingestion, shock, and massive transfusions.

Pathophysiology

The mechanism that initiates and perpetuates the lung injury is not understood. There is a breakdown in the alveolar-capillary barrier with fluid accumulation in the interstitium and alveoli. ARDS has acute and chronic stages. Initially there is capillary congestion and pulmonary edema. Children who do not recover from the acute stage develop fibrosis of the lungs.

Table 45-4 discusses clinical manifestations, therapeutic management, nursing care, and prognosis.

TABLE 45-4 Pulmonary Noninfectious Irritants

	Acute (Adult) Respiratory Distress	Passive Smoking	Smoke Inhalation
Clinical manifestations	Acute, subacute, and chronic phases Pulmonary manifestations may be minimal during acute phase but will move toward respiratory distress (dyspnea, tachypnea, retractions, grunting, cyanosis) May develop severe hypoxemia and, occasionally, hypercapnia It should be noted that there is a primary disease and manifestations of that disease process will also be present	Increased respiratory infections An effect on respiratory function and growth in infants and a small but significant reduction in airway function in older children Possible negative effect on the linear growth of children with cystic fibrosis	Singed nasal hair Cough Hoarseness Hemoptysis Soot in sputum Cyanosis Wheezing Carbon monoxide: Mild—headaches, mild dyspnea, visual changes, confusion Moderate—irritability, diminished judgment, dim vision, nausea Severe—hallucinations, confusion, ataxia, collapse, coma
Therapeutic management	Need to be treated in an intensive care unit (ICU) Treat underlying cause Oxygen/mechanical ventilation Pulse oximetry Maintain cardiac function Stabilize hematocrit Prevent infection	Awareness of problem and preventive teaching Effective programs to prevent smoking in parents and minors	100% oxygen by mask Arterial blood gases Intubation and tracheostomy equipment available Aerosolized bronchodilators Balance fluid therapy between the need for a large volume of fluid and the need to limit fluid to decrease pulmonary edema Prophylactic antimicrobial therapy is controversial
Nursing Care	Monitor respiratory status Monitor blood gas analysis Psychological support of child and parents Monitor urine output, capillary filling, perfusion	Involvement in community projects to designate "no smoking" ordinances in public places School-based prevention programs Education of parents as part of anticipatory guidance of the dangers of smoking, both active and passive Role modeling no smoking	Respiratory assessment Support of pulmonary therapy Psychological support of the child and family as a result of the fear of the trauma of the fire or insult that caused the injury Children who have lost a family member will need long-term psychological support
Prognosis	High mortality, usually more than 50% Those who survive have a good chance of full recovery	Increased numbers of studies have shown the correlation between smoking and respiratory disease; more studies needed to show the long-term effects	Most will return to near-normal pulmonary function, and few will suffer long-term problems associated with the injury

Passive Smoking

Increased attention has been paid to the role of passive smoking in the development of respiratory disease in children. Children with a history of exposure to cigarette smoke have more episodes of airway obstruction; more frequent hospitalizations for respiratory complaints; onset of asthma at an earlier age; and more frequent episodes of otitis media, middle-ear effusion, tonsillectomy, and adenoidectomy than nonexposed children (Ilicali, Keles, Deer, Saun, & Guldiken, 2001). There is increasing evidence that passive smoking increases the incidence of respiratory infections and bronchial hyperresponsiveness (Gurkan, Kiral, Dagli, & Karakoc, 2000). In utero exposure is associated with impaired lung growth and wheezing illnesses, particularly in preschool children (Landau, 2001).

Pathophysiology

Smoke is an irritant that can cause increased airway reactivity and inflammation.

See Table 45-4 for a discussion of clinical manifestations, therapeutic management, nursing care, and prognosis.

Smoke Inhalation

As many as 50% of all fire-related deaths are caused by smoke injuries. The severity of lung injury is related to the nature of the material inhaled, the products of incomplete combustion that are generated, and the child's confinement in a closed space. Besides the noxious gases, fine particles of soot may also be inhaled, which may have toxic gases adsorbed on them or which may cause thermal burns.

Pathophysiology

Because the upper airway has a built-in cooling system, most thermal airway injury is limited to the areas above the larynx. Steam inhalation injury is an exception. Combustion of the materials involved causes a wide variety of noxious gases. These include but are not limited to oxides of sulfur and nitrogen, acetaldehydes, hydrocyanic acid, and carbon monoxide. Exposure to these gases can cause mucosal edema; activation of irritant receptors; necrosis; sloughing of airway mucosa; inspissation (thickening or drying) of sooty debris; and airway obstruction leading to further hypoxemia, atelectasis, and reduced bacterial clearance (Flynn, 2000).

Carbon monoxide poisoning is a complication of smoke inhalation caused when carbon monoxide combines with hemoglobin to form carboxyhemoglobin, causing severe hypoxia.

See Table 45-4 for a discussion of clinical manifestations, therapeutic management, nursing care, and prognosis.

APNEA

Manifestations

Apnea is the cessation of breathing for a period of 20 seconds or longer, or for a shorter period but accompanied by bradycardia or cyanosis. True apnea differs from periodic breathing, which might be seen in premature infants. In periodic breathing, there is a shift from regular rhythmic breathing to brief episodes of apnea. This type of breathing pattern consists of three or more respiratory pauses of longer than 3 seconds, with less than 20 seconds of respiration between pauses. Rarely, periodic breathing is associated with changes in heart rate or color. Periodic breathing is very common in premature infants and decreases as the infant's gestational age increases. The cause is unknown; periodic breathing may be a normal event.

Apparent life-threatening events are sudden episodes characterized by apnea, a color change, a change in muscle tone, choking, or gagging in an infant who otherwise appears healthy. The observer of the event relates the belief that the infant would have died if not for intervention. Apparent life-threatening events most often occur in infants of 37 weeks' gestational age or older while they are sleeping, feeding, or awake. Infants who have experienced such an event are usually hospitalized for observation and testing and are at increased risk for mortality (American Academy of Pediatrics [AAP], Committee on Fetus and Newborn, 2003).

Two categories of true apnea events are apnea of prematurity and infant apnea (Table 45-5).

Diagnostic Evaluation

Tests are selected for the clinical indications and to rule out any underlying condition. Cardiorespiratory and neurophysiologic studies are commonly ordered. These studies include chest radiography, blood chemistry studies, electrocardiography (ECG), and electroencephalography. Pneumocardiography specifically tests for apnea by recording the heart rate and chest wall movements; however, the reliability of the test in predicting apnea has not been well established.

■NURSING CARE
The Infant With Apnea

Assessment

The infant's heart rate and respirations are monitored continuously. The nurse should ascertain that the alarms on the cardiorespiratory monitor are set. Resuscitative equipment should be available.

If an apneic episode is observed, the nurse should record the time and duration of the episode, the skin color change, heart rate, and oxygen saturation. The nurse should also describe what the infant was doing before the episode and any actions the nurse took to stimulate breathing.

Nursing Diagnosis and Planning

The nursing diagnoses and expected outcomes that may be appropriate for the infant with apnea and the family are

- Ineffective Breathing Pattern related to apnea secondary to prematurity of respiratory control mechanisms (premature infant); and related to apnea of known or unknown etiology (term infant).
  Expected Outcome: The infant will have regular breathing patterns, as evidenced by respiratory rate and rhythm within normal limits for age.
- Anxiety (parental) related to the possibility of the infant's death.
  Expected Outcome: The parents will verbalize feelings concerning the infant's periods of apnea.
- Deficient Knowledge (parental) related to unfamiliarity with apnea monitoring equipment and cardiopulmonary resuscitation (CPR).
  Expected Outcome: The parents will learn how to perform infant CPR and how to operate the apnea monitor.

Interventions

The nurse sets the heart rate parameters of the cardiorespiratory monitor according to the infant's age, and the respiratory pause at greater than 15 seconds. Resuscitative equipment should be available, and the nurse should be proficient in using it.

The apneic infant can be stimulated by gently tapping the foot or trunk or turning the infant over. The infant should not be shaken vigorously. If breathing does not resume, institute bag-and-mask ventilation.

Maintain a neutral thermal environment while the infant is hospitalized, and avoid suctioning if possible. Several studies have shown that feeding affects ventilation. Therefore infants should be monitored closely when being fed.

If home apnea monitoring is ordered, the family should be instructed in the use of the monitor and in CPR (Fig. 45-4) (Bennett, 2002). Emphasize to the parents that when the monitor alarm is triggered, they should immediately assess the infant rather than focus on the machine (Box 45-2).

Evaluation

- Does the infant demonstrate normal respiratory rate and rhythm?
- Have the parents verbalized their fears associated with the infant's apnea?
- Have the parents demonstrated the ability to operate monitoring equipment and to perform CPR?

TABLE 45-5 Apnea of Prematurity Compared With Infant Apnea

Etiology and Incidence	Pathophysiology	Therapeutic Management
APNEA OF PREMATURITY		
The most common type of apnea, it occurs in neonates of 24-32 weeks' gestational age, with onset usually within the first week of life. It usually resolves by 38 wk. Although the neonate's age may be related to a higher incidence of sudden infant death syndrome (SIDS), apnea of prematurity is not considered to predict risk.*	It varies among neonates but may be caused by upper airway obstruction, immaturity of central control mechanisms, compliant chest wall, or abnormal response during rapid eye movement (REM) sleep. Apnea often occurs during feeding because of immaturity of breathing, sucking, and swallowing coordination.	Gentle cutaneous stimulation is used to stimulate breathing in neonates with mild apnea (<10 episodes per day with little desaturation). For persistent apnea, use oxygen administration, cardiorespiratory monitor; consider continuous positive airway pressure (CPAP) for neonates with severe apnea. Drug therapy may include caffeine, oral theophylline, or intravenous (IV) aminophylline to increase central respiratory drive and improve CO_2 sensitivity.
INFANT APNEA		
Most infant apnea has no known cause. Underlying conditions such as gastroesophageal reflux, seizures, or hypoglycemia should be ruled out.	Three types: • *Central*—absence of respiratory effort and air movement. • *Obstructive*—apparent respiratory efforts without air movement or sound. • *Mixed*—absence of respiratory effort and nasal air movement followed by resumption of respiratory effort without air movement. Short episodes of apnea are usually central apnea; apnea episodes that last 15 sec or more are usually mixed.	If no underlying disorder is identified, home monitoring with a respiratory stimulant (caffeine, theophylline).

*Bhatt-Mehta, V., & Schumacher, R.E. (2003). Treatment of apnea of prematurity. *Paediatric Drugs, 5*(3), 195-210.

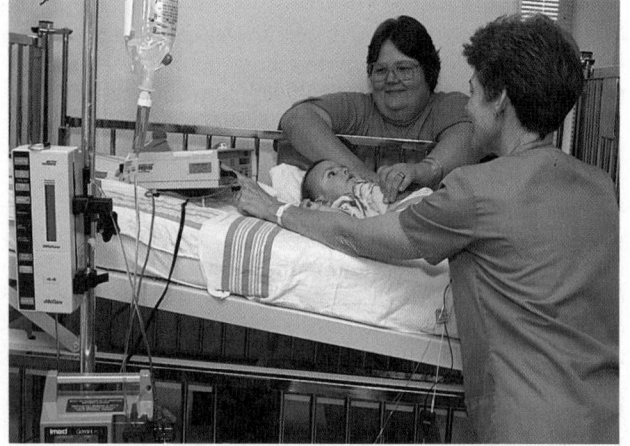

Figure 45-4 Teaching the family about using an apnea monitor and how to respond to alarms is an important element in caring for the child with infant apnea. The nurse must assess the parents' ability to tolerate the stressors of living with a child who is prone to apnea and support them as they deal with these stressors.

SUDDEN INFANT DEATH SYNDROME

Sudden infant death syndrome (SIDS) is defined as the sudden and unexplained death of an infant younger than 1 year. The exact cause is unknown despite a thorough investigation that includes a complete autopsy, examination of the death scene, and review of the clinical history. It is sometimes referred to by the public as *crib death*. SIDS usually occurs during sleep.

Etiology and Incidence

Although numerous theories have been proposed, the cause of SIDS is unknown. Proposed contributing factors include prematurity, brainstem defects, severe infant botulism, infections, reactions to immunizations, and hypersensitivity to cow's milk. Some studies have suggested a connection with lower socioeconomic status, cultural influences, lack of prenatal care, smoking, a sibling with SIDS, and season (winter).

Numerous reports from countries outside the United States have found a significant association between a prone

BOX 45-2
Home Apnea Monitoring

Indications

- The infant is a survivor of an apparent life-threatening event (an event that required administration of cardiopulmonary resuscitation [CPR]).
- The infant is a newborn sibling of two or more infants who have died of sudden infant death syndrome.
- The infant is premature and has symptoms of idiopathic apnea of prematurity but is otherwise ready for hospital discharge.
- The infant has a tracheostomy.
- The infant has sleep apnea syndrome caused by a neurologic disorder, periodic breathing, upper airway abnormality, or idiopathic syndrome.

Conditions

- The parents must be trained to do CPR and understand conditions for calling the health care provider.
- Twenty-four-hour medical and technical (equipment trouble-shooting) coverage is mandatory.
- Parents should maintain a diary specifically describing each episode.

Modified from Hanly, P. (1992). Mechanisms and management of central sleeping apnea. *Lung, 170,* 1017; Brooks, J. (1998). SIDS and ALTE. In V. Chernick, T. Boat, & E. Kendig (Eds.), *Kendig's disorders of the respiratory tract in children* (6th ed., pp. 1166-1172). Philadelphia: Saunders.

---

sleeping position and the incidence of SIDS. Based on this information, in 1992 the American Academy of Pediatrics (AAP) recommended that healthy infants be placed on their sides or backs to sleep, rather than prone. A 2003 update from the American Academy of Pediatrics clearly suggests a strong correlation between the decreased percentage of infants being put to sleep in a prone position and the decreasing incidence of SIDS (AAP, 2003).

Risk factors are also associated with the use of soft bedding. Infants may suffocate by rebreathing CO_2-laden expired air when sleeping face down on soft bedding (Pastore, Guala, & Zaffaroni, 2003).

SIDS occurs most frequently between the 2nd and 4th months of life, with 95% of cases occurring before age 6 months. It is more common in boys, low-birth-weight infants, and infants from lower socioeconomic groups. It occurs more often during the winter months. Native Americans have the highest incidence, followed by African-Americans.

Manifestations

The principal manifestation of SIDS is silent death. The child may be found in any position and may be clutching bedding.

Diagnostic Evaluation

Diagnosis is confirmed through autopsy. A medical history of the infant and family should be taken. The infant is examined for signs of illness or trauma. The death scene is also investigated.

Pathophysiology
of Sudden Infant Death Syndrome

Autopsy findings in infants who have died of sudden infant death syndrome (SIDS) have varied widely. Nonspecific findings such as mild pulmonary edema, vascular congestion, or pulmonary inflammation are common. Other consistent findings include retarded postnatal growth, increased pulmonary arterial smooth muscle, retention of brown fat, brainstem gliosis, and intrathoracic petechiae. Partial upper airway obstruction in association with rebreathing may be an explanation for many SIDS deaths.* No single cause has been identified.

*Brooks, J. (1998). SIDS and ALTE. In V. Chernick, T. Boat, & E. Kendig (Eds.). *Kendig's disorders of the respiratory tract in children* (pp. 1166-1172). Philadelphia: Saunders.

▪NURSING CARE
The Family of the Infant With Sudden Infant Death Syndrome

Assessment

When an infant is brought into the emergency department with suspected SIDS, the family is often confused. If resuscitation was begun at home, they may assume that it was effective and that their infant is alive. Assessment of the family's understanding of the situation is necessary to plan for teaching and support. The nurse should assess the family's emotional status and coping strategies.

The nurse interviews the family in a calm, slow, and nonthreatening manner. Questions should not imply negligence or any involvement in the death. Parents need to be given time to think before they answer questions. Because the parents will be overwhelmed, questions may need to be repeated for clarity.

Nursing Diagnosis and Planning

The nursing diagnoses and expected outcomes that may be appropriate for the family of the infant victim of SIDS are

- Interrupted Family Processes related to death of a child.
  Expected Outcome: The parents and family will verbalize feelings related to the death of the infant.
- Compromised Family Coping related to death of a child.
  Expected Outcomes: The parents and family will identify strengths and accept support of other family members, friends, professionals, and support groups.
- Deficient Knowledge related to not understanding the cause of death.
  Expected Outcome: The parents will verbalize an understanding of the cause of their child's death.

Interventions

The nurse working with a family whose child has died of SIDS should provide calm and compassionate support. The parents are confused about the death and are trying to cope with many emotions. Most parents will experience a combination of guilt, anger, and emotional pain.

A quiet room with dim lighting and a rocking chair should be provided for the family, and someone should remain with them. Assist the family to call family, friends, or clergy. The nurse should accompany the physician when the parents are told their infant is dead. At this time the parents should also be told that the apparent cause of death is SIDS and that nothing could have been done to prevent the death. This information will help minimize feelings of guilt.

Parents should be given the opportunity to say good-bye to their child. Because the parents may not think to ask to see their infant, the nurse should provide this opportunity.

The nurse might say, "Would you like to have some time alone with your baby? We will bring him to you, and you can take as long as you would like to hold him."

The infant should be cleaned and wrapped in a blanket and brought to the parents. Parents who are not given the opportunity to hold their child and say good-bye often regret it later, but parents who do not want time alone with their baby should have their decision respected. The nurse should accept the parents' decision in this matter. Each parent will cope in an individualized way.

The need for an autopsy should be explained. The autopsy will verify the cause of death and confirm for the parents that they did not cause the death.

Before the parents leave the hospital, arrangements for follow-up care should be made. Many hospitals have a team consisting of a social worker, chaplain, and nurse that is called when a suspected SIDS death occurs.

Refer the family to a local SIDS program for information, support, and counseling (American SIDS Institute, 2480 Windy Hill Road, Suite 380, Marietta, GA 30067. Website: www.sids.org). Nurses who are involved in home visiting can encourage the family to communicate their feelings. Siblings should not be overlooked; parents may be so overwhelmed with their own grief that they forget their other children. Another reaction might be to overprotect their other children. The nurse should guide the family in identifying the members' various responses and in treating them at the appropriate developmental level. Children in the family who perhaps resented the new baby may have tremendous guilt feelings. The loss of a sibling may be especially traumatic to a toddler, who does not understand the changes that are taking place in the family. Routines and rituals that are important to the toddler may be disrupted.

Evaluation

- Is the family able to verbalize feelings associated with the death of the child?
- Has the family joined a support group or identified a support system?
- Has the extended family mobilized to support the family?
- Is the family using effective coping skills to work toward an understanding of the child's death?

ASTHMA

Asthma, or reactive airway disease, is a leading cause of acute and chronic illness in children and the most frequent admitting diagnosis in children's hospitals. Despite advances in medical treatment, the incidence and death rate from asthma have increased markedly in recent years.

Etiology

It is unclear why some children's airways are more reactive than others'. It is known, however, that heredity plays a role, because asthma tends to appear in families. Other risk factors include male gender, African-American or Latino ethnic background, crowded living conditions, poverty, prematurity, and exposure to environmental smoke (Federierico & Liu, 2003; Guilbert & Drawiec, 2003).

An asthma episode may be triggered by a variety of stimuli, among them cold air, smoke, fumes, viral infection, stress, exercise, odors, medications (particularly aspirin and non-steroidal antiinflammatory drugs [NSAIDs]), or allergens (Sockrider, 2002). Foods are occasionally the trigger in infants but less commonly in older children.

The immature anatomy of infants and small children predisposes them to increased distress from asthma. Children's smaller, narrower airways and decreased elastic lung recoil make them more prone to airway obstruction. The child's flexible rib cage and underdeveloped chest muscles and diaphragm lead to exhaustion when respiratory effort increases. Although asthma is not actually outgrown, the severity of asthma attacks often decreases as the child gets older because of increased airway size, improved diaphragmatic support, and better clearing of mucus. Asthma is considered a lifelong condition and may become increasingly severe after a period of remission.

Incidence

Since the early 1980s, the incidence of asthma has risen in the United States and other parts of the world. Asthma affects an estimated 6.3 million American children, with approximately 1.5 million of those younger than 5 years (American Academy of Allergy, Asthma, and Immunology, 2003). Asthma is more common among boys than girls until puberty, when the gender difference in incidence equalizes. Asthma is 26% more prevalent in African-American children than in white children (American Lung Association, 2002).

Manifestations

The manifestations of asthma may vary. A child experiencing an asthma episode may have only a dry cough. Wheezing is a classic sign of asthma, but other signs may be present, including shortness of breath, cough, or dyspnea on exertion. Other manifestations may have a sudden or an insidious onset:

- Retractions, nasal flaring, or stridor
- Nonproductive cough (with or without wheezing) that later becomes productive
- Tachypnea, orthopnea
- Restlessness, apprehension, diaphoresis
- Abdominal pain secondary to the strain placed on the abdominal muscles during labored breathing
- A hunched-over sitting position with arms braced (tripod position)
- Fatigue and difficulty performing simple tasks, such as eating, walking, or even talking, because of shortness of breath

Pathophysiology

of Asthma

Asthma is a reversible obstructive airway disease characterized by:

- *Increased airway responsiveness* to a variety of stimuli
- *Bronchospasm* resulting from constriction of bronchial smooth muscle
- *Inflammation* and *edema* of the mucous membranes that line the small airways and the subsequent accumulation of thick secretions in the airways

Immediate Reaction (Early-Phase Response)

Allergens or other trigger substances activate immunoglobulin E (IgE) receptors on sensitized airway mast cells, causing mast cell degranulation and release of chemical mediators (histamine, leukotrienes, prostaglandins). These mediators cause bronchoconstriction shortly after exposure to the trigger; the bronchoconstriction resolves within 1 to 2 hours.

Delayed Reaction (Late-Phase Response)

Chemical mediators attract immune system cells (eosinophils, neutrophils, basophils) to the respiratory tract. Infiltration by these cells and their release of additional inflammatory substances damage the epithelial and smooth muscle cells, causing airway edema, mucous plugging of small airways, and additional inflammation. Bronchoconstriction recurs and can persist for several hours. The airway hyperresponsiveness resulting from this inflammatory process can last several weeks or months.

Late asthmatic responses can occur without a previous early (immediate) response. When asthma is precipitated by nonallergenic stimuli (exercise, cold air), bronchospasm usually lasts less than 1 hour and is not followed by a late response.

During an asthma episode, the mucous membranes lining the bronchioles become edematous and secrete large amounts of thick mucus. As a result, the airways narrow, leading to increased airway resistance and respiratory distress. Because small airways are normally wider on inspiration than expiration, the child is able to inhale but has difficulty exhaling through the narrowed bronchioles. Wheezing can be heard as air is forced through the narrow passages during expiration. Air becomes trapped, causing hyperinflation of the alveoli.

Airway obstruction is more severe in some parts of the lungs than in others, and air flows more easily into areas with the least resistance. The blood that flows to the less-ventilated portions of the lungs is inadequately saturated with oxygen. Thus a mismatch between ventilation and perfusion in poorly ventilated areas of the lung occurs, resulting in incompletely saturated blood entering the systemic circulation and decreased Po_2 levels (hypoxia).

As the child struggles to get enough air, respiratory rate increases (tachypnea). Tachypnea lowers carbon dioxide levels in the blood (hypocapnia). As the child tires from the increased work of breathing, hypoventilation occurs and carbon dioxide levels increase. Increased levels of carbon dioxide in the blood (hypercapnia) during an asthma episode may be a sign of severe airway obstruction and impending respiratory failure.

- A feeling of chest tightness followed by a dry cough, wheezing, and dyspnea
- Worsening of symptoms after the child goes to bed at night because of increased narrowing of the airways at night and pooling of secretions

At the beginning of the asthma episode, wheezing may be heard only with a stethoscope. As the severity of the episode increases, wheezing may be audible to the unaided ear. Children in severe respiratory distress may not demonstrate wheezing because of decreased air movement; decreased wheezing in a child who is not improving clinically may signal an inability to move air. This is referred to as a *silent chest* and is an ominous sign during an asthma episode. With treatment, increased wheezing may actually signal that the child's condition is improving.

Diagnostic Evaluation

Chest radiographs are usually normal except in cases of severe asthma, in which hyperinflation of the airways can be seen. Pulmonary function tests reveal a decreased forced expiratory volume in 1 second (FEV_1), increased residual volume from air trapping, and decreased vital capacity (the maximum amount of air exhaled after a maximum inhalation). Other pulmonary function test results might be altered as well. The peak expiratory flow rate (PEFR) is used to monitor children with chronic asthma. Because asthma can be triggered by gastroesophageal reflux, some children will be evaluated for its presence (see Chapter 43).

Rhinitis, sinusitis, and nasal polyps are often present in children with asthma. Eosinophilia is present in both the blood and the sputum. Skin tests are often performed to identify specific allergens. The RAST may be used to identify specific antigens. Arterial blood gas measurements may be ordered in children having a severe asthma episode because of initial respiratory alkalosis and subsequent metabolic acidosis. Pulse oximetry values provide information about oxygenation.

Therapeutic Management

Acute Asthma Episode

A child who is experiencing an episode of wheezing along with other symptoms of asthma is usually seen at a physician's office or emergency room. First, a bronchodilator, usually a short-acting beta$_2$-adrenergic agonist such as albuterol, is administered by a powered nebulizer or metered-dose inhaler (MDI) as often as every 20 minutes for 1 hour or continuously. Close monitoring of the child's respiratory status after each course of medication assesses resolution of the episode. Beta$_2$-agonists, ipratropium bromide, and corticosteroids remain the most useful therapeutic agents for acute asthma episodes in children (Streetman, Bhatt-Mheta, & Johnson, 2002).

If the child improves, the child can return home with an albuterol prescription and instructions for assessing respiratory status or with instructions for administering albuterol more frequently along with routine asthma medications. If symptoms do not improve or if the asthmatic child's PEFR is less than 70% of baseline, the child should receive a dose of an oral corticosteroid (liquid preparations are available for infants). If symptoms continue to worsen, administration of the bronchodilator every 20 minutes for an additional hour is warranted. Indicators for hospital admission include (Blaisdell et al., 2002):

- PEFR less than 50% of baseline
- Inspiratory and expiratory wheezing
- Tachycardia and tachypnea
- Dyspnea, retractions
- Oxygen saturation 91% or lower after aggressive treatment

Once the child is hospitalized, humidified oxygen is administered at 30%, either by nasal prongs or by facemask, to keep the oxygen saturation at 95% or greater. An IV line delivers fluids and provides venous access for parenteral medications (e.g., methylprednisolone) as ordered. Chest radiography, arterial blood gas determinations, or pulse oximetry may be performed to further evaluate the child's oxygenation status. The child receives a bronchodilator (albuterol) by nebulizer every 1 to 2 hours initially, with the interval between doses increased as the child's condition improves. Ipratropium bromide (Atrovent), an anticholinergic agent, has been found to be an effective bronchodilator when administered along with albuterol in children with severe exacerbations.

Increasingly severe asthma that is unresponsive to vigorous treatment measures is termed *status asthmaticus*. Status asthmaticus is a medical emergency that can cause respiratory failure and death. Hospitalization, usually in an intensive care unit, is indicated. The child is placed on a continuous cardiorespiratory monitor and continuous pulse oximeter. Blood gas and serum electrolyte values are monitored. In addition to the previously discussed measures, the child may receive continuous nebulized albuterol, and ipratropium bromide every 6 hours. If the child's condition does not respond to these medications, oral or intravenous steroids are then administered. Levalbuterol is a relatively new treatment for acute asthma and is delivered via a nebulizer.

Endotracheal intubation with mechanical ventilation may be necessary. Acidosis is corrected with IV administration of sodium bicarbonate. Antibiotics may also be administered to treat concurrent infection (e.g., pneumonia).

Ongoing Asthma

A partnership between the health care provider, parent, and child is necessary for asthma to be managed effectively. Long-term asthma treatment should minimize symptoms, prevent acute asthma episodes, avoid the side effects of therapy, and help the child maintain a normal lifestyle. Children with asthma and their parents need to be taught methods of managing asthma, including environmental control and monitoring symptoms and medication. A resource for parents is the

---

⚠ CRITICAL TO REMEMBER

Emergency Asthma Management

The following symptoms indicate the need for emergency treatment of asthma:

- Worsening wheeze, cough, or shortness of breath
- A peak flow rate that decreases or does not change (even after use of an inhaled beta$_2$-adrenergic agonist) or that is less than 30% to 50% of the child's predicted baseline level or personal best
- Difficulty breathing (the child's chest and neck are pulled in with each breath, or the child hunches over or struggles to breathe)
- Trouble with walking or talking
- Discontinuation of play without the ability to resume activity
- Listlessness and weak cry in an infant; refusal to suck bottle or breast
- Gray or blue lips or fingernails (in which case the child needs emergency treatment *immediately*!)

Modified from Rachelefsky, G.S. (1995). Asthma update: New approaches and partnerships. *Journal of Pediatric Health Care, 9,* 12-21.

Asthma and Allergy Foundation of America, 1125 15th Street, NW, Suite 502, Washington, DC 20005. Website: www.aafa.org.

Environmental Control

Irritants and Allergens. Children with asthma and their parents can decrease the frequency and severity of asthma episodes by recognizing and controlling the triggers that precipitate symptoms. Common environmental irritants include cigarette smoke, smoke from wood-burning stoves and fireplaces, fumes, deodorants, overhumidified air, and perfume. Allergenic triggers, such as animal dander, seasonal pollens, and molds, often cause problems. House dust can be both an irritant and an allergen (Arshad et al., 2003).

The extent of environmental control needed depends on the severity of the asthma. If the asthma is mild, prohibiting smoking in the house and controlling dust with frequent house cleaning may be adequate. If the child continues to have problems after these interventions, additional steps should be taken to minimize environmental triggers.

Immunotherapy (allergy shots) can be helpful in decreasing asthma symptoms caused by specific allergens the child cannot avoid. Immunotherapy is used in conjunction with, not in place of, other asthma therapies.

Exercise. Exercise is a trigger of asthma in most asthmatic children. Exercise-induced asthma may be triggered by rapid breathing of large volumes of cool, dry air (e.g., with mouth breathing during exercise). The symptoms of exercise-induced asthma usually begin after 5 to 10 minutes of exercise and often last from 30 to 60 minutes.

Measures to prevent exercise-induced asthma include:

- Warming the air by breathing through the nose or covering the mouth and nose with a scarf when exercising in cold weather
- Using an inhaled beta$_2$-agonist or cromolyn before exercise

---

BOX 45-3
Monitoring Breathing Capacity Using a Peak Flowmeter

The peak flowmeter is a device used to monitor breathing capacity in the child with asthma. It measures the flow of air in a forced exhalation in liters per minute. Peak flow monitoring can help identify the start of an asthma episode, often before symptoms are evident. To help children monitor their asthma, a zone system can be explained as a traffic light, making it easier for them to identify and understand differences in peak flow values.

Peak Flow Zones
Personal best: _____
Green: All clear—no asthma symptoms are present (80%-100% of personal best).
Yellow: Caution—acute episode may be present (50%-80% of personal best). A temporary increase in medication may be indicated. Asthma may not be under control. Medication may need to be increased.
Red: Medical alert (below 50% of personal best). An immediate bronchodilator should be taken. Practitioner should be notified if measurements do not return immediately to and stay in yellow or green zones.

How To Use a Peak Flowmeter
1. Remove gum or food from the mouth, and stand up.
2. Move the pointer on the meter to zero.
3. Hold the meter horizontally, being sure to keep your fingers away from vent holes and the marker.
4. Relax, and take a few moderately slow, deep breaths. Slowly take the deepest breath possible with your mouth wide open.
5. Hold your breath while placing the mouthpiece on your tongue. Seal your lips tightly around the mouthpiece.
6. Blow out as hard and fast as possible. Give a short, sharp blast—not a slow blow. (The meter records the fastest huff, not the longest.) Note the number by the marker on the numbered scale.
7. Repeat three times. Wait at least 10 seconds between attempts. (Be sure to move the pointer to zero after each try.)
8. Record the highest of the three readings.
9. Ideally, peak flow values are obtained a minimum of once a day, preferably in the morning. Peak flow measurements should be done before and after administration of an inhaled bronchodilator. The number of measurements should be increased during a flare-up.

Modified from National Heart, Lung and Blood Institute (1997, July). *Expert panel report 2: Guidelines for the diagnosis and management of asthma.* Bethesda, MD: Author.

- Practicing techniques to decrease hyperventilation (e.g., progressive muscle relaxation, diaphragmatic breathing)

Because athletics and active play are important parts of a child's life, children with asthma should not be restricted from physical activity. Exercise not only increases physical fitness but also enhances self-esteem and offers valuable opportunities for socialization. Swimming is frequently recommended as an ideal sport for children with asthma because the air is humidified and exhaling underwater prolongs exhalation and increases end-expiratory pressure. Other sports that do not require sustained exertion, such as gymnastics, baseball, and weight lifting, are also well tolerated, and if asthma is well controlled, the child can usually participate in any type of sport.

Infection. Viral respiratory infections are the most frequent triggers of pediatric asthma. It is advisable for children with frequent or severe asthma to avoid exposure to individuals with a viral respiratory infection. Children with asthma also benefit from influenza vaccine.

Emotions. Asthma is not caused by psychosocial problems. Emotional upset, however, can exacerbate asthma symptoms. Laughing, crying, or shouting can act as mechanical triggers of bronchoconstriction. Also, a child with asthma may become angry or frustrated and refuse to take medication or adhere to a treatment regimen. Moreover, anxiety during an episode may cause the child to hyperventilate, aggravating asthma symptoms.

Monitoring Symptoms. Asthma symptoms can best be treated if they are detected early. Children and their parents should be taught the subtle early symptoms of an asthma episode (itchy chest or chin, cough, irritability or tired feeling, increased breathing rate, dry mouth, unusually dark circles under the eyes).

A useful device for monitoring breathing capacity is the peak flowmeter, which measures the flow of air in a forced exhalation in liters per minute. Peak flow monitoring can help identify the start of an asthma episode, often before the child is aware of symptoms. It can also help determine the need for treatment modification. Home monitoring of PEFR may be performed several times a day. The results can be compared with the child's normal predicted level and with results obtained over the preceding several days, providing an objective assessment of respiratory status (Box 45-3). Children with moderate to severe persistent asthma should do daily PEFR monitoring.

Recent studies suggest that parents and children sometimes have difficulty recognizing asthma trouble signs, and even if signs are recognized they do not make appropriate treatment accommodations (Hogan & Wilson, 2003). This observation underscores the need for thorough teaching guidelines for home asthma management, including (Baker, Friedman, & Schmitt, 2002):

- A written asthma plan that includes details of home management and lists indications for seeking physician or emergency room care
- Daily use of a peak flowmeter (in children older than 5 years) to monitor pulmonary status and response to treatment

---

BOX 45-4
Classification of Asthma

Mild Intermittent
- Symptoms less than or equal to twice a week or only with exercise
- Asymptomatic and normal peak expiratory flow rate (PEFR) between episodes; PEFR 80% of predicted rate during exacerbation
- Brief episodes
- Infrequent use of bronchodilator
- Few missed school days
- Rare activity limitation
- Symptoms rarely disturb sleep (less often than twice monthly)

Mild Persistent
- Symptoms more often than twice a week but less than once a day
- Exacerbations may begin to affect activity

Moderate Persistent
- Symptoms occur and bronchodilator used daily; exacerbations two or more times weekly
- More than 9 school days missed per year
- Frequent activity limitation (most days)
- Sleep disturbed by symptoms more than once a week
- PEFR 60% to 80% of predicted

Severe Persistent
- Daily symptoms
- Daily (or almost daily) use of bronchodilator for more than 6 months per year
- Limited physical activity
- Frequent sleep disturbance and exacerbations
- PEFR less than or equal to 60% of predicted

Modified from Kercsmar, C. (1998). Asthma. In V. Chernick, T. Boat, & E. Kendig (Eds.), *Kendig's disorders of the respiratory tract in children* (6th ed., p. 699). Philadelphia: Saunders; National Heart, Lung and Blood Institute. (1997). *Expert panel report 2: Guidelines for the diagnosis and management of asthma.* Bethesda, MD: Author.

- Home initiation of inhaled beta₂-adrenergic agonists, and oral steroids when beta₂-adrenergic agonists are ineffective for resolving symptoms
- Prompt communication with the health care provider for deteriorating respiratory status or reduced response to medication

Medications. Generally, asthma is treated with a combination of medications from two categories: bronchodilators and antiinflammatory agents. The medication regimen is based on the classification of the child's asthma and can be changed at home according to symptoms and peak flowmeter readings (Box 45-4). It is important to differentiate rescue medications (those used for immediate relief of an exacerbation) and routine medications.

Rescue Medications. Some medications used to relieve an asthma episode are described here:

- *Short-acting bronchodilators:* Beta₂-adrenergic agonists, such as albuterol (Ventolin, Proventil), metaproterenol (Alupent), terbutaline (Brethaire), bitolterol (Tornalate), and pirbuterol (Maxair inhaler), relax bronchial smooth muscle and inhibit the release of mediators from mast cells. They are delivered by metered-dose inhalers (MDIs) or by nebulizer three or four times daily if the child is symptomatic or before exercise.
- *Anticholinergic:* Ipratropium bromide is used in combination with beta₂-adrenergic agonists.
- *Mast cell inhibitors:* Cromolyn sodium (Intal), an inhaled NSAID, prevents asthma symptoms by blocking the release of mast cell mediators. It can be given 30 minutes before exposure to triggers. Another antiinflammatory asthma medication, nedrocromil sodium (Tilade), is available for use in children age 12 years or older.
- *Systemic corticosteroids:* Prednisone or prednisolone decreases airway inflammation. They are preferably given in short-burst courses of 5 to 7 days.

Routine Medications. The medications used for long-term, routine control of asthma are the same as those used for relief but are administered in different dosages, depending on the classification of the child's asthma. Several additional medications have become available or are being tested for asthma control:

- *Long-acting bronchodilators:* Sustained-release albuterol, salmeterol (Serevent).
- *Inhaled corticosteroids:* Beclomethasone, triamcinolone, budesonide, and flunisolide deliver topical antiinflammatory action directly to the airway.
- *Leukotriene blockers:* Zafirlukast and Zileuton diminish the mediator action of leukotrienes. They are used only in children older than 12 years.
- *Anti-IgE antibody:* omalizumab (Xolair) for allergic-type moderate to persistent asthma. Approved for use in children older than 12 years (Buhl, 2003).

Children with mild asthma use bronchodilators as needed for symptom relief. Children and families need to be cautioned not to overuse these medications and to notify the health care provider if the medications are needed more than twice a week or more frequently than every 3 to 4 hours during a 12-hour period.

PARENTS
Want to Know

Tips on Using a Nebulizer

1. Use clean hands and a clean area.
2. Take slow, deep breaths through pursed lips to maximize deposition of aerosolized medication in the lungs.
3. Use all the medication in the nebulizer during one treatment. Do not store medication in the nebulizer for later use.
4. The length of the treatment is usually 10 to 15 minutes if the equipment is working properly and the correct amount of medication and diluent are used. If the length of treatments is prolonged, check the nebulizer or the compressor for defects.
5. Rinse the nebulizer in clean water after each treatment. Allow it to air-dry after loosely covering it with a clean paper towel. Once daily, wash the nebulizer in warm, soapy water and then rinse. Disinfect by boiling for 5 minutes in water or place in a dishwasher (temperature must be ≥158° F). Air-dry the equipment. Never store the nebulizer in a closed plastic bag until it is completely dry. Storing wet equipment promotes the growth of mold and bacteria.

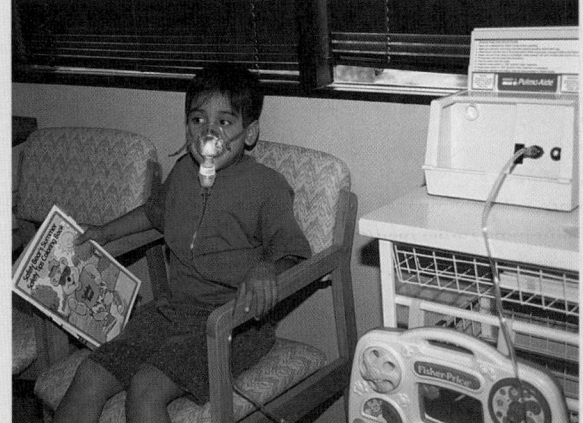

The powered nebulizer delivers a bronchodilator to the child who is having an acute asthma episode. This boy has a viral respiratory infection, which is a common trigger of acute asthma episodes in the pediatric population.

Modified from Brim, S. (1989, Jan.-Feb.). A quick guide for home use of inhalant medications. *Pediatric Nursing, 15*(1), 87-94, by permission of Janetti Publications, Inc. Photo courtesy Parkland Health and Hospital System Community Oriented Primary Care Clinic, Dallas, TX.

THE CHILD
Want to Know

How to Use a Metered-Dose Inhaler

1. Stand up. Shake the inhaler well. Remove the cap.
2. Hold the inhaler upright. Hold the mouthpiece or spacer mouthpiece 1 to 2 inches from your lips, and open your mouth wide.
3. Tilt your head back slightly, and breathe out fully.
4. Place your lips tightly around the mouthpiece, press down on the inhaler, and start to breathe in slowly.
5. Breathe in slowly (3-5 sec), because this allows the medicine to be inhaled more deeply.
6. Hold your breath for as long as possible—up to 10 seconds.
7. Remove the inhaler, and breathe out slowly through your nose.
8. Wait at least 2 minutes, and shake the inhaler again before repeating the dose.
9. Visible mist escaping from your open mouth indicates improper technique. Do not count that try. Relax and repeat.
10. Rinse your mouth with water if desired.

Children with mild to moderate persistent asthma should take daily antiinflammatory medications. The inhaled corticosteroid budesonide allows flexible once-daily dosing and is available for administration in ages 6 months and older (Szefler & Pedersen, 2003). It can take up to 3 weeks of daily dosing to realize a therapeutic effect. In addition, beta₂-adrenergic agonists are used to relieve symptoms. Long-acting bronchodilators or inhaled corticosteroids are also considered. Theophylline may be given to children who do not respond to mast cell inhibitors. PEFR monitoring helps the child with mild to moderate asthma monitor symptoms and pulmonary function. The family is given a written management plan.

Children with persistent severe asthma take daily mast cell inhibitors, inhaled corticosteroids, and long-acting bronchodilators or leukotriene blockers. Ipratropium bromide and oral corticosteroids are considered for management.

Medication Delivery. Inhaled medications are delivered either by nebulizer or by MDI. Both can be used for older and younger children. A spacer attached to an MDI (see Chapter 38) prolongs the medication transit, effectively delivers the medication to the airway instead of the mouth, improves deposition of the medication by 50%, and makes it easier for younger children to use an MDI (Devadason & Le Souef, 2002). If using a spacer, the child attaches the spacer to the outlet of the MDI, closes the lips around the spacer mouthpiece, activates the canister, and then inhales. Dry-powder inhalers (DPIs) require that patients have an inspiratory flow rate of at least 30 L/min, but they are easier to use and do not contain the ozone-damaging chlorofluorocarbons that MDIs use (Anderson, 2001). In addition to the single-dose DPI, a multidose tubular inhaler (for budesonide) and a multidose disk-shaped inhaler (for fluticasone and salmeterol) are now available (O'Connell, 2002).

Text continued p. 1237

Nursing Care Plan

The Child Hospitalized With Asthma

FOCUSED ASSESSMENT

Begin assessment with a thorough history that includes any family history of asthma or allergy as well as past episodes of asthma, allergy, or other respiratory problems. Ask the parents what treatment has been effective in previous asthma episodes. A new case of asthma may begin as a cough without wheezing. The child may have had recurrent bouts of pneumonia or sinusitis.

Assessment during an acute asthma episode should include vital signs and a careful evaluation of respiratory and oxygenation status. Note respiratory rate and effort, the presence or absence of retractions, the use of accessory muscles, nasal flaring, and pulse oximetry values. Level of consciousness is an important indicator of oxygenation and should be assessed carefully. The chest should be carefully auscultated for breath sounds, noting any adventitious sounds or areas of diminished breath sounds. The child should be assessed for neurologic signs of impending respiratory failure (changes in consciousness, increased fatigue, somnolence). As infants and children become more hypoxic, they may not recognize or interact appropriately with their parents. Failure to resist or to cry during painful procedures is an ominous sign.*

Because tachypnea and decreased intake of oral fluids may cause dehydration, hydration status should also be assessed (urine output, status of mucous membranes, presence of tears, skin turgor, weight).

A record of the child's routines and habits should be included in the psychosocial history. Previous hospitalizations should be documented, because a past experience may affect the child's perception of the current illness. An assessment of the family's knowledge of the disease, degree of compliance, and growth and development provides the basis for future teaching.

Nursing Diagnoses

Ineffective Airway Clearance related to bronchospasm and mucosal edema.
Impaired Gas Exchange related to air trapping in the bronchioles.

Expected Outcomes

The child will:
- Be able to clear the airway, as evidenced by a respiratory rate and rhythm appropriate for the child's age, the ability to expectorate mucus, and normal vital signs for age.
- Have improved gas exchange, as evidenced by clear breath sounds, a pulse oximetry value of greater than 95% on room air, no use of accessory muscles, pink mucous membranes and nail beds, and a capillary refill time of less than 2 seconds.

INTERVENTION	RATIONALE
1. Monitor respiratory rate and effort, color, heart rate, and blood pressure every 15 to 30 minutes, with the interval lengthened as the child improves. Auscultate the chest for breath sounds. Monitor arterial blood gas values, pulse oximetry values, and pulmonary function test results. Notify the physician of any significant change (increased respiratory rate and effort, changes in wheezing, retractions, nasal flaring, severe cough, decreased alertness, cyanosis, increased dyspnea, apprehension).	1. Subtle changes in the child's condition may serve as an early warning of increased airway obstruction.
2. Administer humidified oxygen at the ordered flow rate. If the child has chronic carbon dioxide retention, do not exceed 2 L/min.	2. Supplemental oxygen decreases hypoxia secondary to airway edema, mucus, and bronchospasm. Administration of oxygen to a child with chronic carbon dioxide retention may lead to respiratory depression by decreasing the stimulus to breathe.
3. Help the child assume an upright position or position of comfort. The older child may be most comfortable leaning forward on a pillow or over-bed table.	3. An upright position aids in expansion of the lungs and decreases pressure on the diaphragm.
4. Administer medications as ordered, and monitor for effectiveness. Assess whether medications are effectively relieving the child's symptoms. Monitor the child for side effects.	4. Short-acting bronchodilators provide relief fairly quickly. Intravenous (IV) methylprednisolone begins to reduce airway inflammation.

*Bechler-Karsch, A. (1994). Assessment and management of status asthmaticus. *Pediatric Nursing, 20* (3), 217-223.

Nursing Care Plan

The Child Hospitalized With Asthma—cont'd

INTERVENTION	RATIONALE
5. Keep the child on nothing-by-mouth (NPO) status during periods of respiratory distress, as ordered by the physician.	5. Oral intake is contraindicated for the child in respiratory distress because of the risk for aspiration.
6. Maintain an IV line.	6. IV access is necessary for administering medications and fluids.
7. Ensure that respiratory treatments are given as ordered. Assess the child's breath sounds before and after treatments. Encourage the child to cough and deep breathe, especially after treatments. Suction as needed.	7. Breathing treatments help loosen or eliminate secretions and reexpand lung tissue. Mucous plugs can cause atelectasis and alveolar collapse.
8. Ensure that emergency equipment is available (e.g., appropriate-size ventilation bag, endotracheal tubes, laryngoscope, emergency medication).	8. The child's condition can deteriorate rapidly. Immediate resuscitation may be necessary in the event of severe respiratory distress.
9. Keep the child as calm as possible. Offer support during periods of respiratory distress.	9. Anxiety increases bronchospasms.

Evaluation

- Does the child have clear breath sounds with free movement of air?
- Does the child expend minimal respiratory effort?
- Does the child maintain a patent airway?
- Is the respiratory rate within normal limits for age, and is the oxygen saturation greater than 95%?

Nursing Diagnosis

Fatigue related to hypoxia and an increased work of breathing.

Expected Outcome

The child will:

- Exhibit decreased fatigue, as evidenced by less irritability and restlessness, uninterrupted sleep periods, and ability to perform usual activities.

INTERVENTION	RATIONALE
1. Observe the child for signs and symptoms of hypoxia, including restlessness, fatigue, irritability, increased heart rate, and increased respiratory rate.	1. Irritability and agitation may be early signs of hypoxia. Prompt treatment of hypoxia decreases fatigue.
2. Organize nursing care to provide periods of uninterrupted rest and sleep.	2. Periods of quiet decrease stress and promote rest.
3. Encourage the parents' presence, particularly if the child is young.	3. The parents' presence decreases fear and anxiety.
4. Provide for the child's physical comfort. Encourage quiet, age-appropriate play activities as the child's condition improves.	4. Physical and emotional comfort confers a sense of well-being and promotes rest.
5. Implement measures to relieve respiratory distress. Monitor the frequency of nebulized medications.	5. Restlessness, agitation, and inability to sleep are side effects of some asthma medications.

Evaluation

- Is the child able to play or perform usual activities without undue fatigue?

Nursing Diagnosis

Risk for Deficient Fluid Volume related to increased respiratory rate, diaphoresis, and decreased oral intake.

Expected Outcomes

The child will:

- Drink adequate fluid for age and weight.
- Not become dehydrated.

Continued

Nursing Care Plan

The Child Hospitalized With Asthma—cont'd

INTERVENTION	RATIONALE
1. Monitor intake and output, status of mucous membranes, body weight, tearing, and urine specific gravity. Maintain urine specific gravity at 1.002 to 1.030. Monitor electrolyte levels. Observe the child's sputum for color, tenacity, and amount.	1. Rapid respiratory rate, diaphoresis, and increased pulmonary secretions may cause dehydration and increased viscosity of excretions.
2. Maintain intravenous (IV) infusion at the ordered flow rate. Avoid excessive amounts of fluid.	2. Adequate hydration enhances liquefaction of secretions, and thinner secretions are more easily expectorated. Excessive fluids may lead to pulmonary edema.
3. Encourage oral fluids when the respiratory distress has decreased, with the amount consumed being determined by the child's calculated needs. Offer favorite fluids. Provide liquids at the bedside.	3. Oral fluids are contraindicated during acute respiratory distress to minimize the risk for aspiration. Children are most likely to drink fluids if they are offered fluids they like.
4. Offer liquids at room temperature. Avoid milk and milk products.	4. Cold liquids may aggravate bronchospasm. Milk sometimes causes increased coughing and production of mucus.
5. Provide a humidified atmosphere.	5. Humidification helps liquefy secretions and helps maintain hydration.

Evaluation

- Does the child ingest adequate fluid for age and weight?
- Does the child maintain a urine specific gravity of 1.002 to 1.030?
- Does the child maintain pre-illness weight?
- Are moist mucous membranes and good skin turgor present?
- Does the child have urinary output appropriate for age (see Chapter 42)?

Nursing Diagnosis

Anxiety related to hospitalization and respiratory distress.

Expected Outcomes

The child will:
- Exhibit reduced anxiety, as evidenced by a relaxed body position and a decrease in negative behaviors.

The parents will:
- Demonstrate reduced anxiety by verbalizing an accurate knowledge of asthma and participating in the child's care in a calm manner.

INTERVENTION	RATIONALE
1. Teach the child techniques to control panic and anxiety and to slow the breathing rate (e.g., visually imagining staying calm, breathing exercises, pursed-lip breathing, belly breathing).	1. Concentration on such activities during an asthma episode calms the child and decreases the fear of suffocation.
2. Maintain a calm, quiet environment and a reassuring manner. Stay with the child. Provide care efficiently and calmly.	2. The ability to remain calm decreases the child's oxygen demand and work of breathing.
3. Reassure the child that there is someone nearby to assist if breathing difficulties develop. To allay any fears about going to sleep, tell the child that someone will be watching at night. Make the call light available for older children.	3. Calm reassurance by the nurse can decrease the child's fear of suffocation and facilitate rest.
4. Use play therapy.	4. Therapeutic play allows the child to work through fears in a nonthreatening manner.

Nursing Care Plan

The Child Hospitalized With Asthma—cont'd

INTERVENTION	RATIONALE
5. Encourage the parents to stay with the child. Praise the parents for rooming-in and supporting the child.	5. The presence of a familiar person can decrease fear and anxiety.
6. Keep parents informed of treatments, routines, and the child's condition.	6. Reassuring the parents can help calm the child, because parental anxiety is quickly transferred to the child. Frequent and accurate updating of the child's condition reassures parents and decreases fear of the unknown.
7. Encourage expression of feelings by child and parents.	7. Expressing feelings can help relieve stress and guilt.
8. Avoid the use of sedatives.	8. Sedatives may depress respirations.
9. Explain all procedures in an age-appropriate manner.	9. Procedures and an unfamiliar hospital setting may produce anxiety. Explanations decrease fear of the unknown.
10. Facilitate trust by being truthful and acknowledging the discomfort of procedures.	10. Honesty fosters trust.

Evaluation

- Does the child cooperate with and participate in treatment and appear relaxed?
- Does the child obtain adequate rest and sleep?
- Do the parents verbalize decreased anxiety about the hospitalization and the child's condition?

Nursing Diagnosis

Interrupted Family Processes related to the possibility of a chronic illness.

Expected Outcomes

The family will:
- Cope with the child's illness and comply with management in a way that promotes the child's normal growth and development.

INTERVENTION	RATIONALE
1. Provide opportunities for the family to express feelings. Recognize and accept negative feelings about the child and the illness.	1. This nonjudgmental approach helps the family work through fear, guilt, anxiety, and economic problems.
2. Explore previous coping mechanisms used in times of stress.	2. Identification and review of previously successful coping skills can assist the family in dealing with the present crisis.
3. Explain all procedures and treatments.	3. A thorough explanation decreases fear of the unknown and anxiety.
4. Keep parents informed of the child's condition.	4. Knowledge gives parents a sense of control.
5. Arrange for the family to meet with others affected by asthma. Identify available community resources (see Appendix I on Evolve website).	5. Meeting others with asthma can assist with problem solving and provide support.

Evaluation

- Is the family able to provide necessary care?
- Can the family describe how to access helpful resources?

Continued

Nursing Care Plan

The Child Hospitalized With Asthma—cont'd

Nursing Diagnosis

Deficient Knowledge about the disease process and home management related to inexperience with asthma.

Expected Outcomes

The family will:
- Identify asthma triggers.
- Describe home management principles.

INTERVENTION	RATIONALE
1. Determine the child's and parents' understanding of asthma. Explain unfamiliar procedures and equipment at the child's level of understanding. Teach the family about the disease, its triggers, and prescribed medications and treatments.	1. Understanding increases compliance with treatment.
2. Help the family identify precipitating factors (e.g., exercise, infections, allergens, weather changes).	2. An awareness of triggers may decrease future asthma episodes.
3. Explain the role of emotions and stress in the development of asthma symptoms.	3. Stress and emotional upset can trigger bronchospasm.
4. Teach the child and family about the importance of taking medications as prescribed. Assess ability to afford medications. Provide written information and instructions about medications (names, side effects, dosages, times of administration). Teach the family to recognize signs and symptoms that warrant notification of the physician. Reinforce the need to keep follow-up appointments.	4. Knowledge of medications increases compliance with the therapeutic regimen; compliance helps maintain serum drug levels within a therapeutic range.
5. Assist in developing an exercise program for the child. Medication may be needed before exercise. Teach the importance of a healthy lifestyle (regular exercise, adequate fluids and nutrition, rest, prevention of infection).	5. Exercise promotes pulmonary and cardiovascular health and assists the child in leading a normal life.
6. Refer the family to a support group.	6. Meeting with other children and families affected by asthma provides an avenue for expressing feelings and sharing information.
7. Teach self-management of asthma. Teach the necessary skills for home care. Encourage the child to take charge of asthma. The child should know what triggers to avoid, early warning signs of an episode, the correct use of treatment aids (metered-dose inhaler [MDI], dry powder inhaler [DPI], nebulizer, peak flowmeter), as well as proper administration of medications and techniques for stress reduction and relaxation. Encourage the child and family to participate in programs designed to develop effective self-management and decision-making skills.	7. Knowledge of asthma decreases anxiety during acute episodes. The frequency and severity of episodes will be minimized if the child knows the appropriate actions for controlling symptoms. Learning about the condition can help decrease anxiety during episodes and increase the child's ability to take appropriate action to control symptoms. The frequency and severity of asthma episodes will be minimized if the child knows what triggers to avoid, the early warning signs of an episode, and the correct treatment of symptoms.
8. Teach the importance of follow-up care and routine health maintenance, such as keeping immunizations up-to-date.	8. Preventing infection and practicing healthy living habits help decrease asthma triggers.

Evaluation

- Do the child and family verbalize an accurate knowledge of asthma and its treatment?
- Do the child and family keep follow-up appointments?
- Does the child resume normal daily activities?

Nursing Care Plan

The Child With Asthma in the Community Setting

FOCUSED ASSESSMENT

Parents and children usually are successful managing asthma at home with the proper guidance from health care providers in the community. Whether in an outpatient facility or in a school health office, the nurse needs to know how to assess whether a child is experiencing an asthma exacerbation. It is important to obtain information about:

- The child's baseline peak flow reading and the current reading (calculate the percentage of baseline to determine if the child may need immediate intervention)
- Whether the child's respiratory effort has increased and whether the child complains of "feeling tight" or wheezing
- How often the child has taken an inhaled medication over the past 24 hours
- If the child has recently been exposed to an environmental trigger either at home or at school or whether the child has experienced a recent upper respiratory infection
- Whether the child is able to engage in usual activities and whether sleep has been interrupted because of respiratory signs

Nursing Diagnosis

Risk for Suffocation related to the child's response to environmental triggers and allergens.

Expected Outcomes

The child will:
- Avoid possible allergens.

The child and family will be able to:
- Detect signs of an impending asthma episode and implement appropriate interventions.

INTERVENTION	RATIONALE
1. Teach the child and family how to avoid situations that trigger an asthmatic episode.	1. Knowledge about the disease process will decrease possible asthma exacerbations.
2. Review potentially allergenic foods.	2. The child and family will be knowledgeable about specific food items that trigger an asthmatic response.
3. Remove or limit interaction with pets.	3. Removing pets will decrease potential asthma exacerbations because animal dander is a known allergen.
4. Assist the family in obtaining dehumidifier or air conditioner as needed.	4. The proper electronic device for controlling the environment at home for molds and mildew will help minimize exacerbations.
5. Eliminate the child's exposure to second-hand smoke.	5. Second-hand smoke is an irritant, and thus minimizing exposure will minimize exacerbation of asthma symptoms.
6. Teach the child and family to recognize early signs and symptoms of an asthmatic episode.	6. Control an impending episode before it becomes distressful.

Evaluation

- Is the family able to identify potential allergens that trigger episodes in the child?
- Is the family able to avoid or eliminate environmental triggers?
- Can the family and child describe what action they will take in the event of an asthma episode?

Nursing Diagnosis

Ineffective Airway Clearance related to bronchospasm and mucosal edema.

Expected Outcomes

The child will:
- Breathe easily without dyspnea.

The child and family will:
- Be able to use prescribed medications appropriately.

Continued

Nursing Care Plan

The Child With Asthma in the Community Setting—cont'd

INTERVENTION	RATIONALE
1. Review correct use of prescribed medications; write down orders and directions for the family and the school nurse.	1. It is important for the child and family to understand correct use of short-acting bronchodilators versus long-acting bronchodilators versus corticosteroids. Giving the school written directions improves management.
2. Teach proper use of peak flowmeter, nebulizer, MDI, DPI as indicated. Be sure the equipment is available for the child to use in school. Teach proper cleaning and maintenance of equipment.	2. Teaching optimizes the therapeutic benefit of medications as well as compliance.
3. Educate the family about prophylactic treatments when appropriate.	3. Education will minimize the need for rescue medications.
4. Review with the child and family the emergency plan if rescue medications are not effective.	4. Having a plan of action will decrease the family's and child's anxiety.
5. Explain immunotherapy to the child and family if prescribed.	5. Allergy shots are often prescribed in allergic asthma. It is important for the child and family to understand the benefits and reasons for frequent visits.

Evaluation

- Are the child and family able to demonstrate proper use of prescribed devices?
- Are the child and family able to discuss when and how to utilize prescribed medications?
- Does the family keep appointments for immunotherapy?
- Does the family contact the pediatrician and/or access local emergency department when prescribed rescue medications are not effective?
- Does the child know when to visit the school health office if having problems at school?

Nursing Diagnosis

Activity Intolerance related to fatigue and shortness of breath.

Expected Outcome

The child will:
- Be able to participate in normal daily activities, obtain adequate rest and sleep, and participate in physical activity without shortness of breath.

INTERVENTION	RATIONALE
1. Encourage appropriate activities for the child's capabilities, including sports and other school or recreational activities.	1. Participating in activities will promote a sense of well-being and foster the child's independence.
2. Review with the child and family symptoms of difficulty breathing, times to take medication, and a plan for rest periods during the day as needed.	2. The child and family will know when to administer rescue medications as prescribed and/or limit activity.
3. Discuss with the child and family a plan for adequate sleep and rest.	3. Scheduled rest and adequate nighttime sleep will promote health and minimize fatigue.

Evaluation

- Is the child able to participate in normal daily activities?
- Does the child obtain adequate sleep and rest?
- Is the child able to engage in physical activity without excess fatigue?

Nursing Diagnosis

Deficient Knowledge related to unfamiliarity with the pathophysiology of the disease and treatment regimen.

Expected Outcomes

The family and child (if age-appropriate) will:
- Describe the disease process.
- Demonstrate any associated treatment.

Nursing Care Plan

The Child With Asthma in the Community Setting—cont'd

INTERVENTION	RATIONALE
1. Reinforce proper use of medications and prescribed devices; give family members written instructions, and advise them to keep a peak flow diary.	1. Having accurate knowledge will decrease anxiety as well as improve compliance.
2. Encourage verbalization of concerns and fears about diagnosis.	2. Expressing feelings will alleviate anxiety.
3. Reinforce the need to respond to early signs of asthma episode using prescribed medications.	3. When the child and family have accurate knowledge, they will respond with preventive and/or emergency interventions in a timely fashion.
4. Encourage contact with daycare or school personnel about diagnosis and treatment plan.	4. It is important to communicate the plan of care to all individuals caring for the child.
5. Refer the family to appropriate support group.	5. It is helpful to meet with other children and families affected by asthma because they can offer support, suggestions, and information about the practical aspects of caring for a child with asthma.

Evaluation

- Can the family and child, if appropriate, demonstrate use of devices?
- Can the family verbalize the correct use of medications and their side effects?
- Have the family and child responded to early signs of an impending asthma episode in a timely and appropriate manner?

BRONCHOPULMONARY DYSPLASIA

Bronchopulmonary dysplasia (BPD) is a chronic obstructive pulmonary disease that occurs as a result of acute lung injury in some infants who have received supplemental oxygen and mechanical ventilation. BPD is now commonly referred to as *chronic lung disease of infancy* (CLD).

Etiology

Lung immaturity seems to be a key factor in the development of BPD, but many other factors affect its development as well. Genetic predisposition, a family history of atopic disorders, oxygen exposure (which injures immature lungs), positive-pressure ventilation (which stretches lung tissue), neonatal respiratory infection, and inadequate nutrition in the very immature neonate are all risk factors for BPD (Nieves & Chernick, 2002). Infants with BPD often also have patent ductus arteriosus (see Chapter 46). Because lung development varies among infants, gestational age alone does not always predict the development of BPD.

Incidence

BPD is a significant cause of morbidity and mortality among very-low-birth-weight infants (<1000 g) and infants who have survived RDS. It is the most frequently seen chronic lung condition in infants. The current high survival rates of low-birth-weight, preterm infants have resulted in the disorder being seen more often.

Pathophysiology

of Bronchopulmonary Dysplasia

The pressures of mechanical ventilation damage bronchial epithelium. Macrophages and polymorphonuclear inflammatory cells invade the airways, causing airway edema. Alveolar walls become thickened, and fibrotic changes occur in the airways and alveoli. The continued use of oxygen affects the growth and development of lung structures, significantly reducing the number of developing alveoli.

Cystic and atelectatic areas develop in the lungs, predisposing the infant to pulmonary hypertension. Loss of ciliated cells also may occur, which decreases the lungs' ability to remove mucus and leads to mucous plugs, atelectasis, and pneumonia.

Manifestations

Manifestations of BPD include tachycardia and tachypnea related to decreased oxygenation; an increased work of breathing, retractions, and prolonged exhalation with the increased use of abdominal and accessory muscles; pallor associated with chronic hypoxia; and cyanosis and activity intolerance (feeding, handling). Affected infants also exhibit weight loss or poor weight gain related to the increased metabolic workload, hypoxia, and poor feeding; restlessness and irritability related to hypoxia; wheezing (intermittent or chronic) associated with a hyperresponsive airway; and puckering or pursing of the mouth with flaring of the nares (early signs of impending respiratory distress).

Diagnostic Evaluation

The diagnosis is based on clinical manifestations and radiographic abnormalities. Infants with respiratory symptoms that persist beyond 28 days of life, who need supplemental oxygen by 1 to 2 weeks of age and are still oxygen-dependent after 28 days, or who need mechanical ventilation during the first week of life are suspected of having BPD. Chest radiographs may show infiltrates.

Therapeutic Management

Treatment goals for the infant with BPD include maintaining adequate oxygenation to promote growth and development, preventing further lung disease, and promoting healing of the damaged lungs. Treatment consists of oxygen therapy, drug therapy, and nutritional support.

Positive-pressure ventilation should be discontinued as soon as possible. If mechanical ventilation is necessary to maintain life, the lowest possible inflation pressures should be used, together with expiratory times that allow the lung to empty completely. Weaning from the ventilator may be a slow, tedious process, sometimes requiring many months to complete and often interrupted by infections and other problems (Wadlinger, 1999).

Oxygen Therapy

Approximately 10% of infants with BPD will need supplemental oxygen for more than 1 year (Hazinski, 1998). Oxygen can be administered through a hood, tent, facemask, or nasal cannula. Oxygen saturation rates should be monitored closely and should be maintained between 92% and 94%. Many infants are discharged from the hospital while still oxygen-dependent.

Medications

Diuretics and fluid restriction are initiated to treat pulmonary interstitial edema. Furosemide is the most common diuretic used, with some physicians attempting to change to chlorothiazide and spironolactone once enteral feeds are tolerated. Because infants with BPD often experience fluid overload and edema, fluid and electrolyte status should be monitored closely. Supplemental calcium, potassium, and chloride may be indicated for the infant receiving diuretics.

Inhaled bronchodilators, especially albuterol, when given in the early stages of BPD, can lessen airway resistance and decrease the possibility of lung damage. The corticosteroid dexamethasone is often administered during weaning from mechanical ventilation. Careful monitoring during steroid administration is needed, because dexamethasone increases lung compliance, putting the infant at risk for pulmonary barotrauma. Administration of inhaled glucocorticoids early on has been shown to decrease the use of systemic glucocorticoid therapy as well as mechanical ventilation (Jobe & Ikegami, 2001).

Infants with BPD experience frequent infections related to increased susceptibility and exposure to invasive treatments and procedures. After the initial stages of BPD, the risk for infection is probably the greatest risk to survival for these infants. Antibiotics are often needed. Ribavirin may be given to infants with RSV.

Nutrition

The infant needs increased nutritional intake for lung growth and repair beyond that required for normal infant growth. Other factors, such as frequent respiratory exacerbations and feeding problems, also increase caloric needs. A calorie intake of 110 to 150 kcal/kg/day to produce a weight gain of 15 to 30 g/day (Atkinson, 2001) is an appropriate goal. High-calorie formulas (24 or 27 cal/oz) assist with meeting this requirement, especially in infants in whom fluids are restricted. Medium-chain triglyceride (MCT) oil or glucose polymers, if added to the formula, increase the calories per ounce.

Prognosis

Most infants with BPD do improve. The mortality ranges from 10% to 25%; death usually is a result of pulmonary complications. Most infants with BPD will require ongoing therapy at home, and some will develop chronic airway hyperreactivity, which may progress to bronchial asthma. These problems are detected even in adolescents who were chronically oxygen-dependent after premature birth (Greenough, 2000). Many infants with BPD are rehospitalized during the first year of life because of acute respiratory tract infections. Infants have growth retardation and developmental delay for the first 24 to 36 months of life (Abrams, 2001).

Nursing Considerations

Because of their low birth weight and possible RDS, most neonates with BPD are initially cared for in a special care nursery. Nursing intervention before discharge includes meticulous planning for home care, coordinating referrals, and teaching home management.

Home care of the infant with BPD decreases the risk for hospital-acquired infection and reduces health care costs. Care at home also improves social development by encouraging interaction between the child and family.

Preparation for discharge and home care requires a great deal of education and reassurance. Educating the family with a chronically ill or technology-dependent child must begin early with basic care—feeding, bathing, holding, and playing. This care progresses to medical, nursing, and respiratory procedures. The infant may continue to receive supplemental oxygen at home or may have a tracheostomy. Some infants are discharged while they are still ventilator-dependent. Families must be taught the necessary precautions for safe use of oxygen in the home. Before hospital discharge, the nurse contacts emergency services, utility companies, and the telephone company to notify them that a technology-dependent child will be living in their area (Fig. 45-5). Required actions for contacting these services in case of emergency should be reviewed with the family.

Evaluating the family's response to the infant's illness and their coping strategies is critical for optimal home management of the infant with a chronic condition. The nurse should help the family identify physical as well as psychological strengths and weaknesses. Because the care of an infant with BPD can be extraordinarily expensive, the nurse should consider referring the family to social services for access to potential financial assistance.

PARENTS
Want to Know

About Safe Use of Oxygen at Home

Safety Guidelines	Rationale
Secure the oxygen tank in an upright position.	Oxygen tanks are highly explosive. If a horizontally positioned tank explodes, the rapid release of oxygen can catapult it through both animate (human bodies) and inanimate (walls) objects.
Keep oxygen tanks at least 5 feet from heat sources and electrical devices (e.g., space heaters, heating vents, fireplaces, radios, vaporizers).	
Ensure that no one smokes in the room or in the area of the oxygen tank.	Smoking increases the risk for fire, which could cause the tank to explode; escaped oxygen would feed the fire.
Avoid using alcohol-based substances or oil to relieve dryness around your child's mouth (e.g., petroleum jelly, vitamin A & D ointment, baby oil).	Both alcohol and oil are flammable and increase the risk for fire.
Keep a fire extinguisher readily available.	A fire extinguisher may be needed to put out a fire immediately.
Turn off both the volume regulator and the flow regulator when oxygen is not in use.	If the volume regulator is on when the oxygen is turned on, the child might receive a rapid, forceful flow of oxygen in the face that could be frightening and uncomfortable. Oxygen leakage, which might not be detected because oxygen is odorless, can cause a fire.

ELECTRIC COMPANY
REQUEST FOR SPECIAL CONSIDERATION

Date: _____

Name: _____
Address: _____
_____
Phone: _____
Account Number: _____

Attention: Customer Service

Our infant/child, _____ , is under the
care of Dr. _____ at _____
for _____. This condition(s) requires the use of a
cardiorespiratory monitor and/or other life support equipment, specifically:

_____

The necessary equipment selected for home care is equipped with a battery back-up system that will power the equipment in the event of a power failure for a limited period of time. If a power failure occurs, it is imperative to restore service to this home as soon as possible. Please place this home on a priority list for restoration of electric service. If you have advance warning of a temporary interruption in electric service, please notify the parents so alternative arrangements can be made. If you have questions regarding the specifications of the equipment provided, please contact our equipment provider, Pediatric Home Care Associates.

Thank you for your cooperation.

Sincerely yours,

OUR EQUIPMENT PROVIDER IS: _____

Figure 45-5 Example of a letter that can be used to notify the local public service company that a technology-dependent child is living in the service area. (Courtesy Pediatric Home Care Associates, Garfield, NJ. From Barnhart, S.L., & Czervinske, M.P. [1995]. *Perinatal and pediatric respiratory care* [p. 662]. Philadelphia: Saunders.)

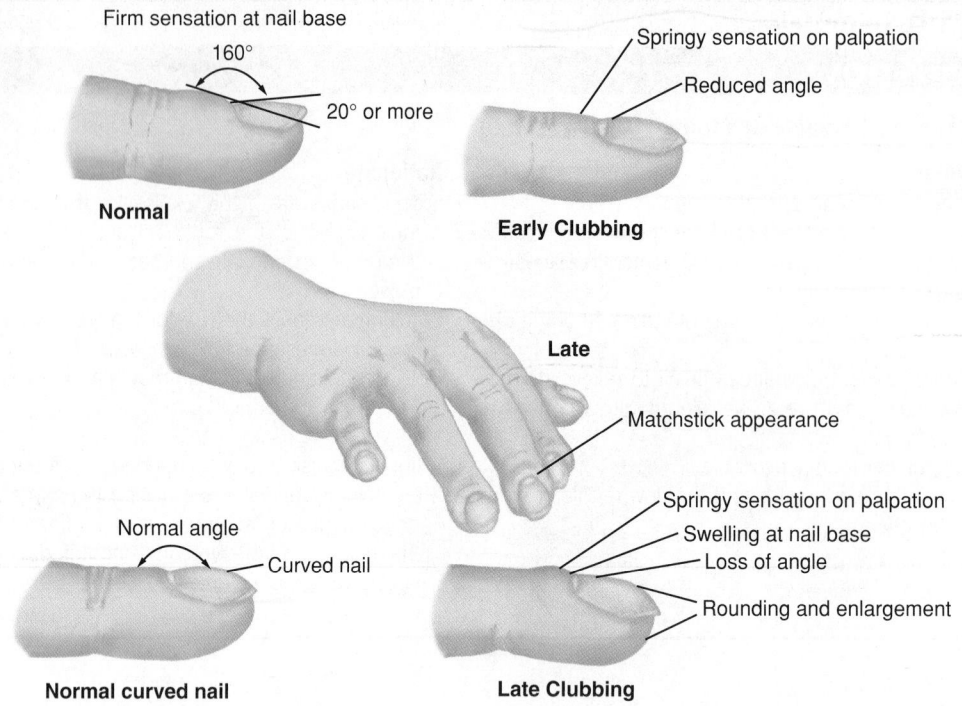

Figure 45-6 Digital clubbing may be an indication of hypoxia, which often occurs in cystic fibrosis and other respiratory disorders.

CYSTIC FIBROSIS

Cystic fibrosis (CF), the most common lethal genetic disease in whites, is a chronic multisystem disorder affecting the exocrine glands. The mucus produced by the exocrine glands (particularly those of the bronchioles, small intestine, and pancreatic and bile ducts) is abnormally thick, causing obstruction of the small passageways of these organs. Although CF is incurable, the life expectancy of affected children has increased dramatically. The median survival age is 33 years, making CF a disease not only of children but also of young adults. The discovery of the mutated gene encoding a defective chloride channel in epithelial cells (named *cystic fibrosis transmembrane conductance regulator [CFTR]*) has improved clinicians' understanding of the disorder's pathophysiology and has significantly aided diagnosis.

Etiology

CF is transmitted as an autosomal recessive trait, which means that both parents must carry the gene for the child to be affected. If both parents carry the CF gene, each pregnancy has a 25% chance of producing an affected child. The CF gene has been localized to the long arm of chromosome 7.

Incidence

The incidence of CF in white children is approximately 1 in 4000 live births (Ratjen & Doring, 2003). The prevalence in African-Americans is considerably lower, and CF rarely affects Latinos or Asians. It is estimated that 1 in 28 white Americans carries the gene for CF. Of all patients with CF in the US, 50% are diagnosed by 6 months of age and 90% by 8 years (Ratjen & Doring, 2003).

Manifestations

Signs and symptoms of CF, the extent of specific organ system involvement, and age at which symptoms begin vary widely among affected children. Symptoms gradually worsen as the disease progresses, and the outcome is eventually fatal.

Respiratory System

Signs and symptoms of respiratory involvement include wheezing and a dry, nonproductive cough (earliest pulmonary manifestations), repeated bouts of pneumonia and bronchitis, and purulent and copious sputum accompanying chronic bacterial infections. The cough at this stage is wet and paroxysmal and may be followed by vomiting. Crackles, wheezes, and diminished breath sounds; accessory muscle use, retractions, hypoxia, and cyanosis; and increased cough, dyspnea, tachypnea, and cyanosis occur as the disease progresses. Emphysema and atelectasis may develop as the airways become increasingly obstructed with secretions; cor pulmonale and congestive heart failure secondary to fibrotic lung changes can be seen in later stages of the disease. Spontaneous pneumothorax or hemoptysis (blood-stained sputum) is seen in later stages as well. Nasal polyps (10%-25% of patients), sinusitis (evident on radiography in nearly 90% of patients), digital clubbing (Fig. 45-6), and a barrel chest (increased anteroposterior chest diameter) are also noted.

Digestive System

Digestive system involvement is marked by steatorrhea (frothy, foul-smelling stools two to three times bulkier than normal) and flatus. Malnutrition and growth failure are evident despite normal caloric intake; deficiencies in fat-soluble vitamins A, D, E, and K are caused by an inability to absorb fats. Vitamin A deficiency may lead to xerophthalmia (abnormal thickening of

Pathophysiology

of Cystic Fibrosis

Cystic fibrosis (CF) affects the exocrine glands throughout the body and causes respiratory, digestive, integumentary, and reproductive dysfunction and damage.

Respiratory System

Abnormally thick, sticky secretions cause obstruction of both the small and large airways. Stasis of secretions from bronchial obstruction provides a medium for bacterial growth. Chronic infection causes the release of toxic chemicals that damage lung tissues and alter host defenses within the airways, thus exacerbating the infection and inflammation. Inflammation may also cause bronchospasm, worsening airway blockage. Because airways dilate on inspiration and constrict on exhalation, air trapping occurs in the peripheral airways narrowed by mucous secretions. Hyperinflation is one of the first findings on chest radiographs of a child with CF. Chronic infection leads to atelectasis and eventual fibrosis and destruction of pulmonary tissue.

As the disease progresses, the lungs of almost all children with CF eventually become colonized with *Pseudomonas aeruginosa,* an organism that most clinicians believe can never be completely eradicated from the respiratory tract but can be controlled with vigorous antibiotic therapy. With chronic respiratory tract infection, impaired oxygen and carbon dioxide exchange causes varying degrees of hypoxia, hypercapnia, and acidosis. Fibrotic lung changes occur as the disease worsens and hypoxia increases. Alveolar hypoxia leads to pulmonary vasoconstriction, increasing pulmonary vascular resistance. Increased pulmonary vascular resistance causes the right side of the heart to work harder to pump blood into the lungs. Enlargement of the right ventricle in response to increased pulmonary resistance (cor pulmonale) results. Congestive heart failure may develop. Pulmonary complications include sinusitis, spontaneous pneumothorax, and hemoptysis. Death in individuals with CF is almost always the result of respiratory failure.

Digestive System

Eighty-five percent of patients with CF have pancreatic involvement. The pancreatic ducts, blocked by thick mucus, are unable to secrete trypsin, amylase, and lipase into the small intestine. Without these digestive enzymes, proteins, carbohydrates, and fats are poorly absorbed. Bowel obstruction from thickened intestinal mucus and pancreatic insufficiency may be present at birth (meconium ileus). The islets of Langerhans in the pancreas are normal in patients with CF, but they may decrease in number as the disease progresses and the pancreas undergoes fibrotic changes. Older children with CF sometimes develop type 1 diabetes mellitus. Abnormalities of the gallbladder are common.

Integumentary System

The sweat glands of children with CF secrete normal amounts of sweat. The levels of sodium and chloride in the sweat, however, are two to five times the normal range.

Reproductive System

Ninety-eight percent of males with CF are sterile because of obstruction of the deferent ducts and seminal vesicles. Females have reduced fertility because of abnormally thick cervical mucus, which impedes sperm penetration of the cervical canal.

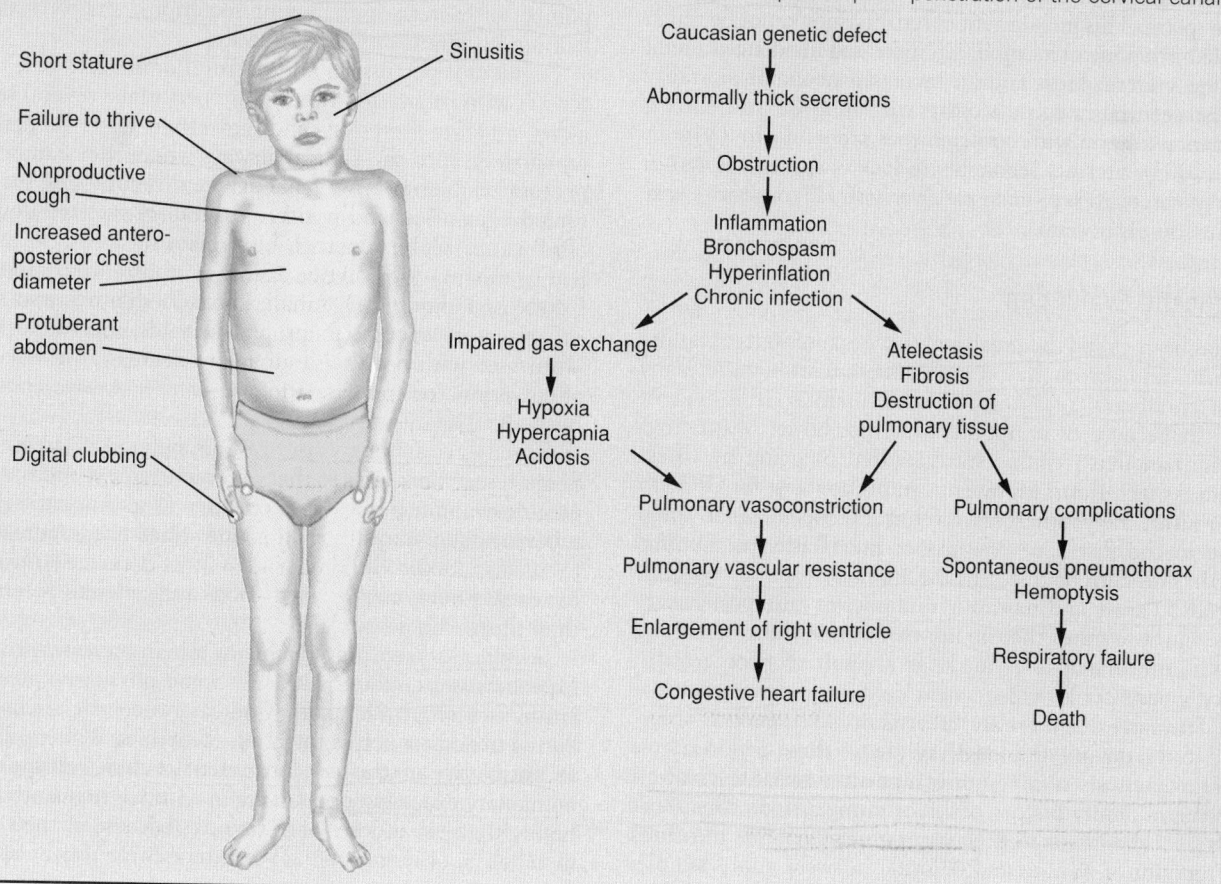

eye tissue), and vitamin K deficiency may result in bleeding, especially in infants. Children with CF are usually thin and underweight, but with adequate treatment most attain normal height. Eighteen percent of children with CF are assigned to less than the 5th percentile for height or weight (Cystic Fibrosis Foundation, 2002). A protuberant abdomen, barrel chest, wasted buttocks, and thin extremities are common.

Meconium ileus in the neonate is the earliest clinical manifestation of CF. Intestinal obstruction later in life, called *meconium ileus equivalent*, may occur and is the result of impacted feces at the ileocecal junction. Rectal prolapse and intussusception may also occur. Liver disease, as manifested by biliary cirrhosis, portal hypertension, and esophageal varices, secondary to obstruction of the bile ducts, is seen in 17% to 25% of CF patients (Feranchak & Sokol, 2001). Diabetes mellitus has evolved as a complication because of increased longevity. The prevalence of diabetes increases with age—at 30 years, 50% of those with CF are diabetic (Moran, 2002).

Exocrine Glands

Abnormally high concentrations of sodium and chloride in sweat are an early sign of CF (mothers often report that their infants taste salty when kissed). The risk for electrolyte imbalance during hot weather is high; infants are especially prone to developing hyponatremia and hypochloremia as well as dehydration. Many children complain of dry mouth and have an increased susceptibility to infection.

Reproductive System

Reproductive system involvement is marked by an average of 2 years' delay in the development of secondary sex characteristics. Females with CF may have difficulty becoming pregnant because of the thick cervical mucus, which acts as a barrier to sperm. This impairment of fertility should not be relied on as a birth control method. An increased incidence of fetal loss and preterm birth and an increased neonatal mortality are also seen, although a woman with mild CF can carry a pregnancy to term with conscientious prenatal care (Virgilis et al., 2003). Sterility secondary to lack of sperm is noted in approximately 98% of male patients with CF; otherwise sexual function is normal.

Diagnostic Evaluation

CF has been called the great imitator because signs of failure to thrive and chronic respiratory infection are signs of many other childhood conditions. In some infants, CF is evident at birth because of symptoms of severe bowel obstruction (meconium ileus) caused by intestinal plugging by thick, tenacious secretions. Many U.S. states now test for CF with the routine newborn screen. Thus the diagnosis is often made in the first 2 to 3 weeks of life (Ratjen & Doring, 2003). The current test uses the immunoreactive trypsinogen (IRT) assay and has a high number of false-positive results. In those states that do not perform newborn screening for CF, the diagnosis is made as a result of poor growth; bulky, greasy stools; and frequent colds or bouts of pneumonia. The early diagnosis and treatment of CF make a difference in the quality and length of life for these children.

The diagnosis of CF requires a positive sweat test as well as either a family history of CF or clinical signs consistent with CF. The sweat test, *pilocarpine iontophoresis*, measures the amount of sodium and chloride in sweat and is simple,

painless, and reliable. It is usually performed twice to ensure accuracy. A chloride level greater than 60 mEq/L is considered to be diagnostic for CF; a level of 40 to 60 mEq/L is suggestive of CF and requires repeating the test. A sample of at least 50 mg of sweat is required for accurate results. Because this amount is difficult to obtain from small infants, the sweat test is usually not reliable in infants younger than 3 weeks.

In addition to the sweat test, the following studies may also be performed: 72-hour fecal fat determination; liver function tests (alanine transaminase [ALT], aspartate transaminase [AST]); fasting blood glucose test; chest radiography; sputum culture (for identification of infective organisms); and pulmonary function tests.

DNA analysis of chorionic villi samples or amniotic fluid testing can establish a diagnosis prenatally. DNA analysis (via buccal smear or blood sample) can also determine whether siblings of the affected child are carriers.

Therapeutic Management

Therapy is individualized for each child and is aimed at preventing and treating pulmonary infections, maintaining optimal nutritional status, and promoting psychological adjustment. Children with CF are cared for at home most of the time. They are hospitalized during acute pulmonary infections, periodically for IV antibiotic treatment and vigorous chest physical therapy (CPT), and for end-stage disease.

Respiratory Problems

Because chronic respiratory infection is a major cause of lung damage in patients with CF, treatment goals are to relieve airway obstruction by mobilizing secretions, to decrease the number of bacteria by removing secretions, and to treat infections by administering antibiotics.

Segmental percussion and postural drainage (see Chapter 37) with inhalation therapy are performed several times a day to loosen secretions and move them from the peripheral airways into the central airways where they can be expectorated. Newer airway management techniques, such as forced exhalation and positive expiratory pressure devices (PEP valve, Flutter device), have been successful in mobilizing mucus. Mucolytic agents (inhaled recombinant DNase or Pulmozyme), inhaled bronchodilators, and anti-inflammatory agents (ibuprofen, steroids, macrolides) are often used with postural drainage to decrease the viscosity of secretions or increase the size of the airways (Jaffe & Bush, 2001).

Exercise is an important part of pulmonary treatment. Some researchers suggest that aerobic exercise, such as jogging or swimming, may be as effective as traditional CPT in relieving pulmonary obstruction and adherence is more likely (Samuels, 2000). Children with CF who exercise regularly have fewer pulmonary exacerbations and generally feel better than those who do not.

Antibiotics have played a major role in increasing the life expectancy of children with CF. Some physicians prescribe antibiotics prophylactically, whereas others use them only during periods of active infection (Smyth & Walters, 2003). IV antibiotics are the usual treatment of choice during acute pulmonary exacerbations. Children with CF frequently need higher-than-usual doses of antibiotics because of their rapid metabolism of these drugs. IV antibiotics are usually administered during hospitalization, but home IV therapy is becoming more widely accepted, offering substantial savings and minimizing disruption of daily activities. Oral or aerosolized antibiotics (Tobramycin Solution for Inhalation [TOBI]) may be used instead of IV therapy.

Steroids are sometimes prescribed when pulmonary symptoms are unresponsive to antibiotics and increased CPT because they decrease inflammation in the lung. Because of the side effects of steroid therapy, including growth retardation and altered glucose tolerance, oral steroids are most often prescribed in short courses of 5 to 7 days (Boat, 2004). High-dose ibuprofen has also been used for its antiinflammatory properties (Konstan & Davis, 2002). Azithromycin has been shown to improve lung function and decrease the need for IV antibiotics in a small study of patients (Equi, Balfour-Lynn, Bush, & Rosenthal, 2002). Oxygen therapy also is used with caution, because many children with CF have chronic carbon dioxide retention and are at risk for oxygen-induced carbon dioxide narcosis.

Digestive Problems

Early in the course of CF, the child may exhibit a huge appetite but not gain weight. Chronic pulmonary infections, an increased work of breathing, and malabsorption place an increased caloric and protein demand on the child with CF. The child's calorie requirements are approximately 150% of the normal recommended daily allowance (RDA). Children with CF are managed with a high-calorie, high-protein diet, pancreatic enzyme replacement therapy, fat-soluble vitamin supplements, and, if nutritional problems are severe, nighttime gastrostomy feedings or total parenteral nutrition. Fats are not restricted unless steatorrhea cannot be controlled by increased pancreatic enzymes.

Infants are sometimes given a predigested formula (Pregestimil, Nutramigen), which is more easily absorbed than regular formula. Formulas may also be concentrated to provide increased calories. For the older child, caloric intake may be increased with food supplements or enteral tube feedings. The administration of growth hormone has had significant improvement in both height velocity and weight gain in children with CF (Hardin, 2002).

Enteric-coated microencapsulated pancreatic enzyme preparations (Ultrase, Creon, Pancrease) are administered with every meal and snack. Enzyme dosage is adjusted according to stool formation: less enzyme with constipation; more enzyme with loose, fatty stools. Bowel obstruction has been reported as being associated with high-dose enzyme replacement (lipase, 6000 U/kg/meal) but recent studies have not supported this belief (Dialer, Hundt, Bertele-Harms, & Harms, 2003). Still, the enzyme dosage should be individualized for each child and kept as low as possible while still maintaining the child's nutritional status. Extra salt is added to the diet in extremely hot weather or when the child exercises vigorously.

■ NURSING CARE

The Child With Cystic Fibrosis

Assessment

The child with CF should be assessed for signs and symptoms in each of the systems usually affected by the disease, as well as for psychosocial adaptation to this chronic condition.

Respiratory Assessment

The child may have had frequent episodes of pneumonia or bronchitis. Auscultate the chest to detect any crackles, wheezes, areas of diminished breath sounds, or a prolonged expiratory phase of respiration. Note signs of long-standing respiratory difficulty, such as barrel chest or digital clubbing. The respiratory status is assessed by noting the rate, depth, and ease of respirations; from the color of the nail beds and mucous membranes; and by pulse oximetry. The characteristics of the child's cough and the color, amount, and quality of sputum should be documented, along with any fever. Exercise tolerance and the child's ability to sleep lying down at night should also be assessed.

Digestive Assessment

The nurse weighs and measures the child, plotting the results on a standardized growth chart. Signs of malabsorption (e.g., steatorrhea; loose, bulky stools; protuberant abdomen with thin extremities) should be noted. A diet history is useful in assessing the child's caloric intake. The use of vitamins and dietary supplements should be recorded. Determining the number and consistency of stools assesses the adequacy of intestinal enzyme replacement. Because ulcers and intestinal obstruction often accompany CF, complaints of abdominal pain, blood in the stools, and constipation should be noted. Use of antacids, H_2-receptor blockers, or antireflux medications should also be assessed.

Reproductive Assessment

Girls should be assessed for vaginal itching or drainage, which may indicate a vaginal infection. Contraception should be discussed with adolescents.

Nursing Diagnosis and Planning

The nursing diagnoses and expected outcomes that often apply to children with CF are

- Ineffective Airway Clearance related to increased pulmonary secretions.

  Expected Outcome: The child will be able to remove secretions from the airway.

- Impaired Gas Exchange related to air trapping within the alveoli secondary to obstruction of the airways by thick mucus.

  Expected Outcome: The child will maintain an oxygen saturation level of greater than 95%.

- Risk for Infection related to tenacious secretions and altered body defenses.

  Expected Outcome: The child will remain free of infection.

- Imbalanced Nutrition: Less Than Body Requirements related to poor intestinal absorption of nutrients.

  Expected Outcomes: The child's nutritional status will improve, and the child will exhibit normal growth; the child's stools will be of normal consistency, frequency, and color.

- Activity Intolerance related to pulmonary congestion and poor absorption of nutrients.

  Expected Outcomes: The child will rest comfortably and will engage in age-appropriate activities.

- Situational Low Self-Esteem related to physical changes from chronic illness.

  Expected Outcome: The child will demonstrate a positive self-concept and feelings of independence, as demonstrated by participating in self-care and in age-appropriate activities.

- Ineffective Coping (individual) and Compromised Family Coping related to chronic illness.
  Expected Outcomes: The child and family will comply with the treatment regimen, will verbalize feelings about the impact of the illness on their lives, and will use available support systems and community resources.
- Anticipatory Grieving related to a potentially fatal diagnosis.
  Expected Outcomes: The child and family will make realistic plans for the future and will be able to discuss feelings about the child's prognosis.

Interventions

Facilitating Airway Clearance and Gas Exchange

Perform CPT two or three times a day and as needed; perform treatments at least 1 hour before or 2 hours after meals to reduce gastrointestinal upset. The child's respiratory status should be determined before and after CPT. Note the child's tolerance of the procedure. Teach "huffing" (forced expiration) to mobilize secretions. The child should take a deep breath and then exhale rapidly while whispering the word "huff." Administer ordered bronchodilators or mucolytics in conjunction with CPT or as ordered. There are now many techniques from which to choose to facilitate airway clearance (Davidson, 2002). These include PEP valve, autogenic drainage, active cycle of breathing, Flutter valve, Acapella, and the ThAIRapy® vest.

To facilitate gas exchange, administer humidified, low-flow (2 L/min or less) oxygen as ordered. The recommended amount of oxygen should not be exceeded because too much oxygen administered to children who are chronically hypoxic can depress respirations. Elevate the head of the bed, or support the child in an upright position, if the child is dyspneic. Be sure to stay with the child during coughing episodes.

Preventing Infection

Children with CF are prone to respiratory infection, especially airway colonization with *Pseudomonas aeruginosa,* and oral or inhaled antibiotic therapy may be routine. IV antibiotics may be required during acute exacerbations. Pay meticulous attention to hygiene measures, especially handwashing, and teach the child and family to do the same. Monitor the child for signs of respiratory infection (fever, chills, increased respirations, dyspnea, cough, purulent secretions, increased WBC count). Advise the family to avoid exposing the child to others who are ill. Children with CF should receive all routine childhood immunizations at ages recommended by the American Academy of Pediatrics (see Appendix D). An annual influenza vaccine also is appropriate, based on recommendations by the Centers for Disease Control and Prevention (CDC).

Providing Optimal Nutrition for Growth

Provide a well-balanced diet that is high in calories, protein, and carbohydrates and that includes the child's favorite foods. Oral or enteral high-calorie supplements can increase the child's calorie intake.

The child needs to take pancreatic enzymes (which come as enteric-coated capsules containing the enzyme beads) as ordered within 30 minutes of eating all meals and snacks. The child should not mix the enzymes with hot or starchy foods because enzymes are inactivated by heat. Most older children can swallow the enteric-coated pancreatic enzyme capsules. For children who cannot swallow capsules, the capsules may be opened to display the beads, which can then be mixed with a small amount of a nonprotein food. Because prolonged contact with enzyme beads may cause excoriation of oral mucosa, wipe off any beads that remain on the child's lips. Advise the family to note the color, consistency, and frequency of the child's stools because enzyme replacement is correlated with the child's bowel elimination pattern (e.g., an acceptable pattern is one or two stools daily in older children and more often in infancy). The enzyme dosage should be increased when high-fat foods are eaten. Administer multivitamins, water-miscible, fat-soluble vitamins, and iron supplements as ordered. Monitor the child's appetite and food intake. Extra salt and fluid are required when the weather is hot.

Promoting Increased Exercise Tolerance

For the child in acute exacerbation, provide rest periods between treatments and organize nursing care to ensure periods of uninterrupted rest. The child's activity level is increased as tolerated. Arrange age-appropriate activities geared to the child's energy level. When the child is feeling well, encourage active play and activities, such as swimming and gymnastics.

Meeting the Child's and Family's Emotional Needs

Encourage the child to express feelings about the chronic illness and its effect on feelings of self-worth. Identifying a support system is especially important for adolescents as they begin to take responsibility for their health (Graetz, Shute, & Sawyer, 2000). Helping the child identify personal strengths and areas of accomplishment will increase the child's self-esteem. Teach parents the importance of fostering independence in their child. As the child grows, encourage discussion about areas of concern, such as dating, sexuality, and peer acceptance. Assist families with the child's transition from pediatric to adult health care providers.

Introducing the family to other families affected by CF can increase problem-solving strategies and facilitate support. Provide information about available community resources, such as the Cystic Fibrosis Foundation and the American Lung Association (see Appendix I on Evolve website). The family also should be encouraged to communicate with personnel at the child's school to ensure coordination of care between home and school.

Although tremendous progress has been made in treating CF, it remains a chronic disease with no cure. Provide the family with honest information about the disease and its prognosis. Refer the family for counseling, and listen if they wish to discuss feelings about the disease, the future, and possible death.

Home Care

Preparation for home care involves teaching family members how to carry out CPT, how to provide breathing treatments, and how to give medications at home. Written instructions should describe the specifics of all aspects of the child's care. Families may need assistance in obtaining home care equipment.

Evaluation

- Does the child exhibit improved breath sounds, oxygen saturation greater than 95% on room air, and stable respiratory status?
- Are the child's body temperature and WBC count within normal limits? Has the sputum amount decreased?
- Is the child growing in height and weight along the normal growth curve?
- Are the child's stools of normal consistency, frequency, and color?
- Is the child able to engage in appropriate physical activity?
- Does the child appear to be developing age-appropriate cognitive, emotional, and social skills and an appropriate level of self-care?
- Does the child demonstrate an attitude of acceptance of self and of the illness?
- Does the family demonstrate appropriate coping strategies, compliance with the child's treatment plan, and the ability to access needed resources?
- Can the parents demonstrate CPT, inhalation therapy, and other treatments to be performed at home?
- Are the child and family able to appropriately express feelings of anger, sadness, and fear without guilt?

TUBERCULOSIS

Tuberculosis (TB) is a reportable contagious disease with a high morbidity and mortality throughout the world. Its incidence was declining until 1985, when it again began to rise. The World Health Organization estimates that there are approximately 8 million new cases of TB each year, with 3 million people dying from this disease (Munoz & Starke, 2004). Left untreated, each person with active TB will infect between 10 and 15 people each year. In the United States, an estimated 15 million people are infected with *Mycobacterium tuberculosis*, but the number of new cases is declining (National Center for HIV, STD, and TB Prevention, 2001).

Etiology

M. *tuberculosis*, an acid-fast bacillus, causes TB. Contamination occurs chiefly through inhalation of droplets from a person with active TB. Droplets produced by coughing and sneezing remain suspended in the air. When they are inhaled, they can reach the bronchioles and alveoli.

The risk for infection by the organism is thought to depend on several physiologic and socioeconomic factors. Most children are infected by a family member, baby-sitter, or other person with whom they have frequent contact (Box 45-5).

BOX 45-5
Risk Factors for the Development of Tuberculosis

- Contact with adults with infectious tuberculosis (TB)
- Chronic illness, immunosuppression, human immunodeficiency virus (HIV) infection
- Malnutrition
- Age (infancy, adolescence)
- Nonwhite racial and ethnic groups; immigration from areas with a high incidence of TB
- Urban, low-income living conditions
- Incarcerated adolescents
- Children in close contact with any of the following groups of adults: HIV-infected persons, users of intravenous (IV) or other street drugs, poor or medically indigent city dwellers, residents of nursing homes, migrant farm workers

---

Pathophysiology

of Tuberculosis

The bacillus multiplies in lung tissue, alveoli, and regional lymph nodes. After an incubation period of 2 to 12 weeks, hypersensitivity develops; at that time, the infected child will test positive on skin tests. Most infected children are asymptomatic at the time of the initial positive skin test result.

The *disease* of tuberculosis (TB) is differentiated from TB *infection* by the presence of clinical manifestations. The risk for developing TB disease is highest in the first 2 years after infection, but many infected children never progress to clinical disease.

The immunologic response of most people is usually strong enough to keep the bacteria from multiplying and spreading. If the host response is adequate, the organism is walled off and the tubercle becomes a healed calcified mass. TB bacilli can remain dormant and cause active disease at a later time if the child's resistance is lowered. If the lesion does not heal and is not walled off, it may continue to enlarge and spread into nearby tissues or it may enter the blood and spread to other sites (middle ear, brain, kidney, bones, joints, skin).

TB disease destroys host tissue. When tubercle bacilli multiply, they may damage tissue so badly that the center of the infected area turns to liquid pus. When this liquid escapes through an airway, it is coughed up as sputum, leaving a tiny hole (cavitation) in the lung. This bacteria-laden sputum is infectious. Children rarely develop active TB with cavitation, in which case they can be infectious to others. Because children with primary pulmonary TB have small lesions and minimal cough, they are not contagious.* The duration of infectivity of treated adults and adolescents depends on the drug susceptibility of the infecting organism and cough frequency. Although infectivity usually lasts only a few weeks after treatment is begun, it may last longer if the person fails to take the prescribed medication or is infected with a resistant strain.

---

*American Academy of Pediatrics, Committee on Infectious Diseases. (2000). *Report of the Committee on Infectious Diseases (2000 Red Book)* (25th ed.). Elk Grove Village, IL: American Academy of Pediatrics.

BOX 45-6
*Definition of a Positive Mantoux
Skin Test in Children*

Area of Induration ≥ 5 mm
- Children in close contact with persons who have known or suspected infectious cases of tuberculosis (TB)
- Children suspected of having TB disease (based on positive chest x-ray findings or clinical manifestations of TB)
- Children with immunosuppressive conditions or human immunodeficiency virus (HIV) infection

Area of Induration ≥ 10 mm
- Children younger than 4 years
- Children with chronic illness (malignant disease, diabetes mellitus, chronic renal failure, malnutrition)
- Children known to have environmental exposure (those born [or with parents born] in regions of the world where TB is highly prevalent; those in close contact with adults who are HIV-infected, homeless, intravenous (IV) drug users, migrant farm workers, nursing home residents, or incarcerated or institutionalized persons)

Induration ≥ 15 mm
- Children 4 years old or older without any risk factors

Modified from American Academy of Pediatrics, Committee on Infectious Diseases. (2000). *Report of the Committee on Infectious Diseases (2000 Red Book)* (25th ed., p. 594.). Elk Grove Village, IL: Author. Used with permission of the American Academy of Pediatrics.

Incidence

Almost 1.3 million cases and 450,000 deaths from TB occur among children each year. More than two thirds of the reported cases in the United States now occur in urban, low-income areas and in nonwhite racial and ethnic groups (AAP, Committee on Infectious Diseases, 2000). In the pediatric population, TB occurs most commonly in infants and adolescents and in children with immunosuppressive conditions. Of particular concern is the increase in multidrug-resistant (MDR) TB. Because this is most often caused by poor adherence to drug therapy, directly observed therapy (DOT) is indicated for anyone being treated for tuberculosis disease (Al-Dossary, Ong, Correa, & Starke, 2002).

Manifestations

Children ages 3 to 15 years are usually asymptomatic, have normal chest radiographs, and can be identified only through a positive skin test. Some children experience malaise, fever, night sweats, a slight cough, weight loss, anorexia, lymphadenopathy, or more specific symptoms related to the site of extrapulmonary infection (e.g., kidneys, brain, bone).

Diagnostic Evaluation

Skin testing is the initial method of screening and testing for TB. In most children, skin testing will become positive 2 to 12 weeks after the initial infection, and once positive, tuber-culin reactivity usually continues throughout life, even with treatment.

Skin testing with 5 tuberculin unit (TU) purified protein derivative (PPD) (Mantoux test) is the preferred method of screening. The PPD is administered by intradermal injection on the forearm. The skin reaction is read by an experienced professional 48 to 72 hours after placement. A 15-mm induration in any child older than 4 years is considered a positive sign of TB. Induration of more than 5 mm suggests TB in children younger than 4 years and in certain populations of children. A negative tuberculin skin test does not rule out TB, particularly in infants (Box 45-6).

Children with positive skin test results undergo follow-up examinations, which include periodic chest radiography and sputum cultures and smears. Because children often swallow sputum rather than expectorate it, gastric washings to obtain swallowed sputum are sometimes done. A thorough history should be obtained, and all contacts of the affected child should be tested for the disease.

Therapeutic Management and Nursing Considerations

It is important to understand the differences between TB exposure, infection, and disease. *Exposure* is recent and significant contact with an individual diagnosed with contagious TB. The skin test is often negative at this point, and the child is asymptomatic. TB *infection* is defined by a positive skin test. The child continues to lack signs and symptoms of TB, and there may be no chest radiograph changes at this time. Prophylactic treatment is instituted to prevent the progression to disease. TB *disease* is defined by chest radiograph changes along with signs and symptoms of disease and a positive skin test.

Tuberculosis Infection

After a chest radiograph is obtained, asymptomatic children with positive tuberculin tests and no previous history of TB receive isoniazid (INH) for 9 months. For children with human immunodeficiency virus (HIV) infection, a minimum of 12 months of treatment is recommended. Children with drug-resistant TB need an individualized treatment regimen. Household contacts (especially children younger than 4 years), immunosuppressed contacts, and contacts who were exposed during the previous 3 months should undergo skin testing and chest radiography. Even if the skin test is negative, asymptomatic contacts should receive INH for at least 12 weeks after contact has been broken until a negative skin test can be confirmed (AAP, Committee on Infectious Diseases, 2000). Reporting cases of TB is required by law in all states in the United States. Nurses should assist in searching for the source case and others infected by the source case.

Bacillus Calmette-Guérin (BCG) vaccine is the only anti-TB vaccine available. Unfortunately, the BCG vaccine varies in the immunity it provides and has resulted in serious reactions. In the United States, it is used mainly for (1) children with negative chest x-ray readings and skin test results who have had repeated exposures to TB and (2) asymptomatic HIV-infected children who are at increased risk for developing TB.

Tuberculosis Disease

A 6-month course of antituberculous medications (INH, rifampin, and pyrazinamide for the first 2 months; INH and rifampin for the next 4 months), optimal nutrition, and preventing exposure to infection, which could further compromise the child's already challenged immune system, are the mainstays of treatment (AAP, Committee on Infectious Diseases, 2000). Most children are treated at home. The nurse needs to emphasize to the family the importance of following the prescribed medication regimen meticulously and for the appropriate length of time, because inappropriate medication dosing contributes to the growth of drug-resistant organisms.

Children with TB may be hospitalized, depending on the severity of the disease, the age of the child, the need for more extensive testing, or the child's family and social environment. Unless the child is acutely ill, bed rest is not required. Isolation usually is not required because children with TB are rarely contagious.

Prevention and Screening

Promptly identifying cases and treating appropriately are the focus of disease prevention (Hoskyns, 2003). Because most children are infected by a family member, the best way to stop transmission of the disease is to identify those who are infected and to provide TB therapy.

Early detection of the disease is accomplished by screening. Children at high risk for TB should be tested annually with the Mantoux test. Annual skin testing of children in low-prevalence areas who have no risk factors is not indicated.

KEY CONCEPTS

- Infants and children younger than 3 years are at increased risk for developing respiratory tract infections because of their immature immune system, smaller airways, and underdeveloped supporting cartilage.
- At birth, the neonate must inflate the lungs, establish continuous breathing, and transfer the gases needed to meet metabolic needs.
- The severity of allergic rhinitis can be decreased through the early identification and treatment of manifestations.
- Respiratory obstruction increases during crying, and stridor increases when the child is supine with the neck flexed.
- The only reliable way to determine whether pharyngitis is viral or bacterial in origin is with a throat culture.
- Manifestations of bleeding after a tonsillectomy include frequent swallowing; restlessness; a fast, thready pulse; and the vomiting of bright-red blood.
- The mucosal edema associated with croup can sometimes be decreased by steam from hot running water in a closed bathroom or a cool humidifier or by taking the child out into the cool, humid night air.
- Children with croup who develop stridor at rest, cyanosis, severe agitation or fatigue, or moderate to severe retractions or who are unable to take oral fluids should be seen in the emergency department.
- The four *D*s of epiglottitis are *d*rooling, *d*ysphagia, *d*ysphoria, and *d*istressed inspiratory efforts.
- Visual examination of the epiglottis is contraindicated if epiglottitis is suspected because the examination tools can provoke laryngospasm and airway obstruction.
- Because respiratory syncytial virus (RSV) infection is highly communicable, during RSV season hospitalized infected children should be placed in contact isolation. Good handwashing should be emphasized and gowns worn when there is a chance that clothing might be soiled.
- Oxygen needs can be decreased in the child in respiratory distress by scheduling nursing care to allow the child periods of rest.
- If a child is aphonic and not breathing, the guidelines for management of an obstructed airway should be followed.
- During an apneic episode, the time and duration of the episode, color change, bradycardia, oxygen saturation, what the infant was doing before the apneic period, and any actions that stimulated breathing should be recorded.
- Healthy infants should be placed on their sides or backs for sleeping to reduce the risk for SIDS.
- When interviewing parents of an infant suspected of dying of SIDS, the nurse should avoid any implication of fault on the part of the parents.
- Asthma is the most common chronic disease of childhood. Asthma is characterized by bronchospasm, edema of the bronchiolar mucous membranes, and increased secretion of mucus in the airways.
- Asthmatic symptoms signaling spasm of the smooth muscle of the bronchi and bronchioles may be triggered by a variety of stimuli, including allergens, cold air, weather changes, infection, exercise, fatigue, and emotional distress.
- Status asthmaticus, or continued severe respiratory distress despite medical treatment, places the child in imminent danger of respiratory arrest and requires immediate hospitalization.
- Nursing care of the child with a severe asthma episode includes administration of inhaled or IV bronchodilators or corticosteroids, as ordered; providing oxygen therapy; providing IV fluids; and assisting with intubation and mechanical ventilation.
- Nursing care of the child with chronic asthma includes administration of prescribed medications and treatments and education of the child and family about medications, how to avoid triggers of asthma symptoms, how to recognize early warning signs of an asthma episode, and measures that can be taken to prevent severe asthma episodes.
- Bronchopulmonary dysplasia (BPD) is a chronic obstructive pulmonary disease characterized by thickening of the alveolar walls and bronchiolar epithelium. BPD occurs primarily in premature and low-birth-weight infants who have been mechanically ventilated with high concentrations of oxygen for prolonged periods.
- Nursing care of the infant with BPD includes supportive interventions to maintain adequate oxygenation and the provision of appropriate stimulation to promote normal growth and development.
- Cystic fibrosis (CF) is an inherited (autosomal recessive), multisystem disorder characterized by widespread dysfunction of the exocrine glands. Abnormal secretion of thick, tenacious mucus causes obstruction and dysfunction of the pancreas, lungs, salivary glands, sweat glands, and reproductive organs.
- Nursing care of the child with CF includes maintaining a patent airway by administering bronchodilators and performing or supervising respiratory treatments, administering antibiotics and pancreatic enzymes, and teaching the child and family about CF and its treatment.
- Nursing care of the child with tuberculosis (TB) includes administering and evaluating TB skin tests and administering anti-TB medications as ordered. The nurse also instructs the child and family about the importance of adequate rest, a nutritionally adequate diet, and compliance with the medication regimen, as well as ways to prevent the transmission of TB infection.

ANSWERS to Critical Thinking Exercise 45-1

1. Children often leave the hospital with pain medication (usually liquid acetaminophen with codeine) ordered to be given as needed (PRN). Ordering the medication this way relies on the parent or caregiver to assess the child's pain before administering the analgesic. Further research is needed to determine how well parents understand and accurately assess their child's pain during the initial postoperative period. In addition, undermedication can be related to the following*:
   - Inadequate doses ordered
   - Parents' fear of overmedication

   - Parents' fear that the child will become addicted to the medication
   - Inadequate instructions for medicating
   - Expectations regarding the amount of pain associated with the procedure
   - Difficulty getting the child to swallow the medication

2. Inadequate pain relief can adversely affect the child's behavior and ability to rest. In the child who has had a tonsillectomy, more serious effects are related to the refusal of fluids. Children who have had tonsils removed can experience moderate to severe postoperative pain. For most effective postoperative progress, pain medication should be administered regularly around-the-clock and not PRN. Nurses should emphasize this to parents before discharge. If the facility allows, a postoperative phone call to the child's home to inquire about the child and remind the parent about continuous pain relief may be helpful.

*Hamers, J.P. & Abu-Saad, H.H. (2002). Children's pain at home following (adeno) tonsillectomy. *European Journal of Pain, 6*(3), 213-219.

REFERENCES and READINGS

Abdel-Rahman, H.A. (2000). Fatal suffocation by rubber balloons in children: Mechanism and prevention. *Forensic Science International, 108*(2), 97-105.

Abrams, S.A. (2001). Chronic pulmonary insufficiency in children and its effect on growth and development. *Journal of Nutrition, 131*(3), 938S-941S.

Al-Dossary, F.S., Ong, L.T., Correa, A.G., & Starke, J.R. (2002). Treatment of childhood tuberculosis with a six month directly observed regimen of only two weeks of daily therapy. *Pediatric Infectious Disease Journal, 21*(2), 91-97.

American Academy of Allergy, Asthma, and Immunology. (2003). *Pediatric asthma, promoting best practice. Guide for managing asthma in children.* Rochester, NY: University of Rochester.

American Academy of Family Physicians, American Academy of Otolaryngology-Head and Neck Surgery, American Academy of Pediatrics Subcommittee on Otitis Media With Effusion. (2004). Otitis media with effusion. *Pediatrics, 113*(5), 1412-1429.

American Academy of Pediatrics (AAP). (1992). *AAP Task Force on Infant Positioning and SIDS.* Elk Grove Village, IL: Author.

American Academy of Pediatrics. (2003). *Positioning & SIDS: Update.* Retrieved on July 31, 2003, from www.aap.org.

American Academy of Pediatrics. (2004). Clinical practice guideline: Diagnosis and management of acute otitis media. *Pediatrics, 113*(5), 1451-1465.

American Academy of Pediatrics, Committee on Fetus and Newborn. (2003). Apnea, sudden infant death syndrome, and home monitoring. *Pediatrics, 111*(4 Pt. 1), 914-917.

American Academy of Pediatrics, Committee on Infectious Diseases. (2000). *Report of the Committee on Infectious Diseases (2000 Red Book)* (25th ed.). Elk Grove Village, IL: American Academy of Pediatrics.

American Lung Association (2002). Epidemiology and Statistics Unit, Best Practice and Program Services. *Trends in asthma morbidity and mortality.* New York: Author.

American Thoracic Society. (2001). *TB is a global problem.* Available on-line: www.thoracic.org.

Anderson, P.J. (2001). Delivery options and devices for aerosolized therapeutics. *Chest, 120*(3 Suppl.), 89S-93S.

Arshad, S., Bateman, B., & Matthews, S. (2003). Primary prevention of asthma and atopy during childhood by allergen avoidance in infancy: a randomised controlled study. *Thorax, 58*(6), 489-493.

Atkinson, S.A. (2001). Special nutritional needs of infants for prevention of and recovery from bronchopulmonary dysplasia. *Journal of Nutrition, 131*(3), 942S-946S.

Baker, V.O., Friedman, J., & Schmitt, R. (2002). Asthma management, part 2: Pharmacologic management. *Journal of School Nursing, 18*(5), 257-269.

Baroody, F.M. (2003). Allergic rhinitis: Broader disease effects and implications for management. *Otolaryngology and Head and Neck Surgery, 128*(5), 616-631.

Barry, P. (2002). Aerosol in bronchiolitis. *Journal of Aerosol Medicine, 15*(2), 109-116.

Bennett, A.D. (2002). Home apnea monitoring for infants. A discussion of primary care issues. *Advance for Nurse Practitioners, 10*(3), 48-53.

Berger, W. (2001). Allergic rhinitis in children. *Current Allergy and Asthma Reports, 1*(6), 498-505.

Bhatt-Mehta, V., & Schumacher, R.E. (2003). Treatment of apnea of prematurity. *Paediatric Drugs, 5*(3), 195-210.

Blaisdell, C.J., Weiss, S.R., Kimes, D.S., Levine, E.R., Myers, M., Timmins, S., & Bollinger, M.E. (2002). Using seasonal variations in asthma hospitalizations in children to predict hospitalization frequency. *Journal of Asthma, 39*(7), 567-575.

Blonshire, S.B. (2000). Pediatric pulmonary function testing. *Respiratory Care Clinics of North America, 6*(1), 27-40.

Boat, T. (2004). Cystic fibrosis. In R. Behrman, R. Kliegman, & H. Jenson (Eds.). *Nelson textbook of pediatrics* (17th ed; pp. 1437-1450). Philadelphia: Saunders.

Bradley, J.S. (2002). Old and new antibiotics for pediatric pneumonia. *Seminars in Respiratory Infections, 17*(1), 57-64.

Brook, I. (2002). Antibacterial therapy for acute group a streptococcal pharyngotonsillitis: Short-course versus traditional 10-day oral regimens. *Paediatric Drugs, 4*(11), 747-754.

Buhl, R. (2003). Omalizumab (Xolair) improves quality of life in adult patients with allergic asthma: A review. *Respiratory Medicine, 97*(2), 123-129.

Castile, R., Filbrun, D., Flucke, R., Franklin, W., & McCoy, K. (2000). Adult-type pulmonary function tests in infants with respiratory disease. *Pediatric Pulmonology, 30*, 215-227.

Centers for Disease Control and Prevention. (1997a). Case definitions for infectious conditions under public health surveillance. *MMWR: Morbidity and Mortality Weekly Report, 46*(RR-10), 1-55.

Centers for Disease Control and Prevention. (1997b). Screening for tuberculosis and tuberculosis infection in high-risk populations: Recommendations of the Advisory Council for the Elimination of Tuberculosis. *MMWR: Morbidity and Mortality Weekly Report, 46*(RR-11), 18-34.

Chernick, V., Boat, T., & Kendig, E. (Eds.). (1998). *Kendig's disorders of the respiratory tract in children* (6th ed.). Philadelphia: Saunders.

Conrad, D., & Jenson, H.B. (2002). Management of acute bacterial rhinosinusitis. *Current Opinion in Pediatrics, 14*(1), 86-90.

Contopoulos-Ioannidis, D.G., Ioannidis, J.P., & Lau, J. (2003). Acute sinusitis in children: Current treatment strategies. *Paediatric Drugs, 5*(2), 71-80.

Cools, F., & Offringa, M. (2000). Neuromuscular paralysis for newborn infants receiving mechanical ventilation. *Cochrane Database of Systematic Reviews, (4)*, CD002773.

Copland, I.B., & Post, M. (2002). Understanding the mechanisms of infant respiratory distress and chronic lung disease. *American Journal of Respiratory Cell & Molecular Biology, 26*(3), 261-265.

Curns, A.T., Holman, R.C., Shay, D.K., Cheek, J.E., Kaufman, S.F., Singleton, R.J., & Anderson, L.J. (2002). Outpatient and hospital visits associated with otitis media among American Indian and Alaska native children younger than 5 years. *Pediatrics, 109*(3), e41-1.

Cystic Fibrosis Foundation. (2002). *Patient registry 2001 annual report.* Bethesda, MD: Cystic Fibrosis Foundation.

Davidson, K.L. (2002). Airway clearance strategies for the pediatric patient. *Respiratory Care, 47*(7), 823-828.

Davis, B., Moon, R., Sachs, H., & Ottolini, M. (1998). Effects of sleep position on infant motor development. *Pediatrics, 102*(5), 1135-1140.

Devadason, S.G., & Le Souef, P.N. (2002). Age-associated factors influencing the efficacy of various forms of aerosol therapy. *Journal of Aerosol Medicine, 15*(3), 343-345.

Dialer, I., Hundt, C., Bertele-Harms, R.M., & Harms, H.K. (2003). Sonographic evaluation of bowel wall thickness in patients with cystic fibrosis. *Journal of Clinical Gastroenterology, 37*(1), 55-60.

Easton, J., Noble, S., & Perry, C.M. (2003). Amoxicillin/clavulanic acid: A review of its use in the management of paediatric patients with acute otitis media. *Drugs, 63*(3), 311-340.

Eigen, H., Rosenstein, B., & Fitzsimmons, S. (1995). A multicenter study of alternate-day prednisone in patients with CF. *Journal of Pediatrics, 126,* 515-523.

Equi, A., Balfour-Lynn, I. M., Bush, A., & Rosenthal, M. (2002). Long term azithromycin in children with cystic fibrosis: A randomized, placebo-controlled crossover trial. *Lancet, 360*(9338), 978-984.

Eren, S., Balci, A.E., Dikici, B., Doblan, M., & Eren, M.N. (2003). Foreign body aspiration in children: Experience of 1160 cases. *Annals of Tropical Paediatrics, 23*(1), 31-37.

Espositio, S., & Principi, N. (2002). Emerging resistance to antibiotics against respiratory bacteria: Impact on therapy of community-acquired pneumonia in children. *Drug Resistance Updates, 5*(2), 73-87.

Federierico, M., & Liu, A. (2003). Overcoming childhood asthma disparities of the inner-city poor. *Pediatric Clinics of North America, 50,* 655-675.

Feranchak, A.P., & Sokol, R.J. (2001). Cholangiocyte biology and cystic fibrosis liver disease. *Seminars in Liver Disease, 21*(4), 471-488.

Fineman, S. (2002). The burden of allergic rhinitis: beyond dollars and cents. *Annals of Allergy, Asthma, and Immunology, 88*(4 suppl. 1), 2-7.

Flynn, C.A., Griffin, G., & Tudiver, F. (2001). Decongestants and antihistamines for acute otitis media in children. *Cochrane Database System Review, (2),* CD001727.

Flynn, M.B. (2000). Identifying and treating inhalation injuries in fire victims. *Nursing, 30*(1 crit care), 32cc1-2, 32cc4, 32cc6-7.

Gallagher, C. (2002). Childhood asthma: tools that help parents manage it. *American Journal of Nursing, 102*(8), 71-83.

Godfrey, S., Bar-Yishay, E., Avital, A., & Springer, C. (2003). What is the role of tests of lung function in the management of infants with lung disease? *Pediatric Pulmonology, 36*(1), 1-9.

Graetz, B.W., Shute, R.H., & Sawyer, M.G. (2000). An Australian study of adolescents with cystic fibrosis: Perceived supportive and non-supportive behaviors from families and friends and psychosocial adjustment. *Journal of Adolescent Health, 26*(1), 64-69.

Greenough, A. (2000). Measuring respiratory outcome. *Seminars in Neonatology, 5*(2), 119-126.

Guilbert, T., & Drawiec, M. (2003). Natural history of asthma. *Pediatric Clinics of North America, 50,* 523-538.

Gunger, A., & Bluestone, C.D. (2001). Antibiotic theory in otitis media. *Current Allergy and Asthma Reports, 1*(4), 364-372.

Gurkan, F., Kiral, A., Dagli, E., & Karakoc, F. (2000). The effect of passive smoking on the development of respiratory syncytial virus bronchiolitis. *European Journal of Epidemiology, 16*(5), 465-468.

Haffner, J., & Schurman, S. (2001). The technology-dependent child. *Pediatric Clinics of North America, 48*(3), 751-764.

Hamers, J.P., & Abu-Saad, H.H. (2002). Children's pain at home following (adeno) tonsillectomy. *European Journal of Pain, 6*(3), 213-219.

Hanafin, S., & Griffiths, P. (2002). Does pacifier use cause ear infections in young children? *British Journal of Pediatrics, 7*(4), 208-211.

Hardin, D.S. (2002). Growth problems and growth hormone treatment in children with cystic fibrosis. *Journal of Pediatric Endocrinology and Metabolism, 15*(Suppl. 2), 731-735.

Hayes, C.S., & Williamson, H. (2001). Management of group A beta-hemolytic streptococcal pharyngitis. *American Family Physician, 63*(8), 1557-1564.

Hazinski, T. (1998). Bronchopulmonary dysplasia. In V. Chernick, T. Boat, & E. Kendig (Eds.). *Kendig's disorders of the respiratory tract in children* (pp. 364-388). Philadelphia: Saunders.

Hegland, A. (1997). Two high-risk infant groups targeted for RSV-IGIV therapy. *AAP News, 13*(2), 1.

Hoberman, A., Marchant, C.D., Kaplan, S.L., & Feldman, S. (2002). Treatment of acute otitis media consensus recommendations. *Clinical Pediatrics, 41*(6), 373-390.

Hogan, M.B., & Wilson N.W. (2003). Asthma in the school-aged child. *Pediatric Annals, 32*(1), 20-25.

Hoskyns, W. (2003). Paediatric tuberculosis. *Postgraduate Medical Journal, 79*(931), 272-278.

Ilicali, O.C., Keles, N., Deer, K., Saun, O.F., & Guldiken, Y. (2001). Evaluation of the effect of passive smoking on otitis media in children by an objective method: Urinary cotinine analysis. *Laryngoscope, 111*(1), 163-167.

Jaffe, A., & Bush, A. (2001). Anti-inflammatory effects of macrolides in lung disease. *Pediatric Pulmonology, 31*(6), 464-473.

Jobe, A., & Ikegami, M. (2001). Prevention of bronchopulmonary dysplasia. *Current Opinion in Pediatrics, 13*(2), 124-129.

Johnson, L.B., Elluru, R.G., & Myer, C.M. (2002). Complications of adenotonsillectomy. *Laryngoscope, 112*(8 Pt. 2), 35-36.

Kercsmar, C. (1998). Asthma. In V. Chernick, T. Boat, & E. Kendig (Eds.), *Kendig's disorders of the respiratory tract in children* (6th ed., p. 699). Philadelphia: Saunders.

Kimpen, J.L. (2001). Management of respiratory syncytial virus infection. *Current Opinion in Infectious Disease, 14*(3), 323-328.

Klein, J.O. (2002). Strategies for decreasing multidrug antibiotic resistance: A role of ototopical agents for treatment of middle ear infections. *American Journal of Managed Care, 8*(14 Suppl.), S345-352.

Konstan, M.W., & Davis, P.B. (2002). Pharmacological approaches for the discovery and development of new anti-inflammatory agents for the treatment of cystic fibrosis. *Advanced Drug Delivery Review, 54*(11), 1409-1423.

Landau, L.I. (2001). Parental smoking: Asthma and wheezing illnesses in infants and children. *Paediatric Respiratory Reviews, 2*(3), 202-206.

Lee, T., Brugge, D., Francis, C., & Fisher, O. (2003). Asthma prevalence among inner-city Asian-American schoolchildren. *Public Health Report, 118*(3), 215-220.

Lima, J.A., & Fischer, G.B. (2002). Foreign body aspiration in children. *Paediatric Respiratory Reviews, 3*(4), 303-307.

Maddern, B.R. (2002). Electrosurgery for tonsillectomy. *Laryngoscope, 112*(8 Pt. 2), 11-13.

Milgrom, H., & Leung, D. (2004). Allergic rhinitis. In R. Behrman, R. Kliegman, & H. Jenson (Eds.). *Nelson textbook of pediatrics* (17th ed.; pp. 759-760). Philadelphia: Saunders.

Moran, A. (2002). Endocrine complications of cystic fibrosis. *Adolescent Medicine State of the Art Reviews, 13*(1), 145-159.

Munoz, F., & Starke, J. (2004). Tuberculosis (Mycobacterium tuberculosis). In R. Behrman, R. Kliegman, & H. Jenson (Eds.). *Nelson textbook of pediatrics* (17th ed.; pp. 956-972). Philadelphia: Saunders.

National Center for HIV, STD, and TB Prevention. (2001, June 12). *U.S. TB cases decline seven percent in 2000, reaching all time low.* Available on-line: www.cdc.gov/nchstp/tb/pubs.

National Heart, Lung and Blood Institute. (1997, July). *Expert panel report 2: Guidelines for the diagnosis and management of asthma.* Bethesda, MD: Author.

Newacheck, P., & Halforn, N. (1998). Prevalence and impact of disabling chronic conditions in childhood. *American Journal of Public Health, 88*(4), 610-615.

Nielsen, L., Meggrid, N., & Dahl, r. (2001). Intranasal corticosteroids for allergic rhinitis: superior relief? *Drugs, 61*(11), 1563-1579.

Nieves, F. F., & Chernick, V. (2002). Bronchopulmonary dysplasia (chronic lung disease of infancy): An update for the pediatrician. *Clinical Pediatrics, 41*(2), 77-85.

O'Connell, E.J. (2002). Efficacy of budesonide in moderate to severe asthma. *Clinical Therapeutics, 24*(6), 887-905.

Ovetchkine, P., & Cohen, R. (2003). Shortened course of antibacterial therapy for acute otitis media. *Paediatric Drugs, 5*(2), 133-140.

Panitch, H.B. (2001). Bronchiolitis in infants. *Current Opinion in Pediatrics, 13*(3), 256-260.

Panitch, H.B. (2003). Respiratory syncytial virus bronchiolitis: Supportive care and therapies designed to overcome airway obstruction. *Pediatric Infectious Disease Journal, 22*(2 Suppl.), S83-87.

Pastore, G., Guala, A., & Zaffaroni, M. (2003). Back to sleep: Risk factors for SIDS as target for public health campaigns. *Journal of Pediatrics, 142*(4), 453-454.

Pelton, S.I. (2002). Acute otitis media in an era of increasing microbial resistance and universal administration of pneumococcal conjugate vaccine. *Pediatric Infectious Disease Journal, 21*(6), 599-604.

Perkins, J.A. (2002). Medical and surgical management of otitis media in children. *Otolaryngologic Clinics of North America, 35*(4), 811-825.

Pichichero, M.E. (2000). Recurrent and persistent otitis media. *Pediatric Infectious Disease Journal, 19*(9), 911-916.

Ratjen, F., & Doring, G. (2003). Cystic fibrosis. *Lancet, 361*(9358), 681-689.

Samuels, S. (2000). Training workshop. Physiotherapy for children with cystic fibrosis. *Pediatric Respiratory Review, 1*(2), 190-196.

Schindler, M. (2002). Do bronchodilators have an effect on bronchiolitis? *Critical Care (London), 6*(2), 111-112.

Schlesinger, C., & Koss, M.N. (2002). Bronchiolitis: Update 2001. *Current Opinion in Pulmonary Medicine, 8*(2), 112-116.

Skoner, D. (2001). Allergic rhinitis: definition, epidemiology, pathophysiology, detection, and diagnosis. *Journal of Allergy and Clinical Immunology, 108*(1 suppl.), S2-S8.

REFERENCES and READINGS

Smyth, A., & Walters, S. (2003). Prophylactic antibiotics for cystic fibrosis. *Cochrane Database of Sytematic Reviews, (3),* CD001912.

Smucny, J.J., Flynn, C.A., Becker, L.A., & Glazier, R.H. (2001). Are beta2-agonists effective treatment for acute bronchitis or acute cough in patients without underlying pulmonary disease? A systematic review. *Journal of Family Practice, 50*(11), 945-951.

Sockrider, M. (2002). Management of asthma in young children. *Current Allergy & Asthma Reports, 2*(6), 453-459.

Sockrider, M. (2003). Asthma prevalence among inner-city Asian American school children. *Public Health Reports, 118*(3), 215-220.

Stone, K.D. (2002). Atopic diseases in children. *Current Opinion in Pediatrics, 14*(5), 634-646.

Streetman, D.D., Bhatt-Mheta, V., & Johnson, C.E. (2002). Management of acute, severe asthma in children. *Annals of Pharmacotherapy, 36*(7-8), 1249-1260.

Stroud, R.H., & Friedman, N.R. (2001). An update on inflammatory disorders of the pediatric airway: Epiglottitis, croup, and tracheitis. *American Journal of Otolaryngology, 22*(4), 268-275.

Suresh, G.K., & Soll, R.F. (2002). Lung surfactants for neonatal respiratory distress syndrome: Animal-derived or synthetic agents? *Paediatric Drugs, 4*(8), 485-492.

Szefler, S.J., & Pedersen, S. (2003). Role of budesonide as maintenance therapy for children with asthma. *Pediatric Pulmonology, 36*(1), 13-21.

Thomas, M., DelMar, C., Glasziou, P. (2000). How effective are treatments other than antibiotics for acute sore throat? *British Journal of General Practice, 50*(459), 817-820.

Thompson, T. (1999). Clinical update, cystic fibrosis: Causes, diagnosis and treatment. *Community Practitioner, 72*(12), 408-409.

Virgilis, D., Rivkin, L., Samueloff, A., Picard, E., Golberg, S., Faber, J., Kerem, E., & Wilschanski, M. (2003). Cystic fibrosis, pregnancy, and recurrent, acute pancreatitis. *Journal of Pediatric Gastroenterology Nutrition, 36*(4), 486-488.

Wadlinger, S. (1999). Case report: Inhaled nitric oxide therapy. *RT: Journal of Respiratory Care Practitioners, 12*(4), 100-101.

WHO annual report on global TB control—summary. *Weekly Epidemiology Record, 78*(15), 122-128.

Wolkoff, L.I., & Narula, P. (2000). Issues in neonatal and pediatric oxygen therapy. *Respiratory Care Clinics of North America, 6*(4), 675-692.

Wright, R.B., Pomerantz, W.J., & Luria, J.W. (2002). New approaches to respiratory infections in children: Bronchiolitis and croup. *Emergency Medicine Clinics of North America, 20*(1), 93-114.

46

The Child with a Cardiovascular Alteration

◆ LEARNING OBJECTIVES

After studying this chapter, you should be able to:

- Describe the anatomy and physiology of the normally functioning heart.
- Describe the major circulatory changes that occur in the fetus during the transition from intrauterine to extrauterine life.
- Discuss specific techniques used in a comprehensive cardiac assessment.
- Explain the various classifications of congenital heart disease, describe their underlying mechanisms, and list the associated congenital cardiac defects.
- Discuss the nursing process used for an infant or child with congestive heart failure.
- Discuss the major physiology and therapeutic management of the child with heart defects that include left-to-right shunting lesions and obstructive or stenotic lesions.
- Discuss the major physiology, therapeutic management, and nursing care of the child with a cyanotic heart defect.
- Discuss the importance of early recognition and treatment of infective endocarditis.
- Describe nursing care of the child with rheumatic fever, Kawasaki disease, or hypertension.
- Explain why high cholesterol is an important health issue for children and adolescents, and describe the assessment and nursing management of children with this problem in the community.
- Explain the effects of childhood obesity on future cardiovascular health.

◆ DEFINITIONS

afterload The amount of force against which the ventricles contract.

angioplasty Procedure that dilates vessels.

cardiomegaly An enlarged heart.

central venous pressure Pressure measured in the right atrium; helpful in determining the amount of circulating blood volume.

chronotropic Affecting the time or rate.

compensation Maintenance of an adequate blood flow without distressing symptoms; accomplished by cardiac and circulatory adjustments, such as tachycardia, cardiac hypertrophy, and increased blood volume from sodium and water retention.

decompensation Inability of the heart to maintain adequate circulation; may be marked by dyspnea, venous engorgement, cyanosis, and edema.

dysrhythmia Disturbance of rhythm.

gradient Difference.

inotropic Affects the force of muscular contractions; can cause a positive or negative effect.

myocardial contractility Ability of myocardial cells and tissues to shorten in response to an appropriate stimulus; force of contraction of the myocardium.

palpitations Sensation of rapid or irregular heartbeat.

preload Amount of stretch of the myocardial fibers before contraction; most easily measured by determining central venous pressure.

pulmonary edema Collection of excessive fluid in the alveoli of the lungs.

pulmonary hypertension Increased pressure in the pulmonary arteries and arterioles.

pulmonary vascular resistance Amount of resistance in the pulmonary vascular bed against which the right ventricle must pump to achieve blood flow to the lungs.

pulmonary venous congestion Increased pulmonary pressure leading to the accumulation of excessive fluid and blood in the pulmonary veins.

regurgitation Abnormal backward flow of blood through a heart valve.

shunt Abnormal blood flow from one part of the circulation to another.

systemic vascular resistance Amount of resistance in the systemic vascular bed against which the left ventricle must pump to achieve cardiac output.

systemic venous congestion Increased systemic venous pressure leading to the accumulation of excessive fluid in the systemic veins.

valvotomy An opening surgically created in a valve.

valvuloplasty Mechanical procedure to open a valve.

REVIEW OF THE HEART AND CIRCULATION

Normal Cardiac Anatomy and Physiology

The heart is a muscular pump divided into four chambers. The two upper chambers are the atria, and the two lower chambers are the ventricles. There are two atrioventricular (AV) valves, the tricuspid valve and the mitral valve. There are two semilunar valves—the pulmonary valve and the aortic valve. In normal blood flow, desaturated venous blood returning from the body flows from the superior vena cava and inferior vena cava into the right atrium. It then moves through the tricuspid valve into the right ventricle and is pumped into the main pulmonary artery and branch pulmonary arteries to the pulmonary circulation (the lungs). In the lungs, carbon dioxide is removed and oxygen added to the blood. This richly oxygen-saturated blood returns from the pulmonary circulation to the left side of the heart via the pulmonary veins and into the left atrium. From the left atrium, it flows through the mitral valve into the left ventricle and is pumped into the aorta and systemic circulation.

Electrical stimulation is required before mechanical contraction of the heart muscle can occur. This electrical stimulation is normally initiated by a group of cells called the *sinus node*, located at the superior vena cava and right atrial junction. The electrical impulse spreads through the atrium to the relay station, the AV node, and is then transmitted to the ventricles through the bundle of His, the bundle-branch system, and finally the Purkinje fibers. The result is rhythmic atrial electrical stimulation and then contraction, followed by ventricular stimulation and contraction. The P wave reflects atrial depolarization, the QRS wave reflects ventricular depolarization, and the T wave reflects ventricular repolarization.

Each cardiac cycle consists of this electrical activity, which produces depolarization and subsequent repolarization of the cardiac muscle—more simply, a heartbeat.

The venous (or right) side of the heart is normally a lower pressure system compared with the higher arterial (or left) side of the heart. The right ventricle has a normal pressure of 25/0 to 25/5 mm Hg and pulmonary artery pressure of 25/10 mm Hg. The left ventricle has a normal pressure in the range of 100/5 mm Hg (age-dependent), and the aorta has a normal pressure of about 100/60 mm Hg (age-dependent). On average, the left-sided pressures are four to five times higher than those on the right side.

In addition, the venous circulation normally has lower oxygen saturations, in the range of 70%. This compares with the arterial circulation, which has a normal range of 95% to 100%. Congenital or acquired malformations or anomalies in any of the cardiac structures may affect blood flow, pressures, and oxygen saturations, thereby altering hemodynamic stability.

Fetal Circulation

Fetal circulation differs from neonatal circulation in three areas: the process of gas exchange, the pressures within the systemic and pulmonary circulations, and the existence of anatomic structures that assist in the delivery of oxygen-rich blood to vital organ systems. In the fetus, oxygenation (gas exchange) takes place at the placenta. Oxygen and nutrients are carried by blood in the umbilical vein, which travels through the fetal liver to the inferior vena cava.

A small amount of blood travels into the hepatic circulation to provide oxygen and nutrients to the hepatic tissue. Liver function is minimal in the fetus, so very little blood supply is required. The remainder of the blood flows into the inferior vena cava through a fetal structure, the *ductus venosus*.

The inferior vena cava empties blood into the right atrium. The trajectory (direction) of the blood flow, as well as the pressure in the right atrium, propels most of this blood through a second fetal structure, the *foramen ovale*, into the left atrium. This richly oxygenated blood travels through the left ventricle into the aorta, feeding the coronary arteries and the brain—the two most oxygen-needy organ systems.

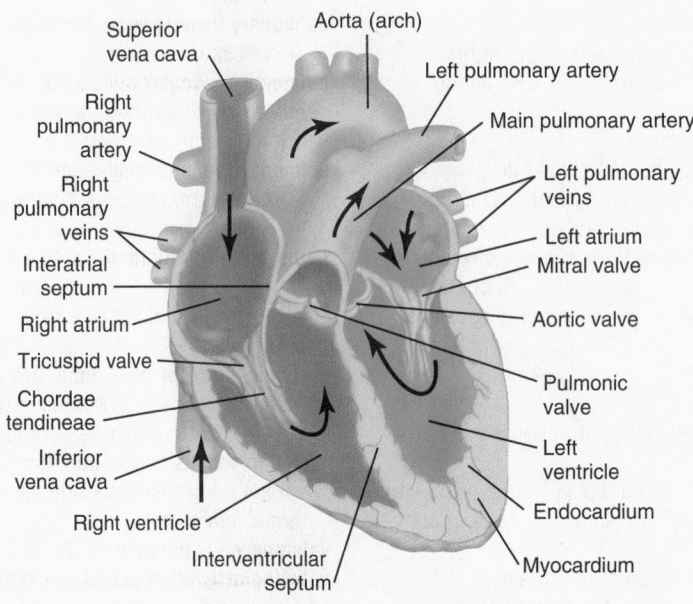

Labels: Superior vena cava; Aorta (arch); Right pulmonary artery; Left pulmonary artery; Main pulmonary artery; Right pulmonary veins; Left pulmonary veins; Interatrial septum; Left atrium; Mitral valve; Right atrium; Aortic valve; Tricuspid valve; Chordae tendineae; Pulmonic valve; Inferior vena cava; Left ventricle; Right ventricle; Endocardium; Interventricular septum; Myocardium

Anatomy of the Heart

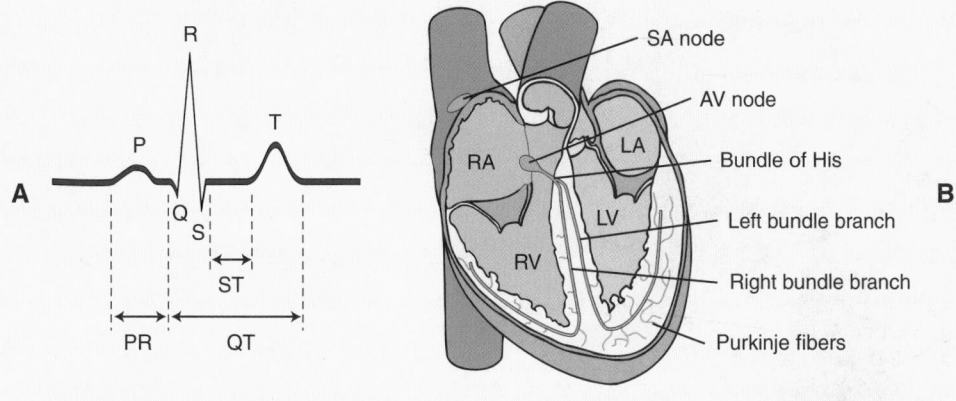

A, Normal heart cycle, represented as an electrocardiographic configuration. **B,** Cardiac electrical conduction system. (Modified from Park, M.K., & Guntheroth, W.G. [1992]. *How to read pediatric ECGs* [3rd ed., p. 1], St. Louis: Mosby.)

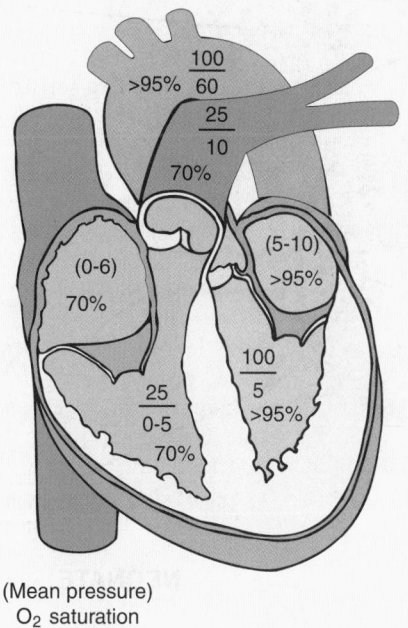

(Mean pressure)
O_2 saturation

Normal pressures (mm Hg) and saturations (%). (Modified from Ko Chiang, L., & Ensor Dunn, A. [2000]. Cardiology. In G.K. Siberry & R. Iannone [Eds.], *The Johns Hopkins Hospital Harriet Lane Handbook* [15th ed., p. 154]. St. Louis: Mosby.)

Blood returning from the upper body enters the right atrium through the superior vena cava. This blood is directed primarily through the tricuspid valve and the right ventricle into the pulmonary artery. Resistance in the pulmonary circulation is very high because the lungs are collapsed and filled with fluid. A very small amount of blood flows through the branch pulmonary arteries to provide oxygen and nutrients to the pulmonary tissue. Most of the blood flows through a third fetal structure, the *ductus arteriosus*, to the descending aorta. This blood is then distributed to the organ systems and tissues in the lower portion of the body and returns to the placenta for gas exchange through two umbilical arteries.

Pediatric Differences in the Heart and Circulation

- The heart and the great vessels develop during the first 3 to 8 weeks of gestation. The fetus is most vulnerable to cardiac malformations during this period.
- Heart sounds in the neonate are higher-pitched and of greater intensity than in the adult, and the pulse rate is higher. Many variations in these parameters are both possible and normal. The intensity of the murmur does not necessarily correlate with the degree and severity of the congenital or acquired heart disease.
- The chest wall of infants and young children is thin because of the relative lack of subcutaneous and muscle tissue. Innocuous murmurs can be auscultated in structurally normal hearts because of the wall thinness.
- Neonatal and infant myocardial muscle is less efficient and has fewer organized myocardial fibers. The neonatal heart is very dependent on calcium, glucose, and volume for optimal cardiac function.
- Neonates and infants are particularly dependent on adequate heart rate and rhythm to maintain their cardiac output because they cannot increase their stroke volume as effectively as the older child or adult (Cardiac output = Stroke volume × Heart rate).
- In a very sick child, the cardiac output should be evaluated as either adequate or inadequate to meet metabolic demands. Shock may be present even when the cardiac output is normal or high.
- Blood pressure is a late indicator of clinical compensation, and hypotension represents decompensated shock.
- Increased pulmonary vascular resistance in the newborn increases pressure on the right side of the heart. This may delay detection of left-to-right shunts in the newborn period because increased right-sided pressure decreases the left-to-right shunting and the intensity of cardiac murmurs. Normally, pulmonary vascular resistance decreases to the adult range over the first 4 to 6 weeks of life. Obvious signs and symptoms of left-to-right shunting may not be present until that time.

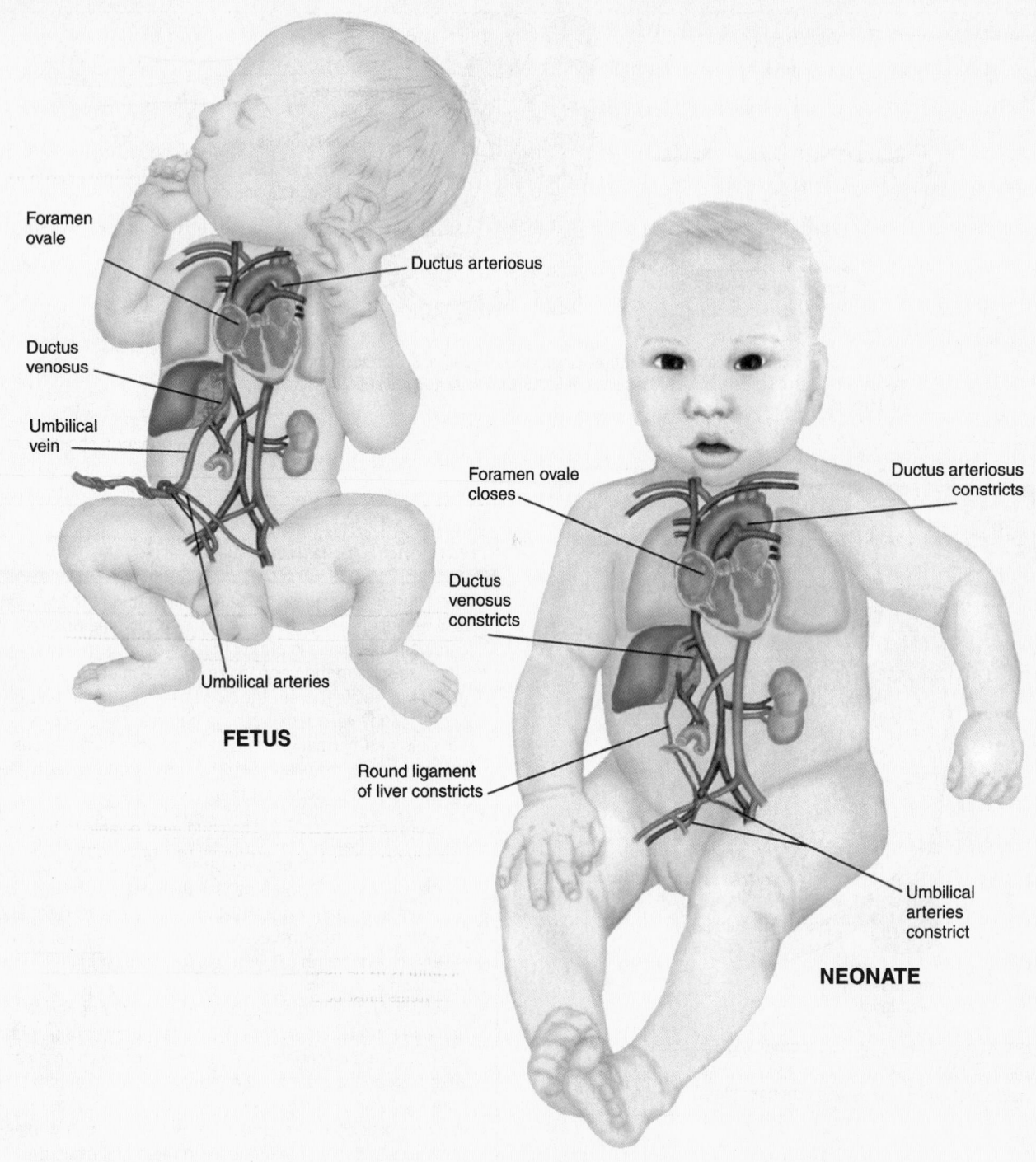

Foramen
ovale

Ductus arteriosus

Ductus
venosus

Umbilical
vein

Umbilical arteries

FETUS

Foramen ovale
closes

Ductus arteriosus
constricts

Ductus
venosus
constricts

Round ligament
of liver constricts

Umbilical
arteries
constrict

NEONATE

Changes in Circulation After Birth

Transitional and Neonatal Circulation

Major changes in the circulatory system occur at birth. With the neonate's first breath, gas exchange is transferred from the placenta to the lungs.

In the normal neonate, the fetal shunts (ductus venosus, ductus arteriosus, foramen ovale) close in response to pressure changes in the systemic and pulmonary circulations and increased blood oxygen content. Pulmonary vascular resistance decreases, and a marked increase in pulmonary blood flow follows. Closure of the ductus arteriosus, along with the increased pulmonary blood flow, enhances left ventricular filling. The increase in systemic arterial pressure as a result of placental closure increases the workload of the left ventricle, and the neonatal heart now functions on its own. The neonatal circulation is now normal. In some neonates, it may take several days for the fetal shunts to close.

Common Diagnostic Tests for Cardiac Disorders

Test	Description	Preparation and Nursing Considerations	Comments
Electrocardiography (ECG)	Provides recording of heart's electrical activity from outside surface of body. Electrodes are placed over the precordium and on the four extremities; the electrodes are attached to lead wires. Lead wires are attached to a machine that records and prints electrical activity.	Best done when the child is quiet and cooperative. Skin should be free of lotions and oils.	Detects chamber enlargement and deviations in axis that may be caused by congenital or acquired heart defects or disease. Displays heart rate and rhythm.
Holter monitor	Continuously records heart rate and rhythm for 24 hours. Electrodes and leads are attached to the child, who wears a compact recorder.	Same as for ECG.	Child or parent records times of activities, symptoms, or other events in a diary to be returned with the monitor. Important that diary be accurately completed.
Chest radiography	Provides x-ray picture of heart and associated organs and structures in the chest cavity.	No specific preparation. Encourage the parent or family member to accompany the child to x-ray department.	Provides information about heart size, blood flow to lungs, sidedness of the stomach, liver, and heart.
Echocardiography	Uses high-frequency sound waves (ultrasound) to generate an image of the heart and associated structures. The study assesses location and relationship of intracardiac and extracardiac structures, cardiac function; measures size of cardiac chambers, valve function, size of septal or other defects; estimates gradients across structures and blood flow direction.	Must be done when the child is quiet and cooperative. If not cooperative, sedation may become necessary.	Methods of echocardiograms: • M-mode • Two-dimensional • Doppler Types of echocardiograms: • Transthoracic • Transesophageal • Directly on cardiac muscle • Fetal
Magnetic resonance imaging (MRI)	A strong magnetic field surrounds the child; the field promotes rotation of nuclei (that normally spin) at predictable speed, allowing visualization of soft tissue, tumors, shunts, myocardial thickness, structure, valve function.	Teaching about the procedure. Nothing-by-mouth (NPO) status for at least 4 hr before procedure if requiring sedation. Assessment for allergy if contrast medium is to be used. All metallic items must be removed.	The child must be able to lie still for up to 1 hr or will require sedation.
Ventilation-perfusion scan (V/Q scan)	Intravenous (IV) injection of isotope, which reveals distribution of pulmonary blood flow and ventilation; assists in quantifying percentage and pattern of pulmonary blood flow.	Requires an IV line for radioisotope injection.	The child must be able to lie still for a short time for the scan.
Pulse oximetry	A bandage probe is attached to a digit; measures oxygen saturation of blood noninvasively.	No specific preparation. The extremity needs to be relatively motion-free for accurate reading. All nail polish must be removed.	If low or high saturation level alarms, validate that the child's heart rate corresponds to the monitor and the expected saturation range for the child's cardiac defect.

CLINICAL REFERENCE ■

Heart disease in children is either congenital or acquired. Congenital heart disease denotes one or more structural abnormalities that develop before birth, although the clinical symptoms may not be present in the newborn period. Acquired heart disease, such as the cardiomyopathies, Kawasaki disease, or acute rheumatic fever, develops after birth and may be seen both in children with normal hearts and in those with congenital heart disease.

The nurse's role includes the astute and vigilant assessment, monitoring, and collaborative treatment of a child with known or potential cardiovascular alterations. Rapid changes in acuity and the rate of decompensation can occur in certain congenital and acquired heart diseases. Thus the skills required of the pediatric nurse must be focused and refined to identify clinically significant changes that may have an impact on this often-complex population.

ASSESSMENT OF THE CHILD WITH A CARDIOVASCULAR ALTERATION

Serious cardiac lesions become symptomatic early in infancy. Remarkable technologic advances in the understanding of the cardiovascular system's function and needs have led to refinements in the tools and techniques for detecting, diagnosing, and treating congenital heart defects. Invasive procedures are now required less for initial diagnosis but rather to obtain more detailed hemodynamic information and for interventional procedures. Nevertheless, no tool or technique replaces obtaining a good history from both the child and the parents and performing a thorough physical examination (Table 46-1).

The cardiac assessment should take place in a quiet and nonthreatening environment with a parent present if possible.

TABLE 46-1 Cardiac Assessment*

Parameter	Assessment Guidelines	Findings and Comments
Health history	Inquire about a family history of congenital heart disease, sudden death, or fetal/infant death. Ask about prenatal care, maternal illnesses, infections, medications taken during pregnancy. Discuss birth history, associated birth defects or genetic anomalies.	There may be an increased incidence of congenital heart disease and dysrhythmias within some families. Chronic maternal illness, perinatal infections, and certain medications have been linked to congenital heart disease. There is an increased incidence of congenital heart disease with certain genetic anomalies or birth defects. Cyanosis, murmur, or other cardiac event present at birth may indicate cardiac disease.
	Discuss feeding difficulties (including decreased intake or increased rest periods during feeding), tachypnea or increased work of breathing, frequency of respiratory infections, poor weight gain, fatigue, exercise intolerance, color changes with crying or Valsalva maneuvers, diaphoresis.	Poor weight gain and failure to thrive are often associated with cardiac disease. Cyanosis may be more prominent with crying or Valsalva maneuvers.
Inspection	Color: Assess skin color in natural light if possible. Pay special attention to oral mucous membranes, nail beds, and conjunctiva, which can reflect central cyanosis. Assess hands, feet, and face. Assess body for differential or demarcated cyanosis or color differences.	Central cyanosis can reflect cardiac or pulmonary alterations. Differential cyanosis may indicate complex heart disease dependent on patent ductus arteriosus blood flow for systemic or pulmonary blood flow. Pallor, mottling, or ruddiness may indicate cardiac disease. Acrocyanosis may be seen in the normal newborn. Clubbing of nail beds may indicate chronic hypoxia. Usually present after 6 months of arterial desaturation (see Fig. 45-6).
	Activity level: Assess child while sitting and lying down. Observe level of activity and position of comfort. Observe for color changes with activity, feeding, or crying. Observe for exercise tolerance, including any respiratory distress or frequent rest.	Lethargy, irritability, or restlessness may indicate poor cardiac function. Squatting may indicate cyanotic heart disease and attempts to improve hypoxia.
	Chest: Assess precordial activity, chest movement (including symmetry), and chest shape (including convex or concave). Assess for sternotomy or thoracotomy incisions.	Point of maximal impulse (PMI) (apical pulse) may be seen in thin children. It is found at the fourth left intercostal space in young children and the fifth intercostal space in children older than 7 years. An active precordium may indicate cardiac disease. A convex chest cavity shape may indicate cardiac disease.
	Respiratory pattern: Observe work of breathing at rest and with activity, including feeding. Look for signs of respiratory alteration or distress. (Tachypnea, retractions, nasal flaring, crackles; grunting and head bobbing are late signs of distress and may indicate impending respiratory failure.)	Increased work of breathing and respiratory difficulty may indicate congestive heart failure.

*A thorough cardiac work-up will often include chest radiography, electrocardiogram (ECG), and echocardiogram.

TABLE **46-1** Cardiac Assessment—cont'd

Parameter	Assessment Guidelines	Findings and Comments
Auscultation	Heart sounds: Auscultate using both bell of stethoscope (for low-pitched sounds) and diaphragm (for high-pitched sounds).	Heart sounds should be synchronous with palpable central or peripheral pulse. Rhythm normally is regular. A normal variation is sinus dysrhythmia when the rhythm can alter and rate can increase with inspiration and decrease with expiration. Ask the older child to briefly hold a breath to allow the nurse to hear more clearly.
	Identify first and second heart sounds.	S_1 is heard best at apex of heart (fourth or fifth intercostal space at left midclavicular line). Correlates with palpable pulse. S_2 is heard best at base (right and left of sternum at second intercostal space).
	Identify additional heart sounds (S_3, S_4). These can be assessed with the child lying supine or on the left side.	S_3 can be heard at the left lower sternal border (LLSB) or apex and can be a normal finding or reflect congestive heart failure. S_4 can be heard at the LLSB or apex and reflects cardiac disease. A gallop is an extra heart sound (S_3 or S_4) and is common in congestive heart failure.
	Identify presence of murmurs, clicks, precordial friction rubs.	Murmurs are caused by turbulent blood flow. Murmurs are described according to location, timing within cardiac cycle, intensity, pitch, and duration. Clicks reflect abnormal valve motion. Precordial friction rubs can reflect pericardial inflammation.
Palpation	Temperature: Compare temperature of trunk with temperature of extremities.	Cooler extremities often indicate poor perfusion because of decreased cardiac output. If room is cold, cool extremities may indicate vasoconstriction to conserve heat.
	Pulses: Compare central and distal pulses.	Peripheral pulses may be diminished if cardiac output is impaired. Causes include congestive heart failure or dehydration.
	Assess pulses in all four extremities.	Weak or absent pulses in the lower extremities may indicate coarctation of the aorta.
	Blood pressure: Assess in all four extremities during initial assessment.	Discrepancies between upper and lower extremity blood pressure may indicate cardiac disease, including coarctation of the aorta.
	Capillary refill: Assess capillary filling in extremities; use fingertips to compress skin.	Normal is less than 2 seconds.
	Chest: With fingertips, locate the PMI.	PMI located farther down than normal may indicate cardiac enlargement.
	Assess for presence of vibratory thrills, heaves or lifts, or friction rubs.	Thrills, described as a palpable murmur, are vibratory in nature. Heaves or lifts are palpable chest wall movement, separate from the PMI, and reflect a hyperactive precordium. Friction rubs, caused by the presence of fluid in the cardiac or pleural space, produce a grating sensation.
	Abdomen: Locate the liver border. It should be at or slightly below the right costal margin in infants and young children.	Normally the border should be firm and smooth. Liver may be boggy with a poorly defined edge and palpable more than 1-2 cm below the right costal margin when congestive heart failure is present.
Percussion	Percussion of the chest provides little useful data in a cardiac assessment.	PMI is a better indicator of heart size.

Assessing Murmurs

Develop a systematic approach to assessing heart sounds with every examination. Abnormal heart sounds will be easier to detect once one can recognize normal. Consider other clinical findings, including anemia and fever, which can intensify a murmur by altering cardiac output.

Organic murmurs reflect an abnormality in the heart structures. Innocent (functional) murmurs do not reflect heart abnormalities but are the sounds made as the blood flows through the structurally normal heart. They can be loud or soft and are often vibratory in quality. Innocent murmurs do not affect growth or well-being and are quite common in children.

Parents know their children best, and they can offer a timeline of events and subtle clinical information that may not be evident on examination. The nurse needs to establish an atmosphere of trust and cooperation—cardiac assessment is best and most easily performed on a cooperative infant or child.

The room should be warm and well-lighted. Natural light from windows will allow the nurse to accurately assess skin color.

The assessment should begin with the least threatening steps—the history and inspection. During the parent interview, the child has the opportunity to observe the interaction between nurse and parent and has time to become comfortable with the nurse's presence. The child should be allowed to participate in the assessment and encouraged to touch and inspect each piece of equipment to be used during the examination.

Assessment progression includes inspection, auscultation, and palpation; each step requires more touching. The nurse must remember to warm the stethoscope used for auscultation, as well as the hands before touching the child's skin. This is particularly important when assessing a resting infant, who may become startled by the cold touch of the hands and stethoscope.

CARDIOVASCULAR DIAGNOSIS

Tests used to diagnose cardiac problems in children have been described previously (see p. 1255). The primary method for describing the existence and extent of cardiac disease in children is cardiac catheterization.

Cardiac Catheterization

Cardiac catheterization is both an invasive diagnostic procedure and an interventional and therapeutic procedure. Catheters are advanced, generally through the femoral vein or artery, into the venous or arterial system and directed into the heart. Data obtained and interventions performed during the procedure include:

- Measurement of oxygen saturations in cardiac chambers and great arteries
- Measurement of pressures in cardiac chambers and great arteries, and determination of gradients
- Evaluation of cardiac output

- Angiography to identify detailed images of structures and blood flow patterns
- Electrophysiologic studies to map the cardiac conduction system and identify the locus of dysrhythmia-producing cells; radiofrequency catheter ablation is used for destruction of these cells
- Corrective or palliative interventional procedures include pulmonary artery or valve and aortic valve balloon angioplasty, stent placement to maintain patency of vessels, balloon/blade septostomy for creation of an atrial septal defect (indicated for certain complex congenital heart defects), and device closure of septal defects or coil embolization of a patent ductus arteriosus or collateral vessels

Complications

Complications may result both during and after the procedure. Potential complications of which the nurse should be aware include dysrhythmias, hemorrhage, vascular damage, vasospasm of the catheterized vessel, thrombus or embolus formation, infection, reaction to the dye, and catheter perforation. Perforation by the catheter of the heart or vessels during the procedure can result in cardiac tamponade and cardiac arrest. Dysrhythmias may be hemodynamically compromising. Vasospasm of the vessel results in poor perfusion to the affected leg. Clot formation at the catheter insertion site may impair perfusion to the affected limb and may shed emboli that may travel anywhere in the vascular system depending on the cardiac anatomy, including the lung or brain. Thrombus formation may occur in the systemic-to-pulmonary artery shunts that provide pulmonary blood flow. Reactions to the dye may be mild (vomiting) or, very rarely, severe (anaphylaxis). Additional minor reactions to the procedure include nausea and vomiting related to anesthetics or sedatives, or pressure ulceration of pressure points related to prolonged immobility and decreased subcutaneous tissue.

Nursing Care

Because impaired peripheral perfusion is a possible consequence of a cardiac catheterization, it is important for the nurse to locate and mark distal pulses prior to the procedure. Marking the location of pulses will assist the nurse with rapid post-procedure assessment.

After the procedure, the child is positioned with the affected leg straight for 4 to 6 hours; infants may be held prone on a parent's lap. Older children remain in bed with the head of the bed raised at only a 20-degree incline. Intravenous (IV) fluid administration continues until the infant or child is taking and retaining adequate amounts of oral fluids.

Vital signs should be obtained frequently (every 5-15 min) for the first hour, with continuous initial monitoring of heart rate, blood pressure, respiratory rate and oxygen saturation, and temperature.

The insertion site dressing should be observed frequently, at least every 5 to 15 minutes, during the early postprocedure hours. Assess for bleeding not only on the dressing but also on sheets. Look under the child to check for pooled blood. Pull back bed linens and remove the infant's diaper (if applicable) to check the perineal area for bleeding under the skin. If bleeding occurs, place a gloved heel of the hand firmly on the insertion site. Apply pressure for at least 10 to 15 minutes, and assess distal perfusion of the extremity. Immediately notify the cardiologist. Assess blood loss and the child's hemodynamic status.

Peripheral perfusion is also monitored. The affected extremity will frequently be mottled in appearance and cooler to touch than the other extremities. Distal pulses should, however, be palpable, although they may be weaker than in the contralateral extremity. Non-palpable distal pulses should be checked using a Doppler. Notify the cardiologist if distal pulses are absent on the affected extremity or the temperature or degree of mottling has changed or the child complains of increasing pain.

Heparin drip infusions are initiated under certain circumstances that may be related to the catheter route or to placement of stents, coils or closure devices.

Children who have undergone a diagnostic cardiac catheterization are often discharged the same day. Children undergoing interventional procedures or electrophysiologic studies may remain hospitalized overnight. The following day, the pressure bandage is removed and is replaced with a Band-Aid. Discharge instructions vary according to the institution but may include:

- Inspecting the catheter insertion site to assess healing or the presence of local infection
- Bathing limited to a shower, sponge bath, or brief tub bath (no soaking) for the first 1 to 3 days after the procedure
- Avoiding strenuous exercise (climbing trees, swimming, contact sports) for up to 1 week after the procedure
- Returning to school on the 3rd day after the procedure for obs.
- Notifying the cardiologist if the child develops a fever above 38.3° C (101° F); bleeding or drainage (pus) from catheter insertion site; or pallor, coolness, or numbness of the affected extremity
- Resuming normal feeding patterns and medication therapy if applicable
- Reviewing the need to continue antibiotic prophylaxis for dental or other specific medical procedures
- Follow-up with a cardiologist at a scheduled visit

CONGENITAL HEART DISEASE

Congenital heart defects are some of the most frequently seen congenital defects in infants and children, with the incidence reported in approximately 1% of pregnancies, and approximately 6 per 1000 live births (Neilson & Robin, 2002). Of the cardiac problems in children, the majority result from congenital heart disease—structural defects within the heart that are present at birth. The precise etiology of congenital heart disease is not known. The majority of cases (~ 90%) are thought to be multifactorial.

Investigations into environmental and genetic causes of congenital heart disease are in progress. The genetic component of congenital heart disease has been investigated more thoroughly than the environmental aspect. Children with certain genetic defects have an extremely high incidence of cardiac disorders, including children with chromosome aberrations, most specifically trisomy 21 (Down syndrome), in which the incidence of congenital heart disease is approximately 50% (Park, 2002). Other children who have an increased risk of having congenital heart disease include girls with *Turner's syndrome* (genetically having only a single X chromosome) and boys with *Klinefelter's variant* (genetically having additional X chromosomes), children with velocardiofacial syndrome (*DiGeorge syndrome*), and children with Marfan syndrome. Some children with nonhereditary conditions, such as fetal alcohol syndrome (25% to 30% incidence) are at increased risk for CHD, as are infants of diabetic mothers (3% to 5%) (Park, 2002).

A family history of congenital heart disease increases the risk for giving birth to a child with congenital heart disease. Siblings of a child with congenital heart disease have a 2% to 3% risk, and the risk may be even higher if one of the parents has a cardiac lesion (Neilson & Robin, 2002).

The current approach to congenital heart disease is to return the child to normal or near-normal anatomy and physiology as soon as possible. Corrective and palliative procedures are now performed earlier in life because of a number of advances in surgical techniques and medical management. In addition, the impact on the natural history of uncorrected, palliated, and corrected defects and the effect on the child's morbidity and mortality are now better understood given the past four to five decades of surgical intervention. Also, there is an increased awareness and understanding of the impact of chronic illness on the child and family.

Classification of Congenital Heart Disease

Congenital cardiac defects can be classified according to structural abnormalities, functional alterations, or both (Table 46-2). Historically, defects were classified according to whether they were acyanotic or cyanotic. This classification is generally imprecise because children who may be acyanotic initially can become cyanotic as an uncorrected lesion worsens cardiac status. Clinical signs of congenital cardiac defects are not always apparent at birth; they can manifest any time during infancy or early childhood. The degree of symptomatology, indications for medical and surgical interventions, and chronicity of condition depend on the diagnosis.

Shunting: Saturation Considerations

Shunting, or blood flow through an abnormal opening in the heart or great vessels, occurs when (1) an abnormal opening or connection is between the cardiac chambers or great arteries, (2) the pressure is higher on one side of the heart compared with the other, and (3) the oxygen saturation is increased or decreased in the normally desaturated or fully saturated blood. It is important to remember that the venous side (often the right side) is normally a low-pressure, desaturated (average 70%) system and the arterial side (often the left side) is normally a high-pressure, fully saturated (95% to 100%) system. The combination of pressure differences and the size of the abnormal opening determine the extent of shunting. Understanding the principles of shunting and normal saturations helps clarify the blood flow direction in congenital heart disease.

Blood Flow Considerations

Normally the amount of blood flow to the lungs through the pulmonary artery is the same as to the systemic circulation through the aorta. This ratio of pulmonary to systemic blood flow is described as the *pulmonary to systemic ratio* (QP/QS ratio), which is usually 1:1. Congenital heart defects have normal, increased, or decreased pulmonary to systemic blood flow ratios. Left-to-right shunts or obstructive lesions have normal or increased pulmonary to systemic blood flow ratios. Right-to-left, or complex, cyanotic lesions may have normal, decreased, or increased pulmonary to systemic blood flow ratios.

TABLE 46-2 Classification of Congenital Heart Disease

Defect	Underlying Mechanism	Examples
Left-to-right shunting lesions (lesions that increase pulmonary blood flow)	Left-sided heart pressures, which normally exceed right-sided pressures, cause saturated blood to shunt through any abnormal opening in the heart, aorta, or pulmonary artery. This left-to-right shunting of blood results in a volume overload in the right side of the heart and in the pulmonary artery; cardiac workload (including ventricular strain, dilation, hypertrophy) increases to manage the additional volume (pressure overload). A "step-up" oxygen saturation (abnormal increase because of the addition of more highly saturated blood), combined with the increased fluid volume in the lungs, results in altered gas exchange. One of the major consequences of left-to-right shunting lesions is congestive heart failure. Other consequences include pulmonary hypertension, pulmonary vascular disease, and frequent upper and lower respiratory infections that can progress to respiratory failure.	Atrial septal defect (ASD) Ventricular septal defect (VSD) Patent ductus arteriosus (PDA) Atrioventricular septal defect (AVSD; endocardial cushion defect)
Obstructive or stenotic lesions, or lesions that decrease cardiac outflow	Stenosis, the narrowing or constriction of an opening, can occur in a valve or vessel constricting or obstructing blood flow through the area. Pressure rises in the area behind the obstruction; blood flow distal to the obstruction may be decreased or absent. Stenotic lesions can occur in the right or left side of the heart; obstruction on the left side of the heart decreases the amount of available blood for systemic perfusion. Physiologic effects of stenotic lesions include increased cardiac workload and ventricular strain, with clinical consequences of congestive heart failure, decreased cardiac output, and pump failure.	Pulmonary stenosis Aortic stenosis Coarctation of the aorta
Cyanotic lesions with decreased pulmonary blood flow	These lesions arise from an error in fetal development that results in hypoplasia (incomplete development), malalignment, or obstruction on the right side of the heart and decrease the amount of blood volume to the lungs. Pulmonary blood flow may rely on having a patent ductus arteriosus. There is a "stepdown" (abnormally decreased) oxygen saturation in the left side of the heart. Physiologically, the child manifests hypoxemia, increased cardiac workload, and ventricular strain. The hypoxemia results in cyanosis (baseline saturations often as low as 75%-85%), and, even with oxygen administration, saturations do not approximate normal. Other clinical findings may include upper respiratory infection, severely limited pulmonary blood flow, and marked exercise intolerance.	Tetralogy of Fallot Tricuspid valve abnormalities Pulmonary atresia with intact ventricular septum
Cyanotic lesions with increased pulmonary blood flow	When the fetal heart fails to develop into separate pulmonary and systemic circulations (so that there is a mixing of saturated and desaturated blood), or when there is a reversal of circulation so that desaturated blood goes to the systemic circulation and saturated blood to the pulmonary circulation, cyanosis occurs. Sometimes classified as mixing lesions, these defects cause increased cardiac workload, ventricular strain, and decreased cardiac output. Usually discovered early in the neonatal period, the infant might appear ruddy or cyanotic, with increased respiratory effort, or, if systemic circulation is compromised, may be dusky or gray and present in cardiogenic shock (see Chapter 34). To support life, these complex cardiac defects may require intervention that allows for mixing of arterial and venous blood.	Truncus arteriosus Hypoplastic left heart syndrome* Transposition of the great arteries

*Also classified as a lesion that decreases cardiac outflow

PHYSIOLOGIC CONSEQUENCES OF CONGENITAL HEART DISEASE IN CHILDREN

Congestive Heart Failure

Congestive heart failure (CHF) is a clinical syndrome that reflects the heart's inability to maintain cardiac output sufficiently to meet the metabolic demands of the body. Heart failure is one of the most frequently seen consequences of congenital heart disease and is often what is diagnosed first in an older infant with a previously undiagnosed congenital cardiac defect. Congestive heart failure results from both hemodynamic and neurohumoral responses in an attempt to compensate for inadequate cardiac output. Symptomatology is related to these responses. In infants and children decreased cardiac output is most often caused by effects of volume overload or pressure overload caused by underlying defects (e.g., large left-to-right shunts or palliated complex defects).

Pediatric CHF can develop from many other etiologies, including congenital and acquired anatomic anomalies (including cardiomyopathies), dysrhythmias, infections (e.g., endocarditis, myocarditis), inborn metabolic disorders, tumors, drugs, and toxins (Balaguru, Artman, & Auslender, 2000).

Manifestations

The clinical manifestations of CHF are related to the degree of hemodynamic and neurohormonal responses. Manifestations include tachycardia and gallop rhythm; tachypnea, increased work of breathing demonstrated by intercostal and subcostal retractions, grunting, nasal flaring, rales, and rarely wheezing or cough; periorbital and facial edema, neck vein distention (in children), hepatomegaly, and splenomegaly; and decreased peripheral perfusion, decreased urine output, diaphoresis, mottling, and cyanosis or pallor. The infant or child may be lethargic, be irritable, or fatigue more easily.

The earliest clinical manifestations of CHF are often subtle. The infant may have mild resting tachypnea and increasing difficulty feeding. Feedings take longer, and less is consumed while expending more energy, resulting in fewer calories being consumed even though metabolic demands are increased. Feedings therefore provide little satisfaction. The infant may appear hungry and irritable soon after a feeding. Over time, the infant fails to gain weight and eventually has failure to thrive.

Diagnostic Evaluation

The diagnosis of CHF is established on the basis of clinical history, physical examination, chest radiographic appearance, electrocardiography (ECG), and echocardiography. Chest x-ray may reveal cardiomegaly and increased pulmonary vascular markings reflecting increased interstitial pulmonary fluid. Laboratory studies that may be indicated to determine the presence of heart failure in children include determinations of arterial blood gas values, serum electrolyte levels, complete blood cell count, sedimentation rate, serum glucose and calcium levels, and urinalysis.

Therapeutic Management

Management of a child with CHF involves correcting the underlying problem as soon as it is feasible to do so. The medical management of CHF is directed toward decreasing cardiac workload and improving cardiac output through the manipulation of the hemodynamics and neurohormonal responses. Supplemental oxygen can be helpful for increasing oxygen saturation, but it should be used with caution in children with left-to-right shunting lesions. Pharmacologic agents used include positive inotropes, diuretics, and angiotensin-converting enzyme (ACE) inhibitors. In addition, optimizing nutritional intake to meet the metabolic demands and improve growth is of paramount importance. Inability to decrease symptoms and achieve weight gain is an indication for surgical intervention.

Initial medication therapy depends on the presenting symptoms. Diuretics and a positive inotropic agent (e.g., digoxin) are used most commonly.

Diuretics are administered to eliminate excess water and sodium through increased urine production, thereby reducing

---

Pathophysiology

of Congestive Heart Failure

In congestive heart failure, hemodynamic and neurohormonal changes occur in response to decreased cardiac output and these changes determine the clinical manifestations. The hemodynamics affected include preload, afterload, contractility, and cardiac output. Cardiac output is the amount of blood ejected with each heart beat. The neurohormonal responses include the stimulation of both the sympathetic nervous system and the renin-angiotensin system. In addition, the chronologic age of the child influences other factors (e.g., cardiac muscle maturity) that affect the manifestations and their management.*

Maintaining blood pressure, blood flow, and oxygen delivery to vital organs is the goal of the compensatory systems. With decreased cardiac output, there is stimulation of the sympathetic nervous system. This initially leads to increased heart rate, contractility, and stroke volume; increased systemic vascular resistance (afterload); and selective peripheral vasoconstriction. Tachycardia, although beneficial to compensate for early congestive heart failure, increases myocardial oxygen consumption, decreases the diastolic filling time and resting phase of the heart, and decreases coronary artery perfusion.†

Decreased cardiac output also causes the renal system to have diminished glomerular filtration rate and decreased renal blood flow. This leads to increased stimulation of the renin-angiotensin-aldosterone system. Sodium and water are reabsorbed, leading to fluid retention and thereby increasing intravascular volume. Initially, this volume retention increases preload and cardiac output. Later, the myocardium becomes more edematous, and ventricular function decreases from volume and pressure overload.

The pulmonary system is also affected by this increased volume, and interstitial edema develops. In addition, myocardial oxygen consumption increases and may exceed the oxygen availability. Finally, myocardial muscle can undergo cellular and muscular mass changes, or hypertrophy. Without intervention, heart failure progresses until the compensatory mechanisms are no longer effective.

*Balaguru D., Artman, M., & Auslender M. (2000). Management of heart failure in children. *Current Problems in Pediatrics, 30*(1), 5-30.
† Bernstein, D. (2004). The cardiovascular system. In R.E. Behrman, R.M. Kliegman, & H. Jenson (Eds.), *Nelson textbook of pediatrics* (17th ed., pp. 1475-1591). Philadelphia: Saunders.

---

systemic and pulmonary congestion. Furosemide is a potent loop diuretic and is frequently the initial diuretic therapy. Another classification of diuretics, the thiazides, acts at the distal renal tubules. These can be less potent than loop diuretics. These drugs cause the kidneys to waste potassium, placing the child at risk for hypokalemia. Potassium-sparing diuretics, such as spironolactone, are weak diuretics. This class of diuretics is often given with loop diuretics or thiazides to decrease the potential for hypokalemia. Potassium supplements can also be given in tandem with diuretics to replace these losses.

Digoxin is a cardiac glycoside that increases cardiac output and improves cardiac effectiveness by several mechanisms. It

PARENTS
Want to Know

About Giving Your Child Digoxin Elixir

Medication: Digoxin (Lanoxin)

Your child's dosage: _____ml twice a day. Your child will be taking this medicine twice a day for several months to years.

What it does: Digoxin (Lanoxin) helps the heart pump blood more efficiently.

What you need to know:

- Digoxin (Lanoxin) is usually given every morning and evening. You may adjust the times to fit your and your child's schedule.
- Give the digoxin 20 to 30 minutes before a feeding. Give it at the same time every day so that it becomes part of your routine.
- The amount of digoxin you give your child must be measured carefully using a syringe, not the dropper provided with the medicine.
- Put a few drops of digoxin in your child's mouth, and let the child swallow it before giving more.
- If you forget to give your child a single dose of digoxin, give the dose when you remember it; then resume your original schedule.
- If your child vomits after taking the digoxin, do not repeat the dose. Resume the digoxin at the next dosage time.
- *If you miss or your child vomits two doses in a row, call the cardiology department.*
- Rarely, children have too much digoxin in their body and can develop vomiting. If your child develops vomiting, call your pediatrician or cardiologist. You will be instructed what to do about your child's dosage.
- Keep the digoxin in a place where children living or playing in your home will not be able to reach.
- If someone accidentally takes the digoxin, call poison control and/or take the person and digoxin bottle to the emergency room.
- Obtain refills at least 1 week before you are out of medicine. Ask for new prescriptions as needed.

Modified and used with permission from Children's Hospital Oakland, Department of Cardiology, Oakland, CA. Developed and revised by Lili Cook, RN, MS, and Sally Higgins, PhD, RN, FAAN.

CRITICAL THINKING EXERCISE 46-1

Lin, a 2-month-old infant, is seen in the pediatrician's office. She has gained 1 lb since birth and has a murmur. She is admitted to the pediatric unit with a diagnosis of congestive heart failure. You will obtain a health history and perform an admission assessment.

1. What specific questions should Lin's parents be asked about her feeding patterns and behavior?
2. What physical assessment findings would you expect in an infant with congestive heart failure?
3. List nursing interventions that would address Lin's nutritional and comfort needs.

! CRITICAL TO REMEMBER

Feeding the Infant or Child With Congestive Heart Failure

Feed the infant or child in a relaxed environment. Time the feedings before multiple other activities to preserve the infant's energy. The infant with congestive heart failure tends to tire easily during feedings. Frequent, small feedings may be less tiring. Holding the infant in an upright position may provide less stomach compression and improve respiratory effort during the feeding. If the child is unable to consume an appropriate amount during a 30-minute feeding period every 3 hours, nasogastric feeding should be considered. Monitor for increased tachypnea, diaphoresis, or feeding intolerance (vomiting). Concentrating formula from the basic level of 20 kcal/oz to 27 kcal/oz can increase caloric intake without increasing the infant's work.

has a positive inotropic effect that strengthens the force of ventricular contractions. It has a negative chronotropic effect that slows the heart rate and, at higher doses, conduction of cardiac impulses through the AV node, allowing the ventricles more time to fill with blood. It also improves blood flow to the kidneys and enhances diuresis.

Obtain a baseline ECG before initiating digoxin. Digoxin may be administered IV or orally. The effectiveness of digoxin depends on achieving and maintaining a therapeutic serum drug level. A loading or digitalizing dose is administered in divided doses over 12 to 18 hours, and maintenance doses are given daily, usually in two divided doses. The range between therapeutic and toxic levels is narrow, with the therapeutic range 0.8 to 2.0 ng/ml (Park, 2002). In order to avoid a falsely elevated serum digoxin level, serum levels should be measured at a minimum of 6 hours from the previous dose of digoxin; measurement in the first 3 to 5 days after digitalizing could also result in elevated results (Park, 2002). Levels are generally obtained when assessing for toxicity or medication adherence. Digoxin levels may be difficult to measure and monitor in preterm infants (Park, 2002). If a child is on digoxin and is having dysrhythmias, a digoxin level should be obtained. Hypokalemia and hypomagnesemia can potentiate digoxin toxicity. In addition, the dose needs to be decreased in children with altered renal function.

Vasodilators, such as captopril or enalapril, may be used to relax vascular smooth muscles and reduce afterload (Bernstein, 2004). This class of vasodilators is called ACE *inhibitors* because they block the conversion of angiotensin I to angiotensin II and reduce vasoconstriction and sodium retention. In addition, ACE inhibitors also decrease norepinephrine release from the sympathetic nervous system (Balaguru, Artman, & Auslender, 2000).

Pulmonary Hypertension

Pulmonary hypertension is defined as an elevated mean pulmonary artery pressure of greater than 20 mm Hg at sea level, compared with the normal of 15 mm Hg (Park, 2002). Initially, in children with significant left-to-right shunting, there is reversible pulmonary vasoconstriction and increased pulmonary blood flow that causes elevated pulmonary artery pressure. Pulmonary vascular disease

Nursing Care Plan

The Child With Congestive Heart Failure

FOCUSED ASSESSMENT

Assessment of the child with congestive heart failure (CHF) includes close monitoring of vital signs and a thorough cardiovascular, pulmonary, nutritional, and fluid status evaluation. Children being medically treated for CHF are often admitted because of worsening symptoms, including failure to thrive. In the newborn period, recognizing the early signs of CHF will expedite timely treatment. The early symptoms of tachycardia, tachypnea, poor feeding, and diaphoresis during feeding, and increased irritability or fatigue should be noted and the physician or nurse practitioner alerted. Strict monitoring of intake and output and daily weights is also important in assessment and management.

Nursing Diagnosis

Decreased Cardiac Output related to congestive heart failure or decreased myocardial function.

Expected Outcome

The child will:
- Have adequate cardiac output, as evidenced by pink or baseline cyanotic (in cyanotic heart disease) mucous membranes and nail beds, a capillary refill time of less than 2 seconds, warm extremities, easily palpable peripheral pulses, adequate urinary output, no edema, appropriate heart rate, and an activity level within the normal limits of the defect.

INTERVENTION	RATIONALE
1. Monitor peripheral perfusion by palpating peripheral pulses, noting temperature, color changes, and capillary refill time.	1. Poor peripheral perfusion is usually evidenced by decreased or absent pulses in the extremities. Color and temperature changes (e.g., cyanosis, coolness, mottling) may be present in all extremities. Prolonged capillary refill time is an additional sign of poor perfusion.
2. Assess if heart rate is appropriate for level of activity.	2. Tachycardia occurs in an attempt to maintain adequate cardiac output.
3. Monitor and document hourly urine output.	3. Altered renal perfusion caused by decreased cardiac output results in decreased urinary output.
4. Maintain a neutral thermal environment; use a warmer bed or isolette for the newborn; treat fever promptly.	4. Episodes of hypothermia or hyperthermia increase oxygen demands and increase the cardiac workload.
5. Time nursing interventions to allow the infant or child rest periods. Anticipate and respond quickly to stressful events, crying, or restlessness.	5. Rest periods reduce cardiac workload. Organizing nursing activities decreases the child's stress and fatigue.
6. Administer digoxin (Lanoxin) as prescribed. Ascertain that the dosage is within safe limits. Count the apical rate for 1 full minute. Check the dosage with a second nurse. Withhold the dose and notify physician if the heart rate is less than 100 beats/min in infants; the heart rate at which the medication should be withheld varies in older children and adolescents. In general, if the withholding pulse rate is not ordered, withhold the medication and call the physician if the pulse rate is progressively decreasing or markedly lower than previous rates. Observe for signs of toxicity (see Parents Want to Know: About Giving Your Child Digoxin Elixir), and monitor for hyperkalemia in the child taking potassium-sparing diuretics.	6. Digoxin is effective within a narrow therapeutic range (0.8-2 ng/ml*) although the pediatric range is not well defined. Safety in dosing is achieved by double-checking the dose and counting the apical heart rate for a full minute. Digoxin toxicity can manifest with slow pulse, vomiting and dysrhythmias.

Evaluation

- Are mucous membranes and nail beds pink or baseline cyanosis?
- Is the capillary refill time less than 2 seconds?
- Are peripheral pulses easily palpated, and is the child alert and active?
- Is the heart rate in the expected range for activity?

* Park, M.K. (2002). *Pediatric cardiology for practitioners* (4th ed.). St. Louis: Mosby.

Continued

Nursing Care Plan

The Child With Congestive Heart Failure—cont'd

Nursing Diagnosis

Excess Fluid Volume related to volume overload and congestive heart failure.

Expected Outcome

The infant or child will:
- Remain free of evidence of fluid overload (e.g., infrequent urination, inappropriate water weight gain, inadequate balance between intake and output, edema [periorbital, hepatomegaly], respiratory distress, poor feeding).

INTERVENTION	RATIONALE
1. Administer diuretics as prescribed, ensuring correct dosage, route, and effectiveness.	1. Diuretics help the body eliminate excess fluid. Their effectiveness is evaluated from the urine output (either by measuring the amount of urine or by weighing diapers), weight, decreasing edema, decreasing respiratory distress, improved feeding.
2. Maintain accurate intake and output records.	2. The fluid intake and output should be about the same. If intake grossly exceeds output, the diuretics may need to be altered, the child may need fluid restriction, or both.
3. Maintain fluid restriction, if ordered.	3. Fluid restriction will decrease pulmonary and liver edema.
4. Using the same scales, weigh the child daily at approximately the same time. Notify the physician of excessive weight gain (>50 g/day in infants; >200 g/day in children).	4. Excess fluid volume is not always overtly visible. Weight changes may indicate fluid retention. Weighing the infant or child on the same scales at the same time each day ensures consistency.
5. Provide skin care and change position frequently.	5. Edematous areas are extremely prone to skin breakdown because of stretching and opacity. Frequent position changes will prevent undesirable pooling of fluid in certain areas.
6. Assess for increased or decreased edema. (In infants and young children, edema is usually periorbital and hepatomegaly; generalized edema in the preoperative patient is extremely rare).	6. Changes in the amount of edema can indicate the effectiveness or ineffectiveness of therapies and interventions.
7. Monitor serum electrolyte levels, especially potassium.	7. Diuretics may stimulate potassium loss.

Evaluation

- Is the child urinating frequently in comparison with age-related norms (see Chapter 42)?
- Is the child edematous?
- Has the child lost or gained weight?
- Are intake and output balanced?

Nursing Diagnosis

Ineffective Breathing Pattern related to pulmonary congestion.

Expected Outcomes

The child will:
- Demonstrate a respiratory rate within normal limits for age and a normal respiratory effort.
- Have satisfactory rest periods.
- Have color that remains pink or baseline cyanosis.

INTERVENTION	RATIONALE
1. Monitor respiratory rate and rhythm, the presence or absence of retractions or nasal flaring, the use of accessory muscles, and the presence or absence of crackles or rhonchi.	1. Infants and children with CHF experience changes in their breathing pattern because of increased fluid retention in the lungs, liver, and other areas of the body.

Nursing Care Plan

The Child With Congestive Heart Failure—cont'd

INTERVENTION	RATIONALE
2. Position the infant or child with the head of the bed elevated 30 to 45 degrees. Avoid clothing that constricts the chest.	2. An elevated position lowers the diaphragm and maximizes chest expansion.
3. Administer oxygen as needed.	3. Supplemental oxygen administration improves oxygen saturation and delivery to tissues. Cautious use of oxygen is indicated in left-to-right shunting lesions because of the effect of oxygen on lowering pulmonary vascular resistance, which can increase pulmonary blood flow and increase the degree of pulmonary congestion and symptoms of CHF.
4. Plan nursing interventions to allow maximum rest for the child. Feed the child when the child is rested. Avoid performing multiple interventions at any one time.	4. Organizing nursing activities decreases the child's fatigue, promotes feeding effort, and conserves metabolic demands.
5. Prevent exposure to individuals with respiratory illnesses. Prevent nosocomial exposures and infections.	5. Respiratory infections with associated congenital heart disease (CHD) can have a severe adverse impact on respiratory stability. Children with CHD are at a higher risk for nosocomial infections.

Evaluation

- Is the child's respiratory rate within normal limits for age?
- Are the child's mucous membranes and nail beds pink or at baseline cyanosis?
- Is the child breathing easily?
- Is the child able to obtain an appropriate amount of rest?

Nursing Diagnosis

Imbalanced Nutrition: Less Than Body Requirements related to increased energy expenditure and increased feeding effort.

Expected Outcome

The infant or child will:

- Demonstrate appropriate weight gain and no significant loss of weight over a short period.

INTERVENTION	RATIONALE
1. Weigh the infant or child daily or before and after each feeding for breastfed infants. Use the same scale.	1. Using the same scale ensures consistency.
2. Feed smaller volumes of concentrated formula (24-27 cal/oz) every 3 hours	2. Increased caloric content of formula increases caloric consumption and enhances weight gain. May require 120 to 150 kcal/kg/day for adequate weight gain.
3. Use a nipple that the infant can comfortably adjust for flow rate and energy to express milk. May need a soft, large-hole nipple.	3. Infants with CHF tire easily. An appropriate nipple for the infant minimizes the level of energy required to express milk at a rate of flow the baby can swallow comfortably. A soft nipple with a large hole may facilitate easy sucking and decrease energy expenditure during feeding.
4. Implement gavage feedings if the infant tires before the recommended amount of feedings is consumed, takes longer than 30 minutes to feed, experiences increased fatigue during or after feeding, or demonstrates poor weight gain on adequate caloric intake.	4. Gavage feedings decrease energy expenditure and allow calories consumed to be used for growth. Can be used in conjunction with timed nipple periods to maintain feeding skills.
5. Time the feedings to allow for adequate rest. Every 3 hours is a frequently used interval.	5. Frequent disturbances increase oxygen consumption. Too frequent feedings disturb rest, whereas less frequent feedings require increased intake, which tires the infant.
6. Monitor for feeding intolerance.	6. May not tolerate concentrated formulas. Also, gastroesophageal reflux may be present.

Continued

Nursing Care Plan

The Child With Congestive Heart Failure—cont'd

Evaluation

- Has the infant or child maintained a steady weight gain?
- Is the feeding pattern stable or changing?
- Is the infant or child tolerating feedings without vomiting or other signs of intolerance?

Nursing Diagnosis

Deficient Knowledge related to anxiety and unfamiliarity with the disease process, treatment, interventions, and home care.

Expected Outcomes

Parents will:
- Describe the cardiac defect and current and future interventions.
- Demonstrate an ability to perform treatments, including medication administration.

INTERVENTION	RATIONALE
1. Determine the parents' readiness to learn, anxiety level, knowledge needed to care for their child, and specific concerns.	1. A baseline assessment of prior knowledge should be considered before developing a teaching plan. Addressing special concerns initially can facilitate parents' comfort level and receptiveness to new knowledge. Decreasing anxiety assists with information processing.
2. Provide brief, factual explanations of the child's defect or any treatments and interventions. Do so frequently.	2. Parents are most likely to retain consistent, repetitive explanations.
3. Allow the parents and child to verbalize feelings and concerns related to hospitalization and caring for the child at home.	3. Hospitalization is a frightening experience. By allowing verbalization of feelings and concerns related to the experience, nurses can assist in allaying fears and addressing concerns. Discussing care at home can also assist in allaying fears and addressing concerns.
4. Teach the parents to administer all necessary cardiac medications and explain their associated actions and potential adverse effects. Provide demonstrations and obtain return demonstrations by parents. Explain the use of oral syringes for accurate measurement of drugs. Provide a daily medication chart (that can be color-coded for specific medications) for children receiving multiple medications. Provide parents with written information (see Parents Want to Know: Giving Your Child Digoxin Elixir).	4. Family members should be taught how to administer all cardiac medications before discharge. This allows for teaching appropriate medication dosage, questions, answers, and evaluation of their home care techniques. Written information provides an adjunct to individual teaching and a reference for the caregiver at home. Written information can be referred to during less stressful times, when it may be more likely to be retained or used as a reference.
5. Assess parents' understanding of instructions through return demonstrations and repeated information. This includes signs and symptoms requiring medical or nursing assessment.	5. Return demonstrations and repeated information validate that learning has occurred and that the parents are competent to provide care.

Evaluation

- Have the parents verbalized adequate and correct knowledge of the diagnosis and interventions?
- Have the parents demonstrated confidence and competence in caregiving activities, including medicine administration?
- Are the parents able to describe conditions that necessitate a call for medical or nursing advice?

occurs when vascular changes lead eventually to vessel wall thickening, severe irreversible vasoconstriction, and vascular obstruction. This severe condition leads to a reversal of the cardiac shunting, becoming right to left (called *Eisenmenger syndrome*), with less blood being pumped to the lungs, so that the child becomes cyanotic even though the defect was previously acyanotic. It is critical to time any surgical intervention before the development of irreversible vascular changes. This information is assessed clinically and in the cardiac catheterization laboratory. Repair of lesions with large left-to-right shunts is generally recommended in the first 3 to 6 months of life.

Pulmonary hypertension has multiple etiologies. In children with congenital heart disease, the causes include pulmonary overcirculation, pulmonary vasoconstriction, and pulmonary vascular disease (Kinsella, Neish, Abman, & Wolfe, 1998). Concurrent risk factors for secondary pulmonary hypertension and pulmonary vascular disease include alveolar hypoxia, pulmonary parenchymal disease, airway obstruction (often seen with Down syndrome), obstructive lesions, large left-to-right shunt lesions, pulmonary venous hypertension, and cyanotic heart disease. Some children have primary pulmonary vascular disease.

Children with large left-to-right shunting lesions, particularly at the ventricular level, have high pulmonary artery pressures but low pulmonary vascular resistance and initially develop congestive heart failure. Management of these children is directed toward treating the CHF. Additionally, they are advised to avoid strenuous exercise and high altitudes. Treatment with vasodilators or oxygen may, or may not, be helpful (Park, 2002). Inhaled nitrous oxide has been shown to be an effective pulmonary vasodilator and is used in the treatment of persistent pulmonary hypertension of the newborn. With early surgical intervention, children with reversible pulmonary hypertension can have a return of normal pulmonary pressures postoperatively. As children develop increasing pulmonary vascular resistance caused by pulmonary vascular changes, they have a higher risk for surgical morbidity and mortality.

Cyanosis

Significant congenital heart disease manifests with central cyanosis (hypoxemia). Cyanosis, a bluish discoloration of the skin, nail beds, and mucous membranes, appears when tissues are deprived of adequate amounts of oxygen. Cyanosis becomes visible when hemoglobin, approximately 5 g/dl blood, circulates unbound to oxygen and the measured oxygen saturation drops below 85%. The degree of cyanosis varies; some children will appear pale and mildly cyanotic, whereas others will be quite dusky. In anemic infants or children, desaturation will be higher before cyanosis is apparent (lower hemoglobin in anemia, so a higher percentage needs to be desaturated before cyanosis is visible). Concurrently, with significant polycythemia, they will appear cyanotic when less desaturated (higher hemoglobin in polycythemia, so a lower percentage needs to be desaturated before cyanosis is visible).

Cardiac lesions produce cyanosis when desaturated blood from the venous system enters the saturated arterial system without passing through the lungs. Cyanosis can occur when (1) blood flow to the lungs is decreased or insufficient or (2) deoxygenated, or desaturated, blood is pumped to the body and a decreased, normal, or increased amount of deoxygenated and oxygenated blood is pumped to the lungs (Grifka, 1999).

The clinical consequences of cyanosis include polycythemia, anemia, clotting abnormalities, hypercyanotic episodes, central nervous system (CNS) injury caused by abscess or embolic events, pulmonary hypertension, and endocarditis. Developmental delay can be related to CNS injury, severe hypoxic events, or chronic illness.

Polycythemia is a compensatory response of the body to chronic hypoxia. The body attempts to improve tissue oxygenation by increasing the oxygen-carrying capacity of the blood—in other words, by producing additional red blood cells (RBCs). Accelerated RBC production increases the viscosity of the blood and crowds the vascular space so there is less room for plasma and clotting factors. Children who are polycythemic are at greater risk for bruising and prolonged bleeding because of decreased specific clotting factors.

Increased blood viscosity makes the peripheral circulation sluggish and places the child at risk for CNS injury from a brain abscess or cerebrovascular accident. Depletion of iron stores may also result, and anemia may develop if iron is not available to participate in hemoglobin formation.

Dehydration can occur rapidly in cyanotic heart disease. Hyperthermia (fever or environmental), poor oral intake, vomiting, and diarrhea can cause acute dehydration. Dehydration can be life-threatening for the child with cyanotic heart disease who is shunt-dependent for pulmonary blood flow. Once the shunt clots off, there is no pulmonary blood flow and the infant or child will develop metabolic acidosis and severe hypoxemia and degenerate to cardiopulmonary arrest.

Hypercyanotic Episode

A serious, clinically significant, and dramatic event seen in children with cyanotic heart disease is the hypercyanotic episode. These events are often called *tet spells* because they frequently occur in children with unrepaired tetralogy of Fallot. The exact cause is unknown, but it is thought that the child experiences acute spasm of the right ventricular outflow tract as a result of agitation or another adverse event that dramatically decreases pulmonary blood flow, causing hypoxia and metabolic acidosis (Bernstein, 2004). These episodes include rapid and deep respirations (tachypnea, hyperpnea), irritability and crying, peripheral vasodilation, increased systemic venous return, increasing cyanosis that can be very severe, and a decrease in the systolic murmur, reflecting decreased pulmonary blood flow (Doyle, Kavanaugh-McHugh, & Graham, 2000). As the child becomes more cyanotic, the child experiences increased tachypnea and hyperpnea, and these increase the degree of right-to-left shunting. The incidence of hypercyanotic spells is not directly related to the degree of baseline desaturation and cyanosis.

Hypercyanotic episodes are seen most frequently in the first year of life and seem to occur mainly in the morning. Often the episode is preceded by crying, feeding, or defecation (Spilman & Furdon, 1998). The infant becomes agitated and may eventually lose consciousness. Although tet spells are usually self-limiting, they can progress to a vicious cycle that can be fatal if not recognized and treated. Frequent or prolonged episodes may lead to diminished cerebral oxygenation and ischemic brain injury.

Treatment of the episode includes calming the infant, placing the infant in the knee-chest position, and administering oxygen. Morphine sulfate is administered to suppress the respiratory center and decrease the degree of hyperpnea (which contributes to vasodilation) (Park, 2002). Potent medications that cause vasoconstriction (e.g., phenylephrine) may be needed to increase systemic vascular resistance, decrease the degree of right-to-left shunting, and force blood into the pulmonary system. Preventing or treating hypovolemia is also an important factor. Ultimately, however, hypercyanotic episodes indicate the need to surgically repair or palliate the defect.

■ NURSING CARE
The Child With Cyanosis

Assessment

The nurse must know the source of pulmonary blood flow when caring for a child with cyanotic heart disease. Infants and children who are shunt-dependent for pulmonary blood flow are at risk for shunt thrombosis (as just detailed). Infants with right-to-left shunts are at risk for air embolus via IV lines.

Evaluation of the child with cyanotic heart disease includes an assessment of baseline cyanosis and general appearance. Assess the level of activity, including irritability. Visible cyanosis is most easily seen in natural light and is evaluated by observing the skin of the central mucous membranes of the mouth and conjunctiva and the nail beds. General skin color is also assessed. Cyanotic children may be smaller than their peers and may demonstrate clubbing, thickening, and flattening of the fingertips and toes as a result of polycythemia (see Fig. 45-7). Oxygen saturations should be obtained and compared with their baseline. Some children with cardiac defects are on lifelong daily antibiotic prophylaxis in addition to subacute bacterial endocarditis (SBE) prophylaxis, and the nurse needs to document this.

The child may become dyspneic during feeding, crying, and other exertional activities and may have difficulty keeping up with peers. Children with cyanosis may experience frequent respiratory infections, may miss more school days, and may, as a result, academically lag behind their classmates although they are often developmentally normal. They are also at greater risk for developing infective endocarditis and need ongoing antibiotic prophylaxis. If the child requires an IV line for hydration or another indication, it is imperative that no air be in the IV system because the risk of systemic air emboli causing a stroke or heart attack is always present.

Nursing Diagnosis and Planning

Nursing diagnoses and expected outcomes typical for the child with cyanosis and the child's family include

- Deficient Knowledge related to inexperience with the management of a child with a life-threatening illness.
  Expected Outcomes: The parents, and child if age-appropriate, will explain the disease process, treatment, and interventions and will demonstrate the ability to perform home care treatments, including medication administration.
- Interrupted Family Processes related to impact of an acute, chronic, and/or life-threatening disease.
  Expected Outcomes: The parents will express positive feelings for their child and for each other and will demonstrate the ability to meet the needs of the child, each other, and other family members.
- Delayed Growth and Development related to altered oxygenation or inadequate cardiac output to meet metabolic needs.
  Expected Outcomes: The child will demonstrate adequate growth according to an optimal growth curve for age and condition and will perform motor, social, and expressive skills typical of age-group within the scope of the child's present capabilities. The parents will describe any developmental delay or deviation and make plans for intervention.

- Ineffective Tissue Perfusion related to hypercyanotic episodes.
  Expected Outcomes: The child will remain free of decreased tissue perfusion, as evidenced by the absence of profound cyanosis and by the child's activity level, affect, respiratory status, and oxygenation all being normal. The parents will list signs and symptoms that would signal the onset of hypercyanotic episodes.
- Risk for Infection related to the presence of infection-promoting conditions created by the underlying defect.
  Expected Outcomes: The child will remain free of endocardial infection. The parents will understand and carry out the ordered antibiotic prophylaxis; and the parents will list when to seek medical attention for fevers.
- Deficient Knowledge related to unfamiliarity with the system complications from increased risk of clotting.
  Expected Outcome: The parents will describe the signs and symptoms to report immediately, including increasing cyanosis, vomiting, diarrhea, and fever (signs of clotting of the pulmonary shunt), and new-onset facial or extremity weakness, slurred speech, clumsiness, or breathing difficulty (signs of a CNS clot).

Interventions

Cyanotic heart disease is usually diagnosed in the newborn period. The initial nursing interventions are directed toward stabilizing the child hemodynamically and preparing the child for medical or surgical intervention. Pulmonary blood flow in cyanotic heart disease may depend on the persistence of the ductus arteriosus. PGE_1, a vasodilator, is often administered IV to maintain ductal patency. The nurse is responsible for monitoring PGE_1 infusion flow and evaluating peripheral perfusion and respiratory status. The nurse assesses IV line patency and inspects IV tubing for the presence of air. The use of an air filter is recommended.

Parental teaching and support at the time of diagnosis are paramount. Parents receive complicated information and are often asked to make important decisions that may affect their child's current therapy and, perhaps, future interventions. Parents need simple yet thorough explanations to help them make informed choices. The nurse may need to repeat the information several times. Help parents identify sources of emotional support, and encourage communication within the family.

Parents of children with cardiovascular disease respond with a variety of reactions. Knowing this, the nurse has a responsibility to educate parents about their child's disease and to stress the importance of the child interacting with the environment as normally as possible. For effective planning and provision of care, the disease must be placed in the context of the family's life.

In the child with cyanosis, careful monitoring of fluid status is necessary to prevent hemoconcentration. Intake and output are closely monitored, and daily weights may be recorded during hospitalization. Teach parents to recognize illnesses that place their child at risk for dehydration and to seek medical attention when their child experiences fluid losses.

Parents have concerns about worsening cyanosis and fear hypercyanotic episodes. Teach parents to recognize events that may trigger an episode and to respond calmly and place the infant in a knee-chest position. Review indications to seek medical care. Remind parents that they do not need to strictly limit their child's physical activity because most cyanotic children will do so themselves (Holt, 1998).

Prevention of infective endocarditis is accomplished through antibiotic prophylaxis. Parents may be given copies of the American Heart Association's guidelines for infective endocarditis prophylaxis.

Children with cyanosis are prone to frequent respiratory infections. Respiratory infections may increase cardiac workload and lead to increased cyanosis and desaturation. Careful handwashing is necessary to reduce the risk of infection. Teach parents to avoid crowded areas and contact between their child and other people with respiratory infections.

Evaluation

- Can the parents, or child if appropriate, describe the cardiac defect and its implications?
- Are the parents able to monitor their child's condition, provide home treatments, administer medications, and support the child's fluid and nutritional needs?
- Are family members appropriately expressing feelings and supporting each other and the child, and can the parents meet the needs of siblings and each other?
- Is the child showing a steady increase in physical growth and attaining age-appropriate developmental milestones?
- Is the child experiencing any change in the level of cyanosis, activity, or respiratory status and oxygenation?
- Can the parents describe signs, symptoms, and management of hypercyanotic episodes?
- Is the child afebrile and free of other signs and symptoms of infection, and can the parents explain the necessity for seeking medical attention for any fevers?
- Are the parents able to list complications related to possible pulmonary shunt or CNS clotting?

LEFT-TO-RIGHT SHUNTING LESIONS

Patent Ductus Arteriosus

Incidence and Pathophysiology. As an isolated lesion, patent ductus arteriosus (PDA) (Fig. 46-1) accounts for 5% to 10% of all congenital heart disease (Park, 2002). In the preterm infant, however, the incidence can be as high as 80%, depending on weight (Driscoll, 1999). PDA can also be present with all other types of congenital heart defects. In certain congenital heart diseases (e.g., tetralogy of Fallot, hypoplastic left heart syndrome), keeping the ductus arteriosus patent is critical to ensure viability through maintaining pulmonary or systemic blood flow.

PDA is caused by failure of the fetal ductus arteriosus to close completely after birth. The stimuli for this closure are the increased oxygen levels in the blood when the infant begins to breathe normally and a decrease in prostaglandin levels after birth. Normally, the ductus arteriosus constricts within 10 to 18 hours of birth (functional closure) (Mullins & Pagotto, 1998) and degenerates to a ligament (anatomic closure) within the first few weeks of life.

Altered Hemodynamics

In utero, the pulmonary vascular resistance is high and the lungs receive only about 5% to 8% of blood flow from the aorta. The blood flows from the pulmonary artery through

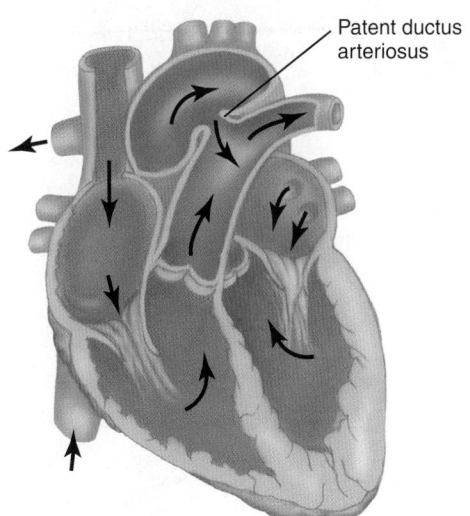

Figure 46-1 Patent ductus arteriosus.

the PDA to the aorta (right-to-left shunting). After birth, the pulmonary vascular resistance drops and the systemic pressure is higher than the pulmonary pressure. Then oxygenated blood from the aorta returns through the PDA to the pulmonary arteries (left-to-right shunting) to the lungs and on to the left atrium and left ventricle. The effects of this altered circulation include increased cardiac workload on the left side of the heart and increased pulmonary blood flow. There can also be decreased systemic blood flow if the PDA is large. The degree of left-to-right shunting depends on the pulmonary vascular resistance, the size and shape of the ductus, and the systemic blood pressure.

Manifestations

The degree of CHF symptoms depends on the amount of left-to-right shunting. Many children can be clinically asymptomatic. The classic murmur is a machinery-like one that can be heard throughout both systole and diastole, called a *continuous murmur*. This murmur may be accompanied by a suprasternal thrill. Continuous "runoff" of the aortic blood flow to the pulmonary arteries produces a widened pulse pressure (increased difference between systolic and low diastolic blood pressures) and bounding pulses. With significant left-to-right shunting, the heart will be enlarged and there will be increased pulmonary vascular markings on chest radiographs. Also, the infant may experience tachypnea, poor feeding and weight gain, frequent respiratory tract infections, fatigue, and diaphoresis.

Preterm infants frequently present with CHF and increased respiratory distress. They may require ventilatory support and intensified medical and surgical interventions.

Therapeutic Management

The symptomatic term newborn is treated with diuretics and digoxin to control CHF. Caloric density may be increased in the formula to improve weight gain. The infant should be given rest periods to conserve energy, placed in a position of comfort to optimize respiratory effort, and monitored for signs and symptoms of increasing CHF. It is important to prevent exposure to others who have respiratory illnesses.

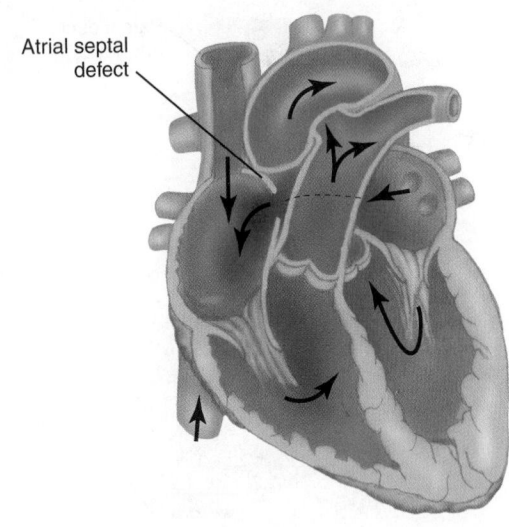

Figure 46-2 Atrial septal defect.

Medical Management. In premature, symptomatic infants, ductal closure may be achieved by the use of indomethacin (Indocin), a prostaglandin inhibitor that promotes ductal constriction. Renal function can be adversely affected and needs to be monitored. Contraindications to therapy may include abnormal renal function, thrombocytopenia, blood in the stool, necrotizing enterocolitis, cerebral intraventricular hemorrhage, or ischemic injury to the intestine (Corbet, 1998).

Interventional Cardiac Catheterization. Nonsurgical closure of ductus arteriosus can be performed during cardiac catheterization and this type of closure has become the corrective measure of choice because it is less invasive than surgical closure and has positive results. A coil is placed that promotes embolization (occlusion) of the ductus arteriosus. Occasionally, closure is incomplete and either additional coil placement or surgical intervention is required. Antibiotics for endocarditis prophylaxis (see p. 1285) continue for 6 months until the coil endothelializes.

Surgical Management. For PDAs that cannot be closed with coils or indomethacin, surgical closure is necessary. Surgical closure is performed through a left thoracotomy. The ductus is ligated (circumferential sutures) or divided (surgically cut and the ends oversewn). Surgery is usually performed within the first year of life in symptomatic term infants who were either not candidates for or not responsive to medical management of CHF. The ductus is also ligated in preterm infants for whom indomethacin therapy is unsuccessful.

The major complication of uncorrected PDA is congestive heart failure. In addition, there is the risk for endocarditis or aneurysm if the PDA persists.

Atrial Septal Defect

Incidence and Pathophysiology
Atrial septal defect (ASD) (Fig. 46-2) accounts for approximately 5% to 10% of all congenital heart disease. It is seen approximately twice as often in females than in males (Park, 2002). This lesion consists of an abnormal opening between the atria. The three types are: (1) ostium secundum, which is located in the middle of the atrial septum (fossa ovalis) and is the most common type seen; (2) ostium primum, which is located low in the atrial septum, results from a defect in endocardial tissue formation, and is often associated with a cleft mitral valve malformation; and (3) sinus venosus, which is located high in the septum close to the superior vena cava and frequently is associated with an anomalous connection of a right-sided pulmonary vein (called *partial anomalous pulmonary venous return [PAPVR]*). Mitral regurgitation is associated with some atrial septal defects.

Altered Hemodynamics
Lower right ventricular *compliance*, which is the ease of ventricular diastolic (relaxation) filling, compared with left ventricular compliance leads to left-to-right shunting at the atrial level through the ASD. This increased blood flow through the ASD leads to an enlarged right atrium and ventricle and increased pulmonary blood flow.

Manifestations
Most infants and children are asymptomatic but, over years to decades, may experience fatigue and dyspnea on exertion. Other symptoms can include palpitations or atrial dysrhythmias. Recurrent respiratory infections can occur when there is a large amount of pulmonary blood flow. A murmur may not be present in infants. The characteristic systolic murmur is produced by increased blood flow across the pulmonary valve. A diastolic murmur is present with large shunts. The second heart sound usually displays fixed splitting. The chest wall may be mildly hyperactive. Congestive heart failure is a rare finding in childhood. It can develop in young adults because of pulmonary vascular disease and decreased right ventricular function after the second decade of life if the lesion is unrepaired. Atrial dysrhythmias have been reported, usually as the result of atrial enlargement. Rarely, stroke or major organ damage can occur because of embolization of a thrombus, air, or other material that is shunted right to left at the atrial level. This is called a *paradoxical embolism*.

Therapeutic Management
The asymptomatic child is followed by the cardiologist. Spontaneous closure can occur in the first years of life for smaller-size secundum ASDs. Elective surgical repair is performed around 2 to 5 years of age. Surgical repair is recommended for all sinus venosus and ostium primum defects. Infective endocarditis prophylaxis should be provided when indicated for 6 months after surgical repair.

Medical Management. Asymptomatic infants with moderate-size secundum ASDs are monitored for spontaneous closure in the first years of life without medication. Symptomatic infants and children are treated with diuretics and digoxin as indicated for CHF. Atrial dysrhythmias are treated with appropriate antidysrhythmics.

Interventional Cardiac Catheterization. Devices to achieve transcatheter closure of ASDs are showing promising results in children with ASD, particularly of the osteum secundum type (Uzark, 2001). The U.S. Food and Drug Administration approved one such device, the Amplatzer Septal Occluder, in 2001. Other devices have been used in human research trials; research is ongoing on a variety of device models.

Surgical Management. Surgical closure using either sutures or a pericardial or prosthetic patch is performed on an elective basis early in childhood. This is an open heart procedure, through a sternal incision, in which cardiopulmonary bypass is used. Mortality rate is less than 2%, with most centers near 0%. For the young adult with ventricular dysfunction or pulmonary hypertension, the risk can be significantly higher.

Surgical complications include sinus node and atrial dysrhythmias (early and late development) and postpericardiotomy syndrome (an inflammatory process with the development of pericardial effusion).

Ventricular Septal Defect *— has more of an impact on life most common one.*

Incidence and Pathophysiology

Ventricular septal defects (VSDs) (Fig. 46-3) account for approximately 15% to 20% of all congenital heart disease (Park, 2002). The type of VSD is based on the location. These types include conoventricular, AV canal type, and muscular (the names have been changing over the past decades because of improved diagnostic tools). VSD is the most common congenital cardiac lesion and is often accompanied by other cardiac defects. The lesion consists of an abnormal opening between the right and left ventricles, which may vary in size from a minuscule hole to complete absence of the septum, resulting in a common ventricle. VSDs that are part of complex lesions are discussed in those sections.

Altered Hemodynamics

The degree of left-to-right shunting through the VSD depends on the size of the defect and the pulmonary vascular resistance compared with the systemic vascular resistance. Pulmonary vascular resistance is high in the newborn, but over the first few weeks of life, the resistance decreases. As this occurs, an increased amount of blood shunts left to right at the VSD level. The pulmonary vascular circulation receives increased pulmonary blood flow. With large defects the pulmonary arteries are exposed to systemic pressures, causing pulmonary hypertension and, over time, progressive pulmonary vascular disease (see "Pulmonary Hypertension" p. 1262).

Manifestations

Signs and symptoms vary with the size of the defect and the presence of associated cardiac lesions. Clinical symptoms are usually not seen at birth because of continued high pulmonary vascular resistance in the newborn. Infants with moderate to large defects will become symptomatic within the first few weeks of life. Children with small defects will remain asymptomatic.

A murmur may not be heard in the newborn. The characteristic murmur is loud and harsh, and can be heard over the entire systole, but the murmur can vary in duration and intensity based on the degree of shunting and the size of the defect. The murmur can have an associated palpable thrill. In children with large defects, a diastolic murmur and a gallop rhythm may be present.

Infants with moderate to large defects may develop CHF that is accompanied by poor feeding and failure to thrive. An associated ASD and/or PDA may increase the symptoms.

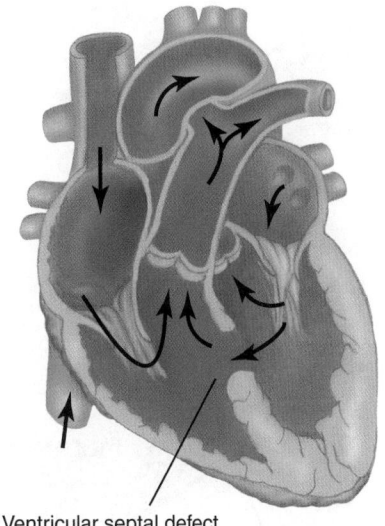

Ventricular septal defect

Figure 46-3 Ventricular septal defect.

Therapeutic Management   *1st yr. during of life*

From 20% to 80% of all VSDs close spontaneously. Most small lesions do not require surgical intervention. Occasionally, there is aortic valve regurgitation related to VSD position near the valve, and even if the defect is small, surgery is indicated to reduce the progression of valve insufficiency (Chang & Jacobs, 1998). Surgical timing is based on the location of the VSD, the symptoms, and the incidence of spontaneous closure of certain types of VSDs. Generally, surgery is in the first year of life. Antibiotic prophylaxis is indicated for all VSDs.

Medical Management. Infants who develop CHF are managed with digoxin, diuretics, and, increasingly, afterload reduction (e.g., ACE inhibitors). Nutritional status is a concern, and supplements are often added to the infant's formula to increase caloric intake. Some infants have such poor energy reserves that they are unable to obtain adequate calories orally. These infants may require nasogastric tube or gastrostomy tube feedings. In addition, decreasing exposure to respiratory infections is very important.

Interventional Cardiac Catheterization. Umbrella devices to close VSDs, similar to those used for ASDs, are presently under investigation.

Surgical Management. Young infants with severe CHF and failure to thrive undergo total repair, with patch closure of the defect, on cardiopulmonary bypass. Children with multiple muscular VSDs, which make complete repair more complicated, may be candidates for pulmonary artery banding. In this palliative procedure, a band is placed around the main pulmonary artery, decreasing pulmonary blood flow, reducing the severity of CHF, and decreasing the risk for pulmonary vascular disease. The current trend is to perform corrective surgery earlier in life, and consequently, pulmonary artery banding is performed less frequently than in the past.

Total correction is accomplished by placing sutures to close small defects or by placing a pericardial or prosthetic patch over moderate and large defects. Both procedures require cardiopulmonary bypass. The surgical approach is usually

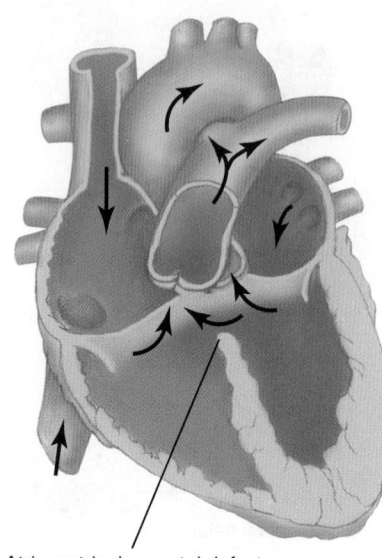

Atrioventricular septal defect

Figure 46-4 Atrioventricular septal defect.

through the right atrium to avoid a right ventricular incision, which could impair the contractility of the ventricle. VSDs just below the pulmonary valve are closed through an incision in the main pulmonary artery. Mortality is 5% to 8%, depending on the age and type of VSD.

Surgical complications include residual VSDs, pulmonary hypertension in the postoperative period, heart block that may require a pacemaker (temporary or permanent), and an abnormal rhythm called *junctional ectopic tachycardia*. In both these dysrhythmias, the atria and ventricles do not conduct in the normal sequence. Cardiac output can be significantly decreased if dysrhythmias are persistent. Postpericardiotomy syndrome can also occur.

Atrioventricular Septal Defect (Endocardial Cushion Defect)

Incidence and Pathophysiology

Atrioventricular septal defects (AVSDs) (Fig. 46-4) account for 2% of all congenital heart disease in live births (Park, 2002). They are often associated with genetic syndromes, with a high incidence in children with Down syndrome. Inappropriate development of the endocardial cushion tissue produces abnormalities in the atrial and ventricular septum and the AV valves (the tricuspid and the mitral valves). The three major classifications of AVSDs are: (1) partial/incomplete, which is marked by an ostium primum ASD, two AV valves with a cleft in the mitral; (2) intermediate or transitional, in which the atrioventricular valve configuration is between two AV valves and a common AV valve, an ASD, and no significant VSD; and (3) complete, marked by a single common AV valve orifice as well as an ASD and VSD. The term *canal* has been used to describe this lesion because the defect creates a large opening in the center of the heart. *Endocardial cushion defect* is another term used to describe this defect.

Altered Hemodynamics

The direction and magnitude of the intracardiac shunting are determined by the combination of defects and the difference between aortic and pulmonary pressures. Partial defects produce left-to-right shunting with increased pulmonary blood flow and the risk of CHF; complete defects produce CHF as a result of greatly increased pulmonary blood flow and have a risk of developing into early pulmonary vascular disease in association with pulmonary hypertension. Also, there can be significant AV valve regurgitation that increases the risk of pulmonary vascular disease. Mixing of oxygenated and unoxygenated blood also occurs in very large defects, along with right-to-left shunting, so mild cyanosis may be seen. The risk of systemic air or thrombus embolization to the systemic circulation is present with right-to-left shunting.

Manifestations

The child with a partial defect may be asymptomatic. A systolic pulmonary flow murmur, however, may be heard. Children with complete AV canal can have no significant murmur as a newborn, with a murmur developing over the first few weeks of life. The symptoms seen in a child with a complete defect depend on the pulmonary artery pressure (presence or absence of pulmonary hypertension) and the size of the septal defects and degree of shunting. CHF will develop when pulmonary pressures are low and there is a large amount of left-to-right shunting. If pulmonary hypertension is present, the child may have borderline normal saturations and be intermittently cyanotic. If there is associated Down syndrome, concurrent airway compromise may be present (e.g., upper airway obstruction, hypoventilation, tracheomalacia), leading to an increased risk of pulmonary hypertension and pulmonary vascular disease.

Therapeutic Management

Medical Management. CHF is treated symptomatically with digoxin, diuretics, and afterload reduction. As in large VSDs, poor feeding and failure to thrive may develop. Nutritional recommendations include increasing caloric density, with the need for nasogastric feedings based on feeding capabilities and weight gain.

Surgical Management. If the child with a partial defect is asymptomatic, an elective surgical repair is planned in later infancy or early childhood. The ostium primum defect is closed with sutures or a prosthetic patch, and the mitral valve cleft is sutured. The infant with a complete defect undergoes surgery preferably around 3 to 4 months of age, depending on the presence of severe CHF or increased pulmonary vascular resistance. Total correction involves closing the atrial and ventricular septal defects and constructing two AV valves from the common valve. If the mitral valve remains severely deficient (mostly regurgitation), a replacement valve may be used (although rarely performed, this is associated with a higher morbidity and mortality). Correction for less symptomatic children is generally at an age older than 3 months but before pulmonary vascular disease develops.

Children with small left or right ventricles may not be candidates for complete repair and may require palliation, such as a Fontan procedure (a surgical procedure that directs venous return directly to the pulmonary artery). Children with Down syndrome have a higher incidence of pulmonary vascular disease, and surgery is performed ideally by 3 to 6 months of age, regardless of the clinical course.

The surgical mortality may be as high as 10% in complete AV canal. For partial AV canal, the risk of mortality is less than 5%. Postoperative complications include those listed for VSDs. In addition, postoperative pulmonary hypertension or significant low cardiac output related to mitral valve regurgitation may develop.

OBSTRUCTIVE OR STENOTIC LESIONS

Pulmonary Stenosis — *narrowing constricted* *pulmonary artery obstructed*

Incidence and Pathophysiology
Isolated pulmonary stenosis occurs in about 10% of congenital heart defects (Blieden, Berant, & Zeevi, 2000) (Fig. 46-5). Obstruction of the right ventricular outflow tract and pulmonary artery tree in combination with other cardiac lesions occurs in 25% to 30% of all congenital heart disease (Blieden, Berant, & Zeevi, 2000). The lesions are marked by narrowing at the entrance to the pulmonary artery, which may be valvular, subvalvular, or supravalvular. The valve may be a normal tricuspid or bicuspid or dysplastic.

Altered Hemodynamics
Resistance to blood flow at the right ventricular outflow tract or valve leads to right ventricular hypertrophy. In severe pulmonary stenosis, right ventricular pressures may be severely elevated and may cause blood to regurgitate through the tricuspid valve into the right atrium, increasing right atrial pressure and forcing the foramen ovale open to allow blood to flow from the right to left atrium. This will lead to systemic desaturation and cyanosis. "Critical" pulmonary stenosis denotes very severe pulmonary stenosis that leads to low cardiac output. Also, in severe forms the right ventricle may be underdeveloped, which will influence the choice of medical and surgical interventions.

Manifestations
Many children are clinically asymptomatic. They present with a systolic ejection murmur that may be accompanied by a palpable thrill. The heart is enlarged on chest radiographs.

Children with moderate to severe pulmonic stenosis may experience exercise intolerance. Severe pulmonary stenosis may manifest with right ventricular failure, CHF, and, if there is right-to-left shunting through the foramen ovale, mild to severe cyanosis.

Therapeutic Management
Medical Management. In the clinically asymptomatic child, cardiac follow-up and appropriate antibiotic prophylaxis are the usual treatment. Over time, children with pulmonic stenosis may develop an increasing pressure gradient across the pulmonary valve. The timing of intervention is based on the gradient across the valve, even if the child is asymptomatic. Severe pulmonary stenosis in the neonate requires emergent intervention, through either balloon dilation or surgical valvotomy. These neonates often require prostaglandin E_1 (PGE_1) infusion to maintain ductus arteriosus patency so that there is a way for a sufficient amount of blood to return to the lungs for oxygenation (see p. 1275 for

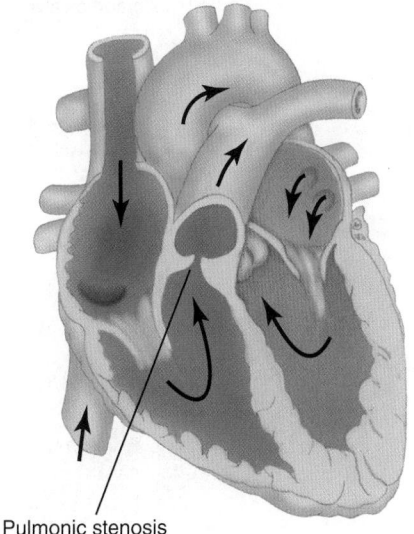

Pulmonic stenosis

Figure 46-5 Pulmonary stenosis.

a discussion of PGE_1). This infusion is often maintained for a certain stabilization period after interventional cardiac catheterization.

Interventional Cardiac Catheterization. Balloon valvuloplasty is often cited as the treatment of choice for isolated valvular pulmonary stenosis (Blieden et al., 2000; Uzark, 2001). Pressure gradients are obtained during the cardiac catheterization. The valve is then dilated, with a goal of significantly decreasing the pressure. There may be some degree of pulmonary regurgitation afterward. It is often very successful and carries a low risk. Mortality rates are higher in the neonate with critical pulmonary stenosis. Reintervention because of continued significant stenosis or recurrent stenosis is sometimes necessary.

Surgical Management. Surgical valvotomy is performed when balloon dilation is unsuccessful or there is associated supravalvular stenosis. The mortality is very low for surgical repair. For neonates with critical pulmonary stenosis who remain dependent on PGE_1 after balloon dilation because of continued significant cyanosis related to subvalvular obstruction or a small right ventricle, surgical placement of a shunt from the aorta to the pulmonary artery may be necessary (called a *systemic-to-pulmonary artery shunt*).

Aortic Stenosis

Incidence and Pathophysiology
Aortic stenosis (Fig. 46-6) accounts for 3% to 8% of all congenital heart disease. It is four times more common in males than females (Neutze, Calder, Gentles, & Wilson, 2000). The level of obstruction to blood flow leaving the left ventricle can be at the valve level, supravalvular, or subvalvular. The majority of children with aortic stenosis have valvular stenosis. Severe aortic stenosis is often diagnosed in the neonatal period or first year of life. These children can be critically ill with CHF and decreased cardiac output. Children diagnosed after 1 to 2 years of age can be mostly asymptomatic with some exercise fatigue. In this lesion, the aortic

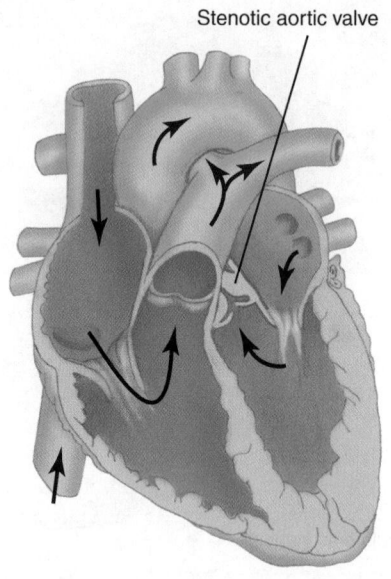

Stenotic aortic valve

Figure 46-6 Aortic stenosis.

valve is thickened and rigid, with some fusion of the commissures (leaflets); the valve frequently is bicuspid.

Altered Hemodynamics

Stenosis creates a pressure gradient across the aortic valve. Left ventricular hypertrophy develops. In children with severe aortic stenosis, cardiac output and myocardial blood supply via the coronary arteries may be diminished. In neonates with critical aortic stenosis, the left ventricle may not be large enough to eject a normal or adequate cardiac output.

Manifestations

Aortic stenosis may be classified as mild, moderate, or severe, depending on the degree of stenosis and the pressure gradient across the aortic valve. The diagnosis may be made with echocardiography or cardiac catheterization.

Very severe aortic stenosis manifests in early infancy and is called *critical aortic stenosis*. The infant exhibits profoundly decreased cardiac output with faint peripheral pulses, poor peripheral perfusion, severe CHF, and feeding difficulties. Older children with severe aortic stenosis may experience chest pain, dizziness, and syncope on exertion. Sudden death has been reported (Fedderly, 1999).

Children with mild to moderate aortic stenosis are frequently clinically asymptomatic and enjoy normal growth and development, although they may manifest ECG abnormalities with strenuous exercise. A systolic ejection murmur, sometimes accompanied by a thrill or an ejection click, is heard on examination. Cardiomegaly is seen on chest radiographs.

Therapeutic Management

Medical Management. Aortic stenosis can increase over time, so ongoing follow-up with the cardiologist is indicated. Treatment with antibiotics for endocarditis prophylaxis is indicated. The timing for intervention is based on the pressure gradient at the valve level, the ventricular function, and symptoms. Physical activity is often limited in this group

of children based on their degree of stenosis and symptoms. Guidelines include the following: if severe aortic stenosis, no competitive sports; if moderate aortic stenosis, restricted strenuous activities and competitive sports; and if mild aortic stenosis, without symptoms or ECG changes, competitive sports may be allowed (Fedderly, 1999).

Interventional Cardiac Catheterization. Aortic balloon valvuloplasty is performed to treat moderate to severe aortic stenosis. Decreasing the stenosis can improve cardiac output, decrease the degree of left ventricular dysfunction and hypertrophy, and reduce the risk of sudden death.

Interventional cardiac catheterization can be performed in neonates as well as older children. It is often performed in an attempt to delay surgical intervention. Complications can include the development of aortic insufficiency, artery damage or thrombosis, and infection.

Surgical Management. Surgical valvotomy may be performed in infants and children with severe aortic stenosis. Many children experience aortic valvular insufficiency and restenosis after either surgical or balloon procedures and may need additional intervention.

For recurrent stenosis or progressive insufficiency, aortic valve replacement may be indicated. This becomes a very complex situation in neonates and younger children. Mechanical aortic valves require warfarin (Coumadin) for anticoagulation to decrease the risk of systemic thrombosis or valve failure because of thrombus. In addition, mechanical valves do not grow with the child and often need to be replaced. There is also an increased risk of endocarditis.

Another approach is the resection of the native aortic valve and reimplantation of the child's own pulmonary valve into the native aortic position. A pulmonary valve from a donor, called a *homograft*, is implanted from the right ventricle to the main pulmonary artery. This is called the *Ross procedure*. It does not require anticoagulation. The newly positioned "aortic" valve will grow with the child. The homograft will require replacement over time, and sometimes the new "aortic" valve will develop insufficiency. The indications for the Ross procedure are still evolving as long-term outcome data become available.

Coarctation of the Aorta

Incidence and Pathophysiology

Coarctation of the aorta (Fig. 46-7) accounts for 8% to 10% of congenital heart disease (Park, 2002). Many children with coarctation of the aorta have a bicuspid aortic valve that may later become stenotic. This lesion consists of localized constriction of the aorta at or near the insertion site of the ductus arteriosus, termed the *juxtaductal region*. This improper development of the aorta creating narrowing of the aortic wall causes obstruction to left ventricular output. This narrowing can be localized to the area opposite the ductus arteriosus or there may be a more extensive area of narrowing. Narrowing increases the afterload and work on the left ventricle. Blood supply is decreased to the abdominal organs.

Altered Hemodynamics

Aortic narrowing impedes systemic blood flow and in severe cases can lead to CHF with low cardiac output as a result of left ventricular failure. Pulmonary congestion or edema can also occur as the left-sided heart pressures increase. Aortic pressure

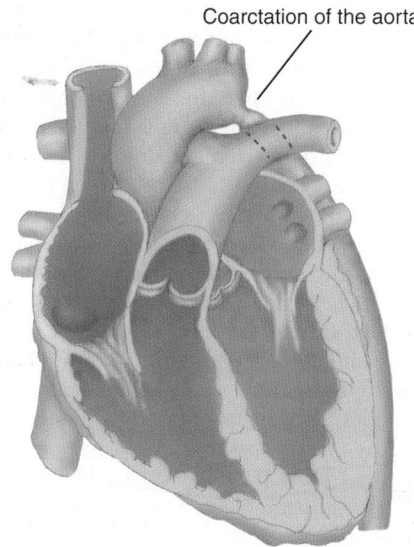

Coarctation of the aorta

Figure 46-7 Coarctation of the aorta.

is high proximal to the constriction and low distal to the constriction. In severe cases, the neonate depends on the ductus arteriosus being patent to provide adequate systemic blood flow (circulation) to the descending aorta and abdominal organs (especially the mesenteric and renal systems). In less severe coarctations, collateral blood vessels develop over time to provide channels for blood flow past the constricted area.

Manifestations

The clinical symptoms seen are directly related to the severity of the constriction and the presence of associated cardiac lesions. In the newborn with severe coarctation of the aorta, the PDA helps maintain systemic blood flow in a reverse direction from normal because aortic pressure is decreased (from the right ventricle to main pulmonary artery to ductus arteriosus to descending aorta). This decreases the workload on the left ventricle. When the ductus closes, signs of poor lower body perfusion, metabolic acidosis, CHF, and shock may develop. The infant may require PGE_1 infusion to maintain ductal patency. If a PDA is present, there may be right-to-left shunting and differential cyanosis (significant differences in color and oxygen saturation between upper and lower body parts) may result. The upper extremity saturations will be higher and reflective of left ventricular outflow and cerebral blood oxygenation. The lower extremity saturations will be lower and reflective of right ventricular outflow and descending aorta oxygenation.

Children who are diagnosed after infancy are frequently asymptomatic. They may be referred to the cardiologist after systolic hypertension (in the upper extremities) is detected on routine screening. The right upper extremity is the preferred location for blood pressure checks because the left subclavian artery can be involved in coarctation and may not accurately reflect hypertension. The classic finding in these children is a disparity in pulses and blood pressures between the upper and lower extremities. Frequently, femoral pulses are weak or absent. The child may describe weakness, tingling in the lower extremities, and muscle cramps on exer-

tion. A systolic murmur may be heard on auscultation and may be accompanied by an ejection click (if there is a bicuspid aortic valve) or thrill.

Therapeutic Management

Treatment of the symptomatic newborn depends on the severity of the coarctation, symptomatology, degree of CHF, and systemic circulation. Treatment of the older child includes hypertension management and corrective interventions.

Medical Management. Medical management of the newborn or infant with CHF includes the use of diuretics, digoxin, or other inotropic medications to improve cardiac output. In addition, the newborn may require PGE_1 infusions to maintain ductal patency and improve perfusion to the lower body.

Interventional Cardiac Catheterization. The use of balloon dilation of the coarctation as a primary intervention remains controversial. Balloon dilation, with possible stent placement, for children who have had a recurrence of coarctation is a well-accepted treatment option. It is a safe procedure, with low morbidity and mortality. Risks include artery thrombosis or damage, tear in the aorta, or inadequate relief of coarctation.

Surgical Management. Surgical intervention for the newborn may require cardiopulmonary bypass through a midline sternotomy incision if an extensive region of the aorta requires reconstruction or if associated intracardiac defects need repair. If the narrowing is discrete, cardiopulmonary bypass may not be needed. Elective surgical repair occurs near the time of diagnosis for significant coarctation of the aorta. The repair is performed through a left thoracotomy. Several surgical techniques are available: end-to-end anastomosis if the constricted area is short; use of a prosthetic patch to widen the constriction; or a subclavian flap in which the left subclavian artery provides the patch. Children undergoing the subclavian flap procedure will no longer have a palpable pulse in their left arm. Blood pressures should not be taken in the left arm.

The mortality after surgical repair of children is less than 1% (Chang & Starnes, 1998). In neonates and infants, the mortality rates can be 13% in isolated coarctation or higher with associated VSDs or other left-sided lesions (Chang & Starnes, 1998).

Renal failure, among other postoperative complications, can increase mortality (Park, 2002). The rate of recurrence of the coarctation is significant, especially in children whose repairs were performed in infancy (Wood, 1998). These children may benefit from balloon dilation performed in the cardiac catheterization laboratory.

CYANOTIC LESIONS WITH DECREASED PULMONARY BLOOD FLOW

Cyanotic lesions permit unoxygenated, or desaturated, blood to enter the systemic circulation. Infants with complex or mixing cyanotic heart lesions who are dependent on having a PDA for all or the majority of their pulmonary or systemic blood flow can become severely symptomatic within the first few days of life as the ductus arteriosus begins to close. They often need emergency management with medical or surgical intervention to survive the neonatal period.

PGE_1 is a potent vasodilating drug that is administered to prevent closure of the ductus or to reopen the ductus arteriosus and restore pulmonary or systemic blood flow. Continuous

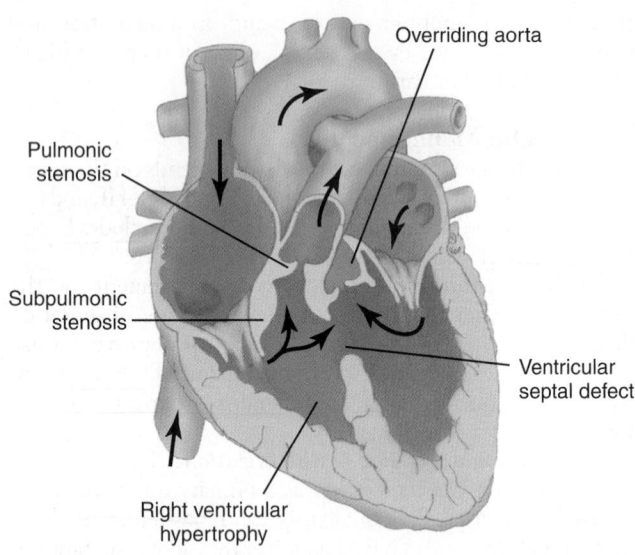

Overriding aorta

Pulmonic
stenosis

Subpulmonic
stenosis

Ventricular
septal defect

Right ventricular
hypertrophy

Figure 46-8 Tetralogy of Fallot.

infusion of the drug may improve arterial oxygen saturation and tissue perfusion, allowing the infant to be stabilized in anticipation of further diagnostic and treatment interventions. It is rapidly metabolized through the pulmonary circulation and excreted through the renal system. It must be infused by continuous IV administration. The major side effect is apnea, and infants frequently require intubation.

Tetralogy of Fallot   *heart is boot shaped b/c (R) ventricle*

Incidence and Pathophysiology   *is hypertrophied*
Tetralogy of Fallot (Fig. 46-8) accounts for 10% of all congenital heart disease and is the most frequently seen cyanotic lesion in older infants and children (Park, 2002). Malalignment of the ventricular septum during fetal development results in the constellation of three of the four characteristics of this lesion: (1) a ventricular septal defect, (2) pulmonary stenosis, and (3) overriding of the aorta (into the right ventricular side instead of over the left ventricle). The fourth characteristic, *right ventricular hypertrophy,* develops secondary to the pulmonary stenosis (also termed *right ventricular outflow tract obstruction*).

usually happen in utero

Altered Hemodynamics
The degree of pulmonary stenosis determines the resistance to blood flow out to the lungs through the pulmonary artery. The ventricular septal defect is usually large, and the pressures in both ventricles are equal. As desaturated blood enters the right ventricle (from the right atrium), it can flow into the pulmonary artery or shunt right to left into the aorta (causing desaturated blood to enter the systemic circulation), depending on the relative resistance of the pulmonary versus the aortic circulation.

Manifestations
The degree of pulmonary stenosis governs the onset and severity of the symptoms. The more severe the pulmonary stenosis, the less pulmonary blood flow, the greater the right-to-left shunting, the more desaturated is the blood and the

more cyanotic is the child. If pulmonary stenosis is mild, there is little or no right-to-left shunting. The saturations can be normal or low normal. This is known as *pink tet.*

Some infants present as cyanotic newborns. When antegrade (forward) pulmonary blood flow is severely impeded because of pulmonary stenosis, blood flow to the lungs depends on a PDA. As the mixed saturated blood enters the aorta, a certain amount will shunt through the ductus arteriosus into the pulmonary arteries, allowing it to be oxygenated. As this structure closes, the newborn becomes profoundly cyanotic.

Other infants become cyanotic over the first few months of life. Initially, they may tire easily, especially with exertion, and may have difficulty feeding and gaining weight before cyanosis develops. In time, these infants may have hypercyanotic episodes, as well as other clinical signs of chronic hypoxemia. Auscultation reveals a harsh systolic murmur, often accompanied by a palpable thrill. The heart is boot-shaped on chest radiographs because of poor development of the pulmonary artery.

Therapeutic Management
The symptomatic newborn (severe desaturation related to decreased pulmonary blood flow or frequent tet spells) frequently needs continuous PGE_1 infusion to maintain ductal patency. Palliative or definitive surgical intervention is necessary in the first days of life.

Medical Management. Older infants need very close monitoring for signs and symptoms of worsening hypoxemia. Illnesses that put them at risk for dehydration must be treated promptly. Hemoglobin levels and hematocrit values may be evaluated to assess for anemia. Close monitoring for hypercyanotic episodes may detect some very subtle and often self-limiting episodes lasting 10 to 15 minutes.

Surgical Management. Choices in surgical management include palliative procedures to increase pulmonary blood flow or a definitive intracardiac repair. Decisions and considerations regarding palliative or definitive repairs include institutional approach, associated anatomic issues such as abnormal coronary arteries, branch pulmonary artery size or stenosis, infant size, and whether pulmonary atresia is also present. Earlier surgical intervention is indicated for increasing or severe cyanosis, significant polycythemia, or hypercyanotic episodes. In recent years, primary repair during infancy has become the treatment of choice at many centers, with surgery scheduled at 2 to 4 months of age for asymptomatic infants (Spray & Wernovsky, 1998) and sooner, if indicated, for certain symptomatic infants. The rationale for early definitive repair is to normalize the physiology sooner and promote normal growth of the pulmonary arteries. Definitive repair requires cardiopulmonary bypass. Postoperative complications include rhythm disturbances (e.g., a narrow complex tachycardia, varying degrees of heart block), residual ventricular septal defect, low cardiac output related to right ventricular dysfunction, residual right ventricular outflow obstruction, and branch pulmonary artery stenosis (Spray & Wernovsky, 1998). Mortality rate for uncomplicated tetralogy of Fallot repair is reported at 2% to 5% (Spray & Wernovsky, 1998).

Some symptomatic newborns are poor candidates for primary repair. These infants may benefit from the lower-risk surgical creation of a systemic-pulmonary artery shunt to increase pulmonary blood flow. The most commonly performed is the modified Blalock-Taussig procedure (Waldman & Wernly, 1999). This usually is not done with the child on cardiopulmonary bypass. The complications are the same as for other thoracotomy incisions. In addition, shunt failure because of thrombosis or clot remains a potential major problem.

Tricuspid Atresia

S₁ only heart sounds
needs to be surgically fixed w/ open heart

Incidence and Pathophysiology

Tricuspid atresia (Fig. 46-9) represents approximately 1% to 3% of all congenital heart disease (Park, 2002). It is the third most common cyanotic cardiac condition. It is a complex lesion with many variations. In this lesion, the tricuspid valve does not develop. An ASD or patent foramen ovale must be present for the fetus or infant to survive. The right ventricle is hypoplastic (underdeveloped). The VSD can be of varying size. The pulmonary artery may be in the normal position or transposed with the aorta. There may be pulmonary stenosis of varying degrees. The newborn may rely on the ductus arteriosus for pulmonary blood flow. The degree of cyanosis and symptoms is related to these multiple factors.

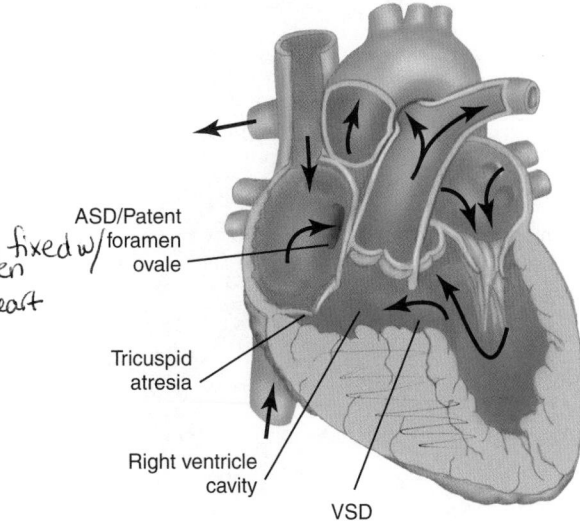

Figure 46-9 Tricuspid atresia.

Altered Hemodynamics

In a common form of tricuspid atresia, the desaturated blood enters the right atrium and is shunted right to left through the patent foramen ovale/ASD into the left atrium, since it cannot flow into the right ventricle because the tricuspid valve is atretic or absent. In the left atrium, the desaturated blood mixes with the saturated blood (returning from the lungs). From the left atrium, it flows through the mitral valve, into the left ventricle. Some of the mixed saturated blood flows out the aorta and to the systemic circulation. Some will flow through the VSD and into the right ventricular chamber, into the pulmonary artery, and to the lungs to become oxygenated.

For children with severe pulmonary stenosis and no VSD or other complex anatomy, the PDA is critical to ensure pulmonary blood flow.

Manifestations

Profound cyanosis may be present in the neonate and is usually visible within the first few hours of life in neonates with decreased pulmonary blood flow. Infants with increased pulmonary blood flow present with milder cyanosis and increasing signs of congestive heart failure. A single first heart sound is present because there is no closure of the tricuspid valve. A systolic murmur of the VSD or a PDA murmur may be heard (if patent).

Therapeutic Management

Medical Management. For infants who depend on the PDA for pulmonary blood flow, continuous PGE₁ infusion is initiated. The infant is stabilized and readied for surgery. The foramen ovale can become restrictive over weeks to months, and the infant may require urgent intervention in the form of a balloon atrial septostomy during cardiac catheterization to allow blood to flow from the right atrium to the left atrium. This is a rare occurrence.

Interventional Cardiac Catheterization. To perform a balloon atrial septostomy, a catheter is inserted into the femoral vein (usually) and advanced into the right atrium

and across the foramen ovale/intraatrial septum. A balloon in this catheter is then inflated, and this balloon is pulled back through the foramen ovale, tearing the septum. If the balloon procedure is not effective, as can happen in infants beyond newborn age, a catheter blade septostomy can be performed to cut the septum (see "Transposition of the Great Arteries," p. 1280).

Surgical Management. The goal of this staged palliative repair is to separate the desaturated and saturated blood, thereby eliminating systemic cyanosis. The equally important goal is to optimize ventricular function, by decreasing the workload (volume overload) on the heart. The child will ultimately have a single ventricle.

The newborn may require a systemic-to-pulmonary artery shunt to provide adequate pulmonary blood flow if significant pulmonary stenosis is present (see discussion under "Tetralogy of Fallot," p. 1276). This is the first procedure in a three-stage effort to palliate this defect.

A connection between the superior vena cava and the pulmonary arteries (bidirectional Glenn procedure) is performed at 4 to 6 months of age, once the pulmonary vascular resistance has decreased to normal pressures. This procedure reduces the volume in the left ventricle because, instead of crossing from the right atrium to the left side of the heart, the desaturated blood flows from the superior vena cava directly into the pulmonary artery and to the lungs. Pulmonary hypertension must be prevented and managed aggressively postoperatively to ensure adequate pulmonary blood flow. In addition, positioning the child with the head of the bed up to encourage passive blood flow to the lungs will help decrease the degree of venous congestion in the upper body. Pleural effusions can develop as the body adjusts to the flow and pressure changes. Occasionally, atrial dysrhythmias are seen.

A third procedure, the Fontan operation, is usually performed between ages 18 months and 6 years. In this procedure, desaturated blood is directly channeled from the inferior vena cava to the pulmonary arteries. The goals with the Fontan procedure are (1) separation of the desaturated venous and saturated arterial blood and (2) volume unloading of the single ventricle. Sometimes, a small connection be-

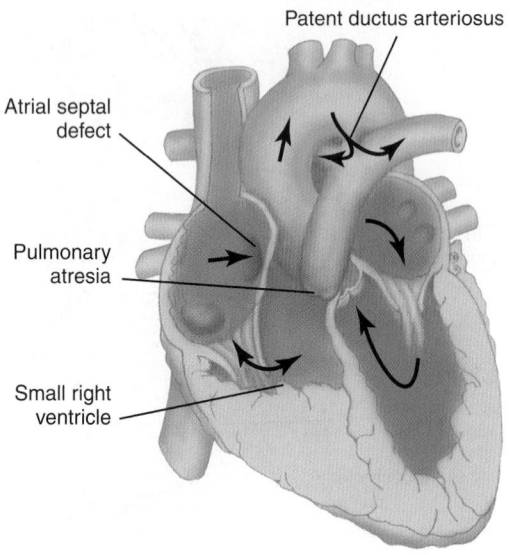

Patent ductus arteriosus

Atrial septal
defect

Pulmonary
atresia

Small right
ventricle

Figure 46-10 Pulmonary atresia.

tween the venous and arterial circulations is maintained, called a *fenestration*. This is placed in case the pressures are slightly higher than normal in the pulmonary arteries so that some desaturated blood can shunt right to left to the systemic circulation until the pulmonary arteries adjust to the new flow and pressures. At a later time, the fenestration may be closed.

Approximately 90% of children survive this procedure (Park, 2002), although postoperative and long-term complications (e.g., systemic venous pressures, pericardial and pleural effusions, supraventricular dysrhythmias) are not unusual.

Pulmonary Atresia With Intact Ventricular Septum
Incidence and Pathophysiology
only have the second heart sound s,
Heart transplant need
The incidence of pulmonary atresia with intact ventricular septum (Fig. 46-10) is less than 1% of cardiac defects seen in infants and children (Park, 2002). The causes of this lesion are the failure of the pulmonary valve to develop, accompanied by hypoplastic development of the pulmonary artery and right ventricle. The tricuspid valve may also be underdeveloped. The right ventricle pressures may be extremely high, and the coronary arteries may also be abnormal.

Altered Hemodynamics
As the blood enters the right ventricle, it cannot flow directly to the pulmonary arteries because of atresia of the pulmonary valve. The blood entering the right ventricle is propelled back through the tricuspid valve into the right atrium and shunted right to left through the foramen ovale to the left atrium. The desaturated and saturated blood mix in the left atrium and flow through the mitral valve and into the left ventricle, where the mixed blood is pumped to the aorta. From the aorta, this mixed saturated blood flows to the body and brain. Oxygenation of the blood occurs through the left-to-right shunting of blood in the aorta through persistent PDA into the pulmonary arteries and to the lungs.

Manifestations
Profound cyanosis is seen during the early neonatal period. Survival depends on the presence of a PDA. On auscultation, the second heart sound (S_2) is single. The patent ductus murmur may be present as a soft systolic murmur or continuous murmur.

Therapeutic Management
Medical Management. The newborn requires continuous PGE_1 infusion to maintain ductal patency. The primary treatment of this lesion is surgical.

Interventional Cardiac Catheterization. As an alternative to surgical intervention, interventional cardiac catheterization with wire and radiofrequency-assisted valvotomy achieves the same objective as surgical valvotomy, but with decreased risk for mortality (approximately 5%). Balloon dilatation of the valve follows the valvotomy (Bernstein, 2004; Park, 2002).

Surgical Management. Early surgical intervention involves pulmonary valvotomy and/or the creation of a systemic-to-pulmonary artery shunt (often a Blalock-Taussig shunt) (Bernstein, 2004; Wernovsky & Hanley, 1998). Valvotomy may encourage growth of the right ventricular chamber. Over time, right-to-left shunting at the atrial level may decrease as the right ventricle increases the amount of blood it pumps to the pulmonary system. If valvotomy is successful, future surgical interventions can include closing the ASD and the systemic-to-pulmonary shunt. The child will no longer be cyanotic. Surgical mortality is approximately 20% after the first procedure and 15% after the second (Park, 2002). If the right ventricle remains very small and cannot pump an adequate amount of blood to the lungs, a bidirectional Glenn procedure (as discussed earlier) or staging to the modified Fontan procedure is performed.

Rarely, very high right ventricle pressures and associated coronary artery abnormalities are contraindications to pulmonary valvotomy because there would be coronary blood flow, myocardial infarction, and ventricular muscle dysfunction. These children are given a systemic-to-pulmonary artery shunt and then staged as for a single ventricle. Sometimes, cardiac transplantation may be indicated for this subgroup of children with pulmonary atresia and intact ventricular septum.

CYANOTIC LESIONS WITH INCREASED PULMONARY BLOOD FLOW

Truncus Arteriosus

Incidence and Pathophysiology
Truncus arteriosus (Fig. 46-11) accounts for approximately 1% of all congenital heart disease (Park, 2002). It is marked by incomplete division of the common great vessel, the truncus arteriosus, which normally divides into the pulmonary artery and pulmonary valve and the aorta and aortic valve during fetal development. This failure in division results in a single large vessel and single valve, which gives rise to the pulmonary, systemic, and coronary circulations. The ventricular septum fails to develop at the same time, and therefore an associated VSD is present. The common truncal arteriosus vessel overrides the VSD and receives blood from both right and left ventricles (Grifka, 1999). There are four classifications of truncus arterio-

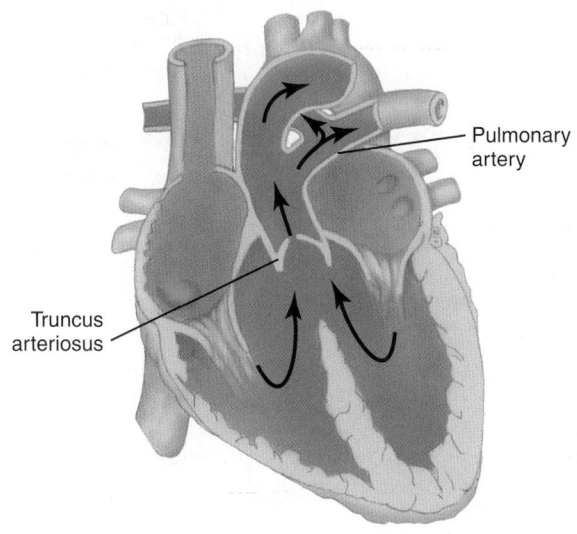

Figure 46-11 Truncus arteriosus.

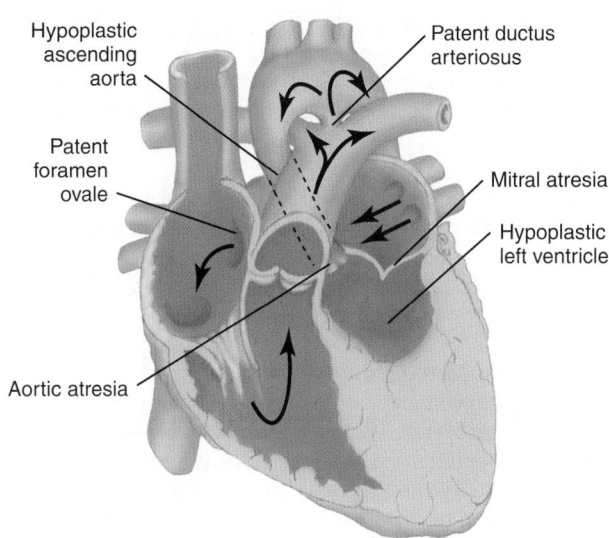

Figure 46-12 Hypoplastic left heart syndrome.

sus related to the site of origin of the pulmonary artery from the common truncal vessel. The truncal valve is not a normal semilunar valve and can be stenotic or regurgitant.

Altered Hemodynamics

Desaturated blood enters the right atrium and flows through the tricuspid valve into the right ventricle. Saturated blood from the left atrium flows through the mitral valve and into the left ventricle. The desaturated and saturated blood mix in the ventricles at the level of the VSD and common ventricular outflow tract. The common great vessel sends this mixed blood to the systemic, pulmonary, and coronary circulations. Oxygen saturation depends on the volume of pulmonary blood flow, related to the pulmonary vascular resistance; the greater this flow, the more symptoms of CHF, decreased cardiac output, and potential for coronary artery ischemia. The ventricles are under pressure and volume overload.

Manifestations

The infant presents, often in the neonatal period, with CHF and some degree of cyanosis. The volume of pulmonary blood flow determines the severity of symptoms. Unrestricted flow to the pulmonary artery results in pulmonary congestion and severe CHF. If undetected, pulmonary vascular disease can develop in early infancy. If pulmonic stenosis is present, pulmonary blood flow is limited and cyanosis increases.

A harsh systolic murmur is heard and may be accompanied by a thrill. A diastolic murmur of truncal valve insufficiency may be heard. The opening of the single truncal valve may produce a click. The infant may also have bounding pulses and a widened pulse pressure because of truncal valve insufficiency.

Therapeutic Management

polycythemia

Medical Management. Medical management is aimed at reducing the effects of CHF and preventing polycythemia. CHF is treated with digoxin and diuretics. Surgical repair is recommended in the neonatal period (Chang & Reddy, 1998). Pulmonary hypertensive crisis can be a significant postoperative complication even by age 3 to 4 months (Chang & Reddy, 1998).

Surgical Management. Newborns who do not respond to early medical management may benefit from pulmonary artery banding; however, known risks and complications are associated with this procedure (Grifka, 1999), and total corrective surgery is preferred.

The corrective repair includes closing the VSD and placement of a conduit from the right ventricle to the pulmonary artery. A valvuloplasty of the truncal valve, which is the neoaortic valve, may be performed to improve valvular competence. Blood flow postoperatively is normal.

Surgical mortality depends on the type of truncus and the extent of the required repair. The mortality risk is higher with truncal valve stenosis or insufficiency or other associated problems. Conduit replacement is necessary as the child grows, and a future truncal valve repair or replacement may be needed. SBE prophylaxis is indicated.

 # 1 priority for Heart transplant list

Hypoplastic Left Heart Syndrome *Don't have left ventricle*

Incidence and Pathophysiology

Hypoplastic left heart syndrome (Fig. 46-12) accounts for 1% of all congenital heart disease (Park, 2002). It is seen more frequently in males than in females. Most infants with untreated hypoplastic left heart syndrome die within the first few months of life (Bernstein, 2004).

Inadequate development of the left side of the heart results in only one effective ventricle. The syndrome may include aortic valve atresia, hypoplasia of the left ventricle, atresia or hypoplasia of the ascending aorta, and mitral valve stenosis or atresia. Most infants have an intact ventricular septum (Fedderly, 1999).

Altered Hemodynamics

Saturated pulmonary venous blood return is unable to flow from the left atrium through the rest of the left side of the heart. It is shunted left to right through a patent foramen ovale into the right atrium, where it mixes with desaturated blood. Mixed saturated blood travels through the right ventricle to the main pulmonary artery. A portion of blood flows to the branch pulmonary arteries and to the lungs. A portion flows from the pulmonary artery through the PDA to the descending aorta. From the aorta this mixed saturated blood provides systemic and coronary blood supply. The coronary blood supply is from retrograde flow in the ascending aorta to the coronary arteries.

Manifestations

Most infants present within the first few days of life with tachypnea and early CHF from increased pulmonary blood flow and, as the ductus arteriosus begins to close, systemic hypoperfusion and shock. The infant appears grayish blue in color, with dyspnea and hypotension.

Therapeutic Management

Management recommendations include options of supportive care only, surgical staged repair, or cardiac transplantation. The management options depend on the facility, team, and country. Over the past 20 years, progress in the stabilization, surgical interventions, and medical management has improved considerably and surgical intervention has become the preferred approach in many centers. Because parents often need to make the choice between the three options very rapidly, they may not be totally prepared to make such an important decision. Parents are likely to be highly anxious, responding to the severity of the child's condition, the prospect that their infant may die, and their own feelings of loss. Because these overwhelming feelings can interfere with effective decision-making, health professionals need to be certain to fully inform the parents about the risks and benefits (both short-term and long-term) of each course of action, allow them the time to evaluate, and respect the parents' decision (Zeigler, 2003).

Medical Management. Emergency management addresses correction of the acid-base and electrolyte imbalances and reestablishment of ductal patency with PGE_1. If the family chooses not to have surgical or transplant intervention, PGE_1 is discontinued and supportive care is provided.

Surgical Management. Two surgical courses are available. Cardiac transplantation, as a single, definitive correction, has been successful, particularly when performed very early. The scarcity of neonatal donor hearts, however, greatly limits the number of infants who may receive transplants, and the prospect of lifelong immunosuppression must be considered (Bernstein, 2004).

A three-stage palliative repair is known as the *Norwood procedure*. The child will have a single ventricle at the completion of the procedure. The stage I Norwood procedure provides unobstructed blood flow from the right ventricle to the main pulmonary artery, which is surgically connected to the ascending aorta making a "neoaorta". This effectively allows the right ventricle to act as the systemic ventricle and the pulmonary artery to act as the aorta. Pulmonary blood flow is supplied through a systemic-to-pulmonary artery surgical shunt. This procedure is performed during the neonatal period.

The second stage, a bidirectional Glenn procedure, is performed at approximately 6 months of age (see "Tricuspid Atresia," p. 1277). The palliation is completed, usually before the child is 6 years of age with a modified Fontan procedure (see "Tricuspid Atresia," p. 1277). Surgical mortality for the staged procedure varies widely among institutions. The 4-year survival after staged repair is greater than 50% (Park, 2002).

Mortality remains a major factor after the stage I Norwood procedure and subsequent stages for single ventricle physiology. Postoperative and long-term complications include hypoxemia, CHF, right ventricular (systemic) dysfunction, pulmonary

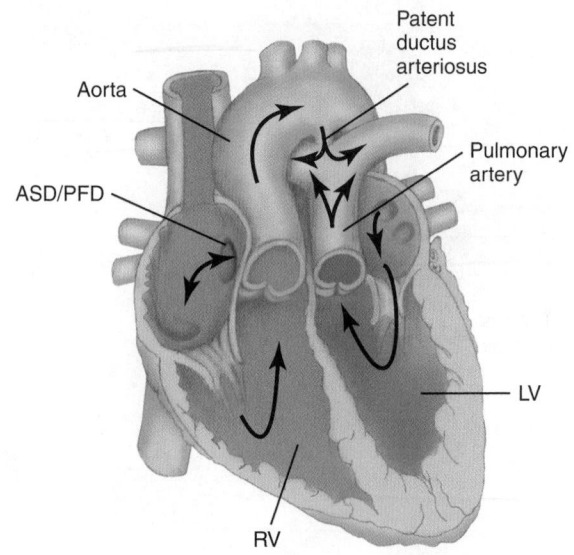

Figure 46-13 Transposition of the great arteries.

artery anomalies, systemic venous hypertension, pleural effusion, protein losing enteropathy, dysrhythmias, endocarditis, and developmental delays (Rosenthal, 2000). There is a risk of ventricle failure later in life.

Transposition of the Great Arteries

2 separate symptoms

Incidence and Pathophysiology

Transposition of the great arteries (Fig. 46-13) accounts for 5% of all congenital heart disease (Bernstein, 2004). It is more common in males than in females. Nearly half of affected children have a coexisting VSD (Bernstein, 2004). Improper septation and rotation of the common truncal vessel in fetal life cause this defect. The right ventricle gives rise to the aorta, and the left ventricle gives rise to the pulmonary artery.

Altered Hemodynamics

In this defect, the pulmonary and systemic circulations exist in parallel. Desaturated systemic venous blood returns to the right atrium, flows into the right ventricle, and pumps the desaturated blood into the aorta and back to the body. Saturated pulmonary venous blood returns to the left atrium (from the lungs), flows into the left ventricle, and is pumped through the pulmonary artery and back through the lungs. Survival depends on mixing of these two circulations through the fetal structures—the foramen ovale and ductus arteriosus. This allows oxygenated blood to be delivered to the body and deoxygenated blood to return to the lungs for oxygenation.

Manifestations

Most newborns with this defect present with cyanosis during the first few hours or days of life. They demonstrate hypoxemia with a minimal response to oxygen administration. If intracardiac mixing is inadequate, they have progressive desaturation and acidosis. They can develop CHF. Prompt diagnosis and treatment are paramount for survival.

Therapeutic Management

Medical Management. A continuous infusion of PGE_1 is begun to maintain ductal patency and support mixing of oxy-

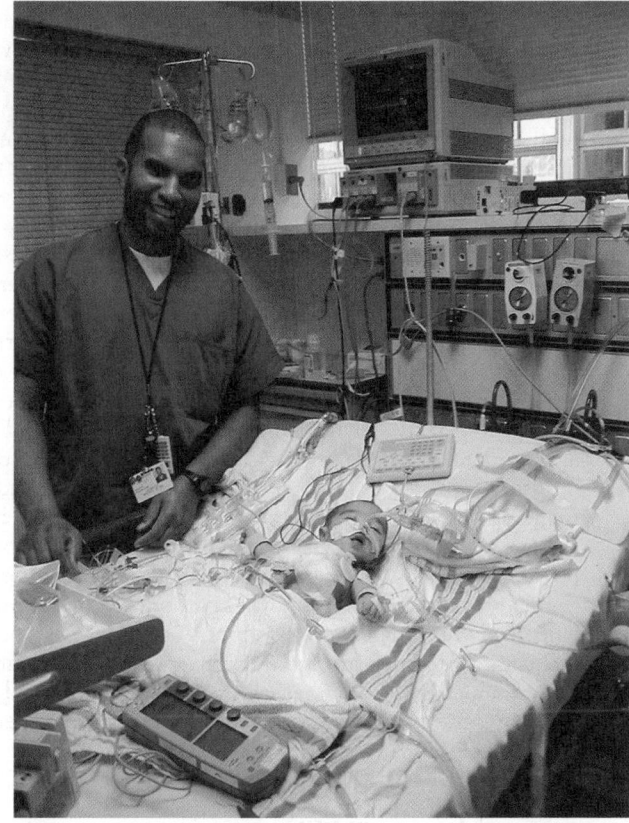

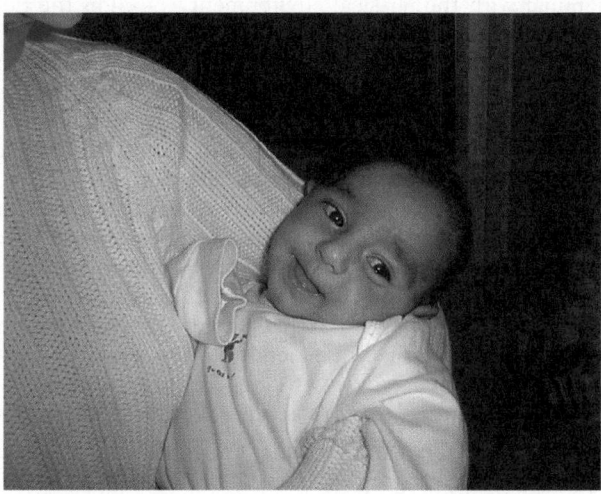

Figure 46-14 A, A preoperative visit to the intensive care unit and other units should be directed at an age-appropriate level for the child and the family before the child undergoes cardiac surgery. The experience prepares the family for the sights and sounds of the unit. **B,** Going home. (Courtesy Children's Hospital Oakland, Oakland, CA.)

genated and unoxygenated blood at the level of the ductus. A Rashkind balloon atrial septostomy via interventional cardiac catheterization may be performed on some infants if there is not adequate intraatrial mixing to enhance mixing of blood. Neonates with a VSD may have improved intracardiac mixing and improved oxygen saturation.

Surgical Management. The current surgical treatment of choice is the arterial switch procedure (Grifka, 1999). This procedure anatomically corrects the defect by placing the pulmonary artery and aorta in their proper anatomic positions over the right ventricle and left ventricle, respectively. The critical component of this surgery is the reimplantation of the coronary arteries in the newly positioned aorta. The arterial switch survival rate is 90% to 95% for uncomplicated lesions (Grifka, 1999). Coronary artery anomalies, associated coarctation, and multiple VSDs can increase mortality. Postoperative complications include low cardiac output related to poor left ventricular function, as well as dysrhythmias related to decreased coronary artery perfusion and myocardial ischemia.

THE CHILD UNDERGOING CARDIAC SURGERY

Most cardiac lesions are amenable to palliative or corrective repair, and the child with significant congenital heart disease will undergo a surgical or interventional catheterization procedure at some point during infancy or childhood. The timing of surgery is dictated by the child's clinical condition, but the trend in recent years is to intervene at an early age. The ultimate goal of intervention is for a two-ventricle repair, with physiologic and anatomic correction to normal or near-normal circulation. Complex lesions may require multiple,

palliated stages with the goal of separating the saturated and desaturated blood, correcting cyanosis, and optimizing pulmonary and cardiac function.

Families anticipate surgery as a means of achieving a more normal lifestyle, but they also experience anxiety about the child's postoperative course and ultimate outcome. The nurse can help both the child and the parents cope with this stressful and traumatic event through support and education.

Preoperative Preparation

Preoperative teaching and preparation expose the child and family to the hospital environment and expected perioperative and postoperative care. The family should receive verbal, written, and visual information that describes the course of events throughout the hospitalization. Interpreter services should be used when indicated. It is important to evaluate the family's understanding of the surgical procedure and its expected outcomes. A multidisciplinary team, including physicians, nurses, child life specialist, and social services, provides a comprehensive approach in the assessment of and interventions for the child and family. Barriers to actual hospitalization (e.g., financial, social, transportation) and discharge can be identified and interventions begun before the actual hospitalization. In addition, identifying positive coping mechanisms and providing anticipatory guidance can help the child and parent be empowered in their understanding and participation in care while the child is hospitalized. In family-centered care the health care team works with the family in caring for the child.

The parents and child should tour the intensive care unit (Fig. 46-14) and other units in which the child will be during the hospitalization. This preparation allows them to become familiar with the physical environment as well as the noise and activity level. The visit should allow time for the family to meet members of the nursing staff and see equipment that will be used in the child's postoperative care. In addition, seeing other families and children who have undergone similar procedures as they progress and recover from the surgical process can be an encouraging experience.

Monitors, ventilators, and tubes should be described and shown to the family. Parents and children should be reminded that invasive monitoring lines, chest tubes, and an endotracheal tube are inserted during surgery while the child is anesthetized, and they should be reassured that these tubes and lines will be removed as soon as the child's condition permits.

The sequence of events surrounding the day of surgery—when and where to arrive and where to wait during the procedure—should be reviewed. Parents should be assured that they will receive updates about their child's condition throughout the procedure and will be permitted to visit soon after the surgery is completed.

Postoperative Management

Postoperative nursing management includes promoting hemodynamic and respiratory stability, preventing and identifying potential complications, providing comfort, ensuring pain assessment and interventions, and providing ongoing educational and emotional support. Early postoperative care in the intensive care unit involves continuous monitoring of vital signs and cardiac output and frequent multisystem assessments. These assessments continue, with decreasing intensity, until discharge.

Cardiac surgical repair is either a closed heart procedure or an open heart procedure. The underlying cardiac defect and anticipated surgical intervention are the determining factors in the type of procedure performed.

In a closed heart surgery, the heart continues to pump and maintain cardiac function during the repair. Some closed heart procedures are repair of a PDA, coarctation of the aorta, and certain aorta-to-pulmonary shunts.

Potential complications include recurrent laryngeal nerve injury with associated vocal cord paralysis, pneumothorax, chylothorax, atelectasis, phrenic nerve injury and associated diaphragm paralysis, bleeding, infection, and rarely death.

Open heart surgery is done with the child on a cardiopulmonary bypass machine. The machine takes over the roles of the lungs and heart—oxygenation and the delivery of blood to the body. Special cannulas are placed in the venous side of the heart, and venous blood is diverted into the bypass circuit. In the circuit, the blood is oxygenated and filtered and returned to the aorta, where it is pumped to the brain and systemic circulation. The principles of hemodilution, hypothermia, and anticoagulation are critical on bypass. In addition, myocardial preservation is critical. The heart is generally not pumping during cardiopulmonary bypass, and all systems are supported. Potential complications from cardiopulmonary bypass include bleeding, stroke, myocardial infarct, dysrhythmias, fluid and electrolyte imbalance, and death. Additional complications include those detailed for closed heart surgery (see previous paragraph). The majority of repairs are done with the child on bypass and include ASD, VSD, tetralogy of Fallot, and atrioventricular canal.

Monitoring Cardiac Output

The child's cardiac output is monitored through the assessment of vital signs and peripheral perfusion. Signs of low cardiac output include tachycardia, coolness and mottling of extremities, diminished peripheral pulses, delayed capillary refill time, hypotension, decreased urine output, metabolic acidosis, and changes in level of consciousness (difficult to assess in a sedated and intubated child). Intracardiac pressure monitoring is also used and assessed.

The components of cardiac output (heart rate times stroke volume) are heart rate, preload, contractility, and afterload. Problems with one or more of these components may develop during the early postoperative period. Changes in heart rate or rhythm affect cardiac function, and antidysrhythmic drugs or temporary cardiac pacing may be instituted to correct transient postoperative rhythm disturbances. Blood loss and leakage of fluid into the interstitial space influence preload. Transfusions of blood products, colloids, and crystalloids are frequently needed to maintain adequate circulating blood volume. Acid-base and electrolyte imbalances, as well as hypoxia, adversely affect contractility. Correction of these abnormalities may improve cardiac function, but most children will need some degree of continuous infusion of inotropic medications to support cardiac output. Changes in systemic and pulmonary vascular resistance influence afterload, and the use of vasodilators, such as nitroprusside, sometimes proves necessary.

Supporting Respiratory Function

During cardiopulmonary bypass, the lungs are not ventilated and expanded, placing the child at risk for postoperative atelectasis. Also, fluid may accumulate in the pleural and interstitial spaces during and after cardiopulmonary bypass. For surgery, the child will be intubated and mechanically ventilated. The child often returns to the intensive care unit intubated.

Airway patency is maintained, in part, through prudent suctioning of the endotracheal tube. The nurse must pay strict attention to oxygen saturation readings (and know the anticipated saturations for the specific cardiac defect and surgical intervention), including during suctioning, to avoid episodes of transient hypoxia. Frequently, the child receives bolus or continuous infusions of sedative medications to help maintain comfort during this time.

Once extubated, the child is encouraged to deep breathe and cough. Incentive spirometry or therapy is often used to enhance lung expansion. Supplemental oxygen is administered initially and then tapered off as the child's condition permits. Pain medication is given before treatments and pulmonary exercises to allow the child to participate with minimal discomfort. The child can be encouraged to splint the chest during coughing by hugging a favorite stuffed animal.

Chest tubes are placed during surgery to evacuate drainage and air and assist with lung reexpansion. These tubes are inserted in either the mediastinal or pleural space, depending on the surgical approach, and are removed when lung reexpansion is confirmed and drainage has ceased.

Initial chest tube drainage is bloody and changes to serosanguineous and then serous over time. Drainage is heaviest during the first 12 to 24 hours postoperatively, and it is measured and color evaluated hourly. Increased chest tube drainage may indicate surgical bleeding or clotting abnormalities and must be strictly monitored and rapidly resolved.

Chest tubes are uncomfortable while in place; they restrict movement and cause discomfort when the child's position is changed. Chest tube removal is a painful experience, and the child should be premedicated with an opiate analgesic before the procedure.

Pulmonary hypertension presents a complicated and potentially life-threatening problem postoperatively. Intensive monitoring of pulmonary status (while intubated and extubated), saturations, and pulmonary artery pressures is indicated. In addition, special precautions before suctioning or other noxious stimuli are indicated while caring for these children.

Maintaining Fluid and Electrolyte Balance

Cardiac surgery and cardiopulmonary bypass affect fluid and electrolyte status. Blood loss and fluid shifts reduce circulating blood volume. Cardiopulmonary bypass stimulates secretion of aldosterone and antidiuretic hormone (ADH), resulting in water and sodium retention and potassium loss (Holt, 1998). Stress can increase calcium deposition in bone, placing the child at risk for hypocalcemia. In addition, administration of blood products can bind circulating calcium and lead to hypocalcemia.

Accurate recording of intake and output monitors fluid balance. Urine output is measured hourly, and weight is often measured daily. Fluid requirements are calculated based on the 24-hour intake and output and child's weight. The child with fluid-volume deficit may require fluid boluses of crystalloid, colloid, or blood, whereas the child with fluid-volume excess may require fluid restriction and diuretic therapy.

Electrolyte imbalances adversely affect cardiac contractility. Serum electrolyte values are determined at regular intervals in the early postoperative period, and IV boluses of calcium or potassium are administered to correct abnormalities. Calcium chloride continuous infusions are often instituted in neonates who have undergone open heart surgery. These medications are delivered through a centrally placed venous line and given according to precise guidelines.

In addition, glucose is a critical factor in maintaining cardiac contractility, especially in the neonate and infant. Monitoring for and treating hypoglycemia are critical.

Promoting Comfort

Postoperative pain management is an important nursing function in the care of the child undergoing cardiac surgery. The experience is frightening to both the child and parents. Parents worry that their child will be in constant, severe pain after the procedure.

PARENTS
Want to Know

About Care After Heart Surgery

Activity
- Resume regular nap and sleep schedules and play activities (infants).
- Omit contact play for several weeks; allow quiet inside and outside play as tolerated. Avoid wrestling, jumping, tugging on arms. Also, avoid sandbox play or swimming until the incision is healed.
- Avoid activities where the child could fall (e.g., riding tricycles or bicycles, swinging, playing on monkey bars or jungle gyms, sliding) for 4 to 6 weeks after hospital discharge.
- Avoid ill contacts.
- Resume regular bedtime (children).
- Avoid large crowds of people for up to 4 to 6 weeks after discharge (including daycare and church), especially during winter months.

Diet
- Resume regular or fortified formula (as instructed) and baby foods (infant).
- Do not give any new foods until after the first checkup (infant).
- Encourage adequate liquid intake.
- Appetite should improve at home.

Incision
- Do not bathe the infant or child until instructed to do so.
- Bathe the infant or child with soap and water in the usual way. Pat the incision, do not rub it while it is healing.
- If the infant drools saliva or formula, cover incision with gauze to prevent excessive moisture.

- Do not use creams, lotions, or powders on incision until it is completely healed and without scabs.
- Report any redness, drainage, or signs of infection at the incision or suture sites.

School
- The child may return to school the 2nd to 3rd week after hospital discharge.
- The child may return to school for half-days for the first few days.
- The child should not participate in physical education until 2 months after the operation.

When to Call the Physician
- Faster, harder breathing than normal when child is at rest.
- Temperature above 100° F (37.7° C).
- New, frequent coughing.
- Turning blue or bluer than normal.
- Any swelling, redness, or drainage of the incision.
- Frequent vomiting or diarrhea.
- Pain worse instead of better.
- Appetite worse than at time of discharge.

Checkup
- An appointment should be made for a 1- to 2-week follow-up at the time of discharge.
- No immunizations should be given for 4 to 6 weeks postoperatively.

Optimal pain management in the initial postoperative period may require the use of a continuous IV infusion of an opiate analgesic, such as morphine sulfate or fentanyl. This infusion is often accompanied by the administration of sedatives and antianxiety agents. In addition, nonsteroidal antiinflammatory agents can be used. This combination of drugs controls pain, relieves anxiety, and allows the child to rest. Scheduled pain medication, along with as-needed (PRN) doses, often provides better pain control than only PRN pain medication.

Once invasive monitoring lines and tubes have been removed, pain control can usually be achieved through the use of oral analgesics. Acetaminophen with or without an opiate additive and/or nonsteroidal antiinflammatory agents are frequently the drugs of choice. The incision site sometimes determines the amount of pain medication the child will need to remain comfortable. A thoracotomy incision usually divides muscle and necessitates spreading of the ribs for exposure; children who have undergone this surgical approach frequently experience more postoperative discomfort than those who have had a midsternotomy incision.

Pain should be assessed frequently throughout the hospitalization. Preverbal children are unable to express their discomfort, and older children may not be able to accurately describe their pain. Pain assessment tools should be used to accurately assess the child's pain. The nurse also must be alert to nonverbal pain behavior, which includes restlessness and irritability, difficulty resting and sleeping, guarding, rigidity, resistance to movement, an increase in heart rate and blood pressure, and disinterest in eating and other activities. Consulting the parents can help the nurse validate the assessment. Parents know their child best and are familiar with their child's response to stressful situations.

Promoting Healing and Recovery

A balance between rest and activity is necessary to promote healing. Children often experience fatigue during their postoperative recovery and may benefit from a planned schedule of progressive activity. Parents should be encouraged to allow their child to gradually resume the preoperative activity level. Regularly scheduled administration of pain medication provides comfort during activity, allows the child to rest, and reduces fatigue and anxiety.

Nutritional intake is monitored, and the child is encouraged to resume normal eating patterns. Infants and children who were in significant CHF preoperatively from large left-to-right shunting lesions may demonstrate improved oral intake even before discharge home. Rarely, diet restrictions are implemented for the older child. These restrictions may be related to long-term anticoagulation with warfarin (Coumadin) or salt restrictions.

ACQUIRED HEART DISEASE

Acquired heart disease encompasses all cardiac conditions that are not present at birth. Children with congenital heart disease may develop acquired cardiac problems, such as dysrhythmias and bacterial endocarditis. Children with structurally normal hearts may be affected by these conditions as well. Some factors that play a role in triggering these problems include genetic tendencies, autoimmune responses, and infection.

Infective Endocarditis

Infective endocarditis (IE) is an inflammation resulting from infection of the cardiac valves and endocardium by a bacterial or occasionally a fungal or viral agent. The infection can occur as the result of procedures such as dental work or surgery to the gastrointestinal tract; however, most cases are not attributable to an invasive procedure. Previously, distinction was made between acute bacterial endocarditis, with a rapid fulminant course of days to weeks, and subacute bacterial endocarditis, with a slow, indolent course of several months' duration. The general term *infective endocarditis* is now more accepted, with further classification based on the organism responsible for the infection.

Etiology

IE in children occurs most commonly in the presence of congenital heart disease. Those with prosthetic heart valves, complex cyanotic heart disease, or surgically constructed systemic-to-pulmonary artery shunts, and those with a previous history of endocarditis are at greatest risk (Park, 2002). At moderate risk are patients with PDA, VSDs, coarctation of the aorta, and bicuspid aortic valves. Acquired valvular disease (e.g., from rheumatic fever) also presents a risk for IE, but the incidence of this is decreasing (Brook, 1999). The bacterial organisms most commonly responsible are gram-positive organisms, including *Streptococcus viridans, Streptococcus pneumoniae, Staphylococcus aureus,* and *Staphylococcus epidermidis.* Occasionally, fungi may be identified on culture (Brook, 1999).

Incidence

The incidence of infective endocarditis is variable depending on the population. The incidence is as high as 10% to 13% in children with unrepaired tetralogy of Fallot and VSD; however, the incidence in children who have undergone complete repair is much lower. The mean age of children with endocarditis has risen over the past several decades as survival has increased because of surgical intervention and the availability of corrective, as opposed to palliative, surgical options. The incidence of IE in neonates has increased over the past decade, probably attributable to the increased survival of at-risk neonates, such as those with congenital heart disease. The long-term use of central venous catheters in immunocompromised children is an additional risk (Brook, 1999). Bernstein (2004) enumerates reasons why endocarditis is still a significant cause of morbidity and mortality, despite the availability of antibiotic prophylaxis:

- Changes in the infecting organisms.
- Lack of health provider knowledge or awareness of the threat of the disease and recommendations for prevention.
- Delay in recognizing that subtle signs and symptoms may suggest the diagnosis.
- Emergence of additional at-risk groups that include IV drug users, survivors of cardiac surgery, children and infants with lowered resistance to infection, and those who require long-term intravascular catheters.

Manifestations

The clinical manifestations of infective endocarditis are highly variable depending on the organism and the host immune response. Some of the most common signs and symp-

Pathophysiology

of Infective Endocarditis

Children with congenital heart defects often have pressure gradients between the structures of their heart. This pressure gradient causes turbulence, which may result in damage or disruption of the endocardium or endothelium. A fibrin clot composed of fibrin and entrapped platelets may form at the site of the disruption. If bacteria are present, this clot may also entrap circulating microorganisms and cause a vegetation to form. The vegetation increases in size as the microorganisms, fibrin, and platelets proliferate within a protective sheath of fibrin. The contained and protected bacteria can quickly destroy the surrounding tissue and valve structures. Because the vegetation is constantly exposed to pressure from blood flow, the vegetation may break off and migrate to other tissues. Particularly dangerous is a cerebral infarct.

Data from Brook, M. (1999). Pediatric bacterial endocarditis treatment and prophylaxis. *Pediatric Clinics of North America, 46*(2), 275-287; Estlow, M.M. (1998). Prevention of infective endocarditis in the pediatric congenital heart population. *Pediatric Nursing, 24*(3), 205-225.

toms are fever (90%); nonspecific complaints of anorexia, nausea, fatigue, and malaise; arthralgias (24%); chest pain (10%); heart failure; petechiae; neurologic impairment as a result of embolic events (20%); and a new or changing heart murmur (25%). Murmurs are present in up to 90% of children with IE, but most have underlying congenital heart disease and have presented with a murmur before the development of endocarditis (Friedman & Starke, 1998).

Diagnostic Evaluation

The diagnosis of bacterial endocarditis is established primarily on the basis of several blood cultures that yield the causative organism. In 90% of cases, the first two blood cultures will be positive if the patient has not received antibiotics (Park, 2002). The visualization of a *vegetation* (an abnormal growth of infected tissue) on echocardiographic studies helps considerably in establishing the diagnosis, but a study that is negative for vegetations does not rule out infective endocarditis. Echocardiography may help identify the subgroup of children who may require early surgical intervention to prevent further hemodynamic compromise or neurologic complications, such as those with large, mobile, left-sided vegetations. Other laboratory tests that may help confirm the diagnosis are an elevated erythrocyte sedimentation rate and C-reactive protein level (Brook, 1999), but the development of AV block suggests extension of disease into the myocardium and can be helpful in identifying another subgroup of children who may benefit from early surgery.

Therapeutic Management

Prevention is the most important therapeutic intervention for infective endocarditis. Children at risk should establish and maintain a good oral hygiene routine to reduce the incidence of periodontal infections. Before any procedure that may increase the risk of introduction of organisms into the

BOX 46-1

Recommendations for Infective Endocarditis Prophylaxis

Defects Requiring Prophylaxis
- Prosthetic cardiac valves
- Previous bacterial endocarditis, even without heart disease
- Most congenital heart malformations
- Acquired valve abnormalities as a result of surgery, heart disease, rheumatic fever
- Hypertrophic cardiomyopathy
- Persistent ventricular septal defect (VSD) despite surgery
- First 6 months after congenital heart disease repair

Defects Not Requiring Prophylaxis
- Isolated ostium secundum atrial septal defect (ASD)
- Beyond first 6 months after ASD, VSD, or patent ductus arteriosus (PDA) repair
- Mitral valve prolapse *without* regurgitation
- Physiologic or functional heart murmurs
- Previous Kawasaki disease *without* valvular dysfunction
- Previous rheumatic fever *without* valvular dysfunction
- Cardiac pacemakers and implanted defibrillators

Procedures Requiring Prophylaxis
- All dental procedures likely to induce gingival or mucosal bleeding, including professional teeth cleaning (not simple adjustment of orthodontic appliances or shedding of deciduous teeth)
- Tonsillectomy and/or adenoidectomy
- Surgical procedures or biopsy involving respiratory or intestinal mucosa
- Incision and drainage of infected tissue
- Genitourinary and gastrointestinal procedures, including most diagnostic and therapeutic procedures that are invasive (sclerotherapy for esophageal varices, esophageal dilation, cystoscopy, urethral dilation, urethral catheterization or surgery if urinary tract infection is present, prostatic surgery)

Modified from Dajani, A.S., Taubert, K.A., & Wilson, W. (1997). Prevention of bacterial endocarditis: Recommendations by the American Heart Association. *JAMA: The Journal of the American Medical Association, 227*(22), 1794-1801. Copyright 1997, American Medical Association.

blood, bacterial endocarditis prophylaxis is recommended. Examples include dental procedures that may induce gingival or mucosal bleeding, as well as certain respiratory, genitourinary, and gastrointestinal procedures. The standard general prophylactic agent is amoxicillin given orally 1 hour before the procedure. Clindamycin is the antibiotic of choice in children allergic to penicillin or amoxicillin (Dajani, Taubert & Wilson, 1997) (Box 46-1).

Treatment for infective endocarditis caused by bacteria invariably includes parenteral administration of antibiotics for 4 to 8 weeks, depending on the pathogen and the clinical circumstances. The prolonged course of antibiotics is necessary because the bacteria are protected from phagocytes and other host defense mechanisms by the deposition of platelets and fibrin that form the vegetation, and the density of bacteria is high (Brook, 1999).

Surgical interventions such as excision of the vegetation or removal of an infected valve may be indicated, particularly in the acute forms of endocarditis such as those caused by *S. aureus* and *S. pneumoniae*. The child should be continuously evaluated for circulatory and neurologic compromise. If compromise is present, the need for surgical intervention should be urgently addressed before the child's condition deteriorates significantly, in order to decrease morbidity and mortality (Brook, 1999).

▪ NURSING CARE
The Child With Infective Endocarditis

Assessment

Assessment of the child with infective endocarditis requires close monitoring of temperature elevations and vital signs. Vital signs should be monitored every 2 to 4 hours, along with a thorough cardiovascular and neurologic assessment. If a heart murmur is present, any change in it should be reported to the physician.

Nursing Diagnosis and Planning

Nursing diagnoses and expected outcomes for the child with infective endocarditis include

■ Ineffective Tissue Perfusion (peripheral and cerebral) related to hemodynamic instability as a result of impaired valvular or myocardial function and effects of a cerebral infarction.
  Expected Outcome: The child will have adequate peripheral tissue perfusion, as evidenced by pink mucous membranes and nail beds, a capillary refill time of less than 2 seconds, strong peripheral pulses, vital signs within normal limits, and adequate cerebral perfusion, as evidenced by mental status and a level of consciousness within normal limits and no evidence of focal neurologic deficits.

■ Hyperthermia related to bacterial infection.
  Expected Outcome: The child will maintain a body temperature that is within normal limits.

■ Acute Pain or Chronic Pain (headaches, arthralgias, myalgias) related to the body's immunologic response.
  Expected Outcome: The pain associated with headaches, arthralgias, and myalgias will be reduced or eliminated.

■ Deficient Knowledge about home care of the child with infective endocarditis related to unfamiliarity of the information.
  Expected Outcomes: The parents will be able to administer medications and monitor the child's condition.

They will explain the need for antibiotic prophylaxis and when it is indicated.

Interventions

The child will need vigilant monitoring of vital signs, peripheral perfusion, and hemodynamic stability. Any change in the vital signs, neurologic status, heart murmur, or tissue perfusion should be immediately reported to the physician. The child's activity level may be diminished, necessitating assistance with activities of daily living. Opportunities for quiet activities, such as reading, watching videos, drawing, and doing puzzles, should be provided.

The child's temperature should be monitored every 2 to 4 hours and plotted on a graph. If the child is receiving an aminoglycoside antibiotic, serum peak and trough levels may be monitored. The nurse must administer the antibiotics at the appropriate time, with trough levels determined before and peak levels determined 1 hour after the dose is administered. Acetaminophen is administered as needed for fever, as ordered by the physician, once the initial blood samples have been drawn for culture. Acetaminophen may also be administered for persistent headaches, arthralgias, and myalgias. Reassure the child and parents that the aches and malaise will resolve.

The child may be discharged home receiving parenteral antibiotic therapy. It is imperative that the parents have access to adequate community resources. The nurse must confirm that they have undergone formal instruction in the use of the IV mode selected (e.g., heparin lock, Port-a-Cath, Hickman catheter, percutaneous line) and the proper administration of antibiotics. Provide reassurance and support to the family and child regarding the extensive and lengthy therapy that will be needed.

Evaluation

- Have the child's vital signs improved?
- Does the child have a capillary refill of less than 2 seconds?
- Does the child have a negative neurologic examination?
- Is the child's body temperature within normal limits?
- Have symptoms of anorexia, malaise, arthralgia, and fever subsided?
- Can the parents return-demonstrate administration of medications and verbalize an understanding of the need and indications for antibiotic prophylaxis?
- Are the parents demonstrating the ability to manage their child's condition at home?

Rheumatic Fever

Rheumatic fever is a diffuse inflammatory condition, most probably of autoimmune origin (see Chapter 41), of the connective tissue, primarily of the heart, joints, subcutaneous tissues, brain, and blood vessels. The most serious complication is rheumatic heart disease, which can result in permanent damage to the cardiac valves, most commonly the mitral and aortic valves.

Etiology

Rheumatic fever characteristically manifests 2 to 6 weeks after an untreated or partially treated group A beta-hemolytic streptococcal infection of the upper respiratory tract. The initial infection may or may not produce symptoms of

Pathophysiology

of Rheumatic Fever

Infection by group A beta-hemolytic streptococci located in the pharyngeal area triggers an abnormal humoral and cell-mediated immunologic response in children who develop rheumatic fever. Immune complexes cross-react with normal tissue in the heart, brain, skin and joints causing inflammation in these sites. The inflammatory response appears particularly intense in connective tissue. Eventually, although the disease is self-limiting, permanent damage to cardiac valve tissue can occur.

Data from Brashers, V. (2002). Alterations of cardiovascular function. In K. McCance & S. Huether (Eds.). *Pathophysiology the biologic basis for disease in adults & children* (4th ed., pp. 1025-1026). St. Louis, MO: Mosby.

Chorea
Involuntary movements of extremities and face–affects speech

Fever
With history of sore throat

Carditis
Inflammation of all parts of the heart, primarily the mitral valves

Abdominal pain
Occurs in some cases

Erythema marginatum
Red skin lesions starting on the trunk and spreading peripherally

Subcutaneous nodules
Small, nontender swellings, often over the joints

Polyarthritis
Tender, painful joints (elbows, knees, ankles, wrists)

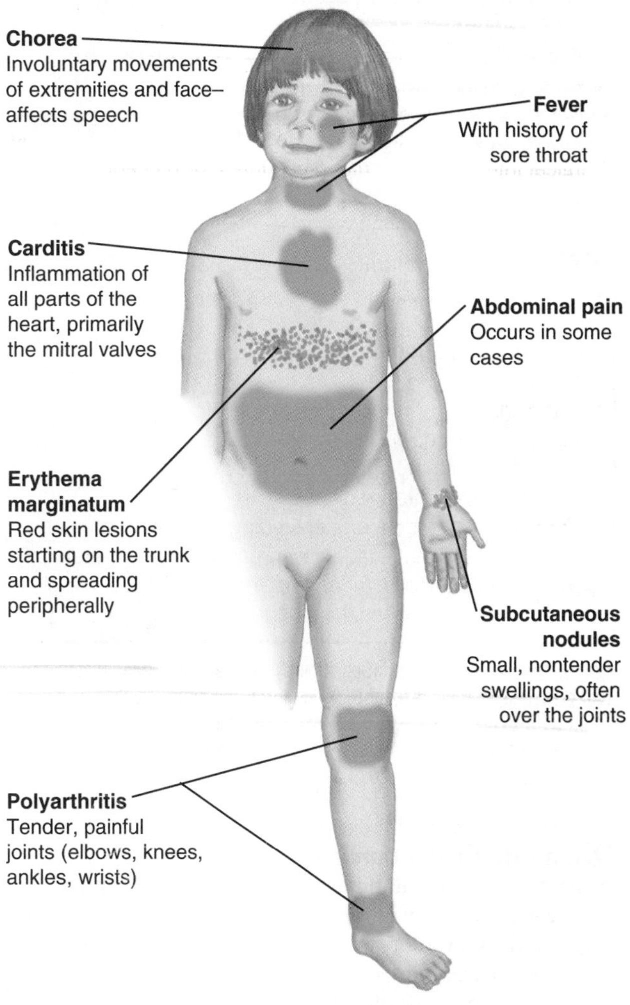

Figure 46-15 Clinical manifestations of rheumatic fever.

pharyngitis. Crowding in inadequate housing seems to be the main risk factor for acquiring streptococcal infections and the resulting rheumatic fever (El-Said, El-Refaee, Sourour, & El-Said, 1998).

Incidence

Rheumatic fever is a disease in transition. Its incidence decreased dramatically in the late 1960s and 1970s but unexpectedly rose in the middle to late 1980s (Todd, 2000). Rheumatic fever is most often seen in susceptible children between the ages of 5 and 15 years, and the annual incidence in the United States is less than 1 per 10,000 (Gerber, 2004). However, it is still the most common cause of heart disease in children in many developing countries. No differences in incidence have been found based on gender or ethnic group, and living conditions are thought to account for varying susceptibilities (El-Said et al., 1998). Rheumatic fever is seasonal in occurrence, with most new cases seen in late winter and spring.

Manifestations

Major manifestations of rheumatic fever include (Fig. 46-15):

- Arthritis—tender, warm, erythematous joints, especially in the large joints, including the elbows, knees, ankles, and wrists; occurs in 75% of rheumatic fever (RF) cases during the acute febrile period (first 1 to 2 weeks of illness). The typical presentation is a migratory polyarthritis, with inflammation moving rapidly from one joint to another and usually lasting less than 1 week for an individual joint before resolving.
- Carditis—inflammation of the endocardium, including the valves, myocardium, and pericardium; may be subclinical and is usually diagnosed by the development of a cardiac murmur, cardiac enlargement or failure, or a pericardial friction rub. Mitral valve involvement is the most frequent manifestation of carditis.
- Chorea—involuntary, purposeless, jerky movements of the legs, arms, and face, with speech impairment as well as emotional lability, caused by CNS involvement in rheumatic fever. Also referred to as *Sydenham's chorea*, it is more common in girls and usually occurs in the absence of

plaques that come off

carditis or polyarthritis. Chorea has a longer latency period of up to 6 months after the initial streptococcal pharyngitis.
- Erythema marginatum—red, painless skin lesions that start as flat or slightly raised macules, usually over the trunk. The erythema spreads at the margins of the lesion with central clearing.
- Subcutaneous nodules—small, nontender lumps, attached to the tendon sheaths of joints and on bony prominences. They occur only rarely in RF and usually are associated with severe carditis.

Although arthritis is the most common manifestation, carditis is by far the most serious and the major cause of morbidity and mortality during both acute and chronic phases of the disease. Cardiac valvular disease is the major long-term consequence of rheumatic fever (Todd, 2000).

Minor criteria that assist in making a diagnosis of RF include a history of previous rheumatic fever; arthralgias (joint pain) without arthritis; fever; elevated acute-phase reactants, including C-reactive protein and erythrocyte sedimentation rate; and first-degree AV block on the ECG.

BOX 46-2
Diagnosis of Acute Rheumatic Fever by the Jones Criteria—1992 Update

Major Manifestations
- Carditis
- Polyarthritis
- Chorea
- Erythema marginatum
- Subcutaneous nodules

Minor Manifestations
- Fever
- Arthralgia
- Elevated erythrocyte sedimentation rate (ESR) or positive C-reactive protein (CRP)
- Prolonged P-R interval

Plus supporting evidence of preceding streptococcal infection: history of recent scarlet fever, positive throat culture for group A streptococcus, increased antistreptolysin O (ASO) titer, or other streptococcal antibodies

From American Heart Association, Council on Cardiovascular Disease in the Young Special Writing Group of the Committee on Rheumatic Fever, Endocarditis, and Kawasaki Disease. (1992). Guidelines for the diagnosis of rheumatic fever: Jones criteria, 1992 update. *JAMA: The Journal of the American Medical Association, 268*(15), 2069-2073.

Diagnostic Evaluation

A diagnosis of rheumatic fever is made using the Jones criteria in the presence of at least two major manifestations or one major and two minor manifestations, plus evidence of a recent streptococcal infection based on at least one of the following diagnostic studies: positive throat culture; antistreptolysin O titer, streptozyme, or anti-DNase B assay; or by a history of scarlet fever (Box 46-2). In children with suspected carditis, a chest radiograph may show enlargement of the heart. An ECG may show rhythm abnormalities or the decreased voltages and ST-T abnormalities associated with myocarditis. An echocardiogram is essential in determining the extent of valvular, myocardial, and pericardial involvement, including the severity of mitral or aortic insufficiency, decreased ventricular function, or pericardial effusions.

Therapeutic Management

The management of rheumatic fever includes eradication of the streptococcal bacteria and treatment of other symptoms, such as joint inflammation, CHF, and chorea. Penicillin is the drug of choice for eradication of streptococcus. Erythromycin may be used in penicillin-allergic children. Once the diagnosis is firmly established, antiinflammatory agents, including aspirin, or corticosteroids in the presence of significant carditis, are administered to speed resolution of the inflammatory process, although neither therapy has been proven to have an effect on the incidence or course of carditis. The duration of therapy is tailored according to the clinical course of the child.

Children who have had rheumatic fever are susceptible to recurrent attacks, risk further cardiac valve damage, and require secondary prophylaxis to prevent recurrence. The child without cardiac complications should receive antibiotic prophylaxis for 5 years or through age 21 to 25 years, whichever

is longer. Those with rheumatic heart disease should continue prophylaxis for at least 10 years and at least until age 40 years. The American Heart Association recommends prophylaxis for life for those who have contact with children who may have group A streptococcus infection, such as teachers, health care workers, and parents of school-age children. Penicillin is the drug of choice, either by monthly intramuscular injection, which is more reliable in terms of adherence, or using an oral dose of 250 mg twice daily.

■NURSING CARE
The Child With Rheumatic Fever

Assessment

Initially, the nurse determines whether the child or any family members have had a sore throat or unexplained fever within the past 2 months. The child should be monitored for cardiac symptoms throughout the course of hospitalization. Temperature, pulse, respiration, and blood pressure are assessed, and the child is observed for signs of carditis, including tachycardia; heart murmur; friction rub; shortness of breath; or edema of the face, abdomen, or ankles. Examination of the joints may reveal very tender elbows, knees, ankles, and wrists, with subcutaneous nodules over extensor surfaces of the joints. Children with rheumatic fever may have red skin lesions on the trunk or rapid, purposeless, involuntary movements (chorea), either on observation or by history.

Nursing Diagnosis and Planning

Nursing diagnoses and expected outcomes for the child with rheumatic fever include
- Deficient Knowledge related to unfamiliarity with medications and activity restrictions.
  Expected Outcome: The child will adhere to the medication regimen and activity restrictions.
- Ineffective Coping related to confinement.
  Expected Outcomes: The child will participate in quiet activities and will maintain social contact.
- Acute Pain related to polyarthritis.
  Expected Outcomes: The child will verbalize an increase in comfort and will indicate a decrease in pain on an age-appropriate pain tool.
- Risk for Injury related to subsequent streptococcal infection.
  Expected Outcomes: The child will inform parents at the first sign of a sore throat, and the family will adhere to antibiotic prophylaxis.

Interventions

The nurse administers antibiotics, analgesics, and antipyretics as ordered and reports to the physician any fever or pain. In addition, children with rheumatic fever require bed rest during the acute febrile stage of the illness and should not return to school while there is clear evidence of rheumatic activity. While the child's activities are restricted, the nurse and family should talk about limiting visitors and arranging for quiet yet enjoyable activities. Family members and friends may provide board and computer games, movies, puzzles, and crafts for the school-age child. Such activities will help minimize activity and cardiac demand. The child may benefit from a daily schedule that includes rest periods interspersed with these diverse activ-

! CRITICAL TO REMEMBER

Streptococcal Prophylaxis for the Child With Rheumatic Fever

Streptococcal prophylaxis is the most important aspect of therapeutic management because damaged valves can become further damaged with repeated infections. This prophylaxis is lifelong if there is actual valve involvement. Intramuscular penicillin, administered monthly, is the drug of choice. Alternatives include oral penicillin taken twice daily or sulfadiazine taken orally once per day; either daily sulfadiazine or erythromycin taken twice a day is appropriate for children who are sensitive to penicillin.

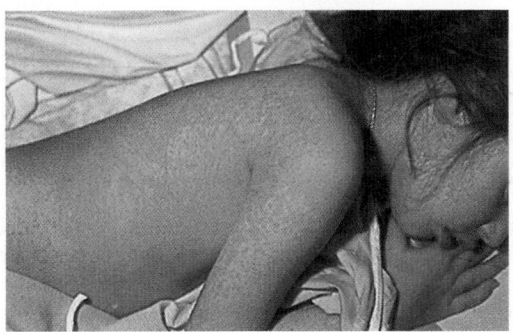

Figure 46-16 Erythematous rash of Kawasaki disease. (From Lookingbill, D.P., & Marks, JG., Jr. (1992). *Principles of dermatology* (2nd ed., p. 223). Philadelphia: Saunders.)

ities and some limited exercise (e.g., passive range-of-motion exercises). An art or play therapist can work with the child who is extremely anxious because of confinement.

Nursing comfort measures include alternating application of heat and cold to affected joints, repositioning, massage, and providing distraction using guided imagery and relaxation. Seizure precautions are warranted if the child is experiencing chorea. At home, parents must practice safety measures. For example, the child who cannot control movements may need to sleep on a mattress on the floor and may need assistance going up and down stairs. The child may be embarrassed by uncontrolled movements, especially in front of peers, and will need reassurance that these symptoms are temporary.

Emphasize to parents the importance of adherence to antibiotic prophylaxis. The family may be allowed to offer an adolescent the choice of monthly injections versus daily oral administration. If the child chooses the oral route, instruct the family about the required dose, frequency of administration, duration, effects, and side effects, as well as potential cardiac complications if the regimen is not followed precisely.

Evaluation

- Is the child taking antibiotics as ordered?
- Is the child following modified bed rest guidelines?
- Is the child playing board games, reading, and visiting with friends as tolerated?
- Has the child verbalized a decrease in pain and indicated decreased pain on an appropriate assessment tool?
- Does the child take antibiotic prophylaxis as ordered and notify the parent if experiencing a sore throat?

Kawasaki Disease

Kawasaki disease, also called *mucocutaneous lymph node syndrome*, is an acute, febrile, exanthematous illness of children with a generalized vasculitis of unknown etiology. Kawasaki disease is a major cause of acquired heart disease in children in the United States. Coronary artery aneurysms are seen in 20% of children with untreated Kawasaki disease (Rowley & Shulman, 2004).

Etiology

The cause of Kawasaki disease remains unknown. However, recent evidence suggests it is an immune-mediated vasculitis triggered by an acute infection or by a bacterial toxin. (See Chapter 41 for a discussion of immune complex disease.)

Pathophysiology

of Kawasaki Disease

An infectious or possibly toxic trigger initiates an immune system response that affects medium-size arteries, especially the coronary arteries. A generalized immune response becomes more specific, with increasing numbers of T lymphocytes and B lymphocytes infiltrating the smooth muscle cells of the vascular walls. The infiltration causes edema and inflammation, which progressively weakens the vascular walls, leading to aneurysms. As the disease progresses, fibrous connective tissue forms at the inflammatory sites, eventually thickening and scarring the vascular walls. These vascular changes, along with the increased platelets that occur as part of the disease process, can cause thrombus formation, myocardial infarction, and death in some children.

Kawasaki disease also has a seasonal component; it is diagnosed most often in late winter and early spring.

Incidence

Kawasaki disease is seen most frequently in children younger than 5 years, with a peak incidence in the United States at 18 to 24 months (Rubin & Cotton, 1998). Kawasaki disease is diagnosed less frequently in children older than 8 years. These older children tend to be diagnosed later in the course of the disease, contributing to a greater morbidity and mortality from coronary artery complications (Momenah et al., 1998). Affected boys outnumber affected girls by at least 1.5 to 1, with an increased incidence in children of Asian ancestry (Rowley & Shulman, 2004).

Manifestations

Kawasaki disease manifests in three phases. The acute stage lasts approximately 10 to 14 days and is characterized by a high fever that persists longer than 5 days. The fever is unresponsive to antibiotic treatment. Clinical signs include bilateral, nonpurulent conjunctivitis; changes in the mucous membranes (i.e., erythema, fissures, and cracking of the lips; strawberry tongue); changes in the peripheral extremities, such as swelling of the hands and feet and erythema of the palms and soles; a generalized erythematous rash (Fig. 46-16); and enlarged cervical lymph nodes. Tachycardia and extreme irritability are also common.

The second or subacute phase lasts from approximately day 15 to day 25. The fever disappears, and most symptoms resolve. The phase is characterized by continued irritability, anorexia, desquamation of the fingers and toes, arthritis and arthralgia, and cardiovascular manifestations, including CHF, dysrhythmias, and the typical coronary aneurysms (Rowley & Shulman, 2004; Rubin & Cotton, 1998).

Coronary aneurysm formation begins early in the second phase. A baseline echocardiogram at diagnosis with repeat studies during week 3 of the illness and again 1 month later will help identify those with coronary artery involvement (Rubin & Cotton, 1998). Severe thrombocytosis occurs during this period and marks the period of highest risk for coronary artery thrombosis in the areas of aneurysm, resulting in myocardial infarction.

The final or convalescent stage begins on day 26 and lasts until the erythrocyte sedimentation rate returns to normal and all signs of illness have disappeared. Deep transverse grooves, called *Beau's lines*, may appear on the child's nails.

Diagnostic Evaluation

Fever of 5 days' duration in conjunction with at least four of the five following primary clinical findings for the acute phase establishes the diagnosis of Kawasaki disease (Rowley & Shulman, 1999; Rowley & Shulman, 2004):

- Bilateral nonpurulent conjunctivitis
- Oral mucosal alterations (e.g., strawberry tongue; pharyngeal erythema; dry, fissured lips)
- Redness of the hands and feet followed by desquamation
- Rash on the trunk
- Cervical lymphadenopathy with large nodes
  AND
- No other known disease process to explain the signs and symptoms

Laboratory data are nonspecific. The white blood cell (WBC) count is elevated during the acute phase, as is the erythrocyte sedimentation rate and C-reactive protein level. There is sterile pyuria. The ECG in the acute phase may demonstrate first-degree heart block. Platelet levels dramatically rise during the subacute phase. Aneurysms are detected with echocardiography.

Therapeutic Management

Therapeutic management is directed toward preventing or reducing the coronary artery damage from Kawasaki disease. High-dose intravenous immune globulin (IVIG) in combination with aspirin has been shown to lower the prevalence of coronary artery abnormalities when given within 10 days of fever onset. At diagnosis, IVIG is given in a dosage of 2 g/kg over a 10- to 12-hour infusion (Rowley & Shulman, 2004). High-dose aspirin therapy is begun at the same time. Initially, the dosage is in the antiinflammatory range of 80 to 100 mg/kg/day in four evenly divided doses until fever resolves. The dosage is then reduced to an antiplatelet aggregation dose of 3 to 5 mg/kg/day once daily and continued through weeks 6 to 8 of the illness. If coronary artery abnormalities are identified, this dosage is continued indefinitely (Rowley & Shulman, 2004). Corticosteroids may be considered if the child is unresponsive to standard therapy.

▪ NURSING CARE
The Child With Kawasaki Disease

Assessment

During the acute phase, the nurse must monitor the child's cardiac status closely, looking for clinical signs and symptoms of heart failure. Changes in pulse, respiration, blood pressure, and color, along with shortness of breath, chest pain, and decreased activity, may suggest cardiac complications. It is important to examine the child's eyes, mouth, and skin for signs of infection and the joints for redness, swelling, and tenderness.

The nurse should determine the parents' anxiety level. Parents are often frightened by how sick the child is and the threat of a possibly devastating outcome. Families appreciate talking about their fears; learning about the cause of the illness, the treatment plan, and the prognosis; and participating in the child's care.

Nursing Diagnosis and Planning

Nursing diagnoses and expected outcomes for the child with Kawasaki disease and the family include

- Risk for Deficient Fluid Volume related to fever.
  Expected Outcome: The child will maintain fluid and electrolyte balance, as evidenced by normal laboratory values and intake and output appropriate for age.
- Acute Pain related to fever, skin manifestations, and joint inflammation.
  Expected Outcomes: The child will rest comfortably, as evidenced by periods of uninterrupted sleep, and will express decreased pain on an age-appropriate pain assessment tool.
- Fear related to changes in the child's behavior and uncertainty about the long-term prognosis.
  Expected Outcome: The parents and child will discuss their fears related to having a serious disease with a long recuperative period.

Interventions

The nurse should administer aspirin with milk or food and infuse IVIG as ordered. During the infusion, it is important to monitor the child's vital signs and any adverse reactions to IVIG, including facial flushing, tightness in the chest, chills, dizziness, nausea, vomiting, diaphoresis, and hypotension. Blood pressure is checked every 15 minutes for the first hour and every 30 minutes thereafter until the infusion is complete. A precipitous fall in blood pressure may occur 30 to 60 minutes after the infusion has begun and is often related to the rate of infusion. The physician will usually lower the prescribed rate of infusion if such a reaction occurs and may order diphenhydramine (Benadryl) and acetaminophen to control side effects. Epinephrine is given for anaphylactic reactions. IVIG may interfere with achieving immunity from live-virus vaccines, so some immunizations (e.g., measles, mumps, rubella, varicella) should be delayed for 11 months after IVIG therapy (American Academy of Pediatrics, 2000).

Nursing care focuses on comfort measures and adequate hydration. The nurse and parents must encourage fluid intake by offering Popsicles or ice to numb affected mucous membranes; giving liquids that are high in calories and low in acid through a straw (avoiding citrus drinks and sodas); and offering favorite foods that are soft and bland. The nurse or family can apply salve to soothe cracked, dry lips.

Sponge baths with tepid water often decrease fever and relieve discomfort from skin manifestations. The child should be handled gently and only when necessary. If itching is severe, the physician should be notified.

Toddlers and preschool children fear hospitalization and body changes, often exhibiting regressive behavior and sleeping poorly. In addition, children with Kawasaki disease also manifest increased irritability during the acute phase. If possible, keep the environment calm by talking in gentle tones, playing soft music, and avoiding bright overhead lights. It may help to line the bed with soft blankets from home. Assure the family that the fever, pain, and irritability will eventually resolve, and praise their hard work in keeping the child comfortable. Because the child's extreme irritability is an area of concern for parents, the nurse should provide support so the parent can take periodic breaks. Discharge instructions should include provisions for a cardiac follow-up examination. Parents' fears can be decreased through an understanding of the disease and treatment.

Evaluation

- Is the child taking adequate amounts of fluid and maintaining electrolyte balance?
- Is the child's urine output appropriate for age (see Chapter 42)?
- Is the child experiencing periods of uninterrupted rest?
- Does the child demonstrate decreased pain on an age-appropriate assessment tool?
- Are the parents able to verbalize their fears and discuss the course of the illness and their commitment to follow-up care?

Hypertension

Secondary HTN related to congenital problem

Hypertension is defined as an average systolic and/or average diastolic blood pressure that exceeds or is equal to the 95th percentile for age and gender, based on measurements obtained on at least three occasions. Normal blood pressure is defined as a systolic and/or diastolic pressure that is less than the 90th percentile for age and gender (see Appendix G).

The two primary categories of hypertension are *primary* (essential or idiopathic) and *secondary* (symptom of underlying disease). Primary hypertension predominates in the older adolescent, whereas secondary causes are overwhelmingly more common in the younger age-groups.

Etiology

Essential hypertension is considered an inherited disorder. In essential hypertension, elevated blood pressure may be a response to environmental stimuli. Affected adults and children exhibit exaggerated blood pressure responses to physical and emotional stresses as compared with normotensive individuals. Some individuals (particularly the African-American population) with essential hypertension are negatively affected by increased levels of dietary sodium (Bartosh & Aronson, 1999).

Height and weight are additional determinations of blood pressure in children. Children with elevated blood pressure are usually taller and heavier than their age-matched peers. Obesity is a common concurrent condition in children with hypertension.

PARENTS Want to Know

About Kawasaki Disease

Review the following at the time of hospital discharge of a child diagnosed as having Kawasaki disease:

- Skin:
  - Rinse with water only.
  - Avoid soaps and lotions.
  - Use salve on the lips.
  - Call the physician for severe itching.
- Temperature:
  - Record the child's temperature in the morning and evening before giving aspirin.
  - Bring the temperature chart to all physician appointments.
- Arthritis:
  - Look for hot, reddened joints.
  - Observe for pain with touch or movement.
  - Elevate affected joints.
  - Call the physician if the child refuses to walk.
- Heart:
  - Offer a low-cholesterol diet.
  - Give aspirin as ordered.
  - Call the physician for bleeding or bruising, color changes, shortness of breath, chest pain, or decreased activity level.
- Personality:
  - Discuss personality changes with household members.
  - Provide support and reassurance.
  - Encourage quiet activities and rest periods.
  - Eliminate stimulation at naptime and bedtime.
  - Play soft music, and use dim lights.
- Anorexia:
  - Offer liquids high in calories but low in acid.
  - Avoid citrus juices and sodas.
  - Give bland foods initially.
  - Prepare favorite dishes.

Modified from Lux, K. M. (1991). New hope for children with Kawasaki disease. *Journal of Pediatric Nursing, 6*, 159-165.

The causes of secondary hypertension in children include various renal and renovascular diseases, coarctation of the aorta, endocrine and metabolic disorders, neurologic disease, and drug-related causes.

Of children with significant blood pressure elevations, 80% to 90% have renal or renovascular disease as the underlying cause. Renal arterial disease is a common etiology in the sick neonate and is usually caused by renal artery thrombosis secondary to the use of umbilical artery catheters or polycythemia. Renal parenchymal diseases, such as glomerulonephritis, obstructive uropathy, and hemolytic uremic syndrome (see Chapter 44), are the most common causes of hypertension in children before adolescence.

Coarctation of the aorta is the primary cardiovascular cause of hypertension. Coarctation should be ruled out early in the course of the evaluation, because this is a treatable

Pathophysiology

of Hypertension

Systolic pressure reflects the stroke volume of the heart, the rate of blood ejected, and the elasticity of the aorta. Diastolic pressure reflects the resting pressure of the arterial system and is affected by the peripheral vascular resistance or the diameter of the arteries and the heart rate. An increase in the heart rate decreases the diastolic or ventricular filling time. Together, these measurements form the arterial blood pressure and provide information about arterial function.

Hypertension, or increased arterial blood pressure over time, may produce cardiac enlargement and subsequent cardiac failure, cerebrovascular disease, renal disease and failure, retinal disease, and accelerated atherosclerosis and coronary heart disease. These effects are seen predominantly with primary or essential hypertension.

cause of hypertension but one that may result in fixed vascular changes if not detected before adolescence. The heart itself is primarily an *end-organ*, in which hypertension can have long-term detrimental effects, as opposed to having any important etiologic role in hypertension. Endocrine causes include pheochromocytoma and congenital adrenal hyperplasia. Diabetes mellitus is frequently complicated by renal involvement and associated hypertension. Increased intracranial pressure from a tumor, trauma, or meningitis will produce acute, severe hypertension and is a medical emergency. Common causes of elevated blood pressure include corticosteroids, oral contraceptives, sympathomimetic drugs (e.g., those found in over-the-counter cold preparations), and cocaine or amphetamine abuse.

Incidence

The prevalence of hypertension is low before adulthood. Studies have reported that screening of well children for hypertension finds less than 1% of school-age children are affected (Sinaiko & Prineas, 1998). The majority of these children have only mild elevations of blood pressure, and those with significant blood pressure elevations often have secondary hypertension. Blood pressure does not appear to differ significantly by racial group in children—a finding different from that in adults (Bartosh & Aronson, 1999); however, because adult hypertension is more prevalent in the African-American and Asian populations, adolescents from these racial groups should be monitored carefully. Children in families who have members with hypertension tend to have higher-than-normal blood pressures (Bartosh & Aronson, 1999).

Manifestations

Children with primary hypertension rarely have clinical evidence of disease; the elevated blood pressure is usually detected on a routine physical examination. High elevations of blood pressure, however, can lead to the following manifestations:

- Essential or primary hypertension—dizziness, headaches, epistaxis, and visual disturbances. Late signs of severe

and/or acute hypertension include neurologic deficits, extremity weakness, and cerebrovascular accidents.

- Secondary hypertension—*Renal:* weight loss or failure to gain weight, facial or pretibial edema, pale mucous membranes, and unilateral or bilateral abdominal mass. *Cardiovascular:* absent or decreased femoral pulses, decreased blood pressure in the lower extremities compared with the upper extremities, cardiomegaly, murmur, and signs and symptoms of CHF.

Diagnostic Evaluation

Differentiating primary from secondary hypertension requires a comprehensive medical history and physical examination. Blood pressure measurements are done on all four extremities and repeated twice if elevated. Blood tests (CBC count; blood urea nitrogen, creatinine, uric acid, and electrolyte levels), urinalysis, echocardiography, ultrasonography of the kidneys, and arteriography can rule out causes of secondary hypertension.

The diagnosis of primary, or essential, hypertension is established primarily by excluding an underlying disease. A hypertensive preadolescent or adolescent with a family history of hypertension is more likely to have primary hypertension as opposed to secondary hypertension. For younger age-groups, secondary causes of hypertension are much more prevalent.

Therapeutic Management

Primary Hypertension. Treatment of primary, or essential, hypertension in the adolescent emphasizes risk factor modification. Lifestyle counseling focuses on non-pharmacologic therapy that includes weight reduction, physical conditioning, dietary modifications, and stress modification. If the non-pharmacologic treatments are maximized, the need for pharmacologic therapy in children with hypertension should be less than 1% (Second Task Force on Blood Pressure Control in Children, 1987).

Weight Reduction. A direct relationship exists between obesity and hypertension in older children and adolescents. This relationship may be caused in part by increased sympathetic nervous system activity. Weight reduction plays an important role in lowering blood pressure. Weight loss requires a program of diet, exercise, and lifestyle changes, and it is often very difficult to achieve significant results in asymptomatic young people. Even so, a modest 5- to 10-lb weight loss can have a positive effect on blood pressure reduction. Because of the long-term nature of primary hypertension, efforts should focus on education regarding a healthy lifestyle and the gradual incorporation of good dietary habits and activity into the patient's everyday life. Success frequently depends on support from health care professionals, nutritionists, and family members.

Physical Conditioning. An exercise program should be initiated in conjunction with a dietary weight reduction plan. Not only does exercise facilitate weight loss but also it lowers blood pressure independently of weight loss. Twenty to thirty minutes of aerobic exercise two or three times per week may result in a consistently lower resting blood pressure. Recently, studies have also suggested that any increase in total physical activity during the day, such as climbing a flight of stairs several times per day instead of using an elevator, can show measurable benefit over months and years.

The most successful approach in children and adolescents is to focus on activities they enjoy and that provide a social outlet, such as organized sports or bike riding. Exercise in which the whole family can participate, such as walking or hiking, is also more likely to be successful in terms of maintaining a consistent lifestyle change. Even though research has not linked hypertension with sudden death in athletes, current recommendations limit participation in competitive sports for children and adolescents with severe hypertension (>99th percentile) until blood pressure is under control (Bartosh & Aronson, 1999).

Dietary Modification. Avoidance of a high-sodium intake is recommended in hypertensive as well as normotensive children and adolescents. The degree of sodium restriction necessary to decrease blood pressure has not been established, but it is recommended that the dietary intake should be not greater than 5 to 6 g/day, or a no-added-salt diet (National Institutes of Health, 1996; Second Task Force on Blood Pressure Control in Children, 1987).

Studies have suggested a relationship between potassium and calcium levels and hypertension. Some researchers believe that adequate dietary potassium and calcium may play a role in reducing blood pressure (Bartosh & Aronson, 1999).

Evidence shows an association between alcohol and hypertension, believed to be related to alterations in the renin-angiotensin system and neurotransmitters. Smoking produces an aldosterone-like hypertension in young people. Therefore avoidance of alcohol and tobacco is recommended.

Relaxation Techniques. Relaxation techniques have resulted in modest reductions in blood pressure in the adult population. Information on efficacy in children is not yet available. The Second Task Force on Blood Pressure Control in Children (1987), however, states that reducing undue environmental stress and providing support for coping with family and school difficulties may be effective strategies for blood pressure modification.

Pharmacologic Treatment. Pharmacologic treatment of primary hypertension may be indicated if there is significant diastolic hypertension, evidence of target organ injury such as left ventricular hypertrophy, and clinical signs or symptoms related to blood pressure elevation. The first-line drugs for children and adolescents are beta-adrenergic receptor blockers; diuretics; and vasodilators, primarily ACE inhibitors.

Secondary Hypertension. Treatment of the underlying process is the focus of therapy in secondary hypertension. If the secondary disease is coarctation of the aorta or renal artery disease, surgery may be indicated. Therapy in patients with renal parenchymal or endocrine pathologic conditions focuses on the disease process. Effective treatment will often result in secondary control of blood pressure.

! CRITICAL TO REMEMBER

Infusing Intravenous Antihypertensive Medications

Intravenous antihypertensive medications must be infused very slowly, and an arterial line must be in place for monitoring. Sudden hypotension may result after initiation of antihypertensive drugs.

■ NURSING CARE
The Child With Hypertension

Assessment

Blood Pressure Screening

Blood pressure screening should be initiated when a child is 3 years old and should continue through adolescence. Blood pressure should be checked at least yearly. The environment should be as quiet as possible, and the child's arm should be supported at the heart level. If an elevated blood pressure is found, measurement should be repeated two more times, allowing a 2- to 3-minute interval between blood pressure checks.

Cuff size is of critical importance. A too-small blood pressure cuff will result in an inappropriately high blood pressure reading. The common practice of using arm length to choose the proper cuff may result in false readings because of the varying heights and weights of children at any particular age. The most accurate and easiest way to choose a cuff is to hold the cuff *lengthwise* up to the arm and ensure that the cuff width is about 1.5 times the width of the arm. This will compensate for a shorter, obese patient, in whom using arm length as a gauge would result in the use of a smaller cuff than is appropriate.

Physical Assessment

Assessment of a child with hypertension includes inspection of the skin to detect evidence of underlying disease, including edema (renal disease) and the presence of café au lait spots (neurofibromatosis) or moon facies (Cushing's syndrome, steroid administration). The pulses should be palpated for symmetry and strength. A child with coarctation of the aorta is likely to have bounding upper extremity pulses and diminished or absent femoral and pedal pulses. The heart and chest are auscultated to determine the heart rate and to detect any heart murmur, gallop, or aortic bruit. The abdomen is auscultated for renal bruits. A neurologic examination is urgently indicated in children with acute, severe hypertension to rule out increased intracranial pressure.

Nursing Diagnosis and Planning

Nursing diagnoses and expected outcomes for the child with hypertension include

- Ineffective Tissue Perfusion (peripheral and cardiovascular) related to elevation in systolic and/or diastolic arterial blood pressure.
   Expected Outcome: The child will maintain normal tissue perfusion with blood pressure at a controlled level (below the 95th percentile for age).
- Ineffective Therapeutic Regimen Management related to excessive demands of dietary restrictions, physical conditioning, and a possible medication regimen.
   Expected Outcomes: The child will describe and will engage in diet, physical conditioning, and medication therapy to lower blood pressure.

Interventions

Nursing interventions focus on education and family support and adherence to the treatment regimen. The nurse may consult a dietitian and collaboratively develop a teaching plan regarding a modified-sodium and weight-reduction diet if ordered. When counseling the family and child about dietary modifications, it is important to include the whole family in making dietary changes to increase motivation and compliance.

If a physical conditioning program is prescribed, physical activities the child enjoys are identified so that they can be incorporated into the plan. Family members and friends are encouraged to join the child in the exercise program. Praise the child for progress in weight loss and increased endurance. Encourage the child to express feelings about any possible problems related to home or school situations. Discuss methods for facilitating relaxation that may be helpful during periods of stress.

The child who is hospitalized with acute, severe hypertension may require medications. Once the child has been stabilized after an acute hypertensive crisis, oral antihypertensive medications will likely be prescribed. During discharge planning, reinforce the importance of adherence with the medication regimen and of periodic follow-up evaluations.

Evaluation

- Does the child maintain blood pressure below the 95th percentile for age?
- Has the child achieved weight loss?
- Is the child adhering to a modified-sodium diet?
- Is the child engaging in regular physical exercise according to the prescribed regimen?
- Is the child complying with the medication regimen?

CARDIOMYOPATHIES

The cardiomyopathies are diseases of the heart muscle in which the cardiac pathologic condition is not secondary to congenital heart disease, coronary artery disease, or other systemic disease. Cardiomyopathy is classified into three types based on the size and function of the ventricles:

- *Dilated:* Decreased contractility and dilation of the ventricles without an increase in wall thickness (hypertrophy). There are congenital or genetic forms, as well as acquired forms caused by infection or toxin exposure.
- *Hypertrophic:* Hypertrophy of the ventricles, generally with improved contractility but impaired ventricular filling because of increased "stiffness" of the ventricular walls. The interior chamber size of the ventricle may be decreased. Considered a genetic disorder.
- *Restrictive:* Impaired ventricular filling usually caused by infiltration of the muscle with abnormal material. The ventricular size and contractility are usually fairly normal. May be congenital or acquired.

Hypertrophic cardiomyopathy (HCM), with an annual incidence in children of 6% (Berger, Dhala, & Friedberg, 1999), is one of the major causes of sudden cardiac death in adolescents. Predicting sudden cardiac death from this cause is difficult, because children with this disorder may have completely normal physical examinations.

The assessment data that best predict whether a child or adolescent may be at risk are a family history of early or sudden cardiac death or a family history of hypertrophic cardiomyopathy (Berger, Dhala, & Friedberg, 1999). If the adolescent is symptomatic, the most frequently seen signs and symptoms include dyspnea or chest pain with exertion, palpitations, presyncope, and syncope. Infants and children may fatigue easily. The thickened left ventricle is poorly compliant (stiff) and has impaired filling, causing pulmonary venous congestion and associated exertional dyspnea and orthopnea (dyspnea when supine). On auscultation, the heart sounds are normal and there is often a systolic murmur at the left sternal border or apex. The murmur will characteristically vary in intensity depending on position or recent exertion.

The ECG may demonstrate left ventricular hypertrophy, deep Q waves, and ST-T abnormalities. Affected individuals should have a Holter monitor test to screen for asymptomatic ventricular dysrhythmias. The chest radiograph may show mild cardiomegaly. The diagnosis is usually established by echocardiogram, often with concentric or localized ventricular hypertrophy, of the left and often the right ventricle.

All children with diagnosed HCM should be restricted from strenuous exertion and competitive sports. Beta blockade or calcium channel blockade (verapamil) is frequently employed, especially in children with obstructive HCM, to decrease ventricular hypercontractility and outflow tract obstruction. Beta blockade is also used as prophylaxis against ventricular dysrhythmias. Prophylactic therapy may be started in asymptomatic children with HCM, especially in the case of a family history of sudden death. SBE prophylaxis is also indicated.

The indications for surgical intervention include children who are symptomatic or who have severe outflow tract obstruction despite medical management. The most common procedure is a septal myomectomy, which is resection of a portion of the left ventricular septum to relieve obstruction. This often results in an improvement in symptoms with low surgical mortality but does not decrease the mortality rate of the disease itself.

A newer intervention is insertion of a pacemaker, which, by depolarizing the ventricle, causes dyssynchronous ventricular contraction and decreased outflow tract obstruction. In addition, children with life-threatening dysrhythmias may be offered an implantable defibrillator pacemaker. The surgical risk of pacemaker and/or defibrillator insertion is much lower than that of myomectomy, and these options are likely to be used increasingly as long-term outcome data become available.

DYSRHYTHMIAS

The identification of a dysrhythmia, a cardiac rhythm disturbance, in childhood is an important finding. The most important aspect is to recognize that a dysrhythmia is present and classify it quickly as life-threatening or non–life-threatening. Assessing the child hemodynamically is a critical factor in determining the interventions. Often, the nurse will note an abnormal rhythm during a child's or adolescent's well examination. Following the assessment of an abnormal or irregular radial pulse measurement, the nurse should obtain an apical pulse, counting for a full minute (if a pulse is present).

Etiology

Cardiac rhythm disturbances have numerous causes. Dysrhythmias may be associated with underlying congenital heart disease or structurally normal hearts. Either an abnor-

Pathophysiology

of Dysrhythmias

Tachydysrhythmias

Primary tachydysrhythmias can originate in either the atria or the ventricles. The most common atrial tachydysrhythmia is supraventricular tachycardia (SVT). SVT is triggered by an atrial ectopic focus (a group of irritable cells somewhere in the atrium) or a reentry circuit (accessory pathway permitting abnormal conduction within the heart). Ventricular tachycardia is uncommon; it is seen in prolonged QT syndrome or in the preoperative or postoperative period in children with underlying structural heart disease.

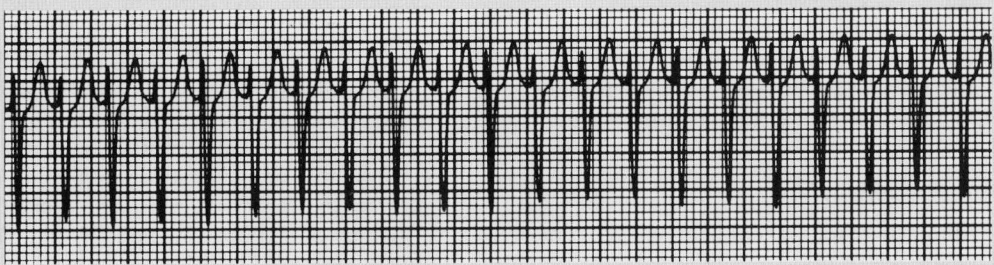

Supraventricular tachycardia. (From Park, M.K., & Guntheroth, W.G. [1992]. *How to read pediatric ECGs* [3rd ed., p. 202]. St. Louis: Mosby.)

Bradydysrhythmias

In children, bradydysrhythmias are most commonly secondary to hypoxia resulting from respiratory failure or arrest. Primary cardiac bradydysrhythmias usually result from damage to the sinus node or the conduction pathway between the atria and the ventricles (AV block).

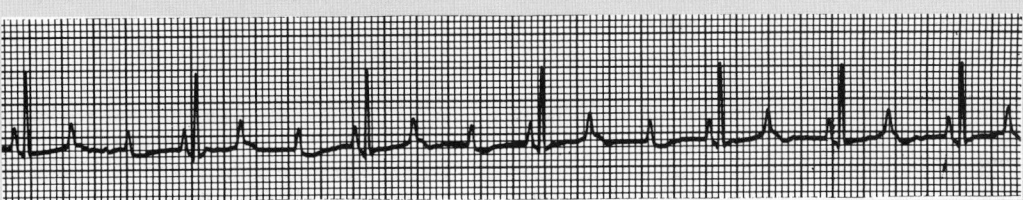

Heart block—two or three P waves for every QRS. Cardiac output is based on the rate of the QRS complexes—ventricular contraction. (From Park, M.K., & Guntheroth, W.G. [1992]. *How to read pediatric ECGs* [3rd ed., p. 210]. St. Louis: Mosby.)

Data from Zeigler, V.L. (1994b). Supraventricular tachycardia in children: A challenge for pediatric nurses. *Journal of Pediatric Nursing, 9*(5), 288-298; Chameides, L., & Hazinski, M.F. (1997). *American Heart Association pediatric advanced life support* (3rd ed., pp. 7.1-7.15). Dallas: American Heart Association.

mal impulse formation or abnormal conduction or a combination of these two factors causes a dysrhythmia. Rhythm disturbances can be classified as tachydysrhythmic (rapid) or bradydysrhythmic (slow) (Dubin, 2004).

Dysrhythmias may be seen in the postoperative period after repair or palliation of a cardiac lesion. Post-surgical dysrhythmias result from injury to the conduction system, edema, ischemia, incision or suture placement, and acid-base or electrolyte imbalances.

Underlying acquired heart disease, such as myocarditis or cardiomyopathy, sometimes produces dysrhythmias. Abnormal electrical pathways in the heart can cause certain dysrhythmias. *Wolff-Parkinson-White (WPW) syndrome* is the most common example. Abnormal electrical repolarization of the heart can cause disturbances such as prolonged QT syndrome, which can result in a life-threatening ventricular tachycardia. This can have a genetic cause. Noncardiac causes of rhythm disturbances include fever, temperature instability, hypoxia, electrolyte and metabolic disturbances, increased intracranial pressure, hypovolemia, cardiac tamponade, and drug therapy or reactions.

Incidence

Dysrhythmias in children are not uncommon, most are not life-threatening, and most appear in children whose hearts are structurally normal (Hanisch, 2001). Supraventricular tachycardia (SVT) is the most common primary symptomatic rhythm disturbance seen in infants and children (Park, 2002).

Manifestations

In tachydysrhythmias and bradydysrhythmias, cardiac output is diminished. The clinical presentation is of low cardiac output syndrome with poor end-organ perfusion. The earliest signs and symptoms may be subtle; later they can be quite dramatic. Clinical manifestations for the infant and toddler may include poor feeding, irritability, lethargy, pale or mottled color, poor peripheral perfusion (diminished pulses, mottling, cool extremities, delayed capillary refill time), decreased urine output, and CHF.

In older children, palpitations, dizziness, syncope, and exercise intolerance may be demonstrated. Tolerance of rhythm disturbances is based on the type of rhythm, underlying cardiac condition, and duration of rhythm and the effect on cardiac output.

In absent rhythms there is no cardiac output. This is a medical emergency. Cardiopulmonary resuscitation (CPR) and medical intervention must be initiated if the child is to survive.

Diagnostic Evaluation

The primary tool for diagnosing pediatric dysrhythmias is the 12-lead ECG. Twenty-four-hour Holter monitoring and transtelephonic monitoring may be useful for documenting intermittent episodes of cardiac rhythm disturbances.

Therapeutic Management

Pediatric rhythm disturbances should be treated as emergencies if they compromise cardiac output or have the potential to degenerate into lethal (collapse) rhythms (e.g., ventricular fibrillation) (Dubin, 2004). Management strategies include drug therapy, radiofrequency ablation, cardioversion, and pacemakers; the choice of treatment is guided by the origin of the dysrhythmia and the clinical consequences.

Fast Pulse Rate

Supraventricular Tachycardia. Supraventricular tachycardia is a narrow QRS tachycardia. This narrow QRS configuration indicates that the impulse begins above the ventricles. Rates can be in the 220 to 300 beats/min range. Children who are asymptomatic and hemodynamically stable can be treated conservatively. Vagal maneuvers may be used to terminate an episode of SVT by eliciting the diving reflex. Immersing the older child's face in ice water stimulates a vagal response that may stop the tachycardia; briefly placing an ice bag or bag of frozen vegetables over the infant's face accomplishes the same result. This should be done only while constantly monitoring the child and with emergency equipment available in case the child has a prolonged slow heart rate while converting back to a normal rhythm.

If vagal maneuvers do not convert the child to a normal rhythm, antidysrhythmics need to be considered. Antidysrhythmic drug therapy may also be successful in suppressing further episodes. Older children who continue to have episodes of SVT may benefit from radiofrequency ablation of the ectopic focus or accessory pathway.

Infants and children who are hemodynamically unstable require emergency intervention. If vascular access is present, the drug adenosine may be given. Adenosine is an effective antidysrhythmic because of its ability to slow conduction through the AV node and, in many cases, successfully terminate episodes of SVT rapidly and safely (Park, 2002). Synchronized cardioversion, however, remains the treatment of choice for the child with profound cardiovascular compromise.

Ventricular Tachycardia. Ventricular tachycardia is a wide complex tachycardia. This indicates that the impulse originates in the ventricle. The emergency management of ventricular tachycardia in unconscious children is synchronized cardioversion. Children with a wide complex tachycardia and no pulse (absent pulse) require CPR until defibrillation is available. Lidocaine, 1 mg/kg, may be administered

before cardioversion, followed by a continuous infusion of the drug to prevent further episodes (Park, 2002). Once the tachycardia has been terminated, underlying causes should be explored.

Slow Pulse Rate

Bradydysrhythmias. Most episodes of bradydysrhythmia during childhood are the result of noncardiac secondary causes. Hypoxia is a major cause of bradycardia in children, and the airway and breathing effort must be assessed in every situation. Airway management, oxygenation, ventilation, and cardiac compressions, if indicated, may successfully resolve the event. The use of epinephrine or atropine (or both) may be indicated if the rhythm has not improved once oxygenation and ventilation have been reestablished.

Primary cardiac bradydysrhythmias include the varying degrees of heart block and junctional or ventricular "escape" rhythms caused by sinus node dysfunction. These dysrhythmias are marked by dissociation between the P wave and the QRS complex, with the asynchrony between the atrial and ventricular contractions. These dysrhythmias may be congenital but are often seen in children who have undergone cardiac surgery. Temporary or permanent cardiac pacing may be necessary to maintain adequate cardiac output.

Absent Rhythms. The classification of absent or collapse rhythms includes asystole, ventricular fibrillation, and pulseless electrical activity. In asystole, electrical cardiac activity is absent. Epinephrine is administered to stimulate cardiac activity. The heart is in electrical standstill, and there is no myocardial activity or cardiac output. The ECG rhythm strip is a "flat line." The emergency management of asystole is CPR and medical management. Epinephrine is administered to stimulate cardiac activity. The drug may be given IV, intraosseously, or through an endotracheal tube.

Ventricular fibrillation is rare in children and frequently the result of underlying cardiac disease. The emergency management of episodes of ventricular fibrillation is defibrillation and CPR. Drugs administered during resuscitation efforts include epinephrine, lidocaine, and other antidysrhythmic agents.

Pulseless electrical activity indicates a hemodynamically compromised state in which cardiac electrical activity is unable to generate effective myocardial contraction and cardiac output. The ECG rhythm strip appears like a normal rhythm. When palpating for a pulse or listening for a heart beat, there

---

! **CRITICAL** **TO REMEMBER**

Dysrhythmias

If a child is having a dysrhythmia, assess responsiveness and remember the ABCs:
- **AIRWAY** assessment
- **BREATHING** assessment
- If no breathing, begin ventilation.
- **CIRCULATION** assessment.
  - —Palpate and auscultate pulses.
  - —If no pulse, begin chest compressions.
  - —If slow pulse, assess the child's tolerance of slow pulse (including perfusion and pulses).
  - —Obtain an electrocardiogram rhythm strip for assessment.

will be none. CPR must be initiated. The underlying cause is usually noncardiac and must be identified and corrected for the child to survive the episode. Causes include severe hypoxia or acidosis, hypovolemia, tension pneumothorax, and cardiac tamponade. Emergency management includes CPR, administration of epinephrine, and discovery and treatment of the underlying cause (Chameides & Hazinski, 1997).

■NURSING CARE
The Child With a Dysrhythmia

Assessment

Children with dysrhythmias require a thorough cardiovascular assessment because they are at risk for developing cardiogenic shock. In a stable or compensated child with a dysrhythmia, it is important to obtain a comprehensive and accurate history of activity tolerance. Older children may have unexplained episodes of dizziness, palpitations, or syncope. Irregular pulse may be noted. Nurses who have been trained to read pediatric ECG rhythm strips may observe signs of a particular dysrhythmia.

Nursing Diagnosis and Planning

Nursing diagnoses and expected outcomes for the child with a dysrhythmia include

■ Decreased Cardiac Output related to decreased ventricular filling or decreased rate of heart contractions.
   Expected Outcome: The child will have pink or baseline cyanotic mucous membranes and nail beds, brisk capillary refill, good-quality pulses, and normal level of consciousness.
■ Risk for Injury related to episodes of syncope.
   Expected Outcome: The child will remain free of injury during any episode of syncope.
■ Deficient Knowledge about care of a child with a potentially fatal condition related to unfamiliarity of the information.
   Expected Outcomes: The family will demonstrate an understanding of medication administration and an ability to identify signs and symptoms indicative of dysrhythmias and will be able to perform CPR.

Interventions

Nursing interventions involve immediate care of the child who is experiencing the dysrhythmia, as well as education of the child and family. The child and family will need information regarding monitoring for future signs and symptoms of dysrhythmias, administering medications as ordered, and appropriate emergency measures to initiate, including CPR, once the child has been discharged from the hospital.

Education of the child and family is imperative for those children with life-threatening dysrhythmias. Teach the child and family how to take a pulse or listen to the heart rate with a stethoscope. Teach the child and family to identify the signs and symptoms of dysrhythmia, including poor feeding, color changes, palpitations, syncope/dizziness, respiratory distress, and fatigue. These signs and symptoms should be reported to the parent or teacher as soon as possible, and medical attention should be sought. Children who take antidysrhythmics at home need to adhere to the prescribed medication schedule closely

and must be careful not to skip any doses. Medic-Alert bracelets should be worn by children who are in preschool or school. Parents and teachers also need to be aware of signs and symptoms that may indicate early appearance of dysrhythmias. All caretakers should complete a formal course in CPR and know how to activate the Emergency Medical Service (EMS) system.

Evaluation

● Are the child's pulses of good quality and mucous membranes pink or baseline cyanosis, and does the child have a normal level of consciousness?
● Has the child remained free of injury related to falling secondary to syncope?
● Have the child, parents, and other caregivers demonstrated an understanding of medications, activity limitations, and the possibility of a life-threatening episode and how to activate the EMS system?
● Have the child and parents demonstrated how to listen to the heart rate with a stethoscope or palpate a pulse?

HIGH CHOLESTEROL IN CHILDREN AND ADOLESCENTS

Preventive cardiology has become increasingly important during childhood and adolescence. Developing heart-healthy habits during these years reduces the risk for coronary artery disease and other cardiovascular problems during adulthood. Several major risk factors during childhood and adolescence appear routinely in the literature. They include (Gidding, 1999):

● Tobacco use
● Dyslipidemia (elevated low-density lipoproteins [LDLs] and cholesterol and decreased high-density lipoproteins [HDLs])
● Hypertension
● Decreased physical activity
● Obesity

More than half of the children in the United States are considered to be obese, and many of the recently updated national health objectives address the issue of obesity and dietary management in children (U.S. Department of Health and Human Services, 2000).

Assessment of Children at Risk

High cholesterol can be genetic or dietary or a combination. Children at risk for high cholesterol should be screened during their developing years. According to guidelines from the National Cholesterol Education Program, the following children older than 2 years should be screened:

● Children whose parents or grandparents developed vascular or cerebrovascular disease or who have been diagnosed with coronary atherosclerosis before the age of 55 years
● Children who have at least one parent with a total cholesterol level greater than or equal to 240 mg/dl
● Children who demonstrate other risk factors and whose parental history is unavailable
● Children or adolescents who have risk factors independent of family history (excessive smoking, decreased exercise, excessive fat intake) (American Academy of Pediatrics, Committee on Nutrition, 1998; Gidding, 1999)

Children with any of these risk factors should be followed with periodic cholesterol level measurements. Children whose total cholesterol measurement is 200 mg/dl or more, or 170 mg/dl or more on two successive measurements, need to have a follow-up fasting lipid profile.

Therapeutic Management

All children older than 2 years can follow a sensible low-fat dietary program. This includes using nonfat or low-fat dairy products, limiting red meat intake, and decreasing the amount of dietary saturated fat (see Chapter 4). The total daily fat intake should be no more than 30% of total calories, with saturated fat being no more than 10% of daily caloric intake. Children with borderline LDL measurements (110 to 129 mg/dl) need to have their food and fat intake carefully monitored by a health professional until cholesterol levels have improved. Children with high LDL measurements (>130 mg/dl) will need a more restrictive diet and comprehensive instruction and monitoring by a registered dietitian (American Academy of Pediatrics, Committee on Nutrition, 1998).

Cholesterol-lowering medications generally are not used in the pediatric population. Medications that bind bile acids in the intestine (cholestyramine, colestipol) are reserved for older children (>10 years old) who have very high LDLs with or without associated risk factors (Gidding, 1999).

Nursing Considerations

The most effective approach to decreasing risk factors during childhood and adolescence appears to be a population-based approach, with ongoing education about risk factors occurring in communities, schools, physicians' offices, and the media. Nurses play an important part in educating parents and children about healthy diets, the importance of regular exercise, and reduction of other risk factors.

KEY CONCEPTS

- With the neonate's first breath, gas exchange is transferred from the placenta to the lungs. The fetal shunts (ductus venosus, ductus arteriosus, foramen ovale) close, and resistance to flow in the pulmonary system decreases as systemic resistance increases. Pulmonary vascular resistance decreases, and a marked increase in pulmonary blood flow follows.
- Stenosis can occur in a valve or a vessel and result in obstruction of blood flow through the area.
- In left-to-right shunts, blood is shunted to the right side of the heart because the pressure is lower on the right side. Oxygenated and unoxygenated blood mix. Systemic saturations are normal.
- Poor weight gain with failure to thrive is a common sign of congestive heart failure.
- Hypercyanotic episodes, or "tet spells," are characterized by increased respiratory rate, depth of respiration, and severe hypoxemia.
- Assessment of the family of a child with a congenital cardiac defect should begin at diagnosis and continue throughout the care of the child.
- Common nursing diagnoses associated with infants with congenital heart defects and their parents include Decreased Cardiac Output,

Imbalanced Nutrition: Less than Body Requirements, Activity Intolerance, Deficient Knowledge, Anxiety, Interrupted Family Processes, Risk for Infection, and Risk for Ineffective Health Maintenance.
- Signs of congestive heart failure include tachycardia, cardiomegaly, gallop rhythm, decreased peripheral perfusion, excessive diaphoresis, weight gain, ascites, liver and spleen enlargement, edema, neck vein distention, dyspnea, rales, tachypnea, intercostal muscular and sternal retractions, and wheezing.
- Measures to decrease the workload on the heart include limiting the time the child is allowed to bottle-feed or breastfeed, elevating the head of the bed, allowing for uninterrupted rest periods, allowing self-limiting activity, and providing oxygen (cautious use with left-to-right shunting lesions) during stressful periods.
- It is imperative to educate parents regarding medications, monitoring for signs and symptoms of congestive heart failure, increasing cyanosis, dehydration, infection, dysrhythmias (when indicated), subacute bacterial endocarditis prophylaxis, decreased nutritional intake, and decreasing ill contacts in the environment as the family is prepared for home discharge with infants or children with

congestive heart failure and congenital heart disease.
- Prophylaxis with penicillin is the most important aspect of therapeutic management for rheumatic fever. Intramuscular injection is the route of choice. Oral medication is an alternative, if given precisely and faithfully.
- In Kawasaki disease, coronary aneurysms may occur about 11 days after the onset of fever.
- Nursing management of a child with Kawasaki disease includes administering intravenous immune globulin and aspirin to reduce the formation of the aneurysms and fever.
- The initial management of children with primary hypertension includes diet modification, reduction of weight (when needed), physical conditioning, and relaxation techniques.
- An appropriate-size blood pressure cuff, two repeat blood pressure readings on all four extremities, and a careful medical history are important in assessment for a diagnosis of hypertension.
- The heart rate is usually faster in infants and children than in adults and decreases with age.
- Population-based education of children and parents is the most effective way to prevent the cardiac consequences of high cholesterol.

ANSWERS to Critical Thinking Exercise 46-1

1. Appropriate questions to ask concerning infant feeding patterns include:
   - How often does she eat?
   - How much does she eat at each feeding?
   - Does she tire easily?
   - Does she require frequent rest periods?
   - Do you notice beads of perspiration on her forehead during feedings?
   - Do you notice any change in her color or respiratory pattern during feedings?
   - Does she raise her eyebrows or wrinkle her forehead during feedings?

2. Some frequently seen physical assessment findings associated with congestive heart failure include tachycardia; tachypnea; increased work of breathing—nasal flaring, grunting, use of accessory muscles; pulmonary congestion, crackles; dry cough; hepatomegaly; distended neck veins; and periorbital, facial, or generalized edema.

3. Nutritional nursing care would include:
   - Finding an appropriate nipple for feeding; may need to enlarge the nipple hole to reduce the energy needed to suck

   - Feeding every 3 hours and allowing rest periods between feedings
   - Increasing the caloric content of the formula
   - May need to provide supplemental feedings through a nasogastric tube
   Comfort measures include allowing rest periods between feedings. Do not overtire infants with multiple interventions at any one time. Place infants and children in a position of comfort, usually with the head of the bed elevated to decrease the work of breathing

REFERENCES and READINGS

American Academy of Pediatrics. (2000). *2000 Red Book: report of the Committee on Infectious Diseases* (25th ed.). Elk Grove Village, IL: Author.

American Academy of Pediatrics. (1987). Report of the Second Task Force on Blood Pressure Control in Children. *Pediatrics, 79*(1), 1-25.

American Academy of Pediatrics, Committee on Nutrition. (1998). Cholesterol in childhood. *Pediatrics, 101*(1), 141-147.

American Academy of Pediatrics, Committee on Sports Medicine and Fitness. (1997). Athletic participation by children and adolescents who have systemic hypertension. *Pediatrics, 99*(4), 637-638.

Balaguru D., Artman, M., & Auslender M. (2000). Management of heart failure in children. *Current Problems in Pediatrics, 30*(1), 5-30.

Barst, R. (1999). Recent advances in the treatment of pediatric pulmonary artery hypertension. *Pediatric Clinics of North America, 46*(2), 331-345.

Bartosh, S., & Aronson, A. (1999). Childhood hypertension: An update on etiology, diagnosis, and treatment. *Pediatric Clinics of North America, 46*(2), 235-252.

Belkengren, R., & Sapala, S. (1997). Pediatric management problems. *Pediatric Nursing, 23*(4), 4094-4095.

Berger, S., Dhala, A., & Friedberg, D. (1999). Sudden cardiac death in infants, children, and adolescents. *Pediatric Clinics of North America, 46*(2), 221-234.

Bernstein, D. (2004). The cardiovascular system. In R.E. Behrman, R.M. Kliegman, & H. Jenson (Eds.), *Nelson textbook of pediatrics* (17th ed., pp. 1475-1591). Philadelphia: Saunders.

Blieden, L.C., Berant, M., & Zeevi, B. (2000). Pulmonic stenosis. In J.H. Moller & J. Hoffman (Eds.), *Pediatric cardiovascular medicine* (pp. 552-566). Philadelphia: Churchill Livingstone.

Brook, M. (1998). The cardiovascular system. In R.E. Behrman & R.M. Kliegman (Eds.), *Nelson's essentials of pediatrics* (3rd ed., pp. 497-544). Philadelphia: Saunders.

Brook, M. (1999). Pediatric bacterial endocarditis: Treatment and prophylaxis. *Pediatric Clinics of North America, 46*(2), 275-288.

Canobbio, M. (2001). Health care issues facing adolescents with congenital heart disease. *Journal of Pediatric Nursing, 16*(5), 363-370.

Carey, L., Nicholson, B., & Fox, R. (2002). Maternal factors related to parenting young children with congenital heart disease. *Journal of Pediatric Nursing, 17*(3), 174-183.

Case, C. (1999). Diagnosis and treatment of pediatric arrhythmias. *Pediatric Clinics of North America, 46*(2), 347-350.

Chameides, L., & Hazinski, M.F. (1997). *American Heart Association pediatric advanced life support* (3rd ed., pp. 7.1-7.15). Dallas: American Heart Association.

Chang, A.C., & Burke, R.P. (1998). Left ventricular outflow tract obstruction. In A.C. Chang, F.L. Hanley, G. Wernovsky, & D.L. Wessel (Eds.), *Pediatric cardiac intensive care* (pp. 233-256). Baltimore: Williams & Wilkins.

Chang, A.C., & Jacobs, J. (1998). Ventricular septal defect. In A.C. Chang, F.L. Hanley, G. Wernovsky, & D.L. Wessel (Eds.), *Pediatric cardiac intensive care* (pp. 212-217). Baltimore: Williams & Wilkins.

Chang, A.C., & Reddy, M. (1998). Truncus arteriosus. In A.C. Chang, F.L. Hanley, G. Wernovsky, & D.L. Wessel (Eds.), *Pediatric cardiac intensive care* (pp. 228-232). Baltimore: Williams & Wilkins.

Chang, A.C., & Starnes V.A. (1998). Coarctation of the aorta. In A.C. Chang, F.L. Hanley, G. Wernovsky, & D.L. Wessel (Eds.), *Pediatric cardiac intensive care* (pp. 247-256). Baltimore: Williams & Wilkins.

Chang, A.C., & Wells, W. (1998). Patent ductus arteriosus. In A.C. Chang, F.L. Hanley, G. Wernovsky, & D.L. Wessel (Eds.), *Pediatric cardiac intensive care* (pp. 203-207). Baltimore: Williams & Wilkins.

Corbet, A. (1998). Medical manipulation of the ductus arteriosus. In A. Garson, Jr., J.T. Bricker, D.J. Fisher, & S.R. Neish (Eds.), *The science and practice of pediatric cardiology* (2nd ed., pp. 2489-2513). Baltimore: Williams & Wilkins.

Dajani, A.S., Taubert, K.A., & Wilson, W. (1997). Prevention of bacterial endocarditis: Recommendations by the American Heart Association. *JAMA: The Journal of the American Medical Association, 227*(22), 1794-1801.

DeJong, M.J. (1998). Infectious endocarditis. *American Journal of Nursing, 98*(5), 34-35.

Dooley, K., & Bishop, L. (2002). Medical management of the cardiac infant and child after surgical discharge. *Critical Care Nursing Quarterly, 25*(3), 98-104.

Doyle, T.P., Kavanaugh-McHugh, A., & Graham, T.P. (2000). Tetralogy of Fallot and pulmonary atresia with ventricular septal defect. In J.H. Moller & J.I. Hoffman (Eds.), *Pediatric cardiovascular medicine* (pp. 391-408). Philadelphia: Churchill Livingstone.

Driscoll, D. (1999). Left-to-right shunt lesions. *Pediatric Clinics of North America, 46*(2), 355-368.

Dubin, A. (2004). Cardiac arrhythmias. In R.E. Behrman, R.M. Kliegman, & H. Jenson (Eds.), *Nelson textbook of pediatrics* (17th ed., pp. 1554-1565). Philadelphia: Saunders.

El-Said, G.M., El-Refaee, M.M., Sorour, K.A., & El-Said, H.G. (1998). Rheumatic fever and rheumatic heart disease. In A. Garson, Jr., J.T. Bricker, D.J. Fisher, & S.R. Neish (Eds.), *The science and practice of pediatric cardiology* (2nd ed., pp. 1691-1724). Baltimore: Williams & Wilkins.

Estlow, M.M. (1998). Prevention of infective endocarditis in the pediatric congenital heart population. *Pediatric Nursing, 24*(3), 205-225.

Fedderly, R.T. (1999). Left ventricular outflow obstruction. *Pediatric Clinics of North America, 46*(2), 369-384.

Fineman, J.R., Black, S.M., & Heymann, M. (2000). Control of pulmonary vasculature. In J.H. Moller & J.I. Hoffman (Eds.), *Pediatric cardiovascular medicine* (pp. 86-94). Philadelphia: Churchill Livingstone.

Freedom R.M. (2000). Pulmonary atresia and intact ventricular septum. In J.H. Moller & J.I. Hoffman (Eds.), *Pediatric cardiovascular medicine* (pp. 442-460). Philadelphia: Churchill Livingstone.

Friedman, R.A., & Starke, J.R. (1998). Infective endocarditis. In A. Garson, Jr., J.T. Bricker, D.J. Fisher, & S.R. Neish (Eds.), *The science and practice of pediatric cardiology* (2nd ed., pp. 1759-1775). Baltimore: Williams & Wilkins.

Fukushige, J., & Nihill, M.R. (1998). Kawasaki disease. In A. Garson, Jr., J.T. Bricker, D.J. Fisher, & S.R. Neish (Eds.), *The science and practice of pediatric cardiology* (2nd ed., pp. 1741-1758). Baltimore: Williams & Wilkins.

Fyfe, D., & Parks, W.J. (2002). Noninvasive diagnostics in congenital heart disease: echocardiography and magnetic resonance imaging. *Critical Care Nursing Quarterly, 25*(3), 26-36.

Gerber, M. (2004). Group A streptococcus. In R.E. Behrman, R.M. Kliegman, & H. Jenson (Eds.), *Nelson textbook of pediatrics* (17th ed., pp. 870-878). Philadelphia: Saunders.

Gidding, S. (1999). Preventive pediatric cardiology: Tobacco, cholesterol, obesity, and physical activity. *Pediatric Clinics of North America, 46*(2), 253-262.

Griffin, K., Elkin, D., & Smith, C. (2003). Academic outcomes in children with congenital heart disease. *Clinical Pediatrics, 42*, 401-409.

Grifka, R.G. (1999). Cyanotic congenital heart disease with increased pulmonary blood flow. *Pediatric Clinics of North America, 46*(2), 405-425.

Hanisch, D. (2001). Pediatric arrhythmias. *Journal of Pediatric Nursing, 16*(5), 351-362.

Hinocki, K.W. (1998). Congenital heart disease: Effects on the family. *Neonatal Network, 7,* 1-10.

Holt, C.F. (1998). Alterations in cardiovascular status. In V.R. Bowden, S.B. Dickey, & C.S. Greenberg (Eds.), *Children and their families: The continuum of care* (pp. 782-862). Philadelphia: Saunders.

Ikemba, C., Kozinetz, C., Feltes, T., Fraser, C., McKenzie, E., Shah, N., & Mott, A. (2002). Internet use in families with children requiring cardiac surgery for congenital heart disease. *Pediatrics, 109*(3), 419-423.

Kinsella, J., Neish, S., Abman, S., & Wolfe, R. (1998). Therapy of pulmonary hypertension. In A. Carson, J. Borcher, D. Fisher, & S. Weish (Eds.). *The science and practice of pediatric cardiology* (2nd ed., pp. 2345-2366). Baltimore: Williams & Wilkins.

Latson, L.A. (2000). Atrial septal defect. In J.H. Moller & J.I. Hoffman (Eds.), *Pediatric cardiovascular medicine* (pp. 311-321). Philadelphia: Churchill Livingstone.

Momenah, T., Sanatani, S., Potts, J., Sandor, G.G., Human, D.G., & Patterson, M.W. (1998). Kawasaki disease in the older child. *Pediatrics, 102*(1), 7-13.

Moody, L.Y. (1997). Pediatric cardiovascular assessment and referral in the primary care setting. *Nurse Practitioner, 22*(1), 120-134.

Mullins, C.E., & Pagotto, L. (1998). Patent ductus arteriosus. In A. Garson Jr., J.T. Bricker, D.J. Fisher, & S.R. Neish, (Eds.), *The science and practice of pediatric cardiology* (2nd ed., pp. 1181-1197). Baltimore: Williams & Wilkins.

National Institutes of Health. (1996). *Update on the task force report (1987) on high blood pressure in children and adolescents: A working group report from the national high blood pressure education program.* Bethesda, MD: Author.

Neilson, D., & Robin, N. (2002). Advances in the genetics of pediatric heart disease. *Contemporary Pediatrics, 19*(1), 85-94.

Neutze, J., Calder, A.L., Gentles, T., & Wilson, N.J. (2000). Aortic stenosis. In J.H. Moller & J.I. Hoffman (Eds.), *Pediatric cardiovascular medicine* (pp. 511-551). Philadelphia: Churchill Livingstone.

Park, M.K. (2002). *Pediatric cardiology for practitioners* (4th ed.). St. Louis: Mosby.

Pelech, A.N. (1998). The cardiac murmur: When to refer? *Pediatric Clinics of North America, 45*(1), 107-122.

REFERENCES and READINGS

Rocchini, A.P. (2000). Coarctation of the aorta and interrupted aortic arch. In J.H. Moller & J.I. Hoffman (Eds.), *Pediatric cardiovascular medicine* (pp. 567-593). Philadelphia: Churchill Livingstone.

Rosenthal, A. (2000). Hypoplastic left heart syndrome. In J.H. Moller & J.I. Hoffman (Eds.), *Pediatric cardiovascular medicine* (pp. 567-593). Philadelphia: Churchill Livingstone.

Rowley, A., & Shulman, S. (1999). Kawasaki syndrome. *Pediatric Clinics of North America, 46*(2), 313-330.

Rowley, A., & Shulman, S. (2004). Kawasaki disease. In R.E. Behrman, R.M. Kliegman, & H. Jenson (Eds.), *Nelson textbook of pediatrics* (17th ed., pp. 823-826). Philadelphia: Saunders.

Rubin, B., & Cotton, D.M. (1998). Kawasaki disease: A dangerous acute childhood illness. *Nurse Practitioner, 23*(2), 34-48.

Second Task Force on Blood Pressure Control in Children. (1987). Report of the Second Task Force on Blood Pressure Control in Children: National Heart, Lung, and Blood Institute—1987. *Pediatrics, 79*(1), 1-25.

Sinaiko, A., & Prineas, R. (1998). Reduction of cardiovascular disease: What is the role of the pediatrician? *Pediatrics, 105*(5), e61.

Smith, P. (2001). Primary care in children with congenital heart disease. *Journal of Pediatric Nursing, 16*(5), 308-319.

Spilman, L.J., & Furdon, S.A. (1998). Recognition, understanding, and current management of cardiac lesions with decreased pulmonary blood flow. *Neonatal Network, 17*(4), 7-18.

Spray, T.L., & Wernovsky, G. (1998). Right ventricular outflow tract obstruction. In A.C. Chang, F.L. Hanley, G. Wernovsky, & D.L. Wessel (Eds.), *Pediatric cardiac intensive care* (pp. 257-265). Baltimore: Williams & Wilkins.

Suddaby, E. (2001). Contemporary thinking for congenital heart disease. *Pediatric Nursing, 27*(3), 233-240.

Talner, N.S. (1998). The physiology of congestive heart failure. In A. Garson, Jr., J.T. Bricker, D.J. Fisher, & S.R. Neish (Eds.), *The science and practice of pediatric cardiology* (2nd ed., pp. 1181-1197). Baltimore: Williams & Wilkins.

Taylor, J.F. (2000). Persistent truncus arteriosus. In J.H. Moller & J.I. Hoffman (Eds.), *Pediatric cardiovascular medicine* (pp. 499-510). Philadelphia: Churchill Livingstone.

Teitel, D.F., & Cassidy, J.W. (1995). Fetal and post-natal circulations: Systemic circulation. In G.C. Emmanouilides, A.J. Moss, & F.H. Adams (Eds.), *Moss and Adams' heart disease in infants, children, and adolescents: Including the fetus and young adult* (5th ed., pp. 47-59). Baltimore: Williams & Wilkins.

Todd, J. (2000). Group A streptococcus. In R.E. Behrman, R.M. Kliegman, & H.B. Jenson (Eds.), *Nelson textbook of pediatrics* (16th ed., p. 808). Philadelphia: Saunders.

U.S. Department of Health and Human Services. (2000). *Healthy People 2010* (Conference edition, in 2 volumes [pp. 19-1–19-43]). Washington, DC: Author.

Uzark, K. (2001). Therapeutic cardiac catheterization for congenital heart disease – a new era in pediatric care. *Journal of Pediatric Nursing, 16*(5), 300-307.

Vessey, J., & O'Sullivan, P. (2000). A study of children's concepts of their internal bodies: A comparison of children with and without congenital heart disease. *Journal of Pediatric Nursing, 15*(5), 292-298.

Waldman, J., & Wernly, J. (1999). Cyanotic congenital heart disease with decreased pulmonary blood flow in children. *Pediatric Clinics of North America, 46*(2), 385-404.

Wernovsky, G., & Hanley, F.L. (1998). Pulmonary atresia with intact ventricular septum/pulmonary stenosis. In A.C. Chang, F.L. Hanley, G. Wernovsky, & D.L. Wessel (Eds.), *Pediatric cardiac intensive care* (pp. 265-270). Baltimore: Williams & Wilkins.

Wood, M.K. (1998). Acyanotic cardiac lesions with normal pulmonary blood flow. *Neonatal Network, 17*(3), 5-11.

Zeigler, V.L. (1994). Supraventricular tachycardia in children: A challenge for pediatric nurses. *Journal of Pediatric Nursing, 9*(5), 288-298.

Zeigler, V.L. (2003). Ethical principles and parental choice: treatment options for neonates with hypoplastic left heart syndrome. *Pediatric Nursing, 29*(1), 65-69.

47

The Child with a Hematologic Alteration

◆ LEARNING OBJECTIVES

After studying this chapter, you should be able to:

- ◎ Describe the anatomy and physiology of the hematopoietic system.
- ◎ Discuss the pediatric differences related to blood and blood formation.
- ◎ Discuss the role of the nurse in the prevention of iron-deficiency anemia.
- ◎ Describe common factors in the care of a child with anemia.

- ◎ Discuss the pathophysiology and therapeutic management of common hematologic alterations.
- ◎ List possible nursing diagnoses for children with hematologic alterations.
- ◎ Describe possible nursing care for children with hematologic alterations.

◆ DEFINITIONS

autoimmune disorder A disorder in which the body launches an immunologic response against itself.

chelation Binding of a metallic ion with a structure so that the ion is inactivated.

erythropoiesis Production of erythrocytes (red blood cells, RBC).

extramedullary Outside the bone marrow.

granulocytes Polymorphonuclear leukocytes (neutrophils, eosinophils, basophils).

hematopoiesis Production of blood cells; normally occurs in the bone marrow but may occur in extramedullary sites.

hemolysis Breakdown of red blood cells.

hemostasis Process of vasoconstriction and coagulation to stop bleeding.

hemosiderosis Focal or general increase in tissue iron stores without associated tissue damage.

pancytopenia A reduction in all types of blood cells.

reticulocyte Immature red blood cell.

reticuloendothelial system The collection of cells, throughout the body, that are capable of phagocytosis.

REVIEW OF THE HEMATOLOGIC SYSTEM

Hematology is the study of the blood and blood-forming tissues. In fetal life, various tissues produce red blood cells (RBCs), but after birth, their production is controlled exclusively by the bone marrow, primarily in the long bones. With age, the more membranous bones of the vertebrae, sternum, and ribs assume RBC production. Age, gender, and the altitude at which a person lives affect the number of RBCs.

Normally, RBCs are biconcave disks that are capable of changing shape as they flow through the microvasculature of the body. They have a fairly uniform size that is determined mainly by the amount of cellular content of substances, primarily hemoglobin. Their function is to transport oxygen to tissues. Essential to this ability to carry oxygen is an appropriate amount of hemoglobin, whose production depends on sufficient amounts of circulating iron. Iron is absorbed from dietary intake by the intestines and stored by the liver in both soluble and insoluble forms, to be used when necessary.

The stimulus for production of RBCs is a decrease in circulating oxygen, which in turn stimulates the kidneys to produce a hormone called *erythropoietin*. Erythropoietin stimulates the production of RBC precursors and causes them to mature rapidly. Disorders of the kidney can affect the individual's ability to produce this hormone and thus can affect RBC production by the bone marrow.

Anemia is a decrease in the number of RBCs reduction in their hemoglobin content, or reduced volume of packed red blood cells. Anemia results from one of two problems: either too rapid a loss of RBCs (via covert or overt bleeding or destruction) or too slow a production of RBCs. Anemias are categorized according to the size of the RBC (macrocytic, microcytic, normocytic) and the content of hemoglobin in the RBC (hypochromic, normochromic).

Polycythemia, which is an increase in the number of RBCs, is less commonly seen than anemia. *Polycythemia* can occur secondary to hypoxia, such as that experienced at high altitude or when oxygen is not sufficiently directed to the tissues, as in cyanotic heart disease.

White blood cells (WBCs), or leukocytes, are formed in the bone marrow and in lymphatic tissue. They assist in the body's ability to distinguish "self" from "nonself." WBCs destroy foreign cells through the processes of phagocytosis and antibody production. Both phagocytes and antibodies destroy foreign cells and tissues perceived by the body as nonself (including, e.g., bacteria, fungi, viruses, parasites, transplanted tissue). WBC disorders result from an altered rate of production of WBCs (lymphocytosis or lymphopenia) or an alteration in function of the cells.

Platelets are the cells that promote hemostasis—the prevention of blood loss. They are formed in the bone marrow from megakaryocytes. Megakaryocytes later fragment into smaller cells known as *platelets*, either in the bone marrow or shortly after release into the systemic circulation. Platelets can circulate in the blood for about 10 days before they die; however, disease, fever, and infection can shorten a platelet's lifetime. Platelet disorders occur when the bone marrow cannot meet the production demands of the body.

Pediatric Hematologic System ●

- The life span of erythrocytes in neonates is shorter than in older infants and children because of increased destruction during rapid growth.
- By 2 months of age, erythropoiesis increases, leading to increased reticulocytes in the blood and a rise in hemoglobin.
- Erythrocytes are produced initially in the marrow of all bones. After 5 years of age, RBC production in the shafts of the long bones (tibia, femur) is reduced, and production ceases in these locations entirely at age 20 years. Hematopoiesis takes place primarily in the marrow of the ribs, sternum, vertebrae, pelvis, skull, clavicle, and scapulas.
- The number of erythrocytes varies according to age. The fetus has a higher oxygen-carrying capacity than an infant because of a considerably higher number of erythrocytes with proportionately elevated hemoglobin and hematocrit value.

after 2-3 days it drops due to volume changes

Types and Functions of White Blood Cells

- **Granulocytes**: Phagocytic cells produced in the bone marrow and found in the circulation.
  - *Neutrophils*: primary defense in bacterial infection; capable of phagocytizing and killing bacteria.
  - *Eosinophils*: influence the inflammatory process, fight parasites and influence allergic hypersensitivity reactions.
  - *Basophils*: activate the inflammatory response; contain histamine; other roles are unclear.
- **Agranulocytes:** Participate in inflammatory and immune reactions.
  - *Monocytes/macrophages*: Phagocytize large cells, including necrotic tissue; they are therefore important in fighting chronic infection.
  - *Lymphocytes:* Found in bone marrow, spleen, thymus, lymph glands, tissues, and circulation.
    * *T cells:* made in the thymus and responsible for cell-mediated immunity.
    * *B cells:* responsible for humoral immunity (antibody production).
    * *Natural killer cells:* Lymphocyte-like cells that can kill certain type of tumor cells and viruses directly

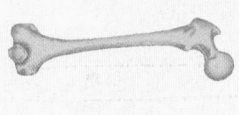

BONE MARROW   Hematopoiesis (red blood cell production) occurs in the bone marrow during the first 5 years of life. Beyond 5 years of age, most red blood cells are produced in the marrow of the ribs, sternum, vertebrae, pelvis, skull, and clavicles.

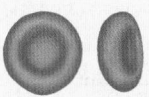

ERYTHROCYTES   Biconcave, anuclear discs that transport oxygen and carbon dioxide. Red blood cell lifetime is 120 days.

LEUKOCYTES   Spherical, nucleated cells

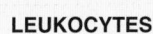

Granulocytes   Phagocytic cells found in bone marrow

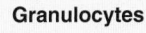

Neutrophils   Nucleated, multi-lobed cells that fight bacteria

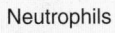

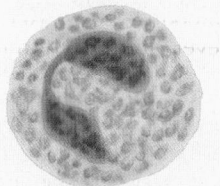

Eosinophils   Nucleated, bilobed cells that fight parasites and respond to allergens

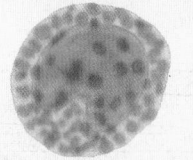

Basophils   Nucleated, lobed cells that secrete heparin and speed fat removal

Lymphocytes   Cells with a spherical or indented nucleus; found in bone marrow, spleen, thymus, and other lymph glands and tissue

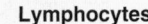

T lymphocytes   T cells made in the thymus, responsible for cell-mediated immunity

B lymphocytes   B cells responsible for humoral immunity

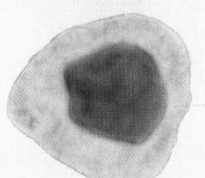

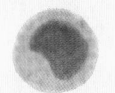

Monocytes   Cells with a U– or kidney–shaped nucleus that phagocytize large cells, including necrotic tissue, therefore having an important role in chronic infection

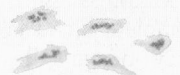

PLATELETS   Cell fragments partially responsible for blood clotting. Lifespan is 10 days.

Review of the Hematologic System

When caring for infants and children with blood disorders, the nurse is challenged in the areas of preventive, acute, and chronic care. Depending on the disorder and the child's condition, care may be provided in the home, outpatient setting, or hospital. It is not unusual for a child to be seen in an outpatient setting (clinic, school), referred to a hospital for diagnosis and stabilization, and returned to the home for maintenance. Genetic counseling may be indicated for children or families with certain types of blood disorders.

Many medications for hematologic disorders can be given at home, including deferoxamine mesylate (Desferal), intravenous (IV) immune globulin (IVIG), IV antibiotics, coagulation factor products, and, in some instances, even blood transfusions. Parents are learning to manage infusion therapy in regard to initiating, monitoring, and discontinuing infusions when appropriate, with guidance from the collaborative efforts of the multidisciplinary health care team.

IRON-DEFICIENCY ANEMIA

Iron deficiency is the most common cause of anemia during infancy, childhood, and adolescence. Iron-deficiency anemia (IDA) may be characterized by mild or marked anemia.

Etiology and Incidence

Several factors can contribute to iron-deficiency anemia, including decreased iron intake, increased iron or blood loss, and periods of increased growth rate.

IDA related to inadequate dietary iron intake is rare before age 4 to 6 months because of the presence of maternal iron stores; it occurs most often in children age 9 to 24 months as iron stores are depleted. Premature infants may develop iron deficiency early in life because they are born with insufficient maternal iron stores (Glader, 2004). Decreased iron intake is often related to the intake of large amounts of cow's milk instead of breast milk or fortified formula and inadequate intake of iron-fortified foods (Glader, 2004). The incidence has dropped in recent years because of increased education about and availability of iron-fortified formula and cereals. Early transition from breast milk or infant formula to cow's milk can precipitate chronic diarrhea with occult intestinal bleeding in children younger than 2 years. This results from exposure to a protein found in cow's milk (Glader, 2004). The rapid growth of infants and children younger than 2-years-old, combined with decreased iron intake further contributes to the increased incidence in this age group.

Adolescents are also at risk for iron-deficiency anemia because they too are experiencing increased growth and often have poor dietary habits. The situation is further complicated by the blood loss at menarche in young women.

Manifestations

The clinical manifestations of iron-deficiency anemia vary with the degree of anemia but may include extreme pallor with porcelain-like skin, pale mucus membranes and conjunctiva, tachycardia, tachypnea, lethargy, fatigue, and irritability. Children with lead poisoning often have associated iron-deficiency anemia.

Pathophysiology

of Iron-Deficiency Anemia

Iron is one of the components necessary for the synthesis of hemoglobin. Without an adequate amount of iron, the bone marrow continues to manufacture red blood cells (RBCs) but their content of hemoglobin is decreased, rendering these RBCs inefficient at carrying oxygen to the tissues. The constellation of clinical signs evident with iron-deficiency anemia results from compromised tissue oxygenation.

The full term neonate is born with enough stored maternal iron to produce adequate amounts of hemoglobin for 4 to 6 months. The average life of an RBC is about 120 days. Thus iron-deficiency anemia is usually not seen in children before age 9 months. (moms iron not theirs yet)

As RBCs undergo *hemolysis*, intracellular iron is released into the circulation for use by the body. Adults are able to use this breakdown of RBCs as a primary source of iron. Children, however, grow very rapidly and expand their circulating blood volume at the same time. Because the breakdown of RBCs in children exceeds their ability to produce new RBCs, and their need for iron to synthesize new hemoglobin for RBC production is increased, children must increase their dietary consumption of iron. The American Academy of Pediatrics recommends routine iron supplementation with iron-fortified formula in non-breastfeeding term and preterm infants, as well as iron salt supplementation for all preterm infants (born before 32 weeks' gestation), who are at greater risk for anemia due to having less stored iron. Iron-fortified cereals are recommended when solids are introduced.

Various factors can contribute to a lack of absorption of iron by the gastrointestinal tract. When cow's milk is introduced into the diet before age 1 year in place of breast milk or formula, infants do not ingest sufficient iron because cow's milk is a poor dietary source of iron. Often the potentially large amount of cow's milk replaces iron-fortified cereals and iron-rich baby food. Although iron from breast milk is well absorbed, it is not a complete source of iron, and dietary iron supplements must be introduced to augment its nutrients when the infant is approximately 4 to 6 months old.

Blood loss from an infant's intestine occurs very slowly and has several causes. The immature intestine may be unable to tolerate the protein in cow's milk or milk-based infant formula. Irritation of the bowel results in hemorrhages of the microvasculature, resulting in blood loss in the stool. Although unusual, parasitic infections can also irritate the intestinal lining, causing slow blood loss.

Diagnostic Evaluation

Any child presenting with anemia should first have a complete history taken, with particular emphasis on assessment of nutritional intake. The results of a complete blood count (CBC) in individuals with iron-deficiency anemia will show low hemoglobin levels (6 to 11 g/dl) and microcytic, hypochromic RBCs, reflected in a decreased mean cell volume (MCV) and decreased mean cell hemoglobin (MCH) (see Appendix H). The reticulocyte count is usually normal or slightly elevated. With these findings, serum ferritin levels

Nursing Care Plan

The Child With Iron-Deficiency Anemia in the Community Setting

FOCUSED ASSESSMENT

Parents may state that their child is more quiet than usual, with an increased desire to be held. In cases of extreme anemia, the parents may report that the child's heart races when the child is held. More often than not, there is a history of introduction to cow's milk before age 12 months, as well as a history of increased milk consumption to the exclusion of solid foods.

On physical examination, the child is pale and appears tired, with mild to severe tachycardia. If the anemia is severe, a heart murmur may be heard; this will disappear as the anemic state is reversed.

Nursing Diagnosis

Imbalanced Nutrition: Less Than Body Requirements related to parents' lack of knowledge of age-appropriate nutritional needs.

Expected Outcome

The parents will:
- Have an understanding of the child's nutritional needs, as evidenced by verbalization of the child's dietary plan, including foods containing appropriate dietary iron.

INTERVENTION	RATIONALE
1. Obtain the child's past and current nutritional history. Instruct the caregiver to continue to give infant iron-fortified formula or breastfeed and give supplementary iron-fortified foods until age 12 months. In a child older than 12 months, milk intake should be decreased to 24 oz/day or less. Per the child's age, suggest intake of liver, dried beans, Cream of Wheat, iron-fortified cereal, apricots, prunes, egg yolks, and leafy, dark-green vegetables (see Parents Want to Know: About Home Care of the Child With Iron-Deficiency Anemia box). Advise the parent to keep a dietary diary.	1. Therapy is based on the child's history. Cow's milk is poorly digested and is not rich in iron. The American Academy of Pediatrics (AAP) recommends continuing breast milk or iron-fortified formula until age 12 months. Decreasing milk intake will encourage the consumption of other iron-rich foods. Iron-fortified formula and food will establish healthier eating habits. Keeping a record of food and fluid intake assists with a dietary evaluation and identifies areas that need additional teaching.
2. Explain the need for iron in the manufacture of red blood cells (RBCs), the effect of iron therapy on laboratory test results, the potential outcome with no intervention, the lack of iron in cow's milk, and iron's effect on the body.	2. Providing explanations of the rationale for therapy can often help improve adherence to therapy.
3. Instruct the caregiver to administer oral iron supplements as ordered by the physician, and allow opportunity to practice technique with assistance. Iron is usually given in three divided doses between meals (see Parents Want to Know: About Home Care of the Child With Iron-Deficiency Anemia box).	3. The immediate need is to increase iron intake beyond that absorbed from formula or food. Do not assume the parents are able to administer iron effectively. Evaluate their technique of medication administration to build their skill and confidence.
• Encourage administration on an empty stomach, with fruit juice, and avoid administration with milk, formula, and cereals.	• An acid stomach environment facilitates absorption. Calcium in milk products binds with iron to decrease iron absorption.
• Instruct the caregiver to administer iron through a straw or medicine dropper placed at the back of the mouth. Brush or wipe teeth after administration.	• Iron temporarily stains teeth.
• Instruct the caregiver to administer vitamin C as ordered, and encourage intake of foods rich in vitamin C.	• Vitamin C increases the absorption of iron by the body.
4. Instruct the caregiver to keep iron supplements (and all medications) out of reach of children.	4. Iron poisoning is possible with overdose. This can be serious and possibly fatal.
5. Instruct the caregiver to comply with follow-up laboratory examinations, including reticulocyte count and hemoglobin level.	5. Reticulocyte count should peak in 5-7 days. It serves as an objective test for determining the parents' degree of compliance with therapy. The hemoglobin level should increase in 4-30 days.*

*Glader, B. (2004). Iron deficiency anemia. In R. Behrman, R. Kliegman, & H. Jenson (Eds.), *Nelson textbook of pediatrics* (17th ed., pp. 1614-1616). Philadelphia: Saunders.

Continued

Nursing Care Plan

The Child With Iron-Deficiency Anemia in the Community Setting—cont'd

INTERVENTION	RATIONALE
6. Instruct the caregiver to expect black stools, and inquire about their presence.	6. The absence of tarry stools may indicate lack of adherence to therapy.
7. Obtain a social services consultation for enrollment in a federal or state social services program if warranted.	7. Poor nutritional habits may be attributable to a lack of resources.

Evaluation

- Does the dietary diary reflect an increase in iron-rich foods in the child's daily meal plan?
- Does the child have normal iron, hemoglobin, and hematocrit levels?
- Do the parents demonstrate adherence to the prescribed therapy and verbalize appropriate questions?
- Has the child experienced a recurrence of iron-deficiency anemia?

PARENTS Want to Know

About Home Care of the Child With Iron-Deficiency Anemia

Dietary Changes

- Provide iron-fortified formula or breast milk with iron-fortified food supplements if the child is younger than 12 months.
- If the child is older than 12 months, limit intake of cow's milk to 24 oz/day or less.
- Increase the child's intake of age-appropriate iron-rich foods, with selections based on the age of the child: liver, dried beans, Cream of Wheat, iron-fortified cereal, apricots and prunes (and other dried fruits), egg yolks, dark-green, leafy vegetables.

Administration of Iron

- Administer iron in three divided doses between meals.
- Give with vitamin C–rich fluids.
- Administer iron through a straw or medicine dropper placed at the back of the mouth, away from the teeth. Brush or wipe off teeth.
- Recognize that iron supplementation causes black, tarry stools.
- Avoid administration of iron with milk or formula and cereal, because iron binds with calcium, thus impeding absorption.

Follow-Up Care

- Keep appointments for follow-up evaluations.
- Expect blood work to be done at follow-up visits.

! CRITICAL TO REMEMBER

Obtaining a Dietary Intake History

Parents may not readily or accurately report their child's dietary intake without being asked specific questions. Ask the parent to begin the dietary history at the time the child awoke yesterday, describing the child's activities and exactly what the child ate. Correlating activities with diet may enable the nurse to obtain a better history and may alert the nurse to feeding patterns for which counseling may be indicated.

CRITICAL THINKING EXERCISE 47-1

Mrs. Anders has brought 18-month-old Jacob to the clinic because he is irritable, running a low-grade fever, and has a cough. In the process of assessing Jacob, you note that he seems lethargic and his skin is very pale. A complete blood cell (CBC) count confirms a diagnosis of iron-deficiency anemia.

1. What do you think Mrs. Anders is most concerned about?
2. What is the nurse's role when a child enters the health care system with an acute illness?
3. What opportunities present when a child is brought to an outpatient setting because of an acute illness?

and serum iron or iron-binding capacity should be assessed. Iron-binding capacity is usually increased secondary to decreased serum iron. Hemoglobin electrophoresis may be done to rule out causes other than iron-deficiency anemia.

Therapeutic Management

Therapy is directed toward increasing the dietary intake of iron and iron supplementation. The absorption of dietary iron-rich foods can be unreliable and will not rapidly provide the body with enough iron to correct the iron deficiency. Therefore affected children are given a daily oral iron preparation (often three times per day) of one of the available ferrous salts (ferrous sulfate, ferrous gluconate, ferrous fumarate), based on the content of elemental iron (dose should be 3 to 6 mg/kg/day [2 to 4 mg/kg/day for premature infants] in three divided doses). Iron therapy is continued for 3 months after the hemoglobin and hematocrit levels return to normal, after which a daily multivitamin with iron can be recommended.

Follow-up monitoring includes a CBC and reticulocyte count. The reticulocyte count should increase within days of the initiation of iron therapy. An increased hemoglobin level can be expected in 4 to 30 days. The response to iron therapy can often be positively predicted, so blood transfusions are rarely indicated to correct iron-deficiency anemia. RBC transfusions are reserved for severe anemia and cardiovascular compromise.

SICKLE-CELL DISEASE

Sickle-cell disease (SCD) is the generic term that refers to a group of genetic disorders characterized by the production of sickle hemoglobin (HbS), chronic hemolytic anemia, and ischemic tissue injury. The more common forms of SCD include homozygous HbSS disease (sickle-cell anemia), HbC disease (sickle C disease), and the sickle beta-thalassemia syndromes. SCD is an inherited, lifelong disease that affects primarily African Americans but can occur also in individuals of Mediterranean, Indian, and Middle Eastern descent. Morbidity and mortality from the severe forms of the disease have decreased as a result of newborn screening for the disease, routine prophylactic penicillin administration, and pneumococcal and *Haemophilus influenzae* vaccines.

Etiology

SCD is a group of hemoglobinopathies in which normal hemoglobin is partially or totally replaced by an abnormal hemoglobin, hemoglobin S (HbS). They are inherited, autosomal recessive conditions (see Chapter 9). If one parent has the HbS trait and the other parent does not, each pregnancy has a 50% risk of having the child inherit the trait. If each parent carries the trait, there is a 25% chance that the child will be unaffected, a 50% chance that the child will carry the trait, and a 25% chance that the child will have the disease. While not a disease in and of itself, the carrier state of SCD—sickle-cell trait—may produce clinical symptoms (e.g., hematuria, bacteriuria) in times of extreme stress, during extremely vigorous exercise, and in high altitudes.

Incidence

SCD affects approximately 1 in 600 African Americans. In 1910 Herrick described the first patient with SCD, and 36 years later, Beet discovered that sickle red blood cells have an increased resistance to malaria. Protection from malaria helps maintain the high prevalence of the sickle gene in areas where malaria is endemic (Fixler & Styles, 2002). Sickle cell trait is found in 8% of African Americans and is prevalent also in persons of Mediterranean, Middle Eastern, Indian, Caribbean, and Central and South American descent (National Institutes of Health, 2002).

Manifestations

All the clinical manifestations of SCD are a result of the obstructions caused by the sickled RBCs and the increased destruction of sickled and normal RBCs caught in microcirculation obstructions. Large amounts of fetal hemoglobin (HbF) present in the first few months of life obscure the presence of HbS, so symptoms of the disease usually do not appear until age 4 to 6 months when the infant begins to manufacture hemoglobin.

The disease affects most organ systems. Delayed growth and puberty are common. The child usually has small stature throughout adolescence but attains normal growth in the early 20s.

The general manifestations of SCD are chronic hemolytic anemia, pallor, jaundice, fatigue, cholelithiasis, delayed growth and puberty, avascular necrosis of the hips and shoul-

ders, renal dysfunction, and retinopathy. However, sickling events may also progress to acute episodic exacerbations known as *sickle-cell crisis*. Infection, dehydration, hypoxia, trauma, or general stress may precipitate a crisis episode. The crisis may take one of three forms: vaso-occlusive, acute sequestration, or aplastic. Repeated vaso-occlusive crises and a virtually continual state of anemia produce long-term problems later in the life of the individual with SCD. Table 47-1 presents the clinical manifestations of SCD.

Diagnostic Evaluation

In the past, many infants died from complications of SCD before being diagnosed. However, newborn screening for SCD has significantly decreased the mortality rate. A laboratory diagnosis of SCD is established on the basis of a CBC, isoelectric focusing, hemoglobin electrophoresis, and high-performance liquid chromatography. Children with SCD have elevated reticulocyte counts because of the chronicity of loss and destruction as a result of the shortened life span of the sickled RBCs. Prenatal diagnosis is an option and is made using chorionic villus sampling at 8 to 10 weeks of gestation or amniocentesis at 15 weeks of gestation.

Therapeutic Management

In SCD, the spleen often does not function properly or has been surgically removed because of complications. Functional or actual asplenia places children and adults with SCD in an immunocompromised state at high risk for infection. Splenic dysfunction can begin at 6 months of age, and those with HbSS may have total dysfunction by age 5 years. Bacterial septicemia is associated with a 30% mortality rate in children younger than 5 years with SCD (Dover & Platt, 2003). The bacteria *Streptococcus pneumoniae* and *H. influenzae* are normally destroyed by the reticuloendothelial system of the spleen, but because children with SCD do not have a properly functioning spleen, they are considered to be more susceptible to infection with these bacteria.

The natural history of splenic dysfunction in children with HbSS places them at higher risk for fulminate septicemia and death during the first 3 years of life than children with HbC. Prophylactic daily penicillin therapy is recommended in all children with suspected or actual diagnosis by age 2 months and is continued until at least age 5 years (American Academy of Pediatrics [AAP], 2000a). Although views regarding the use of penicillin differ, some experts will continue penicillin prophylaxis throughout childhood in high-risk patients with asplenia. The pneumococcal polyvalent vaccine is recommended at age 2 years for children who did not receive it during infancy, with a booster after 3 to 5 years for children age 10 years or younger and for older children who were immunized at least 5 years earlier (AAP, 2000a). *H. influenzae* vaccine is recommended at 2 months of age, as in healthy children, and for all previously unimmunized children with asplenia (AAP, 2000a). Routine immunization against hepatitis B is recommended, particularly in light of possible blood transfusions. Moreover, children with SCD should receive the influenza vaccine annually and immunization against meningococcal disease after age 2 years (AAP, 2000b) secondary to their increased risk for related complications.

A child with SCD and a temperature of 38.5° C (101.3° F) or higher should receive prompt medical evaluation and

Pathophysiology

of Sickle-Cell Disease

The normal red blood cell (RBC) is a smooth, biconcave disk that is capable of changing shape to enable it to flow easily through the microvasculature of the circulation. Under conditions of low oxygen concentration, acidosis, and dehydration, the RBCs in a child with sickle-cell disease (SCD) assume a sickle shape, which prevents them from flowing easily through the smallest blood vessels. Sickled RBCs are stiff and nonpliable. These sickled cells clump together, causing occlusions in the small vessels. With reoxygenation, most of the sickled RBCs resume their normal shape. After repeated sickling and unsickling, however, the cells become irreversibly sickled and their life span is reduced from 120 days to 12 days.

Sickled cells cause microvascular occlusion, leading to tissue ischemia, infarcts, and organ damage. The lungs, spleen, and brain are the organs most seriously affected by the complications of SCD. The normal spleen functions to filter bacteria in the blood. The spleen of a child with SCD does not function properly much beyond age 5 years. The large vessels are also affected, leading to strokes and other vaso-occlusive events.

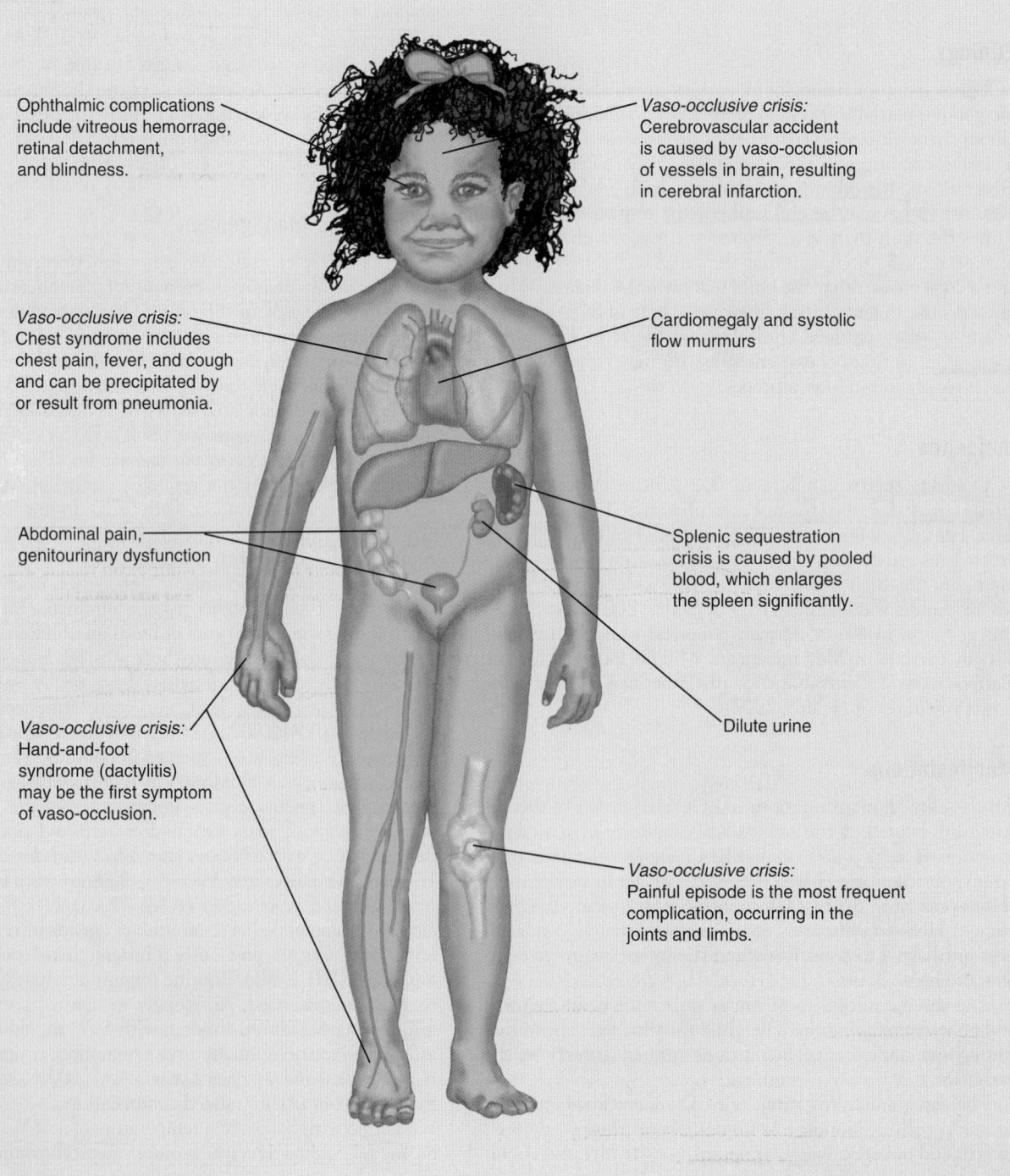

Ophthalmic complications include vitreous hemorrage, retinal detachment, and blindness.

Vaso-occlusive crisis: Cerebrovascular accident is caused by vaso-occlusion of vessels in brain, resulting in cerebral infarction.

Vaso-occlusive crisis: Chest syndrome includes chest pain, fever, and cough and can be precipitated by or result from pneumonia.

Cardiomegaly and systolic flow murmurs

Abdominal pain, genitourinary dysfunction

Splenic sequestration crisis is caused by pooled blood, which enlarges the spleen significantly.

Vaso-occlusive crisis: Hand-and-foot syndrome (dactylitis) may be the first symptom of vaso-occlusion.

Dilute urine

Vaso-occlusive crisis: Painful episode is the most frequent complication, occurring in the joints and limbs.

TABLE **47-1** Clinical Manifestations and Therapeutic Management of Sickle-Cell Disease Complications

Complication	Characterisics	Manifestations	Treatment
VASO-OCCLUSIVE CRISIS			
Painful episode	Most common type of crisis and reason for hospitalization Typically produces bone or joint pain, but pain can occur anywhere Pain may come and go Frequency of pain is individualized Pain is precipitated by infection, cold, stress, acidosis, local or generalized hypoxia	*Mild:* joint or bone pain lasting a few hours *Severe:* joint or bone pain lasting days	Oral analgesics initially and if ineffective, IV opioids (usually morphine), which may be given by either intermittent or continuous infusion Oral or IV NSAIDs Oral and IV hydration Oxygen in hypoxic patients Aggressive incentive spirometry use (10 breaths q2h when awake) Consistent manner to assess subjective experience of pain is essential Use of non-pharmacologic pain management strategies in addition to medications
Acute chest syndrome	Common cause of hospitalization Sometimes confused with pneumonia Can recur	Chest pain, fever, cough, abdominal pain	IV hydration (1-1½ times maintenance), antibiotics, oxygen, RBC transfusion, analgesics
Dactylitis (hand-and-foot syndrome)	Occurs in children ages 6 mo to 4 yr Self-limiting complication	Swelling of hands and/or feet, pain, warmth in affected area	Oral analgesics, hydration (oral or IV), rest
Priapism (persistent erection of the penis)	Occurs if penile blood flow becomes obstructed	Persistent, painful erection	Analgesics; hydration Avoid hot and cold packs If prolonged, transfusion therapy
Cerebrovascular accident	Without treatment, mortality rate of 20%; and 70% of patients experience a recurrence	Hemiparesis or monoparesis, aphasia/dysphasia, seizures, alteration in level of consciousness, vomiting, vision changes, ataxia, headache	Long-term RBC transfusion therapy for indefinite period and possibly chelation therapy May require extensive rehabilitation
ACUTE SEQUESTRATION CRISIS			
	Blood volume pooling in the spleen, causing splenic enlargement Life-threatening condition of hypovolemic shock Usually occurs in children ages 6 mo to 4 yr One episode increases the risk of future occurrences	Decreased hemoglobin level, acutely ill-looking child, pallor, irritability, tachycardia, impressively enlarged spleen, hypovolemic shock	Emergency treatment to restore circulating blood volume with crystalloid and colloid (blood) infusion Chronic transfusion therapy if recurrent Eventual splenectomy in cases of persistent recurrence
APLASTIC CRISIS			
	Profound anemia caused by diminished erythropoiesis Has been observed after parvovirus-like agent exposure	Pallor, lethargy, headache, fainting	RBC transfusions and treatment of symptoms

IV, Intravenous; *NSAIDs,* nonsteroidal antiinflammatory drugs; *RBC,* red blood cell.

treatment because of the overwhelming risk for infectious complications. Fever can be the first sign of bacteremia. Parenteral antibiotics, blood cultures, IV hydration, and general monitoring are the standard of care for children with SCD who have fever. Outpatient therapy with long-acting parenteral antibiotics may be provided in combination with rigorous evaluation and follow-up in those centers with the capabilities to do so. Children who are not eligible for outpatient therapy are those with the following signs and symptoms (and thus they are considered at high risk for sequelae):

- Ill appearance
- Cardiovascular instability
- Age younger than 1 year
- Pulmonary infiltrate
- Prior splenectomy or history of pneumococcal sepsis
- Hemoglobin less than 5 g/dl
- Family's or child's lack of ability to comply with outpatient therapy
- WBC less than 500/mm³ or more than 30,000/mm³
- Dehydration

Nursing Care Plan

The Child With Sickle-Cell Disease

FOCUSED ASSESSMENT

On initial diagnosis, the subjective data usually include parental concern that the child is in pain. The parents may have noticed swelling of the joints, the child's refusal to move an extremity, or the child's crying out when a joint is moved or touched. Fever and irritability may accompany the pain. Parents of a child already diagnosed with sickle-cell disease (SCD) who have been educated about the signs of complications will give a much more detailed history of the present illness that will likely include pain. A nurse familiar with the child can become adept at assessing the severity of that child's condition. The presence of SCD does not eliminate other serious causes of pain.

Despite teenagers' ability to verbalize symptoms, assessment of adolescents who are experiencing pain is a unique challenge. During the developmental time in their life when they most want to fit in with their peer group, teenagers with SCD are different. After the initial pain of an episode has subsided, teens may seek attention from health care providers in an attempt to avoid their peer group, verbalizing continued symptoms that would make them unable to return to their normal activities. Objective data will vary according to the type of painful episodes.

Parents should be taught to assess and report the size of the child's spleen for close monitoring of the child's condition.

Nursing Diagnosis

Ineffective Tissue Perfusion related to red blood cell sickling.

Expected Outcomes

The child will:
- Demonstrate adequate tissue perfusion, as evidenced by palpable peripheral pulses; warm, dry skin; adequate urinary output; and the absence of respiratory distress (oxygen saturation >95%).

The child and family will:
- Verbalize knowledge of treatment regimen, including medications and their actions and possible side effects.

INTERVENTION	RATIONALE
1. Monitor the child's vital signs and respiratory status every 4 hours and as needed.	1. Vital signs and respiratory status are assessed frequently to detect changes in tissue perfusion and respiratory status. Signs of altered perfusion include increased respiratory rate, increased work of breathing, decreased oxygenation saturation, poor color, mottled appearance, prolonged capillary refill time, decreased peripheral pulses, and altered level of consciousness. Change in level of consciousness often indicates poor perfusion or oxygenation of the brain.
2. Monitor pulse oximetry, and administer oxygen to keep saturation >95%.	2. Oxygen saturation levels are monitored with pulse oximetry. Ensuring adequate oxygen can ease the child's work of breathing and facilitate tissue oxygenation. Oxygen does not reverse the sickling process but may prevent more sickling.
3. Ensure adequate hydration by measuring intake and output and administering crystalloids and colloids (red blood cells [RBCs]) as ordered.	3. Measuring intake and output monitors renal function and level of hydration. Transfusions of crystalloids and (nonsickled) RBCs will increase the oxygen-carrying capacity of the blood and decrease the relative amount of sickled cells.
4. Evaluate the child's and family's understanding of SCD and treatment regimen, and provide information or clarification as necessary.	4. Adequate understanding of SCD can increase compliance with preventive measures and prompt interventions during exacerbations and hospitalizations.

Nursing Care Plan

The Child With Sickle-Cell Disease—cont'd

Evaluation

- Are the child's vital signs and oxygen saturation within normal limits?
- Does the child demonstrate palpable peripheral pulses, capillary refill less than 2 seconds, and warmth of extremities?
- Can the child and family return-demonstrate their ability to administer medication and describe possible side effects?
- Have the child and family requested additional information and/or clarification related to treatment?

Nursing Diagnosis

Acute Pain related to vaso-occlusion.

Expected Outcome

The child will:
- Have decreased pain, as evidenced by a lowered score on the selected pain assessment tool.

INTERVENTION	RATIONALE
1. Monitor and record pain every 1-2 hr and more frequently if needed, using a pain assessment tool appropriate for the child's age.	1. Pain can be severe in vaso-occlusive crisis and is relieved for only short periods. An assessment tool that measures the subjective experience of pain is helpful in determining the child's level of discomfort.
2. Administer analgesics as ordered.	2. Analgesics may be administered intermittently, via a patient- or parent-controlled analgesic pump, or by continuous infusion through an intravenous (IV) line.
3. Increase oral fluids, if able to tolerate, or administer fluids IV at a rate that is 1 to 1½ times the maintenance rate.	3. Increased fluid volume reduces the viscosity of the blood, thus alleviating sites of vascular occlusion and preventing further sickling secondary to dehydration.
4. Administer RBCs as ordered.	4. Maintaining an adequate hemoglobin increases oxygen-carrying capacity to aid in further preventing sickling and microvascular ischemia.
5. Incorporate the use of age-appropriate non-pharmacologic pain-relief measures.	5. Comfort measures often help distract the patient from discomfort (see Chapter 39).
6. Perform passive range of motion exercises and avoid exertion	6. Passive ROM promotes circulation without exacerbating fatigue.

Evaluation

- Does the child verbalize or demonstrate decreased pain?
- Does review of the child's pain assessment tool rating show a decrease in discomfort?

Nursing Diagnosis

Risk for Infection related to chronic immunocompromised state.

Expected Outcomes

The child will:
- Remain free from infection, as evidenced by normal vital signs and activity for age.

The child and family will:
- Verbalize signs and symptoms of infection and when to notify the medical team.

INTERVENTION	RATIONALE
1. Monitor vital signs every 4 hr and more frequently as needed. Report any temperature elevations to the physician.	1. Elevated temperature and increased respiratory rate may be signs of infection.
2. Administer antipyretics and antibiotics as ordered.	2. Antibiotics may be given prophylactically because of the high risk for infection. Prompt intervention is critical in children with HbSS and sickle beta-thalassemia during febrile illness.

Continued

Nursing Care Plan

The Child With Sickle-Cell Disease—cont'd

INTERVENTION	RATIONALE
3. Administer penicillin daily as ordered. Administer preventive immunizations to decrease the risk of infection (Pneumovax, meningococcal vaccine, *Haemophilus influenzae* type b [Hib], influenza vaccines).	3. Children are at a high risk for pneumococcal infections and should receive long-term penicillin therapy. The Pneumovax, meningococcal, and Hib vaccines can prevent sepsis, and the influenza vaccine can prevent complications from influenza.
4. Teach the parents signs of infection to watch for, as well as the proper way to obtain the child's temperature. Confirm that the parent has a thermometer.	4. Develop a teaching plan to address signs and symptoms of infection, including when to notify the physician. Do not assume that the parent has a thermometer or knows how to accurately obtain a temperature reading.

Evaluation

- Is the child's body temperature within normal limits?
- Can the child and family describe their plan to identify and respond to signs of infection?

Nursing Diagnosis

Ineffective Coping related to chronic illness.

Expected Outcomes

The child and family will:
- Adhere to the treatment plan and follow-up visits.
- Verbalize feelings about the impact of the illness on their lives.
- Utilize available support systems and community resources.

INTERVENTION	RATIONALE
1. Teach the family the necessity of and rationale for following the treatment as outlined by the health care team.	1. Conscientious adherence to the treatment regimen decreases the frequency of hospitalization and improves the child's health and longevity.
2. Provide written instructions on all aspects of care and complications. Provide the address and phone number of the local chapter of the Sickle Cell Foundation (see Appendix I on Evolve website).	2. Education helps the family gain a sense of control by allowing them to make informed decisions regarding their child's health. Written instructions can be referred to later when the parent is less stressed and is able to comprehend.
3. Listen and encourage the child and family to verbalize their feelings and express their concerns regarding SCD. Answer questions honestly and openly. Encourage consultation with the social work team to provide additional support and referrals as necessary.	3. Identifying concerns and clarifying misconceptions will help the family cope with the stress of chronic illness.
4. Introduce the family to other families of children with SCD.	4. Families of other children with SCD can offer support, suggestions, and strategies for dealing with problems.
5. Provide parents with phone numbers of persons to contact if they have questions or problems. The Sickle Cell Foundation has information on the disease and on support groups in the area.	5. Knowing about resources decreases parents' feelings of frustration and helplessness.

Evaluation

- Are the child and family demonstrating compliance with the treatment plan?
- Do the child and family demonstrate positive coping mechanisms?
- Do the child and family use available resources?
- Is the family able to discuss problems related to caring for a child with a chronic disease?
- Does the child share fears and frustrations related to having SCD?

PARENTS
Want to Know

About Home Care of the Child With Sickle-Cell Disease ✳

- Encourage fluid intake; increase fluid intake in hot weather or when there are other risks for dehydration.
- Expect frequent urination.
- Provide for adequate rest periods.
- Avoid cold, which can increase sickling, and extreme heat which can cause dehydration.
- Avoid known sources of infection.
- Avoid prolonged exposure to the sun.
- Monitor the child's body temperature (know the proper use of a thermometer), and promptly notify the medical team in the event of a fever (avoid antipyretics until discussed with the medical team).
- Administer penicillin daily as ordered.
- Avoid use of aspirin; use acetaminophen or ibuprofen as an alternative.
- Be cautious when traveling with the child to avoid conditions or locations with decreased atmospheric oxygen. *high altitude places*
- Call the primary caregiver if symptoms of infection are evident.
- Know the physician's telephone number.

Opioids and nonsteroidal antiinflammatory drugs (NSAIDs) (i.e., ibuprofen, ketorolac) are the mainstay of analgesic treatment, particularly in combination for painful crises. Morphine is the current opioid of choice, since meperidine (Demerol) is no longer recommended for long-term pain management because of its side effect profile. Opioids provide systemic relief, and the NSAIDS act locally to decrease inflammation at the site of vaso-occlusion and provide analgesia without the potential side effect of respiratory depression. Morphine has been very effective when administered IV and particularly when given in a patient-controlled analgesia (PCA) fashion (see Chapter 39).

The treatment of SCD focuses on prompt diagnosis, education about the disease, prevention of exacerbations, prompt identification of exacerbation, and supportive care during crises (hydration, oxygenation, analgesia, RBC transfusion). Additional therapies currently under investigation include erythrocytapheresis (removal of sickled erythrocytes via an exchange transfusion technique), phenotyping RBCs for transfusion ("tissue typing" blood products that can potentially reduce alloimmunization), and hydroxyurea administration (augments HbF, which interferes with the RBC sickling process).

Research toward a cure continues; especially promising may be gene therapy. Another promising area of research is hematopoietic stem cell transplantation. It has been a successful treatment modality for a limited number of children. Logistical issues are related to candidate selection regarding this potentially curative strategy, as well as ethical issues promoted by some.

Table 47-1 presents the therapeutic management of SCD.

BETA-THALASSEMIA

The thalassemias are a group of inherited disorders characterized by an abnormality in hemoglobin synthesis that results from a reduction in or absence of one of the chains found in normal hemoglobin. These disorders are categorized by the site of the aberrant globin synthesis (e.g., alpha-thalassemia, beta-thalassemia). The thalassemias are found primarily in people of Mediterranean descent, although the disease also has been reported in Asian and African populations. Beta-thalassemia, also known as *thalassemia major* or *Cooley's anemia*, is the most common and severe form of thalassemia.

Etiology and Incidence

Inheritance is through an autosomal recessive pattern. The child who inherits only one gene for beta-thalassemia may have only a mild anemia; hence the term *thalassemia minor*. From 3% to 8% of Americans of Italian or Greek ancestry and 0.5% of African Americans carry a gene for beta-thalassemia (Quirolo & Vichinsky, 2003).

Pathophysiology

of Beta-Thalassemia

The abnormality of the beta-polypeptide chain in hemoglobin synthesis impairs the erythrocytes' ability to carry oxygen. Thalassemia is classified by the degree of imbalance in the globin chain and can be minor, intermediate, or severe.

Typically, during the second 6 months of life, a severe anemia develops. Erythrocytes are *hemolyzed* as they are produced. Because the body's natural response to a reduction in circulating hemoglobin is to try to produce more erythrocytes, the bone marrow begins massive production. Progressive disease constantly stimulates the bone marrow. The body perceives this as an inability to keep up with the need for erythrocytes. As a result, *extramedullary* (outside the bone marrow) sites of production of erythrocytes begin *erythropoiesis*. The result is a chronic state of production and destruction of erythrocytes, with a resulting inadequate amount of normal circulating hemoglobin.

Iron is necessary for the production of hemoglobin and is a by-product of the hemolysis of red blood cells (RBCs). Normally the intestines absorb small amounts of iron. In this disorder, however, the body increases the absorption of iron for some reason. When increased iron absorption is combined with increased iron from the breakdown of RBCs and the increased iron introduced into the circulation by the transfusions necessary to treat thalassemia, *hemosiderosis* occurs, usually during the second decade of life. Hemosiderosis is the deposition of excess amounts of iron in tissue.

The results of excessive erythropoiesis and hemolysis are considerable. The bones become thin and fragile from excessive erythropoiesis. Hepatosplenomegaly occurs as a result of extramedullary erythropoiesis and hemosiderosis. Growth is impaired and puberty delayed. Without proper management, multisystem organ dysfunction ensues.

BOX 47-1
Characteristic Features of a Child With Beta-Thalassemia

Features develop as a consequence of inadequate treatment:
- Frontal bossing (prominent and protruding forehead)
- Maxillary prominence
- Wide-set eyes with a flattened nose
- Hepatosplenomegaly
- Greenish yellow skin tone

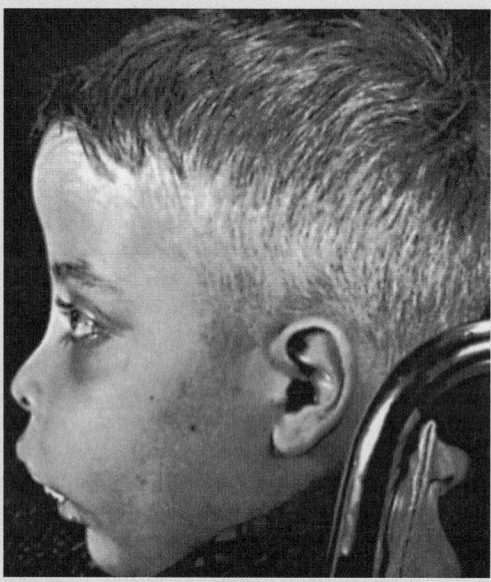

(Photo from Behrman, R.E., Kliegman, R.M., & Arvin, A.M. [Eds.]. [1996]. *Nelson textbook of pediatrics* [15th ed., p. 1402]. Philadelphia: Saunders.)

Manifestations

[handwritten: body increases absorption of iron taking it out of bones and moving it into tissues = big spleen]

The clinical manifestations of beta-thalassemia include pallor, growth and maturation retardation, severe anemia, characteristic facies (enlarged head, frontal and parietal bossing, severe maxillary hyperplasia, malocclusion), hepatosplenomegaly, and a bronze skin tone (Box 47-1).

Diagnostic Evaluation

In addition to a CBC, laboratory testing should include quantification of reticulocyte count, serum iron level, total iron-binding capacity, hemoglobin electrophoresis, and HbA and HbF levels to confirm the diagnosis. The CBC will often reflect microcytic hypochromic erythrocytes. A detailed family history may also reveal a history of anemia and delayed growth and maturation.

Therapeutic Management

The management of beta-thalassemia centers on three techniques: (1) erythrocyte transfusions, (2) chelation therapy, and (3) splenectomy. The use of neocyte transfusions is also being investigated. In neocyte transfusions, units of blood that contain young erythrocytes—neocytes—are preferentially separated out and transfused. Theoretically, administration of neocytes provides erythrocytes with a longer life and increases

the time between transfusions while decreasing the overall amount of transfusion. To prevent the severe side effects and bony changes associated with the disease, the hemoglobin is maintained at approximately 11 g/dl, although this parameter is often individualized.

The major complication of long-term transfusion therapy is hemosiderosis. To prevent organ damage from excessive iron overload, chelation therapy with deferoxamine (Desferal) is instituted. The drug is most effective when given subcutaneously or intravenously. To avoid hospitalizing children who require deferoxamine therapy, it is often administered in the home by continuous subcutaneous infusion (via pump) over an 8- to 12-hour period at night. This approach can preserve some degree of normalcy in lifestyle for the family. Therapy is continued until the iron returns to an acceptable level. This goal can be accomplished within months of initiating chelation therapy. Research continues in developing and improving the efficacy of oral iron chelation agents as well (Vichinsky, 2001).

Splenectomy may be required secondary to sporadic or moderate transfusion therapy, whereas aggressive transfusion therapy may delay the need for splenectomy. Splenectomy is a therapy that should not be considered casually, because susceptibility to infection with *S. pneumoniae*, *H. influenzae*, and *Neisseria meningitidis* increases after splenectomy in children, particularly in those younger than 5 years. Standard therapy for asplenic individuals includes immunizations, prophylactic penicillin, and a high index of suspicion and aggressive antibiotic therapy for febrile illnesses (AAP, 2000a). They should also receive the influenza vaccine annually (AAP, 2000b). When splenectomy occurs, the transfusion requirements often drop moderately to significantly.

Bone marrow transplantation is the only available cure for thalassemia at this time. More than 1000 successful transplants have been performed. Only a small percentage of patients (estimated at 30%) who have a matched donor and low risk factors, however, can undergo this procedure (Lo & Singer, 2002).

■ NURSING CARE
The Child With Beta-Thalassemia

Assessment

Subjective data may include the parents' observation that their child is not as active as other children of the same age. The child may sleep more than other children or want to be held often. The child appears pale, with laboratory values reflecting a microcytic, hypochromic anemia. Clinical symptoms are related to the degree of anemia, ranging from mild to severe.

An older child with the disease or a child who has not received adequate treatment will likely have characteristic facial deformities, including maxillary hyperplasia and malocclusion. These characteristics develop from extramedullary marrow expansion, a result of the marrow's effort to keep up with the demand for RBCs secondary to anemia. Hepatosplenomegaly is usually seen at this time but is not a symptom in infancy.

Nursing Diagnosis and Planning

The nursing diagnoses and expected outcomes that may be appropriate after assessment of the child with beta-thalassemia are

PARENTS
Want to Know

About Home Chelation Therapy

Subcutaneous Route Via Infusion Pump
- Know the technique for placing the subcutaneous needle, medication preparation, and infusion pump operation.
- Check needle security and placement.
- Check pump for proper infusion rate.
- Call the home care, clinic, or physician resource if the site becomes inflamed, red, or painful.
- Know indications for medication and side effects that require health care team notification: hearing loss or ringing in the ears, fever, fever with diarrhea, visual disturbances, allergic reactions, respiratory compromise.

Intravenous Route: Totally Implantable or Tunneled Access Device
- Know the technique for placing access needle or catheter connection, medication preparation, and infusion pump operation.
- Call the home care, clinic, or physician resource if the site becomes inflamed, red, or painful or the specific access device is obstructed.
- Have a list of home care resources for technique assistance, supplies, and problematic pump functioning.
- Know indications for medication and side effects that require health care team notification: hearing loss or ringing in the ears, fever, fever with diarrhea, visual disturbances, allergic reactions, respiratory compromise.

- Ineffective Tissue Perfusion related to anemia.
  Expected Outcome: The child demonstrates adequate tissue perfusion, as evidenced by palpable peripheral pulses; warm dry skin; urinary output appropriate for age; and the absence of cardiorespiratory distress (oxygen saturation >95%).
- Disturbed Body Image related to altered appearance and the perception of having a chronic disease.
  Expected Outcome: The child and family will verbalize feelings related to changes in appearance and the limitations imposed by the disease process.
- Anxiety related to the diagnosis.
  Expected Outcome: The child and family will express feelings about the disorder, lifestyle disruptions as a result of treatment, and possible genetic transmission of the disease.
- Deficient Knowledge related to inadequate information about the disorder.
  Expected Outcome: The child and family will verbalize knowledge of the disorder and its treatment regimen, including medications and their actions and possible side effects.

Interventions

Expect transfusions to begin immediately for an affected child while cardiovascular compromise from the anemia is being assessed. Preparing the child and family for diagnostic procedures will help alleviate fears. Once the diagnosis is made, education should begin. Parents need to understand the importance of proper and ongoing follow-up. The family needs much support as they begin chelation therapy, which is very time-consuming and interferes with family routines. Routinely monitor the family's compliance with therapy. If hematopoietic stem cell transplantation becomes an option, the parents will need referral to a specialty center and will need support from the entire health care team as they contemplate the course of therapy.

If parents are considering having another child, they should be offered genetic counseling. When both parents carry the defective gene, each pregnancy carries a 1 in 4 chance of producing another child with the disease. Genetic counseling should also be made available to the affected child upon reaching maturity. If the affected individual conceives a child with someone who is a carrier of the thalassemia gene, with each pregnancy there is a 2 in 4 chance of producing a child with beta-thalassemia. Techniques for prenatal diagnosis are available and effective (Weatherall, 1997). Referral should be made to the Cooley's Anemia Foundation (see Appendix I on Evolve website).

Evaluation

- Are the child's peripheral pulses palpable and oxygen saturation increased to 95%?
- Is the child's hemoglobin level improving?
- Is the child able to verbalize feelings associated with the treatment or the psychosocial implications of the disease?
- Is the child sharing feelings related to changes in appearance, limitations imposed by the disease, and having a chronic disease?
- Has the family sought genetic counseling?
- Does the family readily verbalize feelings about having a child with beta-thalassemia?
- Has the family sought information and support from the Cooley's Anemia Foundation?

HEMOPHILIA

Hemophilia is a lifelong, hereditary blood disorder with no cure. Until recently, the transfusion of replacement blood factors to prevent or stop episodes of bleeding was associated with the risk of contracting hepatitis or human immunodeficiency virus (HIV) infection because the blood factors were manufactured from pooled human plasma. Advances in pharmacologic therapy have now eliminated that risk.

Until 1952, hemophilia was associated solely with the deficiency of coagulation factor VIII. Since that time, the absence of two additional coagulation factors, factors IX and XI, has been associated with a constellation of symptoms similar to factor VIII deficiency. Congenital deficiencies in these three factors account for approximately 90% to 95% of the bleeding disorders referred to as *hemophilia*.

Etiology and Incidence

Hemophilia is an X-linked autosomal recessive disorder; carrier females pass on the defect to affected males. Women who never produce an affected male child may silently carry the gene for generations, but typically there is a history of hemophilia in the family. Rarely, female offspring are born with the disorder but only if they inherit an

Pathophysiology

of Hemophilia

More than 10 factors in the blood work in sequence to produce blood clotting. Factor VIII, or antihemophilic factor, and factor IX, or plasma thromboplastin component, are the two missing or defective constituents in the blood that cause hemophilia A, or classic hemophilia, and hemophilia B, or Christmas disease. When these factors are missing or defective, blood does not clot as it should. The two disorders are inherited in the same way and have similar manifestations. Normal factor activity is described as a percentage. The percentage of factor activity is closely related to the level of factor in the blood (e.g., 100 units/dl factor equals 100% factor activity). Normal levels of factor VIII and IX are 50% to 150%. The severity of the disease is classified as follows:

- *Severe:* less than 1% factor activity
- *Moderate:* 1% to 5% factor activity
- *Mild:* 6% to 50% factor activity *(get replacement therapy)*

affected gene from their mother and are the offspring of a father with hemophilia.

Manifestations

The disease severity is individual but tends to be familial. Bleeding occurs after surgery or serious trauma in all children with this disease. Bleeding occurs after tissue trauma in children with moderate and severe disease. Bleeding occurs for no apparent reason in children with severe disease. Affected children bruise easily, have episodes of epistaxis, and may experience hematuria. They may also experience bleeding with loss of deciduous teeth, from even minor lacerations, and from injections. Most commonly, bleeding develops in the muscles and joints, especially the knees, for moderate and severe disease (Fig. 47-1). Recurrent bleed-

> **! CRITICAL TO REMEMBER**
>
> **Acetylsalicylic Acid: Contraindication**
>
> Acetylsalicylic acid (ASA) (e.g., aspirin, aspirin-containing products) should not be given to children with factor disorders because it inhibits platelet function. Because some over-the-counter medications may contain acetylsalicylic acid, it is important to read all labels carefully before giving the child the medication.

ing commonly occurs in the same joint for severely affected children. Swelling, pain, bleeding, and stiffness (hemarthrosis) occur.

Diagnostic Evaluation

Hemophilia is sometimes but not always diagnosed after circumcision, at which time prolonged bleeding may be observed. Because the most common sites of bleeding are in the muscles and joints, the diagnosis may be delayed until the toddler years, when the child becomes more active and the disease has an opportunity to manifest itself. By the preschool years, most affected children have experienced an episode of persistent bleeding from a minor traumatic laceration.

A diagnostic work-up for the child with suspected hemophilia includes determining the prothrombin time (PT), partial thromboplastin time (PTT), bleeding time, fibrinogen level, and platelet count; quantitative immunoelectrophoretic assay; and factor VIII and factor IX assays.

Therapeutic Management

The management of hemophilia is very individual and depends on the severity of the illness. Therapy aims to prevent excessive bleeding and tissue damage by supplying the body with the missing or ineffective factors (VIII or IX).

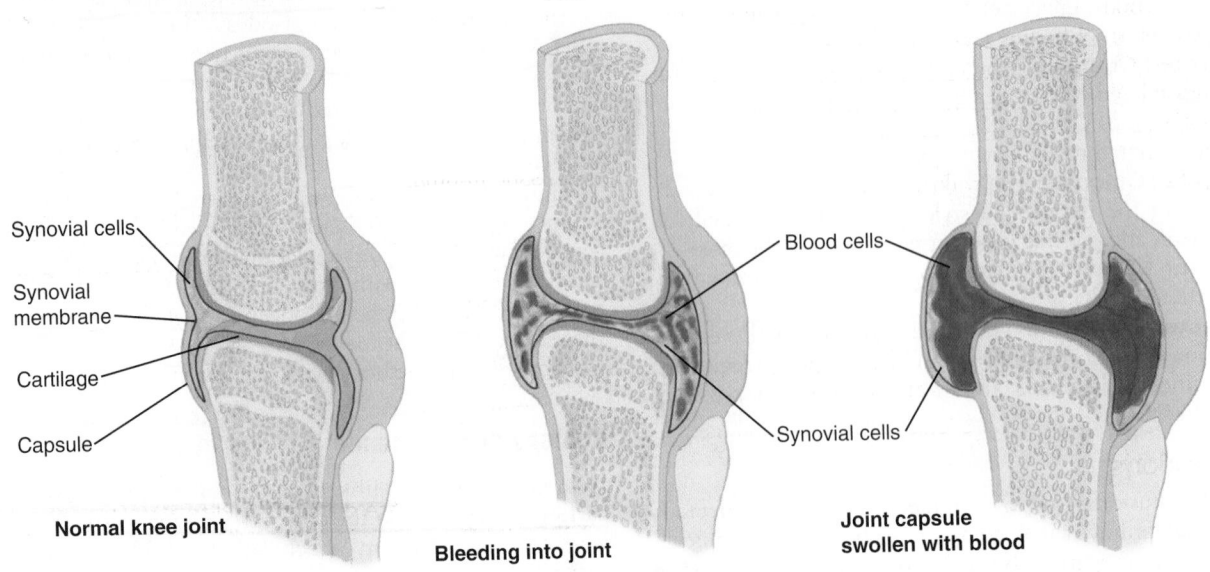

Synovial cells
Synovial membrane
Cartilage
Capsule

Normal knee joint

Blood cells
Synovial cells

Bleeding into joint

Joint capsule swollen with blood

Figure 47-1 Hemarthrosis and joint destruction are characteristic of hemophilia.

Nursing Care Plan

The Child With Hemophilia

FOCUSED ASSESSMENT

In a male neonate, observe the circumcision site or injection sites for prolonged bleeding. Notify the physician if prolonged bleeding is observed.

Be alert to the possibility of hemophilia when the parents of a child just learning to crawl or walk express concern that their child bruises easily on tumbling or falling down. Questions should be asked about previous cuts and scrapes to determine whether the child seemed to need more than the usual amount of pressure application or time for the bleeding to subside. The family should also be asked if there is a family history of bleeding disorders.

Nursing Diagnosis

Risk for Injury related to prolonged bleeding.

Expected Outcome

The child and family will:
- Recognize bleeding resulting from injury and promptly control it to prevent permanent tissue damage.

INTERVENTION	RATIONALE
1. Monitor the area of injury frequently for bleeding over a 24-hour period.	1. Bleeding may be prolonged and, especially in the case of head trauma, may not manifest immediately.
2. Measure the injured joint.	2. Joint measurement provides objective rather than subjective data for future comparisons.
3. In the case of head trauma, assess the child's level of consciousness and note any behavioral changes.	3. Decreased level of consciousness and unusual behaviors are early indicators of increased intracranial pressure secondary to hemorrhage.
4. Apply gentle pressure for 10 to 15 minutes to small superficial wounds, and assess the area for subcutaneous bleeding.	4. Small wounds may ooze blood into the subcutaneous tissue. Pressure facilitates clot formation.
5. Administer factor replacement as ordered.	5. Factor must be reconstituted just before infusion. It may be given as a prophylactic measure even if no bleeding is apparent.
6. Monitor factor levels as ordered.	6. With serious injuries warranting hospitalization, factor levels aid in prescribing dosages and in establishing thresholds for an individual child.
7. If a muscle or joint injury occurs, immobilize, elevate, and apply ice to the affected part, as ordered by the physician.	7. Initial immobilization will help prevent further injury until the bleeding resolves.
8. Offer suggestions for establishing a safe home environment for the child (see Parents Want to Know: About Home Care of the Child With Hemophilia box).	8. A safe home environment will help prevent injuries.
9. Avoid rectal temperature measurement.	9. Rectal temperatures may cause bleeding secondary to tissue trauma.
10. Provide for and expect behaviors consistent with normal growth and development for the child's age.	10. Parents may tend to overprotect or provide special treatment for their child. This unnecessarily limits the child's opportunities for normal psychosocial development and decreases self-esteem.

Evaluation
- Has the child experienced serious bleeding from injury?
- Has the child adhered to the treatment regimen to control injuries?
- Are there long-term complications from injury?

Nursing Diagnosis

Deficient Knowledge related to the need for information about disease diagnosis and treatment.

Expected Outcome

The child and family will:
- Explain the diagnosis.
- Demonstrate adherence to the home care regimen.

Continued

Nursing Care Plan

The Child With Hemophilia—cont'd

INTERVENTION	RATIONALE
1. Assess the child's and family's readiness for learning. Create an environment conducive to learning.	1. The family may need time to adjust to the initial diagnosis before they are ready to be educated. The appropriate setting for an educational session may be away from the child so that parents will be able to focus on the information.
2. On initial diagnosis and with subsequent follow-up visits, spend time with the family explaining the diagnosis, sequelae, and treatment. Offer written literature and educational tapes.	2. Education is ongoing and will need to be reinforced with stressed parents. Explaining the rationale for treatment and the disease's sequelae will help ensure compliance with therapy.
3. Offer encouragement and praise for prompt parental recognition and response to bleeds.	3. Written or taped information can be reviewed later, when comprehension is likely to be improved.
4. Teach techniques for reconstitution and infusion of factor at home. The instruction technique may be for peripheral infusion or infusion via a central venous access line, depending on the child's individual situation (see Parents Want to Know: About Home Care of the Child With Hemophilia box).	4. Praise will reinforce behavior. Parents want to know they are doing the right things for their child.
5. Consider using a topical anesthetic, such as eutectic mixture of local anesthetics (EMLA), when accessing infusion ports or peripheral sites.	5. Parents are taught techniques for accessing the port, infusing the factor, and heparinizing the port. The use of topical anesthetics decreases pain, thus causing less trauma and anxiety.

Evaluation
- Are the child and family able to safely administer factor replacement at home?
- Do the child and family promptly recognize and react to bleeding?

Nursing Diagnosis
Ineffective Coping related to chronic illness and guilt.

Expected Outcomes
The child and family will:
- Adhere to the treatment plan, as evidenced by safety alterations being made in the home and community.
- Utilize available support systems and community resources.

Family members will:
- Verbalize concerns about the impact of the illness on the family.

INTERVENTION	RATIONALE
1. Teach the family the need for safety precautions, reacting cautiously to injury, administering medications properly, and following the treatment plan as outlined by health care providers (see Parents Want to Know: About Home Care of the Child With Hemophilia box).	1. Conscientious adherence to the treatment regimen decreases the potential for long-term complications.
2. Listen to and encourage the child and family to verbalize their feelings and express their concerns regarding hemophilia. Answer questions honestly and openly. Be particularly aware of feelings of guilt expressed by the mother.	2. Identifying concerns and clarifying misconceptions help families cope with the stress of chronic illness.
3. Introduce the family to other families of children with hemophilia.	3. Other families of children with hemophilia can offer support, suggestions, and strategies for coping.

Nursing Care Plan

The Child With Hemophilia—cont'd

INTERVENTION	RATIONALE
4. Provide referral to the National Hemophilia Foundation (see Appendix I on Evolve website).	4. Access to information and assistance can help the family deal with the sometimes overwhelming financial and emotional burdens of caring for a child with hemophilia, especially if complications occur.
5. Explore with the child feelings related to participation in some sports and other restrictions related to having hemophilia.	5. Discussing feelings related to a chronic disease provides an opportunity for the child to explore options and for the nurse to assess the child's needs and coping strategies.

Evaluation

- Does the older child avoid contact sports and participate in other activities, such as swimming?
- Has the family contacted the National Hemophilia Foundation?
- Is the child able to balance increased limitations and normal childhood?

PARENTS *type 1*
Want to Know

About Home Care of the Child With Hemophilia

- Apply gentle, prolonged pressure to superficial wounds until the bleeding has stopped.
- Call the physician in the event of blunt trauma, especially trauma involving the joints.
- Establish an age-appropriate, safe environment:
  —Pad table corners.
  —Pad crib rails.
  —Provide extra joint padding on clothes.
  —Remove items that can tip over or be pulled down on the child.
  —Do not leave a crawling or toddling child unattended.
  —Use a tooth brush with soft bristles and a WaterPik for dental care.
- Instruct older children to avoid contact sports and to take precautions with other sports:
  —Pad the knees and elbows for physical education class.
  —Use protective helmets for any sport in which head injury could occur (e.g., bicycling, skating).
  —Use an electric razor for shaving.
- Call the physician if any head injury occurs.
- Reconstitute and administer factor through an intravenous line or the child's central venous access device.
- If a child has an implantable infusion device, caregivers should understand the following:
  —Site preparation.
  —Sterile technique for insertion of access needle.
  —Technique for verification of needle placement.

can swim

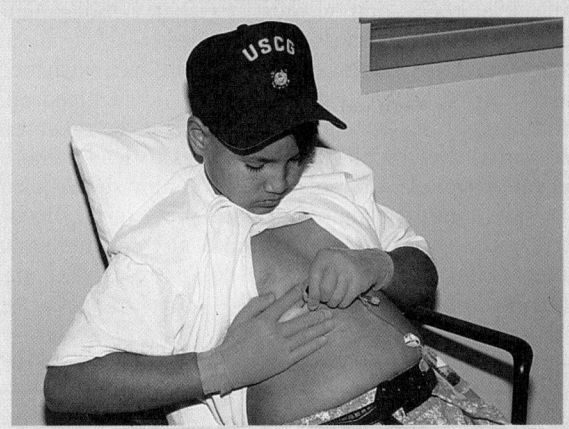

Control of deficient blood clotting in hemophilia requires injection of the missing clotting factors. This young man is injecting his factor into an implanted central venous access port. Sterile technique is essential. (Courtesy the family of Jason Lee Davis.)

  —Administration of factor by IV push.
  —Saline and heparin flush.
  —Removal and proper disposal of needle.
- Keep current with the schedule of immunizations, dental hygiene, and routine well-child care.
- Allow your child to set personal safety limits when possible.
- Provide for normal growth and development opportunities (safe activities, time with other children, limit setting, independence).

Previously, treatment involved transfusions of blood products or administration of freeze-dried products manufactured from blood products. One of the major risks associated with this factor replacement therapy was contracting hepatitis or HIV infection. Because of this risk, manufacturers began to heat-treat the blood factor to reduce the risk of viral transmission. Monoclonal products were then developed and were found to be even safer than the heat-treated products. The most recent development in the treatment of hemophilia is the availability of recombinant antihemophilic factor, which is not derived from human plasma but is produced synthetically from isolation of the gene. Recombinant factor eliminates the risk

---

! CRITICAL TO REMEMBER

Interviewing a Child With Hemophilia

Subjective data gathered for a child known to have hemophilia should include information about recent trauma and initial measures to stop bleeding. An important question is the length of time that pressure had to be applied before the bleeding subsided. Other questions to ask include whether the swelling increased after the surface bleeding stopped and whether swelling and stiffness occurred without apparent trauma.

---

of virus transmission. The freeze-dried product is supplied with sterile water and must be reconstituted before being given intravenously.

Prophylactic therapy is now being started in infants and young children with severe hemophilia to prevent joint problems. Children age 1 to 2 years receive factor replacement on a regular schedule if they develop clinical symptoms. Children with mild hemophilia A may be able to use desmopressin acetate (1-deamino-8-D-arginine vasopressin [DDAVP]) intranasal spray, because of its vasoconstrictor action, to stop bleeding. Children with hemophilias A and B can be given aminocaproic acid (Amicar) or tranexamic acid (Cyclokapron)—oral medications that stabilize oral clots and can also sometimes stop nosebleeds.

Aside from administration of factor, children with hemophilia must try to avoid activities that induce bleeding. For mild hemophilia, special precautions can be taken to protect joints, thereby allowing the child to lead a more normal life. Prophylactic replacement therapy should also be given before surgery and some dental procedures. Bleeding is treated with rest, ice, elevation of the affected part, and compression (also referred to as *RICE: r*est, *i*ce, compression, *e*levation).

VON WILLEBRAND'S DISEASE

Von Willebrand's disease (VWD) is the most commonly inherited bleeding disorder (Hambleton, 2001). At least 20 subtypes of VWD have been identified. Three subtypes are based on the mechanism of bleeding: type I, type IIA, and type IIB.

Etiology

Von Willebrand's disease is an autosomal dominant inherited disorder.

Pathophysiology

Children with VWD have either underproduction of or dysfunction of von Willebrand's protein. The VWD protein is the carrier protein for coagulation factor VIII, and it is also a co-factor for the binding of platelets to damaged endothelial tissue. Clinical features and the need for treatment depend on the severity of the disorder.

Manifestations

The clinical manifestations of VWD include a history of epistaxis, bleeding from the gums, prolonged bleeding from cuts, excessive bleeding after surgery or trauma, and menorrhagia (excessive menstrual bleeding) in females.

Diagnostic Evaluation

A thorough history will ascertain whether the episode of bruising is proportional to the degree of trauma. A family history of bleeding disorders is important.

Laboratory tests may include a bleeding time and PTT, the results of which may be normal. The most clinically useful laboratory test for diagnosing this disorder is the quantitative immunoelectrophoretic assay, which, in the presence of the disease, will reveal a discrepancy in the quantity and function of von Willebrand's factor in the plasma.

Therapeutic Management

Therapy is aimed at replacing the missing or dysfunctional factor in the blood. In the past, cryoprecipitate or fresh frozen plasma was given before surgery or after trauma with excessive bleeding. Presently, this treatment is recommended only if the cryoprecipitate is donated from a well-screened, unaffected family member or a repeat individual donor and the child is not responding to DDAVP.

The treatment of choice is DDAVP, which is administered intravenously or intranasally. The DDAVP products are given for type I and type IIA von Willebrand's disease only (Hambleton, 2001). High-purity (not monoclonal or recombinant) factor VIII products that are specifically known to contain von Willebrand's factor can be used to treat type IIB disease. (Only a minority of currently available factor VIII concentrates actually contain von Willebrand's factor.)

NURSING CARE
The Child With von Willebrand's Disease

Assessment

A careful history detailing episodes of bruising and bleeding is essential. Possible causes of any previous episodes of bleeding, if any can be identified, should also be discussed. Ask how many times the child has experienced a nosebleed, how long the child bleeds from "normal" trauma, and whether there is a history of prolonged bleeding associated with surgery or trauma.

Physical examination usually reveals a normal child except for evidence of bruising greater than expected for the degree of trauma experienced. If the child is being seen after a major bleeding episode, signs of hemorrhage or a decreased hemoglobin level (or both) will be seen.

Nursing Diagnosis and Planning

The nursing diagnoses and expected outcomes that may be appropriate after assessment of the child with von Willebrand's disease are

■ Ineffective Protection related to abnormal clotting.
  Expected Outcome: The child will remain free of life-threatening episodes of hemorrhage.
■ Deficient Knowledge related to the disorder.
  Expected Outcome: The child and family will explain the disorder, its management, and its chronic nature.

Interventions

Education of the family is aimed at producing an understanding of the precautions to take with the child, as well as knowledge of when prophylactic therapy should be given before elective procedures. The child should wear a Medic-Alert tag at all times. The family should be referred to the Hemophilia Foundation for support services (see Appendix I on Evolve website). Avoidance of prescription and over-the-counter medications that affect platelet function, such as aspirin, is also recommended.

The degree of activity limitation will depend on the severity of the disorder. Limitations may include avoidance of contact sports, especially football.

Evaluation

- Are episodes of bleeding minimal and controlled?
- Does the family communicate an understanding of the importance of avoiding medications that affect platelet function and avoiding activities that increase the risk of bleeding?
- Does the family seek appropriate resources for information about the condition and its management?

IMMUNE THROMBOCYTOPENIC PURPURA

Immune thrombocytopenic purpura (ITP) is an acquired hemorrhagic disorder characterized by thrombocytopenia (platelet count <150,000/mm^3), a purpuric rash, normal bone marrow, and the absence of signs of other identifiable causes of thrombocytopenia. It is classified as acute or chronic, with chronic being defined as the persistence of thrombocytopenia for more than 6 months.

Etiology and Incidence

ITP is estimated to be one of the most common acquired bleeding disorders in children. The incidence of symptomatic disease is approximately 3 to 8 per 100,000 children per year. Acute ITP is more prevalent among children younger than 10 years, affects males and females equally, and is more prevalent during the late winter and spring. Chronic ITP affects adolescents more than younger children, with females being affected more frequently than males (Di Paola & Buchanan, 2002). The etiology of ITP is unknown, although in the majority of children it follows a viral illness and is considered to be an autoimmune process.

Pathophysiology

In general, ITP is thought to occur as a result of the destruction of platelets by autoantibodies to glycoproteins normally expressed on platelet membranes. The spleen and other organs of the reticuloendothelial system subsequently destroy these antibody-coated platelets (Chu, Korb, & Sakamoto, 2000).

Manifestations

Clinical manifestations of ITP include the sudden onset of bruising and petechiae, with bleeding involving the mucous membranes and gums, in a child who is in otherwise good health (Fig. 47-2).

Diagnostic Evaluation

The initial diagnostic evaluation should include a thorough history and a CBC, including evaluation of a peripheral blood smear. The history should include information about

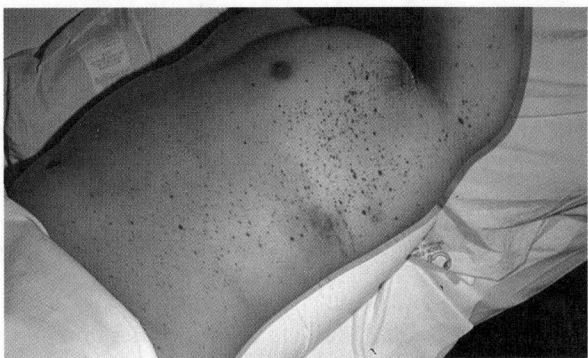

Figure 47-2 Multiple petechiae are characteristic of immune thrombocytopenic purpura. This disorder results in the destruction of circulating platelets and decreased bone marrow production of new platelets. (Courtesy Cook Children's Medical Center, Fort Worth, TX.)

any medications the child has taken that could cause thrombocytopenia, history of recent live virus vaccination, and any instances of illness, especially febrile illness, in the past month. In an affected child, the initial CBC will reveal a low platelet count, often below 50,000/mm^3, but the results will otherwise be normal. The physical examination findings will be normal, aside from the signs of bleeding.

If any data in the history or CBC are suggestive of a diagnosis other than ITP, the physician may obtain a bone marrow aspirate to rule out an oncologic disorder and to determine whether megakaryocytes, the precursors of platelets, are present. Routine bone marrow examination is not warranted in a child with findings consistent with acute ITP.

Physical examination of the affected child reveals bruising and petechiae, the severity of which depends on how low the platelet count is and the child's tolerance of the low platelet count. The spleen and liver are generally normal in size. The greatest risk of a low platelet count is intracranial hemorrhage, so a neurologic assessment is important.

Therapeutic Management

The goal of treatment is to prevent rare, life-threatening bleeding events, such as intracranial bleeding. Additional goals include restoration of the platelet count to above 20,000/mm^3 in children with mucocutaneous bleeding and a reduction in the duration of thrombocytopenia. Treatment is based on the child's presenting condition.

Treatment options have been an intense topic of discussion for years and have divided pediatric hematologists between what have been called *interventionists* and *non-interventionist* (Di Paola, & Buchanan, 2002). Because most cases of ITP are self-limiting, with a normal platelet count returning within 6 months, the non-interventionists recommend no therapy but frequent monitoring of platelet counts and bleeding status (Chu et al., 2000).

Depending on whether the child is an inpatient or outpatient, IV or oral steroids may be administered over a 2- to 4-week period. For unknown reasons, the steroids block the autoimmune destruction of platelets. The other drug that may be used to treat ITP is IV immune globulin (IVIG), administered once daily for 1 to 2 days. Often, the platelet count is dramatically increased after one dose of IVIG. In children with Rh positive blood types (A+, B+, and 0+), IV anti-D immunoglobulin may be used.

ITP is considered to be acute if recovery of a normal platelet count is seen within 6 months. The condition becomes chronic if recovery takes longer than 6 months. Children with chronic ITP may initially respond to steroids with an increase in platelet count, but it will not reach normal levels. These children may go for long periods without experiencing problems with excessive bleeding or a low platelet count; the count will then begin to decline again, at which time steroid therapy should be resumed.

When steroids and IVIG do not control the thrombocytopenia in a child with chronic ITP, a splenectomy may be indicated. Splenectomy will cure most children with chronic ITP because the spleen synthesizes the antiplatelet antibody that results in the destruction of circulating platelets. The risk associated with removal of the spleen is sepsis from those organisms that the spleen's reticuloendothelial system fights. Without the spleen, the body's ability to fight *S. pneumoniae*, *H. influenzae*, and *N. meningitidis* is limited. This limitation is greater in children younger than 5 years, so ITP is managed without splenectomy, if possible, until age 5 years. Platelet transfusions are given in children only when active, uncontrolled bleeding occurs.

■ NURSING CARE
The Child With Immune Thrombocytopenic Purpura

Assessment

Parents usually bring their child to the physician because they have noticed excessive bruising or a "red rash" in the child's mouth or on the child's body. Although this "rash" may look remarkable to a nurse, it often evolves so gradually that it escapes the immediate notice of a parent who sees the child every day. As a result, health care may not be sought until very significant bruising and petechiae, even hematomas, are present.

Affected children usually demonstrate normal activity levels for their age, because they do not "feel bad." Assessment should include observation for signs of any further bruising or bleeding, including epistaxis, hematuria, or blood in the stools, as well as for signs of a decreasing level of consciousness, which could indicate intracranial hemorrhage.

Nursing Diagnosis and Planning

The nursing diagnoses and expected outcomes that may be appropriate after assessment of the child with ITP are

■ Ineffective Protection related to low platelet count.
  Expected Outcome: The child will exhibit no signs of active bleeding or intracranial hemorrhage, as evidenced by pulse and blood pressure within normal limits and an alert and responsive child.
■ Risk for Infection related to chronic use of steroids or splenectomy.
  Expected Outcomes: The family will identify signs of infection and notify the health care team, and the child will respond rapidly to treatment for infection.
■ Deficient Knowledge related to insufficient information about the disorder and its therapeutic management.
  Expected Outcome: The child and family will describe ITP and the treatment plan.

Interventions

The family is referred to a health care center to carry out medical treatments, and the family is educated about ITP and home care.

An IV access line may be established for the purpose of administering IV steroids or IVIG. It can be quite challenging to establish IV access in children with ITP because merely puncturing the skin may result in a hematoma, which may be confused with "blowing" the vein. Careful evaluation of blood return and flushing of the IV catheter with normal saline will confirm proper placement of the catheter.

Restricting the activity of toddlers and young children can be a challenge. Extra-soft-bristle toothbrushes or toothettes should be used for mouth care on all children whose platelet count is less than 20,000/mm³. Until the platelet count returns to normal, activities such as bicycle riding, contact sports, and roller-skating should be curtailed.

Education includes teaching the family about the disease process of ITP; the side effects of steroids and IVIG, if used; the need to restrict the child's activity; and the importance of proper follow-up evaluations. Parents should be instructed regarding the signs and symptoms of infection and actions in the event of signs of fever, because steroids may mask an infection.

Ensure that parents and the child's primary care physician are informed if the child receives IVIG. The American Academy of Pediatrics (AAP) recommends delaying the administration of routine measles immunization for a minimum of 10 months to children who have received immune globulin preparations because they may block the replication of live-virus vaccine immune response (AAP, 2000b).

If the child has had a splenectomy, pneumococcal vaccine or daily penicillin (or both) should be administered. Any

---

PARENTS
Want to Know

About Home Care of the Child With Immune Thrombocytopenic Purpura

- Eliminate participation in high-risk activities, such as contact sports, bicycle riding, roller-skating, and diving, if the child's platelet count is low.
- Avoid medications that can affect platelet function (ibuprofen, aspirin). Be sure to read over-the-counter medication labels to check for these medications, which can be included in combination products, such as cold, flu, and upset stomach remedies.
- Use an extra-soft toothbrush if the platelet count is less than 20,000/mm³.
- Establish an age-appropriate, safe home environment.
- Pad table corners.
- Pad crib rails.
- Offer extra joint padding on clothes.
- For additional resources and information, contact national organizations (e.g., the ITP Society; see Appendix I on Evolve website).

signs and symptoms of infection should be reported immediately to the physician so that proper therapy can be initiated before the infection becomes life-threatening.

Evaluation

- Are the child's vital signs within normal limits?
- Is the child responding in an age-appropriate manner?
- Have areas of ecchymosis and petechiae decreased?
- Does the family verbalize and implement a plan of care that decreases the risk of the child incurring an injury that is likely to cause hemorrhage?
- Does the family respond quickly to early signs of infection by notifying the primary health care provider?

DISSEMINATED INTRAVASCULAR COAGULATION

Disseminated intravascular coagulation (DIC) is an acquired hemorrhagic syndrome characterized by uncontrolled formation and deposition of fibrin thrombi and by the resulting consumption of clotting factors leading to uncontrolled bleeding. In children, DIC occurs without the overwhelming mortality that occurs in adults. The keys to recovery are identification and treatment of the underlying cause of the DIC.

Etiology

DIC is triggered by any factor that causes endothelial damage, liberation of tissue thromboplastin, circulating endotoxins, or immune complexes. In children, the most common causes are trauma, hypoxia, necrotizing enterocolitis, shock, liver disease, overwhelming viral or bacterial infections, and acute promyelocytic leukemia.

Manifestations

Manifestations of DIC involve an insidious onset, corresponding to platelet count and fibrinogen levels. Early indicators include excessive bruising and petechiae, oozing from puncture sites, oozing from sites of mild tissue trauma (e.g., site of insertion of a nasogastric tube), and mild gastrointestinal bleeding. As the disease progresses, manifestations of DIC include purpuric rash, worsening of bleeding, hemoptysis, hypoxemia, oliguria progressing to renal failure, progressive organ failure, and intracranial hemorrhage.

Diagnostic Evaluation

The diagnosis of DIC is confirmed by laboratory testing (Box 47-2).

BOX 47-2

Confirmatory Laboratory Findings in Disseminated Intravascular Coagulation

- Decreased red blood cell (RBC) count
- Low platelet count noted on complete blood cell (CBC) count
- RBC fragments on the smear
- Prolonged prothrombin time
- Decreased fibrinogen level
- Elevated levels of fibrin degradation products (e.g., D dimer)

Therapeutic Management

To control DIC, the clinician must identify and then treat the underlying cause of the condition. Treatment then becomes symptomatic and directed at replenishing consumed coagulation factors. Depleted fibrinogen and other coagulation factors are replaced (e.g., cryoprecipitate, fresh frozen plasma [FFP]) to normalize the PT. RBCs and platelet transfusions can aid in replacing cells lost in hemorrhage. Exchange transfusions may be used in neonates to minimize the excessive fluid volume required by replacing platelets, clotting factors, and RBCs. Vitamin K may also be administered to normalize the PT. The most familiar drug used to dissolve clots is heparin. However, heparin has

---

Pathophysiology

of Disseminated Intravascular Coagulation

Disseminated intravascular coagulation (DIC) is a consumptive disorder caused by abnormal activation of the clotting mechanism, which causes rapid depletion of platelets, prothrombin, and fibrinogen. It is a pathologic syndrome resulting from the formation of thrombin, subsequent activation and consumption of certain coagulant proteins, and the production of fibrin thrombi. DIC manifests with diffuse microvascular coagulation secondary to depletion of clotting factors, resulting in impaired hemostasis.

The pathophysiology of DIC is complicated and often not easily understood, because both excessive bleeding and excessive clotting are occurring at the same time. The syndrome of DIC leads to deposition of platelet and fibrin plugs in the vasculature and the simultaneous depletion of platelets and clotting factor proteins.

The process of blood coagulation follows either an intrinsic or an extrinsic pathway.* Both pathways ultimately lead to the common pathway of prothrombin forming thrombin, which, in the presence of fibrinogen, forms fibrin. Alternately, fibrinolysis (clot destruction) requires the presence of thrombin. During this process, the enzyme *plasmin* lyses fibrin into fragments called *fibrin degradation products (FDPs)*, which interfere with the ability of platelets to adhere to one another. In DIC, initiation of the clotting process is stimulated by endothelial damage or some form of tissue injury. Platelets and clotting factors are subsequently depleted. As clotting is stimulated, the body perceives the need to produce substances to dissolve those clots and there is an increase in the end result of clot lysis, FDPs. The overstimulation of both these normal processes has three major effects on the body:

- Increased, uncontrolled bleeding resulting from the depletion of platelets and clotting factors and overstimulation of the fibrinolytic process
- Anemia caused by the excessive bleeding and the mechanical fragmentation of red blood cells (RBCs)
- Organ damage secondary to the formation of emboli
- Tissue hypoxia leading to tissue necrosis

*Guyton, A.C., & Hall, J.E. (2000). *Textbook of medical physiology* (10th ed.). Philadelphia: Saunders.

a controversial role in the treatment of childhood DIC because it may increase the risk for bleeding.

Nursing Considerations

DIC typically develops in a child who is already hospitalized. The subjective and objective data assessed will depend entirely on the initial illness. The nurse must be cognizant of the patient who is at risk for DIC. Evidence of bleeding at any site of integumentary interruption and at every orifice should be assessed. The nurse also notes any changes in the pattern of vital signs. Adequate tissue perfusion should be confirmed, because normal function of an organ is the end result of sufficient oxygenation of that organ. Children with full clinical manifestations of DIC are typically cared for in an intensive care setting owing to the complex multisystem sequelae and management of DIC.

Any areas of active bleeding should be located promptly and pressure applied, if possible. Continue to monitor the child for overt and covert signs of bleeding. Care should be taken to avoid any unnecessary tissue trauma or injury. IV lines and indwelling tubes should be secured and protected to eliminate the additional trauma caused by reinsertion. Frequent monitoring of vital signs is necessary to identify changing patterns and ensure adequate cardiac output and end-organ perfusion. Laboratory results are also monitored carefully, with particular attention to the trending of values. Medical orders are followed with regard to the administration of medicines, blood products, and treatments, including monitoring the child's tolerance and outcomes. Because hypoxemia and acidosis may actually cause DIC, adequate ventilation must be ensured to prevent or reduce compromised respiratory function.

Because DIC can be life-threatening, the nurse helps parents deal with their anxiety about their child's condition. Being available to answer questions and updating the parents on the child's progress are essential.

The morbidity and mortality of children with DIC depend on the underlying causative condition. With prompt recognition of both the underlying cause and diagnosis of DIC and with proper management of both, these children can have favorable outcomes.

APLASTIC ANEMIA

Aplastic anemia is a condition in which the bone marrow ceases production of the cells it normally manufactures. The result is peripheral *pancytopenia*, a condition in which

Pathophysiology

of Aplastic Anemia

Aplastic anemia is characterized by cessation of hematopoiesis by the bone marrow of granulocytes, erythrocytes, and megakaryocytes. The disease may be classified as mild, moderate, or severe, depending on how low the values are for absolute neutrophil count, platelet count, and absolute reticulocyte count. The diagnosis of severe aplastic anemia requires two of the following anomalies: granulocyte count less than 500/mm^3, platelet count less than 20,000/mm^3, and reticulocyte count below 1% (after correction for hematocrit). In addition, the bone marrow biopsy must contain less than 25% of the normal cellularity.

Adapted from Hord, J. (2004). The acquired pancytopenias. In R. Behrman, R. Kliegman, & H. Jenson (Eds.), *Nelson textbook of pediatrics* (17th ed., pp. 1644-1646). Philadelphia: Saunders.

all formed elements of the blood are simultaneously depressed.

Etiology and Incidence

Aplastic anemia can be congenital or acquired. Several rare, inheritable disorders are characterized by aplastic anemia. The most common of these is Fanconi's anemia. Aplastic anemia can also be acquired, with a number of agents and conditions implicated as the probable cause. These most often include drugs or chemicals and less often radiation exposure, viruses, and immune diseases. Most cases (approximately 70%) of aplastic anemia in children are idiopathic—without an identifiable cause. Aplastic anemia results in a physiologic and anatomic failure of the bone marrow, preventing the development of granulocytes, erythrocytes, and megakaryocytes. Annually, in the United States and Europe, the incidence of aplastic anemia is two cases per million per year. Leukemia, by comparison, has an incidence of 50 cases per million per year (Nathan et al., 2003).

Manifestations

The clinical manifestations of aplastic anemia include petechiae, ecchymosis, pallor, epistaxis, fatigue, tachycardia, anorexia, and infection.

Diagnostic Evaluation

Although the diagnosis of aplastic anemia may be suspected from the child's history and the results of a CBC, bone marrow aspiration and biopsy must be performed to confirm the diagnosis. Biopsy results should reveal the presence or absence of precursors of the mature cells found in a peripheral blood sample. In aplastic anemia, these precursors are notably absent from the marrow sample. This type of marrow is described as *hypocellular* and often contains a predominance of lymphocytes and yellowish fatty tissue.

Therapeutic Management

If the aplastic anemia is determined by history to be acquired, exposure to the causative agent is discontinued immediately. Treatment then is based on symptoms. Platelet and erythrocyte transfusions may be ordered. Granulocyte transfusions are not used routinely because of their short life span in the circulation. When signs and symptoms of infection are suspected or present, antibiotics are administered after appropriate cultures are obtained.

Bone marrow or allogeneic hematopoietic stem cell transplantation remains the treatment of choice for children with severe aplastic anemia for whom a suitable donor has been identified (Young, 2002). (See Chapter 48 for a discussion of hematopoietic stem cell transplantation.) A medication regimen of cyclosporine, antithymocyte globulin (ATG)/antilymphocyte globulin (ALG), and colony-stimulating factors effectively treats acquired aplastic anemia for many children for whom a suitable bone marrow or stem cell donor is not available (Hord, 2004).

NURSING CARE
The Child With Aplastic Anemia

Assessment

The subjective assessment usually elicits parents' observations of bruising immediately after an event that would not normally result in a bruise. For example, an observant parent may have noted petechiae in the child's mouth while assisting the child in brushing the teeth. Information should be elicited about medications recently taken or recent exposures to environmental substances outside the child's usual realm in an effort to determine possible drug- or chemical-related causes for the pancytopenia.

Petechiae, bruising, pallor, lethargy, and tachycardia are the usual abnormal findings and are directly related to the degree of pancytopenia. Otherwise, the results of the physical assessment are usually normal.

Nursing Diagnosis and Planning

The nursing diagnoses and expected outcomes that may be appropriate for the child with aplastic anemia are

- Risk for Infection related to inadequate secondary defenses and/or immunosuppression.
  Expected Outcome: The child remains free from infection, as evidenced by body temperature, neurologic assessment, cardiorespiratory assessment, gastrointestinal status, and genitourinary status in expected range.
- Ineffective Protection related to thrombocytopenia.
  Expected Outcomes: The child will remain free of bleeding episodes and will demonstrate appropriate precautions to prevent or decrease bleeding.
- Ineffective Tissue Perfusion related to anemia.
  Expected Outcome: The child's tissues will be perfused, as evidenced by palpable peripheral pulses, normal capillary refill, urine output appropriate for age, and absent respiratory distress.

- Deficient Knowledge related to incomplete information about the disease process.
  Expected Outcome: The child and family will describe the disease process and its potential complications.

Interventions

Nursing care initially focuses on providing supportive care and preventing any serious physiologic sequelae of pancytopenia. Because of the increased risk of bacterial infection, affected children should be assigned to private rooms and instructed in meticulous handwashing. Precautionary measures should be taken as for any individual with a low platelet count, including no injections; no rectal temperatures, examinations, or medications; use of an extra-soft-bristle toothbrush or toothette; abstinence from any contact sports or activity; and periodic assessment for increased bleeding.

Physicians' orders should be followed with regard to blood transfusions, acquisition of blood cultures, and antibiotic administration. Usually, the platelet count will be maintained at a level greater than 20,000/mm³ to prevent intracranial hemorrhage or signs of active bleeding. The hemoglobin level is typically maintained above 7 g/dl. However, if a child is to receive a hematopoietic stem cell transplant, efforts are made to use blood transfusions only as necessary to avoid possible alloimmunization. If any symptoms of infection are present, blood should be drawn for culture. The need for other cultures will depend on the child's clinical examination.

Antibiotics should be administered immediately to a febrile child with neutropenia, owing to the risk of rapid, overwhelming sepsis. Children who are hospitalized, febrile, and neutropenic should be assessed frequently for signs of septic shock. Assessment includes the quality of peripheral pulses compared with central pulses, extremity temperature, capillary refill time, level of consciousness, and vital signs, as well as examination of cannulation sites or skin breakdown.

Education of the family and child should include information about the disease process and the complications that should be reported promptly to the health care provider. Often, referral is made to a transplant center. If so, intense pretransplant education is indicated. The Aplastic Anemia & MDS International Foundation, Inc. is a good source of information for children, parents, and health care providers (see Appendix I on Evolve website). Follow-up studies should include frequent CBC and physical examinations.

Evaluation

- Is the child afebrile, and do cannulation or other skin sites remain free of redness or swelling?
- Are assessment data related to other body systems within normal ranges?
- Has the child experienced any major bleeding?
- Is the child able to participate in age-appropriate activities without injury?
- Does the child demonstrate palpable peripheral pulses, capillary refill less than 2 seconds, urine output appropriate for age (see Chapter 42), and oxygen saturation more than 95%?
- Has the family received instruction regarding the disease and home care and verbalized an understanding of the information?

KEY CONCEPTS

■ For erythrocytes to carry oxygen there must be an adequate amount of hemoglobin, the level of which depends on sufficient circulating iron.

■ Anemia results from blood loss, decreased production of erythrocytes or hemoglobin, or increased destruction of erythrocytes.

■ Caring for children with blood disorders requires an understanding of the anatomy and physiology of blood and blood-forming tissues, genetics, and the care of children with a chronic disease.

■ The number of erythrocytes varies according to age, gender, and the altitude at which a person lives.

■ Iron-deficiency anemia can largely be prevented by teaching parents the importance of providing iron-fortified formula or breast milk with iron supplementary foods, such as iron-fortified cereal, to children until age 12 months.

■ Morphine is the drug of choice for children with a painful episode associated with sickle-cell disease.

■ Complications associated with sickle-cell anemia can be reduced through early screening; parent/child education; routine immunizations; pneumococcal, meningococcal, and influenza immunizations; penicillin prophylaxis; and early diagnosis and management of complications.

■ Children with decreased platelet counts and factor disorders should not receive aspirin or have their temperature taken rectally. Invasive procedures should be done only when necessary and then only with extreme caution to avoid hemorrhage.

■ Factor prophylaxis is warranted in infants and young children with hemophilia who are at risk for developing joint problems secondary to bleeding.

■ Bleeding associated with hemophilia is treated with rest, ice, elevation, compression, and factor replacement, as necessary.

■ Education of the family about home care for the child with hemophilia should include information on the management of bleeding episodes, environmental safety, administration of medications, health promotion, and normal growth and development.

■ Educating the family of a child with immune thrombocytopenic purpura (ITP) about the need to restrict activity and to provide protection is a major nursing challenge.

■ Treatment of disseminated intravascular coagulation (DIC) is directed toward treating the cause of the condition.

■ Nursing care of the child with aplastic anemia focuses on the prevention of infection secondary to pancytopenia.

ANSWERS to Critical Thinking Exercise 47-1

1. Mrs. Anders is probably most concerned about Jacob's cough and fever. For that reason, the nurse will want to address the acute illness and then approach Mrs. Anders about concerns related to the anemia. Nurses must be sensitive to what parents perceive as priorities and should address those needs, so that the parents will be able to give their attention to other concerns. In this case, even if Jacob has a minor common cold, the nurse can provide Mrs. Anders with information that will make Jacob more comfortable and then approach the treatment of anemia.

2. Although the priority is to take action related to the acute disease, it is also a time to assess the child and to provide preventive care. Some families see health care providers only when a family member is ill. Knowing the severity of the acute illness, the nurse can determine what can be achieved during the visit and what warrants a follow-up.

3. It is an opportunity to start or update a child's health records through assessment of the child and communicating with the parent and the child, if age-appropriate.

Such a visit also provides an opportunity to administer immunizations, if the child is not too ill, and to provide anticipatory guidance related to nutrition, safety, growth and development, and preventive care. For Jacob, the nurse will want to do a thorough nutrition assessment to determine if diet is the causative factor in the anemia. To increase the chance of compliance, a system of tracking children with diseases that need long-term treatment should also be in place.

REFERENCES and READINGS

Ackley, B.M., & Ladwig, G.B. (2002). *Nursing diagnosis handbook: A guide to planning care* (5th ed.). St Louis: Mosby.

Alter, B.P., & Young, N.S. (1998). The bone marrow failure syndrome. In D.G. Nathan & S.H. Orkin (Eds.), *Nathan and Oski's hematology of infancy and childhood* (5th ed.). Philadelphia: Saunders.

American Academy of Pediatrics (AAP), Committee on Infectious Diseases. (2000a). *Active and passive immunization. In report of the Committee on Infectious Diseases: 2000 Red Book* (25th ed., pp. 1-82). Elk Grove Village, IL: American Academy of Pediatrics.

American Academy of Pediatrics, Committee on Infectious Diseases. (2000b). Section III: *Summaries of infectious diseases. In report of the Committee on Infectious Diseases: 2000 Red Book* (25th ed., pp. 161-644). Elk Grove Village, IL: American Academy of Pediatrics.

American Academy of Pediatrics, Committee on Nutrition. (1998). *Pediatrics nutrition handbook* (4th ed.). Elk Grove Village, IL: American Academy of Pediatrics.

Behrman, R.E., Kliegman, R.M., & Jenson, H. (Eds.). (2004). *Nelson textbook of pediatrics* (17th ed.). Philadelphia: Saunders.

Blanchette, V., & Carcao, M. (2000). Approach to the investigation and management of immune thrombocytopenic purpura in children. *Seminars in Hematology, 37,* 299-314.

Bogen, D., Duggan, A., Dover, G., & Wilson, M. (2000). Screening for iron deficiency anemia by dietary history in a high-risk population. *Pediatrics, 105*(6), 1254-1259.

Brinker, D., & Moloney-Harmon, P. (2001). Hematologic critical care problems. In M.A. Curley, J.B. Smith, & P. Moloney-Harmon (Eds.), *Critical care nursing of infants and children* (2nd ed., pp. 821-850). Philadelphia: Saunders.

Carley, A. (2003). Anemia: when is it iron deficiency? *Pediatric Nursing, 29*(2), 127-133.

Chu, Y., Korb, J., & Sakamoto, K. (2000). Idiopathic thrombocytopenic purpura. *Pediatrics in Review, 21*(3), 95-103.

Curley, M.A., Smith, J.B., & Moloney-Harmon, P. (Eds.). (2001). *Critical care nursing of infants and children* (2nd ed.). Philadelphia: Saunders.

Day, S., Brunson, G., Wang, W. (1997). Successful newborn sickle cell trait counseling program using health department nurses. *Pediatric Nursing, 23*(6), 557-561.

Day, S.W., & Wynn, L. (2000). Sickle cell pain and hydroxyurea. *American Journal of Nursing, 100*(11), 34-39.

Di Paola J., & Buchanan, G. (2002). Immune thrombocytopenic purpura. *Pediatric Clinics of North America, 49*(5), 911-928.

Dover, G., & Platt, O. (2003). Sickle cell disease. In D.G. Nathan, S.H. Orkin, A.T. Look, & D.

Ginsburg (Eds.), *Nathan and Oski's hematology of infancy and childhood* (6th ed.). Philadelphia: Saunders.

Fixler, J., & Styles, L. (2002). Sickle cell disease. *Pediatric Clinics of North America, 49*(6), 1193-1210.

Glader, B. (2004). Iron deficiency anemia. In R. Behrman, R. Kliegman, & H. Jenson (Eds.), *Nelson textbook of pediatrics* (17th ed., pp. 1614-1616). Philadelphia: Saunders.

Guyton, A.C., & Hall, J.E. (2000). *Textbook of medical physiology* (10th ed.). Philadelphia: Saunders.

Hambleton J. (2001). Advances in the treatment of von Willebrand Disease. *Seminars in Hematology, 38*(4 Suppl. 9), 7-10.

Hedner, U., Ginsburg, D., Lusher, J., & High, K. (2000) Congenital hemorrhagic disorders: New insights into the pathophysiology and treatment of hemophilia. *American Society of Hematology Education Program Book*, Dec.1-5, 241-265.

Hord, J. (2004). The acquired pancytopenias. In R. Behrman, R. Kliegman, & H. Jenson (Eds.), *Nelson textbook of pediatrics* (17th ed., pp. 1644-1646). Philadelphia: Saunders.

Lo, L., & Singer, S.T. (2002). Thalassemia: Current approach to an old disease. *Pediatric Clinics of North America, 49*(6), 1165-1191.

Mannucci, P.M. (2002). Hemophilia and related bleeding disorders: A story of dismay and success. *American Society of Hematology Education Program Book*, Dec. 6-10, 1-9.

Nathan, D.G., Orkin, S.H., Look, A.T., & Ginsburg, D. (2003). *Nathan & Oski's hematology of infancy and childhood* (6th ed.). Philadelphia: Saunders.

National Institutes of Health, Division of Blood Diseases and Resource. (2002). *The management of sickle cell disease* (NIH Publication No. 02-2117). Bethesda, MD: Author.

Northington, L. (2000). Chronic sorrow in caregivers of school-age children with sickle cell disease: A grounded theory approach. *Issues in Comprehensive Pediatric Nursing, 23*(3), 141-154.

Quirolo K., & Vichinsky E. (2003). Hemoglobin disorders. In R.E. Behrman, R.M. Kliegman, & A. Arvin (Eds.), *Nelson textbook of pediatrics* (17th ed., pp. 1623-1634). Philadelphia: Saunders.

Taketomo, C., Hodding, J., & Kraus, D. (2000). *Pediatric dosage handbook* (7th ed.). Washington, DC: American Pharmaceutical Association.

Vichinsky E. (2001). Consensus document for transfusion-related iron overloads. *Seminars in Hematology, 38* (1 Suppl. 1), 2-4.

Weatherall, D.J. (1997). The thalassaemias. *British Medical Journal, 314*, 1675-1678.

Young, N. (2002). Acquired aplastic anemia. *Annals of Internal Medicine, 136*(7), 534-546.

48

The Child with Cancer

◆ DEFINITIONS

benign Slow-growing cells, often almost normal in appearance, forming a tumor with distinct borders.

blast cells Immature white blood cells, such as lymphoblasts, myeloblasts, or monoblasts.

clean margins Evidence of normal, disease-free tissue in the outermost layer of cells of a surgical sample.

extramedullary Outside the bone marrow.

hematopoiesis The normal formation and development of blood cells in the bone marrow.

hepatosplenomegaly Enlargement of the liver and spleen detected by palpation of the abdomen.

immunosuppression A weakening or cessation of the body's normal immune response.

intrathecal Within the spinal column.

leukokoria Appearance of a whitish reflex or mass in the pupillary area behind the lens of the eye.

lymphadenopathy Swelling of the lymph nodes detected by palpation.

malignant Abnormal cells that have invasive and unregulated growth and the potential to spread to distant locations in the body; life-threatening.

neutropenia Decrease in the number of circulating neutrophils that results in a decreased ability of the body to fight infection.

protocol A systematic plan of care outlining drug therapy and follow-up care based on research in cancer treatment.

thrombocytopenia A reduction in platelet count; places the individual at risk for increased bruising and bleeding.

REVIEW OF CANCER

A *neoplasm* is any tumor that arises from new, abnormal growth. A tumor may be either benign or malignant. The distinguishing feature of cancer is its ability to invade surrounding tissue and spread to distant sites. Cancer cells spread in one of two ways: (1) by *invasion*, in which cells grow in unrestricted disorderly fashion at the site of origin; and (2) by *metastasis*, in which the cells grow in sites other than the site of the primary cancer. The cancerous cells grow progressively. The cells have lost the ability to perform their intended functions because changes in the cell's deoxyribonucleic acid (DNA) cause "wrong" information to be transmitted. As the cancerous cells continue to proliferate, they crowd out normal cells and compress vascular structures and vital organs, which results in symptoms.

Tumor staging is based on the results of diagnostic studies and in some cases surgical examination. Staging describes the extent of disease locally, regionally, and systemically and guides the therapy for most solid tumors. Each tumor has its own specific system of staging, which assists in determining treatment and prognosis.

The cause of most childhood cancers is unknown. It is currently believed that the underlying cause of cancer is genetic. Alterations in normal DNA occur, which predispose the individual to the development of cancer. A small percentage of

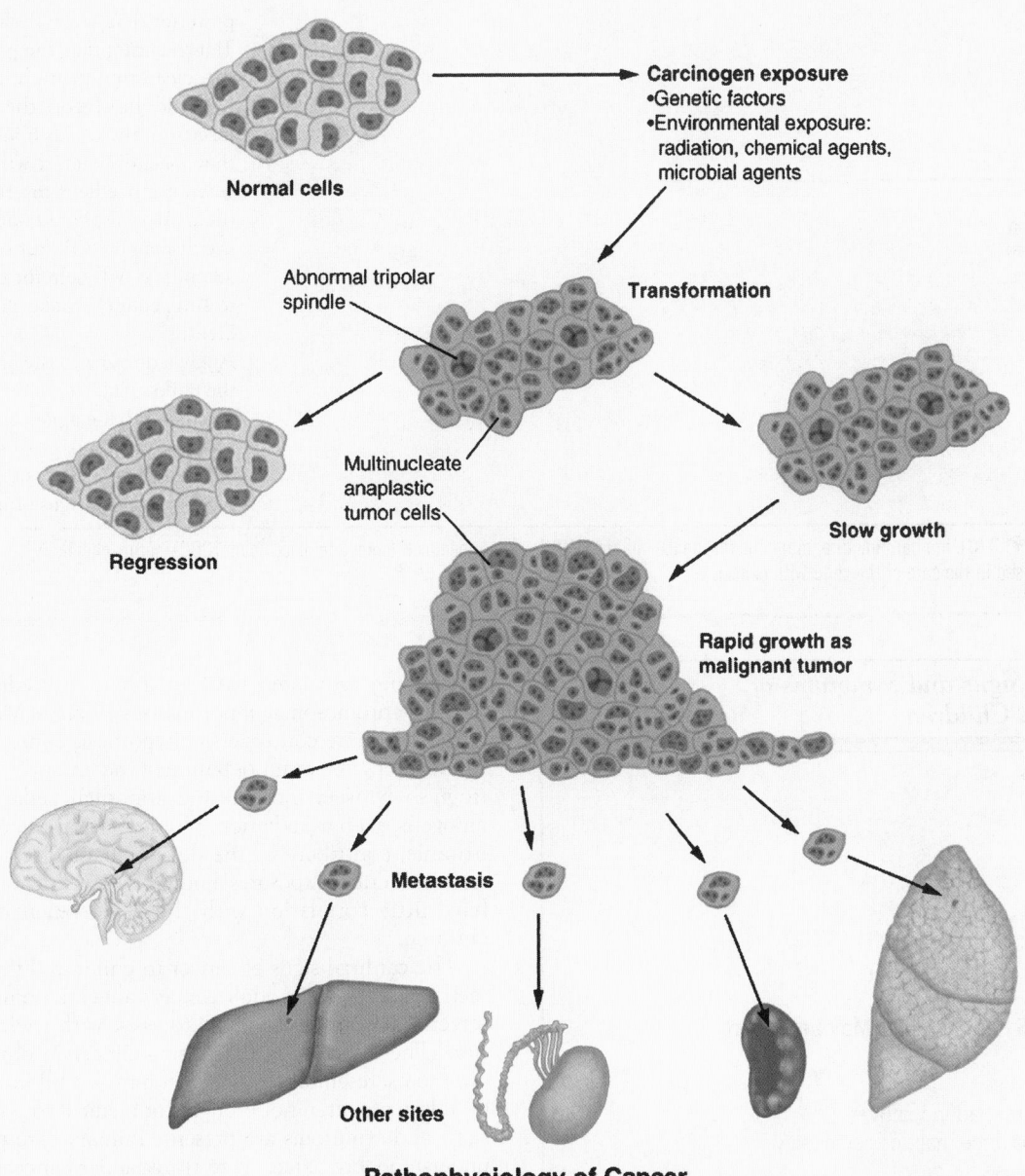

Pathophysiology of Cancer

CLINICAL REFERENCE

Diagnostic Tests and Procedures for Cancer

Test	Description	Purpose	Nursing Considerations
Bone marrow aspiration	Bone marrow is aspirated from the anterior or posterior iliac crests (the tibia is sometimes used in infants).	Pathologic examination of the aspirated material shows the presence, absence, and ratio of cells that are specific to and diagnostic of certain diseases. Some conditions that can be diagnosed are leukemia, specific vitamin deficiencies, neoplastic diseases in which the marrow is invaded by tumor cells, and agranulocytosis.	1. Describe the procedure to the child and parents. Check the signed consent. Allow parents to stay with the child if they wish. 2. Depending on the protocol of the facility, the child may receive a wide range of sedative or anesthetic agents. Some centers use local anesthesia with no systemic sedation; others use a combination of a sedative and an analgesic. 3. The child should be positioned prone with a small pillow under the hips to facilitate access to the posterior iliac crest, the usual site. Tell the child that the physician will clean the site and that it will feel cold. Just before the needle insertion, the child should be told that some discomfort will be felt when the needle is inserted and the marrow aspirated but that the discomfort will last only a few seconds; it will help for the child to sing, count, or take slow, deep breaths. 4. Apply a dressing to the area. If the child's platelet count is below 50,000/mm^3, use a pressure dressing. Monitor vital signs until stable, and monitor the puncture site for bleeding and later for signs of infection.

NOTE: See Chapter 52 (CT, lumbar puncture, magnetic resonance imaging [MRI]); and Appendix H (complete blood count [CBC], serum chemistry, urinalysis) for other common tests used in the care of the child with cancer.

Cardinal Signs and Symptoms of Cancer in Children

Overt Signs
A mass
Purpura
Pallor
Weight loss
Whitish reflex in the eye
Vomiting in early morning
Recurrent or persistent fever

Signs and Symptoms that May be Covert
Bone pain
Headache
Persistent lymphadenopathy
Change in balance, gait, or personality
Fatigue, malaise

cancers are associated with an inherited predisposition related to chromosomal abnormalities (Plon & Malkin, 2002). A second, more controversial hypothesis contends that cancer develops as a result of failure of the immune system to distinguish between normal and abnormal cells. Known carcinogens, such as radiation, physical irritation, and chemical irritants, contribute to the development of cancer. Certain environmental exposures known to cause cancer in adults have little correlation with the development of cancer in children.

The cardinal signs of cancer in children differ from those seen in adults. Most adult cancers are carcinomas, and more screening tools are available to assist with their early detection. The difficulty in diagnosing cancer in children is that symptoms resemble those of common childhood illnesses. Children are often not brought for medical care until obvious signs and symptoms are present. Primary care providers are understandably reluctant to think about cancer as the cause of the child's illness.

Diagnostic Tests and Procedures for Cancer—cont'd

Test	Description	Purpose	Nursing Considerations
Bone scintigraphy	A radio-labeled nucleotide is injected into the bloodstream. This tracer migrates to areas of the body in a predictable pattern.	Pattern of uptake in the axial skeleton is evaluated for variation from normal. Areas of increased uptake indicate increased cellular turnover related to growth, infection, trauma, or tumor activity.	Preparation similar to steps 1 and 2 for bone marrow aspiration. The child will be asked to lie still for 45-60 min to complete testing.
Gallium scan	Similar to bone scintigraphy.	Radiotracer uptake occurs in areas of active Hodgkin's disease; 60%-70% of those with Hodgkin's disease have uptake of this isotope at diagnosis, which can be used as a marker for disease during and after therapy.	Preparation similar to steps 1 and 2 for bone marrow aspiration. The child will be asked to lie still for 45-60 min to complete testing.
Positron emission tomography (PET)	This study combines conventional nuclear medicine techniques with tomography and adds double-photon imaging, which images metabolic activity.	PET scans reveal differences in metabolic processes. Tumor cells have accelerated glycolysis compared with the tissues of origin. PET can be useful for diagnosis, staging, and follow-up monitoring.	Be sure the patient is not pregnant. Younger children may need sedation. Older children should be told about the scan and allowed to see the equipment.
Single-photon emission computed tomography (SPECT)	This study combines the techniques of conventional nuclear medicine imaging with that of computed tomography (CT) using gamma-emitting radioactive isotopes.	SPECT displays a normal organ in axial, parasagittal, and coronal sections.	Same as for PET.

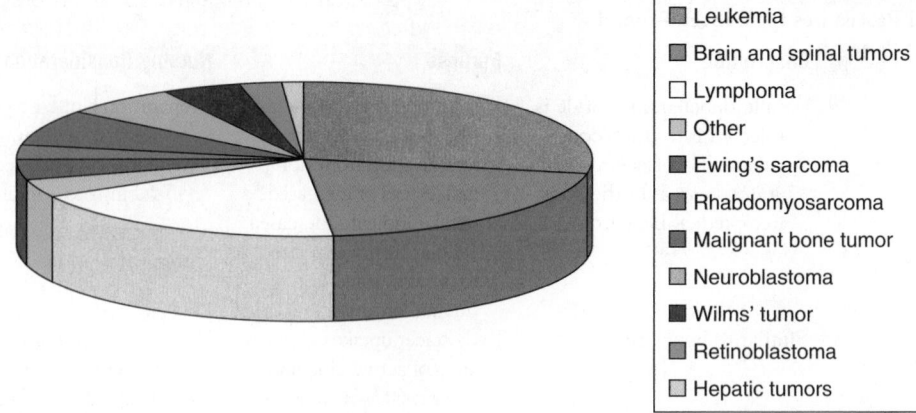

Leukemia
Brain and spinal tumors
Lymphoma
Other
Ewing's sarcoma
Rhabdomyosarcoma
Malignant bone tumor
Neuroblastoma
Wilms' tumor
Retinoblastoma
Hepatic tumors

Figure 48-1 Pie chart depicting incidence of cancers in children.

THE CHILD WITH CANCER

Cancer in children is often difficult to diagnose, and health care providers must be aware of the clinical manifestations that should raise the suspicion of cancer. The signs and symptoms depend on the type of tumor, the extent of the disease, and the child's age. Testing, diagnosis, and initiation of therapy may occur within a very short time period. The diagnosis of cancer can be devastating to both the child and the family. The nurse becomes the informational lifeline for the child and the family as they go through the treatment process.

Incidence

Cancer is uncommon in children; nevertheless, childhood cancer is the second leading cause of death during childhood, following unintentional injuries. Cancer is the leading cause of death from disease in childhood. Fourteen childhood cancers per 100,000 children younger than 15 years and 20 cancers per 100,000 children ages 15 to 19 years are diagnosed each year (Greenlee, Murray, Bolden, & Wingo, 2000). Childhood cancer represents only about 1% of all cancers diagnosed annually. Treatment challenges include minimizing treatment-related side effects while maintaining the child's normal growth and development (Fig. 48-1).

Childhood Cancer and Its Treatment

Children with cancer are treated in a multidisciplinary setting. Pediatric oncology nurses play a prominent role in the care of children with cancer and their families. They support and educate the children and their families as they move through a stressful process. Pediatric oncology nurses are challenged to maintain a high level of technical competence and an ability to provide the psychological support required by the child and family. Working with children with cancer can be an emotional experience. The nurse in this setting must have a support system and be aware of personal limitations.

A great deal of research has been done over the past 30 years to improve the outcome for children with cancer. Current survival rates are attributed to cooperative, systematic research through the Children's Oncology Group (COG) and the International Society for Pediatric Oncology. Each group meets twice a year to develop new protocols and monitor the progress of current protocols; subgroups meet as needed

throughout the year. Protocols direct when drugs are to be given, how frequently, and in what dosages, as well as which diagnostic and follow-up studies are to be done. Research has shown that children have better outcomes if they are treated on a scientifically derived protocol.

Because of the efforts of cooperative pediatric clinical trials, approximately 74% of children diagnosed with cancer will survive 5 years or longer after their diagnosis (Greenlee et al., 2000). It is estimated that there are now more than 100,000 adult survivors of childhood cancer. The marked improvement in childhood cancer survival has placed renewed emphasis on the importance of identifying the long-term sequelae of cancer treatment in children and initiating timely intervention (Friedman & Meadows, 2002).

Even after apparently successful treatment of cancer in children, cancer may recur. A recurrence may occur shortly after therapy has been completed or years later. A second tumor may represent a new (or second) malignancy. Recurrence represents the failure to cure the initial disease, whereas a second cancer is a likely result of the initial treatment. For example, some children with acute lymphocytic leukemia (ALL) develop acute myelocytic leukemia (AML) after therapy is complete. A small number of children with ALL who were treated with radiation to their central nervous system (CNS) may develop brain tumors.

Therapeutic Management

Chemotherapy, surgery, and radiation therapy are the primary treatment modalities for children with cancer. Bone marrow transplantation (BMT), stem cell transplantation, and biologic response modifiers are reserved for a specific subpopulation of children with cancer.

Chemotherapy

Chemotherapy is the use of drugs (antineoplastic agents) to kill cancer cells. Different drugs have different side effect profiles and modes of action. Combinations of drugs known individually to be active against the specific disease are used. Tumors possess the ability to develop resistance to chemotherapy agents, so a variety of active drugs are frequently used. Chemotherapy may be given orally, intravenously, intramuscularly, subcutaneously, or intrathecally (via the spinal column). Depending on the protocol, a child may be hospitalized for chemotherapy, receive it on an outpatient basis, or be treated at home.

The side effects of chemotherapeutic agents represent challenges to caregivers. Chemotherapy nonselectively kills rapidly dividing cells. The cells most often affected include cells of the hematopoietic system, gastrointestinal (GI) tract, and integumentary system (Box 48-1).

The bone marrow cells are one of the rapidly proliferating tissues adversely affected by many chemotherapy agents. Bone marrow production may become suppressed, resulting in neutropenia, anemia, and/or thrombocytopenia. The nadir—the time of the greatest bone marrow suppression—generally occurs 7 to 10 days after chemotherapy administration, depending on the specific agent used. The greatest concern during the period of bone marrow suppression is infection.

Neutropenia places the child with cancer at risk for the development of opportunistic infections. Opportunistic infections are caused by nonpathogenic bacteria and fungi, which, because of compromised immunity, may invade and cause infection. Bacteria, generally present on the skin and within the gut, may invade the bloodstream via a break in the skin, leading to a life-threatening infection. In the presence of markedly decreased white blood cells (WBCs), the usual inflammatory response (erythema, edema, swelling), indicative of an infection, is not present. Fever is frequently the only indication of infection. Health care providers and families must remain acutely aware of elevated body temperature and breaks in the skin during periods of neutropenia.

The GI tract is affected in a number of ways. Chemotherapy represents a noxious stimulus that triggers nausea and vomiting. The treatment of nausea and vomiting was revolutionized in 1992 with the release of the class of non-sedating antiemetic drugs called *5-HT3 serotonin antagonists*. These drugs include ondansetron (Zofran), granisetron (Kytril), and dolasetron (Anzemet). They have been more effective in combating hemotherapy-induced nausea and vomiting than earlier antiemetics.

Anorexia is associated not only with nausea but also with a change in taste experienced by some people in response to certain chemotherapeutic agents. Some children use anorexia as a way to exert what little control they have left after the diagnosis.

Certain chemotherapeutic agents cause sloughing of the mucosal tissue of the GI tract, leading to the development of mucositis and esophagitis. This condition can be painful and can contribute to poor nutrition. Bacteria and yeasts, present as part of the normal digestive process in the mouth and gut, may cross the open skin and be absorbed into the bloodstream. The presence of breaks in the integument may lead to bacterial infections of the blood.

Decreased activity, pain medication, and poor oral intake may contribute to the development of constipation. Certain chemotherapeutic agents may also contribute to constipation. Passage of hard stool may cause abrasion of the delicate mucous membrane of the rectum. The stool is loaded with microorganisms as part of the digestive process. Again, the presence of breaks in the integument may lead to bacterial infections of the blood.

Hair loss has a tremendous psychological effect, especially on the school-age and adolescent population. Some chemotherapeutic agents do not produce hair loss, but most do. Treatment-related fatigue, common in adult cancer patients, is poorly reported in the child and adolescent populations. Other side effects are specific to the agent being used, as well as the dose.

Nurses administering chemotherapeutic agents should be trained by the institution in which they work. Currently, there is no nationally recognized chemotherapy administration certification. Nursing responsibilities and precautions related to chemotherapy administration are detailed in Box 48-2.

Surgery

Surgery is frequently part of cancer therapy for children. The surgery may be limited to a biopsy or be used to remove a solid tumor mass. The purpose of a biopsy is to obtain a small piece of the tumor for microscopic examination. Examination of the tissue by a pathologist confirms the tumor type and influences therapy decisions. Surgery may also be used to debulk or resect a solid tumor mass. In some diseases, the tumor cannot be resected at the beginning of therapy. After the child has received some chemotherapy, the mass may decrease in size and a less extensive surgical procedure may be performed (see Chapter 37 for a discussion of preoperative care).

A central venous catheter is frequently placed to facilitate chemotherapy administration. A central venous catheter is a Silastic tube placed to provide easy access to the venous system; the proximal part of the catheter ends in the large vein just above the heart, the superior vena cava. There are essentially three types of central venous catheters. In an external catheter, the distal portion exits the skin and a tiny Dacron cuff is located under the exit site where the skin will adhere and hold the catheter in place. In an implanted catheter, the distal portion ends in a well, which is placed in the subcutaneous tissue, frequently in the anterior chest wall. A percutaneously (peripherally) inserted central catheter (PICC) is not surgically placed. The proximal tip ends in the same large vein as other catheters, but the distal portion is not tunneled. The catheter is frequently inserted in the antecubital fossa using a technique similar to placement of a peripheral intravenous (IV) catheter.

Radiation Therapy

Radiation may be given curatively to eradicate disease or palliatively in low doses to prevent further growth of a tumor. Total body irradiation given before some BMTs attempts to eradicate microscopic disease and promote bone

BOX 48-1
Common Side Effects of Chemotherapy and Radiation Therapy

Chemotherapeutic drugs and radiation therapy affect normal as well as abnormal cells, primarily cells that divide rapidly, such as cells of the gastrointestinal (GI) tract, hair follicles, and bone marrow. As a result, children undergoing these therapies frequently experience the following.

Chemotherapy Side Effects
Bone marrow suppression
Alopecia
Malaise and fatigue
Nausea
Vomiting
Anorexia
Stomatitis

Radiation Side Effects
Skin reactions
Fatigue
Bone marrow suppression
Nausea
Vomiting
Anorexia
Mucositis

Side Effects of Radiation to the Brain

Acute (During and Shortly After Irradiation)
Brain edema
Transient increase in neurologic symptoms
General radiation side effects listed previously

Subacute (1 to 6 Months After Irradiation)
Somnolence syndrome—pronounced drowsiness, nausea, and malaise (typically 4 to 8 weeks after completing radiation therapy)
Fever
Irritability
Ataxia
Anorexia
Dysphasia

Late Effects (More Than 6 Months After Irradiation)
Morphologic changes—cerebral atrophy, white matter degeneration, necrosis, calcification
Functional changes—encephalopathy, neuropsychological deterioration, focal neurologic deficits
Alopecia within the radiation field

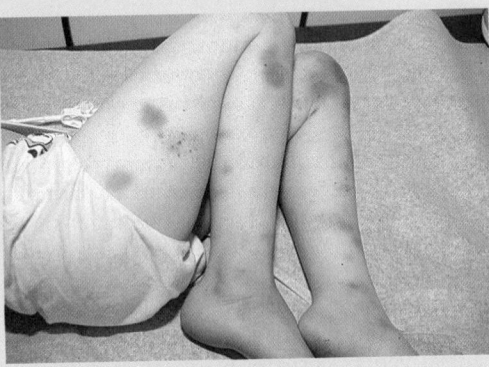

Suppression of the bone marrow because of chemotherapy or radiation therapy reduces the blood counts. Low platelet levels lead to spontaneous bruising, as shown here. Nosebleeds and bleeding of the gums are other consequences. The nurse must make a special effort to observe for bruising in dark-skinned children because it will be more difficult to see.

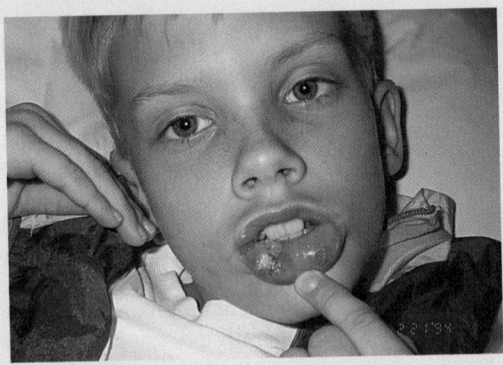

Mucositis (inflammation of the mucous membranes) and mouth ulcers are common side effects of chemotherapeutic drugs. Any mucous membrane can be affected.

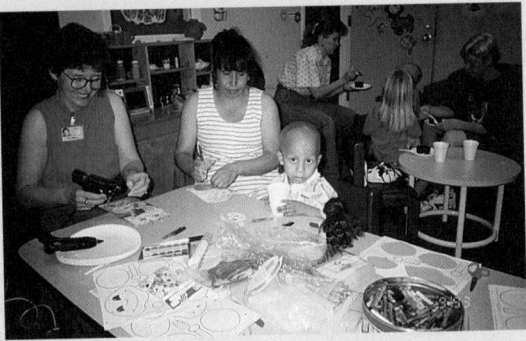

Hair loss is a distressing side effect of cancer treatment. School-age children and adolescents are most likely to feel this distress. Activities such as crafts or play groups help children feel more normal and provide interaction with others in an accepting environment.

Photos courtesy Cook Children's Medical Center, Fort Worth, TX.

BOX 48-2
Nursing Responsibilities and Precautions for Chemotherapy

- Know Occupational Safety and Health Administration (OSHA) guidelines for administration of antineoplastic agents.
- Measure child's height and weight accurately.
- Confirm body surface area (BSA)—calculated in square meters and used to determine dosages.
- Always double-check the ordered dosage against the BSA.
- Always double-check the ordered dosage against protocol recommendations.
- Always double-check the medication against the original physician's order.
- A complete blood count should be obtained within 48 hours preceding administration of chemotherapy.
- The white blood cell and platelet counts need to be at a predetermined level before chemotherapy is given.
- Know the potential side effects of the drugs being administered and appropriate actions to ameliorate those effects.
- Ensure the patency of intravenous (IV) tubing before giving drugs by checking for blood return.
- If using an implantable infusion device, ensure that needle placement is secure and blood returns.
- Vesicants (agents that produce blisters) should be given through a fresh IV site.
- Have emergency drugs available.

---

marrow suppression. Radiation may be given in hyperfractionated doses, in which the daily dose is split into smaller doses given more frequently to minimize side effects and to increase tumor kill by decreasing time for cell repair between doses.

Preparing the child and family for radiation involves education about the process in addition to the side effects. Some institutions provide a pre-radiation tour so the child may experience the room and surroundings before therapy. During the tour, children should be shown the window or monitor through which they will be observed while undergoing radiation alone in the room. Some children need to be sedated for radiation treatments; others can be coached to lie still with the help of child life specialists and parents. The child must lie still for prolonged periods because the radiation oncologist must control the depth and peripheral margins of the radiation site very carefully.

The side effects of radiation are dose and treatment site specific. As with chemotherapy, side effects are a result of radiation's effect on healthy, rapidly dividing cells. The side effects usually appear 7 to 10 days after the initiation of therapy. Acute side effects usually dissipate within days or a few weeks of cessation of the radiation therapy. The decision regarding radiation dose, frequency, and location depends on the purpose of the radiation and the disease process being treated.

Erythema within the radiated area is the most common side effect. Fatigue associated with therapy may necessitate more frequent rest periods than parents are used to their child taking. Anorexia, nausea, and vomiting commonly occur. Radiation therapy will also cause bone marrow suppression, depending on the dose and site of therapy.

Radiation therapy slows the growth of tumors and kills rapidly dividing cells nonselectively. Unfortunately, in a developing child, normal cell development may not be complete when radiation exposure occurs. Radiation therapy to developing brain tissue may alter cognitive potential. In children younger than 3 years, the effect of radiation therapy can be cognitively devastating. Bone growth is altered if radiation therapy is delivered to areas of growth potential, such as facial bones, spine, or growth plates in long bones. The result, many years later, may be skeletal malformations.

The use of radiation as a treatment modality is not without risk. Radiation exposure has been linked to the development of certain types of cancer, and radiation exposure to treat cancer may lead to the development of a second malignancy. It is estimated that approximately 8% of children treated for cancer will develop a second malignancy. A subset of this 8% will be linked to the exposure to radiation as a primary treatment.

Hematopoietic Stem Cell Transplantation

In recent years, the use of hematopoietic stem cell or bone marrow transplantation (BMT) has become accepted therapy for the treatment of several hematologic and oncologic disorders. Transplantation allows extremely high doses of chemotherapy (with or without radiation) to be given without regard for bone marrow recovery, because hematopoiesis will be restored through transplantation.

BMT uses bone marrow to reconstitute the immunologic function of the patient after high-dose chemotherapy. Stem cell transplantation uses a unique immature cell present in the peripheral circulation to restore immunologic function in a similar manner. Stem cells are able to differentiate into any type of hematologic cell.

The healthy bone marrow cells or stem cells are infused into the bloodstream and migrate to the marrow space to replenish the patient's immunologic function. The decision regarding the source of marrow or stem cells depends on the disease process being treated.

Recent advances in the understanding of histocompatibility and advances in supportive care have improved outcomes in allogeneic (matched related or unrelated donor) bone marrow transplants. Autologous (the patient's own harvested stem cells) peripheral blood stem cell transplant is done in certain instances to allow more aggressive chemotherapy than could be safely given without fear of total bone marrow ablation. Peripheral blood stem cells (PBSCs) are then given back to "rescue" and restore hematopoietic function.

Umbilical cord blood is another source of transplanted stem cells. Since it is now possible to electively "bank" or store umbilical cord blood, this source is becoming more significant. Bone marrow from infants has a higher concentration of nucleated cells and probably a higher proportion of marrow repopulating cells than bone marrow from older donors (Guinan, Krance, & Lehmann, 2002). A national or international search for a matched, unrelated donor can be done through the National Marrow Donor Program (NMDP).

In preparation for a transplant, the child begins a regimen of chemotherapy with or without radiation (called *conditioning*). The goal of conditioning is to eradicate any disease from the body with high-dose chemotherapy and radiation therapy. WBC, red blood cell (RBC), and platelet counts begin to drop as the chemotherapy and radiation exert their effects on the bone marrow. When the conditioning phase is over, the child receives the donor marrow or stem cell by IV infusion.

Once the marrow is infused, nursing care focuses on preventing profoundly immunosuppressed children from developing life-threatening infections. The "waiting game" begins for parents and children until the daily complete blood cell count (CBC) begins to show signs of marrow engraftment. The production of WBCs, RBCs, and platelets from the transplantation of normal cells is evidence that the marrow has "engrafted," or been accepted by the body.

Common complications in the days and weeks after a BMT include mucositis, diarrhea, fevers, and nosebleeds. Children receive aggressive nutritional support because most will not be able to take food and fluids as a result of severe mucositis and GI discomfort and diarrhea.

The major problem associated with allogeneic transplants is graft-versus-host disease (GVHD). GVHD is caused when the infused immunocompetent bone marrow recognizes the recipient's tissue as foreign. GVHD may affect numerous organ systems. Children may exhibit a wide variety of symptoms associated with GVHD, such as mild to severely elevated liver enzyme levels, mild to copious diarrhea, and maculopapular skin reactions ranging from rashes to full skin desquamation. Antirejection drugs are given to prevent GVHD from occurring or to lessen its severity.

Transplantation is currently standard therapy for children in first remission with Philadelphia chromosome–positive ALL (a genetically specific type of ALL with a 90% relapse rate), AML, stage IV neuroblastoma, severe aplastic anemia, severe combined immunodeficiency syndrome, and certain other hematologic disorders. Transplantation is also used for children with solid tumors, Hodgkin's disease, and non-Hodgkin's lymphoma resistant to conventional chemotherapy and radiation, as evidenced by their relapse while the child is receiving therapy.

Biologic Response Modifiers

The most recent additions to cancer therapy are the biologic response modifiers. Biologic response modifiers are naturally occurring substances found in small quantities in the body that influence immune system functions (e.g., colony-stimulating factors [CSFs]).

Used to enhance cell recovery, different CSFs work on different types of blood cells to reduce the time and severity of bone marrow suppression. The granulocyte colony-stimulating factors (GCSFs) stimulate WBC recovery. GCSFs may reduce the length of time a child experiences neutropenia by stimulating production of neutrophils, a type of granulocyte. Other CSFs may promote recovery of platelets or RBCs to reduce the need for blood products.

Over the past few years, a number of immune modulating agents have been examined in the laboratory with very few translating into clinically beneficial treatment modalities. Interleukin, a protein that mobilizes the immune response, monoclonal antibodies, interferon, and activated T cell antigens are all in ongoing clinical trials to evaluate their role in the treatment of cancer (Lum, 1999).

LEUKEMIA

Leukemia is the most common form of cancer in children younger than 15 years. Leukemia is caused by proliferation of immature WBCs. Considerable progress in its treatment has been achieved through years of research. Leukemia was uni-formly fatal in the 1960s. Today, children diagnosed with the most common form of leukemia, acute lymphocytic leukemia (ALL), with a disease-free survival rate approaching 85%.

Etiology

The cause of childhood leukemia is unknown. Geographic distribution varies around the world, with leukemia being uncommon in developing countries but more common in industrialized countries. This variation may be correlated with underdiagnosis in developing countries or exposure to agents that may be implicated in the development of leukemia in industrialized countries.

Genetic factors appear to play a significant role in the development of leukemia. When karyotyped, the leukemic cells in more than 90% of children with the disease reveal chromosomal abnormalities (Friebert & Shurin, 1998a). The twin of a child who has had ALL has a slightly higher likelihood of developing the disease than other children. For monozygous twins, the unaffected twin has a 25% risk of developing the disease in the first year after the affected twin is diagnosed. At age 7 years, the unaffected twin's risk drops to that of the general population (Friebert & Shurin, 1998a). Children with Down syndrome have a twenty-fold greater risk of developing leukemia than the general population (Plon & Malkin, 2002). Other less-common preexisting chromosomal abnormalities have been correlated with the development of leukemia.

Exposure to ionizing radiation and certain chemical toxins has been shown to increase the risk of developing leukemia. Leukemia was well documented in both the child and adult survivors of the atomic bomb explosions in Japan during World War II. Chemical exposure to alkylating agents, a drug class used to treat cancer, has been shown to increase the risk of developing AML.

Exposure to pesticides, electromagnetic fields, or parental smoking; parental alcohol use; or parental exposures to occupational chemicals have not demonstrated a relationship to leukemia in childhood. Large epidemiologic studies are ongoing.

Incidence

Leukemia represents 38% of all childhood cancers (Smith & Ries, 2002). Approximately 3000 new cases of childhood leukemia are diagnosed each year in the United States (Margolin, Steuber, & Poplack, 2002). Overall incidence of ALL has been constant for the past 30 years and accounts for 80% of all cases of leukemia, AML accounts for 15% to 20%, and chronic myelocytic leukemia (CML) and other subtypes are relatively rare. The peak incidence occurs between ages 2 and 5 years for ALL. Leukemia is more common in boys than in girls.

Manifestations

Clinical manifestations of leukemia include fever, pallor, excessive bruising, bone or joint pain (usually leg pain), lymphadenopathy, malaise, hepatosplenomegaly, abnormal WBC counts (either lower or higher than normal for age), and mild to profound anemia and thrombocytopenia. The severity of the clinical manifestations varies with the cell type of leukemia and the length of time before diagnosis.

Pathophysiology

of Leukemia

Leukemia most likely arises from a fundamental alteration in the genetic makeup of the white cell. Cells produced from the altered cell have a defect that prevents maturation. These cells tend to replicate quickly, forming immature cells, or blast cells, in the bone marrow, crowding other normal cells produced. The blast cells do not respond properly to the body's feedback mechanism and continue to replicate in great numbers. Blast cells are then released into the peripheral circulation and appear in a complete blood count test.

In leukemia, normal bone marrow is replaced by malignant blast cells. As the blast cells take over the bone marrow, eventually red blood cell (RBC) and platelet production is affected and the child becomes anemic and thrombocytopenic. The symptoms of the disease reflect bone marrow failure and organ infiltration.

In addition to being present in the blood and bone marrow, leukemia cells infiltrate extramedullary sites, most commonly the central nervous system (CNS) and the testicles. Although it is not common to see extramedullary leukemia at time of diagnosis, these are common sites of relapse.

Leukemias are classified by the type of white blood cell (WBC) affected. Broadly, acute leukemias are classified as acute lymphocytic leukemia (ALL) and acute nonlymphocytic leukemia (ANLL). ALL is an abnormality of the lymphocytes. ANLL is a broad term for leukemias not originating from abnormal lymphocytes. Acute myelocytic leukemia (AML) is one such leukemia. AML can be further classified as acute promyelocytic leukemia (APL), acute myelomonocytic leukemia (AMMoL), and acute monocytic leukemia (AMoL). ANLL tends to be less common in children, less responsive to therapy, difficult to treat, and more likely to result in relapse than ALL.

Chronic leukemias are rare in children. The term *chronic* refers to the indolent nature of the disease. Whereas acute leukemias have a rapid onset to detectable disease, chronic leukemias have a slower onset of symptoms.

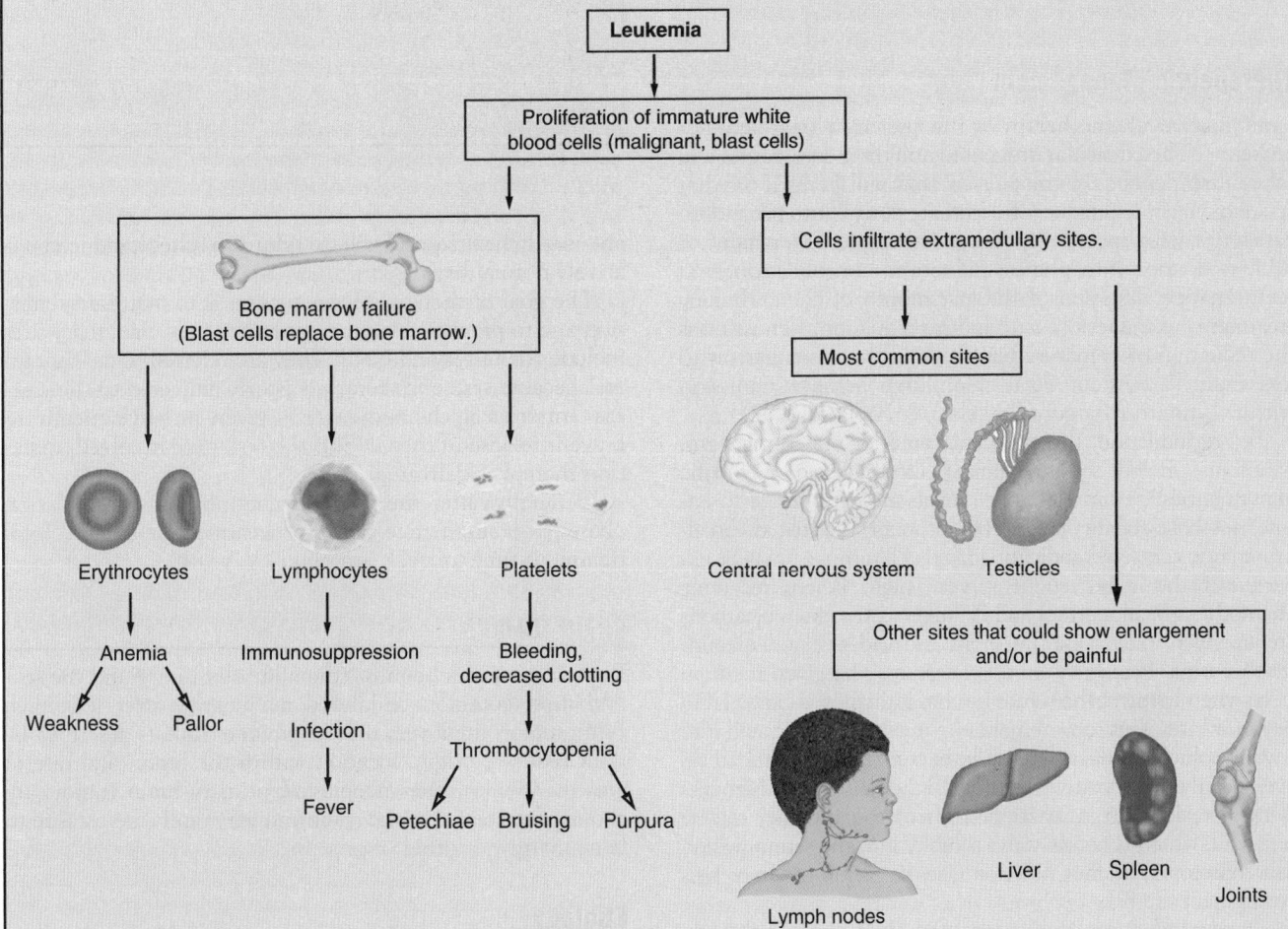

Diagnostic Evaluation

The diagnosis can be strongly suspected from a history of the clinical manifestations and an initial CBC. The confirmatory test for leukemia is microscopic examination of bone marrow obtained by bone marrow aspiration and biopsy. A bone marrow aspirate alone usually provides sufficient material to establish the diagnosis of ALL. A lumbar puncture is also done to look for blast cells in the spinal fluid that are indicative of CNS involvement.

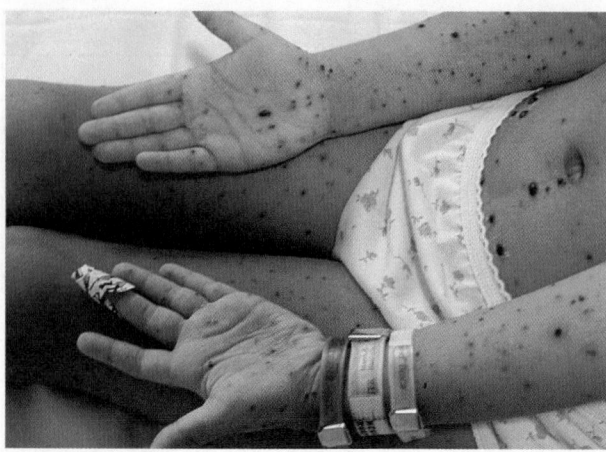

Figure 48-2 Varicella (chickenpox) can be deadly in the immunocompromised child. Thrombocytopenia (low platelet count) associated with chemotherapy can cause the varicella lesions to be hemorrhagic, like those shown here. Secondary infections of the lesions are also common because of low white blood cell (WBC) counts. (Courtesy Cook Children's Medical Center, Hematology-Oncology Clinic, Fort Worth, TX.)

Therapeutic Management

Combination chemotherapy is the preferred treatment for leukemia. The particular drugs used and their dose, route, and scheduling depend on the *protocol* that will be used for that specific type of leukemia. Children are placed into prognostic categories with specifically tailored therapies. Treatment of ALL is divided into phases: induction, consolidation, and maintenance. The aim of the first month of chemotherapy treatment, or induction, is to induce remission. Remission is the reduction of immature blast cells in the bone marrow to less than 5%. About 95% of children achieve remission within 1 month (Margolin, Steuber, & Poplack, 2002).

Before induction, the child is treated for presenting signs, which may include sepsis, anemia, hemorrhage, and metabolic abnormalities. Serum electrolyte levels are determined to ensure metabolic stability before chemotherapy is initiated. An elevated uric acid level, indicating rapid cell turnover, may be expected if the WBC count is very high. Before receiving chemotherapy, allopurinol and IV fluids with sodium bicarbonate are given to decrease the serum uric acid level and alkalinize the urine. Parenteral urate oxidase may be given in situations when lysing of the tumor by chemotherapy is expected to be significant. This recombinant enzyme oxidizes uric acid into a water-soluble product that can be excreted (Lohr, 2002). This is especially important when the WBC count is very high. As WBCs break down in reaction to chemotherapy, they release uric acid, which is poorly water soluble, into the serum, which can compromise kidney function (see discussion of tumor lysis syndrome, p. 1349).

During induction, the hospitalized child receives the first doses of chemotherapy while the response to the drugs is assessed. Remission can be verified within the first 28 days after the initiation of chemotherapy by sequential bone marrow aspirates and lumbar punctures. If a significant number of blast cells are still present, a new and stronger drug regimen is given. The presence of more than 5% blasts in the marrow at day 28 is an ominous sign, indicative of a poorer prognosis.

Once the child is medically stable, most chemotherapy treatment for ALL is given on an outpatient basis. Children

are usually healthy and able to return to school and lead relatively normal lives.

The goal of therapy after remission is to maintain remission and to prevent disease in sanctuary sites. Sanctuary sites include the testes and CNS. They are referred to as "sanctuary" because systemic therapy is poorly delivered to these areas. Intrathecal chemotherapy is given prophylactically to prevent relapse in the CNS. If the testes are involved, radiation therapy is delivered.

Generally, after the initial induction and consolidation phases, a maintenance phase of treatment is begun. Total treatment time for ALL is around 2 1/2 years.

BRAIN TUMORS

Brain tumors are the most common solid tumor and the second most common childhood malignancy after leukemia. Brain tumors are a very diverse group of tumors described by their tissue of origin, location within the brain, and rate of growth. Unlike other neoplasms, primary brain tumors are confined to the brain and spine and very rarely metastasize to bone marrow or other organs.

Etiology

The cause of brain tumors remains unknown. Heredity and environment have both been associated with their development. Several inherited syndromes are associated with the development of brain tumors in children, such as neurofibromatosis and tuberous sclerosis. Additional risk factors include immune system suppression and cranial irradiation. Although it has been suggested that exposure to electromagnetic fields increases a child's risk of developing a brain tumor, no confirming evidence supports this theory (Gurney & Bondy, 2002).

Text continued on p. 1344

Nursing Care Plan

The Child With Leukemia

FOCUSED ASSESSMENT

Subjective data almost always reveal an insidious onset of symptoms. The parents may have recognized the following: their child was less active than normal, had a persistent or recurrent fever of unknown cause, had more bruises than usual, complained of an intermittent stomachache that the parents attributed to school avoidance, or had leg pain attributed to growing pains or laziness. Parents commonly express guilt because they did not recognize anything was wrong with their child sooner, or, if they did notice, the manifestations were so vague they delayed seeking treatment. Psychosocial assessment of the family is ongoing.

Children often present with fever, fatigue, pallor, bruising on the extremities, petechiae in the mouth and sclera, and hepatosplenomegaly. Children with very high white blood cell (WBC) counts or acute myelocytic leukemia (AML) may present with more pronounced manifestations, such as bleeding. The mental and neurologic status of the child is assessed because of the risk of infiltration into the central nervous system (CNS).

Observe both the child's and the parents' reactions to the disease. The emotional maturity of the child and the family will affect how each person copes with the illness and treatment. The child's chronologic age and stage of development as well as previous experience with the health care system are critical factors in the assessment.

Parents who are unable to cope with the disease and who display a high level of anxiety will transfer this anxiety to their child. Children who have had previous negative experiences associated with hospitals, nurses, and physicians may exhibit increased anxiety. Families who have had prior experience with cancer may exhibit increased anxiety and need for support.

Nursing Diagnosis

Risk for Infection related to the immunosuppressed state.

Expected Outcomes

The child will:
- Be free of signs of infection, as evidenced by an afebrile state, no redness of the integument, no redness or swelling at the site of insertion of a central venous catheter, and negative culture results.

The parents and the child will:
- Recognize and verbalize early signs of infection.

INTERVENTION	RATIONALE
1. Monitor vital signs every 4 hr and as necessary if the child is hospitalized. Instruct parents to measure the child's temperature as needed at home (by the oral, axillary, or tympanic routes only).	1. In the presence of markedly decreased WBCs, an elevated temperature may be the only sign of infection. The risk of injury to the fragile mucous membranes is so great that only oral, tympanic, or axillary routes should be used to measure temperatures. Rectal abscesses can easily occur to friable rectal tissue. Temperatures should not be measured rectally. Report a single temperature ≥38.5° C or a temperature of 38.0° C that continues for over 1 hr.
2. Monitor complete blood cell count (CBC) with differential as ordered. Report moderate to severe neutropenia.	2. The risk of infection increases significantly with moderate and severe neutropenia.

Absolute Neutrophil Count (ANC)

(cells/mm³)	Risk
1500-2000	Not significant
1000-1500	Minimal
500-1000	Moderate
<500	Severe

INTERVENTION	RATIONALE
3. Practice proper handwashing, and teach this to the family.	3. Proper handwashing is the best way to prevent the spread of infection.
4. Inspect the child's skin daily for breaks and redness.	4. Some neutropenic children will not produce erythema or purulent drainage. Because pus is made of WBCs, drainage cannot be used as a sign of infection. Skin provides a barrier against infection.
5. Inspect the child's mouth daily for oral ulcers, and inspect the perineum for fissures. Teach older children to do self-examination. No suppositories should be given.	5. The mucous membranes are fragile and easily affected by chemotherapy and irradiation. Mouth ulcers and rectal fissures are common side effects of chemotherapy and radiation therapy and potential sites for bacteria entry because of the impaired mucosa.

Continued

Nursing Care Plan

The Child With Leukemia—cont'd

INTERVENTION	RATIONALE
6. Encourage and monitor regular bowel habits.	6. Decreased activity, altered nutrition, and certain medications may predispose to constipation. The passage of hard stool may traumatize delicate rectal mucous membranes and create a potential site for entry of bacteria.
7. Teach the parents and child meticulous oral hygiene at diagnosis: a. Use a soft-bristle toothbrush or toothettes. b. Perform oral hygiene four times a day. c. If the platelet count is low, use a cotton-tipped applicator, finger cot, or washcloth wrapped around a finger instead of a toothbrush.	7. Preventing dental caries and ulcerations on fragile oral mucosa will help prevent infections.
8. At the first signs of mouth ulcers, begin a mouth care regimen three or four times daily, including an antifungal drug as ordered by the physician. Avoid alcohol-containing mouthwashes.	8. Fungal infections originating from the mouth or gastrointestinal (GI) tract can quickly become disseminated in immunosuppressed children. Over-the-counter mouthwashes may have a high alcohol content and may be drying to oral mucosa, thus increasing the risk of breaking down the protective barrier of the skin.
9. For the hospitalized neutropenic child, fresh flowers or plants are usually not permitted. Do not use humidifiers.	9. Standing water and damp soil harbor *Aspergillus* and *Pseudomonas,* to which these children are very susceptible.
10. Use sterile techniques to change any dressings and intravenous (IV) lines.	10. Because the child with neutropenia is not able to fight infection normally, extra precautions must be taken.
11. The child should not receive live-virus or live bacterial vaccines. Siblings should receive inactivated polio vaccine but may receive live measles-mumps-rubella (MMR) vaccine or varicella vaccine.	11. Live virus is shed in the stool after administration of the polio vaccine. The live MMR vaccine could produce infection in the severely immunocompromised child, but no virus shedding occurs to create a threat if given to the sibling. Exposure to a rash produced by the varicella vaccine does have the potential of causing varicella disease in an immunocompromised child. If rash should occur in a vaccinated sibling, the immunocompromised child should be separated from the sibling until the rash resolves.
12. Keep any child with chickenpox or any child who has been exposed to the virus away from the child with cancer. Inform the teacher of the importance of notifying parents immediately if a case of chickenpox occurs in another child at school. Encourage vaccination of siblings who have not had varicella, to create herd immunity.	12. Immunocompromised patients are unable to fight varicella adequately. Chickenpox can be deadly to the immunocompromised child (see Fig. 48-2). If a child who has not had chickenpox is exposed to someone with varicella, the child should receive varicella-zoster immune globulin within 96 hours of exposure.
13. Obtain specimens for culture as ordered, and monitor the results.	13. Physicians will order blood, urine, stool, and wound cultures as signs appear when the neutropenic child has fever.
14. Administer acetaminophen for fever.	14. Aspirin and ibuprofen given to a child who is thrombocytopenic can cause platelet dysfunction.
15. Administer antibiotics as ordered after culture results are available.	15. Cultures identify the specific organism so that the most effective antibiotic can be given. Appropriate antibiotic treatment should begin promptly.

Evaluation

- Is the child afebrile and free of redness or swelling at insertion sites or other integumentary sites?
- Have the child and parents promptly recognized and responded to warning signs of infection?

Nursing Care Plan

The Child With Leukemia—cont'd

Nursing Diagnosis

Risk for Injury related to thrombocytopenia.

Expected Outcomes

The child will:
- Have no excessive, uncontrolled bleeding.

The parents and child will:
- Understand risk for hemorrhage, as evidenced by safety-proofing the home and by their ability to respond appropriately to bleeding.

INTERVENTION	RATIONALE
1. Apply gentle, firm pressure to any puncture sites. Apply a pressure dressing to sites of bone marrow aspiration.	1. Additional pressure may be needed to stop bleeding if the platelet count is low.
2. If the child is severely thrombocytopenic (platelet count <20,000/mm³), take the following steps: a. Limit any activity that could result in head injury; encourage the child to participate in quiet activities (e.g., reading books, watching videos, coloring). No contact sports are allowed. b. Provide a soft-bristle toothbrush only or toothettes. c. Give stool softeners to prevent straining with constipation. d. Do not use suppositories. e. Check urine and stools for blood. f. Avoid sharp foods such as chips.	2. A decreased platelet count increases the risk for bleeding. There is a potential risk for intracranial hemorrhage.
3. Teach the child how to control nosebleeds and to blow the nose gently.	3. One of the most common sites of bleeding is the nose. Blood loss can be reduced through avoidance of nosebleeds.
4. Evaluate menstrual flow in adolescent girls.	4. Menstrual bleeding can be severe when girls have low platelet counts. Occasionally, hormone therapy is required to inhibit menses.

Evaluation
- Has the child experienced bleeding that could not be controlled?
- Have the parents demonstrated what to do for a nosebleed?
- Have the child or parents promptly recognized and responded to bleeding?

Nursing Diagnosis

Imbalanced Nutrition: Less Than Body Requirements related to nausea and vomiting, mucositis, or taste changes.

Expected Outcomes

The child will:
- Experience no more than 5% weight loss.
- Eat palatable foods that provide appropriate nutrients for growth.

INTERVENTION	RATIONALE
1. Administer antiemetics prophylactically and as needed or as ordered.	1. Antiemetics will decrease or prevent vomiting.
2. When the child is nauseated, offer cool, clear liquids. Offer bland, soft foods at room temperature, served in small portions. Be creative with the liquids and foods offered to make them more interesting and inviting.	2. Cool liquids and foods are soothing and better tolerated than hot ones, and the risk of burning fragile mucosa is eliminated.
3. Offer small, frequent meals of high-protein and high-calorie content. Fortify foods with nutritional supplements. Allow the family to bring favorite foods to the hospital.	3. Small, frequent meals are better tolerated than large ones. Protein promotes tissue healing. High calories are needed for growth. Children are more likely to eat their favorite foods.

Continued

Nursing Care Plan

The Child With Leukemia—cont'd

INTERVENTION	RATIONALE
4. Do not offer favorite foods when the child is nauseated.	4. Foods eaten within hours of nausea will be associated with being sick.
5. Administer ordered mouth analgesics before oral intake.	5. If mouth sores are present, analgesics will increase comfort and provide interest in eating.
6. Monitor daily weight. Keep strict intake and output records. Weigh the infant's diapers.	6. Strict measurement ensures adequate intake and provides an objective assessment to alert the nurse that further interventions may be needed.
7. Involve the child in food selection.	7. Food selection allows the child control over as much as possible and may increase interest and participation in eating.
8. Include a dietitian in the nutritional assessment and evaluation.	8. A dietitian provides specialized input into developing and evaluating nutritional status.

Evaluation

- Did the child experience no more than 5% weight loss, as documented on a growth chart?
- Does the child eat foods that provide appropriate nutrients for growth?

Nursing Diagnosis

Deficient Knowledge related to unfamiliarity with the disease process and treatment plan.

Expected Outcomes

The child and parents will:
- Explain the diagnosis.
- Demonstrate compliance with treatment.

INTERVENTION	RATIONALE
1. Assess the child's and parents' readiness for learning. Create an environment of learning.	1. On initial diagnosis, family members may need time to adjust before they are ready for education. Offer written supporting information.
2. On initial diagnosis and during subsequent follow-up visits, spend time with the family, repeating and explaining the diagnosis, its sequelae, and its treatment. Offer written literature, or offer to tape educational sessions (see Parents Want to Know: About Caring for the Child With Cancer box, p. 1338).	2. Education is ongoing and will need reinforcing with stressed parents. Explaining the treatment rationale and sequelae helps ensure compliance with therapy. Written or taped information can be reviewed later for better absorption.
3. Keep explanations at the family's level of understanding.	3. Vary explanations to meet the family's educational level.
4. Offer encouragement for parents' recognition of danger signs and parents' appropriate use of medical care.	4. Praise reinforces behavior. Parents want to know they are doing the right thing for their child.

Evaluation

- Have the parents and child demonstrated an understanding of the treatment protocols by complying with therapy and seeking appropriate medical care for danger signs?

Nursing Diagnosis

Disturbed Body Image related to hair loss.

Expected Outcomes

The child will:
- Adapt to alopecia, as evidenced by a return to socialization.
- Discuss concerns related to hair loss.

INTERVENTION	RATIONALE
1. Instruct the child and parents on the progression of hair loss and potential changes in color and texture when the hair regrows. Suggest obtaining a wig before hair is lost or bringing a clipping of hair with a recent photograph.	1. Reassure that hair loss is temporary for most cancers, but some cranial irradiation can result in patches of permanent hair loss. Matching a wig to original hair color, texture, and style is easier before hair is lost.

Nursing Care Plan

The Child With Leukemia—cont'd

INTERVENTION	RATIONALE
2. Encourage verbalization of feelings about hair loss. Enlist the help of a child life specialist to engage the child in play therapy.	2. Allowing the child to verbalize concerns about returning to a social environment or school is important. Play therapy is a safe way for the child to express feelings and fears.
3. Discuss ways to minimize the reaction to alopecia by promoting creative solutions, such as hats, wigs, or scarves.	3. Allowing children to create their own headpieces may minimize the negative impact of hair loss.
4. Make visits to the child's classroom.	4. Preparation of classmates for the child's school reentry will lessen classmates' negative reactions, fears, anxiety, and lack of understanding. It will also increase the support they can give the ill child.
5. Encourage a return to school as soon as possible.	5. The sooner the child returns to school, the less likely the child will begin a pattern of absenteeism. If the child returns to school before major body changes take place, the changes may not be so noticeable to the other children, thus decreasing undesirable reactions.

Evaluation

- Is the child involved in prediagnosis social life?
- Has the child discussed hair loss and feelings connected with body image?

Nursing Diagnosis

Ineffective Coping (individual) or Compromised Family Coping related to chronic illness.

Expected Outcomes

The child will:
- Adhere to the treatment plan.

The parents will:
- Verbalize concerns about the impact of the illness on their family.

The child and parents will:
- Use available support systems and community resources.

INTERVENTION	RATIONALE
1. Teach the family the necessity of adhering to the protocol. Teach the warning signs of problems and how to access after-hours emergency care.	1. Conscientious application of the treatment plan increases the chance of a positive outcome.
2. Listen and encourage the child and family to verbalize their feelings and express their concerns. Answer questions honestly and openly.	2. Identifying concerns and clarifying misconceptions will help families cope with the stress of chronic illness.
3. Introduce the family to other families of children with cancer.	3. Other families of children with cancer can offer suggestions and support.
4. Consult social services and a chaplain or appropriate religious figure.	4. The financial and emotional burden of caring for a child with cancer can be overwhelming.
5. Offer a list of local support groups appropriate to the child's age and the family's individual needs.	5. Support groups of individuals in similar situations can provide much comfort and support to the child and the family.

Evaluation

- Is the family adhering to the treatment plan?
- Do the family and child verbalize appropriate concerns and questions?
- Has the family contacted a local support group?

Continued

Nursing Care Plan

The Child With Leukemia—cont'd

Nursing Diagnoses

Acute Pain and Chronic Pain related to the disease process and procedures.

Expected Outcome

The child will:

- Experience decreased discomfort, as evidenced by periods of uninterrupted rest, verbalization of increased comfort, indication of increased comfort on an age-appropriate pain assessment tool, and participation in play activities.

INTERVENTION	RATIONALE
1. Explain procedures to the child in an age-appropriate manner before performing them.	1. Honest explanations build rapport and reduce fear.
2. Monitor for signs and symptoms of pain, such as inactivity for age, increased heart rate or blood pressure, grimacing, verbalization of discomfort, irritability, and crying. Use a developmentally appropriate assessment tool and nonverbal cues to evaluate pain.	2. Younger children will not be able to verbalize pain. Stoic children may not express discomfort. Nurses must watch for physiologic signs of pain.
3. Administer comfort measures as needed, such as positioning, adjusting room temperature, and offering distractions appropriate for age.	3. Comfort measures can decrease the perception of pain and even decrease the amount of analgesic needed.
4. Administer analgesics promptly as ordered. Use topical anesthetics for procedural pain. Ensure analgesia or non-pharmacologic strategies before painful procedures.	4. Analgesics reduce the pain of procedures and of the disease. Delays in analgesic administration can increase anxiety and thus increase pain. Non-pharmacologic interventions can decrease anxiety and decrease pain experienced.
5. Explain the pain-control regimen to the parents and child, as age-appropriate.	5. Parents know their child and can assist the nurse in assessing pain and reporting it promptly.
6. Notify the physician if pain relief is not obtained with the ordered dose of analgesic.	6. Pain tolerance varies greatly among children. Dosage increases may be needed, especially in the child with chronic pain or the dying child.
7. Enlist a child life specialist's help before and during procedures.	7. Child life specialists are trained to use distraction techniques with children and represent a "safe" person for the child to be with during repeated painful procedures.
8. Administer antianxiety drugs as ordered (see Chapter 39 for more information related to pain management in children).	8. Especially in the adolescent, anticipation of a painful procedure may worsen the pain. Giving an antianxiety drug may help calm the child so the procedure is better tolerated.

Evaluation

- Does the child express decreased levels of discomfort, and is this evident on an appropriate pain assessment tool?
- Is the child joining other children in play?

Nursing Diagnosis

Impaired Skin Integrity related to radiation therapy, chemotherapy, and immobility.

Expected Outcome

The child and family will:

- Appropriately manage any problems with skin integrity.

Incidence

In the United States, approximately 2200 children younger than 20 years are diagnosed with brain tumors annually (American Brain Tumor Association [ABTA], 1998). CNS tumors represent 20% of malignancies diagnosed in children (Keating, Goodrich, & Packer, 2001). More than 50% of pediatric CNS tumors develop in the posterior fossa—the lower part of the brain that contains both the cerebellum and the brainstem (Keating et al., 2001).

Manifestations

Manifestations of brain tumors vary with tumor location and the age and development of the child. Symptoms produced by tumors in the posterior fossa include ataxia (unsteady

Nursing Care Plan

The Child With Leukemia—cont'd

INTERVENTION	RATIONALE
1. Assess the child's skin each shift.	1. Skin erythema is common with radiation therapy but should not progress to skin breakdown.
2. Use only approved lotions and creams on the skin, and instruct parents in the same.	2. Some commercial lotions can increase skin irritation and redness.
3. Avoid excessive scrubbing of skin, hot water, and abrasive soaps.	3. Friction may increase skin breakdown. Hot water is uncomfortable to irritated tissue.
4. Offer loose clothing of soft materials.	4. Tight clothing or abrasive fabrics may further irritate the skin.
5. Notify the physician if skin breakdown occurs.	5. Additional orders for therapeutic creams may be needed.
6. If the child is immobile, gently turn and vary the position at least every 2 hours and teach parents to do the same.	6. Immobility may increase pressure on skin and promote breakdown.

Evaluation

■ Has the child's skin remained intact, and can parents describe skin care techniques?

Nursing Diagnosis

Impaired Oral Mucous Membranes related to chemotherapy and radiation therapy.

Expected Outcome

The child will:

■ Show no signs of side effects of treatment, as evidenced by intact oral and rectal mucous membrane.

INTERVENTION	RATIONALE
1. Monitor the child's mouth and anus each shift for ulcers, erythema, or breakdown. Teach the parent or child, if age-appropriate, the same. Report ulcerations to the physician.	1. A breakdown in mucous membranes usually begins with erythema and progresses to ulcerations. Home care should include this assessment for the duration of therapy. Additional medications, mouth rinses, or ointments will be ordered if ulcerations occur.
2. Do not take a rectal temperature in a child undergoing chemotherapy or radiation therapy. Do not take oral temperatures if mouth ulcers are present. Teach parents how to take accurate axillary or tympanic temperatures.	2. The introduction of a thermometer into the rectum or mouth of a child with fragile mucous membranes, no matter how carefully done, can tear tissue.
3. Begin meticulous mouth care, avoiding alcohol-based mouthwashes, several times a day with a soft-bristle toothbrush or toothettes.	3. Frequent mouth care will help remove bacteria from the oral mucosa, decreasing the risk of infection of irritated tissue.
4. If the rectum becomes irritated, begin sitz baths several times a day and after bowel movements.	4. Lukewarm sitz baths keep the perineum clean and soothe irritated tissue.
5. In diaper-wearing children, use only diaper wipes that do not contain alcohol or perfumes. If the perineum is very irritated, use only warm water wipes of the area.	5. Alcohol and perfumes will further irritate the skin and can cause great discomfort. Very few commercial diaper wipes are safe for these children.
6. Offer bland, nonirritating foods and cool liquids.	6. Citrus products may be very painful to an ulcerated mouth, as may spicy foods. Cool liquids are soothing. Ice pops and slushes are usually well tolerated.

Evaluation

■ Has the child exhibited signs of oral mucositis or rectal ulceration?

---

gait), poor coordination of the upper extremities, visual changes (nystagmus, diplopia, strabismus), and occasionally head tilt. Tumors in this location are frequently associated with increased intracranial pressure caused by the tumor mass itself or, more commonly, by the tumor obstructing the normal flow of cerebrospinal fluid (CSF). Increased intracranial pressure (ICP) often causes headaches, vomiting, and lethargy. These symptoms are usually most intense on arising in the morning. Frequently, symptoms of increased ICP are subacute and nonspecific.

Infants may present with irritability, lethargy, poor feeding, increased head circumference, and bulging fontanel. Many younger children demonstrate loss of developmental milestones. School-age children may demonstrate declining academic performance, fatigue, personality changes, and complaints of vague, intermittent headache. Cranial

Pathophysiology

of Brain Tumors

Brain tumors are classified according to cell histology and rate of tumor proliferation. About 50% of pediatric brain tumors are astrocytomas, 25% are medulloblastomas, 11% are brainstem gliomas, and 9% are ependymomas.*

The histology of brain tumors ranges from benign to highly malignant. The impact these tumors have on the brain and the clinical symptoms they produce often have more to do with the tumor size and location than with the aggressiveness of the tumor. The majority of astrocytomas are low-grade or slow-growing; however, if they persist in spite of treatment, they can produce significant neurologic deficits.

Sarcoma
• Arises from soft connective tissue (e.g., pia mater)

Meningioma
• Arises from arachnoidal cells in the meninges, primarily dura

Astrocytoma
• Occurs in cerebral hemispheres or midline structures

Supratentorial ependymona
• Arises from lining tissue of lateral ventricles

Pinealoma
• Arises from suprasellar germ cells supporting or adjacent to the pineal gland

Optic glioma
• Occurs in optic nerve or chiasm

Supratentorial tumors
Above the roof of the cerebellum

Craniopharyngioma
• Occurs adjacent to structure containing pituitary gland

Infratentorial tumors
Below the roof of the cerebellum

Medulloblastoma
• Occurs in cerebellum
• About 25% of brain tumors in children

Brainstem glioma
• Occurs in any portion of brain stem
• About 11% of brain tumors in children

Cerebellar astrocytoma
• Occurs in cerebellum
• Most common brain tumor in children

Infratentorial ependymona
• Occurs in lining tissue of fourth ventricle

Location of brain tumors in children. **Boldface labels** indicate the most frequently occurring tumors in children.

*Heideman, R., Packer, R., Albright, L., Freeman, C., & Rorke, L. (1997). Tumors of the central nervous system. In P.A. Pizzo & D.G. Poplack (Eds.), *Principles and practice of pediatric oncology* (pp. 633-698). Philadelphia: Lippincott-Raven.

! CRITICAL TO REMEMBER

Signs of Brain Tumor in Children

The hallmark symptoms of children with brain tumors are headache and morning vomiting related to the child getting out of bed. The sudden increase in intracranial pressure with the change in position causes the vomiting.

---

nerve deficits and hemiparesis are usually associated with brainstem involvement. Supratentorial tumors characteristically present with headaches, seizures, and/or focal neurologic deficits. Especially with slow-growing tumors, symptoms may be subtle and initially attributed to more common childhood illnesses.

Diagnostic Evaluation

Once a tumor is suspected, magnetic resonance imaging (MRI), computed tomography (CT), single-photon emission computed tomography (SPECT), or positron emission tomography (PET) may be done. MRI is currently the imaging modality most commonly used to evaluate brain tumors. During MRI, the child must lie motionless inside a dark tunnel for approximately 1 hour. This is especially difficult for young children. In general, children younger than 6 years need sedation. A spinal MRI is done to look for metastatic disease in the spine. A CSF sample obtained from lumbar puncture is examined for the presence of tumor cells. In some cases, the tumor produces tumor markers that can be identified in the CSF or blood.

Usually the diagnosis is suspected from the child's signs and symptoms and the location of the tumor (see Fig. 48-3).

Pathologic examination confirms the tissue type and tumor diagnosis. On the rare occasion when the tumor is not surgically accessible, the diagnosis must be made based on location and radiologic evaluation alone.

Therapeutic Management

Initial intervention for a child with a brain tumor is surgery. The goal is to remove as much of the tumor as possible while minimally disturbing the surrounding brain tissue so that the child's neurologic functioning is preserved to the highest degree possible. Complete removal of the tumor is associated with the best prognosis. In the case of a brainstem tumor or optic pathway glioma, the risk to neurologic function outweighs the benefit of resection, so surgery is not done. Depending on the location of the tumor and the extent of surgical resection, a ventriculoperitoneal (VP) shunt may be inserted to relieve the hydrocephalus and the symptoms associated with it (see Chapter 52 for care of the child with a VP shunt). Children with tumors located above the roof of the cerebellum (supratentorial) are at risk for seizures from the tumor itself or from scar tissue formation after surgery. These children are prescribed anticonvulsants with monitoring of therapeutic levels.

Therapy depends on the type of tumor, its location, the amount of residual tumor after surgery, and the child's age. Benign tumors, such as low-grade astrocytomas, require only surgery if the tumor can be completely resected. Often, however, treatment with chemotherapy and radiation therapy is needed as well. Radiation therapy is avoided in children younger than 3 years because of the toxic effects on the developing brain, particularly in very young children (Bestak, 2001). Imaging is performed at intervals to help determine the response to therapy.

Over the past decade, chemotherapy has emerged as treatment for pediatric brain tumors, either in conjunction with radiation therapy or alone (Keating et al., 2001). Prognostic percentages vary with the type of tumor, the amount resected, metastatic spread, age and physical status of the child, and individual response.

■ NURSING CARE
The Child With a Brain Tumor

Assessment

A thorough neurologic examination is paramount for any child diagnosed with a brain tumor. Knowing the location of the tumor will heighten the nurse's understanding of neurologic deficits the child may experience (Fig. 48-3). It is important to obtain a good psychosocial and developmental history, including information regarding the child's neurologic symptoms, achievement of developmental milestones in younger children, and school performance in older children. Children who have insidious loss of vision may have learned to compensate well; excellent nursing skills will be needed to identify vision loss. Consider impaired balance and coordination, brainstem dysfunction, and any loss of vision when assessing the child's safety. The nurse should be especially vigilant of symptoms of increased ICP in children newly diagnosed with a brain tumor, in children in the immediate postoperative period, and in children who have a VP shunt

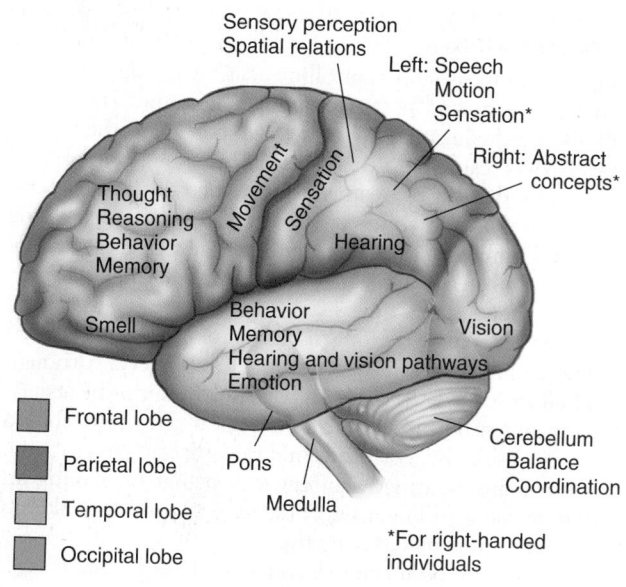

Figure 48-3 Lobes of the brain (for right-handed individuals).

in place. Approximately 50% of children with brain tumors experience seizures at some time during their illness (ABTA, 1998). Seizure precautions should be considered even in the child with no previous history of seizures (see Chapter 52). Depending on the length of time the child has been feeling ill, weight loss and poor nutrition may be present. Assess nutritional status throughout treatment.

Nursing Diagnosis and Planning

The nursing diagnoses and expected outcomes that may be appropriate for the child with a brain tumor and the child's family are

- Acute Pain and Chronic Pain related to increased ICP.
  Expected Outcome: The child will verbalize a decrease in the severity of headaches.
- Risk for Infection related to surgery or immunosuppression after chemotherapy.
  Expected Outcome: The child will remain free from signs of infection, as evidenced by body temperature within normal limits and demonstration of infection prevention measures.
- Anxiety (child and parent) related to the surgery and diagnosis.
  Expected Outcome: The child and parents will exhibit decreased anxiety about the outcomes of surgery and therapy, as evidenced by verbalization of less stress and an ability to problem solve.
- Deficient Knowledge about the disease process related to unfamiliarity with the information.
  Expected Outcome: The parents will describe the disease process and its management.
- Disturbed Body Image related to a shaved head, hair loss, and/or neurologic deficits.
  Expected Outcome: The child will demonstrate appropriate coping techniques for hair loss and changes in coordination or other abilities, as evidenced by maintaining social relationships and statements indicating adaptation to the changed appearance.

Interventions

Nursing care focuses on controlling acute symptoms, preparation for surgery, and postoperative management. The family will also need education and support to cope with the significant anxiety caused by the potential neurologic impact of surgery and the fear of treatment failure and death. Preoperative teaching at the child's developmental level prepares the child and family for the potential outcomes of surgery. The child should be educated about anesthesia and should be prepared to spend some time in the intensive care unit after surgery. (See Chapter 37 for a discussion of preoperative care.)

The child's head will be shaved before surgery. Although every effort is made to shave only as much hair as necessary, shaving may still be traumatic for the child. The nurse should be aware of this and assist the child in verbalizing fears. Some children enjoy wearing a favorite cap or hat or making an outing of going to buy a hat. Prepare the child to wake up with a large dressing covering the head.

In addition to postoperative concerns of pain, hemorrhage, and infection, the nurse must also monitor for signs and symptoms of increased ICP. Increased ICP (see Chapter 52) is a risk in the postoperative period related to cerebral edema, hydrocephalus, or hemorrhage. It can also occur at diagnosis or with recurrent tumor because of pressure from the tumor mass and associated edema or CSF obstruction. A shunt malfunction in any child with a VP shunt may result in hydrocephalus and increased ICP. Check and record vital signs, mental status, and neurologic status frequently when the child returns from surgery. Never place the child in Trendelenburg position because it increases ICP and the risk of bleeding. Symptoms that suggest increased ICP in any child diagnosed with a brain tumor should always be brought to the attention of the physician and generally require evaluation, including an MRI or CT scan.

Many children return from the surgical suite with external ventricular shunts in place that temporarily remove CSF as a means to reduce ICP. The external drains must be maintained at appropriate levels and CSF measured accurately. Normal CSF is colorless; therefore bloody or discolored drainage can be a sign of contamination or bleeding. This should be reported to the physician immediately (Bowden & Greenberg, 2003). Many children require placement of a permanent shunt due to secondary hydrocephalus. (Chapter 52 addresses care of the child with a shunt.)

After the child's condition has been stabilized, assess for functional deficits resulting from surgery or damage to normal brain tissue by the tumor. These deficits are somewhat predictable if the involved area of the brain and the function of that area are known (Box 48-3). If the deficits are significant, rehabilitative therapy may be necessary to help the child regain function. Studies have shown that radiation to the brain can impact cognitive abilities, with more significant deficits in children treated at a younger age (Bestak, 2001). Adequate academic support should always be considered for these children when they return to school.

If radiation therapy is delivered, the side effects of radiation merit special attention, as previously discussed. It is important for families to be aware of its potential side effects and to understand that acute side effects will resolve. Chemotherapy may be delivered on an inpatient or outpatient basis, depending on the intensity, and the nursing care is similar for any child receiving chemotherapy.

BOX 48-3
Potential Functional Deficits Related to a Brain Tumor

After surgery, the child should be assessed for functional deficits in the following areas:
- Gait – look for ataxia, including head control and truncal stability
- Bilateral extremity strength and purposeful movement
- Speech
- Ability to swallow
- Vision and hearing
- Presurgical development task mastery
- Receptive and expressive language

If the deficits are significant, the child may need rehabilitative therapy to regain function.

Evaluation

- Are there both verbal and nonverbal indications of a positive comfort level?
- Does the child's rating on a pain assessment tool indicate decreased pain?
- Has the child remained afebrile, and do the child and family demonstrate infection prevention measures?
- Have the child and family expressed decreased levels of stress and the ability to rely on coping strategies?
- Is the family able to discuss the treatment plan and concerns related to the disease and treatment plan?
- Is the child relating with peers in the same manner as before the diagnosis and hospitalization, and is the child expressing adaptation to the changed appearance?

MALIGNANT LYMPHOMAS

Malignant lymphomas are neoplasms of lymphoid cells, a component of the immune system. Lymphomas represent 24% of childhood cancers in children younger than 20 years, making lymphomas the third most common childhood malignancy (Smith & Ries, 2002). Lymphomas are divided into two main types: non-Hodgkin's lymphoma (NHL) and Hodgkin's lymphoma.

The average annual occurrence of NHL in children younger than 20 years in the United States is 8.9 per million, with incidence higher in the white population versus the African-American population (Gilchrist, 2004). It represents approximately 60% of all lymphomas and 6% of all childhood malignancies. NHL originates from a proliferation of either B or T lymphocytes. The three subtypes of pediatric NHL are (1) small, noncleaved cell (Burkitt's, Burkitt's-like) lymphomas; (2) large cell lymphomas; and (3) lymphoblastic lymphomas.

Hodgkin's lymphoma in 15- to 19-year-olds comprises approximately 15% of all cancers seen in this age group; it accounts for 5% of all cancers seen in children younger than 15 years (Gilchrist, 2004). It represents the remaining 40% of lymphomas. The presence of giant multinucleated cells (Reed-Sternberg cells) is the hallmark of Hodgkin's disease.

The incidence of NHL increases gradually throughout life. Unlike Hodgkins disease, which has a bimodal incidence curve, the incidence of NHL increases with age (Magrath, 2002). Because the incidence of Hodgkin's disease peaks in children 15 years old and older, it accounts for a greater proportion of the lymphomas seen in older children. The incidence of either disease in children younger than 5 years is rare.

Non-Hodgkin's Lymphoma

Non-Hodgkin's lymphomas differ greatly from Hodgkin's disease in their clinical behavior, pathology, mode of metastasis, and responsiveness to therapy. These diseases have a rapid onset with widespread involvement at diagnosis.

Etiology

Viral, immunologic, genetic, and environmental factors may contribute to the development of NHL. Although the exact etiology is unknown, a linkage to the immune system is thought to exist. B cell lymphoma has been associated with the Epstein-Barr virus, which suggests that delayed exposure to infectious agents may play a part (Hudson & Donaldson, 2002). Children with congenital immunodeficiency syndromes or acquired immunodeficiency syndrome (AIDS), as well as those who have undergone organ transplantation and have chronically suppressed immune systems, are at higher risk for developing NHL or other lymphoproliferative disorders (Mueller, 2002).

Manifestations

Symptoms of abdominal disease include abdominal cramping, constipation, pain, anorexia, weight loss, ascites, and obstruction, with vomiting as a late sign. Painless, enlarged lymph nodes are found in the cervical or axillary region and less commonly in the inguinal area. If mediastinal disease is present, cough, respiratory distress, symptoms of bronchitis, and possibly significant tracheal deviation are seen. Bone marrow disease leads to a general decline in health and bone marrow suppression.

Diagnostic Evaluation

In addition to a physical examination looking for enlarged lymph nodes and hepatosplenomegaly, extensive laboratory work will be ordered. Especially with Burkitt's lymphoma, the uric acid level will often be high, indicating a rapid turnover of cells.

A chest radiograph will be obtained to look for mediastinal disease and tracheal deviation. The extent of disease is further evaluated with a CT scan of the chest, abdomen, and pelvis. Bone marrow aspirations and biopsies are done to assess involvement of disease in the marrow. A lumbar puncture is done to assess the CSF for disease. Pathologic findings are confirmed with a lymph node biopsy.

Therapeutic Management

Children with NHL, especially Burkitt's lymphoma, often present in metabolic disarray owing to the rapidity with which the disease progresses. These children are prone to tumor lysis syndrome from the large tumor burden and rapid tumor cell turnover and death. Before chemotherapy can be started, the metabolic state must be rectified.

In children susceptible to tumor lysis syndrome, intensive hydration with an IV fluid containing bicarbonate alkalinizes the urine to help prevent the formation of uric acid crystals,

---

> **! CRITICAL TO REMEMBER**
>
> **Tumor Lysis Syndrome**
>
> In tumor lysis syndrome, the intracellular contents are dumped into the extracellular fluid as the tumor cells are lysed, or killed. Because the intracellular contents are a different electrolyte concentration from extracellular blood volume, electrolytes overload the kidneys and, if the condition is not monitored and treated carefully, cause kidney failure. Tumor lysis syndrome is most common in children with leukemias that present with very high white blood cell (WBC) counts and in children with non-Hodgkin's lymphomas, especially when extensive disease is present.

which damage the kidney. Oral allopurinol is started to decrease the uric acid level. Parenteral urate oxidase may be indicated to further degrade uric acid (Lohr, 2002). With the initiation of chemotherapy, serum electrolyte levels may be checked several times a day to keep a close watch on the child's metabolic state because these tumors respond rapidly to treatment. The urine may turn milky white as the tumor cells are filtered through the kidneys. Children who cannot be hemodynamically monitored on the general unit may be moved to the intensive care unit until metabolically stabilized.

The primary treatment modality for all histologic classifications and stages of NHL involves multiagent chemotherapy. Surgery is used to obtain a diagnostic biopsy. In general, these lymphomas present as generalized disease, making them less amenable to treatment with radiation therapy; irradiation is reserved for emergent situations resulting from CNS disease or compromised airway. Chemotherapy is given over a 6- to 24-month period, depending on the type of lymphoma. Typically, a central venous catheter is placed to assist in delivering chemotherapy drugs. Frequent follow-up visits are made after the completion of treatment because the risk of recurrent disease is greatest immediately after therapy is stopped.

The overall 5-year survival rate for NHL is 77% (Greenlee et al., 2000). Survival rates of children treated for Burkitt's and non-Burkitt's lymphoma are 70% to 80%. Those treated for lymphoblastic lymphoma have disease-free survival rates of 50% to 70% when disease is extensive at diagnosis and 90% when disease is limited. Large cell lymphoma is the most difficult to cure, with 50% to 70% of patients achieving disease-free survival (Gilchrist, 2004).

■ NURSING CARE
The Child With Non-Hodgkin's Lymphoma

Assessment

The parents of children with non-Hodgkin's lymphoma will report an acute onset of symptoms that vary with the type of organ involved. Most parents will state that their children have become very irritable and "just not themselves." Children with metastatic disease often appear very sick. Assess lymph nodes and closely check the respiratory system in a child with mediastinal disease, especially if the trachea is deviated. Signs of tumor lysis syndrome include subtle changes in behavior, such as restlessness and irritability, and changes in the sensorium, which are ominous signs of electrolyte imbalances (hyperuricemia, hyperkalemia, hyperphosphatemia, hypocalcemia).

Nursing Diagnosis and Planning

The nursing diagnoses and expected outcomes that apply to the child with non-Hodgkin's lymphoma and the child's family are

- Ineffective Breathing Pattern related to mediastinal disease.
  Expected Outcome: The child's respiratory status will remain stable, as evidenced by normal breath sounds for age and stable respiratory rate and rhythm.
- Risk for Injury related to electrolyte imbalances secondary to tumor lysis syndrome.
  Expected Outcome: The child will maintain electrolyte balance, as evidenced by a stable metabolic state and urine output appropriate for age.
- Risk for Infection related to the state of immunosuppression.
  Expected Outcome: The child will exhibit no signs and symptoms of infection, as evidenced by normal body temperature.
- Deficient Knowledge related to unfamiliarity with the disease process.
  Expected Outcome: The parents will describe the disease process and its management.

Interventions

Initial nursing care focuses on following the physician's orders for maintaining a stable metabolic state before and during the induction phase of chemotherapy. All children undergoing induction chemotherapy should have intake and output and serum chemistry values strictly monitored. Occasionally, children with Burkitt's lymphoma will need a urinary catheter inserted for measurement of output. If a fever develops, urine and blood should be cultured to rule out an infection. These children may be so sick that their nutritional status needs attention after induction, and many will receive enteral nutritional support. If necessary, hyperalimentation may be given.

Parents will need support because the chemotherapy may initially make the child more ill. Questions should be answered directly and honestly. Time to provide the child with extensive education about therapy may not exist until after the child has begun to recover from the initial chemotherapy.

Consultations with chaplains or other religious figures and social workers may enhance the psychosocial care of these families. Realistic expectations of therapy and of the child's response to therapy will help parents deal rationally with their fears (see pp. 1339-1345 for other related nursing care).

Evaluation

- Has the child's respiratory status remained stable, with normal rate and rhythm and clear breath sounds?
- Is the child's urine output appropriate for age, and are electrolytes within normal range?
- Are the child's vital signs within normal limits?
- Are the parents asking questions about the disease process and the care of their child?

Hodgkin's Disease

Hodgkin's disease has a more indolent course than non-Hodgkin's lymphoma. It frequently presents as localized disease.

> ! **CRITICAL** TO REMEMBER
>
> **Prevention of Urinary Tract Infections in the Immunocompromised Child**
>
> Urinary catheters are used very infrequently in immunocompromised patients because of the risk of introducing organisms into the urinary system.

Etiology

The cause of Hodgkin's disease is unknown. However, the possibility of an infectious agent is being investigated. Herpesvirus 6, cytomegalovirus, and Epstein-Barr virus have been associated with Hodgkin's disease, but the exact relationship remains unknown. There is evidence of *in situ* hybridization of EBV genomes in Reed Sternberg cells and its variants (Hudson & Donaldson, 2002).

Manifestations

Painless, firm, movable adenopathy in the cervical and supraclavicular regions is the most common presentation. Mediastinal involvement, with or without airway obstruction, occurs in two thirds of children. Twenty to thirty percent of children present with constitutional symptoms that include fever, drenching night sweats, and weight loss. Other manifestations are hepatosplenomegaly and fatigue.

Diagnostic Evaluation

Biopsy of an involved lymph node and histologic classification of the tissue confirm the diagnosis. Laboratory tests include a CBC, renal and liver function tests, erythrocyte sedimentation rate (ESR), and serum copper and serum ferritin levels. Elevation of ESR or serum copper or ferritin level may be useful for follow-up evaluation if it correlates with disease activity at diagnosis. A gallium scan is done to look for extent of disease. Gallium is a staging study as well as an excellent disease response marker when the tumor takes up gallium at diagnosis (Hudson & Donaldson, 2002). Chest radiography and CT of the chest, abdomen, and pelvis are done to determine the extent of disease. Bilateral bone marrow aspirations and biopsies are done only if constitutional symptoms are present.

In the past, a surgical staging laparotomy was performed frequently. It is an invasive surgical procedure that involves splenectomy, liver biopsy, and sampling of the retroperitoneal and pelvic nodes and defines the extent of disease more precisely than radiographic studies alone. However, precise staging is less important now that most children receive systemic chemotherapy as part of their treatment. Because of the potential complications, a staging laparotomy is avoided unless the findings would significantly alter therapy (Hudson & Donaldson, 2002).

Some manifestations are of prognostic significance, and staging takes them into account. Children with unexplained weight loss of more than 10% body weight in the preceding 6 months, unexplained fevers above 38° C (100.4° F), and night sweats are considered to have B disease, as opposed to A (asymptomatic) disease. The presence of B symptoms is thought to negatively impact prognosis (Gilchrist, 2004). There are four stages, with stage I having limited disease and the most favorable prognosis.

Pathophysiology

of Hodgkin's Disease

Hodgkin's disease originates in a single lymph node or a group of lymph nodes in the same anatomic region. Hodgkin's disease is characterized by giant multinucleated cells called *Reed-Sternberg cells* that are thought to represent activated B and T lymphocytes (see Chapter 41, Clinical Reference section). Hodgkin's disease spreads predictably from lymph nodes to non-nodal sites, such as the spleen, liver, bone, bone marrow, lungs, and mediastinum.

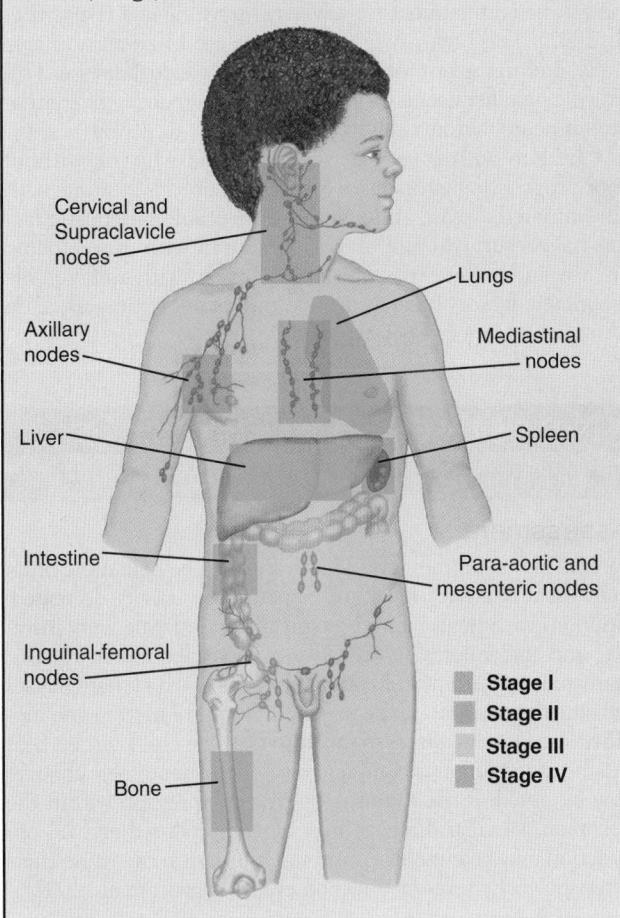

Cervical and Supraclavicle nodes
Lungs
Axillary nodes
Mediastinal nodes
Liver
Spleen
Intestine
Para-aortic and mesenteric nodes
Inguinal-femoral nodes
Bone

Stage I
Stage II
Stage III
Stage IV

Therapeutic Management

Therapy depends on the child's age at diagnosis, disease stage, and histologic type. If the mediastinal disease is expansive, it may compromise respiration. Radiation therapy may be used to shrink the tissue before the child undergoes general anesthesia.

Most children are treated with chemotherapy alone or chemotherapy and low-dose, involved-field radiation therapy. High-dose, extended-field radiation therapy alone may be used if the disease is detected in a single site or in fully grown children where growth and development are not a concern. Long-term survival rates in excess of 90% can be expected with stages I and II disease. For more advanced stages of disease, the long term survival rate is approximately 70% (Gilchrist, 2004).

Nursing Considerations

The onset of Hodgkin's disease is insidious. Frequently, when asked about activity level, children report not noticing any change until it was brought to their attention. Typically, the child noticed lumps around the neck while bathing. Initial assessment of these children includes a thorough lymph node examination. Depending on the presence of the mediastinal disease, the respiratory system should be assessed for a change in status with the child both sitting and lying down.

Initially, the nurse will need to prepare the child for the diagnostic procedures and a surgical biopsy. A central venous catheter may be inserted at the time of diagnosis. In older children, a peripheral IV line may be placed at the time of each chemotherapy treatment to avoid a central venous catheter placement.

At least two thirds of children present with some degree of mediastinal involvement (Hudson & Donaldson, 2002). As with non-Hodgkin's lymphoma, management of the airway is a concern if the child has any mediastinal disease.

A staging laparotomy with splenectomy is generally avoided. If it is required, however, these children need special care. The spleen removes organisms such as *Streptococcus pneumoniae* and *Haemophilus influenzae*. Without the spleen, these organisms can produce fulminant infections. Ideally, children who undergo splenectomy receive a pneumococcal, meningococcal, and *H. influenzae* type B immunization before the procedure. Postoperative care includes assessing for bleeding at dressing sites and administering prophylactic antibiotics.

Induction chemotherapy is begun as soon as the child is stable and staging of disease has been completed. If the airway is compromised, radiation therapy will be given locally to provide immediate relief.

Education includes an explanation of the therapeutic protocol. Questions should be answered honestly. Realistic expectations of response to therapy will help parents deal rationally with their fears. Hodgkin's disease in first remission is treated in the outpatient setting at most centers. The nursing care is similar to that for a child with non-Hodgkin's lymphoma.

NEUROBLASTOMA

Neuroblastoma is the second most common solid tumor of childhood. It is found exclusively in infants and children. Children who present at younger than 12 months may experience spontaneous remission of the disease.

Etiology

The cause of neuroblastoma is unknown. Its prevalence is similar in various countries around the world, suggesting that environmental factors do not cause the disease. There is evidence that a familial form of neuroblastoma may occur; children in families with one or more affected members may be at increased risk for the development of neuroblastoma.

Incidence

Neuroblastoma represents approximately 8% to 10% of all childhood cancers (Brodeur & Maris, 2002). Neuroblastoma occurs at a rate of 8.7 per 1 million children, or 500 to 600 new cases diagnosed each year in the United States. It is more common in boys than in girls and more common in white children than in African-American children. The peak age of presentation is 22 months, with the majority of cases being younger than 5 years. Metastatic disease may be present in the bone marrow, bone, liver, and skin and rarely in the lung or brain (Brodeur & Maris, 2002).

Pathophysiology

Neuroblastoma arises from neural crest cells, which normally develop into the sympathetic nervous system and the adrenal medulla. Cells proliferate and begin to form a solid mass or tumor. These cells are immature and nonfunctional. Typically, the tumor infringes and infiltrates into adjacent normal tissue and organs. Greater understanding of the cellular genetic makeup of this tumor has given researchers insight into prognostic indicators, which help with treatment planning.

Manifestations

The manifestations of neuroblastoma depend on the extent of disease and the location of the tumor. In 65% of cases, a primary abdominal mass and a protuberant, firm abdomen are present (Brodeur & Maris, 2002). Other manifestations include impaired range of motion and mobility, pain and limping, and a large abdominal mass, which can disrupt bowel and bladder function. Chest tumors may produce cough and decreased chest expansion, with respiratory compromise. Compression of the superior vena cava results in facial and periorbital edema. Spinal cord compression may cause inability to walk and impaired bowel and bladder function. Bruising, drooping eyelids, or small pupils may be evident, and possibly opsomyoclonus, or "dancing" eye movements and myoclonic jerks.

Diagnostic Evaluation

The diagnostic work-up includes chest radiography; CT of the chest, abdomen, and pelvis; and skeletal scintigraphy to determine the extent of disease. Bone marrow aspiration and biopsy, usually of both posterior iliac crests, are done to evaluate marrow involvement. Urine catecholamines (homovanillic acid, or HVA; and vanillymandelic acid, or VMA) are elevated in 90% of patients with neuroblastoma. In these patients, serial monitoring of HMA and VMA are helpful as markers during treatment and for follow-up when treatment is complete (Baggott, Kelly, Fochtman, & Foley, 2002).

Definitive diagnosis is made when tissue is obtained by biopsy. Tumor samples are sent to special reference laboratories to look at the genetic makeup of the tumor. The genetic information may reveal the aggressiveness of the tumor and help determine the prognosis and treatment plan.

Therapeutic Management

The treatment of neuroblastoma depends on the presence and extent of metastasis. The International Staging System for Neuroblastoma is used to compare patients. Staging is graded I through IV, with stage I representing localized disease and stage IV distant spread. Staging criteria include the extent and location of metastases, lymph node involvement, and whether the tumor is unilateral or crosses the midline. Early-stage disease (stage I or II) without metastasis may require only surgical excision of the tumor and follow-up evaluations. Children with later-stage (stage IV) disease may undergo surgery to obtain tissue samples or for tumor debulking for pain control.

Age at diagnosis is an important prognostic indicator. Children diagnosed before they are 1 year old have a better prognosis than children diagnosed at a later age. About half of the infants diagnosed with neuroblastoma at younger than 1 year have a less-aggressive tumor type genetically and may be watched carefully or treated with low-dose chemotherapy.

Treatment plans for children with advanced disease (stage III or IV) may include radiation therapy to tumor sites and systemic chemotherapy for several months. Another attempt may be made to resect the tumor after combination chemotherapy has been administered to reduce the tumor size. Peripheral blood stem cell transplant after myeloablative chemotherapy is part of the risk-based treatment for advanced-stage disease (Baggott et al., 2002). This high-risk group may also use 13-*cis*-retinoic acid orally after transplant for possible minimal residual disease. This biologic modifier decreases proliferation and induces differentiation in neuroblastoma cell lines (Matthay et al., 1999).

Children with stage I or II disease and who are without poor prognostic factors have a cure rate of 95%. Infants with disseminated disease and who have favorable prognostic factors have a survival rate of 80%. Children with disseminated disease and infants younger than 1 year with unfavorable prognostic factors have a survival rate of approximately 25% (American Cancer Society, 2003a).

▪ NURSING CARE
The Child With Neuroblastoma

Assessment

Parents may state their child has wanted to be held more often than usual. Activity level and appetite are usually decreased. Children with neuroblastoma typically appear pale, very irritable, and uncomfortable. Because of large abdominal tumors, many present with protuberant abdomens in which hard masses crossing the midline can be palpated. Range of motion and mobility are often impaired, so much so that the child cannot bear weight. If the tumor is compressing a nerve, neurologic changes may be noted. If the tumor is causing compression within the abdomen, vascular drainage may be compromised and GI obstruction may be present. Periorbital infiltration can cause characteristic ecchymosis or "raccoon eyes" (Baggott et al., 2002).

Nursing Diagnosis and Planning

The nursing diagnoses and expected outcomes that may be appropriate for the child with a neuroblastoma and the child's family are

- Acute Pain related to tumor pressure.
  Expected Outcome: The infant will exhibit pain relief, as evidenced by decreased crying and a relaxed body position.
- Anxiety (parents) related to a diagnosis of cancer, surgery, and treatment plan.
  Expected Outcome: The parents will express decreased anxiety about the outcomes of therapy.
- Deficient Knowledge related to unfamiliarity with the disease process and its management.
  Expected Outcome: The parents will describe the disease process and its implications.

Interventions

Nursing care focuses initially on support of family members as they react and adjust to the diagnosis of cancer. The nurse facilitates the educational process to allay fears of the unknown. The initial care of the child includes pain management, both preoperatively and postoperatively. Expect the child with an abdominal tumor to return from surgery with a nasogastric (NG) tube in place. Assess the wound carefully for bleeding and signs of infection. (Postoperative care of the child is discussed in Chapter 37.) With responsive tumors, the child's disposition will improve very quickly.

Bowel habits may be altered because of pain, immobility, medication, surgery, and alteration in nutritional patterns. Children with large abdominal tumors may become obstructed because of tumor compression. The nurse should obtain a history of bowel habits and notify the physician if bowel habits are dramatically altered.

Management of the airway is of concern if the child has any mediastinal disease. Monitor respiratory effort, color, and pulses. Position for comfort.

Evaluation

- Has the infant exhibited decreased crying and irritability?
- Does the infant rest quietly and comfortably in the parent's arms and have uninterrupted periods of rest?
- Are the parents verbalizing their fears and expressing decreased anxiety?
- Are the parents asking questions related to the child's disease and treatment and seeking the support of family and friends?

OSTEOSARCOMA

Osteosarcoma (also called *osteogenic sarcoma*) is the most common primary bone malignancy in children. The symptoms of this disease in its earliest stage are almost always attributed to extremity injury or normal growing pains. Typically, unresolved pain related to trauma brings the tumor to the attention of medical personnel.

Etiology

The cause of osteosarcoma is unknown, although associations have been made between radiation therapy for other diseases and osteosarcoma. Familial tendencies have been seen, suggesting that genetic factors are involved (Link, Gebhardt, & Meyers, 2002).

Incidence

Osteosarcoma represents 7% of all childhood cancers (Smith & Ries, 2002). The incidence of osteosarcoma peaks in the teenage years. The rapid bone growth of the adolescent growth spurt is associated with the development of this tumor. Osteosarcoma occurs at an earlier age in girls than in boys, which corresponds to the earlier maturation of girls. Before adolescence, osteosarcoma is rare. In about 15% to 20% of children, the disease has metastasized at the time of diagnosis, usually to the lungs (Link et al., 2002).

Pathophysiology

Osteosarcoma originates from bone-producing cells, which invade the medullary canal of the bone and form a solid tumor. Incidence is higher in the most rapidly growing bones in adolescents—that is, the distal femur, proximal tibia, and proximal humerus (Link et al., 2002).

Manifestations

Manifestations of osteosarcoma include progressive, insidious, or intermittent pain at the tumor site; a palpable mass; limping, if a weight-bearing limb is affected; progressive, limited range of motion; and eventually pathologic fractures at the tumor site.

Diagnostic Evaluation

Initially, radiographs of the primary site and chest are taken, and then CT or MRI and skeletal scintigraphy are performed. The CT scan includes the chest to search for pulmonary metastases, which helps with staging the disease. A biopsy of the tumor must be performed with great care so that there is no local contamination of tissue by tumor. Laboratory tests include a CBC, chemistry levels, and serum alkaline phosphatase (ALP) and lactate dehydrogenase (LDH) determinations. Higher levels of the enzymes ALP and LDH correlate with a higher probability of treatment failure.

Therapeutic Management

The goals of therapy are to remove the tumor and to prevent the spread of disease. Osteogenic sarcoma is treated with a combination of surgery and chemotherapy. Chemotherapy is administered before and after surgery. Radiation therapy is used only for palliative pain control in advanced-stage disease because osteosarcoma is generally unresponsive to irradiation.

Amputation was once the standard surgical intervention and is still necessary in some cases. Favorable tumor location allows specially trained orthopedic surgeons to perform a complex limb-salvage operation. The affected tissue is removed with the certainty of clean margins, and limb function is preserved. The diseased bone is removed, and either bone grafts or surgically placed orthopedic devices are implanted.

Early research on this disease found that 90% of patients developed recurrent disease after surgery alone. This finding alerted physicians to the presence of microscopic disease. Therefore, after surgery, chemotherapy is continued even if the surgical procedure appears to have been successful. Chemotherapy is aimed at preventing the spread of disease by killing any microscopic tumor cells present anywhere in the body.

The extent of disease at diagnosis, elevated LDH and ALP levels, and tumor necrosis found on surgical resection are the three most significant prognostic indicators. The cure rate is about 80% to 90% for children who respond well to chemotherapy treatment(American Cancer Society, 2003b). The 20% of children with metastatic disease at diagnosis have a substantially poorer outcome.

▪NURSING CARE
The Child With Osteosarcoma

Assessment

Subjective data to be gathered include a history of any injury to the affected limb and a history of discomfort. By the time children with osteosarcomas come to medical attention, they may be in considerable pain from the tumor. Warmth, erythema, and tenderness at the site of tumor are not uncommon. If the swelling is great, the skin may appear shiny and taut, with dilated blood vessels. Lung involvement is usually asymptomatic.

To prepare the child for outcomes of surgery, an assessment of physical activity and sports involvement is essential, as is the psychosocial history. As for any child with cancer, body image changes, especially if the affected limb must be amputated, are of paramount importance. Preoperatively, the nurse should not only assess children's values and fears but also begin the process of preparing children for postoperative lifestyle modifications.

Nursing Diagnosis and Planning

The nursing diagnoses and expected outcomes that may be appropriate for the child with an osteosarcoma and the child's family are

- Acute Pain related to disease process and procedures.
  Expected Outcome: The child will experience decreased pain, as evidenced by verbalization of adequate pain control and decreased pain rating on an age-appropriate pain assessment tool.
- Fear and Anxiety related to the potential loss or impairment of a limb and a diagnosis of cancer.
  Expected Outcome: The child and parents will express decreased fears and anxiety related to the surgery and diagnosis.
- Risk for Infection related to chemotherapy or surgery.
  Expected Outcome: The child will remain free from signs and symptoms of infection, as evidenced by normal body temperature and no redness or purulent drainage from the surgical site.
- Disturbed Body Image related to loss or impairment of a limb.
  Expected Outcome: The child will have a positive body image, as evidenced by a return to appropriate social situations and statements that indicate adaptation to the altered appearance and function.
- Impaired Physical Mobility related to loss or impairment of limb function.
  Expected Outcome: The child will regain maximum mobility, as evidenced by ability to perform activities of daily living.
- Deficient Knowledge related to unfamiliarity with the disease process and anxiety.
  Expected Outcome: The child and parents will describe the disease process and potential postoperative adaptations.

Interventions

Initial care is focused on making the child comfortable. Preoperative teaching is extensive and procedure-specific. If limb salvage is the procedure of choice, the surgeon and nurse will spend considerable time with the family explaining what is to be done. The nurse reinforces the preoperative and postoperative teaching.

In addition to the usual postoperative care, pain, infection, and potential hemorrhage are nursing concerns. The potential for postoperative pneumonia may be greater in the child with pulmonary metastases than in the child without such metastases.

If amputation occurs, phantom limb pain is a temporary condition some children may experience. This sensation of burning, aching, or cramping in the missing limb is most distressing to the child. The child needs to be reassured that the condition is normal. Numerous pharmacologic agents are available to help with postoperative neurogenic pain.

The child who undergoes amputation will be fitted with a permanent prosthesis once the surgical site has thoroughly healed. To begin to mold the stump for that, a temporary prosthesis may be used. A temporary prosthesis enables the child to maintain use and strength of surrounding muscles in preparation for the permanent device. A prosthesis will address the issue of body image disturbance and enable the child to become more quickly independent in activities of daily living. Prepare the child for extensive work with physical therapists to achieve mobility with the prosthesis. Teenagers especially may become discouraged if they expect the prosthesis to enable them to move normally. Prepare them for a limp or for awkward movements with the prosthesis.

Assist the child to verbalize feelings about changes in body image and function. Involve the child in age-appropriate decision-making concerning care. Encourage interaction with other children of the same age who have the same disease (support groups). Provide opportunities for the family to participate in the care of the child and to provide support and encouragement.

Follow-up outpatient visits need to include a careful assessment of psychosocial adjustment. Questions should include the topics of social interactions, school attendance and performance, and behavioral changes.

Evaluation

- Is the child experiencing discomfort related to the surgical procedures?
- Does the pain assessment tool show decreased pain?
- Are the family and child discussing fears related to the disease and treatment?
- Is the child afebrile, and is the surgical site free of redness and purulence?
- Is the child relating with peers?
- Has the child made positive statements indicating beginning adaptation to the physical impairment?
- Is the child readily participating in physical therapy and returning to performing activities of daily living?
- Are the child and family asking questions related to the disease process?
- Do the family and child describe the treatment of the tumor?

EWING'S SARCOMA

Ewing's sarcoma is the second most common bone tumor seen in children. The diagnosis is often challenging to make because this disease mimics infection and may be difficult to differentiate from other malignancies. Ewing's sarcoma may also manifest as a soft tissue mass.

Etiology

The cause of Ewing's sarcoma is unknown. Interestingly, Ewing's sarcoma has not been commonly associated with other preexisting congenital chromosomal abnormalities, suggesting chance rather than biology in the development of this tumor.

Incidence

The incidence of Ewing's sarcoma is 2.1 per 1 million white children per year (Ginsberg, Woo, Johnson, Hicks, & Horowitz, 2002). The disease is very uncommon in African-

American and Asian children. Ewing's sarcoma is rare in children younger than 5 years and adults older than 30 years. The incidence peaks between ages 10 and 20 years.

Pathophysiology

The diagnosis of Ewing's sarcoma is made after all other solid tumors have been excluded. Ewing's sarcoma has no defining characteristics. Like osteosarcoma, this tumor invades the bone and is found most often in the midshaft of long bones, especially the femur, vertebrae, ribs, and pelvic bones. Gross metastasis is uncommon at diagnosis but does occur, most often to the lungs, bones, or bone marrow. As with osteosarcoma, microscopic disease is thought to be present early in the disease process.

Manifestations

Manifestations of Ewing's sarcoma include pain, soft tissue swelling around the affected bone, and fever. If metastatic disease occurs, anorexia, fever, malaise, fatigue, and weight loss are seen. If a vertebral tumor is present, neurologic symptoms will be seen. If a rib tumor is present, respiratory symptoms may be seen.

Diagnostic Evaluation

The diagnostic work-up is the same as for osteosarcoma, and biopsy is necessary to differentiate Ewing's sarcoma from other neoplastic processes.

Therapeutic Management

Treatment begins with chemotherapy to decrease the tumor bulk, followed by surgical resection of the primary tumor. Clinicians debate whether to manage the primary tumor site with surgery or radiation therapy because this tumor is so sensitive to radiation. Consideration is given to the expendability of the bone involved when surgery is a treatment option, versus the potential late effects of radiation. Ribs and the proximal fibula are considered expendable and may be removed to excise the tumor without affecting function. Cure rates exceed 75% in children with small extremity tumors and no metastases (Arndt, 2000). With gross metastasis, the cure rate is dramatically decreased.

Nursing Considerations

Nursing care is similar to that for children with osteosarcomas, with the addition of care for the child receiving radiation therapy.

RHABDOMYOSARCOMA

Rhabdomyosarcoma is a malignancy of muscle, or striated tissue, that most often occurs periorbitally, in the head and neck in younger children, or in the trunk and extremities in older children. Long-term survival rates vary with the child's age, the histologic subtype, and the location of the tumor.

Etiology

Although the exact etiology is unknown, rhabdomyosarcoma has been associated with familial cancer syndromes.

Incidence

Rhabdomyosarcoma is the most common soft tissue malignancy in children and accounts for 5% to 10% of all malignant solid tumors in children (Smith & Ries, 2002). The annual incidence in the United States is estimated at 4.3 cases per 1 million white children and 3.3 cases per 1 million African-American children. Two age-groups predominate: children younger than age 10 years and adolescents (American Cancer Society, 2003c).

Pathophysiology

Four histologic subtypes of rhabdomyosarcoma exist. The embryonal type accounts for 50% to 60% of the tumors and has the best prognosis. About 20% of cases are of the alveolar type, which is found most often in the perineal area, trunk, and extremities and has a less favorable prognosis. Pleomorphic rhabdomyosarcoma is rarely diagnosed, but this subtype seems to have the worst prognosis (Wexler, Crist, & Helman, 2002).

The prognosis depends on several factors other than histologic type. If the tumor is in a location where manifestations appear early, rather than deeply buried in a body cavity, the prognosis is better because the tumor is usually found before it has metastasized. Abnormalities in the DNA content of the tumor cells have prognostic significance. Staging of the tumor is based on whether the tumor was resected completely, was resected with residual microscopic disease, was incompletely resected, or had metastasized to distant sites (McHugh & Boothroyd, 1999). Local failure is more common if the tumor cannot be completely resected.

Manifestations

The manifestations of rhabdomyosarcoma depend on the tumor location. Soft to hard, nontender, relatively immobile masses may be mistaken for a traumatic hematoma. If the lesion is periorbital, visual changes are present; the child may have ptosis, exophthalmos, or proptosis (bulging). Cranial nerve involvement may occur. If the lesion affects an extremity, range of motion will be limited. In the case of pelvic tumors, the function of organs around the tumor is disrupted.

Diagnostic Evaluation

CT, skeletal scintigraphy, and bone marrow aspiration and biopsy are performed to determine the extent of disease. The diagnosis is made after biopsy or attempted surgical resection of the tumor. A decision about treatment is made, depending on the location of the tumor, histologic subtype, and the presence of distant metastases. Laboratory studies include a CBC, urinalysis, and renal and liver function tests.

Therapeutic Management

Rhabdomyosarcoma is treated with chemotherapy, surgery, and radiation therapy. Chemotherapy is used to decrease the tumor bulk and reduce the extent and morbidity of surgery. After surgical removal of the tumor, additional chemotherapy is provided. Like Ewing's sarcoma, microscopic rhabdomyosarcoma is often present at the time of diagnosis. Discontinuation of chemotherapy after removal of the tumor generally results in recurrent disease. Tumor cells not removed by surgery are referred to as *residual disease*. Radiation therapy is used for children who have residual disease or whose tumor was not resectable. About 50% of children with metastatic disease at the time of diagnosis do not achieve lasting remission (Arndt, 2004).

Follow-up care involves periodic CT or MRI studies to assess tumor response to therapy and to monitor any development of disease progression. Most relapses occur within 2 years of diagnosis and during therapy, although relapses have been reported as late as 6 years after diagnosis (Pappo et al., 1997).

Nursing Considerations

Parents may relate that their first indication that something was wrong was a decreased activity level in a young child unable to verbalize pain. If the tumor is more superficially located, parents may have discovered a lump or swelling.

The physical examination findings will depend on the location of the tumor, but typically a soft to hard, nontender mass will be palpated. The surrounding lymph nodes should be palpated for enlargement, which may indicate tumor involvement. The CBC is usually normal unless the tumor has extended into bone marrow, causing a decrease in hemoglobin and platelet values.

Nursing care initially focuses on support of family members as they react and adjust to the diagnosis of cancer. Second, the nurse facilitates the educational process to allay fears of the unknown.

Postoperative care of the biopsy or surgical site involves careful observation for signs of infection, hemorrhage, and edema. If surgery entailed excision of an abdominal or pelvic tumor, the child will return from the surgical suite with an NG tube and possibly drains in place.

WILMS' TUMOR (NEPHROBLASTOMA)

Wilms' tumor, or nephroblastoma, is the most common renal tumor in children. Much research has been done on this disease, and the subsequent changes in therapy have resulted in favorable outcomes. Prognosis is related to stage of disease at diagnosis, histopathologic features of the tumor, and patient age.

Etiology

The cause of Wilms' tumor is unknown. Most Wilms' tumors occur in children with no unusual physical features and no family history of the disease. These are considered sporadic cases. In some cases, however, a genetic predisposition exists. Approximately 1% to 2.5% of children who develop this disease have a familial predisposition. Bilateral disease is more common in familial cases than in sporadic cases. Wilms' tumor has been associated with other congenital anomalies including aniridia (absence of the irises), hemihypertrophy, cryptorchidism, and hypospadias. Wilms' tumor is associated with some other syndromes seen in childhood.

Incidence

Incidence is higher in African-Americans and lower in East Asians. Approximately 400 new cases of Wilms' tumor are diagnosed annually, representing 5% to 6% of childhood cancers (Grundy et al., 2002). The mean age at diagnosis is 2 to 5 years (Jaffe & Huff, 2004). Most children present before 7 years of age. Seven percent of children have bilateral tumors (Jaffe & Huff, 2004).

Pathophysiology

Wilms' tumor arises from the renal parenchyma of the kidney. Categories of Wilms' tumor are based on favorable and unfavorable histologic findings; children with favorable histologic findings (the majority of children with Wilms' tumor) have a more positive prognosis (Jaffe & Huff, 2004). Wilms' tumor may occur in one or both kidneys, although the latter is much less common. At the initial diagnosis, the disease is usually local, but occasionally there are metastases to other organs. The lungs are the most common site of metastasis. As with other tumors, a staging system directs treatment.

Manifestations

The most common clinical presentation of Wilms' tumor is an asymptomatic, mobile, abdominal mass discovered by the parent or primary care provider during a routine physical examination. Additional manifestations include microscopic or gross hematuria, hypertension, abdominal pain, fatigue, anemia, and fever. The lungs are the primary site for distant metastasis.

Diagnostic Evaluation

The diagnosis can be suspected from a good history. Abdominal ultrasonography is the initial study done to detect a solid intrarenal mass. Abdominal CT or MRI, chest radiography, and chest CT are done to further evaluate extent of disease. Laboratory tests include a CBC, electrolyte levels, liver and kidney function tests, and urinalysis. A definitive diagnosis is made at the time of surgery on the basis of pathologic findings.

Therapeutic Management

Treatment for Wilms' tumor consists of surgery and chemotherapy alone or in combination with radiation therapy. In most cases, the tumor can be completely removed by surgical resection at the time of diagnosis. During surgery, the surgeon is careful to prevent spillage of the tumor, which would necessitate more aggressive treatment (Jaffe & Huff, 2004). In a few cases, complete surgical resection is considered too great a risk at the time of diagnosis and only a biopsy is performed to determine pathology. The goal of the initial chemotherapy treatments in these children is to reduce the tumor size before definitive surgery. All children receive chemotherapy after the tumor is surgically removed. Radiation therapy is added to the treatment of larger, more extensive tumors or those with an unfavorable histologic classification.

Survival rates for Wilms' tumor are much better than for many other forms of cancer. Histologic features remain the most important determinant of prognosis. Five-year survival rates exceed 90% for children with favorable histology tumors (American Cancer Society, 2003d).

▪NURSING CARE

The Child With Wilm's Tumor

Assessment

Parents often report that when bathing or dressing their child they noticed the child's stomach seemed swollen. Some parents will state the diapers no longer fit easily around the child's abdomen. More often than not, the child's activity level and appetite have not changed. Except for a palpable abdominal mass that usually does not cross the midline, the child's physical examination is normal.

Nursing Diagnosis and Planning

The nursing diagnoses and expected outcomes that apply to the child with Wilms' tumor and the child's family are
- Anxiety related to surgery with nephrectomy.
  Expected Outcome: The child and parents will express decreased anxiety about the outcome of surgery.
- Risk for Infection related to surgical interventions.
  Expected Outcome: The child will exhibit no signs and symptoms of infection, as evidenced by normal body temperature, intact incision site, and absence of purulent drainage.
- Deficient Knowledge related to unfamiliarity with the disease process and treatment plan.
  Expected Outcome: The child and parents will describe the disease process and treatment plan.
- Risk for Deficient Fluid Volume related to having only one kidney postoperatively.
  Expected Outcome: The child will demonstrate fluid balance, as evidenced by moist mucous membranes, normal electrolyte and urine values, and hourly urine output appropriate for age.

Interventions

Because the child usually feels well, nursing care initially focuses on preoperative teaching of the parents and child. Place a sign on the bed warning against palpating the abdomen. A nephrectomy is a serious surgical procedure, and family members will have anxiety about the child losing a kidney. Nurses must offer support and reassurance.

Postoperatively, monitor the child for GI activity, bowel sounds, stool production, abdominal distention, signs and symptoms of infection, hemorrhage, and changes in blood pressure. Careful assessment of output by the remaining kidney is important. Intake and output are precisely measured and totaled at least every 4 hours. These children will probably return from surgery with an NG tube in place and with an order for replacement IV fluid for the NG drainage. Typically, NG tube output is totaled every 4 hours; that total is divided by 4, and either the resulting number is added to the current IV fluid rate or another IV solution is hung so that the amount lost by NG drainage is replaced over the next 4 hours. The process is repeated until the NG drainage has slowed enough that it does not affect overall fluid and electrolyte balance. The replacement fluid usually contains potassium because gastric contents are potassium-rich. Serum electrolyte levels are checked every 8 to 12 hours during this process.

Once the tumor has been staged, the child is assigned to the appropriate therapeutic protocol. Teaching should center on the sequencing of tests and drugs on that protocol. Support for family members and assessment of their coping skills

---

! CRITICAL TO REMEMBER

Assessing the Child With a Wilms' Tumor

The tumor mass should not be palpated during the assessment because of the risk of rupturing the protective capsule. Excessive manipulation can cause seeding of the tumor and spread of cancerous cells.

---

continue throughout therapy. Therapy for Wilms' tumor is usually accomplished on an outpatient basis.

Evaluation

- Are the parents and child using coping skills and mobilizing support systems?
- Has the child remained afebrile?
- Is the incision site dry and intact and free from redness, swelling, and purulence?
- Does the child have moist mucous membranes, electrolytes and urinalysis within normal limits, and hourly urine output appropriate for age?
- Is the family asking questions and sharing concerns and fears?

RETINOBLASTOMA

Retinoblastoma is a rare, malignant tumor of the embryonic neural retina. This tumor of the eye is found only in children. Observant parents may bring this disease to the attention of the physician when they look at a photograph and see a white reflection (leukokoria) in one of the child's eyes instead of the normal red color when the camera flash is reflected off the retina.

Etiology

Retinoblastoma is thought to result from a sequence of genetic mutations. The majority of these genetic mutations are sporadic, occurring within a single retinal cell that then multiplies to form the tumor. Hereditary, or familial, retinoblastoma occurs in individuals who have a germline mutation present. The mutation places the child at high risk of developing retinoblastoma as well as other associated malignancies. A second mutation occurs in one or more of the retinal cells, which then multiply to form a tumor. Advances in genetic studies of this disease have led to genetic research on other forms of childhood cancer.

Incidence

Retinoblastoma represents 1% to 3% of all pediatric cancers (Baggott et al., 2002). Approximately 80% of cases are diagnosed before age 3 to 4 years (Hurwitz et al., 2002). Forty percent of retinoblastomas are the hereditary form, and 60% are the nonhereditary form. Approximately 21% or less of children 1 year of age or older present with tumors in both eyes (Herzog, 2004).

Pathophysiology

The tumor develops on the retina, growing inward toward the vitreous humor or out toward the subretinal space. Retinoblastoma can develop at a single site or as multiple independent tumors that originate within the globe of the eye. The process of cells breaking off from the main mass and forming additional independent tumors is called *seeding*. There are two forms of retinoblastoma: hereditary and non-hereditary. The hereditary form usually presents as multifocal tumors found in both eyes, whereas the nonhereditary form usually presents as a unifocal tumor present in only one eye (Zhao, Shields, Shields, & Gunduz, 1998). Extension of the tumor down the optic nerve and into the CNS does not often occur in children living in the United States (Herzog, 2004). As with other cancers, a staging system has been developed to standardize descriptions of extent of disease confined to the eye and those tumors that have spread outside the eye and to other parts of the body. This system directs treatment and indicates prognosis.

Manifestations

The most common findings of retinoblastoma are leukokoria and strabismus resulting from vision loss. In general, young children will not complain of vision loss limited to one eye. Manifestations may also include pain, redness, and inflammation of the eye.

Diagnostic Evaluation

Leukokoria or strabismus discovered by the parent or on a routine physical examination results in a referral to an ophthalmologist. A funduscopic examination performed by the ophthalmologist with the child under general anesthesia is the best means of diagnosing and following retinoblastoma. Ultrasound imaging confirms that the retinoblastoma tumors are present and determines their thickness and height. CT or MRI of the eyes, orbits, and brain is performed to evaluate the tumors within the eyes and to search for extraocular spread. Skeletal scintigraphy, bone marrow aspiration and biopsy, and lumbar puncture generally are not necessary unless there is clinical evidence of metastasis (Hurwitz et al., 2002).

Therapeutic Management

The goal of current treatment of retinoblastoma is not only to save the child's life but also to preserve the eye and useful vision when possible (Zhao et al., 1998). Enucleation, or removal of the eye, was standard therapy but is becoming less frequent as nonsurgical therapies improve. Enucleation may be indicated if the child has no chance for useful vision even if the tumor is destroyed. Another indication is failure of nonsurgical treatment. A disadvantage of enucleation in children younger than 3 years is that the orbit ceases to develop normally after the eye is removed and will look increasingly sunken as the child's face continues to grow. When enucleation is performed, the child does not require any further therapy and is followed closely with serial examinations to confirm that there is no tumor recurrence.

External beam radiation therapy is another treatment modality that can be used for multifocal disease. The disadvantages of radiation therapy are cosmetic deformities resulting from abnormal growth of the areas of skull exposed to radiation and a higher risk of secondary malignancies in children with familial retinoblastoma. Cryotherapy or photocoagulation may also be used for very small lesions.

The role of chemotherapy in treating intraocular disease has not been as useful in retinoblastoma because intraocular penetration of systemic drugs is poor and the tumors often develop multi-drug resistance. Multi-agent chemotherapy is used in certain circumstances (Nathan & Orkin, 1998). Chemotherapy is used to treat metastatic disease; however, these children are rarely cured. The long-term survival rate among children with retinoblastoma limited to the eyes is excellent, with a 5-year survival rate of 95% (Herzog, 2004). Retinoblastoma that extends to extraocular sites is associated with a poor prognosis.

▪NURSING CARE
The Child With Retinoblastoma

Assessment

Except for leukokoria (a whitish reflex in the pupillary area), the findings on physical examination may be normal. Assess for strabismus, esotropia, exotropia, or decreased vision. The child may have compensated for loss of vision in one eye; therefore the nurse must be very astute when assessing vision in these children.

Nursing Diagnoses and Planning

The nursing diagnoses and expected outcomes that apply to the child with retinoblastoma and the child's family are

- Anxiety (child and family) related to cancer and enucleation or fear of blindness.
  Expected Outcome: The child and family will express decreased anxiety about outcomes of therapy.
- Disturbed Sensory Perception (visual) related to visual changes caused by the tumor or enucleation.
  Expected Outcome: The child will develop compensatory mechanisms for vision, as evidenced by ability to perform activities of daily living.
- Deficient Knowledge related to unfamiliarity with the disease process and treatment.
  Expected Outcomes: The child and parents will describe the disease process and the treatment plan and will demonstrate use of any prosthetic device, if required.

Interventions

Nursing care initially focuses on support of family members as they react and adjust to the diagnosis of cancer. Second, the nurse facilitates the educational process to allay fears based on unknown factors.

Postoperative care of the enucleated orbit entails careful observations for signs of infection, hemorrhage, and edema. The child will wear a patch over the socket for about 1 week postoperatively. To preserve the shape of the orbit for prosthesis, which will be fitted 5 to 6 weeks after surgery, a conformer is placed in the orbit. Nursing interventions include teaching the parents (and child if old enough) how to remove, clean, and reinsert first the conformer and then the prosthesis.

The nurse can reassure parents that children can generally accommodate for vision in only one eye. It is very important that these children wear protective eye wear during sports or other hazardous activities to protect their remaining eye.

Whatever the extent of involvement by tumor or the treatment modality used, careful follow-up monitoring by retinal examination with the child under anesthesia and by

CT is indicated. Genetic counseling is recommended. If the retinoblastoma is found to be genetically inherited, siblings should be periodically examined, as well as any children the affected child should have.

Children with familial retinoblastoma have a high incidence of developing second malignancies later in life because of the genetic origin of the disease. Although no specific screening is recommended, signs and symptoms should be carefully evaluated with a high index of suspicion.

Evaluation

- Are the child and family verbalizing fears and a decrease in anxiety?
- Is the child able to compensate for loss of vision and continue daily activities?
- Is the child able to relate to peers and family?

- Are the child and family able to describe the disease and the treatment plan and demonstrate proper care of any prosthetic device?

RARE TUMORS OF CHILDHOOD

The most common malignancies of childhood are discussed in this chapter; however, this is not an exhaustive list. Several tumors not mentioned occur infrequently in the pediatric population. These include soft tissue sarcomas, other than rhabdomyosarcoma, primary tumors of the liver (e.g., hepatoblastoma and hepatocellular carcinoma), and gonadal and extragonadal germ cell tumors. Carcinomas, melanomas, and primary cancer of the lungs are a few of the cancers seen in adults that are exceptionally rare in children.

KEY CONCEPTS

- The signs and symptoms of childhood cancer vary according to the child's age, the type of tumor, and the extent of the disease.
- Childhood cancer is difficult to diagnose because most symptoms can be attributed to common childhood illnesses.
- The decision to use allogeneic bone marrow, autologous peripheral blood stem cells, or umbilical cord blood stem cells is made in regard to the disease process being treated and available sources of hematopoietic cells. Increased screening for possible bone marrow donors through the National Marrow Donor Program (NMDP) has greatly increased the donor pool for stem cell transplantation.
- Nursing care of children with bone marrow transplants is complex and focuses on preventing infection until the marrow engrafts

and the children produce their own white blood cells with which to fight infection. All other organ systems must be monitored for GVHD and for toxicities associated with preconditioning chemotherapy and radiation.
- Biologic response modifiers are naturally occurring substances found in the body that influence the immune system.
- Chemotherapy is nonselective in its cytotoxic effect.
- Fatigue is a common side effect of radiation therapy, and the child may need longer or more frequent periods of rest.
- Common nursing diagnoses associated with the child with cancer include Risk for Infection; Imbalanced Nutrition: Less Than Body Requirements; Deficient Knowledge; Ineffective Coping (individual); Compromised Family

Coping; Acute and Chronic Pain; Impaired Skin Integrity; Disturbed Body Image; and Impaired Oral Mucous Membrane.
- The mouth and anus are at increased risk for breakdown in the child receiving chemotherapy or radiation therapy. Temperatures should not be measured rectally, and meticulous mouth and anal care should be given.
- Postoperatively, the child with a brain tumor is at risk for increased intracranial pressure related to edema, hydrocephalus, or hemorrhage. Vital signs and mental and neurologic status are checked frequently.
- The abdomen of a child with a Wilms' tumor should not be palpated because excessive manipulation can cause seeding of the tumor if the protective capsule is ruptured.

ANSWERS to Critical Thinking Exercise 48-1

1. There is a definite difference between complementary and alternative therapies. Complementary therapies are those that are used in addition to conventional treatment and focus mainly on symptom relief. They are proven therapies (based on adequate research) or therapies that are not yet scientifically proven but deemed to be not harmful as adjunctive treatment. Alternative therapies are those designed to replace conventional therapy in the treatment of individuals with cancer.*

2. More and more people are using the Internet for information about various therapies for their specific health condition. The Internet is very accessible; however, there is little control over information published on various websites. In the area of complementary and alternative therapies, any individual or group can publish information on a website;

this information can be inaccurate, scientifically unfounded, and, in some cases, dangerous. As a nurse, you should become familiar with reputable websites that can provide you with the information you need. The following are reputable websites that have information about complementary and alternative therapies:
American Cancer Society: www.cancer.org/
National Cancer Institute: www.nci.nih.gov
National Institutes of Health: www.nih.gov
National Center for Complementary and Alternative Medicine: www.nccam.nih.gov
National Institute of Nursing Research: www.nih.gov/ninr/
Leukemia and Lymphoma Society: www.leukemia.org
Children's Oncology Group: www.childrensoncologygroup.org

3. When assisting families in their thinking about complementary and alternative therapies, health professionals should help them ask themselves the following questions†:
- What are the treatment's claims—cure, relief of symptoms?
- Are the people promoting the claims recognized and well-published experts in the field?
- How did the family find out about the treatment—mass media, scientific journals, word of mouth, local salesperson?
- What are the costs of the therapy?
- Is the therapy widely available within the health care system, or is it available to only a few?
- Will using the therapy delay conventional cancer treatment?

*Cassileth, B. (1999). Evaluating complementary and alternative therapies for cancer patients. *Cancer Journal for Clinicians, 49*(6), 362-375.
†National Center for Complementary and Alternative Medicine (2001). *Considering complementary and alternative therapies.* Available on-line: http://nccam.nih.gov.

REFERENCES and READINGS

American Academy of Pediatrics. (2003). Pickering, L.K. (Ed.). *Red Book: 2003 report of the Committee on Infectious Diseases* (26th ed.). Elk Grove Village, IL: American Academy of Pediatrics.

American Brain Tumor Association (ABTA). (1998). *A primer of brain tumors: A patient's reference manual.* Des Plaines, IL: Author.

American Cancer Society. (2003a). How is neuroblastoma staged? Retrieved June 4, 2004 from www.cancer.org

American Cancer Society. (2003b). How is osteosarcoma treated? Retrieved June 4, 2004 from www.cancer.org

American Cancer Society. (2003c). What are the key statistics for rhabdomyosarcomas? Retrieved June 4, 2004 from www.cancer.org

American Cancer Society. (2003d). What are the key statistics for Wilms' tumor? Retrieved June 4, 2004 from www.cancer.org

Arndt, C. (2000). Neoplasms of bone. In R. Behrman, R. Kliegman, & H. Jenson (Eds.). *Nelson textbook of pediatrics* (16th ed., pp. 1558-1560). Philadelphia: Saunders.

Arndt, C. (2004). Soft tissue sarcomas. In R. Behrman, R. Kliegman, & H. Jenson (Eds.). *Nelson textbook of pediatrics* (17th ed., pp. 1714-1717). Philadelphia, PA: Saunders.

Ater, J. (2004). Neuroblastoma. In R. Behrman, R. Kliegman, & H. Jenson (Eds.). *Nelson textbook of pediatrics* (17th ed., pp. 1709-1711). Philadelphia, PA: Saunders.

Baggott, C.R, Kelly, K.P., Fochtman, D., & Foley, G.V., (2002). *Nursing care of children and adolescents with cancer* (3rd ed.). Philadelphia: Saunders.

Bestak, M. (2001). Epidemiology of brain tumors. In R.F. Keating, J.T. Goodrich, & R.J. Packer (Eds.), *Tumors of the pediatric central nervous system* (pp. 14-21). New York: Thieme Medical Publishers.

Bowden, V., & Greenberg, C. (2003). *Pediatric nursing procedures.* Philadelphia: Lippincott Williams & Wilkins.

Brodeur, G.M., & Maris, J.M. (2002). Neuroblastoma. In P.A. Pizzo & D.G. Poplack (Eds.), *Principles and practice of pediatric oncology* (pp. 895-937). Philadelphia: Lippincott Williams & Wilkins.

Cassileth, B. (1999). Evaluating complementary and alternative therapies for cancer patients. *Cancer Journal for Clinicians, 49*(6), 362-375.

Friebert, S.E., & Shurin, S.B. (1998a). Acute lymphocytic leukemia: Diagnosing acute lymphocytic leukemia in children. *Patient Care, 32*(10), 100.

Friebert, S.E., & Shurin, S.B. (1998b). Acute lymphocytic leukemia: Treatment and ongoing care. *Patient Care, 32*(11), 183.

Friedman, D., & Meadows, A. (2002). Late effects of childhood cancer therapy. *Pediatric Clinics of North America, 49,* 1083-1106.

Gilchrist, G. (2004). Lymphoma. In R. Behrman, R. Kliegman, & H. Jenson (Eds.). *Nelson textbook of pediatrics* (17th ed., pp. 1698-1702). Philadelphia, PA: Saunders.

Ginsberg, J.P., Woo, S.Y., Johnson, M.E., Hicks, M.J., & Horowitz, M.E. (2002). Ewing's sarcoma family of tumors: Ewing's sarcoma of bone and soft tissue and the peripheral primitive neuroectodermal tumors. In P.A. Pizzo & D.G. Poplack (Eds.), *Principles and practice of pediatric*

oncology (pp. 973-1016). Philadelphia: Lippincott Williams & Wilkins.

Greenlee, R., Murray, T., Bolden, S., & Wingo, P. (2000). Cancer statistics, 2000. *CA: a cancer journal for clinicians, 50*(1), 7-33.

Grundy, P., Green, D., Coppes, M., Breslow, N., Ritchey, M., Perlman, E., & Macklis, R. (2002). Renal tumors. In P.A. Pizzo & D.G. Poplack (Eds.), *Principles and practice of pediatric oncology* (pp. 865-893). Philadelphia: Lippincott Williams & Wilkins.

Guinan, E., Krance, R., & Lehmann, L. (2002). Stem cell transplantation in pediatric oncology. In P.A. Pizzo & D.G. Poplack (Eds.), *Principles and practice of pediatric oncology* (pp. 429-451). Philadelphia: Lippincott Williams & Wilkins.

Gurney, J., & Bondy, M. (2002). Epidemiologic research methods and childhood cancer. In P.A. Pizzo & D.G. Poplack (Eds.), *Principles and practice of pediatric oncology* (pp.13-20). Philadelphia: Lippincott Williams & Wilkins.

Heideman, R., Packer, R., Albright, L., Freeman, C., & Rorke, L. (1997). Tumors of the central nervous system. In P.A. Pizzo & D.G. Poplack (Eds.), *Principles and practice of pediatric oncology* (pp. 633-698). Philadelphia: Lippincott-Raven.

Herzog, C. (2004). Retinoblastoma. In R. Behrman, R. Kliegman, & H. Jenson (Eds.). *Nelson textbook of pediatrics* (17th ed., pp. 1722-1723). Philadelphia, PA: Saunders.

Hudson, M., & Donaldson, S. (2002). Hodgkin's disease. In P.A. Pizzo & D.G. Poplack (Eds.), *Principles and practice of pediatric oncology* (pp. 637-660). Philadelphia: Lippincott Williams & Wilkins.

Hurwitz, R.L., Shields, C.L., Shields, J.A., Chevez-Barrios, P., Hurwitz, M.Y., & Chintagumpala, M.M. (2002). Retinoblastoma. In P.A. Pizzo & D.G. Poplack (Eds.), *Principles and practice of pediatric oncology* (pp. 825-846). Philadelphia: Lippincott Williams & Wilkins.

Jaffe, N. & Huff, V. (2004). Neoplasms of the kidney. In R. Behrman, R. Kliegman, & H. Jenson (Eds.). *Nelson textbook of pediatrics* (17th ed., pp. 1711-1714). Philadelphia, PA: Saunders.

Keating, R.F., Goodrich, J.T., & Packer, R.J. (2001). *Tumors of the pediatric central nervous system.* New York: Thieme Medical Publishers.

Kusumakumary, P., Ajithkumar, T., Ratheesan, K., Chellam, V., & Nair, M. (1998). Pattern and outcome of neuroblastoma: A 10 year study. *Indian Pediatrics, 35*(3), 223-229.

Link, M.P., Gebhardt, M.C., & Meyers, P.A. (2002) Osteosarcoma. In P.A. Pizzo & D.G. Poplack (Eds.), *Principles and practice of pediatric oncology* (pp. 1051-1089). Philadelphia: Lippincott Williams & Wilkins.

Lohr, L.K. (2002, Oct.). Rasburicase, a new, recombinant form of urate oxidase, treats hyperuricemia in tumor lysis syndrome In *Hem/Onc today.* Retrieved July 6, 2003, from www.hemonctoday.com.

Lum, L. (1999). T cell-based immunotherapy for cancer: A virtual reality? *CA: a cancer journal for clinicians, 49*(2), 74-100.

Magrath, I.T. (2002). Malignant non-Hodgkins lymphomas in children. In P.A. Pizzo & D.G. Poplack (Eds.), *Principles and practice of pediatric oncology* (pp. 661-705). Philadelphia: Lippincott Williams & Wilkins.

Margolin, J.F., Steuber, C.P., & Poplack, D.G. (2002). Acute lymphoblastic leukemia. In P.A.

Pizzo & D.G. Poplack (Eds.), *Principles and practice of pediatric oncology* (pp. 489-544). Philadelphia: Lippincott Williams & Wilkins.

Matthay, K.K., Villablanca, J.G., Seeger R.C., Stram, D.O., Harris, R.E., Ramsay, N.K., Swift, P., Shimada, H., Black, C.T., Brodeur, G.M., Gerbing, R.B., & Reynolds, C.P. (1999). Treatment of high risk neuroblastoma with intensive chemotherapy, radiotherapy, authologous bone marrow transplantation and 13-cis retinoic acid. *The New England Journal of Medicine, 341,* 1165-1173.

McHugh, K., & Boothroyd, A. (1999). The role of radiology in childhood rhabdomyosarcoma. *Clinical Radiology, 54*(1), 2-10.

Mueller, B.U. (2002). Lymphoproliferative disorders and malignancies related to immunodeficiencies. In P.A. Pizzo & D.G. Poplack (Eds.), *Principles and practice of pediatric oncology* (pp. 707-731). Philadelphia: Lippincott Williams & Wilkins.

Nathan, D.G., & Orkin, S.H. (1998). *Nathan & Oski's hematology of infancy and childhood* (5th ed.). Philadelphia: Saunders.

National Center for Complementary and Alternative Medicine (2001). *Considering complementary and alternative therapies.* Available on-line: http://nccam.nih.gov.

Otto, S.E. (2001). *Oncology nursing* (4th ed.). St. Louis: Mosby.

Pappo, A., Shapiro, D., & Crist, W. (1997). Rhabdomyosarcoma: Biology and treatment. *Pediatric Clinics of North America, 44*(4), 953-972.

Pizzo, P.A., & Poplack, D.G. (2002). *Principles and practice of pediatric oncology* (4th ed.). Philadelphia: Lippincott Williams & Wilkins.

Plon, S.E., & Malkin, D. (2002). Childhood cancer and heredity. In P.A. Pizzo & D.G. Poplack (Eds.), *Principles and practice of pediatric oncology* (pp. 21-44). Philadelphia: Lippincott Williams & Wilkins.

Pratt, C.B. (1998). Use of chemotherapy for retinoblastoma. *Medical and Pediatric Oncology, 31,* 531-533.

Smith, M.A. & Ries, L.A. (2002). Childhood cancer: Incidence, survival and mortality. In P.A. Pizzo & D.G. Poplack (Eds.), *Principles and practice of pediatric oncology* (pp. 1-12). Philadelphia: Lippincott Williams & Wilkins.

Stewart, E., & Cohen, D. (1998). Central nervous system tumors in children. *Seminars in Oncology Nursing, 14*(1), 34-42.

Wexler, L., Crist, W.M., & Helman, L.J. (2002). Rhabdomyosarcoma and the undifferentiated sarcomas. In P.A. Pizzo & D.G. Poplack (Eds.), *Principles and practice of pediatric oncology* (pp. 939-971). Philadelphia: Lippincott Williams & Wilkins.

Wingard, J. (1997). Bone marrow to blood stem cell: Past, present, future. In M.B. Whedon & D. Wujcik (Eds.), *Blood and marrow stem cell transplantation: Principles, practice and nursing insight* (2nd ed., pp. 3-24). Boston: Jones & Bartlett.

Zhao, D., Shields, C.L., Shields, J.A., & Gunduz, K. (1998). New developments in the management of retinoblastoma. *Journal of Ophthalmic Nursing and Technology, 17*(1), 13-18.

49

The Child with an Integumentary Alteration

◆ LEARNING OBJECTIVES

After studying this chapter, you should be able to:

◉ Describe the anatomy and physiology of normal skin.
◉ Contrast characteristics of the newborn's, child's, and adult's skin.
◉ Identify common skin disorders seen in infants and children.
◉ Discuss the manifestations of and treatment for skin disorders such as bacterial, fungal, and viral infections; infestations; inflammatory disorders; acne vulgaris; and insect bites and stings.

◉ Discuss common causes of burns in children and the prevention of burn injuries.
◉ Analyze the implications of burn injuries in children.
◉ Discuss the classifications of depth, extent, and severity of a burn injury.
◉ Describe the therapeutic management and nursing care of children with minor burns.
◉ Apply the nursing process to the care of infants and children with skin disorders.

◆ DEFINITIONS

alopecia Hair loss.
débridement Removal of foreign material and devitalized or contaminated tissue from a traumatic or infected lesion to expose healthy tissue.
desquamation Sloughing of the skin in scales or sheets; can lead to loss of the deeper skin layers.
ecchymosis Discoloration of the skin or mucous membranes caused by leakage of blood into the subcutaneous tissue.
erythema Redness of the skin.
eschar Dark plaque associated with tissue necrosis, which can form an inelastic shell over wounds.
excoriation Scratch or abrasion of the skin.
hydrotherapy Therapy entailing water soaks to clean wounds, which removes old dressings and softens dead tissue for easier removal.

intertrigo Maceration of two closely apposed skin surfaces.
keratosis Overgrowth and thickening of the cornified epithelium.
lichenification Thickening and hardening of the skin with accentuation of skin markings; often the result of chronic scratching.
pediculocide An agent used to destroy lice.
petechiae Tiny, flat, purplish red spots on the skin surface resulting from minute hemorrhages within the dermis.
pruritus Itching.
urticaria (hives) Vascular reaction of the skin characterized by pruritic wheals, often caused by allergy or emotional stress.

REVIEW OF THE INTEGUMENTARY SYSTEM

A knowledge of integumentary structure and function is necessary to understand the changes that occur with disease. There are a number of important differences between the skin of infants and young children and that of adults.

The skin has five major functions: (1) to protect the deeper tissues from injury, drying, and invasion by foreign matter; (2) to regulate temperature; (3) to aid in excretion of water; (4) to aid in production of vitamin D; and (5) to initiate the sensations of touch, pain, heat, and cold.

The skin is composed of two principle layers: the outer *epidermis* and the inner supportive *dermis*. Beneath these layers is the *subcutaneous layer*, which is composed largely of adipose tissue.

The *epidermis* is nonvascular stratified epithelium. It is divided into two major layers. The outermost layer, the *stratum corneum*, is a tough, horny collection of dead keratinized cells that have migrated up from the underlying layers. *Keratin*, a fibrous protein, is also the principal component of nails and hair. Skin cells are constantly being shed and replaced with new cells from the layers below.

The *stratum basale*, or basal cell layer, anchors the epidermis to the dermis. This innermost layer contains melanocytes—the source of melanin, the pigment that gives skin its color. The epidermis is completely replaced every 4 weeks.

The *dermis*, composed of tough connective tissue, contains lymphatics and nerves. The highly vascular dermis nourishes the epidermis.

Appendages from the epidermis—sebaceous glands, sweat glands, and hair follicles—are embedded in the dermis. The sebaceous glands arise from the hair follicles and produce sebum, which lubricates the epidermis and is slightly bacteriostatic. Sebaceous glands are particularly abundant on the face and scalp. Hormones influence their activity, with testosterone increasing secretion and estrogen suppressing it.

There are two types of sweat glands. The *eccrine sweat glands* open directly onto the skin surface and produce sweat, which evaporates to reduce body temperature. Eccrine sweat glands are widely distributed over the body and are functionally mature by two months of age. The *apocrine sweat glands* produce a thick, milky secretion and open onto hair follicles. They are located mainly in the axillary and genital areas and become active during puberty.

Pediatric Differences in the Skin

- The newborn's skin is thinner and more susceptible to irritants and infection than the skin of adults. Handle carefully to avoid skin injury.
- Because the ratio of skin surface area to body volume is greater in infants and small children than in adults, there is a risk of greater absorption through the skin. Therefore topical ointments and other skin preparations should not be used without a physician's order.
- Premature infants have a proportionately greater body surface area than older infants and children, which increases evaporative fluid losses. Full-term infants are born with the ability to sweat in response to heat, although higher temperatures are required to induce sweating relative to adults.
- Eccrine glands do not reach mature function until age 2 or 3 years, making infants and young toddlers less able to regulate body temperature.
- The skin of infants and young children is more susceptible to bacterial infection.
- Immunoglobulin A (IgA), secreted by the epithelial cells of the mucous membranes, does not reach adult levels until age 2 to 5 years. This makes the infant less resistant to organisms, such as those occurring on the hands or other objects the infant might mouth.
- Hormonal changes during adolescence increase sebum production, which contributes to acne vulgaris.

Modified from Rutter, N. (2000). Physiology of the newborn skin. In J. Harper, A. Oranje, & N. Prose (Eds), *Textbook of pediatric dermatology* (pp. 43-47). Oxford: Blackwell Science.

Each hair is composed of a shaft and a root, which lie in a deep cavity of dermal cells called the *hair follicle*. There are several types of hair. *Lanugo* is the fine first hair that covers the body during fetal life and generally disappears before or shortly after birth. It is replaced by fine, nonpigmented *vellus* hair. *Terminal* hair covers all the ordinarily hairy parts of the body and is coarse, long, and pigmented.

The *subcutaneous layer*, composed of fat cells, underlies the dermis. Adipose tissue helps cushion and insulate underlying structures.

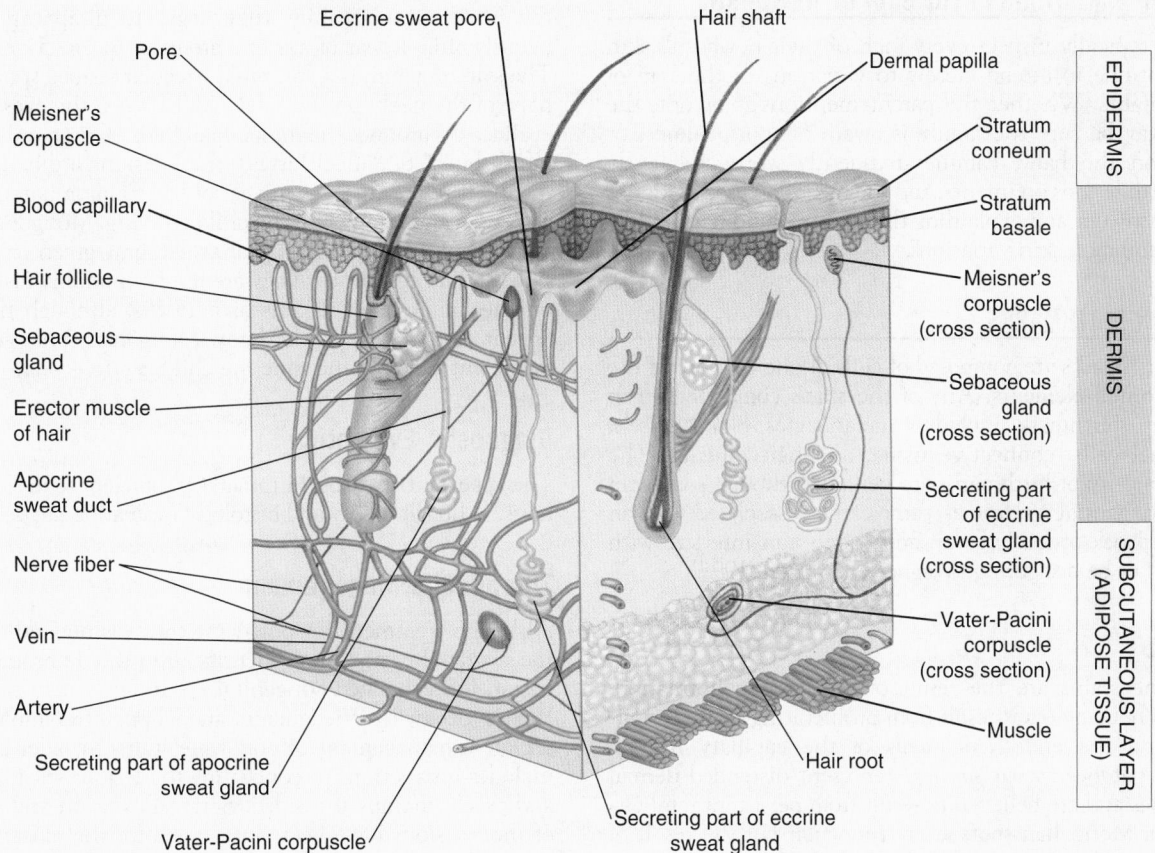

Eccrine sweat pore

Hair shaft

Pore

Meisner's corpuscle

Dermal papilla

Blood capillary

Stratum corneum

Hair follicle

Stratum basale

Sebaceous gland

Meisner's corpuscle (cross section)

Erector muscle of hair

Sebaceous gland (cross section)

Apocrine sweat duct

Secreting part of eccrine sweat gland (cross section)

Nerve fiber

Vein

Vater-Pacini corpuscle (cross section)

Artery

Muscle

Secreting part of apocrine sweat gland

Hair root

Vater-Pacini corpuscle

Secreting part of eccrine sweat gland

EPIDERMIS

DERMIS

SUBCUTANEOUS LAYER (ADIPOSE TISSUE)

The skin is a sensitive indicator of a child's general health. Skin disorders are among the most common health problems in children. They may cause pain, pruritus, or changes in local sensation. Because the skin is visible and its disorders are often disfiguring, skin disorders can cause emotional and psychological stress for the child and family. Whether it is the discomfort and stress produced by an infant's eczema or the emotional upset caused by an adolescent's acne, these disorders can influence the child's psychological and social development.

Nurses caring for children are in a unique position to assess the condition of children's skin and to help children and families cope with skin disorders. Nurses can play an important role by teaching parents and children strategies to maintain healthy skin and prevent future skin problems.

COMMON VARIATIONS IN THE SKIN OF NEWBORNS

Parents typically inspect every inch of their newborn's skin and continue to attend closely to variations in the skin of older infants. Whether the parent mentions it or not, the nurse may be sure the family is aware of spots, bumps, or rashes on the baby. Families frequently worry needlessly about skin lesions on infants, and the nurse can ease anxieties by pointing out and explaining the meaning and natural history of common skin variations.

COMMON BIRTHMARKS

Most birthmarks are composed of cells of one or more of the skin's normal elements. Any of the skin's components can produce a birthmark, including melanocytes, blood vessels, epidermal cells, connective tissue, and hair follicles. The great majority of birthmarks are benign, although some can signal congenital syndromes, some can be associated with an increased risk of malignancy, and others can interfere with function or be disfiguring (Wagner & Hansen, 1995).

Etiology

Port-wine stains are the result of capillary malformation, whereas hemangiomas result from proliferating dilated capillaries and the endothelial cells of the capillary linings. Salmon patches (*nevus simplex*) represent distended dermal capillaries and are believed to result from persistent fetal circulation. Mongolian spots are not vascular but the result of collections of pigment deep in the dermis. They occur as a result of arrested migration of melanocytes from the neural crest to the skin during embryonic development. Café au lait spots, light-brown pigmented areas, can appear anywhere on an infant's body. Six or more of these lesions, if larger than 5 mm in diameter, suggest an underlying disorder, such as neurofibromatosis, Noonan syndrome, and McCune-Albright syndrome (Bolognia, 2000).

Incidence

Vascular birthmarks are extremely common, with most references estimating incidence to occur in at least 20% to 40% of newborns. Port-wine stains occur in 3 in 1000 live births, and about 2.5% of all newborns have hemangiomas. The most common vascular lesion is the salmon patch, which

some references estimate to occur in as many as 40% of newborns. The incidence of mongolian spots is proportional to the depth of the baby's pigmentation. As many as 90% of African-American and Native-American infants are born with mongolian spots, and 70% to 80% of Asian and Latino infants have them. Fewer than 10% of white infants present with mongolian spots.

Manifestations

The port-wine stain is present at birth. At first it is only faintly colored and flat, but it becomes darker as the child grows. In some cases, underlying bone and tissue may enlarge as well. The port-wine stain is permanent, and by middle age, the mark may be dark purple and rough or nodular. Hemangiomas, on the other hand, are not usually visible at birth but appear during the first few weeks of life and then grow during the first year. Generally, they begin to disappear spontaneously after 1 year of age and are gone by age 5 or 6 years. The salmon patch is a flat, pink, irregular-shaped spot on the nape of the neck, on the forehead, between the eyes, on the eyelids, or around the nasolabial folds. Commonly called "stork bites" or "angel kisses," these lesions are benign and usually fade during the first year of life. Salmon patches typically appear darker when the child is crying. Mongolian spots are present at birth and appear as flat, gray-green or blue lesions similar to bruises. They are most commonly distributed on the lumbosacral regions or buttocks, although they can appear on any part of the body. Mongolian spots generally fade completely by the time the child is 3 to 4 years old.

Diagnostic Evaluation

The appearance of most birthmarks is sufficient to make a diagnosis, although biopsy and histologic evaluation are definitive.

Therapeutic Management

Although treatment for port-wine stains is not indicated in the neonatal period, their identification should prompt evaluation for associated congenital syndromes, such as Sturge-Weber, Beckwith-Wiedemann, and Klippel-Trenaunay. Conservative management of port-wine stains in older children includes instructions in concealing the lesions with makeup, and psychotherapy if needed. Surgical excision and grafting of these lesions have been abandoned for the most part because of disfiguring scarring. However, laser therapy has been used on port-wine stains since the 1980s with increasing sophistication and success.

The treatment for hemangiomas includes simple observation as the lesion involutes on its own, pharmacotherapy, surgical excision, radiation, and laser therapy. Active intervention is reserved for hemangiomas that interfere with function, such as those that obstruct the nose, mouth, or eyes or lesions that tend to ulcerate and bleed frequently. Pharmacologic approaches include injection of steroids into the lesion, oral steroids, and topical imiquimod (Martinez, North, & Mihm, 2002). The argon laser tends to relieve the symptoms of ulcerated hemangiomas in a matter of days, and involution typically follows. A rapidly growing, deep hemangioma may be associated with Kasabach-Merritt syndrome, a coagulopathy that results from the collecting of platelets within the hemangioma. This may be life-threatening, and treatment may include hospitalization and treatment with anticoagulants.

Other than education, treatment for salmon patches and mongolian spots is not indicated.

Nursing Considerations

Assess the child's entire body for distribution, size, and shape of lesions. Assess hemangiomas for symptoms such as ulceration or bleeding and for potential to obstruct function. Assess the extent of the parents' knowledge regarding the infant's birthmarks.

Parents are frequently anxious about newborns' skin lesions, and it is not unusual to discover that parents already have acquired misinformation from friends and family members about the meaning and prognosis of birthmarks. Common anxiety-provoking beliefs include the ideas that prominent lesions are malignant or that the mother caused the lesions by careless behaviors during her pregnancy.

The parents should receive a simple, scientific explanation for the skin lesions and instructions regarding usual skin care for newborns. Parents should be made aware of the expected course of their child's lesion, and their expectations should be explored. Parents should be reassured when the lesions are benign and educated thoroughly about what to expect when treatment is indicated.

INFECTIONS OF THE SKIN

Skin infections are common in childhood. Bacteria are normally present on healthy skin. The skin's susceptibility to bacterial infection depends on several factors, including the intactness of the skin, the virulence of the organisms, and the child's immune status.

Children are also susceptible to fungal and viral infections. Unlike bacterial infections, which generally respond fairly quickly to treatment, fungal and viral infections can be more persistent and challenging to treat.

IMPETIGO

Impetigo is the most common bacterial skin infection of childhood. Close contact contributes to the spread of impetigo, which is very contagious. Children in daycare facilities, schools, or camps and adolescent athletes are at increased risk.

Etiology

Impetigo often occurs as a secondary infection from another skin lesion, such as an insect bite. It can be caused by *Staphylococcus aureus*, group A beta-hemolytic streptococci, or a combination of these bacteria. *S. aureus* is the primary pathogen in most cases.

The incubation period is 7 to 10 days. Impetigo is extremely contagious and may spread to other parts of the child's skin or to others who touch the child, use the same towel, or drink from the same glass. Spread of the infection is fostered by poor hygiene, crowded living conditions, and a hot, humid environment. Lesions resolve in 12 to 14 days with treatment.

Incidence

Impetigo occurs most often during hot, humid summer months. Toddlers and preschoolers are most commonly affected, often when recovering from an upper respiratory tract infection.

Manifestations

The primary lesions of impetigo occur in two forms. Bullous impetigo characteristically presents as small vesicles that can progress to bullae. The lesions are initially filled with serous fluid and later become pustular. The bullae rapidly rupture, leaving a shiny, lacquered-appearing lesion surrounded by a scaly rim. Crusted impetigo appears initially as a vesicle or pustule that ruptures to become an erosion with an overlay of honey-colored crust. The erosions bleed easily when crusts are removed (Fig. 49-1). Lesions are mildly pruritic. Scarring is uncommon but may occur if the child picks or scratches

---

PARENTS

Want to Know

About Care of Newborn and Infant Skin

Encourage parents to protect the infant's skin by teaching the following:
- Infants may be bathed and shampooed daily after the umbilical cord has fallen off. Use mild soap and warm water.
- Avoid overbathing, which dries the skin. Do not allow the infant to bathe longer than 10 minutes. Avoid bubble-bath products; they dry and irritate the skin.
- Lotions, creams, and powders are not needed after the bath.
- Change diapers frequently, and clean diaper area with water at each change.
- Remove diapers for short periods during the day while the baby lies on a washable pad, to expose diaper area to air.
- Avoid hot environments and overbundling the baby. Infants do not sweat effectively, and heat results in rashes as well as problems with temperature regulation.
- Do not permit direct exposure to the sun during the first 2 weeks of life, and avoid sun exposure for more than 10 to 15 minutes daily thereafter during early infancy. Babies should wear hats or bonnets and shirts in the sun. Do not use sunscreen on infants younger than 6 months.

Pathophysiology

of Impetigo

Impetigo begins in an area of broken skin, such as an insect bite, scabies, or atopic dermatitis. The break in the skin allows for organism entry. The inflammatory process results in the formation of a pustular lesion. Honey-colored fluid from this lesion becomes crusted. In some children, nasal discharge containing the organism erodes healthy skin above the upper lip, allowing for organism entry.

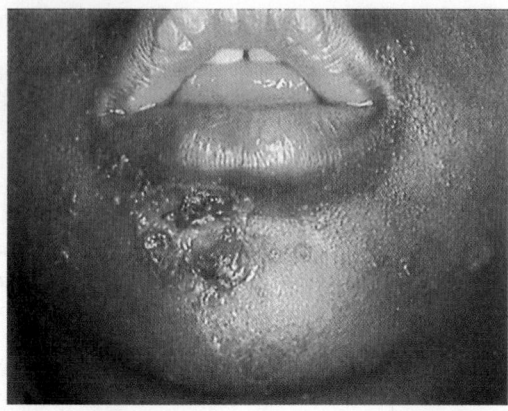

Figure 49-1 Impetigo lesions are usually located around the mouth and nose but may be located on the extremities. (From Hurwitz, S. [1993]. *Clinical pediatric dermatology: A textbook of skin disorders of childhood and adolescence* [2nd ed., p. 280]. Philadelphia: Saunders.)

the lesions. Postinflammatory hyperpigmentation is a frequent sequela in dark-skinned children. The lesions are often located around the mouth and nose but can present on any part of the body.

Diagnostic Evaluation

The characteristic appearance of the lesions usually confirms the diagnosis. A culture is not often done unless the child fails to respond to treatment. If a culture is ordered, the specimen should be obtained from beneath the crust or from the fluid inside the lesions.

Therapeutic Management

Impetigo is treated with topical and oral antibiotics. The lesions should be gently washed three times a day with a warm, soapy washcloth and the crusts soaked and carefully removed. A topical ointment, such as mupirocin (Bactroban) or bacitracin (Baciguent), is then applied to the lesions. Topical therapy lasts 7 to 10 days. Severe cases of impetigo or cases of impetigo around the mouth are treated with oral antibiotics that are effective against both staphylococcal and streptococcal organisms. Impetigo that is extensive is treated with intravenous (IV) antibiotics. Antibiotic treatment of streptococcal impetigo does not prevent glomerulonephritis, but it does hasten healing of the lesions.

Good handwashing and careful hygiene are imperative to prevent spread of the infection and should be emphasized to the child and parents. The child should not attend school or daycare for 24 hours after beginning treatment (American Academy of Pediatrics [AAP], 2000). The school should be notified of the diagnosis.

■ NURSING CARE
The Child With Impetigo

Assessment

Assess the child's skin for the size, distribution, and spread of impetigo lesions. If the child is taking systemic antibiotics, monitor for signs of adverse effects, such as rashes or diarrhea.

> ### ! CRITICAL TO REMEMBER
> **Caring for a Child With Impetigo**
>
> - The child can spread impetigo lesions merely by touching another part of the skin after scratching the infected area.
> - Keep the child's fingernails short, and wash the child's hands frequently with antibacterial soap.
> - Emphasize good handwashing and careful hygiene for the child's entire household.
> - Discourage family members from sharing towels, combs, or eating utensils with the infected child.

If the impetigo is caused by beta-hemolytic streptococci, observe for periorbital edema or blood in the urine, which may signal the development of acute glomerulonephritis.

Nursing Diagnosis and Planning

The nursing diagnoses and expected outcomes that may be appropriate for the child with impetigo and the child's family are

■ Impaired Skin Integrity related to destruction of skin layers secondary to bacterial infection.
   Expected Outcomes: The child will maintain skin integrity, as evidenced by confinement of the infection to the primary site. The area will heal without scarring or further infection.

■ Deficient Knowledge related to unfamiliarity with prevention of spread of infection, care of impetigo lesions, and antibiotic administration.
   Expected Outcomes: The child and family will comply with measures to prevent the spread of infection. The parent will demonstrate care of the lesions and administration of medications.

Interventions

Teach parents to soak the crusts and then wash them off with a warm, soapy washcloth three times a day. Advise them to gently remove the crusts after soaking, taking care not to spread the infection to other parts of the body with the contaminated washcloth. Antibiotic ointment should then be applied to the lesions and the affected areas left open to air. A small amount of bleeding after crust removal is common.

The child should sleep alone and should be bathed daily, alone, with antibacterial soap. The caregiver should wear gloves when caring for the child. Emphasize the importance of administering the full course of topical or systemic antibiotics as prescribed.

Evaluation

- Are the lesions healing, and have they remained confined to the primary site?
- Do the child and family members practice handwashing and other techniques to prevent the spread of infection?
- Do the parents appropriately explain the necessity for administering the full course of treatment?

CELLULITIS

Cellulitis is a bacterial infection of the subcutaneous tissue and the dermis. It is usually associated with a break in the skin. Cellulitis of the head and neck can follow an upper respiratory tract infection, sinusitis, otitis media, or tooth abscess. Cellulitis occurs most commonly in the lower extremities and the buccal (inside the cheek) and periorbital (around the eye) regions. Complications of cellulitis include septic arthritis, meningitis, and brain abscess. Periorbital cellulitis can lead to blindness.

Etiology and Incidence

Streptococcus, S. aureus, and *Haemophilus influenzae* are the most common causes of cellulitis. The incidence of *H. influenzae* cellulitis has decreased since the *H. influenzae* type B (Hib) vaccine was introduced. Cellulitis is most common in children age 2 years and younger.

Pathophysiology

A failure of the body's immune system results in a more extensive invasion of the causative organism. The infection moves from superficial tissue to deeper subcutaneous tissue.

Manifestations

The affected area is red, hot, tender, and indurated. If *H. influenzae* is the suspected organism, the affected area might have a purplish tinge. Edema and purple discoloration of the eyelids and decreased eye movement are present in periorbital cellulitis (see Chapter 55). Lymphangitis is seen, with red "streaking" of the surrounding area and enlarged regional lymph nodes (lymphadenitis). The child usually exhibits fever, malaise, and headache.

Diagnostic Evaluation

Usually a complete blood count (CBC), blood cultures, and culture of the affected area are done. If no drainage is present, the affected area can be aspirated. Orbital cellulitis can be diagnosed by computed tomography (CT) of the orbit.

Therapeutic Management

After an initial intramuscular (IM) or IV dose of an antibiotic, such as ceftriaxone, the child with cellulitis of an extremity is usually treated at home with a 10-day course of oral antibiotics (cephalosporin, cloxacillin, or dicloxacillin) and warm compresses. If the cellulitis involves a joint or the face or if the child shows other signs of acute febrile illness, hospitalization and IV antibiotics are required. Incision and drainage of the affected area may be necessary.

▪ NURSING CARE
The Child With Cellulitis

Assessment

Record the history, and question the parent regarding recent ear infections, dental caries, or trauma to the skin surrounding the affected area. Other pertinent data include when the inflammation started and how rapidly it has progressed. Examine the skin, noting any temperature increase, swelling, redness, and drainage. Assess for fever, pain, guarding, and irritability.

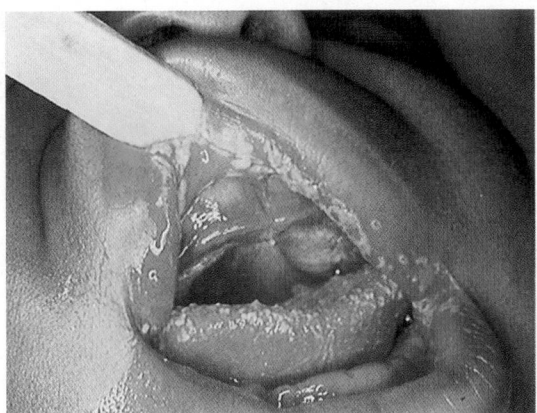

Figure 49-2 White, curdlike plaques of thrush (oral candidiasis, oral moniliasis), a common fungal infection in infants. (From Hurwitz, S. [1993]. *Clinical pediatric dermatology: A textbook of skin disorders of childhood and adolescence* [2nd ed., p. 36]. Philadelphia: Saunders.)

Nursing Diagnosis and Planning

The nursing diagnoses and expected outcomes that may be appropriate for the child with cellulitis and the child's family are
- Impaired Skin Integrity related to bacterial invasion.
  Expected Outcome: The child will exhibit signs of healing, such as decreased redness, decreased swelling, and decreased fever.
- Acute Pain related to soft tissue swelling and inflammation.
  Expected Outcomes: The child will be able to sleep and will demonstrate decreased irritability.
- Deficient Knowledge related to unfamiliarity with the illness and treatment.
  Expected Outcomes: The family will describe measures to prevent the spread of infection, will describe how to administer antibiotics as prescribed, and will demonstrate the ability to carry out treatment measures.

Interventions

The child should rest in bed with the affected extremity elevated and immobilized. Warm, moist soaks applied every 4 hours increase circulation to the infected area, relieve pain, and promote healing. Acetaminophen can be given to control fever and pain. Frequent handwashing is essential to prevent the spread of infection. If the child is hospitalized, IV antibiotics should be administered accurately and on time to maintain a therapeutic blood level. If the child is being treated at home, the parents must understand the importance of administering the entire course of antibiotics as ordered. The child should be carefully monitored for signs of sepsis (increased fever, chills, confusion) and spread of infection.

Evaluation

- Does the child's skin exhibit signs of healing?
- Is the child free from signs of infection and pain?
- Does the parent administer prescribed medications and carry out appropriate home care?

CANDIDIASIS

Thrush (oral candidiasis) (Fig. 49-2) is a superficial fungal infection of the oral mucous membranes that is common in infants. Thrush occurs as a result of overgrowth of *Candida albi-*

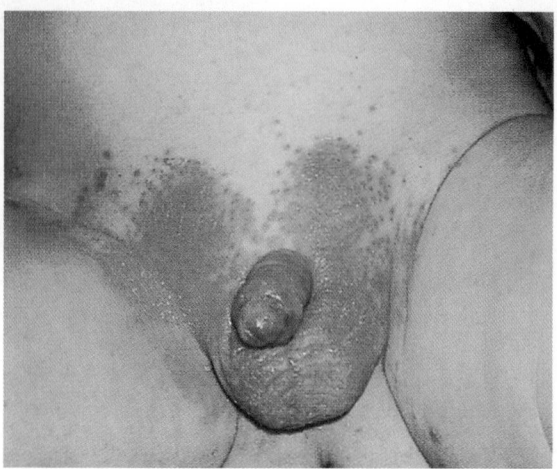

Figure 49-3 Diaper candidiasis. (From Feigin, R.D., & Cherry, J.D. [Eds.]. [1999]. *Textbook of pediatric infectious diseases* [4th ed., p. 728]. Philadelphia: Saunders.)

cans. In addition to oral lesions, the child may exhibit lesions in the diaper area, which are caused by *C. albicans* passing through the intestine. Moisture and heat in the diaper area create an environment favorable to the development of *Candida* dermatitis. Persistent candidiasis suggests that the child might be immunocompromised.

Etiology

A neonate can acquire candidiasis during delivery while passing through an infected vagina. An older infant may develop a fungal overgrowth as a result of immunosuppression, during antibiotic therapy, from exposure to the mother's infected breasts, or from unclean bottles and pacifiers.

Incidence

Candidiasis occurs most often in infants. Predisposing factors in all age-groups include antibiotic therapy, diabetes, and altered immune status.

Manifestations

White, curdlike plaques are noted on the tongue, gums, and buccal mucosa in children with thrush. They can be distinguished from milk curds by the difficulty encountered in removing them and the bleeding of an erythematous base when plaques are removed. A child with severe infection may have difficulty eating. The lesions of diaper dermatitis are usually bright red and coalesced, with some discrete lesions spreading out to the child's abdomen and thighs (Fig. 49-3).

Diagnostic Evaluation

The diagnosis of thrush and candidal diaper dermatitis is made from the clinical appearance of the lesions.

Therapeutic Management

Nystatin oral suspension (100,000 U/ml), swabbed onto the mucous membranes of the mouth, is effective in treating thrush. Because *Candida* is present in the gastrointestinal tract,

oral nystatin also may be ordered to decrease the likelihood of recurrence. Mothers of breastfeeding infants with thrush can paint their nipples with the nystatin solution before nursing. Candidal diaper dermatitis is treated with a topical antifungal agent, such as nystatin or clotrimazole (Lotrimin).

■ NURSING CARE
The Child With Candidiasis

Assessment

Nursing assessment includes obtaining a history of maternal and infant *Candida* infections. Question the mother regarding vaginal itching or discharge or any nipple tenderness or redness. Also discuss methods used to clean bottles and pacifiers. Examine the infant's mouth and diaper area, and assess nutrition and hydration status.

Nursing Diagnosis and Planning

The nursing diagnoses and expected outcomes that may be appropriate for the child with candidiasis and the child's family are

- Impaired Skin Integrity related to the effects of fungal infection.
  Expected Outcome: The infant will exhibit signs of healing lesions, as evidenced by pink, intact mucous membranes or resolution of diaper rash.
- Acute Pain related to oral lesions or skin irritation.
  Expected Outcome: The infant will have reduced discomfort, as evidenced by ability to take feedings without difficulty, decreased fussiness, and improved ability to sleep.
- Deficient Knowledge related to incomplete understanding of the cause of the infection and administration of medication.
  Expected Outcomes: The family will demonstrate methods to prevent spread of infection and will administer the entire course of medication as prescribed.
- Imbalanced Nutrition: Less Than Body Requirements related to mouth irritation and altered taste.
  Expected Outcomes: The infant will accept feedings and will consume appropriate amounts of nutrients.

Interventions

Teach the parent to swab 1 ml of oral nystatin suspension onto the infant's gums and tongue every 6 hours until 3 to 4 days after symptoms have disappeared. Older children can receive up to 4 ml four times a day. Because cotton-tipped applicators tend to absorb the medication, a more effective method of administration is to rub the suspension onto the mucous membranes with a gloved finger. To increase the amount of time the medication is in contact with the mucous membranes, nystatin should be applied after feedings. Alternatively, oral fluconazole may be used for treatment of thrush in infants.

Pacifiers, nipples, and bottles should be thoroughly cleaned to decrease the chance of reinfection. Teach the parents the technique and importance of good handwashing. If the infant is breastfed, the mother's breasts should also be treated with nystatin.

Suggest small, frequent feedings for the infant or child with thrush who is uncomfortable. Cool liquids are soothing to the older child.

For the infant with candidal diaper dermatitis, suggest that the parent apply nystatin or clotrimazole cream. Leaving the diaper area exposed to air reduces the moisture that facilitates fungal growth.

Advise the parent to contact the health care provider if the infant refuses to eat or develops fever or if the candidiasis does not clear with treatment.

Evaluation

- Have the lesions disappeared, leaving intact skin and oral mucous membranes?
- Does the child appear to be comfortable, sleeping well, and less irritable?
- Can the parents demonstrate proper medication administration?
- Is the child increasing the amount of oral intake?

TINEA INFECTION

Tinea is a superficial skin infection caused by a group of fungi known as *dermatophytes*. Tinea infections are designated by the word *tinea* followed by the Latin word for the affected part of the body. Figure 49-4 illustrates various types of tinea infections.

Etiology

Two types of dermatophytes, *Trichophyton* spp. and *Microsporum* spp., cause the majority of tinea infections. *Trichophyton* affects all keratinized tissue, including skin, nails, and hair. *Microsporum* invades the hair.

Tinea infections are transmitted from person to person, by animal contact, or by contact with contaminated fomites (e.g., combs, hats, headrests, pillows). Ninety percent of cases of tinea capitis (fungal infection of the scalp) in the United States are caused by *T. tonsurans*, which is transmitted from person to person (Clayton, 2000). Tinea cruris (fungal infection affecting the groin and scrotal area) is not highly contagious. Poor hygiene, friction from tight clothing, and obesity are predisposing factors. Tinea pedis (athlete's foot) is a fungal infection of toes and feet. It is contagious but rarely develops on healthy, dry skin.

Incidence

Tinea capitis usually occurs in children ages 1 to 10 years, whereas tinea pedis and tinea cruris are most common in adolescent boys. Because a moist environment supports the growth of fungal infections, most tinea infections appear when the weather is hot and humid.

Manifestations

Common manifestations of tinea capitis include erythema and scaling of the scalp, as well as one or more round patches of alopecia that slowly increase in size. Small papules at the base of hair follicles become crusting pustules and red scales. In some cases, thick, broken hairs close to the scalp surface result in patches of "black dot" alopecia. Kerion formation may occur as a result of an inflammatory response to fungal antigens. A kerion is a boggy, fluctuant nodule, typically crusted and studded with pustules. Surrounding lymph nodes may be enlarged.

Tinea corporis, commonly seen on the trunk, face, and extremities, is characterized by ringlike plaques with pale centers and scaly, red margins. Lesions are usually $1/2$ to 1 inch in diameter and mildly pruritic.

Pathophysiology

of Tinea Infection

Tinea infection occurs when the fungus causing tinea invades the hair, the stratum corneum of the skin, or the nails.

In *tinea capitis,* the fungus invades the hair shafts, causing the hairs to become brittle and to break off at the level of the scalp, leaving an area of stubby, black-dotted alopecia. An immune reaction to the fungus may develop in the form of a *kerion,* a boggy, red, tender scalp mass that may contain *Staphylococcus aureus* and is often accompanied by fever and lymphadenopathy. Children with allergies seem to be more susceptible to tinea capitis.

Tinea corporis (ringworm) is a fungal infection of the face, trunk, or extremities. It can be transmitted by humans or by dogs and cats. Most lesions of tinea corporis clear without treatment in several months, but some may become chronic.

Tinea cruris (jock itch) is characterized by an intense inflammatory reaction with severe pruritus.

Tinea pedis (athlete's foot) may become chronic, particularly in adolescents who wear nonventilated athletic shoes. Tinea lesions may become secondarily infected with bacteria or *Candida.*

Manifestations of tinea cruris may include pink papules and scales on the inner thighs, groin, scrotum, and buttocks (but not the penis). Pruritus is also present.

Tinea pedis may produce fine vesiculopustular or scaly lesions on the soles of the feet, between the toes, and under the nails. Peeling, fissures, and maceration appear in severe cases, and pruritus and burning are typically present.

Diagnostic Evaluation

Most tinea infections can be diagnosed from the clinical appearance of the lesions. Fungal cultures or microscopic examination of skin scrapings prepared with potassium hydroxide (KOH) confirms the diagnosis. In the past, tinea infections were diagnosed when the lesions fluoresced under an ultraviolet Wood's light. However, the most common organism causing tinea today, *T. tonsurans*, does not fluoresce. *Microsporum* lesions fluoresce as a bright blue-green.

Therapeutic Management

Tinea Capitis

For treatment to be effective, medication must penetrate the hair follicles. Topical therapy alone is not effective for tinea capitis. Oral griseofulvin for 6 to 8 weeks is the treatment of choice, and the trend is toward the higher end of the dosing range because of an increasing incidence of treatment failures. Because griseofulvin is insoluble in water, its absorption is increased if it is taken with a high-fat meal or with milk. Ketoconazole (Nizoral) or terbinafine (Lamisil) may be prescribed for children who cannot tolerate griseofulvin or who fail to respond to it (Fuller et al., 2001). Ketoconazole is used with caution in children because of the risk of hepatotoxicity when prescribed for long-term therapy. Selenium sulfide shampoo (Selsun Blue) should be used twice per week for 2 weeks to eliminate spores.

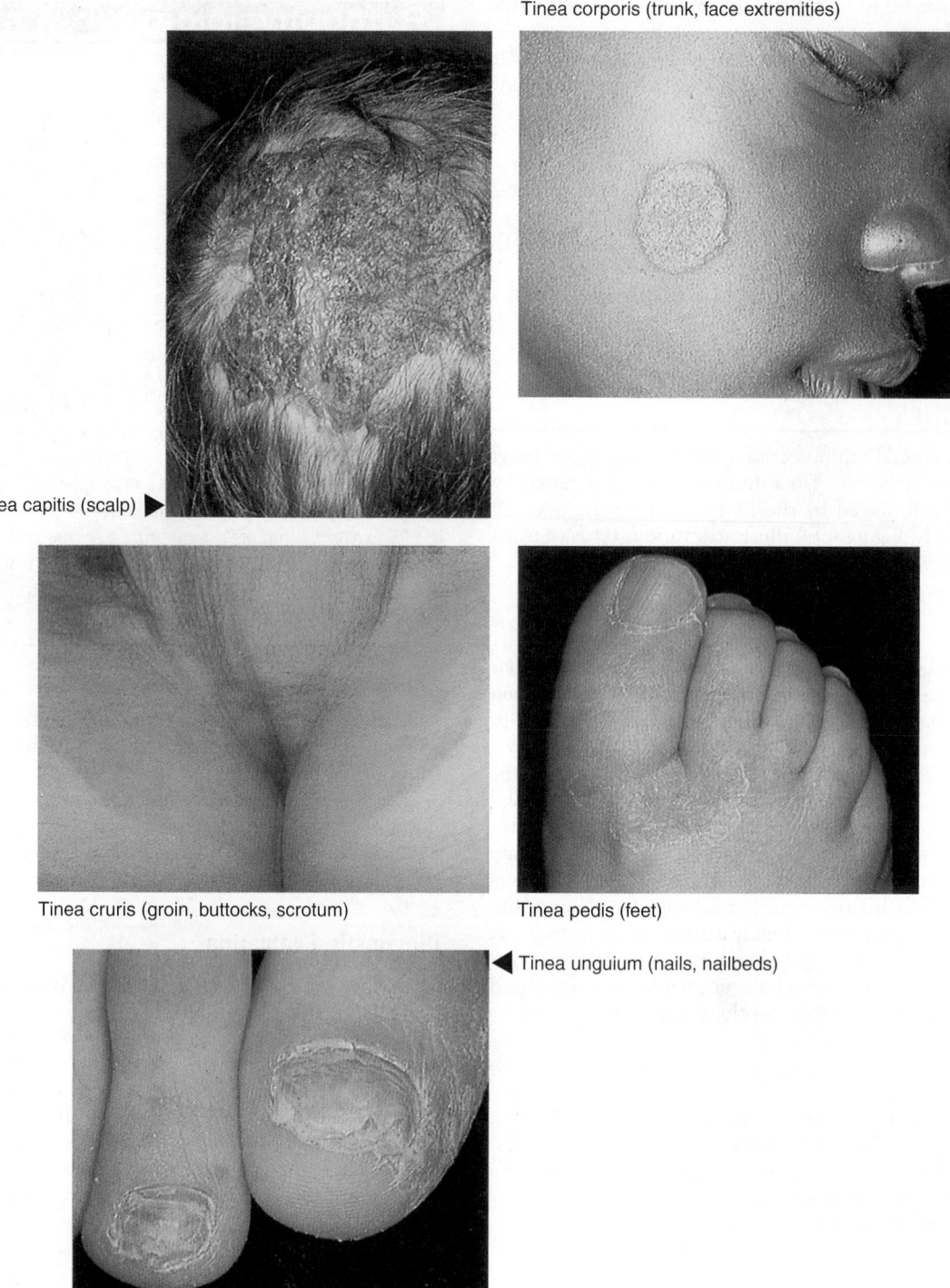

Tinea corporis (trunk, face extremities)

Tinea capitis (scalp) ▶

Tinea cruris (groin, buttocks, scrotum)

Tinea pedis (feet)

◀ Tinea unguium (nails, nailbeds)

Figure 49-4 Tinea (ringworm) is an infection caused by dermatophytes, a group of fungi. Tinea is classified according to the part of the body affected. Five common types of tinea are shown here. (From Hurwitz, S. [1993]. *Clinical pediatric dermatology: A textbook of skin disorders of childhood and adolescence* [2nd ed., pp. 376, 380, 383, 385]. Philadelphia: Saunders.)

Tinea Corporis

Local treatment is usually effective for tinea corporis. Antifungal preparations, such as clotrimazole (Lotrimin) or miconazole (Monistat), can be used three times a day until the lesions have been gone for 1 week. Application of cream should extend 1 inch beyond the lesion borders to prevent spread. Infected pets should be treated as well. The child should avoid close contact with the infected pet. Natural im-

munity develops in animals after 4 months (Schmitt, 1999). Extensive cases of tinea corporis might require systemic antifungal treatment.

Tinea Cruris

Management for tinea cruris is similar to that for tinea corporis. Topical antifungal preparations should be applied twice a day to the lesions and at least 1 inch beyond the borders.

Care should be taken to apply the medication to all creases, and the adolescent should be advised to wear loose clothing.

Tinea Pedis

A prescribed topical antifungal agent, such as clotrimazole (Lotrimin), miconazole (Monistat), or oxiconazole (Oxistat), is applied twice a day until the lesions have been cleared for 1 week. If the lesions do not respond to topical therapy, oral griseofulvin may be given for 1 month or longer, to promote healing. Newer systemic antifungals, such as itraconazole (Sporanox), have demonstrated improved success over a shorter time than griseofulvin, but administration of this medication requires baseline and follow-up liver function tests (Berg & Erickson, 2001). If the affected area is inflamed and oozing, soaking the feet in Burow's solution can promote healing.

▪ NURSING CARE
The Child With a Tinea Infection

Assessment

Obtain a history that includes a description of the skin lesions and possible contacts. Animals with which the child has played should be carefully inspected for ringworm. The child's siblings and playmates should also be examined, because children often share hairbrushes, hats, and barrettes, increasing the spread of infection.

Nursing Diagnosis and Planning

The nursing diagnoses and expected outcomes that may be appropriate for the child with a tinea infection and the child's family are
- Impaired Skin Integrity related to inflammation and excoriation.
  Expected Outcomes: The child will exhibit intact skin over impaired areas. The skin lesions will exhibit progressive healing.
- Impaired Comfort related to pruritic lesions.
  Expected Outcomes: The child will remain calm and will exhibit no evidence of discomfort or pruritus; scratching will decrease.
- Deficient Knowledge of the cause, treatment, and spread of the infection related to lack of information.
  Expected Outcomes: The child and family will verbalize accurate information about the child's skin condition. The child and family will demonstrate behaviors that prevent spread of the fungus. Treatments will be performed correctly.
- Disturbed Body Image related to alopecia or unattractive lesions.
  Expected Outcome: The child will return to or continue with social involvement.

Interventions

Adequate teaching is essential for successful treatment of tinea infection. In addition to teaching therapeutic management techniques specific for the child's particular type of tinea, emphasize to the parent that any prescribed oral medication regimen must be followed meticulously. Tinea infections are sometimes difficult to eradicate; discontinuing medication too soon risks recurrence. Treatment commonly continues for as long as 6 to 8 weeks and may con-

THE CHILD AND PARENTS
Want to Know

About Home Care for a Child or Adolescent With a Tinea Infection

When providing information to the parent or older child with tinea, emphasize the following:
- Keep the infected areas as dry as possible.
- Do not share personal items, such as towels, washcloths, combs, hats, or hair ornaments.
- Athlete's foot: Wash the feet daily, and keep them dry. Nonventilated athletic shoes should dry thoroughly between wearings. Wear heavy cotton socks, and change socks at least twice a day. Talcum powder or antifungal powder applied twice a day might help keep feet dry.
- Jock itch: Keep the groin area dry. Wear loose-fitting cotton underwear. Wash athletic supporters and underwear frequently. Wash the rash each day with plain water, and dry carefully. Do not use soap on the affected area. Avoid scratching.
- Continue to take oral medication as directed, even if the condition has improved. Discontinuing medication too soon can allow the infection to reappear.
- Call your physician if the infection has not cleared up in 4 weeks or if it continues to spread after 1 week of treatment.

tinue for months for difficult infections of fingernails or toenails. It is important to advise the parent and the older child that the child taking griseofulvin must avoid sun exposure because griseofulvin makes the skin more susceptible to a photosensitivity reaction. If the child is taking itraconazole or longer courses of griseofulvin, the parent must ensure that the child undergoes the recommended liver function studies.

Fungus thrives in a warm, moist environment, so it is important to keep infected areas as dry as possible. Teaching proper hygiene is essential for preventing and treating fungal infections. Teach children to avoid sharing personal items, such as combs, hats, and hair ornaments. Children with tinea infections should sleep alone and should not share towels and washcloths with others. Feet should be washed daily and kept dry. Advise children to allow their nonventilated athletic shoes to dry thoroughly between wearings. Heavy cotton socks absorb sweat and keep the feet dry. If tinea pedis is present, the child should change socks at least twice a day and go barefoot or wear sandals as much as possible. Talcum powder or antifungal powder applied twice a day might help keep feet dry. If the child showers at school or at a gym, shower shoes should be worn.

Tinea cruris heals much faster if the groin area is kept dry. Loose-fitting cotton underwear should be worn, and athletic supporters and underwear should be washed frequently. The rash should be washed each day with plain water and carefully dried. Soap should be avoided. Scratching delays healing, so instruct the child to avoid scratching the area. Reassure the young man and his parents that tinea cruris is not associated with sexually transmissible disease.

Instruct parents to call the physician if the infection has not cleared up in 4 weeks or if it continues to spread after 1 week of treatment. Reassure parents that fungal infection is not an indication of poor hygiene or neglect. Avoid expressions of distaste or surprise when caring for children with severe alopecia and/or inflammation. Encourage parents to return the school-age child to school as soon as possible. Children with severe inflammatory tinea capitis may wish to wear a cap or scarf for a time until healing has progressed.

Evaluation

- Does the child have clean, intact skin?
- Is the child comfortable and without pruritus?
- Do the child and parents perform treatments correctly and verbalize ways to prevent the spread of infection?
- Does the child participate in usual social activities?

HERPES SIMPLEX VIRUS INFECTION

Herpes simplex types 1 and 2 (HSV-1, HSV-2) are responsible for a common, contagious, and often recurrent infection of the skin and mucous membranes. This infection can be asymptomatic or symptomatic and extremely painful. A wide spectrum of disease is caused by HSV: the common fever blister or cold sore (herpes labialis); corneal lesions; genital lesions (rare in children); and central nervous system infection.

Pathophysiology

of Herpes Simplex Type 1 Infection

The four types of human herpes viruses are: herpes simplex virus (HSV types 1 and 2); cytomegalovirus (CMV); Epstein-Barr virus (EBV), which causes infectious mononucleosis; and varicella-zoster virus. HSV-1 causes the "oral" type of herpes and usually affects areas above the waist, producing cold sores, fever blisters, and corneal lesions. HSV-2 affects areas below the waist (anal-genital area). However, either type can affect any region of the body. After an initial HSV-1 infection, the virus remains dormant but alive within nerve cells innervating that portion of the skin originally infected. Fever, stress, trauma, sun exposure, menstruation, or immunosuppression can reactivate the virus. When reactivated, the virus migrates to the skin area innervated by the ganglia that harbor it, near the site of the initial infection. The recurrent infection can be symptomatic or asymptomatic, but it is just as contagious as the initial infection. Recurrent infections tend to be less severe than the initial infection.

The immune status of the host determines the severity of HSV infection. HSV-1 infection in the newborn or immunocompromised child can be fatal. HSV-1 is a common cause of viral encephalitis in children.

Herpetic whitlow, a painful HSV-1 infection of the fingers, can be transmitted to a nurse during oral or tracheal care of a child with herpes infection. Thumb-sucking children with oral HSV-1 infection can also develop this condition. Health care personnel with herpetic whitlow should not have patient contact until the infection has healed because the infection is highly contagious.

Etiology

HSV is transmitted by infected body fluids and secretions coming in contact with breaks in the skin or mucous membranes. Delivery through an infected birth canal can cause infection in newborns. HSV can be transmitted by nurses who fail to practice careful handwashing. Children with burns, eczema, or diaper rash or those who are immunosuppressed are particularly susceptible to HSV infection.

Incidence

HSV is widespread. Up to 50% of children have been infected with HSV-1 by 5 years of age (Goodyear, 2000). HSV infections in children are usually caused by HSV-1. Infection with HSV-2, which affects primarily the anal-genital area, is rare before age 14 years. Child sexual abuse should be considered in any child with a genital herpes infection.

Manifestations

Herpes Labialis ("Cold Sore," "Fever Blister")

Prodromal symptoms of herpes labialis are burning, itching, or tingling; these symptoms occur up to several days before lesions appear. Symptoms appear 2 days to 2 weeks after exposure. Lesions appear in clusters of fluid-filled vesicles that ulcerate, dry, and crust within 7 to 14 days (Fig. 49-5). Usually one or two lesions are present on the lips, tongue, gingiva, or buccal mucosa. Pruritus and pain are present. Approximately 85% of active HSV-1 infections are asymptomatic.

Herpetic Gingivostomatitis

Herpes gingivostomatitis is a severe oral infection that affects children younger than 5 years. Vesicles and ulcerations, an edematous throat, and enlarged, painful cervical lymph nodes are seen. Associated signs and symptoms include chills, fever, malaise, bad breath, and drooling.

Herpetic Ocular Infection

Herpetic ocular infection causes irritation and inflammation of the conjunctiva or cornea with associated tearing and photophobia. Vesicles appear on the eyelid and mucous membranes of the eye.

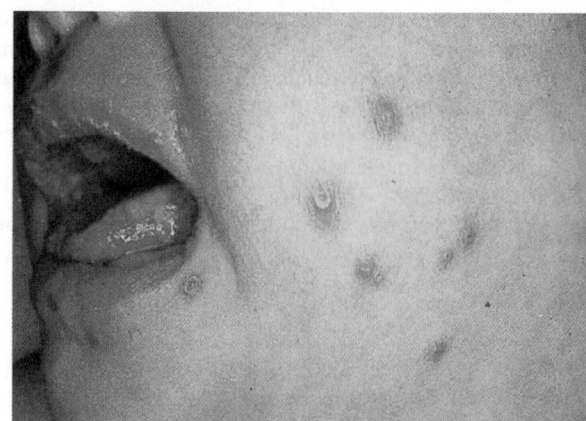

Figure 49-5 Herpes simplex infection in an infant. (From Feigin, R.D., & Cherry, J.D. [Eds.]. [1992]. *Textbook of pediatric infectious diseases* [3rd ed., p. 773]. Philadelphia: Saunders.)

Herpetic Whitlow

Symptoms of herpetic whitlow appear 3 to 7 days after exposure and include vesicles, swelling, pruritus, and severe pain of the affected fingers. Discomfort may continue for weeks after the vesicles have healed.

Diagnostic Evaluation

Clinical manifestations and the child's history can suggest the diagnosis. A Tzanck smear can confirm a herpes infection, but a positive smear cannot differentiate between varicella-zoster virus and HSV-1, and a negative smear does not rule out HSV infection. Tissue culture is a more reliable method of diagnosis.

Therapeutic Management

Treatment is symptomatic. The child with oral HSV-1 infection is usually cared for at home if able to take adequate fluids. If the child becomes dehydrated, IV fluids are needed.

Topical or oral acyclovir (Zovirax), if given early enough in the course of the infection, can reduce the time to recovery. Although there is no cure for HSV-1 infection, acyclovir (Zovirax) given IV may be used in immunocompromised children, neonates, and children with encephalitis or ocular HSV to decrease the severity of the infection.

Antibiotic ointment may be used to treat secondary bacterial infection of lesions. Corticosteroids are contraindicated because they can worsen HSV-1 infection. Oral or rectal acetaminophen, with or without codeine, may be prescribed, and topical anesthetics may be dabbed on lesions to help relieve pain. A prescribed anesthetic mouth rinse of equal parts of diphenhydramine (Benadryl) elixir, Kaopectate, and 2% viscous lidocaine may decrease pain and help the child eat.

▪ NURSING CARE

The Child With a Herpes Simplex Infection

Assessment

Obtain a history, and ask the parent or child about previous HSV infections or contact with an infected person. Examine the skin carefully for lesions. Inspect the eyes for corneal ulcerations and edema, and assess the child's vision for blurring and photophobia. Referral to an ophthalmologist is necessary for suspected ocular HSV infection. For the child with herpes gingivostomatitis, pay particular attention to assessing hydration status.

Nursing Diagnoses and Planning

The nursing diagnoses and expected outcomes that may be appropriate for the child with a herpes simplex infection and the child's family are

▪ Impaired Skin Integrity related to inadequate secondary defenses.
  Expected Outcomes: The child will demonstrate healing of lesions. The child will have no other signs of infection.
▪ Acute Pain related to inflammation and infection.
  Expected Outcome: The child will have minimal pain, as evidenced by adequate fluid intake, decreased verbalization of pain, and decreased restlessness and irritability.

▪ Risk for Infection related to changes in skin integrity.
  Expected Outcome: The child will have no signs of secondary bacterial infection, as evidenced by healing lesions and normal body temperature.
▪ Risk for Deficient Fluid Volume related to painful oral lesions.
  Expected Outcomes: The child will maintain urine output appropriate for age (see Chapter 42) and will exhibit moist mucous membranes and good skin turgor.

Interventions

Children with oral HSV infection may be extremely uncomfortable. Swallowing can cause severe pain, and dehydration is a real danger. Advise parents to contact the physician if the child develops signs of dehydration. Fluid intake is very important, and the child must be encouraged to drink. Most children will accept Popsicles, non-citrus juices, milk, and noncarbonated or "flattened" soft drinks. Frequent small feedings of bland, soft foods can be offered. Reassure parents that a few days without solid food will not harm the child as long as fluid intake is adequate.

To prevent secondary infection, the child's mouth should be rinsed often with normal saline, especially after eating. Oral or rectal acetaminophen with codeine can be given as ordered for pain and fever. Topical anesthetics, such as viscous lidocaine, must be used with caution. Overuse of topical anesthetics in small children can depress the gag reflex and increase the risk of aspiration.

Hospitalized children infected with HSV should be placed on Contact Precautions. The child is considered contagious until the scabs from visible lesions have fallen off. Because scabs do not form on mucous membranes, these lesions are considered contagious until they are completely healed.

All personnel who have contact with the child should follow Standard Precautions and be particularly careful when touching the child near the lesions, during oral care or suctioning, and when handling bed linens or objects that might be contaminated with saliva or secretions from the lesions. Careful handwashing is essential.

Parents should take similar precautions when caring for the child at home to prevent spread of infection. Advise the parents to wash bottles, nipples, toys, eating utensils, and towels in hot, soapy water or in a dishwasher, if available. Family members should not share any of these items with the infected child.

Because the infection can be spread to other parts of the body, the child should not put his or her fingers near the mouth or infected area. Elbow restraints may be necessary for children too young to understand this. The child with HSV-1 infection is usually miserable and needs generous cuddling and comforting.

Evaluation

- Are lesions healed, with no sign of infection spread?
- Does the child demonstrate increased comfort?
- Does the skin remain free of signs of secondary infection (redness, swelling, purulence)?
- Is the child properly hydrated with adequate fluid intake and hourly urine output?
- Can the parent or caregiver describe infection control measures?

Pathophysiology

of Pediculosis

Pediculosis may involve the scalp (pediculosis capitis), the body (pediculosis corporis), and the pubic area and eyelashes (pediculosis pubis). A specific type of louse, each of which has a similar life cycle, causes each of these infestations. All lice pierce the skin and suck blood. Severe itching caused by bites can predispose the child to secondary infection.

Head and pubic lice spend their life cycles on the skin of the human host; body lice live in clothing, coming to the skin only to feed. The female head louse lays eggs (nits) at the base of the hair shaft. The egg is covered with a gelatinous material, which hardens to semi-opaque, tiny, pearly whitish masses that are stuck tight to the hair shaft (see Fig. 49-6). Eggs incubate for about 1 week, and lice reach sexual maturity in about 2 weeks.

Pediculosis pubis is spread through sexual contact. Half of all patients with pediculosis pubis have another sexually transmissible disease, usually gonorrhea.

Lice may spread as long as the lice and nits remain alive on the infested person or belongings. Lice can live only 48 hours off the human host. Nits shed into the environment are capable of hatching for 10 days.

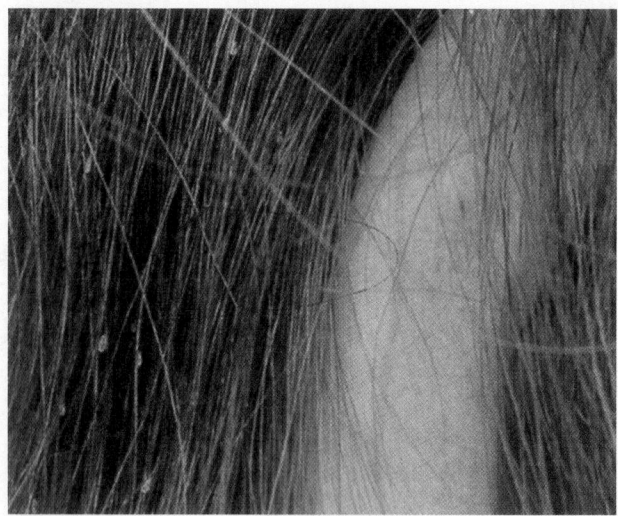

Figure 49-6 Head lice (pediculosis capitis). Note the nits attached to the hair shafts. (From Calen, J., Greer, K.E., Hood, A.F., Paller, A.S., & Swinyer, L.J. [1993]. *Color atlas of dermatology* [p. 373]. Philadelphia: Saunders.)

LICE INFESTATION

Lice are small, blood-sucking insects about 2 to 4 mm in length. Pediculosis (infestation of lice on the scalp or body) is a major problem in schools today. Although pediculosis is not a serious health problem, it causes embarrassment and often elicits an emotional reaction among parents and school personnel.

Etiology

Lice live only on humans and are transmitted by direct contact with infected persons and indirect contact with infested objects (e.g., brushes, hats). Lice cannot jump like fleas, and clean hair is no deterrent to head lice.

Incidence

The American Academy of Pediatrics (AAP) (2002) reports approximately 6 to 12 million cases of head lice each year among children 3 to 12 years of age in the United States. Pediculosis rarely occurs in African-Americans. Girls are affected twice as often as boys. All socioeconomic groups are affected. The peak incidence is in preschool and young school-age children. Pubic lice are usually seen in adolescents or young adults and are generally transmitted by sexual contact.

Manifestations

Pediculosis Capitis (Head Lice)

Nits are visible and are attached firmly to the hair shafts near the scalp. They are tiny, silvery or grayish white specks resembling dandruff but are more difficult to remove. They are commonly found behind the ears and at the nape of the neck. In active infestation, nits are found approximately $1/4$ to $1/2$ inch away from the scalp surface (Fig. 49-6). Adult lice are difficult

to see because of their small size and the fact that they crawl very fast to avoid light. Scattered lesions on the scalp, behind the ears, or on the back of the neck cause intense pruritus. These lesions are often associated with posterior cervical lymph adenopathy. Secondary scalp infection may develop from scratching.

Pediculosis Corporis (Body Lice)

Papular, rose-colored dermatitis, causing intense pruritus, appears on the skin in areas under tight clothing. Nits attach firmly to seams of the child's clothing or bedding.

Pediculosis Pubis (Pubic Lice, Crab Lice)

Pediculosis pubis are lice that can be found in pubic hair, facial hair, and axillae and on the body surface. The presence of pubic lice in the eyebrows or eyelashes of a prepubescent child suggests sexual abuse (Starr, 2000). Pubic lice also cause intense pruritus. *Maculae ceruleae* (blue spots) may be seen on the thighs and trunk in cases of heavy infestation. Dark-brown spots on underwear and sheets are insect waste materials.

Diagnostic Evaluation

The diagnosis of head lice is made by identification of nits or lice on the scalp. The examiner parts the hair with two tongue depressors and moves from side to side and front to back, paying particular attention to the crown, behind the ears, and the nape of the neck. The exposed scalp should be carefully examined under bright light or in a sunny area. A magnifying glass can assist in identification. Unlike dandruff, nits are not easily removed from hair shafts. Pubic lice are diagnosed from a history of symptoms and visual inspection.

Therapeutic Management

Management of the child with pediculosis involves a three-tiered approach: (1) killing the active lice; (2) removing nits; and (3) preventing spread or recurrence by managing the environment.

Killing Active Lice

Approaches to treating pediculosis have changed recently as a result of the development of pediculicide-resistant strains of lice and because prescription lindane (Kwell) can be neurotoxic if absorbed through the skin. Over-the-counter products containing pyrethrins (RID, Triple X, R&C, Pronto) are safe and effective. Because they lack residual activity (i.e., they do not stay in the hair after treatment), treatment with these products must be repeated 1 to 2 weeks after the initial treatment.

An over-the-counter pediculicide, permethrin 1% (Nix), kills head lice and pubic lice and eggs with one application and has residual activity for 10 days. Nix crème rinse is applied to the hair after washing with a conditioner-free shampoo. It is applied as a lotion to pubic hair. Cream rinse and/or lotion should be rinsed out after 10 minutes. The hair should not be shampooed for 24 hours after the treatment. Treatment and testing for other sexually transmissible diseases are required for sexual contacts of a person with pubic lice.

Body lice are treated with a prescription drug or an over-the-counter medication (RID, Pyrinate200, Triple X), following the manufacturer's instructions. Clothing and bedding should be dusted with lindane or other recommended powder and then washed in hot water and dried for 20 minutes at a hot dryer setting.

The pesticide malathion (Ovide) has recently been approved for the treatment of lice as well, but it requires prolonged contact (i.e., 8-10 hr) to be effective. It is also flammable, and families should be cautioned not to use hairdryers or allow the child near fires or heaters while hair is being treated. Some practitioners have had success with systemic trimethoprim-sulfamethoxazole (AAP, 2002), but it is not currently approved by the FDA as a pediculicide.

Removing Nits

Unless the eggs are examined under a microscope, it is nearly impossible to tell whether treated nits have been killed. To ensure that living eggs will not hatch, all nits should be removed from the child's hair with a very-fine-tooth nit comb.

Addressing the Environment

Environmental objects, clothing, and bedding should be treated or washed. It is important to examine and treat family members and others who might be in close contact with the infested child. Meticulous vacuuming of carpets in classrooms with affected children will help prevent continuation of an epidemic.

■ NURSING CARE
The Child With Pediculosis

Assessment

Examine children for lice in an unobtrusive and private manner. In a school setting, classmates should be brought to the school nurse's office and admitted one at a time, rather than being seen together in a general check in a classroom setting. Use disposable tongue depressors or Popsicle sticks to part the hair, and discard these implements between children. Check all family members for the presence of nits or lice.

Assess adolescents with pubic lice for signs of other sexually transmissible diseases, and ask about sexual contacts because they will need treatment as well.

Nursing Diagnosis and Planning

The nursing diagnoses and expected outcomes that may be appropriate for the child with pediculosis and the child's family are

- Acute Pain related to inflammatory response and pruritus.
  Expected Outcomes: The child will rest comfortably and be free of scratching.
- Risk for Infection related to scratching of scalp.
  Expected Outcome: The child will have no signs of secondary bacterial infection, as evidenced by intact skin and normal-size cervical lymph nodes.
- Deficient Knowledge about treatment of lice infestation and the prevention of recurrence related to anxiety or incomplete information.
  Expected Outcomes: The child and/or family will carry out the prescribed treatment. The parent will demonstrate measures taken to prevent reinfestation.
- Risk for Situational Low Self-Esteem related to social stigma associated with lice.
  Expected Outcomes: The child and/or family will verbalize self-acceptance and will engage in usual social activities.

Interventions

Advise parents to carefully follow directions that come with over-the-counter pediculicides or to follow the physician's instructions for using prescription products. Caution parents against applying the medication more frequently than recommended.

Reassure parents that lice infestation does not reflect poor hygiene or low socioeconomic status. Advise them that it is necessary to notify the school nurse if the child is infested.

Teach parents to remove nits by back-combing with a fine-tooth comb. One hour before combing, nits can be loosened with a mixture of half vinegar and half water or a commercial product, such as Clear or Step 2. It is easier to comb the child's hair for nit removal when the hair is damp rather than wet or dry. Lice and nits can be removed from eyelashes by applying petrolatum to the eyelashes twice a day for 8 days. The goal is to remove all nits, leaving none with the potential to hatch. Many schools have a "no nit" policy, which requires that a child be free of all nits before reentry, although such policies are strongly discouraged by the American Academy of Pediatrics (2002).

Advise parents to wash clothing (especially hats and jackets), bedding, and linens in hot water and dry at a hot dryer setting. Dress-up clothes, bicycle helmets, batting helmets, headphones, and similar objects should be treated as well. Items that cannot be washed should be dry-cleaned or sealed in plastic bags and kept in a warm place for 2 to 3 weeks.

Anti-lice sprays used for furniture and other environmental objects should *never* be used on a child. Thorough home cleaning is necessary to remove any remaining lice or nits. Parents should vacuum floors, play areas, and furniture to remove any hairs that might carry live nits. Combs and brushes should be boiled or soaked in anti-lice shampoo or hot water (>140° F) for at least 10 minutes. Routinely teach children not to share hats, combs, or hair ornaments with other children. At school, individually assigned lockers or separate hooks for coats can help inhibit spread of lice.

The child should be rechecked for infestation in 7 to 10 days. Advise parents to call the physician if itching interferes with the child's sleep, if the condition does not clear up after 1 week, or if scalp lesions look infected. The National Pediculosis Association provides information about this disorder (see www.headlice.org or Appendix I on Evolve website).

Evaluation
- Is the child free of infestation, pain, and pruritus?
- Is the skin intact, and does the child exhibit normal cervical lymph nodes?
- Do parents carry out the prescribed treatments?
- Can parents describe measures to prevent the spread of lice to others?
- Do the parents and child realistically describe the cause of pediculosis and continue to engage in usual social activities?

MITE INFESTATION (SCABIES)

Scabies is a contagious condition that has been recognized for many centuries. It results from infestation with *Sarcoptes scabiei*, the "itch mite."

Etiology

Scabies is transmitted by close personal contact with infected persons. Persons who share a bed or live in crowded conditions are likely to transmit scabies to each other. The scabies mite cannot survive for more than 3 days away from human skin. For that reason, transmission of scabies by bedding or clothing is infrequent.

Incidence

Scabies is widespread throughout the United States and is prevalent in many schools. All socioeconomic groups are affected.

Pathophysiology

The female mite burrows into the epidermis, lays her eggs, and dies in the burrow after 4 to 5 weeks. The eggs hatch in 3 to 5 days, and larvae migrate to the skin surface to mature and complete the life cycle. The mites, eggs, and their excrement cause intense pruritus. One of the major complications of scabies is impetigo secondary to scratching.

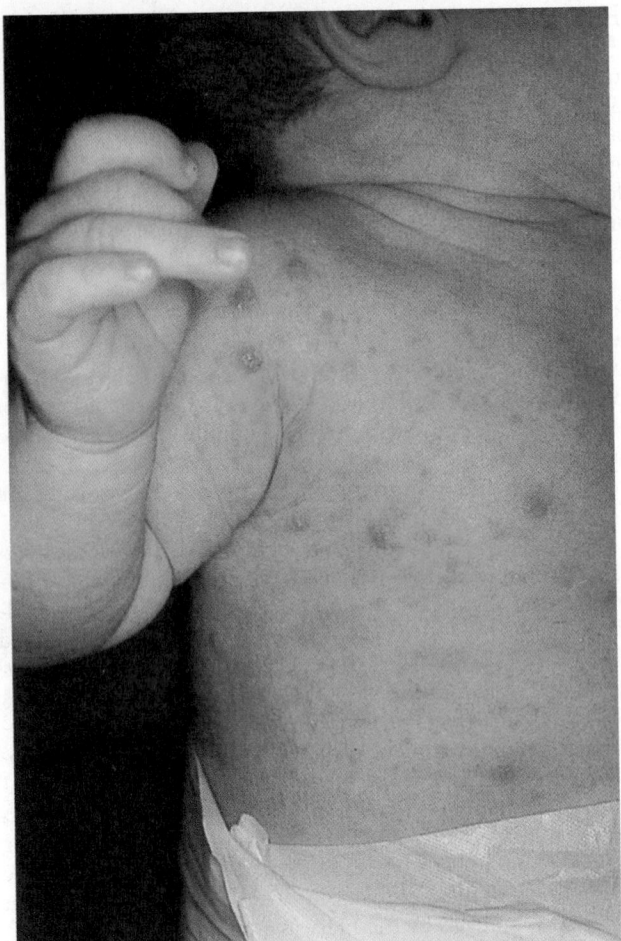

Figure 49-7 Scabies lesions on an infant. (From Calen, J.P., Greer, K.E., Hood, A.F., Paller, A.S., & Swinyer, L.J. [1993]. *Color atlas of dermatology* [p. 301]. Philadelphia: Saunders.)

Manifestations

Intense pruritus occurs, especially at night. Infants may be cranky, sleep fitfully, and rub their hands and feet together. Burrows (fine, grayish, threadlike lines) can be difficult to see because they are usually obscured by secondary changes of excoriation and inflammation. Papules, vesicles, and nodules are common (Fig. 49-7) and are located mainly on the wrists, in the finger webs, on the elbows, in the umbilicus, in the axillae, in the groin, and on the buttocks. In infants, the head, palms, and soles may be affected. Lesions often become secondarily infected from scratching.

Diagnostic Evaluation

The characteristic skin eruption and a history of intense pruritus, especially at night, are suggestive of scabies. The diagnosis is made by microscopic examination of scrapings of the lesions.

Therapeutic Management

Scabies can be treated with topical application of either permethrin 5% (Elimite) or lindane cream (Kwell, Scabene). Because of the risk of neurotoxicity, lindane should not be used in children younger than 2 years or in pregnant women. The medication is applied to the body and head, avoiding the eyes and mouth. The medication must remain on the child for 8 to 14 hours to be effective, so applying it at bedtime is most effective. It is washed off in the morning. Retreatment in 1 week is usually recommended. Pruritus may last for several days to weeks after treatment and can be relieved with corticosteroid cream (e.g., hydrocortisone cream) and oral antihistamines.

Family members, even if asymptomatic, and daycare contacts (except for pregnant women) should also be treated. The child's bedding and clothing should be washed in hot water in a fashion similar to the environmental treatment for pediculosis.

Nursing Considerations

Nursing care of the child and family with scabies is similar to that for pediculosis. Inspect the child's hands, elbows, umbilicus, groin, and buttocks for burrows. Burrows may be difficult to see, however, and complaints of persistent itching may be the only symptom. Evaluate an adolescent with scabies for sexually transmissible disease.

Instruct parents to use the scabicide according to manufacturer's instructions. The lotion is applied all over the child's body, including the soles of the feet, the scalp behind the ears, in intertriginous areas, and under the toenails and fingernails. The lotion should be kept on for the recommended time (4-8 hr for lindane; 8-14 hr for Elimite), and then the child should be bathed. Infants should be clothed during treatment so they will not lick their skin. To minimize absorption and the risk of toxic effects from lindane, the lotion should not be applied for at least $1/2$ hour after bathing and should be applied only to cool, dry skin. Advise the parent that persistent itching after treatment is expected for about 2 weeks and is not a sign of reinfestation or an indication for repeated application.

Scabies is usually cured with one treatment; however, a repeat application in 1 week is recommended. Clothing and bed linen should be dry-cleaned or washed in hot water and dried at a hot dryer setting.

ATOPIC DERMATITIS

Atopic dermatitis, or eczema, is a common chronic, allergic, inflammatory disease of the skin characterized by severe pruritus. Atopic dermatitis can have distressing psychosocial effects on the child and family.

Etiology

The cause of atopic dermatitis is unknown, but the disease is thought to be genetically determined. Contributing factors include an inherited tendency for dry, sensitive skin; allergy; and emotional stress. Most children with atopic dermatitis have a family history of asthma, hay fever, or atopic dermatitis, and up to 80% of children with atopic dermatitis develop asthma or allergic rhinitis (Eichenfield et al., 2003). Although the role of allergy in the etiology of atopic dermatitis is controversial, immunoglobulin E (IgE)–mediated food allergy has been shown to be an exacerbating factor in some children.

Pathophysiology

of Atopic Dermatitis

Atopic dermatitis is an allergic skin condition. The skin of affected children releases twice as much histamine as that of normal children. The high levels of histamine trigger an inflammatory response, resulting in erythema, edema, and intense pruritus. Scratching increases itching, leading to an itch-scratch-itch cycle. Continual scratching and rubbing excoriate and damage the skin. Oozing, weeping, crusting, and cracking lesions develop. The skin of children with atopic dermatitis carries a higher-than-normal colonization of *Staphylococcus aureus,* and secondary infection is common. Impetigo and viral infections (herpes, molluscum contagiosum) occur frequently in these children.

Incidence

Atopic dermatitis is a common condition that affects 9% to 12% of young children (Kristal & Klein, 2000). The condition usually begins in infancy and clears by age 2 or 3 years, although it can persist through adolescence and adulthood. Children who continue to have signs into childhood present a rash pattern that differs from the rash seen during infancy. Atopic dermatitis affects all races. Symptoms tend to be worse during winter months.

Manifestations

During infancy, erythematous areas of oozing and crusting appear first on the cheeks and then on the forehead, scalp, and extensor surfaces of the arms and legs (Fig. 49-8). Papulovesicular rash and scaly, red plaques become excoriated and lichenified. The affected scalp area resembles seborrheic dermatitis, but unlike seborrheic dermatitis, atopic dermatitis is intensely pruritic. Infants begin manifesting symptoms at approximately age 1 to 4 months.

If the condition persists into childhood or adolescence, the skin appears scaly. The flexor surfaces of the wrists, ankles, knees, and elbows are affected, as are the neck creases, the eyelids, and the dorsal surfaces of the hands and feet. There may be acute weeping areas, with or without secondary infection. Chronic lichenification results from persistent scratching.

Children and adolescents with atopic dermatitis more readily experience intense itching, especially in response to sweating or contact with irritating fabrics, such as wool. Emotional upset increases sweating and precipitates itching and scratching. Dry skin is a hallmark of this condition.

Diagnostic Evaluation

The diagnosis is based on the clinical features of intense pruritus, the appearance of the lesions, the pattern of remissions and exacerbations, and a family history of allergy. IgE levels and eosinophils are often elevated. Skin testing for food allergies—usually milk, eggs, wheat, soy, peanuts, and fish—can help identify potential food triggers.

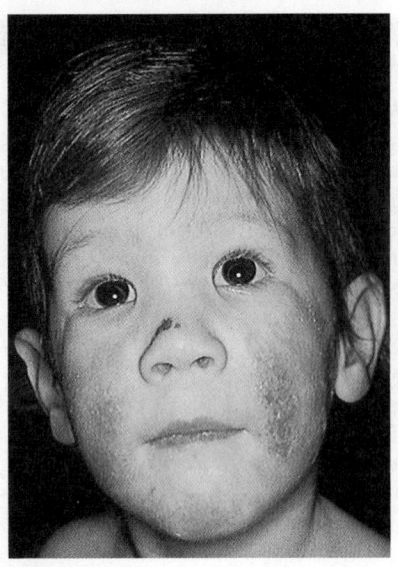

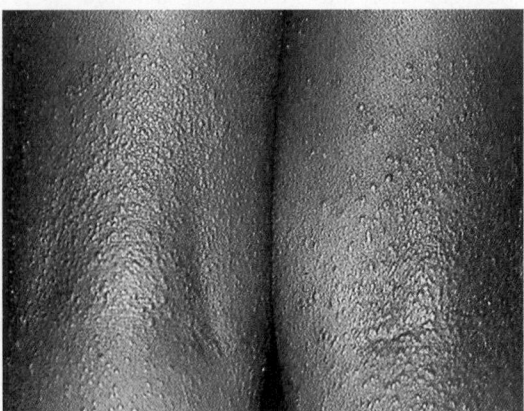

◀ Lesions on cheeks often spread to the forehead, scalp, and extensor surfaces of arms and legs.

Flexor surfaces of wrists, ankles, knees, and elbows may be affected in the childhood form of the disease.

Figure 49-8 Atopic dermatitis, an allergic skin condition, usually begins in infancy and clears by age 2 to 3 years. However, it can continue into childhood. (From Hurwitz, S. [1993]. *Clinical pediatric dermatology: A textbook of skin disorders of childhood and adolescence* [2nd ed., pp. 49, 51]. Philadelphia: Saunders.)

Therapeutic Management

The main goals of treatment are to control itching and scratching, moisturize the skin, prevent secondary infection, and remove irritants and allergens. Control of pruritus includes avoiding environmental triggers, such as overheating, soaps, wool clothing, and other skin irritants. Oral antihistamines, such as hydroxyzine (Atarax), diphenhydramine (Benadryl), and loratadine (Claritin), can be used to help break the "itch-scratch-itch" cycle. Nonsedating antihistamines, such as loratadine, may be preferred for school-age children. Itching is typically more severe at night; thus antihistamines should be given before bedtime. Secondary infection is treated with antibiotic therapy.

Proper skin hydration is essential. Bathing and the use of wet compresses and occlusive creams and ointments are the mainstays of treatment. In humid climates, bathing should be as infrequent as possible, and only lukewarm water and mild, nonperfumed soap (e.g., Purpose, white Dove, Basis) should be used. Emollients such as Eucerin cream or petroleum jelly applied immediately after bathing to damp skin will help the skin retain moisture. Applying the moisturizer while the skin is still damp hydrates the skin. The child who lives in a dry climate should bathe frequently (several times a day), using a hydrophilic agent such as Cetaphil, instead of soap, and should moisturize with a moisturizing ointment or cream immediately after bathing. The child should avoid using lotions that contain alcohol, because these can contribute to skin dryness. Moisturizing the skin is maintenance therapy for atopic dermatitis and should become a daily routine for the child.

Antiinflammatory corticosteroid creams and ointments (Cutivate, Elocon) are prescribed for inflamed or lichenified areas. These creams are more effective when applied after bathing to damp skin. The lowest potency that controls signs should be used, and topical steroids are usually reserved for treatment of episodic flares (Drug Guide).

Topical immunosuppressants, such as tacrolimus and pimecrolimus, may be applied to 100% of the body surface if needed, and may be used for longer periods of time than topical steroids. Topical immunomodulators do not cause skin atrophy, and although they can penetrate the skin enough to suppress local inflammation, they are only minimally absorbed into the circulation. Routine blood studies (to monitor for immunosuppression) of children using tacrolimus and pimecrolimus are not indicated. However, caution should be used in children whose skin integrity suffers widespread damage because immunosuppressives can be absorbed systemically in such cases (Leung & Bieber, 2003; Tharp, 2002).

Identifying and eliminating allergens can be helpful. Allergy-proofing the home might be recommended (see Chapter 45). Because allergy to certain foods is an exacerbating factor in some children, those foods should be eliminated from the diets of sensitive infants. Breastfeeding for the first year is recommended for infants at risk for allergy. Solid foods should not be introduced until the infant is at least 6 months old.

■ NURSING CARE
The Child With Atopic Dermatitis

Assessment

Obtain a thorough history that includes information about allergies in the family. Question parents about any environmental or dietary factors that seem to worsen the child's condition. Determine what treatments have been tried and their effectiveness. Examine skin lesions for type, distribution, and evidence of any secondary infection. Assess the child's comfort level and the family's feelings and coping methods.

Nursing Diagnosis and Planning

The nursing diagnoses and expected outcomes that may be appropriate for the child with atopic dermatitis and the child's family are

■ Impaired Skin Integrity related to environmental and immunologic factors.

Drug Guide

Topical Corticosteroids

Classification: Topical antiinflammatory.

Action: Reduce inflammation by causing vasoconstriction and inhibiting the movement of inflammatory cells from the bloodstream into local tissue.

Indications: Inflammatory skin diseases, such as atopic dermatitis.

Dosage and Route: Topical route; number of applications depends on the child's condition and the potency of the medication. Topical steroids are commonly divided into seven classes, with those of lowest potency assigned to the lowest (seventh) class.

- Class I: Optimized betamethasone dipropionate 0.05% (Diprolene cream or ointment)
- Class II: Triamcinolone acetonide ointment 0.5% (Kenalog); mometasone furoate ointment 0.1% (Elocon)
- Class III: Triamcinolone acetonide ointment 0.1% (Aristocort A); triamcinolone acetonide cream (Aristocort-

HP); fluticasone propionate ointment 0.005% (Cutivate)
- Class IV: Hydrocortisone valerate ointment 0.2% (Westcort); mometasone furoate cream 0.1% (Elocon); desoximetasone cream 0.05% (Topicort-LP)
- Class V: Fluticasone propionate cream 0.05% (Cutivate); hydrocortisone valerate cream 0.2% (Westcort); triamcinolone acetonide cream 0.025% (Aristocort)
- Class VI: Desonide cream 0.05% (DesOwen); alclometasone dipropionate cream 0.05% (Aclovate)
- Class VII: Hydrocortisone cream 0.5%, 1% (Cortizone, Hytone, generic)

Absorption: Better absorbed through the skin immediately after bathing.

Contraindications: Never apply to diaper rashes or chickenpox lesions. Superpotent topical steroids (class I) are rarely used for children. Only low-potency agents should be used on the face.

Precautions: Unless directed by the physician, do not bandage, wrap, or otherwise cover areas being treated with topical steroids. In general, the more potent the medication, the shorter the treatment time will be.

Adverse Reactions: Systemic side effects can occur with short-term use of high-potency topical steroids or with long-term use of lower-potency topicals. Systemic effects include suppression of the hypothalamic-pituitary-adrenal axis, resulting in growth suppression; suppression of immune response; osteoporosis; moon face; and obesity. Locally, thinning of the skin, striae, telangiectasia, atrophy, and purpura can occur.

Nursing Considerations: Advise the parent to apply to the child's skin within 5 minutes of bathing, to meticulously follow the physician's directions for use, and to immediately report any side effects.

Expected Outcome: The child's skin will exhibit decreased evidence of excoriation.

- Acute Pain related to dry skin, secondary infection, and external irritations.
  Expected Outcomes: The child will exhibit reduced skin dryness and irritation. The child will experience minimal pain and pruritus, as evidenced by decreased irritability, absence of scratching, and uninterrupted periods of sleep.

- Risk for Infection related to skin excoriation.
  Expected Outcome: The child will have no signs of secondary bacterial infection, as evidenced by a normal body temperature and absence of purulent drainage.

- Deficient Knowledge about controlling itching, preventing secondary infection, and identifying aggravating factors related to anxiety or incomplete understanding of information.
  Expected Outcomes: The child and family will identify and eliminate allergens and aggravating factors. The family will carry out prescribed treatments correctly. Family members will express any anxiety related to the child's condition.

- Interrupted Family Processes related to the child's pruritus and involved treatment.
  Expected Outcome: The child and family will discuss their feelings and concerns.

Interventions

Care of the child with atopic dermatitis is demanding, and the entire family routine may revolve around the affected child. Parents need support and reassurance as they care for an uncomfortable, often irritable child.

Keeping the child's skin hydrated will help relieve itching. Instruct parents to apply moisturizing creams, such as Eucerin, Nivea, or Vaseline Dermatology Formula, several times a day and immediately after the child is bathed. Reassure parents that moisturizing creams contain no harmful drugs and should be applied whenever the child's skin looks dry. Soaks and cool, wet compresses are soothing and can be applied to remove crusts, reduce inflammation, and dry weeping areas. Provide parents with explicit instructions on the use of soaks and topical medications. Strips of old cotton sheets moistened in lukewarm or cool tap water work well for wet dressings. Wet compresses should not be used for more than 3 days.

Rough clothing can aggravate eczema, particularly wool or other fabrics that cause sweating. Soft cotton or cotton-polyester blends are tolerated best. Undergarments with irritating seams can be turned inside out so that the soft seam is against the skin. Heat and sweating increase pruritus, so instruct parents to be careful not to "bundle up" the child in heavy blankets or clothing. Because detergents and fabric softeners can also aggravate atopic dermatitis, clothes should be washed in mild detergent and rinsed twice.

Advise the parents to keep the child's fingernails clean and short. Cotton gloves or mittens might be needed to prevent excoriation from scratching but should be used with caution, preferably only at night, because overuse could interfere with fine motor development. Lightweight, long-sleeved tops and one-piece outfits discourage scratching.

The child's skin must be kept clean to minimize secondary infection. Avoid using soap. Bath oil or emulsifying ointment can be used as a soap substitute but must be used with caution because these cause both the child and the tub to become slippery. Tepid bath water helps prevent the child from becoming overheated and itchy. Instruct parents to contact the physician at the earliest signs of skin infection (weeping skin, pustules) and to administer topical and oral antibiotics as prescribed.

Children with atopic dermatitis who swim should apply moisturizer before swimming and immediately on exiting the pool. Prolonged immersion in water (more than 20 minutes) can have a drying effect. A humidifier in the child's room during winter months may decrease skin dryness. The child should avoid sun exposure.

Children and families of children with atopic dermatitis exhibit frustration when the condition does not resolve quickly. The parent or child might be concerned about the child's appearance as well as the child's discomfort.

Help parents take control of the child's condition by empowering them with knowledge about therapeutic management. Allowing parents to verbalize frustrations and helping them learn management techniques that do not disrupt family routine are important interventions.

Although studies do not consistently support emotional upset as a direct cause of atopic dermatitis flares, it is helpful to teach an older child stress-reduction techniques to help cope with the frustration and discomfort of the condition. A resource for families of a child with atopic dermatitis is the National Eczema Association for Science and Education.

Evaluation

- Is the child's skin intact and smooth?
- Have itching and pain been reduced?
- Is the child's skin free from redness or purulence that would indicate secondary infection?
- Do parents carry out prescribed treatments correctly?
- Are parents able to demonstrate appropriate coping techniques?
- Can the child demonstrate stress-relief measures to decrease itching?

SEBORRHEIC DERMATITIS

Seborrheic dermatitis, or "cradle cap," is a chronic inflammatory skin condition seen frequently in infants. It often begins in the first 2 to 3 weeks of life and usually disappears by age 12 months. Seborrhea in older children might appear on the face, behind the ears, around the umbilicus, or in any other area with a large number of sebaceous glands. Although its cause is unknown, it appears to be related to sebaceous gland dysfunction.

Seborrheic dermatitis is characterized by nonpruritic, oily, yellow scales that block sweat and sebaceous glands, causing retained secretions and inflammation in affected areas (Fig. 49-9). Confluent erythema might be present in the diaper and intertriginous areas and around the umbilicus (Fig. 49-10). Often, there is overgrowth of normal skin bacteria and yeast, which increases inflammation and leads to secondary infection.

The nurse inspects the infant's scalp or other affected areas for lesions and inflammation and questions parents about the frequency and technique of washing the infant's scalp. Instruct the parents to remove the scales daily by shampooing with a mild baby shampoo or an over-the-counter antiseborrheic shampoo containing sulfur and salicylic acid (Fostex Medicated Cleansing, P&S, Sebulex), selenium, or tar (Neutrogena T/Gel, Polytar). Massaging the scalp with warm mineral oil before shampooing helps loosen scales. Using a fine-tooth comb or a clean, soft-bristle toothbrush during the shampoo also helps loosen scales. Eyelid dermatitis (blepharitis) is treated with warm tap water compresses and cleansing with "no tears" baby shampoo. Care must be taken to keep topical medications out of the infant's eyes.

Teach the parents the importance of good hygiene of the infant's scalp and skin to prevent recurrence. Reassure them that the fontanel is not fragile and will not be damaged by gentle pressure and washing. Advise the parents to contact the physician if the sites become infected. Skin lesions that do not clear with frequent washing can be treated with hydrocortisone cream applied twice a day.

Seborrheic dermatitis of the diaper area is often secondarily infected with *C. albicans* and requires appropriate treat-

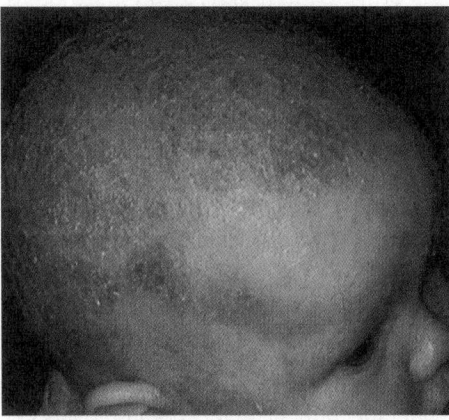

Figure 49-9   "Cradle cap," the most frequent form of seborrheic dermatitis in infants. The condition often begins in the first 2 to 3 weeks of life and usually disappears by age 12 months. (From Hurwitz, S. [1993]. *Clinical pediatric dermatology: A textbook of skin disorders of childhood and adolescence* [2nd ed., p. 17]. Philadelphia: Saunders.)

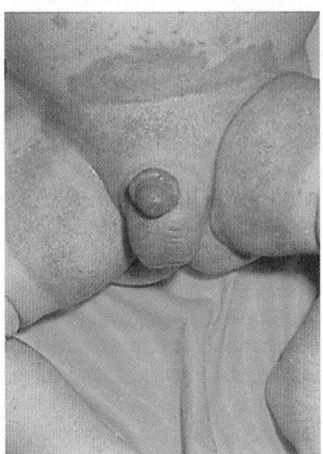

Figure 49-10   Seborrheic diaper dermatitis. (From Moschella, S.L., & Hurley, H.J. [1992]. *Dermatology* [3rd ed., p. 239]. Philadelphia: Saunders.)

ment. Lotions and creams tend to aggravate the condition and should not be used.

CONTACT DERMATITIS

Contact dermatitis is a skin inflammation that results from direct skin-to-irritant contact.

Etiology

Contact dermatitis can be caused by hundreds of substances. Among the most common causes of contact dermatitis are rubber products, clothing dyes, nickel (in jewelry, bra strap hooks, jeans fasteners), and plant oils. Scented or strongly alkaline soaps, skin lotions, cosmetics, and wool clothing also are irritating to many children.

Diaper dermatitis (diaper rash) is a contact dermatitis from irritants such as moisture, friction, and chemical substances. Urine ammonia, formed from the breakdown of urea by fecal bacteria, is extremely irritating to sensitive infant skin. Ammonia alone does not cause skin breakdown. Only skin damaged by infrequent diaper changes and constant urine and feces contact is prone to damage from ammonia in urine. Inadequate fluid intake, heat, and detergents in diapers aggravate the condition.

Incidence

Irritant contact dermatitis is more common in children than allergic contact dermatitis. Diaper rash occurs in about 10% of infants, usually between the ages of 3 and 18 months, although it is most common between ages 6 and 9 months.

Manifestations

Manifestations of irritant contact dermatitis include dry, inflamed, and pruritic skin. The distribution of lesions correlates with the skin surface in contact with the offending agent (e.g., watchband, clothing). Diaper dermatitis begins with erythema in the perianal region and can progress to macules and papules, which form erosions and crusts (Fig. 49-11). Manifestations of allergic contact dermatitis include blistering, weeping lesions over an area of inflamed skin, intense pruritus, and crusted, scaly lesions that heal in 10 to 14 days without treatment. Rhus dermatitis may cause severe systemic reactions.

Diagnostic Evaluation

The characteristic appearance of the lesions and a history of exposure to an irritating substance establish the diagnosis. Skin testing might be performed in children with persistent or recurrent dermatitis.

Therapeutic Management

Discontinuing exposure to the offending agent treats contact dermatitis. The skin should be washed thoroughly if any irritant remains on the skin. Cool compresses of tap water or Burow's solution can soothe weeping, crusting lesions. Steroid cream (e.g., triamcinolone 0.1% or fluocinolone 0.025%) may be applied several times a day after application of compresses. Severe contact dermatitis might require treatment with oral steroids, which should be tapered gradually. Desensitization therapy is usually not effective in managing contact dermatitis.

▪NURSING CARE
The Child With Contact Dermatitis

Assessment

Investigate new or continuing exposure to any potentially irritating substances. Assessment of skin lesions includes noting their distribution and configuration and looking for evidence of pruritus.

For a child with diaper dermatitis, carefully inspect the diaper area, noting the type and extent of lesions. It is important to evaluate the infant's hygiene as well as the parents' knowledge of care related to the infant's skin integrity. Question parents about the type of diapers used, laundering practices, and frequency and method of cleaning

---

Pathophysiology

of Contact Dermatitis

Contact dermatitis is an inflammatory reaction of the skin either caused by direct exposure to an irritant *(irritant contact dermatitis)* or as a result of a delayed hypersensitivity response to an allergen *(allergic contact dermatitis).*

Irritant contact dermatitis can occur in any person who has repeated or prolonged contact with a primary irritant. Examples of primary irritants include citrus juices, detergents, bubble-bath formulations, and urine. Diaper dermatitis is an example of irritant dermatitis that results from prolonged exposure to urine. Teething infants can develop dermatitis on the face and neck folds from drooling.

Allergic contact dermatitis, a delayed hypersensitivity reaction, occurs in susceptible individuals who are sensitized to a substance by a previous exposure to the contact allergen. *Rhus dermatitis* (caused by poison ivy, oak, and sumac), the most common type of allergic contact dermatitis in children, is caused by oleoresins contained in all parts of the plant. Lesions appear several hours to several days after contact.

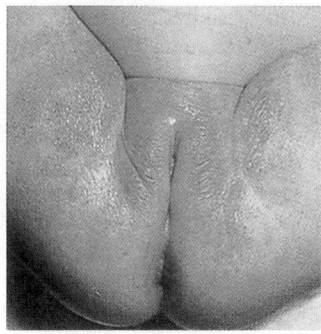

Figure 49-11 Contact diaper dermatitis. (From Moschella, S.L., & Hurley, H.J. [1992]. *Dermatology* [3rd ed., p. 239]. Philadelphia: Saunders.)

the diaper area. Any recent changes in the infant's care, such as new foods, soaps, detergents, or lotions, should be investigated.

Nursing Diagnosis and Planning

The nursing diagnoses and expected outcomes that may be appropriate for the child with contact dermatitis and the child's family are

- Acute Pain related to skin inflammation.
  Expected Outcomes: The child will have reduced skin irritation, as evidenced by decreased excoriation and increased healing. The child will exhibit minimal pain and pruritus, as evidenced by decreased irritability, absence of scratching, and uninterrupted periods of sleep.
- Risk for Infection related to scratching of pruritic lesions.
  Expected Outcome: The child will have no signs of secondary bacterial infection, as evidenced by clear intact skin.
- Deficient Knowledge of management and prevention of future skin inflammation related to incomplete understanding of therapeutic principles.
  Expected Outcomes: The child and family will identify and avoid irritating substances and will carry out prescribed treatments correctly.

Interventions

Nursing care of the child with contact dermatitis is directed toward relieving itching, preventing infection, and identifying and removing offending substances. Cool compresses and tepid Aveeno baths provide some relief from itching. Prescribed topical steroid creams should be applied in a thin layer after moisturizing with wet compresses to relieve inflammation. Antihistamines, such as diphenhydramine (Benadryl) or hydroxyzine (Atarax), also help the child rest. Because overheating increases itching, advise the parents to occupy the child with quiet activities and to keep the room temperature at a comfortable level.

Reassure the parents and child that the lesions are not contagious and cannot be spread to others or to other parts of the body by scratching. Oils from rhus plants (poison ivy, oak, sumac) that adhere to the skin, under the fingernails, and on clothing can cause new lesions if they are not removed with soap and water. Lesions can become secondarily infected, so the skin should be kept clean and every effort should be made to prevent scratching. Instruct the parents to contact the physician if the child develops a fever or if the lesions become purulent.

Contact dermatitis is prevented by avoiding offending substances. Children should be taught to recognize plants of the rhus group. If the child is exposed to these plants, rinse the skin with cool water immediately (within 15 minutes) and wash clothing in hot, soapy water. Oleoresins in the plants can be spread not only by direct contact with the plant but also in the smoke of burning leaves or by touching pets that have contacted the plants.

Avoiding known irritants, such as cosmetics, jewelry, and canvas athletic shoes, can prevent other types of contact dermatitis. Nickel-sensitive children can usually tolerate 14-karat gold or sterling silver jewelry. Pierced earrings should have hypoallergenic or surgical stainless steel posts.

Diaper dermatitis is much easier to prevent than to treat. Successful treatment and prevention of diaper rash, regard-

less of the cause, depend on cleaning the diaper area thoroughly and keeping the skin dry. Prompt, gentle cleaning with water and mild soap (Dove, Neutrogena Baby Soap) after each voiding or defecation rids the skin of ammonia and other irritants and decreases the chance of skin breakdown and infection. Careful attention should be given to skin folds and creases. The parent should pat the skin dry with a soft cloth towel after washing. Air-drying the skin and frequently exposing the skin to air and light promote healing of diaper rash. During bouts of diaper rash, the diaper may be left off during nap times.

A bland, protective ointment (A and D, Desitin, zinc oxide) can be applied to clean, dry, intact skin to help prevent diaper rash. Ointments should not be applied to inflamed areas because they retain moisture. Occlusion increases the risk of systemic absorption of steroid; thus steroid creams are rarely used for diaper dermatitis because the diaper functions as an occlusive dressing.

Frequent diaper changes decrease irritation from urine and feces. Encourage the parents to check the newborn's diaper every hour and the older infant's diaper every 2 hours. Using disposable diapers does not eliminate the need for frequent diaper changes. Although the "wicking" action of disposable diapers pulls moisture away from the skin toward the liner, ammonia and other by-products are left behind on the infant's skin, causing irritation. Rubber or plastic pants increase skin breakdown by holding in moisture and should be used infrequently.

If cloth diapers are laundered at home, the parents should wash them in hot water, using a mild soap and double-rinsing. Soaking diapers before washing in a quaternary ammonium compound (Diaperene) decreases ammonia in the diapers. Using $1/4$ cup of vinegar in the rinse is also helpful.

Advise parents to contact the physician if the rash does not improve in 3 days with treatment, if the rash becomes solid and bright red, if the rash becomes raw or bleeds, if blisters or boils develop, or if the infant develops a fever.

Evaluation

- Is the child's skin intact, with healed lesions and no evidence of pain or pruritus?
- Is the child's skin free from signs of secondary infection?
- Do the parents demonstrate understanding of proper skin and diaper area care?

ACNE VULGARIS

Acne is a disorder of the sebaceous hair follicles. Although acne is generally perceived as a minor disorder, it can cause significant anxiety and emotional pain for the affected adolescent. The disfiguring lesions of acne, although temporary, can lead to physical and emotional scarring.

Etiology

Multiple factors play a role in the development of acne lesions, including abnormal sloughing of skin cells lining the sebaceous hair follicles, overgrowth of normal bacteria, and host factors, such as heredity, hormonal influences, and emotional stress. Foods do not appear to cause or increase

Pathophysiology

of Acne Vulgaris

Acne begins when sebaceous glands, stimulated by androgens at the onset of puberty, enlarge and secrete increased amounts of sebum. The sebaceous glands become plugged and dilated with sebum. When the enlarged gland is open to the skin surface, an open comedo, or blackhead, is formed. The characteristic black color is not a result of poor hygiene but is produced as fatty acids are oxidized on the skin. If the gland does not have an opening, a closed comedo, or whitehead, is formed. Closed comedones are small, nonerythematous papules just beneath the skin surface. Because a closed comedo has only a microscopic opening on the skin surface, pressure from excess sebum and keratin causes the comedo walls to rupture. Fatty acids produced by bacterial action on sebum are released into the surrounding tissues, causing inflammation. If the rupture occurs close to the surface, a pustule is formed. Ruptures deep in the dermis result in cysts and abscesses, which can lead to significant scarring.

Bacteria, particularly *Propionibacterium acnes,* play a role in the development of acne lesions by increasing inflammation and disrupting the integrity of the follicle walls.

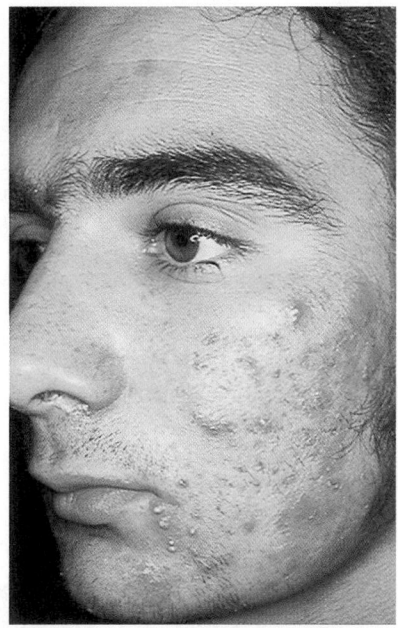

Figure 49-12 An adolescent with acne vulgaris. (From Hurwitz, S. [1993]. *Clinical pediatric dermatology: A textbook of skin disorders of childhood and adolescence* [2nd ed., p. 137]. Philadelphia: Saunders.)

the severity of acne. Acne is unrelated to the general cleanliness of the skin.

Incidence

Acne affects approximately 85% of adolescents. Although acne may begin at any age, it usually develops during puberty and lasts into early adulthood. Acne is more common in boys than in girls. It tends to improve in summer and flare up in winter.

Manifestations and Diagnostic Evaluation

Acne consists of closed whiteheads, blackheads, papules, pustules, nodules, and cysts (Fig. 49-12). Not all adolescents experience all types of acne, and treatment is based on the type experienced. The areas most often affected are the face, neck, back, shoulders, and upper chest. The diagnosis is based on examination of the lesions and the child's history.

Therapeutic Management

The goal of treatment is to prevent scarring and to promote a positive self-image in the adolescent. Treatment must be individualized according to the severity of the condition, the types of lesion present, and the adolescent's gender. Improvement usually begins in 4 to 6 weeks, so the adolescent needs support to keep from feeling discouraged after treatment begins. Three to five months are needed for optimal results.

Topical therapy with a variety of agents is the primary treatment for acne. Commonly used agents include benzoyl peroxide, which reduces fatty acid production and is bactericidal for *Propionibacterium acnes,* and tretinoin (Retin-A), a vitamin A derivative. Tretinoin reduces comedo formation and eliminates the lesions already present. Benzoyl peroxide comes in a gel, cream, lotion, or soap in various strengths. Lower-potency formulas are available over the counter. Tretinoin is available in cream, gel, or liquid form by prescription. Sunscreen should be used with tretinoin to reduce photosensitivity. When applied together to the skin, benzoyl peroxide and tretinoin have a potentially offsetting effect and can reduce the overall effectiveness of each individual agent. For this reason, the physician may order that the two medications be applied on alternate days or that benzoyl peroxide be applied in the morning and tretinoin at bedtime.

Topical antibiotics, such as clindamycin and erythromycin, decrease the number of *P. acnes* organisms in hair follicles and are often used for inflammatory acne. Topical antibiotics are preferred over systemic antibiotics.

Oral antibiotics (tetracycline, minocycline, erythromycin, clindamycin) might be prescribed for adolescents with severe inflammatory acne or those who are unresponsive to topical treatment. Exposure to sunlight should be avoided if tetracycline is used. Oral isotretinoin (Accutane) has dramatically improved the condition of adolescents with severe nodular/cystic acne. This drug suppresses sebum production and sebaceous gland activity. Because of the severity of side effects, isotretinoin is not indicated for all adolescents. Side effects include cataracts, cheilitis, dry skin, pruritus, conjunctivitis, nosebleeds, and depression. In some instances, depression associated with isotretinoin has possibly resulted in suicide (Darmstadt & Sidbury,

2004). Young women who anticipate becoming pregnant should not take isotretinoin because of its teratogenic effects. Sexually active female adolescents should use an effective form of contraception, or combination of contraceptive methods, from 1 month before treatment until 1 month after discontinuing treatment. A negative pregnancy test must be obtained before initiating therapy. Informed consent is recommended for treatment with isotretinoin.

Estrogen may be prescribed for young women who are unresponsive to antibiotic therapy or who cannot take isotretinoin. Some combination (progestin and estrogen) oral contraceptives may also be indicated for acne treatment. Although the dermatologist may mechanically express comedones, the adolescent should be cautioned not to pick or squeeze lesions. Although scars cannot be completely removed, techniques such as dermabrasion, plastic repair, and collagen implants may improve appearance.

■NURSING CARE
The Adolescent With Acne Vulgaris

Assessment

Obtain a history that includes how long acne lesions have been present and the effect of menses, stress, and other aggravating factors on the severity and frequency of the lesions. Investigate acne treatments that have been tried and their effectiveness. Establish how often the adolescent washes the skin and hair and the type of cleansing agents used. Inquire about whether the adolescent uses cosmetics on a regular basis and what types of cosmetics are used. Try to assess the adolescent's understanding of the development and treatment of acne.

Examine the adolescent's face, chest, back, and neck for lesions. The depth of tissue involvement and the presence of pustules, papules, cysts, and scars should be noted. The adolescent's feelings about appearance and self-image should be explored, as well as the effects acne may have had on social functioning.

Nursing Diagnosis and Planning

The nursing diagnoses and expected outcomes that may be appropriate for the adolescent with acne vulgaris are

■ Impaired Skin Integrity related to increased sebaceous gland secretions, hormonal changes, and the action of bacteria on the contents of clogged follicles.
  Expected Outcome: Affected areas will exhibit signs of healing.
■ Risk for Infection related to inflammation of skin lesions.
  Expected Outcome: The adolescent will have no signs of secondary bacterial infection, as evidenced by clear, intact skin.
■ Disturbed Body Image related to appearance of skin lesions.
  Expected Outcomes: The adolescent will verbalize feelings and concerns and will participate in desired social activities.
■ Deficient Knowledge about skin care and treatment regimen related to being too embarrassed to ask questions.

Expected Outcome: The adolescent will carry out the prescribed treatment regimen to control excessive sebaceous gland activity.

Interventions

Because acne is a long-term condition, the affected adolescent needs support and encouragement if the treatment regimen is to be effective. Improvement may take as long as 12 weeks, and exacerbations are common. Although there is no cure for acne, much can be done to control inflammation and reduce scarring.

Explain the cause of acne and the rationale for treatment at the outset, so the adolescent can help plan the treatment regimen. Providing written instructions and involving the adolescent in care can help improve adherence. The treatment must be individualized, but all treatment regimens include measures to reduce oil on the skin. Gently cleaning the face twice a day with mild antibacterial soap and shampooing the hair daily are important facets of care. Warn the adolescent to avoid vigorous scrubbing and picking or squeezing of lesions, which can rupture pilosebaceous ducts and cause secondary infection. Teach the adolescent how to apply topical medications, and caution against overusing these products to speed results. Because oily cosmetics and creams add to the plugging of follicles, only water-based cosmetics should be used.

A healthy lifestyle, including adequate rest, exercise, and a balanced diet, promotes healing of lesions. Explore the adolescent's feelings about appearance and coping mechanisms. Reinforce positive self-image and self-esteem. Concerns and fears should be openly discussed and myths about acne dispelled. Provide parents with needed information about acne to clear up misconceptions and to prevent needless nagging of the adolescent.

Evaluation

- Do the acne lesions exhibit signs of healing without signs of infection?
- Is the adolescent able to express feelings and concerns about possible change in body image?
- Does the adolescent appear confident and assured as the process of healing is occurring?
- Does the adolescent carry out the treatment regimen to control acne and prevent scarring?

MISCELLANEOUS SKIN DISORDERS

There are a number of less common skin disorders of varied causes and manifestations. These disorders, along with their manifestations, management, and special considerations, are listed in Table 49-1.

INSECT BITES OR STINGS

Insects are found almost everywhere, and children often come in contact with them during play. The bites of most insects are not serious, usually causing only itching and mild pain. Severe systemic reactions can occur in sensitized children, however. Approximately 2 million people in the United States are severely allergic to venomous stinging insects. Anaphylaxis from insect stings occurs in 0.5% to 5% of the U.S. population

(Neugat & Miller, 2001) resulting in at least 40 deaths per year (American College of Allergy, Asthma, and Immunology, 1998). Children who are allergic to insect stings should wear identification describing the allergy and outlining appropriate treatment. An emergency kit containing an antihistamine, epinephrine, and a syringe should be kept immediately available for such children. Parents should check the expiration date on the kit and replace it if it is outdated. (See Chapter 41 for a discussion of anaphylactic reactions.)

Arachnids (scorpions, spiders, ticks, mites) are found in areas where children play. Most arachnids are not dangerous or aggressive. In the United States, only one type of scorpion and two types of spiders (black widow, brown recluse) cause life-threatening reactions.

Topical insect repellents are usually safe and effective in preventing insect bites. Repellents containing high concentrations of diethyltoluamide (DEET) should not be used on small children because of the risk of toxic encephalopathy. Such repellents should not be applied near the face, and children should be cautioned not to put their fingers in their mouths when wearing DEET.

The bites and stings of common insects and arachnids are discussed in Table 49-2. The table includes information on manifestations, treatment, and prevention.

TABLE **49-1** Skin Disorders			
Disorder/Etiology	**Manifestations**	**Management**	**Comments**
STEVENS-JOHNSON SYNDROME, ERYTHEMA MULTIFORME			
Acute, sometimes recurrent autoimmune disease. May be triggered by infections or medications, such as sulfonamides or anticonvulsants. New lesions continue to erupt for 2-3 wk, followed by healing during the next 6 wk.	After a prodromal respiratory illness, bullae appear on the lips, mouth, eyes, and genitalia. Fever, chills, malaise, neutropenia, anemia, weakness. Purulent conjunctivitis is common. Skin lesions rupture and may lead to significant fluid loss.	Withdraw the triggering medication. Treatment of skin lesions similar to treatment of extensive burns: aseptic technique, intravenous (IV) fluids, air/fluid bedding, nutritional support, pain management. Give antibiotics for secondary infections. Obtain ophthalmology consultation for eye lesions.	Reassure the child that the skin lesions will disappear. Inform parents about the possibility of recurrence, and encourage them to avoid any implicated medications.
PSORIASIS			
Chronic, inflammatory rash caused by rapid proliferation of keratinocytes. Hereditary predisposition; onset in first 2 decades of life. Remissions and exacerbations; lasts throughout life. Exacerbations associated with stress. Arthritis is sometimes a complication.	Pruritus; erythematous, elevated plaques and silvery scales on the scalp, face, knees, elbows, and gluteal folds. Scales are attached at the center rather than edges and may bleed when removed.	Topical corticosteroids and tar preparations; keratolytic agents. Exposure to ultraviolet light and sunlight. Skin care to prevent secondary infection. Keratolytic agents enhance penetration of topical steroids. Sunlight may cause phototoxic reactions with tar preparations. To prevent tar folliculitis, tar should be applied down an extremity rather than up.	There is no cure for psoriasis. A resource for families of children with psoriasis is in Appendix I on Evolve website.
PITYRIASIS ROSEA			
Acute, inflammatory, self-limited skin disorder. Etiology unknown; may be viral.	Sudden eruption of salmon-pink, irregular patches on trunk and proximal portions of extremities. Symmetric distribution of lesions, "Christmas tree" appearance on back. "Herald patch" precedes rash by 7-10 days.	No treatment required for asymptomatic children. Pruritus can be treated with antipruritic lotions, ultraviolet light, or sunlight.	Child generally feels well. Rash may last 6-12 wk.

Continued

TABLE **49-1**   Skin Disorders—cont'd

Disorder/Etiology	Manifestations	Management	Comments
WARTS			
Skin infection caused by human papillomavirus (HPV). Incubation period is 1-6 mo. Can persist from a few months to 5 or more years.	Painless, hyperkeratotic papule. Begins as a round, flesh-colored papule; later becomes brown or tan with a rough surface. Most common sites: dorsum of hands, fingers, feet, face, genitalia.	Various methods of treatment: daily application of lactic acid and salicylic acid (e.g., Compound W); freezing with liquid nitrogen; topical application of cantharidin for plantar or periungual warts.	Most warts disappear without treatment in 2-3 yr. With treatment, they usually resolve in 2-3 mo. Picking at warts may cause them to spread to other areas of the body. Warts are not highly contagious to other people. Immunocompromised children are more susceptible to warts.
MOLLUSCUM CONTAGIOSUM			
Viral infection of the skin and mucous membranes. Transmitted by skin-to-skin and fomite-to-skin contact. May be transmitted by sexual contact.	Begin as pinpoint papules that increase in size to 2-3 mm or larger. Firm, solid, pink papules changing into soft, waxy, umbilicated papules. Curdlike core of the lesion can be expressed. Most common sites: face, trunk, extremities, oral mucous membranes, conjunctiva, genitalia.	Lesions may be treated with cantharidin, cryotherapy, tretinoin, or imiquimod. Condition usually responds well to treatment. Spontaneous disappearance is common.	Lesions may be spread to other parts of the body and may be transmitted to others. Lesions disappear spontaneously over time. Children with eczema or impaired immunity are at risk for generalized spread of lesions.
FROSTBITE			
Freezing of tissue resulting from exposure to extreme cold. Exposed areas (fingers, toes, nose, cheeks, ears) are most often affected. Cold causes arteriolar vasoconstriction, resulting in tissue anoxia and destruction.	*Early signs:* blanching of skin; stinging sensation followed by numbness and white, mottled appearance. Area feels cold, hard; may be without sensation. *First-degree:* redness and discomfort with return to normal in a few hours. *Second-degree:* redness; blisters and bullae 24-48 hr after rewarming. Pain during rewarming. *Third-degree:* cyanosis and mottling, followed by redness and swelling. Necrosis of epidermis, dermis, and subcutaneous tissue. Sensation is absent. Pain during rewarming. *Fourth-degree:* Complete necrosis with gangrene, possible loss of body part.	Immediately cover affected areas with warm hands and warm clothing. Massaging areas causes further damage and should be avoided. Rapidly rewarm areas by immersion in a warm water bath (90°-106° F) until all frozen tissues are thawed and the skin appears flushed. Pain during thawing can be severe and should be treated with analgesics and sedatives. Severely damaged areas are treated as burns.	Children in cold climates should be taught to prevent frostbite by wearing adequate warm, layered clothing, hat, gloves, and two pairs of socks (one cotton, one wool). Children should be taught to warm themselves when hands or feet begin to sting. Young children should not be allowed to play outside in extremely cold temperatures.
FOREIGN BODIES			
Skin injury caused by penetration of splinters, gravel, cactus spines, bee stingers, glass, or other foreign objects.	Pain, erythema, possible secondary infection. Foreign body may or may not be visible.	Area surrounding foreign body should be washed with soap and water before removal. Superficial splinters can be removed with a needle and tweezers disinfected with alcohol or flame.	Deeply embedded foreign bodies, fishhooks, and other difficult-to-remove objects may require medical attention. Tetanus prophylaxis may be indicated.

TABLE **49-2** Skin Lesions Caused by Insects and Arachnids

Agent and Characteristics	Manifestations	Treatment and Prevention
INSECTS		
Mosquitoes, Fleas, Flies, Gnats Foreign protein in insect's saliva is injected as insect pierces skin to suck blood.	Itching, erythema, small wheal. Allergic reaction may occur.	Apply antipruritic lotions and cool compresses to relieve itching. Give antihistamines if needed for sleep. *Prevention:* Wear insect repellent when contact is anticipated. Treat potential breeding places (standing water for mosquitoes; pets, furniture, yard for fleas).
Hymenoptera (Bees, Wasps, Hornets, Yellow Jackets, Fire Ants) Venom is injected through a stinger.	Histamine and foreign proteins in venom cause local reaction of pain, swelling, redness, and itching. Systemic allergic reactions may be manifested by nausea, generalized edema, respiratory distress, and shock.	Carefully remove stinger by scraping it out horizontally. Avoid squeezing stinger, because more venom will be released. Wash with soap and water. Paste made of powdered meat tenderizer and water is soothing. Apply ice and analgesics for discomfort, antihistamines for itching. For a systemic allergic reaction, give epinephrine and corticosteroids immediately; transport to emergency facility. Children allergic to hymenoptera should wear medical identification. *Prevention:* Treat known hives or nests. Avoid wearing colorful clothing and perfumes when outside.
ARACHNIDS		
Brown Recluse ("Fiddle Back") Spider Yellowish to reddish brown with a violin-shaped mark on its back. Venom injected by fangs. Bites only when threatened. Lives in dark, protected areas (woodpiles, basements, closets, trash heaps).	Mild stinging at time of bite. Within 2-8 hr, area around bite becomes painful and erythema develops, followed by a blister. Venom is necrotoxic. Edema, redness, and purpura may involve entire limb. Central portion of lesion develops an indurated wheal that progresses to deep, sloughing ulcer in 7-14 days. Ulcer often does not heal for several months. Usually results in a scar.	Immobilize and elevate affected extremity. Cool compresses, analgesics, tetanus prophylaxis. Observe for secondary infection. Skin graft may be necessary for large ulcers. No antivenin available. *Prevention:* Avoid areas inhabited by spiders.
Black Widow Spider Shiny black with a red hourglass-shaped mark on abdomen. Female's venom is very poisonous to humans. Males do not bite. Female builds irregular web in dark, sheltered spots and aggressively defends eggs.	Bite may be painless initially. Within 1 hr pain develops at site. Severe muscle pains and numbness spread from bite, and puncture site becomes red, swollen, and pruritic. Neurotoxic venom enters the bloodstream within 1 hr, causing dizziness, headache, nausea, vomiting, cramps, tremors, and rapid, shallow respirations. Shock and renal failure may develop in young children.	Hospitalization for children. Antivenin if no allergy to horse serum. Supportive care, including IV calcium gluconate, morphine, muscle relaxants. Tetanus prophylaxis. *Prevention:* Avoid areas infested by spiders (woodpiles, outhouses).
Ticks Brown or gray; live in fields, pastures, woods. Feed on blood of humans, dogs, livestock, or deer. Larvae feed on rodents. Tick buries head and mouthparts in the skin to suck blood.	Bites may cause local reactions or, rarely, systemic reactions (tick fever, tick paralysis). Ticks can transmit Lyme disease, Rocky Mountain spotted fever, Q fever, tularemia.	*Methods to remove ticks:* Remove with tweezers as close to the skin as possible, taking care to remove head. If mouthparts remain, remove with sterile needle. Wash site with soap and water. There is some evidence that prompt removal of ticks decreases chance of transmission of disease. *Prevention:* Wear long sleeves and pants and use insect repellent when walking in tick-infested areas. Inspect clothing and hair for ticks after walking through fields or woods.

Continued

TABLE **49-2** Skin Lesions Caused by Insects and Arachnids—cont'd

Agent and Characteristics	Manifestations	Treatment and Prevention
ARACHNIDS—cont'd		
Scorpions		
Most scorpions are not dangerous. They rarely attack humans unless accidentally disturbed or stepped on. If disturbed, they inflict a painful sting. One type (found in Arizona), *Centruroides sculpturatus*, is extremely poisonous, and its sting can be fatal. Scorpions are found mainly in the southwestern United States. Scorpions hide by day in basements, garages, closets, crevices. Some varieties burrow and hide in gravel or children's sandboxes.	Sting is extremely painful. Local reaction of swelling at puncture site. Some species cause systemic reactions: tachycardia, hypertension, dysrhythmias, irritability, seizures, pulmonary edema, coma. Fatal reactions most often occur in children younger than 3 yr.	Ice packs and tourniquet applied proximal to the site slow the spread of venom. Wound should not be excised. Topical steroids and antihistamines are used to relieve symptoms. For severe reactions, provide supportive care for pain, shock, seizures. Narcotic analgesics act synergistically with scorpion venom and are contraindicated. Antivenin is given for systemic reactions (available from the Antivenom Production Laboratory, Arizona State University). *Prevention:* Wear shoes to prevent stepping on scorpions. Inspect shoes and clothing before dressing. Apply creosote to garages, basements.
Chiggers (Harvest Mites)		
Live in tall grass and underbrush; burrow into hair follicles and skin pores to feed.	Tend to concentrate in warm areas where clothing is snug (underwear elastic). Cause erythematous papules and intense itching.	Antipruritic agents. Prevention of secondary infection. *Prevention:* Insect repellent on clothing, ankles, legs.

BOX 49-1
Pediatric Differences in the Effects of Burn Injury

- Very young children who have been severely burned have a higher mortality rate than older children and adults with comparable burns.
- Because a child's skin is thinner than that of an adult, lower burn temperatures and shorter exposure to heat or chemicals can cause a more severe burn.
- A larger body surface area as compared with that of adults places severely burned children at increased risk for fluid and heat loss. Children are also at increased risk for dehydration and metabolic acidosis secondary to diarrhea, evaporative water loss, and increased fluid requirements.
- The higher proportion of body fluid to mass in children increases the risk of cardiovascular problems because of their less-effective cardiovascular response to changing intravascular volume.
- Burns involving more than 10% total body surface area (TBSA) require a form of fluid resuscitation.
- Infants and children are at increased risk for protein and calorie deficiency because they have smaller muscle mass and lower body fat than adults. If they are not eating and their metabolism is increased, their protein and calorie needs will not be met.
- Hypertrophic scarring is more severe, and scar maturation is prolonged.
- An immature immune system means an increased risk of infection for infants and young children.
- A delay in growth may follow extensive burns.
- In children, Curling (gastroduodenal) ulcer occurs in the 3rd or 4th week after a burn, which is later than in adults.

Modified from U.S. Department of Health and Human Services. (2000). *Healthy People 2010* (conference edition, in two volumes). Washington, D.C.: Author.

BURN INJURIES

Burn injury may involve a small, painful area that hurts until healing occurs, or it may involve most of a child's body, with resulting severe trauma or death. Infants and toddlers are at greatest risk for sustaining burns because they depend totally on others for safety.

Recovery from a major burn injury requires many months, and the child's appearance might be altered for life. Caring for a burned child entails a multidisciplinary approach with a focus on the child and the family. Nursing care involves treating the physical injury and its psychological effects on the child and family members. The challenges of burn nursing begin with acute burn care but continue through the rehabilitation phase until the child is restored to optimal function (Box 49-1).

Etiology

Burn injuries in children can be unintentional or intentional. In children younger than 5 years, unintentional burns are likely to occur as a result of environmental situations that are not controlled by caretakers. The young child's curiosity and increasing mobility contribute to the risk (Table 49-3). A child can start a fire by playing with matches (Fig. 49-13) or flammable materials near open fires, or a child might be the victim of a house fire while sleeping or might be unintentionally scalded or electrocuted (Fig. 49-14). (See Chapters 5 through 8 for a discussion of safety.) Either neglectful supervision or purposeful abuse can cause intentional burns.

The extent of the injury determines whether the problem is local or systemic. Other factors, such as the location of the burned area, whether it is an electrical injury, whether there is a concurrent inhalation injury or trauma, and whether there is a preexisting medical disease, contribute to morbidity and mortality. Morbidity and mortality are higher in children who have been burned than in adults.

TABLE **49-3** Age-Related Risks for Burn Injury

Age	Injury Type	Risk Factors
<5 yr	Flame	Playing with matches and cigarette lighters
		Playing with fires in fireplaces, barbecue pits, trash fires
	Scald	Kitchen injury from tipping scalding liquids
		Bathtub scalds associated with lack of supervision or child abuse
		Most pediatric burn patients are infants and toddlers younger than 3 yr burned by scalding liquids
5-10 yr	Flame	Boys at increased risk
		Often associated with fire play and risk-taking behaviors
	Scald	Girls at increased risk
		Likely to occur at home in kitchen or bathroom
Adolescent	Flame	Injury associated with male peer-group activities involving gasoline or other flammable products
		Gasoline sniffing possibly involved
		Rarely occurs in female adolescents except in house fires or automobile accidents
	Electrical	Occurs most often in male adolescents involved in dare-type behaviors, such as climbing utility poles or antennas
		In rural areas, may be associated with moving irrigation pipes that touch an electrical source

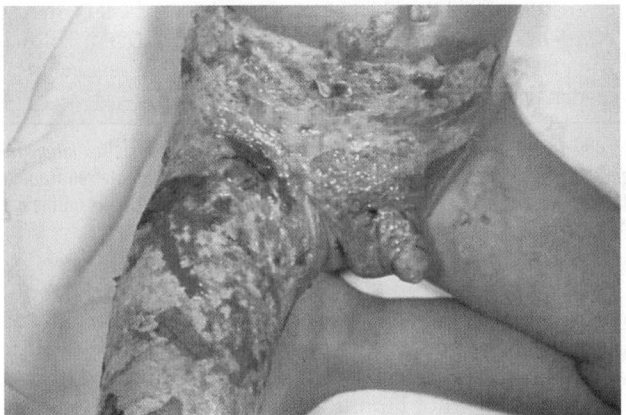

Figure 49-13 These burns were sustained when the child's pajamas caught fire while he was playing with matches. (From Cosman, B. [1973]. *Management of the burned patient.* New York: MEDCOM.)

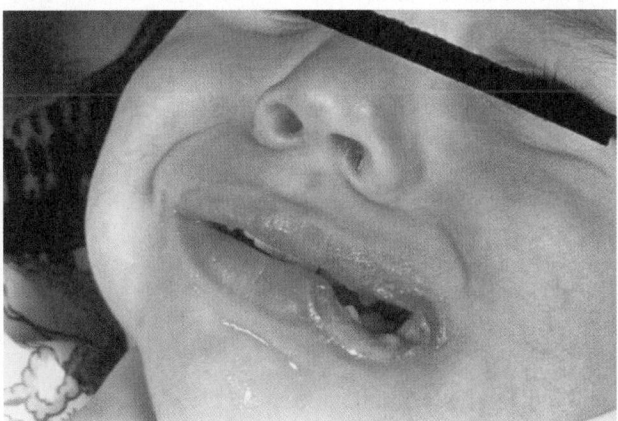

Figure 49-14 These burns were sustained when the child sucked on an electrical socket. (From Cosman, B. [1973]. *Management of the burned patient.* New York: MEDCOM.)

Incidence

Fire and burn injuries are the fifth leading cause of unintentional deaths in children ages 1 to 14 years in the United States (National SAFEKIDS Campaign, 2004). In children younger than 4 years, 66% of burns result from scalds and 14% from flame injury (Dickerson, Gordon, & Walter, 1998). The rest of the burn injuries have electrical and chemical causes. Approximately 18% of burn injuries are related to child abuse (Antoon & Donovan, 2000).

Most children with severe burns are treated in burn centers. The American Burn Association has outlined criteria for referral to a burn center (Box 49-2).

Pathophysiology

Burn injuries are described using three parameters: depth of tissue damage, extent of injury, and severity. The combination of these factors determines referral and therapeutic management decisions.

Depth of Burn Injury

Depth of burn injury describes local tissue damage and is largely a factor of the duration of exposure and the temperature or destructive potential of the agent causing the damage. Depth of injury is classified as superficial (first-degree), partial-thickness (second-degree), or full-thickness (third-degree) (Table 49-4).

Partial-thickness thermal, chemical, or electrical injury to the skin interferes with the skin's ability to carry out its normal physiologic functions of protection from infection or injury and preservation of fluid balance and temperature regulation. In addition, deep tissue injury damages sensory nerve endings and local circulatory patterns and adversely affects the skin's ability to regenerate or synthesize vitamin D.

Extent of Burn Injury

The extent of injury refers to the percent of total body surface area (TBSA) burned. The standard "rule of nines" used in adults gives an inaccurate estimate for children because of the differences in body proportion between children and

THE CHILD AND PARENTS
Want to Know

About Measures to Prevent and Initially Manage a Burn

Prevention
- Have periodic fire drills to teach your children how to evacuate the house in the event of a fire.
- Place child identification stickers, which can be obtained from most fire departments, on the outside of the bedroom door and in one window of each child's bedroom.
- Identify two or more exits from each room and a location to meet outside the house. Emphasize to your children that they should not return to the house under any circumstances, even if another family member or pet remains in the house.
- Be sure your child understands "stop, drop, and roll" as a measure to stop the burning process.
- Be sure to keep all matches and lighters out of reach. Check electrical cords regularly. Use outlet covers if children younger than 5 years are in the house.
- Check smoke detectors regularly, and keep them clean. Replace the batteries regularly if they are battery operated.
- To reduce the number of scald burns, turn the hot water heater thermostat down to 120° F.
- Turn pot handles in, and use back burners on the stove whenever possible.
- Do not set a child on your lap while you are drinking a hot liquid.
- Keep your children away from outdoor grills and indoor wood- or coal-burning stoves. Keep older infants from crawling near floor heating grates.

Initial Emergency Burn Management
- Apply cool compresses, or submerge minor burns in cool water, not ice.
- To prevent scalding, remove clothing soaked with hot water as quickly as possible.
- Contact the physician for any child with a burn that has blistered.
- Cover a child who has a major burn with a clean sheet while waiting for emergency personnel.
- Do not try to remove clothing that is adhering to burned skin.

BOX 49-2
Burn Center Referral Criteria

The following injuries have been identified as those requiring referral to a burn center. Children with these burns should be treated in a specialized burn facility after initial assessment and stabilization in an emergency department.
- Burns of more than 10% total body surface area (TBSA)
- Second- and third-degree burns with serious threat of functional or cosmetic impairment that involve the face, hands, feet, genitalia, perineum, and major joints
- Electrical burns, including lightning injury
- Chemical burns with serious threat of functional or cosmetic impairment
- Inhalation injury with burn injury
- Home situations that may not facilitate adequate care
- Co-existing trauma, such as fractures, smoke inhalation, or head trauma

Stabilization in Preparation for Transfer
Once the decision has been made to transfer a burned child, it is essential that the child be properly stabilized before the transfer process. Infants with burns exceeding 10% of TBSA and children with burns exceeding 15% of TBSA require immediate fluid resuscitation.

Modified from Deitch, E., & Rutan, R. (2001). *The challenges of children: The first 48 hours.* Chicago: The American Burn Association; Committee on Trauma. (1999). *Resources for optimal care of the injured patient* (Ch. 14). Chicago: American College of Surgeons.

---

adults. Many burn facilities use the Lund and Browder chart, which is a body surface chart corrected for age (Fig. 49-15). Another method estimates burn percentage by calculating the complete palmar surface of the child's hand and assumes the area of the palmar surface equals 1% of the TBSA. In fact, the palm is somewhat smaller, about 0.70% to 0.87% of TBSA in children, so this method overestimates the extent of injury but is convenient for children or small or irregular burns (Amirsheybani, 2001; Berry, Evison, & Roberts, 2001).

Severity of Burn Injury
Severity of burn injury is determined by the degree to which the skin's physiologic functions are disrupted beyond the body's normal ability to respond with compensatory mecha-

nisms. Burn injuries are classified as minor, moderate uncomplicated, and major. The severity of burn injury is related to a combination of factors. These include age, medical history, extent and depth of burn, special care of the body area involved (e.g., face, hands), and the presence of concomitant trauma, such as fractures or head injury, sustained at the time of the burn. Burn severity relates to the child's eventual morbidity or mortality status.

Manifestations

Table 49-5 lists the clinical manifestations associated with burns of different severity.

Therapeutic Management

Superficial Burn Injuries
The most common cause of a superficial (epidermal layer only) burn is sunburn. Although uncomfortable, sunburn rarely requires intensive burn treatment. Cool compresses and application of soothing topical lotions (especially those containing aloe) or mild topical corticosteroids (Starr, 2000) provide symptomatic treatment. If the discomfort is disturbing the child's sleep, acetaminophen or ibuprofen can provide relief.

Preventing sunburn is especially important in children because frequent sunburn causes long-term damage to the skin. Children who are susceptible to sunburn are also susceptible to the later development of melanoma and non-melanoma skin cancers (Hornung, 2000; Kennedy, Bajdik, Willemze, De Gruijl, & Bouwes Bavinek, 2003). Children should avoid sun

TABLE **49-4** Depth of Burn Injury

	Superficial (First Degree)	Partial-Thickness (Second-degree)		Full-Thickness (Third Degree)
		Superficial	Deep	
Morphology	Destruction of epidermis; physiologic functions remain intact	Destruction of epidermis and some dermis	Destruction of epidermis and dermis	Destruction of epidermis, dermis, underlying tissue; may include fascia, muscle, tendon, bone
Blister formation	After 24 hr (e.g., from sunburn)	Within minutes; thin-walled, fluid-filled	May or may not appear as fluid-filled blisters; often they are flat, dehydrated, and like tissue paper; body fluids lost through burn tissue must be replaced	Rare; may appear as a tissue paper–like layer that is flat and dehydrated
Appearance	Peels after 24-48 hr	Red to pale ivory, moist surface	Mottled, waxy white, dry surface	White, cherry red, or black
Healing time	3-7 days	7-21 days if no infection develops	30 days to several months if no infection; if infected, this type of burn may convert to full-thickness	Will not heal; skin grafting required; very small areas may heal from edges after a period of weeks
Patient reaction	Moderate discomfort, pain; chills; nausea; vomiting	May cause considerable pain	Severe pain on exposure to air or water because nerve endings are intact	No pain in area of full-thickness burn because nerve endings are destroyed; surrounding areas of lesser depth are painful
Scarring	None	Minimal; influenced by genetic predisposition	Greatest because the slow healing of these burns increases scar tissue; scar formation influenced by genetic predisposition	Autograft scarring is minimized by early excision and grafting; scar formation influenced by genetic predisposition

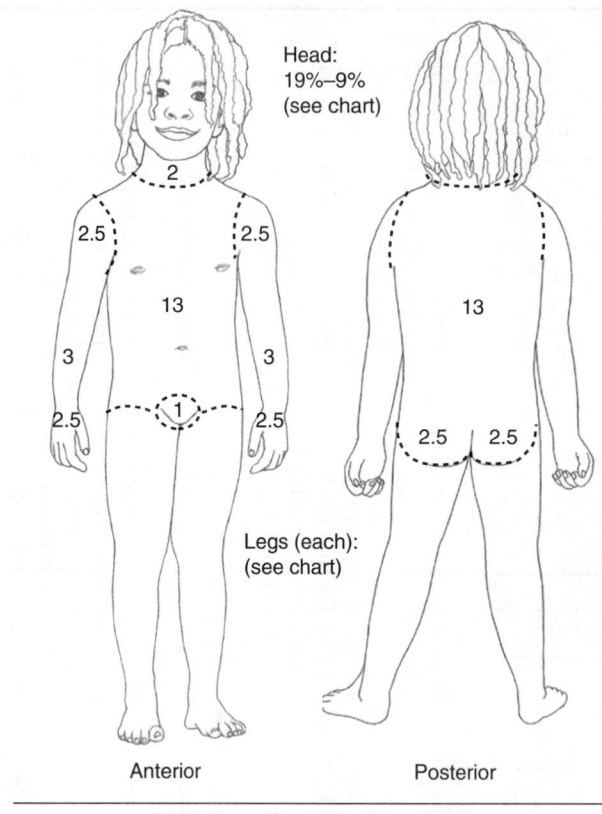

Head:
19%–9%
(see chart)

Legs (each):
(see chart)

Anterior   Posterior

Child Burn Size Estimation Table
(percent total body surface area)

Age in Years

	< 1yr	1	5	10	15	Adult
Head	19	17	13	11	9	7
Neck	2	2	2	2	2	2
Ant Trunk	13	13	13	13	13	13
Post Trunk	13	13	13	13	13	13
Buttock	2.5	2.5	2.5	2.5	2.5	2.5
Genitalia	1	1	1	1	1	1
Upper arm	2.5	2.5	2.5	2.5	2.5	2.5
Lower arm	3	3	3	3	3	3
Hand	2.5	2.5	2.5	2.5	2.5	2.5
Thigh	5.5	6.5	8	8.5	9	9.5
Leg	5	5	5.5	6	6.5	7
Foot	3.5	3.5	3.5	3.5	3.5	3.5

Figure 49-15 Calculating total body surface area (TBSA) burned in children. The standard "rule of nines" and standard body surface charts must be adapted because of the difference in body proportions between adults and children. (From Deitch, E., & Rutan, R. [2001]. *The challenges of children: The first 48 hours.* Chicago: American Burn Association.)

exposure, especially between the hours of 10 AM and 3 PM during the summer. During sun exposure, parents should apply to the child's skin an appropriate ultraviolet A and ultraviolet B protective sunscreen with a sun protection factor (SPF) greater than 15. Hats and shirts are also desirable. Waterproof sunscreens are available for children who like to run in and out of the water, but frequent applications of sunscreen are still desirable. Sunscreen is contraindicated for infants younger than 6 months. Parents should keep infants in the shade, away from reflecting sun rays.

Minor Partial-Thickness Burn Injuries

In general, children with a minor burn injury are treated as outpatients in a physician's office, clinic, or hospital physical therapy department unless the extent of injury warrants hospital admission. Therapy is aimed at promoting wound healing, preventing infection, and providing pain relief. Burn wound care requires aseptic technique. Because anaerobic and aerobic bacteria can grow at the interface between burned and healthy tissue, tetanus toxoid is given to children whose immunizations are not up-to-date.

TABLE **49-5** Classification of Severity of Burn Injury in Children

Type of Injury	Clinical Manifestations
MINOR	
Partial-thickness burn of <10% of total body surface area (TBSA)	Localized pain and blister formation in the area of injury; white or black full-thickness injury
Full-thickness burn of <2% of TBSA that does not involve special care areas (eyes, ears, face, hands, feet, perineum, joints)	No systemic effects
Excludes electrical injury, inhalation injury, concurrent trauma, all poor-risk children (e.g., those of extremely young age or with concurrent disease)	Little or no scarring, except in areas of full-thickness injury
MODERATE, UNCOMPLICATED	
Partial-thickness burns of 10%-20% of TBSA	Open wound that is a potential source of infection and a site for loss of fluids and electrolytes
Full-thickness burns of <10% of TBSA that do not involve special care areas	Pain that may interfere with routines of daily living
Excludes electrical injury, inhalation injury, concurrent trauma, all poor-risk children (e.g., those of extremely young age or with concurrent disease)	Wound healing rate influenced by nutritional status
	Possible scarring in areas of partial- and full-thickness injuries
MAJOR	
Partial-thickness burns of >20% of TBSA	Life-threatening injuries with risk for severe complications and death
All full-thickness burns of ≥10% of TBSA	Volatile hospital course characterized by periods of relative physiologic stability followed, within hours, by life-threatening emergencies, such as shock
All burns involving eyes, ears, face, hands, feet, perineum, or joints	Repeated operative procedures for skin grafting that are accompanied by major blood loss requiring multiple transfusions
All inhalation injury, electrical injury, concurrent trauma, all poor-risk patients	Potential risk for infection, either of the burn wound or related to pulmonary complications or systemic sepsis, until wound closure is achieved over 80% of the TBSA
	Much higher mortality associated with burn injury accompanied by inhalation injury than with burn injury alone

Wound Cleaning. Burn wounds receive care at least daily until closure is achieved. After old dressings are removed, the burned skin is cleaned with sterile saline or mild soap and water. If the child is hospitalized, hydrotherapy (Fig. 49-16) can be used to remove old dressings and clean the wound and the child. During this cleaning process, the child can perform active range-of-motion exercises. Hydrotherapy can be done in a tank, tub, or shower. Some facilities use disposable plastic liners to prevent contamination between uses. Hydrotherapy should last no longer than 20 minutes to prevent electrolyte loss (through skin into water, secondary to osmosis). The room temperature is kept warm, and the child is covered and dried immediately after the procedure.

Débridement. Débridement is the removal of dead material within a wound to promote healing. In a burn injury, there is necrosis of skin and subcutaneous tissue. The burned tissue is called *eschar*. Eschar releases chemical mediators that stimulate leukocytes to digest debris, but this also damages capillaries and skin elements. Necrotic tissue within a wound prolongs inflammation and slows healing and epidermal coverage.

Initial débridement might be performed in the office, emergency department, or hydrotherapy treatment room. The burned area is débrided of loose debris and necrotic tissue. Blisters usually are left intact and débrided only after they open (Brady, 2000b; Kumar, 1999). Old creams and ointments must be removed as part of the débridement, and loose tissue is trimmed around the burned area.

Application of Antimicrobial Agents and Dressings. Topical antibacterial agents (Table 49-6) are placed on burn wounds to penetrate the eschar and to control bacterial growth in and around the burn wound. Silver sulfadiazine (Silvadene) is the most commonly used topical agent, but it is not typically used on the face or on electrical burns. Facial burns are covered with a light layer of antimicrobial ointment. Mafenide (Sulfamylon) is the topical agent of choice for burns to the ear or electrical burns because of its deep penetration into the eschar. Mafenide should not be applied to the face.

After application of the topical antibacterial agent, a dressing usually is applied. Depending on the burn care protocol, dressings are changed one to three times a day. Because exposed nerve endings can cause significant pain, wound assessment and care should be done as quickly as possible. Narcotic or non-narcotic pain medications are administered 20 to 30 minutes before dressing changes to ensure maximum pain control at the time of the procedure. The child life specialist can assist with teaching the child how to use non-pharmacologic pain-relief techniques.

Besides pain control, measures to maintain the child's core body temperature, minimize shivering, and conserve energy also must be implemented as part of wound care activities. To the degree possible, the child's capacity for self-care should be optimized. Allowing the child to remove dressings provides a measure of control.

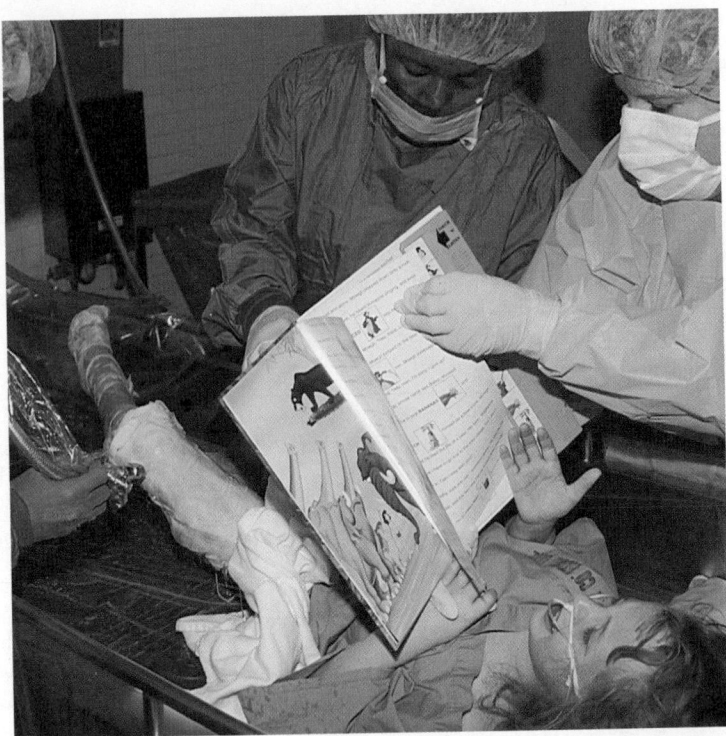

Figure 49-16 Burn dressings can be changed in the hydrotherapy room. The room is kept warm because children who have been burned have poor body temperature control. The child life therapist reads a book to the child to distract her from the discomfort associated with the procedure. (Courtesy Parkland Health and Hospital System, Dallas, TX.)

TABLE **49-6** Topical Antimicrobial Agents Commonly Used for Burns

Agent	Advantages	Side Effects and Disadvantages	Nursing Considerations
Silver nitrate solution	Effective against most gram-positive and some gram-negative organisms	Hyponatremia, hypokalemia, hypochloremia Decreased penetration of eschar Not effective against established infection Requires large, bulky dressings that limit mobility	0.5% solution in distilled water applied to wet dressing every 2 hr Dressing changes twice daily Can cause staining of linens and clothing and interferes with accurate wound assessment
Mafenide acetate cream (Sulfamylon)	Effective against a wide range of gram-positive and gram-negative organisms Rapid penetration through eschar (improved effectiveness in established infections) Permits open treatment of wound, thus increasing mobility	Painful on application May cause hypersensitivity reaction in 5%-7% of patients Associated with acid-base alteration (metabolic acidosis)	Applied to cleansed wound 1 or 2 times per day Treated area usually left open; a light dressing may be used Must be completely removed before reapplication Check sensitivity to sulfonamides
Silver sulfadiazine cream (Silvadene)	Effective against a wide range of gram-positive and gram-negative organisms Soothing on application Moderate eschar penetration Absorbed slowly, reducing the possibility of nephrotoxicity	May cause hypersensitivity reaction in 5%-7% of patients Associated with initial decrease in leukocyte count (transient)	Applied to cleansed wound 1 or 2 times per day Wound may be left open or covered with light dressing Check sensitivity to sulfonamides Must remove all medication before reapplication

Aseptic technique is used during dressing changes. After dressings are applied to burn wounds, isolation is not necessary and the child does not need to be restricted to a room or to an area of the hospital.

Depending on the depth and extent of the burn, the physician might choose to cover the area with a biologic or synthetic dressing to reduce the chance of infection, provide pain relief, reduce evaporative fluid and heat loss, and promote healing. Such dressings are best used for partial-thickness burns. Commonly used biologic dressings include human skin, pig skin, and fresh human amniotic membrane (from the placenta). Synthetic dressings include plastic films, hydrocolloids, hydrogels, and collagen-impregnated dressings. The major risk associated with these dressings is infection; thus the wound must be clean and dry before dressing application.

Nursing Care Plan

The Child With a Minor Partial-Thickness Burn

FOCUSED ASSESSMENT

In the first few seconds after the arrival of a child who has been burned, the severity of the burn is determined. If the burn is of minor severity, care focuses on pain management and wound care. Children with burns of moderate uncomplicated severity may need fluid resuscitation. Take vital signs, paying special attention to the child's body temperature. Without skin, the burned child, especially if very young, rapidly loses heat to the atmosphere and is at risk for hypothermia. The child should be awake, alert, and oriented unless some condition other than an uncomplicated burn injury exists.

Assessment for pain intensity takes place on a scheduled basis, and interventions to control pain are implemented as needed. Assess the wound with each dressing change, and document any signs of decreased circulation or infection. Assessment also includes range-of-motion abilities and the frequency and effectiveness of any physical therapy treatments. It is important to assess the child's ability to assume independent activities, particularly when the burn affects the child's extremities. Young children tend to protect injuries, so the child might need encouragement to move appropriately. Children with minor partial-thickness burns may be managed completely on an outpatient basis, with parents bringing the child daily to the physician's office for burn assessment, débridement, and dressing changes.

Nursing Diagnosis

Impaired Skin Integrity related to thermal injury.

Expected Outcome

The burn will:
- Heal without infection, as evidenced by normal temperature, normal granulating tissue, and restoration of the epithelial layer.

INTERVENTION	RATIONALE
1. Clean and débride the wound daily, and apply antimicrobial ointments and dressings as ordered. Observe and assess the site, and record findings.	1. Infection can be prevented by removing bacterial contamination, exudate, and previously applied medication.
2. Maintain aseptic technique for wound care by wearing protective gear and practicing meticulous handwashing techniques.	2. An open skin surface allows for organism entry.
3. Promote adequate fluid and nutritional intake. Offer, or encourage the parent to offer, high-calorie, high-protein meals and snacks. Provide foods that the child likes. Arrange the timing of meals so that they do not immediately precede or follow painful or distressing events.	3. Healing occurs only in the presence of a positive nitrogen balance. The child's protein and calorie needs are elevated because of increased metabolism and catabolism.
4. Perform active and passive range-of-motion exercises of the affected parts of the child's body; this can be done at the time of dressing change and between dressing changes.	4. Use of the burned area promotes edema reabsorption and prevents contracture deformity.
5. Make sure that the child's tetanus toxoid immunizations are current.	5. Anaerobic bacteria can cause infection at the interface between the burn wound and healthy tissue.
6. Monitor the child for signs and symptoms of infection: changes in sensorium, hypothermia, fever, or a change in wound appearance (drainage, odor). Obtain specimens for culture if ordered.	6. Early detection of infection will ensure prompt treatment.
7. Administer vitamins and minerals (vitamins A, B, C and iron, zinc) as ordered, or encourage the parent to do so.	7. Vitamin and mineral supplements facilitate wound healing and epithelialization.
8. Instruct the child and parents to keep the healed burn wound out of the sun for at least 1 year.	8. Burned skin is more sensitive to sunlight, which increases the risk of sunburn.

Evaluation

- Does the burn wound show signs of progressive healing?
- Is the tissue pink and free from exudate?
- Is the child free of fever and other signs of infection?

Continued

Nursing Care Plan

The Child With a Minor Partial-Thickness Burn—cont'd

Nursing Diagnosis

Acute Pain related to thermal injury and related procedures.

Expected Outcomes

The child will:
- Describe decreased pain on an age-appropriate pain assessment tool, except during procedures and physical therapy.
- Exhibit age-appropriate behaviors, adequate nutritional intake, and appropriate sleep patterns.

INTERVENTION	RATIONALE
1. Determine the child's pain level using an age-appropriate assessment tool (see Chapter 39).	1. The child's developmental stage affects response to pain, and the child's response to various pain assessment tools is related to developmental level.
2. Administer pain-relief measures and medication on a scheduled basis, rather than on demand. Premedicate the child at least 20 to 30 minutes before painful procedures, and advise the parent to do the same before the physician visit.	2. The fact that burns hurt is irrefutable, so there is no need to wait until pain is behaviorally indicated before administering medication.
3. Minimize the time spent on wound manipulation and exposure.	3. Exposure of the burned area to air or water causes pain because the nerve endings are exposed. Dressing changes should be done as quickly as possible to minimize pain.
4. Use non-pharmacologic pain reduction measures (see Chapter 39).	4. Distraction, relaxation techniques, therapeutic touch, and other measures may help alleviate pain.
5. Perform passive and active range-of-motion exercises. Be careful that dressings are applied so as to preserve function of body parts.	5. Exercise, although painful in the acute stage, reduces the likelihood of contracture formation and increases functional ability.

Evaluation
- Except during times of direct wound care and physical therapy, is the child pain-free, as evidenced by decreased pain assessment score and normal sleep, play, and eating patterns?
- Is the child able to cooperate with dressing changes and range-of-motion exercises?

Nursing Diagnosis

Risk for Deficient Fluid Volume related to fluid shifts into burned tissue.

Expected Outcome

The child will:
- Maintain normal fluid and electrolyte balance, as evidenced by intake and output measurements and serum electrolyte values within normal ranges, moist mucous membranes, and good skin turgor on unaffected area.

INTERVENTION	RATIONALE
1. Administer fluids orally or intravenously (IV) as ordered.	1. Fluids help maintain capillary circulation to the viable skin appendages and general circulation to the vital organs. Fluid replacement continues until wound coverage is achieved.
2. Instruct the parents to monitor the child's intake and output frequently.	2. Close monitoring is necessary to determine whether fluid resuscitation is necessary or adequate. Fluid intake sufficient to produce age-appropriate hourly urine output (see Chapter 42) ensures adequate tissue perfusion.
3. Weigh the hospitalized child daily.	3. Weight is an accurate measurement of hydration status. Increasing weight indicates fluid overload.
4. Monitor laboratory values for elevated electrolyte or hemoglobin levels.	4. Early identification of abnormal laboratory values permits early treatment of fluid-volume imbalances.

Evaluation
- Is the child voiding adequate urine output for age (see Chapter 42)?
- Are serum electrolyte values within normal ranges?
- Does the child appear well hydrated with moist mucous membranes and good skin turgor?
- Does the child take fluids well?

Nursing Care Plan

The Child With a Minor Partial-Thickness Burn—cont'd

Nursing Diagnosis

Risk for Infection related to scratching of healing tissue.

Expected Outcomes

The child will:
- Not complain of itching.
- Express understanding of the danger of scratching healing tissue.

INTERVENTION	RATIONALE
1. Administer antihistamines as ordered.	1. Itching persists for several months after burns heal, as new nerve endings and dermal elements reestablish themselves. Antihistamines such as diphenhydramine hydrochloride (Benadryl) reduce itching.
2. Apply soothing lotions, such as Nivea or Eucerin, to healing skin.	2. These lotions reduce dryness, which is a factor contributing to itching.
3. Keep the child's hands clean at all times and the fingernails cut short. Encourage the child not to scratch or rub healing skin.	3. These actions reduce the risk of impairing skin integrity.

Evaluation
- Is the child's skin intact and healing as expected?
- Is itching reduced?

Nursing Diagnosis

Disturbed Body Image related to altered appearance of the healing burn.

Expected Outcomes

The child will:
- Reenter previous social settings and will express a feeling of comfort in these areas.
- Discuss feelings about others' reactions to the change in appearance.

The family will:
- Provide emotional support for the child.

INTERVENTION	RATIONALE
1. Encourage the child to verbalize feelings about appearance and about returning to school.	1. Identifying the child's concerns and anxieties is the first step in developing effective coping strategies.
2. Provide honest answers to the child's questions regarding appearance.	2. Honesty builds trust and helps the child develop realistic expectations.
3. Encourage the family's involvement in the child's care (See Parents Want to Know: About Home Care for a Child With Burns box).	3. Family involvement provides support for the child and decreases the child's feelings of separation from significant others.
4. Encourage the child to provide age-appropriate self-care.	4. Participating in self-care helps increase self-esteem.
5. Identify support systems and coping mechanisms used in previous times of stress or crisis.	5. Strategies that were previously effective can be mobilized to aid the child and family through a stressful period.
6. Engage the assistance of a child life specialist to work with the child to identify feelings.	6. Children can often best express feelings through play and art.
7. Discuss ways in which the child can "cover up" any disfigurement through clothing and makeup.	7. Cosmetics can decrease or minimize the disfigurement.
8. Visit the child's school before the child's return, or remain in contact with the school nurse.	8. Visiting the school will prepare the child's classmates for the changes in the child's appearance and engage them in making the reentry a positive experience through acceptance. If visiting is not possible, the school nurse can assist the child with the transition to school.

Evaluation
- Does the child express a desire to reengage social contacts?
- Is the child able to express fears related to the reactions of others?
- Does the family support the child emotionally and encourage the child to express feelings?

PARENTS
Want to Know

About Home Care for a Child With Burns

Often it is the parents' responsibility to care for the burn wound at home, supported by daily visits to the office or clinic for débridement and wound assessment.

Parents will need to know the following to adequately care for the child:
- Type of cleaning method used to remove old antimicrobial ointment
- Where to obtain the topical ointment and dressing supplies
- How often to visit the office or clinic (the nurse provides the telephone number and a list of scheduled appointments)

Teach the parents the following:
- Use principles of aseptic technique. Use sterile gloves and applicators, and know where to obtain these supplies. Know how to put on the gloves; give a return demonstration.
- Give the child medication for pain (if needed) 20 to 30 minutes before changing the dressing. Enlist other family members to provide distraction or to help hold the child.
- Wash the area with mild soap and tepid water or sterile saline. The old dressing can be soaked in tepid water to loosen it and decrease the discomfort of its removal.
- Apply the prescribed ointment and a light gauze dressing. Cover the area with a tubular net bandage if possible rather than wrapping with flexible gauze.
- Recognize signs and symptoms of infection, provide adequate fluids, and be sure the child's nutritional needs are met.
- Encourage the child in activities appropriate for age and development.
- Keep follow-up appointments.

CONDITIONS ASSOCIATED WITH MAJOR BURN INJURIES

For a child with a major burn injury, initial assessment and care focus on the ABCs—establishing and maintaining the child's *a*irway, *b*reathing, and *c*irculation. After an airway and IV access have been established, a catheter is inserted into the bladder to begin hourly urine output measurements and a nasogastric tube is inserted into the stomach to prevent aspiration.

Burn shock is a hypovolemic condition that develops after a burn injury that affects more than 15% to 20% of TBSA in children. Mechanisms of burn shock are not well understood, but the sequence of major burn injury followed by massive capillary leakage of circulating fluid into the surrounding tissues is well recognized.

Within minutes of a major burn injury, all the capillaries in the circulatory system, not just those in the area of the burn, lose their capillary seal, resulting in leakage of intravascular body fluid into the interstitial spaces. Erythrocytes and leukocytes remain in the circulation and produce an elevated hematocrit and leukocyte count. The process of burn shock continues for approximately 24 to 48 hours, at which time the capillary seal is restored.

Treatment for burn shock is aimed at supporting the child through the period of hypovolemic shock until capillary integrity is restored. To maintain adequate circulating volume, isotonic IV fluids are administered at a rate greater than the rate of fluid loss. Many formulas can be used to calculate the rate of fluid administration. The specific formula is determined by the burn unit or health care facility. In general, the amount of fluid replacement in children is calculated using body surface area (a function of height and weight). Half of the calculated fluid amount is given over the first 8 hours after the burn, and the remaining half is given over the next 16 hours (Deitch & Rutan, 2001).

Because urine output reflects end-organ tissue perfusion, IV fluids are administered at a rate sufficient to maintain the child's urine output at a value appropriate for age (see Chapter 42). Inadequate urine output during burn shock is usually the result of insufficient administration of resuscitative fluids. Renal failure is not an expected component of burn shock if an adequate volume of IV fluids is being administered for burn shock resuscitation. It should be recognized that burn shock fluid resuscitation formulas are guidelines; individual children may need more fluids during the first 24 hours after the burn.

Table 49-7 lists additional physiologic effects caused by moderate to major burns. Once a child with a moderate or major burn has been stabilized, the child usually is transferred to a burn center for specialized care.

CONDITIONS ASSOCIATED WITH ELECTRICAL INJURY

Electrical injury is a major injury that often results in instant death, because the electrical current disrupts the electrical rhythm of the heart. The child who does not die instantly is at risk for four major complications during the acute phase:

- Cardiac arrest or dysrhythmia
- Tissue damage
- Myoglobinuria (globulin from muscle serum appearing in the urine)
- Metabolic acidosis

Cardiac Arrest or Dysrhythmia

The immediate risk is cardiac arrest or dysrhythmia secondary to damage to the heart's electrical conduction system. If cardiac arrest occurs, standard cardiac life support measures are initiated (see Chapter 34).

Tissue Damage

The electrical current follows the path of least resistance through the body. Entering through the skin, electricity causes heat damage to the skin layers, bone, nerves, tendons, and blood vessels. The heat of the electrical current coagulates blood vessels and leaves the affected area without blood supply. Gangrene develops in necrotic tissue unless it is removed. Amputation is necessary in more than 90% of children sustaining electrical injuries. The location of the damage depends on the child's position and exposure. Electricity may enter one hand and exit from the other, for example, or it may travel through the body and exit from one or both legs. The greatest damage occurs at the entrance and exit sites.

Myoglobinuria

Myoglobinuria develops from release into the blood of products found in normal muscle; the release can be occasioned by electrical injury. Myoglobin is a large molecule that can

TABLE **49-7** Body System Alterations After Moderate to Severe Burns

System/Alteration	Cause	Management
RESPIRATORY		
Upper airway tissue injury with respiratory distress, possible obstruction	Edema from inhalation of superheated air	Establish adequate airway, provide moist mist with oxygen as needed
Lower airway tissue injury	Inhalation of smoke	Give oxygen as needed, place child in a head-elevated position, intubate with ventilatory support if necessary
Carbon monoxide inhalation, hypoxia	End products of combustion	Give 100% oxygen by mask; intubate and provide ventilatory support if necessary
Limited chest expansion	Circumferential burns	Escharotomy
CARDIOVASCULAR		
Fluid volume deficit with decreased cardiac output; tachycardia	Fluid shifts from vascular to interstitial compartment; massive leaking of fluid through the burn wound	Provide fluid and electrolyte replacement with or without colloids; goal is to achieve urinary output appropriate for age and good capillary refill
Initial vasodilation, then vasoconstriction	Compensatory mechanism to preserve fluid volume and prevent shock	
Edema, compartment syndrome	Increased fluid in interstitial spaces	
Elevated hemoglobin, hematocrit	Hemoconcentration caused by fluid loss	
Increase followed by decrease in serum potassium	Release of destroyed tissue cells into extracellular space	
Decreased serum sodium	Trapped in edema fluids	
GASTROINTESTINAL		
Gastric dilation, paralytic ileus	Decreased perfusion to gastrointestinal (GI) tract as a result of hypovolemia	Restore fluid and electrolyte balance
Thirst	Hypovolemia	
RENAL		
Oliguria, elevated blood urea nitrogen and creatinine values	Reduced circulation to kidneys	Adequate fluid resuscitation
Risk for acute tubular necrosis	Obstruction of renal tubules	
METABOLIC		
Increased metabolic rate with elevated body temperature and massive evaporative heat loss	Insult of open wound	Provide caloric requirements 2 or 3 times basal requirements; provide high-protein diet or protein supplements; tube feed or use parenteral nutrition as necessary; provide vitamin C and vitamin A supplements
Catecholamine release	Burn stress; increased temperature and metabolic rate	
Hyperglycemia	Mobilization of glucagon and decreased insulin production	
HEMATOLOGIC		
Decreased hematocrit follows initial hematocrit increase (from hemoconcentration)	Increased red blood cell (RBC) hemolysis, decreased RBC production, blood loss from wound care	Packed RBC transfusion for low hematocrit
Coagulation disorders	Decreased platelet count and serum clotting factors	
Increased immature neutrophils to digest products of injury	Depletion of mature neutrophils	
High risk for infection, wound sepsis, septic shock (disorientation, fever, diminished bowel sounds are first signs, temperature falls below normal as body's resistance to infection decreases)	Open wound; altered protective mechanisms; decreased circulation to the skin	Burn excision and débridement followed by application of topical antimicrobial agents; may need biologic or synthetic skin coverings, graft
PAIN		
	Tissue injury exposing nerve endings; edema; burn treatments	Meticulous pain management both round-the-clock and before treatments

mechanically obstruct the renal tubules and lead to acute tubular necrosis unless large amounts of IV fluid are administered to flush the myoglobin out of the kidney. Osmotic diuretics may be administered to promote increased urine volume. IV fluid is administered at a rate that maintains urine output at 2 ml/kg/hr until the myoglobinuria resolves.

Metabolic Acidosis

Metabolic acidosis follows electrical injury because of the associated cellular destruction and hypovolemic shock. Ringer's lactate, the fluid used for fluid resuscitation, contains sufficient bicarbonate to manage the acidosis that accompanies burn shock but not enough to correct that associated with shock following electrical injury (i.e., pathophysiologic hypovolemic shock, not a "shock" from the electrical current).

Other Complications

The four complications just described usually resolve within 24 hours after injury. Other complications that follow electrical injury include loss of short-term memory and altered emotional states. Children can usually remember events up to the time of injury, including the names of family members and their own address, telephone number, and personal information, but they are unable to recall more recent events. This loss of memory can be distressing to the child and frustrating to the family. For example, the child may be unable to remember visits by the family and so may feel abandoned by them. It is difficult for the child to follow instructions because of the inability to retain instructions, and this may lead to difficulty in planning care. Altered emotional states may include an absence of affect and blank stares or the opposite type of emotional response—manic behavior, hyperactivity, swearing, physical violence, and feelings of paranoia. Emotional responses usually become normal after about 1 week but may persist longer in some children. The electrical injury need not be to the head for these altered states to occur.

The long-term sequelae of electrical injury may include neurologic deficits, amputations, and ocular cataracts. Ocular cataracts may occur in one or both eyes at varying times from 3 months to 18 months after injury. In the very young child, changes in visual acuity may not be noticed; therefore regular eye examinations should be scheduled every 3 months for the first year after injury.

KEY CONCEPTS

- The functions of the skin include protection, thermoregulation, excretion, production of vitamin D, and sensation.
- The skin comprises two layers—the outer epidermis and the inner supportive dermis. The dermis contains blood vessels, nerves, and sweat glands. Beneath these layers is subcutaneous tissue, which attaches the dermis to the underlying structures.
- Developmental differences cause the skin of infants and children to be more susceptible to external irritants and infection than adults' skin.
- Impetigo, the most common skin infection of childhood, is highly contagious. Nursing care includes administration of topical or oral antibiotics and education regarding good handwashing and careful hygiene to prevent spread of infection.
- Because the fungus that causes tinea thrives where it is moist and warm, infected areas should be kept as dry as possible. Proper hygiene should be taught and maintained to minimize the spread of infection.
- Herpes simplex virus is transmitted by infected body fluids coming in contact with breaks in the skin or mucous membranes. Careful handwashing and attention to hygiene decrease the risk of spreading infection.
- Preventing reinfestation is a primary goal in the treatment of pediculosis and scabies.
- Nursing care for the child with eczema includes frequent skin moisturizing and cautioning against the use of clothing, fabrics, or soaps that might irritate the skin. Identifying and eliminating allergens may be helpful.
- Diaper dermatitis is much easier to prevent than to treat. Successful treatment and prevention of diaper rash entail thorough cleansing of the diaper area and keeping the skin dry.
- Nursing care of the adolescent with acne includes teaching about regular, gentle cleansing of the skin, applying topical medications, and encouraging a healthy lifestyle with adequate rest, exercise, and a balanced diet. The nurse must be sensitive to the effect of acne on the adolescent's self-image.
- Insect bites and stings can cause severe systemic reactions in a sensitized child.
- Young children are at increased risk for burn injuries because they are curious, mobile, and totally dependent on their caretakers for safety.
- The extent of a burn injury (depth, severity) determines whether the child will experience a local or a systemic reaction.
- The depth of a burn injury is classified as superficial (first-degree), partial-thickness (second-degree), or full-thickness (third-degree).
- In comparison with adults, children who sustain burn injuries are at increased risk for fluid and heat loss, hypertrophic scarring, cardiovascular problems, infection, and protein and calorie deficiency.
- In calculating the total body surface area (TBSA) burned, a body surface chart that is corrected for age should be used.
- A minor burn wound should be cleaned with mild soap and water, débrided of loose debris and tissue, and covered with an antimicrobial ointment and a sterile dressing.
- After stabilization, a child with a major burn is cared for in a burn treatment center because of multiple body system complications.

ANSWERS to Critical Thinking Exercise 49-1

1. The nurse should first ask the mother what symptoms, if any, the child is experiencing. If the child is symptomatic with pruritus and visible nits or lice, treatment failure is a possibility. The nurse needs to ask what pediculicide was used, whether nits were fully combed out, whether family members were treated, and what environmental measures were taken to prevent reinfestation in the home. If the parent has followed the instructions meticulously, the nurse needs to explore other areas. Because of the child's age, the nurse needs to question whether the mother has treated her daughter's dress-up clothes and hair ornaments as well as the usual bedding, clothing, combs, brushes, and furniture. The parent should review her child's other contacts as well, such as neighborhood playmates or church play groups. If it appears the management has been thorough, the child may

have developed pediculicide-resistant lice and will need a different treatment.

2. If the child is not symptomatic, the school official may be seeing dead nits in the child's hair. The nurse needs to ask the mother about the treatment used and whether all the nits were removed. Removing nits is es-

pecially difficult in preschool children because it is time-consuming and these young children find sitting still that long difficult. Also, many preschool girls have long hair, which can prolong the process. The nurse should advise the mother to remove all the nits and check her child regularly to be sure

that all the nits are gone. The nurse can give the mother suggestions about the most effective method of nit removal and encourage the mother to be persistent. Positive reassurance and encouragement are most important.

REFERENCES and READINGS

American Academy of Pediatrics (AAP). (2000). *Red Book 2000: Report of the Committee on Infectious Diseases*. Elk Grove Village, IL: Author.

American Academy of Pediatrics. (2002). Head lice: Clinical report. *Pediatrics, 110,* 638-643.

American College of Allergy, Asthma, and Immunology. (1998). Insect sting allergies pose serious risk. Author. Retrieved June 1, 2003, from www.allergy.mcg.edu/news/insects.html.

Amirsheybani, H.R. (2001). The natural history of the growth of the hand: Hand area as a percentage of body surface area. *Plastic Reconstructive Surgery, 107,* 726-733.

Antoon, A., & Donovan, M. (2000). Burn injuries. In R. Behrman, R. Kliegman, & H. Jenson (Eds.), *Nelson textbook of pediatrics* (16th ed., pp. 287-294). Philadelphia: Saunders.

Barret, J.P., & Herndon, D.N. (2001). *Color atlas of burn care.* Philadelphia: Saunders.

Berg, D., & Erickson, P. (2001). Fungal skin infections in children. *Postgraduate Medicine, 110,* 83-89.

Berry, M.G., Evison, D., & Roberts, A.H.N. (2001). The influence of body mass index on burn surface area estimated from the area of the hand. *Burns, 27,* 591-594.

Bolognia, J.L. (2000). Disorders of hypopigmentation and hyperpigmentation. In J. Harper, A. Oranje, & N. Prose (Eds.), *Textbook of pediatric dermatology* (pp. 837-880). Oxford: Blackwell Science.

Brady, M. (2000a). Atopic disorders and rheumatic diseases. In C. Burns, M. Brady, A. Dunn, & N. Starr (Eds.), *Pediatric primary care: A handbook for nurse practitioners* (pp. 625-660). Philadelphia: Saunders.

Brady, M. (2000b). Common injuries. In C. Burns, M. Brady, A. Dunn, & N. Starr (Eds.), *Pediatric primary care: A handbook for nurse practitioners* (pp. 1230-1259). Philadelphia: Saunders.

Centers for Disease Control and Prevention. (1997). Recommended framework for presenting injury mortality data. *MMWR Recommended Reports: Morbidity and Mortality Weekly Report, 46*(RR-14), 11.

Clayton, Y.M. (2000). Superficial fungal Infections. In J. Harper, A. Oranje, & N. Prose (Eds.), *Textbook of pediatric dermatology* (pp. 447-473). Oxford: Blackwell Science.

Darmstadt, G., & Sidbury, R. (2004). The skin. In R. Behrman, R. Kliegman, & H. Jenson (Eds.), *Nelson textbook of pediatrics* (17th ed., pp. 2243-2246). Philadelphia, PA: Saunders.

Deitch, E., & Rutan, R. (2001). *The challenges of children: The first 48 hours.* Chicago: American Burn Association.

Dickerson, P., Gordon, M., & Walter, P. (1998). Burns. In M. Slota (Ed.), *Core curriculum for pediatric critical care nursing* (pp. 652-675). Philadelphia, PA: Saunders.

Dohil, M., Baugh, W., & Eichenfield, L. (2000). Vascular and pigmented birthmarks. *Pediatric Clinics of North America, 47*(4), 783-811.

Eichenfield, L.F., Hanifin, J.M., Beck, L.A., Lemanske, R.F. Jr., Sampson, H.A., Weiss, S.T., & Leung, D.Y. (2003). Atopic dermatitis and asthma: Parallels in the evolution of treatment. *Pediatrics, 111,* 608-616.

Farhat, D.W. (2000). Arachnidism. *Topics in Emergency Medicine, 22,* 1-15.

Fuller, L.C., Smith, C.H., Cerio, R., Marsden, R.A., Midgley, G., Beard, A.L., Higgins, E.M., & Hay, R.J. (2001). A randomised comparison of 4 weeks of terbinafine vs. 8 weeks of griseofulvin for the treatment of tinea capitis. *British Journal of Dermatology, 144*(2), 321-327.

Goodyear, H. (2000). Herpes simplex virus infections. In J. Harper, A. Oranje, & N. Prose (Eds.), *Textbook of pediatric dermatology* (pp. 321-329). Oxford: Blackwell Science.

Greco, L.K. (2000). Hymenoptera stings. *Topics in Emergency Medicine, 22,* 37-43.

Hainer, B.L. (2003). Dermatophyte infections. *American Family Physician, 67,* 101-108.

Hornung, R. (2000). Photoprotection. In J. Harper, A. Oranje, & N. Prose (Eds.), *Textbook of pediatric dermatology* (pp. 921-934). Oxford: Blackwell Science.

Kennedy, C., Bajdik, C.D., Willemze, R., De Gruijl, F.R., & Bouwes Bavinek, J.N. (2003). The influence of painful sunburns and lifetime sun exposure in the risk of actinic keratoses, seborrheic warts, melanocytic nevi, atypical nevi, and skin cancer. *Journal of Investigative Dermatology, 120*(6), 1087-1093.

Kristal, L., & Klein, P. (2000). Atopic dermatitis in infants and children. *Pediatric Clinics of North America, 47*(4), 877-896.

Krowchuk, D. (2000). Managing acne in adolescents. *Pediatric Clinics of North America, 47*(4), 841-858.

Kumar, V. (1999). Burns in childhood. In F. Burg, E. Wald, J. Ingelfinger, & R. Polin (Eds.), *Gellis and Kagan's current pediatric therapy* (16th ed., pp. 1171-1172). Philadelphia: Saunders.

Leung, D.Y.M., & Bieber, T. (2003). Atopic dermatitis. *The Lancet, 361,* 151-160.

Lewis, A.M. (1999). Managing common pediatric emergencies. *Nursing 1999, 29*(1). Available online: www.springnet.com/content/nursing/9901.

Martinez, I.S., North, P.E., & Mihm, M.C. (2002). Infantile hemangioma: Clinical resolution with

5% imiquimod cream. *Archives of Dermatology, 138,* 881-884.

National SAFE KIDS Campaign (NSKC). (2004). *Residential fire injury fact sheet.* Washington, DC: Author.

Neugut, A.I., & Miller, R.L. (2001). Anaphylaxis in the United States: An investigation into its epidemiology. *Archives of Internal Medicine, 161,* 2046-2047.

Paller, A. (1999). Vascular nevi. In R. Dershewitz (Ed.), *Ambulatory pediatric care* (pp. 432-435). Philadelphia: Lippincott-Raven.

Palmieri, T.L., & Greenhalgh, D.G. (2002). Topical treatment of pediatric patients with burns. *American Journal of Clinical Dermatology, 3,* 526-534.

Resnick, S.D. (2000). Staphylococcal and streptococcal skin infections: Toxin mediated syndromes. In J. Harper, A. Oranje, & N. Prose (Eds.), *Textbook of pediatric dermatology* (pp. 369-383). Oxford: Blackwell Science.

Russell, J.J. (2000). Topical treatment for acne. *American Family Physician, 61,* 357-366.

Schmitt, B.D. (1999). *Instructions for pediatric patients.* Philadelphia: Saunders.

Seigfred, E.C., & Shah, P.Y. (1999). Skin care practices in the neonatal nursery: A clinical survey. *Journal of Perinatology, 19,* 31-39.

Starr, N.B. (2000). Dermatological diseases. In C. Burns, M. Brady, A. Dunn, & N. Starr (Eds.), *Pediatric primary care: A handbook for nurse practitioners* (pp. 1059-1133). Philadelphia: Saunders.

Stulberg, D.L., & Hutchinson, A.G. (2003). Molluscum contagiosum and warts. *American Family Physician, 67*(6), 1233-1240.

Tharp, M.D. (2002). Calcineurin inhibitors. *Dermatologic Therapy, 15*(4), 325-332.

Torrelo, A. (2002). What's new in the treatment of viral warts in children? *Pediatric Dermatology, 19,* 191-199.

Wagner, A.M., & Hansen, R.C. (1995). Neonatal skin and skin disorders. In Schachner, L.A., & Hansen, R.C. (Eds.), *Pediatric dermatology* (pp. 263-346). New York: Churchill Livingstone.

Weinstein, A., & Berman, B. (2002). Topical treatment of common superficial tinea infections. *American Family Physician, 65,* 2095-2102.

Weston, W. (2000). Erythema multiforme, Stevens-Johnson syndrome and toxic-epidermal necrolysis. In J. Harper, A. Oranje, & N. Prose (Eds.), *Textbook of pediatric dermatology* (pp. 628-636). Oxford: Blackwell Science.

Weston, W., & Bruckner, A. (2000). Allergic contact dermatitis. *Pediatric Clinics of North America, 47*(4), 897-908.

50

The Child with a
Musculoskeletal Alteration

◆ LEARNING OBJECTIVES

After studying this chapter, you should be able to:

◎ Describe the anatomy and physiology of an infant's and young child's musculoskeletal system.
◎ Describe the pathology, etiology, manifestations, diagnostic evaluation, and therapeutic management of common musculoskeletal alterations seen in infants and children.
◎ Select relevant criteria to determine the etiology and diagnosis of common musculoskeletal alterations.

◎ State appropriate nursing diagnoses for the child with alterations in musculoskeletal function.
◎ Identify characteristic behaviors that indicate alterations in musculoskeletal function.
◎ Summarize the treatment modalities used to manage the child with musculoskeletal alterations.
◎ Design, implement, and evaluate appropriate nursing interventions for the child with altered musculoskeletal function.

◆ DEFINITIONS

abduction Movement of a limb away from the midline of the body.

adduction Movement of a limb toward the midline of the body.

ankylosis Condition in which a joint is stiff or difficult to move.

arthroscopic surgery (arthroscopy) Surgical procedure in which a lighted tubular scope is inserted into a joint to diagnose or treat traumatic soft tissue injury.

autologous blood transfusion Transfusion of one's own, previously harvested blood.

avascular necrosis Tissue damage secondary to inadequate blood supply.

callus Tissue that joins fractured bone ends or repairs damaged bone; begins as cartilaginous tissue and becomes hardened through osteoblastic activity.

crepitus A grating sensation at a fracture site that occurs when the ends of a broken bone move against each other.

dislocation Displacement of a bone from its normal articulation within a joint.

dysplasia Abnormal development of tissue.

eversion Turned away from the midline.

external fixation Placement of pins, screws, or bars through bone and soft tissue to immobilize or correct a deformity.

external rotation Turning outward, or laterally, within a joint.

internal fixation Placement of instruments (wires, pins, rods, screws) inside the body to immobilize parts.

internal rotation Turning inward, or medially, within a joint.

inversion Turning toward the midline.

orthoses Braces, external supports, or artificial limbs made by a specialist to meet individual needs.

ossification The process of forming bone from osseous tissue or cartilage.

osteoblasts Mesodermal cells whose activity produces bone.

osteoclasts Cells found in bones that absorb and remove old bony tissue.

osteotomy Surgical cutting of bone.

paresthesia Sensation of numbness and tingling.

plantar flexion Bending toward the sole of the foot.

polydactyly Extra fingers or toes.

pseudarthrosis Failure of the bones to fuse.

reduction Repositioning of bone fragments into normal alignment followed by application of a device or mechanism that will maintain alignment of bone until healing occurs.

subluxation Partial dislocation of a joint.

superior mesenteric artery syndrome A condition resembling intestinal obstruction caused by reduced blood supply to a segment of the mesentery.

syndactyly Fusion or webbing of two or more fingers or toes.

valgum Abnormal position of a limb in which it is bent away from the midline of the body.

varum Abnormal position of the limb in which it is bent toward the midline of the body.

REVIEW OF THE MUSCULOSKELETAL SYSTEM

Bones, joints, muscles, and cartilaginous tissues make up the musculoskeletal system. To understand alterations in musculoskeletal function, it is first necessary to understand normal musculoskeletal structure and function as well as patterns of growth and development.

Skeletal System

The bony skeleton provides a surface for the attachment of muscles, tendons, and ligaments. The pulling action on individual bones makes it possible for us to move. The human skeletal system consists of 206 bones, which are classified as long bones (e.g., humerus, radius), short bones (e.g., carpals, tarsals), flat bones (e.g., ribs), irregular bones (e.g., vertebrae), and sesamoid bones (e.g., kneecaps).

Each long bone consists of a diaphysis (shaft) with an epiphysis (secondary ossification center) at each end. The muscles attach here and are responsible for joint stability. The metaphysis, or wide portion of the bone, is responsible for growth. The metaphysis consists of cartilage and actively produces bone through osteoblastic activity. Periosteum, a vascular connective tissue, covers the bone. The medullary cavity is located in the center of the diaphysis.

Articular System

The joints, which are composed of connective tissue and cartilage, connect bones to one another and enable great freedom of movement. Joints are classified by their degree of movement: *synarthrotic*, or immovable (e.g., the skull); *amphiarthrotic*, or slightly movable (e.g., the symphysis); and *di-*

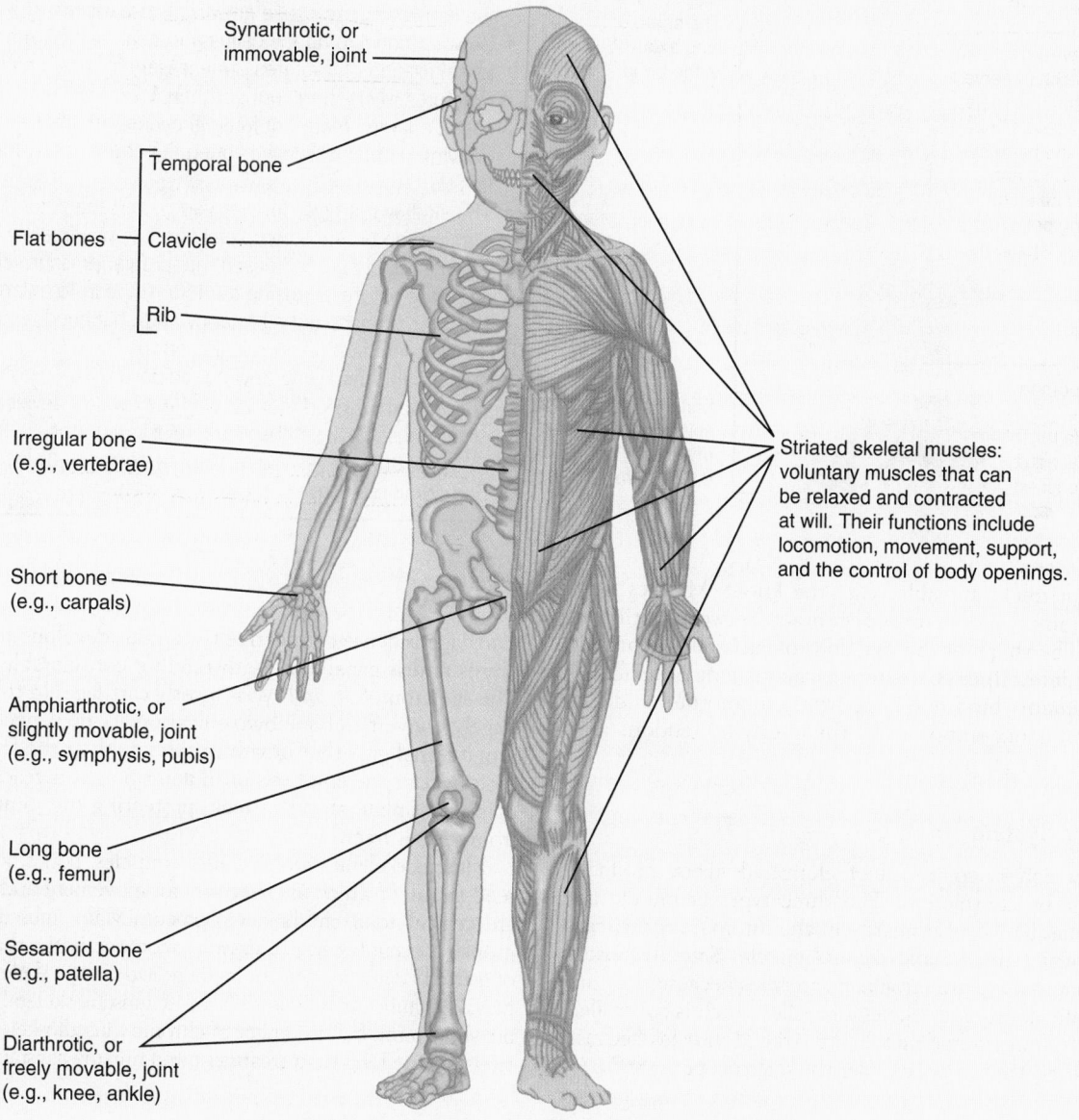

Anatomy of the Musculoskeletal System

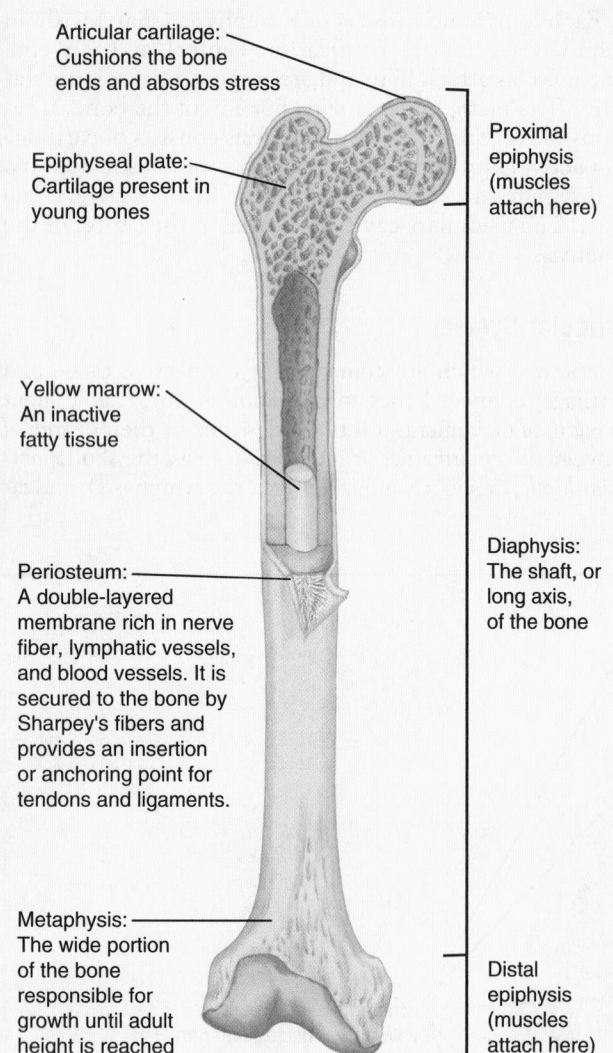

Articular cartilage: Cushions the bone ends and absorbs stress

Epiphyseal plate: Cartilage present in young bones

Yellow marrow: An inactive fatty tissue

Periosteum: A double-layered membrane rich in nerve fiber, lymphatic vessels, and blood vessels. It is secured to the bone by Sharpey's fibers and provides an insertion or anchoring point for tendons and ligaments.

Metaphysis: The wide portion of the bone responsible for growth until adult height is reached

Proximal epiphysis (muscles attach here)

Diaphysis: The shaft, or long axis, of the bone

Distal epiphysis (muscles attach here)

Pediatric Differences in the Musculoskeletal System

- Muscle tissue is almost completely developed at birth. Growth occurs because of an increase in size rather than number of the muscle fibers.
- In the fetus, bony tissue begins to develop as closely packed connective tissue. Connective tissue is replaced by cartilage, and cartilage is replaced by mineral salts, which give rise to solid bone. The infant's bones are only 65% ossified at 8 months of age and are neither as firm nor as brittle as those of the older child.
- New bony tissue is produced during periods of growth. The rate of growth varies at different ages. Skeletal growth is stimulated by pituitary growth hormone. Growth of the long bones occurs at the epiphyses, which are located at the ends of the bones and separated from the main portion of the bone by cartilage during the period of growth. Injury to the epiphyses can cause growth disturbances.
- Growing bones produce callus and heal quickly, making internal fixation of fractures unnecessary in most children. Fractures in children younger than 1 year are unusual because a large amount of force is necessary; abuse or underlying pathophysiology is often the cause of fractures in infants.
- The skull is not rigid during infancy, and the sutures of the cranium do not fuse completely until approximately 16 to 18 months of age. Increased intracranial pressure can separate the sutures, causing the infant's head to enlarge.
- Postural changes during infancy and childhood result from the development of neurologic control, bone and muscle growth, and the laying down of adipose tissue. Postural changes are a good indication of the level of development of the musculoskeletal and neurologic systems.
- Because soft tissues are resilient in children, dislocations and sprains are less common than in adults.

arthrotic, or freely movable (e.g., the knee). Muscles help stabilize joints and maintain contact between articular surfaces. The shape of the two ends of each muscle and of the joint determines the extent of movement or articulation. Ligaments bind one bone firmly to another, and the joints are further stabilized by the overlying tendons and muscles.

Muscular System

Muscle, which is composed of elongated fibers, produces movement by contraction. The three types of muscle are smooth muscle, found primarily in the internal organs; cardiac, or heart, muscle; and skeletal muscle. Smooth muscle and cardiac muscle are *involuntary* muscles because they are not willfully controlled. Skeletal muscle, which is controlled voluntarily, and cardiac muscle are striated muscles because of their striped appearance under the microscope.

Cartilage

Cartilage is dense connective tissue that develops at the epiphysis and is capable of withstanding considerable tension. The skeleton of an embryo is mostly cartilage. In time it will largely convert to bone by ossification. Bone is necessary for longitudinal growth. Growth in the length of the long bones continues at the epiphysis until adult height is reached. The epiphyseal plate absorbs shock, protecting the joint surfaces from serious fractures.

Musculoskeletal problems affect muscles, bones, joints, and tendons, all of which are necessary for movement and therefore are critical to a child's development. Many musculoskeletal problems occur because of vigorous motor activities that are part of a child's daily life, but the rapid growth of the skeletal system plays a significant role as well. Most musculoskeletal problems are short term, but a number of chronic musculoskeletal conditions require long-term treatment and nursing assistance.

Common Diagnostic and Laboratory Tests and Procedures for Musculoskeletal Disorders in Children

Test	Purpose and Description	Nursing Implications
Radiography (x-ray)	For detection of abnormalities or to determine bone age. X-rays (gamma radiation) pass through the body, reach the film on the other side of the body, and turn the film black. Areas filled with air appear dark on the film. Different densities of tissue absorb various amounts of radiation. The four densities of x-ray: Air: blackish Fat: dark gray Water: lighter gray Bone: whitish	Food and fluids are not usually restricted. Clothing and jewelry should be removed; a paper or cloth gown is worn. Young children may require immobilization. Adequate preparation is essential to ensure cooperation.
Arthrography	To evaluate suspected joint damage, such as tears of cartilage. Dye is injected into the joint—usually the knee; sometimes the shoulder or other joint.	Performed with the child under local anesthesia. Check for allergies to iodine. May have mild to moderate discomfort after the procedure. Joint should rest for about 12 hr; compression dressing may be applied after procedure to reduce swelling.
Radionuclide scintigraphy (bone scan)	To detect tumors, infection, inflammation. Radioactive material given intravenous (IV). In 2-4 hr, the entire body is scanned—front and back.	Young children need sedation. Encourage fluids 2-4 hr before the test to ensure the child is well hydrated and to quickly eliminate radioactive material not absorbed by the bones. Child must void before the scan so that the pelvic bones can be seen.
Computed tomography (CT)	To visualize anatomic details. Narrow-beam x-rays are used to scan an area in successive layers. A computer processes readings and converts them to a picture shown on a screen, which is stored on disks. A three-dimensional cross section of body parts is shown.	Although the procedure is painless, it may be frightening. The child must remain still during procedure, so young children need sedation. Contrast medium may or may not be used. Tell the child the machine looks and sounds like a clothes dryer or washing machine. Remove clothing and jewelry.
Magnetic resonance imaging (MRI)	Clearly defines organ structures; shows changes in tissue, such as edema, blood flow patterns, infarcts. Demonstrates marrow, bone and soft tissue tumors, structure of muscles, ligaments, bones. Huge magnet and radio waves create an energy field that can be translated into a visual image. Child is placed on a moving stretcher, which is pushed into the large cylinder that contains the magnet. A variety of noises will be heard during the procedure.	Food and fluids are not restricted. Study is not done in children with metal implants, pacemakers, or prostheses. Procedure may take 1 hr or more, so young children need sedation. The child should void before procedure. Adequate preparation, relaxation techniques, and parental presence decrease fear and feelings of claustrophobia. Use of a music headset may promote relaxation.
Arthroscopy	To image the inside of a joint for diagnosis of injury or minor surgical repairs. Normally, arthrography is performed before arthroscopy. Fiberoptic endoscope is inserted to examine interior of joint.	Requires local or general anesthesia. The child must be on nothing-by-mouth (NPO) status for 8 hr before the test if general anesthesia is used; NPO status recommendations for local anesthesia vary with the practitioner. Prepare the child for postoperative dressings, altered mobility, pain. Assess for infection. Prophylactic antibiotics may be ordered. Use ice bags postoperatively to reduce swelling.
Joint aspiration	Fluid is withdrawn for analysis, usually to detect infection or to relieve pain.	Requires local anesthesia. Prepare the child for some discomfort during and after procedure.

Continued

Common Diagnostic and Laboratory Tests and Procedures for Musculoskeletal Disorders in Children—cont'd

Test	Purpose and Description	Nursing Implications
Ultrasound	To demonstrate body tissue structure or for wave-form analysis of Doppler studies. Doppler probe is held over the skin surface or in a body cavity to produce an ultrasound beam in the tissues. Echoes reflected from the tissues are transformed by computer into a visual image or audible sounds (Doppler).	Noninvasive; food and fluid are not restricted, except in small infants, who may be on NPO status for 2-3 hr before the procedure so they can eat during the test.
Alkaline phosphatase (ALP)	ALP is an enzyme found mainly in bone, liver, placenta, kidney; levels may be elevated in bone disease, fractures, trauma, or liver disease and during periods of rapid growth. Determinations may be ordered to differentiate between bone and liver problems.	Nonfasting
Creatine kinase (CK)	CK is an enzyme found in heart and skeletal muscle; the CK assay is a specific test for cardiac and muscle damage. Levels are elevated in trauma, myocardial infarction, muscular dystrophy. Determinations may be ordered to differentiate between cardiac (MB) and skeletal (MM) CK.	Nonfasting
Rheumatoid factor (RF)	Rheumatoid factors are antibodies that may be responsible for the destructive changes associated with rheumatoid arthritis. A positive RF supports the possible diagnosis of juvenile arthritis (JA).	Nonfasting
C-reactive protein (CRP)	CRP is a protein that appears in blood because of an inflammatory process. It is not seen in healthy people. The measurement is nonspecific, merely indicating the presence of inflammation.	Nonfasting
Erythrocyte sedimentation rate (ESR)	ESR is the rate at which erythrocytes settle out of unclotted blood, measured in millimeters per hour. Inflammation and necrotic problems cause an elevation in ESR levels.	Nonfasting

CASTS, TRACTION, AND OTHER IMMOBILIZING DEVICES

Immobilizing a bone or joint helps achieve and maintain a more functional position or rests an affected area during bone healing. Because many musculoskeletal problems require the application of an immobilizing device, the nurse needs to understand general principles of care.

Casts

A cast provides support and maintains anatomic position for bone healing or correction of a deformity. Casts may also be used to ensure compliance with treatment protocols. Materials most frequently used for casting are synthetic materials, such as fiberglass, or plaster of Paris. Plaster of Paris is a heavier material that molds easily to the extremity and is less expensive than synthetic materials. However, plaster takes 24 hours or more to dry. Plaster of Paris is not water-resistant; when wet, a cast made of plaster of Paris will begin to disintegrate.

Synthetic casts are more expensive, but they dry quickly and are lighter weight and water-resistant (Fig. 50-1). They also come in varied colors and patterns that appeal to young children. Should a synthetic cast become wet, inadequate airflow under the cast prevents thorough drying of the skin, and damp skin is more susceptible to skin breakdown. Also, synthetic casts do not mold well to the body and are not recommended for young children or those with serious fractures.

Most casts are applied on an outpatient basis. The type of the fracture or injury and the amount of weight bearing the extremity can tolerate dictate the size of the cast. Short or long leg or arm casts are generally used for fractures of the upper and lower limbs. Fractures of the hip and knee may require a body, or *spica*, cast.

Equipment needed for cast application includes:

- Tubular gauze (stockinette)
- Cotton under-cast padding material (e.g., Webril)
- Casting material (rolls or strips)
- Water

The tubular gauze is placed over the extremity to be casted, and the limb is held in the appropriate position. After applying a thin layer of under-cast padding and soaking the casting material in water, the physician or other trained personnel applies the strips over the padding material, bringing the end of the padding material and stockinette over the end of the casting material and under the last casting strip to provide a smooth, padded, edge. A chemical reaction between the casting material and the water will cause a feeling of warmth as the cast is applied.

Traction

Effective immobilization may be achieved also through the use of traction. Traction is a pull or force exerted on one part of the body; in treatment, traction may be applied to the spine, pelvis, or long bones of the upper and lower extremities. The angle formed by the placement of the pulley on the bed frame and the angle of the involved joint determine the direction of the pull or force.

Once the direction of the pull or force has been determined, it is important to direct the traction along the long axis of the bone. Traction can be applied to the skin or the

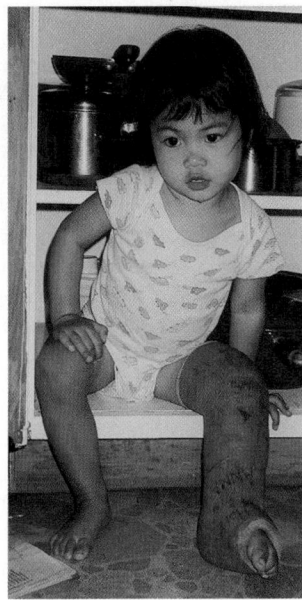

Figure 50-1 Child in a synthetic cast.

bone. Some traction, such as halo femoral traction used for spinal problems, exerts a force without the use of weights.

An opposing pull or force (countertraction) must be provided at the same time if the traction is to be effective. Countertraction results in a two-way pull that maintains alignment of the affected extremity. The child's weight is usually sufficient to provide the countertraction. If body weight is not sufficient, additional weights may be used. Depending on the age of the child, restraining devices may be needed to maintain countertraction.

The part of the bed that holds the traction apparatus is tilted or elevated, thereby assisting with countertraction. For example, if the leg were being placed in traction, the foot of the bed would be elevated. Otherwise, the child would slide in the direction of the traction, disrupting the alignment of the extremity and reducing the effectiveness of treatment. Also, the mattress should be firm and a foot board or foot plate may be necessary to keep the extremity in the correct position.

The disadvantages of traction include the need for hospitalization and prolonged immobility. Currently, early casting and percutaneous pinning are replacing the use of traction for some musculoskeletal conditions.

Traction can be described as either *continuous* or *intermittent*. Continuous traction exerts a constant pull and is used for fractures and dislocations. Intermittent traction provides a periodic pull or force and is used for contractures, low back pain, or muscle spasm. *The nurse should always assume that traction is continuous unless the physician states otherwise*. The removal of traction that was intended to be continuous could prove harmful to the child and result in poor healing. The nursing care plan should always reflect the frequency and amount of time intermittent traction may be removed. When removing the traction apparatus, the nurse must use the hands to maintain manual traction and pull on the body part.

Traction may also be described as *running* or *balanced*. Running, or straight, traction exerts a pull on the affected part without balanced support from a sling or splint. The child's weight provides the countertraction. Balanced, or suspension,

BOX 50-1
Types of Skin Traction

Buck's Extension

Purpose: Used to treat some fractures, hip disorders, contractures, and muscle spasms.

Description: Continuous or intermittent boot or circular wrap is applied to the skin. Traction is applied to boot or wrap. Rolled towels are placed on the external surface of the knee to prevent external rotation of the affected leg. Unless otherwise ordered, the mattress should be flexed at the knee (20-30 degrees) to maintain a neutral hip.*

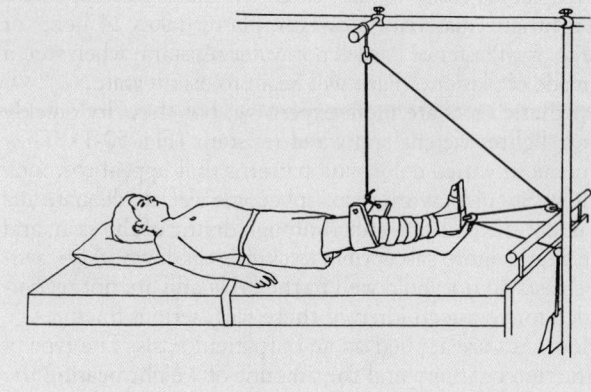

Buck's extension

Russell Traction

Purpose: Used to stabilize fractured femurs until callus forms.

Description: Continuous traction. Knee slightly flexed and supported with sling. Trapeze overhead may be used by child for repositioning and upper extremity muscle integrity.

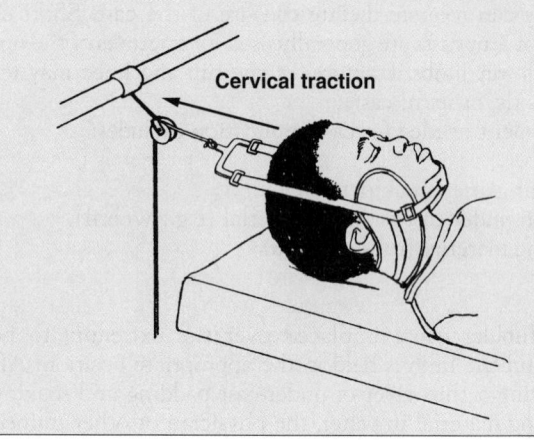

Cervical Traction

Purpose: Used to treat muscle or nerve irritation of shoulders and upper arms.

Description: May be continuous or intermittent. Maintains the head in extension via a halter: front straps fit under the chin; rear straps rest at base of skull. Spreader bar equalizes force of pull. Elevating the head of the bed 20 to 30 degrees helps maintain alignment.

Cervical traction

*Byrne, T. (1999). The setup and care of a patient in Buck's traction. *Orthopaedic Nursing, 18*(2), 79-83.

---

traction also exerts a pull on the affected part, but the extremity is supported by a sling or splint. Countertraction is provided through the use of weights and pulleys attached to the sling or splint. When balanced traction is applied, the pull remains constant, even when the child moves. The countertraction offsets any movement and results in fewer problems with immobility. Both balanced and running traction may be applied to either the skin or bone.

Skin Traction

Skin traction (Box 50-1) exerts force directly on the body surface. It is noninvasive and well tolerated and does not require anesthesia. Skin traction is most effective with children who weigh less than 30 lb or are younger than 2 to 3 years. It can be applied to the pelvis, spine, or extremities (usually the long bones). Skin traction is preferred for

conditions in which invasive procedures are contraindicated, such as hemarthrosis (collection of blood in the joint) as a result of hemophilia. Foam rubber straps, adhesive moleskin, or cloth belts are applied to the skin and then attached to the weights and pulleys. Sometimes an elastic bandage is wrapped around the skin to hold the traction apparatus in place. If skin traction to the lower leg is needed, a foam rubber or fabric boot may be used; the fit should be secure.

The effectiveness of skin traction is determined by the amount of pull that can be placed on the extremity. For this reason, skin traction is not appropriate if the child has a skin infection, an open wound, or extensive tissue damage. Skin breakdown may also develop. Spraying the intact skin with tincture of benzoin before the traction is applied may protect against skin irritation.

If the traction has not been set up correctly, neurovascular impairment may occur. Hyperextension of the knee and elastic bandages that have been wrapped too tightly are the most common causes of this problem. A thorough assessment of the traction apparatus as well as the extremity should be conducted at least once each shift as a preventive measure.

Skeletal Traction

Skeletal traction (Box 50-2 and Fig. 50-2) exerts greater force than skin traction and can be physiologically tolerated for longer periods. Traction is maintained via a metal device that is inserted into the bone. This is accomplished by introducing a Kirschner wire or Steinmann pin into the bone or Crutchfield tongs into the skull.

The fracture site determines the insertion site of these stainless steel wires, pins, or tongs. Common sites for skeletal traction include the skull, the proximal end of the ulna, and the distal end of the femur, as well as the tibia and heel. Internal fixation is common in skeletal traction. It helps maintain correct alignment of the bony fragments and assists in proper healing. General anesthesia is required for internal fixation.

The most serious complication associated with skeletal traction is *osteomyelitis*, an infection involving the bone. Organisms gain access to the bone systemically or through the opening created by the metal pins or wires used for traction. Osteomyelitis may also occur with any open fracture. Clinical manifestations include complaints of localized pain, swelling, warmth, tenderness, or unusual odor. An elevated temperature may accompany the symptoms. To decrease the risk of infection at the pin sites, many facilities have an institutional protocol for frequent pin site care (once per day or more often). This procedure involves inspecting each site for signs of infection (e.g., tenting or pulling around the pin, redness at the site, purulent drainage), cleaning the skin around pin sites with one of various cleansing solutions (e.g., half- or full-strength hydrogen peroxide, povidone-iodine solution, chlorhexidine gluconate, plain normal saline, soap and water), often followed by application of an antibiotic ointment and a gauze pad.

Skeletal traction is always continuous. If the force of the traction were altered, the muscles would contract and fracture alignment would be disrupted. The tissues around the fracture could also be injured.

External Fixation Devices

External fixation devices, such as the Ilizarov external fixator (Fig. 50-3), consist of pins or wires inserted through skin, soft tissue, and bone and secured on the outer limb surface to a rigid metal frame. The external fixator provides distraction, keeping the bone ends separated and in alignment so healing can occur. In this way, the fixator acts like traction, except that, unlike traction, it allows the child to be somewhat mobile during the healing process. In fact, external fixation devices are becoming so common in the treatment of fractures that traction is infrequently used. Because the screws of the external fixator pass through the skin to anchor in the bone, meticulous assessment of entry sites for signs of inflammation, infection, or loose pins is necessary. Pin care usually is recommended to prevent infection; in this instance, it is similar to pin care for children in traction. To prevent injury to the other limb or to others, sharp protrusions from the fixator need to be adequately covered. General anesthesia is necessary for removal of external fixation devices.

Nursing Considerations

Before application of an immobilizing device, assess the child's and parent's knowledge about the procedure. Also assess the child's skin, and note the presence of any bruises or abrasions that might be covered by the device.

✳ *Neurovascular Status*

After the device is applied, perform a neurovascular assessment (CSM—**c**irculation, **s**ensation, and **m**otion) at least every 1 to 2 hours during the first 48 hours. Assess the strength of the pulse distal to the site, and compare it with the pulse in the uninvolved extremity. A sluggish capillary refill time usually indicates neurovascular impairment.

Signs of circulatory impairment include coldness, pallor, blueness of the extremity, swelling, loss of motion, and numbness and tingling of the extremity. Touch the child's foot to assess for temperature; ask the child to move fingers or toes. Paresthesia, or numbness and tingling, can be assessed by touching the fingers or toes and noting any decrease or loss of feeling. Paresthesia is of serious concern because paralysis can result if the problem is not corrected. Report a child's complaints of a pins-and-needles sensation or of the extremity "feeling asleep."

Because young children are not always able to describe a feeling or sensation, avoid questions such as "Do you feel this?" Asking a child to wiggle the fingers or toes is an appropriate way to determine motor impairment.

Immobility

Children in immobilizing devices are subject to the consequences of immobility. Immobility can affect several body systems. Appropriate assessment and intervention can prevent adverse effects (Table 50-1).

⚠ CRITICAL TO REMEMBER

The Child in a Cast or Traction

Tissue ischemia and nerve damage are serious complications that may accompany immobilization in a cast or traction. Skin color and temperature, movement and sensation of the extremity, quality of pulses, and capillary refill time of the extremity are related to neurovascular status and should be assessed carefully; problems must be handled quickly to prevent permanent disabilities.

The five *P*'s of vascular impairment can be used as a guide when assessing neurovascular problems:

*P*ain
*P*allor
*P*ulselessness
*P*aresthesia
*P*aralysis

Pain or a burning sensation unrelieved by analgesia or nursing interventions may indicate tissue ischemia. Prompt intervention is crucial if neurovascular impairment is to be prevented. This type of complaint must be referred to the physician.

BOX 50-2
Types of Skeletal Traction

Crutchfield Tongs

Purpose: To stabilize fractures or displaced vertebrae in cervical and thoracic areas.

Description: Tongs are inserted on either side of the head through drill holes. The center of the curved metal bar must extend along the same planes as the spinal cord. Traction pull is always along the axis of the spine. The child must maintain straight body alignment.

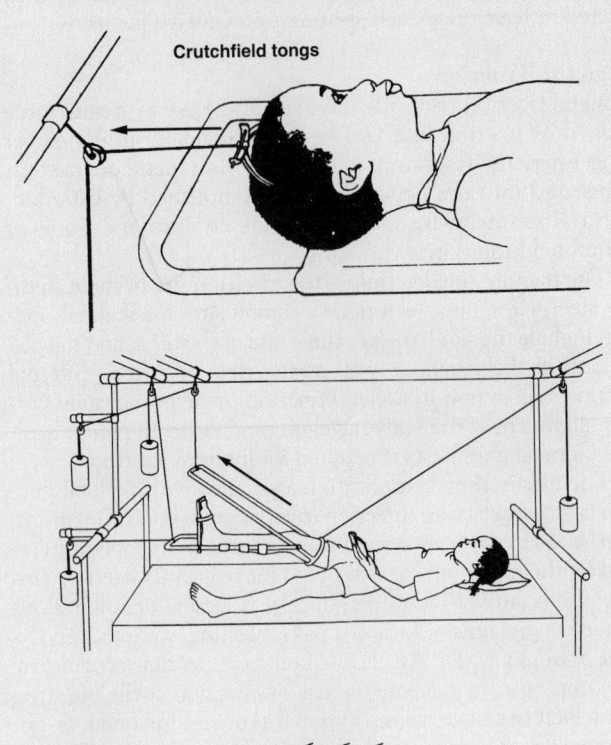

Crutchfield tongs

Balanced Suspension

Purpose: Suspends and immobilizes a leg without applying traction to the body.

Description: May be applied to a hip, tibia, fibula, or femur. The leg is supported by a Pearson attachment and a Thomas splint. A Thomas splint is a padded ring that fits around the upper leg; a Pearson attachment meets the Thomas splint at the knee and supports the lower leg. A canvas sling may be used to further support the lower leg.

90/90 Femoral Traction

Purpose: Most commonly used traction for complicated fractures of the femur; most effective in children older than 6 years. Within 2 to 3 weeks, callus formation is sufficient to allow application of a spica cast.

Description: A pin or wire is inserted through the distal femur; the lower leg may be casted.

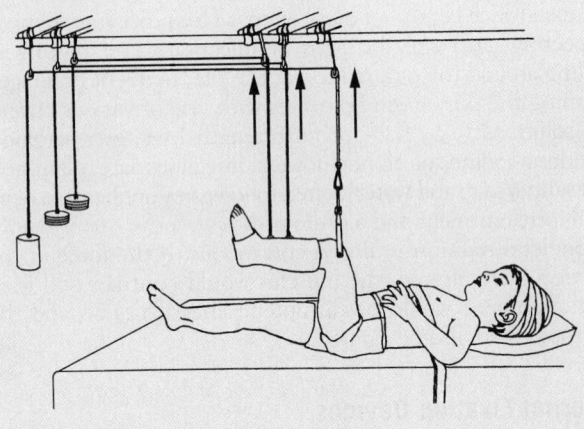

Dunlop Traction

Purpose: Used to treat supracondylar fractures of the humerus.

Description: A pin is inserted through the distal humeral fragments. The elbow is flexed at a 90-degree angle with the forearm in neutral position.

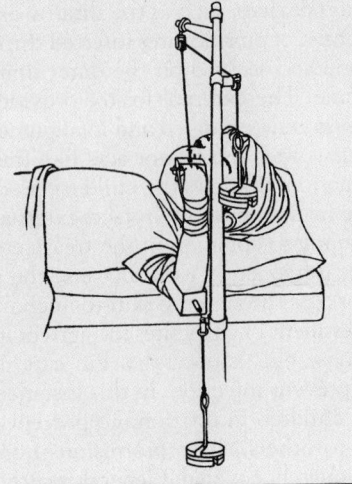

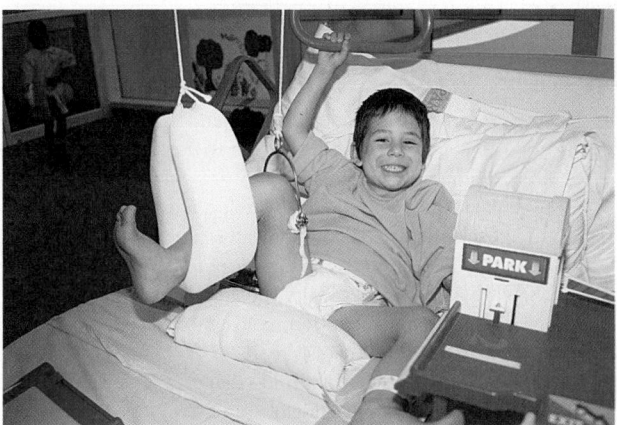

Figure 50-2 Skeletal traction is used to reduce and immobilize fractures and allows greater pull than would be possible with skin traction. Osteomyelitis may be a serious complication because skeletal traction is invasive. (Courtesy Parkland Health and Hospital System, Dallas, TX.)

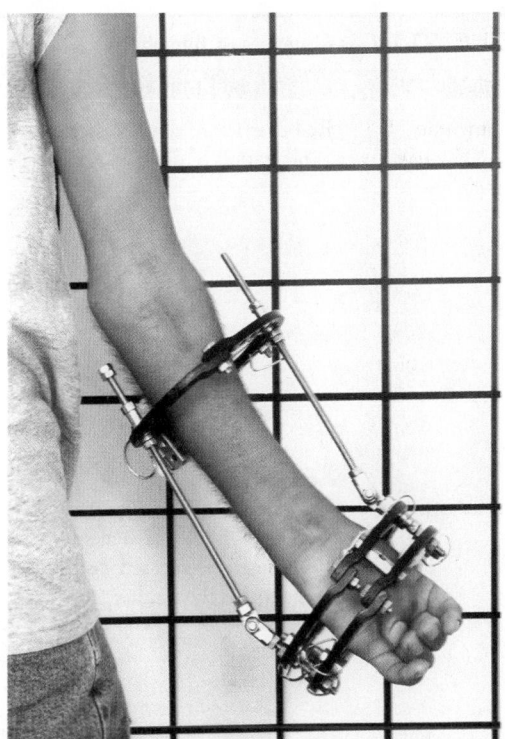

Figure 50-3 Ilizarov external fixator. (Courtesy Shriners Hospitals for Children, Houston, TX.)

PARENTS AND CHILD
Want to Know

About Home Care for the Child in a Cast

Check the edges of the cast as follows:
- If they appear rough or are irritating the skin, "petal" the cast by overlapping moleskin or adhesive tape (1-2 inches in width; 3-4 inches in length with one rounded edge) around the cast edges.

To assist with drying the cast, do the following:
- Place your child on a firm mattress.
- Support the cast and adjacent joints with pillows.
- For a plaster cast, reposition every 2 to 4 hours to ensure thorough drying.
- Lift the cast using the palms of your hands.
- You may direct a fan toward the cast to facilitate drying.
- Once dry, the cast should sound hollow and be cool to the touch.

Swelling generally peaks within 24 to 48 hours. To prevent problems, do the following:
- Apply bagged ice to the casted area (be sure to keep melting ice from touching the cast or leaking underneath).
- Elevate the extremity with pillows.
- Apply pressure to the child's nail bed, and count how long it takes for the color to return (it should take no longer than 2 seconds). Repeat every 2 to 3 hours for the first 24 to 48 hours.
- The casted extremity should be the same color and temperature as the other extremity.
- Check each finger or toe for sensation and movement several times each day for 2 days.

Protect the cast as follows:
- If the child is permitted to bathe or shower, be sure to cover the cast with plastic and waterproof tape to keep the cast dry.
- Do not put anything inside the cast. Keep small toys and sharp objects away from the cast. Supervise your child during mealtimes, so the child does not get food underneath the cast.

Contact the physician if any of the following occurs:
- The cast feels warm or hot or has an unusual smell.
- Any drainage or blood suddenly appears on the cast.
- Your child complains of pain, burning, numbness, or tingling; the extremity changes color or temperature; or any swelling persists.

When it is time for the cast to be removed, do the following:
- Explain the cast removal to your child. The cast cutter works by vibrations that create heat and a tickling feeling on the skin. It sometimes sounds loud, so you need to provide reassurance if your child is afraid of loud noises.
- Allow time for the child to adjust to the cast cutter. Ask the technician or physician if your child can examine the cast cutter and see how it works ahead of time. Sometimes children are allowed to remove a doll's cast with supervision.
- Once the cast is removed, the skin will be dry and flaky. Wash the area with warm water and soap.
- The extremity will be stiff for a while and will look smaller because the muscles have not been used. It may need to be supported with a sling. Normal movement will correct the stiffness.

TABLE 50-1 Consequences of Immobility

System Affected	Assessment Criteria	Nursing Diagnosis	Intervention
Integumentary	Red or irritated skin, presence of ulceration or drainage	Impaired Skin Integrity	Reposition the child every 2 hr and as needed; encourage the child in traction to use a trapeze to facilitate movement.
			Use an eggcrate-type or sheepskin mattress under the back and lower legs; use water-filled gloves under the heels to prevent skin breakdown.
			Wash and thoroughly dry the areas twice a day; refrain from using lotion, powder, or talc because they can retain moisture.
			Change the untrained child's diapers frequently to prevent skin breakdown.
			Examine and record the child's skin condition once per shift.
Gastrointestinal	Decrease in number or consistency of bowel movements because of decreased gastrointestinal (GI) motility	Constipation	Monitor bowel sounds, abdominal distention, elimination pattern; be sure to know the child's normal pattern, usual stool consistency, words used for defecation.
			Provide a diet high in roughage and fiber, and increase fluid intake with foods and fluids the child likes.
			Position the child as upright as possible during defecation; administer stool softeners or mild laxatives if needed.
Respiratory	Decreased or altered respirations, shortness of breath, lying supine for prolonged periods, decreased breath sounds, adventitious breath sounds	Ineffective Breathing Pattern	Monitor respiratory status at least once per shift.
			Encourage coughing and deep breathing through the use of games, such as blowing bubbles, pinwheels, or magic tricks; older children can use an incentive spirometer.
			Reposition every 2 hr and as needed.
Genitourinary	Decreased urinary output from stasis or retention, concentrated or foul-smelling urine	Impaired Urinary Elimination	Maintain hydration levels that are age-appropriate.
			Offer juices (cranberry, apple) and acid-ash foods (cereal, meats) that will acidify the urine.
			Monitor the child's urinary output.

Special Considerations for the Child in Traction

Children who are placed in traction are hospitalized from several days to weeks, depending on the underlying condition. Effective traction prevents movement of the affected limb and maintains skeletal alignment during healing. The correct amount of weight is necessary to maintain bone position. After checking with the physician's order that the correct weight is applied, be sure that all weights are hanging free and are not touching the floor or bed and that all ropes are appropriately on the pulleys. Elevate the head or foot of the bed as indicated to maintain countertraction. It may be necessary to draw a line on the child's bed sheet and ask the parents to keep the child above that line. An older child can pull on an overhead trapeze to maintain proper position and alignment.

Home Care

Most children are discharged home shortly after a cast application. See The Parents and Child Want to Know box for basic principles for caring for a child in a cast at home. Care for children discharged with an external fixator may involve frequent neurovascular assessments and, possibly, pin site care. It is most important that parents describe how to care for the cast or fixator, when they need to contact their physician, and

how to contact any needed resources in the community (e.g., physical therapy, occupational therapy, school district personnel). The nurse can also help the parents select appropriate clothing and adaptive devices, if appropriate. Encourage the parents to promote the child's self-care whenever possible.

LIMB DEFECTS

Limb defects are common in children and are a concern for parents. Most alterations of arms and legs are mild variations of normal posturing, but some are severe anomalies or abnormalities.

Etiology and Incidence

Limb defects result from birth anomalies and sometimes from trauma. These defects take many forms, including webbing (*syndactyly*) or extra digits (fingers or toes; *polydactyly*); congenital absence of all or part of an extremity; *genu valgum* (knock-knees) and *genu varum* (bowlegs); and clubfoot. Bowlegs are common in sturdily built infants and toddlers (Fig. 50-4). This condition is also associated with tibial torsion, a normal variation in toddlers. Knock-knees

TABLE **50-1** Consequences of Immobility—cont'd

System Affected	Assessment Criteria	Nursing Diagnosis	Intervention
Musculoskeletal	Reduced strength and joint mobility, loss of muscle tone and potential for increased muscle atrophy, limited range of motion	Impaired Physical Mobility	Test muscle strength and joint mobility every shift and as needed. Encourage active range-of-motion and stretching exercises of unaffected extremities as appropriate. Plan age-appropriate activities that require the use of unaffected extremities. Provide foods high in protein and calcium. Use elastic stockings or thromboembolitic disease (TED) hose to promote venous return and decrease circulatory stasis.
	Developmental regression, irritability, anxiety, excessive dependence on others, passive behavior	Powerlessness	Recognize the child's need to regress in response to the immobility; assist the child to regain prior developmental stages when ready. Explain all routines and procedures to the child and parents, and encourage them to participate in care. Provide the opportunity for therapeutic play—bean bags, foam balls, modeling clay, paints, remote-control toys (give the feeling of mobility and control), puppet play, story telling, role playing. Allow the child to use age-appropriate dishes and cups, clothing from home (may have to be adapted to fit over an immobilizing device), transitional object, night light. Determine and follow the child's usual routine. Encourage the school-age child and adolescent to keep up with school work and keep in contact with peers. Frequently provide a change in environment—move the bed to take advantage of a different view; move the bed into the playroom. Allow the child some autonomy in decision making.

are often seen in the preschool-age group. The structure and function of congenitally malformed limbs can be improved with therapy, but the affected limbs seldom become normal.

Trauma to or infection of an extremity may result in a variety of difficulties. Leg-length discrepancy can be a result of trauma, infection, or radiation therapy, because the unaffected limb continues to grow.

Pathophysiology

Mild limb defects most frequently occur secondary to extrinsic pressure, such as *in utero* positioning, or to the sitting and sleeping postures of young children. Heredity may also play a part in mild limb defects. These disorders are usually cosmetic, although occasionally function is altered as well. They tend to correct as the child grows.

Diagnostic Evaluation

Severe congenital defects are readily apparent at birth. Mild defects and deformities that develop over time are usually identified by parents or school nurses and are evaluated by specialized

clinicians. Radiographs may be necessary to fully evaluate limb defects and assist with developing a treatment plan.

Therapeutic Management

Mild limb deformities often resolve without treatment. Exercises, splints, special shoes, or casts may be prescribed. Surgical intervention may be required for severe deformities to release tendons, reposition bones, reconstruct parts, retard growth of an extremity, or augment growth of a limb. In some situations, long-term immobility of an extremity is necessary using casts or external fixation. Orthoses or physical therapy may be prescribed for specific needs.

Nursing Considerations

Nursing care varies with the defect and its treatment. Parents may need reassurance about the outcome of their child's therapy. The nurse should reinforce the principles of therapy, teach parents to carry out treatments at home, and encourage parents to persist with the treatment regimen even if the child does not like it. For example, exercises, special appliances, or braces may require daily use. Children in casts will

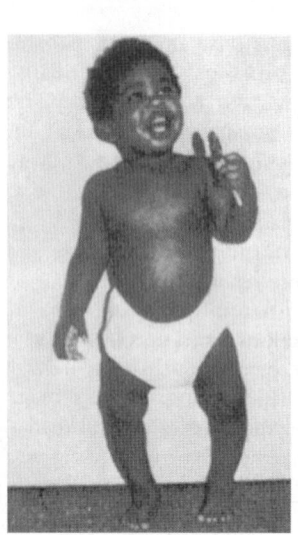
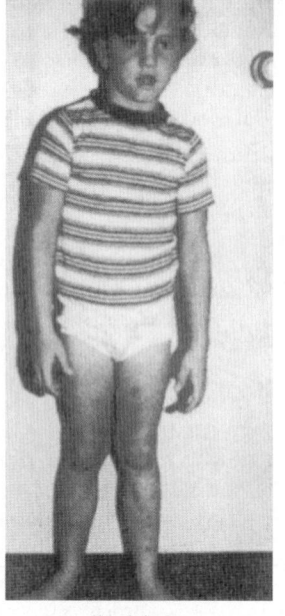

Bowlegs   Knock-knees

Figure 50-4 In the child with genu varum, or bowlegs, there is a persistent space between the knees when the ankles are together. Genu varum is a normal finding for 1 year after the child begins walking. In the child with genu valgum, or knock-knees, there is a space between the ankles when the knees are together. To remember the terminology, link the *r*'s and *g*'s: genu va*r*um—knees apa*r*t; genu val*g*um—knees to*g*ether. (From McKade, W. [1977, Nov.]. Bowlegs and knock-knees. *Pediatric Clinics of North America, 24*[4], 831.)

require specialized home care. Parents may be referred to an orthotist for construction of a device to assist with the child's function or mobility. Periodic follow-up is often necessary to reinforce correct use of appliances and care of the skin.

CLUBFOOT

Clubfoot is a congenital malformation of the lower extremity that affects the lower leg, ankle, and foot.

Etiology and Incidence

Clubfoot shows a genetic predisposition and a multifactorial etiology. Children with certain neuromuscular disorders, such as myelomeningocele, are especially at risk, as are children who have siblings with the disorder. Clubfoot occurs in 1.2 of 1000 births in the United States (Alexander, Ackman, & Kuo, 1999; Cummings, Davidson, Armstrong, & Lehman, 2002). Boys are more commonly affected than girls, in a 2:1 ratio. The prevalence is higher in Pacific Islanders (Cummings, Davidson, Armstrong, & Lehman, 2002).

Manifestations and Diagnostic Evaluation

The clinical manifestations of clubfoot include a plantar-flexed foot, with an inverted heel and adducted forefoot (Fig. 50-5), unilateral or bilateral defect, and a rigid limb that cannot be manipulated into a neutral position. Clubfoot is distinguished from *metatarsus adductus*, a nonrigid medial deviation of the

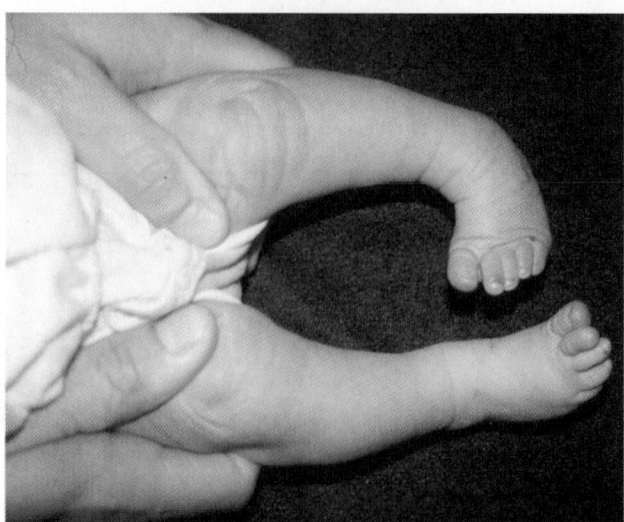

Figure 50-5 An infant with left clubfoot. Note the positional difference between the two feet.

forefoot. Clubfoot is readily apparent on clinical examination at birth. Radiographic imaging may be helpful for classifying the extent of the deformity.

Therapeutic Management

Treatment for clubfoot is started as soon after birth as possible. The goal of treatment is to gently stretch tightened ligaments and tendons and return the foot to a maximum anatomic position. Serial stretching, manipulation, and casting are performed at least weekly. If sufficient correction is not achieved in 3 to 6 months, surgery followed by casting is usually indicated. Some malformations respond readily to treatment; other, more severe forms respond less well to even vigorous and prolonged therapy. Although early treatment may result in a foot that appears normal, recurrence is common. For this reason, long-term follow-up, until the child reaches skeletal maturity, is essential because further treatment may be indicated. Even with aggressive treatment, the foot is seldom completely normal. Lifelong atrophy of the calf is common, and the affected foot is usually smaller than the other (Alexander, Ackman, & Kuo, 1999).

Treatment for infants with metatarsus adductus, however, usually involves passive stretching exercises. Parents are instructed to perform these exercises several times a day in conjunction with some aspect of the infant's care routine, such as at each feeding or when diapers are changed. Occasionally a brace, a cast, or straight-last shoes may be needed. Many children outgrow this deformity with little treatment.

Nursing Considerations

Nursing interventions are related to the stage of treatment. Initially, parents need help understanding clubfoot and the possible treatments and outcomes. They also may need help acknowledging their disappointment in having a less-than-perfect baby. The nurse can encourage parents to discuss and recognize each other's unique strategies for coping. Long-

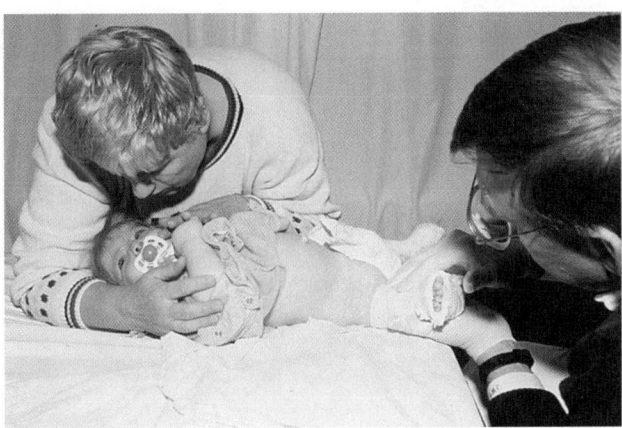

Figure 50-6 In the infant with clubfoot, serial manipulation and casting are started as soon after birth as possible to take advantage of the natural pliability of the neonate's connective tissue. Long-term casting with frequent cast changes places great responsibility on the parents. (Courtesy Cook Children's Medical Center, Fort Worth, TX.)

term casting with frequent cast changes places great responsibility on the parents (Fig. 50-6). The nurse should assess the parents' ability to adequately monitor the child for complications and pursue long-term follow-up.

If surgery is needed, the nurse oversees pain management in the immediate postoperative period. Initially, an intravenous (IV) analgesic is used, with progression to an oral analgesic, such as codeine, and then to non-aspirin-containing, nonnarcotic analgesics. Elevate the child's feet postoperatively, and apply ice bags to reduce swelling and pain. Assess the neurovascular status of the toes at least every 1 to 2 hours in the immediate postoperative period. Parents will need help positioning the infant for comfortable feeding.

The nurse also teaches parents how to keep the cast clean and dry at home. Parents should be taught how to bathe and diaper the infant without soiling or wetting the cast. When casts are changed on an outpatient basis, parents need to learn how to assess the child's neurovascular status and when to seek help.

The nurse may refer the family to the local visiting nurse agency. Because clubfoot can recur, all children with this condition require interval follow-up until they reach skeletal maturity.

DEVELOPMENTAL DYSPLASIA OF THE HIP

Developmental dysplasia of the hip has traditionally been known as *congenital dislocation of the hip*. Developmental dysplasia of the hip is a condition in which the head of the femur (ball) is improperly seated in the acetabulum (hip socket) of the pelvis. Hip dysplasia varies in severity from very mild to severe dislocation. Developmental dysplasia of the hip can be present at birth (congenital), but in some children it develops after birth—hence the term *developmental*.

Etiology

Developmental dysplasia of the hip appears to be multifactorial in origin. Genetic factors and prenatal and postnatal positioning seem to be implicated. Laxity of the ligaments holding the femur head within the acetabulum may be an underlying predisposing factor. A most significant predisposing factor is a family history of the disorder (French & Dietz, 1999).

Incidence

The incidence of developmental dysplasia of the hip varies greatly among people of different races. It is less common in African-American and Asian infants and more common in Native Americans. It is most common in whites, in girls, and in first-born infants. It is marked by a familial tendency. The condition is associated with breech deliveries. The overall incidence is difficult to determine because it varies with age and the severity of the problem (Harcke, 1999).

Manifestations

The manifestations of developmental dysplasia of the hip vary according to age. In neonates, laxity of the ligaments around the hip allows the femoral head to be displaced from the acetabulum on manipulation. Infants beyond the newborn period exhibit asymmetry of the gluteal skinfolds when the infant is lying and the legs are extended against the examining table (or when the infant is held upright with the legs dangling). There is a limited range of motion in the affected hip, as well as asymmetric abduction when the child is placed supine with the knees and hips flexed. The femur on the affected side appears to be short. The walking child displays minimal to pronounced variations in gait, with lurching toward the affected side.

Diagnostic Evaluation

Because of the complexities of diagnosis, a well-trained nurse or physician should screen for developmental dysplasia at birth and during each routine infant well-child visit.

The diagnosis of developmental dysplasia of the hip in the neonate can be very difficult to make because the signs and symptoms may be very subtle. In affected newborns, the hip joints appear lax rather than completely dislocated. Ortolani and Barlow tests (see Chapter 22) can assess subluxation or laxity, but the results are not diagnostically valid after the infant is 1 month old (Harcke, 1999). Radiography is not useful in the neonate because bony ossification is not complete, but it can be diagnostic in an older infant. Ultrasonography, best done when the infant is 4 to 6 weeks old, is now used to assist with the diagnosis of developmental dysplasia of the hip (French & Dietz, 1999). Computed tomography (CT) and magnetic resonance imaging (MRI) may also be helpful, but use of these studies is limited.

In the older infant, the physical signs of developmental dysplasia of the hip are different. The symptoms change from lax ligaments to contractures and stiffness in the affected hip joint or joints. Limited abduction on the affected side or sides is a major diagnostic sign. Any abnormalities in an older child's gait need to be carefully evaluated as possible signs of the condition. Radiography is more useful in establishing the diagnosis in older infants and children than in very young infants.

Bilateral dysplasia is always more difficult to identify than unilateral dysplasia because there is no normal hip that can be used for comparison. Interestingly, many unstable hips resolve spontaneously. If untreated, only about 20% will settle into a dislocated position.

Pathophysiology

of Developmental Dysplasia of the Hip

In the normal infant hip, the head of the femur is well seated in the acetabulum (hip socket) and is stable. Developmental dysplasia of the hip occurs in varying degrees, ranging from instability of the hip joint to frank dislocation, as defined below:

- *Instability of the hip* is the appropriate term when the head of the femur is located in the acetabulum but may be subluxated (partially dislocated) or even dislocated with manual manipulation.

- *Subluxation of the hip* occurs when the head of the femur is positioned under the edge of the acetabulum. It is not well seated in the acetabulum, yet neither is it completely dislocated.

- *Dislocation of the hip* occurs when the head of the femur lies outside the acetabulum. It can occur as a late stage of developmental dysplasia of the hip, or it can occur in children with certain neuromuscular disorders.

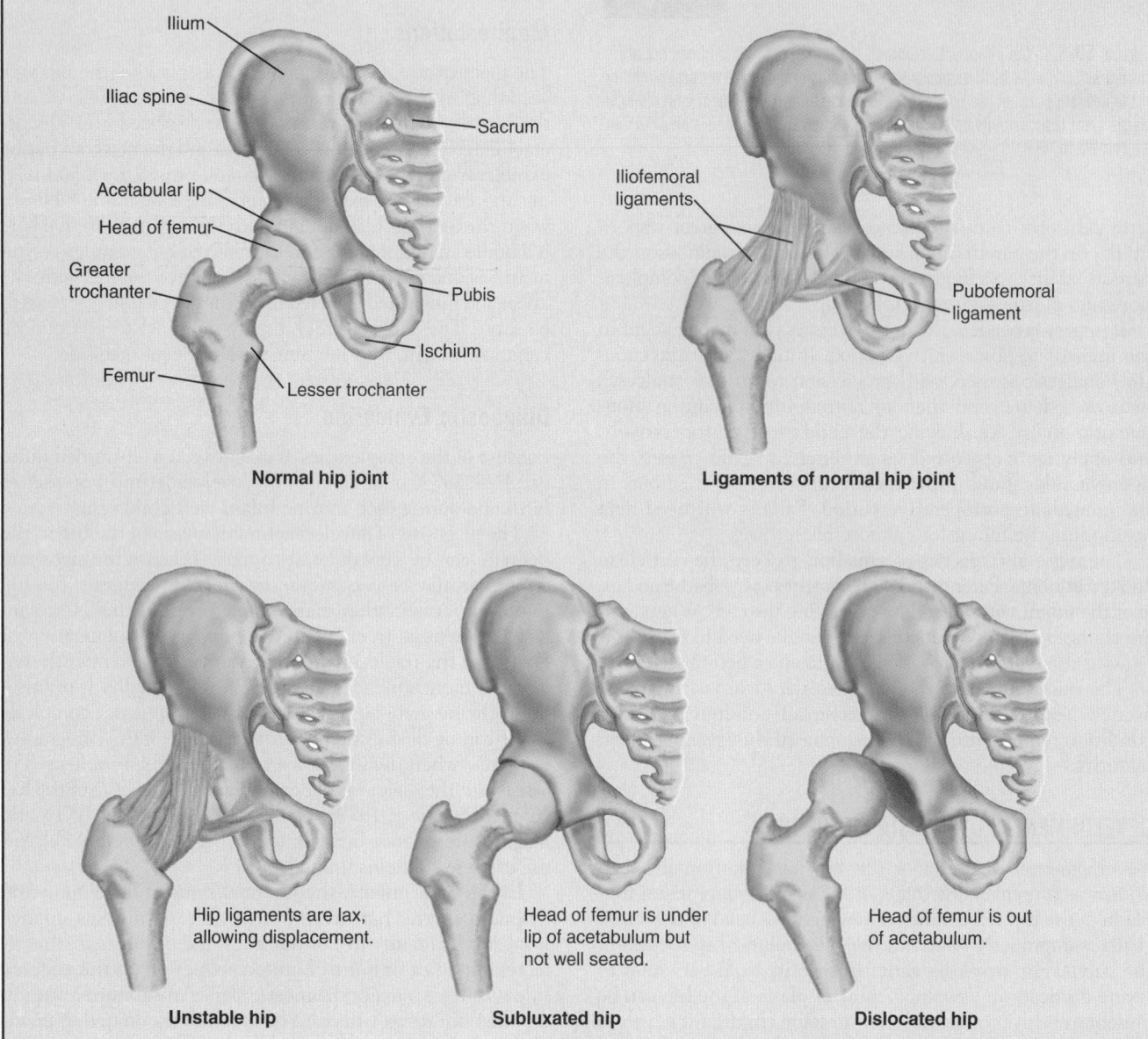

Normal hip joint

Ilium
Iliac spine
Sacrum
Acetabular lip
Head of femur
Greater trochanter
Pubis
Ischium
Femur
Lesser trochanter

Ligaments of normal hip joint

Iliofemoral ligaments
Pubofemoral ligament

Hip ligaments are lax, allowing displacement.

Unstable hip

Head of femur is under lip of acetabulum but not well seated.

Subluxated hip

Head of femur is out of acetabulum.

Dislocated hip

Therapeutic Management

Early diagnosis and treatment of developmental dysplasia of the hip are important to maximize the likelihood of a successful outcome. Treatment depends on the age of the child at the time of diagnosis and on the severity of the dysplasia.

Because the musculoskeletal development of the neonate is immature, early diagnosis and successful treatment of developmental dysplasia of the hip can result in a normal or near-normal hip.

In the neonatal period, treatment involves splinting the hips with a Pavlik harness to maintain flexion and abduction

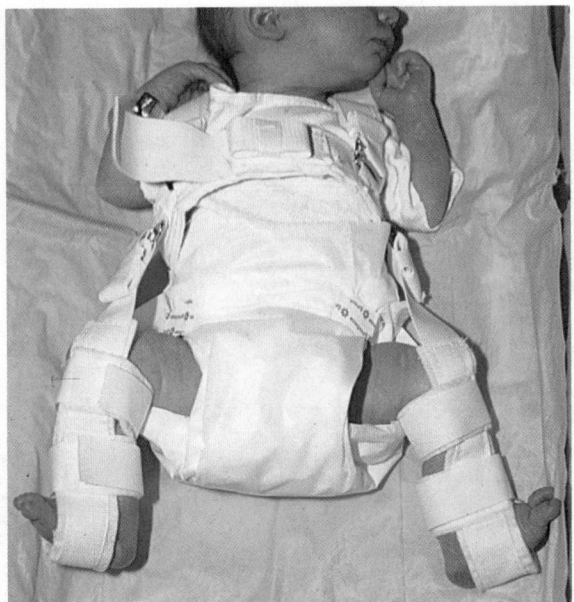

Figure 50-7 An infant in a Pavlik harness to treat developmental dysplasia of the hip.

and external rotation. The Pavlik harness consists of chest and shoulder straps and foot stirrups (Fig. 50-7). Initially, the harness is worn continuously. Positioning in the harness promotes development of a functional hip socket and a well-formed femoral head. This splinting may be the only treatment necessary to allow the hip to mold and grow normally. Hips that remain unstable become progressively deformed as the skeleton matures, resulting in functional disability. Parents must be taught the proper use of the harness, because improper positioning of the infant's hip can cause interruption of the blood supply to the head of the femur, resulting in *avascular necrosis* (tissue damage secondary to an inadequate blood supply). In addition, skin care, techniques for holding and feeding, and the importance of vigilant follow-up must be emphasized.

Treatment is more complicated when the condition is diagnosed after the newborn period. Traction or surgery to release muscles and tendons is usually necessary to allow adequate control of the hip joint. Positioning and immobilization in a spica cast follow the procedure. For profoundly affected children, traction is often followed by *osteotomy* (surgical cutting of the bone) and repositioning of the femur. After surgery, long-term immobilization in a spica cast is necessary until healing is achieved. Radiographs show the progress achieved with treatment. Follow-up monitoring is essential, because the treatment may have to be modified.

▪ NURSING CARE
The Child With Developmental Dysplasia of the Hip

Assessment
All infants should be assessed for developmental dysplasia of the hip during routine neonatal and well-child visits to ensure prompt diagnosis and treatment. Assessment procedures are complex and vary with the age of the child. Once the di-

agnosis is established, nursing assessment is directed to the parents' knowledge level, their anxiety and coping abilities, and ensuring that the treatment regimen is followed.

Because the needs of children with musculoskeletal disorders are often long-term, parents usually have a good understanding of their child's progress. Questions such as "What concerns do you have about your child's progress today?" or "How are you doing at home?" acknowledge that the parents' feelings and ideas are valued and important. Information generated by such questions can become the focus for assessment and further intervention.

Monitor the skin integrity of an infant in a Pavlik harness or cast. When surgery becomes necessary, nursing priorities shift to an assessment of lower extremity circulation and pain.

Nursing Diagnosis and Planning
The nursing diagnoses and expected outcomes that may be appropriate for the child with developmental dysplasia of the hip and the child's family are

■ Deficient Knowledge about the diagnosis of developmental dysplasia of the hip and its treatment related to unfamiliarity with the child's condition.
   Expected Outcomes: The parents will demonstrate the therapeutic and safe use of a Pavlik harness. The parents will describe and demonstrate how to care for their child in a spica cast. The parents can describe adverse effects and complications of treatment.
■ Anxiety (parental) related to having a less-than-perfect child and the need to provide complex care for an extended period.
   Expected Outcome: The parents will feel less anxious, as evidenced by being able to describe developmental dysplasia of the hip and its treatment in lay terms to other family members; carry out treatment regimens, demonstrating increased self-confidence in the care of their child; treat the child as normally as possible; and interact with health care providers and others in a calm and friendly manner.
■ Risk for Impaired Skin Integrity related to skin chafing by the Pavlik harness or cast.
   Expected Outcomes: The child's skin will remain clear and free from lesions. On follow-up visits, the cast will be reasonably clean and dry and the child's skin will be clear and intact, without abrasions or sores.
■ Ineffective Tissue Perfusion (lower extremities) related to impaired circulation secondary to surgery or casting.
   Expected Outcome: The circulation to the child's feet and toes will remain adequate.
■ Risk for Injury related to difficult positioning of a child in infant-carrying devices (infant seats, strollers, car seats).
   Expected Outcomes: The child will be safe from falls and will be adequately restrained when traveling in an automobile.
■ Deficient Knowledge about home care related to depth of presented information.
   Expected Outcomes: The family will successfully manage treatment at home, as evidenced by correctly demonstrating harness or cast care, facilitating normal developmental milestones, and engaging in appropriate follow-up. The parents will describe age-appropriate home adaptations for the child.

Caring for Nicole, a Child in a Spica Cast

Four-year-old Nicole is immobilized in a spica cast after hip surgery. She receives intravenous (IV) morphine for pain. The therapies imposed by surgery and casting can lead to complications of respiration, elimination, skin breakdown, nutrition, and boredom. These potential complications, along with Nicole's growth and developmental needs, present challenges to her parents and the nurses caring for her.

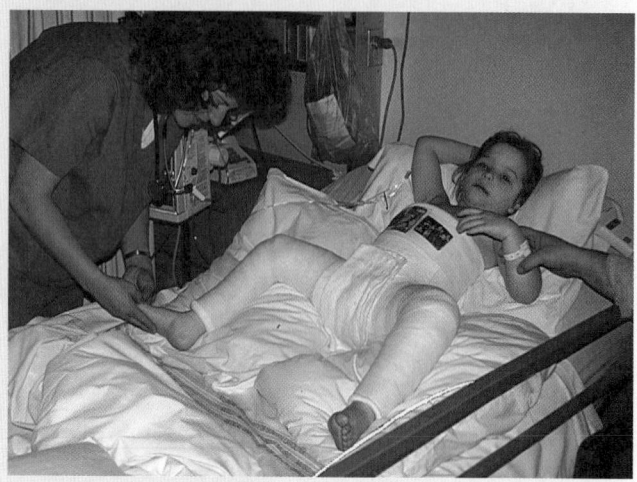

Nicole is positioned to her level of comfort with pillows at her back. A folded pillow under each leg keeps her heels from pressing against the mattress, thereby preventing pressure points. If Nicole were a few years younger, she would not be able to tell her caregivers where to place pillows for comfort or if her heels or toes were hurting or bent. Particular attention to potential pressure points is necessary with preverbal children.

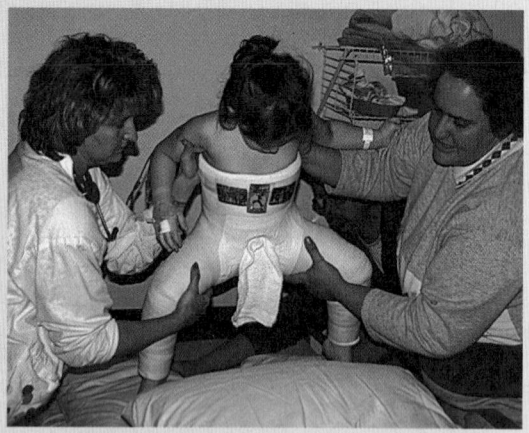

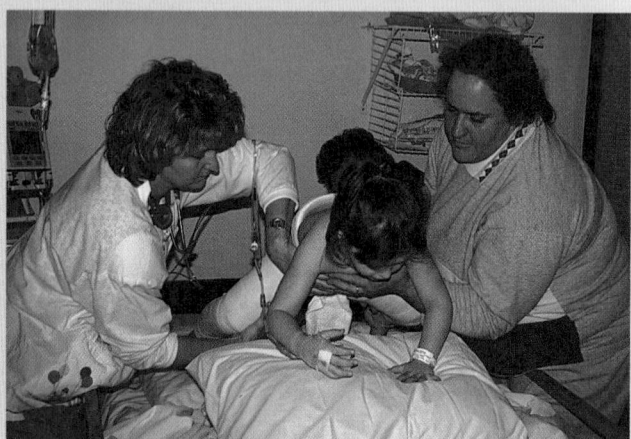

Three people are needed to turn Nicole: two to lift and turn her and a third to reposition pillows. Nicole is repositioned every 2 hours to prevent respiratory stasis. The crossbar between the legs of a spica cast (not present on this cast) should not be used as a handle when lifting the child. Once the child is feeling better and develops trust that she will not be dropped, repositioning is less frightening for her.

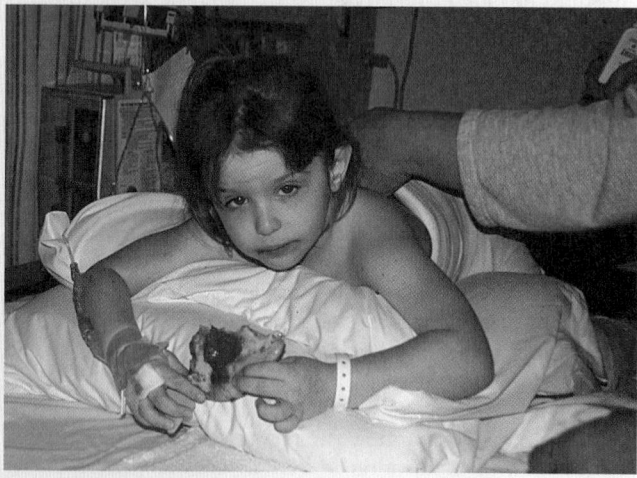

When prone, Nicole has a pillow under her chest to keep her face off the mattress and to allow her head mobility. A pillow under each leg keeps her feet and toes free. The prone position provides independence and increases Nicole's perception of control. To prevent aspiration, Nicole eats in a prone position. Because independence and autonomy are important to children, every opportunity to enhance the child's independence should be encouraged. Food should be served in bite-size pieces; finger foods may be preferred. Straws are used for liquids. The child should not be left unattended while eating.

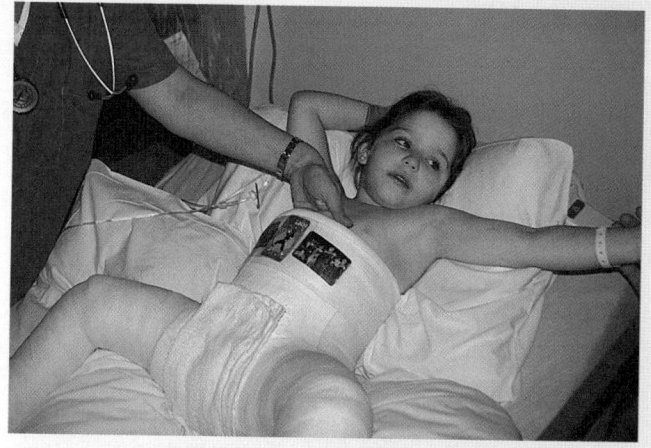

Nicole's nurse assesses her respiratory status. The cast must allow adequate room for respiratory excursion. Note that the nurse is able to fit several fingers under the edge of the cast around Nicole's chest.

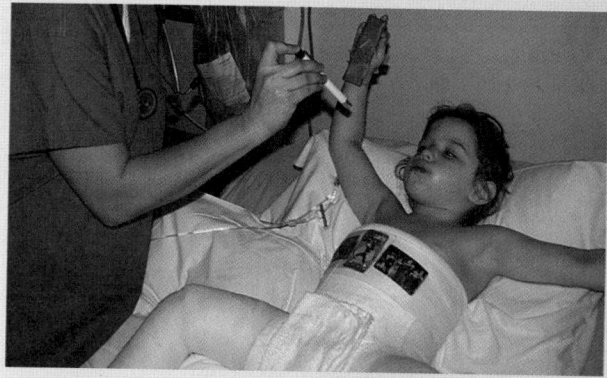

Respiratory assessment is performed at least every 8 hours. Deep breathing should be accomplished every 2 to 4 hours in the immediate postoperative period. Here the nurse asks Nicole to "blow out the light." Pinwheels, soap bubbles, and other tricks may be used to encourage deep breathing. In young children, crying provides the exercise of deep breathing.

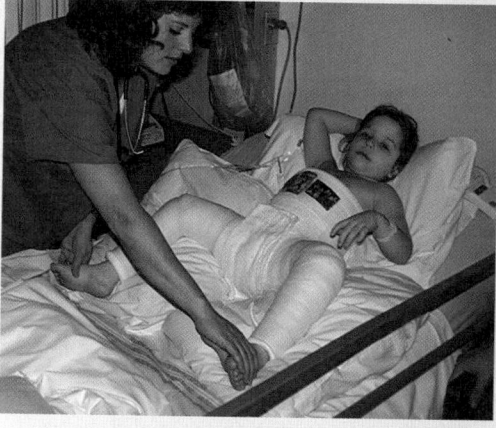

The nurse performs neurologic checks to ensure the adequacy of circulation and sensation in Nicole's feet. The nurse assesses bilaterally for color, temperature, sensation, swelling, and pulses.

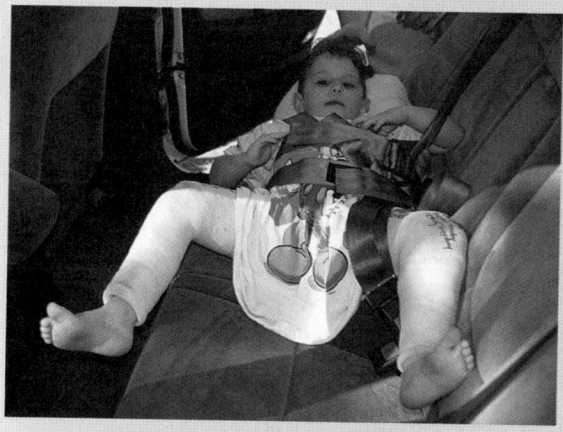

After Nicole is discharged from the hospital, her safety on the trip home is ensured by a special car seat restraint available for children in spica casts. Whenever she travels in the car, Nicole is secured safely with this restraint.

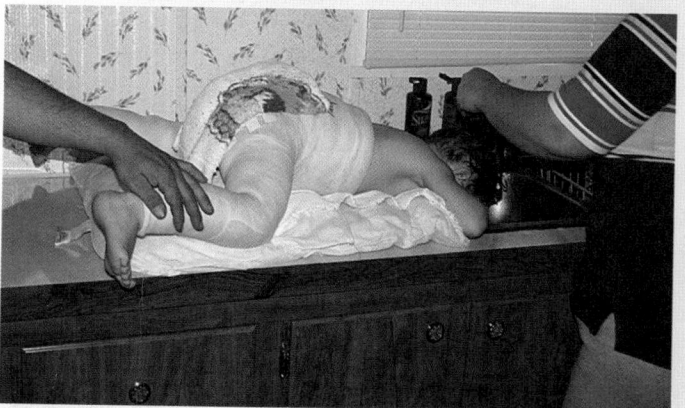

Before Nicole's discharge, her parents were instructed in body mechanics to prevent injury when lifting and turning Nicole in her heavy cast. At home, Nicole's mother washes her hair at the kitchen sink. Towels are used for comfort and to prevent water from running under the cast. Nicole is never left unattended on the kitchen counter or in other high places. To prevent burning Nicole, her mother is careful to check the water temperature.

Continued

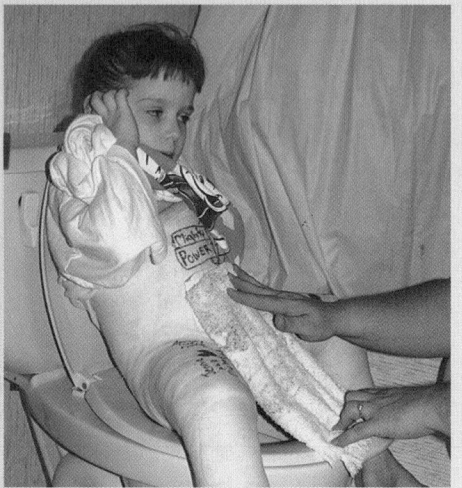

Nicole's mother has devised a system for using the toilet at home. Keeping Nicole in an upright position prevents soiling of the cast. Attention to bowel function is important, because constipation is a potential problem. Increased dietary fiber and fluid intake, including prune juice, are usually adequate to promote regularity.

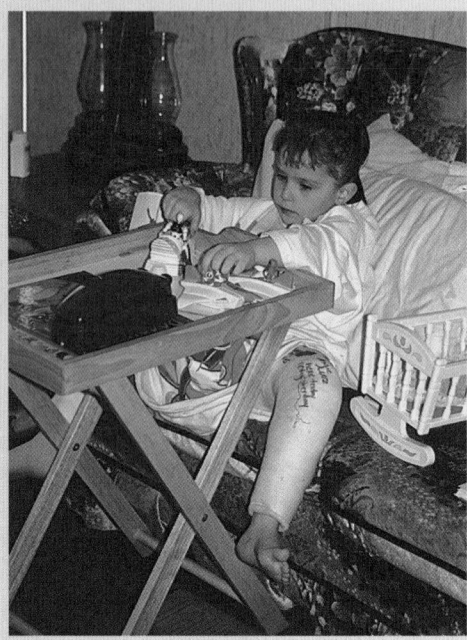

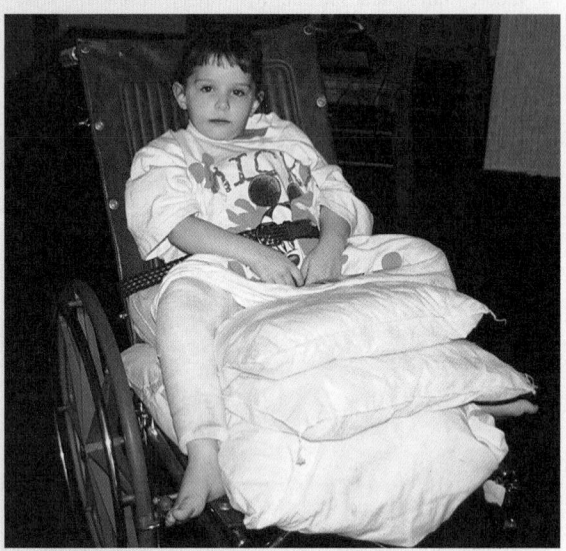

Nicole is usually dressed in large T-shirts, which are soft, absorbent, and easy to put on and take off. Although Nicole is continent, a disposable diaper is taped under her perineal area in place of underpants. Clothing may be adapted with Velcro closures. Socks are used when needed to keep Nicole's feet warm.

Age-appropriate activities help the immobilized child pass the time and can challenge and enhance development. Dolls, books, and coloring interest Nicole. At home, Nicole prefers to sit on the edge of the couch. She is never left alone and is old enough to request assistance if she feels herself sliding.

With pillows for positioning and comfort, Nicole uses a wheelchair for mobility. A younger child in a spica cast may be placed in a wagon padded with pillows. Children in wheelchairs and wagons should be strapped in to prevent falls. A child in a spica cast may also be placed on a blanket on the floor in an area of activity. This effort decreases the child's sense of isolation by increasing interactions with family members and friends.

Photos courtesy of Judy Gross and Children's Hospital, Orthopediatric Unit, Medical University of South Carolina, Charleston, SC.

Interventions

Teaching About the Pavlik Harness

Demonstrate and teach the parents the proper care and application of the Pavlik harness, including how to position and fasten the chest halter. Place the child's leg and foot into the stirrup and straps, and connect the straps to the halter. Because the requirements for harness use may change during therapy, teaching, demonstration, and return demonstration are essential at every visit. Harness straps should be secure enough to keep the child's hips flexed, without being tight. The harness should be worn 23 hours per day and should be removed only according to the physician's recommendation. The hips and buttocks should be carefully supported if the infant is out of the harness. Encourage the parents to hold and cuddle the infant as much as possible. An infant in a Pavlik harness can be fed in the usual positions, with the parent carefully supporting the lower extremities during the feeding.

Teach parents to protect the child's skin and legs under the harness. A long T-shirt ("onesie") under the halter reduces harness rubbing. The use of long socks and cotton padding (e.g., Webril) around the shoulder straps is helpful. The diaper should go on under the harness as well. Teach the parents to inspect the child's skin frequently for reddened or irritated areas and to reposition the child frequently.

Teaching About Spica Cast Care

Caring for a child in a spica cast is similar to caring for a child in any other type of cast (discussed previously), with some additional adaptations. Because the cast covers the entire lower half of the child's body, with the exception of the perineal opening, managing the child's elimination is a challenge. Excess urine can trickle under the cast, irritating and macerating the skin, resisting drying, and becoming malodorous. Advise the family to tuck a disposable diaper underneath the cast edges at the circular perineal opening; alternatively, sheet plastic is tucked under the cast opening and brought over the cast edge to the outside. Tuck sanitary napkins under the plastic, and cover with a disposable diaper. Elevating the head of the bed helps urine and feces drain downward and away from the cast.

Monitor the child's neurovascular status frequently, and teach the family the signs of neurovascular compromise. Fever, wound drainage, and discomfort may be signs of infection and should be reported promptly. Teach the family ways to provide environmental and developmental stimulation (e.g., by moving the child to different areas during the day, placing the child's bed near a window, placing appropriate toys within reach, providing age-appropriate activities). Explain the importance of feeding the child a diet high in fluids, calories, calcium, protein, and fiber. Instruct the parents about ways to dress their child to accommodate climate, style, and other needs (e.g., by fitting socks over the toes of the cast, using Velcro closures on pants and shorts, using clothing made of stretch fabrics). Give the parents the name and telephone number of an easily accessible health care provider in case questions arise at home.

Alleviating Anxiety

Communicate information to parents in a clear, kind, and straightforward manner because complex or ambiguous messages raise anxiety. Adjust teaching to accommodate parents' need for information and support. Reduce waiting time during follow-up visits, and express interest in the child and parents. Providing reliable, respectful, and empathetic care builds trust and reduces stress.

Preventing Injury

Assume a proactive role, and advise parents of the potential for injury and the importance of taking safety precautions. Most infant-carrying devices are not suitable or safe for infants in spica casts. Assist parents in identifying strategies for transporting their infant in a safe and comfortable manner, including the use of a car seat that can accommodate the wide leg spread caused by the spica cast. During waking hours, suggest placing the child on an open area of the floor that has been covered with a blanket, as an alternative to an infant seat. Remind parents that the child must not be left unattended; infants and young children often develop a surprising ability to move, despite the restrictions imposed by a cast.

Evaluation

- Do the parents demonstrate the use of the Pavlik harness or spica cast in a safe and therapeutic manner?
- Can the parents describe adverse effects or complications of treatment?
- Can the parents describe developmental dysplasia of the hip and its treatment in lay terms to other family members, carry out the prescribed therapy to the greatest extent possible, and treat the child as a normal developing child?
- Do the parents and child appear calm and able to participate in care?
- Do the parents seek recommended health care and keep follow-up appointments?
- Is the child's skin clear and free of lesions or breakdown?
- Are the child's toes warm and pink, with capillary refill less than 2 seconds; can the child move the toes freely?
- Does the child remain injury-free?
- Can the parents describe home care adaptations, and are these appropriate for the child's developmental level?

LEGG-CALVÉ-PERTHES DISEASE

Legg-Calvé-Perthes disease, also known as *osteochondritis deformans juvenilis* or *coxa plana*, is a self-limiting disorder in which there is avascular necrosis of the femoral head. The child suffers from a painful limp that is exacerbated by activities such as walking or running.

Etiology

Although the cause of Legg-Calvé-Perthes disease is unknown, it is widely accepted to be a disorder of growth. Children with Legg-Calvé-Perthes disease are usually of shorter-than-average height; many of these children were low-birth-weight infants as well (<2.5 kg [5.5 lb]). Some children have demonstrated a deficiency in components of growth factor (Shah, 2002).

Incidence

The incidence of Legg-Calvé-Perthes disease is approximately 1 in 20,000. It is more likely to occur in boys than in girls (Dyment, 1999), and in boys it occurs most frequently between ages 4 and 8 years, with an average age at onset of

Pathophysiology

of Legg-Calvé-Perthes Disease

A disturbance in the blood supply to the femoral epiphysis results in avascular necrosis of the femoral head. The most serious problem associated with Legg-Calvé-Perthes disease is the risk of permanent deformity. If the femoral head protrudes outside the acetabulum and the healing process within the femoral head is incomplete, over time the femoral head will flatten and take on a misshapen appearance. This could lead to later problems with arthritis.

The disorder is considered to be self-limiting and is classified by the extent of femoral head involvement and by disease stage. The disorder usually progresses through five stages over 1 to 2 years.

During *stage 1*, the epiphysis begins to show the results of ischemia. Synovitis produces stiffness and pain. Necrosis begins; radiographs show a reduction in size and increased density of the femoral head. Once necrosis occurs (*stage 2*), the bone weakens and dies, causing collapse of the femoral head. *Stage 3* is the fragmentation stage, in which avascular bone is reabsorbed. Healing occurs as new bone is formed. During the reossification stage, *stage 4,* the femoral head and neck begin to re-form. *Stage 5*, or the stage of reconstitution, results in final healing.*

*Thompson, G.H. (2004). Bone and joint disorders. In R. Behrman, R. Kliegman, & H. Jenson (Eds.), *Nelson textbook of pediatrics* (17th ed., pp. 2251-2297). Philadelphia: Saunders.

approximately 6 years. Unilateral hip involvement is more common than bilateral involvement. This disease is rare in African-Americans and Asians.

Manifestations

Manifestations of Legg-Calvé-Perthes disease include complaints of hip, thigh, or knee soreness or stiffness; the pain may be intermittent. A painful limp, quadriceps muscle atrophy, and pain of insidious onset may also be present.

Diagnostic Evaluation

The diagnosis is made by radiographic examination. A bone scan or MRI study may reveal necrosis and irregularity of the femoral head. However, in the vast majority of cases, plain radiographs of the femoral head will disclose the condition.

Therapeutic Management

Treatment goals include maintaining the spherical shape of the femoral head as it regenerates and reducing the risk of permanent stiffness and degenerative arthritis. Close clinical and radiographic monitoring is appropriate for children diagnosed at younger than 6 years (Thompson, 2004). For children diagnosed at older than 6 years or for those whose femoral head has come out of the acetabulum, treatment is containment of the femoral head in the acetabulum through nonsurgical or surgical means (Thompson, 2004). The femoral head is maintained in the acetabulum and protected from the stress of weight bearing during the healing process. In addition, synovitis should be

reduced to improve range of motion. Some physicians, however, do not believe that weight bearing is harmful as long as the femur remains in the acetabulum.

Because Legg-Calvé-Perthes disease is first identified from the child's complaints of a painful, stiff hip joint, the physician may recommend non–weight bearing, range-of-motion exercises and bed rest. If improvement is not seen within 7 to 10 days and the child is still unable to abduct the hip, alternative methods of treatment are considered.

For children with severe necrosis, the femoral head is abducted and internally rotated in relation to the acetabulum through some type of containment device that uses the acetabulum to maintain the spherical shape of the femoral head. Containment prevents the acetabulum from rubbing against the weakened portion of the femoral head and creating a flat shape. Methods of containment usually include bracing or surgical intervention.

The position of the femoral head is maintained in the acetabulum by abducting the leg. The child wears an abduction brace for approximately 18 months, or until reossification is evident. Some abduction braces allow the child to be ambulatory without crutches.

Surgical procedures include an osteotomy, which places the femur more securely into the acetabulum, or an innominate osteotomy, which rotates the acetabulum to completely cover the femoral head. Many physicians recommend surgical intervention because it reduces treatment time and eliminates problems with adherence to treatment.

▪ NURSING CARE
The Child With Legg-Calvé-Perthes Disease

Assessment

Assessment of a child with Legg-Calvé-Perthes disease reveals loss of internal hip rotation and limited abduction. The nurse should determine how long the child has been limping, as well as the pattern, timing, and severity of the pain. The pain may be referred to the thigh or knee. The child will describe the pain as increasing with activity and decreasing with rest. Physical examination of the extremity may reveal muscle wasting of the thigh and buttock—a reflection of disuse. Shortening of the extremity on the affected side indicates collapse of the femoral head.

Nursing Diagnosis and Planning

The nursing diagnoses and expected outcomes that may be appropriate following assessment of the child with Legg-Calvé-Perthes disease are

- Impaired Physical Mobility related to the disease process and activity restrictions.
  Expected Outcomes: The child will maintain mobility and strength of all unaffected joints, tolerate activity restrictions, and cooperate with the treatment regimen.
- Risk for Impaired Skin Integrity related to skin contact with the brace.
  Expected Outcomes: The child's skin will remain free of chafing, redness, and irritation. The parents will describe and carry out appropriate skin care.
- Disturbed Body Image related to wearing a corrective brace.
  Expected Outcomes: The child will exhibit age-appropriate behaviors and adjustment to the altered

mobility imposed by the brace. The child will appropriately express any frustrations or decrease in self-esteem.

■ Deficient Knowledge about the condition and home management related to insufficient prior information.
  Expected Outcomes: The parents will provide safe home care, will demonstrate the correct use of the brace or crutches, will perform neurovascular assessments, and will provide age-appropriate activities for their child.

Interventions

Facilitating Appropriate Activity

Activity restrictions are one of the most problematic areas in the care of a child with Legg-Calvé-Perthes disease. The child may become frustrated and angry when unable to meet the physical and social demands of peers. Initially, the child may appear to adjust to the lifestyle restrictions, but the nurse must be alert to subtle indicators of rebelliousness and uncooperative behavior. Other children will adapt quickly to the appliance they wear and demonstrate incredible activity levels. Do not construe a child's refusal to comply with treatment regimens as maladaptive behavior. The demand to keep up with their peers is sometimes so great that children are simply unable to make cognitively appropriate choices regarding their health.

Returning to school with a brace poses unique problems as well. The school nurse and the child's teacher should be involved in the discharge planning because it is important that the child participate in as many school-related activities as possible. Acknowledging the child's mobility limitations and working with school officials to identify appropriate alternatives will ensure a successful school reentry. Emphasizing hobbies and other creative activities provides ways for the child to excel and feel a sense of accomplishment.

Teaching Home Management

Because the child will receive the greater part of care as an outpatient, nursing care should focus on home care and management of the appliance selected for therapy. Parents will need information concerning the purpose, application, and care of the appliance. The family must clearly understand the issue of adherence and the role it will play in the healing process. Parents will need to learn how to perform neurovascular assessments. Also, the nurse should help parents identify safety issues regarding the child's mobility when wearing the brace. The physical therapist and occupational therapist are important resources for the parents.

The purpose of any brace used to treat Legg-Calvé-Perthes disease is to distribute the child's weight to the ischial tuberosities. Because of its design, the appliance places additional stress on the child's skin. Advise the parent to assess the child's skin condition frequently and identify any friction areas. Teach parents to check bony prominences; any reddened area on the skin that persists longer than 20 to 30 minutes demands immediate attention.

Mild soaps (Dove, Cetaphil) should be used during bathing. Do not use moisturizers on pressure areas; if lotion or moisturizers are used elsewhere on the skin, teach parents to wipe the excess off to prevent skin breakdown. Bony prominences should not be massaged. Place protective foam or transparent dressings over susceptible areas. If appropriate, protective cotton clothing may be worn under the brace, but keep the clothing as free from wrinkles as possible.

Evaluation

- Does the child exhibit normal joint and muscular integrity, and does the child cooperate with the treatment regimen?
- Is the child's skin intact, smooth, clear, and free from pressure areas?
- Can parents demonstrate skin care associated with an orthopedic appliance?
- Does the child participate in age-appropriate peer and school-related activities, within activity limitations?
- Can the child appropriately express frustration or feelings about being different?
- Are the parents able to provide developmentally appropriate activities for their child?
- Can the parents describe and demonstrate brace care and neurovascular assessments?

SLIPPED CAPITAL FEMORAL EPIPHYSIS

Slipped capital femoral epiphysis (SCFE) is a condition that affects the upper (capital) femoral growth plate. It is a hip disorder related to times of rapid growth, particularly during adolescence.

Etiology and Incidence

The cause of slipped capital femoral epiphysis is unknown. Slippage appears to be related to increased stress on the proximal femur at a time when the epiphyseal plate is thinning in preparation for eventual closure. The weakness of the growth plate may be related to adolescent hormonal imbalance and is seen most frequently in adolescents who are short and heavy for their age but have not yet developed secondary sex characteristics. SCFE also can occur in adolescents who are tall and thin, subsequent to a recent growth spurt (Thompson, 2004).

The incidence of SCFE is approximately 2 per 100,000 (Dyment, 1999). The average age at onset is 12 years for girls and 13½ years for boys (Shah, 2002), but boys are affected twice as frequently as girls. There may be an increased incidence in families. The majority of affected adolescents exceed the 95th percentile for weight and the 90th percentile for height. Although initially the condition is unilateral, approximately 25% become bilateral.

Pathophysiology

The epiphyseal plate begins to thin in response to hormonal influences during adolescence. Eventually the plate closes completely, when the adolescent has reached skeletal maturity. Increased body weight and height place more stress on the epiphyses, causing a relative displacement (slip) of the femoral neck from the femoral head; the epiphyseal movement appears to be in a posterior and inferior direction. In most instances, the slippage occurs gradually.

Manifestations and Diagnostic Evaluation

The classic manifestations of SCFE include a limp, gait disturbance, and pain. The pain usually is in the groin, thigh, or knee; it is intermittent and worse with activity. The leg often is externally rotated. Because the adolescent often presents with knee pain, hip involvement may be overlooked. Presenting symptoms along with characteristic growth signs suggest the diagnosis, so hip disease should be ruled out in adolescents who present with knee pain. Radiographs confirm the diagnosis. Radiographs are obtained with the legs in a frog-leg position.

Therapeutic Management and Nursing Considerations

Treatment is usually internal fixation: a pin or screw inserted across the growth plate secures the femoral head and prevents further slippage. More severe slips may require reconstruction of the femoral head, followed by pinning.

As soon as the diagnosis is made, the adolescent is admitted to the hospital and placed on bed rest to prevent exacerbation of the slip. Often Buck's extension is used preoperatively to relieve muscle spasms and keep the hip in alignment. Postoperatively, the adolescent uses crutches with partial weight bearing for 4 to 6 weeks. The screw or pin may be removed after several years.

The nurse should assess adolescents for slipped capital femoral epiphysis any time an adolescent complains of knee or thigh pain. Interventions are similar to those for any child in traction or undergoing surgery. Postoperatively, the adolescent needs to be taught isometric exercises and crutch walking. Weight control may be an issue; the overweight adolescent needs to learn to develop good nutritional habits and avoid high-calorie foods. Referral to a dietitian may be helpful. Provide the adolescent and parent with written instructions before discharge.

FRACTURES

Although fractures are not always serious, they are important because they may lead to life-threatening complications. A fracture is a break or disruption in a bone's continuity. Generally, fractures occur when excessive or traumatic force exceeds the strength of the bone.

Etiology

Fractures in children usually result from increased mobility and inadequate or immature motor and cognitive skills. They may result from trauma (e.g., falls, motor vehicle crashes, sports injuries, child abuse) or bone diseases that result in abnormally fragile bones (e.g., osteogenesis imperfecta).

An understanding of growth and development is helpful when assessing trauma in specific age-groups. For example, fractures in infancy are generally rare because of the cartilaginous quality of the skeleton. Fractures in infants are usually the result of trauma during birth or nonaccidental trauma. Therefore fractures in infants warrant further investigation to rule out the possibility of child abuse.

Accidental injury is the leading cause of death in children of all ages (see Chapter 34). Trauma, probably the most ominous threat to children today, frequently causes fractures. Traumatic musculoskeletal injuries are among the most frequently seen injuries in hospital emergency rooms (Walls, 2002).

The other major cause of children's fractures is falls. Because children attempt to protect themselves, the outstretched arm receives the full force of the fall (Fig. 50-8). This type of fall can affect every part of that outstretched arm (wrist, elbow, shoulder). A supracondylar humeral fracture, an elbow fracture com-

---

CRITICAL THINKING EXERCISE 50-1

Children often come to the ambulatory care setting complaining of hip or knee pain and walking with a limp. Compare and contrast the three common hip disorders in children.

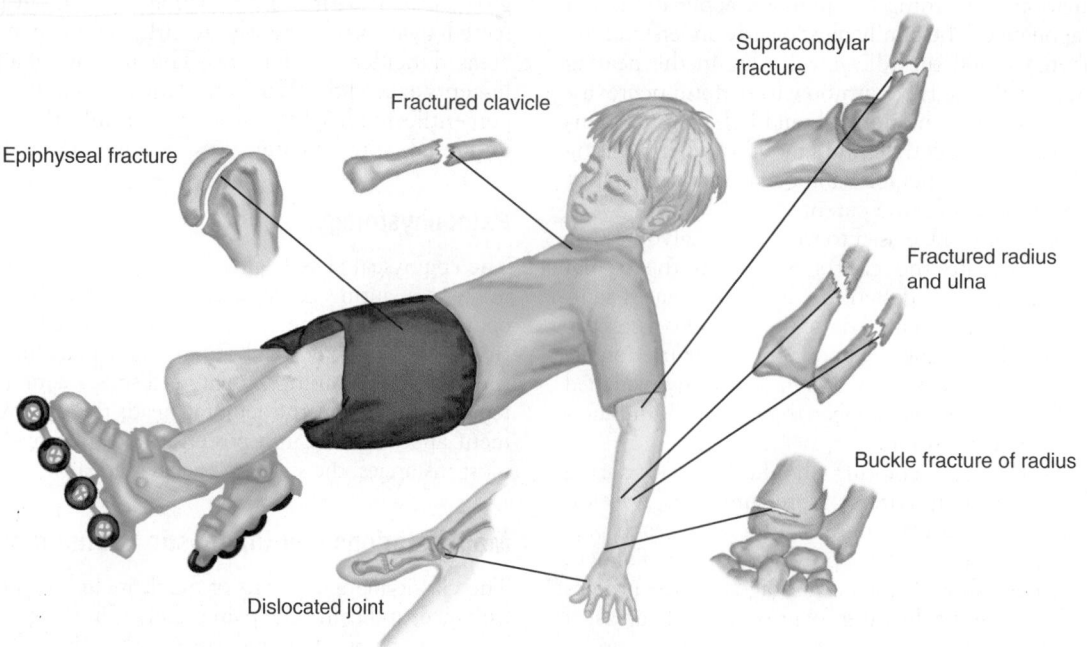

Figure 50-8 Upper extremity fractures in children often occur when the child attempts to break a fall with an outstretched arm.

monly seen with this type of fall, is a serious injury because it may lead to circulatory impairment, cellular necrosis, and ischemic contracture (Volkmann's contracture).

A fractured clavicle can occur at any age. Lack of movement or a pseudoparalysis of the upper arm may be the only sign in an infant who has sustained a fractured clavicle during birth. An older child will complain of pain and will experience a swelling on the clavicle at the point of the fracture.

Regardless of the cause of the fracture, it is important to remember that a child with an uncomplicated fracture should not present with signs of shock. If shock is evident, more than likely a more serious problem exists and a thorough assessment is required.

Incidence

Because the daily actions of children include numerous gross motor activities that place them at risk for injuries, fractures are common during childhood and adolescence.

Children between ages 5 and 9 years are most likely to experience fractures, particularly of the hip and femur, related to motor vehicle crashes (see Chapter 34). The most common sites of fractures in children are the ulna, clavicle, tibia, and femur. Epiphyseal fractures are also common in children. A severe epiphyseal fracture can interfere with bone growth.

Manifestations

The signs and symptoms of a fracture vary with the location, type, and cause of the injury. General manifestations include pain or tenderness at the site, immobility or decreased range of motion, deformity of the extremity, and edema. Other signs and symptoms include crepitus, ecchymosis, erythema, muscle spasm, and inability to bear weight.

Diagnostic Evaluation

Local signs and symptoms of a fracture are not always present, which may make assessment of a fracture difficult. Radiography of the skeleton is the most effective tool for determining the type and location of a fracture. Often a radiograph of the unaffected extremity is obtained for comparison purposes, especially when the physician is trying to determine whether a line on the radiograph represents a fracture or merely an epiphyseal line. Because the periosteum of children's bones is thicker and stronger than that of adults, it is less likely to displace at the fracture site. Consequently, the fracture may not be visible on radiographs until healing begins. Radiographs are also obtained after fracture reduction and during the healing process to assess progress.

Therapeutic Management

The key to healing is correct fracture reduction and retention. *Reduction* is the repositioning of the bone fragments into normal alignment. *Retention* entails the application of a device or mechanism that maintains alignment until healing occurs.

Reduction Methods

Fractures are treated by either closed or open reduction. Closed reduction is accomplished by manual alignment of the fragments followed by immobilization. Simple or closed fractures are treated by closed reduction. Hospitalization is seldom necessary for closed reduction, and most of these fractures heal without complications.

Open reduction entails the surgical insertion of internal fixation devices, such as rods, wires, or pins, that help maintain alignment while healing occurs. External fixation devices may also be used to lengthen bones and correct angular deformities

Pathophysiology

of Fractures

When a fracture occurs, the break in the continuity of the bone results in bone fragmentation and injury to the surrounding tissues. Torn blood vessels cause bleeding from the bone and tissues around the bone fragments. As blood clots at the site, fibrin strands provide a network for healing. Osteoblasts begin forming in immense numbers almost immediately after the injury. This increased osteoblastic activity results in the formation of new bone matrix between the bone fragments. Calcium salts are deposited in the new bone matrix, forming a *callus*. The callus is responsible for stability and support of the fracture while healing occurs. Gradually the callus is formed into new bone. Remodeling, or correction of an injury at the fracture site through the buildup of callus, occurs more rapidly in growing children.

Fractures are referred to as *simple* or *compound*. A fracture that is *simple* (closed) is characterized as intact with no breaks in the skin. If wounds accompany a simple fracture, they are usually superficial or unrelated to the fracture. The nurse should never assume, however, that a simple fracture does not warrant close assessment. It is quite possible that other problems associated with the injury exist. For example, if hemorrhage occurs, it would be internal.

A systemic risk associated with fractures, especially multiple fractures or femur fractures, is emboli. Emboli can form from postinjury bleeding with clotting or from fat droplets, shed from the fractured bone marrow (fat embolism), that enter the circulatory system and travel to the lungs or brain.

Fractures in which the skin, subcutaneous tissue, or muscle has been disrupted are called *compound* (open) fractures. Infection is a risk with this type of fracture because organisms can enter the fracture site through the wound. Children with compound fractures are at risk for blood loss secondary to external hemorrhage.

Epiphyseal injuries occur when a break or fracture occurs between the shaft of the bone and epiphyseal plate. In a growing bone, the region of least resistance to stress is the area between the metaphysis and the cartilaginous epiphyseal plate. The amount of growth arrest associated with an epiphyseal injury is determined by the extent of the damage to the epiphyseal plate. If the germinal cells remain with the epiphysis and appear uninjured, healing is rapid and growth is seldom affected. If the germinal layer is destroyed, however, growth disturbances will occur. The Salter-Harris classification system classifies epiphyseal growth-plate injuries and their associated risk of growth disturbance.

Continued

Pathophysiology

of Fractures—cont'd

Pediatric fractures are seldom complete breaks. Rather, children's bones tend to bend or buckle because of increased flexibility. This flexibility is due to a thicker periosteum and increased amounts of immature bone.

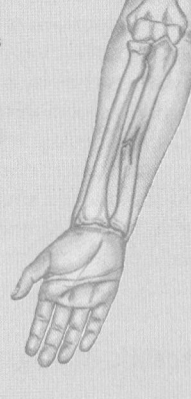

Greenstick

Break occurs through the periosteum on one side of the bone while only bowing or buckling on the other side. Seen most frequently in forearm.

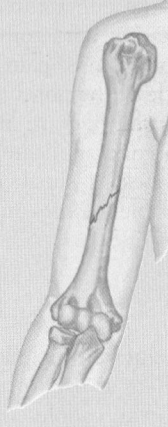

Spiral

Twisted or circular break that affects the length rather than the width. Seen frequently in child abuse.

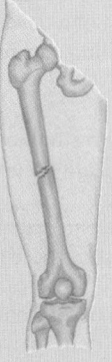

Oblique

Diagonal or slanting break that occurs between the horizontal and perpendicular planes of the bone.

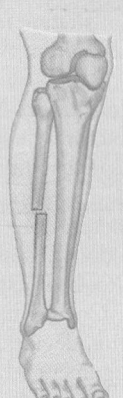

Transverse

Break or fracture line occurs at right angles to the long axis of the bone.

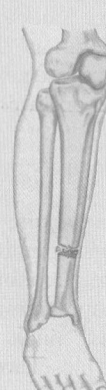

Comminuted

Bone is splintered into pieces. This is a rare occurrence in children.

Physeal growth plate injuries: Salter-Harris classification. Epiphyseal fractures are common in children.

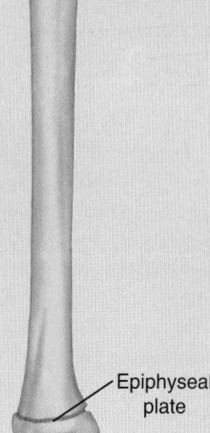

Epiphyseal plate

Epiphyseal plate

Type I

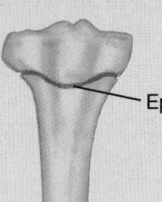

Epiphysis is completely separated from the metaphysis without fracture.

Type II

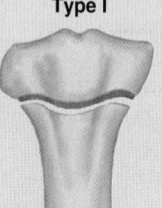

Transverse fracture extends through the separated epiphyseal plate, producing triangular break.

Type III

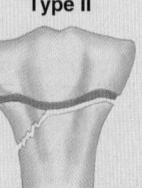

Fracture extends through part of the epiphyseal plate into the joint.

Type IV

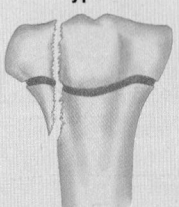

Fracture extends through the epiphyseal plate and through the metaphysis.

Type V

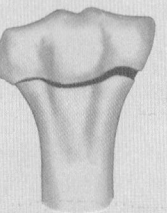

Epiphyseal plate is crushed, causing cell death in growth plate.

that involve bone and soft tissue. External fixators allow for periodic changes in alignment and length of the bone. When open reduction is employed, hospitalization is required and the child is monitored for postoperative complications. Complications after open reduction include delayed healing and nonunion. Infections may also interfere with recovery. Close assessment by the health care team as well as strict adherence to sterile technique during dressing changes can decrease the risk of postoperative problems and promote healing.

Retention

Once the fracture is aligned, it is imperative to protect the fracture site as well as maintain position of the fragments. This is accomplished through the application of a cast or, in certain situations, traction, which effectively immobilizes the area while healing occurs.

Nursing Considerations

Initial Trauma Assessment

Nursing assessment of the child with a traumatic fracture should begin with a thorough assessment of the child's airway, breathing, and circulation (see Chapter 34). Once this is done, obtain a history of the circumstances surrounding the fracture. Determining the cause of any fracture is important because nonaccidental trauma may be involved. Both a complete history of how the fracture occurred and physical findings are important if child abuse is suspected.

Examine the fracture site for bruising, skin lacerations, and swelling. Generally the child will favor the extremity, even to the point of cradling or supporting it. Often the child will complain of numbness and tingling distal to the fracture site. Movement may be limited. The area of the fracture is important to determine because growth plate injuries are not always evident on radiographs.

Assessing and Managing Fat Embolism

A serious complication of orthopedic trauma is fat embolism, which occurs most often after crush injuries and fractures of long bones (Walls, 2002). Although the etiology of fat embolism is unclear, particles of fat escape from the fracture site, are carried through the circulatory system, and lodge in the lung capillaries, causing severe respiratory distress with hypoxemia and respiratory acidosis. The child may also exhibit altered consciousness, cardiac signs, and thrombocytopenia (Hager & Brncick, 1998). Rarely, fat emboli can lodge in the small capillaries in the brain (Walls, 2002). Clinical manifestations of fat embolism usually begin in the first 3 days after trauma.

Minimal movement of fractured extremities can prevent fat embolism. Treatment includes volume resuscitation, respiratory support, and adequate oxygenation.

Assessing and Managing Compartment Syndrome

Serious complications, such as nerve compression, circulatory impairment, or compartment syndrome, can result from swelling caused by trauma or an immobilizing device. The muscles and nerves of the upper and lower extremities are enclosed in compartments that are surrounded by tough, inelastic fascia. Compartment syndrome occurs when swelling causes pressure within this closed space to rise. The increased pressure compromises circulation to the muscles and nerves within the compartment and can result in paralysis and necrosis of tissues.

Signs of compartment syndrome include severe pain, often unrelieved by analgesics, and signs of neurovascular impairment. Compartment syndrome is not uncommon in forearm fractures; therefore assess the quality of the radial pulse and the child's ability to extend the fingers. If extending the fingers produces pain, notify the physician. When assessing a complaint of pain, make a distinction between pain related to the fracture and burning sensations distal to the fracture. Pain associated with compartment syndrome usually is described as more intense than would be expected from the severity of the injury, and it does not remit with analgesics. In addition, assess for pallor, paresthesia, and pulselessness (see Critical to Remember: The Child in a Cast or Traction box).

Diagnosis is by compartmental pressure measurement; a pressure measurement of 20 mm Hg or more can result in injury (Day, 1999). If compartment syndrome is suspected, the nurse should immediately elevate the extremity only to the level of the child's heart, administer pain medication as ordered, and notify the physician (Walls, 2002).

Children who sustain fractures are treated with casts or traction. For this reason, nursing diagnoses, planning, intervention, and evaluation are the same as for any child in a cast or traction.

SOFT TISSUE INJURIES: SPRAINS, STRAINS, AND CONTUSIONS

Soft tissue injuries are common among children. They are usually the result of accidents during play or athletic activities.

Etiology

Sprains occur as a result of trauma to a joint in which ligaments are stretched or partially or completely torn. Anterior cruciate ligament (ACL) tears are one of the most common types of knee injury, especially in athletes. *Strains*, also known as *pulls*, *tears*, or *ruptures*, result from an excessive stretch of muscle. *Contusions* occur when soft tissue, muscle, or subcutaneous tissues are damaged. Sprains and contusions frequently accompany each other. *Dislocations* occur when a joint is disrupted in such a way that articulating surfaces are no longer in contact.

Incidence

Sprains are not frequently seen in young children because of their poorly developed epiphyseal plate. A twisting or turning injury will more likely result in a fracture than a sprain because the epiphyseal plate is weaker. Sprains and strains are more common in adolescents and are frequently the result of athletic injuries. Sports-related trauma is a primary cause of orthopedic injury in adolescents (Metzl, 2002). In general, sprains and contusions are more likely to occur with more physical or violent sports activities, such as football, wrestling, gymnastics, soccer, running, and cheerleading.

Manifestations and Diagnostic Evaluation

Manifestations of soft tissue injuries include pain, swelling, localized tenderness, limited range of motion, poor weight bearing, and a pop or snapping sound (sprain). The diagnosis is

> **⚠ CRITICAL TO REMEMBER**
>
> **The Child With a Soft Tissue Injury**
>
> The first 6 to 12 hours after soft tissue injury are the most important in controlling swelling and reducing muscle damage. Treatment of soft tissue injuries is summarized in the acronyms *RICE* and *ICES:*
>
> **R** = Rest
> **I** = Ice
> **C** = Compression
> **E** = Elevation
>
> **I** = Ice
> **C** = Compression
> **E** = Elevation
> **S** = Support

based on the clinical picture. An x-ray examination, however, may be ordered to rule out a fracture. An MRI or arthroscopy might be necessary to diagnose knee ligament tears.

Therapeutic Management

Control of swelling and the prevention of further injury are paramount with sprains and contusions. Swelling can inhibit healing by keeping the ligament ends apart and increasing fibrous scarring. The earlier that treatment is initiated, the less severe the swelling and immobility become.

The injured area should be wrapped immediately with a thin layer of elastic bandage or elastic wrap to support the joint and control the swelling. To reduce the swelling, ice is applied to the injured area, with additional wrap used to secure the ice. Ice should be applied for no longer than 20 minutes every 1 to 4 hours, even though the effects of the ice can last as long as 5 to 6 hours. Ice is used for several days. Nonsteroidal antiinflammatory drugs (NSAIDs) alleviate pain and reduce inflammation.

For more severe soft tissue injury, the child should avoid weight bearing for 3 days; crutches may be necessary to be sure the child does not bear weight. An *air cast,* which is a plastic, air-filled pressure cuff, may be used over the elastic wrap to support the joint and reduce swelling; the child will use the air cast for several weeks while the joint is healing. When the swelling and pain have diminished, the child can begin stretching and isometric exercises to improve joint stability.

Immobilization of the injured joint and cold application are generally very effective in the treatment of incomplete ligament tears. A complete rupture could require surgery to prevent excessive scar formation and long-term joint stability problems. Application of a cast or splint for 4 to 5 weeks may also be necessary, especially for knee injuries.

Nursing Considerations

One of the major nursing functions when assessing a sprain is to determine the severity of the injury. Assess the child for neurovascular impairment as well as for diminished range of motion. The initial examination may reveal localized tenderness over the injured joint as well as limited joint mobility.

Analgesics, such as ibuprofen or acetaminophen, are appropriate for pain management. Distraction as well as age-appropriate play activities can be very effective in managing a child's pain.

The nurse needs to keep the extremity elevated above the heart. This position enhances venous return and aids in reducing the swelling. Pillows placed beneath the extremity will provide support as well as comfort. When applying the elastic wrap, assess neurovascular status because it is possible to apply the wrap too tightly.

For the child who has undergone surgery for any type of knee ligament reconstruction, the nurse can expect to see immediate postoperative use of a cold compression cuff and a *continuous passive motion* (CPM) *machine*—a machine that continuously moves the knee joint in flexion and extension. Nursing measures involve regular emptying and refilling of the cuff to maintain the cold temperature. The nurse must also check the settings on the CPM machine to be sure they match the ordered degree of flexion and extension. Pain control is most important.

Stretching and strengthening exercises are helpful in maintaining joint and muscle integrity. These exercises are done passively at first. As healing progresses, teach the child active stretching and strengthening exercises. Asking parents for a return demonstration helps evaluate the effectiveness of teaching. Physical therapy referrals may be helpful as well.

The amount of time needed for healing is determined by the severity of the injury. Weight bearing is increased gradually as the pain subsides. More severe injuries may require partial weight-bearing exercises, with full weight bearing introduced once the swelling has resolved. Sports activities may be restricted for 3 to 8 weeks.

Review the principles of rest, support, and the application of ice with the parents and child. If wraps, splints, or air casts are used, teach the parents and child how to assess neurovascular status. If crutches are required, review the principles of crutch walking with both the parents and the child. Make sure all family members understand activity and sports restrictions. Discuss follow-up appointments and the importance of adhering to activity restrictions until the injury has healed and the child has been cleared for sports.

OSGOOD-SCHLATTER DISEASE

The classic picture of Osgood-Schlatter disease is bilateral knee pain that is exacerbated by running, jumping, or climbing stairs in a very active adolescent boy or girl who is involved in sports activities. The child will point to the tibial tubercle as the site of pain.

Etiology, Incidence, and Pathophysiology

The etiology of Osgood-Schlatter disease is believed to be related to repetitive stress from sports-related activities, combined with overuse of immature muscles and tendons over an extended period and an imbalance in the strength of the quadriceps muscle during adolescent growth. Osgood-Schlatter disease occurs in boys and girls between ages 8 and 16 years, although it is more common in boys. Usually both knees are involved.

During the adolescent growth spurt, overuse trauma causes inflammation in the tibial tubercle at the tendon insertion site. This causes tendinitis of the distal infrapatellar tendon. Without treatment, the tubercle enlarges and can cause later functional and cosmetic problems.

Manifestations and Diagnostic Evaluation

Osgood-Schlatter disease is characterized by the insidious onset of knee pain and tenderness, followed by swelling of the tibial tubercle and difficulty with weight bearing. The diagnosis is based on the clinical picture and radiographic examination.

Therapeutic Management

Treatment is conservative because the disorder is usually self-limiting. Avoiding activities such as kneeling, bicycling, and running provides adequate pain control. In some cases the physician may suggest wrapping the affected knee with elastic bandages. This limits knee flexion, reduces swelling, and provides time for healing. Physical therapy for quadriceps stretching and strengthening might be required.

In severe cases, ice, heat, and NSAIDs are helpful. A knee immobilizer or casting with the knee in full extension may be necessary to decrease pain in the child with severe pain. Activity may be restricted for 6 weeks or more. Improvement generally is seen within 6 to 8 weeks, and the problem disappears once growth stops.

Nursing Considerations

As Osgood-Schlatter disease develops in response to repetitive stress from sports-related activities, the nurse should obtain a thorough history of the child's activities. Examine the knee for pain, tenderness, and swelling over the proximal tibia.

Pain that is aggravated by activities that require kneeling, running, or climbing stairs is an important feature of this disease. Inability to shift from a squatting position to a standing position without experiencing pain is highly significant. When asked to identify the area that hurts, the child will point to the tibial tubercle.

Nurses working with school-age children and adolescents should have a clear understanding of Osgood-Schlatter disease so that a simple complaint of knee pain is not overlooked or incorrectly diagnosed, resulting in more serious problems later. The restrictions placed on the child's activity may interfere with the healthy development of peer relationships and self-esteem. Missing school or sports-related activities, limited interactions with peers, or even the need for special arrangements to participate in a peer-related activity contribute to the child's sense of isolation and alienation. Continued contact with peers is important to help the child achieve age-appropriate developmental tasks.

Because prevention of sports-related injuries should be the primary concern among all those involved in youth athletic participation, the school nurse should provide injury prevention education to all children involved in athletics. The school nurse should work with teachers and coaches as well, giving them the information they need to recognize and prevent overuse syndromes.

Reassure parents that the child will outgrow this problem. Although Osgood-Schlatter disease is self-limiting, activity restrictions must be clearly understood by the parents. Before the child resumes athletics, the parents and child should discuss the advisability of such activities with their physician. Hamstring stretching exercises may be helpful, but frequently physical therapy is required. This can prove to be expensive.

OSTEOGENESIS IMPERFECTA

Etiology

Osteogenesis imperfecta, also known as *brittle bone disease*, is a disorder inherited through an autosomal dominant inheritance pattern and characterized by connective tissue and bone defects. Depending on the type of inheritance pattern, the child's symptoms will be more or less severe. Osteogenesis imperfecta affects 1 in 10,000 to 20,000 infants (Marini, 2004; Marlowe, 2002).

Manifestations

In the most common type of osteogenesis imperfecta (type 1), the child experiences osteoporosis, excessive bone fragility, blue sclerae, discolored teeth, and deafness by age 20 to 30 years as a result of problems with bony ear structures. The child's skin may appear transparent. Eventual adult height is shorter than average. By far, the most common sign is frequent fractures. Sometimes the excessive number of old fractures can cause health care personnel unfamiliar with the disease to suspect child abuse, but new genetic testing methods can identify with 90% accuracy those infants and children who have osteogenesis imperfecta (Marlowe, 2002).

Diagnostic Evaluation

Clinical evaluation is very helpful in diagnosing osteogenesis imperfecta, with x-ray films identifying current or healed fractures. Biochemical studies of collagen structure confirm the diagnosis; children with osteogenesis imperfecta may also demonstrate elevated alkaline phosphatase levels in infancy (Marini, 2004). Genetic testing may be ordered to rule out other hereditary problems as well as to advise the parents on the risk of the disease for other children.

Therapeutic Management

Treatment goals include maintaining the integrity of the musculoskeletal system and preventing fractures. Various approaches, including traction, casting, fixation, and other orthopedic stabilizing methods, are used. Physical and occupational

---

Pathophysiology

of Osteogenesis Imperfecta

In osteogenesis imperfecta, there is a biochemical defect in the synthesis of collagen. Because collagen is an essential component of connective tissue, the abnormal collagen results in the incomplete development of bones, teeth, ligaments, and sclerae. Bones are brittle and extremely fragile, and they fracture easily.

therapy are helpful adjuncts. Intravenous infusions of biphosphonate medications have demonstrated increased bone density, decreased pain, facilitated height achievement in prepubertal children, and enhanced ambulation (Astrom & Soderhall, 2002).

Nursing Considerations

The child with osteogenesis imperfecta has a history of multiple fractures and delayed growth. The extremities may have an angular deformity secondary to old fractures. On examination, the nurse may note deformities of the leg and kyphoscoliosis. The child will appear short because of compression fractures of the spine, and joint mobility will be unusual because of relaxed ligaments. The child's teeth may appear discolored because of abnormal enamel. Too often, because of the child's appearance, people assume that the child is cognitively impaired. Children with osteogenesis imperfecta have normal or above-normal intelligence.

There is no cure for osteogenesis imperfecta; therefore providing care for a child with this disease requires attention to detail and the use of anticipatory guidance.

Identifying mobility issues that affect the child's functioning is important. Highest priority is given to preventing fractures and maintaining muscle and joint integrity. Gentle turning, passive range-of-motion exercises, daily skin care, and thorough assessment of high-stress areas of the body are necessary to protect the child from fractures and related complications.

Excessive weight gain can place undue stress on the musculoskeletal system. Maintaining optimal physiologic functioning is critical if the complications of osteogenesis imperfecta are to be avoided. Instruct parents about nutritional guidelines that support healthy growth and development, including emphasizing high-calcium foods. If necessary, calcium, magnesium, and vitamin supplements may be added to the diet.

Because each child is different, responses to the disease will vary. Coping with a chronic illness (see Chapter 36) that involves repeated hospitalizations and restricted mobility places incredible stress on the child and family. Learning how to accept the illness and how to adapt to the demands of the disease while meeting the needs of the family stresses the parents' ability to cope. The nurse needs to become aware of family dynamics, determine how the illness is affecting the family system, and assess the effectiveness of current coping strategies. Once this is done, appropriate interventions should be developed to address problematic areas.

Parents may need assistance with dressing and bathing the child. Clothing may have to be altered to allow for ease in dressing and undressing. If the child is to be discharged with a cast, the nurse should review the principles of cast care and assessment of neurovascular status. Because of the risk of accidental fractures, the nurse should review the principles of safety during play and normal activities. A home referral may be appropriate to assist the family in the transition from hospital to home.

OSTEOMYELITIS

Osteomyelitis is a bacterial infection of the bone that involves the cortex or marrow cavity. It is classified as *acute* or *chronic*. Osteomyelitis is considered chronic if the infection persists longer than 1 month or does not respond to the initial antibiotic protocol. Regardless of advances in antibiotic treatment, osteomyelitis is a serious problem that can be very difficult to diagnose and, if inadequately treated, results in high morbidity.

Etiology

Bacteria infiltrate the bone through endogenous routes (e.g., skin or respiratory infections, abscessed teeth, acute otitis media) or exogenous routes (e.g., injury, surgical procedures). The infection is usually the result of vascular spread of the bacteria. Osteomyelitis also may occur as a result of direct entry (open fracture) or injury to surrounding soft tissues (cellulitis). External fixation devices and skeletal traction can lead to osteomyelitis. Although strict adherence to aseptic techniques and frequent assessments of pin sites have greatly controlled this problem, the development of osteomyelitis can be a serious deterrent to successful healing.

The most common causative organism in all ages is *Staphylococcus aureus. Streptococcus pyogenes, Haemophilus influenzae* (in unimmunized infants), and *Escherichia coli* and group B streptococci (in neonates) also are responsible for osteomyelitis. In children older than 6 years, a *Pseudomonas aeruginosa* infection, which is associated with a puncture wound through an athletic shoe, is the most common cause (Lampe, 2004). The most common causative organism for osteomyelitis in children with sickle cell anemia is *Salmonella*.

Pathophysiology

of Osteomyelitis

Osteomyelitis occurs most frequently in the metaphyseal region of the long bones, especially the femur or tibia. Bacteria enter the metaphysis via small capillaries, and the inflammatory process begins. A preceding trauma can cause rupture of these capillaries, providing a medium for bacterial growth. Pus forms, and because it cannot move from the metaphyseal area into a joint, it spreads toward the medullary canal as well as the cortex of the bone. Pus accumulates under the periosteum and displaces it, causing it to separate and form an abscess.*

The underlying blood supply is interrupted, which causes necrotic tissue to form *(sequestrum)*. New bone *(involucrum)* develops around the sequestrum, and the inflammatory process continues, causing further damage to surrounding bone tissue.†

Large sections of sequestrum may eventually become honeycombed with cavities or sinuses that contain infective material. These cavities are so effectively walled off that antibiotic therapy may not be successful. Thus it is possible for osteomyelitis to recur in a chronic form.

---

*Lampe, R. (2004). Osteomyelitis and suppurative arthritis. In R. Behrman, R. Kliegman, & H. Jenson (Eds.), *Nelson textbook of pediatrics* (17th ed., pp. 2297-2302). Philadelphia, PA: Saunders.
†Hansen, M. (1998). *Pathophysiology: Foundations of disease and clinical intervention* (Ch. 34). Philadelphia: Saunders.

Incidence

Osteomyelitis occurs in young children, most often children younger than 5 years. Boys are affected at least two times as often as girls (Lampe, 2004). Although osteomyelitis is more likely to occur during growth spurts, the age-groups typically affected are preschoolers and adolescents.

Manifestations

The manifestations of osteomyelitis in infants can be vague and nonspecific, such as fever, irritability, and feeding difficulties. Some infants demonstrate signs of sepsis. In the older child the major signs and symptoms include pain, warmth, and tenderness localized over the site of infection; favoring the affected extremity; erythema; limited range of motion; and systemic manifestations, such as fever and lethargy. Septic arthritis in an adjacent joint may precede or be concurrent with osteomyelitis (Perlman, Patzakis, Kumar, & Holtom, 2000).

Diagnostic Evaluation

Imaging studies, such as radiography, ultrasonography, radionuclide bone scans, MRI, and CT scans diagnose and monitor the progress of osteomyelitis. Laboratory evidence of an infectious process, such as elevated erythrocyte sedimentation rate (ESR) or leukocytosis, is nonspecific for osteomyelitis. The physician may choose to aspirate the affected area to obtain fluid for culture and sensitivity.

Therapeutic Management

Once a culture has been done and the organism's sensitivity to antibiotics determined, antibiotic treatment is initiated. Controversy exists regarding the length of time required for antibiotic therapy, the need for IV versus oral antibiotics, and the role of bactericidal antibiotics and therapeutic blood levels. Nevertheless, it is generally recommended that therapy for osteomyelitis requires high-dose parenteral therapy, preferably through a peripherally inserted central catheter (PICC). The organism involved dictates the type of antibiotic and the length of treatment. With some children, parenteral antibiotics can be changed to large-dose oral antibiotics after at least 1 week of therapy (Lampe, 2004).

Because the antibiotics are administered over an extended period and high-dose therapy may be necessary to obtain the desired outcome, assessing the child's response to the antibiotics is an integral part of the treatment protocol. Peak and trough serum antibiotic levels are monitored closely. Renal and hepatic function should be monitored and blood cell counts done frequently to determine bone marrow activity. Children receiving aminoglycosides should be assessed periodically for side effects, such as ototoxicity and nephrotoxicity.

To limit the spread of infection and to promote healing, the child is placed on complete bed rest. The extremity may be immobilized with a splint or bivalved cast. After several days of healing, physical therapy with passive range of motion exercises usually is indicated to prevent contractures (Lampe, 2004). Surgical intervention may be necessary if an abscess is present or if the infection fails to respond to antibiotics. Invasive procedures include draining the abscess, débriding necrotic tissue, and performing a sequestrectomy (removal of the sequestrum). Osteomyelitis of the proximal femur generally requires some type of surgical decompression because septic arthritis of the hip may accompany this infection. Aseptic technique is critical after any type of orthopedic surgery because a secondary infection could inhibit the healing process.

▪ NURSING CARE

The Child With Osteomyelitis

Assessment

Although it may be difficult for parents to recall every injury their child has experienced, a thorough history of recent falls or traumas is helpful in determining the source of the infection. The nurse should carefully examine the affected area and note any pain, tenderness, erythema, or swelling. Usually the child will appear to protect the extremity, even tensing adjacent muscles and demonstrating reluctance to straighten or move the extremity.

Nursing Diagnosis and Planning

The nursing diagnoses and expected outcomes that may be appropriate following assessment of the child with osteomyelitis are

- Risk for Injury related to complications of antibiotic therapy.
  Expected Outcomes: The parenteral insertion site will remain patent and free from signs of infection. The parents will properly store and administer the ordered antibiotics and will properly dispose of IV equipment.
- Acute Pain related to the infectious process.
  Expected Outcome: The child will experience a decrease in pain, as evidenced by a decreased score on an appropriate pain assessment tool.
- Impaired Physical Mobility related to the infectious process and activity restrictions.
  Expected Outcomes: The child will exhibit full range of motion of the unaffected extremities and will participate in self-care.
- Delayed Growth and Development related to immobility and activity restrictions.
  Expected Outcomes: The child will exhibit age-appropriate growth and developmental behavior. The parents will provide developmentally appropriate activities for their child.
- Deficient Knowledge about home management of long-term antibiotic therapy related to unfamiliarity with the procedures.
  Expected Outcomes: The parents will demonstrate the correct administration of antibiotics, will verbalize reportable adverse effects, and will identify any other concerns or issues regarding home care.

Interventions

Chart the child's neurovascular and pain status at least every 8 hours and more often if indicated. Because any movement of the involved extremity will be accompanied by discomfort, the extremity should be immobilized and supported with pillows. When moving or turning is necessary, ask the child what the most comfortable way to achieve position changes is. If the child is preverbal or not able to explain, the nurse should consult the parents. During the acute phase, the pain may be quite severe and the nurse should premedicate the child with an analgesic before any repositioning.

Administering Intravenous Antibiotics

Because it is important to maintain a long-term IV site for antibiotic administration, the nurse carefully and frequently monitors the site for signs of complications (see Chapter 38) and flushes the line according to facility protocol.

The nurse should have a thorough knowledge of the antibiotic being given. This includes calculating dosage based on body weight or surface area, reviewing side and adverse effects, and determining if therapeutic blood levels are required. If the level of drug in the patient's blood exceeds the therapeutic range, the antibiotic should be withheld and the physician notified. Notify the physician also if the level is below the therapeutic level.

Because the child will probably be receiving multiple antibiotics, compatibility is important. Allergies and any problems the parents may have encountered during previous antibiotic administration should be noted. Periodically, the nurse should review current laboratory data to ensure adequate liver and kidney function. A complete blood cell count (CBC) and ESR should be measured on a regular basis to evaluate the child's response to treatment.

Providing Wound Care

Standard Precautions should be maintained at all times. Sterile technique and appropriate removal of soiled materials should be strictly enforced. Children with surgical wounds or drains need close monitoring. Drainage should be measured as accurately as possible and recorded at the end of the shift. The color and consistency of the drainage and any unusual odor should be noted in the nurses' notes. A description of the wound should also be included.

Maintaining Activity Limitations

Bed rest or non–weight bearing is very important to prevent spread of the infection. Returning the child to full weight bearing and self-care activities is determined by the child's response to treatment and the physician's assessment of the healing process.

Actions to prevent consequences of immobility have been discussed previously. Immobility can diminish the child's appetite. Meeting the child's nutritional needs is essential to facilitate growth and development and to assist with the healing process. The child should receive a diet high in calories and protein. Frequent small meals and food that has been brought from home are helpful in stimulating the child's appetite.

Teaching Home Management

If the child is to receive IV antibiotic therapy at home, teach the parents how to set up the medication and how to ensure the infusion is being administered safely. Plan the teaching to fit the parents' schedule, and pay particular attention to signs of frustration or anxiety. Repetitive questions, poor eye contact, and nervous gestures are indicators that anxiety may be interfering with the parents' ability to retain information. Allow parents to express feelings of concern, and give them positive feedback as they learn procedures. A return demonstration is the most effective way to evaluate teaching effectiveness. Make a home care referral to assist the family with the IV infusions.

Occasionally, children who have had a favorable clinical response to IV antibiotics will be discharged with a course of oral antibiotics. It is imperative to discuss adherence to the medication regimen with the parents. Emphasize the importance of follow-up care. A referral to a home care agency would be appropriate.

Promoting Optimal Development

Developmental issues need to be addressed by the nurse. If the child is to remain at home with restricted activity, the family must clearly understand how the restrictions aid the healing process. Discuss age-appropriate activities that will maintain current developmental levels. If the child is exhibiting any residual fears or concerns related to hospitalization, therapeutic play activities may be needed. School-age children need to continue with their schoolwork and maintain contact with their friends. Advise and arrange for tutoring as soon as possible. Resources available to home-bound children should be explored with the parents.

Evaluation

- Is the peripheral insertion site free from redness or swelling, and does the antibiotic infuse well?
- Can the parents describe and demonstrate proper antibiotic administration and disposal of associated equipment?
- Does the child indicate decreased pain on an appropriate pain assessment scale?
- Can the child exhibit full range of motion of unaffected extremities?
- Does the child participate in self-care?
- Do the parents provide developmentally appropriate activities for their child within activity restrictions?
- Does the child exhibit any signs of developmental regression?
- Can the parents demonstrate all procedures needed for home care?

JUVENILE ARTHRITIS

Juvenile arthritis (JA), formerly known as *juvenile rheumatoid arthritis*, is an autoimmune inflammatory disease with no known cause. The term *juvenile rheumatoid arthritis* is misleading because it implies a positive rheumatoid factor (RF+), which is not always present in children with the disease. Because arthritis in children can appear in a number of different forms, each with a different treatment protocol and prognosis, the more accurate term is *juvenile arthritis*.

Regardless of which term is used, there is overwhelming consensus that this is a multisystem disorder that affects the body's connective tissue. It is characterized by joint swelling with limited range of motion, accompanied by pain, tenderness, and inflammation usually of multiple joints. For diagnostic purposes, the symptoms must be present for 6 weeks or more.

Juvenile arthritis, one of the more common chronic diseases in children, is the leading cause of blindness and disability in children. Juvenile arthritis is not a childhood version of rheumatoid arthritis. Rather, the onset and course of the disease are very clearly defined. The prognosis is considered good, but success is influenced by how well the child's growth and developmental needs are integrated into the treatment plan.

Pathophysiology

of Juvenile Arthritis

The synovial joints are the primary structures involved in this rheumatic process. Normally, synovial joints are movable and contain synovium, a highly vascular tissue that produces a clear, viscous synovial fluid that nourishes and lubricates articular cartilage. In juvenile arthritis, immune complexes in blood and synovial tissue initiate the inflammatory response, producing inflammatory cytokines. Phagocytosis and accumulation of immune complexes cause chronic inflammation and joint destruction.

As the synovium becomes inflamed, excessive fluid is produced. Unlike normal synovial fluid, this fluid is thin and watery. The synovium swells, and thickened villi and nodules protrude into the joint cavity. Pannus formation occurs over the articular cartilage.

Periarticular structures outside the joint may also become involved. With further deterioration, the articular cartilage and contiguous bone become eroded and are destroyed.

Etiology

Despite extensive research, the cause of juvenile arthritis remains unknown. Infection, trauma, and emotional stress, frequently cited as factors that may trigger the autoimmune response, occur with such frequency in all children that a relationship is difficult to demonstrate. Genetic factors called *human leukocyte antigens* (HLAs) are believed to play a role in the development of juvenile arthritis (Woo & Wedderburn, 1998).

Incidence

Juvenile arthritis affects approximately 30 to 50 in 100,000 children in the United States (Ilowite, 2002). It occurs before age 16 years, although in most cases the onset is between the toddler and the adolescent years. Juvenile arthritis seldom occurs before age 6 months and is more than twice as likely to occur in girls than in boys. Approximately 30% of children with juvenile arthritis experience moderate to severe functional limitations over the long term (Ilowite, 2002).

Manifestations

Intermittent joint pain that lasts longer than 6 weeks in one or more joints suggests juvenile arthritis. The joints may appear painful, stiff, swollen, warm to the touch (no redness), and with limited range of motion. Stiffness is worse in the morning or after a prolonged period of rest. This is referred to as the "gel phenomenon" because the joints seem to gel in place. Table 50-2 lists associated signs and symptoms of the juvenile arthritis subtypes. Uveitis, or inflammation of the eye structures in the uveal tract, can cause blindness.

relationship b/w juvenile arthritis and blindness

Diagnostic Evaluation

The early diagnosis of juvenile arthritis relies on recognizing the several modes of onset and incidence patterns. The character, frequency, and severity of the systemic and articular manifestations are also critical to the diagnosis. Rheumatoid factor (RF), antinuclear antibodies (ANA), an elevated ESR, and C-reactive protein (CRP) may or may not be present, according to the type of juvenile arthritis. Certain types of juvenile arthritis are specific HLA antigen-positive. Uveitis is diagnosed by slit lamp examination.

Therapeutic Management

Therapeutic management is supportive and directed toward preserving joint function, controlling the inflammatory process, minimizing deformity, and reducing the impact of the disease on the child's development. Drug therapy, physical and occupational therapy, family education regarding home care, and developmental interventions are the treatments of choice. It is important to remember that none of these treatment modalities is curative. When they are used appropriately, however, synovitis can be reduced, mobility increased, and the child's growth and developmental needs addressed appropriately.

Drug Therapy

The major groups of drugs used to suppress the inflammatory process and control pain are the NSAIDs, such as ibuprofen, naproxen sodium (Naprosyn), tolmetin sodium (Tolectin), and aspirin. For children who do not respond well to NSAIDs and who have severe disease, the slower-acting anti-rheumatic drugs (SAARDs), such as hydroxychloroquine, gold salts, or penicillamine, can be given alone or in conjunction with the NSAIDs. Corticosteroid (e.g., prednisone) use is limited in the treatment of juvenile arthritis. Despite antiinflammatory properties, corticosteroid use neither cures juvenile arthritis nor prevents long-term joint damage. Moreover, the chronic side effects that frequently occur can be problematic for children (see Chapter 41). Indications for use are limited to life-threatening complications of juvenile arthritis, such as pericarditis, profound anemia, and vasculitis.

Immunosuppressive and cytotoxic agents (e.g., cyclophosphamides, chlorambucil) have been effective in the treatment of certain children with juvenile arthritis. Disease-modifying anti-rheumatic drugs (DMARDs), such as methotrexate, sulfasalazine, and etanercept, are being used more frequently as second-line drugs because of their effectiveness and relatively few side effects (Ilowite, 2002; Miller & Cassidy, 2004). Newer experimental drugs, such as monoclonal antibodies and COX-2 inhibitors, are in clinical trials and demonstrate promise for treating JA (Ilowite, 2002).

Physical and Occupational Therapies

By controlling the synovitis of juvenile arthritis, drug therapy plays a role in preventing additional musculoskeletal problems. Preserving muscle integrity and joint mobility is equally important. Juvenile arthritis places the child at risk for impaired mobility, contractures, and altered growth and development.

Rehabilitation is designed to prevent such problems from occurring. A program of rest, proper positioning, and exercises (strengthening, active and passive range-of-motion, resistive exercises) has been developed by occupational and physical therapists. To ensure cooperation when developing an exercise program, the therapist considers the child's interests as well as school and extracurricular activities.

TABLE 50-2 Major Types of Juvenile Arthritis

Type	Incidence	Gender Affected	Age	Joints Affected	Other Manifestations	Laboratory Values	Prognosis
Systemic	10%-20%	Males and females equally affected	Any	Few to multiple	High fever (especially in the evening), chills, rash on trunk and extremities, enlarged liver and lymph nodes, pericarditis/pleuritis, leukocytosis, abdominal pain, anemia, arthralgias before arthritis begins	↑WBC; ↓Hct; ↑ESR; ↑CRP; RF negative; ANA negative	Approximately 20% develop chronic joint disease
Polyarticular, rheumatoid factor positive	5%; may be familial	90% girls	>8 yr old	Any or multiple large and small joints, upper and lower extremities, symmetric pattern	Rapid, severe course; rheumatoid nodules (palpable near elbows); low fever; slight anemia	↑ESR, RF positive	Early joint erosion, with many having permanent disability
Polyarticular, rheumatoid factor negative	20%-30%	70%-75% girls	Early childhood; school age	Multiple large and small joints	Arthritis persists, loss of bone mass, small percentage with iridocyclitis, growth disturbances, low fever, malaise, anorexia, anemia	↑ESR, RF negative	Small percentage have joint damage
Pauciarticular oligoarthritis	40%-55%; may be familial	Girls: 20%-35% will develop a polyarticular course after approximately 3 yr	Early childhood	Knees, ankles, elbows (fewer than four joints), asymmetric pattern	Chronic uveitis with occasional loss of vision, malaise, low fever, slight anemia; slightly enlarged liver, spleen, lymph nodes during active disease	HLA-DR5 antigen positive ANA positive	Those with polyarticular course have more severe functional problems
		Boys: many develop spondyloarthropathies	Late childhood	Large joints of lower extremities, hips, spine	Small percentage have acute uveitis	HLA-B27 antigen positive	

Modified from Schulte, B., Price D., & James, S. (1997). *Thompson's pediatric nursing: An introductory text* (p. 344). Philadelphia: Saunders.
WBC, White blood cell count; *Hct,* hematocrit; *ESR,* erythrocyte sedimentation rate; *CRP,* C-reactive protein; *RF,* rheumatoid factor; *ANA,* antinuclear antibody; *HLA,* human leukocyte antigen.

To maximize the effectiveness of the exercise program, the strengths and limitations of the child's joints must be thoroughly evaluated. With this information, an individualized exercise program can be developed. Swimming is an excellent exercise for the child. The warmth of the water coupled with the mild resistance it provides makes swimming the perfect medium for strengthening and range-of-motion exercises while protecting the joint.

Children are naturally active, and children with juvenile arthritis are no different. Activity helps maintain normal muscle and joint integrity. During remissions of the disease, the youthful activity level assists with maintaining muscle strength. During painful exacerbations of the disease, however, the child's natural reaction is to rest the painful joint. Inactivity could lead to muscle wasting and flexion deformity. Hot or cold packs, splinting, and positioning the affected joint in a neutral position help reduce the pain during painful episodes. Although resting the extremity is appropriate, it is important to begin simple isometric or tensing exercises as soon as the child is able. These exercises are appropriate during exacerbations of the disease because they do not involve joint movement.

Besides physical and occupational therapy, several other treatment modalities have proved effective. Ultrasound, cold, and electrical stimulation assist in controlling the child's pain and increasing joint mobility. Heat also helps reduce joint stiffness and muscle spasm because the fibrous tissue found in joints and tendons yields better to stretching when it is heated. Examples of heat therapies are hot baths, whirlpools, Hydrocollator packs, and paraffin baths.

Surgical Treatment

Surgical intervention is considered when the child or adolescent is having problems with joint contractures and unequal growth of extremities. This type of treatment can range from diagnostic procedures, such as arthroscopic examination or open biopsy, to soft tissue release (*tenotomy*) for contractures. Surgery to correct leg-length discrepancies as well as arthroplasty and joint replacement may also be necessary.

■ NURSING CARE
The Child With Juvenile Arthritis

Assessment

Most children with juvenile arthritis are managed successfully at home, and hospital admission is not needed. The nursing assessment focuses on the status of the affected joints, the physical restrictions placed on the child, the level and intensity of the pain, and the child's and family's response to the disease process.

Examine affected joints for warmth, tenderness, pain, and limited range of motion. Because children are not always able to clearly identify the problem, be alert for irritability, guarding of the painful joints, or refusal to bear weight. The child may limp or favor the extremity.

Pain is a major component of this disease. Attempt to determine the intensity and severity of the pain. It is important to remember that the nonverbal child cannot report pain. The parent may describe the child as very fussy and irritable in the morning. The young child may be reluctant to walk and want to be carried. Help the family determine what activities increase the pain as well as what the child does when the pain starts. Explore with the child methods that may relieve the pain and whether they are effective.

Assess joint stiffness as well as the duration of the stiffness and the child's description of how difficult it is to move around after periods of inactivity. Assess the child for any indication of systemic involvement, such as a history of temperature elevations, especially in the late afternoon or evening, and determine whether a rash occurs with the fever. Anorexia, weight loss, and failure to grow may be the first indicators that something is wrong. The parent may report that the child is not sleeping at night or may simply describe the child as irritable and fussy. Lethargy and malaise may also occur.

During the physical examination, assess for lymphadenopathy, hepatosplenomegaly, and visual problems. Uveitis will be apparent only on slit lamp examination. An accurate height and weight should be obtained and, if possible, past growth parameters should be plotted on a growth chart to determine any alterations in growth. Cardiac and respiratory system assessments provide baseline information that will allow early detection of pericarditis and pleuritis.

Nursing Diagnosis and Planning

The nursing diagnoses and expected outcomes that may be appropriate to the child with juvenile arthritis and the child's family are

- Chronic Pain related to the inflammatory process.
  Expected Outcome: The child's pain will decrease, as evidenced by increased participation in usual activities and verbal report of decreased pain.
- Impaired Physical Mobility related to inflammation of the joint and associated muscle weakness.
  Expected Outcomes: As a result of appropriate activity and an ongoing exercise program, the child's joints will remain mobile. The child will correctly use any appropriate adaptive equipment to accomplish activities of daily living (ADL) and participate in a regular exercise program. The child will show no signs of the hazards of immobility.
- Delayed Growth and Development related to activity intolerance.
  Expected Outcomes: The child will exhibit age-appropriate behaviors. The parents will support and maintain appropriate developmental activities for their child.
- Disturbed Body Image related to activity intolerance.
  Expected Outcomes: The child will maintain relationships with peers and will participate in age-appropriate activities when able.
- Deficient Knowledge about the care and treatment of juvenile arthritis related to unfamiliarity with the condition.
  Expected Outcome: The parents will demonstrate safe home care and adherence to the treatment regimen and the prescribed exercise program.

Interventions
Managing Pain

Teach parents to identify both verbal and nonverbal pain indicators. Nonverbal cues are more difficult to recognize but may include restlessness, withdrawal, decreased attention span, increased crying, and decreased sleep. Maintaining a therapeutic blood level of pain medication is the most effective way to ensure maximum comfort. The nurse needs to teach parents the side effects of the prescribed medications and advise that most

Drug Guide

Naproxen, Naproxen Sodium

Classification: Nonsteroidal antiinflammatory drug (NSAID).

Action: Unknown; reduces inflammation and fever possibly by inhibiting prostaglandin synthesis.

Indication: Juvenile arthritis.

Dosage and Route: 10 mg/kg/day orally in two divided doses; medication comes in tablet or liquid suspension (125 mg/5 ml).

Absorption: Absorbed rapidly from the gastrointestinal tract with peak action in 1 to 4 hours.

Excretion: Effects last approximately 7 hours; eliminated primarily by the kidneys.

Contraindications: Contraindicated in any child who has experienced an allergic reaction to this drug or similar drugs or in children who present with a syndrome of asthma, rhinitis, and nasal polyps; naproxen should not be administered concurrently with naproxen sodium.

Precautions: Can prolong bleeding time, alter liver functions, and contribute to renal toxicity. Use cautiously if the child is also taking methotrexate, aspirin, anticoagulants, probenecid, or steroids.

Adverse Reactions: Primarily gastrointestinal irritation (gastrointestinal ulceration with bleeding from prolonged use); edema; headache, drowsiness, or dizziness; tinnitus; pruritus or skin rash; risk for renal failure.

Nursing Considerations: Monitor closely for adverse reactions, particularly if the child is receiving long-term therapy. Advise the child to take the medication with food or milk to minimize gastrointestinal upset. Be aware that antiinflammatory medications can mask signs of infection. Teach the child and family signs of gastrointestinal bleeding.

NSAIDs should be given with food or milk to prevent gastrointestinal irritation (see Drug Guide: Naproxen).

Because some medications used to treat juvenile arthritis cause immunosuppression, teach parents to recognize the signs of immunosuppression and notify the physician as appropriate. Some childhood immunizations may need to be postponed. Because the combination of aspirin and viral infection can predispose the child to Reye's syndrome (see Chapter 52), aspirin should be discontinued if the child is experiencing a viral illness. As long as the child is not immunosuppressed, administer varicella and influenza vaccines to prevent these viral infections.

Non-pharmacologic pain-relief measures, such as diversion, splinting, heat or cold application, imagery, and meditation, can be useful for some children. Remind parents to continue encouraging isometric exercises.

Promoting Mobility

Teach positioning of inflamed joints, appropriate application of heat or cold, and how to support and protect the affected joints. Emphasize that isometric exercises and passive range-of-motion exercises will prevent contractures and deformities. Assist the family to identify when the child's condition has exacerbated.

Assist the parents to learn the exercise program. Be sure that the program is developmentally appropriate and fun for the child. Teach the parents how to assess joint mobility and to maintain correct body alignment. The child might need elastic stockings if prolonged inactivity is expected.

Discuss with the parent and child age-appropriate play activities that involve the unaffected extremities; aerobic activities, such as swimming, will prevent stasis of respiratory secretions. The child will need more time than average to begin morning activities. Teach the parents to allow plenty of time for the child to awaken, take a warm shower or bath, and relieve morning joint stiffness. Keeping the child's room or bed warm is important. Administering the medication with a snack first thing in the morning and allowing the medication to take effect before the child arises help reduce pain.

Facilitating Emotional and Social Development

Acknowledge the child's and family's anxiety, and allow family members to express concerns. Encourage expressive therapeutic activities, such as pounding boards, bean bag throws, clay, painting, story composing, and doll play. Therapeutic play provides a safe and effective mechanism for reducing the stress of immobility. The nurse should recognize that age, gender, and self-concept play a role in a child's adjustment to chronic illness. Use anticipatory guidance to assist the child in developing coping mechanisms that will foster the development of optimism and a sense of personal competence.

Communicate with the school nurse about scheduling necessary rest periods for the child during the school day. The child might enjoy a short period of quiet activity in the school health office if allowed to bring a friend. School nurses can help the child's daily transition to school by communicating with teachers about the child's needs.

Assisting the child to identify strengths and areas of accomplishments increases self-esteem. Identify creative hobbies or activities that will enhance the child's sense of self-worth.

Family Education

As part of the multidisciplinary approach, the nurse must take an active part in helping the parents and child learn how to cope with and adapt to the limitations of the disease. This includes referring them from the outset to sources of accurate information about the condition and its associated care. Information should be in a variety of media and appropriate for the child's developmental level. The Arthritis Foundation (see Appendix I on Evolve website) can provide information to parents and children. Parents and children also are concerned that other children and parents understand juvenile arthritis (Barlow, Shaw, & Harrison, 1999). Increased understanding by others will increase the affected child's ability to maintain a normal, developmentally appropriate lifestyle.

Because the greater part of the child's care will take place in the home, the success of the therapeutic plan will be determined by the parents. Planning begins as soon as possible in the course of the illness. The parents should be involved in as many nursing activities as possible. This will

TABLE **50-3** Muscular Dystrophies of Childhood

Type	Onset and Progression	Inheritance and Incidence	Clinical Manifestations
Duchenne	Onset: 1-4 yr Rapidly progressive; loss of walking by 9-10 yr; death in late teens from respiratory failure, heart failure, pneumonia	X-linked recessive Most common hereditary neuromuscular disease; affects all races Incidence: 1 in 3000 male infants	Progressive generalized weakness and muscle wasting affecting limb and trunk muscles first; calves often enlarged; waddling gait; lordosis; cardiomyopathy; Gowers' maneuver; mental retardation common
Myotonic (Steinert disease)	Onset: in severe neonatal form: weakness at birth, may have paralysis of diaphragm If child survives early weeks of life, steady improvement in motor function over the first decade, usually developing ability to walk; often survive to late adulthood	Autosomal dominant Incidence: 1 in 30,000 births	In the severe neonatal form, hypotonia and weakness are evident at birth; others may appear normal at birth; mild weakness in first few years, with progressive wasting of distal muscles; myotonia worsened by cold, fatigue, stress; mental retardation in about half of cases
Becker	Onset: 5-10 yr Slowly progressive; maintain walking past early teens; life span into third decade	X-linked recessive Incidence: 1 in 20,000 births	Almost identical to Duchenne but less severe; child is mobile until late teens; normal intelligence
Congenital	Onset: birth Typically slow but variable; many do not attain walking; shortened life span	Autosomal recessive Incidence: Rare	Generalized muscle weakness with possible joint deformities; hypotonia; mental retardation and seizures common in types with central nervous system (CNS) disease
Facioscapulohumeral (FSH, or Landouzy-Dejerine disease)	Onset: first decade Slowly progressive loss of walking in later life; variable life expectancy; disease may span many decades	Autosomal dominant or recessive Incidence: 3-10 per million births	Earliest and most severe weakness occurs in facial and shoulder girdle muscles; may be unable to close eyes completely during sleep; progressive disability, leading to inability to walk; may be mild, causing minimal disability
Scapuloperoneal or scapulohumeral (Emery-Dreifuss)	Onset: middle childhood to early teens Progression is very slow; many survive to late adulthood	X-linked recessive Incidence: Rare	Contractures of elbows and ankles develop early; shoulder muscles become wasted; slowly progressive, with eventual cardiac abnormality

reduce their anxiety and increase their sense of control over a very frightening situation. Provide verbal and written instructions, and use return demonstrations to ensure parental understanding of procedures. Coordinate referrals and physical therapy with the child's and parents' routines and schedules.

Encourage the parents to provide a diet high in fiber, protein, and calcium and an adequate fluid intake. If the child experiences anorexia or pain while eating, consider smaller, more frequent high-calorie foods.

Emphasize regular visits to the ophthalmologist to prevent complications from uveitis. In general, children with juvenile arthritis should undergo slit lamp examinations every 6 months; children with pauciarticular juvenile arthritis should be seen more frequently (O'Neil, 1998).

Evaluation

- Does the child experience pain control, as evidenced by report of decreased pain, increased sleep, decreased restlessness and irritability, and increased participation in age-appropriate activities?
- Is the child free from joint inflammation, and does the child demonstrate age-appropriate range of motion and muscle strength?

- During an exacerbation, is the child able to accept activity restrictions and participate in the exercise program?
- Is the child free from respiratory problems or other problems associated with immobility?
- Is the child able to perform self-care activities appropriate for age?
- Do the parents demonstrate the ability to facilitate the child's growth and development within the limitations posed by the child's disease?
- Does the child demonstrate age-appropriate behaviors, increased social interactions with friends, and appropriate adaptation to school?
- Are the parents able to articulate and demonstrate solutions to care problems encountered in the home?

MUSCULAR DYSTROPHIES

Muscular dystrophies are a group of progressively degenerative, inherited diseases that affect the muscle cells of specific muscle groups, causing weakness and atrophy. They vary in pattern of inheritance and age at onset, but most are identified in early childhood and are characterized by progressive muscle weakness (Table 50-3). Duchenne muscular dystrophy is the most common of several forms of muscular dystrophy.

Etiology

Muscular dystrophies are inherited in various genetic patterns. Duchenne muscular dystrophy is a gender-linked recessive disorder, and therefore it affects only males. Females are carriers and pass the defect on to their male children.

Incidence

Duchenne muscular dystrophy occurs in 1 in 3000 male children. Spontaneous mutations are responsible for 30% or more of those affected; therefore many of these children have no family history of the disorder. Other forms of muscular dystrophy are less common, with varying patterns of inheritance.

Pathophysiology

Over time, muscle fibers degenerate and are replaced by fat and connective tissue. Progressive weakness and wasting of symmetric groups of skeletal muscles result in increasing disability and deformity.

Manifestations

Progressive, symmetric muscle wasting and weakness without loss of sensation first appear after walking is achieved (usually 3 to 7 years). The child must use Gowers' maneuver to rise from the floor (child puts hands on knees and moves the hands up legs until standing erect). The child has a waddling, wide-based gait. The muscles of the pelvis and shoulders are most often affected in Duchenne muscular dystrophy. The calf muscles are characteristically weak but hypertrophied. Increasing disability and deformities include hip and knee contractures, foot deformities, scoliosis, and lordosis; walking ability (in Duchenne muscular dystrophy) is lost by age 9 to 12 years. Associated signs and symptoms include moderate obesity, decreased intelligent quotient (IQ), cardiomyopathy, and shortened life span. Cardiopulmonary complications are the most common cause of death.

Diagnostic Evaluation

Children with a positive family history are especially at risk for muscular dystrophy and should be monitored for clinical symptoms, which generally do not appear until the preschool years. Serum creatine kinase (CK) levels are elevated in the early stages of the disease and then decrease as muscle bulk decreases. Electromyography and muscle biopsy may also assist with the diagnosis. The gene locus for Duchenne muscular dystrophy has been identified, which makes it easier to determine whether a woman is a carrier.

Therapeutic Management

The therapeutic management of the child with a muscular dystrophy is aimed at maintaining ambulation and independence for as long as possible as muscle weakness progresses. Contractures further reduce mobility and independence. Surgery, bracing, and physical therapy contribute to keeping the child as mobile as possible. Later, therapy is directed toward maximizing sitting capabilities, respiratory function, and self-care. Preventing obesity to facilitate mobility and care is a priority. Prompt attention to infection, especially of the respiratory tract, is essential.

Nursing Considerations

Where there is a family history of muscular dystrophy, infants and young children need to be monitored carefully for its occurrence. When a diagnosis is made, nursing interventions can become a major source of support for these children and their families. The family's ability to cope with chronic illness and the poor prognosis of muscular dystrophy needs to be assessed. Over time, the child's mobility and self-care abilities should be monitored to ensure independence for as long as possible. The potential for weight gain and respiratory tract infection and the adequacy of support systems must be regularly assessed.

Nursing interventions for the child with muscular dystrophy include coordinating a variety of health care services. Anticipating the child's future needs requires a sensitive yet knowledgeable approach. Maintenance of activity and self-care functions is important to the child and the family, and independence must be fostered, within the limits of safety. Activities such as swimming that promote range of motion and mobility for as long as possible are helpful. As the disease progresses and movement is increasingly restricted, the nurse can suggest activities that take less energy but keep the child involved with peers.

Because children in the late stages of muscular dystrophy have difficulty moving, the nurse and family should assist with position changes every 2 hours to prevent injury to the skin and other tissues from prolonged pressure. Adequate fluid intake must be encouraged to prevent urine stasis. A bowel regimen, including stool softeners or laxatives, may be necessary.

The home environment, including bathing and toileting facilities, may need to be modified to allow wheelchair mobility. Creative approaches to clothing can simplify dressing while meeting the needs of a child trying to fit in with peers.

Specific suggestions about dietary modifications to control weight may be necessary. The nurse can educate families about how to make dietary changes without making food a source of controversy. To reduce the chance of life-threatening respiratory infections, the child needs to be protected from children with respiratory and contagious diseases. As disability progresses, pulmonary hygiene and respiratory exercises are needed to maintain respiratory function.

Regular monitoring by a multispecialty team helps meet the varying needs of the child and family as the child's condition changes. Therapy is individualized to address the specific needs of the child. Genetic screening and counseling are recommended for parents and siblings of children with muscular dystrophy.

Parents must be taught how to perform basic nursing tasks and referred to agencies that can assist with home care and equipment, such as a motorized wheelchair. Extended family and support groups, such as the Muscular Dystrophy Association of America (see Appendix I on Evolve website), can provide needed emotional support and specific assistance as parental energies are exhausted. In addition, the needs of the grieving family should be addressed.

SCOLIOSIS

Although scoliosis is defined as lateral curvature of the spine, structural scoliosis is in fact a three-dimensional deformity involving rotation of the vertebral bodies. The forces of a curved spine on the structure of the body cause the rib cage to become misshapen. The body develops a compensatory curve to maintain posture and balance. Scoliotic curves are measured in degrees: a curve of 10 to 20 degrees is a slight curve; a curve of more than 40 degrees usually requires surgery; and a curve of more than 80 degrees compromises respiratory function and is considered severe. Nonstructural scoliosis, which does not involve rotational or muscular deformity, can result from poor posture, increased weight bearing on one shoulder (e.g., from carrying a heavy book bag), and other conditions that cause the child to lean in one direction. Nonstructural scoliosis is treated by correcting the underlying contributing factor.

Etiology

Most cases of scoliosis can be classified into three major categories, which offer some insight into the causes of the disorder. *Idiopathic scoliosis* is the predominant form of scoliosis. Although there is no recognizable cause for idiopathic scoliosis, the disease appears to have a genetic component. Most cases of idiopathic scoliosis occur in adolescent girls and tend to progress more rapidly during growth spurts, such as the period immediately preceding menarche. Idiopathic scoliosis can also occur in other age-groups.

Congenital scoliosis is another major category of scoliosis. It is the result of vertebral abnormalities, such as hemivertebra or vertebral bars, and is associated with other congenital anomalies.

A third category of scoliosis is *neuromuscular scoliosis*. This type of scoliosis is relatively common in individuals with certain neuromuscular conditions, such as cerebral palsy, muscular dystrophy, paraplegia, or quadriplegia.

Scoliosis may also develop in children with certain other disorders, such as osteogenesis imperfecta, juvenile arthritis, and spinal cord tumors, and it may occur secondary to radiation therapy.

Incidence

The incidence of scoliosis varies with the cause. Idiopathic scoliosis is a common disorder, affecting approximately 10% of the population. Most cases of idiopathic scoliosis are of no clinical significance and go undetected. Idiopathic scoliosis is most common in females and in families in which another member is affected. The incidence of congenital scoliosis is variable. It is believed to be caused by a variety of factors and is also asso-

ciated with certain other congenital anomalies. Scoliosis is relatively common in children with neuromuscular disorders.

Manifestations

The clinical manifestations of scoliosis include a visible curve of the spine (Fig. 50-9), a rib hump when the child is bending forward, an asymmetric rib cage, and uneven shoulder or pelvic heights and prominence of the scapula or hip. There is a difference in the space between the arms and the trunk when the child is standing, as well as an apparent leg-length discrepancy. In severe cases, the child's vital capacity is reduced (see Chapter 33 for a discussion of screening for scoliosis).

Diagnostic Evaluation

Scoliosis may be detected at any time during childhood or adolescence. It is often first discovered during routine screening for scoliosis either at school or a physician's office. Clinical manifestations should lead to more thorough assessment of the spine. Radiographic examination of the thorax will confirm the diagnosis and add information to be considered in planning treatment. In addition, children with disorders commonly associated with scoliosis should be monitored for the development of spinal deformity.

Therapeutic Management

The treatment of scoliosis is complex. Depending on the extent of the curve, the child's age and projected growth, and presence of associated complications, treatment options include regular and periodic observation with radiographic evaluation, bracing, or spinal fusion surgery. Although mild curvatures may never progress to the point that treatment is warranted, the curvature can become increasingly pronounced, which is why children must be examined regularly over the long term.

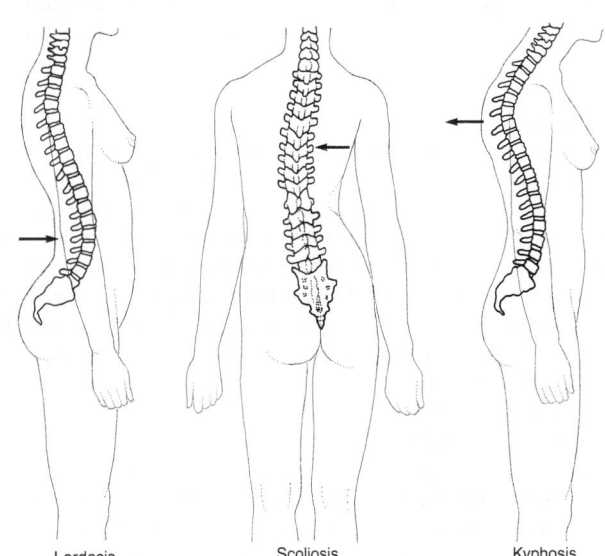

Figure 50-9 Most spinal abnormalities in children are abnormal curvatures. In *scoliosis*, the spine curves laterally and the vertebrae rotate, pulling the ribs along. *Kyphosis* is a front-to-back rounding, usually of the thoracic spine; it is often accompanied by scoliosis. *Lordosis* is an exaggerated concave curvature of the spine, usually in the lumbar area. (From Ignatavicius, D.D., Workman, M.L., & Mishler, M.A. [1995]. *Medical surgical nursing: A nursing process approach* [2nd ed., p. 1399]. Philadelphia: Saunders.)

Pathophysiology

of Scoliosis

Muscle weakness on one side of the spinal column results in shortening of the muscles and ligaments on the opposite side. These tight ligaments cause the spinal column to curve, compressing the vertebrae on that side into a concave curve. The compression of the vertebrae causes an imbalance in bone production during growth, which exacerbates the progression of the curvature.*

Spinal curvatures are measured in degrees through use of a procedure called the *Cobb method*, which measures the angle between two lines drawn from the top and bottom vertebrae on the curve. A *scoliometer* is a small screening device that approximates a spinal curve during screening.

*Hansen, M. (1998). *Pathophysiology: Foundations of disease and clinical intervention* (Ch. 34). Philadelphia: Saunders.

Bracing

In the past, bracing was used extensively in the treatment of scoliosis, and it may still be used today to stabilize some curves (those <40 degrees). Bracing will not resolve an existing curve, but theoretically it may reduce the progression of the curve during growth (Thompson, 2004). If used, the brace must be worn 18 to 23 hours per day. The child's skin needs to be meticulously monitored for signs of breakdown.

Surgery

Spinal fusion is used to treat severe scoliosis. Because fusion results in cessation of growth of the fused vertebrae, it is delayed for as long as possible to allow maximum skeletal growth. Many new surgical techniques have shown improved outcomes while decreasing the length of hospitalization. Most surgical techniques rely on some form of internal instrumentation—rods or wires—that corrects the deformity (curve) and holds the spine immobile during the long healing period. Operations are usually accomplished through incisions in the back (for posterior fusion); some surgeons prefer the anterior thoracic approach. An iliac bone graft can be used for the fusion.

Significant blood loss may occur during spinal fusion procedures, and replacement of blood is frequently necessary. Because spinal fusion for scoliosis is a planned procedure, children are often able to donate their own blood in the weeks preceding the surgery for use at the time of surgery. Such autologous blood transfusions have become common in response to the human immunodeficiency virus (HIV) epidemic.

Prognosis

With close monitoring and follow-up, the treatment outcomes for idiopathic scoliosis are excellent. The older the child is at the time of surgery, the more successful the ultimate result is likely to be. The prognosis for congenital scoliosis is variable and depends on the underlying defect. The treatment of scoliosis in children with neuromuscular disorders is a challenge, and outcomes are variable. These children must be monitored for an indefinite period for the possibility of curve progression.

Complications

A variety of complications can occur during treatment for scoliosis. Braces can cause skin irritation and even pressure sores. Neurologic damage can result from mechanical injury during surgery or from stretching of the spinal column during correction. Although electronic monitoring (somatosensory evoked potentials) during surgery helps reduce the possibility of spinal cord damage intraoperatively, postoperative sensation and motor function are the only definitive indicators of neurologic function.

Another complication in the surgical treatment of scoliosis is superior mesenteric artery syndrome. This disorder is caused by mechanical changes in the position of the patient's abdominal contents, resulting from lengthening of the body. It results in a syndrome of emesis and abdominal distention similar to that occurring with intestinal obstruction or paralytic ileus; therefore postoperative vomiting warrants attention. Fluid or electrolyte imbalances can also occur in the postoperative period, as can atelectasis and sluggish bowel function. Superficial or deep wound infection also is possible. The major long-term complication of spinal fusion is *pseudarthrosis*, or failure of one or more segments of the spine to fuse.

ADOLESCENTS AND PARENTS
Want to Know

About Home Care for the Adolescent in an Orthoplast Jacket or Brace

- Follow your physician's directions about applying and wearing time for your brace. Different braces have different methods of application, but all should fit comfortably and snugly once applied. It is important also to ask whether the brace should be applied in a lying or standing position. You might need a helper to get you into the brace. If you have had surgery, do not bend or twist while you are out of the brace.
- Always wear a 100%-cotton, preferably seamless, T-shirt under the brace to protect your skin, and be sure to pull down on the shirt to remove all wrinkles once the brace is applied. Your bra should be worn under the T-shirt unless the physician has directed otherwise; underpants and remaining clothes can go over the brace once it is on.
- Proper skin care is most important to prevent soreness or raw skin. Wash the skin that is covered by the brace once or twice a day, according to your physician's directions. Before you wash your skin, examine it closely for pink or red areas. Notify the orthopedic nurse or physician if skin areas appear raw.
- After washing, dry the skin thoroughly and put on a clean T-shirt. Avoid using creams, lotions, or powders under the brace because they can soften the skin. If your skin is particularly dry, consult with the orthopedic nurse or physician about approaches for this problem.
- Clean the inside and outside of the brace daily with mild soap and water; rinse and let dry for 20 to 30 minutes. Do not use a warm hair dryer or leave your brace anywhere warm because the plastic can soften and lose its shape.
- Notify your physician if any of the following occur: signs of an infected incision (redness, drainage, fever) if you have had surgery; numbness or tingling of your arms, legs, or feet; cracks or breaks in the brace; skin problems; any respiratory problems.

Modified from *Brace Care* and from *Instructions for Wearing Your Boston Brace.* Children's Hospital, Boston, Division 10 North and Orthopaedic Clinic.

KYPHOSIS

Kyphosis is defined as a front-to-back rounding of the thoracic spine. Mild kyphosis occurs normally and in varying amounts. It may be a postural deviation related to self-consciousness that is manifested by round shoulders. Although kyphosis usually occurs in the thoracic area, it can occur in other areas of the spine, and it becomes especially problematic when it progresses uncontrollably and results in neurologic damage or reduced respiratory function. Kyphosis is often accompanied by scoliosis, although the reverse is not necessarily true.

Etiology and Incidence

Kyphosis can occur as a postural defect (idiopathic), as a result of structural abnormalities of the vertebral bodies of the spine, or secondary to certain neuromuscular disorders (e.g.,

Text continued on p. 1444

Nursing Care Plan

The Adolescent With Scoliosis in the Community Setting

FOCUSED ASSESSMENT

Nurses are involved with routine screening of children and adolescents for scoliosis in acute care settings, in outpatient settings, and in schools. School nurses screen children for scoliosis, beginning in the fourth or fifth grade, although scoliosis usually does not become apparent until during the adolescent growth spurt. For adolescents who have been diagnosed but are not undergoing treatment, periodic reassessment is necessary to monitor possible progression of the curve. For those undergoing treatment, assessment focuses on determining the adolescent's and parents' level of knowledge about scoliosis, any body image concerns, any anxiety about the various treatment modalities, and whether the adolescent is cooperative with prescribed treatments.

Examine the child or adolescent for any of the following: uneven scapulae, shoulders, and hips and other lack of symmetry in various postural positions (see Chapter 33). Ask about any family history of scoliosis. It is important for the school nurse to be sure the family has followed up on any referral for medical evaluation of scoliosis and to assess whether family members understand the course of treatment. Other assessment factors include whether the adolescent properly wears any corrective device and whether there appear to be any body image concerns or concerns regarding appropriate activities.

Nursing Diagnosis

Deficient Knowledge about natural history of scoliosis and the treatment modalities available.

Expected Outcome

The adolescent and family will:
- Demonstrate knowledge acquisition, as evidenced by explaining what has been taught about scoliosis, including the reasons for therapy, demonstrating the skills taught (e.g., performance of prescribed exercise or brace care), asking appropriate questions that indicate a knowledge of scoliosis and its treatment (e.g., "Will I be able to play basketball?"), and following through with needed therapy at school and at home.

INTERVENTION	RATIONALE
1. Determine the adolescent's and family's knowledge level about scoliosis and treatment modalities.	1. Teaching needs to begin at the adolescent's level of understanding.
2. Teach the adolescent and family about scoliosis, its signs and symptoms, progression, and treatment.	2. Knowledge and understanding increase motivation and compliance with treatment while reducing anxiety.
3. Identify the adolescent's and parents' areas of concern (e.g., activity restriction, outcomes of therapy).	3. Teaching will be most effective if it is directed at the individual's needs.
4. Select instructional methods that are appropriate to the adolescent's developmental level (audiovisuals, pamphlets, talking with affected peers). Include the parents in the teaching.	4. Learning styles vary with individual interest, developmental level, and abilities. Including the parents in teaching increases their confidence level and improves consistency of care.
5. Explain the reasons for the various interventions (e.g., exercise regimen, brace), and emphasize that adherence to the treatment will give the most desirable results.	5. Adolescents are more cooperative in the treatment if they know the reason for interventions.
6. Have the adolescent (or parents) demonstrate specific skills (e.g., brace application, skin care, daily exercises). See Adolescent and Parents Want to Know: About Home Care for the Adolescent in an Orthoplast Jacket or Brace box.	6. Demonstration allows the nurse to evaluate learning and encourages the adolescent to gain confidence in the ability to perform the appropriate skills.

Evaluation

- Can the adolescent and family describe the natural history of scoliosis treatment prescribed?
- Can the adolescent and family demonstrate correct application of the brace (if required), proper skin care, or prescribed exercise regimen?
- Does the adolescent obtain information by asking appropriate questions of health care personnel?
- Does the adolescent follow the prescribed therapy?

Nursing Diagnosis

Disturbed Body Image related to having a postural deformity, to bracing, or to any activity limitation.

Continued

Nursing Care Plan

The Adolescent With Scoliosis in the Community Setting—cont'd

Expected Outcome

The adolescent will:
- Demonstrate adjustment to changes in physical appearance or function, as evidenced by stated confidence in abilities (academic, physical, social) and willingness to try different strategies to enhance appearance.

INTERVENTION	RATIONALE
1. Assist the teen to talk about the diagnosis, treatment, and feelings about the experience.	1. This allows assessment of perceptions and provides opportunities to clarify misconceptions and to vent feelings.
2. Engage the adolescent in conversation that focuses on body perception.	2. This allows the nurse to provide emotional support and may ease anxiety.
For example, "Some girls I have known who have had to wear a brace have been anxious about whether they will be able to find attractive clothes to fit over the brace. If this is a concern of yours, maybe we can explore some strategies together."	
3. Encourage the adolescent to discuss experiences with friends.	3. Friends are likely to be very supportive and helpful if they share a knowledge of the disorder.
4. Provide information about the disorder and the treatment. Assist the adolescent to consider a school or recreational activity that can be mastered and create a sense of accomplishment.	4. This helps the adolescent gain a sense of control over the experience.
5. Provide privacy to the greatest extent possible for any adolescent who needs to adjust the brace or perform skin care during the school day.	5. Children and teens are very modest.

Evaluation
- Does the adolescent express confidence in academic, physical, and social activities?
- Is the adolescent able to discuss creative strategies for dress or physical adaptations?

Nursing Care Plan

The Adolescent Undergoing a Spinal Fusion

FOCUSED ASSESSMENT

Preoperatively, adolescents can experience anxiety and fear about the surgical procedure, anticipated care postoperatively, and the hospital experience. They are concerned about pain, the physical experience of the operative site, postoperative activity limitations, and altered appearance. In the immediate postoperative period, adolescents are closely assessed to determine the neurologic status of the lower extremities, as well as to evaluate pain, fluid status, bleeding, and return of bowel function. It is also imperative to assess respiratory status, especially if the anterior/thoracic approach has been used and the adolescent has a chest tube. Most adolescents are cared for in the intensive care unit (ICU) for several days postoperatively.

As the adolescent stabilizes postoperatively, continue previous assessments, along with wound healing, ease of mobility, and nutritional status. Before discharge, assess the adolescent's and family's understanding of home and follow-up care. An Orthoplast jacket (brace) may be used postoperatively with some adolescents. It is not unusual for adolescents to be discharged from the hospital by the 5th postoperative day. Because the treatment of scoliosis is a long-term process that can affect an adolescent for most of the growing years, close monitoring is important to ensure positive outcomes.

Nursing Care Plan

The Adolescent Undergoing a Spinal Fusion—cont'd

Nursing Diagnosis

Anxiety (preoperative) related to impending surgery.

Expected Outcome

The adolescent will:

■ Reduce anxiety, as evidenced by seeking information about the surgery and postoperative care and by identifying and using effective coping mechanisms to address it.

INTERVENTION	RATIONALE
1. Determine whether the adolescent is anxious about surgery.	1. The adolescent may not be anxious or may be hiding anxiety.
2. Initiate a conversation with the adolescent about how anxiety makes one feel and how anxiety is a normal response to anticipated surgery.	2. The adolescent may need permission to discuss anxiety and may require assistance verbalizing feelings. Adolescents need to be assured that they are normal.

For example, "Many girls facing surgery are nervous about what it will be like to have this operation. Perhaps you would like to know more about what it will be like."

INTERVENTION	RATIONALE
3. Assist the adolescent with identifying positive and effective means for resolving anxiety (e.g., talking with a friend, exercising or engaging in other activities, practicing relaxation techniques).	3. In role modeling for the adolescent and discussing various possibilities for coping, the nurse allows the adolescent to find a comfortable means for expressing feelings.
4. Identify and discourage negative behaviors associated with anxiety (e.g., verbal outbursts, physical aggression, withdrawal).	4. The adolescent needs to understand that there are acceptable and unacceptable ways to express one's feelings.

Try telling the adolescent, "It's OK and normal to be anxious about surgery. This is hard for your parents, too. Let's talk about ways you might let your parents know how you are feeling."

INTERVENTION	RATIONALE
5. Reassure the adolescent about specific fears ("Can my parents be with me?" "Will I get a shot?" "Will I have a huge scar?").	5. Reassurance and conversation may help to resolve some fears.
6. Determine the adolescent's need for specific information, particularly about postoperative care.	6. Fears about the unknown may be reduced by increasing knowledge.

7. Explain the reason for the various postoperative interventions:
  • ICU care for the first several days
  • Neurovascular checks every 1 to 2 hours for the first 24 hours and every 4 hours thereafter
  • Turning by log-rolling every 2 hours
  • Deep breathing and use of incentive spirometer (chest tube if anterior approach is used)
  • Wound dressing (if applicable)
  • Brace application and skin care
	7. Adolescents are more cooperative in the postoperative period if they know the reason for interventions.

8. Have the adolescent (or parents and adolescent) demonstrate specific skills (e.g., coughing, recumbent log-rolling).	8. This allows the nurse to evaluate learning and allows the adolescent to gain confidence in being able to perform the maneuver; confidence in managing care decreases anxiety.
9. Encourage the adolescent to ask questions and discuss concerns. Correct any inaccurate information.	9. Verbalizing concerns helps clarify misperceptions and decreases anxiety.

Continued

Nursing Care Plan

The Adolescent Undergoing a Spinal Fusion—cont'd

Evaluation

- Does the adolescent seek information about the surgery and its postoperative course?
- Is the adolescent able to talk about anxiety or fears with parents, friends, or the nurse?
- Can the adolescent use appropriate techniques to reduce anxiety?

Nursing Diagnosis

Acute Pain related to the operative procedure.

Expected Outcomes

The adolescent will:

- Indicate decreasing amounts of pain, as measured on a pain scale.
- Appear calm and relaxed.
- Participate in postoperative activities.

INTERVENTION	RATIONALE
1. Frequently monitor the adolescent's pain level using an appropriate pain rating scale in the postoperative period. (Statements of pain, anxiety, an inability to cough, hyperalertness, reluctance or refusal to move, and/or sweating may indicate pain.)	1. Adolescents may be unable or unwilling to verbalize their pain.
2. Provide prescribed analgesics in a timely manner (children usually receive patient-controlled analgesia [PCA] morphine or epidural analgesia for several days).	2. Appropriate and timely use of analgesics provides optimal control of pain. Epidural analgesia provides more constant pain relief and prevents peaks and valleys of pain.
3. Assist family members in understanding the adolescent's experience and interventions.	3. When parents understand and can participate in the adolescent's care, they can provide appropriate support.
4. Explore alternative means for relieving pain (using anxiety-reducing techniques, dimming the room lights, reducing stimuli, playing music, therapeutic touching).	4. Alternative therapy may be very effective.
5. Determine response to pain-relief measures, and communicate with the physician about possible adjustments if needed. (Also refer to Chapter 39 for a thorough discussion of the nursing care of pain in children and teenagers.)	5. Adjustments may be necessary to achieve optimal pain relief.

Evaluation

- Can the adolescent use a pain scale to rate pain?
- Does the adolescent appear calm and relaxed?
- Is the adolescent able to participate in postoperative activities?

---

myelomeningocele) or to other factors (e.g., tumors, surgery, radiation therapy).

Postural kyphosis is found in about 4% of otherwise healthy adolescents. The incidence of kyphosis that occurs secondary to other conditions and disorders and that is severe enough to treat is variable.

Manifestations

The clinical manifestations of kyphosis include a visually appreciable humpback or convex deformity that predominantly affects the thoracic area but may involve a lower portion of the spine (see Fig. 50-9).

Diagnostic Evaluation

The diagnosis of kyphosis is relatively easy to establish from visual examination of the spine. It is often associated with other conditions, necessitating a comprehensive analysis of its cause.

Therapeutic Management and Nursing Considerations

Exercises may be recommended for mild postural curves. The treatment for severe kyphosis is similar to the treatment for scoliosis. Because the two conditions are often found in the same child, treatment is directed toward both conditions. In children who have not yet reached skeletal maturity and

Nursing Care Plan

The Adolescent Undergoing a Spinal Fusion—cont'd

Nursing Diagnosis

Deficient Knowledge about home care related to unfamiliarity with information about spinal fusion.

Expected Outcome

The family and adolescent will:

- Successfully manage treatment at home, as evidenced by demonstrating procedures, accessing appropriate community resources, and keeping follow-up appointments.

INTERVENTION	RATIONALE
1. Teach the family and adolescent the correct technique for wound care (dressing or adhesive strips) and the signs of a wound infection (redness, swelling, drainage, fever). Discuss the importance of a well-balanced diet.	1. Proper wound care and good nutrition promote healing and decrease the chance of infection.
2. Discuss activity restrictions. (Usually, these adolescents cannot ride a bike, use roller blades, ski, participate in sports or gym, mow the lawn, or lift more than 10 lb.) Show the adolescent how to perform activities without twisting or bending at the waist.	2. Home care instructions for activity are important to reduce the possibility of complications. Activity restrictions are usually maintained for 6 to 9 months, depending on the type of surgery and the physician.
3. Instruct the family and child to be alert for unfavorable signs, such as skin breakdown, pain, numbness or tingling in the extremities, or difficulty breathing, and inform them about problems that can be anticipated.	3. Home care instructions reduce the possibility of complications.
4. Provide the name and telephone number of an easily accessible health care provider in case questions arise at home. Inform the family about community resources available, including resources for tutoring. Referral to national scoliosis associations (see Appendix I on Evolve website) may be helpful.	4. Access to a health care provider and/or community resources decreases anxiety and improves compliance with treatment.
5. Before discharge, schedule a follow-up appointment. Emphasize the importance of keeping appointments.	5. Periodic evaluation is important to recovery.

Evaluation

- Can the family demonstrate the procedures necessary to care for the adolescent at home?
- Is the family aware of sources of help, if needed?
- Does the family keep follow-up appointments?

---

whose curves are flexible, casting or bracing may be attempted first. For complex progressive curves, spinal fusion frequently becomes necessary.

Nursing care of the child with kyphosis, including home care, is based on the same principles as outlined for scoliosis management.

LORDOSIS

Lordosis is an exaggerated concave curvature of the spine, usually in the lumbar area, where a mild concave curve is normal. Occasionally it occurs in other areas of the spine, in which case it is not considered normal because it can compress vital organs, such as the heart and lungs, and may require immediate intervention.

Etiology and Incidence

Lumbar lordosis by itself is usually not severe enough to cause concern. It may, however, occur secondary to other defects, such as hip flexion contracture, muscular dystrophy, obesity, or developmental dysplasia of the hip. Lordosis is a frequent complication of myelomeningocele and several other neuromuscular disorders (see Chapter 52).

The incidence of lordosis is variable and depends on the presence of associated conditions.

Manifestations and Diagnostic Evaluation

The clinical manifestations of lordosis include an exaggerated concave curve in the lumbar area, pain in the lower back, and an accompanying defect, such as developmental dysplasia of the hip, hip flexion contracture, or obesity.

A diagnosis of lordosis is confirmed by physical examination and radiographic studies.

Therapeutic Management and Nursing Considerations

Treatment for lordosis depends on its cause, but treatment modalities are based on the principles outlined for scoliosis management.

The nursing care for children with lordosis, including home care, is similar to that outlined for children with scoliosis. In addition, accompanying disorders must be monitored and treated concurrently.

KEY CONCEPTS

- Musculoskeletal problems are frequently caused by trauma. Therefore nursing assessment should always begin with the child's airway, breathing, and circulation.
- The cause of the musculoskeletal injury must be determined because nonaccidental trauma or child abuse may be involved.
- The neurovascular assessment of a child in traction or a cast includes assessment of skin color, capillary refill time, temperature, and sensation in the extremity. The quality of the pulse distal to the site should also be evaluated and compared with that of the uninvolved extremity.
- When evaluating neurovascular status, remember to assess for the five *P*s of ischemia—*p*ain, *p*allor, *p*ulselessness, *p*aresthesia, and *p*aralysis.
- Commonly seen musculoskeletal developmental disorders include clubfoot, developmental dysplasia of the hip, Legg-Calvé-Perthes disease, and slipped capital femoral epiphysis. Each often requires splinting, traction, bracing, casting, or a combination of these.
- Treatment for Legg-Calvé-Perthes disease maintains the femoral head in the acetabulum and protects the hip from the stress of weight bearing during the healing process.
- Nursing outcomes for the child with Legg-Calvé-Perthes disease include adherence to activity restrictions, facilitating home care and

management of the appliance selected for treatment, and promoting age-appropriate cognitive and emotional development.
- In an open fracture (marked by a wound or break in the skin), the possibility of infection is increased.
- Treatment of fractures involves repositioning the bone fragments (reduction) and applying a cast or traction to maintain alignment (retention) until healing occurs.
- Treatment for Osgood-Schlatter disease is conservative and involves limiting activities that require bending or kneeling. These restrictions may interfere with the achievement of developmental milestones and may result in isolation and alienation.
- Nursing care of the child with Osgood-Schlatter disease involves promoting adherence to treatment recommendations, reassuring the child that the problem is self-limiting, and assisting the child to achieve age-appropriate developmental tasks.
- Osteogenesis imperfecta places the child at risk for pathologic fractures, bony deformities caused by bending and bowing of softened bones, and kyphoscoliosis.
- Nursing outcomes for the child with osteogenesis imperfecta include keeping the child free from injury, the development of healthy coping behaviors, and the maintenance of developmental integrity.

- Nursing care of the child with osteomyelitis includes assessment and documentation of the child's status, support and immobilization of the extremity, administration of antibiotics without iatrogenic injury, and careful monitoring of the infusion equipment and IV site.
- Therapeutic management of juvenile arthritis is supportive and directed toward preserving joint function, controlling the inflammatory process, minimizing deformity, and reducing the impact of the disease on the child's development.
- Nursing outcomes for a child with juvenile arthritis include keeping the child free from injury, controlling pain, enhancing physical mobility, and promoting age-appropriate developmental behaviors.
- Nursing outcomes for a child with muscular dystrophy include maintaining physical activity, promoting respiratory function, managing weight, and reducing the impact of the disease on the child's development.
- Scoliosis, kyphosis, and lordosis are spinal abnormalities that require long-term assessment and management. Each has the potential for altering a child's body image, so nursing interventions must address emotional as well as physical consequences of these disorders.

ANSWER to Critical Thinking Exercise 50-1

The following summary compares the three common hip disorders.

	Developmental Dysplasia of the Hip	Legg-Calvé-Perthes Disease	Slipped Capital Femoral Epiphysis
Age at onset	Infancy, early childhood	Preschool, young school age	Adolescence
Manifestations	Hip instability, as evidenced by positive Barlow and/or Ortolani signs; limp or waddling gait in the older child; limited abduction on affected side	Presence of synovitis and necrosis on x-rays; limp; intermittent knee or hip soreness; child small for age; limited internal rotation and abduction on affected side	Radiographic demonstration of slippage; limp; intermittent knee or thigh pain that worsens with exercise; child large for age; external rotation of the affected leg

Joint synovitis, or septic hip, is a condition that can span age-groups. Hip pain and joint limitation are prominent manifestations. Pain is of more acute onset and may be accompanied by fever and laboratory signs of inflammation.

REFERENCES and READINGS

Alexander, M., Ackman, J., & Kuo, K. (1999). Congenital idiopathic club foot. *Orthopaedic Nursing, 18*(4), 47-58.

American Academy of Pediatrics. (1998). In-line skating injuries in children and adolescents. *Pediatrics, 101*(4), 720-722.

American Academy of Family Physicians. (1999). Infant hip problems. *American Family Physician, 60*(1), 187-188.

American Academy of Family Physicians. (1998). Slipped capital femoral epiphysis. *American Family Physician, 57*(9), 2148-2150.

Anderson, B. (1999). *Office orthopedics for primary care diagnosis and treatment* (2nd ed.). Philadelphia: Saunders.

Anderson, S. (2002). Lower extremity injuries in youth sports. *Pediatric Clinics of North America, 49*, 627-641.

Arnold, T., & Shelbourne, K.D. (2000). A perioperative rehabilitation program for anterior cruciate ligament surgery. *The Physician and Sportsmedicine, 28*(1), 31-44.

Astrom, E., & Soderhall, S. (2002). Beneficial effect of long term intravenous biphosphonate treatment of osteogenesis imperfecta. *Archives of Disease in Childhood, 86*(5), 356-365.

Barlow, J., Shaw, K., & Harrison, K. (1999). Consulting the "experts": Children's and parents' perceptions of psycho-educational interventions in the context of juvenile chronic arthritis. *Health Education Research, 14*(5), 597-610.

Barlow, T.G. (1962). Early diagnosis and treatment of congenital dislocation of the hip. *Journal of Bone and Joint Surgery, 44B*(2), 292-301.

Bernardo, L.M. (2001). Evidence-based practice for pin site care in injured children. *Orthopaedic Nursing, 20*(5), 29-35.

Byrne, T. (1999). The setup and care of a patient in Buck's traction. *Orthopaedic Nursing, 18*(2), 79-83.

Cantu, R., & Mueller, F. (1999). Fatalities and catastrophic injuries in high school and college sports, 1982-1997. *The Physician and Sportsmedicine, 27*(8), 35-48.

Corbett, J. (1998). Laboratory tests and diagnostic procedures in orthopedic nursing practice. *Nursing Clinics of North America, 33*(4), 685-700.

Cummings, J., Davidson, R., Armstrong, P., & Lehman, W. (2002). Congenital clubfoot. *Journal of Bone and Joint Surgery, 84*(2), 290-309.

Day, M. (1999). Compartment syndrome. *Nursing 1999, 29*(6), 33.

DiFazio, R. (2003). Creating a halo traction wheelchair resource manual: Using the EBP approach. *Journal of Pediatric Nursing, 18*(2), 148-152.

DiFiori, J. (1999). Overuse injuries in children and adolescents. *The Physician and Sportsmedicine, 27*(1), 75-89.

Dyment, P. (1999). The hip. In F. Burg, J. Ingelfinger, E. Wald, & R. Polin (Eds.). *Gellis & Kagan's current pediatric therapy* (16th ed., pp. 934-936). Philadelphia, PA: Saunders.

Fernbach, S. (1998). Common orthopedic problems of the newborn. *Nursing Clinics of North America, 33*(4), 583-594.

French, L., & Dietz, F. (1999). Screening for developmental dysplasia of the hip. *American Family Physician, 60*(1), 177-183.

Green, M., Haggerty, R., & Weitzman, M. (1999). *Ambulatory pediatrics* (5th ed.). Philadelphia: Saunders.

Green, N., & Swiontkowski, M. (1998). *Skeletal trauma in children* (2nd ed.). Philadelphia: Saunders.

Hager, C., & Brncick, N. (1998). Fat embolism syndrome: A complication of orthopaedic trauma. *Orthopaedic Nursing, 17*(2), 41-58.

Hansen, M. (1998). *Pathophysiology: Foundations of disease and clinical intervention* (Ch. 34). Philadelphia: Saunders.

Harcke, H. (1999). Developmental dysplasia of the hip: A spectrum of abnormality. *Pediatrics, 103*(1), 152-153.

Hart, K., & Kester, K. (1999). Supracondylar fractures in children. *Orthopaedic Nursing, 18*(3), 23-27.

Hixon, A., & Gibbs, L. (2000). Osteochondritis dissecans: A diagnosis not to miss. *American Family Physician, 61*(1), 151-156.

Ilowite, N. (2002). Current treatment of juvenile rheumatoid arthritis. *Pediatrics, 109*(1), 109-115.

Kautz, S., & Skaggs, D. (1998). Getting an angle on spinal deformities. *Contemporary Pediatrics, 15*(9), 111-118.

Kester, K. (1997). Epidural pain management for the pediatric spinal fusion patient. *Orthopaedic Nursing, 16*(6), 55-62.

Lampe, R. (2004). Osteomyelitis and suppurative arthritis. In R. Behrman, R. Kliegman, & H. Jenson (Eds.), *Nelson textbook of pediatrics* (17th ed., pp. 2297-2302). Philadelphia: Saunders.

Lee, K.C., & Huie, G. (1999). Slipped capital femoral epiphysis. *Physician Assistant, 23*(2), 47, 50, 53-56.

Lewis, A.M. (1999). Orthopedic and vascular emergencies. *Nursing 1999, 29*(12), 54-56.

Loder, R. (1998). Slipped capital femoral epiphysis. *American Family Physician, 57*(9), 2135-2142.

Luke, A., & Micheli, L. (1999). Sports injuries: Emergency assessment and field-side care. *Pediatric Review, 20*(9), 291-301.

Macias, C., Bothner, J., & Wiebe, R. (1998). A comparison of supination/flexion to hyperpronation in the reduction of radial head subluxations. *Pediatrics, 102*(1), e10.

Mangini, M. (1998). Physical assessment of the musculoskeletal system. *Nursing Clinics of North America, 33*(4), 643-652.

Marini, J. (2004). Osteogenesis imperfecta. In R. Behrman, R. Kliegman, & H. Jenson (Eds.), *Nelson textbook of pediatrics* (17th ed., pp. 2336-2338). Philadelphia, PA: Saunders.

Marlowe, A. (2002). Testing for osteogenesis imperfecta in cases of suspected non-accidental injury. *Journal of Medical Genetics, 39*(6), 382-387.

McKenzie, L. (1999). In search of a standard for pin site care. *Orthopaedic Nursing, 18*(2), 73-78.

Metzl, J. (2002). Expectations of pediatric sport participation among pediatricians, patients, and

parents. *Pediatric Clinics of North America, 49*, 497-504.

Miller, M., & Cassidy, J. (2004). Juvenile rheumatoid arthritis. In R. Behrman, R. Kliegman, & H. Jenson (Eds.), *Nelson textbook of pediatrics* (17th ed., pp. 799-805). Philadelphia: Saunders.

O'Neil, K. (1998). Juvenile arthritis. In L. Finberg (Ed.), *Saunders manual of pediatric practice*. Philadelphia: Saunders.

Patterson, M. (1999). Prevention: The only cure for pediatric trauma. *Orthopaedic Nursing, 18*(4), 16-20.

Perlman, M., Patzakis, M., Kumar, P., & Holtom, P. (2000). The incidence of joint involvement with adjacent osteomyelitis in pediatric patients. *Journal of Pediatric Orthopedics, 20*(1), 40-43.

Randolph, C. (1998). Considerations for the orthopedic nurse in diagnosis and treatment of adolescent sports injuries. *Nursing Clinics of North America, 33*(4), 615-628.

Ryu, R., & Fan, R. (1998). Adolescent and pediatric sports injuries. *Pediatric Clinics of North America, 45*(6), 1601-1635.

Santy, J. (2000). Nursing the patient with an external fixator. *Nursing Standard, 14*(31), 47-52.

Sarnat, H. (2004). Neuromuscular disorders. In R. Behrman, R. Kliegman, & H. Jenson (Eds.), *Nelson textbook of pediatrics* (17th ed., pp. 2060-2064). Philadelphia: Saunders.

Schwend, R., & Geiger, J. (1998). Outpatient pediatric orthopedics. *Pediatric Clinics of North America, 45*(4), 943-971.

Shah, S. (2002). The hip. In F. Burg, J. Ingelfinger, R. Polin, & A. Gershon (Eds.). *Gellis & Kagan's current pediatric therapy* (17th ed., p. 844). Philadelphia: Saunders.

Shaw, B., Gerardi, J., & Hennrikus, W. (1999). How to avoid orthopedic pitfalls in children. *Patient Care, 33*(4), 95-106.

Slowikowski, R., & Flaherty, S. (2000). Epidural analgesia for postoperative orthopaedic pain. *Orthopaedic Nursing, 19*(1), 23-33.

Sprague, J. (1998). Cast syndrome: The superior mesenteric artery syndrome. *Orthopaedic Nursing, 17*(4), 12-17.

Sydell, W. (1999). Care of patients in casts. *Nursing Standard, 14*(8), 55.

Theophilopoulos, E., & Barrett, D. (1998). Get a grip on the pediatric hip. *Contemporary Pediatrics, 15*(11), 43-50.

Thompson, G.H. (2004). Bone and joint disorders. In R. Behrman, R. Kliegman, & H. Jenson (Eds.), *Nelson textbook of pediatrics* (17th ed., pp. 2251-2297). Philadelphia: Saunders.

Walls, M. (2002). Orthopedic trauma. *RN, 65*(7), 52-57.

Woo, P., & Wedderburn, L.R. (1998). Juvenile chronic arthritis. *Lancet, 351*, 969-973.

51

The Child with an Endocrine or Metabolic Alteration

LEARNING OBJECTIVES

After studying this chapter, you should be able to:

◎ List the major hormones of the endocrine system.
◎ Describe negative feedback.
◎ Discuss nursing strategies to improve cooperation with medication administration.
◎ Discuss and describe endocrine problems seen in the neonate.
◎ Describe the signs and symptoms of hypothyroidism versus hyperthyroidism.
◎ Compare and contrast the relationship between diabetes insipidus and syndrome of inappropriate antidiuretic hormone as they relate to fluid and electrolyte balance.
◎ Describe the psychosocial issues concerning children with precocious puberty.

◎ Identify the role of insulin in the metabolism of carbohydrates, fats, and proteins in both the fasting and postprandial states.
◎ Compare and contrast type 1 diabetes mellitus and type 2 diabetes mellitus.
◎ Identify management goals and nursing implications of insulin therapy, diet therapy, exercise, self-monitoring of blood glucose, and urine ketone monitoring in the management of the child with type 1 diabetes.
◎ Describe the signs, symptoms, causes, and treatment of hypoglycemia and hyperglycemia in the child with diabetes.
◎ Identify the pathophysiology of diabetic ketoacidosis, and describe the management and nursing care of the child in diabetic ketoacidosis.

DEFINITIONS

beta cells Specialized cells in the pancreas that manufacture and secrete insulin; thought to be the target of the autoimmune destructive process of type 1 diabetes mellitus.

diabetic ketoacidosis (DKA) Metabolic consequence of severe insulin deficiency; marked by hyperglycemia, acidosis, and ketosis.

euthyroid Normal thyroid function.

gland An organ or structure that secretes a substance or hormone to be used in another part of the body.

glucagon A hormone produced by the alpha cells of the pancreas; counteracts the action of insulin by converting liver stores of glycogen to blood glucose, resulting in an elevation of the blood glucose concentration.

glucose The substrate of choice for cellular energy; the breakdown product of stored glycogen or dietary carbohydrate.

glycosuria Glucose in urine that occurs when the blood glucose level exceeds the renal threshold and glucose "spills" into the urine.

glycosylated hemoglobin A laboratory test used to evaluate long-term blood glucose control by measuring glycosylation (glucose attachment to a protein) of a portion of the hemoglobin molecule in red blood cells; offers a 3-month average of blood glucose control.

honeymoon phase An early stage of diabetes characterized by residual endogenous insulin production that results in a lower need for exogenous insulin to maintain normal blood glucose.

hormone A chemical substance produced by one gland or tissue and transported by the blood to other tissues or organs, where it causes a specific effect.

hyperglycemia Blood glucose in a diabetic child above the target range; in a nondiabetic child, fasting blood glucose of 110 mg/dl or higher.

hyperkalemia Elevated serum potassium above the range for age.

hypoglycemia Blood glucose levels below 70 mg/dl.

hypothalamus Portion of the brain that secretes releasing factors to the pituitary gland for the maintenance of endocrine and metabolic activities.

idiopathic For unknown reasons.

ketone, ketoacid An acid produced in response to starvation (in the diabetic child a result of insulin deficiency); produced from fat stores, which can be used for energy by some tissues when glucose is unavailable.

Kussmaul respiration Deep, rapid respiration seen with DKA, in which carbon dioxide (CO_2) is expelled as a respiratory compensation for acidosis; also described as *air hunger*.

pituitary An endocrine gland attached to the base of the brain that secretes numerous hormones including thyroid-stimulating hormone (TSH), growth hormone (GH), adrenocorticotropic hormone (ACTH), antidiuretic hormone (ADH), prolactin, luteinizing hormone (LH), and follicle-stimulating hormone (FSH).

REVIEW OF THE ENDOCRINE SYSTEM

The endocrine system comprises various tissues that produce and secrete chemicals called *hormones*. The hormones stimulate and regulate the actions of other tissues—the target tissues.

The endocrine system and the autonomic nervous system function in tandem to regulate growth, metabolism, and reproduction. The hypothalamic-pituitary axis controls their activities. The autonomic nervous system reacts to a stimulus, transmitting its message to the hypothalamus. In turn, the hypothalamus manufactures and secretes the appropriate hormonal factors. These are transmitted to the anterior pituitary gland, which then stimulates or inhibits the release of the involved hormones.

The principle of feedback control is involved in hormone production and secretion. In negative feedback, increasing levels of a specific hormone begin to inhibit the system responsible for releasing that hormone. As the hormonal secretion rises, there is a corresponding decrease in secretion and production of its stimulating hormone. Conversely, when there is too little circulating hormone, the target gland is stimulated to secrete additional hormone.

The pituitary gland is composed of an anterior lobe and a posterior lobe. The anterior lobe secretes adrenocorticotropic hormone (ACTH), thyroid-stimulating hormone (TSH), follicle-stimulating hormone (FSH), luteinizing hormone (LH), growth hormone (GH), and prolactin. Four of these hormones (ACTH, TSH, LH, FSH) in turn stimulate their target glands to secrete the appropriate specific hormones.

Pediatric Differences in the Endocrine System

- The endocrine system is less developed at birth than any other body system.
- Hormonal control of many body functions is lacking until 12 to 18 months of age. As a result, infants might manifest imbalances in concentration of fluids, electrolytes, amino acids, glucose, and trace substances.

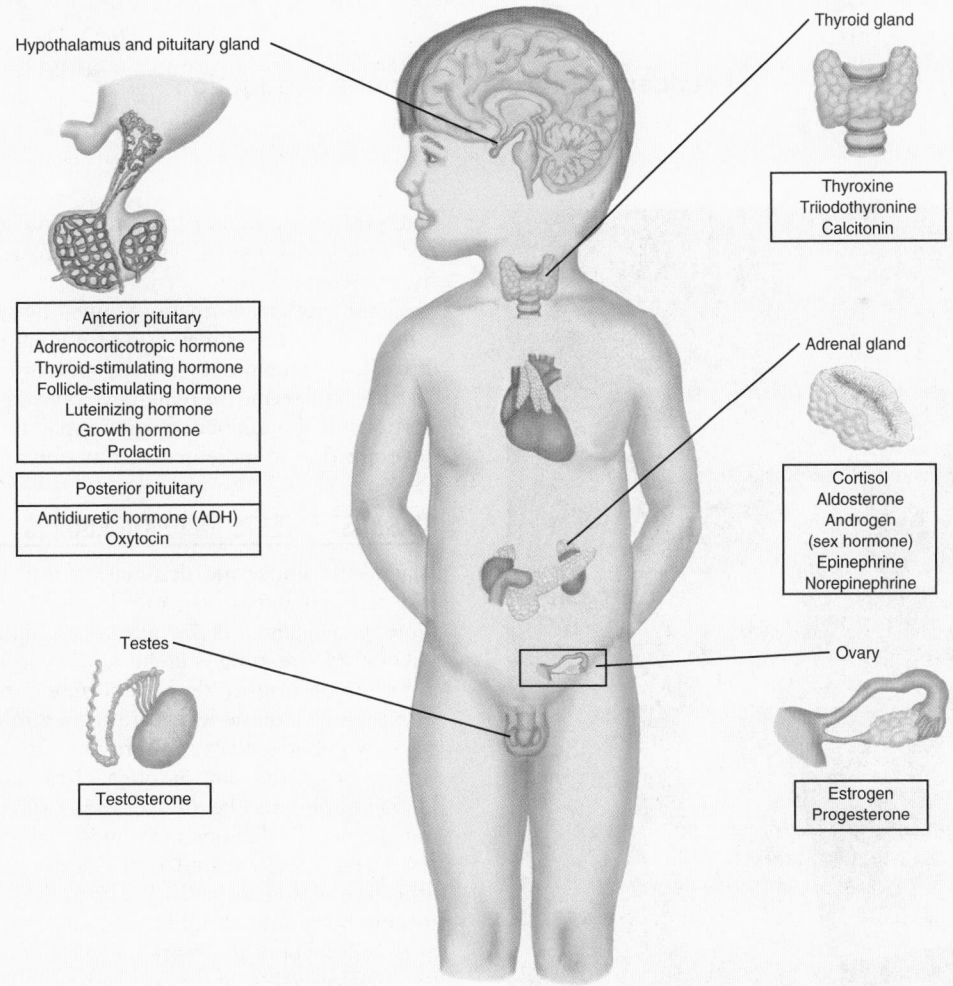

Anatomy of the Endocrine System

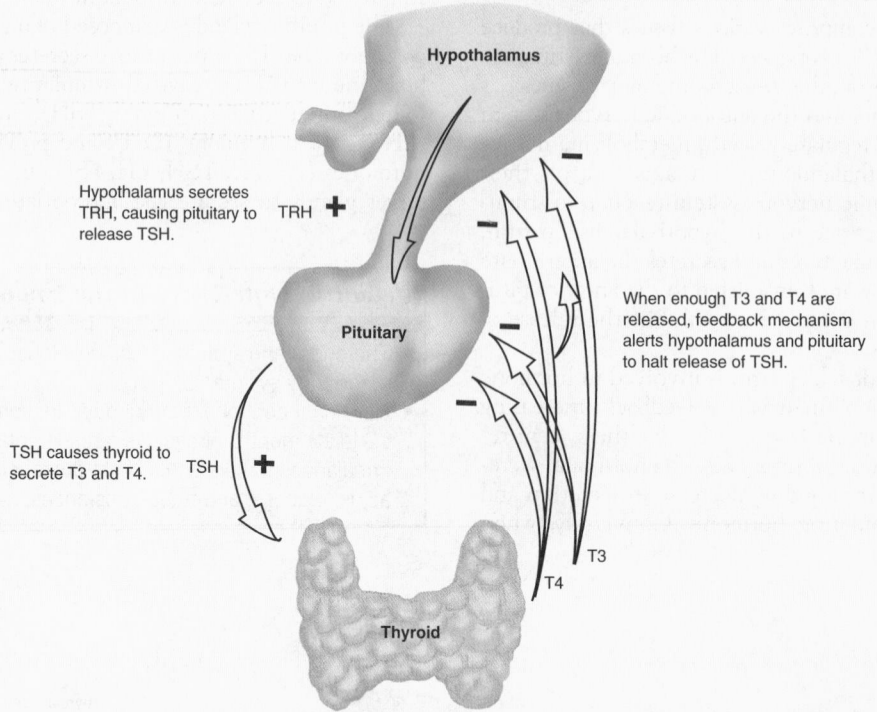

Hypothalamus secretes TRH, causing pituitary to release TSH.

TRH **+**

When enough T3 and T4 are released, feedback mechanism alerts hypothalamus and pituitary to halt release of TSH.

TSH causes thyroid to secrete T3 and T4.

TSH **+**

Feedback Control in Hormone Production

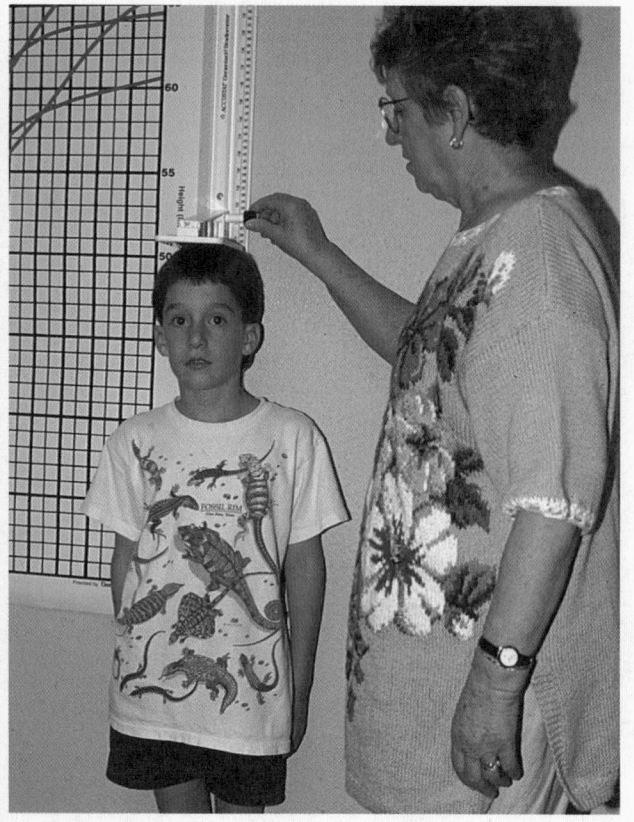

The posterior pituitary lobe stores and releases antidiuretic hormone (ADH) and oxytocin, which are synthesized by the hypothalamus.

Congenital malformations, infections, neoplastic or autoimmune processes may disrupt normal endocrine function at the hypothalamus, pituitary gland, or target gland.

Fetal endocrine systems develop and function *in utero*. Portions of the endocrine system may be immature at birth but transition to more mature function after delivery.

DIAGNOSTIC TESTS AND PROCEDURES

Diagnosing endocrine dysfunction usually involves laboratory testing. Serum hormone levels are measured to determine if the amounts are adequate, deficient, or excessive. Laboratory screening is useful for diagnosis of disease as well as for monitoring children on hormone therapy.

Normal hormone levels are related to the child's age and stage of puberty. Because hormones are secreted at various times during the day or on a circadian rhythm, random blood samples may be difficult to interpret. Stimulation testing frequently demonstrates more accurate and definitive test results. With stimulation testing, a releasing factor or other agent is given to trigger the release or inhibition of a specific hormone. Serial blood sampling identifies the peak or trough level of the hormone, aiding in more accurate interpretation. A list of the common stimulation studies is provided in the table.

Common Laboratory and Diagnostic Tests of Endocrine Function

Test	Description	Normal Findings	Indications	Preparation and Nursing Considerations
Growth hormone (GH) test	An agent (e.g., insulin, arginine, clonidine) is given to stimulate release of GH.	One or more peak levels of GH >7-10 ng/ml.	Evaluate GH production. Identify GH deficiency.	Time specific; specimens must be drawn accurately. NPO after midnight. Notify physician if hypoglycemia or hypotension develops.
Cortrosyn test	Cortrosyn (ACTH) is given after baseline laboratory values have been obtained and 1 hr later. Tests adrenal gland's ability to function.	Cortisol should rise at least double the baseline. Cortisol <18 mcg/dl suggests adrenal insufficiency.	Evaluate adrenal production of cortisol. Identify infants with congenital adrenal hyperplasia.	Time specific; laboratory samples must be drawn before and 1 hr after Cortrosyn.
Factrel (gonadorelin) test	GnRH is administered IV or subcutaneously to test the pituitary-ovarian axis for central precocious puberty.	For IV test, <4-fold to 5-fold rise in LH is observed. For subcutaneous test, LH rises <8 ng/ml.	Evaluate for central precocious puberty. Identify premature thelarche.	Time specific; specimens must be drawn accurately. IV test with serial sampling of LH, FSH. Subcutaneous test with one laboratory sample drawn at 40 min.
Water deprivation test	Child deprived of water and fluids for 7-8 hr.	Decreased urine output. Increased urine specific gravity. Normal serum sodium and osmolality.	Confirm diagnosis of diabetes insipidus.	Strict monitoring of serum sodium and serum and urine osmolality. Weigh child before, during, and after test. Stop test if significant weight loss or change in vital signs or neurologic status develops.
hCG test	Intramuscular hCG is administered serially to stimulate testicular production of testosterone. Allows test for conversion of testosterone to DHT. Tests function of undescended testes.	Low levels of testosterone and DHT in prelaboratory samples. Elevated levels of both testosterone and DHT—compare with known standards.	Confirm testicular insufficiency. Confirm 5-α-reductase deficiency. Undescended testes may descend.	Time specific; draw samples before and after hCG. Monitor for testicular descent and increase in phallic length.

NPO, Nothing by mouth; *ACTH*, adrenocorticotropic hormone; *GnRH*, gonadotropin-releasing hormone; *IV*, intravenously; *LH*, luteinizing hormone; *FSH*, follicle-stimulating hormone. *hCG*, human chorionic gonadotropin; *DHT*, dihydrotestosterone.

Other diagnostic tests include radiography and imaging techniques. Bone age radiographs can determine bone maturation, and from this, growth potential can be determined. Computed tomography (CT) scans and magnetic resonance imaging (MRI) are used to determine the presence of tumors or congenital malformations affecting the hypothalamus, pituitary, or target glands.

Accurate measurements of height and weight are essential when assessing the child for endocrine function. Evaluation of sexual development according to Tanner stages is also a part of the diagnostic work-up (see Chapter 8). Developmental milestones and school performance should also be monitored because delays might be associated with endocrine disorders.

CLINICAL REFERENCE

Pediatric endocrine disorders are generally managed in the outpatient setting. Most endocrine disorders are chronic conditions requiring long-term nursing management. The nurse assumes a role of both educator and advocate for the child. Also important for the care of children with chronic medical problems is a careful psychosocial evaluation on a regular basis.

PHENYLKETONURIA

Phenylketonuria (PKU) is a genetic metabolic disorder that results in central nervous system (CNS) damage from toxic levels of phenylalanine in the blood. In PKU, there is a deficiency of phenylalanine hydroxylase, the enzyme needed to convert phenylalanine to tyrosine.

Etiology

PKU is an autosomal recessive disorder and is manifested only in the homozygote (individual who inherited two identical genes for a specific trait). With both parents carrying the recessive gene, each pregnancy has a 25% chance that the child will have PKU.

Incidence

PKU occurs in approximately 1 in 10,000 to 25,000 births in the United States (Glass, 1999). It is more prevalent in some European countries.

Manifestations

The underlying metabolic alterations begin to have an immediate effect on the infant, although signs may not be apparent until the infant is approximately 3 months old. The first sign may be digestive problems with vomiting. These infants also may experience musty or mousy odor to the urine, infantile eczema, hypertonia, and hyperactive behavior. Older children may have hypopigmentation of the hair, skin, and irises, and they are commonly blond with light blue eyes. Mental retardation is a long-term consequence of untreated PKU.

Pathophysiology

of Phenylketonuria

Phenylketonuria (PKU) refers to a group of biochemical diseases associated with enzymatic blocks in the conversion of the essential amino acid *phenylalanine* to *tyrosine*. Classic PKU consists of the absence of the enzyme *phenylalanine hydroxylase*. This deficiency results in the toxic accumulation of phenylalanine in the bloodstream after the ingestion of protein containing phenylalanine. Phenylalanine can adversely affect the myelinization process in central nervous system (CNS) development. Most of that process takes place during the first decade of life. Mental retardation occurs and will progress if treatment is not implemented.

Diagnostic Evaluation

Routine neonatal screening for PKU is mandatory in all 50 states of the United States. With early postpartum discharge, screening is often performed at less than 2 days of age because of the concern that the infant will be lost to follow-up. Because the test depends on the accumulation of phenylalanine, screening done before the 3rd day of life has a higher risk of a false-negative outcome. For this reason, testing should be done after the infant is 48 hours old, or, if done earlier, the test should be repeated at several days of age. Small quantities of blood are collected on filter paper cards. Screening is done using bacterial inhibition (Guthrie test) or chromatographic or fluorometric assays. A positive result is not diagnostic but indicates which infants should be evaluated further. PKU is characterized by serum phenylalanine levels greater than 20 mg/dl (normal level <2 mg/dl) (Rezvani, 2000).

Therapeutic Management

Treatment should be instituted as soon as the diagnosis is confirmed because the best results are obtained with early treatment. Infants and children with PKU are treated with a special diet that restricts phenylalanine intake. Phenylalanine tolerance varies according to the infant and the severity of the enzyme deficiency. The goal of therapy is to keep the serum phenylalanine level at 2 to 6 mg/dl in infants and young children and 2 to 15 mg/dl in children older than 12 years. It is important to limit phenylalanine intake while providing enough to meet the body's growth requirement of this essential amino acid. Dietary management must be started early in neonatal life because the untreated infant will show evidence of CNS damage by several weeks of age. Recent results of long-term studies done on adults who discontinued the restricted diet in middle childhood have suggested that these people experience a decrease in mental function that can occur years after discontinuing the diet. For this reason, a recent National Institutes of Health (NIH) Consensus Panel (2000) has recommended lifelong dietary restrictions.

Another consideration is women with the disorder who become pregnant. Adolescent girls require counseling about fetal risks, which can include mental deficiency, microcephaly, retarded growth, seizures, and an increased incidence of structural defects. The goal is to control phenylalanine levels before conception and maintain strict control during the pregnancy.

Nursing Considerations

Although a family history of PKU would alert the caregiver to an infant at risk, most infants with PKU are not identified at birth. Neonatal symptoms are usually not present. A screening test, part of the newborn screen done in all states, is the first diagnostic procedure. Newborn screenings usually include testing for PKU and congenital hypothyroidism as well as any other screening tests mandated by local and state public health departments, such as sickle cell trait, galactosemia, or maple syrup urine disease. A positive screening result requires further diagnostic evaluation to verify the diagnosis.

A low-phenylalanine diet is begun immediately. The infant is fed with low-phenylalanine formula, and as foods are introduced, the child must follow a protein-restricted diet. The child avoids high-protein foods, such as meats, fish, eggs, cheese, milk, and legumes. Because protein is also present in grains, low-protein breads, cereals, and pastas are used. Dietary staples are vegetables, fruits, and starches. To avoid the consequences of insufficient protein for growth, children with PKU may take a phenylalanine-free protein supplement. The growth pattern and neurobehavior of the affected child must be followed.

Follow-up is provided for all infants if the initial screening result is abnormal. The nurse assists with referral to a genetic center that is capable of diagnosing and treating the infant. Phenylalanine requirements change rapidly in the first months of life. Encourage parental adherence with monitoring requirements for the infant diagnosed with PKU. Rigid regimens for diet control will not be successful unless the family accepts the changes required. Assist the family in dealing with lifestyle changes by initiating referrals as needed (e.g., to social service agencies, registered dietitian, support groups). On-line support groups and chat rooms provide helpful ideas for adapting recipes; specialized cookbooks are also available.

Encourage the parents to express their feelings about the infant's diagnosis and the risk of PKU in future children. Assist family members in recognizing the problems caused by the disease, and help them identify strategies for dealing with the stress of having a child with a chronic illness. Physical measurements and neurologic and intellectual development should be documented through standardized testing. If good control is established early, normal infant growth and development should occur.

INBORN ERRORS OF METABOLISM

Rarely, infants are born with other genetically transmitted metabolic disease (Table 51-1). It is important for nurses to create a climate in which parents can express their feelings not only about the lifelong care of their child but also about concerns for future pregnancies. Families with affected infants are referred to genetic counseling centers. Many of these infants are identified through universal newborn screening or screening specific for at-risk infants. Additional nursing care is related specifically to the disorder but is similar to that for the child with PKU.

CONGENITAL ADRENAL HYPERPLASIA

Congenital adrenal hyperplasia (CAH) is a group of disorders in which the adrenal gland is not able to manufacture adequate glucocorticoid and, while working to make glucocorticoid, produces excess androgens. CAH is caused by a defect in the enzymatic pathway of adrenal steroid production. Diminished glucocorticoid production prompts increased ACTH production, further increasing adrenal androgen excess.

TABLE 51-1 Inborn Errors of Metabolism

Condition	Description	Management
Galactosemia	A deficiency of galactose-1-phosphate uridylyl-transferase prevents the conversion of galactose to glucose in lactose digestion. Infants cannot properly digest milk or sugar. Although rare (1 in 60,000 to 80,000 live births), infants exhibit intrauterine growth retardation, hypoglycemia, liver damage, cataracts, and infections. The urine contains reducing substances. Vomiting and diarrhea occur after feedings.	The child is on a lifelong lactose-restricted diet and close monitoring for and treatment of infections. If untreated, the infant usually dies; infants who have been treated may experience developmental or learning deficits. The condition is genetically transmitted through an autosomal recessive inheritance pattern; referral to a genetic counseling center is warranted.
Maple syrup urine disease	This is a very rare (1 in 250,000 to 300,000 live births) autosomal recessive inherited condition that affects metabolism of certain amino acids. Buildup of acids causes ketoacidosis, which appears 48-72 hr after birth. The infant is lethargic and can experience poor feeding, vomiting, weight loss, seizures, and loss of reflexes. The urine smells like maple syrup.	Dialysis is needed to reduce accumulated acids. The child must be on a lifelong low-protein, limited–amino acid diet. If untreated, the child can die quickly; children who have been treated can experience neurologic deficits. Referral to a genetic counseling center is warranted.
Tay-Sachs disease	A genetic condition that affects primarily infants in the Ashkenazi Jewish population. It is caused by an abnormal buildup of gangliosides (normal constituents in nerve synapse membrane) in the neurons. After a 6-mo period of relatively normal development, the infant begins to demonstrate developmental delay and progressive neurologic deterioration. The infant usually exhibits macrocephaly, seizures, blindness, and deafness; death occurs during early childhood.	Management is symptomatic and supportive to the child and family. Referral to a genetic counseling center is essential.

Data from Haslam, R. (2000). The nervous system. In R. Behrman, R. Kliegman, & H. Jenson (Eds.), *Nelson textbook of pediatrics* (16th ed., p. 1850). Philadelphia: Saunders; Glass, S. (1999). Genetic screening. In P. Thureen, J. Deacon, P. O'Neill, & J. Hernandez (Eds.), *Assessment and care of the well newborn* (pp. 216-217). Philadelphia: Saunders.

Mineralocorticoid production may be normal or low. Infants with diminished mineralocorticoid production will waste salt through the kidneys, resulting in a "salt-wasting" crisis. Salt-wasting crisis results in hypovolemia, low serum sodium levels, and hyperkalemia. Several enzymatic defects have been identified, the most common being 21-hydroxylase deficiency. CAH is an autosomal recessive condition.

Manifestations

CAH is marked by ambiguous genitalia of the newborn female infant; postnatal virilization in both genders; and salt-wasting crisis (first few weeks of life) with low serum sodium, high serum potassium, hypovolemia, and hypotensive crisis. Simple virilizing CAH is not associated with a salt-wasting crisis and presents with a muscular body, advanced bone age, and premature pubic hair. Typically, this form presents later in infancy or early childhood. Untreated or poorly treated CAH can result in an advanced bone age with ultimate adult short stature. A milder form of CAH, 3-beta-hydroxysteroid dehydrogenase (3β-HSD), may present in childhood or adolescence with hirsutism, menstrual irregularities, or delayed menses.

Diagnostic Evaluation

The finding of ambiguous genitalia in the newborn infant should raise the possibility of CAH. The diagnosis is confirmed by elevated values of 17-hydroxyprogesterone, a glucocorticoid precursor. CAH is a part of newborn screening in many states. Appropriate evaluation including electrolytes, CO_2, and physical examination may avert a salt-wasting crisis. Serum sodium levels in the infant suspected of CAH will be low, with elevated serum potassium. Serum renin levels in this setting will be elevated, indicating mineralocorticoid deficiency. A karyotype to determine genetic gender may be indicated, depending on the degree of genital ambiguity.

Therapeutic Management

Treatment for the child with CAH involves lifelong glucocorticoid therapy. Oral glucocorticoid (hydrocortisone acetate, cortisone acetate) dosage is prescribed based on body size and is given two or three times per day in either liquid suspension or tablet form. For children with salt-wasting CAH, mineralocorticoid replacement is required. Fludrocortisone acetate (Florinef) is prescribed to be taken once or twice daily. Therapy is evaluated with serum electrolytes, 17-hydroxyprogesterone levels, and renin levels if mineralocorticoid replacement therapy is required. Special sick-day instructions should be provided to the family. The glucocorticoid dosage is usually doubled or tripled when the child is ill, has a broken bone, or is undergoing a surgical procedure. Bone age radiographs are performed yearly to assess skeletal maturity; poor adherence or undertreatment results in advanced bone age and will decrease final height.

Nursing Considerations

All newborn girls should be assessed for ambiguous genitalia: fused labia, enlarged clitoris, or migration of urethral opening. Infant boys with unexplained dehydration and low serum

---

! CRITICAL TO REMEMBER

Congenital Adrenal Hyperplasia

- Children with salt-wasting congenital adrenal hyperplasia (CAH) require glucocorticoid replacement to survive.
- In the event of significant stress, such as fever, broken bone, or surgery, children with CAH will require "stress dose" medical therapy.
- If the child with CAH develops vomiting, the glucocorticoid must be administered parenterally.
- Mineralocorticoid therapy is required in salt-wasting CAH.
- Occasionally, supplemental sodium may also be required.

---

sodium should be considered to have adrenal insufficiency, requiring careful assessment of fluid and electrolyte status.

Infant girls with ambiguous genitalia might require reconstructive surgery. Depending on degree of virilization, surgical correction may be recommended in infancy or in early puberty. If appropriate, reassure parents that the infant has appropriate internal structures and that external structures can be corrected surgically. Allow them to express any concerns, and encourage parent-infant attachment.

Assess older children receiving glucocorticoid replacement therapy for growth and signs of early puberty. Noncompliance can cause early virilization, increased growth velocity, diminished final adult height, and menstrual irregularities in girls. Blood pressure monitoring is important for children receiving mineralocorticoid replacement therapy.

Instruct parents about replacement hormone administration and the timing of medication. Develop a plan for sickday dosage of medication. The infant with salt-wasting CAH may require salt supplements; the family needs instruction on preparation of the supplement.

Follow-up evaluations with the endocrinologist are scheduled every 2 to 3 months in infancy and every 4 to 6 months in the older child. Parents of the child with CAH should be referred to a genetics counselor if planning more pregnancies, because future children are at risk for CAH. *In utero* treatment is available to prevent virilization of the female fetus. This eliminates the need for surgical correction of ambiguous genitalia in the affected female infant.

Encourage the adolescent to assume increasing responsibility for medication administration. Emphasize the importance of adherence. Surgical genital reconstruction and vaginal dilation may be required in the adolescent years. Careful explanations of procedures reassure affected adolescents that they are "normal."

CONGENITAL HYPOTHYROIDISM

Congenital hypothyroidism is a condition in which the thyroid gland does not produce sufficient thyroid hormone to meet the body's metabolic needs. The condition is present from birth and, if not treated, can lead to mental retardation.

Etiology

Congenital hypothyroidism is caused by an absent (aplastic), underdeveloped, or ectopic thyroid gland. This group of congenital defects is referred to as *thyroid dysgenesis*. For unknown reasons, the fetal thyroid gland fails to develop properly or fails to migrate to the appropriate location. Other rare causes are hypothalamic or pituitary disorders in which TSH is insufficient to stimulate the thyroid gland. Biochemical defects in thyroid hormone production also cause congenital hypothyroidism. Maternal intake of medications such as propylthiouracil (PTU) during pregnancy to control maternal hyperthyroidism can cause transient hypothyroidism in the infant. Transfer of maternal antibodies to the fetus may also cause transient hypothyroidism (LaFranchi, 2002).

Incidence

Congenital hypothyroidism secondary to thyroid dysgenesis occurs in 1 in 4000 live births. Biochemical defects in thyroid hormone production occur in 1 of 30,000 live births. Hypothalamic-pituitary hypothyroidism occurs in 1 in 30,000 to 100,000 live births (LaFranchi, 2002). Because untreated hypothyroidism causes mental retardation, all states have mandatory newborn screening programs to diagnose hypothyroidism before symptoms occur. Early detection and treatment favor increased intellectual function. Most occurrences are spontaneous, with a smaller percentage having a genetic (autosomal recessive) inheritance that results in defective thyroxine synthesis (LaFranchi, 2004).

Manifestations

The infant with congenital hypothyroidism may display the following signs (Fig. 51-1): skin mottling, a large fontanel, a large tongue, hypotonia, slow reflexes, and a distended abdomen. Other signs and symptoms include prolonged jaundice, lethargy, constipation, feeding problems, coldness to touch, umbilical hernia, hoarse cry, and excessive sleeping. The infant with congenital hypothyroidism may have none of these signs or symptoms; screening is essential to recognize these infants.

Pathophysiology

of Congenital Hypothyroidism

The thyroid gland is a butterfly-shaped gland located in front of the neck. Thyroid-stimulating hormone (TSH), secreted by the pituitary, induces the thyroid to produce thyroxine (T_4) and triiodothyronine (T_3). The thyroid traps iodine and produces T_4, which is essential for normal growth and development, especially brain development, in the first 2 years of life. Immediately after delivery, TSH increases dramatically, likely related to the stress of the birth process. Within the first week of life, the TSH level gradually falls.

Underdevelopment of the thyroid gland or a hypothalamic or pituitary disorder causes inadequate production of T_4, which is essential for brain development. If not treated, this can cause mental retardation in the developing child. An infant with congenital hypothyroidism has an elevated TSH and a low T_4.

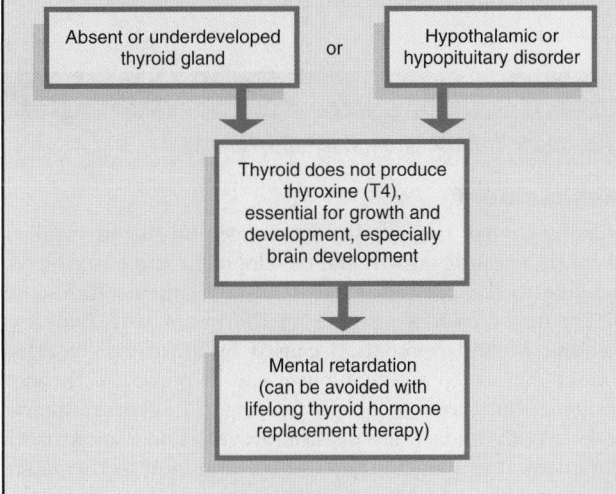

Absent or underdeveloped thyroid gland — **or** — Hypothalamic or hypopituitary disorder

↓

Thyroid does not produce thyroxine (T4), essential for growth and development, especially brain development

↓

Mental retardation (can be avoided with lifelong thyroid hormone replacement therapy)

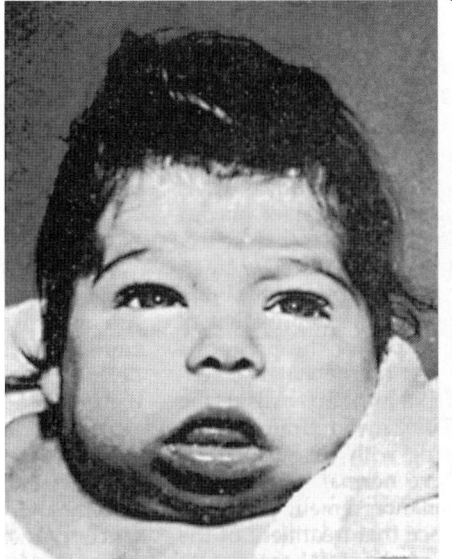

◄ Untreated congenital hypothyroidism in a 6-month-old infant

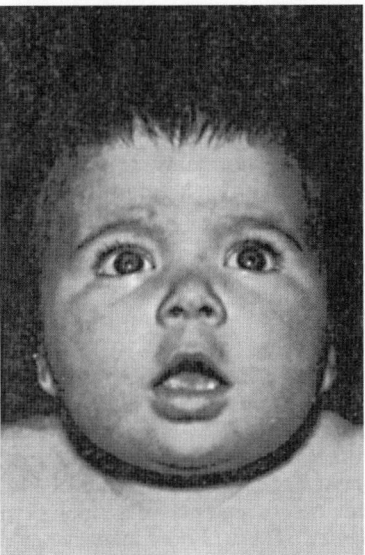

Four months after treatment ▶

Figure 51-1 A, This untreated 6-month-old infant with congenital hypothyroidism fed poorly and was constipated. She was very lethargic and had no social smile and no head control. Note her puffy face, large tongue, dull expression, and hirsute forehead. **B,** The same infant 4 months after treatment. Note the decreased facial puffiness, decreased hirsutism of the forehead, and an alert appearance. Newborn screening for hypothyroidism is important because treatment should begin in the first weeks of life to prevent mental retardation and other problems. Treatment consists of lifelong thyroid hormone replacement. (From Behrman, R.E., Kliegman, R.M., & Arvin, A.M. [1996]. *Nelson textbook of pediatrics* [15th ed., p. 1592]. Philadelphia: Saunders.)

Diagnostic Evaluation

Congenital hypothyroidism is usually diagnosed by newborn screening. Ideally, testing should be done at 2 to 6 days of age. Tests done sooner than 48 hours after delivery may be falsely interpreted because of the rise in TSH immediately after birth as part of the normal newborn transition.

Thyroid scans can identify any functioning thyroid tissue. Treatment should never be delayed while waiting for scan results.

Therapeutic Management

Treatment of children with congenital hypothyroidism consists of lifelong thyroid hormone replacement, usually in the form of levothyroxine. It is given as a single daily oral dose that varies with body size. The dosage is titrated to maintain TSH in a normal range and maintain T_4 in the upper half of the normal range (LaFranchi, 2002).

■ NURSING CARE
The Infant With Congenital Hypothyroidism

Assessment

Nursing care of the infant with congenital hypothyroidism involves assessing growth and development and ensuring adherence to the prescribed medication regimen. Nurses can play a major role in recognizing the infant with hypothyroidism. Mental retardation caused by untreated hypothyroidism cannot be reversed, but it can be prevented through early identification and proper treatment. In general, infants with hypothyroidism are evaluated every 1 to 2 months for the first year of life and then every 3 to 6 months thereafter. The nurse should obtain accurate measurements of height, weight, and head circumference at each visit. Frequent developmental assessment is also essential.

Nursing Diagnosis and Planning

The nursing diagnoses and expected outcomes that may be appropriate for the infant with congenital hypothyroidism and the infant's parents are

■ Deficient Knowledge related to unfamiliarity with the congenital disorder.
   Expected Outcomes: The parents will demonstrate the ability to monitor their infant for signs and symptoms of hypothyroidism and hyperthyroidism; will verbalize an understanding of normal growth and developmental milestones; will give thyroid medication properly; and will discuss the child's lifelong needs and routine.
■ Delayed Growth and Development related to disease process.
   Expected Outcome: As a result of appropriately managed disease, the infant will demonstrate growth and developmental milestones appropriate for age.
■ Ineffective Thermoregulation related to decreased basal metabolic rate.
   Expected Outcome: As a result of disease management, the infant will maintain a temperature within normal range.

Interventions

Instruct family members on the importance of medication adherence. Emphasize that the medication is necessary for the child's growth, especially for the rapidly developing brain.

! CRITICAL TO REMEMBER
The Child With Congenital Hypothyroidism

- Untreated hypothyroidism leads to mental retardation.
- Thyroxine (T_4) and thyroid-stimulating hormone (TSH) levels vary with age, but any infant with a low T_4 and a TSH value exceeding 40 mU/L is considered to have primary hypothyroidism until proven otherwise.*

*From American Academy of Pediatrics, & American Thyroid Association. (1993). Newborn screening for congenital hypothyroidism: Recommended guidelines. *Pediatrics, 91*(6), 1203-1209.

Teach the family how and when to administer the medication. Levothyroxine is given orally as a single daily dose. The medication can be dissolved in a small amount of water and given by syringe or placed into the nipple of a baby bottle along with a small amount of formula. Warn the caregiver not to dissolve the medication in a large amount of formula because, if the formula is unfinished, the infant will not receive the full dosage. When the infant is older, the medication can be given in a spoonful of cereal or baby food. If the infant or child vomits within 1 hour of taking medication, the dose should be readministered. Frequently missed doses can lead to developmental delays and poor growth.

Also, teach the parents the signs and symptoms of both hypothyroidism and hyperthyroidism and when to notify the physician if symptoms occur. Hyperthyroidism can develop in infants receiving too much medication. Parents need to be taught to count their child's pulse and to notify their health care provider if the rate is greater than the recommended parameter.

Because hypothyroidism is a lifelong condition, school-age children and teenagers should be made aware of the importance of taking their medication and of keeping regular follow-up appointments with the physician.

Evaluation

- Have the parents demonstrated ability to monitor the child's signs and symptoms, recognize growth and developmental problems, administer the medication, and discuss the child's lifelong needs and routines?
- Is the child developing appropriately for age according to growth charts and Denver Developmental Screening Test (DDST) scores?
- Does the child have normal results on thyroid function tests?
- Is the child's body temperature within normal limits?

ACQUIRED HYPOTHYROIDISM

Hypothyroidism is a condition in which the thyroid gland produces an inadequate amount of thyroid hormone to meet the body's metabolic needs.

Etiology

Hashimoto's thyroiditis, a common cause of acquired hypothyroidism, is usually associated with a goiter. It is an autoimmune process. Other causes of acquired hypothyroidism include surgical thyroidectomy, radioactive iodine therapy for hyperthyroidism, radiation therapy for malignancies, and excessive iodine ingestion. Less frequently, decreased TSH secretion by the pituitary gland or decreased thyrotropin-releasing hormone (TRH) secretion by the hypothalamus causes hypothyroidism.

Autoimmune thyroiditis is the most common cause of acquired hypothyroidism in children and adolescents. It often occurs in families with a history of thyroid disease. Other family members may have positive thyroid antibodies. Thyroiditis is more common in girls.

Pathophysiology

Circulating autoantibodies known as *thyroid-blocking immunoglobulins* decrease thyroid gland production of T_3 and T_4. These antibodies bind at the TSH receptor sites on the thyroid gland, resulting in decreased thyroid hormone production. The cause of antibody production is unknown.

In contrast to congenital hypothyroidism, adverse effects from hypothyroidism acquired after 2 to 3 years of age are often reversible. Goiter, an enlarged thyroid gland, occurs in response to increased TSH secretion, autoimmune attack of the thyroid gland, or goitrogens.

Manifestations

Clinical manifestations of hypothyroidism include goiter (one lobe frequently larger than the other); dry, thick skin; coarse, dull hair; fatigue; cold intolerance; constipation; weight gain; decreased linear growth; edema of face, eyes, and hands; and irregular or delayed menses.

Diagnostic Evaluation

An elevated TSH and low T_4 are diagnostic of hypothyroidism. Elevated TSH is the most sensitive indicator of primary hypothyroidism.

Thyroiditis is diagnosed by the presence of circulating thyroid antibodies and is usually associated with a firm goiter. Initially, TSH is elevated with normal T_4, although T_4 decreases over time. With secondary or tertiary hypothyroidism, TSH is not elevated; therefore TRH stimulation testing is usually required for diagnosis.

Therapeutic Management

Management of the child with hypothyroidism involves thyroid hormone replacement, usually with levothyroxine. Dosage varies according to the child's age and weight and is given as a single daily dose. The dose is titrated to maintain T_4 in the upper half of the normal range and to maintain TSH in the normal range for age.

▪ NURSING CARE
The Child With Acquired Hypothyroidism

Assessment

Care of the child with acquired hypothyroidism includes assessing response to treatment and adherence to the medication regimen. With treatment, the goiter should decrease in size. Signs and symptoms of hypothyroidism should also re-

solve with adequate thyroid hormone replacement. Monitoring height, weight, and performance on the DDST at each visit assesses the child's growth and development. The nurse should monitor school performance as well and maintain contact with the school nurse.

Nursing Diagnosis and Planning

The nursing diagnoses and expected outcomes that may be appropriate for a child with acquired hypothyroidism are

- Constipation related to decreased basal metabolic rate secondary to hypothyroidism.
  Expected Outcome: The child will maintain regular bowel movements of normal consistency as basal metabolic rate improves.
- Activity Intolerance related to fatigue.
  Expected Outcome: The child will maintain normal energy levels for age, as evidenced by the ability to exercise at the same level as peers.
- Disturbed Body Image related to weight gain/obesity.
  Expected Outcomes: The child will verbalize feelings about body changes and will accept reassurances that changes will resolve with treatment.
- Ineffective Thermoregulation related to decreased basal metabolic rate secondary to hypothyroidism.
  Expected Outcome: As a result of appropriate disease management, the child will maintain normal body temperature.

Interventions

Parents and school-age children or older should be instructed on the correct dose and timing of thyroid medication. Thyroid hormone levels are usually checked every 3 to 6 months. Laboratory values within the normal range indicate good response to therapy. Instruct parents on the signs and symptoms of hypothyroidism and hyperthyroidism and to notify the physician if symptoms occur. Reassure the child that signs such as constipation, fatigue, and weight gain will resolve as the medication becomes effective.

Evaluation

- Has the child maintained regular bowel movements of normal consistency?
- Can the child tolerate exercise at the same level as peers?
- Does the child express feelings related to body changes and accept reassurances that problems will resolve?
- Has the child maintained normal body temperature?

HYPERTHYROIDISM (GRAVES' DISEASE)

Graves' disease is an autoimmune condition in which excessive thyroid hormones are produced by an enlarged thyroid gland. It is the most common cause of hyperthyroidism in children.

Incidence

The incidence of Graves' disease in children is approximately 1 in 5000, with girls being five times more likely than boys to acquire the condition. Peak age for acquiring the condition is between 11 and 15 years (LaFranchi, 2004). There may also be a familial tendency toward Graves' disease. Children with autoimmune disease are at risk for other autoimmune disorders. Neonatal Graves' disease is associated with maternal hyperthyroidism and is relatively uncommon.

BOX 51-1
Hypothyroidism Versus Hyperthyroidism

Hypothyroidism	Hyperthyroidism
• Fatigue	• Nervousness, anxiety
• Constipation	• Diarrhea
• Cold intolerance	• Heat intolerance
• Weight gain	• Weight loss
• Dry, thick skin	• Smooth, velvety skin
• Edema of face, eyes, hands	• Prominent eyes
• Decreased growth	• Accelerated linear growth
• Decreased activity and energy	• Emotional lability
• Muscle hypertrophy (pseudodystrophy)	• Muscle weakness
• Decreased heart rate	• Increased heart rate
• Delayed skeletal maturation	• High blood pressure
• Delayed puberty	• Tremor
	• Increased appetite

Pathophysiology

Circulating autoantibodies known as *thyroid-stimulating immunoglobulins (TSIs)* stimulate the thyroid gland to make T_3 and T_4. These antibodies bind to the TSH receptor sites on the thyroid gland, resulting in excessive thyroid hormone production. The cause of antibody production is unknown. In newborns, maternal TSI is transferred through the placenta to the fetus. TSI binds to the TSH receptor, causing neonatal hyperthyroidism.

Manifestations

The following manifestations are common in Graves' disease: goiter, increased appetite, weight loss, nervousness, diarrhea, increased perspiration, heat intolerance, increased heart rate, muscle weakness, palpitations, tremors, exophthalmos, poor attention span, and behavior or school problems (Box 51-1). In the neonate, irritability, tachycardia, hypertension, voracious appetite with poor weight gain, flushing, prominent eyes, and thyroid enlargement are major signs. These are self-limiting, but cardiac failure and death can occur if the signs are unrecognized or poorly treated.

Diagnostic Evaluation

Elevated serum T_4 levels and suppressed TSH levels, associated with symptoms of hyperthyroidism, suggest Graves' disease. Autoantibodies to thyroid tissue usually are positive. Thyroid uptake of radioactive iodine is increased.

Therapeutic Management

The three approaches to the management of Graves' disease are antithyroid drug therapy, radioactive iodine, or surgery. Antithyroid drug therapy with propylthiouracil or methimazole is the treatment of choice for childhood hyperthyroidism. These drugs act by blocking thyroid hormone production by the thyroid gland. The medications usually are given three times per day, and they lower thyroid hormone levels in several weeks. Minor adverse effects include arthralgia, skin rash, pruritus, and gastric intolerance. Major

! CRITICAL TO REMEMBER
Autoimmune Thyroid Disorders

- Treatment for Graves' disease may be medical (antithyroid medications) or ablative (radioactive iodine or surgery).
- Adherence to medical therapy is problematic because of the requirement for twice-daily or three-times-daily dosing for protracted periods (2-3 years).
- Goiter may be present with either hypothyroidism or hyperthyroidism.
- Autoimmune thyroiditis resulting in either hypothyroidism or hyperthyroidism may be permanent or transient.

adverse effects may include neutropenia, hepatotoxicity, and hypothyroidism.

A second approach to management is oral radioactive iodine treatment. Radioactive iodine (^{131}I) is given as an oral solution. With this therapy, the radioactive iodine is absorbed and concentrated by the thyroid gland, destroying the thyroid tissue in approximately 6 to 18 weeks. Hyperthyroid symptoms may intensify briefly after treatment. Hypothyroidism can result once the thyroid gland is radiated, necessitating thyroid replacement therapy.

Subtotal or partial thyroidectomy, the surgical removal of thyroid gland tissue, is the third form of management. Lugol's solution (potassium iodide), given 10 to 14 days before surgery, decreases the gland's vascularity. Surgery carries the risk of injury to the parathyroid glands, resulting in hypocalcemia. Calcium levels are monitored after surgery.

Recurrence of hyperthyroidism is uncommon but possible. There is also a 60% to 80% chance for development of hypothyroidism, which can be treated with thyroid replacement therapy.

Follow-up evaluations correlate with response to therapy. As thyroid functions normalize, follow-up endocrine evaluations are recommended once or twice per year.

■ NURSING CARE
The Child With Hyperthyroidism

Assessment

The treatment goals consist of normalizing thyroid hormone levels, alleviating symptoms of hyperthyroidism, and decreasing the goiter. The nurse should assess for adherence with medical therapy. Determine that the family understands that medical therapy might take several weeks to decrease thyroid hormone action. Propranolol, a beta-adrenergic blocker, may be prescribed to decrease adrenergic symptoms (tachycardia, heat intolerance, tremor) until the antithyroid medication is effective. Monitor the child for signs of adrenergic symptoms.

A child being treated with propylthiouracil has an increased risk of neutropenia and hepatotoxicity; regular blood counts and liver function studies are done to assess these risks. Assess the child for fever, joint pain, edema, rash, or excessive bruising. A child who acquires a fever or sore throat while receiving propylthiouracil should be evaluated by a physician. A complete blood count should be obtained.

Nursing Diagnosis and Planning

The nursing diagnoses and expected outcomes that may be appropriate for a child with hyperthyroidism are

- Ineffective Therapeutic Regimen Management related to nonadherence with medication.
  Expected Outcome: The child will adhere to the medication regimen, as evidenced by normal thyroid hormone levels.
- Diarrhea related to increased basal metabolic rate secondary to hyperthyroidism.
  Expected Outcomes: The child will be euthyroid, as evidenced by normal results on thyroid function tests; the child will have normal bowel movements.
- Risk for Activity Intolerance related to loss of muscle mass from increased basal metabolic rate secondary to hyperthyroidism.
  Expected Outcome: The child will be able to exercise at the same level as peers as basal metabolic rate returns to normal.
- Disturbed Sleep Pattern related to increased metabolic rate secondary to hyperthyroidism.
  Expected Outcome: The child will gain appropriate amounts of sleep for age as basal metabolic rate returns to normal.
- Ineffective Thermoregulation related to increased basal metabolic rate secondary to hyperthyroidism.
  Expected Outcome: The child will regain normal body temperature as basal metabolic rate returns to normal.

Interventions

The antithyroid drugs *propylthiouracil* and *methimazole* are usually given two or three times per day. This regimen may be difficult for some children to follow. Advise the use of pill dispensers and a watch with an alarm to remind the child to take the medication at specific times. The endocrinologist should evaluate the child and monitor thyroid function every 2 to 4 months while the child is undergoing treatment. Normal values for thyroid function tests and alleviation of symptoms indicate good response to therapy.

Once the child is euthyroid and asymptomatic, the child should be evaluated once or twice a year. Medical therapy may be tapered after 2 to 3 years to evaluate for remission. Contact sports should be limited while the child is being treated, to decrease the possibility of damage to the liver.

Evaluation

- Does the child have normal results on thyroid function tests?
- Has the basal metabolic rate returned to normal?
- Does the child demonstrate normal bowel movements?
- Is the child able to exercise at an age-appropriate level?
- Does the child obtain an appropriate amount of sleep?
- Has the child maintained a normal body temperature?

DIABETES INSIPIDUS

Diabetes insipidus is an inability to concentrate urine because of a deficiency of vasopressin, also known as *antidiuretic hormone* (ADH).

Etiology

Diabetes insipidus commonly results from head trauma, tumors, or infection in the area of the hypothalamus. The most common type of tumor involving the hypothalamus that causes diabetes insipidus is craniopharyngioma.

Cranial radiation for treatment of tumors also may lead to ADH deficiency. Other causes include infections of the CNS, such as meningitis or encephalitis, and congenital malformations, such as septo-optic dysplasia or isolated pituitary malformation or ectopy. It may also be idiopathic.

Incidence

Head trauma and surgical resection of suprasellar tumors account for most cases of diabetes insipidus. Permanent diabetes insipidus develops in approximately 50% of children who have sustained trauma to the sella turcica. Transient or permanent diabetes insipidus is related to the percentage of damage to the vasopressin neurons (Breault & Majzoub, 2004).

Manifestations

Increased urination (polyuria) and excessive thirst (polydipsia) are the classic manifestations of diabetes insipidus. Other signs and symptoms include nocturia and dehydration.

Diagnostic Evaluation

Diagnostic criteria include polyuria with associated hypernatremia (>150 mEq/L) and low urine specific gravity (<1.005) in the absence of hyperglycemia. Urine should be checked for glucose to rule out hyperglycemia as a cause of increased urine output.

A water deprivation test may also be necessary to confirm the diagnosis. In this 7- to 8-hour procedure, the child is deprived of all fluid intake. A normal response is decreased urine output with a high urine specific gravity and no change in serum sodium. In diabetes insipidus, when fluid is restricted, the child continues to have large amounts of dilute urine, evidenced by low urine specific gravity. The serum sodium level also increases. To ensure the child's safety, this test is done in a hospital setting with frequent monitoring of serum sodium, hematocrit, and osmolality. Urine osmolality and output are also measured. The child is weighed at the beginning, middle, and conclusion of the water deprivation test. Water deprivation should be stopped if the child loses 3% to 5% of baseline body weight, becomes dehydrated, or demonstrates a significant change in vital signs or neurologic status.

Therapeutic Management

Treatment involves maintaining fluid balance and administering synthetic vasopressin (1-deamino-8-D-arginine vasopressin [DDAVP]). The dose of DDAVP ranges from 5 to 30 mcg/day (intranasal) or 2-4 mcg/day (IV/sc), divided into one to two doses. It is administered either intranasally, through a soft, flexible tube (rhinal tube) or metered spray, or by subcutaneous injection. The concentration of intranasal DDAVP is 100 mcg/ml; the concentration of subcutaneous DDAVP is 4 mcg/ml. The oral form of DDAVP is used primarily for nocturnal enuresis. It has also been used in the treatment of diabetes insipidus.

Dosage is individualized based on the child's age, size, urine output, and urine specific gravity. The subcutaneous dose is 10% of the intranasal dose. The duration of action varies from 8 to 24 hours. Doses are timed so that before the next dose, the child is allowed to have mildly increased urination. This helps prevent overtreatment and water retention. Parents are often taught to measure urine specific gravity at home to monitor effectiveness of treatment.

Pathophysiology

of Diabetes Insipidus

Antidiuretic hormone (ADH) is produced in the hypothalamus, transported through the pituitary stalk, and stored in the posterior pituitary. It is carried through the blood to the kidneys, where it acts on the distal tubules and collecting ducts to increase reabsorption of free water, thereby concentrating urine and decreasing urinary output.

ADH is under the control of osmoreceptors in the anterior pituitary. These osmoreceptors operate on a negative-feedback system based on serum osmolality, particularly sodium concentration. When the osmolality is low, production of ADH decreases, causing increased urine output and normalizing osmolality; conversely, when osmolality is increased, ADH production increases, causing water retention and decreasing urine output. In diabetes insipidus, a deficiency of ADH makes the body unable to conserve water, which results in large volumes of dilute urine. Loss of free water leads to an increase in serum sodium concentration. If the child has an intact thirst center, increasing oral intake might compensate for the large fluid loss. If the thirst drive is not intact or the child is unable to drink enough, the child may become dehydrated and have a high serum sodium level.

A child with an intact thirst center is able to self-regulate fluid needs and intake. If the child is not able to recognize thirst because of head trauma or surgery, the physician may prescribe a 24-hour fluid requirement.

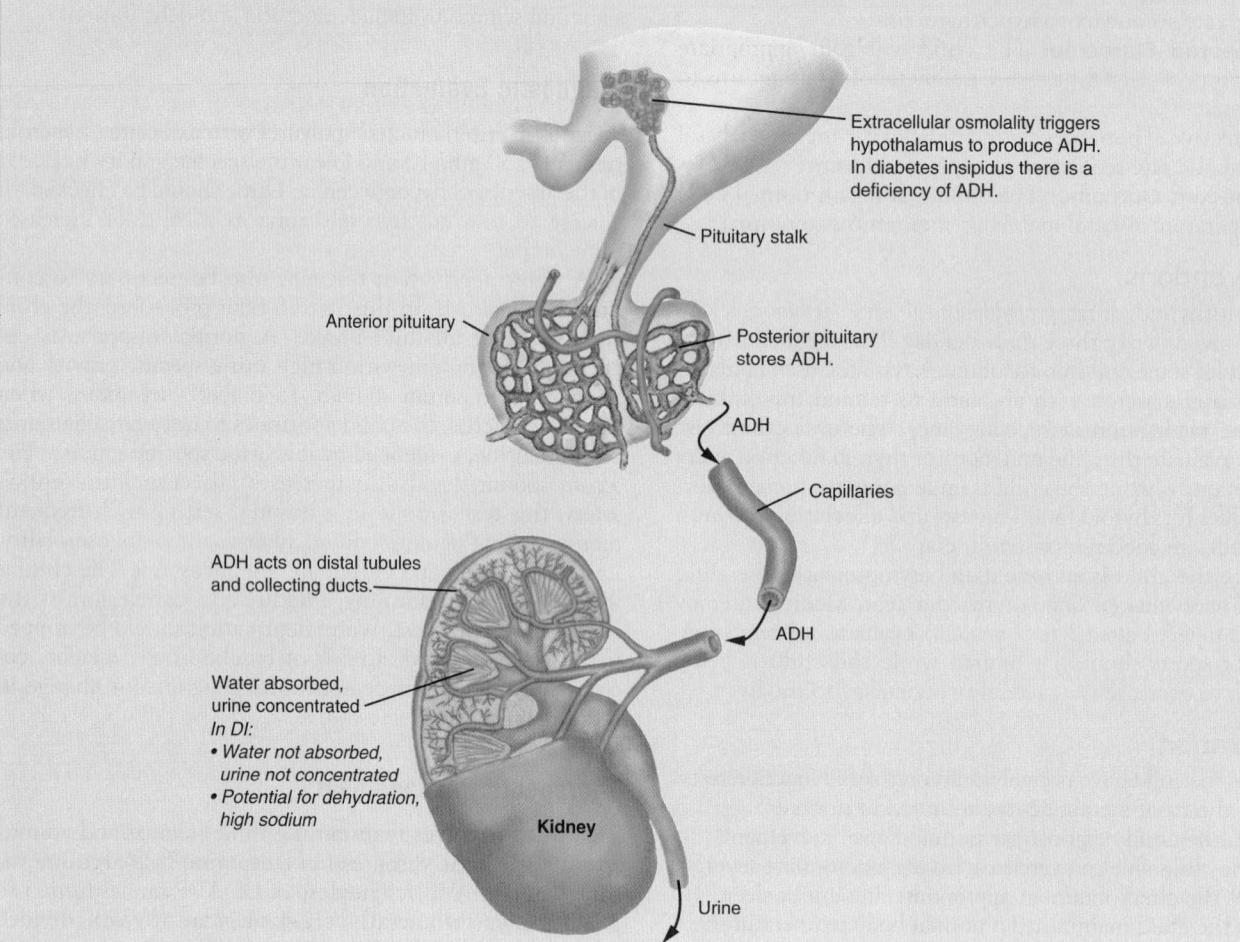

Extracellular osmolality triggers hypothalamus to produce ADH. In diabetes insipidus there is a deficiency of ADH.

Pituitary stalk

Anterior pituitary

Posterior pituitary stores ADH.

ADH

Capillaries

ADH

ADH acts on distal tubules and collecting ducts.

Water absorbed, urine concentrated
In DI:
• *Water not absorbed, urine not concentrated*
• *Potential for dehydration, high sodium*

Kidney

Urine

Nursing Considerations

Nursing care involves assessing the parents' and child's understanding of diabetes insipidus. Educate the family about the basic pathophysiology of water metabolism and the cause of diabetes insipidus. Include a description of signs and symptoms. Instruct the parents about signs and symptoms indicating the need for DDAVP (increased thirst, polyuria, dehydration) as well as signs and symptoms of excessive DDAVP (decreased urine output, headaches, water retention).

Teach the family the proper administration of DDAVP, and observe a return demonstration of medication administration. If appropriate, instruct the family in using a refractometer to measure urine specific gravity. The child should wear a Medic-Alert bracelet noting the diagnosis of diabetes insipidus. The child's teachers need to be aware of the diagnosis and must allow the child free access to water and toilet facilities. Advise the family to watch the child closely for signs of dehydration.

BOX 51-2
Diabetes Insipidus Versus Syndrome of Inappropriate Antidiuretic Hormone (SIADH)

Diabetes Insipidus (High and Dry)	SIADH (Low and Wet)
• Increased urination	• Decreased urination
• Increased thirst	• Hypertension
• Nocturia	• Weight gain
• Dehydration	• Fluid retention
• Hypernatremia	• Hyponatremia
• Urine specific gravity <1.005	• Urine specific gravity >1.030
• Elevated serum osmolality (>300 mOsm/kg)	• Decreased serum osmolality (<280 mOsm/kg)
• Decreased urine osmolality	• Increased urine osmolality

SYNDROME OF INAPPROPRIATE ANTIDIURETIC HORMONE

The syndrome of inappropriate antidiuretic hormone (SIADH) results from excessive production or release of ADH, or vasopressin.

Etiology

Childhood SIADH usually is caused by disorders affecting the CNS, including infections (e.g., meningitis), head trauma, and brain tumors (see Chapter 52). SIADH is rare in children and is usually related to an underlying cause. Surgery for brain tumors may cause the child to experience transient SIADH. Often, a triple response occurs after surgery. Initially the child has diabetes insipidus, then the child experiences temporary SIADH, and finally the child returns to diabetes insipidus (Victorina, Rydstedt, & Sowers, 2002). SIADH is usually transient and resolves when the underlying condition is corrected.

Manifestations

Manifestations that occur with SIADH include decreased urine output, increased urine specific gravity, fluid retention, weight gain, hyponatremia, and increased urine osmolality (Box 51-2).

Diagnostic Evaluation

SIADH should be suspected in children with CNS involvement, such as infections or head trauma, who have decreased urine output despite adequate intake. Laboratory diagnosis includes evidence of hyponatremia, hypochloremia, and low serum osmolality. Urine osmolality is usually greater than serum osmolality. Urine specific gravity is more than 1.030. Adrenal, thyroid, and renal function studies can rule out other causes of hyponatremia.

Therapeutic Management

Initial treatment is correction of the underlying cause. The physician orders fluid restriction to correct hyponatremia.

A child with severe hyponatremia may need IV infusion of sodium chloride. Drug therapy usually is not indicated for transient SIADH. Medications such as lithium and demeclocycline block the action of ADH at the renal collecting tubules and have been used in the management of chronic SIADH (Box 51-3).

Nursing Considerations

The nurse should assess the child with SIADH for signs and symptoms of fluid overload, including edema, weight gain, urine specific gravity more than 1.030, and dilutional hyponatremia. If the child is hyponatremic, monitor neurologic status by assessing level of consciousness and observing for headache, irritability, or seizures.

The child with fluid overload is at risk for injury related to seizures caused by hyponatremia. Interventions are directed toward maintaining fluid balance and preventing injury. Assess the child's hydration and neurologic status every 2 to 4 hours. Carefully maintain strict fluid restrictions, and document intake and output. Weigh the child daily to monitor fluid retention.

The child may have difficulty complying with the fluid restrictions. Explain to the child and parents the need for limited

Pathophysiology

of Syndrome of Inappropriate Antidiuretic Hormone

Excessive antidiuretic hormone results in the kidney reabsorbing too much free water. This causes decreased output of concentrated urine, evidenced by a high urine specific gravity (>1.030). The excess water also causes an expanded fluid volume and a low serum sodium level. Once the sodium level falls below 125 mEq/L, the child can become symptomatic and experience anorexia, nausea, weakness, weight gain, confusion, irritability, and seizures.

BOX 51-3
Signs of Hyponatremia

Mild (Early)	Moderate	Severe
Anorexia	Confusion	Seizures
Nausea	Lethargy	Coma
Headache	Irritability	
Vomiting	Altered level of consciousness	

> ## ! CRITICAL TO REMEMBER
>
> ### Syndrome of Inappropriate Antidiuretic Hormone
>
> - Syndrome of inappropriate antidiuretic hormone (SIADH) is characterized by low serum sodium (<125 mEq/L) and high urine specific gravity as well as decreased serum osmolality and increased urine osmolality.
> - Seizures may develop with hyponatremia.
> - Treatment depends on strict fluid restriction to maintain serum sodium in a near-normal range. Strict measurements of intake and output are critical to evaluation and management of the patient with SIADH.

fluids and that the restriction is temporary. The nurse may give the child hard sugarless candies or apply wet washcloths to help keep mucous membranes moist.

Diet for the child with hyponatremia should include foods with high-sodium content because extra sodium can help correct this problem. Keep in mind, however, that salty foods such as chips might make the child thirsty.

Closely monitor serum electrolyte levels as ordered by the physician. Alert the physician immediately to any change in neurologic status. Because severe hyponatremia can cause seizures, initiate seizure precautions if the serum sodium level drops below 125 mEq/L.

Evaluation of the child with SIADH should address a balanced intake and output, stable weight, and normal serum sodium levels. Urine specific gravity should be maintained between 1.010 and 1.020.

PRECOCIOUS PUBERTY

Precocious puberty refers to early onset of puberty. Traditionally, this has been viewed as the onset of puberty before 8 years of age in girls and before 9 years of age in boys. It is defined as the premature appearance of secondary sexual characteristics, accelerated growth rate, and advanced bone maturation. The major consequence of precocious puberty is rapid bone growth, which causes early growth-plate fusion and ultimately short stature in adulthood.

Recently, as the age of normal pubertal maturation has been noted to be declining, the Lawson Wilkins Pediatric Endocrine Society has proposed that there is no need to look for a pathologic cause of puberty when breasts or pubic hair develops in white girls older than 7 years or in African-American girls older than 6 years. Exceptions to this recommendation should be considered when (1) the progression of puberty is unusually rapid, with bone age more than 2 years ahead of chronologic age, and predicted height is less than 150 cm (59 inches); (2) there are new CNS findings, such as headaches, seizures, or focal neurologic deficits; or (3) puberty is having adverse emotional effects (Kaplowitz & Oberfield, 1999).

Etiology

Central, or true, precocious puberty can be idiopathic or caused by CNS tumors (most commonly hamartomas), head trauma, or cranial radiation. Peripheral causes include abnormalities or tumors of the adrenal glands, ovaries, or testes.

Congenital adrenal hyperplasia, a genetic disorder of the adrenal pathway, is the most common cause of peripheral precocious puberty. McCune-Albright syndrome may cause early puberty in girls and boys; the genetic disorder *familial testotoxicosis* causes early puberty in boys.

Incidence

Precocious puberty occurs more frequently in girls than in boys; approximately 70% of cases are idiopathic, although boys have a higher incidence of CNS lesions. Both boys and girls can have hypothalamic hamartomas.

Manifestations

Manifestations of precocious puberty reflect gender differences:

Girls	Boys
Breast development	Testicular enlargement
Pubic hair	Penile enlargement
Axillary hair	Pubic hair
Enlargement of vagina, uterus, and ovaries	Facial hair
Acne	Acne
Growth spurt	Adult body odor
Adult body odor	Deepening of voice
Onset of menstrual periods	Moodiness
Moodiness	

Diagnostic Evaluation

Diagnosis of precocious puberty begins with a thorough history, including onset of sexual characteristics, and a physical examination. Blood tests are then necessary to evaluate for elevated levels of LH, FSH, testosterone, and estrogen. Unfortunately, because these hormones are released in small bursts during the day, random samples may not be adequate.

The gonadotropin-releasing hormone (GnRH) stimulation test is a more accurate and definitive test to determine the role of the pituitary gland during early puberty. Synthetic GnRH is administered IV or subcutaneously to stimulate the release of LH and FSH from the pituitary gland. Serial samples of LH and FSH are then obtained over a 2-hour period after IV administration. With subcutaneous administration, a single sample of LH and FSH may be obtained with the use of an ultrasensitive assay (Lawson & Cohen, 1999). Before the onset of puberty, the FSH peak is higher than the LH peak. With the onset of puberty, the LH peak is higher than the FSH peak.

Radiographic studies also support the diagnosis of precocious puberty. Radiographs of the wrist determine bone age and maturation and can assist in predicting final adult height. Skull radiographs screen for CNS lesions, although CT scans and MRI are more accurate in visualizing tumors. Abdominal ultrasound and pelvic ultrasound are beneficial in diagnosing adrenal and ovarian tumors or cysts. Pelvic ultrasound also provides evidence of pubertal changes in the uterus and ovaries. Finally, isolated pubic hair development and elevated androgen hormone levels suggest an adrenal origin for premature sexual hair growth.

Pathophysiology

of Precocious Puberty

Puberty occurs when the hypothalamus releases gonadotropin-releasing hormone (GnRH). This stimulates the pituitary gland to release luteinizing hormone (LH) and follicle-stimulating hormone (FSH). In girls, FSH stimulates formation of ovarian follicles to produce estrogen. Estrogen is necessary for the development of secondary sexual characteristics, such as breast development and maturation of the vagina and labia. LH is involved in the process of ovulation. In boys, FSH triggers the testes to support the development of sperm. LH stimulates the production of testosterone, which is necessary for the development of sexual characteristics and sperm production. Puberty development is classified according to Tanner stages 1 through

5 (see Chapter 8). The adrenal glands produce the hormone *dehydroepiandrosterone (DHEA),* which causes pubic and axillary hair growth. During puberty, there is also an increase in growth rate, or a "growth spurt," in which a child grows an average of 4 to 6 inches per year.

In precocious puberty, the sex hormones that accelerate growth also cause the bone plates to close early. Bone usually fuses at 14 years of age for girls and 17 years for boys. With true precocious puberty, children have hormonal changes that mimic the onset of normal puberty. These hormonal changes may be central, arising from the hypothalamus, or peripheral, arising from the ovaries, testes, or adrenal glands.

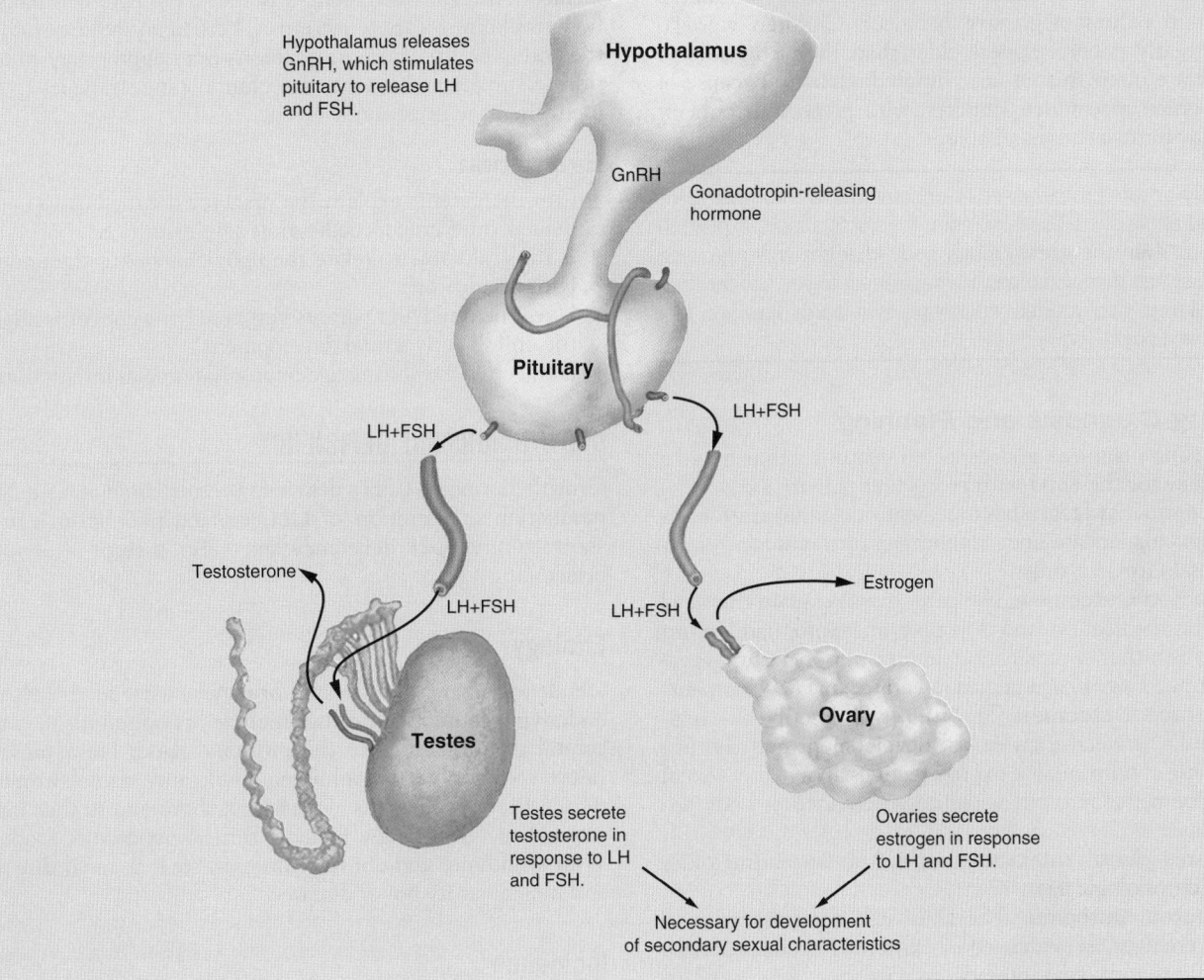

Hypothalamus releases GnRH, which stimulates pituitary to release LH and FSH.

Hypothalamus

GnRH

Gonadotropin-releasing hormone

Pituitary

LH+FSH

LH+FSH

Testosterone

LH+FSH

LH+FSH

Estrogen

Testes

Ovary

Testes secrete testosterone in response to LH and FSH.

Ovaries secrete estrogen in response to LH and FSH.

Necessary for development of secondary sexual characteristics

Therapeutic Management

Treatment of the child with precocious puberty aims to stop or reverse the development of secondary sexual characteristics and to maximize adult height. Current therapy for central precocious puberty involves administration of a GnRH agonist, or blocker. GnRH blockers inhibit the binding of GnRH to the pituitary gland, causing decreased production of the pubertal hormones and slowing or reversing sexual development.

Several commercially available GnRH agonists can be administered either intranasally or by a monthly intramuscular injection. Once therapy is initiated, GnRH secretion is suppressed within 2 to 4 weeks. The accelerated growth rate and bone maturation will slow, and some secondary sexual characteristics will regress within the first year of treatment. Nonadherence with medication therapy, such as missed or delayed administration of injections, can promote pubertal changes rather than suppress puberty.

No evidence suggests that GnRH agonist therapy interferes with the child's reproduction in the future. Once therapy is discontinued, pubertal progression resumes. For children with peripheral precocious puberty, treatment is aimed at correcting the underlying cause.

■NURSING CARE
The Child With Precocious Puberty

Assessment

Nursing care of the child with precocious puberty addresses the physical and behavioral changes associated with puberty. A nurse working with these children may note that they feel more comfortable around older children rather than peers their own age. They often experience teasing about their bodies and may limit social activities, such as swimming. Boys often exhibit aggressive behavior. Children who go through early puberty appear older than their chronologic age and are often treated accordingly by adults. Because of their mature appearance, children with precocious puberty are at greater risk for sexual abuse.

If a child appears embarrassed or uncomfortable when being interviewed about sexual development, the nurse should explain to the child: "Everyone goes through body changes when growing up; it's just that these changes are happening to you sooner than most children. Can you tell me in your own words how you feel about your body?"

Nursing Diagnosis and Planning

The nursing diagnoses and expected outcomes that may be appropriate for the child with precocious puberty are

■ Deficient Knowledge about medication administration related to inadequate understanding of intramuscular or intranasal GnRH agonist.
   Expected Outcomes: The parents will explain the need for the medication and will give an appropriate return demonstration of medication administration technique.
■ Disturbed Body Image related to early sexual development.
   Expected Outcomes: The child will describe the relationship between early sexual development and the underlying condition, will express feelings about early sexual development, and will verbalize acceptance of body appearance.
■ Impaired Social Interaction related to appearing older than chronologic age.
   Expected Outcome: The child will adjust socially to body changes, as evidenced by exhibiting age-appropriate behaviors and social interactions.

Interventions

Many parents may not be comfortable with their child's early development. The nurse assists with explaining the stages of puberty and each stage's associated behavioral changes. The nurse teaches parents that the child is experiencing normal changes at an earlier time than expected.

Explanations given to the child should be geared to chronologic age. The nurse can direct the parent to books that explain sexual maturation in terms the child can under-

---

! CRITICAL TO REMEMBER
Precocious Puberty

- Children with precocious puberty appear older than their chronologic age. Although they tend to be treated as older children, they should be treated according to their chronologic age.
- Other children often tease children with precocious puberty.
- Children with precocious puberty are at increased risk of child abuse because of their more mature appearance.
- Precocious puberty may present in infancy or childhood.

---

stand. Psychological counseling might be necessary to help the family deal with the sensitive issues of sexuality.

The nurse also teaches the family about the prescribed medication regimen. In some instances, the parent is taught how to administer the injections. These might be stressful for the young child. The nurse demonstrates appropriate injection technique and teaches the child coping strategies to be used when the injection is given.

Evaluation

- Can the parents explain the need for the medication and demonstrate proper medication administration?
- Is the child able to relate the body changes to the underlying condition?
- Have the child and parents verbalized any concerns about the child's early sexual development?
- Is the child exhibiting age-appropriate social interactions?

GROWTH HORMONE DEFICIENCY

Growth hormone (GH) deficiency results from inadequate production or secretion of GH, causing poor growth and short stature. GH deficiency may also present as hypoglycemia.

Etiology

GH deficiency may be isolated or may be associated with an underlying cause. Such causes include hypopituitarism, congenital malformations of the pituitary gland, brain tumors (most commonly craniopharyngioma), and cranial irradiation. Other disorders associated with short stature that may respond to GH therapy include Turner's syndrome, Prader-Willi syndrome, and chronic illnesses, such as renal disease and inflammatory bowel disease.

Incidence

The incidence of GH deficiency is at least 1 in 3480 children in the United States. A survey of 48,000 Scottish school children indicated an incidence of at least 1 in 4000 (Rosenfeld, 1996).

Manifestations

These manifestations are typical of GH deficiency: height less than 5th percentile for age and gender, diminished growth rate (less than two standard deviations from the mean for age and

Pathophysiology

of Growth Hormone Deficiency

Growth hormone (GH), thyroxine, cortisol, and sex hormones all influence growth. The hypothalamus secretes GH-releasing factor, which stimulates the pituitary gland to release GH. This hormone is secreted in pulses, with increased secretion during the night. In the presence of hypoglycemia, GH is secreted to counteract insulin and raise the blood glucose level. Many children with GH deficiency may present with hypoglycemia.

Most children with short stature have constitutional growth delay. Children with short stature or poor growth rates may also be deficient in other hormones. Normal thyroid function is essential for growth; therefore hypothyroidism may also present with short stature. Sex hormones are required for the growth spurt and sexual maturation that occurs with puberty. Children lacking more than one hormone produced by the pituitary gland are referred to as having *hypopituitarism*. Rate of growth and final adult height depend on factors such as family heights, nutrition, and general health. Any child growing less than 5 cm per year should be referred to an endocrinologist for further evaluation.

---

gender), immature or cherubic facies, delayed puberty, hypoglycemia, diminished muscle mass and relatively increased adiposity, and micropenis (associated with hypopituitarism).

Diagnostic Evaluation

Diagnosis of GH deficiency begins with careful measurements of growth over an extended period (usually 6-12 mo). Height should be measured on a consistent scale, preferably with a calibrated stadiometer.

Initial screening involves thyroid function tests, electrolytes, blood urea nitrogen (BUN), creatinine, complete blood count, insulin-like growth factor 1 (IGF-1; formerly somatomedin-C) and IGF binding proteins (IGFBP-3) (indirect measures of GH production), and a bone age radiograph. Normal thyroid function is essential for adequate growth; thyroid studies are essential when evaluating for short stature. Complete blood count and other specific blood screening for any systemic or chronic illness should be done. Electrolytes and renal function studies eliminate primary kidney dysfunction as a cause of poor growth.

Because GH is normally secreted in pulses throughout the day and night, stimulation testing is necessary to confirm the diagnosis of GH deficiency. Agents used in provocative testing to stimulate GH production include insulin, arginine, clonidine, glucagon, and levodopa (L-dopa). Once the stimulating agent is given, serial GH levels are drawn. Although diagnostic criteria vary, most clinicians accept a GH level below 10 ng/ml as indicative of GH deficiency. Generally, two positive tests are required for diagnosis.

Therapeutic Management

A child with GH deficiency requires replacement therapy. Synthetic GH comes in a powdered form that must be diluted for administration or a premixed liquid form. It is given as a subcutaneous injection six or seven times per week, usually at bedtime. An alternative form of administration is a subcutaneous deposition of time-release GH, designed to last 2 to 4 weeks. Dosage ranges from 0.18 to 0.3 mg/kg/wk, depending on the child's age, pubertal stage, and response to therapy (Parks, 2004; Wilson et al., 2003). Once diluted, GH must be stored at 36° to 46° F. Treatment is usually considered effective if the child exhibits a height increase of 2 cm/yr over the pretreatment growth rate. The earlier treatment is initiated, the greater the child's height potential. Treatment is continued until the child's growth plates close or the child reaches an acceptable height or predicted final height. GH should not be administered to a child with short stature who does not demonstrate GH deficiency. Administering GH to these children may cause an initial height spurt but does not appreciably affect the child's adult height and may be associated with complications, such as testicular dysfunction, after therapy (Allen, 1999; Bertelloni et al., 1999).

▪NURSING CARE
The Child With Growth Hormone Deficiency

Assessment

Nursing care of the child with GH deficiency includes assessment of family attitudes and perceptions. Parental attitudes regarding the child's size can influence the child's self-esteem. Assess the child's attitude about height. Are height and growth issues voiced more by the parent or by the child? If parents place excessive emphasis on height, the child may be more self-conscious or demonstrate low self-esteem. Height issues might affect a child's psychosocial adjustment, as demonstrated by poor school performance and lack of involvement in extracurricular activities. Often, short children appear younger and are often treated as such by adults, or they may be teased by their peers.

When assessing a child with short stature, the nurse should ask the child if height causes any problems at school. For example, the nurse might ask, "Have you ever been teased or been in any fights at school because of your height?"

Once the child is receiving therapy, the nurse should assess adherence with the medication regimen, injection technique, and medication preparation and storage. These should be reviewed periodically and with each dosage change. As children with this problem mature, they might elect to learn to self-administer injections.

Nursing Diagnosis and Planning

The nursing diagnoses and expected outcomes that may be appropriate for the child with GH deficiency are
- Delayed Growth and Development related to GH deficiency.
   Expected Outcomes: The child will receive and respond to treatment, as evidenced by increased growth rate.
- Disturbed Body Image related to short stature.
   Expected Outcome: The child will demonstrate acceptance of body image, as evidenced by verbalization of acceptance of ultimate growth.

! CRITICAL TO REMEMBER

Criteria for Suspecting Growth Hormone Deficiency

- Consistently poor growth (<5 cm/yr)
- Growth rate more than two standard deviations below the mean for age
- Downward deviation from the previous growth curve

CRITICAL THINKING EXERCISE 51-1

Periodically, the media have drawn attention to the use of growth hormone. Parents of young teenage boys often are concerned about their child's present and eventual height. Boys who are significantly shorter than their peers during early adolescence can experience altered self-esteem.

How should a nurse respond if parents ask whether giving growth hormone to their short son will increase his eventual height?

- Situational Low Self-Esteem related to short stature.
  Expected Outcome: The child will accept short stature, as evidenced by verbalizing appropriate feelings of self-esteem.
- Ineffective Family Therapeutic Regimen Management related to nonadherence with daily injection.
  Expected Outcome: The child and parents will adhere to the injection schedule, as evidenced by appropriate record keeping and the child's steady growth.

Interventions

The nurse reassures the child and parents that adherence to the injections will improve growth rate. It is also helpful to remind children that the injections are temporary and are helping them to grow. Keeping a growth chart at home and needing larger clothing sizes are physical signs the child can use to monitor growth. These indicators also assist with adherence.

The nurse has an important role in educating children and families about the proper dilution and administration of the GH. Demonstrate injection technique to the caregiver, and request a return demonstration.

Effectiveness of therapy is evaluated by growth rate. Children are evaluated approximately every 3 to 4 months by an endocrinologist. Accurate measurements of height are essential to evaluate efficacy. Using a growth chart helps identify growth velocity. Therapy is continued until the child reaches an acceptable adult height or there is radiographic evidence of growth-plate fusion.

Evaluation

- Has the child exhibited increased growth rate?
- Does the child verbalize feelings regarding body image and self-esteem?
- Do the child and family adhere to injection schedule?

DIABETES MELLITUS

Evidence has been accumulating that demonstrates a worldwide increase in the incidence of type 1 diabetes mellitus, with incidence rising specifically in areas where type I dia-

betes was previously low (Alemzadeh & Wyatt, 2004; Sullivan-Bolyai, Deatrick, Gruppuso, Tamborlane, & Grey, 2002). This trend to a steadily increased incidence of type 1 diabetes extends back for 30 years (Onkamo, Vaananen, Karvonen, & Tuomilehto, 1999). Additionally, children are developing type I diabetes at an earlier age. The incidence of type 2 diabetes has also risen in children.

Type 1 Diabetes Mellitus

Type 1 diabetes mellitus results when the pancreas is unable to produce and secrete insulin. This form of diabetes, the most common childhood endocrine disorder, presents challenges in the areas of teaching, management, and adherence. Because of recent changes in the health care delivery system, meeting the needs associated with management of type 1 diabetes mellitus has become more complicated. Unless the newly diagnosed child is in diabetic ketoacidosis (DKA), the child may not be hospitalized. The nurse must develop a plan of care that involves family education, in either an inpatient or outpatient setting. Including the family in the child's care and support must be part of planning and implementation of nursing care. Because type 1 diabetes mellitus is a chronic disease, see Chapter 36 for a discussion of that aspect of care.

Type 2 Diabetes Mellitus

Type 2 diabetes is an emerging problem in the pediatric population. Type 2 diabetes in children is characterized by production of excess insulin, but the cells are not able to utilize it properly. These youths tend to be obese, similar to adults with type 2 diabetes (Dabelea, Pettitt, Jones, & Arslanian, 1999).

Etiology

Type 1 diabetes mellitus results from an autoimmune process that causes the destruction of the insulin-secreting cells of the pancreas. A genetic predisposition plus an environmental or viral trigger are thought to initiate the autoimmune destructive process. Current research focuses on identifying specific genes that may affect a person's susceptibility to type 1 diabetes mellitus, as well as exploring methods of interrupting or preventing the autoimmune response in susceptible people (first-degree relatives of a diabetic person). At this time, no prevention or cure is available; however, several different means of islet cell transplantation are being explored and are quite promising.

Recently, another etiology for some individuals with insulin-dependent diabetes has been identified. A viral infiltration of the pancreas that appears to directly destroy beta cells results in insulinopenia and therefore diabetes. This form of diabetes is clinically indistinguishable from autoimmune diabetes, but these individuals will have no markers of autoimmunity in the blood. It has been termed *type 1B* (Imagawa, Hanafusa, Miyagawa, & Matsuzawa, 2000).

Incidence

The incidence of type 1 diabetes mellitus in the United States is 1.7 in 1000 people, with approximately 13,000 new cases diagnosed every year (American Diabetes Association, 1999). This incidence decreases to 5 per 100,000 for the population older than 20 years. The risk of diabetes increases to 1 in 20 if the person has a first-degree relative (parent, sibling) with type 1 diabetes mellitus, and it increases to 1 in 3 if an identical twin has the disease. The average age of onset is during the early school-age period and again in early adolescence.

The peak incidence of type 2 diabetes occurs with the onset of puberty. The exact incidence is unknown in the pediatric population; however, type 2 diabetes is clearly on the rise in this population (Dabelea et al., 1999). Children as young as 3 years have been diagnosed with type 2 diabetes. Type 2 diabetes is more common in certain populations, including American Indians, African-Americans, Latinos, and individuals with Asian ancestry. It tends to be more common in females than in males (Dabelea et al., 1999).

Manifestations

The classic initial signs of hyperglycemia, known as the "three **P**'s," are **p**olyuria (or enuresis in a toilet-trained child), **p**olydipsia, and **p**olyphagia. The child experiences weight loss (despite increased food intake), fatigue, and blurred vision.

If the condition progresses without intervention, the child can exhibit the following signs of ketoacidosis: nausea and vomiting, abdominal pain, acetone (fruity) odor to breath, dehydration, increasing lethargy, Kussmaul respirations, and coma.

Children who receive insulin for treatment of type 1 diabetes mellitus can experience hypoglycemia. Table 51-3 compares hypoglycemia, hyperglycemia, and ketoacidosis.

Children with type 2 diabetes are typically overweight and have a darkening of the skin around the neck (acanthosis nigricans). This may also be found in the groin, axillae, antecubital fossa, or dorsum of the hand and is a marker for

Pathophysiology

of Type 1 Diabetes Mellitus

Glucose is the primary source of energy for body cells. Any extra glucose taken in by the body can be stored as glycogen, in muscle or liver cells or the form of fatty tissues. Glucose can be extracted from glycogen for periods of fasting (e.g., overnight). Once glycogen stores have been depleted, new glucose (gluco-neogenesis) is made from amino acids released from muscle into the bloodstream. The energy for gluconeogenesis is supplied by the breakdown of stored fats.

Insulin, a hormone, is secreted by the beta cells of the pancreas. Its main function is to regulate the blood glucose level by

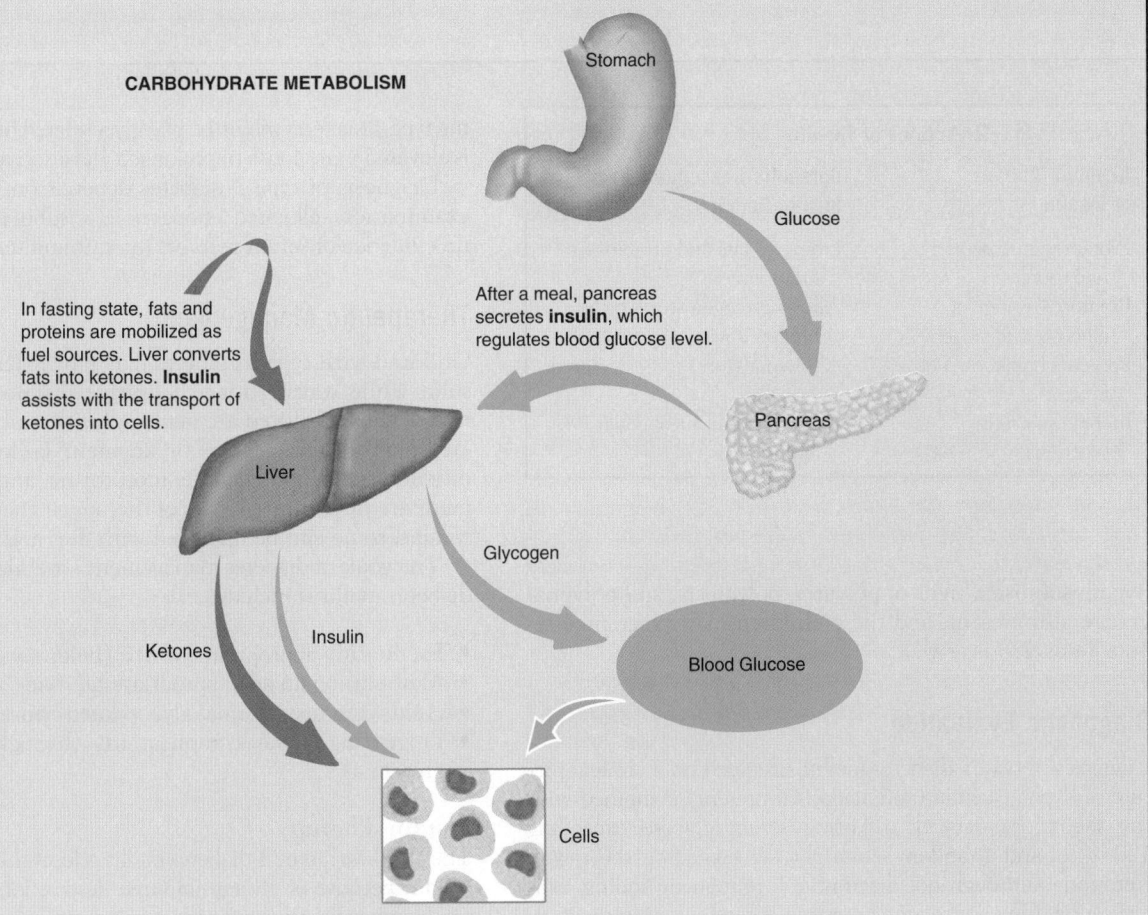

CARBOHYDRATE METABOLISM

Stomach

Glucose

In fasting state, fats and proteins are mobilized as fuel sources. Liver converts fats into ketones. **Insulin** assists with the transport of ketones into cells.

After a meal, pancreas secretes **insulin**, which regulates blood glucose level.

Pancreas

Liver

Glycogen

Ketones

Insulin

Blood Glucose

Cells

Continued

Pathophysiology

of Type 1 Diabetes Mellitus—cont'd

controlling the rate of glucose uptake by cells. Little or no insulin is secreted by the beta cells when a person is in the fasting state; greater quantities are secreted after the person has eaten a meal. In the fasting state, with relatively small quantities of available insulin, the body mobilizes fats and proteins to be used as fuel sources. The liver then converts the fats into ketoacids, or ketones. With the assistance of insulin, ketones are transported into the cells and are used as an alternative source of fuel for cellular energy. This process ensures an energy source during long periods of fasting. Not all cells in the body are capable of utilizing ketone bodies and require glucose as their primary fuel (see Table 51-2).

In the absence of insulin, the metabolism of fats, proteins, and carbohydrates is impaired. Glucose is unable to move into the intracellular space, resulting in hyperglycemia. As blood glucose levels exceed the renal threshold, glucose is "spilled" into the urine through osmotic diuresis, resulting in polyuria. Excessive thirst follows in response to fluid loss. Fatigue, hunger, and weight loss also accompany the onset of type 1 diabetes mellitus because cellular starvation continues in the absence of insulin.

Ketones (ketoacids), manufactured by the liver from adipose tissue, are produced in response to cellular starvation. In the absence of insulin, ketones are also unavailable to the cell for nourishment. Increasing blood levels of ketones (ketonemia) result in ketoacidosis.

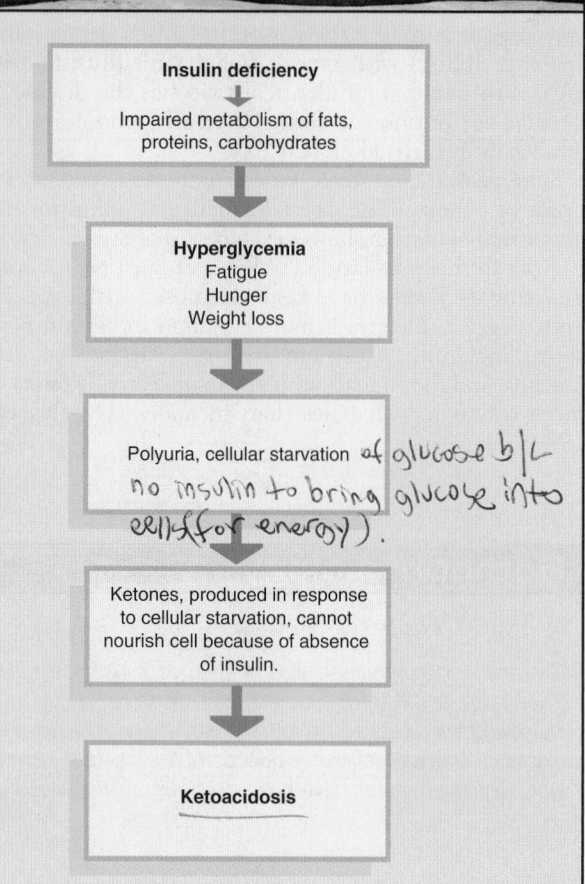

TABLE 51-2 Actions of Insulin	
Anabolic Actions of Insulin	**Catabolic Consequences of Insulin Deficit**
Promotes glucose as a fuel source.	Promotes fats and proteins as fuel sources.
Promotes storage of glucose as glycogen.	Allows glycogen stores to be broken down.
Prevents breakdown of fat stores.	Allows fat stores to be depleted.
Increases protein synthesis.	Allows protein breakdown into amino acids.

hyperinsulinism. Signs of polyuria, polydipsia, and polyphagia are also present, and these children may experience severe ketoacidosis as well.

Diagnostic Evaluation

Diagnosis of type 1 diabetes mellitus is based on a clinical picture of hyperglycemia (and acidosis if present) combined with the laboratory data of a fasting serum glucose exceeding 120 mg/dl and a random serum glucose exceeding 160 mg/dl. Ketonuria, although not diagnostic, is a frequent finding, as is glycosuria. Glucose tolerance testing is rarely used in diagnos-

ing type 1 diabetes mellitus. The glycosylated hemoglobin value is elevated in response to prolonged elevations of blood glucose.

Diagnosis of type 2 diabetes depends on careful physical examination, elevated endogenous insulin production, and no evidence of serum markers for autoimmunity.

Therapeutic Management

Children with type 2 diabetes may have been started on insulin while waiting for a definitive diagnosis. Once diagnosed, these children are managed with oral agents that decrease insulin resistance or augment endogenous insulin production. Blood glucose monitoring and diet management are important aspects of therapy. If these children lose weight, some can be managed with diet and exercise alone.

The goals of diabetes management for children with type 1 diabetes mellitus include:

- Facilitating appropriate growth (height, weight)
- Maintaining an age-appropriate lifestyle
- Achieving near-normal glycosylated hemoglobin
- Preventing acute complications (hypoglycemia, hyperglycemia)

Insulin Therapy

The child with type 1 diabetes mellitus loses the ability to make insulin because of an autoimmune destruction of the insulin-producing cells, the beta cells. Symptoms of hyperglycemia be-

TABLE **51-3** Comparison of Hypoglycemia, Hyperglycemia, and Ketoacidosis

Descriptor	HYPOGLYCEMIA	Hyperglycemia	Ketoacidosis
Onset	Rapid	Slow	Slow
Signs and symptoms	*Adrenergic signs:* Trembling Sweating Tachycardia Pallor Clammy skin	Increased urination Increased thirst Fatigue Weight loss (gradual, over several weeks) Blurred vision	*Hyperglycemia signs plus:* Abdominal pain Chest pain Kussmaul respirations Nausea and vomiting Acetone (fruity) breath odor *Signs and symptoms of dehydration:* Dry lips and mucous membranes Sunken eyes Sudden weight loss Decreased urination
Alterations in sensorium	*Neuroglycopenic symptoms:* Personality change Irritability Drunken behavior Slurred speech Decreased level of consciousness to total loss of consciousness Seizure activity	Emotional lability Headache Hunger	Increasing lethargy Decreasing level of consciousness Coma
Laboratory data	Blood glucose <70 mg/dl	Blood glucose >160 mg/dl	Blood glucose >300 mg/dl Urinary ketones positive Serum pH <7.25 Serum ketones positive
Causes	Too much insulin Excessive activity without eating extra carbohydrates Missed or delayed meal	Excessive intake of carbohydrate Little or no exercise Inadequate amount of insulin Increased stress, either emotional or physical	Inadequate amount of insulin Excessive stress
Treatment	15 g of carbohydrate *For loss of consciousness or seizure activity:* Glucagon subcutaneous (SQ) or intramuscular (IM) Intravenous (IV) glucose	Insulin Exercise Increased oral fluids	IV fluids IV insulin Electrolyte replacement Generalized supportive care

come evident when most of the beta cells are destroyed. After initiation of insulin therapy, the child may experience a "honeymoon" phase, characterized by hypoglycemia and a decreasing need for insulin. This may last from a few weeks to 1 year or longer. It is important to prepare the child and family for the possibility of a honeymoon phase, both to avoid the misconception that the diabetes is "going away" and to provide instruction on recognition and treatment of hypoglycemia.

The goal of insulin therapy is to replace the insulin the child is no longer able to make. Synthetic human insulin, made by recombinant deoxyribonucleic acid (DNA) technology, is free of animal impurities and is recommended for children. Previously, insulin was derived from bovine and porcine pancreatic extracts. Oral hypoglycemic agents, although useful in the treatment of type 2 diabetes, are not effective in the treatment of type 1 diabetes.

TABLE **51-4** Insulin Action by Type (Humulin)

Type	Onset	Peak	Duration
Lispro/Aspart	10-15 min	30-90 min	3 hr
Regular	30-60 min	2-3 hr	3-6 hr
NPH or Lente	2-4 hr	4-10 hr	10-16 hr
Glargine	——	——	24 hr

The choice of insulin types and schedule of injections is based on the child's needs (Table 51-4). Daily self-monitoring of blood glucose aids in defining insulin requirements. The child in the honeymoon phase needs less insulin than the

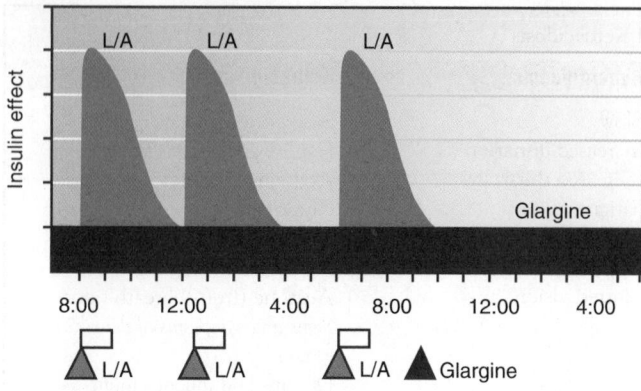

Figure 51-2 Peak action of insulin injections is timed to correspond with the child's usual meal and snack times to minimize the chance of hypoglycemia. (From Alemzadeh, R., & Wyatt, D. [2004]. Diabetes mellitus in children. In R. Behrman, R. Kliegman, & H. Jensen [Eds.]. *Nelson textbook of pediatrics* [p. 1956, A]. Philadelphia: Saunders.)

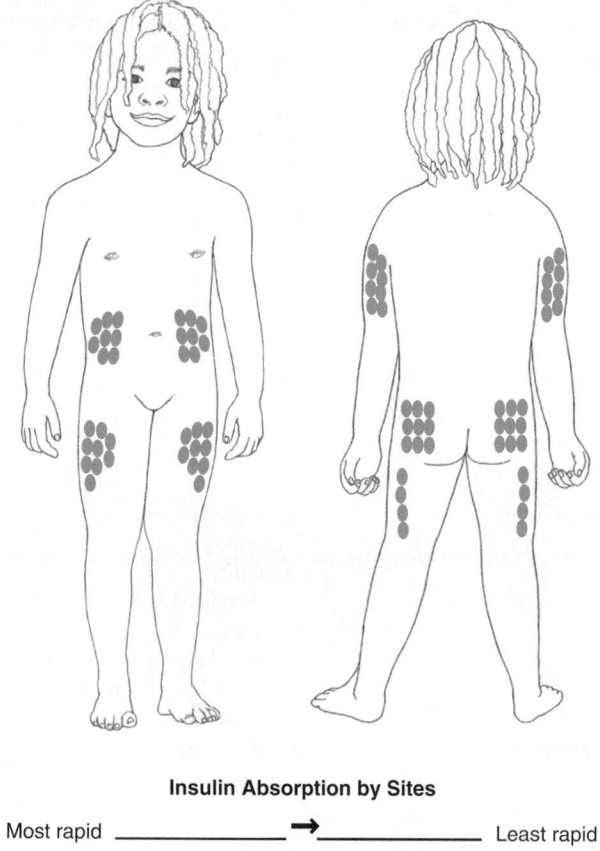

Insulin Absorption by Sites

Most rapid _____ ➡ _____ Least rapid

Abdomen ➡ Arms ➡ Hips ➡ Thighs

Figure 51-3 Subcutaneous insulin injection sites most commonly used are illustrated here, although almost any area on the body may be used. Sites are rotated on a daily basis to help prevent the formation of fatty lumps, which absorb insulin poorly. However, because the rate of absorption varies by site (*see chart*), the child is advised to rotate sites within the same general area (e.g., arm, thigh) for a period of 2 to 3 weeks before changing to another area. This will help decrease variations in absorption from day to day. (Chart modified from Albisser, A.M., & Sperlich, M. [1993]. Adjusting insulins. *Diabetes Educator, 18*[3], 211-227.)

child who makes no endogenous insulin. The pubertal child requires larger insulin dosages.

Schedule. The Diabetes Control and Complications Trial Research Group concluded that long-term diabetic complications can be minimized by intensive treatment (Tamborlane & Ahern, 1997). This treatment, defined as administration of insulin by three or more injections a day of a combination long-acting basal and rapid-acting bolus (multiple daily injection [MDI]) or continuously by insulin pump (continuous subcutaneous insulin infusion [CSII]), mimics physiologic delivery of insulin. The injection schedule is individually prescribed according to the child's glycemic targets and may consist of an intermediate-acting insulin combined with rapid-acting insulin injected before breakfast, rapid-acting insulin injected before the evening meal, and intermediate-acting insulin injected before bed. The peak actions of these insulins are timed to correspond to the child's usual mealtimes and snack times to minimize the possibility of hypoglycemia. More recent studies have suggested that glargine (Lantus), given in the evening as the basal insulin and complemented during the day by a rapid-acting insulin (lispro or aspart) when the child eats carbohydrates, provides improved glycemic control (Bloomgarden, 2002) (Fig. 51-2).

Administration. Because insulin is a protein and would be digested if taken orally, it is given parenterally. Insulin is administered by subcutaneous injection into the adipose tissue over large muscle masses: the back of the arms, the top and outer portion of the thighs, the abdomen, and the hip (Fig. 51-3). To avoid injecting into the muscle or vascular space, use a 45-degree angle of injection with the $^{1}/_{2}$-inch needle or a 90-degree angle with the $^{5}/_{16}$-inch needle. Rotation of injection sites helps prevent adipose hypertrophy (fatty lumps), which absorb insulin poorly. Various injection sites absorb insulin at slightly different rates. Absorption is also affected by the amount of exercise the underlying muscle engages in and by body temperature. To help decrease day-to-day variations in absorption, the child should use one location within a major site for the morning injection; then rotate to another location within the

site for the evening injection; and a third location for the bedtime injection.

Insulin can be administered by an insulin syringe, air injector, or insulin pump. Disposable syringes are to be used only one time and then safely discarded (with the syringe placed in a puncture-resistant, opaque container before placing in the trash).

The air injector uses compressed air to deposit the insulin within the fatty tissue, without the use of a needle. The child or family must learn to use the device correctly: load insulin, adjust pressure settings to avoid intramuscular delivery, and clean properly.

The insulin pump is a device that provides a continuous infusion of rapid-acting insulin. The device comprises a computer, a reservoir of rapid-acting insulin, and thin tubing, through which the insulin is delivered by a small needle inserted into the abdomen. A continuous basal rate of insulin infusion is maintained, and bolus dosages are infused as determined by blood glucose testing. The pump most closely mimics physiologic delivery of insulin and provides a more flexible lifestyle. This option may appeal to adolescents, but the candidate for insulin pump therapy must be willing to meticulously measure blood glucose throughout the day (and, often, at night as well) to avoid hypoglycemia and to respond to hyperglycemia. Dietary recommendations are different for children or adolescents using an insulin pump and are based on carbohydrate counting (American Diabetes Association, 1999; Olohan & Zappitelli, 2003).

Nutrition Therapy

The goal of nutrition therapy is to promote normal growth, encourage good nutrition, prevent complications, and maintain near-normal blood glucose levels. Because the insulin dosage is balanced with food intake, the diet plan should stress a consistent intake, particularly of carbohydrate food products. The diet therapy chosen should be easy to understand and should help the child and family learn to make healthy food choices. The meal plan is based on the child's diet history. As the child grows, the meal plan is tailored to meet changing dietary needs.

Exercise

Exercise is an important aspect of diabetes management. Exercise enhances the action of insulin in lowering blood glucose levels. The child with diabetes should be encouraged to participate in age-appropriate sports. Early enjoyment of a sport or activity can promote a lifelong active lifestyle. Because exercise lowers glucose levels, the child must be taught how to prevent hypoglycemia. The child should try to schedule activities to avoid exercising when an insulin dose is peaking. Maintaining proper hydration while exercising is very important.

Teach the family to add extra snacks of 15 to 30 g carbohydrate for each 45 to 60 minutes of exercise. Coaches and teammates should be taught how to recognize and treat hypoglycemia. Delayed or nocturnal hypoglycemia can occur after strenuous activity. Additional carbohydrate might be required after exercise to maintain blood glucose levels. The child should always wear Medic-Alert identification.

Blood Glucose Monitoring

Self-monitoring of blood glucose provides an objective tool to assist with diabetes control. Monitoring is recommended before meals and before the bedtime snack. More frequent monitoring may be used during prolonged exercise, during an illness, or if nighttime hypoglycemia is suspected.

Blood glucose goals must be tailored to the abilities of the family and the age of the child. Goals for the infant or toddler are usually liberalized to aid in preventing severe hypoglycemia. Preprandial blood glucose goals are as follows:

- Nondiabetic: 70 to 110 mg/dl
- Children with type 1 diabetes mellitus: 80 to 180 mg/dl
- Infants and toddlers with type I diabetes mellitus: 80 to 200 mg/dl

The identified goals are a target range; not all glucose levels fall in this range, even in the child with excellent diabetes control.

> ## ⚠ CRITICAL TO REMEMBER
>
> ### Managing the Child With Type 1 Diabetes Mellitus
>
> **Insulin**
> - Store insulin in a cool, dry place. Do not freeze or expose to excessive heat or agitation.
> - Check the expiration date on the vial before using.
> - Once opened, date the vial and discard as recommended.
> - When mixing two different types of insulin, inject the appropriate amount of air into both vials and then withdraw the short-acting (clear) insulin first.
>
> **Nutrition**
> - Meals and snacks are balanced with insulin action.
> - Both the timing of the meal or snack and the amount of food are important in avoiding hyperglycemia or hypoglycemia.
> - Adherence to a daily schedule that maintains a consistent food intake combined with consistent insulin injections aids in achieving metabolic control.
>
> **Exercise**
> - Avoid exercising during insulin peak.
> - Add extra 15- to 30-g carbohydrate snacks for each 45 to 60 minutes of exercise.
>
> **Blood Glucose Monitoring**
> - Record blood glucose results in a diary.
> - A 3- to 4-day alteration in glucose levels requires an adjustment of insulin dose.

Glucose test results should be recorded in a glucose diary or record book. Patterns or trends in blood glucose levels outside the target range indicate a need to adjust the insulin dose. Three or four days of a consistent pattern of glucose values (e.g., 200 mg/dl before the evening meal for 3 consecutive days) indicate a need to increase the appropriate insulin. The health care team may provide the family with guidelines for increasing insulin dose based on blood glucose patterns.

Blood glucose meters are accurate only if used according to manufacturers' recommendations. Regardless of the brand selected, quality control procedures must be performed as recommended. Test supplies must be stored according to manufacturers' specifications and discarded when outdated. (Procedure 37-6, p. 951, shows the finger stick method for obtaining a small blood sample.)

Developmental Issues

Infant and Toddler. The infant or toddler with type 1 diabetes poses special challenges for diabetes management. The burden of management falls on the parents or other caregivers. Achieving consistency in dietary intake with the infant can be quite difficult. Inconsistent intake, particularly of carbohydrates, contributes to blood glucose variability. Food control issues can easily become a battleground between the child and the parent. A diet strategy

TABLE 51-5 Examples of Delegation of Diabetes Tasks (With Supervision)

Developmental Characteristics	Diabetes Task	Diet Task
TODDLER OR PRESCHOOLER		
Likes rituals Finicky eater Not yet able to understand need for insulin	Chooses and cleans finger for puncture Helps by holding still for injection Identifies a word or phrase to describe a feeling of hypoglycemia	Helps by choosing foods
SCHOOL-AGE CHILD		
Present-oriented Spending large amounts of time away from parents Begins to develop self-concept	Performs finger puncture and blood glucose test Chooses injection site according to rotation schedule Pushes plunger on insulin syringe after the needle is inserted by parent or gives own injection Performs ketone test	Recognizes need to eat on time to avoid hypoglycemia Knows treatment for hypoglycemia
EARLY ADOLESCENT		
Looks to peer group for identity Needs to conform to peer-group norms Increased risk-taking behaviors	Records blood glucose values in diary Draws up insulin with supervision Performs insulin injection	Knows meal plan Can choose correct foods for snack Adds extra snack for increased activity
MIDDLE OR LATE ADOLESCENT		
Future-oriented Wants to take charge of life Able to recognize consequences of behaviors and choices Emotional separation from parents	Draws up and injects insulin Looks for patterns in blood glucose values Recognizes when to test for ketones Initiates treatment for ketones (fluids)	Can plan meals and snacks based on meal plan Can choose appropriate foods at a party

that stresses carbohydrate consistency rather than specific food groups offers more flexibility than a structured meal plan.

Allow the toddler to participate in making food choices (from perhaps two or three options) to offer the child a sense of control. The signs and symptoms of hypoglycemia are difficult to recognize in the infant or might be mistaken for the toddler's temper tantrum. The glucose goals for this age-group are liberalized to avoid episodes of severe hypoglycemia.

Establishing rituals and routines helps the toddler feel more in control. Encourage a parent to have a specific place to perform the blood test and a special place to keep supplies. Toddlers feel more in control if they are able to predict and participate in diabetes activities (Table 51-5).

Preschooler. The preschool years are characterized by increasing motor maturity, a widening social circle, and magical thinking. The preschooler can understand simple explanations regarding diabetes. Such explanations help to allay fears that the diabetes was caused by the child being "bad." Play therapy using dolls and diabetes equipment helps the preschooler express concerns regarding injections and finger sticks.

The preschooler has a more predictable appetite than the toddler and is frequently willing to try new foods. Nonetheless, supervision is necessary to ensure that meals and snacks are eaten, especially if the child is in a daycare setting with many distractions.

The preschooler may be able to identify the feelings associated with hypoglycemia. Use the child's description as a code word for the onset of hypoglycemia symptoms. Preschoolers' preference for high-energy activities puts them at risk for hypoglycemia. The caregiver should be prepared with readily available carbohydrate foods as well as emergency medications.

School-Age Child. The school-age child and family face the challenge of incorporating diabetes care within a busy school day. To avoid singling out the child, the diabetes care should be as unobtrusive as possible while still maintaining a safe environment for the child. The family should communicate with school personnel about the child's diabetes. A school nurse or health aide should be identified to supervise prelunch blood glucose monitoring, to assist with insulin injections, and to educate other school personnel in recognizing and treating hypoglycemia. Schools vary on the availability of nursing services. Parents may have to work with school personnel to identify appropriate staff to supervise their child's diabetes care.

Planning ahead for field trips, school parties, and athletic events allows the child with diabetes to participate safely in age-appropriate activities. For example, the child who has soccer practice three afternoons per week needs to plan how to prevent hypoglycemia during practice.

Adolescent. The developmental milestones of the adolescent are often in conflict with the recommendations for achieving diabetes control. The young adolescent is concerned with body image and peer group acceptance and is moving away from the family for support and identity. Clothing, diet, lifestyle, and speech are areas in which the early adolescent strives to conform to peers.

The midadolescent is open to risk-taking behaviors and is more openly challenging of parental authority. By late adolescence, the person becomes more future-oriented, with behaviors based more on abstract morals and less on peer group demands.

These normally recognized milestones become dilemmas when diabetes control is affected. Missed injections, omitted blood tests, irregular meals, and dietary splurges are frequent complaints of parents of diabetic adolescents.

Parents and their adolescents must accept that diabetes responsibility increasingly shifts to the adolescent. Encourage parents to work as partners with the adolescent to achieve diabetes control. Identify what is important to the adolescent, and use that information as a tool to motivate adherence. The adoles-

cent is not motivated by predictions of complications in the distant future. Rather, motivation should focus on issues important to the adolescent: personal appearance, athletic ability, strength and muscle mass, endurance, or ideal weight.

Delegating Diabetes Responsibilities

Children with diabetes are functionally able to perform diabetes skills far sooner than they can cognitively understand the implications of the activity or consequences of omitting the activity. Transfer of responsibility should be on a step-by-step basis, according to the child's cognitive understanding and functional abilities. Diabetes responsibilities shift from full parental responsibility to a partnership between parent and child and then to the acceptance of responsibility by the young adult. Delegating diabetes responsibility at an inappropriate age results in poor diabetes control and frequent bouts of DKA. The importance of ongoing parental support and supervision cannot be overemphasized.

Text continued on p. 1479

FAMILIES
Want to Know

About Home Management of Type 1 Diabetes Mellitus

The child and family are understandably overwhelmed with questions and fears about the diagnosis. Encourage all family members to participate. Choose a comfortable location subject to few interruptions. Provide appropriate literature and materials for family members. Videotapes, booklets, and pamphlets should be developmentally appropriate. Educational materials for the parents should also match the parents' literacy skills.

The family needs to know the following. The accompanying checklist of outcomes evaluates level of understanding.
• General information about type 1 diabetes mellitus
• How to administer and store insulin
• How to monitor blood glucose levels, using the equipment properly
• Signs and management of hypoglycemic episodes
• Signs and management of hyperglycemia
• Strategies for when the child is ill
• Nutrition and exercise principles
• Potential long-term complications
• Available resources for emotional and physical support

All family members should be given the opportunity to practice skills taught. Practicing procedures on themselves or each other helps allay family fears and allows the child to supervise as a family member performs the procedure. Help develop problem-solving skills by using various scenarios that encourage decision-making. Because education is an ongoing process, the family needs a contact person to whom they can turn for advice and support.

Outcomes

General Information
The child and family will be able to:
1. Describe the action of insulin in the body.
2. Describe the characteristics of type 1 versus type 2 diabetes.

3. Identify three factors that can be used to control blood glucose levels.

Medication Therapy
The child and family will be able to:
1. Name the child's insulin, and identify the onset, peak, and duration of action.
2. State the storage recommendations for insulin.
3. State the recommended expiration date of the insulin.
4. Demonstrate accurate syringe preparation for a single type of insulin.
5. Demonstrate syringe preparation using two types of insulin.
6. Demonstrate subcutaneous insulin injection technique.
7. Identify insulin injection sites, and describe a pattern of rotation.
8. Identify a plan for safe syringe disposal.
9. Identify recommended insulin dosages and injection times.

Home Glucose Monitoring
The child and family will be able to:
1. Identify nondiabetic blood glucose levels and target goals for good glucose control.
2. Demonstrate the use, calibration, control testing, and cleaning of the blood glucose monitor.
3. Identify a plan for recording blood glucose values.

Hypoglycemia
The child and family will be able to:
1. Identify the signs and symptoms of a hypoglycemic reaction.
2. Describe appropriate treatment for both a mild and a severe hypoglycemic reaction.
3. Identify three potential causes of a hypoglycemic reaction.
4. Identify the importance of medical emergency identification.
5. Describe typical blood glucose trends during the honeymoon phase.

Continued

FAMILIES
Want to Know

About Home Management of Type 1 Diabetes Mellitus—cont'd

Hyperglycemia/Sick Day

The child and family will be able to:

1. Identify the signs and symptoms of hyperglycemia.
2. Identify strategies to control hyperglycemia.
3. Describe the possible effects of stress or illness on diabetes control.
4. Demonstrate the procedure for ketone (urine, serum) testing.
5. State when to test for ketones.
6. State basic treatment for ketones.
7. Describe the signs and symptoms requiring physician or other health care team contact.

Exercise

The child and family will be able to:

1. State the effect of exercise on blood glucose levels.
2. State the benefits and precautions for exercise.
3. Identify the relationship of diet, exercise, and insulin to blood glucose control.

4. Generate a home schedule that identifies mealtimes, blood test times, and insulin injection times.

Complications

The child and family will be able to:

1. Identify the role of glucose control in the prevention or delay of diabetes-related complications.
2. Identify appropriate health care follow-up for the child with diabetes.

Psychological Adjustment and Family Involvement

The child and family will be able to create a plan for the entire family to participate in diabetes care and management.

Community Resources

The child and family will be able to identify available community resources for ongoing diabetes education and support.

When other parts of the treatment regimen have become familiar, ▶ the injections can be taught. Initially, self-injecting insulin will be scary for the school-age child. It is usually advisable to start with the parent inserting the needle and the child pushing the plunger. The child can then progress to performing self-injection.

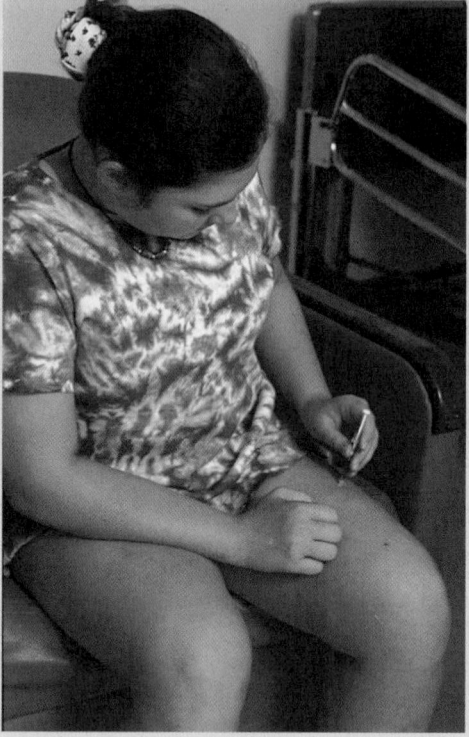

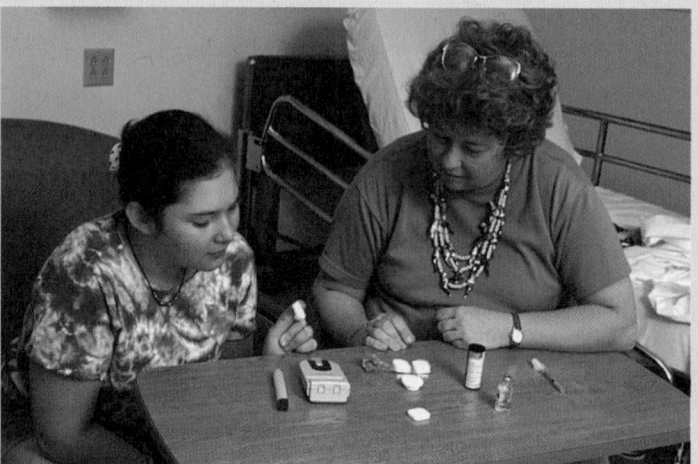

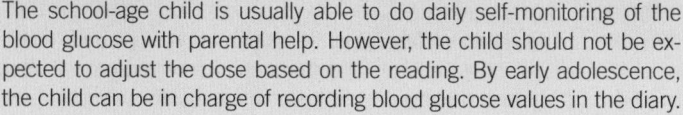

The school-age child is usually able to do daily self-monitoring of the blood glucose with parental help. However, the child should not be expected to adjust the dose based on the reading. By early adolescence, the child can be in charge of recording blood glucose values in the diary.

Nursing Care Plan

The Child With Type 1 Diabetes Mellitus in the Community Setting

FOCUSED ASSESSMENT

Nursing assessment of the child diagnosed with type 1 diabetes mellitus begins with a careful history. Most children with diabetes are identified on a routine well visit, or the child may exhibit signs on a visit to the school nurse. Identify signs and symptoms of hyperglycemia—the three *P*'s (*p*olydipsia, *p*olyuria, and *p*olyphagia). Daytime polydipsia and polyuria may not worry a parent, but enuresis or accidents in the previously toilet-trained child and nighttime requests for water spark concern. New-onset diabetes is frequently overlooked in light of specific symptoms. A urinary tract infection might be suspected based on urinary frequency. An infective process frequently accompanies the onset of diabetes but is not the cause of the diabetes. The stress associated with an infection can compromise the function of the remaining insulin-secreting cells. A history of weight loss or fatigue is also a common parental observation. Nausea and vomiting are present in the child who is acidotic. Ask about other medications used. Glucocorticoids and some chemotherapeutic agents can cause hyperglycemia.

Physical assessment should include signs and symptoms of dehydration: dry mucous membranes, flushed skin, acute weight change, absence of tearing, or poor skin turgor. Identify the time of most recent voiding. Oliguria is a significant finding in the assessment of dehydration.

If the child is admitted to the hospital, assess for signs and symptoms of acidosis: abdominal pain, nausea and vomiting (which also contribute to dehydration), Kussmaul respirations coupled with a fruity breath odor, or decreasing level of consciousness (LOC). Ongoing assessment of the child in acidosis should include vital signs, LOC, and intake and output. Vital signs and LOC should be monitored frequently until stable.

Assess the family's knowledge of diabetes. For the newly diagnosed child, prepare the family to participate in a diabetes education program to learn home care skills. Encourage parents to arrange for time away from work and school to participate. Assess the family's ability to cope with the diagnosis of a chronic disease. Identify usual methods of coping with stress and usual support systems. Explore the availability of financial resources to meet the child's health care needs.

Nursing Diagnosis

Deficient Knowledge related to unfamiliarity with home care needs of the child with type 1 diabetes mellitus.

Expected Outcome

The child and family will:
■ Be able to successfully manage diabetes, as evidenced by demonstration of skills and verbalization of concepts necessary for home care.

INTERVENTION	RATIONALE
1. Identify barriers to learning that might hinder the family's ability to learn home care information. Barriers could include issues such as language fluency, literacy, employment pressures, and childcare. These issues should be addressed before initiating education.	1. Identifying and addressing these issues optimize the learning ability of the family. For example, provide appropriate written materials for the person with low literacy skills or a different native language.
2. Identify learning objectives with the family.	2. A written list of specific objectives helps the family prioritize education, as well as provides a sense of accomplishment as learning objectives are met.
3. Present information at a developmentally appropriate level for the child.	3. The child must cognitively understand diabetes. More advanced information can be presented as the child matures.

Continued

Nursing Care Plan

The Child With Type 1 Diabetes Mellitus in the Community Setting—cont'd

Evaluation

- Can the child and family successfully manage care, as evidenced by return demonstrations of skills necessary to provide home care?
- Are the child and family able to describe principles of diabetes management?

Nursing Diagnosis

Interrupted Family Processes related to the chronic health care needs of a child with type 1 diabetes mellitus.

Expected Outcome

The family will:

- Cope with caring for a child with diabetes, as evidenced by recognizing and identifying stresses and constructing strategies for dealing with the stress of a chronic disease.

INTERVENTION	RATIONALE
1. Assist the family to identify age-appropriate diabetes skills for the child's and the parent's responsibilities.	1. Delegation of responsibilities should occur as the child is both able to perform the skill and able to understand the implications of the skill. Parental support and supervision are essential for all children for successful home management of diabetes.
2. Assist the child and family to identify behaviors that the child recognizes as supportive; for example, all family members follow the child's meal plan, avoid having sweets in the home, offer to record blood glucose levels in the diary for the child, or recognize and praise the child's attempts at adherence.	2. Discussions of family support help involve all family members in the child's care, as well as give the child the opportunity to identify supportive behaviors. Adaptation is enhanced by focusing on the strengths of the child and family.
3. Identify community support systems available for the family, such as summer diabetes camp and age-specific support groups, parent support group, or participation in fund-raising activities in a local diabetes community group.	3. Community resources offer a variety of opportunities for support, as well as an alternative to relying solely on family coping skills (see Appendix I on Evolve website). Activities for the diabetic child can build motivation and self-esteem.
4. Identify a "vacation" plan in which the major caregiver can take a break from diabetes responsibilities. This might include ongoing, day-to-day responsibility of diabetes management shared among parents, siblings, and others or temporarily sharing one aspect of the management.	4. Taking responsibility for diabetes control is very stressful and demanding. Sharing responsibilities among family members helps prevent burnout, discouragement, and frustration.

Evaluation

- Can the child and family verbalize a plan for sharing diabetes responsibility?

Nursing Diagnosis

Imbalanced Nutrition: Less Than Body Requirements related to insulin deficit.

Expected Outcomes

The family and child will:

- Maximize nutritional status, as evidenced by demonstrating the ability to use insulin therapy, diet therapy, and glucose self-monitoring.

The child will:

- Be in nutritional balance, as evidenced by appropriate glucose levels and absence of hyperglycemia and hypoglycemia.

INTERVENTION	RATIONALE
1. Teach the family the action of food (carbohydrates, fats, proteins) on blood glucose level: carbohydrates raise blood glucose levels; fats and proteins have minimal effects on glucose levels.	1. Understanding the relationship of food to blood glucose levels will help the family recognize the rationale for adhering to the diabetic diet.

Nursing Care Plan

The Child With Type 1 Diabetes Mellitus in the Community Setting—cont'd

INTERVENTION	RATIONALE
2. Together with the family, develop an eating schedule that includes times for blood glucose testing, medication, meals, and snacks.	2. Consistency in timing of meals and snacks in relation to insulin injections is essential. Encouraging child and family input into this aspect of planning will impart a sense of control as well as promote adherence.
3. Ask the child to identify favorite foods, and demonstrate how to incorporate these into the meal plan.	3. Most foods can be incorporated into the meal plan, even if only in small amounts. Allowing small amounts of favorite treats can encourage adherence.
4. Observe whether the child's hunger is satisfied on the prescribed diet. Instruct the child and parent to notify the dietitian if the meal plan forces the child to overeat or if the child is persistently hungry. Use an appropriate growth chart to track the child's height and weight with respect to age.	4. The meal plan is tailored to the child and the child's activity level. Nutritional needs vary with age as well as with variations in activity level. For example, a morning gym class may require that the child add a midmorning snack.
5. Discuss the relationship between insulin, food (carbohydrate), and exercise. Identify ideal blood glucose goals for the child. Present a sample situation in which the blood glucose is out of the ideal range, and encourage the family to identify possible options using diet, insulin, and/or exercise to more closely attain the blood glucose goal.	5. Diet, exercise, and insulin therapy are the tools of diabetes management. This exercise will develop problem-solving skills within the family and provide a sense of competency.
6. Instruct the family to plan 3 or 4 days of menus based on the meal plan. Both the type of food as well as the amount of food should be included.	6. This exercise will help the family demonstrate understanding of the diet instructions.

Evaluation

- Do the child and family demonstrate appropriate insulin administration, diet therapy, and glucose monitoring?
- Is the child's height and weight appropriate for age compared with growth chart percentiles?
- Is the child free of episodes of severe hypoglycemia or hyperglycemia?

Nursing Diagnosis

Risk for Injury related to hypoglycemia or hyperglycemia.

Expected Outcomes

The child will:
- Remain injury-free as a result of appropriate recognition and management of hypoglycemia or hyperglycemia.

Family members will:
- Demonstrate knowledge of the signs, symptoms, and treatment of hypoglycemia and hyperglycemia and will initiate appropriate treatment.

INTERVENTION	RATIONALE
For hypoglycemia (blood glucose below 70 mg/dl)	
1. Teach the child and family to recognize the signs and symptoms of hypoglycemia (see Table 51-3). School personnel should also be involved in teaching. The school nurse, if available, can play a key role in the care of a child with diabetes.	1. Signs and symptoms of hypoglycemia should prompt the child or parent to test the blood glucose level. Some children do not display adrenergic signs of hypoglycemia. Neuroglycopenic signs (altered sensorium) may be the only clues to hypoglycemia in these children. These signs are very hard for the child to recognize but can be observed by a parent or teacher. Blood glucose goals for this child may need to be modified to prevent hypoglycemic unawareness.

Continued

Nursing Care Plan

The Child With Type 1 Diabetes Mellitus in the Community Setting—cont'd

INTERVENTION	RATIONALE
2. Treat hypoglycemia promptly with 15 g of easily digested carbohydrate. If symptoms are not relieved (or blood glucose level is not above 80 mg/dl) in 15 minutes, repeat the treatment. If the hypoglycemia occurs during the night, treat with 30 g carbohydrate: 15 g simple carbohydrate and 15 g complex carbohydrate with protein. Examples of 15 g of carbohydrate include 4 oz of real fruit juice, 6 oz of regular soda, 6 Life Savers, or a commercial glucose product.	2. Prompt treatment reduces the possibility of a severe reaction. Candy bars, donuts, and cookies are poor treatment choices because of their high fat content, which can delay carbohydrate digestion. The child could also interpret these treats as a reward for hypoglycemia.
3. Help the child and family identify strategies to prevent hypoglycemia based on its common causes: missed or delayed meal, excess insulin, extra exercise without increasing carbohydrate intake. Encourage the family to teach the signs and symptoms of hypoglycemia and necessary treatment to school personnel and daycare workers. Help the child prepare to explain hypoglycemia to friends. Compile a diabetes box for school and daycare. The box should contain carbohydrates for treating hypoglycemia as well as written information. Instruct the child to wear Medic-Alert identification at all times.	3. Many episodes of hypoglycemia can be avoided by careful planning and anticipating potential situations that could result in hypoglycemia. Instruction about the signs, symptoms, and treatment of hypoglycemia is essential information to be shared with people caring for the child. Hypoglycemia is a potential emergency that requires prompt recognition and treatment.
4. Teach the parents how to treat severe hypoglycemia. For the unconscious child or the child having a seizure, a small amount of glucose gel (cake frosting or honey will also work) can be rubbed on the inner cheek and gums. Avoid placing a large amount of gel in the mouth because the child could choke. Glucagon (available by prescription as *Glucagon Emergency Kit* from Eli Lilly Co.) can be injected subcutaneously or intramuscularly. Inject 1 mg for the child weighing over 50 lb (22.75 kg) or 20 to 30 mcg/kg for children weighing less than 50 lb (22.75 kg). The onset of action is 10 to 15 minutes. Position the unconscious child on the side. Once conscious, the child needs a large snack to replace lost glycogen stores.	4. The unconscious child or the child having a seizure requires prompt treatment. Glucagon is a pancreatic hormone that opposes the action of insulin and promotes the conversion of liver glycogen to blood glucose. The child is positioned on the side to prevent aspiration. Both severe hypoglycemia and glucagon administration can result in nausea with vomiting.

BOX 51-4
Sick-Day Rules for the Child with Type 1 Diabetes Mellitus

1. Always give the insulin injection, even if the child does not have an appetite. If you believe that the child will become hypoglycemic with the usual dose, contact the physician or nurse educator for specific instructions. If ordered, use sliding-scale rapid-acting insulin for hyperglycemia every 3 to 4 hours.
2. Test blood glucose level at least every 4 hours and more often for persistent hypoglycemia or hyperglycemia.
3. Test for urine ketones with each voiding. Notify the physician or nurse educator if moderate or large amounts of urine ketones are present. Additional regular insulin may be ordered.
4. Encourage calorie-free liquids. If ketones are present, liquids are essential to aid in clearing.
5. Follow the child's usual meal plan. If the child has a poor appetite, a sick-day diet consisting of simple carbohydrates can be substituted. Try to replace the usual grams of carbohydrate with simple carbohydrate foods.
6. Encourage rest, especially if urine ketones are present. Exercising while ketones are present results in increased ketone formation.
7. Notify the physician or nurse educator of:
   - Nausea and vomiting
   - Fruity odor to the breath
   - Deep, rapid respirations
   - Decreasing level of consciousness
   - Moderate or high urine ketones
   - Persistent hyperglycemia

Nursing Care Plan

The Child With Type 1 Diabetes Mellitus in the Community Setting—cont'd

INTERVENTION	RATIONALE
For hyperglycemia (blood glucose higher than target range)	
1. Teach the family to recognize potential causes of hyperglycemia: inadequate insulin, increased dietary intake, decreased exercise, stress response (either emotional or physical stress [e.g., illness]).	1. Anticipating situations that might result in hyperglycemia can help the family plan for such events. The signs and symptoms of hypoglycemia and hyperglycemia can be difficult to distinguish from one another. Test blood glucose before treating to verify glucose level. If testing is impossible, treat for hypoglycemia.
2. Instruct family on sick-day diabetes management, including when and how to test for urine ketones. Identify a home treatment plan for ketones, and identify precautions for vomiting (see Box 51-4).	2. Testing for ketones when ill or when blood glucose is 250 mg/dl or higher aids in detecting insulin deficit. Ketones are treated with (calorie-free) fluids and additional rapid-acting insulin as ordered by the physician. Nausea with vomiting leads to dehydration and cannot be treated with oral fluids. The physician must be notified if the child is vomiting.
3. Identify strategies to prevent or treat hyperglycemia.	3. Consistency in diet, exercise, and insulin injection times aids in preventing hyperglycemia. Persistent hyperglycemia may indicate a need for an insulin dosage adjustment. The growing child needs periodic increases in baseline insulin dosages.

Evaluation

- Does the child remain injury-free?
- Are the child and family able to correctly recognize and promptly treat hypoglycemia and hyperglycemia?

DIABETIC KETOACIDOSIS

Diabetic ketoacidosis (DKA) is the metabolic consequence of a severe insulin deficit.

Etiology

DKA results from an absolute or relative insulin deficit. In the younger diabetic child, the most common cause is insulin resistance, such as a stress response initiated by an infection. In the adolescent, the most common cause is one or more missed insulin injections.

Manifestations

Table 51-3 lists signs and symptoms of DKA, which include abdominal and chest pain, nausea and vomiting, fruity breath, decreased level of consciousness (LOC), Kussmaul respirations, and symptoms of dehydration.

Diagnostic Evaluation

Diabetic ketoacidosis is confirmed by the following test results:

- Blood glucose: elevated
- Arterial or venous pH: low
- Urine ketones: large
- Serum ketones (beta-hydroxybutyric acid, acetone): elevated
- Serum potassium: elevated, normal, or low
- Serum phosphorus: low
- White blood cell count (WBC): elevated secondary to stress demargination (higher with infection)
- Serum CO_2: low

Nursing Care Plan

The Child in Diabetic Ketoacidosis

FOCUSED ASSESSMENT

Assessment of the child in diabetic ketoacidosis (DKA) includes assessing the child's level of consciousness, hydration status, respiratory status, and weight. If the child has a known history of type 1 diabetes mellitus, obtain the following data:

- Most recent blood glucose values
- History of urinary ketones and the steps taken to manage ketones at home
- Usual insulin dosages and the time and amount of the most recent injection
- Time of last meal and amount of food eaten
- Identification of the family member usually given the responsibility for injections and blood tests
- The family's understanding of the daily management of diabetes
- Usual sick-day management plan

Nursing Diagnosis

Deficient Fluid Volume related to abnormal fluid losses through diuresis and emesis.

Expected Outcome

The child will:
- Be safely rehydrated, as evidenced by normal weight, good skin turgor, appropriate urine output for age, and moist mucous membranes.

INTERVENTION	RATIONALE
1. Determine the child's hydration status, evaluating weight, skin turgor, mucous membranes, and urine output.	1. This identifies baseline hydration status. A comparison of the child's usual weight with the admission weight provides an estimation of percent body fluid loss.
2. Encourage calorie-free fluids if the child is not nauseated. Initiate intravenous (IV) fluids as ordered. Normal saline is the initial fluid used, followed by half-normal saline.	2. Rehydration is the initial step in resolving DKA. If acidosis has resulted in nausea and vomiting, IV fluids are required. Fluid losses occur primarily from the osmotic diuresis occurring with hyperglycemia. Emesis can also contribute to fluid loss. Normal saline is the initial IV rehydration fluid. Although normally a hypertonic solution compared with blood, it is isotonic to hypotonic in states of dehydration.
3. Maintain strict intake and output monitoring.	3. Accurate intake and output records are essential in calculating rehydration status.
4. Observe for edema or pulmonary congestion during rehydration.	4. These signs indicate overhydration.
5. Weigh on arrival and frequently during rehydration (every 8 hr may be appropriate).	5. A comparison of the admission weight with the child's usual weight provides an indication of hydration status. Follow-up weights provide ongoing assessment.

Evaluation

- Is the child safely rehydrated, as evidenced by normal weight, urine output appropriate for age, good skin turgor, and moist mucous membranes?

Nursing Diagnosis

Risk for Injury from altered acid-base balance leading to ketone production and acidosis related to lack of insulin.

Expected Outcome

The child will:
- Experience a resolution of ketosis and acidosis, as evidenced by laboratory results and clinical assessment.

Nursing Care Plan

The Child in Diabetic Ketoacidosis—cont'd

INTERVENTION	RATIONALE
1. Test all urine samples for the presence of ketones. Monitor the child's breath for acetone. Observe respirations to identify Kussmaul respirations.	1. The presence of urinary ketones indicates possible acidosis. Serum ketone analysis, or beta-hydroxybutyric acid, is a direct measurement of ketone activity. The liver produces three ketoacids: beta-hydroxybutyric acid, acetoacetate, and acetone. Acetone, the weakest of the acids, is expelled and can be assessed as a fruity smell to the child's breath. High acid levels trigger a rapid and deep respiration (Kussmaul respirations) in an effort to remove excessive acetone.
2. Encourage calorie-free fluids if the child is able to drink. If ordered, begin IV fluids.	2. Fluids are essential in flushing ketones as well as in maintaining hydration. In severe dehydration, the osmotic pull of the blood glucose helps hold fluid in the bloodstream, thus preventing circulatory shock. Insulin is not given until rehydration has begun to diminish the risk of circulatory shock.
3. Initiate IV insulin therapy as ordered. Prime the IV tubing according to institution protocol.	3. Insulin therapy is initiated after rehydration has begun. A continuous IV infusion of Regular insulin is titrated to keep blood glucose in a safe range while avoiding hypoglycemia. Insulin therapy inhibits the production of ketones. Subcutaneous insulin is not an appropriate therapy for the dehydrated child. With dehydration, peripheral vessels constrict, resulting in poor absorption and distribution of the insulin. Insulin adheres to the plastic of the IV bag and tubing, and it is not known whether this affects therapy. Some clinicians recommend priming the IV tubing with the insulin solution and flushing with a fresh solution before delivery. This technique saturates the binding sites of the plastic and provides nonfluctuating insulin delivery.
4. Monitor blood glucose frequently.	4. IV insulin acts rapidly. A continuous infusion of insulin could quickly result in hypoglycemia.
5. Provide glucose-containing IV fluids as ordered.	5. Insulin is needed to inhibit ketone formation. Even though blood glucose values may be in an acceptable range, the insulin infusion must continue until the serum ketones are cleared. To prevent hypoglycemia, glucose is added to the saline hydration solutions.

Evaluation

■ Within 24 hours of admission, does the child display any evidence of ketosis (ketonuria, fruity breath, elevated blood glucose)?

Nursing Diagnosis

Risk for Injury related to electrolyte imbalance from emesis and acidosis.

Expected Outcome

The child will:

■ Remain free from adverse consequences of electrolyte abnormalities, as evidenced by normal serum sodium and potassium values.

Continued

Nursing Care Plan

The Child in Diabetic Ketoacidosis—cont'd

INTERVENTION	RATIONALE
1. Monitor potassium levels closely, looking for signs and symptoms of hyperkalemia, including bradycardia, muscle weakness, hyperreflexia, and respiratory arrest. Also monitor for symptoms of hypokalemia, including muscle weakness, fatigue, hypotension, and hyporeflexia.	1. During acidosis, potassium moves out of the cell and into the intravascular spaces. Intravascular potassium is lost through diuresis. Initially, serum potassium levels may appear in an acceptable range, but this does not reflect the lost intracellular potassium. As rehydration and correction of acidosis begin, potassium moves back into the cells, resulting in lower serum levels. Serum potassium levels are obtained frequently (every 1-2 hr initially) during treatment of DKA to adequately assess potassium needs. (See Chapter 42 for further discussion.)
2. Use cardiac monitor to determine abnormal electrocardiogram resulting from altered potassium levels. Hypokalemia produces prolonged ST segment; notched, flat, or inverted T waves; and dysrhythmias. Hyperkalemia produces flattened P wave or peaked T wave and ventricular fibrillation.	2. Hypokalemia or hyperkalemia can cause a medical emergency, requiring rapid response.
3. After verifying urine output, initiate potassium therapy as ordered. If the child is anuric, notify the physician and do not give potassium.	3. Renal failure can result from severe dehydration. If the child is anuric, potassium is retained, causing abnormal serum levels. Replacement therapy must be done cautiously.

Evaluation

- Does the child maintain a stable fluid and electrolyte balance, with serum sodium and potassium levels within normal limits?

Nursing Diagnosis

Risk for Injury related to cerebral edema from resolving DKA.

Expected Outcome

The child will:
- Remain free from adverse consequences of cerebral edema, as evidenced by appropriate level of consciousness, pupils equal and reacting to light, and absence of headache.

INTERVENTION	RATIONALE
1. Observe the child frequently for signs of cerebral edema: complaints of headache; decreasing level of consciousness; or unequal, fixed, or dilated pupils. Notify physician of any changes from the baseline assessment.	1. Cerebral edema is a complication of resolving DKA that can result in brain damage or death. The causes are unclear but may be related to overhydration; rapid fluid shifts, particularly into the cerebral intracellular space; and electrolyte imbalance. Frequent neurologic checks aid in prompt recognition and prevention of neurologic deficits.
2. Monitor blood glucose values frequently (hourly) when IV insulin is being infused.	2. Blood glucose values should not drop more than 50 to 100 mg/dl to prevent rapid osmotic shifts. As the serum glucose approaches the mid-200s, glucose will be added to the IV fluids. Blood glucose levels are maintained in the mid-200s for the duration of the IV insulin therapy.

Nursing Care Plan

The Child in Diabetic Ketoacidosis—cont'd

Evaluation

- Is the child alert, with equal pupils and without complaints of headache?

Nursing Diagnosis

Deficient Knowledge related to unfamiliarity with home management during sick days.

Expected Outcome

The family will:

- Demonstrate knowledge of home care, as evidenced by promptly recognizing and responding to situations requiring sick-day management.

INTERVENTION	RATIONALE
1. Teach the family how and when to test for urine ketones; that is, when blood glucose level exceeds 250 mg/dl or when the child is ill.	1. Ketones are formed in response to insulin deficit. Either high glucose values or illness could be associated with insulin deficit.
2. Instruct family about sick-day management.	2. Stress, either from an infection or the environment, can cause hyperglycemia and uncontrolled diabetes. Early recognition and treatment of ketones can prevent acute complications.
3. Identify situations requiring the family to contact the diabetes health care team, including nausea with vomiting, high levels of urine ketones, procedures requiring nothing-by-mouth (NPO) status, and signs of acidosis.	3. Early intervention is essential in preventing acidosis and its sequelae. The family can initiate outpatient management of ketones with direction from the diabetes team.
4. Provide the child and family with telephone numbers of appropriate health care professionals for questions on sick-day management.	4. The child and family should know whom to call and how to reach the appropriate health care professional for guidance during sick days.
5. Frequent bouts of DKA require evaluation of home care knowledge, compliance with recommended regimen, home supervision, and coping skills.	5. Frequent episodes of DKA may reflect poor compliance, poor understanding of home care needs, inappropriate or absent parental supervision, or depression. A team approach (including nurse educator, nutritionist, social worker, psychologist, physician) can address many of these issues.

Evaluation

- Can the child and family promptly recognize and respond appropriately to situations requiring sick-day management?
- Is the child able to prevent DKA?

LONG-TERM HEALTH CARE NEEDS FOR THE CHILD WITH TYPE 1 DIABETES MELLITUS

Serious complications are associated with long-term diabetes: retinopathy, nephropathy, neuropathy, and cardiovascular disease. Studies have demonstrated that strict metabolic control of diabetes may decrease the onset or severity of complications. A team approach to diabetes management can best provide the tools to achieve metabolic control. The team includes the physician specialist, nurse educator, dietitian, and behavioral specialist. Regular checkups and telephone contact with the diabetes team are essential to address the needs of the growing child.

Routine health care for the child with diabetes should also include yearly dental and ophthalmologic evaluations, as well as prophylactic interventions, such as influenza vaccinations. Other referral sources should be used as specific needs are identified.

Diabetes research is aimed at preventing diabetes and finding a cure after diagnosis. Multiple immune intervention strategies are being identified and tested, and islet cell transplantation research holds promise for a cure.

KEY CONCEPTS

- The six major hormones of the endocrine system are adrenocorticotropic hormone (ACTH), thyroid-stimulating hormone (TSH), follicle-stimulating hormone (FSH), luteinizing hormone (LH), growth hormone (GH), and prolactin.

- The pituitary gland stimulates target organs to produce specific hormones. When sufficient hormone is produced, the gland signals the pituitary to stop stimulation. This mechanism is referred to as *negative feedback.*

- To improve compliance with daily medications, the nurse may suggest using pill dispensers or a watch with an alarm as a reminder to take medication at specific times.

- A variety of metabolic conditions, most of which are genetically transmitted, can affect newborns; many require long-term dietary management and referral of the family to a genetic counseling center.

- Congenital adrenal hyperplasia (CAH) should be considered in any neonate with unusual-appearing genitalia.

- Signs and symptoms of hypothyroidism include fatigue; constipation; cold intolerance; weight gain; dry, thick skin; edema; and poor growth. Signs and symptoms of hyperthyroidism include nervousness; diarrhea; heat intolerance; weight loss; smooth, velvety skin; exophthalmos; and increased appetite.

- Diabetes insipidus is an inability to concentrate urine because of deficiency of antidiuretic hormone. Diabetes insipidus is characterized by polyuria, dehydration, increased serum sodium, and a low urine specific gravity. In comparison, syndrome of inappropriate antidiuretic hormone (SIADH) results from excessive production of antidiuretic hormone. This is evidenced by decreased urine output, increased urine specific gravity, and decreased serum sodium.

- Psychosocial issues concerning children with precocious puberty include self-consciousness about their bodies, being treated as older than their chronologic age, and aggressive behavior by boys.

- In the absence of insulin, the metabolism of fats, proteins, and carbohydrates is impaired and glucose is unable to move into the intracellular space, resulting in hyperglycemia.

- Both type 1 diabetes mellitus and type 2 diabetes mellitus involve abnormal carbohydrate metabolism; but risks related to age of onset, body size, gender, ethnic background, and treatments differ for the two types of diabetes.

- The goals of diabetes management are to maintain appropriate height and weight, maintain an age-appropriate lifestyle, maintain near-normal glycosylated hemoglobin, and prevent acute complications of hypoglycemia and hyperglycemia.

- Common nursing diagnoses associated with type 1 diabetes mellitus include Deficient Knowledge, Interrupted Family Processes, Imbalanced Nutrition: More or Less Than Body Requirements, and Risk for Injury related to hypoglycemia and hyperglycemia.

- Teaching needs associated with home management of type 1 diabetes mellitus are related to the disease process, medication, home glucose monitoring, hypoglycemia, hyperglycemia, exercise, complications, and support services.

- There are adrenergic and neuroglycopenic clinical manifestations of hypoglycemia. Hypoglycemia should be treated with 15 g of easily digested carbohydrate.

- Hyperglycemia is caused by an inadequate amount of insulin, increased dietary intake, decreased amount of exercise, or a response to emotional or physical stress. Persistent hyperglycemia may indicate a need for an insulin dosage adjustment.

- Nursing diagnoses related to care of the child in diabetic ketoacidosis (DKA) include Deficient Fluid Volume, Risk for Injury related to altered acid-base balance, Risk for Injury related to electrolyte imbalance, Risk for Injury related to cerebral edema, and Deficient Knowledge.

ANSWERS to Critical Thinking Exercise 51-1

Signs of growth hormone (GH) deficiency or another underlying disorder affecting growth are related to the rate of the child's growth, not to the height measurement itself. If, over a period of 6 to 12 months of careful growth measurement, the child demonstrates a marked downward deviation from a previous growth rate along with other signs of GH deficiency, the child needs to be referred for diagnostic evaluation.

Children grow and mature at varying rates, depending on genetic and environmental factors. Many boys do not begin their growth spurts until the late teen years but still attain an adequate adult height. Some children have a familial tendency toward short stature not related to any underlying disorder. One way of estimating a child's eventual adult height (within 2-3 inches) is to add the mother's and father's heights (in inches) and divide by 2. To this, add 2½ inches (for boys), or subtract 2½ inches (for girls). Emphasize to a worried parent that administration of GH will not help a child who does not have a true GH deficiency.

REFERENCES and READINGS

Allen, D.B. (1999). Short stature. In F. Burg, E. Wald, J. Ingelfinger, & R. Polin (Eds.), *Gellis & Kagan's current pediatric therapy* (16th ed., pp. 733-734). Philadelphia: Saunders.

Alemzadeh, R., & Wyatt, D. (2004). Diabetes mellitus in children. In R. Behrman, R. Kliegmen, & H. Jenson (Eds.). *Nelson textbook of pediatrics* (17th ed., pp. 1947-1971). Philadelphia, PA: Saunders.

American Academy of Pediatrics, & American Thyroid Association. (1993). Newborn screening for congenital hypothyroidism: Recommended guidelines. *Pediatrics, 91*(6), 1203-1209.

American Diabetes Association. (2004). 2004 clinical practice recommendations (Electronic Version). *Diabetes Care, 27*(Supplement 1), S1-S142. Retrieved July 20, 2004 from www.diabetes.org.

American Diabetes Association. (1999). Clinical practice recommendations 1999. *Diabetes Care, 22*(Suppl. 1). Available on-line: www. diabetes.org/diabetescare/supplementl99/.

Bertelloni, S., Baroncelli, G.I., Viacava, P., Massimetti, M., Simi, P., & Saggese, G. (1999). Can growth hormone treatment in boys without growth hormone deficiency impair testicular function? *Journal of Pediatrics, 135*(3), 278-279.

Bloomgarden, Z. (2002). Treatment issues in type 1 diabetes. *Diabetes Care, 25*(1), 230-236.

Chase, H.P. (2002). *Understanding diabetes* (10th ed.). Denver, CO: The Guild of the Children's Diabetes Foundation at Denver.

Breault, D., & Majzoub, J. (2004). Diabetes insipidus. In R. Behrman, R. Kliegmen, & H. Jenson (Eds.). *Nelson textbook of pediatrics* (17th ed., pp. 1853-1855). Philadelphia, PA: Saunders.

Caffrey, R. (2003). Diabetes under control: are all syringes created equal? *American Journal of Nursing, 103*(6), 46-49.

Critical care: A quick check of the endocrine system. (1998). *Nursing, 28*(7), 12-13, 32.

Dabelea, D., Pettitt, D.J., Jones, K.L., & Arslanian, S.A. (1999). Type 2 diabetes mellitus in minority children and adolescents: An emerging problem. *Endocrinology and Metabolism Clinics of North America, 28*(4), 709-729.

Delamater, A. (2002). Working with children who have type 1 diabetes mellitus. *Practical Psychology* for *Diabetes Clinicians* (pp.127-137). Alexandria, Virginia: American Diabetes Association.

Glass, S. (1999). Genetic screening. In P. Thureen, J. Deacon, P. O'Neill, & J. Hernandez (Eds.), *Assessment and care of the well newborn* (pp. 214-215). Philadelphia: Saunders.

Grey, M., Boland, E.A., Davidson, M., Yu, C., & Tamborlane, W.V. (1999). Coping skills training for youths with diabetes on intensive therapy. *Applied Nursing Research, 12*(l), 3-12.

Harrell, G.B., & Murray, P.D. (1998). Diagnosis and management of congenital hypothyroidism. *Journal of Perinatal and Neonatal Nursing, 2*(4), 75-85.

Imagawa, A., Hanafusa, T., Miyagawa, J., & Matsuzawa, Y. (2000). A novel subtype of type 1 diabetes mellitus characterized by a rapid onset and an absence of diabetes-related antibodies. Osaka IDDM Study Group. *New England Journal of Medicine, 342*(5), 301-307.

Kaplowitz, P.B., & Oberfield, S.E. (1999). Reexamination of the age limit for defining when puberty is precocious in girls in the United States: Implications for evaluation and treatment. Drug and Therapeutics and Executive Committees of the Lawson Wilkins Pediatric Endocrine Society. *Pediatrics, 104*, 936-941.

Kaufman, F., Heluorson, M., & Lohry, J. (2001). *Putting your diabetes on the pump.* Alexandria, VA: American Diabetes Association.

Kyngas, H., Hentinen, M., & Barlow, J. (1998). Adolescents' perceptions of physicians, nurses, parents and friends: Help or hindrance in compliance with diabetes self-care? *Journal of Advances in Nursing, 27*(4), 760-769.

LaFranchi, S. (2002). Newborn thyroid disorders and screening. In Lavin, N. (Ed.). *Manual of endocrinology and metabolism* (3rd ed., pp. 422-438). Philadelphia: Lippincott.

LaFranchi, S. (2004). Disorders of the thyroid gland. In R. Behrman, R. Kliegmen, & H. Jenson (Eds.). *Nelson textbook of pediatrics* (17th ed., pp. 1870-1887). Philadelphia, PA: Saunders.

Lawson, M.L., & Cohen, N. (1999) A single sample luteinizing hormone (LH)–releasing hormone (LHRH) stimulation test for monitoring LH suppression in children with precocious puberty receiving LHRH agonists. *Journal of Clinical Endocrinology and Metabolism, 84*(12), 4536-4540.

Lee, Peter (2002). Precocious, early and delayed female pubertal development. In Lavin, N. (Ed.). *Manual of endocrinology and metabolism* (3rd ed., pp. 210-222). Philadelphia: Lippincott.

Leonard, B., Skay, C., & Rheinberger, M. (1998). Self-management development in children and adolescents with diabetes: The role of maternal self-efficacy and conflict. *Journal of Pediatric Nursing, 13*(4), 224-233.

Levine, L. (2002). Congenital adrenal hyperplasia. In Lavin, N. (Ed.) *Manual of endocrinology and metabolism* (3rd ed., pp.147-162). Philadelphia: Lippincott.

National Institutes of Health. (2000, Oct. 18). NIH Consensus Panel recommends comprehensive approach to life long care for PKU. Available on-line: www.nichd.nih.gov.

Olohan, K., & Zappitelli, D. (2003). The insulin pump. *American Journal of Nursing, 103*(4), 48-56.

Onkamo, P., Vaananen S., Karvonen, M., & Tuomilehto, J. (1999). Worldwide increase in incidence of type 1 diabetes: The analysis of the data on published incidence trends. *Diabetologia, 42*(12), 1395-1403.

Parks, J. (2004). Hypopituitarism. In R. Behrman, R. Kliegmen, & H. Jenson (Eds.). *Nelson textbook of pediatrics* (17th ed., pp. 1847-1852). Philadelphia, PA: Saunders.

Rezvani, I. (2000). Defects in metabolism of amino acids. In R. Behrman, R. Kliegman, & H. Jenson (Eds.). *Nelson textbook of pediatrics* (16th ed., pp. 344-345). Philadelphia: Saunders.

Rosenfield, R. (1996). Disorders of growth hormone and insulin-like growth factor secretion and action. In M. Sperling (Ed.), *Pediatric endocrinology* (pp. 117-169). Philadelphia: Saunders.

Sperling, M.A. (2002). Hypoglycemia in infants and children. In Lavin, N. (Ed.) *Manual of endocrinology and metabolism* (3rd ed., pp. 472-478). Philadelphia: Lippincott.

Sullivan-Bolyai, S., Deatrick, J., Gruppuso, P., Tamborlane, W., & Grey, M. (2002). Mothers' experiences raising young children with type 1 diabetes. *Journal for Specialists in Pediatric Nursing: JSPN, 7*(3), 93-103.

Sullivan-Bolyai, S., Deatrick, J., Gruppuso, P., Tamborlane, W., & Grey, M. (2003). Constant vigilance: mothers' work parenting young children with type I diabetes. *Journal of Pediatric Nursing, 18*(1), 21-29.

Tamborlane, W.V., & Ahern, J. (1997). Implications of the diabetes control and complications trial. *Pediatric Clinics of North America, 44*(2), 285-300.

Townsend, S. (1999a). Approach to the infant at risk for hypoglycemia. In P. Thureen, J. Deacon, P. O'Neill, & J. Hernandez (Eds.), *Assessment and care of the well newborn* (pp. 267-271). Philadelphia: Saunders.

Townsend, S. (1999b). The large-for-gestational-age and small-for-gestational-age infant. In P. Thureen, J. Deacon, P. O'Neill, & J. Hernandez (Eds), *Assessment and care of the well newborn* (pp. 272-283). Philadelphia: Saunders.

Victorina, W., Rydstedt, L, & Sowers, J. (2002). Clinical disorders of vasopressin. In N. Lavin (Ed) *Manual of endocrinology and metabolism* (3rd ed., pp. 68-82). Philadelphia: Lippincott.

Wilson, T., et al. (2003). Update of guidelines for the use of growth hormone in children: the Lawson Wilkins Pediatric Society Drug and Therapeutics Committee. *Journal of Pediatrics, 143*(4), 415-421.

52

The Child with a Neurologic Alteration

DEFINITIONS

Arnold-Chiari malformation Abnormalities of the fourth ventricle, lower cerebellum, and brainstem; often associated with myelomeningocele.

autoregulation The unique ability of the cerebral arteries to maintain a steady blood flow during changes in blood pressure and perfusion by adjusting their diameter in response to alterations in cerebral perfusion pressure.

basal ganglia A major communication and sorting area for messages to and from the cerebral hemispheres, composed of masses of gray matter; controls movement and participates in emotion and cognition.

battle sign Bruising or hemorrhage over the mastoid.

blood-brain barrier The separation between brain tissue and blood; it is very selective and normally permeable only to glucose, water, carbon dioxide, and some chemicals and drugs.

brainstem Structure connected to the cerebral hemispheres by thick bunches of nerve fibers; all nerve fibers traverse through the brainstem from the hemispheres to the cerebellum and spinal cord.

cerebral cortex Gray matter of the cerebrum where the higher functions of thinking occur.

cerebral herniation Shift of brain tissue sideways, under the falx cerebri, or downward, causing severe neurologic dysfunction.

cerebral perfusion pressure (CPP) The difference between mean arterial blood pressure and intracranial pressure.

Cushing's response Late sign of increased intracranial pressure; includes increased blood pressure, widened pulse pressure, decreased heart rate, and decreased or irregular respiratory rate.

decerebrate (extension) posture Abnormal extension of the upper extremities with internal rotation of the upper arms and wrists; lower extremities will extend with some internal rotation.

decorticate (flexion) posture Abnormal flexion of the upper extremities and extension of the lower extremities.

extrapyramidal tract Descending pathway of the motor neurons concerned with involuntary or unconscious skeletal muscle coordination and reflex control of coordination.

glia cells Cells composing the support tissue that nourishes and protects the neurons.

Monro-Kellie doctrine Theory describing the compensatory mechanism of the cranial contents to maintain a steady volume and pressure.

myelinization Formation of the proteolipid coating of the nerves that facilitates conduction of impulses.

papilledema Edema of the optic disc.

pyramidal tract Descending pathway of the upper motor neuron concerned with voluntary movement.

REVIEW OF THE CENTRAL NERVOUS SYSTEM

Embryologic Development

The nervous system is one of the first systems to form *in utero*. By the 4th week of gestation, the neural tube has closed at the anterior end to form the brain and at the posterior end to form the spinal cord.

During the 2nd month of gestation the brain becomes the prominent body structure. It grows rapidly and continues to grow until around the 5th year of life. There appear to be two periods of rapid brain cell growth during gestation. Between the 15th and 20th weeks of gestation, the number of neurons increases significantly. At 30 weeks, the number of neurons increases again, continuing through 1 year of age. Appropriate prenatal care during periods of rapid neuronal increase can prevent developmental neurologic deficits.

The Myelin Sheath

Myelin is the fatty substance that surrounds the nerves of both the central and the peripheral nervous systems. The myelin begins to form at about the 16th week of gestation. Myelin in-sulates the nerves and helps conduct electrical impulses. Co-ordination of fine and gross motor skills progresses with the deposition of the myelin sheath. Nerve fibers can conduct impulses in the absence of myelin; however, the impulses travel more slowly. Gross motor skills develop before fine motor skills, as coordination and control advance throughout childhood. The myelin sheath can be destroyed by disease, drugs, and the aging process.

The Neural System

The neural system develops multiple connections among the areas of the brain that control specific functions, including vision, hearing, motor function, sensation, coordination, and speech. Each function is under the control of a specific area of the brain. The right half, or hemisphere, of the brain controls the left side of the body and is concerned with the social aspects of perception, intuition, and experience. The left hemisphere controls the right side of the body and is largely concerned with language acquisition and use and logical, verbal reasoning.

The neonate's neurologic system functions at a subcortical level. Spinal cord reflexes, such as sucking and cardiorespiratory

CLINICAL REFERENCE

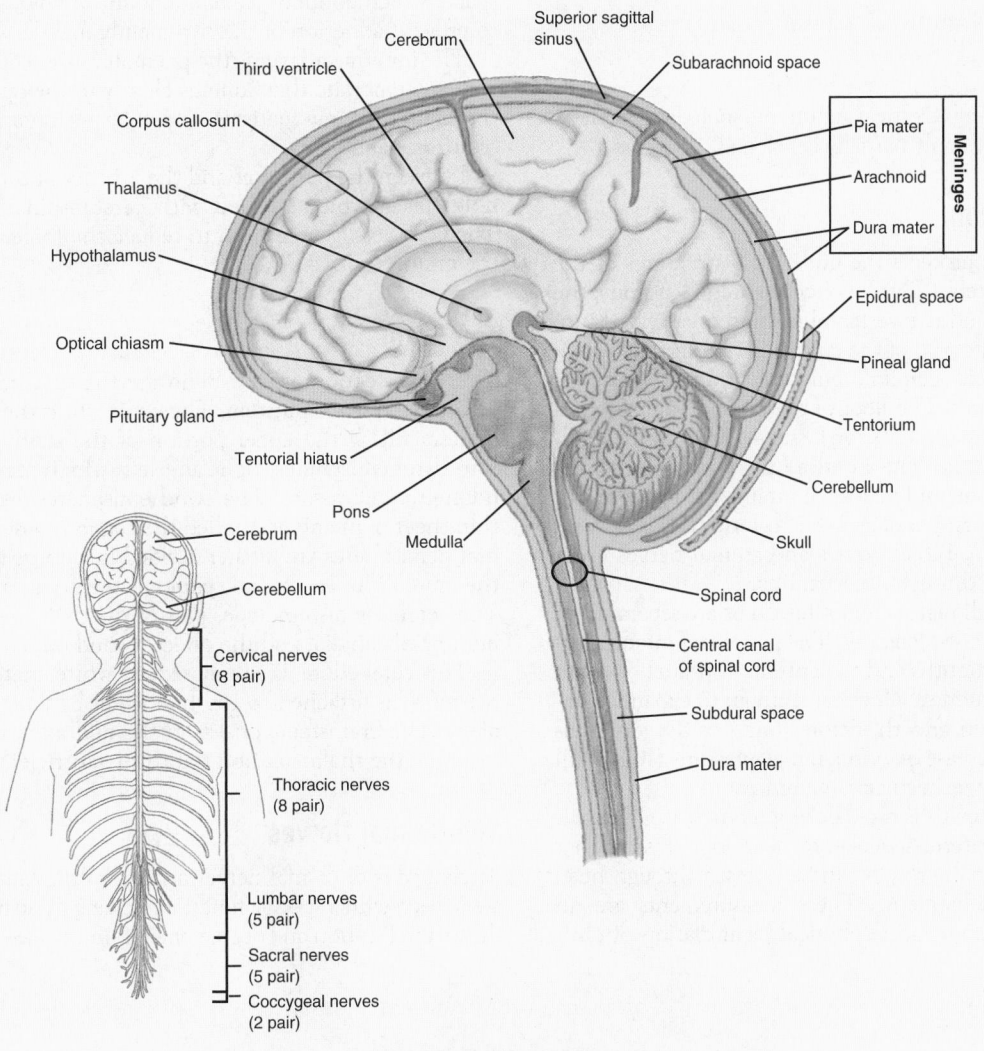

Anatomy of the Central Nervous System

Pediatric Differences in the Central Nervous System

- The brain constitutes 12% of a newborn's body weight, in contrast to only 2% of an adult's body weight.
- The brain of a term infant is two-thirds the weight of an adult's brain. By age 1 year, it weighs 80% as much as an adult's brain, and by age 6 years, it weighs approximately 90% as much as an adult's brain.
- An infant has about 50 ml of cerebrospinal fluid, compared with 150 ml in an adult.
- The peripheral nerves are not completely myelinated by birth. As myelinization progresses, so do the child's coordination and fine muscle movements.
- The head circumference in a term infant is 34 to 35 cm. By age 6 months the head circumference is 44 cm, and by age 12 months it is 47 cm.
- Papilledema rarely occurs in infancy because of the open fontanels and sutures, which can expand with increased intracranial pressure.
- The primitive reflexes of Moro, grasp, and rooting, present at birth, disappear at various times during the first 5 months. These primitive reflexes may reappear with neurologic disease.

functions, are present. Cortical functions, including memory and coordination, are only partially developed.

The Axial Skeleton

The axial skeleton protects the underlying structures of the central nervous system (CNS). For convenience of study, the bones of the skull and the vertebral column are divided into regions that form the wall of the cranial cavity and the spinal column. The frontal, occipital, temporal, and parietal bones form the cranial vault. The floor of the cranial vault is composed of three compartments, or fossae—the anterior, middle, and posterior fossae. The anterior fossa houses the frontal lobes of the brain, the middle fossa contains the upper brainstem and the pituitary gland, and the posterior fossa contains the lower brainstem. Blood vessels and cranial nerves enter and leave the skull through the foramina.

At birth, the skull plates are not fused but are separated by nonossified spaces called *fontanels*. The posterior fontanel usually fuses by age 2 months and the anterior fontanel by 16 to 18 months. The fontanels allow the cranium to expand in response to rapid brain growth. Before fusion of the fontanels and sutures, an increase in intracranial pressure (ICP) will produce an increase in head circumference.

Because brain growth is rapid during infancy, it is difficult to predict the long-term sequelae of neurologic insults that occur to infants. Brain growth can be assessed through head circumference measurements. These measurements are an important part of the routine physical examination of chil-

dren and should be plotted on a growth chart. Insufficient or excessive head and brain growth could indicate a potential neurologic problem. Premature closing of the fontanels or sutures can cause massive neurologic damage, and continued evaluation by the physician will be needed.

The Meninges

The meninges are the membranes that surround the brain and spinal column. The outer layer is the dura mater, a fibrous connective tissue structure containing many blood vessels and fibroblast-like cells that secrete collagen to produce a tough, protective membrane (Martin, 2003). The dura mater consists of two layers having outer and inner meningeal components. Between the periosteum of the bone and the dura mater lies the epidural space. Sheets of dura also extend downward and inward to form partitions within the cranium. The falx cerebri separates the cerebral hemispheres, and the falx cerebelli separates the cerebellar hemispheres.

The *tentorium* is a tentlike structure that separates the cerebellum from the occipital lobe of the cerebrum. The large gap through which the brainstem passes is the tentorial hiatus.

The middle meningeal layer is the arachnoid, a delicate, avascular, weblike, serous membrane loosely covering the brain. Between the arachnoid and the dura lies the subdural space, which contains a small amount of fluid, just sufficient to prevent adhesion of the two membranes.

The innermost layer is the pia mater. It is a delicate, transparent membrane that adheres closely to the outer surface of the brain. The pia mater is a vascular membrane, consisting of arteries and veins.

Between the pia mater and the arachnoid is the subarachnoid space, which is filled with cerebrospinal fluid (CSF). The CSF acts as a cushion to reduce the force of trauma on the brain.

The Brain

The three sections of the brain are the cerebrum, the cerebellum, and the brainstem. The cerebrum is the largest component, filling the upper portion of the skull. It is divided into two hemispheres, right and left, which are separated by a longitudinal fissure. The two hemispheres are joined by a thin sheet of membrane called the *corpus callosum*. The cerebral hemispheres are further divided into lobes in relation to the cranial bones: frontal, parietal, temporal, and occipital. The cerebrum also includes part of the thalamus, hypothalamus, basal ganglia, and the olfactory and optic nerves.

The cerebellum is composed of white matter and gray matter. It is attached to the brainstem by paired bundles of fibers. The brainstem consists of the midbrain, the pons, the medulla, the thalamus, and the third ventricle.

The Cranial Nerves

Twelve pairs of cranial nerves arise from the brain and brainstem, each with a specific function. Testing these nerves can indicate the location and degree of CNS injury (see Chapter 33).

Cerebrospinal Fluid Analysis in Children: Normal Findings			
Parameter Evaluated	Neonate Preterm	Neonate Full Term	Child Older than 6 Months
White blood cells (per mm³)	≤25	≤7	≤5
Protein (mg/dl)	<150	<170	<40
Glucose (mg/dl)	>30	>60	>40
Red blood cells (per mm³)	>1000	<800	<5
Pressure (mm Hg)	50-80	50-80	100-280

The Spinal Cord

The spinal cord is described as segmented into the cervical, thoracic, lumbar, and sacral regions. The spinal nerves are named for their corresponding vertebral segments.

The spinal cord transmits signals to and from the brain and responds to local sensory information through automatic motor responses called *reflexes*. The simplest type of spinal cord response is the reflex arc. Sensation is transmitted to the spinal cord from a sensory nerve fiber. It synapses with a motor neuron in the same cord segment, causing a muscle or tendon contraction in the corresponding motor nerve. Deep tendon reflexes are examples of the reflex arc.

Sensory innervation occurs as sensory nerves carrying body sensations enter the spinal cord on the dorsal surface. Most sensory fibers for pain and temperature ascend to the brain by way of lateral spinal tracts. Sensory fibers for touch and pressure ascend through anterior tracts. Almost all sensory fibers pass through the thalamus, where the perceptions of touch, pressure, and temperature are interpreted. Perceptions of texture, size, and weight are interpreted in the cortex.

Motor nerves are stimulated to respond after the brain receives a signal from a sensory nerve. The motor nerves cross over to the *contralateral* (opposite) side of the spinal cord from which they originate and then exit on the ventral surface of the spinal cord. The side of the body contralateral to the injured side of the brain will be the side affected by injury.

Functional differences exist between the upper and lower motor neurons. The outcome of a spinal cord injury is affected by the site of the injury. An injury between the brain and the dendrites (the nerve fibers that carry impulses toward the cell body) will render the brain incapable of signaling the muscle cells to cease responding reflexively, and the muscle will become contracted, or spastic. If the injury is to a section of the nerve between the muscle and axons (the nerve fibers that carry impulses away from the cell body), the muscles will become incapable of responding reflexively, causing them to become flaccid.

Cerebrospinal Fluid

CSF is a clear liquid produced in the choroid plexus of the ventricles. The CSF aids in protecting the brain, spinal cord, and meninges by acting as a watery cushion surrounding them, to absorb the shocks to which they are exposed. It is reabsorbed through the arachnoid villi into the venous sinuses.

Cerebrospinal Fluid Analysis: Findings in Pathologic Conditions					
Condition	Appearance	Pressure	Cells	Protein	Glucose/ Other
Traumatic tap	Bloody; supernatant fluid clear	Normal	Any red blood cells	4 mg/dl rise per 5000 red cells	NA
Acute bacterial meningitis	Cloudy to milky or xanthochromatic	Usually elevated	Polymorphonuclear cells: 100/mm³ or more	100-500 mg/dl	Decreased compared with blood
Viral meningitis	Clear	Normal or increased	Zero to a few hundred per mm³, mostly leukocytes	50-200 mg/dl	Normal
Encephalitis	Clear, colorless	Normal or slightly increased	Normal or increased	50-200 mg/dl	<40 mg/dl
Subdural hematoma	Yellow to clear, colorless	Increased	Normal	Normal or increased	Normal
Diabetic coma	Clear, colorless	Decreased	Normal	Normal or slightly increased	May be 200-300 mg/dl
Guillain-Barré syndrome	Clear	Normal	<10 white blood cells	More than 2× normal	Normal

NA, Not applicable.

CLINICAL REFERENCE ■

Common Diagnostic Tests and Procedures for Neurologic Disorders in Children

Test	Description	Purpose	Nursing Considerations
Computed tomography (CT) scan	Produces computer image of horizontal and vertical cross sections of brain at any axis.	Identifies abnormal tissue and structures, such as in brain tumor, bleeding, or hydrocephalus.	An IV line may need to be inserted if contrast medium is used. Notify the radiologist if the child is allergic to iodine. The child may be sedated if necessary.
Angiography	After IV contrast dye is injected, a clear image of the vessels is obtained because the computer eliminates all tissue that has not been infused by the contrast dye.	Shows vascular abnormalities.	May be NPO. Notify the radiologist if the child is allergic to iodine. Obtain signed permission form. There are restrictions on activity after the test.
Echoencephalography	Echoes from ultrasonic waves are recorded as they reflect off various surfaces of the skull.	Identifies abnormal structure, position, and function.	Painless procedure. No preparation.
Electroencephalography (EEG)	Electrodes placed on the scalp conduct and amplify electrical activity; electrical potential of the brain is measured and recorded.	Identifies abnormal electrical brain discharges, such as in seizures.	Child may have regular diet or fluids but no caffeine or stimulants. Hair should be clean. May include sleep EEG; in this case, child should be sleep-deprived the night before test. Tell the child the procedure is painless.
Long-term video (EEG)	Continuous EEG with video of physical symptoms. Process can last 24 hr to several days.	Clinical events can be recorded and played back for in-depth review, as well as correlated with the presence of abnormal electrical activity.	Electrodes are secured with a skin glue. Electrode sites should be evaluated and documented every shift. Child will have to stay in a small area during testing. Age-appropriate toys and activities should be available for child.
Lumbar puncture (LP)	CSF pressure is measured and a specimen obtained as a needle is inserted into the subarachnoid space between L3 and L4.	Measures pressure, and analysis of CSF identifies infections. Procedure may be used to administer medications.	Obtain signed consent. Instruct the child to lie on the side with the knees up to chest. After the procedure, the child lies flat. If not fluid-restricted, encourage PO fluids after the procedure.
Magnetic resonance imaging (MRI)	Produces computer images of the brain by means of radiofrequency emissions from certain elements.	Demonstrates morphologic features of tissue and structures with degree of detail not achievable by other methods.	The procedure is painless, but the child may be sedated if necessary. Inform child that loud clicking noises will be heard. The child's head will be restrained.
Nuclear brain scan (single photon emission computed tomography [SPECT])	A radioactive substance is injected IV (the amount of the substance is measured and recorded). Abnormal uptake indicates abnormal tissue or structure.	Identifies focal brain lesions and demonstrates CSF pathways.	The child needs to remain still during the test. An IV line is needed.

IV, Intravenous; *NPO,* nothing by mouth; *CSF,* cerebrospinal fluid; *PO,* by mouth.

Cerebral Blood Flow

The internal carotid arteries supply blood to all parts of the brain. Approximately 17% of cardiac output and 20% of body oxygen are transported to the brain. The brain requires approximately 10 times the oxygen used by the rest of the body.

Cerebral blood flow (CBF) is controlled by *cerebral perfusion pressure* (CPP), which is the difference between the mean arterial blood pressure (MBP) and ICP.

Autoregulation, or self-regulation, is a unique physiologic ability. It allows cerebral arteries to change diameter in response to changes in the CPP. The cerebral vessels can maintain a steady blood flow to the brain during alterations in blood pressure and perfusion. However, autoregulation fails when the limits of cerebrovascular dilation are reached.

Autoregulation may be impaired as a result of trauma or ischemia. It is influenced significantly by changes in PaO_2 and $PaCO_2$. An increase in $PaCO_2$ (above 40 mm Hg) produces cerebral vasodilation and an increase in cerebral blood flow. A decrease in $PaCO_2$ (25 to 30 mm Hg) causes cerebral vasoconstriction and thus reduces blood flow to the brain. Alterations in PaO_2 between 80 and 100 mm Hg have little effect on cerebral blood flow, although hypoxia will dramatically increase cerebral blood flow.

Teaching for a Lumbar Puncture

If the child is old enough to understand, explain the following:

- The child will need to lie on the side with body bent and knees and chin touching. Explain that you will help hold the child in that position by "hugging" the knees to the chin. If there is time, allow the child to practice the position. (An infant can be in a side-lying position or a sitting position with the infant facing you and your thumbs across the infant's scapulae; steady the infant's head against your body.)
- Tell the child that the physician will wash the back with a cool liquid. After that, the child might feel a "pinch" or "sting" as the needle is inserted. In some instances, EMLA cream (see Chapter 38) may be used as a topical anesthetic. It is important that the child remain still.
- Encourage the child to relax, sing, take deep breaths, or use guided imagery throughout the procedure to help decrease anxiety. The collection of cerebrospinal fluid (CSF) samples and pressure measurement usually takes several minutes. When the needle is withdrawn, the child will feel light pressure and the application of a small dressing.

Remember to

- Monitor the child's cardiorespiratory status throughout the procedure.
- Assist the parents to comfort the child during and after the procedure.

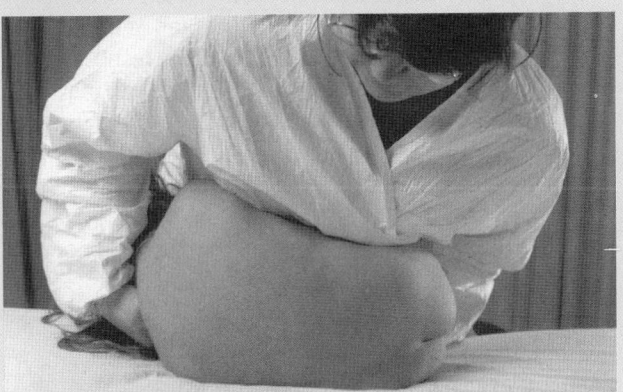

For the lumbar puncture: Place one hand farther down, under the child's neck. Your forearm moves behind the child's head to support the neck. Place the other arm farther under the child's upper thighs, and curl the body by bringing the knees up to the head. Note that this nurse's weight is supported on the edge of the gurney, and the nurse leans slightly over the child, controlling the arms and legs. Because direct visibility of the child's respiratory status is limited in this position, a cardiorespiratory monitor must be on the child, or another nurse should be at the bedside.
(Photo courtesy Cook Children's Medical Center, Fort Worth, TX. © Bob Lukeman, photographer.)

EMLA, Eutectic mixture of local anesthetics.

are of the child with neurologic problems requires knowledge of neuroanatomy, neurophysiology, and normal growth and development. The nurse plays an important role in the early recognition of pediatric neurologic problems, some of which have the potential for devastating long-term outcomes. The nurse assesses the child's condition by comparing the child's normal behavior with current behavior. The family is an invaluable source of information about the child's normal behavior and how current behavior deviates from that norm. The child and the family need support and understanding because the child's illness represents a crisis in their lives. The family's ability to respond and influence the child's coping mechanisms will directly influence the recovery and adaptation process.

Many conditions of the nervous system share common assessment data, diagnoses, and interventions. Principles of nursing care for the child with a nervous system disorder can be applied to a variety of situations.

Nursing Care Plan

The Child With a Nervous System Disorder

FOCUSED ASSESSMENT

Begin the neurologic assessment by testing the child's level of consciousness using the Glasgow Coma Scale (GCS) modified for children, cerebral function, cerebellar function, and orientation. Note the child's mood and behavior. Compare the results with normal developmental milestones (see Chapters 5 through 8). Observe the child's interaction with the family and the environment for additional data. Note lethargy, drowsiness, hyperactivity, tremors, or jitteriness.

Assess balance, coordination, and motor skills by observing the child's behaviors, particularly while the child is dressing or playing. Coordination can be assessed by the finger-to-nose test or by observing the child throw a ball, handle a pencil, or use rapidly alternating movements. Observe the child's walking gait for hemiplegia, scissors gait, or an abnormally wide-spaced gait. Observe and record the child's muscle development, strength, and tone. Test deep tendon reflexes and range of motion of all joints. Check the sensory function of the face, trunk, arms, and legs. Test both sides of the child for vibration, superficial tactile sensation, superficial pain, and temperature.

Nursing Diagnosis

Ineffective Tissue Perfusion (cerebral) related to alteration of arterial or venous blood flow, cerebral infarction, hemorrhage, hematoma, increased intracranial pressure (ICP), cerebral edema, seizures, hypoventilation, or increased cerebral metabolism.

Expected Outcomes

The child will:
- Have improved cerebral perfusion, as evidenced by no cranial nerve deficits, improved or normal level of consciousness, vital signs in baseline normal, and GCS score within normal limits.
- Demonstrate appropriate behavior or thought patterns for age.

INTERVENTION	RATIONALE
1. Determine the child's baseline age and developmental level.	1. Baseline age and developmental level will help the nurse gauge changes in neurologic status.
2. Perform a baseline neurologic and level of consciousness (LOC) assessment, and measure vital signs on admission.	2. Changes in neurologic signs can indicate deterioration or improvement in status. Changes are compared with baseline.
3. Monitor factors that may further increase cerebral edema and ICP (hypoxia, fever, seizures, hypotension, hypercapnia).	3. Monitoring these factors allows for correction of conditions that increase ICP and keeps cerebral metabolic needs to a minimum.
4. Maintain head of bed at a 30- to 45-degree angle.	4. Venous outflow drainage of the brain is facilitated by gravity.
5. Avoid the prone position, neck flexion, or hip flexion.	5. All these positions tend to increase ICP. Lying flat in bed increases ICP. Neck flexion kinks the jugular vein where venous drainage occurs. Hip flexion can increase intraabdominal or intrathoracic pressure, thus increasing ICP.
6. Organize nursing care around periods of low ICP.	6. Nursing care, such as suctioning, bathing, and repositioning, increases ICP.
7. Monitor pupil size and reactivity every hour as needed or as ordered.	7. An increase in pupil size and inactivity might indicate an increase in ICP.

Nursing Care Plan

The Child With a Nervous System Disorder—cont'd

INTERVENTION	RATIONALE
8. Measure head circumference daily or as needed, and record on growth chart if age-appropriate.	8. If fontanels are open, cranial expansion takes place when the cerebrospinal fluid (CSF) is under pressure.
9. Palpate the anterior fontanel every shift if age-appropriate.	9. An increase in fontanel size and tenseness may indicate an increase in CSF accumulation.
10. Palpate the cranial suture lines every shift if age-appropriate.	10. The cranial sutures may separate with an increase in CSF volume or pressure.
11. Observe the infant for irritability, lethargy, feeding intolerance, and decreasing GSC score.	11. All are signs of increasing ICP and deteriorating neurologic status.
12. Place emergency equipment (oxygen, suction, bag-valve-mask) near the child's room or at the bedside.	12. Increased ICP can cause apnea and may lead to cardiopulmonary arrest.

Evaluation

- Does the child demonstrate an improved LOC?
- Are vital signs within normal limits?
- Does the child show intact cranial nerve function, an optimum level on the GCS, and behavior and thought patterns appropriate for age?

Nursing Diagnosis

Imbalanced Nutrition: Less Than Body Requirements related to restricted intake, neurologic impairment, swallowing or chewing difficulty, risk for aspiration, nausea, or vomiting.

Expected Outcome

The child will:

- Have adequate nutritional intake, as evidenced by maintaining stable or normal weight for age and height; exhibiting normal serum proteins, moist mucous membranes, and adequate urine output; and being free of nausea and vomiting.

INTERVENTION	RATIONALE
1. Determine the child's level of consciousness before giving liquids.	1. A decreased level of consciousness increases the risk of aspiration with swallowing.
2. Weigh the child daily on the same scale, at the same time of day, and in the same clothes. Record on a growth chart.	2. Changes in weight indicate alterations in fluid balance and nutritional status. Being consistent with timing and type of clothing enhances accurate comparison. The nurse should weigh only if the procedure does not increase ICP.
3. Monitor skin turgor, mucous membranes, eye orbits, urine output, urine specific gravity, and serum and urine electrolyte values.	3. These are indicators of fluid and electrolyte status.
4. Consult a registered dietitian.	4. The dietitian will advise how best to meet metabolic demands and plan the most efficient way to get calories.
5. Position the child or infant upright after feedings. If the child is old enough and the ICP is not elevated, the head should be slightly flexed and facing forward. Arms should be positioned forward with feet placed on a firm surface.	5. Proper positioning will decrease the risk of aspiration, enhance comfort, prevent contractures, and provide for safety while feeding.
6. Verify placement of any oral or nasogastric tube before tube feedings are initiated.	6. Incorrect placement of a nasogastric tube will result in placing feedings into the lungs (see Chapter 37).
7. Provide a flexible feeding schedule with small feedings of favorite foods.	7. These techniques facilitate digestion and the ability to maintain adequate caloric intake.
8. Minimize handling around feeding times.	8. Minimal handling during feeding decreases the likelihood of vomiting and aspiration.
9. If swallowing is impaired, assist the child with chewing by holding the child's chin and jaw.	9. Swallowing may be facilitated by this method, because it keeps the child's head stabilized in an appropriate anatomic position.
10. Obtain order to medicate for nausea and vomiting if necessary.	10. The child will be more likely to tolerate feedings when nausea is controlled.

Continued

Nursing Care Plan

The Child With a Nervous System Disorder—cont'd

Evaluation

- Does the child show normal growth for age, with no weight loss?
- Does the child have age-appropriate caloric intake daily?
- Does the child have proper hydration with moist mucous membranes and age-appropriate urine output for age?
- Is the child free from nausea and vomiting?

Nursing Diagnosis

Risk for Impaired Skin Integrity related to neuromuscular impairment, decreased level of consciousness, inadequate physical activity, immobility, or improper fluid or nutritional intake.

Expected Outcome

The child's skin will:

- Remain intact and free from pressure breakdown.

INTERVENTION	RATIONALE
1. Use an eggcrate-type mattress or special flotation mattress to protect bony prominences. Reposition every 2 hr and as needed. Check for redness and pressure areas.	1. The child with a depressed LOC may not be active, and immobility can cause skin breakdown.
2. Observe skin condition every 2 hr with the repositioning of the child or infant.	2. Prolonged pressure on the skin will quickly lead to its breakdown.
3. Avoid putting temperature probes, cardiac monitor leads, or excessive tape over a shunt site.	3. Irritation from adhesives will contribute to skin breakdown and possible infection.
4. Encourage parents or caregivers to participate in passive range-of-motion exercises for the child if appropriate.	4. Participating in the child's care enhances the parents' control and the child's sense of well-being. Passive range-of-motion exercises provide emotional and physical support for the child and increase the child's activity.
5. If braces or splints are used, assess the skin before and after the splints or assistive devices are put on and taken off.	5. Correct application of braces will minimize pressure points and reduce skin breakdown.
6. Implement a daily skin care regimen. Teach parents or family to check skin frequently.	6. Bathing, moisturizing, and inspecting the skin will preserve skin integrity.

Evaluation

- Does the child have intact, clean, dry skin without pressure areas or sores?

Nursing Diagnosis

Anxiety (parental) related to change in the child's health status, threat to self-concept, behavior changes, possible injury, social isolation, seizures, neurologic impairment, or lack of privacy.

Expected Outcome

The parents will:

- Demonstrate management of anxiety, as evidenced by maintaining social and personal relationships, verbalizing relaxation, verbalizing feelings about the child's neurologic impairment, and demonstrating effective coping skills.

INTERVENTION	RATIONALE
1. Keep the parents informed of the child's progress, prognosis, and plan of care. Encourage parents to talk about concerns and ask questions. Allow parents to make decisions where possible.	1. Control over any event in the child's care helps the parents feel they are part of the caregiving team and will lessen their anxiety.
2. Encourage parents to participate actively in activities of daily living (e.g., oral hygiene, bathing, feeding).	2. Touching the child and actively participating in the child's care lower parental anxiety.

Nursing Care Plan

The Child With a Nervous System Disorder—cont'd

INTERVENTION	RATIONALE
3. Orient the parents to hospital routine, and refer to clergy, social worker, and other team members.	3. A familiar environment is less threatening and will enable the family to better deal with the child's condition and prognosis.
4. Encourage rooming-in when possible.	4. Rooming-in will involve the parents more in the child's care, make them part of the health care team, and decrease the child's anxiety.
5. Assist with anxiety-reduction techniques, such as relaxation techniques, music, and guided imagery.	5. Such techniques facilitate coping and stress reduction.

Evaluation

- Are the parents able to discuss concerns and fears?
- Do the parents plan with the team for the child's future and participate in decision making?
- Are the parents able to state reduced feelings of anxiety?
- Do the parents demonstrate coping and problem-solving skills?

Nursing Diagnosis

Deficient Knowledge related to unfamiliarity with infectious process, disease process, medication regimen, dietary or fluid needs, measures for prevention, or chronic illness of a child or infant.

Expected Outcomes

The child and parents will:
- Verbalize and demonstrate an understanding of the child's disease process, as evidenced by stating age-appropriate, realistic factors about the child's condition, listing factors to decrease neurologic deficits and measures to prevent further occurrences of illness, and demonstrating medication administration and nutritional adaptations.

INTERVENTION	RATIONALE
1. Allow time for teaching. If the child is to undergo surgery, do preoperative teaching for the parents as well.	1. Teaching answers questions and reinforces information given to the parents by the physician. It includes the parents in the learning experience.
2. Determine the parents' understanding of the child's disability, including the child's need for physical, speech, or occupational therapy.	2. Parents need to understand the intellectual and physical abilities and disabilities of their child to give informed consent or reinforce the need for therapies.
3. Put parents in touch with community support groups.	3. Support can be gained by seeing or hearing how others coped with similar situations.
4. Supply the parents with telephone numbers to call for needed information once they are home.	4. Health care workers can help parents feel in touch and educate them at the same time by discussing the child's condition on the telephone.
5. Teach the parents important signs and symptoms of the child's condition, side effects of medications, and when to call the physician or nurse. Provide written instructions.	5. The parents need to state important signs and symptoms that indicate a change in the child's condition and be aware of when to seek medical attention. Anxiety reduces learning and attention span. A written copy of signs and symptoms provides an ongoing resource that can be referred to later.
6. Review the signs and symptoms of wound infection.	6. Until the surgical incision is healed, the risk of infection is present.
7. Review with the parents the signs and symptoms of urinary tract retention or infection.	7. Because of retention and reflux, the child might be at risk for urinary tract infections.

Evaluation

- Can the parents discuss the child's care appropriately?
- Are the parents able to list situations in which the child should be seen by the physician or nurse?
- Do the parents know how to contact community support?
- Can the parents demonstrate required adaptation?

INCREASED INTRACRANIAL PRESSURE

Increased intracranial pressure (ICP) reflects the pressure exerted by the blood, brain, cerebrospinal fluid (CSF), and any other space-occupying fluid or mass. Increased ICP results from a disturbance in autoregulation and is defined as pressure sustained at 20 mm Hg or higher.

Etiology

Alterations in the brain can result from a space-occupying lesion, such as a brain tumor or hematoma. The brain can swell as a result of head trauma, infection, or a hypoxic episode. Overproduction of fluid, malabsorption of fluid, or a communication problem within the system can disrupt CSF dynamics.

Manifestations

Signs and symptoms of increased ICP differ according to the child's developmental level (Box 52-1).

Level of Consciousness

Children with increased ICP often have an altered level of consciousness. The Glasgow Coma Scale (GCS) is a standardized scale that, in a modified form, is frequently used to assess level of consciousness in infants and children. It consists of a three-part assessment: eye opening, verbal response, and motor response (Table 52-1). Each level of response is assigned a number value. When the assessment of each response is complete, the scores are totaled, providing an objective measure of the child's level of consciousness. The total numeric scores range from 15, indicating no change in level of consciousness, to 3, indicating a deep coma and poor prognosis.

Behavior

Changes in the child's normal behavior pattern may be an important early sign of increased ICP. Parents often are the first to notice a change in the child's behavior; therefore a parent's comment that "he isn't acting like himself" should be taken seriously. The child who no longer recognizes parents, cannot follow commands, or has minimal response to pain is

Pathophysiology

of Increased Intracranial Pressure

The major pathophysiologic changes associated with increased intracranial pressure (ICP) result from alterations in the brain, cerebrospinal fluid (CSF) dynamics, and cerebral blood flow. To maintain cerebral pressure and volume within normal range, changes in one or more of the contents of the cranium must be compensated for by changes in the others; this is referred to as the *Monro-Kellie doctrine.*

Compensatory mechanisms include a reduction in CSF production, an increase in CSF absorption, and a reduction in cerebral mass as a result of fluid displacement. Once the limits of compensation are reached, any further increase in volume or pressure will cause a sudden increase in ICP and an associated decline in the child's clinical status. Ultimately, increased ICP will compromise cerebral perfusion and produce shifting of brain tissue, causing herniation. The consequences of herniation depend on its severity and location.

There are four types of herniation. *Transtentorial herniation* occurs when part of the brain herniates downward and around the tentorium cerebelli. It may be unilateral or bilateral and may involve anterior or posterior portions of the brain. If a large amount of tissue is involved, it may cause death because vital brain structures are compressed and become unable to perform their functions.

Temporal lobe herniation, or uncal herniation, refers to a shifting of the temporal lobe laterally across the tentorial notch. This produces compression of the third cranial nerve and ipsilateral pupil dilation. If pressure continues to rise, flaccid paralysis, pupil dilation, pupil fixation, and death will result.

Tonsillar herniation occurs when the cerebellar tonsils herniate through the foramen magnum. The child will develop nuchal rigidity, shoulder or arm numbness, and changes in heart and respiratory rates and patterns. Arnold-Chiari malformation, a condition sometimes associated with hydrocephalus, includes herniation of the cerebellar tonsils.

Brainstem herniation through the foramen magnum results in death as a result of compression of vital cardiorespiratory centers.

Infants are somewhat able to compensate for increasing ICP because their cranial sutures remain open. Craniosynostosis is premature closure of the cranial sutures. This abnormal skull development causes an abnormally shaped skull. In some cases, craniectomy is needed to manage the increased ICP.

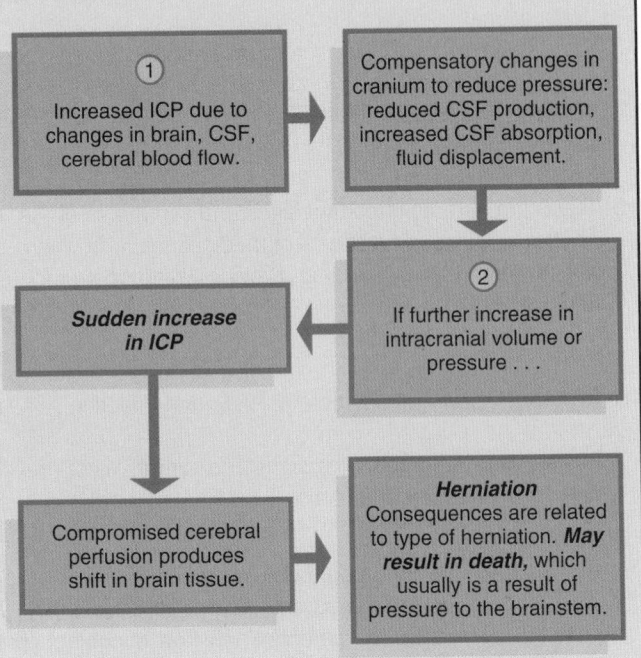

! CRITICAL TO REMEMBER

Standard Terms for Level of Consciousness

Level of consciousness should be described by the nurse using standard terminology:

- Full consciousness: awake, alert, oriented, interacts with environment
- Confused: lacks ability to think clearly and rapidly
- Disoriented: lacks ability to recognize place or person
- Lethargic: awakens easily but exhibits limited responsiveness
- Obtunded: sleeps unless aroused, and once aroused has limited interaction with the environment
- Stupor: requires considerable stimulation to arouse
- Coma: vigorous stimulation produces no motor or verbal response

BOX 52-1
Developmental Manifestations of Increased Intracranial Pressure

Infant
- Poor feeding or vomiting
- Irritability or restlessness
- Lethargy
- Bulging fontanel
- High-pitched cry
- Increased head circumference
- Separation of cranial sutures
- Distended scalp veins
- Eyes deviated downward ("setting-sun" sign)
- Increased or decreased response to pain

Child
- Headache
- Diplopia
- Mood swings
- Slurred speech
- Papilledema (after 48 hours)
- Altered level of consciousness
- Nausea and vomiting, especially in the morning

deteriorating. Decreased responsiveness to painful stimuli is a significant sign of alteration in level of consciousness.

Pupil Evaluation

As ICP rises, compression of the third cranial nerve occurs, resulting in pupil dilation with sluggish or absent constriction in response to light. A fixed dilated pupil is an ominous sign in an unconscious child. This suggests a herniation of the center section of the brain (also known as a *transtentorial herniation*).

Motor Function

The child with increased ICP will exhibit changes in motor function. Purposeful movement will decrease, and abnormal posturing may be observed. *Flexion posturing* refers to flexion of the upper extremities (elbows, wrists) and extension of the lower extremities. Plantar flexion of the feet may also be

TABLE 52-1 Glasgow Coma Scale Modified for Children

Child	Infant
EYES	
4 Opens eyes spontaneously	Opens eyes spontaneously
3 Opens eyes to speech	Opens eyes to speech
2 Opens eyes to pain	Opens eyes to pain
1 No response	No response
_____ = Score (Eyes)	
MOTOR	
6 Obeys commands	Spontaneous movements
5 Localizes	Withdraws to touch
4 Withdraws	Withdraws to pain
3 Flexion	Flexion (decorticate)
2 Extension	Extension (decerebrate)
1 No response	No response
_____ = Score (Motor)	
VERBAL	
5 Oriented	Coos and babbles
4 Confused	Irritable cry
3 Inappropriate words	Cries to pain
2 Incomprehensible words	Moans to pain
1 No response	No response
_____ = Score (Verbal)	
_____ = Total Score (Eyes, Motor, Verbal) Scores will range from 3 to 15.	

Reprinted from James, H.E., Anas, N.G., & Perkin, R.M. (1985). *Brain insults in infants and children.* Orlando, FL: Grune & Stratton.

Flexion Posturing

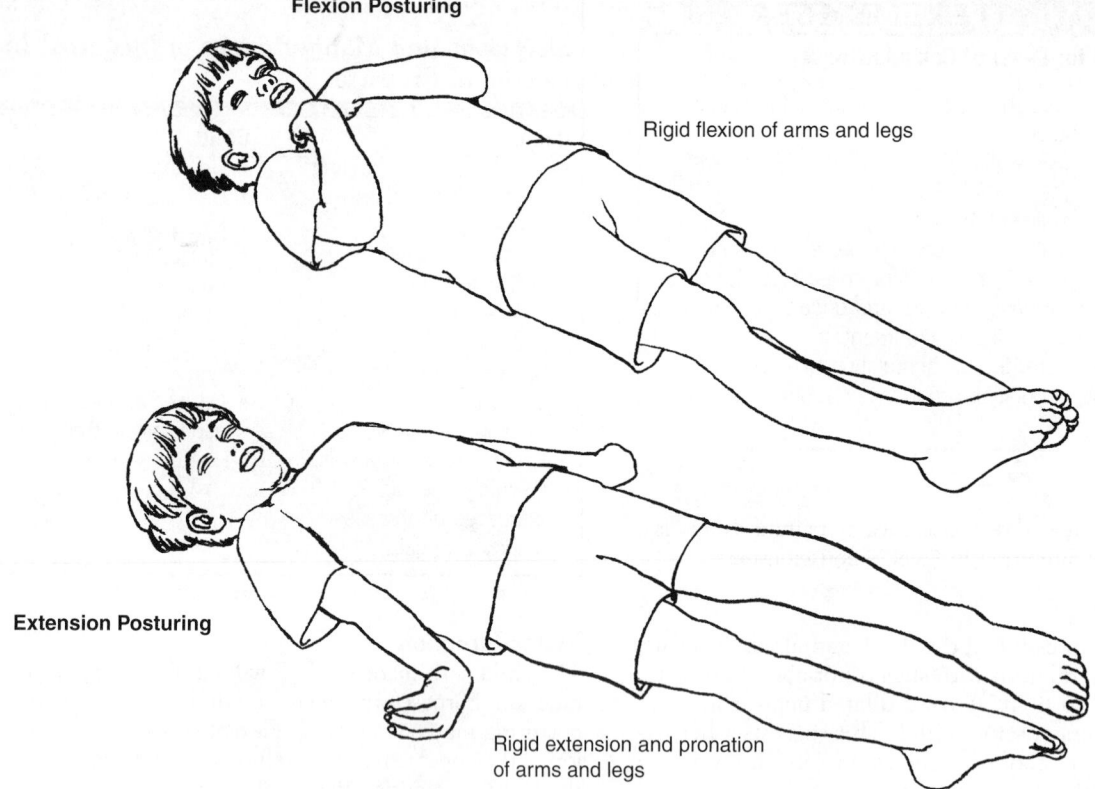

Rigid flexion of arms and legs

Extension Posturing

Rigid extension and pronation
of arms and legs

Figure 52-1 Decorticate (flexion) and decerebrate (extension) posturing.

observed. This type of posturing implies an injury to the cerebral hemispheres. *Extension posturing* involves extension of the upper extremities with internal rotation of the upper arm and wrist. The lower extremities will extend, with some internal rotation noted at the knees and feet. This type of posturing indicates damage to more areas of the brain, such as the diencephalon, midbrain, or pons. The progression from decorticate to decerebrate posturing usually indicates deteriorating neurologic function and warrants physician notification (Fig. 52-1). Flaccid paralysis indicates further deterioration in the child's condition.

Vital Signs

Temperature elevation may occur in children with increased ICP. *Cushing's response*, which consists of an increased systolic blood pressure with widening pulse pressure, bradycardia, and a change in respiratory rate and pattern, is usually apparent just before or at the time of brainstem herniation. This usually indicates an alteration in brainstem perfusion, with the body attempting to improve cerebral blood flow by increasing blood pressure. In children, Cushing's response is a late sign of increased ICP.

As ICP rises, the child's baseline respiratory pattern may change, exhibiting Cheyne-Stokes respiration, central neurogenic hyperventilation, or apneustic breathing. *Cheyne-Stokes respiration* refers to a pattern of breathing characterized by increasing rate and depth and then decreasing rate and depth with a pause of variable length. The cycle will be repeated again and again. *Central neurogenic hyperventilation* is identified by a rapid rate despite normal arterial blood gas

values. This type of breathing pattern usually indicates midbrain or pontine involvement. *Apneustic breathing* occurs when the child demonstrates prolonged inspiration and expiration. As Cushing's response occurs, the child will develop apnea.

Late signs of increased ICP include tachycardia that leads to bradycardia, apnea, systolic hypertension, widening pulse pressure, and decorticate or decerebrate posturing.

Diagnostic Evaluation and Therapeutic Management

Diagnostic tests for increased ICP include computed tomography (CT), magnetic resonance imaging (MRI), lumbar puncture, serum and urine electrolytes, arterial blood gas determinations, a complete blood count (CBC), electroencephalography (EEG), and radiography. Normal blood gas levels are PaO_2 above 80 mm Hg and $PaCO_2$ below 45 mm Hg in a child with normal ICP. Passive hyperventilation may be an initial treatment for the child with increased ICP because it lowers the $PaCO_2$, causing cerebral vasoconstriction and decreased fluid. The goal of hyperventilation is to achieve a $PaCO_2$ between 30 and 35 mm Hg (Dias, 2004).

The management of increased ICP is directed toward treating its underlying cause, reducing the volume of the CSF, preserving cerebral metabolic function, and avoiding situations that increase ICP.

The head of the child's bed should be elevated 30 degrees. The child may be given an osmotic diuretic (e.g., mannitol) or dexamethasone.

Nursing Care Plan

The Child With Increased Intracranial Pressure

FOCUSED ASSESSMENT

Assessment of the child with increased intracranial pressure (ICP) requires astute clinical observation. The assessment parameters are those common to all children with an underlying neurologic problem. The nurse should focus special attention on level of consciousness, behavior, pupil status, cranial nerve function, motor function, reflexes, and vital signs. Overt signs and symptoms may not occur until the ICP is significantly elevated and the child's condition is deteriorating rapidly.

Because the child's neurologic status directs nursing intervention, meticulous and ongoing assessment of neurologic status is required. The nurse should monitor and document a baseline level of consciousness, using the modified Glasgow Coma Scale (GCS) and observing the child's interactions with others. Pupils are evaluated to detect increasing ICP. Pupils are described according to size, equality, and reaction to light. When evaluating pupils, be aware that some medications can affect pupillary reactions; for example, atropine will cause the pupils not to react to light.

Measure vital signs regularly, every 15 minutes to 2 hours, depending on the child's status. Particular attention should be given to careful measurement of blood pressure, pulse, and respiratory rate. Significant changes in vital signs should be reported immediately. Because elevated temperatures can increase ICP, initiating measures to decrease elevated temperatures (>40° C [>104° F]) will be a priority in care.

Information about the child's normal behavior should be obtained from the parents or primary caregivers. Serial observations are made to assess changes in the child's condition. ICP monitoring devices may be used to measure pressure (see Box 52-2).

Nursing Diagnosis

Risk for Infection related to invasive monitoring lines and procedures.

Expected Outcome

The child will:
- Remain free from infection, as evidenced by being afebrile and having a normal white blood cell (WBC) count, no evidence of meningitis or pneumonia, no cerebrospinal fluid (CSF) drainage or purulent drainage, and no urinary tract infection.

INTERVENTION	RATIONALE
1. Maintain strict asepsis when manipulating ventriculostomy drainage system.	1. Asepsis helps prevent an infection of the catheter site and CSF.
2. Monitor invasive sites for redness or drainage.	2. These are signs of infection.
3. Monitor temperature, WBC count, appearance on chest radiographs, and urinalysis results for signs of infection.	3. Steroids given to decrease ICP may mask infection and decrease immunity to infectious organisms.
4. Use aseptic technique with a Foley catheter.	4. Children on bed rest or who are immobilized are prone to urinary tract infection.

Evaluation

- Is the child's temperature within normal limits?
- Is the child free from other signs of infection?

Nursing Diagnosis

Deficient Fluid Volume related to restricted intake, inability to swallow, and change in mental status.

Expected Outcome

The child will:
- Maintain fluid and electrolyte balance, as evidenced by moist mucous membranes, serum osmolality and electrolyte values within normal limits for age, and intake and output normal for age.

INTERVENTION	RATIONALE
1. Monitor intake and output and urine specific gravity. Notify physician of a urine output <1 ml/kg/hr or >2 ml/kg/hr.	1. Syndrome of inappropriate antidiuretic hormone (SIADH) or diabetes insipidus can occur with stress, surgery, brain dysfunction, or some medications. SIADH often occurs as a sequela to increased ICP (see Chapter 51).

Continued

Nursing Care Plan

The Child With Increased Intracranial Pressure—cont'd

INTERVENTION	RATIONALE
2. Administer fluids within fluid restrictions.	2. Fluid restriction aids in decreasing extracellular fluid volume, which in turn decreases ICP.
3. Administer medications as ordered.	3. Osmotic and loop diuretics (mannitol, furosemide) will decrease cerebral edema by increasing fluid excretion.
4. Monitor serum sodium, electrolytes, and serum osmolality.	4. These levels indicate fluid status and help identify measures to take to keep electrolytes in balance. Hyponatremia will cause cerebral edema.

Evaluation

■ Does the child demonstrate appropriate fluid balance and normal electrolyte levels?
■ Is urinary output appropriate for age (see Chapter 42)?

BOX 52-2
Instruments for Monitoring Increased Intracranial Pressure

Subarachnoid Bolt
The end of the bolt is placed in the subarachnoid space. The top of the bolt is attached to a transducer to conduct a waveform to the monitor. The neurosurgeon adjusts the transducer to produce a waveform on the monitor.

Intraventricular Catheter
The catheter is placed in the lateral ventricle or subarachnoid space. The catheter provides a method for measuring pressure as well as a conduit to drain off extra fluid into the drainage bag. The manometer and drainage bag are part of a sterile closed system.

SPINA BIFIDA

Spina bifida is a congenital neural tube defect in which there is incomplete closure of the vertebrae and neural tube during fetal development. Spina bifida is classified as spina bifida occulta and spina bifida cystica (Fig. 52-2). Spina bifida occulta usually occurs between the L5 and S1 vertebrae, with failure of the vertebrae to completely fuse. The child may have no sensory or motor defects. The only clinical manifestation that may appear is a dimple, a small tuft of hair, a hemangioma, or a lipoma in the lower lumbar or sacral area. These defects may be detected accidentally on routine radiographs.

Spina bifida cystica results in incomplete closure of the vertebrae and neural tube, evidenced by a saclike protrusion in the lumbar or sacral area with varying degrees of nervous tissue involvement. Spina bifida cystica is further described as meningocele, myelomeningocele, lipomeningocele, and lipomyelomeningocele. Meningocele is a saclike protrusion filled with spinal fluid and meninges. The most severe form of meningocele is myelomeningocele, in which the sac is filled with spinal fluid, meninges, nerve roots, and spinal cord. Nearly 80% of infants with myelomeningocele develop hydrocephalus as a result of a type II Chiari malformation (Arnold-Chiari malformation) (Haslam, 2000).

Pathophysiology
of Spina Bifida

During the 4th week of gestation (days 24 to 28), ventral induction of the neural tube fails to occur. The degree of impairment corresponds to the level of the defect on the spinal cord and the size of the defect. Ninety percent of spinal cord lesions are at or below the L2 vertebra. The lesion results in paralysis, partial paralysis, or varying sensory defects. Clubfeet, scoliosis, and contracture and dislocation of the hips may also be associated with the defect. Associated malformations include hydrocephalus and Arnold-Chiari malformation.

Etiology and Incidence

The cause of spina bifida is unknown in most cases. Evidence suggests that there may be a genetic predisposition. Maternal folic acid deficiency has been strongly linked to neural tube defects. Daily consumption of 0.4 mg folic acid by all women of childbearing age is recommended. Evidence of a viral origin has prompted research, but other than folic acid, no cause or preventive measures have been identified.

The incidence of myelomeningocele is 1 to 5 in 1000 live births. Geographic locations of incidence vary within the United States and worldwide (Haslam, 2000).

Manifestations

In addition to the appearance of the lesion, manifestations relate to the degree of deficit, which is determined by the level of the lesion (Fig. 52-3).

T12:	Flaccid lower extremities, decreased sensation, and bowel and bladder incontinence
L1 to L3:	Hip flexion, flail feet
L2 to L4:	Hip adduction
L3 to S2:	Hip adduction, hip extension, knee flexion
S3 and below:	No motor impairment
Sacral roots:	Plantar flexion

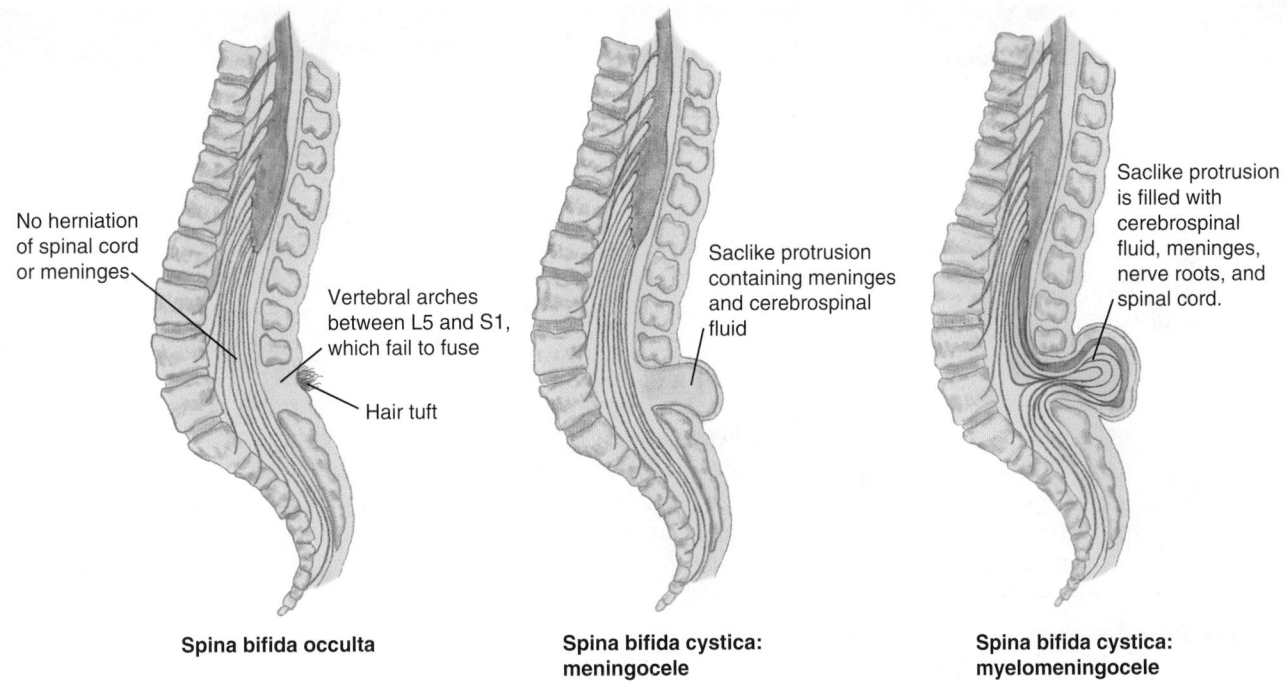

No herniation
of spinal cord
or meninges

Vertebral arches
between L5 and S1,
which fail to fuse

Hair tuft

Saclike protrusion
containing meninges
and cerebrospinal
fluid

Saclike protrusion
is filled with
cerebrospinal
fluid, meninges,
nerve roots, and
spinal cord.

Spina bifida occulta

**Spina bifida cystica:
meningocele**

**Spina bifida cystica:
myelomeningocele**

Figure 52-2 Three forms of spina bifida.

Children with spina bifida are at high risk for developing latex allergies because of frequent exposure to latex during catheterizations and multiple operations. Latex allergy is estimated to occur in 18% to 60% of children with spina bifida. Allergic reactions can range from mild signs and symptoms to anaphylactic shock. Children should be tested for latex allergy, and precautions should be taken from birth to decrease exposures. The nurse should check equipment for latex and choose non-latex alternatives.

Diagnostic Evaluation

Diagnostic tests include determining alpha-fetoprotein (AFP) levels in blood at 16 to 18 weeks of gestation. If the AFP screen is elevated, amniocentesis and fetal ultrasound are performed. After delivery, a CT scan or myelography may be done.

Therapeutic Management

Prenatal microsurgical closure of the myelomeningocele, performed at approximately 19 to 25 weeks' gestation, shows promise for reducing the severity of Chiari II malformations and incidence of hydrocephalus (Kaufman, 2004). Risks associated with antenatal surgery include premature birth, with its associated consequences and possible fetal death. Maternal risks (e.g., abruptio placenta, uterine rupture) are directly related to the hysterotomy (Kaufman, 2004).

Immediate surgical closure decreases the risk of infection, morbidity, and mortality. Other benefits are improved prognosis without further cord deterioration and earlier and easier physical handling and bonding.

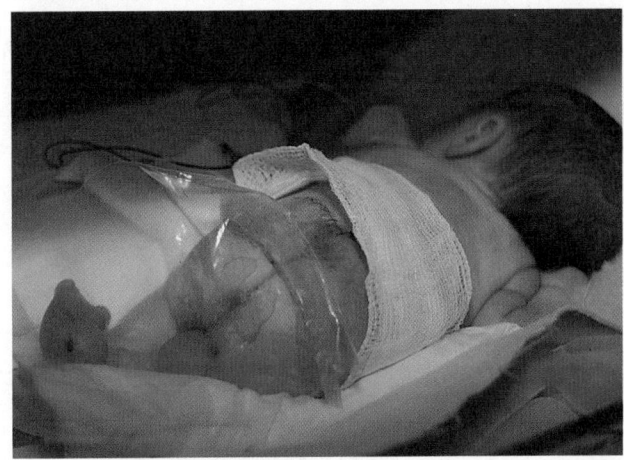

Figure 52-3 This infant has a repaired myelomeningocele. Note the left clubfoot. This deformity often accompanies the defect because normal intrauterine movement does not occur in the fetus with spina bifida, interfering with the development of the extremities. The legs are flaccid, and normal neonatal flexion is absent. The infant is also incontinent, dribbling stool and urine constantly. Hydrocephalus also commonly accompanies these neural tube defects. (Courtesy Parkland Health & Hospital System, Dallas, TX.)

The child will need lifelong management of neurologic, orthopedic, and urinary problems and is best managed in a multispecialty outpatient setting. Urodynamic studies are performed early, and a bladder-emptying program is initiated, with close monitoring of the child's infection status. In most instances, the child will require orthopedic bracing and possibly orthopedic surgery to maximize the child's mobility.

Nursing Care Plan

The Child With Spina Bifida

FOCUSED ASSESSMENT

The saclike protrusion of the meningocele should be assessed and the lesion measured. The nurse should measure the infant's head circumference and regularly palpate the anterior fontanel for fullness.

Continuous baseline and neurologic assessment is necessary. Assess the infant's overall tone, taking special note of spontaneous movement of the extremities. The motor examination is done with the infant at rest, using painful stimuli from the torso downward. Observe for voluntary movement below the level of the lesion.

The infant is at risk for infection before the sac is closed. Therefore the infant's temperature must be monitored every 1 to 2 hours. Note signs of infection along with irritability, lethargy, or nuchal rigidity. A sterile saline dressing is placed over the sac to maintain the moisture of the sac and its contents. A risk of infection remains, however, and the dressing needs to be changed on a regular schedule or whenever soiled. Record the appearance of the sac and contents with each dressing change.

Other assessments and nursing care are similar to those discussed earlier for any child with a neurologic problem. Because children with spina bifida have multisystem, long-term problems, the nurse needs to do ongoing assessments of the child's emotional needs and coping skills. Communication with the school nurse may be required.

Nursing Diagnosis

Risk for Infection related to the open sac and the operative procedure.

Expected Outcomes

Preoperatively, the child will:
- Remain free of infection, as evidenced by the absence of drainage from the sac, normal white blood cell (WBC) count, absence of signs of meningeal irritation, and normal temperature.

Postoperatively, the child will
- Be free of infection, as evidenced by remaining afebrile; maintaining a WBC count within normal limits; and exhibiting no redness, swelling, or purulent drainage from the incision site.

INTERVENTION	RATIONALE
1. Monitor vital signs and WBC count. Observe the sac or incision site for redness and clear or purulent drainage.	1. These are signs of infection that need to be documented and reported to the physician.
2. Perform regular neurologic checks, including palpating the fontanel.	2. Altered neurologic signs, irritability, and full fontanel are signs of meningeal infection.
3. Maintain sterile dressings over the sac or incision site.	3. Sterile dressings will facilitate healing and decrease the risk of infection.

Evaluation

- Does the infant's sac remain intact preoperatively?
- Is the infant infection-free (afebrile, normal WBC count, calm, able to eat)?
- Does the incision site appear intact and without redness or drainage?

Nursing Diagnosis

Risk for Impaired Skin Integrity related to neurologic motor deficits.

Expected Outcome

The child will:
- Have intact skin, as evidenced by absence of pressure areas or ulcerations.

INTERVENTION	RATIONALE
1. Use a special mattress or pad for the infant's bed. Preoperatively, place the infant in a prone or side-lying position with a small blanket or diaper roll under the ankles and between the knees.	1. Special bedding can help alleviate pressure points caused by the required preoperative prone position. Placing rolls helps maintain anatomic position of the feet and hips.
2. Assess the infant's skin, and reposition frequently. Leave the diaper under the infant; do not fasten. Change a soiled diaper immediately, and clean the diaper area when soiled.	2. Keeping the infant's diaper open will facilitate frequent cleaning of the perineal area because oozing of stool and dribbling of urine may occur. Keeping the area clean and dry reduces skin breakdown.

Nursing Care Plan

The Child With Spina Bifida—cont'd

INTERVENTION	RATIONALE
3. Use stoma adhesive on each side of the sac to anchor the dressing; consult the stoma therapist if needed.	3. Frequent dressing changes can irritate the skin, and the potential for irritation will be less if the tape is stuck to the stoma adhesive. The stoma therapist may make special recommendations for neonatal skin needs.
4. Teach the parents to routinely check the child's skin for pressure areas, particularly if the child requires bracing or other orthopedic support as the child grows.	4. Because the child has sensory as well as motor deficits, the child may not be able to feel abnormal pressure. Pressure spots from orthopedic appliances can contribute to skin breakdown.

Evaluation

- Does the infant exhibit any signs of skin breakdown?
- Are the perineal area, incision site, and buttocks clean and dry?
- Do the parents and older child perform regular skin checks for abnormal pressure areas?

Nursing Diagnosis

Impaired Physical Mobility related to neuromuscular impairment.

Expected Outcome

The child will:
- Maximize mobility by learning to use appropriate mobilization devices and by maximizing opportunities to be mobile.
- Achieve developmental milestones within the limits of the motor impairment.

The child will:
- Demonstrate proper application of any orthopedic devices.

INTERVENTION	RATIONALE
1. Determine and record physical impairments and abilities. Note the activities in which the child can participate, and encourage as much activity as tolerated.	1. This documentation notes advances or regression in activities or the child's abilities. Encouraging activity maintains muscle tone.
2. Maintain splints, braces, and casts. Use wheelchairs, walkers, and other assistive devices as needed. Teach parents how to apply the devices and perform routine skin care (see Chapter 50).	2. These aids may be used for proper alignment and to decrease contractures. Other devices may increase independence and mobility.
3. Ensure that the child attends physical therapy sessions and participates fully. Encourage self-care.	3. Therapy and self-care help prevent contractures, encourage independence, and increase self-esteem.
4. Refer the family to the Spina Bifida Association (see Appendix I on Evolve website).	4. Support groups can help families cope with the stresses of a chronic condition.

Evaluation

- Does the child enjoy mobility as desired and as allowed by impairments?
- Do the parents demonstrate proper use and application of orthopedic devices and encourage occupational and physical therapy?
- Do the parents facilitate the child's maximum development?

Nursing Diagnosis

Impaired Urinary Elimination related to the neuromuscular deficit.

Expected Outcome

The child will:
- Be free of urinary tract infections (UTIs), as evidenced by urine that is clear, odor-free, and sterile.

INTERVENTION	RATIONALE
1. Observe urinary stream, and teach the parents to observe for any dribbling of urine. Give the parents written instructions on how to administer any ordered medications (antispasmodics, antibiotics).	1. Urinary dribbling indicates interrupted innervation to the bladder. Antispasmodics act on the smooth muscle of the bladder, allowing for increased bladder capacity. Antibiotics are given to treat UTIs.

Continued

Nursing Care Plan

The Child With Spina Bifida—cont'd

INTERVENTION	RATIONALE
2. Offer adequate fluids.	2. Good hydration will help prevent UTIs.
3. Teach and maintain regular toilet habits. Teach the parents and child how to perform intermittent clean catheterization if necessary. Emphasize use of a latex-free catheter.	3. Regular toilet habits facilitate complete and regular emptying of the bladder and help prevent urine retention and UTIs. If catheterization is necessary, it is usually done every 2-4 hr while the child is awake. Children with spina bifida have a high incidence of allergies to latex and rubber products. Because of this only latex-free products should be used with these children.
4. Check urinary frequency, input and output, and specific gravity. Teach the parents to observe the color, clarity, and odor of the urine. Encourage follow-up with urine cultures if ordered.	4. These values may be initial indicators of urinary pattern alteration. The child will not experience urinary urgency or painful urination because of neurologic sensory deficits; observation of the urine is essential to recognize a developing UTI.

Evaluation

- Has the child established regular voiding or catheterization patterns?
- Are the urinalysis and urine cultures normal?

Nursing Diagnosis

Constipation related to sensory deficit and neurologic impairment.

Expected Outcome

The child will:
- Be free of constipation or impaction, as evidenced by regular bowel movements and soft stool.

INTERVENTION	RATIONALE
1. Observe and record the infant's or child's anal tone and pattern of bowel movements.	1. Absence of rectal sphincter tone indicates abnormal bowel function; noting the pattern will alert caregivers to implement a bowel program.
2. Monitor for abdominal distention, vomiting, and poor feeding.	2. These signs may indicate constipation.
3. Develop a bowel program in cooperation with the parents: give a suppository before breakfast and have the child sit on toilet after breakfast. May need to stimulate the anal sphincter.	3. A bowel program will ensure elimination needs are met.
4. Consult a registered dietitian to be sure the diet provides adequate fluid and fiber.	4. Fluid and fiber facilitate softer stools and easier passage.

Evaluation

- Is the child free of constipation or impaction, as evidenced by regular bowel movements?

HYDROCEPHALUS

Hydrocephalus develops as a result of an imbalance between the production and absorption of CSF. As excess CSF accumulates in the ventricular system, the ventricles become dilated and the brain is compressed against the skull. This results in enlargement of the skull if the sutures are open; it results in signs and symptoms of increased ICP if the sutures are fused.

Etiology

Hydrocephalus may be congenital, acquired, or of unknown etiology. In infancy, hydrocephalus is most often congenital or related to prematurity. Congenital hydrocephalus results from developmental defects, such as Arnold-Chiari malformations, congenital arachnoid cysts, congenital tumors, or aqueductal stenosis. In premature infants, neonatal meningitis or subarachnoid hemorrhage may result in hydrocephalus.

Pathophysiology

of Hydrocephalus

Cerebrospinal fluid (CSF) is produced primarily by the choroid plexus, which lines the lateral ventricles. CSF circulates through the ventricular system and flows into the subarachnoid space around the brain and the spinal cord. It is then reabsorbed within the subarachnoid spaces.

Hydrocephalus results when there is either (1) impaired absorption of CSF within the subarachnoid space *(communicating hydrocephalus)* or (2) obstruction of CSF flow within the ventricles that prevents CSF from circulating around the spinal cord and the subarachnoid space *(noncommunicating hydrocephalus)*. Hydrocephalus may rarely be caused by overproduction of CSF because of a tumor of the choroid plexus.

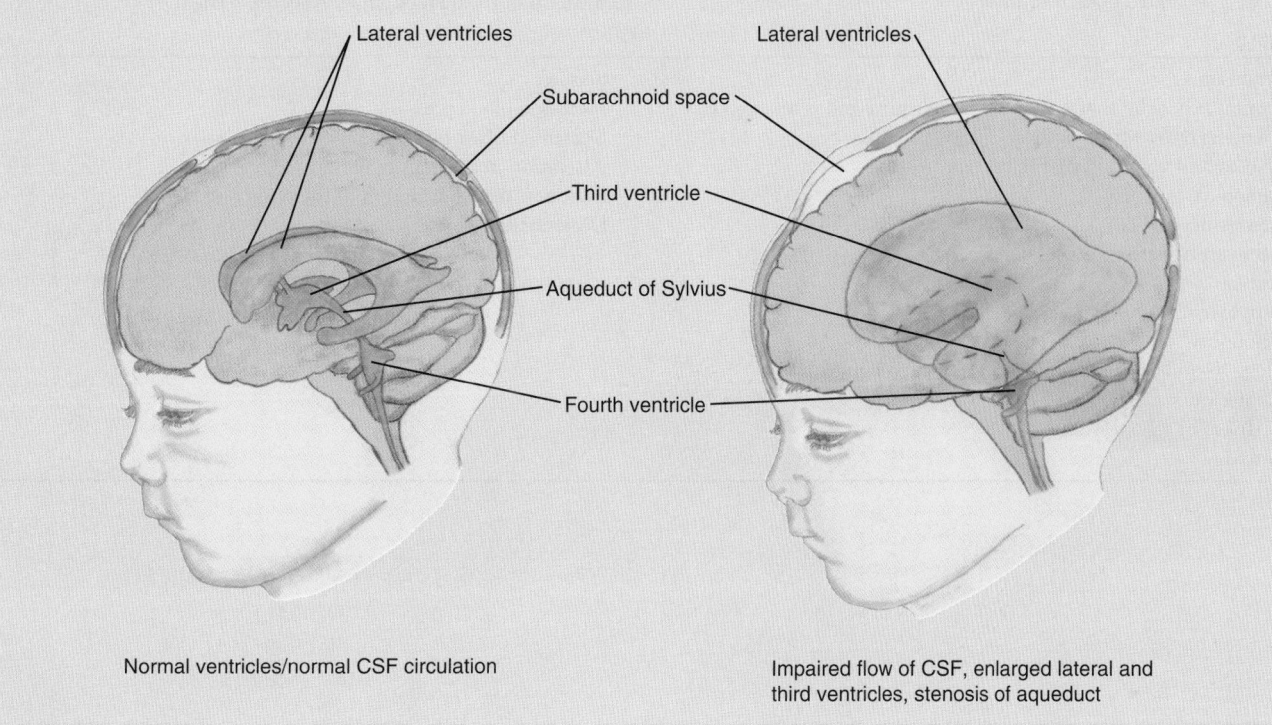

Normal ventricles/normal CSF circulation

Impaired flow of CSF, enlarged lateral and third ventricles, stenosis of aqueduct

Hydrocephalus is often associated with myelomeningocele. Intrauterine infection and perinatal hemorrhage cause hydrocephalus in some infants. In older children, hydrocephalus is usually acquired as a complication of meningitis, tumor, or hemorrhage.

Incidence

The incidence of hydrocephalus in infancy is 1.2 in 1000 births (Garton & Piatt, 2004). The incidence of hydrocephalus with spina bifida is considered to be 3 to 4 in 1000 births. Obstructive, or noncommunicating, hydrocephalus accounts for 99% of all cases of hydrocephalus in children.

Manifestations and Diagnostic Evaluation

Because of anatomic differences between infants and children, manifestations of hydrocephalus differ according to developmental stage (Table 52-2).

Diagnostic tests for hydrocephalus include serial measurements of head circumference, CT, MRI, and lumbar puncture.

Therapeutic Management

Therapy is aimed at preventing further CSF accumulation and reducing disability and death. The objective is to bypass the blockage and drain the fluid from the ventricles to an area where it may be reabsorbed into the circulation. A *ventriculoperitoneal shunt,* or tube leading from the ventricles out of the skull and passing under the skin to the peritoneal cavity, accomplishes this (Fig. 52-4). An alternative shunt, the *ventriculoatrial shunt,* which is used in older children, drains the fluid from the ventricles to the right atrium of the heart.

The shunt may need to be revised as the child grows. Long-term follow-up is essential. The child may exhibit mild learning problems and may have accelerated pubertal development (Haslam, 2000).

TABLE 52-2 Early and Late Manifestations of Hydrocephalus

Early	Late
INFANT	
Rapid head growth—increase in head circumference above the normal growth curve	Setting-sun sign: sclera visible above the iris
Full, bulging anterior fontanel	Frontal bone enlargement, or bossing
Irritability	Vomiting; difficulty swallowing or feeding
Poor feeding	Increased blood pressure, decreased heart rate
Distended, prominent scalp veins	Altered respiratory pattern
Widely separated cranial sutures	Shrill, high-pitched cry
	Sluggish or unequal pupillary response to light
CHILD	
Strabismus	Seizures
Frontal headache that occurs in the morning and is relieved by emesis or by sitting upright	Increased blood pressure
Nausea and vomiting that may be projectile	Decreased heart rate
Diplopia	Alteration in respiratory pattern
Restlessness	Blindness from herniation of the optic disc
Behavior or personality changes	Decerebrate rigidity
Ataxia	
Papilledema	
Irritability	
Sluggish and unequal pupillary response to light	
Confusion	
Changes in school work	
Lethargy	

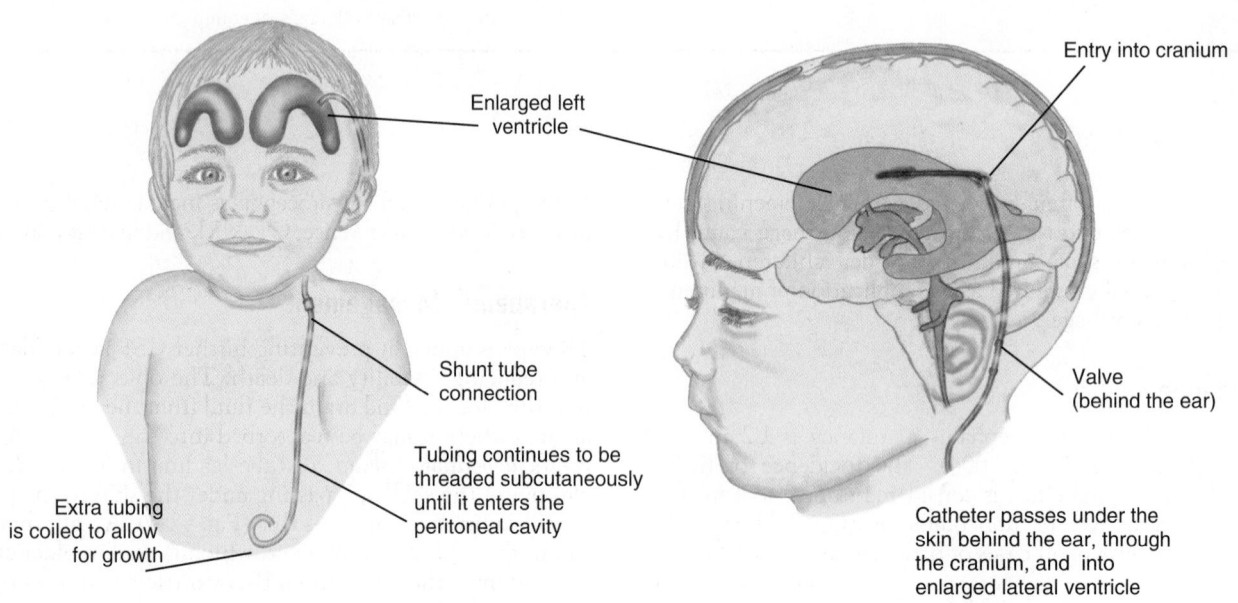

Entry into cranium

Enlarged left ventricle

Shunt tube connection

Tubing continues to be threaded subcutaneously until it enters the peritoneal cavity

Extra tubing is coiled to allow for growth

Valve (behind the ear)

Catheter passes under the skin behind the ear, through the cranium, and into enlarged lateral ventricle

Figure 52-4 A ventriculoperitoneal shunt is implanted in the child with hydrocephalus to prevent excess accumulation of cerebrospinal fluid (CSF) in the ventricles. The tubing diverts the CSF from the ventricles into the peritoneal cavity, where it is reabsorbed. Nursing care of the child with a ventricular shunt includes monitoring for infection and pain, administering antibiotics and pain medications as ordered, and teaching the family how to change dressings and how to recognize shunt problems.

Nursing Care Plan

The Child With Hydrocephalus

FOCUSED ASSESSMENT

When an infant is born with hydrocephalus, signs may be apparent at birth or signs of an obstruction may appear over the next few months. The first sign may be an abnormal head circumference or a head circumference that is increasing at a rate greater than the expected percentile. The parent may notice and report increased irritability or other neurologic signs.

If the child is older, any change in level of consciousness, personality, interaction with the environment, or sleep patterns or any delays in developmental milestones need to be explored with the parents. Note complaints of headache that may be relieved when the child sits upright and vomiting of unexplained origin. If the child has a history of vomiting, hydration status also should be assessed.

Postoperatively, the infant's head circumference should be measured daily or more frequently, depending on the infant's condition, and should be recorded and plotted on a graph. To facilitate accuracy when different personnel take the measurement, make a pen mark on the scalp where the tape measure is placed. The tape measure is usually placed just above the top of the ears and around the head, around the midforehead and the most prominent portion of the occiput.

Palpate the infant's anterior fontanel for size, bulging and tenseness, and palpate the cranial sutures for separation. The fontanel is assessed with the baby sitting upright and quiet. It may bulge or pulsate if the infant is crying.

Observe the infant's behavior when the fontanel is full or tense. Ask the parent if the baby is irritable or lethargic or if any change in feeding behavior has been noticed. Ask if the infant has had any seizures. Vital signs are assessed to identify any changes from the infant's baseline measurements.

Nursing Diagnosis

Risk for Infection related to surgical shunt placement.

Expected Outcomes

The child will:
- Remain free of infection, as evidenced by a normal temperature; a clean, dry suture line; toleration of feedings; and no signs of increased intracranial pressure (ICP).

The parents will:
- Demonstrate infection control measures.

INTERVENTION	RATIONALE
1. Monitor temperature every 1-2 hr and as needed. Observe for decreased level of consciousness and vomiting. Also monitor for swelling or redness along the shunt tract.	1. These are the first signs of an infection.
2. Observe head, abdominal, and chest dressings for drainage. Test drainage for glucose with a Dextrostix, or check for a halo sign on gauze.	2. Drainage could be cerebrospinal fluid (CSF), indicating a route for infection to reach the brain. CSF contains glucose and makes a halo on gauze.
3. Position the child off the shunt site so that no weight is placed on the valve for the first 2 days.	3. Careful placement prevents skin breakdown and reduces the risk of infection.
4. Administer intravenous (IV) antibiotics as ordered, and monitor serum levels to prevent subtherapeutic or toxic levels.	4. *Staphylococcus epidermidis* infection is the major complication of shunts.
5. Teach the parents the dressing change technique, and show them how to recognize shunt infection.	5. Parents need to know how to care for their child at home and when to seek medical attention.

Evaluation

- Does the child have a normal body temperature?
- Does the child have a clean, dry suture site?
- Can the parent demonstrate dressing changes using aseptic technique and state the signs of infection?

Nursing Diagnosis

Acute Pain related to operative procedure.

Continued

Nursing Care Plan

The Child With Hydrocephalus—cont'd

Expected Outcome

The child will:
- Exhibit pain relief, as evidenced by stable vital signs, sleeping restfully, playing whenever possible, and verbalizing decreased pain.

INTERVENTION	RATIONALE
1. Determine child's pain level, activity, and irritability, and give pain medications as needed. Administer analgesics (e.g., codeine) as ordered if needed.	1. Pain relief will help decrease crying, ICP, and metabolic demands. Codeine does not interfere with the child's level of consciousness.
2. Hold, cuddle, and distract the child. Teach therapeutic play to family members and caregivers.	2. Non-pharmacologic methods of pain management also decrease ICP.

Evaluation

- Are the child's vital signs normal for age?
- Does the child smile and interact with the caregivers?
- Does the older child express pain relief or choose a lower value on a pain assessment scale?

Nursing Diagnosis

Deficient Knowledge (parental) related to unfamiliarity with home care and signs and symptoms of shunt malfunction or complications.

Expected Outcome

The parents will:
- Have an understanding of care of their child, as evidenced by an ability to demonstrate assessment of the child's level of consciousness, describe signs of infection, and discuss the shunt's purpose and function.

INTERVENTION	RATIONALE
1. Determine the parents' knowledge of changes in the child's level of consciousness. Begin teaching at their level of understanding.	1. Parents need to understand that shunt malfunction will cause increased ICP.
2. Teach the parents to observe the child for abdominal distention or discomfort.*	2. Shunt placement may cause a paralytic ileus or peritonitis.
3. Teach the parents to observe for poor feeding, nausea or vomiting, elevated temperature, and skin redness or tenderness and report these to the physician.	3. These are all signs of an infection.
4. Teach parents safety measures for use in home care, playing, and the car (padded seats).	4. It is important to provide anticipatory guidance for the growing child.
5. Emphasize the importance of neurosurgical follow-up care.	5. The shunt may need revision as the child grows.

Evaluation

- Can the parents verbalize an understanding of how to assess level of consciousness and signs of infection?
- Can the parents discuss care of the child with a shunt?
- Are the parents able to describe signs of shunt malfunction?

*Williams, D.G., Hayes, J., & McCool, S. (1996). Shunt infections in children: Presentation and management. *Journal of Neuroscience Nursing, 28*(3), 155-162.

A surgical procedure, endoscopic third ventriculostomy, has been used with increasing success in older children (>2 years) with obstructive hydrocephalus. For this procedure, the surgeon creates a small burr hole in the skull, through which an endoscope is passed. The third ventricle is visualized and a small opening is created in its floor. This allows the CSF to bypass the fourth ventricle and return to circulation where it is reabsorbed. The procedure is successful approximately 50% of the time (Ohm, 1998) and reduces the need for a permanent mechanical shunt.

CEREBRAL PALSY

Cerebral palsy, also known as *static encephalopathy*, is a chronic, nonprogressive disorder of posture and movement. It is characterized by difficulty in controlling the muscles be-

Factors Associated With Cerebral Palsy

Prenatal
- Maternal diabetes
- Rh or ABO incompatibility
- Rubella in the first trimester
- Genetic causes
- Intrauterine ischemic event
- Toxoplasmosis
- Cytomegalovirus
- Congenital brain abnormality

Perinatal
- Asphyxia
- Low birth weight
- Prematurity
- Precipitous delivery
- Pregnancy-induced hypertension
- Birth trauma
- Anoxia
- Prolonged labor
- Perinatal metabolic condition (diabetes)
- Intracranial hemorrhage

Postnatal
- Infections
- Trauma
- Stroke
- Poisoning

cause of an abnormality in the extrapyramidal or pyramidal motor system (motor cortex, basal ganglia, cerebellum).

Etiology and Incidence

The damage to the motor system can occur prenatally, perinatally, or postnatally (Box 52-3). Approximately 2 in 1000 live births in the United States result in a child with cerebral palsy.

Manifestations

The manifestations of cerebral palsy may vary, and one or more of the following may be observed in any one child: persistence of primitive reflexes, delayed gross motor development, and lack of progression through the developmental milestones. Abnormal posturing with inability to maintain normal posture and balance may be present, as well as spasticity or uncontrollable movements in the extremities. Also documented are disturbances of gait (particularly ataxia and toe walking), seizures, attention deficit disorder, sensory impairment, failure of automatic reactions (equilibrium), and speech and swallowing impairments.

Diagnostic Evaluation and Therapeutic Management

Diagnostic tests include EEG, CT or MRI, electrolyte levels, metabolic work-up, and a thorough neurologic examination. Persistent primitive reflexes are seen, as are abnormal muscle tone and posture and abnormal motor development.

The goal of managing the child with cerebral palsy is early recognition and intervention to maximize the child's abilities. Cerebral palsy often is not diagnosed before the child is 2 years old. Through repetition, new brain pathways develop through alternative receptor sites to achieve proper motor function. The child may be intellectually intact, but this may be overlooked because of the child's physical limitations. Intrathecal Baclofen via an infusion pump can be used to treat severe spasticity in children with cerebral palsy. Baclofen is a skeletal muscle relaxant. Close monitoring of the child for infection and the pump for malfunction is required (Johnston, 2004).

A multidisciplinary health care team approach is necessary to meet the many needs of the child with cerebral palsy. The team includes the child and family, a pediatrician, neurologist, orthopedic surgeon, nurse, speech and hearing therapist, social worker, occupational therapist, physical therapist, and educators.

Pathophysiology

of Cerebral Palsy

A number of neuromuscular disabilities are associated with cerebral palsy. The alteration in voluntary muscular control is related to a cerebral insult. The area of the brain that has been injured determines the type of neuromuscular disability.

The five classifications of cerebral palsy are: dyskinetic, spastic, ataxic, rigid, and mixed. *Dyskinetic (athetoid) palsy* refers to an injury in the basal ganglia. Slow, writhing, uncontrolled, involuntary movements involving all extremities characterize this type.

Spastic cerebral palsy is the most common type. The affected area of the brain is the cortex. Spastic cerebral palsy is characterized by increased deep tendon reflexes, hypertonia, flexion, and sometimes contractures. The child's muscles are very tense, and any stimulus may cause a sudden jerking movement. The child has to make a conscious effort to relax. Scissors gait, hip flexion with adduction and internal rotation, or toe walking because of tight heel cords may be present.

In *ataxic cerebral palsy*, the affected area of the brain is the cerebellum. This type of cerebral palsy is characterized by a loss of coordination, equilibrium, and kinesthetic sense. Overall, the child appears clumsy.

Rigid (tremor, atonic) cerebral palsy is relatively rare in children. The child has rigidity of both flexor and extensor muscles. In a child with tremors, the tremors are apparent both at rest and during movement. The prognosis for a child with this type of cerebral palsy is poor because of associated deformities and lack of active movement.

Approximately half of children with cerebral palsy have some degree of mental retardation and other disabilities. Other than epilepsy and mental retardation, learning problems, poor attention span, hyperactivity, hearing or visual loss, and emotional problems may be seen. Gastroesophageal reflux may be a problem (see Chapter 43). There is a high expenditure of calories with the intense movements, and difficulty feeding leads to a calorie deficit.

Nursing Care Plan

The Child With Cerebral Palsy in the Community Setting

FOCUSED ASSESSMENT

The most important component of assessment is identifying the condition. The infant identified to be at risk is then monitored for irritability, feeding difficulties, delayed development, poor motor development, abnormal posturing, persistence of primitive reflexes, ataxic gait, and poor muscle tone. Assessing the child's response to therapy is important. Monitoring and documenting progress or lack of progress are just as important as identifying problems.

The nurse needs to be aware of normal growth and development, with special attention to developmental milestones, as delay in reaching these milestones may be a key indicator of cerebral palsy.

School and community nurses are in the best position to work with families and children with cerebral palsy. Many of these children will need both learning and physical adaptations as they enter school. For the most part, children with cerebral palsy are educated in the regular school program with assistive devices, such as communication boards or computers. The school nurse regularly assesses these children, because the nurse may be part of an educational team that develops an individual learning plan for the child.

Nursing Diagnosis

Impaired Physical Mobility related to spasticity and muscle weakness.

Expected Outcomes

The child will:
- Maximize ability for movement, as evidenced by freedom from contractures or injuries and no complications from immobility.

The parents will:
- Demonstrate how to do the child's exercises and will notify the school nurse if there are any changes in the child's plan.

INTERVENTION	RATIONALE
1. Reinforce physical therapy exercises to strengthen and help coordination of muscles. These exercises may have to be performed in the school setting.	1. Early intervention and consistent therapy will facilitate proper posture and circumvent the development of contractures.
2. Encourage parents to be active in the child's daily physical and occupational therapy.	2. Active involvement in the child's care empowers the parents.
3. Observe and record the child's response to physical therapy.	3. Changes in therapy may be made in a timely fashion for a higher degree of success.
4. Determine the need for special equipment for reading, writing, eating, and mobility. Convey this information to the school evaluation team.	4. The use of special equipment will improve the chance for successful self-care. Incorporating this into the child's education plan will maximize learning potential.

Evaluation

- Have the child's joints remained mobile and free from contractures?
- Does the child demonstrate improved mobility and self-care?
- Can the parents demonstrate physical therapy techniques used for their child?
- Have the parents notified the school about any changes in the child's plan of care?

Nursing Diagnosis

Delayed Growth and Development related to neuromuscular impairment.

Expected Outcome

The child will:
- Maximize potential for meeting growth and development milestones, as evidenced by participation in family, social, and school activities.

Nursing Care Plan

The Child With Cerebral Palsy in the Community Setting—cont'd

INTERVENTION	RATIONALE
1. Monitor the child's developmental level and intelligence. Administer the Denver Developmental Screening Test (see Chapter 4) if needed.	1. The child with cerebral palsy should be given opportunities to learn and should be exposed to new experiences to maximize developmental progress.
2. Encourage early intervention and participation in school programs. Refer for early intervention community programs.	2. Interventions by multidisciplinary groups will maximize the child's potential for learning.
3. Communicate and interact with the child at the child's functional level, not chronologic age.	3. A child with normal intelligence can understand age-appropriate communication and speech, but a child with decreased intelligence might have a different cognitive understanding than age would indicate.

Evaluation

- Do the parents encourage social and developmental activities that maximize the child's potential?
- Does the child attend public school and play with peers whenever possible?
- Does the child participate in physical, speech, and occupational therapy at school?

Nursing Diagnosis

Risk for Injury related to spasticity, uncontrolled muscle movements, or seizures.

Expected Outcomes

The child will:
- Have a safe environment, as evidenced by freedom from injuries.

The parents will:
- Describe ways to adapt the child's environment to maximize safety.

INTERVENTION	RATIONALE
1. Teach the family principles for providing a safe environment (e.g., remove sharp objects and toys, pad sharp furniture edges).	1. Providing a safe environment will reduce the risk of injury.
2. Have the child wear a protective helmet and pads if the child falls frequently.	2. A helmet protects against head injury.
3. If the child is hospitalized, implement bedside seizure precautions. (Do not pad the rails with pillows.)	3. Keeping suction, oxygen, and airway equipment at the bedside and padding the side rails help prevent injury and allow for resuscitation of the child if necessary. Pillows should not be used as pads because they may cause suffocation.
4. Provide safe toys that are appropriate for age and developmental level.	4. No sharp, very small, or easily shattered toys should be allowed for the child who may fall because of erratic movements.
5. Position the child upright after meals.	5. An upright position prevents aspiration secondary to gastroesophageal reflux.

Evaluation

- Does the child remain free from injury?
- Do the parents demonstrate safety measures for the child?
- Have the parents adapted the child's environment to be safe and secure?

Nursing Diagnosis

Impaired Verbal Communication related to neuromuscular impairment and difficulty with articulation.

Continued

Nursing Care Plan

The Child With Cerebral Palsy in the Community Setting—cont'd

Expected Outcome

The child will:
- Maximize communication ability, as evidenced by appropriately expressing needs and developing methods for communicating with others.

INTERVENTION	RATIONALE
1. Use flash cards and talking boards to facilitate communication.	1. Teaching aids help reinforce language and speech development and increase self-esteem.
2. Refer the child to a speech therapist.	2. Early intervention will maximize speech capabilities.
3. Encourage and reinforce speech therapy techniques, nonverbal methods of communication, proper feeding techniques, and jaw control.	3. These techniques facilitate communication and decrease the child's frustration at not being understood. They also facilitate the goals of speech therapy.
4. Encourage parents to convey in detail the child's communication techniques any time the child is in a new situation.	4. Sharing the child's communication techniques helps the child adjust to new situations.

Evaluation

- Does the child participate in groups using appropriate communication?
- Does the child use various methods to communicate?
- Do the parents allow time for the child to respond to questions and conversations?
- Have the parents learned the same communication method that the child uses?

HEAD INJURY

Head injury refers to the pathologic result of any mechanical force to the scalp, skull, meninges, or brain.

Types of Head Injuries

Types of head injury include:

- *Closed head injury:* nonpenetrating injury to the head in which there is no break in the integrity of the barrier between the outside environment and the intracranial cavity
- *Open head injury:* penetrating injury to the head in which there is a break in the integrity of the barrier (skull, meninges) between the outside environment and the intracranial cavity; infection will be a major concern
- *Coup injury:* cerebral injury sustained directly below the site of impact
- *Contrecoup injury:* cerebral injury sustained in the region or pole opposite the site of impact; caused by the rapid movements of the semisolid brain within the cranial vault
- *Missile injury:* penetrating injury of the skull or brain, most often caused by a bullet
- *Impalement injury:* penetrating injury caused by a pierce to the scalp, skull, or brain with something sharp

Skull Fractures

Skull fractures include the following types:

- *Linear:* straight-line fracture; dura not involved
- *Depressed:* bone pressing downward, indented

- *Basilar:* fracture of the base of the skull; symptoms are Battle's sign, raccoon eyes, rhinorrhea, otorrhea, and hemotympanum (blood behind the eardrum)
- *Comminuted:* fragmentation of the bone into many pieces or a multiple fracture line

Contusion

Contusions are petechial hemorrhages along the superficial aspects of the brain. They may occur at the site of impact or in association with a lesion remote from the site of direct impact.

Concussion

A concussion is a transient and reversible neuronal dysfunction, with instantaneous loss of awareness and responsiveness.

Intracranial Hemorrhage

Intracranial hemorrhages include two types:

Epidural: blood accumulates between the dura and the skull; arterial damage is the usual type of injury, and therefore the hemorrhage develops rapidly.

Subdural: blood accumulates between the dura and the cerebrum; a subdural hemorrhage can be acute or chronic (Fig. 52-5).

Incidence

Multiple trauma is the leading cause of death in children beyond infancy. Approximately 250,000 children are hospitalized yearly in the United States for evaluation and treatment

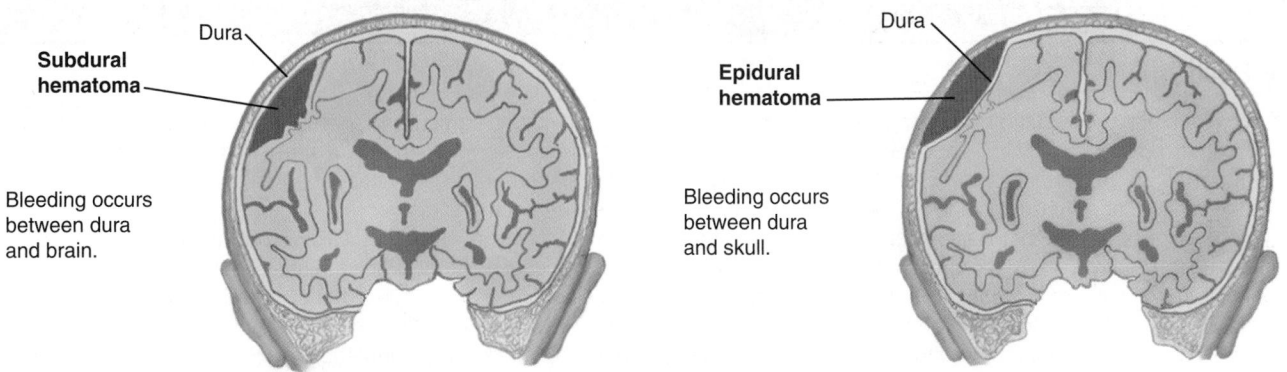

Figure 52-5 Subdural and epidural hematomas are the two most common cranial hematomas; one or the other occurs in 6% to 7% of head-injured children. A *subdural hematoma* is often caused when the head strikes an immovable object. However, in an infant a subdural hematoma may result from aggressive shaking (a form of child abuse); retinal hemorrhage is also a classic sign of shaking injury in infants. With *epidural hematoma,* a rapid decline in neurologic function may occur 4 to 8 hours after a brief period of lucidity. If untreated, the increased intracranial pressure (ICP) can cause death in a short time.

of a head injury (Quayle, 1999). Common causes of head injuries include motor vehicle crashes, bicycle collisions, falls, sports injuries, beatings, and gunshot wounds.

Manifestations

Head injuries are classified as minor, moderate, or severe as correlated with the Glasgow Coma Scale. Minor head injuries exhibit the following manifestations: possible change in level of consciousness, transient period of confusion, irritability, vomiting, somnolence, and headache (GCS score of 13 to 15). Moderate to severe head injuries are marked by altered mental states, changes in vital signs, signs of increased ICP, retinal hemorrhage, hemiparesis, and papilledema (Box 52-4).

Diagnostic Evaluation

A complete history of the event helps determine the mechanism of injury and whether the child lost consciousness. Spinal radiographs are obtained to ascertain there is no cervical spinal cord injury; radiographs are followed by a complete neurologic examination. Any indication of increased ICP is quickly reported to the physician. CT or MRI is the most precise study with which to diagnose the specific kind of head injury sustained. A scalp hematoma in an infant suggests underlying skull fracture; skull radiography is recommended for these children (Quayle, 1999).

Therapeutic Management

Initial management of the child with a head injury includes assessing ventilatory function, neurologic status, and any other injuries present (see Chapter 34). Interventions to maintain vital functions are provided until all injuries are determined. Increased ICP or seizures may develop in a child with a head injury. The long-term outcome of a head injury is related to the child's GCS score.

BOX 52-4
Classification of Severity of Head Injuries Based on Glasgow Coma Scale

Minor Head Injury (Score of 13 to 15)
- Possible headache and cognitive deficits (especially affecting memory)
- Possible stress intolerance

Moderate Head Injury (Score of 9 to 12)
- Headache, memory deficits, cognitive deficits, difficulty with activities of daily living; occasionally results in death

Severe Head Injury (Score of 3 to 8)
- Posttrauma syndromes and cognitive, emotional, motor, and sensory deficits caused by irreversible brain injury
- Long-term care or support in the community usually needed
- Occasionally results in death

Nursing Considerations

Initial assessment of the child with a head injury includes the ABCs—evaluation of **a**irway, **b**reathing, and **c**irculation (see Chapter 34). The child's neck is immobilized as special attention is given to the cervical spine. Obtain and record baseline vital signs, and obtain further signs as indicated by the child's clinical condition. A complete history and comprehensive neurologic examination should be completed. Assess the child's level of consciousness (with the Glasgow Coma Scale), pupil size, and pupil reactivity to light.

Test cranial nerve function to identify deficits resulting from the injury and to monitor for increased ICP. The clinical signs and symptoms of increased ICP, with or without actual measurement of the ICP, will determine both the child's clinical status and the medical and nursing interventions. Nasotracheal suctioning is contraindicated in a child with a

Pathophysiology

of Head Injury

The cranium is a rigid structure that contains blood, brain tissue, and cerebrospinal fluid (CSF). The pressure exerted by these components on the cranium is between 4 and 15 mm Hg. According to the Monro-Kellie doctrine, an increase in one of these components must be accompanied by a decrease in one of the others to maintain intracranial pressure (ICP) within normal range. Cerebral function depends on adequate delivery of nutrients, such as oxygen, glucose, and other substrates; an abnormal increase in ICP will interfere with the balance and delivery of these nutrients.

Head injuries are either primary or secondary. *Primary head injuries* are those in which damage is sustained at the time of injury; *secondary head injuries* refer to the consequences of the

primary injury, particularly increased ICP. The severity of the injury depends on the amount of stress to the cranium and brain. Head injuries include concussions, contusions, lacerations, fractures, and hematomas.

Motor vehicle collisions, falls, sports injuries, child abuse, and neglect cause most head injuries in children. *Acceleration-deceleration* is the term used to describe the mechanism of injury. The shearing force of the initial impact moves the brain forward, followed by a countering, backward movement of the brain in the skull. The shearing force produces bruising, tearing, and bleeding. Shaken baby syndrome, a type of child abuse, may result in epidural hematomas and retinal hemorrhages (see Chapter 53).

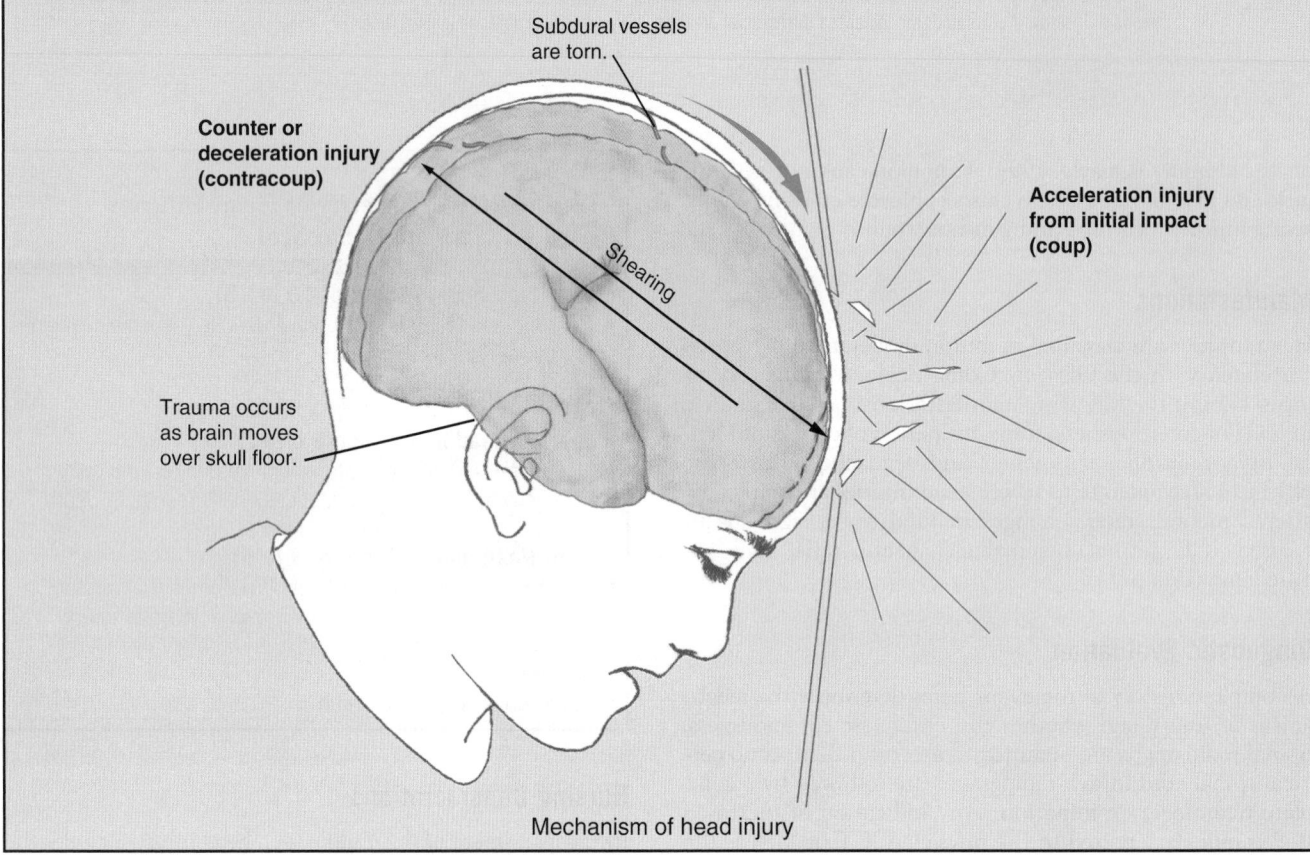

Subdural vessels are torn.

Counter or deceleration injury (contracoup)

Shearing

Acceleration injury from initial impact (coup)

Trauma occurs as brain moves over skull floor.

Mechanism of head injury

basilar skull fracture; because of the nature of the injury, the suction catheter could be introduced into the brain.

The child with a head injury can experience a postinjury alteration in antidiuretic hormone (ADH). Possibly as a result of injury to the hypothalamus or posterior pituitary, the child can exhibit signs of excess ADH (syndrome of inappropriate antidiuretic hormone [SIADH]) or deficit of ADH (diabetes insipidus) (see Chapter 51). Any child with a head injury needs to be assessed for fluid and electrolyte alteration.

Nursing care of the child with a head injury is similar to nursing care of any child with increased ICP, with the additional attention to fluid and electrolyte balance. The nurse carefully monitors any intravenous (IV) and oral fluid intake and determines and records hourly fluid output. If the child

develops SIADH, fluids may be restricted to reduce the risk of increasing ICP from cerebral edema. Fluid restriction is a nursing challenge because it involves the cooperation of parents and others involved in the child's care. Placing a sign at the child's bedside alerts others. Be sure to choose fluids the child likes and distribute the allocated amounts over the course of the child's waking hours.

If the child is discharged from the emergency room, written instructions should be given to parents.

SPINAL CORD INJURY

Spinal cord injury can result from any trauma or injury to the spinal cord or to its vascular supply or venous drainage.

PARENTS
Want to Know

About Guidelines for the Child With a Head Injury

Apply ice to the child's head to prevent swelling. Clean any scrapes or cuts with soap and water. Encourage the child to rest, and limit foods if the child is vomiting. You will need to watch the child carefully for 2 days. For 2 nights, awaken the child once at your bedtime and once 4 hours later. Check that the child becomes alert and can answer questions appropriately.

Call the physician immediately after the injury if the child:

- Has bleeding that does not stop after pressure has been applied for 10 minutes
- Needs sutures
- Is younger than 1 year
- Had a seizure after the head injury
- Was unconscious or confused
- Has a severe headache or vomiting

- Has slurred speech or blurred vision
- Has blood or watery fluid coming from the ear or nose
- Has unequal pupils or crossed eyes
- Has difficulty walking or crawling or weakness in the arms
- Has other symptoms that concern you

POSTCONCUSSION SYNDROME

Some children who have had a head injury can experience an aftereffect called *postconcussion syndrome*. If your child has this condition, your child may be upset easily and may be irritable if tired or stressed. Memory problems are common, as are learning difficulties, double vision, dizziness, headaches, fatigue, and light sensitivity. These symptoms may last many months.

Data from Schmitt, B.D. (1999). *Instructions for pediatric patients* (2nd ed., p. 138). Philadelphia: Saunders.

Etiology

Spinal cord injuries in children are usually caused by motor vehicle crashes, falls, diving accidents, sports injuries, gunshot or knife wounds, or attempted suicide. In the infant, a common cause of spinal cord injury is intentional, aggressive shaking by an older person.

Incidence

Although spinal cord injuries are less common in children than in adults, 75% of spinal cord injuries in children occur in the cervical spine, between the occiput and C3. Young children are more susceptible to upper spinal cord injury because of the larger head size in relation to body size. As the child grows older, the site of the spinal cord injury moves distally.

Manifestations

Manifestations of spinal cord injury include loss of some or all movement or sensation below the level of injury, respiratory depression or apnea, hypotension and bradycardia, hypothermia, and neck pain.

Diagnostic Evaluation

After the nurse takes the history of the injury and performs a complete neurologic examination, the extent of the spinal cord injury will be determined with radiography or MRI. The extent of the motor or sensory deficit may resolve somewhat as spinal shock resolves.

Therapeutic Management

Treatment includes steroid therapy, which may be administered within 8 hours of the injury as a bolus of 30 mg/kg followed by a continuous infusion of 5.4 mg/kg/hr for 23 hours. Until permanent surgical stabilization can be performed, other treatments including halo traction (Fig. 52-6) and Gardner-Wells tongs, may be used as a temporary stabilization method.

Pathophysiology

of Spinal Cord Injury

Spinal cord injuries occur in children when vertebral bodies are fractured or subluxation of the vertebra occurs. Subluxation results in malalignment of contiguous vertebrae, so that the spinal cord is compressed. The cord may be crushed, stretched beyond tolerance, or completely divided. All neurons carrying sensations from those parts of the body below the lesion are unable to pass their message on to the brain. A severe cord injury will cause complete paralysis and complete loss of sensation below the severed level.

Flaccid paralysis of the affected limbs immediately follows a spinal cord injury. Paralysis is caused by spinal shock, which can last 3 weeks or more. The flaccidity changes to spasticity when the spinal shock resolves.

▪NURSING CARE
The Child With a Spinal Cord Injury

Assessment

The spine must be immobilized before any attempt is made to move the child. The airway is assessed immediately, and if intubation is necessary, it is done without hyperextending the neck (see Chapter 34). Next, assess circulation, keeping in mind that hypotension may be a result of either hypovolemia or neurologic shock. Bradycardia and hypothermia may ensue. Attempt to maintain the body temperature and keep the child well oxygenated.

The neurologic assessment includes evaluating mobility, sensation, and reflexes. The injury may be complete or incomplete. In a complete spinal cord injury, the cord is completely severed and there is no spinal innervation below the injury. With an incomplete spinal cord injury, the cord has some function remaining. The neurologic assessment is ongoing and carefully documented so that changes can be dealt with in a timely fashion. The child is then assessed for trauma to other systems.

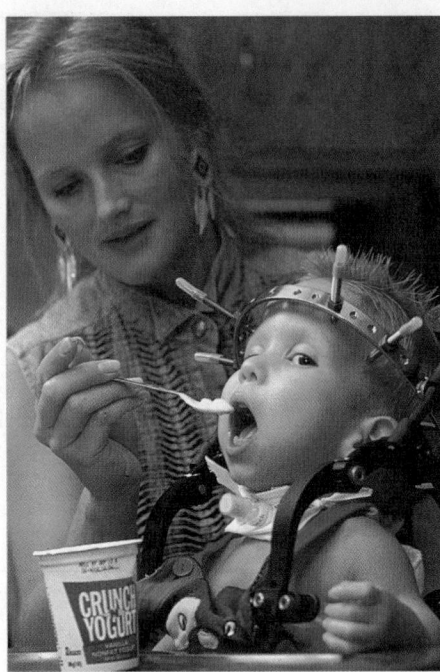

Figure 52-6 Children who have injuries or birth defects that involve the upper spine may be placed in halo traction to stabilize the spine and prevent added nerve damage. Spinal cord injury is a catastrophic event for the child and family, who will need intense nursing support and education as well as referral to support groups. (Courtesy Cook Children's Medical Center, Fort Worth, TX.)

Nursing Diagnoses and Planning

The nursing diagnoses and expected outcomes that may be appropriate following assessment of the child with spinal cord injury are

- Ineffective Breathing Pattern related to weakness or paralysis of respiratory muscles following spinal cord injury.
  Expected Outcome: The child will not experience respiratory distress, as evidenced by arterial blood gas values within normal limits, stable vital signs, and motor and sensory function.
- Risk for Impaired Skin Integrity related to immobility.
  Expected Outcome: The child will maintain skin integrity, as evidenced by intact skin and absence of breakdown.
- Anxiety related to having a child with an acute condition.
  Expected Outcome: The child and parents will experience decreased anxiety, as evidenced by an ability to verbalize what the spinal cord injury means to them.
- Interrupted Family Processes related to having a child with an acute and chronic injury.
  Expected Outcome: The parents will show signs of adapting to their child's injury, as evidenced by participating in the child's care and seeking appropriate support within the community.
- Impaired Physical Mobility related to neuromuscular impairment.
  Expected Outcome: The child will maximize potential for improvement of mobility, as evidenced by involvement in physical therapy and occupational therapy.

Interventions

The goal of nursing care is to minimize the potential for further injury, prevent the sequelae of immobility, and promote maximal spinal cord recovery. The spinal cord is immobilized with the use of tongs or halo traction. The child will remain in traction for several weeks (see Chapter 50). The nurse is responsible for maintaining proper alignment by monitoring the status of the traction every 1 to 2 hours. Towels and rolls can be useful to help position the child. The nurse should perform a motor and sensory assessment after each change of position (see Chapter 33).

If the child's situation becomes unstable, surgical stabilization may become necessary. Progressive neurologic deterioration is the major indicator for surgery.

The child who is immobilized and neurologically impaired is at risk for respiratory complications as a result of muscle weakness and immobility. Respiratory status and pulse oximetry readings are assessed and recorded every 1 to 2 hours. Supplemental oxygen may be indicated. Nebulizer, incentive spirometry, and intermittent positive-pressure breathing (IPPB) may be ordered. Some children may need a tracheostomy and mechanical ventilation if the respiratory muscles are involved or if weaning from the ventilator is slow and difficult to accomplish.

The nurse assesses perfusion by monitoring vital signs, color, skin temperature, and intake and output. Because of bladder muscle weakness or paralysis, an indwelling urinary catheter facilitates bladder emptying and accurate measurement of intake and output, which is monitored hourly. If alterations in perfusion occur, the child will receive crystalloids by bolus infusion. Vasopressors, such as dopamine and dobutamine, may also be used.

The child with a spinal cord injury may have a problem with body temperature control and so should be warmed or cooled as appropriate. If the child has an elevated temperature, samples of wound material and blood are obtained for culture. Sputum cultures may be necessary. Antipyretic and broad-spectrum antibiotic therapy is initiated after the specimens are sent to the laboratory.

The child may have a nasogastric tube in place. The nurse will maintain tube patency and monitor and record drainage. The pH of the gastric fluid may be tested and the child treated with antacids, sucralfate (Carafate), or histamine blockers. The child is at risk for stress ulcers and gastrointestinal hemorrhage. A bowel regimen will be initiated and maintained to prevent impaction. Bowel training includes ingestion of a high-fiber diet (when the child is able to eat), the use of stool softeners, and increased water intake. While the indwelling catheter is in place, care is taken to prevent infection. Intermittent catheterization may eventually be initiated if necessary.

Inspect the child's skin frequently, and administer skin care each time the child is repositioned. Pressure on the bony prominences is minimized with the use of special mattresses and padding.

Adequate nutrition is essential to the healing process. Caloric intake is monitored, and the child may receive nutrition by oral intake, tube feeding, or total parenteral nutrition. A good indicator of a favorable response to the nutrition is timely healing of wounds.

Spinal cord injury is a catastrophic event. The lives of the child and family have been suddenly and permanently altered. They will need intense assistance and support. These goals can be achieved through therapeutic play, promotion of independent functioning, referral to a multidisciplinary rehabilitation team, referral to support groups, and thorough discharge planning and home care teaching.

Evaluation

- Are body functions (respiration, elimination, muscle strength) maintained as normally as possible?
- Is the child's skin intact and free from breakdown?

BOX 52-5
International Classification of Seizures

Generalized Seizures

Onset starts at any age. Clinical features indicate involvement of both cerebral hemispheres. Consciousness is impaired.

Tonic-Clonic Seizures

Formerly called *grand mal seizures,* tonic-clonic seizures cause an abrupt arrest of activity and impairment of consciousness. The *tonic phase* consists of a sustained, generalized stiffening of muscles, including the diaphragm, lasting a few seconds. The *clonic phase* is symmetric and rhythmic, consisting of alternating contraction and relaxation of major muscle groups. This phase usually ends spontaneously in less than 5 minutes. Respirations are irregular and may be stridulous. Sphincter incontinence may or may not be present. The tonic-clonic seizure is followed by a variable period of confusion, lethargy, and sleep (postictal phase).

Atonic Seizures

Atonic seizures cause an abrupt loss of postural tone, impairment of consciousness, confusion, lethargy, and sleep.

Myoclonic Seizures

Myoclonic seizures are brief, random contractions of a muscle group. They can occur on both sides of the body and may occur singly or in clusters. Impairment of consciousness might occur during myoclonic seizures. Onset can occur as early as age 2 months, but myoclonic seizures are more frequently seen in school-age children or adolescents than in very young children. Myoclonic seizures that occur during infancy are called *infantile spasms;* those that occur during adolescence are called *juvenile myoclonic epilepsy.*

Absence Seizures

Formerly called *petit mal seizures,* absence seizures are very brief episodes of altered consciousness. There is no muscle activity except for eyelid fluttering, twitching, or head bobbing.

The child has a blank facial expression. Absence seizures last only 5 to 10 seconds, but they may occur one after another several times per day. The onset of absence seizures usually does not occur before age 5 years. Children usually outgrow absence seizures during adolescence.

Partial Seizures

Onset starts at any age. The clinical features suggest that only a limited functional area in one hemisphere of the brain is involved, and therefore symptoms are seen on only one side of the body. Partial seizures begin focally but may become generalized when the electrical impulses are passed across the corpus callosum to the other hemisphere. Partial seizures are further divided into those with or without change in level of consciousness.

Simple Partial Seizures

Simple partial seizures consist of motor, autonomic, or sensory symptoms. There is no change in level of consciousness with simple partial seizures. Symptoms may include an odd taste in the mouth or odd smell, abdominal discomfort, unexplained feelings of fear or dread, or motor movements. This type of seizure may last 20 seconds to several minutes.

Complex Partial Seizures

Complex partial seizures may begin with or without an aura and with or without a simple partial seizure. Symptoms include impaired consciousness; transient staring; altered mental status; and feelings of unreality, detachment, and disrupted memory. There may be distortions of perception or hallucinations, teeth grinding, lip smacking, chewing, swallowing, scratching, or pulling at shirt buttons. Tonic-clonic movements of one side of the body may also be seen. The average duration of a complex partial seizure is 1 to 2 minutes. A complex partial seizure is followed by a variable period of confusion, lethargy, and sleep.

Modified from Haslam, R. (2000). Seizures in childhood. In R. Behrman, R. Kliegman, & H. Jenson (Eds.), *Nelson textbook of pediatrics* (16th ed.). Philadelphia: Saunders.

- Do the child and parents verbalize feelings and emotions about the injury and the prognosis?
- Do the parents demonstrate ability to provide physical and emotional support for the child?
- Has the child's neurologic function improved?

SEIZURE DISORDERS

A seizure consists of brief paroxysmal behavior that is caused by excessive abnormal discharge of neurons. Epilepsy is marked by recurrent seizure activity that does not occur in association with an acute illness. The two types of seizures are: partial (focal) and generalized. Partial seizures occur in one part of the brain and may or may not alter consciousness. Generalized seizures occur over the entire brain and do alter consciousness.

Etiology

Seizures are symptomatic of altered neuronal activity in the CNS. Seizures can occur for many reasons and are categorized as *primary* or *secondary*. Primary seizures occur in the absence of any underlying brain structural abnormality. Primary seizures are linked to genetic predisposition and include febrile seizures, absence seizures,

and benign seizures of the newborn. Secondary, or symptomatic, seizures are usually provoked by some temporary or permanent structural or metabolic abnormality. Cerebral lesions, malformations, metabolic disorders, acquired causes (e.g., anoxia, trauma, stroke), infections, degenerative disorders, and toxic disturbances are linked to secondary seizures. Approximately 50% of childhood seizures are idiopathic, meaning they have no known cause.

Incidence

Approximately 3% to 5% of all children younger than 18 years experience a seizure (Haslam, 2000). An estimated 3% to 4% of children age 6 months to 3 years will have a febrile seizure. Sixty percent of children with epilepsy experience the onset of seizures before 18 years of age. Neonatal seizures occur in approximately 20% of preterm infants.

Pathophysiology

During a seizure, there are excessive, self-limiting neuronal discharges. The result of these discharges is activation of associated motor or sensory organs. The extent of the seizure depends on the location and extent of the abnormal neuronal discharges. The brain consists of millions of nerve cells; electrical impulses are sent through many of these cells by means of neurotransmitters. When numerous nerve cells fire abnormally at the same time, a seizure may result.

Manifestations

There are many types of seizures. The International Classification of Seizures is used to divide seizures into two groups: generalized and partial. In addition, some other types of seizures are seen in children (Box 52-5).

Febrile seizures are generally seen in young children. Only about one third of these children ever have another seizure, and about 3% of this group of children develop epilepsy. The height and rapidity of temperature elevation seem to be factors in precipitating febrile seizures. The temperature is usually elevated above 38.8° C (102° F). The seizure activity occurs during the temperature rise rather than after prolonged elevation. Simple febrile seizures are familial and probably transmitted by autosomal dominant inheritance (Fenichel, 2001). Ninety percent of febrile seizures occur as a result of fever caused by otitis media, pharyngitis, and adenitis. The family of a child who experiences a febrile seizure should be given information about these seizures and instructed what to do if another seizure occurs.

Neonatal seizures are usually caused by an underlying pathologic process. The most frequent cause of neonatal seizures is perinatal asphyxia leading to hypoxic-ischemic encephalopathy, which accounts for as many as 65% of neonatal seizures. Another 15% of cases can be attributed to intracranial hemorrhage. Other causes include metabolic disturbances, meningitis, cerebral infarcts, drug withdrawal, hyperthermia, hypoglycemia, sodium and potassium imbalances, congenital anomalies of the CNS, and inherited syndromes.

The mechanism of neonatal seizures is not clearly understood. Possible explanations include an excess of excitatory neurotransmitter compared with inhibitory neurotransmitter, altered permeability of the neuronal membrane inhibiting

---

! CRITICAL TO REMEMBER

Observations and Nursing Care During a Seizure

- As the seizure begins, look at your watch or a clock. It is important to be able to describe how long seizure activity lasts.
- Protect the child from injury by loosening clothing at the neck and turning the child gently onto the side. Do not restrain the child or insert any object into the child's mouth.
- Carefully observe where the seizure begins, its progression, and how it ends.
- Be able to describe any preceding or accompanying sensory or motor manifestations.
- When the seizure is over, allow the child to rest if she or he desires. Record the child's behavior before, during, and after the seizure and the approximate duration of the seizure.
- In neonates, if the movement can be initiated by a stimulus, such as touch, it is probably a tremor. If it cannot be stopped or controlled with gentle restraint or passive flexion, it is probably a seizure.

---

sodium movement, and an imbalance between depolarization and repolarization of the neurons. Because of the overall anatomic and physiologic immaturity of the nervous system in the neonate, well-organized generalized seizures are rare.

Because of the lack of myelinization of fiber tracts, neonates do not experience the same type of tonic-clonic seizure that an older child experiences. Seizures in neonates may produce subtle signs, such as sustained eye opening, tonic horizontal deviation of the eyes, blinking or eyelid fluttering, sucking, smacking, drooling, tongue thrusting, pedaling movements of the legs, swimming movements of the arms, and apnea. These manifestations are more common in preterm infants and infants with hypoxic-ischemic encephalopathy. Neonatal seizures also can be focal, tonic, or myoclonic, with jerking movements of the extremities.

PARENTS
Want to Know

About Guidelines for the Child or Adolescent Taking Seizure Medication

- Oral care is very important for children taking phenytoin (Dilantin), because phenytoin can cause gum problems. Your child should brush and floss after every meal, using a soft brush. Take your child to the dentist every 3 to 6 months for a checkup and teeth cleaning.
- Once your child has started taking the medication, blood levels should be monitored to determine that the medication has reached and maintained a therapeutic level and to monitor for a toxic level. In addition, other blood tests may be needed to be sure the medication is not harming the liver or blood cells. Blood levels should be measured periodically as your physician recommends, if a seizure occurs, or if side effects are noticed.
- If your child is taking valproic acid, be alert for any signs of unusual bleeding or bruising. Valproic acid can affect the

- platelets (cells that help the blood clot) and cause the platelet counts to drop.
- Be sure your child does not suddenly stop taking antiepileptic medications without discussing it with a physician or nurse. Suddenly stopping medications can cause the child to have a seizure or status epilepticus.
- Some states require a driver to be seizure-free for 6 to 12 months to obtain a driver's license. If your child is of driving age, discuss this with your health care provider.
- Birth control pills might be less effective while taking antiepileptic medications. If sexually active, your adolescent should consult a nurse or physician for additional forms of birth control.
- Alcohol, marijuana, and street drugs will lower the seizure threshold. It is best to avoid or limit these drugs.

TABLE **52-3** Common Seizure Medications

Drug Name	Seizure Type	Side Effects	Nursing Implications
Carbamazepine (Tegretol)	Partial or generalized	Sedation, cognitive deficits, behavior outbursts	Watch for change in behavior or decrease in school grades. Child should not be given erythromycin; will cause increase in drug level.
Felbamate (Felbatol)	Partial	Nausea and vomiting, weight loss, anorexia, agitation and aggression, aplastic anemia, liver failure	Shake oral suspension well.
Ethosuximide (Zarontin)	Generalized	Nausea and vomiting, lethargy	Observe for excessive drowsiness. Take with food.
Lamotrigine (Lamictal)	Generalized or partial	Rash (increased risk of rash exists in children with previous reaction to any drug or to another antiepileptic drug), dizziness, headache, double vision, nausea and vomiting, ataxia	Not affected by food absorption.
Gabapentin (Neurontin)	Partial	Drowsiness, dizziness, nystagmus, nausea and vomiting, ataxia	Dosage must be adjusted for renal function.
Levetiracetam (Keppra)	Partial	Sleepiness, weakness, headache, infection	Monitor for side effects and frequency of seizures. Monitor for renal dysfunction
Phenobarbital	Generalized or partial	Sedation, cognitive deficits, behavior outbursts	Watch for excessive drowsiness, changes in school grades, and respiratory depression.
Phenytoin (Dilantin)	Partial, generalized, or status	Lethargy, nystagmus, ataxia, allergic reactions, hypertrophic gums, hirsutism	Teach good oral care to decrease gum hypertrophy. Intravenous (IV) form must be given in normal saline and filtered.
Topiramate (Topamax)	Partial	Fatigue, nervousness, decreased attention, anorexia, renal stones, tremor	Affects levels of other epilepsy medications. Keep children well-hydrated to decrease chances of renal stones.
Tiagabine (Gabatril)	Partial	Lethargy, sedation, double vision, ataxia	Monitor for generalized weakness.
Valproic acid (Depakene)	Generalized	Nausea and vomiting, tremor, weight gain, hair loss, thrombocytopenia, liver failure	Do not crush or cut pills/sprinkles—can cause stomach ulcers. Take with food.
Oxcarbazepine (Trileptal)	Partial	Fatigue, headache, dizziness, double vision, unsteadiness, nausea and vomiting.	Interacts with other seizure medications. Levels of other medications should be monitored.

Diagnostic Evaluation

The child's health history and family history are important parts of the initial work-up. A thorough description of the child's behavior before, during, and after the seizure activity is important to delineate the type of seizure. Video recording and EEG monitoring will help identify the seizure. Serum electrolyte determinations, CBC, blood glucose determination, lumbar puncture, and other laboratory tests can help uncover metabolic causes. CT and MRI will indicate trauma, tumor, or congenital malformation. In neonates, several other laboratory tests may be included, such as *t*oxoplasmosis, *o*ther agents, *r*ubella, *c*ytomegalovirus, and *h*erpes simplex virus (TORCH) titers, to exclude congenital viral infections, as well as amino acid and organic acid studies to exclude inborn errors of metabolism.

Therapeutic Management

The basic tenet of treatment for the child with seizures is to treat the whole child. The goals are to identify and correct the cause of the seizure, eliminate the seizure with a minimum of side effects and using the least amount of medication, and normalize the child's and family's lives (Table 52-3).

Stimulating the vagal nerve via a device implanted in the chest wall, has been found, in some cases, to reduce seizure occurrence through a presently unknown mechanism (Lee & Adelson, 2004). It has few side effects and can decrease the need for pharmacologic intervention.

Nursing Care Plan

The Child With a Seizure Disorder in the Community Setting

FOCUSED ASSESSMENT

A detailed history that includes the prenatal, perinatal, and neonatal periods is important in determining factors precipitating seizure activity. Pathologic precipitating factors include hypoxia, cerebral trauma, high fever, lead poisoning, metabolic disorders, brain tumors, birth trauma, and central nervous system (CNS) infections. Nonpathologic factors include overhydration, oversedation, drug abuse, sleep deprivation, antihistamine drug use, alcohol intoxication, and family history.

Seizures often are not witnessed by the health care professional. Ask the parents about the child's age at onset of the seizure activity, time of onset, precipitating events, and the child's behavior before and after the seizure. Ask the parents to describe the seizures, including the child's behaviors during the seizure, how the seizure progresses, how long it lasts, and the child's behavior after the seizures.

The child is given a comprehensive physical examination with special emphasis on the neurologic system. Parameters include assessment of behavior, motor skills, and developmental level. The child's and family's emotional response to the seizure disorder is assessed at this time.

The school nurse may be called to a classroom to manage a child who is having a seizure. If the child is known to have had seizures in the past, it is important for the school nurse to have appropriate information in the child's record and to communicate that information, if necessary, to the child's teacher. Accurate observation in the school setting can assist with seizure management.

Nursing Diagnosis

Risk for Injury related to seizure activity.

Expected Outcomes

The child will:
- Remain free from injury through the use of appropriate injury prevention strategies.

The parents and older child will:
- Discuss seizure prevention and demonstrate first aid for seizures.

INTERVENTION	RATIONALE
1. If the child is hospitalized, institute seizure precautions: padded side rails, bed in low position, suction and airway at bedside. At home, place the child on a soft surface if not in bed. Remove sharp objects, and keep furniture out of the way.	1. These actions modify the environment to make it safer for the child during the seizure.
2. Do not put anything into the child's mouth during a seizure.	2. Forcing something into the child's mouth may injure the child's mouth, gums, or teeth.
3. During a seizure, advise the parent or teacher to place the child on the side in a lateral position. Do not restrain the child. Loosen clothing around the child's neck.	3. Positioning the child on the side will prevent aspiration, because saliva will drain out the corner of the child's mouth. Restraints could cause injury to the child. The nurse or family may gently guide or protect the child's movements and may suction the child's mouth after the seizure is over if suction is available.
4. Record and advise the parent to record the time of seizures, precipitating factors, types of behavior observed during the seizure, bladder or bowel incontinence, and frequency of seizures.	4. These observations help pinpoint the focus of the seizure and will help the physician treat the seizure correctly.
5. Stay with the child.	5. Staying with the child reduces the risk of injury and allows for observation and documentation of the seizure.
6. If the seizure lasts longer than 5 minutes, notify a physician.	6. Medication may need to be administered to stop prolonged seizures. Remember that the main side effect of diazepam (Valium) and lorazepam (Ativan) is respiratory depression.

Evaluation

- Does the child remain injury-free?
- Do the child and family implement injury-prevention strategies?
- Do the parents monitor the seizure and record vital information?
- Can the parents demonstrate first aid for seizures?

Nursing Care Plan

The Child With a Seizure Disorder in the Community Setting—cont'd

Nursing Diagnosis

Deficient Knowledge related to the need for information about how to manage a child with a seizure disorder.

Expected Outcome

The child and parents will:
- Seek information about the child's management and describe how to meet the child's physical, emotional, and educational needs.

INTERVENTION	RATIONALE
1. Determine the child's and parent's educational needs.	1. Determining educational needs provides baseline information to develop a teaching plan.
2. Provide an individual teaching plan for the child and parents for handling seizures.	2. An individualized teaching plan ensures that what is needed by the child and parents will be taught.
3. Explore actual and potential problems that may arise and interfere with treatment.	3. Exploring possible problems facilitates adjustment and normalizes life; it also provides anticipatory guidance.
4. Measure outcomes of education to ensure that learning has taken place and is facilitating acceptance.	4. Evaluation of teaching is an ongoing process to ensure continued learning.
5. Refer to an epilepsy support group. (See Appendix I on Evolve website for a list of resource organizations.)	5. Social support is helpful for some families and may promote adjustment to lifestyle changes.
6. Educate the child and parents about the medication regimen (see Parents Want to Know: About Guidelines for the Child or Adolescent Taking Seizure Medication box, p. 1518). Emphasize the importance of complying with medical treatment.	6. The goal of pharmacologic management is to raise the seizure threshold, thus preventing seizures.
7. Identify the side effects of the medication and when medical attention should be sought.	7. Knowledge of what is expected and normal will facilitate proper use and adherence with medication.
8. Point out the hazards of nonadherence with medications. Encourage the parents and child not to discontinue medications even if the child is seizure-free.	8. Nonadherence will affect the serum levels of anticonvulsants and may cause a seizure to occur.
9. Emphasize to the child and parents the importance of regular medical evaluation and follow-up, including measurement of blood levels of the medication and evaluating for toxicity or side effects.	9. Regular medical follow-up facilitates maintenance of appropriate therapeutic blood levels of anticonvulsants and identification of side effects of medication.
10. Inform the parent about the need for a Medic-Alert bracelet for the child.	10. Medic-Alert bracelets alert others to the child's condition in an emergency. If the child has a seizure in a public place, the bracelet will inform passersby of what to do for the child.
11. Encourage the family to find alternative activities besides contact sports for the child. The child should avoid swimming or climbing alone. Identify the child's strengths—not what the child *cannot* do.	11. Appropriate activities will reduce the risk of injury while promoting a positive self-image.
12. Encourage verbalization of fears and concerns about having seizures.	12. This therapeutic communication may identify issues that need to be addressed.
13. Teach the child and parent to educate other family members, friends, and teachers about seizures. Advise the family to provide necessary information to the school nurse.	13. Accurate information reduces the stigma associated with epilepsy.

Evaluation

- Does the child discuss having seizures, fears and concerns about seizures, and life with them?
- Does the child participate in the medical regimen by discussing medication side effects and dosage?
- Does the child demonstrate a positive self-image?
- Does the family administer anticonvulsants safely and appropriately and know when to call the physician?

STATUS EPILEPTICUS

Status epilepticus is a pediatric emergency. It is marked by prolonged seizure activity, in the form of either a single seizure lasting 30 minutes or more or recurrent seizures lasting more than 30 minutes with no return to a normal level of consciousness between seizures (Hanhan, Fiallos, & Orlowski, 1999). Any seizure lasting 10 minutes or more can suggest pending status and should be treated as such. The most common form of status epilepticus is generalized status, which has the highest potential for complications and possible death.

Etiology

The causes of status epilepticus are many. Acute CNS injury from head trauma, meningitis, or electrolyte imbalance frequently precipitates status epilepticus. The condition can also be caused by toxins and specific medications. Other causes are chronic CNS injury and sudden withdrawal from anticonvulsants.

Incidence

Status epilepticus occurs in 5% to 10% of children with epilepsy. The most common form in children younger than 3 years is febrile status epilepticus.

Pathophysiology

Status epilepticus is caused by the random discharge of large numbers of neurons firing abnormally. The discharges cause abnormal repetitive motor activity. In the CNS, the metabolic rate increases, glucose stores are depleted, and oxygen consumption increases. If cerebral metabolic demands are not met, these changes cause neuronal injury. Prolonged seizures cause lactic acidosis, an altered blood-brain barrier, and increased ICP.

Manifestations

See the International Classification of Seizures in Box 52-5.

Diagnostic Evaluation

Diagnostic laboratory tests should include blood glucose, arterial blood gases, electrolytes, anticonvulsant drug levels, a toxicology screen, and possibly lumbar puncture. Results may be similar to those of the child with increased ICP.

Therapeutic Management

Generalized tonic-clonic status epilepticus is a medical emergency. Treatment consists of maintaining optimal respiratory and hemodynamic function and identifying and treating the causes of the seizure activity. Diazepam (Valium) or lorazepam (Ativan) is given IV. If IV access cannot be obtained, medication can be given orally or rectally. Clorazepate dipotassium (Tranxene) can be given orally for cluster seizures. Fosphenytoin (Cerebyx) or phenobarbital may be given IV as a second round of drugs if diazepam or lorazepam does not stop the seizures. The intramuscular route is not used because it is unpredictable.

! CRITICAL TO REMEMBER

Drug Therapy for Generalized Tonic-Clonic Status Epilepticus

Generalized tonic-clonic status epilepticus is a medical emergency. Intravenous (IV) diazepam (Valium) or lorazepam (Ativan) is given. IV diazepam must be given directly into the vein (not the tubing, because it interacts with plastic) at a rate no greater than 1 mg/min. It should not be mixed with other drugs or solutions, and it can be diluted only with normal saline. Resuscitation equipment should be at the bedside and the child's respirations closely monitored during IV administration.

▪ NURSING CARE
The Child With Status Epilepticus

Assessment

On arrival at the hospital, the child will exhibit seizure activity and have unstable vital signs. Along with general seizure precautions, this child requires rapid assessment and vigorous supportive therapy. Supportive measures include assessing and maintaining a patent airway and administering oxygen. IV hydration and drug therapy are initiated to arrest the seizure activity.

Nursing Diagnoses and Planning

The nursing diagnoses and expected outcomes that may apply to the child with status epilepticus are
- Impaired Gas Exchange related to decreased respirations associated with seizures.
  Expected Outcome: The child will remain free from respiratory distress, as evidenced by pulse oxygen saturation remaining at or above 95%.
- Ineffective Breathing Pattern related to loss of muscle control associated with seizures.
  Expected Outcome: The child will maintain a normal breathing pattern, as evidenced by pulse oxygen saturation remaining at or above 95% and respiratory rate within normal range.
- Ineffective Airway Clearance related to possible aspiration during seizure.
  Expected Outcome: The child's airways will be clear, as evidenced by clear breath sounds.
- Ineffective Cerebral Tissue Perfusion related to lactic acidosis with prolonged seizure activity.
  Expected Outcome: The child will reestablish tissue perfusion, as evidenced by a return to normal levels of consciousness.

Interventions and Evaluation

The child will initially require meticulous airway establishment and maintenance. Take frequent vital signs, and perform neurologic checks. Once the child is stable, nursing interventions and evaluation are similar to those described for the child with epilepsy.

MENINGITIS

Meningitis is the most common infectious process affecting the CNS. It can occur as a primary disease or as a result of complications of neurosurgery, trauma, systemic infection, or sinus or ear infections. A wide variety of bacteria and viruses can be responsible for the primary infection. Earlier diagnosis and improved antibiotic therapy have reduced the mortality and incidence of complications from bacterial meningitis.

Etiology

The primary organisms responsible for causing bacterial meningitis vary according to age. Among children ages 2 months to 12 years, three pathogens seem to be the most prevalent: *Haemophilus influenzae* type B, *Neisseria meningitidis,* and *Streptococcus pneumoniae* cause 95% of cases of purulent meningitis in this age-group. Tuberculous meningitis also is becoming more common in this age-group. These types of meningitis usually result from extension of a localized infection, such as otitis media, sinusitis, pharyngitis, or pneumonia, into the CSF. The organisms primarily responsible for neonatal meningitis are group B streptococci and *Escherichia coli.*

Organisms also may be introduced directly after an injury in which the skin is broken and communication between skin, sinuses, and CSF occurs. Entry may occur in association with a lumbar puncture, skull fracture, or surgery.

Meningococcal meningitis caused by *Neisseria* usually occurs in older children and adolescents. Because it is transmitted primarily by droplet infection, the risk increases as the number of contacts increases.

Viral meningitis is associated with viruses such as mumps, paramyxoviruses, herpesviruses, and enteroviruses. In rare cases, protozoa or fungi are the infecting organisms. These types of meningitis are seen most frequently in children with acquired immunodeficiency syndrome (AIDS).

Incidence

Meningitis most commonly affects children between ages 1 month and 5 years, but it can occur at any age. Boys are affected more frequently than girls, and risk factors increase where individuals are in close contact with one another (e.g., daycare centers, college dormitories, large families in small dwellings). Incidence is higher among African-American children than among white children. The incidence of *H. influenzae* type B infection related to meningitis has declined rapidly with the immunization of infants.

Manifestations

Signs and symptoms of meningitis vary according to the age of the child and the duration of the preceding illness. There is no single hallmark sign or symptom.

The clinical signs of meningitis in the neonate include poor feeding; poor sucking; vomiting; diarrhea; poor muscle tone; poor cry; hypothermia or hyperthermia; apnea; seizures; sepsis; disseminated intravascular coagulation (DIC); a full, tense, and bulging fontanel; and lethargy.

Clinical signs of meningitis in the infant and child include fever, poor feeding, vomiting, irritability, seizures, a high-pitched cry, a bulging anterior fontanel, and lethargy. In the neonate, infant, and young child, the symptoms of meningitis are frequently vague and nonspecific.

Early clinical signs of meningitis in children and adolescents include severe headache, photophobia, nuchal rigidity, fever, altered level of consciousness (lethargy, irritability), decreased appetite, vomiting, diarrhea, agitation, and drowsi-

Pathophysiology

of Meningitis

Meningitis is an inflammation of the meninges of the brain that results from a pathogen entering the central nervous system (CNS) and causing a toxic response. As the process continues, increased intracranial pressure (ICP) develops, along with subdural empyema. If the infection spreads to the ventricles, edema and tissue scarring around the ventricle cause obstruction of the cerebrospinal fluid (CSF) and subsequent hydrocephalus.

This process can happen very rapidly as CSF is an excellent growth medium for bacteria because it contains nutrient substances, such as protein and glucose. Leukocytes are unable to function as a defense mechanism in the fluid environment of the CSF. Leukocytes require a tissue surface to destroy bacteria, so there is little defense to stop the growth of bacteria, and they can multiply quickly.

As the infection spreads farther into brain tissue, changes occur in the permeability of capillaries and blood vessels in the dura mater. These changes lead to increased passage of albumin and water into the subdural space, with a subsequent accumulation of protein and fluid. This results in an additional increase in ICP.

The most common neurologic sequelae of meningitis are hearing loss, mental retardation, seizures, visual impairment, and behavioral problems. Other complications include cranial nerve dysfunction, brain abscess, and the syndrome of inappropriate antidiuretic hormone (SIADH). Meningococcemia, a fulminating manifestation of *Neisseria meningitides* infection that manifests with petechiae and purpura and signs of viral-type illness, can proceed in a matter of a few hours to adrenal insufficiency (Waterhouse-Friedrickson syndrome) and septic shock.*

*Woods, C. (2004). *Neisseria meningitides* (Meningococcus). In R. Behrman, R. Kliegman, & H. Jenson (Eds.). *Nelson textbook of pediatrics* (17th ed., pp. 896-899). Philadelphia, PA: Saunders.

ness. Muscle or joint pain and purpura may be noted. Kernig's sign (pain with extension of leg and knee; Fig. 52-7) and Brudzinski's sign (flexion of head causing flexion of hips and knees; Fig. 52-7) are often exhibited. In addition, petechial or purpuric rash (meningococcal infection) may be observed.

Late clinical signs of meningitis in children and adolescents include changes in level of consciousness and seizures.

Diagnostic Evaluation

The diagnosis is made by testing CSF obtained by lumbar puncture. Findings usually include increased CSF pressure, cloudy CSF (in the case of bacterial meningitis), high protein concentration, and low glucose level. Blood cultures may be done, and nose and throat cultures are occasionally helpful if the CSF is negative.

Therapeutic Management

Acute bacterial meningitis is a medical emergency requiring early recognition and prompt, aggressive management. The child is placed in a private room on Droplet Transmission Pre-

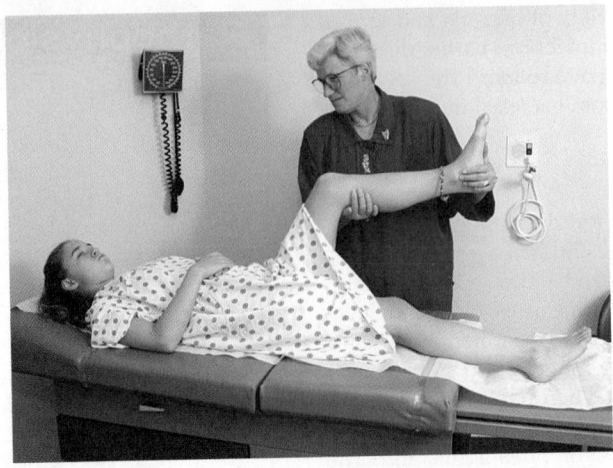

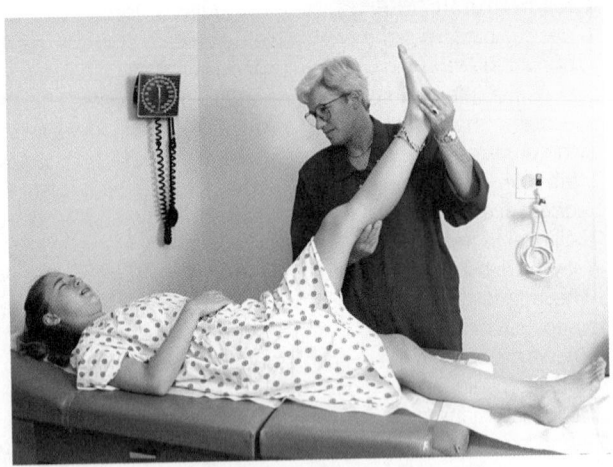

Kernig's Sign
The child can easily extend the leg when in the supine position. However, when the thigh is flexed toward the abdomen, pain prevents complete extension of the leg.

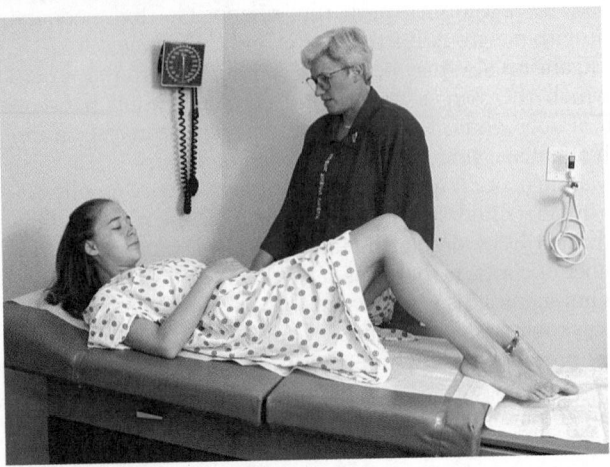

Brudzinski's Sign
In the supine position, the child bends her head toward her chest. (In a younger child, the nurse can bend the child's head.) This action usually produces involuntary hip and knee flexion in the child with meningitis.

Figure 52-7 As part of the assessment for meningitis, the nurse can attempt to elicit Kernig's sign and Brudzinski's sign. Both are early signs of meningitis in children and adolescents. (Courtesy Parkland Health & Hospital System, Dallas, TX.)

cautions, and these are maintained for at least 24 hours after antibiotics are given. Prompt initiation and uninterrupted IV administration of appropriate antibiotics are essential in cases of suspected bacterial meningitis. Treatment is started before the causative organism is identified because cultures may take up to 3 days to yield results. It is vital to start antibiotics early because delay could be fatal. Antibiotic therapy is based on the age of the child, the pathogen most frequently encountered in that age-group, and the initial appearance of the CSF. If IV access is difficult to achieve, the first dose of antibiotics should be administered intramuscularly.

Treatment for neonatal bacterial meningitis consists of ampicillin and an aminoglycoside or a third-generation cephalosporin. For older children and adolescents, the treatment of choice is ampicillin and penicillin G. The initial antibiotic must be a broad-spectrum drug to cover most of the suspected pathogens. When the culture and sensitivity test results are available, treatment regimens may have to be changed. The treatment for viral meningitis is symptomatic and supportive, usually with complete recovery. Current recommendations are that prospective college students receive meningococcal vaccine before college entry to prevent meningococcal meningitis.

▪NURSING CARE
The Child With Meningitis

Assessment
The information from the history and physical examination will provide baseline data, along with a complete neurologic assessment that includes evaluating for the presence or absence of headaches, photophobia, hearing loss, seizure activity, changes in level of consciousness, changes in pupil reactions and size, nuchal rigidity, and muscle flaccidity. Personality changes and irritability may be noted. It is also important to note any abnormal changes in food and fluid intake, nausea, vomiting, or loss of appetite. The nurse should review the history for recent immunizations or recent illnesses, such as upper respiratory tract infections, otitis media, surgery, skull fracture, or previous lumbar puncture.

! CRITICAL TO REMEMBER

Guidelines for the Child With Meningitis

- The close contacts of the child with *Haemophilus influenzae* infection need prophylactic treatment with rifampin.
- Anyone who spent at least 4 hours with the child in the 5 to 7 days preceding the child's hospitalization with *H. influenzae* needs prophylactic treatment if not already immunized.
- All close contacts of children with *Neisseria meningitidis* need prophylactic treatment, regardless of age or immunization status.
- Rifampin colors the urine and sweat red-orange and will stain contact lenses.

CRITICAL THINKING EXERCISE 52-1

Pediatric nurses in the community often are in a position to answer questions about childhood illnesses. Recently, parents of high school children received a notice from the school nurse that a male student had been diagnosed with meningococcal meningitis. The nurse recommended that parents should be watchful but not overly concerned. Her letter advised parents to watch their children for 2 weeks and call the physician at any sign of illness.
1. Is this course of action prudent?
2. If so, why? If not, why not?

Early recognition and treatment of complications can substantially reduce the morbidity and mortality. Thorough knowledge of the disease process is important, and assessments must be complete, frequent, and alert to any changes in the child's condition. Assessment of peak and trough antibiotic levels is important to prevent ototoxicity from aminoglycosides.

Nursing Diagnosis and Planning

Nursing diagnoses that apply to the child with meningitis include those common to other neurologic disorders. Care related to these nursing diagnoses is detailed on pp. 1492-1496. The nursing diagnosis specific to the child with meningitis and family is

■ Deficient Knowledge related to seriousness of meningitis, possible residual neurologic deficits, home management, and prophylaxis.

Expected Outcome: The parent's level of understanding of meningitis will increase, as evidenced by an ability to discuss the disease process and possible sequelae, treatment, home management, and possible implications for spread of the disease.

Interventions

Discuss the disease process and prognosis with the parents after assessing their existing knowledge. It is important to teach the family about the possible complications and sequelae of meningitis. Discuss the importance of follow-up care.

It is necessary to provide prophylaxis for the ill child's close contacts. Ask the parents to identify others exposed to meningitis, and refer them for treatment. Close contacts should not wait for signs of meningitis to develop but should seek prompt medical attention because they may be incubating the infection.

Instruct the parents about prescribed medications and treatments. Document instructions, and request a return demonstration by parents or caregiver. The parents will be anxious and grieving about the child's illness and outcome; learning will be difficult. To be sure the parents have learned, watch them perform the necessary procedures.

Complications of meningitis can include hydrocephalus, vision and hearing loss, delayed growth and development, seizures, subdural effusions, and cranial nerve palsy.

Evaluation

- Can the parents demonstrate the ability to administer the child's treatments and medications?
- Do the parents discuss the disease and treatments?
- Have the parents referred close contacts for treatment?

GUILLAIN-BARRÉ SYNDROME (POSTINFECTIOUS POLYNEURITIS)

Guillain-Barré syndrome (GBS) is a progressive motor weakness in association with an infection. The illness may have originated as an upper respiratory infection, possibly viral in nature, such as rubella, enterovirus, Epstein-Barr virus, cytomegalovirus (CMV), mycoplasma, or varicella. The syndrome may also occur as a toxic response to immunizations. If the cause is unknown, it may be related to an autoimmune or inflammatory response, which produces demyelinization of the motor and sometimes sensory nerves.

Incidence

GBS affects approximately 1 to 1.5 people in 100,000 per year worldwide. It affects all ages, including infants. It occurs moderately more often in males.

Pathophysiology

The most prominent feature of GBS is the infiltration of lymphocytes in peripheral nerves, causing inflammation. Initially, the myelin sheath becomes edematous; as further inflammation takes place, segmental demyelinization occurs. This process takes place along the membrane surrounding the Schwann cells. As the inflammatory process continues, myelin loss increases and results in axonal degeneration.

Manifestations

- *Limb paresthesias and/or pain*, including numbness, tingling, and weakness of the lower extremities with an ascending loss of deep tendon reflexes leading to a flaccid paralysis.
- *Autonomic instability*, including blood pressure fluctuations, cardiac dysrhythmias, postural hypotension, and urinary and bowel incontinence.
- *Cranial nerve dysfunction* may occur, such as facial nerve paralysis; dysphagia; and poor cough, gag, and swallow reflexes. If this occurs, respiratory function will be impaired.
- *Respiratory failure* results from the progressive motor paralysis of the intercostal and phrenic nerves. Respiratory failure may occur in 15% to 25% of patients with GBS.
- *Neuromuscular impairment* (bilateral ascending weakness or paralysis) usually progresses upward from the feet to the head and is reversed as healing takes place.

Diagnostic Evaluation

Bilateral ascending weakness or paralysis following an upper respiratory infection by 1 or 2 weeks is a diagnostic indication. The paralysis can affect the respiratory muscles quickly. The CSF may demonstrate high protein levels.

Therapeutic Management

Children with rapidly progressing paralysis are treated with IV immunoglobulin (IVIG) for several days (Sarnat, 2000). Medical management of the child with GBS is supportive, with attention given to the neurologic, respiratory, and cardiovascular systems. Special attention to respiratory support is needed, because most deaths are attributed to respiratory failure. Plasmapheresis may be beneficial, as may steroids or immunosuppressive medications (Sarnat, 2000).

▪NURSING CARE
The Child With Guillain-Barré Syndrome

Assessment

A complete history and physical examination are important to determine the presence of an antecedent viral illness and to establish baseline clinical status. Special attention is given to the respiratory and neurologic systems. Respiratory assessment should take place frequently because of the risk of respiratory compromise and the need for prompt action should the child's respiratory status deteriorate. Major assessment parameters include respiratory rate, chest excursion, energy expended to breathe, and breath sounds. Pulse oximetry assesses adequate gas exchange. Daily pulmonary function testing may be necessary. The frequency of neurologic assessment depends on the child's clinical condition. Neurologic parameters include cranial nerve function, motor capabilities, sensory perception, and deep tendon reflexes.

Nursing Diagnosis and Planning

The nursing diagnoses and expected outcomes that may be appropriate following assessment of the child with Guillain-Barré syndrome are

- Ineffective Breathing Pattern related to neuromuscular impairment.
  Expected Outcome: The child will remain free from respiratory distress, as evidenced by clear bilateral breath sounds, good chest expansion, and normal tidal volume.
- Decreased Cardiac Output related to autonomic instability.
  Expected Outcome: The child will maintain cardiac output, as evidenced by brisk capillary refill, normal urine output, good pulses in all extremities, and no dysrhythmias.
- Risk for Impaired Skin Integrity related to immobility with paralysis.
  Expected Outcome: The child will maintain skin integrity, as evidenced by no skin breakdown or pressure sores.
- Impaired Verbal Communication related to neuromuscular impairment.
  Expected Outcome: The child will maintain ability to communicate, as evidenced by demonstration of new ways to communicate using available muscles, such as eye blinks or eye movements.

- Impaired Urinary Elimination related to paralysis.
  Expected Outcome: The child will have urinary elimination needs met, as evidenced by an empty bladder, no urinary tract infection or distention of the abdomen, and urine output within normal limits for age (see Chapter 42).
- Anxiety related to increasing ascending paralysis.
  Expected Outcome: The child will display decreased anxiety, as evidenced by an ability to calmly interact with caregivers and have decreased fretful periods and increased restful periods.
- Deficient Knowledge related to anxiety about disease progression and home care.
  Expected Outcome: The child and parents will have increased knowledge of the disease and treatment, as evidenced by an ability to make plans about discharge care and to discuss the illness and possible complications.
- Interrupted Family Processes related to having a child with a prolonged illness.
  Expected Outcome: The parents will use coping strategies to adjust to their child's illness, as evidenced by discussing support systems and changes in the family.

Interventions

The goals of nursing care for the child with GBS are to achieve optimal neurologic function with an emphasis on maintaining independence in activities of daily living and to facilitate a recovery without complication.

Treatment is largely supportive with a focus on assessing and monitoring the child's clinical status and preventing or minimizing complications. The nurse must be able to recognize changes in the child's condition and intervene in a timely and effective manner.

Initially, the nurse must provide respiratory support if the respiratory system becomes compromised and muscles weaken and become flaccid. Resuscitation and ventilatory support may be needed; the appropriate emergency equipment and personnel should be at hand. Anticipate deterioration in respiratory status. Emergency equipment, such as a bag-valve-mask device, oxygen, suction, endotracheal tubes, laryngoscope, blade, and stylet, should be at the bedside.

Interruption in the autonomic nervous system reflexes can cause circulatory changes, resulting in dysrhythmias, hypotension, dizziness, and night sweats. Early detection of neurologic changes is made by serial assessments, and prompt action should be taken to correct problems and prevent complications.

The child with GBS is at an increased risk for developing complications associated with immobility. Maintaining skin integrity is a priority. Frequent turning and repositioning, attention to pressure points, and use of special mattresses are all important steps to take to prevent skin breakdown. Managing incontinence also will help prevent skin breakdown. To prevent contractures, physical and occupational therapy must be initiated as part of the child's daily routine. Range of motion, self-help exercises, correct alignment, and application of splints and braces are part of the child's daily care.

Anticipate loss of motor function, and initiate preventive nursing measures, such as passive range of motion, turning, and repositioning at least every 2 hours. Chest physiotherapy should be done every 2 to 4 hours.

The risk of pulmonary embolus as a result of deep vein thrombosis is always a threat. Frequent turning and repositioning, with special attention to positioning the child's legs to alleviate pressure on the dorsal aspect of the knees, are essential. Anticoagulant therapy may be initiated; if so, the nurse should monitor clotting times and watch for any signs of bleeding.

As cranial nerve function is altered and interference with gag and swallow occurs, nutrition becomes an important issue. Adequate caloric intake is essential to prevent catabolism. Alternative methods of providing nutrition must be employed. The physician may consider nasogastric, nasojejunostomy, or gastrostomy feedings. The nurse monitors the type and amount of feeding, tube placement and patency, and tolerance of feedings, as evidenced by residuals, abdominal distention, stools, and weight gain. Total parenteral nutrition is also an option. This is usually reserved for the acute or critical phase of the illness or for the child who does not tolerate alternative methods of nutritional support.

The progression of the disease is unpredictable, the loss of function is frightening, and the recovery time varies from months to years. The long-term implications for nursing care are easily identified. The child and family will require a great deal of emotional support. Full recovery from GBS is possible. The uncertainty of the progression of the disease can contribute to the child's and family's anxiety. Keep them well-informed, and answer their questions. Questions that the nurse cannot answer should be referred to the appropriate health care member. Encourage verbalization of feelings concerning the illness and hospitalization, and support and validate the feelings of the family and child.

Foster the child's positive development during the illness by normalizing the situation as much as possible. As the child's clinical condition worsens and dependency on the parents increases, encourage control by offering choices and encouraging decision making when appropriate. Contact the child's teacher for continuation of studies and communication with school friends.

Support the role of the parent as the primary caregiver by facilitating parent participation. Help the parent support the child. If the child's clinical condition deteriorates enough to warrant transfer to a critical care unit, prepare the family for the move. Initiate telephone contact with the receiving nurse to establish a relationship before transfer to lessen the family's anxiety.

If possible, a physician or nurse orientation to the critical care unit will help the family deal with the stress of the transfer. Compassionate and competent health care team members can optimize the child's recovery.

Evaluation

- Does the child demonstrate normal respiratory function?
- Is the child able to communicate needs?
- Has the child's neurologic status returned to normal?
- Is the child's skin intact?
- Do the parents participate in and discuss the child's care?

NEUROLOGIC CONDITIONS REQUIRING CRITICAL CARE

A number of neurologic conditions, including encephalitis, Reye's syndrome, botulism, and tetanus, require critical nursing care. Children with these conditions are frequently admitted to hospital critical care units where the care is specialized (Table 52-4).

	TABLE 52-4 Neurologic Conditions Requiring Critical Care			
Condition	**Pathophysiology, Etiology, and Incidence**	**Manifestations**	**Therapeutic Management**	**Nursing Considerations**
Encephalitis	Inflammation caused by infection or toxin and resulting in cerebral edema and neurologic dysfunction. Numerous agents are causative. Peak incidence is in middle to late childhood.	Headache, irritability, lethargy, altered level of consciousness, nuchal rigidity, seizures, fever, malaise, dizziness, nausea and vomiting, ataxia, sensory disturbances.	Diagnosed by lumbar puncture and CSF culture; EEG alterations are not unusual. Care includes hospitalization and monitoring for increased ICP. Medication: cephalosporin or acyclovir (depending on causative agent), anticonvulsants.	Care is similar to that for any child with increased ICP. Care also includes fever management with antipyretics and tepid baths; pharmacologic and non-pharmacologic headache relief measures; maintenance of fluid and electrolyte balance; providing support to anxious family members; assisting the family to manage any long-term neurologic deficits; and facilitating grieving for the family of a child with a poor prognosis.

CSF, Cerebrospinal fluid; *EEG,* electroencephalogram; *ICP,* intracranial pressure; *IV,* intravenous; *CNS,* central nervous system.

Continued

TABLE **52-4** Neurologic Conditions Requiring Critical Care—cont'd

Condition	Pathophysiology, Etiology, and Incidence	Manifestations	Therapeutic Management	Nursing Considerations
Reye's syndrome	Exposure to viral agent or toxin in at-risk children leads to liver cell damage with rising serum ammonia levels. The toxic serum ammonia levels result in cerebral dysfunction (encephalopathy, cerebral edema), fluid and electrolyte and acid-base imbalances, and coagulopathies. The average age at onset is 6-7 years. Reye's syndrome might be related to administration of aspirin to children with viral disease.	Antecedent viral infection; malaise, nausea, vomiting, progressive neurologic deterioration. Laboratory tests: elevated serum ammonia levels, liver dysfunction on biopsy, hypoglycemia, altered coagulation times, increased ICP with respiratory dysfunction. Reye's syndrome is clinically staged from I (lethargy) to V (coma with flaccidity/decerebrate posturing), according to degree of altered consciousness.	Care includes hospitalization for monitoring of neurologic status, increasing ICP, hydration and acid-base balance, and cardiorespiratory status.	Care is similar to that for any child with increasing ICP, with the potential addition of mechanical respiratory support. Accurate, continuous monitoring of neurologic and cardiorespiratory status is essential because the child's condition can deteriorate suddenly. Fluid replacement is achieved with IV hypertonic solutions if ICP is not increased. Protect the child from coagulopathy-related injury.
Botulism	Food poisoning caused by *Clostridium botulinum* toxin. The source is honey (in infants) or improperly sterilized canned foods.	CNS symptoms 12-36 hr after ingestion: weakness, headache, double vision, vomiting, difficulty talking, respiratory paralysis, decreased deep tendon reflexes, impaired gag reflex.	Care is supportive and includes respiratory support and administering antitoxin. Recovery after treatment takes an average of 1 mo.	Advise parents not to give infants honey or syrup in their milk or water. Educate the public about proper food preparation techniques.
Tetanus (lockjaw)	Caused by endotoxin produced by the anaerobic, spore-forming, gram-positive bacillus *Clostridium tetani*. Entry sites include puncture wounds, burns, lacerations, and compound fractures. The incubation period is 3 days to 3 weeks.	Painful muscular rigidity of masseter and neck muscles, facial spasms, dysphagia, laryngospasm, severe pain, respiratory arrest.	Care includes ventilatory and respiratory support. Medication: diazepam (Valium) or lorazepam (Ativan) for seizures; tetanus immune globulin.	Assess the child's ventilatory and neurologic status, and provide respiratory support as needed. Provide fluids and electrolytes; seizure precautions; quiet environment. Educate the child and family about immunizations.

HEADACHES

Headaches are a common complaint in children of all ages. Seventy-five percent of all children will suffer a significant headache before age 15 years (Winner, 1997).

Etiology

The three primary sources of recurrent headache are vascular, tension-related, and increased ICP (Box 52-6).

Incidence

Migraine (vascular) headaches occur in close to 5% of children. Tension-type headaches are seen in about 15% of children, and 30% experience non-migrainous headaches (Singh & Roach, 1998). Migraine in preadolescents is equally prevalent in males and females, but in adolescents the prevalence greatly increases for females. A family history of headache is noted in a majority of these cases.

Manifestations

Headaches related to increased ICP were addressed in the earlier discussion about increased ICP.

Migraine

Symptoms range from mild episodes, in which case the child may continue with daily activities, to episodes that force the child to go to a quiet, dark room. In some cases, an aura may occur before the headache begins. The aura may include seeing flashing lights; smelling specific odors;

BOX 52-6
Etiology of Recurrent Headache

Vascular Headache
- Migraine
- Arteriovenous malformations

Tension-Type Headache
- Stress

Headache Caused by Increased Intracranial Pressure
- Space-occupying lesion
- Idiopathic intracranial hypertension (pseudotumor cerebri)

Other Causes
- Systemic diseases
- Sinusitis
- Ocular diseases
- Temporomandibular joint disease

Data from Singh, B.V., & Roach, E.S. (1998). Diagnosis and management of headaches in children. *Pediatrics in Review, 19*(4), 132-135.

blurry, double, or lost vision; and tingling in the arms or legs. Once the headache begins, the most common symptoms include throbbing pain, typically on one side of the head, nausea and vomiting, irritability, abdominal pain, photophobia, and phonophobia. The pain can last from minutes to several hours.

Tension-Type Headaches

The pain associated with tension-type headaches is usually more generalized than that of a migraine. The child may describe the pain as a bandlike tightness or pressure, tight neck muscles, or soreness of the scalp. Nausea is rare, but fatigue and dizziness are common. These headaches may last for days or weeks but usually do not interfere with the child's regular activities.

Diagnostic Evaluation

The child's blood pressure should be evaluated, and the child's head size should be measured (for evidence of chronically increased ICP). A detailed neurologic examination should be performed, with special attention given to auscultating for a bruit in the head (suggesting an arteriovenous malformation), assessing mental status, and examining both optic discs for papilledema. CT or MRI may be performed in children with chronic headaches or those with abnormalities found on the neurologic examination.

■ NURSING CARE
The Child With Headaches

Assessment

A detailed history of the child's headache and preheadache events is important to determine precipitating factors. A social history of the child and family may identify triggering stressors (e.g., divorce; move to a new school; loss of a family member, friend, or pet). The child should receive a comprehensive physical examination with emphasis on the neurologic system.

Nursing Diagnosis and Planning

Nursing diagnoses that may apply to a child with a headache and the child's family include those common to other neurologic disorders

- Acute Pain or Chronic Pain related to underlying contributing factors.
  Expected Outcome: The child will experience decreased pain related to headaches, as evidenced by an ability to identify triggering factors and demonstrate appropriate non-pharmacologic approaches.
- Deficient Knowledge related to unfamiliarity about management of a child with a headache and the child's medication regimen.
  Expected Outcome: The child and parents will discuss headaches and educational needs.
- Risk for Injury related to headache symptoms (change in vision, dizziness).
  Expected Outcome: The child will have risk for injury reduced, as evidenced by parents verbalizing a safety plan for the child during the headache and describing the medication regimen.

Interventions

Certain factors may trigger the onset of a headache. Triggers may include stress, food, menstruation, visual stimuli, fatigue, and certain medications. The child and family need to be educated about lifestyle changes that will lower stress and about avoiding other triggers. Keeping a diary of the child's headaches and preheadache events will aid in identifying the triggers specific for the child.

For mild or infrequent migraines and tension headaches, common analgesics, such as acetaminophen or ibuprofen, may be effective. For a more severe migraine, treatment may include naproxen, metoclopramide, or combination drugs containing sympathomimetic drugs, sedatives, serotonin agonists (sumatriptan, zolmitriptan), and analgesics. If children have two or more severe migraine headaches per month, they may need daily prophylactic medication. Commonly used prophylactic medications include amitriptyline and propranolol. Psychological evaluation followed by relaxation therapy, counseling, and biofeedback therapy may be helpful for some children.

The nursing care for a child with headaches is acute and long-term. Acute management includes placing the child in a dark, quiet environment and administering medication. Long-term management focuses on education about and elimination of trigger factors, stress relief measures, and medication administration.

Evaluation

- Can the child and parents describe the management of headache and the medication regimen?
- Do the child and parents understand the need for following a safety plan to prevent injury during headache and medication?
- Are the child and parents learning to eliminate headache trigger factors?
- Can the child demonstrate and benefit from relaxation therapy and biofeedback?

KEY CONCEPTS

- The central nervous system (CNS) is composed of the brain and spinal cord, which are protected by bony coverings (skull, vertebral column). The skull has several bones that are not fused at birth and do not fuse until 12 to 18 months of life. The brain and spinal cord are also covered by the meninges, a fibrous connective tissue structure that contains many blood vessels.
- Cerebrospinal fluid (CSF) surrounds the brain and spinal cord. The brain consists of the cerebrum, cerebellum, and brainstem.
- The peripheral nervous system consists of 12 pairs of cranial nerves and 31 pairs of spinal nerves. The autonomic nervous system consists of the sympathetic and parasympathetic systems, which are in control of the body's automatic functions.
- The physiologic process of autoregulation helps the body regulate blood flow. When autoregulation fails to change vascular diameter in response to changes in cerebral perfusion pressure, cerebrovascular dilation is impaired and cerebral blood flow decreases.
- Hypercapnia or hypoxia leads to cerebral dilation and increased intracranial pressure (ICP). Hypocapnia leads to cerebral arterial constriction and decreased ICP.
- An infant's brain is two-thirds the size of an adult's brain. The brain grows to 80% of adult size by age 1 year.
- Head circumference can change in the infant and young child, but the head of the adolescent and adult is unyielding. This change has implications for head circumference measurement for growth and development in the infant and young child.
- The spinal cord, cranial nerves, and peripheral nerves get longer during childhood; the spinal cord terminates at L3 in the newborn and L1 to L2 in the adult.
- Myelinization of nerves begins in the 3rd month of gestation and is completed in adolescence, as demonstrated by progressive development and coordination.
- Neurologic changes may be more subtle in the infant or child than in the adult and may be indicated by irritability or poor feeding behaviors.
- The neurologic examination assesses level of consciousness, pupil size and reaction to light, cranial nerve function, motor and sensory functions, respiratory status and function, vital signs, and head circumference.
- Different seizure types are treated with specific anticonvulsants to achieve optimal seizure control. Anticonvulsants have many side effects, which may include blood dyscrasias, liver damage, weight gain, abdominal discomfort, gum hypertrophy, and cosmetic changes. The complete blood count (CBC) and liver enzyme levels should be determined routinely.
- When anticonvulsants are given intravenously (IV), the most common side effect is respiratory depression. Mannitol and furosemide (Lasix) are diuretics that are used to help decrease ICP. Their effect is monitored with serum electrolyte levels and serum osmolality.
- Cerebral edema is decreased by hyperoxygenating and hyperventilating the child, administering diuretics, elevating the head of the bed 30 to 45 degrees, keeping the child in good alignment so that venous drainage is not impaired, and reducing agitation and noxious stimuli.
- Abnormal posturing is an ominous neurologic sign. Flexion (decorticate) posturing refers to flexion of the upper extremities, arms, hands, and wrists. The child's legs are extended.
- Flexion indicates cortical damage. Extension (decerebrate) posturing refers to extended arms that are inwardly rotated and extended legs. Extension indicates damage to a greater area of the brain, theoretically extending to the brainstem.
- Impaired absorption of cerebral spinal fluid (CSF) in the arachnoid villi secondary to meningitis or subarachnoid hemorrhage is referred to as *communicating hydrocephalus*. Blockage of the flow of CSF through the ventricular system, most commonly related to tumor or developmental defect, is referred to as *noncommunicating hydrocephalus*. Changes in the brain include enlarged ventricles and increased ICP. If the cranial sutures are not ossified, the head circumference will be abnormally large.
- Teaching for the child with a neurologic deficit and the child's family is begun after the child's and family's needs have been assessed. The family's grieving may be verbalized; emotions and fears should be expressed and validated. The nurse reinforces information that has been supplied by other members of the health care team.
- The nurse encourages parents in their caregiving efforts, when appropriate; assists the family in setting realistic goals for the child; and identifies support systems and refers to community agencies.
- The nurse has family members demonstrate skills necessary for home care and encourages therapeutic play, which can promote peer contact, when possible and appropriate. The nurse provides incentives for accomplishments and points out the child's positive qualities and coping mechanisms.

ANSWERS to Critical Thinking Exercise 52-1

1. The course of action is a prudent one. It is often difficult to alert large numbers of people and at the same time not create panic. Although meningococcal meningitis can be serious in children, it is not so highly communicable that prophylaxis for the entire school would be required. For high school students, it is generally not necessary to provide prophylaxis, even to classmates. The illness is transmitted through close or intimate contact and through contact with the ill person's oral secretions. Family members and other close personal contacts should receive rifampin or ceftriaxone prophylaxis.

2. If the student were in preschool or in a daycare setting, the risk of coming in contact with oral secretions would be higher. Kissing or sharing eating utensils can transmit the illness, so prophylaxis should be considered for the teen's girlfriend. Also, if the ill teen is a member of a sports team, prophylaxis should be considered for the other members of the team because they share water bottles during practices and games. The parents of the other students should know the signs of meningitis and be given criteria for when to call their physician. Immunization against meningococcal meningitis is available. It should be considered for college-bound students.

REFERENCES and READINGS

Bedford, H. (2001). Prevention, treatment and outcomes of bacterial meningitis in childhood. *Professional Nurse, 17*(2), 100-102.

Berkowitz, C.D. (2000). *Pediatrics: A primary care approach*. Philadelphia: Saunders.

Bral, E.E. (1999). Migraine in children. *American Journal of Nursing, 99*(11), 35-41.

Burg, F.D., Ingelfinger, J.R., Wald, E.R., & Polin, R.A. (1999). *Gellis and Kagan's current pediatric therapy*. Philadelphia: Saunders.

Burns, C.E., Barber, N., Brady, M.A., & Dunn, A.M. (1996). *Pediatric primary care: A handbook for nurse practitioners*. Philadelphia: Saunders.

Celand, R.T. (1998). Diagnosing pediatric epilepsy: An update for the primary care clinician. *Nurse Practitioner, 23*(3), 69.

Curley, M.A.Q., & Moloney-Harmon, P.A. (2001). *Critical care nursing of infants and children*. St. Louis, Mosby.

DeVeber, G., Roach, E.S., Riela, A.R., & Wizhitzer, M. (2000). Stroke in children; Recognition, treatment, and future directions. *Seminar of Pediatric Neurology, 7*(4), 309-317.

Dias, M. (2004). Traumatic brain and spinal cord injury. *Pediatric Clinics of North America, 51*(2), 271-304.

Fecht-Gramley, M.E. (1995). Emergency pediatric head trauma. *American Journal of Nursing, 95*, 54.

Fenichel, G.M. (2001). *Clinical pediatric neurology: A signs and symptoms approach*. Philadelphia: Saunders.

Finnell, R.H., Gould, A., & Spiegelstein, O. (2003). Pathobiology and genetics of neural tube defects. *Epilepsia, 44*(Suppl. 3), 14-23.

Fox, J.A. (2002). *Primary health care of infants, children, and adolescents*. St Louis: Mosby.

Frey, L., & Hauser, W.A. (2003). Epidemiology of neural tube defects. *Epilepsia, 44*(Suppl. 3), 4-13.

Garton, H., & Piatt, J. (2004). Hydrocephalus. *Pediatric Clinics of North America, 51*(2), 305-326.

Hanhan, V., Fiallos, M., & Orlowski, J. (1999). Status epilepticus. *Pediatric Clinics of North America, 48*(3), 683-694.

Haslam, R. (2000). The nervous system. In R. Behrman, R. Kliegman, & H. Jenson (Eds.), *Nelson textbook of pediatrics* (16th ed., pp. 1793-1866). Philadelphia: Saunders.

Jarrar, R.G, & Buchhalter, J.R. (2003). Therapeutics in pediatric epilepsy, part 1: The new antiepileptic drugs and the ketogenic diet. *Mayo Clinic Proceedings, 78*(3), 359-370.

Johnston, M. (2004). Encephalopathies. In R. Behrman, R. Kliegman, & H. Jenson (Eds.). *Nelson textbook of pediatrics* (17th ed., pp. 2023-2028). Philadelphia, PA: Saunders.

Kamienski, M. (2003). Reye syndrome. *American Journal of Nursing, 103*(7), 54-57.

Kaufman, B. (2004). Neural tube defects. *Pediatric Clinics of North America, 51*(2), 389-420.

Lawton, K.H., Meyers, M., & Donahue, E.M. (1997). Current practices and advances in pediatric neurosurgery. *Nursing Clinics of North America, 32*(1), 73-96.

Lee, J., & Adelson, D. (2004). Neurosurgical management of pediatric epilepsy. *Pediatric Clinics of North America, 51*(2), 441-456.

Levine, M.D., Carey, W.B., & Crocker, A.C. (1999). *Developmental-behavioral pediatrics*. Philadelphia: Saunders.

Lewis, D.W. (2002). Headaches in children and adolescents. *American Family Physician, 65*(4), 625-632.

Martin, J.H. (2003). *Neuroanatomy: Text and atlas* (2nd ed.). Stamford, CT: Appleton & Lange.

Mitcho, K., & Yanko, J.R. (1999). Acute care management of spinal cord injuries. *Critical Care Nursing Quarterly, 22*(2), 60-79.

Ohm, B. (1998). Endoscopic third ventriculostomy for obstructive hydrocephalus. Retrieved June 6, 2004 from www.neurosurg.wisc.edu

Palmer, J. (2000). Management of raised intracranial pressure in children. *Intensive Critical Care Nursing, 16*(5), 319-327.

Pena, C. (2003). Emergency: seizure. *American Journal of Nursing, 103*(11), 73-81.

Pierre-Louis, S.J. (2000). New drugs: Which should be included in the formulary? Epilepsy: New drugs should be included. *Archives of Neurology, 57*(2), 272-273.

Pope, W. (1998). External ventriculostomy: A practical application for the acute care nurse. *Journal of Neuroscience Nursing, 30*(3), 185-190.

Quayle, K. (1999). Minor head injury in the pediatric patient. *Pediatric Clinics of North America, 46*(6), 1189-1199.

Reuter, D., & Brownstein, D. (2002). Common emergent pediatric neurologic problems. *Emergency Medical Clinics of North America, 20*(1), 155-176.

Roddy, S.P., Cohn, S., Moller, B., Duncan, S., Gosche, J., & Seashore, J. (1998). Minimal head trauma in children revisited: Is routine hospitalization required? *Pediatrics, 101*(4), 575-577.

Sarnat, H. (2000). Guillain-Barré syndrome. In R. Behrman, R. Kliegman, & H. Jenson (Eds.), *Nelson textbook of pediatrics* (16th ed., pp. 1892-1893). Philadelphia: Saunders.

Schmitt, B.D. (1999). *Instructions for pediatric patients* (2nd ed.). Philadelphia: Saunders.

Singh, B.V., & Roach, E.S. (1998). Diagnosis and management of headaches in children. *Pediatrics in Review, 19*(4), 132-135.

Vernon-Levett, P. (1998). Neurologic system. In M. Slota (Ed.), *Core curriculum for pediatric critical care nursing* (pp. 274-359). Philadelphia: Saunders.

Williams, D.G., Hayes, J., & McCool, S. (1996). Shunt infections in children: Presentation and management. *Journal of Neuroscience Nursing, 28*(3), 155-162.

Winner, P.K. (1997). Headaches in children: When is a complete diagnostic workup indicated? *Postgraduate Medicine, 101*(5), 81-85.

53

The Child with a Psychosocial Disorder

◆ DEFINITIONS

abuse Intentional physical injury or a nonaccidental act of omission by a parent or person responsible for the care of a child; may include physical injury, sexual molestation, neglect, or emotional injury.

co-morbidity The simultaneous co-occurrence of two different but interactive conditions in a single individual.

double message A verbal message that contradicts the underlying tone or meaning of the message.

substance abuse Excessive or inappropriate use of medication to modify mood or behavior or in a manner that results in social, occupational, psychological, or physical problems or in a situation that creates a physical hazard.

substance addiction Physical or psychological dependence on a substance, with continued use even when it is known to impair cognitive or social functioning.

substance dependence A physical or psychological craving for a chemical substance, the cessation of which causes withdrawal symptoms.

suicide Voluntary and intentional cessation of one's life.

suicide attempt Any actions taken by an individual toward self that will result in death if not interrupted.

suicide gesture A suicide attempt that is undertaken primarily to get attention rather than to actually take one's life; nonetheless, it is still considered a serious behavior.

suicide threat A statement or behavior that usually occurs before overt suicidal activity.

violence The use of extreme force or a destructive action that results in injury, discordance, or outrage; engaging in sudden intense activity to the point of loss of control.

OVERVIEW OF CHILDHOOD PSYCHOPATHOLOGY

Neurobiologic, family, and sociocultural factors can contribute to the development of psychosocial disorders in children. Neurobiologic factors are briefly reviewed here; family, social, and cultural factors are discussed in the text in conjunction with the various disorders presented.

Neurobiologic Factors

For disorders with a psychological basis, the primary organ involved is the brain, together with chemicals produced and used by the brain to initiate specific actions. These actions include memory, learning, attention and concentration, mood, and cognition. Because the brain develops throughout childhood, significant changes in the anatomy and physiology of the brain also occur. The most significant changes affecting psychosocial development include myelinization,

---

> ### *Psychosocial Disorders Typically Manifested in Childhood*
>
> - Mental retardation (see Chapter 54)
> - Pervasive developmental disorders, autistic disorder
> - Learning disorders: reading, arithmetic, other skills
> - Disruptive behavior disorders: attention-deficit hyperactivity disorder, conduct disorder, oppositional defiant disorder
> - Anxiety disorders: separation anxiety disorder, posttraumatic stress disorder, phobias, obsessive-compulsive disorder
> - Mood disorders: depression, bipolar disorder
> - Eating disorders: anorexia nervosa, bulimia nervosa, pica, obesity, rumination disorder of infancy
> - Tic disorders: Tourette's disorder, chronic motor or vocal tics, transient tics
> - Elimination disorders: functional encopresis, functional enuresis (see Chapters 43 and 44)
> - Communication disorders: receptive or expressive language disorders, cluttering, stuttering, elective mutism

Data from American Psychiatric Association. (2000). *Diagnostic and statistical manual of mental disorders* (4th ed., Text Revision). Washington, DC: Author.

---

growth of new tissue, and extension of the neural system throughout the brain. (See p. 1488 for a review of brain anatomy and physiology.)

The brain increases in tissue mass and size throughout childhood and adolescence. The increase in the size of the brain results in an increased potential for memory and complex cognitive reasoning, as well as the capacity to learn new skills and acquire new information. Cognitive development proceeds from the simple to the complex and from the concrete to the abstract.

The effect of brain damage depends on several factors. One of the most significant factors is the maturational stage of the brain at the time the damage occurs. Early damage spares more language functions but may cause changes in all subsequent areas of development related to the specific area of the brain that is injured. Another factor is the length of time the brain tissue is impaired (as a result of swelling, hemorrhage, or tissue destruction). Finally, the specific area of the brain that is damaged may determine the specific areas of deficit. One factor that is not directly related to actual tissue damage but is clearly related to effects on behavior is the individual's perception of an experience, which is encoded in the brain's memory system and used as a basis for later behaviors.

Manifestations of Psychopathology

Psychosocial disorders are responses to stress and may be manifested as disturbances in feeling (e.g., depression, anxiety), in body functions (e.g., encopresis, enuresis), in behavior (e.g., conduct disturbance, school avoidance, passive-aggressive behaviors), or in performance (learning problems). The manner in which an individual responds to stress depends on multiple factors.

Individual Responses to Stress

Factors that influence responses to stress include:

- Temperament
- Developmental level
- The nature and duration of the stress
- Past experiences
- Coping and adaptive abilities of the family

Mental Status Examination of Children

- Appearance: dress, gestures, posture, tics, other repetitive movements; physical presentation, such as age, stature, race, age-appropriate behaviors
- Ability to attend to task
- Mood or affect: predominant feelings, mood fluctuations, mood congruence with verbalizations
- Manner of relating to the examiner: exploration of the child's understanding of the purpose of the interview, approach or avoidance behaviors, use of play materials available, verbalizations
- Intellectual skills: problem-solving abilities, conceptualization of causality, body image, memory, judgment, general fund of knowledge, insight (findings are compared with developmental norms)
- Capacity for imaginative thinking and play
- Sensorimotor development: fine and gross motor skills, symmetry and coordination of movement, hand and eye dominance, right-left discrimination
- Perceptions and thought content: presence or absence of suicidal-homicidal ideation, intent, plan; delusions or illusions; hallucinations
- Speech: fluency, tone, volume, age appropriateness

Common Laboratory and Diagnostic Tests for Psychosocial Disorders in Children and Adolescents

- *Urine Tests:* Used to assess specific drugs excreted by the kidneys
- *Blood and Serum Tests:* Used to assess the long-term effects of malnutrition, evidence of specific drugs or ingested chemicals, and the potency of selected pharmacotherapeutic agents prescribed for symptom reduction
- *Radiographs of the Skull and Long Bones:* Frequently used to identify current and previous fractures, which are common signs of physical abuse
- *Genital and Anal Examinations:* Performed by a physician and used, together with slides of secretions, to help determine whether sexual abuse has occurred
- *Measurement of Subcutaneous Tissue:* May be ordered if physical neglect associated with malnutrition is suspected

Diagnostic Evaluation

Diagnosing psychosocial disturbance in a child is difficult for several reasons. First, young children normally exhibit a wide range of emotional and social behaviors. Even through adolescence, the individual is maturing and developing in terms of coping skills, attitudinal responses, and perspective. During childhood, behavioral responses to various situations are markedly inconsistent and unpredictable. Also, during examinations, both the child and the adolescent are markedly affected by their relationship and level of comfort with the examiner and by the setting. Finally, children and adolescents are affected and shaped by their relationships with parents and other social figures. For a thorough assessment of psychosocial disorders, a structured mental status examination of the child must be completed. Various laboratory and diagnostic tests may also be appropriate. The results of these tests will help determine whether pharmacologic and psychological interventions may be effective.

Nurses caring for children encounter a number of disorders and conditions that are best viewed as psychosocial disorders, because they involve primarily the way in which the child or adolescent relates to others and copes with stress. Most psychosocial disorders have a familial or biologic predisposition that may be triggered if the environment is demanding or unsupportive. Physical stressors, such as birth defects, physical injuries, and chronic illness, may produce psychosocial disorders. Emotional stressors, such as inconsistent or contradictory child-rearing practices, marital conflict, or neglect, may also contribute to psychiatric disorder development. Some psychosocial disorders, such as fragile X syndrome, are inheritable disorders. Other disorders are related primarily to an inaccurate or inappropriate relationship between the child and significant others in the social environment. Research consistently shows that psychosocial disorders are caused by a combination of predisposing or inherent factors and environmental or interactional factors.

ANXIETY AND DEPRESSION

Mood or affective disturbances in children and adolescents are generally of two types: *anxiety* or *depression*. It is difficult to differentiate between anxiety and depressive disorders in children for several reasons. In children and adolescents, the behavioral presentation of both disorders may be similar. For example, the child who is anxious may be withdrawn, tearful, unwilling to engage in play, or prone to acting aggressively toward others. These same symptoms typically occur in children who are depressed. Moreover, it is often difficult to differentiate between normal mood changes secondary to normal developmental maturation and adaptation and abnormal, persistent mood disturbances. Generally, however, mood disturbance is more intense and persistent and interferes with social relations and daily functioning. Finally, the child or adolescent can have both anxiety and depression.

Anxiety Disorders

Anxiety is one of the most common categories of psychopathology in childhood. Anxiety is expected and normal in children at specific times in development. For example, infants and children up to preschool age often show intense distress at times of separation from their parents or family members (see Chapter 35). It is not uncommon for young children to have short-lived fears related to darkness, storms, animals, and imaginary situations. Whereas school-age children typically express anxiety or fear of body harm or potentially real worries (e.g., thunder, lightning), adolescents may exhibit anxiety regarding social situations and acceptance. When worry and distress become overwhelming and begin to interfere with daily functioning, anxiety becomes pathologic and warrants serious intervention.

Separation Anxiety and School Refusal

The essential feature of separation anxiety is disabling anxiety about being apart from one's parents or an attachment figure or away from home (American Academy of Child and Adolescent Psychiatry, 1997). It may develop spontaneously or under stress (e.g., in temporal relation to a move or a death in the family) and may last for several years, waxing and waning. Children with separation anxiety frequently fear that if they are apart from their parents, harm will come to the parent or themselves. Separation anxiety occurs in approximately 4% of children and young adults (American Psychiatric Association, 2000).

Persistent reluctance or refusal to go to school or elsewhere may be the primary reason families seek intervention. Unlike truants, who are relatively fearless and avoid school to pursue other interests, children with separation anxiety stay home or attempt to remain with their parents. The child may complain of physical symptoms, cry, plead, or even exhibit panic symptoms shortly before the time for school approaches, but the symptoms subside after the child is allowed to stay home, only to reappear the next morning. Sometimes the child may simply refuse to leave the home.

School refusal may also be related to a *social phobia*, whereby individuals avoid social or performance situations to such a degree that their daily routine is affected (e.g., by refusing to participate in physical education exercises or by failing to raise their hands to ask a question in class). School refusal is discussed also in Chapter 7.

Other Anxiety Disorders

In addition to separation anxiety, anxiety disorders present as other specific disorders. Anxiety may be so intense that the child experiences a sense of panic, in which case the disorder may be termed *panic disorder*. One type of panic disorder that follows a specific and terrifying event is *posttraumatic stress disorder*. Symptoms of this disorder include intense fear, helplessness, or horror, along with physiologic symptoms of increased arousal. The individual demonstrates persistent avoidance of stimuli associated with the traumatic event. This disorder is frequently seen in children who have been sexually or physically abused. Obsessive-compulsive disorder may manifest in children as it does in adults as intrusive, unwanted thoughts that create mounting tension that is relieved only by repetitive, compulsive actions. These acts are designed to relieve the anxiety that the child usually realizes is irrational.

Depressive Disorders

Depressive disorders are also varied and are specified according to the intensity or duration of depressive symptoms or the particular behaviors displayed by the individual. Children or adolescents who exhibit a depressed or irritable mood for at least 1 year meet the criteria for *dysthymic disorder*. If the child experiences chronic, fluctuating mood disturbances between depressive lows and highs characterized by bizarre ideations or grandiose delusions for 1 year, *cyclothymic disorder* or *bipolar mood disorder* may be diagnosed. If the clinical presentation includes a 2-week (or longer) episode of depressed or irritable mood in addition to disturbances in appetite, sleep, psychomotor activity, energy, or self-esteem, the child meets the criteria for *major depressive disorder*. A psychiatric nursing text should be consulted for more detailed information about these specific disorders.

Psychophysiology

Research supports the view that both anxiety and depression have a biologic basis. Among the biochemical agents that appear to modulate mood are monoamines, including catecholamines and indolamines, and neurotransmitters, such as norepinephrine, serotonin, and acetylcholine. The limbic region in the brain is considered to be the seat of emotions, and chemical or physical alterations in this region have been found to affect mood as well as some other characteristics, such as energy, self-valuation, and sleep patterns.

Etiology

Affective disorders have been shown to have a genetic basis. Having a first-degree relative with an anxiety or depressive disorder may predict an increased risk of the disorder in offspring. A family history of suicide or depression (particularly parental) is a significant risk factor (Pataki, 2000).

Psychosocial theories emphasize the importance of the interaction within the family system, behavioral patterns of the individual, and interpersonal factors in the development of depression. There is evidence that children and adolescents with a history of verbal, physical, or sexual abuse, frequent separation from or loss of loved ones, drug use, incarceration, pregnancy, lower socioeconomic status, homosexuality, chronic illness, behavioral disorders, and dysfunctional families are more likely than peers with healthy family patterns to develop anxiety or depressive disorders (Sadock & Sadock, 2003; Shelton, 2000).

Incidence

Current epidemiologic information about anxiety disorders indicates that separation anxiety occurs in 3%, social phobia in 1%, panic disorder in 0.6%, and generalized anxiety disorder in 3.7% of school-age children (Sadock & Sadock, 2003).

The incidence of major depression and dysthymic disorder is estimated at 1% in preschoolers, 2% in school-age children, and 6% in adolescents (Rushton, Forcier, & Schectman, 2002). Bipolar disorder occurs in approximately 1% of adolescents, but hypomania, a low grade mania, is seen in 10%. Retrospective studies have suggested a higher incidence with bipolar disorder developing in 20% to 40% of children and adolescents with initial presentations of depressive disorders, attention deficit hyperactivity disorder, and anxiety disorders (American Academy of Child and Adolescent Psychiatry, 1998).

Manifestations

The clinical manifestations of anxiety or depressive disorders include sad or irritable mood, diminished interest in daily activities, significant weight loss or gain, insomnia or hypersomnia, psychomotor agitation or retardation, and fatigue or loss of energy. Feelings of worthlessness, hopelessness, or excessive guilt, as well as diminished ability to think or concentrate, are exhibited. Somatic complaints, such as recurrent abdominal pain or headaches, with no physical cause are common. Recurrent thoughts of death or suicide are sometimes reported.

Therapeutic Management

Antidepressants, particularly selective serotonin reuptake inhibitors (SSRIs), are frequently prescribed for anxiety and depressive disorders. The most effective treatment, however, combines medication and the child's and family's ex-

ploration of situations and environmental factors that are related to the child's symptoms. Individual therapy and family therapy are essential for children with suicidal ideation or persistent mood disturbances. It is common for both anxiety disorders and mood disorders to recur. Social skills training or group therapy may be most helpful for social anxiety. School phobia is treated by insisting that the child attend school, offering interventions during school time to reduce anxiety symptoms, and refusing to pick up the child from school, even if the child insists. This form of intervention is a type of desensitization therapy. Other strategies for decreasing anxiety or depressive symptoms include relaxation therapy, distraction strategies, self-talk, or cognitive strategies, as well as support from adults or friends who are safe and reassuring.

■ NURSING CARE
The Child With Anxiety or Depression

Assessment

A thorough history should be obtained from the child and the family. Initially it may be necessary to interview the child with the parents present, but once the child becomes more comfortable with the nurse, time alone with the child should be offered. The interview should cover both the child's moods and events related to those moods; physiologic symptoms; patterns of daily activities; identification of stressors; and information about the duration, frequency, and intensity of symptoms. Suicidal ideation or plans should be assessed by asking both direct and indirect questions.

Questions about the family environment should seek to identify those with whom the child relates most easily as well as family interaction patterns. It is important to explore any family history of mood disturbance, as well as other emotional problems or substance abuse problems.

Several self-reporting instruments and interview schedules are available for the specific assessment of anxiety and depression. They are used to assess and quantify progress or regression of treatment.

Nursing Diagnosis and Planning

The nursing diagnoses and expected outcomes that apply to the child with anxiety or depression are

- Ineffective Coping related to loss of energy, sleep disturbance, biochemical imbalance, or loss of control.
  Expected Outcome: The child will display adaptive ability, as evidenced by an ability to attend to activities of daily living.
- Situational Low Self-Esteem related to cognitive distortions, inability to manage daily events, and a sense of hopelessness or guilt.
  Expected Outcome: The child will experience increased self-esteem, as evidenced by verbalization of an increase in self-confidence and an increase in positive feelings about self.
- Risk for Self-Directed Violence related to suicidal ideation, guilt, or hopelessness.
  Expected Outcome: The child will have a decreased risk for self-directed violence, as evidenced by verbalizing a decrease in the frequency or severity of depressed or anxious moods.

- Disturbed Sleep Pattern related to anxiety, depression, and inactivity.
  Expected Outcome: The child will exhibit appropriate sleep patterns, as evidenced by expressing feelings of being well-rested, showing no signs of sleep deprivation (e.g., irritability, lethargy, restlessness), and showing no signs of excessive sleeping.

Interventions

The nurse is part of a team that offers support for the entire family while exploring the factors that contribute to the emotional distress in the child. The nurse should identify specific changes in the environment and interaction patterns that could support a sense of control and positive regard for the child. Privacy and space for the child or family members to discuss their feelings as treatment progresses should be made available on a regular basis.

If the child needs hospitalization, admission will generally be to a psychiatric unit where specialized nursing is available. Mood disturbances often are identified on pediatric units, in outpatient clinics, or in school systems. Educating parents and teachers about depression and anxiety in childhood is an important service for nurses to provide to the community.

Evaluation

- Does the child exhibit an energy level that allows for interactions, play, and work?
- Does the child seem interested in people and events?
- Does the child communicate positive statements about self?
- Does the child report feeling happier, less sad, or less upset?
- Does the child exhibit normal patterns of eating and sleeping?

SUICIDE

Suicide is the third leading cause of death among adolescents between 15 and 19 years old and the fourth among children 10 to 14 years old (U.S. Department of Health and Human Services [U.S. DHHS], 2000b). Parents often underestimate the severity of warning signs, particularly depression, substance abuse, or other psychological disorders, until a child actually attempts suicide or succeeds. Risk factors for suicide are depression, a family history of psychiatric disorders (especially depression and suicide), and previous attempts. Other significant risk factors are chronic medical illness, family violence, substance abuse, poor impulse control, poor school performance, homosexuality, and access to firearms in the household (Gould, Greenberg, Velting, & Shaffer, 2003).

Psychopathology

Most adolescent suicide attempts are impulsive; however, any verbalization or gesture of suicide should be taken very seriously. It is estimated that two thirds of adolescents who attempt suicide have high intent and a strong wish to die. The motive may be a desire to influence others, gain attention, communicate love or anger, or escape a difficult or painful situation.

The development of a concept of mortality and death follows the general principles of the development of cognitive and affective abilities, from the concrete to the abstract. Up to age 6 years, it is unlikely that a child has any realistic concept of death or looks for it in an active way. Children as young as 3 years, however, have tried to commit suicide and

! CRITICAL TO REMEMBER
Threats of Suicide
A suicide gesture or threat should *never* be ignored. The child should be encouraged to discuss the thought specifically to determine if there is a plan and the lethality of the plan. Help should be obtained from qualified health professionals.

apparently understood what they were doing. Between ages 6 and 8 years, children abandon an egocentric view and discover that death is one of many events out of an individual's control. From age 9 years on, the child begins to view death as inevitable and universal.

Etiology

Underlying depression, poor self-concept, and hopelessness appear to be the most significant factors contributing to suicide, regardless of age or gender. Long-standing family dysfunction is generally present, with emotional detachment and isolation among family members. The suicide victim is typically a vulnerable individual who, under stress, seeks and finds a way to die. The individual is for some reason unable to elicit adequate adult support to stop the suicide process.

Incidence

Estimates of the prevalence of suicidal *ideation* are 19% in males and 23% in females. The prevalence of *suicide attempts* is 5% in males and 13% in females. For completed suicides, the male-to-female ratio is 7:1 (National Institute of Mental Health [NIMH], 2001). The higher incidence of completed suicides in males may be related to the more violent methods of suicide used by boys. It is also common for suicides to occur in a cluster within a community.

Of significant importance, gay and lesbian youths are two to three times more likely to attempt suicide than their heterosexual peers. Suicide is the leading cause of death in this group. Approximately 40% consider suicide and one third report at least one attempt (Russell & Joyner, 2001; D'Augelli, Hershberger, & Pilkington, 2001).

Manifestations and Risk Factors

The risk of suicide should be considered if the following are present:

- Suicidal clues, such as cryptic verbal messages, giving away personal items, and changes in expected patterns of behaviors (e.g., sudden calmness in a normally anxious teenager)
- Specific statements about suicide or self-harm
- Preoccupation with death, often manifested by an interest in death themes in literature and art
- Frequent risk-taking or self-abusive behaviors
- Use of alcohol or drugs to cope
- Overwhelming sense of guilt or shame
- Obsessional self-doubt
- Open signs of mental illness manifested as delusions or hallucinations

- Significant change or a major life event that is internally disruptive
- History of physical or sexual abuse
- Homosexuality, especially if the teen discovers same-gender orientation early in adolescence, experiences violence because of homosexual identity, or is rejected by family members as a result of sexual orientation

Therapeutic Management

Suicide prevention is viewed as the most significant mental health contribution and is promoted at local, state, and federal levels. Prevention is offered through multimedia educational presentations in schools, through support groups at local mental health centers, through community emphasis on stress reduction, through social affiliations, and through networking with support systems.

Screening for depression, both at school and in the health care system, is one of the most significant prevention strategies. Most individuals who commit suicide have offered at least veiled information about their suicidal ideation or feelings of despair to classmates, teachers, or health care providers.

After a child's suicide, counseling services must be provided to family members and the child's immediate friends. It is important that these services be offered quickly, preferably within the first 24 hours after the suicide, and that counselors remain available for 1 year after the event. Grieving and emotional adjustments often take several months and may peak around the anniversary of the suicide event.

Children or adolescents with persistent suicidal ideation should undergo a thorough psychiatric evaluation by a mental health professional. The child may need pharmacotherapeutic agents, such as antidepressants or antipsychotic medications. The use of medications in children and adolescents at risk for suicide requires close monitoring and medications should be distributed in small doses because they could be used in a suicide attempt or act.

■NURSING CARE

The Child or Adolescent at Risk for Suicide

Assessment

The risk of suicide is best assessed using a systematic approach to behaviors, attitudes, and risk factors. Several instruments have been developed to assess lethality and potentiality, which lessens the likelihood of overlooking contributing factors. The instruments are similar and explore risk factors, stressors, lethality of method, coping mechanisms, and support systems. Subtle symptoms of depression or anxiety, such as decreased energy or persistent restlessness, should also be considered. It is important to explore thought content and organization, awareness and expression of feelings, perceived level and types of stress, perceived availability of support resources, prior suicidal behaviors, and medical status (Box 53-1).

Nursing Diagnosis and Planning

The nursing diagnoses and expected outcomes that apply to the child or adolescent at risk for suicide and the family are

■ Risk for Self-Directed Violence related to a desire to end emotional pain, to solicit the attention of others, or to avoid responsibility.

BOX 53-1
Questions to Assess Suicide Potential

1. Have you ever thought of trying to hurt yourself? How might you do this?
2. Have you ever thought of killing yourself? How might you do this?
3. Have you known anyone who has committed suicide? When did this occur? What was it like for you?
4. Do you have access to firearms or knives?
5. Do you ever do things to deliberately place yourself in danger, such as driving when you are drunk or playing Russian roulette with a gun?
6. Have you ever told anyone about wanting to kill yourself?
7. Have you ever been hospitalized for suicidal behavior?
8. How do you feel right now?

Expected Outcome: The child or adolescent will indicate a decrease in the risk for self-directed violence, as evidenced by an ability to use effective communication techniques to express needs and feelings and verbalize that there are solutions to problems.

■ Situational Low Self-Esteem or Chronic Low Self-Esteem related to a perception of failure and hopelessness about the ability to change self or circumstances.
Expected Outcome: The child or adolescent will experience increased self-esteem, as evidenced by verbalization of ability to change self or circumstances.

■ Anxiety related to current or anticipated events.
Expected Outcome: The child or adolescent will have decreased anxiety, as evidenced by recognition of own anxiety and use of effective coping mechanisms.

■ Interrupted Family Processes related to relational disturbance or possible abuse or neglect.
Expected Outcome: The child or adolescent and family will stabilize family systems, as evidenced by mobilization of support systems in an effective manner to reduce the likelihood of another suicide decision.

■ Ineffective Coping related to a sense of despair or limited availability of support.
Expected Outcome: The child or adolescent and family will cope with the situation, as evidenced by development of a suicide prevention plan.

Interventions

The approach to therapy should be empathic and nonjudgmental to decrease the child's or adolescent's sense of isolation and rejection. The nurse should adopt a voice and demeanor that are clear, direct, and supportive. Being emotionally and physically available, offering opportunities to discuss feelings and the suicidal event, and removing potentially harmful objects will help protect the youth from self-injury.

The nurse should suggest different coping strategies, such as choosing alternative activities when impulses arise and remaining near other people. The nurse can help the child identify specific feelings and effective ways to manage those feelings. It is important for the nurse to assess how closely a child needs to be monitored throughout the day, realizing that the potential for self-harm fluctuates.

To allow a balance between the need to explore personal issues and the need for social support, anticipatory guidance related to grieving for families of suicidal or potentially suicidal individuals is best provided on both an individual and a group basis. Grieving will occur even if the suicide attempt was unsuccessful. Individual and family therapy will also provide an opportunity to explore contributory factors that can be altered to reduce the suicide potential. Working with the parents, together with other therapeutic team members, will help the parents regain their ability to assist their child and manage the home environment. It is important to increase the adult-child interactions, thereby decreasing the risk of another suicide attempt.

Prevention of suicide is an essential role for the school nurse, especially nurses at the middle or high school level. It is imperative that school nurses educate school personnel about recognizing the subtle signs of an impending suicide attempt so intervention can occur. Included in ongoing education should be whom to contact if a teacher or other school worker suspects a child is considering suicide, who will interview and evaluate the child, and what personnel will notify the family. Often, schools have professional teams that perform the evaluation and make appropriate referrals. Suicide prevention and incidence reduction are two of the national goals described in *Healthy People 2010* (U.S. DHHS, 2000b).

Evaluation

- Is the child or adolescent able to identify times when suicidal potential is greatest and to seek help during these times?
- Does the child or adolescent participate in activities that reduce feelings of despair and hopelessness?
- Does the child or adolescent display evidence of positive self-esteem through positive self-statements or ability to describe how circumstances can be changed?
- Has the child or adolescent verbalized a decrease in anxiety?
- Is the family able to identify warning signs of suicidal risk?
- Do family members support one another, and can the family identify community resources to assist?
- Has the child or adolescent developed coping mechanisms and effective problem solving?
- Has the family developed a suicide prevention plan?

EATING DISORDERS: ANOREXIA NERVOSA AND BULIMIA NERVOSA

Eating disorder is a general term that encompasses anorexia nervosa, bulimia nervosa, pica, binge eating disorder, obesity (discussed in Chapter 7), and rumination disorders. Anorexia nervosa and bulimia nervosa are the two most common eating disorders in children. Anorexia and bulimia have overlapping features and similar underlying mechanisms, which supports viewing these disorders as a continuum.

Anorexia nervosa is characterized by a deliberate refusal to maintain adequate body weight, a distorted body image, and amenorrhea (in females). The term *anorexia* is a misnomer, because the individual rarely experiences loss of appetite. Weight loss can be extremely dramatic. *Bulimia nervosa* is characterized by recurrent episodes of binge eating; a sense of lack of control over eating binges; self-induced vomiting or excessive use of laxatives, diuretics, or emetics to prevent weight gain; excessive exercise to prevent weight gain; and a persistent overconcern with body image although body image is usually not distorted. Children and adolescents with eating disorders typically report shame and guilt about many life experiences, but especially eating.

Individuals with severe eating disorders, particularly anorexia nervosa, have a mortality rate up to 20% from complications of the disorder or from suicide (U.S. DHHS, 2000b). Treatment resistance is very high in individuals with anorexia and bulimia, because all of their psychological and sociologic experiences are framed by their body image and self-esteem and because of secondary gains such as attention, admiration, envy, and control over others through eating patterns. Unfortunately, in addition to the eating disorder, about 50% of these children and adolescents also meet criteria for other serious psychiatric disorders, such as major depression or a personality disorder.

Ritualistic behaviors are common in these children and adolescents, particularly around issues of food. For example, the child or adolescent may eat only at a particular time of day, eat foods only in a certain order, or insist on washing all foods before eating them. The rituals are often an attempt to control the portions, fat content, or nutrients ingested. The rituals also serve to enhance the individual's sense of control over food or dietary intake.

Children or adolescents with anorexia will go to extreme measures to prevent others from becoming aware of the weight loss or lack of food intake. They may ingest large amounts of water or insert heavy objects in the vaginal cavity before weighing to give the impression of weight gain. The child or adolescent with either anorexia or bulimia may eat in front of people and then go to the bathroom to purge after the meal.

Etiology

Disordered eating emerges from multiple risk factors including biological, social, and psychological factors. One of the most salient factors appears to be enmeshed family relationships in which the child is considered to be an extension of the parent or is viewed as a means of meeting the parent's needs rather than being allowed to develop as an autonomous individual. The disorder is more common among sisters and mothers of those with the disorder than in the general population, suggesting some familial predisposition.

The development and severity of the individual's risk for eating disorders appear to be related to the child's response to biologic maturity and to the psychological and social demands of sexual development. Other significant risk factors are earlier pubertal maturation and higher body fat, depressive tendencies, concurrent psychological disturbance, alterations in brain neurotransmitters, subsequent eating problems, cultural expectations to be thin, and the individual's pervasive sense of ineffectiveness (Sadock & Sadock, 2003).

Individuals with eating disorders usually have a family history of affective disorders. The family dynamics for males with anorexia are reported to include poor father-son relationships, with the father typifying the strong, cultural image, and a mother who is overinvolved, overprotective, and overdependent on the mother-son relationship.

Incidence

Bulimia nervosa appears to be more prevalent than anorexia nervosa, with as many as 2% to 8% of the female adolescent population reporting symptoms. For girls between the ages of

Pathophysiology

of Eating Disorders

Frequently, impaired carbohydrate metabolism in the hypo-thalamic-pituitary axis is noted in individuals with an eating disorder. The conversion of thyroxine (T_4) to triiodothyronine (T_3) is inadequate. Phosphate concentrations are inadequate, especially in patients with severe anorexia complicated by bulimic episodes. Individuals with eating disorders commonly experience hypokalemia, hypochloremia, hyponatremia, alkalosis, dental enamel erosion, parotid and salivary gland enlargement, decreased transferrin levels, and malabsorption complications.

12 and 18 years, the reported incidence of eating disorders of some type is approximately 1 in 1000. Eating disorders are rarer in boys; only 1 in 10 individuals with an eating disorder is male.

Manifestations

Anorexia Nervosa

The hallmark of anorexia nervosa is the refusal to maintain a body weight that exceeds the minimal weight recommended for height (15% below expected weight). Intense preoccupation with and unrelenting fear of obesity and a disturbed body image (weight, size, or shape) that is obviously contrary to reality (Fig. 53-1) are also observed. Other clinical manifestations in females include at least three missed menstrual periods (primary or secondary amenorrhea); a misperception of internal and external stimuli, particularly food-related cues such as hunger; overwhelming feelings of ineffectiveness and inadequacy; lanugo, dry or flaky skin, and dull, brittle hair; and fatigue and muscle wasting.

Boys with eating disorders demonstrate many behavior patterns similar to girls' behavior patterns, including weight loss through excessive dieting, compulsive activities, and purging, to get strong or to develop an athletic build (rather than to be thin, as reported by females).

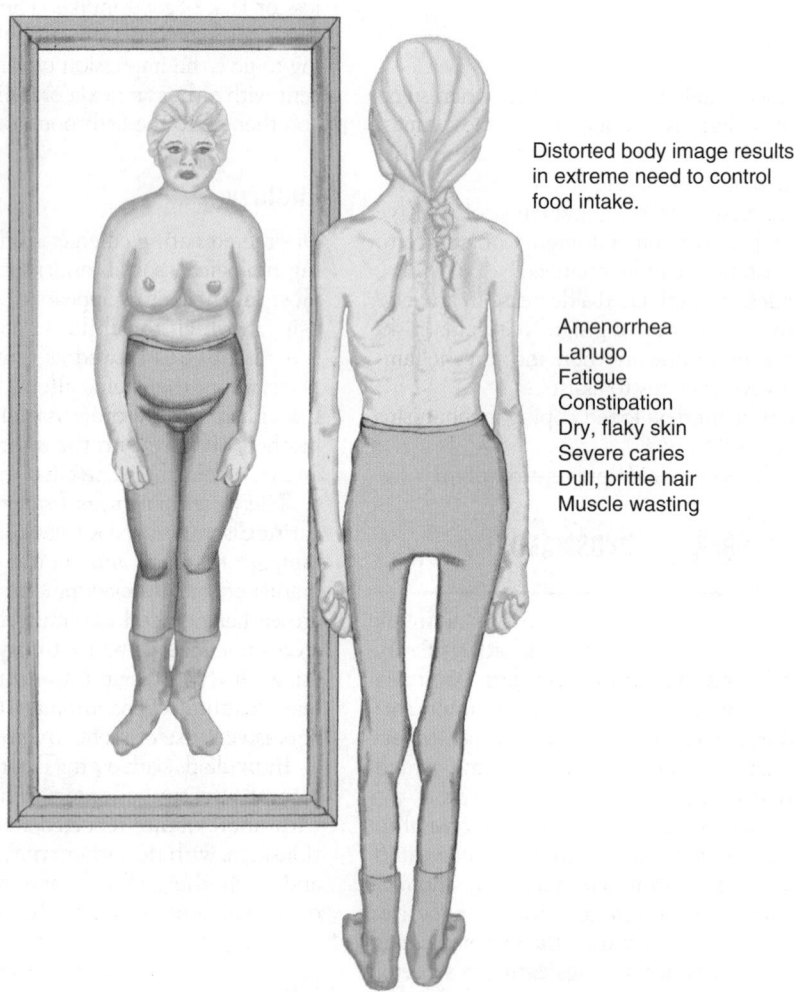

Distorted body image results in extreme need to control food intake.

Amenorrhea
Lanugo
Fatigue
Constipation
Dry, flaky skin
Severe caries
Dull, brittle hair
Muscle wasting

Figure 53-1 In anorexia nervosa, the adolescent refuses to maintain adequate body weight, partly because of a distorted body image: she perceives herself as overweight when in fact she is below minimum weight.

Bulimia Nervosa

The clinical manifestations associated with bulimia nervosa include recurrent episodes of binge eating; a sense of lack of control over eating behaviors during binges; and strategies that prevent weight gain (self-induced vomiting; use of laxatives, diuretics, or emetics; fasting; vigorous and excessive exercise). A minimum of two binge eating episodes per week for at least 3 months and persistent overconcern with body shape and weight are also common factors. These individuals are also at increased risk for tooth erosion secondary to the effects of acidic content on the teeth from the subsequent vomiting. Some children and adolescents with bulimia use excessive exercise along with bingeing and purging to control weight. Unlike children and adolescents with anorexia, those with bulimia are mostly within normal weight percentiles.

Diagnostic Evaluation

An electrocardiogram and chest radiograph are typically obtained if symptoms of bradycardia, hypotension, or hypothermia are noted. Complete liver and renal function tests, thyroid function tests, and serum electrolyte studies are usually included in the medical work-up.

Therapeutic Management

The treatment of eating disorders initially focuses on the secondary effects of self-induced vomiting, excessive use of diuretics and laxatives, and insufficient nutrients to sustain the function of body systems. Electrolyte levels and body chemistry values should be stabilized to prevent sustained damage to body systems, especially the cardiac, respiratory, and gastrointestinal systems. Adequate caloric intake is the next major goal of treatment and often requires strict monitoring to prevent sabotage of medical treatment. Ongoing intensive and highly individualized therapy helps the adolescent cope with complex issues. Finally, alteration of misperceptions about body image and a reorientation to issues of control and self-management are necessary. Follow-up therapy for the individual and family is indicated for a period of several months to 3 years.

■ NURSING CARE
The Child or Adolescent With an Eating Disorder

Assessment

Children and adolescents with eating disorders typically have varying degrees of mistrust, ambivalence, and denial. It is generally better if the assessment is conducted in a structured and concrete manner (rather than as an open-ended exploration), with an emphasis placed on alliance building and periodic review of the assessment process for the child or adolescent. Determining motivations for changing behaviors is crucial, and motives should be assessed for each specific behavior (i.e., weight gain, induced vomiting, altered self-perception of body). A mental status examination should also be included, because the side effects of restrictive dieting can impair cognitive functioning and perpetuate affective disturbances. Any history of self-injury should be noted. The nurse should assist the child or adolescent in gaining an understanding of impulse control problems and ritualistic and compulsive behaviors.

The medical history and physical assessment should be comprehensive, focusing on any medically based illness that mimics an eating disorder or exists concomitantly. Psychological assessment of body image and identification of problems, substance abuse, and social support systems used by the child or adolescent are important components of the assessment. A family history of eating disorders or other psychiatric illnesses should be noted. Family dynamics, including level or quality of interaction, support, discipline, and differentiation of members, should be explored in depth. Previous treatment attempts and coping strategies should also be identified.

School nurses or nurses in community settings are in an optimal position for recognizing children and adolescents with eating disorders. They become familiar with students they see on a regular basis and can readily assess changes in weight, emotional status, or behaviors. Once considered an adolescent problem, eating disorders are occurring in much younger children, so nurses in elementary schools need to be aware of the early signs. Awareness programs organized by school nurses often facilitate inquiries from children who might not normally speak about their eating problems or concerns about weight.

Nursing Diagnosis and Planning

The nursing diagnoses and expected outcomes that apply to the child or adolescent with an eating disorder are

- Imbalanced Nutrition: Less Than Body Requirements related to inadequate intake, malabsorption from extended periods of starvation, or distorted body image.
  Expected Outcome: The child or adolescent will meet daily nutritional requirements, as evidenced by sufficient weight gain or maintenance of an adequate weight to sustain systemic homeostasis and physiologic health.
- Anxiety, Fear, or Powerlessness related to weight gain, sense of inadequacy, and lack of control over body and self.
  Expected Outcome: The child or adolescent will experience decreased anxiety, fear, and powerlessness, as evidenced by demonstration of the ability to seek help with anxiety management and demonstration of improved coping strategies, including open expression of feelings.
- Risk for Activity Intolerance or Disturbed Sleep Pattern related to fatigue, depression, and an excessive drive to exercise and expend energy.
  Expected Outcome: The child or adolescent will have adequate rest, as evidenced by an ability to establish improved sleeping and activity patterns with a corresponding improvement in affect, energy, and sense of well-being.
- Deficient Fluid Volume related to excessive use of diuretics or laxatives and/or inadequate fiber and fluid intake.
  Expected Outcome: The child or adolescent will maintain fluid and electrolyte balance, as evidenced by electrolyte levels within normal limits, normal skin turgor, and moist mucous membranes.

Interventions

Children and adolescents with severe eating disorders may need to be hospitalized to achieve physiologic stability. These children are then generally transferred to a day treatment program. Care focuses on restructuring cognitive perceptions, reducing opportunities to engage in ritualistic and self-injurious behaviors, and reestablishing physiologic homeostasis. The programs typically include interventions that enlist the adolescent's cooperation in a refeeding program. Nutritional consultation is provided to facilitate gradual weight gain. Intake and output, weight gain, vital signs, laboratory values, electrolyte status, and cardiac status are carefully monitored.

Support in exploring refeeding sensations of fullness, bloating, and delayed gastric emptying and help tolerating these feelings and body sensations are important. The nurse and child or adolescent jointly participate in monitoring affect, mood, and potential for suicide. They also agree to a contract specifying necessary interventions to ensure safety, as well as to monitor daily food intake and feelings. These interventions may take the form of interacting with the staff at regular intervals or agreeing to approach the staff if suicidal ideation is present. The nurse will need to validate the adolescent's feelings of ambivalence, fear, and powerlessness. If hyperalimentation or nasogastric tube feedings are needed for adequate nutritional intake, the nurse should support the child or adolescent and monitor feedings. Finally, the nurse should provide educational information about the short-term and long-term effects of starvation.

The nurse is likely to participate in providing or supporting psychological treatments, such as individual, group, and family therapy sessions. Especially in the early phase of treatment, the child or adolescent may be very resistant to efforts to increase nutritional intake and may resort to denial, trickery, or manipulation to prevent a weight increase or thwart adherence to dietary regimens. It may be necessary to observe the child or adolescent after meals to prevent episodes of purging.

The family should be informed and involved in treatment goals and progress. Participation in family therapy is generally a required part of the treatment plan, because the cause may be directly related to family interactional patterns. The nurse should support the family in voicing concerns while encouraging them to view the adolescent as having an independent identity and sense of control.

Evaluation

- Does the child or adolescent demonstrate an increase in food consumption adequate to sustain growth and developmental needs?
- Has the child or adolescent reduced bingeing or purging activities?
- Can the child or adolescent demonstrate a positive alteration in self-perceptions and body image, as evidenced by verbalizing an increased sense of self-control and decreased anxiety about the present and the future?
- Does the child or adolescent demonstrate a decrease in ambivalence and mistrust about self and significant others?
- Does the child or adolescent show increased energy and display appropriate affect?
- Are electrolyte levels within normal limits, and are mucous membranes moist?

ATTENTION-DEFICIT HYPERACTIVITY DISORDER

Attention-deficit hyperactivity disorder (ADHD) is the most common chronic behavioral disorder of children. ADHD is associated with significant problems in three areas: (1) attention and concentration, (2) impulse control, and (3) overactivity. Over the years, it has variously been called *posten-*

cephalitic behavior disorder, restlessness syndrome, hyperkinetic impulse disorder, minimal brain dysfunction, and *hyperactive child syndrome.* There is evidence based on neuroimaging, neurophysiologic, and neurochemical data that developmental failure in brain circuitry underlies the impulsivity and hyperactivity, or poor response regulation and inhibition (Myers, Eisenhauer, & Ryan, 2003).

Referrals for ADHD may be made by parents or teachers. Of concern are not only the primary symptoms, which often result in frequent injuries, poor scholastic performance, and low performance motivation, but also the associated symptoms, which may include anxiety or depression, aggressiveness toward peers, and antisocial or oppositional defiance toward authority figures.

A single child affected with ADHD may exhibit wide variations in response to the environment. For example, a child with ADHD is likely to perform poorly on a highly complex task. If the structure is rigid or if behavior is severely restricted, the child with ADHD becomes increasingly frustrated and distinguishable from unaffected children. If instructions are repeated frequently or if the task is novel or unfamiliar, the child's performance tends to improve. Immediate reinforcement is very important because these children require much higher rates of reinforcement than their same-age peers. Fatigue may also affect the degree to which ADHD symptoms are exhibited.

Etiology

ADHD occurs more commonly in first-degree biologic relatives of people with the disorder than in the general population, which suggests a genetic predisposition for the disorder. Other central nervous system (CNS) abnormalities, such as the presence of neurotoxins and epilepsy, or other neurologic disorders are thought to be predisposing factors, although fewer than 5% of children with ADHD have definitive neurologic findings. Chaotic or abusive environments may predispose to the appearance of ADHD.

Incidence

Estimates of the incidence of ADHD range from 1% to 20%, but the general consensus is that 4% to 12% of children are affected with ADHD. Symptoms generally occur early in childhood, with the mean age at onset 3 or 4 years; however,

Pathophysiology

of Attention-Deficit Hyperactivity Disorder

Inconclusive but consistent evidence indicates that the basis of attention-deficit hyperactivity disorder (ADHD) is a sluggish or underreactive neurologic, electrophysiologic response to stimulation. Prefrontal and limbic system connections in the brain are viewed as the likely locations for neurologic functional abnormalities. Hypotheses have been made that dopaminergic and noradrenergic function plays a central role, since medications addressing these neurotransmitters are effective in treatment. This information suggests that higher levels of norepinephrine and lower levels of epinephrine activity seen in children with ADHD may play a role.

medication treatment may not be started until the child is in a structured school setting (Sadock & Sadock, 2003). In epidemiologic studies, the male-to-female ratio is approximately 3:1 among non-referred children displaying ADHD symptoms. Aggressive and antisocial behaviors are thought to explain the higher rate of referrals of boys.

Manifestations

Children with ADHD can typically exhibit clusters of signs and symptoms that are primarily inattentive, primarily impulsive/hyperactive, or a combination. Signs usually must be present for at least 6 months, have occurred before the age of 7 years, be present in two or more settings (e.g., home, school, recreation, church), not be associated with another mental or developmental disorder, and significantly impair at least one level of functioning (academic, social, occupational) (American Psychiatric Association, 2000). Even though the American Psychiatric Association calls this disorder *ADHD*, not all children with the disorder exhibit hyperactivity, although most demonstrate a degree of impulsivity.

According to the American Psychiatric Association (2000), to be diagnosed with ADHD, a child must exhibit six or more of the hallmark behaviors included below under *Inattention* and *Impulsivity/hyperactivity*:

- *Inattention:* carelessness, inattention to details, difficulty attending to work or games, does not listen, poor follow-through with instructions or does not complete tasks, difficulty with organization skills, avoidance of tasks that require mental effort, misplaces equipment or supplies necessary to complete tasks, easily distracted, forgetful
- *Impulsivity/hyperactivity:* fidgets with hands, feet, or hair; unable to remain in a seat for extended periods; runs and climbs excessively in inappropriate settings; difficulty in engaging in quiet activities; mostly "on the go"; talks excessively; blurts out questions or answers; cannot await a turn; interrupts conversations

ADHD can also be associated with other disorders, such as motor disorders, oppositional defiant disorder, mood disorders, and anxiety disorders. Children with ADHD often have diagnosed learning disability (Leslie, 2002).

Diagnostic Evaluation

Although high-resolution magnetic resonance imaging (MRI) and blood and urine studies of metabolites of brain neurotransmitters have been performed in individuals with ADHD, none of these tests has provided consistent information. The diagnosis of ADHD is currently established on the basis of reports by the child, parent, and teacher. The behaviors and symptoms of ADHD must be present in two of three areas—home, school, or social situations—to support the diagnosis. These reports are coupled with psychological assessments conducted while the child is completing tasks requiring vigilance, attention, and concentration, as well as those involving delayed gratification. Clinical interviews may be coupled with clinical trials of psychopharmacologic agents, such as methylphenidate (Ritalin), dextroamphetamine (Dexedrine), or amphetamine/dextroamphetamine (Adderall), to determine the child's behavioral response.

Therapeutic Management

The goal of therapeutic management is to reduce the frequency and intensity of unsocialized behaviors. This requires achieving a balance between the child's temperament and environmental demands, expectancies, and supports. Therefore treatment interventions must be targeted at enhancing the child's capabilities and self-esteem. Expectations that may be appropriate for a child without ADHD—"he should be able to sit still in school for 40 minutes," or "she should be able to handle 1 hour of homework"—may need to be modified for the child with ADHD. In every case, the nurse should work with the parents to modify the environment and develop strategies that foster competencies in the child. Most clinicians combine psychopharmacotherapy with behavior-oriented family therapy to achieve alterations in the child's internal functioning and external environment. Stimulant medications commonly used as part of the treatment plan include methylphenidate (Ritalin), dextroamphetamine (Dexedrine), and amphetamine/dextroamphetamine (Adderall). Newer time-released formulas of methylphenidate (Concerta, Ritalin LA, and Metadate ER) and amphetamine/dextroamphetamine (Adderall XR) are advantageous for the once-a-day dosing, thereby eliminating midday trips to the nurse's office. Atomoxetine (Strattera) a non-stimulant medication, has also been used with success in the treatment of ADHD. Medication treatment is most effective when used in conjunction with behavior and psychosocial therapy.

Some parents and professionals prefer more conservative approaches to the treatment of ADHD, such as dietary changes. Even though researchers continue to debate whether food additives and sugars have significant clinical influences on most children with ADHD, the general consensus is that they do not. Medication is typically administered during the school day, but it has become increasingly recognized that attention, concentration, and alertness are needed for any learning task, such as learning to play baseball or learning to drive a car. The side effects and potency of the medications used to treat ADHD often make parents and physicians hesitant to administer medications other than during critical learning periods.

▪ NURSING CARE
The Child With Attention-Deficit Hyperactivity Disorder

Assessment

The nurse should document the parent's description of the typical behavior of the child playing alone and with other children, during mealtimes, and while the parent is on the telephone or occupied with chores. The length of time it takes the child to bathe or dress and how often the child becomes distracted during these tasks are also explored. These behaviors are then compared with those exhibited when the child is engaged in highly stimulating activities and activities with frequent feedback, such as video and computer games. The child's behavior is also compared during novel versus routine activities.

The child's developmental and family history are explored in detail, with the nurse noting the age at which the child began to exhibit independent behaviors, such as walking, getting out of bed alone, and exploring the environment. It is not uncommon for children with ADHD to explore the environment at an early age, with only limited need to return to the caregiver for support or approval. Family members diagnosed with ADHD or who exhibit similar behaviors are noted. Parents should be given self-report inventories, such as the Child Behavior Checklist, Conners Teacher Rating Scale—Revised, or the Attention-Deficit/Hyperactivity Disorder (ADHD) Rating Scale, to complete and return to the appropriate professional.

Observation within the home or school setting is likely to generate the most valid information, because the clinic environment may be unfamiliar and, by the nature of the disorder, may inhibit the child's natural tendency to explore, become distracted, or display limited motivation in task completion.

Nursing Diagnosis and Planning

The nursing diagnoses and expected outcomes that apply to the child with ADHD and the child's family are

- Impaired Social Interaction related to impulsivity, poor self-management skills, and aggressive behaviors.
  Expected Outcomes: The child will experience an improvement in social interactions, as evidenced by improvement in impulse control and an ability to sustain attention on tasks. The child will relate in a more positive way with peers.
- Risk for Injury related to impulsivity, limited judgment skills, or excessive need for mobility and stimulation.
  Expected Outcome: The child will remain safe from injury, as evidenced by a decrease in injuries and implementation of a plan to prevent injuries.
- Compromised Family Coping or Disabled Family Coping related to the need for consistent and close supervision of the child, the child's hyperactivity, or social stigma of having a child with impulsive or aggressive behaviors.
  Expected Outcome: The family will mobilize coping strategies, as evidenced by an ability to discuss the child's needs and to plan to provide the needed support.
- Deficient Knowledge related to perceptions that the child is willfully defiant or disobedient in following directions or in testing limits.
  Expected Outcome: The family will increase knowledge related to their child's condition, as evidenced by a willingness to discuss the child's condition and display an understanding of the condition and its treatment.

Interventions

The primary nursing intervention for the child with ADHD is to teach the family about the disorder. Emphasis is placed on reducing the parents' blame and guilt about the child's problems and altering their perceptions that the child intentionally misbehaves or lacks motivation to learn or achieve. Teaching demonstrates ways to provide frequent positive reinforcement. Also, instruction about medications is important for both parents and child, as well as the adaptations in environment that are needed to allow the child to practice new skills.

The nurse may facilitate communication between the family and the school about ways to accommodate the child's shortened attention span and increased need for mobility and frequent breaks. Often cognitive-behavioral therapy, provided by a specially trained professional, is helpful in identifying specific exercises that can reduce bothersome traits. Support groups for parents can help families cope with the

child with ADHD and modify their interactions with and expectations of the child.

Ordinarily, positive effects of medication are seen within 1 to 2 weeks when medication is taken as prescribed. It is common for the family to observe a rapid change in the child's behavior and experience relief as manifestations subside. Ongoing support is required because this disorder is lifelong and progress in self-control and behavioral patterns is usually slow. Parents may need to be actively involved in dispensing medication, even through adolescence, because children fluctuate in their willingness to adhere to therapy. Affected children also may have difficulty remembering to take the medication because of the attentional deficits characteristic of the disorder.

Evaluation

- Does the child adhere to the cognitive and pharmacologic strategies designed to increase self-control, as evidenced by a decrease in impulsivity and increase in attention to task?
- Does the child complete school assignments in less time than formerly, with less distractibility?
- Does the child demonstrate increased skill in peer relations, as evidenced by fewer conflicts and more frequent positive statements to and about peers?
- Does the family provide a safe and supportive environment within the home, as evidenced by adequate supervision and opportunities for meeting the child's mobility needs in a safe manner?
- Does the family demonstrate acceptance of the child and the special needs of the child?
- Does the family demonstrate an increased acceptance of the child's condition as a medical problem, rather than a social or behavioral problem?
- Does the family comply with the medication regimen?

SUBSTANCE ABUSE

Chemical agents that are typically abused by children and adolescents include alcohol, hallucinogens, sedatives, analgesics, anxiolytics, steroids, inhalants, and stimulants. The substance abused depends on its availability and cost, as well as on social influences and parental behaviors or tolerance of drug use. Most professionals differentiate between *substance abuse* and *substance addiction*. However, the basic treatment concerns are similar. Substance abuse is generally considered to increase over time.

Etiology

Productive analysis of substance abuse considers risk factors, which include social, personal, and familial factors. Substance abuse and substance dependence tend to cluster in

---

! CRITICAL TO REMEMBER

Risks for Substance Abuse

Family systems that are closed to outsiders, that have a history of psychiatric disturbance, including substance abuse, or that have poor communication skills are at risk for creating an environment in which substance abuse in youth occurs.

TABLE 53-1 Commonly Abused Drugs and Their Effects

Drug	Expected Behaviors and Effects	Special Considerations
Tobacco	Chronic cough, wheezing, increased phlegm production, atherosclerosis	Considered a gateway drug; initial use usually begins in elementary school
Alcohol	Amount-related effects include euphoria followed by depression or hostility, decreased inhibitions, impaired judgment, incoordination, and slurred speech	Considered a gateway drug; easily accessible
Marijuana	Relaxation, mild euphoria, loss of inhibition, decreased motivation, red eyes, dry mouth	Considered a gateway drug
Opiates	Euphoria, elation, pain relief, detachment and apathy, drowsiness, constricted pupils, constipation, slurred speech, impaired judgment	Long-term apathy about self, often leading to physical malnutrition and dehydration; criminal behaviors associated with obtaining drugs likely to occur; infections at injection sites common
Barbiturates	Similar to those associated with alcohol	Often used in conjunction with stimulants; may have a paradoxical effect of hyperactivity in children
Amphetamines	Euphoria, hyperactivity, agitation, irritability, insomnia, weight loss, tachycardia, hypertension	May have a paradoxical effect of depression in children
Cocaine	Euphoria, elation, agitation, hyperactivity, irritability, pressured speech, grandiosity, tachycardia, hypertension, diaphoresis, anorexia, weight loss, insomnia	Psychotic behavior possible if the dose is large; can be fatal if combined with other drugs
Hallucinogens (lysergic acid diethylamide [LSD]; methylenedioxymethamphetamine [MDMA, "ecstasy"])	Distorted perceptions, heightened awareness, hallucinations, illusions, depersonalization, dilated pupils, hypertension, increased salivation	Psychotic behaviors, panic flashbacks long after drug use ceases, self-destructive behaviors
Phencyclidine hydrochloride (PCP)	Euphoria, distorted perceptions, agitation, violence, antisocial behaviors, hypertension, increased salivation, increased pain response	Panic, irrational behaviors, psychosis

families, with clinical evidence of genetic influences. For alcohol, as for most other drugs, there also is some evidence that substance abuse often represents the child's or adolescent's attempt to cope with anxiety generated by impaired social skills, low self-esteem, poor interpersonal relationships, or lack of adaptive behaviors. Some psychosocial disorders, such as ADHD, depression, and conduct disorder, are associated with an increased risk of substance abuse.

Incidence

Great variation exists in the types of substances abused across gender and age (Table 53-1). Typically, boys consume alcohol more than girls do. Female junior high school students are increasing their use of tobacco, whereas tobacco use by their male counterparts has remained consistent.

The National Institute on Drug Abuse has tracked illicit drug use and attitudes toward drug use in middle and high school students since 1975. Each fall, the updated results of the Monitoring the Future Survey are released. According to the 2002 results, the trend of use of marijuana, club drugs, cigarettes, and alcohol has been declining since 1998 (National Institute of Drug Abuse [NIDA], 2002).

Illicit drug use, including alcohol and tobacco, remains high despite reports of declining use among adolescents. Marijuana use among adolescents in 2001 was 14.6% to 30.3%. Cocaine usage was 2.3% to 5%. Heroin use was at 1%. Nonmedical use of pain medication such as Vicodin was between 2% and 10%, and tobacco use was 31% to 58%. Club drugs such as methylenedioxymethamphetamine (MDMA ["ecstasy"]), nitrite inhalants ("poppers"), and gamma-hydroxybutyrate (GHB ["ice"]) remain popular among this age-group (NIDA, 2002). It is estimated that 90% of adolescents have tried alcohol by the time they reach adulthood. The earlier an individual begins to use alcohol, the more likely dependence will develop (U.S. DHHS, 2000b). Experimentation with marijuana, the most widely used illicit drug, is reported in nearly one fourth of 8th-graders and approximately one half of 12th-graders. Research consistently supports the hypothesis that drug use progresses from beer or wine to cigarettes or hard liquor and then marijuana, followed by other illicit drugs. These substances are sometimes referred to as *gateway substances.* Substance use is strongly associated with other risk behaviors in adolescence, such as unintentional injuries and unprotected sexual encounters (Box 53-2).

Public awareness and emphasis on treatment and prevention seem to be working, even though they had very limited impact on teenagers in the 1990s. Reducing substance abuse is a national health goal identified in *Healthy People 2010* (U.S. DHHS, 2000b). An awareness of the possibility of substance

BOX 53-2
Phases of Substance Abuse

Phase 1: Experimentation
The drug is taken to see what it does or to appease peers.

Phase 2: Early Drug Use
A specific drug or various drugs are used with some regularity for their pleasurable effects or to reduce anxiety. Social use of drugs typically falls into this category.

Phase 3: True Drug Addiction
Drugs are used regularly, and physical dependence begins if it is characteristic of the drug. Social functioning revolves around a drug focus.

Phase 4: Severe Drug Addiction
The physical condition of the addicted child or adolescent deteriorates. All activities are related to obtaining or using the drug, with isolation from nondrug culture.

---

abuse is the responsibility of the parent, teacher, and health professional. Knowing the clinical behavioral manifestations of substance abuse is essential, and much information is readily available to adults interested in prevention and early identification.

Manifestations

The clinical manifestations of substance abuse are marked by increased antisocial behavior as the desire for social conformity and acceptance decreases and the need for the substance increases. Behaviors that may indicate substance abuse problems include irregular school attendance, low grades or poor school performance, aggressive or rebellious behavior, excessive dependence on peer influence, and deterioration of relationships with family members or former friends. Rapid or extreme changes in behavior or mood and loss of interest in hobbies, sports, or other favorite activities are often observed. Lack of parental support and supervision, as well as changes in eating or sleeping patterns that increase as manipulative behaviors increase, especially those that are related to the need to acquire desired substances, may also be involved.

Pathophysiology

of Substance Abuse

The primary effect of substance abuse is on the brain and residually on the rest of the body. The actual action depends on the type of substance used, because substances act in accordance with their specific chemical composition. For example, alcohol affects the entire brain by decreasing its responsiveness.

! CRITICAL TO REMEMBER
Relapse Among Substance Abusers

Substance abusers' rates of refusal to adhere to therapeutic recommendations, together with resulting relapses, are quite high. More than 60% of those completing a course of treatment continue to abuse substances throughout their lifetimes.

Therapeutic Management

Treatment in a center specifically designed for substance abuse is recommended and includes individual, group, and family therapy. Participation in Alcoholics Anonymous or Narcotics Anonymous is advocated. These organizations also offer support groups geared toward helping family members with programs that promote alterations in the family system to decrease the likelihood of relapse.

▪NURSING CARE
The Child or Adolescent With a Substance Abuse Problem

Assessment

Physical assessment should include evaluation of the child's or adolescent's respiration rate, heart rate, blood pressure, activity level (hyperactive, hypoactive), mood, affect, judgment, speech, sensory responses, and memory. A thorough history of current and past drug use should be obtained. A family and social history, a medical history, and a legal history (e.g., past and current charges related to substance abuse) should be obtained.

Nursing Diagnosis and Planning

The nursing diagnoses and expected outcomes that apply to the child or adolescent with a substance abuse problem are

- Disturbed Thought Processes related to the specific effects of the particular substance involved.
  Expected Outcome: The child or adolescent will exhibit behaviors indicative of the absence of substance abuse, as evidenced by the ability to maintain orientation to time, place, and person.
- Disturbed Sensory Perception related to the specific effects of the particular substance involved.
  Expected Outcome: The child or adolescent will remain free from experiencing sensory changes, as evidenced by the absence of falls or other injuries.
- Anxiety related to a decrease in sense of control over self or the environment.
  Expected Outcome: The child or adolescent will experience decreased anxiety, as evidenced by verbalization of increased feelings of self-worth and the ability to change behavior.
- Ineffective Coping related to limited development of effective social interactions and problem-solving skills.
  Expected Outcome: The child or adolescent will increase ability to interact socially and to problem solve, as evidenced by an ability to identify current stressors leading to substance use or abuse.

- Impaired Social Interaction related to anxiety or limited social skills.

  Expected Outcome: The child or adolescent will begin to develop healthy social skills, as evidenced by an ability to identify alternative activities, people, and social situations that discourage substance abuse.

- Situational Low Self-Esteem or Chronic Low Self-Esteem related to limited social skills, ineffective coping skills, or a poor sense of self-management.

  Expected Outcome: The child or adolescent will increase self-esteem, as evidenced by replacing substance abuse with more appropriate social skills and developing meaningful relationships with non-abusing peers and family members.

Interventions

The nurse's responsibilities in caring for children or adolescents with substance abuse problems depend on the severity of the abuse and the treatment goals. If the nurse is the first to encounter the abuse, notification of the family and referrals for treatment should be initiated. If the youth has been identified as a substance abuser and referred to a treatment facility, the nurse's primary responsibility will be to stabilize the child's or adolescent's physiologic status and support recommendations for treatment. Explaining the expectations and the types of services offered is important, because most treatment programs increase child or adolescent and family responsibilities over time.

Initially, maintaining safety and an optimal level of physical comfort is necessary, especially if detoxification is required. This includes close observation, removal of any potentially dangerous items, and monitoring vital signs. Being readily available to discuss thoughts, concerns, and perceptions is important to create an emotional sense of safety. Additional interventions include educating the child or adolescent and family members about necessary laboratory tests and providing ongoing information about the nature of substance abuse.

Another significant nursing intervention is to assist the child or adolescent and family in developing social support systems and refer them to appropriate resources that can offer additional support as they make long-term changes in their social and emotional patterns of relating. It is also essential to help the youth assume responsibility for the substance abuse problem, rather than passing the blame on to others. Providing emotional support for the youth and family as they develop insight into their behaviors and the need for changes is important because these changes are often difficult to effect.

The relapse rate among youthful substance abusers is extremely high, and success in a short-term treatment program is not necessarily an indicator of long-term control. The incidence of relapse is generally reduced if the child and family maintain active, long-term involvement in support groups, such as Alcoholics Anonymous, Ala-Teen, Ala-Tot, and Narcotics Anonymous. Tough Love support groups for parents may also be beneficial in providing counsel and support.

Evaluation

- Has the child or adolescent remained substance-free and been oriented to time and place?
- Has the child or adolescent remained injury-free secondary to sensory or perceptual changes?
- Is the child or adolescent able to identify stressors and use appropriate coping mechanisms?
- Has the child or adolescent assumed responsibility for changing behaviors related to the substance abuse?
- Is the child or adolescent participating in daily activities?
- Does the child or adolescent show improvement in peer and family relationships?
- Does the child or adolescent demonstrate an increased sense of self-confidence?

CHILDHOOD PHYSICAL AND EMOTIONAL ABUSE AND NEGLECT

Child abuse includes emotional abuse, physical abuse, and neglect, as well as sexual exploitation or molestation by caretakers or other individuals.

Etiology

Family dysfunction underlies most forms of child abuse. The family profile varies with the type of abuse, although it is not uncommon for multiple types of abuse to exist in a single family. Generally, the dysfunctional family dynamics are multigenerational and involve both parents (Box 53-3).

Socioeconomic factors also appear to influence the incidence and etiology of child abuse, with increased child abuse observed during periods of economic hardship or external stress. The typical perpetrator is a direct relative of the child, usually the parent (87%) or primary caretaker, is younger than 40 years (80%), and is female (60%) (U.S. DHHS, 2000a). Often this individual has limited coping skills and was abused as a child or teenager. The typical profile of an abused child is more difficult to determine. Some research indicates that the typical abused child is younger than 5 years, often has mild physical abnormalities, is developmentally or physically delayed, has a difficult temperament, or reminds the abuser of someone else. A parent is 100 times more likely to kill a stepchild than a biologic child.

BOX 53-3
Characteristics of the Abusive Family

- Isolation from community and social groups
- Intense competition for emotional resources within the family, such as affection, attention, and nurturance
- Low levels of differentiation among family members
- Low trust for outsiders and family members
- Unpredictable and unstable family environment
- Conflict resolution generally achieved through aggression or power struggle between family members
- Present focus and crisis-oriented actions for immediate gratification
- Communication often characterized by mixed or double messages, threats, or a focus on nonverbal communication rather than direct verbalization
- Family roles that are typically fixed and traditional, with rigid rules
- Frequent domination by a single family member who maintains control through manipulation, intimidation, deceit, and aggression

Incidence

Physical and Emotional Abuse and Neglect

Child abuse reports to child protective services have increased. This increase has been attributed to the public's, teachers', and clinicians' increased awareness and willingness to report, rather than to an actual increase in prevalence. In 2001, 56.5% of reports to child protective services nationwide were made by professionals (U.S. DHHS, 2003).

In 2001, slightly fewer than 1 million children were identified as victims of substantiated abuse or neglect. Of those identified, 59.2% suffered from neglect; 18.6% were physically abused; 9.6% were victims of sexual abuse; and 6.8% were abused emotionally. The national rate of victimization is 12.4 in 1000 children (U.S. DHHS, 2003).

Approximately 1300 children died from maltreatment in 2001. Eighty-five percent were younger than 6 years and 41% were younger than 1 year when they died (U.S. DHHS, 2003).

Sexual Abuse

Victims of sexual abuse are usually between 6 and 9 years old at the onset of the abuse. The accepted ratio of three females to every male, however, may represent less than the actual incidence for boys.

Manifestations

Physical Indicators of Abuse

Physical indicators of abuse include unexplained bruises or welts that appear in various stages of healing, often in clustered patterns that reflect the shapes of the articles used to inflict injury, and unexplained burns, especially on the soles, palms, back, or buttocks; immersion burns may be seen (sock-like, glovelike, or doughnut-shaped) on buttocks or genitalia (Fig. 53-2). Other signs may include infected burns, which indicate a delay in seeking treatment, and bald patches on the scalp. Unexplained fractures of the skull, nose, or facial structures or multiple or spiral fractures or dislocations, as well as numerous fractures in various stages of healing, are also significant.

Behavioral Indicators of Abuse

Behavioral indicators of abuse include a child's wariness in response to adult contact, apprehension when others cry or lack of crying when approached by a stranger or examiner, and fear of parents or of going home. Extreme aggressiveness or withdrawal, vacant or frozen stares, monosyllabic responses to questions, and lying very still when surveying surroundings may be observed. A capacity to engage only in superficial relationships, manipulative behaviors to get attention, inappropriate or precocious maturity, and indiscriminate seeking of attention may also be reactions to abusive situations.

Physical Indicators of Neglect

Children experiencing neglect will probably show inadequate weight gain for age, poor growth pattern, and failure to thrive. They may exhibit constant hunger, poor hygiene, wasting of subcutaneous tissue, and bald patches on the scalp, and they may be dressed in clothes that are not seasonally suitable (e.g., no coat or shoes in winter). Reports of lack of supervision for long periods, permission to engage in unsafe activities, or abandonment may also accompany a neglected child.

Behavioral Indicators of Neglect

A child who begs or steals food, has inconsistent school attendance or comes very early and stays very late at school, or is constantly fatigued or listless in class may be exhibiting the effects of neglect. Other behavioral indicators of neglect include assuming adult responsibilities or roles, alcohol or substance abuse, and delinquency.

Physical Indicators of Emotional Abuse

Children who have been emotionally abused may exhibit speech disorders, lags in physical development, failure to thrive, or hyperactive and disruptive behaviors.

Behavioral Indicators of Emotional Abuse

Behavioral indicators of emotional abuse may include habit disorders (sucking, biting, rocking), conduct or learning disorders, or overly adaptive or compliant behaviors (withdrawal, aggression). Neurotic traits, including sleep disorders, inhibition of play, and unusual fearfulness, as well as psychoneurotic reactions, such as hysteria, obsession, compulsions, phobias, and hypochondriasis, are also observed. Suicide attempts may also indicate emotional abuse.

Physical Indicators of Sexual Abuse

The sexually abused child may exhibit difficulty walking or sitting; torn, stained, or bloody underclothing; pain, swelling, or itching of genitalia; and pain on urination. Additional physical signs include bruises, bleeding, or lacerations involving the external genitalia, vagina, or anal area, and vaginal or penile discharge. Sexually transmitted disease, poor sphincter tone, and excessive masturbation may also be present.

Behavioral Indicators of Sexual Abuse

The sexually abused child may demonstrate an unwillingness to change clothes or participate in gym activities; withdrawal, fantasy, or infantile behavior; or bizarre, sophisticated, or unusual sexual behavior or knowledge. Promiscuity, poor peer relations, delinquency, running away, depression, or suicidal ideation, gestures, or attempts are often observed. These behaviors may coincide with aggression, a change in school performance, or sleep disturbances or nightmares. In addition, eating disturbances (obesity, anorexia, bulimia), self-destructive behaviors (substance abuse, self-mutilation), and sexual acting out toward a younger child are sometimes present.

Children often cope with sexual victimization through an accommodation syndrome, in which the coping mechanisms become the child's normal behaviors in response to an abnormal event. There is nothing the child can do to prevent the abuse. The initial strategy involves secrecy because the child realizes the situation lacks social acceptance. This awareness dominates the child's sense of self, and the child experiences a great deal of guilt. The guilt may be intensified by the child's ambivalence about pleasure that may be experienced during the event. The secrecy is typically reinforced by threats that the child, the perpetrator, or another loved one will "get into trouble."

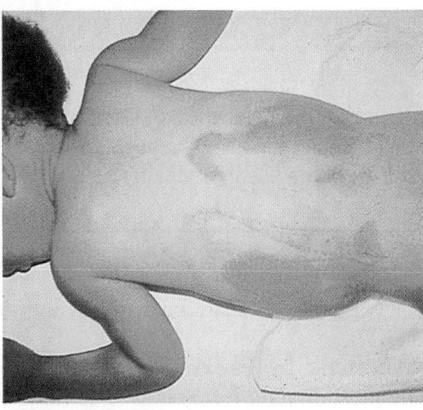

Intentional distribution of bruises—All four surfaces of the mid-body are involved, but there are no bruises on arms and legs.

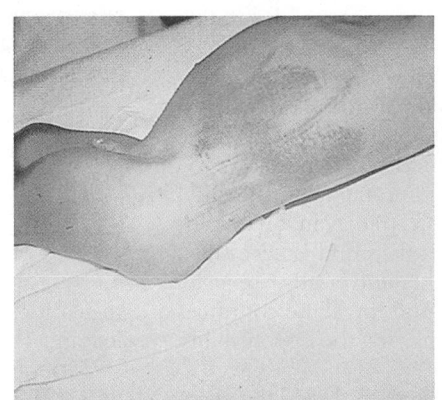

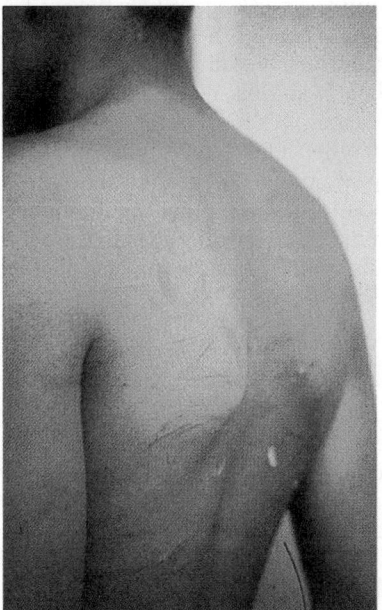

Pattern of injury—Linear scars of various ages indicate repeated abuse using a switch or whip. The loop pattern on the boy's anterior torso is consistent with a looped electrical cord used as a whip.

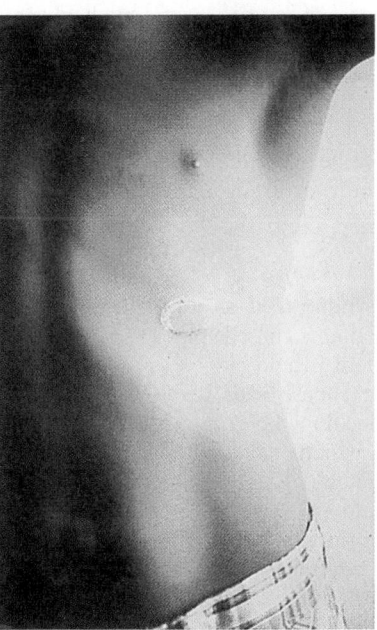

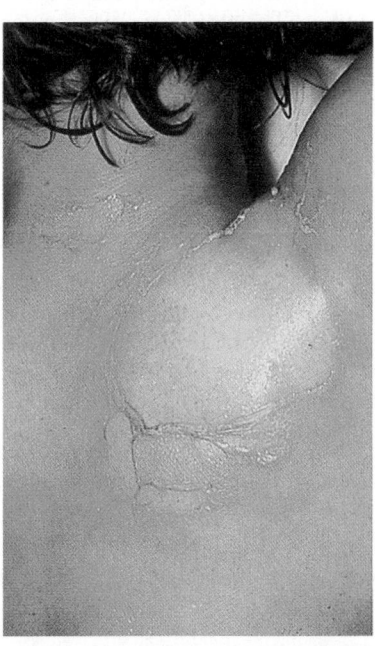

Scald burn of shoulder and neck—The typical distribution of a scald burn in a toddler. This type of injury occurs when a toddler pulls a cup of coffee or pan of water off a stove.

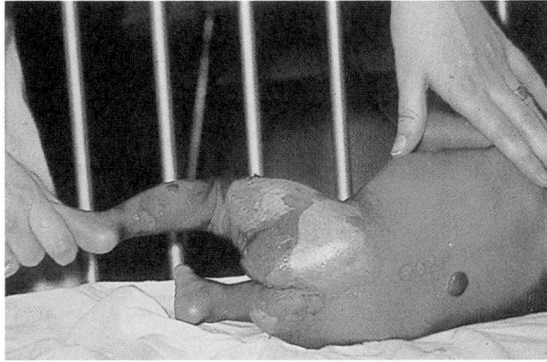

Intentional immersion scald—Involvement of virtually the entire posterior surface of the legs indicates that the legs were held under scalding water; even an infant this young would flex the knees to avoid the hot water.

Figure 53-2 Physical signs of child abuse. The nurse should be alert for the typical behavioral indicators of abuse. (Courtesy Barbara Tenney, M.D. From Henry, M.C., & Stapleton, E.R. [1992]. *EMT: Prehospital care* [p. 675]. Philadelphia: Saunders.)

The second behavioral response arises from the child's sense of helplessness. The child feels responsible for holding the family system together and feels isolated from peers because of shame and guilt, so the child plays possum, pretending to be asleep or unaffected by the sexual abuse. This is the child's attempt to manage the intrusion experienced.

To cope with an enduring sense of entrapment, the child takes responsibility for the abuse. This strategy involves minimizing the pain, because as long as the child is accessible, the molestation continues. Almost universally, sexually abused children believe that the reason the abuse continues is because they are bad, rather than placing the responsibility on the perpetrator.

Sexually abused children often dissociate during the abuse to avoid feelings or physical pain. Frequently the child will make veiled attempts at disclosure or will delay disclosure to keep the abuse secret and avoid the risk of alienating significant others. The child fears that the consequences of revealing the abuse will be worse than keeping the secret. In fact, most sexually abused children keep the abuse secret throughout their lives, unless there is some intervention from outside the abusive system. Finally, the sexually abused child typically retracts the revelation of abuse once it has been made, out of fear of ridicule, retaliation, attending court, or losing contact with a loved one.

Other Specific Abusive Situations

Shaken Baby Syndrome. Shaken baby syndrome is a widely recognized form of physical child abuse that is caused by vigorous shaking of the infant while the infant is held by the extremities or shoulders. This type of physical abuse leads to whiplash-induced intracranial and retinal bleeding. There is generally no external sign of head trauma, which makes this syndrome difficult to detect. The most common trigger of severe shaking is crying, especially if the child is colicky. Shaken baby syndrome should be considered in infants who present with failure to thrive, seizures, apnea, respiratory irregularities, coma, or vomiting associated with drowsiness or lethargy (Usinski, 2002).

Munchausen Syndrome by Proxy. Munchausen syndrome by proxy is the most difficult form of child abuse to diagnose. It is often inflicted by the mother or primary caretaker. The caretaker falsifies illness in the child through simulation or production of illness and then takes the child for medical care, claiming no knowledge of how the child became ill. The most common reasons these caretakers give for seeking medical treatment are bleeding, seizures, CNS depression, apnea, diarrhea, vomiting, fever, and rash. Long-term mortality in these cases is as high as 10% to 15%. Under the supervision of other adults, the child exhibits no symptoms and may appear normal and healthy. The parent's behavior reflects a serious disturbance that requires specialized psychiatric treatment and removal of the child from the parent's care. A multidisciplinary team is the best approach to diagnosing this disorder (Bennet, 2000).

> **⚠ CRITICAL TO REMEMBER**
>
> **Denial of Abuse**
>
> It is common for the abuser, the noninvolved parent, and the child to deny the abuse. Each may deny the event, awareness of the event, impact of the event, or any responsibility for the event.

FAILURE TO THRIVE

Most clinicians agree that failure to thrive is not an actual diagnosis but rather a term that describes a cluster of concurrent symptoms. In practice, if a child's weight falls below the 5th percentile or drops more than two major percentile groups or if the average daily growth gain in grams is less than normal values, the child is considered to be at risk for failure to thrive and a more thorough evaluation is warranted.

Etiology

Nonorganic failure to thrive is thought to be caused by multiple factors, including poverty, maternal depression, poor social support systems, poor bonding or maladaptive interactions between the child and mother, and irritable, resistant-to-touch infant. A maladaptive parent-infant relationship, in which the parent displays impaired skills in reading or responding to the infant's cues, is the most commonly observed risk factor for nonorganic failure to thrive. The infant has difficulty eliciting attention and appropriate care, often becoming irritable or stiff, or exhibits feeding difficulties. These symptoms are difficult for new parents to manage, resulting in parental anxiety and difficulty in bonding emotionally with the infant (Sirotnak, 2003).

Incidence

From 1% to 5% of hospitalized infants are listed as being admitted for failure to thrive; however, these estimates of occurrence may be low. It is estimated that 10% of children seen in the primary care setting have symptoms of failure to thrive (Bassali & Benjamin, 2002). Although failure to thrive occurs in children of all social classes, a disproportionate number of these children are from low-income families.

CRITICAL THINKING EXERCISE 53-1

Matthew, age 2 years, is brought to the emergency department by his mother, Ms. Jackson, and her boyfriend. Ms. Jackson tells the nurse that Matthew has been crying and holding his arm since she picked him up at the baby-sitter's earlier in the evening. On further questioning, Ms. Jackson states that "Matthew is all boy. You have to watch him every minute or he is into something. He is constantly climbing and falling."

On examination, the nurse notes several bruises on Matthew's right leg and right arm. He also has a small abrasion on his nose. Ms. Jackson is holding Matthew and seems concerned, as does her boyfriend. Matthew quiets when his mother holds him and drifts off to sleep. Ms. Jackson's boyfriend leaves the room and returns with a snack for both Matthew and Ms. Jackson. He offers to hold Matthew.

1. What are some of the possible reasons Matthew is crying and holding his arm? Support your assumptions with rationales.
2. If the nurse suspects child abuse, what added assessments should be performed?
3. What legal responsibility does the nurse have in cases of suspected child abuse?

Nursing Care Plan

The Abused Child

FOCUSED ASSESSMENT

The nurse should conduct a thorough evaluation for skin integrity, including examination of the scalp, bottoms of the hands and feet, front and back of the trunk, and genitalia. A baseline measurement of height and weight should be obtained, along with documentation of the birth weight for infants. An assessment of the child's anxiety level, ability to relate to the examiner, and emotional tone is also crucial. In addition, an assessment of the family support system, including patterns of interaction, belief systems, and social support systems, should be conducted.

During the physical assessment, information about bruises, injuries, and sexual abuse should be requested in a non-emotional, matter-of-fact manner with particular attention to the child's need for privacy and dignity. Comments made by the child should be written down verbatim, because disclosure of abuse is often subtle and this information may be used in legal proceedings at a later time. Assessment should include an account of written or verbal contact with teachers, relatives (including both parents, siblings, and grandparents), and others who have been involved with the child over an extended period.

Trust may be enhanced by answering questions directly and specifically, assuming a nonjudgmental and supportive stance throughout all interactions, and acting as an advocate for the holistic care of the child as well as of the family. Recognition of the child's low self-esteem, feelings of inadequacy, and fear will enable the nurse to relate in a manner that is supportive. The child will need encouragement to make self-care decisions and to discuss thoughts and feelings that may have been repressed to survive the trauma (Fig. 53-3). The child may also feel affection for the perpetrator and believe that the abuse is a necessary part of the relationship.

When sexual abuse is suspected, the child and parent should be interviewed in the same manner as described for physical abuse. The nurse should observe for clinical manifestations of sexual abuse in a manner that provides dignity and respect for both the child and the parent. Assessment tools are available that identify

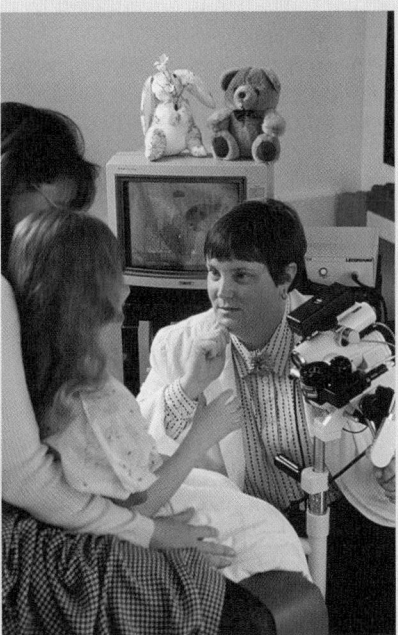

Drawings may help to identify the abused child and assist in therapy. Art can also help the child express what cannot be expressed in words.

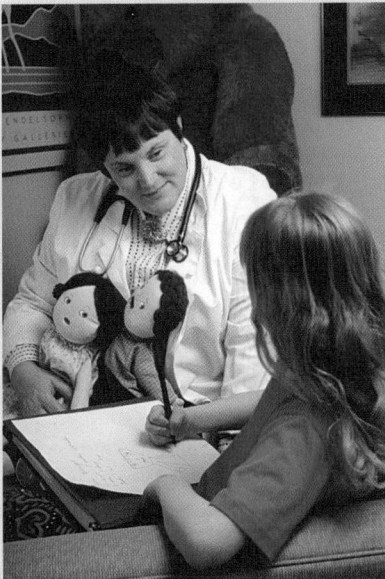

◀ Note the communication techniques designed to reassure the child and give the child some power. The little girl is not immediately positioned for a genital examination. The physician first sits to talk with the child at her eye level and makes eye contact with her.

Figure 53-3 Disclosure of abuse may be slow because the child often has difficulty trusting any adult. Identification of sexual abuse requires particular sensitivity, because physical examination of the child's genitalia to detect signs of injury or sexually transmitted disease can be frightening for the child, who associates handling of the genitalia with pain or shame. Anatomically correct dolls are often used in the assessment of abuse within a family. These dolls help children express what they cannot express in words; young children in particular have a limited vocabulary to use when describing the events that have occurred. (Courtesy Cook Children's Medical Center, Fort Worth, TX.)

Continued

Nursing Care Plan

The Abused Child—cont'd

behaviors typical of the child who has been sexually abused. Nurses are considered to be mandated reporters and therefore *must* report any *suspected* child abuse to the appropriate authorities.

Nursing Diagnosis

Impaired Parenting related to immaturity, lack of knowledge, apathy on the part of parental caregivers, or limited or negative past parenting experience.

Expected Outcome

The family will:

- Exhibit appropriate parenting skills, as evidenced by expressing an understanding of positive parenting models and responding to the child's needs in a timely and appropriate manner.

INTERVENTION	RATIONALE
1. Assess the parents' strengths and weaknesses, normal coping mechanisms, and the presence or absence of support systems. Special attention should be paid to: • Expectations with regard to the child • Comforting behaviors • Response to the child • General knowledge about the child	1. To provide optimal care for the child, involvement of the family is crucial. By understanding the needs of the family, the nurse can develop a plan of care, including referral to appropriate supportive agencies.
2. Discuss with the parents the parenting they received as children.	2. Parenting is a learned behavior.
3. Observe the parents' interactions with the child.	3. Although parents may verbalize a positive relationship with their child, observation of actual interactions provides a more realistic view of the parent-child relationship.
4. Provide an accepting environment.	4. Communication is encouraged by demonstrating acceptance.
5. Provide information for parents regarding normal growth and development.	5. Parents who are abusers often have unrealistic expectations of their children, in part because of their lack of knowledge regarding growth and development.
6. Include role modeling as a method of teaching parenting.	6. By observing the way the nurse touches and talks to the child in an affirming manner, the parents can observe firsthand the child's response to positive parenting-type skills.
7. Devote part of the time spent with the child and family to focusing on the child's positive attributes.	7. Parents' negative perceptions of the child, which may be based on their own life experiences, can be altered by viewing the child through another's eyes.
You might say "You are such a pretty little girl," or "Look at that wonderful smile."	
8. Encourage the parents to participate in the care of the child. Reinforce positive behaviors.	8. Strategies that encourage and reinforce positive parental participation in child care build self-esteem and confidence in parenting skills.

Evaluation

- Do the parents interact appropriately with the child through verbal, physical, and visual contact?
- Have the parents verbalized an understanding of normal growth and development?
- Do the parents make positive statements about the child?
- Do the parents bring the child in for follow-up visits?

Nursing Diagnosis

Fear and/or Powerlessness related to the possible outcomes of disclosure, sense of shame, and possible loss of family.

Expected Outcomes

The child will:

- Verbalize the source of fear.
- Express feelings related to shame and fear of loss of family.

Nursing Care Plan

The Abused Child—cont'd

INTERVENTION	RATIONALE
1. Reassure the child in regard to personal safety.	1. Verbal reassurance can provide a sense of security.
2. Identify specific strategies the child can use to maintain a sense of stability (i.e., stay with a trusted adult, refuse to answer intrusive questions, limit exposure to adults who are not trusted).	2. By providing some viable options, the nurse can help the child begin to gain a sense of control over the experience.
3. Acknowledge the child's fear.	3. Acknowledgment helps the child identify feelings and opens up new areas of communication.
4. Spend time with the child. Use both verbal and nonverbal forms of communication.	4. Actions of support provide comfort and encourage verbalization of feelings.
5. Offer choices, when available, regarding activities of daily living, recreation time, and time with other children and adults.	5. Being offered choices gives the child a sense of control and diminishes feelings of powerlessness.

Evaluation

■ Does the child participate in play activities?
■ Has the child verbalized specific fears related to abuse and disclosure?
■ Has the child verbalized fears related to being removed from the family?

Nursing Diagnosis

Deficient Knowledge about the child's realistic developmental abilities, how to access external support resources, or ways to manage internal and external stressors related to past inexperience with parenting.

Expected Outcomes

The family will:
■ Increase knowledge related to growth and development, as evidenced by verbalization of an understanding of the child's developmental and emotional needs in a framework that is oriented to the child's welfare.
■ Identify support systems.

INTERVENTION	RATIONALE
1. Determine the parents' knowledge of child growth and development.	1. A baseline assessment must be done to develop a plan of care.
2. Serve as a role model for positive parenting skills.	2. Learning can be enhanced through observing the application of parenting skills, which is more effective than listening to a lecture.
3. Assist the family in identifying stressors and the support systems and resources that may help decrease the parents' stress level.	3. If the parents' level of stress is decreased, the risk of abuse is decreased.
4. Refer the family to pertinent support groups, such as Parents Anonymous.	4. Lack of support and isolation are common among abusive families. A support group may decrease isolation.
5. Involve the parents in the care of the child.	5. Participation in care will provide opportunities for positive reinforcement, teaching, and increased emotional attachment to the child.
6. Provide education in the following areas: • Growth and development • Nutrition • Care related to activities of daily living • Routine well-child care • Manifestations of illness • Need for care and loving	6. Education in parenting skills may decrease unrealistic expectations, increase awareness of the needs of children, and increase the chances of positive parenting. Parents may not have had positive parenting role models as children.
7. Provide a consistent caregiver from among the nursing staff.	7. Consistency of care increases the child's feelings of trust and security and provides increased opportunities for the child to verbalize feelings.

Continued

Nursing Care Plan

The Abused Child—cont'd

Evaluation

- Can the parents describe normal child growth and development and developmental expectations?
- Have the parents joined a support group?

Nursing Diagnosis

Risk for Injury related to a family with a history of physical abuse, physical neglect, emotional abuse, or sexual abuse.

Expected Outcome

Injury related to abuse will:

- Cease, as evidenced by the child remaining free from physical or psychological injury and neglect.

INTERVENTION	RATIONALE
1. Assess the child's physical and mental status.	1. All children should undergo a thorough physical assessment on presentation to the health care setting and should be assessed for bruises, burns, scars, and other signs of abuse. Children may enter the health care system for reasons other than injury.
2. Observe the interactions between child and family.	2. Subtle signs of abuse may be detected in the way the child interacts with the abuser and other adults.
3. Obtain a thorough history.	3. Frequent presentation of the child for injuries or signs of healed injuries may indicate a pattern of abuse.
4. Use a nonthreatening, nonjudgmental manner when interacting with the child's parents.	4. By building a trusting relationship with the parents, the nurse can help the child. If the parents become suspicious or alienated, they may deny the child access to health care. They will become defensive and will not be open to teaching.
5. Report all cases in which abuse is suspected.	5. All 50 states require health care professionals to report all cases of suspected abuse.
6. Assist in removing children from an unsafe environment.	6. Suspected abuse should be evaluated immediately so that the child can be removed to an environment that is safe, thereby preventing further injury.
7. Document the following: • Results of the child's physical assessment • Observations of interactions between the child and family and between the child and other adults, as well as the child's reaction to hospitalization or the health care setting • Direct comments made by the child and the family that pertain to the child or the child's injury • Child's developmental level	7. Objective documentation is essential in all cases of suspected abuse.
8. If the child is removed from the home, provide the child and family with support and opportunities to verbalize feelings. Play therapy may be used effectively with children.	8. Children who are removed from the custody of their parents will grieve their loss. Parents will need support in dealing with guilt and loss.

Evaluation

- Does the child remain free of inflicted injury?
- Has the child been placed in a safe environment?
- Has the child verbalized feelings regarding placement outside the home?
- Has the family sought psychological counseling?

Pathophysiology

of Failure to Thrive

Three types of failure to thrive are typically described: organic, nonorganic, and mixed.

Organic failure to thrive is marked by failure to gain weight secondary to physical factors. These physical factors may be a specific physiologic impairment, such as a congenital heart defect, gastrointestinal disorder, or endocrine disorder. Alternatively, the physical factor may be a chronic infection, a central nervous system abnormality, a chromosomal disorder, or a metabolic disorder. Organic failure to thrive is a sign of possible human immunodeficiency virus (HIV) infection in an infant (see Chapter 41).

Nonorganic failure to thrive is a diagnosis applied in the absence of a history contributing to, or physical or laboratory findings suggestive of, an organic disease capable of causing failure to gain weight. Generally, environmental factors influence a child's intake or use of calories. This form of the disorder is commonly believed to result from a complex interactive pattern between the infant and the primary caregivers.

Mixed failure to thrive is caused by a combination of organic and inorganic factors. The initial problem may be physical, such as respiratory distress, which limits effective suckling. This difficulty in turn interferes with the caregiver's sense of adequacy

and ability to provide nurturing care to the infant. The infant becomes more irritable and difficult to manage, further increasing the caregiver's sense of inadequacy.

Persistent failure to gain weight is considered to originate with malnutrition. The long-term effects of undernutrition, regardless of the cause, may include secondary immune system dysfunction, deficiencies in micronutrients, and developmental delays in all major areas. Associated immune system dysfunctions include reductions in complement, secretory immunoglobulin A (IgA), and T cell function. Affected children may have repeated gastrointestinal or respiratory infections, with each episode raising the child's caloric needs and lowering intake, resulting in even greater vulnerability. Micronutrient deficiencies often complicate undernutrition by causing anemia and rickets. Iron and calcium deficiencies tend to increase lead absorption, which can lead to constipation, abdominal pain, or anorexia. Zinc deficiency impairs growth directly and can also interfere with taste bud function. Chronic undernutrition in the first 2 years of life can result in limited brain size, a reduction in neuronal number, and decreased synaptic complexity. Acquired microcephaly may persist even when somatic growth recovers.

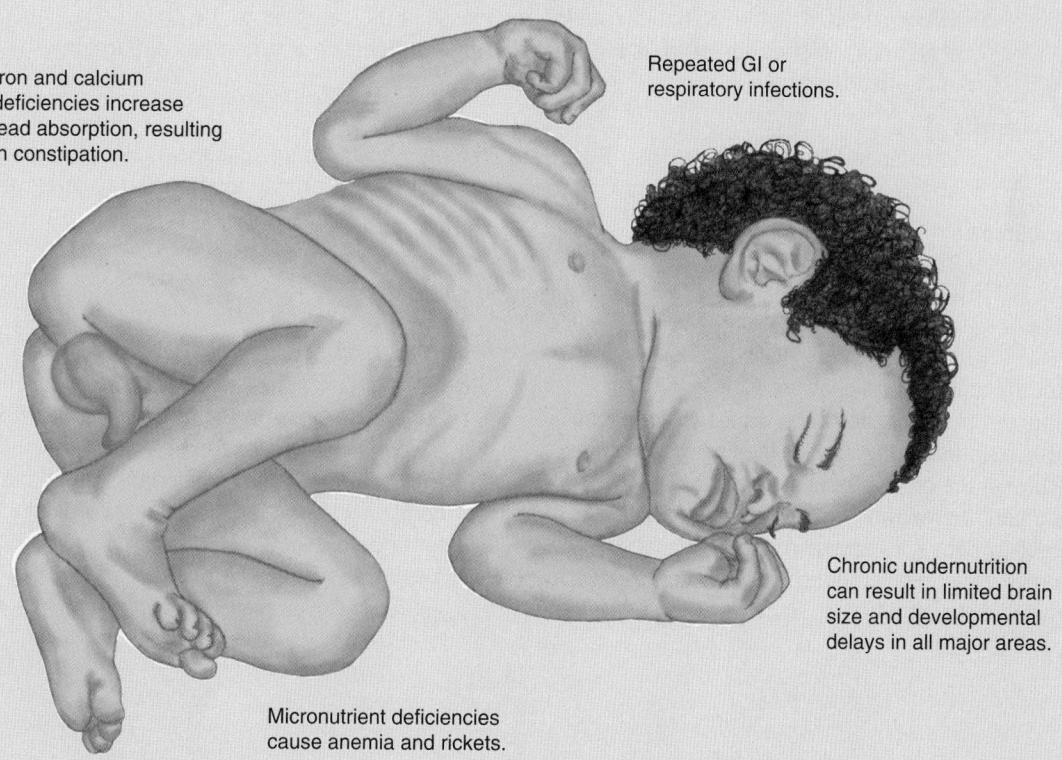

Failure to thrive

Iron and calcium deficiencies increase lead absorption, resulting in constipation.

Repeated GI or respiratory infections.

Chronic undernutrition can result in limited brain size and developmental delays in all major areas.

Micronutrient deficiencies cause anemia and rickets.

Nursing Care Plan

The Child Who Is Failing to Thrive

FOCUSED ASSESSMENT

The initial assessment should include a complete history of the presenting problem, with an emphasis on age at onset, recent changes in the child's routines (e.g., travel out of the country), and attendance at large daycare centers or shelter-type living environments. The nurse should also obtain information about any chronic nasal obstruction, episodes of bronchitis or wheezing, or other respiratory difficulties. Information about stool frequency, consistency, and any discomfort associated with excretion should be documented. A thorough dietary history should include all drinks, meals, and snacks consumed by the child, as well as where, when, how, and by whom the child is typically fed. The nurse should explore possible reasons for low intake, such as recurrent infections or medical complications of earlier episodes of malnutrition (Box 53-4). Common dietary patterns may be overlooked if the dietary history is not carefully investigated.

The physical examination should focus especially on the skin, hair, nails, and mucous membranes of the child to identify signs of malnutrition. Also, the nurse should look for lesions that could interfere with eating, such as dental caries, tongue enlargement, mandibular hypoplasia, unrecognized submucosal cleft palate, or tonsillar hypertrophy.

The nurse should complete a thorough psychosocial history that focuses on income, family (dis)organization, social isolation, stress factors, support systems, and family psychopathology, such as maternal depression, family violence, or alcoholism. It is important to ask about the availability of food, especially around the time of arrival of a paycheck or other forms of income. Finally, the psychosocial history should include questions about facilities for storing and preparing food.

Assessment of infant-parent interactions should focus on the ways in which the child is held and fed, how eye contact is initiated and maintained, and the facial expressions of both the child and the caregiver during interactions. Observations of various kinds of interactions are also important and should include play, talk, and touch by both the child and caregiver, as well as the other's reaction to these attempts to engage in interaction. The nurse should note the responses of the caregiver to the child's cues, such as when the child cries, reaches out, or looks toward the caregiver. A feeling of synchrony or harmony should be sensed in the interaction.

Nursing Diagnosis

Imbalanced Nutrition: Less Than Body Requirements related to insufficient intake of calories, incomplete absorption of nutrients, impaired interactions with caregivers, or inadequate care by caregivers.

Expected Outcome

The child's caloric intake will:
- Increase, as evidenced by an increase in physical growth.

INTERVENTION	RATIONALE
1. Monitor the child's nutritional status: • Document physical alterations, especially changes in physical status during or after feedings. • Document the child's feeding patterns. • Document the nature of parent-child interactions, especially before, during, and after feedings. 2. Encourage the caregiver to discuss both positive and negative feelings about care, procedures, and interactions with the child.	1. Fatigue, colic, or respiratory distress may indicate an underlying cause of the disorder. Subtle deficits may have a significant bearing on nutritional intake. Psychological components revealed in the context of interactions may be the most significant indicators of the cause for undernutrition. 2. The caregiver may be unaware of some of the underlying feelings that may be affecting the infant-caregiver relationship.

Nursing Care Plan

The Child Who Is Failing to Thrive—cont'd

INTERVENTION	RATIONALE
3. Increase the child's caloric intake by feeding the child on demand or increasing intake as tolerated, offering high-protein snacks between meals, offering small portions of a wide variety of food at mealtimes, teaching the child healthy mealtime behaviors (decrease distractions, make mealtime pleasurable), planning naps or rest periods, and intervening in the event of fretfulness or crying.	3. The child's intake must be greater than the caloric expenditure.
4. Monitor the child's intake and output.	4. Fluid loss may affect daily weight patterns.
5. Weight should be measured daily at the same time, using the same scales, and with the child dressed in the same amount of clothing each time.	5. This approach reduces the effect of various factors that influence weight measurements.
6. Provide a consistent caregiver from the nursing staff.	6. This strategy increases trust and provides the child with an adult who anticipates needs, thus decreasing the child's level of frustration.

Evaluation

- Is the child attaining developmental milestones?
- Does the child eat the food offered?
- Do the parents participate in feeding the child?
- Does the child's physical growth show an increase?

Nursing Diagnosis

Deficient Knowledge related to lack of experience and of positive parenting training.

Expected Outcome

Knowledge related to parenting will:

- Increase, as evidenced by caregiver holding and maintaining eye contact with the child and participating in feeding the child and by expression by the parents of realistic expectations of the child based on the child's developmental needs.

INTERVENTION	RATIONALE
1. Provide instruction in child care, being sure to model appropriate adult-child interactions. Include techniques for holding, touching, and feeding the child.	1. Instruction, coupled with modeling and practice, will facilitate integration of information.
2. Exhibit a positive attitude toward the parents.	2. Acceptance increases trust and fosters openness to learning.
3. Provide information regarding normal growth and development.	3. Parents may lack an understanding of normal growth and development and may have unrealistic expectations of the child.
4. Provide for rooming-in with the child.	4. This arrangement allows the nurse to observe parent-child interactions and provide further teaching if necessary.
5. Teach the parents ways to increase the child's caloric intake and to minimize the control issues associated with mealtimes (See Parents Want to Know: About Effective Feeding Practices box, p. 1558).	5. Lack of previous experience and knowledge may result in ineffective parenting skills.

Evaluation

- Have the parents been observed interacting appropriately with the child during meals?
- Do the parents verbalize an openness to learning new techniques of feeding?
- Are the parents holding and touching the child?
- Have the parents asked appropriate questions related to parenting?

Common Reasons for Inadequate Nutritional Intake in Infants and Children

- Overdilution of formula
- Large quantities of cereal or baby food in bottles
- Excessive intake of fluids other than formula or milk
- Selection of foods with inappropriate texture for infant's stage of development
- Infrequent feedings, especially in children who are temperamentally quiet or undemanding
- No set feeding times
- No highchair
- Frequent small sips from a bottle (grazing)
- Distractions during feedings (television, social interactions)
- Struggles over feeding between caregiver and child

Manifestations and Risk Factors

Physical Indicators

Physical indicators of failure to thrive include weight below the 5th percentile, a sudden or rapid deceleration in the growth curve, delay in reaching developmental milestones, and decreased muscle mass. Muscle hypotonia, abdominal distention, generalized weakness, and cachexia (general ill health and malnutrition) are additional signs.

Behavioral Indicators

Behavioral indicators of failure to thrive include avoidance of eye contact, avoidance of physical touch, intense watchfulness, and sleep disturbances. Lack of age-appropriate stranger anxiety, inappropriate lack of preference for one's own parents, and disturbed affect (e.g., apathy, extreme irritability, extreme compliance) may also be observed. Repetitive self-stimulating behaviors, such as rocking, head banging, intense sucking, intense chewing on fingers or hands, and head rolling, are also seen.

Diagnostic Evaluation

The differential diagnosis is generally made by a multidisciplinary team whose initial task is to search for an organic cause of the growth failure. If no cause is identified, the approach is to diagnose by response. Nutrition and nurturing are provided in a consistent manner, and if the infant gains the expected weight, nonorganic failure to thrive is considered to be the appropriate diagnosis.

Therapeutic Management

Treatment provides nutritional therapy to increase the child's caloric intake. The goal is for the child to grow at two to three times the average rate for age. Daily multivitamin supplements with minerals are often prescribed to ensure that specific nutritional deficiencies do not occur in the course of rapid growth. Caloric enrichment of food is essential, and formula may be concentrated in titrated amounts up to 24 calories per ounce. Greater concentrations can lead to diarrhea and dehydration.

PARENTS
Want to Know

About Effective Feeding Practices

Almost all children at one time or another do not eat as well as parents would like. If you are concerned about your child's eating, these guidelines may help:

- Children do well with schedules. Try to maintain consistent mealtimes and snack times each day.
- Children need to eat often, not constantly. Offer something every 2 to 3 hours, allowing three meals and two or three snacks per day.
- Make sure your child can easily reach the food served. Use a highchair, telephone books, or small table. Be certain the child is safely secured.
- Allow children to feed themselves. Try very small amounts at first. Offer seconds later. Expect messiness, and prepare in advance for easy cleanup (use bibs, newspapers under the highchair, or whatever works for you). If you are worried that little food actually gets into the child's mouth, use two spoons: one for the baby to control, and one for you to use for feeding.
- Do not force-feed, bribe, or cajole! These approaches will backfire.

- Do not worry if your child wants to eat the same food every day; many children are like that. Variety is not important to a toddler's nutrition. What matters is the total caloric and protein intake.
- At mealtimes, offer solids first. Liquids are filling and provide fewer calories.
- Limit the amount of juice, water, and carbonated drinks consumed. Offer milk or formula instead.
- Offer foods that are easy for your child to handle. Finger foods, such as Cheerios, French fries, slices of banana, and peas, are ideal. Make sure pieces are small to avoid the child's choking.
- For more calories per bite, add margarine, mayonnaise, gravies, and grated cheese to foods. For snacks, use peanut butter, cheese, pudding, bananas, or dried fruit.
- Limit the consumption of junk foods, such as soda, chips, and candy. They take up valuable space in the stomach without providing nutrients.
- Eat with your child or allow your child to eat with others, so that meals and snacks can be fun.

Modified from Frank, D.A., Silva, M., & Needlman, R. (1993, Feb.). Failure to thrive: Mystery, myth, and method. *Contemporary Pediatrics, 10,* 121.

KEY CONCEPTS

- In children and adolescents, the behavioral manifestations of anxiety and depression may be similar. Individuals with both diagnoses may be withdrawn, tearful, unwilling to engage in play, and aggressive toward others.
- It is difficult to differentiate between normal mood changes secondary to developmental maturation and abnormal, persistent mood disturbances.
- Separation anxiety and school avoidance need to be addressed if the problem becomes persistent or debilitating. Such anxiety is characterized by excessive fear, even panic, of being away from the parent or home.
- A suicide gesture or statement should never be ignored.
- Protecting a child or adolescent from inflicting harm to self involves being emotionally and physically available, offering opportunities to discuss feelings and the suicidal event, and removing potentially harmful objects.
- Support for grieving families of suicidal or potentially suicidal individuals is best provided on both an individual and a group basis to allow exploration of personal issues and social support.
- Anorexia nervosa is characterized by a deliberate refusal to maintain adequate body weight, a distorted body image, and amenorrhea (in female patients).
- One common factor among children with an eating disorder is a family system in which the individual is considered to be an exten-

sion of the parent or serves as a means of meeting the parents' needs, rather than being allowed to develop as an autonomous individual. The mother tends to be overprotective, lacking in empathy, and overly invested in the daily activities of the child. The father is often emotionally distant from the mother and the child.

- The focus of care for an adolescent with an eating disorder involves restructuring cognitive perceptions, reducing opportunities for engaging in ritualistic and self-injurious behaviors, and reestablishing physiologic homeostasis.
- During the early treatment phase of eating disorders, it may be necessary to observe the adolescent after meals to prevent episodes of purging.
- Attention-deficit hyperactivity disorder (ADHD) is a developmental disorder characterized by developmentally inappropriate degrees of inattention, overactivity, and impulsivity.
- Support groups are important in assisting families to cope with and modify expectations and interactions involving the child with ADHD.
- Educating the family about ADHD is a crucial component of caring for the child with this disorder.
- Low grades, irregular school attendance, aggressive or rebellious behavior, deteriorating relationships with family members or former friends, rapid or extreme changes in behaviors or mood, and loss of interest in hobbies,

sports, or other activities are some common signs of substance abuse.

- An individual with a substance abuse problem, together with the family, should receive help in developing social support systems, with referral to appropriate resources that can offer additional support as they attempt to make long-term changes in their social and emotional patterns of relating.
- Child abuse tends to increase during times of economic hardship or external stress. Abusive families are often isolated, lack a support system, exhibit low levels of trust, resolve conflict through aggression, assume fixed and traditional roles within the family, and establish rigid rules.
- All suspected child abuse must be reported to the appropriate authorities.
- Abusive parents often have unrealistic expectations of their children, which may relate to lack of knowledge of normal growth and development.
- Role modeling positive parenting skills is an effective intervention in the care of the child who has been abused.
- The assessment of infant-parent interactions in cases of nonorganic failure to thrive should include observation of the ways in which the child is held and fed, how eye contact is initiated and maintained, and the facial expressions of both the child and the caregiver during interactions.

ANSWERS to Critical Thinking Exercise 53-1

1. Matthew may have fallen while at the baby-sitter's or even at home and either sprained or fractured his arm. Two-year-olds are curious and also like to climb. Children get frequent scrapes and bruises at this age. Because of the injured arm, bruises, and abrasion, physical abuse is also a possibility.
2. Matthew should be assessed for other bruises in various stages of healing or clustered in patterns reflecting the shape of a hand or an article that may have caused the bruise. The nurse must determine if the injury matches the description of the cause. The nurse should also check for records of

other emergency department visits for injuries or signs of old fractures on Matthew's radiographs. In addition, the nurse should gather information about the baby-sitter: Has any other injury occurred while Matthew was in the sitter's care? What explanation did the sitter give for Matthew's behavior when his mother picked him up? During the interview, the nurse should observe both Ms. Jackson and her boyfriend to assess their relationship with Matthew. Do they comfort him? Do they respond to his needs? Do they seem overly concerned about the injury? Matthew's behavior is not

typical of an abused child. He seeks comfort from his parent and does not appear apathetic. If, at the end of the interview, history, assessment, and diagnostic testing, it is determined that an adult did not inflict the injury, the nurse should use the opportunity to explore ways that the injury could have been prevented. The roles of mother, baby-sitter, and boyfriend should be incorporated into the discussion.
3. If the nurse suspects child abuse, it must be reported to child protective services.

REFERENCES and READINGS

American Academy of Child and Adolescent Psychiatry. (1997). Practice parameters for the assessment and treatment of children and adolescents with anxiety disorders. *Journal of the American Academy of Child and Adolescent Psychiatry, 36*(Suppl. 10), 69S-84S.

American Academy of Child and Adolescent Psychiatry. (1998). Practice parameters for the assessment and treatment of children and adolescents with depressive disorders. *Journal of the American Academy of Child and Adolescent Psychiatry, 37*(Suppl. 10), 63S-83S.

American Psychiatric Association. (2000). *Diagnostic and statistical manual of mental disorders* (4th ed., Text Revision.). Washington, DC: Author.

Bassali, R. & Benjamin, J. (2002). *Failure to thrive* [on-line]. Available at www.emedicine.com/ped/topic738.htm#target6.

REFERENCES and READINGS

Bennett, K. (2000). Munchausen syndrome by proxy abuse. *Journal of Child Health Care, 4,* 163-166.

D'Augelli, A.R., Hershberger, S.L., & Pilkington, N.W. (2001). Suicidality patterns and sexual orientation–related factors among lesbian, gay, and bisexual youths. *Suicide & Life-Threatening Behavior, 31*(3), 250-264.

Gould, M.S., Greenberg, T., Velting, D.M., & Shaffer, D. (2003). Youth suicide risk and preventive interventions: A review of the past 10 years. *Journal of the American Academy of Child and Adolescent Psychiatry, 42*(4), 386-405.

Leslie, L. (2002). The role of primary care physicians in attention deficit/ hyperactivity disorder. *Pediatric Annals, 31*(8), 475-484.

Meyers, S., Eisenhauer, N., & Ryan, M. (2003). ADHD: It is real and it can be treated. *The Clinical Advisor: A Forum for Nurse Practitioners, 6*(3), 15-25.

National Institute of Drug Abuse (NIDA). (2002). *Monitoring the future study* [on-line]. Available at www.nida.nih.gov.

National Institute of Mental Health (NIMH). (2001, Jan.). *In harm's way: Suicide in America* [on-line]. Available at www.nimh.nih.gov/publicat/harmaway.cfm.

Pataki, C. (2000). Mood disorders and suicide in children and adolescents. In B.J. Saddock & V.A. Saddock (Eds.), *Kaplan and Saddock's comprehensive textbook of psychiatry* (pp. 2740-2757). Philadelphia: Lippincott.

Rushton, J.L., Forcier, M., & Schectman, R.M. (2002). Epidemiology of depressive symptoms in the National Longitudinal Study of Adolescent Health. *Journal of the American Academy of Child and Adolescent Psychiatry, 41*(2), 199-205.

Russell, S.T., & Joyner, K. (2001). Adolescent sexual orientation and suicide risk: Evidence from a national study. *American Journal of Public Health, 91*(8), 1276-1281.

Sadock, B., & Sadock, V.A. (2003). *Kaplan and Sadock's synopsis of psychiatry: Behavioral sciences/clinical psychiatry* (9th ed.) Philadelphia: Lippincott Williams & Wilkins.

Schuckit, M.A. (2000). Alcohol related disorders. In B.J. Sadock & V.A. Sadock (Eds.), *Comprehensive textbook of psychiatry* (pp. 953-971). Lippincott Williams & Wilkins.

Shelton, D. (2000). Child mental health policy. *Journal of Pediatric Nursing, 15,* 115-118.

Sirotnak, A.P. (2003). *Child abuse and neglect: Failure to thrive* [on-line]. Available at www.emedicine.com/ped/topic2647.htm.

Steward, D.K., & Garvin, B.J. (1997). Nonorganic failure to thrive: A theoretical approach. *Journal of Pediatric Nursing, 12*(6), 342-347.

U.S. Department of Health and Human Services (U.S. DHHS). (2000a). *Child maltreatment 1998: Reports from the states to the national child abuse and neglect data system.* Washington, DC: U.S. Government Printing Office.

U.S. Department of Health and Human Services (U.S. DHHS). (2000b). *Healthy People 2010* (Conference edition, in 2 volumes). Washington, DC: Author.

U.S. Department of Health and Human Services (U.S. DHHS), Administration on Children, Youth and Families. (2003). *Child welfare outcomes 2002: Annual report.* Washington, DC: U.S. Government Printing Office.

Usinski, R. (2002). Shaken baby syndrome: Fundamental question. *British Journal of Neurosurgery 16*(3), 217-219.

The Child with a Cognitive Impairment

After studying this chapter, you should be able to:

◎ Define the concepts of cognitive impairment, mental retardation, and developmental disability.
◎ Identify the various causes of mental retardation.
◎ Identify specific tools used in assessing the presence and degree of mental retardation.
◎ Identify educational and support resources for families with a child who is mentally retarded or developmentally delayed.
◎ Develop appropriate nursing strategies for supporting the family and child with mental retardation or developmental delay.
◎ Develop nursing strategies for families caring for a child with Down syndrome.

◎ Identify behavioral characteristics and appropriate nursing actions when working with a child with fragile X syndrome.
◎ Identify the basic diagnostic criteria for autism.
◎ Explain the ways autism differs from other types of pervasive developmental disorders.
◎ Identify the major considerations in working with the family of an autistic child.
◎ Develop home care interventions appropriate to the family's abilities and the developmental needs of a child with a cognitive disability.

◆ **DEFINITIONS**

co-morbidity The occurrence of two or more different disorders in the same individual; children with cognitive impairments often have coexisting psychiatric disorders.

echolalia Stereotyped repetition of another person's words or phrases.

functional age The age equivalent at which the child is actually able to perform specific self-care or relational tasks; for example, the child may be 6 years old chronologically but only able to perform skills representative of children 4 years old, and thus the child's functional age is 4 years.

intelligence The innate capacity of the individual; what individuals can do relative to learning, thinking, and problem solv-

ing; results obtained on intelligence tests that measure specific skills, such as verbal, nonverbal, or mechanical abilities.

mutation Variation in a gene that affects its function.

pervasive developmental disorders (PDDs) Infant and childhood disorders characterized by severe and pervasive impairment in several areas of development in a manner distinctly deviant from the individual's developmental level or mental age (American Psychiatric Association, 2000).

premutation Gene alteration that is generally not associated with symptoms, but could be inherited as a full mutation.

Common Diagnostic Tests for Cognitive Disorders

Test	Description	Normal Findings	Indications	Nursing Implications
Vision Test	Assessment of vision, ocular pressure, and structural defects	Normal vision, normal structures	Children with Down syndrome; 40%-45% have refractive errors, cataracts, or other visual problems.	Explain pupil dilation. Provide protective eyewear following the examinations.
Hearing Test	Assessment of perception of sound frequency and volume	Normal hearing range	Children with Down syndrome; 70%-80% have hearing defects. Children with autism and pervasive developmental disorder (PDD); often appear to have defective hearing, despite normal hearing function, so hearing tests should be conducted.	Explain the test in simple terms. The test may require that the child wear a headphone, which may be difficult to tolerate.
Thyroid Studies	Blood serum tests to determine thyroid levels—serum thyroxine	Ages 1-3 yr: 6.8-13.5 mcg/dl Ages 3-10 yr: 5.5-12.8 mcg/dl Puberty to adulthood: 4.2-13.0 mcg/dl	Children with Down syndrome; slowed growth rates are common.	These studies should not be performed within 7 days of a radionuclide scan.
Adaptive Behavior Scales*	Assessment of language, motor, social, and self-care skills	Age-expected skills within 1 standard deviation (SD) from the mean	Children with suspected developmental delays.	Explain the test and how results will be interpreted.
IQ Tests†	Assessment of cognitive abilities	Age-normal skills within 1½ SD from the mean	Children with suspected developmental delays.	Explain the test and how results will be interpreted.
Bone Roentgenography	Assessment of bone plates and joint spaces	Age-expected bone age	Children with Down syndrome; decreased growth rate is common.	The child must be motionless during the study.
Brain Sonography	Ultrasonogram of cranium	Normal position of brain's midline structures and normal blood flow velocity, no hemorrhages	Microcephaly or macrocephaly, misshapen cranium, family history of hydrocephaly.	The child must be supine. Any jewelry or metal objects should be removed from the child's head. The child may need sedation or may need to be restrained, because this procedure takes 1 hr to complete. Explain to the child that the test is not painful. Keep the child warm during the procedure.

*Adaptive behavior scales include the American Association on Mental Retardation (AAMR) test, the Minnesota Child Development Inventory Profile (MCDI), the Denver Developmental Screening Test (DDST-II), the Wechsler Preschool and Primary Scale of Intelligence (WPPSI), the Wechsler Intelligence Scale for Children (WISC-III), and the Wechsler Adult Intelligence Scale—Revised (WAIS-R).
†IQ tests include the Bayley Scales (birth to 3 yr), the Stanford-Binet Scale (2 yr and older), the WPPSI (3-6 yr), the WISC-III (6-16 yr), and the WAIS-R (16 yr and older).

Common Diagnostic Tests for Cognitive Disorders—cont'd

Test	Description	Normal Findings	Indications	Nursing Implications
Genetic Analysis	Cytogenic bonding, culture media analysis	Normal findings for gene product analysis	Suspected genetic or neoplastic disorders.	Allow the child an opportunity to ask questions and express concerns about the possible results and implications of the testing.
Computed Tomography (CT)	Special noninvasive radiographic technique that images brain tissue in very thin sections	No blood clots, tumors, or infections	Impaired development, such as microcephaly; family history of central nervous system malformations; possible tumors or subdural hematomas.	The child may need to be sedated or restrained and will need to assume supine position. CT scans require the use of contrast medium and so require informed consent.
Magnetic Resonance Imaging (MRI)	Noninvasive method used to create images corresponding to density of tissue	Normal anatomy and physiology of the brain and spinal column	Same as for CT.	The test requires informed consent. Remove metal or magnetic objects from the child before the study. Sedation of the child is usually required.
Positron Emission Tomography (PET)	Noninvasive means of comparing cerebral brain flow and metabolic changes; used to localize seizure foci, visualize brain hemodynamics, and study brain pharmacology using radioisotopes	Normal metabolism of glucose in brain, normal blood flow and electrical activity	Seizures, hydrocephaly, evidence of cerebral dysfunction.	The test requires informed consent. The child will need to be sedated. Liquids may be limited before the procedure. If not in diapers, the child will need to void before the procedure. Parents may be able to remain with the child during the procedure

CLINICAL REFERENCE ■

Children with cognitive impairments have significant impairments in measured intelligence and adaptive behavior. Cognitive impairments can result from malformations of the brain and central nervous system, injury, infections, anoxia, or poisoning, or the cause may be unknown. Specific disabilities are differentiated on the basis of an assessment of language, cognition, academic ability, self-help skills, social behaviors, and motor performance.

A cognitive impairment may be classified as a general delay, such as in mental retardation, or as a part of a larger constellation of failures in skill acquisition, such as in pervasive developmental disorders (PDDs). There is considerable overlap within several cognitive-related disorders. For example, children with autism, a specific disorder classified as a PDD, are often moderately or severely mentally retarded.

The family of a child with a cognitive impairment must cope with frequent and exceptionally high demands. The family is confronted with serious medical and environmental issues that rarely seem to be solved, only managed. Independence and self-management should be emphasized throughout childhood and adolescence so that, as the individual reaches adulthood, the possibility of independent living and gainful employment can be maximized.

The nurse is an integral part of the multidisciplinary team that manages the care of a child with a cognitive impairment. The nurse is involved in early assessment of the child, support of the family, assistance with self-care training and behavioral training, referral to support services, and providing the necessary nursing care for other disabilities the child may have. School and community nurses need a broad range of knowledge to support children who have multiple cognitive and physical disabilities.

TERMINOLOGY

The terminology associated with cognitive impairment differs according to the context of the setting in which the child is seen. Nurses encounter children with cognitive impairments in the hospital and community. The medical interpretation of cognitive impairment might differ from the legal interpretation; implications for nursing care will vary accordingly.

Cognitive Impairment

Cognitive impairment is a general term that denotes limitations in intellectual and functional abilities. Intelligence is a difficult concept, defined in a number of ways. The nurse needs to determine the meaning of the word as it is used by the professional and by the parent. Often, the child's intelligence quotient (IQ) has little meaning for the parent, so the nurse may need to explain its meaning and purpose. *Mental age* and *functional age* are terms often used to compare a child's mental ability with the expected mental or functional abilities of other children of the same chronologic age. Mental age gives some information about the level of cognitive understanding. For example, if an individual has a mental age of 5 years, the nurse's explanations need to be simple and specific, regardless of the individual's chronologic age. If the individual has a mental age of 12 years, however, the nurse's explanations can provide more description and detail and can require some degree of inductive reasoning.

Functional age does not include the individual's life experience or functioning in adaptive skills. For example, an adult with a functional age of 12 years does not "have the mind of a 12-year-old" because that individual may have been affected by environmental experiences, such as job training and group living situations.

Mental Retardation

The term *mental retardation* is often misunderstood and considered derogatory because some believe the definition relates only to low IQ measurements and to the perception that mentally retarded people cannot learn self-care (American Academy of Child and Adolescent Psychiatry, 1995). Although mentally retarded persons may have below-normal cognitive and adaptive functioning, with support, many can be educated, learn to hold a job, and independently accomplish some self-care activities.

Mental retardation is not diagnosed unless the following conditions have been met (American Psychiatric Association, 2000; American Association on Mental Retardation, 2001):

- Manifests before age 18 years
- Includes significant subaverage general intellectual functioning
- Concurrent deficits in two or more adaptive areas, such as communication, home living, community use, health and safety, leisure, self-care, social skills, self-direction, functional academics, and work

Other terms used to describe individuals with mental retardation are *developmentally disabled, mentally handicapped,* and *mentally deficient.* The term applied usually reflects more the discipline of the professional assigning the diagnostic label rather than manifestations.

When standardized tests of intelligence are used, subaverage general intellectual functioning refers to an IQ score of 70 or below. Adaptive functioning refers to effective coping with common life demands, as well as the ability to maintain acceptable community standards of personal independence expected of individuals of the same age-group, sociocultural background, and community setting.

The American Association on Mental Retardation (AAMR), the leading professional organization in the area of mental retardation, has proposed that the subaverage intellectual functioning score definition be modified to include individuals with an intellectual functioning score of 70 to 75. The AAMR emphasizes that the assessment of mental retardation be done within a cultural and environmental context and with a focus on the individual's adaptive strengths and supports (American Association on Mental Retardation, 2001).

Developmental Disability

Developmental disability is a term that has implications more for legal, administrative, and educational spheres than in medical or nursing diagnosis and treatment. The U.S. government, in its attempt to provide equal rights for all disabled individuals, has defined a developmental disability as having the following components (Developmental Disabilities Assistance and Bill of Rights Act of 2000, 2000):

- Severe and chronic disability that is attributable to mental or physical impairment or a combination of both.
- The impairment must be present before the individual turns 22 years old.
- The impairment is likely to continue, reflecting the need for lifelong individual services or supports.
- There must be substantial functional limitations in three or more areas, such as self-care, receptive and expressive language, learning, mobility, self-direction, capacity for independent living, or economic self-sufficiency.

The definition of developmental disability encompasses children with mental retardation, sensory deficits (hearing, vision, speech), orthopedic problems, and conditions such as cerebral palsy and PDDs.

Provisions in law that affect individuals with various disabilities have implications for nurses working in community or school settings. The Education for All Handicapped Children Act (EAHCA, PL 94-142) passed in 1975 required that states provide an education for all disabled children ages 3 to 21 years that is free and appropriate and in the least restrictive environment. Although the terminology has changed, this means that developmentally disabled children should be included in a regular classroom with their nondisabled peers. In 1990, this act was renamed the Individuals With Disabilities Education Act, and it was reapproved in 1997.

PL 99-457, signed into law in 1986, provided for early intervention for younger children. Early childhood intervention programs, such as Head Start, are ensured for any child with mental or physical disability from birth to age 3 years, at which time the public school system becomes involved.

As a result of these legislative efforts, each disabled child must have a written individualized education program (IEP) that outlines specialized instruction and services the school system will provide. The child's parents and school personnel design this after the school conducts an educational assessment. School nurses often sit on teams that design the IEP, giving expert advice about classroom adaptations or medical services needed for these children. When working with these families, the nurse may need to serve as a resource for helping families locate advocacy services for their children.

COGNITIVE IMPAIRMENT

Etiology

Cognitive impairment may be the result of congenital or early environmental factors such as maternal substance abuse or lack of stimulation in early childhood. It may also be secondary to head injury, asphyxia, intracranial hemorrhage, infections, poisoning, or the presence or treatment of a brain tumor. Mental retardation has more than 350 known causes, but its specific cause is unknown in nearly half of all cases. New etiologies are being identified, and underlying mechanisms of known causes are becoming more clearly understood.

As medical technology advances, a medical basis for cognitive and adaptive impairments is found in an increasing proportion of cognitively impaired children. Often the cause is a subtle but nonetheless significant biologic factor, such as minor chromosomal abnormalities, rare genetic syndromes,

---

> **BOX 54-1**
> *Causes of Cognitive Impairment*
>
> **Hereditary Origin (5%)**
> *Inborn errors of metabolism:* galactosemia, Tay-Sachs disease, phenylketonuria
> *Hereditary syndromes:* muscular dystrophy, tuberous sclerosis, neurofibromatosis
> *Chromosomal aberrations:* Down syndrome, fragile X syndrome
> *Familial retardation of probable polygenic origin*
>
> **Early Embryonic Alterations (30%–35%)**
> *Sporadic chromosomal changes:* Down syndrome
> *Multiple congenital anomalies:* congenital hypothyroidism
> *Prenatal influence syndrome:* intrauterine infections, drugs, human immunodeficiency virus (HIV), unknown forces
> *Intrauterine infections:* congenital rubella, toxoplasmosis, herpes
>
> **Early Intrauterine or Neonatal Alterations (10%–15%)**
> *Fetal malnutrition:* placental insufficiency, pregnancy-induced hypertension, drug addiction, maternal uterine cancer, multiple pregnancy
> *Neonatal conditions:* prematurity, neonatal asphyxia, hyperbilirubinemia, hypoglycemia, central nervous system hemorrhage, ABO incompatibilities
>
> **Acquired Childhood Conditions or Diseases (3%–5%)**
> *Complications of infections:* meningitis, encephalitis, pertussis, varicella
> *Lead poisoning*
> *Cranial trauma*
> *Cerebral tumors*
> *Cardiac arrest*
> *Asphyxiation*
>
> **Environmental Problems and Behavioral Syndromes (20%)**
> *Psychosocial deprivation*
> *Parental neurosis, psychosis, character disorder*
> *Childhood psychosis, autism, other pervasive developmental disorders*
>
> **Unknown Causes (30%–35%)**

Data from American Psychiatric Association. (2000). *Diagnostic and statistical manual of mental disorders* (4th ed., Text Revision). Washington, DC: Author; King, B.H., State, M.W., Shah, B., Davanzo, P.O., & Dykens, E. (1997). Mental retardation: A review of the past 10 years, part 1. *Journal of the American Academy of Child and Adolescent Psychiatry, 36*(12), 1656-1663.

subclinical lead intoxication, nutritional deficiencies, or exposure to numerous prenatal risks or trauma. Evidence suggests that early neurodevelopmental functioning and later neurologic integrity and intellectual ability are strongly associated. Low socioeconomic status and related factors have also been consistently reported as influencing cognitive function (Box 54-1).

BOX 54-2
Problems Related to Cognitive Impairment

Mild
Self-esteem issues related to presence or absence of physical features, largely determined by the cause of the cognitive disability
Social isolation and loneliness
Depression

Severe
Self-injury
Fecal smearing
Tearing of personal clothes and objects
Severe temper tantrums
Disrobing

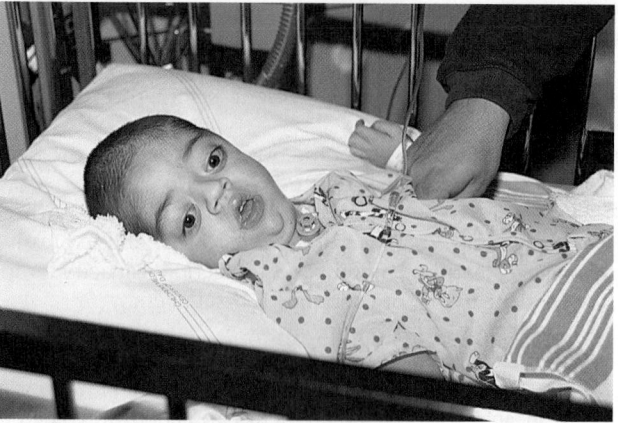

Figure 54-1 Children with cognitive impairments may have other dysfunctions as well. The family of a child with a cognitive impairment often experiences ongoing grieving because the child does not meet their expectations. This child has Marshall-Smith syndrome, which does not appear to be hereditary. His bones ossified unusually early, necessitating a craniotomy to allow greater brain development. He has a tracheostomy because of respiratory difficulties associated with an abnormally developed larynx. A gastrostomy button facilitates his nutrition. (Courtesy Children's Medical Center, Dallas, TX.)

Incidence

Cognitive impairments occur in 1% to 3% of the general population. Among those diagnosed with mental retardation, 85% display only mild cognitive impairment, 10% are classified as moderately mentally retarded, 3% to 4% are severely mentally retarded, and 1% to 2% are profoundly mentally retarded. This distribution has clinical significance in that most families are able to care for mildly to moderately impaired children and adolescents at home.

Because a diagnosis of mental retardation and other developmental disabilities is based on adaptive behavior as well as intellectual functioning, the epidemiology varies throughout the life cycle. An increased incidence of retardation is reported in the early school years, and then the incidence declines in late adolescence as the children leave the formal education setting and are assimilated into the adult world. Most cognitively impaired individuals are able to marry (often to individuals with normal intellectual functioning), maintain employment, and have satisfying relationships.

Psychiatric co-morbidity is common in people with cognitive impairment. For example, prevalence estimates for mental disorders and mental retardation are up to 60% to 70%, but the incidence is lower in children and adolescents compared with adults with mental retardation (Sadock & Sadock, 2003). Brain malfunctions that cause cognitive impairments frequently affect those areas of the brain that monitor emotional states. The most frequent accompanying diagnoses include disruptive behavioral disorders, depression, and atypical psychosis (Khan, Osinowo, & Pary, 2002).

There appears to be a significant relationship between developmental disabilities and child abuse. Children with developmental disabilities are two to three times more likely to be abused or neglected compared with their nondisabled counterparts (Sullivan & Knutson, 2000). Possible reasons for this strong relationship are the intense stress experienced by families of disabled children, parental isolation, and unrealistic expectations for the child's performance because of a lack of knowledge about normal growth and development.

Evidence also suggests that abuse can result in developmental disabilities or physically disabling conditions. Despite available funding and support groups, families of children with developmental delays often feel isolated from supportive services and report that professionals have limited understanding of their children's needs. These factors further perpetuate the sense of helplessness and lack of control in these family systems.

Manifestations

The cardinal sign of cognitive impairment or developmental disability is delayed achievement of developmental milestones. Specific congenital malformations often result in specific clinical manifestations. Also, the severity of the impairment affects the types and frequency of problem behaviors (Box 54-2).

In addition to general clinical manifestations based on the degree of impairment, many syndromes are characterized by particular features that are helpful in determining the cause of the cognitive impairment. The two most common genetic disorders in which cognitive impairment is a central feature are Down syndrome and fragile X syndrome.

Many disabilities associated with cognitive impairment can further limit a child's adaptive skills. These include cerebral palsy, visual deficits, seizure disorders, communication deficits, feeding problems, PDDs, failure to thrive, and attention-deficit hyperactivity disorder. Speech and language development are often profoundly affected. Depending on the condition, seizure disorders frequently develop as the child matures.

Although children who are cognitively impaired can be generally healthy, the presence of associated disabilities may place these children at increased risk for illness (Fig. 54-1). For example, if a child who is cognitively impaired also has

BOX 54-3
Expected Skills According to IQ Scores

Normal Intelligence (IQ 85-115)
Age-normal skills across all domains

Borderline Mental Retardation (IQ 71-84)
Early milestones achieved
Likely to be noticed when school performance is monitored
Vocational skills adequate for competitive employment

Mild Mental Retardation (IQ 50-55 to ~70)
Slight delay in achieving developmental milestones
No alteration in sequence of skill acquisition
Likely to require special education services with an emphasis on vocational and self-maintenance skills
Able to form and maintain adult relationships

Moderate Mental Retardation (IQ 35-40 to 50-55)
Noticeable delay in motor and speech development
Early and persistent training in self-care required
Supervision required for complex activities or problem solving

Severe Mental Retardation (IQ 20-25 to 35-40)
Marked delay in all motor skills
Limited expressive speech, even though some receptive language skills may be present
Constant supervision required

Profound Mental Retardation (IQ <20-25)
May be able to walk
May have primitive speech
Constant supervision required

Modified from American Psychiatric Association. (2000). *Diagnostic and statistical manual of mental disorders* (4th ed., Text Revision). Washington, DC: Author; Batshaw, M.L. (2001). *When your child has a disability.* (2nd ed.). Baltimore: Paul H. Brookes Publishing.
IQ, Intelligence quotient.

cerebral palsy, the risk for gastroesophageal reflux and aspiration pneumonia is high. Motor or swallowing problems may result in inadequate oral intake or insufficient weight gain.

Diagnostic Evaluation

Diagnostic evaluations may be performed *in utero*, during the neonatal period, or after the child fails to achieve expected developmental milestones. Tests may be general or specific for the neurologic or cognitive area in question. Several neuropsychological tests assess the child's current level of functioning and help the clinician anticipate persistent cognitive impairments. These tests—which may involve pencil-and-paper tasks, motor tasks, sensory tasks, or some degree of cognitive processing—help determine both the severity and type of cognitive impairment (Box 54-3). Learning disabilities are often identified using some of these same instruments, and many are available through the school system. Nurses also can learn to administer developmental screening tools, such as the

Denver Developmental Screening Test II (DDST-II) (see Chapter 4 and Appendix F).

Often, a diagnosis of mental retardation is not made until the child enters school and experiences significant academic failure, prompting formal psychological testing. Routine assessment of development during pediatric visits, however, is the best method of early detection.

Therapeutic Management

General Strategies

Medical strategies are directed toward preventing and treating infections, correcting structural deformities, and treating associated behaviors, such as aggressiveness. Corrective measures might include congenital heart surgery for malformations, inserting tympanostomy tubes, or placing splints on joints that are hypotonic and hyperextended. Frequently, antibiotics are given prophylactically to reduce the likelihood of infections. The treatment of behavioral difficulties and psychosocial disturbances may involve administration of medications.

Therapeutic management depends largely on community and educational resources. Obtaining services for these children, however, requires multidisciplinary efforts and strong advocacy on the part of both parents and professionals. Reduction in the occurrence of developmental disabilities is a national priority identified in *Healthy People 2010* (U.S. Department of Health and Human Services [U.S. DHHS], 2000). Adequate prenatal care is of primary importance. An additional priority related to children with disabilities is increasing the percentage of time children with disabilities spend in regular school programs (U.S. DHHS, 2000).

Safety Challenges

Children who are cognitively impaired are, by definition, less capable of managing environmental challenges than their peers who are unimpaired. Because of impaired functioning, injuries are generally more common in these children than in same-age peers. Among preschool-age children, however, injuries are less common in those with cognitive impairment, because the parents of these children are very protective and the children have less exposure to risk.

Table 54-1 presents some safety issues to be taught in the home and in the community. Although the learning needs of children who are cognitively impaired are similar to those of children without disabilities, children with cognitive impairments may need prolonged teaching, more demonstration during teaching, frequent verbal and visual reminders, and more practice.

> **! CRITICAL TO REMEMBER**
> **Safety for the Child With a Cognitive Impairment**
>
> Safety is a persistent concern of parents, teachers, and health professionals caring for children who are cognitively impaired. The child's maturation in anticipating danger, in problem solving, and in judgment is generally impaired across the life span. Children with motor disabilities are often unable to perform skills in ways that foster safety.

TABLE **54-1** Safety Concerns for Developmentally Delayed or Impaired Children

Site of Concern	Possible Injury	Education and Training Issues
HOME		
Kitchen	Burns Poisoning	*Preschool age:* preventive education (i.e., instruct not to touch hot stove, not to ingest toxic substances) *Elementary school age:* safe use of equipment, basic safety *High school age:* cooking safety, emergency precautions
Bathroom	Falls Burns Cuts	*Elementary school age:* tub safety, precautions on wet floors *High school age:* safe use of hair care equipment, shaving utensils, and similar objects
General		*Preschool and elementary school age:* avoidance of electrical outlets, safe passage around objects
Outdoors	Animal bites Poisoning Abduction	*Preschool age:* staying within boundaries, appropriate response to strange animals and people, safe use of equipment, avoidance of ingestion of berries *Elementary school age:* stranger safety, bicycle safety, traffic safety, water safety
YARD OR PLAYGROUND		
Vehicles	Cuts Falls Serious injury	*Preschool and elementary school age:* seatbelt use, keeping hands in car *High school age:* traffic safety

Nursing Care Plan

The Child With a Cognitive Impairment in the Community Setting

FOCUSED ASSESSMENT: THE CHILD

Assess cognitive skills and level of adaptive functioning, keeping in mind age-expected abilities that can be used as a standard for comparison (see Chapters 5 through 8). Life experiences also affect a child's abilities. Children who have had limited exposure to social rules and limited opportunities for thinking about their experiences will talk and act differently from children who have had more practice in these areas. Alternating between questions and demonstrations may be helpful in maintaining the child's interest in the assessment.

Look directly at the child, and speak in a direct and simple yet noncondescending manner. Ask the child for as much of the necessary information as possible rather than relying solely on the parents to provide the information. As the child speaks, attend to the child's level of communication, skill in using words to communicate, and ability to follow one-step commands or more complicated requests.

FOCUSED ASSESSMENT: THE FAMILY

Assess the family's level of functioning, particularly available coping skills and the family's awareness of and involvement in addressing the child's needs. The child may come from a home where the parents have below-average intellectual functioning; or the parents may be young and lack understanding of development, making them less aware of their child's abilities and functional deficits. Explore the family's social and financial resources in a manner that is informative but respectful of privacy. A matter-of-fact approach is helpful in assessing how the family meets the basic needs of each member and manages the exceptional medical, psychological, educational, and social needs of the child who is cognitively impaired. This part of the assessment may be lengthy because it may be necessary to assist the family in seeking long-term assistance for meeting the child's needs.

The family's interaction patterns and situational coping skills should be assessed on an ongoing basis. Families with developmentally disabled children experience grief much as do families of children with other chronic illnesses (see Chapter 36), particularly when there is no known cause for the disability. During the grief process, the family becomes preoccupied with the child's disabilities and symptoms, and then the family begins to identify the child's strengths and resources and moves toward a sense of integration and homeostasis. This process is repeated with each new developmental stage or situational setback, such as surgery or illness.

An interdisciplinary approach is critical for the effective management of children with cognitive impairments. The team generally includes physicians, nurses, psychologists, speech and language pathologists, educational and recreational professionals, and possibly physical therapists and occupational therapists. In addition to nursing care, the family may be referred for genetic counseling and supportive psychotherapy. The assessment should identify the need for other team members or auxiliary services. Long-term services may include respite care, in-home services, parent training, and support groups.

Nursing Care Plan

The Child With a Cognitive Impairment in the Community Setting—cont'd

Nursing Diagnosis

Risk for Injury related to level of self-care skills and inability to anticipate danger.

Expected Outcome

The parent and child will:
- Describe and avoid unsafe situations that lead to self-injury or unintentional injury.

INTERVENTION	RATIONALE
1. Provide anticipatory guidance relative to the child's specific developmental abilities.	1. Parents may not be able to anticipate the child's cognitive or functional level accurately, particularly if the parents are inexperienced or have limited cognitive skills themselves.
2. Keep safety rails up on hospital beds and on the bed at home if the child is predisposed to falling or roaming at night. Provide child-size furniture, and select age- and skill-related play equipment.	2. These strategies help prevent accidental falls, because these children are accident-prone and have limited ability to assess the environment for safety.
3. Give simple explanations about unsafe areas in the environment. Use the child's cognitive level as a key to what the child can understand or the degree of unsupervised freedom that can safely be allowed.	3. Young or cognitively delayed individuals can understand concrete explanations.

Evaluation

- Can the parent or child describe unsafe situations?
- Has the child remained safe and not sustained any injury?

Nursing Diagnosis

Deficient Knowledge (family members) related to unfamiliarity with the cause and likely outcomes of the child's cognitive disabilities, available support systems, or information about sexuality, vocational options, leisure skills, and so on.

Expected Outcomes

The family will:
- Describe and plan for the child's special needs.
- Access and use personal and community resources to increase the child's ability to develop personal skills for appropriate social, leisure, and vocational abilities.

INTERVENTION	RATIONALE
1. Provide information that is simple, concrete, and solution-focused.	1. Stress may impair the family's adaptive coping skills.
2. Explain any medical terms without assuming that the family knows the terminology. Give explanations to both the child and the parents. Use demonstrations and therapeutic play. If the child is hospitalized, communicate information about the child's cognitive and functional level to other team members.	2. The child may have a limited capacity to understand words but may be able to understand a demonstration.
3. Select skills that enhance self-care and socially appropriate behaviors. As the child reaches puberty, provide simple information about sexuality and physical changes. Support training in leisure skills.	3. Education that is practical and functional for the child's mental and chronologic age fosters self-esteem, compliance, and cooperation.
4. Identify for the parents local and national resources for the home care, education, and training of cognitively impaired individuals.	4. Additional services will be needed as the child grows or needs more specialized training. Families may have to find out-of-home placement if the child's disability is severe or destructive to the family.
5. Provide parents with anticipatory guidance about developmental milestones and anticipated skills, including safety, sexuality, skills that can be expected, and behavioral changes throughout the developmental process.	5. Parents may have unrealistic expectations or expect too little from the child.

Continued

Nursing Care Plan

The Child With a Cognitive Impairment in the Community Setting—cont'd

Evaluation

- Has the family made progress in describing and planning for the child's special needs?
- Has the family used the resources available in the community to maximize the child's abilities?

Nursing Diagnosis

Impaired Social Interaction related to an inability to initiate and maintain social relationships.

Expected Outcomes

The child will:
- Develop positive relationships with family and peers.
- Have solitary leisure skills.

INTERVENTION	RATIONALE
1. Encourage the parents to support the child in participating in group activities that promote peer interactions (e.g., Special Olympics, special camps) (Fig. 54-2). The family will arrange social activities with other children (e.g., visiting the park with friends, inviting friends to the home to play).	1. To accommodate to social expectations and demands, children who are cognitively impaired or developmentally disabled need to be exposed to children who are not impaired as well as to children with similar handicaps.
2. Encourage the parents to participate in interactive activities, such as reading books and playing, on a regular basis.	2. Families are likely to limit interactions because the child offers reduced reinforcements in social situations.

Evaluation

- Has the child demonstrated a sense of pleasure in social interactions with family members and with other individuals within the child's social sphere?

Nursing Diagnosis

Compromised Family Coping or Disabled Family Coping related to excessive emotional and financial strain on family members caring for an individual who is cognitively impaired, lack of acceptance by society, or an extended grieving process associated with diagnosis of a child with a chronic disability.

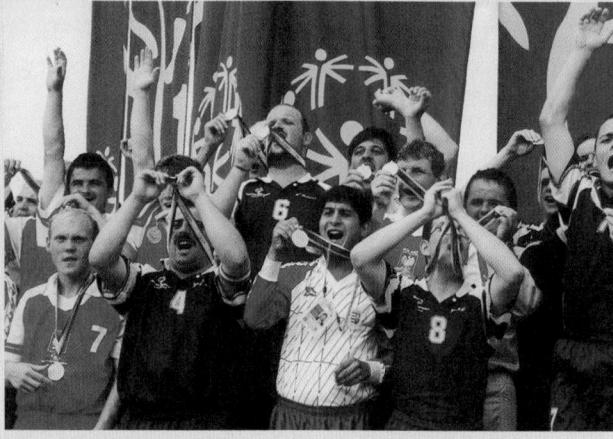

Figure 54-2 Special Olympics International is the largest recreational program in the world for people with mental retardation. With more than 1 million athletes in 125 countries, Special Olympics offers opportunities for social interaction with peers and assists children who are mentally retarded in reaching their maximum potential. (Courtesy Special Olympics, Inc.)

DOWN SYNDROME

The most common genetic disorder causing moderate to severe mental retardation is Down syndrome (trisomy 21). The assessment and nursing interventions for the child who is cognitively impaired is applicable to these individuals. Additional considerations, however, apply to those identified as having Down syndrome.

Depending on the severity of the symptoms, the most common experience is for parents to rear the child at home until early adulthood, after which group home placement is an option. Supported employment is encouraged, and parents are typically advised to initiate vocational training in elementary school. The partnership of parents and professionals is vital in managing the symptoms and in providing the comprehensive services that are needed.

Nursing Care Plan

The Child With a Cognitive Impairment in the Community Setting—cont'd

Expected Outcomes

The family will:

- Integrate the child in the family system in a manner that facilitates maximum growth and maturity.
- Express self-satisfaction in their family management.
- Demonstrate social acceptance within the community.

INTERVENTION	RATIONALE
1. Provide anticipatory and ongoing support for the grieving process. Parents should be told the diagnosis and needed information as quickly as possible. This information should be given when both parents or supportive family members are available. Information may need to be explained in different ways (orally, in writing, with videos) to help parents grasp the meaning of the diagnosis.	1. Families typically experience a cycle of grieving that is repeated when milestones are not reached or when the child experiences an illness or a change in behavior.
2. Assist in identifying appropriate resources for social interactions and social training (e.g., early intervention programs, special education programs, recreational programs for developmentally disabled children).	2. Individuals who are mildly or moderately impaired often experience loneliness and depression as a result of insufficient stimulation and social contact. Such programs can assist the child in reaching maximum potential.
3. Identify and refer the family to appropriate community resources for both emotional support and family and child education. The nurse may need to act as an advocate and referral center (about support groups, education consultants, home health agencies).	3. The grieving process and the need to accommodate to the child's skill level are ongoing; families often feel isolated and helpless in locating necessary resources.
4. Assist family members in identifying realistic short- and long-term goals for the child and themselves. Encourage the family to express feelings and concerns; provide hope when appropriate.	4. Stress, grieving, and limited knowledge may impair the family's ability to set reasonable goals itself.
5. Educate the parents in monitoring the child for alterations in health status. Help the family recognize nonverbal signs of discomfort.	5. The child may be unable to verbalize pain typically associated with ear infections, colds, or major illnesses.
6. Assist family members in exploring their choices for home care, a group home, or a residential facility.	6. Families may hesitate to discuss care options out of fear of being perceived as uncaring or unable to provide home care.

Evaluation

- Does the family integrate the child in the family system in a manner that facilitates growth and maturity to the greatest degree possible?
- Does the family seek medical attention when needed and use several resources to meet the child's social, emotional, educational, and medical needs?
- Is the family able to meet financial responsibilities?
- Does the family participate in social activities outside the family?

Services required throughout the life span include education and vocational training, transitional services, respite care, social services, financial supplements, psychotherapy, and preventive or corrective medical care (Box 54-4). This array of needed services may be overwhelming to the family, and the potential for frustration on the part of both the parents and the professional team is high. Communication and coordination of services are considered primary tasks for each team member (Fig. 54-3).

Etiology

Although the specific cause is unknown, late maternal age has been consistently identified as one of the most significant factors associated with Down syndrome. The risk of a 35-year-old woman bearing a child with trisomy 21 is 1 in 250. By age 48 years, the risk increases to 1 in 11. As a result of early screening for women who are at high risk for having

BOX 54-4
Medical Conditions Associated with Down Syndrome

Conditions Frequently Identified During the Neonatal Period
- Cardiac conditions:
  —Endocardial cushion defect
  —Tetralogy of Fallot
  —Atrial septal defects
  —Patent ductus arteriosus
  —Ventricular septal defects
- Gastrointestinal conditions:
  —Tracheoesophageal fistula
  —Pyloric stenosis
  —Imperforate anus
  —Duodenal atresia
  —Aganglionic megacolon (Hirschsprung's disease)
- Congenital cataracts
- Hypothyroidism
- Dysplastic hips
- Leukemia-like conditions

Conditions Frequently Identified During Childhood
- Endocrine disorders:
  —Decreased growth
  —Obesity secondary to overeating, underexercise, or undetected hypothyroidism
  —Thyroid dysfunction
  —Infertility (male)
  —Alopecia
  —Thin hair

- Sensitive skin and propensity for rashes
- Ophthalmic problems, such as myopia, strabismus, nystagmus, cataracts, blepharitis, and keratoconus
- Chronic serous otitis media
- Hematologic abnormalities:
  —Subtle immune deficiencies
  —Acute nonlymphoblastic leukemia
  —Acute lymphoblastic leukemia
- Craniofacial defects:
  —Malocclusions
  —Delayed tooth eruption
  —Periodontal disease and gingivitis
  —Bruxism
  —Sinusitis and rhinitis
  —Sleep apnea secondary to cranial malformations
- Musculoskeletal abnormalities:
  —Hypotonia
  —Joint laxity and dislocations
  —Atlantoaxial subluxation or dislocation
- Sensory deficits
- Seizure disorders
- Psychiatric disorders, particularly adjustment reaction disorders, anxiety disorders, depression, behavior disorders, dementia
- Pervasive developmental disorders

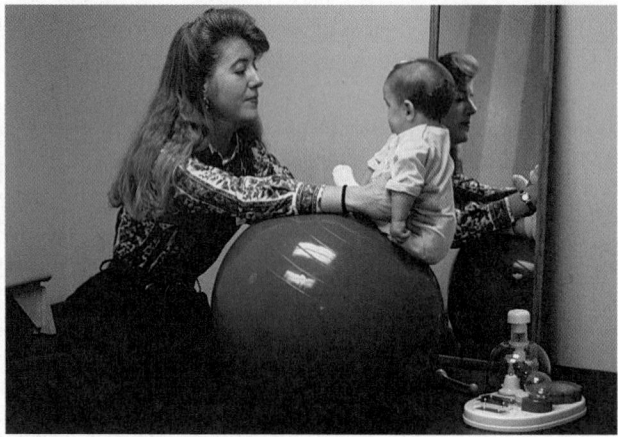

Figure 54-3 Children with delayed motor or cognitive function, whether temporary or pervasive, benefit from early and vigorous therapy to help them reach their maximum development. (Courtesy Cook Children's Medical Center, Fort Worth, TX.)

a child with Down syndrome, most of these children are now born to women younger than 35 years (75%-80% of affected children).

Several chromosomal alterations that result in Down syndrome have been identified. In 97% of Down syndrome cases, *nondisjunction*, a failure of the chromosomes to separate normally during meiosis, occurs. The remaining 3% result from *translocation*, a fusion of two chromosomes, usually 21 and 15,

resulting in a total of 46 chromosomes despite the extra chromosome 21. Translocator carrier parents are at increased risk of producing multiple offspring with Down syndrome (King, Hodapp, & Dykens, 2000).

Incidence

In the United States, more than 300,000 individuals have Down syndrome, with up to 10,000 new cases occurring each year. This syndrome accounts for one third of all cases of moderate to severe mental retardation. The prevalence of Down syndrome is 1 in 800 live births (Leshin, 2003). Affected boys outnumber girls 1.3:1.0. As a result of increased prenatal diagnosis, approximately 40% of fetuses with Down syndrome in women age 35 years or older are now aborted voluntarily. This trend has resulted in a recent decrease in the birth rate of children with Down syndrome.

Manifestations

More than 100 signs describe Down syndrome, including:

- Brachycephaly (disproportionate shortness of the head)
- Flat profile
- Upward-slanted palpebral fissures
- Inner epicanthal folds
- Wide, flat nasal bridge
- Speckled irises
- Narrow, high-arched palate

Pathophysiology

of Down Syndrome

Trisomy 21, or Down syndrome, occurs when three representatives of chromosome 21 are present instead of the usual two. There is some evidence that a particular region of chromosome 21 is responsible for the facial features, heart defects, mental retardation, and dermatologic changes. Many of the malformations in this disorder result from incomplete rather than abnormal embryogenesis. Examples include malformations of the atrioventricular canal, tracheoesophageal fistula, and imperforate anus. Alterations in neurotransmitters, particularly in the cholinergic system, are responsible for the premature aging and Alzheimer's-type dementia that are common in individuals with Down syndrome.

A number of medical problems in the newborn period can seriously compromise health and survival. If the child survives these complications, a number of less serious difficulties are generally encountered in childhood.

- Protruding tongue
- Small, short ears, which may be low-set
- Delayed teeth eruption and frequently poor alignment

Body features associated with Down syndrome include:

- Short stature
- Short, broad hands
- Simian line (single transverse palmar crease)
- Clinodactyly (in-curved little finger)
- Broad, stubby feet with plantar crease
- Wide gap between first and second toes
- Short, broad neck
- Likelihood of diastasis recti abdominis and umbilical hernia
- Small penis in males, bulbous vulva in females
- Dry skin with tendency to crack and fissure
- Hyperextensibility of joints and hypotonicity of muscles
- Atlantoaxial instability (i.e., at the first and second cervical vertebrae) in 15% of children with Down syndrome

Down syndrome is associated with intellectual, language, and social dysfunctions, including:

- Mild to severe mental retardation, with intellectual abilities that continue to decline with age
- Onset of Alzheimer's-type dementia with increasing age
- Language development characterized by particular difficulty with grammar but general strength in pragmatic language (social usage) (pragmatic language includes such skills as maintaining the conversation on a specific topic and taking turns during conversation)
- Social skills that surpass expected skills based on intellectual capacity
- Social skills and adaptive self-care skills that decline with age
- A limited ability to use the environmental cues available (i.e., infrequent scanning and use of only a few referential cues, such as eye contact with the primary caregiver, which often results in an inability to extract the information needed to draw conclusions)

- Blunted affect
- Fewer disruptive behaviors than with other chromosomal disorders

Diagnostic Evaluation

Down syndrome is usually evident at birth because of the characteristic prominent features, although if the diagnosis is questionable, chromosomal analysis is conducted. Other diagnostic tests are conducted on the basis of the associated features, such as nasopharyngeal abnormalities or cardiac defects.

To rule out associated disorders and to detect frequently encountered difficulties, clinicians recommend that the child be monitored frequently throughout the first 12 months of life, with an emphasis on gastrointestinal and cardiac symptoms. The diagnosis often requires a full cardiac work-up initially and an electrocardiogram at the end of the first year. In the 2nd to 4th years of life, the medical emphasis is on sleep and behavioral difficulties, along with annual thyroid screening and ophthalmologic assessment. Generally, the child is referred for dental assessments at 24 months and should be reevaluated medically and behaviorally at least annually throughout childhood.

Therapeutic Management

The management of Down syndrome is manifestation-specific, because there is no cure for the disorder. Surgery to correct cardiac abnormalities, gastrointestinal malformations, and craniofacial deviations has been used to prolong life, alleviate discomfort, and decrease the likelihood of further medical complications. Neck radiography should be performed before participating in any sports because of the risk of children with Down syndrome having atlantoaxial instability.

▪NURSING CARE

The Child With Down Syndrome

Assessment

Neonatal assessment is crucial in diagnosing Down syndrome on the basis of physiologic characteristics (see Chapter 22). Assessment for Down syndrome is based on family history, especially the mother's age. If Down syndrome is suspected or already confirmed on the basis of earlier genetic testing, serum alpha-fetoprotein levels, or amniotic fluid samples, an assessment is conducted to determine the severity of the manifestations and the family's ability to cope with and accommodate the needs of the infant. Assessment for mental retardation is also appropriate for the child with Down syndrome.

A thorough physical examination should be conducted, including hearing and vision examinations. Children with Down syndrome are at increased risk for hearing deficits and refractive errors or cataracts.

If a child with Down syndrome is hospitalized for surgical repair, infections, or injury, assess the child's typical coping patterns to support strategies already in place. Children with Down syndrome prefer routine and consistency, so an assessment of their daily routine is important; include times and habits related to mealtimes, bathing, and order of dressing.

Assessing the child's understanding of language and ability to communicate is important to provide information that the child can understand. Knowing the child's words for specific body functions, such as voiding, defecating, or sleeping, will allow for greater comfort for the hospitalized child. It is important to assess the child's learning abilities before initiating any education or procedure-related play.

The child's motor skills are assessed to determine what procedures will be necessary to ensure the child's safety. Children with Down syndrome often are awkward and somewhat uncoordinated, which increases the likelihood of their falling. Self-stimulating behaviors (e.g., picking at the arm) need to be identified, because they are often used as coping strategies but may also be self-injurious. Sensory deficits, such as vision or hearing difficulties, should be identified as part of the routine assessment. Such deficits can be detected by closely observing as the child reaches for objects, by listening to conversation, or by speaking the child's name. The child with Down syndrome, however, may respond to sensory stimuli less noticeably than unimpaired children or may respond with dulled affect, even if hearing or vision deficits are not present.

Health care professionals may forget the importance of discussing normal aspects of the child with parents. For example, the nurse may state, "Billy has the most beautiful eyes. They seem to light up when he sees someone he knows."

An environmental assessment will help determine whether it is conducive to safety and provides sufficient stimulation. Affected children frequently do not seek out stimulation and may need encouragement through colors, sound, and motion. An assessment of social behaviors is also important and should include play, social judgment skills, and social interest in the environment. The child may demonstrate inappropriate behaviors similar to those associated with severe mental retardation. Moreover, the child's natural curiosity may be diminished as a result of fear or frustration. Nursing care of the child with Down syndrome is similar to that for any child with a cognitive impairment with some specific additions.

Nursing Diagnosis and Planning

The nursing diagnoses and expected outcomes that are appropriate for the child with Down syndrome and the child's family are

- Impaired Parenting related to the child's delayed development, physical appearance, and medical complications.
  Expected Outcome: The family will demonstrate satisfying and supportive relationships that meet the physical and emotional needs of each family member.
- Self-Care Deficit (Bathing/Hygiene, Dressing/Grooming, Feeding, Toileting) related to cognitive immaturity.
  Expected Outcome: The child will demonstrate the ability to independently meet needs related to bathing/hygiene, dressing/grooming, feeding, and toileting.
- Delayed Growth and Development related to poor sucking abilities or mouth deformities, flaccid facial muscles, or other abnormalities.
  Expected Outcomes: The child will maximize progress toward attaining developmental milestones and will demonstrate appropriate and measurable growth during childhood.

Interventions

When the child is a neonate, the parents will need assistance and support to accept the child's diagnosis and appropriately plan for the child's care. The nurse assists the parents to identify positive features and behaviors in the child; looking at the child's strengths from the beginning reduces the likelihood that parents will see the child negatively as the child does not attain milestones along with others of the same chronologic age.

The nurse helps the parents explore options for fluid and calorie intake. Breastfeeding may not be possible if the child's muscle tone or sucking reflex is immature, although some children with Down syndrome can breastfeed adequately. As the child develops, special bottles or adaptive utensils may assist the child with feeding. Refer the parents for nutritional counseling as needed. Provide resources for behavioral training to encourage intake of new foods or the acquisition of new skills.

Children with Down syndrome like routine, and changes in routine often result in excessive frustration and decreased coping abilities. When the child is hospitalized, the nurse must try to keep the child's environment and routine as close to the home routine as possible; providing important details on the child's written care plan ensures consistency. Remember that the child's plan of care is based on the child's cognitive and adaptive abilities, rather than on chronologic age, and the child's skills may be age-appropriate in some areas but markedly delayed in others. Observe the child for signs of readiness to learn a new task (reaching for a cup, attempting to dress), and encourage self-care whenever possible. The child's level of coordination, muscle strength, and dexterity may not allow the child to zip, button, or feed self in the usual way, so adaptive tools may be needed.

As the child grows, advise the parents to encourage participation in recreational activities that the child can manage. Be sure to advise them that the child will need to have neck radiography before participating in any active sports program.

Evaluation

- Have the child and family demonstrated positive and mutually satisfying interactions?
- Are the parents able to identify the child's strengths and positive attributes?
- Do the parents state an interest and willingness to help the child learn new skills through demonstration, repetition, and much positive feedback?
- Does the child demonstrate continued development and a sense of competence in self-care skills?
- Does the child demonstrate steady progress toward attaining developmental milestones and appropriate measurable growth?

FRAGILE X SYNDROME

Fragile X syndrome is the most common inherited cause of mental retardation. It accounts for 10% to 12% of all mental retardation in males. The disorder usually does not manifest as mental retardation in females, but a female carrier normally passes the fragile X chromosome to the offspring. This syndrome has a unique profile of behavioral and cognitive patterns.

Pathophysiology

of Fragile X Syndrome

Fragile X syndrome is caused by an underlying single gene defect. There is an abnormality in the *FMR1* (fragile X mental retardation) gene in all affected individuals. There are excessive repetitions of the nucleotide CGG DNA sequences in affected individuals.

Etiology

The gene that causes fragile X syndrome is located on the X chromosome. Typically, a female child receiving the X chromosome that has a fragile site will become a carrier and will be mildly affected, if at all. The female may continue to pass on the abnormal X chromosome. A male, however, will usually exhibit the full effects if he receives the abnormal gene. Transmission occurs through carrier mothers and not through an unaffected "carrier" father.

Incidence

Fragile X syndrome affects approximately 1 in 1000 male children and 1 in 2000 female children (King, Hodapp, & Dykens, 2000). As many as 1 in 259 females carry the fragile X gene, either as a premutation or as a full mutation (Dykens, Hodapp, & Finucane, 2000). In general, only males exhibit the full effects of the X-linked recessive disorder because their single X chromosome has the abnormal gene. Approximately 50% to 70% of females with the full genetic mutation manifest cognitive impairments, usually with borderline to mild mental retardation.

Manifestations

Physical features associated with fragile X syndrome include:

- Facial dysmorphism, with large or prominent ears and a long, narrow face; a head circumference that may be disproportionate to height and weight; lowered epicanthal folds; and prominent nasal alae (cartilaginous flap on outer side of each nostril)
- Postpubertal macroorchidism
- Flat feet
- Lax ankles
- Hyperextensible fingers
- Extremely soft and smooth skin
- Mitral valve prolapse (common)

Intellectual, language, and social dysfunctions associated with fragile X syndrome include the following characteristics (King, Hodapp, & Dykens, 2000):

- Autistic-like behaviors, such as gaze avoidance, hand flapping, echolalia, and abnormal speech patterns
- Hyperkinetic behaviors, including restlessness, agitation, and attention deficits
- Hand biting

- Sensory motor integration deficits, such as poor coordination, motor planning deficits, and tactile defensiveness
- *In boys:* cognitive deficits in the moderate to severe range, strengths in visual memory but weaknesses in auditory processing abilities and abstract reasoning, improved performance with simultaneous rather than sequential processing, language delays, perseveration, tangential speech, and other communicative disorders
- *In girls:* generally only mild cognitive deficits but with many variations
- High degree of disruptive behaviors, including temper tantrums, self-injurious behaviors, extreme agitation
- Progressive dementia

Diagnostic Evaluation

Deoxyribonucleic acid (DNA) testing is the definitive method of diagnosing fragile X syndrome. Identification of the *FMR1* gene mutation allows diagnosis in both carriers and those affected. Individuals with mental retardation of unknown cause or learning disabilities, together with manifestations of fragile X syndrome, should be considered for fragile X testing.

Therapeutic Management

Treatment is provided through various types of therapy. Special education, vocational programs, and behavioral management classes are important to overall development. Speech and language evaluation and therapy are generally prescribed during the first year of life and are made available on an ongoing basis. Sensorimotor integration therapy may be offered to enhance motor planning, joint stability, coordination, and integration of visual, auditory, and tactile information. Sensorimotor therapy is considered to be the intervention of choice for these children with learning disabilities.

Nursing Considerations

The nursing care of individuals with fragile X syndrome is similar to care for any child with a cognitive impairment but with specific attention to the behavioral and cognitive difficulties presented by the individual child. The plan should include a multidisciplinary team approach to assessment. Anticipatory guidance should be provided, with a review of the support groups and services available. Special education services will be necessary to address the child's specific cognitive and academic difficulties, as well as to foster continued skill development and to reduce the stress created in the typical educational setting. Remediation services should include behavioral interventions specific to the child's needs, speech and language assistance, and possibly occupational and physical therapy to address visual-motor and motor skill deficits. Family members of individuals with fragile X syndrome should receive genetic counseling and testing.

Assessment for other related abnormalities, such as cleft palate, foot deformities, hip dislocations and other conditions involving joint hyperextensibility, hernias, and hypertonia, should also be performed. Seizures occur in 17% to 50% of these children, so medications and educating the family about seizure disorders may be warranted.

AUTISM

Autism is the most severe condition classified as a pervasive developmental disorder (PDD) by the American Psychiatric Association (2000). PDDs are disorders characterized by "severe and pervasive impairment in several areas of development: reciprocal social interaction skills, communication skills, or the presence of stereotyped behavior, interests, and activities" (American Psychiatric Association, 2000, p. 69). Typically, these conditions are evident in the first 12 months of life, but they may be overlooked if gross motor skills are progressing normally. Frequently they occur concurrently with a diverse group of other medical conditions. Other conditions included in this category are Rett syndrome and childhood thought disorders, formerly known as *childhood schizophrenia, symbiotic psychosis,* and *childhood psychosis.* Autism is the most severe of these disorders, but it is not the most frequently encountered disorder among PDDs.

There is no evidence that autism can be cured, so treatment is generally lifelong and is characterized by varying degrees of success. Children with IQs of less than 50 generally remain cognitively stable. In those with IQs above 50, the outcome varies, depending on education and early treatment. Research indicates that language functions rather than social behaviors can be used most successfully to predict short-term outcomes. The early onset of social symptoms does not necessarily indicate greater severity of symptoms, lower intelligence, or insecure attachments.

Etiology

The cause of autism is unknown, but it is believed that the disorder can be caused by a wide range of prenatal, perinatal, and postnatal conditions, including maternal rubella, untreated phenylketonuria, tuberous sclerosis, anoxia during birth, encephalitis, seizures, and fragile X syndrome (Sadock & Sadock, 2003). It was once believed that family child-rearing practices and parental personality characteristics influenced the development of autism, but no controlled studies confirm this view. Because siblings are more likely to develop the disorder than children in the general population, genetic factors are believed to play a role. Recently there has been some publicity in the lay literature about a possible connection between autism and the measles-mumps-rubella (MMR) vaccine. The American Academy of Pediatrics, after comprehensive review, has issued a statement that available evidence does not support this connection (Halsey & Hyman, 2001).

Incidence

Autism affects 10 to 15 children in 10,000 and is four to five times more common in boys than in girls. No differences in incidence have been correlated with race, socioeconomic level, or culture.

Manifestations

Autism is a severely incapacitating, lifelong developmental disability that is characterized by a qualitative impairment in four developmental areas:

- Disturbance in the rate and appearance of physical, social, and language skills

- Abnormal responses of the body sensations
- Thinking capacity, but with absent or delayed speech and language
- Abnormal ways of relating to people, objects, and events

A child may have a vast vocabulary yet have no comprehension of the meaning of the words. Another child may be able to solve intricate mathematical problems but not be able to make change from a dollar. Children may seem oblivious to the sound of their own names but may come running into the room at the sound of a truck. Generally, they show a fixed, unchanging response to a particular stimulus. Self-stimulation is common and generally involves repetition of a particularly pleasing sensory stimulus, such as twirling a toy or rubbing the top of the head. The autistic child typically repeats an act, such as fingering an object or continuously spinning around, rather than responding to a new stimulus.

Apparently, interest is limited by nature, rather than by choice, to an extremely narrow range. The child with autism generally overreacts to any change within the environment. Often, autistic children do not have a typical sense of personal space and so may touch others on the face or stand face to face, with noses touching, even when encountering a total stranger.

Autism is usually apparent to parents before age 3 years, although a period of apparently normal development may be followed by rapid deterioration. There is a wide range in the degree of impairment produced. Autism shares some similarities with the characteristic presentation of what has been called *childhood schizophrenia* and *mental retardation* but with definitive differences. These differences are outlined in Table 54-2. Seventy-five percent of autistic individuals are cognitively impaired. A few individuals with autism also have an extremely developed skill in a particular area, such as music or mathematics. These individuals are sometimes known as *idiot savants* because they have both a severe cognitive impairment and an extraordinary cognitive skill or expertise.

The child with autism exhibits the following behaviors and characteristics (American Psychiatric Association, 2000).

Social behaviors associated with autism include:

- Marked lack of awareness of the existence or feelings of others (e.g., individual ignores emotions of others)
- Lack of or abnormal amount of comfort-seeking at times of distress (e.g., individual does not show pain when hurt)
- Lack of or abnormal imitation of others' actions
- Lack of or abnormal social play (generally plays alone or involves others only as mere objects)
- Gross impairment in social peer relationships (appears not to want or need friends)

The child with autism typically exhibits the following language characteristics:

- Lack of or impaired verbal communication and abnormalities in the production of speech (inappropriate volume, pitch, rate, rhythm, or intonation, such as a monotone voice or echolalia)
- Markedly abnormal nonverbal communication (i.e., the child uses no gestures or behavioral cues)
- Absence of imaginative play (no imitative or dramatic role playing)

TABLE **54-2** Differential Diagnosis of Autism, Mental Retardation, and Schizophrenia

Autism	Mental Retardation
Peaked skill profile	Flat skill profile
Lack of imitative skills	Imitation skills and gesturing
Nonsocial behaviors with little initiation	Social behavior, initiation of social contact
Abnormal communication and language	Limited language ability but sufficient for communication
Development of seizures possible during adolescence	Usually no seizures, Alzheimer's-type dementia in adulthood

Autism	Schizophrenia
Onset before age 30 mo	Onset during pubescence or adolescence
No remissions	Remissions and relapses
Hallucinations and delusions rare	Hallucinations and delusions common
Absence of thought disorder	Thought disorder
No family history of schizophrenia	Family history of schizophrenia
Self-stimulating behaviors	Odd behavior but no self-stimulating behaviors
Medications of limited use	Medications often helpful in reducing symptoms

- Impaired interactive speech and communication (the child does not allow for the normal give-and-take of conversation and tends to become preoccupied with a given subject or word out of context with the conversation)

The child with autism also exhibits a restricted behavioral repertoire, including:

- Stereotyped body movements (e.g., spinning around, head banging, "flapping," rocking)
- Persistent preoccupation with characteristics of objects (smell, taste, texture) or an abnormal attachment to objects (e.g., piece of string, picture of a whale)
- Marked distress over a minor change in the environment (e.g., exhibiting tantrums when a light is turned on, refusing to look at a teacher who is wearing a new dress)
- Unreasonable insistence on routine (e.g., following a schedule exactly to the minute or second, refusal to attend an assembly during a scheduled mathematics class)
- Self-injurious behaviors (e.g., biting, picking at skin, scratching eyes)
- Marked restriction in range of interests (e.g., may repeatedly align objects and cannot be diverted from doing so)

Diagnostic Evaluation

A diagnosis of autism is usually established on the basis of manifestations. Often, the family is interviewed initially, followed by observation of the child alone, with the parent, and interacting with the examiner or others in the environment. Interviews are coupled with observations and clinician's rating scales. The onset of characteristic delays or of abnormal functioning must occur before age 3 years.

Therapeutic Management

Early identification of autism is essential. Treatment generally entails placement in an environment that facilitates interaction and promotes replacement of stereotypical behaviors with more normal behaviors. Behavioral methods are typically used. Autistic people have a normal life span; con-

CRITICAL THINKING EXERCISE 54-1

You are a nurse working in a clinic and doing a health assessment on a 9-month-old infant. As you provide the parent with information about the measles-mumps-rubella (MMR) vaccine, which the baby would expect to receive at the 1-year well visit, the parent expresses concern that he has heard that the MMR vaccine causes autism.
1. What will be your response to this parent?
2. What kind of information can you give the parent to assist him evaluate information he reads or hears about through the lay media?

sequently, they require significant financial resources for treatment and supervision.

Because of the severity of the social impairment and the ineffectiveness of normal environmental interventions, affected children are usually referred to special programs designed to offer stimulation, modify stereotypical behaviors, or establish routines for teaching as soon as the disorder has been identified. Programs usually focus on safety precautions for self-injurious behaviors, such as head banging, and the promotion of communication. Facilitative communication through the use of picture boards or keyboards is controversial but has been used in many educational settings to help these children interact with their environment.

■NURSING CARE
The Child With Autism

Assessment

Because there are no classic physical features that highlight autism, the nurse must assess the child with possible autism as if no physical or cognitive impairments are present. This is done before establishing a diagnosis. The primary characteristic of autism is lack of social interaction and awareness. For this reason, if the child is very young, the nurse who interacts only with the child's parents is unlikely to be aware of the child's degree of social disengagement. If the child has already been diagnosed as having autism and the purpose of assessment is to determine the severity of the disorder—or the assessment occurs before a procedure or hospitalization—it is performed in the same manner as with any normal child. The nurse, however, will quickly become aware of the child's social detachment or lack of language as the assessment continues.

A systematic exploration of the child's skills and comparison with developmental norms are essential. For the staff nurse, this process may include evaluating the child's ability to feed self, dress, and toilet. The assessment should include the child's interactive patterns and verbalization skills. It is important to note the child's motor skills also, because these have major implications for safety and self-care. For initial, generalized screening, the DDST-II may be helpful (see Chapter 4 and Appendix F). A family history of autism or other mental disorders, family coping skills, and available social support systems should also be assessed.

Nursing Diagnosis and Planning

The nursing diagnoses and expected outcomes that may be appropriate following assessment of the child with autism are

- Risk for Injury related to an inability to anticipate danger, a tendency for self-mutilation, and sensory perceptual deficits.

   Expected Outcome: The child's safety will be ensured, as evidenced by maintaining integrity of skin and avoiding self-injury or accidental injury.

- Impaired Social Interaction related to an inability to initiate and maintain social relationships and to limited verbal skills.

   Expected Outcomes: The child will demonstrate improvement in communication skills and will begin to show appropriate interaction with others.

- Disturbed Thought Processes related to an inability to perceive self or others accurately and to cognitive and perceptual dysfunction.

   Expected Outcomes: The child will show progress in developing an interest in surroundings and the ability to acknowledge others in the environment; will demonstrate orientation to person, place, and time; and will perform activities of daily living appropriate to this orientation.

Interventions

When working with autistic children in the hospital setting, the nurse needs to work closely with the family to determine the child's routines, habits, and preferences. The nurse

should write down any specific cues that will help the child remain oriented to the environment and will facilitate tolerance to change. For example, the nursing staff should be limited to as few individuals as possible. The child may need to perform toileting and self-care activities in a particular order. The child may need an environmental cue, such as stroking a favorite blanket, before being able to move from one activity to the next. The nurse can generally evaluate the child's tolerance of the situation by monitoring signs of anxiety or emotional comfort, as evidenced by such behaviors as attending or observing the nurse in the room or demonstrating a willingness to participate in self-care.

The nurse must work closely with the family to determine the specific ways in which the child communicates. The child may use sign language or pictures to specify needs if no verbal skills are developed. Children with autism are often reluctant to initiate or sustain direct eye contact, so the nurse may interpret this behavior as meaning that the child is not listening or is unaware of what is being said. In addition, the child may answer questions after several minutes' delay. The nurse should identify these behaviors, allow extra time, and be alert to differences in communication styles. Children with autism generally understand much more language than they are able to use expressively.

The child who demonstrates a tendency for head banging may need a helmet or side rolls. Wrist restraints may be necessary if the child is unable to remain in the bed at night. The nurse should help the parents understand and explain to their child any safety precautions that are unfamiliar to the child. The presence of a parent or older sibling is almost always necessary when an autistic child is hospitalized. Evaluating the child for safety is an ongoing nursing function. Reducing the adjustment demands for the child may be necessary if the nurse recognizes behaviors indicating stress or anxiety.

Evaluation

- Has the child remained free of injury?
- Has the child developed a way to communicate needs?
- Does the child demonstrate an interest in surroundings?
- Does the child acknowledge the presence of others in the environment?

! CRITICAL TO REMEMBER

Maintaining Routine for the Child With Autism

Children with autism often are unable to tolerate even the slightest change in routine and may become withdrawn, self-abusive, or violent if their routines are altered.

KEY CONCEPTS

- Children with a cognitive deficit experience limitations in social interactions, use of language for self-expression, and self-care abilities. If these limitations are severe, the child will need the lifelong care of mature, caring adults.

- Children with cognitive deficits have many normal needs, including the need for positive attention and opportunities for self-discovery

and growth. The nurse needs to work closely with the family to identify the child's specific patterns of interacting with the environment. This is done by asking relevant, clear questions about how the child communicates and perceives experiences.

- The nurse should consider that families with a cognitively impaired child experience re-

peated stress and grief as the child continues to fail to reach developmental expectations.

- The nurse can be most helpful by offering family members an opportunity to discuss feelings and by identifying resources to help meet the child's needs. The nurse may act as an advocate for the parents in the school system and the community.

- Mental retardation may be the result of congenital or early environmental factors, or it may occur secondary to head injury, asphyxia, intracranial hemorrhage, infections, poisoning, or the presence or treatment of a brain tumor.
- *Developmental disability* is a legal term that encompasses mental retardation and other cognitive impairments.
- Several neuropsychological tests are available to assess levels of mental retardation. The best method of early detection is by assessing development during routine pediatric preventive care visits.
- Parents of children with cognitive deficits should be provided with anticipatory guidance relative to their child's developmental abilities.

- Changes in routine can frustrate the child with Down syndrome.
- The family of a child with Down syndrome may need assistance in identifying and obtaining adaptive tools for dressing, bathing, and eating.
- The family of a child with Down syndrome should be encouraged and assisted in helping the child learn new skills through demonstration, repetition, and positive feedback.
- Children with fragile X syndrome exhibit autistic-like behaviors, such as gaze avoidance, hand flapping, echolalia, and abnormal speech patterns. In addition, affected children have poor coordination, hyperkinetic behaviors, and cognitive deficits that are moderate to severe.

- Autism is characterized by an impairment in the rate and appearance of physical, social, and language skills; abnormal responses of the body sensations; thinking capacity, but with absent or delayed speech and language; and abnormal ways of relating to people, objects, and events.
- Autism shares similarities with childhood schizophrenia and mental retardation, but there are definitive differences.
- When working with children with autism, the nurse needs to work with the family to determine the child's routines, habits, and preferences.

ANSWERS to Critical Thinking Exercise 54-1

1. Both television and newspaper articles have suggested that MMR vaccine is related to the onset of autism. These reports were based on some non-epidemiologic studies done in Europe that reported inconsistent data. You can reassure the parent that the American Academy of Pediatrics convened a special panel to examine the available evidence and determined that the evidence does not support a causative relationship between MMR and autism.

2. It is important for the nurse to know how to advise parents and others about obtaining accurate information about health issues. Often, the media report on "newsworthy" issues, based on only one study or on a piece of research that has not been appropriately peer-reviewed. You can suggest to parents that they do the following:
   - Look at whether the information comes from a reliable, peer-reviewed, scientific source and preferably from several sources finding the same results.
   - Note whether the results have been found in humans and not just in animals.
   - Assess whether the risk is large or small by putting the numbers in a format you understand (e.g., 1 in 100, 1%), and try to understand if the number given is a single number or if it is within a range of numbers.
   - Look at the risk compared with other known risks.
   - Access information from your health care provider, your local health department, government sources, libraries, and reputable Internet websites (websites of official organizations).

Data from Harvard School of Public Health, Center for Risk Analysis. (1999). *Health insight: A consumer's guide to taking charge of health information.* Boston: Author.

REFERENCES and READINGS

American Academy of Child and Adolescent Psychiatry. (1995). *Facts for families #23: Children who are mentally retarded.* Washington, DC: Author.

American Association on Mental Retardation. (2001). *Fact sheet: What is mental retardation.* Available on-line at www.aamr.org.

American Psychiatric Association. (2000). *Diagnostic and statistical manual of mental disorders* (4th ed., Text Revision). Washington, DC: Author.

Batshaw, M. (2001). *When your child has a disability* (2nd ed.). Baltimore: Paul H. Brookes Publishing.

Developmental Disabilities Assistance and Bill of Rights Act of 2000 (PL 106-402). Passed by the U.S. Congress on 10/30/2000.

Dykens, E., Hodapp, R.M., & Finucane, M.S. (2000). *Genetic and mental retardation syndromes: A new look at behavior and interventions.* Baltimore: Paul H. Brookes Publishing.

Halsey, N., & Hyman, S. (2001). Measles-mumps-rubella vaccine and autistic spectrum disorder: Report from the new challenges in childhood immunizations conference convened in Oak Brook, IL, June 12-13, 2000. *Pediatrics, 107*(5), e84.

Khan, S., Osinowo, T., & Pary, R.J. (2002). Down syndrome and major depressive disorder: A review. *Mental Health Aspects of Developmental Disabilities, 5*(2), 46-52.

King, B.H., Hodapp, R.M., & Dykens, E.M. (2000). Mental retardation. In B.J. Saddock & V.A. Saddock (Eds.), *Kaplan and Saddock's comprehensive textbook of psychiatry* (pp. 2587-2613). Philadelphia: Lippincott.

Leshin, L. (2003). *Down syndrome health issues: News and information for parents and health professionals.* Available online at www.ds-health.com/.

Sadock, B., & Sadock, V.A. (2003). *Kaplan and Sadock's synopsis of psychiatry: Behavioral sciences/clinical psychiatry* (9th ed.). Philadelphia: Lippincott Williams & Wilkins.

Sullivan, P.M., & Knutson, J.F. (2000). Maltreatment and disabilities: A population-based epidemiological study. *Child Abuse & Neglect, 24,* 1257-1274.

U.S. Department of Health and Human Services (U.S. DHHS). (2000). *Healthy People 2010* (Conference edition, in 2 volumes). Washington, DC: Author.

55

The Child with a Sensory Alteration

◆ LEARNING OBJECTIVES

After studying this chapter, you should be able to:

- Describe the structure and function of the eye and ear.
- Describe the specific information required in a health history for a child with potential sensory deficits.
- Define the nurse's role in assessing for sensory deficits.
- Describe specific nursing care for children with health problems affecting the eye and ear.
- Describe how alterations in the sensory organs affect the child's ability to communicate.
- Identify potential growth and development interruptions that may occur with problems affecting the sensory organs.

◆ DEFINITIONS

amblyopia Reduced visual acuity not correctable by refractive means and not attributable to structural or pathologic ocular anomalies.

astigmatism Abnormal curvature of the cornea or the lens.

cataract A loss of transparency of the crystalline lens or its capsule.

central hearing loss Result of damage to the conduction system between the brainstem and cerebral cortex.

concomitant strabismus Not of paralytic origin; remains constant for all directions of gaze.

conductive hearing loss Reversible loss caused by damage, inflammation, or obstruction to outer or middle ear; sound is prevented from progressing across middle ear.

congenital (infantile) glaucoma Increased intraocular fluid pressure that occurs during first 3 years of life because of a defect in the drainage network of the eye.

diplopia Double vision.

hyperopia Farsightedness; close vision is abnormal.

hyphema A hemorrhage or sanguineous exudate in the anterior chamber of the eye.

mixed hearing loss Combination of conductive and sensorineural loss.

myopia Nearsightedness; distance vision is abnormal.

nonconcomitant strabismus Angle of deviation varying with direction of gaze because of paralysis or paresis of one or more extraocular muscles.

nystagmus Involuntary eye movements that make the eyes appear to be darting back and forth.

ophthalmia neonatorum Conjunctivitis noted in the first few weeks of life, usually gonococcal or chlamydial.

refractive error Light rays passing through eye structures come into focus at an inappropriate location relative to the retina.

secondary glaucoma Increased intraocular fluid pressure that occurs after 3 years of age and may be the result of disease or surgery.

sensorineural hearing loss Result of damage or malformation of the middle ear or auditory nerve; hearing loss is usually permanent.

strabismus "Squint," "cross-eyes"; a condition in which the eyes are not straight because of lack of coordination of the extraocular muscles; most often caused by muscle imbalance or paralysis of the extraocular muscles but may also result from conditions such as a brain tumor, myasthenia gravis, or infection.

subconjunctival hemorrhages Bleeding situated beneath the conjunctiva; in children, most frequent cause is trauma or severe coughing or sneezing episodes (Valsalva maneuvers); also caused by infection with *Streptococcus pneumoniae* and *Haemophilus influenzae*.

visual accommodation Ability to focus on distant and near objects.

visual acuity Clarity of vision; visual acuity is tested through use of vision charts, and results are compared with what a person with normal vision can see at a distance of 20 feet (see Chapter 33).

REVIEW OF THE EYE

Structure and Function

The eye is attached to the skull by six accessory muscles. These are used to move the eye to achieve vision. Ciliary muscles function to alter the shape of the eye to provide focus and accommodation at various distances. Cranial nerves II, III, IV, V, and VI all affect the eye.

The orb, or eye, is made up of several parts. The cornea is the clear area located in the front of the eye, where light enters the eye. The cornea and sclera (white outer covering) make up the eye's outer layer. The middle layer is composed of the choroid (vascular lining), the lens (a clear structure that changes shape to allow accommodation of light on the retina), and the iris (the colored muscular ring located behind the cornea that expands or contracts to control the amount of light entering the eye). The inner layer of the eye is known as the *retina*. This area contains the rods and cones. These receive light impulses and transmit them through the optic nerve (cranial nerve II) to the brain. The macula contains the greatest concentration of nerve endings. The cornea and lens focus light onto the macula. The optic disc is the area where the optic nerve enters the eye.

Neonatal Development

The eyes begin to develop at approximately 22 days' gestation. The critical period for development is considered to be 22 to 50 days. Congenital abnormalities appear to be caused by either genetic or environmental factors or by a combination of the two. The eye is especially sensitive to teratogens, in particular to infections such as cytomegalovirus and rubella.

REVIEW OF THE EAR

Structure and Function

The ear is divided into three parts: the outer ear, the middle ear, and the inner ear. The outer ear includes the auricle and external ear canal. It is separated from the middle ear by the tympanic membrane (eardrum). The tympanic membrane vibrates to conduct sound waves to the middle ear. The middle ear contains the bones of hearing—the malleus (hammer), incus (anvil), and stapes (stirrup). These bones conduct sound waves from the tympanic membrane to the inner ear. The inner ear contains the nerve endings that conduct sound impulses to the brain. These are located in a snail-shaped chamber (the cochlea) that is filled with fluid. The inner ear also controls balance. The eustachian tube connects the middle ear with the nasopharynx. It functions to allow fluids to drain into the nasopharynx and to assist in equalizing pressure between the outer ear and the middle ear.

Neonatal Development

The ear begins to develop during the 3rd week of gestation. The critical period for the development of the ear is between 4 and 6 weeks' gestation. Like the eye, the ear is very sensitive to teratogens. It is innervated by the acoustic nerve (cranial nerve VIII). Congenital deafness appears to be largely the result of genetic factors.

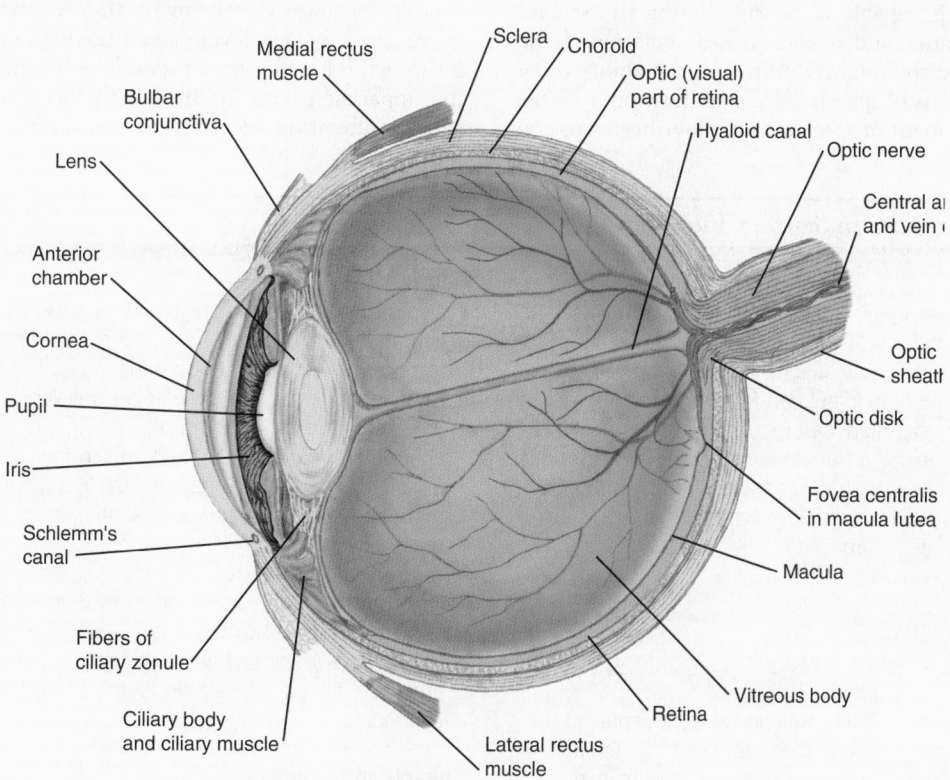

Anatomy of the Eye

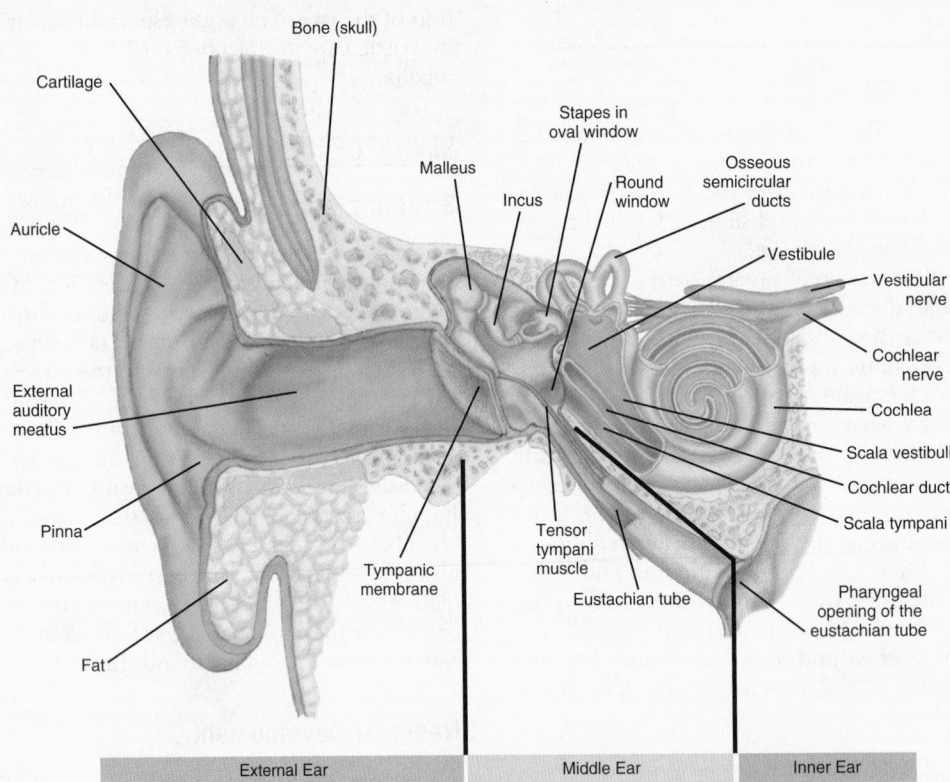

Bone (skull)

Cartilage

Stapes in
oval window

Malleus

Auricle

Incus

Round
window

Osseous
semicircular
ducts

Vestibule

Vestibular
nerve

Cochlear
nerve

Cochlea

External
auditory
meatus

Scala vestibuli

Cochlear duct

Scala tympani

Pinna

Tensor
tympani
muscle

Pharyngeal
opening of the
eustachian tube

Tympanic
membrane

Eustachian tube

Fat

| External Ear | Middle Ear | Inner Ear |

Anatomy of the Ear

SPEECH DEVELOPMENT

Because the fetus is capable of hearing during the second trimester of pregnancy and is able to hear voices and the mother's heart beat, the infant is born with the ability to be sensitive to variations of speech. Adequate hearing is essential for the development of speech. The infant begins to coo and vocalize quite early (birth to 4 months). Babbling begins at approximately 4 to 6 months. Babbling is followed by receptive language development (understanding words) and expressive language development (saying words; see Chapters 5 through 8 for specifics of speech development). Any hearing impairment can interfere with speech development, as can any alteration affecting the oral cavity.

Pediatric Differences in Sensory Function

Vision
- Development of the eye is not complete at birth, but the newborn is able to fixate, follow an object to midline, and react to a change in intensity of light.
- By 3 months of age, the infant can follow moving objects; by 4 months of age, the infant can recognize familiar objects.
- Binocularity, the ability to fixate on one visual field with both eyes, is not present at birth but is established by 6 months of age. Frequent eye crossing after 6 months of age is abnormal and indicates strabismus.
- Visual acuity changes with age:

4 months	20/50 to 20/80
1 year	20/40 to 20/70
4 years	20/30 to 20/40
5 years	20/20 to 20/30

- Lacrimal glands are not fully developed at birth. Tears are not often present with crying until after 1 to 3 months. Temporary obstruction of lacrimal ducts may cause overflow of tears.
- The size of the orbits doubles by the time the child is 1 year of age and doubles again by 6 years. Eye growth is completed at 10 to 12 years of age.

Hearing
- Development of the ear begins during the 3rd week of gestation and is complete by the 3rd month of embryonic life. Infection or other insult to the fetus during this time can cause irreparable damage to the ear. Ear development occurs at the same time as kidney development, so malformation in one system may indicate problems in the other.
- An infant as young as 3 days is able to distinguish between familiar and unfamiliar sounds and can recognize the mother's voice. The infant can distinguish between frequently heard words and other words (nonsense language) by 1 year.
- Basic auditory skills are in place by 3 years of age. Hearing can be evaluated by audiometry testing by this age.
- Infants and young children have shorter, more horizontal, and more flaccid eustachian tubes, predisposing them to otitis media.

Speech and Language
- Infants can imitate sounds heard by 3 to 5 months of age.
- Verbal dialogue similar to an adult's is noted by approximately 6 months of age.

Because a child learns so much through the senses, deficits in hearing and vision can have profound effects on development. Appropriate screening and early interventions are crucial. Early identification of vision and hearing deficits allows for early intervention—either correction or the provision of adaptive measures, so that the child's "normal" growth and development may be preserved. Because a child cannot report sensory deficits, nurses must assess carefully for alterations in vision or hearing.

U.S. legislation, PL 94-142 (the Education for All Handicapped Children Act) was passed in 1975 and subsequently updated as the Individuals With Disabilities Education Act (see Chapter 54); it provides for special education services for children with severe sensory deficits. It is important to identify children who might be eligible for special educational services at a young age so their education can be maximized.

The health history of a child with a potential sensory deficit is essentially the same for any child (see Chapter 33) but should include some additional pieces of information:

- Thorough prenatal history
- Growth and developmental history
- Past history of any infections (including treatment, because many medications can cause sensory deficits)
- Previous trauma to the eye or ear
- Changes noted in behavior (e.g., rubbing the eyes, turning up the volume on the television, decreased attention span)
- Changes in appearance (e.g., red, inflamed eyes; drainage from the eye or ear)
- Physical complaints (e.g., complaints of ear or eye pain, headache, nausea and vomiting)

After carefully reviewing the health history, the nurse performs a thorough physical examination using age-appropriate measures of vision and hearing acuity (see Chapter 33).

DISORDERS OF THE EYE

The nurse has a very important role in the prevention and early detection of eye problems. All children should have vision screening done at well visits and according to the following schedule (Committee on Practice and Ambulatory Medicine, 2003):

BOX 55-1
Signs and Symptoms of Potential Vision Problems

- Inability to fix both eyes on an object and follow the track of a moving object with both eyes
- Persistent discharge from one or both eyes, especially accompanied by redness of the sclera
- Excessive tearing, especially when accompanied by itchiness or pain
- Cloudiness or white areas in the pupil
- Deviation of the iris in an inward or outward direction (crossing)
- Head tilting or closing one eye to see
- Squinting
- Complaints of headache or blurred or double vision
- The need to sit close to a television or blackboard to see
- Holding reading material close to the eyes
- Excessive fatigue with visual concentration

- At birth—external and internal appearance for structural abnormalities, red reflex, fixation
- Age 3 to 6 months—fixation and ability to follow, alignment (corneal light reflex, photo screening)
- Age birth to 3 years—all of the above with ocular history
- Age 3 years and older—all of the above plus visual acuity, using developmentally appropriate charts (Allen chart, picture chart, tumbling E) and ophthalmoscopy

Refer children who fail structural or vision screening for complete ophthalmologic evaluation. Careful attention to behavior and appearance changes as well as physical complaints assists in the early detection and treatment of eye disorders (Box 55-1). Children who have any symptoms should be referred for further evaluation.

Nursing Considerations for the Child With a Refractive Error

Refractive errors cause vision disturbances from alterations in the path of light rays through the eye. They usually result from an abnormally shaped orb; the orb may be flattened or

---

! CRITICAL TO REMEMBER
Vision Screening

- Thoroughly explain the procedure to the child before beginning. If using a picture chart, show the child the pictures and ask the child to identify them. Children might have different names for the same picture. If using a machine to test the child's vision, demonstrate in advance how it works.
- Take the child to a quiet, nondistracting area that has been marked for the appropriate distance from the chart.
- Have the child cover one eye. Use a colorful, opaque cover that completely blocks the child's vision. The parent can help hold the cover in place.
- Point to a picture (letter, number) on a line that the child can probably see readily, and move to smaller lines. Vary the direction (left to right, right to left) to reduce the likelihood that the child is memorizing the symbols.
- Give positive feedback. Perform the test as quickly as possible because small children lose interest quickly.
- Test both eyes. Refer for further evaluation if there is a discrepancy of two lines or if the child tests in the abnormal range on two successive screenings.

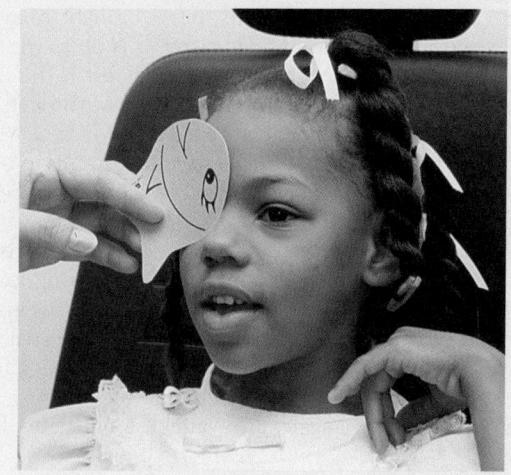

TABLE **55-1** Types of Refractive Disorders

Refractive Error	Description	Clinical Manifestations	Treatment
Myopia	Nearsightedness Ability to see close objects more clearly than those at a distance Caused by the image focusing in front of the retina	Difficulty seeing the blackboard or television clearly Decreased interest in activities requiring distance vision Squinting, head tilting, holding books close to eyes Decreased attention span, poor school performance	Treated with biconcave lenses New lenses may be required every 1-2 yr as the child grows
Hyperopia	Farsightedness Ability to see distant objects more clearly than those close up Caused by the image focusing beyond the retina	Most children are normally hyperopic until approximately 7 years of age but are able to accommodate to see clearly Strabismus or amblyopia may develop from prolonged hyperopia	Most young children with hyperopia need no correction If correction is required, convex lenses are used
Astigmatism	Unequal curvature of the cornea or the lens, causing light rays to bend in different directions May coexist with myopia or hyperopia	Mild astigmatism may be asymptomatic Manifestations may be similar to myopia	Treated with special lenses to compensate for the unequal curvature of the cornea

elongated (Table 55-1). Refractive errors are often discovered when a child squints or frowns or moves objects so that they are more easily seen. A teacher or complaints from the child may also alert parents. *Legal blindness* is defined as a correction of 20/200 or worse in the better eye or a visual field of 20 degrees or less.

Nurses should assess children's vision at every well-child visit, particularly during the preschool years. Visual acuity can be reliably tested in a cooperative child as young as 3 years. When testing visual acuity, the nurse needs to remember that a vision discrepancy of two lines or more on the vision chart, even if one eye tests normal, is cause for referral. A child with this discrepancy could have *anisometropia*, or a large refractive discrepancy between eyes. If not corrected, this condition can lead to amblyopia.

School nurses routinely test children's vision, and in fact, annual vision screening is offered to children throughout the United States. School nurses have used various methods of notifying families of children who fail a school vision screening (e.g., telephone call to parents, letter brought home by the child, letter mailed home). However, it is up to the parent to follow through with a visit to a specialist if the child fails the vision screen. Parents who fail to follow through cite lack of time and lack of financial resources (Mark & Mark, 1999). These findings make it imperative that nurses in other settings ask for details about the child's vision and previous vision testing.

Corrective lenses are used to improve the child's vision. Glasses should be impact-resistant and have spring-loaded frames that are less likely to be bent or warped. Fitting glasses to an infant or young child can be challenging; the goal is to choose shatter-resistant lenses in a type of frame that can be closely fitted to prevent easy dislodging during activity. Special prescription sports goggles are available for athletes. Both gas-permeable and soft contact lenses provide an alternative for children old enough and responsible enough to care for contacts independently.

The nurse needs to teach parents and children about appropriate care of corrective lenses and should educate parents and children about recognizing and intervening with vision problems early.

Nursing Considerations for the Child With Color Deficiency

Color "blindness," or color deficiency, occurs in 8% of the population and affects primarily boys. It affects the ability to distinguish between colors within certain groups, such as red, blue, and green.

Testing should be done if the clinician suspects a problem (i.e., a suspected optic nerve or retinal dysfunction) or the family has a history of color deficiency. Testing is routine in preschool boys. The most common detection test is the pseudoisochromatic (color confusion) test, in which color plates include patterns that are hidden to a person with a color deficit. Pseudoisochromatic plates are also available for children who cannot yet read. If a problem is detected, more sophisticated testing may be necessary to determine the exact type of color deficiency. Although color deficiency has no cure, certain types of tints used in contact lenses and glasses can help the child discriminate color differences.

Because color deficiency cannot be cured, nursing care focuses on adaptive and supportive measures. Encourage parents to have children tested if there is a family history of color deficiency or if the nurse suspects the child is having trouble distinguishing colors.

Parent and child education is very important for the child with color deficiency. Teaching should focus on alternative ways to discriminate the deficient colors. For the older child who can dress without assistance, clothes can be labeled or organized consistently in the closet and bureau so that items can be coordinated easily.

Safety is a major concern for the color-deficient child. For example, the child who cannot distinguish red and green must learn another way to distinguish traffic signals and other warning lights. Finally, anticipatory guidance is sometimes related to appropriate career choices. For example, color deficiency might prohibit an adult from becoming a pilot, police officer, or firefighter.

Nursing Considerations for the Child With a Blocked Lacrimal Duct

A blocked lacrimal (tear) duct is characterized by excessive tearing (epiphora) and crusting, or "matter," on the eyelids on awakening. Parents may also note a small mass just below the inner aspect of the eye. Treatment usually consists of massaging the duct. If the duct remains blocked despite massaging or remains blocked after 1 year of age, surgical opening of the duct is indicated.

The nurse should carefully assess the mucoid drainage. In a noninfected duct, the drainage is usually white or clear. If the duct has become infected, however, the drainage may be green or yellow. If the drainage suggests an infected duct, antibiotic eye drops or ointment is indicated.

The nurse teaches the parent about the proper technique for lacrimal massage. This process involves washing hands thoroughly and placing the index finger over the lacrimal duct (at the inner aspect of the eye by the bridge of the nose) and "milking," or gently massaging, the duct in an upward motion. Emphasize that massaging down the nasal bone has very little effect on the duct because the lacrimal system is intraosseous and unaffected by massage over bone. Other teaching includes monitoring for signs and symptoms of infection.

Nursing Considerations for the Child With Strabismus

Strabismus is a condition in which the eyes are not aligned because of lack of coordination of the extraocular muscles. It is present in 4% of children younger than 4 years (Mills, 1999). Strabismus is most often caused by muscle imbalance or paralysis of the extraocular muscles but may also result from conditions such as a brain tumor, myasthenia gravis, or infection. Infants and children with strabismus often have a close relative with the condition; other contributing factors include genetic abnormalities, neuromuscular disease, exposure to teratogens, and trauma (Ticho, 2003). The type of deviation noted defines strabismus (Box 55-2). When assessing infants for strabismus, the nurse needs to remember that strabismus is normal in the young infant but should not be present after approximately 3 months of age.

When both eyes are unable to focus simultaneously, the brain suppresses the image from the deviating eye to avoid double vision (diplopia). Amblyopia ("lazy eye"), or decreased vision in the deviated eye, can develop if strabismus is not treated early. Amblyopia can also accompany other eye conditions, such as congenital cataract and severe refractive error. If untreated amblyopia occurs in a child younger than 4 years (the critical period for development of the visual cortex), permanent loss of vision in the deviated eye can result. Because the child loses binocular vision, depth perception may also be impaired. Early detection and treatment of strabismus or other underlying cause of amblyopia are essential to prevent loss of vision.

The corneal light reflex test, simultaneous red reflex test, cover-uncover test, and the alternate-cover tests (see Chapter 33) are used in the diagnosis of strabismus. The nurse may suspect strabismus when the child complains of frequent headaches, squints, or tilts the head to see. The parent might suspect something is wrong when a flash photograph of the child reveals unequal "red eye." Children with family members with strabismus should be regularly assessed for development of the condition.

Treatment of strabismus may include special corrective lenses, vision therapy, surgery, or pharmacologic therapy. If the deviation is caused by hyperopia, corrective lenses are indicated to correct vision. Eyeglasses with specially ground prism power may also be indicated. These glasses correct vision in the affected eye so that the brain receives the same image from both eyes.

Botulinum toxin (Botox) was approved in 1989 by the U.S. Food and Drug Administration as an alternative to surgery in some cases. The toxin is injected into the eye muscle and produces temporary paralysis. This condition allows the muscles opposite the paralyzed muscle to straighten the eye. With successful treatment, the correction remains after the medication wears off (in approximately 2 months). The most common side effect is a drooping eyelid (ptosis), which usually resolves spontaneously.

BOX 55-2
Types of Strabismus

Comitant Strabismus: Most common type of strabismus in children. Constant deviation in all fields of gaze; not associated with eye muscle paralysis. All extraocular muscles function but are not coordinated. Child has difficulty seeing at close range and often squints. Accommodative nonparalytic strabismus may develop between 2 and 4 years of age as a result of a large refractive error.

Paralytic Strabismus: Caused by a weakness or paralysis of one or more of the extraocular muscles. Usually involves dysfunction of one or more cranial nerves involved with ocular movement. The eye appears crossed when turned in the direction of the affected muscle. May cause headache, poor coordination. Diplopia may cause child to close one eye or tilt head.

Esotropia (Convergent): The eye turns inward; most common type of strabismus in infants. May occur with hyperopia as the eyes compensate for the refractive error by overconvergence.

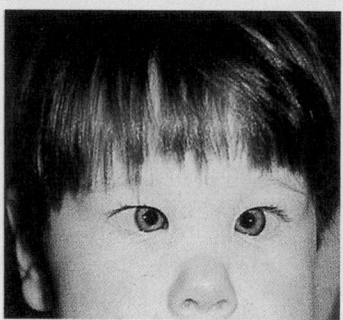

Infant with early-onset esotropia. The deviation may not be apparent until age 3 or 4 months.

Exotropia (Divergent): The eyes turn away from the midline; occurs most often when the child attempts to focus on a distant object. May be present at birth.

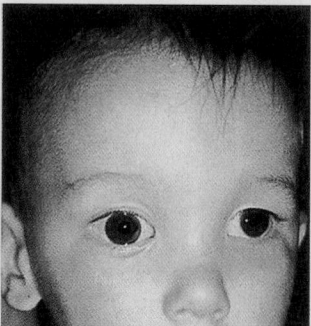

Child with left exotropia. Most exodeviations in childhood are intermittent.

Pseudostrabismus: Not a true strabismus. The eyes appear to deviate inward but are actually in alignment. Facial features, such as epicanthal folds and a broad, flat nasal bridge, can give the appearance of misalignment.

Phoria: A tendency for the eye to deviate. More evident during times of stress, fatigue, or illness.

Tropia: A continuous or intermittent misalignment of the eye.

Photographs from Albert, D.M., & Jakobiec, F.A. (Eds.). (1994). *Principles and practice of ophthalmology* (pp. 2731, 2733). Philadelphia: Saunders.

Surgery may be indicated to realign the weakened muscles in a child with strabismus. It is most often indicated when amblyopia is present and should be performed before the child is 2 years of age. The stronger eye may be patched before surgery to treat any existing amblyopia, but surgery can be done before the amblyopia treatment begins (Bacal & Hertle, 1998). Surgery may be required only on the weakened eye or on both eyes. More than one surgery may be necessary. During the surgery, small incisions are made and the weakened muscles are tightened.

If the child is to have a surgical correction, the nurse should prepare the child and parents before surgery for what to expect after surgery and should provide information about dressing changes, eye drops, corrective lenses, and any other postoperative treatments that may be required. Interventions are similar to those for any child having eye surgery (see p. 1591).

Patching is used primarily to correct amblyopia and is used mostly during the preschool years when the visual cortex is developing. In this treatment, the normal eye is patched so that the child is forced to use the weaker eye. The schedule for patching is individualized; a common regimen is an initial patching for a period equal to 1 week for every year of the child's age (Jockin, 2002). Depending on the severity of the

amblyopia, the child may need to wear the patch for nearly 24 hours each day (Mittleman, 2003). The patching regimen is prescribed by the ophthalmologist.

Cooperation with the patching regimen is essential. Teaching should explain the reasons for patching or corrective lenses, the expected results of wearing the patch or lens, correctly placing the patch, the number of hours per day the patch or lens is to be worn, and the expected length of treatment. The child needs to understand that wearing the patch or lens is not negotiable. The nurse often must teach parents strategies for dealing with resistant behaviors.

Nursing Considerations for the Child With Glaucoma

Glaucoma is a condition in which the intraocular fluid pressure of the eye is increased. This pressure increase, if left untreated, leads to atrophy of the optic disc and, ultimately, blindness.

There are several types of glaucoma in children. Congenital and infantile glaucomas occur during the first 3 years of life and are caused by a defect in the drainage network of the eye. *Secondary glaucoma* refers to disease that occurs

PARENTS
Want to Know

Information About Eye Patching

- Your child will need to wear the eye patch for the exact time your physician has prescribed. Not complying with the full wearing time could interfere with the treatment.
- Prescribed patching will not harm your child's stronger eye but will force the muscles of the weaker eye to be used.
- Apply the patch directly to your child's face, being sure to cover the whole eye. Do not leave any openings through which the child can peek.
- If your child wears eyeglasses as well, put the glasses on over the patch.
- It can be frustrating for the child to have to wear the patch. Try to be patient, understanding, and supportive. It is essential that patching be nonnegotiable. Find decorative patches, or put your own decoration on the patch. Praise your child frequently for cooperating with the treatment.

after 3 years of age and may be the result of inherited disease (juvenile glaucoma) or may be acquired from infection, trauma, or cataract removal (acquired glaucoma) (Kipp, 2003).

Clinical signs of glaucoma include excessive tearing, light sensitivity, blepharospasm (muscle spasm causing involuntary closing of the eyelid), and enlargement of the globe and cornea. Parents often note excessive tearing or corneal haziness caused by edema and bring the child in for clinical evaluation. The child may also be brought to the practitioner for what appears to be conjunctivitis, or pinkeye.

Physical examination includes an assessment of visual acuity, measurement of intraocular pressure (tonometry), assessment of corneal diameter and clarity, and an examination of the retina to assess for optic nerve cupping. Any infant with a visible iris diameter greater than 10.5 mm should be evaluated. If retinal edema is present, the light reflex is diffuse. Because young children may not be able to cooperate during an examination, they are often sedated. Intraocular pressure should be measured only under light sedation, however, because deeper sedation may alter readings (either high or low, depending on the agent used).

The preferred treatment for childhood glaucoma is surgery. Medications to clear the cornea may be used before surgery to allow better visibility. Surgery should be done as soon as possible after diagnosis to prevent loss (or further loss) of vision. The goal of surgery is to increase the outflow of the aqueous humor from the anterior chamber. Medications, such as cholinergic agents, beta-adrenergic blocking agents, or adrenergic agents, may be indicated after surgery to maintain a low intraocular pressure.

Prognosis varies from child to child. The earlier the glaucoma develops, the poorer the prognosis, because infants and children with early-onset glaucoma usually have defects in the development of the anterior chamber of the eye that occurred during fetal development (Kipp, 2003). In general, with prompt treatment, most children attain appropriate vi-

sion. Decreased vision may result from damage to the optic nerve, opacity of the cornea or lens, or amblyopia resulting from refractive errors. Children with glaucoma must be followed closely over the long term to quickly identify any rise in intraocular pressure.

Nursing interventions are similar to those for any child having eye surgery. Postoperative nursing care includes monitoring for signs and symptoms of increased intraocular pressure (pain, nausea and vomiting, increased inflammation) and administering any ordered medications, such as miotic eye drops (used to constrict the pupils) and antibiotic ointments or eye drops. If the child's eyes are patched, the nurse pays special attention to the resulting sensory deficits. The nurse also considers safety to be an issue when eyes are patched.

Parent education is essential to maintain the appropriate intraocular pressure and prevent complications (including blindness). Education includes the use of any prescribed medications, patching, and any other measures designed to correct refractive errors. The importance of returning for follow-up care should be emphasized. The child and caregivers should also be taught signs and symptoms of increasing intraocular pressure. Any signs of increasing intraocular pressure or infection should be reported immediately to the ophthalmologist.

Nursing Considerations for the Child With a Cataract

A cataract is an opacity, or loss of transparency, of the lens. Causes include an inherited tendency (usually an autosomal dominant trait), infection (e.g., rubella), trauma, or a metabolic imbalance. Cloudiness of the lens may be noted during examination in the newborn nursery (indicated by a white instead of red reflex) or by parents. Ophthalmoscopy may reveal a dark spot in the lens. Parents may note that the infant exhibits visual inattentiveness and come in for an evaluation. Other clinical signs include nystagmus and strabismus.

The cataract alters vision because it does not allow a sharp, clear image to be formed on the retina. Early intervention (before 3 months of age) for the infant born with cataracts is crucial to allow vision to develop normally (Levin, 2003).

Treatment for cataracts is the surgical removal of the opaque lens. The resultant hyperopia is then dealt with using a contact lens or an intraocular lens implant. Glasses may also be used to correct the resultant vision problem.

Amblyopia may also be present. In this case, the normal eye may be patched after surgery to develop the weakened eye.

Postoperative interventions are directed toward avoiding increased intraocular pressure. Measures include preventing coughing, straining, vomiting, and touching the operative site. A patch and "hard shield" are usually in place after surgery to prevent injury to the operative site. To prevent edema and pressure on the site, the nurse should elevate the head of the bed slightly and should position the child so that the affected eye is not in a dependent position. Monitor the child for signs and symptoms of infection (fever, drainage, redness). Medications, including antibiotics, mydriatics, and steroids, may be used after surgery.

Postoperative teaching includes how to insert, remove, and care for the child's contact lens. Parents need to be taught the signs and symptoms of infection and increasing intraocular pressure. To provide visual stimulation to the affected eye and prevent further loss of vision, the importance of complying with the patching regimen should also be emphasized. Finally, the nurse teaches the importance of returning for follow-up visits to ensure that the lens fits correctly, the vision correction is appropriate, and there are no signs and symptoms of complications.

Nursing Considerations for the Child With an Eye Infection

Conjunctivitis

Conjunctivitis (pinkeye) is an inflammation of the conjunctiva (the clear, membranous lining of the lid and sclera). Signs and symptoms of conjunctivitis may include itching, burning, light sensitivity (photophobia), "scratchy" eyelids, redness, edema, and discharge. It is caused usually by either allergy or infection. Accurate diagnosis before treatment is important because inappropriate treatment can lead to complications.

Conjunctivitis noted in the first few weeks of life is called *ophthalmia neonatorum*. In infants, conjunctivitis occurring in the first 24 hours of life is usually caused by chemical irritation from infection prophylaxis administered soon after birth. Either infection or a blocked lacrimal duct can cause conjunctivitis that occurs after the first 24 hours. Infants acquire infection during birth (from passing through the birth canal) or after birth. *Chlamydia* is responsible for most eye infections noted in infants (Hammerschlag, 2004). Medical treatment should be directed at the cause of the infection. Antibiotic or antiviral eye drops or ointments are most often used to treat infectious conjunctivitis. If *Chlamydia* is the cause, however, systemic antibiotics (e.g., erythromycin) are also used to prevent pneumonia.

Conjunctivitis in older children may have a variety of etiologies, including bacteria, viruses, allergy, infection, and trauma. Organisms most frequently implicated in bacterial conjunctivitis include *Haemophilus influenzae* and *Streptococcus pneumoniae*, although with the introduction of *H. influenzae* type B (Hib) vaccine, *H. influenzae* has decreased as a major cause. As with the infant, treatment depends on the cause. The nurse obtains a detailed history to help determine the cause. Infection should be suspected if the child has recently been exposed to another person with conjunctivitis or has had an upper respiratory infection. Itching often identifies the cause as an allergic response. Although children with allergic conjunctivitis exhibit redness of the conjunctiva, they usually do not manifest the type of thick discharge seen in bacterial conjunctivitis.

Chlamydial conjunctivitis is rare in children older than 3 years. It may be suspected, however, in a sexually active adolescent with persistent conjunctivitis. A diagnosis of chlamydial conjunctivitis in an older child who is not sexually active should signal the health care provider to assess the child for possible sexual abuse.

Medical management depends on the cause of the conjunctivitis. If the cause is infection, antibiotic or antiviral eye drops or ointment may be prescribed. If allergies are suspected, antihistamines, either oral or in the form of eye drops, may be indicated. In severe cases of allergic conjunctivitis, steroid eye drops and cromolyn sodium eye drops may be helpful. The steroid eye drops are tapered over approximately 7 days. Because steroids can worsen the severity of many infections, they are used with caution and only for a short time. Used over the long term, steroids can exacerbate glaucoma and contribute to cataract development.

Teach parents to keep the child's eye clean and to administer any prescribed medications (see Chapter 37). The parent can gently remove crusted material from the eye with a cotton ball soaked in warm water. Teach the parent to wipe the eye from the inner to the outer aspect and to wash the hands and use a new cotton ball for the other eye. Because bacterial or viral conjunctivitis is extremely contagious, the nurse teaches infection control measures. These include good handwashing and not sharing towels and washcloths. Bottles of eye medication should never be shared with another person. The tip of the dropper or ointment tube should not touch the child's eye or eyelid during administration. The child should also be kept home from school or daycare until 24 hours after antibiotics are started.

Preventing injury from rubbing the eye is also important. Mittens may be used for infants. These may be fashioned from bootie-type socks or may be commercially made mittens. Distraction and constant reminding are recommended for toddlers and older children. If the child wears contact lenses, advise discontinuing them until the infection has completely cleared. Securing new contact lenses eliminates the chance of reinfection from contaminated contact lenses and also lessens the risk of a corneal ulceration. Eye makeup should also be discarded and replaced, because the chance of reinfecting eyes from contaminated makeup is high. Mascara should be replaced routinely at least every 3 months.

If the conjunctivitis is allergic in origin, cool compresses and dark glasses may also help lessen the irritation and photophobia. If cromolyn sodium eye drops are prescribed, parents should be taught to begin using them *before* the allergy season because they need several weeks to reach full effectiveness. Ophthalmic nonsteroidal antiinflammatory preparations may also be helpful.

Orbital Cellulitis

Orbital cellulitis is caused by an infection of the soft tissues of the orbit. It may occur as a result of trauma or, more commonly, an infection of the ethmoid sinus. Clinical signs and symptoms include severe eyelid edema, erythema, and an anteriorly displaced eye. The child is febrile and has an elevated white blood cell count. Orbital cellulitis can be distinguished from periorbital cellulitis, inflammation of the tissue surrounding the orbit, which usually results from trauma (Givner as cited in Sadovsky, 2003).

Treatment for orbital cellulitis includes intravenous antibiotics after appropriate cultures have been taken. If the area is painful, analgesics might also be prescribed. Children with orbital cellulitis need to be admitted to the hospital for observation and treatment because of the potential for rapid progression into systemic disease. Left untreated, the infection causing the orbital cellulitis can spread to the optic nerve and then directly to the brain, causing meningitis.

Nursing care involves administering prescribed medications and monitoring the child receiving intravenous therapy. The child should also be carefully monitored for signs and symptoms that the infection is spreading. This includes a thorough neurologic assessment. Finally, the nurse assesses the child's pain status frequently. Hot packs four times a day and prescribed analgesics as ordered can relieve pain.

Corneal Ulcer

Corneal ulcers are usually caused by ocular infection secondary to trauma. Signs and symptoms include pain, tearing, purulent discharge, and blurred vision. Besides trauma, risk factors for corneal ulceration include extended wearing of soft contact lenses, surgical procedures, and viral infection in the eye (usually herpesvirus type 1). Corneal ulcerations may be a sign of underlying systemic disease. If not properly and aggressively treated, corneal ulcerations can cause corneal scarring and blindness.

Treatment includes aggressive topical antibiotic therapy with a broad-spectrum antibiotic until cultures return. Treatment is started with a potent new generation of fluoroquinolones: ciprofloxacin, ofloxacin, and norfloxacin. Topical antiviral preparations are used for ulcers caused by viral infection.

The nurse teaches the parent about administration of any prescribed medications and the cause and prevention of future ulcerations. The parent needs to discourage the child from rubbing the eyes (which can worsen the injury). The child who wears contact lenses should avoid wearing them until the ulceration and infection are completely healed. Any lenses worn during the episode should be discarded.

Nursing Considerations for the Child With Eye Trauma

Corneal Abrasion

Corneal abrasions usually result from a scraping or tearing of the cornea by foreign bodies, contact lenses, paper, and fingernails. The child may present with light sensitivity, pain, excessive tearing, and decreased vision. The abrasion is diagnosed by instilling a fluorescein dye in the eye and examining the eye under a blue filtered light (Wood's lamp) to highlight the injury. If foreign bodies remain in the eye, they should be removed.

If the abrasion is small, treatment may consist only of the instillation of antibiotic ointment four times a day for 1 to 2 days with a follow-up evaluation to check healing. Larger abrasions require patching for 24 hours. Referral to an ophthalmologist should be considered with any eye injury, but particularly for a large abrasion or with the suspicion of a penetrating injury. Many authorities now recommend no patching unless the wound is very large. If patched, the eye should be examined in 24 hours. Failure to treat an abrasion can result in loss of visual acuity or permanent scarring and opacity of the cornea.

Parent education is very important in caring for the child with a corneal abrasion. Because an abrasion increases the risk of infection, parents should be taught the importance of administering ophthalmic antibiotics as prescribed. The child should not rub the eye because rubbing can worsen an abrasion. If the eye is patched, advise the parents not to remove the patch for 24 hours, even to instill ointment. Keeping the patch in place prevents further damage to the eye from blinking. The nurse also reinforces injury prevention, especially wearing safety goggles during sports and other activities, such as woodworking.

Subconjunctival Hemorrhage

Subconjunctival hemorrhages present as red areas beneath the conjunctiva. They are often the result of Valsalva maneuvers, such as coughing, vomiting, or straining. Subconjunctival hemorrhages resolve on their own within 2 to 3 weeks and require no treatment. Although they often appear worse than they are, they may be associated with other ocular or physical problems and should be evaluated.

Because these hemorrhages resolve spontaneously, care is aimed at reassurance. Parents should be told that the hemorrhage will appear to grow larger in the first few days because of the effects of gravity.

Hyphema

A hyphema is a hemorrhage resulting from a blow or penetrating injury to the eye. Symptoms include a recent history of injury, pain, light sensitivity, decreased vision, the presence of floaters, and excessive tearing. The child is usually sleepy. If there is no known history of injury, the child should be assessed for a bleeding disorder, anticoagulant therapy, renal or hepatic disease, retinoblastoma, or child abuse. Children with sickle cell disease are prone to hyphema. An examination of the eye reveals blood in the anterior chamber (between the cornea and iris) of the eye. Traumatic hyphema usually fills less than one third of the anterior chamber.

Recommendations for management vary. Any penetrating eye injury is an emergency, requiring rapid referral to an ophthalmologist and treatment to prevent blindness. At the scene of the injury, the eye should be covered immediately with a sterile dressing and an eye shield (manufactured rigid eye shield, Styrofoam or plastic cup); do not instill any type of eye drops without orders from an ophthalmologist. Maintain minimal movement of the child's head until the child is seen by a physician (Olitsky & Nelson, 2000; Rodriguez, 2003).

Treatment for hyphema usually includes hospitalization, bed rest, sedation, and patching of both eyes. Because of the risk of a rebleed between the 3rd and 5th days, bed rest and patching are often recommended (Hertle & Roy, 2002) for at least that length of time. Medications, such as steroid eye drops, antifibrinolytic eye drops (tranexamic acid is best for pediatric use), antiglaucoma medications, and cycloplegic eye drops (atropine), may also be used.

Careful assessment is required for the child with a hyphema. Assess the eye frequently for a secondary hemorrhage, or rebleed. This condition is characterized by an increase in size of the hyphema, with bright-red "new" blood noted over the existing clot. Children who rebleed have a poorer long-term prognosis for vision because acute or chronic glaucoma can be a consequence. The child should also be monitored for signs and symptoms of increasing intraocular pressure (pain, nausea and vomiting, increased inflammation). The child should be monitored closely for side effects of medications, which will vary according to the prescribed therapy.

CHILDREN
Want to Know

How to Prevent Eye Injuries While Participating in Sports

- High-risk sports include those in which no eye protection is worn, such as boxing and martial arts, or those with a rapidly moving ball, bat, or puck.
- The highest percentage of injuries is seen in basketball and baseball.
- Wear protective eye wear, such as goggles and face shields, when possible.
- Wear goggles under helmets and with hockey masks.
- Always remove orthodontic headgear when playing sports.

Modified from Catalano, R.A. (1993). Eye injuries and prevention. *Pediatric Clinics of North America, 40,* 827-839.

The child is usually restricted to bed rest with bathroom privileges. Elevating the head of the bed 30 to 40 degrees helps settle the hyphema in the inferior anterior chamber angle. Television viewing may or may not be allowed, and reading and other close-up activities are usually forbidden. Therefore boredom is a problem for most children. Offer diversional activities that do not involve reading or straining the eyes, such as music and books on tape. If both eyes are patched, the nurse orients the child to the environment and provides for safety.

Discharge teaching includes use of prescribed home medications, patching regimen (the eye is usually patched at night for 2 weeks after discharge), and prevention of further injury. The child's eye should be protected with a shield if an eye patch is worn at night. The child can usually return to all normal activities several weeks after the injury. Eye protection is recommended for all children who participate in sports or other high-risk activities, but lifelong use of protective eye wear is recommended for the child who experiences hyphema. The nurse should also emphasize the importance of follow-up because the child is at risk for complications such as glaucoma and cataracts.

Splash Injury

Splash injury can occur any time infective, hot, or corrosive liquid splashes into a child's eye; burns of the eye constitute an ocular emergency. Burns may occur from any number of common household items, such as bleach, ammonia, drain opener, and oven cleaner.

Initial care of the child with a splash injury to the eyes focuses on immediate irrigation with water or saline to prevent further injury. In a chemical splash, if the chemical is alkaline, the irrigation may continue for several hours because the damaging action of alkaloids may be prolonged. If the burn is mild, irrigate for at least 30 minutes, using at least 2 L of irrigant; if the burn is severe, continue irrigating for 2 to 4 hours or with at least 10 L of irrigant (Olitsky & Nelson, 2004). The cornea may appear cloudy after an alkali burn. Irrigation of a frightened child's eyes can be very difficult and painful. Helping the child lean over a water fountain that is spraying upward makes the task easier.

! CRITICAL TO REMEMBER

Working With a Child Who Has a Visual Impairment

- Orient the child to the hospital environment on admission. Orientation can be done by walking the child around the room and identifying objects, such as the bed, bathroom, doorways, windows, and chairs.
- Never touch the child without identifying yourself and explaining what you plan to do.
- When describing objects or the environment to a child who is blind or visually impaired, use familiar terms. For example, if the child is older and recently blinded, you may be able to use color when describing objects. If the child has been blind since birth, color has no meaning. It is also useful to describe how many steps away something is or the placement of eating utensils on a tray. Remember that parents are often the best source for communication.
- Identify noises for the child because children who are visually impaired or blind often have difficulty in establishing the source of a noise.
- Orient the child frequently to time and place. Confusion can be frightening.
- Keep all items in the room in the same location and order. Changing the order or spacing of objects may cause confusion or lead to injury.
- Provide detailed explanations and allow the child to progress through care in steps to learn the order.
- As with any child, allow as much control over the situation as possible.
- Supervise the child, and counsel parents to supervise the child as needed.

Further treatment may include referral to an ophthalmologist for topical steroids, medications to dilate the pupils and decrease the risk of adhesions, antibiotic ointment, and patching. Oral antibiotics and analgesics may also be indicated. Nursing care focuses on prescribed medical treatments, comfort measures, and injury prevention (particularly if both of the child's eyes are patched).

Discharge teaching focuses not only on the prescribed medical treatments but also on the importance of adherence with long-term follow-up and injury prevention. Follow-up care includes monitoring visual acuity and monitoring for side effects, such as increased intraocular pressure and cataracts.

EYE SURGERY

Several eye disorders seen in infancy and childhood require surgical correction. Any surgical procedure is stressful for the child and family. Eye surgery is particularly stressful because the child's visual fields or acuity may be greatly reduced or absent for a period. If both eyes are affected, the child's ability to maneuver and perform activities of daily living independently is also affected.

The nurse should pay special attention to education. If the child is going home with patches, drops, or any other procedure that must be performed, the family needs to know how to perform this care and should also know the safety precautions involved.

Nursing Care Plan

The Child Having Eye Surgery

FOCUSED ASSESSMENT

Assessment of the child and family begins with determining their understanding of the planned surgical procedure and why this is necessary. This includes assessing their knowledge of the care that will be necessary after discharge, as well as any changes to expect. These might include home schooling if both eyes are affected. Understanding of safety principles should also be addressed at admission and should be reinforced during the child's hospitalization. Finally, the nurse assesses understanding of any special adaptations for procedures and begins teaching at the time of admission.

Nursing Diagnosis

Disturbed Sensory Perception (visual impairment) related to eye patching or surgical procedure.

Expected Outcomes

The child and family will:
- Describe any anticipated temporary vision changes.
- Demonstrate familiarity with the surroundings and with associated sights and sounds.

The child will:
- Remain alert and oriented to time and place.

INTERVENTION	RATIONALE
1. Prepare the child and family before surgery for any changes expected in vision, including blurred vision or patched eyes.	1. Preoperative preparation allows the child and family to know what to expect, thus lessening anxiety.
2. Before surgery, orient the child and family to the surroundings, including the recovery room and hospital room. Describe any unfamiliar sounds the child might experience; have the child close the eyes and listen.	2. Preoperative orientation to surroundings allows the child a feeling of familiarity during the postoperative period.
3. Provide reality orientation (time, day) for the child during the postoperative period, especially if vision is impaired or eyes are patched.	3. Providing a sense of time passage and orienting to day and night prevent the child from becoming disoriented and confused.
4. Provide emotional support, and allow expression of feelings of anger and frustration, often through play therapy and therapeutic communication.	4. Allowing the child and family to express their fears and frustrations in a "healthy" manner provides an appropriate outlet and encourages the use of other senses.

Evaluation

- Can the child and family describe expected temporary postoperative vision changes?
- Can the child describe the hospital and room environment and its associated sounds?
- Does the child remain alert and oriented to time and place?

Nursing Diagnosis

Risk for Injury related to increased intraocular pressure resulting from bleeding, edema, hematoma, postoperative vomiting.

Expected Outcome

The child will:
- Remain free from injury (increased intraocular pressure, bleeding) through appropriate management of postoperative eye care, crying, nausea, and vomiting.

INTERVENTION	RATIONALE
1. Fully orient the child to surroundings, and ensure that unsafe objects are removed from the environment.	1. Orienting the child to the environment and ensuring that the environment is safe prevent falls and other injuries when the child is out of bed.
2. Ensure that the child wears eye patches or shields as ordered.	2. Eye patches and shields are often prescribed to prevent any further injury to the eye.
3. Encourage the parents to remain with the child and prevent the child from rubbing the eyes. Restraints are used as a last resort to prevent injury. Encourage the parent to keep side rails up at all times.	3. Rubbing the eyes can damage the surgical site. If restraints are needed, elbow restraints provide protection without total restriction.

Continued

Nursing Care Plan

The Child Having Eye Surgery—cont'd

INTERVENTION	RATIONALE
4. Monitor for signs and symptoms of increased intraocular pressure. Give ordered antiemetics if the child is nauseous. Administer intravenous fluids until the child is stable.	4. Increasing intraocular pressure can damage the eye and seriously impair vision. Vomiting can increase intraocular pressure.
5. Approach the child in a calm and soothing manner. Assign personnel whom the child has met and trusts. Encourage the parent to soothe the child who is crying.	5. Avoidance of crying postoperatively reduces the risk for increasing intraocular pressure. Assigning the child to a familiar nurse will reduce fear and anxiety that might lead to crying.

Evaluation

- Does the child remain free of physical injury?
- Is the child's intraocular pressure within normal limits?
- Is the child free from crying, nausea, or vomiting?

Nursing Diagnosis

Risk for Infection related to surgical incision.

Expected Outcome

The child will:

- Remain free from infection, as evidenced by normal temperature and absence of discharge and excessive tearing or edema.

INTERVENTION	RATIONALE
1. Monitor the child for signs and symptoms of infection, including redness, drainage, fever, and excessive tearing or edema.	1. These are physical signs that a postoperative infection is developing in the eye.
2. Administer antibiotic therapy as ordered.	2. Antibiotics may be used as prophylaxis against infection.

Evaluation

- Is the child free from fever, redness, edema, or excessive eye drainage?

Nursing Diagnosis

Acute Pain related to surgical procedure.

Expected Outcome

The child will:

- Experience minimal discomfort during the postoperative period, as evidenced by acceptable pain scale rating, normal vital signs, and participation in approved quiet activities.

INTERVENTION	RATIONALE
1. Monitor the child frequently (every 2-4 hr while awake) for pain using an age-appropriate pain scale. Monitor physiologic signs of pain in the young child (increased pulse, restlessness, inability to sleep, inability to play).	1. Pain can increase anxiety and restlessness that could lead to increased intraocular pressure. The young child who would ordinarily use a visual scale to rate pain is unable to do so if eyes are patched.
2. Administer pain medications as ordered.	2. Pain control decreases the child's need to rub or touch the eyes, which can cause trauma to the surgical site.
3. Provide non-pharmacologic pain-relief measures, such as ice pack and moist heat, as indicated. Use distraction techniques frequently (music, stories).	3. Non-pharmacologic pain-relief measures can replace or augment pharmacologic measures. Verbal distraction techniques can decrease pain and take the child's mind away from the bandages.

Evaluation

- Does the child express relief of pain using an age-appropriate pain scale?
- Are the child's vital signs within normal limits, and can the child participate appropriately in approved quiet activities?

HEARING LOSS IN CHILDREN

Etiology

Damage to, or impairment of, any part of the ear can cause hearing loss. Four types of hearing loss have been identified: conductive, sensorineural, mixed, and central. Each has a different treatment regimen and response to intervention (Box 55-3).

Incidence

The incidence of newborns diagnosed with significant hearing loss is 1 to 6 newborns in 1000 (Cunningham & Cox, 2003). As many as 14.9% of children 6 to 19 years of age experience slight hearing loss, particularly at the upper and lower frequencies (Nisak et al., 1998).

Diagnostic Evaluation

Evidence suggests that infants with hearing loss who have been identified and treated before 6 months of age have a better prognosis than those for whom treatment has been delayed. Using risk criteria for screening infants for hearing loss helps identify only approximately 50% of infants affected (Box 55-4). The Joint Committee on Infant Hearing has recommended that all infants be screened before 1 month of age, that hearing loss be identified before 3 months of age, and that intervention occur before 6 months of age (American Academy of Pediatrics [AAP], 2000). Many states in the United States have passed legislation making newborn hearing screening mandatory.

Hearing screening for infants is challenging because of their inability to give accurate behavioral cues indicating intact hearing. Historically, assessing hearing in the newborn or young infant often relied on eliciting a startle reflex with a loud noise. It is difficult, however, to be certain that the response is actually caused by the sound itself. Two hearing screening tests can accurately identify infants with hearing deficits: the auditory brainstem response and the evoked otoacoustic emissions test (Box 55-5). Newer equipment has made it possible for these tests to be completed quickly and accurately in the hospital nursery. Both tests have a pass/refer option. If the infant fails after two tries (2 weeks apart), referral to an audiologist for more accurate testing is required. More sophisticated testing, such as visual reinforcement audiometry or conditioned-play audiometry, is done by audiologists.

Hearing testing in the older child (3 years and older) is done by play audiometry (e.g., the child performs a play activity when the sound is heard) or conventional audiometry (Cunningham & Cox, 2003). The child is presented tones of varying frequencies at a standard volume (usually 20 decibels [dB]). A quick screening test done in a physician's office with a hand-held audiometer tests frequencies of 500, 1000, 2000, and 4000 hertz (Hz). If the child fails the screening, particularly at lower frequencies and the lower volume, a tympanogram might indicate middle ear effusion (see Chapter 45). The problem with office audiometric screening is that it can miss hearing loss at higher frequencies, which is usually sensorineural. When doing audiometry screening of children, therefore, the nurse should perform the test in a quiet environment and determine ahead of time what signal the child will use to indicate hearing the tone.

Therapeutic Management

The goals of identification and management of infants and children with hearing loss are directed toward maximizing language development and preventing later problems with school performance and social interaction. Treatment of

---

BOX 55-3
Types and Etiology of Hearing Loss

Conductive: Outer or middle ear affected by damage, inflammation, or obstruction. Sound conduction is prevented from progressing from the outer ear to the inner ear. May be the result of excessive cerumen (wax), foreign bodies, perforated tympanic membrane, or otitis media (with or without effusion). Hearing loss is often temporary and reversible.

Sensorineural: Result of damage or malformation of structures of the inner ear and/or auditory nerve. May be the result of infection (meningitis or intrauterine), heredity, exposure to loud noise, ototoxic medications, or prematurity. Meningitis causes 6% to 13% of acquired hearing loss in children.* Hearing loss is usually permanent.

Mixed: Combination of conductive and sensorineural loss. Conductive loss is often reversible, whereas sensorineural loss is not.

Central: Result of damage to the conduction system between the auditory nervous system and cerebral cortex. May be the result of trauma, neurovascular changes, or brain tumors. May cause difficulty in differentiation of sounds, auditory memory.

*Roizen, N. (1999). Etiology of hearing loss in children. *Pediatric Clinics of North America, 46,* 49-64.

Pathophysiology
of Hearing Loss

Adequate hearing depends on intact auditory structures and quality of sound. Sound is described in terms that combine volume (expressed in decibels [dB]) and pitch, or frequencies (expressed in hertz [Hz]). Normal speech ranges in volume between 10 and 60 dB. Normal hearing ranges from -10 to +15 dB at a variety of frequencies. Most people can hear frequencies between 10 and 20,000 Hz but are particularly sensitive to sounds between 1000 and 2000 Hz.* Hearing loss is categorized as follows:

Slight: Failure to hear at 16 to 25 dB
Mild: Failure to hear at 26 to 40 dB
Moderate: Failure to hear at 41 to 55 dB
Moderately severe: Failure to hear at 56 to 70 dB
Severe: Failure to hear at 71 to 90 dB
Profound: Failure to hear at more than 90 dB

A child with moderate hearing loss has difficulty hearing speech beyond a distance of 3 to 5 feet.* This deficit obviously poses problems for children who have not been identified as having a hearing loss and miss most of what a teacher says in a classroom.

Modified from Joint Committee on Infant Hearing. (1994).1994 Position statement. *ASHA, 36*(12), 38-41.
*Nash, D., Schochat, E., Rozycki, A., & Musiek, F. (1997). When loud noises hurt. *Contemporary Pediatrics, 14*(6), 97-109.

BOX 55-4
Risk Factors Indicating the Need for Hearing Screening

Neonates (Birth–28 Days)
- Family history of inherited sensorineural hearing loss
- Intrauterine infections, such as rubella, cytomegalovirus, and toxoplasmosis
- Craniofacial abnormalities
- Birth weight below 1.5 kg (3.3 lb)
- Hyperbilirubinemia requiring exchange transfusion
- Ototoxic medications given in multiple courses or with loop diuretics
- Bacterial meningitis
- Apgar scores of 0 to 4 at 1 minute or 0 to 6 at 5 minutes
- Mechanical ventilation for 5 or more days
- Any findings associated with a syndrome that includes hearing loss

Infants (29 Days–2 Years) Developing Certain Conditions Associated with Hearing Loss
- Hearing, speech, language, or developmental delay
- Infections associated with sensorineural hearing loss
- Head trauma resulting in loss of consciousness or skull fracture

- Any findings associated with a syndrome that includes hearing loss
- Ototoxic medications given in multiple courses or with loop diuretics
- Recurrent otitis media with effusion lasting at least 3 months

Infants (29 Days–3 Years) Needing Periodic Hearing Screening
Sensorineural
- Family history of inherited sensorineural hearing loss
- Intrauterine infections, such as rubella, cytomegalovirus, and toxoplasmosis
- Neurofibromatosis type II or other neurodegenerative disorder

Conductive
- Recurrent otitis media with effusion lasting at least 3 months
- Anything that affects eustachian tube function
- Neurodegenerative disorders

Data from Joint Committee on Infant Hearing. (1994). 1994 position statement. *ASHA* 36(12):38-41.

BOX 55-5
Hearing Tests Used for Infants

Auditory Brainstem Response
- Electrodes, which record brainwave activity, are placed on the infant's head.
- Foam-padded earphones are placed over the ears.
- The earphones sound a click at a 35-dB volume.
- The resulting brainwave measurement is compared with the brainwave measurement from a normal infant.
- More accurate testing can be done with more electrodes and clicks of varying intensities. The auditory brainstem response does not test hearing directly but tests the function of the auditory system and hearing sensitivity in the middle- to high-frequency ranges.*
- The test takes 10 to 60 minutes to administer, depending on the underlying testing objective.

Evoked Otoacoustic Emissions
- This test assesses the integrity of the inner ear structures by recording sounds (otoacoustic emissions) that are generated by the inner ear. It cannot assess the degree of hearing loss but can assess whether hearing is present.
- An ear probe, which contains a sound transmitter and microphone, is attached to a computer and placed in the ear.
- Click sounds evoke the emissions, which are displayed on the computer screen.
- Emissions are present in infants who can hear at 20 dB but not present in infants who hear only at 35 to 45 dB (mild to moderate hearing loss).*
- The test takes approximately 5 minutes to administer.

*Folsom, R., & Diefendorf, A. (1999). Physiologic and behavioral approaches to pediatric hearing assessment. *Pediatric Clinics of North America, 46,* 107-120.

---

hearing loss depends on the type of loss. Conductive hearing loss is managed by medical or surgical correction of the underlying problem (otitis, cerumen).

Sensorineural hearing loss, which is seldom reversible, requires a different approach. Hearing aids are often recommended for these children. The type of aid chosen depends on the specific needs of the child. The aid should provide the best acoustics and be cosmetically appropriate. For example, an adolescent seldom chooses a body-type hearing aid if an ear-level aid (one inserted into the ear canal) suffices. The four types of hearing aids most commonly used for pediatric patients are the behind-the-ear, the ear-level (in the ear), the eyeglass (aids attached to the temples of eyeglass frames), and the body (a box with wires connected to an ear mold). Infants and young children often do better with ear-level hearing aids. Infants diagnosed with hearing loss need to begin wearing hearing aids as soon as possible to help facilitate language development.

Cochlear implants offer new options for children with sensorineural hearing loss, even those with some residual hearing. The implant is a small electronic device surgically implanted in the cochlea. It delivers electrical stimulation to the inner ear, causing nerve impulses to travel to the brain, where they are interpreted as normal sound. The implant improves communication, but commitment to rehabilitative efforts and proper use and maintenance of the device by the family and child are essential for success (Francis & Niparko, 2003).

Nursing Considerations for the Child With Hearing Loss

Assess the child's hearing at each well-child visit and with any complaint specific to ears, including otitis media (see Chapter 45). Note an infant's response to bells, rattles, clapping of hands, or horns held approximately 12 inches from the ear. Older children can be asked to repeat whispered words or phrases or listen for a ticking watch. Begin audiometry testing at 3 years of age or younger in a cooperative child.

Assess language skill development. Deaf infants babble like hearing infants until approximately 5 to 6 months of age, when babbling is noted to cease in children who are deaf. The nurse also questions parents about the child's attention span, disruptive behavior, and other behaviors, such as increasing the volume on the television. If the child appears to have hearing loss or is lagging behind in developmental milestones, refer for further evaluation by an audiologist and ear, nose, and throat specialist.

When caring for a child who is hearing-impaired, the nurse should do the following:

- If the child has a hearing aid, encourage its use. Make sure it is in place before beginning to speak.
- Look directly in the child's face. To enhance lip reading, have the child's complete attention before beginning to speak.
- Speak clearly. Slow speech slightly. Do not speak loudly.
- Eliminate background noise.
- Use visual aids to assist communication. These include pictures, hands, and written messages for older children.
- If the child uses American Sign Language to communicate, have a diagram of commonly used words readily available. Use an interpreter for more complex discussions.

An important nursing responsibility is to educate parents about preventable hearing loss. Mild sensorineural hearing loss can occur from exposure to loud noises, such as from firecrackers, firearms, loud infant squeak toys, outdoor yard equipment, boat and snowmobile motors, and rock music. People exposed to loud sounds over long periods need to wear protective ear coverings (e.g., ear plugs, mufflers). Advise teens to decrease exposure to loud rock music and to turn music volume down, especially when listening through earphones. Children with hearing loss may need speech therapy; referral to a speech therapist or early intervention program should occur as soon as possible.

LANGUAGE DISORDERS

Until 10 to 12 months of age, a child is considered prelingual. The sounds the child makes have no direct meaning or connection to future language. They are, instead, practice of a learned skill. Before approximately 6 months of age, infants make few sounds other than crying. At approximately 4 to 6 months of age, however, they enter the babbling phase. These are the cooing, happy sounds that an infant makes

when content. The first words appear at approximately 10 to 12 months of age. First sentences appear at approximately 18 months of age. By 2 years of age, most children have at least a 50-word spoken vocabulary.

Girls have more rapid language development until approximately 3 years of age, when the difference disappears. By adolescence, however, girls again show superior verbal skills. Although a relationship exists between developmental delay and verbal skills, the relationship between language development and intelligence is unclear. There seems to be no scientific evidence that a child who talks early is brighter than one who does not. Children who talk very early do appear, however, to be bright, whereas those who talk extremely late appear to have some developmental delay.

Language disorders in the child are usually of two types. The first is the inability to comprehend (receptive disorder). The second is a disorder in which the child cannot express thoughts through speech (expressive disorder). Receptive disorders result from some type of central nervous system failure or hearing deficit. This may be the result of trauma, a congenital malformation, or other failure of language development. This child cannot express symbols and abstract ideas in clearly spoken words or in a logical manner.

Expressive disorders are most often of three types. The first is a disorder of the voice. This is an alteration in the pitch and intonation that may result from a medical condition, such as a cleft palate. The second is a defect of articulation, or the way in which words are pronounced. This is the most common type of speech defect and may be related to neuromuscular disease or to structural abnormalities of the nose, throat, and mouth. It may also be idiopathic. Finally, fluency disorders interrupt the flow of normal speech. Included in this category are lisping and stuttering. If stuttering persists after 5 years of age, the child should receive appropriate referrals for speech evaluation (Fig. 55-1).

As with screens for hearing loss, the nurse should assess the child's communication patterns with each well-child visit. Any problems should be noted and referrals made to provide appropriate intervention as soon as possible. Encourage parents to take measures to encourage speech and prevent speech problems.

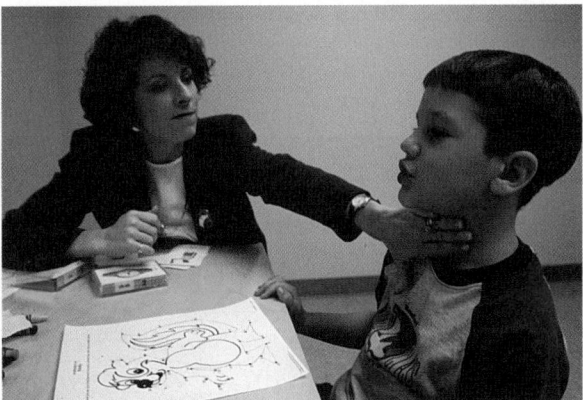

Figure 55-1 Expressive speech disorders include disorders of voice, articulation, and fluency. A speech therapist works with the child to help the child speak more clearly and be better understood. Early intervention is very important to correct speech disorders. The nurse should therefore assess speech patterns during each health screening visit. Referrals should be made for any problems noted. (Courtesy Cook Children's Medical Center, Fort Worth, TX.)

PARENTS Want to Know

How to Encourage Language Development

Talk

Talking to your child is necessary for language development. Because children usually imitate what they hear, how much you talk to your child, what you say, and how you say it affect how much and how well your child talks.

Look

Look directly at your child's face, and wait until your child pays attention before you begin talking.

Control distance

Be sure that you are close to your child when you talk (no farther than 5 feet). The younger the child, the more important it is to be close.

Loudness

Talk slightly louder than you normally do. To remove background noise, turn off the radio, television, dishwasher.

Be a good speech model

• Describe daily activities to your child as they occur.
• Expand what your child says. For example, if your child points and says "car," you say, "Oh, you want the car."
• Add new information. You might add, "That car is little."
• Build vocabulary. Make teaching new words and concepts a natural part of every day's activities. For example, use new words while shopping, taking a walk, or washing dishes.
• Repeat your child's words using adult pronunciation.

Play and talk

Set aside some times throughout each day for play time for just you and your child. Play can be looking at books, exploring toys, singing songs, coloring, and so on. Talk to your child during these activities, keeping the conversation at your child's level.

Read

Begin reading to your child at a young age (younger than 12 months). Ask a librarian for books that are right for your child's age. Reading can be a calming-down activity that promotes closeness between you and your child. Reading provides another opportunity to teach and review words and ideas. Some children enjoy looking at pictures in magazines and catalogs.

Do not wait

Your child should have the following skills by these ages:
• 18 months: 3-word vocabulary
• 2 years: 25- to 30-word vocabulary and several 2-word sentences
• 2½ years: at least a 50-word vocabulary and 2-word sentences consistently

If your child does not have these skills, tell your physician. A referral to an audiologist and speech pathologist may be indicated. Hearing and language testing may lead to a better understanding of your child's language development.

From Northern, J.L., & Downs, M.P. (1991). *Hearing in children* (4th ed., pp. 26-27). Baltimore: Williams & Wilkins. Modified from *Suggestions for parents*, Noel Matkin, PhD.

KEY CONCEPTS

■ Anything that alters a child's sensory perception can adversely affect growth and development.

■ Sense organs develop very early and are sensitive to teratogens. Any interference with development can result in later sensory alteration.

■ Special care should be taken when caring for the child with sensory alterations. Orientation to a new environment is critical in preventing stress and possible injury.

■ Most screenings for sensory alterations are noninvasive and relatively painless.

■ Parent education and support are critical in assisting the child with sensory alteration to develop as normally as possible.

■ Early intervention and special school supports for the child with sensory alterations allow for more normal growth and development.

■ Health teaching should include injury prevention.

ANSWERS to Critical Thinking Exercise 55-1

With any new program, it is important to look at the cost/benefit ratio. The benefits of this program cannot be argued. The costs can be high, but the increased initial cost could decrease later costs associated with intervention, rehabilitation, and emotional stress for the child and family.

Advantages:
• With this program, the approximately 1 to 4 in 1000 infants who are deaf at birth might be identified early enough to begin intervention.

• Deafness in the newborn is difficult to diagnose by behavior alone because responding to loud noises with a startle or blink might be related more to vibration than actual hearing.
• Delayed diagnosis compromises language development and future school performance.
• Only 50% of infants with deafness are identified under the risk referral criteria currently recommended.
• Diagnosis and intervention before the infant is 6 months old greatly improve outcomes.

Disadvantages:
• Equipment to do valid testing on newborns is expensive.
• Not all institutions could afford to implement a program without some monetary assistance.
• Depending on the test used, additional personnel might be required.
• Follow-up by the parent cannot be mandated. Tracking those who do not follow up could require additional personnel and paper work.

REFERENCES and READINGS

Allegretti, C. (2002). The effects of a cochlear implant on the family of a hearing-impaired child [Electronic version]. *Pediatric Nursing, 28*(6), 614-621.

American Academy of Pediatrics (AAP). (2000). Year 2000 position statement: Principles and guidelines for early hearing detection and intervention programs. *Pediatrics, 106*(4), 798-817.

American Academy of Pediatrics. (2002). Use of photoscreening for children's vision screening. *Pediatrics, 109*(3), 524-525.

Bacal, D., & Hertle, R. (1998). Don't be lazy about looking for amblyopia. *Contemporary Pediatrics, 15*(6), 99-107.

Bacal, D., Rousta, S., & Hertle, R. (1999). Why early vision screening matters. *Contemporary Pediatrics, 16*, 155-163.

Brookhouser, P., Beauchaine, K., & Osberger, M. (1999). Management of the child with sensorineural hearing loss. *Pediatric Clinics of North America, 46*, 121-141.

Cheng, K. (2001). When to prescribe glasses for young children. *Review of Ophthalmology, 8*(10), 70-75.

Coats, D., Carothers, T., Brady-McCreery, K., & Paysse, E. (2004). Ocular infectious diseases. In R. Feigin, J. Cherry, G. Demmler, & S. Kaplan (Eds.). *Textbook of pediatric infectious disease* (5th ed., pp.787-807). Philadelphia: Saunders.

Committee on Practice and Ambulatory Medicine. (2003). Eye examination in infants, children, and young adults by pediatricians [Electronic version]. *Pediatrics, 111*(4), 902-907.

Cunningham, M., & Cox, E. (2003). Hearing assessment in infants and children: Recommendations beyond neonatal screening. *Pediatrics, 111*(2), 436-441.

Curnyn, K., & Kaufman, L. (2003). The eye examination in the pediatrician's office. *Pediatric Clinics of North America, 50*, 25-40.

Downey, D., Mraz, R., Knott, J., Knutson, C., Holte, L., & VanDyke, D. (2002). Diagnosis and evaluation of children who are not talking [Electronic version]. *Infants & Young Children, 15*(1), 38-49.

Finitzo, T., & Crumley, W. (1999). The role of the pediatrician in hearing loss. *Pediatric Clinics of North America, 46*, 15-34.

Flax, J., & Rapin, I. (1998). Evaluating children with delayed speech and language. *Contemporary Pediatrics, 15*(10), 164-172.

Folsom, R., & Diefendorf, A. (1999). Physiologic and behavioral approaches to pediatric hearing assessment. *Pediatric Clinics of North America, 46*, 107-120.

Francis, H., & Niparko, J. (2003). Cochlear implantation update. *Pediatric Clinics of North America, 50*, 341-361.

Greenwald, M. (2003). Refractive abnormalities in childhood. *Pediatric Clinics of North America, 50*, 197-212.

Hammerschlag, M. (2004). Chlamydia infections. In R. Feigin, J. Cherry., G. Demmler, & S. Kaplan (Eds.). *Textbook of pediatric infectious diseases* (5th ed., pp. 2482-2486). Philadelphia: Saunders.

Hertle, R., & Roy, C. (2002). Uveitis and hyphema. In F. Burg, J. Ingelfinger, R. Polin, & A. Gershon (Eds.), *Gellis and Kagan's current pediatric therapy* (17th ed., pp. 908-910). Philadelphia: Saunders.

Jockin, Y. (2002). Strabismus and amblyopia. In F. Burg, J. Ingelfinger, R. Polin, & A. Gershon (Eds.), *Gellis and Kagan's current pediatric therapy* (17th ed., pp. 915-916). Philadelphia: Saunders.

Johnson, A. (2002). Update on newborn hearing screening programs [Electronic version]. *Pediatric Nursing, 28*(3), 267-271.

Joint Committee on Infant Hearing. (1994). 1994 position statement. *ASHA, 36*(12), 38-41.

Kipp, M. (2003). Childhood glaucoma. *Pediatric Clinics of North America, 50*, 89-104.

Levin, A. (2003). Congenital eye anomalies. *Pediatric Clinics of North America, 50*, 55-76.

Mark, H., & Mark, T. (1999). Parental reasons for non-response following a referral in school vision screening. *Journal of School Health, 69*(1), 35-37.

McCartney, P. (1999). Newborn hearing screening: What nurses think. *MCN: The American Journal of Maternal/Child Nursing, 24*, 48.

Mills, M. (1999). The eye in childhood. *American Family Physician, 60*(3), 906-915.

Mittleman, D. (2003). Amblyopia. *Pediatric Clinics of North America, 50*, 189-196.

Nash, D., Schochat, E., Rozycki, A., & Musiek, F. (1997). When loud noises hurt. *Contemporary Pediatrics, 14*(6), 97-109.

Nisak, A., Kieszak, S., Holmes, A., Esteban, E., Rubin, C., & Brody, D. (1998). Prevalence of hearing loss among children 6 to 19 years of age: The third national health and nutrition examination survey. *JAMA: The Journal of the American Medical Association, 279*, 1071-1075.

Olitsky, S., & Nelson, L. (2000). Disorders of the eye. In R. Behrman, R. Kliegman, & H. Jenson (Eds.), *Nelson textbook of pediatrics* (16th ed., pp. 1895-1937). Philadelphia: Saunders.

Olitsky, S., & Nelson, L. (2004). Disorders of the eye. In R. Behrman, R. Kliegman, & H. Jenson (Eds.), *Nelson textbook of pediatrics* (17th ed., pp. 2083-2126). Philadelphia: Saunders.

Robinson, B., Bobier, W., Martin, E., & Bryant, L. (1999). Preschool vision screening program. *American Journal of Public Health, 89*, 193-197.

Rodriguez, J. (2003). Prevention and treatment of common eye injuries in sports [Electronic version]. *American Family Physician, 67*(7), 1481-1489.

Roizen, N. (1999). Etiology of hearing loss in children. *Pediatric Clinics of North America, 46*, 49-64.

Sadovsky, R. (2003). Distinguishing periorbital from orbital cellulites. *American Family Physician, 67*(6), 1349-1350.

Stein, L. (1999). Factors influencing the efficacy of universal newborn hearing screening. *Pediatric Clinics of North America, 46*, 95-105.

Ticho, B. (2003). Strabismus. *Pediatric Clinics of North America, 50*, 173-188.

Tomaski, S., & Grundfast, K. (1999). A stepwise approach to the diagnosis and treatment of hereditary hearing loss. *Pediatric Clinics of North America, 46*, 35-48.

Wilson, M. (2002). Cornea. In F. Burg, J. Ingelfinger, R. Polin, & A. Gershon (Eds.), *Gellis and Kagan's current pediatric therapy* (17th ed., pp. 906-908). Philadelphia: Saunders.

Wittman-Price, R., & Pope, K. (2002). Universal newborn hearing screening. *American Journal of Nursing, 102*(11), 71-77.

APPENDIX A

Laboratory Values in Pregnant and Nonpregnant Women and in the Newborn

Laboratory Values in Pregnant and Nonpregnant Women

Value	Nonpregnancy	Pregnancy
Blood volume, total	55-80 ml/kg	Increases 40-50%
Plasma volume	30-45 ml/kg	Increases 50% (1200-1300 ml above nonpregnancy levels)
Red blood cell mass	20-35 ml/kg	Increases 25-33% (average total increase of 250-450 ml)
Red blood cell count	4.2-5.4 million/mm³	Decreases slightly due to hemodilution
Hemoglobin	12-16 g/dl	At least 11 g/dl during first and third trimesters, at least 10.5 in second trimester
Hematocrit, packed cell volume	37-47%	>33%
White blood cell count	5000-10,000/mm³	5000-12,000/mm³ Rises during labor and early postpartum
Platelets	150,000-400,000/mm³	150,000-400,000/mm³ or slight decrease
Prothrombin time	11-12.5 sec	Slight decrease but remains within normal limits
Activated partial thromboplastin time	21-35 sec	Slight decrease but remains within normal limits
Glucose, serum		
Fasting	65-110 mg/dl	≤95 mg/dl
Postprandial	<140 mg/dl	<140 mg/dl
Creatinine, serum	0.5-1.1 mg/dl	Decreased, ≤8 mg/dl
Creatinine clearance, urine	87-107 ml/min	110-180 ml/min
Fibrinogen	200-400 mg/dl	300-600 mg/dl

Data from Blackburn, S.T. (2003). *Maternal, fetal, & neonatal physiology* (2nd ed.). Philadelphia: Saunders; Cunningham, F.G., Gant, N.F., Leveno, K.J., Gilstrap, L.C., Hauth, J.C., & Wenstrom, K.D. (2001). *Williams obstetrics* (21st ed.). New York: McGraw-Hill; Fischbach, F. (2000). *A manual of laboratory and diagnostic tests* (6th ed.). Philadelphia: Lippincott; Gordon, M.C. (2002). Maternal physiology in pregnancy. In S.G. Gabbe, J.R. Niebyl, & J.L. Simpson (Eds.), *Obstetrics: Normal and problem pregnancies* (4th ed.). Philadelphia: Churchill Livingstone; Moore, T.R. (2004). Diabetes in pregnancy. In R.K. Creasy & R. Resnik (Eds.), *Maternal-fetal medicine: Principles and practice* (5th ed.). Philadelphia: Saunders; and Pagana, K.D. & Pagana, T.J. (2002). *Mosby's manual of diagnostic and laboratory tests* (2nd ed.). St. Louis: Mosby.

Laboratory Values in the Newborn

Test, Specimen, and Unit of Measurement	Age	Normal Ranges
Erythrocyte (RBC or red blood cell) count, whole blood (million/mm³)	Cord	3.9-5.5
	1-3 days	4-6.6
	1 wk	3.9-6.3
	1 mo	3-5.4
Hemoglobin, whole blood (g/dl)	1-3 days (capillary)	14.5-22.5
	2 mo	9-14
Hematocrit, whole blood (%)	1 day (capillary)	48-69
	2 days	48-75
	3 days	44-72
	2 mo	28-42
White blood cell count, whole blood (thousand/mm³)	Birth	9-30
	24 hr	9.4-34
	1 mo	5-19.5
White blood cell differential count, whole blood (%)		
Myelocytes		0
Neutrophils ("bands")		3-5
Neutrophils ("segs")		54-62
Lymphocytes		25-33
Monocytes		3-7
Eosinophils		1-3
Basophils		0-0.75
Platelet count, whole blood (thousand/mm³)	Newborn	84-478
	>1 wk	150-400
Glucose, serum (mg/dl)	Cord	45-96
	Newborn at 1 day	40-60
	Newborn, >1 day	50-90
Calcium, serum (mg/dl)	Cord	9-11.5
	Newborn	
	3-24 hr	9-10.6
	24-48 hr	7-12
	4-7 days	9-10.9
Magnesium, plasma (mg/dl)	Newborn 0-6 days	1.2-2.6

		Normal Ranges	
		Preterm	Full-Term
Bilirubin, total serum (mg/dl)	Cord	<2	<2
	0-1 day	<8	<6
	1-2 days	<12	<8
	2-5 days	<16	<12
	>5 days	<20	<10
Bilirubin, direct (conjugated) serum (mg/dl)		0-0.2	0-0.2

Adapted from Nicholson, J.F., & Pesce, M.A. (2004). Reference ranges for laboratory tests and procedures. In R.E. Behrman, R.M. Kliegman, & H.B. Jenson (Eds.), *Nelson textbook of pediatrics* (17th ed., pp. 2396-2427). Philadelphia: Saunders.

APPENDIX B

Use of Drug Preparations During Pregnancy and Breastfeeding

FOOD AND DRUG ADMINISTRATION PREGNANCY RISK CATEGORIES

The U.S. Food and Drug Administration (FDA) has assigned pregnancy risk categories to many drugs on the basis of their known relative safety or danger to the fetus and on the basis of whether safer alternative drugs exist. Depending on fetal effects or nearness of births, drugs may carry different risk categories at different points during pregnancy. For many drugs, little is known about the fetal risk. FDA categories are as follows:

A: No evidence of risk to the fetus exists.
B: Animal reproduction studies have not demonstrated a risk to the fetus. No adequate and well-controlled studies have been done in pregnant women.
C: Animal reproduction studies have shown an adverse effect on the fetus but no adequate, well-controlled studies have been done in humans. Potential benefits may warrant use of the drug in pregnant women despite fetal risks. Or, animal studies show adverse effect on fetus but human studies with pregnant women have not demonstrated a risk to the fetus in any trimester of pregnancy.

D: There is positive evidence of human fetal risk based on adverse reaction data, but potential benefits may warrant use of the drug in pregnant women despite fetal risks. Essentially, no safer alternatives to the drug are available.
X: There is positive evidence of human fetal risk based on animal or human studies and/or adverse reaction data. The risks of using the drug in pregnant women clearly outweigh potential benefits. Safer alternatives to these drugs may be available.

DRUG USE DURING LACTATION

The effects of many drugs, when used during lactation, have not been studied. In general, if a drug is safe for use in infants, it is probably safe for the lactating woman to take. Other drugs are known not to be excreted in breast milk or excreted in an inactive form or very low concentrations. Modifying the time of maternal ingestion may reduce transfer of the drug to the infant. Some drugs are undesirable because they suppress lactation, which is a problem primarily in the earliest stages of breastfeeding.

Maternal use of social and illicit drugs during pregnancy or breastfeeding are discussed in Chapters 25 and 30.

Drug	Use During Pregnancy	Use During Breastfeeding
AMEBICIDES		
Metronidazole (Flagyl)	*Risk category* B. Previous concerns about teratogenic effects on the fetus have not been supported (CDC, 2002). Treatment of choice for trichomoniasis but may also be chosen as part of drug regimen for inflammatory bowel disease or postpartum endometriosis.	Breastfeeding may be discontinued for 12 to 24 hr during single-dose treatment of mother. However, few known adverse infant effects.

Drug	Use During Pregnancy	Use During Breastfeeding
ANALGESICS		
Aspirin	*Risk category C (D in third trimester).* Has been linked to fetal gastroschisis and small intestine atresia.	Single doses not associated with risk to breastfeeding infant. Greater potential risk if mother requires higher doses for disorders such as arthritis.
Acetaminophen (Tylenol, Datril, Tempra)	*Risk category B.* Problems have not been documented, but drug crosses placenta in low concentrations. Maximum dosage 4 g/day. Drug often combined with other medications and should be considered when determining the maximum daily dose received.	Safe. Very small amounts secreted into breast milk.
Opiate analgesics Butorphanol (Stadol), fentanyl (Sublimaze), hydrocodone (Lortab, Vicodin), hydromorphone (Dilaudid), meperidine (Demerol), morphine, nalbuphine (Nubain), oxycodone (Percocet, Tylox, Percodan)	*Most are risk category B or C.* Neonatal respiratory depression is the most significant adverse effect when large amounts of opiates are used during labor, making them a *category D* at this time. Neonatal withdrawal may occur if the woman is addicted to an opiate drug.	Most narcotics given briefly and in therapeutic doses are compatible with breastfeeding, including intrathecal (before epidural catheter removal) morphine given postoperatively. Prolonged infant sedation during the early postpartum period may occur with maternal meperidine analgesia.
Nonsteroidal antiinflammatory drugs (NSAIDs) Fenoprofen (Nalfon), flurbiprofen (Ansaid), ibuprofen (Advil, Motrin, Nuprin), indomethacin (Indocin), ketoprofen (Actron, Orudis), naproxen (Aleve, Anaprox)	*Risk category B or C; category D in third trimester.* May prolong pregnancy or labor because of antiprostaglandin effects. Indomethacin associated with premature closure of ductus arteriosus or oligohydramnios in fetus but may be given in limited doses to stop preterm labor or reduce excess amniotic fluid in hydramnios.	Ibuprofen, indomethacin, and naproxen are American Academy of Pediatrics (AAP) approved. All should be used cautiously owing to potential for infant bleeding. Indomethacin has been used for treatment of neonatal patent ductus arteriosus.
COX-2 inhibitors Celecoxib (Celebrex), rofecoxib (Vioxx), valdecoxib (Bextra)	*Risk category C.* Associated with oligohydramnios and constriction of the ductus arteriosus.	No adverse effects reported via milk. Observe for infant gastrointestinal (GI) cramping, diarrhea.
Migraine agents Almotriptan (Axert), frovatriptan (Frovan), naratriptan (Amerge), rizatriptan (Maxalt), sumatriptan (Imitrex)	*Risk category C.* Minimal well-controlled studies about fetal safety during pregnancy.	No identified pediatric concerns via breast milk but caution recommended. Pumping and discarding milk for 24 hr after medication administration prevent transfer to infant.
ANTIALLERGIC		
Antihistamines (See middle column for drugs.)	*Risk category B.* Chlorpheniramine (Chlor-Trimeton), clemastine (Contac, Tavist), diphenhydramine (Benadryl), loratadine (Claritin), meclizine (Antivert, Dramamine). *Risk category C.* Astemizole (Hismanal), brompheniramine (Dimetane), phenylephrine (Neo-Synephrine), terfenadine (Seldane), triprolidine (Alleract).	All should be used with caution. Most are safe but may cause infant drowsiness. If these adverse effects occur, a different drug may be tried. Clemastine noted by AAP to be given with caution due to one case of infant irritability, refusal to feed, neurologic symptoms, seizures, and a high-pitched cry.
ANTIASTHMATIC DRUGS (See also *Decongestants, Hormones, Corticosteroids other than inhalers*)		
Corticosteroid inhalers Beclomethasone (Beclovent, Vanceril); triamcinolone (Aristacort, Azmacort, Nasacort)	*Risk category C*	Safety in lactation not fully known but none reported following breast milk.
Nonsteroidal antiinflammatory asthma medications Cromolyn (Intal, NasalCrom, Opticrom); nedocromil (Alocril, Miraze)	*Risk category B*	Minimal oral absorption. No reported adverse effects via milk.

Continued

Drug	Use During Pregnancy	Use During Breastfeeding
ANTIASTHMATIC DRUGS		
Epinephrine (Adrenalin, Sus-Phrine, Primatene)	*Risk category* C. To treat bronchospasm in acute asthma attack.	Observe for brief infant stimulation after maternal drug use.
Montelukast (Singulair); zafirlukast (Accolate); zyleuton (Zyflo)	*Risk categories* B (zafirlukast, montelukast) and C (zyleuton)	No reported problems via breast milk; little published experience.
Metaproterenol (Alupent)	*Risk category* C. May inhibit uterine contractions.	Unknown if secreted in milk; use cautiously.
ANTICOAGULANTS		
Enoxaparin (Lovenox)	*Risk category* B. Not interchangeable with heparin.	Unlikely to produce clinically relevant levels in breast milk due to molecular size.
Heparin	*Risk category* C	Not excreted in breast milk
Warfarin (Coumadin)	*Risk category* X. Known teratogen that should be used during pregnancy only if the benefits outweigh risks. Associated with central nervous system (CNS) and facial malformations, mental retardation, prenatal growth deficiency, and other fetal defects.	Small amounts secreted in milk. Infant bleeding abnormalities may result. Avoiding breastfeeding during therapy may be recommended.
ANTICONVULSANTS		
Carbamazepine (Tegretol); oxcarbazepine (Trileptal)	*Risk category* C. Associated with craniofacial abnormalities, underdeveloped fingernails, neural tube defects, and developmental delay.	Small amounts secreted in breast milk; accumulation does not seem to occur. Observe infant for sedation.
Clonazepam (Klonopin)	*Risk category* D. No firm evidence that clonazepam is teratogenic. Infant after birth may display mild sedation, hypotonia, poor sucking.	Enters breast milk in a possibly relevant quantity.
Magnesium sulfate	*Risk category* A during early pregnancy. Infants exposed to magnesium sulfate 2 hr before birth may exhibit respiratory depression, hypotonic muscle tone, depressed reflexes, hypocalcemia, or cardiac dysrhythmias. Although infant risks exist when used during labor, complications of preeclampsia and eclampsia are greater.	Milk levels return to normal about 24 hr after drug is stopped.
Phenobarbital	*Risk category* D. Fetal addiction with subsequent withdrawal is possible but rare at dose levels used for seizure control. Abnormalities similar to those seen in infants exposed to carbamazepine, phenytoin, and valproic acid have been reported.	Infant serum levels approximately one-third of adult levels. Psychomotor delay and sedation possible.
Fosphenytoin (Cerebyx); phenytoin (Dilantin)	*Risk category* D. Few studies of fosphenytoin. Phenytoin's risk for fetal malformations, specifically congenital heart defects and cleft palate, is double that of the general population.	Methemoglobinemia, drowsiness, and poor sucking have been reported. Most studies do not suggest problems.
Primidone (Mysoline)	*Risk category* D	Drug and its metabolites are secreted into breast milk. Has been associated with neonatal sedation.
Topiramate (Topamax)	*Risk category* C	No studies available. Use with caution.
Valproic acid (Depakene)	*Risk category* D. Associated with neural tube defects, craniofacial, cardiac, and hand abnormalities.	Secreted in small amounts. May cause drowsiness. Used for treatment of infant seizures.

Drug	Use During Pregnancy	Use During Breastfeeding
ANTIDIABETIC AGENTS		
Insulin	*Risk category* B. Insulin is the drug of choice during pregnancy because it does not cross placenta.	Orally ingested insulin would be destroyed in infant's gastrointestinal tract.
Oral hypoglycemic agents Metformin (Glucophage); nateglinide (Starlix); pioglitazone (Actos); repaglinide (Prandin); rosiglitazone (Avandia)	*Risk category* B for metformin and C for remaining drugs.	Safety not established for most oral hypoglycemics. Observe for infant hypoglycemia if used.
ANTIFUNGALS		
Fluconazole (Diflucan), miconazole (Monistat), nystatin (Mycostatin), terconazole (Terazol)	*Risk category* C	Fluconazole excreted in breast milk at levels similar to the mother's plasma level. Most considered safe if ingested in breast milk.
ANTIHYPERTENSIVES (See also *Diuretics*)		
Angiotensin-converting enzyme inhibitors Benazepril (Lotensin), captopril (Capoten), enalapril (Vasotec), fosinopril (Monopril), lisinopril (Prinivil, Zestril), quinapril (Accupril), ramipril (Altace), trandolapril (Mavik)	*Risk category* D (primarily second and third trimesters). Renal dysplasia leading to oligohydramnios may result in pulmonary hypotension and death after birth.	Observe for infant hypotension. Less safety data available for newer agents.
Beta-adrenergic blockers Acebutolol (Monitan, Sectral), atenolol (Tenormin), betaxolol (Kerlone), labetalol (Normodyne), metoprolol (Lopressor, Toprol), nadolol (Corgard), penbutolol (Levatol), pindolol (Viskin), propranolol (Inderal)	*Risk categories* C (labetalol, metoprolol, nadolol, penbutalol, and propranolol) and D (acebutolol, atenolol). *Risk category* B for pindolol. Possible fetal or neonatal effects include intrauterine growth restriction, neonatal hypotension, bradycardia, transient tachypnea, respiratory depression, and hypoglycemia.	Acebutalol, labetalol, metoprolol, nadolol, and propranolol considered safe. Less known about other drugs. Observe infant for possible effects listed in Use During Pregnancy column.
Calcium channel blockers Amlodipine (Norvasc), diltiazem (Cardizem), nicardipine (Cardene), nifedipine (Adalat, Procardia), verapamil (Calan, Isoptin)	*Risk category* C. May benefit fetus by reducing resistance to placental blood flow. Nifedipine and verapamil may be given to reduce preterm contractions, prolonging pregnancy.	Diltiazem, nifedipine, verapamil generally considered safe although diltiazem levels in breast milk may reach maternal serum levels. Less known about other drugs listed.
Centrally acting antihypertensives Clonidine (Catapres), guanabenz (Wytensin), guanadrel (Hylorel), guanfacine (Tenex), methyldopa (Aldomet)	*Risk categories* B (guanadrel, guanfacine, methyldopa) and C (clonidine, guanabenz). Methyldopa is an accepted antihypertensive drug during first trimester of pregnancy.	Methyldopa is considered safe. Little information about effects of the other centrally acting antihypertensive drugs on lactation. Observe infant for hypotension.
Vasodilators Hydralazine (Apresoline), minoxidil (Loniten), nitroprusside (Nipride, Nitropress)	*Risk category* C. Hydralazine is drug of choice for serious hypertension during pregnancy. Nitroprusside given in carefully titrated doses to control severe hypertension during pregnancy.	Hydralazine considered safe but less is known about minoxidil use. Nitroprusside is a concern because of the drug's conversion to a potentially toxic thiocyanate metabolite.

Continued

Drug	Use During Pregnancy	Use During Breastfeeding
ANTIMICROBIALS		
Aminoglycosides Gentamicin (Garamycin), streptomycin, tobramycin (Tobrex, Nebcin)	*Risk category C or D.* Associated with hearing loss and renal toxicity.	Most drugs in this class are considered safe because minimal amounts are secreted in breast milk and the drugs are poorly absorbed if orally ingested. Observe for changes in the GI flora.
Macrolides Azithromycin (Zithromax), clarithromycin (Biaxin), erythromycin (EES, Erythrocin, Ilotycin)	*Risk category B*	Appear to be safe. Drugs available in pediatric preparations.
Cephalosporins (first- through fourth-generation drugs)	*Risk category B*	Most are considered safe for breastfeeding.
Chloramphenicol (Chloromycetin)	*Risk category D.* Not recommended for use near term because it is associated with neonatal "gray baby syndrome" (rapid respiration, ashen and pale color, poor feeding, abdominal distention, vasomotor collapse, death).	Generally unsafe in breastfeeding mothers due to potential toxicity and "gray baby syndrome" risk for newborns.
Fluoroquinolones Ciprofloxacin (Cipro), levofloxacin (Levaquin), norfloxacin (Chibroxin), ofloxacin (Floxin)	*Risk category C.* Animal studies have shown skeletal abnormalities.	Potentially hazardous. Ofloxacin and ciprofloxacin reach breast milk concentrations similar to or higher than maternal plasma. Less known about other drugs. Observe infant for diarrhea.
Nitrofurantoin (Furadantin, Macrodantin)	*Risk category B.* Crosses placenta. Reassuring animal studies and no evidence of being a teratogenic drug.	Should avoid if infant is younger than 1 mo. Risk for hemolytic anemia if infant has an enzyme (G-6-PD) deficiency.
Penicillins Amoxicillin (Amoxil), ampicillin (Omnipen, Polycillin), penicillin G	*Risk category B.* No reported adverse fetal effects. Penicillins combined with beta-lactamase inhibitors (amoxicillin/clavulanate [Augmentin]), ticarcillin/clavulanate [Timentin], and ampicillin/sulbactram [Unasyn]) also are *risk category B.*	Low concentrations of penicillins in breast milk, including those combined with beta-lactamase inhibitors. Observe for infant diarrhea or candidiasis.
Sulfonamides Sulfadiazine (Coptin), sulfamethoxazole (Gantanol), sulfisoxazole (Gantrisin)	*Risk category C*	AAP recommends caution in use of breast milk if infant has jaundice or G-6-PD deficiency and in the ill or preterm infant.
Tetracycline	*Risk category D.* Can interfere with tooth enamel formation and cause discolored teeth. Prenatal exposure does not affect permanent teeth.	Thought to be compatible with breastfeeding. Oral ingestion appears to be safe although few well-controlled studies exist.
Vancomycin (Vancocin)	*Risk category B.* Used for maternal methicillin-resistant *Staphylococcus aureus* infections and prophylaxis to prevent endocarditis.	Thought to be safe because oral absorption by breastfeeding infant is minimal.
ANTIRETROVIRAL AGENTS		
Nucleoside reverse transcriptase inhibitors (NRTIs) Abacavir (ABC, Ziagen), didanosine (ddI, Videx), amivudine (3TC, Epivir), stavudine (d4T, Zerit), tenovir DF (Viread, TDF), zalcitabine (ddC, Hivid), zidovudine (ZDV, Retrovir)	*Risk category B* (didanosine) or C (abacavir, lamivudine, stavudine, tenovir DF, zalcitabine, zidovudine). Zidovudine is recommended for HIV-seropositive women to reduce risk for perinatal transmission of the virus.	Breastfeeding not recommended due to possibility of HIV transmission to infant.

Drug	Use During Pregnancy	Use During Breastfeeding
ANTIRETROVIRAL AGENTS—cont'd		
Nonnucleotide reverse transcriptase inhibitors (NNRTIs) Delavirdine (DLV, Rescriptor), efavirenz (Sustiva, EFV), nevirapine (NVP, Viramune)	Risk category C. For efavirenz, category C in first trimester and category D in second and third trimesters.	Breastfeeding not recommended due to possibility of HIV transmission to infant.
Fusion inhibitors Enfuviritide (Fuzeon, T-20)	Risk category B	Breastfeeding not recommended due to possibility of HIV transmission to infant.
Protease inhibitors (PIs) Amprenavir (Agenerase), indinavir (Crixivan), nelfinavir (Viracept), ritonavir (Norvir), saquinavir (Invirase)	Risk categories B (nelfinavir, ritonavir, saquinavir) and C (amprenavir, indinavir).	Breastfeeding not recommended due to possibility of HIV transmission to infant.
ANTITUBERCULOSIS AGENTS (See also *Antimicrobials*)		
Ethambutol (Myambutol)	Risk category B. No evidence of increased abnormalities.	Small amounts of ethambutol are excreted into breast milk.
Isoniazid (INH)	Risk category C.	Scant drug levels found in breast milk. Observe infant for hepatitis, vision changes.
Pyrazinamide	Risk category C. No adverse experience with this widely-prescribed agent.	None reported in breast milk.
Rifampin (Rifadin)	Risk category C	Trace amounts excreted in breast milk.
ANTITUSSIVES AND EXPECTORANTS		
Dextromethorphan (Robitussin-DM)	Risk category C	No reported adverse effects.
Guaifenesin (Robitussin)	Risk category C. Usefulness as an expectorant is questionable.	No reported adverse effects.
ANTIVIRAL AGENTS		
Genital herpes infection Acyclovir (Avirax, Zovirax), foscarnet (Foscavir), valacyclovir (Valtrex)	Risk categories B (acyclovir) and C (foscarnet, valacyclovir).	Few reported toxicities except foscarnet associated with higher milk levels than other drugs. Wash topical drug from area before nursing and consult with physician about breastfeeding safety if lesion is present on nipple.
Ribavirin (Virazole)	Risk category X. Administered by aerosol, usually to young children only. Women who are pregnant or may become pregnant should avoid exposure.	Drug is most often given to young children hospitalized with respiratory syncytial virus (RSV), so transfer to breast milk is not likely.
CARDIAC MEDICATIONS		
Antiarrhythmics for serious arrhythmias Amiodarone (Cardarone, Pacerone), bretylium (Bretylol)	Risk category C (bretylium) or D (amiodarone). May reduce uterine blood flow. Possible neurotoxic effects of amiodarone.	Used for life-threatening arrhythmias; woman unlikely to be nursing.
Digitoxin (Crystodigin), digoxin (Lanoxin)	Risk category C. Has been used to treat fetal cardiac arrhythmias.	Digoxin considered safe but less known about digitoxin safety.
Lidocaine (used as antiarrhythmics) (Xylocaine)	Risk category B	Lidocaine considered safe for breastfeeding.
DECONGESTANTS		
Ephedrine, epinephrine (EpiPen, Sus-Phrine)	Risk category C. Ephedrine is commonly used to support blood pressure during epidural or subarachnoid block during intrapartum period.	Acute, one-time use of ephedrine or epinephrine is likely to be safe. Breastfeeding not recommended if regularly used by mother.

Continued

Drug	Use During Pregnancy	Use During Breastfeeding
DECONGESTANTS—cont'd		
Nasal sprays Oxymetazoline (Afrin, Coricidin, Dristan), phenylephrine (Neo-Synephrine), phenylpropanolamine (Kleer, Propan)	*Risk category* C. Avoid during third trimester.	Minimal amounts secreted in milk (oxymetazole and phenylephrine). Less information about phenylpropanolamine in milk secretion.
Pseudoephedrine (Sufedrine)	*Risk category* C. Avoid during first trimester because fetus may have higher risk for gastroschisis or small intestinal atresia.	Generally considered safe for breastfeeding if used occasionally rather than chronically.
DIURETICS		
Carbonic anhydrase inhibitors Acetazolamide (Diamox), methazolamide (Neptazane)	*Risk category* C	Acetazolamide is considered safe. Safety of methazolamide unknown.
Loop diuretics Ethacrynic acid (Edecrin), furosemide (Lasix), torsemide (Demadex)	*Risk category* B (ethacrynic acid) or C (furosemide and torsemide).	Few well-controlled studies; effects probably minimal. Maternal use could suppress lactation.
Potassium-sparing diuretics Amiloride (Midamor, spironolactone (Aldactone), triamterene (Dyrenium)	*Risk category* B (amiloride, triamterene) or D (spironolactone).	Amiloride concentrated in breast milk. Few studies of triamterene. Spironolactone considered safe by AAP.
Thiazide diuretics Chlorothiazide, hydrochlorothiazide (HydroDIURIL)	*Risk category* D. Decreased intravascular volume may reduce uteroplacental perfusion and result in growth retardation. Metabolic disturbances and thrombocytopenia may occur in mother and fetus.	Considered safe during lactation.
Thiazide-like diuretics Chlorthalidone (Hygroton), indapamide (Lozide, Lozol), metolazone (Mykrox, Zaroxolyn)	*Risk category* B	Chlorthalidone safe during lactation by AAP but may reduce milk supply.
HORMONES		
Corticosteroids Beclomethasone (Vanceril, Beclovent), betamethasone (Celestone), cortisone (Cortone), examethasone (Decadron), prednisolone (Delta-Cortef, Prelone), prednisone (Deltasone)	*Risk category* C. Prednisone or prednisolone (category C) is common for asthmatic woman who needs steroids. Betamethasone and dexamethasone are used to accelerate maturation of fetal lungs if preterm delivery is likely.	Prednisone and prednisolone compatible with breastfeeding. Delay nursing 4 hr after dose to reduce transfer to infant. Remove from nipples prior to nursing if applied topically.
Clomiphene citrate (Clomid)	*Risk category* X. Questionable association with neural tube defects. Drug is discontinued after pregnancy is achieved.	Unlikely to be given during lactation because the drug is for infertility treatment.
Danazol (Danocrine)	*Risk category* X. May cause virilization of female fetus.	Breastfeeding not advised.
Estrogens (Azumon, Conjugen, Ovest, Premarin)	*Risk category* X. No indication for estrogens during pregnancy. Diethylstilbestrol (DES) is associated with development of vaginal cancer in female offspring during adolescence or adulthood.	Try to delay drug until breastfeeding is firmly established.
Estradiol (Alora, Climara, Estrace, Estraderm, Estring, Fempatch, Vivelle)	*Risk category* X. Contraceptives; not indicated during pregnancy.	Safe during lactation. Early use sometimes reduces milk volume secreted.
Estrogen-progestin combinations	*Risk category* X. Most often used for menopausal symptoms in women having a uterus. Doses much higher than those for oral contraceptives and are associated with masculinization of the female fetus' genitalia.	Ideally, avoid until lactation is well established for best quantity and quality of breast milk.
Progesterone (Gesterol 50, Lutolin-S, Progestagect-50, Prometrium, Crinone)	*Risk category* D. Most often given for amenorrhea, hormone replacement therapy, infertility (luteal phase support only during pregnancy).	Generally considered safe when breastfeeding.

Drug	Use During Pregnancy	Use During Breastfeeding
PSYCHOACTIVE DRUGS		
Benzodiazepines Alprazolam (Xanax), chlordiazepoxide (Librium, Libritabs), clonazepam (Klonopin), diazepam (Valium), flurazepam (Dalmane), lorazepam (Ativan), midazolam (Versed), oxazepam (Serax), temazepam (Restoril), triazolam (Halcion)	Most are *risk category D.* Some reports of mild facial abnormalities and developmental delay, but no conclusive studies. Use during the third trimester may slow the infant's neurologic development and result in sedation after birth. Midazolam is primarily used as a brief maternal perioperative sedative. The following sedative-hypnotic drugs in this class are *risk category* X: flurazepam, temazepam, and triazolam.	Potentially hazardous due to the long half-lives of many drugs in this class and the potential development of dependence. Few reported adverse effects, but observe infant for sedation, poor feeding.
Anxiolytics Meprobamate (Equanil, Miltown)	*Risk category D.* Has been associated with cardiac malformations.	Concentrations in milk are higher than in maternal serum. Observe for infant sedation.
Antipsychotics Lithium (Eskalith, Lithobid)	*Risk category D.* Slightly increased risk for cardiac abnormalities.	Infant blood concentration of lithium reaches 30% to 40% of the mother's concentration. Infant drug levels should be evaluated. T-wave abnormalities and decreased muscle tone have been noted.
Phenothiazines Chlorpromazine (Thorazine), prochlorperazine (Compazine), thioridazine (Mellaril)	*Risk category C.* Risk of malformations is uncertain but these are probably safe for use in humans. Alcohol may increase CNS depression. Taking other drugs with phenothiazines may alter serum levels of one or more of the drugs taken.	Neonatal hypoglycemia has been reported with chlorpromazine. Less known about breastfeeding effects of maternal prochlorperazine and thioridazine.
MAO (monoamine oxidase) inhibitors Phenelzine (Nardil), tranylcypromine (Parnate)	*Risk category C.* Documented interactions between opioids and MAO inhibitors. Potential risks if taken near the time other drugs were taken. Consult a detailed drug guide. Little documentation of fetal effects.	Few published reports related to entry of these MAO inhibitor drugs into breast milk.
Tricyclic antidepressants Amitriptyline (Elavil), amoxapine (Asendin), clomipramine (Anafranil), desipramine (Norpramin), doxepin (Adepin, Sinequan), imipramine (Tofranil), nortriptyline (Aventyl, Pamelor), protriptyline (Vivactil)	*Risk category C* for most tricyclics but *D* for imipramine and nortriptyline. Several studies have shown that tricyclic antidepressant use during pregnancy is most likely not teratogenic	Few contraindications for most tricyclic antidepressants. Infant apnea and drowsiness during maternal doxepin intake have been described with maternal doxepin intake.
Selective serotonin-reuptake inhibitors Citalopram (Celexa), escitalopram (Lexapro), fluoxetine (Prozac), fluvoxamine (Luvox), paroxetine (Paxil), sertraline (Zoloft)	Most *risk category C*; sertraline is *risk category B*.	Most considered safe for breastfeeding infant. Citalopram and escitalopram have been associated with excessive somnolence, decreased intake, and infant weight loss.
Other psychoactive drugs Buproprion (Wellbutrin), mirtazapine, (Remeron), nefazodone (Serzone), trazodone (Desyrel), venlafaxine (Effexor)	*Risk category C* except for buproprion (*risk category B*).	Few reports on breast milk safety for infant for most drugs. No AAP contraindications for buproprion or trazodone. Observe infant for sedation.
THYROID DRUGS		
Antithyroids Methimazole (Tapazole), propylthiouracil (PTU)	*Risk category D.* May result in neonatal goiter or hypothyroidism, although uncommon at usual therapeutic doses. Methimazole has possible association with scalp defects. PTU is drug of choice during pregnancy.	Approved by AAP. Neonatal thyroid function apparently unaffected by maternal treatment.
Potassium iodide (SSKI, Thyro-Block)	*Risk category D.* Long-term exposure may produce fetal thyroid enlargement or hypothyroidism.	May cause rash or suppress infant's thyroid function. Dose should not be higher than RDA (recommended daily allowance).

Continued

Drug	Use During Pregnancy	Use During Breastfeeding
THYROID DRUGS—cont'd		
Thyroid replacement hormone: levothyroxine (Levoxyl, Synthroid)	*Risk category A.* Crosses placenta only to limited extent.	Apparently safe during breastfeeding.
VITAMINS AND RETINOIDS		
Retinoids: isotretinoin (Accutane)	*Risk category X.* Related to vitamin A. Associated with severe fetal malformations (microcephaly, ear abnormalities, cardiac defects, central nervous system abnormalities).	Contraindicated for use during breastfeeding because of severe fetal effects.
Vitamin A	*Risk category A* at doses no higher than 6000 units/day (safety of doses above 6000 units/day not established). Excess intake may lead to abnormalities noted for isotretinoin.	Breast milk usually supplies sufficient vitamin A to infant. Mother should not take more than 6000 units per day.
Vitamin D	*Risk category A (risk category D* at doses above RDA). Excess intake associated with malformations, including aortic stenosis, facial abnormalities, and mental retardation.	AAP approved. Infant serum level assessment recommended if mother taking a therapeutic dose.
MISCELLANEOUS DRUGS		
Nicotine gum; nicotine transdermal	*Risk category C* (nicotine gum) or *D* (transdermal nicotine). *Risk category X* if used in overdose. Stopping nicotine intake by ceasing smoking lowers complications such as preterm birth.	Lactation safe, although passed into breast milk. Infant exposure to passive environmental nicotine smoke is not considered safe, however.

REFERENCES and READINGS

American Academy of Pediatrics and American College of Obstetricians and Gynecologists. (2002). *Guidelines for perinatal care* (5th ed.). Elk Grove Village, IL, and Washington, DC: The Academy.

American Academy of Pediatrics Committee on Drugs (2001). Transfer of drugs and other chemicals into human milk. *Pediatrics, 108*(3), 776-789.

American Academy of Pediatrics Committee on Drugs (2000). Use of psychoactive medications during pregnancy and possible effects on the fetus and newborn (RE9866). *Pediatrics, 105*(4), 880-887.

Andres, R.L. (2004). Effects of therapeutic, diagnostic, and environmental agents and exposure to social and illicit drugs. In R.K. Creasy, R. Resnik, & J.D. Iams (Eds.), *Maternal-fetal medicine: Principles and practice* (5th ed.). Philadelphia: W.B. Saunders.

Blanchard, D.G., & Shabetai, R. (2004). Cardiac diseases. In R.K. Creasy, R. Resnik, & J.D. Iams (Eds.), *Maternal-fetal medicine: Principles and practice* (5th ed., pp. 281-314). Philadelphia: W.B. Saunders.

Centers for Disease Control and Prevention (CDC). (2002). Sexually transmitted diseases treatment guidelines. *Morbidity and Mortality Weekly Report, 51*(RR-6).

Cunningham, F.G., Gant, N.F., Leveno, K.J., Gilstrap, L.C., Hauth, J.C., & Wenstrom, K.D. (2001). *Williams obstetrics* (21st ed.). New York: McGraw-Hill.

Gal, P., & Reed, M.D. (2004). Medications. In R.E. Behrman, R.M. Kliegman, & H.B. Jenson (Eds.), *Nelson's textbook of pediatrics* (17th ed., pp. 2432-2501). Philadelphia: W.B. Saunders.

Gibbs, R.S., Sweet, R.L., & Duff, W.P. (2004). Maternal and fetal infectious disorders. In R.K. Creasy, R. Resnik & J.D. Iams (Eds.), *Maternal-fetal medicine: Principles and practice* (5th ed., pp. 741-801). Philadelphia: W.B. Saunders.

Harkness, R., & Bratman, S. (2003). *Mosby's handbook of drug-herb and drug-supplement interactions.* St. Louis: Mosby.

Hale, T.W. (2004). *Medications and mothers' milk* (11th ed.). Amarillo, TX: Pharmasoft Medical Publishing.

Lawrence, R.M., & Lawrence, R.A. (2004). The breast and the physiology of lactation. In R.K. Creasy, R. Resnik, & J.D. Iams (Eds.), *Maternal-fetal medicine: Principles and practice* (5th ed., pp. 135-153). Philadelphia: W.B. Saunders.

Minkoff, H.L. (2004). Human immunodeficiency virus. In R.K. Creasy, R. Resnik, & J.D. Iams (Eds.), *Maternal-fetal medicine: Principles and practice* (5th ed., pp. 803-814). Philadelphia: W.B. Saunders.

Novey, D.W. (2000). *Clinician's complete reference to complementary & alternative medicine.* St. Louis: Mosby.

Skidmore-Roth, L. (2004). *Mosby's handbook of herbs & natural supplements* (2nd ed.). St. Louis: Mosby.

Skidmore-Roth, L. (2004). *Mosby's nursing drug reference.* St. Louis: Mosby.

Tiran, D., & Mack, S. (2000). *Complementary therapies for pregnancy and childbirth* (2nd ed.). Edinburgh: Ballière-Tindall.

U.S. Department of Health and Human Services. (2004). *AIDS info: Approved medications to treat HIV infection.* Retrieved April 1, 2004, from *http://aidsinfo.nih.gov/other/FDAApproved_HIV_012004.asp.*

Weiner, C.P. & Buhimschi, C. (2004). *Drugs for pregnant and lactating women.* New York: Churchill Livingstone.

APPENDIX C

Recommendations for Preventive
Pediatric Health Care

Recommendations for Preventive Pediatric Health Care (RE9535)

Committee on Practice and Ambulatory Medicine

Each child and family is unique; therefore, these **Recommendations for Preventive Pediatric Health Care** are designed for the care of children who are receiving competent parenting, have no manifestations of any important health problems, and are growing and developing in satisfactory fashion. **Additional visits may become necessary** if circumstances suggest variations from normal.

These guidelines represent a consensus by the Committee on Practice and Ambulatory Medicine in consultation with national committees and sections of the American Academy of Pediatrics. The Committee emphasizes the great importance of **continuity of care** in comprehensive health supervision and the need to avoid **fragmentation of care.**

AGE[5]	PRENATAL[1]	NEWBORN[2]	2-4d[3]	By 1mo	2mo	4mo	6mo	9mo	12mo	15mo	18mo	24mo	3y	4y	5y	6y	8y	10y	11y	12y	13y	14y	15y	16y	17y	18y	19y	20y	21y
HISTORY Initial/Interval	●	●	●	●	●	●	●	●	●	●	●	●	●	●	●	●	●	●	●	●	●	●	●	●	●	●	●	●	●
MEASUREMENTS Height and Weight		●	●	●	●	●	●	●	●	●	●	●	●	●	●	●	●	●	●	●	●	●	●	●	●	●	●	●	●
Head Circumference		●	●	●	●	●	●	●	●	●																			
Blood Pressure													●	●	●	●	●	●	●	●	●	●	●	●	●	●	●	●	●
SENSORY SCREENING Vision		S	S	S	S	S	S	S	S	S	S	S	O[6]	O	O	O	O	O	S	O	S	S	O	S	S	O	S	S	S
Hearing		O[7]	S	S	S	S	S	S	S	S	S	S	S	O	O	O	O	O	S	O	S	S	O	S	S	O	S	S	S
DEVELOPMENTAL/ BEHAVIORAL ASSESSMENT[8]		●	●	●	●	●	●	●	●	●	●	●	●	●	●	●	●	●	●	●	●	●	●	●	●	●	●	●	●
PHYSICAL EXAMINATION[9]		●	●	●	●	●	●	●	●	●	●	●	●	●	●	●	●	●	●	●	●	●	●	●	●	●	●	●	●
PROCEDURES-GENERAL[10] Hereditary/Metabolic Screening[11]		◀––––▶																											
Immunization[12]		●		●	●	●	●	●	◀▲▶		▲			◀▲▶	▲				●				●	15					●
Hematocrit or Hemoglobin[13]							★	★			★	★	★	★	★	★	★	★	★	★	★	★	★	★	★	★	★	★	★
Urinalysis		●																											
PROCEDURES-PATIENTS AT RISK Lead Screening[16]							★	★	★	★	★	★	★	★	★	★	★	★	★	★	★	★	★	★	★	★	★	★	★
Tuberculin Test[17]							★		★		★	★	★	★	★	★	★	★	★	★	★	★	★	★	★	★	★	★	★
Cholesterol Screening[18]															★	★	★	★	★	★	★	★	★	★	★	★	★	★	★
STD Screening[19]																			★	★	★	★	★	★	★	★	★	★	★
Pelvic Exam[20]																			◀–––––––20–––––––▶										★
ANTICIPATORY GUIDANCE[21] Injury Prevention[22]		●	●	●	●	●	●	●	●	●	●	●	●	●	●	●	●	●	●	●	●	●	●	●	●	●	●	●	●
Violence Prevention[23]		●	●	●	●	●	●	●	●	●	●	●	●	●	●	●	●	●	●	●	●	●	●	●	●	●	●	●	●
Sleep Positioning Counseling[24]		●	●	●	●	●	●																						
Nutrition Counseling[25]		●	●	●	●	●	●	●	●	●	●	●	●	●	●	●	●	●	●	●	●	●	●	●	●	●	●	●	●
DENTAL REFERRAL[26]													◀––––▶																

Key:	● = to be performed	★ = to be performed for patients at risk
	S = subjective, by history	O = objective, by a standard testing method
	◀–––▶ = the range during which a service may be provided, with the dot indicating the preferred age.	

1. A prenatal visit is recommended for parents who are at high risk, for first-time parents, and for those who request a conference. The prenatal visit should include anticipatory guidance, pertinent medical history, and a discussion of benefits of breastfeeding and planned method of feeding per AAP statement "The Prenatal Visit" (1996).
2. Every infant should have a newborn evaluation after birth. Breastfeeding should be encouraged and instruction and support offered. Every breastfeeding infant should have an evaluation 48-72 hours after discharge from the hospital to include weight, formal breastfeeding evaluation, encouragement, and instruction as recommended in the AAP statement "Breastfeeding and the Use of Human Milk" (1997).
3. For newborns discharged in less than 48 hours after delivery per AAP statement "Hospital Stay for Healthy Term Newborns" (1995).
4. Developmental, psychosocial, and chronic disease issues for children and adolescents may require frequent counseling and treatment visits separate from preventive care visits.
5. If a child comes under care for the first time at any point on the schedule, or if any items are not accomplished at the suggested age, the schedule should be brought up to date at the earliest possible time.
6. If the patient is uncooperative, rescreen within 6 months.
7. All newborns should be screened per the AAP Task Force on Newborn and Infant Hearing statement, "Newborn and Infant Hearing Loss: Detection and Intervention" (1999).
8. By history and appropriate physical examination; if suspicious, by specific developmental testing. Parenting skills should be fostered at every visit.
9. At each visit, a complete physical examination is essential, with infant totally unclothed, older child undressed and suitably draped.
10. These may be modified, depending upon entry point into schedule and individual need.
11. Metabolic screening (eg, thyroid, hemoglobinopathies, PKU, galactosemia) should be done according to state law.
12. Schedule(s) per the Committee on Infectious Diseases, published annually in the January edition of *Pediatrics*. Every visit should be an opportunity to update and complete a child's immunizations.
13. See AAP *Pediatric Nutrition Handbook* (1998) for a discussion of universal and selective screening options. Consider earlier screening for high-risk infants (eg, premature infants and low birth weight infants). See also "Recommendations to Prevent and Control Iron Deficiency in the United States. *MMWR*. 1998;47 (RR-3):1-29.
14. All menstruating adolescents should be screened annually.
15. Conduct dipstick urinalysis for leukocytes annually for sexually active male and female adolescents.
16. For children at risk of lead exposure consult the AAP statement "Screening for Elevated Blood Levels" (1998). Additionally, screening should be done in accordance with state law where applicable.
17. TB testing per recommendations of the Committee on Infectious Diseases, published in the current edition of *Red Book: Report of the Committee on Infectious Diseases*. Testing should be done upon recognition of high-risk factors.
18. Cholesterol screening for high-risk patients per AAP statement "Cholesterol in Childhood" (1998). If family history cannot be ascertained and other risk factors are present, screening should be at the discretion of the physician.
19. All sexually active patients should be screened for sexually transmitted diseases (STDs).
20. All sexually active females should have a pelvic examination and routine pap smear should be offered as part of preventive health maintenance between the ages of 18 and 21 years.
21. Age-appropriate discussion and counseling should be an integral part of each visit for care per the AAP *Guidelines for Health Supervision III* (1998).
22. From birth to age 12, refer to the AAP injury prevention program (TIPP*) as described in *A Guide to Safety Counseling in Office Practice* (1994).
23. Violence prevention and management for all patients per AAP statement "The Role of the Pediatrician in Youth Violence Prevention in Clinical Practice and at the Community Level" (1999).
24. Parents and caregivers should be advised to place healthy infants on their backs when putting them to sleep. Side positioning is a reasonable alternative but carries a slightly higher risk of SIDS. Consult the AAP statement "Positioning and Sudden Infant Death Syndrome (SIDS): Update" (1996).
25. Age-appropriate nutrition counseling should be an integral part of each visit per the AAP *Handbook of Nutrition* (1998).
26. Earlier initial dental examinations may be appropriate for some children. Subsequent examinations as prescribed by dentist.

American Academy of Pediatrics

APPENDIX D

Recommended Childhood
Immunizations

Recommended Childhood and Adolescent Immunization Schedule
United States • July–December 2004

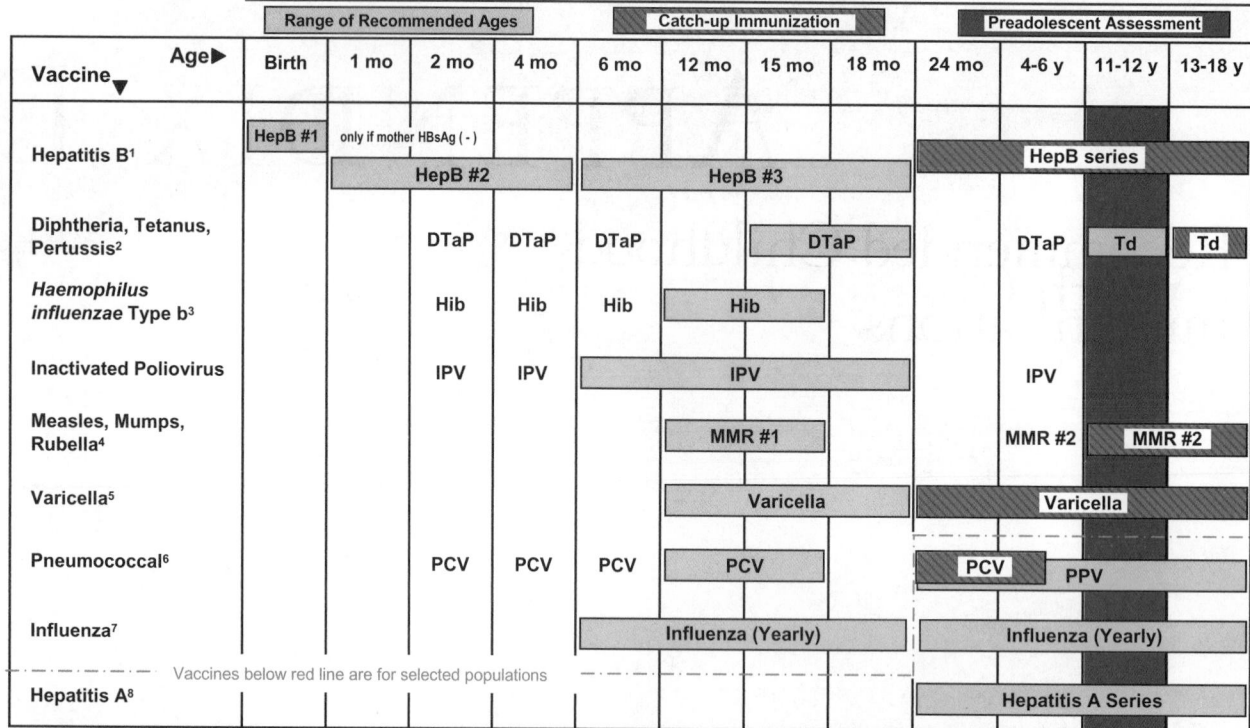

Vaccine ▼ / Age ▶	Birth	1 mo	2 mo	4 mo	6 mo	12 mo	15 mo	18 mo	24 mo	4-6 y	11-12 y	13-18 y
					Range of Recommended Ages			Catch-up Immunization			Preadolescent Assessment	
Hepatitis B[1]	HepB #1	only if mother HBsAg (-)									HepB series	
			HepB #2			HepB #3						
Diphtheria, Tetanus, Pertussis[2]			DTaP	DTaP	DTaP		DTaP			DTaP	Td	Td
Haemophilus influenzae Type b[3]			Hib	Hib	Hib	Hib						
Inactivated Poliovirus			IPV	IPV		IPV				IPV		
Measles, Mumps, Rubella[4]						MMR #1				MMR #2		MMR #2
Varicella[5]						Varicella					Varicella	
Pneumococcal[6]			PCV	PCV	PCV	PCV				PCV	PPV	
Influenza[7]						Influenza (Yearly)					Influenza (Yearly)	
Vaccines below red line are for selected populations												
Hepatitis A[8]										Hepatitis A Series		

This schedule indicates the recommended ages for routine administration of currently licensed childhood vaccines, as of April 1, 2004, for children through age 18 years. Any dose not given at the recommended age should be given at any subsequent visit when indicated and feasible. ▨Indicates age groups that warrant special effort to administer those vaccines not previously given. Additional vaccines may be licensed and recommended during the year. Licensed combination vaccines may be used whenever any components of the combination are indicated and the vaccineís other components are not contraindicated. Providers should consult the manufacturers' package inserts for detailed recommendations. Clinically significant adverse events that follow immunization should be reported to the Vaccine Adverse Event Reporting System (VAERS). Guidance about how to obtain and complete a VAERS form can be found on the Internet: www.vaers.org or by calling 800-822-7967.

1. Hepatitis B (HepB) vaccine. All infants should receive the first dose of hepatitis B vaccine soon after birth and before hospital discharge; the first dose may also be given by age 2 months if the infantís mother is hepatitis B surface antigen (HBsAg) negative. Only monovalent HepB can be used for the birth dose. Monovalent or combination vaccine containing HepB may be used to complete the series. Four doses of vaccine may be administered when a birth dose is given. The second dose should be given at least 4 weeks after the first dose, except for combination vaccines which cannot be administered before age 6 weeks. The third dose should be given at least 16 weeks after the first dose and at least 8 weeks after the second dose. The last dose in the vaccination series (third or fourth dose) should not be administered before age 24 weeks.

Infants born to HBsAg-positive mothers should receive HepB and 0.5 mL of Hepatitis B Immune Globulin (HBIG) within 12 hours of birth at separate sites. The second dose is recommended at age 1–2 months. The last dose in the immunization series should not be administered before age 24 weeks. These infants should be tested for HBsAg and antibody to HBsAg (anti-HBs) at age 9–15 months.

Infants born to mothers whose HBsAg status is unknown should receive the first dose of the HepB series within 12 hours of birth. Maternal blood should be drawn as soon as possible to determine the mother's HBsAg status; if the HBsAg test is positive, the infant should receive HBIG as soon as possible (no later than age 1 week). The second dose is recommended at age 1–2 months. The last dose in the immunization series should not be administered before age 24 weeks.

2. Diphtheria and tetanus toxoids and acellular pertussis (DTaP) vaccine. The fourth dose of DTaP may be administered as early as age 12 months, provided 6 months have elapsed since the third dose and the child is unlikely to return at age 15–18 months. The final dose in the series should be given at age ≥4 years. **Tetanus and diphtheria toxoids (Td)** is recommended at age 11–12 years if at least 5 years have elapsed since the last dose of tetanus and diphtheria toxoid-containing vaccine. Subsequent routine Td boosters are recommended every 10 years.

3. Haemophilus influenzae type b (Hib) conjugate vaccine. Three Hib conjugate vaccines are licensed for infant use. If PRP-OMP (PedvaxHIB or ComVax [Merck]) is administered at ages 2 and 4 months, a dose at age 6 months is not required. DTaP/Hib combination products should not be used for primary immunization in infants at ages 2, 4 or 6 months but can be used as boosters following any Hib vaccine. The final dose in the series should be given at age ≥12 months.

4. Measles, mumps, and rubella vaccine (MMR). The second dose of MMR is recommended routinely at age 4–6 years but may be administered during any visit, provided at least 4 weeks have elapsed since the first dose and both doses are administered beginning at or after age 12 months. Those who have not previously received the second dose should complete the schedule by the visit at age 11–12 years.

5. Varicella vaccine. Varicella vaccine is recommended at any visit at or after age 12 months for susceptible children (i.e., those who lack a reliable history of chickenpox). Susceptible persons age ≥13 years should receive 2 doses, given at least 4 weeks apart.

6. Pneumococcal vaccine. The heptavalent **pneumococcal conjugate vaccine (PCV)** is recommended for all children age 2–23 months. It is also recommended for certain children age 24–59 months. The final dose in the series should be given at age >12 months. **Pneumococcal polysaccharide vaccine (PPV)** is recommended in addition to PCV for certain high-risk groups. See *MMWR* 2000;49(RR-9):1-35.

7. Influenza vaccine. Influenza vaccine is recommended annually for children aged ≥6 months with certain risk factors (including but not limited to asthma, cardiac disease, sickle cell disease, HIV, and diabetes), healthcare workers, and other persons (including household members) in close contact with persons in groups at high risk (see *MMWR* 2004;53;[RR-6]:1-40) and can be administered to all others wishing to obtain immunity. In addition, healthy children aged 6–23 months and close contacts of healthy children aged 0–23 months are recommended to receive influenza vaccine, because children in this age group are at substantially increased risk for influenza-related hospitalizations. For healthy persons aged 5–49 years, the intranasally administered live, attenuated influenza vaccine (LAIV) is an acceptable alternative to the intramuscular trivalent inactivated influenza vaccine (TIV). See *MMWR* 2004;53;[RR-6]:1-40. Children receiving TIV should be administered a dosage appropriate for their age (0.25 mL if 6–35 months or 0.5 mL if ≥3 years). Children aged ≤8 years who are receiving influenza vaccine for the first time should receive 2 doses (separated by at least 4 weeks for TIV and at least 6 weeks for LAIV).

8. Hepatitis A vaccine. Hepatitis A vaccine is recommended for children and adolescents in selected states and regions and for certain high-risk groups; consult your local public health authority. Children and adolescents in these states, regions, and high-risk groups who have not been immunized against hepatitis A can begin the hepatitis A immunization series during any visit. The 2 doses in the series should be administered at least 6 months apart. See *MMWR* 1999;48(RR-12):1-37.

For additional information about vaccines, including precautions and contraindications for immunization and vaccine shortages, please visit the National Immunization Program Web site at www.cdc.gov/nip/ or call the National Immunization Information Hotline at 800-232-2522 (English) or 800-232-0233 (Spanish).

Approved by the Advisory Committee on Immunization Practices (www.cdc.gov/nip/acip), the American Academy of Pediatrics (www.aap.org), and the American Academy of Family Physicians (www.aafp.org).

APPENDIX E

Growth Charts

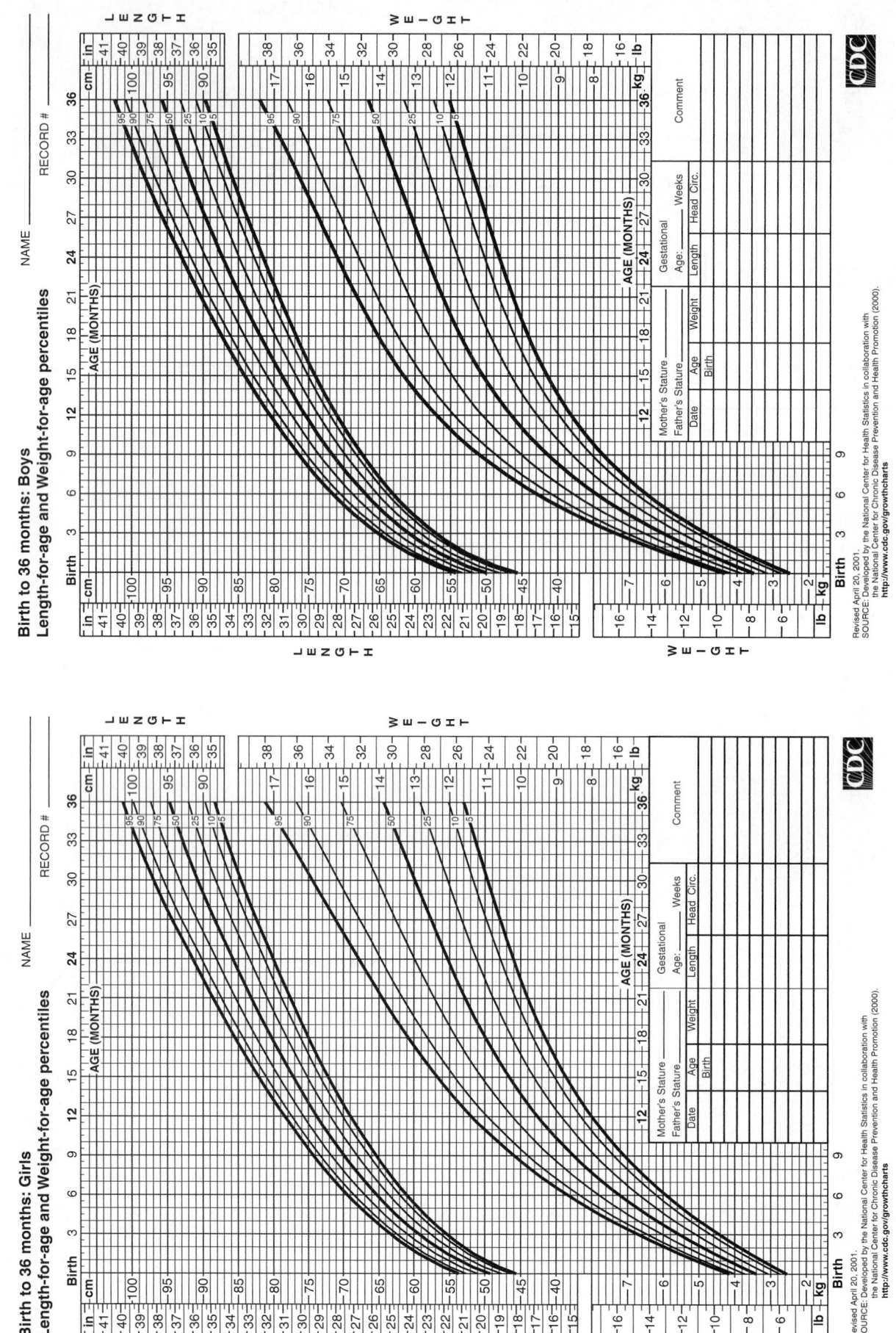

Birth to 36 months: Boys
Length-for-age and Weight-for-age percentiles

NAME _____ RECORD # _____

Revised April 20, 2001.
SOURCE: Developed by the National Center for Health Statistics in collaboration with
the National Center for Chronic Disease Prevention and Health Promotion (2000).
http://www.cdc.gov/growthcharts

Birth to 36 months: Girls
Length-for-age and Weight-for-age percentiles

NAME _____ RECORD # _____

Revised April 20, 2001.
SOURCE: Developed by the National Center for Health Statistics in collaboration with
the National Center for Chronic Disease Prevention and Health Promotion (2000).
http://www.cdc.gov/growthcharts

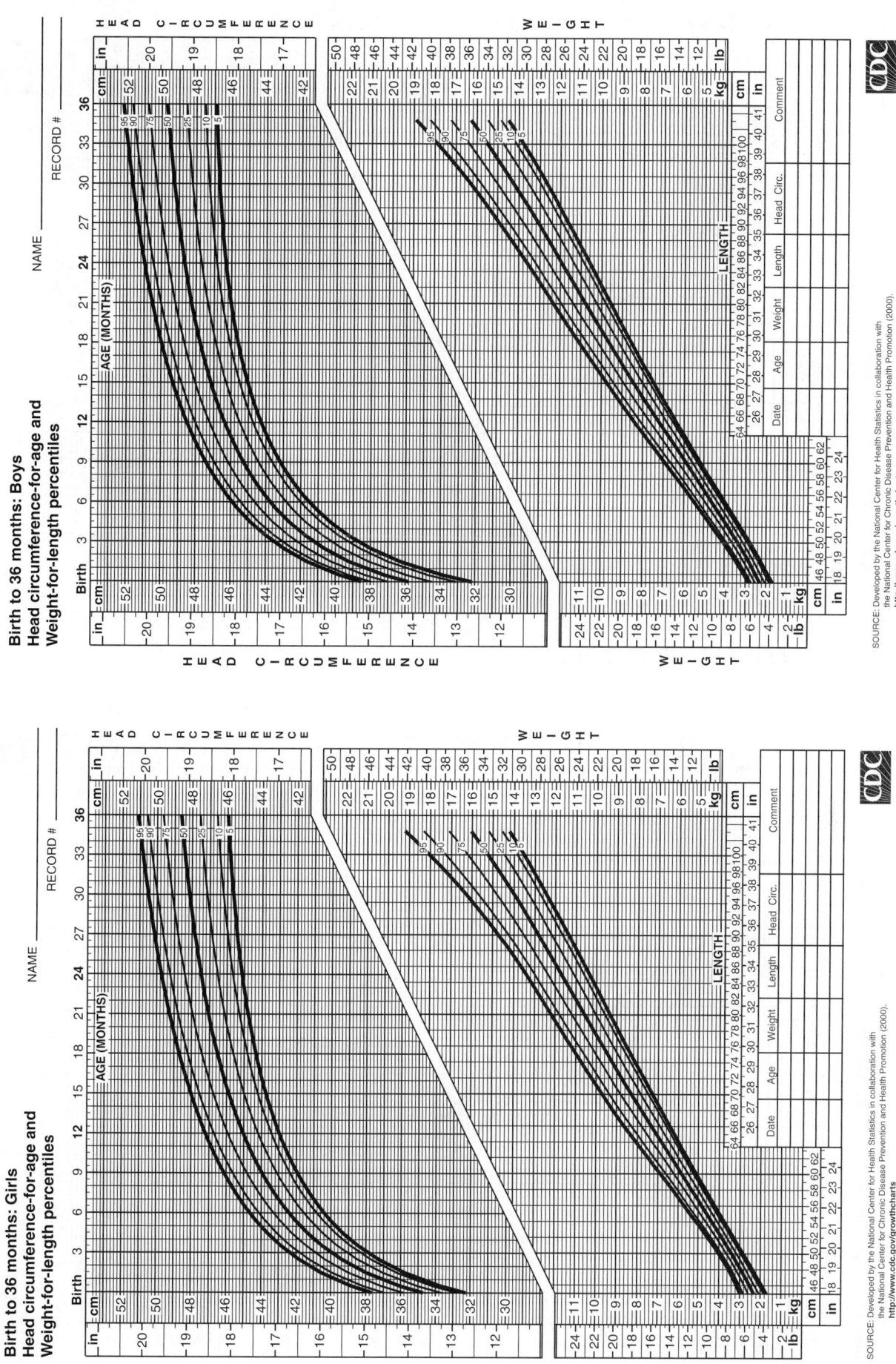

Birth to 36 months: Boys
Head circumference-for-age and
Weight-for-length percentiles

NAME

RECORD #

SOURCE: Developed by the National Center for Health Statistics in collaboration with
the National Center for Chronic Disease Prevention and Health Promotion (2000).
http://www.cdc.gov/growthcharts

Birth to 36 months: Girls
Head circumference-for-age and
Weight-for-length percentiles

NAME

RECORD #

SOURCE: Developed by the National Center for Health Statistics in collaboration with
the National Center for Chronic Disease Prevention and Health Promotion (2000).
http://www.cdc.gov/growthcharts

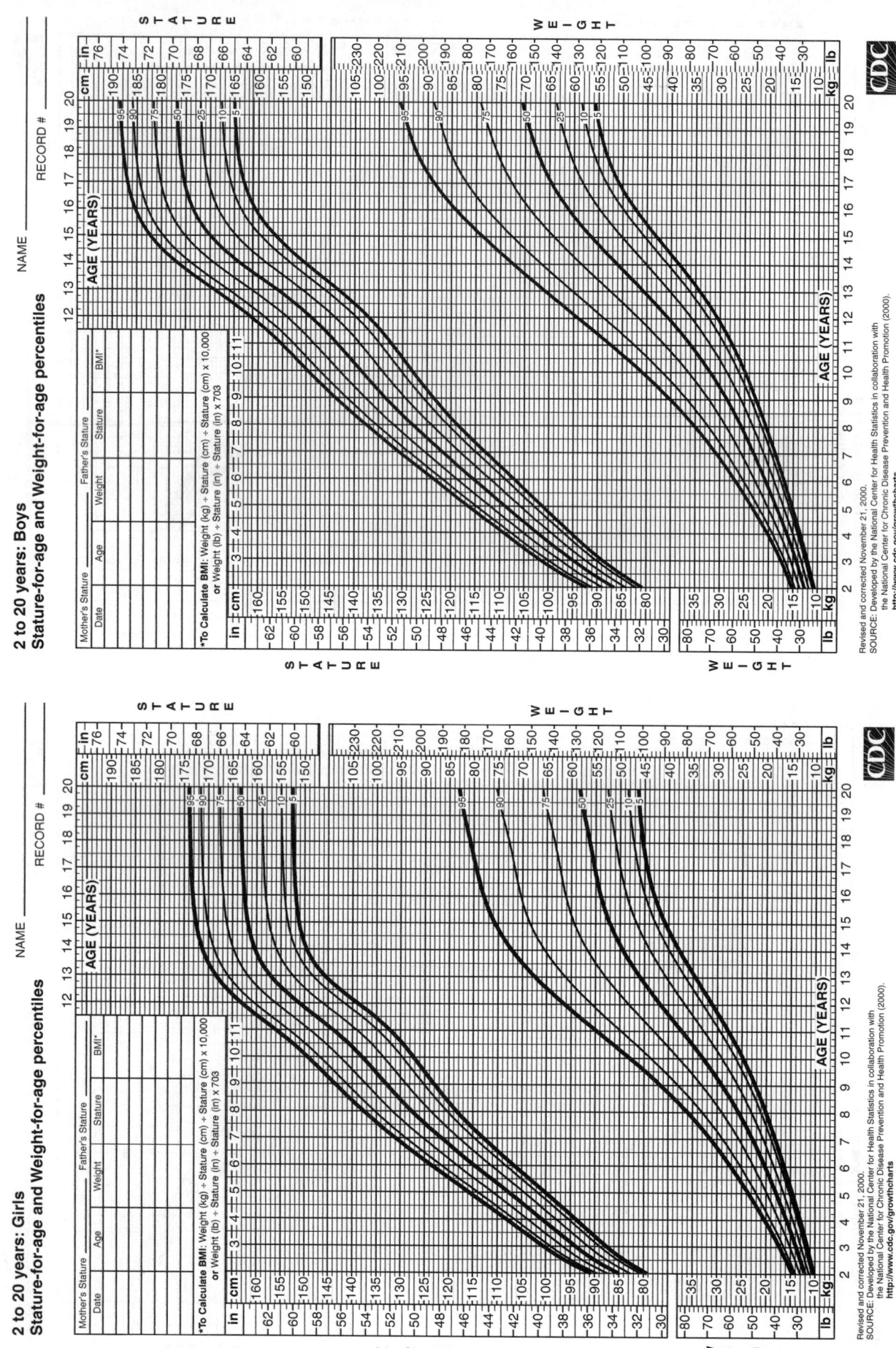

2 to 20 years: Boys
Stature-for-age and Weight-for-age percentiles

NAME _____   RECORD # _____

Revised and corrected November 21, 2000.
SOURCE: Developed by the National Center for Health Statistics in collaboration with
the National Center for Chronic Disease Prevention and Health Promotion (2000).
http://www.cdc.gov/growthcharts

2 to 20 years: Girls
Stature-for-age and Weight-for-age percentiles

NAME _____   RECORD # _____

Revised and corrected November 21, 2000.
SOURCE: Developed by the National Center for Health Statistics in collaboration with
the National Center for Chronic Disease Prevention and Health Promotion (2000).
http://www.cdc.gov/growthcharts

2 to 20 years: Girls
Body mass index-for-age percentiles

NAME _____   RECORD # _____

Date	Age	Weight	Stature	BMI*	Comments

*To Calculate BMI: Weight (kg) ÷ Stature (cm) ÷ Stature (cm) × 10,000
or Weight (lb) ÷ Stature (in) ÷ Stature (in) × 703

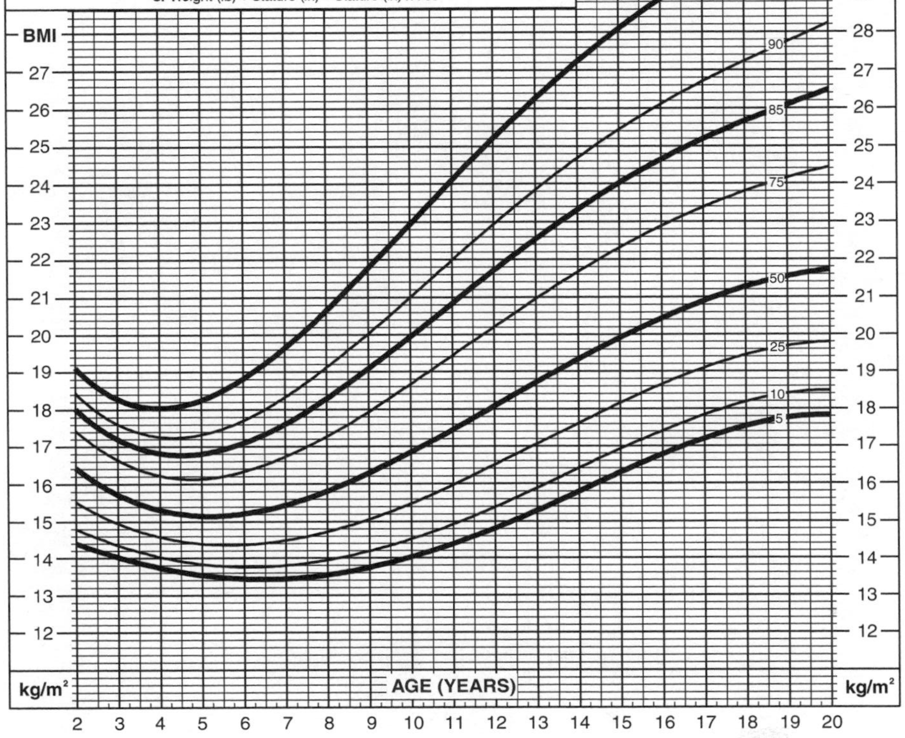

SOURCE: Developed by the National Center for Health Statistics in collaboration with
the National Center for Chronic Disease Prevention and Health Promotion (2000).
http://www.cdc.gov/growthcharts

2 to 20 years: Boys
Body mass index-for-age percentiles

NAME _____   RECORD # _____

Date	Age	Weight	Stature	BMI*	Comments

*To Calculate BMI: Weight (kg) ÷ Stature (cm) ÷ Stature (cm) × 10,000
or Weight (lb) ÷ Stature (in) ÷ Stature (in) × 703

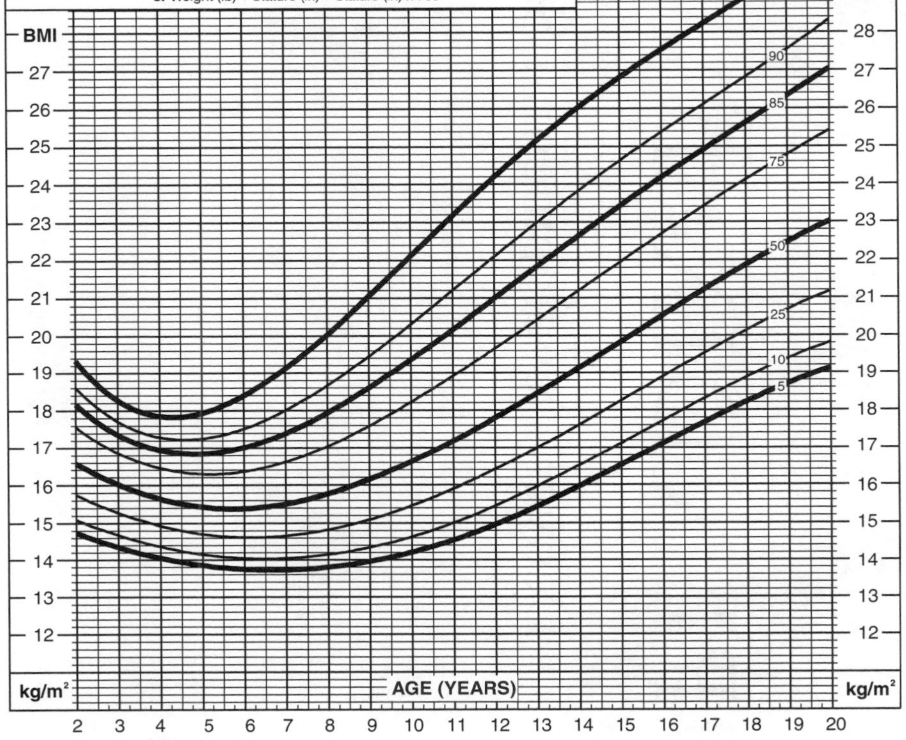

SOURCE: Developed by the National Center for Health Statistics in collaboration with
the National Center for Chronic Disease Prevention and Health Promotion (2000).
http://www.cdc.gov/growthcharts

APPENDIX F

Denver Developmental Screening Test II

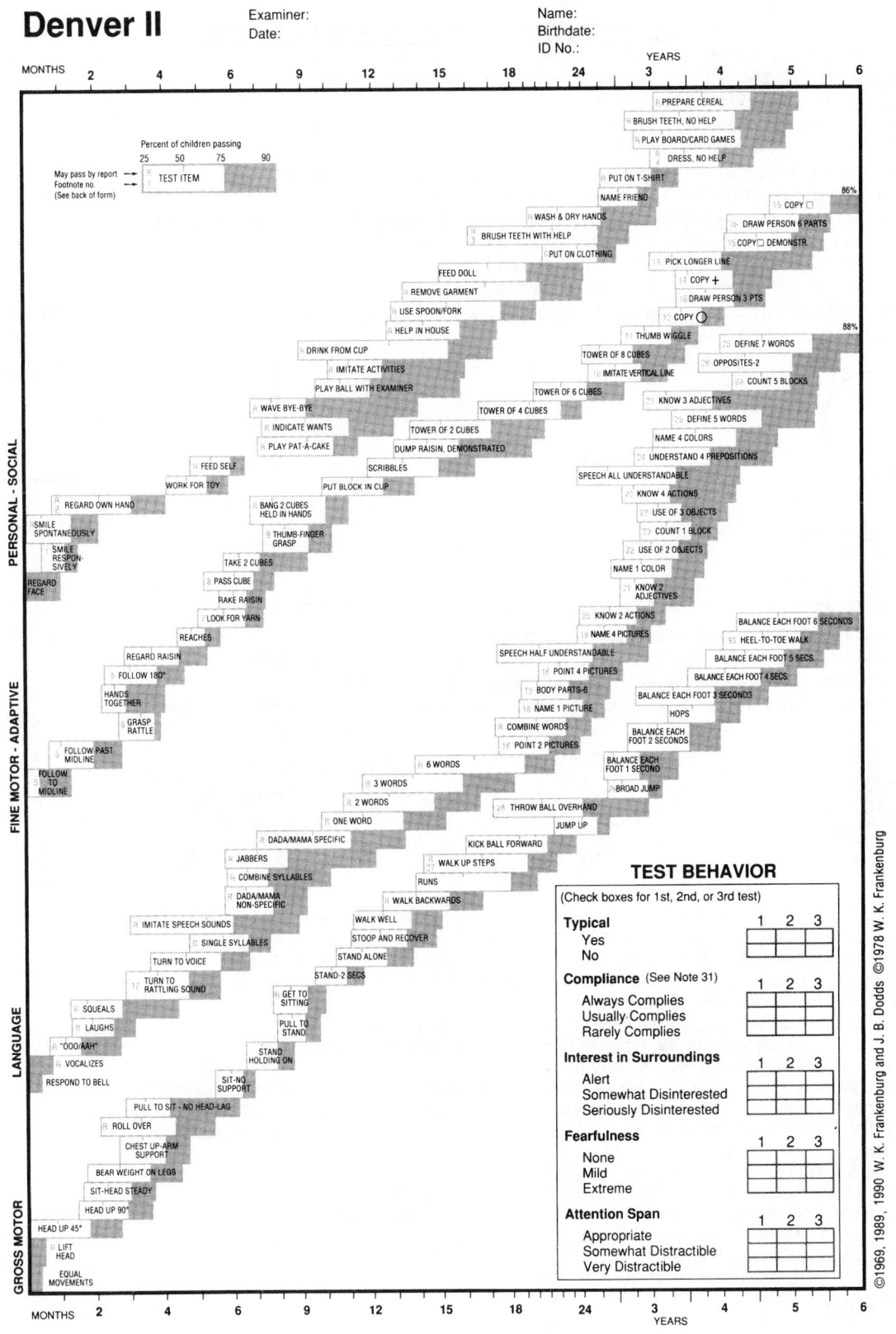

DIRECTIONS FOR ADMINISTRATION

1. Try to get child to smile by smiling, talking or waving. Do not touch him/her.
2. Child must stare at hand several seconds.
3. Parent may help guide toothbrush and put toothpaste on brush.
4. Child does not have to be able to tie shoes or button/zip in the back.
5. Move yarn slowly in an arc from one side to the other, about 8" above child's face.
6. Pass if child grasps rattle when it is touched to the backs or tips of fingers.
7. Pass if child tries to see where yarn went. Yarn should be dropped quickly from sight from tester's hand without arm movement.
8. Child must transfer cube from hand to hand without help of body, mouth, or table.
9. Pass if child picks up raisin with any part of thumb and finger.
10. Line can vary only 30 degrees or less from tester's line.
11. Make a fist with thumb pointing upward and wiggle only the thumb. Pass if child imitates and does not move any fingers other than the thumb.

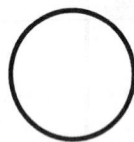

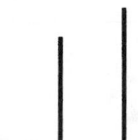

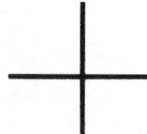

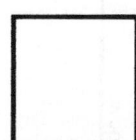

12. Pass any enclosed form. Fail continuous round motions.
13. Which line is longer? (Not bigger.) Turn paper upside down and repeat. (pass 3 of 3 or 5 of 6)
14. Pass any lines crossing near midpoint.
15. Have child copy first. If failed, demonstrate.

When giving items 12, 14, and 15, do not name the forms. Do not demonstrate 12 and 14.

16. When scoring, each pair (2 arms, 2 legs, etc.) counts as one part.
17. Place one cube in cup and shake gently near child's ear, but out of sight. Repeat for other ear.
18. Point to picture and have child name it. (No credit is given for sounds only.)
    If less than 4 pictures are named correctly, have child point to picture as each is named by tester.

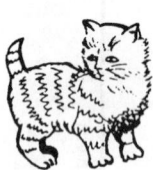 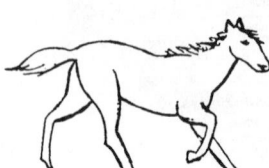 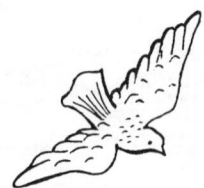 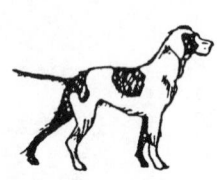 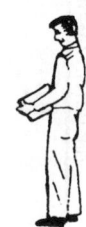

19. Using doll, tell child: Show me the nose, eyes, ears, mouth, hands, feet, tummy, hair. Pass 6 of 8.
20. Using pictures, ask child: Which one flies?... says meow?... talks?... barks?... gallops? Pass 2 of 5, 4 of 5.
21. Ask child: What do you do when you are cold?... tired?... hungry?   Pass 2 of 3, 3 of 3.
22. Ask child: What do you do with a cup? What is a chair used for? What is a pencil used for?
    Action words must be included in answers.
23. Pass if child correctly places and says how many blocks are on paper. (1, 5).
24. Tell child: Put block **on** table; **under** table; **in front of** me, **behind** me. Pass 4 of 4.
    (Do not help child by pointing, moving head or eyes.)
25. Ask child: What is a ball?... lake?... desk?... house?... banana?... curtain?... fence?... ceiling? Pass if defined in terms of use, shape, what it is made of, or general category (such as banana is fruit, not just yellow). Pass 5 of 8, 7 of 8.
26. Ask child: If a horse is big, a mouse is __? If fire is hot, ice is __? If the sun shines during the day, the moon shines during the __? Pass 2 of 3.
27. Child may use wall or rail only, not person. May not crawl.
28. Child must throw ball overhand 3 feet to within arm's reach of tester.
29. Child must perform standing broad jump over width of test sheet (8 1/2 inches).
30. Tell child to walk forward, ⟳⟳⟳⟳➤ heel within 1 inch of toe. Tester may demonstrate.
    Child must walk 4 consecutive steps.
31. In the second year, half of normal children are non-compliant.

OBSERVATIONS:

```
DENVER ARTICULATION SCREENING EXAM
  for children 2 1/2 to 6 years of age

Instructions:  Have child repeat each word after
you.  Circle the underlined sounds that he pro-
nounces correctly.  Total correct sounds is the
Raw Score.  Use charts on reverse side to score
results.
```

NAME

HOSP. NO.

ADDRESS

Date: _____   Child's Age:_____ Examiner: _____   Raw Score:_____

Percentile:_____   Intelligibility:_____   Result:_____

1. table	6. zipper	11. sock	16. wagon	21. leaf
2. shirt	7. grapes	12. vacuum	17. gum	22. carrot
3. door	8. flag	13. yarn	18. house	
4. trunk	9. thumb	14. mother	19. pencil	
5. jumping	10. toothbrush	15. twinkle	20. fish	

Intelligibility: (circle one)   1. Easy to understand   3. Nct understandable
                                2. Understandable 1/2   4. Can't evaluate
                                      the time.

Comments:

Date: _____   Child's Age:_____ Examiner:_____   Raw Score _____

Percentile:_____   Intelligibility:_____   Result:_____

1. table	6. zipper	11. sock	16. wagon	21. leaf
2. shirt	7. grapes	12. vacuum	17. gum	22. carrot
3. door	8. flag	13. yarn	18. house	
4. trunk	9. thumb	14. mother	19. pencil	
5. jumping	10. toothbrush	15. twinkle	20. fish	

Intelligibility: (circle one)   1. Easy to understand   3. Not understandable
                                2. Understandable 1/2   4. Can't evaluate
                                      the time.

Comments:

Date: _____   Child's Age: _____   Examiner:_____   Raw Score_____

Percentile: _____   Intelligibility:_____   Result:_____

1. table	6. zipper	11. sock	16. wagon	21. leaf
2. shirt	7. grapes	12. vacuum	17. gum	22. carrot
3. door	8. flag	13. yarn	18. house	
4. trunk	9. thumb	14. mother	19. pencil	
5. jumping	10. toothbrush	15. twinkle	20. fish	

Intelligibility: (circle one)   1. Easy to understand   3. Not understandable
                                2. Understandable 1/2   4. Can't evaluate
                                      the time.

To score DASE words: Note raw score for child's performance. Match raw score line (extreme left of chart) with column representing child's age (to the closest *previous* age group). Where raw score line and age column meet denotes percentile rank of child's performance when compared with other children that age. Percentiles above heavy line are *abnormal,* below heavy line are *normal.*

PERCENTILE RANK

Raw Score	2.5 yr	3.0 yr	3.5 yr	4.0 yr	4.5 yr	5.0 yr	5.5 yr	6 yr
2	1							
3	2							
4	5							
5	9							
6	16							
7	23							
8	31	2						
9	37	4	1					
10	42	6	2					
11	48	7	4					
12	54	9	6	1	1			
13	58	12	9	2	3	1	1	
14	62	17	11	5	4	2	2	
15	68	23	15	9	5	3	2	
16	75	31	19	12	5	4	3	
17	79	38	25	15	6	6	4	
18	83	46	31	19	8	7	4	
19	86	51	38	24	10	9	5	1
20	89	58	45	30	12	11	7	3
21	92	65	52	36	15	15	9	4
22	94	72	58	43	18	19	12	5
23	96	77	63	50	22	24	15	7
24	97	82	70	58	29	29	20	15
25	99	87	78	66	36	34	26	17
26	99	91	84	75	46	43	34	24
27		94	89	82	57	54	44	34
28		96	94	88	70	68	59	47
29		98	98	94	84	84	77	68
30		100	100	100	100	100	100	100

To score intelligibility:

	NORMAL	ABNORMAL
2.5 years	Understandable half of the time or easy to understand	Not understandable
3 years and older	Easy to understand	Understandable half of the time or not understandable

Test result: 1. Normal on DASE and intelligibility = *normal*
2. Abnormal on DASE or intelligibility = *abnormal**

* If abnormal on initial screening, rescreen within 2 weeks. If abnormal again, child should be referred for complete speech evaluation.

APPENDIX G

Blood Pressure Levels for the 90th and 95th Percentile for Children*

A Guide to Evaluating Blood Pressure in Girls

Age (yr)	BP Percentiles†	Systolic BP (mm Hg) Height Percentiles*							Diastolic BP (mm Hg) Height Percentiles*						
		5th	10th	25th	50th	75th	90th	95th	5th	10th	25th	50th	75th	90th	95th
1	90th	97	98	99	100	102	103	104	53	53	53	54	55	56	56
	95th	101	102	103	104	105	107	107	57	57	57	58	59	60	60
2	90th	99	99	100	102	103	104	105	57	57	58	58	59	60	61
	95th	102	103	104	105	107	108	109	61	61	62	62	63	64	65
3	90th	100	100	102	103	104	105	106	61	61	61	62	63	63	64
	95th	104	104	105	107	108	109	110	65	65	65	66	67	67	68
4	90th	101	102	103	104	106	107	108	63	63	64	65	65	66	67
	95th	105	106	107	108	109	111	111	67	67	68	69	69	70	71
5	90th	103	103	104	106	107	108	109	65	66	66	67	68	68	69
	95th	107	107	108	110	111	112	113	69	70	70	71	72	72	73
6	90th	104	105	106	107	109	110	111	67	67	68	69	69	70	71
	95th	108	109	110	111	112	114	114	71	71	72	73	73	74	75
7	90th	106	107	108	109	110	112	112	69	69	69	70	71	72	72
	95th	110	110	112	113	114	115	116	73	73	73	74	75	76	76
8	90th	108	109	110	111	112	113	114	70	70	71	71	72	73	74
	95th	112	112	113	115	116	117	118	74	74	75	75	76	77	78
9	90th	110	110	112	113	114	115	116	71	72	72	73	74	74	75
	95th	114	114	115	117	118	119	120	75	76	76	77	78	78	79
10	90th	112	112	114	115	116	117	118	73	73	73	74	75	76	76
	95th	116	116	117	119	120	121	122	77	77	77	78	79	80	80
11	90th	114	114	116	117	118	119	120	74	74	75	75	76	77	77
	95th	118	118	119	121	122	123	124	78	78	79	79	80	81	81
12	90th	116	116	118	119	120	121	122	75	75	76	76	77	78	78
	95th	120	120	121	123	124	125	126	79	79	80	80	81	82	82
13	90th	118	118	119	121	122	123	124	76	76	77	78	78	79	80
	95th	121	122	123	125	126	127	128	80	80	81	82	82	83	84
14	90th	119	120	121	122	124	125	126	77	77	78	79	79	80	81
	95th	123	124	125	126	128	129	130	81	81	82	83	83	84	85
15	90th	121	121	122	124	125	126	127	78	78	79	79	80	81	82
	95th	124	125	126	128	129	130	131	82	82	83	83	84	85	86
16	90th	122	122	123	125	126	127	128	79	79	79	80	81	82	82
	95th	125	126	127	128	130	131	132	83	83	83	84	85	86	86
17	90th	122	123	124	125	126	128	128	79	79	79	80	81	82	82
	95th	126	126	127	129	130	131	132	83	83	83	84	85	86	86

*Height percentile determined by standard growth curves; †blood pressure (BP) percentile determined by a single measure.

Source: *Update on the Task Force Report (1987) on High Blood Pressure in Children and Adolescents: A Working Group Report from the National High Blood Pressure Education Program,* NIH Publication No. 96-3790, September 1996.

*By age, gender, and height. Systolic and diastolic blood pressure readings below the 90th percentile are considered to be within normal range.

A Guide to Evaluating Blood Pressure in Boys

Age (yr)	BP Percentiles†	Systolic BP (mm Hg) Height Percentiles*							Diastolic BP (mm Hg) Height Percentiles*						
		5th	10th	25th	50th	75th	90th	95th	5th	10th	25th	50th	75th	90th	95th
1	90th	94	95	97	98	100	102	102	50	51	52	53	54	54	55
	95th	98	99	101	102	104	106	106	55	55	56	57	58	59	59
2	90th	98	99	100	102	104	105	106	55	55	56	57	58	59	59
	95th	101	102	104	106	108	109	110	59	59	60	61	62	63	63
3	90th	100	101	103	105	107	108	109	59	59	60	61	62	63	63
	95th	104	105	107	109	111	112	113	63	63	64	65	66	67	67
4	90th	102	103	105	107	109	110	111	62	62	63	64	65	66	66
	95th	106	107	109	111	113	114	115	66	67	67	68	69	70	71
5	90th	104	105	106	108	110	112	112	65	65	66	67	68	69	69
	95th	108	109	110	112	114	115	116	69	70	70	71	72	73	74
6	90th	105	106	108	110	111	113	114	67	68	69	70	70	71	72
	95th	109	110	112	114	115	117	117	72	72	73	74	75	76	76
7	90th	106	107	109	111	113	114	115	69	70	71	72	72	73	74
	95th	110	111	113	115	116	118	119	74	74	75	76	77	78	78
8	90th	107	108	110	112	114	115	116	71	71	72	73	74	75	75
	95th	111	112	114	116	118	119	120	75	76	76	77	78	79	80
9	90th	109	110	112	113	115	117	117	72	73	73	74	75	76	77
	95th	113	114	116	117	119	121	121	76	77	78	79	80	80	81
10	90th	110	112	113	115	117	118	119	73	74	74	75	76	77	78
	95th	114	115	117	119	121	122	123	77	78	79	80	80	81	82
11	90th	112	113	115	117	119	120	121	74	74	75	76	77	78	78
	95th	116	117	119	121	123	124	125	78	79	79	80	81	82	83
12	90th	115	116	117	119	121	123	123	75	75	76	77	78	78	79
	95th	119	120	121	123	125	126	127	79	79	80	81	82	83	83
13	90th	117	118	120	122	124	125	126	75	76	76	77	78	79	80
	95th	121	122	124	126	128	129	130	79	80	81	82	83	83	84
14	90th	120	121	123	125	126	128	128	76	76	77	78	79	80	80
	95th	124	125	127	128	130	132	132	80	81	81	82	83	84	85
15	90th	123	124	125	127	129	131	131	77	77	78	79	80	81	81
	95th	127	128	129	131	133	134	135	81	82	83	83	84	85	86
16	90th	125	126	128	130	132	133	134	79	79	80	81	82	82	83
	95th	129	130	132	134	136	137	138	83	83	84	85	86	87	87
17	90th	128	129	131	133	134	136	136	81	81	82	83	84	85	85
	95th	132	133	135	136	138	140	140	85	85	86	87	88	89	89

*Height percentile determined by standard growth curves; †blood pressure (BP) percentile determined by a single measure.
Source: *Update on the Task Force Report (1987) on High Blood Pressure in Children and Adolescents: A Working Group Report from the National High Blood Pressure Education Program*, NIH Publication No. 96-3790, September 1996.

APPENDIX H

Common Pediatric Laboratory Tests and Normal Values

To conserve space, the following common abbreviations are used.

Abbreviations

Ab	absorbance
AU	arbitrary unit
CKBB	brain isoenzyme of creatine kinase
CKMB	heart isoenzyme of creatine kinase
d	diem, day, days
F	female
g	gram
hr	hour, hours
Hb	hemoglobin
HbCO	carboxyhemoglobin
IU	International Unit of hormone activity
L	liter
M	male
MCV	mean corpuscular volume
MEq/L	milliequivalents per liter
min	minute, minutes
mm³	cubic millimeter; equivalent to microliter (μl)
mm Hg	millimeters of mercury
mo	month, months
mol	mole
mOsm	milliosmole
MW	relative molecular weight
N	nitrogen
Pa	pascal
pc	postprandial
RBC	red blood cell(s); erythrocyte(s)
RT	room temperature
s	second, seconds
U	International Unit of enzyme activity
vol	volume
WBC	white blood cell(s)
wk	week, weeks
yr	year, years

Symbols

>	greater than
≥	greater than or equal to
<	less than
≤	less than or equal to
±	plus or minus
~	approximately
≅	approximately equal to

Abbreviations for Specimens

S	serum
P	plasma
(H)	heparin
(LiH)	lithium heparin
(E)	EDTA
(C)	citrate
(O)	oxalate
W	whole blood
U	urine
F	feces
CSF	cerebrospinal fluid
AF	amniotic fluid
(NaC)	sodium citrate
(NH₄H)	ammonium heparinate

Key to Comments

30°, 37°	temperature of enzymatic analysis (Celsius)
a	colorimetry
b	Ektachem, proprietary analytic system of Johnson & Johnson Clinical Diagnostics, Inc.
c	enzyme-amplified immunoassay
d	values obtained are significantly method dependent
e	nephelometry
f	cation-exchange chromatography
g	values in older males higher than those in older females
h	ion-selective electrode
i	fluorescence polarization
j	enzymatic assay

Prefixes Denoting Decimal Factors

Prefix	Symbol	Factor	Prefix	Symbol	Factor
mega	M	10^6	milli	m	10^{-3}
kilo	k	10^3	micro	μ	10^{-6}
hecto	h	10^2	nano	n	10^{-9}
deka	da	10^1	pico	p	10^{-12}
deci	d	10^{-1}	femto	f	10^{-15}
centi	c	10^{-2}			

Modified from Behrman, R.E., Kliegman, R.M., & Jenson, H. (2000). *Nelson textbook of pediatrics* (16th ed., pp. 2184-2224). Philadelphia: Saunders.

Therapeutic and Toxic Ranges (Peak and Trough) of Antibiotics

Antibiotic	Specimen	Peak Therapeutic (mg/L)	Peak Toxic (mg/L)	Trough Therapeutic (mg/L)	Trough Toxic (mg/L)	Factor
Amikacin	S	20-40	>40	5-10	>10	×1.708
Chloramphenicol	S	10-20	>25	5-10	>10	×3.095
Gentamicin	S	6-10	>12	0.5-2.0	>2.0	×2.064
Netilmicin	S	6-10	>12	0.5-2.0	>2	×2.103
Tobramycin	S	6-10	>12	0.5-2.0	>2	×2.139
Vancomycin	S	30-40	>60	5-10	>20	×0.303

Common Laboratory Tests and Normal Values

Test	Specimen	Reference Range (Conventional Units)	Factor	Reference Range, International Units (SI)	Comments
Acetaminophen	S, P (H, E)	Therapeutic concentration 10-30 mcg/ml; Toxic concentration >200 mcg/ml	× 6.62	66-200 µmol/L; >1300 µmol/L	i z
Activated partial thromboplastin time (APTT)	P (C)	25-35 s; Infant: <90 s		25-35 s; Infant: <90 s	
Adrenocorticotropic hormone (ACTH)	P (H)	Cord blood 130-160 pg/ml; 1-7 d postnatal 100-140 pg/ml; Adult 0800 hr 25-100 pg/ml; 1800 hr <50 pg/ml	× 1	130-160 mcg/L; 100-140 mcg/L; 25-100 mcg/L; <50 mcg/L	
Alanine aminotransferase (ALT, SGPT)	S	0-5 d 6-50 U/L; 1-19 yr 5-45 U/L	× 1	6-50 U/L; 5-45 U/L	37° b h
Albumin	P	Premature 1 d 1.8-3.0 g/dl; Full-term <6 d 2.5-3.4 g/dl; <5 yr 3.9-5.0 g/dl; 5-19 yr 4.0-5.3 g/dl	× 10	18-30 g/L; 25-34 g/L; 39-50 g/L; 40-53 g/L	
	U	4-16 yr 3.35-15.3 mg/24 hr/1.73 m²			c
Ammonia nitrogen	CSF	10-30 mg/dl		100-300 mg/L	
	S, P (LiH)	Neonate 90-150 mcg N/dl; 0-2 wk 79-129 mcg N/dl; >1 mo 29-70 mcg N/dl; Thereafter 15-45 mcg N/dl; 1-90 d 59-202 mcg N/dl; 3 mo-3 yr 48-195 mcg N/dl	× 0.714	64-107 µmol/L; 56-92 µmol/L; 21-50 µmol/L; 11-32 µmol/L; 42-144 µmol/L; 34-139 µmol/L	j f
	U	500-1200 mg N/24 hr	× 0.0714	36-86 mmol/d	
Amphetamine	S, P (H, E)	Therapeutic concentration 20-30 ng/ml; Toxic concentration >200 ng/ml	× 7.396	150-220 nmol/L; >1500 nmol/L	
Antistreptolysin-O titer (ASO titer)	S	≤166 Todd units; 170-330 Todd units in school-age children			
Base excess	W (H)	Neonate (−10)-(−2) mmol/L; Infant (−7)-(−1) mmol/L; Child (−4)-(+2) mmol/L; Thereafter (−3)-(+3) mmol/L		(−10)-(−2) mmol/L; (−7)-(−1) mmol/L; (−4)-(+2) mmol/L; (−3)-(+3) mmol/L	
Bicarbonate	S, P	Arterial 21-28 mmol/L; Venous 22-29 mmol/L		21-28 mmol/L; 22-29 mmol/L	
Bilirubin	S, P				

Bilirubin

		PREMATURE (mg/dl)	FULL-TERM (mg/dl)	Factor	PREMATURE (µmol/L)	FULL-TERM (µmol/L)
Total	S	Cord blood <2.0	<2.0	× 17.10	<34	<34
		0-1 d <8.0	<6.0		<137	<103
		1-2 d <12.0	<8.0		<205	<137
		2-5 d <16.0	<12.0		<274	<205
		>5 d <2.0	0.2-1.0		<34	3.4-17.1

Continued

Common Laboratory Tests and Normal Values—cont'd

Test	Specimen	Reference Range (Conventional Units)	Factor	Reference Range, International Units (SI)	Comments
	U	Negative		Negative	
	AF	28 wk <0.075 mg/dl	×17.10	<1.3 µmol/L	
		(or Ab450 <0.048)		(or Ab450 <0.048)	
		40 wk <0.025 mg/dl		<0.43 µmol/L	
		(or Ab450 <0.02)		(or Ab450 <0.02)	
Conjugated	S	0-0.2 mg/dl	×17.10	0-3.4 µmol/L	
Bleeding time (BBT)					
Ivy		Normal 2-7 min		Normal 2-7 min	
		Borderline 7-11 min		Borderline 7-11 min	
Simplate (G-D)		2.75-8 min		2.75-8 min	
Blood volume	W (H)	M 52-83 ml/kg	×0.001	M 0.052-0.083 L/kg	
		F 50-75 ml/kg		F 0.050-0.075 L/kg	
C-reactive protein	S	Cord blood 52-1330 ng/ml	×1	52-1330 mcg/L	c
		2-12 yr 67-1800 ng/ml		67-1800 mcg/L	
Calcium, ionized (Ca)	S, P (H), W (H)	Cord blood 5.0-6.0 mg/dl	×0.25	1.25-1.50 mmol/L	
		Neonate			
		3-24 hr 4.3-5.1 mg/dl		1.07-1.27 mmol/L	
		24-48 hr 4.0-4.7 mg/dl		1.00-1.17 mmol/L	
		Thereafter 4.8-4.92 mg/dl, or		1.12-1.23 mmol/L	
		2.24-2.46 mEq/L		1.12-1.23 mmol/L	
Calcium, total	S	Cord blood 9.0-11.5 mg/dl	×0.25	2.25-2.88 mmol/L	
		Neonate			
		3-24 hr 9.0-10.6 mg/dl		2.3-2.65 mmol/L	
		24-48 hr 7.0-12.0 mg/dl		1.75-3.0 mmol/L	
		4-7 d 9.0-10.9 mg/dl		2.25-2.73 mmol/L	
		Child 8.8-10.8 mg/dl		2.2-2.70 mmol/L	
		Thereafter 8.4-10.2 mg/dl		2.1-2.55 mmol/L	
	U	Ca in diet			
		Ca-free 5-40 mg/24 hr	×0.025	0.13-1.0 mmol/24 hr	
		Low to average 50-150 mg/24 hr		1.25-3.8 mmol/24 hr	
Carbon dioxide	W (H)	Neonate 27-40 mm Hg	×0.1333	3.6-5.3 kPa	
Partial pressure (P_{CO_2})		Infant 27-41 mm Hg		3.6-5.5 kPa	
		Thereafter			
		M 35-48 mm Hg		4.7-6.4 kPa	
		F 32-45 mm Hg		4.3-6.0 kPa	
Total (tCO_2)	S, P (H)	Cord blood 14-22 mmol/L	×1	14-22 mmol/L	
		Premature 14-27 mmol/L		14-27 mmol/L	
		Neonate 13-22 mmol/L		13-22 mmol/L	
		Infant 20-28 mmol/L		20-28 mmol/L	
		Child 20-28 mmol/L		20-28 mmol/L	
		Thereafter 23-30 mmol/L		23-30 mmol/L	
Carbon monoxide	W (E)	Nonsmokers <2% HbCO	×0.01	HbCO fraction <0.02	
		Smokers <10%		<0.10	
		Lethal >50%		>0.5	

Test	Specimen	Reference Range (Conventional Units)		Factor	Reference Range, International Units (SI)	Comments
Cerebrospinal fluid						
Pressure	CSF	70-180 mm H$_2$O		× 0.001	70-180 mm H$_2$O	
Volume	CSF	Child 60-100 ml		× 0.001	Child 0.06-0.10 L	
		Adult 100-160 ml			Adult 0.1-0.16 L	
Chloral hydrate	S	As trichloroethanol		× 6.694		
		Therapeutic concentration	2-12 mcg/ml		13-80 µmol/L	
		Toxic concentration	>20 mcg/ml		>134 µmol/L	
Chloride	S, P (H)	Cord blood	96-104 mmol/L	× 1	96-104 mmol/L	
		Neonate	97-110 mmol/L		97-110 mmol/L	
		Thereafter	98-106 mmol/L		98-106 mmol/L	
	CSF	Infant	118-132 mmol/L	× 1	118-132 mmol/L	
	U	Infant	2-10 mmol/24 hr	× 1	2-10 mmol/24 hr	
		Child	15-40 mmol/24 hr		15-40 mmol/24 hr	
		Thereafter	110-250 mmol/24 hr (varies greatly with Cl intake)		110-250 mmol/24 hr	
	Sweat	Normal	<40 mmol/L	× 1	<40 mmol/L	
		Borderline	45-60 mmol/L		45-60 mmol/L	
		Cystic fibrosis	>60 mmol/L		>60 mmol/L	
Cholesterol, total	S	1-3 yr	45-182 mg/dl	× 0.0259	1.15-4.70 mmol/L	j
	S	4-6 yr	109-189 mg/dl	× 0.0259	2.80-4.80 mmol/L	
Clotting time, Lee-White, 37° C	W	Glass tubes	5-8 min (5-15 min at RT)		Glass tubes	5-8 min (5-15 min at RT)
		Silicone tubes	About 30 min prolonged		Silicone tubes	About 30 min prolonged
Creatine kinase	S	Cord blood	70-380 U/L	× 1	70-380 U/L	30° g
		5-8 hr	214-1175 U/L		214-1175 U/L	
		24-33 hr	130-1200 U/L		130-1200 U/L	
		72-100 hr	87-725 U/L		87-725 U/L	
		Adult	5-130 U/L		5-130 U/L	
Creatine kinase isoenzymes	S		**CKMB (%)**	**CKBB (%)**		
		Cord blood	0.3-3.1	0.3-10.5		
		5-8 hr	1.7-7.9	3.6-13.4		
		24-33 hr	1.8-5.0	2.3-8.6		
		72-100 hr	1.4-5.4	5.1-13.3		
		Adult	0-2	0		
Creatinine, plasma Jaffe, kinetic, or enzymatic	S, P	Cord blood	0.6-1.2 mg/dl	× 88.4	53-106 µmol/L	
		Neonate	0.3-1.0 mg/dl		27-88 µmol/L	
		Infant	0.2-0.4 mg/dl		18-35 µmol/L	
		Child	0.3-0.7 mg/dl		27-62 µmol/L	
		Adolescent	0.5-1.0 mg/dl		44-88 µmol/L	
		Adult				
		M	0.6-1.2 mg/dl		53-106 µmol/L	
		F	0.5-1.1 mg/dl		44-97 µmol/L	

Continued

Common Laboratory Tests and Normal Values—cont'd

Test	Specimen	Reference Range (Conventional Units)	Factor	Reference Range, International Units (SI)	Comments
Jaffe, manual	S, P	0.8-1.5 mg/dl	× 88.4	70-133 µmol/L	
	AF	>2.0 mg/dl	× 88.4	>180 µmol/L	d b
Creatinine, urinary	U		× 8.84		
		Premature 8.1-15.0 mg/kg/24 hr		72-133 µmol/kg/24 hr	
		Full-term 10.4-19.7 mg/kg/24 hr		92-174 µmol/kg/24 hr	
		1.5-7 yr 10-15 mg/kg/24 hr		88-133 µmol/kg/24 hr	
		7-15 yr 5.2-41 mg/kg/24 hr		46-362 µmol/kg/24 hr	
Creatinine clearance (endogenous)	S, P, U	Neonate 40-65 ml/min/1.73 m²			
		<40 yr			
		M 97-137 ml/min/1.73 m²			
		F 88-128 ml/min/1.73 m²			
		Decreases ~6.5 ml/min/decade			
Diazepam	S, P (H, E) at trough	Therapeutic concentration 100-1000 ng/ml	× 3.512	350-3500 nmol/L	
		Toxic concentration >5000 ng/ml		>17,500 nmol/L	
Digoxin	S, P (H, E) (12-hr post)	Therapeutic concentration	× 1.281		ic
		CHF 0.8-1.5 ng/ml		1.0-1.9 nmol/L	
		Arrhythmias 1.5-2.0 ng/ml		1.9-2.6 nmol/L	
		Toxic concentration			
		Child >2.5 ng/ml		>3.2 nmol/L	
		Adult >3.0 ng/ml		>3.8 nmol/L	
Eosinophil count	W (E, H) capillary	50-350 cells/mm³ (µl)	× 10⁶	50-350 × 10⁶ cells/L	
Erythrocyte count (RBC) count	W (E)	MILLIONS OF CELLS/mm³ (µl)	× 1	× 10¹² CELLS/L	
		Cord blood 3.9-5.5		3.9-5.5	
		1-3 d (capillary) 4.0-6.6		4.0-6.6	
		1 wk 3.9-6.3		3.9-6.3	
		2 wk 3.6-6.2		3.6-6.2	
		1 mo 3.0-5.4		3.0-5.4	
		2 mo 2.7-4.9		2.7-4.9	
		3-6 mo 3.1-4.5		3.1-4.5	
		0.5-2 yr 3.7-5.3		3.7-5.3	
		2-6 yr 3.9-5.3		3.9-5.3	
		6-12 yr 4.0-5.2		4.0-5.2	
		12-18 yr			
		M 4.5-5.3		4.5-5.3	
		F 4.1-5.1		4.1-5.1	
		18-49 yr			
		M 4.5-5.9		4.5-5.9	
		F 4.0-5.2		4.0-5.2	
Erythrocyte sedimentation rate (ESR) Westergren, modified	W (E)	Child 0-10 mm/hr		0-10 mm/hr	

Test	Specimen	Reference Range (Conventional Units)		Factor	Reference Range, International Units (SI)		Comments
Wintrobe		Adult					
		M <50 yr	0-15 mm/hr		0-15 mm/hr		
		F <50 yr	0.20 mm/hr		0-20 mm/hr		
		Child	0-13 mm/hr		0-13 mm/hr		
		Adult					
		M	0.9 mm/hr		0-9 mm/hr		
		F	0-20 mm/hr		0-20 mm/hr		
Fat, fecal	F (72 hr)		41-54%		41-54 AU		
		Infant, breast-fed	<1 g/24 hr	× 1	<1 g/24 hr		
		0-6 yr	<2 g/24 hr		<2 g/24 hr		
		Adult					
		Normal diet	<7 g/24 hr		<7 g/24 hr		
		Fat-free diet	<4 g/24 hr		<4 g/24 hr		
		COEFFICIENT OF FAT ABSORPTION (%)			**ABSORBED FRACTION**		
		Infant		× 0.01			
		Breast-fed	>93		>0.93		
		Formula-fed	>83		>0.83		
		>1 yr	≥95		≥0.95		
α-Fetoprotein (AFP)	S maternal	**PREGNANCY (wk)**	**MEDIAN (ng/ml)**		**MEDIAN (mcg/L)**		
		15	34	× 1	34		
		16	38		38		
		17	44		44		
		18	49		49		
		19	56.5		56.5		
		20	66		66		
	AF		**MEAN (mcg/ml)**				
		15	13.5 ± 3.42				
		16	11.7 ± 3.38				
		17	10.3 ± 3.03				
		18	9.5 ± 3.22				
		19	7.1 ± 2.86				
		20	5.0 ± 2.45				
Fibrinogen	P (NaCl)	Neonate	125-300 mg/dl	× 0.01	1.25-3.00 g/L		
		Adult	200-400 mg/dl		2.00-4.00 g/L		
Galactose	S	Neonate	0-20 mg/dl	× 0.0555	0-1.11 mmol/L		
	P	5 mo-17 yr	0.0-0.5 mg/dl		0.0-0.03 mmol/L		
	U	Neonate	≤60 mg/dl	× 0.0555	≤3.33 mmol/L		
		Thereafter	14 mg/24 hr	× 0.00555	<0.08 mmol/24 hr		
Glucose	S	Cord blood	45-96 mg/dl	× 0.0555	2.5-5.3 mmol/L		j
		Neonate					
		1 d	40-60 mg/dl		2.2-3.3 mmol/L		
		>1 d	50-90 mg/dl		2.8-5.0 mmol/L		
		Child	60-100 mg/dl		3.3-5.5 mmol/L		
		Adult	70-105 mg/dl		3.9-5.8 mmol/L		

Continued

Common Laboratory Tests and Normal Values—cont'd

Test	Specimen	Reference Range (Conventional Units)	Factor	Reference Range, International Units (SI)	Comments
Quantitative, enzymatic	W (H)	Adult 65-95 mg/dl	× 5.55	3.6-5.3 mmol/L	
	CSF	Adult 40-70 mg/dl		2.2-3.9 mmol/L	
	U	<0.5 g/24 hr		<2.8 mmol/24 hr	
Qualitative	U	Negative		Negative	
Glucose, 2 hr pc	S	<120 mg/dl	× 0.0555	<6.7 mmol/L	
Glucose tolerance test (GTT), oral	S	(For diabetes, see Glucose tolerance test, oral)			
Adult dose: 75 g		**NORMAL (mg/dl)** / **DIABETIC (mg/dl)**	× 0.0555	**NORMAL (mmol/L)** / **DIABETIC (mmol/L)**	
Child dose: 1.75 g/kg of ideal weight up to maximum of 75 g		Fasting 70-105 / >115		3.9-5.8 / >6.4	
		60 min 120-170 / ≥200		6.7-9.4 / ≥11	
		90 min 100-140 / ≥200		5.6-7.8 / ≥11	
		120 min 70-120 / ≥140		3.9-6.7 / ≥7.8	
Growth hormone (hGH) somatotropin	S, P (E, H)	Neonate 5-23 ng/ml	× 1	5-53 mcg/L	
		1 d 5-27 ng/ml		5-27 mcg/L	
		1 wk 1-12 mo 2-10 ng/ml		2-10 mcg/L	
	Fasting, at rest	Child <0.7-6 ng/ml		<0.7-6 mcg/L	
		Adult <0.7-6 ng/ml		<0.7-6 mcg/L	
Hematocrit (HCT, Hct)	W (E)	**PERCENT PACKED RED CELLS (VOL. RED CELLS/VOL. WHOLE BLOOD CELLS × 100) (%)**	× 0.01	**VOLUME FRACTION (VOL. RED CELLS/VOL. WHOLE BLOOD)**	
Calculated from MCV and RBC (electronic displacement or laser)		1 d (capillary) 48-69		0.48-0.69	
		2 d 48-75		0.48-0.75	
		3 d 44-72		0.44-0.72	
		2 mo 28-42		0.28-0.42	
		6-12 yr 35-45		0.35-0.45	
		12-18 yr M 37-49		0.37-0.49	
		F 36-46		0.36-0.46	
		18-49 yr M 41-53		0.41-0.53	
		F 36-46		0.36-0.46	
Hemoglobin (Hb)	W (E)	1-3 d (capillary) 14.5-22.5 g/dl	× 0.155	2.25-3.49 mmol/L	MW Hb = 64,500
		2 mo 9.0-14.0 g/dl		1.40-2.17 mmol/L	
		6-12 yr 11.5-15.5 g/dl		1.78-2.40 mmol/L	
		12-18 yr M 13.0-16.0 g/dl		2.02-2.48 mmol/L	
		F 12.0-16.0 g/dl		1.86-2.48 mmol/L	
		18-49 yr M 13.5-17.5 g/dl		2.09-2.27 mmol/L	
		F 12.0-16.0 g/dl		1.86-2.48 mmol/L	

Test	Specimen	Reference Range (Conventional Units)	Factor	Reference Range, International Units (SI)	Comments
Hemoglobin A	P (H)	<10 mg/dl	× 0.155	<1.55 µmol/L	
		<3 mg/dl with butterfly setup and 18-gauge needle		<0.47 µmol/L with butterfly setup and 18-gauge needle	
Hemoglobin F	U	Negative		Negative	
Alkali denaturation	W (E, C, H)	>95%	× 0.01	Fraction of hemoglobin >0.95	
	W (E)	1 d — 63-92% HbF	× 0.01	0.62-0.92 mass fraction	
		5 d — 65-88% HbF		0.65-0.88 mass fraction	
		3 wk — 55-85% HbF		0.55-0.85 mass fraction	
		6-9 wk — 31-75% HbF		0.31-0.75 mass fraction	
		3-4 mo — <2-59% HbF		<0.02-0.59 mass fraction	
		6 mo — <2-9% HbF		<0.02-0.09 mass fraction	
		Adult — <2% HbF		<0.02 mass fraction	
Immunoglobulin A (IgA)	S	Cord blood — 1.4-3.6 mg/dl	× 10	14-36 mg/L	e
		1-3 mo — 1.3-53 mg/dl		13-530 mg/L	
		4-6 mo — 4.4-84 mg/dl		44-840 mg/L	
		7 mo-1 yr — 11-106 mg/dl		110-1060 mg/L	
		2-5 yr — 14-159 mg/dl		140-1590 mg/L	
		6-10 yr — 33-236 mg/dl		330-2360 mg/L	
		Adult — 70-312 mg/dl		700-3120 mg/L	
Immunoglobulin D (IgD)	S	Neonate — None detected		None detected	
		Thereafter — 0-8 mg/dl	× 10	0-80 mg/L	
Immunoglobulin E (IgE)	S	M — 0-230 IU/ml	× 1	0-230 kIU/L	
		F — 0-170 IU/ml		0-170 kIU/L	
Immunoglobulin G (IgG)	S	Cord blood — 636-1606 mg/dl	× 0.01	6.36-16.06 g/L	e
		1 mo — 251-906 mg/dl		2.51-9.06 g/L	
		2-4 mo — 176-601 mg/dl		1.76-6.01 g/L	
		5-12 mo — 172-1069 mg/dl		1.72-10.69 g/L	
		1-5 yr — 345-1236 mg/dl		3.45-12.36 g/L	
		6-10 yr — 608-1572 mg/dl		6.08-15.72 g/L	
		Adult — 639-1349 mg/dl		6.39-13.49 g/L	
Immunoglobulin M (IgM)	S	Cord blood — 6.3-25 mg/dl	× 10	63-250 mg/L	e
		1-4 mo — 17-105 mg/dl		170-1050 mg/L	
		5-9 mo — 33-126 mg/dl		300-1260 mg/L	
		10 mo-1 yr — 41-173 mg/dl		410-1730 mg/L	
		2-8 yr — 43-207 mg/dl		430-2070 mg/L	
		9-10 yr — 52-242 mg/dl		520-2420 mg/L	
		Adult — 56-352 mg/dl		560-3520 mg/L	
Iron	S	Neonate — 100-250 mcg/dl	× 0.179	17.90-44.75 µmol/L	
		Infant — 40-100 mcg/dl		7.16-17.90 µmol/L	
		Child — 50-120 mcg/dl		8.95-21.48 µmol/L	
		Thereafter			
		M — 50-160 mcg/dl		8.95-28.64 µmol/L	
		F — 40-150 mcg/dl		7.16-26.85 µmol/L	
		Intoxicated child — 280-2550 mcg/dl		50.12-456.5 µmol/L	
		Fatally poisoned child — >1800 mcg/dl		>322.2 µmol/L	

Continued

Common Laboratory Tests and Normal Values—cont'd

Test	Specimen	Reference Range (Conventional Units)	Factor	Reference Range, International Units (SI)	Comments
Iron-binding capacity, total (TIBC)	S	Infant: 100-400 mcg/dl; Thereafter: 250-400 mcg/dl	× 0.179	17.90-71.60 μmol/L; 44.75-71.60 μmol/L	
17-Ketogenic steroids (17-KGS)	U	0-1 yr: <1.0 mg/24 hr; 1-10 yr: <5 mg/24 hr; 11-14 yr: <12 mg/24 hr; Thereafter: M 5-23 mg/24 hr, F 3-15 mg/24 hr	× 3.467	<3.5 μmol/24 hr; <17 μmol/24 hr; <42 μmol/24 hr; 17-80 μmol/24 hr; 10-52 μmol/24 hr	{ Conversion based on dehydroepiandrosterone, MW 288
Ketone bodies Qualitative	S	Negative		Negative	
	U	Negative		Negative	
Quantitative	S	0.5-3.0 mg/dl	× 10	5-30 mg/L	
LDL-cholesterol (LDLC)	S, P (E)	M (mg/dl) / F (mg/dl): Cord blood 10-50 / 10-50; 1-9 yr 60-140 / 60-150; 10-19 yr 50-170 / 50-170; 20-29 yr 60-175 / 60-160; 30-39 yr 80-190 / 70-170; 40-49 yr 90-205 / 80-190; Recommended (desirable) range for adults <1300 mg/dl	× 0.0259	M (mmol/L) / F (mmol/L): 0.26-1.30 / 0.26-1.30; 1.55-3.63 / 1.55-3.89; 1.30-4.40 / 1.30-4.40; 1.55-4.53 / 1.55-4.14; 2.07-4.92 / 1.81-4.40; 2.33-5.31 / 2.07-4.92; 1.68-4.53 mmol/L	
Lead	W (H)	Child <10 mg/dl; Adult <40 mcg/dl; Acceptable for industrial exposure <60 mcg/dl; Toxic ≥100 mcg/dl	× 0.0483	<0.48 μmol/L; <1.93 μmol/L; <2.90 μmol/L; ≥4.83 μmol/L	
	U (24-hr)	<80 mcg/dl	× 0.00483	<0.39 μmol/L	
Leukocyte count (WBC)	W (E)	× 1000 cells/mm³ (μl): Birth 9.0-30.0; 24 hr 9.4-34.0; 1 mo 5.0-19.5; 1-3 yr 6.0-17.5; 4-7 yr 5.5-15.5; 8-13 yr 4.5-13.5; Adult 4.5-11.0		× 10⁹ cells/L: 9.0-30.0; 9.4-34.0; 5.0-19.5; 6.0-17.5; 5.5-15.5; 4.5-13.5; 4.5-11.0	
Leukocyte differential Myelocytes Neutrophils—"bands" Neutrophils—"segs" Lymphocytes Monocytes Eosinophils Basophils	W (E)	0; 3%-5%; 54%-62%; 25%-33%; 3%-7%; 1%-3%; 0%-0.75%	× 0.01	0; 0.03-0.05 number fraction; 0.54-0.62 number fraction; 0.25-0.33 number fraction; 0.03-0.07 number fraction; 0.01-0.03 number fraction; 0-0.0075 number fraction	

Test	Specimen	Reference Range (Conventional Units)	Factor	Reference Range, International Units (SI)	Comments
Mean corpuscular hemoglobin concentration (MCHC)	W (E)	Birth 31-37 pg/cell	× 0.0155	0.48-0.57 fmol/cell	
		1-3 d (capillary) 31-37 pg/cell		0.48-0.57 fmol/cell	
		1 wk-1 mo 28-40 pg/cell		0.43-0.62 fmol/cell	
		2 mo 26-34 pg/cell		0.40-0.53 fmol/cell	
		3-6 mo 25-35 pg/cell		0.39-0.54 fmol/cell	
		0.5-2 yr 23-31 pg/cell		0.36-0.48 fmol/cell	
		2-6 yr 24-30 pg/cell		0.37-0.47 fmol/cell	
		6-12 yr 25-33 pg/cell		0.39-0.51 fmol/cell	
		12-18 yr 25-35 pg/cell		0.39-0.54 fmol/cell	
		18-49 yr 26-34 pg/cell		0.40-0.53 fmol/cell	
Mean corpuscular hemoglobin	W (E)	**PERCENTAGE HB/CELL OR G HB/DL RBC**	× 0.155	**MMOL HB/L RBC**	
		Birth 30-36		4.65-5.58	
		1-3 d (capillary) 29-37		4.50-5.74	
		1-2 wk 28-38		4.34-5.89	
		1-2 mo 29-37		4.50-5.74	
		3 mo-2 yr 30-36		4.65-5.58	
		2-18 yr 31-37		4.81-5.74	
		>18 yr 31-37		4.81-5.74	
Mean corpuscular volume (MCV)	W (E)	1-3 d (capillary) 95-121 μm³	× 1	95-121 fl	
		0.5-2 yr 70-86 μm³		70-86 fl	
		6-12 yr 77-95 μm³		77-95 fl	
		12-18 yr			
		M 78-98 μm³		78-98 fl	
		F 78-102 μm³		78-102 fl	
		18-49 yr			
		M 80-100 μm³		80-100 fl	
		F 80-100 μm³		80-100 fl	
Occult blood	F	Negative (>2 ml blood/24 hr in ~ 100-200 g stool)		Negative	
	U	Negative		Negative	
Osmolality	S	Child and adult 275-295 mOsm/kg H₂O			
	U	50-1400 mOsm/kg H₂O, depending on fluid intake. After 12 hr of fluid restriction, normal range is >850 mOsm/kg H₂O			
	U (24-hr)	300-900 mOsm/kg H₂O			
Oxygen, partial pressure of (PO₂)	W (H), arterial	Birth 8-24 mm Hg	× 0.133	1.1-3.2 kPa	
		5-10 min 33-75 mm Hg		4.4-10.0 kPa	
		30 min 31-85 mm Hg		4.1-11.3 kPa	
		>1 hr 55-80 mm Hg		7.3-10.6 kPa	
		1 d 54-95 mm Hg		7.2-12.6 kPa	
		Thereafter (decreases with age) 83-108 mm Hg		11-14.4 kPa	

Continued

Common Laboratory Tests and Normal Values—cont'd

Test	Specimen	Reference Range (Conventional Units)	Factor	Reference Range, International Units (SI)	Comments
Oxygen saturation	W (H), arterial	Neonate 85%-90% Thereafter 95%-99%	× 0.01	0.85-0.90 Saturated fraction 0.95-0.99 Saturated fraction	
Partial thromboplastin time (PTT) Nonactivated	W (NaCl)	60-85 s (Platelin)		60-85 s	
Activated		25-35 s (differs with method)		25-35 s	
Phenobarbital	S, P (H, E) at trough	Therapeutic concentration 15-40 mcg/ml Toxic concentration Slowness, ataxia, nystagmus 35-80 mcg/ml Coma With reflexes 65-117 mcg/ml Without reflexes >100 mcg/ml	× 4.306	65-170 µmol/L 150-345 µmol/L 280-504 µmol/L >430 µmol/L	i c
Phenylalanine	S	Premature 2.0-7.5 mg/dl Neonate 1.2-3.4 mg/dl Thereafter 0.8-1.8 mg/dl	× 60.54	120-450 µmol/L 70-210 µmol/L 50-110 µmol/L	
	U	10 d-2 wk 1-2 mg/24 hr 3-12 yr 4-18 mg/24 hr Thereafter Trace-17 mg/24 hr	× 6.054	6-12 µmol/24 hr 24-110 µmol/24 hr Trace-103 µmol/24 hr	
Plasma volume	P (H)	M 25-43 ml/kg F 28-45 ml/kg	× 0.001	M 0.025-0.043 L/kg F 0.028-0.045 L/kg	
Platelet count (thrombocyte count)	W (E)	Neonate 84-478 × 10³/mm³ (µl) (after 1 wk same as adult) Adult 150-400 × 10³/mm³ (µl)	× 10⁶	84-478 × 10⁹/L 150-400 × 10⁹/L	h
Potassium	S	<2 mo 3.0-7.0 mmol/L 2-12 mo 3.5-6.0 mmol/L >12 mo 3.5-5.0 mmol/L	× 1	3.0-7.0 mmol/L 3.5-6.0 mmol/L 3.5-6.0 mmol/L 3.5-4.5 mmol/L	Increased by hemolysis Serum values systematically higher than plasma values
	P (H)				
	U (24-hr)	2.5-125 mmol/L (varies with diet)		2.5-125 mmol/L (varies with diet)	
Protein Total	S	Premature 4.3-7.6 g/dl Neonate 4.6-7.4 g/dl 1-7 yr 6.1-7.9 g/dl 8-12 yr 6.4-8.1 g/dl 13-19 yr 6.6-8.2 g/dl	× 10	43-76 g/L 46-74 g/L 61-79 g/L 64-81 g/L 66-82 g/L	
Total urinary	U (24-hr)	1-14 mg/dl 50-80 mg/24 hr (at rest) <250 mg/24 hr after intense exercise	× 10	10-140 mg/L 50-80 mg/24 hr (at rest) <250 mg/24 hr after intense exercise	
Total protein (column)	CSF	Lumbar 8-32 mg/dl	× 10	80-320 mg/L	

Test	Specimen	Reference Range (Conventional Units)	Factor	Reference Range, International Units (SI)	Comments
Prothrombin time (PT)					
One-stage (quick)	W (NaC)	In general, 11-15 s (varies with type of thrombo- plastin)		11-15 s	
		Neonate: prolonged by 2-3 s		Neonate: prolonged by 2-3 s	
Two-stage modi- fied (Ware and Seegers)	W (NaC)	18-22 s		18-22 s	
RBC count: see Erythrocyte count					
Red cell volume	W (H)	M	× 0.001	0.020-0.036 L/kg	
		20-36 ml/kg			
		F		0.019-0.031 L/kg	
		19-31 ml/kg			
Reticulocyte count	W (E, H, O)	Adults 0.5%-1.5% of erythrocytes,	× 0.01	0.005-0.015 number fraction	
		or 25,000-75,000/mm³ (µl)	× 10⁶	25,000-75,000 × 10⁶/L	
	W (capillary)	0.4%-6.0%	× 0.01	0.004-0.060 number fraction	
		1 d		<0.001-0.013 number fraction	
		7 d <0.1%-1.3%		<0.001-0.012 number fraction	
		1-4 wk <1.0%-1.2%		<0.001-0.024 number fraction	
		5-6 wk <0.1%-2.4%		0.001-0.029 number fraction	
		7-8 wk 0.1%-2.9%		<0.001-0.026 number fraction	
		9-10 wk <0.1%-2.6%		0.001-0.013 number fraction	
		11-12 wk 0.1%-1.3%			
Salicylate	S, P (H, E) at trough	Therapeutic concentration	× 0.0724	1.1-2.2 mmol/L	
		15-30 mg/dl			
		Toxic concentration		>2.2 mmol/L	
		>30 mg/dl			
Sedimentation rate: see Erythrocyte sedimentation rate					
Sickle cell tests					
Sodium meta- bisulfite	W (E, H, O)	Negative		Negative	
Dithionite test	W (E, H, O)	Negative			
Sodium	S, P (LiH, NH₄H)	Neonate 134-146 mmol/L	× 1	134-146 mmol/L	
		Infant 139-146 mmol/L		139-146 mmol/L	
		Child 138-145 mmol/L		138-146 mmol/L	
		Thereafter 136-146 mmol/L		136-148 mmol/L	
	U (24-hr)	40-220 mmol		40-220 mmol	
		(depending on diet)			
	Sweat	Normal	× 1	<40 mmol/L	
		<40 mmol/L			
		Indeterminate		45-60 mmol/L	
		45-60 mmol/L			
		Cystic fibrosis		>60 mmol/L	
		>60 mmol/L			
Specific gravity	U	Adult		1.002-1.030	
		1.002-1.030			
		After 12-hr fluid restriction		>1.025	
		>1.025			
	U (24-hr)	1.015-1.025			
Theophylline	S, P (H, E)	Therapeutic concentration, bronchodilator	× 5.550	56-110 µmol/L	ij
		10-20 mcg/ml			

Continued

Common Laboratory Tests and Normal Values—cont'd

Test	Specimen	Reference Range (Conventional Units)	Factor	Reference Range, International Units (SI)	Comments
		Premature apnea 5-10 mcg/ml		28-56 µmol/L	
		Toxic concentration >20 mcg/ml		>110 µmol/L	
Thrombin time	W (NaC)	Control time ± 2 s when control is 9-13 s		Control time ± 2 s when control is 9-13 s	
Thyroxine Total	S	Full-term infant	× 12.8700		
		1-3 d 8.2-19.9 mcg/dl		106-256 nmol/L	
		1 wk 6.0-15.9 mcg/dl		77-205 nmol/L	
		1-12 mo 6.1-14.9 mcg/dl		79-192 nmol/L	
		Prepubertal child			
		1-3 yr 6.8-13.5 mcg/dl		88-174 nmol/L	
		3-10 yr 5.5-12.8 mcg/dl		71-165 nmol/L	
		Pubertal children and adults 4.2-13.0 mcg/dl		54-167 nmol/L	
Free	S	Neonate 3 d 2.0-4.9 ng/dl	× 12.87	26-631 pmol/L	
		Infant 1-12 mo 0.9-2.6 ng/dl		12-33 pmol/L	
		Prepubertal child 0.8-2.2 ng/dl		10-28 pmol/L	
		Pubertal children and adults 0.8-2.3 ng/dl		10-30 pmol/L	
Thyroxine, total	W	Neonatal screen (filter paper) 6.2-2.2 mcg/dl			
Tourniquet test		<5-10 petechiae in 2.5-cm circle on forearm (halfway between systolic and diastolic); pressure maintained for 5 min		<5-10 petechiae in 2.5-cm circle on forearm (halfway between systolic and diastolic); pressure maintained for 5 min	
		0-8 petechiae in 6-cm circle (50 mm Hg for 15 min)		0-8 petechiae in 6-cm circle (50 mm Hg for 15 min)	
		10-20 petechiae in 5-cm circle (80 mm Hg)		10-20 petechiae in 5-cm circle (80 mm Hg)	
Triglycerides	S after ≥12-hr fast	**M (mg/dl)** **F (mg/dl)**	× 0.01	**M (g/L)** **F (g/L)**	
		Cord blood 10-98 10-98		0.10-0.98 0.10-0.98	
		0-5 yr 30-86 32-99		0.30-0.86 0.32-0.99	
		6-11 yr 31-108 35-114		0.31-1.08 0.35-1.14	
		12-15 yr 36-138 41-138		0.36-1.38 0.41-1.38	
		16-19 yr 40-163 40-128		0.40-1.63 0.40-1.28	
		20-29 yr 44-185 40-128		0.44-1.85 0.40-1.28	
		Adults: Recommended (desirable) levels		Adults: Recommended (desirable) levels	
		M 40-160 mg/dl		M 0.40-1.60 g/L	
		F 35-135 mg/dl		F 0.35-1.35 g/L	
Urea nitrogen	S, P	Cord blood 21-40 mg/dl	× 0.357	7.5-14.3 mmol urea/L	
		Premature (1 wk) 3-25 mg/dl		1.1-9 mmol urea/L	
		Neonate 3-12 mg/dl		1.1-4.3 mmol urea/L	
		Infant/child 5-18 mg/dl		1.8-6.4 mmol urea/L	
		Thereafter 7-18 mg/dl		2.5-6.4 mmol urea/L	
Urine, volume	U (24-hr)	Neonate 50-300 ml/24 hr	× 0.001	0.050-0.300 L/24 hr	
		Infant 350-550 ml/24 hr		0.350-0.550 L/24 hr	
		Child 500-1000 ml/24 hr		0.500-1.000 L/24 hr	
		Adolescent 700-1400 ml/24 hr		0.700-1.400 L/24 hr	
		Thereafter			
		M 800-1800 ml/24 hr		0.800-1.800 L/24 hr	
		F 600-1600 ml/24 hr		0.600-1.600 L/24 hr	
		(varies with intake and other factors)			

WBC: see Leuko-

INDEX

Normal Vital Signs by Age

Age	Temperature* Fahrenheit	Temperature* Celsius	Pulse Rate (beats/min)	Respiratory Rate (breaths/min)	Blood Pressure (mm Hg)
Newborn	96.8-99 (axillary)	36-37.2 (axillary)	120-160	30-60	Systolic: 60-99† Diastolic: 30-62
4 Years	97.5-98.6 (axillary)	36.4-37 (axillary)	80-125	20-30	Girls: Systolic: 101-111 Diastolic: 63-71 Boys: Systolic: 102-115 Diastolic: 62-71
10 Years	97.5-98.6 (oral)	36.4-37 (oral)	70-110‡	16-22	Girls: Systolic: 112-122 Diastolic: 73-80 Boys: Systolic: 110-123 Diastolic: 73-82
16 Years	97.5-98.6 (oral)	36.4-37 (oral)	55-90	15-20	Girls: Systolic: 120-130 Diastolic: 79-86 Boys: Systolic: 125-130 Diastolic: 79-87

*The normal range of the child's temperature will depend on the measuring method used. Temperatures exhibit circadian rhythms at all ages.
†Taken with Doppler.
‡After age 12 years, a boy's pulse is 5 beats/min slower than a girl's.

Temperature Equivalents: Celsius and Fahrenheit

Celsius	Fahrenheit	Celsius	Fahrenheit
34.0	93.2	38.4	101.1
34.2	93.6	38.6	101.4
34.4	93.9	38.8	101.8
34.6	94.3	39.0	102.2
34.8	94.6	39.2	102.5
35.0	95.0	39.4	102.9
35.2	95.4	39.6	103.2
35.4	95.7	39.8	103.6
35.6	96.1	40.0	104.0
35.8	96.4	40.2	104.3
36.0	96.8	40.4	104.7
36.2	97.1	40.6	105.1
36.4	97.5	40.8	105.4
36.6	97.8	41.0	105.8
36.8	98.2	41.2	106.1
		41.4	106.5
37.0	98.6	41.6	106.8
		41.8	107.2
37.2	98.9	42.0	107.6
37.4	99.3	42.2	108.0
37.6	99.6	42.4	108.3
37.8	100.0	42.6	108.7
38.0	100.4	42.8	109.0
38.2	100.7		

Conversion formulas:
Fahrenheit to Celsius ($°F - 32$) $\times$ (5/9) = $°C$
Celsius to Fahrenheit ($°C$) $\times$ (9/5) + 32 = $°F$